CARDIAC SURGERY IN THE ADULT

CARDIAC SURGERY IN THE ADULT

Fifth Edition

Lawrence H. Cohn, MD

Virginia and James Hubbard Professor of Cardiac Surgery
Harvard Medical School
Division of Cardiac Surgery
Brigham and Women's Hospital
Boston, Massachusetts

David H. Adams, MD

Cardiac Surgeon-in-Chief, Mount Sinai Health System
Marie-Josée and Henry R. Kravis Professor and Chairman
Department of Cardiovascular Surgery
Icahn School of Medicine at Mount Sinai and The Mount Sinai Hospital
New York, New York

McGraw Hill Education

New York   Chicago   San Francisco   Athens   London   Madrid   Mexico City
Milan   New Delhi   Singapore   Sydney   Toronto

Cardiac Surgery in the Adult, Fifth Edition

Copyright © 2018 by McGraw-Hill Education. All rights reserved. Printed in China. Except as permitted under the United States Copyright Act of 1976, no part of this publication may be reproduced or distributed in any form or by any means, or stored in a database or retrieval system, without the prior written permission of the publisher.

Previous editions copyright © 2012, 2008, 2003, 1997 by The McGraw-Hill Companies, Inc.

4 5 6 7 8 9   DSS   22 21

ISBN 978-0-07-184487-1
MHID 0-07-184487-2

This book was set in Adobe Garamond Pro by Cenveo® Publisher Services.
The editors were Brian Belval and Christie Naglieri.
The production supervisor was Catherine H. Saggese.
Project management was provided by Anupriya Tyagi, Cenveo Publisher Services.

Library of Congress Cataloging-in-Publication Data

Names: Cohn, Lawrence H., 1937- , editor.
Title: Cardiac surgery in the adult / [edited by] Lawrence H. Cohn.
Description: Fifth edition. | New York : McGraw Hill Education, [2016] |
   Includes bibliographical references and index.
Identifiers: LCCN 2015046542| ISBN 9780071844871 (hardcover) |
   ISBN 0071844872 (hardcover)
Subjects: | MESH: Cardiac Surgical Procedures | Cardiovascular
   Diseases—surgery | Adult
Classification: LCC RD598 | NLM WG 169 | DDC 617.4/12—dc23 LC record available
   at http://lccn.loc.gov/2015046542

McGraw-Hill are available at special quantity discounts to use as premiums and sales promotions, or for use in corporate training programs. To contact a representative please visit the Contact Us pages at www.mhprofessional.com.

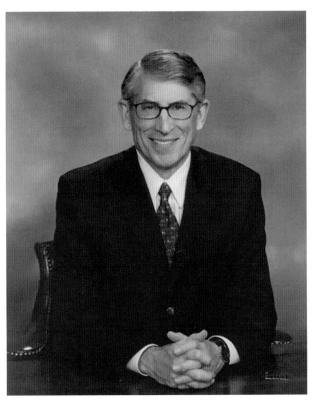

Lawrence H. Cohn, MD

The 5th edition of *Cardiac Surgery in the Adult* is dedicated to Dr. Lawrence Cohn, Emeritus Chief of the Division of Cardiac Surgery at Brigham and Women's Hospital and Virginia and James Hubbard Professor of Cardiac Surgery at Harvard Medical School, who sadly passed away unexpectedly during the final stages of preparation of this latest edition of "his" reference textbook. Dr. Cohn leaves a legacy of excellence seldom seen in academic surgery, and he will be sorely missed by all of us who knew him, and especially those of us lucky enough to have been mentored by him. Dr. Cohn received his training in cardiothoracic surgery under the tutelage of Dr. Norman Shumway at Stanford University, and after completing his fellowship in 1971 he joined the staff of the Peter Bent Brigham Hospital in Boston. Over the next 45 years he was the driving force behind the success of the Harvard program, and became the Chief of the Division of Cardiac Surgery in 1986. A clinical cardiac surgeon first and foremost, Dr. Cohn performed over 11,000 open heart procedures during his career, and was best known for his pioneering and international leadership in minimally invasive valve surgery. His academic contributions included over 500 peer-reviewed publications, 100 book chapters, and 750 invited lectures on virtually all topics in cardiac surgery, but perhaps his greatest academic legacy was his editorship of the 2nd, 3rd, and 4th editions of *Cardiac Surgery in the Adult*, which under his vision became the most widely referenced international textbook in adult cardiac surgery. During his career Dr. Cohn earned the highest awards and honors a cardiac surgeon could possibly achieve, serving as the 79th President of the American Association for Thoracic Surgery, receiving an honorary Masters of Medicine from Harvard, and receiving the American Heart Association's Paul Dudley White Award, among numerous others. He would claim his greatest honor, however, was the opportunity to train over 200 residents and fellows from all over the world, many of whom went on to become Division Chiefs, Department Chairs, and leaders in the specialty. His American Association for Thoracic Surgery presidential address "What the Cardiothoracic Surgeon of the 21st Century Ought to Be" personifies the essence of what made him one of the masters of cardiac surgery who will be remembered by generations to come. Through leadership by example in all phases of his career, his unwavering commitment to the individual patient was the foundation of all of his accomplishments, and few surgeons have had such a profound impact on our specialty. Dr. Cohn was my teacher, mentor, and friend, and it was an honor to be asked by his wife of 55 years, Roberta, to assume the role of Co-Editor to complete this 5th edition of his textbook. Dr. Cohn left footprints too large to fill, but with the help of the many authors who contributed chapters and the publisher's leadership, we now present this peer tribute to one of the greatest cardiac surgeons of all time.

David H. Adams, MD

CONTENTS

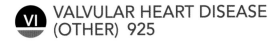

CONTRIBUTORS

Kevin D. Accola, MD
Director, Valve Center of Excellence
Florida Hospital Cardiovascular Institute
Cardiovascular Surgeons, PA
Orlando, Florida

David H. Adams, MD
Cardiac Surgeon-in-Chief, Mount Sinai Health System
Marie-Josée and Henry R. Kravis Professor and Chairman
Department of Cardiovascular Surgery
Icahn School of Medicine at Mount Sinai and
 The Mount Sinai Hospital
New York, New York

Jatin Anand, MD
Duke University Medical Center
Durham, North Carolina

Robert H. Anderson, BSc, MD, FRCPath
Visiting Professorial Fellow
Institute of Genetic Medicine
Newcastle University
Newcastle-upon-Tyne
United Kingdom

Sary Aranki, MD
Associate Professor of Surgery
Brigham and Women's Hospital
Harvard Medical School
Boston, Massachusetts

Mani Arsalan, MD
Department Cardiac Surgery
Kerckhoff Heart Center
Bad Nauheim, Germany
The Heart Hospital Baylor Plano
Plano, Texas

John G. Augoustides, MD, FASE, FAHA
Professor
Cardiovascular and Thoracic Section
Department of Anesthesiology and Critical Care
Perelman School of Medicine
University of Pennsylvania
Philadelphia, Pennsylvania

Agnes Azimzadeh, PhD
Associate Professor
Department of Surgery
University of Maryland School of Medicine
Baltimore, Maryland

Frank A. Baciewicz, Jr., MD
Professor and Chief
Division of Cardiothoracic Surgery
Wayne State University
Harper University Hospital/Karmanos Cancer Center
Detroit, Michigan

Andrew C. W. Baldwin, MD
Clinical Fellow in Cardiothoracic Transplant
Texas Heart Institute
Houston, Texas
Resident in General Surgery
Yale School of Medicine
New Haven, Connecticut

Joseph E. Bavaria, MD
Roberts-Measey Professor and Vice-Chief
Department of Cardiovascular Surgery
Hospital of the University of Pennsylvania
Philadelphia, Pennsylvania

Peyman Benharash, MD
Assistant Professor in-Residence
Division of Cardiac Surgery
Department of Surgery
David Geffen School of Medicine at UCLA
Los Angeles, California

David P. Bichell, MD
Cornelius Vanderbilt Chair in Surgery
Chief, Pediatric Cardiac Surgery
Vanderbilt University
Monroe Carell Jr. Children's Hospital
Nashville, Tennessee

Steven F. Bolling, MD
The University of Michigan Hospitals
Department of Cardiac Surgery
Cardiovascular Center
Ann Arbor, Michigan

Chase R. Brown, MD
Cardiothoracic Surgery
Department of Cardiovascular Surgery
Hospital of the University of Pennsylvania
Philadelphia, Pennsylvania

Nicolas A. Brozzi, MD
Department of Cardiothoracic Surgery
Cleveland Clinic Florida
Weston, Florida

Anna Brzezinski, MD
Medical Student (M2)
University of Illinois at Chicago
Chicago, Illinois

Redmond P. Burke, MD
Chief, Division of Cardiovascular and Thoracic Surgery
Miami Children's Hospital
Miami, Florida

Clay M. Burnett, MD
Florida Hospital Cardiovascular Institute
Orlando, Florida

John G. Byrne, MD
Hospital Corporation of America
Houston, Texas

Javier G. Castillo, MD
Assistant Professor
Department of Cardiovascular Surgery
The Mount Sinai Medical Center
New York, New York

Edward P. Chen, MD
Director of Thoracic Aortic Surgery
Associate Professor
Division of Cardiothoracic Surgery
Emory University School of Medicine
Atlanta, Georgia

Frederick Y. Chen, MD, PhD
Associate Surgeon
Director, Cardiac Surgery Research Laboratory
Division of Cardiac Surgery
Brigham and Women's Hospital
Associate Professor of Surgery
Harvard Medical School
Boston, Massachusetts

Jason S. Chinitz, MD, FACC, FHRS
Director, Cardiac Electrophysiology
Assistant Professor, Hofstra Northwell School of Medicine
Southside Hospital
Bayshore, New York

W. Randolph Chitwood, Jr, MD, FACS, FRCS (Eng)
Emeritus Professor and Chairman
Department of Surgery
Founder—East Carolina Heart Institute
Brody School of Medicine
East Carolina University
Greenville, North Carolina

George T. Christakis, MD, FRCS(C)
Professor, Department of Surgery
Division of Cardiac Surgery, Schulich Heart Centre
Sunnybrook Health Sciences Centre
Director, Undergraduate Medical Education
University of Toronto
Ontario, Canada

William E. Cohn, MD, FACS, FACCP
Professor of Surgery
Director of Surgical Innovation
Baylor College of Medicine
Director of Minimally Invasive Surgical Technology
Texas Heart Institute
Houston, Texas

Lawrence H. Cohn, MD*
Emeritus Virginia and James Hubbard Professor
Harvard Medical School
Division of Cardiac Surgery
Brigham and Women's Hospital
Boston, Massachusetts
*Deceased

Jeffrey B. Cooper, PhD
Professor of Anesthesia
Department of Anesthesia, Critical Care, and Pain Medicine
Harvard Medical School
Massachusetts General Hospital
Executive Director Emeritus and Senior Fellow
Center for Medical Simulation
Boston, Massachusetts

Joseph S. Coselli, MD
Professor and Chief of the Division of Cardiothoracic Surgery
Vice Chair, Michael E. DeBakey Department of Surgery
Baylor College of Medicine
Chief of the Section of Adult Cardiac Surgery
Texas Heart Institute
Houston, Texas

Kim I. de la Cruz, MD, FACS
Assistant Professor
Division of Cardiothoracic Surgery
Michael E. DeBakey Department of Surgery
Baylor College of Medicine, and Clinical Staff
Texas Heart Institute
Houston, Texas

William C. Culp, Jr., MD
Professor
Scott & White Hospital
Department of Anesthesiology
The Texas A&M University System Health Science
 Center College of Medicine
Bryan, Texas

Michael D'Ambra, MD
Associate Professor of Anesthesia
Harvard Medical School
Boston, Massachusetts

Ralph J. Damiano, Jr., MD
Evarts A. Graham Professor of Surgery
Chief, Division of Cardiothoracic Surgery
Co-Chair, Heart & Vascular Center
Washington University School of Medicine
St. Louis, Missouri

Tirone E. David, MD
Professor of Surgery
University of Toronto
Toronto, Ontario, Canada

Piroze M. Davierwala, MD
Department of Cardiac Surgery
Heart Center Leipzig
Leipzig, Germany

Andreas R. de Biasi, MD
Research Fellow
Department of Cardiothoracic Surgery
Weill Cornell Medical College
New York-Presbyterian Hospital
New York, New York

William J. DeBois, CCP, MBA
Chief Perfusionist and Director
Department of Perioperative Services
New York-Presbyterian Hospital
Weill Cornell Medical Center
New York, New York

Mario Deng, MD, FACC, FESC
Professor of Medicine
Advanced Heart Failure/Mechanical Support/Heart Transplant
David Geffen School of Medicine at UCLA
Ronald Reagan UCLA Medical Center
Los Angeles, California

Nimesh D. Desai, MD, PhD, FRCSC, FAHA
Co-Director, Aortic and Vascular Center of Excellence
Director, Thoracic Aortic Surgery Research Program
Assistant Professor, Division of Cardiovascular Surgery
Hospital of the University of Pennsylvania
Philadelphia, Pennsylvania

J. Michael DiMaio, MD
The Heart Hospital Baylor Plano
Plano, Texas

Robert E. Eckart, DO
Heart Specialists of Sarasota
Sarasota, Florida

Fred H. Edwards, MD
Emeritus Professor of Surgery
University of Florida
Jacksonville, Florida

Julius I. Ejiofor, MD
Division of Cardiac Surgery
Brigham and Women's Hospital
Harvard Medical School
Boston, Massachusetts

Robert J. Emery, BS, MMS
Medical University Medical School
Philadelphia, Pennsylvania

Robert W. Emery, MD
Director Emeritus, Cardiovascular and Thoracic Surgery
HealthEast Care System
St Joseph's Hospital
St Paul, Minnesota

Laurence M. Epstein, MD
Professor of Medicine
Harvard Medical School
Chief, Arrhythmia Service
Brigham and Women's Hospital
Boston, Massachusetts

James I. Fann, MD
Professor
Department of Cardiothoracic Surgery
Stanford University
Stanford, California

Eric N. Feins, MD
Division of Cardiac Surgery
Department of Surgery
Massachusetts General Hospital
Boston, Massachusetts

Victor A. Ferraris, MD, PhD
Tyler Gill Professor of Surgery
Division of Cardiothoracic Surgery
University of Kentucky Chandler Medical Center
Lexington, Kentucky

O.H. Frazier, MD
Professor of Surgery
Michael E. DeBakey Department of Surgery
Baylor College of Medicine
Chief of the Center for Cardiac Support
Texas Heart Institute
Houston, Texas

Courtney J. Gemmato, MD
Resident in Cardiothoracic Surgery
Texas Heart Institute
Baylor College of Medicine
Houston, Texas

Ravi K. Ghanta, MD
Assistant Professor of Surgery
Department of Surgery
University of Virginia
Charlottesville, Virginia

Andreas A. Giannopoulos, MD
Research Fellow
Applied Imaging Science Laboratory
Brigham and Women's Hospital
Harvard Medical School
Boston, Massachusetts

A. Marc Gillinov, MD
The Judith Dion Pyle Chair in Heart Valve Research
Department of Thoracic and Cardiovascular Surgery
Cleveland Clinic
Cleveland, Ohio

Donald D. Glower, MD
Professor of Surgery
Duke University Medical Center
Durham, North Carolina

Danielle Gottlieb Sen, MS, MD, MPH
Assistant Professor of Surgery
Pediatric Cardiovascular Surgery
Children's Hospital of New Orleans/LSU Health Science Center
New Orleans, Louisiana

Roberta A. Gottlieb, MD
Director, Molecular Cardiobiology
Dorothy and E. Phillip Lyon Chair in Molecular Cardiology in honor of Clarence M. Agress MD
Research Scientist, Heart Institute
Los Angeles, California

Bartley P. Griffith, MD
The Thomas E. and Alice Marie Hales
Distinguished Professor in Transplantation
Executive Director, Program in Lung Healing
University of Maryland School of Medicine
Baltimore, Maryland

Wendy Gross, MD
Assistant Professor of Anesthesia
Department of Anesthesiology, Perioperative and Pain Medicine
Brigham and Women's Hospital
Harvard Medical School
Boston, Massachusetts

Michael E. Halkos, MD, MSc, FACS, FACC
Associate Professor of Surgery
Division of Cardiothoracic Surgery
Scientific Director, Cardiothoracic Center for Clinical Research
Associate Program Director
Thoracic Surgery Residency Program
Atlanta, Georgia

John W. Hammon, MD
Professor of Surgery, Emeritus
Department of Cardiothoracic Surgery
Wake Forest University School of Medicine
Winston-Salem, North Carolina

Matthew C. Henn, MS, MD
Cardiac Surgery Research Fellow
Washington University School of Medicine
St. Louis, Missouri

David M. Holzhey, MD
Department of Cardiac Surgery
Heart Center Leipzig
Leipzig, Germany

Syed T. Hussain, MD
Assistant Professor of Surgery
Department of Thoracic & Cardiovascular Surgery
Cleveland Clinic
Cleveland, Ohio

John S. Ikonomidis, MD, PhD
Professor of Surgery
Chief, Division of Cardiothoracic Surgery
University of North Carolina at Chapel Hill
Chapel Hill, North Carolina

Neil B. Ingels, Jr., PhD
Consulting Professor
Department of Cardiothoracic Surgery
Stanford University School of Medicine
Stanford, California

O. Wayne Isom, MD
The Terry Allen Kramer Professor of Cardiothoracic Surgery
Chairman, Department of Cardiothoracic Surgery
Cardiothoracic Surgeon-in-Chief
Weill Cornell Medical College
New York-Presbyterian Hospital
New York, New York

M. Salik Jahania, MD
Associate Professor of Surgery
Cardiothoracic Surgery
Wayne State University
Detroit, Michigan

Stuart W. Jamieson, MD, FRCS, FACS
Endowed Chair and Distinguished Professor
Dean, Cardiovascular Affairs
University of California
San Diego, California

Tsuyoshi Kaneko, MD
Division of Cardiac Surgery
Brigham and Women's Hospital
Boston, Massachusetts

Hanjo Ko, MD
Assistant Professor
Department of Anesthesiology and Critical Care
University of Pennsylvania Health System
Philadelphia, Pennsylvania

Marijan Koprivanac, MD, MS
Resident, Department of General surgery
Cleveland Clinic
Research Fellow
Department of Cardiothoracic Surgery, Cleveland Clinic
Clinical Instructor, Case Western University
Cleveland, Ohio

Irving L. Kron, MD
S. Hurt Watts Professor and Chair
Department of Surgery
University of Virginia
Charlottesville, Virginia

Michael H. Kwon, MD
Research Fellow, Brigham and Women's Hospital
Clinical Fellow in Surgery (EXT), Harvard Medical School
Boston, Massachusetts

Marzia Leacche, MD
Spectrum Health
Meijer Heart Center
Grand Rapids, Michigan

Lawrence Lee, MD
Clinical Fellow in Surgery
Harvard Medical School
Resident in Cardiothoracic Surgery
Brigham and Women's Hospital
Boston, Massachusetts

Lawrence S. Lee, MD
Assistant Professor of Surgery
Division of Cardiothoracic Surgery
University of Tennessee Graduate School of Medicine
Knoxville, Tennessee

Scott A. LeMaire, MD
Professor and Director of Research
Division of Cardiothoracic Surgery
Michael E. DeBakey Department of Surgery
Baylor College of Medicine, and Cardiovascular Surgery Staff
Texas Heart Institute
Houston, Texas

Bradley G. Leshnower, MD
Assistant Professor of Surgery
Division of Cardiothoracic Surgery
Emory University School of Medicine
Atlanta, Georgia

Jerrold H. Levy, MD, FAHA, FCCM
Professor of Anesthesiology
Associate Professor of Surgery
Co-Director Cardiothoracic Intensive Care Unit
Duke University School of Medicine
Durham, North Carolina

Dan Loberman, MD
Division of Cardiac Surgery
Brigham and Women's Hospital
Harvard Medical school
Boston, Massachusetts

Bruce W. Lytle, MD
Director of Strategic Operations
The Heart Hospital Baylor-Plano
Dallas, Texas

Michael Mack, MD
The Heart Hospital Baylor Plano
Plano, Texas

Michael M. Madani, MD
Professor and Chief
Division of Cardiovascular and Thoracic Surgery
University of California, San Diego
La Jolla, California

Hari R. Mallidi, MD
BWH Thoracic and Cardiac Surgery
Co-Director, Program in Heart and Lung Transplant and MCS
Surgical Director of Lung Transplant and Pulmonary
  Vascular Disease
Senior Surgeon, Collaborative Center for Advanced Heart Failure
Executive Director, BWH ECMO Program
Boston, Massachusetts

Jeremiah T. Martin, MBBCh, FRCSI
Assistant Professor of Surgery
University of Kentucky Chandler Medical Center
Lexington, Kentucky

John E. Mayer, Jr., MD
Senior Associate in Cardiac Surgery
Childrens Hospital, Boston
Professor of Surgery
Harvard Medical School
Department of Cardiac Surgery
Children's Hospital
Boston, Massachusetts

Edwin C. McGee, Jr., MD
Thoracic and Cardiovascular Surgery
Professor
Director, Heart Transplant & Ventricular Assist Device Program
Loyola Medicine
Maywood, Illinois

Mandeep R. Mehra, MD
Professor of Medicine
Harvard Medical School
Medical Director
Heart and Vascular Center
Brigham and Women's Hospital
Boston, Massachusetts

Spencer J. Melby, MD
Associate Professor of Surgery
Department of Surgery
Division of Cardiothoracic Surgery
Washington University in St. Louis and Barnes Jewish Hospital
St. Louis, Missouri

Robert M. Mentzer, Jr., MD
Professor of Medicine and Surgery
Cedars-Sinai Heart Institute
Cedars-Sinai Medical Center
Los Angeles, California

Carlos M. Mery, MD, MPH
Assistant Professor of Surgery and Pediatrics
Department of Surgery
Texas Children's Hospital/Baylor College of Medicine
Houston, Texas

Bret A. Mettler, MD
Assistant Professor in Surgery
Vanderbilt University
Monroe Carell Jr. Children's Hospital
Nashville, Tennessee

Stephanie L. Mick, MD
Cardiac Surgery, Surgical Director of Transcatheter Valve Insertion Program
Department of Thoracic and Cardiovascular Surgery,
Heart and Vascular Institute
Cleveland Clinic
Cleveland, Ohio

Tomislav Mihaljevic, MD
Professor of Surgery
Cleveland Clinic Lerner College of Medicine
Cleveland, Ohio
Chief Executive Officer
Cleveland Clinic Abu Dhabi
Abu Dhabi, United Arab Emirates

Michael R. Mill, MD
Professor
Departments of Surgery and Pediatrics
University of North Carolina
Chapel Hill, North Carolina

D. Craig Miller, MD
Thelma and Henry Doelger Professor of Cardiovascular Surgery
Dept. of Cardiothoracic Surgery
Stanford University School of Medicine
Falk CV Research Building
Stanford, California

R. Scott Mitchell, MD
Professor Emeritus
Department of Cardiothoracic Surgery
Stanford University School of Medicine
Falk Cardiovascular Research Building
Stanford, California
Attending Surgeon
Division of Cardiac Surgery
V.A. Hospital Palo Alto
Palo Alto, California

Annette Mizuguchi, MD
Assistant Professor of Anesthesia
Department of Anesthesiology, Perioperative and Pain Medicine
Brigham and Women's Hospital
Harvard Medical School
Boston, Massachusetts

Nader Moazami, MD
Thoracic and Cardiovascular Surgery
Cleveland Clinic
Cleveland, Ohio

Susan D. Moffatt-Bruce, MD, PhD
Associate Professor, Division of Thoracic Surgery
Department of Surgery
Ohio State University
Wexner Medical Center
Columbus, Ohio

Friedrich-Wilhelm Mohr, MD, PhD
Professor of Cardiac Surgery
University of Leipzig
Medical Director Heart Center Leipzig
Director Department of Cardiac Surgery
Heart Center Leipzig
Leipzig, Germany

L. Wiley Nifong, MD
Division of Cardiothoracic Surgery
Department of Cardiovascular Sciences
East Carolina Heart Institute
Brody School of Medicine at East Carolina University
Greenville, North Carolina

Patrick T. O'Gara, MD
Watkins Family Distinguished Chair in Cardiology
Brigham and Women's Hospital
Professor of Medicine
Harvard Medical School
Boston, Massachusetts

Robert F. Padera, MD, PhD
Associate Pathologist
Department of Pathology
Brigham and Women's Hospital
Assistant Professor of Pathology
Harvard Medical School
Boston, Massachusetts

Prakash A. Patel, MD
Assistant Professor
Cardiovascular and Thoracic Section
Department of Anesthesiology and Critical Care
Perelman School of Medicine
University of Pennsylvania
Philadelphia, Pennsylvania

Gösta B. Pettersson, MD, PhD
Professor of Surgery
Vice Chairman
Department of Thoracic and Cardiovascular Surgery
Cleveland Clinic
Cleveland, Ohio

Michael H. Picard, MD
Professor of Medicine
Harvard Medical School
Director, Echocardiography
Massachusetts General Hospital
Boston, Massachusetts

Paul A. Pirundini, MD
Chief, Cardiac Surgery
Cape Cod Hospital
Hyannis, Massachusetts
Associate Surgeon
Brigham and Women's Hospital
Boston, Massachusetts

Ourania Preventza, MD
Associate Professor of Surgery
Division of Cardiothoracic Surgery
Michael E DeBakey Department of Surgery
Baylor College of Surgery
Attending Cardiac and Endovascular Surgeon
Texas Heart Institute
Baylor St Luke's Medical Center
Houston, Texas

John D. Puskas, MD
Chair, Cardiovascular Surgery
Mount Sinai St. Luke's, Mount Sinai Beth Israel, and
  Mount Sinai West
New York, New York

T. Konrad Rajab, MD
Clinical Fellow in Surgery
Harvard Medical School
Resident in Cardiothoracic Surgery
Brigham and Women's Hospital
Boston, Massachusetts

Basel Ramlawi, MD, FACC, FACS
Chairman, Heart & Vascular Center
Director, Advanced Valve & Aortic Center Valley Health System
Winchester, Virginia

James G. Ramsay, MD
Professor Anesthesiology
Director of Cardiothoracic Intensive Care Unit
University of California
San Francisco, California

James D. Rawn, MD
Director, Cardiac Surgery Intensive Care Unit
Instructor in Surgery, Harvard Medical School
Cardiac Surgery
Boston, Massachusetts

Michael J. Reardon, MD, FACS, FACC
Professor of Cardiothoracic Surgery
Allison Family Distinguished Chair of Cardiovascular Research
Department of Cardiovascular Surgery
Houston Methodist DeBakey Heart & Vascular center
Houston, Texas

Kent Rehfeldt, MD, FASE
Associate Professor of Anesthesiology
Mayo Clinic
Rochester, Minnesota

Robert C. Robbins, MD
President and CEO
Texas Medical Center
Houston, Texas

Barbara Robinson, MD, MS, FACS, FAHA, FACC
Division of Cardiothoracic Surgery
Department of Cardiovascular Sciences
East Carolina Heart Institute
Brody School of Medicine at East Carolina University
Greenville, North Carolina

Matthew A. Romano, MD
Assistant Professor
Department of Cardiac Surgery
University of Michigan
Ann Arbor, Michigan

Christian T. Ruff, MD, MPH
Assistant Professor of Medicine
Cardiovascular Medicine Division
Brigham and Women's Hospital
Harvard Medical School
Boston, Massachusetts

Frank J. Rybicki, MD, PhD
Professor, Chair and Chief, Department of Radiology
The University of Ottawa
Faculty of Medicine and The Ottawa Hospital
Ottawa, Ontario, Canada

Arash Salemi, MD
Associate Professor of Cardiothoracic Surgery
Department of Cardiothoracic Surgery
Weill Cornell Medical College
New York-Presbyterian Hospital
New York, New York

Edward B. Savage, MD
Clinical Professor
Cleveland Clinic Lerner College of Medicine
Chairman
Department of Cardiothoracic Surgery
Director
Heart and Vascular Institute
Cleveland Clinic Florida
Weston, Florida

Hartzell Schaff, MD
Professor of Surgery, College of Medicine
Department of Cardiovascular Surgery
Mayo Clinic
Rochester, Minnesota

Frederick J. Schoen, MD, PhD
Executive Vice Chairman
Department of Pathology
Brigham and Women's Hospital
Professor of Pathology and Health Sciences and Technology (HST),
Harvard Medical School
Boston, Massachusetts

Claudio J. Schonholz, MD
Department of Surgery, Division of Cardiothoracic Surgery
Department of Radiology, Division of Interventional Radiology
Medical University of South Carolina
Charleston, South Carolina

Jacob N. Schroder, MD
Assistant Professor of Surgery
Co-Director, Cardiothoracic Intensive Care Unit
Duke University School of Medicine
Durham, North Carolina

Pinak Shah, MD
Associate Professor of Medicine
Division of Cardiology
Department of Medicine
Brigham and Women's Hospital
Harvard Medical School
Boston, Massachusetts

Prem S. Shekar, MD
Assistant Professor of Surgery
Harvard Medical School
Chief, Division of Cardiac Surgery
Brigham and Women's Hospital
Boston, Massachusetts

Richard J. Shemin, MD
Robert and Kelly Day Professor and Chief
Division of Cardiac Surgery
Vice Chairman, Department of Surgery
Co-director, Cardiovascular Center at UCLA
David Geffen School of Medicine at UCLA
Los Angeles, California

Stanton K. Shernan, MD, FAHA, FASE
Professor of Anesthesia
Department of Anesthesiology, Perioperative and Pain Medicine
Brigham and Women's Hospital
Harvard Medical School
Boston, Massachusetts

Tarang Sheth, MD, FRCPC
Cardiovascular Radiologist
Director of Cardiac CT and MR
Department of Diagnostic Imaging
Trillium Health Partners
Mississauga, Ontario, Canada

Deane E. Smith III, MD
Assistant Professor of Cardiothoracic Surgery
NYU School of Medicine
New York, New York

Philip J. Spencer, MD
Department of Surgery
Massachusetts General Hospital
Boston, Massachusetts

Michelle D. Spotnitz, MD
Cardiologist
EHE International
New York, New York

Henry M. Spotnitz, MD
George H. Humphreys, II, Professor of Surgery
Department of Surgery
Columbia University
New York, New York

Paul Stelzer, MD
Professor
Department of Cardiovascular Surgery
Icahn School of Medicine at Mount Sinai
New York, New York

Larry W. Stephenson, MD
Professor Emeritus
Ford Webber Professor of Surgery
Department of Surgery
Wayne State University
Detroit, Michigan

Thoralf M. Sundt, MD
Edward D. Churchill Professor of Surgery
Harvard Medical School
Chief, Division of Cardiac Surgery
Massachusetts General Hospital
Boston, Massachusetts

Rakesh Mark Suri, MD, D.Phil
Cleveland Clinic Foundation
Department of Thoracic and Cardiovascular Surgery
Cleveland, Ohio

Lars G. Svensson, MD, PhD
Chairman, Heart and Vascular Institute
Cleveland Clinic
Cleveland, Ohio

Vakhtang Tchantchaleishvili, MD
Cardiothoracic Surgery
University of Rochester Medical Center
Rochester, New York

Usha Tedrow, MD
Assistant Professor of Medicine
Division of Cardiology
Department of Medicine
Brigham and Women's Hospital
Harvard Medical School
Boston, Massachusetts

Eliza P. Teo, MBBS
Clinical and Research Fellow in Medicine
Massachusetts General Hospital
Research Fellow
Harvard Medical School
Boston, Massachusetts

Tom P. Theruvath, MD, PhD
Department of Surgery, Division of Cardiothoracic Surgery
Department of Radiology, Division of Interventional Radiology
Medical University of South Carolina
Charleston, South Carolina

George Tolis, Jr., MD
Assistant Professor of Surgery
Harvard Medical School
Boston, Massachusetts

Robin Varghese, MD, MS, FRCSC
Associate Professor
Department of Cardiovascular Surgery
Icahn School of Medicine at Mount Sinai
New York, New York

Subodh Verma, MD, PhD, FRCSC
Cardiac Surgeon
St Michael's Hospital
Professor of Surgery & Pharmacology and Toxicology
University of Toronto
Canada Research Chair in Atherosclerosis
Toronto, Ontario

Rochus K. Voeller, MD
Cardiovascular Surgeon
Fairview Health System
Fairview Southdale Hospital
Edina, Minnesota

Jennifer D. Walker, MD
Professor and Chief
Division of Cardiac Surgery
Surgical Director
Heart & Vascular Center of Excellence
UMass Memorial Medical Center
Worcester, Massachusetts

Toni B. Walzer, MD, FACOG
Assistant Professor, Part-Time, of Obstetrics, Gynecology, and
Reproductive Biology
Harvard Medical School
Department of Obstetrics and Gynecology
Brigham and Women's Hospital
Assistant in Healthcare Education
Department of Anesthesia, Critical Care, and Pain Medicine
Massachusetts General Hospital
Director, Labor and Delivery Program
Center for Medical Simulation
Boston, Massachusetts

James T. Willerson, MD, FACC
President and Medical Director
Texas Heart Institute
Houston, Texas

Mathew R. Williams, MD
Associate Professor of Cardiothoracic Surgery & Medicine
Chief, Division of Adult Cardiac Surgery
Director, CVI Structural Heart Program
Director, Interventional Cardiology
NYU School of Medicine
New York, New York

James M. Wilson, MD
Director, Cardiology Education
Texas Heart Institute
Houston, Texas

Maroun Yammine, MD
Division of Cardiac Surgery
Brigham and Women's Hospital
Boston, Massachusetts

Bobby Yanagawa, MD, PhD, FRCSC
Assistant Professor
Division of Cardiac Surgery
St Michael's Hospital
Toronto, Canada

Farhang Yazdchi, MD, MS
Clinical Fellow in Surgery (EXT)
Brigham and Women's Hospital Surgery
Brigham and Women's Hospital
Cardiac Surgery
Boston, Massachusetts

FUNDAMENTALS

History of Cardiac Surgery

Larry W. Stephenson • Frank A. Baciewicz, Jr.

The development of major surgery was retarded for centuries by a lack of knowledge and technology. Significantly, the general anesthetics ether and chloroform were not developed until the middle of the nineteenth century. These agents made major surgical operations possible, which created an interest in repairing wounds to the heart, leading some investigators in Europe to conduct studies in the animal laboratory on the repair of heart wounds. The first simple operations in humans for heart wounds soon were reported in the medical literature.

HEART WOUNDS

On July 10, 1893, Dr. Daniel Hale Williams (Fig. 1-1), a surgeon from Chicago, successfully operated on a 24-year-old man who had been stabbed in the heart during a fight. The stab wound was slightly to the left of the sternum and dead center over the heart. Initially, the wound was thought to be superficial, but during the night the patient experienced persistent bleeding, pain, and pronounced symptoms of shock. Williams opened the patient's chest and tied off an artery and vein that had been injured inside the chest wall, likely causing the blood loss. Then he noticed a tear in the pericardium and a puncture wound to the heart "about one-tenth of an inch in length."[1]

The wound in the right ventricle was not bleeding, so Williams did not place a stitch through the heart wound. He did, however, stitch closed the hole in the pericardium. Williams reported this case 4 years later.[1] This operation, which is referred to frequently, is probably the first successful surgery involving a documented stab wound to the heart. At the time Williams' surgery was considered bold and daring, and although he did not actually place a stitch through the wound in the heart, his treatment seems to have been appropriate. Under the circumstances, he most likely saved the patient's life.

A few years after Williams' case, a couple of other surgeons actually sutured heart wounds, but the patients did not survive. Dr. Ludwig Rehn (Fig. 1-2), a surgeon in Frankfurt, Germany, performed what many consider the first successful heart operation.[2] On September 7, 1896, a 22-year-old man was stabbed in the heart and collapsed. The police found him pale, covered with cold sweat, and extremely short of breath. His pulse was irregular and his clothes were soaked with blood. By September 9, his condition was worsening, as shown in Dr. Rehn's case notes:

> Pulse weaker, increasing cardiac dullness on percussion, respiration 76, further deterioration during the day, diagnostic tap reveals dark blood. Patient appears moribund. Diagnosis: increasing hemothorax. I decided to operate entering the chest through the left fourth intercostal space, there is massive blood in the pleural cavity. The mammary artery is not injured. There is continuous bleeding from a hole in the pericardium. This opening is enlarged. The heart is exposed. Old blood and clots are emptied. There is a 1.5 cm gaping right ventricular wound. Bleeding is controlled with finger pressure. …
>
> I decided to suture the heart wound. I used a small intestinal needle and silk suture. The suture was tied in diastole. Bleeding diminished remarkably with the third suture, all bleeding was controlled. The pulse improved. The pleural cavity was irrigated. Pleura and pericardium were drained with iodoform gauze. The incision was approximated, heart rate and respiratory rate decreased and pulse improved postoperatively.
>
> … Today the patient is cured. He looks very good. His heart action is regular. I have not allowed him to work physically hard. This proves the feasibility of cardiac suture repair without a doubt! *I hope this will lead to more investigation regarding surgery of the heart. This may save many lives.*

Ten years after Rehn's initial repair, he had accumulated a series of 124 cases with a mortality of only 60%, quite a feat at that time.[3]

Dr. Luther Hill was the first American to report the successful repair of a cardiac wound, in a 13-year-old boy who was a victim of multiple stab wounds.[4] When the first doctor arrived, the boy was in profound shock. The doctor remembered that Dr. Luther Hill had spoken on the subject of repair of cardiac wounds at a local medical society meeting in Montgomery, Alabama. With the consent of the boy's parents, Dr. Hill was summoned. He arrived sometime after midnight with six other physicians. One was his brother. The surgery

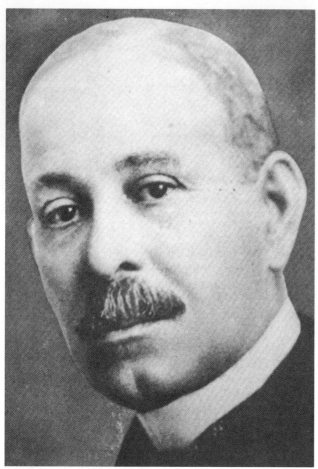

FIGURE 1-1 Daniel Hale Williams, a surgeon from Chicago, who successfully operated on a patient with a wound to the chest involving the pericardium and the heart. (Reproduced with permission from Organ CH Jr., Kosiba MM: *The Century of the Black Surgeons: A USA Experience.* Norman, OK: Transcript Press, 1937; p 312.)

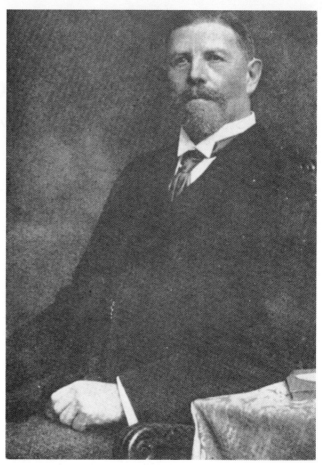

FIGURE 1-2 Ludwig Rehn, a surgeon from Frankfurt, Germany, who performed the first successful suture of a human heart wound. (Reproduced with permission from Mead R: *A History of Thoracic Surgery.* Springfield: Charles C Thomas; 1961.)

took place on the patient's kitchen table in a rundown shack. Lighting was provided by two kerosene lamps borrowed from neighbors. One physician administered chloroform anesthesia. The boy was suffering from cardiac tamponade as a result of a stab wound to the left ventricle. The stab wound to the ventricle was repaired with two catgut sutures. Although the early postoperative course was stormy, the boy made a complete recovery. That patient, Henry Myrick, eventually moved to Chicago, where, in 1942, at the age of 53, he got into a heated argument and was stabbed in the heart again, very close to the original stab wound. This time, Henry was not as lucky and died from the wound.

Another milestone in cardiac surgery for trauma occurred during World War II when Dwight Harken, then a U.S. Army surgeon, removed 134 missiles from the mediastinum, including 55 from the pericardium and 13 from cardiac chambers, without a death.[5] It is hard to imagine this type of elective (and semielective) surgery taking place without sophisticated indwelling pulmonary artery catheters, blood banks, and electronic monitoring equipment.

Rapid blood infusion consisted of pumping air into glass bottles of blood.

OPERATIVE MANAGEMENT OF PULMONARY EMBOLI

Martin Kirschner reported the first patient who recovered fully after undergoing pulmonary embolectomy in 1924.[6] In 1937, John Gibbon estimated that nine of 142 patients who had undergone the procedure worldwide left the hospital alive.[7] These dismal results were a stimulus for Gibbon to start work on a pump oxygenator that could maintain the circulation during pulmonary embolectomy. Sharp was the first to perform pulmonary embolectomy using cardiopulmonary bypass, in 1962.[8]

SURGERY OF THE PERICARDIUM

Pericardial resection was introduced independently by Rehn[9] and Sauerbruch.[10] Since Rehn's report, there have been few advances in the surgical treatment of constrictive pericarditis.

Some operations are now performed with the aid of cardiopulmonary bypass. In certain situations, radical pericardiectomy that removes most of the pericardium posterior to the phrenic nerves is done.

CATHETERIZATION OF THE RIGHT SIDE OF THE HEART

Although cardiac catheterization is not considered heart surgery, it is an invasive procedure, and some catheter procedures have replaced heart operations. Werner Forssmann is credited with the first heart catheterization. He performed the procedure on himself and reported it in *Klrinische Wochenschrift*.[11] In 1956 Forssmann shared the Nobel Prize in Physiology or Medicine with Andre F. Cournand and Dickenson W. Richards, Jr. His 1929 paper states, "One often hesitates to use intercardiac injections promptly, and often, time is wasted with other measures. This is why I kept looking for a different, safer access to the cardiac chambers: the catheterization of the right heart via the venous system."

In this report by Forssmann, a photograph of the x-ray taken of Forssmann with the catheter in his own heart is presented. Forssmann, in that same report, goes on to present the first clinical application of the central venous catheter for a patient in shock with generalized peritonitis. Forssmann concludes his paper by stating, "I also want to mention that this method allows new options for metabolic studies and studies about cardiac physiology."

In a 1951 lecture Forssmann discussed the tremendous resistance he faced during his initial experiments.[12] "Such methods are good for a circus, but not for a respected hospital" was the answer to his request to pursue physiologic studies using cardiac catheterization. His progressive ideas pushed him into the position of an outsider with ideas too crazy to give him a clinical position. Klein applied cardiac catheterization for cardiac output determinations using the Fick method a half year after Forssmann's first report.[13] In 1930, Forssmann described his experiments with catheter cardiac angiography.[14] Further use of this new methodology had to wait until Cournand's work in the 1940s.

HEART VALVE SURGERY BEFORE THE ERA OF CARDIOPULMONARY BYPASS

The first clinical attempt to open a stenotic valve was carried out by Theodore Tuffier on July 13, 1912.[15] Tuffier used his finger to reach the stenotic aortic valve. He was able to dilate the valve supposedly by pushing the invaginated aortic wall through the stenotic valve. The patient recovered, but one must be skeptical as to what was accomplished. Russell Brock attempted to dilate calcified aortic valves in humans in the late 1940s by passing an instrument through the valve from the innominate or another artery.[16] His results were poor, and he abandoned the approach. During the next several years, Brock[17] and Bailey and colleagues[18] used different dilators and various approaches to dilate stenotic aortic valves in patients. Mortality for these procedures, which was often done in conjunction with mitral commissurotomy, was high.

Elliott Cutler worked for 2 years on a mitral valvulotomy procedure in the laboratory. His first patient underwent successful valvulotomy on May 20, 1923, using a tetrasomy knife.[19] Unfortunately, most of Cutler's subsequent patients died because he created too much regurgitation with his valvulotome, and he soon gave up the operation.

In Charles Bailey's 1949 paper entitled, "The Surgical Treatment of Mitral Stenosis," he states, "After 1929 no more surgical attempts [on mitral stenosis] were made until 1945. Dr. Dwight Harken, Dr. Horace Smithy, and the author recently made operative attempts to improve mitral stenosis. Our clinical experience with the surgery of the mitral valves has been five cases to date." He then describes his five patients, four of whom died and only one of whom lived a long life.[20,21]

A few days after Bailey's success, on June 16 in Boston, Dr. Dwight Harken successfully performed his first valvulotomy for mitral stenosis.[22]

The first successful pulmonary valvulotomy was performed by Thomas Holmes Sellers on December 4, 1947.[23]

Charles Hufnagel reported a series of 23 patients starting September 1952 who had operation for aortic insufficiency.[24] There were four deaths among the first 10 patients and two deaths among the next 13. Hufnagel's caged-ball valve, which used multiple-point fixation rings to secure the apparatus to the descending aorta, was the only surgical treatment for aortic valvular incompetence until the advent of cardiopulmonary bypass and the development of heart valves that could be sewn into the aortic annulus position.

CONGENITAL CARDIAC SURGERY BEFORE THE HEART-LUNG MACHINE ERA

Congenital cardiac surgery began when John Strieder at Massachusetts General Hospital first successfully interrupted a ductus on March 6, 1937. The patient was septic and died on the fourth postoperative day. At autopsy, vegetations filled the pulmonary artery down to the valve.[25] On August 16, 1938, Robert Gross, at Boston Children's Hospital, operated on a 7-year-old girl with dyspnea after moderate exercise.[26] The ductus was ligated and the patient made an uneventful recovery.

Modifications of the ductus operation soon followed. In 1944, Dr. Gross reported a technique for dividing the ductus successfully. The next major congenital lesion to be overcome was coarctation of the aorta. Dr. Clarence Crafoord, in Stockholm, Sweden, successfully resected a coarctation of the aorta in a 12-year-old boy on October 19, 1944.[27] Twelve days later he successfully resected the coarctation of a 27-year-old patient. Dr. Gross first operated on a 5-year-old boy with this condition on June 28, 1945.[28] After he excised the coarctation and rejoined the aorta, the patient's heart stopped suddenly. The patient died in the operating room. One week later, however, Dr. Gross operated on a second patient, a 12-year-old girl. This patient's operation was successful. Dr. Gross had been unaware of Dr. Crafoord's successful surgery several months previously, probably because of World War II.

In 1945, Dr. Gross reported the first successful case of surgical relief for tracheal obstruction from a vascular ring.[29] In the 5 years that followed Gross's first successful operation, he reported 40 more cases.

The famous Blalock-Taussig operation also was first reported in 1945. The first patient was a 15-month-old girl with a clinical diagnosis of tetralogy of Fallot with a severe pulmonary stenosis.[30] At age 8 months, the baby had her first cyanotic spell, which occurred after eating. Dr. Helen Taussig, the cardiologist, followed the child for 3 months, and during that time, cyanosis increased, and the child failed to gain weight. The operation was performed by Dr. Alfred Blalock at Johns Hopkins University on November 29, 1944. The left subclavian artery was anastomosed to the left pulmonary artery in an end-to-side fashion. The postoperative course was described as stormy; the patient was discharged 2 months postoperatively. Two additional successful cases were done within 3 months of that first patient.

Thus, within a 7-year period, three congenital cardiovascular defects, patent ductus arteriosus, coarctation of the aorta, and vascular ring, were attacked surgically and treated successfully. However, the introduction of the Blalock-Taussig shunt probably was the most powerful stimulus to the development of cardiac surgery because this operation palliated a complex intracardiac lesion and focused attention on the pathophysiology of cardiac disease.

Anomalous coronary artery in which the left coronary artery communicates with the pulmonary artery was the next surgical conquest. The surgery was performed on July 22, 1946, and was reported by Gunnar Biorck and Clarence Crafoord.[31] The anomalous coronary artery was identified and doubly ligated. The patient made an uneventful recovery.

Muller[32] reported successful surgical treatment of transposition of the pulmonary veins in 1951, but the operation addressed a partial form of the anomaly. Later in the 1950s, Gott, Varco, Lillehei, and Cooley reported successful operative variations for anomalous pulmonary veins.

Another of Gross's pioneering surgical procedures was surgical closure of an aortopulmonary window on May 22, 1948.[33] Cooley and colleagues[34] were the first to report on the use of cardiopulmonary bypass to repair this defect and converted a difficult and hazardous procedure into a relatively straightforward one.

Glenn[35] reported the first successful clinical application of the cavopulmonary anastomosis in the United States in 1958 for what has been termed the *Glenn shunt*. Similar work was done in Russia during the 1950s by several investigators. On January 3, 1957, Galankin,[36] a Russian surgeon, performed a cavopulmonary anastomosis in a 16-year-old patient with tetralogy of Fallot. The patient made a good recovery with significant improvement in exercise tolerance and cyanosis.

THE DEVELOPMENT OF CARDIOPULMONARY BYPASS

The development of the heart-lung machine made repair of intracardiac lesions possible. To bypass the heart, one needs a basic understanding of the physiology of the circulation, a method of preventing the blood from clotting, a mechanism to pump blood, and finally, a method to ventilate the blood.

One of the key requirements of the heart-lung machine was anticoagulation. Heparin was discovered in 1915 by a medical student, Jay McLean, working in the laboratory of Dr. William Howell, a physiologist at Johns Hopkins.[37]

John Gibbon contributed more to the success of the development of the heart-lung machine than anyone else.

Gibbon's work on the heart-lung machine took place over 20 years in laboratories at Massachusetts General Hospital, the University of Pennsylvania, and Thomas Jefferson University. In 1937, Gibbon reported the first successful demonstration that life could be maintained by an artificial heart and lung and that the native heart and lungs could resume function. Unfortunately, only three animals recovered adequate cardiorespiratory function after total pulmonary artery occlusion and bypass, and even they died a few hours later.[38] Gibbon's work was interrupted by World War II; afterward, he resumed his work at Thomas Jefferson Medical College in Philadelphia (Table 1-1).

Forest Dodrill and colleagues used the mechanical blood pump they developed with General Motors on a 41-year-old man[43] (Fig. 1-3). The machine was used to substitute for the left ventricle for 50 minutes while a surgical procedure was carried out to repair the mitral valve; the patient's own lungs were used to oxygenate the blood. This, the first clinically successful total left-sided heart bypass in a human, was performed on July 3, 1952, and followed from Dodrill's experimental work with a mechanical pump for univentricular, biventricular, or cardiopulmonary bypass. Although Dodrill and colleagues had used their pump with an oxygenator for total heart bypass in animals,[54] they felt that left-sided heart bypass was the most practical method for their first clinical case.

Later, on October 21, 1952, Dodrill and colleagues used their machine in a 16-year-old boy with congenital pulmonary stenosis to perform a pulmonary valvuloplasty under direct vision; this was the first successful right-sided heart bypass.[44] Between July 1952 and December 1954, Dodrill performed approximately 13 clinical operations on the heart and thoracic aorta using the Dodrill—General Motors machine, with at least five hospital survivors.[55] Although he used this machine with an oxygenator in the animal laboratory, he did not start using an oxygenator with the Dodrill—General Motors mechanical heart clinically until early 1955.

Hypothermia was another method to stop the heart and allow it to be opened.[44]

John Lewis closed an atrial septal defect (ASD) in a 5-year-old girl on September 2, 1952 using a hypothermic technique.[44]

⊙ TABLE 1-1: Twilight Zone: Clinical Status of Open-Heart Surgery, 1951–1955

1951	*April 6:* Clarence Dennis at the University of Minnesota used a heart-lung machine to repair an ostium primum or AV canal defect in a 5-year-old girl. Patient could not be weaned from cardiopulmonary bypass.[39]
	May 31: Dennis attempted to close an atrial septal defect using heart-lung machine in a 2-year-old girl who died intraoperatively of a massive air embolus.[40]
	August 7: Achille Mario Digliotti at the University of Turino, Italy, used a heart-lung machine of his own design to partially support the circulation (flow at 1 L/min for 20 minutes) while he resected a large mediastinal tumor compressing the right side of the heart.[41] The cannulation was through the right axillary vein and artery. The patient survived. This was the first successful clinical use of a heart-lung machine, but the machine was not used as an adjunct to heart surgery.
1952	*February* (1952 or 1953 John Gibbon; see February 1953)
	March: John Gibbon used his heart-lung machine for right-sided heart bypass only while surgeon Frank Allbritten at Pennsylvania Hospital, Philadelphia, operated to remove a large clot or myxomatous tumor suspected by angiography.[42] No tumor or clot was found. The patient died of heart failure in the operating room shortly after discontinuing right-sided heart bypass.
	April 3: Helmsworth in Cincinnati used a pump oxygenator of his own design connecting it in a veno-veno bypass mode to temporarily treat a patient with end-stage lung disease. The patients symptoms improved but recurred shortly after bypass was discontinued.[60]
	July 3: Dodrill used the Dodrill-GMR pump to bypass the left side of the heart while he repaired a mitral valve.[43] The patient survived. This was the first successful use of a mechanical pump for total substitution of the left ventricle in a human being.
	September 2: John Lewis, at the University of Minnesota, closed an atrial septal defect under direct vision in a 5-year-old girl. The patient survived. This was the first successful clinical heart surgery procedure using total-body hypothermia. A mechanical pump and an oxygenator were not used. Others, including Dodrill, soon followed, using total-body hypothermia techniques to close atrial septal defects (ASDs) and perform pulmonary valvulotomies. By 1954, Lewis reported on 11 ASD closures using hypothermia with two hospital deaths.[44] He also operated on two patients with ventricular septal defect (VSD) in early 1954 using this technique. Both resulted in intraoperative deaths.
	October 21: Dodrill performed pulmonary valvulotomy under direct vision using Dodrill-GMR pump to bypass the right atrium, ventricle, and main pulmonary artery.[45] The patient survived.
	Although Dr. William Mustard in Toronto would describe a type of "corrective" surgical procedure for transposition of the great arteries (TGA) in 1964, which, in fact, for many years, would become the most popular form of surgical correction of TGA, his early results with this lesion were not good. In 1952, he used a mechanical pump coupled to the lung that had just been removed from a monkey to oxygenate the blood in seven children while attempts were made to correct their TGA defect.[46] There were no survivors.
1953	*February* (or 1952): Gibbon at Jefferson Hospital in Philadelphia operated to close an ASD. No ASD was found. The patient died intraoperatively. Autopsy showed a large patent ductus arteriosus.[47]
	May 6: Gibbon used his heart-lung machine to close an ASD in an 18-year-old woman with symptoms of heart failure.[47,57] The patient survived the operation and became the first patient to undergo successful open-heart surgery using a heart-lung machine.
	July: Gibbon used the heart-lung machine on two 5-year-old girls to close atrial septal defects.[47] Both died intraoperatively. Gibbon was extremely distressed and declared a moratorium on further cardiac surgery at Jefferson Medical School until more work could be done to solve problems related to heart-lung bypass. These were probably the last heart operation he performed using the heart-lung machine.
1954	*March 26:* C. Walton Lillehei and associates at the University of Minnesota closed a VSD under direct vision in a 15-month-old boy using a technique to support the circulation that they called *controlled cross-circulation*. An adult (usually a parent) with the same blood type was used more or less as the heart-lung machine. The adult's femoral artery and vein were connected with tubing and a pump to the patient's circulation. The adult's heart and lungs were oxygenated and supported the circulation while the child's heart defect was corrected. The first patient died 11 days postoperatively from pneumonia, but six of their next seven patients survived.[48] Between March 1954 and the end of 1955, 45 heart operations were performed by Lillehei on children using this technique before it was phased out. Although controlled cross-circulation was a short-lived technique, it was an important stepping stone in the development of open-heart surgery.
	July: Clarence Crafoord and associates at the Karolinska Institute in Stockholm, Sweden, used a heart-lung machine of their own design coupled with total-body hypothermia (patient was initially submerged in an ice-water bath) to remove a large atrial myxoma in a 40-year-old woman.[49] She survived.
1955	*March 22:* John Kirklin at the Mayo Clinic used a heart-lung machine similar to Gibbon's, but with modifications his team had worked out over 2 years in the research laboratory, to successfully close a VSD in a 5-year-old patient. By May of 1955, they had operated on eight children with various types of VSDs, and four were hospital survivors. This was the first successful series of patients (ie, more than one) to undergo heart surgery using a heart-lung machine.[50]
	May 13: Lillehei and colleagues began using a heart-lung machine of their own design to correct intracardiac defects. By May of 1956, their series included 80 patients.[48] Initially they used their heart-lung machine for lower-risk patients and used controlled cross-circulation, with which they were more familiar, for the higher-risk patients. Starting in March 1955, they also tried other techniques in patients to oxygenate blood during heart surgery, such as canine lung, but with generally poor results.[48]

(Continued)

TABLE 1-1: Twilight Zone: Clinical Status of Open-Heart Surgery, 1951–1955 (*Continued*)

1955	Dodrill had been performing heart operations with the GM heart pump since 1952 and used the patient's own lungs to oxygenate the blood. Early in the year 1955, he attempted repairs of VSDs in two patients using the heart pump, but with a mechanical oxygenator of his team's design both died. On December 1, he closed a VSD in a 3-year-old girl using his heart-lung machine. She survived. In May 1956 at the annual meeting of the American Association for Thoracic Surgery, he reported on six children with VSDs, including one with tetralogy of Fallot, who had undergone open-heart surgery using his heart-lung machine. All survived at least 48 hours postoperatively.[51] Three were hospital survivors, including the patient with tetralogy of Fallot.
	June 30: Clarence Dennis, who had moved from the University of Minnesota to the State University of New York, successfully closed an ASD in a girl using a heart-lung machine of his own design.[52]
	Mustard successfully repaired a VSD and dilated the pulmonary valve in a 9-month-old with a diagnosis of tetralogy of Fallot using a mechanical pump and a monkey lung to oxygenate the blood.[53] He did not give the date in 1955, but the patient is listed as Human Case 7. Unfortunately, in the same report, cases 1–6 and 8–15 operated on between 1951 and the end of 1955 with various congenital heart defects did not survive the surgery using the pump and monkey lung, nor did another seven children in 1952, all with TGA (see timeline for 1952) using the same bypass technique.

Note: This list is not all-inclusive but likely includes most of the historically significant clinical open-heart events in which a blood pump was used to support the circulation during this period. (A twilight zone can mean an ill-defined area between two distinct conditions, such as the area between darkness and light.)

The use of systemic hypothermia for open intracardiac surgery was relatively short-lived; after the heart-lung machine was introduced clinically, it appeared that deep hypothermia was obsolete. However, during the 1960s it became apparent that operative results in infants under 1 year of age using cardiopulmonary bypass were poor. In 1967, Hikasa and colleagues,[56] from Kyoto, Japan, published an article that reintroduced profound hypothermia for cardiac surgery in infants and used the heart-lung machine for rewarming. Their technique involved surface cooling to 20°C, cardiac

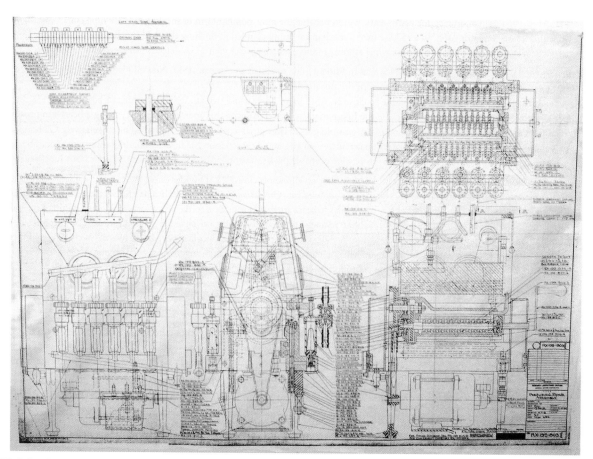

FIGURE 1-3 Blueprints by General Motors engineers of the Dodrill-GMR mechanical heart. (Used with permission from Calvin Hughes.)

surgery during circulatory arrest for 15 to 75 minutes, and rewarming with cardiopulmonary bypass. At the same time, other groups reported using profound hypothermia with circulatory arrest in infants with the heart-lung machine for cooling and rewarming. Results were much improved, and subsequently the technique also was applied for resection of aortic arch aneurysms.

After World War II, John Gibbon resumed his research. He eventually met Thomas Watson, chairman of the board of the International Business Machines (IBM) Corporation. Watson was fascinated by Gibbon's research and promised help. Soon afterward, six IBM engineers arrived and built a machine that was similar to Gibbon's earlier machine, which contained a rotating vertical cylinder oxygenator and a modified DeBakey rotary pump. Gibbon operated on a 15-month-old girl with severe congestive heart failure (CHF). The preoperative diagnosis was ASD, but at operation, none was found. She died, and a huge patent ductus was found at autopsy. The next patient was an 18-year-old girl with CHF owing to an ASD. This defect was closed successfully on May 6, 1953, with the Gibbon-IBM heart-lung machine.

The patient recovered, and several months later the defect was confirmed closed at cardiac catheterization.[57] Unfortunately, Gibbon's next two patients did not survive intracardiac procedures when the heart-lung machine was used. These failures distressed Dr. Gibbon, who declared a 1-year moratorium for the heart-lung machine until more work could be done to solve the problems causing the deaths.

During this period, C. Walton Lillehei and colleagues at the University of Minnesota studied a technique called *controlled cross-circulation*.[58] With this technique, the circulation of one dog was used temporarily to support that of a second dog while the second dog's heart was stopped temporarily and opened. After a simulated repair in the second dog, the animals were disconnected and allowed to recover.

Lillehei and colleagues[58] used their technique at the University of Minnesota to correct a ventricular septal defect (VSD) in a 12-month-old infant on March 26, 1954 (Fig. 1-4). Either a parent or a close relative with the same blood type was connected to the child's circulation. In Lillehei's first clinical case, the patient made an uneventful recovery until death on the eleventh postoperative day from a

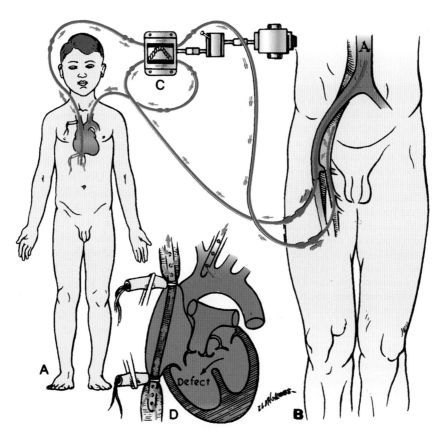

FIGURE 1-4 A depiction of the method of direct-vision intracardiac surgery using extracorporeal circulation by controlled cross-circulation. (A) The patient, showing sites of arterial and venous cannulations. (B) The donor, showing sites of arterial and venous (superficial femoral and great saphenous) cannulations. (C) The Sigma motor pump controlling precisely the reciprocal exchange of blood between the patient and donor. (D) Close-up of the patient's heart, showing the vena caval catheter positioned to draw venous blood from both the superior and inferior venae cavae during the cardiac bypass interval. The arterial blood from the donor circulated to the patient's body through the catheter that was inserted into the left subclavian artery. (Reproduced with permission from Lillehei CW, Cohen M, Warden HE, et al: The results of direct vision closure of ventricular septal defects in eight patients by means of controlled cross circulation, *Surg Gynecol Obstet.* 1955 Oct;101(4):446-466.)

rapidly progressing tracheal bronchitis. At autopsy, the VSD was closed, and the respiratory infection was confirmed as the cause of death. Two weeks later, the second and third patients had VSDs closed by the same technique 3 days apart. Both remained long-term survivors with normal hemodynamics confirmed by cardiac catheterization.

In 1955, Lillehei and colleagues[59] published a report of 32 patients that included repairs of VSDs, tetralogy of Fallot, and atrioventricularis communis defects. By May of 1955, the blood pump used for systemic cross-circulation by Lillehei and colleagues was coupled with a bubble oxygenator developed by Drs. DeWall and Lillehei, and cross-circulation was soon abandoned after use in 45 patients during 1954 and 1955. Although its clinical use was short-lived, cross-circulation was an important steppingstone in the development of cardiac surgery.

Meanwhile, at the Mayo Clinic only 90 miles away, John W. Kirklin and colleagues launched their open-heart program on March 5, 1955.[50] They used a heart-lung machine based on the Gibbon-IBM machine but with their own modifications. Kirklin wrote:[61]

> We investigated and visited the groups working intensively with the mechanical pump oxygenators. We visited Dr. Gibbon in his laboratories in Philadelphia, and Dr. Forest Dodrill in Detroit, among others. The Gibbon pump oxygenator had been developed and made by the International Business Machine Corporation and looked quite a bit like a computer. Dr. Dodrill's heart-lung machine had been developed and built for him by General Motors and it looked a great deal like a car engine. We came home, reflected and decided to try to persuade the Mayo Clinic to let us build a pump oxygenator similar to the Gibbon machine, but somewhat different. We already had had about a year's experience in the animal laboratory with David Donald using a simple pump and bubble oxygenator when we set about very early in 1953, the laborious task of building a Mayo-Gibbon pump oxygenator and continuing the laboratory research.
>
> Most people were very discouraged with the laboratory progress. The American Heart Association and the National Institutes of Health had stopped funding any projects for the study of heart-lung machines, because it was felt that the problem was physiologically insurmountable. David Donald and I undertook a series of laboratory experiments lasting about 1½ years during which time the engineering shops at the Mayo Clinic constructed a pump oxygenator based on the Gibbon model.
>
> … In the winter of 1954 and 1955 we had nine surviving dogs out of 10 cardiopulmonary bypass runs. With my wonderful colleague and pediatric cardiologist, Jim DuShane, we had earlier selected eight patients for intracardiac repair. Two had to be put off because two babies with very serious congenital heart disease came along and we decided to fit them into the schedule. We had determined to do all eight patients even if the first seven died. All of this was planned with the knowledge and approval of the governance of the Mayo Clinic. Our plan was then to return to the laboratory and spend the next 6 to 12 months solving the problems that had arisen in the first planned clinical trial of a pump oxygenator. … We did our first open-heart operation on a Tuesday in March 1955.

Kirklin continued:[61]

> Four of our first eight patients survived, but the press of the clinical work prevented our ever being able to return to the laboratory with the force that we had planned. By now, Walt Lillehei and I were on parallel, but intertwined paths.

By the end of 1956, many university groups around the world had launched into open-heart programs. Currently, it is estimated that more than 1 million cardiac operations are performed each year worldwide with use of the heart-lung machine. In most cases, the operative mortality is quite low, approaching 1% for some operations. Little thought is given to the courageous pioneers in the 1950s whose monumental contributions made all this possible.

Extracorporeal Life Support

Extracorporeal life support (ECLS) is an extension of cardiopulmonary bypass. Cardiopulmonary bypass was limited initially to no more than 6 hours. The development of membrane oxygenators in the 1960s permitted longer support. Donald Hill and colleagues in 1972 treated a 24-year-old man who developed shock lung after blunt trauma.[62] The patient was supported for 75 hours using a heart-lung machine with a membrane oxygenator, cannulated via the femoral vein and artery. The patient was weaned and recovered. Hill's second patient was supported for 5 days and recovered. This led to a randomized trial supported by the National Institutes of Health to determine the efficacy of this therapy for adults with respiratory failure. The study was conducted from 1972 to 1975 and showed no significant difference in survival between patients managed by ECLS (9.5%) and those who received conventional ventilatory therapy (8.3%).[63] Because of these results, most U.S. centers abandoned efforts to support adult patients using ECLS, also known as *extracorporeal membrane oxygenation* (ECMO).

One participant in the adult trial decided to study neonates. The usual causes of neonatal respiratory failure have in common abnormal postnatal blood shunts known as *persistent fetal circulation* (PFC). This is a temporary, reversible phenomenon. In 1976, Bartlett and colleagues at the University of Michigan were the first to treat a neonate successfully using ECLS. More than 8000 neonatal patients have been treated using ECLS worldwide, with a survival rate of 82% (ELSO registry data).

MYOCARDIAL PROTECTION

Melrose and colleagues[64] in 1955 presented the first experimental study describing induced arrest by potassium-based cardioplegia. Blood cardioplegia was used "to preserve myocardial energy stores at the onset of cardiac ischemia." Unfortunately, the Melrose solution proved to be toxic to the myocardium, and as a result cardioplegia was not used widely for several years.

Gay and Ebert[65] and Tyres and colleagues[66] demonstrated that cardioplegia with lower potassium concentrations was safe. Studies by Kirsch and colleagues,[67] Bretschneider and colleagues,[68] and Hearse and colleagues[69] demonstrated the effectiveness of cardioplegia with other constituents and renewed interest in this technique. Gay and Ebert in 1973 demonstrated a significant reduction in myocardial oxygen consumption during potassium-induced arrest when compared with that of the fibrillating heart.[65] They also showed that the problems in the use of the Melrose solution in the early days of cardiac surgery probably were caused by its hyperosmolar properties and perhaps not the high potassium concentration.

In a 1978 publication by Follette and colleagues,[70] the technique of blood cardioplegia was reintroduced. In experimental and clinical studies, these authors demonstrated that hypothermic, intermittent blood cardioplegia provided better myocardial protection than normothermic, continuous coronary perfusion and/or hypothermic, intermittent blood perfusion without cardioplegia solution. The composition of the best cardioplegia solution remains controversial, and new formulations, methods of delivery, and recommended temperatures continue to evolve.

EVOLUTION OF CONGENITAL CARDIAC SURGERY DURING THE ERA OF CARDIOPULMONARY BYPASS

With the advent of cardiopulmonary bypass using either the cross-circulation technique of Lillehei and colleagues or the version of the mechanical heart-lung machine used by Kirklin and colleagues, the two groups led the way for intracardiac repairs for many of the commonly occurring congenital heart defects. Because of the morbidity associated with the heart-lung machine, palliative operations also were developed to improve circulatory physiology without directly addressing the anatomic pathology. These palliative operations included the Blalock-Taussig subclavian–pulmonary arterial shunt[30] with modifications by Potts and colleagues[71] and Waterston,[72] the Blalock-Hanlon operation to create an ASD,[73] and the Galankin-Glenn superior vena cava–right pulmonary arterial shunt.[35,36]

As the safety of cardiopulmonary bypass improved steadily, surgeons addressed more and more complex abnormalities of the heart in younger and younger patients. Some of the milestones in the development of operations to correct congenital heart defects using cardiopulmonary bypass appear in Table 1-2.

VALVULAR SURGERY: CARDIOPULMONARY BYPASS ERA

Cardiac valve repair or replacement under direct vision awaited the development of the heart-lung machine. The first successful aortic valve replacement (AVR) in the subcoronary position was performed by Dr. Dwight Harken and associates.[91] A caged-ball valve was used. Many of the techniques described in Harken's 1960 report are similar to those used today for AVR.

That same year, Starr and Edwards[92] successfully replaced the mitral valve using a caged-ball valve of their own design.

By 1967, nearly 2000 Starr-Edwards valves had been implanted, and the caged-ball-valve prosthesis was established as the standard against which all other mechanical prostheses would be compared.

In 1964, Starr and colleagues reported 13 patients who had undergone multiple valve replacement.[93] One patient had the aortic, mitral, and tricuspid valves replaced on February 21, 1963. Cartwright and colleagues, however, on November 1, 1961, were the first to replace both the aortic and mitral valves successfully with ball-valve prostheses that they had developed.[94] Knott-Craig and colleagues,[95] from the Mayo Clinic, successfully replaced all four heart valves in a patient with carcinoid involvement.

In 1961, Andrew Morrow and Edwin Brockenbrough[96] reported a treatment for idiopathic hypertrophic subaortic stenosis by resecting a portion of the thickened ventricular septum. They referred to this as *subaortic ventriculomyotomy*. They gave credit to William Cleland and H.H. Bentall in London, who had encountered this condition unexpectedly at operation and resected a small portion of the ventricular mass. The patient improved, but no postoperative hemodynamic studies had been reported. The subaortic ventriculomyotomy became the standard surgical treatment for this cardiac anomaly, although in some patients systolic anterior motion (SAM) of the anterior leaflet of the mitral valve necessitates mitral valve replacement with a low-profile mechanical valve.

An aortic homograft valve was used clinically for the first time by Heimbecker and colleagues in Toronto for replacement of the mitral valve in one patient and an aortic valve in another.[97] Survival was short, 1 day in one patient and 1 month in the other. Donald Ross reported on the first successful aortic valve placement with an aortic valve homograft.[98] He used a technique of subcoronary implantation developed in the laboratory by Carlos Duran and Alfred Gunning in Oxford.

The technique of AVR with a pulmonary autograft described initially by Ross in 1967 is advocated by some groups for younger patients who require AVR.[99] An aortic or pulmonary valve homograft is used to replace the pulmonary valve that has been transferred to the aortic position.

Other autogenous materials that have been used to manufacture valve prostheses include pericardium, fasciae latae, and dura mater. In the 1960s, Binet and colleagues[100] began to develop and test tissue valves. In 1964, Duran and Gunning in England replaced an aortic valve in a patient using a xenograft porcine aortic valve. Early results with formaldehyde-fixed xenografts were good,[100] but in a few years these valves began to fail because of tissue degeneration and calcification.[101] Carpentier and colleagues revitalized interest in xenograft valves by fixating porcine valves with glutaraldehyde. Carpentier also mounted his valves on a stent to produce a bioprosthesis. Carpentier-Edwards porcine valves and Hancock and Angell-Shiley bioprostheses became popular and were implanted in large numbers of patients.[102,103]

With the development of cardiopulmonary bypass, valves could be approached under direct vision, and for the first

⬤ TABLE 1-2: First Successful Intracardiac Repairs Using Cardiopulmonary Bypass or Cross-Circulation

Lesion	Year	Reference	Comment
Atrial septal defect	1953	Gibbon[57]	May 6, 1953
Ventricular septal defect	1954	Lillehei et al[58]	Cross-circulation
Complete atrioventricular canal	1954	Lillehei et al[59]	Cross-circulation
Tetralogy of Fallot	1954	Lillehei et al[58]	Cross-circulation
Tetralogy of Fallot	1955	Kirklin[50]	Cardiopulmonary bypass (CPB)
Total anomalous pulmonary veins	1956	Burroughs and Kirklin[74]	
Congenital aneurysm sinus of Valsalva	1956	McGoon et al[75]	
Congenital aortic stenosis	1956	Ellis and Kirklin[76]	First direct visual correction
Aortopulmonary window	1957	Cooley et al[77]	First closure using CPB
Double outlet right ventricle	1957	Kirklin et al[78]	Extemporarily devised correction
Corrected transposition great arteries	1957	Anderson et al[79]	
Transposition of great arteries: atrial switch	1959	Senning[80]	Physiologic total correction
Coronary arteriovenous fistula	1959	Swan et al[81]	
Ebstein's anomaly	1964	Hardy et al[82]	Repair of atrialized tricuspid valve
Tetralogy with pulmonary atresia	1966	Ross and Somerville[83]	Used aortic allograft
Truncus arteriosus	1967	McGoon et al[84]	Used aortic allograft
Tricuspid atresia	1968	Fontan and Baudet[85]	Physiologic correction
Single ventricle	1970	Horiuchi et al[86]	
Subaortic tunnel stenosis	1975	Konno et al[87]	
Transposition of great arteries: arterial switch	1975	Jatene et al[88]	Anatomic correction
Hypoplastic left heart syndrome	1983	Norwood et al[89]	Two-stage operation
Pediatric heart transplantation	1985	Bailey et al[90]	

time, mitral insufficiency could be attacked by reparative techniques. Techniques for mitral annuloplasty were described by Wooler and colleagues,[104] Reed and colleagues,[105] and Kay and colleagues.[106] The next step forward was development of annuloplasty rings by Carpentier and Duran. In the 1970s, few groups were involved in valve repairs. Slowly, techniques evolved, were tested clinically, and were followed over the years. Carpentier led the field by establishing the importance of careful analysis of valve pathology, describing in detail several techniques of valve repair, and reporting good results after early and late follow-up, especially with concomitant use of annuloplasty rings.[107]

From 1966 to 1968, a small epidemic of infective endocarditis in Detroit among heroin addicts broke out. Patients were dying of intractable gram-negative tricuspid valve endocarditis, often caused by *Pseudomonas aeruginosa*. Long-term antibiotic administration in combination with tricuspid valve replacement was 100% fatal. Starting in 1970, Arbulu operated on 55 patients; in 53, the tricuspid valve was removed without replacing it.[108,109] At 25 years, the actuarial survival is 61%.

Alan Cribier in Rouen France was first to successfully perform a transcatheter aortic valve insertion in a patient on

April 16, 2002.[110] Prospective clinical trials soon followed, which demonstrated that percutaneous aortic valve insertion improved 1 year survival compared to medically treated patients with critical aortic stenosis, and that this procedure had similar 30-day and 1-year mortalities when compared to the standard surgical procedure. There was, however, an increased rate of stroke/transient ischemic attack (TIA) with percutaneous approach.[111, 112]

CORONARY ARTERY SURGERY

Selective coronary angiography was developed by Sones and Shirey at the Cleveland Clinic and reported in their 1962 classic paper entitled, "Cine Coronary Arteriography."[113] They used a catheter to inject contrast material directly into the coronary artery ostia. This technique gave a major impetus to direct revascularization of obstructed coronary arteries.

From 1960 to 1967, several sporadic instances of coronary grafting were reported. All were isolated cases and, for uncertain reasons, were not reproduced. None had an impact on the development of coronary surgery. Dr. Robert H. Goetz performed what appears to be the first clearly documented coronary artery bypass operation in a human, which was successful. The surgery took place at Van Etten Hospital in New York City on May 2, 1960.[114] He operated on a 38-year-old man who was severely symptomatic and used a nonsuture technique to connect the right internal mammary artery to a right coronary artery. It took him 17 seconds to join the two arteries using a hollow metal tube. The right internal mammary artery–coronary artery connection was confirmed patent by angiography performed on the 14th postoperative day. The patient remained asymptomatic for about a year and then developed recurrent angina and died of a myocardial infarction on June 23, 1961. Goetz was severely criticized by his medical and surgical colleagues for this procedure, although he had performed it successfully many times in the animal laboratory. He never attempted another coronary bypass operation in a human.

Another example involved a case of autogenous saphenous vein bypass grafting performed on November 23, 1964, in a 42-year-old man who was scheduled to have endarterectomy of his left coronary artery.[115] Because the lesion involved the entire bifurcation, endarterectomy with venous patch graft was abandoned as too hazardous. The authors, Garrett, Dennis, and DeBakey, however, did not report this case until 1973. The patient was alive at that time, and angiograms showed the vein graft to be patent.

Shumaker[116] credits Longmire with the first internal mammary–coronary artery anastomosis. "It was almost surely Longmire, long-time chairman at UCLA, and his associate, Jack Cannon, who first performed an anastomosis between the internal mammary artery and a coronary branch, probably in early 1958."

The reference that Shumaker gives for this quotation from Longmire is a personal communication to Shumaker in 1990, which was 32 years after the fact!

As early as 1952, Vladimir Demikhov, the renowned Soviet surgeon, was anastomosing the internal mammary artery to the left coronary artery in dogs.[117] In 1967, at the height of the Cold War, a Soviet surgeon from Leningrad, V. I. Kolessov, reported his experience with mammary artery–coronary artery anastomoses for the treatment of angina pectoris in six patients in an American surgical journal.[118] The first patient in that series was done in 1964. Operations were performed through a left thoracotomy without extracorporeal circulation or preoperative coronary angiography. The following year, Green and colleagues[119] and Bailey and Hirose[120] separately published reports in which the internal mammary artery was used for coronary artery bypass in patients.

Rene Favalaro from the Cleveland Clinic used saphenous vein for bypassing coronary obstructions.[121] Favalaro's 1968 article focused on 15 patients, who were part of a larger series of 180 patients who had undergone the Vineberg procedure. In these 15 patients with occlusion of the proximal right coronary artery, an interpositional graft of saphenous vein also was placed between the ascending aorta and the right coronary artery distal to the blockage. The right coronary artery was divided, and the vein graft was anastomosed end to end. Favalaro states that this procedure was done because of the unfavorable results with pericardial patch reconstruction

of the coronary artery. In an addendum to that paper, 55 patients were added, 52 for segmental occlusion of the right coronary and 3 others for circumflex disease.

The contributions by Favalaro, Kolessov, Green and colleagues, and Bailey and Hirose all were important, but arguably the official start of coronary bypass surgery as we know it today happened in 1969 when W. Dudley Johnson and coworkers from Milwaukee reported their series of 301 patients who had undergone various operations for coronary artery disease (CAD) since February of 1967.[122] In that report, the authors presented their results with direct coronary artery surgery during a 19-month period. They state:

> After two initial and successful patch grafts, the vein bypass technique has been used exclusively. Early results were so encouraging that last summer the vein graft technique was expanded and used to all major branches. Vein grafts to the left side of the arteries run from the aorta over the pulmonary artery and down to the appropriate coronary vessel. Right-sided grafts run along the atrioventricular groove and also attach directly to the aorta. There is almost no limit of potential (coronary) arteries to use. Veins can be sutured to the distal anterior descending or even to posterior marginal branches. Double vein grafts are now used in more than 40% of patients and can be used to any combination of arteries.

Johnson goes on to say:

> Our experience indicates that five factors are important to direct surgery. One: Do not limit grafts to proximal portions of large arteries. ... Two: Do not work with diseased arteries. Vein grafts can be made as long as necessary and should be inserted into distal normal arteries. Three: Always do end-to-side anastomoses. ... Four: Always work on a dry, quiet field. Consistently successful fine vessel anastomoses cannot be done on a moving, bloody target. ... Five: Do not allow the hematocrit to fall below 35.

In discussing Dr. Johnson's presentation, Dr. Frank Spencer commented:

> I would like to congratulate Dr. Johnson very heartily. We may have heard a milestone in cardiac surgery today. Because for years, pathologists, cardiologists, and many surgeons have repeatedly stated that the pattern of coronary artery disease is so extensive that direct anastomosis can be done in only 5 to 7% of patients. If the exciting data by Dr. Johnson remain valid and the grafts remain patent over a long period of time, a total revision of thinking will be required regarding the feasibility of direct arterial surgery for CAD.[122]

The direct anastomosis between the internal mammary artery and the coronary artery was not as popular initially as the vein-graft technique; however, owing to the persistence of Drs. Green, Loop, Grondin, and others, internal mammary artery grafts eventually became the conduit of choice when their superior long-term patency became known.[123]

Andreas Gruntzig working in Zurich, Switzerland, was the first to successfully dilate a stenotic coronary artery in a patient, percutaneously and used a balloon-tip catheter he had developed. The procedure was performed on September 16, 1977, on a 38-year-old woman with an 85% stenosis of the left anterior descending coronary artery. In 1979, he reported on the first 50 patients to undergo percutaneous transluminal coronary angioplasty (PTCA).[124] However despite the almost instant popularity of this procedure in the Western world, it was soon found that the restenosis rate was relatively high when compared with that of coronary bypass surgery, and there was also risk of sudden closure of the artery in the area that had been dilated.

Research in the animal laboratory with stents was carried out in the hope of solving these problems.

Jacque Puel in Toulouse, France, and shortly afterward, Ulrich Sigwart in Lausanne, Switzerland, were first to implant stents in patient's coronary arteries in the spring of 1986.[125–128] Although stents improved the results of PTCA and significantly decreased the incidence of acute coronary closure, the long-term patency rates in general were not as good as those in coronary bypass surgery. Therefore, stents that were impregnated with drugs or other chemicals were developed, which would be slowly released with hopes of decreasing the restenosis rate. Clinical trials with these drug-eluting types of stents began in 2003 and indicate they are associated with a decrease in restenosis rates.

Denton Cooley and colleagues made two important contributions to the surgery for ischemic heart disease.[129] In 1956, with the use of cardiopulmonary bypass, they were the first to repair a ruptured interventricular septum following acute myocardial infarction. The patient did well initially but died of complications 6 weeks after the operation. Cooley and colleagues also were the first to report the resection of a left ventricular aneurysm with the use of cardiopulmonary bypass.[130]

ARRHYTHMIC SURGERY

Cobb and colleagues at Duke University developed the first successful surgical treatment for cardiac arrhythmias.[131] A 32-year-old fisherman was referred for symptomatic episodes of atrial tachycardia that caused CHF. On May 2, 1968, after epicardial mapping, a 5- to 6-cm cut was made extending from the base of the right atrial appendage to the right border of the right atrium during cardiopulmonary bypass. The incision transected the conduction pathway between the atrium and ventricle. Subsequent epicardial mapping indicated eradication of the pathway. Six weeks after the operation, heart size had decreased and lung fields had cleared. The patient eventually returned to work.

A year earlier, Dr. Dwight McGoon at the Mayo Clinic closed an ASD in a patient who also had Wolff-Parkinson-White (WPW) syndrome.[132] At operation, Dr. Birchell mapped the epicardium of the heart and localized the accessory pathway to the right atrioventricular groove. Lidocaine was injected into the site, and the delta wave disappeared immediately. Unfortunately, conduction across the pathway reappeared a few hours later. This probably was the first attempt to treat the WPW syndrome surgically. As a result of knowledge gained from the surgical treatment for WPW syndrome, more than 95% of all refractory clinical cases now are treated successfully by nonsurgical means.[132]

Ross and colleagues[133] in Sydney, Australia, and Cox and colleagues[134] in St. Louis, Missouri, used cryosurgical treatment of atrial ventricular node re-entry tachycardia. Subsequently, James L. Cox, after years of laboratory research, developed the Maze operation for atrial fibrillation.[135] That technique, with his subsequent modifications, is now known as the *Cox Maze procedure* and has become the world standard with which other techniques used to treat atrial fibrillation, either surgically or with catheters, are compared.[136]

Guiraudon and colleagues,[136] from Paris, reported their results with an encircling endomyocardial ventriculotomy for the treatment of malignant ventricular arrhythmias. The following year, in 1979, Josephson and colleagues[137] described a more specific procedure for treatment of malignant ventricular arrhythmias. After endocardial mapping, the endocardial source of the arrhythmia was excised. Although the Guiraudon technique usually isolated the source of the arrhythmia, the incision also devascularized healthy myocardium and was associated with high mortality. Endocardial resection was safer and more efficacious and became the basis of all approaches for the treatment of ischemic ventricular tachycardia.[137]

Stimulated by the death of a close personal friend from ventricular arrhythmias, Dr. Mirowski developed a prototype defibrillator over a 3-month period in 1969. In 1980, Mirowski and colleagues described three successful cases using their implantable myocardial stimulator at Johns Hopkins.[138]

Soon a version of Mirowski's defibrillator was commercially available. Initially centers implanting them were part of the clinical trials being conducted and required Food and Drug Administration (FDA) approval. The chest needed to be opened to place the relatively large electrodes directly on the ventricles. The battery used to power the device and generate the electrical shock was also large and was usually placed in the abdominal wall. Within 10 years, smaller, more advanced ventricular leads were developed and inserted percutaneously through the venous system. The battery was made much smaller in size. During the 1990s, clinical trials were conducted, which showed the automatic implantable cardiac defibrillators decreased mortality when compared to medically treated patients in subsets of patients prone to ventricular tachycardia and fibrillation. As a result of these findings, the use of these devices has increased significantly.[139, 140]

PACEMAKERS

In 1952, Paul Zoll applied electric shocks 2 ms in duration that were transmitted through the chest wall at frequencies from 25 to 60 per minute and increased the intensity of the shock until ventricular responses were observed. However, after 25 minutes of intermittent stimulation the patient died, although many subsequent patients recovered.[141] The next step came when Lillehei and colleagues reported a series of patients who had external pacing after open-heart surgery during the 1950s.[142] The field of open-heart surgery gave a major impetus to the development of pacemakers because there was a high incidence of heart block following many intracardiac repairs. The major difference between Zoll's pacing and that of Lillehei and colleagues was that Zoll used external electrodes placed on the chest wall, whereas Lillehei and colleagues attached electrodes directly to the heart at operation. Lillehei and colleagues used a relatively small external pacemaker to stimulate the heart and much less electric current. This form of heart pacing was better tolerated by the patient and was a more efficient way to stimulate the heart. The survival rate of Lillehei's patients with surgically induced heart block was improved significantly.

During this period, progress was made toward a totally implantable pacemaker. Elmquist and Senning[143] developed a pacer battery that was small enough for an epigastric pocket with electrodes connected to the heart. They implanted the unit in a patient with atrioventricular block in 1958. Just before implantation, the patient had 20 to 30 cardiac arrests a day. The first pacemaker that was implanted functioned only 8 hours; the second pacemaker implanted in the same patient had better success. The patient survived until January 2002 and had many additional pacemakers. Chardack and colleagues are perhaps better known for their development of the totally implantable pacemaker.[144] In 1961, they reported a series of 15 patients who had pacemakers that they had developed implanted.

Early implantable pacemakers were fixed-rate, asynchronous devices that delivered an impulse independent of the underlying cardiac rhythm. During the past 40 years, enormous progress has been made in the field of pacing technology. The number of individuals with artificial pacemakers is unknown; however, estimates indicate that approximately 500,000 Americans are living with a pacemaker and that each year another 100,000 or more patients require permanent pacemakers in the United States.

HEART, HEART-LUNG, AND LUNG TRANSPLANTATION

Alexis Carrel and Charles Guthrie reported transplantation of the heart and lungs while at the University of Chicago in 1905.[145] The heart of a small dog was transplanted into the neck of a larger one by anastomosing the caudad ends of the jugular vein and carotid artery to the aorta and pulmonary artery. The animal was not anticoagulated, and the experiment ended about 2 hours after circulation was established because of blood clot in the cavities of the transplanted heart.

Vladimir Demikhov, from Russia, described more than 20 different techniques for heart transplantation in 1950.[146] He also published various techniques for heart and lung transplantation. He was even able to perform an orthotopic heart transplant in a dog before the heart-lung machine was developed. This was accomplished by placing the donor heart above the dog's own heart, and then with a series of tubes and connections, he rerouted the blood from one heart to the other until he had the donor heart functioning in the appropriate position and the native heart removed. One of his dogs climbed the steps of the Kremlin on the sixth postoperative day but died shortly afterward of rejection.

Richard Lower and Norman Shumway established the technique for heart transplantation as it is performed today.[147] Preservation of the cuff of recipient left and right atria with part of the atrial septum was described earlier by Brock[148] in England and Demikhov[117] in Russia,[149] but it became popular only after Shumway and Lower reported it in their 1960 paper.

The first attempt at human heart transplantation was made by Hardy and colleagues[150] at the University of Mississippi. Because no human donor organ was available at the time, a large chimpanzee's heart was used; however, it was unable to support the circulation because of hyperacute rejection.

The first human-to-human heart transplant occurred on December 3, 1967, in Capetown, South Africa.[151] The surgical team, headed by Christiaan Barnard, transplanted the heart of a donor who had been certified dead after the electrocardiogram showed no activity for 5 minutes into a 54-year-old man whose heart was irreparably damaged by repeated myocardial infarctions. The second human heart transplant using a human donor was performed on a child 3 days after the first on December 6, 1967, by Adrian Kantrowitz in Brooklyn, New York. Dr. Kantrowitz's patient died of a bleeding complication within the first 24 hours.[152] Barnard's patient, Lewis Washkansky, died on the 18th postoperative day. At autopsy, the heart appeared normal, and there was no evidence of chronic liver congestion, but bilateral pneumonia was present, possibly owing to severe myeloid depression from immunosuppression.[153]

On January 2, 1968, Barnard performed a second heart transplant on Phillip Blaiberg, 12 days after Washkansky's death.[154] Blaiberg was discharged from the hospital and became a celebrity during the several months he lived after the transplant. Blaiberg's procedure indicated that a heart transplant was an option for humans suffering from end-stage heart disease. Within a year of Barnard's first heart transplant, 99 heart transplants had been performed by cardiac surgeons around the world. However, by the end of 1968, most groups abandoned heart transplantation because of the extremely high mortality related to rejection. Shumway and Lower, Barnard, and a few others persevered both clinically and in the laboratory. Their efforts in discovering better drugs for immunosuppression eventually established heart transplantation as we know it today.

A clinical trial of heart-lung transplantation was commenced at Stanford University in 1981 by Reitz and colleagues.[155] Their first patient was treated with a combination of cyclosporine and azathioprine. The patient was discharged from the hospital in good condition and was well more than 5 years after the transplant.

The current success with heart, heart-lung, and lung transplantation is related in part to the discovery of cyclosporine by workers at the Sandoz Laboratory in Basel, Switzerland, in 1970. In December of 1980, cyclosporine was introduced at Stanford for cardiac transplantation. The incidence of rejection was not reduced, nor was the incidence of infection. However, these two major complications of cardiac transplantation were less severe when cyclosporine was used. Availability of cyclosporine stimulated many new programs across the United States in the mid-1980s.

The first human lung transplant was performed by Hardy and colleagues[156] at the University of Mississippi on June 11, 1964. The patient died on the 17th postoperative day. In 1971, a Belgian surgeon, Fritz Derom, achieved a 10-month survival in a patient with pulmonary silicosis.[157]

Much of the credit, however, for the success of lung transplantation belongs to the Toronto group, whose efforts were headed by Joel Cooper. Their successes were based on laboratory experimentation and the discovery of cyclosporine. After losing an early patient to bronchial anastomotic dehiscence in 1978, the group substituted cyclosporine for cortisone and wrapped the bronchial suture line with a pedicle of omentum. They also developed a comprehensive preoperative preparation program that increased the strength and nutritional status of the recipients. In 1986, Cooper and associates presented their first two successful patients, who had returned to normal activities and were alive 14 and 26 months after operation.[158]

HEART ASSIST AND ARTIFICIAL HEARTS

In 1963, Kantrowitz and colleagues reported the first use of the intra-aortic balloon pump (IABP) in three patients.[159] All were in cardiogenic shock but improved during balloon pumping. One survived to leave the hospital.

In 1963, Liotta and colleagues reported a 42-year-old man who had a stenotic aortic valve replaced but suffered a cardiac arrest the following morning.[160] The patient was resuscitated but developed severe ventricular failure. An artificial intrathoracic circulatory pump was implanted. The patient's pulmonary edema cleared, but he died 4 days later with the pump working continuously. In 1966, the same group used a newer intrathoracic pump to support another patient who could not be weaned from cardiopulmonary bypass. This pump maintained the circulation. The patient eventually died before the pump could be removed.[161] Later that year, the same group used a left ventricular assist device (LVAD) in a woman who could not be weaned from cardiopulmonary bypass after double valve replacement.[162] After 10 days of circulatory assistance, the patient was weaned successfully from the device and recovered. This woman was probably the first patient to be weaned from an assist device and leave the hospital.

The first human application of a totally artificial heart was by Denton Cooley and colleagues as a "bridge" to transplantation.[163] They implanted a totally artificial heart in a patient who could not be weaned from cardiopulmonary bypass. After 64 hours of artificial heart support, heart transplantation was performed, but the patient died of *Pseudomonas* pneumonia 32 hours after transplantation. The first two patients bridged successfully to transplantation were reported

at almost the same time and in the same location by different groups. On September 5, 1984, in San Francisco,[164] Donald Hill implanted a Pierce-Donachy LVAD in a patient in cardiogenic shock. The patient received a successful transplant 2 days later and was discharged subsequently. The assist device used by Hill was developed at Pennsylvania State University by Pierce and Donachy. Phillip Oyer and colleagues at Stanford University placed an electrically driven Novacor LVAD in a patient in cardiogenic shock on September 7, 1984.[165] The patient was transplanted successfully and survived beyond 3 years. The device used by the Stanford group was developed by Peer Portner.

The first implantation of a permanent totally artificial heart (Jarvik-7) was performed by DeVries and colleagues at the University of Utah in 1982.[166] By 1985, they had implanted the Jarvik in four patients, and one survived for 620 days after implantation. This initial clinical experience was based heavily on the work of Kolff and colleagues.

THORACIC AORTA SURGERY

Alexis Carrel was responsible for one of the great surgical advances of the twentieth century: techniques for suturing and transplanting blood vessels.[167] Although Carrel initially developed his methods of blood vessel anastomosis in Lyon, France, his work with Charles Guthrie in Chicago led to many major advances in vascular, cardiac, and transplantation surgery. In a short period of time, these investigators perfected techniques for blood vessel anastomoses and transposition of arterial and venous segments using both fresh and frozen grafts. After leaving Chicago, Carrel continued to expand his work on blood vessels and organ transplantation and in 1912 received the Nobel Prize. Interestingly, Carrel's work did not receive immediate clinical application.

Rudolph Matas pioneered clinical vascular surgery. Matas' work took place before drugs were available to prevent blood clotting, before antibiotics, and without reliable blood vessel substitutes.[168] Matas performed 620 vascular operations between 1888 and 1940. Only 101 of these were attempts to repair arteries; most involved ligation. Matas developed three variations of his well-known endoaneurysmorrhaphy procedure. The most advanced was to reconstruct the wall of the blood vessel from within while using a rubber tube as a stent.

Vascular surgery advanced tentatively during World War II as traumatic injuries to major blood vessels were repaired in some soldiers with results significantly better than with the standard treatment of ligation.[169] The successful treatment of coarctation of the aorta by Crafoord and Gross added a major boost to the reconstructive surgery of arteries.

Shumaker reported the excision of a small descending thoracic aortic aneurysm with reanastomosis of the aorta in 1948.[170] Swan and colleagues[171] repaired a complex aneurysmal coarctation and used aortic homograft for reconstruction in 1950. Gross[172] reported a series of similar cases using homograft replacement. In 1951, DuBost and colleagues[173] in Paris resected an intra-abdominal aortic aneurysm with homograft replacement.

In 1953, Henry Bahnson,[174] from Johns Hopkins, successfully resected six saccular aneurysms of the aorta in eight patients. In the same year, DeBakey and Cooley[175] reported a 46-year-old man who had resection of a huge aneurysm of the descending thoracic aorta that measured approximately 20 cm in length and in greatest diameter. The aneurysm was resected and replaced with an aortic homograft approximately 15 cm in length.

During the Korean War, the arterial homograft and autogenous vein graft were used to reconstruct battlefield arterial injuries and reduce the overall amputation rate to 11.1%[176] compared with the rate of 49.6% reported in World War II. Although the vein autograft remains the first-choice peripheral vascular conduit today, the arterial homograft was superseded by the development of synthetic vascular grafts by Arthur Voorhees at Columbia University in 1952. Voorhees and colleagues developed Vinyon-N cloth tubes to substitute for diseased arterial segments.[177]

Another advance in aortic surgery appeared in 1955 when DeBakey and colleagues[178] reported six cases of aortic dissection treated by aggressive surgery. Because mortality of operation for acute dissections remained high, Myron Wheat Jr. introduced medical therapy for the disease.[179]

During the late 1950s, the Houston group, consisting of Michael DeBakey, Denton Cooley, Stanley Crawford, and their other associates, systematically developed operations for resection and graft replacement of the ascending aorta,[180] descending aorta, and thoracoabdominal aorta.[181] Cardiopulmonary bypass was used for the ascending aortic resections. The high risk of paraplegia highlighted a major complication of thoracoabdominal aortic resections. The Houston group was the first to resect an aortic arch with the use of cardiopulmonary bypass in 1957 and replace the arch with a reconstituted aortic arch homograph.[182] More interesting is that Cooley and colleagues, using great ingenuity, resected a large aortic arch aneurysm that also involved a portion of the descending aorta in a 49-year-old patient on June 24, 1955. The surgery was done, without the use of cardiopulmonary bypass, by first sewing in a temporary graft from the ascending aorta to the distal descending aorta and sewing in two more temporary limbs off that graft, which were anastomosed to the left and right carotid arteries, while the aneurysm was resected and a permanent graft was placed.[183]

In 1968, Bentall and De Bono[184] introduced replacement of the ascending aorta and aortic valve with reanastomoses of the coronary ostia to the replacement graft. They described the composite-graft technique for replacement of the ascending aorta with reimplantation of the coronary arteries into the composite Dacron graft containing the prosthetic aortic valve. As mentioned, Cooley and DeBakey were the first to replace the supracoronary ascending aorta in 1956. In 1963, Starr and colleagues[185] reported replacing the supracoronary ascending aorta and the aortic valve at the same sitting. The technique of fashioning "buttons" of aortic tissue adjacent to the coronary ostia and then incorporating these buttons into the aortic graft along with the AVR was described by Wheat and colleagues[186] in 1964. Bentall and De Bono incorporated the aortic prosthesis into the tube graft and used the Wheat technique for implanting the coronary arteries into the composite graft.

Since the early 1990s, stents also have been used for the treatment of aneurysms in both the descending aorta and the abdominal aortas.[187, 188]

The first thoracic stent placed in a patient's thoracic aorta was performed to treat a false aneurysm after a coarctation of the aorta repair.[189] The procedure was carried out at Stanford University Hospital in July 1992 by Michael Drake and D. Craig Miller. Since then, the indications for using thoracic stent grafts have gradually expanded and include transected aortas, aneurysms, penetrating atherosclerotic ulcers, and intramural hematomas of the descending aorta. The long-term follow-up with these stents still needs to be better defined.[190–193]

REFERENCES

1. Williams DH: Stab wound of the heart, pericardium—Suture of the pericardium—Recovery—Patient alive three years afterward. *Med Rec* 1897;1.
2. Rehn L: On penetrating cardiac injuries and cardiac suturing. *Arch Klin Chir* 1897;55:315.
3. Rehn L: Zur chirurgie des herzens und des herzbeutels. *Arch Klin Chir* 1907;83:723. Quoted from Beck CS: Wounds of the heart: the technic of suture. *Arch Surg* 1926;13:212.
4. Hill LL: A report of a case of successful suturing of the heart, and table of thirty seven other cases of suturing by different operators with various terminations, and the conclusions drawn. *Med Rec* 1902;2:846.
5. Harken DE: Foreign bodies in and in relation to the thoracic blood vessels and heart: I. Techniques for approaching and removing foreign bodies from the chambers of the heart. *Surg Gynecol Obstet* 1946;83:117.
6. Kirschner M: Ein durch die Trendelenburgische operation geheiter fall von embolie der art. pulmonalis. *Arch Klin Chir* 1924;133:312.
7. Gibbon JH: Artificial maintenance of circulation during experimental occlusion of pulmonary artery. *Arch Surg* 1937;34:1105.
8. Sharp EH: Pulmonary embolectomy: successful removal of a massive pulmonary embolus with the support of cardiopulmonary bypass. Case report. *Ann Surg* 1962;156:1.
9. Rehn I: Zur experimentellen pathologie des herzbeutels. *Verh Dtsch Ges Chir* 1913;42:339.
10. Sauerbruch R: *Die Chirurgie der Brustorgane*, Vol. II. Berlin, 1925.
11. Forssmann W: Catheterization of the right heart. *Klin Wochenshr* 1929;8:2085.
12. Forssmann W: 21 jahre herzkatheterung, rueckblick and ausschau. *Verh Dtsch Ges Kreislaufforschung* 1951;17:1.
13. Klein O: Zur bestimmung des zirkulatorischen minutenvoumnens beim menschen nach dem fisckschen prinzip. *Meunsch Med Wochenschr* 1930;77:1311.
14. Forssmann W: Ueber kontrastdarstellung der hoehlen des lebenden rechten herzens und der lungenschlagader. *Muensch Med Wochenschr* 1931;78:489.
15. Tuffier T: Etat actuel de la chirurgie intrathoracique. *Trans Int Congr Med 1913* (London, 1914), 7; *Surgery* 1914;2:249.
16. Brock RC: The arterial route to the aortic and pulmonary valves: the mitral route to the aortic valves. *Guys Hosp Rep* 1950;99:236.
17. Brock, Sir Russell: Aortic subvalvular stenosis: surgical treatment. *Guys Hosp Rep* 1957;106:221.
18. Bailey CP, Bolton HE, Nichols HT, et al: Commissurotomy for rheumatic aortic stenosis. *Circulation* 1954;9:22.
19. Cutler EC, Levine SA: Cardiotomy and valvulotomy for mitral stenosis. *Boston Med Surg J* 1923;188:1023.
20. Bailey CP: The surgical treatment of mitral stenosis. *Dis Chest* 1949;15:377.
21. Naef AP: *The Story of Thoracic Surgery*. New York, Hogrefe & Huber, 1990.

22. Harken DE, Ellis LB, Ware PF, Norman LR: The surgical treatment of mitral stenosis stent I. Valvuloplasty. *New Engl J Med* 1948;239:804.

23. Sellers TH: Surgery of pulmonary stenosis: a case in which the pulmonary valve was successfully divided. *Lancet* 1948;1:988.

24. Hufnagel CA, Harvey WP, Rabil PJ, et al: Surgical correction of aortic insufficiency. *Surgery* 1954;35:673.

25. Graybiel A, Strieder JW, Boyer NH: An attempt to obliterate the patent ductus in a patient with subacute endarteritis. *Am Heart J* 1938;15:621.

26. Gross RE, Hubbard JH: Surgical ligation of a patent ductus arteriosus: report of first successful case. *JAMA* 1939;112:729.

27. Crafoord C, Nylin G: Congenital coarctation of the aorta and its surgical treatment. *J Thorac Cardiovasc Surg* 1945;14:347.

28. Gross RE: Surgical correction for coarctation of the aorta. *Surgery* 1945;18:673.

29. Gross RE: Surgical relief for tracheal obstruction from a vascular ring. *New Engl J Med* 1945;233:586.

30. Blalock A, Taussig HB: The surgical treatment of malformations of the heart in which there is pulmonary stenosis or pulmonary atresia. *JAMA* 1945;128:189.

31. Biorck G, Crafoord C: Arteriovenous aneurysm on the pulmonary artery simulating patent ductus arteriosus botalli. *Thorax* 1947;2:65.

32. Muller WH Jr: The surgical treatment of the transposition of the pulmonary veins. *Ann Surg* 1951;134:683.

33. Gross RE: Surgical closure of an aortic septal defect. *Circulation* 1952;5:858.

34. Cooley DA, McNamara DR, Latson JR: Aorticopulmonary septal defect: diagnosis and surgical treatment. *Surgery* 1957;42:101.

35. Glenn WWL: Circulatory bypass of the right side of the hearts: IV. Shunt between superior vena cava and distal right pulmonary artery—report of clinical application. *NEJM* 1958;259:117.

36. Galankin NK: Proposition and technique of cavopulmonary anastomosis. *Exp Biol (Russia)* 1957;5:33.

37. Johnson SL: *The History of Cardiac Surgery, 1896–1955.* Baltimore, Johns Hopkins Press, 1970, pp. 121-122.

38. Gibbon JH Jr: Artificial maintenance of circulation during experimental occlusion of the pulmonary artery. *Arch Surg* 1937;34:1105.

39. Dennis C, Spreng DS, Nelson GE, et al: Development of a pump oxygenator to replace the heart and lungs: an apparatus applicable to human patients, and application to one case. *Ann Surg* 1951;134:709.

40. Miller CW: *King of Hearts: The True Story of the Maverick Who Pioneered Open Heart Surgery.* New York, Random House, 2000.

41. Digliotti AM: Clinical use of the artificial circulation with a note on intra-arterial transfusion. *Bull Johns Hopkins Hosp* 1952;90:131.

42. Schumaker HB Jr: *A Dream of the Heart.* Santa Barbara, CA, Fithian Press, 1999.

43. Dodrill FD, Hill E, Gerisch RA: Temporary mechanical substitute for the left ventricle in man. *JAMA* 1952;150:642.

44. Lewis FJ, Taufic M: Closure of atrial septal defects with the aid of hypothermia: experimental accomplishments and the report of one successful case. *Surgery* 1953;33:52.

45. Dodrill FD, Hill E, Gerisch RA, Johnson A: Pulmonary valvuloplasty under direct vision using the mechanical heart for a complete bypass of the right heart in a patient with congenital pulmonary stenosis. *J Thorac Surg* 1953;25:584.

46. Mustard WT, Chute AL, Keith JD, et al: A surgical approach to transposition of the great vessels with extracorporeal circuit. *Surgery* 1953;6:39.

47. Romaine-Davis A: *John Gibbon and His Heart-Lung Machine.* Philadelphia, University of Pennsylvania Press, 1991.

48. Lillehei CW: Overview: Section III: Cardiopulmonary bypass and myocardial protection, in Stephenson LW, Ruggiero R (eds): *Heart Surgery Classics.* Boston, Adams Publishing Group, 1994;p 121.

49. Radegram K: The early history of open-heart surgery in Stockholm. *J Cardiac Surg* 2003;18:564.

50. Kirklin JW, DuShane JW, Patrick RT, et al: Intracardiac surgery with the aid of a mechanical pump-oxygenator system (Gibbon type): report of eight cases. *Mayo Clin Proc* 1955;30:201.

51. Dodrill FD, Marshall N, Nyboer J, et al: The use of the heart-lung apparatus in human cardiac surgery. *J Thorac Surg* 1957;1:60.

52. Acierno LJ: *The History of Cardiology.* New York, Parthenon, 1994.

53. Mustard WT, Thomson JA: Clinical experience with the artificial heart lung preparation. *Can Med Assoc J* 1957;76:265.

54. Dodrill FD, Hill E, Gerisch RA: Some physiologic aspects of the artificial heart problem. *J Thorac Surg* 1952;24:134.

55. Stephenson LW: Forest Dewey Dodrill—Heart surgery pioneer, part II. *J Cardiac Surg* 2002;17:247.

56. Hikasa Y, Shirotani H, Satomura K, et al: Open-heart surgery in infants with the aid of hypothermic anesthesia. *Arch Jpn Chir* 1967;36:495.

57. Gibbon JH Jr: Application of a mechanical heart and lung apparatus to cardiac surgery. *Minn Med* 1954;37:171.

58. Lillehei CW, Cohen M, Warden HE, et al: The results of direct vision closure of ventricular septal defects in eight patients by means of controlled cross circulation. *Surg Gynecol Obstet* 1955;101:446.

59. Lillehei CW, Cohen M, Warden HE, et al: The direct vision intracardiac correction of congenital anomalies by controlled cross circulation. *Surgery* 1955;38:11.

60. Helmsworth JA, Clark LC Jr, Kaplan S, et al: Clinical use of extracorporeal oxygenation with oxygenator-pump. *JAMA* 1952;1(5):50.

61. Kirklin JW: The middle 1950s and C. Walton Lillehei. *J Thorac Cardiovasc Surg* 1989;98:822.

62. Hill JD, O'Brien TG, Murray JJ, et al: Prolonged extracorporeal oxygenation for acute posttraumatic respiratory failure (shock-lung syndrome): use of the Bramston membrane lung. *New Engl J Med* 1972;286:629.

63. Zapol WM, Snider MT, Hill JD, et al: Extracorporeal membrane oxygenation in severe acute respiratory failure: a randomized, prospective study. *JAMA* 1979;242:2193.

64. Melrose DG, Dreyer B, Bentall MB, Baker JBE: Elective cardiac arrest. *Lancet* 1955;2:21.

65. Gay WA Jr, Ebert PA: Functional, metabolic, and morphologic effects of potassium-induced cardioplegia. *Surgery* 1973;74:284.

66. Tyers GFO, Todd GJ, Niebauer IM, et al: The mechanism of myocardial damage following potassium-induced (Melrose) cardioplegia. *Surgery* 1978;78:45.

67. Kirsch U, Rodewald G, Kalmar P: Induced ischemic arrest. *J Thorac Cardiovasc Surg* 1972;63:121.

68. Bretschneider HJ, Hubner G, Knoll D, et al: Myocardial resistance and tolerance to ischemia: physiological and biochemical basis. *J Cardiovasc Surg* 1975;16:241.

69. Hearse DJ, Stewart DA, Braimbridge MV, et al: Cellular protection during myocardial ischemia. *Circulation* 1976;16:241.

70. Follette DM, Mulder DG, Maloney JV, Buckberg GD: Advantages of blood cardioplegia over continuous coronary perfusion or intermittent ischemia. *J Thorac Cardiovasc Surg* 1978;76:604.

71. Potts WJ, Smith S, Gibson S: Anastomosis of the aorta to a pulmonary artery. *JAMA* 1946;132:627.

72. Waterston DJ: Treatment of Fallot's tetralogy in children under one year of age. *Rozhl Chir* 1962;41:181.

73. Blalock A, Hanlon CR: The surgical treatment of complete transposition of the aorta and the pulmonary artery. *Surg Gynecol Obstet* 1950;90:1.

74. Burroughs JT, Kirklin JW: Complete correction of total anomalous pulmonary venous correction: report of three cases. *Mayo Clin Proc* 1956;31:182.

75. McGoon DC, Edwards JE, Kirklin JW: Surgical treatment of ruptured aneurysm of aortic sinus. *Ann Surg* 1958;147:387.

76. Ellis FH Jr, Kirklin JW: Congenital valvular aortic stenosis: anatomic findings and surgical techniques. *J Thorac Cardiovasc Surg* 1962;43:199.

77. Cooley DA, McNamara DG, Jatson JR: Aortico-pulmonary septal defect: diagnosis and surgical treatment. *Surgery* 1957;42:101.

78. Kirklin JW, Harp RA, McGoon DC: Surgical treatment of origin of both vessels from right ventricle including cases of pulmonary stenosis. *J Thorac Cardiovasc Surg* 1964;48:1026.

79. Anderson RC, Lillehei CW, Jester RG: Corrected transposition of the great vessels of the heart. *Pediatrics* 1957;20:626.

80. Senning A: Surgical correction of transposition of the great vessels. *Surgery* 1959;45:966.

81. Swan H, Wilson JH, Woodwork G, Blount SE: Surgical obliteration of a coronary artery fistula to the right ventricle. *Arch Surg* 1959;79:820.

82. Hardy KL, May IA, Webster CA, Kimball KG: Ebstein's anomaly: a functional concept and successful definitive repair. *J Thorac Cardiovasc Surg* 1964;48:927.

83. Ross DN, Somerville J: Correction of pulmonary atresia with a homograft aortic valve. *Lancet* 1966;2:1446.

84. McGoon DC, Rastelli GC, Ongley PA: An operation for the correction of truncus arteriosus. *JAMA* 1968;205:59.

85. Fontan F, Baudet E: Surgical repair of tricuspid atresia. *Thorax* 1971;26:240.

86. Horiuchi T, Abe T, Okada Y, et al: Feasibility of total correction for single ventricle: a report of total correction in a six-year-old girl. *Jpn J Thorac Surg* 1970;23:434 (in Japanese).

87. Konno S, Iami Y, Iida Y, et al: A new method for prosthetic valve replacement in congenital aortic stenosis associated with hypoplasia of the aortic valve ring. *J Thorac Cardiovasc Surg* 1975;70:909.

88. Jatene AD, Fontes VF, Paulista PP, et al: Anatomic correction of transposition of the great vessel. *J Thorac Cardiovasc Surg* 1976;72:364.

89. Norwood WI, Lang P, Hansen DD: Physiologic repair of aortic atresia-hypoplastic left heart syndrome. *New Engl J Med* 1983;308:23.

90. Bailey LL, Gundry SR, Razzouk AJ, et al: Bless the babies: one hundred fifteen late survivors of heart transplantation during the first year of life. *J Thorac Cardiovasc Surg* 1993;105:805.

91. Harken DE, Soroff HS, Taylor WJ, et al: Partial and complete pros-theses in aortic insufficiency. *J Thorac Cardiovasc Surg* 1960;40:744.

92. Starr A, Edwards ML: Mitral replacement: clinical experience with a ball-valve prosthesis. *Ann Surg* 1961;154:726.

93. Starr A, Edwards LM, McCord CW, et al: Multiple valve replacement. *Circulation* 1964;29:30.

94. Cartwright RS, Giacobine JW, Ratan RS, et al: Combined aortic and mitral valve replacement. *J Thorac Cardiovasc Surg* 1963;45:35.

95. Knott-Craig CJ, Schaff HV, Mullany CJ, et al: Carcinoid disease of the heart: surgical management of ten patients. *J Thorac Cardiovasc Surg* 1992;104:475.

96. Morrow AG, Brockenbrough EC: Surgical treatment of idiopathic hypertrophic subaortic stenosis: technic and hemodynamic results of subaortic ventriculomyotomy. *Ann Surg* 1961;154:181.

97. Heimbecker RO, Baird RJ, Lajos RJ, et al: Homograft replacement of the human valve: a preliminary report. *Can Med Assoc J* 1962;86:805.

98. Ross DN: Homograft replacement of the aortic valve. *Lancet* 1962;2:487.

99. Ross DN: Replacement of aortic and mitral valves with a pulmonary autograft. *Lancet* 1967;2:956.

100. Binet JP, Carpentier A, Langlois J, et al: Implantation de valves hetero-genes dans le traitement des cardiopathies aortiques. *C R Acad Sci Paris* 1965;261:5733.

101. Binet JP, Planche C, Weiss M: Heterograft replacement of the aortic valve, in Ionescu MI, Ross DN, Wooler GH (eds): *Biological Tissue in Heart Valve Replacement*. London, Butterworth, 1971;p 409.

102. Carpentier A: Principles of tissue valve transplantation, in Ionescu MI, Ross DN, Wooler GH (eds): *Biological Tissue in Heart Valve Replacement*. London, Butterworth, 1971;p 49.

103. Kaiser GA, Hancock WD, Lukban SB, Litwak RS: Clinical use of a new design stented xenograft heart valve prosthesis. *Surg Forum* 1969;20:137.

104. Wooler GH, Nixon PG, Grimshaw VA, et al: Experiences with the repair of the mitral valve in mitral incompetence. *Thorax* 1962;17:49.

105. Reed GE, Tice DA, Clause RH: A symmetric, exaggerated mitral annu-loplasty: repair of mitral insufficiency with hemodynamic predictability. *J Thorac Cardiovasc Surg* 1965;49:752.

106. Kay JH, Zubiate T, Mendez MA, et al: Mitral valve repair for significant mitral insufficiency. *Am Heart J* 1978;96:243.

107. Carpentier A: Cardiac valve surgery: the French correction. *J Thorac Cardiovasc Surg* 1983;86:23.

108. Arbulu A, Thoms NW, Chiscano A, Wilson RF: Total tricuspid valvulec-tomy without replacement in the treatment of *Pseudomonas* endocarditis. *Surg Forum* 1971;22:162.

109. Arbulu A, Holmes RJ, Asfaw I: Surgical treatment of intractable right-sided infective endocarditis in drug addicts: 25 years' experience. *J Heart Valve Dis* 1993;2:129.

110. Cribier A, Eltchaninoff H, Bash A, et al: Percutaneous transcatheter implantation of an aortic valve prosthesis for calcific aortic stenosis. *Circulation* 2002;106(24):3006–3008.

111. Cribier A, Eltchaninoff H, Tron C, Bauer F, Agatiello C, et al: Early experience with percutaneous transcatheter implantation of heart valve prosthesis for the treatment of end-stage inoperable patients with calcific aortic stenosis. *J Am Coll Cardiol* 2004;43(4):698–703.

112. Walther T, Simon P, Dewey T, et al: Transapical minimally inva-sive aortic valve implantation: multicenter experience. *Circulation* 2007;116(11 Suppl):1240–1245.

113. Sones FM, Shirey EK: Cine coronary arteriography. *Mod Concepts Car-diovasc Dis* 1962;31:735.

114. Konstantinov IE: Robert H. Goetz: The surgeon who performed the first successful clinical coronary artery bypass operation. *Ann Thorac Surg* 2000;69:1966.

115. Garrett EH, Dennis EW, DeBakey ME: Aortocoronary bypass with saphenous vein grafts: seven-year follow-up. *JAMA* 1973;223:792.

116. Shumaker HB Jr: *The Evolution of Cardiac Surgery*. Indianapolis, Indiana University Press, 1992.

117. Demikhov VP: *Experimental Transplantation of Vital Organs*. Authorized translation from the Russian by Basil Haigh. New York, Consultants Bureau, 1962.

118. Kolessov VI: Mammary artery–coronary artery anastomosis as a method of treatment for angina pectoris. *J Thorac Cardiovasc Surg* 1967;54:535.

119. Green GE, Stertzer SH, Reppert EH: Coronary arterial bypass grafts. *Ann Thorac Surg* 1968;5:443.

120. Bailey CP, Hirose T: Successful internal mammary–coronary arterial anas-tomosis using a minivascular suturing technic. *Int Surg* 1968;49:416.

121. Favalaro RG: Saphenous vein autograft replacement of severe segmental coronary artery occlusion. *Ann Thorac Surg* 1968;5:334.

122. Johnson WD, Flemma RJ, Lepley D Jr, Ellison EH: Extended treatment of severe coronary artery disease: a total surgical approach. *Ann Surg* 1969;171:460.

123. Loop FD, Lytle BW, Cosgrove DM, et al: Influence of the internal-mam-mary-artery graft on 10-year survival and other cardiac events. *New Engl J Med* 1986;314:1.

124. Grüntzig AR, Senning A, Siegenthaler WE: Nonoperative dilation of coronary-artery stenosis percutaneous transluminal coronary angio-plasty. *New Engl J Med* 1979;301:217.

125. Ruygorok PN, Serruys PW: Intracoronary stenting, *Circulation* 1996;94:882–890.

126. King SB 3rd, Barnhard HX, Kosniski AS, et al: Angioplasty or surgery for multivessel coronary artery disease: comparison of eligible registry and randomized patient in the EAST trial and influence of treatment selections on outcomes. Emory angioplasty versus surgery trial investiga-tors. *Am J Cardiol* 1997;79:1453.

127. Hannan EL, Racz MJ, McCallister BD, et al: A comparison of three-year survival after coronary artery bypass graft surgery and percutameous transluminal coronary angioplasty. *J Am Coll Cardiol* 1999;33:63.

128. Hannan EL, Racz MJ, Walford G, et al: Long-term outcomes of cor-onary artery bypass grafting versus stent implantation. *N Engl J Med* 2005;352:2174.

129. Cooley DA, Belmonte BA, Zeis LB, Schnur S: Surgical repair of rup-tured interventricular septum following acute myocardial infarction. *Surgery* 1957;41:930.

130. Cooley DA, Henly WS, Amad KH, Chapman DW: Ventricular aneu-rysm following myocardial infarction: results of surgical treatment. *Ann Surg* 1959;150:595.

131. Cobb FR, Blumenshein SD, Sealy WC, et al: Successful surgery inter-ruption of the bundle of Kent in a patient with Wolff-Parkinson-White syndrome. *Circulation* 1968;38:1018.

132. Cox JL: Arrhythmia surgery, in Stephenson LW, Ruggiero R (eds): *Heart Surgery Classics*. Boston, Adams, 1994;p 258.

133. Ross DL, Johnson DC, Denniss AR, et al: Curative surgery for atrioven-tricular junctional (AV node) reentrant tachycardia. *J Am Coll Cardiol* 1985;6:1383.

134. Cox JL, Holman WL, Cain ME: Cryosurgical treatment of atrioven-tricular node reentrant tachycardia. *Circulation* 1987;76:1329.

135. Cox JL: The surgical treatment of atrial fibrillation, IV surgical tech-nique. *J Thorac Cardiovasc Surg* 1991;101:584.

136. Guiraudon G, Fontaine G, Frank R, et al: Encircling endocardial ven-triculotomy: a new surgical treatment for life-threatening ventricular tachycardias resistant to medical treatment following myocardial infarc-tion. *Ann Thorac Surg* 1978;26:438.

137. Josephson ME, Harken AH, Horowitz LN: Endocardial excision: a new surgical technique for the treatment of recurrent ventricular tachycardia. *Circulation* 1979;60:1430.

138. Mirowski M, Reid PR, Mower MM, et al: Termination of malignant ventricular arrhythmias with an implanted automatic defibrillator in human beings. *N Engl J Med* 1980;303:322.

139. Myerburg RJ, Reddy V, Castellanos A: Indications for implantable car-dioverter defibrillators based on evidence and judgement. *J Am Coll Car-diol* 2009;54:747.

140. Epstein AE: Update on primary prevention implantable cardioverter defibrillator therapy. *Curr Cardiol Rep* 2009;11:335.

141. Zoll PM: Resuscitation of the heart in ventricular standstill by external electrical stimulation. *N Engl J Med* 1952;247:768.

142. Lillehei CW, Gott VL, Hodges PC Jr, et al: Transistor pacemaker for treatment of complete atrioventricular dissociation. *JAMA* 1960;172:2006.

143. Elmquist R, Senning A: Implantable pacemaker for the heart, in Smyth CN (ed): *Medical Electronics: Proceedings of the Second International Conference on Medical Electronics, Paris, June, 1959.* London, Iliffe & Sons, 1960.

144. Chardack WM, Gage AA, Greatbatch W: Correction of complete heart block by a self-contained and subcutaneously implanted pacemaker: clinical experience with 15 patients. *J Thorac Cardiovasc Surg* 1961;42:814.

145. Carrel A, Guthrie CC: The transplantation of vein and organs. *Am J Med* 1905;10:101.

146. Demikhov VP: Experimental transplantation of an additional heart in the dog. *Bull Exp Biol Med (Russia)* 1950;1:241.

147. Lower RR, Shumway NE: Studies on orthotopic homotransplantation of the canine heart. *Surg Forum* 1960;11:18.

148. Brock R: Heart excision and replacement. *Guys Hosp Rep* 1959;108:285.

149. Spencer F: Intellectual creativity in thoracic surgeons. *J Thorac Cardiovasc Surg* 1983;86:172.

150. Hardy JD, Chavez CM, Hurrus FD, et al: Heart transplantation in man and report of a case. *JAMA* 1964;188:1132.

151. Barnard CN: A human cardiac transplant: an interim report of a successful operation performed at Groote Schuur Hospital, Cape Town. *South Afr Med J* 1967;41:1271.

152. Kantrowitz A: Heart, heart-lung and lung transplantation, in Stephenson LW, Ruggiero R (eds): *Heart Surgery Classics.* Boston, Adams, 1994;p 314.

153. Thomson G: Provisional report on the autopsy of LW. *South Afr Med J* 1967;41:1277.

154. Ruggiero R: Commentary on Barnard CN: a human cardiac transplant: an interim report of a successful operation performed at Groote Schuur Hospital, Cape Town. *South Afr Med J* 1967;41:1271; In Stephenson LW, Ruggiero R (eds): *Heart Surgery Classics.* Boston, Adams, 1994;p 327.

155. Reitz BA, Wallwork JL, Hunt SA, et al: Heart-lung transplantation: Successful therapy for patients with pulmonary vascular disease. *N Engl J Med* 1982;306:557.

156. Hardy JD, Webb WR, Dalton ML Jr, Walker GR Jr: Lung homotransplantation in man: report of the initial case. *JAMA* 1963;286:1065.

157. Derom F, Barbier F, Ringoir S, et al: Ten-month survival after lung homotransplantation in man. *J Thorac Cardiovasc Surg* 1971;61:835.

158. Cooper JD, Ginsberg RJ, Goldberg M, et al: Unilateral lung transplantation for pulmonary fibrosis. *N Engl J Med* 1986;314:1140.

159. Kantrowitz A, Tjonneland S, Freed PS, et al: Initial clinical experience with intra-aortic balloon pumping in cardiogenic shock. *JAMA* 1968;203:135.

160. Liotta D, Hall W, Henly WS, et al: Prolonged assisted circulation during and after cardiac or aortic surgery: prolonged partial left ventricular bypass by means of intracorporeal circulation. *Am J Cardiol* 1963;12:399.

161. Shumaker HB Jr: *The Evolution of Cardiac Surgery.* Bloomington, University Press, 1992.

162. DeBakey ME: Left ventricular heart assist devices, in Stephenson LW, Ruggiero R (eds): *Heart Surgery Classics.* Boston, Adams, 1994.

163. Cooley DA, Liotta D, Hallman GL, et al: Orthotopic cardiac prosthesis for two-staged cardiac replacement. *Am J Cardiol* 1969;24:723.

164. Hill JD, Farrar DJ, Hershon JJ, et al: Use of a prosthetic ventricle as a bridge to cardiac transplantation for postinfarction cardiogenic shock. *N Engl J Med* 1986;314:626.

165. Starnes VA, Ayer PE, Portner PM, et al: Isolated left ventricular assist as bridge to cardiac transplantation. *J Thorac Cardiovasc Surg* 1988;96:62.

166. DeVries WC, Anderson JL, Joyce LD, et al: Clinical use of total artificial heart. *N Engl J Med* 1984;310:273.

167. Edwards WS, Edwards PD: *Alexis Carrel: Visionary Surgeon.* Springfield, IL, Charles C Thomas, 1974.

168. Acierno LJ: *The History of Cardiology.* New York, Parthenon, 1994.

169. DeBakey ME, Simeone FA: Battle injuries of the arteries in World War II. *Am J Surg* 1946;123:534.

170. Shumaker HB: Surgical cure of innominate aneurysm: report of a case with comments on the applicability of surgical measures. *Surgery* 1947;22:739.

171. Swan HC, Maaske M, Johnson M, Grover R: Arterial homografts: II. Resection of thoracic aneurysm using a stored human arterial transplant. *Arch Surg* 1950;61:732.

172. Gross RE: Treatment of certain aortic coarctations by homologous grafts: a report of nineteen cases. *Ann Surg* 1951;134:753.

173. DuBost C, Allary M, Oeconomos N: Resection of an aneurysm of the abdominal aorta: reestablishment of the continuity by a preserved human arterial graft, with results after five months. *Arch Surg* 1952;62:405.

174. Bahnson HT: Definitive treatment of saccular aneurysms of the aorta with excision of sac and aortic suture. *Surg Gynecol Obstet* 1953;96:383.

175. DeBakey ME, Cooley DA: Successful resection of aneurysm of thoracic aorta and replacement by graft. *JAMA* 1953;152:673.

176. Hughes CW: Acute vascular trauma in Korean War casualties. *Surg Gynecol Obstet* 1954;99:91.

177. Voorhees AB Jr, Janetzky A III, Blakemore AH: The use of tubes constructed from Vinyon-N cloth in bridging defects. *Ann Surg* 1952;135:332.

178. DeBakey ME, Cooley DA, Creech O Jr: Surgical consideration of dissecting aneurysm of the aorta. *Ann Surg* 1955;142:586.

179. Wheat MW Jr, Palmer RF, Bartley TD, Seelman RC: Treatment of dissecting aneurysms of the aorta without surgery. *J Thorac Cardiovasc Surg* 1965;50:364.

180. Cooley DA, DeBakey ME: Resection of entire ascending aorta in fusiform aneurysm using cardiac bypass. *JAMA* 1956;162:1158.

181. DeBakey ME, Creech O Jr, Morris GC Jr: Aneurysm of the thoracoabdominal aorta involving the celiac superior mesenteric, and renal arteries: report of four cases treated by resection and homo-graft replacement. *Ann Surg* 1956;144:549.

182. DeBakey ME, Crawford ES, Cooley DA, Morris GC Jr: Successful resection of fusiform aneurysm of aortic arch with replacement by homograft. *Surg Gynecol Obstet* 1957;105:657.

183. Cooley DA, Mahaffey DE, DeBakey ME: Total excision of the aortic arch for aneurysm. *Surg Gynecol Obstet* 1955;101:667.

184. Bentall H, De Bono A: A technique for complete replacement of the ascending aorta. *Thorax* 1968;23:338.

185. Starr A, Edwards WL, McCord MD, et al: Aortic replacement. *Circulation* 1963;27:779.

186. Wheat MW Jr, Wilson JR, Bartley TD: Successful replacement of the entire ascending aorta and aortic valve. *JAMA* 1964;188:717.

187. Miller C: Stent-grafts: avoiding major aortic surgery, in Stephenson LW (ed): *State of the Heart: The Practical Guide to Your Heart and Heart Surgery.* Fort Lauderdale, Write Stuff, 1999;p 230.

188. Parodi JC, Palmaz JC, Barone HD: Transfemoral intraluminal graft implantation for abdominal aortic aneurysms. *Ann Vasc Surg* 1991;5:491.

189. Michael Drake MD, Craig Miller DC, et al: Transluminal Placement of endovascular stent/grafts for the treatment of descending thoracic aortic aneurysms. *N Engl J Med* 1994;1729–1734.

190. Andrassy J, Weidenhagen R, Meimarakis G, et al: Stent versus open surgery for acute and chronic traumatic injury of the thoracic aorta: a single-center experience. *J Trauma* 2006;60(4):765–771; discussion 771–762.

191. Ott MC, Stewart TC, Lawlor DK, Gray DK, Forbes TL: Management of blunt thoracic aortic injuries: endovascular stents versus open repair. *J. Trauma* 2004;56(3):565–570.

192. Gleason TG: Thoracic aortic stent grafting: is it ready for prime time? *J Thorac Cardiovasc Surg* 2006;131:16.

193. Ricco J-B, Cau J, Marchant D, et al: Stent-graft repair for thoracic aortic disease: results of an independent nationwide study in France from 1999 to 2001. *J Thorac Cardiovasc Surg* 2006;131:131.

Surgical Anatomy of the Heart

Michael R. Mill • Robert H. Anderson • Lawrence H. Cohn

A thorough knowledge of the anatomy of the heart is a prerequisite for the successful completion of the myriad procedures performed by the cardiothoracic surgeon. This chapter describes the normal anatomy of the heart, including its position and relationship to other thoracic organs. It also describes the incisions used to expose the heart for various operations and discusses in detail the cardiac chambers and valves, coronary arteries and veins, and the important but surgically invisible conduction tissues.

OVERVIEW

Location of the Heart Relative to Surrounding Structures

The overall shape of the heart is that of a three-sided pyramid located in the middle mediastinum (Fig. 2-1). When viewed from the heart's apex, the three sides of the ventricular mass are readily apparent (Fig. 2-2). Two of the edges are named. The *acute margin* lies inferiorly and describes a sharp angle between the sternocostal and diaphragmatic surfaces. The *obtuse margin* lies superiorly and is much more diffuse. The posterior margin is unnamed but is also diffuse in its transition.

One-third of the cardiac mass lies to the right of the midline and two-thirds to the left. The long axis of the heart is oriented from the left epigastrium to the right shoulder. The short axis, which corresponds to the plane of the atrioventricular groove, is oblique and is oriented closer to the vertical than the horizontal plane (see Fig. 2-1).

Anteriorly, the heart is covered by the sternum and the costal cartilages of the third, fourth, and fifth ribs. The lungs contact the lateral surfaces of the heart, whereas the heart abuts onto the pulmonary hila posteriorly. The right lung overlies the right surface of the heart and reaches to the midline. In contrast, the left lung retracts from the midline in the area of the cardiac notch. The heart has an extensive diaphragmatic surface inferiorly. Posteriorly, the heart lies on the esophagus and the tracheal bifurcation and bronchi that extend into the lung. The sternum lies anteriorly and provides rigid protection to the heart during blunt trauma and is aided by the cushioning effects of the lungs.

The Pericardium and Its Reflections

The heart lies within the pericardium, which is attached to the walls of the great vessels and the diaphragm. The pericardium can be visualized best as a bag into which the heart has been placed apex first. The inner layer, in direct contact with the heart, is the *visceral epicardium*, which encases the heart and extends several centimeters back onto the walls of the great vessels. The outer layer forms the *parietal pericardium*, which lines the inner surface of the tough fibrous pericardial sack. A thin film of lubricating fluid lies within the pericardial cavity between the two serous layers. Two identifiable recesses lie within the pericardium and are lined by the serous layer. The first is the *transverse sinus*, which is delineated anteriorly by the posterior surface of the aorta and pulmonary trunk and posteriorly by the anterior surface of the interatrial groove. The second is the *oblique sinus*, a cul-de-sac located behind the left atrium, delineated by serous pericardial reflections from the pulmonary veins and the inferior vena cava.

Mediastinal Nerves and Their Relationships to the Heart

The vagus and phrenic nerves descend through the mediastinum in close relationship to the heart (Fig. 2-3). They enter through the thoracic inlet, with the phrenic nerve located anteriorly on the surface of the anterior scalene muscle and lying just posterior to the internal thoracic artery (internal mammary artery) at the thoracic inlet. In this position, the phrenic nerve is vulnerable to injury during dissection and preparation of the internal thoracic artery for use in coronary arterial bypass grafting. On the right side, the phrenic nerve courses on the lateral surface of the superior vena cava, again in harm's way during dissection for venous cannulation for cardiopulmonary bypass. The nerve then descends anterior to the pulmonary hilum before reflecting onto the

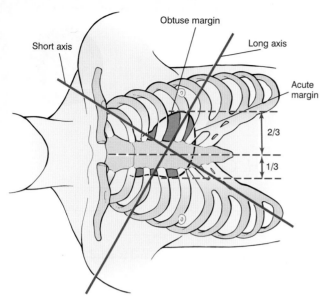

FIGURE 2-1 This diagram shows the heart within the middle mediastinum with the patient supine on the operating table. The long axis lies parallel to the interventricular septum, whereas the short axis is perpendicular to the long axis at the level of the atrioventricular valves.

right diaphragm, where it branches to provide its innervation. In the presence of a left-sided superior vena cava, the left phrenic nerve is applied directly to its lateral surface. The nerve passes anterior to the pulmonary hilum and eventually branches on the surface of the diaphragm. The vagus nerves enter the thorax posterior to the phrenic nerves and course along the carotid arteries. On the right side, the vagus gives off the recurrent laryngeal nerve that passes around the right

subclavian artery before ascending out of the thoracic cavity. The right vagus nerve continues posterior to the pulmonary hilum, gives off branches of the right pulmonary plexus, and exits the thorax along the esophagus. On the left, the vagus nerve crosses the aortic arch, where it gives off the recurrent laryngeal branch. The recurrent nerve passes around the arterial ligament before ascending in the tracheoesophageal groove. The vagus nerve continues posterior to the pulmonary hilum, gives rise to the left pulmonary plexus, and then continues inferiorly out of the thorax along the esophagus. A delicate nerve trunk known as the *subclavian loop* carries fibers from the stellate ganglion to the eye and head. This branch is located adjacent to the subclavian arteries bilaterally. Excessive dissection of the subclavian artery during shunt procedures may injure these nerve roots and cause Horner syndrome.

SURGICAL INCISIONS

Median Sternotomy

The most common approach for operations on the heart and aortic arch is the median sternotomy. The skin incision is made from the jugular notch to just below the xiphoid process. The subcutaneous tissues and presternal fascia are incised to expose the periostium of the sternum. The sternum is divided longitudinally in the midline. After placement of a sternal spreader, the thymic fat pad is divided up to the level of the brachiocephalic vein. An avascular midline plane is identified easily but is crossed by a few thymic veins that are divided between fine silk ties or hemoclips. Either the left or right or, occasionally, both lobes of the thymus gland are removed in infants and young children to improve exposure

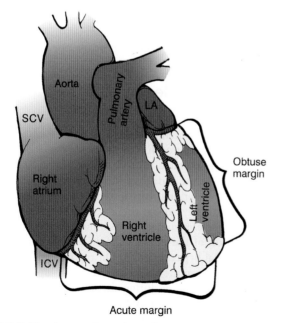

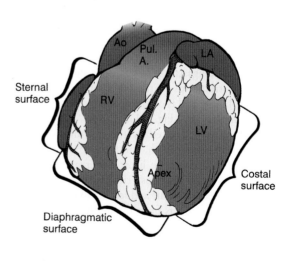

FIGURE 2-2 This diagram shows the surfaces and margins of the heart as viewed anteriorly with the patient supine on the operating table (*left*) and as viewed from the cardiac apex (*right*).

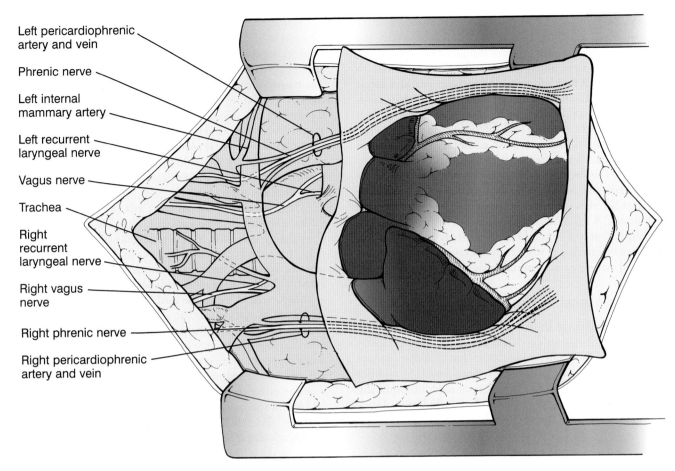

Left pericardiophrenic
artery and vein

Phrenic nerve

Left internal
mammary artery

Left recurrent
laryngeal nerve

Vagus nerve

Trachea

Right
recurrent
laryngeal nerve

Right vagus
nerve

Right phrenic nerve

Right pericardiophrenic
artery and vein

FIGURE 2-3 Diagram of the heart in relation to the vagus and phrenic nerves as viewed through a median sternotomy.

and minimize compression on extracardiac conduits. If a portion of the thymus gland is removed, excessive traction may result in injury to the phrenic nerve. The pericardium is opened anteriorly to expose the heart. Through this incision, operations within any chamber of the heart or on the surface of the heart and operations involving the proximal aorta, pulmonary trunk, and their primary branches can be performed. Extension of the superior extent of the incision into the neck along the anterior border of the right sternocleidomastoid muscle provides further exposure of the aortic arch and its branches for procedures involving these structures. Exposure of the proximal descending thoracic aorta is facilitated by a perpendicular extension of the incision through the third intercostal space.

Bilateral Transverse Thoracosternotomy (Clamshell Incision)

The bilateral transverse thoracosternotomy (clamshell incision) is an alternative incision for exposure of the pleural spaces and heart. This incision may be made through either the fourth or fifth intercostal space, depending on the intended procedure. After identifying the appropriate interspace, a bilateral sub-mammary incision is made. The incision is extended down

through the pectoralis major muscles to enter the hemithoraces through the appropriate intercostal space. The right and left internal thoracic arteries are dissected and ligated proximally and distally prior to transverse division of the sternum. Electrocautery dissection of the pleural reflections behind the sternum allows full exposure of both hemithoraces and the entire mediastinum. Bilateral chest spreaders are placed to maintain exposure. Morse or Haight retractors are particularly suitable with this incision. The pericardium may be opened anteriorly to allow access to the heart for intracardiac procedures. When required, standard cannulation for cardiopulmonary bypass is achieved easily. This incision is popular for bilateral sequential double-lung transplants and heart-lung transplants because of enhanced exposure of the apical pleural spaces. When made in the fourth intercostal space, the incision is useful for access to the ascending aorta, aortic arch, and descending thoracic aorta.

Anterolateral Thoracotomy

The right side of the heart can be exposed through a right anterolateral thoracotomy. The patient is positioned supine, with the right chest elevated to approximately 30 degrees by a roll beneath the shoulder. An anterolateral thoracotomy incision can be made that can be extended across the midline by transversely dividing the sternum if necessary. With the lung retracted posteriorly, the pericardium can be opened just anterior to the right phrenic nerve and pulmonary hilum to expose the right and left atria. The incision provides access to both the tricuspid and mitral valves and the right coronary artery. Cannulation may be performed in the ascending aorta and the superior and inferior venae cavae. Aortic cross-clamping, administration of cardioplegia, and removal of air from the heart after cardiotomy are difficult with this approach. This incision is particularly useful nonetheless for performance of the Blalock-Hanlon atrial septectomy or valve replacement after a previous procedure through a median sternotomy. A left anterolateral thoracotomy performed in a similar fashion to that on the right side may be used for isolated bypass grafting of the circumflex coronary artery or for left-sided exposure of the mitral valve.

Posterolateral Thoracotomy

A left posterolateral thoracotomy is used for procedures involving the distal aortic arch and descending thoracic aorta. With left thoracotomy, cannulation for cardiopulmonary bypass must be done through the femoral vessels. A number of variations of these incisions have been used for minimally invasive cardiac surgical procedures. These include partial sternotomies, parasternal incisions, and limited thoracotomies.

RELATIONSHIP OF THE CARDIAC CHAMBERS AND GREAT ARTERIES

The surgical anatomy of the heart is best understood when the position of the cardiac chambers and great vessels is known in relation to the cardiac silhouette. The atrioventricular junction is oriented obliquely, lying much closer to the vertical than to the horizontal plane. This plane can be viewed from its atrial aspect (Fig. 2-4) if the atrial mass and great arteries are removed by a parallel cut just above the junction. The tricuspid and pulmonary valves are widely separated by the inner curvature of the heart lined by the transverse sinus. Conversely, the mitral and aortic valves lie adjacent to one another, with fibrous continuity of their leaflets. The aortic valve occupies a central position, wedged between the tricuspid and pulmonary valves. Indeed, there is fibrous continuity between the leaflets of the aortic and tricuspid valves through the central fibrous body.

With careful study of this short axis, several basic rules of cardiac anatomy become apparent. First, the atrial chambers lie to the right of their corresponding ventricles. Second, the right atrium and ventricle lie anterior to their left-sided counterparts. The septal structures between them are obliquely oriented. Third, by virtue of its wedged position, the aortic valve is directly related to all the cardiac chambers. Several other significant features of cardiac anatomy can be learned from the short-axis section. The position of the aortic valve minimizes the area of septum where the mitral and tricuspid valves attach opposite to each other. Because the tricuspid valve is attached to the septum further toward the ventricular apex than the mitral valve, it seems that a muscular atrioventricular septum interposes between the right atrium and the left ventricle. We now know that a continuation of the inferior atrioventricular groove interposes between the atrial and ventricular walls in this area, so that it is a sandwich rather than a true septum, with the fibro-adipose tissue of the atrioventricular groove forming the "meat" in the sandwich. The central fibrous body, where the leaflets of the aortic, mitral, and tricuspid valves all converge, lies cephalad and anterior to the muscular atrioventricular sandwich. The central fibrous body is the main component of the fibrous skeleton of the heart

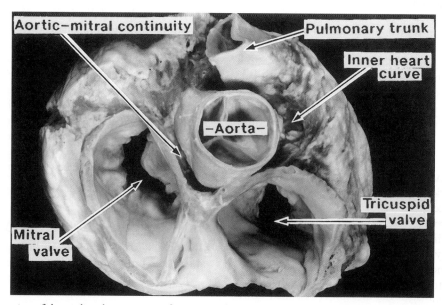

FIGURE 2-4 This dissection of the cardiac short axis, seen from its atrial aspect, reveals the relationships of the cardiac valves.

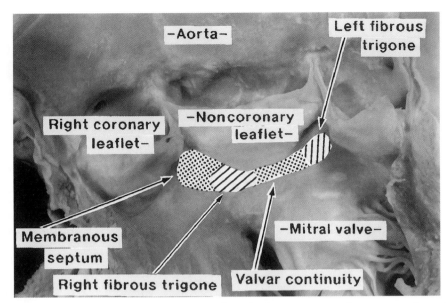

FIGURE 2-5 This view of the left ventricular outflow tract, as seen from the front in anatomical orientation, shows the limited extent of the fibrous skeleton of the heart.

and is made up in part by the right fibrous trigone, a thickening of the right side of the area of fibrous continuity between the aortic and mitral valves, and in part by the membranous septum, the fibrous partition between the left ventricular outflow tract and the right-sided heart chambers (Fig. 2-5). The membranous septum itself is divided into two parts by the septal leaflet of the tricuspid valve, which is directly attached across it (Fig. 2-6). Thus the membranous septum has an atrioventricular component between the right atrium and left ventricle, as well as an interventricular component. Removal of the noncoronary leaflet of the aortic valve demonstrates the significance of the wedged position of the left ventricular outflow tract in relation to the other cardiac chambers. The subaortic region separates the mitral orifice from the ventricular septum; this separation influences the position of the atrioventricular conduction tissues and the position of the leaflets and tension apparatus of the mitral valve (Fig. 2-7).

THE RIGHT ATRIUM AND TRICUSPID VALVE

Appendage, Vestibule, and Venous Component

The right atrium has three basic parts: the appendage, the vestibule, and the venous component (Fig. 2-8). Externally, the right atrium is divided into the appendage and the venous component, which receives the systemic venous return. The junction of the appendage and the venous component is identified by a prominent groove, the *terminal groove*. This corresponds internally to the location of the terminal crest. The right atrial appendage has the shape of a blunt triangle, with a wide junction to the venous component across the terminal groove. The appendage also has an extensive junction with the vestibule of the right atrium; the latter structure is

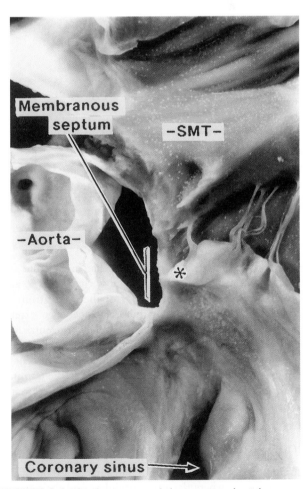

FIGURE 2-6 This dissection, made by removing the right coronary sinus of the aortic valve, shows how the septal leaflet of the tricuspid valve (*asterisk*) divides the membranous septum into its atrioventricular and interventricular components. SMT = septomarginal trabeculation.

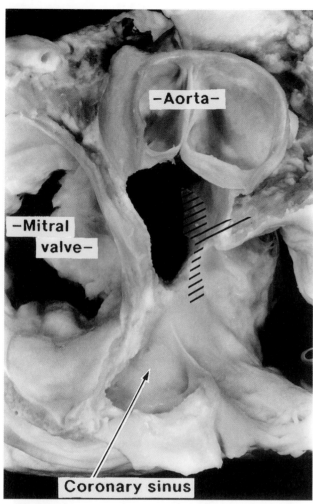

FIGURE 2-7 This dissection, made by removing the noncoronary aortic sinus (compare with Figs. 2-4 and 2-6), shows the approximate location of the atrioventricular conduction axis (*hatched area*) and the relationship of the mitral valve to the ventricular septum.

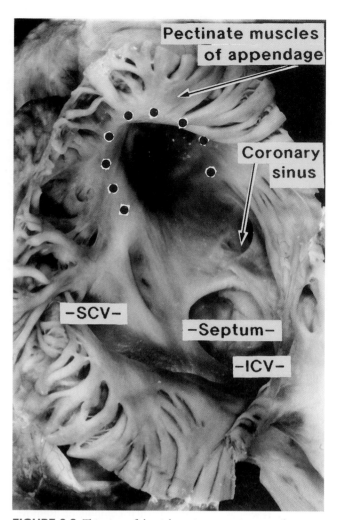

FIGURE 2-8 This view of the right atrium, seen in surgical orientation, shows the pectinate muscles lining the appendage, the smooth vestibule (*circles*) surrounding the orifice of the tricuspid valve, and the superior vena cava (SCV), inferior vena cava (ICV), and coronary sinus joining the smooth-walled venous component. Note the prominent rim enclosing the oval fossa, which is the true atrial septum (see Fig. 2-11).

the smooth-walled atrial myocardium that inserts into the leaflets of the tricuspid valve. The most characteristic and constant feature of the morphology of the right atrium is that the pectinate muscles within the appendage extend around the entire parietal margin of the atrioventricular junction (Fig. 2-9). These muscles originate as parallel fibers that course at right angles from the terminal crest. The venous component of the right atrium extends between the terminal groove and the interatrial groove. It receives the superior and inferior venae cavae and the coronary sinus.

Sinus Node

The sinus node lies at the anterior and superior extent of the terminal groove, where the atrial appendage and the superior vena cava are juxtaposed. The node is a spindle-shaped structure that usually lies to the right or lateral to the superior cavoatrial junction (Fig. 2-10). In approximately 10% of

cases, the node is draped across the cavoatrial junction in horseshoe fashion.[1]

The blood supply to the sinus node is from a prominent nodal artery that is a branch of the right coronary artery in approximately 55% of individuals and a branch of the circumflex artery in the remainder. Regardless of its artery of origin, the nodal artery usually courses along the anterior interatrial groove toward the superior cavoatrial junction, frequently within the atrial myocardium. At the cavoatrial junction, its course becomes variable and may circle either anteriorly or posteriorly or, rarely, both anteriorly and posteriorly around the cavoatrial junction to enter the node. Uncommonly, the artery arises more distally from the right coronary artery and courses laterally across the atrial appendage. This places it at risk of injury during a standard right atriotomy. The artery also may arise distally from the circumflex artery to cross the

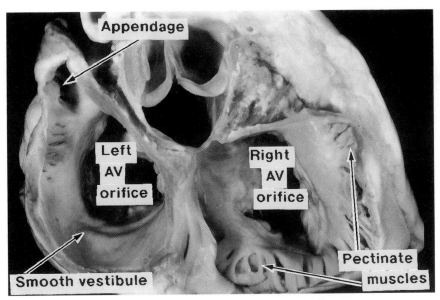

FIGURE 2-9 This dissection of the short axis of the heart (compare with Fig. 2-4) shows how the pectinate muscles extend around the parietal margin of the tricuspid valve. In the left atrium, the pectinate muscles are confined within the tubular left atrial appendage, leaving the smooth vestibule around the mitral valve confluent with the pulmonary venous component of the left atrium.

dome of the left atrium, where it is at risk of injury when using a superior approach to the mitral valve. Incisions in either the right or left atrial chambers always should be made with this anatomical variability in mind. In our experience, these vessels can be identified by careful gross inspection, and prompt modification of surgical incisions can be made accordingly.

Atrial Septum

The most common incision into the right atrium is made into the atrial appendage parallel and anterior to the terminal groove. Opening the atrium through this incision confirms that the terminal groove is the external marking of the prominent terminal crest. Anteriorly and superiorly, the crest curves in front of the orifice of the superior vena cava to become continuous with the so-called septum secundum, which, in reality, is the superior rim of the oval fossa. When the right atrium is inspected through this incision, there appears to be an extensive septal surface between the tricuspid valve and the orifices of the venae cavae. This septal surface includes the opening of the oval fossa and the orifice of the coronary sinus. The apparent extent of the septum is spurious because the true septum between the atrial chambers is virtually confined to the oval fossa[2,3] (Fig. 2-11). The superior rim of the fossa, although often referred to as the *septum secundum*, is an extensive infolding between the venous component of the right atrium and the right pulmonary veins. The inferior rim is directly continuous with the so-called sinus septum that separates the orifices of the inferior caval vein and the coronary sinus (Fig. 2-12).

The atrial wall surrounding the mouth of the coronary sinus is continuous anteriorly and superiorly with the atrial component of the atrioventricular muscular sandwich. Removing the floor of the coronary sinus reveals the anterior extension of the atrioventricular groove in this region. The inferior component of the anterior rim of the oval fossa is a true septal structure. It is continuous superiorly with the anterior atrial wall overlying the aortic root. Thus dissection outside the limited margins of the oval fossa will penetrate the heart to the outside rather than provide access to the left atrium via the septum.

Atrioventricular Septum and Node: Triangle of Koch

In addition to the sinus node, another major area of surgical significance is occupied by the atrioventricular node. This structure lies within the triangle of Koch, which is demarcated by the tendon of Todaro, the septal leaflet of the tricuspid valve, and the orifice of the coronary sinus (Fig. 2-13). The floor of the triangle of Koch is made up of the atrial wall of the atrioventricular muscular sandwich. The tendon of Todaro is a fibrous structure formed by the junction of the eustachian valve and thebesian valve (the valves of the inferior vena cava and the coronary sinus, respectively). The entire atrial component of the atrioventricular conduction tissues is contained within the triangle of Koch, which must be avoided to prevent surgical damage to atrioventricular conduction. The atrioventricular bundle (of His) penetrates directly at the apex of the triangle of Koch before it continues to branch on the crest of the ventricular septum (Fig. 2-14). The key to avoiding atrial arrhythmias is careful preservation of the sinus and atrioventricular nodes and their blood supply.

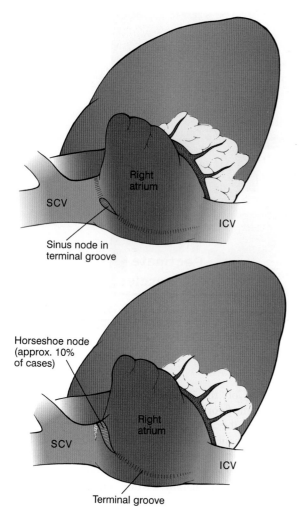

FIGURE 2-10 This diagram shows the location of the sinus node at the superior cavoatrial junction. The node usually lies to the right (*lateral*) side of the junction but may be draped in horseshoe fashion across the anterior aspect of the junction. ICV = inferior vena cava; SCV = superior vena cava.

No advantage is gained in attempting to preserve nonexistent tracts of specialized atrial conduction tissue, although it makes sense to avoid prominent muscle bundles where parallel orientation of atrial myocardial fibers favors preferential conduction (Fig. 2-15).

Tricuspid Valve

The vestibule of the right atrium converges into the tricuspid valve. The three leaflets reflect their anatomical location, being septal, anterosuperior, and inferior (or mural). The leaflets join together over three prominent zones of apposition; the peripheral ends of these zones usually are described as *commissures*. The leaflets are tethered at the commissures by fan-shaped cords arising from prominent papillary muscles. The anteroseptal commissure is supported by the medial papillary muscle. The major leaflets of the valve extend from this

position in anterosuperior and septal directions. The third leaflet is less well defined. The anteroinferior commissure is usually supported by the prominent anterior papillary muscle. Often, however, it is not possible to identify a specific inferior papillary muscle supporting the inferoseptal commissure. Thus the inferior leaflet may seem duplicated. There is no well-formed collagenous annulus for the tricuspid valve. Instead, the atrioventricular groove more or less folds directly into the tricuspid valvar leaflets at the vestibule, and the atrial and ventricular myocardial masses are separated almost exclusively by the fibrofatty tissue of the groove. The entire parietal attachment of the tricuspid valve usually is encircled by the right coronary artery running within the atrioventricular groove.

THE LEFT ATRIUM AND MITRAL VALVE

Appendage, Vestibule, and Venous Component

Like the right atrium, the left atrium has three basic components: the appendage, the vestibule, and the venous component (Fig. 2-16). It also possesses a large smooth walled-body, which represents the larger part of the atrial component of the developing heart tube. Unlike the right atrium, the venous component is considerably larger than the appendage and has a narrow junction with it that is not marked by a terminal groove or crest. There also is an important difference between the relationship of the appendage and vestibule between the left and right atria. As shown, the pectinate muscles within the right atrial appendage extend all around the parietal margin of the vestibule. In contrast, the left atrial appendage has a limited junction with the vestibule, and the pectinate muscles are located almost exclusively within the appendage (see Fig. 2-8). The larger part of the vestibule that supports and inserts directly into the mural leaflet of the mitral valve is directly continuous with the smooth atrial wall of the pulmonary venous component.

Because the left atrium is posterior to and tethered by the four pulmonary veins, the chamber is relatively inaccessible. Surgeons use several approaches to gain access. The most common is an incision just to the right of and parallel to the interatrial groove, anterior to the right pulmonary veins. This incision can be carried beneath both the superior and inferior venae cavae parallel to the interatrial groove to provide wide access to the left atrium. A second approach is through the dome of the left atrium. If the aorta is pulled anteriorly and to the left, an extensive trough may be seen between the right and left atrial appendages. An incision through this trough, between the pulmonary veins of the upper lobes, provides direct access to the left atrium. When this incision is made, it is important to remember the location of the sinus node artery, which may course along the roof of the left atrium if it arises from the circumflex artery. The left atrium also can be reached via a right atrial incision and an opening in the atrial septum.

When the interior of the left atrium is visualized, the small size of the mouth of the left atrial appendage is apparent.

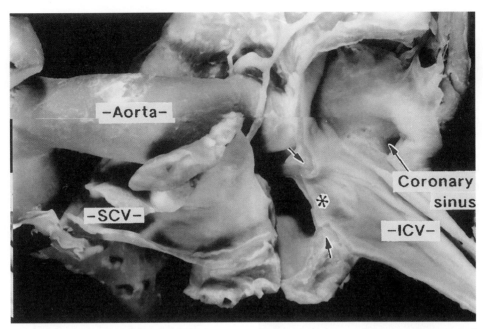

FIGURE 2-11 This transection across the middle of the oval fossa (*asterisk*) shows how the so-called septum secundum, the rim of the fossa, is made up of the infolded atrial walls (*arrows*). ICV = inferior vena cava; SCV = superior vena cava.

It lies to the left of the mitral orifice as viewed by the surgeon. The majority of the pulmonary venous atrium usually is located inferiorly away from the operative field. The vestibule of the mitral orifice dominates the operative view. The septal surface is located anteriorly, with the true septum relatively inferior (Fig. 2-17).

Mitral Valve

The mitral valve is supported by two prominent papillary muscles located in supero-lateral and infero-septal positions. The two leaflets of the mitral valve have markedly different appearances (Fig. 2-18). The aortic (or anterior) leaflet is short and relatively square, and guards approximately one-third of the circumference of the valvar orifice. This leaflet is in fibrous continuity with the aortic valve and, because of this, is best referred to as the *aortic leaflet* because it is neither strictly anterior nor superior in position. The other leaflet is much shallower but guards approximately two-thirds of the circumference of the mitral orifice. Because it is connected to the parietal part of the atrioventricular junction, it is most accurately termed the *mural leaflet* but often is termed the *posterior leaflet*. It is divided into a number of subunits that fold against the

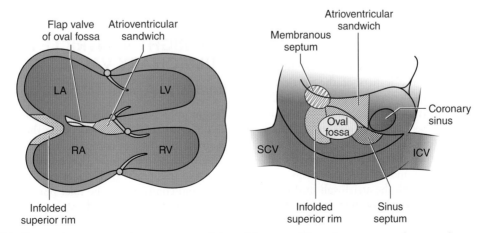

FIGURE 2-12 This diagram demonstrates the components of the atrial septum. The only true septum between the two atria is confined to the area of the oval fossa. ICV = inferior vena cava; SCV = superior vena cava.

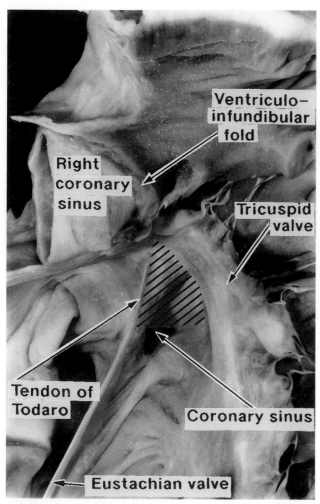

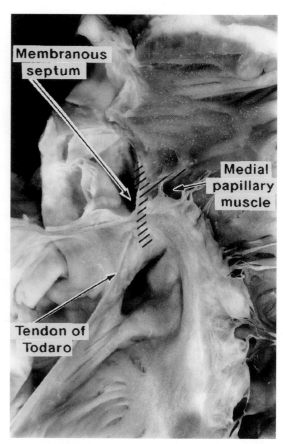

FIGURE 2-14 Further dissection of the heart shown in Fig. 2-13 reveals that a line joining the apex of the triangle of Koch to the medial papillary muscle marks the location of the atrioventricular conduction axis.

FIGURE 2-13 This dissection, made by removing part of the subpulmonary infundibulum, shows the location of the triangle of Koch (*shaded area*).

aortic leaflet when the valve is closed. Although generally there are three, there may be as many as five or six scallops in the mural leaflet.

Unlike the tricuspid valve, the mitral valve leaflets are supported by a rather dense collagenous annulus, although it may take the form of a sheet rather than a cord. This annulus usually extends parietally from the fibrous trigones, the greatly thickened areas at either end of the area of fibrous continuity between the leaflets of the aortic and mitral valves (see Fig. 2-6). The area of the valvar orifice related to the right fibrous trigone and central fibrous body is most vulnerable with respect to the atrioventricular node and penetrating bundle (see Fig. 2-7). The midportion of the aortic leaflet of the mitral valve is related to the commissure between the noncoronary and left coronary cusps of the aortic valve. An incision through the atrial wall in this area may be extended into the subaortic outflow tract and may be useful for enlarging the aortic annulus during replacement of the aortic valve (Fig. 2-19). The circumflex coronary artery is adjacent to the left half of the mural leaflet,

whereas the coronary sinus is adjacent to the right half of the mural leaflet (Fig. 2-20). These structures can be damaged during excessive dissection or by excessively deep placement of sutures during replacement or repair of the mitral valve. When the circumflex artery is dominant, the entire attachment of the mural leaflet may be intimately related to this artery (Fig. 2-21).

THE RIGHT VENTRICLE AND PULMONARY VALVE

Inlet and Apical Trabecular Portions

The morphology of both the right and left ventricles can be understood best by subdividing the ventricles into three anatomically distinct components: the inlet, apical trabecular, and outlet portions.[2] This classification is more helpful than the traditional division of the right ventricle into the sinus and conus parts. The inlet portion of the right ventricle surrounds the tricuspid valve and its tension apparatus. A distinguishing feature of the tricuspid valve is the direct attachment of its septal leaflet. The apical trabecular portion of the right ventricle extends out to the apex. Here, the wall

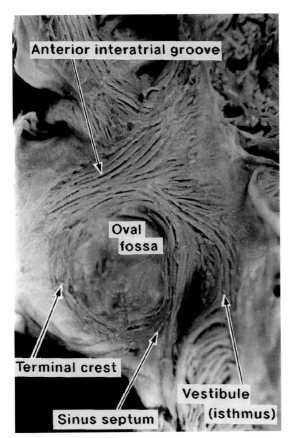

FIGURE 2-15 This dissection, made by careful removal of the right atrial endocardium, shows the ordered arrangement of myocardial fibers in the prominent muscle bundles that underscore preferential conduction. There are *no* insulated tracts running within the internodal atrial myocardium. (Used with permission from Prof. Damian Sanchez-Quintana.)

of the ventricle is quite thin and vulnerable to perforation by cardiac catheters and pacemaker electrodes.

Outlet Portion and Pulmonary Valve

The outlet portion of the right ventricle consists of the infundibulum, a circumferential muscular structure that supports the leaflets of the pulmonary valve. Because of the semilunar shape of the pulmonary valvar leaflets, this valve does not have an annulus in the traditional sense of a ringlike attachment. The leaflets have semilunar attachments that cross the musculoarterial junction in a corresponding semilunar fashion (Fig. 2-22). Therefore, instead of a single annulus, three rings can be distinguished anatomically in relation to the pulmonary valve. Superiorly, the sinotubular ridge of the pulmonary trunk marks the level of peripheral apposition of the leaflets (the commissures). A second ring exists at the ventriculoarterial junction. A third ring can be constructed by joining together the basal attachments of the three leaflets to the infundibular muscle. None of these rings, however, corresponds to the attachments of the leaflets, which must be semilunar to permit the valve to open and close competently. In fact, these semilunar attachments, which mark the hemodynamic ventriculoarterial junction, extend from the first ring, across the second, down to the third, and back in each cusp (Fig. 2-23).

Supraventricular Crest and Pulmonary Infundibulum

A distinguishing feature of the right ventricle is a prominent muscular shelf, the supraventricular crest, which separates the

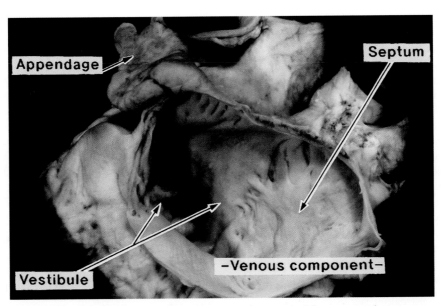

FIGURE 2-16 Like the right atrium, the left atrium (seen here in anatomical orientation) has an appendage, a venous component, and a vestibule. It is separated from the right atrium by the septum.

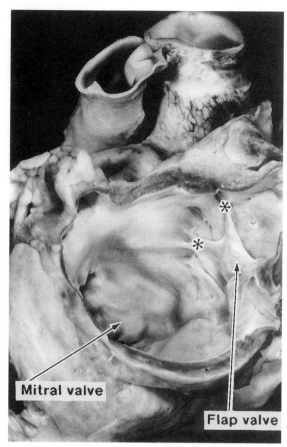

FIGURE 2-17 This view of the opened left atrium shows how the septal aspect is dominated by the flap valve, which is attached by its horns (*asterisks*) to the infolded atrial groove.

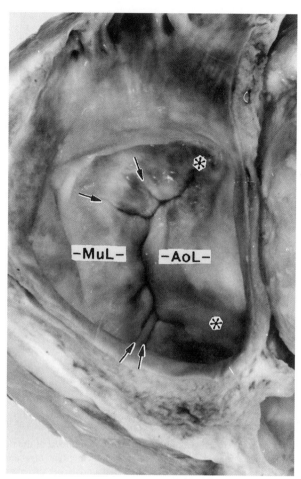

FIGURE 2-18 This view of the opened left atrium shows the leaflets of the mitral valve in closed position. There is a concave zone of apposition between them (*between asterisks*) with several slits seen in the mural leaflet (MuL). Note the limited extent of the aortic leaflet (AoL) in terms of its circumferential attachments.

tricuspid and pulmonary valves (Fig. 2-24). In reality, this muscular ridge is the posterior part of the subpulmonary muscular infundibulum that supports the leaflets of the pulmonary valve. In other words, it is part of the inner curve of the heart. Incisions through the supraventricular crest run into the transverse septum and may jeopardize the right coronary artery. Although this area is often considered the outlet component of the interventricular septum, in fact the entire subpulmonary infundibulum, including the ventriculoinfundibular fold, can be removed without entering the left ventricular cavity. This is possible because the leaflets of the pulmonary and aortic valves are supported on separate sleeves of right and left ventricular outlet muscles. There is an extensive external tissue plane between the walls of the aorta and the pulmonary trunk (Fig. 2-25), and the leaflets of the pulmonary and aortic valves have markedly different levels of attachments within their respective ventricles. This feature enables enucleation of the pulmonary valve, including its basal attachments within the infundibulum, during the Ross procedure without creating a ventricular septal defect. When the infundibulum is removed from the right ventricle, the insertion of the supraventricular crest between the limbs of the septomarginal trabeculation is visible (Fig. 2-26). This

trabeculation is a prominent muscle column that divides superiorly into anterior and posterior limbs. The anterior limb runs superiorly into the infundibulum and supports the leaflets of the pulmonary valve. The posterior limb extends backward beneath the ventricular septum and runs into the inlet portion of the ventricle. The medial papillary muscle arises from this posterior limb. The body of the septomarginal trabeculation runs to the apex of the ventricle, where it divides into smaller trabeculations. Two of these trabeculations may be particularly prominent. One becomes the anterior papillary muscle, and the other crosses the ventricular cavity as the moderator band (Fig. 2-27).

THE LEFT VENTRICLE AND AORTIC VALVE

Inlet and Apical Trabecular Portions

The left ventricle can be subdivided into three components, similar to the right ventricle. The inlet component surrounds

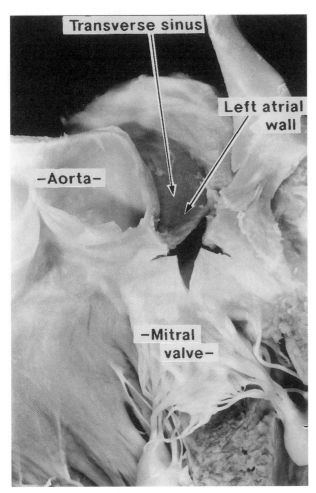

FIGURE 2-19 This dissection simulates the incision made through the aortic-mitral fibrous curtain to enlarge the orificial diameter of the subaortic outflow tract in a normal heart.

and is limited by the mitral valve and its tension apparatus. The two papillary muscles occupy superolateral and inferoseptal positions and are positioned rather close to each other. The leaflets of the mitral valve have no direct septal attachments because the deep posterior diverticulum of the left ventricular outflow tract displaces the aortic leaflet away from the inlet septum. The apical trabecular component of the left ventricle extends to the apex, where the myocardium is surprisingly thin. The trabeculations of the left ventricle are quite fine compared with those of the right ventricle (Fig. 2-28). This characteristic is useful for defining ventricular morphology on diagnostic ventriculograms.

Outlet Portion

The outlet component supports the aortic valve and consists of both muscular and fibrous portions. This is in contrast to the infundibulum of the right ventricle, which consists entirely of muscle. The septal portion of the left ventricular outflow tract, although primarily muscular, also includes the membranous portion of the ventricular septum. The posterior quadrant of the outflow tract consists of an extensive fibrous curtain that extends from the fibrous skeleton of the heart across the aortic leaflet of the mitral valve and supports the leaflets of the aortic valve in the area of aortomitral continuity (see Fig. 2-5). The lateral quadrant of the outflow tract again is muscular and consists of the lateral margin of the inner curvature of the heart, delineated externally by the transverse sinus. The left bundle of the cardiac conduction system enters the left ventricular outflow tract posterior to the membranous septum and immediately beneath the commissure between the right and noncoronary leaflets of the aortic valve. After traveling a short distance down the septum, the left bundle divides into anterior, septal, and posterior divisions.

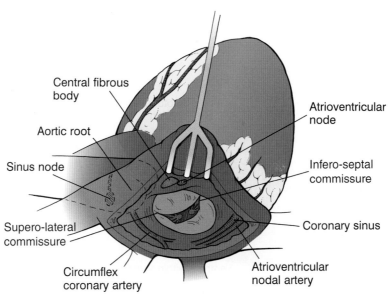

FIGURE 2-20 This diagram depicts the mitral valve in relationship to its surrounding structures as viewed through a left atriotomy.

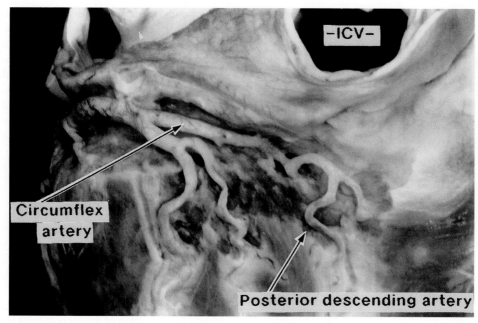

FIGURE 2-21 The extensive course of a dominant circumflex artery within the left atrioventricular groove shown in anatomic orientation. ICV = inferior vena cava.

Aortic Valve

The aortic valve is a semilunar valve that is quite similar morphologically to the pulmonary valve. Likewise, it does not have a discrete annulus. Because of its central location, the aortic valve is related to each of the cardiac chambers and valves (see Fig. 2-4). A thorough knowledge of these relationships is essential to understanding aortic valve pathology and many congenital cardiac malformations.

The aortic valve consists primarily of three semilunar leaflets. As with the pulmonary valve, attachments of the leaflets extend across the ventriculoarterial junction in a curvilinear fashion. Each leaflet therefore has attachments to the aorta

and within the left ventricle (Fig. 2-29). Behind each leaflet, the aortic wall bulges outward to form the sinuses of Valsalva. The leaflets themselves meet centrally along a line of coaptation, at the center of which is a thickened nodule called the *nodule of Arantius*. Peripherally, adjacent to the commissures, the line of coaptation is thinner and normally may contain small perforations. During systole the leaflets are thrust upward and away from the center of the aortic lumen, whereas during diastole they fall passively into the center of the aorta. With normal valvar morphology, all three leaflets meet along lines of coaptation and support the column of blood within the aorta to prevent regurgitation into the ventricle. Two of the three aortic sinuses give rise to coronary

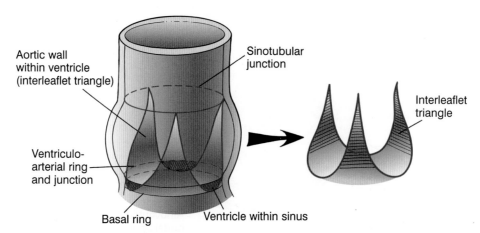

FIGURE 2-22 The semilunar valves do not have an annulus in the traditional sense. Rather, three rings can be identified anatomically, at the (1) sinotubular junction, (2) musculoarterial junction, and (3) base of the sinuses within the ventricle.

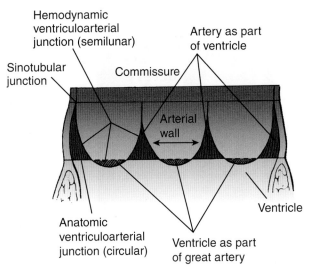

FIGURE 2-23 The hemodynamic ventriculoarterial junction of the semilunar valves extends from the sinotubular junction across the anatomical ventriculoarterial junction to the basal ring and back in each leaflet (see Fig. 2-22). This creates a portion of ventricle as part of the great artery in each sinus and a triangle of artery as part of the ventricle between each leaflet.

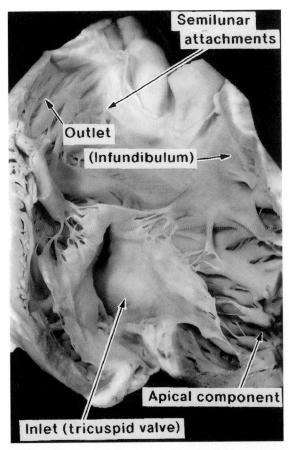

FIGURE 2-24 View of the opened right ventricle, in anatomical orientation, showing its three component parts and the semilunar attachments of the pulmonary valve. These are supported by the supraventricular crest.

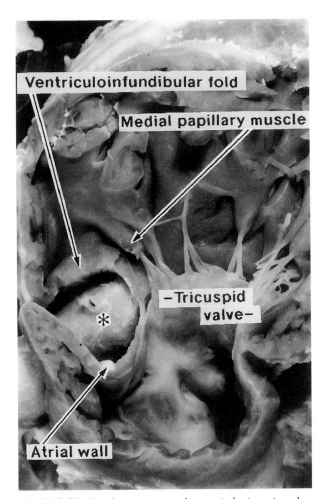

FIGURE 2-25 This dissection, viewed in surgical orientation, shows how the greater part of the supraventricular crest is formed by the freestanding subpulmonary infundibulum in relation to the right coronary aortic sinus (*asterisk*).

arteries, from which arise their designations as *right, left,* and *noncoronary sinuses.*

By sequentially following the line of attachment of each leaflet, the relationship of the aortic valve to its surrounding structures can be clearly understood. Beginning posteriorly, the commissure between the noncoronary and left coronary leaflets is positioned along the area of aortomitral valvar continuity. The fibrous subaortic curtain is beneath this commissure (see Fig. 2-29). To the right of this commissure, the noncoronary leaflet is attached above the posterior diverticulum of the left ventricular outflow tract. Here, the valve is related to the right atrial wall. As the attachment of the noncoronary leaflet ascends from its nadir toward the commissure between the noncoronary and right coronary leaflets, the line of attachment is directly above the portion of the atrial septum containing the atrioventricular node. The commissure between the noncoronary and right coronary leaflets is located directly above the penetrating atrioventricular bundle and the membranous ventricular septum (Fig. 2-30). The attachment of the right coronary leaflet then descends

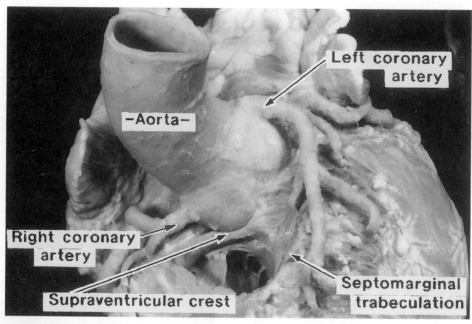

FIGURE 2-26 Removal of the freestanding subpulmonary infundibulum reveals the insertion of the supraventricular crest between the limbs of the septomarginal trabeculation and shows the aortic origin of the coronary arteries (anatomical orientation).

across the central fibrous body before ascending to the commissure between the right and left coronary leaflets. Immediately beneath this commissure, the wall of the aorta forms the uppermost part of the subaortic outflow. An incision through this area passes into the space between the facing surfaces of the aorta and pulmonary trunk (see Fig. 2-30). As the facing left and right leaflets descend from this commissure, they

are attached to the outlet muscular component of the left ventricle. Only a small part of this area in the normal heart is a true outlet septum because both pulmonary and aortic valves are supported on their own sleeves of myocardium. Thus, although the outlet components of the right and left ventricles face each other, an incision below the aortic valve enters low into the infundibulum of the right ventricle. As

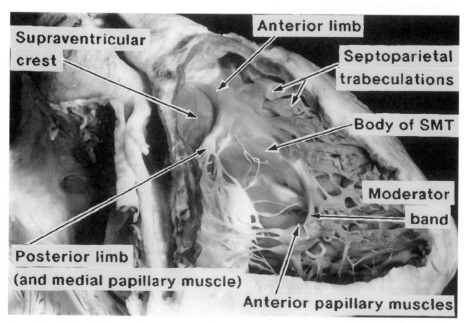

FIGURE 2-27 This dissection of the right ventricle, in anatomical orientation, shows the relations of supraventricular crest and septomarginal (SMT) and septoparietal trabeculations.

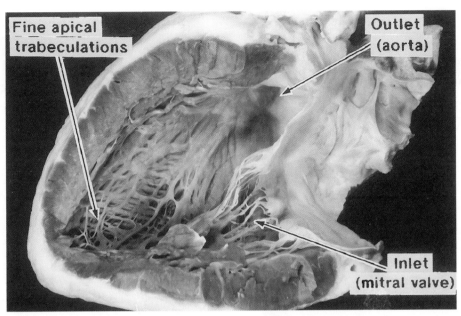

FIGURE 2-28 This dissection of the left ventricle shows its component parts and characteristically fine apical trabeculations (anatomical orientation).

the lateral part of the left coronary leaflet descends from the facing commissure to the base of the sinus, it becomes the only part of the aortic valve that is not intimately related to another cardiac chamber.

Knowledge of the anatomy of the aortic valve and its relationship to surrounding structures is important to successful replacement of the aortic valve, particularly when

enlargement of the aortic root is required. The Konno-Rastan aortoventriculoplasty involves opening and enlarging the anterior portion of the subaortic region.[4,5] The incisions for this procedure begin with an anterior longitudinal aortotomy that extends through the commissure between the right and left coronary leaflets. Anteriorly, the incision is extended across the base of the infundibulum. The differential level of

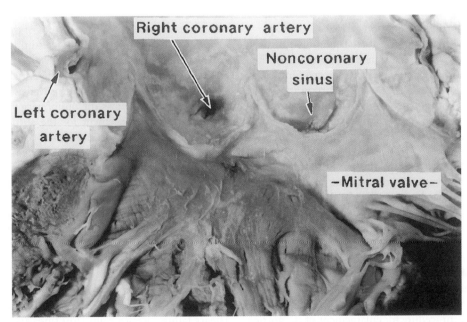

FIGURE 2-29 This dissection in anatomic orientation, made by removing the aortic valvar leaflets, emphasizes the semilunar nature of the hinge points (see Figs. 2-22 and 2-23). Note the relationship to the mitral valve (see Fig. 2-5).

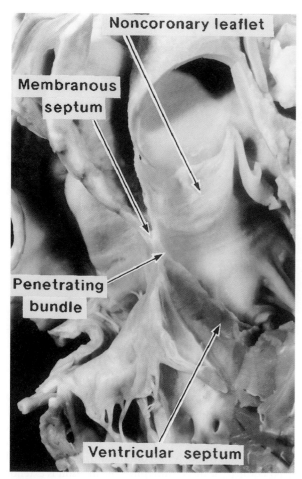

FIGURE 2-30 Dissection made by removing the right and part of the left aortic sinuses to show the relations of the fibrous triangle between the right and noncoronary aortic leaflets (anatomical orientation).

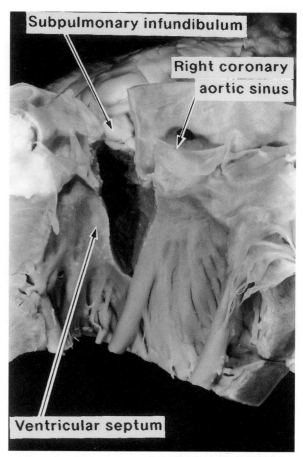

FIGURE 2-31 This incision, made in a normal heart, simulates the Konno-Rastan procedure for enlargement of the aortic root.

attachment of the aortic and pulmonary valve leaflets permits this incision without damage to the pulmonary valve (Fig. 2-31). Posteriorly, the incision extends through the most medial portion of the supraventricular crest into the left ventricular outflow tract. By closing the resulting ventricular septal defect with a patch, the aortic outflow tract is widened to allow implantation of a larger valve prosthesis. A second patch is used to close the defect in the right ventricular outflow tract.

Alternative methods to enlarge the aortic outflow tract involve incisions in the region of aortomitral continuity. In the Manouguian procedure (see Fig. 2-19), a curvilinear aortotomy is extended posteriorly through the commissure between the left and noncoronary leaflets down to and occasionally into the aortic leaflet of the mitral valve.[6] A patch is used to augment the incision posteriorly. When the posterior diverticulum of the outflow tract is fully developed, this incision can be made without entering other cardiac chambers, although not uncommonly the roof of the left atrium is opened. The Nicks procedure for enlargement of the aortic

root involves an aortotomy that passes through the middle of the noncoronary leaflet into the fibrous subaortic curtain and may be extended into the aortic leaflet of the mitral valve.[7] This incision also may open the roof of the left atrium. When these techniques are used, any resulting defect in the left atrium must be closed carefully.

As discussed previously, the differential level of attachment of aortic and pulmonary valves, as well as the muscular nature of their support, allows the pulmonary valve to be harvested and used as a replacement for the aortic valve in the Ross procedure.[8,9] This procedure can be combined with the incisions of the Konno-Rastan aortoventriculoplasty to repair left ventricular outflow tract obstructions in young children with a viable autograft that has potential for growth and avoids the need for anticoagulation.

Accurate understanding of left ventricular outflow tract anatomy is also important in the treatment of aortic valvar endocarditis.[10,11] Because of the central position of the aortic valve relative to the other valves and cardiac chambers (see Fig. 2-4), abscess formation can produce fistulas between the aorta and any of the four chambers of the heart. Therefore, patients may present with findings of left-sided heart failure, left-to-right shunting, and/or complete heart block in addition to the usual signs of sepsis and systemic embolization.

THE CORONARY ARTERIES[12-14]

The right and left coronary arteries originate behind their respective aortic valvar leaflets (see Fig. 2-26). The orifices usually are located in the upper third of the sinuses of Valsalva, although individual hearts may vary markedly. Because of the oblique plane of the aortic valve, the orifice of the left coronary artery is superior and posterior to that of the right coronary artery. The coronary arterial tree is divided into three segments; two (the left anterior descending artery and the circumflex artery) arise from a common stem. The third segment is the right coronary artery. The dominance of the coronary circulation (right vs left) usually refers to the artery from which the inferior interventricular artery originates, not the absolute mass of myocardium perfused by the left or right coronary artery. Right dominance occurs in 85 to 90% of normal individuals. Left dominance occurs slightly more frequently in males than in females.

Main Stem of the Left Coronary Artery

The main stem of the left coronary artery courses from the left sinus of Valsalva anteriorly, inferiorly, and to the left between the pulmonary trunk and the left atrial appendage (Fig. 2-32). Typically, it is 10 to 20 mm in length, but can extend to a length of 40 mm. The left main stem can be absent, with separate orifices in the sinus of Valsalva for its two primary branches (1% of patients). The main stem divides into two major arteries of nearly equal diameter, the left anterior descending artery and the circumflex artery.

Left Anterior Descending Artery

The left anterior descending (or interventricular) coronary artery continues directly from the bifurcation of the left main stem, coursing anteriorly and inferiorly in the anterior interventricular groove to the apex of the heart (Fig. 2-33). Its branches include the diagonals, the septal perforators, and the right ventricular branches. The diagonals, which may be two to six in number, course along the anterolateral wall of the left ventricle and supply this portion of the myocardium. The first diagonal generally is the largest and may arise from the bifurcation of the left main stem (formerly known as the *intermediate artery*). The septal perforators branch perpendicularly into the ventricular septum. Typically, there are three to five septal perforators; the initial one is the largest and commonly originates just beyond the take-off of the first diagonal. This perpendicular orientation is a useful marker for identification of the left anterior descending artery on coronary angiograms. The septal perforators supply blood to the anterior two-thirds of the ventricular septum. Right ventricular branches, which may not always be present, supply blood to the anterior surface of the right ventricle. In approximately 4% of hearts, the left anterior descending artery bifurcates proximally and continues as two parallel vessels of approximately equal size down the anterior interventricular groove. Occasionally, the artery

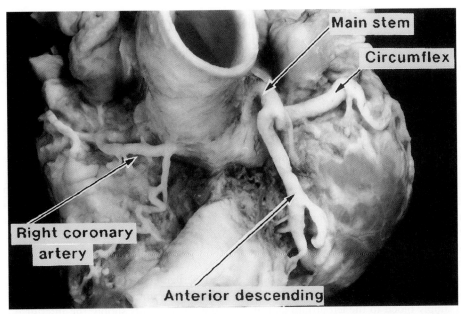

FIGURE 2-32 The short extent of the main stem of the left coronary artery is seen before it branches into the circumflex and anterior descending arteries. Note the small right coronary artery in this heart, in which the circumflex artery was dominant (see Fig. 2-21).

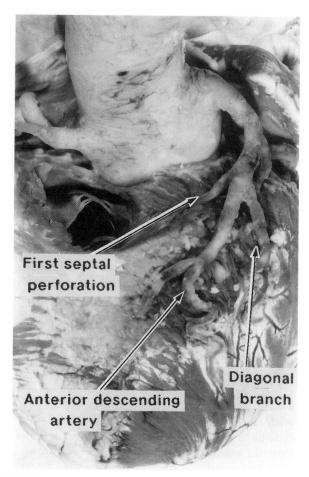

FIGURE 2-33 The important branches of the anterior descending artery are the first septal perforating and diagonal arteries.

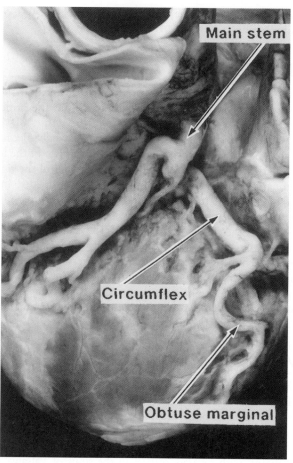

FIGURE 2-34 The important branches of the circumflex artery, seen in anatomical orientation.

wraps around the apex of the left ventricle to feed the distal portion of the posterior interventricular groove. Rarely, it extends along the entire length of the posterior groove to replace the inferior interventricular artery.

Circumflex Artery

The left circumflex coronary artery arises from the left main coronary artery roughly at a right angle to the anterior interventricular branch. It courses along the left atrioventricular groove and in 85 to 95% of patients terminates near the obtuse margin of the left ventricle (Fig. 2-34). In 10 to 15% of patients, it continues around the atrioventricular groove to the crux of the heart to give rise to the inferior interventricular artery (left dominance; see Fig. 2-21). The primary branches of the left circumflex coronary artery are the obtuse marginals. They supply blood to the lateral aspect of the left ventricular myocardium, including the posteromedial papillary muscle. Additional branches supply blood to the left atrium and, in 40 to 50% of hearts, the sinus node. When the circumflex coronary artery supplies the inferior interventricular artery, it also supplies the atrioventricular node.

Right Coronary Artery

The right coronary artery courses from the aorta anteriorly and laterally before descending in the right atrioventricular groove and curving posteriorly at the acute margin of the right ventricle (Fig. 2-35). In 85 to 90% of hearts, the right coronary artery crosses the crux, where it makes a characteristic U-turn before bifurcating into the inferior interventricular artery and the right posterolateral artery. In 50 to 60% of hearts, the artery to the sinus node arises from the proximal portion of the right coronary artery. The blood supply to the atrioventricular node (in patients with right-dominant circulation) arises from the midportion of the U-shaped segment. The inferior interventricular artery, usually described incorrectly as being posterior and descending, runs along the inferior interventricular groove, extending for a variable distance toward the apex of the heart. It gives off perpendicular branches, the inferior septal perforators, that course anteriorly in the ventricular septum. Typically, these perforators supply the inferior one-third of the ventricular septal myocardium.

The right posterolateral artery gives rise to a variable number of branches that supply the posterior surface of the left

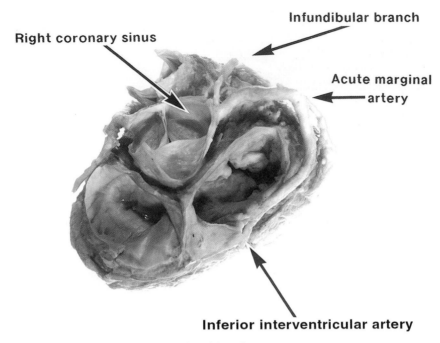

Right coronary sinus

Infundibular branch

Acute marginal artery

Inferior interventricular artery

FIGURE 2-35 This dissection shows the relationships and branches of the right coronary artery.

ventricle. The circulation of the posteroinferior portion of the left ventricular myocardium is quite variable. It may consist of branches of the right coronary artery, the circumflex artery, or both. The acute marginal arteries branch from the right coronary artery along the acute margin of the heart, before its bifurcation at the crux. These marginals supply the anterior free wall of the right ventricle. In 10 to 20% of hearts, one of these acute marginal arteries courses across the diaphragmatic surface of the right ventricle to reach the distal ventricular septum. The right coronary artery supplies important collaterals to the left anterior descending artery through its septal perforators. In addition, its infundibular (or conus) branch, which arises from the proximal portion of the right coronary artery, courses anteriorly over the base of the ventricular infundibulum and may serve as a collateral to the anterior descending artery. Kugel's artery is an anastomotic vessel between the proximal right coronary and the circumflex coronary artery that also can provide a branch that runs through the base of the atrial septum to the crux of the heart, where it supplies collateral circulation to the atrioventricular node.[15]

THE CORONARY VEINS[14]

A complex network of veins drains the coronary circulation. An extensive degree of collateralization among these veins and the coronary arteries and the paucity of valves within coronary veins enable the use of retrograde coronary sinus cardioplegia for intraoperative myocardial protection. The venous circulation can be divided into three systems: the coronary sinus and its tributaries, the anterior right ventricular veins, and the thebesian veins.

Coronary Sinus and Its Tributaries

The coronary sinus predominantly drains the left ventricle and receives approximately 85% of coronary venous blood. It lies within the posterior atrioventricular groove and empties into the right atrium at the lateral border of the triangle of Koch (Fig. 2-36). The orifice of the coronary sinus is guarded by the crescent-shaped thebesian valve. The named tributaries of the coronary sinus include the anterior interventricular vein, which courses parallel to the left anterior descending coronary artery. Adjacent to the bifurcation of the left main stem, the anterior interventricular vein courses leftward in the atrioventricular groove, where it is referred to as the *great cardiac vein*. It receives blood from the marginal and posterior left ventricular branches before becoming the coronary sinus at the origin of the oblique vein (of Marshall) at the posterior margin of the left atrium. The inferior interventricular vein, or *middle cardiac vein*, arises at the apex, courses parallel to the inferior interventricular artery, and extends proximally to the crux. Here, this vein drains directly either into the right atrium or into the coronary sinus just prior to its orifice. The *small cardiac vein* runs inferiorly through the right atrioventricular groove.

Anterior Right Ventricular Veins

The anterior right ventricular veins travel across the right ventricular surface to the right atrioventricular groove, where they enter directly into either the right atrium or coalesce to form the small cardiac vein. As indicated, this vein travels down the right atrioventricular groove, around the acute margin,

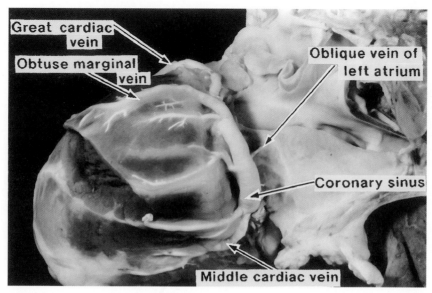

FIGURE 2-36 The coronary veins on the diaphragmatic surface of the heart, seen in anatomical orientation, have been emphasized by filling them with sealant. The tributaries of the coronary sinus are well demonstrated. Note that, strictly speaking, the sinus does not begin until the oblique vein enters the great cardiac vein.

and enters into the right atrium directly or joins the coronary sinus just proximal to its orifice.

Thebesian Veins

The thebesian veins are small venous tributaries that drain directly into the cardiac chambers. They exist primarily in the right atrium and right ventricle.

REFERENCES

1. Anderson KR, Ho SY, Anderson RH: The location and vascular supply of the sinus node in the human heart. *Br Heart J* 1979; 41:28.
2. Wilcox BR, Anderson RH: *Surgical Anatomy of the Heart.* New York, Raven Press, 1985.
3. Sweeney LJ, Rosenquist GC: The normal anatomy of the atrial septum in the human heart. *Am Heart J* 1979; 98:194.
4. Konno S, Imai Y, Iida Y, et al: A new method for prosthetic valve replacement in congenital aortic stenosis associated with hypoplasia of the aortic valve ring. *J Thorac Cardiovasc Surg* 1975; 70:909.
5. Rastan H, Koncz J: Aortoventriculoplasty: a new technique for the treatment of left ventricular outflow tract obstruction. *J Thorac Cardiovasc Surg* 1976; 71:920.
6. Manouguian S, Seybold-Epting W: Patch enlargement of the aortic valve ring by extending the aortic incision into the anterior mitral leaflet: new operative technique. *J Thorac Cardiovasc Surg* 1979; 78:402.
7. Nicks R, Cartmill T, Berstein L: Hypoplasia of the aortic root. *Thorax* 1970; 25:339.
8. Ross DN: Replacement of aortic and mitral valve with a pulmonary autograft. *Lancet* 1967; 2:956.
9. Oury JH, Angell WW, Eddy AC, Cleveland JC: Pulmonary autograft: past, present, and future. *J Heart Valve Dis* 1993; 2:365.
10. Wilcox BR, Murray GF, Starek PJK: The long-term outlook for valve replacement in active endocarditis. *J Thorac Cardiovasc Surg* 1977; 74:860.
11. Frantz PT, Murray GF, Wilcox BR: Surgical management of left ventriculaaortic discontinuity complicating bacterial endocarditis. *Ann Thorac Surg* 1980; 29:1.
12. Anderson RH, Becker AE: *Cardiac Anatomy.* London, Churchill Livingstone, 1980.
13. Kirklin JW, Barratt-Boyes BG: Anatomy, dimensions, and terminology, in Kirklin JW, Barratt-Boyes BG (eds): *Cardiac Surgery,* 2nd ed. New York, Churchill Livingstone, 1993; p 3.
14. Schlant RC, Silverman ME: Anatomy of the heart, in Hurst JW, Logue RB, Rachley CE, et al (eds): *The Heart,* 6th ed. New York, McGraw-Hill, 1986; p 16.
15. Kugel MA: Anatomical studies on the coronary arteries and their branches: I. Arteria anastomotica auricularis magna. *Am Heart J* 1927; 3:260.

Cardiac Surgical Physiology

Edward B. Savage • Nicolas A. Brozzi

A cardiac surgical procedure is the most acute application of basic dynamic physiology that exists in medical care. Basic physiologic concepts of electromechanical activation and association, loading conditions, inotropy, etc all affect a successful outcome. Working knowledge of these fundamental concepts is imperative to maintain and return a patient to normal function. The purpose of this chapter is to present a manageable outline of cardiac physiology that can be used in daily practice, as a framework against which pathologic processes can be measured, assessed, and treated.

CELLULAR COMPONENTS AND CELLULAR ACTIVATION

The heart beats continuously based on the unique features of its component cells. A cardiac cycle begins when spontaneous depolarization of a pacemaker cell initiates an action potential. This electrical activity is transmitted to atrial muscle cells and to the conduction system which transmits the electrical activity to the ventricle. Activation is dependent on components of the cell membrane and cell which induce and maintain the ion currents that promote and spread electrical activation.

The activity of cells in the heart is triggered by an action potential. An action potential is a cyclical activation of the cell comprised of a rapid change in the membrane potential (the electrical gradient across the cell membrane) and subsequent return to a resting membrane potential. This process is dependent on a selectively permeable cell membrane and proteins that actively and passively direct ion passage across the cell membrane. The specific components of the myocyte action potential are detailed in Figure 3-3. The myocyte action potential is characterized by a rapid initial depolarization mediated by fast channels (sodium channels), then a plateau phase mediated by slow channels (calcium channels). Further details of this process are introduced as their components are described.

The Sarcolemma

The cardiac cell is surrounded by a membrane (plasmalemma or more specific to a muscle cell, sarcolemma). The structural components of the sarcolemma allow for the origination and then the conduction of an electrical signal through the heart with subsequent initiation of the excitation-contraction coupling process. The sarcolemma also participates in the regulation of excitation, contraction, and intracellular metabolism in response to neuronal and chemical stimulation.

THE PHOSPHOLIPID BILAYER

The sarcolemma is a phospholipid bilayer that provides a barrier between the extracellular compartment and the intracellular compartment or cytosol. The sarcolemma, which is only two molecules thick, consists of phospholipids and cholesterol aligned so that the lipid, or the hydrophobic, portion of the molecule is on the inside of the membrane, and the hydrophilic portion of the molecule is on the outside (Figure 3-1). The phospholipid bilayer provides a fluid barrier that is particularly *impermeable to the diffusion of ions*. Small lipid-soluble molecules such as oxygen and carbon dioxide diffuse easily through the membrane. The water molecule, although insoluble in the membrane, is small enough that it diffuses easily through the membrane (or through pores in the membrane). Other, slightly larger molecules (sodium, chloride, potassium, calcium) cannot easily diffuse through the lipid bilayer and require specialized channels for transport.[1,2]

The specialized ion-transport systems within the sarcolemma consist of membrane-spanning proteins that float in and penetrate through the lipid bilayer. These proteins are associated with three different types of ion transport: (1) diffusion through transmembrane channels that can be opened or closed (gated) in response to electrical (voltage-gated) or chemical (ligand-gated) stimuli; (2) exchange of one ion for another by attachment to binding sites for transmission in response to an electrochemical gradient; and (3) active (energy-dependent) transport of ions against an electrochemical gradient.

Other proteins located in the sarcolemma serve as receptors for neuronal or chemical control of cellular processes.

ION CHANNELS

Most of the voltage-gated channels consist of four subunits that surround the water-filled pore through which ions cross

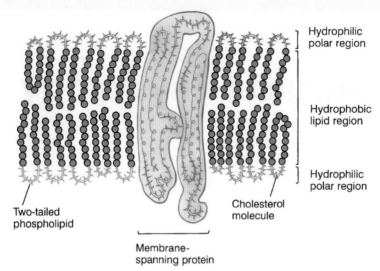

FIGURE 3-1 The sarcolemma is a bilayer in which phospholipid and cholesterol molecules are arranged with hydrophobic domains within the membrane and hydrophilic domains facing outward. The membrane-spanning protein shown here is similar to many ion channels, with six hydrophobic alpha-helices spanning the membrane and surrounding a central channel.

the membrane. A schematic diagram of an ion channel is shown in Figure 3-2. Each channel contains a selectivity filter that allows the passage of particular ions based upon pore size and electrical charge, and an activation gate regulated by conformational changes induced by either a voltage-sensitive or a ligand-binding region of the protein. Many channels also have an inactivation gate.[1,3]

Voltage-Gated Sodium Channels

The voltage-gated sodium channel is prominent in most electrically excitable muscle and nerve cells. Energy-dependent pumps and other ions create a large concentration gradient of positive sodium ions (142 mEq/L outside, 10 mEq/L inside) and a large electrical gradient (−70 to −90 millivolts (mV) from outside to inside) across the cell membrane. Both gradients favor the influx of sodium. This passive influx is termed an inward current. The inward current of sodium ions begins to depolarize (reduce the

electrical gradient) across the sarcolemma. When the membrane potential is raised to between −70 and −50 mV, the activation gate of the sodium channel opens. Sodium ions rapidly rush into the cell depolarizing the sarcolemmal membrane. The inactivation gate of the sodium channel begins to close at the same voltage, with a built-in time delay, so the sodium channel is open for only a few milliseconds. Because these channels open and close so quickly, they are called fast channels. The inactivation gate of the sodium channel remains closed until the cell is repolarized to the resting negative membrane potential.[4,5]

Voltage-Gated Calcium Channels

There are two important calcium channels. The type T (transient)-calcium channels open as the membrane potential rises to −60 to −50 mV, and then close quickly. These T-calcium channels are important in early depolarization, especially in atrial pacemaker cells.

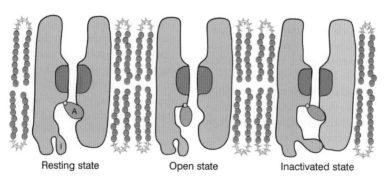

FIGURE 3-2 A voltage-gated sodium channel is schematically depicted. The shaded region is the selectivity filter. *A* represents the activation gate, and *I* represents the inactivation gate. At rest, the inactivation gate is open and the activation gate is closed. As the transmembrane potential rises from −80 to −60 mV, the activation gate opens, and sodium ions pass through the channel. Within a few milliseconds, the inactivation gate closes. Once the cell repolarizes the resting ion channel returns to the resting state.

The second major calcium channel, type L (long-lasting) channel, a slow channel, leads to an inward (depolarizing) current that is slowly inactivated and therefore prolonged. These channels open at a less negative potential (–30 to –20 mV). Once open, the prolonged inward calcium current (Figure 3-3) sustains the action potential. This increase in cytosolic calcium begins the excitation-contraction sequence. Beta-receptor stimulation induces conformational changes in the channel, resulting in an increased influx of calcium ions and an associated increase in the strength of sarcomere contraction. This effect is attenuated by stimulation of acetylcholine and adenosine receptors.[6,7]

Potassium Channels

A variety of potassium channels, both voltage- and ligand-gated, are present in cardiac cells. Three voltage-gated potassium channels moderate the delayed rectifier current which repolarizes the cell membrane (Figure 3-3).[8]

Several ligand-gated potassium channels have been identified. Acetylcholine and adenosine-activated potassium channels are time-independent, and lead to hyperpolarization in pacemaker and nodal cells, thereby delaying spontaneous depolarization. A calcium-activated potassium channel opens in the presence of high levels of cytosolic calcium and probably enhances the delayed rectifier current, leading to early termination of the action potential. An adenosine triphosphate (ATP)-sensitive potassium channel is closed in the metabolically normal myocyte, but is opened in the metabolically starved myocyte in which ATP stores have been depleted, leading to hyperpolarization of the cell, thereby retarding depolarization and contraction.

ENERGY-DEPENDENT ION PUMPS

Sodium-potassium atp-dependent pump.
The sodium-potassium pump uses the energy obtained from the hydrolysis of ATP to move three Na[+] ions out of the cell and two K[+] ions into the cell, each against its respective concentration gradient. Since there is a net outward current (three Na[+] ions for two K[+] ions), the pump contributes about 10 mV to the resting membrane potential. The activity of the pump is strongly stimulated by attachment of sodium to its binding site. The Na[+]-K[+] adenosine triphosphatase, Na[+]-K[+] (ATPase), has a very high affinity for ATP, so that the pump continues to function even if ATP levels are reduced.

Atp-dependent calcium pump.
The ATP-dependent calcium pump transports calcium out of the cell against a strong concentration gradient. This action represents a net outward current, but the magnitude of this current is quite small because the bulk of calcium transferred out of the cell occurs with sodium-calcium exchange (described in the following). The cytosolic protein, calmodulin, can complex with calcium and facilitate the action of the pump; thus, increased intracellular calcium levels stimulate the pump.[9,10]

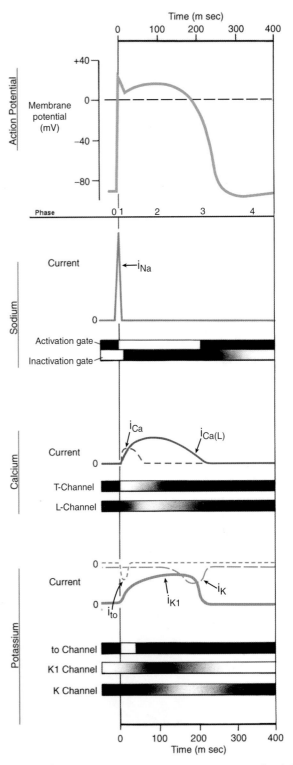

FIGURE 3-3 A typical ventricular myocyte action potential and the ion currents contributing to it are schematically represented. Inward (depolarizing) currents are depicted as positive, and outward (repolarizing) currents are depicted as negative. The horizontal filled bars show the state of the gate of the ion channel (white = open; black = closed; shaded = partially open). In the case of the sodium channel, both the activation and inactivation gates are shown (Ca = calcium; i = current; K = potassium; Na = sodium).

ION EXCHANGERS

Sodium-calcium exchanger. Multiple proteins that traverse the membrane allow ion exchanges using the potential energy of the electrochemical gradient which favors the influx of sodium. The sodium-calcium exchanger exchanges three extracellular sodium ions for one intracellular calcium ion, leading to a net single positive charge transported into the cell with each exchange. The exchange system is sensitive to the concentration of sodium and calcium on both sides of the membrane, and to the membrane potential. If external sodium concentrations decrease, the driving force for removal of calcium from the cell is decreased, leading to an increase in cytosolic calcium (and a consequent increase in contraction). Thus, hyponatremia can increase cardiac contractility. If the intracellular sodium concentration increases, as occurs with ischemia, the gradient for sodium influx is reduced, and the pump slows down or actually reverses, extruding sodium in exchange for an influx of calcium. This mechanism may be central to the accumulation of calcium during ischemia. The sodium-calcium exchange mechanism has a maximum exchange rate that is some 30 times higher than the sarcolemmal ATP-dependent calcium pump and is the primary mechanism for removal of excess cytosolic calcium.[7]

Sodium-hydrogen exchanger. The sodium-hydrogen exchanger extrudes one intracellular hydrogen ion in exchange for one extracellular sodium ion, and is electrically neutral. This pump prevents intracellular acidification. Acidification (eg, during ischemia) increases the affinity of the pump for H^+ ions, promoting the removal of H^+ preserving intracellular pH at the expense of sodium accumulation. The accumulation of sodium ions may then trigger reversal of the sodium-calcium exchange pump to favor the accumulation of calcium within the cell. This is a possible mechanism underlying injury or cell death during ischemia-reperfusion.

INTRACELLULAR COMMUNICATION PATHWAYS

To allow concurrent activation of all the myofibrils in the muscle cell, the electrical activation signal must be rapidly and evenly spread through all portions of the cell. This is accomplished through the t-tubules, and the subsarcolemmal cisternae and sarcotubular network of the sarcoplasmic reticulum.

Transverse tubules (T-tubules). The basic contractile unit in a muscle cell is the sarcomere. Sarcomeres are joined together in the myofibril at the z-lines. A system of transverse tubules (t-tubules) extends the sarcolemma into the interior of the cardiac cell (Figure 3-4). These tubules are perpendicular to the sarcomere, near the z-lines, extending the extracellular space close to the contractile proteins. The transverse tubules contain the calcium channels, which are in close relationship to the foot proteins of the subsarcolemmal cisternae.

Sarcoplasmic reticulum. The sarcoplasmic reticulum is a membrane network within the cytoplasm of the cell surrounding the myofibrils. The primary function of the sarcoplasmic reticulum is excitation-contraction coupling by sudden release of calcium to stimulate the contraction proteins and then rapid removal of this calcium to allow relaxation of the contractile elements. The subsarcolemmal cisternae and the

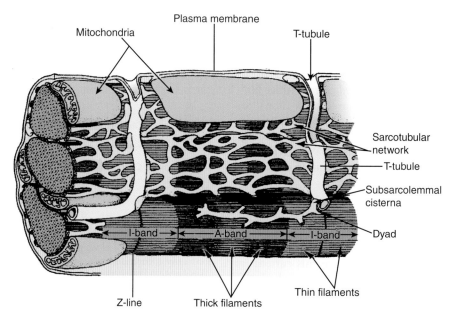

FIGURE 3-4 Myocyte anatomy. (Reproduced with permission from Katz AM: *Physiology of the Heart*, 4th ed. Philadelphia, Lippincott Williams & Wilkins; 2006.)

sarcotubular network are the two portions of the sarcoplasmic reticulum that mediate this process.

The subsarcolemmal cisternae are near the sarcolemma and the t-tubules. Foot proteins are found in the membrane of the sarcoplasmic reticulum, with a large protein component extending into the gap between the subsarcolemmal cisternae and the sarcolemma of the t-tubule. The foot proteins respond to the release of calcium by opening a calcium channel, which allows the release of a much larger quantity of calcium from the subsarcolemmal cisternae. This is "calcium-triggered" calcium release with calcium transported across the sarcolemma, leading to calcium release from the subsarcolemmal cisternae. The magnitude of calcium release from the subsarcolemmal cisternae appears to be related to the magnitude of the trigger. The calcium channels then close and the calcium is returned to the sarcoplasmic reticulum by an ATP-dependent calcium pump located in the sarcotubular network.[1,10] The sarcotubular network is the portion of the sarcoplasmic reticulum that surrounds the contractile elements of the sarcomere (Figure 3-5).

Regulation of calcium transport by the cardiac sarcoplasmic reticulum occurs primarily at the site of the calcium pump. A calcium-calmodulin complex phosphorylates the pump to stimulate pump activity. Reduced ATP availability will slow pump function. Phospholamban inhibits the basal rate of calcium transport by the calcium pump. This inhibition is reversed when phospholamban is phosphorylated by a cyclic AMP-or calcium-calmodulin–dependent protein kinase. This is a very important mechanism for beta-adrenergic regulation; cyclic AMP levels increase with activation of the beta-adrenergic receptor. As phospholamban is phosphorylated, there is accelerated calcium turnover and increased sensitivity of the calcium pump, which facilitates uptake of calcium from the cytosol and relaxation of the heart. Phosphorylation of phospholamban does not affect the sarcolemmal calcium pump, thereby tending to favor retention of calcium within the cell (increasing the calcium content of the sarcoplasmic reticulum at the expense of calcium removed from the cell through the sarcolemma). This might lead to an increased pulse of calcium within the cell, thereby favoring increased contractility.[7,10] Phosphorylation of phospholamban, in the presence of intracellular calcium, stimulates calcium uptake to protect the heart from calcium overload.

In this ionic milieu, the importance of intracellular pH maintenance should be stressed. Regulation of intracellular pH is complex and beyond the scope of this text, but a few simple principles are important to review. Reduced intracellular pH diminishes the amount of calcium released from

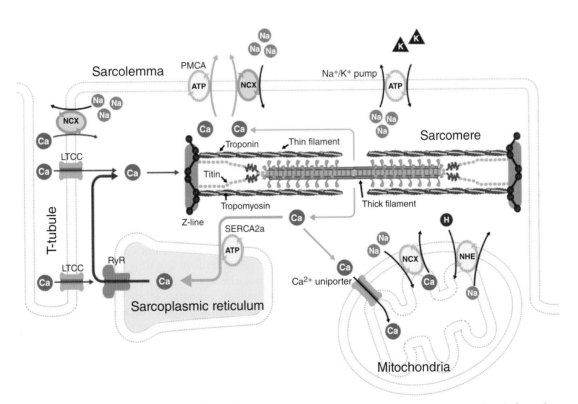

FIGURE 3-5 Anatomy of the cardiac sarcomere. Ca^{2+} influx during excitation provokes the release of additional Ca^{2+} from the sarcoplasmic reticulum (SR). The Ca^{2+} binds to troponin on the thin filaments triggering sarcomeric contraction (systole). The Ca^{2+} is then removed from the cytosol through uptake into the SR and extracellular extrusion allowing sarcomere relaxation (diastole). (Reproduced with permission from Kobirumaki-Shimozawa F, Inoue T, Shintani SA, et al: Cardiac thin filament regulation and the Frank-Starling mechanism, *J Physiol Sci.* 2014 Jul;64(4):221-232.)

the sarcoplasmic reticulum and reduces the responsiveness of myofilaments to calcium. Elevation of the pH will have the opposite effect. The clinical relevance of this observation cannot be overstressed.

ELECTRICAL ACTIVATION OF THE HEART

Normal Cardiac Rhythm

THE RESTING MEMBRANE POTENTIAL

The state of the cardiac cell is determined by a balance of forces based on electrical and chemical gradients. At rest (during diastole), the cardiac cell is polarized. The electrical potential across the sarcolemma is primarily determined by the concentration gradient of potassium across the membrane. This gradient is established by the sodium-potassium pump. However, once this pump shuts off, the steady state is determined by the balance of electrical and chemical forces. The sarcolemma is impermeable to some ions, permeable to others, and selectively permeable to others. Steady-state properties of a mixture of ions of variable permeabilities across a membrane are described by the Gibbs-Donnan equilibrium.[11] The sarcolemma prevents the diffusion of large anions (eg, proteins and organic phosphates). At rest, the sarcolemma is relatively permeable to potassium ions because of the open state of most potassium channels, but less permeable to sodium. The concentration gradient established by the sodium-potassium pump promotes the efflux of potassium ions across the sarcolemma. The outward flow of positive ions is counterbalanced by the increasing electronegativity of the interior of the cell owing to the impermeant anions. A Gibbs-Donnan equilibrium is established such that the electronegativity of the cell interior retards potassium-ion efflux to the same degree that the concentration gradient favors K^+ efflux. At equilibrium, the forces balance with an intracellular potassium concentration of 135 mM and extra-cellular concentration of 4 mM and a predicted resting membrane potential of −94 mV. The actual resting membrane potential is measured at about −90 mV because of smaller contributions from the current of other less permeable ions (eg, sodium and calcium). However, the potassium current is the main determinant of the resting membrane potential.[12]

THE ACTION POTENTIAL

The action potential represents the triggered response to a stimulus derived either internally (slow depolarizing ionic currents) or externally (depolarization of adjacent cells). A typical fast-response action potential which occurs in atrial and ventricular myocytes and special conduction fibers is depicted in Fig. 3-3. As the transmembrane potential decreases to approximately −65 mV, the "fast" sodium channels open. These channels remain open for a few milliseconds when the inactivation gate of the "fast" sodium channel closes. The large gradient of sodium ions promotes rapid influx, depolarizing the cell to a slightly positive transmembrane potential:

phase 0 of the action potential. A transient potassium current (i_{to}) causes a very early repolarization (phase 1) of the action potential, but this fast channel closes quickly. The plateau of the action potential (phase 2) is sustained at a neutral or slightly positive level by an inward flowing calcium current, first from the transient calcium channel and second through the long-lasting calcium channel. The plateau is also sustained by a decrease in the outward potassium current (i_{K1}). With time, the long-lasting calcium channels begin to close, and the repolarizing potassium current (i_K, the delayed rectifier current) leads to the initiation of phase 3 of the action potential. As repolarization progresses, the stronger first potassium current (i_{K1}) dominates, leading to full repolarization of the membrane to the resting negative potential. During the bulk of the depolarized interval (phase 4) the first potassium current predominates in myocytes.

REFRACTORY PERIOD

The sodium channels cannot respond to a second wave of depolarization until the inactivation gates are reopened (by repolarization during phase 3). As a result, the membrane is refractory to the propagation of a second impulse during this time interval, referred to as the absolute refractory period. As the membrane is repolarized during early phase 3 of the action potential, and some of the sodium channels have been reactivated, a short interval exists during which only very strong impulses can activate the cell, which is termed the relative refractory period. A drug that acts to speed up the inactivation gate will shorten both the absolute and the relative refractory periods.[1,13,14]

SPONTANEOUS DEPOLARIZATION

The action potential of the slow response cells of the nodal tissue (sinoatrial node, or SA node, and atrioventricular node, or AV node) differs from that in the fast-response cells, as shown in Figure 3-6. The rapid upstroke of phase 0 is less prominent due to the absence of fast Na^+ channels. Phase 1 is absent, as there is no rapid inward potassium current. In addition, the plateau phase (phase 2) is abbreviated because of the lack of a sustained active Na^+ inward current, and the lack of sustained calcium current. The repolarization phase (phase 3) leads to a resting phase (phase 4) that begins to depolarize again, as opposed to the relatively stable resting membrane potential of myocytes. The slowly depolarizing phase 4 resting potential is called the diastolic depolarization current, or the pacemaker potential. Continued depolarization of the membrane potential ultimately reduces it to the threshold potential that stimulates another action potential. This diastolic depolarization potential is the mechanism of automaticity in cardiac pacemaker cells. Diastolic depolarization is caused by the concerted and net actions of: (1) a decrease in the outward K^+ current during early diastole (phase 4); (2) persistence of the slow inward Ca^{2+} current; and (3) an increasing inward Na^+ current during diastole. The inward Na^+ current most likely predominates in nodal and conduction tissue. The slope of the diastolic

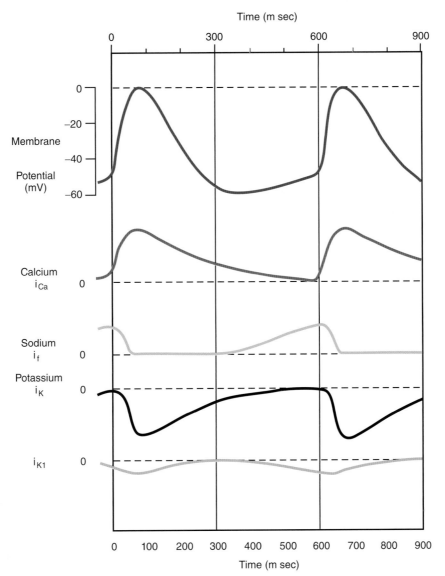

FIGURE 3-6 The membrane potential of a spontaneously depolarizing cell of the sinoatrial node, and the ion currents contributing to it. Inward (depolarizing) currents are depicted as positive, and outward (repolarizing) currents are depicted as negative (Ca = calcium; i = current; K = potassium; Na = sodium).

depolarization determines the rate of action-potential generation in the pacemaker cells, and is the primary mechanism determining heart rate. Of all the cardiac cells, the fastest rate of depolarization is in the SA node, and action potentials are generated at a rate of 70 to 80 per minute. The AV node is a slower rate of depolarization, at 40 to 60 times per minute. The ventricular myocytes are the slowest, at 30 to 40 times per minute. Once a depolarization is initiated in a pacemaker cell and propagated, it will depolarize the remainder of the heart in a synchronized and sequential manner. The heart rate can be altered by changing the slope of the diastolic depolarization (eg, acetylcholine decreases the slope and heart rate; beta-adrenergic agonists increase the slope and heart rate). If the slope is unchanged, hyperpolarization (more negative resting potential) or raising the

threshold potential will increase the time to reach threshold, thus decreasing the heart rate.

PROPAGATION OF THE ACTION POTENTIAL

Each myocyte is mechanically anchored and electrically connected to the next myocyte by an intercalated disc at the end of the cell. These discs contain gap junctions that facilitate flow of charged molecules from one cell to the next. These pores are composed of a protein, connexin. Permeability through the cardiac gap junction is increased by both ATP- and cyclic AMP-dependent kinases. This allows the gap junctions to close if ATP levels fall, thereby reducing electrical and presumably mechanical activity, which is essential in limiting cell death when one region of the heart is damaged. It also allows conduction to increase when cyclic AMP increases in response to adrenergic stimulation.

After spontaneous depolarization occurs in the pacemaker cells of the SA node, the action potential is conducted throughout the heart. Special electrical pathways facilitate this conduction. Three internodal paths exist through the atrium between the SA node and the AV node. After traversing the AV node, the action potential is propagated rapidly through the bundle of His and into the Purkinje fibers located on the endocardium of the left and right ventricles. Rapid conduction through the atrium causes contraction of most of the atrial muscle synchronously (within 60 to 90 ms).Similarly, the rapid conduction of the signal throughout the ventricle leads to synchronous contraction of the bulk of the ventricular myocardium (within 60 ms). The delay in the propagation of the action potential through the AV node by 120 to 140 ms allows the atria to complete contraction before the ventricles contract. Slow conduction in the AV node is related to a relatively higher internal resistance because of a small number of gap junctions between cells, and slowly rising action potentials.

Abnormal Cardiac Rhythm

ABERRANT PACEMAKER FOCI

Normally the SA node spontaneously depolarizes first, such that the cardiac beat originates from this primary pacemaker site. If the SA node is damaged or slowed by vagal stimulation or drugs (eg, acetylcholine), ectopic pacemakers in the atrium, AV node, or the His-Purkinje system can take over. Occasionally, aberrant foci in the heart spontaneously depolarize, thereby leading to aberrant or "premature" contractions from the atrium or the ventricle. These contractions ordinarily do not interfere with the normal depolarization of the heart.

REENTRY ARRHYTHMIAS

Reentry arrhythmias are perhaps the most common dangerous cardiac rhythm. Ordinarily, the action potential depolarizes the entire atrium or the entire ventricle in a short enough time interval so that all of the muscle is refractory to further stimulation at the same time. A reentry arrhythmia is caused by propagation of an action potential through the heart in a "circus" movement. For reentry to occur there must be a unidirectional block (transient or permanent) to action potential propagation. Additionally, the effective refractory period of the reentered region must be shorter that the propagation time around the loop.[12] For example, if a portion of the previously depolarized myocardium has repolarized before the propagation of the action potential is completed throughout the atrium or ventricle, then that action potential can continue its propagation into this repolarized muscle. Such an event generally requires either dramatic slowing of conduction of the action potential, a long conduction pathway, or a shortened refractory period (Figure 3-7). All of these situations occur clinically. Ischemia slows the sodium-potassium pump, which decreases the resting membrane potential and slows

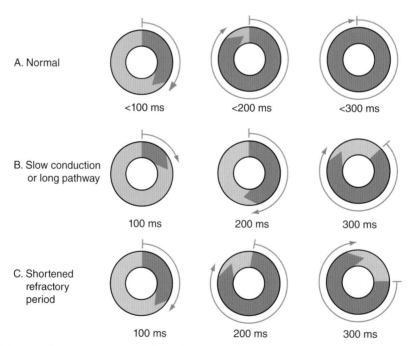

FIGURE 3-7 Three conditions predisposing to reentry or "circus" pathways for action potential propagation are shown. Muscle that is refractory to action potential propagation is shown as black. Normally, as the action potential travels through the atrium or ventricle, all the muscle is depolarized sufficiently that the action potential encounters no more nonrefractory muscle and stops (*A*). If there is slowed conduction speed or a long pathway (*B*), the action potential may find repolarized (nonrefractory) muscle and continue in a circular path. Similarly, a shortened refractory period (*C*) may lead to rapid repolarization and predispose to a reentry and continuation of the action potential.

propagation of the action potential. Hyperkalemia decreases the resting membrane potential, which increases excitability and inactivates the sodium-potassium pump, slowing propagation of the action potential. Progressive atrial dilation creates a long conduction pathway around the atrium. Adrenergic stimulation shortens the refractory period.

A special type of reentry arrhythmia occurs in Wolff-Parkinson-White syndrome in which an accessory pathway electrically connects the atrium and the ventricle. This accessory pathway can complete a circular electrical pathway between the atrium and the ventricle. Conduction is unidirectional across the AV node and the accessory pathway creates a loop that has a propagation time that is greater than the AV node refractory period, resulting in supraventricular tachycardia. In an alternative situation, because the accessory pathway does not have the inherent delay and refractory period of the AV node, rapid atrial tachycardias can be conducted in a 1:1 manner across the accessory pathway, leading to ventricular rates as fast as 300 beats per minute.

REGULATION OF CELLULAR FUNCTION

Types of Receptors and Second Messengers

Numerous types of receptors are involved in regulating cardiovascular function. They include G-protein (GTP-binding proteins) coupled receptors, enzyme-linked receptors, ion channel-linked receptors, and nuclear receptors. Other ligands, such as nitric oxide, bind directly to their intracellular target.[15] G-protein–coupled receptors are the most important. Ligand binding activates the synthesis of intracellular second messengers, protein kinases, and voltage-gated potassium channels.[16] The most important second messenger is cyclic AMP, which transmits the response to sympathetic stimulation. Cyclic AMP is produced from ATP by adenylyl cyclase and broken down to AMP by phosphodiesterases. Cyclic AMP production is promoted by sympathetic and inhibited by parasympathetic stimulation. Another second messenger, cyclic guanosine monophosphate (GMP) is similarly produced, in response to nitric oxide and natriuretic peptides, by guanylyl cyclase and broken down by phosphodiesterases and opposes the actions of cyclic AMP.[17] These and other second messengers activate signaling enzymes within the cell such as protein kinases.

Innervation of the Heart

Sympathetic fibers originate from the fourth and fifth thoracic spinal cord regions. Parasympathetic innervation derives through the vagus nerve connecting to the SA and AV nodes, atria, and blood vessels. Stretch receptors located in the atria and ventricles provide feedback to the central nervous system. Atrial natriuretic peptide, (similar to B-type natriuretic peptide which is clinically measured) is secreted by atrial myocytes in response to stretch and promotes natriuresis, diuresis,

and smooth muscle relaxation. Stretch receptors on the posterior and inferior ventricular wall can trigger parasympathetic stimulation and inhibit sympathetic activity, leading to bradycardia and conduction block (von Bezold-Jarisch reflex).[18]

PARASYMPATHETIC REGULATION

The parasympathetic nervous system is particularly important in control of the SA node. Acetylcholine released by the nerve endings of the parasympathetic system stimulates muscarinic receptors in the heart. The activated receptors produce an intracellular stimulatory G-protein that opens acetylcholine gated potassium channels. An increased outward (repolarizing) flow of potassium leads to hyperpolarization of the SA node cells. Stimulation of the muscarinic receptors also inhibits the formation of cyclic AMP, inhibiting the opening of calcium channels. A decreased inward flow of calcium, combined with an increased outward flow of potassium, leads to slowing of the spontaneous diastolic depolarization of the SA node cells (Figure 3-6). A similar effect in the AV node leads to slowing of conduction through the AV node.[1]

SYMPATHETIC STIMULATION AND BLOCKADE

Sympathetic or adrenergic receptors in the heart affect heart rate, contractility, conduction velocity, and automaticity; and in the peripheral vasculature they affect smooth muscle contraction and relaxation. Alpha-adrenergic receptors cause vasoconstriction. There are two types of beta-adrenergic receptors: the beta$_1$-adrenergic receptors, which predominate in the heart, and the beta$_2$-adrenergic receptors, which are present in blood vessels and promote relaxation. The number of beta receptors per unit area (receptor density) of the sarcolemma can be upregulated or downregulated in response to various stimuli. Receptor sensitivity can also change depending on ambient conditions and variable stimuli.[19] Cardiopulmonary bypass and ischemia cause downregulation of cardiac beta receptors. Acidemia causes desensitization of beta receptors. This is important in the perioperative period when acidemia can reduce cardiac contractility, systemic vascular tone, and the response to inotropic agents.

The beta$_1$-adrenergic receptor couples with adenylyl cyclase (Figure 3-8). When the receptor site is occupied by an adrenergic agonist, a stimulatory G-protein is formed, which combines with GTP. This activated G-protein–GTP complex then promotes the activity of adenylyl cyclase, leading to the formation of cyclic AMP from ATP. The G-protein–GTP complex and the cyclic AMP actively promote calcium channel opening. The increased tendency for calcium channels to open during beta$_1$-receptor stimulation increases cytosolic calcium and leads to a number of physiologic effects: (1) A positive chronotropic (heart rate) effect whereby the heart rate, conduction, and contraction velocity increase and the action potential is shortened, leading to a shortening of systole; (2) a positive dromotropic (conduction velocity) effect of accelerated conduction through the AV node; and (3) a positive inotropic (contractility) effect. Increased activity of the sarcoplasmic reticulum calcium pump (more rapid calcium

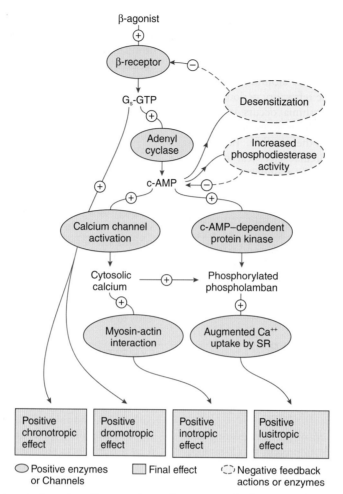

β-agonist

β-receptor

Desensitization

Gs-GTP

Adenyl
cyclase

Increased
phosphodiesterase
activity

c-AMP

Calcium channel
activation

c-AMP–dependent
protein kinase

Cytosolic
calcium

Phosphorylated
phospholamban

Myosin-actin
interaction

Augmented Ca++
uptake by SR

Positive
chronotropic
effect

Positive
dromotropic
effect

Positive
inotropic
effect

Positive
lusitropic
effect

Positive enzymes
or Channels

Final effect

Negative feedback
actions or enzymes

FIGURE 3-8 Adrenergic stimulation via the action of beta agonists on beta receptors leads to a cascade of events in the myocyte, some of which are shown here. Note that an increase in cyclic AMP causes the activation of two inhibitory pathways, retarding excessively sustained adrenergic stimulation (cyclic AMP = cyclic adenosine monophosphate; Gs = stimulatory G-protein; GTP = guanosine triphosphate; SR = sarcoplasmic reticulum).

uptake) leads to more rapid relaxation, which facilitates ventricular filling; (4) a positive lusitropic (relaxation) effect.[20]

Two negative feedback systems diminish the response to beta agonists when stimulation is repetitive or persistent (tachyphylaxis). Increased cyclic AMP leads to: (1) increased phosphorylation of beta receptors leading to downregulation; and (2) increased activity of phosphodiesterase, the enzyme that degrades cyclic AMP. Acidosis will inhibit many steps in the sympathetic activation cascade, impairing contractility.

The activity spectrum of adrenergic receptors forms the basis of many therapeutic interventions; perioperatively to support cardiac function, and chronically to reduce mortality from myocardial infarction and treat congestive heart failure. The selectivity of the agonists and antagonists allows adaptation for various clinical scenarios. Some examples are detailed in Table 3-1.

Reduction in inotropy, lusitropy, chronotropy, and dromotropy by beta blockade will reduce myocardial oxygen consumption contributing to many of its beneficial effects. As beta blockade will lead to upregulation of sarcolemmal

receptors, sudden cessation of beta blockade may cause a temporarily enhanced (and potentially dangerous) sensitivity to adrenergic stimulation.

PHOSPHODIESTERASE INHIBITION

Cyclic AMP plays a central role in the regulation of the cardiac cell. Cytosolic levels of cyclic AMP are also increased by activation of receptors other than beta receptors (ie, for histamine, dopamine, glucagon), and are decreased by inhibitory G-proteins produced by stimulation of muscarinic receptors by acetylcholine and by stimulation of adenosine receptors. Referring to Figure 3-8, one negative feedback response to the increase in cyclic AMP is an increase in phosphodiesterase, which breaks down cyclic AMP. Phosphodiesterase inhibitors (amrinone, milrinone) inhibit the breakdown of cyclic AMP and thereby increase its level in the cytosol. Their effect is synergistic to that of beta agonists. Because they do not stimulate the production

TABLE 3-1: Adrenergic Agonists and Antagonists Correlating Selective Activity with Clinical Usage

	Drug	Alpha	Beta$_1$	Beta$_2$	Clinical Usage
Agonists	Epinephrine	Y	Y	Y	Low cardiac output, hypotension
	Norepinephrine	Y	Y		Hypotension
	Phenylephrine	Y			Hypotension
	Dobutamine		Y		Low cardiac output
	Dopamine	Y	Y		Low cardiac output, hypotension
	Isoproterenol		Y	Y	Bradycardia, low cardiac output, pulmonary hypertension
Antagonists (beta-blockers)	Metoprolol		Y		Tachycardia, hypertension, MI, angina
	Atenolol		Y		Tachycardia, hypertension, MI, angina
	Esmolol		Y		Tachycardia, hypertension, MI, angina
	Carvedilol	Y (alpha-1)	Y	Y	Congestive heart failure

of the G-protein–GTP complex, they have a lesser effect on calcium channel activation, and therefore less of the troublesome positive chronotropic and dromotropic effects of beta-adrenergic stimulation.[21]

ADENOSINE RECEPTORS

There are four types of adenosine receptors. Adenosine receptors are linked to inhibitory and stimulatory G-proteins and various kinases. Activation of adenosine A$_1$ receptors leads to inhibition of cyclic AMP production, inhibition of the slow calcium channel, and opening of an adenosine-activated ATP-sensitive potassium (K$_{ATP}$) channel. This leads to hyperpolarization, which delays conduction through the AV node and slows the ventricular response to atrial tachycardia.[1,22] Pretreatment with adenosine confers a cardioprotective effect during ischemia and can inhibit the inflammatory responses initiated by ischemia and reperfusion.[22]

Other Regulators of Hemodynamic Function

Angiotensin II is a vasoconstrictor and reduces renal fluid excretion. It is the final effector of the renin-angiotensin-aldosterone system. Renin, secreted by the juxtaglomerular apparatus in the kidney, splits angiotensin I from angiotensinogen, produced by the liver. Angiotensin I is converted to angiotensin II by the angiotensin-converting enzyme (ACE or kininase II, the target of ACE inhibitors) mainly in the lungs. Angiotensin II acts by causing: (1) vasoconstriction to increase systemic vascular resistance; and (2) stimulation of the adrenal cortex to secrete aldosterone, which increases fluid volume and thus cardiac output. Through both actions, angiotensin II modifies blood pressure. Angiotensin II receptor blockers (ARBs) directly inhibit angiotensin II subtype IA receptors.

The endothelins (ETs) have multiple effects. When bound to ET-A receptors they cause vasoconstriction, increased contractility, and proliferation. When bound to ET-B receptors they stimulate the release of nitric oxide and prostacyclin and have a vasodilatory effect.[23]

Bradykinins, acting through their receptors, cause vasodilation. Arginine vasopressin promotes reabsorption of water by the kidney and has a vasoconstrictor effect. Natriuretic peptides, released in response to atrial distension, promote diuresis and arteriolar dilatation.

Nitric oxide (NO) plays an essential role in cardiac excitation-contraction coupling. NO can regulate Ca^{2+} entry into the cardiomyocyte, and the release of NO in specific subcellular compartments can influence Ca^{2+} release from the sarcoplasmic reticulum. NO influences the contractile kinetics of the myofilaments, ensuring that Ca^{2+} homeostasis is closely matched with the activity of the contractile machinery and allowing for dynamic adjustments during the systolic and diastolic phase. Through the stimulus of cyclic-GMP production, low amounts of NO can increase contractility but higher doses attenuate cardiomyocyte contraction.[17,24,25] Changes in cardiac NO production by nitric oxide synthase impact responses to heart failure, diabetes, atrial fibrillation and ischemia reperfusion states.[26] Inhaled NO administered at low concentrations causes pulmonary arterial dilatation, reduces chronotropy, and has a positive inotropic effect.[27]

CONTRACTION OF CARDIAC MUSCLE
Molecular Level (The Sarcomere)

The primary contractile unit of all muscle cells is the sarcomere (Figs. 3-4 and 3-5). Sarcomeres are connected end to end at the z-line to form myofibrils. The myocyte contains numerous myofibrils arranged in parallel. A portion of a sarcomere is schematically depicted in Figure 3-9. Actin polymerizes to form the thin filaments that are anchored at the z-line. Myosin polymerizes to form the thick filaments of the sarcomere. Myosin consists of a tail of two "heavy" chains

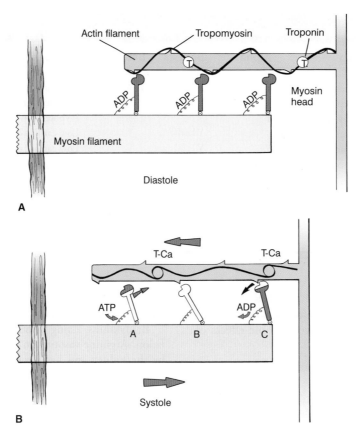

FIGURE 3-9 The interaction of actin and myosin filaments converts chemical energy into mechanical movement. In diastole, the active sites on the actin filament are covered by tropomyosin. When calcium combines with troponin, the tropomyosin is pulled away from the actin active sites, allowing the energized myosin heads (depicted in solid black and cocked at right angles to the filament) to engage and sweep the actin filament along. The myosin heads are de-energized in this process. Myosin ATPase re-cocks (re-energizes) the head by utilizing the energy derived from the hydrolysis of ATP. In systole, a de-energizing head (*C*), a de-energized head (*B*), and a re-energizing head (*A*) are shown.

intertwined to form a helix, forming the rigid backbone of the thick filament. The globular head of myosin is attached to the heavy chain backbone by a mobile hinge and projects outward. Myosin connects with the z-line via an elastic fiber made of titin. Titin is like a spring impacting passive elasticity. The globular myosin head is an ATPase with a binding site for actin. Actin binds to the myosin globular head activating the myosin ATPase to hydrolyze ATP. This leads to a conformational change in the myosin that pulls the filament (Figure 3-9B).

Two proteins modulate the interaction of actin and myosin: troponin and tropomyosin. Troponin ("T" in Figure 3-9A) is composed of three units: Tn-C, the regulatory calcium binding unit; Tn-T, which binds the troponin complex to tropomyosin; and Tn-I, which facilitates interruption of actin-myosin interaction by tropomyosin. Associated with each troponin complex is tropomyosin, a filamentous protein composed of two tightly coiled chains that lie in the groove formed by the two intertwined filaments of actin. In the absence of calcium, Tn-I is tightly bound to actin so that tropomyosin blocks the binding of myosin to actin. When calcium binds to troponinC, Tn-I becomes unbound, the tropomyosin moves to expose the myosin binding site on

actin, thereby allowing cross-bridge formation between actin and myosin. Tn-C has several regulatory sites that are affected by phosphorylation in response to hormonal and other stimuli, to alter the sensitivity and degree of force generation. Acidosis will reduce contractile force through an allosteric affect because of protons binding to Tn-I, and reducing affinity of calcium binding sites.[28]

During diastole, Ca^{2+} is unavailable to bind troponin C and the myosin binding site on actin is blocked. Depolarization leads to an influx of calcium ions and the subsequent "calcium-triggered, calcium release" increases the intracellular Ca^{2+} levels by approximately two orders of magnitude (from 10^{-7} M in diastole to 10^{-5} M in systole). This provides sufficient calcium to bind to troponin C, which causes a conformational change in the troponin molecule, removing the inhibitory effect of troponin I-tropomyosin, allowing actin-myosin cross-bridge formation (Figure 3-9A). Cross-bridge formation activates the myosin ATPase and initiates the conformational change in the myosin "hinge" drawing the z-lines closer together (Figure 3-9B). Adenosine diphosphate (ADP) and P_i are released. ATP binds to the myosin head, allowing dissociation from the actin and realigning the myosin globular head, preparing it to repeat the process. This process cycles until the end of muscular contraction is signaled by the reduction in intracellular calcium levels by sequestration into the sarcoplasmic reticulum.

The strength of the myocardial contraction is primarily mediated by the degree to which actin-binding sites are exposed. This depends on the affinity of troponin for calcium and the availability of calcium ions. The initial calcium ion influx is altered by cyclic AMP, stimulatory and inhibitory G-proteins, and acetylcholine. The magnitude of the calcium trigger determines the magnitude of the cytosolic calcium release from the sarcoplasmic reticulum. The rate of uptake of calcium from the cytosol is altered by cyclic AMP (Figure 3-8). Cyclic AMP can phosphorylate a portion of the troponin molecule, facilitating the rapid release of calcium, increasing the rate of relaxation of the actin-myosin complex.[7,29]

The Cytoskeleton

Cytoskeletal elements include microfilaments composed of actin, intermediate filaments composed of desmin, and micro-tubules made of tubulin.[30] The cytoskeleton maintains cellular anatomy, transmits developed tension, and links adjacent myocytes. It also has a role in intracellular signaling. Cardiac myocytes are mechanically linked through the intercalated discs by the fascia adherens and desmosomes.[31] Sarcomere tension is transmitted through actin microfilaments to the fascia adherens of the intercalated discs. Intermediate filaments of adjacent cells are linked through desmosomes.

Regulation of the Strength of Contraction by Initial Sarcomere Length

In cardiac muscle, the strength of contraction is related to resting sarcomere length (see also the Frank-Starling relationship in the following). Maximal contraction force occurs when the resting sarcomere length is between 2 and 2.4 μm. At this length, there is optimal overlap of the actin and myosin maximizing the number of actin-myosin cross-bridges. Force declines at a greater sarcomere length, with decreased overlap of actin and myosin. In the heart, a decrease in contractility related to decreased overlap of the filaments does not seem to occur clinically, as the resting length of the cardiac sarcomere rarely exceeds 2.2 to 2.4 μm. Once this length is reached, a stiff parallel elastic element prevents further dilation. If chamber dilation does occur, it appears to be primarily through slippage of fibers or myofibers rather than stretching of sarcomeres.[1] Stretching the myocardium increases contractility by increasing the sensitivity of troponin C to calcium. This length-dependent sensitivity to calcium is an important part of the ascending limb of the Starling curve observed in the intact ventricle. Two known factors that contribute to control of length-dependent activation are: (1) conformational changes in the lattice of titin fibers and (2) thin filament "on-off" equilibrium regulated by protein kinase A and protein kinase C.[32]

THE PUMP

Microscopic Architecture

Each myocyte is surrounded by a connective tissue framework called the endomysium. Groups of myocytes are joined within the perimysium, and the entire muscle within the epimysium. Muscle bundles are anchored in the fibrous skeleton at the base of the heart. Muscle bundles spiral around the cavity in overlapping patterns.

Macroscopic Architecture

The geometry of each ventricle is adapted to the function required of it. The left ventricle, which must eject against high pressure, is conical in shape with inlet and outlet adjacent at the base of the cone. Cavity volume is reduced during systole by a combination of concentric contraction and wall thickening, the latter predominating. The right ventricle wraps around the left ventricle, its cavity is crescent shaped with separated points of inflow and outflow. Cavity reduction is primarily a result of concentric contraction of the right ventricular free wall against the septum.

Mechanics

CLINICALLY MEASUREABLE PHYSIOLOGIC PARAMETERS

Cardiac surgeons can assess the function of the heart in a number of ways. Aortic, pulmonary artery, pulmonary capillary wedge, and central venous pressures can be measured directly. Cardiac output can be estimated using thermodilution or based on oxygen saturation measurements. From these direct measurements, other parameters can be derived—although less accurate because of the cumulative error of the measured parameters inherent in the calculation—such as pulmonary and systemic vascular resistance, and ventricular stroke work. Ejection fraction—defined as stroke volume/end-diastolic volume—can be estimated by echocardiography and ventriculography, but is subject to change based on loading conditions, heart rate, and degree of contractility. Although clinically useful, these parameters do not directly measure contractility.

THE FRANK-STARLING RELATIONSHIP

Within physiologic limits, the heart functions as a sump pump. The heart has an intrinsic ability to increase systolic force in response to a rise in ventricular filling. The more the heart is filled during diastole, the greater the quantity of blood that will be pumped out of the heart during systole. Under normal circumstances, the heart pumps all the blood that comes back to it without excessive elevation of venous pressures. In the normal heart, as ventricular filling is increased, the strength of ventricular contraction increases. The influence of sarcomere length on the force of contraction is called the Frank-Starling relationship. This relationship for the left ventricle is depicted in Figure 3-10. Also depicted

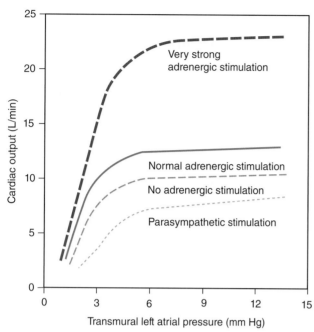

FIGURE 3-10 Starling curves for the left ventricle. The influence of four different states of neurohumoral stimulation on global ventricular performance is shown.

in Figure 3-10 are two other states, a condition of normal adrenergic stimulation and a condition of maximal adrenergic stimulation. Force is increased for the same resting conditions by adrenergic stimulation; this is a positive inotropic effect.

PRELOAD: DIASTOLIC DISTENSIBILITY AND COMPLIANCE

Preload is the load placed on a resting muscle that stretches it to its functional length. In the heart, preload references the volume of blood in the cavity immediately prior to contraction (at end-diastole) because volume determines the degree of stretch imposed on the resting sarcomere. As volume cannot be easily assessed clinically, pressure is used as a surrogate; thus, the concept of preload is represented as the filling pressure of a chamber. The relationship between the end-diastolic pressure and the end-diastolic volume is complex. Several different diastolic pressure-volume relationships are shown in Figure 3-12 (green line). As end-diastolic volume increases, and the heart stretches, the end-diastolic pressure also increases. The compliance, or distensibility of the ventricle, is defined as the change in volume divided by the change in pressure. Conversely, the stiffness of the ventricle is the reciprocal of compliance, or the change in pressure divided by the change in volume.

A number of factors affect the diastolic pressure-volume relationship. A fibrotic heart, a hypertrophied heart, or an aging heart becomes increasingly stiff (Figure 3-12C and Figure 3-12E). In the case of fibrosis, this increasing stiffness is related to the development of a greater collagen network. In

the case of hypertrophy, this increased stiffness is related both to stiffening of the noncontractile components of the heart and also to impaired relaxation of the heart. Relaxation is an active, energy-requiring process. This process is accelerated by catecholamine stimulation, but is impaired by ischemia, hypothyroidism, and chronic congestive heart failure. Examination of the diastolic pressure-volume curves in Figure 3-12 reveals the importance of changes in diastolic distensibility in pathologic cardiac conditions.

AFTERLOAD: VASCULAR IMPEDANCE

The afterload of an isolated muscle is the tension against which it contracts. In simplest terms, for the heart, the afterload is determined by the pressure against which the ventricle must eject. The greater the afterload, the more mechanical energy that must be imparted to the blood mass (potential energy) to begin ejection. In addition to the potential energy imparted to the ejected blood by a change in pressure, the contracting left ventricle generates kinetic energy which overcomes the compliance of the distensible aorta and systemic arterial tree to move the blood into the arterial system. The energy necessary for this flow to occur is relatively small (potential energy >> kinetic energy). Resistance, which equals the change in pressure divided by cardiac output, reflects the potential energy imparted to blood. To accurately describe the forces overcome to eject blood from the ventricle, the compliance of the vascular system and kinetic energy imparted must also be considered: the impedance of the vascular system (commonly, but less accurately referred to as aortic impedance). Compliance reflects the capacity of the vascular system to accept the volume of ejected blood. When the vascular system is very compliant, resistance ≈ impedance. As compliance decreases (eg, with arteriosclerosis), resistance is less than impedance.[33] The interaction of resistance and compliance define the dicrotic notch, marking end-systole, closure of the aortic valve, on the aortic pressure tracing (Figure 3-11).

THE CARDIAC CYCLE

Multiple parameters of the cardiac cycle are represented in Figure 3-11. By convention the cardiac cycle begins at end-diastole (ED), just prior to electrical activation of the ventricle. As the heart contracts, intracavitary pressure closes the mitral valve, then rapidly increases until the systemic diastolic pressure is reached (isovolumic contraction) and the aortic valve opens. Ejection begins and the intracavitary pressure continues to rise then fall as the ventricular volume decreases (ejection). When ejection ceases and the aortic valve closes, intracavitary pressure decreases rapidly until the mitral valve opens (isovolumic relaxation). Once the mitral valve opens, the ventricle fills rapidly, then more slowly as the intracavitary pressure slightly increases from distension prior to atrial systole (diastolic filling phase). The completion of atrial systole is the end of ventricular diastole. Atrial systole serves to increase the preload of the ventricle at a given systemic venous pressure.

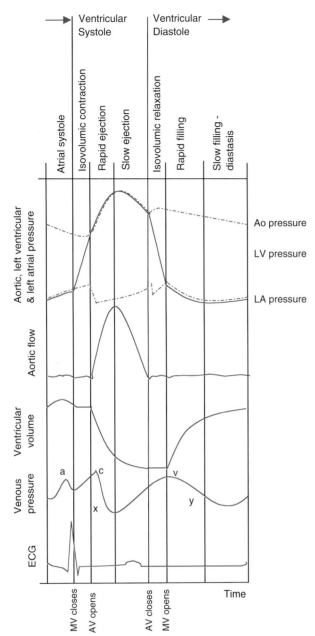

FIGURE 3-11 Temporal correlation of left atrial and ventricular, aortic, and systemic venous pressures, aortic flow, left ventricular volume, and surface electrocardiogram.

A conceptual understanding of the venous pressure changes is important in diagnosing certain pathologic processes. The right atrial pressure is easily measured and pulmonary capillary wedge pressure is reflective of left atrial pressure. The "a" wave corresponds to atrial systole as pressure increases at end-diastole to complete ventricular filling. The "c" wave reflects pressure pushing the atrioventricular (AV) valve back into the atrium as the ventricular pressure rises then falls during systole. The "x" descent results from atrial relaxation and downward displacement of the AV valve with

ventricular emptying. The "v" wave reflects the increasing atrial pressure from filling before the AV valve opens. The "y" descent is caused by rapid emptying of the atrium after the AV valve opens. Characteristic changes in these waveforms are used to diagnose and differentiate constrictive and restrictive processes, as discussed elsewhere in the text. A prominent left atrial "v" wave suggests mitral regurgitation.

VENTRICULAR PRESSURE-VOLUME RELATIONSHIPS

The function of the heart can be described and quantified based on the relative intraventricular pressure and volume during the cardiac cycle (Figure 3-12). Based on this relationship, various measures can be derived to assess cardiac performance. The ventricular pressure-volume relationship derives from the Frank-Starling relationship of sarcomere length and peak developed force: The force and extent of contraction (stroke volume) is a function of end-diastolic length (volume).

End-diastole (ED) is represented at the lower right corner of the loop in Figure 3-12A. The pressure-volume loop then successively tracks changes through isovolumic contraction (up to the upper right corner); ejection (left to the upper left corner, which represents end-systole [ES]); isovolumic relaxation (down to the bottom left corner); then filling (right to the lower right corner). Descriptive data to assess ventricular function are derived from the end-systolic pressure-volume point located in the upper left corner of the loop, and end-diastolic pressure-volume point located in the lower right corner of the loop. The area within the pressure-volume loop represents the internal work of the chamber.

CONTRACTILITY

The term contractility (inotropic state) refers to the intrinsic performance of the ventricle for a given preload, afterload, and heart rate. Otherwise stated, contractility refers to all the factors that impact cardiac performance independent of the acute effects of preload, afterload, and heart rate. In the purest sense, at a level of constant contractility, increased preload will increase cardiac output and stroke volume; increased afterload will decrease cardiac output and stroke volume; and increased heart rate (assuming adequate time for complete diastolic filling) will increase cardiac output without changing stroke volume. Although the inotropic state impacts cardiac output, it is difficult to quantify in clinically useful terms. For research purposes, the pressure-volume relationship can be used to quantify contractility by deriving the end-systolic pressure-volume relationship (ESPVR): contractility is reflected in the slope (E_{ES}) and volume axis intercept (V_0) of the ESPVR (Figure 3-13). Holding afterload and heart rate constant, a series of pressure-volume loops are inscribed during transient preload reduction induced by temporary vena caval occlusion; the area of the loops decreases and the loops are shifted to the left. The progressive pressure-volume points at end systole are then linearized to derive the ESPVR. Within

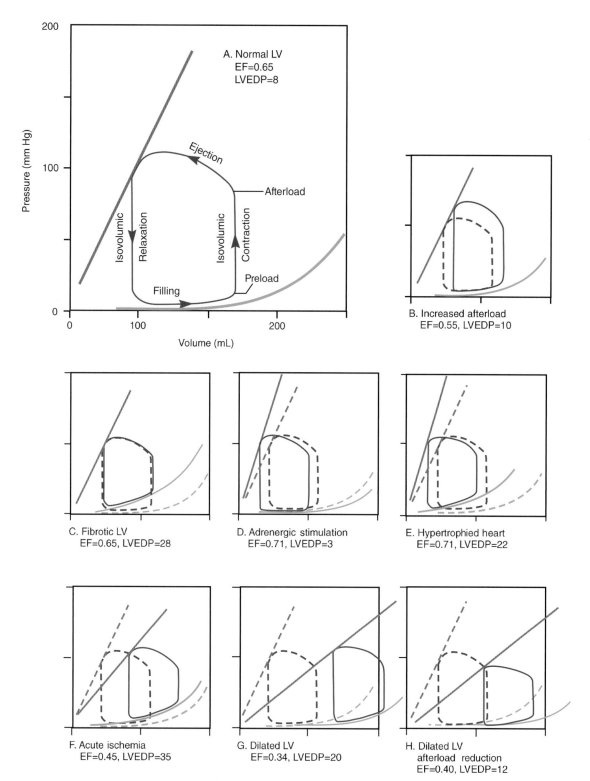

FIGURE 3-12 Left ventricular pressure-volume curves for various physiologic and pathologic conditions. (Detailed descriptions are in the text.) The bold curved line at the bottom of each loop series represents the diastolic pressure-volume relationship. The straight line located on the upper left side of each loop series is the end-systolic pressure-volume relationship. The stroke volume for each curve has been arbitrarily set at 75 mL. Systolic aortic pressure is 115 mm Hg in all curves except *B* (increased afterload, systolic pressure 140 mm Hg) and *H* (reduced afterload, systolic pressure 90 mm Hg) (EF = ejection fraction; LV = left ventricle; LVEDP = left ventricular end-diastolic pressure), in mm Hg.

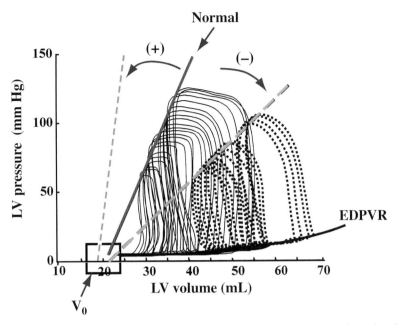

FIGURE 3-13 Two series of declining left ventricular pressure-volume loops generated during transient bicaval occlusion. Loops were generated in normal left ventricles (normal) and after 30 minutes of global normothermic ischemia and subsequent reperfusion (*dashed lines*). The end-systolic pressure-volume points from each series are connected by a line generated by linear regression. The end-diastolic pressure-volume relationship indicating chamber stiffness (inverse of compliance) is generated by fitting the end-diastolic point from each loop to an exponential curve. The volume axis intercept (V_0) is shown in the inset. A negative inotropic effect (ie, ischemia-reperfusion) is characterized by a decrease in the ESPVR slope, while a positive inotropic state is characterized by an increase in ESPVR slope. Notice that the V_0 for these conditions are in close proximity (*inset*). In some cases, a negative inotropic state is associated with a decrease in slope and an increase in V_0.

a clinical range of systolic pressures (80 to 120 mm Hg), the end-systolic pressure-volume line is largely linear. An increase in inotropic state of the left ventricle is expressed as an increase in E_{ES} and sometimes a decrease in V_0. Conversely, a decrease in inotropic state is expressed as a decrease in E_{ES} and sometimes an increase in V_0 (Figure 3-13). As the ESPVR describes systolic function, the end-diastolic pressure volume relationship (EDPVR) (Figure 3-13) describes ventricular diastolic compliance (more specifically, the inverse of the slope of the EDPVR is compliance) a measure of lusitropy. The EDPVR is impacted by calcium uptake, ease of dissociation of contractile proteins, the cytoskeleton, ventricular wall thickness, and the pericardium.

Pressure-volume loops can be used to analyze various physiologic situations. Increased afterload (Figure 3-12B) moves the end-systolic pressure-volume point slightly upward and to the right. If stroke volume is maintained, end-diastolic volume must increase. Thus, though contractility is unchanged, ejection fraction is slightly decreased. Figure 3-12C shows the effect of a decrease in ventricular compliance (increased EDPVR) such as may result from hypertrophy, fibrosis, or cardiac tamponade. Systolic function is maintained (E_{ES} and V_0 are unchanged), and stroke volume and ejection fraction can be maintained but require an increased end-diastolic pressure. The positive inotropic (increased E_{ES}) and lusitropic (decreased EDPVR) effects

of adrenergic stimulation (Figure 3-12D), at constant stroke volume, shift the pressure-volume loop to the left, and increase the ejection fraction. In the hypertrophied heart (Figure 3-12E), in contrast to Figure 3-12C, diastolic compliance is decreased and systolic contractility is increased. A constant stroke volume leads to an increase in end-diastolic filling pressure and decreased end-diastolic volume. The pressure-volume loop shifts to the left with an increase in ejection fraction. The ability of the hypertrophied heart to increase stroke volume is limited. Acute ischemia (Figure 3-12F) decreases diastolic compliance (increases EDPVR) and contractility. The pressure-volume loop shifts to the right and up to maintain stroke volume, consistent with the clinical observation of an acute decrease in ejection fraction and increase in left ventricular filling pressure. In the dilated heart of chronic congestive heart failure (Figure 3-12G), the pressure-volume loop is shifted to the right. Note that the slope of the diastolic pressure-volume curve (EDPVR) changes little; rather the curve shifts to the right. The end-diastolic pressure is not increased because of a change in compliance; instead, to maintain stroke volume, the pressure-volume loop has moved upward on the compliance curve. Contrast this with the fibrotic process discussed in the preceding. The effect of afterload reduction on the chronically failing heart from Figure 3-12G is demonstrated in Figure 3-12H. Note that the ESPVR, EDPVR, and

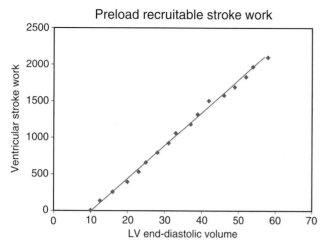

FIGURE 3-14 Plot of hypothetical measurement of preload recruitable stroke work.

stroke volume are unchanged. The pressure volume loop has moved back to the left, decreasing both the degree of chamber dilatation, end-diastolic pressure, and ejection fraction. A positive inotropic agent would shift the ESPVR line to the left (toward the dashed line), and the degree of dilatation would be reduced and both stroke volume and ejection fraction would be increased. It is important to remember that these relationships are idealized and may not completely reflect true clinical responses. For example, reduced diastolic dilatation from afterload reduction could return the ventricle to a state of improved intrinsic contractility. Despite these interactions, the pure concepts discussed here are very helpful in understanding the response of the heart to clinical interventions.

Another index of contractility, perhaps less influenced by other parameters, is the preload recruitable stroke work (PRSW) relationship. Stroke work is the area of the pressure-volume loop. For each pressure-volume loop derived by vena caval occlusion, the stroke work is plotted relative to its end-diastolic volume[34] (Figure 3-14). The slope of the derived linear relationship is a measure of contractility independent (within physiologic ranges) of preload and afterload. The PRSW relationship reflects overall performance of the left ventricle, combining systolic and diastolic components.[35]

CLINICAL INDICES OF CONTRACTILITY

Clearly, from the preceding discussion, the degree of contractility can be assessed, but unlike blood pressure, an ideal number or range to describe it cannot be derived. Because ESPVR and PRSW are unique for each ventricle, these parameters more accurately measure changes in contractility. The greatest impediment to the clinical application of the ESPVR and PRSW is the difficulty measuring ventricular volume and inducing preload reduction to derive the pressure-volume loops. More easily measurable indices of contractility have been actively sought.

Ejection fraction is used by many clinicians as a measure of contractility. However, as noted in the discussion of Figure 3-12, ejection fraction is influenced by preload and afterload alterations without any change in contractility. Depending on loading conditions, hearts with a lower ejection fraction can produce a greater cardiac output. Although roughly indicative of cardiac reserve, ejection fraction is an inconsistent marker for overall cardiac function perioperatively but is a useful, gross measure of cardiac reserve.

MYOCARDIAL WALL STRESS

The left ventricle is a pressurized, irregularly shaped chamber. During systole, wall stress develops to overcome afterload and eject the blood. The pressure within the chamber and the geometry of the ventricle determine the tension in the wall. A model of the ventricle as a cylinder can be used to examine the effects of chamber size and wall thickness on wall stress. In this model, circumferential stress is based on the law of Laplace:

$$\sigma \mu \frac{Pr}{w}$$

where σ is wall stress ($\approx$ tension), P is transmural pressure, r is radius, and w is wall thickness. This relationship has several important clinical implications. Wall tension must be balanced by the energy available. The only nutrient nearly completely extracted from the blood by the heart is oxygen and wall tension is the primary determinant of oxygen consumption. In one scenario, the heart can compensate for changes in wall stress. If systolic pressure within the ventricle is chronically increased (aortic stenosis or systemic hypertension), then compensatory hypertrophy or thickening of the ventricular wall can return systolic wall stress close to normal. However, as detailed in Figure 3-12E, the price paid is that end-diastolic pressures must be higher.

In another scenario, the function of a heart that has dilated for other reasons is further compromised by the relationship between wall stress and oxygen consumption. As a result of or to compensate for systolic failure, the ventricle will dilate. The increased diastolic diameter proportionally increases wall stress and oxygen consumption. The ability of the heart to increase cardiac output in response to exercise will be limited, leading to symptoms.

Right Ventricular Physiology

The left and right ventricles are anatomically partnered, sharing the septum, and physiologically partnered by the serial flow of blood. Changes affecting one chamber can impact the other. Many of the physiologic aspects discussed previously are easily adapted to the left ventricle because of its conical shape and axial symmetry. The right ventricular geometry is more complex since it wraps around the left ventricle and the chamber is crescent shaped in the axial plane. Though the septum contributes to right ventricular ejection most of the decrease in chamber volume during systole is due to free wall contraction. The thinner right ventricular free wall and conus have one-sixth the muscle mass of the left ventricle. The right ventricle functions under lower pressure conditions and operates at volumes slightly greater than the left ventricle. The right ventricular end-diastolic volume is greater than that of the left ventricle. Likewise right ventricular ejection fraction is lower. The lower limit of normal for the right ventricle ranges from 40 to 45%.

The pulmonary circulation determines right ventricular afterload. The pulmonary vascular bed is a highly compliant, low-pressure, low-resistance system. Pulmonary vascular resistance is impacted by hypoxia (vasoconstriction), hypercarbia (vasoconstriction), nitric oxide (vasodilation), prostaglandins (vasodilation), and endothelins (vasoconstriction).

Ventricular Interdependence

Functionally, the cardiac ventricles can be viewed as two hydraulic pumps in series, one coupled to a highly compliant pulmonary vasculature and the other matched to a less compliant systemic circulation. However, the ventricles have common structural elements and are contained within the non-compliant pericardium. The right ventricle, in particular, relies on the left ventricle to maintain its functional geometry. This anatomic and functional arrangement creates direct and serial interactions between the two chambers when an acute or chronic hemodynamic perturbation impacts either ventricle. Acute changes in ventricular interaction can include a shift of the septum towards one chamber in response to sudden volume overload; and enlargement of one chamber impacting diastolic filling of the other in the confined pericardial space. Clinical examples include: (1) massive right ventricular distension and reduced left ventricular filling in the setting of an acute pulmonary embolus; and (2) right ventricular dysfunction after left ventricular assist device implant due to septal shift and changes in right ventricular cavity geometry.

ENERGETICS

Chemical Fuels

Nearly all chemical energy used by the heart is generated by oxidative phosphorylation. Anaerobic metabolism is very limited because anaerobic enzymes are not present in sufficient concentrations. The major fuels for the myocardium are carbohydrates (glucose and lactate) and free fatty acids. When sufficient oxygen is present, these fuels are used to generate ATP. Most of the ATP used by the heart (60 to 70%) is expended in the cyclic contraction of the muscle. Ten to fifteen percent is required for maintaining the concentration gradients across the cell membrane; the rest is used in the constant uptake and release of calcium by mitochondria, the breakdown and regeneration of glycogen, and the synthesis of triglycerides.

The heart is quite flexible in the aerobic state in its use of fuels. In the fasting state, lipids may account for 70% of the fuel used by the heart. When present in adequate amounts, fatty acids will inhibit use of glucose by the heart.[36] After a high carbohydrate meal, blood glucose and insulin levels are high and free fatty acids are low, and glucose accounts for close to 100% of the metabolism. During exercise, elevated lactate levels inhibit the uptake of free fatty acids and carbohydrates, mostly lactate, can account for up to 70% of the metabolism.[37]

Whatever the fuel source, oxygen is necessary for its efficient utilization. In the absence of oxygen, there are two mechanisms to provide ATP, glycolysis and conversion of phosphate stored in creatine phosphate, since free fatty acids and the by-products of glycolysis cannot be metabolized. Glycolysis is very inefficient—for 1 mol of glucose, 2 mol of ATP are produced by anaerobic glycolysis, compared with 38 moles of ATP with aerobic metabolism. Phosphate stored in creatine phosphate can convert ADP to ATP, but this is not stored in significant amounts.

The availability of ADP is the primary determinant of the rate of oxidative phosphorylation. With ischemia and hypoxia, ATP breaks down to ADP and subsequently to AMP, adenosine, and inosine. The nucleoside building blocks of ATP, adenosine, inosine, and hypoxanthine are lost from the ischemic myocardium. If oxygen is restored, ATP levels can be partially restored rapidly by salvage pathways with inosine, hypoxanthine, or inosine monophosphate. However, de novo synthesis of ATP is also required and can take hours or even days to restore significant ATP levels. Glycolysis becomes the primary, albeit inefficient source of ATP with ischemia; this leads to an increase in lactate. The increase in lactate and inorganic phosphate causes acidosis. Acidosis slows glycolysis by reducing the activity of 6-phosphofructo-1-kinase, the rate-limiting enzyme in the glycolytic pathway.[38] The excess protons compete with calcium-binding sites, interfering with contraction and relaxation. Nevertheless, ATP generated by glycolysis maintains cell viability. Glucose, insulin, and potassium support glycolysis and may be the source of the benefit of administering this combination after an ischemic insult.[39]

Determinants of Oxygen Consumption

Because nearly all the energy used by the heart is generated by oxidative metabolism, the rate of oxygen consumption ($M\dot{V}O_2$) is indicative of the metabolic rate of the heart:

$$M\dot{V}O_2 = \frac{CaO_2 - CvO_2}{CBF}/Mass$$

where $M\dot{V}O_2$ is myocardial oxygen consumption, CaO_2 is arterial oxygen content in mL O_2/100mL blood, CvO_2 is coronary venous oxygen content in mL O_2/100 mL blood, CBF is coronary blood flow in mL/min. Because the bulk of the energy is expended on contraction, changes in the rate of oxygen consumption of the heart are directly related to changes in the contraction cycle and workload. Energy utilization can be increased by an increase in cardiac workload or a decrease in the efficiency of conversion of chemical to mechanical energy.

Minute work of the heart is the product of heart rate, stroke volume, and developed pressure. A change in each of these factors alters oxygen demand; however, minute work is not the direct determinant of oxygen consumption. The primary determinant of oxygen demand is the wall tension or stress developed in each cardiac cycle. Indeed, during the period of isovolumic contraction, energy is expended by the heart without the delivery of any kinetic energy to the blood.[40] The energetic cost of ejecting blood from the ventricular chamber is approximately 20 to 30% of that required for isovolumic contraction. To restate this simply, the principal determinant of the cardiac energy requirement is the pressure against which blood is ejected and the volume ejected at that pressure. An increase in afterload requires greater energy than an increase in volume ejected. Oxygen consumption is also increased as the heart dilates and begins ejection from a greater diastolic volume.

Cardiac efficiency relates oxygen consumption to cardiac work. Hence, cardiac efficiency = work/M$\dot{V}$O$_2$. The overall efficiency of the heart ranges from 5 to 40%, depending on the type of work (pressure versus volume versus velocity) performed.[41-44] The low efficiency of the heart is caused by the expenditure of a predominant portion of the oxygen consumed in generating pressure and stretching internal elastic components of the myocardium during isovolumic systole (a form of internal work). The velocity of shortening, affected in part by the inotropic state of the myocardium, also is not factored into the work equation, but contributes significantly to oxygen consumption. Dilation of the ventricle reduces efficiency because as cavity size increases the reduction in wall stress with ejection is decreased.

Following cardiac surgery, cardiac efficiency generally decreases because of the increase in M$\dot{V}$O$_2$ relative to the cardiac work performed. The additional oxygen consumed may result from an increase in basal metabolism and/or an increase in the cost of the excitation-contraction process, or inefficiencies of ATP production at the mitochondrial level.

A clear understanding of the role of wall tension and its relation to oxygen demand is essential in cardiac surgery. Excessive systemic pressure may place inordinate energy demands on a compromised ventricle. An intra-aortic balloon pump may shift the energy balance by reducing afterload and improving coronary blood flow. Ventricular distension during the weaning process after removal of the aortic cross-clamp, or with heart failure may create wall stress that outstrips the capacity to deliver oxygen to the myocardium. In the failing heart, where stroke volume is reduced, cardiac output is maintained by increasing heart rate, which increases the percentage of time that the myocardial wall stress is elevated, reduces

the time when diastolic blood flow occurs, and creates an imbalance between oxygen demand and delivery.

FUNCTIONAL RESPONSES TO METABOLIC DEMANDS[45]

There are three distinct responses to altered metabolic demands. Two are responses to acute short-term alterations; the third is a response to chronic alterations in metabolic demands.

Acute Physiologic Responses

These responses consist of intrinsic physiologic adaptations to acute changes in hemodynamics and metabolic demands. Generally, these responses are regulated by changes in end-diastolic volume mediated by changes in preload and afterload. Beat-to-beat responses to changes in end-diastolic volume are important to equalizing the output of the ventricles.

Alterations of Biochemical Functions

Contractility (inotropy) and relaxation (lusitropy) change in response to altered metabolic demands. These are principally mediated by alterations in calcium fluxes in the myocyte.[46] The principal determinant of calcium concentration is the flux across the sarcoplasmic reticulum membrane. The fluxes are determined by the amount of calcium in the sarcoplasmic reticulum and the amount of calcium crossing the plasma membrane to stimulate calcium release. Reduced ATP levels inhibit calcium release and uptake. Enzymatic phosphorylation of myosin can increase the rate of cross-bridge cycling, and phosphorylation of troponin I facilitates relaxation.[47] Acidosis reduces contraction and relaxation by inhibiting many calcium pumps, channels, and exchangers.[48]

Altered Gene Expression

Chronic changes in metabolic demands will provoke proliferative responses leading to altered gene expression. These include changes in the types of myosin and actin and changes in the number of membrane channels and pumps.

CORONARY BLOOD FLOW
Normal Coronary Blood Flow

Resting coronary blood flow is slightly less than 1 mL per gram of heart muscle per minute. This blood flow is delivered to the heart through large epicardial conductance vessels and then into the myocardium by penetrating arteries leading to a plexus of capillaries. The bulk of the resistance to coronary flow is in the penetrating arterioles (20 to 120 μm in size). Because the heart is metabolically very active, there is a high density of capillaries such that there is approximately one capillary for every myocyte, with an intercapillary distance at rest of approximately 17 μm. Capillary density is greater in subendocardial myocardium compared with subepicardial tissue. When there is an increased myocardial oxygen demand, myocardial blood flow can increase to three or four times the normal (coronary flow reserve). This is accomplished by vasodilation of the resistance vessels and recruitment of additional capillaries (many of which are closed in the resting state). Capillary recruitment is important in decreasing the intercapillary distance and the distance that oxygen and nutrients must diffuse through the myocardium.

The blood flow pattern from a coronary artery perfusing the left ventricle, measured by flow probe, is phasic in nature, with greater blood flow occurring in diastole than in systole.[49] The cyclic contraction and relaxation of the left ventricle produces this phasic blood flow pattern by extravascular compression of the arteries and intramyocardial microvessels during systole. There is a gradient in these systolic extravascular compressive forces, being greater than or equal to intracavitary pressure in the subendocardial tissue, and decreasing toward the subepicardial tissue. Measurement of transmural blood flow distribution during systole shows that subepicardial vessels are preferentially perfused, whereas subendocardial vessels are significantly hypoperfused. Toward the end of systole, blood flow actually reverses in the epicardial surface vessels.[50] Hence, the subendocardial myocardium is perfused primarily during diastole, whereas subepicardial myocardium is perfused during both systole and diastole. A greater capillary density per square millimeter in the subendocardium compared with the subepicardial tissue facilitates the distribution of blood flow to the inner layer of myocardium.[51] The subendocardium is at greater risk of dysfunction, tissue injury, and necrosis during any reduction in perfusion. This is related to: (1) the greater systolic compressive forces; (2) the smaller flow reserve resulting from a greater degree of vasodilation; and (3) the greater regional oxygen demands owing to wall tension and segmental shortening. If end-diastolic pressure is elevated to 25, 30, or 35 mm Hg, then there is diastolic as well as systolic compression of the subendocardial vasculature. Flow to the subepicardium is effectively autoregulated as long as the pressure in the distal coronary artery is above approximately 40 mm Hg. Flow to the subendocardium, however, is effectively autoregulated only down to a mean distal coronary artery pressure of approximately 60 to 70 mm Hg. Below that level, local coronary flow reserve in the subendocardium is exhausted, and local blood flow decreases linearly with decreases in distal coronary artery pressure. Subendocardial perfusion is further compromised by pathologic processes that increase wall thickness and systolic and diastolic wall tension. Aortic regurgitation particularly threatens the subendocardium, because systemic diastolic arterial pressure is reduced and intraventricular systolic and diastolic pressures are elevated.[49,52]

In contrast to the phasic nature of blood flow in the left coronary artery, blood flow in the right coronary artery is relatively constant during the cardiac cycle. The constancy of blood flow is related to the lower intramural pressures and the near absence of extravascular compressive forces in the right ventricle compared with the left ventricle.

Control of Coronary Blood Flow

Coronary blood flow is tightly coupled to the metabolic needs of the heart. Under normal conditions, 70% of the oxygen available in coronary arterial blood is extracted, near the physiologic maximum. Any increase in oxygen delivery comes mostly from an increase in blood flow. To maximize efficiency, local coronary blood flow is precisely controlled by a balance of vasodilator and vasoconstrictor mechanisms, including: (1) a metabolic vasodilator system; (2) aneurogenic control system; and (3) the vascular endothelium.[53] Blood flow is controlled by moment-to-moment adjustment of coronary tone of the resistance vessels, that is, arterioles and precapillary sphincters.

The metabolic vasodilator mechanism responds rapidly when local blood flow is insufficient to meet metabolic demand. The primary mediator is adenosine generated within the myocyte and released into the interstitial compartment. Adenosine relaxes arteriolar smooth muscle cells by activation of A_2 receptors. Adenosine is formed when the oxygen supply cannot sustain the rapid rephosphorylation of ADP to ATP. Once sufficient oxygen is supplied to the myocardium, less adenosine is formed. Adenosine is therefore the coupling agent between oxygen demand and supply. Other local vasodilators that influence coronary blood flow are carbon dioxide, lactic acid, and histamine.

The sympathetic nervous system acts through alpha receptors (vasoconstriction) and beta receptors (vasodilation). There are direct innervations of the large conductance vessels and lesser direct innervations of the smaller resistance vessels. Sympathetic receptors on the smooth muscle cells of the resistance vessels respond to humoral catecholamines. Alpha receptors predominate over beta receptors such that when norepinephrine is released from the sympathetic nerve endings, vasoconstriction ordinarily occurs.

Endothelium-dependent regulation of coronary artery blood flow is a dynamic balance between vasodilating and vasoconstricting factors. Vasodilators include nitric oxide (NO) synthesized from L-arginine by endothelial nitric oxide synthase, and endothelially released adenosine. The principal vasoconstrictor is the endothelially derived constricting peptide endothelin-1. Other vasoconstrictors include angiotensin II and superoxide free radical.[54] NO is dominant in the local regulation of coronary arterial tone. NO is released by the coronary vascular endothelium by both soluble factors (acetylcholine, adenosine, and ATP) and mechanical signals (shear stress and pulsatile stress secondary to increased intraluminal blood flow). If the endothelium is intact, acetylcholine from the sympathetic nerves causes vasodilation through generation of NO. If the endothelium is not functionally intact, acetylcholine causes vasoconstriction by direct stimulation of the vascular smooth muscle. NO is a potent inhibitor of platelet aggregation and neutrophil function (superoxide generation, adherence, and migration), which has implications in the anti-inflammatory response to ischemia-reperfusion and cardiopulmonary bypass.

Endothelin-1 interacts principally with specific endothelin receptors, ET_A, on vascular smooth muscle, and causes smooth muscle vasoconstriction. Endothelin-1 counteracts the vasodilator effects of endogenous adenosine, NO, and prostacyclin (PGI_2). Endothelin-1 is rapidly synthesized in the vascular endothelium, particularly during ischemia, hypoxia, and other stress conditions, where it acts in a paracrine fashion. ET-1 has a short half-life (4 to 7 minutes), which exceeds that of adenosine (8 to12 seconds) and NO (microseconds). However, the avid binding of ET-1 to ET_A receptors prolongs its effects beyond its half-life. Human coronary arteries demonstrate abundant endothelin-1 binding sites, suggesting that ET-1 has an important role in the control of coronary blood flow in humans.[55] The levels of ET-1 have been observed to increase with myocardial ischemia-reperfusion and after cardiac surgery.

Under ordinary circumstances the metabolic vasodilator system is the dominant force acting on the resistance vessels. For example, the increased metabolic activity caused by sympathetic stimulation leads to vasodilation of the coronary arterioles through the metabolic system, despite a direct vasoconstriction effect of norepinephrine.[56-58]

Coronary artery blood flow is also determined by perfusion pressure. However, in the coronary vasculature blood flow can remain constant over a range of perfusion pressures. The control mechanisms described allow autoregulation of blood flow adjusting vascular resistance to match blood flow requirements. The autoregulatory "plateau" occurs between approximately 60 and 120 mm Hg perfusion pressure. If distal coronary artery perfusion pressure is reduced by a critical stenosis or hypotension, vasodilator capacity will be exhausted and coronary blood flow will decrease, following a linear relationship with perfusion pressure. Because the subendocardial region of the left ventricle has a lower coronary vascular reserve, maximal dilation is reached in this region before the subepicardial tissue, and a preferential hypoperfusion of the subendocardial tissue results.

Hemodynamic Effect of Coronary Artery Stenosis

Surgically treatable atherosclerotic disease primarily affects the large conductance vessels of the heart. The hemodynamic effect of a stenosis is determined by Poiseuille's law, which describes the resistance of a viscous fluid to laminar flow through a cylindrical tube; specifically:

$$Q = \frac{\pi(\Delta P)}{8\eta} \cdot \frac{r^4}{l}$$

where Q is the flow, ΔP is the pressure change, η is the viscosity, r is the radius, and l is the length of the resistance segment. Resistance (pressure change/flow):

$$R = \frac{(\Delta P)}{Q} = \frac{8\eta}{\pi} \cdot \frac{l}{r^4}$$

is inversely proportional to the *fourth* power of the radius and directly proportional to the length of the narrowing. Therefore, a small change in diameter has a magnified effect on vascular resistance (Table 3-2). Conductance vessels are sufficiently large that a 50% reduction in the diameter of the vessel has minimal hemodynamic effect. A 60% reduction in the diameter of the vessel has only a very small hemodynamic effect. As the stenosis progresses beyond 60%, small decreases in diameter have significant effects on blood flow. For a given segment length, an 80% stenosis has a resistance that is 16 times greater a 60% stenosis. For a 90% stenosis, the resistance is 256 times greater than for a 60% stenosis.[59] Furthermore, for successive stenoses in the same vessel the resistance is additive. An additional factor in resistance to flow is turbulence. Stenotic lesions can cause conversion from laminar to turbulent flow.[60] With laminar flow the pressure drop is proportional to flow rate Q; with turbulent flow pressure drop is

TABLE 3-2: Effect of Degree and Length of Stenosis on Resistance to Flow Based on Poiseuille's Law

% Stenosis of a 1-cm-diameter vessel	Radius (in cm)	Proportional resistance for various segment lengths (cm)		
		0.25 cm	1 cm	2 cm
0	0.5	1	4	8
50	0.25	16	64	128
60	0.2	39	156	313
70	0.15	123	494	988
80	0.1	625	2500	5000
90	0.05	10000	40000	80000
Proportional increase in resistance 80% versus 60% stenosis				16
Proportional increase in resistance 90% versus 60% stenosis				256

The value for a reference vessel of length 0.25 cm with 0% stenosis (in the box) is set to 1 for comparison.

proportional to Q^2. For all of these reasons, patients who have had a small progression in the degree of coronary stenosis may experience a rapid acceleration of symptoms.

Atherosclerosis also alters normal vascular regulatory mechanisms. The endothelium is often destroyed or damaged, so vasoconstrictor mechanisms are relatively unopposed by the impaired vasodilator mechanism; constriction is exaggerated and responses to stimuli that require dilatation are blunted.[61]

As noted, when a stenosis is less than 60%, little change is flow is noted. This is due to compensation by the coronary flow reserve of the resistance vessels distal to the stenotic conductance vessel. As resistance to flow is additive, a decrease in distal resistance will balance an increase in proximal resistance and flow will be unchanged. As flow reserve decreases, any stimulus that increases myocardial oxygen demand (such a tachycardia, hypertension, or exercise) cannot be met by dilation of the distal vasculature, and myocardial ischemia results.[53]

In the human, coronary arterial vessels are end vessels with little collateral flow between major branches except in pathologic situations. With sudden coronary occlusion, although there is usually modest collateral flow through very small vessels (20 to 200 μm in size), this flow is generally insufficient to maintain cellular viability. Collateral flow gradually begins to increase over the next 8 to 24 hours, doubling by about the third day after total occlusion. Collateral blood flow development appears to be nearly complete after 1 month, restoring normal or nearly normal resting flow to the surviving myocardium in the ischemic region. Previous ischemic events or gradually developing stenoses can lead to larger preexisting collaterals in the human heart. The presence of these pre-existing collaterals has been shown to be important in the prevention of ischemic damage if coronary occlusion should occur.[62]

Endothelial Dysfunction

As previously noted, nitric oxide, adenosine, and endothelin-1 are synthesized and released by the endothelium.[63,64] Ischemia-reperfusion, hypertension, diabetes, and hypercholesterolemia can impair generation of NO and vasoconstriction may predominate, mediated by the relative overexpression of endothelin-1. Reperfusion after temporary myocardial ischemia is one situation in which NO production may be impaired, leading to a vicious cycle in which the vasodilator reserve of the resistance vessels is reduced with a consequent and progressive "low-flow" or "no-flow" phenomenon. The coronary vascular NO system may also be impaired in some cases after coronary artery bypass surgery.

The endothelium helps prevent cell-cell interactions between blood-borne inflammatory cells (ie, leukocytes and platelets) that initiate a local or systemic inflammatory reaction. Inflammatory cascades occur with sepsis, ischemia-reperfusion, and cardiopulmonary bypass. Under normal conditions, the vascular endothelium resists interaction with neutrophils and platelets by tonically releasing adenosine and NO, which have potent antineutrophil and platelet inhibitory

effects. Damage to the endothelium lowers the resistance to neutrophil adhesion. Neutrophils can damage the endothelium by adhesion to its surface, and subsequent release of oxygen radicals and proteases. This amplifies the inflammatory response and decreases the tonic generation and release of adenosine and NO, which then permits further interaction with activated inflammatory cells. The products released by activated neutrophils have downstream physiologic consequences on other tissues, notably the heart, including increasing vascular permeability, creating blood flow defects (no-reflow phenomenon), and promoting the pathogenesis of necrosis and apoptosis.[65]

The triggers of these inflammatory reactions in the heart include cytokines (IL-1, IL-6, IL-8), complement fragments (C3a, C5a, membrane attack complex), oxygen radicals, and thrombin, which upregulate adhesion molecules expressed on both inflammatory cells (CD11a/CD18) and endothelium (P-selectin, E-selectin, and intercellular adhesion molecule-1 (ICAM-1)). The release of cytokines and complement fragments during cardiopulmonary bypass activates the vascular endothelium on a systemic basis, which contributes to the inflammatory response to cardiopulmonary bypass.[66] Both adenosine and NO have been used therapeutically to reduce the inflammatory responses to cardiopulmonary bypass, and to reduce ischemic-reperfusion injury and endothelial damage.[67,68]

The Sequelae of Myocardial Hypoperfusion: Infarction, Myocardial Stunning, and Myocardial Hibernation

As oxygen delivery is reduced, contraction strength decreases rapidly (within 8 to 10 heart beats). This is seen acutely in response to ischemia and is rapidly reversed with reperfusion. If the extent of reduction of coronary blood flow is severe, mild-to-moderate abnormalities in cellular homeostasis occur. Reduced cellular levels of ATP lead to a loss of adenine nucleotides from the cell. If the reduction in coronary flow is sustained, progressive loss of adenine nucleotides and the elevation of intracellular and intramitochondrial calcium may lead to cellular death and subsequent necrosis. Increased intramitochondrial calcium uncouples oxidative phosphorylation, creating a vicious cycle.[69] If the myocyte is reperfused before subcellular organelles are irreversibly damaged, the myocyte may slowly recover. A period of days is necessary for full recovery of myocyte ATP levels as adenine nucleotides must be resynthesized. During this time contractile processes are impaired. This impairment is related to reversible damage to the contractile proteins such that their responsiveness to cytosolic levels of calcium is diminished. The magnitude of the cytosolic pulse of calcium with each heartbeat appears to be nearly normal, but the magnitude of the consequent contraction is greatly reduced. Over a period of 1 to 2 weeks this myocardium gradually recovers. This viable but dysfunctional myocardium is called stunned myocardium.[70-72]

With chronic hypoperfusion, oxygen delivery is at a reduced level but above the level required for cell viability. This can cause a chronic hypocontractile state known as hibernation. Hibernation appears to be associated with a decrease in the magnitude of the pulse of calcium involved in the excitation-contraction process such that the calcium levels developed within the cytosol during each heartbeat are inadequate for effective contraction to occur. Histologic examination shows islets in the subendocardium where there is a loss of contractile proteins, sarcoplasmic reticulum, and alterations of other subcellular structures.[73,74] With reperfusion, hibernating myocardium can very quickly resume normal and effective contraction, though complete recovery may be delayed for several months.[70,75-77] This is of particular importance for patients with poor ventricular function but viable heart muscle.[78]

Reperfusion of acutely ischemic myocardium may cause further cellular damage and necrosis rather than lead to immediate recovery. The etiology of reperfusion injury is multifactorial. Damaged endothelium in the reperfused region fails to prevent adhesion and activation of leukocytes and platelets. Oxygen-free radicals are released. Derangement of the ATP-dependent sodium-potassium pump disrupts cell volume regulation with consequent leakage of water into the cell, explosive cell swelling, and rupture of the cell membrane. Techniques applied to reduce reperfusion injury, minimize adverse sequelae, and preserve myocytes include leukocyte depletion or inactivation, prevention of endothelial activation, free radical scavenging, reperfusion with solutions low in calcium content, and reperfusion with hyperosmolar solutions.[79,80] Both adenosine and low-dose NO are potent cardioprotective agents that attenuate neutrophil-mediated damage, infarction, and apoptosis.[81]

The metabolic changes that occur with ischemia-reperfusion represent a complex system of adaptive mechanisms that allow the myocyte to survive despite a temporary reduction in oxygen delivery. These adaptive mechanisms may be triggered by a very brief coronary occlusion (as short as 5 minutes) such that the negative sequelae of a subsequent prolonged coronary occlusion are greatly minimized. This phenomenon has been called ischemic preconditioning. A coronary occlusion that might cause as much as 40% myocyte death in a region subjected to prolonged ischemia may be reduced to only 10% myocyte death if the prolonged period of ischemia is preceded by a 5-minute interval of "preconditioning" coronary occlusion.[79,82,83]

PHYSIOLOGY OF HEART FAILURE

Definition and Classification

Heart failure is the inability of the heart to deliver adequate blood to the tissues to meet end-organ metabolic needs at rest or during mild to moderate exercise. Processes that cause heart failure can impair systolic function (the ability to contract and empty) or diastolic function (the ability to relax and

fill) or both. The acute and chronic stages of a myocardial infarction involving a large area of the left ventricle cause systolic heart failure. The acute loss of contractile function compromises the ability of the ventricle to maintain a normal stroke volume (Figure 3-12F). As the infarction heals, the adaptive response of ventricular dilation reduces the heart's systolic functional reserve. Cardiomyopathies affect the myocardium globally leading to reduced systolic function. Long-standing valvular insufficiency alters ventricular geometry and muscular function leading to ventricular failure. In all these examples, the left ventricle dilates, which causes the pressure-volume relationship of the left ventricle to shift to the right (Figure 3-12G). In these situations, the diastolic portion of the pressure-volume curves is not greatly changed. However, the global systolic performance of the heart (ie, the ability to pump blood) maybe inadequate to meet even resting needs.[84,85]

Diastolic failure may occur without an impairment of systolic contractility if the myocardium becomes fibrotic or hypertrophied, or if there is an external constraint on filling such as with pericardial tamponade.[86] Increased stiffness of the left ventricular myocardium is associated with an excessive upward shift in the diastolic pressure-volume curve (Figure 3-12C and Figure 3-12E). The most common cause of increased myocardial stiffness is chronic hypertension with consequent left ventricular hypertrophy and diastolic stiffness (related both to myocyte hypertrophy and increased fibrosis of the ventricle).[87,88]

It should be noted from these examples that although one process may predominate, most patients with heart failure manifest both systolic and diastolic dysfunction.

Early Cardiac and Systemic Sequelae of Heart Failure

The adaptive homeostatic reactions of the body leading to heart failure depend on the duration of the ongoing pathologic process. When cardiac function acutely deteriorates and cardiac output diminishes, neurohumoral reflexes attempt to restore both cardiac output and blood pressure. Activation of the sympathetic adrenergic system in the heart and in the peripheral vasculature causes systemic vasoconstriction and increases heart rate and contractility. A variety of mediators formed during this adaptive stage, including norepinephrine, angiotensin II, vasopressin, B-type natriuretic peptic, and endothelin, not only promote renal retention of salt and water leading to volume expansion but also cause vasoconstriction. Aldosterone output is increased, conserving sodium. The concerted responses of the adrenergic system and the renin-angiotensin system alter the primary determinants of stroke volume and cardiac output—preload, afterload, and contractility. The heart responds to loss of systolic function by progressively dilating. This dilation leads to preservation of stroke volume by Frank-Starling mechanisms but increased stroke volume is achieved at the expense of ejection fraction, as shown in Figure 3-12G, as a right shift in the pressure-volume relationship of the left ventricle with an increase in end-diastolic volume (and pressure). In addition to a global dilation response, acute alterations in cardiac geometry may occur early after a large myocardial infarction, with thinning of the left ventricular wall in the region of the infarct as well as expansion of overall left ventricular cavity size. As volume expansion occurs, production of the cardiac atrial natriuretic peptide is increased, which tends to prevent excessive sodium retention and inhibit activation of the renin-angiotensin and aldosterone systems.[89-93]

Cardiac and Systemic Maladaptive Consequences of Chronic Heart Failure

The acute phase response is initially beneficial but becomes maladaptive and contributes to long-term problems in patients with heart failure (Figure 3-15). In the latter stages of heart failure, the kidneys tend to retain sodium and become hyporesponsive to atrial natriuretic peptide and B-type natriuretic peptide.[90] Desensitization of beta-adrenergic receptors is a consequence of sustained stimulation with a reduced response to elevated circulating catecholamine levels.[19]

Left ventricular dilation is caused by hypertrophy of the myocytes as well as lengthening of the myocytes as sarcomeres are added. However, there is significant slippage of myofibrils leading to dilation without an increase in the number of myocytes. Progressive dilation of the heart leads to an increase in oxygen consumption during systole. Ventricular remodeling leads to progressive fibrosis.

Angiotensin and aldosterone stimulate collagen formulation and proliferation of fibroblasts in the heart, leading to an increase in the ratio of interstitial tissue to myocardial tissue in the noninfarcted regions of the heart.[94] The impact of aldosterone has been documented by the effectiveness of aldosterone receptor antagonists in improving the morbidity and mortality of patients with heart failure.[95]

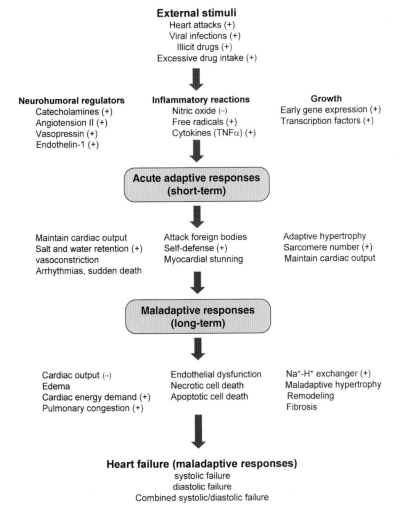

FIGURE 3-15 Pathophysiology of heart failure from stimulus (etiology) to acute adaptive and chronic maladaptive responses. (+) Indicates positive stimulation; (–) indicates negative factors that tend to reduce stimulation of heart failure.

The progressive fibrosis leads to increased diastolic stiffness which limits diastolic filling and increase end-diastolic pressure. Fibrosis and increased ventricular size predispose to reentry ventricular arrhythmias that are a common cause of death in the late stages of heart failure.[96] Hence, heart failure progresses as a result of a vicious cycle of left ventricular dilatation and remodeling, responses that decrease cardiac performance further.

Evidence has accumulated over the past decade that suggests endothelial dysfunction, release of cytokines, and apoptotic cell death may participate in the development of heart failure as a maladaptive reaction (Figure 3-15). Reduced availability of nitric oxide and increased production of vasoconstrictor agents such as endothelin and angiotensin II has been reported in failing hearts.[97] Heart failure is often accompanied by changes in the endogenous antioxidant defense mechanisms of the heart as well as evidence of oxidative injury to the myocardium. Cytokines, released from systemic and local inflammatory responses in the failing heart, directly activate inflammatory cells to release superoxide radicals and cause endothelial dysfunction by augmenting inflammatory cell-endothelial cell interactions. Cytokines may also directly induce necrotic and apoptotic myocyte cell death.[98]

Cardiac secretion of B-type natriuretic peptide (BNP) has been shown to be increased with heart failure. BNP is a cardiac neurohormone released as preproBNP that is enzymatically cleaved to N-terminal-proBNP and BNP upon ventricular myocyte stretch. The physiologic effects of BNP include natriuresis, vasodilation and neurohumoral changes. Measurement of plasma BNP is a useful and cost-effective marker for heart failure.[99] Other factors rather than stretch may stimulate BNP release including fibrosis, arrhythmias, ischemia, endothelial dysfunction, and cardiac hypertrophy.

ACKNOWLEDGMENTS

The authors would like to acknowledge the work of the authors of this chapter in the 2nd edition, Jakob Vinten-Johansen, Zhi-Qing Zhao, and Robert A. Guyton. The current revision was based on the solid foundation they had prepared.

REFERENCES

1. Opie LH. Fuels: carbohydrates and lipids, in Swynghedauw B, Taegtmeyer H, Ruegg JC, Carmeliet E (eds): *The Heart: Physiology and Metabolism*. New York, Raven Press, 1991, p 208.
2. Katz AM: Regulation of cardiac contraction and relaxation, in Willerson JT, Cohn JN (eds): *Cardiovascular Medicine*. New York, Churchill Livingstone, 1995; p 790.
3. Andersen OS, Koeppe RE: Molecular determinants of channel function. *Physiol Rev* 1992; 72:S89-158.
4. Catterall WA: Cellular and molecular biology of voltage-gated sodium channels. *Physiol Rev* 1992; 72:S15-48.
5. Levitan IB: Modulation of ion channels by protein phosphorylation and dephosphorylation. *Annu Rev Physiol* 1994; 56:193-212.
6. McDonald TF, Pelzer S, Trautwein, et al: Regulation and modulation of calcium channels in cardiac, skeletal, and smooth muscle cells. *Physiol Rev* 1994; 74:365-507.
7. Barry WH, Bridge JHB: Intracellular calcium homeostasis in cardiac myocytes. *Circulation* 1993; 87:1806-1815.
8. Pallotta BS, Wagoner PK: Voltage-dependent potassium channels since Hodgkin and Huxley. *Physiol Rev* 1992; 72:S49-67.
9. Horisberger JD, Lemas V, Kraehenbuhl JP, Rossier BC: Structure-function relationship of Na, K-ATPase. *Annu Rev Physiol* 1991; 53:565-584.
10. Pozzan T, Rizzuto R, Volpe P, Meldolesi J: Molecular and cellular physiology of intracellular calcium stores. *Physiol Rev* 1994; 74:595-636.
11. Kutchai HC: Ionic equalibria and resting membrane potentials, in Berne RM, Levy MV, Koeppen BM, Stanton BA (eds): *Physiology*. St. Louis, Mosby, 2004; pp 23-26.
12. Levy MN: Electrical activity of the heart, in Berne RM, Levy MV, Koeppen BM, Stanton BA (eds): *Physiology*. St. Louis, Mosby, 2004; pp 276-277.
13. Coraboeuf E, Nargeot J: Electrophysiology of human cardiac cells. *Cardiovasc Res* 1993; 27:1713-1725.
14. Naccarelli GV: Recognition and physiologic treatment of cardiac arrhythmias and conduction disturbances, in Willerson JT, Cohn JN (eds): *Cardiovascular Medicine*. New York, Churchill Livingstone, 1995; p 1282.
15. Katz AM: *Physiology of the Heart*, 4th ed. Philadelphia, Lippincott Williams & Wilkins, 2006; p 217.
16. Katz AM: *Physiology of the Heart*, 4th ed. Philadelphia, Lippincott Williams & Wilkins, 2006; p 220.
17. Katz AM: *Physiology of the Heart*, 4th ed. Philadelphia, Lippincott Williams & Wilkins, 2006; p 227.
18. Katz AM: *Physiology of the Heart*, 4th ed. Philadelphia, Lippincott Williams & Wilkins, 2006; p 538.
19. Homcy CJ, Vatner ST, Vatner DE: Beta-adrenergic receptor regulation in the heart in pathophysiologic states: abnormal adrenergic responsiveness in cardiac disease. *Annu Rev Physiol* 1991; 53:137-159.
20. Feldman AM: Classification of positive inotropic agents. *J Am Coll Cardiol* 1993; 22:1223-1237.
21. Honerjager P: Pharmacology of bipyridine phosphodiesterase III inhibitors. *Am Heart J* 1991; 1939-1944.
22. Vinten-Johansen J, Zhao Z, Corvera JS, et al: Adenosine in myocardial protection in on-pump and off-pump cardiac surgery. *Ann Thorac Surg* 2003; 75:S691-699.
23. Hynynen MM, Khalil RA: The vascular endothelin system in hypertension—Recent patents and discoveries. *Recent Pat Cardiovasc Drug Discov* 2006; 1:95-108.
24. Brady AJ, Warren JB, Poole-Wilson PA, et al: Nitric oxide attenuates cardiac myocyte contraction. *Am J Physiol* 1993; 265:H176-82.
25. Rastaldo R, Pagliaro P, Cappello S, et al: Nitric oxide and cardiac function. *Life Sci* 2007; 81:779-793.
26. Simon JN, Duglan D, Casadei B, et al: Nitric oxide synthase regulation of cardiac excitation-contraction coupling in health and disease. *J Mol Cell Cardiol* 2014; 73:80-91.
27. Katz AM: *Physiology of the Heart*, 4th ed. Philadelphia, Lippincott Williams & Wilkins, 2006; p 241.
28. Parsons B, Szczesna D, Zhao J, Van Slooten G, Kerrick WG, Putkey JA, Potter JD: The effect of pH on the Ca^{2+} affinity of the Ca^{2+} regulatory sites of skeletal and cardiac troponin C in skinned muscle fibres. *J Muscle Res Cell Motil* 1997; 18:599-609.
29. Ebashi S: Excitation-contraction coupling and the mechanism of muscle contraction. *Annu Rev Physiol* 1991; 53:1-16.
30. Katz AM: *Physiology of the Heart*, 4th ed. Philadelphia, Lippincott Williams & Wilkins, 2006; p 128.
31. Perriard JC, Hirschy A, Ehler E: Dilated cardiomyopathy: a disease of the intercalated disc? *Trends Cardiovasc Med* 2003; 13:30-38.
32. Kobirumaki-Shimozawa F, Inoue T, Shintani SA, et al: Cardiac thin filament regulation and the Frank-Starling mechanism. *J Physiol Sci* 2014; 64:221-232.
33. Briand M, Dumesnil JG, Kadem L, et al: Reduced systemic arterial compliance impacts significantly on left ventricular afterload and function in aortic stenosis: implications for diagnosis and treatment. *J Am Coll Cardiol* 2005; 46:291-298.
34. Glower DD, Spratt JA, Snow ND, et al: Linearity of the Frank-Starling relationship in the intact heart: the concept of preload recruitable stroke work. *Circulation* 1985; 71:994-1009.

35. Feneley MP, Skelton TN, Kisslo KB, Davis JW, Bashore TM, Rankin JS: Comparison of preload recruitable stroke work, end-systolic pressure-volume and dP/dtmax-end-diastolic volume relations as indexes of left ventricular contractile performance in patients undergoing routine cardiac catheterization. *J Amer Coll Cardiol* 1992; 19:1522-1530.

36. Katz AM: *Physiology of the Heart*, 4th ed. Philadelphia, Lippincott Williams & Wilkins, 2006; p 74.

37. Taegtmeyer H: Myocardial metabolism, in Willerson JT, Cohn JN (eds): *Cardiovascular Medicine.* New York, Churchill Livingstone, 1995; p 752.

38. Hollidge-Horvat MG, Parolin ML, Wong D, Jones NL, Heigenhauser GJ: Effect of induced metabolic acidosis on human skeletal muscle metabolism during exercise. *Am J Physiol* 199; 277:E647-658.

39. Apstein CS: The benefits of glucose-insulin-potassium for acute myocardial infarction (and some concerns). *J Am Coll Cardiol* 2003; 42:792-795.

40. Indolfi C, Ross J: The role of heart rate in myocardial ischemia and infarction: implications of myocardial perfusion-contraction matching. *Prog Cardiovasc Dis* 1993; 36:61-74.

41. Carden DL, Young JA, Granger DN: Pulmonary microvascular injury after intestinal ischemia-reperfusion: role of P-selectin. *J Appl Physiol* 1993; 75:2529-2534.

42. Luscinskas FW, Brock AF, Arnaout MA, Gimbrone MA: Endothelial-leukocyte adhesion molecule-1-dependent and leukocyte (CD11/CD18)-dependent mechanisms contribute to polymorphonuclear leukocyte adhesion to cytokine-activated human vascular endothelium. *J Immunol* 1989; 142:2257-2263.

43. Li J, Bukoski RD: Endothelium-dependent relaxation of hypertensive resistance arteries is not impaired under all conditions. *Circ Res* 1993; 72:290-296.

44. Johnston WE, Robertie PG, Dudas LM, Kon ND, Vinten-Johansen J: Heart rate-right ventricular stroke volume relation with myocardial revascularization. *Ann Thorac Surg* 1991; 52:797-804.

45. Katz AM: *Physiology of the Heart*, 4th ed. Philadelphia, Lippincott Williams & Wilkins, 2006; p 282.

46. Katz AM: *Physiology of the Heart*, 4th ed. Philadelphia, Lippincott Williams & Wilkins, 2006; p 297.

47. Katz AM: *Physiology of the Heart*, 4th ed. Philadelphia, Lippincott Williams & Wilkins, 2006; p 302.

48. Katz AM: *Physiology of the Heart*, 4th ed. Philadelphia, Lippincott Williams & Wilkins, 2006; p 304.

49. Beyar R: Myocardial mechanics and coronary flow dynamics, in Sideman S, Beyar R (eds): *Interactive Phenomena in the Cardiac System.* New York, Plenum Press, 1993; p 125.

50. Yamada H, Yoneyama F, Satoh K, et al: Comparison of the effects of the novel vasodilator FK409 with those of nitroglycerin in isolated coronary artery of the dog. *Br J Pharmacol* 1991; 103:1713-1718.

51. Vinten-Johansen J, Weiss HR: Regional O$_2$ consumption in canine left ventricular myocardium in experimental acute aortic valvular insufficiency. *Cardiovasc Res* 1981; 15:305-312.

52. Guyton RA, McClenathan JH, Newman GE, Michaelis LL: Significance of subendocardial S-T segment elevation caused by coronary stenosis in the dog. Epicarial S-T segment depression, local ischemia and subsequent necrosis. *Am J Cardiol* 1977; 40:373-380.

53. Bradley AJ, Alpert JS: Coronary flow reserve. *Am Heart J* 1991; 1116-1128.

54. Stewart DJ, Pohl U, Bassenge E: Free radicals inhibit endothelium-dependent dilation in the coronary resistance bed. *Am J Physiol Heart Circ Physiol* 1988; 255:H765-H769.

55. Hou M, Chen Y, Traverse JH, Li Y, Barsoum M, Bache RJ: ET-A receptor activity restrains coronary blood flow in the failing heart. *J Cardiovasc Pharmacol* 2004; 43:764-769.

56. Umans JG, Levi R: Nitric oxide in the regulation of blood flow and arterial pressure. *Annu Rev Physiol.* 1995; 57:771-790.

57. Gross SS, Wolin MS: Nitric oxide: pathophysiological mechanisms [review]. *Annu Rev Physiol* 1995; 57:737-769.

58. Highsmith RF, Blackburn K, Schmidt DJ: Endothelin and calcium dynamics in vascular smooth muscle. *Annu Rev Physiol* 1992; 54:257-277.

59. Katritsis D, Choi MJ, Webb-Peploe MM: Assessment of the hemodynamic significance of coronary artery stenosis: theoretical considerations and clinical measurements. *Prog Cardiovasc Dis* 1991; 34:69-88.

60. Levy MN: Hemodynamics, in Berne RM, Levy MV, Koeppen BM, Stanton BA (eds): *Physiology.* St. Louis, Mosby; 2004; pp 341-354.

61. Cohn PF: Mechanisms of myocardial ischemia. *Am J Cardiol* 1992; 70:14G-18G.

62. Charney R, Cohen M: The role of the coronary collateral circulation in limiting myocardial ischemia and infarct size. *Am Heart J* 1993; 126:937-945.

63. Meredith IT, Anderson TJ, Uehata A, Yeung AC, Selwyn AP, Ganz P: Role of endothelium in ischemic coronary syndromes. *Am J Cardiol* 1993; 72:27C-32C.

64. Harrison DG: Endothelial dysfunction in the coronary microcirculation: a new clinical entity or an experimental finding? [editorial; comment]. *J Clin Invest* 1993; 91:1-2.

65. Jordan JE, Zhao Z-Q, Vinten-Johansen J: The role of neutrophils in myocardial ischemia-reperfusion injury. *Cardiovasc Res* 1999; 43:860-878.

66. Boyle EM, Pohlman TH, Johnson MC, Verrier ED: Endothelial cell injury in cardiovascular surgery: the systemic inflammatory response. *Ann Thorac Surg* 1997; 63:277-284.

67. Vinten-Johansen J, Thourani VH, Ronson RS, et al: Broad spectrum cardioprotection with adenosine. *Ann Thorac Surg* 1999; 68:1942-1948.

68. Vinten-Johansen J, Sato H, Zhao Z-Q: The role of nitric oxide and NO-donor agents in myocardial protection from surgical ischemic-reperfusion injury. *Int J Cardiol* 1995; 50:273-281.

69. Katz AM: *Physiology of the Heart*, 4th ed. Philadelphia, Lippincott Williams & Wilkins, 2006; p 73.

70. Marban E: Myocardial stunning and hibernation: the physiology behind the colloquialisms [review]. *Circulation* 1991; 83:681-688.

71. Kusuoka H, Marban E: Cellular mechanisms of myocardial stunning [review]. *Annu Rev Physiol* 1992; 54:243-256.

72. Ross J: Left ventricular function after coronary artery reperfusion. *Am J Cardiol* 1993; 72:91G-97G.

73. Flemeng W, Suy R, Schwarz F, et al: Ultrastructural correlates of left ventricular contraction abnormalities in patients with chronic ischemic heart disease: determinants of reversible segmental asynergy postrevascularization surgery. *Am Heart J* 1981; 102:846-857.

74. Borgers M, Thoné F, Wouters L, Ausma J, Shivalkar B, Flameng W: Structural correlates of regional myocardial dysfunction in patients with critical coronary artery stenosis: chronic hibernation? *Cardiovasc Pathol* 1993; 2:237-245.

75. Vanoverschelde JL, Melin JA, Depré C, Borgers M, Dion R, Wijns W: Time-course of functional recovery of hibernating myocardium after coronary revascularization. *Circulation* 1994; 90(Suppl):I-378.

76. Ross J: Myocardial perfusion-contraction matching implications for coronary heart disease and hibernation. *Circulation* 1991; 83:1076-1083.

77. Guth BD, Schulz R, Heusch G: Time course and mechanisms of contractile dysfunction during acute myocardial ischemia. *Circulation* 1993; 87:IV35-42.

78. Wijns W, Vatner SF, Camici PG: Hibernating Myocardium. *N Engl J Med* 1998; 339:173-181.

79. Granger DN, Korthuis RJ: Physiologic mechanisms of postischemic tissue injury. *Annu Rev Physiol* 1995; 57:311-332.

80. Vinten-Johansen J, Thourani VH: Myocardial protection: an overview. *J Extra Corpor Tech* 2000; 32:38-48.

81. Vinten-Johansen J, Zhao Z-Q, Sato H: Reduction in surgical ischemic-reperfusion injury with adenosine and nitric oxide therapy. *Ann Thorac Surg* 1995; 60:852-857.

82. Kloner RA, Yellon D: Does ischemic preconditioning occur in patients? *J Am Coll Cardiol* 1994; 24:1133-1142.

83. Carroll R, Yellon DM: Myocardial adaptation to ischemia—the preconditioning phenomenon. *Int J Cardiol* 1999; 68:S93-101.

84. Gaasch WH: Diagnosis and treatment of heart failure based on left ventricular systolic or diastolic dysfunction. *JAMA* 1994; 271:1276-1280.

85. Goldsmith SR, Dick C: Differentiating systolic from diastolic heart failure: pathophysiologic and therapeutic considerations. *Am J Med* 1993; 95:645-655.

86. Kass DA, Bronzwaer JG, Paulus WJ: What mechanisms underlie diastolic dysfunction in heart failure? *Circ Res* 2004; 94:1533-1542.

87. Litwin SE, Grossman W: Diastolic dysfunctions a cause of heart failure. *J Am Coll Cardiol* 1993; 22:49A-55A.

88. Bonow RO, Udelson JE: Left ventricular diastolic dysfunction as a cause of congestive heart failure. Mechanisms and management. *Ann Intern Med* 1992; 117:502-510.

89. Brandt RR, Wright RS, Redfield, Burnett JC: Atrial natriuretic in heart failure. *J Am Coll Cardiol* 1993; 22:86A-92A.

90. Floras JS: Clinical aspects of sympathetic activation and parasympathetic withdrawal in heart failure. *J Am Coll Cardiol* 1993; 22:72A-84A.

91. Pfeffer MA: Left ventricular remodeling after acute myocardial infarction. *Annu Rev Med* 1995; 46:455-466.

92. Komuro I, Yazaki I: Control of cardiac gene expression by mechanical stress. *Annu Rev Physiol* 1993; 55:55-75.

93. Schwartz K, Chassagne C, Boheler K: The molecular biology of heart failure. *J Am Coll Cardiol* 1993; 22:30A-33A.

94. Pfeffer JM, Fischer TA, Pfeffer MA: Angiotensin-converting enzyme inhibition and ventricular remodeling after myocardial infarction. *Annu Rev Physiol* 1995; 57:805-826.

95. Nolan PE: Integrating traditional and emerging treatment options in heart failure. *Am J Health Syst Pharm* 2004; 61(Suppl 2):S14-22.

96. Weber KT, Brilla CG: Pathological hypertrophy and cardiac interstitium. Fibrosis and rennin-angiotensin-aldosterone system. *Circulation* 1991; 83:1849-1865.

97. Treasure CB, Alexander RW: The dysfunctional endothelium in heart failure. *J Am Coll Cardiol* 1993; 22:129A-134A.

98. Zhao Z-Q, Velez DA, Wang N-P, et al: Progressively developed myocardial apoptotic cell death during late phase of reperfusion. *Apoptosis* 2001; 6:279-290.

99. Gallagher MJ, McCullough PA: The emerging role of natriuretic peptides in the diagnosis and treatment of decompensated heart failure. *Curr Heart Fail Rep* 2004; 1:129-135.

Cardiac Surgical Pharmacology

Jerrold H. Levy • Jacob N. Schroder • James G. Ramsay

Clinical pharmacology associated with cardiac surgery is an important part of patient management. Patients in the perioperative period receive multiple therapeutic agents that affect cardiovascular and pulmonary functions. This chapter summarizes the pharmacology of the agents commonly used for treating the primary physiologic disturbances associated with cardiac surgery, hemodynamic instability, respiratory insufficiency, and alterations of hemostasis. For cardiovascular drugs, the common theme is that pharmacologic effects are produced by intracellular ion fluxes.

Several basic subcellular/molecular pathways are important in cardiovascular pharmacology, as shown in Fig. 4-1. The action potential in myocardial cells is a reflection of ion fluxes across the cell membrane, especially Na^+, K^+, and Ca^{2+}.[1,2] Numerous drugs used to control heart rate and rhythm act by altering Na^+ (eg, lidocaine and procainamide), K^+ (eg, amiodarone, ibutilide, and sotalol), or Ca^{2+} (eg, diltiazem) currents. Calcium also has a dominant effect on the inotropic state but by highly specialized intracellular mechanisms.[3,4]

Myocardial contractility is a manifestation of the interaction of actin and myosin, with conversion of chemical energy from adenosine triphosphate (ATP) hydrolysis into mechanical energy. The interaction of actin and myosin in myocytes is inhibited by the associated protein tropomyosin. This inhibition is "disinhibited" by intracellular calcium. A similar situation occurs in vascular smooth muscle, where the interaction of actin and myosin (leading to vasoconstriction) is modulated by the protein calmodulin, which requires calcium as a cofactor. Thus intracellular calcium has a "tonic" effect in both the myocardium and vascular smooth muscle.

Numerous drugs used perioperatively alter intracellular calcium.[3,4]

Catecholamines (eg, norepinephrine, epinephrine, and dobutamine) with beta1 agonist activity regulate intramyocyte calcium levels via the nucleotide cyclic adenosine monophosphate (cyclic AMP) (Fig. 4-2). Beta agonists bind to receptors on the cell surface that are coupled to the intracellular enzyme adenylate cyclase via the stimulatory transmembrane GTP-binding protein. This leads to increased cyclic AMP synthesis, and cyclic AMP, in turn, acts as a second messenger for a series of intracellular reactions resulting in higher levels of intracellular calcium during systole. Less well known is that drugs with only alpha-adrenergic agonist activity also may increase intracellular Ca^{2+} levels, although by a different mechanism.[5,6] Although under investigation, the probable basis for the inotropic effect of alpha-adrenergic drugs is the stimulation of phospholipase C, which catalyzes hydrolysis of phosphatidyl inositol to diacylglycerol and inositol triphosphate (see Fig. 4-2). Both of these compounds increase the sensitivity of the myofilament to calcium, whereas inositol triphosphate stimulates the release of calcium from its intracellular storage site, the sarcoplasmic reticulum. There is still some debate about the mechanism for the inotropic effect of alpha-adrenergic agonists and its significance for the acute pharmacologic manipulation of contractility, but there is little debate about the importance of this mechanism in vascular smooth muscle, where the increase in intracellular calcium stimulated by alpha-adrenergic agonists can increase smooth muscle tone significantly. However, intracellular calcium in vascular smooth muscle is also controlled by cyclic nucleotides.[7,8] In contrast to the myocyte, in vascular smooth muscle, cyclic AMP has a primary effect of stimulating the uptake of calcium into intracellular storage sites, decreasing its availability (Fig. 4-3). Thus drugs that stimulate cyclic AMP production (beta agonists) or inhibit its breakdown (phosphodiesterase inhibitors) will cause vasodilation. In addition, cyclic guanosine monophosphate (cyclic GMP) also increases intracellular calcium storage (see Fig. 4-3), decreasing its availability for modulating the interaction of actin and myosin. Several commonly used pharmacologic agents act via cyclic GMP. For example, nitric oxide stimulates the enzyme guanylate cyclase, increasing cyclic GMP levels. Drugs such as nitroglycerin and sodium nitroprusside achieve their effect by producing nitric oxide as a metabolic product. Vasodilation is also produced by "cross-talk" between K^+ and Ca^{2+} fluxes. Decreased levels of ATP, acidosis, and elevated tissue lactate levels increase the permeability of the ATP-sensitive K^+ channel. This increased permeability results in hyperpolarization of the cell membrane that inhibits the entry of Ca^{2+} into the cell. This results in decreased vascular tone.

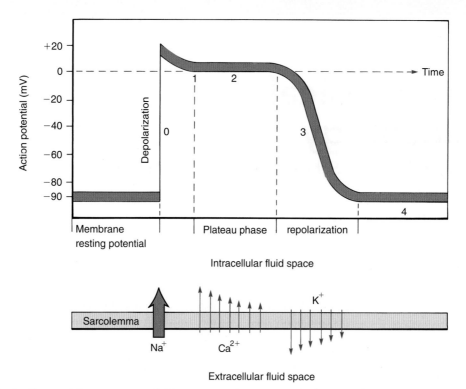

FIGURE 4-1 Cardiac ion fluxes and the action potential. The resting membrane potential is largely a reflection of the intercellular/intracellular potassium gradient. Depolarization of the membrane during phase 4 triggers an initial fast sodium channel with overshoot (phase 0) followed by recovery (phase 1) to a plateau (phase 2) maintained by an inward calcium flux and then repolarization owing to an outward potassium flux (phase 3).

The simplistic overview of pathways of cardiac pharmacology as summarized in Figs. 4-1 through 4-3 also suggests the primary cause of difficulty in the clinical use of the drugs discussed in this chapter. The mechanisms of action for control of heart rate and rhythm, contractility, and vascular tone are interrelated. For example, beta-adrenergic agonists not only increase intracellular calcium to increase contractility, but they also alter K^+ currents, leading to tachycardia. Catecholamines not only have beta-adrenergic agonist activity, with inotropic and chronotropic effects, but they also possess alpha-agonist activity, leading to increased intracellular calcium in vascular smooth muscle and vasoconstriction. Phosphodiesterase (PDE) inhibitors like milrinone not only increase contractility by increasing cyclic AMP in the myocyte, but they also cause vasodilation by increasing cyclic AMP in the vasculature. The interplay of the various mechanisms means the clinical art of cardiac surgical pharmacology lies as much in selecting drugs for their side effects as for their primary therapeutic effects.

ANTIARRHYTHMICS

Arrhythmias are common in the cardiac surgical period. A stable cardiac rhythm requires depolarization and repolarization in a spatially and temporally coordinated manner, and dysrhythmias may occur when this coordination is disturbed. The mechanisms for arrhythmias can be divided into abnormal impulse initiation, abnormal impulse conduction, and

combinations of both.[9,10] Abnormal impulse initiation occurs as a result of increased automaticity (spontaneous depolarization of tissue that does not normally have pacemaking activity) or as a result of triggered activity from abnormal conduction after depolarizations during phase 3 or 4 of the action potential. Abnormal conduction often involves reentry phenomena, with recurrent depolarization around a circuit owing to unilateral conduction block in ischemic or damaged myocardium and retrograde activation by an alternate pathway through normal tissue. In this simplistic view, it is logical that dysrhythmias could be suppressed by slowing the conduction velocity of ectopic foci, allowing normal pacemaker cells to control heart rate, or by prolonging the action potential duration (and hence refractory period) to block conduction into a limb of a reentry circuit.

A scheme proposed originally by Vaughan Williams and modified subsequently[11,12] is used often to classify antidysrhythmic agents, and although alternative schemes describing specific channel-blocking characteristics have been proposed and may be more logical,[13] this discussion is organized using the Vaughan Williams system of four major drug categories. In this scheme, class I agents are those with local anesthetic properties that block Na^+ channels, class II drugs are beta-blocking agents, class III drugs prolong action potential duration, and class IV drugs are calcium entry blockers. Amiodarone is discussed in detail owing to its expanding role in treating both supraventricular and ventricular arrhythmias and because its use has replaced

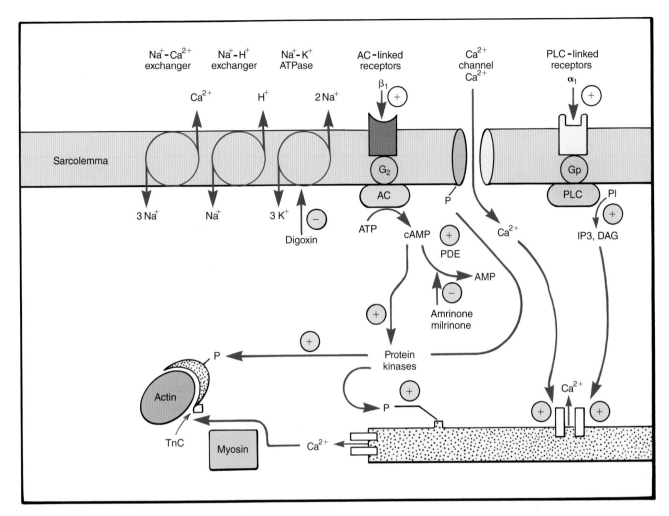

FIGURE 4-2 Mediators of cardiac contractility. Myocardial contractility is a manifestation of the interaction of actin and myosin, which is facilitated by the binding of calcium to troponin C (TnC). Intercellular calcium levels are controlled by direct flux across the membrane, by cyclic AMP, and by inositol triphosphate (IP_3) and diacylglycerol (DAG) produced by the action of phospholipase C (PLC). The synthesis of cyclic AMP is catalyzed by adenylate cyclase (AC), which is activated by binding of agonist to the beta-adrenergic receptor, and its breakdown is catalyzed by phosphodiesterase (PDE), which is inhibited by amrinone and milrinone. The action of PLC is activated by binding of agonist to the alpha-adrenergic receptor.

many of the previously used agents. Because of the efficacy of intravenous amiodarone and its recommendations in Advanced Cardiac Life Support (ACLS) guidelines, many of the older drugs used in cardiac surgery have a historical perspective and are considered briefly.

Class I Agents

Although each of the class I agents blocks Na^+ channels, they may be subclassified based on electrophysiologic differences. These differences can be explained, to some extent, by consideration of the kinetics of the interaction of the drug and the Na^+ channel.[14,15] Class I drugs bind most avidly to open (phase 0 of the action potential; see Fig. 4-1) or inactivated (phase 2) Na^+ channels. Dissociation from the channel occurs during the resting (phase 4) state. If the time constant for dissociation is long in comparison with the diastolic interval

(corresponding to phase 4), the drug will accumulate in the channel to reach a steady state, slowing conduction in normal tissue. This occurs with class Ia (eg, procainamide, quinidine, and disopyramide) and class Ic (eg, encainide, flecainide, and propafenone) drugs. In contrast, for the class Ib drugs (eg, lidocaine and mexiletine), the time constant for dissociation from the Na^+ channel is short, the drug does not accumulate in the channel, and conduction velocity is affected minimally. However, in ischemic tissue, the depolarized state is more persistent, leading to greater accumulation of agent in the Na^+ channel and slowing of conduction in the damaged myocardium.

Procainamide is a class Ia drug that has various electrophysiologic effects.[16] Administration may be limited by the side effects of hypotension and decreased cardiac output.[17,18] The loading dose is 20 to 30 mg/min, up to 17 mg/kg, and should be followed by an intravenous infusion of 20 to

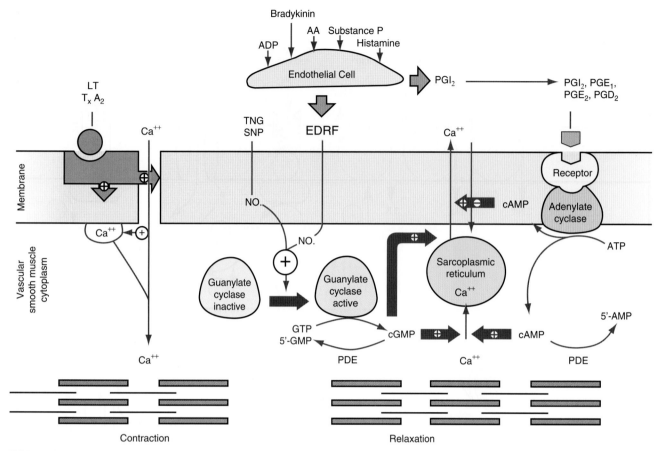

FIGURE 4-3 Mediators of vascular tone. Cyclic AMP and cyclic GMP increase the uptake of calcium into cellular storage sites in vascular smooth muscle, leading to vasodilation. The synthesis of cyclic GMP is catalyzed by guanylate cyclase, which is activated by nitric oxide (NO), which, in turn, is produced by nitroglycerin (NTG) and sodium nitroprusside (SNP). Excessive vasodilation often is a reflection of other endogenous mediators such as prostaglandins (PGI_2, PGE_1, PGE_2, and PGD_2) and thromboxane A_2 (Tx A_2). Several mediators, such as arachidonic acid (AA), bradykinin, histamine, and substance P, stimulate the release of endothelium-derived relaxing factor (EDRF), which is identified with NO. (Reproduced with permission from Levy JH: *Anaphylactic Reactions in Anesthesia and Intensive Care*, 2nd ed. Boston, Butterworth-Heinemann, 1992.)

80 mg/kg per minute. Because procainamide prolongs action potential duration, widening of the QRS complex often heralds a potential overdose. The elimination of procainamide involves hepatic metabolism, acetylation to a metabolite with antiarrhythmic and toxic side effects, and renal elimination of this metabolite. Thus the infusion rate for patients with significant hepatic or renal disease should be at the lower end of this range.

Class Ib drugs include what is probably the best-known antiarrhythmic agent, lidocaine. As noted, lidocaine is a Na^+ channel blocker that has little effect on conduction velocity in normal tissue but slows conduction in ischemic myocardium.[14,15] Other electrophysiologic effects include a decrease in action potential duration but a small increase in the ratio of effective refractory period to action potential duration. The exact role of these electrophysiologic effects on arrhythmia suppression is unclear. Lidocaine has no significant effects on atrial tissue, and it is not recommended for therapy in shock-resistant ventricular tachycardia/fibrillation (VT/VF) in the recent *Guidelines for Emergency Cardiovascular Care*.[19] After an initial bolus dose of 1 to 1.5 mg/kg of

lidocaine, plasma levels decrease rapidly owing to redistribution to muscle, fat, etc. Effective plasma concentrations are maintained only by following the bolus dose with an infusion of 20 to 50 mg/kg per minute.[20] Elimination occurs via hepatic metabolism to active metabolites that are cleared by the kidneys. Consequently, the dose should be reduced by approximately 50% in patients with liver or kidney disease. The primary toxic effects are associated with the central nervous system (CNS), and a lidocaine overdose may cause drowsiness, depressed level of consciousness, or seizures in very high doses. Negative inotropic or hypotensive effects are less pronounced than with most other antiarrhythmics. The other class Ib drugs likely to be encountered in the perioperative period are the oral agents tocainide and mexiletine, which have effects similar to lidocaine.[15]

The class Ic agents, including flecainide, encainide, and propafenone, markedly decrease conduction velocity.[20,21] The Cardiac Arrhythmia Suppression Trial (CAST) study[20,21] of moricizine found that although ventricular arrhythmias were suppressed, the incidence of sudden death was greater than with placebo with encainide and flecainide, and these drugs are not in wide use. Propafenone is available for oral use in the United States, but IV form is available in Europe. The usual adult dose is 150 to 300 mg orally every 8 hours. It has beta-blocking (with resulting negative inotropic effects) as well as Na$^+$ channel-blocking activity; lengthens the PR, QRS, and QT duration; and may be used to treat both atrial and ventricular dysrhythmias.[15]

Class II Agents

Beta-receptor-blocking agents are another important group of antiarrhythmic (denoted class II in the Vaughan Williams scheme). However, because of their use as antihypertensive as well as antiarrhythmic agents, they are discussed elsewhere in this chapter, and we will move on to consider bretylium, amiodarone, and sotalol, the class III agents in the Vaughan Williams scheme. These drugs have a number of complex ion channel-blocking effects, but possibly the most important activity is K$^+$ channel blockade.[22] Because the flux of K$^+$ out of the myocyte is responsible for repolarization, an important electrophysiologic effect of class III drugs is prolongation of the action potential.[23]

Class III Agents

Ibutilide, dofetilide, sotalol, and bretylium are class III agents. Intravenous ibutilide and oral dofetilide are approved for the treatment of atrial fibrillation (AF) but carry the risk of torsades de pointes.[24,25] Sotalol is a nonselective beta-blocker that also has K$^+$ channel-blocking activity.[26] In the United States, it is now available for IV and previously for oral administration. The approved indication is for treating life-threatening ventricular arrhythmias, although it is effective against atrial arrhythmias as well. Bretylium is no longer available or recommended in the most recent American Heart Association (AHA) *Guidelines for Emergency Cardiovascular Care*.[19]

Class IV Agents

Calcium entry blockers (class IV in the Vaughan Williams scheme), including verapamil and diltiazem, are antiarrhythmics. In sinoatrial (SA) and atrioventricular (AV) nodal tissues, Ca^{2+} channels contribute significantly to phase 0 depolarization, and the AV nodal refractory period is prolonged by Ca^{2+} entry blockade.[27,28]

This explains the effectiveness of verapamil and diltiazem in treating supraventricular arrhythmias. It is also clear why these drugs are negative inotropes. Both verapamil and diltiazem are effective in slowing the ventricular response to AF, flutter, and paroxysmal supraventricular tachycardia (SVT) and in converting to sinus rhythm.[29-31] Verapamil has greater negative inotrope effects than diltiazem; therefore, it is used rarely for supraventricular arrhythmias. The intravenous dose of diltiazem is 0.25 mg/kg, with a second dose of 0.35 mg/kg if the response is inadequate after 15 minutes. The loading dose should be followed by an infusion of 5 to 15 mg/h. Intravenous diltiazem, although useful for rate control, has been replaced by intravenous amiodarone in clinical therapy of SVT and prophylaxis (see Amiodarone).

Other Drugs

One of the difficulties of classifying antiarrhythmics by the Vaughan Williams classification is that not all drugs can be incorporated into this scheme. Three examples are digoxin, adenosine, and magnesium, each of which has important uses in the perioperative period.

Digoxin inhibits the Na$^+$, K$^+$-ATPase pump, leading to decreased intracellular K$^+$, a less negative resting membrane potential, increased slope of phase 4 depolarization, and decreased conduction velocity. These direct effects, however, usually are dominated by indirect effects, including inhibition of reflex responses to congestive heart failure (HF) and a vagotonic effect.[10,32] The net effect is greatest at the AV node, where conduction is slowed and the refractory period is increased, explaining the effectiveness of digoxin in slowing the ventricular response to AF. The major disadvantages of digoxin are the relatively slow onset of action and many side effects, including proarrhythmia effects, and it is now used rarely for rate control in acute AF because of the advent of IV amiodarone and diltiazem.

Adenosine is an endogenous nucleoside that has an electrophysiologic effect similar to that of acetylcholine. Adenosine decreases AV node conductivity, and its primary antiarrhythmic effect is to break AV nodal reentrant tachycardia.[33] An intravenous dose of 100 to 200 μg/kg is the treatment of choice for paroxysmal SVT. Adverse effects, such as bronchospasm, are short-lived because its plasma half-life is so short (1 to 2 seconds). This short half-life makes it ideal for treating reentry dysrhythmia, in which transient interruption can fully suppress the dysrhythmia.

Appropriate acid-base status and electrolyte balance are important because electrolyte imbalance can perturb the membrane potential, leading to arrhythmia generation, as can altered acid-base status, by effects on K$^+$ concentrations and sympathetic tone. Therapy for dysrhythmia should include correction of acid-base and electrolyte imbalances. Magnesium supplementation should be considered.[34] Magnesium deficiency is common in the perioperative period, and magnesium administration has been shown to decrease the incidence of postoperative dysrhythmia.[35]

Amiodarone

Intravenous amiodarone has become one of the most administered intravenous antiarrhythmics used in cardiac surgery because of its broad spectrum of efficacy. Amiodarone was developed originally as an antianginal agent because of its vasodilating effects, including coronary vasodilation.[36] It has various ion channel-blocking activities.[10,29,36] The resulting electrophysiologic effects are complex, and there are differences in acute intravenous and chronic oral administration. Acute intravenous administration can produce decreases in heart rate and blood pressure, but there are minimal changes in QRS duration or QT interval. After chronic use, there may be significant bradycardia and increases in action potential duration in AV nodal and ventricular tissue, with increased QRS duration and QT interval.[37-39]

Pharmacokinetics

Amiodarone is a complex highly lipophilic drug that undergoes variable absorption (35 to 65%) after oral administration and is taken up extensively by multiple tissues with interindividual variation and complex pharmacokinetics.[38-40] The short initial context-sensitive half-life after intravenous administration represents drug redistribution. The true elimination half-life for amiodarone is extremely long, up to 40 to 60 days. Because of the huge volume of distribution (~60 L/kg) and a long duration of action, an active metabolite loading period of several months may be required before reaching steady-state tissue concentrations. Further, in life-threatening arrhythmias, intravenous loading often is starting to establish initial plasma levels. Measuring amiodarone plasma concentrations is not useful owing to the complex pharmacokinetics and the metabolites of the parent drug. Plasma concentrations greater than 2.5 mg/L have been associated with an increased risk of toxicity. The optimal dose of amiodarone has not been well characterized and may vary depending on the specific arrhythmias treated. Further, there may be differences in dose requirements for therapy of supraventricular and ventricular arrhythmias.[37-40]

Because of these distinctive pharmacokinetic properties, steady-state plasma levels are achieved slowly. Oral administration for a typical adult consists of a loading regimen of 80 to 1600 mg/d (in two or three doses) for 10 days, 600 to 800 mg/d for 4 to 6 weeks, and then maintenance doses of 200 to 600 mg/d. For intravenous loading, specific studies will be reviewed, but the recommended dosing is 150 mg given over 10 minutes for acute therapy in an adult, followed first by a secondary loading infusion of 60 mg/h for 6 hours and then by a maintenance infusion of 30 mg/h to achieve a 1000 mg/d dosing.[37-40]

Electrophysiology

The electrophysiologic actions of amiodarone are complex and incompletely understood. Amiodarone produces all four effects according to the Vaughan Williams classification. It also has been shown to have use-dependent class I activity, inhibition of the inward sodium currents, and class II activity.[10] The antiadrenergic effect of amiodarone, however, is different from that of beta-blocker drugs because it is noncompetitive and additive to the effect of beta-blockers. Amiodarone depresses SA node automaticity, which slows the heart rate and conduction and increases refractoriness of the AV node, properties useful in managing supraventricular arrhythmia. Its class III activity results in increases in atrial and ventricular refractoriness and prolongation of the QTc interval. The effects of oral amiodarone on SA and AV nodal function are maximal within 2 weeks, whereas the effects on ventricular tachycardia (VT) and ventricular refractoriness emerge more gradually during oral therapy, becoming maximal after 10 weeks or more.

Indications

The primary indication for amiodarone is VT or fibrillation.[40-48] It is also effective for the treatment of atrial dysrhythmias and in treating AF (see Atrial Fibrillation).

Side Effects

Although there are numerous adverse reactions to amiodarone, they occur with long-term oral administration and are rarely associated with acute intravenous administration. The most serious is pulmonary toxicity, which has not been reported with acute administration in a perioperative setting. Some case series have reported an increased risk of marked bradycardia and hypotension immediately after cardiac surgery in patients already on amiodarone at the time of surgery.[49,50] Other case-control studies, however, have not reproduced this finding.[51] None of the placebo-controlled trials of prophylactic amiodarone for perioperative atrial fibrillation prevention report adverse cardiovascular effects, although bradycardia and hypotension are known side effects.[52-56] Case reports and case series of postoperative acute pulmonary toxicity are similarly lacking in the rigor of randomized, controlled methodology.

PHARMACOLOGIC THERAPY OF SPECIFIC ARRHYTHMIAS

Ventricular Tachyarrhythmias

Intravenous amiodarone is approved for rapid control of recurrent VT or VF. Three randomized controlled trials of patients with recurrent in-hospital, hemodynamically unstable VT or VF with two or more episodes within the past 24 hours who failed to respond to or were intolerant of lidocaine, procainamide, and (in two of the trials) bretylium have been reported.[42,44,46] Patients were critically ill with ischemic cardiovascular disease, 25% were on a mechanical ventilator or intraaortic balloon pump before enrollment, and 10% were undergoing cardiopulmonary resuscitation at the time of enrollment. One study compared three doses of IV amiodarone: 525, 1050, and 2100 mg/d.[44] Because of the use of investigator-initiated intermittent open-label amiodarone boluses for recurrent VT, the actual mean amiodarone doses received by the three groups were 742, 1175, and 1921 mg/d. There was no statistically significant difference in the number of patients without VT/VF recurrence during the 1-day study period: 32 of 86 (41%), 36 of 92 (45%), and 42 of 92 (53%) for the low-, medium-, and high-dose groups, respectively. The number of supplemental 150-mg bolus infusions of amiodarone given by blinded investigators was statistically significantly less in those randomized to higher doses of amiodarone.

A wider range of amiodarone doses (125, 500, and 1000 mg/d) was evaluated by Sheinman and colleagues, including a low dose that was expected to be subtherapeutic.[46] This stronger study design, however, also was confounded by open-label bolus amiodarone injections given by study investigators. There was, however, a trend toward a relationship between intended amiodarone dose and VT/VF recurrence rate (p = .067). After adjustment for baseline imbalances, the median 24-hour recurrence rates of VT/VF, from lowest to highest doses, were 1.68, 0.96, and 0.48 events per 24 hours.

The third study compared two intravenous amiodarone doses (125 and 1000 mg/d) with bretylium (2500 mg/d).[42] Once again, the target amiodarone dose ratio of 8:1 was compressed to 1.8:1 because of open-label boluses. There was no significant difference in the primary outcome, which was median VT/VF recurrence rate over 24 hours. For low-dose amiodarone, high-dose amiodarone, and bretylium, these rates were 1.68, 0.48, and 0.96 events per 24 hours, respectively (p = .237). There was no difference between high-dose amiodarone and bretylium; however, more than 50% of patients had crossed over from bretylium to amiodarone by 16 hours.

The failure of these studies to provide clear evidence of amiodarone efficacy may be related to the "active-control study design" used, a lack of adequate statistical power, high rates of supplemental amiodarone boluses, and high cross-over rates. Nonetheless, these studies provide some evidence that IV amiodarone (1 g/d) is moderately effective during a 24-hour period against VT and VF.

Sustained Monomorphic Ventricular Tachycardia and Wide QRS Tachycardia

Although the most effective and rapid treatment of any hemodynamically unstable sustained ventricular tachyarrhythmia is electrical cardioversion or defibrillation, intravenous antiarrhythmic drugs can be used for arrhythmia termination if the VT is hemodynamically stable. The *Guidelines for Emergency Cardiovascular Care*[19] has removed the former recommendation of lidocaine and adenosine use in stable wide QRS tachycardia, now labeled as "acceptable" but not primarily recommended (lidocaine) or not recommended (adenosine). Intravenous procainamide and sotalol are effective, based on randomized but small studies;[10] amiodarone is also considered acceptable.[19]

Shock-Resistant Ventricular Fibrillation

The *Guidelines for Emergency Cardiovascular Care* recommends at least three shocks and epinephrine or vasopressin before any antiarrhythmic drug are administered.[10,19] No large-scale controlled, randomized studies have demonstrated efficacy for lidocaine, bretylium, or procainamide in shock-resistant VF,[10,19] and lidocaine and bretylium are no longer recommended in this setting.[19] Two pivotal studies have been reported recently studying the efficacy of agents in acute shock-resistant cardiac arrest.

The Amiodarone in the Out-of-Hospital Resuscitation of Refractory Sustained Ventricular Tachycardia (ARREST) study was randomized, double blind, and placebo controlled. The ARREST study in 504 patients showed that amiodarone 300 mg administered in a single intravenous bolus significantly improves survival to hospital admission in cardiac arrest still in VT or VF after three direct-current shocks (44% vs 34%; p < .03).[43] Although the highest survival rate to hospital admission (79%) was achieved when the amiodarone was given within 4 to 16 minutes of dispatch, there was no significant difference in the proportional improvement in the amiodarone group compared with the placebo group when drug administration was delayed (up to 55 minutes). Amiodarone also had the highest efficacy in patients (21% of all study patients) who had a return of spontaneous circulation before drug administration (survival to hospital admission increased to 64% from 41% in the placebo group). Among patients with no return of spontaneous circulation, amiodarone only slightly improved outcome (38% vs 33%).

Dorian performed a randomized trial comparing intravenous lidocaine with intravenous amiodarone as an adjunct to defibrillation in victims of out-of-hospital cardiac arrest.[48] Patients were enrolled if they had out-of-hospital ventricular fibrillation resistant to three shocks, intravenous epinephrine, and a further shock or if they had recurrent ventricular fibrillation after initially successful defibrillation. They were randomly assigned in a double-blind manner to receive intravenous amiodarone plus lidocaine placebo or intravenous lidocaine plus amiodarone placebo. The primary end point was the proportion of patients who survived to be admitted to the hospital. In total, 347 patients (mean age 67 ± 14 years) were enrolled. The mean interval between the time at which paramedics were dispatched to the scene of the cardiac arrest and the time of their arrival was 7 ± 3 minutes, and the mean interval from dispatch to drug administration was 25 ± 8 minutes. After treatment with amiodarone, 22.8% of 180 patients survived to hospital admission compared with 12.0% of 167 patients treated with lidocaine (p = .009). Among patients for whom the time from dispatch to the administration of the drug was equal to or less than the median time (24 minutes), 27.7% of those given amiodarone and 15.3% of those given lidocaine survived to hospital admission (p = .05). The authors concluded that compared with lidocaine, amiodarone leads to substantially higher rates of survival to hospital admission in patients with shock-resistant out-of-hospital ventricular fibrillation.

Supraventricular Arrhythmias

A supraventricular arrhythmia is any tachyarrhythmia that requires atrial or AV junctional tissue for initiation and maintenance. It may arise from reentry caused by unidirectional conduction block in one region of the heart and slow conduction in another, from enhanced automaticity akin to that seen in normal pacemaker cells of the sinus node and in latent pacemaker cells elsewhere in the heart, or from triggered activity, a novel type of abnormally enhanced impulse initiation caused by membrane currents that can be activated and inactivated by premature stimulation or rapid pacing.[56-58] Pharmacologic approaches to treating supraventricular arrhythmias, including AF, atrial flutter, atrial tachycardia, AV reentrant tachycardia, and AV nodal reentrant tachycardia, continue to evolve.[56-60] Because AF is perhaps the most common arrhythmia after cardiac surgery, this condition is emphasized in detail.

Atrial Fibrillation

Atrial fibrillation is a common complication of cardiac surgery that increases the length of stay in the hospital with resulting increases in health-care resource utilization.[56-61] Advanced age, previous AF, and valvular heart operations are the most consistently identified risk factors for this arrhythmia. Because efforts to terminate AF after its initiation are problematic, current interests are directed at therapies to prevent postoperative AF. Most studies suggest that prophylaxis with antiarrhythmic compounds can decrease the incidence of AF, length of hospital stay, and cost significantly. Class III antiarrhythmic drugs (eg, sotalol and ibutilide) also may be effective but potentially pose the risk of drug-induced polymorphic VT (torsades de pointes). Newer intravenous agents including vernakalant were investigated but in the current Food and Drug Administration (FDA) era of drug safety concerns, antiarrhythmic agents are difficult to get approved. Defining which subpopulations benefit most from such therapy is important as older and more critically ill patients undergo surgery. Intravenous sotalol is currently available in the United States.

Amiodarone is also an effective approach for prophylactic therapy of AF. Intravenous amiodarone is an important consideration because loading with oral therapy is often not feasible in part owing to the time required. There also may be added benefits of prophylactic therapies in high-risk patients, especially those prone to ventricular arrhythmias (ie, patients with preexisting HF).

Two studies deserve mention regarding prophylaxis with amiodarone. To determine if IV amiodarone would prevent AF and decrease hospital stay after cardiac surgery, Daoud and colleagues assessed preoperative prophylaxis in 124 patients who were given either oral amiodarone (64 patients) or placebo (60 patients) for a minimum of 7 days before elective cardiac surgery.[62] Therapy consisted of 600 mg amiodarone per day for 7 days and then 200 mg/d until the day of discharge from the hospital. The preoperative total dose of amiodarone was 4.8 ± 0.96 g over 13 ± 7 days. Postoperative AF occurred in 16 of the 64 patients in the amiodarone group (25%) and 32 of the 60 patients in the placebo group (53%). Patients in the amiodarone group were hospitalized for significantly fewer days than were patients in the placebo group (6.5 ± 2.6 vs 7.9 ± 4.3 days; $p = .04$). Total hospitalization costs were significantly less for the amiodarone group than those for the placebo group ($\$18,375 \pm \$13,863$ vs $\$26,491 \pm \$23,837$; $p = .03$). Guarnieri and colleagues evaluated 300 patients randomized in a double-blind fashion to IV amiodarone (1 g/d for 2 days) versus placebo immediately after open-heart surgery.[54] The primary end points of the trial were incidence of AF and length of hospital stay. AF occurred in 67 of 142 (47%) patients on placebo versus 56 of 158 (35%) on amiodarone ($p = .01$). Length of hospital stay for the placebo group was 8.2 ± 6.2 days, and 7.6 ± 5.9 days for the amiodarone group. Low-dose IV amiodarone was safe and effective in reducing the incidence of AF after heart surgery but did not significantly alter length of hospital stay.

In summary, AF is a frequent complication of cardiac surgery. Many cases can be prevented with appropriate prophylactic therapy. Beta-adrenergic blockers should be administered to most patients without contraindication. Prophylactic amiodarone should be considered in patients at high risk for postoperative AF. The lack of data on cost-benefits and cost-efficiency in some studies may reflect the lack of higher-risk patients in the study. Patients who are poor candidates for beta-blockade may not tolerate sotalol, whereas amiodarone does not have this limitation. Additional studies also need to be performed to better assess the role of prophylactic therapy in off-pump cardiac surgery.

INOTROPIC AGENTS

Some depression of myocardial function is common after cardiac surgery.[63-65] The etiology is multifactorial—preexisting disease, incomplete repair or revascularization, myocardial edema, postischemic dysfunction, reperfusion injury, etc—and usually is reversible. Adequate cardiac output usually can be maintained by exploiting the Starling curve with higher preload, but often the cardiac function curve is flattened, and it is necessary to use inotropic agents to maintain adequate organ perfusion.

The molecular basis for the contractile property of the heart is the interaction of the proteins actin and myosin, in which chemical energy (in the form of ATP) is converted into mechanical energy. In the relaxed state (diastole), the interaction of actin and myosin is inhibited by tropomyosin, a protein associated with the actin-myosin complex. With the onset of systole, Ca^{2+} enters the myocyte (during phase 1 of the action potential). This influx of Ca^{2+} triggers the release of much larger amounts of Ca^{2+} from the sarcoplasmic reticulum. The binding of Ca^{2+} to the C subunit of the protein troponin interrupts inhibition of the actin-myosin interaction by tropomyosin, facilitating the hydrolysis of ATP with the generation of a mechanical force. With repolarization of the myocyte and completion of systole, Ca^{2+} is taken back up into the sarcoplasmic reticulum, allowing tropomyosin to again inhibit the interaction of actin and myosin with consequent relaxation of contractile force. Thus inotropic action is mediated by intracellular Ca^{2+}.[66] A novel drug, levosimendan, currently under clinical development in the United States but approved in several countries, increases the sensitivity of the contractile apparatus to Ca^{2+},[67] whereas the positive inotropic agents available for clinical use achieve their end by increasing intracellular Ca^{2+} levels.

The first drug to be considered is simply Ca^{2+} itself. In general, administration of calcium will increase the inotropic state of the myocardium when measured by load-independent methods, but it also will increase vascular tone (afterload) and impair diastolic function. In addition, the effects of calcium on myocardial performance depend on the plasma Ca^{2+} concentration. Ca^{2+} plays important roles in cellular function, and the intracellular Ca^{2+} concentration is highly regulated by membrane ion channels and intracellular organelles.[68,69] If the extracellular Ca^{2+} concentration is normal, administration of Ca^{2+} will have little effect on the intracellular level and less pronounced hemodynamic effects. On the other hand, if the ionized plasma calcium concentration is low, exogenous calcium administration may increase cardiac output and blood pressure.[70] It also should be realized that even with normal plasma Ca^{2+} concentrations, administration of Ca^{2+} may increase vascular tone, leading to increased blood pressure but no change in cardiac output. This increased afterload, as well as the deleterious effects on diastolic function, may be the basis of the observation that Ca^{2+} administration can blunt the response to epinephrine.[71] Routine use of Ca^{2+} at the end of bypass should be tempered by the realization that Ca^{2+} may have little effect on cardiac output while increasing systemic vascular resistance, although this in itself may be of importance. If there is evidence of myocardial ischemia, Ca^{2+} administration may be deleterious because it may exacerbate both coronary spasm and the pathways, leading to cellular injury.[72,73]

Digoxin, although not effective as acute therapy for low-cardiac-output syndrome in the perioperative period, nevertheless well illustrates the role of intracellular Ca^{2+}. Digoxin functions by inhibiting Na^+, K^+-ATPase, which is responsible for the exchange of intracellular Na^+ with extracellular K^+.[3,4] It is thus responsible for maintaining the intracellular/extracellular K^+ and Na^+ gradients. When it is inhibited, intracellular Na^+ levels increase. The increased intracellular Na^+ is an increased chemical potential for driving the Ca^{2+}/Na^+ exchanger, an ion exchange mechanism in which intracellular Na^+ is removed from the cell in exchange for Ca^{2+}. The net effect is an increase in intracellular Ca^{2+} with an enhancement of the inotropic state.

The most commonly used positive inotropic agents are the beta-adrenergic agonists. The $beta_1$ receptor is part of a complex consisting of the receptor on the outer surface of the cell membrane and membrane-spanning G proteins (so named because they bind GTP), which in turn stimulate adenylate cyclase on the inner surface of the membrane, catalyzing the formation cyclic adenosine monophosphate (cyclic AMP). The inotropic state is modulated by cyclic AMP via its catalysis of phosphorylation reactions by protein kinase A. These phosphorylation reactions "open" Ca^{2+} channels on the cell membrane and lead to greater release and uptake of Ca^{2+} from the sarcoplasmic reticulum.[3,4]

There are many drugs that stimulate $beta_1$ receptors and have a positive inotropic effect, including epinephrine, norepinephrine, dopamine, isoproterenol, and dobutamine, the most commonly used catecholamines in the perioperative period. Although there are differences in their binding at the $beta_1$ receptor, the most important differences between the various catecholamines are their relative effects on alpha- and $beta_2$ adrenergic receptors. In general, alpha receptor stimulation on the peripheral vasculature causes vasoconstriction, whereas $beta_2$ receptor stimulation leads to vasodilation (see the discussion elsewhere in this chapter). For some time it was believed that $beta_2$ and alpha receptors were found only in the peripheral vasculature, as well as in a few other organs, but not in the myocardium. However, alpha receptors are also found in the myocardium and mediate a positive inotropic effect.[5,6] The mechanism for this positive inotropic effect is probably the stimulation of phospholipase C, leading to hydrolysis of phosphatidyl inositol to diacylglycerol and inositol triphosphate, compounds that increase Ca^{2+} release from the sarcoplasmic reticulum and increase myofilament sensitivity to Ca^{2+}. It is also possible that alpha-adrenergic agents increase intracellular Ca^{2+} by prolonging action potential duration by inhibition of outward K^+ currents during repolarization or by activating the Na^+/H^+ exchange mechanism, increasing intracellular pH and increasing myofilament sensitivity to Ca^{2+}. Just as the exact mechanism is uncertain, the exact role of alpha-adrenergic stimulation in control of the inotropic state is unclear, although it is apparent that onset of the effect is slower than that of $beta_1$ stimulation.

Besides the discovery of alpha receptors in the myocardium, $beta_2$ receptors are present in the myocardium.[74] The fraction of $beta_2$ receptors (compared with $beta_1$ receptors) is increased in chronic HF, possibly explaining the efficacy of drugs with $beta_2$ activity in this setting. This phenomenon is part of the general observation of $beta_1$ receptor downregulation (decrease in receptor density) and desensitization (uncoupling of effect from receptor binding) that is observed in chronic HF.[75] Interestingly, it has been demonstrated in a dog model that this same phenomenon occurs with cardiopulmonary bypass (CPB).[76] In this situation, a newer class of drugs, the phosphodiesterase inhibitors, may be of benefit. These drugs, typified by the agents available in the United States, amrinone and milrinone, increase cyclic AMP levels independently of the beta receptor by selectively inhibiting the myocardial enzyme responsible for the breakdown of cyclic AMP.[3,4]

In clinical use, selection of a particular inotropic agent usually is based more on its side effects than its direct inotropic properties. Of the commonly used catecholamines, norepinephrine has alpha and $beta_1$ but little $beta_2$ activity and is both an inotrope and a vasopressor. Epinephrine and dopamine are mixed agonists with alpha, $beta_1$, and $beta_2$ activities. At lower doses, they are primarily inotropes and not vasopressors, although vasopressor effects become more pronounced at higher doses. This is especially true for dopamine, which achieves effects at higher doses by stimulating the release of norepinephrine.[77] Dobutamine is a more selective $beta_1$ agonist, in contrast to isoproterenol, which is a mixed beta agonist. Selection of a drug depends on the particular hemodynamic problem at hand. For example, a patient with depressed myocardial function in the presence of profound vasodilation may require a drug with both positive inotropic and vasopressor effects, whereas a patient who is vasoconstricted may benefit from some other choice. Recent studies report that in patients with myocardial infarction (MI) who develop cardiogenic shock, dopamine increases mortality compared to norepinephrine.[78,79] On the basis of multiple considerations, we recommend an empiric approach to selecting inotropic agents with careful monitoring of the response to the drug and selection of the agent that achieves the desired effect.

Clinical experience suggests that phosphodiesterase inhibitors are effective when catecholamines do not produce an acceptable cardiac output. Milrinone is the phosphodiesterease most used, and amrinone is no longer available. Enoximone, a similar agent with different pharmacokinetic properties, was used in Europe but not available in the United States. All agents increase contractility with minimal effect on heart rate, and both are vasodilators. There is significant venodilation, as well as pulmonary and systemic vasodilation, and maintaining adequate preload is important in avoiding hypotension.[80-82] Administering the loading dose over 15 to 30 minutes may also attenuate possible hypotension, or alternately starting an infusion alone without loading is an alternative method. Plasma levels drop rapidly after a loading dose because of redistribution, and the loading dose should be followed immediately by a continuous infusion.[82-84] Because of their longer half-lives, it is rather more difficult to readily titrate plasma levels than with catecholamines (which have plasma half-lives of a few minutes).

Phosphodiesterase inhibitors, specifically milrinone, facilitate separation from CPB with biventricular dysfunction and are used for treating low-cardiac-output syndrome after cardiac surgery.[82-86] Doolan and colleagues also demonstrated that milrinone, in comparison with placebo, significantly facilitated separation of high-risk patients from CPB.[87] Despite the extensive use of pharmacologic therapy, there are no convincing data to support a distinct inotropic or vasodilator drug-based therapy as a superior solution to treat biventricular dysfunction and/or potentially reduce mortality in hemodynamically unstable patients with cardiogenic shock or low cardiac output, especially complicating an acute MI.[88]

Levosimendan

Levosimendan is a class of drugs known as *calcium sensitizers*. The molecule is a pyridazinone-dinitrile derivative with additional action on ATP-sensitive potassium channels.[67,89,90] Levosimendan is used intravenously for treating decompensated HF because it increases contractility and produces anti-stunning effects without increasing myocardial intracellular calcium concentrations or prolonging myocardial relaxation. Levosimendan also causes coronary and systemic vasodilation. In patients with HF, IV levosimendan reduced worsening HF or death significantly. IV levosimendan significantly also increased cardiac output and decreased filling pressure in decompensated HF in large, double-blind, randomized trials and after cardiac surgery in smaller trials. Levosimendan

is well tolerated without arrhythmogenicity. In addition to sensitizing troponin to intracellular calcium, levosimendan inhibits phosphodiesterase III and open ATP-sensitive potassium channels (K_{ATP}), which may produce vasodilation. Unlike currently available intravenous inotropes, levosimendan does not increase myocardial oxygen use and has been used effectively in beta-blocked patients. Levosimendan does not impair ventricular relaxation. Clinical studies have demonstrated short-term hemodynamic benefits of levosimendan over both placebo and dobutamine. Although large-scale, long-term morbidity and mortality data are scarce, the Levosimendan Infusion versus Dobutamine in Severe Low-Output Heart Failure (LIDO) study suggested a mortality benefit of levosimendan over dobutamine. Clinical studies comparing levosimendan with other positive inotropes, namely, milrinone, are lacking. Currently, this agent is being evaluated in a clinical trial in North America for patients with left ventricular dysfunction undergoing CPB (https://clinicaltrials.gov/ct2/show/NCT02025621?term=levosimendan&rank=14).

Clinical Trials

Despite their common use after cardiac surgery, there have been relatively few comparative studies of inotropic agents in the perioperative period. In 1978, Steen reported the hemodynamic effects of epinephrine, dobutamine, and epinephrine immediately after separation from CPB.[91] The largest mean increase in cardiac index was achieved with dopamine at 15 mcg/kg per minute. However, it should be noted that the only epinephrine dose studied was 0.04 mcg/kg per minute. In a later comparison of dopamine and dobutamine, Salomon concluded that dobutamine produced more consistent increases in cardiac index, although the hemodynamic differences were small, and all patients had good cardiac indices at the onset of the study.[92] Fowler also found insignificant differences in the hemodynamic effects of dobutamine and dopamine, although they reported that coronary flow increased more in proportion to myocardial oxygen consumption with dobutamine.[93] Although neither of these groups reported significant increases in heart rate for either dopamine or dobutamine, clinical experience has been otherwise. This is supported by a study by Sethna, who found that the increase in cardiac index with dobutamine occurs simply because of increased heart rate, although they found that myocardial oxygen was maintained.[94] Butterworth subsequently demonstrated that the older and much cheaper agent, epinephrine, effectively increased stroke volume without as great an increase in heart rate as dobutamine.[95] More recently, Feneck compared dobutamine and milrinone and found them to be equally effective in treating low-cardiac-output syndrome after cardiac surgery.[96] This study was a comparison of two drugs, and the investigators emphasized that the most efficacious therapy is probably a combination of drugs. In particular, phosphodiesterase inhibitors require the synthesis of cyclic AMP to be effective, and thus use of a combination of a beta$_1$-adrenergic agonist and a phosphodiesterase inhibitor would be predicted to be more effective than either agent alone.

Finally, while global hemodynamic goals (ie, heart rate, blood pressure, filling pressures, and cardiac output) may be achieved with inotropic agents, this does not guarantee adequate regional perfusion, in particular renal and mesenteric perfusion. So far there have been few investigations of regional perfusion after cardiac surgery. There has been more interest in regional (especially mesenteric) perfusion in the critical care medicine literature, and some of the studies may be relevant to postoperative care of the cardiac surgical patient. Two studies have indicated that epinephrine may impair splanchnic perfusion, especially in comparison with combining norepinephrine and dobutamine.[97,98] Norepinephrine alone has variable effects on splanchnic blood flow in septic shock,[99] although adding dobutamine can improve splanchnic perfusion significantly when blood pressure is supported with norepinephrine.[98] Low-dose dopamine improves splanchnic blood flow,[100] but there is evidence that dopamine in higher doses impairs gastric perfusion.[101] The relevance of these studies of septic patients for the cardiac surgical patient is unclear, although there are similarities between the inflammatory responses to CPB and to sepsis.

VASOPRESSORS

CPB often is characterized by derangements of vascular tone. Sometimes CPB induces elevations in endogenous catecholamines, as well as other mediators, such as serotonin and arginine vasopressin (AVP), leading to vasoconstriction. However, more often CPB is characterized by a systemic inflammatory response, with a cascade of cytokine and inflammatory mediator release and profound vasodilation. The pathophysiology has a striking resemblance to that of sepsis or an anaphylactic reaction. Further, vasodilation after cardiac surgery may be exacerbated by the preoperative use of angiotensin-converting enzyme (ACE) inhibitors and post-CPB use of milrinone.

The mechanisms of vasodilatory shock have been reviewed previously.[102] Vascular tone is modulated by intracellular Ca^{2+}, which binds calmodulin. The Ca^{2+}-calmodulin complex activates myosin light-chain kinase, which catalyzes the phosphorylation of myosin to facilitate the interaction with actin. Conversely, intracellular cyclic GMP activates myosin phosphatase (also via a kinase-mediated phosphorylation of myosin phosphatase), which dephosphorylates myosin and inhibits the interaction of actin and myosin. A primary mediator of vasodilatory shock is nitric oxide (NO), which is induced by cytokine cascades. NO activates guanylate cyclase, with resulting loss of vascular tone. Another mechanism of vasodilation that may be particularly relevant to prolonged CPB is activation of ATP-sensitive potassium (K_{ATP}) channels. These channels are activated by decreases in cellular ATP or increases in hydrogen ion or lactate. All these could result from the abnormal perfusion associated with CPB and/or hypothermia. Increases in potassium channel conductance result in hyperpolarization of the vascular smooth muscle membrane, which decreases Ca^{2+} flux into the cell, leading to decreased vascular tone. A third mechanism of vasodilatory shock that also may be particularly relevant to cardiac surgery

is deficiency of vasopressin. As noted earlier, CPB often induces the release of vasopressin, and this may contribute to the excessive vasoconstriction sometimes seen after CPB. However, it has been observed in several experimental models of shock that the initially high levels of vasopressin decrease as shock persists, leading some investigators to suggest that vasopressin stores are limited and are depleted by the initial response to hypotension.

Excessive vasodilation during shock usually is treated with catecholamines, most typically phenylephrine, dopamine, epinephrine, or norepinephrine.[103] Although catecholamines produce both alpha- and beta-adrenergic effects, alpha$_1$-adrenergic receptor stimulation produces vasoconstriction. As noted, stimulation of these receptors activates membrane phospholipase C, which in turn hydrolyzes phosphatidylinositol 4,5-diphosphate.[7] This leads to the subsequent generation of two second messengers, including diacyl glycerol and inositol triphosphate. Both these second messengers increase cytosolic Ca^{2+} by different mechanisms, which include facilitating release of calcium from the sarcoplasmic reticulum and potentially increasing the calcium sensitivity of the contractile proteins in vascular smooth muscle.

Mediator-induced vasodilation often is poorly responsive to catecholamines,[103] and the most potent pressor among catecholamines, norepinephrine, is required frequently. Some clinicians are concerned about renal, hepatic, and mesenteric function during norepinephrine administration. However, in septic patients, norepinephrine can improve renal function,[102-107] and there is evidence that it may improve mesenteric perfusion as well.[108] Given the hemodynamic similarities between septic patients and some patients at the end of CPB, these results often are extrapolated to the cardiac surgical patient but have not been confirmed by a systematic study. In some cases of profound vasodilatory shock, even norepinephrine is inadequate to restore systemic blood pressure. In this situation, low doses of vasopressin may be useful. Argenziano[109] studied 40 patients with vasodilatory shock (defined as a mean arterial blood pressure of less than 70 mm Hg with a cardiac index greater than 2.5 L/m^2 per minute) after cardiac surgery. AVP levels were inappropriately low in this group of patients, and low-dose vasopressin infusion (≤0.1 U/min) effectively restored blood pressure and reduced norepinephrine requirements without significantly changing cardiac index. These observations were similar to an earlier report of the use of vasopressin in vasodilatory septic shock.[110] Vasopressin also has been reported to be useful in treating milrinone-induced hypotension.[111] In this latter report, vasopressin was reported to increase urine output, presumably via glomerular efferent arteriole constriction. However, the overall effects on renal function are unclear. In addition, there are still important unanswered questions about vasopressin and mesenteric perfusion. Although vasopressin effectively may restore blood pressure in vasodilatory shock, it must be remembered that in physiologic concentrations it is a mesenteric vasoconstrictor, and mesenteric hypoperfusion may be a factor in developing sepsis and multiorgan dysfunction syndrome.

VASODILATORS

Different pharmacologic approaches are available to produce vasodilation (Table 4-1). Potential therapeutic approaches include (1) blockade of alpha$_1$-adrenergic receptors, ganglionic transmission, and calcium channel receptors; (2) stimulation of central alpha$_2$-adrenergic receptors or vascular guanylate cyclase and adenylate cyclase; and (3) inhibition of phosphodiesterase enzymes and ACEs.[112] Adenosine in low concentrations is also a potent vasodilator with a short half-life, but it is used, as noted earlier, for its ability to inhibit AV conduction. Losartan, a novel angiotensin II (AII) antagonist, has just been released for treating hypertension but is not available for intravenous use.

Stimulation of Adenylate Cyclase (Cyclic AMP)

Prostacyclin, prostaglandin E$_1$, and isoproterenol increase cyclic nucleotide formation (eg, adenosine-3′,5′-monophosphate and cyclic AMP) in vascular smooth muscle to produce calcium mobilization out of vascular smooth muscle. Inhibiting the breakdown of cyclic AMP by phosphodiesterase also will increase cyclic AMP.[112] Increasing cyclic AMP in vascular smooth muscle facilitates calcium uptake by intracellular storage sites, thus decreasing calcium available for contraction. The net effect of increasing calcium uptake is to produce vascular smooth muscle relaxation and hence vasodilation. However, most catecholamines with beta$_2$-adrenergic activity (eg, isoproterenol) and phosphodiesterase inhibitors have positive inotropic and other side effects that include tachycardia, glycogenolysis, and kaluresis.[113] Prostaglandins (ie, prostacyclin and prostaglandin E$_1$) are potent inhibitors of platelet aggregation and activation. Catecholamines with beta$_2$-adrenergic activity, phosphodiesterase inhibitors, and prostaglandin E$_1$ and prostacyclin have been used to vasodilate the pulmonary circulation in patients with pulmonary hypertension and right ventricular failure (see Table 4-1).[113]

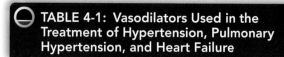

TABLE 4-1: Vasodilators Used in the Treatment of Hypertension, Pulmonary Hypertension, and Heart Failure

Angiotensin-converting enzyme inhibitors
Angiotensin II antagonists
Alpha$_1$-adrenergic antagonists (prazosin)
Alpha$_2$-adrenergic agonists (clonidine)
Endothelin antagonists
Nitrates
Nitric oxide
Hydralazine
Phosphodiesterase inhibitors (milrinone, sildenafil)
Prostacyclin, PGE$_1$
Calcium channel blockers
Dihydropyridine agents (clevidipine, nicardipine, amlodipine)

Nitrates, Nitrovasodilators, and Stimulation of Guanylyl Cyclase (Cyclic GMP)

The vascular endothelium modulates vascular relaxation by releasing both nitric oxide and prostacyclin.[114-116] Inflammatory mediators also can stimulate the vascular endothelium to release excessive amounts of endothelium-derived relaxing factor (EDRF, or nitric oxide), which activates guanylyl cyclase to generate cyclic GMP.[89,90] Nitrates and sodium nitroprusside, however, generate nitric oxide directly, independent of vascular endothelium.[115,116] The active form of any nitrovasodilator is nitric oxide (NO), in which the nitrogen is in a +2 oxidation state. For any nitrovasodilator to be active, it first must be converted to NO. For nitroprusside, this is easily accomplished because nitrogen is in a +3 oxidation state, with the nitric oxide molecule bound to the charged iron molecule in an unstable manner, allowing nitroprusside to readily donate its nitric oxide moiety. For nitroglycerin, nitrogen molecules exist in a +5 oxidation state, and thus they must undergo significant metabolic transformations before they are converted to an active molecule. Nitroglycerin is a selective coronary vasodilator and does not produce coronary steal compared with nitroprusside because the small intracoronary resistance vessels, those less than 100 μm thick, lack whatever metabolic transformation pathway is required to convert nitroglycerin into its active form of nitric oxide.[115,116] Chronic nitrate therapy can produce tolerance through different mechanisms.[114-118] Sodium nitroprusside and nitroglycerin are effective vasodilators that produce venodilation that contributes significantly to the labile hemodynamic state.[114] Intravenous volume administration often is required with nitroprusside owing to the relative intravascular hypovolemia.

Dihydropyridine Calcium Channel Blockers

Dihydropyridine calcium channel blockers are direct arterial vasodilators.[119] Nifedipine was the first dihydropyridine calcium channel blocker, and intravenous forms studied in cardiac surgery include clevidipine, isradipine, and nicardipine. These agents are selective arterial vasodilators that have no effects on the vascular capacitance bed, AV nodal conduction, or negative inotropic effects.[120-125] Clevidipine and nicardipine are available in the United States and offer novel and important therapeutic options to treat perioperative hypertension following cardiac surgery. Also, intravenous dihydropyridines can be used to treat acute hypertension that occurs during the perioperative period (ie, intubation, extubation, CPB-induced hypertension, and aortic cross-clamping) and postoperative hypertension.

Phosphodiesterase Inhibitors

Two major classes of phosphodiesterase inhibitors are currently available for use. Milrinone is a prototypic type III inhibitor that is cyclic AMP specific, as previously described, and produces both positive inotropic effects and vasodilation.[126] When administered to patients with ventricular dysfunction, milrinone increases cardiac output, venodilates, vasodilates, and is a pulmonary vasodilator. Sildenafil is a type V-specific inhibitor that is cyclic GMP specific and is a pulmonary and systemic vasodilator without a primary inotropic response, although isotypes for phosphodiesterases exist. Because of their unique mechanisms of vasodilation, these agents are especially useful for patients with acute pulmonary vasoconstriction and right ventricular dysfunction. Multiple forms of the drug are available including bipyridines (eg, amrinone and milrinone), imidazolones (eg, enoximone), and methylxanthines (eg, aminophylline), and sildenafil. Papaverine, a benzyl isoquinolinium derivative isolated from opium, is a nonspecific phosphodiesterase inhibitor and vasodilator used by cardiac surgeons for its ability to dilate the internal mammary artery.[126]

Angiotensin-Converting Enzyme Inhibitors

ACE inhibitors have growing use in managing HF, and more patients are receiving these drugs. The ACE inhibitors prevent the conversion of angiotensin I to angiotensin II by inhibiting an enzyme called *kininase* in the pulmonary and systemic vascular endothelium. This enzyme is also important for the metabolism of bradykinin, a potent endogenous vasodilator, and for release of EDRF. Although there are little data in the literature regarding the preoperative management of patients receiving these drugs, withholding them on the day of surgery has been our clinical practice based on their potential to produce excessive vasodilation during CPB. Although Tuman was unable to find any difference in blood pressure during CPB in patients receiving ACE inhibitors, contact activation during CPB has the ability to generate bradykinin and thus amplify the potential for vasodilation. The vasoconstrictor requirements were increased after bypass in his study.

Angiotensin II-Receptor Blockers

ACE inhibitors may not be tolerated in some patients owing to cough (common) and angioedema (rare). Inhibition of kininase II by ACE inhibitors leads to bradykinin accumulation in the lungs and vasculature, causing cough and vasodilation. Alternative treatment with angiotensin II-receptor blockers (ARBs) may be associated less frequently with these side effects because ARBs do not affect kinin metabolism. Six ARBs are currently available for antihypertensive therapy in the United States: losartan (Cozaar), valsartan (Diovan), irbesartan (Avapro), candesartan (Atacand), eprosartan (Teveten), and telmisartan (Micardis). Mortality in chronic HF is related to activation of the autonomic nervous and renin-angiotensin systems, and ACE inhibitor therapy seems to attenuate progression of myocardial dysfunction and remodeling. ACE inhibitors do not completely block angiotensin II (A-II) production,[127] and may even increase circulating A-II levels in patients with HF. It was thought initially that ARBs might offer advantages over ACE inhibitors for heart failure therapy in terms of tolerability and more complete A-II blockade. Although ARBs were better tolerated, all-cause mortality and the number of sudden deaths or resuscitated cardiac arrests were not different when losartan (Cozaar) and captopril (Capoten) were compared in patients (>60 years of age, New York Heart Association (NYHA) classes II to IV, left-ventricular ejection fraction (LVEF) <40%).[128] Perioperative hypotension may be encountered in ARB-treated patients as well as ACE inhibitor-treated patients, and increased inotropic support may be required.

BETA-ADRENERGIC RECEPTOR BLOCKERS

Not surprisingly, most of the effects observed after administration of a beta-adrenergic receptor blocker reflect the reduced responsiveness of tissues containing beta-adrenergic receptors to catecholamines present in the vicinity of those receptors. Hence the intensity of the effects of beta-blockers depends on both the dose of the blocker and the receptor concentrations of catecholamines, primarily epinephrine and norepinephrine. In fact, a purely competitive interaction of beta-blockers and catecholamines can be demonstrated in normal human volunteers as well as in isolated tissues studied in the laboratory. The presence of disease and other types of drugs modifies the responses to beta-blockers observed in patients, but the underlying competitive interaction is still operative. The key to successful use of beta-adrenergic receptor blockers is to titrate the dose to the desired degree of effect and to remember that excessive effects from larger than necessary doses of beta-adrenergic receptor blockers can be overcome by (1) administering a catecholamine to compete at the blocked receptors; and/or (2) administering other types of drugs to reduce the activity of counterbalancing autonomic mechanisms that are unopposed in the presence of beta-receptor blockade. An example of the latter is propranolol-induced bradycardia, which reflects the increased dominance of the vagal cholinergic mechanism on cardiac nodal tissue. Excessive bradycardia may be relieved by administering atropine to block the cholinergic receptors, which are also located in the SA and AV nodes (see Table 4-2).

Knowledge of the type, location, and action of beta receptor is fundamental to understanding and predicting effects of beta-adrenergic receptor-blocking drugs[129] (see Table 4-2). Beta-adrenergic receptor blockers are competitive inhibitors; hence, the intensity of blockade depends on both the dose of the drug and the receptor concentrations of catecholamines, primarily epinephrine and norepinephrine.

Beta-adrenergic receptor antagonists (blockers) include many drugs (Table 4-3) that typically are classified by their relative selectivity for beta$_1$ and beta$_2$ receptors (ie, cardioselective or nonselective), the presence or absence of agonist activity, membrane-stabilizing properties, alpha-receptor-blocking efficacy, and various pharmacokinetic features (eg, lipid solubility, oral bioavailability, and elimination half-time).[129] The

TABLE 4-2: Location and Actions of Beta-Adrenergic Receptors

Tissue	Receptor	Action	Opposing Actions
Heart			
Sinus and AV nodes	1	↑ Automaticity	Cholinergic receptors
Conduction pathways	1	↑ Conduction velocity	Cholinergic receptors
		↑ Automaticity	Cholinergic receptors
Myofibrils	1	↑ Contractility	—
		↑ Automaticity	—
Vascular smooth muscle (arterial, venous)	2	Vasodilation	Alpha-adrenergic receptors
Bronchial smooth muscle	2	Bronchodilation	Cholinergic receptors
Kidneys	1	↑ Renin release (juxtaglomerular cells)	Alpha$_1$-adrenergic receptors
Liver	2	↑ Glucose metabolism	Alpha$_1$-adrenergic receptors
		↑ Lipolysis	
Fat/adipose tissue	3	↑ Lipolysis	—
Skeletal muscle	2	↑ Potassium uptake glycogenolysis	—
Eye, ciliary muscle	2	Relaxation	Cholinergic receptors
GI tract	2	↑ Motility	Cholinergic receptors
Gallbladder	2	Relaxation	Cholinergic receptors
Urinary bladder detrussor muscle	2	Relaxation	Cholinergic receptors
Uterus	2	Relaxation	Oxytocin
Platelets	2	↓ Aggregation	Alpha$_2$-adrenergic receptors (aggregation)

practitioner must realize that the selectivity of individual drugs for beta$_1$ and beta$_2$ receptors is relative, not absolute. For example, the risk of inducing bronchospasm with a beta$_1$-adrenergic (cardioselective) blocker (eg, esmolol or metoprolol) may be relatively less than that with a nonselective blockers (eg, propranolol); however, the risk is still present.

Acute Myocardial Infarction

Earlier clinical trials of intravenous beta-adrenergic blockers in the early phases of acute myocardial infarction suggest they decrease mortality. Following myocardial infarction, chronic oral beta-blocking agents reduce the incidence of recurrent myocardial infarction (see Table 4-3).[130]

Supraventricular Tachycardias and Ventricular Dysrhythmias

Beta-adrenergic blocking agents are Vaughan Williams class II antidysrhythmics that primarily block cardiac responses to catecholamines. Metoprolol and esmolol are used commonly for this indication. Beta-blocking agents decrease spontaneous depolarization in the SA and AV nodes, decrease automaticity in Purkinje fibers, increase AV nodal refractoriness, increase threshold for fibrillation (but not for depolarization), and decrease ventricular slow responses that depend on catecholamines. Amiodarone, a class III agent, also exerts noncompetitive alpha- and beta-adrenergic blockade, which may contribute its antidysrhythmic and antihypertensive actions. Sotalol is another class III antidysrhythmic with nonselective

beta-blocking action. Beta-adrenergic blocking agents also decrease intramyocardial conduction in ischemic tissue and reduce the risks of dysrhythmias to the extent that they decrease myocardial ischemia.

TABLE 4-3: Beta-Adrenergic Receptors Blockers

Generic Name	Trade Name	Dosage Forms	Beta$_1$-Selective
Acebutolol	Sectral	PO	Yes
Atenolol	Tenormin	IV, PO	Yes
Betaxolol	Kerlone	PO	Yes
Bisoprolol	Zebeta	PO	Yes
Esmolol	Brevibloc	IV	Yes
Metoprolol	Lopressor, Toprol-XL	IV, PO	Yes
Carvedilol*	Coreg	PO	No
Carteolol	Cartrol	PO	No
Labetalol*	Normodyne, Trandate	IV, PO	No
Nadolol	Corgard	PO	No
Penbutolol	Levatol	PO	No
Pindolol	Visken	PO	No
Propranolol	Inderal	IV, PO	No
Sotalol	Betapace	PO	No
Timolol	Blocadren	PO	No

*Alpha$_1$: beta-adrenergic blocking ratio; carvedilol 1:10, labetalol 1:3 (oral)/1:7 (IV).

Hypertension

Hypertension, if not treated, is a major risk factor for myocardial infarction, stroke, renal failure and death, and patients often present for cardiac surgery with poorly controlled blood pressure (BP) management. The recently published recommendations of Eighth Joint National Committee (JNC 8) provide an evidence-based approach to recommend treatment thresholds, goals and specific therapy for management of hypertension, and have been liberalized since the last report.[131] They recommend treating patients aged >60 years with <150/90 mm Hg whereas younger patients 30 to 59 years to a diastolic goal of <90 mm Hg, and in younger patients a BP of <140/90 mm Hg, whether or not they have diabetes or chronic kidney disease (CKD). They suggest initiating therapy with an ACE inhibitor, angiotensin receptor blocker, calcium channel blocker, or thiazide-type diuretic in the nonblack hypertensive population, including those with diabetes. In the black hypertensive population, a calcium channel blocker or thiazide-type diuretic is recommended as initial therapy. There is moderate evidence to support initial or add-on antihypertensive therapy with an ACE inhibitor or angiotensin receptor blocker in persons with CKD to improve kidney outcomes. Of note, they emphasize the importance of clinical judgment as a critical component.[131,132]

Hypertenisve Emergencies and Urgencies

Hypertensive emergencies/crises include multiple clinical presentations where uncontrolled hypertension leads to progressive or impending end-organ dysfunction requiring BP to be lowered aggressively over minutes to hours. Neurologic end-organ dysfunction due to uncontrolled hypertension includes encephalopathy, cerebral vascular infarction, subarachnoid hemorrhage, and/or intracranial hemorrhage. Cardiovascular end-organ injury includes myocardial ischemia and/or infarction, acute HF, pulmonary edema, and/or aortic dissection. Other organ systems may also be affected by uncontrolled hypertension, which may lead to acute renal failure/insufficiency, eclampsia, or coagulopathy. In hypertensive emergencies, intravenous therapy with specific BP titration is the cornerstone of therapy.

Hypertensive urgencies are seen in a clinical setting where patients present asymptomatically with high blood pressures that should be treated but with oral therapies, restarting on their medications or therapy initiated with care to avoid overshoot and hypotenstion. Hypertensive urgencies are common in cardiac surgery where BP is maintained at specific arbitrary levels based on concerns about bleeding and/or suture line disruption.

Acute Dissecting Aortic Aneurysm

The primary goal in managing dissecting aneurysms is to reduce stress on the dissected aortic wall by reducing the systolic acceleration of blood flow. Beta-blockers reduce cardiac inotropy and ventricular ejection fraction. They also may limit reflex sympathetic responses to vasodilators used to control systemic arterial pressure.

Pheochromocytoma

The presence of catecholamine-secreting tissue is tantamount to the continuous or intermittent infusion of a varying mixture of norepinephrine and epinephrine. It is absolutely essential that virtually complete alpha-adrenergic receptor blockade be established prior to administering the beta-blocker to prevent exacerbation of hypertensive episodes by unopposed alpha-adrenergic receptor activity in vascular smooth muscle.

Chronic Heart Failure

It is now understood that activation of the autonomic nervous system (ANS) and renin-angiotensin system (RAS) as compensatory mechanisms for the failing heart actually may contribute to deterioration of myocardial function. Mortality in chronic HF seems related to activation of ANS and RAS. Progression of myocardial dysfunction and remodeling may be attenuated by the use of beta-blocking agents and ACE inhibitors. Carvedilol (Coreg) is a beta-blocker approved by the FDA to treat patients with HF. It has an alpha$_1$- and nonselective beta-blocking activity (alpha:beta = 1:10). It is contraindicated in severe decompensated HF and asthma. In patients with AF and left-sided HF treated with carvedilol, improved ejection fraction, and a trend toward a decreased incidence of death and chronic HF hospitalization were observed in a retrospective analysis of a US carvedilol study. There are several ongoing clinical trials with carvedilol, metoprolol (Toprol), and bisoprolol (Zebeta). The results of these studies may provide answers as to which beta-blocking agent would be most successful in the treatment of specific patient populations.

Other Indications

The other clinical applications of beta-adrenergic receptor blockers listed in Table 4-4 are based on largely symptomatic treatment or empirical trials of beta-adrenergic antagonists.

Side Effects and Toxicity

The most obvious and immediate signs of a toxic overdose of a beta-adrenergic receptor blocker are hypotension, bradycardia, congestive HF, decreased AV conduction, and a widened QRS complex on the electrocardiogram. Treatment is aimed at blocking the cholinergic receptor responses to vagal nerve activity (eg, atropine) and administering a sympathomimetic to compete with the beta-blockers at adrenergic receptors. In patients with asthma and chronic obstructive pulmonary disease (COPD), beta-blockers may cause bronchospasm. Beta-blockers may increase levels of plasma triglycerides and reduce levels of high-density lipoprotein (HDL) cholesterol. Rarely, beta-blockers may mask the symptoms of hypoglycemia in

> ### TABLE 4-4: Clinical Applications of Beta-Adrenergic Receptor Blockers
>
> Angina pectoris
> Acute myocardial infarction (prophylaxis)
> Supraventricular tachycardia
> Ventricular dysrhythmias
> Hypertension (usually in combination with other drugs)
> Pheochromocytoma (after alpha-receptor blockade is established)
> Acute dissecting aortic aneurysm
> Hyperthyroidism
> Hypertrophic obstructive cardiomyopathy (IHSS)
> Dilated cardiomyopathy (selected patients)
> Migraine prophylaxis
> Acute panic attack
> Alcohol withdrawal syndrome
> Glaucoma (topically)

diabetic patients. Other side effects include mental depression, physical fatigue, altered sleep patterns, sexual dysfunction, and gastrointestinal symptoms, including indigestion, constipation, and diarrhea (see Table 4-4).

Drug Interactions

Pharmacokinetic drug interactions include reduced gastrointestinal absorption of the beta-blocker (eg, aluminum-containing antacids and cholestyramine), increased biotransformation of the beta-blocker (eg, phenytoin, phenobarbital, rifampin, and smoking), and increased bioavailability owing to decreased biotransformation (eg, cimetidine and hydralazine). Pharmacodynamic interactions include an additive effect with calcium channel blockers to decrease conduction in the heart and a reduced antihypertensive effect of beta-blockers when administered with some of the nonsteroidal anti-inflammatory drugs (NSAIDs).

DIURETICS

Diuretics are drugs that act directly on the kidneys to increase urine volume and produce a net loss of solute (principally sodium and other electrolytes) and water. Diuretics and beta-blockers are initial drugs of choice for uncomplicated hypertension in patients younger than 65 years.[132] The currently available diuretic drugs have a number of other uses in medicine (eg, glaucoma and increased intracranial pressure). The principal indications for the use of diuretics by intravenous administration in the perioperative period are to: (1) increase urine flow in oliguria; (2) reduce intravascular volume in patients at risk for acute HF from excessive fluid administration or acute HF; and (3) mobilize edema.

Renal function depends on adequate renal perfusion to maintain the integrity of renal cells and provide the hydrostatic pressure that produces glomerular filtration. There are no drugs that act directly on the renal glomerulus to affect glomerular filtration rate (GFR). In the normal adult human of average size, GFR averages 125 mL/min and urine production approximates 1 mL/min. In other words, 99% of the glomerular filtrate is reabsorbed. Diuretics act primarily on specific segments of the renal tubule to alter reabsorption of electrolytes, principally sodium, and water.

There are two basic mechanisms behind the renal tubular reabsorption of sodium. First, sodium is extruded from the tubular cell into peritubular fluid primarily by active transport of the sodium ion, which reflects the action of the Na^+, K^+ ATPase pump, as well as the bicarbonate reabsorption mechanism (see the following). This extrusion of sodium creates an electrochemical gradient that causes diffusion of sodium from the tubular lumen into the tubular cell. Second, sodium moves from the glomerular filtrate in the tubular fluid into the peritubular fluid by several different mechanisms. The most important quantitatively is the sodium electrochemical gradient created by the active extrusion of sodium from the tubular cell into the peritubular fluid. In addition, sodium is coupled with organic solutes and phosphate ions, exchanged for hydrogen ions diffusing from the tubular cell into the tubular lumen, and coupled to the transfer of a chloride ion or a combination of potassium and two chloride ions (Na^+-K^+-$2Cl^-$ cotransport) from the tubular fluid into the tubular cell. Diuretics are classified by their principal site of action in the nephron and by the primary mechanism of their natriuretic effect (Table 4-5).

Osmotic Diuretics

Mannitol is the principal example of this type of diuretic, which is used for two primary indications: (1) prophylaxis and early treatment of acute renal failure that is characterized by a decrease in GFR leading to a decreased urine volume and an increase in the concentration of toxic substances in the renal tubular fluid; and (2) enhancing the actions of other diuretics by retaining water and solutes in the tubular lumen, thereby providing the substrate for the action of other types of diuretics. Normally, 80% of the glomerular filtrate is reabsorbed isosmotically in the proximal tubules. By its osmotic effect, mannitol limits the reabsorption of water and dilutes the proximal tubular fluid. This reduces the electrochemical gradient for sodium and limits its reabsorption so that more is delivered to the distal portions of the nephron. Mannitol produces a prostaglandin-mediated increase in renal blood flow that partially washes out the medullary hypertonicity, which is essential for the countercurrent mechanism promoting the reabsorption of water in the late distal tubules and collecting system under the influence of antidiuretic hormone (ADH). Mannitol is used often (25 to 50 g) as part of the priming solution of CPB for the above-mentioned indications. The principal toxicity of mannitol is acute expansion of the extracellular fluid volume leading to HF in the patient with compromised cardiac function (see Table 4-5).

TABLE 4-5: Classification of Diuretics

Site of Action	Mechanism	
Osmotic	Proximal convoluted and late proximal for Na$^+$ diffusion from tubular fluid into tubular cell	↓ Electrochemical gradient
	Late proximal tubule	↓ Gradient for Cl$^-$ (accompanying Na$^+$ diffusion)
	Thick ascending loop of Henle	↓ Na$^+$-K$^+$-2Cl$^-$ cotransport
Carbonic	Proximal convoluted tubule anhydrase inhibitors	↓ Na$^+$-H$^+$ exchange
Thiazides	Distal convoluted tubule	↓ Na$^+$-Cl$^-$ cotransport
High-ceiling loop diuretics	Thick ascending loop of Henle	↓ Na$^+$-K$^+$-2Cl$^-$ cotransport
Potassium-sparing diuretics	Late distal tubule and collecting duct	↓ Electrogenic Na$^+$ entry into cells (driving force for K$^+$ secretion)

High-Ceiling (Loop) Diuretics

Furosemide (Lasix), bumetanide (Bumex), and ethacrynic acid (Edecrin) are three chemically dissimilar compounds that have the same primary diuretic mechanism of action. They act on the tubular epithelial cell in the thick ascending loop of Henle to inhibit the Na$^+$-K$^+$-2Cl$^-$ cotransport mechanism. Their peak diuretic effect is far greater than that of the other diuretics currently available. Administered intravenously, they have a rapid onset and relatively short duration of action, the latter reflecting both the pharmacokinetics of the drugs and the body's compensatory mechanisms to the consequences of diuresis.

These three diuretics increase renal blood flow without increasing GFR and redistribute blood flow from the medulla to the cortex and within the renal cortex. These changes in renal blood flow are also short-lived, reflecting the reduced extracellular fluid volume resulting from diuresis. Minor actions, including carbonic anhydrase inhibition by furosemide and bumetanide and actions on the proximal tubule and on sites distal to the ascending limb, remain controversial. All three of the loop diuretics increase the release of renin and prostaglandin, and indomethacin blunts the release as well as the augmentation in renal blood flow and natriuresis. All three of the loop diuretics produce an acute increase in venous capacitance for a brief period of time after the first intravenous dose is administered, and this effect is also blocked by indomethacin.

Potassium, magnesium, and calcium excretion is increased in proportion to the increase in sodium excretion. In addition, there is augmentation of titratable acid and ammonia excretion by the distal tubules leading to metabolic alkalosis, which is also produced by contraction of the extracellular volume. Hyperuricemia can occur but usually is of little physiologic significance. The nephrotoxicity of cephaloridine, and possibly other cephalosporins, is increased. A rare but serious side effect of the loop diuretics is deafness, which may reflect electrolyte changes in the endolymph.

Because of their high degree of efficacy, prompt onset, and relatively short duration of action, the high-ceiling or loop diuretics are favored for intravenous administration in the perioperative period to treat the three principal problems cited earlier. Dosage requirements vary considerably among patients. Some may only require furosemide 3 to 5 mg (IV) to produce a good diuresis. And for some patients, the less potent benzothiazides may be sufficient.

Benzothiazides

Hydrochlorothiazide (HCTZ) is the prototype of more than a dozen currently available diuretics in this class. Although the drugs differ in potency, they all act by the same mechanism of action and have the same maximum efficacy. All are actively secreted into the tubular lumen by tubular cells and act in the early distal tubules to decrease the electroneutral Na$^+$-Cl$^-$ cotransport reabsorption of sodium. Their moderate efficacy probably reflects the fact that more than 90% of the filtrated sodium is reabsorbed before reaching the distal tubules. Their action is enhanced by their combined administration with an osmotic diuretic such as mannitol. The benziothiazides increase urine volume and the excretion of sodium, chloride, and potassium. The decreased reabsorption of potassium reflects the higher rate of urine flow through the distal tubule (diminished reabsorption time).

This class of diuretics produces the least disturbance of extracellular fluid composition, reflecting their moderate efficacy as diuretics and perhaps suggesting their usefulness when a moderate degree of diuretic effect is indicated. Their principal side effects include hyperuricemia, decreased calcium excretion, and enhanced magnesium loss. Hyperglycemia can occur and reflects multiple variables. With prolonged use and development of a contracted extracellular fluid volume, urine formation decreases (ie, tolerance develops to their diuretic actions). These agents also have a direct action on the renal vasculature to decrease GFR.

Carbonic Anhydrase Inhibitors

Acetazolamide (Diamox) is the only diuretic of this class available for intravenous administration. Its use is directed primarily toward alkalinization of urine in the presence of metabolic alkalosis, which is a common consequence of prolonged diuretic therapy. It acts in the proximal convoluted tubule to inhibit carbonic anhydrase in the brush border of the tubular epithelium, thereby reducing the destruction of bicarbonate ions (ie, conversion to CO_2 that diffuses into the tubular cell). The carbonic anhydrase enzyme in the cytoplasm of the tubular cell is also inhibited, and as a consequence, conversion of CO_2 to carbonic acid is reduced markedly, as is the availability of hydrogen ions for the Na-H exchange mechanism. Hence the reabsorption of both sodium and bicarbonate in the proximal tubules is diminished. However, more than half the bicarbonate is reabsorbed in more distal segments of the nephron, thereby limiting the overall efficacy of this class of diuretics.

Potassium-Sparing Diuretics

Spironolactone (Aldactone) is a competitive antagonist of aldosterone. Spironolactone binds to the cytoplasmic aldosterone receptor and prevents its conformational change to the active form, thereby aborting the synthesis of active transport proteins in the late distal tubules and collecting system in which the reabsorption of sodium and secretion of potassium are reduced.

Triamterene (Dyrenium) and amiloride (Midamor) are potassium-sparing diuretics with a mechanism of action independent of the mineralocorticoids. They have a moderate natriuretic effect leading to an increased excretion of sodium and chloride with little change or a slight increase in potassium excretion when the latter is low. When potassium secretion is high, they produce a sharp reduction in the electrogenic entry of sodium ions into the distal tubular cells and thereby reduce the electrical potential that is the driving force for potassium secretion.

Both types of potassium-sparing diuretics are used primarily in combination with other diuretics to reduce potassium loss. Their principal side effect is hyperkalemia. It is appropriate to limit the intake of potassium when using this type of diuretic. It is also appropriate to use this type of diuretic cautiously in patients taking ACE inhibitors, which decrease aldosterone formation and consequently increase serum potassium concentrations.

Other Measures to Enhance Urine Output and Mobilization of Edema Fluid

The infusion of albumin (5–25% solutions) or other plasma volume expanders (eg, hetastarch) is often employed in an attempt to draw water and its accompanying electrolytes (ie, edema fluid) osmotically from the tissues into the circulating blood and thereby enhance their delivery to the kidneys for excretion. In the presence of a reduced circulating blood volume, this approach seems to be a logical method to increase the circulating blood volume and renal perfusion. The limiting feature of this approach to enhancing diuresis relates to the fact that the osmotic effect of albumin and plasma expanders is transient because they can diffuse (at a rate slower than water) from blood through capillary membranes into tissue. The albumin or plasma expander then tends to hold water and its accompanying electrolytes in tissue (ie, rebound edema). The same limiting feature applies to osmotic diuretics such as mannitol, which may transiently draw water and its accompanying electrolytes from tissues into the circulating blood for delivery to the kidneys, where the mannitol passes through the glomerulus and delays the reabsorption of water and its accompanying electrolytes from the proximal tubular fluid. Although this mechanism may enhance the actions of other diuretics, it is a transient effect that is limited by the diffusion of mannitol from blood into tissues with the production of rebound edema.

Dopamine, at doses from 1 to 3 µg/kg per minute, has been used conventionally to support mesenteric and renal perfusion as "renal dose dopamine." Vasodilation at low doses is mediated via vascular dopamine 1 (D_1) receptors in coronary, mesenteric, and renal vascular beds. By activating adenyl cyclase and raising intracellular concentrations of cyclic AMP, D_1-receptor agonists cause vasodilatation. There are also dopamine 2 (D_2) receptors that antagonize D_1-receptor stimulation. Fenoldopam (Corlopam), a parenteral D_1-receptor-specific agonist, is also available as a therapy. However, there are no data supporting its use to improve renal function other than by increasing cardiac output, and it also increases the risk of postoperative AF.[133] Infusion of fenoldopam (0.1 to 0.3 µg/kg per minute) causes an increase in GFR, renal blood flow, and Na^+ excretion.

Clinical trials of dopamine failed to show improvement in renal function, which probably is a result of the nonspecificity of dopamine. As a catecholamine and a precursor in the metabolic synthesis of norepinephrine and epinephrine, dopamine has inotropic and chronotropic effects on the heart. The inotropic effect is mediated by beta₁-adrenergic receptors and usually requires infusion rates higher than those able to produce enhanced renal perfusion and diuresis. However, there are varied pharmacokinetic responses to dopamine infusion even in healthy subjects; therefore, the use of a "renal dose" dopamine regimen may not always result in the desirable effects. Stimulation of catecholamine receptors and D_2 receptors antagonizes the effects of D_1-receptor stimulation. Current data do not consistently demonstrate improved renal outcomes with use of the D_1-receptor-specific agonist fenoldopam.

HERBAL MEDICINE

A large number of Americans take herbal remedies for their health. Most of these herbal therapies are not supported by clear scientific evidence and are not under rigorous control by the FDA.[134-136] Patients who take alternative remedies may not necessarily disclose this information to their physicians.[135] There are increasing concerns regarding serious drug interactions between herbal therapy and prescribed medication.

⊖ TABLE 4-6: Commonly Used Herbal Remedies

Name	Common Uses	Side Effects/Drug Interactions
Cayenne (paprika)	Muscle spasm, GI disorders	Skin ulcers/blistering Hypothermia
Echinacea	Common cold, antitussive, urinary tract infections	May cause hepatotoxicity May decrease effects of steroids and cyclosporine
Ephedra (Mahuang)	Antitussive, bacteriostatic	Enhanced sympathomimetic effects with guanethidine or monoamine oxidase inhibitor (MAOI) Arrhythmias with halothane or digoxin Hypertension with oxytocin
Feverfew	Migraine, antipyretic	Platelet inhibition, rebound headache, aphthous ulcers, GI irritation
Garlic	Lipid-lowering, antihypertensive antithrombotic	May potentiate warfarin
Ginger	Antinauseant, antispasmodic	May potentiate aspirin and warfarin
Ginkgo	Improve circulation	May potentiate aspirin and warfarin
Ginseng	Adaptogenic, enhance energy level, antioxidant	Ginseng abuse syndrome: sleepiness, hypertonia, edema May cause mania in patients on phenelzine May decrease effects of warfarin Postmenopausal bleeding Mastalgia
Goldenseal	Diuretic, anti-inflammatory, laxative, hemostatic	Overdose may cause paralysis; aquaretic (no sodium excretion); may worsen edema/hypertension
Kava-kava	Anxiolytic	Potentiates barbiturates and benzodiazepines Potentiates ethanol May increase suicide risk in depression
Licorice	Antitussive, gastric ulcers	High blood pressure, hypokalemia, and edema
Saw palmetto	Benign prostatic hypertrophy, antiandrogenic	Additive effects with other hormone replacement therapy (eg, HRT)
St. John's wort	Antidepressant, anxiolytic	Possible interaction with MAOIs Decreases metabolism of fentanyl and ondansetron
Valerian	Mild sedative, anxiolytic	Potentiates barbiturates and benzodiazepines

Some of the most common herbal remedies and drug interactions are summarized in Table 4-6.

AIRWAY MANAGEMENT

Airway management in cardiovascular surgical patients is important because patients often present with coexisting conditions that may complicate endotracheal intubation. For example, a patient with morbid obesity and sleep apnea may require awake intubation with a fiberoptic bronchoscope, or a history of smoking and COPD may make the patient susceptible to rapid desaturation and/or bronchospasm. Airway management in the perioperative period is a primary responsibility of the anesthesiologist, but the surgeon becomes involved in the absence of the anesthesiologist or in assisting the anesthesiologist in difficult situations. Airway management involves instrumentation and mechanics (not discussed here) and employs pharmacologic approaches to overcome pathophysiologic problems contributing to airway obstruction and to facilitate manipulation and instrumentation of the airway. Pharmacologic agents are considered at the end of this section.

Five major challenges may be encountered in airway management. Each of these is described succinctly below to facilitate understanding of the roles that drugs play in meeting the challenges. The five challenges are (1) overcoming airway obstruction, (2) preventing pulmonary aspiration, (3) performing endotracheal intubation, (4) maintaining intermittent positive-pressure ventilation (IPPV), and (5) reestablishing spontaneous ventilation and airway protective reflexes.

Airway Obstruction

Obstruction to gas flow can occur from the entry of a foreign object (including food) into the airway and as a result of pathophysiologic processes involving airway structures (eg, trauma and edema). In the anesthetized or comatose patient, the loss of muscle tone can allow otherwise normal tissues (eg, tongue and epiglottis) to collapse into the airway and cause obstruction. The first measure in relieving such obstructions involves manipulation of the head and jaw, insertion of an artificial nasal or oral airway device, and evacuation of obstructing objects and substances (eg, blood, secretions, or food particles). Except for drugs used to facilitate endotracheal intubation (see the following), the only drug useful to improve gas flow through a narrowed airway is a mixture of helium and oxygen (Heliox), which has a much reduced viscosity resulting in reduced resistance to gas flow.

Aspiration

The upper airway (above the larynx/epiglottis) is a shared porthole to the lungs (gas exchange) and gastrointestinal tract (fluids and nutrition). Passive regurgitation or active vomiting resulting in accumulation of gastric contents in the pharynx places the patient at risk of pulmonary aspiration, especially under circumstances in which airway reflexes (eg, glottic closure and coughing) and voluntary avoidance maneuvers are suppressed (eg, anesthesia or coma). Particulate matter can obstruct the tracheobronchial tree, and acidic fluid (pH < 2.5) can injure the lung parenchyma. The resulting pneumonitis can cause significant morbidity (eg, acute respiratory distress syndrome) and has a high mortality rate. Preoperative restriction of fluids and food (NPO status) does not guarantee the absence of aspiration risks. Similarly, the advance placement of a nasogastric or orogastric tube may serve to reduce intragastric pressure but does not guarantee complete removal of gastric contents. Nevertheless, both NPO orders and the insertion of a nasogastric or orogastric tube under some circumstances are worthwhile measures to reduce the risks of pulmonary aspiration. In some circumstances, the deliberate induction of vomiting in a conscious patient may be indicated, but this is done rarely and almost never involves the use of an emetic drug. In fact, more often antiemetic drugs are employed to reduce the risks of vomiting during airway manipulation and induction of anesthesia.

Drug therapy to reduce the risks of pulmonary aspiration is focused on decreasing the quantity and acidity of gastric contents and on facilitating endotracheal intubation (see the following). Nonparticulate antacids (eg, sodium citrate [Bicitra]) are used to neutralize the acidity of gastric fluids. Drugs to reduce gastric acid production include H_2-receptor blockers (eg, cimetidine [Tagamet], ranitidine [Zantac], famotidine [Pepcid]), and inhibitors of gastric parietal cell hydrogen-potassium ATPase (proton pump inhibitors, eg, omeprazole [Prilosec], lansoprazole [Prevacid], and esomeprazole [Nexium]). Metoclopramide [Reglan] enhances gastric emptying and increases gastroesophageal sphincter tone. Cisapride [Propulsid] also increases gastrointestinal motility via the release of acetylcholine at the myenteric plexus.

Antiemetic drugs are used more commonly in the postoperative period and include several different drug classes: anticholinergics (eg, scopolamine [Transderm Scop]), antihistamines (eg, hydroxyzine [Vistaril] and promethazine [Phenergan]), and antidopaminergics (eg, droperidol [Inapsine] and prochlorperazine [Compazine]). Antidopaminergic agents may cause extrapyramidal side effects in elderly patients. More costly but effective alternatives include the use of antiserotinergics (eg, ondansetron [Zofran] and dolasetron [Anzemet]).

Endotracheal Intubation

Drugs are employed for three purposes in facilitating endotracheal intubation: (1) to improve visualization of the larynx during laryngoscopy; (2) to prevent closure of the larynx; and (3) to facilitate manipulation of the head and jaw.

For bronchoscopy, laryngoscopy, or fiberoptic endotracheal intubation, the reflex responses to airway manipulation can be suppressed by several different methods alone or in combination. Topical anesthesia (2 or 4% lidocaine spray) can be used to anesthetize the mucosal surfaces of the nose, oral cavity, pharynx, and epiglottis. Atomized local anesthetic can be inhaled to anesthetize the mucosa below the vocal cords. The subglottic mucosa also can be anesthetized topically by injecting local anesthetic into the tracheal lumen through the cricothyroid membrane. A bilateral superior laryngeal nerve block eliminates sensory input from mechanical contact or irritation of the larynx above the vocal cords. It must be remembered that anesthesia of the mucosal surfaces to obtund airway reflexes compromises the reflex-protective mechanisms of the airway and increases the patient's vulnerability to aspiration of substances from the pharynx. Improvement of visualization of the larynx includes decreasing salivation and tracheal bronchial secretions by administration of an anticholinergic drug (eg, glycopyrrolate), reducing mucosal swelling by topical administration of a vasoconstrictor (eg, phenylephrine), and minimizing bleeding owing to mucosal erosion by instrumentation, which also is minimized by topical vasoconstrictors. The use of steroids in minimizing acute inflammatory responses in the airway may have some delayed benefit, but steroids usually are not indicated just before intubation.

Systemic drugs, usually administered intravenously, can be used to obtund the cough reflex. Intravenous lidocaine (1 to 2 mg/kg) transiently obtunds the cough reflex without affecting spontaneous ventilation to any significant degree. The risks of CNS stimulation and seizure-like activity have to be kept in mind and can be reduced by the prior administration of an intravenous barbiturate or benzodiazepine in small doses. Intravenous opioids are effective in suppressing cough reflexes, but the doses required impair spontaneous ventilation to the point of apnea. A combination of an intravenous opioid and a major tranquilizer (eg, neuroleptic analgesia) allows the patient to tolerate an endotracheal tube with much smaller doses of the opioid and less embarrassment of spontaneous ventilation. Small doses of opioids are also useful in obtunding airway reflexes during general anesthesia provided by either intravenous (eg, thiopental) or inhaled anesthetics (eg, isoflurane). Not only do the opioids obtund the cough reflex that results in closure of the larynx, but they also are useful in limiting the autonomic sympathetic response to endotracheal intubation that typically leads to hypertension and tachycardia.

Skeletal muscle relaxants are used most commonly in conjunction with a general anesthetic to allow manipulation of the head and jaw and prevent reflex closure of the larynx. Of course, they also render the patient apneic, and two procedures are used commonly to maintain oxygenation of the patient's blood. First, the patient breathes 100% oxygen by mask while still awake to eliminate nitrogen from the lungs, and then a rapid-sequence administration of an intravenous anesthetic (eg, thiopental) is followed immediately by a rapid-acting neuromuscular blocker (eg, succinylcholine or rocuronium), and cricoid pressure is applied (Sellick maneuver). As soon as the muscle relaxation is apparent (30 to 90 seconds), laryngoscopy is performed, an endotracheal tube is inserted, the tracheal tube cuff is inflated, and the position of the tube in the trachea is verified. Second, when there is minimal risk of pulmonary aspiration (eg, presumed empty stomach), the patient is anesthetized and paralyzed while ventilation is supported by intermittent positive pressure delivered via a face mask. At the appropriate time, laryngoscopy is performed and the endotracheal tube is inserted.

Normalizing Pulmonary Function during Positive-Pressure Ventilation

Once an endotracheal tube is in place, it is common practice in the operating room to maintain general anesthesia and partial muscular paralysis in order to facilitate positive-pressure ventilation and continued toleration of the endotracheal tube by the patient. Postoperatively, in the post-anesthesia care unit (PACU) and intensive care unit (ICU), general anesthesia and partial muscular paralysis may be continued if prolonged positive-pressure ventilation is anticipated, or sedatives may be administered by intravenous infusion to allow toleration of the endotracheal tube in anticipation of recovery of spontaneous ventilation and tracheal extubation.

Three other problems are encountered in the patient whose ventilation is supported mechanically by an endotracheal tube: (1) poor ventilatory compliance; (2) bronchoconstriction; and (3) impaired gas exchange. Poor ventilatory compliance can reflect limited compliance of the chest wall and diaphragm, limited compliance of the lungs per se, or both. Deepening general anesthesia and administration of a skeletal muscle relaxant can be used to reduce intercostal and diaphragmatic muscle tone, but they obviously cannot improve the chest cavity compliance that is fixed by disease (eg, scoliosis or emphysema).

Poor lung compliance may reflect pulmonary interstitial edema, consolidation, bronchial obstruction (eg, mucus plugs), bronchoconstriction, or compression of the lung by intrathoracic substances (eg, pneumothorax, hemothorax, or tumor mass). Treatment of these involves drug therapy of HF and infection and procedures such as bronchoscopy and thoracentesis.

Bronchoconstriction may exist chronically (eg, asthma or reactive airways disease), and these conditions can be exacerbated by the collection of tracheobronchial secretions in the presence of an endotracheal tube, which reduces the effectiveness of coughing in clearing the airway. Occasionally bronchoconstriction can be induced by mechanical stimulation of the airway by an endotracheal tube or other object in an otherwise normal patient. Drug treatment is focused on reducing bronchial smooth muscle tone (eg, beta$_2$ sympathomimetic or anticholinergic agents), minimizing tracheal bronchial secretions, and decreasing sensory input from the tracheal bronchial tree (eg, topical anesthetic, deeper general anesthesia, intravenous lidocaine, or an opioid). Acute treatment of bronchoconstriction may involve any combination of the following: (1) an aerosolized beta$_2$ sympathomimetic and/or anticholinergic agent; and (2) systemic intravenous administration of a beta$_2$ sympathomimetic agent, a phosphodiesterase inhibitor (eg, theophylline salts [aminophylline]), and/or an anticholinergic agent.

Intravenous steroids are indicated in severe bronchoconstriction, especially in asthmatic patients, for whom they have been effective in the past. With the administration of 100% oxygen, blood oxygenation usually is not the main problem in patients with bronchoconstriction; the progressive development of hypercarbia and the trapping of air in lung parenchyma reduce ventilatory compliance and increase intrathoracic pressure. These, in turn, reduce venous return and may cause a tamponade-like impairment of cardiac function.

Impaired alveolar-capillary membrane gas exchange can result from alveolar pulmonary edema (treated by diuretics, inotropes, and vasodilators), decreased pulmonary perfusion (treated by inotropes and vasodilators), and lung consolidation (antibiotic therapy for infection).

Restoration of Spontaneous Ventilation and Airway Protective Mechanisms

The anesthesiologist attempts to tailor the anesthetic plan according to postoperative expectations for the patient. In the relatively healthy patient for whom tracheal extubation can be anticipated in the operating room, the goal is to have the patient breathing spontaneously with airway reflexes intact and the patient arousable to command immediately on completion of the operation. The challenge for the anesthesiologist is to maintain satisfactory general anesthesia through the entire course of the operation and yet have the patient sufficiently recovered from anesthetic drugs, including hypnotics and opioids, shortly after conclusion of the operation. If this is not possible, then the patient is transferred to the PACU to allow additional time for elimination of drugs that depress spontaneous ventilation and cough reflexes. Another possibility is to administer antagonists to opioids (eg, naloxone) and benzodiazepines (eg, flumazenil), but this approach risks sudden awakening, pain, and uncontrolled autonomic sympathetic activity leading to undesirable hemodynamic changes. And there is the risk of recurrent ventilatory depression because it is difficult to match the doses of the antagonists to the residual amounts of anesthetic drugs. On the other hand, it is fairly routine for the effects of neuromuscular blockers to be antagonized by administration of an anticholinesterase (eg, neostigmine) in combination with an anticholinergic agent (eg, atropine) to limit the autonomic cholinergic side effects of the anticholinesterase.

When the expectation is for maintenance of mechanical ventilation for some time in the postoperative period, then the patient's tolerance of the endotracheal tube is facilitated by the persistent effect of residual anesthetic drugs subsequently supplemented by administration of intravenous hypnotics (eg, propofol) and opioids (eg, fentanyl or morphine). These agents can be associated with side effects, including respiratory depression, especially when they are used concurrently. Dexmedetomidine (Precedex), an alpha$_2$-adrenergic agonist, may offer advantages for sedation during weaning from mechanical ventilation because it provides sedation, pain relief, anxiety reduction, stable respiratory rates, and predictable cardiovascular responses. Dexmedetomidine facilitates patient comfort, compliance, and comprehension by offering sedation with the ability to rouse patients. This "arousability" allows patients to remain sedated yet communicate with health-care workers.

When the appropriate time comes to have the patient take over his or her own ventilation completely, these sedative and analgesic drugs are weaned to a level allowing satisfactory maintenance of blood oxygenation and carbon dioxide removal, easy arousal of the patient, and at least partial restoration of airway reflex mechanisms.

Pharmacology Related to Airway and Lung Management

Cardiac surgical patients are usually kept intubated and ventilated at the end of surgery, and ventilator support is withdrawn in the ICU. Sedative drugs are required to facilitate this transfer from operating room to intensive care, and while the patient is ventilated. Some patients require continued ventilation because of primary pulmonary disease, underlying cardiac disease and/or perioperative complications. Others may require medications to treat bronchospasm or airway obstruction, or to facilitate reintubation if they develop respiratory failure once extubated.

Sedative Medications to Facilitate Mechanical Ventilation

PROPOFOL

The medications used in cardiac surgery patients are the same as those used in other mechanically ventilated patients. A common approach is to use propofol, an intravenous anesthetic/sedative agent that is rapidly eliminated by the liver

and therefore facilitates rapid awakening. This drug is not water soluble so is supplied in a lipid emulsion; for short-term infusions (less than a day or two) lipid accumulation is not an issue, but triglyceride levels should be measured if the drug is given in high doses, especially at the same time as intravenous feeding. The hemodynamic effects of propofol are mostly a result of vasodilation, both arterial and venous, as well as the usual "withdrawal of sympathetic tone," which occurs when anxious, stressed patients are sedated. In addition there is a mild bradycardia and blunted heart rate response to hypotension, and a mild negative inotropic effect usually not relevant at clinical doses. The clinical dose range for sedation is 25 to 75 µg/kg per minute but must be titrated.

Benzodiazepines

Benzodiazepines are also used to facilitate mechanical ventilation, commonly midazolam (Versed) or lorazepam (Ativan). These drugs do not have the vasodilating effects of propofol, are good amnestic agents, but have a major disadvantage in that awakening is less predictable and more often prolonged, especially with lorazepam. In addition, these drugs appear to be more associated with postoperative delirium than other sedative drugs. Despite these problems, benzodiazepines are useful in the sedation of severely hypotensive patients requiring vasoconstrictor support. They have minimal, if any, direct cardiovascular effects, but withdrawal of sympathetic tone can lead to hypotension. Midazolam is usually administered as a continuous infusion of 1 to 4 mg/h, while lorazepam is most often given by intermittent dosing of 1 to 2 mg every 4 to 6 hours.

Dexmedetomidine

A relatively new addition to the sedative drug family is dexmedetomidine (Precedex), a centrally acting alpha$_2$ agonist. This drug is the same class as clonidine, but has a much greater affinity for the alpha receptor. Not surprisingly, the most common hemodynamic effect, which sometimes limits its use, is bradycardia and hypotension. This drug can be used as a single agent to facilitate transfer from the operating room (OR) to the ICU and the period of ventilator weaning and extubation. The major advantage of dexmedetomidine is that it does not affect ventilatory drive and patients can usually be aroused while receiving the drug. It also has a significant analgesic component, different from propofol or the benzodiazepines. The usual infusion rate of dexmedetomidine is 0.2 to 0.7 µg/kg per hour, preceded by a loading dose of 1 µg/kg over 20 to 30 minutes. The loading dose can be reduced or not given if hemodynamics warrant.

Opioids

The main reason patients need sedation during mechanical ventilation is to tolerate the presence of a transoral tracheal tube. In addition to general discomfort, there is continuous airway stimulation by the foreign object. To blunt airway reflexes as well as to treat postoperative pain, it is useful to add an opioid drug to whichever sedative agent the patient is receiving. For early postoperative awakening (ie, in the first hours), this is less of an issue as there is usually residual opioid effect from drugs given intraoperatively; however, patients will need additional opioid as they awaken and experience pain. For patients ventilated overnight or longer, use of opioid drugs will have these same benefits and likely result in a reduced need for the sedative drug. Fentanyl is a commonly used drug in this setting, partly because it has a rapid onset of action and relatively rapid recovery if dosing is not prolonged. Infusions of 1 to 4 μg/kg per hour are used. Alternatively intermittent dosing with 1 to 4 mg morphine or 0.5 to 1 mg hydromorphone (Dilaudid) every 1 to 4 hours may be employed.

Medications Used to Facilitate Urgent Tracheal Intubation

Patients in extremis (eg, during cardiac or respiratory arrest) rarely require medications to facilitate intubation. In decompensating patients who are fully or partially conscious, challenges may include agitation, resistance to opening the mouth, and/or closed vocal cords when intubation is attempted. In some patients small doses of sedative/opioid medications with a rapid onset such as midazolam and fentanyl, respectively, are adequate; in others an anesthetic induction agent such as propofol or etomidate can be used, with or without a paralytic drug. The disadvantage to propofol is hypotension caused by vasodilation, as referred to in the preceding. This drug should be used in incremental doses, 10 to 20 mg at time, until a dose of 1 to 2 mg/kg has been given. Etomidate has no direct cardiovascular effects and is usually given in a dose of 0.15 to 0.3 mg/kg. This drug has an unusual side effect of impairing steroid synthesis and has been associated with adrenal insufficiency in critically ill patients when given by infusion. In addition, many patients experience unusual movements as this drug is administered. In general, the use of paralytic drugs is discouraged unless there is an anesthesiology provider or someone skilled in the use of these drugs and airway management present.

Succinylcholine is the most rapidly acting paralytic agent with an onset of 30 to 60 seconds and is given in a dose of 1 mg/kg. This depolarizing agent causes potassium release and must be avoided in hyperkalemic patients. It causes stimulation of muscarinic and nicotinic receptors, an increase in serum catecholamines, and many different, usually mild, dysrhythmias have been reported. Alternatively, rocuronium in a dose of 0.5 mg/kg can be given, but 60 to 90 seconds are required for adequate paralysis. Rocuronium in this dose has no cardiovascular effect. If an anesthetic induction agent and/or a neuromuscular blocking agent are being considered, an important issue is the possibility of aspiration of stomach contents. In an urgent situation the risk of this is reduced if the drugs are administered in rapid sequence with an assistant providing cricoid pressure (to occlude the esophagus), and manual ventilation is minimized until the tube is in place.

Drugs to Treat Airway Pathology: Stridor/Edema, Bronchospasm, Secretions

Fluid overload, prolonged positioning with the head dependent, or superior vena cava obstruction may all lead to edema of the upper airway. Alternatively, trauma from intubation or other devices in the oropharynx (eg, transesophageal echocardiography [TEE] probe) may cause glottis edema. There may be edema below the cords resulting from presence of the endotracheal tube/cuff. The common treatments for airway narrowing resulting from edema are: (1) use of a mixture of helium/oxygen; (2) inhaled racemic epinephrine; (3) diuretics and head-up position; and (4) a brief course of dexamethasone (IV).

Helium/Oxygen. Helium with oxygen (Heliox) is supplied as an 80:20 mix. Helium is less dense than nitrogen, facilitating laminar rather than turbulent flow through a narrowed airway. If a patient cannot tolerate the relatively low concentration of oxygen (20%), then additional oxygen will need to be administered. Although the greatest benefit is provided by 80% helium, concentrations of 40 to 50% provide some benefit.

Racemic Epinephrine. Racemic epinephrine is supplied as 1% solution and administered through an aerosol mask in a dose of 2.5 mL to cause vasoconstriction and reduced airway edema. Absorption of epinephrine can cause tachycardia and hypertension.

Diuretics and Dexamethasone. Specific diuretic drugs are discussed in the preceding; when a rapid effect is desired, then usually a loop diuretic such as furosemide is employed. Although this may not specifically treat airway edema, the combination of elevated head and diuresis will reduce edema in the upper body. Dexamethasone is used as part of the "steroids for anything that swells" philosophy. There is little evidence of efficacy of corticosteroids in this setting; dexamethasone is used to avoid the mineralocorticoid effect of other potent intravenous steroid preparations. The usual dose is 8 mg followed by 4 mg every 6 hours for four to eight doses.

Bronchodilators and Mucolytics. A summary of bronchodilator and mucolytic drugs is given in Table 4-7. In the cardiac surgical patient, wheezing is more likely because of fluid overload or left ventricular failure than primary bronchospastic disease, but inhaled bronchodilators may give some relief while treatment of the primary disorder is being instituted (eg, diuresis or administration of an inotropic drug). In order of preference, inhaled beta agonists, anticholinergic agents, and intravenous steroids are used.[137] All three

TABLE 4-7: Inhaled Bronchodilators and Mucolytics

	Drug	Mechanism	Dosage	Frequency
Bronchodilators	Albuterol	Beta$_2$ agonist	2.5 mg/3 mL	Q 4-6 h[*]
	Levalbuterol	Beta$_2$ agonist	0.63-1.25 mg/3 mL	Q 6 h
	Ipratropium	Anticholinergic	0.5 mg/3 mL	Q 4-6 h
Mucolytic	Dornase alpha	Cleaves DNA	2.5 mg/3 cc	Q 12 h

*May be given more frequently.

may be indicated. Beta agonists relax smooth muscle in the airways and usually have the most rapid therapeutic effect. In the acute setting aerosolized drug via a facemask is more effective than metered-dose inhalers. It should be noted that management of chronic asthma focuses on inhaled anti-inflammatory agents, but these drugs are not helpful in the acute setting, such as postoperatively. The presence of tenacious secretions should prompt consideration of an inhaled mucolytic such as dornase/DNAse (Pulmozyme). *N*-acetylcysteine (Mucomyst) is another mucolytic but may cause airway irritation so should not be given in the setting of acute bronchospasm. See the table for dosages of these drugs (see Table 4-7).

REFERENCES

1. Lynch C III: Cellular electrophysiology of the heart, in Lynch C III (ed): *Cellular Cardiac Electrophysiology: Perioperative Considerations.* Philadelphia, Lippincott, 1994; p 1.
2. Katz AM: Cardiac ion channels. *N Engl J Med* 1993; 328:1244.
3. Colucci WS, Wright RF, Braunwald E: New positive inotropic agents in the treatment of heart failure, part I. *N Engl J Med* 1986; 314:290.
4. Colucci WS, Wright RF, Braunwald E: New positive inotropic agents in the treatment of heart failure, part II. *N Engl J Med* 1986; 314:349.
5. Terzic A, Puceat M, Vassort G, Vogel SM: Cardiac alpha$_1$ adrenoreceptors: an overview. *Pharmacol Rev* 1993; 45:147.
6. Berridge MJ: Inositol lipids and calcium signaling. *Proc R Soc Lond (Biol)* 1988; 234:359.
7. Lucchesi BR: Role of calcium on excitation-coupling in cardiac and vascular smooth muscle. *Circulation* 1978; 8:IV-1.
8. Kukovertz WR, Poch G, Holzmann S: Cyclic nucleotides and relaxation of vascular smooth muscle, in Vanhoutte PM, Leusen I (eds): *Vasodilation.* New York, Raven Press, 1981; p 339.
9. Singh BN, Sarma JS: Mechanisms of action of antiarrhythmic drugs relative to the origin and perpetuation of cardiac arrhythmias. *J Cardiovasc Pharmacol Ther* 2001; 6:69.
10. Pinter A, Dorian P: Intravenous antiarrhythmic agents. *Curr Opin Cardiol* 2001; 16:17.
11. Roden DM: Antiarrhythmic drugs: from mechanisms to clinical practice. *Heart* 2000; 84:339.
12. Vaughan Williams EM: A classification of antiarrhythmic agents reassessed after a decade of new drugs. *J Clin Pharmacol* 1984; 24:129.
13. The Task Force of the Working Group on Arrhythmias of the European Society of Cardiology: The "Sicilian gambit": a new approach to the classification of antiarrhythmic drugs based on their actions on arrhythmic mechanisms. *Eur Heart J* 1991; 12:1112.
14. Hondeghem LM: Antiarrhythmic agents: modulated receptor applications. *Circulation* 1987; 75:514.
15. Zipes DP, Camm AJ, Borggrefe M, et al: ACC/AHA/ESC 2006 Guidelines for Management of Patients with Ventricular Arrhythmias and the Prevention of Sudden Cardiac Death: a report of the American College of Cardiology/American Heart Association Task Force and the European Society of Cardiology Committee for Practice Guidelines (writing committee to develop Guidelines for Management of Patients With Ventricular Arrhythmias and the Prevention of Sudden Cardiac Death): developed in collaboration with the European Heart Rhythm Association and the Heart Rhythm Society. *Circulation* 2006; 114:e385.
16. Hoffman BF, Rosen MR, Wit AL: Electrophysiology and pharmacology of cardiac arrhythmias: VII. Cardiac effects of quinidine and procainamide. *Am Heart J* 1975; 90:117.
17. Giardenia EG, Heissenbuttel RH, Bigger JT Jr: Intermittent intravenous procaine amide to treat ventricular arrhythmias: correlation of plasma concentration with effect on arrhythmia, electrocardiogram, and blood pressure. *Ann Intern Med* 1973; 78:183.
18. Stiell IG, Wells GA, Field B, et al: Advanced cardiac life support in out-of-hospital cardiac arrest. *N Engl J Med* 2004; 351:647.
19. The 2010 American Heart Association Guidelines for Cardiopulmonary Resuscitation and Emergency Cardiovascular Care. *Circulation* 2010; 122:S639.
20. Cardiac Arrhythmia Suppression Trial (CAST) Investigators: Preliminary report, effect of encainide and flecainide on mortality in a randomized trial of arrhythmia suppression after myocardial infarction. *N Engl J Med* 1989; 321:406.
21. Echt DS, Liebson PR, Mitchell LB, et al: Mortality and morbidity in patients receiving encainide, flecainide or placebo: the cardiac arrhythmia suppression trial. *N Engl J Med* 1991; 324:781.
22. Escande D, Henry P: Potassium channels as pharmacologic targets in cardiovascular medicine. *Eur Heart J* 1993; 14:2.
23. Singh BN: Arrhythmia control by prolonging repolarization: the concept and its potential therapeutic impact. *Eur Heart J* 1993; 14:14.
24. Kudenchuk PJ: Advanced cardiac life support antiarrhythmic drugs. *Cardiol Clin* 2002; 20:79.
25. Balser JR: Perioperative arrhythmias: incidence, risk assessment, evaluation, and management. *Card Electrophysiol Rev* 2002; 6:96.
26. Mahmarian JJ, Verani MS, Pratt CM: Hemodynamic effects of intravenous and oral sotalol. *Am J Cardiol* 1990; 65:28A.
27. Levy JH, Huraux C, Nordlander M: Treatment of perioperative hypertension, in Epstein M (ed): *Calcium Antagonists in Clinical Medicine.* Philadelphia, Hanley and Belfus, 1997; p 345.
28. Conti VR, Ware DL: Cardiac arrhythmias in cardiothoracic surgery. *Chest Surg Clin North Am* 2002; 12:439.
29. Waxman HL, Myerburg RJ, Appel R, Sung RJ: Verapamil for control of ventricular rate in paroxysmal supraventricular tachycardia and atrial fibrillation or flutter: a double-blind randomized cross-over study. *Ann Intern Med* 1981; 94:1.
30. Salerno DM, Dias VC, Kleiger RE, et al: Efficacy and safety of intravenous diltiazem for treatment of atrial fibrillation and atrial flutter: the DiltiazemAtrial Fibrillation/Flutter Study Group. *Am J Cardiol* 1989; 63:1046.
31. Ellenbogen KA, Dias VC, Plumb VJ, et al: A placebo-controlled trial of continuous intravenous diltiazem infusion for 24-hour heart rate control during atrial fibrillation and atrial flutter: a multi-center study. *J Am Coll Cardiol* 1991; 18:891.
32. Smith TW, Antman EM, Friedman PL, et al: Digitalis glycosides: mechanisms and manifestations of toxicity, part I. *Prog Cardiovasc Dis* 1984; 26:413.
33. DiMarco JP, Sellers TD, Berne RM, et al: Adenosine: electrophysiological effects and therapeutic use for terminating paroxysmal supraventricular tachycardia. *Circulation* 1983; 68:1254.

34. Hollifield JW: Potassium and magnesium abnormalities: diuretics and arrhythmias in hypertension. *Am J Med* 1984; 77:28.

35. England MR, Gordon G, Salem M, Chernow B: Magnesium administration and dysrhythmia after cardiac surgery: a placebo-controlled, double-blind, randomized trial. *JAMA* 1992; 268:2395.

36. Singh BN, Vaughan Williams EM: The effect of amiodarone, a new antianginal drug, on cardiac muscle. *Br J Pharmacol* 1970; 39:657.

37. Connolly SJ: Evidence-based analysis of amiodarone efficacy and safety. *Circulation* 1999; 100:2025.

38. Chow MS: Intravenous amiodarone: pharmacology, pharmacokinetics, and clinical use. *Ann Pharmacother* 1996; 30:637.

39. Mitchell LB, Wyse G, Gillis AM, Duff HJ: Electropharmacology of amiodarone therapy initiation. *Circulation* 1989; 80:34.

40. Holt DW, Tucker GT, Jackson PR, Storey GCA: Amiodarone pharmacokinetics. *Am Heart J* 1983; 106:840.

41. Fogoros RN, Anderson KP, Winkle RA, et al: Amiodarone: clinical efficacy and toxicity in 96 patients with recurrent, drug-refractory arrhythmias. *Circulation* 1983; 68:88.

42. Kowey PR, Levine JH, Herre JM, et al: Randomized, double-blind comparison of intravenous amiodarone and bretylium in the treatment of patients with recurrent, hemodynamically destabilizing ventricular tachycardia or fibrillation. *Circulation* 1995; 92:3255.

43. Kudenchuk PJ, Cobb LA, Copass MK, et al: Amiodarone for resuscitation after out-of-hospital cardiac arrest due to ventricular fibrillation. *N Engl J Med* 1999; 341:871.

44. Levine JH, Massumi A, Scheinman MM, et al: Intravenous amiodarone for recurrent sustained hypotensive ventricular tachyarrhythmias. Intravenous Amiodarone Multicenter Trial Group. *J Am Coll Cardiol* 1996; 27:67.

45. Morady F, Sauve MJ, Malone P, et al: Long-term efficacy and toxicity of high-dose amiodarone therapy for ventricular tachycardia or ventricular fibrillation. *Am J Cardiol* 1983; 52:975.

46. Scheinman MM, Levine JH, Cannom DS, et al: Dose-ranging study of intravenous amiodarone in patients with life-threatening ventricular tachyarrhythmias. *Circulation* 1995; 92:3264.

47. Scheinman MM, Winkle RA, Platia EV, et al: Intravenous amiodarone for recurrent sustained hypotensive ventricular tachyarrhythmias. *J Am Coll Cardiol* 1996; 27:67.

48. Dorian P, Cass D, Schwartz B, et al: Amiodarone as compared with lidocaine for shock-resistant ventricular fibrillation. *N Engl J Med* 2002; 346:884.

49. Kupferschmid JP, Rosengart TK, McIntosh CL, et al: Amiodarone-induced complications after cardiac operation for obstructive hypertrophic cardiomyopathy. *Ann Thorac Surg* 1989; 48:359.

50. Rady MY, Ryan T, Starr NJ: Preoperative therapy with amiodarone and the incidence of acute organ dysfunction after cardiac surgery. *Anesth Analg* 1997; 85:489.

51. Daoud EG, Strickberger SA, Man KC, et al: Preoperative amiodarone as prophylaxis against atrial fibrillation after heart surgery. *N Engl J Med* 1997; 337:1785.

52. Dorge H, Schoendube FA, Schoberer M, et al: Intraoperative amiodarone as prophylaxis against atrial fibrillation after coronary operations. *Ann Thorac Surg* 2000; 69:1358.

53. Giri S, White CM, Dunn AB, et al: Oral amiodarone for prevention of atrial fibrillation after open-heart surgery, the Atrial Fibrillation Suppression Trial (AFIST): a randomised, placebo-controlled trial. *Lancet* 2001; 357:830.

54. Guarnieri T, Nolan S, Gottlieb SO, et al: Intravenous amiodarone for the prevention of atrial fibrillation after open-heart surgery: the amiodarone reduction in coronary heart (ARCH) trial. *J Am Coll Cardiol* 1999; 34:343.

55. Lee SH, Chang CM, Lu MJ, et al: Intravenous amiodarone for prevention of atrial fibrillation after coronary artery bypass grafting. *Ann Thorac Surg* 2000; 70:157.

56. Carlson MD: How to manage atrial fibrillation: an update on recent clinical trials. *Cardiol Rev* 2001; 9:60.

57. Fuster V, Ryden LE, Asinger RN, et al: ACC/AHA/ESC guidelines for the management of patients with atrial fibrillation: executive summary. *Circulation* 2001; 104:2118.

58. Maisel WH, Rawn JD, Stevenson WG: Atrial fibrillation after cardiac surgery. *Ann Intern Med* 2001; 135:1061.

59. Hogue CW Jr., Hyder ML: Atrial fibrillation after cardiac operation: risks, mechanisms, and treatment. *Ann Thorac Surg* 2000; 69:300.

60. Reddy P, Richerson M, Freeman-Bosco L, et al: Cost-effectiveness of amiodarone for prophylaxis of atrial fibrillation in coronary artery bypass surgery. *Am J Health Syst Pharm* 1999; 56:2211.

61. Reiffel JA: Drug choices in the treatment of atrial fibrillation. *Am J Cardiol* 2000; 85:12D.

62. Daoud EG, Strickberger SA, Man KC, et al: Preoperative amiodarone as prophylaxis against atrial fibrillation after heart surgery. *N Engl J Med* 1997; 337:1785.

63. Gray R, Maddahi J, Berman D, et al: Scintigraphic and hemodynamic demonstration of transient left ventricular dysfunction immediately after uncomplicated coronary artery bypass grafting. *J Thorac Cardiovasc Surg* 1979; 77:504.

64. Mangano DT: Biventricular function after myocardial revascularization in humans: deterioration and recovery patterns during the first 24 hours. *Anesthesiology* 1985; 62:571.

65. Breisblatt WM, Stein K, Wolfe CJ, et al: Acute myocardial dysfunction and recovery: a common occurrence after coronary bypass surgery. *J Am Coll Cardiol* 1990; 15:1261.

66. Fabiato A, Fabiato F: Calcium and cardiac excitation-contraction coupling. *Ann Rev Physiol* 1979; 41:473.

67. Figgitt DP, Gillies PS, Goa KL: Levosimendan. *Drugs* 2001; 61:613.

68. Doggrell SA, Brown L: Present and future pharmacotherapy for heart failure. *Exp Opin Pharmacother* 2002; 3:915.

69. Endoh M: Mechanism of action of Ca^2 sensitizers—update 2001. *Cardiovasc Drugs Ther* 2001; 15:397.

70. Drop LJ, Geffin GA, O'Keefe DD, et al: Relation between ionized calcium concentration and ventricular pump performance in the dog under hemodynamically controlled conditions. *Am J Cardiol* 1981; 47:1041.

71. Zaloga GP, Strickland RA, Butterworth JF, et al: Calcium attenuates epinephrine's β-adrenergic effects in postoperative heart surgery patients. *Circulation* 1990; 81:196.

72. Engelman RM, Hadji-Rousou I, Breyer RH, et al: Rebound vasospasm after coronary revascularization in association with calcium antagonist withdrawal. *Ann Thorac Surg* 1984; 37:469.

73. Cheung JY, Bonventre JV, Malis CD, Leaf A: Calcium and ischemic injury. *N Engl J Med* 1986; 314:1670.

74. Del Monte F, Kaumann AJ, Poole-Wilson PA, et al: Coexistence of functioning β₁- and β₂-adrenoreceptors in single myocytes from human ventricle. *Circulation* 1993; 88:854.

75. Bristow MR, Ginsburg R, Minobe W, et al: Decreased catecholamine sensitivity and β-adrenergic receptor density in failing human hearts. *N Engl J Med* 1982; 307:205.

76. Schwinn DA, Leone BJ, Spahn DR, et al: Desensitization of myocardial β-adrenergic receptors during cardiopulmonary bypass: evidence for early uncoupling and late down-regulation. *Circulation* 1991; 84:2559.

77. Port JD, Gilbert EM, Larabee P, et al: Neurotransmitter depletion compromises the ability of indirect acting amines to provide inotropic support in the failing human heart. *Circulation* 1990; 81:929.

78. De Backer D, Biston P, Devriendt J, et al: SOAP II Investigators. Comparison of dopamine and norepinephrine in the treatment of shock. *N Engl J Med* 2010; 362(9):779-789.

79. Levy JH: Treating shock—old drugs, new ideas. *N Engl J Med* 2010; 362(9):841-843.

80. Prielipp RC, Butterworth JF 4th, Zaloga GP, et al: Effects of amrinone on cardiac index, venous oxygen saturation and venous admixture in patients recovering from cardiac surgery. *Chest* 1991; 99:820.

81. Levy JH, Bailey JM: Amrinone: its effects on vascular resistance and capacitance in human subjects. *Chest* 1994; 105:62.

82. Levy JH, Bailey JM, Deeb GM: Intravenous milrinone in cardiac surgery. *Ann Thorac Surg* 2002; 73:325.

83. Bailey JM, Levy JH, Kikura M, et al: Pharmacokinetics of intravenous milrinone in patients undergoing cardiac surgery. *Anesthesiology* 1994; 81:616.

84. Feneck RO: Effects of variable dose in patients with low cardiac output after cardiac surgery. European Multicenter Trial Group. *Am Heart J* 1991; 121:1995.

85. Kikura M, Levy JH, Michelsen LG, et al: The effect of milrinone on hemodynamics and left ventricular function after emergence from cardio-pulmonary bypass. *Anesth Analg* 1997; 85:16.

86. Butterworth JF 4th, Hines RL, Royster RL, James RL: A pharmacokinetic and pharmacodynamic evaluation of milrinone in adults undergoing cardiac surgery. *Anesth Analg* 1995; 81:783.

87. Doolan LA, Jones EF, Kalman J, et al: A placebo-controlled trial verifying the efficacy of milrinone in weaning high-risk patients from cardiopulmonary bypass. *J Cardiothorac Vasc Anesth* 1997; 11:37.

88. Unverzagt S, Wachsmuth L, Hirsch K, et al: Inotropic agents and vasodilator strategies for acute myocardial infarction complicated by cardiogenic shock or low cardiac output syndrome. *Cochrane Database Syst Rev.* 2014 Jan 2 (ePub).

89. Follath F, Cleland JG, Just H, et al: Efficacy and safety of intravenous levosimendan compared with dobutamine in severe low-output heart failure (the LIDO study): a randomised double-blind trial. *Lancet* 2002; 360:196.

90. Slawsky MT, Colucci WS, Gottlieb SS, et al: Acute hemodynamic and clinical effects of levosimendan in patients with severe heart failure. *Circulation* 2000; 102:2222.

91. Steen H, Tinker JH, Pluth JR, et al: Efficacy of dopamine, dobutamine, and epinephrine during emergence from cardiopulmonary bypass in man. *Circulation* 1978; 57:378.

92. Salomon NW, Plachetka JR, Copeland JG: Comparison of dopamine and dobutamine following coronary artery bypass grafting. *Ann Thorac Surg* 1981; 3:48.

93. Fowler MB, Alderman EL, Oesterle SN, et al: Dobutamine and dopamine after cardiac surgery: greater augmentation of myocardial blood flow with dobutamine. *Circulation* 1984; 70:1103.

94. Sethna DH, Gray RJ, Moffit EA, et al: Dobutamine and cardiac oxygen balance in patients following myocardial revascularization. *Anesth Analg* 1982; 61:917.

95. Butterworth JF 4th, Prielipp RC, Royster RL, et al: Dobutamine increases heart rate more than epinephrine in patients recovering from aortocoronary bypass surgery. *J Cardiothorac Vasc Anesth* 1992; 6:535.

96. Feneck RO, Sherry KM, Withington S, et al: Comparison of the hemodynamic effects of milrinone with dobutamine in patients after cardiac surgery. *J Cardiothorac Vasc Anesth* 2001; 15:306.

97. Meier-Hellmann A, Reinhart K, Bredle DL, et al: Epinephrine impairs splanchnic perfusion in septic shock. *Crit Care Med* 1997; 25:399.

98. Levy B, Bollaert PE, Charpentier C, et al: Comparison of norepinephrine and dobutamine to epinephrine for hemodynamics, lactate metabolism, and gastric tonometric variables in septic shock: a prospective, randomized study. *Intensive Care Med* 1997; 23:282.

99. Ruokonen E, Takala J, Kari A, et al: Regional blood flow and oxygen transport in septic shock. *Crit Care Med* 1993; 21:1296.

100. Meier-Hellmann A, Bredle DL, Specht M, et al: The effects of low-dose dopamine on splanchnic blood flow and oxygen utilization in patients with septic shock. *Intensive Care Med* 1997; 23:31.

101. Marik PE, Mohedin M: The contrasting effects of dopamine and norepinephrine on systemic and splanchnic oxygen utilization in hyperdynamic sepsis. *JAMA* 1994; 272:1354.

102. Landry DW, Oliver JA: The pathogenesis of vasodilatory shock. *N Engl J Med* 2001; 345:588.

103. Levy JH: *Anaphylactic Reactions in Anesthesia and Intensive Care*, 2nd ed. Boston, Butterworth-Heinemann, 1992.

104. Desjars P, Pinaud M, Potel G, et al: A reappraisal of norepinephrine in human septic shock. *Crit Care Med* 1987; 15:134.

105. Meadows D, Edwards JD, Wilkins RG, Nightingale P: Reversal of intractable septic shock with norepinephrine therapy. *Crit Care Med* 1998; 16:663.

106. Hesselvik JF, Broden B: Low dose norepinephrine in patient with septic shock and oliguria: effects on afterload, urine flow, and oxygen transport. *Crit Care Med* 1989; 17:179.

107. Martin C, Eon B, Saux P, et al: Renal effects of norepinephrine used to treat septic shock patients. *Crit Care Med* 1990; 18:282.

108. Marik PE, Mohedin M: The contrasting effects of dopamine and norepinephrine on systemic and splanchnic oxygen utilization in hyperdynamic sepsis. *JAMA* 1994; 272:1354.

109. Argenziano M, Chen JM, Choudhri AF, et al: Management of vasodilatory shock after cardiac surgery: identification of predisposing factors and use of a novel pressor agent. *J Thorac Cardiovasc Surg* 1998; 116:973.

110. Landry DW, Levin HR, Gallant EM, et al: Vasopressin deficiency in vasodilatory septic shock. *Crit Care Med* 1997; 25:1279.

111. Gold JA, Cullinane S, Chen J, et al: Vasopressin as an alternative to norepinephrine in the treatment of milrinone-induced hypotension. *Crit Care Med* 2000; 28:249.

112. Levy JH: The ideal agent for perioperative hypertension. *Acta Anaesth Scand* 1993; 37:20.

113. Huraux C, Makita T, Montes F, Szlam F: A comparative evaluation of the effects of multiple vasodilators on human internal mammary artery. *Anesthesiology* 1998; 88:1654.

114. Harrison DG, Bates JN: The nitrovasodilators: new ideas about old drugs. *Circulation* 1993; 87:1461.

115. Anderson TJ, Meredith IT, Ganz P, et al: Nitric oxide and nitrovasodilators: similarities, differences and potential interactions. *J Am Coll Cardiol* 1994; 24:555.

116. Harrison DG, Kurz MA, Quillen JE, et al: Normal and pathophysiologic considerations of endothelial regulation of vascular tone and their relevance to nitrate therapy. *Am J Cardiol* 1992; 70:11B.

117. Munzel T, Giaid A, Kurz S, Harrison DG: Evidence for a role of endothelin 1 and protein kinase C in nitrate tolerance. *Proc Natl Acad Sci USA* 1995; 92:5244.

118. Munzel T, Sayegh H, Freeman, Harrison DG: Evidence for enhanced vascular superoxide anion production in tolerance: a novel mechanism underlying tolerance and cross-tolerance. *J Clin Invest* 1995; 95:187.

119. Fleckenstein A: Specific pharmacology of calcium in the myocardium, cardiac pacemakers and vascular smooth muscle. *Annu Rev Pharmacol* 1977; 17:149.

120. Begon C, Dartayet B, Edouard A, et al: Intravenous nicardipine for treatment of intraoperative hypertension during abdominal surgery. *J Cardiothorac Anesth* 1989; 3:707.

121. Cheung DG, Gasster JL, Neutel JM, Weber MA: Acute pharmacokinetic and hemodynamic effects of intravenous bolus dosing of nicardipine. *Am Heart J* 1990; 119:438.

122. David D, Dubois C, Loria Y: Comparison of nicardipine and sodium nitroprusside in the treatment of paroxysmal hypertension following aortocoronary bypass surgery. *J Cardiothorac Vasc Anesth* 1991; 5:357.

123. Lambert CR, Grady T, Hashimi W, et al: Hemodynamic and angiographic comparison of intravenous nitroglycerin and nicardipine mainly in subjects without coronary artery disease. *Am J Cardiol* 1993; 71:420.

124. Singh BN, Josephson MA: Clinical pharmacology, pharmacokinetics, and hemodynamic effects of nicardipine. *Am Heart J* 1990; 119:427A.

125. Leslie J, Brister N, Levy JH, et al: Treatment of postoperative hypertension after coronary artery bypass surgery: double-blind comparison of intravenous isradipine and sodium nitroprusside. *Circulation* 1994; 90:II256.

126. Huraux C, Makita T, Montes F, et al: A comparative evaluation of the effects of multiple vasodilators on human internal mammary artery. *Anesthesiology* 1998; 88:1654.

127. Dzau VJ, Sasamura H, Hein L: Heterogeneity of angiotensin synthetic pathways and receptor subtypes: physiological and pharmacological implications. *J Hypertens* 1993; 11:S13.

128. Granger CB, Ertl G, Kuch J, et al: Randomized trial of candesartan cilexetil in the treatment of patients with congestive heart failure and a history of intolerance to angiotensin-converting enzyme inhibitors. *Am Heart J* 2000; 139:609.

129. Lefkowitz RH, Hoffman BB, Taylor P: Neurotransmission: the autonomic and somatic motor nervous system, in Hardman JL, Molinoff PB, Ruddon RW, Gilman AG (eds): *The Pharmacological Basis of Therapeutics.* New York, McGraw-Hill, 1996; p 110.

130. Fleisher LA, Beckman JA, Brown KA, et al: 2009 ACCF/AHA focused update on perioperative beta blockade incorporated into the ACC/AHA 2007 guidelines on perioperative cardiovascular evaluation and care for noncardiac surgery: a report of the American college of cardiology foundation/American Heart Association task force on practice guidelines. *Circulation* 2009; 120:e169-276.

131. James PA, Oparil S, Carter BL, et al: 2014 evidence-based guideline for the management of high blood pressure in adults: report from the panel members appointed to the Eighth Joint National Committee (JNC 8). *JAMA* 2014; 5;311(5):507-520.

132. Volpe M, Tocci G: 2007 ESH/ESC Guidelines for the management of hypertension, from theory to practice: global cardiovascular risk concept. *J Hypertens* 2009; 27(Suppl 3):S3.

133. Argalious M, Motta P, Khandwala F, et al: "Renal dose" dopamine is associated with the risk of new-onset atrial fibrillation after cardiac surgery. *Crit Care Med* 2005; 33(6):1327-1332.

134. Eisenberg DM, Davis RB, Ettner SL, et al: Trends in alternative medicine use in the United States, 1990–1997: results of a follow-up national survey. *JAMA* 1998; 280:1569.

135. Ang-Lee MK, Moss J, Yuan CS: Herbal medicines and perioperative care. *JAMA* 2001; 286:208.

136. American Society of Anesthesiologists: *What You Should Know About Your Patients' Use of Herbal Medicines*. Available at: www.asahq.org/ProfInfo/herb/herbbro.html.

137. National Heart Blood and Lung Institute, Expert Panel Report 3 (EPR3): *Guidelines for the Diagnosis and Management of Asthma*. http://www.nhlbi.nih.gov/guidelines/asthma/gdln.htm; 2007, pp 248-249.

Cardiovascular Pathology

Frederick J. Schoen • Robert F. Padera

5

Cardiovascular pathology defines the morphology and mechanisms of cardiovascular disease in individual patients and patient cohorts, both along the natural history of a disease and following surgery and interventions. The data derived through cardiovascular pathology thereby facilitate evidence-based choices among surgical or catheter-based interventional options and optimize short- and long-term patient management. Beyond implicit clinical benefit for individual patients, the discipline of cardiovascular pathology is a cornerstone of modern cardiovascular research and the preclinical development and clinical implementation of innovative drugs, devices, and other therapeutic options.

This chapter summarizes pathologic anatomy, clinicopathologic correlations, and pathophysiologic mechanisms in the various forms of structural heart disease most relevant to surgery and catheter-based interventions used to diagnose and treat the major forms of acquired structural cardiovascular disease. In view of space limitations, several important areas (eg, aortic disease) are necessarily omitted from discussion and others (eg, cardiac assist and replacement devices) are focused on details not covered elsewhere in this book. Moreover, although we have not included the key considerations herein, we are mindful that the number of adults with congenital heart disease is increasing rapidly and that they have unique and important clinical and pathologic concerns.[1,2]

MYOCARDIAL RESPONSE TO INCREASED WORK AND MYOCARDIAL DISEASE

Myocardial Hypertrophy

Hypertrophy is the compensatory response of the cardiac muscle (the *myocardium*), to increased work (Fig. 5-1).[3] This structural and functional adaptation accompanies nearly all forms of heart disease, and its consequences often dominate the clinical picture. Hypertrophy induces an increase in the overall mass and size of the heart that reflects an increased size of individual myocytes largely through addition of contractile elements (the *sarcomeres*) and associated cell and tissue elements. Substantial and functionally beneficial augmentation of myocyte number (*hyperplasia*) in response to stress or injury has not been demonstrated in the adult heart.

The pattern of hypertrophy reflects the nature of the stimulus (see Fig. 5-1B). Pressure overload (eg, in systemic hypertension or aortic stenosis) induces an increased ventricular mass, increased wall thickness, and increased ratio of wall thickness to cavity radius without dilation. In contrast, volume overload (eg, in aortic or mitral regurgitation, myocardial infarction, or dilated cardiomyopathy) promotes hypertrophy accompanied by chamber dilation, in which both ventricular radius and total mass are increased. The chamber wall is affected globally by the increased chamber pressure of hypertension, the pressure or volume overload of valvular heart disease, and in dilated cardiomyopathy. In contrast, the ischemic myocyte necrosis and loss of contractile tissue myocardial infarction induce hypertrophy only in non-infarcted regions of myocardium. The terms *concentric*, *eccentric*, and *compensatory* have previously been used to describe pressure, volume, and ischemic injury-related hypertrophy, respectively.

The constellation of changes that occur regionally following myocardial infarction, or more globally in pressure and volume overload, is called *ventricular remodeling*.[4] At a cell level, pressure overload promotes augmentation of cell width via parallel addition of sarcomeres; in contrast, volume overload and/or dilation stimulate augmentation of both cell width and length via both parallel and series addition of sarcomeres.

Hypertrophic changes initially increase the efficiency of the heart, enhance function, and are thereby adaptive. However, when these changes are excessive and prolonged, they may ultimately become deleterious and contribute to cardiac failure via several mechanisms. Because the vasculature does not proliferate and blood flow is not augmented commensurate with increased cardiac mass, hypertrophied myocardium is vulnerable to ischemic damage. Moreover, myocardial fibrous tissue is often increased. Also important are the molecular changes that accompany and likely mediate enhanced function in hypertrophied hearts, and which may subsequently

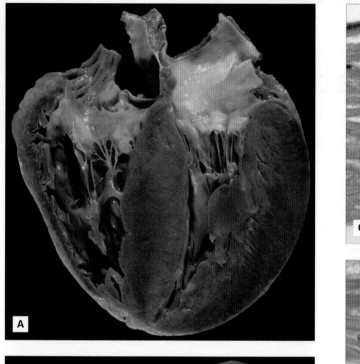

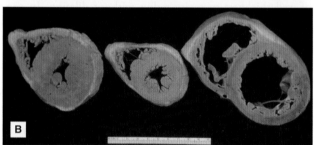

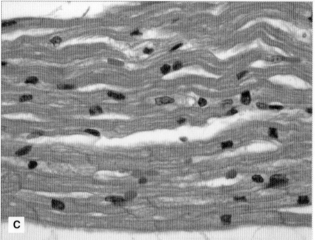

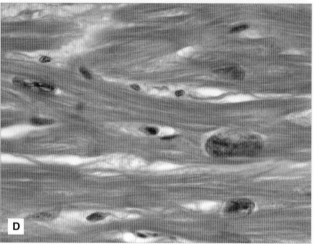

FIGURE 5-1 Summary of the gross and microscopic changes in cardiac hypertrophy. (A) Gross photo of heart with hypertrophy caused by aortic stenosis. The wall of the left ventricle is thick and the chamber is not dilated. The left ventricle is on the lower right in this apical four-chamber view of the heart. (B) Altered cardiac configuration in left ventricular hypertrophy without and with dilation, viewed in transverse heart sections. Compared with a normal heart (*center of this panel*), a pressure overloaded heart, caused for example by aortic valve stenosis (*left*), has increased mass and a thick left ventricular wall, whereas a volume overloaded heart, caused for example by mitral valve regurgita-tion, is both hypertrophied and dilated (*right*), having increased mass with a near normal or diminished wall thickness. (C) Photomicrograph of normal myocardium. (D) Photomicrograph of hypertrophied myocardium at same magnification as (C), showing large cells with enlarged. ([B] Reproduced with permission from Allen HD, Gutgesell HP, Clark EB, et al: *Moss and Adams' Heart Disease in Infants, Children, and Adoles-cents: Including the Fetus and Young Adults.* 6th ed. Philadelphia: Lippincott Williams & Wilkins; 2001. [C and D] Reproduced with permission from Kumar V, Fausto N, Abbas A, et al: *Robbins/Cotran Pathologic Basis of Disease*, 8th ed. Philadelphia, WB Saunders, 2010.)

promote development of heart failure. For example, hypertro-phy induces a gene expression profile in cardiac myocytes that is similar to that of proliferating cells generally and particu-larly that of fetal cardiac myocytes during development. Dif-ferentially expressed proteins may be less functional and/or more or less abundant than normal. Hypertrophied and/or failing myocardium also may have a mechanical disadvan-tage engendered by altered chamber configuration, impaired energetics, reduced adrenergic responsiveness, decreased calcium availability, impaired mitochondrial function, microcirculatory spasm, and apoptosis of cardiac myocytes.

Novel therapeutic strategies for heart failure treatment based on molecular mechanisms are under investigation.[5]

Owing to the totality of the changes described above, cardiac hypertrophy comprises a tenuous balance. The adaptive changes may be overwhelmed by potentially del-eterious quantitative or qualitative alterations in structure, function, and biochemistry/gene expression, including car-diac configuration, metabolic requirements of an enlarged muscle mass, protein synthesis, decreased capillary/myocyte ratio, fibrosis, microvascular spasm, cell loss, and impaired contractile mechanisms. Hypertrophy also decreases

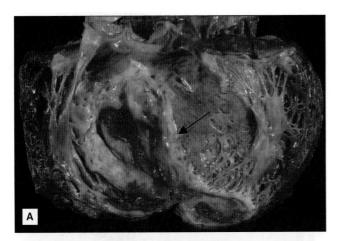

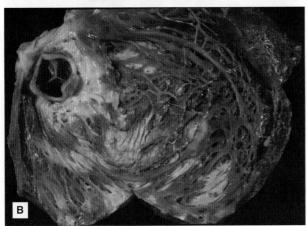

FIGURE 5-2 Cardiac failure necessitating heart transplantation. (A) Ischemic heart disease, with a large anteroapical-septal myocardial infarct (with mural thrombus) noted to the left of center of the photo (*arrow*). (B) Four years following mitral valve replacement with a porcine bioprosthesis for congenital deformity causing mitral regurgitation. ([A] Reproduced with permission from Schoen FJ: *Interventional and Surgical Cardiovascular Pathology: Clinical Correlations and Basic Principles.* Philadelphia: Saunders; 1989.)

myocardial compliance and may thereby hinder diastolic filling. In addition, hypertrophy is an independent risk factor for cardiac mortality and morbidity, especially sudden death.[6]

Heart failure can occur with pressure or volume overload of many causes, owing to both regional and global lesions (Fig. 5-2). Although left ventricular hypertrophy (as measured by left ventricular size and mass) regresses in many cases following removal of the stimulus, the extent of resolution in an individual is unpredictable, and the processes by which recovery of the hypertrophied or failing heart (often termed reverse remodeling occur) are uncertain.[7] Moreover, progressive cardiac failure may ensue following cardiac surgery and despite revascularization or hemodynamic adjustment, by structural repair (see Fig. 5-2B). In addition, the markedly increased cardiac muscle mass in a hypertrophied heart may compromise intraoperative myocardial preservation.

Cardiomyopathies

Cardiomyopathies are diseases in which the primary cardiovascular abnormality is in the myocardium. A *primary cardiomyopathy* comprises a condition solely or predominantly confined to heart muscle, whereas a *secondary cardiomyopathy* (often called *specific heart muscle disease*) implies myocardial involvement as a feature of a generalized systemic or multisystem disorder, such as amyloidosis and hemochromatosis, other infiltrative and storage diseases, drug and other toxic reactions, sarcoidosis, various autoimmune and collagen vascular diseases, or neuromuscular/neurologic disorders (eg, Duchenne-Becker muscular dystrophy). Genetic causes of primary cardiomyopathy include hypertrophic cardiomyopathy (HCM), arrhythmogenic right ventricular cardiomyopathy (ARVC), left ventricular noncompaction, the ion channel disorders (eg, long QT and Brugada syndromes), and some cases of dilated cardiomyopathy.[8] Acquired causes include myocarditis (inflammatory cardiomyopathy), and stress-provoked (takotsubo), tachycardia-induced, and peripartum cardiomyopathy. Although ischemic heart disease, valvular heart disease, and hypertensive heart disease can lead to a clinical practice resembling dilated cardiomyopathy, the terms *ischemic cardiomyopathy, valvular cardiomyopathy*, and *hypertensive cardiomyopathy* are discouraged because these conditions more likely reflect compensatory and remodeling changes induced by another cardiovascular abnormality. In contrast to the atherosclerotic coronary arterial disease that underlies most cases of ischemic heart disease, the epicardial coronary arteries are usually free of significant obstructions in patients with a cardiomyopathy.

In some cases (eg, myocarditis, sarcoidosis, amyloidosis, and hemochromatosis) the cause of a cardiomyopathy may be revealed by light and/or electron microscopic examination of a sample of myocardium obtained by endomyocardial biopsy, and other conditions such as ARVC and HCM have characteristic gross and microscopic features demonstrated at the time of transplantation or autopsy (but not generally by endomyocardial biopsy). In endomyocardial biopsy, also used in the management of the ongoing surveillance of cardiac transplant recipients,[9] a bioptome is inserted into either the right internal jugular or femoral vein and advanced under fluoroscopic or echocardiographic guidance through the tricuspid valve, to the apical aspect of the right side of the ventricular septum, yielding 1- to 3-mm fragments of myocardium.

The common variants of cardiomyopathy are illustrated in Fig. 5-3.

Dilated Cardiomyopathy

Dilated cardiomyopathy is characterized by cardiomegaly usually two to three times of normal weight, and four-chamber dilation (see Fig. 5-3A). The primary functional abnormality in dilated cardiomyopathy is impairment of left ventricular systolic function. Mural thrombi are sometimes

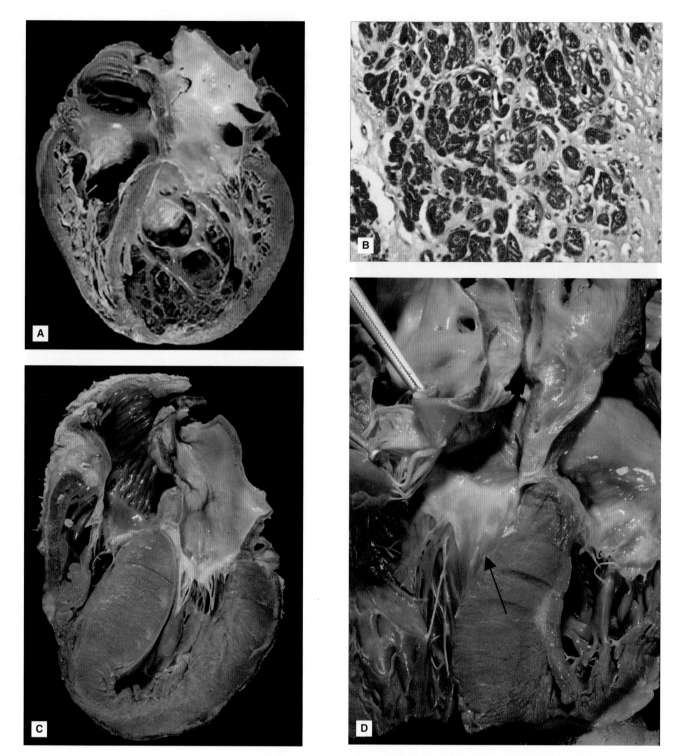

FIGURE 5-3 Cardiomyopathies. (A and B) Dilated cardiomyopathy. (A) Gross photo showing four-chamber dilation and hypertrophy. (B) Photomicrograph of myocardium in dilated cardiomyopathy, demonstrating irregular hypertrophy and interstitial fibrosis. (C-F) Hypertrophic cardiomyopathy. (C) Gross photo, showing septal muscle bulging into the left ventricular outflow tract. In the gross photo shown in (D) the anterior mitral leaflet has been moved away from the septum to reveal a fibrous endocardial plaque, caused by systolic anterior motion (see text). In (A) and (C), the LV is on the right side of the photo; in (D) the LV is on the left. (E) Gross photo of left ventricular outflow tract of patient with extensive fibrosis owing to remote surgical septal myotomy/myectomy. (F) Photomicrograph of myocardium in hypertrophic cardiomyopathy demonstrating myofiber disarray, with marked hypertrophy, abnormal branching of myocytes, and interstitial fibrosis. (G and H) Arrhythmogenic right ventricular cardiomyopathy. (G) Gross photograph, showing dilation of the right ventricle (on the right) and near transmural replacement of the right ventricular free-wall myocardium by fat and fibrosis. (H) Photomicrograph of the right ventricular free wall in arrythmogenic right ventricular cardiomyopathy, demonstrating focal transmural replacement of myocardium by fibrosis and fat. Fibrosis (collagen) is blue in the Masson trichrome stain in parts (B), (F), and (H).

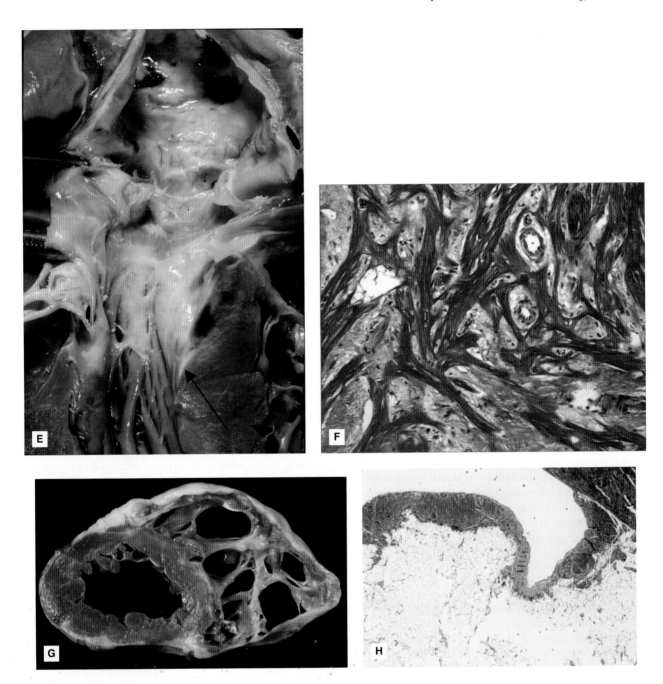

FIGURE 5-3 *(Continued)*

present predominantly in the left ventricle, and are a potential source of thromboemboli. The histologic changes in dilated cardiomyopathy, comprising myocyte hypertrophy and interstitial fibrosis, are nonspecific and indistinguishable from those in failing muscle in ischemic or valvular heart disease (see Fig. 5-3B). Moreover, the severity of the morphologic changes does not necessarily correlate with the severity of dysfunction or the patient's prognosis.

Dilated cardiomyopathy has a genetic and often familial basis in approximately 25 to 50% of cases, and our knowledge of the relevant molecular biology is increasing rapidly.[10]

Mutations most commonly involve genes encoding proteins of the cardiac myocyte cytoskeleton and sarcomere. Alcoholism, pregnancy-associated nutritional deficiency, and myocarditis can yield a dilated phenotype.[11]

Hypertrophic Cardiomyopathy

Hypertrophic cardiomyopathy is characterized macroscopically by massive myocardial hypertrophy, usually without dilation (see Fig. 5-3C), and often with disproportionate thickening of the ventricular septum relative to the free wall of the left ventricle (ratio > 1.3) (termed *asymmetric septal hypertrophy*). In some patients, the basal septum is markedly thickened at the level of the mitral valve, and the outflow of the left ventricle may be narrowed during systole, yielding dynamic left ventricular outflow tract obstruction. In such cases, contact between the left ventricular outflow tract and the anterior mitral leaflet during ventricular systole (observed by echocardiography as *systolic anterior motion* of the mitral valve) results in outflow tract endocardial thickening, in a configuration that mirrors the anterior leaflet of the mitral valve (see Fig. 5-3D). The most important microscopic features in HCM include (1) disorganized myocytes and contractile elements within cells (*myofiber disarray*); (2) extreme myocyte hypertrophy, with myocyte diameters frequently more than 40 μm (normal approximately 15 to 20 μm); and (3) interstitial and replacement fibrosis (see Fig. 5-3F).

Hypertrophic cardiomyopathy usually has a genetic basis.[12] In many patients the disease is familial; remaining cases are sporadic. Over 1500 mutations have been identified in at least 11 genes; almost all occur in genes for sarcomeric proteins, most commonly β-myosin heavy chain and myosin-binding protein C. Occasional cases mimicking HCM are a result of deposition (eg, Fabry's disease).

The clinical course of HCM is variable. Complications include atrial fibrillation with potential mural thrombus formation and embolization, infective endocarditis of the mitral valve, intractable cardiac failure, and sudden death. End-stage heart failure can be accompanied by cardiac dilation. Sudden death is common, with risk related to the degree of hypertrophy and specific gene mutations. Reduced stroke volume results from decreased diastolic filling of the massively hypertrophied left ventricle. Patients with left ventricular obstruction may benefit from septal reduction by surgical myotomy/myectomy or chemical ablation.[13]

Restrictive Cardiomyopathy

Restrictive cardiomyopathy comprises a pathophysiologically heterogeneous spectrum of conditions characterized by heart failure with preserved ejection fraction and previously called *diastolic dysfunction*; many of the potential causes are functional and are potentiated by aging, obesity, and hypertension.[14] Biatrial dilation may be prominent. Structural disorders that interfere with ventricular filling can cause restrictive cardiomyopathy physiology (eg, eosinophilic endomyocardial disease, amyloidosis, storage diseases such as Fabry's disease, or postirradiation fibrosis, constrictive pericarditis, and HCM). Distinct morphologic patterns may be revealed by endomyocardial biopsy.

Arrhythmogenic Right Ventricular Cardiomyopathy

Arrhythmogenic right ventricular cardiomyopathy is characterized by a dilated right ventricular chamber and severely thinned right ventricular wall, with extensive fatty infiltration, loss of myocytes with compensatory myocyte hypertrophy, and interstitial fibrosis (see Fig. 5-3G-H).[15] Clinical features include right-sided heart failure and arrhythmias. Arrhythmias are often brought on by exertion, and this condition is associated with sudden death in athletes. ARVC may be associated with mutations in several genes involved in cell-cell adhesion and in intracellular signaling.

CORONARY ARTERY AND ISCHEMIC HEART DISEASE

Myocardial ischemia occurs when perfusion via coronary flow is inadequate to meet metabolic needs, thus interfering with both the cellular delivery of oxygen and nutrients to cardiac myocytes, and the removal of waste products. Myocardial ischemia most often results from obstruction or narrowing of a coronary artery secondary to atherosclerosis. Nonatherosclerotic epicardial coronary artery obstructions can also occur in autoimmune diseases (eg, systemic lupus erythematosus and rheumatoid arthritis), progressive systemic sclerosis (scleroderma), vasculitis (eg, Buerger disease and Kawasaki disease), fibromuscular dysplasia, and as a result of dissection, spasm, embolism, or some drugs such as cocaine. Obstruction of small intramural coronary arteries occurs in diabetes, Fabry's disease, and amyloidosis, and in cardiac allografts (see later). Decreased coronary flow leading to global hypoperfusion and myocardial ischemia can occur during cardiopulmonary bypass. Ischemia can also result from increased cardiac demand secondary to exercise, tachycardia, hyperthyroidism, or ventricular hypertrophy and/or dilation. Moreover, the effects of ischemia are potentiated when oxygen supply is decreased secondary to anemia, hypoxia, or cardiac failure.

Atherosclerosis

Atherosclerosis is a chronic, progressive, multifocal disease of the vessel wall, beginning in the intima, whose characteristic lesion is the atheroma or plaque that forms through intimal thickening (mediated predominantly by smooth muscle cell proliferation and matrix production) and lipid accumulation (mediated primarily by insudation of lipid into the arterial wall).[16] Atherosclerosis primarily affects the large elastic arteries and large- and medium-sized muscular arteries of the systemic circulation, particularly near branches, sharp curvatures, and bifurcations. Coronary arterial atherosclerosis involves especially the epicardial branches of the left anterior descending (LAD) and circumflex arteries, and the right coronary diffusely, but generally not their intramural branches. Most atheromas in the coronary arteries are segmental and eccentric, with plaque-free segments longitudinally and circumferentially. In early lesions, the plaque bulges outward at the expense of the media with the arterial lumen remaining circular in cross-section at essentially the same original diameter (ie, the vessel wall outer diameter enlarges, a process termed *vascular remodeling*).[17]

Although veins are usually spared from atherosclerosis, venous grafts interposed within branches of the arterial system (such as aorto-coronary bypass grafts created from saphenous vein) frequently develop intimal thickening and ultimately atherosclerosis, with obstructions or aneurysms. Paradoxically, some arteries used as arterial grafts, including the internal mammary artery (IMA), are largely spared.

Pathogenesis

The prevailing theory of lesion formation in atherosclerosis centers on interactions among arterial wall endothelial and vascular smooth muscle cells, circulating monocytes, platelets, and plasma lipoproteins. A key contributor to atherosclerosis is endothelial cell injury induced by chronic hypercholesterolemia, homocystinemia, chemicals in cigarette smoke, viruses, localized hemodynamic forces, systemic hypertension, hyperglycemia, or the local effects of cytokines. These factors cause phenotypic and hence functional changes in endothelial cells, called *endothelial dysfunction*.[18] Endothelial dysfunction causes (1) vasoconstriction owing to decreased production of the vasodilator nitric oxide; (2) increased permeability to lipoproteins; (3) expression of tissue factor leading to thrombosis; and (4) expression of certain injury-induced adhesion molecules leading to adherence of platelets and inflammatory cells.

Progression from an early, subendothelial lesion (called a *fatty streak*) to a complex atheromatous plaque involves the following processes: (1) monocytes adhere to endothelial cells, migrate into the subendothelial space, and transform into tissue macrophages; (2) smooth muscle cells migrate from the media into the intima, proliferate, and secrete collagen and other extracellular matrix (ECM) constituents; (3) lipids accumulate via phagocytosis in macrophages (forming foam cells) and smooth muscle cells, as well as extracellularly; (4) lipoproteins are oxidized in the vessel wall leading to generation of potent biologic stimuli such as chemoattractants and cytotoxins; (5) persistent chronic inflammation; (6) cellular necrosis with release of intracellular lipids (mostly cholesterol esters); and often (7) calcification. Mature atherosclerotic plaques consist of a central core of lipid, cholesterol crystals, macrophages, smooth muscle cells, foam cells, and lymphocytes along with necrotic debris, separated from the lumen by a fibrous cap rich in collagen.

Clinical manifestations of advanced coronary arterial atherosclerosis occur through encroachment of the lumen leading to progressive stenosis, or to acute plaque disruption with thrombosis (see the following). In the absence of significant coronary blockages, myocardial perfusion is adequate at rest, and compensatory vasodilation provides flow reserve that is more than sufficient to accommodate increased metabolic demand during vigorous exertion. When the coronary luminal cross-sectional area is decreased by approximately 75%, blood flow becomes limited during exertion; with 90% reduction, coronary flow may be inadequate at rest. However, occlusions that develop slowly may stimulate the formation of collateral vessels that protect against distal myocardial ischemia. Aneurysms may form secondary to atherosclerosis as a result

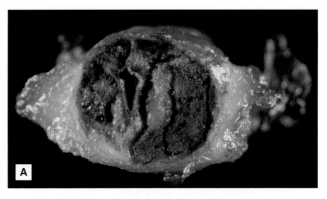

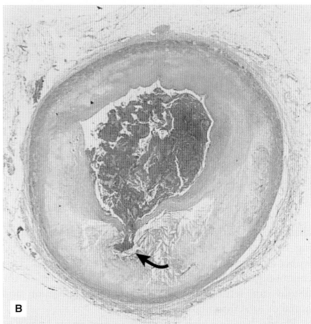

FIGURE 5-4 Acute plaque rupture with superimposed thrombus complicating coronary arterial atherosclerosis and triggering fatal myocardial infarction. (A) Gross photo. (B) Photomicrograph. (The arrow demonstrates the site of plaque rupture.) ([B] Reproduced with permission from Schoen FJ: *Interventional and Surgical Cardiovascular Pathology: Clinical Correlations and Basic Principles.* Philadelphia: Saunders; 1989.)

of destruction of the media beneath a plaque, a process most common in the aorta and other large vessels (where plaque does not easily cause obstruction). The natural history, morphologic features, key pathogenetic events, and clinical complications of atherosclerosis are summarized in Figs. 5-4 and 5-5.

Role of Acute Plaque Change

The onset and prognosis of ischemic heart disease are not well predicted by the angiographically determined extent and severity of luminal obstructions.[19] The conversion of chronic stable angina or an asymptomatic state to an *acute coronary syndrome* (ie, myocardial infarction, unstable angina, and sudden coronary death) is dependent on dynamic vascular

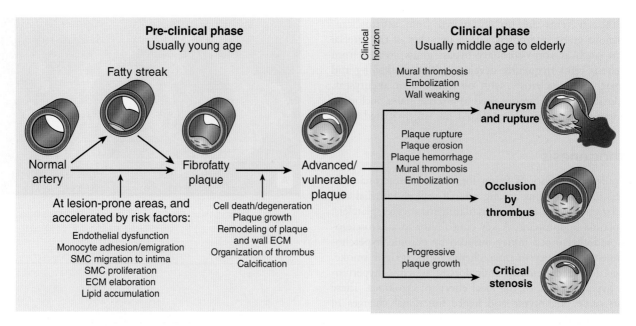

FIGURE 5-5 Schematic diagram summarizing the morphology, pathogenesis, and complications of atherosclerosis. Plaques usually develop slowly and insidiously over many years, beginning in childhood or shortly thereafter and exerting clinical effect in middle age or later. As described in the text, lesions may progress from a fatty streak to a fibrous plaque and then to plaque complications that lead to disease. ECM = extracellular matrix; SMC = smooth muscle cell. (Reproduced with permission from Kumar V, Fausto N, Abbas A, et al: *Robbins/Cotran Pathologic Basis of Disease*, 8th ed. Philadelphia, WB Saunders, 2010.)

changes, such as fracture or rupture of the fibrous cap, exposing deep plaque constituents, and subsequent thrombus, wither occlusive, or partial, sometimes with emboli. Less commonly, the change is erosion and/or ulceration of the fibrous cap, setting the stage for platelet aggregation and mural or total thrombosis.

Plaques having a high propensity to rupture are known as *vulnerable plaques*. Such lesions (1) have a thin collagenous fibrous cap and few smooth muscle cells (the cells that produce collagenous matrix); (2) contain many macrophages producing matrix metalloproteinases (MMP) (enzymes that degrade the collagen that ordinarily lends strength to the fibrous cap); and (3) contain large areas of foam cells, extracellular lipid and necrotic debris. Inflammation may contribute to coronary thrombosis by altering the balance between prothrombotic and fibrinolytic properties of the endothelium. There is evidence that lipid lowering by diet or drugs such as statins (HMG CoA reductase inhibitors) reduces accumulation of macrophages expressing matrix-degrading enzymes and thereby stabilizes plaque by increasing the thickness and strength of the fibrous cap.[20]

Vulnerable plaques without significant obstruction can be clinically important. Indeed, pathologic and clinical studies show that plaques that rupture and lead to coronary occlusion often produced only mild to moderate luminal stenosis (and often no symptoms) prior to acute plaque change. Thus, there is great interest in identifying vulnerable plaques in individuals at a potentially therapeutic stage. Calcification of the coronary arteries detected noninvasively by electron beam computed tomography predicts the extent

of atherosclerotic disease overall but does not predict plaque instability. The most relevant features of plaque structure can be evaluated using intravascular ultrasound, optical coherence tomography (OCT), and potentially noninvasive molecular imaging.[21]

The events that trigger abrupt changes in plaque configuration and superimposed thrombosis and the efficacy and safety of interventional therapies depend on influences both intrinsic (eg, structure and composition, as described above) and extrinsic (eg, blood pressure, vasospasm, and platelet reactivity) to the plaque.[22,23] Potential outcomes for ruptured plaques include progression to thrombotic occlusion, non-occlusive thrombosis, healing at the site of plaque erosion, atheroembolization or thromboembolization, organization of mural thrombus causing (plaque progression), and organization of the occlusive mass with recanalization.

The clinical manifestations of ischemic heart disease most frequently reflect the downstream effects of a complex and dynamic interaction among fixed atherosclerotic narrowing of the epicardial coronary arteries, plaque vulnerability, intraluminal thrombosis overlying a ruptured or fissured atherosclerotic plaque, platelet aggregation, vasospasm, and the responses of the myocardium to ischemia.

Progression of Ischemic Myocardial Injury

The changes in the myocardium following the onset of myocardial ischemia are sequential and the cellular consequences are primarily determined by the severity and duration of

TABLE 5-1: Approximate Time of Onset and Recognition of Key Features of Ischemic Myocardial Injury

Event/process	Time of onset
Onset of anaerobic metabolism	Within seconds
Loss of contractility	<2 min
ATP* reduced	
to 50% of normal	10 min
to 10% of normal	40 min
Irreversible cell injury	20-40 min
Microvascular injury	>1 h

Pathologic feature	Time of recognition
Ultrastructural features of reversible injury	5-10 min
Ultrastructural features of irreversible damage	20-40 min
Wavy fibers	1-3 h
Staining defect with tetrazolium dye	2-3 h
Classic histologic features of necrosis	6-12 h
Gross alterations	12-24 h

*ATP = adenosine triphosphate.

flow deprivation (Table 5-1). Within seconds of onset, ischemia induces a transition from aerobic metabolism to anaerobic glycolysis in cardiac myocytes, leading to inadequate production of high-energy phosphates such as ATP, and the accumulation of metabolites such as lactic acid, causing intracellular acidosis. Myocardial function is exquisitely sensitive to these biochemical consequences, with total loss of contraction within 2 minutes in severe ischemia. Nevertheless, ischemic changes in an individual cell are not immediately lethal, and short duration injury is potentially reversible. Irreversible injury of cardiac myocytes marked by cell membrane structural defects occurs only after 20 to 40 minutes within the most severely ischemic area (Fig. 5-6). Lethal injury to clusters of cells owing to severe prolonged ischemia causes *myocardial infarction*.

Within the region of myocardium vulnerable to die if ischemia is not relieved in a timely manner (termed the *area at risk*), loss of perfusion is not uniform and not all cells in the area at risk are equally affected. The most severely affected myocytes, and therefore the first to become necrotic, reside in the subendocardium and in the papillary muscles furthest from lateral regions of noncompromised circulation and adequate perfusion. Thus, if uninterrupted ischemia progresses, there is a *wavefront* of cell death outward from the mid-subendocardial region, eventually encompassing the lateral borders and less severely ischemic subepicardial and peripheral regions of the area at risk. In myocardial infarction, approximately 50% of the area at risk becomes necrotic in approximately 3 to 4 hours. The final transmural extent of an infarct is generally established within 6 to 12 hours. The key principle is that if perfusion is restored prior to the onset of irreversible changes, cell death can be prevented. Thus, restoration of flow to a severely ischemic area via therapeutic intervention (such as percutaneous coronary intervention [PCI] with stent placement) can alter the outcome, depending on the interval between the onset of ischemia and restoration of blood flow (*reperfusion*).[24]

Necrosis existing less than 6 or more hours before patient death is not visible by routine gross or microscopic pathologic analysis of a cardiac specimen at autopsy. However, in a patient who died at least 2 to 3 hours following the onset of gross infarction, the presence of a necrotic region may be detected as a staining defect with triphenyl tetrazolium chloride (TTC), a dye that turns viable myocardium a brick-red color on reaction of the dye with intact myocardial dehydrogenases.[25] The earliest observable microscopic features of infarction are intense eosinophilia, nuclear pyknosis, and loss of myocytes in clusters; some may be stretched and wavy. Short-term ischemia

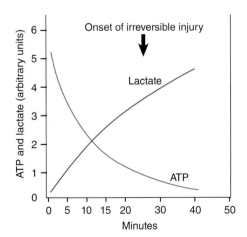
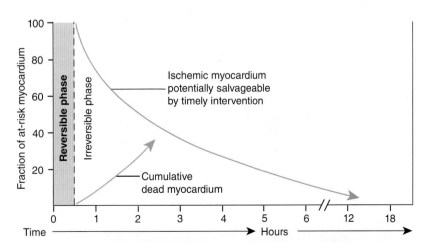

FIGURE 5-6 Temporal sequence of early biochemical findings and progression of necrosis after onset of severe myocardial ischemia. *Left panel:* Early changes include loss of ATP and accumulation of lactate. *Right panel:* Myocardial injury is potentially reversible for approximately 20 minutes after the onset of even the most severe ischemia. Thereafter, progressive loss of viability occurs, which is complete by 6 to 12 hours. The benefits of reperfusion are greatest when it is achieved early; progressively smaller benefit is accrued when reperfusion is delayed.

without necrosis cannot be reliably demonstrated by pathologic examination.

Tissue repair following myocardial infarction. The inflammation and repair sequence in response to myocardial cell death follows a largely stereotyped sequence similar to tissue repair following injury at extracardiac sites. The inflammatory reaction is characterized by early exudation of polymorphonuclear leukocytes, seen after 6 to 12 hours and maximal within 1 to 3 days. Subsequently (3 to 5 days), the infiltrate consists predominantly of macrophages that remove the necrotic tissue. Collagen production accompanied by neovascularization begins approximately 7 to 10 days at the margins of preserved tissue. The gross appearance reflects the progressive microscopic changes described above (Fig. 5-7). Ultimately, the infarcted tissue is replaced by dense collagenous scar, which is fully mature by about 6 to 8 weeks. Healing of myocardial infarction may be altered by reperfusion (see the following), mechanical stress, sex, and neurohumoral and other factors such as immunosuppressive drugs.[26]

Although cardiac myocytes are traditionally thought incapable of regeneration, a growing body of evidence suggests that regeneration of cardiac myocytes can occur under certain circumstances, including at the viable borders of myocardial infarcts.[27] Whether this capacity for renewal can be harnessed to therapeutic advantage is not yet known (discussed later in this chapter).

Effects of Reperfusion

Reperfusion of an ischemic zone occurring before the onset of irreversible injury (recall, approximately 20 to 30 minutes) prevents infarction. Reperfusion later (ie, following some cell death) may limit infarct size through salvage of myocytes located outside the leading edge of the "wavefront," provided that these myocytes are only reversibly injured at the time reperfusion occurs.[28] Thus, the potential for recovery of viable tissue decreases with increasing severity and duration of ischemia (see Fig. 5-6). Owing to the typical progression of ischemic injury, reperfusion 3 to 4 hours following onset of ischemia is considered the practical limit for significant myocardial salvage, and 90 minutes ("door to balloon time") is the present clinical goal in PCI.[29]

Reperfused previously ischemic myocardium often has hemorrhage (owing to microvascular damage; see the following) and necrotic myocytes with transverse eosinophilic lines (called *contraction bands*) that represent hypercontracted sarcomeres (Fig. 5-8) caused by ischemic cell membrane damage followed by a massive cellular influx of calcium derived from the restored blood flow. Microvascular occlusions (resulting from endothelial or interstitial edema and/or plugging by platelet or neutrophil aggregates) may inhibit the reperfusion of damaged regions (*no-reflow phenomenon*).[30] Moreover, reperfusion itself may damage some of the ischemic but still viable myocytes that were not irreversibly injured (called *reperfusion injury*), and arrhythmias may occur.[31] In reperfusion after severe global ischemia (eg, during cardiac surgery), the left ventricle may undergo a massive tetanic contraction (*stone heart syndrome*).[32]

MYOCARDIAL STUNNING, HIBERNATION, AND PRECONDITIONING

Although reperfusion may salvage ischemic but not necrotic myocardium, metabolic and functional recovery is usually not instantaneous; indeed, reversible postischemic myocardial dysfunction (called *myocardial stunning*) may persist for hours to days following brief periods of ischemia.[33] Myocardial stunning may also occur in the setting of PCI, cardiopulmonary bypass, or ischemia related to unstable angina or stress.

Regions of viable myocardium with chronically reduced coronary blood flow may have impaired function (termed *hibernating myocardium*).[34,35] Myocardial hibernation is characterized by (1) persistent wall motion abnormality, (2) low myocardial blood flow, and (3) evidence of viability in at least some of the affected areas. Contractile function of hibernating myocardium can improve if blood flow returns toward normal or if oxygen demand is reduced. Correction of this abnormality is likely responsible for the reversal of long-standing defects in ventricular wall motion observed following coronary bypass graft surgery or PCI. Morphologically,

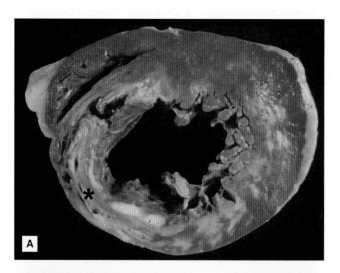

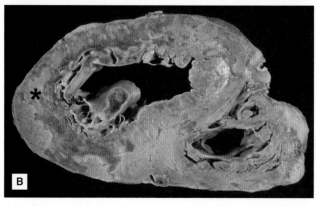

FIGURE 5-7 Gross photos of healing myocardial infarcts (A) approximately 3 to 4 days, (B) approximately 2 weeks. Asterisk highlights area of damage in each case.

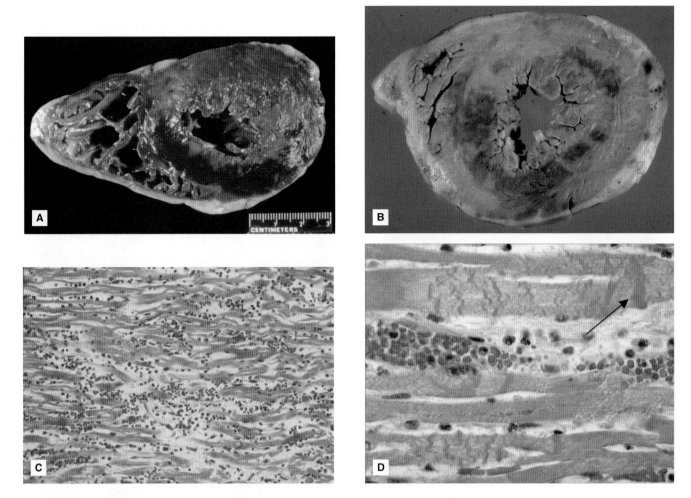

FIGURE 5-8 Reperfusion following severe myocardial ischemia. (A) Large, densely hemorrhagic anteroseptal acute myocardial infarct from patient treated by intracoronary thrombolysis for left anterior descending (LAD) artery thrombus, approximately 4 hours following onset. (B) Subendocardial circumferential hemorrhagic acute myocardial necrosis occurring perioperatively in cardiac valve replacement. (C) Photomicrograph of hemorrhagic myocardial necrosis. (D) High-power photomicrograph demonstrating contraction bands (*arrow*). Hematoxylin and eosin 375×.

sublethal chronic ischemic injury often manifests as myocyte vacuolization, particularly in the subendocardium.[36]

Adaptation to short-term transient ischemia (ie, duration insufficient to cause cell death) may induce tolerance against subsequent, more severe ischemic insults (*ischemic preconditioning*).[37] Thus, short (eg, 5-minute) periods of cardiac ischemia followed by reperfusion can protect myocardium against injury during a prolonged period of subsequent ischemia. Understanding the yet uncertain mechanisms of this protection could lead to targets for "preemptive" pharmacologic stimulation of these pathways.

Myocardial Infarction and Its Complications

Coronary atherosclerosis with acute plaque rupture and superimposed thrombosis often results in a *transmural* (Q-wave) myocardial infarct, in which ischemic necrosis involves at least half and usually a nearly full thickness of the ventricular wall in the distribution of the involved artery. In contrast, a *subendocardial* (nontransmural, non–Q-wave) infarct constitutes an area of ischemic necrosis that is limited to the inner third to half of the ventricular wall, which can occur in the setting of episodic hypotension, global ischemia, or hypoxemia, or from interruption by reperfusion of the evolution of a transmural infarct. Subendocardial infarction associated with diffuse stenosing coronary atherosclerosis can be multifocal, extending laterally beyond the perfusion territory of a single coronary artery.

The short-term in-hospital mortality rate from acute myocardial infarction has declined from nearly 30% in the 1950s and 1960s to 7% or less today, especially for patients who receive aggressive reperfusion/revascularization and pharmacologic therapy.[38] However, half of all deaths from myocardial infarction occur within the first hour after the onset of symptoms, potentially before a victim can reach the hospital. Poor prognostic factors include advanced age, female sex, diabetes mellitus, and a previous myocardial infarction. Left ventricular function and the extent of obstructive lesions in vessels perfusing viable myocardium are the most important prognostic factors.

Important complications of myocardial infarction include ventricular dysfunction, cardiogenic shock, arrhythmias, cardiac rupture, infarct extension and expansion, papillary muscle dysfunction, right ventricular involvement, ventricular aneurysm, pericarditis, and systemic arterial embolism; the cardiac rupture syndromes and ventricular aneurysm are illustrated in Fig. 5-9. Outcome after myocardial infarction depends on infarct size, location, and transmurality. Patients with transmural anterior infarcts are at greatest risk for regional dilation and mural thrombi and have a worse clinical

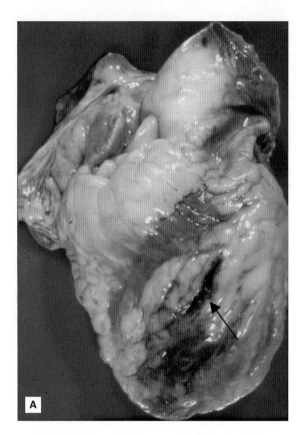

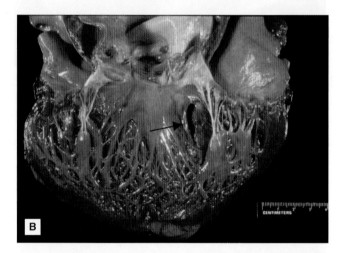

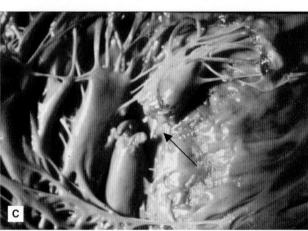

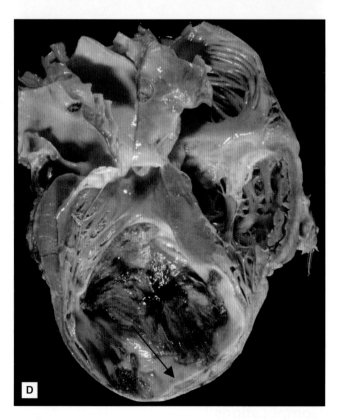

FIGURE 5-9 Cardiac rupture syndromes and ventricular aneurysm following myocardial infarction. (A) Anterior myocardial rupture (*arrow*). (B) Rupture of the ventricular septum (*arrow*). (C) Rupture of a necrotic papillary muscle (*arrow*). (D) Large left ventricular aneurysm, with thin fibrotic wall (*arrow*) and mural thrombus.

course than those with inferior-posterior infarcts. In contrast, inferior-posterior infarcts are more likely to have serious conduction blocks and right ventricular involvement.

Myocardial infarcts produce functional abnormalities approximately proportional to their size. Large infarcts have a higher probability of cardiogenic shock and congestive heart failure. Nonfunctional scar tissue resulting from previous infarcts and areas of stunned or hibernating myocardium may also contribute to overall ventricular dysfunction. Cardiogenic shock following myocardial infarction generally indicates a large infarct (often > 40% of the left ventricle). The high mortality of myocardial dysfunction and cardiogenic shock has been alleviated somewhat by the use of ventricular assist devices (VADs) to bridge patients through phases of prolonged reversible ischemic dysfunction.

Although many patients have cardiac rhythm abnormalities following myocardial infarction, the conduction system is involved by necrosis or inflammation only in a minority, and heart block following myocardial infarction usually is transient. Tachyarrhythmias usually originate owing to electrically unstable ischemic or necrotic myocardium, often at the edge of an infarct. However, autopsy studies of sudden death victims and clinical studies of resuscitated survivors of cardiac arrest show that only a minority of patients with ischemia-induced malignant ventricular arrhythmias develop a full-blown acute myocardial infarction.

Cardiac rupture syndromes comprise three entities (see Fig. 5-9A-C): (1) rupture of the ventricular free wall (most common), usually with hemopericardium and cardiac tamponade; (2) rupture of the ventricular septum (less common), leading to an acquired ventricular septal defect with a left-to-right shunt; and (3) papillary muscle rupture (least common), resulting in the acute onset of severe mitral regurgitation. Ruptures tend to occur relatively early following infarction with as many as 25% presenting within 24 hours (mean interval 4 to 5 days), most commonly through the lateral free wall. Acute free wall ruptures usually are rapidly fatal; repair is rarely possible.[39] Rarely, a rupture is contained as a hematoma communicating with the ventricular cavity (*false aneurysm*); this is an unstable situation and the false aneurysm may eventually rupture.

Postinfarction septal ruptures with acute ventricular septal defect are of two types: (1) single or multiple sharply localized, jagged, linear passageways that connect the ventricular chambers (simple type), usually involving the anteroapical aspect of the septum; and (2) defects that tunnel serpiginously through the septum to a somewhat distant opening on the right side (complex type), usually involving the basal inferoseptal wall.[40] In complex lesions, the tract may extend into regions remote from the site of the infarct, such as the right ventricular free wall. Without surgery, the prognosis is poor for patients with infarct-related ventricular septal defects.

Papillary muscles are particularly vulnerable to ischemic injury and rupture, particularly the posterior medial papillary muscle, and rupture can occur later than other rupture syndromes (as late as 1 month after myocardial infarction). Because tendinous cords arise from the heads of the papillary muscles and cords from each are distributed to both valve leaflets, interference with the structure or function of either papillary muscle can result in dysfunction of both mitral valve leaflets and resultant mitral regurgitation (see later).

Isolated right ventricular infarction and involvement of the right ventricle by extension of a posteroseptal infarct can have important functional consequences, including right ventricular failure with or without tricuspid regurgitation and arrhythmias.

Infarct *extension* is characterized by incremental new or recurrent necrosis in the same distribution as a completed recent infarct. Extension most often occurs along the lateral and subepicardial borders of a recent infarct, and histologically appears younger than the previously necrotic myocardium. In contrast, infarct *expansion* is a disproportionate thinning and dilation of the infarcted region which does not lead to additional necrotic myocardium per se, but may promote both further ischemia and intracardiac mural thrombus formation. The increase in ventricular volume caused by regional dilation increases the wall stress and thereby the workload of noninfarcted myocardium. Infarct expansion is often the substrate for late aneurysm formation and increases morbidity and mortality.

Ventricular aneurysms are large scars that paradoxically bulge during ventricular systole and often result from healing of a large transmural infarct that undergoes expansion (see Fig. 5-9D).[41] Although frequently as thin as 1 mm, ventricular aneurysms rarely rupture owing to their walls of tough fibrous or fibrocalcific tissue. Hypertrophied myocardial remnants as well as necrotic but inadequately healed myocardium often are present in aneurysm walls and mural thrombus is common.

Ventricular remodeling comprises the collective structural changes that occur in both the necrotic zone and uninvolved areas of the heart, including left ventricular dilation, wall thinning by infarct expansion, compensatory hypertrophy of noninfarcted myocardium, and potentially late aneurysm formation.[42] Congestive heart failure secondary to coronary artery disease (CAD) occurs when the overall function of viable myocardium can no longer maintain an adequate cardiac output or regions of hyperfunctioning residual myocardium suffer additional ischemic episodes.

Revascularization

Revascularization early after acute myocardial infarction is rationalized as follows: (1) prolonged thrombotic occlusion of a coronary artery causes transmural infarction; (2) the extent of necrosis during an evolving myocardial infarction progresses as a wavefront and becomes complete only 6 to 12 hours or more following coronary occlusion (see Fig. 5-6); (3) both early- and long-term mortality following acute myocardial infarction correlate strongly with the amount of residual functioning myocardium; and (4) early reperfusion rescues some jeopardized myocardium.[43] Thus, the benefits of revascularization depend on and are assessed by the amount of myocardium salvaged, recovery of left ventricular function, and resultant reduction in mortality. These clinical end points are largely determined by the time interval between onset of symptoms and successful reflow, and the degree of residual stenosis of the infarct vessel. Spontaneous recanalization via endogenous thrombolysis can be beneficial to left ventricular function but occurs in only a small percentage of patients within the critical interval.

Percutaneous Coronary Intervention

Percutaneous coronary intervention can restore blood flow through a diseased portion of the coronary circulation obstructed by atherosclerotic plaque and/or thrombotic deposits, and in obstructions in saphenous vein grafts, IMA grafts, and occasionally, coronary arteries in transplanted hearts.

PERCUTANEOUS TRANSLUMINAL CORONARY ANGIOPLASTY

In percutaneous transluminal coronary angioplasty (PTCA), the plaque splits at its weakest point and enlargement of the lumen occurs by plaque fracture (the predominant mechanism); and by embolization, compression, redistribution of the plaque contents, and overall mechanical expansion of the vessel wall can also occur.[44] The split extends to the intimal-medial border and often into the media, is accompanied by variable circumferential and longitudinal medial dissection, and can induce a flap that impinges on the lumen. These changes can result in local flow abnormalities and generation of new, thrombogenic blood-contacting surfaces (to some extent similar to what is observed with spontaneously disrupted plaque) and contribute to the propensity for acute thrombotic closure.

The long-term success of PTCA is limited by the development of progressive restenosis, which occurs in 30 to 50% of patients, most frequently within the first 4 to 6 months.[45] Although vessel wall recoil and organization of thrombus likely contribute, the major process leading to restenosis is excessive medial smooth muscle migration to the intima, proliferation, and secretion of abundant ECM as a response to angioplasty-induced injury.

Although not widely used today, coronary atherectomy of primary or restenosis lesions mechanically can remove obstructive tissue by excision.[46] Deep arterial resection, including medial and even adventitial elements, occurs frequently but has not been associated with acute symptomatic complications. The morphology of arterial vessel healing after directional or rotational atherectomy is similar to that following angioplasty.

STENTS

Stents are expandable tubes of metallic or polymeric mesh that are used to split open the vessel wall at the site of balloon angioplasty and thereby mitigate the negative sequelae of PTCA.[47] Stents preserve luminal patency and provide a larger and more regular lumen by acting as a scaffold to support the disrupted vascular wall and minimize flow disruption and thrombus formation. Placement of a stent yields outcomes superior to angioplasty alone in vessels greater than 3 mm in diameter, chronic total occlusions, stenotic vein grafts, restenotic lesions after angioplasty alone, and in patients with myocardial infarction.[48]

Stent technology has undergone a rapid evolution, including sequentially: (1) bare-metal stents (BMS); and (2) drug-eluting stents (DES), both used extensively in clinical interventional cardiology; and more recently (3) completely resorbable/biodegradable stents (RBS). Bare-metal stents for coronary implantation are short tubular segments of metal mesh composed of balloon-expandable 316L stainless steel or nickel-titanium alloy (Nitinol) that range from approximately 2.5 to 3.5 mm in diameter and approximately 1 to 3 cm in length. Development has focused on permitting stents to become more flexible and more easily delivered and deployed, allowing the treatment of a greater number and variety of lesions.

Key stent complications are thrombosis, usually occurring early, and late proliferative restenosis (Fig. 5-10). Thrombotic occlusion, occurring in 1 to 3% of patients within 7 to 10 days of the procedure (see Fig. 5-10A), has largely been overcome by aggressive multidrug treatment with antiplatelet agents such as clopidogrel, aspirin, and glycoprotein IIb/IIIa inhibitors. The major long-term complication of bare-metal stenting is in-stent restenosis, which occurs in 50% of patients within 6 months.[49] The causes of stent thrombosis and restenosis are complex and are largely owing to stent-tissue interactions, damage to the endothelial lining, and stretching of the vessel wall, which stimulate inflammation and adherence and accumulation of platelets and fibrin.[50] Stent wires may eventually become completely embedded in an endothelium-lined intimal fibrosis layer composed of smooth muscle cells in a collagen matrix (see Fig. 5-10B). This tissue may thicken secondary to the release of growth factors, chemotactic factors, and inflammatory mediators from platelets and other inflammatory cells that result in proliferation of smooth muscle cells and increased production of ECM molecules, narrowing the lumen and resulting in restenosis.

Drug-eluting stents, which impart the controlled release of drugs from durable polymers to the vessel wall, effectively inhibit in-stent restenosis.[51,52] The drugs used most widely are rapamycin (sirolimus)[53] and paclitaxel[54] in the Cypher (Cordis) and Taxus (Boston Scientific) stents, respectively. Rapamycin, a drug used for immunosuppression in solid organ transplant recipients, inhibits proliferation, migration, and growth of smooth muscle cells and ECM synthesis. Paclitaxel, a drug used in the chemotherapeutic regimens for several types of cancer, also has similar anti-smooth muscle cell activities. These drugs are embedded in a polymer matrix (such as a copolymer of poly-*n*-butyl methacrylate and polyethylene-vinyl acetate or a gelatin-chondroitin sulfate coacervate film) that is coated onto the stent. However, stent thrombosis emerged as a major safety concern with DES early after their adoption in clinical practice, requiring prolonged dual antiplatelet therapy.[55] Pathological examination of clinical specimens and animal studies have suggested that these DES were associated with DES-induced inhibition of stent endothelialization and delayed arterial healing and polymer hypersensitivity reactions resulting in chronic inflammation that contributed to stent thrombosis. Recently, DES have

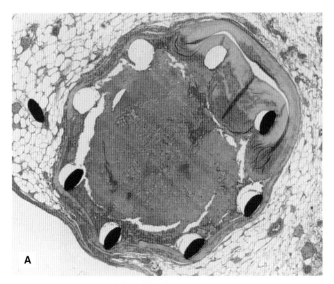

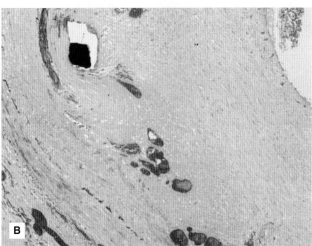

FIGURE 5-10 Stent pathology. (A) Thrombosis. H&E stain. (B) Thickened proliferative neointima separating the stent wires (*black structure*) from the lumen, with bare metal coronary artery stent implanted long term. Movat stain. (Reproduced with permission from Silver MD, Gotlieb AI, Schoen FJ: *Cardiovascular Pathology*, 3rd ed. Philadelphia: Churchill Livingstone/Elsevier; 2001.)

been developed to overcome these issues with improved stent designs and construction and the use of biocompatible polymers.[56]

In contrast to the permanent presence of a foreign body in BMS and DES, RBS provide a scaffold and then ultimately disappear by resorption of foreign scaffold material that may potentiate a thrombotic event, permit more versatility in subsequent therapies, and not interfere with the diagnostic evaluation by noninvasive imaging such as cardiac magnetic resonance and CT.[57,58] Several RBS are in development or in clinical trials. The key challenge is to balance biomechanics (strength, deliverability, and lesion crossing), potential for side-branch occlusion (owing to thicker struts), durability

and biocompatibility, and to control the kinetics of stent degradation at a rate appropriate to maintain mechanical strength to limit recoil.

Coronary Artery Bypass Graft Surgery

Coronary artery bypass graft (CABG) surgery improves survival in patients with significant left main CAD, three-vessel (and possibly two-vessel) disease, or reduced ventricular function, and prolongs and improves the quality of life in patients with left main equivalent disease (proximal LAD and proximal left circumflex), but does not protect them from the risk of subsequent myocardial infarction.[59] The principal mechanism for these benefits is thought to be the restoration of blood flow to hibernating myocardium.

The hospital mortality rate for CABG surgery is approximately 1% in low-risk patients, with fewer than 3% of patients suffering perioperative myocardial infarction. The most consistent predictors of mortality after CABG are urgency of operation, age, prior cardiac surgery, female sex, low left ventricular ejection fraction, degree of left main stenosis, and number of vessels with significant stenoses. The most common mode of early death after CABG is acute cardiac failure leading to low output or arrhythmias, owing to myocardial necrosis (often with features of reperfusion described in the preceding), postischemic dysfunction of viable myocardium, or a metabolic cause, such as hypokalemia.

Early thrombotic occlusion of the graft vessel may occur, usually potentiated by inadequate distal run-off from extremely small and/or atherosclerotic distal native coronaries. Additional factors may include atherosclerosis, arterial branching or dissection of blood into the graft or native vessel at the anastomotic site, or distortion of a graft that is too short or too long for the intended bypass. In some cases, thrombosis occurring early postoperatively involves only the distal portion of the graft, suggesting that early graft thrombosis was initiated at the distal anastomosis. Most patients who die early after CABG have patent grafts.

The patency of saphenous vein grafts is reported as 60% at 10 years; occlusion results from (with increasing postoperative interval) thrombosis, progressive intimal thickening, and/or obstructive atherosclerosis.[60] Between 1 month and approximately 1 year, graft stenosis is usually caused by intimal hyperplasia with excessive smooth muscle proliferation and ECM production (similar to that seen in restenosis following angioplasty and stenting). Atherosclerosis becomes the predominant mechanism in graft occlusion beyond 1 to 3 years after CABG, and earliest in those patients with the most significant atherosclerotic risk factors. Plaques in grafts often have poorly developed fibrous caps with large necrotic cores and can develop secondary dystrophic calcific deposits that extend to the lumen (Fig. 5-11); thus, the potential for disruption, aneurysmal dilation, and embolization of atherosclerotic lesions in vein grafts exceeds that for native coronary atherosclerotic lesions, and balloon angioplasty, stenting or intraoperative manipulation of grafts may potentiate atheroembolism.

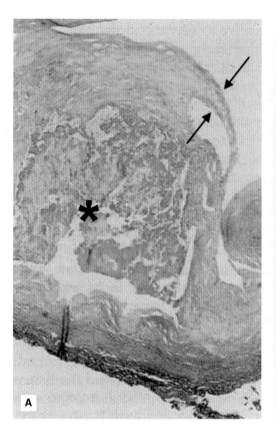
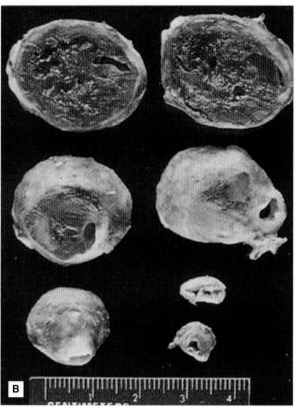

FIGURE 5-11 Atherosclerosis of saphenous vein bypass graft. (A) Fibrous cap (*between arrows*) is attenuated over the necrotic core (*large asterisk*). Lumen is at upper right. (B) Saphenous vein graft aneurysm. Hematoxylin and eosin (A) 100×; Gross photo. Verhoff von Giesen stain (for elastin) 10×. ([A] Reproduced with permission from Schoen FJ: *Interventional and Surgical Cardiovascular Pathology: Clinical Correlations and Basic Principles.* Philadelphia: Saunders; 1989. [B] Reproduced with permission from Liang BT, Antman EM, Taus R, et al: Atherosclerotic aneurysms of aortocoronary vein grafts, *Am J Cardiol.* 1988 Jan 1;61(1):185-188.)

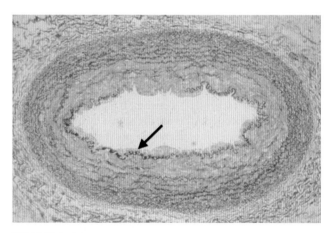

FIGURE 5-12 Internal mammary artery as coronary artery bypass graft removed 13 years following surgery, demonstrating near-normal morphology, including an intact internal elastic lamina (*arrow*) Verhoff von Giesen stain (for elastin, *black*) 60×. (Reproduced with permission from Schoen FJ: *Interventional and Surgical Cardiovascular Pathology: Clinical Correlations and Basic Principles.* Philadelphia: Saunders; 1989.)

In contrast to saphenous vein grafts, IMA grafts have greater than 90% patency at 10 years (Fig. 5-12).[61] Multiple factors likely contribute to the remarkably higher long-term patency of IMA grafts compared with vein grafts. Although free saphenous vein grafts sustain disruption of their vasa vasora and nerves, endothelial damage, medial ischemia, and acutely increased internal pressure, an IMA graft generally has minimal preexisting atherosclerosis and requires minimal surgical manipulation, maintains its nutrient blood supply, is adapted to arterial pressures, needs no proximal anastomosis, and has an artery-to-artery distal anastomosis. Graft and recipient vessel have comparable sizes with the IMA but are disparate (graft substantially larger) with saphenous vein. The advent of off-pump and minimally invasive coronary artery bypass grafting has stimulated efforts to facilitate sutureless anastomosis of the graft to the aorta.[62]

Although advances in medical therapy and PCI have contributed to fewer CABGs performed each year, challenges remain and new technologies are under consideration to make the procedure safer and more efficacious.[63]

For example, patients needing revascularization have a much more complicated combination of disease processes and many of the patients have extensive CAD with prior attempts at revascularization. The future of coronary artery bypass grafting may benefit from smaller incisions and potentially robotic endoscopic CABG, facilitated by novel anastomotic devices and intraoperative determination of graft patency. Hybrid surgical/catheterization suites that allow for simultaneous staged CABG and PCI are currently under development.

VALVULAR HEART DISEASE

Normal valve function requires structural integrity and coordinated interactions among multiple anatomical components. For the atrioventricular valves (mitral and tricuspid), these elements include leaflets, commissures, annulus, tendinous cords (chordae tendineae), papillary muscles, and the atrial and ventricular myocardium. For the semilunar valves (aortic and pulmonary), the key structures are the cusps, commissures, and their respective supporting structures in the aortic and pulmonary roots.

The anatomy of the mitral and aortic valves is illustrated in Fig. 5-13.

Mitral Valve

The mitral valve (see Fig. 5-13A) has two leaflets: the anterior (also called septal, or aortic) leaflet, roughly triangular and deep, with the base inserting on approximately one-third of the annulus, and the posterior (also called mural or ventricular) leaflet, more shallow than the anterior and attached to about two-thirds of the annulus. The posterior leaflet typically has distinct scallops that are designated P1, P2, and P3, respectively, beginning from the anterolateral toward the posteromedial commissure. The mitral leaflets have a combined area approximately twice that of the annulus; apposition during systole occurs over approximately 50% of the depth of the posterior leaflet and 30% that of the anterior leaflet. Each leaflet receives tendinous cords from both anterior and posterior papillary muscles. The mitral valve orifice is D-shaped, with the flat anteromedial portion comprising the subaortic attachment of the anterior mitral leaflet. This part of the annulus is fibrous and noncontractile; in contrast, the posterolateral portion of the annulus is muscular and contracts during systole to asymmetrically reduce the area of the orifice. The edges of the mitral leaflets are held in or below the plane of the orifice by the tendinous cords, which themselves are pulled from below by the contracting papillary muscles during systole. This serves to draw the leaflets to closure and maintain competence. The posterior leaflet, with its more delicate structure and shorter annulus-to-free-edge dimension than the anterior, is more prone to postinflammatory fibrous retraction and deformation owing to myxomatous degeneration. The orifice of the tricuspid valve is larger and less distinct than that of the mitral; its three leaflets (anterior, posterior, and septal) are larger and thinner than those of the mitral valve.

Aortic Valve

The aortic valve has structural complexity at several levels.[64] The three aortic valve cusps (left, right, and noncoronary) attach to the aortic wall in a semilunar fashion, ascending to the commissures and descending to the base of each cusp (see Fig. 5-13B). Commissures are spaced approximately 120 degrees apart and occupy the three points of the annular crown, representing the sites of separation between adjacent cusps. Behind the valve cusps are dilated pockets of aortic root, called the sinuses of Valsalva. The right and left coronary arteries arise from orifices behind the right and left cusps, respectively. At the midpoint of the free edge of each cusp is a fibrous nodule called the nodule of Arantius. A thin, crescent-shaped portion of the cusp on either side of the nodule, termed the lunula, defines the surfaces of apposition of the cusps when the valve is closed (approximately 40% of the separating area). The lunular tissue does not contribute to separate aortic from ventricular blood during diastole. Thus, fenestrations (holes) near the free edges commonly occur as a small (<2 mm in diameter), developmental, or degenerative abnormality and have no functional significance. In contrast, defects in the portion of the cusp below the lunula are associated with functional incompetence; such holes also suggest previous or active infection. When the aortic valve is closed during diastole, there is a back pressure on the cusps of approximately 80 mm Hg. The pulmonary valve cusps and surrounding tissues have architectural similarity to but are more delicate than those of the corresponding aortic components, and lack coronary arterial origins.

All four cardiac valves have a similar microscopically inhomogeneous architecture, consisting of well-defined tissue layers in the plane of the cusp. Using the aortic valve as the paradigm (see Fig. 5-13C), beneath the valvular endothelium, on the inflow side the *ventricularis* faces the left ventricular chamber and is enriched in radially aligned elastic fibers, which enable the cusps to have minimal surface area when the valve is open but stretch during diastole to form a large coaptation area. The *spongiosa* is centrally located and is composed of loosely arranged collagen and abundant proteoglycans. This layer has negligible structural strength, but accommodates relative movement between layers during the cardiac cycle and absorbs shock during closure. The *fibrosa* provides structural integrity and mechanical stability through a dense aggregate of circumferentially aligned, densely packed collagen fibers, largely arranged parallel to the cuspal free edge. Normal human aortic and pulmonary valve cusps have few blood vessels; they are sufficiently thin to be perfused from the surrounding blood. In contrast, the mitral and tricuspid leaflets contain a few capillaries in their most basal thirds.

Best developed in aortic valve, key specializations facilitating valve function include crimp of collagen fibers along

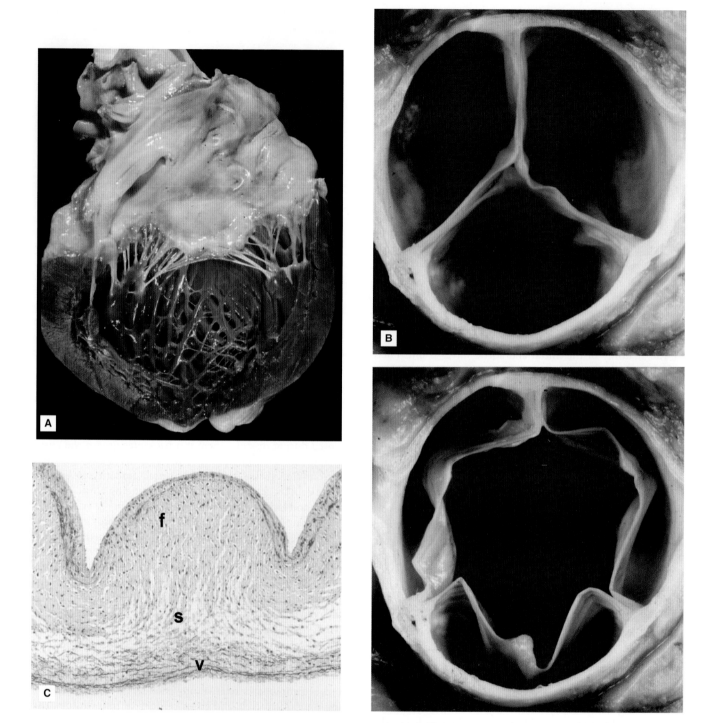

FIGURE 5-13 Normal mitral and aortic valves. In (A), opened left ventricle of the normal heart, demonstrating mitral valve and components of the mitral apparatus. (B) Aortic valve viewed from distal aspect in open (*bottom*) and closed (*top*) phases. (C) Normal aortic valve histology, demonstrating layered structure, including the fibrosa (f), spongiosa (s), and ventricularis (v) layers. The inflow surface is at bottom. Verhoeff van Giesen (stain for elastin, *black*) 150×. ([A] Reproduced with permission from Schoen FJ: *Interventional and Surgical Cardiovascular Pathology: Clinical Correlations and Basic Principles.* Philadelphia: Saunders; 1989. [B and C] Reproduced with permission from Silver MD, Gotlieb AI, Schoen FJ: *Cardiovascular Pathology*, 3rd ed. New York: Churchill Livingstone/Elsevier; 2001.)

their length, bundles of collagen in the fibrous layer oriented toward the commissures, and grossly visible corrugations; these allow cusps to be extremely soft and pliable when unloaded in systole, but taut and stiff when stretched in diastole. Moreover, the orientation of connective tissue and other architectural elements is nonrandom in the plane of the cusp, yielding greater compliance in the radial than circumferential direction. The fibrous network within the cusps effectively transfers the stresses of the closed phase to the annulus and aortic wall. This minimizes sagging of the cusp centers, preserves maximum coaptation, and prevents regurgitation. Additionally, for the mitral valve, the subvalvular apparatus including tendinous cords and papillary muscles is a critical mechanism of valve competency.

Valvular Cell Biology

Recent studies have fostered an emerging picture of how valves form embryologically, mature in the fetus, and function, adapt, maintain homeostasis, and change throughout life. These essential relationships facilitate an understanding of valve pathology and mechanisms of disease, foster the development of improved tissue heart valve substitutes, and inform innovative approaches to heart valve repair and regeneration.[65]

During normal development of the heart, the heart tube undergoes looping, following which the valve cusps/leaflets originate from mesenchymal outgrowths known as endocardial cushions.[66] A subset of endothelial cells in the cushion-forming area, driven by a complex array of signals from the underlying myocardium, changes their phenotype to mesenchymal cells and migrates into the acellular ECM called cardiac jelly. Likely regulated by TGF-β and vascular endothelial growth factor (VEGF), the transformation of endocardial cells to mesenchymal cells is termed trans-differentiation or *endothelial-to-mesenchymal transformation* (EMT). Changes in cell phenotype and ECM remodeling continue throughout human fetal and postnatal development, and throughout life, leading to ongoing changes in properties, as evidenced by increasing valve stiffness with increasing age.[67,68]

Two types of cells are present in the aortic valve: endothelial cells located superficially and interstitial cells located deep to the surface. Aortic valve endothelial cells (VECs) have a different phenotype than endothelial cells in the adjacent aorta and elsewhere,[69,70] but the implications of these differences are not yet known. The second cell type comprises the valvular interstitial cells (VICs), which have variable properties of fibroblasts, smooth muscle cells, and myofibroblasts. VICs maintain the valvular ECM, the key determinant of valve durability. To maintain integrity and pliability throughout life, the valve cusps and leaflets must undergo ongoing physiologic remodeling that entails synthesis, degradation, and reorganization of its ECM, which depends on matrix-degrading enzymes such as MMP. Although VICs are predominantly fibroblast-like in normal valves, they can become activated when exposed to environmental (ie, mechanical and chemical) stimulation and assume a myofibroblast-like phenotype that mediates connective tissue remodeling.

Pathologic Anatomy of Valvular Heart Disease

Cardiac valve operations utilizing replacement or repair usually are undertaken for dysfunction caused by calcification, fibrosis, fusion, retraction, perforation, rupture, stretching, infection, dilation, or congenital malformations of the valve leaflets/cusps or associated structures. Valvular stenosis, defined as inhibition of forward flow secondary to obstruction caused by failure of a valve to open completely, is almost always caused by a cuspal abnormality that induces a chronic disease process. In contrast, valvular insufficiency, defined as reverse flow caused by failure of a valve to close completely, may result from intrinsic disease of the cusps/leaflets and/or damage to or distortion of the supporting structures (eg, the aorta, mitral annulus, chordae tendineae, papillary muscles, and ventricular free wall). Thus, regurgitation can appear either precipitously, as with cordal rupture, or gradually, as with leaflet scarring and retraction. Both stenosis and insufficiency can coexist in a single valve. The most commonly encountered types of valvular heart disease are illustrated in Figs. 5-14 and 5-15.

Calcific Aortic Valve Stenosis

Aortic stenosis (AS) is the most common valvular heart disease in Western countries and has serious consequences.[71] The prevalence of AS increases with age, reaching about 3% after the age of 75 in the United States. Thus, the global burden of AS is expected to double within the next 50 years as life expectancy lengthens. The limited available understanding of AS mechanisms and pathobiology has precluded development of effective noninvasive medical treatments.[72] Symptomatic severe AS not treated promptly by corrective surgery has a high mortality as well as high and accelerating symptom burden.

Calcific AS, the most frequent valvular abnormality requiring surgery, is usually the consequence of calcium phosphate deposition in either an anatomically normal aortic valve or in a congenitally bicuspid valve (see Fig. 5-14A,B).[73] Stenotic, previously normal tricuspid valves present primarily with calcific aortic valve disease in the seventh to ninth decades of life, while congenitally bicuspid valves with superimposed calcification generally become symptomatic earlier (usually sixth to seventh decades).[74]

Calcific AS is characterized by heaped-up, calcified masses initiated in the cuspal fibrosa at the points of maximal cusp flexion (the margins of attachment); they protrude distally from the aortic aspect into the sinuses of Valsalva, inhibiting cuspal opening. However, the ventricular surfaces of the cusps usually remain smooth (see Fig. 5-14C). The calcification process generally does not involve the free cuspal edges, appreciable commissural fusion is absent, and the mitral valve generally is uninvolved. Calcified material resembling bone is

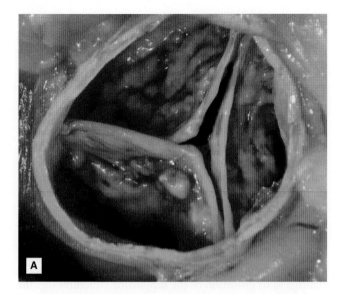

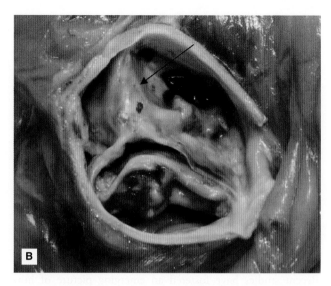

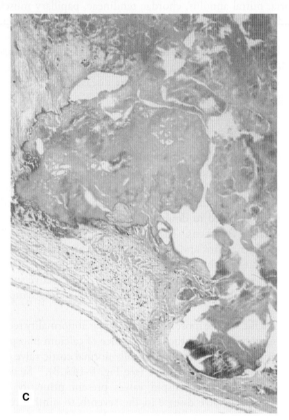

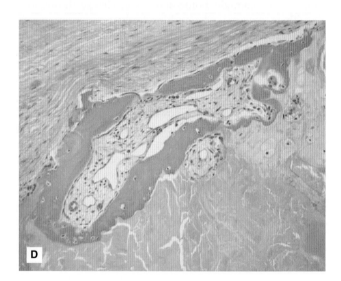

FIGURE 5-14 Calcific aortic valve stenosis. (A) Calcific aortic valve disease causing aortic stenosis in an elderly patient, characterized by mineral deposits at basal aspect of cusps. (B) Calcification of congenitally bicuspid aortic valve, having two unequal cusps, the larger with a central raphe (*arrow*). (C and D) Photomicrographs of calcific deposits in calcific aortic valve disease. Hematoxylin and eosin 15×. Calcific aortic valve stenosis. (C) Nearly transmural deposits with only thin uninvolved cusp on inflow surface (at bottom). (D) Bone formation (osseous metaplasia).

often present (see Fig. 5-14D). Aortic valve *sclerosis* comprises a common, earlier, and hemodynamically less significant stage of the calcification process. Nevertheless, aortic sclerosis is associated with an approximately 50% increase in the risk of death from cardiovascular causes, even in the absence of hemodynamically significant obstruction of left ventricular outflow.[75]

Aortic stenosis induces a pressure gradient across the valve, which may reach 75 to 100 mg Hg in severe cases, necessitating a left ventricular pressure of 200 mg Hg or more to expel blood. Consequently, cardiac output is maintained by the development of pressure-overload left ventricular hypertrophy. The onset of symptoms such as angina, syncope, or heart failure in AS heralds the exhaustion of compensatory cardiac hyperfunction and carries a poor prognosis if not treated by aortic valve replacement (AVR).[76] Other complications of calcific AS include embolization that may occur spontaneously or during interventional procedures,

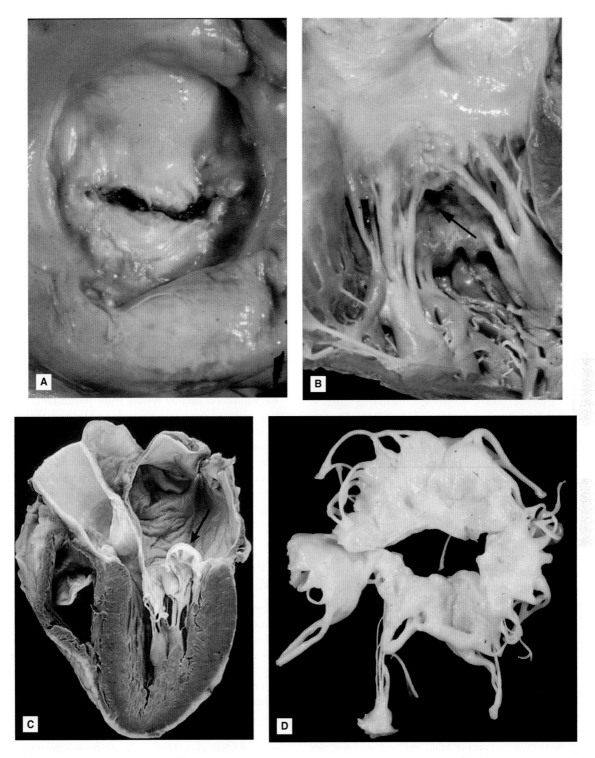

FIGURE 5-15 Etiologies of mitral valvular disease. (A and B) Rheumatic valve disease. (A) Atrial view and (B) subvalvular aspect of valve from patient with rheumatic mitral stenosis. The valvular changes are severe, including diffuse leaflet fibrosis and commissural fusion and ulceration of the free edges of the valve, as well as prominent subvalvular involvement with distortion (*arrow* in [*B*]). (C and D) Myxomatous degeneration of the mitral valve. In (C) there is prolapse into the left atrium of a redundant posterior leaflet (*arrow*). (D) Surgically resected, markedly redundant myxomatous valve. ([A and B] Reproduced with permission from Schoen FJ: *Interventional and Surgical Cardiovascular Pathology: Clinical Correlations and Basic Principles.* Philadelphia: Saunders; 1989.)

hemolysis, infective endocarditis, and extension of the calcific deposits into the ventricular septum causing conduction abnormalities.

Aortic valve calcification has been traditionally considered a wholly degenerative, dystrophic, and passive process. However, recent studies suggest active regulation of calcification in aortic valves, with mechanisms that include inflammation, lipid infiltration, and phenotypic modulation of VIC to an osteoblastic phenotype,[77] and risk factors overlapping with those of arterial atherosclerosis. Similarities to atherosclerosis have stimulated interest in the possibility that statin drugs may decrease the rate of AS progression; however, benefit of statins for AS has not been supported by clinical studies.[78]

Congenitally Bicuspid Aortic Valve

Bicuspid aortic valve (BAV) typically has two cusps of unequal size, with the larger (conjoined) cusp having a midline raphe, representing an incomplete separation or congenital fusion of two cusps. Less frequently, the cusps are of equal size (see Fig. 5-14B). Neither stenotic nor symptomatic at birth or throughout early life, BAV are predisposed to accelerated calcification; ultimately, almost all become stenotic. Aortic pathology, including dilation and/or dissection, commonly accompanies BAV. Despite a prevalence of approximately 1%,[79] BAV and other congenital valve abnormalities underlie over two-thirds of AS in children and almost 50% in adults. Infrequently, BAV become purely incompetent, or complicated by infective endocarditis, even when the valve is hemodynamically normal. Only rarely is an uncomplicated BAV encountered incidentally at autopsy.

Recent studies have confirmed previous reports of familial clustering of BAV and left ventricular outflow tract obstruction malformations, and their association with other cardiovascular malformations.[80] For example, mutations in the signaling and transcriptional regulator NOTCH1 caused a spectrum of developmental aortic valve abnormalities and severe calcification in two families with nonsyndromic familial aortic valve disease.[81]

Mitral Annular Calcification

Calcific deposits also can develop in the ring (annulus) of the mitral valve of elderly individuals, especially women. Although generally asymptomatic, the calcific nodules may lead to regurgitation by interference with systolic contraction of the mitral valve ring or, very rarely, stenosis by impairing mobility of the mitral leaflets during opening. Occasionally, the calcium deposits may penetrate sufficiently deeply to impinge on the atrioventricular conduction system to produce arrhythmias (and rarely sudden death). Patients with mitral annular calcification have an increased risk of stroke, and the calcific nodules, especially if ulcerated, can be the nidus for thrombotic deposits or infective endocarditis. Mitral annular calcification can also mimic a left ventricular neoplasm.

Rheumatic Heart Disease

Rheumatic fever is an acute, often recurrent, inflammatory disease that generally follows a pharyngeal infection with group A beta-hemolytic streptococci, principally in children. In the past several decades, rheumatic fever and rheumatic heart disease have declined markedly but not disappeared in the United States and other developed countries. Evidence strongly suggests that rheumatic fever is the result of an immune response to streptococcal antigens, inciting either a cross-reaction to tissue antigens or a streptococcal-induced autoimmune reaction to normal tissue antigens.[82]

Chronic rheumatic heart disease most frequently affects the mitral and to a lesser extent the aortic and/or the tricuspid valves. Usually dominated by mitral stenosis,[83] chronic rheumatic valve disease is characterized by fibrous or fibrocalcific thickening of leaflets and tendinous cords, and commissural and chordal fusion (see Fig. 5-15A and B). Stenosis results from leaflet and chordal fibrous thickening and commissural fusion, with or without secondary calcification. Regurgitation usually results from postinflammatory scarring-induced retraction of cords and leaflets. Combinations of lesions may yield valves that are both stenotic and regurgitant. Although considered the pathognomonic inflammatory myocardial lesions in acute rheumatic fever, Aschoff nodules are found infrequently in myocardium sampled at autopsy or at valve replacement surgery, most likely reflecting the extended interval from acute disease to critical functional impairment.

Degeneration of the Mitral Valve (Mitral Valve Prolapse)

Degenerative mitral valve disease (mitral valve prolapse) causes chronic, pure, isolated mitral regurgitation by leaflet stretching and prolapse into the left atrium and occasionally cordal rupture.[84] Owing to improved imaging technology and large community studies, a prevalence of mitral valve prolapse (MVP) of approximately 2% has been established. Potentially serious complications include progressive congestive heart failure, infective endocarditis, stroke, or other manifestation of thromboembolism, sudden death, or atrial fibrillation. Mitral valve prolapse is the most common indication for mitral valve repair or replacement.

In MVP, one or both mitral leaflets are enlarged, redundant, or floppy and will prolapse or balloon back into the left atrium during ventricular systole (see Fig. 5-15C). The three characteristic anatomic changes in MVP are: (1) intercordal ballooning (hooding) of the mitral leaflets or portions thereof (most frequently involving the posterior leaflet), sometimes accompanied by elongated, thinned, or ruptured cords;

(2) rubbery diffuse leaflet thickening that hinders adequate coaptation and interdigitation of leaflet tissue during valve closure; and (3) annular dilation, with diameters and circumferences that may exceed 3.5 and 11.0 cm, respectively (see Fig. 5-15D). Pathologic mitral annular enlargement predominates in and may be confined to the posterior leaflet, because the anterior leaflet is firmly anchored by the fibrous tissue at the aortic valve and is far less distensible. The key microscopic change is myxomatous degeneration with attenuation or focal disruption of the fibrous layer of the valve, weakening the leaflet. Focal or diffuse thickening of the spongy layer by proteoglycan deposition gives the tissue an edematous, blue appearance on microscopy (called *myxomatous* by pathologists).[85] Concomitant involvement of the tricuspid valve is present in some cases, and the aortic and pulmonary valves are rarely affected.

Secondary changes may occur, including (1) fibrous thickening along both surfaces of the valve leaflets; (2) linear thickening of the subjacent mural endocardium of the left ventricle as a consequence of friction-induced injury by cordal hamstringing of the prolapsing leaflets; (3) thrombi on the atrial surfaces of the leaflets, particularly in the recesses behind the ballooned leaflet segments; (4) calcification along the base of the posterior mitral leaflet; and (5) cordal thickening and fusion that can resemble postrheumatic disease.

Although the pathogenesis of mitral valve degeneration is uncertain, this valvular abnormality is a common feature of Marfan's syndrome and occasionally other hereditary connective tissue disorders such as Ehlers-Danlos syndrome, suggesting an analogous connective tissue defect. In heritable disorders of connective tissue, including Marfan's syndrome, MVP is usually associated with mutations in fibrillin-1 (FBN-1); recent evidence also has implicated abnormal TGF-β signaling (similar to the aortic abnormalities in the pathogenesis of Marfan's syndrome and related disorders).[86] Although it is unlikely that more than 1 to 2% of patients with MVP have an identifiable connective tissue disorder, studies utilizing genetic linkage analysis have mapped families with autosomal dominant MVP to specific chromosomal abnormalities, several of which involve genes that could be involved in valvular tissue remodeling.

Ischemic Mitral Regurgitation

In ischemic mitral regurgitation (IMR), also called functional mitral regurgitation, myocardial structure and function are altered by ischemic injury; in contrast to degenerative valve disease, the leaflets are intrinsically normal.[87] Present in many patients with CAD, IMR worsens prognosis following myocardial infarction, with reduced survival directly related to the severity of the regurgitation. Mechanisms of IMR include an ischemic papillary muscle that fails to tighten the cords during systole, and fibrotic, shortened papillary muscle that fixes the chordae deeply within the ventricle. Nevertheless, papillary muscle dysfunction alone is generally insufficient

to produce IMR, and regional dysfunction and dilation with an increasing spherical shape of the left ventricle, which pulls the papillary muscles down and away from the center of the chamber, usually contributes. Although there is substantial interest in developing surgical and/or percutaneous approaches to the repair of IMR,[88,89] the degree to which correcting IMR improves survival and/or symptoms remains uncertain.[90,91]

Carcinoid and Drug-Induced Valve Disease

Patients with the carcinoid syndrome often develop plaque-like intimal thickenings of the endocardium of the tricuspid valve, right ventricular outflow tract, and pulmonary valve superimposed on otherwise unaltered endocardium.[92] The left side of the heart is usually unaffected. These lesions are related to elaboration by carcinoid tumors (most often primary in the gut) of bioactive products, including serotonin, which cause valvular endothelial cell proliferation but are inactivated by passage through the lung.

Left-sided but similar valve lesions have been reported to complicate the administration of fenfluramine and phentermine (fen-phen), appetite suppressants used for the treatment of obesity, which may affect systemic serotonin metabolism (see Fig. 5-15E).[93] Typical diet drug-associated plaques have proliferation of myofibroblast-like cells in a myxoid stroma. Similar left-sided plaques may be found in patients who receive methysergide or ergotamine therapy for migraine headaches; these serotonin analogs are metabolized to serotonin as they pass through the pulmonary vasculature. Moreover, drug-related valve disease has been reported in patients taking pergolide mesylate, an ergot-derived dopamine receptor agonist used to treat Parkinson's disease and restless leg syndrome.[94]

Infective Endocarditis

Infective endocarditis is characterized by colonization or invasion of the heart valves, mural endocardium, aorta, aneurysmal sacs, or other blood vessels, by a microbiologic agent, leading to the formation of friable vegetations laden with organisms, fibrin, and inflammatory cells (Fig. 5-16).[95] Although virtually any type of microbiologic agent can cause infective endocarditis, most cases are bacterial.

The clinical classification into acute and subacute forms is based on the severity and tempo of the disease, virulence of the infecting microorganism, and presence of underlying cardiac disease. *Acute endocarditis* is a destructive infection by a highly virulent organism, often involving a previously normal heart valve, and leading to death within days to weeks in more than 50% of patients if left untreated. In contrast, in a more indolent lesion, called *subacute endocarditis*, organisms of low virulence cause infection on previously deformed valves; in this situation, the infection may pursue a protracted

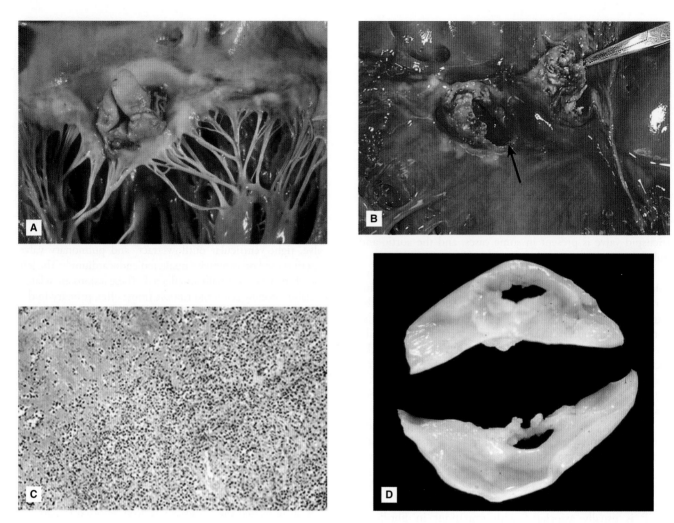

FIGURE 5-16 Infective (bacterial) endocarditis. (A) Endocarditis of mitral valve with damage to the anterior mitral leaflet. (B) Acute endocarditis of congenitally bicuspid aortic valve (caused by *Staphylococcus aureus*), with large vegetation, causing extensive cuspal destruction and ring abscess (*arrow*). (C) Photomicrograph of vegetation, showing extensive acute inflammatory cells and fibrin. Bacterial organisms were demonstrated by tissue Gram stain. (D) Healed endocarditis, demonstrating aortic valvular destruction but no active vegetations on a congenitally bicuspid aortic valve. ([B] Reproduced with permission from Schoen FJ: *Interventional and Surgical Cardiovascular Pathology: Clinical Correlations and Basic Principles.* Philadelphia: Saunders; 1989. [C] Reproduced with permission from Schoen FJ. Surgical pathology of removed natural and prosthetic heart valves, *Hum Pathol.* 1987 Jun;18(6):558-567.)

course of weeks to months during which the infection may be undetected and untreated.

Staphylococcus aureus is the leading cause of acute endocarditis and produces necrotizing, ulcerative, invasive, and highly destructive valvular infections. The subacute form is usually caused by *Streptococcus viridans*. Cardiac abnormalities, such as chronic rheumatic heart disease, congenital heart disease (particularly anomalies that have small shunts or tight stenoses creating high-velocity jet streams), degenerative mitral valves, BAVs, and artificial valves and their sewing rings predispose to endocarditis. In intravenous drug abusers, left-sided lesions predominate, but right-sided valves are commonly affected. In about 5 to 20% of all cases of endocarditis, no organism can be isolated from the blood (*culture-negative endocarditis*), often because of prior antibiotic therapy or organisms difficult to culture.[96]

The modified Duke criteria provide a standardized assessment of patients with suspected infective endocarditis that integrates factors predisposing patients to the development of infective endocarditis, blood-culture evidence of infection, echocardiographic findings, and clinical and laboratory information.[97] The previously important clinical findings of petechiae, subungual hemorrhages, Janeway's lesions, Osler's nodes, and Roth's spots in the eyes (secondary to retinal microemboli) have now become uncommon owing to the shortened clinical course of the disease as a result of antibiotic therapy.

The complications of endocarditis include valvular insufficiency (rarely stenosis), abscess of the valve annulus (*ring abscess*), suppurative pericarditis, and embolization. With appropriate antibiotic therapy, vegetations may undergo healing, with progressive sterilization, organization, fibrosis, and

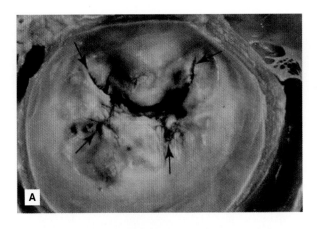
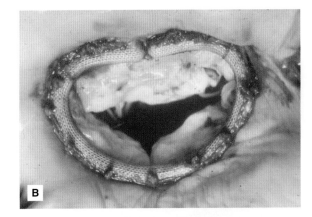
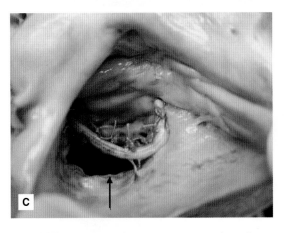
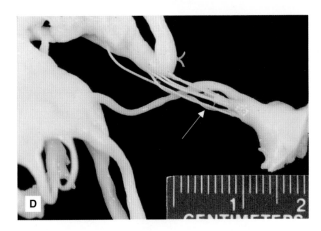

FIGURE 5-17 Open surgical reconstructive procedures for mitral valve disease. (A) Mitral commissurotomy in mitral stenosis; incised commissures are indicated by arrows. (B) Mitral valve repair with annuloplasty ring. (C) Dehiscence of mitral annuloplasty ring (*arrow*). (D) ePTFE suture replacement (*arrow*) of ruptured cord in myxomatous mitral valve. ([A] Reproduced with permission from Schoen FJ. Surgical pathology of removed natural and prosthetic heart valves, *Hum Pathol.* 1987 Jun;18(6):558-67. [C] Used with permission from William A. Muller, MD, PhD, Northwestern University School of Medicine, Chicago.)

occasionally calcification. Cusp or leaflet perforation, cordal rupture, or fistula formation from a ring abscess into an adjacent cardiac chamber or great vessel can cause regurgitation. Ring abscesses are generally associated with virulent organisms, and a relatively high mortality rate.

Valve Reconstruction and Repair

Reconstructive procedures to repair mitral insufficiency of various etiologies and to minimize the severity of rheumatic mitral stenosis are now highly effective and commonplace.[98] Reconstructive therapy of selected patients with aortic insufficiency (AI) and aortic dilation may also be done in some cases,[99] but repair of AS has been notably more challenging. The major advantage of repair over replacement relates to the elimination of both prosthesis-related complications and the need for chronic anticoagulation therapy. Other reported advantages include a lower hospital mortality, better long-term function owing to the ability to maintain the continuity of the mitral apparatus, and a lower rate

of postoperative endocarditis. Figures 5-17 and 5-18 illustrate the pathologic anatomy of various open and catheter-based mitral valve reconstruction procedures. Figure 5-19 illustrates a key difficulty of surgical repairs for AS, in that the cuspal calcification extends nearly to the inflow surface (recall Fig.14-C).

Mitral Stenosis

Commissurotomy may be employed in the operative repair of some stenotic mitral valves in which fibrosis and shortening of both cords and leaflets have markedly decreased leaflet mobility and area. Factors that compromise the late functional results of or technically prevent mitral commissurotomy and thereby necessitate valve replacement include (1) left ventricular dysfunction; (2) pulmonary venous hypertension and right-sided cardiac factors, including right ventricular failure, tricuspid regurgitation, or a combination of these; (3) systemic embolization; (4) coexistent cardiac disorders, such as coronary artery or aortic valve diseases;

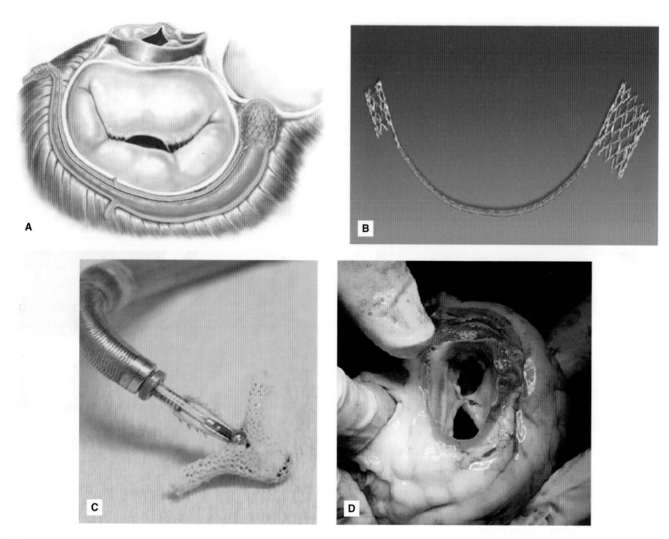

FIGURE 5-18 Percutaneous correction of mitral regurgitation. (A) Schematic approach utilizing the proximity of the coronary sinus to the posterior mitral annulus to effect a simulated annuloplasty. Diagram showing the relationship of the coronary sinus and the posterior leaflet of the mitral valve. A remodeling device is seen within the coronary sinus. (B) The Monarc device consists of two anchoring stents with a bridge connector that shortens approximately 25% over the space of weeks with the intention of reducing the dimensions of the mitral annulus. Percutaneous correction of mitral regurgitation. (C and D) Edge-to-edge approximation of the anterior and posterior leaflets of the mitral valve is achieved by deployment of clip (Evalve mitral clip device) that is analogous to an Alfieri stitch, thereby creating a double orifice with improved leaflet coaptation. (Reproduced with permission from McManus BM, Braunwald E: *Atlas of Cardiovascular Pathology for the Clinician.* Philadelphia: Current Medicine; 2008.)

(5) residual or progressive mitral valve disease, including valve restenosis, residual (unrelieved) stenosis, or regurgitation induced at operation; (6) advanced leaflet (especially commissural) calcification; (7) subvalvar (predominantly chordal) fibrotic changes; and (8) significant regurgitation owing to retraction.

Percutaneous balloon mitral valvuloplasty has been used to treat mitral stenosis for over two decades, with excellent success in patients with suitable valvular and subvalvular morphology.[100] However, because balloon valvuloplasty largely involves separation of the fused leaflets at the commissures, this procedure is also unlikely to provide significant benefit to patients with the valve features summarized in the preceding that obviate surgical commissurotomy.

Mitral Regurgitation

Reconstructive techniques are widely used to repair mitral valves with nonrheumatic mitral regurgitation.[101-103] Structural defects responsible for chronic mitral regurgitation include (1) dilation of the mitral annulus; (2) leaflet prolapse into the left atrium with or without elongation or rupture of chordae tendineae; (3) redundancy and deformity of leaflets; (4) leaflet perforations or defects; and (5) restricted leaflet motion as a result of commissural fusion in an opened position, and leaflet retraction, or chordal shortening or thickening.

Following surgical resection of excess anterior or posterior leaflet tissue in valves with redundancy, annuloplasty with or without a prosthetic ring is used to reduce the annulus

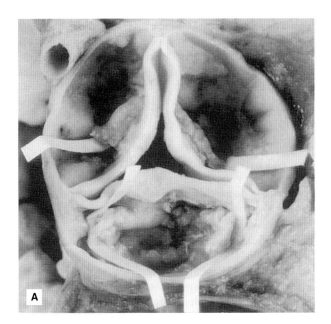

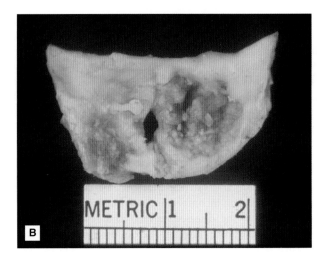

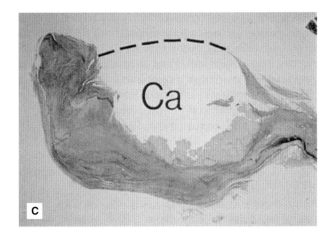

FIGURE 5-19 Reconstructive procedures for aortic stenosis. (A) Aortic valve balloon valvuloplasty for degenerative calcific aortic stenosis, demonstrating fractures of nodular deposits of calcifications highlighted by tapes. [B and C] Operative decalcification of the aortic valve. (B) Aortic valve after operative mechanical decalcification demonstrating perforated cusp. (C) Low-power photomicrograph of cross-section of aortic valve cusp after decalcification with lithotripter. Weigert elastic stain. Ca = calcium. ([A] Reproduced with permission from Silver MD, Gotlieb AI, Schoen FJ: *Cardiovascular Pathology*, 3rd ed. New York: Churchill Livingstone/Elsevier; 2001. [B and C] Reproduced with permission from Schoen FJ: *Interventional and Surgical Cardiovascular Pathology: Clinical Correlations and Basic Principles*. Philadelphia: Saunders; 1989.)

dimension to correspond to the amount of leaflet tissue available. Edge-to-edge (Alfieri stitch) mitral valve repair has also been used.[104] Tissue substitutes such as glutaraldehyde-pretreated xenograft or autologous pericardium can be used to repair or enlarge leaflets. Ruptured or elongated cords may be repaired by shortening or replacement with pericardial tissue or thick suture material.

Percutaneous approaches currently being evaluated for mitral regurgitation attempt to emulate one or more of the components of surgical mitral valve repair, including annular reduction and edge-to-edge mitral leaflet apposition.[105-107] However, leaflet resection and cordal modification cannot be easily done via catheter, and there is considerable anatomical variability of the coronary sinus.[108] Percutaneous approaches considered include implantation of a device in the coronary sinus, left atrium (or both), or by device placement behind the posterolateral leaflet of the mitral valve (see Fig. 5-18A and B). The goal is to plicate or straighten the posterior mitral annulus. Additional annuloplasty approaches, presently in preclinical testing, include a suture annuloplasty from the

ventricular side of the mitral annulus, thermal modification of the annulus to obtain shrinkage, and a percutaneous ventricular restraint system that attempts to reshape the left ventricle. Another catheter-based approach uses an edge-to-edge clip prosthesis simulating the edge-to-edge surgical (Alfieri stitch) repair in which the midportions of the anterior and posterior mitral leaflets are clipped together (see Fig. 5-18C and D).[109,110]

Aortic Stenosis

In balloon dilation of calcific AS, individual functional responses vary considerably and data suggest a modest early incremental benefit, high early mortality, and high early restenosis rate owing to recoil of stretched tissue. Improvement derives from commissural separation, fracture of calcific deposits, and stretching of the valve cusps (see Fig. 5-19A). The major complications include cerebrovascular accident secondary to embolism, massive regurgitation owing to valve trauma, and cardiac perforation with tamponade. Fractured calcific nodules can themselves prove dangerous.[111] In pediatric cases in which the cusps are generally pliable, cuspal stretching, tearing, or avulsion may also occur.

In calcific AS, the calcific deposits arise deep in the valve fibrous layer (see Fig. 5-14C). Their removal by sharp dissection or ultrasonic debridement generally removes a considerable fraction of the valve substance, resulting in severe compromise of mechanical integrity (see Fig. 5-19B and C).[112]

Valve Replacement

Severe symptomatic valvular heart disease other than pure mitral stenosis or incompetence is most frequently treated by excision of the diseased valve(s) and replacement by a functional substitute. Five key factors determine the results of valve replacement in an individual patient: (1) technical aspects of the procedure; (2) intraoperative myocardial ischemic injury; (3) irreversible and chronic structural alterations in the heart and lungs secondary to the valvular abnormality; (4) coexistent obstructive CAD; and (5) valve prosthesis reliability and host-tissue interactions.

Cardiac valvular substitutes are of two types, mechanical and biologic tissue (Fig. 5-20 and Table 5-2).[113,114] Prostheses function passively, responding to pressure and flow changes within the heart. Mechanical valves are composed of nonphysiologic biomaterials and employ a rigid, mobile occluder (composed of pyrolytic carbon in contemporary valves), in a metallic cage (cobalt-chrome or titanium alloy) as in the Bjork-Shiley, Hall-Medtronic, or Omniscience valves, or two carbon hemidisks in a carbon housing (as in the St. Jude Medical, CarboMedics CPHV, and On-X prostheses). Pyrolytic carbon has high strength and fatigue and wear resistance and good thromboresistance. Tissue valves resemble natural semilunar valves, with pseudoanatomical central flow and biological material. In the past decade, innovations in tissue valve technologies and design have expanded indications for their use. Contemporary utilization of bioprosthetic tissue valves is estimated to be about 80% of all aortic and 69% of all mitral substitute heart valves.[115,116] Most tissue valves are bioprosthetic xenografts fabricated from porcine aortic valve or bovine pericardium, which have been preserved in a dilute glutaraldehyde solution, and a small percentage are cryopreserved allografts.

In a recent compilation of risk models of isolated valve surgery by the Society for Thoracic Surgeons, the overall mortality was 3.4% (3.2% aortic and 5.7% mitral) and varied strongly with case mix.[117] The majority of early deaths are caused by hemorrhage, pulmonary failure, low cardiac output, and sudden death with or without myocardial necrosis or documented arrhythmias. Potential complications related to mitral valve insertion include hemorrhagic disruption and dissection of the atrioventricular groove, perforation or entrapment of the left circumflex coronary artery by a suture, and pseudoaneurysm or rupture of the left ventricular free wall.

Improvement in late outcome has occurred predominantly from earlier referral of patients for valve replacement, decreased intraoperative myocardial damage, improved surgical technique, and improved valve prostheses. Following valve replacement with currently used devices, the probability of 5-year survival is about 80% and of 10-year survival about 70%, depending on overall functional state, preoperative left ventricular function, left ventricular and left atrial size, and extent and severity of CAD.

Substitute Valve-Related Complications

Although early prosthetic valve–associated complications are unusual, prosthetic valve–associated pathology becomes an important consideration beyond the early postoperative period. Late death following valve replacement results predominantly from either cardiovascular pathology unrelated to the substitute valve or prosthesis-associated complications. In the few randomized studies comparing mechanical prosthetic and bioprosthetic valves several decades ago (comprising Bjork-Shiley mechanical and porcine aortic bioprosthetic valves), approximately 60% or more patients had an important device-related complication within 10 years postoperatively. Moreover, long-term survival was better among patients with a mechanical valve, but with an increased risk of bleeding.[118,119] Valve-related complications frequently necessitate reoperation, now accounting for approximately 10 to 15% of all valve procedures, and they may cause death. Four categories of valve-related complications are most important: thromboembolism and related problems, infection, structural dysfunction (ie, failure or degeneration of the biomaterials comprising a prosthesis), and nonstructural dysfunction (ie, miscellaneous complications and modes of failure not encompassed in the previous groups) (Table 5-3).[120]

THROMBOSIS AND THROMBOEMBOLISM

Thromboembolic complications are the major valve-related cause of mortality and morbidity after replacement with mechanical valves, and patients receiving them require lifetime chronic therapeutic anticoagulation with warfarin derivatives.[121,122] Thrombotic deposits on a prosthetic valve can immobilize the occluder(s) or cusps, or shed emboli (Fig. 5-21). Owing to biologic material and central flow, tissue valves are less thrombogenic than mechanical valves; their recipients generally do not require long-term anticoagulation in the absence of another specific indication, such as atrial fibrillation. Nevertheless, the rate of thromboembolism in patients with mechanical valves on anticoagulation is not widely different from that in patients with bioprosthetic valves without anticoagulation (2 to 4% per year). Chronic oral anticoagulation also carries a risk of hemorrhage. Anticoagulation is particularly difficult to manage in pregnant women.[123] The risk of thromboembolism is potentiated by preoperative or postoperative cardiac functional impairment.

"Virchow's triad" of factors promoting thrombosis (surface thrombogenicity, hypercoagulability, and locally static blood flow) largely predicts the relative propensity toward and locations of thrombotic deposits.[124] For example, with caged-ball prostheses, thrombi form distal to the poppet at the cage apex. Tilting disk prostheses are particularly susceptible to

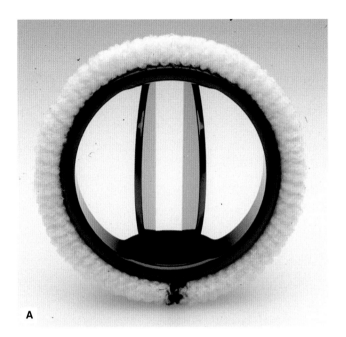

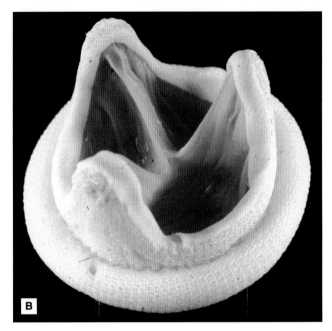

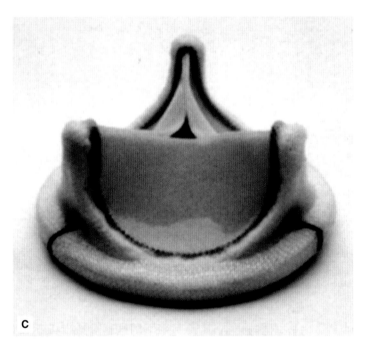

FIGURE 5-20 Photographs of the widely used types of heart valve substitutes. (A) Bileaflet tilting disk mechanical heart valve (St. Jude Medical, St. Jude Medical Inc., St. Paul, MN). (B) Porcine aortic valve bioprosthesis (Hancock, Medtronic Heart Valves, Santa Ana, CA). (C) Bovine pericardial bioprosthesis (Carpentier-Edwards, Edwards Life Sciences, Santa Ana, CA). (Reproduced with permission from Silver MD, Gotlieb AI, Schoen FJ: *Cardiovascular Pathology*, 3rd ed. New York: Churchill Livingstone/Elsevier; 2001.)

total thrombotic occlusion or shedding emboli from small thrombi, with the thrombotic deposits generally initiated in a flow stagnation zone in the minor orifice of the outflow region of the prosthesis. In contrast, bileaflet tilting disk valves are most vulnerable to thrombus formation near the hinges where the leaflets insert into the housing (see Fig. 5-21A). Late thrombosis of a bioprosthetic valve is marked by large

thrombotic deposits in one or more of the prosthetic sinuses of Valsalva (see Fig. 5-21B), and no causal underlying cuspal pathology can usually be demonstrated by pathologic studies. Some valve thromboemboli, especially early postoperatively with any valve type, are thought to be initiated at the valve sewing cuff before it is healed, thus providing a rationale for early antithrombotic therapy for all types.

TABLE 5-2: Types and Characteristics of Representative Types of Substitute Heart Valves*

Valve type	Model(s)	Hemodynamics	Freedom from thrombosis/ thromboembolism	Durability
Mechanical				
Caged ball	Starr-Edwards	+[§]	+	+ + +
Single tilting disk	Bjork-Shiley			
	Hall-Medtronic	+ +	+ +	+ + +[†]
	Omnicarbon			
Bileaflet tilting disk	St. Jude Medical	+ + +	+ + +	+ + +[‡]
	Carbomedics			
	Edwards-Duromedics			
Tissue				
Heterograft/ xenograft bioprostheses	Carpentier-Edwards (porcine and bovine pericardial)	+ +	+ + +	+ +
	Hancock (porcine) Ionescu-Shiley (bovine pericardial)			
	Mitroflow (bovine pericardial)			
Homograft/allograft	Cryopreserved human aortic/pulmonary valve	+ + + +	+ + + +	+ +

*Presently or previously.
[†]Except Bjork-Shiley 60°/70° convexo-concave valve (see text).
[‡]Except previous model of Edwards-Duromedics valve (see text).
[§]Performance criteria: + = least favorable to + + + + = most favorable.
Data from Vongpatanasin, et al.

 TABLE 5-3: Complications of Substitute Heart Valves

Generic	Specific
Thrombotic limitations	Thrombosis
	Thromboembolism
	Anticoagulation-related hemorrhage
Infection	Prosthetic valve endocarditis
Structural dysfunction (intrinsic)	Wear
	Fracture
	Poppet escape
	Cuspal tear
	Calcification
	Commisural region dehiscence
Nonstructural dysfunction (most extrinsic)	Pannus (tissue overgrowth)
	Entrapment by suture or tissue
	Paravalvular leak
	Disproportion
	Hemolytic anemia
	Noise

Modified with permission from Schoen FJ, Levy RJ, Piehler HR: *Pathological considerations in replacement cardiac valves, Cardiovasc Pathol.* 1992 Jan-Mar;1(1):29-52.

Although platelet deposition dominates initial blood-surface interaction, and prosthetic valve thromboembolism correlates strongly with altered platelet function, antiplatelet therapy alone is generally considered insufficient to adequately prevent thromboembolism. The lack of vascular tissue adjacent to thrombi that form on bioprosthetic or mechanical valves retards their histologic organization and may prolong the susceptibility to embolization as well as render the age of such thrombi difficult to determine microscopically. Nevertheless, this feature has permitted thrombolytic therapy to be an option in some cases.[125]

PROSTHETIC VALVE ENDOCARDITIS

Prosthetic valve infective endocarditis (Fig. 5-22) occurs in 3 to 6% of recipients of substitute valves.[126] Infection can occur early or late. The microbial etiology of early prosthetic valve endocarditis (<60 days postoperative) is dominated by *Staphylococcus epidermidis* and *S. aureus*, even though prophylactic regimens used today target these microorganisms. The clinical course of early prosthetic valve endocarditis tends to be fulminant. In the generally less virulent late endocarditis, a source of infection and/or bacteremia can often be found; the most frequent initiators are dental procedures, urologic infections and interventions, and indwelling catheters. The most common organisms in these late infections are *S. epidermidis, S. aureus, S. viridans,* and enterococci. Rates of infection of bioprostheses and mechanical valves are similar, and

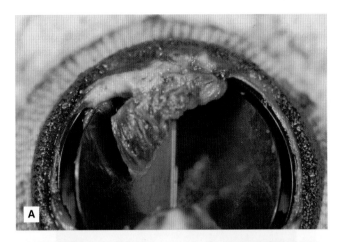

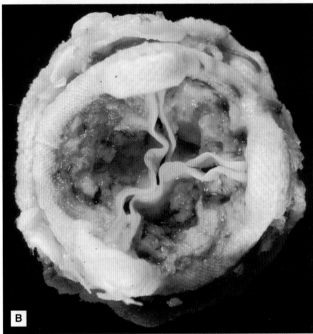

FIGURE 5-21 Thrombotic occlusion of substitute heart valves. (A) Bileaflet tilting disk prosthesis, with thrombus initiated in the region of the pivot guard, causing near-total occluder immobility. (B) Porcine bioprosthesis, with thrombus filling the bioprosthetic sinuses of Valsalva. ([A] Reproduced with permission from Buchart EG, Bodnar E: *Thrombosis, Embolism, and Bleeding.* London: ICR Publishers; 1992. [B] Reproduced with permission from Schoen FJ, Hobson CE: Anatomic analysis of removed prosthetic heart valves: causes of failure of 33 mechanical valves and 58 bioprostheses, 1980 to 1983, *Hum Pathol.* 1985 Jun;16(6):549-559.)

previous endocarditis on a natural or substitute valve markedly increases the risk.

Infections associated with mechanical prosthetic valves and some with bioprosthetic valves are localized to the prosthesis-tissue junction at the sewing ring, and accompanied by tissue destruction around the prosthesis (see Fig. 5-22A). This comprises a ring abscess, with potential paraprosthetic leak, dehiscence, fistula formation, or heart block caused by

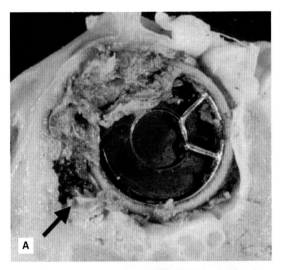

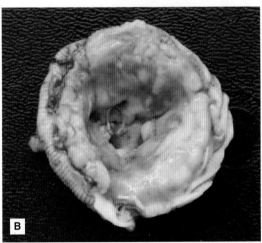

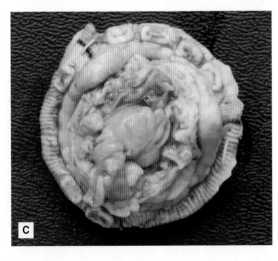

FIGURE 5-22 Prosthetic valve endocarditis. (A) Endocarditis with large ring abscess (*arrow*) observed from ventricular surface of aortic Bjork-Shiley tilting disk prosthesis in patient who died suddenly. Ring abscess impinged on proximal atrioventricular conduction system. (B and C) Bioprosthetic valve endocarditis viewed from inflow (B) and outflow (C) aspects. (Reproduced with permission from Schoen FJ: Cardiac valve prostheses: pathological and bioengineering considerations, *J Card Surg.* 1987 Mar;2(1):65-108.)

conduction system damage. Bioprosthetic valve infections may also involve, and are occasionally limited to, the cuspal tissue, sometimes causing secondary cuspal tearing or perforation with valve incompetence or obstruction (see Fig. 5-22 B and C). Surgical reintervention usually is indicated for large highly mobile vegetations or cerebral thromboembolic episodes, or persistent ring abscess.

STRUCTURAL VALVE DYSFUNCTION

Prosthetic valve dysfunction owing to materials degradation can necessitate reoperation or cause prosthesis-associated death

(Fig. 5-23). Durability considerations vary widely for mechanical valves and bioprostheses, specific types of each, different models of a particular prosthesis (utilizing different materials or having different design features), and even for the same model prosthesis placed in the aortic rather than the mitral site. Mechanical valve structural failure is often catastrophic and may be life threatening; in contrast, bioprosthetic valve failure generally causes progressive symptomatic deterioration.

Fractures of metallic carbon components (disks or housing) are unusual in most contemporary bileaflet tilting disk mechanical valves[127] (see Fig. 5-23A). Historically, however,

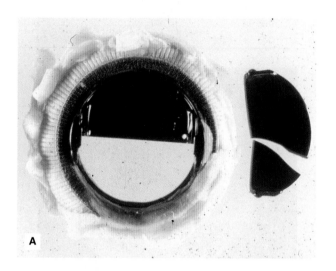
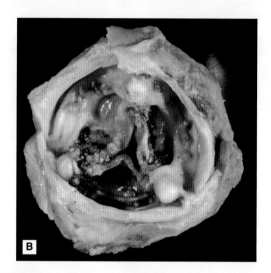
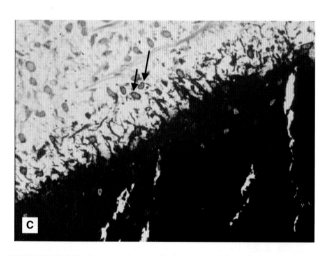
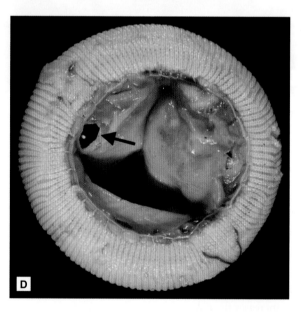

FIGURE 5-23 Structural valve dysfunction. (A) Disk fracture and escape in a Hemex-Duramedics heart valve prosthesis. (B and C) Porcine valve primary tissue failure owing to calcification with severe stenosis. (B) Gross photograph. (C) Photomicrograph demonstrating predominant site of calcification in cells of the residual porcine valve matrix (*arrows*). (D) Clinical porcine bioprosthesis with noncalcific tear of one cusp (*arrow*). ([A] Reproduced with permission from Schoen FJ, Levy RJ, Piehler HR: Pathological considerations in replacement cardiac valves, *Cardiovasc Pathol.* 1992 Jan-Mar;1(1):29-52. [B] Reproduced with permission from Schoen FJ, et al: Long-term failure rate and morphologic correlations in porcine bioprosthetic heart valves, *Am J Cardiol.* 1983 Mar 15;51(6):957-964. [C] Reproduced with permission from Silver MD, Gotlieb AI, Schoen FJ: *Cardiovascular Pathology*, 3rd ed. New York: Churchill Livingstone/Elsevier; 2001.)

durability failures of mechanical valves were not uncommon. For example, of approximately 86,000 Bjork-Shiley 60- and 70-degree convexo-concave heart valves implanted, a cluster of more than 500 cases has been reported in which the two attachment points of the welded outlet strut fractured because of metal fatigue, leading to disk escape and often death.[128]

In contrast, structural dysfunction of tissue valves continues to be the major cause of failure of the most widely used bioprostheses (flexible-stent-mounted, glutaraldehyde-preserved porcine aortic valves, and bovine pericardial valves) (see Fig. 5-23B-D).[129] Long-term data on the first several decades of bioprosthetic valves (1970s through almost 2000) indicate that 50% of bioprosthetic mitral or AVRs require replacement within 15 to 20 years following implantation, because of structural dysfunction manifested as primary tissue failure. Cuspal mineralization is the key mechanism, causing stenosis, and secondary tears can cause regurgitation. Noncalcific structural damage owing to collagen fiber disruption (independent of calcification) also contributes to bioprosthetic heart valve failure.[130] Calcific deposits are usually localized to cuspal tissue (*intrinsic calcification*), but calcific deposits extrinsic to the cusps may occur in thrombi or endocarditic vegetations. Calcification is markedly accelerated in younger patients, with children and adolescents having an especially accelerated course. Bovine pericardial valves can also suffer calcification and tearing, with abrasion of the pericardial tissue an important contributing factor in some designs.[131]

The morphology and determinants of calcification of bioprosthetic valve tissue have been widely studied. The process is initiated primarily within residual membranes and organelles of the nonviable connective tissue cells that have been devitalized by glutaraldehyde pretreatment procedures, and involves reaction of calcium-containing extracellular fluid with membrane-associated phosphorus. The pathologic changes in bioprosthetic valves that occur following implantation are largely rationalized on the basis of changes induced by the preservation and manufacture of a bioprosthesis, including (1) denudation of surface cells, including endothelial cells in porcine aortic valves, and mesothelial cells in bovine pericardium; (2) loss of viability of the interstitial cells; and (3) locking of the cuspal microstructure in a static geometry.[129]

NONSTRUCTURAL DYSFUNCTION

Nonstructural dysfunction of substitute heart valves are illustrated in Fig. 5-24. Paravalvular defects may be clinically inconsequential may aggravate hemolysis or may cause heart failure through regurgitation. Early paravalvular leaks may be related to suture knot failure, inadequate suture placement, or separation of sutures from a pathologic annulus in endocarditis with ring abscess, myxomatous valvular degeneration, or calcified valvular annulus as in calcific AS or mitral annular calcification. Late small paravalvular leaks usually are caused by tissue retraction from the sewing ring between sutures during healing. Small paravalvular defects are difficult to locate by surgical or pathologic examination (see Fig. 5-24A).

Extrinsic factors can mediate late prosthetic valve stenosis or regurgitation, including a large mitral annular calcific

nodule, septal hypertrophy, exuberant overgrowth of fibrous tissue (see Fig. 5-24B and C), interference by retained valve remnants (such as a retained posterior mitral leaflet or components of the submitral apparatus; see Fig. 5-24D), or unraveled, long, or looped sutures or knots (see Fig. 5-24E). With bioprosthetic valves, cuspal motion can be restricted by sutures looped around stents, and suture ends cut too long may erode into or perforate a bioprosthetic valve cusp.

Valvular Allografts/Homografts

Aortic or pulmonary valves (with or without associated vascular conduits) transplanted from one individual to another have exceptionally good hemodynamic profiles, a low incidence of thromboembolic complications without chronic anticoagulation, and a low reinfection rate following valve replacement for endocarditis.[132] Contemporary cryopreserved allografts, in which freezing is performed with protection from crystallization by dimethyl-sulfoxide and storage until use at −196°C in liquid nitrogen, have demonstrated freedom from degeneration and durability equal to or better than those of conventional porcine bioprosthetic valves.

Morphologic changes are summarized in Fig. 5-25. Cryopreserved human allograft heart valves/conduits show gross changes of conduit calcification and cuspal stretching (see Fig. 5-25A and B). Microscopically, there is progressive loss of normal structural demarcations and cells beginning in days. Long-term explants are devoid of both surface endothelium and deep connective tissue cells; they have minimal inflammatory cellularity (Fig. 5-25C).[133] Despite the widely discussed hypothesis that human allograft valve failure can be attributed to an immunological process, the available evidence supports purely degenerative mechanisms.

Pulmonary Valvular Autografts

Often called the *Ross operation* in recognition of its originator, Sir Donald Ross, pulmonary autograft replacement of the aortic valve yields excellent hemodynamic performance, avoids anticoagulation, and carries a low risk of thromboembolism.[134] Explanted pulmonary autograft cusps show (1) near-normal trilaminar structure; (2) near-normal collagen architecture; (3) viable endothelium and interstitial cells; (4) usual outflow surface corrugations; (5) sparse inflammatory cells; and (6) absence of calcification and thrombus (see Fig. 5-25C).[135] However, the arterial walls show considerable transmural damage (probably perioperative ischemic injury caused by disruption of vasa vasorum) with scaring and loss of medial smooth muscle cells and elastin. The early necrosis and healing with probable resultant loss of strength/elasticity of the aortic wall may potentiate late aortic root dilation.[136,137]

Stentless Porcine Aortic Valve Bioprostheses

Nonstented (stentless) porcine aortic valve bioprostheses consist of glutaraldehyde-pretreated pig aortic root and valve cusps that have no supporting stent.[138] The most widely used models,

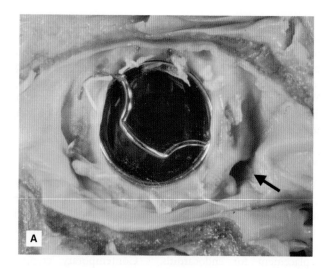

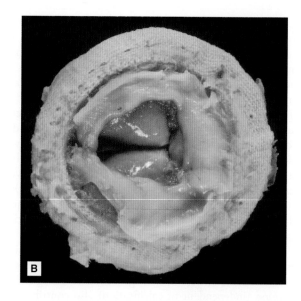

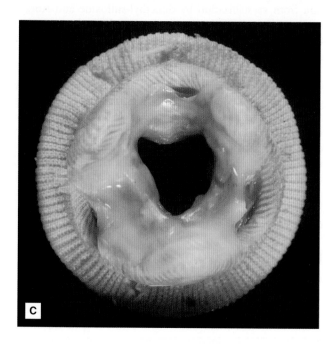

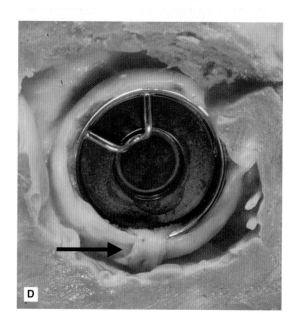

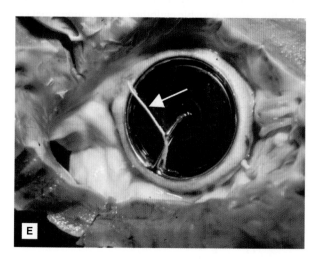

FIGURE 5-24 Nonstructural dysfunction of prosthetic heart valves. (A) Paravalvular leak adjacent to mitral valve prosthesis (*arrow*). (B) Tissue overgrowth compromising inflow orifice of porcine bioprosthesis. (C) Tissue overgrowth incorporating and resultant retraction and obliteration of bioprosthetic valve cusps. (D) Immobility of tilting disk leaflet by impingement of retained component of submitral apparatus (*arrow*) that had moved through orifice late following mitral valve replacement surgery. (E) Suture (*arrow*) looped around central strut of a Hall-Medtronic tilting disk valve causing disk immobility. ([A and C] Reproduced with permission from Schoen FJ, Gimbrone MA: *Cardiovascular Pathology: Clinicopathologic Correlations and Pathogenetic Mechanisms.* Philadelphia: Williams & Wilkins; 1995. [B] Reproduced with permission from Schoen FJ, Levy RJ, Piehler HR: Pathological considerations in replacement cardiac valves, *Cardiovasc Pathol.* 1992 Jan-Mar;1(1):29-52. [D] Reproduced with permission from Silver MD, Gotlieb AI, Schoen FJ: *Cardiovascular Pathology,* 3rd ed. New York: Churchill Livingstone/Elsevier; 2001. [E] Used with permission from the Chief Medical Examiner, New York City.)

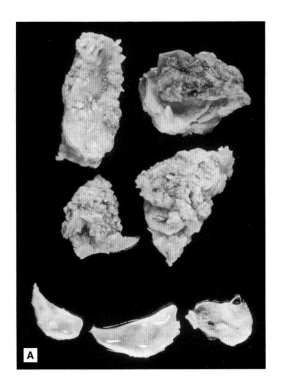

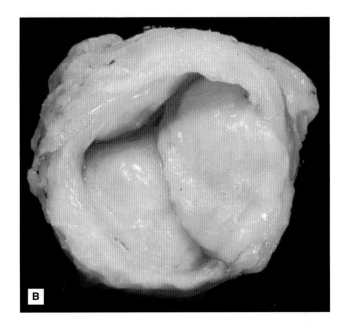

Autograft valves   Homograft valves

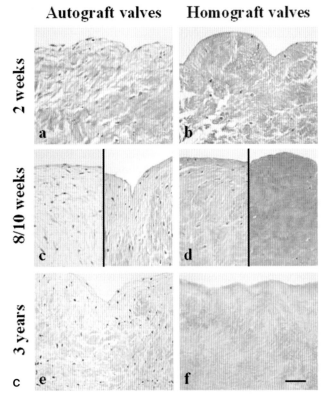

FIGURE 5-25 Morphology of valve allografts (homografts) valve and pulmonary valve autografts. (A) Gross photograph of pulmonary valve allograft removed following 7 years for conduit stenosis in a child. The pulmonary arterial wall is heavily calcified but the cusps are not. (B) Gross appearance of cryopreserved aortic valve allograft removed at 3 years for aortic insufficiency. (C) Comparative morphologic features of autografts and homografts obtained from the same patients. Autograft valves had near-normal structure and cellular population (a, c, e), in contrast, homografts from the same patients (b, d, f) had a progressive collagen hyalinization and loss of cellularity. Bar = 200 μm ×400. (Reproduced with permission from Rabkin-Aikawa E, Aikawa M, Farber M, et al: Clinical pulmonary autograft valves: pathological evidence of adaptive remodeling in the aortic site, *J Thorac Cardiovasc Surg.* 2004 Oct;128(4):552-561.)

St. Jude Medical Toronto SPV (St. Jude Medical Inc., St. Paul, MN), Medtronic Freestyle (Medtronic Heart Valves, Santa Ana, CA), and Edwards Prima (Edwards Life Sciences, Irvine, CA), bioprostheses differ slightly in overall configuration, details of glutaraldehyde fixation conditions, and anticalcification pretreatment. The principal advantage of a stentless porcine aortic valve is that it generally allows for the implantation of a larger bioprosthesis (than stented) in any given aortic root, which is hypothesized to enhance hemodynamics and thereby regression of hypertrophy and patient survival.[139]

The available evidence suggests that the durability of stentless bioprostheses is comparable with that of contemporary stented bioprostheses. However, nonstented porcine aortic valves have greater portions of aortic wall exposed to blood than in currently used stented valves, and calcification of the aortic wall and inflammation at the junction of aortic wall within the recipient's tissue, are potentially deleterious, owing to the large area of this interface. Calcification of the wall portion of a stentless valve could stiffen the root, cause nodular calcific obstruction potentiate wall rupture, or provide a nidus for emboli. Analyses of explanted nonstented valves show pannus and tissue degeneration, manifest as tears and cuspal calcification, but not substantial aortic wall calcification.[140,141]

Catheter-Based Valve Implantation

New catheter techniques for inserting foldable prosthetic valves within stenotic aortic and pulmonary valves, and for emulating surgical repair of regurgitant mitral valves are in various stages of preclinical development and clinical use.[142,143] Presently, catheter-based, percutaneous or transapical valve replacement is most widely used in patients with severe AS disease deemed otherwise inoperable as a bridge to valve replacement in patients in whom surgery needs to be delayed or has excessive risk, in repair of failed bioprosthetic valves, and in congenital heart disease, in which percutaneous pulmonary valve replacement may find a distinct niche to obviate the morbidity of reoperation to replace malfunctioning pulmonary conduits.

Catheter-based valve implantation uses a device that has two components: (1) an outer stentlike structure and (2) leaflets; these two components together constitute a functioning valvular prosthesis. Representative designs are illustrated in Fig. 5-26. The stent holds open a valve annulus or segment of a prosthetic conduit, resists recoil, provides the means for seating of the prosthesis in the annulus or vessel, and supports the valve leaflets.

Valves designed for catheter-based implantation generally consist of biologic tissue such as bovine, equine, or porcine pericardium (for aortic valve implantation) and bovine jugular venous valves (for pulmonary conduit implantation) mounted within a collapsible stent. The stents can be made from self-expandable or shape-memory materials such as nickel-titanium alloys (eg, Nitinol), or from balloon-expandable materials such as stainless steel, platinum-iridium, or other alloys. For a balloon-expandable device the delivery strategy involves collapsing the device over a balloon and placing it within a catheter-based sheath. The catheter containing the device can be inserted into the femoral artery (or vein) for right-sided valves.

The Medtronic Melody transcatheter pulmonary valve is composed of a balloon expandable platinum-iridium alloy stent that houses a segment of bovine jugular vein containing its native venous valve. The Melody was designed to be used in children or young adults with congenital heart disease who have received surgically implanted right ventricular outflow tract conduits that are failing because of either stenosis or regurgitation.

Catheter-based stent-mounted prosthetic valves present novel challenges. Valved stents are significantly larger than most existing percutaneous cardiac catheters and devices, and are presently on the order of 22 to 24 Fr. In the aortic position, there is the potential to impede coronary flow, or interfere with anterior mitral leaflet mobility or the conduction system or the native diseased leaflets. Stent architecture may also preclude future catheter access to the coronaries for possible interventions. Secure seating without paravalvular leaks within the aortic annulus or a pulmonary conduit and long-term durability of both the stent and the valve tissue are also major considerations.

Transcatheter Aortic Valve Implantation

Transcatheter aortic valve implantation (TAVI), first performed in humans in 2002, is accomplished through peripheral arterial access, is a less invasive alternative to conventional AVR, and extends the opportunity for effective mechanical correction to a potentially large population of otherwise untreatable individuals.[144,145] Approximately 65,000 AVRs are done in the United States each year. It is estimated that at least 30% of patients with severe symptomatic AS are inoperable.[146] Previously, incumbent surgical valve manufacturers offered no effective surgical intervention suitable for these patients.

Clinical experience with TAVI is growing rapidly, with an estimated 200,000+ TAVI procedures performed worldwide to date. Randomized and observational clinical trials comparing TAVI to classical open surgical AVR suggest that survival following TAVI in high-risk patients is equivalent to or better than that of AVR at 1 to 2 years.[147-149] TAVI has rapidly become the new standard of care for many patients with symptomatic AS who would otherwise be deemed inoperable or have high risk for surgery.

For repair of AS, the device is passed from the femoral artery retrograde up the aorta to the aortic valve and deployed between the cusps of the calcified aortic valve, pushing the diseased cusps out of the way. Alternatively, in patients with significant atherosclerotic disease of the femoral artery and/or aorta, the device can be deployed in an antegrade fashion through a minimally invasive surgical approach exposing the apex of the left ventricle (transapical implantation). The valve is inserted within the diseased native aortic valve, unlike surgical AVR that removes the native valve, and without the use of cardiopulmonary bypass. Access is obtained either through a peripheral artery (femoral or subclavian) or directly through the aorta or left ventricular apex. Once located at the level of the aortic valve, the device requires balloon dilatation or self-expands (if fabricated from a shape memory alloy such as Nitinol). The patient's native aortic valve is not removed (as in AVR) but rather is pushed aside to the periphery of

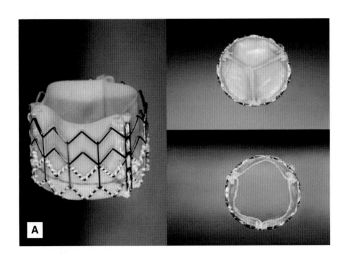

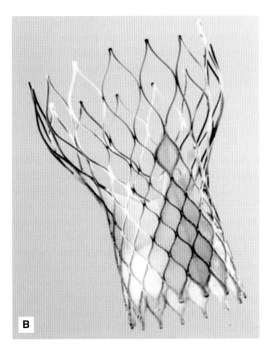

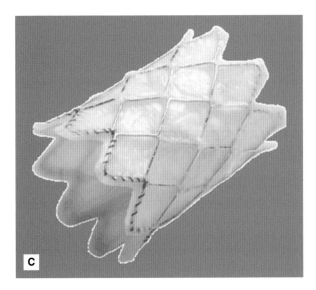

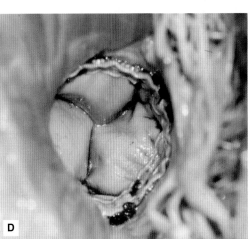

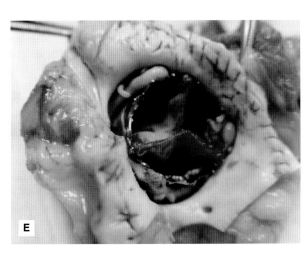

FIGURE 5-26 Transcatheter valves. (A) The Cribier-Edwards/Sapien valve consists of three equine pericardial leaflets fixed to a balloon-expandable steel stent. It is hand crimped over a delivery balloon prior to deployment. (B) The CoreValve system is constructed of porcine pericardium attached to a self-expanding nickel-titanium alloy (nitinol) stent. The ventricular portion has a high radial force to compress the native valve. The midportion is tapered to avoid interference with the coronary arteries. The aortic portion is flared to provide additional fixation against the wall of the ascending aorta. (C) The Melody pulmonary valve is constructed from a bovine jugular venous valve attached with sutures to a platinum-iridium alloy stent. Its use is primarily in failed surgically constructed right ventricular to pulmonary artery conduits in the pediatric population. (D) Postmortem photograph from a patient who died following percutaneous valve implantation. The valve prosthesis can be seen to be fully expanded within the left ventricular outflow tract with good leaflet coaptation. The interventricular septum can be seen to the left and the anterior leaflet of the mitral valve to the right. (E) Specimen from a patient who had a valve-in-valve procedure. (Reproduced with permission from McManus BM, Braunwald E: *Atlas of Cardiovascular Pathology for the Clinician.* Philadelphia: Current Medicine; 2008.)

the annulus, and compressed against the aortic root. During TAVI, delivery, positioning, and permanent fixation in the optimal location are guided by fluoroscopy and echocardiography are critical to procedural success. These devices may also play a role in the treatment of surgically implanted bioprosthetic valves that are failing because of stenosis or regurgitation in a so-called "valve-in-valve" application, in which a new valve is placed via catheter into the lumen of the existing valve (see Fig. 5-26E).

The design of the devices used in TAVI is necessarily different than that of conventional substitute heart valves. Valves used in TAVI generally consist of a bioprosthetic tissue valve, typically fabricated from bovine pericardium, mounted on a compressible metallic stent (Fig. 5-26). Complications have been observed in approximately one-third of patients and may include vascular injury, paravalvular leak, and stroke.[150]

Several devices are currently in various stages of development and clinical use in the aortic and pulmonary position. The two transcatheter aortic valves with the largest clinical experience are the Edwards SAPIEN device (Fig. 5-26A) and the CoreValve system (Fig. 5-26B).[151,152] The SAPIEN device is composed of a balloon expandable stainless steel stent that houses a bovine pericardial valve. The stent has a low profile and is designed to be placed in the subcoronary position. There is a polymer skirt circumferentially attached to the stent to reduce paravalvular leaks. The CoreValve device is composed of a self-expandable Nitinol stent that houses a porcine pericardial trileaflet valve. The CoreValve stent is longer and is meant to be placed in the left ventricular outflow tract extending into the aortic root. These devices have been approved by the US Food and Drug Administration (FDA) and other regulatory bodies abroad.

There have been a number of clinical trials from different countries, including randomized trials comparing transcatheter aortic valve replacement to classical AVR . The consensus of these studies is that TAVI is not inferior to classical AVR in terms of procedure "success" and short-term morbidity and mortality. Long-term survival is primarily limited by comorbidities in this elderly group of patients—death is often due to severe renal, pulmonary, or nonvalvular heart disease.

Aortic insufficiency, while uncommon after classical AVR, is common after TAVI, and is usually due to paravalvular leaks. Repositionable valves may be beneficial in lowering procedural complications. Vascular events are the most common complications of the procedure and contribute to procedural mortality. The resulting vascular injury may lead to significant bleeding requiring transfusion and even death. As smaller, lower-profile systems are developed, vascular injuries leading to significant blood loss are expected to occur less frequently. A rise in creatinine following TAVR has been reported in 5 to 28% of cases. However, renal function often improves with the increase in cardiac output. Elderly patients that are candidates for TAVI generally have some degree of atherosclerotic CAD. The presence of severe CAD increases procedural risks and must be dealt with before the procedure. The coronary ostia can be blocked by the device. The risk is dependent on the site of placement of the device and anatomic factors, such as unusually heavy calcification of the

aortic valve or aortic root, or low coronary ostia. The conduction system passes through the interventricular septum immediately below the aortic valve. Hence, injury to this region during valve placement may cause partial or complete heart block. New-onset bundle branch block following TAVI has been reported in up to 45% of patients, according to early reports. TAVI is commonly associated with some myocardial injury, as assessed by CK-MB and cTnT release. Myocardial injury, judged by elevated cardiac biomarkers, is inversely correlated to improvement in ejection fraction and directly proportional to postprocedural cardiac mortality. Stroke during or after TAVI may occur from thromboemboli, aortic injury (eg, dissection or atheroemboli), hypotension, hemorrhage, or dislodgement of calcific fragments during valvuloplasty. Given that TAVI is intended for individuals who are poor surgical candidates, it is not surprising that many have comorbidities that increase the risk of thrombosis and stroke. Not surprisingly, individuals most at risk include those with a history of atrial fibrillation, severe diastolic dysfunction, and/or left atrial or ventricular hypertrophy.

Transcatheter heart valves (THVs) are susceptible to failure modes typical to those of surgical bioprostheses and unique to their specific design.[153] A recent review found 87 published cases of TAVI failure. Similar to surgical bioprosthetic heart valve failure, prosthetic valve endocarditis, structural valve failure due to leaflet calcification thrombosis were the most frequent complications THV embolization and THV compression occurred in multiple cases following cardiopulmonary resuscitation (CPR).

CARDIAC REPLACEMENT AND MECHANICAL ASSIST

Cardiac Transplantation

Cardiac transplantation provides long-term survival and improved quality of life for many individuals with end-stage cardiac failure that is refractory to optimal medical management.[154] The current 1-year survival is approximately 90% and 5-year survival is about 70%.[155] The most common indications for cardiac transplantation, accounting for 90% of the adult recipients, are idiopathic cardiomyopathy and end-stage ischemic heart disease; other recipients have congenital, other myocardial, or valvular heart disease. Retransplantation is a viable option for patients with failing allografts, and rates of retransplantation have been rising recently.

Hearts explanted at the time of transplantation may also have previously undiagnosed conditions and unexpected findings.[156] Some of these findings are important for patient management, as certain diseases responsible for failure of the native heart such as amyloidosis, sarcoidosis, giant cell myocarditis, and Chagas disease may recur in the transplanted heart. Making a specific diagnosis of a genetic condition such as HCM or ARVC at the time of explant has important implications for the family members. The most frequent unexpected finding in the explanted heart is eosinophilic or hypersensitivity myocarditis, seen in 7 to 20% of explants and characterized by a focal or diffuse mixed inflammatory infiltrate, rich in eosinophils, and generally associated with minimal myocyte necrosis. In virtually all cases, the hypersensitivity is a response to one or more of the many heart failure medications taken by transplant candidates, including dobutamine. Recipients of heart transplants undergo surveillance endomyocardial biopsies on an institution-specific schedule, which typically evolves from weekly during the early postoperative period, to biweekly until 3 to 6 months, and then approximately one to four times annually, or at any time when there is a change in clinical state. Histologic findings of rejection frequently precede clinical signs and symptoms of acute rejection. Optimal biopsy interpretation requires four or more pieces of myocardial tissue; descriptions of technical details and potential tissue artifacts are available.[157]

The major sources of mortality and morbidity in the first few post transplant years are perioperative ischemic injury/graft failure, infection, and multisystem organ failure, while malignancy, graft vasculopathy, and renal failure dominate after 3 to 5 years posttransplant. Because of the success of surveillance endomyocardial biopsies and current effective immunosuppressive therapies, acute cellular rejection is an uncommon cause of death in the modern era.[155]

Early Ischemic Injury

Ischemic injury can originate from the ischemia that accompanies procurement and implantation of the donor heart. Several time intervals are potentially important: (1) the donor interval between brain death and heart removal, perhaps partially related to terminal administration of pressor agents or the release of norepinephrine and cytokines associated with brain death; (2) the interval of warm ischemia between donor cardiectomy to cold storage; (3) the interval during cold transport; and (4) the interval during rewarming, trimming, and implantation. Hypertrophy and coronary obstructions in the donor heart tend to promote ischemia, whereas decreased tissue temperature and cardioplegic arrest mitigate against ischemic injury. As in other situations of transient myocardial ischemia, frank necrosis, or prolonged

ischemic dysfunction of viable myocardium or both may be present. Myocardial injury can cause low cardiac output in the perioperative period.

Perioperative myocardial ischemic injury may be detectable in endomyocardial biopsies. Owing to the anti-inflammatory effects of immunosuppressive therapy, the histologic progression of healing of myocardial necrosis in transplanted hearts may be delayed (Fig. 5-27). Therefore, the repair phase of perioperative myocardial necrosis frequently confounds the diagnosis of rejection in the first postoperative month, and in some cases, for as long as 6 weeks. Late ischemic necrosis suggests occlusive graft vasculopathy (see the following).

Rejection

Improved immunosuppressive regimens in heart transplant patients have substantially decreased the incidence and severity of rejection episodes. Hyperacute rejection occurs rarely, most often when a major blood group incompatibility exists between donor and recipient, and acute rejection is unusual earlier than 2 to 4 weeks postoperatively. Although acute rejection episodes occur largely in the first several months after transplantation, rejection can occur years postoperatively, rationalizing the practice of many transplant centers to continue late surveillance biopsies at late but widely spaced intervals.

Acute cellular rejection is characterized histologically by an inflammatory cell infiltrate, with or without damage to cardiac myocytes; in late stages, vascular injury may become prominent (Fig. 5-28). The current International Society for Heart and Lung Transplantation (ISHLT) grading system for acute cellular rejection, revised (denoted by "R") in 2004 from the 1990 version, is: Grade 0R—no rejection (no change from 1990), Grade 1R—mild rejection (1990 grades 1A, 1B, and 2), Grade 2R—moderate rejection (1990 grade 3A), and Grade 3R—severe rejection (1990 grades 3B and 4).[158] The 1990 and 2004 formulations are compared in Table 5-4. The past decade has seen tremendous progress in the recognition, understanding, and diagnosis of acute antibody-mediated rejection (AMR). AMR was originally recognized as a

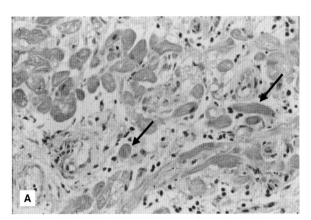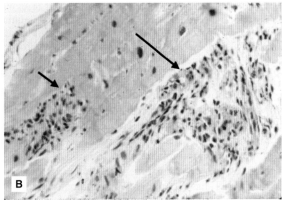

FIGURE 5-27 Perioperative ischemic myocardial injury demonstrated on endomyocardial biopsy. (A) Coagulative myocyte necrosis (*arrows*). (B) Healing perioperative ischemic injury with predominantly interstitial inflammatory response (*arrows*), not encroaching on and clearly separated from adjacent viable myocytes. The infiltrate consists of a mixture of polymorphonuclear leukocytes, macrophages, lymphocytes, and plasma cells. Hematoxylin and eosin, 200×.

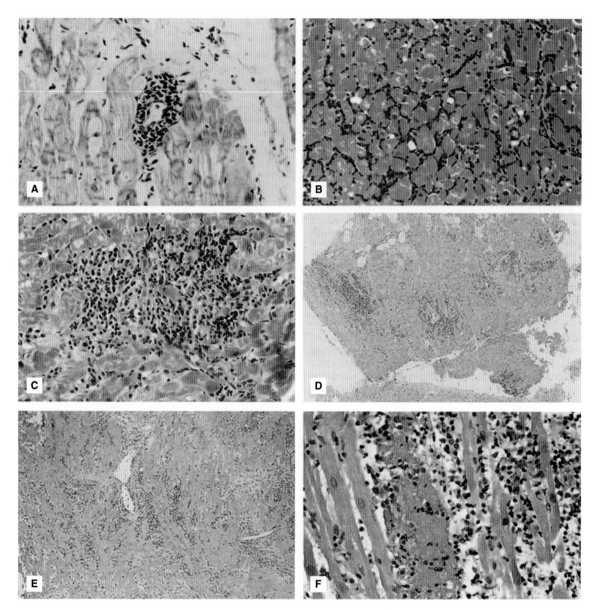

FIGURE 5-28 Histologic features of cardiac transplant rejection, designated as International Society for Heart and Lung Transplantation (ISHLT), 2004 Formulation, grades of rejection. (A-C) Grade 1R (mild). Focal perivascular lymphocytic and diffuse interstitial lymphocytic infiltrate without damage to adjacent myocytes, and up to one focus of dense lymphocytic infiltrate with associated myocyte damage, respectively. (D) Grade 2R (moderate). Multiple foci of dense lymphocytic infiltrates with associated myocyte damage and intervening areas of uninvolved myocardium. (E and F) Grade 3R (severe). Diffuse infiltrate with associated myocyte damage and polymorphous infiltrate with extensive myocyte damage, edema, and hemorrhage, respectively. (H&E stain). (Reproduced with permission from Silver MD, Gotlieb AI, Schoen FJ: *Cardiovascular Pathology*, 3rd ed. New York: Churchill Livingstone/Elsevier; 2001.)

clinicopathologic entity characterized by (1) cardiac dysfunction in the absence of cellular rejection or ischemic injury; (2) histologic features of interstitial edema, endothelial cell swelling, and intravascular macrophages on endomyocardial biopsy; (3) positive immunoperoxidase staining for C4d; and (4) the presence of circulating antidonor antibodies. Recently, the ISHLT has recommended pathologic grading of AMR in the following manner: pAMR0—no histologic changes of AMR and negative immunopathologic (eg, C4d) staining, pAMR1 (H+)—histologic changes consistent with AMR but immunopathologic studies are negative, pAMR1

(I+)—no histologic changes of AMR but immunopathologic studies are positive, pAMR2—pathologic AMR with histologic changes and positive immunopathologic studies, pAMR3—severe pathologic AMR with histologic changes, positive immunopathologic studies and marked edema, interstitial hemorrhage, capillary fragmentation, endothelial cell damage, and mixed interstitial inflammation.[159] AMR most often is diagnosed in sensitized patients (including those with previous transplantation, transfusion or pregnancy, and previous ventricular assist device use) and is associated with worse graft survival. Evidence is mounting that

TABLE 5-4: ISHLT Standardized Cardiac Biopsy Grading of Acute Cellular Rejection: Clinicopathologic Comparison of 1990 and 2004 Formulations

Rejection level	Histologic findings	Rejection grade 1990	Rejection grade 2004	Clinical response
None	Normal	0	0R	No change
Mild	Lymphocytic inflammation ± one focus of myocyte damage	1A, 1B, 2	1R	No/minimal change to chronic immunosuppressive regimen
Moderate	Lymphocytic inflammation + multiple foci of myocyte damage	3A	2R	Steroid bolus ± change in chronic immunosuppressive regimen
Severe	Lymphocytic inflammation + diffuse myocyte damage ± vascular injury	3B, 4	3R	Aggressive therapy (eg, steroids ± monoclonal antibodies [OKT3])

ISHLT = International Society for Heart and Lung Transplantation.

episodes of AMR predispose to the earlier development of allograft coronary disease. Although the optimal therapeutic strategy is still under debate, most transplant centers will use plasmapheresis to treat AMR with impaired cardiac function. Findings in surveillance endomyocardial biopsies that must be distinguished from rejection include lymphoid infiltrates either confined to the endocardium or extending into the underlying myocardium and often accompanied by myocyte damage (so-called Quilty lesions, which have no known clinical significance), old biopsy sites, and healing ischemic injury either in the perioperative period or resulting from graft vasculopathy. Lymphoproliferative disorders and infections also may be seen in biopsies.

Infection

The immunosuppressive therapy required in all heart transplant recipients confers an increased risk of infection with bacterial, fungal, protozoan, and viral pathogens, with cytomegalovirus (CMV) and *Toxoplasma gondii* remaining common opportunistic infections in this setting. Prophylaxis is typically given to patients at high risk of primary CMV infection (donor seropositive, recipient seronegative). Viral and parasitic infections can present a challenge in endomyocardial biopsies as the multifocal lymphocytic infiltrates with occasional necrosis seen with these infections can mimic rejection.

Graft Vasculopathy (Graft Coronary Disease)

Graft vasculopathy is the major limitation to long-term graft and recipient survival following heart transplantation.[160] Up to 50% of recipients have angiographically evident disease 5 years after transplantation, whereas intravascular ultrasound identifies graft vasculopathy in 75% of patients at 3 years posttransplant. However, graft vasculopathy may become significant at any time and can progress at variable rates. We have encountered graft coronary disease in several patients as early as 6 to 12 months postoperatively at the Brigham and Women's Hospital.

Graft vasculopathy (Fig. 5-29) occurs diffusely and ultimately involves both intramyocardial and epicardial allograft vessels, potentially leading to myocardial infarction, arrhythmias, congestive heart failure, or sudden death. Although this process has been called "accelerated atherosclerosis," the morphology of the obstructive lesion of graft vasculopathy is distinct from that of typical atherosclerosis (Table 5-5).

The vessels involved have concentric occlusions characterized by marked intimal proliferation of myofibroblasts and smooth muscle cells with deposition of collagen, ECM, and lipid (see Fig. 5-29A and B). Lymphocytic infiltration varies from almost none to quite prominent. The internal elastic lamina often is almost completely intact, with only focal fragmentation. The resulting myocardial pathology includes subendocardial myocyte vacuolization (indicative of sublethal ischemic injury) and myocardial coagulation necrosis (indicative of infarction).

Evidence suggests that chronic allogenic immune response to the transplant and nonimmunologic factors mediate the vascular injury.[161] Conventional risk factors of atherosclerosis (eg, hyperlipidemia, diabetes, advanced age), pre- or peritransplant injuries, infection, innate immunity, T-cell-mediated immunity, and B-cell-mediated immunity via production of donor specific antibodies have been associated with increased and accelerated graft vasculopathy, likely acting in concert with each other. There is no apparent difference in the frequency with which graft vasculopathy develops in patients who were transplanted for end-stage CAD versus idiopathic cardiomyopathy.

Early diagnosis of graft vasculopathy is limited by the lack of clinical symptoms of ischemia in the denervated allograft, by the relative insensitivity of coronary angiography, which frequently underestimates the extent and severity of this diffuse disease, and by the exclusive or predominant involvement of small intramyocardial vessels. Histologic changes of chronic ischemia such as subendothelial myocyte vacuolization can be seen on surveillance biopsies as evidence of myocardial ischemia and may suggest graft vasculopathy (see Fig. 5-29C and D). Obstructive vascular lesions are not usually amenable to PCI or coronary artery bypass grafting

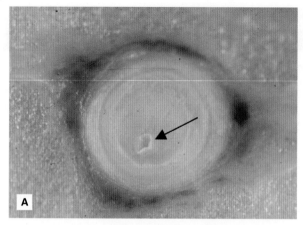

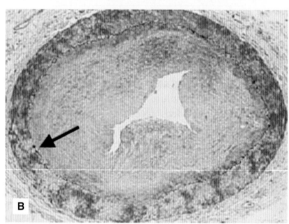

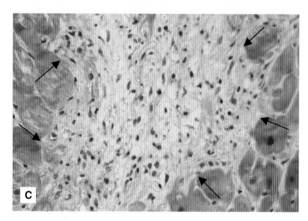

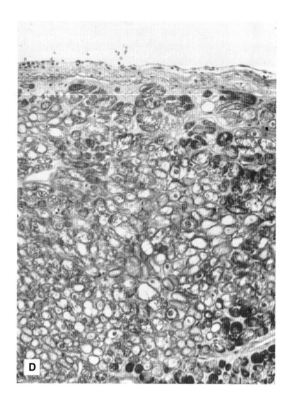

FIGURE 5-29 Gross and microscopic features of graft disease and graft arteriosclerosis–induced myocardial pathology in heart transplant recipients. (A) Gross photograph of transverse cross-section of heart from patient who died of graft arteriosclerosis. Severe concentric stenosis of an epicardial coronary is apparent with only a pinhole lumen (*arrow*). (B) Histologic appearance of graft arteriosclerosis as low-power photomicrograph of vessel cross-section, demonstrating severe, near-complete, and predominantly concentric intimal proliferation with nearly intact internal elastic lamina (*arrow*). Verhoff-van Gieson stain (for elastin) 60×. Gross and microscopic features of graft coronary disease and graft arteriosclerosis–induced myocardial pathology in heart transplant recipients. (C) Myocardial microinfarct indicative of disease of small intramural arteries (*outlined by arrows*) Hematoxylin and eosin and (D) subendocardial myocyte vacuolization indicative of severe chronic ischemia. Trichrome stain, 375×. ([B] Reproduced with permission from Salomon RN, Hughes CWH, Schoen FJ, et al: Human coronary transplantation-associated arteriosclerosis: evidence for a chronic immune reaction to activated graft endothelial cells, *Am J Pathol.* 1991 Apr;138(4):791-798.)

because of their diffuse distribution. Retransplantation is the only effective therapy for most cases of established graft atherosclerosis.

Posttransplant Lymphoproliferative Disorders

Posttransplant lymphoproliferative disorders (PTLDs) are a well-recognized and serious complication of the high-intensity long-term immunosuppressive therapy required to prevent rejection in cardiac allografts. PTLD occurs in approximately

2% of cardiac allograft recipients. Several factors increase the risk of PTLD, including pretransplant Epstein-Barr virus (EBV) seronegativity (10- to 75-fold increase), young recipient age, and CMV infection or mismatching (donor-positive, recipient-negative).[162]

Posttransplant lymphoproliferative disorders can present as an infectious mononucleosis-like illness or with localized solid tumor masses, especially in extranodal sites (eg, heart, lungs, gastrointestinal tract). The vast majority (>90%) of PTLDs derive from the B-cell lineage and are associated with EBV infection, although T- or NK-cell origin and late-arising

⬤ **TABLE 5-5: Characteristics of Graft Arteriosclerosis versus Typical Atherosclerosis**

Graft arteriosclerosis	Typical atherosclerosis
Rapid onset (months to years)	Slow onset (many years)
Risk factors uncertain	Hypertension, lipids, smoking, etc
Usually silent/congestive heart failure, sudden death	Chest pain, etc
Diffuse	Focal
Epicardial/intramural	Epicardial
Concentric	Eccentric
Lesions rarely locally complicated	Lesions often locally complicated
Smooth muscle cells, macrophages, lymphocytes	Smooth muscle cells, macrophages, foam cells
Primary immunologic mechanism(s)	Complicated stimuli
Difficult to treat; retransplant usually only option	Revascularization by angioplasty, stents, aortocoronary bypass

Reproduced with permission from Schoen FJ, Libby P: Cardiac transplant graft arteriosclerosis, *Trends Cardiovasc Med.* 1991 Jul-Aug;1(5):216-223.

EBV-negative lymphoid malignancies have been described. There is strong evidence that the lesions progress from polyclonal B-cell hyperplasias (early lesions) to lymphomas (monomorphic PTLDs) in a short period of time, in association with the appearance of cytogenetic abnormalities. Therapy centers on a stepwise approach of antiviral treatment and reduction in immunosuppression, and then progression to lymphoma chemotherapy.

Cardiac Assist Devices and Total Artificial Hearts

Continuing and increasing discrepancy between the number of available donor hearts and therefore transplants performed (2500 annually in the United States) and the number of patients in the terminal phase of heart failure and refractory to medical management (estimated at 250,000 to 500,000 in the United States, and rising) has prompted efforts in the development of VADs, total artificial hearts, and other therapies.

Mechanical cardiac assist devices and artificial hearts have traditionally been used in two settings: for ventricular augmentation sufficient to permit a patient to survive postcardiotomy or postinfarction cardiogenic shock while ventricular recovery is occurring, and as a bridge to transplantation when ventricular recovery is not expected and the goal is hemodynamic support until a suitable donor organ is located. More recently, left ventricular assist devices (LVADs) have been shown to provide long-term cardiac support with survival and quality-of-life improvement over optimal medical therapy in patients with end-stage congestive heart failure who are not candidates for transplantation. LVADs are also being investigated as a "bridge-to-recovery" in patients with congestive heart failure to induce reverse ventricular remodeling leading to an improvement in cardiac function that would eventually allow device removal. Many types of pumps are currently under development or in clinical use as ventricular assist devices.[163] Mechanical devices that entirely replace the native heart are currently in use or under development as bridge to transplant (SynCardia Total Artificial Heart)[164] or as destination therapy (Abiomed AbioCor).[165]

The major complications of cardiac assist devices are hemorrhage, thrombosis/thromboembolism, infection, and interactions with host tissue (Fig. 5-30).[166] Hemorrhage continues to be a problem in device recipients, although the risk of major hemorrhage has been decreasing with improved devices, therapies, patient selection, and surgical methods. Many factors predispose to perioperative hemorrhage, including (1) coagulopathy secondary to hepatic dysfunction, poor nutritional status, and antibiotic therapy; (2) platelet dysfunction and thrombocytopenia secondary to cardiopulmonary bypass; and (3) the extensive nature of the required surgery.

Nonthrombogenic blood-contacting surfaces are essential for a clinically useful cardiac assist device or artificial heart. Indeed, thromboembolism occurred in most patients having long-term implantation of the Jarvik-7 artificial heart and is a major design consideration for current devices. The current generation of continuous flow LVADs is carefully designed to minimize thrombosis, but oral anticoagulation is still required. The incidence of pump thrombosis in the continuous axial flow HeartMate II LVAD (see Fig 5-30A) appears to have been increasing,[167] and is currently the subject of intense debate and research. Thrombi also may form outside the LVAD, often in association with crevices and voids, and in areas of disturbed blood flow such as near connections of conduits and other components to the native heart (see Fig. 5-30B).[168] Accounting for significant morbidity and mortality following the prolonged use of cardiac assist devices, infection can occur either within the device or associated with percutaneous drive lines (see Fig. 5-30C). Susceptibility to infection is potentiated by not only the usual prosthesis-associated factors (see later), but also by the multisystem organ damage from the underlying disease, the periprosthetic culture medium provided by postoperative hemorrhage, and by prolonged hospitalization with the associated risk of nosocomial infections. Assist device-associated infections are often resistant to antibiotic therapy and host defenses, but are generally considered not an absolute contraindication to subsequent cardiac transplantation. Novel device designs, including alternative sites for driveline placement and the elimination of the driveline altogether with transcutaneous energy transmission technology, may play a role in further decreasing infection.

Left ventricular assist device implantation can allow for reverse remodeling (see below), resulting in a decrease of the size of the left ventricular chamber. Therefore, an LVAD inflow cannula may end up contacting cardiac structures in the now-smaller left ventricular chamber that it was nowhere near at the time of implantation into a dilated ventricle. This can lead to inflow obstruction (see Fig. 5-30D), acquired

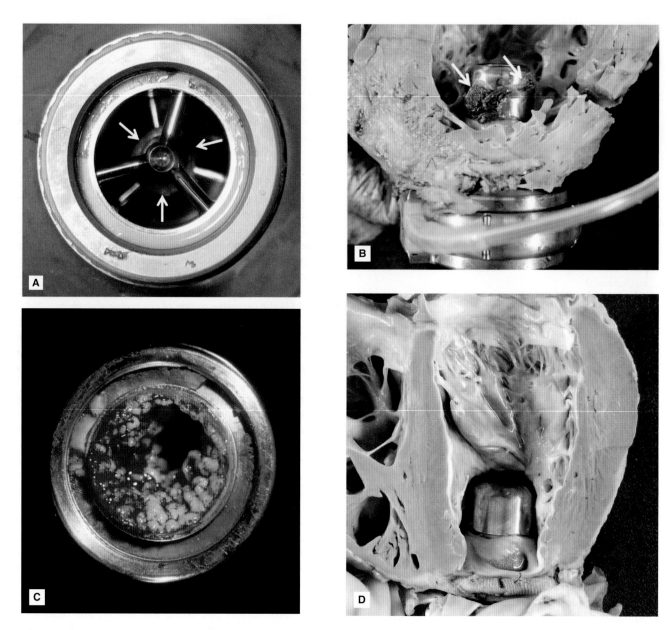

FIGURE 5-30 Complications of left ventricular assist devices (LVADs). (A) Circumferential thrombus (*arrows*) on the inflow bearing of the impeller of a Thoratec HeartMate II LVAD. (B) Thrombus (*arrows*) on the outer aspect of the inflow cannula of a HeartWare HVAD within the left ventricular cavity. (C) Fungal infection in LVAD outflow graft. (D) Inflow cannula of a HeartWare HVAD impinging on the posterior left ventricular wall resulting in obstruction. (Reproduced with permission from Silver MD, Gotlieb AI, Schoen FJ: *Cardiovascular Pathology*, 3rd ed. New York: Churchill Livingstone/Elsevier; 2001.)

ventricular septal defect, myocardial hemorrhage, and potential arrhythmias. Other complications include hemolysis, pannus formation around anastomotic sites, calcification, and device malfunction. There is evidence that patients on LVADs are more likely to develop allosensitization, which can pose a significant risk to posttransplantation outcome in the bridge-to-transplant patients.[169] These complications not only have significant morbidity and can be fatal, but they may make a previously suitable patient ineligible for future transplantation.

Long-term LVADs are primarily used as a bridge to transplantation because cardiac transplantation currently offers a better long-term outlook for most patients. In a subset of patients, support by LVAD results in improved cardiac function, with heart transplantation no longer necessary even after removal of the LVAD (bridge to recovery). Left ventricular assist device support is now recognized to offer potential for myocardial recovery, a favorable outcome that is further enhanced by combination with pharmacologic therapy. LVADs lead to lowered cardiac pressure and volume overload in the myocardium followed by decreased ventricular wall tension, reduced cardiomyocyte hypertrophy, improved coronary perfusion, and decreased chronic ischemia.

To what extent recovery of myocardial function can occur during VAD implantation is uncertain. Many pathophysiologic changes occur during the progression to end-stage heart failure, ranging from the subcellular (eg, abnormal mitochondrial function and calcium metabolism) to the organ and system level (eg, ventricular dilation, decreased ejection fraction, and neurohormonal changes), leading to the signs and symptoms of congestive failure. Implantation of an LVAD can reverse many of these changes (*reverse remodeling*), leading to increased cardiac output, decreased ventricular end-diastolic volume, and normalization of neurohormonal status such that a small fraction of patients can be weaned from the device without the need for subsequent cardiac transplantation. Current research focuses on the mechanisms of cardiac recovery, identification of patients who could achieve recovery, and specifics such as the timing and duration of therapy; a key goal is to identify potential predictors and novel therapeutic targets capable of enhancing myocardial repair.[170]

ARRHYTHMIAS

Arrhythmias generally occur as a result of disorders of electrical impulse formation, disorders of electrical impulse conduction, or a combination of the two. The underlying anatomic substrates for arrhythmogenesis are many. Many cardiomyopathies can present with arrhythmias, including those with genetic (eg, HCM, ARVC, and the ion channelopathies), mixed (eg, dilated cardiomyopathy), and acquired (eg, myocarditis, sarcoidosis and amyloidosis) etiologies. A common cause of arrhythmias and sudden death (especially in the older adult population) is ischemic heart disease, both in patients with and without a prior myocardial infarction. Myocardial hypertrophy and fibrosis of any etiology (eg, secondary to valvular heart disease, hypertension, or a remote infarction) also can provide the anatomical and functional substrate for the development of an arrhythmia. These underlying processes and pathologic anatomy increase the risk of spontaneous lethal arrhythmias in the setting of acute initiating events such as acute ischemia, neurohormonal activation, changes in electrolytes, and other metabolic stressors.[171]

Treatments for arrhythmias and their complications include pharmacologic therapy, device therapy[172,173] (eg, pacemakers, defibrillators), and ablation therapy.

Pacemakers and Implantable Cardioverter-Defibrillators

Modern cardiac pacing is achieved by a system of interconnected components consisting of (1) a pulse generator that includes a power source and electric circuitry to initiate the electric stimulus and to sense normal activity; (2) one or more electrically insulated conductors leading from the pulse generator to the heart, with a bipolar electrode at the distal end of each; and (3) a tissue, or blood and tissue, interface between electrode and adjacent stimulatable myocardial cells, which is of critical importance in the proper functioning of the pacemaker. Typically, a layer of nonexcitable fibrous tissue forms around the tip of the electrode. This fibrosis may be induced by the electrode itself or may result from myocardial scarring from some other cause, most commonly a healed myocardial infarction. The thickness of this nonexcitable tissue between the electrode and excitable tissue determines the stimulus threshold, or the strength of the pacing stimulus required to initiate myocyte depolarization, and thus the amount of energy required from the pacemaker. Attempts to reduce the thickness of this layer (thereby extending battery life) include improved lead designs[174] with active fixation and the use of slow, local release of corticosteroids from the lead tip. Implantable cardioverter-defibrillators (ICDs) are used in the treatment of patients who have life-threatening ventricular arrhythmias that are refractory to medical management and unsuitable for other surgical or ablative therapy, and have similar components to the pacemaker described in the preceding. These devices sense arrhythmias that can lead to sudden death and deliver therapy in the form of rapid ventricular pacing and/or a defibrillation current to terminate the dysrhythmic episode. ICDs also must overcome the barrier posed by the interfacial fibrosis at the electrode tip.

Complications from the use of pacemakers include lead displacement, vascular or cardiac perforation leading to hemothorax, pneumothorax or tamponade, lead entrapment, infection, erosion of the device into adjacent tissues owing to pressure necrosis, rotation of the device within the pocket, thrombosis and/or thromboembolism, and lead fracture, in addition to malfunction of the device itself. If the lead needs to be extracted for chronic infection or device-related defects, damage to the myocardium and/or tricuspid valve may occur secondary to encasement of the lead in fibrous tissue. Similar complications affect ICDs, with additional considerations being the consequences of repeated defibrillations on the myocardium and vascular structures, including myocardial necrosis, and the risk of oversensing (with resultant unnecessary shocks) or undersensing (with resultant sudden death). Increased attention has been paid of late to malfunctioning ICDs because of electrical flaws in a specific model that resulted in failure to terminate fatal arrhythmias.[175]

Ablation

Ablation involves the directed destruction of arrhythmogenic myocardium, accessory pathways, or conduction system structures to control or cure a variety of arrhythmias, including atrial flutter and fibrillation, ventricular tachycardias, and paroxysmal supraventricular tachycardias that are refractory to medical management.[176,177] Ablation can be carried out as part of a surgical procedure, or through percutaneous catheter means. Electrophysiologic (EP) studies can be used to (1) provide information on the type and location of rhythm disturbance, (2) terminate a tachycardia by electrical stimulation, (3) evaluate the effects of therapy, (4) ablate myocardium involved in the tachycardia, and (5) identify patients at risk for sudden cardiac death.

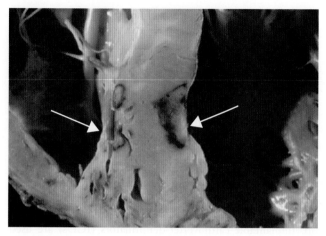

FIGURE 5-31 Site of ablation of arrhythmogenic focus by radiofrequency ablation (*arrows*).

Radiofrequency ablation acutely produces coagulation necrosis within the myocardium directly underneath the source tip, eliminating the source or pathway of the arrhythmia. The characteristic histologic changes include loss of myocyte striations, loss or pyknosis of nuclei, hypereosinophilia, and contraction bands. The edge of the fresh lesion is often hemorrhagic with interstitial edema (Fig. 5-31) and inflammation. The area undergoes the usual progression of healing similar to that in an infarct, with an early neutrophilic infiltrate, followed by macrophages to handle the necrotic debris, followed by granulation tissue formation and eventual scarring. Through the use of irrigated, cooled catheters, the lesions can penetrate deeply into the myocardium. Techniques using other forms of energy, including cryoablation, microwave, and lasers, have been used to create lesions in the myocardium for the treatment of arrhythmias.

NEOPLASTIC HEART DISEASE

Although metastatic tumors to the heart are present in 1 to 3% of patients dying of cancer, primary tumors of the heart are unusual.[178,179] The most common tumors, in descending order of frequency, are: myxomas, lipomas, papillary fibroelastomas, angiomas, fibromas, and rhabdomyomas, all benign and accounting for approximately 80% of primary tumors of the adult heart. The remaining 20% are malignant tumors, including angiosarcomas, other sarcomas, and lymphomas. Many cardiac tumors have a genetic basis.

The most frequent cardiac tumors are illustrated in Fig. 5-32.

Myxoma

Myxomas are the most common primary tumor of the heart in adults, accounting for about 50% of all benign cardiac tumors. They typically arise in the left atrium (80%) along the interatrial septum near the fossa ovalis. Occasionally, myxomas arise in the right atrium (15%), the ventricles (3–4%),

or valves. These tumors arise more frequently in women and usually present between the ages of 50 and 70 years. Sporadic cases of myxoma are almost always single, whereas familial tumors can be multiple and present at an earlier age.

Myxomas range from small (<1 cm) to large (up to 10 cm) and form sessile or pedunculated masses that vary from globular and hard lesions mottled with hemorrhage to soft, translucent, papillary, or villous lesions having a myxoid and friable appearance (see Fig. 5-32A). The pedunculated form frequently is sufficiently mobile to move into or sometimes through the ipsilateral atrioventricular valve annulus during ventricular diastole, causing intermittent and often position-dependent obstruction. Sometimes, such mobility exerts a wrecking ball effect, causing damage to and secondary fibrotic thickening of the valve leaflets.

Clinical manifestations are most often determined by tumor size and location; some myxomas are incidentally detected in patients undergoing echocardiography for other indications, whereas others may present with sudden death. Symptoms are generally a consequence of valvular obstruction, obstruction of pulmonary or systemic venous return, embolization, or a syndrome of constitutional symptoms. Intracardiac obstruction may mimic the presentation of mitral or tricuspid stenosis with dyspnea, pulmonary edema, and right-sided heart failure. Fragmentation of a left-sided tumor with embolization may mimic the presentation of infective endocarditis with transient ischemic attacks, strokes, and cutaneous lesions; emboli from right-sided lesions may present as pulmonary hypertension. Constitutional symptoms such as fever, erythematous rash, weight loss, and arthralgias may result from the release of the acute-phase reactant interleukin-6 from the tumor leading to these inflammatory and autoimmune manifestations. Echocardiography, including transesophageal echocardiography, provides a means to non-invasively identify the masses and their location, attachment, and mobility. Surgical removal usually is curative with excellent short- and long-term prognosis. Rarely, the neoplasm recurs months to years later, usually secondary to incomplete removal of the stalk.

The Carney complex is a multiple neoplasia syndrome featuring cardiac and cutaneous myxomas, endocrine and neural tumors, as well as pigmented skin and mucosal lesions. Previously described cardiac myxoma syndromes such as LAMB (lentigines, atrial myxoma, mucocutaneous myxomas, and blue nevi) and NAME (nevi, atrial myxomas, mucinosis of the skin, and endocrine overactivity) are now encompassed by the Carney complex. The Carney complex is inherited as an autosomal dominant trait, and is associated with mutations in the PRKAR1α gene encoding the R1α regulatory subunit of cyclic AMP–dependent protein kinase A.

Histologically, myxomas are composed of stellate or globular cells (myxoma cells), often in formed structures that variably resemble poorly formed glands or vessels, endothelial cells, macrophages, mature or immature smooth muscle cells, and a variety of intermediate forms embedded within an abundant acid mucopolysaccharide matrix and covered by endothelium. Although it had long been questioned whether

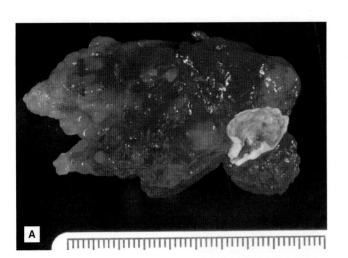

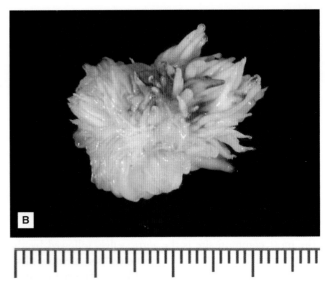

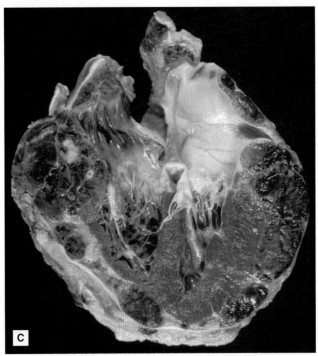

FIGURE 5-32 Gross features of primary cardiac tumors. (A) Resected left atrial myxoma, as irregular polypoid, gelatinous friable mass. The resection margin that surrounds the proximal portion of the stalk is at right. (B) Papillary fibroelastoma. Gross photograph demonstrating resemblance of this lesion to a sea anemone, with papillary fronds. (C) Massive pericardial angiosarcoma, subepicardial and with deep myocardial invasion at multiple sites. ([C] Reproduced with permission from Schoen FJ: *Interventional and Surgical Cardiovascular Pathology: Clinical Correlations and Basic Principles.* Philadelphia: Saunders; 1989.)

cardiac myxomas were neoplasms, hamartomas, or organized thrombi, it is now widely believed that they represent benign neoplasia. These tumors are thought to arise from remnants of subendocardial vasoformative reserve cells or multipotential primitive mesenchymal cells, which can differentiate along multiple lineages, giving rise to the mixture of cells present within these tumors.

Other Cardiac Tumors and Tumor-like Conditions

Cardiac lipomas are discrete masses that are typically epicardial, but may occur anywhere within the myocardium or pericardium. Most are clinically silent, but some may cause symptoms secondary to arrhythmias, pericardial effusion, intracardiac obstruction, or compression of coronary arteries. Magnetic resonance imaging is useful in the diagnosis of adipocytic lesions because of its ability to identify fatty tissues. Histologically, these tumors are composed of mature adipocytes, identical to lipomas elsewhere. A separate, non-neoplastic condition called lipomatous hypertrophy of the interatrial septum is characterized by accumulation of unencapsulated adipose tissue in the interatrial septum that can lead to arrhythmias. Histologically, this tissue is composed of a mixture of mature and immature adipose tissue and cardiac myocytes, in contrast to the pure mature adipose tissue of a proper lipoma.

Papillary fibroelastomas[180] are usually solitary and located on the valves, particularly the ventricular surfaces of semilunar valves and the atrial surfaces of atrioventricular valves. The most common site is the aortic valve, followed by the mitral valve. They constitute a distinctive "sea anemone–like" cluster of hair-like projections up to 1 cm or more in length, and can mimic valvular vegetations echocardiographically (see Fig. 5-32B).[181] Histologically, they are composed of a dense core of irregular elastic fibers, coated with myxoid connective tissue, and lined by endothelium. They may contain focal platelet-fibrin thrombus and serve as a source for embolization, commonly to cerebral or coronary arteries. Surgical excision is recommended to eliminate these embolic events. Although classified with neoplasms, fibroelastomas may represent organized thrombi, similar to the much smaller, usually trivial, whisker-like Lambl's excrescences that are frequently found on the aortic valves of older individuals.

Rhabdomyomas comprise the most frequent primary tumor of the heart in infants and children.[182] They are usually multiple and involve the ventricular myocardium on either side of the heart. They consist of gray-white myocardial masses up to several centimeters in diameter that may protrude into the ventricular or atrial chambers, causing functional obstruction. These tumors tend to spontaneously regress, so surgery is usually reserved for patients with severe hemodynamic disturbances or arrhythmias refractory to medical management. Most cardiac rhabdomyomas occur in patients with tuberous sclerosis, the clinical features of which also include infantile spasms, skin lesions (hypopigmentation, shagreen patch, subcutaneous nodules), retinal lesions, and angiomyolipomas. This disease, in its familial form, exhibits autosomal dominant inheritance, but about half the cases are sporadic owing to new mutations. Histologically, rhabdomyomas contain characteristic "spider cells," which are large, myofibril-containing, rounded, or polygonal cells with numerous glycogen-laden vacuoles separated by strands of cytoplasm running from the plasma membrane to the centrally located nucleus.

Cardiac fibromas, although also occurring predominantly in children and presenting with heart failure or arrhythmias, or incidentally, differ from rhabdomyomas in being solitary lesions that may show calcification on a routine chest radiograph.[183] Fibromas are white, whorled masses that are typically ventricular. There is an increased risk of cardiac fibromas in patients with Gorlin's syndrome (nevoid basal cell carcinoma syndrome),[184] an autosomal dominant disorder characterized by skin lesions, odontogenic keratocysts of the jaw, and skeletal abnormalities. Histologically, fibromas consist of fibroblasts showing minimal atypia and collagen with the degree of cellularity decreasing with increasing age of the patient at presentation. Although they are grossly well circumscribed, there is usually an infiltrating margin histologically. Calcification and elastin fibers are not uncommon in these lesions.

Sarcomas, with angiosarcomas, undifferentiated sarcomas, and rhabdomyosarcomas being the most common, are not distinctive from their counterparts in other locations. They tend to involve the right side of the heart, especially the right atrioventricular groove (see Fig. 5-32C). The clinical course is rapidly progressive as a result of local infiltration with intracavity obstruction and early metastatic events.

Peculiar microscopic-sized cellular tissue fragments have been noted incidentally as part of endomyocardial biopsy or surgically removed tissue specimens, either free-floating or loosely attached to a valvular or endocardial mass.[185] Termed mesothelial/monocytic incidental cardiac excrescences (MICE), they appear histologically largely as clusters and ribbons of mesothelial cells and entrapped erythrocytes and leukocytes, embedded within a fibrin mesh. These "masses" are considered artifacts of no clinical significance formed by compaction of mesothelial strips (likely from the pericardium) or other tissue debris and fibrin, which are transported via catheters or around an operative site on a cardiotomy suction tip.

BIOMATERIALS AND TISSUE ENGINEERING

Biomaterials are synthetic or modified biologic materials that are used in implanted or extracorporeal medical devices to augment or replace body structures and functions.[186,187] Biomaterials include polymers, metals, ceramics, carbons, processed collagen, and chemically treated animal or human tissues, the latter exemplified by glutaraldehyde-preserved heart valves and pericardium. Biomaterials in medical devices interact with the surrounding tissues. The first generation of biomedical materials (eg, metals used for early valve substitutes) was generally designed to be inert; the goal was to reduce the host inflammatory responses to the implanted material. By the mid-1980s, a second generation of technology, comprising *bioactive* biomaterials, was emerging that could interact with the host in a beneficial manner (eg, biodegradable polymer sutures, drug delivery systems, textured bladder surfaces in ventricular assist devices). In the recent past, with a greater understanding of material-tissue interactions at the cellular and molecular levels, materials are being designed to stimulate specific cellular and tissue responses at the molecular level.[188,189] These materials are intended to be *regenerative*, and to yield functional tissue and organs, in approaches called *tissue engineering* (discussed later).

Biomaterial-tissue interactions comprise effects of both the implant on the host tissues and the host on the implant,

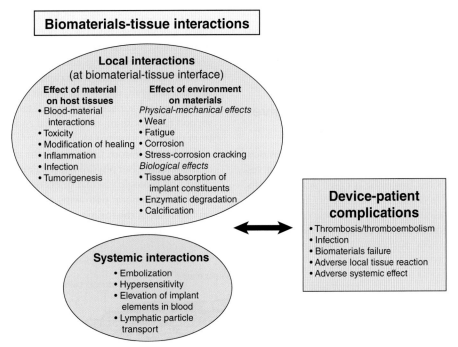

FIGURE 5-33 Overview of potential interactions of biomaterials with tissue, comprising local, distant, and systemic effects of the biomaterial on the host tissue, as well as the physical and biologic effects of the environment on the materials and the device. These interactions comprise the pathophysiologic basis for device complications and failure modes. (Modified with permission from Ratner BD, Hoffman AS, Schoen FJ, et al: *Biomaterials Science: An Introduction to Materials in Medicine,* 2nd ed. Orlando: Elsevier; 2004.)

and are important in mediating prosthetic device complications (Fig. 5-33).[190] These interactions have local and potentially systemic consequences. Complications of cardiovascular medical devices, irrespective of anatomical site of implantation, can be grouped into six major categories: (1) thrombosis and thromboembolism; (2) device-associated infection; (3) exuberant or defective healing; (4) biomaterials failure (eg, degeneration, fracture); (5) adverse local tissue interaction (eg, toxicity, hemolysis); and (6) adverse effects distant from the intended site of the device (eg, biomaterials/device embolism/migration, systemic hypersensitivity).

Blood-Surface Interaction

Thromboembolic complications of cardiovascular devices cause significant mortality and morbidity. Thrombotic deposits can impede the function of a prosthetic heart valve, vascular graft, or blood pump, or cause distal emboli. As in the cardiovascular system in general, surface thrombogenicity, hypercoagulability, and locally static blood flow (called *Virchow's triad*), present individually or in combination, determine both the relative propensity toward thrombus formation and the location of thrombotic deposits with specific devices. No known synthetic or modified biologic surface is as thromboresistant as the normal, unperturbed endothelium. Like a blood vessel denuded of endothelium, foreign materials on contact with blood spontaneously and rapidly (within seconds) absorb a film of plasma components, primarily protein, followed by platelet adhesion.[191]

If conditions of relatively static flow are present, macroscopic thrombus can ensue. The specific physical and chemical characteristics of materials that regulate the outcomes of blood-surface interaction are incompletely understood.

Coagulation proteins, complement products, other proteins, and platelets are activated, damaged, and consumed by blood-material interactions. The clinical approach to control of thrombosis in cardiovascular devices is generally through systemic anticoagulants, particularly Coumadin (warfarin) or antiplatelet agents. Coumadin inhibits thrombin formation but does not inhibit platelet-mediated thrombosis and induces a risk of hemorrhage. Coumadin is also teratogenic, causing a risk of fetal malformations in pregnant women. Hemolysis (damage to red blood cells) in implants and extracorporeal circulatory systems can results from both cell-surface contact and turbulence-induced shear forces.

Tissue-Biomaterials Interaction

Synthetic biomaterials elicit a *foreign body reaction*, a special form of nonimmune inflammatory response with an infiltrate predominantly composed of macrophages.[192,193] For most biomaterials implanted into solid tissue, encapsulation by a relatively thin fibrous tissue capsule (composed of collagen and fibroblasts) resembling a scar ultimately occurs, often with a fine capillary network at its junction with normal tissue. Ongoing mild chronic inflammation associated with this fibrous capsule is common with clinical implants.

Although immunologic reactions have been proposed rarely for synthetic biomaterial-tissue interactions,[194] and antibodies can be elicited by implantation of some materials in finely pulverized form, proven clinical cardiovascular device failure owing to immunologic reactivity is rare.

Healing of a Vascular Graft, Heart Valve Sewing Cuff, or Endovascular Stent

Healing of a vascular graft, heart valve sewing cuff, or endovascular stent derives principally from overgrowth from the host vessel across anastomotic sites; this tissue is called *pannus*. Grafts, fabrics, and stents used as cardiovascular implants heal primarily by ingrowth of endothelium and smooth muscle cells from the cut edges of the adjacent artery, and contact points with vessels

and/or myocardium; where endothelium is present, the tissue is called a *neointima*. Additional potential mechanisms of endothelialization include (1) tissue ingrowth through the fabric of a graft with interstices large enough to permit ingrowth of fibrovascular elements arising from capillaries extending from outside to inside the graft, which may permit endothelial cells to migrate to the luminal surface at a large distance from the anastomosis; and (2) deposition of functional endothelial cell progenitors from the circulating blood.[195]

Exuberant fibrous tissue can occur at a vascular anastomosis as an overactive but physiologic repair response (Fig. 5-34). Synthetic and biologic vascular grafts often fail because of generalized or anastomotic narrowing mediated by connective tissue proliferation in the intima, and heart valve prostheses can have excessive pannus that occludes the orifice. Intimal hyperplasia

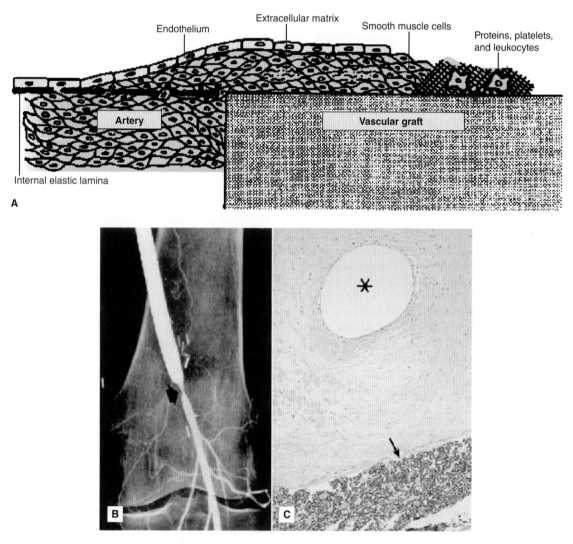

FIGURE 5-34 Vascular graft healing. (A) Schematic diagram of pannus formation, the major mode of graft healing with currently available vascular grafts. Smooth muscle cells migrate from the media to the intima of the adjacent artery and extend over and proliferate on the graft surface. The thin smooth muscle cell layer is covered by a proliferating layer of endothelial cells. (B and C) Anastomotic hyperplasia at the distal anastomosis of synthetic femoropopliteal graft. (B) Angiogram demonstrating constriction of distal graft anastomosis (*arrow*). (C) Photomicrograph demonstrating Gore-Tex graft (*arrow*) with prominent intimal proliferation and very small residual lumen (*asterisk*). (Reproduced with permission from Schoen FJ: *Interventional and Surgical Cardiovascular Pathology: Clinical Correlations and Basic Principles.* Philadelphia: Saunders; 1989.)

results primarily from smooth muscle cell migration, proliferation, and ECM elaboration following and possibly mediated by acute or ongoing endothelial cell injury. Important contributing factors include (1) surface thrombogenesis; (2) delayed or incomplete endothelialization of the fabric; (3) disturbed flow across the anastomosis; and (4) mechanical "mismatch" at the junction of implant and host tissues.

Diminished healing also is clinically important in certain circumstances, such as periprosthetic leak associated with heart valve prostheses. Moreover, markedly diminished endothelialization owing to toxicity of the cytostatic agents, paclitaxel and sirolimus, has been implicated in late thrombosis of drug-eluting coronary stents. For uncertain reasons, humans have a limited ability to completely endothelialize cardiovascular prostheses beyond a zone near an anastomosis, typically 10 to 15 mm, thereby allowing healing of intracardiac fabric patches and prosthetic valve sewing rings, but not long vascular grafts. Thus, except adjacent to an anastomosis of a vascular graft, a compacted platelet-fibrin aggregate (*pseudointima*) comprises the inner lining, even after long-term implantation. Because firm adherence of such linings to the underlying graft may be impossible, dislodgment of the lining and formation of a flap-valve can occur and cause obstruction.[196] Current research focuses on novel vascular graft materials that enhance endothelial cell attachment, grafts, and other implants preseeded with unmodified or genetically engineered endothelial cells, attempts to block smooth muscle cell proliferation, and engineered tissue vascular grafts (see the following).[197]

Infection

Infection is a common complication of implanted prosthetic devices and a frequent source of morbidity and mortality.[198,199] Early implant infections (<1 to 2 months postoperatively) most likely result from intraoperative contamination or early postoperative wound infection. In contrast, late infections generally occur by a hematogenous route, and can be initiated by bacteremia induced by therapeutic dental, gastrointestinal, or genitourinary procedures. Antibiotics given prophylactically at the time of device implantation and shortly before subsequent diagnostic and therapeutic procedures may protect against implant infection.

The presence of a foreign body potentiates infection in several ways. Microorganisms may inadvertently be introduced into deep tissue locations by contamination at device implantation, bypassing natural barriers against infection. Some devices, such as current left ventricular assist devices, require a percutaneous driveline, providing a continuous potential means of entry for microorganisms. Infections associated with medical devices are characterized microbiologically by a high prevalence of organisms capable of forming protective biofilms (ie, a multicellular consortium of microbial cells that is irreversibly associated with a material surface and enclosed in a self-produced ECM composed primarily of polysaccharides),[200] including gram-positive bacteria such as *S. epidermidis, S. aureus, Enterococcus faecalis,* and *S. viridans,* gram-negative bacteria such as *Escherichia coli* and *Pseudomonas*

aeruginosa, and fungi such as *Candida albicans.* Some of these organisms, especially *S. epidermidis* and *S. viridans,* are of relatively low virulence in the absence of a foreign body, but are frequent causes of medical device infection. The production of a *biofilm* by an organism is protective against the humoral and cellular immune response of the host[201] and inhibits the penetration and effectiveness of opsonizing antibodies, inflammatory cells, and antibiotics. Moreover, vasculature may be diminished and there may be necrotic tissue in the vicinity of an implant. Consequently, an implant-associated infection often persists until the device is removed.

Tissue Engineering and Cardiovascular Regeneration

Tissue engineering comprises therapeutic approaches that use endogenous or exogenously delivered living cells together with natural materials or synthetic polymers to develop or regenerate functional tissues.[202-204] In the most widely used generic strategy to engineering tissues, cells are initially seeded on a synthetic polymer scaffold (usually a bioresorbable polymer in a porous configuration) or natural material (such as collagen, decellularized tissue, or otherwise chemically treated tissue), in the desired geometry for the engineered tissue, and a tissue is matured in vitro. The in vitro phase is done in a vessel (a *bioreactor*), containing a metabolically and mechanically supportive environment with growth media. The cells, which may be either fully differentiated or stem cells, proliferate and an elaborate ECM is created in the form of a "new" tissue (the *construct).* In the second step, the construct is implanted in vivo into the appropriate anatomical location. Following implantation remodeling of the construct in vivo is intended to recapitulate normal functional architecture of an organ or tissue. Another collection of methods uses the in vivo environment as the bioreactor and thereby aims to recruit endogenous cells to build tissues from within. Key processes occurring during the in vitro and in vivo phases of tissue formation and maturation are: (1) cell proliferation, sorting, and differentiation; (2) ECM production and organization; (3) degradation of the scaffold; and (4) remodeling and potentially growth of the tissue.

The principles and processes of tissue engineering have been applied to vascular grafts, myocardium, and heart valves, as discussed next.

Engineered Vascular Grafts

Tissue-engineered vascular grafts blood vessels of small caliber are actively being investigated.[205-207] Vascular cells have been applied onto tubular resorbable polymer scaffolds and matured in vitro in a bioreactor prior to in vivo implantation.[208] Exposure to pulsatile physical forces during tissue formation generally enhances graft properties; pulsed grafts are thicker, have greater suture retention, and higher cell and collagen density than nonpulsed engineered grafts, and have a histologic appearance similar to that of native arteries. Other investigators have fabricated mechanically sound engineered tissue vascular grafts by constructing a cohesive cellular sheet of smooth muscle cells, rolling this sheet to form the vessel media, analogous to a jelly roll, wrapping a sheet of human fibroblasts around the media to serve as an adventitia, and seeding endothelial cells in the lumen.[209] Vessel "equivalents" composed of collagen and cultured bovine fibroblasts, and smooth muscle and endothelial cells have been investigated, but despite reinforcement with a Dacron mesh, such grafts have been unable to withstand burst strengths for in vivo applications.[210] Another approach to vascular graft engineering utilizes naturally derived matrices with or without cell repopulation prior to implantation.[211] Vascular grafts fabricated from small intestine submucosa used as experimental vascular grafts in dogs were reported to be completely endothelialized and histologically similar to arteries.[212,213]

Another approach to vascular tissue engineering extends the concept of Sparks' silicone mandril-grown graft used clinically in the 1970s, in which a collagenous fibrous capsule tube was formed around an implanted cylindrical foreign body (silicone mandril) adjacent to a diseased vessel; the mandril was subsequently removed yielding an autologous tissue tube that could be anastomosed to the vessels proximal and distal to an obstruction.[214] However, owing to the variability of the quality of tissue generated in older patients in areas of circulatory insufficiency, such vascular replacements often developed aneurysms when used clinically. Grafts grown as the reactive tissue that forms around silicone tubing inserted into the peritoneal cavity of rats, rabbits, and dogs, everted (so that a mesothelial cell lined surface become the blood-contacting surface), and grafted into the carotid artery of the same animal remained patent up to 4 months.[215]

Initial clinical studies of tissue-engineered blood vessels as pulmonary artery segments and hemodialysis access grafts have been reported.[216,217] Clinically employed conventional ePTFE vascular grafts have been seeded with endothelial cells at the time of implantation, yielding reportedly better outcomes than unseeded grafts.[218-224]

Regeneration of Cardiac Tissue

The adult heart responds to mechanical overload by hypertrophy (increase in cell size) and to severe ischemic or other injury by cell death (see earlier). Functional increase in cardiac myocyte number by cell regeneration or hyperplasia has generally not been considered possible. Nevertheless, several lines of research raise enthusiasm that clinically important cardiac regeneration and/or engineered cardiac tissue may indeed be possible.

Recent evidence suggests that myocyte regeneration and death occur physiologically, and that these cellular processes are enhanced in pathologic states, challenging the dogma that the heart as a postmitotic organ. Some investigators believe that heart homeostasis may be regulated by a stem cell compartment in the heart characterized by multipotent cardiac stem cells having the ability to acquire the distinct cell lineages of the myocardium. In this view, humans are capable of regenerating myocytes and coronary vessels throughout life

and have the capacity to adapt to increases in pressure and volume loads.[225] Moreover, adult bone marrow cells may be able to differentiate into cells beyond their own tissue boundary and create cardiomyocytes and coronary vessels. Myocardial tissue generated from cells, scaffolds, and bioreactors has been encouraging with respect to construct survival, vascularization, and integration, but significant and sustained functional improvement has yet to be demonstrated.[226,227] Application of cyclic mechanical stretch and electrical signals have been shown to enhance cell differentiation and force of contraction.[228]

Animal experiments and some early-phase clinical trials lend credence to the notion that cell-based cardiac repair may be an achievable therapeutic target, including (1) the possibility that the heart may have endogenous mechanisms of repair; (2) cell-based therapies in which fetal or adult cardiomyocytes, skeletal myoblasts or nonmuscle stem or differentiated cells are injected into the heart; and (3) experimental generation of functional myocardium by cell-scaffold-bioreactor tissue engineering approaches yielding a prosthetic myocardial patch.[229-231] Clinical trials have used cells derived from skeletal muscle and bone marrow, and basic researchers are investigating sources of new cardiomyocytes, such as resident myocardial progenitors and embryonic stem cells to achieve structural and functional integration of the graft with the host myocardium. Nevertheless, the most appropriate form of cellular therapy for myocardial injury remains to be identified. Moreover, and it remains unclear at present whether the beneficial effects observed in some studies are a result of functional and electrically integrated myocytes (the ideal), enhancement of angiogenesis owing to a local and nonspecific inflammatory reaction at the site of injection, or a "paracrine" effect, whereby transplanted cells produce growth factors, cytokines, and other local signaling molecules that are beneficial to the infarct through neovascularization and/or scar remodeling.

Tissue-Engineered Heart Valves

Recent scientific and technological progress has stimulated the goal of generating a living valve replacement that would obviate the complications of conventional valve replacement, adapt to changing environmental conditions in the recipient, and potentially grow with a growing patient.[232-235] The long-term success of a tissue-engineered (living) valve replacement will depend on the ability of its living cellular components (particularly VIC) to assume normal function with the capacity to repair structural injury, remodel the ECM, and potentially grow.

Tissue-engineered heart valves (TEHV) grown as valved conduits from autologous cells (either vascular wall cells or bone marrow–derived mesenchymal stem cells) seeded on biodegradable synthetic polymers grown in vitro have functioned in the pulmonary circulation of growing lambs for up to 5 months.[236,237] In some studies, these grafts evolved in vivo to a specialized layered structure that resembled that of native semilunar valve. Pulmonary vascular walls fabricated from vascular wall cells and biodegradable polymer and implanted into very young lambs enlarged proportionally to overall animal growth over a 2-year period.[238]

To eliminate the need for in vitro cell seeding and culture steps, an alternative tissue engineering strategy has used a scaffold of either decellularized naturally derived biomaterial (such as animal or human allograft valve, decellularized sheep intestinal submucosa [SIS]), or a porous polymer matrix implanted without prior seeding but with the intent of harnessing intrinsic circulating cells to populate and potentially remodel the scaffold.[239] Tissue-derived scaffolds must possess desirable three-dimensional architecture, mechanical properties, and potential adhesion/migration sites for cell attachment and ingrowth. Nevertheless, decellularized porcine valves implanted in humans had a strong inflammatory response and suffered structural failure.[240] Work is also being done on cell-seeded, engineered tissue valves for transcatheter implantation.[241]

Translation of heart valve tissue engineering and regenerative medicine from the laboratory to the clinical realm has exciting potential but also formidable challenges and uncertainties. Key hurdles include selection and validation of suitable animal models, development of guidelines for characterization and assurance of the quality of an in vitro fabricated TEHV for human implantation, and strategies to understand, monitor, and potentially control patient-to-patient variability in wound healing and tissue remodeling in vivo.

DISCLOSURE

Frederick J. Schoen is or has been a consultant to CardAQ, Celxcel, Corazon, Cordis, Direct Flow Medical, Ethicon, Edwards Lifesciences, Gore, Medtronic, NeoGraft, Pi-R-Square/PiCardia, Sadra Medical/Boston Scientific, Sorin Medical, St. Jude Medical, Sulzer Carbomedics, Symetis, Syncardia, Thoratec, and Xeltis in the past 5 years.

Robert Padera is or has been a consultant to Atria, Direct Flow, Du Pont, Medtronic, Mitral Solutions, Mitralign, Sadra, Sorin, St. Jude, and Transmedics.

REFERENCES

1. Avila P, Mercier LA, Dore A, et al: Adult congenital heart disease: a growing epidemic. *Can J Cardiol* 2014; 30:S410.
2. Schoen FJ, Edwards WD: Pathology of cardiovascular interventions, including endovascular therapies, revascularization, vascular replacement, cardiac assist/replacement, arrhythmia control and repaired congenital heart disease, in Silver MD, Gotlieb AI, Schoen FJ (eds): *Cardiovascular Pathology*, 3rd ed. Philadelphia, Churchill Livingstone, 2001; p 678.
3. Schoen FJ, Mitchell RN: The heart, in Kumar V, Abbas A, Aster J (eds): *Robbins and Cotran Pathologic Basis of Disease*. 9th ed. Philadelphia, WB Saunders, 2015; p 523.
4. Opie LH, Commerford PJ, Gersh BJ, Pfeffer MA: Controversies in ventricular remodeling. *Lancet* 2006; 367:356.
5. Braunwald E: The war against heart failure: the Lancet lecture. *Lancet* 2015; 385:812.
6. Gosse P: Left ventricular hypertrophy as a predictor of cardiovascular risk. *J Hypertens Suppl* 2005; 23:S37.
7. Mann DL, Barger PM, Burkhoff D: Myocardial recovery and the failing heart. *J Am Coll Cardiol* 2012; 60:2465.
8. Teekakirikul P, Kelly MA, Rehm HL, Lakdawala NK, Funke BH: Molecular genetics and clinical genetic testing in the postgenomic era. *J Mol Diagn* 2013; 15:158.
9. Stone JR: Diagnostic biopsies of the native heart. *Surgical Pathology* 2012; 5:401.
10. McNally EM, Golbus JR, Puckelwartz MJ: Genetic mutations and mechanisms in dilated cardiomyopathy. *J Clin Invest* 2013; 123:19.
11. Cooper LT Jr: Myocarditis. *N Engl J Med* 2009; 360:1526.
12. Maron BJ, Ommen SR, Semsarian C, Spirito P, Olivotto I, Maron MS: Hypertrophic cardiomyopathy. Present and future, with translation into contemporary cardiovascular medicine. *J Am Coll Cardiol* 2014; 64:83.
13. Said SM, Dearani JA, Ommen SR, Schaff HV: New treatment strategies for hypertrophic obstructive cardiomyopathy. Surgical treatment of hypertrophic cardiomyopathy. *Expert Rev Cardiovasc Ther* 2013; 11:617.
14. Borlaug BA: The pathophysiology of heart failure with preserved ejection fraction. *Nat Rev Cardiol* 2014; 11:507.
15. Iyer VR, Chin AJ: Arrhythmogenic right ventricular cardiomyopathy/dysplasia (ARVC/D). *Am J Med Genet C Semin Med Genet* 2013; 163C:185.
16. Libby P, Theroux P: Pathophysiology of coronary artery disease. *Circulation* 2005; 111:3481.
17. Schoenhagen P, Ziada KM, Vince DG, et al: Arterial remodeling and coronary artery disease. The concept of "dilated" versus "obstructive" coronary atherosclerosis. *J Am Coll Cardiol* 2001; 38:297.
18. Mitchell RN: Blood vessels, in Kumar V, Abbas A, Aster J (eds): *Robbins and Cotran Pathologic Basis of Disease*, 9th ed. Philadelphia, WB Saunders, 2015; p 483.
19. Naghavi M, Libby P, Falk E, et al: From vulnerable plaque to vulnerable patient. A call for new definitions and risk management strategies. Parts 1 and 2. *Circulation* 2003; 108:1664 and 1772.
20. Libby P, Tabas I, Fredman G, Fisher EA: Inflammation and its resolution as determinants of acute coronary syndromes. *Circ Res* 2014; 114:1867.
21. Tomey MI, Narula J, Kovacic JC: Advances in the understanding of plaque composition and treatment options: year in review. *J Am Coll Cardiol* 2014; 63:1604.
22. Slager CJ, Wentzel JJ, Gijsen FJ, et al: The role of shear stress in the generation of rupture-prone vulnerable plaques. *Nat Clin Pract Cardiovasc Med* 2005; 2:401.
23. Kolodgie FD, Burke AP, Farb A: The thin-cap fibroatheroma. A type of vulnerable plaque: the major precursor lesion to acute coronary syndromes. *Curr Opin Cardiol* 2001; 16:285.
24. Yellon DM, Hausenloy DJ: Myocardial reperfusion injury. *NEJM* 2007; 357:1121.
25. Vargas SO, Sampson BA, Schoen FJ: Pathologic detection of early myocardial infarction. A critical review of the evolution and usefulness of modern techniques. *Mod Pathol* 1999; 12:635.
26. Ertl G, Frantz S: Healing after myocardial infarction. *Cardiovasc Res* 2005; 66:22.
27. Beltrami AP, Urbanek K, Kajstura J, et al: Evidence that cardiac myocytes divide after myocardial infarction. *N Engl J Med* 2001; 344:1750.
28. Faxon DP: Early reperfusion strategies after acute ST-segment elevation myocardial infarction. The importance of timing. *Nat Clin Pract Cardiovasc Med* 2005; 2:22.
29. Menees DS, Peterson ED, Wang Y, et al: Door-to-balloon time and mortality among patients undergoing primary PCI. *N Engl J Med* 2013; 369:901.
30. Alfayoumi F, Srinivasan V, Geller M, Gradman A: The no-reflow phenomenon. Epidemiology, pathophysiology, and therapeutic approach. *Rev Cardiovasc Med* 2005; 6:72.
31. Bainey KR, Armstrong PW: Clinical perspectives on reperfusion injury in acute myocardial infarction. *Am Heart J* 2014; 167:637.
32. Hutchins GM, Silverman KJ: Pathology of the stone heart syndrome. Massive myocardial contraction band necrosis and widely patent coronary arteries. *Am J Pathol* 1979; 95:745.
33. Camici PG, Prasad SK, Rimoldi OE: Stunning, hibernation, and assessment of myocardial viability. *Circulation* 2008; 117:103.
34. Alman KC: Noninvasive assessment myocardial viability: current status and future directions. *J Nucl Cardiol* 2013; 20:618.
35. Grover S, Srinivasan G, Selvanayagam JB: Evaluation of myocardial viability with cardiac magnetic resonance imaging. *Prog Cardiovasc Dis* 2011; 54:204.

36. Winters GL, Schoen FJ: Graft arteriosclerosis-induced myocardial pathology in heart transplant recipients. Predictive value of endomyocardial biopsy. *J Heart Lung Transplant* 1997; 16:985.

37. Ovize M, Thibault H, Przyklenk: Myocardial conditioning: opportunities for clinical translation. *Circ Res* 2013; 113:439.

38. Nabel EG, Braunwald E: A tale of coronary artery disease and myocardial infarctions. *N Engl J Med* 2012; 366:54.

39. McMullan MH, Maples MD, Kilgore TL Jr, et al: Surgical experience with left ventricular free wall rupture. *Ann Thorac Surg* 2001; 71:1894.

40. Birnbaum Y, Fishbein MC, Blanche C, et al: Ventricular septal rupture after acute myocardial infarction. *N Engl J Med* 2002; 347:1426.

41. Antunes MJ, Antunes PE: Left-ventricular aneurysms. From disease to repair. *Expert Rev Cardiovasc Ther* 2005; 3:285.

42. Cohn JN, Ferrari R, Sharpe N: Cardiac remodeling—concepts and clinical implications: a consensus paper from an international forum on cardiac remodeling. *J Am Coll Cardiol* 2000; 35:569.

43. Antman EM, Braunwald E: ST-elevation myocardial infarction. Pathology, pathophysiological and clinical feature, in Libby P, Bonow RD, Mann DL, Zipes DD (eds): *Braunwald's Heart Disease. A Textbook of Cardiovascular Medicine*, 8th ed. Philadelphia, WB Saunders, 2008; p 1207.

44. Landau C, Lange RA, Hillis LD: Percutaneous transluminal coronary angioplasty. *N Engl J Med* 1994; 330:981.

45. Haudenschild CC: Pathobiology of restenosis after angioplasty. *Am J Med* 1993; 94(Suppl):40.

46. Tomey MI, Kini AS, Sharma SK: Current status of rotational artherectomy. *JACC Cardiac Interv* 2014; 7:345.

47. Daemen J, Serruys PW: Drug-eluting stent update 2007: Part I. A survey of current and future generation drug-eluting stents: meaningful advances or more of the same? Part II: Unsettled issues. *Circulation* 2007; 116:316 and 961.

48. Agostoni P, Valgimigli M, Biondi-Zoccai GG, et al: Clinical effectiveness of bare-metal stenting compared with balloon angioplasty in total coronary occlusions: insights from a systematic overview of randomized trials in light of the drug-eluting stent era. *Am Heart J* 2006; 151:682.

49. Farb A, Sangiorgi G, Carter AJ, et al: Pathology of acute and chronic coronary stenting in humans. *Circulation* 1999; 99:44.

50. Welt FG, Rogers C: Inflammation and restenosis in the stent era. *Arterioscler Thromb Vasc Biol* 2002; 22:1769.

51. Nakazawa G, Finn AV, Kolodgie FD, Virmani R: A review of current devices and a look at new technology. Drug eluting stents. *Expert Rev Med Dev* 2009; 6:33.

52. Kukreja N, Onuma Y, Daemen J, Serruys PW: The future of drug-eluting stents. *Pharmacol Res* 2008; 57:171.

53. Sousa JE, Costa MA, Sousa AG, et al: Two-year angiographic and intravascular ultrasound follow-up after implantation of sirolimus-eluting stents in human coronary arteries. *Circulation* 2003; 107:381.

54. Ong AT, Serruys PW: An overview of research in drug-eluting stents. *Nat Clin Pract Cardiovasc Med* 2005; 2:647.

55. Holmes DR, Kereiakes DJ, Laskey WK, et al: Thrombosis and drug-eluting stents: an objective appraisal. *J Am Coll Cardiol* 2007; 50:109.

56. Palmerini T, Biondi-Zoccai G, Della Riva D, et al: Stent thrombosis with drug-eluting stents: is the paradigm shifting? *J Am Coll Cardiol* 2013; 62:1915.

57. Wiebe J, Nef HM, Hamm CW: Current status of bioresorbable scaffolds in the treatment of coronary artery disease. *J Am Coll Cardiol* 2014; 64:2541.

58. Iqbal J, Onuma Y, Ormiston J, et al: Bioresorbable scaffolds: rationale, current status, challenges, and future. *Eur Heart J* 2014; 35:765.

59. Opie LH, Commerford PJ, Gersh BJ: Controversies in stable coronary artery disease. *Lancet* 2006; 367:69.

60. Schachner T: Pharmacologic inhibition of vein graft neointimal hyperplasia. *J Thorac Cardiovasc Surg* 2006; 131:1065.

61. Loop FD, Lytle BW, Cosgrove DM, et al: Influence of the internal-mammary-artery graft on 10-year survival and other cardiac events. *N Engl J Med* 1986; 314:1.

62. Falk V, Walther T, Gummert JF: Anastomotic devices for coronary artery bypass grafting. *Expert Rev Med Dev* 2005; 2:223.

63. Diodato M, Chedrawy EG: Coronary artery bypass graft surgery: the past, present, and future of myocardial revascularisation. *Surg Res Pract* 2014; 2014:726158.

64. Ho SY: Structure and anatomy of the aortic root. *Eur J Echocardiogr* 2009; 10:i3.

65. Schoen FJ: Evolving concepts of cardiac valve dynamics. The continuum of development, functional structure, pathology and tissue engineering. *Circulation* 2008; 118:1864.

66. Combs MD, Yutzey KE: Heart valve development. Regulatory networks in development and disease. *Circ Res* 2009; 105:408.

67. Aikawa E, Whittaker P, Farber M, et al: Human semilunar cardiac valve remodeling by activated cells from fetus to adult. *Circulation* 2006; 113:1344.

68. Christie GW, Barratt-Boyes BG: Age-dependent changes in the radial stretch of human aortic valve leaflets determined by biaxial testing. *Ann Thorac Surg* 1995; 60(S1):156.

69. Davies PF, Passerini AG, Simmons GA: Aortic valve. Turning over a new leaf(let) in endothelial phenotypic heterogeneity. *Arterioscler Thromb Vasc Biol* 2004; 24:1331.

70. Simmons CA, Grant GR, Manduchi E, Davies PF: Spatial heterogeneity of endothelial phenotypes correlates with side-specific vulnerability to calcification in normal porcine aortic valves. *Circ Res* 2005; 96:792.

71. Carabello BA, Paulus WJ: Aortic stenosis. *Lancet* 2009; 373:956-966.

72. Rajamannan NM, Evans FJ, Aikawa E, et al: Calcific aortic valve disease: not simply a degenerative process. A Review and Agenda for Research from the National Heart and Lung and Blood Institute Aortic Stenosis Working Group. *Circulation* 2011; 124:1783-1791.

73. Carabello BA, Paulus WJ: Aortic stenosis. *Lancet* 2009; 363:956.

74. Roberts WC, Ko JM: Frequency by decades of unicuspid, bicuspid, and tricuspid aortic valves in adults having isolated aortic valve replacement for aortic stenosis, with or without associated aortic regurgitation. *Circulation* 2005; 111:920.

75. Otto CM, Lind BK, Kitzman DW, et al: Association of aortic-valve sclerosis with cardiovascular mortality and morbidity in the elderly. *N Engl J Med* 1999; 341:142.

76. Lindman BR, Bonow RO, Otto CM: Current management of calcific aortic stenosis. *Circ Res* 2013; 113:223.

77. O'Brien KD: Pathogenesis of calcific aortic valve disease. A disease process comes of age (and a good deal more). *Arterioscler Thromb Vasc Biol* 2006; 26:1721.

78. Rajamannan NM: Calcific aortic stenosis. Lessons learned from experimental and clinical studies. *Arterioscler Thromb Vasc Biol* 2009; 29:162.

79. Fedak PW, Verma S, David TE, et al: Clinical and pathophysiological implications of a bicuspid aortic valve. *Circulation* 2002; 106:900.

80. Cripe L, Andelfinger G, Martin LJ, et al: Bicuspid aortic valve is heritable. *J Am Coll Cardiol* 2004; 44:138.

81. Garg V, Muth AN, Ransom JF, et al: Mutations in NOTCH1 cause aortic valve disease. *Nature* 2005; 437:270.

82. Bryant PA, Robins-Browne R, Carapetis JR, Curtis N: Some of the people, some of the time. Susceptibility to acute rheumatic fever. *Circulation* 2009; 119:742.

83. Chandrashekhar Y, Westaby S, Narula J: Mitral stenosis. *Lancet* 2009; 374:1271.

84. Hayek E, Gring CN, Griffin BP: Mitral valve prolapse. *Lancet* 2005; 365:507.

85. Rabkin E, Aikawa M, Stone JR, et al: Activated interstitial myofibroblasts express catabolic enzymes and mediate matrix remodeling in myxomatous heart valves. *Circulation* 2001; 104:2525.

86. Gelb BD: Marfan's syndrome and related disorders—more tightly connected than we thought. *N Engl J Med* 2006; 355:841.

87. Badiwala MV, Verma S, Rao V: Surgical management of ischemic mitral regurgitation. *Circulation* 2009; 120:1287.

88. Marwick TH, Lancellotti P, Pierard L: Ischemic mitral regurgitation. Mechanisms and diagnosis. *Heart* 2009; 95:1711.

89. Boyd JH: Ischemic mitral regurgitation. *Circ J* 2013; 77:1952.

90. Chan KM, Punjabi PP, Flather M, et al: Coronary artery bypass surgery with or without mitral valve annuloplasty in moderate functional ischemic mitral regurgitation: final results of the Randomized Ischemic Mitral Evaluation (RIME) trial. *Circulation* 2012; 126:2502.

91. Hung JW: Ischemic (functional) mitral regurgitation. *Cardiol Clin* 2013; 31:231.

92. Fox DJ, Khattar RS: Carcinoid heart disease. Presentation, diagnosis, and management. *Heart* 2004; 90:1224.

93. Bhattacharyya S, Schapira AH, Mikhailidis DP, Davar J: Drug-induced fibrotic valvular heart disease. *Lancet* 2009; 374:577.

94. Zadikoff C, Rochon P, Lang A: Cardiac valvulopathy associated with pergolide use. *Can J Neurol Sci* 2006; 33:27.

95. Haldar SM, O'Gara PT: Infective endocarditis: diagnosis and management. *Nat Clin Pract Cardiovasc Med* 2006; 3:310.

96. Werner M, Andersson R, Olaison L, Hogevik H: A clinical study of culture-negative endocarditis. *Medicine* 2003; 82:263.

97. Bashore TM, Cabell C, Fowler V Jr: Update on infective endocarditis. *Curr Probl Cardiol* 2006; 31:274.

98. Biegel R, Wunderlich NC, Kar S, Siegel RJ: The evolution of percutaneous mitral valve repair therapy: lessons learned and implications for patient selection. *J Am Coll Cardiol* 2014; 64:2688.

99. Boodhwani M, El Khoury G: Aortic valve repair: indications and outcomes. *Curr Cardiol Rep* 2014; 16:490.

100. Nobuyoshi M, Arita T, Shirai S, et al: Percutaneous balloon mitral valvuloplasty: a review. *Circulation* 2009; 119:e211.

101. Carabello BA: The current therapy for mitral regurgitation. *J Am Coll Cardiol* 2008; 52:319.

102. Enriquez-Sarano M, Akins CW, Vahanian A: Mitral regurgitation. *Lancet* 2009; 373:1382.

103. Bouma W, van der Horst IC, Wijdh-den Hamer IJ, et al: Chronic ischaemic mitral regurgitation: current treatment results and new mechanism-based surgical approaches. *Eur J Cardiothorac Surg* 2010; 37:170.

104. Kherani AR, Cheema FH, Casher J, et al: Edge-to-edge mitral valve repair. The Columbia Presbyterian experience. *Ann Thorac Surg* 2004; 78:73.

105. Feldman T, Cilingiroglu M: Percutaneous leaflet repair and annuloplasty for mitral regurgitation. *J Am Coll Cardiol* 2011; 57:529.

106. Al-Atassi T, Malas T, Mesana T, Chan V: Mitral valve interventions in heart failure. *Curr Opin Cardiol* 2014; 29:192.

107. Mack M: Percutaneous mitral valve therapy. When? Which patients? *Curr Opin Cardiol* 2009; 24:125.

108. Maselli D, Guarracino F, Chiaramonti F, et al: Percutaneous mitral annuloplasty. An anatomic study of human coronary sinus and its relation with mitral valve annulus and coronary arteries. *Circulation* 2006; 114:377.

109. Maisano F, La Canna G, Colombo A, Alfieri O: The evolution from surgery to percutaneous mitral valve interventions. *J Am Coll Cardiol* 2011; 58:2174.

110. Munkholm-Larsen S, Wan B, Tian DH, et al: A systematic review on the safety and efficacy of percutaneous edge-to-edge mitral valve repair with the MitraClip system for high surgical risk candidates. *Heart* 2014; 100:473.

111. Treasure CB, Schoen FJ, Treseler PA, et al: Leaflet entrapment causing acute severe aortic insufficiency during balloon aortic valvuloplasty. *Clin Cardiol* 1989; 12:405.

112. Schoen FJ, Edwards WD: Valvular heart disease. General principles and stenosis, in Silver MD, Gotlieb AI, Schoen FJ (eds): *Cardiovascular Pathology*, 3rd ed. Philadelphia, WB Saunders, 2001; p 402.

113. Huh J, Bakaeen F: Heart valve replacement: which valve for which patient? *Curr Cardiol Rep* 2006; 8:109.

114. Kidane AG, Burriesci G, Cornejo P, et al: Current developments and future prospects for heart valve replacement therapy. *J Biomed Mater Res B Appl Biomater* 2009; 88:290.

115. Brown JM, O'Brien SM, Wu C, et al: Isolated aortic valve replacement in North America comprising 108,687 patients in 10 years: changes in risks, valve types, and outcomes in the Society of Thoracic Surgeons National Database. *J Thorac Cardiovasc Surg* 2009; 137:82.

116. Gammie JS, Sheng S, Griffith BP, et al: Trends in mitral valve surgery in the United States: results from the Society of Thoracic Surgeons Adult Cardiac Surgery Database. *Ann Thorac Surg* 2009; 87:1431.

117. O'Brien SM, Shahian DM, Filardo G, et al: The Society of Thoracic Surgeons 2008 cardiac surgery risk models: Part 2—isolated valve surgery. *Ann Thorac Surg* 2009; 88:S23.

118. Hammermeister KE, Sethi GK, Henderson WG, et al: Outcomes 15 years after valve replacement with a mechanical versus a bioprosthetic valve. Final report of the Veterans Affairs randomized trial. *J Am Coll Cardiol* 2000; 36:1152.

119. Oxenham H, Bloomfield P, Wheatley DJ, et al: Twenty year comparison of a Bjork-Shiley mechanical heart valve with porcine bioprostheses. *Heart* 2003; 89:715.

120. Akins CW, Miller DC, Turina MI, et al: Guidelines for reporting mortality and morbidity after cardiac valve interventions. *Ann Thorac Surg* 2008; 85:1490.

121. Sun JC, Davidson MJ, Lamy A, Eikelboom JW: Antithrombotic management of patients with prosthetic heart valves: current evidence and future trends. *Lancet* 2009; 374:565.

122. Butchart EG: Antithrombotic management in patients with prosthetic valve: a comparison of American and European guidelines. *Heart* 2009; 95:430.

123. Elkayam U, Bitar F: Valvular heart disease and pregnancy. Part II: prosthetic valves. *J Am Coll Cardiol* 2005; 46:403.

124. Bennett PC, Silverman SH, Gill PS, Lip GY: Peripheral arterial disease and Virchow's triad. *Thromb Haemost* 2009; 101:1032.

125. Lengyel M, Horstkotte D, Voller H, et al: Recommendations for the management of prosthetic valve thrombosis. *J Heart Valve Dis* 2005; 14:567.

126. Habib G, Thuny F, Avierinos JF: Prosthetic valve endocarditis: current approach and therapeutic options. *Prog Cardiovasc Dis* 2008; 50:274.

127. Odell JA, Durandt J, Shama DM, Vythilingum S: Spontaneous embolization of a St. Jude prosthetic mitral valve leaflet. *Ann Thorac Surg* 1985; 39:569.

128. Blot WJ, Ibrahim MA, Ivey TD, et al: Twenty-five-year experience with the Björk-Shiley convexoconcave heart valve. A continuing clinical concern. *Circulation* 2005; 111:2850.

129. Schoen FJ, Levy RJ: Calcification of tissue heart valve substitutes. Progress toward understanding and prevention. *Ann Thorac Surg* 2005; 79:1072.

130. Sacks MS, Schoen FJ: Collagen fiber disruption occurs independent of calcification in clinically explanted bioprosthetic heart valves. *J Biomed Mater Res* 2002; 62:359.

131. Hilbert SL, Ferrans VJ, McAllister HA, et al: Ionescu-Shiley bovine pericardial bioprostheses. Histologic and ultrastructural studies. *Am J Pathol* 1992; 140:1195.

132. O'Brien MF, Harrocks S, Stafford EG, et al: The homograft aortic valve. A 29-year, 99.3% follow up of 1,022 valve replacements. *J Heart Valve Dis* 2001; 10:334.

133. Mitchell RN, Jonas RA, Schoen FJ: Pathology of explanted cryopreserved allograft heart valves. Comparison with aortic valves from orthotopic heart transplants. *J Thorac Cardiovasc Surg* 1998; 115:118.

134. Botha CA: The Ross operation. Utilization of the patient's own pulmonary valve as a replacement device for the diseased aortic valve. *Expert Rev Cardiovasc Ther* 2005; 3:1017.

135. Rabkin-Aikawa E, Aikawa M, Farber M, et al: Clinical pulmonary autograft valves. Pathologic evidence of adaptive remodeling in the aortic site. *J Thorac Cardiovasc Surg* 2004; 128:552.

136. Elkins RC, Thompson DM, Lane MM, et al: Ross operation: 16-year experience. *J Thoracic Cardiovasc Surg* 2008; 136:623.

137. Takkenberg JJ, Klieverik LM, Schoof PH, et al: The Ross procedure: a systematic review and meta-analysis. *Circulation* 2009; 119:222.

138. Luciani GB, Santini F, Mazzucco A: Autografts, homografts, and xenografts: overview of stentless aortic valve surgery. *J Cardiovasc Med* 2007; 8:91.

139. Borger MA, Carson SM, Ivanov J, et al: Stentless aortic valves are hemodynamically superior to stented valves during mid-term follow-up. A large retrospective study. *Ann Thorac Surg* 2005; 80:2180.

140. Fyfe BS, Schoen FJ: Pathologic analysis of non-stented Freestyle™ aortic root bioprostheses treated with amino oleic acid (AOA). *Sem Thorac Cardiovasc Surg* 1999; 11:151.

141. Butany J, Collins MJ, Nair V, et al: Morphological findings in explanted Toronto stentless porcine valves. *Cardiovasc Pathol* 2006; 15:41.

142. Vahanian A, Alfieri OR, Al-Attar N, et al: Transcatheter valve implantation for patients with aortic stenosis: a position statement from the European Association of Cardio-Thoracic Surgery (EACTS) and the European Society of Cardiology (ESC), in collaboration with the European Association of percutaneous Cardiovascular Interventions (EAPCI). *Eur J Cardiothorac Surg* 2008; 34:1.

143. Rahimtoola SH: The year in valvular heart disease. *J Am Coll Cardol* 2009; 53:1894.

144. Rodés-Cabau J: Transcatheter aortic valve implantation: current and future approaches. *Nat Rev Cardiol* 2012; 9:15.

145. Généreux P, Head SJ, Wood DA, et al. Transcatheter aortic valve implantation 10-year anniversary: review of current evidence and clinical implications. *Eur Heart J* 2012; 33:2388.

146. Leon MB, Smith CR, Mack M, et al. Transcatheter aortic-valve implantation for aortic stenosis in patients who cannot undergo surgery. *N Engl J Med* 2010; 363:1597.

147. Kodali SK, Williams MR, Smith CR, et al: Two-year outcomes after transcatheter or surgical aortic-valve replacement. *N Engl J Med* 2012; 366:1686.

148. Chiang YP, Chikwe J, Moskowitz AJ, Itagaki S, Adams DH, Egorova NN: Survival and long-term outcomes following bioprosthetic vs mechanical aortic valve replacement in patients aged 50 to 69 years. *JAMA* 2014; 312:1323.

149. Tice JA, Sellke FW, Schaff HV: Transcatheter aortic valve replacement in patients with severe aortic stenosis who are at high risk for surgical complications: summary assessment of the California Technology Assessment Forum. *J Thorac Cardiovasc Surg* 2014; 148:482.

150. Fassa AA, Himbert D, Vahanian A: Mechanisms and management of TAVR-related complications. *Nat Rev Cardiol* 2013; 10:685-695.

151. Zajarias A, Cribier AG: Outcomes and safety of percutaneous aortic valve replacement. *J Am Coll Cardiol* 2009; 53:1829.

152. Webb JG, Altwegg L, Boone RH, et al: Transcatheter aortic valve implantation. Impact on clinical and valve-related outcomes. *Circulation* 2009; 119:3009.

153. Mylotte D, Andalib A, Theriault-Lauzier P, et al: Transcatheter heart valve failure: a systematic review. *Eur Heart J* 2015; 36:1306.

154. Alraies MC, Eckman P: Adult heart transplant: indications and outcomes. *J Thorac Dis* 2014; 6:1120.

155. Lund LH, Edwards LB, Kucheryavaya AY, et al: The registry of the international society for heart and lung transplantation: thirty-first official adult heart transplant report—2014; focus theme: retransplantation. *J Heart Lung Transplant* 2014; 33:996.

156. Sampson BA: Examination of the cardiac explant, in Winters GL (ed): *Current Concepts in Cardiovascular Pathology.* Philadelphia, WB Saunders, 2012; p 485.

157. Winters GL: Cardiac transplant biopsies, in Winters GL (ed): *Current Concepts in Cardiovascular Pathology.* Philadelphia, WB Saunders, 2012; p 371.

158. Stewart S, Winters GL, Fishbein MC, et al: Revision of the 1990 working formulation for the standardization of nomenclature in the diagnosis of heart rejection. *J Heart Lung Transplant* 2005; 24:1710.

159. Berry GJ, Burke MM, Andersen C, et al: The 2013 International Society for Heart and Lung Transplantation working formulation for the standardization of nomenclature in the pathologic diagnosis of antibody-mediated rejection in heart transplantation. *J Heart Lung Transplant* 2013; 32:1147.

160. Mitchell RN: Graft vascular disease: immune response meets the vessel wall. *Ann Rev Pathol* 2009; 4:19.

161. Pober JS, Jane-wit D, Qin L, et al: Interacting mechanisms in the pathogenesis of cardiac allograft vasculopathy. *Arterioscler Thromb Vasc Biol* 2014; 34:1609.

162. Vesgo G, Hajdu M, Sevestyen A: Lymphoproliferative disorders after solid organ transplantation—classification, incidence, risk factors, early detection and treatment options. *Pathol Oncol Res* 2011; 17:443.

163. Caccamo M, Eckman P, John R: Current state of ventricular assist devices. *Curr Heart Fail Rep* 2011; 8:91.

164. Torregrossa G, Morshuis M, Varghese R, et al: Results with SynCardia total artificial heart beyond 1 year. *ASAIO J* 2014; 60:626.

165. Frazier OH, Dowling RD, Gray LA, et al: The total artificial heart: where we stand. *Cardiology* 2004; 101:117.

166. Padera RF: Pathology of cardiac assist devices, in McManus B, Braunwald E (eds): *Atlas of Cardiovascular Pathology.* Philadelphia, Current Medicine, 2008; p 257.

167. Starling RC, Moazami N, Silvestry SC, et al: Unexpected abrupt increase in left ventricular assist device thrombosis. *N Engl J Med* 2014; 370:33.

168. Strickland KC, Watkins JC, Couper GS, et al: Thrombus around the redesigned HeartWare HVAD inflow cannula: a pathologic series. *J Heart Lung Transplant* 2016, PMID 27021277 [Epub].

169. Itescu S, John R: Interactions between the recipient immune system and the left ventricular assist device surface. Immunological and clinical implications. *Ann Thorac Surg* 2003; 75:S58.

170. Ibrahim M, Yacoub M: Bridge to recovery and weaning protocols. *Heart Fail Clin* 2014; 10:S47. Felkin LE, Lara-Pezzi E, George R, et al: Expression of extracellular matrix genes during myocardial recovery from heart failure after left ventricular assist device support. *J Heart Lung Transplant* 2009; 28:117.

171. Saffitz JE: The pathology of sudden cardiac death in patients with ischemic heart disease—arrhythmology for anatomic pathologists. *Cardiovasc Pathol* 2005; 14:195.

172. Vardas PE, Simantirakis EN, Kanoupakis EM: New developments in cardiac pacemakers. *Circulation* 2013; 127:2343.

173. Goldberger Z, Lampert R: Implantable cardioverter-defibrillators: expanding indications and technologies: *JAMA* 2006; 295:809.

174. Kistler PM, Liew G, Mond HG: Long-term performance of active-fixation pacing leads. A prospective study. *Pacing Clin Electrophysiol* 2006; 29:226.

175. Steinbrook R: The controversy over Guidant's implantable defibrillators. *NEJM* 2005; 353:221.

176. Andrade JG, Rivard L, Macle L: The past, the present, and the future of cardiac arrhythmia ablation. *Can J Cardiol* 2014; 30:S431.

177. Yamada T, Kay GN: Optimal ablation strategies for different types of ventricular tachycardias. *Nat Rev Cardiol* 2012; 9:512.

178. Sabatine MS, Colucci WS, Schoen FJ: Primary tumors of the heart, in Zipes DD, Libby P, Bonow RD, Braunwald E (eds): *Braunwald's Heart Disease. A Textbook of Cardiovascular Medicine,* 7th ed. Philadelphia, WB Saunders, 2004; p 1807.

179. Reardon MJ, Walkes JC, Benjamin R: Therapy insight: malignant primary cardiac tumors. *Nat Clin Pract Cardiovasc Med* 2006; 3:548.

180. Gowda RM, Khan IA, Nair CK, et al: Cardiac papillary fibroelastoma. A comprehensive analysis of 725 cases. *Am Heart J* 2003; 146:404.

181. Howard RA, Aldea GS, Shapira OM, et al: Papillary fibroelastoma. Increasing recognition of a surgical disease. *Ann Thorac Surg* 1999; 68:1881.

182. Isaacs H Jr: Fetal and neonatal cardiac tumors. *Pediatr Cardiol* 2004; 25:252.

183. Cho JM, Danielson GK, Puga FJ, et al: Surgical resection of ventricular cardiac fibromas. Early and late results. *Ann Thorac Surg* 2003; 76:1929.

184. Bossert T, Walther T, Vondrys D, et al: Cardiac fibroma as an inherited manifestation of nevoid basal-cell carcinoma syndrome. *Tex Heart Inst J* 2006; 33:88.

185. Lin CY, Tsai FC, Fang BR: Mesothelial/monocytic incidental cardiac excrescences of the heart. Case report and literature review. *Int J Clin Pract Suppl* 2005; 147:23.

186. Ratner BD, Hoffman S, Schoen FJ, et al: *Biomaterials Science. An Introduction to Materials in Medicine,* 2nd ed. San Diego, Academic Press, 2004.

187. Langer R, Tirrell DA: Designing materials for biology and medicine. *Nature* 2004; 428:487.

188. Hench LL, Polak JM: Third-generation biomedical materials. *Science* 2002; 295:1014.

189. Lutolf MP, Hubbell JA: Synthetic biomaterials as instructive extracellular microenvironments for morphogenesis in tissue engineering. *Nat Biotechnol* 2005; 23:47.

190. Schoen FJ: Introduction to host reactions to biomaterials and their evaluation, in Ratner BD, Hoffman AS, Schoen FJ, et al (eds): *Biomaterials Science. An Introduction to Materials in Medicine,* 2nd ed. San Diego, Academic Press, 2004; p 293.

191. Hanson SR: Blood coagulation and blood-materials interactions, in Ratner BD, Hoffman AS, Schoen FJ, Lemons JE (eds): *Biomaterials Science. An Introduction to Materials in Medicine,* 2nd ed. Orlando, Academic Press, 2004; p 332.

192. Anderson JM: Inflammation, wound healing and the foreign body response. Perspectives and possibilities in biomaterials science, in Ratner BD, Hoffman AS, Schoen FJ (eds): *Biomaterials Science. An Introduction to Materials in Medicine,* 2nd ed. Orlando, Academic Press, 2004; p 296.

193. Tang L, Hu W: Molecular determinants of biocompatibility. *Expert Rev Med Dev* 2005; 2:493.

194. Mitchell RN: Innate and adaptive immunity. The immune response to foreign materials. Perspectives and possibilities in biomaterials science, in Ratner BD, Hoffman AS, Schoen FJ, Lemons JE (eds): *Biomaterials Science. An Introduction to Materials in Medicine,* 2nd ed. Orlando, Academic Press, 2004; 304.

195. Sata M: Role of circulating vascular progenitors in angiogenesis, vascular healing, and pulmonary hypertension: lessons from animal models. *Arterioscler Thromb Vasc Biol* 2006; 26:1008.

196. DiDonato RM, Danielson GK, McGoon DC, et al: Left ventricle-aortic conduits in pediatric patients. *J Thorac Cardiovasc Surg* 1984; 88:82.

197. Xue L, Greisler HP: Biomaterials in the development and future of vascular grafts. *J Vasc Surg* 2003; 37:472.

198. Darouiche RO: Treatment of infections associated with surgical implants. *NEJM* 2004; 350:1422.

199. Vinh DC, Embil JM: Device related infections: a review. *J Long Term Eff Med Implants* 2005; 15:467.

200. Costerson JW, Cook G, Shirtliff M, et al: Biofilms, biomaterials and device-related infections, in Ratner BD, Hoffman AS, Schoen FJ, et al (eds): *Biomaterials Science. An Introduction to Materials in Medicine*, 2nd ed. San Diego, Elsevier Academic Press, 2004; p 345.

201. Conlan RM, Costerson JW: Biofilms. Survival mechanisms of clinically relevant microorganisms. *Clin Microbiol Rev* 2002; 15:167.

202. Vacanti JP, Langer R: Tissue engineering. The design and fabrication of living replacement devices for surgical reconstruction and transplantation. *Lancet* 1999; 354:SI32.

203. Fuchs JR, Nasseri BA, Vacanti JP: Tissue engineering. A 21st century solution to surgical reconstruction. *Ann Thorac Surg* 2001; 72:577.

204. Rabkin E, Schoen FJ: Cardiovascular tissue engineering. *Cardiovasc Pathol* 2002; 11:305.

205. Peck M, Gebhart D, Dusserre N, et al: The evolution of vascular tissue engineering and current state of the art. *Cells Tissues Organs* 2012; 195:144.

206. Kurobe H, Maxfield MW, Breuer CK, et al: Concise review: tissue-engineered vascular grafts for cardiac surgery: past, present, and future. *Stem Cells Transl Med* 2012; 1:566.

207. Patterson JT, Gilliland T, Maxfield MW, et al: Tissue-engineered vascular grafts for use in the treatment of congenital heart disease: from the bench to the clinic and back again. *Regen Med* 2012; 7:409.

208. Gong Z, NIklason LE: Blood vessels engineered from human cells. *Trends Cardiovasc Med* 2006; 16:153.

209. L'Heureux N, Paquet S, Labbe R, et al: A completely biological tissue-engineered human blood vessel. *FASEB J* 1998; 12:447.

210. Weinberg CB, Bell E: A blood vessel model constructed from collagen and cultured vascular cells. *Science* 1986; 231:397.

211. Kaushall S, Amiel GE, Gulesarian KJ, et al: Functional small diameter neovessels using endothelial progenitor cells expanded ex-vivo. *Nature Med* 2001; 7:1035.

212. Lantz GC, Badylak SF, Hiles MC, et al: Small intestine submucosa as a vascular graft. A review. *J Invest Surg* 1993; 3:297.

213. Badylak SF: Decellularized allogeneic and xenogeneic tissue as a bioscaffold for regenerative medicine: factors that influence the host response. *Ann Biomed Eng* 2014; 42:1517.

214. Sparks CH: Silicone mandril method for growing reinforced autogenous femoro-popliteal artery graft in situ. *Ann Surg* 1973; 177:293.

215. Hoenig MR, Campbell GR, Rolfe BE, Campbell JH: Tissue-engineered blood vessels. Alternative to autologous grafts? *Arterioscler Thromb Vasc Biol* 2005; 25:1128.

216. Shin'oka T, Imai Y, Ikada Y: Transplantation of a tissue-engineered pulmonary artery. *NEJM* 2001; 344:532.

217. McAllister MC, Maruszewski M, Garrido SA, et al: Effectiveness of haemodialysis access with an autologous tissue-engineered vascular graft: a multicentre cohort study. *Lancet* 2009; 373:1440.

218. Meinhart JG, Deutsch M, Fischlein T, et al: Clinical autologous in vitro endothelialization of 153 infrainguinal ePTFE grafts. *Ann Thorac Surg* 2001; 71:S327.

219. Vunjak-Novakovic G, Tandon N, Godier A, et al: Challenges in cardiac tissue engineering. *Tissue Eng Part B Rev* 2010; 16:169.

220. Mummery CL, Davis RP, Krieger JE: Challenges in using stem cells for cardiac repair. *Sci Transl Med* 2010; 2:27.

221. Yi BA, Mummery CL, Chien KR: Direct cardiomyocyte reprogramming: a new direction for cardiovascular regenerative medicine. *Cold Spring Harb Perspect Med* 2013; 3:a014050.

222. Tulloch NL, Murry CE: Trends in cardiovascular engineering: organizing the human heart. *Trends Cardiovasc Med* 2013; 23:282.

223. Zhoa Y, Feric NT, Thavandiran N, et al: The role of tissue engineering and biomaterials in cardiac regenerative medicine. *Can J Cardiol* 2014; 30:1307.

224. Laflamme MA, Murry CE: Heart regeneration. *Nature* 2011; 473:326.

225. Anversa P, Leri A, Kajstura J: Cardiac regeneration. *J Am Coll Cardiol* 2006; 47:1769.

226. Cohen S, Leor J: Rebuilding broken hearts. Biologists and engineers working together in the fledgling field of tissue engineering are within reach of one of their greatest goals. Constructing a living human heart patch. *Sci Am* 2004; 291:44.

227. Zimmerman WH, Didie M, Doker S, et al: Heart muscle engineering. An update on cardiac muscle replacement therapy. *Cardiovasc Res* 2006; 71:419.

228. Radisic M, Park H, Shing H, et al: Functional assembly of engineered myocardium by electrical stimulation of cardiac myocytes cultured on scaffolds. *Proc Natl Acad Sci USA* 2004; 101:18129.

229. Dimmeler S, Zeiher AM, Schneider MD: Unchain my heart. The scientific foundations of cardiac repair. *J Clin Invest* 2005; 115:572.

230. Laflamme MA, Murry CE: Regenerating the heart. *Nat Biotechnol* 2005; 23:845.

231. Fukuda K, Yuasa S: Stem cells as a source of regenerative cardiomyocytes. *Circ Res* 2006; 98:1002.

232. Schoen FJ: Heart valve tissue engineering: quo vadis? *Curr Opin Biotechnol* 2011; 22:698.

233. Rippel RA, Ghanbari H, Seifalian AM: Tissue-engineered heart valve; future of cardiac surgery. *World J Surg* 2012; 36:1581.

234. Bouten CV, Driessen-Mol A, Baaijens FP: In situ heart valve tissue engineering: simple devices, smart materials, complex knowledge. *Expert Rev Med Devices* 2012; 9:453.

235. Emmert MY, Weber B, Falk V, Hoerstrup SP: Transcatheter tissue engineered heart valves. *Expert Rev Med Devices* 2014; 11:15.

236. Hoerstrup SP, Sodian R, Daebritz S, et al: Functional living trileaflet heart valves grown in-vitro. *Circulation* 2000; 102:III44-9.

237. Rabkin E, Hoerstrup SP, Aikawa M, et al: Evolution of cell phenotype and extracellular matrix in tissue-engineered heart valves during in-vitro maturation and in-vivo remodeling. *J Heart Valve Dis* 2002; 11:1.

238. Hoerstrup SP, Cummings I, Lachat M, et al: Functional growth in tissue engineered living vascular grafts. Follow up at 100 weeks in a large animal model. *Circulation* 2006; 114:159.

239. Matheny RG, Hutchison ML, Dryden PE, et al: Porcine small intestine submucosa as a pulmonary valve leaflet substitute. *J Heart Valve Dis* 2000; 9:769.

240. Simon P, Kasimir MT, Seebacher G, et al: Early failure of the tissue engineered porcine heart valve SYNERGRAFT in pediatric patients. *Eur J Cardiothorac Surg* 2003; 23:1002.

241. Driessen-Mol A, Emmert MY, Dijkman PE, et al: Transcatheter implantation of homologous "off-the-shelf" tissue-engineered heart valves with self-repair capacity: long-term functionality and rapid in vivo remodeling in sheep. *J Am Coll Cardiol* 2014; 63:1329.

Computed Tomography of the Adult Cardiac Surgery Patient: Principles and Applications

6

Andreas A. Giannopoulos • Frank J. Rybicki • Tarang Sheth • Frederick Y. Chen

Advances in computed tomography (CT) technology have revolutionized the diagnosis of cardiovascular disease. CT has dramatically reduced, and for some clinical scenarios eliminated, the need for additional testing such as diagnostic arterial catheterization. In the process, CT has become invaluable in cardiac diagnosis and surgical planning.

CT is based on an x-ray source and detector system mounted on the "CT gantry" that rotates around the patient. Major technology advances have enabled CT to image the beating heart, and routine CT at Brigham and Women's Hospital (BWH) has noninvasively excluded coronary artery disease in one heart beat (Fig. 6-1) for over 7 years.[1] However, the role of CT extends far beyond the coronary arteries alone. Using roughly the same CT acquisition strategies, native coronary imaging can be extended to coronary bypass grafts, the beating myocardium, valve motion, the ventricles and ventricular outflow tracks, and cardiac lesions.

In order to understand the clinical contribution of CT and to avoid pitfalls in image interpretation, it is essential for the surgeon to appreciate the basic principles of CT used in cardiac imaging. This chapter is divided into two parts. The first part describes the technical considerations for cardiac CT. By understanding each component, the surgeon will be better able to distinguish image artifacts from pathology. The second part reviews those CT examinations that are most frequently performed in the noninvasive cardiovascular imaging program at BWH, detailing the strengths and limitations of each exam.

PART 1. CARDIAC CT PROTOCOLS

Most advances in cardiac CT, for example in coronary CT angiography (CTA), have focused on the development of protocols consistent with the rapid incremental technology improvements. One of the major technological advances has been the incorporation of multiple elements into the CT detector system, called Multi-Detector CT (MDCT). MDCT is synonymous with multislice CT. Since all modern scanners have multiple detectors, the semantics can and should be eliminated; this chapter simply uses "CT" to describe the technology.

Data from each of CT detector is used to reconstruct an axial slice perpendicular to the long axis, or z-axis, of the patient. The width of the detectors determines the minimum slice thickness and thus the ability to resolve small anatomic detail (spatial resolution) of the scanner. Thinner slices yield superior spatial resolution; however, comparing two scanners that produce the same number of slices, the scanner with thinner slices will have less z-axis (ie, craniocaudal) coverage per gantry rotation and thus will have a longer scan time. To date, the minimum detector width and largest number of detector rows is 0.5 mm and 320, respectively.[2,3] This yields 16 cm (0.5 mm × 320) z-axis coverage per gantry rotation, and thus the entire heart can be imaged with data acquired over a single R-R interval.

TEMPORAL RESOLUTION

Successful cardiac imaging by any modality relies on the ability of the hardware to produce motion-free images or, in other words, to image faster than the heart beats. Because it requires that the gantry be rotated around the patient, CT is inherently slower than digital subtraction angiography (DSA) where each frame corresponds to a single projection image. As described below, CT has become faster so that cardiac CT is now being routinely performed.

Temporal resolution is the metric that measures imaging speed. For a CT scanner with a single photon source, the temporal resolution is one half of the CT gantry rotation time.

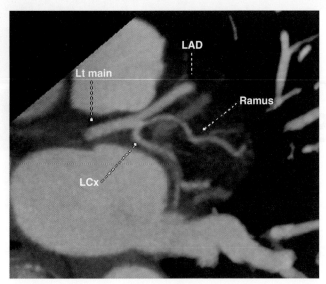

FIGURE 6-1 Selected coronary computed tomography angiography (CTA) image of the proximal left coronary arterial system in a patient scheduled for isolated mitral valve surgery. Using the protocol detailed in this chapter, CT demonstrated normal coronary arteries in this patient, eliminating the need for arterial catheterization.

This is because image reconstruction requires CT data acquired from one half (180°) of a complete gantry rotation. All manufacturers have gantry rotation times on order of 300 ms or less. Using this gantry rotation time as an example, an electrocardiogram (ECG)-gated cardiac image can be reconstructed (using single-segment reconstruction, described below) with CT data acquired over 150 ms of the cardiac cycle. Thus, the reconstructed images inherently display the average of the cardiac motion over the roughly 150 ms during which the data was acquired. This is how ECG gating enables cardiac CT. Without gating, cardiac images are nondiagnostic because the reconstruction "averages" the motion over the entire R-R interval, for example, over 1000 ms for a patient with a heart rate of 60 beats per minute.

There are important strategies to improve temporal resolution. The first uses two independent x-ray CT sources and two independent (64 or greater slice) detector systems built into the CT gantry.[4] The second x-ray source is positioned 90° from the first x-ray source, and the second detection system is positioned 90° from the first detection system. With respect to temporal resolution, the practical consequence of this CT configuration is that 180° of gantry rotation can be achieved in half the time (eg, 75 ms as opposed to 150 ms). This halves the temporal resolution (to 75 ms), and thus for this "dual-source" CT configuration, motion is averaged over only 75 ms. Another strategy uses both X-ray CT source-detector systems to sample the entire heart within a single R-R interval by rapidly moving the patient through the scanner.[5] Both implementations have technical advantages and disadvantages that are beyond the scope of this chapter. However, cardiac imaging in a single heart beat can be achieved using the same heart rate control as noted below.

For single-source scanners, temporal resolution can be improved by adopting a so-called "multisegment" image reconstruction. The difference between single-segment and multisegment reconstruction is that in the former, 180° of data is acquired from a single heart beat, while multisegment reconstruction uses several heart beats to obtain the one half gantry CT data. For example, in a two-segment reconstruction, two heart beats are used to generate a single axial slice, and thus the temporal resolution is halved. Similarly, if four heart beats are used (four-segment reconstruction), only 45° of data are used from each heart beat. This yields a fourfold reduction in the effective temporal resolution, making it theoretically possible to perform high spatial resolution cardiac CT in patients with a rapid (eg, >70 beats per minute) heart rate. However, since multiple heart beats are used to fill the 180° of gantry rotation necessary for the reconstruction, stable periodicity of the heart is essential. When beat-to-beat variations in heart rate occur, image quality is degraded significantly. In our experience, multisegment reconstruction works well in patients with high heart rates who are being studied for clinical indications where the highest image quality may not be required (eg, studies of graft patency or pericardial calcification). For more demanding applications (eg, native coronary CTA) we still routinely employ beta-blockade for heart rates >60 beats per minute.

BETA-BLOCKADE FOR HEART RATE CONTROL

As suggested above, beta-blockade is an important component of most coronary-based CT examinations. As the temporal resolution of cardiac CT improves, the dependence on lowering the heart rate will naturally be mitigated. However, the speed of all CT scanners is inferior to coronary catheterization, and thus beta-blockade is recommended for the large majority of patients in whom it is safe. In our experience, many surgical patients have standing orders for beta-blockers as part of their medical therapy, and image quality is excellent. When this is not the case, either oral and/or IV metoprolol is routinely administered.

ECG GATING

ECG gating refers to the simultaneous acquisition of both the patient's ECG tracing and CT data. By acquiring both pieces of information, CT images can be reconstructed using only a short temporal segment of the R-R interval. Each segment is named by its "phase" in the cardiac cycle; the common nomenclature is to name the percentage of a specific phase with respect to its position in the R-R interval. For example, reconstruction of 20 (equally spaced) phases would be named as 0%, 5%, 10%, ..., 95%. The period in which the heart has the least motion is usually (but not always) in mid-diastole, near 75%. Thus, the CT exposure (and subsequent patient radiation level) can be lowered by limiting the exposure to a small part of the R-R interval where coronary motion is expected to be a minimum. This is termed "prospective" ECG gating since the reconstruction phase and width is determined prospectively. The disadvantage of this approach is that cine loops of the entire R-R interval cannot be reconstructed because a complete data set is not acquired throughout the R-R interval. If this is desired, the so-called "retrospective" ECG gating can be used, at the expense of higher radiation levels.

For patients who require imaging of bypass grafts, it is important to note that periodic displacement of both saphenous vein grafts (SVG), radial grafts, and internal mammary artery (IMA) grafts is far less than the motion of the native coronary arteries. Thus, for these vessels, a single reconstruction at mid-diastole is usually sufficient (Fig. 6-2), and prospective ECG gating is routinely used. However, the benefits of lower radiation in this population are relatively moot, since the latent period for a radiation-induced malignancy

is roughly a decade for blood tumors and significantly longer for solid tumors. Patients under consideration for repeat bypass surgery typically have a shorter life expectancy based on cardiac status. Thus, it is *essential* that the surgeon not only recognizes that motion has degraded image quality, but also realizes that additional reconstructions, and even repeat imaging, *can and should* be performed. If the entire course of the graft is not clear to the surgeon at a single cardiac phase, it is almost always the case that another phase will yield motion-free depiction of the graft segment that was poorly seen. Open communication between the radiologist and the surgeon for every case has eliminated this pitfall and ensures that the maximum amount of imaging data is incorporated into presurgical planning.

In cine CT, such as imaging the aortic valve over the entire R-R interval, images are acquired with retrospective ECG gating and subsequently reconstructed throughout the cardiac cycle and then played, in cine mode, to demonstrate function.

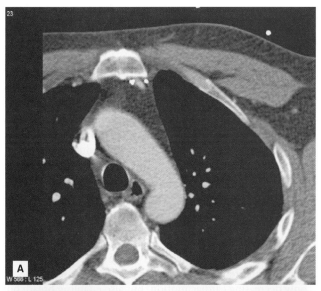

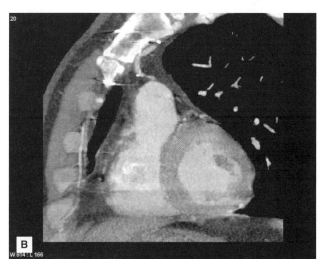

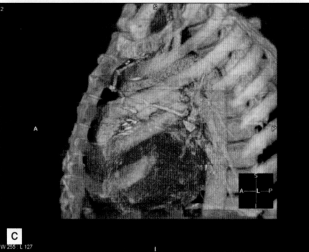

FIGURE 6-2 ECG-gated CT images from a single reconstruction at mid-diastole for a patient scheduled for redo CABG. The patient is status post-LIMA to LAD coronary bypass grafting. (A) Axial image demonstrates the LIMA graft coursing between two staples and adherent to the posterior table of the sternum. (B) Multiplanar reformatting is now performed routinely to detect and illustrate cases where repeat thoracotomy through the sternal incision is likely to damage a patent LIMA graft. An alternate surgical approach was required for this patient. (C) Selected image from a three-dimensional (3D) volume rendering again demonstrates the course of the graft. Volume rendering fully surveys the thoracic landmarks and is useful for spatial relationships and the communication of important findings.

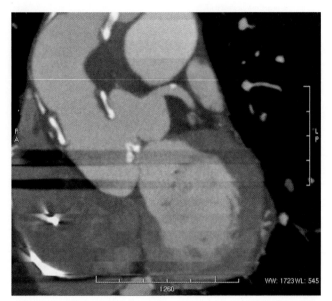

FIGURE 6-3 ECG-gated CT image through the left ventricle and the aortic valve in a patient status post aortic root repair. Note the pacemaker (*right heart wires*); magnetic resonance imaging (MRI) was contraindicated. The repair is well visualized and without complication, with only mild aortic valve calcification (cine images showed a tricuspid valve with no significant stenosis). This image also demonstrates a punctate calcified plaque along the superior course of the proximal left main coronary artery, without a significant stenosis.

Each individual image (Fig. 6-3) offers an outstanding assessment of the aortic valve and root structure. Cine CT can also be used to assess ventricular-wall motion. In comparison with magnetic resonance imaging (MRI), the reference standard for global- and regional-wall motion abnormalities, CT often has inferior temporal resolution. However, it is important to emphasize that cine CT does not require a separate image acquisition. The entire CT data set (coronary, valve, myocardium, and pericardium) is acquired in a single breath hold; cine CT is simply part of the image postprocessing.

For surgical patients, CT has the distinct advantage over MR, in that it is by far the best imaging modality to identify and quantify calcification. Also, the most common contraindications for cardiac CT (eg, impaired renal function as measured by glomerular filtration rate or alternatively by serum creatinine) differ from those for MR (pacemaker), and thus CT can often be used for patients who cannot have MR. As noted above, single heart beat cardiac CT is now a clinical reality, with an entire cardiac acquisition in approximately one second.[1] In addition to the fact that patient radiation is decreased, multiple scans can be performed with the same injection of iodinated contrast material, creating the opportunity for a host of additional studies including myocardial perfusion[6-10] that are, at present, largely in the domain of cardiac MR and nuclear cardiology.

PATIENT IRRADIATION

Because ECG gating is required, ascending aorta and cardiac CT delivers more patient irradiation than CT of any other body part. While details regarding cardiac CT dosimetry are beyond the scope of this chapter, discussions regarding CT dose must be based on sound principles. The radiation risk most commonly quoted relates to the probability that the CT scan will result in the development of a fatal radiation-induced neoplasm.[11] Human data for radiation at this low level (the level delivered in ECG-gated cardiac CT) is very sparse; all anecdotal reports support a long latency period as described above. For this reason, patients should be separated into two groups: those with a life expectancy of roughly 10 to 15 years or less, and those with a longer life expectancy. In the former group, the only dose consideration is whether the radiation could cause a skin burn (the only short-term complication of any consequence). X-ray skin burns are extremely uncommon, particularly in CT (even for ECG-gated studies), and typically result from multiple exams repeated at short-term intervals. Thus, for this subset of patients, *radiation dose should not be a consideration* in determining a modality for cardiac imaging. For those patients for whom radiation is an important consideration, prospective ECG gating should be used. X-ray current modulation is standardly used to lower the radiation dose. The tube current (expressed as the mA) is modulated over the course of the cardiac cycle so that the desired (high) diagnostic current is delivered only in diastole. The patient dose is decreased because the tube current is reduced for the remainder of the cardiac cycle. While current modulation is helpful in many cases (eg, pediatric patients), the decision to use it should be made after consultation between surgeon and radiologist because the potential drawbacks are significant. Most importantly, when current modulation is used, images reconstructed during phases with low tube current are relatively noisy because less tube current is used to generate them.

SCANNING PARAMETERS

The *scan time* refers to the time required to complete the CT acquisition along the z-axis of the patient. As described above, better temporal resolution decreases the scan time, not only decreasing cardiac motion, but also enabling breath hold CT. This is important in cardiac CT because in comparison to nongated CT, ECG gating not only increases patient radiation but also increases the scan time.

In practical terms, a 64-slice ECG-gated cardiac CT scan (craniocaudal, or z-axis imaging over ~15 cm) can be performed in roughly 10 seconds, versus 20 to 25 seconds with a 16-slice scanner. One great benefit of wide area detector CT is faster (single heart beat) scans. If this option is not available, increasing the thickness of the detectors increases the z-axis coverage per rotation and thus decreases the scan time. For example, in a patient that cannot perform the breath hold, using thicker detectors (eg, 1 mm thickness as opposed to 0.5 mm thickness) will decrease the scan time by providing more z-axis coverage per rotation. However, routinely increasing the width of the detectors for cardiac applications is undesirable since it degrades the *spatial resolution* of the examination. In general, spatial resolution refers to the ability to differentiate small detail in an image. This is essential component to coronary imaging since the diameter of the proximal coronary arteries are on the order of 3 to 4 mm. Substitution of 0.5 mm reconstructed images with 1 mm images thus impacts the ability to see detail that may be required for accurate diagnoses. Routine consultation between the surgeon and radiologist is essential to best understand and optimize the tradeoff between scan time and slice thickness. For example, imaging of the myocardium and aorta almost never requires submillimeter slices, because the pathology is larger. Thus, for dyspneic patients who require only imaging of the ascending aorta, thicker slices should be used to cut the scan time.

The scanning parameters that primarily determine the number of photons used to create a CT image are termed "mAs," or milliamperes-seconds and "kV," or kilovolts. The former represents the X-ray tube current; the latter refers to the voltage applied within the tube. For the surgeon, choosing the best numbers (typical values are 550 to 700 effective mAs, 120 kV) is far less important than understanding the fact that modern cardiac CT pushes the limits of technology, and thus creates tradeoffs with respect to the x-ray CT source. The source generates photons that are either attenuated by the patient or reach the detectors. When more photons reach the detectors, the image quality is higher because there is less noise. The decision to image with thinner slices (eg, 0.5 mm as opposed to 1 mm) means that fewer photons reach the detector; thus, thinner slices have more noise. This is especially important in obese patients because their increased body mass absorbs more photons than thin patients. For the same effective mAs and kV, images of obese patients can be dramatically degraded by greater image noise.

If there were no limit to the number of photons that an X-ray CT source could produce, the solution would be to simply increase the number of photons (and the radiation dose) until image noise was satisfactory. Unfortunately, because the X-ray CT tube heats excessively when pushed to its maximum, there is a limit to the number of photons that can be produced. This is why image noise becomes problematic with thin slice imaging of obese patients. When this is the case, consultation between the surgeon and radiologist is important because diagnostic images can often be obtained by increasing the image thickness, scanning a smaller z-axis field of view (FOV), or both. The latter can be particularly useful if the examination can be tailored to the most important structure. Scanning a smaller z-axis means that more photons can be generated and used before the X-ray CT tube reaches its heat limit.

On the other hand, whenever possible, the z-axis FOV should be generous, as unexpected pathology can extend in both cranially and caudally. For example, an ECG-gated cardiac and ascending aorta examination to evaluate extension of the intimal flap into the coronary arteries can reveal extension into the great vessels. Also, scanning must allow for variations in the FOV induced by breath holding. As a general rule, for scanning the native coronaries alone, the superior border of the FOV is set at the axial slice corresponding to the top of the carina. This is typically 2 to 3 cm superior to the origin of the left main coronary artery. The inferior border should scan through the entire inferior wall of the heart and should include several slices of the liver to account for cardiac displacement during breath holding. For bypass graft imaging, the superior border of the FOV must include the subclavian arteries and the origin of both IMAs.

CONTRAST MATERIAL

Most CT examinations are performed with iodinated contrast material. The exceptions are scans performed solely for the assessment of cardiac and aortic calcification, plus imaging of the aorta and great vessels for aneurysm size measurements alone. Contrast is administered from a peripheral vein, typically with a dual injection system. This injector has two reservoirs to inject contrast followed by saline. For coronary imaging, the contrast and saline delivery are timed so that the left heart, aorta, and coronary arteries are enhanced with contrast while the right heart is filled with saline. The use and the timing of the saline are essential parts of the examinations because artifacts that limit interpretation of the RCA will be induced if the right heart and central veins are densely enhanced with contrast (as opposed to saline).

PART 2. APPLICATIONS IN CARDIAC SURGICAL PATIENTS

CORONARY DISEASE

Native Coronary CTA

One of the most common clinical indications for cardiac CT is to evaluate the native coronary arteries for stenosis (Figs. 6-4 to 6-7). Numerous validation studies have evaluated cardiac CT for this purpose.[12-25] In these studies, data are typically reported on a per coronary artery segment basis, comparing CTA and DSA. A significant stenosis is generally defined as >50%, determined by quantitative coronary angiography. Data are also analyzed on a per patient basis regarding the value of CTA in ruling-in or excluding CAD. Literature to date reports on patient populations with a relatively high prevalence of CAD (ie, patients already scheduled for DSA). Among the most consistent findings is a very high negative predictive value (NPV) of coronary CTA when performed with 64 or greater detector row scanners. The data and our experience with 320 row scanners suggest a very high NPV, arguing that cardiac CTA can effectively exclude CAD in patients with low to intermediate pretest probability of disease. Furthermore, noncontrast CTA for evaluation of coronary calcium score, an independent predictor of adverse cardiac events and all-cause mortality, is considered to be appropriate for intermediate-risk patients as well as for low-risk patients with family history of premature CAD.[26-28]

Consequently, CTA has become increasingly useful for the cardiac surgeon in managing patients scheduled for noncoronary cardiac surgery. If the clinical suspicion is low, but not

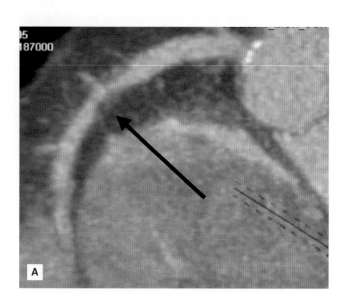

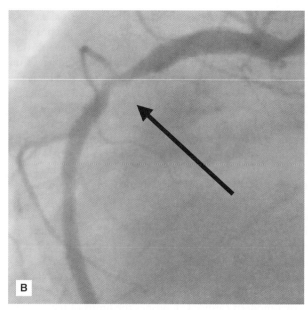

FIGURE 6-4 Proximal RCA 50% stenosis diagnosed by coronary CT angiography and confirmed by conventional angiography. Double oblique maximum intensity projection image (4 mm thick) through proximal RCA (A) and LAO projection still image from conventional angiogram (B) demonstrate a segment of approximately 50% stenosis (*arrows*).

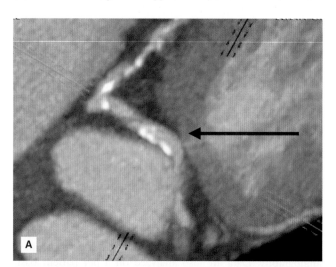

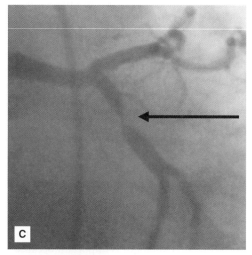

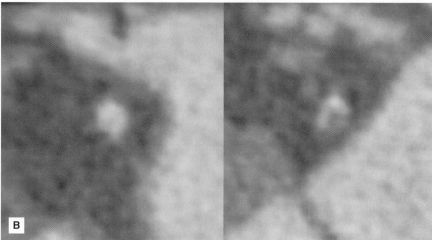

Proximal reference   Lesion

FIGURE 6-5 Proximal left circumflex greater than 50% stenosis diagnosed by coronary CT angiography and confirmed by conventional angiography. Double oblique maximum intensity projection image (4 mm thick) through proximal LCX (A) demonstrates a segment of calcified and noncalcified plaque with significant luminal narrowing (*arrow*). Finding is confirmed by true vessel short axis multiplanar reformatted images through the proximal reference (B-left) and the lesion (B-right) which demonstrate minimal residual lumen at the level of the lesion. AP-Caudal projection still image from conventional angiogram (C) confirms a greater than 50% in the proximal LCX (*arrow*).

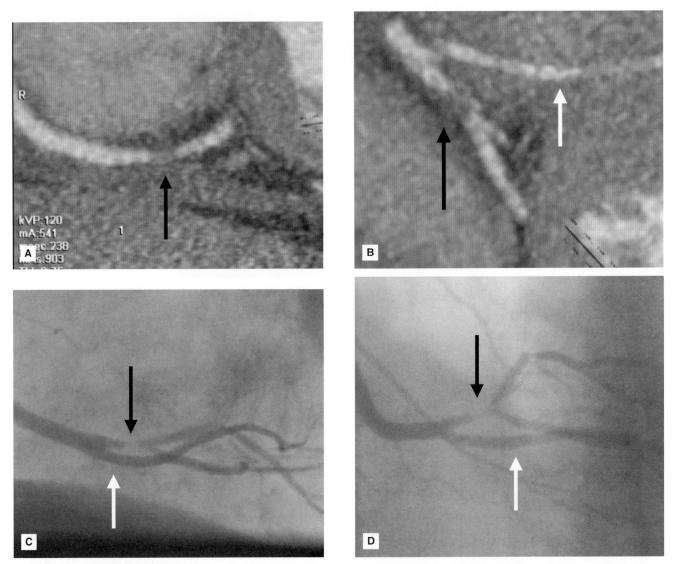

FIGURE 6-6 Right coronary artery greater than 50% stenosis diagnosed by CT and confirmed by conventional angiography. Double oblique maximum intensity projection images (4 mm thick) through ongoing RCA at 90° angles (A, B) demonstrate a segment of noncalcified plaque with nonvisualization of lumen (*black arrows*). The PIV is also partially demonstrated (*white arrow*). Finding is confirmed by LAO (C) and AP-cranial (D) projection still images conventional angiogram (*black arrow*). The PIV is also seen (*white arrow*).

insignificant, CTA affords the surgeon a method of assessing coronary disease without subjecting the patient to femoral arterial puncture with its known complications. For example, patients undergoing isolated mitral valve surgery for degenerative, myxomatous disease have a low prevalence of CAD, making CTA an ideal alternative to conventional angiography to exclude significant CAD. When the CT protocol described in Part 1 is followed, high-quality imaging is *routine*, and when CTA excludes CAD, surgeons have increased confidence in using CTA alone. Follow-up with DSA can be reserved for those patients who might benefit from catheter-based intervention.

Current guidelines from all major societies support the use of cardiac CT for evaluation of low- to intermediate-risk patients while also being appropriate even for the high-risk CAD patients.[28-32]

CORONARY ARTERY BYPASS GRAFT CTA—REOPERATIVE SURGERY

Cardiac CT provides the cardiac surgeon with a noninvasive method to assess graft patency after coronary artery bypass graft (CABG). Studies using early 16 detector row CT scanners suggest 100% sensitivity and specificity for identifying occluded versus patent grafts,[33-35] with benefits from advanced image postprocessing tools.[36] In similar fashion, 64- and 320-slice CTA have demonstrated good diagnostic accuracy in the evaluation of significant venous or arterial

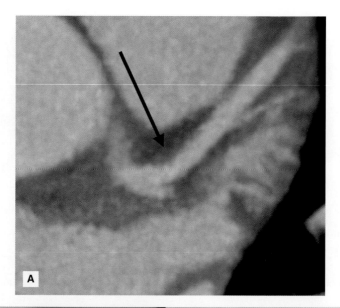

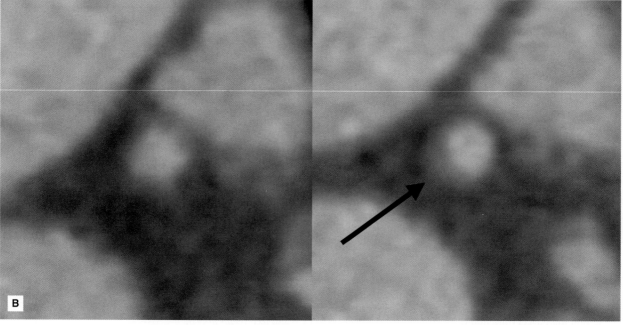

Proximal reference   Lesion

FIGURE 6-7 Proximal LAD less than 50% stenosis diagnosed by coronary CT angiography. Double oblique maximum intensity projection image (4 mm thick) through proximal LAD (A) demonstrates a segment of noncalcified plaque that is not associated with any significant luminal narrowing (*arrow*). True vessel short axis multiplanar reformatted images through the lesion (B-right) and through proximal reference segment (B-left) confirm minimal luminal narrowing. Low-density (ie, noncalcified) plaque with positive vessel remodeling is seen (*arrow*). This case highlights the ability of CTA to detect early stages of subclinical atherosclerosis. This lesion would presumably not have been detected at a conventional angiogram.

grafts stenosis, nongrafted, and recipient vessels.[37,38] The additional prognostic value of CTA helps enable long-term risk stratification of CABG patients.[39] In clinical practice, this application is of value in the evaluation of the symptomatic patient in the early postoperative period in whom graft failure is being considered (Fig. 6-8). It is particularly useful for the demonstration of graft patency in patients with a remote surgical history and unknown graft anatomy prior to DSA, and in patients in whom conventional angiography fails to demonstrate a known graft (Fig. 6-9). In the reoperative setting, such data has virtually revolutionized surgical decision-making and planning prior to surgery in patients who have already undergone CABG. Knowledge of anatomic placement of prior grafts, cannulation sites, and previous incisions

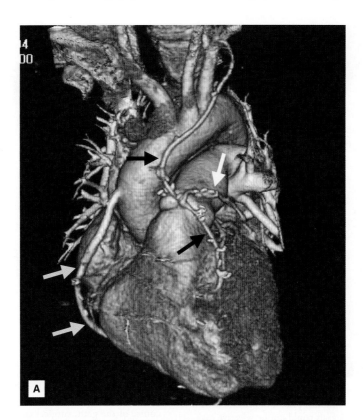

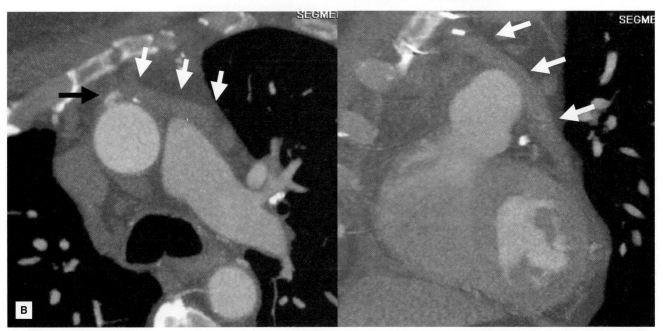

FIGURE 6-8 (A) Postoperative cardiac CT performed for evaluation of graft patency. Three-dimensional volume-rendered image demonstrates patent LIMA to LAD (*black arrows*), T-graft RIMA to obtuse marginal (*white arrows*), and SVG to RCA (*grey arrows*). This study was obtained in a patient 1-day follow off-pump coronary artery bypass grafting. The patient had developed recurrent chest pain and an elevated troponin. Cardiac CT ruled out early graft failure as a cause for the patient's presentation. (B) Companion case in a different patient. Oblique multiplanar reformatted images demonstrate an acutely occluded saphenous vein graft to obtuse marginal. Note the patent graft stump (*black arrow*) and thrombosed graft body (*white arrows*).

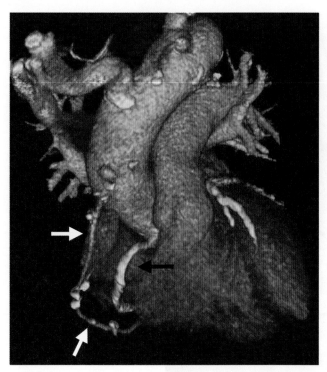

FIGURE 6-9 Cardiac CT performed to evaluate possible radial graft occlusion. The patient had surgery 1 month prior and presented with recurrent angina. The radial to RCA graft could not be selective catheterized at conventional angiography and was also not seen at aortic root injection. Three-dimensional volume-rendered image demonstrates patent radial graft (*white arrows*) to RCA (*black arrow*). The anastomosis is not seen on this orientation.

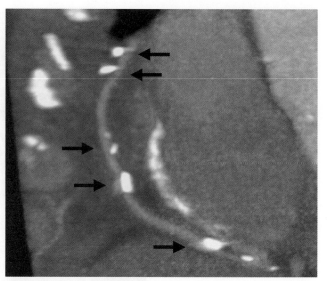

FIGURE 6-10 Surgical clip artifacts can limit cardiac CT evaluation of coronary bypass grafts. Double oblique maximum intensity projection image (10 mm thick) demonstrates multiple surgical clips placed along the length of a radial to PIV graft (*black arrows*). Artifact from these metallic clips can partially or completely obscure the adjacent vessel lumen precluding evaluation of these segments for the presence or absence of stenosis. Although CT can unequivocally demonstrate graft patency based on the delivery of contrast throughout the entire course of the graft, surgical clip artifact usually does not allow complete graft evaluation to rule out graft stenosis.

have impacted properative planning of the reoperative cardiac surgery patient.

Patients with recurrent angina after bypass surgery may have developed stenosis or occlusion in bypass grafts, or may have progression of native coronary disease. In these patients, CTA can be more limited. For example, exclusion of significant stenosis in a graft may be problematic due to metallic surgical clips that cause artifact (Fig. 6-10). Moreover, native CAD in these patients is often advanced and heavily calcified. A large volume of calcium may result in an uninterpretable study for many segments of the native coronaries (Fig. 6-11). CTA for plaque assessment in such patients may not be definitive; consequently conventional angiography may be preferred in this population.[40] CTA is increasingly useful for patients with less calcification and less metal artifact.

In the research context, graft patency is an important outcome in the evaluation of different surgical techniques. Randomized controlled trials utilizing conventional angiography for assessment of graft patency typically demonstrate a 10 to 20% rate of noncompliance. This noncompliance is at least partly attributable to the invasive nature of the test.[41-43] Cardiac CT is an attractive, noninvasive, and very accurate method to assess graft patency for clinical trials, again obviating a traditional arterial puncture with its risks and known

complications. Cardiac CT may also be used for routine postoperative control of grafts following implementation of a new surgical technique in a local center practice (Fig. 6-12). However, to our knowledge, there are no published guidelines for appropriate use of cardiac CT in patients status post CABG.

REOPERATIVE SURGERY

Reoperative cardiac surgery with live coronary grafts after previous CABG represents one of the most difficult problems in cardiac surgery. Reoperative sternotomy is challenging secondary to adhesions, loss of tissue planes, and the potential for injury to patent grafts, the aorta, and the right ventricle. Injury to a patent left internal thoracic artery graft to the left anterior descending artery (LAD) is associated with a mortality of 50%.[44,45] Cardiac CT has been revolutionary in precisely defining the relationship of important structures (including the aorta, right ventricle, and live grafts) to the midline and sternum for reentry planning (Fig. 6-13). At BWH, every reoperative surgery includes a preoperative CTA with z-axis coverage to include all grafts and the entire course of the IMAs. Preoperative identification of all structures at risk is mandatory, and different, specific operative approaches always remain in consideration.[46] Experience suggests that preoperative cardiac CT will lead to a modification in surgical strategy for 1 in 5 patients undergoing re-do cardiac surgery.[36] For example, if CT demonstrates a patent left internal

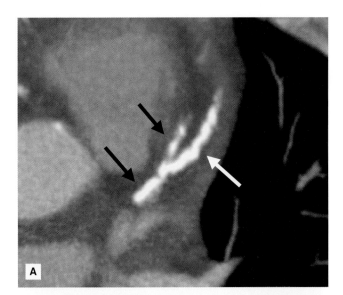

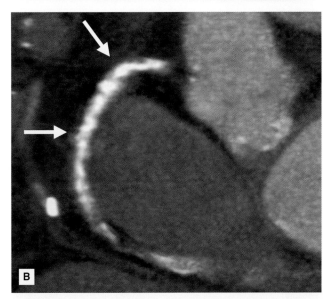

FIGURE 6-11 Cardiac CT is often limited in its evaluation of native coronary arteries in the postcoronary artery bypass graft patient due to the presence of advanced and heavily calcified coronary atherosclerosis. Double oblique maximum intensity projection image (4 mm) demonstrates (A) the proximal LAD (*black arrows*) and a large first diagonal branch (*white arrow*) and (B) the proximal right coronary artery (*white arrows*). The white areas are very high attenuation and represent calcification. All vessel segments demonstrated are heavily calcified. The extent of calcification completely obscures the vessel lumen and presence or absence of stenosis cannot be reliably assessed.

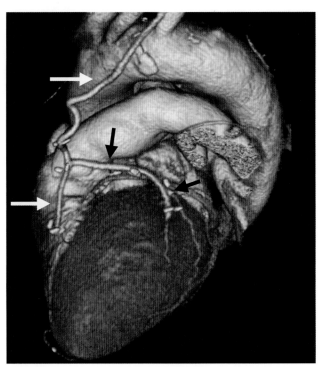

FIGURE 6-12 Cardiac CT obtained for postoperative graft control in patient who underwent MVST. Three-dimensional volume-rendered image demonstrates patent LIMA to LAD (*white arrows*) and radial T-graft to obtuse marginal (*black arrows*).

mammary artery (LIMA) is close to the midline or a right ventricle directly adherent to the posterior table of the sternum, cardiopulmonary bypass is instituted prior to reentry. Definition of live grafts with respect to their proximal placement of the aorta is instrumental in determining, *before the operation*, the precise manner in which those grafts will be handled. For example, in reoperative surgery for conventional

aortic valve replacement (AVR) in the setting of live grafts, CTA allows the surgeon to plan preoperatively whether or not those grafts will have to be divided in carrying out the aortotomy for the AVR. As described above, CT also allows the cardiac surgeon to preoperatively plan the precise location of the aortotomy itself.

Minimally Invasive Surgery Coronary Artery Bypass Grafting (MIDCAB)

Minimally invasive coronary artery bypass surgery is becoming an alternative to open surgery. With limited intraoperative access for direct visualization, aspects of coronary artery anatomy such as vessel diameter, extent of calcification, and the presence of intramyocardial segments become even more important to define preoperatively (Fig. 6-14). In addition, 3D models that combine visualization of a partially transparent thoracic cage over mediastinal structures allow the surgeon to obtain detailed preoperative understanding of the patient's cardiothoracic anatomy (Fig. 6-15). Preoperative CT has demonstrated usefulness for MIDCAB[47] and totally endoscopic coronary artery bypass surgery,[48] whereas postoperative CT has been utilized for graft patency evaluation in a prospective study.[49] CT is also expected to become invaluable for procedures such as multivessel small thoracotomy coronary revascularization.

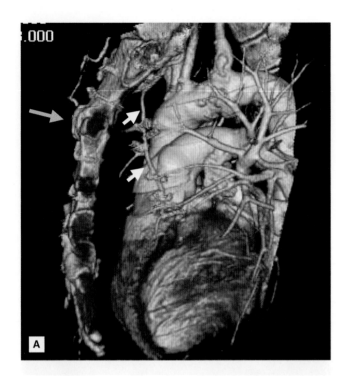

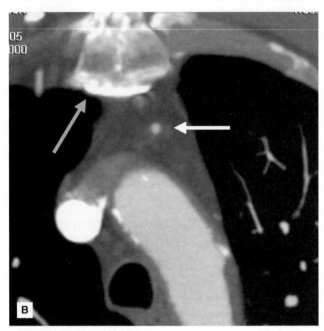

FIGURE 6-13 Planning for reoperative coronary artery bypass grafting. Laterally orientated 3D volume-rendered image (A) from a patient who had previously undergone left internal mammary artery (LIMA) coronary bypass grafting. The LIMA (*white arrows*) is grafted to the left anterior descending coronary artery. Note the relatively large distance between the grafted LIMA and the sternum (*grey arrow*). Axial image (B) clearly shows the LIMA graft (*white arrow*) to be clear of midline and well posterior to the sternum (*grey arrow*). Since the most common surgical approach in a redo CABG is repeat thoracotomy through the sternal incision, this study demonstrates that surgical revascularization through sternal reentry has no significant risk of damage to the patent LIMA graft.

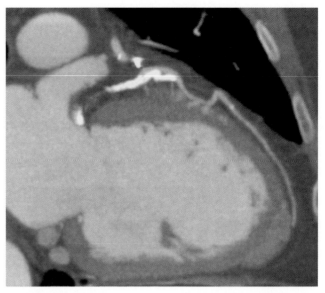

FIGURE 6-14 Preoperative planning for minimally invasive cardiac surgery (MIDCAB). Two chamber plane maximum intensity projection image (6 mm thick) demonstrates the LAD. A segment of heavy calcification is identified in the proximal vessel (*black arrow*), this corresponds to the site of the stenotic lesion. No significant calcification is present in the remainder of the vessel. Immediately beyond the calcified segment an intramyocardial segment is present (*white arrows*).

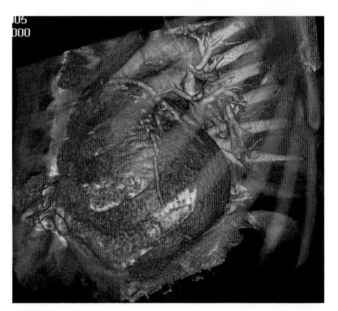

FIGURE 6-15 Preoperative planning for minimally invasive cardiac surgery (MIDCAB). Specialized display protocols for 3D volume-rendered images can be used to provide combined visualization of a semi-transparent thoracic cage and underlying cardiac and mediastinal structures. These models can be rotated and viewed from any angle or degree of magnification. With cardiac CT, 3D localization of target vessels, accessibility from proposed incision site, and position of LV apex with respect to chest wall can all be understood preoperatively.

CARDIAC VALVES

In patients with suspected valve dysfunction based on echo-cardiography, cine CT from retrospective ECG gating as described in Part 1 provides valuable additional data. As noted earlier, reconstruction is performed for all phases of the cardiac cycle, and the reformatted data can be played in a cine loop. This has relevance in assessment in native, bio-prosthetic, and mechanical aortic valves. Recent experience suggests an excellent correlation between planimetric valves areas obtained by CT, MRI and transesophageal echocardiography (TEE).[50] Consequently, CT can be used as an alternate modality for evaluation of aortic valve area. This is relevant if trans-thoracic echocardiography (TTE) is of poor technical quality or discrepant with a clinically expected result. Since patients may be evaluated with CT for concomitant aortic aneurysm or CAD prior to aortic valve surgery, valve area may be obtained from CT with no additional scanning and only a small amount of image postprocessing. CT can be used in correlation with valve area as determined with echocardiography (Fig. 6-16).

Postoperative evaluation of bioprosthetic valves may also be conducted using CT scanning. Although echocardiography determined trans-valvular gradients are the reference standard for determination of "effective" orifice area, CT provides a useful correlative modality—particularly when the echo is technically challenging or discordant with clinical findings. In patients with unexpectedly high gradients post-valve implantation, increasing use of CT will provide more information to guide management (Fig. 6-17). In patients with suspected bioprosthetic valve endocarditis, CT can be an invaluable modality to delineate para-valvular and valvular sequela of the infection (Fig. 6-18).

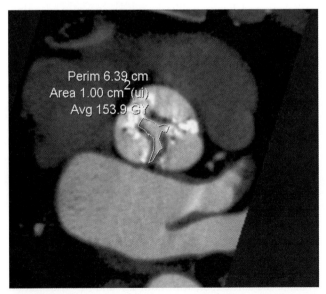

FIGURE 6-16 Reformatted CT angiography through the aortic valve shows calcification and stenosis with a valve area of 1.00 cm^2 measured by direct planimetry.

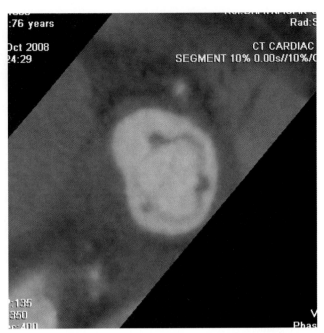

FIGURE 6-17 Seventy-seven-year-old man with a #23 Medtronic Mosaic valve. The patient developed shortness of breath approximately 1 year following surgery. Echocardiography which demonstrated a peak gradient of 78 mm Hg; the effective orifice area was reported at 0.9 cm^2. Subsequent cardiac CT showed a normal valve area of 1.7 cm^2, providing reassurance to both patient and surgeon.

Cardiac CT also permits high-resolution functional evaluation of mechanical aortic valve prostheses without artifact (Fig. 6-19). CT can be readily incorporated to evaluate valve dysfunction, measure opening angles, and to elucidate the underlying cause of valve failure. Figure 6-20 illustrates correlation between CT and surgical specimen in a mechanical aortic valve patient with restricted opening angle and elevated gradients. CT readily made the preoperative diagnosis of pannus in-growth.

Trascatheter Aortic Valve Replacement (TAVR)

Although cardiac CT is traditionally a second line imaging modality for the evaluation of aortic valve disease, it holds a key role in preintervention planning for TAVR.[51,52] Contrast-enhanced CTA is considered by appropriateness criteria guidelines as reference standard for both aortic valve plane planning as well as for supravalvular aorta and iliofemoral system planning.[53] The volumetric data and high spatial resolution afforded by CT makes it ideal for accurate 3D measurements of the aortic annulus, the aortic root, and the ascending aorta; precise measurements of the aortic annulus are particularly important in choosing the appropriate prosthesis size (Fig. 6-21). There is a potential risk that the native valve leaflets will be displaced superiorly during prosthetic valve placement, potentially blocking the coronary artery

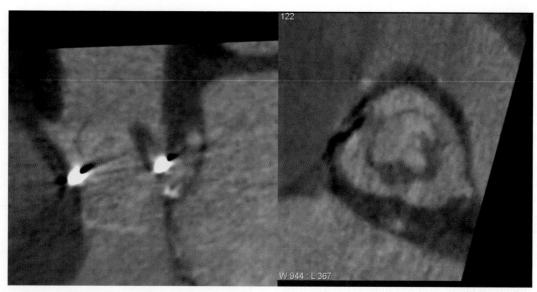

FIGURE 6-18 Patient with clinically suspected bioprosthetic valve endocarditis. Left image shows a pseudoaneurysm originating below the aortic valve ring and exerting mass effect on the adjacent left atrial wall. The right image shows nodular thickening of the aortic valve leaflets consistent with vegetations.

ostia. This risk can be assessed from the CT images by measuring the coronary ostia heights from the leaflet hinge points as well as the leaflet lengths. The optimal fluoroscopic projections, oriented to the aortic valve plane, can also be identified by CT, allowing for improved periprocedural planning.

For TAVR planning, additional CTA images of the abdomen and pelvis enables evaluation of candidate peripheral access vessels, including diameter, distribution of calcification, tortuosity, and angulation. This information is important given the large size of the introducer sheath and delivery catheter used for TAVR.

Although postintervention evaluation of TAVR requires a multidisciplinary imaging approach (MR, TEE, TTE), potential complications can be readily identified with CTA.[54] CT findings correlated with findings from echocardiography allow for excellent assessment of both the postoperative aortic root as well as functional information in patients with paravalvular leak or infection. We note that despite the critical role for CT in TAVR planning, to our knowledge there are no published guidelines for appropriate use of CT for postprocedural TAVR assessment.

AORTA AND GREAT VESSELS

Surgery of the aortic root, the ascending aorta, the arch, and the descending aorta is becoming increasingly commonplace as the population ages. CT has been used for many years to assess the thoracic aorta and is considered to be the currently preferred imaging modality.[55] Non-ECG-gated CT is highly accurate in the assessment of the aortic arch and descending thoracic aorta since they are not subject to significant cardiac motion. However, ECG-gating cardiac CT adds motion-free imaging of the aortic root, aortic arch, and ascending aorta. Gated cardiac CTA is particularly useful for measuring

the true short-axis diameters of the aorta in assessing aortic aneurysmal growth and decision making regarding intervention. As supported by appropriateness criteria guidelines[56] and without question from a clinical perspective, any surgery involving the aorta (whether the root, the arch, the ascending, or the descending portion) requires preoperative and postoperative CTA for surgical decision-making and follow-up.

Noncontrast CTA for Cross-Clamping

The superior imaging of ECG-gated CTA better defines the pathology and hence facilitates the preoperative planning. For example, noncontrast CTA is by far the best imaging modality to clearly define aortic calcification. If portions of the aorta are calcified on CTA, then aortic cross clamping and cannulation for cardiopulmonary bypass at those sites are contraindicated in order to avoid embolic phenomenon and stroke. Studies have supported the routine use of noncontrast enhanced CTA for identifying ascending aortic calcification and selecting the optimal surgery strategy in patients with aortic stenosis or hemodialysis.[57,58] Preoperative cardiopulmonary bypass strategy and myocardial protection are often critically altered by preoperative CTA. At BWH, the majority of elderly patients increasingly undergo noncontrast CT to assess aortic calcifications.

Aortic Aneurysm

As with calcification, CT is the most accurate modality to evaluate the aortic root, with both 2D and 3D visualization (Fig. 6-22). Not only can the aortic root be sized from multiple imaging planes, but also the exact location of the aneurysmal pathology with respect to the valve and sinotubular junction can often be defined.[59] This assessment is critical

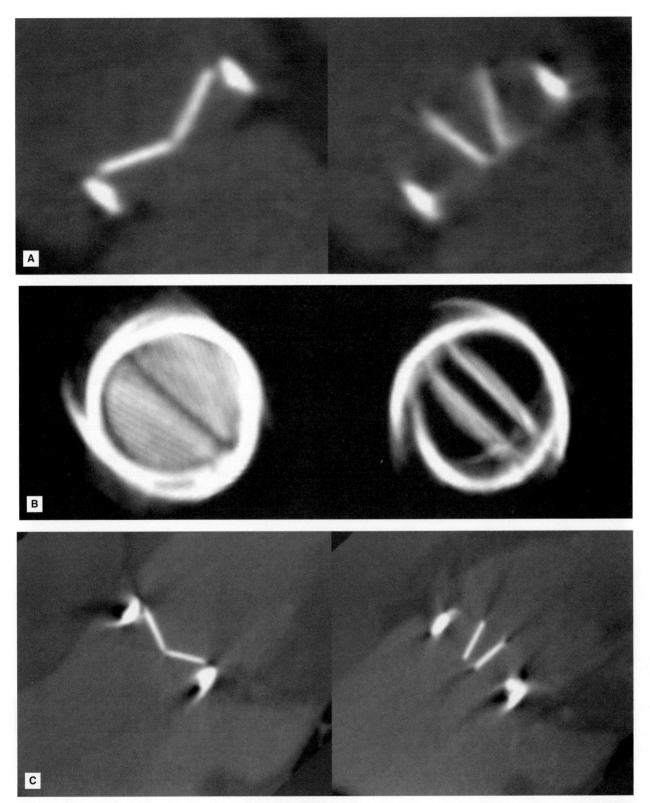

FIGURE 6-19 Evaluation of mechanical valve function with cardiac CT. Coronal oblique multiplanar reformatted images (A) demonstrate closed and open positions of mechanical AVR in a patient with suspected valve dysfunction based on echo-Doppler. Axial oblique slab maximum intensity projection images (B) demonstrate closed and open position of mechanical AVR in a patient in atrial fibrillation at the time of cardiac CT. Although image quality is degraded by arrhythmia, optimization of the dataset with ECG-editing can result in diagnostic quality images. Four-chamber oblique multiplanar reformatted images (C) demonstrate closed and open positions of a mechanical MVR. Images can be generated over the cardiac cycle and displayed in a cine movie format to allow dynamic evaluation of valve function. Since the study is performed with contrast, thrombus or perivalvular abscess can also be identified if present.

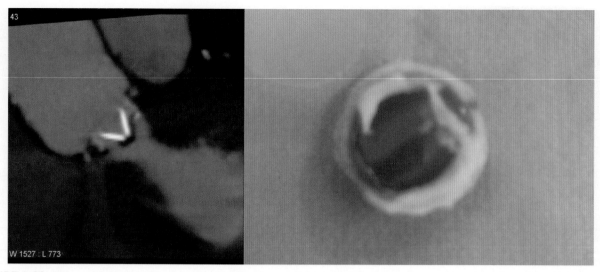

FIGURE 6-20 Patient with mechanical aortic valve. Low density material restricting leaflet opening on the undersurface of the valve is suspicious for pannus in-growth causing restricted opening angle (*left*). Photograph of explant (*right*) demonstrates the pannus with high correlation with presurgical imaging.

for preoperative decision-making and surgical planning. In patients with ascending aortic aneurysm, if the aortic root is determined to be aneurysmal near the coronary ostia, surgical decision-making changes from a simple tube graft repair for the aneurysm to a much more complex composite root repair with coronary reimplantation. Three-dimensional volume rendering optimally depicts other aortic root pathologies such as coronary anomalies or a sinus of Valsalva aneurysm (Fig. 6-23). In patients with a sinus of Valsalva aneurysm, as opposed to a root aneurysm, CT alters surgical strategy for repair.

For known ascending aortic aneurysms that do not meet size criteria for surgery, CTA is excellent to periodically assess size or change. For those patients who require surgery, CTA

with 3D volume-rendered images provides the surgeon with preoperative visualization of aneurysm size and extent. The extension of an ascending aortic aneurysm into the arch can be demonstrated and, as mentioned above, the expected location of aortic cross-clamping can be determined preoperatively (Fig. 6-24). The location of normal aorta distally and the extent of arch involvement will preoperatively determine the arterial cardiopulmonary bypass cannulation site as well as the need for concomitant arch repair, circulatory arrest, or selective antegrade perfusion. Selective antegrade cerebral perfusion itself is dependent on intact right axillary and innominate arteries, and CTA is optimal for defining this anatomy. Since the success of a procedure can be compromised by unexpected intraoperative

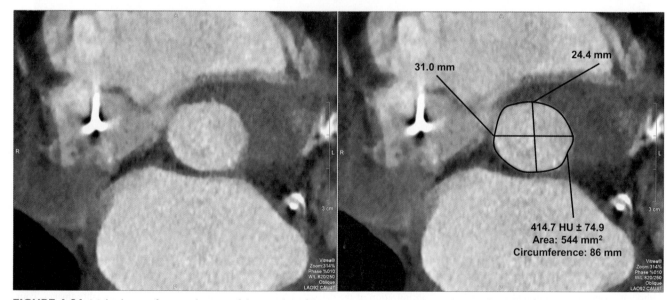

FIGURE 6-21 Multiplanar reformatted image of the annulus of the aorta in a patient under evaluation for TAVR. The right-hand image shows the routine annotation for measuring the annular area and dimensions in both short and long axis. Measurements are used for to determine the best sizing before the procedure.

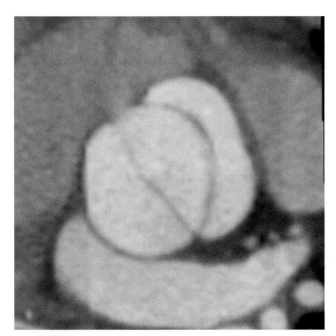

FIGURE 6-22 Demonstration of aortic root and aortic valve. Axial oblique multiplanar reformatted image from a systolic dataset demonstrates an open bicuspid aortic valve. Note the precise definition of the aortic wall, free from the cardiac motion related artifacts that are present at conventional thoracic CT scanning. Aortic root size measurements are highly accurate due to lack of motion artifacts and the high spatial resolution of the cardiac CT scanning (<0.5 mm).

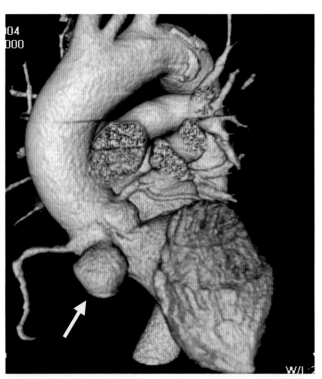

FIGURE 6-23 Cardiac CT provides optimal visualization of complex aortic root pathology. Prior echocardiogram suggested the entire aortic root to be aneurysmal at greater than 4.5 cm. Three-dimensional volume-rendered image from cardiac CT demonstrates a 2.6 cm sinus of Valsalva aneurysm arising off of the right coronary sinus (*white arrow*). The remainder of aortic root is normal.

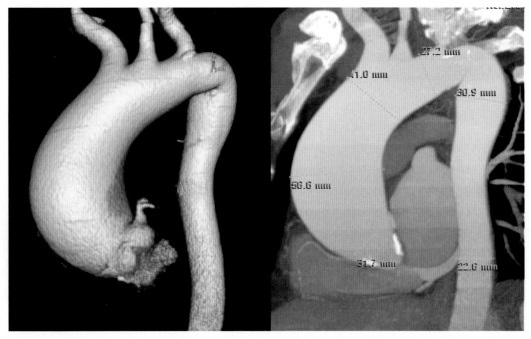

FIGURE 6-24 Comprehensive evaluation of ascending aortic aneurysm for preoperative planning. On the left, 3D volume-rendered image demonstrates an aneurysmal ascending aorta. Sagittal oblique maximum intensity projection image (20 mm thick) can be used to demonstrate aortic size measurements. The aneurysm can be seen to extend into the aortic arch. As the entire ascending aorta and proximal arch needed to be replaced, cross-clamping could not occur proximal to the innominate in this patient and would have to occur in the mid-distal arch altering the surgical risk of the procedure.

findings, CT has contributed enormously to surgical planning by defining anatomy that would not be preoperatively visualized with any other imaging modality.

Aortic Dissection and Aortic Intramural Hematoma (AIH)

CTA enjoys a sensitivity and specificity of almost 100% for detection of aortic dissection and intramural hematoma, thus allowing the surgeon to understand the extent of the intimal flap.[56] In particular, ECG-gated CT offers information regarding dissection of the ascending aorta (the proximal extent of the dissection flap and its relationship to the coronary arteries and the aortic valve) that was not available before gating was routinely performed. In addition, motion-free images obtained with ECG gating allow for definitive exclusion of type A dissection (Fig. 6-25). The location of the true and false lumen is critical in the preoperative planning,

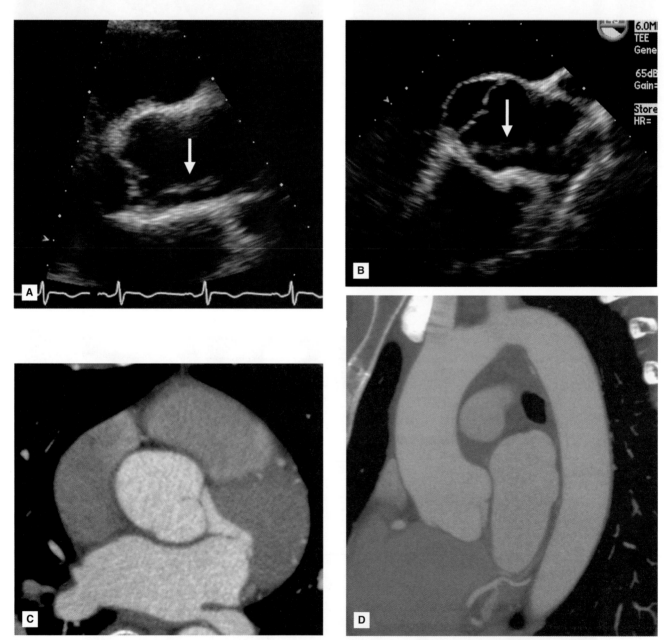

FIGURE 6-25 Although multiple modalities may be used for evaluation of the aortic root, cardiac CT is the gold standard for all pathology of the aorta, including the exclusion and characterization of type A dissection. Parasternal long-axis image from trans-thoracic echocardiogram (A) demonstrates a linear area of echogenicity (*white arrow*) above the noncoronary cusp of the aortic valve concerning for an intimal flap. The finding was detected incidentally in a patient with recent stroke and possible PFO. Subsequent trans-esophageal echocardiogram (B) again demonstrated the finding. Axial image from cardiac CT scan (C) provides excellent visualization of the aortic root and definitively excludes the present of an intimal flap. Sagittal oblique maximum intensity projection image (D) demonstrates aortic root and ascending aorta to be normal. No further evaluation is needed. Echocardiographic findings were presumed to be from artifact.

the operative sequence, and the extent of repair. For example, in dissection of the descending aorta, end-organ perfusion is assessed by demonstrating contrast enhancement of individual organs and related compromise of the celiac, superior mesenteric, inferior mesenteric or renal arteries. As is the case for a nonsurgical aneurysm, if a descending thoracic aortic dissection is stable and to be followed expectantly, CTA remains the reference standard for periodic assessment. Emergency nonenhanced CT, followed by CT contrast-enhanced angiography is the guideline endorsed recommendation,[60] in particular when IMH or aortic dissection are suspected. Contrast-enhanced CTA is the appropriate,[61] definitive test in patients with suspicion of aortic dissection.

Traumatic Aortic Injury

For patients with suspected trauma of the aorta and the great vessels contrast-enhanced CT is the guideline-endorsed[60,62] reference standard. Almost all polytrauma diagnostic algorithms include a combination of chest radiography plus CTA for initial patient evaluation. The sensitivity and specificity of CT are close to 100% and it is the only imaging modality that has NPV of 100%.[63,64]

Aside direct visualization of traumatic aortic injury, CT allows for simultaneous imaging of indirect signs including widened mediastinum, pulmonary contusion, left scapula fracture, hemothorax, and pseudoaneurysm of the aortic wall (Fig. 6-26).[65]

Pulmonary Embolism

Growing evidence from recent studies and known societies guidelines[66,67] support CT pulmonary angiography (CTPA) as the first-line imaging test to confirm or exclude the clinical suspicion of acute pulmonary embolism (PE).[68] Combined with careful clinical assessment and specific biomarkers (D-Dimers, NT-pro-BNP, Troponin I), CTPA can further guide management in patients of low to moderate risk. Right ventricular dysfunction as demonstrated by an enlarged RV diameter,[69,70] abnormal position of interventricular septum and inferior vena cava contrast reflux, provides aside to diagnostic assistance, prognostic value and may predict adverse outcomes and patient mortality (Fig. 6-27).[71]

HEART FAILURE

Heart transplantation is the definitive therapy for end-stage heart failure whereas left ventricular assist devices (LVAD) represent a bridge to transplantation, a destination therapy, or a bridge to recovery.[72,73] Complications can appear either acutely or gradually. Aside providing important anatomical information preoperationally, CT can be utilized for the assessment of proper device function and the early identification of complications. Since this patient population often has impaired renal function, iodinated contrast-induced nephrotoxicity is an important risk that should be carefully considered in discussion between the surgeon and radiologist. Scans

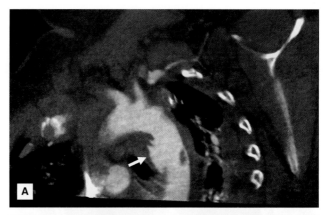

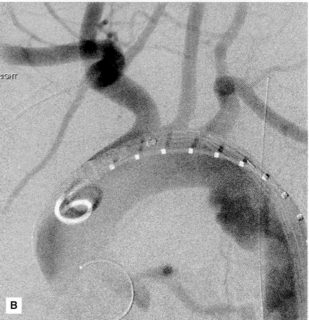

FIGURE 6-26 Patient status post motor vehicle accident. (A) Multiplanar reformatted image demonstrates traumatic aortic injury with a contained pseudoaneurysm (*arrow*) at the level of the ligamentumarteriosum. (B) Image from conventional angiography were obtained at intervention. The modern diagnosis and exclusion of traumatic injury of the aorta rests almost entirely on CT.

can sometimes be performed with a reduced iodine load with satisfactory image quality.

Implantable Devices for Heart Failure

For patients with implantable cardiac devices, ECG-gated cardiac CT is feasible, accurate, and enhances the diagnostic evaluation of suspected LVAD dysfunction, further modifying management.[74,75]

For LVAD assessment, CT is superior to echocardiography that has limited imaging depth and coverage volume with regards to the limited acoustic window and acoustic shadowing.[76] Common complications such as in-device-thrombus formation, hemorrhage, cannula/driveline obstruction, pericardium tamponade, or infections can be recognized; the

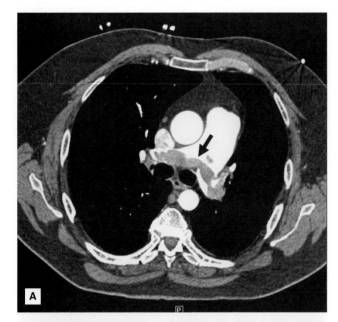

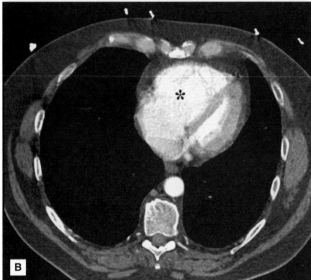

FIGURE 6-27 Patient with acute hypoxia. (A) Saddle pulmonary embolus (*arrow*) demonstrated by a large contrast (*white*) filling defect. Note the enlargement of the main pulmonary artery and (B) relative enlargement of the RV (*) with respect to the LV. This finding strongly suggests right heart strain.

orientation of the device can be assessed using multiplanar reformatted images (Fig. 6-28).[77]

The diagnosis of tamponade in patients with LAVD almost entirely relies on CT, and common findings include inferior vena cava dilatation, right ventricle compression, and contrast material reflux into the azygos vein.[77] Peridevice presence of gas or fluid accumulation are indicative of infections, and given the contraindication of MR, cardiac CT is considered to be the test of choice to evaluate for mycotic pseudoaneurysm.[78] CT is recommended by guidelines[79] for visualization of the native heart and LVAD components and may be valuable when other imaging modalities have not been revealing.

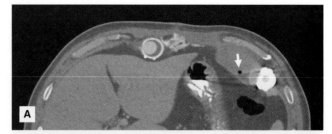

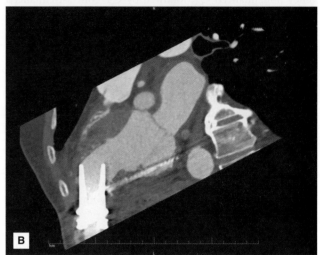

FIGURE 6-28 Heart failure patient status post VAD placement. (A) Axial image demonstrates a fluid attenuation lesion containing a punctate amount of gas (*arrow*) at the level of the ventricular insertion. (B) Reformatted image shows the orientation of the ventricular insertion pointed superiorly to the long axis of the left ventricle with impingement on the anterior heart.

In patients with implantable pacemakers and defibrillators, ECG-gated CT with multiplanar reformatting is useful for identifying late (>1 month postimplantation) lead malposition, and in conjunction with echocardiography findings can evaluate possible cardiac perforation.[80]

Heart Transplantation

The role of cardiac CT is secondary for the diagnosis of acute transplantation complications, namely acute cardiac allograft rejection, as echocardiography and MR are used as the first-line imaging modalities.[81] Coronary allograft vasculopathy (CAV) affects almost half of the transplant recipients and represents one of the major mortality causes. CTA offers a reliable diagnostic tool alternative to the traditionally used interventional coronary angiography (ICA) and intravascular ultrasound. By offering an excellent NPV in relation to reference ICA, CT can be utilized as a noninvasive approach, thereby minimizing invasive procedures.[82, 83] Important limitation is the inability to adequately visualize distal coronary vasculature with a diameter of <1.5 mm where early CAV is usually recognized. Cardiac CT can exclude significant CAV within the larger, major coronary segments that may be suitable for stenting.[84]

VARIOUS

Imaging of the Pericardium

In patients with clinically suspected constrictive pericarditis, cardiac MR or CT can be used to confirm and measure pericardial thickening. In comparison with MR, CT far better demonstrates the presence and extent of calcification as well as the localization and characterization of pericardial effusion, cysts, or masses. This may be of value in confirming chronic calcific pericardial thickening, supporting the diagnosis of constrictive pericarditis (Fig. 6-29). In these cases, 3D volume rendering illustrates regional localization and distribution of pericardial abnormality; CT is an outstanding preoperative planning tool prior to pericardial stripping (Fig. 6-30). Furthermore, retrospectively ECG-gated studies can guide functional evaluation of septal bounce or pericardial tethering.[85]

Primary or metastatic pericardial masses are rare. CT and MRI offer additional information on the localization and sizing, detection of calcification, and tissue characterizations (presence of blood, thrombus, or fat). Usual image findings include contrast enhancement and high-signal intensity T2W images in CT and MR, respectively. Uncommon lesions such as pericardium cysts and diverticula have typical appearance on CT as well-circumscribed, thin-walled fluid collection most frequently found in the right cardiophrenic angle.

Cardiac Masses

Cardiac MRI is the preferred modality for high spatial resolution cross-sectional imaging to evaluate cardiac and pericardial masses. However, CT may be desired, and potentially required, if the mass is known to extend into the mediastinum, chest wall, or lung, or if the patient has a contraindication to MRI. CT also evaluates extra-cardiac thoracic structures with high spatial resolution; thus, it can define the full extent of disease (Fig. 6-31). CT is also useful as a single follow-up examination in patients with metastases to the heart and lungs because it avoids the need for periodic assessment with both conventional chest CT and cardiac MRI. Fat-containing lesions are very amenable to evaluation by CT, since these low attenuation lesions have a characteristic appearance, appearing black relative to water (Fig. 6-32).

Cardiac Infections

Infective endocarditis (IE) may involve native or prosthetic cardiac valves. The diagnosis is typically suggested on clinical assessment. However, imaging confirms the clinical suspicion and demonstrates cardiac valve vegetations, paravalvular abscesses, complications, and further identifying and grading heart failure. ECG-gated CT in IE may be appropriate by guidelines,[86,87] depending on the clinical presentation, and is complimentary to echocardiography (TTE and TEE) for the evaluation of suspected paravalvular and myocardial abscesses, pseudoaneurysms and infections of prosthetic heart valves (Fig. 6-33). CTA may be appropriate, again depending on the clinical scenario, for identifying the coronary arteries origin prior to surgery.[87] Vegetations smaller than 1 cm are hard to detect with CT (NPV = 55.5%).

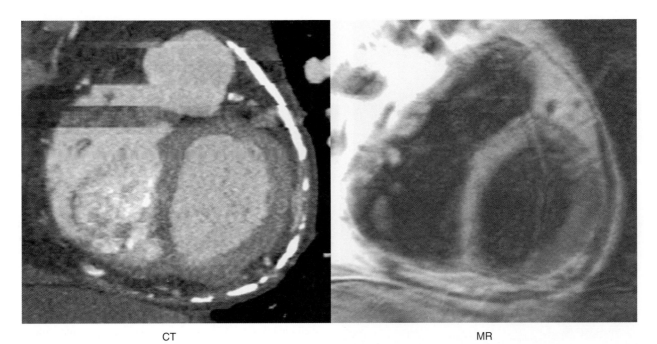

CT   MR

FIGURE 6-29 Calcific constrictive pericarditis. Short axis multiplanar reformatted image from cardiac CT demonstrates extensive thickening and calcification involving left-sided pericardium. In the appropriate clinical setting, these findings would support the diagnosis of constrictive pericarditis. Short axis double inversion recovery fast spin echo image from cardiac MR in the same patient also shows abnormal pericardial thickening, but is insensitive to calcification.

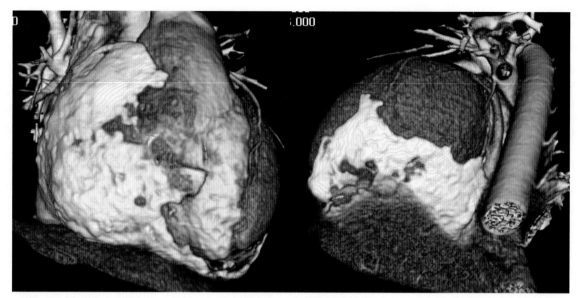

FIGURE 6-30 Preoperative evaluation of chronic calcific pericardial thickening prior to pericardial stripping. Three-dimensional volume-rendered images from cardiac CT demonstrate extensive regional pericardial calcification (*white areas*). This includes over the RVOT, right ventricle, right atrium, and entire inferior wall extending inferolaterally. Anterior and anterolateral pericardium was normal.

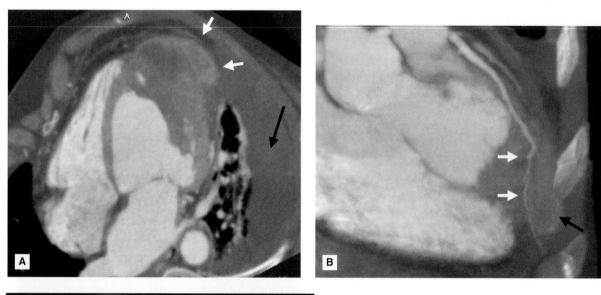

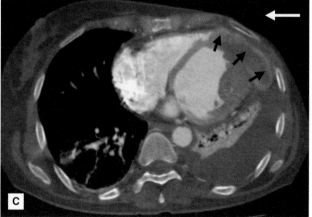

FIGURE 6-31 Cardiac CT of undifferentiated LV sarcoma performed to evaluate cardiac and extra-cardiac extent of disease. Four chamber multiplanar reformatted image (A) demonstrates invasive myocardial mass centered on the lateral wall beginning at the mid-ventricular level with extension to involve the base of both papillary muscles and distal circumferential involvement of the LV apex. Large epicardial component is noted intimate with pericardium (*white arrows*). There is no evidence of chest wall invasion. Left pleural effusion is seen (*black arrow*). Sagittal oblique maximum intensity projection image (B) (12 mm thick) shows encasement but patency of the LAD (*black arrow*) by tumor (*white arrows*) at the LV apex over a 2.5 cm length. Full field of view axial image (C) shows LV mass without gross chest wall invasion (*black arrows*), evidence of prior mastectomy (*white arrow*), and left pleural effusion.

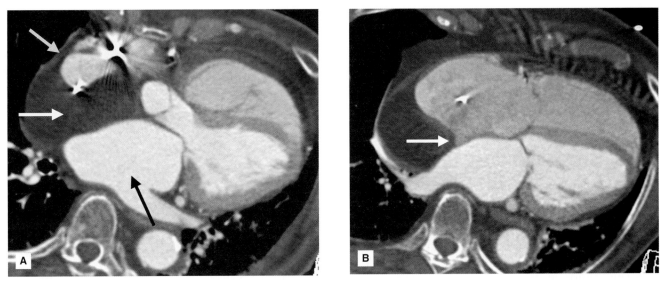

FIGURE 6-32 Lipomatous hypertrophy of the interatrial septum. Oblique axial multiplanar reformatted image (A) demonstrates a low attenuation mass (*white arrow*) insinuated between SVC (*grey arrow*) and left atrium (*black arrow*). Second more caudal image (B) demonstrates characteristic sparing of the fossa ovalis (*white arrow*). This lesion is nonencapsulated and can be quite extensive as in this case. Note presence of leads from pacemaker which precluded an MR study.

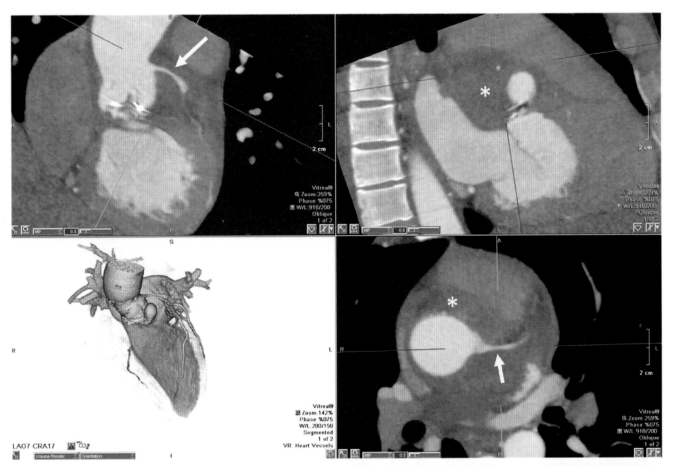

FIGURE 6-33 Intravenous drug user who presented with fever of unknown origin. The four panels of the CT images demonstrate complex fluid (*) at the level of the aortic root, consistent with abscess (confirmed by sampling). The three orthogonal images (*upper panels and lower right panel*) show the relationship with the elongated and narrowed left main coronary artery (*arrow*). The bottom left pane shows a 3D volume rendering that can be viewed at any angle for interventional planning.

Additional imaging utilizing CT or MRI in acute infectious pericarditis can be considered for association with clinical findings and echocardiography in complicated cases. Noncalcified pericardial thickening along with contrast enhancement of visceral and parietal surfaces of the pericardial sac are common findings. CT provides information on the nature of the effusion fluid by distinguishing between exudative versus transudative fluid (usually <10 HU), or hematomas.

CT VERSUS MRI OF THE HEART

Throughout this chapter, comparisons between CT and MRI have illustrated the strengths and limitations of each. Both modalities give the surgeon valuable pre- and postoperative information. While the modality best suited for specific clinical indications evolves with the technology, at present certain generalizations can be made. Cardiac CT is invaluable in reoperative cardiac surgery as it offers higher quality noninvasive angiography of native coronary arteries and bypass grafts. Since 3D volume rendering with CT has higher quality and better spatial resolution, it is preferred for preoperative planning for reoperative CABG or minimally invasive cardiac surgery. All calcifications are poorly seen on MRI and superbly seen with CT, and thus CT is far superior in demonstrating coronary, myocardial, pericardial, and valvular calcifications. The same is true for mechanical valve prostheses; because of large areas of artifact on MR images, functional evaluation is only possible with CT. Finally, all patients with a surgical problem of the aorta require evaluation with CT.

The strengths of MRI include high temporal resolution, greater blood-myocardial image contrast, multiparametric functional evaluation, and techniques for myocardial tissue characterization. In addition, cardiac MRI is invaluable in assessing myocardial function, contractility, and actual tissue perfusion and viability. For these reasons, MRI remains the reference standard to assess biventricular volumes, function, and myocardial mass. A variety of MRI pulse sequences can accurately delineate areas of chronic myocardial infarction, identify certain specific cardiomyopathies, and confirm the presence of neoplasm. With the use of parallel imaging techniques to increase the speed of the MRI acquisition, very high temporal resolution (20–30 ms) can be obtained to study bioprosthetic and native valve function. In addition, measurements of flow parameters through a vessel cross-section can be used to, for example, accurately quantify valvular regurgitant lesions.

One distinct advantage of MRI over CT is that MRI delivers no patient radiation. As detailed in Part 1, the radiation exposure in ECG-gated CT is higher than that for CT of any other body part. In younger patients, who typically have less comorbid disease and may require multiple follow-up examinations over years or decades, MRI should be used when possible.

Dramatic progress in CT technology has enabled advanced cardiac imaging for cardiac surgery patients. CT has rapidly demonstrated broad ranging applicability, and in particular CT has revolutionized the preoperative assessment of patients

for reoperative surgery. Understanding the technical considerations will allow the surgeon to appreciate the inherent strengths and weaknesses of cardiac CT and to optimally communicate with the radiologist. This, in turn, will result in the best quality diagnostic examination in the vast majority of cardiac surgery patients.

REFERENCES

1. Rybicki FJ, Otero HJ, Steigner ML, et al: Initial evaluation of coronary images from 320-detector row computed tomography. *Int J Cardiovasc Imaging* 2008; 24:535-546.
2. Steigner ML, Otero HJ, Cai T, et al: Narrowing the phase window width in prospectively ECG-gated single heart beat 320-detector row coronary CT angiography. *Int J Cardiovasc Imaging* 2009; 25:85-90.
3. Chen MY, Shanbhag SM, Arai AE: Submillisievert median radiation dose for coronary angiography with a second-generation 320-detector row CT scanner in 107 consecutive patients. *Radiology* 2013; 267:76-85.
4. Flohr TG, McCollough CH, Bruder H, et al: First performance evaluation of a dual-source CT (DSCT) system. *Eur Radiol* 2006; 16:256-268.
5. Achenbach S, Marwan M, Schepis T, et al: High-pitch spiral acquisition: a new scan mode for coronary CT angiography. *J Cardiovasc Comput Tomogr* 2009; 3:117-121.
6. Vavere AL, Simon GG, George RT, et al: Diagnostic performance of combined noninvasive coronary angiography and myocardial perfusion imaging using 320 row detector computed tomography: design and implementation of the CORE320 multicenter, multinational diagnostic study. *J Cardiovasc Comput Tomogr* 2011; 5:370-381.
7. George RT, Arbab-Zadeh A, Cerci RJ, et al: Diagnostic performance of combined noninvasive coronary angiography and myocardial perfusion imaging using 320-MDCT: the CT angiography and perfusion methods of the CORE320 multicenter multinational diagnostic study. *AJR Am J Roentgenol* 2011; 197:829-837.
8. Rochitte CE, George RT, Chen MY, et al: Computed tomography angiography and perfusion to assess coronary artery stenosis causing perfusion defects by single photon emission computed tomography: the CORE320 study. *Eur Heart J* 2014; 35:1120-1130.
9. Rybicki FJ, Mather RT, Kumamaru KK, et al: Comprehensive assessment of radiation dose estimates for the CORE320 study. *AJR Am J Roentgenol* 2015; 204:W27-W36.
10. Kishi S, Magalhaes TA, George RT, et al: Relationship of left ventricular mass to coronary atherosclerosis and myocardial ischaemia: the CORE320 multicenter study. *Eur Heart J Cardiovasc Imaging* 2015; 16:166-176.
11. Shu KM, MacKenzie JD, Smith JB, et al: Lowering the thyroid dose in screening examinations of the cervical spine. *Emerg Radiol* 2006; 12:133-136.
12. Hoffmann MH, Shi H, Schmitz BL, et al: Noninvasive coronary angiography with multislice computed tomography. *JAMA* 2005; 293:2471-2478.
13. Garcia MJ, Lessick J, Hoffmann MH: Accuracy of 16-row multidetector computed tomography for the assessment of coronary artery stenosis. *JAMA* 2006; 296:403-411.
14. Turkvatan A, Biyikoglu SF, Buyukbayraktar F, Olcer T, Cumhur T, Duru E: Clinical value of 16-slice multidetector computed tomography in symptomatic patients with suspected coronary artery disease. *Acta Radiol* 2008; 49:400-408.
15. Hausleiter J, Meyer T, Hadamitzky M, et al: Non-invasive coronary computed tomographic angiography for patients with suspected coronary artery disease: the Coronary Angiography by Computed Tomography with the Use of a Submillimeter resolution (CACTUS) trial. *Eur Heart J* 2007; 28:3034-3041.
16. Marano R, De Cobelli F, Floriani I, et al: Italian multicenter, prospective study to evaluate the negative predictive value of 16- and 64-slice MDCT imaging in patients scheduled for coronary angiography (NIMISCAD-Non Invasive Multicenter Italian Study for Coronary Artery Disease). *Eur Radiol* 2009; 19:1114-1123.
17. Shabestari AA, Abdi S, Akhlaghpoor S, et al: Diagnostic performance of 64-channel multislice computed tomography in assessment of significant coronary artery disease in symptomatic subjects. *Am J Cardiol* 2007; 99:1656-1661.

18. Cademartiri F, Maffei E, Notarangelo F, et al: 64-slice computed tomography coronary angiography: diagnostic accuracy in the real world. *Radiol Med* 2008; 113:163-180.

19. Budoff MJ, Dowe D, Jollis JG, et al: Diagnostic performance of 64-multidetector row coronary computed tomographic angiography for evaluation of coronary artery stenosis in individuals without known coronary artery disease: results from the prospective multicenter ACCURACY (Assessment by Coronary Computed Tomographic Angiography of Individuals Undergoing Invasive Coronary Angiography) trial. *J Am Coll Cardiol* 2008; 52:1724-1732.

20. Miller JM, Rochitte CE, Dewey M, et al: Diagnostic performance of coronary angiography by 64-row CT. *N Engl J Med.* 2008; 359:2324-2336.

21. Meijboom WB, Meijs MF, Schuijf JD, et al: Diagnostic accuracy of 64-slice computed tomography coronary angiography: a prospective, multicenter, multivendor study. *J Am Coll Cardiol* 2008; 52:2135-2144.

22. Bettencourt N, Rocha J, Carvalho M, et al: Multislice computed tomography in the exclusion of coronary artery disease in patients with presurgical valve disease. *Circ Cardiovasc Imaging* 2009; 2:306-313.

23. Gouya H, Varenne O, Trinquart L, et al: Coronary artery stenosis in high-risk patients: 64-section CT and coronary angiography—prospective study and analysis of discordance. *Radiology* 2009; 252:377-385.

24. Maffei E, Palumbo A, Martini C, Meijboom W, Tedeschi C, Spagnolo P, et al: Diagnostic accuracy of 64-slice computed tomography coronary angiography in a large population of patients without revascularisation: registry data and review of multicentre trials. *Radiol Med* 2010; 115:368-384.

25. Dewey M, Zimmermann E, Deissenrieder F, et al: Noninvasive coronary angiography by 320-row computed tomography with lower radiation exposure and maintained diagnostic accuracy: comparison of results with cardiac catheterization in a head-to-head pilot investigation. *Circulation* 2009; 120:867-875.

26. Montalescot G, Sechtem U, Achenbach S, et al: ESC guidelines on the management of stable coronary artery disease. *Eur Heart J* 2013; 34:2949-3003.

27. Greenland P, Alpert JS, Beller GA, et al: 2010 ACCF/AHA Guideline for assessment of cardiovascular risk in asymptomatic adults: A report of the American College of Cardiology Foundation/American Heart Association Task Force on practice guidelines developed in collaboration with the American Society of Echocardiography, American Society of Nuclear Cardiology, Society of Atherosclerosis Imaging and Prevention, Society for Cardiovascular Angiography and Interventions, Society of Cardiovascular Computed Tomography, and Society for Cardiovascular Magnetic Resonance. *J Am Coll Cardiol* 56:e50-e103.

28. Mark DB, Berman DS, Budoff MJ, et al: ACCF/ACR/AHA/NASCI/SAIP/SCAI/SCCT 2010. Expert consensus document on coronary computed tomographic angiography: a report of the American College of Cardiology Foundation Task Force on expert consensus documents. *J Am Coll Cardiol.* 2010; 55:2663-2699.

29. Perrone-Filardi P, Achenbach S, Möhlenkamp S, et al: Cardiac computed tomography and myocardial perfusion scintigraphy for risk stratification in asymptomatic individuals without known cardiovascular disease: a position statement of the Working Group on Nuclear Cardiology and Cardiac CT of the European Society of Cardiology. *Eur Heart J* 2011; 32:1986-1993.

30. Hoffmann U, Venkatesh V, White RD, et al: ACR Appropriateness Criteria* acute nonspecific chest pain—low probability of coronary artery disease. *J Am Coll Radiol* 9:745-750.

31. Earls JP, White RD, Woodard PK, et al: ACR Appropriateness Criteria* chronic chest pain—high probability of coronary artery disease. *J Am Coll Radiol* 8:679-686.

32. Woodard PK, White RD, Abbara S, et al: ACR Appropriateness Criteria* chronic chest pain—low to intermediate probability of coronary artery disease. *J Am Coll Radiol* 10:329-334.

33. Schlosser T, Konorza T, Hunold P, Kuhl H, Schmermund A, Barkhausen J: Noninvasive visualization of coronary artery bypass grafts using 16-detector row computed tomography. *J Am Coll Cardiol* 2004; 44:1224-1229.

34. Martuscelli E, Romagnoli A, D'Eliseo A, et al: Evaluation of venous and arterial conduit patency by 16-slice spiral computed tomography. *Circulation* 2004; 110:3234-3238.

35. Chiurlia E, Menozzi M, Ratti C, Romagnoli R and Modena MG: Follow-up of coronary artery bypass graft patency by multislice computed tomography. *Am J Cardiol* 2005; 95:1094-1097.

36. Gasparovic H, Rybicki FJ, Millstine J, et al: Three dimensional computed tomographic imaging in planning the surgical approach for redo cardiac surgery after coronary revascularization. *Eur J Cardiothorac Surg* 2005; 28:244-249.

37. de Graaf FR, Schuijf JD, van Velzen JE, et al: Diagnostic accuracy of 320-row multidetector computed tomography coronary angiography in the non-invasive evaluation of significant coronary artery disease. *Eur Radiol* 2011; 21:2285-2296.

38. Weustink AC, Nieman K, Pugliese F, et al: Diagnostic accuracy of computed tomography angiography in patients after bypass grafting: comparison with invasive coronary angiography. *JACC: Cardiovasc Imaging* 2009; 2:816-824.

39. Mushtaq S, Andreini D, Pontone G, et al: Prognostic value of coronary CTA in coronary bypass patients: a long-term follow-up study. *JACC: Cardiovasc Imaging* 2014; 7:580-589.

40. Mollet NR, Cademartiri F: Computed tomography assessment of coronary bypass grafts: ready to replace conventional angiography? *Int J Cardiovasc Imaging* 2005; 21:453-454.

41. Puskas JD, Williams WH, Mahoney EM, et al: Off-pump vs conventional coronary artery bypass grafting: early and 1-year graft patency, cost, and quality-of-life outcomes: a randomized trial. *JAMA* 2004; 291:1841-1849.

42. Khan NE, De Souza A, Mister R, et al: A randomized comparison of off-pump and on-pump multivessel coronary-artery bypass surgery. *N Engl J Med* 2004; 350:21-28.

43. Collins P, Webb CM, Chong CF, Moat NE: Radial artery versus saphenous vein patency randomized trial: five-year angiographic follow-up. *Circulation* 2008; 117:2859-2864.

44. Elami A, Laks H, Merin G: Technique for reoperative median sternotomy in the presence of a patent left internal mammary artery graft. *J Cardiovasc Surg* 1994; 9:123-127.

45. Steimle CN, Bolling SF: Outcome of reoperative valve surgery via right thoracotomy. *Circulation* 1996; 94:II126-128.

46. Aviram G, Sharony R, Kramer A, et al: Modification of surgical planning based on cardiac multidetector computed tomography in reoperative heart surgery. *Ann Thorac Surg* 2005; 79:589-595.

47. Caimmi PP, Fossaceca R, Lanfranchi M, et al: Cardiac angio-CT scan for planning MIDCAB. *Heart Surg Forum* 2004; 7:E113-E116.

48. Herzog C, Dogan S, Diebold T, et al: Multi-detector row CT versus coronary angiography: preoperative evaluation before totally endoscopic coronary artery bypass grafting. *Radiology* 2003; 229:200-208.

49. Ruel M, Shariff MA, Lapierre H, et al: Results of the minimally invasive coronary artery bypass grafting angiographic patency study. *J Thorac Cardiovasc Surg* 2014; 147:203-209.

50. Pouleur AC, le Polain de Waroux JB, Pasquet A, Vanoverschelde JL, Gerber BL: Aortic valve area assessment: multidetector CT compared with cine MR imaging and transthoracic and transesophageal echocardiography. *Radiology* 2007; 244:745-754.

51. Svensson LG, Adams DH, Bonow RO, et al: Aortic Valve and Ascending Aorta Guidelines for Management and Quality Measures. *Ann Thorac Surg* 2013; 95:S1-S66.

52. Wake N, Kumamaru K, Prior R, Rybicki FJ, Steigner ML: Computed tomography angiography for transcatheter aortic valve replacement. *Radiol Technol* 2013; 84:326-340.

53. Dill KE, George E, Abbara S, et al: ACR appropriateness criteria imaging for transcatheter aortic valve replacement. *J Am Coll Radiol* 2013; 10:957-965.

54. Salgado RA, Budde RPJ, Leiner T, et al: Transcatheter aortic valve replacement: postoperative CT findings of Sapien and CoreValve transcatheter heart valves. *RadioGraphics* 2014; 34:1517-1536.

55. Goldstein SA, Evangelista A, Abbara S, et al: Multimodality imaging of diseases of the thoracic aorta in adults: from the American Society of Echocardiography and the European Association of cardiovascular imaging. *J Am Soc Echocardiogr* 28:119-182.

56. Kalva SP, Dill KE, Bandyk DF, et al: ACR Appropriateness Criteria® nontraumatic aortic disease. *J Thorac Imaging* 2014; 29:W85-W88.

57. Nishi H, Mitsuno M, Ryomoto M, Miyamoto Y: Comprehensive approach for clamping severely calcified ascending aorta using computed tomography. *Interactive Cardiovasc Thorac Surg* 2010; 10:18-20.

58. Nishi H, Mitsuno M, Tanaka H, Ryomoto M, Fukui S and Miyamoto Y: Who needs preoperative routine chest computed tomography for prevention of stroke in cardiac surgery? *Interactive Cardiovasc Thorac Surg* 2010; 11:30-33.

59. Buckley O, Rybicki FJ, Gerson DS, et al: Imaging features of intramural hematoma of the aorta. *Int J Cardiovasc Imaging* 26:65-76.

60. Erbel R, Aboyans V, Boileau C, et al: 2014 ESC Guidelines on the diagnosis and treatment of aortic diseases. *Eur Heart J* 2014; 35:2873-2926.
61. National Guideline Clearinghouse. Guideline summary: ACR appropriateness criteria-acute chest pain-suspected aortic dissection. 2014.
62. Demehri S, Rybicki F, Desjardins B, et al: ACR Appropriateness Criteria* blunt chest trauma—suspected aortic injury. *Emerg Radiol* 2012; 19:287-292.
63. Scaglione M, Pinto A, Pinto F, Romano L, Ragozzino A, Grassi R: Role of contrast-enhanced helical CT in the evaluation of acute thoracic aortic injuries after blunt chest trauma. *Eur Radiol* 2001; 11:2444-2448.
64. Mirvis SE, Shanmuganathan K, Miller BH, White CS, Turney SZ: Traumatic aortic injury: diagnosis with contrast-enhanced thoracic CT—five-year experience at a major trauma center. *Radiology* 1996; 200:413-422.
65. Mosquera V, Marini M, Muñiz J, et al: Traumatic aortic injury score (TRAINS): an easy and simple score for early detection of traumatic aortic injuries in major trauma patients with associated blunt chest trauma. *Intensive Care Med* 2012; 38:1487-1496.
66. Bettmann MA, White RD, Woodard PK, et al: ACR Appropriateness Criteria* acute chest pain—suspected pulmonary embolism. *J Thorac Imaging* 2012; 27:W28-W31.
67. Konstantinides SV, Torbicki A, Agnelli G, et al: 2014 ESC Guidelines on the diagnosis and management of acute pulmonary embolism. *Eur Heart J* 2014; 35:3033-3073.
68. Hunsaker AR, Lu MT, Goldhaber SZ, Rybicki FJ: Imaging in acute pulmonary embolism with special clinical scenarios. *Circ Cardiovasc Imaging* 2010; 3:491-500.
69. Kumamaru KK, Hunsaker AR, Wake N, et al: The variability in prognostic values of right ventricular-to-left ventricular diameter ratios derived from different measurement methods on computed tomography pulmonary angiography: a patient outcome study. *J Thorac Imaging* 2012; 27:331-336.
70. Lu MT, Demehri S, Cai T, et al: Axial and reformatted four-chamber right ventricle-to-left ventricle diameter ratios on pulmonary CT angiography as predictors of death after acute pulmonary embolism. *AJR Am J Roentgenol* 2012; 198:1353-1360.
71. Kang DK, Thilo C, Schoepf UJ, et al: CT signs of right ventricular dysfunction: prognostic role in acute pulmonary embolism. *JACC: Cardiovasc Imag* 2011; 4:841-849.
72. Rose EA, Gelijns AC, Moskowitz AJ, et al: Long-term use of a left ventricular assist device for end-stage heart failure. *N Engl J Med* 2001; 345:1435-1443.
73. Birks EJ, Tansley PD, Hardy J, et al: Left ventricular assist device and drug therapy for the reversal of heart failure. *N Engl J Med* 2006; 355:1873-1884.
74. Acharya D, Singh S, Tallaj JA, et al: Use of gated cardiac computed tomography angiography in the assessment of left ventricular assist device dysfunction. *ASAIO J* 2011; 57:32-37.
75. Raman SV, Sahu A, Merchant AZ, Louis LBIV, Firstenberg MS, Sun B: Noninvasive assessment of left ventricular assist devices with cardiovascular computed tomography and impact on management. *J Heart Lung Transplant* 29:79-85.
76. Mak G, Truong Q: Cardiac CT: imaging of and through cardiac devices. *Curr Cardiovasc Imaging Rep* 2012; 5:328-336.
77. Carr CM, Jacob J, Park SJ, Karon BL, Williamson EE, Araoz PA: CT of left ventricular assist devices. *RadioGraphics* 2010; 30:429-444.
78. Hannan MM, Husain S, Mattner F, et al: Working formulation for the standardization of definitions of infections in patients using ventricular assist devices. *J Heart Lung Transplant* 2011;30:375-384.
79. Feldman D, Pamboukian SV, Teuteberg JJ, et al: The 2013 International Society for Heart and Lung Transplantation Guidelines for mechanical circulatory support: executive summary. *J Heart Lung Transplant* 32:157-187.
80. Pang BJ, Lui EH, Joshi SB, et al: Pacing and Implantable Cardioverter Defibrillator Lead Perforation as Assessed by Multiplanar Reformatted ECG-Gated Cardiac Computed Tomography and Clinical Correlates. *Pacing Clini Electrophysiol* 2014; 37:537-545.
81. Miller CA, Fildes JE, Ray SG, et al: Non-invasive approaches for the diagnosis of acute cardiac allograft rejection. *Heart* 2013; 99:445-453.
82. Wever-Pinzon O, Romero J, Kelesidis I, et al: Coronary computed tomography angiography for the detection of cardiac allograft vasculopathy: a meta-analysis of prospective trials. *J Am Coll Cardiol* 2014; 63:1992-2004.
83. Kobashigawa J: Coronary computed tomography angiography: is it time to replace the conventional coronary angiogram in heart transplant patients? *J Am Coll Cardiol* 2014; 63:2005-2006.
84. Pollack A, Nazif T, Mancini D, Weisz G: Detection and imaging of cardiac allograft vasculopathy. *JACC: Cardiovasc Imaging* 2013; 6:613-623.
85. Klein AL, Abbara S, Agler DA, et al: American Society of Echocardiography Clinical Recommendations for Multimodality Cardiovascular Imaging of Patients with Pericardial Disease. *J Am Soc Echocardiogr* 2013; 26:965-1012.e15.
86. Nishimura RA, Otto CM, Bonow RO, et al: 2014 AHA/ACC guideline for the management of patients with valvular heart disease. *J Thorac Cardiovasc Surg* 2014; 148:e1-e132.
87. National Guideline Clearinghouse. ACR Appropriateness Criteria-suspected infective endocarditis. 2014.

7

Risk Assessment and Performance Improvement in Cardiac Surgery

Victor A. Ferraris • Fred H. Edwards • Jeremiah T. Martin

Assessing risk to improve outcomes is not a new principle. Formal assessment of patient care to improve outcomes dates back millennia. While it may be hard to establish an exact beginning, there are historical times and iconoclastic health-care providers who stand out as important contributors to the modern concepts of quality assessment and performance improvement. At least six individuals stand out as iconoclasts in the field of performance improvement in surgery (Table 7-1). From the practice-changing observational studies of medieval surgeons like Albucasis and Trotula to the twentieth century insistence on evidence-based studies and randomized controlled trials (RCTs) by Archie Cochrane, many individuals served as champions of performance improvement using the tools of their times. The six people outlined in Table 7-1 had exceptional effects on differentiating good from bad outcomes and on implementing process improvements that benefit our patients today. Each of these six shared a common life experience. At some time in their careers, they were outcasts among their peers. Their peers, and in some cases the public, chastised them for stating the obvious. Thankfully, they persisted despite these unpopular reactions. Reading the historical accounts of these six individuals reminds one that today's public resistance to straightforward observations is a long-standing perpetual obstacle that surgical leaders overcame.

ASSESSMENT OF CARDIAC OPERATIONS

Measures of Successful Operations

PERFORMANCE MEASURES—OUTCOMES, STRUCTURE, AND PROCESS

In the early 1960s, Donabedian suggested that quality in health care is defined as improvement in patient status after accounting for the patient's severity of illness, presence of comorbidity, and the medical services received.[1] He further proposed that quality could best be measured by considering three domains: structure, process, and outcome. Only

recently has the notion of measuring health-care quality using this Donabedian framework been accepted and implemented. In 2000, the Institute of Medicine (IOM) issued a report that was highly critical of the US health-care system, suggesting that between 50,000 and 90,000 unnecessary deaths occur yearly because of errors in the health-care system.[2] The IOM reports created a heightened awareness of more global aspects of quality. For most of the history of cardiac surgery an outcome measure, operative mortality, defined surgical quality. After the IOM report appeared, change occurred, and other aspects of Donabedian's framework surfaced to measure quality. In addition to operative mortality, health-care quality measurement gave way to a broader analysis that included additional performance measures including *operative morbidity, processes of care, and structural measures of care.* The Joint Commission on Accreditation of Healthcare Organizations (formerly JCAHO now officially called The Joint Commission) proposed the following definitions of important quality measures:

- **Performance measure**—A quantitative entity that provides an indication of an organization's or surgeon's performance in relation to a specified process or outcome.
- **Outcome measure**—A measure that indicates the results of process measures. Examples are operative mortality, the frequency of postoperative mediastinitis, renal failure, and myocardial infarction.
- **Process measure**—A measure that focuses on a process leading to a certain outcome. Intrinsic in this definition is a scientific basis for believing that the process will increase the probability of achieving a desired outcome. Examples include the rate of internal mammary artery (IMA) use in coronary artery bypass graft (CABG) patients or the fraction of CABG patients placed on anti-platelet agents postoperatively.
- **Structural measure**—A measure that assesses whether an appropriate number, type, and distribution of medical personnel, equipment, and/or facilities are in place to deliver optimal health care. Examples include enrollment in a national database, adequate intensive care unit (ICU) facilities, or procedural volume.

TABLE 7-1: Shaping the Quality of Surgical Care Over Millennia

Health-care Provider (Surgeon, Midwife, or Nurse)	Time Period	Contributions
Albucasis of Andalusia	Around 900 A.D.	• Most frequently cited surgical author of the middle ages.[121] • Greatest contribution to medicine is the *Kitab al-Tasrif*, a thirty-volume encyclopedia of medical practices. • Instrumental in *transforming medicine from "philosophy" to an actual discipline.* Met with great resistance from peers who favored less invasive interventions. • May be the "father of modern surgery" because of his insistence on *observational studies, proper training, and use of operative techniques.* • Firsts include—description of ectopic pregnancy; hereditary nature of hemophilia; performance of bowel surgery; use of surgical instruments for procedures including breast surgery, urethral exam, tooth implant, stone removal (kidney, bladder, and gall bladder), important advances in pharmacology (prepared medicines by sublimation and distillation).
Trota of Salerno	Around 1200 A.D.	• Advised women on conception, menstruation, pregnancy, caesarian sections, and childbirth as a female faculty member of the Medical School of Salerno. • Wrote a textbook that impacted practice for 300-400 years.[122] • Her radical ideas on conception shocked the medical and social community. Based on *observational studies,* Trotula believed that not only women, but men, both have physiologic and anatomic defects that cause conception difficulties. • Defined the *concept of "laudable pus"* for wound abscess drainage.
Angelique du Coudrey of France	Mid 1700s	• As a practicing midwife, Mme du Coudray violated the majority of standards demanded of midwives; she had no children of her own, was not married, and believed in the organization and training of midwives.[123] • In 1759, Mme du Coudray released the first edition of her midwifery manual *Abrege de L'art des Accouchements* that ultimately updated the textbook of Trotula of Salerno. • Trained more than 40,000 midwives in France and dramatically improved the newborn infant mortality rate. By 1780, *two-thirds of the midwives in France were Madame du Coudray's pupils.* • Designed child-bearing machines/models for *simulation training* of vaginal delivery.[124]
John Hunter (England)	Late 1700s	• Premier anatomist/surgeon of his time. Insisted that *diseases were caused by anatomic abnormality* not abstract explanations of illness like "humors" or "spirits."[125] • Outspoken critic of many medications claiming to cure common diseases of the times (eg, gonorrhea). Devised an experiment to test the effect of pills made of bread to show that gonorrhea "mostly cured itself." One of the first records of the *placebo effect.* • Impact of Hunter's anatomic explanations carried forward to modern day (eg, Hunter's canal.) • Friends included Benjamin Franklin, Edward Jenner, Lord Byron, Casanova, and Adam Smith. List of enemies probably equally as distinguished.
Florence Nightingale (England)	Early 1800s	• Battlefield nurse in Crimean War. *Elevated nursing to honorable profession.* Famous quote: "*It may seem a strange principle to enunciate as the very first requirement in a Hospital that it should do the sick no harm.*"[126] • Troubled by observation that hospitalized patients in London hospitals died at higher rates than those in rural hospitals or treated at home. • Studied *epidemiology of hospital deaths.* Introduced *quality improvement* projects that included better sanitation, less crowding, and location of hospitals at a distance from crowded cities. • Observed that some patients admitted to urban hospitals were sicker than others and were more likely to die—beginning of *risk assessment.*
Ernest Amory Codman (United States)	Early 1900s	• Classmate of Harvey Cushing—together they instituted *intraoperative records* to document complications. • Passionate about *outcome analysis*—claimed that most adverse outcomes were the "surgeons' fault." Believed in *"End Result Idea."* • Founded his own hospital after being dismissed from Mass General. Became very unpopular because of his insistence on surgeon-related causes of adverse outcomes. • Co-*founder of the American College of Surgeons* and ultimately the precursor of the *Joint Commission, the ACS tumor registry, and National Trauma Databank.*[127]

(Continued)

TABLE 7-1: Shaping the Quality of Surgical Care Over Millennia (*Continued*)

Health-care Provider (Surgeon, Midwife, or Nurse)	Time Period	Contributions
Archie Cochrane (Scotland)	Mid-twentieth Century	• Volunteered with the International Brigade, Spanish Civil War. Branded as a "Tortyskite" and "socialist" because of insistence on a National Health Service. • Captain, Royal Army Medical Corps. Taken prisoner of war in June 1941 in Crete. • POW medical officer in various German POW camps. Developed questions about the best treatment of TB that triggered his *insistence on randomized trials.* • Strong advocate of *randomized controlled trials* to provide actionable evidence to support evidence-based interventions. • 1960-1974: Director, Medical Research Council Epidemiology Research Unit, Cardiff, Wales. • Published *Effectiveness and Efficiency—Random Reflections on Health Services* that summarized rationale for evidence-based medicine. • Driving force behind the creation of the *Cochrane Collaboration* that serves as the repository of RCT's and systematic reviews today.

Data from Quality Performance Measures. The Society of Thoracic Surgeons.

Birkmeyer and coworkers outlined advantages and disadvantages associated with each of these three specific types of performance measures.[3] The fact that *structural measures* can be readily tabulated in an inexpensive manner using administrative data is a distinct advantage. On the other hand, many structural measures do not lend themselves to alteration. Particularly in smaller hospitals, there may be no way to increase procedural volume or to introduce costly ICU design changes in an attempt to improve their performance on structural measures. Attempts to alter structure might even have adverse consequences (eg, unnecessary operations, costly and unnecessary new beds). Links between health-care quality and *process measures* exist and they are usually actionable on a practical level. Their major disadvantage lies in the fact that their linkage to outcomes may be weak. Although *outcome measures* are the most important endpoint for patients, inadequate sample size and lack of appropriate risk-adjustment limit accurate assessment of these outcomes.

Several national organizations develop and evaluate performance measures. Perhaps the most visible of these is the *National Quality Forum (NQF)*, a public-private collaborative organization that uses a process of exhaustive, evidence-based scrutiny of candidate measures to determine their relevance to both patients and healthcare providers. The NQF considers whether candidate measures can be assessed accurately and whether actionable interventions can improve performance for these measures. Because of this scrutiny, NQF-endorsed measures have a high level of national credibility (Table 7-2).

PATIENT SATISFACTION—PATIENT-REPORTED OUTCOMES

Other outcomes following cardiac procedures, such as patient satisfaction and health-related quality of life, are less well studied but extremely important in the assessment of performance. Meeting or exceeding patients' expectations is a major goal of the health-care system. While all recognize the importance of performing safe surgery, one must also acknowledge that a safe operation with minimal patient benefit is to be avoided. The growing importance of patient-reported outcomes (PRO) also reflects the increasing prevalence of chronic disease in our aging population. The goal of therapeutic interventions is often to relieve symptoms and to improve quality of life, rather than cure a disease and prolong survival. This is especially important in selecting elderly patients for cardiac operations. Recent studies suggest that CABG results in excellent health-related quality of life 10 to 15 years following operation in most patients,[4] and that this benefit extends to those patients older than 80 years of age.[5] Future research into patient-perceived performance assessment is inevitable given the aging of populations in the developed countries.

Statistical models to adjust for patient risk are essential to determine the probability of procedural outcomes. Traditionally, risk models predict the probability of death or other postprocedural complications such as stroke, infection, or renal failure. These traditional models are clearly important to assess procedural risk, but the safety of an operation is only part of the decision-making process as to whether to recommend a given procedure. Patient benefit must be considered as well. Just because one can do a procedure safely does not mean it should be done—if it affords the patient only minimal benefit, then the patient has received poor treatment.

Patient benefit can be represented by using appropriate metrics other than procedural mortality and morbidity. PRO can be objectively determined from a variety of published scoring protocols. These scores can be considered to be an objective measure of patient benefit. In turn, the scores provide information necessary to develop statistical models that

TABLE 7-2: National Quality Forum (NQF) Endorsed National Standards for Cardiac Surgery for 2014*

NQF endorsed adult cardiac surgery measures

Composite Measure

1. STS CABG Composite Score composed of six outcome measures and five process measures.

Outcome Measures

2. Risk-Adjusted Deep Sternal Wound Infection Rate.
3. Risk-Adjusted Operative Mortality for Aortic Valve Replacement (AVR).
4. Risk-Adjusted Operative Mortality for AVR + CABG Surgery.
5. Risk-Adjusted Operative Mortality for CABG.
6. Risk-Adjusted Operative Mortality for Mitral Valve (MV) Repair.
7. Risk-Adjusted Operative Mortality for MV Repair + CABG Surgery.
8. Risk-Adjusted Operative Mortality for MV Replacement.
9. Risk-Adjusted Operative Mortality for MV Replacement + CABG.
10. Risk-Adjusted Postoperative Renal Failure.
11. Risk-Adjusted Prolonged Intubation (Ventilation).
12. Risk-Adjusted Stroke/Cerebrovascular Accident.
13. Risk-Adjusted Surgical Re-exploration.

Process Measures

14. Anti-Lipid Treatment at Discharge.
15. Anti-Platelet Medication at Discharge.
16. Beta Blockade at Discharge.
17. Duration of Antibiotic Prophylaxis for Cardiac Surgery Patients.
18. Preoperative Beta Blockade.
19. Selection of Antibiotic Prophylaxis for Cardiac Surgery Patients.
20. Use of Internal Mammary Artery in CABG.

Structural Measure

21. Participation in a Systematic Database for Cardiac Surgery.

*http://www.sts.org/quality-research-patient-safety/quality/quality-performance-measures.

predict the probability of PRO scores, in much the same way that traditional models predict the probability of procedural complications. The results of these models should serve as a meaningful measure of predicted patient benefit. Clinical registries are now collecting data that will permit an objective estimate of both patient risk and patient benefit. Statistical risk models should soon be available to predict not only procedural mortality and major non-fatal complications, but also the probability of patient benefit.

COMPOSITE MEASURES THAT REFLECT PROCESS, STRUCTURE, AND OUTCOME DOMAINS

The best approach to assessing surgical quality is uncertain. Operative mortality for most cardiac procedures is low and performance assessment requires large patient numbers to discriminate between hospitals and providers. For this reason other measures surface for performance assessment. There is growing interest in the use of *composite measures* to assess provider and hospital performance. Composite measures combine multiple quality indicators into a single score and can include outcome, structural, and process measures in various combinations. Evidence suggests that composite variables that incorporate multiple outcome measures as well as structural and process performance measures are better reflections of quality than are individual outcomes alone.[6] Examples of composite performance measures used for quality assessment include indices that combine ICU care variables with outcome measures,[7] and those that combine process of care variables with outcome variables and structural variables.[8,9]

Certain outcome variables may reflect multiple domains of performance. One such measure is *failure-to-rescue*, usually defined as the mortality rate for a subset of patients who experience postoperative complications. Studies suggest that failure-to-rescue rates depend on structural measures (eg, advanced ICU capabilities and presence of residency training), processes of care, and traditional morbidity outcome measures.[10,11] While traditional outcome measures such as operative mortality are thought to be mostly dependent on patient-related risk factors, it appears that failure-to-rescue rates reflect a different part of the care continuum, specifically the intensive care arena. Some consider failure-to-rescue rates to be primarily a structural measure focused on nursing care and ICU staffing. There are multiple contributions to failure-to-rescue rates, thereby qualifying this variable as a composite performance measure. Several studies are underway to determine the ability of this variable to identify and stratify quality performers.

The development of composite measures is statistically complex. The composite metric is very dependent on the statistical approach used to combine the component variables.[8] Despite the complexities of creating composite measures, increased reliance on composite measures of quality is inevitable, and efforts at improving the reliability and predictive accuracy are underway.

TOOLS OF PERFORMANCE ASSESSMENT

Basic Statistical Treatment of Outcome Data

RECAP, RELATE, AND REGRESS

Analysis of cardiac surgical results is purpose-driven. Use of statistics follows the purpose for which data were gathered. There are three broad uses of statistics for analysis of cardiac surgical outcomes. Perhaps the most basic use of statistics is to *recap or summarize information* about a patient group. Certain reports can only document surgical outcomes in a few patients because of the rarity of disease or limited ability to sample patient populations. A single estimate of an outcome in a limited population may be misleading. In order to acknowledge the inaccuracy of a single estimate of a limited population, statistical measures describe this imprecision. Multiple statistical terms describe this uncertainty, including *sample, mean, standard deviation, interquartile range, confidence interval, and standard error.*

More commonly, statistics serve to *relate or compare attributes of two or more groups.* Comparisons between groups require comparisons between known reference distributions (eg, chi-square and t-distribution) and the data sample distribution. Differences between these two distributions allow calculation of a probability that there really is a difference between the sample and the reference distribution. This probability has different names including *p*-value or alpha (α) level. The most commonly used test for comparisons of two numeric variables is the Student's t-test. The t-test makes use of the symmetry of the t-distribution of a sample and compares the *t* statistic calculated from each of the two group's t-distributions with critical values. The astute reader quickly realizes that the statistical formulation of the t-test requires *computer support as the workhorse that does the calculations.* In fact, very few statistical tests do not rely on computer-intensive calculations. Reliance on computers to calculate *p*-values, and to perform statistical tests in general, provides opportunity for misuse or inaccurate use of both simple and complex statistics.[12] Misuse of the simplest statistical tests is common, and has been for many years.[13-15] It behooves the surgeon who evaluates the literature or who performs statistical analyses to understand the principles and application of various statistical tests used for comparing two or more groups.[12]

Comparing the outcomes between two groups based on several characteristics of each group considered simultaneously requires multivariable analysis. *Multivariate regression analysis* provides a means of accounting for multiple independent variables (also called risk factors) that predict the dependent (also called outcome) variable. The result of multivariate regression is called a "model," a slightly counter-intuitive term. Regression models allow assignment of a regression coefficient to each predictor variable that roughly corresponds to the variable contribution to outcome prediction. Again, computer software does the work; investigators do the interpretation.

OUTCOME MODELS

There is a multitude of regression models available for analysis of cardiac surgical data. Perhaps the most common is *logistic regression.* Logistic regression models are a means of analyzing independent variables that predict a *dichotomous outcome* (eg, death, renal failure, and mediastinitis).

Regression models provide *risk-adjusted assessment* of outcomes that is often used for *performance assessment* across groups of providers. For example, logistic regression models provide a population probability (value between zero and one) of an outcome based on multiple independent predictor variables. These probabilities are called risk-adjusted probabilities and can be defined as the predicted population outcome or *expected outcome.* Individual members of the population have an *observed outcome.* The ratio of observed outcome to predicted outcome is called *O/E ratio*, and reflects a measure of individual provider performance. There are multiple ways to assess adequacy of regression models, especially logistic regression. Hosmer and coauthors provide a particularly comprehensive, yet practical, description of regression model assessment.[16] The O/E ratio for an individual provider may give a rough estimate of risk-adjusted performance, but this measure alone does not strictly determine clinical competence or quality of care. *Cumulative sum (CUSUM) analysis* calculates provider O/E ratios over time and allows a graphical picture of performance that avoids point estimates.

LATE TIME-RELATED EVENTS

Cardiac surgeons are frequently concerned about events that occur late following operations. Special statistical methods are used to determine the long-term status of patients following operative procedures.

The most common way to estimate time-related benefit employs the *Kaplan-Meier method.* This method provides an estimate of survival (or some other later time-dependent event) probability before all patients in the cohort experience the late event. This method assumes that patients who are alive at the time of analysis have the same risk of future death as those who have already died. The graphical representation of the Kaplan-Meier model gives a survival curve and allows comparisons between survival rates associated with different interventions (eg, two different valve types). The *log-rank statistic* is used most often to compare Kaplan-Meier survival curves.

At any point in time, an individual patient has a risk of experiencing the designated endpoint. This risk of reaching the endpoint is known as the *hazard.* If death is the selected endpoint, then the hazard is the risk of dying at any point in time. The *cumulative hazard function* is the negative logarithm of the Kaplan-Meier estimated survival obtained from the survival curve.

Surgeons are often interested in the multiple factors that predict long-term survival. These factors are typically the clinical risk factors for a patient population or the type of intervention performed. *Cox regression models* provide a multivariable analysis of predictors of survival using the hazard function. Using the results of Cox models, one can calculate a *hazard ratio* (HR), which adjusts for clinical factors in the process of providing a comparison of survival for two interventions at a given time. For example, to compare the survival of CABG against the survival of percutaneous coronary intervention (PCI) at a specified time after the procedure, one could determine the HR comparing the two procedures. The HR provides the relative risk of death of CABG versus PCI for risk-adjusted populations at a given point in time. This method assumes that the hazard function is constant over time; hence the proper name *Cox proportional hazards regression.* When survival curves intersect at some point in time, the proportional hazards assumption is not met and one should then use other metrics such as the risk ratio.

Risk Adjustment and Comorbidity

MEASURES OF COMORBIDITY

Essential for the assessment of the success of cardiac operations is the ability to arrange patients according to their severity of illness. Comorbid illness in patients with cardiac disease is common. Various measures of comorbidity compile patients' risk factors into a single variable that reflects global comorbidity (Table 7-3). The comorbidity indices in Table 7-3 adjust for the incremental risk associated with specific preoperative factors variously known as risk factors, risk predictors, comorbidities, or covariates. The comorbidity systems listed in Table 7-3 are in constant evolution and use of these indices often extends to populations that include cardiac surgical patients, despite the fact that none of the indices are derived from patients undergoing cardiac procedures.

Table 7-3 compares commonly used comorbidity measures. The Charlson Index, the CIRS, the ICED, and the Kaplan Index are valid and reliable measures of comorbidity as measured in certain specific patient populations, but

not in patients undergoing cardiac operations.[17] The other comorbidity measures in Table 7-3 do not have sufficient data to assess their validity and reliability and are probably less useful than the four validated measures. There are many limitations of comorbidity indices, and they are not applied widely in studies of efficacy or medical effectiveness for cardiac operations.

RISK ADJUSTMENT SYSTEMS FOR CARDIAC OPERATIONS

Comorbidity indices, and risk factors in general, make up the variables that generate regression models that are used for risk adjustment. Most risk-adjustment models share several common features. First, the risk factors or comorbidities in the model are associated with a specific outcome. Second, if the goal is to measure provider performance, the risk factors include only patient characteristics (not hospital, physician, or regional characteristics) present prior to surgery.[18] Third, a sufficient number of patients must have the risk factor, and

---

⬤ TABLE 7-3: Characteristics and Study Populations of Commonly Used Comorbidity Indices

Comorbidity Index	Variables in the Index	Weights Used to Compute Index	Final Index Score	Population Used to Derive Index
Charlson Index	19 comorbid conditions	Relative risk for each comorbid condition derived from logistic regression of mortality	Sum of weights	Cancer patients, heart disease, pneumonia, elective noncardiac operations, amputees.
CIRS	13 body systems	Score from 0 to 4 for each body system	Sum of weights	Elderly patients many institutionalized for long-term care.
ICED	14 disease categories and 10 functional categories	Score of 1 to 5 for disease categories and 1 to 3 for functional categories	Scoring algorithm that sums up disease and functional scores to arrive at values from 1 to 4	Total hip replacements and nursing home patients.
Kaplan Index	Two categories—vascular or nonvascular disease	Graded 0 through 3 for each category	Most severe condition. Two grade 2 are ranked as grade 3	Diabetes and breast cancer.
BOD Index	59 diseases	0 through 4 for each disease	Sum of weights	Long-stay nursing home patients.
Cornoni-Huntley Index	3 categories	1—No comorbidity 2—Impaired hearing or vision 3—Heart disease, stroke or diabetes 4—Both 2 and 3	Graded 1 through 4	Hypertensive population and age > 75 years.
Disease Count	Number of diseases present based on ICD-9 codes	Sum number of diseases	Maximum score based on number of diseases	Breast cancer, MI, HIV, asthma, appendicitis, low back pain, pneumonia, diabetes, abdominal hernia.
Shwartz Index	21 comorbidities	Relative risks from model that predicts medical costs	Sum of relative risks for each comorbidity	Stroke, lung disease, heart disease, prostate cancer, hip fracture, and low back pain.

Adapted with permission from de Groot V, Beckerman H, Lankhorst GJ, Bouter LM: How to measure comorbidity. A critical review of available methods, *J Clin Epidemiol* 2003 Mar;56(3):221-229.

a sufficient number must experience the adverse outcome, in order to construct an accurate risk model. Finally, it is necessary to define the period of observation for the outcomes of interest (eg, in-hospital, 30-day mortality, or both). Table 7-4 lists risk-adjustment models used to define quality or performance based on clinical outcome measures (eg, risk of death or other adverse clinical outcomes). In addition, two of the risk adjustment models shown in Table 7-4 (the Pennsylvania Cardiac Surgery Reporting System and the Canadian Provincial Adult Cardiac Care Network of Ontario) assess risk based on resource utilization (eg, hospital length-of-stay and cost) as well as on clinical outcome measures.[19,20] Of the risk models listed in Table 7-4, only one, the APACHE III system, computes a risk score independent of patient diagnosis.[21] All of the others in the table are diagnosis-specific systems that use only patients with particular diagnoses in computing risk scores.

Once developed from a reference population, each of the risk stratification models shown in Table 7-4 is validated in some way. There are too many individual patient and procedural differences, many of them unknown or unmeasured, to allow completely accurate validated preoperative risk assessment. The most important reason that risk-adjustment methods fail to completely predict individual outcomes is that the data set used to derive the risk score comes from retrospective, observational data that contain inherent *selection bias*, that is patients were given a certain treatment that resulted in a particular outcome because a clinician had a selection bias about what treatment that particular patient should receive. In *observational datasets*, patients are not allocated to a given treatment in a randomized manner. In addition, clinician bias may not reflect evidence-based data. Methods are available that attempt to overcome some of these limitations of observational data. These methods include use of *propensity matching* and *"bootstrap" variable selection*.[22,23] Observational datasets are much more readily available and represent "real-world" treatment and outcomes compared to RCTs. An

TABLE 7-4: Examples of Risk Adjustment Models Used for Patients Undergoing Cardiac Surgical Procedures

Severity System	Data Source	Classification Approach	Outcomes Measured
APACHE III	Values of 17 physiologic parameters and other clinical information	Integer scores from 0 to 299 measured within 24 hours of ICU admission	In-hospital death
Pennsylvania	Clinical findings collected at time of admission	Probability of in-hospital death ranging from 0 to 1 based on logistic regression model and MediQual's Atlas™ admission severity score	In-hospital death and cost of procedure
New York	Condition specific clinical variables from discharge record	Probability of in-hospital death ranging from 0 to 1 based on logistic regression model	In-hospital death
Society for Thoracic Surgeons	Condition-specific clinical variables from discharge record	Originally used Bayesian algorithm to assign patient to risk interval (percent mortality interval). More recently used logistic and hierarchical regression methods	In-hospital death and morbidity
EuroSCORE	Condition specific clinical variables from discharge record	Additive logistic regression model with scores based on presence or absence of important risk factors	30-day and in-hospital mortality
Veterans Administration	Condition-specific clinical variables measured 30 days after operation	Logistic regression model used to assign patient to risk interval (percent mortality interval)	In-hospital death and morbidity
Canadian	Condition specific clinical variables entered at time of referral for cardiac surgery	Range of scores from 0 to 16 based on logistic regression odds ratio for six key risk factors	In-hospital mortality, ICU stay and postoperative length of stay
Northern New England	Condition specific clinical variables and comorbidity index entered from discharge record	Scoring system based on logistic regression coefficients used to calculate probability of operative mortality from 7 clinical variables and 1 comorbidity index	In-hospital mortality

Abbreviations: Pennsylvania = Pennsylvania Cost Containment Committee for Cardiac Surgery; New York = New York State Department of Health Cardiac Surgery Reporting System; Society for Thoracic Surgeons = Society of Thoracic Surgeons Adult Cardiac Surgery Risk Model; Veterans Administration = Veterans Administration Cardiac Surgery Risk Assessment Program; Canadian = Ontario Ministry of Health Provincial Adult Cardiac Care Network; Northern New England = Northern New England Cardiovascular Disease Study Group.

excellent review of the subtleties of evaluating the quality of risk-adjustment methods is given in the book by Iezzoni and this reference is recommended to the interested reader.[24]

Within the last decade the Society of Thoracic Surgeons (STS) published the most comprehensive set of cardiac surgery risk models yet available. Twenty-seven risk models encompassed nine endpoints for each of three major groups of cardiac procedures (isolated CABG, isolated valve, and valve + CABG).[25-27] These risk models provide the framework for measurement of risk-adjusted outcomes for cardiac operations and, ultimately, for performance assessment of individual cardiac programs or for individual providers. The NQF has endorsed most of the STS risk adjustment models for use in determining cardiac surgery quality measures (see Table 7-2).

Ideally, differences in risk-adjusted outcomes are due to differences in quality of care, but *caution is necessary in the interpretation of provider differences based on differences derived from risk adjustment models.* One study simulated the mortality experience for a hypothetical set of hospitals assuming perfect risk adjustment and with prior perfect knowledge of poor quality providers.[28] These authors used various simulation models, including Monte Carlo simulation, and found that under all reasonable assumptions, sensitivity for determining poor provider quality was less than 20% and the predictive error for determining high outliers was greater than 50%. Much of the observed mortality rate differences between high outliers and nonoutliers were attributable to random variation. Park and coauthors suggest that providers identified as high outliers using conventional risk adjustment methods do not provide lower quality care than do nonoutliers, and that most of the outcome differences are due to random variations.[29]

Performance of Risk Adjustment Models

Many risk stratification models for cardiac operations are used to assess surgical performance. Before a risk model and its component risk factors are used to evaluate provider performance, these models are tested for accuracy. Many patient variables are candidate risk factors for operative mortality following coronary revascularization. Examples include serum blood urea nitrogen (BUN), cachexia, oxygen delivery, HIV, case volume, low hematocrit on bypass, the diameter of the coronary artery, and resident involvement in the operation. On the surface, these variables seem like valid risk factors, but many are not. All putative risk factors should be subjected to rigorous scrutiny. Tests of risk model prediction including regression diagnostics (eg, *receiver operating characteristics (ROC) curves* and *cross-validation studies*) performed on the models included in Tables 7-4 suggest that the models are good, but not perfect, at predicting outcomes. In statistical terms this may mean that all of the variability in outcome measurement is not explained by the set of risk factors included in the regression models. Hence, it is possible that inclusion of new putative risk factors in the regression equations may improve the validity and precision of the models. New regression models, and new risk factors, must

be scrutinized and tested with regression diagnostics before acceptance. However, it is uncertain whether inclusion of many more risk factors will significantly improve the quality and predictive ability of regression models, and there is an ongoing tension between parsimonious models and robust models that contain many variables. For example, the STS risk stratification model described in Table 7-4 includes many predictor variables, while the Toronto risk adjustment model includes only five predictor variables. Yet the regression diagnostics for these two models are similar, suggesting that both models have equal precision and predictive capabilities for identifying outcome measures. Studies show that much of the predictive ability of risk models is contained in a relatively small number of risk factors.[30,31] Other studies suggest that the limiting factor in the accuracy of current risk models may be a failure to understand and account for all the important factors related to risk.[32] Additionally, risk models are useful for predicting the average outcome for a population of patients with specific risk factors, but not necessarily accurate for predicting the outcome for a specific patient. Further work needs to be done, both to explain the differences in risk factors seen between the various risk models and to determine which models are best suited for studies of quality improvement and performance assessment.

Study Designs to Compare Outcomes

RANDOMIZED CONTROL TRIALS

After World War II, there was a rapid expansion of therapeutic options, especially drugs, for treatment of previously untreatable acute and chronic diseases. With the advent of this new drug therapy came the introduction of RCTs to define the efficacy of various drug regimens. Archie Cochrane, a Scottish pulmonary medicine specialist, championed RCTs as the most reliable means of deciding on optimal treatment (Fig. 7-1). He suggested that RCTs were the best means of identifying interventions that have a causal influence on

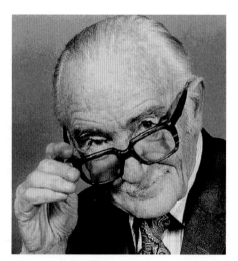

FIGURE 7-1 Portrait of Archie Cochrane and significant life events and accomplishments. (Used with permission from the Cochrane Collaboration.)

outcomes. His efforts eventually led to the creation of the Cochrane Collaboration, a repository for works of evidence-based medicine (EBM). He is arguably the father of EBM and is largely responsible for the current preeminence of RCTs as the "holy grail" of decisions about treatment options. RCTs provide the best evidence to decide about surgical treatment options for cardiac diseases, as well as providing the best means of identifying cause and effect relationships. The impact of Cochrane's insistence on wide dissemination of published high-quality evidence, including RCTs, and summaries of RCTs and observational data including *meta-analyses and systematic reviews* (collectively referred to as EBM publications), is felt today, even more than in previous decades. In 2014, a Pub Med search identified 27 EBM publications concerning various treatment options related to cardiac operations and associated diseases.

NONRANDOMIZED COMPARISONS FOR CAUSAL INFERENCE

Not every question about cardiac operations can be answered by RCTs. For many reasons the majority of the published cardiac surgical studies are *observational studies*, not RCTs. In nearly all observational studies, there may be *selection bias*. Patients underwent a treatment for nonrandom reasons. The nonrandom nature of observational studies mandates statistical methods to account for variables (usually preoperative variables) that affect the outcome (typically operative mortality and/or morbidity). Shortly after the creation of the Cochrane Collaboration in the 1970s, publications suggested that observational studies may weight outcomes in favor of new therapies, much more so than RCTs that address the same comparisons.[33] Almost 20 years later reassessment of the value of nonrandomized comparisons suggested that well-done observational studies using carefully selected controls (either *cohort or case-control designs*) do not overestimate treatment benefit.[34]

There are multiple ways to address bias in observational studies. Perhaps the most widely used technique involves careful matching of treatment and control groups using various statistical techniques, the most popular method being *propensity score matching*.[35] The propensity score is constructed in as robust a manner as possible given the population variables. Typically logistic regression with all preoperative independent variables forced into the regression equation is used to compute the propensity score for comparison of two groups.[36] Matching control and experimental groups based on their propensity scores (ie, probability of a given outcome based on the logistic regression-derived probability) provides a "pseudo-randomized" group from the total population. Comparisons using carefully matched groups approximate RCTs in most cases.[34]

STUDY DESIGN: THE TENSION BETWEEN RANDOMIZED TRIALS AND OBSERVATIONAL STUDIES

There are clear advantages and disadvantages associated with both RCT and observational studies. Because of the absence of confounding and selection bias, the RCT remains the "gold standard" for comparing results. RCTs focus on relatively small, highly select populations that may have little in common with patients typically seen in practice. Small sample size often precludes meaningful subgroup analysis and statistical analyses may be underpowered. RCTs are also quite costly and so time-consuming that results may often be outdated by the time they are reported. On the other hand, observational studies usually involve large populations of "real-world" patients. Subgroup cohorts with adequately powered statistical analysis are commonly seen in observational studies. Since these studies often use registry data, they can be carried out in a timely fashion with minimal expense. Cohort balancing using propensity scoring techniques and other statistical approaches provides useful comparisons that can approximate RCTs, but careful matching techniques for group comparisons never completely rule out bias or confounding.

GOALS OF CARDIAC SURGICAL PERFORMANCE ASSESSMENT

Using Quality Assessments to Create Guidelines

One goal of assessment of cardiac procedures is to define best practices. Wide dissemination of global assessment of cardiac operations can provide evidence that helps surgeons know the best alternative for surgical treatment of cardiovascular disorders. Recognizing the difficulties in defining "best practices" for a given illness, professional organizations opted to promote practice guidelines or "suggested therapy" for cardiac surgical diseases.[37,38] These *practice guidelines* represent a compilation of available published evidence, including randomized trials and observational studies. For example, the practice guideline for CABG is available for both practitioners and the lay public on the Internet (http://circ.ahajournals.org/content/124/23/e652.full.pdf+html).

Guidelines are a list of recommendations that have varying support in the literature. The strength of a guideline recommendation is often graded by class and by level of evidence used to support the class of recommendation. A typical rating scheme used by the STS Workforce on Evidence Based Surgery and by the Joint American College of Cardiology/American Heart Association Task Force on Practice Guidelines has three classes of recommendations as follows:

- Class I—Conditions for which there is evidence and/or general agreement that a given procedure or treatment is beneficial, useful, and effective.
- Class II—Conditions for which there is conflicting evidence and/or a divergence of opinion about the usefulness/efficacy of a procedure or treatment.
- Class IIa—Weight of evidence/opinion is in favor of usefulness/efficacy.
- Class IIb—Usefulness/efficacy is less well established by evidence/opinion.
- Class III—Conditions for which there is evidence and/or general agreement that a procedure/treatment is not useful/effective and in some cases may be harmful.

Evidence supporting the various classes of recommendations ranges from high-quality RCTs to consensus opinion of experts. Three categories describe the level of evidence used to arrive at the Class of Recommendation:

- Level A—Data derived from multiple randomized clinical trials or meta-analyses.
- Level B—Data derived from a single randomized trial or nonrandomized studies.
- Level C—Consensus opinion of experts, case studies, or standard-of-care.

Guidelines, derived from assessment of cardiac operations, provide surgeons with accepted evidence-based standards of care that most would agree upon, with an ultimate goal of limiting deviations from accepted standards.

Other Goals of Performance Assessment (Cost Containment and Altering Physician Practices)

Financial factors are a major force behind health-care reform. America's health-care costs amount to 15 to 20% of the gross national product and this figure is rising at an unsustainable rate. Institutions who pay for health care are demanding change, and these demands are fueled by studies that suggest that 20 to 30% of care is inappropriate with services both underused and overused compared to evidence-based practice standards.[39] This resulted in a shift in emphasis, with health-care costs being emphasized on equal footing with clinical outcomes of care. Sometimes health-care costs and clinical outcomes are combined into a metric that reflects *health-care value* for service rendered.

Variations in physician practice distort the allocation of health-care funds in an inappropriate way. Research suggests that there is a 17-year lag time between medical discovery and when most patients benefit from the discovery. The failure on the part of some surgeons to implement innovation has a huge cost in terms of morbidity and mortality.[40] Solutions to this problem involve altering physician practice patterns to be consistent with best available evidence, something that is difficult to achieve.[41]

Rewarding High Performers ("Pay for Performance")

Many believe that additional incentives for quality improvement can be obtained by linking quality scores to reimbursement.[42] This concept, commonly called *pay-for-performance (P4P)* or *value-based purchasing*, is supported by a variety of organizations. Effective performance-based payments show positive results in private industrial applications and, in spite of the absence of convincing evidence, there is widespread belief that similar results can be obtained in medicine. P4P is particularly popular among third party payers. Historically payment was based on the number and the complexity of services provided to patients, but with P4P, some portion of payment is determined by the quality rather than the quantity of services. It remains to be seen whether reimbursement incentives will lead to meaningful improvements in quality of care.

There are several reimbursement models associated with P4P, the most common of which is the *tournament model.* In the tournament approach, there are unequivocal winners and losers. Top performers get bonuses which come from reduced payments to the lower performers. Although popular because of its simplicity, this budget-neutral approach in which one "robs Peter to pay Paul," penalizes precisely the group which most needs financial resources for improvement.[43] Regardless of the mode of implementation, it is obvious that performance measures are destined to be an important and intrinsic part of the surgical milieu in the upcoming years.

Problems with Assessing Quality of Care—Underuse, Misuse, and Overuse

Assessing the quality of cardiac care is a worthy goal of measuring performance. However, this goal is elusive and hard to define. A major problem arises in attaining this goal because uniform definitions of quality of care are not available. Performance measures are a means of assessing cardiac surgical performance. A logical construct from measuring performance standards is that providers who do not meet the performance standards outlined by these measures are guilty of *misuse* of health-care resources. But there are other indices of health-care quality not covered by these measures, including *appropriateness of care* and *disparities in care* (eg, women and minorities often receiving substandard care). Inappropriate use of procedures is often referred to as *overuse*, and failure to provide indicated care as *underuse*. Both are found in treatment of cardiovascular diseases. For example, there is substantial geographic variation in the rates at which patients with cardiovascular diseases undergo diagnostic procedures, with little, if any, evidence that these variations affect survival or improved outcome. In one study, coronary angiography was performed in 45% of patients after acute myocardial infarction for patients in Texas compared to 30% for patients in New York State.[44] Another study showed large variations in care delivered to patients having cardiac operations.[45] Among six Veteran's Administration Medical Centers that treated very similar patients, there were large differences in the percentage of elective, urgent, and emergent cases, ranging from 58 to 96% elective, 3 to 31% urgent, and 1 to 8% emergent.[45] There was also a tenfold difference in the preoperative use of intra-aortic balloon counterpulsation for control of unstable angina, varying from 0.8 to 10.6%.[45] Similar variations in physician-specific practices exist for mitral valve procedures, carotid endarterectomy and for blood transfusion during cardiac procedures.[46-48] This variation in clinical practice may reflect uncertainty about the efficacy of available interventions or differences in practitioners' clinical judgment.

While wide differences in the use of cardiac interventions initially fueled charges of overuse in certain areas;[49] further evaluations suggest that underuse of indicated cardiac interventions (either PCI or CABG) may be a cause of this variation.[50,51] Whether caused by underuse or overuse of cardiovascular services, regional variations in resource utilization suggest that a rigorous definition of the "correct" treatment of acute myocardial infarction, as in other cardiovascular disease states, is elusive and the definition of quality of care for such patients is imperfect. Regional variations in cardiovascular care delivery are only a few of the examples of *unclear best practices*. Age, gender, race, community size, patient preference, and hospital characteristics influence utilization of diagnostic and operative interventions without much evidence that these factors should direct the appropriate treatment for various cardiac disorders.[52] While measures that define performance assessment may be a way to judge quality of care among providers, much more work needs to be done to define best practices and to limit practice variations before performance measures accurately reflect quality of care.

TYPES OF ASSESSMENT OF CARDIAC PROCEDURES

Assessment Using Operative Mortality

By far, the bulk of available experience with outcome assessment in cardiothoracic surgery deals with operative mortality, particularly in patients undergoing operative coronary revascularization (CABG). Table 7-5 is a partial list of risk models used to assess operative mortality in patients undergoing coronary revascularization. Risk stratification models like those shown in Table 7-5 evaluate mortality outcomes in CABG patients, because mortality is such an unequivocal endpoint of greatest interest to patients and is recorded with high accuracy. For the diagnosis of ischemic heart disease having operative repair, Table 7-5 lists the significant risk factors found to be important for each of the various risk stratification systems. The definition of operative mortality varies among the different systems (either 30-day mortality and/or in-hospital mortality), but the risk factors identified by each of the stratification schemes in Table 7-5 show many similarities. Regression diagnostics validated each of the models in Table 7-5; hence, there is some justification for using any of the risk stratification methods both in preoperative assessment of patients undergoing CABG and in assessing provider performance (either physicians or hospitals). Using the risk models in Table 7-5 for performance assessment of surgeons or hospitals must be done with caution, since, as described previously, risk models are imperfect. Results indicating that a provider is a statistical outlier should always be corroborated by clinical review, and preferably with constructive quality improvement initiatives.

There are many critical features of any risk-adjustment algorithm that must be considered when determining its suitability for profiling provider performance. Daley provides a summary of the key features that are necessary to validate any risk adjustment model.[53] Differences in risk-adjusted mortalities across providers may reflect differences in the process and structure of care,[54] rather than simple outcome assessment, an issue that needs further study.

Assessment Using Postoperative Morbidity and Resource Utilization

Patients with non-fatal outcomes following operations for ischemic heart disease make up more than 95% of the pool of patients undergoing operation. Obviously all non-fatal operative results are not equivalent. Patients who experience renal failure requiring lifelong dialysis, or a serious sternal wound infection, have not had the same result as a patient who leaves the hospital with no major complications, as occurs in about 85% of patients entered in the STS Database. The complications occurring in surviving patients range from serious organ system dysfunction to minor limitation or dissatisfaction with life style, and account for a significant fraction of the cost of the procedures. We estimate that as much as 40% of the yearly hospital costs for CABG are consumed by 10 to 15% of the patients who have serious complications after operation.[10,55] This is an example of a statistical principle called the *Pareto principle* and also suggests that reducing morbidity in *high-risk* cardiac surgical patients has significant impact on cost reduction.

A great deal of information exists on non-fatal complications after cardiac operations. Several large databases identify risk factors for both non-fatal morbidity and increased resource utilization. Table 7-6 is a summary of some of the risk factors identified by available risk stratification models that are associated with either serious postoperative morbidity or increased resource utilization as measures of undesirable outcomes.

For many years, operative mortality was the sole criterion for a successful CABG procedure. This concept gave way to a broader focus on the entire hospitalization associated with CABG. There is universal agreement that non-fatal complications play a central role in the assessment of CABG quality, but many morbidity outcomes are relatively difficult to define and track. Risk adjustment is particularly difficult because of the fact that risk factors for most complications are not well-established. The low frequency of some complications also creates statistical challenges.

Shroyer and coworkers used part of the large national experience captured in the *STS Database* to examine five important postoperative CABG complications: stroke, renal failure, reoperation within 24 hours after CABG, prolonged (>24 hours) postoperative ventilation, and mediastinitis.[56] Revised morbidity models using contemporary statistical approaches followed this landmark study by Shroyer and coworkers.[26,57,58] In 2009, the STS morbidity risk models were updated using data from 2002 to 2006, with specific models for isolated CABG, isolated valve, and combined CABG + valve procedures. Given the contemporary data and large reference populations, these risk models will undoubtedly play an important role in future attempts at performance assessment.

Patient Satisfaction as an Outcome

Patients' assessment of surgical outcome is an alternate means of judging performance. There are several difficulties with

TABLE 7-5: Published Variables Used in Risk Assessment Models to Predict Coronary Bypass Surgical Mortality

Risk Model	STS	NYS	Canada	USA	VA	Australia	Canada2	NNE	Japan
Number of Patients	774,881	174,210	57,187	50,357	13,368	12,712	12,003	3654	24,704
No. of Risk Factors	29	29	16	13	6	9	5	9	17
Age	X	X	X		X	X	X	X	X
Gender	X	X	X	X	X		X		
Surgical urgency	X	X		X	X	X		X	X
Ejection fraction	X	X	X		X		X	X	X
Renal dysfunction	X	X	X	X				X	X
Creatinine	X								
Previous CABG	X	X		X				X	X
NYHA class		X	X	X		X			X
Left main disease	X	X	X					X	
Diseased coronary vessels	X	X	X		X				
Peripheral vascular disease	X	X		X		X			
Diabetes mellitus	X	X	X		X				
Cerebrovascular disease	X	X		X		X			X
Intraop/postop variables				X			X		
Myocardial infarction	X	X	X	X					
Body size	X	X	X						
Preoperative IABP	X	X	X			X			
Cardiogenic shock/unstable	X	X	X					X	X
COPD	X	X	X						X
PTCA	X	X		X					
Angina	X		X				X		
Intravenous nitrates		X				X			
Arrhythmias		X							X
History of heart operation	X		X			X			
Hemodynamic instability	X	X							
Charlson comorbidity score								X	
Dialysis dependence	X	X	X						X
Valvular heart disease	X								X
Pulmonary hypertension		X							
Diuretics		X				X			
Systemic hypertension	X								
Serum albumin									
Race	X	X							
Previous CHF	X							X	X
Myocardial infarction timing	X	X							
Cardiac index									
LV end-diastolic pressure									
CVA timing	X	X							
Liver disease				X					
Neoplasia/Metastatic disease				X					
Ventricular aneurysm				X					
Steroids/Antiplatelet drugs/other drugs	X	X							X

Reproduced with permission from Grunkemeier GL, Zerr KJ, Jin R: Cardiac surgery report cards: making the grade. Ann Thorac Surg. 2001 Dec;72(6):1845-1848.

TABLE 7-6: Risk Factors Associated with Either Increased Length of Stay (L) or Increased Incidence of Organ Failure Morbidity (M) or Both (L/M) Following Coronary Revascularization

Risk Factor	STS[56]	STS Updated[27]	Boston[128]	Albany[55]	VA[129]	Canada[130]
Demographics						
Advanced age	M	M	L		M	L
Low preoperative red blood cell volume	M			L/M		
Race		M				
Female gender	M	M				L
Disease-specific diagnoses						
CHF	M	M	L	L/M	M	
Concomitant valve disease	M	M			M	L
Reoperation	M	M			M	L
LV dysfunction (ejection fraction)	M	M				L
Surgical priority	M	M			M	L
3-Vessel disease		M				
IABP preop	M	M	L			
Active endocarditis					M	
Left-main disease		M				
Preoperative atrial fibrillation		M				
Comorbid conditions						
Obesity		M	L			
Renal dysfunction	M	M	L	L	M	
Diabetes		M				
Peripheral vascular disease	M	M		L	M	
Chronic obstructive lung disease	M	M		L		
Cerebrovascular disease	M	M		L/M		
Hypertension	M	M		L/M		
Immunosuppression		M				

Abbreviations: CHF = congestive heart failure; LV = left ventricular; IABP = intra-aortic balloon pump.

measurement of PRO, and consequently cardiothoracic surgeons are not deeply involved with systematic measurements of patient satisfaction after operation. Considerable research deals with instruments that measure patient satisfaction. At least two of these instruments, the *Short-Form Health Survey or SF-36*[59] and the *San Jose Medical Group's Patient Satisfaction Measure*,[60] are used to monitor patient satisfaction over time. The current status of these and other measures of patient satisfaction does not allow accurate comparisons among providers, because the quality of the data generated by these measures is poor. These instruments are characterized by low response rates, inadequate sampling, infrequent use, and unavailability of satisfactory benchmarks. Nonetheless, available evidence indicates that feedback on patient satisfaction data to physicians may impact physician practices.[61] Managed care organizations and hospitals use PRO measures to compare institutions and individual providers.

Risk stratification methodology can identify patients who are optimal candidates for coronary revascularization based on quality of life and functional status considerations. Multivariate risk factors associated with unimproved postoperative quality of life after CABG include female gender,[62] patients with depressive disorders,[63] and operations complicated by sternal wound infection.[64] One comparative study found no difference between patients older than 65 years and those younger than or equal to 65 with regard to quality of life outcomes after cardiac operations (symptoms, cardiac functional class, activities of daily living, and emotional and social functioning).[65] This study identified a direct relationship between clinical severity and quality of life indicators, since patients with less comorbid conditions and better preoperative functional status had better quality of life indicators six months after operation than those with significant comorbidities. In contrast, Rumsfeld and coworkers found that improvement in the self-reported quality of life (from Form SF-36) was more likely in patients who had relatively poor health status before CABG compared to those who had relatively good preoperative health status.[66] Interestingly, these same authors found that poor preoperative self-reported quality of life indicator was an independent predictor of operative mortality following CABG.[67] These findings suggest that the risks of patient dissatisfaction after CABG are poorly understood but may be dependent on preoperative comorbid factors as well as on the indications for, and technical complexities of, the operation itself. At present, there is no well-established risk model to identify patients who are likely to report dissatisfaction with operative intervention following CABG.

USING DATA TO IMPROVE PERFORMANCE—CASE STUDIES

Management Philosophy and Performance Assessment

American health care made almost unbelievable strides in the last 100 years. We are at the brink of being able to treat disease at the genotypic molecular level. Further, cardiac surgeons treat patients considered inoperable as recently as a decade ago. Yet almost no one is happy with the health-care system. It costs too much, excludes many, is inefficient, and is ignorant about its own effectiveness. A similar state of confusion existed with Japanese industry after World War II. Out of the confusion and crisis of post–World War II, Japan became a monolith of efficiency. Two major architects of this transformation were an American statistician, W. Edwards Deming,

and a Romanian-American theoretician, J. M. Juran. They led the way in establishing and implementing certain principles of management and efficiency based on quality. Their efforts are recognized in Japan by the annual awarding of the *Deming Prizes* in recognition of achievements in attaining high quality. Deming's and Juran's books are some of the classics of quality management in industry.[68,69]

Deming's and Juran's management philosophy are sometimes referred to as *total quality management* or *TQM*. The amazing turn-around in Japanese industry led many organizations to embrace and modify the principles of TQM, including organizations involved in delivery and assessment of health care. Table 7-7 outlines the key features of TQM. A TQM project starts from critical observations. For example, excessive blood transfusion after operation may result in increased morbidity, including disease transmission, increased infection risk, and increased cost. Tools such as *flow diagrams* that document all of the steps in the process are used in a TQM project (eg, steps involved in the blood transfusion process after CABG). A logical starting point for efforts to improve the quality of the blood transfusion process would be to focus on a high-risk subset of patients who consume a disproportionate amount of blood resources. An Italian

---

⬤ TABLE 7-7: Principles of Total Quality Management (TQM) Applied to Health Care

Principle	Explanation
Health-care delivery is a process.	The purpose of a process is to *add value* to the input of the process. Each person in an organization is part of one or more processes.
Quality defects arise from problems with the process.	Former reliance on quotas, numerical goals, and discipline of workers is unlikely to improve quality, since these measures imply that workers are at fault and that quality will get better if workers do better. The problem is with the process not with the worker. Quality improvement involves "driving out fear" on the part of the worker, and breaking down barriers between departments so that everyone may work effectively as a team for the organization.
Customer-supplier relationships are the most important aspect of quality.	A *customer is anyone who depends on the organization*. The goal of quality improvement is to improve constantly and to establish a long-term relationship of loyalty and trust between customer (patient) and supplier (health-care organization) and, thereby, meet the needs of the patient. The competitive advantage for an organization that can better meet the needs of the customer is obvious. The organization will gain market share, reduce costs, and waste less effort in activities that do not add value for patients.
Understand the causes of variability.	Failure to *understand variation in critical processes* within the organization is the cause of many serious quality problems. Unpredictable processes are flawed and are difficult to study and assess. Managers must understand the difference between random (or common-cause) variation and special variation in a given outcome.
Develop new organizational structures.	*Managers are leaders not enforcers*. Eliminate management by objective numerical goals. Remove barriers that rob workers of their right to pride of workmanship. Empower everybody in the organization to achieve the transformation to a quality product.
Focus on the most "vital few" processes.	This is known as the *Pareto principle* (first devised by Juran) and states that whenever a number of individual factors contribute to an outcome, relatively few of those items account for the bulk of the effect. By focusing on the "vital few," the greatest reward for effort will occur.
Quality reduces cost.	*Poor quality is costly*. Malpractice suits, excessive use of costly laboratory tests, and unnecessarily long hospital stay, are examples of costly poor quality. The premise that it is too costly to implement quality control is incorrect.
Statistics and scientific thinking are the foundation of quality.	Managers must make decisions based on *accurate data*, using *scientific methods*. Not only managers, but all members of the organization, utilize the scientific method for improving processes as part of their normal daily activity.

economist, Vilfredo Pareto, made the observation that a relatively few factors account for the majority of the outcomes of a complex process. This has been termed the *Pareto Principle*, also known as the *"80-20 rule."* Juran was one of the first to apply this principle to manufacturing in the United States and Japan.[69] In medicine, this principle is commonly used to point out that most of the observed complications come from a small part of the overall patient population. Applying the Pareto Principle, one should logically focus attention not on the entire population, but rather on that small population associated with the majority of the problem. A graphical method of identifying the spectrum of outcomes in a process is included in most statistics programs, and is termed a Pareto diagram. Figure 7-2 is an example of a Pareto diagram for blood product transfusion in cardiac operations. Figure 7-2 suggests that about 20% of the patients consume 80% of the blood products transfused following cardiac procedures. Substantial savings in cost and morbidity should result by focusing on decreasing the amount of blood transfusion in these 20% "high-end" users. For TQM purposes, strategies can be devised and tested to decrease blood product consumption in the high-risk subset, and ultimately, monitors are set up to measure the effectiveness of the new strategies. Other tools of TQM such as data sampling strategies and use of control charts play an important role in the process.

One example of using the principles of TQM to improve patient care is to isolate high-risk subsets obtained from population-based risk models. These retrospective risk models (ie, effectiveness studies) are examined to define key elements of the processes of care that contribute to outcomes. The key components of the process are then used as test interventions to improve outcome in high-risk subsets using RCTs (ie, efficacy studies). For example, a population-based risk model of postoperative blood transfusion revealed that the following factors were significantly associated with excessive blood transfusion (defined as more than 4 units of blood products after CABG): (1) template bleeding time, (2) red blood cell volume, (3) cardiopulmonary bypass time, and (4) advanced age.[70] Based on these retrospective effectiveness studies, investigators hypothesized that process improvement interventions aimed at reducing blood transfusion after CABG would most likely benefit high-risk patients with prolonged bleeding time and low red blood cell volume. A prospective clinical trial tested this hypothesis using two components of the blood conservation process, platelet-rich plasma saving and normovolemic hemodilution, in patients undergoing CABG. Results showed that these two blood conservation interventions reduced bleeding and blood transfusion only in the high-risk subset of patients.[71] These studies imply that more costly interventions such as use of platelet-rich plasma savers are more efficacious in high-risk patients, with the high-risk subset defined by risk stratification methodologies. This approach of using observational risk adjustment models to devise and test hypotheses using efficacy studies is a valuable use of risk assessment models and embodies principles of TQM.

A limitation of any outcomes-based quality improvement project is that knowing outcomes does not necessarily provide the answer to producing better outcomes, rather, it requires the elements of TQM to make meaningful advances. The principles of TQM, including transparent self-assessment and identification of process deficits, are the foundations of quality improvement. Participating in databases like the STS Adult Cardiac Surgery database or the American College of Surgeons National Surgical Quality Improvement Project database does not guarantee adequate performance assessment and quality improvement.[72,73] Leadership, educational tools, EBM guidelines, practice standards, and benchmarking of improvement processes are important, and essential, additions to outcomes measurement for quality improvement.

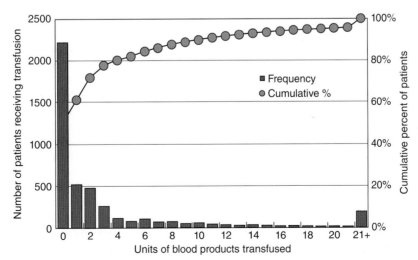

FIGURE 7-2 Pareto diagram of blood transfusion in 4457 patients undergoing cardiac procedures over a 4 year period. (Reproduced with permission from Ferraris VA, Ferraris SP, Saha SP, et al.: Perioperative blood transfusion and blood conservation in cardiac surgery: the Society of Thoracic Surgeons and The Society of Cardiovascular Anesthesiologists clinical practice guideline, *Ann Thorac Surg* 2007 May;83(5 Suppl):S27-86.)

STS Database and Quality Improvement—Transparent Risk Assessment

The *STS* recognized a compelling need for a national standard in cardiac surgery as early as 1986 with the creation of an STS committee to develop a national database of cardiac surgery. This committee gathered and analyzed data in order to establish a national standard of care in cardiac surgery. The *STS Database* is a voluntary registry that currently collects perioperative patient data from more than 90% of cardiac centers in the United States. Individual participant sites enter extensive clinical data on each patient undergoing cardiac surgery. This information is harvested quarterly and aggregated at the *Duke Clinical Research Institute* (DCRI). The data are analyzed and reports, which include *benchmark data* and risk-adjusted outcomes, are provided to each site. This reporting process allows sites to pinpoint areas in need of improvement so that tailored quality assessment and performance improvement programs can be developed. The database has numerous important practical applications that allow performance assessment and document workload.

The STS database allows accurate determination of thoracic surgeons' workload. Much of the recommendations for surgeon reimbursement stems from the *American Medical Association/Specialty Society Relative Value Scale Update Committee, or RUC* (rhymes with "truck") for short. The RUC's recommendations to the Centers for Medicare and Medicaid Services (CMS) influence the relative values assigned to physician services and, as a result, how much physicians are paid. STS data allows monitoring of trends in the patient profile of cardiac surgery patients over the years. This kind of information impacts negotiations with RUC. Deliberations with the RUC were traditionally based on small surveys but the use of STS data allowed a more accurate presentation of objective information that provides a truly fair and meaningful workload analysis.[74]

The STS database reporting and feedback process to individual sites produced impressive *performance improvements in surgical outcomes*. Database information showed a progressive increase in CABG operative risk from 1993 to 2008. In spite of this risk increase, the observed operative mortality steadily declined from over 4% to approximately 2% during this period. Improvements in process measures like use of the IMA in CABG accompanied these impressive advances in outcome measures.

Peer-Directed Outcomes Assessment

A superb example of a TQM-based approach to improving cardiac surgery quality is the Northern New England Cardiovascular Study Group (NNECVDSG). Founded in 1987, this voluntary consortium of clinicians, scientists, and administrators represents cardiac surgery programs in Northern New England. Its mission is to study and improve the quality of cardiovascular care provided to patients through the use of systematic data collection and feedback. Shortly after its formation, this group developed and validated a logistic risk

model to account for case mix differences across its member institutions.[75] Using this model, the group analyzed CABG outcomes for 3055 patients operated upon at five medical centers in Maine, New Hampshire and Vermont between July 1987 and April 1989.[76] Overall unadjusted CABG mortality was 4.3% but this varied substantially among centers (3.1 to 6.3%). Even after case-mix adjustment, significant variability persisted among medical centers ($p = 0.021$) and surgeons ($p = 0.025$). In 1990, the NNECVDSG initiated a regional intervention aimed at reducing both absolute CABG mortality and inter-institutional variability.[76] The three major components of this TQM approach included feedback of outcomes data, training in continuous quality improvement techniques, and site visits to each program. During the latter, visitors from each discipline focused on the practice of their counterparts at the host institutions. Numerous changes were implemented as a result of these site visits including technical aspects, processes of care, personnel organization and training, decision-making, and methods of evaluating care. Following these interventions, observed mortality declined to less than expected in all categories of patient acuity.

Following publication of these landmark papers, the Northern New England consortium continued to grow in size, and their registry forms the basis for numerous publications aimed at improving the care of cardiac surgical patients. Their publications cover a wide range of topics including the impact of preoperative variables on hospital and long-term mortality, the optimal conduct of cardiopulmonary perfusion, the prevention of specific postoperative complications, on-pump versus off pump CABG operations, and modes of death following CABG.[77-79] Over two decades since its inception, the NNECVDSG serves at the "poster child" of efforts to improve cardiac surgery quality through voluntary, confidential, and collaborative TQM.

CONTROVERSIES IN THE ASSESSMENT OF PERFORMANCE

Dangers of Outcome Assessment

After the introduction of provider report cards in New York and Pennsylvania in the early 1990s, studies emerged suggesting that providers were changing their practice patterns in response to public reporting. The release of risk-adjusted data may alienate providers and result in the sickest patients having less accessibility to care. This may have happened in New York State[80] and in other regions where risk-adjusted mortality and cost data were released to the public.

Of even more concern is the selection bias that may exist in managed care Health Maintenance Organization (HMO) enrollment. Morgan and coworkers suggested that Medicare HMOs benefit from the selective enrollment of healthier Medicare recipients and the dis-enrollment or outright rejection of sicker beneficiaries.[81] This form of separation of patients into unfavorable or favorable risk categories is a direct result of risk assessment and may be an unintended consequence of performance assessment methodology. This type of discrimination undermines the effectiveness and appropriateness of care. Omoigui and colleagues addressed this issue in a report about the effect of publication of surgeon-specific report cards in New York state.[82] These authors concluded that surgeons in that state were less willing to operate on high-risk patients. Patients in New York state were subsequently transferred in disproportionately large numbers to the Cleveland Clinic, where both their expected and observed adverse outcomes exceeded those of other referral areas without report cards. Although some public figures challenged this "outmigration" phenomenon, additional studies in New York and Pennsylvania suggest that the concept of risk aversion may have some validity.[83,84] Subsequent and more comprehensive analyses of CABG public reporting in New York state could not document any systematic exclusion of high-risk patients from CABG operations, and showed that the severity of illness and comorbidities of operated patients actually increased over the years.[85,86] There may be some degree of risk aversion in public reporting environments, and this could result in denial of care to the high-risk patients that might benefit most from intervention. Others suggest that it may redirect such patients to the most experienced providers, which could be a more positive result.[87]

Validity and Reliability of Assessment Methods

ACCURACY OF DATABASES—ADMINISTRATIVE VERSUS CLINICAL DATA

Perhaps the most important tool of any outcome assessment endeavor is a database that is made up of a representative sample of the study group of interest. The accuracy of the data elements in any such database cannot be overemphasized. Factors such as the source of data, the outcome of interest, the methods used for data collection, standardized definitions of the data elements, data reliability checking, and the time frame of data collection are essential features that must be considered when either constructing a new database or deciding about using an existing database.[88]

Data obtained from *claims or administrative databases* are less reliable than those obtained from *clinical databases*. Because claims data are generated for the collection of bills, their clinical accuracy is inadequate and it is likely that these databases overestimate complications for billing purposes. They may incorrectly classify some surgical procedures, and this in turn may result in erroneous and misleading outcomes results.[89,90] Furthermore, claims data underestimate the effects of comorbid illness and contain major deficiencies in important prognostic variables for CABG, such as left ventricular function and number of diseased vessels. The Duke Databank for Cardiovascular Disease found major discrepancies between clinical and claims databases, with claims data failing to identify more than half of the patients with important comorbid conditions such as congestive heart failure (CHF), cerebrovascular disease, and angina.[91] The quality of databases used to generate comparisons cannot be overemphasized.

Health-care experts recognize the shortcomings of claims or administrative databases. The primary reason for continued reliance on these types of data sources is their ease of use and readily available access. Current information suggests that discharge coding accuracy is the major problem in the use of administrative databases for outcomes comparisons. Recent reviews found that coding accuracy improved with renewed emphasis on accuracy.[92] It is likely that the low cost and ready availability of administrative data will continue and even increase as health-care resources are ratcheted down.

LOGISTIC REGRESSION AND HIERARCHICAL REGRESSION MODELS

One of the most common yet controversial applications of logistic regression models is provider profiling, sometimes mandated by governmental organizations,[93,94] in which case the results are usually published as report cards and made available to the public. The statistical methodology previously used to develop most such report cards is straightforward. The probability of mortality for each of a provider's patients during a given time period is estimated using logistic regression or some other multivariate method based on a large database containing multiple surgeons' patients. These probabilities are aggregated to determine a particular provider's expected mortality, or E. The observed mortality, O, is simply the counted number of operative deaths. An *O/E ratio* has a value close to one if the performance is what would be predicted from the model. Ratios significantly greater than 1.0 imply worse than expected performance, and ratios significantly less than 1.0 suggest better than expected performance. Often, the O/E ratios are multiplied by the population unadjusted mortality rate to obtain the *risk-adjusted mortality ratio* (RAMR).

Statisticians realize that, although intuitively appealing, it is not ideal to aggregate patient-level data to make inferences about providers using logistic regression.[93] Assessing operative mortality among hospitals and among surgeons is inherently multilevel. Multiple levels exist that may alter operative mortality, including surgeons, hospitals, referring physicians, etc. In such situations simply aggregating between levels may lead to erroneous conclusions. Multilevel or *hierarchical models* are available for such situations. These models address most of the major concerns regarding the use of standard logistic regression models. Hierarchical models "shrink" the observed mortality rates of lower volume providers toward the mean of the overall population of providers, a way of borrowing strength or pooling the data from multiple levels of hospitals and providers. The resulting estimates are more accurate and stable. Standard logistic models do not accurately partition the multiple levels of variability (between and within providers), which is one of the central questions to be answered by profiling. Hierarchical models correctly partition this variability and account for sample size variation and compensate for multiple comparisons. Numerous studies investigated the difference in the results of provider profiling obtained from traditional logistic regression versus hierarchical modeling. For example, Goldstein and Spiegelhalter compared a hierarchical model of operative mortality of surgeons in New York state to a traditional single level logistic model, and found reduced number of surgeon outliers using the hierarchical models.[95] A logical objection to the use of hierarchical models is that, by reducing the chance of false outlier identification, it may also reduce the sensitivity to detect true outliers. Ultimately, this tradeoff is a health policy and regulatory decision.[93] Hierarchical models are complex and require not only extensive computer resources but also close planning and oversight by a statistician experienced in these methods. Most investigators regard them as the best model for multi-level comparisons, and hierarchical modeling is used both by the state of Massachusetts and by the STS for the development of provider profiles.

The Downside of Performance Assessment

COST AND IMPERFECTION

Collecting risk-adjusted data for performance assessment and quality improvement adds to the administrative costs of the health-care system. It is estimated that 20% of health-care costs ($150–$180 billion/year) are spent on the administration of health care.[96] The costs of implementing a risk-adjustment system are substantial. Additional costs are incurred in implementing quality measures that are suggested by risk-stratification methodology. A disturbing notion is that the costs of performance assessment may outweigh the payers' willingness to pay for these benefits. For example, Iowa hospitals estimated that they spent $2.5 million annually to gather MedisGroups severity data that was mandated by the state. Because of the cost, the state abandoned this mandate and concluded that neither consumers nor purchasers used the data anyway.[97] Similarly, reports suggest that public release of quality indicators neither improves composite hospital performance nor changes consumer behavior.[98,99] It is possible that quality improvement may cost rather than save money; although one of the principles of TQM (often quoted by Deming) is that the least expensive means to accomplish a task (eg, deliver health care) is the means that employs the highest quality in the process. Ultimately, improved quality will be cost-efficient, but start-up costs may be daunting. In order to be cost-effective, any cost savings realized from performance assessment must be factored into the total costs of gathering risk-adjusted data and implementing performance improvement. Further, given the considerable costs of a single serious complication, such as stroke, dialysis-dependent renal failure, or a sternal infection, the cost savings of avoiding these complications using performance assessment and quality improvement programs may be substantial.

INTERPRETATION OF RISK-ADJUSTED OUTCOMES

One of the least well understood aspects of performance report cards is the correct interpretation of risk-adjusted or risk-standardized outcomes, which are derived by comparing observed outcomes with those predicted by statistical risk models. There is a tendency by the public, by insurance companies, and by government officials to regard Risk-Adjusted Mortality Ratios (eg, O/E ratios) and Risk-adjusted or Standardized Mortality Rates as the ultimate metric of provider performance. Compared to unadjusted rates these are certainly superior approaches, but their limitations must be recognized. First, all risk models are only approximations of reality, and they cannot adjust for all possible combinations of risk factors. These models are useful for predicting population average outcomes given a particular patient mix, but they are less useful for predicting the outcome for specific patients and providers. Second, even if there were perfect risk adjustment, the results for a particular provider must be correctly interpreted. The risk-standardized or risk-adjusted mortality for a hospital reflects its performance for its specific patient case mix, compared to what would have been expected had these same patients been cared for by an average provider in the reference population. Because *indirect* rather than *direct standardization* is used for virtually all risk models used in profiling, it may not be appropriate to directly compare the risk-adjusted results of one institution with those of another. The risk-adjusted mortality of a small community hospital is based largely on a low-risk population. Even though it is adjusted, it cannot be compared directly to the risk-adjusted rate of a quaternary referral center, which is based largely on a population of patients that the community program rarely if ever sees. In this extreme example, these two hospitals may have virtually no types of patients in common, and even though their rates are adjusted they should not be directly compared with one another.

RANKING PROVIDERS—LEAGUE TABLES VERSUS FUNNEL PLOTS

There is a problem with report cards of provider results that appear in the lay press and on the Internet. Most report cards rank providers in the form of *league tables*, similar to tables used in sports to rank teams or individuals. League tables always have someone on top and someone on the bottom. In general, the public does not understand that there is no meaningful difference for the vast majority of names published in league tables of cardiac surgeons' performance.[100] The limited sample size of any individual surgeon or hospital leads to wide fluctuation in outcomes over time. Reporting of one surgeon as being better (ie, higher in the league table) than another is inaccurate and probably unethical. Spiegelhalter addressed this concern and suggested better options for reporting surgeons' and hospitals' results.[101] He advocated *funnel plots* as a far better alternative than league tables to report provider outcomes. A funnel plot is a plot of individual surgeons' volume (x-axis) versus risk-adjusted mortality (y-axis) with population confidence intervals. The plot allows immediate identification of outliers (ie, providers outside the confidence intervals) and gives the viewer an estimate of the larger uncertainties (ie, increased confidence intervals) of risk-adjusted mortality of low-volume providers compared to high-volume providers. The limits of uncertainty (ie, *control limits*) form a funnel around the provider outcome. The United Kingdom Central Cardiac Audit Database (http://www.ic.nhs.uk/services/national-clinical-audit-support-programme-ncasp/

heart-disease/adult-cardiac-surgery) and the STS Congenital Heart Surgery Database Report use funnel plots to identify outliers.[100]

FUTURE DIRECTIONS

Effectiveness, Appropriateness, Guidelines, and Standards

EFFECTIVENESS VERSUS SAFETY

Since the IOM report on medical errors that appeared in 2000,[2] reducing medical errors both by physicians and by hospitals garnered significant resources. Since then, several authors suggested that the culture of safety in hospitals is unchanged.[102,103] Brennan and coauthors point out that the IOM distinguishes safety from effectiveness. *Effectiveness* is defined as an evidence-based intervention that improves quality, whereas *safety* encompasses a much narrower definition of limiting accidental injury.[102] These authors suggest redirection of health-care goals toward effectiveness interventions and away from accident reduction interventions. An important advantage of focus on effectiveness is the ease with which effectiveness outcomes can be measured compared to safety outcomes. There is some evidence that focus on evidence-based interventions (eg, providing aspirin to cardiac patients when they leave the hospital) improves the effectiveness of treatment with secondary benefit of reducing errors.[104] Furthermore, there is still a reluctance to deal transparently with medical mistakes and identifying problems with safety may be difficult. Health-care providers may not spend significantly increased resources on safety and error management largely because the return on this type of investment is very hard to measure. On the other hand, quality improvement efforts based on evidence of effectiveness are likely to be more readily embraced and may save more lives than will safety-related interventions that lack an evidence base.[102]

PRACTICE GUIDELINES AND APPROPRIATENESS CRITERIA

An important part of implementing effectiveness of care is knowing what evidence-based interventions represent best practice. *Practice guidelines provide evidence-based recommendations* for cardiovascular interventions and serve as a template for effectiveness.[37] Professional societies attempted to enhance adherence to evidence-based practice guidelines by introducing *appropriateness criteria*. Appropriateness criteria are lists of appropriate indications for interventions in common clinical scenarios based on available evidence. They document indications for drug or device intervention with a scale metric. For example, the AHA/ACC/STS Joint Task Force generated appropriateness criteria for coronary revascularization that used a scale of 1 to 10.[105] Values of 7 through 10 indicated that coronary revascularization is appropriate for patients with a particular set of risk factors. Scores of 1 to 3 indicate revascularization is inappropriate and unlikely to improve health outcomes or survival. The mid-range scores

(4–6) suggests that improvement in survival or other health-care outcomes with coronary revascularization is uncertain. The aim of appropriateness criteria is to guide physician decision making toward use of evidence-based interventions. It is likely that expansion of the appropriateness criteria concept will occur.

GUIDELINES VERSUS STANDARDS

Practice guidelines gained a hallowed position in the hierarchy of evidence starting with Archie Cochrane in the 1950s (see Fig. 7-1). Cochrane championed RCTs as a means of testing medical hypotheses in order to make decisions about best treatment for diseases. His work ultimately led to establishment of the Cochrane Collaboration and the Cochrane Library, a repository of RCTs, meta-analyses, and systematic reviews. Cochrane is arguably the father of EBM, although his definition of EBM in the 1960s was much narrower than the current definition. Today's definition of EBM encompasses practice guidelines that reflect available evidence. The basic principles of EBM are that decisions about medical care should be based on research and that these research recommendations should be ranked based on specific norms (ie, the level of evidence).

Several pieces of evidence suggest that adherence to guidelines and incorporation into clinical practice is suboptimal.[106-108] For example, blood conservation guidelines for cardiac surgery developed by the STS were circulated widely and are among the most cited articles in the thoracic surgery literature.[37] Nonetheless, wide variation in the transfusion of blood products in patients having a standard operation for coronary revascularization persists.[109] A Physician Consortium of the American Medical Association and The Joint Commission identified transfusion as one of the five most overused procedures in the United States (http://www.jointcommission.org/overuse_summit/).

There are many reasons for guideline nonadherence,[106] but it is apparent that implementation strategies need to accompany evidence-based recommendations and dissemination. Professional organizations recognize the limits of guideline development and take a different approach to implementation of evidence-based recommendations. These implementation strategies have various names like standardized practice design, standardized EBM protocol, evidence-based algorithm, decision aids, or perhaps most euphemistically, "organizational recommendations." Collectively implementation strategies define a term called *practice standards*. Standards are a means of operationalizing EBM and practice guidelines. For example, the Society for the Advancement of Blood Management (SABM) recognized the limitations of blood management guidelines as a means of improving transfusion practice. SABM developed blood management practice standards to address this problem. This organization defined twelve patient blood management standards that operationalize blood conservation guidelines and provide a roadmap for the creation of an infrastructure that leads to implementation of evidence-based guidelines. Simply stated, *standards allow conversion of guidelines into bedside practice*. Accompanying the standards are hard outcome measures that are monitored by multidisciplinary teams. The efforts that go into creating standards parallel the rigor accompanying development of guidelines. While guidelines reflect available evidence, standards indicate how to implement EBM and monitor the success of those efforts in a continuing cycle of implementation and measurement. The introduction of practice standards guides quality assessment, and their increased use is virtually assured given the changing health-care environment.

Human Factors Research and Performance Assessment

Surgeons make errors in the operating room. The causes of these errors and their ultimate impact on outcomes are an important measure of performance. Human factors are responsible for many errors that affect performance. Human factors research is concerned primarily with the performance of one or more persons in a task-oriented environment interacting with equipment, other people, or both. Structured observation of surgeons by experts in human factor analysis can provide performance assessment and improve outcomes.[110] The airline industry had success in limiting errors by instituting human factor analysis of pilots during simulated flight. This industry is used as a model of successful implementation of error avoidance behavior and process improvement.[111] Several authors report application of these same principles of human factors analysis to pediatric cardiac operations with some success.[112,113] They employed self-assessment questionnaires and human factors researchers who observed behavior in the operating room, an approach similar to the quality improvement steps used in the airline industry. These studies highlight the important role of human factors in adverse surgical outcomes. More importantly, they found that appropriate behavioral responses in the operating room can mitigate potentially harmful events during operation. Such studies emphasize that human factors are associated with outcomes, both good and bad. Behavior modification and process improvement that involves human factor analysis hold promise for error reduction in cardiac surgery.

Public Reporting and Provider Accountability

Today there is an unprecedented call for accountability and public reporting. That call comes from consumer groups and insurers as it has in the past, but today it is coming from governmental organizations including the US Congress as well. There is now federal legislative force mandating the collection and the release of this information. The Centers for Medicare and Medicaid Services (CMS), for example, made it quite clear that their upcoming "pay for performance" programs will include mandated public reporting of data.

The World Wide Web provides ready access to a wide variety of medical facts, particularly concerning cardiothoracic surgery. Simple Internet searches provide the public with literature reviews of cardiac procedures, the results of randomized trials, new innovations, and surgeon and hospital-specific

outcomes. This ready public access will undoubtedly increase. There is limited external scrutiny or validation of many of the information sources. Most information available on these sites is accepted at face value by the public and quality control of the information sources is limited to self-imposed efforts on the part of the website authors. The *Agency for Healthcare Research and Quality (AHRQ)* attempted to empower the public to critically evaluate the various web-based sources of health-care information in order to limit the spread of misinformation. The success of the AHRQ efforts is uncertain but becomes extremely critical as the amount of health-care information available on the web skyrockets.

The goal of public reporting of performance is to empower consumers to seek optimal care and to modify provider practices to improve outcomes. The ability of public reporting of performance to accomplish these goals is uncertain. Evidence suggests that public reporting does not accomplish any of these stated goals. A Cochrane Review found that public release of performance data neither changes consumer behavior nor improves care.[99] Despite shortcomings associated with web-based public information sources, the national cry for public reporting continues unabated. Recognizing the inevitability of this national movement, the *STS* initiated a project to develop a *public reporting* format that contains clinical data that is meaningful, audited, totally transparent and clinically relevant both for physicians and for the public. In collaboration with *Consumers Union*, the STS began publishing the composite CABG performance measures for those program participants that agreed to do so.[114,115] This information appeared in *Consumer's Report* and was one of the most widely read issues of this magazine ever (http://www.consumerreports.org/cro/2011/08/looking-for-a-heart-surgeon/index.htm). There is obvious public interest in information transparency about cardiac operations. The uncertainty is how, or if, the public changes behavior in response to this publically available information. This type of partnership may well become the paradigm for other professional organizations as they manage public reporting. Public reporting of cardiac surgical outcomes provides transparency and has public appeal.

Information Management: Electronic Medical Records

Medical records are an invaluable source of information about patient risk factors and outcomes. Inevitably computer applications are applied to medical records. Pilot studies assessed the importance of *computerized medical records* in a variety of clinical situations. Perhaps the most important example of successful implementation of computerized medical records lies within the *Veterans Health Affairs (VHA)* medical system in the United States.[116] Over a 20 year period the VHA system of hospitals completed a dramatic conversion from problematic, fragmented care to a nationally recognized health-care delivery system.[116] This transformation was aided, if not completely caused by, the implementation of a costly but highly successful computerized medical record system.

Iezzoni pointed out the difficulties with computerized medical records and suggests that they may not adequately reflect the importance of chronic disability while at the same time prolonging the time that physicians spend documenting care into the computer system.[117] Yet the advantages of reduced medical errors, improved efficiency, and expanded access to medical information all overshadow most objections to implementation of an electronic information system.

Legislation passed by Congress allocates health-care reforms that include an investment of $50 billion to promote *health information technology*.[118] Further, in its economic recovery package, the Obama administration will spend $19 billion to accelerate the use of computerized medical records in doctors' offices (http://www.nytimes.com/2009/03/01/business/01unbox.html). Medical experts agree that electronic patient records, when used wisely, can help curb costs and improve care. Pending legislation indicates that physicians will be paid a bonus only for the "meaningful use" of digital records, although the government has not yet defined that term precisely. The new legislation also calls for creation of "regional health I.T. extension centers" to help doctors in small office practices use electronic records. It is apparent that the need for data about large groups of patients exists, especially for managed care and capitation initiatives. It is reasonable to expect that efforts to computerize medical records will expand. Applications of electronic medical records that may be available in the future for cardiothoracic surgeons include monitoring of patient outcomes, supporting clinical decision making, and real-time tracking of resource utilization.

Computer applications were applied to the electronic medical record in hopes of minimizing physician errors in ordering. *Computerized physician order entry* (CPOE) is one of these applications that monitors and offers suggestions when physicians' orders do not meet a predesigned computer algorithm. CPOE is viewed as a quality indicator and private employer-based organizations used the presence of CPOE to judge whether hospitals should be part of their preferred network (http://www.leapfroggroup.org/). One of these private groups is the *Leapfrog Group* and an initial survey by this Group in 2001 found that only 3.3% of responding hospitals currently had CPOE systems in place (http://www.ctsnet.org/reuters/reutersarticle.cfm?article=19325). In New York State, several large corporations and health-care insurers agreed to pay hospitals that meet the CPOE standards a bonus on all health-care billings submitted. Other computer-based safety initiatives that involve the electronic medical record are likely to surface in the future. The impact of these innovations on the quality of health care is untested and any benefit remains to be proven.

The success of information technology used to reduce medical errors is mixed. Innovations that employ monitoring of electronic medical records may reduce errors.[119] However, with the increasing implementation of commercial CPOE systems in various settings of care, evidence suggests that some implementation approaches may not achieve previously published results or may actually cause new errors or even harm.[120] Much work needs to be done before computer-aided methods lead to medical error reduction but the future will see more efforts of this type made. The increasing role of CPOE systems in health care invites much more scrutiny about the effectiveness of these systems in actual practice.

REFERENCES

1. Donabedian A, Bashshur R: *An introduction to quality assurance in health care*. Oxford, New York, Oxford University Press, 2003.
2. Kohn LT, Corrigan J, Donaldson MS, Institute of Medicine (US). Committee on Quality of Health Care in America. *To err is human: building a safer health system*. Washington, D.C., National Academy Press. 2000.
3. Birkmeyer JD, Dimick JB, Birkmeyer NJ: Measuring the quality of surgical care: structure, process, or outcomes? *J Am Coll Surg* 2004; 198:626-632.
4. Herlitz J, Brandrup-Wognsen G, Evander MH, et al: Quality of life 15 years after coronary artery bypass grafting. *Coron Artery Dis* 2009; 20:363-369.
5. Krane M, Bauernschmitt R, Hiebinger A, et al: Cardiac reoperation in patients aged 80 years and older. *Ann Thorac Surg* 2009; 87:1379-1385.
6. Dimick JB, Staiger DO, Osborne NH, Nicholas LH, Birkmeyer JD: Composite measures for rating hospital quality with major surgery. *Health Serv Res* 2012; 47:1861-1879.
7. Coulson TG, Bailey M, Reid CM, et al: Acute Risk Change for Cardiothoracic Admissions to Intensive Care (ARCTIC index): a new measure of quality in cardiac surgery. *J Thorac Cardiovasc Surg* 2014; 148:3076-3081. e3071.
8. O'Brien SM, Shahian DM, DeLong ER, et al: Quality measurement in adult cardiac surgery: part 2—Statistical considerations in composite measure scoring and provider rating. *Ann Thorac Surg* 2007; 83: S13-S26.
9. Shahian DM, He X, Jacobs JP, et al: The STS AVR+CABG composite score: a report of the STS Quality Measurement Task Force. *Ann Thorac Surg* 2014; 97:1604-1609.
10. Ferraris VA, Bolanos M, Martin JT, Mahan A, Saha SP: Identification of patients with postoperative complications who are at risk for failure to rescue. *JAMA surgery* 2014; 149:1103-1108.
11. Wakeam E, Asafu-Adjei D, Ashley SW, Cooper Z, Weissman JS: The association of intensivists with failure-to-rescue rates in outlier hospitals: results of a national survey of intensive care unit organizational characteristics. *J Crit Care* 2014; 29:930-935.
12. Ferraris VA, Ferraris SP: Assessing the medical literature: let the buyer beware. *Ann Thorac Surg* 2003; 76:4-11.
13. Glantz SA: It is all in the numbers. *J Am Coll Cardiol* 1993; 21:835-837.
14. Bhandari M, Devereaux PJ, Li P, et al: Misuse of baseline comparison tests and subgroup analyses in surgical trials. *Clin Orthop Relat Res* 2006; 447:247-251.
15. Gandhi R, Smith HN, Mahomed NN, Rizek R, Bhandari M: Incorrect use of the student t test in randomized trials of bilateral hip and knee arthroplasty patients. *J Arthroplasty* 2011; 26:811-816.
16. Hosmer DW, Lemeshow S, Sturdivant RX: *Applied logistic regression*. 3rd edn. Hoboken, Wiley, 2013.
17. de Groot V, Beckerman H, Lankhorst GJ, Bouter LM: How to measure comorbidity. A critical review of available methods. *J Clin Epidemiol* 2003; 56:221-229.
18. Kozower BD, Ailawadi G, Jones DR, et al: Predicted risk of mortality models: surgeons need to understand limitations of the University HealthSystem Consortium models. *J Am Coll Surg* 2009; 209: 551-556.
19. Steen PM, Brewster AC, Bradbury RC, Estabrook E, Young JA: Predicted probabilities of hospital death as a measure of admission severity of illness. *Inquiry* 1993; 30:128-141.
20. Tu JV, Wu K: The improving outcomes of coronary artery bypass graft surgery in Ontario, 1981 to 1995. *Cmaj* 1998; 159:221-227.
21. Knaus WA, Wagner DP, Draper EA, et al: The APACHE III prognostic system. Risk prediction of hospital mortality for critically ill hospitalized adults. *Chest* 1991; 100:1619-1636.
22. Blackstone EH: Breaking down barriers: helpful breakthrough statistical methods you need to understand better. *J Thorac Cardiovasc Surg* 2001; 122:430-439.

23. Koch CG, Khandwala F, Nussmeier N, Blackstone EH: Gender and outcomes after coronary artery bypass grafting: a propensity-matched comparison. *J Thorac Cardiovasc Surg* 2003; 126:2032-2043.

24. Iezzoni LI: *Risk adjustment for measuring health outcomes.* 4th ed. Chicago, Ill: Health Administration Press, AUPHA, 2013.

25. O'Brien SM, Shahian DM, Filardo G, et al: The Society of Thoracic Surgeons 2008 cardiac surgery risk models: part 2—isolated valve surgery. *Ann Thorac Surg* 2009; 88:S23-S42.

26. Shahian DM, O'Brien SM, Filardo G, et al: The Society of Thoracic Surgeons 2008 cardiac surgery risk models: part 3—valve plus coronary artery bypass grafting surgery. *Ann Thorac Surg* 2009; 88:S43-S62.

27. Shahian DM, O'Brien SM, Filardo G, et al: The Society of Thoracic Surgeons 2008 cardiac surgery risk models: part 1—coronary artery bypass grafting surgery. *Ann Thorac Surg* 2009; 88:S2-S22.

28. Zalkind DL, Eastaugh SR: Mortality rates as an indicator of hospital quality. *Hosp Health Serv Adm* 1997; 42:3-15.

29. Park RE, Brook RH, Kosecoff J, et al: Explaining variations in hospital death rates. Randomness, severity of illness, quality of care. *JAMA* 1990; 264:484-490.

30. Tu JV, Sykora K, Naylor CD: Assessing the outcomes of coronary artery bypass graft surgery: how many risk factors are enough? Steering Committee of the Cardiac Care Network of Ontario. *J Am Coll Cardiol* 1997; 30:1317-1323.

31. Jones RH, Hannan EL, Hammermeister KE, et al: Identification of preoperative variables needed for risk adjustment of short-term mortality after coronary artery bypass graft surgery. The Working Group Panel on the Cooperative CABG Database Project. *J Am Coll Cardiol* 1996; 28:1478-1487.

32. Lippmann RP, Shahian DM: Coronary artery bypass risk prediction using neural networks. *Ann Thorac Surg* 1997; 63:1635-1643.

33. Sacks H, Chalmers TC, Smith H, Jr: Randomized versus historical controls for clinical trials. *Am J Med* 1982; 72:233-240.

34. Concato J, Shah N, Horwitz RI: Randomized, controlled trials, observational studies, and the hierarchy of research designs. *N Engl J Med* 2000; 342:1887-1892.

35. Rosenbaum PR, Rubin DB: The Central Role of the Propensity Score in Observational Studies for Causal Effects. In: Rubin DB, ed. *Matched Sampling for Causal Effects.* Cambridge University Press, 2008; pp 170-192.

36. Blackstone EH: Comparing apples and oranges. *J Thorac Cardiovasc Surg* 2002; 123:8-15.

37. Ferraris VA, Brown JR, Despotis GJ, et al: 2011 update to the Society of Thoracic Surgeons and the Society of Cardiovascular Anesthesiologists blood conservation clinical practice guidelines. *Ann Thorac Surg* 2011; 91:944-982.

38. Hillis LD, Smith PK, Anderson JL, et al: 2011 ACCF/AHA Guideline for Coronary Artery Bypass Graft Surgery: A Report of the American College of Cardiology Foundation/American Heart Association Task Force on Practice Guidelines. *Circulation,* 2011; 124(23):2610-2642.

39. Barbour G: The role of outcomes data in health care reform. *Ann Thorac Surg* 1994; 58:1881-1884.

40. Lenfant C: Shattuck lecture—clinical research to clinical practice—lost in translation? *N Engl J Med* 2003; 349:868-874.

41. Heffner JE: Altering physician behavior to improve clinical performance. *Topics in health information management* 2001; 22:1-9.

42. Casale AS, Paulus RA, Selna MJ, et al: "ProvenCareSM": a provider-driven pay-for-performance program for acute episodic cardiac surgical care. *Ann Surg* 2007; 246:613-621; discussion 621-613.

43. Karve AM, Ou FS, Lytle BL, Peterson ED: Potential unintended financial consequences of pay-for-performance on the quality of care for minority patients. *Am Heart J* 2008; 155:571-576.

44. Guadagnoli E, Hauptman PJ, Ayanian JZ, Pashos CL, McNeil BJ, Cleary PD: Variation in the use of cardiac procedures after acute myocardial infarction. *N Engl J Med* 1995; 333:573-578.

45. Tobler HG, Sethi GK, Grover FL, et al: Variations in processes and structures of cardiac surgery practice. *Med Care* 1995; 33:OS43-58.

46. Maddux FW, Dickinson TA, Rilla D, et al: Institutional variability of intraoperative red blood cell utilization in coronary artery bypass graft surgery. *Am J Med Qual* 2009; 24:403-411.

47. Magner D, Mirocha J, Gewertz BL: Regional variation in the utilization of carotid endarterectomy. *J Vasc Surg* 2009; 49:893-901; discussion 901.

48. Harris KM, Pastorius CA, Duval S, et al: Practice variation among cardiovascular physicians in management of patients with mitral regurgitation. *Am J Cardiol* 2009; 103:255-261.

49. Schneider EC, Leape LL, Weissman JS, Piana RN, Gatsonis C, Epstein AM: Racial differences in cardiac revascularization rates: does "overuse" explain higher rates among white patients? *Ann Int Med* 2001; 135:328-337.

50. Philbin EF, McCullough PA, DiSalvo TG, Dec GW, Jenkins PL, Weaver WD: Underuse of invasive procedures among Medicaid patients with acute myocardial infarction. *Am J Public Health* 2001; 91:1082-1088.

51. Filardo G, Maggioni AP, Mura G, et al: The consequences of under-use of coronary revascularization; results of a cohort study in Northern Italy. *European Heart Journal* 2001; 22:654-662.

52. Alter DA, Austin PC, Tu JV, Canadian Cardiovascular Outcomes Research T: Community factors, hospital characteristics and inter-regional outcome variations following acute myocardial infarction in Canada. *Can J Cardiol* 2005; 21:247-255.

53. Daley J: Validity of risk-adjustment methods. In: Iezzoni L, ed. *Risk Adjustment for Measuring Health Care Outcomes.* Ann Arbor, Health Administration Press, 1994; p 239.

54. Daley J: Validity of risk-adjustment methods. In: Iezzoni LI, ed. *Risk adjustment for measuring healthcare outcomes.* Chicago, Health Administration Press, 1997; pp 331-363.

55. Ferraris VA, Ferraris SP: Risk factors for postoperative morbidity. *J Thorac Cardiovasc Surg* 1996; 111:731-738; discussion 738-741.

56. Shroyer AL, Coombs LP, Peterson ED, et al: The Society of Thoracic Surgeons: 30-day operative mortality and morbidity risk models. *Ann Thorac Surg* 2003; 75:1856-1864; discussion 1864-1855.

57. O'Brien SM, Shahian DM, Filardo G, et al: The Society of Thoracic Surgeons 2008 cardiac surgery risk models: part 2—isolated valve surgery. *Ann Thorac Surg* 2009; 88:S23-S42.

58. Shahian DM, O'Brien SM, Filardo G, et al: The Society of Thoracic Surgeons 2008 cardiac surgery risk models: part 1—coronary artery bypass grafting surgery. *Ann Thorac Surg* 2009; 88:S2-S22.

59. Ware JE Jr, Sherbourne CD: The MOS 36-item short-form health survey (SF-36). I. Conceptual framework and item selection. *Med Care* 1992; 30:473-483.

60. Lee T: *Evaluating the Quality of Cardiovascular Care: A Primer* Bethesda, American College of Cardiology Press, 1995.

61. Cope DW, Linn LS, Leake BD, Barrett PA: Modification of residents' behavior by preceptor feedback of patient satisfaction. *J Gen Int Med* 1986; 1:394-398.

62. Peric V, Borzanovic M, Stolic R, et al: Quality of life in patients related to gender differences before and after coronary artery bypass surgery. *Interact Cardiovasc Thorac Surg* 2010; 10:232-238.

63. Tully PJ, Baker RA, Turnbull DA, Winefield HR, Knight JL: Negative emotions and quality of life six months after cardiac surgery: the dominant role of depression not anxiety symptoms. *J Behavioral Med* 2009; 32:510-522.

64. Jideus L, Liss A, Stahle E: Patients with sternal wound infection after cardiac surgery do not improve their quality of life. *Scand Cardiovasc J* 2009; 43:194-200.

65. Guadagnoli E, Ayanian JZ, Cleary PD: Comparison of patient-reported outcomes after elective coronary artery bypass grafting in patients aged greater than or equal to and less than 65 years. *Am J Cardiol* 1992; 70:60-64.

66. Rumsfeld JS, Magid DJ, O'Brien M, et al: Changes in health-related quality of life following coronary artery bypass graft surgery. *Ann Thorac Surg* 2001; 72:2026-2032.

67. Rumsfeld JS, MaWhinney S, McCarthy M, et al: Health-related quality of life as a predictor of mortality following coronary artery bypass graft surgery. Participants of the Department of Veterans Affairs Cooperative Study Group on Processes, Structures, and Outcomes of Care in Cardiac Surgery. *JAMA* 1999; 281:1298-1303.

68. Deming WE: *Out of the Crisis.* Cambridge, MA.: Massachusetts Institute of Technology Center for Advanced Engineering Study, 1986.

69. Juran JM: *A History of Managing for Quality: The Evolution, Trends, and Future Directions of Managing for Quality* Milwaukee, ASQC Quality Press, 1995.

70. Ferraris VA, Gildengorin V: Predictors of excessive blood use after coronary artery bypass grafting. A multivariate analysis. *J Thorac Cardiovasc Surg* 1989; 98:492-497.

71. Ferraris VA, Berry WR, Klingman RR: Comparison of blood reinfusion techniques used during coronary artery bypass grafting. *Ann Thorac Surg* 1993; 56:433-439; discussion 440.

72. Maggard-Gibbons M: The use of report cards and outcome measurements to improve the safety of surgical care: the American College of

Surgeons National Surgical Quality Improvement Program. *BMJ Qual Saf* 2014; 23:589-599.

73. Etzioni DA, Wasif N, Dueck AC, et al: Association of hospital participation in a surgical outcomes monitoring program with inpatient complications and mortality. *JAMA* 2015; 313:505-511.

74. Smith PK, Mayer JE Jr, Kanter KR, et al: Physician payment for 2007: a description of the process by which major changes in valuation of cardiothoracic surgical procedures occurred. *Ann Thorac Surg* 2007; 83:12-20.

75. O'Connor GT, Plume SK, Olmstead EM, et al: Multivariate prediction of in-hospital mortality associated with coronary artery bypass graft surgery. Northern New England Cardiovascular Disease Study Group. *Circulation* 1992; 85:2110-2118.

76. O'Connor GT, Plume SK, Olmstead EM, et al: A regional intervention to improve the hospital mortality associated with coronary artery bypass graft surgery. The Northern New England Cardiovascular Disease Study Group. *JAMA* 1996; 275:841-846.

77. Birkmeyer NJ, Charlesworth DC, Hernandez F, et al: Obesity and risk of adverse outcomes associated with coronary artery bypass surgery. Northern New England Cardiovascular Disease Study Group. *Circulation* 1998; 97:1689-1694.

78. Braxton JH, Marrin CA, McGrath PD, et al: 10-year follow-up of patients with and without mediastinitis. *Semin Thorac Cardiovasc Surg* 2004; 16:70-76.

79. Hernandez F, Cohn WE, Baribeau YR, et al: In-hospital outcomes of off-pump versus on-pump coronary artery bypass procedures: a multicenter experience. *Ann Thorac Surg* 2001; 72:1528-1533; discussion 1533-1524.

80. Green J, Wintfeld N: Report cards on cardiac-surgeons—assessing New-York States approach. *N Engl J Med* 1995; 332:1229-1232.

81. Morgan RO, Virnig BA, DeVito CA, Persily NA: The Medicare-HMO revolving door—the healthy go in and the sick go out. *N Engl J Med* 1997; 337:169-175.

82. Omoigui NA, Annan K, Brown K, Miller D, Cosgrove D, Loop F: Potential explanation for decreased Cabg related mortality in New-York-State—outmigration to Ohio. *Circulation* 1994; 90:93.

83. Schneider EC, Epstein AM: Use of public performance reports: a survey of patients undergoing cardiac surgery. *JAMA* 1998; 279:1638-1642.

84. Dranove D, Kessler D, McClellan M, Satterthwaite M: Is more information better? The effects of "Report cards" on health care providers. *J Polit Econ* 2003; 111:555-588.

85. Mehta SR, Yusuf S, Peters RJ, et al: Effects of pretreatment with clopidogrel and aspirin followed by long-term therapy in patients undergoing percutaneous coronary intervention: the PCI-CURE study. *Lancet* 2001; 358:527-533.

86. Hannan EL, Chassin MR: Publicly reporting quality information. *JAMA* 2005; 293:2999-3000.

87. Glance LG, Dick A, Mukamel DB, Li Y, Osler TM: Are high-quality cardiac surgeons less likely to operate on high-risk patients compared to low-quality surgeons? Evidence from New York State. *Health Serv Res* 2008; 43:300-312.

88. Daley J: Criteria by which to evaluate risk-adjusted outcomes programs in cardiac surgery. *Ann Thorac Surg* 1994; 58:1827-1835.

89. Shahian DM, Edwards FH, Ferraris VA, et al: Quality measurement in adult cardiac surgery: part 1—Conceptual framework and measure selection. *Ann Thorac Surg* 2007; 83:S3-12.

90. Iezzoni LI: Using administrative data to study persons with disabilities. *Milbank Q* 2002; 80:347-379.

91. Jollis JG, Ancukiewicz M, DeLong ER, Pryor DB, Muhlbaier LH, Mark DB: Discordance of databases designed for claims payment versus clinical information systems. Implications for outcomes research. *An Int Med* 1993; 119:844-850.

92. Burns EM, Rigby E, Mamidanna R, et al: Systematic review of discharge coding accuracy. *J Public Health* 2012; 34:138-148.

93. Shahian DM, Torchiana DF, Normand SL: Implementation of a cardiac surgery report card: lessons from the Massachusetts experience. *Ann Thorac Surg* 2005; 80:1146-1150.

94. Hannan EL, Kilburn H, Racz M, Shields E, Chassin MR: Improving the outcomes of coronary artery bypass surgery in New York State. *JAMA* 1994; 271:761-766.

95. Goldstein H, Spiegelhalter DJ: League tables and their limitations: statistical issues in comparisons of institutional performance (with discussion). *J R Stat Soc (Series A)* 1996; 159:385-443.

96. Woolhandler S, Himmelstein DU: Costs of care and administration at for-profit and other hospitals in the United States. *N Engl J Med* 1997; 336:769-774.

97. Anonymous: Iowa: classic test of a future concept. *Med Outcomes Guidelines Alert* 1995; 8.

98. Tu JV, Donovan LR, Lee DS, et al: Effectiveness of public report cards for improving the quality of cardiac care: the EFFECT study: a randomized trial. *JAMA* 2009; 302:2330-2337.

99. Ketelaar NA, Faber MJ, Flottorp S, Rygh LH, Deane KH, Eccles MP: Public release of performance data in changing the behaviour of healthcare consumers, professionals or organisations. *Cochrane Database of Systematic Reviews (Online).* 2011:CD004538.

100. Jacobs JP, Cerfolio RJ, Sade RM: The ethics of transparency: publication of cardiothoracic surgical outcomes in the lay press. *Ann Thorac Surg* 2009; 87:679-686.

101. Spiegelhalter DJ: Funnel plots for comparing institutional performance. *Stat Med* 2005; 24:1185-1202.

102. Brennan TA, Gawande A, Thomas E, Studdert D: Accidental deaths, saved lives, and improved quality. *N Engl J Med* 2005; 353:1405-1409.

103. Leape LL, Berwick DM: Five years after To Err Is Human: what have we learned? *JAMA* 2005; 293:2384-2390.

104. Kolata G: Program coaxes hospitals to see treatments under their Noses *New York Times on the web.* New York, N.Y. December 25, 2004.

105. Patel MR, Dehmer GJ, Hirshfeld JW, Smith PK, Spertus JA: ACCF/SCAI/STS/AATS/AHA/ASNC 2009 Appropriateness Criteria for Coronary Revascularization: A Report of the American College of Cardiology Foundation Appropriateness Criteria Task Force, Society for Cardiovascular Angiography and Interventions, Society of Thoracic Surgeons, American Association for Thoracic Surgery, American Heart Association, and the American Society of Nuclear Cardiology: Endorsed by the American Society of Echocardiography, the Heart Failure Society of America, and the Society of Cardiovascular Computed Tomography. *Circulation.* 2009; 119:1330-1352.

106. McDonnell Norms G: Enhancing the use of clinical guidelines: a social norms perspective. *J Am Coll Surg* 2006; 202:826-836.

107. Leape LL, Weissman JS, Schneider EC, Piana RN, Gatsonis C, Epstein AM: Adherence to practice guidelines: the role of specialty society guidelines. *Am Heart J* 2003; 145:19-26.

108. Likosky DS, FitzGerald DC, Groom RC, et al: Effect of the Perioperative Blood Transfusion and Blood Conservation in Cardiac Surgery Clinical Practice Guidelines of the Society of Thoracic Surgeons and the Society of Cardiovascular Anesthesiologists upon Clinical Practices. *Anesthesia Analgesia* 2010; 111:316-323.

109. McQuilten ZK, Andrianopoulos N, Wood EM, et al: Transfusion practice varies widely in cardiac surgery: results from a national registry. *J Thorac Cardiovasc Surg* 2014; 147:1684-1690. e1681.

110. Carthey J: The role of structured observational research in health care. *Qual Saf Health Care* 2003; 12 Suppl 2:ii13-ii16.

111. Richardson WC, Berwick DM, Bisgard JC, et al: The Institute of Medicine Report on Medical Errors: misunderstanding can do harm. Quality Health Care Am Committee. 2000; E42.

112. de_Leval MR, Carthey J, Wright DJ, Farewell VT, Reason JT: Human factors and cardiac surgery: a multicenter study. *J Thorac Cardiovasc Surg* 2000; 119:661-672.

113. Hickey EJ, Nosikova Y, Pham-Hung E, et al: National Aeronautics and Space Administration "threat and error" model applied to pediatric cardiac surgery: error cycles precede approximately 85% of patient deaths. *J Thorac Cardiovasc Surg* 2015; 149:496-507. e494.

114. Shahian DM, Edwards FH, Jacobs JP, et al: Public reporting of cardiac surgery performance: part 1—history, rationale, consequences. *Ann Thorac Surg* 2011; 92:S2-S11.

115. Shahian DM, He X, Jacobs JP, et al: The Society of Thoracic Surgeons Isolated Aortic Valve Replacement (AVR) Composite Score: a report of the STS Quality Measurement Task Force. *Ann Thorac Surg* 2012; 94:2166-2171.

116. Longman P: *Best care anywhere: why VA health care would work better for everyone.* 3rd ed. San Francisco, Berrett-Koehler Publishers, 2012.

117. Iezzoni L: Measuring the severity of illness and case mix, in Goldfield N ND (ed.): *Providing Quality Care: The Challenge to Clinicians.* Philadelphia, American College of Physicians, 1989; 70-105.

118. D'Avolio LW: Electronic medical records at a crossroads: impetus for change or missed opportunity? *JAMA* 2009; 302:1109-1111.

119. Langdorf MI, Fox JC, Marwah RS, Montague BJ, Hart MM: Physician versus computer knowledge of potential drug interactions in the emergency department. *Acad Emerg Med* 2000; 7:1321-1329.

120. Classen DC, Avery AJ, Bates DW: Evaluation and certification of computerized provider order entry systems. *J Am Med Inform Assoc* 2007; 14:48-55.
121. Amr SS, Tbakhi A: Abu Al Qasim Al Zahrawi (Albucasis): pioneer of modern surgery. *Ann Saudi Med* 2007; 27:220-221.
122. Ferraris ZA, Ferraris VA: The women of Salerno: contribution to the origins of surgery from medieval Italy. *Ann Thorac Surg* 1997; 64:1855-1857.
123. Beal J: Madame Angelique le Boursier du Coudray: a midwife of enlightenment France. *Midwifery today with international midwife* 2013:29.
124. Moran ME: Enlightenment via simulation: "crone-ology's" first woman. *J Endourol* 2010; 24:5-8.
125. Moore WA: *The Knife Man: The Extraordinary Life and Times of John Hunter, Father of Modern Surgery.* New York: Broadway Books, Westminster, Random House [Distributor], 2005.
126. Cohen IB: Florence Nightingale. *Scientific American* 1984; 250:128-137.
127. Warshaw AL: Presidential address: achieving our personal best—Back to the future of the American College of Surgeons. *Bull Am Coll Surg* 2014; 99:9-18.
128. Lahey SJ, Borlase BC, Lavin PT, Levitsky S: Preoperative risk factors that predict hospital length of stay in coronary artery bypass patients > 60 years old. *Circulation* 1992; 86:II181-II185.
129. Hammermeister KE, Johnson R, Marshall G, Grover FL: Continuous assessment and improvement in quality of care. A model from the Department of Veterans Affairs Cardiac Surgery. *Ann Surg* 1994; 219:281-290.
130. Tu JV, Jaglal SB, Naylor CD: Multicenter validation of a risk index for mortality, intensive care unit stay, and overall hospital length of stay after cardiac surgery. Steering Committee of the Provincial Adult Cardiac Care Network of Ontario. *Circulation* 1995; 91:677-684.

Simulation in Cardiac Surgery

Jennifer D. Walker • Philip J. Spencer • Toni B. Walzer • Jeffrey B. Cooper

Of the many developments in cardiothoracic surgery, the introduction of a broad spectrum of simulation techniques for education and training of students and residents as well as ongoing faculty training are among the most exciting and critical for the continued advancement of the specialty. There are increasing demands for safety during training, for training to be more effective and efficient, and have minimal impact on the process of patient care. The productivity of training for physicians has advanced in many ways; simulation is one approach to teaching that offers solutions to challenges in training in general and especially in cardiac surgery. In this chapter, we describe a spectrum of simulation technologies and techniques that are being applied to address these challenges. We also address approaches to using simulation to its greatest effect and speculate about future technologies and applications and how they will be integrated into education at all levels of experience.

BACKGROUND

Simulation has been described as a "technique, not a technology, to replace or guide real experiences with guided experiences that evoke or replicate substantial aspects of the real world in a fully interactive manner."[1] The roots of simulation in medicine can be traced back for centuries. More recent applications in the 1960s and 1970s for training in specific tasks include the Sim One for teaching in anesthesia residency, Resusci Anne for training in cardiac life support, and Harvey for teaching about cardiology to medical students.[2] The more modern era of simulation began in earnest in the late 1980s with the development of more realistic mannequins for teaching basic skills and management of crises in anesthesia. Surgeons have long used various forms of simulation, from tying knots on paperclips placed in clay to cadavers and animals. The first use of a model simulator was introduced by Howard in 1868 in which a mannequin was created to teach hernia repair.[3] But, more technology-based forms of task trainers for various surgical and procedural skills appeared beginning in the late 1980s.[2]

For many reasons, the use of simulation is growing in all of healthcare, and specifically in cardiac surgery. Ziv and colleagues described the adoption of simulation in surgical training as an ethical imperative noting patient safety as their cause.[4] With patients having increased acuity, practicing outside of the operating room is critical for mastering tasks to quickly develop critical skills without exposing patients to increased risk. Practice via simulation has been shown to increase speed for completion of coronary anastomosis[5] as well as increase speed and accuracy of mitral valve annuloplasty.[6] Through deliberate practice (rehearsing a task or behavior repeatedly), simulation provides the ability to advance the mastery of some skills more quickly, reducing operating time related to training. Simulation is also the preferred modality to improve teamwork and communication and to practice emergencies not frequently seen during training. It enables surgeons and teams to work out complex problems in a nonthreatening setting and apply the lessons to urgent and emergent situations.

Surgical simulation may provide an important modality for measuring proficiency for certification, recertification, or for judging appropriateness of clinical advancement within a training program. For example, a particular task such as anastomosis of one small vessel to another has many components that can be evaluated for simple tasks such as instrument use, suture handling, and tissue handling. The same tasks can be integrated into a more complex scenario on a higher fidelity simulator; for example, rather than sewing a simple anastomosis, anastomoses may be incorporated into a beating-heart coronary artery bypass graft (CABG) on the simulator. Graft measurement, appropriateness of anastamotic site, vessel opening, and preparation can be evaluated. In addition, these tasks can be incorporated into the entire bypass procedure for more advanced learning as training progresses.

Simulation education has gained significant traction in cardiac anesthesia training as well. Bruppacher and colleagues performed a randomized controlled trial in which anesthesia residents were randomized to simulation training and no simulation training for cardiopulmonary bypass weaning.[7] The residents were evaluated using an internally validated

207

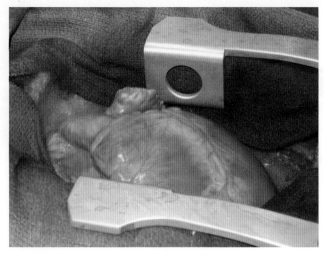

FIGURE 8-1 Porcine heart in Ramphal Simulator.

scoring system administered by blinded attending anesthesiologists before and after simulation training. The residents who underwent two hours of simulation training improved significantly more than the residents who underwent two hours of didactic instruction.

The most exciting advancement in cardiac surgical simulation training occurred in 2005 when Ramphal created a relatively high realism porcine beating-heart model to address the shortage of cardiac surgery cases being afforded to residents in training in Jamaica[8] (Figs. 8-1 and 8-2). The simulator was adapted by a leadership group in cardiothoracic surgery in the United States and incorporated into focused programs to advance simulation-based learning. The Thoracic Surgery Foundation for Research and Education's (TSFRE) annual Boot Camp conference and "Senior Tour" are sponsored by the Thoracic Surgery Directors' Association and the American Board of Thoracic Surgery and the Joint Counsel on Thoracic Surgical Education (JTSE).[9] The three-day, well-orchestrated simulation curriculum has been conducted since

2008 and provides focused learning for first-year cardiothoracic residents with feedback and standardized evaluations. Standardized evaluation of first-year residents participating in the "Boot Camp" consistently show improvement in time to complete basic cardiothoracic techniques as well as accuracy.[10,11]

Creating a successful cardiac simulation program requires understanding and application of the principles of adult learning. In 1993, Reznick[12,13] described the process of adults learning surgery and the relationship between the trainee and expert instructor. He referenced key educational literature describing Kopta's three stages of adult learning, perception, integration, and automatation[14] as well as Collins' framework for the apprenticeship model characterizing the roles the teacher plays as the student progresses from novice to expert.[15] Those principles are applied to how we approach simulation-based training in all aspects. We next present the current state of how this is done for training in basic skills, what specific procedures currently can be simulated, and what existing simulators are available for cardiac and thoracic surgery.

BASIC SKILLS TRAINING

For cardiothoracic surgery, simulation training begins with teaching of component tasks, starting at the most basic level and combining those into multiple tasks and then full procedures. A consortium of six hospitals (Massachusetts General Hospital, University of North Carolina Chapel Hill, Johns Hopkins, University of Rochester, Stanford University, Vanderbilt University, and University of Washington) developed a 7-week syllabus, broken down into multiple key concepts and procedures consisting of cardiopulmonary bypass (Fig. 8-3), CABG (Figs. 8-4 to 8-7), valve replacement (Figs. 8-8 to 8-10), air embolism, and acute intraoperative aortic dissection (Fig. 8-11). First, fundamentals of cardiopulmonary bypass are taught step by step, including cannulation of the aorta, right atrium, and cardioplegia perfusion with repetitive practice on a perfused porcine heart. Concomitant

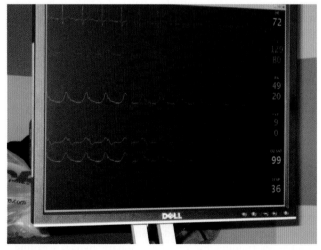

FIGURE 8-2 Anesthesia monitor during simulation with the Ramphal Simulator.

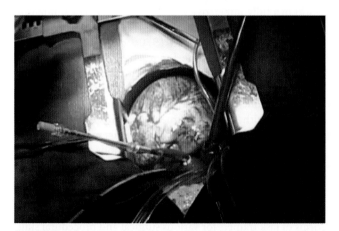

FIGURE 8-3 Porcine heart in the Ramphal Simulator cannulated for cardiopulmonary bypass.

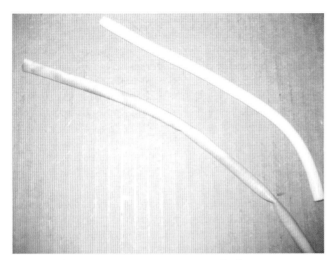

FIGURE 8-4 Synthetic artery and vein grafts for coronary artery bypass simulation.

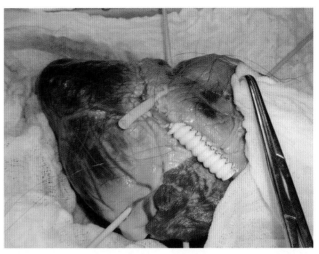

FIGURE 8-7 "Dry" porcine heart with synthetic grafts simulating didstal anastomosis for CABG.

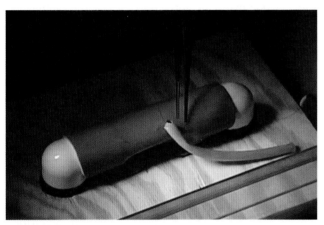

FIGURE 8-5 Synthetic graft anastomosis to synthetic aorta to simulate the proximal anastomosis of coronary artery bypass graft.

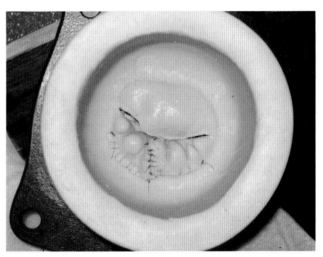

FIGURE 8-8 Mitral valve repair on Chamberlain Group synthetic mitral valve model.

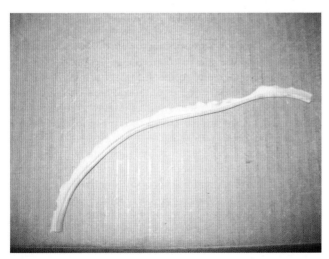

FIGURE 8-6 Chamberlain Group synthetic internal thoracic artery for use in coronary artery bypass graft simulation.

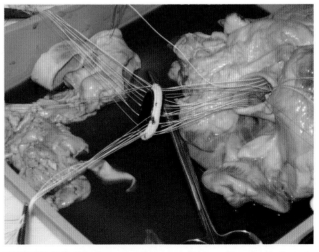

FIGURE 8-9 "Dry" porcine heart simulation of mechanical aortic valve repair.

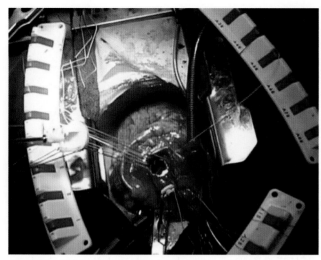

FIGURE 8-10 Simulation of mechanical aortic valve repair on Ramphal beating heart simulator.

with learning the technical aspects of these tasks is a memorization and understanding of the concept of initiating and weaning from cardiopulmonary bypass. The component tasks are then combined with the knowledge base on a higher fidelity model after practicing on the dry porcine heart. The student then integrates these steps using a beating-heart model to fully cannulate, institute bypass, arrest the heart, wean from bypass, and decannulate. The trainee is assessed in a standardized fashion by the expert instructor. The same process of moving from simpler tasks with low-fidelity models to more sophisticated and integrated tasks on higher fidelity simulators is conducted for the five components of the curriculum.

Deliberate practice prepares trainees to apply the basic principles of cardiac surgery to more complicated groupings of tasks. In the CABG component of the curriculum, the resident performs large and small vessel anastomoses, first on a component simulator and later on a porcine heart. The

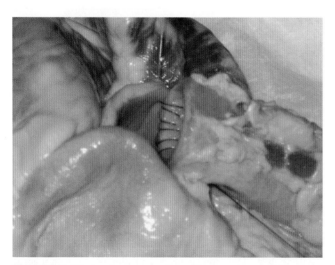

FIGURE 8-11 Aortic anastomosis on "dry" porcine model.

trainee will later combine the steps to perform a full coronary bypass operation on the beating-heart simulator. This process is repeated with the basics of aortic valve surgery. That training begins by teaching the resident about the anatomy of the aortic valve and root and exposing it in the anatomic dissection on the porcine heart. The resident will next practice excising the valve, placing sutures in the annulus repetitively, ultimately seating and tying in all different types of valves until they become proficient. Once this task is mastered, it is incorporated with the previously mastered bypass skills to perform an aortic valve replacement on the beating-heart simulator.

In a similar fashion, mitral valve surgery can be learned. After these basic techniques have been practiced repeatedly, more advanced teaching that incorporates team training and dealing with emergencies can be simulated.

The training via simulation can include creating a plan, implementing that plan with the team in a dry model, and then carrying it out on the beating heart simulator. As noted above, specific emergencies that have been vetted on a simulator include managing aortic dissection at the cannulation site, managing massive air embolism and problems that can occur when weaning off cardiopulmonary bypass, for example, right heart failure, kinked or twisted grafts that can be too long or too short, leaks around the valve, and aortic root dissection. Simulation training is reaching beyond OR-based procedures to bedside invasive resuscitation and surgery.

In cardiac surgery, research has demonstrated that a model neck-cannulation trainer can improve trainee's ability to cannulate the neck vessels for extracorporeal membranous oxygenation (ECMO) resuscitation.[16] Chan and colleagues used a similar model but included a full pediatric intensive care unit (PICU) team in their ECMO training and evaluation.[17] These were not evaluated by assessing participants' skills during the cannulation of a live patient, however. Simulation is also being used to train perfusionists. Morris and Pybus describe a simulated (Orpheus) perfusion machine that can be used for training in the operating room or in a simulation center.[18] Lansdowne and colleagues describe using the same simulator for training perfusionists and respiratory therapists on ECMO management.[19] A new, exciting, and different use of simulation is 3-D printing for operative planning.[20-22] Valverde and colleagues used magnetic resonance imaging (MRI) and angiography to design a 3-D-printed model to plan endovascular stenting of an aortic arch coarctation in a 15-year-old boy.[23] Costello and colleagues even used 3-D printing as an educational model to train residents on ventricular septal defect (VSD) repair.[24]

Trainees can also be led to assimilate hemodynamic information and practice communication skills with other personnel, including anesthesiologists, perfusionists, and nurses. While basic skills can be taught in a laboratory setting, teamwork skills can be taught in a high-realism operating room setting. This multimodal approach, with the gradation from low technology to high fidelity makes a rich environment not only for teaching but also for performance evaluation (see below).

SIMULATORS

In order to accomplish the teaching goals discussed above, many simulators have been developed over the years. These include full mannequin simulators, part task trainers, and virtual reality systems.[25] These are used in various forms to meet the specific training objectives. For training on specific cardiac surgical tasks, various forms of models of the heart and blood vessels have been developed. Virtual reality simulators generally are most useful for laparoscopic procedures. In cardiac surgery, mannequin simulators are mostly used as part of an overall cardiac surgical operating room environment, especially for team training and can also be used for practice of an entirely new procedure.

For training in cardiac surgical procedures, part task trainers have been developed to enable practice on a range of tasks from the most simple and to some more complex. Some of the most realistic cardiac surgery simulation tools have come from the Chamberlain group [Great Barrington Massachusetts] (Figs. 8-4, 8-6, and 8-8). Limbs and Things [Savannah Georgia] and the Wet Lab facility in the United Kingdom (Fig. 8-12) have all been instrumental in providing synthetic and tissue-based simulators. Despite the simulators that are available, many tasks that are required in cardiac surgery do not fit into a typical commercial simulation product. As a result, porcine hearts have become the mainstay for teaching cannulation and many of the other elements of cardiac surgery such as CABG and valve replacement and repair mentioned above. As shown in the accompanying figures, much work has been done to develop perfused pig heart models to more realistically simulate the cannulation scenarios (Figs. 8-1, 8-3, and 8-10).

There is now a 25-year history of using simulation for training in communication and other teamwork skills.[2,26] Generally, this has involved the use of full-body, mannequin simulators of varying degrees of realism and fidelity. The early work of Gaba and colleagues has been widely disseminated and such mannequin simulators are used in thousands of

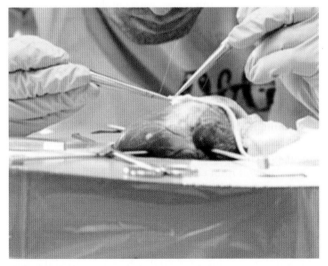

FIGURE 8-12 Disposable Wet Lab station. (Used with permission from Wetlab Ltd.)

centers around the world. The mannequins typically have the features that are needed to simulate many of the characteristics of patient physiology during surgical procedures, for example, audio of a beating heart, respiration, pulses, blinking eyes, and constricting pupils. Placed in a realistic operating room setting, complete with all surgical, anesthesia, nursing, and other paraphernalia, the mannequins enable creation of a setting that is realistic enough to engage teams of operating room professionals into scenarios that mimic many types of critical events that occur during surgical procedures (Fig. 8-13). The mannequins can be enhanced by incorporation of cardiac surgical anatomy and bypass, allowing simulation of an entire procedure and are especially useful for team training and practice for emergencies (see section below) (Fig. 8-14).

SIMULATION AND TEAMWORK TRAINING IN CARDIAC SURGERY

The importance of teamwork to patient safety and efficiency is now well recognized in healthcare.[27] It has been more than two decades since anesthesiologist David Gaba and colleagues brought Crew Resource Management principles from aviation to healthcare and developed a training program he called Anesthesia Crisis Resource Management (ACRM) to teach anesthesiologists to handle critical events in the OR.[26,28] ACRM recognizes that anesthesiology has many similarities to aviation. The environment of the OR, including all of the professionals who work there, is complex and dynamic requiring effective coordination of skills and resources for safe patient care. Similar to aviation, a majority of incidents and accidents in anesthesia involved some level of human error despite technical expertise.[28] There is similar evidence that the same is true for surgery in general and cardiac surgery in particular.[29,30]

The patient safety movement is giving increasing attention to improving team performance in delivery of care. Healthcare professionals from different disciplines and professions must coordinate their activities to make patient care safe and efficient. Those working in a healthcare team, including in cardiac surgery, typically have diverse educational backgrounds and have different experience and perspectives; and they are rarely trained together. Simon and colleagues were the first to demonstrate that formal teamwork training can lead to improvement in staff attitudes toward teamwork, quality of teamwork, and a significant reduction in observed clinical errors in teamwork-trained emergency departments.[31] Despite recognition of the importance of teamwork and existence of teamwork programs, there does not yet seem to be deep penetration or routine training for healthcare professional teams. Interprofessional training in general is lacking in healthcare.[32]

The complexity of medical care is a challenge to the effective communication and teamwork essential for the delivery of high quality and safe patient care. Poor communication and poor teamwork have been shown to be one of the major

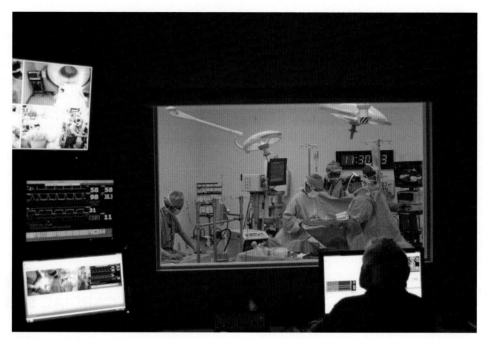

FIGURE 8-13 Simulated operating room viewed from control room.

contributors to adverse events.[33] Communication failures are the leading cause of inadvertent patient harm. Teamwork failures in the operating room have been linked to a higher risk of complications and death.[33] The clinicians providing care had very different views of what was expected to happen; they did not share the same mental model and often did not have an environment to speak up when there were safety concerns. Even the most skilled, experienced, and highly motivated clinicians have performance limitations and will make mistakes. Effective communication can help prevent these mistakes from becoming consequential and harming patients.[34]

The practice of surgery is an area of major risk for malpractice insurers. Root-cause analysis of claims from the Harvard-affiliated malpractice insurer Controlled Risk

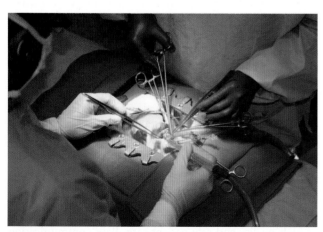

FIGURE 8-14 Simulated cardiac surgical field.

Insurance Company, Risk Management Foundation (CRICO/RMF) and other major insurers show that errors in surgical care most commonly occurred in the operating room. Communication breakdowns were the second most common factors identified in contributing to error, after technical performance.[35]

A growing body of evidence links teamwork in surgery to improved outcomes.[36] Elements of the Surgical Safety Checklist can be used as an actual briefing to enhance teamwork. Voicing one's name, role, and concerns not only gets the entire team on the same page but makes the environment more open for any team member to speak up throughout the case. This struggle over speaking up in a clinical domain is consistent with research in the organizational behavior domain.[37] Interviews with employees have shown that they perceived risks of speaking up to be personal and immediate, whereas they were uncertain of the benefit of sharing their ideas. There was a powerful protective instinct that inhibited speech; employees played it safe by keeping quiet.[38] People have difficulty in speaking up across a hierarchical gradient; such gradients exist in the operating room environment.

Communication breakdowns and lapses in teamwork are a leading cause of errors in the operating room resulting in preventable patient harm, second only to technical errors. Analyses from closed claims from both the American Society of Anesthesiologists and the American College of Surgeons found poor communication both inside and outside the operating room to be a significant cause of preventable adverse events. Technical errors were significantly more likely to be deemed preventable if they were also accompanied by communication failures.[39,40] Studies have supported the concept that interventions designed to improve teamwork and communication may have beneficial effects on technical performance and patient outcome.[41]

Risk management data for CRICO/RMF has shown that the anesthesiologists' already good malpractice profile improved, since the anesthesia staff began participating in Anesthesia Crisis Resource Management training.[42] Encouraged by their success, CRICO/RMF promoted simulation-based team training as a risk control strategy for obstetrical providers. CRICO/RMF later concluded that formal training in communication and teamwork for obstetric clinicians could ultimately mitigate or prevent adverse perinatal events. An interprofessional simulation-based team-training course for obstetric clinicians was systematically designed as advocated by Salas and Cannon-Bowers and modeled after the successful ACRM training. Risk management data from CRICO/RMF has shown that the number of claims has been trending down in the Harvard-affiliated institutions' obstetric departments since their faculty obstetricians and midwives have participated in this course. As a result of this trend, CRICO continues to offer a significant reduction in malpractice insurance premiums to obstetricians and certified nurse midwives who participate in this training.[43,44]

Arriaga and colleagues note that there is a growing call for simulation team training programs with the entire operating room teams on a large scale.[45] They described a standardized multicenter high-fidelity simulation-based team-training pilot program. This program was developed with the interprofessional make-up of the team in mind, ensuring that it was clinically relevant to all of the participants. Simulation scenarios that had been used effectively to train anesthesiologists were adapted to include tasks for the surgeons, nurses, and other professions on the operating room team. Surgical props and models were used to keep the surgeons engaged (Fig. 8-14). Ninety-two percent of participants found the scenarios to be realistic, appropriately challenging, and clinically relevant toward providing safer care.[45] Debriefing of the cases was done by faculty who received training in giving feedback in a direct, clear, and respectful way that was supportive and consistent with "debriefing with good judgment."[46] They found that, despite the simulated crises with chaotic operative environments, more than 96% of participants were comfortable being open and honest with each other in the debriefing. Surgeons commented on the value of improving their communication skills and anesthesiologists and nurses on their desire to improve assertiveness. The vast majority of participants believed the course had a meaningful impact on their approach to clinical practice.

Cardiac surgery is a particularly stressful and intense environment which requires effective teamwork and communication for resolution of acute events and prevention of adverse outcomes. Cardiac surgery operating room teams are generally large interprofessional teams with established hierarchy and requiring seamless coordination. The procedures can be technically challenging and emergencies are common. There can be many challenges with complex bypass equipment, multiple drug infusions, and lack of standardization allowing for individual surgeon's preferences for equipment and cardioplegia. Communication is even more essential with complicated patients and the interruption of continuity of care with work hour limitations.

Stevens and colleagues sought to provide a comprehensive program to sharpen performance of experienced cardiac surgical teams in acute crisis management.[47] They developed and implemented a program of simulation-based training with high enough realism, including a bypass simulator, to engage an entire cardiac surgery team, including surgeon, anesthesiologist, nurses, perfusionists, and physician assistants. Realistic simulated scenarios engaged the team in critical events that elicited teamwork skills, including effective leadership of event management and specific communication skills. As is always done in such training, the simulated cases were each followed by a debriefing by trained facilitators. Critical elements of information sharing in the cardiac surgical environment were identified and ways to optimize their interpersonal communication and team response were discussed. The program also included an interactive, four-hour workshop for the entire hospital cardiac surgical service.[47]

Based on perceptions of the participants, this program was judged to have positive impact within the cardiac surgical service. Focus group participants noted feeling that patient care had improved as a result of this training. The surgeons interviewed reported that they were conducting briefings and other participants described desirable teamwork behavior changes prompted by the program. Eighty-two percent of participants recommended repeat simulation training every 6 to 12 months. The interactive workshop participants identified speaking up about critical information and interprofessional information-sharing as the areas of highest priority.

Involving the full operating room team in teamwork training has presented challenges including logistical and financial barriers. While simulations for operating room professionals have been conducted for many years, the inclusion of practicing surgeons appears still to be rare. Where OR teamwork training is conducted, the role of the surgeon is often played by a member of the team who is of a different profession. Indeed, the use of simulation-based training for surgery to date has been on acquisition of technical skills for surgeons. Less importance is given to the nontechnical skills of communication, leadership, and teamwork. Despite these challenges and small sample size of studies that include attending surgeons, the results suggest a significant positive impact on team performance.[48] As a result of the perceived success of surgical teamwork training pilot programs, CRICO/RMF expanded its malpractice insurance premium incentive program to include surgeons in high-risk specialties. Cardiac and other surgeons participating once every two years in a six-hour simulation-based training with a full operating room team qualify for a ten percent lower annual premium.[a]

---

[a]Personal communication, William Berry, MD.

SIMULATION AS AN EVALUATION TOOL

While simulation has predominantly been used in cardiac surgery as a method for training cardiothoracic surgical residents, simulation also holds the potential to be used as a standardized evaluation tool. This would provide objective criteria for certifying trainees as possessing the competence required to operate independently. In 1997, Martin and colleagues validated the Objective Structured Assessment of Technical Skills for general surgery skills.[49] In 2013, de Montbrun and colleagues validated a similar tool to assess technical competence for colorectal surgical skills.[50] Methods for using simulators to assess task-specific competency for coronary anastomoses, mitral valve surgery, and perfusion management are currently being developed and tested[5,6,51] (Tables 8-1 and 8-2). In 2013, Lee et al. evaluated the Joint Council on Thoracic Surgery Education Coronary Artery Assessment Tool for interrater reliability.[52] The JTSE tool for coronary anastomosis consists of 13 assessment parameters, which are scored on a Likert scale from 1 (poor) to 5 (outstanding). Lee had 10 attending-level surgeons ranging from 2 to 33 years of practice watch videos of a medical student, a resident, a fellow, and two attending surgeons operate on a low-fidelity simulator, high-fidelity simulator, and in a human CABG. The study reported high interrater reliability and internal consistency for this scoring system suggesting it may be useful for assessing trainee's competence for coronary anastomosis.[52] Currently, however, no assessment tools have been validated as a standard assessment tool in cardiothoracic surgery.

FUTURE DIRECTIONS

Ericsson presented evidence that achievement of expert performance in challenging professional domains requires on the order of 10,000 hours of deliberate practice, including mentoring via a coach.[53] Modern clinical residents do not complete their training with nearly 10,000 hours of operating time, not to mention deliberate practice time, and it is doubtful they ever could. Simulation has the promise of offering the opportunity to acquire more deliberate practice particularly in technical skills both during training and throughout a lifetime of surgical practice. Furthermore, because of both safety and efficiency demands, the modern resident should enter the operating room coached on basic skills prior to first being involved in direct patient care. Training programs are moving in that direction, but much more needs to be done before all aspects of pre-training can be accomplished, especially for challenging technical tasks and even more so for all of the areas of surgical care that involve judgments before and during an actual procedure.

This chapter has described a number of the current simulation paradigms available in cardiothoracic training from synthetic to tissue-based, from low- to high-fidelity. However, we are far from a systematic curriculum utilizing these tools. Future training programs will need to develop a training paradigm where residents spend time in simulation with a coach prior to entering the operating room. Baker and colleagues suggested one possible method to design such a curriculum in 2012.[54] Training should begin on low-fidelity simulators where interns and junior residents can learn basic suture

TABLE 8-1: Components of Performance Rating Scores

1. Graft orientation (proper orientation for toe-heel, appropriate start and end points)	1	2	3	4	5
2. Bite appropriate (entry and exit points, number of punctures, even and consistent distance from edge)	1	2	3	4	5
3. Spacing appropriate (even spacing, consistent distance from previous bite, too close vs too far)	1	2	3	4	5
4. Use of Castroviejo needle holder (finger placement, instrument rotation, facility, needle placement, pronation and supination, proper linger and hand motion, lack of wrist motion)	1	2	3	4	5
5. Use of forceps (facility, band mot ion, assist needle placement, appropriate traction on tissue)	1	2	3	4	5
6. Needle angles (proper angle relative to tissue and needle bolder, consider depth of field, anticipating subsequent angles)	1	2	3	4	5
7. Needle transfer (needle placement and preparation from stitch to stitch, use of instrument and band to mount needle)	1	2	3	4	5
8. Suture management/tension (too loose vs too tight, use tension to assist exposure, avoid entanglement)	1	2	3	4	5
9. Knot tying (adequate tension, facility, linger and hand follow for deep knots)	1	2	3	4	5

Scores: 1, excellent. Able to accomplish goal without hesitation, showing excellent progress and flow; 2, good, able to accomplish goal deliberately, with minimal hesitation, showing good progress and flow; 3, average, able to accomplish goal with hesitation. Discontinuous progress and flow; 4, below average, able to partially accomplish goal with hesitation; 5, poor, unable to accomplish goal, marked hesitation (adapted from the Objective Structured Assessment of Technical Skill[3]).
Reproduced with permission from Fann JI, Caffarelli AD, Georgette G, et al: Improvement in coronary anastomosis with cardiac surgery simulation, *J Thorac Cardiovasc Surg* 2008 Dec;136(6):1486-1491.

TABLE 8-2: Mean Performance Rating Scores Comparing Scores Before and After Practice

	Anastomosis Task Station		Beating-heart Model	
	Before	After	Before	After
1. Graft orientation	2.1 ± 1.5	1.4 ± 0.8	1.8 ± 1.1	1.4 ± 0.7
2. Bite appropriate	2.0 ± 1.0	1.5 ± 0.8	1.7 ± 0.8	1.3 ± 0.7
3. Spacing appropriate	1.9 ± 0.9	1.4 ± 0.7	1.7 ± 0.8	1.3 ± 0.7
4. Castroviejo needle holder use	2.0 ± 1.4	1.7 ± 1.0	1.8 ± 1.0	1.6 ± 1.3
5. Use of forceps	2.2 ± 1.1	2.0 ± 1.3	2.1 ± 1.0	1.6 ± 0.9
6. Needle angles	1.8 ± 1.0	1.4 ± 0.7	1.8 ± 0.9	1.5 ± 1.1
7. Needle transfer	2.2 ± 1.1	1.6 ± 0.9	2.1 ± 1.2	1.6 ± 1.2
8. Suture management/ tension	2.2 ± 1.2	1.4 ± 0.7	1.8 ± 0.9	1.3 ± 0.7
9. Knot tying	1.6 ± 0.9	1.4 ± 0.7	1.8 ± 0.9	1.4 ± 0.7

Data are expressed as means ± standard deviation.
Reproduced with permission from Fann JI, Caffarelli AD, Georgette G, et al: Improvement in coronary anastomosis with cardiac surgery simulation, *J Thorac Cardiovasc Surg* 2008 Dec;136(6):1486-1491.

techniques and knot tying progressing to high-fidelity simulation such as the synthetic-beating heart simulator where they can practice aortic cannulation and coronary anastomoses.[54] We expect that competency-based training programs such as described by Ferguson et al. for orthopedic surgery will become more widely used throughout surgery and rely heavily on all of the various forms of simulation.[55]

Simulation for team training likewise is at the early stages of integration into surgical practice. For all types of simulation and other experiential training outside of the direct patient care setting, there is a substantial economic and cultural barrier. The current apprenticeship form of training does not easily accommodate simulation since it requires removing the training from patient-care-related activities, which of course have their own value in developing expertise and are challenged by increasing complexity of care, the need for sub-specialization, and work-hour restrictions.

Another area of utility for cardiac surgical simulation will be for introducing new technologies into the flow of established operations. Opening of a new operating room or suite of rooms, introducing a new type of procedure or new technologies can benefit from conducting simulations before initial utilization. This has been done for numerous other healthcare domains, but we are not aware of a specific published application in cardiac surgical care.[56,57]

Currently, most simulator technologies have a limited repertoire of patient pathology and variations from the normal distribution of anatomy aberrations. And, there are few simulation tools designed to develop judgment for pre- and intra-procedure decision-making. Thus, for the advances above to be achieved, much more technically accurate and biologically diverse simulations must be developed. The increasing use of 3-D printing of patient-specific, anatomically correct organ and body area by combining 3-D imaging and using 3-D printing to build a simulated surgical site is also likely to gain more widespread use and will further enable optimization of surgical approach, practice in performing a complex, atypical procedure and team training required to do that safely and efficiently.

We expect that simulation in all its various forms will be increasingly applied in cardiac surgery as the technology advances and as innovation responds to the demands for greater safety and process efficiency.

REFERENCES

1. Gaba DM: The future vision of simulation in health care. *Qual Saf Health Care* 2004; 13(Suppl 1):i2-10.
2. Cooper JB, Taqueti VR: A brief history of the development of mannequin simulators for clinical education and training. *Qual Saf Health Care* 2004; 13(Suppl 1)i11-18.
3. Owen H: Early use of simulation in medical education. *Simul Healthc* 2012; 7:102-116.
4. Ziv A, Wolpe PR, Small SD, Glick S: Simulation-based medical education: an ethical imperative. *Acad Med* 2003; 78:783-788.
5. Fann JI, Caffarelli AD, Georgette G, et al: Improvement in coronary anastomosis with cardiac surgery simulation. *J Thorac Cardiovasc Surg* 2008; 136:1486-1491.
6. Joyce DL, Dhillon TS, Caffarelli AD, et al: Simulation and skills training in mitral valve surgery. *J Thorac Cardiovasc Surg* 2011; 141:107-112.
7. Bruppacher HR, Alam SK, LeBlanc VR, et al: Simulation-based training improves physicians' performance in patient care in high-stakes clinical setting of cardiac surgery. *Anesthesiology* 2010; 112:985-992.
8. Ramphal PS, Coore DN, Craven MP, et al: A high fidelity tissue-based cardiac surgical simulator. *Eur J Cardiothorac Surg* 2005; 27:910-916.
9. Fann JI, Feins RH, Hicks GL Jr, Nesbitt JC, Hammon JW, Crawford FA, Jr: Evaluation of simulation training in cardiothoracic surgery: the Senior Tour perspective. *J Thorac Cardiovasc Surg* 2012; 143:264-272.
10. Macfie RC, Webel AD, Nesbitt JC, Fann JI, Hicks GL, Feins RH: "Boot camp" simulator training in open hilar dissection in early cardiothoracic surgical residency. *Ann Thorac Surg* 2014; 97:161-166.
11. Fann JI, Calhoon JH, Carpenter AJ, et al: Simulation in coronary artery anastomosis early in cardiothoracic surgical residency training: the Boot Camp experience. *J Thorac Cardiovasc Surg* 2010; 139:1275-1281.
12. Reznick RK: Teaching and testing technical skills. *Am J Surg* 1993; 165:358-361.

13. Reznick RK, MacRae H: Teaching surgical skills—changes in the wind. *N Engl J Med* 2006; 355:2664-2669.

14. Kopta JA: An approach to the evaluation of operative skills. *Surgery* 1971; 70:297-303.

15. Collins A, Brown JS, Newman SE: Cognitive apprenticeship: teaching the crafts of reading, writing, and mathematics, in Resnick LB (ed.) *Knowing, Learning, and Instruction: Essays in Honor of Robert Glaser* Hillsdale, Lawrence Erlbaum Associates, 1989; 41.

16. Allan CK, Pigula F, Bacha EA, et al: An extracorporeal membrane oxygenation cannulation curriculum featuring a novel integrated skills trainer leads to improved performance among pediatric cardiac surgery trainees. *Simul Healthc* 2013; 8:221-228.

17. Chan SY, Figueroa M, Spentzas T, Powell A, Holloway R, Shah S: Prospective assessment of novice learners in a simulation-based extracorporeal membrane oxygenation (ECMO) education program. *Pediatr Cardiol* 2013; 34:543-552.

18. Morris RW, Pybus DA: "Orpheus" cardiopulmonary bypass simulation system. *J Extra Corpor Technol* 2007; 39:228-233.

19. Lansdowne W, Machin D, Grant DJ: Development of the orpheus perfusion simulator for use in high-fidelity extracorporeal membrane oxygenation simulation. *J Extra Corpor Technol* 2012; 44:250-255.

20. Schmauss D, Juchem G, Weber S, Gerber N, Hagl C, Sodian R: Three-dimensional printing for perioperative planning of complex aortic arch surgery. *Ann Thorac Surg* 2014; 97:2160-2163.

21. Schmauss D, Haeberle S, Hagl C, Sodian R: Three-dimensional printing in cardiac surgery and interventional cardiology: a single-centre experience. *Eur J Cardiothorac Surg* 2015; 47:1044-1052.

22. Olivieri LJ, Krieger A, Loke YH, Nath DS, Kim PC, Sable CA: Three-dimensional printing of intracardiac defects from three-dimensional echocardiographic images: feasibility and relative accuracy. *J Am Soc Echocardiogr* 2015; 28:392-397.

23. Valverde I, Gomez G, Coserria JF, et al: 3D printed models for planning endovascular stenting in transverse aortic arch hypoplasia. *Catheter Cardiovasc Interv* 2015; 85:1006-1012.

24. Costello JP, Olivieri LJ, Krieger A, et al: Utilizing three-dimensional printing technology to assess the feasibility of high-fidelity synthetic ventricular septal defect models for simulation in medical education. *World J Pediatr Congenit Heart Surg* 2014; 5:421-426.

25. Riley RH: *A Manual of Simulation in Healthcare*, 1st ed. New York, Oxford University Press, 2008.

26. Gaba D, Fish K, Howard S: *Crisis Management in Anesthesiology*. Philadelphia, Churchill Livingstone, 1994.

27. Kohn LT, Corrigan JM, Donaldson MSe: *To Err is Human: Building a Safer Healthcare System*. Washington, DC, National Academy Press, 1999.

28. Howard SK, Gaba DM, Fish KJ, Yang G, Sarnquist FH: Anesthesia crisis resource management training: teaching anesthesiologists to handle critical incidents. *Aviat Space Environ Med* 1992; 63:763-770.

29. Carthey J, de Leval MR, Reason JT: The human factor in cardiac surgery: errors and near misses in a high technology medical domain. *Ann Thorac Surg* 2001; 72:300-305.

30. de Leval MR, Carthey J, Wright DJ, Farewell VT, Reason JT: Human factors and cardiac surgery: a multicenter study. *J Thorac Cardiovasc Surg* 2000; 119:661-672.

31. Morey JC, Simon R, Jay GD, et al: Error reduction and performance improvement in the emergency department through formal teamwork training: evaluation results of the MedTeams project. *Health Serv Res* 2002; 37:1553-1581.

32. Robertson J, Bandali K: Bridging the gap: enhancing interprofessional education using simulation. *J Interprof Care* 2008; 22:499-508.

33. Mazzocco K, Petitti DB, Fong KT, et al: Surgical team behaviors and patient outcomes. *Am J Surg* 2009; 197(5):678-685.

34. Leonard M, Graham S, Bonacum D: The human factor: the critical importance of effective teamwork and communication in providing safe care. *Qual Saf Health Care* 2004; 13(Suppl 1):i85-90.

35. Rogers SO Jr, Gawande AA, Kwaan M, et al: Analysis of surgical errors in closed malpractice claims at 4 liability insurers. *Surgery* 2006; 140:25-33.

36. Haynes AB, Weiser TG, Berry WR, et al: A surgical safety checklist to reduce morbidity and mortality in a global population. *N Engl J Med* 2009; 360:491-499.

37. Carroll JS, Rudolph RJ, Hatakenaka S: Learning from Experience in High-Hazard Organizations. *Res Organ Beh* 2002;24:87-137.

38. Detert JR, Edmondson AC: Why employees are afraid to speak up. *Har Bus Rev* 2007; 85.

39. Griffen FD, Stephens LS, Alexander JB, et al: Violations of behavioral practices revealed in closed claims reviews. *Ann Surg* 2008; 248:468-474.

40. Davies JM, Posner KL, Lee LA, Cheney FW, Domino KB: Liability associated with obstetric anesthesia: a closed claims analysis. *Anesthesiology* 2009; 110:131-139.

41. Catchpole K, Mishra A, Handa A, McCulloch P: Teamwork and error in the operating room: analysis of skills and roles. *Ann Surg* 2008; 247:699-706.

42. Hanscom R: Medical simulation from an insurer's perspective. *Acad Emerg Med* 2008; 15:984-987.

43. Salas E, Cannon-Bowers J. Design training systematically, in E Locke (ed.): *The Blackwell Handbook of Principles of Organizational Behavior*, Vol. 1. Hoboken, Blackwell Publishers, 2000; pp 43-59.

44. Gardner R, Walzer TB, Simon R, Raemer DB: Obstetric simulation as a risk control strategy: course design and evaluation. *Simul Healthc* 2008; 3:119-127.

45. Arriaga AF, Gawande AA, Raemer DB, et al: Pilot testing of a model for insurer-driven, large-scale multicenter simulation training for operating room teams. *Ann Surg* 2014; 259:403-410.

46. Rudolph JW, Simon R, Dufresne RL, Raemer DB: There's no such thing as "nonjudgmental" debriefing: a theory and method for debriefing with good judgment. *Simul Healthc* 2006; 1:49-55.

47. Stevens LM, Cooper JB, Raemer DB, et al: Educational program in crisis management for cardiac surgery teams including high realism simulation. *J Thorac Cardiovasc Surg* 2012; 144:17-24.

48. Aggarwal R, Undre S, Moorthy K, Vincent C, Darzi A: The simulated operating theatre: comprehensive training for surgical teams. *Qual Saf Health Care* 2004; 13(Suppl 1):i27-32.

49. Martin JA, Regehr G, Reznick R, et al: Objective structured assessment of technical skill (OSATS) for surgical residents. *Br J Surg* 1997; 84:273-278.

50. de Montbrun SL, Roberts PL, Lowry AC, et al: A novel approach to assessing technical competence of colorectal surgery residents: the development and evaluation of the Colorectal Objective Structured Assessment of Technical Skill (COSATS). *Ann Surg* 2013; 258:1001-1006.

51. Hicks GL Jr, Gangemi J, Angona RE Jr, Ramphal PS, Feins RH, Fann JI: Cardiopulmonary bypass simulation at the Boot Camp. *J Thorac Cardiovasc Surg* 2011; 141:284-292.

52. Lee R, Enter D, Lou X, et al: The Joint Council on Thoracic Surgery Education coronary artery assessment tool has high interrater reliability. *Ann Thorac Surg* 2013; 95:2064-2069; discussion 2069-2070.

53. Ericsson KA, Krampe RT, Tesch-Romer Clemens: The role of Deliberate Practice in the Acquisition of Expert Performance. *Psychol Rev* 1993; 100:363-406.

54. Baker CJ, Sinha R, Sullivan ME: Development of a cardiac surgery simulation curriculum: from needs assessment results to practical implementation. *J Thorac Cardiovasc Surg* 2012; 144:7-16.

55. Ferguson PC, Kraemer W, Nousiainen M, et al: Three-year experience with an innovative, modular competency-based curriculum for orthopaedic training. *J Bone Joint Surg Am* 2013; 95:e166.

56. Nielsen DS, Dieckmann P, Mohr M, Mitchell AU, Ostergaard D: Augmenting health care failure modes and effects analysis with simulation. *Simul Healthc* 2014; 9:48-55.

57. Ventre KM, Barry JS, Davis D, et al: Using in situ simulation to evaluate operational readiness of a children's hospital-based obstetrics unit. *Simul Healthc* 2014; 9:102-111.

The Integrated Cardiovascular Center

T. Konrad Rajab • Lawrence Lee • Vakhtang Tchantchaleishvili • Mandeep R. Mehra • John G. Byrne

Cardiovascular care is the diagnosis, treatment, and prevention of cardiovascular disease. Cardiovascular disease includes pathology of the heart and the peripheral vasculature. It remains the number one killer in the United States. The 2010 overall rate of death attributable to cardiovascular disease was 235.5 per 100,000. On the basis of this death rate, more than 2150 Americans die of cardiovascular disease each day, which corresponds to 1 death every 40 seconds. However, the death rate attributable to cardiovascular disease has declined by 31% from 2000 to 2010.[1] The reasons for this include progress in preventive medicine as well as better treatment of risk markers like hypertension and hyperlipidemia, timely application of reperfusion therapy for acute myocardial infarction and better access to cardiovascular operations and procedures. This has correlated with a dramatic increase in the volume of cardiovascular care. For example, there were approximately 6,000,000 inpatient cardiovascular operations and procedures in 2000, which increased by 25% to approximately 7,500,000 inpatient cardiovascular operations and procedures in 2010.[1] As a result of these trends, cardiovascular care comes at a larger cost to society. The total direct and indirect costs of cardiovascular disease and stroke in the United States in 2010 were estimated at $315.4 billion.[1]

EVOLUTION OF CARDIOVASCULAR SUBSPECIALTIES

Cardiovascular care is provided by a number of different cardiovascular subspecialties. This includes cardiac surgeons, cardiovascular physicians, interventional cardiologists, interventional and noninterventional radiologists, vascular surgeons, cardiovascular anesthesiologists, critical care specialists, and primary care physicians. Each of these subspecialties has evolved from very different historical roots. For example, cardiac surgery emerged from general surgery during the Second World War, when Dwight Harken successfully removed foreign bodies in and around the heart of some 130 injured soldiers.[2] In contrast, interventional cardiology emerged from radiology when Dr. Charles Dotter performed the first-ever angioplasty procedure in a leg artery at the Oregon Health and Science University in Oregon[3] and, building on his work, Dr. Andreas Gruentzig performed the first balloon angioplasty procedure on a coronary artery.[4] Similarly, each of the other subspecialties that contribute to cardiovascular care has evolved from distinct historical roots. As a result of these different historic roots, providers of cardiovascular care were originally organized in separate medical school departments according to the patient populations that their disciples historically served and the instruments that were historically used in their clinical practice.

EVOLUTION OF CARDIOVASCULAR CENTERS

The departments of early medical schools were initially formed by individual professors and their assistants. Subsequent expansion of the departments increased their organizational complexity but they continued to operate as separate units under the leadership of autonomous chairmen.[5] Advances in medical research in the twentieth century resulted in the emergence of departmental subspecialists who predominantly treated one specific organ. Consequently, many medical school departments established divisions that focused on particular organ systems.[5] As the divisions became ever more specialized, the clinical interests of individual divisions of separate departments began to overlap more with each other than with the rest of their respective departments. In particular, the emergence of cardiac surgery as a subspecialty resulted in a symbiotic relationship between cardiac surgeons and cardiologists.[5] Moreover, cardiac surgeons and cardiologists increasingly relied on specialized cardiovascular radiologists and cardiovascular anesthesiologists. Over time, these relationships between the cardiovascular subspecialties evolved into formal associations and eventually dedicated cardiovascular centers were formed. These cardiovascular centers allowed physicians of different subspecialties to cooperate at an unprecedented level to optimally orchestrate the cardiovascular care of their patients.

ADVANTAGES OF PROVIDING CARDIOVASCULAR CARE IN CARDIOVASCULAR CENTERS

Cardiovascular centers that integrate multiple cardiovascular subspecialties provide a number of important advantages. Firstly, integrated cardiovascular centers improve the clinical care for patients. For example, clinical care is improved by increasing patient volume. The relationship between patient volume and quality of care has been demonstrated in many areas of cardiovascular care. For example, a large body of evidence shows that increasing procedural volumes in cardiac surgery results in improved quality with decreased complication rates. Moreover, there is evidence that increased surgeon volume results in improved quality of care.[6] Therefore professional organizations have recommended that cardiac surgery programs performing fewer than 125 coronary artery bypass graft (CABG) procedures annually consider affiliation with high-volume tertiary centers.[7] A similar relationship between volume and quality of care exist in interventional cardiology. Among hospitals in the United States that have full interventional capabilities, a higher volume of angioplasty procedures was found to be associated with a lower mortality rate among patients undergoing primary angioplasty.[8] On the basis of this and other studies, professional organizations recommended that patients with ST elevation myocardial infarction undergo primary angioplasty by cardiac catheterization laboratories performing at least 36 primary angioplasties as well as at least 200 total angioplasties per year.[9] Integrated cardiovascular centers are ideally suited to deliver such high procedural numbers by concentrating cardiovascular care in dedicated centers, attracting referrals, co-marketing, and by sharing patients among the physicians. Higher quality of care can also be delivered by building up specialized expertise within narrow boundaries, multidisciplinary management of patients, and co-locating services. Finally, a substantial clinical research effort facilitates participation in multicenter trials that give patients access to the latest clinical treatment modalities.

Secondly, integrated cardiovascular centers improve the efficiency of patient flow pathways. This allows coordination of hospital visits to minimize intrusion in the patients' lives. For example, preoperative tests such as echocardiography, cardiac catheterization, and evaluation by cardiac anesthesia can occur on the least number of visits possible. Besides enhancing the patients' satisfaction with their care, the cost of cardiovascular care to society is reduced by minimizing time off work and allowing patients to participate in other activities.

Finally, integrated cardiovascular centers provide improved efficiency in practice management and reduced expenses. For example, an audit of the merger of a five-physician vascular surgery group, its noninvasive laboratory, and a three-physician interventional radiology group showed that integrating these cardiovascular subspecialties into a single center resulted in increased efficiencies that allowed the total expenses of the merged group to fall by 13% compared with the 12-month period that immediately preceded the merger.[10]

THE INTEGRATED CARDIOVASCULAR CENTER OF THE FUTURE

In the future, the advantages provided by cardiovascular centers will be maximized by full integration at the level of clinical care, education, and research. Integration of clinical care will result in multidisciplinary management at all levels of patient care. This will include multidisciplinary outpatient clinics, conferences, in-patient rounds, and procedures. For example, outpatient clinics for cardiac surgery, cardiology, and preoperative cardiovascular anesthesia will ideally be located in the same physical space and coordinated at the same time. One model could involve clinicians sharing a centralized physician work-space and patients being seen in designated clinic cubicles. This means that patients could be seen by physicians from different subspecialties without having to leave their designated cubicle. Physicians could see their patients together with other providers from different subspecialties at the same time, or sequentially based on the complexity and needs of individual patients. In practice, this may involve taking a joined preoperative history and physical examination by anesthesia and cardiac surgery mid-level providers. Cardiologists and cardiac surgeons could engage in a joined discussion with patients regarding the risks and benefits of the multimodality treatment options, which might include medical management, interventional management, or surgery. Finally, an integrated electronic medical record would minimize redundancy and increase efficiency.

Similarly, interpretation of cardiovascular studies by cardiologists and radiologists will take place in a shared reading room to pool the expertise of the providers. For example, cardiologists could contribute their clinical knowledge and their understanding of cardiovascular pathophysiology, whereas radiologists could offer imaging and information technology expertise.

Multidisciplinary conferences that benefit from the joint expertise of cardiac surgeons, cardiologists, and cardiovascular anesthesiologists include high-risk preoperative conferences for example. During these conferences each specialty can contribute toward an accurate assessment of the overall risk and benefit ratio of different treatment modalities for high-risk patients.

Finally, integration of clinical care will mean that procedures will increasingly take place in shared treatment spaces. The prime example for this is the hybrid operating room. Hybrid operating rooms have the usual features of an operating room with additional cardiac catheterization and endovascular capabilities (Fig. 9-1). This creates a shared work-space where cardiac surgeons, interventional cardiologists, and vascular surgeons can cooperate during joined procedures. Combining the tools of the catheterization laboratory and operating room greatly enhances the options available to surgeons and cardiologists to treat complex patients. One example is hybrid coronary revascularization wherein a left internal mammary artery graft is placed on the left anterior descending (LAD) artery either by minimally invasive or open technique and combined with percutaneous intervention of

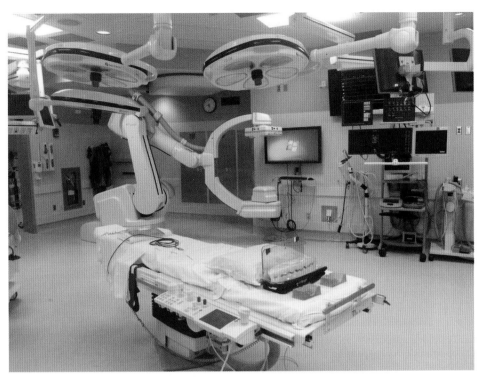

FIGURE 9-1 A hybrid operating room combines the usual features of an operating room with additional cardiac catheterization and endovascular capabilities.

non-LAD vessels.[11] Another example is minimally invasive valve surgery combined with percutaneous intervention to coronary lesions in order to convert high-risk valve and CABG operations into a low-risk isolated minimally invasive valve procedures. Yet, other possibilities include hybrid endomyocardial and epicardial arrhythmia procedures[12] and hybrid open and endovascular approaches for the descending thoracic aorta and pathologies of the aortic arch and distal ascending aorta.[13] Finally, the hybrid operating rooms represent an optimal setting for transcatheter aortic valve replacement.[14] This has already resulted in a new paradigm, the Hybrid Paradigm, where providers of the different cardiovascular subspecialties consider themselves cardiovascular proceduralists.

From the close clinical collaboration between the cardiovascular subspecialties follows that education and training need to be integrated in order to create a common culture and knowledge base. For example, free standing cardiothoracic surgery and vascular surgery residencies are evolving that allow better integration of the cardiovascular subspecialties during training than previous models which depended on general surgery training. For example, residents of a free-standing cardiothoracic surgery residency may rotate with cardiology during their early years of training. Another example is a TAVR fellowship that involves mandatory training with interventionalists in the catheterization suite. Conversely, cardiology fellows subspecializing in heart failure frequently accompany the cardiac surgery teams during heart procurements and are observers in the operating room during recipient implant procedures. Finally, the integration

of cardiovascular centers will allow trainees to participate in more related cases that are not part of their primary specialty.[10]

Research will also be facilitated by integrated cardiovascular centers that attract a critical mass of multidisciplinary research teams focusing on cardiovascular disease. In particular, center will provide organized leadership and the ability to distribute research activity at the level of subgroups. Faculty will also benefit from the close interaction with researchers outside of their divisions. Research support structures that can be custom focused on cardiovascular research include a wide range of areas from basic science core facilities to statistical support, specialized research grant administrators, and maintenance of an institutional clinical outcomes database. Multidisciplinary cardiovascular research conferences, common cafeteria, and leisure space will also facilitate the exchange of ideas between subspecialties. Ideally, integrated cardiovascular centers will participate in basic, translational, and clinical outcomes research focusing on cardiovascular disease since all of these fields benefit from a concentration of cardiovascular knowledge and clinical experience (Fig. 9-2).

In addition, there are specific advantages for each level of research. At the level of basic research, the differences between cardiovascular subspecialties nearly disappear. As a result, integrated cardiovascular centers offer ideal conditions for pooling and conducting such research. At the level of translational research there is also a convergence of interests since cutting edge translational research frequently involves multidisciplinary fields that transcend conventional departmental boundaries. Since basic and translational research

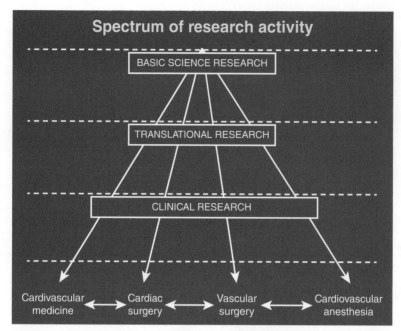

FIGURE 9-2 Integrated cardiovascular centers participate in basic science research, translational research, and clinical outcomes research. At each level there are different opportunities for cooperation between the cardiovascular subspecialties.

is often dependent on large amount of funding, integrated cardiovascular centers will be able to provide laboratories with common small and large animal spaces and provide shared equipment which would otherwise be too expensive for individual departments. Large multidisciplinary laboratories can be set up in cardiovascular centers which would otherwise be hard to assemble or maintain. The larger size of cardiovascular centers will also make it easier to bring in additional multidisciplinary expertise such as stem cell experts, tissue engineering, mechanical and bioengineering, valve hemodynamics, and 3D printed modeling capabilities that can contribute to research efforts of different cardiovascular subspecialties. Finally, clinical outcomes research is more efficient because follow-up of patients involves multiple specialties which can each contribute relevant data to a jointly maintained database.

In summary, the cardiovascular center of the future will be a multidisciplinary and collaborative entity encompassing clinical care, education, and research. This structure has the potential to improve quality of care, reduce costs, improve training, and accelerate research.

REFERENCES

1. Go AS, Mozaffarian D, Roger VL, et al: American Heart Association Statistics Committee and Stroke Statistics Subcommittee. Heart disease and stroke statistics—2014 update: a report from the American Heart Association. *Circulation* 2014; 129:e28-e292.
2. Harken DE: Foreign bodies in, and in relation to, the thoracic blood vessels and heart; techniques for approaching and removing foreign bodies from the chambers of the heart. *Surg Gynecol Obstet* 1946; 83:117-125.
3. Dotter CT, Judkins MP: Transluminal treatment of arteriosclerotic obstruction description of a new technic and a preliminary report of its application. *Circulation* 1964; 30:654-670.
4. Grüntzig A, Siegenthaler W: Die perkutane transluminale Rekanalisation chronischer Arterienverschlüsse mit einer neuen Dilatationstechnik. G. Witzstrock; 1977.
5. Braunwald E: Departments, divisions and centers in the evolution of medical schools. *Am J Med* 2006; 119:457-462.
6. Birkmeyer JD, Stukel TA, Siewers AE, Goodney PP, Wennberg DE, Lucas FL: Surgeon volume and operative mortality in the United States. *N Engl J Med* 2003; 349:2117-2127.
7. Hillis LD, Smith PK, Anderson JL, et al: American College of Cardiology Foundation/American Heart Association Task Force on Practice Guidelines. 2011 ACCF/AHA guideline for coronary artery bypass graft surgery: executive summary: a report of the American College of Cardiology Foundation/American Heart Association Task Force on Practice Guidelines. *J Thorac Cardiovasc Surg* 2012; 143:4-34.
8. Canto JG, Every NR, Magid DJ, et al: The volume of primary angioplasty procedures and survival after acute myocardial infarction. National Registry of Myocardial Infarction 2 Investigators. *N Engl J Med* 2000; 342:1573-1580.
9. Antman EM, Anbe DT, Armstrong PW, et al: American College of Cardiology, American Heart Association Task Force on Practice Guidelines, Canadian Cardiovascular Society. ACC/AHA guidelines for the management of patients with ST-elevation myocardial infarction: a report of the American College of Cardiology/American Heart Association Task Force on Practice Guidelines (Committee to Revise the 1999 Guidelines for the Management of Patients with Acute Myocardial Infarction). *Circulation* 2004; 110:e82-292.
10. Ouriel K, Green RM, Waldman D, Greenberg RK, Shortell CK, Illig K: A model for merging vascular surgery and interventional radiology: clinical and economical implications. *J Vasc Surg* 1998; 28:1006-1013.
11. Zhao DX, Leacche M, Balaguer JM, et al: Routine intraoperative completion angiography after coronary artery bypass grafting and 1-stop hybrid revascularization: results from a fully integrated hybrid catheterization laboratory/operating room. *J Am Coll Cardiol* 2009; 53:232-241.
12. Byrne JG, Leacche M, Vaughan DE, Zhao DX: Hybrid cardiovascular procedures. *JACC Cardiovasc Interv* 2008; 1:459-468.
13. Nollert G, Wich S: Planning a cardiovascular hybrid operating room: the technical point of view. In: the heart surgery forum. Carden Jennings, 2009; pp E125-E130.
14. Walther T, Dewey T, Borger MA, et al: Transapical aortic valve implantation: step by step. *Ann Thorac Surg* 2009; 87:276-283.

PERIOPERATIVE/ INTRAOPERATIVE CARE

10

Preoperative Evaluation for Cardiac Surgery

Christian T. Ruff • Patrick T. O'Gara

Advances in surgical techniques and improved patient outcomes have enabled the application of cardiac surgery in patient populations previously considered ineligible for an intervention of this magnitude. The decision to intervene surgically, as well as the type of intervention best suited to the patient, should be based on an individual risk-benefit analysis. The risks of the procedure, including major morbidities and short- and intermediate-term mortality, must be weighed against the expected benefits with respect to longevity, symptom relief, and improved functional capacity. This chapter reviews the essential information that the cardiologist and surgeon must collect and review to evaluate a patient for cardiac surgery (Table 10-1). This information includes patient and disease characteristics as well as surgical considerations that can be integrated into scoring systems that provide a semiquantitative risk assessment. With the ever-evolving complexity of patients requiring specialized cardiovascular care, the refinement of surgical techniques, and the emergence of less invasive alternatives for high-risk patients, it has become apparent that there are important limitations to these scores in that they do not adequately account for procedure-specific impediments, major organ system compromise, and patient frailty. In addition, there has been recognition that risk assessment must occur in a framework of shared decision making that ensures that patients and their families have a thorough understanding of the relative risks and benefits of the various treatment options and, most importantly, that their wishes and preferences are respected in the therapeutic plan. There has been increasing recognition that a Heart Team approach that draws on the strength of multidisciplinary participation in decision making may be ideally suited to meet this challenge.

RISK ASSESSMENT

Patient Characteristics and Conditions

AGE

The volume of cardiac surgical procedures in the elderly continues to increase as life expectancy improves and the benefits of surgery outweigh the risks in appropriately selected individuals. While perioperative mortality rates do not vary significantly by age, mortality 1 year after surgery is generally higher in patients over 75 years of age, compared with those who are younger.[1] Octagenarians have nearly double the mortality rate compared with younger patients (4.1 vs 2.3%) and more than 60% of octogenarians have at least one nonfatal postoperative complication.[2,3] The most frequent complications include the need for prolonged ventilatory support in intensive care units, reoperation for bleeding and pneumonia—all resulting in longer hospital stays.[3] A higher proportion of complications occur in elderly patients with low body weight ((body mass index) BMI < 23).[4] With improved surgical techniques and careful patient selection, nonagenarians can safely undergo cardiac surgery with a 95% 30-day survival and 93% survival to hospital discharge.[5-7]

GENDER

Some but not all epidemiologic studies suggest that female gender is an independent predictor of postoperative morbidity and mortality.[8-10] Gender differences are present in both traditional coronary artery bypass graft (CABG) and off-pump surgery.[11] Several large retrospective cohort studies of patients undergoing CABG found that women had higher mortality rates than men even after adjusting for comorbidities and confounding factors, including body surface area.[8,9] Possible explanations for worse outcomes in women include smaller coronary arteries (which might enhance the technical difficulty of performing anastomoses and limit graft flow), differences in referral for surgery (ie, women being referred at later disease stages), and gender differences in self-reported outcomes.[12] Data suggest that benefit in terms of QOL after cardiac surgery is similar for men and women.[13]

RACE

Although crude post-CABG mortality rates differ significantly by race, data suggest that after controlling for patient and hospital variables, these differences are small.[14,15] However, in the United States, self-reported black race is associated

TABLE 10-1: Risk Assessment Combining STS Risk Estimate, Frailty, Major Organ System Dysfunction, and Procedure-Specific Impediments

	Low Risk (Must Meet ALL Criteria in This Column)	Intermediate Risk (Any 1 Criterion in This Column)	High Risk (Any 1 Criterion in This Column)	Prohibitive Risk (Any 1 Criterion in This Column)
STS PROM*	<4%	4–8%	>8%	Predicted risk with surgery of death or major morbidity
	AND	OR	OR	
Frailty†	None	1 Index (mild)	≥2 Indices	(all-cause) >50% at 1 year
	AND	OR	(moderate to severe) OR	OR
Major organ system compromise not to be improved postoperatively‡	None	1 Organ system	No more than 2 organ system	≥3 Organ systems
	AND	OR	OR	OR
Procedure-specific impediment§	None	Possible procedure-specific impediment	Possible procedure-specific impediment	Severe procedure-specific impediment

*Use of the STS PROM to predict risk in a given institution with reasonable reliability is appropriate only if institutional outcomes are within 1 standard deviation of STS average observed/expected ratio for the procedure in question.
†Seven frailty indices: Katz Activities of Daily Living (independence in feeding, bathing, dressing, transferring, toileting, and urinary continence) and independence in ambulation (no walking aid or assist required or 5-m walk in <6 s). Other scoring systems can be applied to calculate no, mild-, or moderate-to-severe frailty.
‡Examples of major organ system compromise: Cardiac-severe LV systolic or diastolic dysfunction or RV dysfunction, fixed pulmonary hypertension; CKD stage 3 or worse; pulmonary dysfunction with FEV1 < 50% or DLCO₂ < 50% of predicted; CNS dysfunction (dementia, Alzheimer's disease, Parkinson's disease, OVA with persistent physical limitation); GI dysfunction—Crohn's disease, ulcerative colitis, nutritional impairment, or serum albumin < 3.0; cancer-active malignancy; and liver-any history of cirrhosis, variceal bleeding, or elevated INR in the absence of VKA therapy.
§Examples: Tracheostomy present, heavily calcified ascending aorta, chest malformation, arterial coronary graft adherent to posterior chest wall, or radiation damage.
CKD, chronic kidney disease; CNS, central nervous system; CVA, stroke; DLCO₂, diffusion capacity for carbon dioxide; FEV1, forced expiratory volume in 1 s; GI, gastro-intestinal; INR, international normalized ratio; LV, left ventricular; PROM, predicted risk of mortality; RV, right ventricular; STS, Society of Thoracic Surgeons; and VKA, vitamin K antagonist.
(Reproduced with permission from Nishimura RA, Otto CM, Bonow RO, et al: 2014 AHA/ACC guideline for the management of patients with valvular heart disease: a report of the American College of Cardiology/American Heart Association Task Force on Practice Guidelines, *Am Coll Cardiol* 2014 Jun 10;63(22):e57-e185.)

with an increased risk of postoperative complications, including prolonged ventilatory support, length of stay, reoperation for bleeding, and postoperative renal failure.[16]

DIABETES

Patients with diabetes have significantly worse outcomes following cardiac surgery.[17-19] Studies have shown diabetes to be an independent predictor of in-hospital mortality after CABG although emerging evidence indicates that the severity of diabetes, specifically target organ damage, may be important in risk stratification.[20,21] Postoperative mortality does not differ significantly between nondiabetic and diabetic patients without diabetic sequelae, though diabetic patients with vascular disease and/or renal failure have an increased risk of mortality.[21] Patients with insulin-dependent type II diabetes in particular are at increased risk of major postoperative complications including renal failure, deep sternal wound infection, and prolonged hospital stay.[22,23] Strict perioperative glucose control has been shown to lower operative mortality and the incidence of mediastinitis.[24,25] Off-pump surgery also appears to decrease postoperative morbidity in diabetic patients.[26]

RENAL FUNCTION

Renal dysfunction is common in patients undergoing cardiac surgery. Approximately half of patients undergoing CABG have at least mild renal dysfunction and one quarter have at

least moderate renal dysfunction.[27] There is a graded increase in operative mortality and morbidity with worsening preoperative renal function.[27-29] Renal insufficiency is associated with greater risk of both 30-day (odds ratio, OR = 3.7) and 1-year mortality (OR = 4.6).[30] Even mild renal dysfunction (serum creatinine 1.47–2.25 mg/dL) is associated with increased rates of operative and long-term mortality, need for postoperative dialysis, and postoperative stroke.[31]

Renoprotective drugs, such as fenoldopam and N-acetylcysteine, have no effect on the deterioration of renal function in high-risk patients.[32,33] Off-pump CABG (OP CABG) is associated with a lower prevalence of the need for postoperative renal replacement therapy; larger studies are needed to determine if this correlates with improved outcomes.[34]

PULMONARY FUNCTION

It is well established that patients with compromised pulmonary function, predominantly due to chronic obstructive pulmonary disease (COPD), have a higher mortality and increased incidence of postoperative complications including arrhythmias, reintubation, pneumonia, prolonged intensive care unit (ICU) length of stay (LOS), and increased LOS.[35,36] Postoperative respiratory failure is a common complication (14.8% in a New York State database) with a higher incidence (14.8%) in combined CABG and valve operations.[37] Optimizing respiratory status prior to surgery, including smoking cessation, antibiotics for pneumonia, and treatment of COPD flares with bronchodilator therapy and steroids is a critical part of preoperative management.[38] There is evidence that intensive inspiratory muscle training prevents postoperative pulmonary complications in high-risk patients.[39]

Surgical Considerations

REOPERATION

Hospital mortality among patients undergoing reoperative cardiac surgery has traditionally been higher than among patients undergoing primary operation.[40-42] This is likely due to the higher-risk profile of patients undergoing reoperation (older, more extensive vascular and coronary disease, multiple comorbidities) and the demanding surgical aspects including sternal reentry, pericardial adhesions, in situ arterial grafts and diseased saphenous vein grafts.[43]

Despite these factors, hospital mortality rates associated with coronary reoperation have decreased with greater surgical experience and now approach those observed with primary CABG.[43,44] With careful preoperative risk evaluation and surgical management, reoperation can be performed safely.

PRIOR RADIATION

Patients receiving thoracic radiation for treatment of malignancies before cardiac surgery have poorer short- and long-term outcomes.[45,46] Thoracic radiation exposure is heterogeneous with respect to different malignancies and there is a gradient of risk.

A study dividing patients undergoing cardiac surgery into three levels of radiation exposure: extensive (Hodgkin's disease, thymoma, and testicular cancer), variable (non-Hodgkin's lymphoma and lung cancer), and tangential (breast cancer), demonstrated that patients with extensive radiation exposure had longer radiation-to-operation interval, poorer pulmonary function, and more severe aortic regurgitation, diastolic dysfunction and left main coronary stenosis.[47] Hospital deaths (13% vs 8.6% vs 2.4%) and respiratory complications (24% vs 20% vs 9.6%) were higher after more extensive radiation and 4-year survival was poorer (64% vs 57% vs 80%).

SURGICAL COMPLEXITY AND TECHNIQUE

It is important to consider the type of cardiac surgical procedure (CABG, valve, or combined) as well as the surgical technique (on-pump, off-pump, minimally invasive, robotic, and hybrid) when providing preoperative risk assessment as mortality and morbidity risks may vary.

Valve surgeries generally have a higher complication rate than isolated CABG, and combined surgeries have the highest risk (Fig. 10-1). Participants in the Society of Thoracic Surgeons National Adult Cardiac Surgery Database collected data between 2002 and 2006 on more than 3.6 million procedures.[48-50] They reported 30-day mortality and a composite end point of mortality and major in-hospital morbidity including stroke, renal failure, prolonged ventilation, deep sternal wound infection, and reoperation. CABG mortality was 2.3% with a 14.4% rate for the combined end point of mortality and major morbidity.[48] Isolated valve procedures had higher mortality rates, including 3.2% for aortic valve replacement (AVR), 5.7% for mitral valve replacement (MVR), and 1.6% for mitral valve repair (MVP).[49] Combined mortality and major morbidity was also higher for valve surgery at 18.3% (AVR 17.4%, MVR 26.7%, MVP 12.7%). Combined CABG and valve procedures had the highest mortality rate at 6.8% (AVR + CABG 5.6%, MVR + CABG 11.6%, and MVP + CABG 7.4%) with a combined mortality and major morbidity of 30.1% (AVR + CABG 26.3%, MVR + CABG 43.2%, and MVP + CABG 33.5%).[50]

Minimally invasive surgical techniques can be divided by approach and use of cardiopulmonary bypass (CBP). The use of alternatives to standard median sternotomy has been increasingly adopted in surgical centers for performance of both CABG and valve procedures. The potential benefits of minimally invasive surgery are earlier extubation, reduced

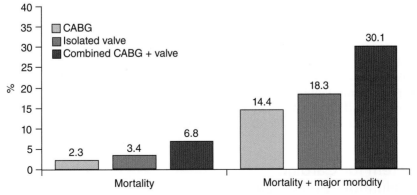

FIGURE 10-1 Thirty-day mortality and a composite end point of mortality and major in-hospital morbidity (stroke, renal failure, prolonged ventilation, deep sternal wound infection, and reoperation) from the Society of Thoracic Surgeons National Adult Cardiac Surgery Database (STS NCD).[48-50] CABG = coronary artery bypass graft surgery.

discomfort, lower rates of wound infection, less blood loss, and shorter recovery times.[51]

Off-pump CABG is performed with stabilization devices to reduce motion of target vessels while anastomoses are performed without CBP. Current surgical approaches to valve surgery require CBP and cardioplegic arrest. Meta-analyses of observational and randomized trials of OP CABG versus on-pump CABG have not demonstrated a clear advantage of OP CABG with respect to mortality or morbidity.[52,53] Postoperative complications with OP CABG generally show consistent reductions in postoperative AF, blood loss, wound infections and myocardial injury with nonsignificant trends toward lower death, myocardial infarction (MI) and stroke.[53-55] The benefits of OP CABG are particularly notable in the elderly and in patients with heavily calcified aortas.[54]

There have been continued advances in optics, instrumentation and perfusion technology that have facilitated use of totally endoscopic robotic cardiac surgery.[56] This technology has been applied to many cardiac surgical procedures, in particular MVP and totally endoscopic coronary artery bypass grafting (TECAB). Short-term results are promising in some series but long-term studies are lacking and a steep learning curve characterizes the early phase of application.

Simultaneous "hybrid" percutaneous coronary intervention with drug-eluting stents and minimally invasive surgical bypass grafting procedures in a specially designed operating suite (hybrid OR) are also gaining more widespread acceptance. Hybrid procedures require close cooperation between surgical and interventional teams. Although there are limited data available, hybrid patients have similar angiographic vessel patency and major adverse cardiac events (MACE) at six months with shorter hospital lengths of stay, intubation times and less blood loss despite aggressive antiplatelet therapy.[57]

RISK SCORES

Preoperative risk assessment has important implications not only for individual patient well-being but as a qualitative tool to serve as a reference standard to compare outcomes among surgeons, institutions, or assessment of new procedures and techniques. There are numerous risk stratification scores and systems that have been developed from large databases to quantify the mortality and morbidity risks of cardiac surgery. Both patient and surgical factors are considered preoperatively and assessed for their ability to predict postoperative complications. This section will focus on two of the most widely used risk scoring systems: European System for Cardiac Operative Risk Evaluation (EuroSCORE) and Society for Thoracic Surgeons (STS) risk estimate (Table 10-2).

The European System for Cardiac Operative Risk Evaluation (EuroSCORE)

The EuroSCORE, initially published in 1999, is the most rigorously evaluated scoring system in cardiac surgery.[58]

TABLE 10-2: Comparison of Preoperative Risk Factors for Risk Stratification Models

Preoperative Risk Factor	EuroSCORE	STS
Age	X	X
Gender	X	X
Race	X	X
Weight/BSA		X
IABP/inotropes		X
LV function	X	X
Renal disease	X	X
Lung disease	X	X
PVD	X	X
Diabetes		X
Neurologic dysfunction	X	X
Active endocarditis	X	
UA or recent MI	X	X
Previous cardiac surgery	X	X
Combined surgery	X	X
Aortic involvement	X	X
Valve surgery	X	X
Emergency surgery	X	X

The score is calculated by assessing 17 risk factors (patient, cardiac, and operation) known to affect outcome. There are two available methods: the original additive model and the more recent logistic model.[59,60] Studies have indicated that the additive model overestimates mortality in low-risk patients and underestimates mortality in high-risk patients.[60-62] The logistic model was designed to address these issues but there is still concern that this model overestimates mortality in many risk groups.[60] The logistic EuroSCORE is more accurate at predicting mortality in combined CABG and valve surgery.[63] The EuroSCORE calculator is available online (www.euroscore.org).

Society for Thoracic Surgeons Score

The STS has an extensive database with an online calculator (www.sts.org). Compared with the EuroSCORE calculator more extensive data entry is required to calculate an STS score. Models have been developed and revised for CABG, valve surgery, and combined procedures.[48-50] These models include mortality as well as multiple morbidity end points including stroke, renal failure, prolonged ventilation, deep sternal wound infection, and prolonged postoperative stay. Studies demonstrate that STS score showed similar discriminative capability and predictive performance compared with EuroSCORE and other risk algorithms.[64,65]

All risk models share important limitations. Preoperative risk factors included in the model can change significantly over time, leading to substantial under- or overestimation of postoperative risk.[66] Caution should also be used when interpreting the results of a model with respect to an individual patient's risk. The models are derived from large databases and do not include important considerations for an individual's specific risk profile such as surgeon experience and comorbidities not incorporated in the model's derivation. These models also do not capture patient frailty, which has been increasingly shown to have a decisive influence on procedural outcomes.

FRAILTY

Frailty is a syndrome that reflects a state of decreased physiological reserve and vulnerability to stressors.[67,68] The prevalence of frailty ranges from 10 to 60%, depending on the cardiovascular burden of the population as well as the specific frailty measures and thresholds utilized for its assessment.[69,70] Following surgery, or any other physiologic stressor, frail patients are at a marked risk for clinical decompensation, procedural complications, prolonged recovery, functional decline, disability, and mortality.[71] The emerging biology of frailty implicates systemic dysregulation of the immune, hormonal, and endocrine systems resulting in up-regulation of inflammatory cytokines, decreased testosterone levels, and insulin resistance.[72-78] The subsequent catabolic state that ensues precipitates a progressive decline in muscle mass and strength (sarcopenia).[79]

Many tools have been developed to measure frailty.[80] Most tools focus on 1 or more of the 5 core domains that define the frailty phenotype: slowness, weakness, low physical activity, exhaustion, and shrinking. Slowness is measured by a comfortable-pace gait speed test, weakness by a maximal handgrip strength test (using a dynamometer), and other domains by questionnaire or more specialized instruments. These domains may be considered individually or combined into a variety of scales (Table 10-3). The Fried scale and the Short Physical Performance Battery (SPPB) are two of the most frequently utilized and cited scores.[81-83] Although in contrast to these multi-item assessments, single measures of

TABLE 10-3: Recommended Frailty Assessment Tools

Domain	Tool(s)	Operational Definition	Common Cutoffs for Frailty
Slowness	5-m gait speed test	Patient is positioned behind start line and asked to walk at a comfortable pace past 5-m finish line; cue to trigger stopwatch is first footfall after start line and first footfall after finish line; repeated 3 times and averaged	Slow: <0.83 m/s (>6 s) Very slow: <0.65 m/s (>7.7 s) Extremely slow: <0.50 m/s (>10 s)
Weakness	Handgrip strength test	Patient is asked to squeeze a handgrip dynamometer as hard as possible; repeated 3 times (once with each hand and then with strongest hand); maximum value is recorded	Men: <30 kg Women: <20 kg
	Knee extensor strength test	Patient is seated on the dynamometer machine and asked to extend his/her knee against resistance; maximum isotonic force is recorded	Frailty cutoffs not yet established
Low physical activity	Physical activity questionnaire	Many questionnaires have been validated; those that provide a measure of activity in kcal/week are recommended (eg, Minnesota Leisure Time Activity, PASE, Paffenbarger Physical Activity Questionnaire)	Men: <383 kcal/week Women: <270 kcal/week
	Portable accelerometer	Patient is asked to wear a portable accelerometer for a period of 1 to 7 days; total kcal expenditure is recorded	Frailty cutoffs not yet established
Exhaustion	CES-D questionnaire	Patient is asked 2 questions: How often in the past week did you feel like everything you did was an effort?/like you could not get going? (often [ie, ≥3 days] or not often [ie, 0-2 days])	Positive if often is the answer to either question
	Anergia questionnaire	Patient is asked 7 questions pertaining to lack of energy over the past month	Positive if major criterion "sits around a lot for lack of energy" + any 2 of 6 minor criteria
Shrinking	Weight loss	Self-reported or measured unintentional weight change not due to dieting or exercise	≥10 lbs in past year
	Appendicular muscle mass	Measured muscle mass in arms and legs using a dual-energy x-ray absorptiometry scan	Frailty cutoffs not yet established; general cutoffs >2 SD from controls Men: ≤7.23 kg/height in m² Women: ≤5.67 kg/height in m²
	Serum albumin	Measured serum albumin	≤3.3 g/dl

(Reproduced with permission from Afilalo J, Alexander KP, Mack MJ, et al: Frailty assessment in the cardiovascular care of older adults, *J Am Coll Cardiol* 2014 Mar 4; 63(8):747-762.)

frailty such as the 5-m gait speed, and to a lesser extent hand-grip strength, often out perform the more elaborate and time-consuming scales.[84-86]

The Frailty ABCs (Frailty Assessment Before Cardiac Surgery) prospective study showed that slow 5-m gait speed was associated with a threefold increase in postoperative mortality or major morbidity and provided incremental value above the STS risk score.[87] Patients with slow gait speed and a high-risk score had a 43% incidence of mortality/major morbidity, whereas those with normal gait speed and a low- to intermediate-risk score had a 6% incidence. Additional studies have demonstrated that preoperative frailty is associated with postoperative mortality at 30 days and 1 to 2 years.[88-90]

HEART TEAM

The concept of the "Heart Team" originated from two randomized trials comparing percutaneous and surgical strategies in patients with coronary artery disease and aortic stenosis: SYNTAX (Synergy between PCI with Taxus and Cardiac Surgery) and PARTNER (Placement of Aortic Transcatheter Valves).[91-93] In these trials, the Heart Team was composed of an interventional cardiologist and a cardiovascular surgeon but membership has expanded in many centers to include specialists from imaging, neurology, pulmonology, anesthesia, geriatrics, palliative care, social work, information technology, administration, and finance.[94] The Heart Team approach is central to the care of high-risk or prohibitive surgical risk patients with severe aortic stenosis. It has a Class I recommendation from American and European valve guidelines and is required for reimbursement for transcatheter AVR in the United States.[95,96]

The goal of this collaborative approach in patients with aortic stenosis is to improve outcomes by optimization of patient selection, utilization of synergistic procedural skill sets, standardization of intra- and post-procedural care pathways, and establishment of post-discharge follow-up.[97] An additional focus is to deliver more patient-centered care, through processes such as shared decision making (SDM).[95,96] With the obvious broad applicability of the Heart Team approach to many of the surgical and percutaneous decisions that patients with advanced heart disease face, it will be critical to focus health services research on the key metrics of patient-centered outcomes, clinician outcomes, and health system outcomes in order to advance our care delivery to our highest risk patients (Table 10-4).

SHARED DECISION MAKING

Clinicians often think that patients do not want to take an active role in decision making and that patients prefer their clinicians to make decisions on their behalf.[98,99] This sentiment does not appear to be reflective of patients' attitudes regarding their roles in health care decisions. Studies have found that the vast majority patients (~70%) prefer a shared role in which both they and their clinicians contribute equally

TABLE 10-4: Potential Outcomes of Effective Heart Team Interventions

	Patient	Clinician	Health System
Improved knowledge	X	X	
Reduced decisional conflict	X		
Greater satisfaction (with care delivery process)	X	X	
Involvement in shared decision making	X	X	
Improved quality of life (functional status [patient] or workplace [clinician])	X	X	
Expanded clinical and procedural skill set		X	
Reduction in variability both in access and outcome			X
Greater adherence to guidelines			X
Lower readmission rates			X
Shorter length of stay			X
Faster time to decision			X
Lower cost			X
Improved care coordination and communication			X

(Reproduced with permission from Coylewright M, Mack MJ, Holmes DR Jr, et al: A call for an evidence-based approach to the Heart Team for patients with severe aortic stenosis, *J Am Coll Cardiol* 2015 Apr 14;65(14):1472-1480.)

to treatment decisions.[100] Health policy has firmly embraced SDM and there is recent advocacy for SDM in cardiovascular clinical practice guidelines.[98,101,102]

One of the biggest challenges remains the logistics of incorporating SDM into routine clinical practice. A helpful first step is to identify and review the various tools and resources available. Three comprehensive publically available resources include Ottawa Decision Aids Repository (available at http://decisionaid.ohri.ca/decaids.html), the Mayo Shared Decision Making Resource Center (available at http://shareddecisions.mayoclinic.org/), and a repository of Option Grids (available at http://www.optiongrid.org/). A key component of SDM beyond just the dissemination and discussion of "facts" is the emphasis placed on developing a therapeutic relationship with the patient to allow him/her to feel comfortable expressing an informed preference.[97]

FUTILITY

Advances in surgical and minimally invasive techniques, as well as coordinated multidisciplinary perioperative care, have successfully extended treatment options to patients previously thought to be too high risk due to advanced age, frailty, and burden of comorbidities. However, there are many patients who are unlikely to benefit from a procedure even if it can be performed successfully. Therapeutic futility has been defined as a lack of medical efficacy—when the therapy is unlikely to produce its intended clinical result, as judged by the physician; or lack of a meaningful survival, as judged by the personal values of the patient.[103,104]

This issue of how to assess futility and incorporate it into the dialogue between patients and caregivers has become increasingly important with the emergence of transcatheter aortic valve replacement (TAVR) as a less invasive alternative to surgical valve replacement.[92,93,105] TAVR is a transformative innovation that has extended treatment to numerous patients with severe aortic stenosis who previously were not referred for or were denied surgical treatment.[103] However, clinical experience demonstrates that some patients die soon after the procedure or have little improvement in QOL or functional status.[106,107] The decision regarding futility is one of the most challenging in medicine and surgery and should be made collaboratively by the care team with the patient. As the ability to distinguish patients who will benefit from therapy from those who will not continue to evolve, it is important to emphasize to patients and families not only that decisions not to offer invasive treatment do not equate with abandonment of care but also that continued efforts will be made to promote patient goals and well-being.[103]

REFERENCES

1. Conaway DG, House J, Bandt K, Hayden L, Borkon AM, Spertus JA: The elderly: health status benefits and recovery of function one year after coronary artery bypass surgery. *J Am Coll Cardiol* 2003; 42:1421-1426.
2. Weissman C: Pulmonary complications after cardiac surgery. *Semin Cardiothorac Vasc Anesth* 2004; 8:185-211.
3. Barnett SD, Halpin LS, Speir AM, et al: Postoperative complications among octogenarians after cardiovascular surgery. *Ann Thorac Surg* 2003; 76:726-731.
4. Maurer MS, Luchsinger JA, Wellner R, Kukuy E, Edwards NM: The effect of body mass index on complications from cardiac surgery in the oldest old. *J Am Geriatr Soc* 2002; 50:988-994.
5. Kurlansky PA, Williams DB, Traad EA, et al: Arterial grafting results in reduced operative mortality and enhanced long-term quality of life in octogenarians. *Ann Thorac Surg* 2003; 76:418-26; discussion 427.
6. Matsuura K, Kobayashi J, Tagusari O, et al: Off-pump coronary artery bypass grafting using only arterial grafts in elderly patients. *Ann Thorac Surg* 2005; 80:144-148.
7. Bacchetta MD, Ko W, Girardi LN, et al: Outcomes of cardiac surgery in nonagenarians: a 10-year experience. *Ann Thorac Surg* 2003; 75:1215-1220.
8. Guru V, Fremes SE, Austin PC, Blackstone EH, Tu JV: Gender differences in outcomes after hospital discharge from coronary artery bypass grafting. *Circulation* 2006; 113:507-516.
9. Blankstein R, Ward RP, Arnsdorf M, Jones B, Lou Y, Pine M: Female gender is an independent predictor of operative mortality after coronary artery bypass graft surgery: contemporary analysis of 31 midwestern hospitals. *Circulation* 2005; 112:I323-327.
10. Toumpoulis IK, Anagnostopoulos CE, Balaram SK, et al: Assessment of independent predictors for long-term mortality between women and men after coronary artery bypass grafting: are women different from men? *J Thorac Cardiovasc Surg* 2006; 131:343-351.
11. Emmert MY, Salzberg SP, Seifert B, et al: Despite modern off-pump coronary artery bypass grafting women fare worse than men. *Interact CardioVasc Thorac Surg* 2010; 10(5):737-741.
12. Vaccarino V, Lin ZQ, Kasl SV, et al: Sex differences in health status after coronary artery bypass surgery. *Circulation* 2003; 108:2642-2647.
13. Falcoz PE, Chocron S, Laluc F, et al: Gender analysis after elective open heart surgery: a two-year comparative study of quality of life. *Ann Thorac Surg* 2006; 81:1637-1643.
14. Lucas FL, Stukel TA, Morris AM, Siewers AE, Birkmeyer JD: Race and surgical mortality in the United States. *Ann Surg* 2006; 243:281-286.
15. Zacharias A, Schwann TA, Riordan CJ, Durham SJ, Shah A, Habib RH: Operative and late coronary artery bypass grafting outcomes in matched African-American versus Caucasian patients: evidence of a late survival-medicaid association. *J Am Coll Cardiol* 2005; 46:1526-1535.
16. Taylor NE, O'Brien S, Edwards FH, Peterson ED, Bridges CR: Relationship between race and mortality and morbidity after valve replacement surgery. *Circulation* 2005; 111:1305-1312.
17. Eagle KA, Guyton RA, Davidoff R, et al: ACC/AHA 2004 guideline update for coronary artery bypass graft surgery: a report of the American college of Cardiology/American heart association task force on practice guidelines (committee to update the 1999 guidelines for coronary artery bypass graft surgery). *Circulation* 2004; 110:e340-437.
18. Mangano CM, Diamondstone LS, Ramsay JG, Aggarwal A, Herskowitz A, Mangano DT: Renal dysfunction after myocardial revascularization: risk factors, adverse outcomes, and hospital resource utilization. The Multicenter Study of Perioperative Ischemia Research Group. *Ann Intern Med* 1998; 128:194-203.
19. Charlesworth DC, Likosky DS, Marrin CA, et al: Development and validation of a prediction model for strokes after coronary artery bypass grafting. *Ann Thorac Surg* 2003; 76:436-443.
20. Clough RA, Leavitt BJ, Morton JR, et al: The effect of comorbid illness on mortality outcomes in cardiac surgery. *Arch Surg* 2002; 137:428-432; discussion 432-433.
21. Leavitt BJ, Sheppard L, Maloney C, et al: Effect of diabetes and associated conditions on long-term survival after coronary artery bypass graft surgery. *Circulation* 2004; 110(11 Suppl1):II41-II44.
22. Luciani N, Nasso G, Gaudino M, et al: Coronary artery bypass grafting in type II diabetic patients: a comparison between insulin-dependent and non-insulin-dependent patients at short- and mid-term follow-up. *Ann Thorac Surg* 2003; 76:1149-1154.
23. Kubal C, Srinivasan AK, Grayson AD, Fabri BM, Chalmers JA: Effect of risk-adjusted diabetes on mortality and morbidity after coronary artery bypass surgery. *Ann Thorac Surg* 2005; 79:1570-1576.
24. Furnary AP, Gao G, Grunkemeier GL, et al: Continuous insulin infusion reduces mortality in patients with diabetes undergoing coronary artery bypass grafting. *J Thorac Cardiovasc Surg* 2003; 125:1007-1021.
25. Furnary AP, Zerr KJ, Grunkemeier GL, Starr A: Continuous intravenous insulin infusion reduces the incidence of deep sternal wound infection in diabetic patients after cardiac surgical procedures. *Ann Thorac Surg* 1999; 67:352-360; discussion 360-362.
26. Srinivasan AK, Grayson AD, Fabri BM: On-pump versus off-pump coronary artery bypass grafting in diabetic patients: a propensity score analysis. *Ann Thorac Surg* 2004; 78:1604-1609.
27. Cooper WA, O'Brien SM, Thourani VH, et al: Impact of renal dysfunction on outcomes of coronary artery bypass surgery: results from the society of thoracic surgeons national adult cardiac database. *Circulation* 2006; 113:1063-1070.
28. Wang F, Dupuis JY, Nathan H, Williams K: An analysis of the association between preoperative renal dysfunction and outcome in cardiac surgery: estimated creatinine clearance or plasma creatinine level as measures of renal function. *Chest* 2003; 124:1852-1862.
29. Hillis GS, Zehr KJ, Williams AW, et al: Outcome of patients with low ejection fraction undergoing coronary artery bypass grafting: renal function and mortality after 3.8 years. *Circulation* 2006; 114(1 Suppl):I414-I419.
30. Lok CE, Austin PC, Wang H, Tu JV: Impact of renal insufficiency on short- and long-term outcomes after cardiac surgery. *Am Heart J* 2004; 148:430-438.
31. Zakeri R, Freemantle N, Barnett V, et al: Relation between mild renal dysfunction and outcomes after coronary artery bypass grafting. *Circulation* 2005; 112(9 Suppl):I270-I275.
32. Bove T, Landoni G, Calabro MG, et al: Renoprotective action of fenoldopam in high-risk patients undergoing cardiac surgery: a prospective, double-blind, randomized clinical trial. *Circulation* 2005; 111:3230-3235.
33. Burns KE, Chu MW, Novick RJ, et al: Perioperative N-acetylcysteine to prevent renal dysfunction in high-risk patients undergoing cabg surgery: a randomized controlled trial. *JAMA* 2005; 294:342-350.
34. Bucerius J, Gummert JF, Walther T, et al: On-pump versus off-pump coronary artery bypass grafting: impact on postoperative renal failure requiring renal replacement therapy. *Ann Thorac Surg* 2004; 77:1250-1256.

35. Cohen A, Katz M, Katz R, Hauptman E, Schachner A: Chronic obstructive pulmonary disease in patients undergoing coronary artery bypass grafting. *J Thorac Cardiovasc Surg* 1995; 109:574-581.

36. Fuster RG, Argudo JA, Albarova OG, et al: Prognostic value of chronic obstructive pulmonary disease in coronary artery bypass grafting. *Eur J Cardiothorac Surg* 2006; 29:202-209.

37. Filsoufi F, Rahmanian PB, Castillo JG, Chikwe J, Adams DH: Predictors and early and late outcomes of respiratory failure in contemporary cardiac surgery. *Chest* 2008; 133:713-721.

38. Weisberg AD, Weisberg EL, Wilson JM, Collard CD: Preoperative evaluation and preparation of the patient for cardiac surgery. *Med Clin North Am* 2009; 93:979-994.

39. Hulzebos EH, Helders PJ, Favie NJ, et al: Preoperative intensive inspiratory muscle training to prevent postoperative pulmonary complications in high-risk patients undergoing CABG surgery: a randomized clinical trial. *JAMA* 2006; 296:1851-1857.

40. Edwards FH, Clark RE, Schwartz M: Coronary artery bypass grafting: The society of thoracic surgeons national database experience. *Ann Thorac Surg* 1994; 57:12-19.

41. He GW, Acuff TE, Ryan WH, He YH, Mack MJ: Determinants of operative mortality in reoperative coronary artery bypass grafting. *J Thorac Cardiovasc Surg* 1995; 110:971-978.

42. Noyez L, van Eck FM: Long-term cardiac survival after reoperative coronary artery bypass grafting. *Eur J Cardiothorac Surg* 2004; 25:59-64.

43. Sabik JF, Blackstone EH, Houghtaling PL, Walts PA, Lytle BW: Is reoperation still a risk factor in coronary artery bypass surgery? *Ann Thorac Surg* 2005; 80:1719-1727.

44. Davierwala PM, Maganti M, Yau TM: Decreasing significance of left ventricular dysfunction and reoperative surgery in predicting coronary artery bypass grafting-associated mortality: a twelve-year study. *J Thorac Cardiovasc Surg* 2003; 126:1335-1344.

45. Handa N, McGregor CG, Danielson GK, et al: Valvular heart operation in patients with previous mediastinal radiation therapy. *Ann Thorac Surg* 2001; 71:1880-1884.

46. Handa N, McGregor CG, Danielson GK, et al: Coronary artery bypass grafting in patients with previous mediastinal radiation therapy. *J Thorac Cardiovasc Surg* 1999; 117:1136-1142.

47. Chang ASY, Smedira NG, Chang CL, et al: Cardiac surgery after mediastinal radiation: extent of exposure influences outcome. *J Thorac Cardiovasc Surg* 2007; 133:404-413.e3.

48. Shahian DM, O'Brien SM, Filardo G, et al: The society of thoracic surgeons 2008 cardiac surgery risk models: Part 1—Coronary artery bypass grafting surgery. *Ann Thorac Surg* 2009; 88:S2-S22.

49. O'Brien SM, Shahian DM, Filardo G, et al: The society of thoracic surgeons 2008 cardiac surgery risk models: Part 2—Isolated valve surgery. *Ann Thorac Surg* 2009; 88:S23-S42.

50. Shahian DM, O'Brien SM, Filardo G, et al: The society of thoracic surgeons 2008 cardiac surgery risk models: Part 3—Valve plus coronary artery bypass grafting surgery. *Ann Thorac Surg* 2009; 88:S43-S62.

51. Verma S, Fedak PW, Weisel RD, et al: Off-pump coronary artery bypass surgery: fundamentals for the clinical cardiologist. *Circulation* 2004; 109:1206-1211.

52. Parolari A, Alamanni F, Polvani G, et al: Meta-analysis of randomized trials comparing off-pump with on-pump coronary artery bypass graft patency. *Ann Thorac Surg* 2005; 80:2121-2125.

53. Wijeysundera DN, Beattie WS, Djaiani G, et al: Off-pump coronary artery surgery for reducing mortality and morbidity: meta-analysis of randomized and observational studies. *J Am Coll Cardiol* 2005; 46:872-882.

54. Sellke FW, DiMaio JM, Caplan LR, et al: Comparing on-pump and off-pump coronary artery bypass grafting: numerous studies but few conclusions: a scientific statement from the American heart association council on cardiovascular surgery and anesthesia in collaboration with the interdisciplinary working group on quality of care and outcomes research. *Circulation* 2005; 111:2858-2864.

55. Puskas JD, Williams WH, Duke PG, et al: Off-pump coronary artery bypass grafting provides complete revascularization with reduced myocardial injury, transfusion requirements, and length of stay: a prospective randomized comparison of two hundred unselected patients undergoing off-pump versus conventional coronary artery bypass grafting. *J Thorac Cardiovasc Surg* 2003; 125:797-808.

56. Mehta Rodriguez E, Chitwood WR, Jr: Robot-assisted cardiac surgery. *Interact CardioVasc Thorac Surg* 2009; 9:500-505.

57. Reicher B, Poston RS, Mehra MR, et al: Simultaneous "hybrid" percutaneous coronary intervention and minimally invasive surgical bypass grafting: feasibility, safety, and clinical outcomes. *Am Heart J* 2008; 155:661-667.

58. Nashef SA, Roques F, Michel P, Gauducheau E, Lemeshow S, Salamon R: European system for cardiac operative risk evaluation (EuroSCORE). *Eur J Cardiothorac Surg* 1999; 16:9-13.

59. Roques F, Michel P, Goldstone AR, Nashef SA: The logistic EuroSCORE. *Eur Heart J* 2003; 24:881-882.

60. Bhatti F, Grayson AD, Grotte G, et al: The logistic EuroSCORE in cardiac surgery: how well does it predict operative risk? *Heart* 2006; 92:1817-1820.

61. Zingone B, Pappalardo A, Dreas L: Logistic versus additive EuroSCORE. A comparative assessment of the two models in an independent population sample. *Eur J Cardiothorac Surg* 2004; 26:1134-1140.

62. Keogh BE: Logistic, additive or historical: is EuroSCORE an appropriate model for comparing individual surgeons' performance? *Heart* 2006; 92:1715-1716.

63. Karthik S, Srinivasan AK, Grayson AD, et al: Limitations of additive EuroSCORE for measuring risk stratified mortality in combined coronary and valve surgery. *Eur J Cardiothorac Surg* 2004; 26:318-322.

64. Nilsson J, Algotsson L, Hoglund P, Luhrs C, Brandt J: Early mortality in coronary bypass surgery: the EuroSCORE versus the society of thoracic surgeons risk algorithm. *Ann Thorac Surg* 2004; 77:1235-1239; discussion 1239-1240.

65. Granton J, Cheng D: Risk stratification models for cardiac surgery. *Seminars in Cardiothoracic and Vascular Anesthesia.* 2008; 12:167-174.

66. Gao D, Grunwald GK, Rumsfeld JS, Schooley L, MacKenzie T, Shroyer AL: Time-varying risk factors for long-term mortality after coronary artery bypass graft surgery. *Ann Thorac Surg* 2006; 81:793-799.

67. Afilalo J, Alexander KP, Mack MJ, et al: Frailty assessment in the cardiovascular care of older adults. *J Am Coll Cardiol* 2014; 63:747-762.

68. Bergman H, Ferrucci L, Guralnik J, et al: Frailty: an emerging research and clinical paradigm—issues and controversies. *J Gerontol A Biol Sci Med Sci* 2007; 62:731-737.

69. Afilalo J, Karunananthan S, Eisenberg MJ, Alexander KP, Bergman H: Role of frailty in patients with cardiovascular disease. *Am J Cardiol* 2009; 103:1616-1621.

70. Collard RM, Boter H, Schoevers RA, Oude Voshaar RC: Prevalence of frailty in community-dwelling older persons: a systematic review. *J Am Geriatr Soc* 2012; 60:1487-1492.

71. Shamliyan T, Talley KM, Ramakrishnan R, Kane RL: Association of frailty with survival: a systematic literature review. *Ageing Res Rev* 2013; 12:719-736.

72. Fulop T, Larbi A, Witkowski JM, et al: Aging, frailty and age-related diseases. *Biogerontology* 2010; 11:547-563.

73. Walston J, McBurnie MA, Newman A, et al: Frailty and activation of the inflammation and coagulation systems with and without clinical comorbidities: results from the cardiovascular health study. *Arch Intern Med* 2002; 162:2333-2341.

74. Cesari M, Penninx BW, Pahor M, et al: Inflammatory markers and physical performance in older persons: the InCHIANTI study. *J Gerontol A Biol Sci Med Sci* 2004; 59:242-248.

75. Schaap LA, Pluijm SM, Deeg DJ, et al: Higher inflammatory marker levels in older persons: associations with 5-year change in muscle mass and muscle strength. *J Gerontol A Biol Sci Med Sci* 2009; 64:1183-1189.

76. Travison TG, Nguyen AH, Naganathan V, et al: Changes in reproductive hormone concentrations predict the prevalence and progression of the frailty syndrome in older men: the concord health and ageing in men project. *J Clin Endocrinol Metab* 2011; 96:2464-2474.

77. Schaap LA, Pluijm SM, Deeg DJ, et al: Low testosterone levels and decline in physical performance and muscle strength in older men: findings from two prospective cohort studies. *Clin Endocrinol (Oxf)* 2008; 68:42-50.

78. Barzilay JI, Blaum C, Moore T, et al: Insulin resistance and inflammation as precursors of frailty: the cardiovascular health study. *Arch Intern Med* 2007; 167:635-641.

79. Boirie Y: Physiopathological mechanism of sarcopenia. *J Nutr Health Aging* 2009; 13:717-723.

80. de Vries NM, Staal JB, van Ravensberg CD, Hobbelen JS, Olde Rikkert MG, Nijhuis-van der Sanden MW: Outcome instruments to measure frailty: a systematic review. *Ageing Res Rev* 2011; 10:104-114.

81. Fried LP, Tangen CM, Walston J, et al: Frailty in older adults: evidence for a phenotype. *J Gerontol A Biol Sci Med Sci* 2001; 56:M146-156.

82. Guralnik JM, Simonsick EM, Ferrucci L, et al: A short physical performance battery assessing lower extremity function: association with self-reported disability and prediction of mortality and nursing home admission. *J Gerontol* 1994; 49:M85-94.

83. Guralnik JM, Ferrucci L, Simonsick EM, Salive ME, Wallace RB: Lower-extremity function in persons over the age of 70 years as a predictor of subsequent disability. *N Engl J Med* 1995; 332:556-561.

84. Abellan van Kan G, Rolland Y, Andrieu S, et al: Gait speed at usual pace as a predictor of adverse outcomes in community-dwelling older people an international academy on nutrition and aging (IANA) task force. *J Nutr Health Aging* 2009; 13:881-889.

85. Dumurgier J, Elbaz A, Ducimetiere P, Tavernier B, Alperovitch A, Tzourio C: Slow walking speed and cardiovascular death in well functioning older adults: prospective cohort study. *BMJ* 2009; 339:b4460.

86. Ling CH, Taekema D, de Craen AJ, Gussekloo J, Westendorp RG, Maier AB: Handgrip strength and mortality in the oldest old population: the leiden 85-plus study. *CMAJ* 2010; 182:429-435.

87. Afilalo J, Eisenberg MJ, Morin JF, et al: Gait speed as an incremental predictor of mortality and major morbidity in elderly patients undergoing cardiac surgery. *J Am Coll Cardiol* 2010; 56:1668-1676.

88. Lee DH, Buth KJ, Martin BJ, Yip AM, Hirsch GM: Frail patients are at increased risk for mortality and prolonged institutional care after cardiac surgery. *Circulation* 2010; 121:973-978.

89. Sundermann S, Dademasch A, Praetorius J, et al: Comprehensive assessment of frailty for elderly high-risk patients undergoing cardiac surgery. *Eur J Cardiothorac Surg* 2011; 39:33-37.

90. Sundermann S, Dademasch A, Rastan A, et al: One-year follow-up of patients undergoing elective cardiac surgery assessed with the comprehensive assessment of frailty test and its simplified form. *Interact Cardiovasc Thorac Surg* 2011; 13:119-123; discussion 123.

91. Serruys PW, Morice MC, Kappetein AP, et al: Percutaneous coronary intervention versus coronary-artery bypass grafting for severe coronary artery disease. *N Engl J Med* 2009; 360:961-972.

92. Leon MB, Smith CR, Mack M, et al: Transcatheter aortic-valve implantation for aortic stenosis in patients who cannot undergo surgery. *N Engl J Med* 2010; 363:1597-1607.

93. Smith CR, Leon MB, Mack MJ, et al: Transcatheter versus surgical aortic-valve replacement in high-risk patients. *N Engl J Med* 2011; 364:2187-2198.

94. Bhattacharyya S, Pavitt C, Lloyd G, Chambers JB: British Heart Valve Society. Prevalence & composition of heart valve multi-disciplinary teams within a national health system. *Int J Cardiol* 2014; 177:1120-1121.

95. Nishimura RA, Otto CM, Bonow RO, et al: 2014 AHA/ACC guideline for the management of patients with valvular heart disease: Executive summary: a report of the American College of Cardiology/American Heart Association Task Force on practice guidelines. *J Am Coll Cardiol* 2014; 63:2438-2488.

96. Vahanian A, Alfieri O, Andreotti F, et al: Guidelines on the management of valvular heart disease (version 2012): the joint task force on the management of valvular heart disease of the European Society of Cardiology (ESC) and the European Association for Cardio-thoracic Surgery (EACTS). *Eur J Cardiothorac Surg* 2012; 42:S1-44.

97. Coylewright M, Mack MJ, Holmes DR Jr, O'Gara PT: A call for an evidence-based approach to the heart team for patients with severe aortic stenosis. *J Am Coll Cardiol* 2015; 65:1472-1480.

98. Hess EP, Coylewright M, Frosch DL, Shah ND: Implementation of shared decision making in cardiovascular care: past, present, and future. *Circ Cardiovasc Qual Outcomes* 2014; 7:797-803.

99. Silvia KA, Ozanne EM, Sepucha KR: Implementing breast cancer decision aids in community sites: barriers and resources. *Health Expect* 2008; 11:46-53.

100. Adams JR, Elwyn G, Legare F, Frosch DL: Communicating with physicians about medical decisions: a reluctance to disagree. *Arch Intern Med* 2012; 172:1184-1186.

101. Allen LA, Stevenson LW, Grady KL, et al: Decision making in advanced heart failure: a scientific statement from the American Heart Association. *Circulation* 2012; 125:1928-1952.

102. Patel MR, Dehmer GJ, Hirshfeld JW, et al: ACCF/SCAI/STS/AATS/AHA/ASNC 2009 appropriateness criteria for coronary revascularization: a report by the American College of Cardiology Foundation Appropriateness Criteria Task Force, Society for Cardiovascular Angiography and Interventions, Society of Thoracic Surgeons, American Association for Thoracic Surgery, American Heart Association, and the American Society of Nuclear Cardiology endorsed by the American Society of Echocardiography, the Heart Failure Society of America, and the Society of Cardiovascular Computed Tomography. *J Am Coll Cardiol* 2009; 53:530-553.

103. Lindman BR, Alexander KP, O'Gara PT, Afilalo J: Futility, benefit, and transcatheter aortic valve replacement. *JACC Cardiovasc Interv* 2014; 7:707-716.

104. American Thoracic Society: Withholding and withdrawing life-sustaining therapy. *Ann Intern Med* 1991; 115:478-485.

105. Holmes DR Jr, Mack MJ, Kaul S, et al: 2012 ACCF/AATS/SCAI/STS expert consensus document on transcatheter aortic valve replacement: developed in collaboration with the American Heart Association, American Society of Echocardiography, European Association for Cardio-thoracic Surgery, Heart Failure Society of America, Mended Hearts, Society of Cardiovascular Anesthesiologists, Society of Cardiovascular Computed Tomography, and Society for Cardiovascular Magnetic Resonance. *J Thorac Cardiovasc Surg* 2012; 144:e29-84.

106. Reynolds MR, Magnuson EA, Lei Y, et al: Health-related quality of life after transcatheter aortic valve replacement in inoperable patients with severe aortic stenosis. *Circulation* 2011; 124:1964-1972.

107. Reynolds MR, Magnuson EA, Wang K, et al: Health-related quality of life after transcatheter or surgical aortic valve replacement in high-risk patients with severe aortic stenosis: results from the PARTNER (Placement of AoRTic TraNscathetER Valve) Trial (Cohort A). *J Am Coll Cardiol* 2012; 60:548-558.

Cardiac Anesthesia

11

*John G. Augoustides • William C. Culp • Wendy Gross
• Annette Mizuguchi • Prakash A. Patel • Kent Rehfeldt
• Pinak Shah • Usha Tedrow • Stanton K. Shernan*

CORONARY REVASCULARIZATION

Coronary Artery Disease, Surgical Revascularization, and Myocardial Oxygen Supply: Demand

Heart disease is the leading cause of death in the United States, accounting for 600,000 fatalities annually.[1] Coronary artery disease (CAD) is a complex and multifactorial process, primarily characterized by the progressive and silent accumulation of atherosclerotic plaques, fibrous materials, and inflammatory mediators within the coronary arteries, potentially leading to obstruction of flow and resultant myocardial hypoperfusion.[2] Manifestations of this disease tend to present in males 40 years and older and in females 50 years and older. Risk factors include a strong family history of the disease, hypercholesterolemia, hypertension, diabetes, obesity, and smoking. If left untreated, CAD can lead to angina, heart failure, arrhythmias, and sudden death. Although medical therapy and percutaneous coronary interventions are often mainstay treatments for milder forms of the disease and most single- and double-vessel lesions, the gold standard for most multi-vessel lesions remains surgical revascularization.[3,4]

Anesthesiologists should be acutely aware of the heightened risks of myocardial ischemia for patients during revascularization surgery due to their obstructed coronary vessels and the critical dependence on oxidative phosphorylation for cardiac energy production. Myocardial oxygen supply is the product of arterial oxygen content and coronary blood flow.

$$O_2 \text{ content} = [(1.34)(\text{hemoglobin concentration})$$
$$(\% \text{ oxygen saturation}) + (0.003)(PaO_2)]$$

Maximizing oxygen release at the tissue level involves maintaining high hemoglobin concentration, high oxygen saturation, warm temperature, and increased 2,3-diphosphoglycerate. The myocardium tends to maximally extract oxygen from its blood supply while at rest, and therefore, can only increase myocardial oxygen delivery during stress by increasing coronary blood flow. If this flow is obstructed by CAD, then the risk of myocardial ischemia is greatly increased.

Coronary artery blood flow is proportional to coronary perfusion pressure (CPP), where

$$CPP = (\text{aortic diastolic blood pressure}) -$$
$$(\text{left ventricular end-diastolic pressure})$$

and is inversely proportional to coronary vascular resistance. Normal coronary arteries have autoregulated flow at CPPs between 50 and 150 mm Hg. Coronary vascular resistance is determined by hormonal and metabolic factors, the autonomic nervous system, endothelial modulation, and in diseased vessels, by atherosclerotic plaques. Left ventricular (LV) endocardial blood flow occurs entirely during diastole, when the vast majority of the remaining myocardium is oxygenated (Fig. 11-1). Therefore, the anesthesiologist attempting to maximize CPP and oxygen supply should target normal to increased diastolic blood pressure, low left ventricular end-diastolic pressure (LVEDP), and a slow heart rate to maximize time during diastole. Additionally, myocardial oxygen demand can be minimized by avoiding tachycardia, minimizing LVEDP, reducing chamber size, and reducing contractility. This general principle of optimizing myocardial oxygen supply while minimizing demand should be an over-reaching goal for the anesthesiologist caring for a patient undergoing coronary revascularization surgery.[5,6]

Preoperative Considerations

When evaluating a patient prior to a coronary revascularization procedure, the anesthesiologist should be mindful of the anesthetic goals common to all surgeries: providing amnesia, analgesia, and a quiet surgical field while ensuring optimal myocardial oxygen supply and demand to minimize ischemic risk. In addition, the anesthesiologist should provide optimal hemodynamic control to optimize cardiac performance, and be prepared to help guide the surgery while rapidly diagnosing cardiac complications, often by using advanced noninvasive and invasive hemodynamic monitors including transesophageal echocardiography (TEE).

Initial preoperative patient assessment should include a comprehensive history and physical examination focused on

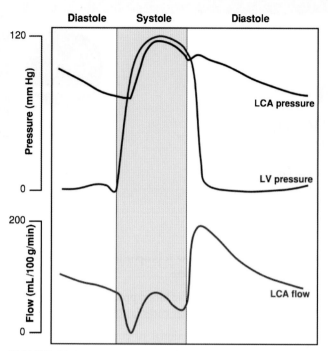

Diastole   Systole   Diastole

FIGURE 11-1 Wiggers diagram depicting relationship of left coronary artery pressure and flow with the phase of the cardiac cycle. Note that left coronary flow occurs primarily during ventricular diastole, even though the head pressure of the vessel is higher during systole. This is due to the high transmural ventricular pressure during systole, and the relatively low pressure in diastole as the myocardium relaxes, as governed by the coronary perfusion equation: CPP=DBP-LVEDP, where CPP=coronary pressure, DBP=diastolic blood pressure, and LVEDP=left ventricular end diastolic pressure. LCA=left coronary artery, LV=left ventricle. (Reproduced with permission from Lee J, Smith NP: The multi-scale modelling of coronary blood flow, *Ann Biomed Eng* 2012 Nov;40(11):2399-2413.)

the cardiac and pulmonary systems, along with a standard airway examination. Though direct laryngoscopy is routinely used to facilitate tracheal intubation, a predicted difficult airway may prompt alternative intubation strategies. A thorough review of the medical record is in order, with careful attention to patient medications, laboratory studies (complete blood count, electrolytes, creatinine, troponin, B-type natriuretic peptide, coagulation panels, blood cross matches), electrocardiogram, carotid ultrasound studies, chest radiograph, cardiac stress tests, cardiac catheterization, and echocardiography reports. The anesthesiologist should be aware of the coronary anatomy and lesions, along with any invasive pressure measurements as described by the catheterization report. Close review of any preoperative echocardiography studies is essential to assess both systolic and diastolic ventricular function and to examine the cardiac valves.

A comprehensive preoperative assessment is important to determine the perioperative risk. The two most widely used risk stratification tools are the Society of Thoracic Surgeons (STS) Risk Calculator and EuroSCORE II, each based on large historical patient databases. These formulae use sophisticated mathematical modeling techniques to allow the user to

determine predicted mortality and other complications based on a variety of entered criteria, including age, gender, ejection fraction, urgency of surgery, renal function, and other variables. Risk assessment calculators can be valuable preoperative planning tools for the patient, surgeon, and anesthesiologist, and their use should be considered prior to each case.[7,8]

While concluding the preoperative visit, the anesthesiologist should ensure informed consent and provide the opportunity for any patient questions to be answered. The anesthesiologist's visit itself is a powerful means to allay patient fears and helps address patient and family members' concerns.[9] Additionally, the anesthesiologist should consider any premedications to administer, include anxiolytics as necessary. Beta-blocker medications are recommended preoperatively to reduce the risk of postoperative atrial fibrillation, myocardial ischemia, and mortality. Statins should be administered unless contraindicated to reduce the rate of myocardial ischemia, graft atherosclerosis, and mortality.[10,11] In general, antihypertensives should be continued on the day of surgery, while use of angiotensin-converting enzyme inhibitors and angiotensin II receptor antagonists is associated with intraoperative hypotension and remains controversial. The use of antiplatelet and anticoagulation agents should be discussed with the surgeon.[12]

Finally, the anesthesiologist should have an active preoperative meeting with the surgeon and the surgical team, as necessary, in order to facilitate the procedure and minimize complications. Checklist and protocol-driven processes have demonstrated reduced complications and improved mortality.[13] Cardiac anesthesiologists with formal fellowship training and skill in TEE are recommended to provide care for high-risk patients.[14]

Monitoring

A vigilant cardiac anesthesiologist is the best single monitor for patients undergoing revascularization procedures. Standard American Society of Anesthesiology monitors should also be used, including FiO_2 monitor, pulse oximeter, end-tidal CO_2 monitor, continuous electrocardiogram, noninvasive blood pressure monitor, and a temperature measurement device. In addition to these standard monitors, a urinary catheter often with bladder thermistor, an arterial catheter most commonly placed in the radial artery, and a central venous catheter are all used routinely. Central venous catheter placement using real-time ultrasound guidance is safer than using an anatomic-guided approach, and is the recommended technique when available.[15]

The risk of intraoperative awareness is increased during cardiac surgery due to the lower use of volatile anesthetics and increased hemodynamic instability in comparison to noncardiac surgery.[16] Processed electroencephalograms, such as the bispectral index (BIS) monitor, have been used to detect inadequate patient amnesia with recent meta-analysis data suggesting that their use reduces the risk of intraoperative awareness in high-risk patients with an odds ratio of 0.24.[17] Although this risk reduction is not universally found[18] and the use of the BIS remains controversial, the National Institute for Health and Clinical Excellence recommends "the use of electroencephalography-based depth of anesthesia monitors…during any type of general anesthesia in patients considered at higher risk."[19]

The technique of near-infrared spectroscopy allows for cerebral regional oxygen saturation to be measured using skin sensors placed on the scalp. Low cerebral tissue oxygen values are associated with increased long-term surgical risk and can also detect cerebral hypoperfusion states caused by problems with bypass cannulae, emboli, and obstruction of cerebral vessels. Cerebral oximetry is often used with aortic surgery involving circulatory arrest, and less commonly with isolated coronary artery bypass grafting (CABG) procedures.[20] Cerebral oximetry has yet to be clearly demonstrated to be beneficial in high-quality randomized intervention trials, and its use remains controversial.[21,22]

The pulmonary artery catheter (PAC) is frequently used during revascularization procedures as a means of measuring cardiac output via thermodilution and directly measuring pulmonary artery pressures. Additionally, LVEDP, as a marker of LV preload, can often be inferred from the pulmonary artery occlusion pressure or the pulmonary artery diastolic pressure. The use of a PAC is not without risk however, and it has been associated with rare but often lethal complications including pulmonary artery rupture. PAC use for revascularization surgery became widespread by the 1980s but its current use is declining due to the proliferation of less-invasive cardiac output monitoring devices, TEE, and some data which fails to demonstrate an association with improved outcome.[23,24] Even so, PACs remain popular with more than two-thirds of anesthesiologists reporting that they use this catheter more than 75% of the time in cases requiring cardiopulmonary bypass (CPB).[25] The perioperative use of a PAC remains recommended in patients with cardiogenic shock (Class I indication), hemodynamic instability (Class IIa), and its use may be reasonable in stable patients undergoing revascularization procedures (Class IIb).[26]

TEE has become a routine monitor during cardiac surgery, and has been shown to have a significant favorable influence on intraoperative surgical management and outcomes.[27] Current practice guidelines recommend that unless contraindicated, TEE be used for all valvular heart procedures and should be considered in CABG surgeries.[28] Recent global survey data suggest that TEE is used in 61 to 69% of isolated CABG procedures.[29] In addition to serving as the gold standard for valve evaluation, TEE can be used to monitor volume status, ventricular function, and gauge regional-wall motion patterns to detect and assess myocardial ischemia—all useful assessments during revascularization surgery.[29]

Anesthetic Techniques and Agents

Historically, general anesthesia was commonly induced and maintained with high-dose fentanyl (50 to 100 mcg/kg) and pancuronium (Table 11-1). This high-dose opiate technique purportedly avoided myocardial depression associated with other anesthetic agents while providing stable hemodynamics and effective blunting of surgical stresses.[30] In the 1990s, efforts at cost reduction spurred the evolution of "fast-track" cardiac anesthetic techniques using volatile anesthetics and low-dose opiates, with early extubation and reducing ICU stays as primary goals. Fast-track techniques have subsequently been demonstrated to be as safe as historical anesthetics in low- and medium-risk patients.[31] Around the same time, the concept of ischemic and pharmacological preconditioning was described, whereby certain maneuvers or pharmacologic agents including volatile anesthetics could minimize the extent of myocardial damage to subsequent myocardial ischemia.[32] As a result, contemporary approaches to coronary revascularization surgery commonly involve induction with thiopental, propofol, etomidate, or midazolam, followed by a balanced anesthetic technique employing a volatile anesthetic (ie, isoflurane, desflurane, or sevoflurane) as its primary component. The volatile anesthetic is accompanied by a low-dose semisynthetic opiate (ie, fentanyl, sufentanil, or remifentanil) and a paralyzing agent. There is no significant difference in extubation times between fentanyl, sufentanil, and remifentanil using fast-track protocols.[33] The use of a volatile anesthetic, and therefore induction of pharmacologic preconditioning, has now become a more common standard anesthetic approach. Meta-analyses suggest that cardiac surgery mortality is reduced when using a volatile anesthetic as compared to a propofol-based intravenous anesthetic, with an odds ratio of 0.51 in favor of volatile anesthetics.[34] Xenon is a promising inhalational anesthetic agent that purports to improve recovery from myocardial stunning, preserve hemodynamic control, and provide neuroprotective qualities. Early trials have been favorable, but its use remains experimental.[35]

Neuroaxial techniques are occasionally used during revascularization surgery. However, systemic heparinization increases the concern of epidural hematoma and resultant spinal cord injury thereby limiting their use, although the actual incidence of this complication is very low.[36] Preoperative intrathecal opiate injection and continuous thoracic epidural local anesthetics can provide good analgesia and facilitate recovery; however, current data do not demonstrate a reduction in the risk of mortality, myocardial infarction, or neurological complications as compared to general anesthetic alone.[37] Awake cardiac surgery is performed in a very small number of centers using thoracic epidural anesthesia and may offer rapid recovery benefits in select patients.[38]

Hemodynamic Optimization

Patients undergoing coronary revascularization frequently develop hypotension and/or low cardiac output, particularly following CPB. Risk factors for low cardiac output syndrome include renal disease, significant regional-wall motion abnormalities, CABG with mitral valve (MV) surgery, reoperation, moderate-to-severe mitral regurgitation (MR), prolonged aortic cross clamp time, left ventricular ejection fraction (LVEF) < 40%, cardiac index < 2.5 L/min/m^2, and LVEDP ≥ 20 mm Hg.[39,40] Strict attention to

TABLE 11-1: General Anesthetic Regimens

	Agent	Dose	Notes
High-dose opiate technique			
	Fentanyl	50-100 mcg/kg load	Technique now less commonly used due to increased risk of delayed extubation, increased risk of intraoperative awareness, and lack of ischemic preconditioning volatile anesthetic.
	Pancuronium	0.1 mg/kg load, then 0.01 mg/kg as needed	Mild tachycardic effect may help offset bradycardia associated with high opiate technique. Must reduce dose in renal impairment.
Fast-track balanced anesthetic			Routinely used.
Induction	Propofol	1-3 mg/kg	
IV induction agent	Thiopental	3-5 mg/kg	
	Etomidate	0.2-0.4 mg/kg	Associated with adrenal suppression.
	Midazolam	0.05-0.15 mg/kg	
Maintenance			
Opiates	Fentanyl	10-20 mcg/kg	Typically given as initial load during induction, with intermittent boluses as necessary.
	Sufentanil	0.5-2.0 mcg/kg	Typically given as initial load, with intermittent boluses or infusion as necessary.
	Remifentanil	0.05-1.0 mcg/kg/min	Administer long-acting analgesics prior to discontinuing remifentanil.
Volatile anesthetic	Isoflurane	MAC 1.13%	Titrate to effect, target 1 MAC for ischemic preconditioning.
	Sevoflurane	MAC 2.05%	Titrate to effect, target 1 MAC for ischemic preconditioning.
	Desflurane	MAC 7.25 %	Titrate to effect, target 1 MAC for ischemic preconditioning.
Paralytic	Rocuronium	0.6 mg/kg load, then 0.15 mg/kg as needed	
	Vecuronium	0.1 mg/kg load, then 0.01 mg/kg as needed	
	cis-Atracurium	0.15-0.20 mg/kg load, then 0.02 mg/kg as needed	Safe for renal failure patients.
Total IV anesthetic			
	Propofol	50-150 mcg/kg/min	Combine with opiate and paralytics as above. Lacks benefit of volatile anesthetic-mediated ischemic preconditioning. Likely increased mortality when compared to volatile anesthetic-based technique.

hemodynamic monitors coupled with a command of cardiac physiology and pharmacology will aid the anesthesiologist in maintaining adequate systemic perfusion. Markers of inadequate systemic perfusion include low cardiac index, hypotension, oliguria, metabolic acidosis, increased base deficit, and elevated serum lactate.

The anesthesiologist is tasked with preventing, diagnosing, and treating inadequate systemic perfusion, and implementing an algorithmic approach may help direct therapy (Fig. 11-2). By using a combination of traditional hemodynamic monitors, invasive and noninvasive cardiac output monitoring devices, dynamic indexes, changes in end-tidal carbon dioxide, arterial blood gas analysis, and echocardiography, systemic perfusion can be assessed and treatment adjusted. A number of vasoactive medications are available and their use should be individualized based on each patient's hemodynamic needs (Table 11-2). A recent addition is levosimendan, a novel inotrope that increases troponin C affinity to calcium without increasing myocardial oxygen consumption or impairing ventricular relaxation, while also exerting pharmacologic preconditioning effects by opening mitochondrial K_{ATP} channels. Levosimendan

Cardiac physiology flowchart

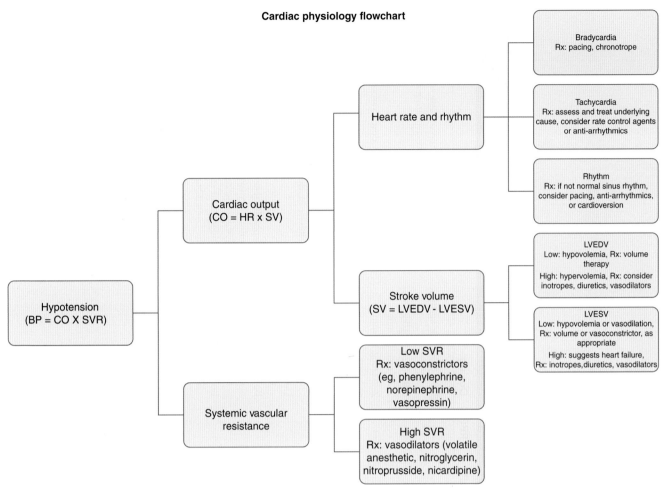

FIGURE 11-2 Algorithm for diagnosing, preventing, and treating inadequate systemic perfusion. (Data from Johnston WE: Applied Cardiac Physiology. *ASA Refresher Courses in Anesthesiology*, 2012;40(1):73-79.)

is recommended for treatment of acute heart failure in Europe[41] and has shown mortality benefits when compared to dobutamine, but is not yet available in the United States. If after optimizing volume status and maximizing pharmacologic support the patient remains hypoperfused, then mechanical assist devices should be considered.[42] The intra-aortic balloon pump (IABP) is well established and technically easiest to place; however its efficacy has been recently questioned.[43] In centers trained in their use, ventricular assist devices (VAD) and extra-corporeal membranous oxygenators (ECMO) may confer a survival benefit and should be considered.

Overview of Procedural Considerations

The anesthetic care of a patient undergoing CABG is a complex, multi-step process. After the anesthesiologist completes a thorough preoperative evaluation, a large bore peripheral IV is placed followed by an arterial catheter, usually placed in the radial artery. Anxiolytics are routinely administered in the preoperative area. In the operating room, standard ASA monitors are applied, and intravenous induction and tracheal intubation are performed, most commonly with a fast-track approach (Table 11-1), targeting early extubation unless contraindicated. A central venous catheter is then placed if not placed prior to induction, often with PAC. Then, the patient is positioned and draped for surgery while a TEE is performed and results are discussed with the surgeon. Prior to incision, an antifibrinolytic is commonly administered (eg, aminocaproic acid, tranexamic acid) to reduce perioperative bleeding. Antibiotics (typically vancomycin and cefuroxime) are given as infection prophylaxis. Anesthetic depth is adjusted to match changes in surgical stimulation with attention to hemodynamic control and myocardial oxygen supply/demand optimization. Heparin is administered several minutes prior to bypass cannulae placement (usually 300 to 400 units/kg), and its effect confirmed by measuring an activated clotting time (ACT) value of 480 seconds or greater prior to initiating bypass. Inadequate ACT values must prompt action by the anesthesiologist to determine the cause and achieve proper

TABLE 11-2: Vasoactive Agents

	a	β1	β2	V₁	HR	CO	SVR	MAP	RBF	Dosing	Notes
Epinephrine	+	++	++	0	++	++	+/−	+	−−	0.01-0.20 mcg/kg/min	May give up to 1 mg intravenously at a time during hemodynamic collapse, repeating as necessary.
Norepinephrine	+++	++	0	0	++	−	+++	+++	−−−	0.01-0.20 mcg/kg/min	
Dopamine	++	++	+	0	+	+++	+	+	+++	2-20 mcg/kg/min	Mild vasodilation at low doses, vasoconstriction at higher doses.
Dobutamine	0	+++	+	0	+	+++	0	+	++	2-20 mcg/kg/min	
Isoproterenol	0	+++	+++	0	+++	+++	−−	+/−	−	0.01-0.07 mcg/kg/min	Use generally limited to heart transplants.
Ephedrine	++	+	+	0	++	++	+	++	−−	10-25 mg SIVP	Marked tachyphylaxis. Not used as infusion.
Phenylephrine	+++	0	0	0	−	−	+++	+++	−−−	50-100 mcg SIVP, 0.3-10 mcg/kg/min	Routinely used to treat mild vasodilation. Causes reflexive bradycardia.
Vasopressin	0	0	0	+++	0	0	+++	+++	−	Up to 40 units IV bolus, 0.01-0.1 units/min	
Milrinone	0	0	0	0	+	+++	−−	−−	−	Bolus up to 50 mcg/kg over 10-30 min, then 0.125-0.75 mcg/kg/min	Phosphodiesterase inhibitor. May be effective for pulmonary hypertension and right ventricular dysfunction can cause systemic hypotension.
Levosimendan	0	0	0	0	+	++	−	−	+	Bolus 12-24 mcg/kg over 10 min, 0.05-0.3 mcg/kg/min	Inodilator and calcium sensitizer, not available in the United States.

Data from Stoelting RK, Hillier SC: *Pharmacology and Physiology in Anesthetic Practice*, 4th ed. Philadelphia, Lippincott Williams and Wilkins; 2005 and Overgaard CB, Dzavik V: Inotropes and vasopressors: review of physiology and clinical use in cardiovascular disease, *Circulation* 2008 Sep 2;118(10):1047-1056.
Heart rate (HR), cardiac output (CO), systemic vascular resistance (SVR), mean arterial pressure (MAP), renal blood flow (RBF). No effect (0), minimal increase (+), moderate increase (++), marked increase (+++), minimal decrease (−), moderate decrease (−−), marked decrease (−−−).

anticoagulation before initiating CPB. The surgeon and perfusionist should be kept notified of the ACT values and any difficulties in anticoagulation. Heparin resistance may require treatment with fresh frozen plasma or antithrombin III concentrate to achieve adequate heparin effect.

After heparinization, the surgeon places an arterial cannula and a venous cannula. Upon initiation of CPB, mechanical ventilation is stopped, the heart is arrested, and revascularization is performed. During this time, volatile anesthetic is typically administered via the bypass circuit by the perfusionist under the anesthesiologist's and surgeon's direction. ACT, hematocrit, arterial blood gases, and blood sugar should be checked periodically during CPB, and any aberrations treated. Serum glucose levels > 180 mg/dL should be treated with insulin infusion.

After the revascularization is complete, the patient should be weaned from bypass. The anesthesiologist should anticipate bypass separation and be prepared, following a standardized routine. Separation preparation steps include: ensuring function of intravascular catheters, ensuring adequate depth of anesthesia, assessing for intracardiac air with TEE, ensuring that core temperature ≥ 36°C, performing a lung recruitment maneuver, and resuming normal ventilation. Establishing an adequate cardiac rhythm and rate, generally 80 to 100 beats per minute may require a pacemaker. Normalizing electrolytes, treating anemia, and preparing vasoactive medications are also important considerations. Though most patients will have adequate cardiac function with a ventricular pacemaker lead, some patients dependent on active atrial contraction for ventricular filling (eg, severe diastolic dysfunction) will require atrial pacing. Biventricular pacing may improve cardiac output to a small degree, which may be clinically important in patients with severe cardiac dysfunction. The actual process of separation requires intense focus and frequent communication amongst the surgeon, anesthesiologist, and perfusionist, and therefore should be conducted in a quiet, "sterile cockpit" environment.[44]

Once the anesthesiologist, surgeon, and perfusionist are prepared to wean from CPB, the anesthesiologist should work to ensure systemic perfusion and cardiac performance by optimizing heart rate and rhythm, infusing volume from the CPB machine to achieve normovolemia, adjusting afterload with vasodilators or vasopressors as necessary, and optimizing contractility with inotropes as needed. This dynamic process occurs while gradually reducing CPB machine flows to minimal support, at which point cardiac function is reassessed, and then pump flow is stopped completely. If cardiac function is not adequate, then steps to correct this are taken prior to separation.

Immediately after separation, the heart is assessed for adequate function, particularly for markers of ischemia (eg, wall motion abnormalities, worsened ventricular function, inadequate graft flow), valvular abnormalities, and for preload, afterload, and contractility. Frequently, adjustments in volume therapy and vasoactive medicines are made, guided primarily by TEE and hemodynamic monitors. After achieving sufficient hemodynamic parameters generally targeting SBP

100 to 120 mm Hg, and a CI ≥ 2.2 L/min/m², protamine is slowly given prior to the bypass cannulae being removed.

Following separation, the anesthesiologist must remain vigilant and continue to control and optimize patient hemodynamics. Hemostasis should be assessed by examining the surgical field, measuring ACT and heparin concentration, and in certain cases with thromboelastography. Cardiac output should be measured again after chest closure and support adjusted as necessary. Transfer to the ICU should conclude with a detailed, clear handoff to the ICU team in order to minimize communication failures.

Surgical coronary revascularization can also be performed on a beating heart without CPB, and is termed "off-pump" coronary artery bypass (OPCAB). OPCAB typically utilizes a heart stabilization device that isolates a localized region of surgical interest immobile while allowing the rest of the heart to beat. OPCAB became popularized in the late 1990s and early 2000s, eventually becoming the surgical approach for nearly one-third of coronary revascularizations in the United States. OPCAB purported to reduce the surgical inflammatory stress response, mortality, stroke, cognitive dysfunction, and kidney injury. However, recent meta-analyses suggest that there is no significant difference in cognitive dysfunction between OPCAB and CABG,[45] and that all-cause mortality in OPCAB (3.7%) was slightly higher than CABG (3.1%).[46] Furthermore, the need for subsequent revascularization may be higher in OPCAB.[47] As a result, the use of beating heart techniques in the United States is declining.

The OPCAB lends itself to fast-track anesthetic regimens, and in some centers, this is augmented with thoracic epidural analgesia. Heparinization protocols for OPCAB are variable, though many surgeons target ACT values of 300 seconds. Ischemic preconditioning techniques should definitely be considered, given that transient ischemia is likely during the grafting procedure. Surgical exposure may lead to marked alterations in the heart's position within the chest, potentially dramatically impacting cardiac output. The anesthesiologist should be prepared to monitor systemic perfusion most commonly with TEE and continuous cardiac output monitors, and treat hypoperfusion with volume and inotropes as necessary. Occasionally, despite hemodynamic optimization, adequate perfusion cannot be maintained, necessitating conversion to an on-pump procedure. As a result, a perfusionist and CPB machine should be available during OPCAB.

Minimally invasive approaches to coronary revascularization, either on- or off-pump are becoming more common, and involve either a shorter sternotomy incision or any of various small thoracotomies for access to the coronary arteries. Robotic-assisted techniques allow for remote surgical access via small incisions or ports into the chest cavity. The anesthesiologist must communicate with the surgeon preoperatively to discuss the operative strategy and plan accordingly. Often, lung isolation with a double-lumen endotracheal tube or bronchial blocker facilitates surgical visualization. Anesthesiologists should also be prepared to aggressively avoid hypothermia and ensure that external defibrillator pads are placed due to the limited direct access to the heart.[48]

VALVE SURGERY

The perioperative care of patients with valvular heart disease creates a considerable challenge for anesthesiologists, surgeons, and intensivists. A great deal of challenge stems from the wide diversity of pathophysiologic derangements found in these patients. This diversity can, in part, be appreciated by comparing representative LV pressure-volume loops for the different left-sided valvular lesions (Fig. 11-3). Clearly, there are significant and important distinctions in end-diastolic LV volume, intracavitary pressure, and stroke volume. However, not only do the major valvular lesions differ from one another in terms of adaptive ventricular responses and hemodynamic profiles, but patients with the same valvular lesion may present with entirely different degrees of symptomatology and hemodynamic compromise depending on the clinical situation and time course over which the valve pathology develops. Again, LV pressure-volume loops illustrate this concept. The patient who develops acute, severe aortic regurgitation (AR) due to endocarditis will present with notably different LV filling volumes and pressures when compared to a patient with a similar regurgitant fraction whose AR develops gradually due to progressive aortic root dilatation (Fig. 11-4). Clinical management must be appropriately adapted.

Another complicating factor in the management of patients with valvular heart disease is the frequent occurrence of multiple valvular lesions in the same patient. General hemodynamic goals for patients with left-sided valve pathology can be easily summarized (Table 11-3). However, not uncommonly, two valve lesions coexist in which hemodynamic goals are opposite. For example, selecting an ideal heart rate for the patient with aortic stenosis (AS) becomes more difficult in the setting of concomitant MR. In these situations, the physician either determines which lesion contributes most to the patient's symptoms, signs, and hemodynamic profile or

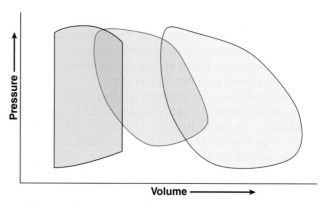

FIGURE 11-4 Representative left ventricular pressure-volume loops comparing a normal ventricle (black) to a patient with acute aortic regurgitation (orange) and chronic aortic regurgitation (purple).

chooses a management strategy that represents a compromise between competing goals.

Although the spectrum of valvular heart disease encompasses a wide variety of hemodynamic findings and adaptive ventricular responses, the natural history of many valve disorders often follows a similar general course. During the initial development of valvular stenosis or regurgitation, the patient remains asymptomatic. Ventricular remodeling serves to normalize indices such as wall tension or stroke volume. Atrial enlargement may mitigate increases in pulmonary or systemic venous pressure. Eventually, following a variable latent period, adaptive responses fail leading to the elevation of cardiac filling pressures, exhaustion of preload reserve, and declining cardiac output. Signs and symptoms of congestive heart failure (CHF) develop or evidence of ventricular dysfunction manifests during imaging studies prompting surgical intervention. The optimal timing of surgical intervention for valvular heart disease continues to evolve, guided by clinical investigations and expert consensus.[49]

Aortic Stenosis

Aortic stenosis represents the most common valve disorder in the United States.[50] Two reasons help explain this observation. First, a congenital bicuspid aortic valve (AV), which has an increased tendency to become stenotic over time, is found in 1 to 2% of the population. Second, risk factors for degenerative calcification of a trileaflet AV such as hyperlipidemia,

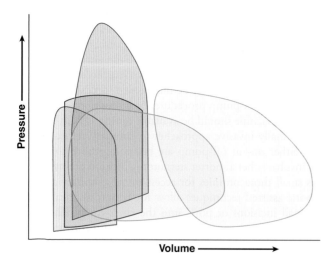

FIGURE 11-3 Representative left ventricular pressure-volume loops depicting a normal ventricle (black), mitral stenosis (blue), aortic stenosis (red), mitral regurgitation (green), and aortic regurgitation (yellow).

⊖ TABLE 11-3: Hemodynamic Goals for Patients with Valvular Heart Disease

	Preload	Afterload	Heart Rate
Aortic stenosis	↑	↑	n/↓
Aortic regurgitation	↑	↓	↑
Mitral stenosis	n/↑	↑	↓
Mitral regurgitation	0	↓	↑

hypertension, smoking, and advanced age are also common. Obstruction to outflow creates abnormal systolic pressure (P) within the LV cavity, which in turn, increases wall tension (T) according to the law of Laplace:

$$T = \frac{PR}{2h}$$

where R represents the radius of the ventricular cavity and h represents myocardial wall thickness. Increases in wall thickness by the process of concentric myocyte hypertrophy serve to normalize wall tension, although this remodeling invariably leads to diastolic dysfunction and creates the setting for oxygen supply and demand mismatch. Thus both LV outflow restriction and the pathophysiology of concentric hypertrophy guide perioperative management. For example, tachycardia is particularly deleterious. Increased heart rates disproportionately encroach on diastolic filling and coronary perfusion time in a ventricle where myocardial relaxation is delayed. At the same time, tachycardia increases myocardial oxygen consumption. Elevated end-diastolic pressures in an LV with reduced compliance limit coronary perfusion to subendocardial regions of the hypertrophied myocardium. Reduced LV compliance also makes the LV more dependent on atrial contraction for diastolic filling and atrial fibrillation may be poorly tolerated. Synchronized cardioversion should be employed early in the patient with severe AS who develops atrial fibrillation with signs of low cardiac output.

The anesthesiologist must consider the pathophysiology of outflow obstruction as well as consequences of concentric LV hypertrophy when selecting a perioperative management plan. Since patients with severe AS are very sensitive to anesthetic-induced decreases in preload and afterload, an arterial line is often placed prior to induction to allow early recognition of blood pressure changes and response to treatment. The choice of induction agent is probably not as important as adherence to key hemodynamic goals that include the maintenance of preload and afterload along with a heart rate in the low to normal range. Hypotension is treated promptly, usually with an α-adrenergic agonist. Opioids such as fentanyl are often included in a balanced anesthetic induction and maintenance regimen since they tend to lower heart rate and minimally impact myocardial contractility. High-dose opioid anesthetic regimens, more popular in preceding decades, provide hemodynamic stability but may hamper early postoperative extubation. Drugs that increase heart rate, such as ketamine or pancuronium, should be used cautiously or in conjunction with vagotonic agents such as opioids. However, while avoidance of tachycardia represents an important perioperative goal, anesthesiologists must also avoid severe bradycardia.[51] In patients with AS, flow across the AV limited and cardiac output declines with heart rates less than 50 beats per minute. When treating bradycardia, drugs such as β-adrenergic agonists or anticholinergics should be titrated carefully to avoid overshoot and the development of tachycardia.[51] Atrial or atrio-ventricular pacing represents an attractive option for

the cardiac surgical patient since it allows precise titration of heart rate.

In addition to an arterial line, central venous access along with a PAC is generally selected for patient undergoing aortic valve replacement (AVR). Central venous access is desirable for the administration of vasoactive medications although central venous pressure (CVP) does not accurately reflect LV filling pressures in patients with severe AS. Likewise, the pulmonary capillary wedge pressure (PCWP) also does not provide a reliable assessment of LV filling in the setting of AS and reduced ventricular compliance. Measuring end-diastolic LV cavity area with TEE provides a more accurate reflection of preload compared with PAC-derived measurements.[51] Nonetheless, despite the limited ability to assess preload and the small risk of arrhythmia during insertion, the PAC offers several advantages including the opportunity to track cardiac output, measure pulmonary artery (PA) pressure, and serve as a conduit for a temporary pacing wire.

Aortic Regurgitation

Aortic regurgitation (AR) leads to significant volume overloading of the LV and when chronic, the pressure-volume loop shifts farther to the right than for any other valvular lesion (Fig. 11-3). The eccentric LV hypertrophy and chamber dilatation that develop in the setting of chronic AR serve to normalize wall tension and accommodate very large end-diastolic volumes without significant increases in end-diastolic pressure. Patients may remain asymptomatic for years, though eventually compensatory changes are exhausted and in the face of progressively larger ventricular volumes, LV systolic function declines. In cases of acute severe AR, compensatory LV changes are not present. End-diastolic pressure rises quickly and may reach aortic diastolic pressure. In such cases, the combination of a low aortic diastolic pressure and a high LV end-diastolic pressure limit CPP, creating the potential for ischemia.

The hemodynamic goals for patients with severe AR differ from those used to manage AS patients. When the regurgitant fractions exceed 60%, maintenance of cardiac output requires an increase in heart rate.[51] A faster heart rate also reduces the diastolic period available for regurgitant flow into the LV. Avoidance of opioid-induced bradycardia along with the use of a muscle relaxant that increases heart rate such as pancuronium may prove useful. A reduction in afterload promotes forward flow. Propofol, which reduces afterload and displays minimal effects on myocardial contractility at usual clinical doses, represents a reasonable option for the induction of anesthesia.[52] Additional afterload reduction in the form of vasodilators such as sodium nitroprusside may be selected. Because the LV may be severely dilated and LV systolic may be depressed even in asymptomatic patients,[51] inotropic support should be readily available. Agents with β-adrenergic agonist activity, such as dobutamine along with phosphodiesterase inhibitors such as milrinone, increase myocardial contractility while favoring a reduction in afterload.

The hemodynamic monitors chosen for patients with severe AR undergoing AVR are similar to those selected for patients with AS. Intra-arterial pressure monitoring, central venous cannulation, and PAC placement are generally used together with intraoperative TEE. As in the case of AS, the measurement of PCWP may not accurately reflect LV filling, particularly in the case of severe, acute AR where the rapid rise of LV end-diastolic pressure may promote closure of the MV in late diastole. However, many anesthesiologists find the ability to obtain serial measurements of cardiac output to be beneficial. Furthermore, a PAC provides an easy route by which a pacing lead may be placed prior to sternal opening, facilitating the maintenance of an elevated heart rate.

Mitral Stenosis

Rheumatic disease accounts for most cases of acquired mitral stenosis (MS) in developed countries. Patients with rheumatic MV disease may remain asymptomatic for many years as the left atrium (LA) progressively dilates. Symptoms develop when severe MS limits LV filling and cardiac output. Alternatively, patients with moderate MS may become symptomatic during periods of increased transvalvular flow such as pregnancy or conditions associated with tachycardia.[51] As shown in the simplified Gorlin equation, for a given valve area, when transvalvular flow increases, the pressure gradient also rises.

$$\text{Valve area} = \frac{\text{Flow}}{\sqrt{\text{Pressure gradient}}}$$

Rising LA pressure promotes pulmonary venous congestion and leads to feelings of dyspnea. Over time, pulmonary hypertension develops which may, in turn, lead to right ventricular (RV) enlargement, RV systolic dysfunction, and functional tricuspid regurgitation (TR). A major goal in the perioperative care of patients with severe MS is the identification and quantification of RV impairment.

The anesthetic management of patients with severe MS undergoing MV replacement is guided by several principles. First, tachycardia, which shortens diastolic LV filling time and increases LA pressure, should be treated promptly. The judicious use of preoperative sedation may ameliorate anxiety-induced tachycardia although excess sedation promotes hypoventilation with the attendant risk of increased pulmonary vascular resistance. A number of different agents may be chosen to reduce heart rate including calcium channel blockers, β-blockers, or amiodarone. Atrial fibrillation is commonly found in patients in this patient group and is generally tolerated provided the ventricular rate is controlled. Therefore, unlike patients with severe AS who develop atrial fibrillation, the immediate focus in patients with MS should be to maintain a low to normal ventricular rate rather than conversion to sinus rhythm. Second, because LV filling is already impaired by the stenotic MV, additional reductions in preload caused by anesthesia or blood loss should be carefully corrected. Vasodilation resulting from inhaled or intravenous anesthetics may be treated with incremental doses of an α-adrenergic

agonist or vasopressin, ideally while monitoring PA pressures. Surgical blood loss should be replaced though overly zealous fluid administration should be avoided to prevent pulmonary vascular congestion and further RV impairment. While the PCWP does not reflect LV end-diastolic pressures in the setting of severe MS, display of PA pressures and serial measurement of cardiac output may be useful in guiding fluid administration. A third principle in the management of these patients involves control of PA pressures and augmentation of the RV systolic function. Because of the aforementioned need to maintain preload, the use of systemic vasodilators, though they may reduce PA pressure, may be poorly tolerated in this group. Instead, a select pulmonary vasodilator such as inhaled prostaglandin or nitric oxide should be considered for those with pulmonary hypertension and RV dysfunction. Additionally, arterial blood gas management is essential. The avoidance of hypoxia together with mild hyperventilation, combine to reduce pulmonary vascular resistance.

Following MVR with normalization of left-sided preload, LV systolic performance is expected to improve. However in a subset of patients, LV systolic performance may be impaired following valve replacement. Possible causes include rheumatic endocarditis or an unfavorable position of the ventricular septum in the setting of pulmonary hypertension and RV enlargement.[51] Intraoperative TEE readily detects abnormalities of ventricular septal position and RV dysfunction in addition to providing a qualitative and quantitative assessment of LV systolic performance. Inotropic support may be required.

Mitral Regurgitation

Mitral regurgitation shares some similarities with AR. Both conditions increase the preload of the LV and over time, eccentric hypertrophy develops. Like those with AR, patients with MR may remain asymptomatic for long periods. Similar to AR patients, those with MR present for surgery with a spectrum of clinical and imaging findings. The patient with MV prolapse who is followed with serial echocardiograms over a decade differs in important ways from the patient with acute, severe MR due to papillary muscle rupture. The former may well remain asymptomatic or minimally symptomatic and be referred for surgery due to abnormalities in LV size or function, while the latter is likely to present in heart failure with florid pulmonary edema and require intra-aortic balloon pump support preoperatively.

In patients with chronic MR, the contractile appearance of the LV in MR patients often improves initially in response to preload augmentation according to the Frank-Starling principle. Furthermore, the ejection of large quantities of blood into the low pressure LA leads to increases in the calculated ejection fraction although forward cardiac output may decline. An LVEF < 60% identifies reduced systolic performance in patients with severe MR and represents an indication for surgery.[49,53] Physicians have also recognized that an early decline in LVEF following MV surgery for MR is common. Although sometimes considered an inevitable consequence of MV surgery for MR, significant reductions in LV function postoperatively associated with an ejection fraction < 40% may identify a group at increased risk for premature death.[54] Several reasons have been postulated to explain reduced LV systolic performance following MV surgery, including reduced preload and ischemic cross-clamp injury[55] as well as unrecognized, preexisting systolic dysfunction.[54] Impaired preoperative LV systolic impairment may be underappreciated by echocardiography.[56] Several risk factors identify patients with MR who are at increased risk for low ejection fraction following mitral surgery, including preoperative pulmonary hypertension, preoperative atrial fibrillation, and a preoperative LV end-systolic diameter > 36 mm which confers a 6.5-fold increased risk of having a postoperative LVEF < 40%.[54,55] By assessing preoperative risks factors, anesthesiologists and surgeons can better prepare for the possible use of pharmacologic and mechanical circulatory support after MV surgery. Inotropic agents such as epinephrine and milrinone should be available. Early consideration should be given to placement of an IABP if hemodynamic compromise is refractory to drug therapy.

Hemodynamic goals for patients with severe MR include a reduction in the regurgitant fraction with augmentation of forward flow. For those patients with longstanding MR and pulmonary hypertension, support of the RV is also important. Providing that LV systolic function is not severely impaired, most patients tolerate an intravenous induction of anesthesia. Agents such as propofol reduce afterload and promote forward flow. Bradycardia is avoided since lower heart rates facilitate greater LV filling and distention. Inhalation agents are good choices for the maintenance of anesthesia as they also provide vasodilatation and may increase heart rate slightly. In patients with chronic MR, the LA is usually dilated. Atrial fibrillation may be present but is generally well tolerated since LV filling is unimpeded.

Robotic and Minimally Invasive Mitral Valve Surgery

The popularity of robotic and other minimally invasive approaches to MV surgery continues to grow. Advantages of these approaches include reduced time to extubation, shortened hospital length of stay, lower blood product transfusion rates, and improved postoperative respiratory function.[57,58] The use of robotic and minimally invasive techniques necessitates changes in anesthetic management. These changes include the need for one-lung ventilation, the percutaneous placement of cannulae for CPB and retrograde cardioplegia, the expanded use of TEE (Table 11-4), and altered strategies for defibrillation. Smaller incisions and reduced need for opioid medications also create the potential for more rapid extubation and the expanded use of regional anesthesia.

Both thoracoscopic and robotic mitral repair utilize a small working incision and additional port access in the right chest. This approach requires deflation of the right lung. Either a double-lumen endotracheal tube or a bronchial blocker may be used to facilitate the operation.[59] Oxygen desaturation associated with one-lung ventilation is particularly problematic

TABLE 11-4: Uses of Transesophageal Echocardiography During Robotic Mitral Valve Surgery

- Assess valvular heart disease
- Assess valve repair/replacement
- Detection of additional findings (eg, patent foramen ovale)
- Guide cannulation
  - Femoral venous/inferior vena cava
  - Internal jugular/superior vena cava
  - Coronary sinus cardioplegia line
  - Endo-aortic balloon
  - Pulmonary artery vent
- Monitor cardioplegia delivery

following CPB and may be treated by the application of continuous positive airway pressure (CPAP) to the nonventilated right lung, the use of positive end-expiratory pressure (PEEP) with the left lung, or intermittent two-lung ventilation.[60]

Cannulation for CPB for these operations usually consists of femoral arterial and venous access with or without supplementary venous drainage in the form of a vent line in the pulmonary artery or a superior vena cava cannula placed percutaneously from the right internal jugular vein. Surgeon preference and institutional experience guide the cannulation strategy. Intraoperative TEE is used to verify the position of the guidewire and femoral venous cannula. Inadvertent placement of a femoral venous guidewire across a patent foramen ovale is possible and should prompt redirection (Fig. 11-5). Supplementary venous drainage from the main pulmonary artery can be accomplished by means of a specialized endovent, the tip of which should be located in the main PA, near the bifurcation (Fig. 11-6A). Again, intraoperative TEE is used to ensure proper placement. TEE imaging can be difficult in these cases requiring the placement of multiple lines in the right heart (Fig. 11-6B).

Aortic cross clamping and cardioplegia administration can be accomplished by several different mechanisms. An endo-aortic balloon may be advanced from the femoral artery into the ascending aorta where inflation serves to isolate the aortic root and facilitate antegrade cardioplegia delivery from the end of the delivery catheter. A percutaneous coronary sinus catheter may also be placed via the right internal jugular vein using TEE or fluoroscopic guidance to allow for the administration of retrograde cardioplegia. Lastly, an antegrade cardioplegia and vent line may be placed via a parasternal stab incision, a strategy similar to many open cardiac operations (Fig. 11-7A). In this last scenario, a long transthoracic aortic cross-clamp is used via a small lateral thoracic incision. The position of this cardioplegia line (Fig. 11-7B) and subsequent cardioplegia delivery (Fig. 11-7C) can be monitored with TEE.

Small incisions preclude the use of internal paddles for defibrillation and cardioversion in robotic MV surgery. Instead, external patches are applied in an anterior-posterior orientation on the left chest.[61] Should defibrillation prove difficult,

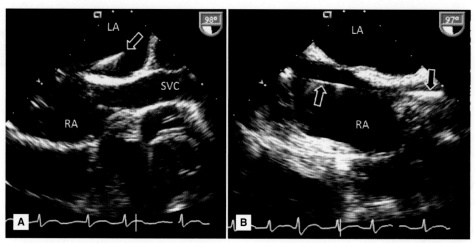

FIGURE 11-5 Transesophageal echocardiographic images showing a guidewire inserted via the femoral vein crossing a patent foramen ovale (A) before being redirected into the superior vena cava (B).

consideration should be given to inflating the right lung to improve electrical impedance.[59]

Minimally invasive mitral surgery facilitates rapid extubation, particularly when regional anesthesia is used.[57] Multiple regional anesthetic techniques have been used in these cases including intrathecal opioid administration, intercostal nerve block, and paravertebral nerve block. The use of preoperative paravertebral nerve block together with a limited opioid dosing strategy was shown to facilitate extubation in the operating room following robotic mitral repair in approximately 90% of cases in one study.[57]

Tricuspid Regurgitation

Tricuspid regurgitation (TR) found in patients presenting for cardiac surgery is most often functional in nature and occurs secondary to left-sided valve disease, pulmonary hypertension, or RV dysfunction. As such, the anesthetic management of these patients is usually dictated by the primary condition. However, patients may present with TR due to isolated, organic tricuspid valve (TV) disease. Examples include endocarditis, carcinoid valvulopathy, trauma, or pacemaker-induced valve dysfunction.

General hemodynamic goals for patients with severe TR include support of RV contractility, maintenance of a mildly elevated heart rate, and reduction of RV afterload by reducing pulmonary vascular resistance. Phosphodiesterase inhibitors such as milrinone may augment RV contractility while reducing RV afterload. Dobutamine and isoproterenol represent other possible options. As in cases of pulmonary hypertension or RV systolic dysfunction, careful attention to arterial blood gas values provides an important nonpharmacologic means by which the anesthesiologist can manipulate pulmonary vascular resistance.

In addition to direct arterial pressure monitoring, CVP monitoring is nearly always used for patients undergoing TV surgery even though CVP is a poor indicator of RV filling in the setting of severe TR. Although it may be difficult to advance in the face of severe TR, consideration can be given to PAC placement especially if TV repair or replacement with a tissue prosthesis is contemplated. A PAC facilitates assessment of pulmonary vascular resistance and thermodilutional cardiac output measurement becomes more feasible following TV surgery. The measurement of cardiac output by arterial waveform analysis provides the anesthesiologist with a reasonable alternative to placement of a PAC. These devices can be connected to any invasive arterial monitoring line. Early comparative studies with thermodilutional techniques were disappointing though the updated software in newer models may deliver more robust results.[62,63] The use of TEE can be invaluable in assessing not only valvular pathology but RV function as well. An additional important use of TEE in isolated TV surgery is the identification of intracardiac shunts since in the absence of shunting, CPB without a cross clamp becomes feasible.

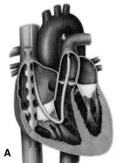
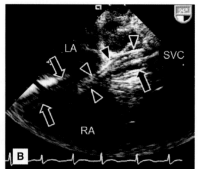

FIGURE 11-6 (A) A potential venous cannulation strategy for robotic mitral valve repair using a multi-orificed cannula inserted via the femoral vein and positioned with its tip in the superior vena cava along with supplemental drainage provided by a vent placed percutaneously into the pulmonary artery. (B) Transesophageal echocardiogram demonstrating a venous cannula in the right atrium and superior vena cava (*arrows*) along with a pulmonary artery vent (*arrowheads*).

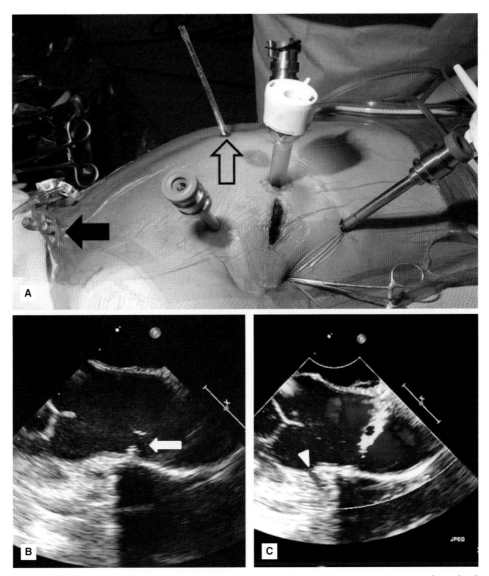

FIGURE 11-7 (A) Surgical site photo of a patient undergoing robotic mitral valve repair. A percutaneous antegrade cardioplegia line is seen (*open arrow*) along with a right internal jugular vein introducer sheath (*solid arrow*) used facilitate placement of a percutaneous superior vena cava cannula. (B) Transesophageal echocardiogram demonstrating the tip of the percutaneous antegrade cardioplegia line in the proximal ascending aorta (*arrow*). (C) Antegrade cardioplegia administration via a percutaneously placed line.

THORACIC AORTIC SURGERY

The spectrum of diseases of the thoracic aorta may be classified according to pathology, etiology, timing, clinical presentation, location, and management options.[64-66] Thorough preoperative assessment including a comprehensive history and physical exam, review of preoperative imaging studies, and patient stability all play a role in determining whether the patient can be treated medically with continued surveillance, or surgically with definitive intervention.[64-66] When surgery is warranted, the urgency and planned surgical approach to repair significantly influence the anesthetic plan. Factors such as the cannulation strategy for CPB, the need for temporary cessation of blood flow, and anticipated methods for organ protection determine the optimal anesthetic technique and monitoring

choices during thoracic aortic surgery. While routine monitoring involved in all cardiac surgery patients applies to aortic surgery as well, the anesthesiologist must further individualize management to the patient's disease and the surgeon's operative approach. Hemodynamic goals, especially blood pressure management, can be significantly different from those of the cardiac surgical patient presenting for nonaortic surgery. Maintaining organ perfusion and protecting major organs, specifically those subjected to periods of ischemia, is crucial in allowing for optimal outcomes. Additional monitoring to detect and treat end-organ ischemia is another factor in procedural success. Furthermore, complex thoracic aortic surgery associated with prolonged procedure times and hypothermia frequently results in postoperative coagulopathy that can be effectively managed with anticipation of bleeding and transfusion requirements. In addition, reliance on intraoperative TEE in guiding the operation, managing isolated single-lung ventilation to allow for adequate surgical exposure, and placement of lumbar cerebrospinal (CSF) drainage catheters are also essential aspects of the operation that give the cardiac anesthesiologist a key role in the surgical treatment of thoracic aortic disease. Recent multi-disciplinary guidelines for thoracic aortic diseases include evidence-based recommendations regarding anesthetic techniques and intraoperative monitoring.[64-66] This review of anesthetic and monitoring considerations for thoracic aortic surgery will be presented in the following three sections: (1) aortic root/ascending aorta; (2) aortic arch; and (3) descending thoracic aorta.

Aortic Root and Ascending Aorta

Surgical intervention for the aortic root and ascending aorta may be isolated to these aortic segments or may continue distally into the arch and beyond. Surgery for ascending aorta pathology above the root may often involve partial reconstruction of the aortic arch as well.[67] When isolated to the level of the aortic root, the aortic arch may not be included in the surgical intervention. Typically, surgical indications for ascending aortic intervention include dissection, intramural hematoma, and aneurysm.[64-67] Factors such as patient age, connective tissue disorder, family history, and bicuspid aortic valve must all be taken into account when finalizing the surgical plan.[64-67]

The surgical approach to these cases is via a midline sternotomy, and therefore, patients will be positioned supine with both arms tucked and padded at their sides. Along with a balanced general endotracheal anesthetic, these patients typically have an arterial line and PAC placed for hemodynamic monitoring. The maintenance of normotensive blood pressure is suitable for patients with chronic aortic disease. When presenting for elective surgery, preoperative antihypertensive therapy should be titrated to achieve a blood pressure less than 140/90 mm Hg or less than 130/80 mm Hg in patients with diabetes or chronic renal disease (Class I recommendation; Level B evidence).[64,65] Preoperative therapy may even be titrated in known aortic aneurysm patients to achieve the lowest possible blood pressure that is tolerated without adverse effects (Class IIa recommendation; Level B evidence).[64,65] In acute pathologies of the ascending aorta such as dissection, more aggressive treatment to a systolic pressure of 100 to 120 mm Hg is recommended since aortic rupture is a major concern in this phase.[64,65] This strict control of systolic blood pressure is typically achieved with adequate anesthetic depth, titrated analgesia with opioids such as fentanyl and morphine, and vasodilator therapy with agents such as beta-blockers, nitroprusside, nicardipine, or morphine. Intravenous beta-blockade is typically avoided in the settings of significant aortic regurgitation and/or cardiac tamponade since cardiac output in these presentations remains rate-dependent.[64,65,68] Since acute aortic dissection is dynamic and progressive, patients may become acutely hemodynamically unstable, emphasizing the importance for not only being

prepared for these scenarios, but also the importance of a prompt anesthetic induction to minimize delays and control patient anxiety and hypertension.

Anesthetic induction should involve a smooth intravenous induction with adequate anesthetic depth and blood pressure control for laryngoscopy and endotracheal intubation. If presenting emergently, concerns for a full stomach should lead to a 'modified' rapid sequence induction, where cricoid pressure is applied but gentle mask ventilation is used prior to endotracheal intubation. The choice of a left or right radial arterial line depends on disease extent and cannulation strategy. High-quality communication between all members of the operating room team streamlines this process. Indications for a left radial arterial line include innominate disease, and planned right axillary arterial cannulation. A right radial arterial line is often indicated for monitoring of cerebral perfusion pressure in antegrade cerebral perfusion during periods of systemic circulatory arrest.[69-71] The institutional practices for cannulation and monitoring will often determine preferences for which side is chosen. This may include a requirement for bilateral upper extremity arterial lines.

TEE is reasonable in all open surgical repairs of the thoracic aorta, unless a specific contraindication to its use exists (Class IIa recommendation; Level B evidence).[65] When used specifically for the ascending aorta or root surgery, there is a strong consensus that TEE is particularly suited for aortic imaging in unstable patients with suspected acute aortic syndromes.[64,65] TEE can also verify the aortic diagnosis, interrogate the aortic valve comprehensively, and confirm important aortic diameters.[64-66,72] Precise measurements of the aortic root diameters can provide data to guide decision making about whether to replace or spare the root, depending on the clinical scenario (Fig. 11-8).[65-67] Similarly, TEE can be used to assess the extent of proximal dissection within the root and whether the dissection flap crosses the AV to cause AR (Fig. 11-9). This information can provide data to guide the surgical plan for the aortic valve.[73,74] In addition to identifying the presence of a pericardial effusion with or without tamponade, the origin of the primary tear, the extent of the dissection, and regional wall motion abnormalities from coronary dissection, TEE can also guide the surgeon's successful placement of the arterial inflow cannula when direct central cannulation through the dissection is chosen.[75] In this scenario, the echocardiographer must identify the true lumen on TEE with certainty in order to verify correct wire placement (Fig. 11-10).[75] Checking for appropriate flow in the true lumen after initiation of CPB can then further verify adequate cannula location. In addition to assessment of the thoracic aorta, TEE also serves to exclude other cardiac pathology and evaluate the surgical repair and ventricular function after CPB. In the setting of aortic root replacement with coronary reimplantation, TEE can analyze ventricular wall motion after CPB to verify adequate blood flow. While the indications described above are more specific to ascending aorta pathology, TEE plays a similar role in open aortic arch and descending aorta surgical procedures. In addition to TEE, intraoperative monitoring of the carotid arteries with

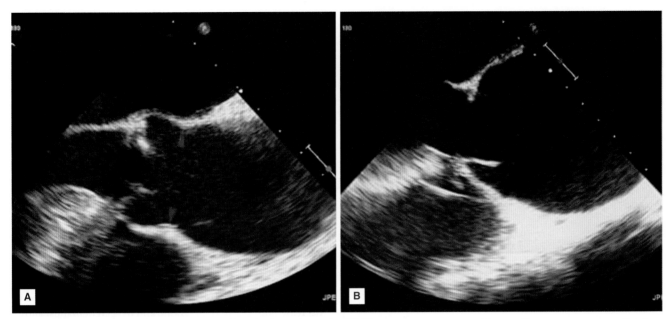

FIGURE 11-8 Aortic valve long-axis transesophageal echocardiography (TEE) views in two patients with ascending aorta aneurysms. The benefits of TEE in aortic surgery include the ability to quantify dilation, as well as identify structural integrity of the aortic valve and root. Panel A demonstrates definition of the sinotubular junction (*arrowheads*), while Panel B demonstrates effacement requiring root replacement.

ultrasound can be beneficial in aortic dissection to confirm bilateral carotid flow prior to CPB, while on CPB, and after cross-clamping. In this scenario, brachiocephalic malperfusion may result from factors such as retrograde arterial perfusion, loss of flow through intimal fenestrations, and loss of pulsatile flow.[76] If detected, changes in cannulation site and/or intimal fenestration can restore normal cerebral perfusion.[76]

While midline sternotomy with CPB is the typical operative plan for ascending aorta pathology, endovascular approaches in patients deemed too high risk for open repair have been performed with success.[77,78] Transapical access allows antegrade stenting of the ascending aorta with verification of wire placement and assistance with stent positioning provided by TEE (Fig. 11-11).[78] Just as in transapical

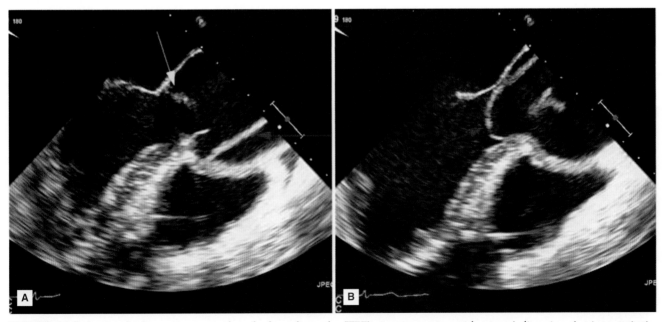

FIGURE 11-9 Aortic valve long-axis transesophageal echocardiography (TEE) views in a patient with a type A dissection. Aortic regurgitation may not necessarily be due to structural valve disease. TEE demonstrates that in systole (Panel A), the dissection flap (*red arrow*) extends into the root, but it is above the aortic valve (*yellow arrow*). During diastole (Panel B), the dissection flap (*red arrow*) prolapses across the aortic valve, thus preventing adequate coaptation of the valve leaflets.

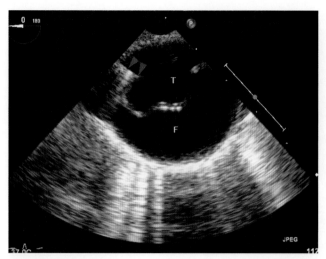

FIGURE 11-10 The role of transesophageal echocardiography (TEE) is again demonstrated in a patient undergoing a Type A dissection repair. Central aortic cannulation was performed over a wire placed into the distal ascending aorta. TEE of the proximal descending aorta confirms that the wire (*arrowheads*) is indeed in the true (T) lumen. TEE is also valuable in guiding venous wire and cannula placement.

transcatheter AVR, the anesthetic plan should anticipate the need for rapid ventricular pacing for stent deployment and should include appropriate resuscitative measures for hemodynamic recovery after pacing.[79]

Aortic Arch

The decision to include the aortic arch in the operative plan depends on the pathology and extent of disease.[64-66,80] Although a hemiarch is often appropriate, total aortic arch replacement may be required in the setting of extensive arch disease.[64-66] Furthermore, the advent and expansion of hybrid aortic arch procedures will likely lead to a drift towards endovascular adjuncts in high-risk patients.[64-66,81] Direct

arch replacement typically requires temporary cessation of systemic blood flow to allow for arch reconstruction, with greater periods of hypothermic circulatory arrest frequently required for total arch replacement. Although hypothermic circulatory arrest is an established classic technique, it still carries the risk of neurological complications.[82] Therefore, neuroprotective strategies must be incorporated into the anesthetic and surgical plans to decrease risk to the patient (Class 1 recommendation; Level B evidence).[64,65] Although there are several neuroprotective options available, there still exists marked variation in the conduct of hypothermic circulatory arrest, including choice of cerebral protection strategies and preferred neuromonitoring techniques.[83,84]

NEUROPROTECTION DURING ADULT AORTIC ARCH REPAIR

The high metabolic rate of the brain makes it particularly susceptible to ischemic injury during periods of circulatory arrest.[85] To mitigate this ischemia, hypothermia is utilized to decrease both cerebral metabolic and oxygen demands, allowing for increased periods of circulatory arrest.[85] The degree of hypothermia utilized for aortic arch repair has recently been defined by international consensus into four levels: profound, deep, moderate, and mild (Table 11-5).[85] The optimal level of hypothermia for aortic arch repair has recently been under scrutiny.[85] The requirement for profound or deep hypothermic circulatory arrest has recently been questioned due to concerns about the increased risks of coagulopathy, inflammatory response, and end-organ dysfunction.[82-85] The increasing utilization of cerebral perfusion adjuncts, such as retrograde cerebral perfusion (RCP) or selective antegrade cerebral perfusion (ACP), have enabled moderate degrees of hypothermia to be increasingly chosen for aortic arch procedures with successful outcomes.[82,85-87] The conduct of RCP involves retrograde perfusion through the superior vena cava cannula to achieve a CVP of 15 to 20 mm Hg, typically monitored at the level of the right internal jugular vein.[88] Although RCP with deep hypothermic circulatory arrest provides excellent

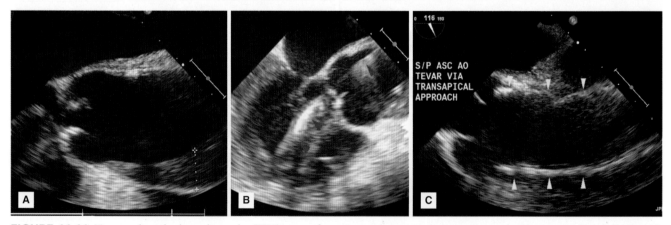

FIGURE 11-11 Transesophageal echocardiography (TEE) views of a patient with an ascending aorta intramural hematoma (Panel A). Considered too high risk for sternotomy and cardiopulmonary bypass, an endovascular approach via the left ventricular apex was chosen. TEE demonstrates wire access (*red arrowheads*) across the aortic valve (Panel B) before stent deployment (*yellow arrowheads*) into the proximal ascending aorta (Panel C).

TABLE 11-5: Consensus Classification of Hypothermia in Aortic Arch Surgery

Level of Hypothermia	Nasopharyngeal Temperature
Profound hypothermia	≤14°C
Deep hypothermia	14.1-20.0°C
Moderate hypothermia	20.1-28.0°C
Mild hypothermia	28.1-34.0°C

outcomes for aortic arch repair with short reconstruction times, the amount of perfusate that actually provides metabolic substrate to support brain metabolic function during RCP remains low.[88,89]

The emerging contemporary paradigm for adult aortic arch repair is the utilization of moderate hypothermia with ACP since this guarantees cerebral perfusion, extends the duration of time for aortic arch reconstruction, and avoids the morbidity of deeper levels of hypothermia.[82,84-87] ACP can be performed either in a unilateral fashion with a cannula in the right axillary artery or innominate artery, or in a bilateral fashion with cannulas in both the innominate and left carotid arteries. Although ACP can be unilateral or bilateral, recent trials both in elective and emergent adult aortic arch repair suggest that unilateral ACP at adequate pressure with appropriate neuromonitoring is safe, effective, and straightforward.[90-92] Perfusion during ACP is often titrated to maintain flows in the range of 10 to 15 mL/kg, a right radial artery pressure of approximately 50 to 60 mm Hg, and a baseline neuromonitoring profile.[93] The final selection of both the degree of hypothermia and type of cerebral perfusion adjunct will depend on factors such as the patient, the aortic arch pathology, surgical preferences, and institutional practices. Despite the significant variability, it is reasonable to use the perfusion management strategy that is best suited to the team and institution (Class IIa Recommendation; Level B Evidence).[65]

In addition to these perfusion strategies for neuroprotection, pharmacologic agents are also often employed.[83,84] Thiopental or propofol may be given at doses to cause burst suppression.[93] Corticosteroids, magnesium, and lidocaine are also popular for their potential neuroprotective benefit.[83,84,94,95] Recent analysis from a large adult European registry has suggested that steroids may decrease the stroke rate after aortic arch reconstruction.[95] There is currently no strong evidence to guide the choice of pharmacologic agents for improving neurologic outcomes after thoracic aortic surgery. Therefore, the use of these agents should be considered an adjunct to hypothermia. Further trials are required to identify best practices in this area.

NEUROMONITORING DURING ADULT AORTIC ARCH REPAIR

Neuroprotective strategies during aortic arch repair such as hypothermia, cerebral perfusion adjuncts, and appropriate pharmacology do not guarantee prevention of postoperative neurologic injury. Furthermore, general anesthesia precludes a full neurological examination during the procedure. Intraoperative neurophysiologic monitoring remains important for early detection of possible neurologic injury and for assessment of adequate perfusion. The ability to identify impending injury can also allow for earlier intervention to prevent permanent injury. The use of intraoperative monitors can certainly help guide therapy, but the decision to use such monitoring will depend on individual patient needs, institutional resources, the urgency of the procedure, and the perfusion techniques being used (Class IIa Recommendation; Level B Evidence).[65] Furthermore, while these monitors provide valuable information intraoperatively, there are no large, randomized controlled trials that provide conclusive evidence that these monitors decrease neurologic injury after adult aortic arch repair.

Electroencephalography (EEG) measures spontaneous electrical brain activity via electrodes placed in a standardized fashion on the scalp. The electrical activity is amplified and displayed on a monitor as a continuous EEG signal. During the use of deep hypothermic circulatory arrest, gradual slowing of the EEG occurs until electrocortical silence is achieved with continued lower temperatures (Fig. 11-12).[96] Therefore, the degree of hypothermia needed for neuroprotection can be determined by EEG silence as a marker of brain temperature and metabolic suppression.[88,96,97] Without EEG, simply cooling to a target temperature such as 18 degrees Celsius may not provide adequate cerebral metabolic suppression since this approach does not guarantee EEG silence in 100% of patients.[96,97] EEG is also a useful monitor to detect seizures and ischemia during thoracic aortic surgery.[98,99] Since anesthetic agents can attenuate EEG amplitude and frequencies, high-quality communication between all intraoperative team members can minimize anesthetic interference with the EEG recordings for optimal neuromonitoring at all phases of the procedure. During systemic rewarming, the return of the EEG signal to baseline suggests neurologic injury did not occur as a result of the arch repair or unintended brain hyperthermia.[97,100]

An increase in jugular bulb venous oxygen saturation monitored via an oximetric catheter has also been utilized for guiding temperature-induced cerebral metabolic suppression.[101] Although jugular bulb saturation > 95% suggests cerebral metabolic suppression, routine jugular bulb saturation monitoring has not enhanced the neuroprotective effects of hypothermia.[101] As an alternative, near-infrared spectrophotometry (NIRS) offers noninvasive measurement of cerebral oxygen saturation.[83,84,93] A further advantage of NIRS over EEG is its ability to continue monitoring cerebral perfusion status after EEG silence has occurred. However, NIRS only provides a focal assessment due to small sample size of brain tissue being monitored, and therefore, it may not detect ischemia in other brain regions.[102] Similar to pulse oximetry, the NIRS device is based on different absorption characteristics of oxygenated and deoxygenated hemoglobin, as measured from two adhesive pads placed over the frontal lobes.[102] Cerebral oximetry values typically increase during deliberate hypothermia since cerebral oxygen demand decreases.

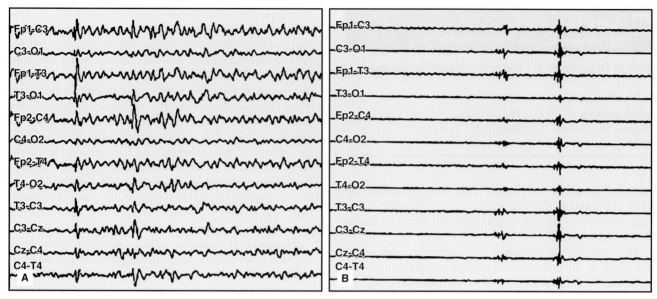

FIGURE 11-12 Electroencephalography (EEG) obtained during a case of ascending aorta and hemiarch replacement using deep hypothermic circulatory arrest. As the patient is progressively cooled, amplitude and frequency decrease from baseline (Panel A) until EEG silence (Panel B) is obtained (approximately 18°C in this patient). Note the signal artifact in Panel B.

During periods of cerebral ischemia such as circulatory arrest, decreases from the baseline cerebral oximetry values suggest inadequate perfusion.[102] Whether RCP or ACP is being employed, perfusion pressures via RCP cannulas or ACP cannulas can be adjusted to seek an improvement in NIRS values. Similarly, when unilateral ACP is being employed, a drop in the contralateral NIRS monitor suggests inadequate contralateral hemispheric perfusion due to an incomplete circle of Willis or due to inadequate ACP flow. Increasing ACP unilateral flow and/or instituting bilateral ACP typically restore the NIRS values to baseline, which may correlate with better perioperative neurologic outcomes.[103,104] While the use of NIRS is becoming more standard in the conduct of adult aortic arch repair, further trials are required to delineate best practices with this novel technology.[102]

Descending Thoracic Aorta

The main diseases of the descending thoracic aorta and/or the thoracoabdominal aorta that require surgical intervention are aneurysm and dissection.[64-66] The repair options include open replacement, thoracic endovascular aortic repair (TEVAR) and hybrid procedures that involve both techniques.[105] The anesthetic plan for descending thoracic aorta repair must be tailored according to the surgical approach, with a major goal for all surgical techniques to prevent distal ischemic injury to the visceral organs and the spinal cord. This ischemia can occur during the repair itself when flow may be intermittently occluded or due to loss of aortic branches. To prevent organ injury and neurologic deficit, emphasis should be placed on strategies to minimize ischemia, as well as quickly identify and treat ischemia.

OPEN SURGICAL REPAIR

Access for open repair of the descending thoracic aorta is achieved by a left thoracotomy with the patient in the right lateral decubitus position. When the disease process extends into the abdominal aorta, an extensive thoracoabdominal incision is indicated for retroperitoneal access to the abdominal aorta.[106] In addition to full invasive monitoring, it is preferable to have a femoral arterial line to monitor lower body perfusion. To allow for adequate visualization in the left chest, a left-sided double-lumen endotracheal tube is typically utilized for selective collapse of the left lung, although at times, aneurysmal compression of the left main bronchus may require downsizing or a switch to a bronchial blocker for effective lung separation. In addition to allowing good exposure, lung isolation also reduces the need for pulmonary retraction and may decrease unintended pulmonary contusions.[65] At the conclusion of the operation, the decision to exchange the endotracheal tube for a single-lumen endotracheal tube should be made after a thorough evaluation for airway edema and bleeding. A single-lumen tube is usually desired to allow for better pulmonary hygiene; however, routine exchange to a single-lumen tube is not recommended when significant upper airway edema or hemorrhage is present (Class III Recommendation; Level C Evidence).[65]

Prevention of postoperative spinal cord ischemia remains a major goal for descending aortic surgery (Table 11-6).[107] When an open repair is performed, various strategies are possible to maintain distal aortic and spinal cord perfusion. These surgical options will only be briefly discussed here, allowing for a focus on nonsurgical adjuncts and neuromonitoring. A simple aortic cross-clamp technique has been used with success when clamp time is minimized, but it does not allow

TABLE 11-6: Strategies for Spinal Cord Protection During Descending Thoracic Aortic Repair

Gott shunt	Augmentation of mean arterial pressure
Partial left heart bypass	Decrease CSF pressure via CSF drainage
CPB with DHCA	Reattachment of intercostal arteries
Systemic hypothermia	Somatosensory evoked potentials
Steroid administration	Motor evoked potentials

CPB, cardiopulmonary bypass; DHCA, deep hypothermic circulatory arrest; CSF, cerebrospinal fluid.

for organ protection during the ischemic period.[107] Prolonged cross clamp can be detrimental to organ function, especially when >30 minutes.[107] Distal perfusion using left heart bypass can be achieved with drainage of oxygenated blood from the left atrium being returned to a femoral artery after going through a perfusion circuit.[106,107] Modifications based on the presence or absence of an oxygenator dictate anticoagulation requirements. This technique has the benefit of maintaining spinal cord, mesenteric, and renal perfusion, while simultaneously allowing for a degree of proximal hypertension to maintain additional spinal cord perfusion via the vertebral artery.[106,107] Left heart bypass can also keep the LV unloaded in situations of extreme proximal hypertension. Alternatively, the surgeon can choose full CPB with hypothermic circulatory arrest to complete the repair when the distal aortic arch requires intervention.[107,108]

An additional strategy to potentially provide spinal cord protection from ischemia includes the use of mild to moderate systemic hypothermia (Class IIa Recommendation; Level B Evidence).[65,106,107] Hypothermia not only decreases metabolic demands, but it also attenuates the inflammatory response during reperfusion. As mentioned above, administration of steroids for neuroprotection is frequently practiced to potentially reduce spinal cord edema, but clear evidence for benefit remains uncertain (Class IIb Recommendation; Level B Evidence).[65,106,107] The augmentation of spinal cord perfusion is also an important perioperative technique for neuroprotection (Class IIa Evidence; Level B Evidence).[65,106,107] Spinal cord perfusion pressure is equal to the difference between the mean arterial pressure and the cerebrospinal fluid (CSF) pressure. Systemic vasoconstrictors such as phenylephrine, norepinephrine, and/or vasopressin to increase the mean arterial pressure can effectively treat spinal cord ischemia, and gradual continued augmentation should be continued if ischemia persists.[106,107] It is important to keep in mind that cardiac output augmentation with inotropes may also be necessary to improve oxygen delivery. The second option for spinal cord perfusion pressure augmentation is CSF drainage via a lumbar CSF drain. CSF drainage is recommended in all patients at high risk for spinal cord ischemia (Class IIa Recommendation; Level B Evidence).[66,108] Both randomized trials and

meta-analyses have demonstrated that CSF drainage results in decreased postoperative paraplegia after open thoracic aortic surgery.[107] Drainage of CSF should aim for a lumbar CSF pressure of 10 mm Hg, without causing rapid drainage that can result in intracranial hypotension.[107] Although preoperative placement of these catheters is common, postoperative placement may be indicated in patients with spinal cord ischemia. Like all neuraxial invasive techniques, the coagulation status of the patient should be normalized prior to instrumentation to avoid hematoma formation. Further reported complications from CSF drainage catheters include retained catheter fragments, spinal headaches, nerve palsy, and meningitis.[107] A surgical option for augmenting spinal cord perfusion is reimplantation of intercostal and segmental branches to the new aortic graft or occlusion of large vessels that backbleed to prevent arterial steal.[107]

As equally important as it is to treat spinal cord ischemia is the ability to detect ischemia.[106-108] Early detection can allow for intervention to take place before permanent, irreversible ischemic damage occurs. Postoperatively, serial neurologic examinations can be performed on the patient that has recovered from general anesthesia.[107] This is not an option, however, for the anesthetized patient in the operating room that is undergoing an open repair. Therefore, the use of neurophysiological monitoring of the spinal cord is advocated when feasible (Class IIb Recommendation; Level B Evidence).[65]

The use of somatosensory evoked potentials (SSEPs) and motor evoked potentials (MEPs) allow the surgeon and anesthesiologist to respond quickly to changes seen from baseline recordings. SSEPs are performed by placing stimulating electrodes on peripheral nerves in both upper and lower extremities. Stimulation is then conducted via the posterior and lateral columns of the spinal cord to the cerebral cortex. SSEPs can influence blood pressure and CSF management, but they can also guide the need for further reimplantation of segmental vessels.[107] The advantage of SSEPs is that the signal is less affected by anesthetics and paralytic agents. However, anterior spinal cord ischemia can still occur without a change in SSEPs. While more complex, the use of MEPs is occasionally advocated because they rely on stimulation of the motor cortex with signals conducted through the anterior column of the spinal cord. Although more sensitive than SSEPs, MEP signal is also more influenced by anesthetic and paralytic agents.[107-109] The choice of SSEPs or MEPs is often also dependent on institutional culture and resources. Interpretation should be performed and guided by trained team that often includes a neurologist. It is essential to keep in mind that changes in SSEP or MEP signals from baseline are not necessarily caused by spinal cord ischemia (Fig. 11-13).[107-110] Hypothermia can cause global signal attenuation.[110] Similarly, interruption of lower extremity blood flow from infrarenal vascular clamping can also cause signal attenuation. The site of signal attenuation along the neural pathway can determine whether central or peripheral malperfusion has occurred. Close communication between the neuromonitoring team and the rest of the intraoperative team is essential to

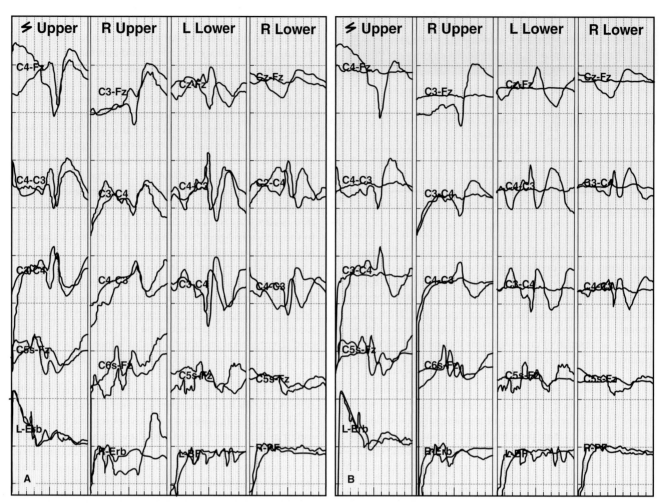

FIGURE 11-13 Somatosensory evoked potentials (SSEPs) are obtained from all four extremities in a patient undergoing open descending aorta repair. Overlapping signal in Panel A suggests similarity to baseline readings, while global loss of signal in Panel B (obtained at 24°C) is likely due to hypothermia and not spinal cord ischemia.

ensure appropriate and timely detection of and intervention for significant events.[107-110]

ENDOVASCULAR REPAIR

Endovascular intervention for descending thoracic aortic disease has significantly increased.[64-66] In addition to being far less invasive and allowing for quicker recovery, TEVAR may also reduce perioperative complications.[64-66,107,111] Similar to open repair, the principles of preventing, detecting, and treating spinal cord and organ ischemia remain important, although the risk of spinal cord ischemia in TEVAR is significantly lower.[107] Risk factors for spinal cord ischemia in this setting include a long segment of aortic coverage (eg, left subclavian to celiac arteries) and patients with prior aortic repair.[107] Although the adjuncts of neuromonitoring and CSF drainage are not routine in TEVAR, they are strongly considered in elective patients with risk factors.[107] Significant attenuation of evoked potentials in this setting merit interventions such as permissive hypertension and CSF drainage, as outlined earlier.

During TEVAR, the patient remains supine with both arms tucked at the sides. For general anesthesia, a single-lumen endotracheal tube suffices since lung isolation is not required. A radial arterial line and typically large-bore central venous access are also obtained. Tracheal extubation is a reasonable goal for uncomplicated interventions. This allows for a quick neurologic examination to rule out any potential ischemia that may have occurred. Alternatively, either regional or local anesthesia may be options, depending on institutional practice and case specifics.[112] A continuous epidural infusion can allow for patient comfort, as well as continuous detection of neurologic function. However, it is imperative to differentiate the effects of neuraxial blockade by local anesthetics from true spinal cord malperfusion. Although not routinely performed, TEE is reasonable in endovascular aortic repair for monitoring, procedural guidance, and/or graft leak detection (Class IIa Evidence; Level B Evidence).[65] Comprehensive TEE can assist with quantifying vessel caliber, locating guidewires, as well as postdeployment assessment of cardiac function and interrogation of the aorta.

Involvement of the distal arch may require a very proximal landing zone for the TEVAR stent. In some instances, coverage of the left subclavian artery may be warranted and unavoidable in emergent situations. While an argument can be made to monitor left radial arterial pressure for this scenario, a right radial arterial line is more practical if preoperative revascularization has not been performed. In more elective cases of TEVAR, a prior staged procedure can include either transposition of the left subclavian to the left common carotid artery or a left carotid-subclavian bypass.[113-115] This revascularization option is now being endorsed when feasible due to recent meta-analysis that suggests an increased risk of arm ischemia, stroke, and spinal cord injury.[113-115]

HEART FAILURE SURGERY

Despite maximal goal-directed medical therapy, a subset of patients with chronic CHF will develop advanced stages of disease.[116] For these patients who progressively deteriorate despite optimal goal-directed medical therapy, interventions including implantable defibrillator device or cardiac resynchronization therapy and surgical therapy including revascularization, valve, ventricular restoration and remodeling surgery, or mechanical circulatory support (VADs, heart transplantation) may be warranted.[116].

Anesthetic Management of the Patient with Heart Failure

Anesthetizing patients with advanced CHF can be challenging as they commonly have the following findings consistent with poor functional reserve: severe symptoms at rest or with minimal exertion; episodes of fluid retention and/or peripheral hypoperfusion; objective evidence of severe cardiac dysfunction (ie, LVEF < 30%, restrictive mitral inflow pattern by Doppler echocardiography, elevated LV and/or RV filling pressures, elevated B-type natriuretic peptides); evidence of systemic organ injury (ie, renal and hepatic dysfunction); severe impairment of functional capacity; and history of multiple hospitalizations for CHF in the prior six months.[117] Hyponatremia with serum sodium < 133 mEq/L is also relatively common and is associated with worse outcomes.[118]

Preoperative evaluation includes an assessment of the level of the patient's dependency on cardiovascular support with medications and devices. Heart failure patients are medically managed with a variety of medications that have significant perioperative implications.[119] Hypotension with induction and maintenance of anesthesia is common among patients taking angiotensin-converting enzyme inhibitors (ACE-I), angiotensin-receptor blockers, milrinone, and nesiritide because all of these drugs can cause significant vasodilation.[120,121] Perioperative hypotension associated with angiotensin-receptor blockers may require the administration of vasopressin because it may be refractory to phenylephrine or ephedrine.[122]

Heart failure patients are often fully anticoagulated at the time of urgent or emergent surgery because they are taking prophylactic agents to attenuate the development of venous thromboembolic disease due to reduced cardiac output, increased systemic venous pressure, and chemical changes promoting blood clotting. As such, they may require aggressive perioperative warfarin reversal. However, instead of volume-loading patients with fresh-frozen plasma, other therapies including vitamin K and/or four-factor prothrombin complex concentrates (ie, plasma-derived concentrates of vitamin K-dependent clotting factors II, VII, IX, X, protein C and S) may be required perioperatively.[123] Of note, most prothrombin complex concentrates contain varying amounts of heparin and are therefore contraindicated in patients with heparin-induced thrombocytopenia (HIT).[124] Furthermore, many patients have had prior cardiac surgery and will need blood products (irradiated and cytomegalovirus-negative) immediately available in the operating room at the time of induction of anesthesia.

Assessment of antiarrhythmic devices and implantable cardioverter-defibrillator includes interrogation and reprogramming to a mode that is not affected by electrocautery. External defibrillator pads need to be placed and the defibrillator function temporarily deactivated.[125] Appropriate arterial and venous lines are placed before induction of anesthesia. Depending on the patient characteristics and the presence of a nonpulsatile VAD, arterial line placement may be difficult and may require ultrasound guided placement. If a patient does not already have a PAC, one can be placed before or after induction of anesthesia. Of note, placing a PAC in a patient with a VAD can be challenging and may have to be placed under fluoroscopic guidance in the catheter laboratory or in the operating room. Floating a PAC across the tricuspid valve is sometimes difficult and for the patient undergoing heart transplantation, the catheter tip needs to be withdrawn into the superior vena cava. In this position, the infusion ports are outside of the vein in the sheath, making them unavailable for use until the catheter is reintroduced into the correct position after the donor heart is transplanted.

Induction and maintenance of anesthesia in CHF patients with marginal reserve requires diligent titration of medications in order to maintain acceptable organ perfusion, while avoiding arrhythmias and hypotension. A balanced anesthetic is usually provided by administering a combination of narcotics, muscle relaxants, and intravenous and/or inhalational anesthetic agents with judicious use of vasopressors and inotropes. Anticoagulation for CPB is usually achieved with heparin, but because heart failure patients are often exposed to heparin, they may have antibodies, and direct thrombin inhibitors may need to be administered instead.[126,127]

Weaning from CPB can be challenging and intraoperative TEE can be useful in guiding patient care. As heart failure patients often have preexisting pulmonary hypertension or RV dysfunction, they are more likely to develop post-bypass right heart failure. Vigilance in prevention and early detection of post-bypass RV failure is important[128] (Table 11-7).

> ### TABLE 11-7: Management of Right Ventricular Failure After Cardiac Surgery
>
> **Optimization of RV rate and rhythm**
> a. Maintain sinus rhythm to maintain optimal filling of a hypertrophied, dilated right ventricle: consider pacing, early cardioversion
> b. Because of associated TR, higher heart rates may be desirable (80-100 beats/min) to reduce end-diastolic volume but if there is significant RV ischemia, excessive tachycardia may not be tolerated
>
> **Optimize RV filling**
> a. When CVP is low, the RV may be "coping" and an elevated CVP may imply a failing RV with or without TR
> b. Although past teachings encouraged volume loading the RV to increase pulmonary blood flow and cardiac output, injudicious volume loading can result in acute RV distention resulting in RV failure
>
> **Maintain RV coronary perfusion pressure**
> a. Inotropic support
>
> **Reduce pulmonary vascular resistance**
> a. Optimize ventilation strategies
> b. Avoid acidosis and hyperinflation of the lungs
> c. Inhaled pulmonary vasodilators (nitric oxide, prostacyclin, iloprost, and milrinone)
>
> **Surgical Management**
> a. RVAD
> b. ECMO

ECMO, extra-corporeal membranous oxygenators; RV, right ventricle; TR, tricuspid regurgitation; CVP, central venous pressure; RVAD, right ventricular assist device.

Anesthetic Management for the Heart Transplantation

Heart transplantation is the gold standard for treatment of end-stage heart failure. The 1-year and 5-year survival after heart transplantation is 81% and 69% respectively, with a median survival of 11 years for all recipients, and 14 years for those surviving the first year after transplantation (www.ishlt.org/registries).[129] Cardiomyopathy (55%) and chronic ischemic heart disease (36%) are the leading underlying cause of heart failure among heart transplant recipients for whom the median adult recipient age is 54 years while the proportion of patients transplanted at extremes of ages continues to increase.[129] Not surprisingly, close to half of the recipients have undergone previous cardiac surgery, 35% have a VAD, most commonly for the LV, and 7% have an IABP. Although 1.1% of transplant recipients were on preoperative extracorporeal membrane oxygenation (ECMO), this number has increased from 0.3% in the mid-1990s.[127]

Heart transplantation occurs urgently or emergently and requires close coordination with the harvesting team to minimize ischemic time. As close to half of the patients have had prior sternotomy, blood availability and cannulation strategies need to be confirmed. In addition to the usual antibiotic prophylaxis, immunosuppressive medications need to be administered. Inotropic medications, IABP, or other

mechanical assistance are maintained until institution of CPB.[130] TEE is useful in assessing the native heart. Pretransplant TEE evaluation includes an assessment of the presence of intracardiac thrombus and degree of atheromatous plaque at cannulation sites.

Heart failure patients are at increased risk for developing HIT. Thus it is important to ascertain that heparin use is acceptable. Otherwise, alternative anticoagulation with direct thrombin inhibitors or preoperative plasmapheresis to reduce HIT antibodies may be necessary.[126,127] Patients who are sensitized with preformed anti-human leukocyte antigen antibodies against donor antigens are at increased risk for acute or hyperacute rejection as well as transplant vasculopathy.[131] Antibodies are common among patients presenting for a second transplant.[131] Various densensitization modalities may need to be employed (plasmapheresis, immunoglobulin, rituximab, and bortezomib), and some of the therapies may require pretreatment with acetaminophen, diphenhydramine, and corticosteroids to prevent cytokine release syndrome.[132]

Weaning from CPB can be challenging as post-bypass contractility can often be marginal or poor. Certain donor heart characteristics may predispose the recipient to poor prognosis after heart transplantation (Table 11-8). After weaning from CPB, right heart failure can develop and in extreme cases, primary graft failure can occur.[133] Careful TEE evaluation and titration of inotropes and ventilator strategies aimed at reducing pulmonary vascular resistance and use of inhaled epoprostenol or other selective inhaled pulmonary vasodilators can facilitate weaning from CPB. Occasionally, patients may develop RV failure requiring temporary support with a VAD or ECMO.[134,135]

Anesthetic Considerations for Ventricular Assist Device Implantation

Mechanical circulatory support, including the use of VADs and the total artificial heart, is another therapeutic option for the advanced stage heart failure patient.[116] Similar to heart transplant recipients, patients eligible for VAD placement have marginal reserve and require careful titration of anesthetic drugs to induce and maintain anesthesia. Many of these patients require significant preoperative inotropic support, which often must be maintained throughout the operative course. Up to 40% of patients undergoing VAD implantation have profound vasoplegia and may require vasopressin and methylene blue administration.[136,137] The goal of perioperative fluid management is to maintain intravascular volume to facilitate left VAD (LVAD) function without creating RV dysfunction.[138] Blood transfusions are avoided if possible to prevent sensitization for future heart transplantation. Because infection is a major cause of death, VAD patients often receive multiple prophylactic antibiotics.

The key to successful LVAD implantation lies in preventing RV failure, which occurs in 25 to 50% of recipients.[139] Ventricular interdependence plays an important role in the development of post-LVAD failure of the RV. Because of the anatomic proximity of the RV to the LV, changes in LV

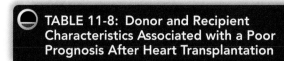

TABLE 11-8: Donor and Recipient Characteristics Associated with a Poor Prognosis After Heart Transplantation

Donor heart characteristics

Donor age
    Increased age is associated with higher risk at 1-year and long-term mortality (12)

Presence of LVH
    LVH > 14 mm associated with lower survival in recipients (33)

Gender mismatches (34)

Donor cause of death (35)
    Intracranial bleed associated with transplant vasculopathy

Donor history of coronary artery disease
    Can cause early and late graft failure (37)

Recipient characteristics

Obesity (BMI > 30 kg/m² or percent ideal body weight > 140%)

Associated with > 5-year mortality rates and shorter time to high-grade acute rejection (7)

Ischemic time* > 210 min

Associated with increase in acute graft failure in 1-year and 5-year mortality rates (17)

Presence of donor-specific antibodies (DSA)
    Increases risk for acute or hyperacute rejection and transplant vasculopathy (38)

Elevated pulmonary vascular resistance

Pretransplant RVAD only, ECMO, extracorporeal LVAD**, TAH (32)
    Associated with poor graft survival

---

*Ischemic time:donor aortic cross-clamp to removal of recipient aortic cross-clamp.

**Pretransplant implantable LVAD dependence was not shown to be associated with decreased graft survival.

References are shown in parenthesis. LVH, left ventricular hypertrophy; BMI, body mass index; RVAD, right ventricular assist device; ECMO, extracorporeal membrane oxygenation; LVAD, left ventricular assist device; TAH, total artificial heart.

---

volume can result in immediate changes to RV pressure and volume and vice versa. Monitoring the position of the septum in the immediate post-CPB period is crucial since >50% of RV function is dependent on proper septal function.[128]

Studies have shown that a functioning LVAD can decrease RV afterload, increase RV compliance, and decrease RV contractility.[140] When the LV is completely decompressed, global RV contractility can be impaired secondary to the leftward shift of the interventricular septum. Nonetheless, RV myocardial efficiency and power output are maintained through a decrease in RV afterload and increase in RV preload.[140] However, with preexisting right heart dysfunction, anatomic ventricular interaction is accentuated causing a greater decrease in RV contractility which can ultimately lead to RV failure.[128]

In order to maintain midline position of the interventricular and interatrial septum, LVAD flows, volume status, RV function, degree of tricuspid regurgitation (TR) as well as other hemodynamic variables (CVP, pulmonary artery pressures, left atrial pressures, and mean blood pressure) may need to be carefully adjusted. LVAD flows may also need to be decreased to prevent increased venous return from overwhelming the functional capacity of the RV. Other treatment principals in preventing or mitigating RV failure need to be considered as well, including (1) maintaining sinus rhythm in order to optimize filling of a hypertrophied or dilated RV; (2) avoiding acute RV distension by overzealous volume loading; (3) maintaining RV CPP and RV inotropic therapy; (4) maintaining RV geometry; and (5) reducing pulmonary vascular resistance[128] (Table 11-7). In severe RV failure, RVAD placement may be necessary.

Although several preoperative risk factors for post-LVAD failure of the RV have been identified, the occurrence of RV failure is largely unpredictable.[138] Therefore, in addition to utilizing ventilator strategies to decrease pulmonary vascular resistance by avoiding PEEP, hypoxia, hypercarbia, and acidosis, nonselectively inhaled pulmonary vasodilators (nitric oxide, epoprostenol) at the time of weaning from bypass may be utilized.

Pre-LVAD implant intraoperative TEE evaluation includes assessment for thrombus in the apex where the inflow cannula will be inserted; evaluation for atherosclerosis of the ascending aorta where the outflow graft will be placed; evaluation for atrial septal defects or patent foramen ovale as significant right-to-left shunting post-LVAD implantation can lead to severe hypoxemia; determining the degree of AR as valve replacement or surgical closure may be required in the presence of moderate or severe AR; and a thorough evaluation of RV function.

TEE is also valuable in assisting the surgeon with the position of inflow and outflow cannulae. The LVAD inflow cannula is usually placed in the apex for destination therapy and bridge-to-transplant, and in the left atrium for those who with a previous ventriculoplasty procedure or in those with an anticipated quick recovery. Ideally, the LV inflow cannula should be angled toward the MV in alignment with the LV inflow tract, while not abutting any wall.[141] The outflow graft in the proximal ascending aorta can sometimes be difficult to visualize by TEE. The tip of an RVAD inflow cannula is ideally oriented in the middle of the right atrium away from the atrial septum and tricuspid valve. The outflow cannula is usually placed in the pulmonary artery, 1.5 to 2 cm beyond the annulus.

The development of smaller VADs has enabled the increasing use of minimally invasive implant strategies, including off-pump procedures. Transthoracic echocardiography (TTE) and TEE are helpful in assisting placement of the inflow cannula via a small thoracotomy or subcostal incision.[142]

Total Artificial Heart

Total artificial heart (TAH) implantation is relatively rare and involves only 2.3% of all device implants.[143] Several management issues specific to the TAH (SynCardia, Inc., Tucson, AZ; formerly known as CardioWest) have significant clinical implications.[144] Anesthetic management of other total artificial heart devices that are not yet FDA-approved is not discussed in this section.

During TAH implantation, the native cardiac ventricles and arterioventricular valves are removed and in its place, an orthotopic pneumatic pulsatile device consisting of two separate artificial ventricles is implanted. Each ventricle has two single-tilting mechanical valves mounted on the housing of the artificial ventricle. Several advantages of a TAH include the ability to pump at high flow rates (>9 L/min at maximal stroke volume of 70 mL) with filling pressures of 8 to 15 mm Hg. Common indications that favor TAH versus biventricular assist device include severe myopathies that result in biventricular hypertrophy with small intraventricular chamber size, failed Fontan, failed cardiac transplantation, myocardial infarction with related ischemic cardiomyopathy resulting in intractable biventricular failure with postinfarct ventricular septal defects (VSD), large LV apical aneurysm or LV thrombus, and severe AV pathology including AR or mechanical valve prosthesis.[144]

When placing a perioperative central venous line, the tip of the central venous catheter must not extend into the right atrium, as central venous catheter entrapment in the right TAH mechanical inflow valve can result in fatal TAH malfunction.[145] Thus, placement of a PAC should not be attempted in these patients after TAH implantation. Although weaning from CPB is generally not an issue, some patients may require vasopressors to treat vasoplegia. Inotropes are not needed in these patients. Assessing adequate de-airing can be challenging because the TAH air diaphragms that drive blood out of the ventricles appear similar to intracardiac air. Thus, de-airing relies on repeated evaluation for air in the atria, pulmonary veins, ascending aorta, and main pulmonary artery.[146]

Cardiac tamponade in the classical sense of RV diastolic compression after TAH implantation cannot occur because of the rigid construction of the artificial ventricles. However, "tamponade" due to compression or kinking of the vena cavae (IVC compression more common than SVC) and/or pulmonary veins (left pulmonary vein compression more common than the right) can occur. Therefore, while the native heart is in place, baseline TEE of the vena cava and pulmonary veins may be useful for enabling identification and evaluation of kinking after TAH implantation.[146]

Peak Doppler flow velocities ≥ 1.1 m/s in patients following radiofrequency ablation for atrial fibrillation have been associated with pulmonary vein stenosis.[147] Although peak velocities > 2 m/s have been associated with no apparent hemodynamic consequences after TAH implantation, more studies are necessary to determine acceptable peak values.[146] In the meantime, establishing baseline post-TAH implant pulmonary vein flow velocities may provide a helpful comparison in the future when other signs of hypoperfusion point to possible kinking of the pulmonary veins.

ELECTROPHYSIOLOGY AND CARDIAC CATHETERIZATION LABS

As technology advances and the population ages, medical interventions and surgical treatments converge, while target patient populations combine as complexity and acuity rise.

Our ability to treat conditions once outside the penumbra of "traditional" surgical and medical care continues to grow. As diagnosis and interventions become more specialized and sophisticated, the broadened scope of our medical horizon necessitates the integration of related disciplines, particularly in the case of interconnected specialties. Nowhere is this more pressing than in cardiovascular medicine. For cardiac surgeons, cardiac anesthesiologists, electrophysiologists, and interventional cardiologists, it is increasingly necessary that we understand the essential framework of each other's medical thought process and practice in order to optimize the care we provide and the therapeutic interventions we offer.[155]

Electrophysiology Lab

In a relatively short period of time, electrophysiology (EP) procedures have developed from largely diagnostic studies to complex, lifesaving interventions. Patients are more complex than ever, and demand for devices and procedures is high. Successful treatments and long-term survival of previously tenuous cardiovascular medicine patients has broadened the target population. Similarly, cardiac surgery patients often benefit from therapeutic interventions in the EP lab.

DEVICES FOR THE MANAGEMENT OF DYSRHYTHMIAS

Pacemakers.   Bradycardia at the level of the sinus node or AV node, either spontaneous or as a result of cardiac medications or surgeries, can be treated with pacemakers.[156] These devices deliver electrical impulses that depolarize myocardial cells near the lead tip and propagate into the contiguous myocardium. Pacemakers can be programmed in many ways. Pulse delivery sequences depend on how the pacemaker is programmed. Single-chamber transvenous pacemakers have a lead in the atrium or in the ventricle. Dual-chamber transvenous pacemakers typically have leads in both the right atrium and ventricle. Pacemakers capable of biventricular pacing have ventricular leads that can pace both the RV and LV. These devices are usually placed within the EP laboratory and require minimal to moderate sedation for the patient. Occasionally in the case of very frail patients, only local anesthesia is used. If the patient has psychiatric, neurological, neuromuscular, or other disorders, which preclude the use of nurse-administered sedative agents, anesthesiologists can provide deeper sedation or general anesthesia with other intravenous agents or volatile anesthetics. Surgically placed epicardial pacemakers may have electrodes that pace the heart overlying the right atrium, RV or LV. Patients often come to the EP lab with surgically implanted epicardial wires for hookup to a pacemaker, which is subsequently placed by an electrophysiologist. When necessary, hybrid surgical and transvenous systems can be created for patients with prohibitive anatomy, including those with tricuspid valve replacement, congenital heart disease or occluded vessels. Standard programmed modes for pacemaker operation are included in Table 11-9.[157]

⬤ TABLE 11-9: Pacemaker Modes[7]

North American Society of Pacing and Electrophysiology (NASPE) and British Pacing and Electrophysiology Group (BPEG) code describing pacemaker function

Position	I	II	III	IV	V
Category	Chambers paced	Chambers sensed	Response to sensing	Programmability, rate modulation	Multisite pacing*
Letters used	O—None	O—None	O—None	O—None	O—None
	A—Atrium	A—Atrium	T—Triggered	R—Rate modulation	A—Atrium
	V—Ventricle	V—Ventricle	I—Inhibit		V—Ventricle
	D—Dual (atrium and ventricle)	D—Dual (atrium and ventricle	D—Dual (triggered and inhibited)		D—Dual (atrium and ventricle)

*Not commonly used in reference to pacemaker modes.

Single-chamber pacemakers are typically programmed to pace in the cardiac chamber where the electrode is attached, only when bradycardia occurs in that chamber. For example, a single-chamber ventricular pacemaker programmed in the VVI mode with a lower rate limit of 60 bpm in a patient with atrial fibrillation and slow ventricular response will only pace when the patient's heart rate goes below 60 bpm. In contrast, a dual-chamber pacemaker programmed in the DDD mode with a lower rate limit of 60 bpm will pace the atrium if the atrial rate falls below 60 bpm but will also pace the ventricle if the programmed AV interval has elapsed. Therefore, a normally functioning dual-chamber pacemaker may at times pace the atrium, the ventricle, or both cardiac chambers.

In response to development of a rapid atrial rhythm such as atrial fibrillation, a device may "mode switch" which means that the device would switch from a tracking mode such as DDD to a nontracking mode such as VVI or DDI in response to rapidly detected atrial rates. The "mode switch" option prevents the device from inappropriate rapid pacing the ventricle when a rapid rhythm occurs in the atrium. Cardiac surgeons and cardiac anesthesiologists need to be aware of pacemaker settings both in the operating room and after surgery. A patient in the operating room with a pacemaker may develop a rapid ventricular rate in response to a rapid atrial rate on induction of anesthesia or insertion of an invasive line if "mode-switch" is not enabled. Atrial fibrillation can commonly occur after cardiac surgery as well. This can be particularly problematic for those with pacemakers without "mode-switch" who do not tolerate rapid rates, such as patients with hypertrophic obstructive cardiomyopathy.

ICDs. Implantable cardioverter defibrillators (ICDs) have the capability of treating rapid ventricular arrhythmias to prevent sudden death. They have pacing functions that are much the same as electronic pacemakers. In the past, patients required separate pacemaker and defibrillator units implanted in order to achieve dual-chamber pacemaker function with concomitant defibrillator capability. However, modern devices are capable of the majority of pacemaker and defibrillator functions simultaneously. ICD leads differ from pacing leads in that there is a coil present on defibrillator leads that

participates in the shocking circuit. ICDs detect ventricular arrhythmias via a small bipolar electrode at the tip of the lead. Detection rates for ventricular arrhythmia are set by the operator via a radiofrequency communication link. ICDs have two ways of responding to ventricular arrhythmia. They can be programmed to deliver antitachycardia pacing or ATP, which will deliver a burst of pacing to the ventricle slightly faster than the cycle length of the ventricular tachycardia. ATP offers the possibility of terminating the arrhythmia without delivering a potentially painful shock to the patient. If ATP is unsuccessful or if the arrhythmia is rapid enough to exceed programmed parameters, the device can also deliver a shock to terminate the tachycardia. ICDs can be implanted in the EP lab with the same anesthetic regimens as pacemakers. If patients requiring ICDs are clinically fragile they may benefit from anesthesiology oversight.

Both pacemakers and ICDs can provide Cardiac Resynchronization Therapy. In patients with low ejection fraction > 35% and ventricular dysynchrony, pacing of both ventricles simultaneously can improve heart failure symptoms. Patients who come to the EP lab for an upgrade or implantation of a device for this purpose frequently manifest the clinical signs of chronic low perfusion. Sedation regimens must be tailored to these individuals and/or anesthesiology backup may be needed.

Electrocautery can produce electromagnetic interference that can alter the appropriate function of both pacemakers and ICDs. This can be a significant problem in the operating room. Electrocautery "noise" can initiate pacemaker failure. In the case of ICDs, electrocautery "noise" can cause inappropriate detection of ventricular arrhythmia and inappropriate delivery of shocks. Both pacemakers and ICDs have their function altered in response to magnet application. This is achieved by a reed switch which moves in response to magnet application and then returns to its original position after the magnet is removed. Pacemakers respond to magnet application by pacing in an asynchronous mode (AOO, VOO, or DOO) at a rate which is related to the remaining battery life. For ICDs, the effect of magnet application is to turn off detection for ventricular arrhythmias. No effect on pacing occurs. If a patient with an ICD is pacemaker dependent, their device may require reprogramming in addition to magnet application for safe performance of a surgical procedure involving electrocautery.

ELECTROPHYSIOLOGY STUDIES AND ABLATION PROCEDURES

Common indications for electrophysiology study include risk stratification for sudden death, determination of cause of syncope, diagnosis and treatment of supraventricular tachycardias, as well as diagnosis and treatment of idiopathic ventricular tachycardias. Standard electrophysiology studies are typically performed under light conscious sedation, though in the pediatric population these are sometimes performed under general anesthesia. EP studies typically require femoral vein access, occasionally bilateral. Arterial access or transseptal puncture is performed to reach left-sided structures. In an electrophysiology study, solid multi-electrode catheters are used to measure electrical impulses during sinus rhythm and arrhythmia from stereotyped locations, including the right atrium, the RV, and the His bundle. For supraventricular tachycardia ablation, a catheter is often also positioned in the coronary sinus. Radiofrequency energy is the most commonly used ablation modality, though cryoablation is also used.

Catheter Ablation of Atrial Fibrillation.

Atrial fibrillation is the most common sustained cardiac arrhythmia. It is the most common contributor to cerebrovascular accident in the United States. Risk factors for developing atrial fibrillation include older age, hypertension, valvular heart disease, cardiomyopathy, obesity, sleep apnea, and CAD. There are also metabolic causes including hyperthyroidism and acute alcohol intoxication. Other diseases or conditions that cause cardiac irritation such as pericardial status or pneumonia can play a role. In 1998 Dr. Haïssaguerre and colleagues showed that atrial fibrillation in patients with paroxysmal atrial fibrillation and frequent atrial ectopy had rapid firing from myocardial sleeves around pulmonary veins that could initiate atrial fibrillation.[158] It is now understood that many patients with atrial fibrillation have at least a contribution from these myocardial sleeves in the pulmonary veins which remain a primary target for typical atrial fibrillation ablation. For patients with more persistent atrial fibrillation, other areas are also targeted, including some lines of ablation such as the roof, mitral isthmus, in an attempt to mimic the results of the Cox MAZE procedure.

Success rates for catheter ablation of atrial fibrillation are in the 80% range for patients with normal hearts, and paroxysmal atrial fibrillation. For patients with low ejection fractions or heart failure, success rates are closer to 50 to 70%. The procedure is improving with better anticoagulation and ablation techniques. Complications are in the 1 to 2% range and include a risk of stroke, myocardial infarction, tamponade, atrial esophageal fistula, pulmonary vein stenosis, pericarditis, and phrenic nerve injury. Many centers utilize esophageal temperature monitoring to avoid esophageal injury during ablation which can be life-threatening. Phrenic nerve injury can also occur during the procedure. Pacing is used to identify the phrenic nerve and avoid injury. Ablation for atrial fibrillation is usually performed under general anesthesia. Multiple anesthetic protocols can be used, but paralysis must be avoided in order to avoid obscuring phrenic nerve injury. Anesthetic regimens should involve short acting agents since pain after the procedure is minimal and can usually be managed with nonsteroidals. Because these procedures can be long, patients often experience discomfort from lying on a hard table for long periods of time. Common comorbidities among patients with atrial fibrillation include obesity and sleep apnea, although many are otherwise healthy. Intubation and extubation require care and expertise. Care must be taken to avoid coughing at the end of the procedure to minimize potential disruption of femoral access sites and retroperitoneal bleeding.[159]

Ventricular Tachycardia Ablation in Structural Heart Disease.

Ventricular tachycardia (VT) in structural heart disease is a highly morbid condition that is associated with inappropriate device discharges, and life-threatening VT storm.[160] Successful catheter ablation can eliminate the need for toxic antiarrhythmic drugs, and can be life-saving particularly in VT storm. Ventricular tachycardia in the setting of structural heart disease is usually the result of reentry circuits which form around regions of scar tissue. Electro-anatomic barriers to conduction due to dense fibrosis form in zones of slow conduction. Patients with scar-related VT can have ischemic heart disease due to myocardial infarction which may be remote. Cardiomyopathies due to sarcoidosis, Chagas disease, idiopathic cardiomyopathy, or viral cardiomyopathy occur as well. All of these conditions have other systemic effects as well. Scar-related VT due to prior cardiac surgery is also seen often after repair of congenital heart disease such as Tetralogy of Fallot.

Catheter ablation of scar-related VT requires thorough preoperative preparation and planning. Interdisciplinary discussion is critical because the patients can be quite tenuous. Anesthesiologists, electrophysiologists, and cardiac surgeons should be aware of the potential for possible untoward events. Echocardiography is used to screen for mobile LV thrombus. Heart failure regimens are optimized. Screening for residual ischemic heart disease is often performed. These patients are also often complex and have many comorbidities. Planning is necessary for intraprocedural and postprocedural management of other concomitant disease, including vascular, pulmonary, and renal disease. This type of ablation is typically done under general anesthesia. Often vasoactive agents are needed, and induction of anesthesia requires planning for potential arrhythmia management during airway manipulation. Invasive lines may be required prior to induction of the arrhythmia so that hemodynamic and fluid management can be optimized. If the patient's ventricular function is severely compromised, adjuvant inotropic, intra-aortic balloon pumping or percutaneous LVADs may be needed.[159] Anesthesiologist and electrophysiologists should both be involved in making planning decisions including when and how to decide on admission to ICU, postprocedure ventilation, and extubation parameters. A plan for the approach to the ventricles is made and should be discussed with all team members. The LV can be accessed via a retrograde aortic or transseptal approach. Epicardialsubxiphoid percutaneous puncture is often also employed. For patients in whom neither of these approaches is possible, surgical approaches to the epicardium as well as transcoronary alcohol approaches can be utilized.[158] The procedure itself usually consists of identification of the relevant scar substrate, induction of the clinical arrhythmia, confirmation of the location of the VT circuit by pacing, and ablation of the slow conduction areas.

Structural Heart Disease in the Cardiac Catheterization Laboratory

The breadth of structural heart conditions now amenable to treatment in the Cardiac Catheterization Laboratory has expanded enormously in the past decade. This is a direct result of both technological advancement and an age-related increase in the size of target patient populations. Not only is the prevalence of age-related disease on the increase, but the long-term survival of surgically treated patients and congenital heart disease patients makes the advent of nonsurgical interventions preferable in a group where surgical options may be limited.

CLOSURE OF PATENT FORAMEN OVALE

Patent foramen ovale (PFO) is a common condition estimated to be present in 25% of the population. However, the vast majority of patients with PFO have no related clinical issues. Clinical conditions that may arise as a result of the present of a PFO include paradoxical embolism resulting in neurological injury, myocardial infarction, renal or mesenteric infarction, or limb ischemia. A PFO may also result in abnormal right to left shunting in patients with alterations in chest anatomy associated with kyphoscoliosis or after surgery resulting in positional hypoxemia also known as platypnea-orthodeoxia syndrome. At the present time, there is no FDA approved indication for PFO closure as clinical trials in patients with neurological events have not definitively shown benefit.[161,162] However, PFO closure is still performed in specific patients who experience neurological events or in patients with platypnea-orthodeoxia syndrome.

PFO closure requires femoral venous access for device delivery. Ultrasound guidance is required and can be achieved by intracardiac ultrasound (ICE) or TEE. If ICE is used, a second femoral venous access site is required for the delivery of the catheter. If TEE is to be utilized, patients are usually placed under general anesthesia for airway protection and comfort during the procedure. Patients undergoing PFO closure usually do not experience hemodynamic compromise, and short-acting anesthetics are advisable since post-op intubation is not usually required. The decision to use ICE versus TEE depends on comfort level of the implanting physician with either modality. ICE does have the advantage of not requiring general anesthesia and allowing the implanting

physician to control image acquisition. TEE has the advantage of greater breadth of visualization of cardiac structures.

The procedure usually does not require hemodynamic assessment as these defects are not hemodynamically significant and usually do not result in left to right shunting. The defect is crossed using any of a variety of catheters and a stiff wire is delivered to the left upper pulmonary vein. The delivery sheath is then advanced to the left atrium and the device is delivered attached to a delivery catheter. The left atrial side of the device is opened, the device pulled back to the intra-atrial septum, and then the right atrial side of the device is deployed. Once the position is confirmed by fluoroscopy and echocardiography, the device is released from the delivery cable. At the present time, there are no FDA approved devices for PFO closure. Devices that can be used for this purpose include the St. Jude Cribriform Septal Occluded (St. Jude Medical, Minneapolis, MN) or the Gore Helix septal occluder (Gore, Newark, DE).

ATRIAL SEPTAL DEFECT

Atrial septal defect (ASD) is a much less common condition than PFO. The adult with ASD is referred for closure if they demonstrate symptoms of dyspnea or exercise intolerance, or they have evidence of right heart volume overload due to left to right shunt which is usually detected by enlargement of right heart structures on echocardiography. Percutaneous closure of ASD is the treatment of choice for ostium secundum defects. Ostium primum and sinus venosus defects require surgical closure as placement of a septal occluder device may impinge on vital adjacent structures.

Like PFO closure, ASD closure can be performed using ICE or TEE. Echocardiography is vital for device sizing. Once femoral access is obtained, right heart catheterization is performed to assess hemodynamics and shunt fraction across the defect. The defect is then crossed and occluded with a sizing balloon until color flow across the defect ceases. The waist of this balloon is then measured on echo for estimation of defect size and device size selection. Echocardiography is also vital for device placement and ensuring proper position of the device prior to releasing it from the delivery system and to ensure that nearby structures including the MV, tricuspid valve, inferior/superior vena cava have not been compromised by the placement of the device. General anesthesia is commonly utilized for these cases. Because patients develop right heart volume overload, close hemodynamic monitoring during the case is necessary. Arrhythmias are not uncommon in this population. Short-acting anesthetics are preferred, post-op intubation is usually not required. At the present time, there are two devices approved for ASD closure, the Amplatzer Atrial Septal Occluder (ASO) (St. Jude Medical, Minneapolis, MN) and the Gore Helix septal occluder (Gore, Newark, DE).

VENTRICULAR SEPTAL DEFECT

Ventricular septal defect can be congenital or acquired. Adult cardiac catheterization labs more typically see acquired VSD in the setting of ventricular septal rupture after myocardial infarction or as a result of trauma. Acquired VSD closure in the catheterization lab can be a very challenging procedure. Patients are critically ill, often decompensated and require intubation. In most cases, the percutaneous option is a salvage procedure. Patients with acute rupture are felt to be poor candidates for surgical repair. VSD closure requires accessing and crossing the defect which can be difficult. Precise visualization can be challenging as collateral structures are often disrupted and hard to identify. TEE guidance may be required for three-dimensional visualization. Venous access can be obtained from the right internal jugular approach or right femoral approach if the defect is to be crossed from the right heart. If the defect is to be crossed from the left heart, some operators choose to take the transseptal approach to left heart access and defect crossing. Once the defect is crossed, a wire is advanced to the other side of the circulation, and the wire is snared from an alternative access site, usually the femoral artery. The wire is retracted out of the sheath and secured, allowing the wire to serve as a rail for device delivery, which can be challenging given the tortuosity involved. There is no ideal device for acquired VSD closure and the device chosen is generally based on the location and perceived shape of the device. Closure of congenital defects is generally an elective procedure with similar techniques used for defect crossing and device delivery. A variety of VSD occluders are available for this purpose.

Anesthetic management during traumatic VSD repair can be complex and extremely demanding. It involves hemodynamic compensation during manipulation required to place and deploy the closure device. Oxygenation may be an issue and patients can present in shock. For closure, more than one device may be required because the integrity of the diseased tissue is poor. Procedures can be long. Vasoactive agents are commonly needed, and post-op intubation is usually required. Although the incision of an open heart procedure is not needed, the circulatory status of the patient is usually severely compromised and the cardiac tissue is in suboptimal condition.

PARA-VALVULAR LEAK

Patients with significant para-valvular leak (PVL) of mitral or aortic valve prostheses who are not candidates for repeat cardiac surgery are referred to the catheterization laboratory for attempt at closure of the defect. These can be the most challenging procedures due to complexities involved in crossing the defect, delivering a closure device, and obtaining a reasonable seal of the defect with the device.

PVL closure is elective. However, patients can be compromised by their pathology. Given the potential length of the procedure as well as the importance of TEE guidance, patients usually receive general endotracheal anesthesia. Three-dimensional TEE has become an important adjunct to this procedure as it allows the operator to see where the defect is along the sewing ring of the valve, and to accurately direct guidewires across the defect. Mitral prosthesis defects are approached by obtaining transseptal access to the left atrium, and crossing the defect into the LV. Aortic prosthesis defects are approached retrograde by gaining access in the femoral artery and crossing from aorta to LV. Once the defect is crossed, the guidewire is snared and externalized via an arterial sheath. The wire is secured and serves as a rail over which a delivery catheter can be delivered. The defect is sized with a balloon and an appropriately sized occluder device is placed across the defect. A variety of closure devices can be used to cross the defect and occlude it. There is no ideal closure device for this purpose as these defects are generally crescentic and irregularly shaped. Post-device closure assessment with TEE is vital to assess residual leak and need for further devices as well as to ensure that prosthetic valve function is not hampered by the presence of the closure device.

AORTIC VALVE DISEASE

As the population ages, a greater number of patients are presenting with severe, symptomatic AS. Once a patient with severe AS becomes symptomatic, there is a rapid decline in functional status and development of congestive heart failure. If not corrected, the condition will ultimately be lethal within several years. Surgical AVR is the standard of care for severe AS; however, transcatheter aortic valve replacement (TAVR) is now an option for some patients. Based on recent clinical trials, TAVR is now indicated for patients who are deemed inoperable or high risk for standard surgical AVR. High risk is defined as having a Society of Thoracic Surgeons risk score of >8%.[163-166] There are several possible routes of access for TAVR with the preferred route being transfemoral access. However, in patients with inadequate femoral access, alternative routes can be considered, including trans-apical, direct trans-aortic, and subclavian access. Depending on the institution and route of access, TAVR can be performed in the catheterization lab or a hybrid catheterization laboratory/operating room.

In patients who are in need for urgent or emergent aortic valve intervention but are not acutely candidates for surgery or TAVR, balloon aortic valvuloplasty (BAV) may be performed to relieve the obstruction across the aortic valve and improve hemodynamics allowing the patient to recover from their acute illness. The durability of the result is limited, however, and if deemed appropriate candidates, these patients will go to need definitive aortic valve therapy.

Most TAVR procedures are performed under general anesthesia with TEE guidance; however there is a growing experience with performing transfemoral procedures under heavy sedation and TTE assessment. Given the potential for acute instability, however, these procedures are virtually uniformly performed in collaboration with anesthesia independent of the method of sedation. Echocardiography is not critical for guidance of the device placement but is necessary post-device placement to assess for complications including PVL, valve dysfunction, and pericardial effusion. For transfemoral TAVR, careful femoral access is critical as the delivery sheaths used for the procedure range in size from 14Fr to 20Fr depending on the device and size of device used. Once the diseased valve is crossed with a guidewire, a balloon dilation of the valve may be performed depending on the device that will be used. The device is then deployed using fluoroscopic guidance and aortography.

There are two devices approved for TAVR at this time, the Sapien XT device (Edwards Lifesciences, Irvine, CA) and the CoreValve device (Medtronic, Minneapolis, MN). The Sapien XT device is a balloon expandable device. Once positioned, rapid pacing is initiated to essentially cease cardiac output and ensure valve stability during deployment. The CoreValve device is a self-expanding prosthesis that is positioned across the valve and opened by "de-sheathing" the valve in position. Rapid pacing may be utilized during the most critical portion of delivery but usually at rates of 110 beats per minute.

TEE is performed to determine if placement is appropriate and to assess PVL. Findings may guide operators to perform an additional balloon dilation to reduce PVL or perhaps consider the placement of a second device.[167] At the conclusion of the procedure, the delivery sheath is removed and the access site closed, usually with a suture-mediated closure device that is deployed in the artery prior to sheath delivery. For patients who have insufficient transfemoral access for TAVR, alternative access sites can be used. The Sapien XT device can be delivered via a direct trans-aortic approach or a trans-apical approach. The CoreValve device can be delivered via a direct trans-aortic approach or a subclavian approach. Each of these alternative access sites require surgical access and are therefore performed under general anesthesia in a hybrid catheterization laboratory/operating room suite.

MITRAL VALVE DISEASE

The treatment of choice for rheumatic MS is balloon mitral valvotomy (BMV) in appropriate patients. Suitability for BMV is based on the degree of leaflet mobility, leaflet calcification, subvalvular apparatus calcification, and degree of MR. Successful BMV has a long-term outcome that is similar to surgical repair; however it is not a commonly performed procedure in developed nations as the incidence of rheumatic fever is low. BMV for rheumatic MS can be performed under conscious sedation, as echocardiography is not usually required for the performance for this procedure. However, some operators prefer the use of general anesthesia and TEE for the procedure and it may be required in patients with respiratory compromise. TEE allows for direct visualization of the intra-atrial septum during the transseptal puncture. TEE also allows for direct assessment of post-BMV MR. The procedure requires femoral vein access for balloon catheter delivery and femoral arterial access for placement of a pigtail catheter in the LV to allow for simultaneous left atrium/ventricle pressure measurement to assess the trans-mitral gradient post-BMV. Transseptal puncture is performed and the appropriately sized balloon is advanced across the septum and MV. The balloon is inflated and then removed. Gradients are then measured to assess adequacy of the result.

The Mitra-Clip (Abbott Vascular, Santa Clara, CA) is FDA approved for patients with severe symptomatic degenerative MR who are deemed high risk or inoperable for surgical MV

repair/replacement.[168] This procedure requires general anesthesia and TEE guidance. The clip is usually placed on the middle anterior (A2) and posterior (P2) segments of the MV, thereby mimicking the effect provided by an Alfieri stitch of the MV, although more than one clip may be necessary. Transseptal puncture is first performed for left atrial access. The device is then delivered into the left atrium and across the MV for echo-guided deployment.

Potential Complications

EP LAB

Any procedure which involves the introduction of wires into the heart or great vessels incurs a risk of perforation of those structures. RV perforation can occur during pacemaker implantation as well as during radiofrequency ablation. Extraction of any hardware can cause perforation as well. Retroperitoneal hematomas can also occur, as well as pneumothoraces. Vigilance is essential on the part of electrophysiologists, anesthesiologists, and consulting surgeons. It is important to remember that some EP labs are located at a distance from the operating rooms, and transport of a rapidly decompensating patient can be difficult.

CARDIAC CATHETERIZATION LAB

Unique risks associated with PFO/ASD closure include device malposition and/or embolization. Given the small size of most PFOs, this is a very rare complication. While also rare with ASD closure, there is a higher risk of this complication with very large defects or defects with deficient rims of atrial tissue that may not allow the device to hold onto the intra-atrial septum. Once the device is deployed, it is still retrievable if positioning or sizing is not satisfactory. Careful TEE assessment is warranted to ensure proper device seating and maintenance of integrity of nearby structures, including the mitral/tricuspid valves, coronary sinus, and vena cavae. If device embolization occurs, the device can generally be retrieved using percutaneous techniques. Rarely, however, surgical extraction may be required. Other complications include air embolism resulting in temporary coronary ischemia. Vascular complications are uncommon when access involves only venous structures.

Patients referred for acquired VSD/PVL closure are usually acutely or chronically ill with multiple comorbidities and are usually already deemed poor surgical candidates prior to referral for the procedure. Their comorbidities increase their risk for complications associated with the procedure and anesthesia. The transseptal puncture is one potential complication point of the procedure. An inappropriately performed puncture may result in aortic perforation or pericardial effusion. The risk of these complications is reduced with echocardiographic guidance. Device embolization is a risk of both of these procedures. Like with PFO/ASD devices, they can be retrieved using percutaneous techniques. In the event of inability to retrieve, these patients will likely not be candidates for surgical retrieval.

There are several points of risk during TAVR. For transfemoral TAVR, careful and safe femoral access is critical due to the size of the sheaths that will be used for the procedure. An inappropriate puncture site can increase the risk of retroperitoneal hematoma or inability to close the access site at the conclusion of the procedure. Attempts to place a delivery sheath in a femoral/iliac of borderline size could result in arterial dissection, or rupture which can be fatal. Both sheath insertion and removal are critical points for complications. During balloon valvuloplasty and valve deployment, patients can experience severe hemodynamic impairment. Since the Sapien XT requires deployment during rapid pacing, recovery of heart rate and contractile function can be compromised if the patient has poor cardiac reserve or severe un-revascularized coronary artery disease. The CoreValve procedure also results in brief severe hypotension during the point where the native aortic valve is obstructed and the prosthetic aortic valve has not fully opened. Annular rupture has been reported with both devices. Risk factors for annular rupture include severe LV outflow tract calcium, device over-sizing, and balloon post-dilation. Annular rupture will likely be immediately fatal with little time for surgical repair. However, contained rupture can occur and the decision to proceed to operative repair needs to be made in real-time with the cardiac surgeon involved in the case. Para-valvular leak after valve deployment needs to be assessed carefully with TEE/TTE, aortography, and/or hemodynamics. Trace and mild PVL is generally of no concern. But moderate to severe leak can occur in up to 10% of cases. Treatment of these leaks usually requires additional post-dilation or the placement of a second prosthesis. PVL rarely results in acute hemodynamic issues, but may limit the benefit of the TAVR. Moderate to severe PVL is associated with worse long-term mortality after TAVR. It is prudent to assess for the presence of a pericardial effusion post-TAVR as perforation can occur following temporary pacemaker placement.

REFERENCES

1. Murphy SL, Xu JQ, Kochanek KD: Deaths: final data for 2010. *Natl Vital Stat Rep* 2013; 61:1-17.
2. Sayols-Baixeras S, Lluís-Ganella C, Lucas G, Elosua R: Pathogenesis of coronary artery disease: focus on genetic risk factors and identification of genetic variants. *Appl Clin Genet* 2014; 7:15-32.
3. Serruys PW, Morice MC, Kappetein AP, et al: Percutaneous coronary intervention versus coronary artery bypass grafting for severe coronary artery disease. *N Engl J Med* 2009; 360:960-972.
4. Weintraub WS, Grau-Sepulveda MV, Weiss JM, et al: Comparative effectiveness of revascularization strategies. *N Engl J Med* 2012; 366:1467-1476.
5. Ardehali A, Ports TA: Myocardial oxygen supply and demand. *Chest* 1990; 98:699-705.
6. Hoffman JI, Buckberg GD: The myocardial oxygen supply: demand index revisited. *J Am Heart Assoc* 2014; 3:e000285.
7. Shahian DM, O'Brien SM, Sheng S, et al: Predictors of long-term survival after coronary artery bypass grafting surgery: results from the Society of Thoracic Surgeons Adult Cardiac Surgery Database (The ASCERT Study). *Circulation* 2012; 125:1491-1500.
8. Chalmers J, Pullan M, Fabri B, et al: Validation of EuroSCORE II in a modern cohort of patients undergoing cardiac surgery. *Eur J Cardio-Thorac Surg* 2013; 43:688-694.
9. Egbert LD, Battit GE, Turndorf H, Beecher HK: The value of the preoperative visit by an anesthetist: a study of doctor-patient rapport. *JAMA* 1963; 185:553-555.
10. Collard CD, Body SC, Shernan SK, et al: Preoperative statin therapy is associated with reduced cardiac mortality after coronary artery bypass graft surgery. *J Thorac Cardiovasc Surg* 2006; 132:392-400.
11. Kuhn EW, Likopoulus OJ, Stange S, et al: Preoperative statin therapy in cardiac surgery: a meta-analysis of 90,000 patients. *Eur J Cardiothorac Surg* 2014; 45:17-26.
12. Windecker S, Kolh P, Alfonso F, et al: 2014 ESC/EACTS guidelines on myocardial revascularization. *Eur Heart J* 2014; 35:2541-2619.
13. Neily J, Mills PD, Young-Xu Y, et al: Association between implementation of a medical team training program and surgical mortality. *JAMA* 2010; 304:1693-1700.
14. Hillis LD, Smith PK, Anderson JL, et al: 2011 ACCF/AHA Guideline for Coronary Artery Bypass Surgery. *J Am Coll Cardiol* 2011; 58:e123-210.
15. Guidance on the use of ultrasound locating devices for placing central venous catheters. National Institute for Health and Clinical Excellence Technology Appraisals TA49. 2002. www.nice.org.uk/guidance/ta49.
16. Pandit JJ, Andrade J, Bogod DG, et al: The 5th National Audit Project (NAP5) on accidental awareness during general anaesthesia: summary of main findings and risk factors. *Anaesthesia* 2014; 69:1089-1101.
17. Punjaswadwong Y, Phongchiewboon A, Bunchungmongkol N: Bispectral index for improving anesthetic delivery and postoperative recovery. *Cochrane Database Syst Rev* 2014; 6:1-101.
18. Avidan MS, Jacobsohn E, Glick D, et al: Prevention of intraoperative awareness in a high-risk surgical population. *N Engl J Med* 2011; 365:591-600.
19. Depth of anaesthesia monitors-bispectral index (BIS), E-Entropy, and Narcotrend-Compact M. National Institute for Health and Clinical Excellence Diagnostics Guidance 6, 2012. www.nice.org.uk/dg6.
20. Zacharias DG, Lilly K, Shaw CL, et al: Survey of the clinical assessment and utility of near-infrared cerebral oximetry in cardiac surgery. *J Cardiothorac Vasc Anesth* 2014; 28:308-316.
21. Vernick WJ, Gutsche JT: Pro: cerebral oximetry should be a routine monitor during cardiac surgery. *J Cardiothorac Vasc Anesth* 2013; 27:385-389.
22. Gregory A, Kohl BA: Con: near-infrared spectroscopy has not proven its clinical utility as a standard monitor in cardiac surgery. *J Cardiothorac Vasc Anesth* 2013; 27:390-394.
23. Barnett CF, Vaduganathan M, Lan G, et al: Critical reappraisal of pulmonary artery catheterization and invasive hemodynamic assessment in acute heart failure. *Expert Rev Cardiovasc Ther* 2013; 11:417-424.
24. Schwann NM, Hillel Z, Hoeft A, et al: Lack of effectiveness of the pulmonary artery catheter in cardiac surgery. *Anesth Analg* 2011; 113:994-1002.
25. Judge O, Fuhai J, Fleming N, Liu H: Current use of the pulmonary artery catheter in cardiac surgery: a survey study. *J Cardiothorac Vasc Anesth*. 2015; 29(1):69-75.
26. Hillis LD, Smith PK, Anderson JL, et al: 2011 ACCF/AHA Guideline for Coronary Artery Bypass Surgery. *J Am Coll Cardiol* 2011; 58:e123-210.
27. Eltzschig HK, Rosenberger P, Löffler M, et al: Impact of intraoperative transesophageal echocardiography on surgical decisions in 12,566 patients undergoing cardiac surgery. *Ann Thorac Surg* 2008; 85:845-853.
28. Thys DM, Abel MD, Brooker RF, et al: Practice guidelines for perioperative transesophageal echocardiography: an updated report by the American Society of Anesthesiologists and the Society of Cardiovascular Anesthesiologists Task Force on Transesophageal Echocardiography. *Anesthesiology* 2010; 112:1-13.
29. Dobbs HA, Bennett-Guerrero E, White W, et al: Multinational institutional survey on patterns of intraoperative transesophageal echocardiography use in adult surgery. *J Cardiothorac Vasc Anesth* 2014; 28:54-63.
30. Bovill JG, Sebel PS, Stanley TH: Opioid analgesics in anesthesia: with special reference to their use in cardiovascular anesthesia. *Anesthesiology* 1984; 61:731-755.
31. Zhu F, Lee A, Chee YE: Fast-track cardiac care for adult cardiac surgical patients. *The Cochrane Collab* 2012; 10:1-1-72.
32. Murry CE, Jennings RB, Reimer KA: Preconditioning with ischemia: a delay of lethal cell injury in ischemic myocardium. *Circulation* 1986; 74:1124-1136.

33. Engoren M, Luther G, Fenn-Buderer N: A comparison of fentanyl, sufentanil, and remifentanil for fast-track cardiac anesthesia. *Anesth Analg* 2001; 93:859-864.

34. Landoni G, Greco T, Biondi-Zoccai G: Anaesthetic drugs and survival: a Bayesian network meta-analysis of randomized trails in cardiac surgery. *Br J Anaesth* 2013; 111:886-896.

35. Stoppe C, Fahlenkamp AV, Rex S, et al: Feasibility and safety of xenon compared with sevoflurane in coronary surgical patients: a randomized controlled pilot study. *Br J Anaesth* 2013; 111:406-416.

36. Hemmerling TM, Cyr S, Terrasini N: Epidural catheterization in cardiac surgery: the 2012 risk assessment. *Ann Card Anaesth* 2013; 16:169-177.

37. Svircevic V, Passier MM, Nierich AP, et al: Epidural analgesia for cardiac surgery. *Cochrane Database Syst Rev* 2013; 6:CD006715.

38. Chakravarthy M: Future of awake cardiac surgery. *J Cardiothorac Vasc Anesth* 2014; 28:771-777.

39. Ahmed I, House CM, Nelson WB: Predictors of inotrope use in patients undergoing concomitant coronary artery bypass graft (CABG) and aortic valve replacement (AVR) surgeries at separation from cardiopulmonary bypass (CPB). *J Cardiothorac Surg* 2009; 4:24.

40. McKinlay KH, Schinderle DB, Swaminathan M, et al: Predictors of inotrope use during separation from cardiopulmonary bypass. *J Cardiothorac Vasc Anesth* 2004; 18:404-408.

41. McMurray JJ, Adamopoulos S, Anker SD, et al: European Society of Cardiology Guidelines for the diagnosis and treatment of acute and chronic heart failure 2012. *Eur Heart J* 2012; 33:1787-1847.

42. Licker M, Diaper J, Cartier V, et al: Clinical review: management of weaning from cardiopulmonary bypass after cardiac surgery. *Ann Card Anaesth* 2012; 15:206-223.

43. Thiele H, Zeymer U, Neumann FJ, et al: Intraaortic balloon support for myocardial infarction with cardiogenic shock (SHOCK II Trial). *New Engl J Med* 2012; 367:1287-1296.

44. Wadhera RK, Parker SH, Burkhart HM, et al: Is the "sterile cockpit" concept applicable to cardiovascular surgery critical intervals or critical events? The impact of protocol-driven communication during cardiopulmonary bypass. *J Thor Cardiovasc Surg* 2010; 139:312-319.

45. Kennedy ED, Choy KC, Alston RP, et al: Cognitive outcome after on- and off-pump coronary artery grafting surgery: a systematic review and meta-analysis. *J Cardiothorac Vasc Anesth* 2013; 27:253-265.

46. Møller CH, Penninga L, Wetterslev J, et al: Off-pump versus on-pump coronary artery bypass grafting for ischaemic heart disease. *Cochrane Database Syst Rev*, 2012, 3. Art. No. CD007224.

47. Takagi H, Mizuno Y, Niwa M, et al: A meta-analysis of randomized trials for repeat revascularization following off-pump versus on-pump coronary artery bypass grafting. *Interact Cardiovasc Thorac Surg* 2013; 17:878-880.

48. Deshpande SP, Fitzpatrick M, Lehr EJ: Totally endoscopic robotic coronary artery bypass surgery. *Curr Opin Anesthesiol* 2014; 27:49-56.

49. Bonow RO: Chronic mitral regurgitation and aortic regurgitation: Have indications for surgery changed? *J Am Coll Card* 2013; 61:693-701.

50. Lund O: Preoperative risk evaluation and stratification of long-term survival after valve replacement for aortic stenosis: reasons for earlier operative interventions. *Circulation* 1990; 82:124-139.

51. Mittnacht AJC, Fanshawe M, Konstadt S: Anesthetic considerations in the patient with valvular heart disease undergoing noncardiac surgery. *Semin Cardiothorac Vasc Anesth* 2008; 12:33-59.

52. Sprung J, Ogletree-Hughes ML, McConnell BK, et al: The effects of propofol on the contractility of failing and nonfailing human heart muscles. *Anesth Analg.* 2001; 93:550-559.

53. Nishimura RA, Otto CM, Bonow RO, et al: 2014 AHA/ACC guidelines for the management of patients with valvular heart disease: executive summary: a report of the American College of Cardiology/American Heart Association Task Force on Practice Guidelines. *Circulation* 2014; 129:2440-2492.

54. Quintana E, Suri RM, Thalji NM, et al: Left ventricular dysfunction after mitral valve repair—the fallacy of "normal" preoperative myocardial function. *J Thorac Cardiovasc Surg* 2014; 148:2752-2760.

55. Varghese R, Itagaki S, Anyanwu AC, et al: Predicting early left ventricular dysfunction after mitral valve reconstruction: the effect of atrial fibrillation and pulmonary hypertension. *J Thorac Cardiovasc Surg* 2014; 148:422-427.

56. Witkowski TG, Thomas JD, Delgado V, et al: Changes in left ventricular function after mitral valve repair for severe organic mitral regurgitation. *Ann Thor Surg* 2012; 93:754-760.

57. Rodrigues ES, Lynch JJ, Suri RM, et al: Robotic mitral valve repair: a review of anesthetic management of the first 200 patients. *J Cardiothor Vasc Anesth* 2014; 28:64-68.

58. Suri RM, Antiel RM, Burkhart HM, et al: Quality of life after early mitral valve repair using conventional and robotic approaches. *Ann Thorac Surg* 2012; 93:761-769.

59. Rehfeldt KH, Mauermann WJ, Burkhart HM, et al: Robot-assisted mitral valve repair. *J Cardiothorac Vasc Anesth* 2011; 25:721-730.

60. Kottenberg-Assenmacher E, Kamler M, Peters J: Minimally invasive endoscopic Port-Access intracardiac surgery with one-lung ventilation: impact on gas exchange and anaesthesia resources. *Anaesthesia* 2007; 62:231-238.

61. Tewari P: Cardioversion during closed chest robotic surgery: relevance of pad position. *Anesth Analg* 2007; 105:542-543.

62. Mayer J, Boldt J, Schollhorn T, et al: Semi-invasive monitoring of cardiac output by a new device using arterial pressure waveform analysis: a comparison with intermittent pulmonary artery thermodilution in patients undergoing cardiac surgery. *Br J Anaesth* 2007; 98:176-182.

63. Mayer J, Suttner S: Cardiac output derived from arterial pressure waveform. *Curr Opin Anesth* 2009; 22:804-808.

64. Erbel R, Aboyans V, Boileau C, et al: 2014 ESC guideline on the diagnosis and treatment of aortic diseases: document covering acute and chronic aortic diseases of the thoracic and abdominal aorta of the adult. The Task Force for the Diagnosis and Treatment of Aortic Diseases of the European Society of Cardiology. *Eur Heart J* 2014; 35:2873-2926.

65. Hiratzka LF, Bakris GL, Beckman JA, et al: 2010 ACCF/AHA/AATS/ ACR/ASA/SCA/SCAI/SIR/STS/SVM guidelines for the diagnosis and management of patients with thoracic aortic disease. *Circulation* 2010; 121:e266-e369.

66. Boodhwani M, Andelfinger G, Leipsic J, et al: Canadian Cardiovascular Society position statement on the management of thoracic aortic disease. *Can J Cardiol* 2014; 30:577-589.

67. Svensson LG, Adams DH, Bonow RO, et al: Aortic valve and ascending aorta guidelines for management and quality measures. *Ann Thorac Surg* 2013; 95(6 Suppl):S1-S66.

68. Bond DM, Milne B, Pym J, et al: Cardiac tamponade complicating anaesthetic induction for repair of ascending aortic dissection. *Can J Anaesth* 1987; 34(3):291-293.

69. Unal M, Yilmaz O, Akar I, et al: Brachiocephalic artery cannulation in proximal aortic surgery that requires circulatory arrest. *Tex Heart Inst J* 2014; 41(6):596-600.

70. Augoustides JG, Desai ND, Szeto WY, et al: Innominate artery cannulation: the Toronto technique for antegrade cerebral perfusion in aortic arch reconstruction—a clinical trial opportunity for the International Aortic Arch Surgery Study Group. *J Thorac Cardiovasc Surg* 2014; 148:2924-2926.

71. Augoustides JG, Harris H, Pochettino A: Direct innominate artery cannulation in acute type A dissection and severe thoracic aortic atheroma. *J Cardiothorac Vasc Anesth* 2007; 21:727-729.

72. Thys DM, Abel MD, Brooker RF, et al: Practice guidelines for perioperative transesophageal echocardiography: an updated report by the American Society of Anesthesiologists and the Society of Cardiovascular Anesthesiologists task force on transesophageal echocardiography. *Anesthesiology* 2010; 112:1084-1096.

73. Saczkowski R, Malas T, Mesana T, et al: Aortic valve preservation and repair in acute Type A aortic dissection. *Eur J Cardiothorac Surg* 2014; 45:e220-226.

74. Augoustides JG, Szeto WY, Bavaria JE: Advance sin aortic valve repair: focus on the functional approach, clinical outcomes, and the central role of echocardiography. *J Cardiothorac Vasc Anesth*. 2010; 24:1016-1020.

75. Frederick JR, Yang E, Trubelja A, et al: Ascending aortic cannulation in acute type A dissection repair. *Ann Thorac Surg* 2013; 95:1808-1811.

76. Augoustides JG, Kohl BA, Harris H, et al: Color-flow Doppler recognition of intraoperative brachiocephalic malperfusion during operative repair of acute Type A aortic dissection: utility of transcutaneous carotid artery ultrasound scanning. *J Cardiothorac Vasc Anesth* 2007; 21:81-84.

77. Lu Q, Feng J, Zhou J, et al: Endovascular repair of ascending aortic dissection: a novel treatment option for patients judged unfit for direct surgical repair. *J Am Coll Cardiol* 2013; 61:1917-1924.

78. Szeto WY, Moser WG, Desai ND, et al: Transapical deployment of endovascular thoracic aortic stent graft for an ascending aortic pseudoaneurysm. *Ann Thorac Surg* 2010; 89:616-618.

79. Cobey FC, Ferreira RG, Naseem TM, et al: Anesthetic and perioperative considerations for transapical transcatheter aortic valve replacement. *J Cardiothorac Vasc Anesth* 2014; 28:1087-1099.

80. Augoustides JG, Szeto WY, Desai ND, et al: Classification of acute type A dissection: focus on clinical presentation and extent. *Eur J Cardiothorac Surg* 2011; 39:519-522.

81. Bavaria JE, Milewski RK, Baker J, et al: Classic hybrid evolving approach to distal arch aneurysms: towards the zone zero solution. *J Thorac Cardiovasc Surg* 2010; 140:S77-S80.

82. Gutsche JT, Ghadimi K, Patel PA, et al: New frontiers in aortic therapy: focus on deep hypothermic circulatory arrest. *J Cardiothorac Vasc Anesth.* 2014; 29:1171-1175.

83. Augoustides JG, Patel P, Ghadimi K, et al: Current conduct of deep hypothermic circulatory arrest in China. *HSR Proc Intensive Care Cardiovasc Anesth* 2013; 5:25-32.

84. Gutsche JT, Feinman J, Silvay G, et al: Practice variations in the conduct of hypothermic circulatory arrest for adult aortic arch repair: focus on an emerging European paradigm. *Heart Lung Vessel* 2014; 6:43-51.

85. Yan TD, Bannon PG, Bavaria J, et al: Consensus on hypothermia in aortic arch surgery. *Ann Cardiothorac Surg* 2013; 2:163-168.

86. Tian DH, Wan B, Bannon PG, et al: A meta-analysis of deep hypothermic circulatory arrest versus moderate hypothermic circulatory arrest with selective antegrade cerebral perfusion. *Ann Cardiothorac Surg* 2013; 2:148-158.

87. Comas GM, Leshnower BG, Halkos ME, et al: Acute type a dissection: impact of antegrade cerebral perfusion under moderate hypothermia. *Ann Thorac Surg* 2013; 96:2135-2141.

88. Appoo JJ, Augoustides JG, Pochettino A, et al: Perioperative outcome in adults undergoing elective deep hypothermic circulatory arrest with retrograde cerebral perfusion in proximal aortic arch repair: evaluation of protocol-based care. *J Cardiothorac Vasc Anesth* 2006; 20:3-7.

89. Milewski RK, Pacini D, Moser GW, et al: Retrograde and antegrade cerebral perfusion: results in short elective arch reconstructive times. *Ann Thorac Surg* 2010; 89:1448-1457.

90. Preventza O, Simpson KH, Cooley DA, et al: Unilateral versus bilateral cerebral perfusion for acute type A aortic dissection. *Ann Thorac Surg* 2015; 99:80-87.

91. Zierer A, Risteski P, El-Sayed Ahmad A, et al: The impact of unilateral versus bilateral antegrade cerebral perfusion on surgical outcomes after aortic arch replacement: a propensity-matched analysis. *J Thorac Cardiovasc Surg* 2014; 147:1212-1217.

92. Okita Y, Miyata H, Motomura N, et al: A study of brain protection during total arch replacement comparing antegrade cerebral perfusion versus hypothermic circulatory arrest, with or without retrograde cerebral perfusion: analysis based on the Japan Adult Cardiovascular Surgery Database. *J Thorac Cardiovasc Surg* 2014; [Epub ahead of print].

93. De Paulis R, Czerny M, Weltert L, et al: Current trends in cannulation and neuroprotection during surgery of the aortic arch in Europe. *Eur J Cardiothorac Surg* 2014; [Epub ahead of print].

94. Dewhurst AT, Moore SJ, Libasn JB: Pharmacological agents as cerebral protectants during deep hypothermic circulatory arrest in adult thoracic aortic surgery: a survey of current practice. *Anaesthesia* 2002; 57:1016-1021.

95. Kruger T, Hoffmann I, Blettner M, et al: Intraoperative neuroprotective drugs without beneficial effects? Results of the German Registry for Acute Aortic Dissection Type A (GERAADA). *Eur J Cardiothorac Surg* 2013; 44:939-946.

96. Stecker MM, Cheung AT, Pochettino A, et al: Deep hypothermic circulatory arrest—I: effects of cooling on electroencephalogram and evoked potentials. *Ann Thorac Surg* 2001; 71:14-21.

97. Stecker MM, Cheung AT, Pochettino A, et al: Deep hypothermic circulatory arrest—II: changes in electroencephalogram and evoked potentials during rewarming. *Ann Thorac Surg* 2001; 71:22-28.

98. Cheung AT, Weiss SJ, Kent G, et al: Intraoperative seizures in cardiac surgical patients undergoing deep hypothermic circulatory arrest monitored with EEG. *Anesthesiology* 2001; 94:1143-1147.

99. Bavaria JE, Brinster DR, Gorman RC, et al: Advances in the treatment of acute type A dissection: an integrated approach. *Ann Thorac Surg* 2002; 74:S1848-S1852.

100. Shann KG, Likosky DS, Murkin JM, et al: An evidence-based review of the practice of cardiopulmonary bypass in adults: a focus on neurologic injury, glycemic control, hemodilution, and the inflammatory response. *J Thorac Cardiovasc Surg* 2006; 132:283-290.

101. Reich DL, Horn LM, Hossain S, et al: Using jugular bulb oxyhemoglobin saturation to guide onset of deep hypothermic circulatory arrest does not affect post-operative neuropsychological function. *Eur J Cardiothorac Surg* 2004; 25:401-406.

102. Steppan J, Hogue CW Jr: Cerebral and tissue oximetry. *Best Pract Res Clin Anaesthesiol* 2014; 28:429-439.

103. Olsson C, Thelin S: Regional cerebral saturation monitoring with near-infrared spectroscopy during selective antegrade cerebral perfusion: diagnostic performance and relationship to postoperative stroke. *J Thorac Cardiovasc Surg* 2006; 131:371-379.

104. Shirasaka T, Okada K, Kano H, et al: New indicator of postoperative delayed awakening after total aortic arch replacement. *Eur J Cardiothorac Surg* 2015; 47:101-105.

105. Andritsos M, Desai ND, Grewal A, et al: Innovations in aortic disease management: the descending aorta. *J Cardiothorac Vasc Anesth* 2010; 24:523-529.

106. Frederick JR, Woo YJ: Thoracoabdominal aortic aneurysm. *Ann Cardiothorac Surg* 2012; 1:277-285.

107. Augoustides JG, Stone ME, Drenger B: Novel approaches to spinal cord protection during thoracoabdominal aortic interventions. *Curr Opin Anaesthesiol* 2014; 27:98-105.

108. Fabbro M, Gregory A, Gutsche JT, et al: Case 11-2014. Successful open repair of an extensive descending thoracic aortic aneurysm in a complex patient. *J Cardiothorac Vasc Anesth* 2014; 28:1397-1402.

109. Dong CC, MacDonald DB, Janusz MT: Intraoperative spinal cord monitoring during descending thoracic and thoracoabdominal aneurysm surgery. *Ann Thorac Surg* 2002; 74:S1873-S1876.

110. Sloan TB, Edmonds HL, Koht A: Intraoperative electrophysiologic monitoring in aortic surgery. *J Cardiothorac Vasc Anesth* 2013; 27:1364-1373.

111. Cheng D, Martin J, Shennib H, et al: Endovascular aortic repair versus open surgical repair for descending thoracic aortic disease a systematic review and meta-analysis of comparative studies. *J Am Coll Cardiol* 2010; 55:986-1001.

112. Hogendorn W, Schlosser FJ, Muhs BE, et al: Surgical and anesthetic considerations for the endovascular treatment of ruptured descending thoracic aortic aneurysms. *Curr Opin Anaesthesiol* 2014; 27:12-20.

113. Matsumura JS, Lee WA, Mitchell RS, et al: The Society for Vascular Surgery practice guidelines: management of the left subclavian artery with thoracic endovascular aortic repair. *J Vasc Surg* 2009; 50:1155-1158.

114. Rizvi AZ, Murad MH, Fairman RM, et al: The effect of left subclavian artery coverage on morbidity and mortality in patients undergoing endovascular thoracic aortic interventions: a systematic review and meta-analysis. *J Vasc Surg* 2009; 50:1159-1169.

115. Cooper DG, Walsh SR, Sadat U, et al: Neurological complications after left subclavian artery coverage during thoracic endovascular aortic repair: a systematic review and meta-analysis. *J Vasc Surg* 2009; 49:1594-1601.

116. Yancy CW, Jessup M, Bozkurt B, et al: 2013 ACCF/AHA guideline for the management of heart failure: a report of the American College of Cardiology Foundation/American Heart Association Task Force on Practice Guidelines. *J Am Coll Cardiol* 2013; 62:e147-239.

117. Mehra MR, Kobashigawa J, Starling R, et al: Listing criteria for heart transplantation: International Society for Heart and Lung Transplantation guidelines for the care of cardiac transplant candidates—2006. *J Heart Lung Transplant* 2006; 25:1024-1042.

118. Gheorghiade M, Abraham WT, Albert NM, et al: Relationship between admission serum sodium concentration and clinical outcomes in patients hospitalized for heart failure: an analysis from the OPTIMIZE-HF registry. *Eur Heart J* 2007; 28:980-988.

119. Groban L, Butterworth J: Perioperative management of chronic heart failure. *Anesth Analg* 2006; 103:557-575.

120. Coriat P, Richer C, Douraki T, et al: Influence of chronic angiotensin-converting enzyme inhibition on anesthetic induction. *Anesthesiology* 1994; 81:299-307.

121. Ryckwaert F, Colson P: Hemodynamic effects of anesthesia in patients with ischemic heart failure chronically treated with angiotensin-converting enzyme inhibitors. *Anesth Analg* 1997; 84:945-949.

122. Brabant SM, Bertrand M, Eyraud D, et al: The hemodynamic effects of anesthetic induction in vascular surgical patients chronically treated with angiotensin II receptor antagonists. *Anesth Analg* 1999; 89:1388-1392.

123. Song HK, Tibayan FA, Kahl EA, et al: Safety and efficacy of prothrombin complex concentrates for the treatment of coagulopathy after cardiac surgery. *J Thorac Cardiovasc Surg* 2014; 147:1036-1040.

124. Gorlinger K, Shore-Lesserson L, Dirkmann D, et al: Management of hemorrhage in cardiothoracic surgery. *J Cardiothorac Vasc Anesth* 2013; 27:S20-34.

125. American Society of A. Practice advisory for the perioperative management of patients with cardiac implantable electronic devices: pacemakers and implantable cardioverter-defibrillators: an updated report by the American Society of Anesthesiologists Task Force on perioperative management of patients with cardiac implantable electronic devices. *Anesthesiology* 2011; 114:247-261.

126. Warkentin TE, Greinacher A, Koster A, Lincoff AM: Treatment and prevention of heparin-induced thrombocytopenia: American College of Chest Physicians Evidence-Based Clinical Practice Guidelines (8th edn). *Chest* 2008; 133:340S-80S.

127. Levy JH, Tanaka KA, Hursting MJ: Reducing thrombotic complications in the perioperative setting: an update on heparin-induced thrombocytopenia. *Anesth Analg* 2007; 105:570-582.

128. Strumpher J, Jacobsohn E: Pulmonary hypertension and right ventricular dysfunction: physiology and perioperative management. *J Cardiothorac Vasc Anesth* 2011; 25:687-704.

129. Lund LH, Edwards LB, Kucheryavaya AY, et al: The Registry of the International Society for Heart and Lung Transplantation: Thirty-first Official Adult Heart Transplant Report-2014; Focus Theme: Retransplantation. *J Heart Lung Transplant* 2014; 33:996-1008.

130. Fischer S, Glas KE: A review of cardiac transplantation. *Anesthesiol Clin* 2013; 31:383-403.

131. Tambur AR, Pamboukian SV, Costanzo MR, et al: The presence of HLA-directed antibodies after heart transplantation is associated with poor allograft outcome. *Transplantation* 2005; 80:1019-1025.

132. Anand J, H RM: The state of the art in heart transplantation. *Semin Thorac Cardiovasc Surg* 2013; 25:64-69.

133. Russo MJ, Iribarne A, Hong KN, et al: Factors associated with primary graft failure after heart transplantation. *Transplantation* 2010; 90:444-450.

134. Kapur NK, Paruchuri V, Jagannathan A, et al: Mechanical circulatory support for right ventricular failure. *JACC Heart Failure* 2013; 1:127-134.

135. Taghavi S, Zuckermann A, Ankersmit J, et al: Extracorporeal membrane oxygenation is superior to right ventricular assist device for acute right ventricular failure after heart transplantation. *Ann Thorac Surg* 2004; 78:1644-1649.

136. Lavigne D: Vasopressin and methylene blue: alternate therapies in vasodilatory shock. *Semin Cardiothorac Vasc Anesth* 2010; 14:186-189.

137. Levin MA, Lin HM, Castillo JG, et al: Early on-cardiopulmonary bypass hypotension and other factors associated with vasoplegic syndrome. *Circulation* 2009; 120:1664-1671.

138. Feussner M, Mukherjee C, Garbade J, Ender J: Anaesthesia for patients undergoing ventricular assist-device implantation. *Best Pract Res Clin Anaesth* 2012; 26:167-177.

139. Meineri M, Van Rensburg AE, Vegas A: Right ventricular failure after LVAD implantation: prevention and treatment. *Best Pract Res Clin Anaesth* 2012; 26:217-229.

140. Santamore WP, Gray LA Jr: Left ventricular contributions to right ventricular systolic function during LVAD support. *Ann Thorac Surg* 1996; 61:350-356.

141. Catena E, Tasca G: Role of echocardiography in the perioperative management of mechanical circulatory assistance. *Best Pract Res Clin Anaesth* 2012; 26:199-216.

142. Haberl T, Riebandt J, Mahr S, et al: Viennese approach to minimize the invasiveness of ventricular assist device implantationdagger. *Eur J Cardiothorac Surg* 2014; 46:991-996; discussion 6.

143. Kirklin JK, Naftel DC, Kormos RL, et al: Fifth INTERMACS annual report: risk factor analysis from more than 6,000 mechanical circulatory support patients. *J Heart Lung Transplant* 2013; 32:141-156.

144. Copeland JG, Smith RG, Arabia FA, et al: Cardiac replacement with a total artificial heart as a bridge to transplantation. *N Engl J Med* 2004; 351:859-867.

145. Zimmerman H, Coehlo-Anderson R, Slepian M, et al: Device malfunction of the CardioWest total artificial heart secondary to catheter entrapment of the tricuspid valve. *ASAIO J* 2010; 56:481-482.

146. Mizuguchi KA, Padera RF Jr, Kowalczyk A, et al: Transesophageal echocardiography imaging of the total artificial heart. *Anesth Analg* 2013; 117:780-784.

147. Obeid AI, Carlson RJ: Evaluation of pulmonary vein stenosis by transesophageal echocardiography. *J Am Soc Echocardiogr* 1995; 8:888-896.

148. Lund LH, Edwards LB, Kucheryavaya AY, et al: The Registry of the International Society for Heart and Lung Transplantation: Thirtieth Official Adult Heart Transplant Report—2013; focus theme: age. *J Heart Lung Transplant* 2013; 32:951-964.

149. Kuppahally SS, Valantine HA, Weisshaar D, et al: Outcome in cardiac recipients of donor hearts with increased left ventricular wall thickness. *Am J Transplant* 2007; 7:2388-2395.

150. Weiss ES, Allen JG, Patel ND, et al: The impact of donor-recipient sex matching on survival after orthotopic heart transplantation: analysis of 18 000 transplants in the modern era. *Circ Heart Failure* 2009; 2:401-408.

151. Yamani MH, Erinc K, Starling RC, et al: Donor intracranial bleeding is associated with advanced transplant coronary vasculopathy: evidence from intravascular ultrasound. *Transplant Proc* 2004; 36:2564-2566.

152. Senanayake EL, Singh H, Ranasinghe AM, Mascaro J: A perilous course following myocardial infarction: ischaemic ventricular septal defect in a transplanted heart. *Interactive Cardiovasc Thorac Surg* 2014; 19:526-528.

153. Lietz K, John R, Burke EA, et al: Pretransplant cachexia and morbid obesity are predictors of increased mortality after heart transplantation. *Transplantation* 2001; 72:277-283.

154. Hong KN, Iribarne A, Worku B, et al: Who is the high-risk recipient? Predicting mortality after heart transplant using pretransplant donor and recipient risk factors. *Ann Thorac Surg* 2011; 92:520-527; discussion 7.

155. Gross WL: Hybrid Procedures: Integrated Care and Teamwork: the Rashomon Effect in Cardiovascular Medicine, Anesthesia and Analgesia Case Reports: November 1, 2014, Vol. 3, No. 9.

156. Epstein AE, DiMarco JP, Ellenbogen KA, et al: ACC/AHA/HRS 2008 guidelines for device-based therapy of cardiac rhythm abnormalities. *Circulation* 2008; 117:350-408.

157. Bernstein AD, Daubert JC, Fletcher RD, et al: The revised NASPE/BPEG generic code for antibradycardia, adaptive-rate, and multisite pacing. North American Society of Pacing and Electrophysiology/British Pacing and Electrophysiology Group. *Pacing Clin Electrophysiol* 2002; 25:260-264.

158. Haissaguerre M, Jais P, Shah DC, et al: Spontaneous initiation of atrial fibrillation by ectopic beats originating in the pulmonary veins. *N Engl J Med* 1998; 339:659-66.

159. Gross WL, Faillace R, Shook DC, et al: New challenges for anesthesiologists outside of the operating room—the cardiac catheterization and electrophysiology Laboratories in Anesthesia Outside of the Operating Room: Oxford University Press, NY, 2011.

160. Allot EM, Stevenson WG, Almendral-Garrote JM, Bogun F: EHRA/HRS expert consensus on catheter ablation of ventricular arrhythmias. *Europace* 2009; 11:771-817.

161. Furlan AJ, Reisman M, Massaro J, et al: Closure or medical therapy for cryptogenic stroke with patent foramen ovale. *N Engl J Med* 2012; 366:991-999.

162. Carroll JD, Saver JL, Thaler DE: Closure of patent foramen ovale versus medical therapy after cryptogenic stroke. *N Engl J Med* 2013; 368:1092-1100.

163. Leon MB, Smith CR, Mack M, et al: Transcatheter aortic valve implantation in patients who cannot undergo surgery. *N Engl J Med* 2010; 363:1597-1607.

164. Smith CR, Leon MB, Mack M, et al: Transcatheter vs. surgical aortic valve replacement in high risk patients. *N Engl J Med* 2011; 364:2187.

165. Popma JJ, Adams DH, Reardon MJ, et al: Transcatheter aortic valve replacement using a self-expanding bioprosthesis in patients with severe aortic stenosis at extreme risk for surgery. *J Am Coll Cardiol* 2014; 63.

166. Adams DH, Popma JJ, Reardon MJ, et al: Transcatheter aortic valve replacement with a self-expanding prosthesis. *N Engl J Med* 2014;

167. Khalique O, Williams M, et al: Predicting paravalvular regurgitation following transcatheter valve replacement: utility of a novel three-dimensional echocardiographic measurements of the annulus. *J Am Soc Echocardiogr* 2013; 26:1043-1052.

Feldman T, Foster E, Glower DG, et al: Percutaneous repair or surgery for mitral regurgitation. *N Engl J Med* 2011; 364:1395-1406.

12

Echocardiography in Cardiac Surgery

Eliza P. Teo • Michael H. Picard • Hanjo Ko • Michael N. D'Ambra

INTRODUCTION

Echocardiography plays an important role in cardiac surgery by defining myocardial structure, function, and intracardiac blood flow velocities. Preoperatively, transthoracic and transesophageal echocardiography with color and spectral Doppler identify, quantify, and characterize cardiac disease and support decision making in terms of surgical timing and choices. Intraoperative transesophageal echocardiography (TEE) provides high-fidelity assessment of underlying pathophysiology, guides beating heart procedures in real time, supports surgical planning, and, allows for timely assessment of the results of surgical procedures. Furthermore, TEE can be critical in the early postoperative period to elucidate various etiologies of perioperative hemodynamic instability, allowing surgeons and intensivists to identify and manage complications accurately and efficiently. Lastly, transthoracic echocardiography (TTE) is often employed to evaluate and monitor long-term surgical results due to its noninvasive nature.

It is important that surgeons appreciate the potential and the limitations of perioperative ultrasound to provide case-specific predictors and intraoperative procedural guidance to improve surgical outcomes and facilitate incorporation of new technologies into current practice.

The goals of this chapter are to provide a framework for understanding the technique, and its indications for use. We summarize American Society of Echocardiography/Society of Cardiovascular Anesthiologists (ASE/SCA) guidelines for the surgical use of epicardial ultrasound, which can supplement or substitute for intraoperative TEE when TEE is contraindicated. Finally, we outline expectations that surgeons should have for intraoperative TEE images and interpretations.

BASIC PRINCIPLES

Echocardiographic images are constructed by transmitting high-frequency sound waves into the chest from a transducer composed of piezo-electric crystals. These waves reflect off cardiac structures, and the returning signals are received by the same transducer. By knowing when the signal was sent, the speed of the sound in the tissue, and the time it takes for the reflected signal to return to the transducer, the position of the structure responsible for the reflection can be calculated. An image from these signals can thus be created. The quality of the image relies on many factors, including the media through which the sound is traveling, the orientation of the structures in relation to the ultrasound beam, and the composition of the structure. Sound travels incredibly well through water and blood, reasonably well through tissue, but poorly through air. Therefore, the media through which the sound travels will determine the strength of the returning signal. When the ultrasound beam reflects off various portions of the heart, the signal is scattered in various directions such that some never return to the transducer. For this reason, structures that are perpendicular to the ultrasound beam and reflect stronger signals back to the transducer produce images of the most accuracy. On the other hand, strong reflectors such as calcified valvular leaflets will result in a bright picture but they also inevitably create imaging artifacts. The fact that sound transmitted from a TEE transducer has less distance to travel (which means less signal lost to scatter) and mainly travels through muscle and blood (and rarely air) explains why the quality of TEE images is usually better than TTE imaging.

Echocardiographic displays include M-mode, two-dimensional (2D) and three-dimensional (3D) imaging. The M-mode echocardiogram has superior temporal resolution and can be thought of as a display of the motion of a single cut through the heart over time. It is now used primarily to quantify the timing of intracardiac events. Two-dimensional echocardiography provides a display with better spatial resolution and excellent temporal resolution. Three-dimensional echocardiography provides the best display of the spatial relationships of various structures and flow patterns, and its resolution continues to improve.

Blood flow velocities are assessed by the Doppler principle. The wavelength of sound reflecting off moving blood particles will be shorter if blood is moving toward the transducer and longer, if moving away. By quantifying this change in frequency of the ultrasound beam, one can determine the blood velocity and direction. This calculation, however, is influenced by the angle between the ultrasound beam and the blood flow such that as this angle increases, the calculated velocity is lower and less accurate. Thus the goal is to keep alignment of the beam as parallel to the blood flow as possible. As blood travels through a restrictive or stenotic region at a constant flow, its velocity will increase and the pressure gradient can be calculated from the simplified Bernoulli Equation (Δpressure = 4 × velocity^2). The peak and mean pressure gradients are calculated from spectral Doppler techniques. Pulse wave (PW) Doppler has excellent spatial resolution, allowing the identification of the specific locations of flow disturbances such as obstructions or leaks. Continuous wave (CW) Doppler has excellent velocity resolution and identifies the highest velocity along the path of the ultrasound beam (which is assumed to occur at the narrowest region). Color-flow mapping displays the velocities and directions of flow determined by Doppler. This technique is valuable to identify and quantify regurgitation. However, it must be remembered that the color display of a regurgitant jet represents the velocity of the blood disturbed by the regurgitation and is *not* the volume of regurgitation as one would see on an angiogram. The color display of these jets is influenced by various echocardiography machine settings.

Doppler quantitation of velocities is dependent on one's hemodynamic profiles, and since these conditions are often different during anesthesia (compared to preoperative resting state), the pressure gradients obtained by spectral Doppler and the color Doppler display of regurgitant jets may differ significantly from preoperative assessments. Thus the decision to operate should be based on preoperative values.

Finally, the echocardiographic views of the heart required to assess different pathologies as well as the necessary components of a perioperative TEE have been established by expert consensus and serve as a roadmap to understand the basic TEE.[1]

SAFETY OF INTRAOPERATIVE TRANSESOPHAGEAL ECHOCARDIOGRAPHY

While TTE has some roles in the operating room, the dominant ultrasound modality for perioperative imaging is TEE. It has been in use in the operating room for over 30 years and has an excellent safety record. The incidence of complications in 7200 intraoperative TEEs performed at the Brigham and Women's Hospital was 0.2%, and no intraoperative TEE-associated mortality was noted. The most common complication was odynophagia severe enough to warrant esophagogastroduodenoscopy (0.1%) and this was followed by acute upper gastrointestinal hemorrhage (0.03% including esophageal tear but not esophageal perforation), dental injury (0.03%), arterial desaturation due to malpositioning of endotracheal tube (0.03%), and esophageal perforation (0.01%). Unsuccessful TEE probe insertion occurred in 0.18% of cases and contraindications to TEE were noted in 0.5%.[2] A small study has reported a higher rate of major upper gastrointestinal complications at 1.2% in patients undergoing intraoperative TEE with a significant proportion of the injury manifesting greater than 24 hours after the procedure.[3] Reported TEE complication rate in pediatric

cardiac surgical patients is higher at 2.4%.[4] As a reference, an older study of the complication rates in over 10,000 TEEs performed on conscious patients outside of the operating room reported an event rate similar to that of adult intraoperative patients (0.18%) however the types of complications differed and included one death.[5]

An important way to reduce complications, especially esophageal and gastric injury, is to prospectively recognize those patients who are at risk and avoid TEE in those with extensive esophageal and gastric diseases. Another key principle is to balance risk and benefit ratio carefully such that TEE is only performed when its benefits outweigh its risks.[6] Absolute contraindications to TEE include perforated viscous, prior esophagectomy, and esophagogastrectomy. Relative contraindications to TEE include those with oropharyngeal cancer, preexisting esophageal pathologies (including varices, strictures, diverticula, esophagitis, Mallory-Weiss tears, radiation injury), and gastrointestinal pathologies (such as recent upper gastrointestinal hemorrhage, gastric ulcer or symptomatic hiatal hernia).[7]

TRAINING AND QUALITY

Both cardiology and anesthesiology specialty and subspecialty societies have outlined recommendations for appropriate training required prior to independent performance of intraoperative TEE such as a minimum number of studies to maintain proficiency along with other benchmarks to guarantee imaging quality and practitioners' ability to interpret findings accurately.[8–12] Some surgeons have taken part in these training and certification programs, and many Cardiothoracic (CT) surgical training programs are including imaging skills-training in the curriculum.

SURGICAL USE OF EPICARDIAL ULTRASOUND

Epiaortic

The cardiac surgical use of ultrasound in most practices is limited to epiaortic scanning prior to aortic cannulation. Evidence is strong that routine use, coupled with alterations in surgical approach in the setting of significant atheromatous changes, reduces morbid neurological outcomes.[82] The Society of Cardiovascular Anesthesiologists (SCA)/American Society of Echocardiography (ASE) Guidelines suggest measuring (1) maximal plaque height/thickness; (2) location of the maximal plaque within the ascending aorta; and (3) presence of mobile components in each of the three ascending aortic short axis segments and for the aortic arch.[80,81] Figure 12-1 shows the guideline views. "Mid" is usually the aortic cross-clamp site, "distal" is usually the cannulation site.

Epicardial

In addition to epiaortic scanning, the epicardial probe can be utilized to supplement intraoperative TEE assessment.

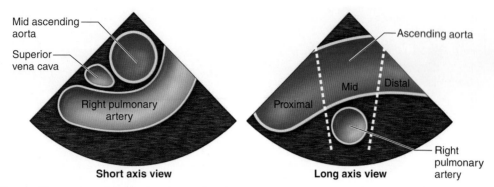

FIGURE 12-1 Short and long axis graphic of epiaortic scanning views.

The ASE guidelines assist surgeons in developing expertise in obtaining meaningful images when TEE is contraindicated. Figures 12-2 through 12-8 demonstrate the recommended views, which can be obtained in a setting of a median sternotomy incision. These ASE views serve as a general suggestion to help develop a user-dependent approach that is tailored to best suit each surgeon's individual practice.

It is suggested that surgeons take a few moments when they have the ultrasound probe in the surgical field to practice obtaining these standard ASE images. In the situation of a critical need for intraoperative ultrasound imaging when TEE is contraindicated (noted above in the section Safety of Intraoperative Transesophageal Echocardiography), a standard epicardial probe can be used if there is a full sternotomy. If there is a minimally invasive incision, placing the TEE probe in a sterile sheath filled with ultrasound gel can also provide excellent epicardial images of all structures from almost any small incision, which allows access to the pericardial space. However, in order for this to be most successful, the surgeon should practice along with the assistance of the echocardiographer as a team to obtain useful views—with the echocardiographer manipulating the controls and the surgeon manipulating the TEE probe over the heart. The same locations used in the ASE epicardial guidelines can be used, but relevant views can be obtained from many locations in the pericardial space.

THE DIAGNOSIS OF INTRACARDIAC AIR AFTER OPEN HEART SURGERY

Once the heart is closed and begins to beat at the end of cardiopulmonary bypass, pockets of air are often present in the left heart and the ascending aorta. Air can change locations quickly. The ability to precisely locate and evacuate air decreases the time from cross-clamp removal to successful weaning from cardiopulmonary bypass and decreases short- and long-term morbidity. Thus it behooves the surgeon to

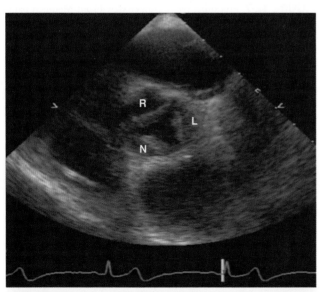

FIGURE 12-2 Epicardial aortic valve short-axis (SAX) view (TTE parasternal AV short-axis equivalent). With the transducer orientation marker facing toward the left shoulder, place the transducer over the aortic valve (AV) groove directly over the AV.

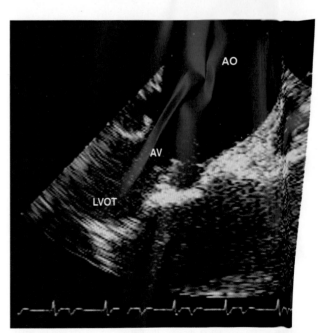

FIGURE 12-3 Epicardial AV long-axis view (TTE Suprasternal long-axis equivalent). With the transducer orientation marker facing toward the right shoulder, place the transducer over the base of the ascending aorta.

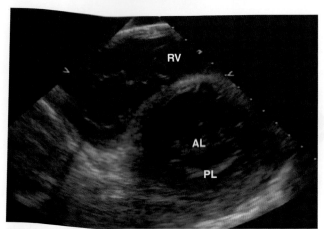

FIGURE 12-4 Epicardial left ventricular (LV) basal SAX view (TTE modified parasternal mitral valve basal SAX equivalent). With the transducer orientation marker facing the left shoulder, place the transducer over the body of the right ventricle (RV). View RV with tricuspid valve and LV with mitral anterior (AL) and posterior (PL) leaflets in short axis.

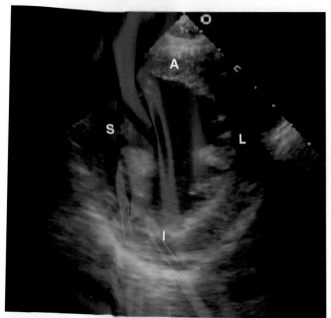

FIGURE 12-5 Epicardial LV mid-SAX view (TTE parasternal LV mid-SAX equivalent). With the transducer orientation marker facing the left shoulder, place the probe over the mid-left anterior descending artery (LAD). A=anterior, S=septal, L=lateral, and I= inferior.

understand how ultrasound imaging can guide this process. The specific views most likely to elucidate air pockets are the left atrial dome view, left and right superior pulmonary vein views, left atrial appendage view, and LV apex and LV septal wall views. Figure 12-9 shows all of these views from the TEE window, but information can also be obtained by the surgeon using the epicardial probe in the event that TEE is not available.

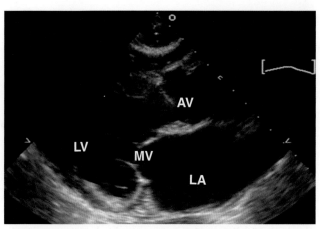

FIGURE 12-6 Epicardial LV long-axis (LAX) view (TTE parasternal LAX equivalent). With the transducer orientation marker facing the right shoulder, place the probe over the mid-right ventricular outflow tract (RVOT).

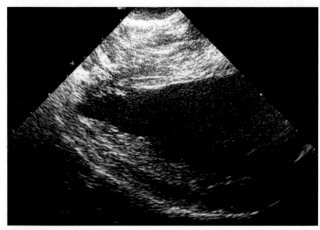

FIGURE 12-7 Epicardial two-chamber view (TTE Modified parasternal LAX equivalent). With the transducer orientation marker facing the right shoulder, place the probe over the mid-LAD artery.

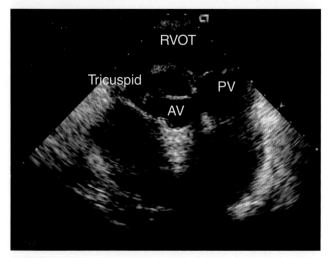

FIGURE 12-8 Epicardial RV outflow tract view (TTE parasternal SAX equivalent). With the transducer orientation marker facing the left shoulder, place the probe over the RVOT.

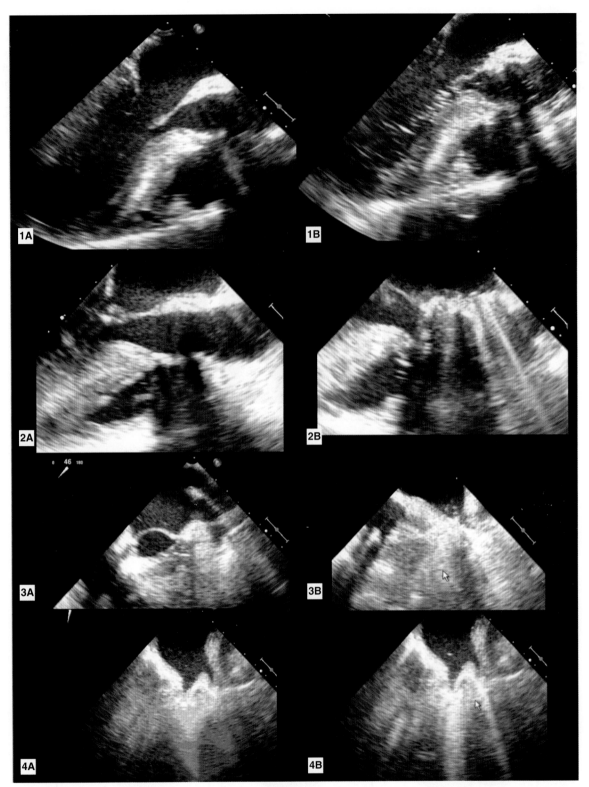

FIGURE 12-9 Diagnosis of intracardiac air at the end of cardiopulmonary bypass—common air locations. The "A" panels show the anatomy without air, and the "B" panels show the same views with air present. Panel 1 is 120 Mid esophageal long axis (120°) with air in the LVOT, Panel 2 shows dome of the LA with air behind the aortic valve in the LA, Panel 3 is a view of the L superior pulmonary vein, and Panel 4 is the right superior pulmonary vein with two comet tail artifacts indicating air in both branches of the vein.

USE OF ECHOCARDIOGRAPHY IN PREOPERATIVE ASSESSMENT OF SPECIFIC CARDIAC DISEASES

Coronary Artery Disease

Echocardiography diagnoses the presence of ischemic heart disease by demonstrating resting LV wall motion abnormalities or inducing new regional wall dysfunction with stress modalities.

The ASE recommends a 16-segment model for the assessment and description of segmental LV wall motion.[13] This model divides the LV basal and mid-ventricular short axis views in a clockwise fashion into anterior, anterolateral, lateral, inferolateral, inferior, inferoseptal and anteroseptal segments. The apex is divided into anterior, lateral, inferior and septal segments (Fig. 12-10). A 17-segment model also exists where there is an additional apical cap to assess myocardial perfusion.

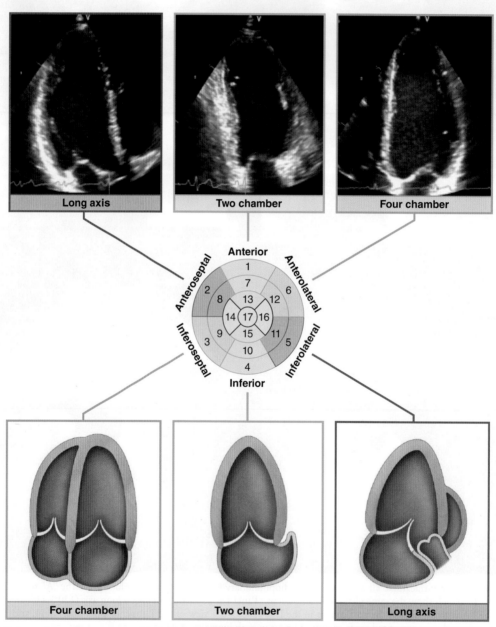

FIGURE 12-10 Echocardiography segments of the left ventricle. Orientation of the apical four-chamber, apical two chamber and apical long axis views in relation to the bull's eye display of the LV segments. (Reproduced with permission from Lang RM, Badano LP, Mor-Avi V, et al: Recommendations for cardiac chamber quantification by echocardiography in adults: an update from the American Society of Echocardiography and the European Association of Cardiovascular Imaging, *J Am Soc Echocardiogr* 2015 Jan;28(1):1-39.)

To assess wall motion, each segment is evaluated in multiple views and reported to be (1) normal or hyperkinetic (normal or enhanced wall thickening), (2) hypokinetic (reduced thickening), (3) akinetic (absent or negligible thickening), or (4) dyskinetic (systolic thinning or bulging).[13]

Resting regional hypokinesis is indicative of ischemia or infarction in a specific coronary artery distribution that supplies the particular segment. Myocardial infarction with scar appears as a thin, highly reflective or bright, akinetic segment. An aneurysm is a thin dyskinetic segment that has a distorted diastolic shape and bulges outward in systole.

STRESS ECHOCARDIOGRAPHY

Stress echocardiography diagnoses and localizes obstructive coronary artery disease (CAD) and is performed with exercise or pharmacological agents. Exercise with supine bicycle or treadmill is physiologic and always preferred to pharmacological stress testing. Patients unable to exercise may be stressed with inotropic drugs (dobutamine), vasodilator agents (adenosine or dipyridamole) or a combination of these. Stress echocardiography has a specificity of 76% and sensitivity of 88%, which are comparable to nuclear stress modalities.[14]

In a normal stress test, there is a hyperdynamic response with an increase in left ventricular ejection fraction (LVEF), decrease in LV cavity size, and absence of new regional wall motion abnormalities. A positive stress test demonstrates new inducible wall motion abnormality in the ischemic segment with stress. Decreases in global LVEF and LV dilatation suggest the presence of severe obstructive CAD such as multivessel CAD or severe left main stenosis.[15]

Intravenous echocardiographic contrast agents can be used to enhance endocardial definition, hence increasing the sensitivity of stress echocardiography for the diagnosis of ischemic heart disease.

MYOCARDIAL VIABILITY

Low-dose dobutamine stress echocardiography is utilized to identify viable myocardium that is stunned or hibernating, and has the potential to recover after revascularization. Viable segments are hypokinetic at rest and typically demonstrate a "biphasic response" with an initial improvement of myocardial contractility with low-dose dobutamine infusion (2.5 to 10 mcg/kg/min). However, at higher doses of dobutamine (20 to 40 mcg/kg/min), the segmental wall motion deteriorates and appears similar or worse than at rest. There is a strong association between myocardial viability on noninvasive testing and improved survival after revascularization in patients with chronic CAD and LV dysfunction.[16] An area that fails to augment is indicative of a nonviable segment or scar.

MECHANICAL COMPLICATIONS OF ISCHEMIC HEART DISEASE

Patients with acute myocardial infarction who develop hemodynamic instability should have an echocardiogram as soon as possible to differentiate mechanical complications that require urgent surgical intervention, from cardiogenic shock secondary to primary 'pump' failure.

RUPTURE OF LEFT VENTRICULAR FREE WALL AND PSEUDOANEURYSM

Rupture of the LV free wall is the second leading cause of in-hospital death, after cardiogenic shock in the setting of an acute myocardial infarction. It is usually associated with a first transmural (usually large anterior) infarct, but not infrequently it can also occur in a small area of lateral necrosis. Acute rupture is catastrophic and rapidly fatal, with death ensuing from cardiac tamponade and pulseless electrical activity. Subacute rupture is a gradual and incomplete rupture of the infarcted area with slow or repetitive bleeding into the pericardial sac causing hemopericardium, which typically occurs through small intramyocardial communications.[17] This leads to a moderate to large pericardial effusion, with or without features of tamponade. Often thrombus forms in the myocardial channels that communicate with the pericardial space, which prevents continued rupture. Thrombus in the pericardial space can be observed as a mass of echoes.

A postmyocardial infarction (post-MI) LV pseudoaneurysm is a rupture of the ventricular free wall contained by local pericardial adhesions or organized thrombus. Echocardiography identifies a narrow neck of the pseudoaneurysm and often spectral and color Doppler imaging shows flow through the communication between the LV and the pericardium.

VENTRICULAR SEPTAL RUPTURE (VSR)

Post myocardial infarction VSRs are uncommon but associated are with high mortality and usually occur in a large transmural, index infarct. Approximately 50 to 66% of postinfarction VSRs occur in anterior infarctions with the rest seen in inferior infarctions.[18,19] A VSR after an anterior MI most often occurs in the distal 1/3 of the septum whereas an inferior MI is associated with rupture of the basal inferior septum. Off-axis 2D and color Doppler imaging are useful, especially to demonstrate the RV exit site (Fig. 12-11). The size of the defect and the pressure difference between the ventricles determine the amount of shunting, which in turns influences mortality. Three-dimensional echocardiography can visualize the defect *en face* to demonstrate the precise location of the rupture and provide size measurements. This can be helpful in determining the suitability of percutaneous device versus surgical closure.[20]

ACUTE MITRAL REGURGITATION (MR)

Acute mitral regurgitation (MR) in the setting of infarction is caused by papillary muscle infarction or rupture. It is usually associated with an inferior infarct as the posteromedial papillary muscle has a single blood supply from the posterior descending artery, whereas the anterolateral papillary muscle has dual blood supply from the left anterior descending artery and the left circumflex artery. Two-dimensional echocardiography demonstrates a flail segment of the mitral valve. The ruptured head of the papillary muscle or corresponding

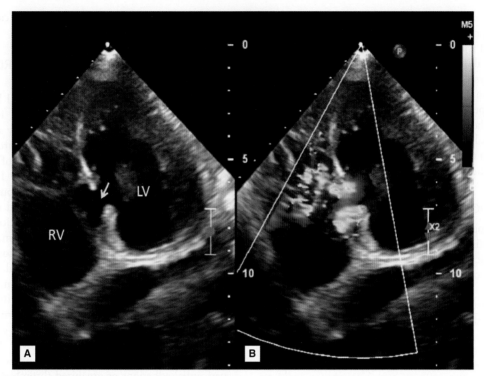

FIGURE 12-11 Post MI ventricular septal rupture. (A) Transthoracic echocardiographic off axis apical four-chamber view displaying the RV exit site of the VSR at the mid-septum. (B) Color Doppler displaying left to right shunting across the VSR in systole. RV = right ventricle, VSR = ventricular septal rupture.

chords may be seen moving randomly within the LV cavity (Fig. 12-12).

Color Doppler can underestimate the severity of acute MR. Due to rapid equalization of left atrial (LA) and LV pressures, coupled with tachycardia and the usually small LA size, the MR jet area can be of short duration and appear deceptively small. Assessment by vena contracta width remains

reliable in this setting. Pulmonary venous systolic flow reversal is a feature which supports the presence of acute severe MR.[21] Assessment with TEE can provide a more definitive diagnosis.

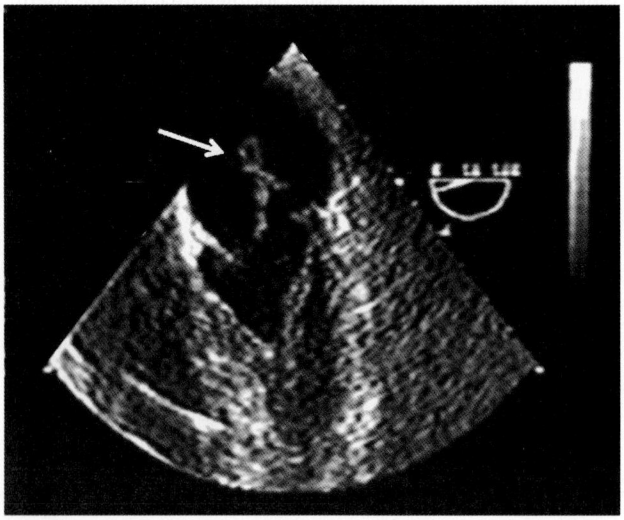

RIGHT VENTRICULAR INFARCTION

Echocardiography is a valuable diagnostic test for RV infarction. The most common features of RV infarction include inferior MI and hemodynamic compromise, often associated with jugular distension and absence of pulmonary edema. RV involvement is associated with higher mortality, arrhythmias, shock and mechanical complications.[22] Echocardiographic signs of RV infarction include RV dilatation and decreased RV free wall function. Impaired function is demonstrated by reduced tricuspid annular plane systolic excursion (TAPSE < 17 mm), and decreased tricuspid annular systolic velocity measured by Doppler tissue imaging (S' velocity < 9.5 cm/s).[13,23] Signs of elevated right atrial (RA) pressure include a dilated inferior vena cava (IVC) that does not collapse >50% on inspiration or bowing of the interatrial septum towards the left.

Mitral Valve Disease

Echocardiography of the mitral valve (MV) includes evaluation of the valvular leaflets, mechanism and grading of severity of mitral stenosis (MS) and mitral regurgitation (MR), and assessment of the effects on the LA and LV. Specifically

FIGURE 12-12 Papillary muscle rupture. Transesophageal echocardiographic four-chamber view of a ruptured papillary muscle head in the left atrium (*arrow*).

this includes 2D imaging of leaflet thickness, coaptation geometry and area, LA size, LV size and function, spectral and color Doppler, valvular gradients, valvular area, and RV systolic pressure (RVSP).

Mitral Regurgitation

ETIOLOGY OF MR

MR can be classified into organic (primary) or functional (secondary). Organic MR is caused by intrinsic valvular disease whereas functional MR occurs as a result of regional or global left ventricular remodeling.

ORGANIC (PRIMARY) MR

The most common cause of MR in the industrialized world is degenerative MV disease. The spectrum of conditions ranges from fibroelastic deficiency causing isolated prolapsed segments due to chordal rupture, to extensive myxomatous disease affecting all segments of the valvular leaflets. The former is most often seen in the older population whilst the latter in younger patients.

Mitral valve prolapse (MVP) is defined by displacement of the body of the leaflets by more than 2 mm behind the annular plane, measured in a long axis view (parasternal or apical views). Due to the saddle shape of the normal mitral annulus with its lowest points anteriorly and posteriorly, assessment in the apical four-chamber view which depicts the medial and lateral MV annulus is not recommended as this can lead to a false diagnosis of MVP.[24]

Flail leaflet is a common sequel of myxomatous disease and occurs due to ruptured chordae. The posterior leaflet (usually middle or P2 scallop) is predominantly affected, resulting in anteriorly directed MR. On echocardiography, the flail portion of the leaflet will exhibit excessive motion and the leaflet tip is displaced into the LA beyond the mitral annular plane (Fig. 12-13).

Other less common causes of primary MR include rheumatic heart disease, infective endocarditis, mitral valve cleft (in conjunction with a partial atrioventricular septal defect, or rarely in isolation), connective tissue diseases, and radiation induced heart disease. Of note, rheumatic mitral regurgitation is caused by commissural thickening, leaflet motion restriction, and loss of central coaptation. This is often accompanied by a degree of stenosis.

ACUTE MR

Acute MR can be assessed by echocardiography and occurs due to disruption of the MV complex. Leaflet destruction or perforation occurs in infective endocarditis. Chordal rupture can be associated with endocarditis, but is more often seen in degenerative mitral valve disease. Papillary muscle dysfunction (rupture or ischemia) occurs with MI (usually the inferior territory). Due to the acute nature of the MR, the LV and LA sizes are often normal. LV systolic function is normal or hyperdynamic, except when the acute MR is due to myocardial ischemia.

FUNCTIONAL (SECONDARY) MR

In functional (or secondary) MR, the mitral valve leaflets and subvalvular apparatus are structurally normal. The MR occurs as a result of LV remodeling from previous infarction or nonischemic cardiomyopathy. Regional or global LV dilatation and remodeling leads to displacement of the papillary muscles, stretching of chordae and subsequent leaflet tethering. The coaptation zone of the mitral valve leaflets is displaced apically and there is incomplete closure of the mitral valve. Dilation of the mitral annulus also contributes to functional MR (Fig. 12-14).

Regional infarction (particularly of the inferoposterior territory) and subsequent local remodeling leads to unbalanced tethering forces that cause asymmetric closure of the valvular

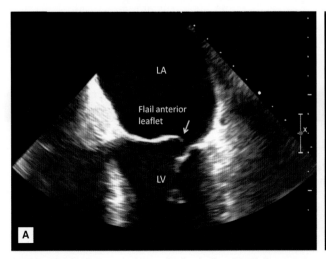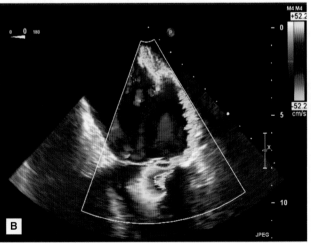

FIGURE 12-13 Flail anterior mitral valve leaflet. (A) Flail anterior mitral valve leaflet displayed on mid-esophageal TEE view with transducer angled at 0°. The leaflet tip is noted to extend into the LA cavity with a large coaptation gaps. (B) This results in severe posterolaterally directed MR.

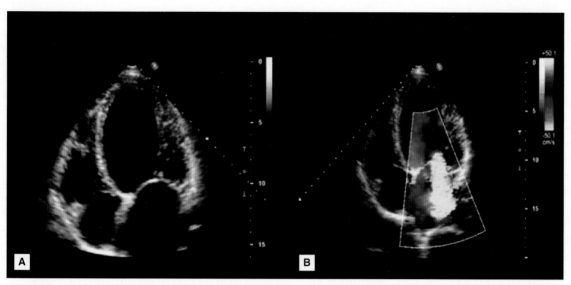

FIGURE 12-14 Incomplete closure of the mitral valve on apical four-chamber TTE. (A) There is global left ventricular dilation resulting in displaced papillary muscles. The mitral valve leaflets are pulled apically resulting in incomplete closure of the mitral valve. (B) Large central jet of mitral regurgitation.

leaflets. In such cases, the anterior leaflet tip may appear to prolapse relative to the tethered posterior leaflet, resulting in a posteriorly directed MR jet. In patients who develop diffuse LV dysfunction and global LV dilation either from ischemic or nonischemic causes, the papillary muscle displacement is more symmetric and the resultant MR is centrally directed.

Carpentier has developed a functional classification to reflect the pathological changes based on leaflet motion that caused MR: normal, excessive, restricted diastolic and restricted systolic motion.[25] (Table 12-1) Both TTE and TEE can be used to identify these patterns.

ECHOCARDIOGRAPHIC ASSESSMENT OF SEVERITY OF MR

The timing for intervention in MR is largely driven by symptoms and the impact of the volume load on LV size and function. Thus, accurate assessment of the severity of MR and the associated hemodynamic consequences is critical. Typical methods and supporting parameters are shown in Table 12-2.

Assessment of severity requires the integration of both qualitative and quantitative methods to minimize the effect of technical or measurement errors. For example, the severity of MR by color Doppler can be influenced by blood pressure, and MR can appear less severe during TEE compared to TTE, especially when lowered blood pressure is secondary to sedation or general anesthesia.

COLOR FLOW DOPPLER

Assessment of the regurgitant jet size and extent into the LA by color flow Doppler is the easiest and most common way to qualitatively assess the severity of MR. Generally speaking, an MR jet area >40% of the LA is consistent with severe MR.[21] However, this method is dependent on multiple hemodynamic and technical factors. For example, the driving blood pressure, machine settings such as gain or velocity scale, and regurgitant jet direction will all influence the appearance of the regurgitant jet area. When it comes to regurgitant jet direction, if MR jets are directed towards the wall of the

TABLE 12-1: Mechanism and Etiology of MR (Carpentier's Classification)

Organic MR		Functional MR	
Normal leaflet motion (Type I)	**Excessive leaflet motion (Type II)**	**Restricted diastolic leaflet motion (Type IIIa)**	**Restricted systolic leaflet motion (Type IIIb)**
• Perforation (endocarditis) • Mitral annular calcification • Mitral annular dilatation • Mitral valve cleft (anterior more common)	• Myxomatous mitral valve disease (most common) • Chordal rupture flail leaflet • Papillary muscle dysfunction	• Rheumatic valve • Drugs (diet pills, ergot) • Radiation heart disease	• Ischemic heart disease (IHD) • Dilated cardiomyopathy

TABLE 12-2: Echocardiographic Methods of Assessment of MR

Semi-quantitative
- Vena contracta
- Jet area/extent

Quantitative: proximal isovelocity surface area (PISA) method
- Effective regurgitant orifice area (EROA)
- Regurgitant volume
- Regurgitant fraction

Supportive
- Pulmonary venous velocity profile
- Continuous wave Doppler velocity profile density
- Transmitral E wave maximum velocity
- LA size
- Pulmonary artery or RV systolic pressure
- LV size and systolic function

LA (ie, eccentric MR jets), then jet energy (velocity) is lost and eccentric MR jets would appear smaller on screen when compared to central MR jets despite similar regurgitant volumes.[26] Color flow should be used to diagnose presence of MR, but quantitative measures should be utilized when more than a small central MR jet is present to avoid this problem.

VENA CONTRACTA WIDTH

The vena contracta is the region of the jet as it exits the regurgitant orifice. When quantified it is an indirect measure of the effective regurgitant orifice area (EROA) and this measurement is less subject to the factors affecting display of the color jet area. The VC is typically measured at the narrowest portion of the MR jet just beyond the coaptation line (Fig. 12-15). When measured as a linear dimension, it is assumed that the regurgitant orifice area is circular; however

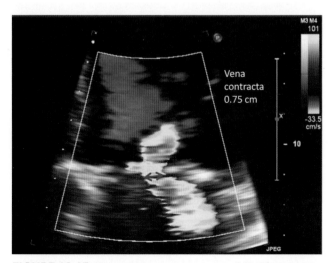

FIGURE 12-15 Vena contracta measurement in MR. The vena contracta is measured at the narrowest portion of the MR jet just beyond the coaptation line (*red double-headed arrow*). A measurement greater than 7 mm is consistent with severe MR.

VC has been found to often be elliptical in functional MR. A VC of >7 mm is consistent with severe MR. Intermediate values (3 to 7 mm) need confirmation by other quantitative methods.

FLOW CONVERGENCE/PROXIMAL ISOVELOCITY SURFACE AREA

Quantitative parameters that assess MR severity include EROA, regurgitant volume (R Vol) and regurgitant fraction. These can be calculated by the proximal isovelocity surface area (PISA) method with echocardiography.

This method relies on the fact that the regurgitant flow at the regurgitant orifice is equal to the product of the cross-section area ($CSA = 2\pi r^2$) of the flow and the peak velocity of the flow (peak MR vel). By adjusting the Nyquist limit (the velocity at which the signal is aliased) towards the direction of the regurgitant jet, a flow convergence zone in the LV with radius r can be depicted and measured.

Assuming that the flow converges onto the regurgitant orifice in an axis-symmetric fashion, the flow of this zone can be identified as $2\pi r^2 \times$ aliasing velocity (V_a) and will also be equal to the flow through the valve. This can be expressed as the product of the EROA and the peak velocity of the MR CW Doppler profile. Rearranging this continuity of flow relation yields:

$$EROA = (2\pi r^2 \times V_a)/\text{peak MR vel}$$

Since stroke volume is quantified as the product of the cross-sectional area and the velocity time integral of the CW MR velocity profile (VTI_{MR}), the regurgitant volume (R Vol) is expressed as

$$R\ Vol\ (cc) = EROA\ (cm^2) \times VTI_{MR}\ (cm)$$

Qualitatively, the presence of flow convergence on TTE at a Nyquist limit of 50 to 60 cm/s should alert the surgeon to the presence of significant MR and prompt an assessment by quantitative method. The two-dimensional isovelocity surface area (2D PISA) approach is performed in either the four- or three-chamber view (Fig. 12-16).

OTHER ECHOCARDIOGRAPHIC METHODS TO QUANTIFY MR

The regurgitant fraction can be calculated from stroke volume calculations if there is no aortic regurgitation present. The regurgitant fraction is the ratio of the volume of MR to the mitral inflow stroke volume. The volume of MR is the difference between the mitral inflow stroke volume and the aortic outflow stroke volume. The stroke volumes are calculated as the product of cross-sectional area (CSA) and velocity time integral (VTI) of flow. Thus, the volume of MR is the difference between (1) the product of the cross-sectional area of the mitral annulus and the VTI at the mitral annulus and (2) the product of the cross-sectional area of the left ventricular outflow tract (LVOT) and the VTI at the LVOT.

Direct measurement of the EROA by 3D planimetry of the vena contracta is feasible, does not require geometric or flow assumptions, and may improve the accuracy of MR grading when compared to the 2D PISA method.[27] However, due to technical limitations such as spatial resolution, 3D

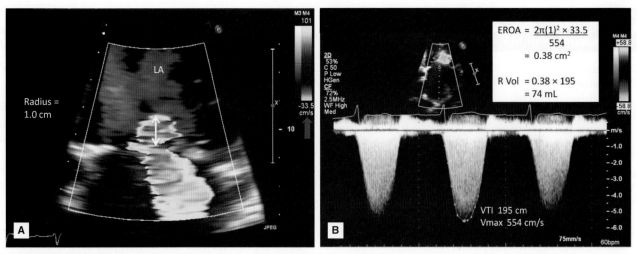

FIGURE 12-16 PISA method to quantify the severity of MR. (A) Measurement of the radius of the flow convergence zone (*double-headed arrow*). The Nyquist limit baseline is shifted in the direction of the MR jet (*red arrow*). (B) The maximum velocity and VTI of the MR jet is measured from the continuous wave Doppler jet profile.

color Doppler to date is used only in TEE and mainly for research applications.

OTHER SUPPORTIVE PARAMETERS

Adjunctive parameters help consolidate determination of the severity of MR when there is discrepancy between the quantified degree of MR and the clinical context.

Systolic reversal of flow in pulmonary veins as assessed by pulse wave Doppler is a reliable marker of severe MR. Blunting alone of systolic flow can accompany mitral regurgitation of increasing severity, but this phenomenon also occurs in atrial fibrillation, increasing age and diastolic dysfunction or other causes of elevated left atrial pressure. Therefore blunting of the pulmonary venous systolic flow lacks specificity for severe MR.

MR of increasing severity leads to increased transmitral forward flow in early diastole, reflected by an elevated E velocity. In the absence of mitral stenosis (MS), a peak E velocity of >1.5 m/s is suggestive of severe MR, whereas the presence of a dominant A wave excludes it. This feature however lacks specificity since anything that raises LA pressure can lead to increased E velocity.

Severe MR produces a dense CW Doppler signal intensity. The CW display of MR velocity can demonstrate a "cut-off" sign, appearing more triangular than parabolic (reflecting the effect of the MR on LA pressure). It may be difficult to capture the full envelope of the MR jet in eccentrically directed MR despite the relatively dense velocity signal.

ECHOCARDIOGRAPHIC QUANTIFICATION OF SEVERE MR

The quantification of severity in functional MR can be difficult. In patients with *functional* MR, adverse outcomes are associated with a smaller calculated EROA compared to *organic* MR. Functional MR will progress due to associated progressive LV systolic dysfunction from the underlying myopathic process and adverse remodeling. There is also

an underestimation of EROA by the 2D echocardiography derived flow convergence method due to the fact that the regurgitant orifice may not be circular. Hence, the threshold to define severe functional MR is lower than that used for organic MR. An EROA ≥ 40 mm² or R Vol ≥ 60 mL indicates severe organic MR while an EROA ≥ 20 mm² or R Vol ≥ 30 mL identifies patients at risk of increased cardiovascular events with functional MR (Table 12-3).[28]

HEMODYNAMIC CONSEQUENCES AND PROGNOSTIC FACTORS OF SEVERE MR

In order to maintain forward stroke volume in chronic significant MR, the LV end diastolic volume increases in response to volume overload. This, in turn, leads to an increased LVEF.

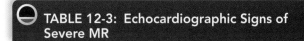

TABLE 12-3: Echocardiographic Signs of Severe MR

- Central jet of MR > 40% LA or holosystolic eccentric jet
- ERO ≥ 0.4 cm² (organic MR), ≥ 0.2 cm² (functional MR)
- Vena contracta ≥ 0.7 cm
- Regurgitant volume ≥ 60 mL (organic MR), ≥ 30 mL (functional MR)
- Regurgitant fraction ≥ 50%
- Systolic flow reversal of the pulmonary veins
- Peak E velocity > 1.5 m/s (in absence of mitral stenosis)
- Moderate-to-severe LA enlargement
- LV enlargement (LVESD > 40 mm)
- Pulmonary hypertension

(Data from Lancellotti P, Tribouilloy C, Hagendorff A, et al: Recommendations for the echocardiographic assessment of native valvular regurgitation: an executive summary from the European Association of Cardiovascular Imaging, *Eur Heart J Cardiovasc Imaging* 2013 Jul;14(7):611-644; Nishimura RA, Otto CM, Bonow RO, et al: 2014 AHA/ACC guideline for the management of patients with valvular heart disease: a report of the American College of Cardiology/American Heart Association Task Force on Practice Guidelines, *J Am Coll Cardiol* 2014 Jun 10;63(22):e57-e185.)

A "normal" LVEF in MR is approximately 70%. Over time, as LV contractility declines, the LV end systolic volume also increases, leading to a reduction in LVEF. Once the LVEF declines below 60%, or when the LV end systolic dimension is >40 mm, this suggests the onset of LV dysfunction, even though the LVEF is still in the normal range. LA dilation also occurs with MR of significant severity (except in acute MR), and therefore the presence of LA dilation suggests chronicity.

In primary MR, negative prognostic features include presence of symptoms, onset of LV dysfunction, pulmonary hypertension (pulmonary artery systolic pressure >50 mm Hg) and onset of new atrial fibrillation.[29,30] Thus these findings are triggers for mitral valve surgery in the 2014 American Heart Association (AHA)/American College of Cardiology (ACC) guidelines (Fig. 12-17).

Mitral valve surgery is a Class I recommendation for chronic severe primary MR and LV dysfunction: LVEF > 30% in symptomatic patients, and LVEF 30 to 60% +/− left ventricular end-systolic diameter (LVESD) ≥ 40 mm in asymptomatic patients. In asymptomatic nonrheumatic MR, a resting pulmonary artery systolic pressure (PASP) of >50 mm Hg or new onset atrial fibrillation (AF) is a Class IIa indication for mitral valve repair.

TEE IN MITRAL REGURGITATION

TTE alone is often helpful in determining the etiology of MR. TEE enables a more detailed and precise anatomic assessment of the mitral valve and should be utilized in more complex lesions or when further anatomic information is required about the mitral valve complex to assist in surgical planning. The proximity of the TEE probe to the mitral valve and the higher imaging frequency result in much improved resolution, which provides a more accurate and higher quality assessment of the vena contracta and PISA. Interrogation of flow in all four pulmonary veins is generally feasible with TEE.

TEE is also particularly useful in infective endocarditis where other potential infected structures can be fully assessed. Three-dimensional echocardiography is widely used as it displays the *en face* "surgeon's view" of the mitral valve and enables direct visualization of mitral valve pathology.

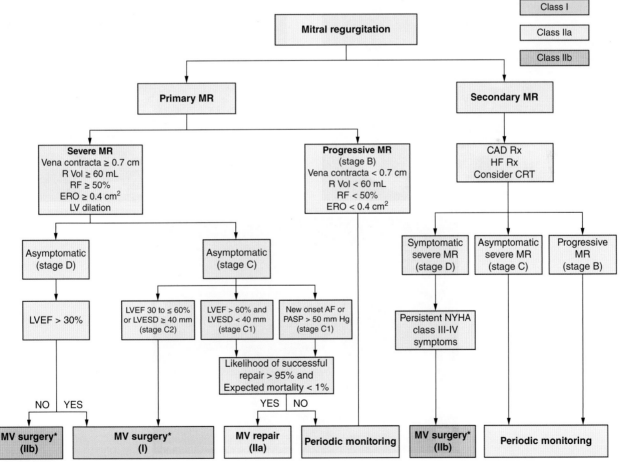

FIGURE 12-17 AHA algorithm for MR. (Reproduced with permission from Nishimura RA, Otto CM, Bonow RO, et al: 2014 AHA/ACC guideline for the management of patients with valvular heart disease: a report of the American College of Cardiology/American Heart Association Task Force on Practice Guidelines, *J Am Coll Cardiol* 2014 Jun 10;63(22):e57-e185.)

EXERCISE ECHOCARDIOGRAPHY IN MITRAL REGURGITATION

Exercise echocardiography may prove helpful when symptoms or degree of LV and LA enlargement are out of proportion to the magnitude of MR on a resting TTE. Worsening MR severity, marked increase in pulmonary arterial pressure (PASP > 60 mm Hg during exercise), impaired exercise ability and symptoms during exercise echocardiography identify patients who may benefit from early surgery.[28]

Mitral Stenosis

The majority of cases of mitral stenosis (MS) are due to rheumatic heart disease. Other less common causes include functional stenosis from severe mitral annular calcification, LA myxoma, congenital mitral stenosis (parachute mitral valve), drug induced valvulopathy, and systemic lupus erythematosus (SLE).

ECHOCARDIOGRAPHIC FEATURES

Rheumatic MS has classic appearances on echocardiography. Thickening of leaflet tips with relative sparing of the midportion and fusion of the commissures leads to a doming or "hockey stick" appearance of the length of the anterior leaflet in diastole, which is best seen in the parasternal long axis view. The posterior leaflet is also thickened and restricted in motion. Commissural thickening and fusion is best appreciated in the short axis view. The subvalvular apparatus, mainly the chordae tendinae, are also thickened and may demonstrate calcification and fusion (Fig. 12-18).

Significant mitral annular calcification is seen in the elderly population. When the annular calcification is bulky enough to reduce the annular area or it extends onto the mitral valve leaflets reducing their excursion, increased diastolic gradients, particular during atrial contraction, are noted across the mitral valve. In these cases, the reduced orifice is most often at the base of the mitral leaflets as opposed to the leaflet tips,

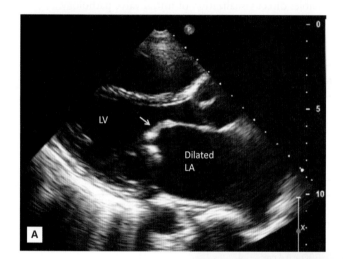

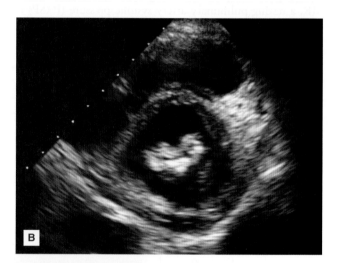

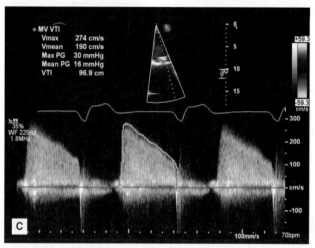

FIGURE 12-18 Mitral stenosis. (A) On parasternal long axis TTE, doming of the anterior mitral valve leaflet results in a "hockey stick deformity" with calcified leaflet tips, causing mitral stenosis. The left atrium is dilated. (B) Planimetry of the mitral valve orifice is performed in the parasternal short axis view. (C) Continuous wave Doppler spectral pattern showing the peak and mean gradients across the stenotic mitral valve. A mean gradient of 16 mm Hg is consistent with severe mitral stenosis.

and the pressure half-time method used to calculate valve area for rheumatic MS cannot be reliably applied.

ASSESSMENT OF SEVERITY OF MITRAL STENOSIS

Anatomic Assessment. The normal MV area (MVA) in adults is 4 to 5 cm². The 2014 AHA/ACC guidelines for valvular heart disease define a MVA of ≤1.5 cm² as severe MS and <1 cm² as very severe MS.[31] This area can be measured directly from echocardiographic images by planimetry in the short axis view. Care must be taken to ensure that the planimetry is performed at the level of the leaflet tips where the orifice is narrowest during the time point where this orifice is the largest in early diastole. Three-dimensional (3D) echocardiography permits proper alignment of the leaflet tips to ensure the most accurate measurement of the MVA.[32]

Doppler Assessment. The mean transmitral gradient is the single-most important factor in describing the severity of MS (mild < 5 mm Hg, moderate 5 to 10 mm Hg, severe >10 mm Hg).[33]

The mean and peak gradients are easily obtained from the mitral inflow CW Doppler signal. However, these measurements are also influenced by heart rate, loading conditions, and stroke volume. With tachycardia, there is reduced diastolic filling time, which leads to an elevation in mean gradient.

The most common Doppler method to calculate MVA is the pressure half-time in milliseconds (PHT), which is the time required for the transmitral pressure gradient to decay to half its value. It has a linear relationship with the MVA; the more severe the MS, the longer the pressure half-time:

$$MVA\ (cm^2) = 220/PHT\ (ms)$$

The constant of 220 is the net compliance constant and is derived empirically in a group of patients with mitral stenosis. Although easy to obtain, PHT measurements can be unreliable in tachycardia or atrial fibrillation (average of 5 beats recommended). PHT is also significantly affected by decreased LV compliance, which results in more rapid equilibration of LA and LV pressures in diastole, leading to a shorter PHT and overestimation of the MVA if the constant of 220 is utilized. For this reason, MVA by PHT can be less reliable in patients with advancing age, hypertension, diabetes, and aortic stenosis. Also in the hours immediately following balloon mitral valvuloplasty, the net compliance constant is not accurately represented by the constant of 220.

MVA by the continuity method can be measured in the absence of MR or aortic regurgitation (AR):

$$MVA = SV_{LVOT}/VTI_{MS}$$

The PISA method, which requires an angle correction to account for the funnel shape of the accelerating mitral valve inflow in MS, is seldom used in clinical practice.

Transesophageal Echocardiography in Mitral Stenosis. A high-quality TTE is often sufficient for the diagnosis and quantification of mitral stenosis. TEE however has incremental value for assessment of associated left atrial body or appendage thrombus, or if TTE images of the valve are suboptimal.

Severe MS. Severe MS is defined by a series of echocardiographic variables. These include: a mitral valve area < 1.5 cm², a mean gradient > 10 mm Hg, a diastolic pressure half time ≥ 150 ms and an RV systolic pressure > 50 mm Hg.

Mitral Stenosis Valve Morphology Score. Percutaneous mitral balloon valvuloplasty (PMBV) is considered first-line therapy when intervention is indicated in mitral stenosis. Mitral valve surgery is generally reserved for patients who are unsuitable candidates for or fail PMBV. Features favoring surgical interventions include moderate-to-severe MR, extensive leaflet and subvalvular thickening, fibrosis and calcification.

The valvular morphology or Wilkins' score is most commonly used in TTE to assess four components of the mitral valve and the summed score describes suitability for PMBV (Table 12-4).[34] A Wilkins' score of >8 and/or presence of moderate MR suggests that the valve will have a low probability of PMBV success and a surgical approach is advisable.

● TABLE 12-4: Wilkins' Score to Assess Suitability for Percutaneous Mitral Balloon Valvuloplasty

Grade	Leaflet mobility	Subvalvular thickening	Leaflet thickening	Leaflet calcification
1	Highly mobile, only restricted leaflet tips	Minimal thickening just below the MV leaflets	Leaflet thickness 4 to 5 mm	Single area of increased echo brightness
2	Leaflet mid and base have normal mobility	Thickening up to 1/3 of chordal length	Mid-leaflets normal, thickening margins 5 to 8 mm	Scattered areas of brightness confined to leaflet margins
3	Valve continues to move forward in diastole, mainly from the base	Thickening extending to distal 1/3 of chords	Entire leaflet thickening 5 to 8 mm	Brightness extending into midportions of leaflets
4	No or minimal forward movement of the leaflets in diastole	Extensive thickening of all chordal structures	Thickening of all leaflet tissue 8 to 10 mm	Extensive brightness throughout much of the tissue

(Adapted with permission from Wilkins GT, Weyman AE, Abascal VM, et al: Percutaneous balloon dilatation of the mitral valve: an analysis of echocardiographic variables related to outcome and the mechanism of dilatation, *Br Heart J* 1988 Oct;60(4):299-308.)

Stress Echocardiography in Mitral Stenosis. The 2014 AHA/ACC guidelines recommend exercise testing with Doppler to evaluate the response of the mean mitral gradient and pulmonary artery pressure in patients with MS when there is a discrepancy between resting Doppler echocardiographic findings and clinical symptoms or signs.[31] Intervention can be considered if there is a rise in right ventricular systolic pressure to >60 to 70 mm Hg with exercise.

Aortic Valve Disease

AORTIC STENOSIS

Echocardiographic imaging of the stenotic aortic valve includes assessment of the valvular leaflet morphology, motion and thickness, description of the presence and location of calcification, measurement of the aortic root and ascending aorta, as well as quantification of LV function and wall thickness. This is followed by Doppler assessment of the severity of stenosis and the presence or absence of concomitant aortic regurgitation.

Etiology. The most common causes of aortic stenosis (AS) in the developed world are degenerative calcification of a trileaflet valve, or accelerated calcification of a bicuspid valve. Rheumatic AS is more prevalent in the developing world.

A bicuspid aortic valve affects approximately one percent of the population. The most common form involves fusion of the right and left coronary cusps (70–86%) with commissures observed in a horizontal position. This is followed by fusion of the right and noncoronary cusps (~12%) with commissures seen in the vertical orientation.[35] Fusion of the left and noncoronary cusps is seen rarely. The diagnosis of bicuspid valve is made in the short axis view in systole where an elliptical orifice formed by two unequally sized leaflets is present. However, when a raphe (fusion line of two leaflets) is present, the diastolic echocardiographic image may mimic the presence of a third leaflet. In the long axis view, the bicuspid aortic valve demonstrates an asymmetric closure line, systolic doming and, often, diastolic prolapse of the valvular leaflets. Since aortopathy is associated with bicuspid aortic valve, assessment of the aortic root and ascending aorta dimensions is necessary. Unicuspid and quadricuspid valves are rare causes of AS. Unicuspid valves usually have a posteriorly positioned commissure.[36]

Rheumatic AS results in commissural fusion and a narrowed triangular systolic orifice. Calcification is most prominent along the edges of the cusps. Aortic regurgitation and mitral involvement are common associations with rheumatic AS.

Subvalvular and Supravalvular Obstruction. Subvalvular and supravalvular AS are identified by 2D echocardiography and further characterized by Doppler velocity. Subvalvular obstruction may be fixed or dynamic. The former is seen in the form of a congenital discrete membrane or muscle band in the LVOT and the peak velocity typically occurs in mid-systole. A common cause of dynamic obstruction is hypertrophic obstructive cardiomyopathy, where the obstruction usually occurs later in systole. In such cases, the CW Doppler systolic velocity profile appears late peaking or "dagger" shaped. Supravalvular obstruction is rare and typically a congenital condition. It is seen in adults as a recurrent or persistent discrete constriction at the superior aspect of the sinuses of Valsalva, or as a diffuse narrowing of the ascending aorta.[37]

Assessment of Severity of Aortic Stenosis by Echocardiography. Doppler methods to assess the hemodynamic severity of aortic stenosis include the maximum transvalvular velocity (V_{max}) and calculation of the peak and mean pressure gradients. The aortic valve area (AVA) is typically calculated by the continuity equation.[33]

Maximum Velocity and Gradients. The maximum transvalvular velocity is measured using CW Doppler. The velocities across the aortic valve are assessed from multiple transducer positions including apical, suprasternal, and right parasternal locations to ensure that the highest velocity is recorded. Velocities from three beats are averaged in sinus rhythm and at least five beats in irregular rhythms. Postextra systolic beats are not measured. In more severe obstruction, the maximum velocity occurs later in systole and the CW Doppler profile assumes a more rounded shape, reflecting a higher gradient throughout systole.

The peak instantaneous gradient is calculated using the simplified Bernoulli equation:

$$\Delta P = 4(V_{max})^2$$

The mean gradient is typically calculated using a measurement program on the echocardiography machine, which averages the instantaneous gradients over the ejection period.

Aortic Valve Area (AVA). A normal AVA is 3 to 4 cm² and one definition of severe AS is an AVA less than 1 cm². The AVA can be indexed to BSA, with a value ≤0.6 cm²/m² considered severe AS in children, adolescents, and small adults (BSA < 1.5 m², BMI < 22).[33] Indexing to BSA is less applicable to obese patients.

The AVA is calculated based on the concept of continuity of flow: the stroke volume (SV) ejected through the LVOT is equal to the SV that passes though the stenotic aortic valve (Fig. 12-19).

Stroke volume is the product of the VTI of the Doppler-derived flow velocity profile and the CSA of the structure at the level the velocity profile is obtained:

$$SV = CSA \times VTI$$

Continuity of flow is represented by

$$SV_{AV} = SV_{LVOT} \text{ or } CSA_{AV} \times VTI_{AV} = CSA_{LVOT} \times VTI_{LVOT}$$

Solving for the AVA (CSA_{AV}) yields:

$$AVA = (CSA_{LVOT} \times VTI_{LVOT})/VTI_{AV}$$

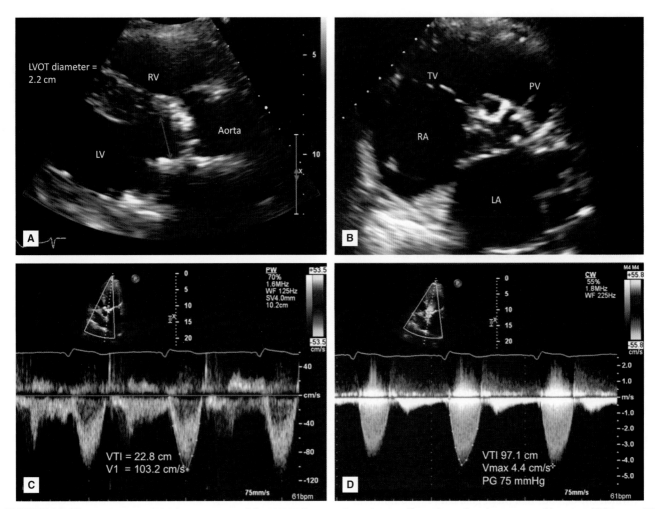

FIGURE 12-19 Aortic stenosis. (A) Measurement of the LVOT diameter (arrow) is usually performed in the parasternal long axis TTE view. (B) Morphology of the aortic valve is determined in the parasternal short axis TTE view. This image shows a calcified trileaflet aortic valve with severe stenosis. (C) Pulse wave Doppler profile with the cursor placed in the LVOT in the apical five-chamber view to obtain the VTI. (D) Continuous wave Doppler profile across the aortic valve reveals a maximum velocity of 4.4 m/s, consistent with severe stenosis. Calculation of the aortic valve area: $CSA_{LVOT} = \pi(2.2/2)^2 = 3.8$ cm^2. AVA $= 3.8 \times 22.8/97.1 = 0.89$ cm^2.

The CSA of the LVOT is assumed to be circular and calculated using the equation for area of a circle:

$$CSA_{LVOT} = \pi(D/2)^2$$

where D is diameter of the LVOT measured in early systole. Of note, often the peak velocity is substituted for the VTI.

Accurate measurement of the LVOT diameter is of utmost importance. Since this parameter is squared for the calculation of the CSA_{LVOT}, deviations in measurement lead to significant errors in the AVA. For example, an under- or over-estimation of a 2-cm LVOT diameter by 5% (1 mm) will result in a 10% error in the LVOT area and AVA. Other potential errors include inaccurate measurement of LVOT or peak AV flow velocity profile when obtained at a nonparallel intercept angle, and failure to interrogate maximum AV velocity from multiple windows to obtain the highest velocity.

One approach that reduces potential sources of error related to inaccurate measurement of the LVOT diameter is to remove the CSA from the equation. The dimensionless index expresses the size of the valvular effective orifice area as a proportion of the CSA_{LVOT}. This index can be calculated using a peak velocity ratio[33] or VTI ratio:

Dimensionless index $= V_{LVOT}/V_{AV}$ or VTI_{LVOT}/VTI_{AV}

A dimensionless index of ≤ 0.25 indicates severe stenosis, corresponding to a valvular area 25% of the normal.[38]

AVA by planimetry is not routinely performed as it can be technically challenging to identify the minimum orifice area at the valvular tips, particularly when extensive calcification is present. Moreover, it is the effective orifice area rather than the anatomic orifice area that is the primary predictor of outcome in severe AS. However, during intra-operative TEE when it may be difficult to obtain accurate LVOT and AV velocities, planimetry can be used as a measure of stenosis.[39]

The 2014 AHA/ACC guidelines classify symptomatic severe AS into three groups: severe high-gradient AS, low

⬤ TABLE 12-5: Classifications of Severe AS

Severe high gradient AS (classical AS)	• AVA ≤ 1 cm² (or AVAi < 0.6 cm²/m²) but may be larger with mixed AS/AR • Or aortic V_{max} ≥ 4 m/s • Or mean gradient ≥ 40 mm Hg
Low flow low gradient AS with reduced LVEF (LVEF < 50%)	• AVA ≤ 1 cm² with resting aortic V_{max} <4 m/s or resting mean gradient <40 mm Hg • Or with dobutamine inotropic stimulation to increase stroke volume, the resultant is AVA ≤ 1 cm² with V_{max} ≥ 4 m/s
Low gradient AS with normal LVEF (paradoxical low flow AS)	• AVA ≤ 1 cm² with V_{max} < 4 m/s or mean gradient < 40 mm Hg • Indexed AVA ≤ 0.6 cm²/m² and • Stroke volume index < 35 mL/m² • Measured when patient is normotensive (systolic BP < 140 mm Hg)

flow low gradient (LFLG) severe AS with reduced LVEF, and low-gradient severe AS with normal LVEF (or paradoxical low flow AS).[31] Echocardiographic definitions for each class are shown in Table 12-5.

Identification of Severe Aortic Stenosis by Echocardiography.

The traditionally well-accepted definition of severe AS is based on the natural history of AS without surgical intervention. Prognosis was shown to be poor with V_{max} > 4 m/s, which corresponds to a mean gradient of > 40 mm Hg.[40] The prognosis of patients was also poorer when AVA < 1 cm².[41] These patients are classified as severe high-gradient AS.

However, a proportion of patients with severe AS have a low velocity and pressure gradient, that is, V_{max} < 4 m/s and mean gradient < 40 mm Hg, despite a calculated AVA of <1 cm². This typically occurs in the setting of decreased LVEF and SV. It is estimated that 5 to 10% of patients with severe AS have LFLG severe AS related to a decrease in LVEF. These patients typically have a dilated LV with markedly decreased LV systolic function due to concurrent ischemic heart disease, other cardiomyopathy and/or secondary to chronic pressure overload from the AS.[42] It is important to ascertain that the calculated low AVA is due to true severe AS, as opposed to pseudo-AS as the former benefits from AVR. In both situations, there is low flow due to the low LVEF, resulting in low V_{max} and low mean transvalvular gradient. In the latter condition, the aortic valve is only mildly or moderately stenotic; however the "weak" LV is unable to generate high enough flow to allow full excursion of the valve leaflets. Therefore, the AVA appears erroneously low. As discussed above, when there is a discrepancy between velocity/gradient and valvular area, it is important to make sure the proper LVOT measurement was used in the AVA calculation.

Low dose dobutamine combined with echocardiography is useful in distinguishing true severe LFLG AS with reduced LVEF from pseudo-severe AS.[43] Patients with pseudo-severe AS will demonstrate an increase in AVA with only a modest increase in transaortic velocity or gradient as transaortic stroke volume increases with the dobutamine infusion. In contrast, patients with true severe AS will have a fixed valve area even with an increase in LV contractility and transaortic flow rate. Severe AS on low dose dobutamine stress echocardiography is defined as a maximum velocity of ≥4.0 m/s with a valve area of ≤1.0 cm² at any point during the test protocol.[33]

Dobutamine stress echo also identifies a subgroup of patients who have a "lack of contractile reserve" by failing to show a 20% increase in stroke volume with dobutamine. This subgroup of patients has a poor prognosis with either medical or surgical therapy.[44]

Low Gradient AS with Normal LVEF.

Low gradient AS with normal LVEF (also known as paradoxical LFLG AS) was first described in 2007.[45] These patients have severe AS defined by an indexed AVA ≤0.6 cm², but paradoxically lower than expected transvalvular gradients due to low stroke volume despite preserved LVEF (>50%). This entity is found in approximately 10 to 25% of patients with severe AS.[42] They consist primarily of elderly women with more pronounced concentric LV hypertrophy resulting in a small LV cavity size and reduced stroke volume (<35 mL/m²). The LV end diastolic diameter is generally <47 mm, and end diastolic volume indexed for BSA < 55 mL/m².[46] Such patients often have signs of diastolic dysfunction with restrictive physiology and decrease in LV compliance and filling.

Identification of this entity is important as patients with symptomatic low-gradient AS with normal LVEF have a poorer prognosis compared with patients with high-gradient severe AS if treated medically rather than surgically.[47] Before this diagnosis is considered, it is important to exclude errors in the component measurements used to calculate aortic valve area (LVOT size, or LVOT and aortic flows).

Hemodynamic Effect on LV.

Echocardiography is useful in assessing the LV response to chronic pressure overload that results in LV hypertrophy. LV systolic function and volumes can be estimated by 2D and 3D echocardiography. Diastolic dysfunction often accompanies LV hypertrophy and is particularly pronounced in low-gradient AS with normal LVEF. Mitral E/e′ > 15, MV E wave deceleration time < 150 ms and a transmitral E/A ratio > 2.5 suggests a restrictive filling pattern.[48] Estimation of pulmonary systolic pressure is obtained from the peak tricuspid regurgitation (TR) velocity using the simplified Bernoulli equation.

Diagnostic Pitfalls with Echocardiography.

Maximum velocity and transvalvular gradients are dependent on LV function and flow. Hence, conditions affecting flow can influence the values of these parameters. For instance, when there is coexisting significant AR, the maximum transvalvular velocity and mean gradient will be higher for a given valvular area because of the high transaortic systolic flow rate.

In the presence of severe MR, transaortic flow rate may be low resulting in a low gradient even when severe AS is present. Valvular area calculations, however, remain accurate.

Use of TEE. TEE allows high-fidelity assessment of the geometry and the height of valvular leaflets relative to one another. This level of detail is not well seen on TTE. The CSA_{LVOT} can also be obtained via 3D multi-planar reconstruction to reduce errors when using the continuity equation to calculation the AVA. TEE is also superior to TTE in obtaining precise measurements of the aortic root and ascending aorta, thus supporting surgical planning for aortic valve repair and guidance in the use of transapical or transcatheter AVR.

The 2014 AHA/ACC guidelines employ multiple echocardiographic parameters discussed above as part of the algorithm to determine the timing for an aortic valve replacement for severe AS (Fig. 12-20).

AORTIC REGURGITATION

Echocardiography provides diagnostic information about the mechanism of aortic regurgitation (AR), assessment of severity of AR, hemodynamic effect of resultant volume overload on the LV, and the morphology and dimensions of the aortic root.

Etiology of Aortic Regurgitation by Echocardiography. Echocardiography can differentiate whether AR occurs as a result of leaflet abnormality, or aortic root dilatation that prevents complete leaflet coaptation. Specifically, echocardiography can identify leaflet abnormalities such as bicuspid aortic valve, degenerative leaflet calcifications, infective endocarditis, and rheumatic thickening. Likewise, dilation of the aortic annulus, sinuses of Valsalva, sinotubular junction, and ascending aorta can be easily quantified with echocardiography. Some causes of aortic dilation include long-standing hypertension, Marfan's syndrome, connective tissue disorders, and aortitis.

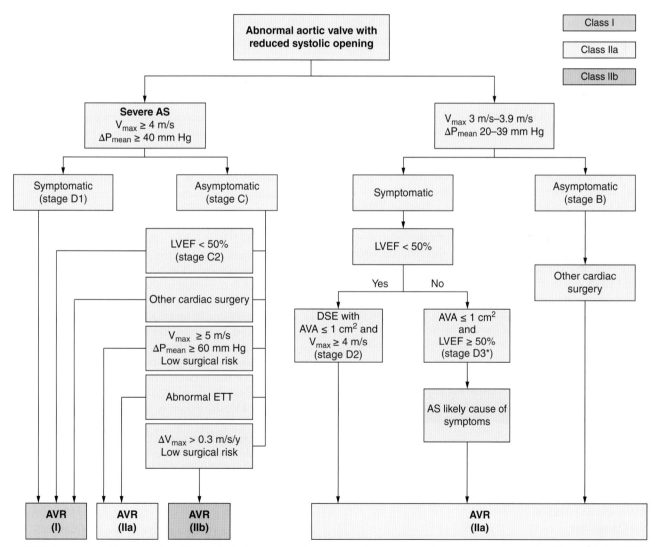

*AVR should be considered with stage D3 AS only if valve obstruction is the most likely cause of symptoms, stroke volume index is <35 mL/m², indexed AVA is ≤0.6 cm²/m², and data are recorded when the patient is normotensive (systolic BP <140 mm Hg).

FIGURE 12-20 AHA/ACC guidelines: Algorithm for management of AS. (Reproduced with permission from Nishimura RA, Otto CM, Bonow RO, et al: 2014 AHA/ACC guideline for the management of patients with valvular heart disease: a report of the American College of Cardiology/American Heart Association Task Force on Practice Guidelines, *J Am Coll Cardiol* 2014 Jun 10;63(22):e57-e185.)

The echocardiographic description of bicuspid aortic valve was discussed earlier under aortic stenosis. Since aortopathy is associated with bicuspid aortic valve, assessment of the aortic root and ascending aorta dimensions are important.

In degenerative calcific AR, the central portions of the cusps are calcified and there is no commissural fusion. In rheumatic AR, in contrast, there is commissural fusion, and the calcification and diffuse thickening of the leaflets at the leaflet free edges result in leaflet retraction and central AR.

Echocardiographic Assessment of AR Severity.
Assessing the severity of AR requires integration of qualitative and quantitative echocardiographic measures, similar to the assessment of MR (Table 12-6).[21]

Color flow imaging is the easiest method to provide a visual estimate of the degree of AR. However, this method is subject to many limitations. Color jet size and length are influenced by the aortic to LV diastolic pressure gradient and LV compliance. Thus, it can poorly correlate with the severity of AR. Jets directed towards the anterior mitral valve leaflet or septum may appear narrow. Jet area and size are often overestimated in the apical views, and for this reason, they are best assessed in the parasternal long axis views due to better axial resolution. The ratio of the proximal jet width (measured from the long axis view) to the diameter of the LV outflow tract of >65% is consistent with severe AR[49] (Fig. 12-21).

The vena contracta width is the narrowest flow diameter at the level of the aortic valve. This is measured in the parasternal long axis view and provides an indirect measure of the EROA. A vena contracta of 6 mm at a Nyquist limit of –60 cm/s correlates with severe AR.[50]

The EROA is an ideal parameter for the assessment and follow up of AR. As discussed for MR, this requires assessment of the flow convergence zone. It is very challenging to derive EROA due to difficulty obtaining high-quality images of the flow convergence zone. Where feasible, the apical five-chamber view is recommended for central regurgitant jets, whereas in eccentric jets, the parasternal long axis view is used. An EROA ≥ 30 mm² or regurgitant volume ≥ 60 mL

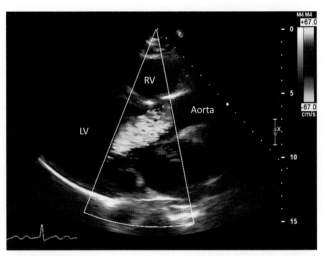

FIGURE 12-21 Aortic regurgitation. Color Doppler parasternal long axis TTE view displays aortic regurgitant jet that fills the entire left ventricular outflow tract, consistent with severe aortic regurgitation.

indicates severe AR.[31] Measurement of this parameter is less common than for MR.

Brief aortic diastolic flow reversal is observed in the aorta in normal studies as measured by pulse wave Doppler in the proximal descending aorta (just distal to the origin of the subclavian artery). In severe AR, there is holodiastolic flow with an end diastolic velocity typically >20 cm/s.[51]

The density of the CW jet in comparison to the antegrade flow provides an estimate of the volume of regurgitation; however, it can be difficult to distinguish moderate from severe regurgitation based on CW jet density alone. CW Doppler of the AR jet is best obtained from the five-chamber view. Eccentrically directed jets may be better obtained from the right parasternal window.

The rate of deceleration of the diastolic regurgitant velocity and the PHT reflect the rate of equalization of aortic and LV diastolic pressure. In severe acute AR, there is rapid equalization resulting in a short PHT. A PHT < 200 ms is consistent with severe AR, whereas >500 ms is consistent with mild AR. However, this parameter is influenced by chamber compliance and pressure. The PHT can be shortened by elevated LV diastolic pressure, or lengthened and normalized with chronic LV adaptations to the severe AR.

Hemodynamic Effects on the LV.
The LV dilates in response to the chronic volume overload of AR and assumes a more spherical shape. LV mass increases, although the increase in wall thickness is modest. Deterioration of LV systolic function is a late and possibly irreversible finding. However, patients with severe LV dysfunction (LVEF ≤ 35%) and severe AR still experience a mortality benefit from AVR.[52]

In the 2014 AHA/ACC guidelines, aortic valve replacement is indicated when LV systolic dysfunction (LVEF < 50%) is present (Class I) and is reasonable with severe LV dilation (LVESD > 50 mm or indexed LVESD indexed > 25 mm/m²) with normal LV systolic function (LVEF ≥ 50%) (Class IIa).

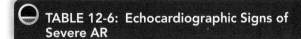

TABLE 12-6: Echocardiographic Signs of Severe AR

Qualitative
- Holodiastolic flow reversal in descending aorta (end-diastolic velocity > 20 cm/s)
- Large central jet (jet width to LVOT diameter ratio > 65%)
- Dense CW signal of AR jet
- Left ventricular dilatation

Semi-Quantitative
- VC width > 6 mm
- Pressure half-time < 200 ms

Quantitative
- EROA ≥ 30 mm²
- Regurgitant Vol ≥ 60 mL

Acute AR. The most common causes of acute AR are infective endocarditis and aortic dissection. The specificity and sensitivity of TTE for the diagnosis of aortic dissection are only 80% and 60% respectively, whereas TEE has a specificity and sensitivity of 95 to 100% and 98 to 100%.[53] Infective endocarditis causes aortic regurgitation via leaflet perforation, destruction, and malcoaptation due to mechanical effects of vegetations on the leaflet tips.

The primary difference in acute and chronic AR on echocardiography is the LV. In chronic AR, the LV has had time to remodel and dilate. Sudden volume overload in acute AR is poorly tolerated by the normally sized LV and this leads to a rapid rise in LV diastolic pressure and pulmonary edema. Due to the rapid equalization of aortic and LV diastolic pressures, the CW velocity profile of the acute AR jet demonstrates a steep slope with a short pressure half-time of <200 ms and pulse wave Doppler of the descending aorta demonstrates no end diastolic velocity. Markedly elevated LV diastolic pressures are indicated by short deceleration time on the mitral inflow and premature closure of the mitral valve on M-mode echocardiography.

TEE in AR. TEE is utilized for assessing the aortic root and ascending aorta dimensions when aortic dissection is suspected and for obtaining precise measurements in the surgical planning phase of aortic valve repair. A magnified view of the aortic valve can provide a cleaner vena contracta measurement than on TTE. Other Doppler assessments are better obtained from TTE due to difficulty obtaining TEE views where the ultrasound beam is parallel to the jet direction. But in the operating room, transgastric TEE can come close to being "on axis" in the LVOT. Also 3D TEE datasets can be manipulated in near real time to obtain perfect alignment and some systems allow reassessment of Doppler information in postanalysis. Also TEE is particularly useful in infective endocarditis to identify vegetations and abscess formation not seen as well on TEE.

Timing of AVR for AR Based on Echocardiographic Parameters. The 2014 AHA/ACC valvular heart disease guidelines utilize echocardiographic parameters in the algorithm for the timing of aortic valve replacement for severe AR. The algorithm is shown in Fig. 12-22.

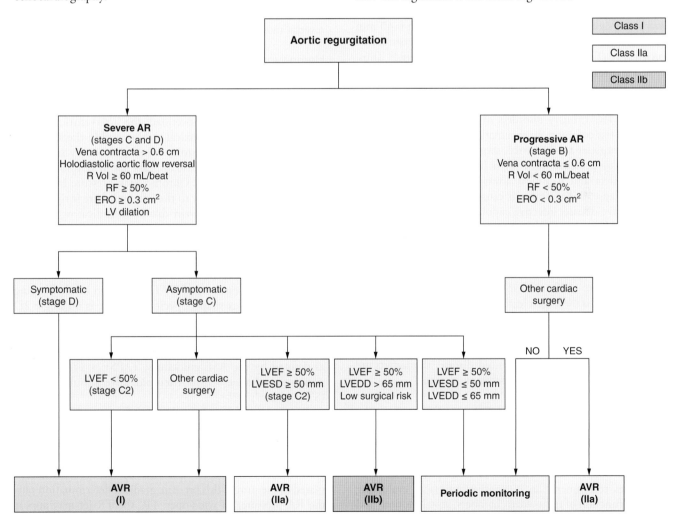

FIGURE 12-22 AR algorithm. (Reproduced with permission from Nishimura RA, Otto CM, Bonow RO, et al: 2014 AHA/ACC guideline for the management of patients with valvular heart disease: a report of the American College of Cardiology/American Heart Association Task Force on Practice Guidelines, *J Am Coll Cardiol* 2014 Jun 10;63(22):e57-e185.)

Tricuspid Valve Disorders

TRICUSPID REGURGITATION

Echocardiographic assessment of TR provides information on valvular morphology, severity of TR, hemodynamic effects on right-sided chambers and significance of left-sided disease. This requires a combination of 2D and Doppler methods to assess leaflet structure and function including thickness, coaptation geometry, gradients, annular dilation, presence of masses, RV size and function, and RV systolic pressure (RVSP).

Functional TR. The most common cause of TR is functional, where the leaflets are structurally normal and regurgitation is caused by incomplete leaflet coaptation due to annular dilatation and leaflet tethering. Any condition that causes RV dilatation and systolic dysfunction can lead to functional TR. The most common causes are left-sided heart disease particularly mitral and aortic valve diseases. Other etiologies include atriopathy related to atrial fibrillation and pulmonary conditions causing pulmonary hypertension. Normal tricuspid valve annulus diameter measured in diastole in the four-chamber view is 28 ± 5 mm. A diastolic annulus > 34 mm is a marker of significant TR. Severe annular dilatation (>40 mm or >21 mm/m²) indicates an increased risk of persistent or progressive TR after isolated mitral valve surgery.[54] Thus, efforts are now focused on identifying patients early who will benefit from tricuspid valve (TV) interventions.

Primary TR. *Primary* disorders of the tricuspid apparatus are much less common. In rheumatic disease, the leaflets and papillary muscles are thickened, shortened and retracted. Tricuspid valve prolapse most often involves the anterior and septal leaflets and is almost always associated with mitral valve prolapse. A flail leaflet is caused by ruptured chordae, degenerative disease, infective endocarditis, trauma, or it can be iatrogenic from central lines, intravalvular pacemaker leads or during endomyocardial biopsies. Intracardiac device leads can also interfere with coaptation if there is impingement of the valvular leaflets.[55] With Ebstein's anomaly, the tricuspid valve leaflets are malformed: in the most common form, the anterior leaflet is the largest leaflet and the posterior and septal leaflets are vestigial and arise posteriorly and apically. Carcinoid disease affects the tricuspid and pulmonary valves. These leaflets appear short, thickened, and fibrotic with restricted motion. In severe cases of carcinoid disease, the leaflets are nonmobile, resulting in wide-open regurgitation.

Assessment of Severity by Echocardiography. The standards for determining the severity of TR are less robust than for MR with limited studies to validate quantitative measures for TR. The European Association of Echocardiography/American Society of Echocardiography (EAE/ASE) guidelines recommend an integrative approach: evaluating size and function of right-sided chambers, septal motion, and various Doppler parameters (Table 12-7).[21,28]

The following parameters are consistent with severe TR: (1) a jet area > 10 cm² (caveat being that the severity

---

◑ TABLE 12-7: Echocardiographic Signs of Severe TR

- Vena contracta width > 0.7 cm
- CW jet density and contour: dense, triangular with early peak ("cut-off" sign)
- EROA ≥ 40 mm²
- Regurgitant volume ≥ 45 mL
- Central jet area > 10 cm²
- Hepatic vein flow: systolic flow reversal
- Tricuspid inflow: E wave dominant (≥1 cm/s)
- Dilated RV, RA and IVC with decreased respirophasic variation
- Interventricular septal flattening in diastole (RV volume overload)

---

of eccentrically directed regurgitant jets may be underestimated); (2) a vena contracta of ≥7 mm;[56] (3) EROA ≥ 40 mm² or regurgitant volume of ≥ 45 mL[57] (although the flow convergence method is rarely used in clinical practice); (4) continuous wave Doppler of the TR jet is dense and complete, and can appear truncated with a triangular contour due to an early peak velocity (cut-off sign); and (5) systolic flow reversal in the hepatic veins (sensitivity of 80%).[6]

Hemodynamic Consequences of TR: Echocardiographic Assessment. Chronic significant TR causes volume overload of the right-sided chambers, which subsequently leads to RV dilatation and failure, and elevated PASP. With RV volume overload, the interventricular septum demonstrates paradoxical motion and in the short axis view, appears flat in diastole. When pulmonary hypertension ensues, the septum also appears flat in systole as a sign of RV pressure overload. Chronic back pressure causes the interatrial septum to bow to the left, and there is right atrial (RA), IVC and hepatic vein dilatation indicating elevated RA pressure.

Impaired RV function has a negative impact on survival outcomes after tricuspid valve surgery[7] and intervention should ideally be performed before RV dysfunction occurs.[58] The assessment of RV function can be challenging due to its complex shape. Specifically, there is no single 2D imaging plane in which the inflow, apical and outflow views of the RV can be imaged simultaneously. Normal RV function can be defined by many echocardiographic parameters as defined by the ASE guidelines: TAPSE > 17 mm, fractional area change >35%, tricuspid valve annular velocity (S') >9.5 cm/s.[13,23]

Estimation of RVSP is obtained from the TR jet peak velocity using the simplified Bernoulli equation (pressure = 4 × velocity²). The velocity of the TR jet itself is not equal to the severity of TR, but rather it is related to the peak systolic gradient between the RV and RA. The RVSP is then estimated as the sum of this pressure gradient determination plus the RA pressure. In wide-open TR, the TR jet may appear less turbulent, with a low jet velocity (<2 m/s) due to rapid equalization of RA and RV pressures. In this scenario the simplified Bernoulli method may underestimate RVSP.

Important Echocardiographic Parameters for Timing of TV Surgery. Severe TR is associated with poor prognosis independent of LV and RV function, RV size and age.[59] TR is most often seen in left-sided disease, particularly mitral or aortic pathologies. The 2014 AHA/ACC guidelines recommend tricuspid valve surgery for patients with severe TR undergoing left-sided valve surgery (Class I).[31] Mild or moderate degrees of TR can progress in up to 25% of patients if left untreated at the time of left-sided valve surgery. Thus, tricuspid valve repair can be beneficial for patients with at least mild functional TR when undergoing left-sided valve surgery, if there is: (1) tricuspid annular dilatation (>40 mm diameter or 21 mm/m^2 indexed to body surface area), (2) prior evidence of right-heart failure (Class IIa); or (3) pulmonary hypertension present (Class IIb).[31] The risk factors for progression of TR include dilated tricuspid annulus (>40 mm diastolic diameter or 21 mm/m^2), degree of RV dysfunction, pulmonary artery hypertension, AF, intra-annular RV pacemaker, or implantable cardioverter-defibrillator leads. Reoperation for severe isolated tricuspid regurgitation after left-sided valve surgery is associated with significant perioperative mortality.

TEE in TR. TEE is seldom required in the preoperative assessment of TR but is useful in infective endocarditis and when assessing for interference of intracardiac device leads on the valve leaflet function. Transgastric views can demonstrate the tricuspid valve in short axis, which is a view not readily seen on TTE, and a transgastric 120° view provides a highly reliable tricuspid annulus measurement for assessing the need for tricuspid repair. Also Doppler analysis of the flow direction in the anterior hepatic vein provides very precise data about the presence of systolic reversal of hepatic vein flow, an important indicator of severe TR.

Prosthetic Valves

Echocardiography with Doppler is the method of choice for the noninvasive evaluation of prosthetic function. Echocardiographic assessment of prosthetic valves includes 2D imaging of the valve, its leaflets and its overall seating, assessment of valvular hemodynamics including transvalvular velocities and gradients, identification and quantification of valvular stenosis or regurgitation; and evaluation of cardiac chamber sizes, left ventricular systolic function and pulmonary artery pressures.

The basic Doppler principles applied to native valves to assess gradients and calculate for effective orifice area (EOA) are also used for prosthetic valves. Different models and sizes of prosthetic valves have different gradients and EOA.[60] The expected ranges of normal gradients and EOA for different types of valves in different valvular positions have been reported and are available in guidelines and other documents.[60]

Peak instantaneous pressure gradient is calculated by the simplified Bernoulli equation as previously described (see the Aortic Stenosis section). The EOA of the prosthetic aortic valve is calculated from the continuity equation, similar to native stenotic aortic valves. For prosthetic aortic valves, it is also reasonable to use the dimensionless velocity index (DVI) to assess for stenosis. The DVI is the ratio of the velocity in the LVOT measured by pulse wave (PW) Doppler to the velocity through the aortic prosthesis measured by CW Doppler. A DVI <0.25 suggests significant valve obstruction if accompanied by an acceleration time > 100 ms (which is the time from transvalvular flow onset to maximum velocity).[60]

The continuity equation can also be applied (in the absence of significant MR or AR) for the mitral valve but is not as frequently used. When applied it is:

$$\text{MV area} = \text{CSA}_{\text{MVannulus}} \times \frac{\text{VTI}_{\text{MVannulus}}}{\text{VTI}_{\text{MV}}}$$

The PHT technique used to quantify the area of native stenotic mitral valves can be used to monitor prosthetic mitral valve function. Prolongation of the PHT when compared to baseline is a reliable indication of obstruction. DVI is increased in mitral prosthetic stenosis or regurgitation. In this scenario, the PHT can help differentiate between the two. A PHT of >200 ms is most consistent with stenosis, whereas a PHT < 130 ms, especially with an elevated peak E wave velocity, suggests regurgitation.[60]

A small degree of regurgitation occurs with virtually all types of mechanical prostheses and can be detected by color Doppler. These jets are normally brief and of low intensity with little penetration into the LA.[61] These "washing jets" are thought to prevent thrombus formation on the edges of the occluders and also reduce friction that might impede rapid valve opening.

PROSTHETIC VALVULAR DYSFUNCTION

The main causes of prosthetic valvular dysfunction requiring surgery are prosthetic valve obstruction manifested by moderate-to-severe stenosis, degeneration manifested by moderate-to-severe central valvular regurgitation, or significant paravalvular regurgitation. Obstructions are most commonly caused by thrombosis, vegetation, pannus or fibrous ingrowth. Degeneration most commonly is due to aging of bioprosthetic leaflets or effects of endocarditis while paravalvular leaks most often are associated with infection.

PROSTHETIC VALVULAR OBSTRUCTION

Almost all prosthetic valves have an EOA that is smaller than the native orifice area. Comparison with the baseline postoperative echocardiogram or with established normal values for valves of that specific type and size is particularly helpful for detection of significant prosthetic valvular obstruction.[60]

Mechanical valvular obstruction or stenosis occurs as a result of thrombus deposition or pannus formation, which interferes with normal leaflet occluder motion. Obstruction may not be obvious on 2D TTE imaging, but is suspected when there is a significant increase in pressure gradient. TEE is the primary means to confirm prosthetic valvular obstruction and identify its causes, particularly for the mitral valve (Fig. 12-23). It can be difficult to differentiate a thrombus

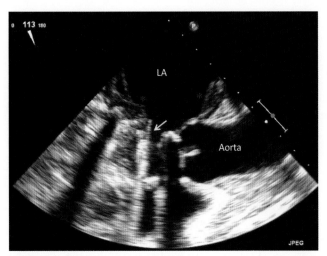

FIGURE 12-23 Mechanical mitral prosthetic valve obstruction. TEE midesophageal long axis view of a thrombosed bileaflet mitral prosthesis. Only one leaflet opens in diastole (*arrow*). The other leaflet is obstructed by thrombus, that is also seen on the left atrial wall (*). LA = left atrium.

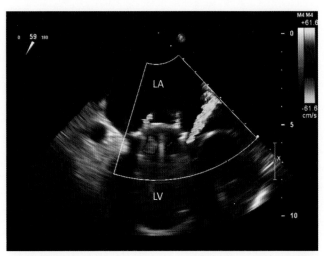

FIGURE 12-24 Mitral paravalvular leak. Mid-esophageal TEE of a mechanical bileaflet mitral prosthesis at transducer angle of 60°. Two physiological washing jets are seen at the periphery of the discs. A large paravalvular leak is noted outside the lateral aspect of the sewing ring. LA = left atrium, LV = left ventricle.

from a pannus on echocardiography. However, a thrombus is usually larger, has a "softer" ultrasound appearance similar to myocardium and may demonstrate mobile elements. Large thrombi (>1 cm in length or 0.8 cm² in area) have a 2.4-fold higher rate of complications per 1 cm² increase in size.[62] Pannus formation is more common in aortic prostheses.[60] For a bioprosthetic valve, fibrosis and calcification of leaflets are the most common causes for obstruction.

Patient prosthesis mismatch (PPM) occurs when the EOA of the prosthesis is too small for the patient's body size and stroke volume requirements, resulting in abnormally high gradients. Most studies have focused on the aortic prosthesis. PPM is considered mild (and therefore not clinically significant) if the indexed EOA of the aortic prosthesis is >0.85 cm²/m², moderate if >0.65 to ≤0.85 cm²/m², and severe if ≤0.65 cm²/m².[63]

PROSTHETIC VALVE PATHOLOGIC REGURGITATION

Pathological regurgitation of a mechanical prosthetic valve is typically due to a paravalvular leak. Paravalvular regurgitation that occurs soon after surgery is usually due to technical factors or infective endocarditis. Late paravalvular regurgitation is almost always due to infective endocarditis, causing suture dehiscence. Significant dehiscence can result in rocking or independent motion of the prosthesis. Occasionally thrombus or pannus formation limits normal occluder closure resulting in significant central valvular regurgitation.

For bioprostheses, pathologic central regurgitation usually occurs as a result of leaflet degeneration and/or calcification. The causes of paravalvular regurgitation are similar to that of mechanical prostheses.

Detection of regurgitation by TTE is challenging for mitral and tricuspid valves due to acoustic shadowing and reverberation artifacts from the prostheses that can obscure

evidence of the Doppler regurgitation signal in the atria. Localization of paravalvular regurgitation may be difficult and can only be diagnosed if the flow is visualized around the outside of the sewing ring. Multiplanar TEE is particular helpful in these situations (Fig. 12-24). Real-time 3D TEE with color Doppler can facilitate the location and quantify the extent of prosthetic regurgitation by visualizing the regurgitant orifice area *en face* from the perspective of the chamber receiving the regurgitation.

Indications for surgical intervention of significant prosthetic valve regurgitation are the same as indications for native regurgitation of the aortic or mitral valve. Specifically, this includes echocardiographic evidence of LV dysfunction including low LVEF or progressive LV dilation.[31]

For a discussion of echocardiographic imaging of infective endocarditis of prosthetic valves, see the section on Infective Endocarditis below.

TTE VERSUS TEE IMAGING OF THE PROSTHETIC VALVES

TTE detects prosthetic valve dysfunction through quantitation of the severity of stenosis and regurgitation by Doppler techniques. TTE also allows assessment of LV size and systolic function, LA size, right heart function and estimation of pulmonary pressures. However, with its better image quality and structure resolution, TEE is superior to determine the actual mechanism of prosthetic valvular dysfunction in addition to providing the same information that TTE is capable of. But in the presence of multiple mechanical prostheses, either method may be limited by echo shadowing from one of the devices, and a combination of both may provide the most complete information. In the operating room this may mean combining TEE with epicardial views.

Infective Endocarditis

Echocardiography plays a pivotal role in the diagnosis of infective endocarditis (IE), identifying underlying predisposing conditions, detecting complications, characterizing the hemodynamic severity of valvular lesions, and assessing ventricular function and pulmonary pressures.

The hallmark of IE on echocardiography is the identification of new vegetations. New or worsening valvular regurgitation, abscess and new partial dehiscence of a prosthetic valve are also important echocardiographic features.[64] A vegetation is defined echocardiographically as a mass that exhibits a motion pattern that is independent of the structure it is attached to, such as a valve or implanted intracardiac device. The sensitivity of TTE for the detection of vegetations ranges from 50 to 90%, depending on the quality of images, the location of the lesion, and the size of the lesion. TEE has far superior sensitivity at 90 to 100%.[31] Identification of vegetations may be difficult in the presence of preexisting lesions (degenerative calcified valves, mitral valve prolapse, prosthetic valves), if the vegetations are small or already embolized.

COMPLICATIONS IDENTIFIED BY ECHOCARDIOGRAPHY

Valvular regurgitation is the most common complication of native valve endocarditis. It can arise from multiple mechanisms: coaptation failure from vegetation interference, leaflet destruction and perforation, or flail leaflet from ruptured chords.

Paravalvular abscess generally affects the aortic valve around the aortic root and can spread to the intervalvular fibrosa and anterior leaflet of the mitral valve. On echocardiography, an abscess is seen as a nonhomogeneous paravalvular thickening often with lucent spaces within it. The abscess can drain into a cardiac cavity and it may appear on echocardiography as a pseudoaneurysm (Fig. 12-25). With color Doppler, the pulsatile flow can be recorded into and out of this echo-free space. Fistula formation is more rare and visualized as a communication between two neighboring cavities through a perforation. The pattern and timing of the flow in the fistula with color Doppler is a function of the relative pressures between the two cavities. Spread of infection into the pericardial space can result in purulent pericarditis. It is difficult using echocardiography to distinguish purulent pericarditis from a sterile inflammatory pericardial effusion; so, the diagnosis is generally made based on clinical findings.

Systemic embolization of the vegetation or portions of the vegetation are a frequent and life-threatening complication. Echocardiographic features of the vegetation that correlate with embolization include large size (>10 mm for left sided lesions and 20 mm for right sided lesions) and excessive mobility especially when associated with the anterior leaflet of the mitral valve.[65,66] Worse prognosis is seen in vegetations >15 mm, increasing vegetation size despite antibiotic therapy, multiple sites of involvement, and extension to extra-valvular structures.[67]

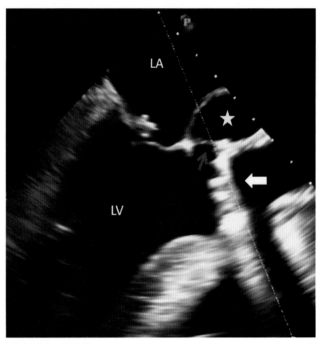

FIGURE 12-25 Prosthetic valve pseudoaneurysm. TEE midesophageal long axis view showing a dehisced mechanical aortic valve (*white arrow*) with pseudoaneurysm formation (star) as a complication of an aortic root abscess. There is communication between the LVOT and the pseudoaneurysm (*red arrow*). LA = left atrium, LV = left ventricle.

PROSTHETIC VALVE ENDOCARDITIS (PVE)

PVE has a lower incidence of vegetations (especially mechanical prostheses) and a higher incidence of annular abscesses and other paravalvular complications. Infection usually involves the region between the sewing ring and the annulus in PVE, leading to abscess formation that can progress to dehiscence, pseudoaneurysms, and fistulae. Echocardiographic features of valve dehiscence include paravalvular regurgitation, and excessive rocking motion of the valve. In bioprosthetic PVE, vegetations can also be seen on the leaflets, which can lead to perforation. Infrequently, large vegetations can cause prosthetic valve obstruction.

TTE and TEE have complementary roles in PVE. TEE is superior for detecting annular abscesses, and smaller vegetations. However, owing to acoustic shadowing from the valve, the anterior portion of the aortic valve and the LV side of the MV prosthesis are not as well seen on TEE and can be better assessed on TTE.[68] Assessment of hemodynamic severity of regurgitation is most often better assessed by TTE. Assessment of Doppler-derived aortic valve pressure gradients is typically better with TTE due to better alignment of the Doppler interrogation with flow.

The 2014 AHA/ACC guidelines for the management of valvular heart disease recommend early surgery during initial hospitalization for valve dysfunction causing heart failure, left-sided IE due to *Staphylococcus aureus*, fungal or highly resistant organism, heart block, annular or aortic abscess, and destructive penetrating lesions (Class I, level of evidence C).

Surgery is recommended in relapsing PVE without other source for portal of infection (Class I, Level of evidence B). Early surgery may be considered in mobile vegetations with a dimension larger than 10 mm (Class IIb, Level of evidence B). Early surgery is reasonable in patients with recurrent emboli and persistent vegetations despite appropriate antibiotic therapy (Class IIa, Level of evidence B).[31]

Diseases of the Aorta

The thoracic aorta can be visualized almost in its entirety by echocardiography. TTE routinely assesses the aortic root and proximal ascending aorta in the parasternal view whereas the aortic arch and its three major branches are seen in the suprasternal view. TEE can depict all portions of the thoracic aorta with high resolution except for a small "blind spot". This blind spot is in the distal ascending aorta just before the innominate artery, and is due to interposition of the right bronchus and trachea between the heart and esophagus. The descending aorta is easily seen from the left subclavian artery to the celiac trunk either in its short or long axis.

AORTIC ANEURYSMS

Aortic root and ascending aorta aneurysms are well seen on echocardiography with reproducible and accurate measurements. Arch and descending aorta aneurysms, however, are better quantified by CT or magnetic resonance imaging (MRI). Since treatment guidelines are based on size, it must be understood that measurements by echocardiography are slightly smaller when compared to CT and MRI. The reason for this is that with echocardiography the measurements of the aorta are typically inner edge to inner edge (internal diameter) while with CT and MRI the outer edge to outer edge (external diameter) is measured.[69] Sinus of Valsalva aneurysms typically affect the right sinus. These are seen protruding into the right atrium in the short axis view and appear like a mobile, "windsock" structure.

ACUTE AORTIC SYNDROMES

The diagnosis of acute aortic syndromes requires speed and accuracy due to the high mortality of these conditions and thus the need for rapid triage to appropriate treatment. TEE has similar diagnostic accuracy to CT and MRI.[70] Additional advantages are absence of radiation, the ability to be performed on unstable patients at the bedside without needing transfer to the imaging equipment, and no need for intravenous contrast whose use is a relative contraindication for patients with renal dysfunction. However, sedation and a fasting state are typically required. Although TEE is the technique of choice, TTE can be utilized initially in the immediate setting to not only diagnose the presence of dissection, but also to assess LV function, the presence of AR and pericardial effusion. A negative TTE does not exclude dissection and another imaging modality must be utilized if clinical suspicion is high. The specificity and sensitivity of TTE for the diagnosis of aortic root dissection are only 80% and 60%

respectively, whereas TEE has a specificity and sensitivity of 95 to 100% and 98 to 100%.[53]

Dissection typically occurs in the setting of aortic dilation. The diagnosis on echocardiography is made by identification of an intimal flap, which divides the aorta into true and false lumens. The true lumen is usually smaller than the false lumen, expands in systole and reveals systolic antegrade flow by Doppler. The false lumen is filled with slow moving blood and *in situ* thrombosis can be present. The points of entry and exit can often be identified by color Doppler.

Reverberation artifacts in a dilated ascending aorta are common and reported to be present in 44 to 55% of studies.[71] While these can be mistaken for a dissection flap they exhibit different characteristics. A dissection flap has independent mobility (low amplitude, high frequency), whereas an artifact moves in parallel motion with the aortic wall (higher amplitude, lower frequency). M-mode echo is often used to display these motion characteristics. Color flow imaging is useful in demonstrating separation of flow by the dissection flap, whereas flow will move through an artifact.

Intramural hematoma occurs as a result of hemorrhage within the medial layer of the aortic wall, with no communication between the media and true lumen. On echocardiographic cross-sectional views this appears as a crescent thickening of the aortic wall. The inner margin is smooth and displacement of intimal calcification due to accumulation of blood within the aortic wall can be seen. In contrast, a penetrating aortic ulcer has a crater-like distortion of the aortic wall, which is often associated with extensive atheroma.[72] A thrombus, represented by soft irregular echoes, often fills the ulceration.

COMPLICATIONS OF AORTIC DISSECTION DETECTED BY ECHOCARDIOGRAPHY

Aortic regurgitation (AR) is a common complication in aortic dissection, occurring in approximately 40 to 76% of patients.[73] Multiple mechanisms account for this and they can be diagnosed by TEE. These include dilation of the aortic root and annulus, disruption of the valvular cusps or annulus, loss of support of the cusps due to extension of the dissection into the aortic root, or prolapse of the intimal flap through the aortic valve leaflets into the LVOT[73] (Fig. 12-26). Identification of the mechanism of AR helps in determining if the aortic valve can be spared at the time of dissection repair.

Pericardial tamponade is observed in <20% of patients with ascending aorta dissection and associated with doubling of mortality.[74] Presence of a pericardial effusion suggests rupture of the aorta has occurred and is associated with poor prognosis. However, the effusion may be secondary solely to inflammation. Determining etiology of the pericardial effusion by echocardiography is often not possible.

During TEE depiction of dissection, the origins of the coronary arteries and extra-aortic arch vessels should be demonstrated to determine the extent of the dissection and whether these vessels are supplied by the true or false lumen. The ostia of the coronary arteries are best seen in a short view of the aortic sinuses of Valsalva. The right coronary artery

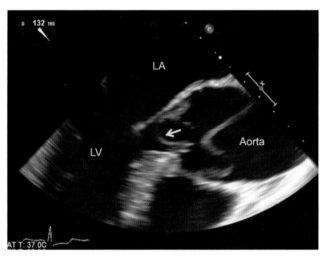

FIGURE 12-26 Aortic root dissection. Aortic root and ascending aorta dissection depicted in this TEE mid-esophageal long axis view. Two dissection flaps are seen: one flap in the aortic root prolapses across the aortic valve in diastole (*arrow*). The ascending aorta is dilated.

is most frequently involved and the presence of a new LV inferior wall motion abnormality can be used as indirect or supporting evidence of this occurrence. On TEE, the origins of the left subclavian and left common carotid arteries are usually easily visualized in an upper esophageal view either in a short axis view or an off-axis view of the aortic arch. However, the origin of the innominate artery is more challenging to visualize on TEE and the suprasternal view of the aortic arch on TTE may be superior for depicting it.

COARCTATION OF AORTA

Coarctation of the aorta is diagnosed on TTE from the suprasternal view. A discrete narrowing of the proximal descending aorta is seen, corresponding with increased turbulence and high velocities detected by Doppler imaging in region of coarctation. In the presence of a hemodynamically significant coarctation, the Doppler display of blood flow in the abdominal aorta persists into diastole in contrast to the normal flow limited to systole.

Pericardial Disease

CARDIAC TAMPONADE

Transthoracic echocardiography is the best diagnostic modality to demonstrate the presence of a pericardial effusion and its hemodynamic significance. In most cases of cardiac tamponade, a moderate-to-large size effusion is present. However, tamponade can occur even in small effusions that have accumulated rapidly in the setting of a normal or noncompliant pericardium. In this situation there is a rapid acute rise in intrapericardial pressure. The sizes of pericardial effusions are typically quantified subjectively: small effusions are generally 50 to 100 mL, moderate 100 to 500 mL, and large greater than 500 mL.

Echocardiographic signs of cardiac tamponade include imaging signs of increased pericardial pressure and Doppler signs of exaggerated respiratory variation in intracardiac flows. Inversion of the RA free wall during ventricular systole (atrial diastole) that persists for greater than one-third of the cardiac cycle is nearly 100% sensitive and is specific for tamponade.[75] Inversion of the RV outflow tract or free wall of the RV in early diastole occurs next; however, this sign may be delayed or absent in the presence of pulmonary hypertension or RV hypertrophy. RV collapse is more specific but less sensitive than RA inversion (Fig. 12-27). With hemodynamically more severe tamponade the duration of diastolic RV wall collapse increases and the sensitivity of this feature increases. Left atrial collapse is a less common but an accurate sign for tamponade. Left ventricular collapse is rare since a higher pericardial pressure is required to distort the thicker LV walls but it can be observed in regional tamponade, which can occur with perioperative or postoperative bleeding.

As the intrapericardial pressure rises during the development of cardiac tamponade, exaggerated respiratory variation in the early mitral and tricuspid inflow (E wave) velocity is noted by pulse wave Doppler. During inspiration, the tricuspid E wave peak velocity increases >60% and the mitral E wave peak velocity decreases by 30%, whereas in expiration, the mitral E velocity increases >30%.[76] These findings reflect the influence of intrathoracic pressure on intracardiac filling as intrapericardial pressure rises. This variation in flow will be reversed during positive pressure ventilation.[77] Dilated inferior vena cava and hepatic veins typically indicate elevated right atrial pressures.

Regional cardiac tamponade, that is tamponade of only a portion of the heart but resulting in systemic hemodynamic affects, is most often noted after cardiac surgery, periocardiotomy, or myocardial infarction. A localized effusion or hematoma that compresses selective cardiac chambers may be

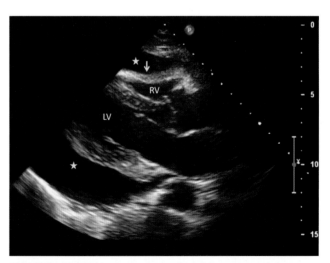

FIGURE 12-27 Cardiac tamponade. TTE parasternal long axis view of a pericardial effusion (star). The anterior portion of the effusion is causing diastolic right ventricular compression (*arrow*) consistent with tamponade.

difficult to visualize on TTE and typically requires a TEE. The Doppler alterations in intracardiac flow may be noted on the TTE in this setting but with a reduced frequency compared to tamponade due to circumferential effusions. Cardiac tamponade seen in the postoperative period can be early (<24 hours), or late (>5 to 7 days). Early tamponade is typically related to surgical bleeding. In this situation, the right-sided chambers, particularly the RA, are usually compressed; however a posterior hematoma may compress the left atrium or LV.[77]

CONSTRICTIVE PERICARDITIS

In the United States and Europe, the most common causes for constrictive pericarditis are postcardiac surgery, idiopathic or secondary to nonspecific viral pericarditis. Other causes include tuberculous pericarditis, radiation pericarditis, and collagen vascular disease.[78]

Typical echocardiographic features include septal motion abnormalities, biatrial enlargement, and alterations in early diastolic mitral inflow. There are two types of septal wall motion abnormalities noted in constrictive pericarditis. The first is called the septal bounce. It is a subtle, early diastolic flutter that is noted on every cardiac cycle. This sign reflects an exaggeration in the difference in timing of passive filling of the right and left ventricles that occurs due to ventricular interdependence. The second septal wall motion abnormality is a brisk movement of the interventricular septum towards the LV in inspiration, followed by a brisk rebound back towards the RV in expiration. This occurs due to an exaggeration in the diastolic ventricular pressure differences induced with respiration. Moderate biatrial enlargement reflects the chronicity of the increase in atrial pressures. A restrictive transmitral pulse wave Doppler filling pattern is observed which is characterized by high early diastolic E velocity, reduced atrial A wave (E/A ratio > 2.5), and short E wave deceleration time (<160 ms).[48,76] This pattern reflects the increase in LA pressure and the reduced filling (due to early equilibration of LA and LV diastolic pressure) from pericardial constraint. Pulse wave Doppler shows a decrease >25% in the mitral inflow velocity and a >40% increase in tricuspid inflow velocity with the first beat of inspiration.[76,4] This variation in flow reflects the fact that the intracardiac pressures are isolated from the intrathoracic pressures due to the thickened pericardium. Thus, as intrathoracic pressure decreases with inspiration, the LA and LV diastolic pressures do not also decrease to the same magnitude and thus flow into the left heart from the pulmonary circulation is reduced. This pattern will be reversed for patients on positive pressure ventilation. The mitral annular motion and velocity assessed by tissue Doppler is normal or elevated (>7 cm/s). In contrast to normal subjects, the lateral annular velocity is lower than septal annular velocity, reflecting tethering of the lateral free wall to the thickened pericardium. The inferior vena cava and hepatic veins are usually dilated indicating elevated right atrial pressure. Prominent diastolic flow reversal in the hepatic veins is a classic finding in pericardial constriction. Some of

the Doppler signs of constrictive pericarditis can be difficult to differentiate from those noted with restrictive cardiomyopathy since that process is also associated with elevated LA pressure and early diastolic pressure equilibration (restrictive filling). However, in restrictive cardiomyopathy the respiratory variation in the Doppler pattern is not present.[79]

Perioperative ECHO Guidance

The cardiac surgeon should develop a pattern of close communication with the echocardiographer, especially in the intraoperative setting. It is important to integrate imaging information into cardiac surgical practice and be willing to change the plan based on the ultrasound data. The surgeon can enhance outcomes by developing and communicating expectations for ultrasound data specific to the operation being performed. Based on data, the echocardiographer should be expected to make predictions which can help the surgeon to choose appropriate surgical techniques to optimize outcomes.[83] Examples of specific data elements and predictions are listed in Table 12-8.

In demanding operations such as aortic and mitral valve repair, communication between surgeon and echocardiographer is ideally a two-way street. The intraoperative

TABLE 12-8: Perioperative ECHO Guidance

Operation	Expected measurements	Echo-based predictions
Mitral repair	Mechanism of MR	Ring or band size
	Leaflet heights	SAM potential
	Distance from Cx coronary to P1 annulus	Size of prosthesis if repair fails
	Coaptation depth potential	Potential for
	Quantitation of tethering	Cx coronary
	LA size	damage
	LV size	
	Mitral inflow gradient	
	MR quantitation	
	Assessment of AL to LVOT	
Mitral replacement	Same as Mitral repair	Potential for Strut SAM
Aortic repair	Mechanism of AI	Potential to
	Annulus diameter	shorten A2 and
	Diameter of Sinuses of Valsalva	create MR
	Diameter of sinotubular junction	
	Quantitation of aortic regurgitation	
	Quantitation of AV systolic gradient	
Tricuspid repair	Mechanism of TR	Ring or band size
	Annulus dimensions	

echocardiographer can use 3D images to enhance communication in terms of structure and function, and can base predictions on precise 3D TEE measurements. The surgeon can provide feedback to the imaging physician by using a head camera or field camera to share the anatomy and the performed operation.

The, modern cardiac surgeon should prepare himself or herself not only to understand ultrasound data, but also to acquire the skill to generate high-quality ultrasound images via an epicardial ultrasound probe in cases where TEE is not possible. Creating a culture of shared information promotes steep and continuous learning curves on both sides of the ether screen, supports the introduction of new technologies and devices, and can only improve patient outcomes.

REFERENCES

1. Reeves ST, Finley AC, Skubas NJ, et al: Basic perioperative transesophageal echocardiography examination: a consensus statement of the American Society of Echocardiography and the Society of Cardiovascular Anesthesiologists. *J Am Soc Echocardiogr* 2013; 26(5):443-456.
2. Kallmeyer IJ, Collard CD, Fox JA, Body SC, Shernan SK: The safety of intraoperative transesophageal echocardiography: a case series of 7200 cardiac surgical patients. *Anesth Analg* 2001; 92(5):1126-1130.
3. Lennon MJ, Gibbs NM, Weightman WM, Leber J, Ee HC, Yusoff IF: Transesophageal echocardiography-related gastrointestinal complications in cardiac surgical patients. *J Cardiothorac Vasc Anesth* 2005; 19(2):141-145.
4. Stevenson JG: Incidence of complications in pediatric transesophageal echocardiography: experience in 1650 cases. *J Am Soc Echocardiogr* 1999; 12(6):527-532.
5. Daniel WG, Erbel R, Kasper W, et al: Safety of transesophageal echocardiography. A multicenter survey of 10,419 examinations. *Circulation* 1991; 83(3):817-821.
6. American Society of Anesthesiologists and Society of Cardiovascular Anesthesiologists Task Force on Transesophageal Echocardiography: Practice guidelines for perioperative transesophageal echocardiography. an updated report by the American Society of Anesthesiologists and the Society of Cardiovascular Anesthesiologists task force on transesophageal echocardiography. *Anesthesiology* 2010; 112(5):1084-1096.
7. Hilberath JN, Oakes DA, Shernan SK, Bulwer BE, D'Ambra MN, Eltzschig HK: Safety of transesophageal echocardiography. *J Am Soc Echocardiogr* 2010; 23(11):1115-1127; quiz 1220-1221.
8. Cahalan MK, Stewart W, Pearlman A, et al: American Society of Echocardiography and Society of Cardiovascular Anesthesiologists task force guidelines for training in perioperative echocardiography. *J Am Soc Echocardiogr* 2002; 15(6):647-652.
9. Cardiovascular Section of the Canadian Anesthesiologists' Society, Canadian Society of Echocardiography, Beique F, et al: Canadian guidelines for training in adult perioperative transesophageal echocardiography. Recommendations of the cardiovascular section of the Canadian Anesthesiologists' Society and the Canadian Society of Echocardiography. *Can J Cardiol* 2006; 22(12):1015-1027.
10. Quinones MA, Douglas PS, Foster E, et al: ACC/AHA clinical competence statement on echocardiography: a report of the American College of Cardiology/American Heart Association/American College of Physicians-American Society of Internal Medicine task force on clinical competence. *J Am Soc Echocardiogr* 2003; 16(4):379-402.
11. Picard MH, Adams D, Bierig SM, et al: American Society of Echocardiography recommendations for quality echocardiography laboratory operations. *J Am Soc Echocardiogr* 2011; 24(1):1-10.
12. Mathew JP, Glas K, Troianos CA, et al: American Society of Echocardiography/Society of Cardiovascular Anesthesiologists recommendations and guidelines for continuous quality improvement in perioperative echocardiography. *J Am Soc Echocardiogr* 2006; 19(11):1303-1313.
13. Lang RM, Badano LP, Mor-Avi V, et al: Recommendations for cardiac chamber quantification by echocardiography in adults: an update from the American Society of Echocardiography and the European Association of Cardiovascular Imaging. *J Am Soc Echocardiogr* 2015; 28(1):1-39.e14.
14. Garber A, Solomon N: Cost-effectiveness of alternative test strategies for the diagnosis of coronary artery disease. *Ann Intern Med* 1999; 130(9):719-728.
15. Yao SS, Shah A, Bangalore S, Chaudhry FA: Transient ischemic left ventricular cavity dilation is a significant predictor of severe and extensive coronary artery disease and adverse outcome in patients undergoing stress echocardiography. *J Am Soc Echocardiogr* 2007; 20(4):352-358.
16. Allman KC, Shaw LJ, Hachamovitch R, Udelson JE: Myocardial viability testing and impact of revascularization on prognosis in patients with coronary artery disease and left ventricular dysfunction: a meta-analysis. *J Am Coll Cardiol* 2002; 39(7):1151-1158.
17. Purcaro A, Costantini C, Ciampani N, et al: Diagnostic criteria and management of subacute ventricular free wall rupture complicating acute myocardial infarction. *Am J Cardiol* 1997; 80(4):397-405.
18. Menon V, Webb JG, Hillis LD, et al: Outcome and profile of ventricular septal rupture with cardiogenic shock after myocardial infarction: a report from the SHOCK trial registry. *J Am College Cardiol* 2000; 36(3s1):1110-1116.
19. Calvert PA, Cockburn J, Wynne D, et al: Percutaneous closure of postinfarction ventricular septal defect: in-hospital outcomes and long-term follow-up of UK experience. *Circulation* 2014; 129(23):2395-2402.
20. Charakida M, Qureshi S, Simpson JM: 3D echocardiography for planning and guidance of interventional closure of VSD. *JACC: Cardiovasc Imaging* 2013; 6(1):120-123.
21. Zoghbi WA, Enriquez-Sarano M, Foster E, et al: Recommendations for evaluation of the severity of native valvular regurgitation with two-dimensional and Doppler echocardiography. *J Am Soc Echocardiogr* 2003; 16(7):777-802.
22. Mehta SR, Eikelboom JW, Natarajan MK, et al: Impact of right ventricular involvement on mortality and morbidity in patients with inferior myocardial infarction 1. *J Am College Cardiol* 2001; 37(1):37-43.
23. Rudski LG, Lai WW, Afilalo J, et al: Guidelines for the echocardiographic assessment of the right heart in adults: a report from the American Society of Echocardiography endorsed by the European Association of Echocardiography, a registered branch of the European Society of Cardiology, and the Canadian Society of Echocardiography. *J Am Soc Echocardiogr* 2010; 23(7):685-713; quiz 786-788.
24. Levine RA, Handschumacher MD, Sanfilippo AJ, et al: Three-dimensional echocardiographic reconstruction of the mitral valve, with implications for the diagnosis of mitral valve prolapse. *Circulation* 1989; 80(3):589-598.
25. Carpentier A: Cardiac valve surgery—the "French correction": *J Thorac Cardiovasc Surg* 1983; 86(3):323-337.
26. Chen CG, Thomas JD, Anconina J, et al: Impact of impinging wall jet on color Doppler quantification of mitral regurgitation. *Circulation* 1991; 84(2):712-720.
27. Zeng X, Levine RA, Hua L, et al: Diagnostic value of vena contracta area in the quantification of mitral regurgitation severity by color Doppler 3D echocardiography. *Circ Cardiovasc Imaging* 2011; 4(5):506-513.
28. Lancellotti P, Tribouilloy C, Hagendorff A, et al: Recommendations for the echocardiographic assessment of native valvular regurgitation: an executive summary from the European Association of Cardiovascular Imaging. *Eur Heart J—Cardiovas Imaging* 2013; 14(7):611-644. doi: 10.1093/ehjci/jet105.
29. Ghoreishi M, Evans CF, DeFilippi CR, et al: Pulmonary hypertension adversely affects short- and long-term survival after mitral valve operation for mitral regurgitation: implications for timing of surgery. *J Thorac Cardiovasc Surg* 2011; 142(6):1439-1452.
30. Ngaage DL, Schaff HV, Mullany CJ, et al: Influence of preoperative atrial fibrillation on late results of mitral repair: is concomitant ablation justified? *Ann Thorac Surg* 2007; 84(2):434-442; discussion 442-443.
31. Nishimura RA, Otto CM, Bonow RO, et al: 2014 AHA/ACC guidelines for the management of patients with valvular heart disease. A report of the American College of Cardiology/American Heart Association task force on practice guidelines. *J Am College Cardiol* 2014; 63(22):e57-e185.
32. Schlosshan D, Aggarwal G, Mathur G, Allan R, Cranney G: Real-time 3D transesophageal echocardiography for the evaluation of rheumatic mitral stenosis. *JACC Cardiovasc Imaging* 2011; 4(6):580-588.
33. Baumgartner H, Hung J, Bermejo J, et al: Echocardiographic assessment of valve stenosis: EAE/ASE recommendations for clinical practice. *J Am Soc Echocardiogr* 2009; 22(1):1-23; quiz 101-102.

34. Wilkins GT, Weyman AE, Abascal VM, Block PC, Palacios IF: Percutaneous balloon dilatation of the mitral valve: an analysis of echocardiographic variables related to outcome and the mechanism of dilatation. *Br Heart J* 1988; 60(4):299-308.

35. Sabet HY, Edwards WD, Tazelaar HD, Daly RC: Congenitally bicuspid aortic valves: a surgical pathology study of 542 cases (1991 through 1996) and a literature review of 2,715 additional cases. *Mayo Clin Proc* 1999; 74(1):14-26.

36. Chu JW, Picard MH, Agnihotri AK, Fitzsimons MG: Diagnosis of congenital unicuspid aortic valve in adult population: the value and limitation of transesophageal echocardiography. *Echocardiography* 2010; 27(9):1107-1112.

37. Flaker G, Teske D, Kilman J, Hosier D, Wooley C: Supravalvular aortic stenosis. A 20-year clinical perspective and experience with patch aortoplasty. *Am J Cardiol* 1983; 51(2):256-260.

38. Oh JK, Taliercio CP, Holmes DR, Jr, et al: Prediction of the severity of aortic stenosis by doppler aortic valve area determination: prospective doppler-catheterization correlation in 100 patients. *J Am Coll Cardiol* 1988; 11(6):1227-1234.

39. Foster GP, Weissman NJ, Picard MH, Fitzpatrick PJ, Shubrooks SJ, Jr, Zarich SW: Determination of aortic valve area in valvular aortic stenosis by direct measurement using intracardiac echocardiography: a comparison with the gorlin and continuity equations. *J Am Coll Cardiol* 1996; 27(2):392-398.

40. Otto CM, Burwash IG, Legget ME, et al: Prospective study of asymptomatic valvular aortic stenosis. Clinical, echocardiographic, and exercise predictors of outcome. *Circulation* 1997; 95(9):2262-2270.

41. Malouf J, Le Tourneau T, Pellikka P, et al: Aortic valve stenosis in community medical practice: determinants of outcome and implications for aortic valve replacement. *J Thorac Cardiovasc Surg* 2012; 144(6):1421-1427.

42. Pibarot P, Dumesnil JG: Low-flow, low-gradient aortic stenosis with normal and depressed left ventricular ejection fraction. *J Am Coll Cardiol* 2012; 60(19):1845-1853.

43. deFilippi CR, Willett DL, Brickner ME, et al: Usefulness of dobutamine echocardiography in distinguishing severe from nonsevere valvular aortic stenosis in patients with depressed left ventricular function and low transvalvular gradients. *Am J Cardiol* 1995; 75(2):191-194.

44. Monin JL, Monchi M, Gest V, Duval-Moulin AM, Dubois-Rande JL, Gueret P: Aortic stenosis with severe left ventricular dysfunction and low transvalvular pressure gradients: risk stratification by low-dose dobutamine echocardiography. *J Am Coll Cardiol* 2001; 37(8):2101-2107.

45. Hachicha Z, Dumesnil JG, Bogaty P, Pibarot P: Paradoxical low-flow, low-gradient severe aortic stenosis despite preserved ejection fraction is associated with higher afterload and reduced survival. *Circulation* 2007; 115(22):2856-2864.

46. Dumesnil JG, Pibarot P: Low-flow, low-gradient severe aortic stenosis in patients with normal ejection fraction. *Curr Opin Cardiol* 2013; 28(5):524-530.

47. Clavel MA, Dumesnil JG, Capoulade R, Mathieu P, Senechal M, Pibarot P: Outcome of patients with aortic stenosis, small valve area, and low-flow, low-gradient despite preserved left ventricular ejection fraction. *J Am Coll Cardiol* 2012; 60(14):1259-1267.

48. Nagueh SF, Appleton CP, Gillebert TC, et al: Recommendations for the evaluation of left ventricular diastolic function by echocardiography. *J Am Soc Echocardiogr* 2009; 22(2):107-133.

49. Perry GJ, Helmcke F, Nanda NC, Byard C, Soto B: Evaluation of aortic insufficiency by Doppler color flow mapping. *J Am Coll Cardiol* 1987; 9(4):952-959.

50. Tribouilloy CM, Enriquez-Sarano M, Bailey KR, Seward JB, Tajik AJ: Assessment of severity of aortic regurgitation using the width of the vena contracta: a clinical color Doppler imaging study. *Circulation* 2000; 102(5):558-564.

51. Tribouilloy C, Avinee P, Shen WF, Rey JL, Slama M, Lesbre JP: End diastolic flow velocity just beneath the aortic isthmus assessed by pulsed Doppler echocardiography: a new predictor of the aortic regurgitant fraction. *Br Heart J* 1991; 65(1):37-40.

52. Kamath AR, Varadarajan P, Turk R, et al: Survival in patients with severe aortic regurgitation and severe left ventricular dysfunction is improved by aortic valve replacement: results from a cohort of 166 patients with an ejection fraction = 35%. *Circulation* 2009; 120(11 suppl 1):S134-S138.

53. Nienaber CA, von Kodolitsch Y, Nicolas V, et al: The diagnosis of thoracic aortic dissection by noninvasive imaging procedures. *N Engl J Med* 1993; 328(1):1-9.

54. Benedetto U, Melina G, Angeloni E, et al: Prophylactic tricuspid annuloplasty in patients with dilated tricuspid annulus undergoing mitral valve surgery. *J Thorac Cardiovasc Surg* 2012; 143(3):632-638.

55. Mediratta A, Addetia K, Yamat M, et al: 3D echocardiographic location of implantable device leads and mechanism of associated tricuspid regurgitation. *JACC: Cardiovascular Imaging* 2014; 7(4):337-347.

56. Tribouilloy CM, Enriquez-Sarano M, Bailey KR, Tajik AJ, Seward JB: Quantification of tricuspid regurgitation by measuring the width of the vena contracta with Doppler color flow imaging: a clinical study. *J Am Coll Cardiol* 2000; 36(2):472-478.

57. Gonzalez-Vilchez F, Zarauza J, Vazquez de Prada JA, et al: Assessment of tricuspid regurgitation by Doppler color flow imaging: angiographic correlation. *Int J Cardiol* 1994; 44(3):275-283.

58. Kim YJ, Kwon DA, Kim HK, et al: Determinants of surgical outcome in patients with isolated tricuspid regurgitation. *Circulation* 2009; 120(17):1672-1678.

59. Nath J, Foster E, Heidenreich PA: Impact of tricuspid regurgitation on long-term survival. *J Am Coll Cardiol* 2004; 43(3):405-409.

60. Zoghbi WA, Chambers JB, Dumesnil JG, et al: Recommendations for evaluation of prosthetic valves with echocardiography and Doppler ultrasound: a report from the American Society of Echocardiography's guidelines and standards committee and the task force on prosthetic valves, developed in conjunction with the American College of Cardiology Cardiovascular Imaging Committee, Cardiac Imaging Committee of the American Heart Association, the European Association of Echocardiography, a registered branch of the European Society of Cardiology, the Japanese Society of Echocardiography and the Canadian Society of Echocardiography, endorsed by the American College of Cardiology Foundation, American Heart Association, European Association of Echocardiography, a registered branch of the European Society of Cardiology, the Japanese Society of Echocardiography, and Canadian Society of Echocardiography. *J Am Soc Echocardiogr* 2009; 22(9):975-1014; quiz 1082-1084.

61. Flachskampf FA, O'Shea JP, Griffin BP, Guerrero L, Weyman AE, Thomas JD: Patterns of normal transvalvular regurgitation in mechanical valve prostheses. *J Am Coll Cardiol* 1991; 18(6):1493-1498.

62. Tong AT, Roudaut R, Ozkan M, et al: Transesophageal echocardiography improves risk assessment of thrombolysis of prosthetic valve thrombosis: results of the international PRO-TEE registry. *J Am Coll Cardiol* 2004; 43(1):77-84.

63. Blais C, Dumesnil JG, Baillot R, Simard S, Doyle D, Pibarot P: Impact of valve prosthesis-patient mismatch on short-term mortality after aortic valve replacement. *Circulation* 2003; 108(8):983-988.

64. Li JS, Sexton DJ, Mick N, et al: Proposed modifications to the Duke criteria for the diagnosis of infective endocarditis. *Clin Infect Dis* 2000; 30(4):633-638.

65. Sanfilippo AJ, Picard MH, Newell JB, et al: Echocardiographic assessment of patients with infectious endocarditis: prediction of risk for complications. *J Am Coll Cardiol* 1991; 18(5):1191-1199.

66. Hecht SR, Berger M: Right-sided endocarditis in intravenous drug users. prognostic features in 102 episodes. *Ann Intern Med* 1992; 117(7):560-566.

67. Thuny F, Di Salvo G, Belliard O, et al: Risk of embolism and death in infective endocarditis: prognostic value of echocardiography: a prospective multicenter study. *Circulation* 2005; 112(1):69-75.

68. Baddour LM, Wilson WR, Bayer AS, et al: Infective endocarditis: diagnosis, antimicrobial therapy, and management of complications: a statement for healthcare professionals from the Committee on Rheumatic Fever, Endocarditis, and Kawasaki Disease, Council on Cardiovascular Disease in the Young, and the Councils on Clinical Cardiology, Stroke, and Cardiovascular Surgery and Anesthesia, American Heart Association: endorsed by the Infectious Diseases Society of America. *Circulation* 2005; 111(23):e394-e434.

69. Hiratzka LF, Bakris GL, Beckman JA, et al: 2010 ACCF/AHA/AATS/ACR/ASA/SCA/SCAI/SIR/STS/SVM guidelines for the diagnosis and management of patients with thoracic aortic disease: executive summary. A report of the American College of Cardiology Foundation/American Heart Association Task Force on Practice Guidelines, American Association for Thoracic Surgery, American College of Radiology, American Stroke Association, Society of Cardiovascular Anesthesiologists, Society for Cardiovascular Angiography and Interventions, Society of Interventional Radiology, Society of Thoracic Surgeons, and Society for Vascular Medicine. *Catheter Cardiovasc Interv* 2010; 76(2):E43-E86.

70. Shiga T, Wajima Z, Apfel CC, Inoue T, Ohe Y: Diagnostic accuracy of transesophageal echocardiography, helical computed tomography, and magnetic resonance imaging for suspected thoracic aortic dissection: systematic review and meta-analysis. *Arch Intern Med* 2006; 166(13):1350-1356.

71. Evangelista A, Garcia-del-Castillo H, Gonzalez-Alujas T, et al: Diagnosis of ascending aortic dissection by transesophageal echocardiography: utility of M-mode in recognizing artifacts. *J Am Coll Cardiol* 1996; 27(1):102-107.

72. Vilacosta I, San Roman JA, Aragoncillo P, et al: Penetrating atherosclerotic aortic ulcer: documentation by transesophageal echocardiography. *J Am Coll Cardiol* 1998; 32(1):83-89.

73. Erbel R, Aboyans V, Boileau C, et al: 2014 ESC guidelines on the diagnosis and treatment of aortic diseases: document covering acute and chronic aortic diseases of the thoracic and abdominal aorta of the adult. The task force for the diagnosis and treatment of aortic diseases of the European Society of Cardiology (ESC). *Eur Heart J* 2014; 35(41):2873-2926.

74. Gilon D, Mehta RH, Oh JK, et al: Characteristics and in-hospital outcomes of patients with cardiac tamponade complicating type A acute aortic dissection. *Am J Cardiol* 2009; 103(7):1029-1031.

75. Gillam LD, Guyer DE, Gibson TC, King ME, Marshall JE, Weyman AE: Hydrodynamic compression of the right atrium: a new echocardiographic sign of cardiac tamponade. *Circulation* 1983; 68(2):294-301.

76. Klein AL, Abbara S, Agler DA, et al: American Society of Echocardiography clinical recommendations for multimodality cardiovascular imaging of patients with pericardial disease: endorsed by the Society for Cardiovascular Magnetic Resonance and Society of Cardiovascular Computed Tomography. *J Am Soc Echocardiogr* 2013; 26(9):965-1012.e15.

77. Faehnrich JA, Noone RB Jr, White WD, et al: Effects of positive-pressure ventilation, pericardial effusion, and cardiac tamponade on respiratory variation in transmitral flow velocities. *J Cardiothorac Vasc Anesth* 2003; 17(1):45-50.

78. Bertog SC, Thambidorai SK, Parakh K, et al: Constrictive pericarditis: etiology and cause-specific survival after pericardiectomy. *J Am Coll Cardiol* 2004; 43(8):1445-1452.

79. Hatle LK, Appleton CP, Popp RL: Differentiation of constrictive pericarditis and restrictive cardiomyopathy by Doppler echocardiography. *Circulation* 1989; 79(2):357-370.

80. Kathryn E. Glas et al: Guidelines for the Performance of a Comprehensive Intraoperative Epiaortic Ultrasonographic Examination: recommendations of the American Society of Echocardiography and the Society of Cardiovascular Anesthesiologists; Endorsed by the Society of Thoracic Surgeons. *J Am Soc Echocardiogr* 2007; 1227-1235.

81. Reeves ST, Glas KE, Eltzschig H, et al: Guidelines for performing a comprehensive epicardial echocardiography examination: recommendations of the American Society of Echocardiography and the Society of Cardiovascular Anesthesiologists. *Anesth Analg* 2007;105(1):22-8.

82. Allyn JW1, Lennon PF, Siegle JH, Quinn RD, D'Ambra MN: The use of epicardial echocardiography as an adjunct to transesophageal echocardiography for the detection of pulmonary embolism. *Anesth Analg* 2006; 102(3):729-730.

83. Myers PO, Khalpey Z, Maloney AM, Brinster DR, D'Ambra MN, Cohn LH: Edge-to-edge repair for prevention and treatment of mitral valve systolic anterior motion. *J Thorac Cardiovasc Surg* 2013; 146(4):836-840. doi: 10.1016/j.jtcvs.2012.07.051. Epub 2012 Sep 11.

Extracorporeal Circulation

13

John W. Hammon • Michael H. Hines

Cardiopulmonary bypass (CPB) for support during cardiac surgery is unique because blood exposed to foreign, non-endothelial cell surfaces is collected and continuously recirculated throughout the body. This contact with synthetic surfaces within the perfusion circuit, as well as open tissue surfaces within the wound, triggers a defense reaction that involves at least five plasma protein systems and five types of circulating blood cells. This inflammatory response to CPB initiates a powerful thrombotic stimulus and the production, release, and circulation of vasoactive and cytotoxic substances that affect every organ and tissue within the body. Because of this, open-heart surgery (OHS) using CPB is essentially not possible without anticoagulation, usually with heparin; thus the inflammatory response to CPB involves the consequences of exposing *heparinized* blood to foreign surfaces, not lined with endothelial cells.

Although the inflammatory response has been well characterized, the development of a nonthrombogenic artificial surface that would allow heparin-free circulatory support has not yet occurred. This chapter summarizes the application of extracorporeal circulation in adult cardiac surgery, and is divided into three sections. The first section describes the components and operation of perfusion systems and related special topics. The issues of thrombosis and bleeding are addressed in the second section, whereas the humoral response to CPB, including the reaction of blood elements and the inflammatory response are presented later in this chapter. The final section deals with organ damage as a consequence of extracorporeal perfusion (ECP).

PERFUSION SYSTEMS

During CPB for cardiac surgery, blood is typically drained by gravity into the venous reservoir of the heart-lung machine via cannulas placed in the superior vena cava (SVC) and inferior vena cava (IVC) or a single cannula placed in the right atrium. Specialized cannulas can also be placed into the lower IVC through a femoral approach. Blood from the reservoir is then pumped through a hollow fiber oxygenator,

and after appropriate gas exchange takes place, into the systemic arterial system through a cannula placed in the distal ascending aorta, the femoral artery, or the axillary artery (Fig. 13-1). This basic ECP system can be adapted to provide partial or total circulatory and respiratory support or partial support for the left or right heart or for the lungs separately.

The complete heart-lung machine includes many additional components (Fig. 13-2).[1] Most manufacturers consolidate a *hollow-fiber oxygenator, venous reservoir*, and *heat exchanger* into a single unit. A *microfilter-bubble trap* is added to the arterial outflow. Depending on the operation, various suction systems can be used to return blood from the surgical field, cardiac chambers, and/or the aorta, directly back into the cardiotomy reservoir, through a *microfilter and then into* the venous reservoir. Increasing evidence of the potential harmful effects of returning fat and lipid particles from the field into directly into the circulation, have increasingly led surgeons to preferentially use a *cell saver system to collect and wash shed blood within the surgical field*, and return the blood to the patient or circuit as packed red cells. In addition to adjusting pump flow, partially occluding *clamps* on venous and arterial lines allow additional regulation of venous drainage and flow. Access ports for sampling and *sensors* for monitoring pressures, temperatures, oxygen saturation, blood gases, and pH are included within most CPB systems. A separate pump and circuit for the administration of *cardioplegic* solutions at controlled composition, rate, and temperature is usually included in the system. An ultrafilter can be easily added within the circuit for the removal of excess fluid, electrolytes, and some inflammatory mediators, or simply for hemoconcentration.

Venous Cannulation and Drainage

PRINCIPLES OF VENOUS DRAINAGE

Venous blood usually enters the circuit by gravity or siphonage into a venous reservoir placed 40 to 70 cm below the level of the heart. The amount of drainage is determined by central venous pressure, the height differential and any resistance within the system (cannulas, tubing, and connectors).

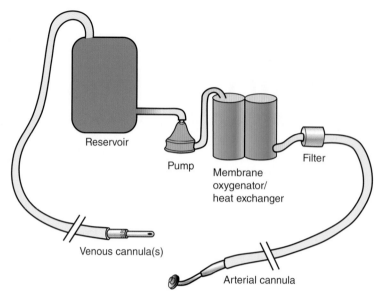

FIGURE 13-1 Basic cardiopulmonary bypass circuit with membrane oxygenator and centrifugal pump.

Successful drainage is dependent on a continuous column of blood or fluid and the absence of air within the system. Central venous pressure is determined by intravascular volume and venous compliance, which is influenced by medications, sympathetic tone, and anesthesia. Inadequate blood volume or excessive siphon pressure may cause compliant venous or atrial walls to collapse against cannular intake openings to produce "chattering" or "fluttering." This phenomenon is corrected by adding volume to the system (circuit and/or patient), or partially occluding the venous line near the inlet to decrease the negative pressure.

VENOUS CANNULAS AND CANNULATION

Most venous cannulas are made out of flexible plastic, which may be stiffened with wire reinforcement to prevent kinking. Cannula tips may be straight or angled and often are constructed of thin, rigid plastic or metal. Cannula sizes are selected based on patient size and weight, anticipated flow rate, and an index of catheter flow characteristics and resistance (provided by the manufacturer), as well as size of the vessel to be cannulated. For an average adult with 60-cm negative siphon pressure, a 30-French cannula in the SVC, and 34 French in the IVC or a single 42-French cavoatrial catheter almost always provides excellent venous drainage. Thin metal tipped right angle cannulas allow placement of smaller diameter cannulas with equal flow characterisitcs, and assist with insertion directly into the vena cavae. Catheters are typically inserted through purse-string guarded incisions in the right atrial appendage, lateral atrial wall, or directly in the SVC and IVC.

Three basic approaches for central venous cannulation are used: bicaval, single atrial, or cavoatrial ("two-stage") (Fig. 13-3). *Bicaval cannulation* and caval tourniquets are

necessary to prevent bleeding into the field, and air entry into the system when the right heart is entered during CPB. Because of coronary sinus return, caval tourniquets should not be tightened without decompressing the right atrium if the heart is not still ejecting. Bicaval cannulation without caval snares is sometimes preferred to facilitate venous return during exposure of the left atrium and mitral valve.

Single venous cannulation is adequate for most aortic valve and coronary artery surgery; however, usually a cavoatrial cannula ("two-stage") is employed (Fig. 13-3B). Introduced via the right atrial appendage, the narrowed distal end is guided into the IVC, leaving the wider proximal portion with multiple side holes to rest within the mid-right atrium. This tends to provide better venous drainage than a single cannula; however, proper positioning is critical.[2] Care must be taken with both a single and two-stage cannula as elevation of the heart may kink the superior cavoatrial junction, decreasing venous return, and potentially, and more importantly, impeding venous outflow from the cerebral circulation.

Venous cannulation can also be accomplished via the femoral or iliac veins through an open or percutaneous technique. This technique is frequently employed in emergency situations, where central venous cannulation may be difficult (as in complex redo sternotomies[3]) or for cardiopulmonary support when a thoracotomy is the approach of choice, as in descending aortic procedures, or redo mitral valve operations. It is also valuable in the support of critically ill or unstable patients prior to the induction of anesthesia, and for applications of CPB that do not require a chest incision. Adequate venous drainage requires the use of larger cannulas (up to 28 French), with the drainage ports either within the intrahepatic IVC or in the right atrium. Transesophageal echocardiography (TEE) can be particularly helpful in assuring proper placement of these cannulas. Specially designed

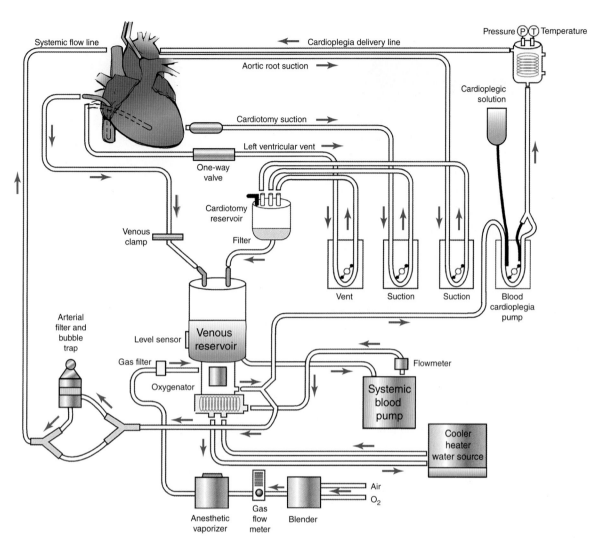

FIGURE 13-2 Diagram of a typical cardiopulmonary bypass circuit with vent, field suction, aortic root suction, and cardioplegic system. Blood is drained from a single "two-stage" catheter into the venous reservoir, which is part of the membrane oxygenator/heat exchanger unit. Venous blood exits the unit and is pumped through the heat exchanger and then the oxygenator. Arterialized blood exits the oxygenator and passes through a filter/bubble trap to the aortic cannula, which is usually placed in the ascending aorta. Blood aspirated from vents and suction systems enters a separate cardiotomy reservoir, which contains a microfilter, before entering the venous reservoir. The cardioplegic system is fed by a spur from the arterial line to which the cardioplegic solution is added and is pumped through a separate heat exchanger into the antegrade or retrograde catheters. Oxygenator gases and water for the heat exchanger are supplied by independent sources.

commercially manufactured long, ultrathin, wire-reinforced catheters are available for this purpose. With recent advances in minimally invasive thoracic surgery, longer two stage cannulas which can be inserted percutaneously via the femoral veins and guided superiorly into the SVC and RA have been developed and are now readily available.

PERSISTENT LEFT SUPERIOR VENA CAVA

A persistent left SVC (PLSVC) is present in 0.3 to 0.5% of the general population and usually drains into the coronary sinus; however, in about 10% of cases it drains into the left atrium.[4] Although more common in association with other congenital defects, it can be seen as an isolated anomaly, and should be suspected when the (left) innominate vein is small

or absent, or when a large coronary sinus (or the PLSVC itself) is seen on baseline TEE.[5]

A PLSVC may complicate the delivery of retrograde cardioplegia or entry into the right heart.[6] If an adequate-sized innominate vein is present (30% of patients), the PLSVC can simply be occluded during CPB, assuming the ostium of the coronary sinus is present, and the coronary venous drainage is not dependent on the PLSVC.[7] If the right SVC is absent (approximately 20% of patients with PLSVC), the left cava cannot be occluded and should be drained. With a normal right SVC (RSVC), but an innominate vein that is absent (40% of patients) or small (about 33%), occlusion of the PLSVC may cause venous hypertension and possible cerebral injury. Although division of the innominate vein during redo-sternotomy or complex surgery such as transplantation

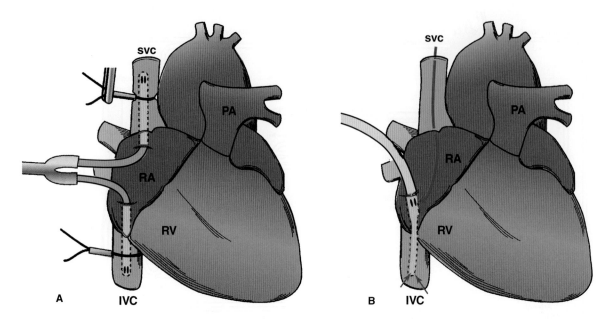

FIGURE 13-3 Placement of venous cannulas. (A) Cannulation of both cavae from incisions in the right atrium. (B) Cannulation using the "two-stage cannula." Blood in the right atrium is captured by vents in the expanded shoulder several inches from the narrower IVC catheter tip.

has been shown to be safe, occlusion of the PLSVC during CPB relies on drainage of the cerebral venous return by the contralateral system, and so special attention must be paid to assure adequate RSVC cannula size, and prevent any kinking of the RSVC. In circumstances in which retrograde cardioplegia is required (severe aortic insufficiency) in the presence of a PLSVC, the retrograde cardioplegia cannula can be directly inserted into the coronary sinus and secured with a pursestring around the orifice of the coronary sinus, and with temporary snaring of the PLSVC, successful retrograde cardioplegia can be delivered.

AUGMENTED OR ASSISTED VENOUS RETURN

Negative pressure can be applied to the venous line to provide assisted venous drainage (AVD) using either a roller or a centrifugal pump system,[8] or by applying a regulated vacuum to a closed hard-shell venous reservoir (vacuum-assisted venous drainage, VAVD).[9] This may permit use of smaller diameter catheters[10] and may be helpful when long, peripheral catheters are used. However augmented negative pressure in the venous line increases the risk of aspirating gross or microscopic air and causing cerebral injury,[11,12] hemolysis, or aspiration of air into the blood phase of hollow fiber oxygenators. Conversely, positive pressure in the venous reservoir can cause air to enter the venous lines and the right heart.[13] These potential complications require special safety monitors and devices and adherence to detailed protocols when using AVD techniques.[13,14]

COMPLICATIONS ASSOCIATED WITH VENOUS CANNULATION AND DRAINAGE

Atrial arrhythmias, bleeding from atrial or vena caval tears, air embolization, venous injury, or obstruction owing to catheter

malposition, reversing arterial and venous lines, and unexpected decannulation can all occur during the conduct of cannulation for CPB. Encircling the vena cavae for snaring may lacerate branches or nearby vessels (eg, right pulmonary artery), or injure the vena cava itself. All of these injuries are more likely in the presence of previous surgery, and need to be recognized and corrected early to assure the proper conduct of CPB and minimize additional complications. During cannulation for minimally invasive procedures where placement is more "blind" than with direct open cannulation techniques, the use of ultrasound and TEE may help guide placement of the various cannulas and potentially prevent very serious complications.

Either before or after CPB, cannulas still in place may compromise venous return to the right atrium. The venous cannulas in the SVC or the superior caval tape may displace or compromise central venous or pulmonary arterial monitoring catheters. Conversely, monitoring catheters may compromise the function of caval tapes, allowing air to enter the venous lines between the cannulas and the catheters or sheaths.

During the conduct of the operation itself, any intracardiac catheter may be trapped by sutures, which may impede removal before or after the wound is closed. Any connection between the atmosphere and cannula intake ports may entrain air to produce an air lock or gaseous microembolism. AVD increases the risk of air entrainment.[15] Finally, improperly placed pursestring sutures may obstruct a cava when tied, particularly in the SVC.[16]

CAUSES OF LOW VENOUS RETURN

Low venous pressure, hypovolemia, drug- or anesthetic-induced venous dilatation, inadequate differential height between the heart and the reservoir, inadequate cannula size, cannula obstruction or kinking, "air-lock," and excessive flow resistance in the drainage system are all possible causes of impaired or inadequate venous return. These can usually be prevented or quickly corrected through close attention to detail, keeping the venous lines visible within the field when possible, and perhaps most importantly, frequent and detailed communication between surgeon and perfusionist. In addition to contributing to inadequate antegrade flow from the pump, partial obstruction of the venous line may lead to right ventricular distention and impair contractility off CPB.

Arterial Cannulation

ARTERIAL CANNULAS

The tip of the arterial cannula is usually the narrowest part of the perfusion system and may produce high pressure differentials, jets, turbulence, and cavitation at the required flows for CPB, particularly if the arterial catheters are small. Most arterial catheters are rated by a performance index, which relates external diameter, flow, and pressure differential.[17] High-velocity jets may damage the aortic wall, dislodge atheroemboli, produce dissections, disturb flow to nearby vessels, and cause cavitation and hemolysis. Pressure differences that exceed 100 mm Hg cause excessive hemolysis and protein denaturation.[18] Weinstein[19] attributed a predominance of left-sided stroke after cardiac surgery to the "sand-blasting" effect of end-hole aortic cannulas directing debris into the left carotid artery. Available aortic catheters with only side ports[20] are designed to minimize jet effects and better distribute arch vessel perfusion and pressure[21] and may be associated with fewer strokes.[19]

Recently a dual-stream aortic perfusion catheter has been developed that features an inflatable horizontal streaming baffle that is designed to protect the arch vessels from atherosclerotic and other emboli and permits selective cerebral hypothermia.[22] Another novel aortic cannula features a side port that deploys a 120-μm mesh filter to remove particulate emboli beyond the ascending aorta.[23] Although this catheter may increase the pressure gradient by 50%,[24] it has been shown to remove an average of eight emboli in 99% of 243 patients studied, and reduce the incidence of cerebral injuries below an expected rate.[25]

CONNECTION TO THE PATIENT

Anatomical sites available for arterial inflow include the proximal aorta, innominate artery and distal arch, femoral, external iliac, axillary, and subclavian arteries. Cannulation can be direct by arterial puncture within a pursestring, through a side graft anastomosed to an arterial vessel, or percutaneous, although usually only in emergency situations. The choice is influenced by the planned operation[26] and distribution of atherosclerotic disease.[27]

ATHEROSCLEROSIS OF THE ASCENDING AORTA

Dislodgement of atheromatous debris from the aortic wall from manipulation,[28] cross-clamping, or the sand-blasting effect of the cannula jet is a major cause of perioperative stroke[29] as well as a risk factor for aortic dissection[30] and postoperative renal dysfunction.[31] Simple palpation has been shown to be sensitive and accurate for detecting severe atherosclerosis than epiaortic ultrasonic scanning.[28,32] Although some have advocated for its use, even TEE views of the middle and distal ascending aorta are often inadequate.[32,33] Epiaortic scanning is now the preferred method of screening in all patients with a history of transient ischemic attack, stroke, severe peripheral vascular disease, palpable calcification in the ascending aorta, calcified aortic knob on chest radiograph, age older than 50 to 60 years, or TEE findings of moderate aortic atherosclerosis.[28] A calcified aorta ("porcelain aorta"), which occurs in 1.2 to 4.3% of patients,[34] is another indication for relocation of the aortic cannula.[35] Alternative sites include the distal aortic arch[34] along with the innominate, axillary-subclavian, or femoral arteries.

ASCENDING AORTIC CANNULATION

The distal ascending aorta is the most common cannulation site because of easy access, and few complications. The cannula is usually placed through a small stab wound within one or two concentric pursestring sutures that are then snared to secure the cannula and provide hemostasis. Risk of dissection may be reduced by avoiding cannulation into the hypertensive aorta, and many surgeons choose to transiently reduce the systemic pressure below 100 mm Hg. The observation of pulsatile back bleeding into the cannula confirms that the tip is within the lumen of the aorta, and then the cannula should be positioned to direct flow to the mid-transverse aorta. The use of a long catheter with the tip placed beyond the left subclavian artery has also been reported.[36] Proper cannula placement is critical[21] and is confirmed by noting pulsatile pressure in the aortic line monitor and equivalent pressure in the radial artery. The cannula must be properly secured in place to prevent inadvertant dislodgement during the conduct of the operation.

Complications include difficult insertion; bleeding; tearing of the aortic wall; intramural or malposition of the cannula tip (in or against the aortic wall, toward the valve, or in an arch vessel)[37]; atheromatous emboli; failure to remove all air from the arterial line after connection; injury to the aortic back wall; high line pressure, indicating obstruction to flow; inadequate or excessive cerebral perfusion[38]; inadvertent decannulation; and aortic dissection.[39] It is essential to monitor aortic line and radial artery pressures and carefully observe the aorta for possible cannula-related complications particularly during the initiation of CPB as well as during the placement of aortic clamps. Asymmetric cooling of the face or neck may suggest a problem with cerebral perfusion. Late bleeding and infected or noninfected false aneurysms are delayed complications of aortic cannulation.

Aortic dissection occurs in 0.01 to 0.09% of aortic cannulations[30,40] and is more common in patients with aortic root disease. Early signs of aortic dissection include discoloration beneath the adventia near the cannulation site, an increase in arterial line pressure, or a sharp reduction in return to the venous reservoir. TEE may be helpful in confirming the diagnosis,[41] but prompt action is necessary to limit the dissection and maintain perfusion. The cannula must be promptly transferred to a peripheral artery or uninvolved distal aorta. Blood pressure should be controlled pharmacologically and perfusion cooling to temperatures less than 20°C initiated. During hypothermic circulatory arrest, the aorta is opened at the original site of cannulation and repaired by direct suture, patch, or circumferential graft.[40] When recognized early, survival rates range from 66 to 85%, but when undiscovered until late during of after the operation, survival is approximately 50%.

CANNULATION OF THE FEMORAL OR ILIAC ARTERY

These vessels are usually the first alternative to aortic cannulation, but may be the primary choice for rapid initiation of CPB for severe bleeding, cardiac arrest, acute intraoperative dissection, or severe shock. It is also a common first choice for limited access cardiac surgery, as well as in selected reoperative patients.[3] Femoral or iliac cannulation limits cannula size but the retrograde distribution of blood flow is similar to antegrade flow.[42] Percutaneous cannulation kits are available for emergency femoral access, and many surgeons also use these long wire reinforced peripheral arterial cannulas with an open Seldinger technique, inserting the cannula through a pursestring in the femoral or iliac vessel by direct cutdown. This may reduce some of the complications of open insertion of large short cannluas, and simplifies cannula removal and arterial repair. Femoral cannulation may be associated with many complications,[3] including tears, dissection, late stenosis or thrombosis, bleeding, lymphatic collection or drainage, groin infection, and cerebral and coronary atheroembolism. In patients with prior aortic dissections, retrograde femoral perfusion may create a malperfusion situation; thus, some surgeons recommend alternative cannulation sites for these patients.[43] Ischemic complications of the distal leg may occur during prolonged (3- to 6-hour) retrograde perfusions,[44,45] unless perfusion is provided to the distal vessel. This may be provided by a small Y catheter in the distal vessel[45] or a side graft sutured to the artery.[46]

Retrograde arterial dissection is the most serious complication of femoral or iliac arterial cannulation and may extend to the aortic root or cause retroperitoneal hemorrhage with an incidence of around 1% or less,[47] and is associated with a mortality of about 50%. This complication is more common in patients greater than 40 years, and in those with significantly diseased arteries. The diagnosis is similar to an aortic cannula dissection and may be confirmed by TEE of the descending thoracic aorta.[41] Antegrade perfusion in the true lumen must be immediately resumed by either the heart itself or cannulation in the distal aorta or axillary-subclavian artery. It is not always necessary to repair the dissected ascending aorta unless it progresses proximally to involve the aortic root.[47]

OTHER SITES FOR ARTERIAL CANNULATION

The axillary-subclavian artery has been increasingly used for cannulation.[48,49] Advantages include freedom from atherosclerosis, antegrade flow into the arch vessels, and protection of the arm and hand by collateral flow. Because of these advantages and the dangers of retrograde perfusion in patients with aortic dissection, some surgeons prefer this cannulation site over femoral access for these patients.[49] Brachial plexus injury and axillary artery thrombosis are reported complications.[48] The axillary artery is approached through a subclavicular incision, whereas the intrathoracic subclavian artery may be cannulated through a thoracotomy.[50]

Occasionally the innominate artery may be cannulated through a pursestring suture without obstructing flow to the right carotid artery by using a 7- or 8-French cannula.[26] The ascending aorta can also be cannulated by passing a cannula through the aortic valve from the left ventricular apex.[51] Coselli and Crawford[52] also describe retrograde perfusion through a graft sewn to the abdominal aorta.

Venous Reservoir

The venous reservoir serves as volume reservoir during CPB and particularly with the body exsanguination of deep hypothermic circulatory arrest. It is placed immediately before the arterial pump when a membrane oxygenator is used (see Fig. 13-1). This reservoir serves as a high-capacitance (ie, low-pressure) receiving chamber for venous return, facilitates gravity drainage, is a venous bubble trap, provides access for drugs, fluids, or blood, and increases the storage capacity for the perfusion system. As much as 1 to 3 L of blood may be translocated from patient to circuit when full CPB is initiated. The venous reservoir also provides several seconds of reaction time if venous return is suddenly decreased or interrupted.

Reservoirs may be rigid (hard) plastic canisters ("open" types) or soft, collapsible plastic bags ("closed" types). The rigid canisters facilitate volume measurements and management of venous air, often have larger capacity, are easier to prime, permit suction for VAVD, and may be less expensive. Some hardshell venous reservoirs incorporate macrofilters and microfilters and can serve as cardiotomy reservoirs to receive vented blood.

Disadvantages include the use of silicon antifoam compounds, which may produce microemboli,[53] and increased activation of blood elements.[54] Soft bag reservoirs eliminate the blood-gas interface and by collapsing reduce the risk of pumping massive air emboli if venous return is suddenly interrupted.

Interest in miniaturization of the circuit has peaked over recent years in an effort to reduce priming volumes and the need for transfusion with its associated consequences as discussed later in this chapter. A variety of these devices are now available. However as with all "advances", there are associated disadvantages, primarily the loss of a safety margin of circuit blood volume for continued perfusion should there be a sudden interruption in venous return.

Oxygenators

Membrane oxygenators imitate the natural lung by interspersing a thin membrane of microporous polypropylene or polymethylpentene (0.3- to 0.8-μm pores), or silicone rubber between the gas and blood phases. Compared with previously used bubble oxygenators, membrane oxygenators are safer, produce less particulate and gaseous microemboli,[55] are less reactive to blood elements, and allow superior control of blood gases.[56] With microporous membranes, plasma-filled pores prevent gas entering blood, but facilitate transfer of both oxygen and CO_2. Because oxygen is poorly diffusible in plasma, blood must be spread as a thin film (approximately 100 μm) over a large area with high differential gas pressures between compartments to achieve oxygenation. Areas of turbulence and secondary flow enhance diffusion of oxygen within blood and thereby improve oxyhemoglobin saturation.[57] Carbon dioxide is highly diffusible in plasma and easily exits the blood compartment despite small differential pressures across the membrane.

The most popular design uses sheaves of hollow fibers (120-200 μm) connected to inlet and outlet manifolds within a hard-shell jacket (Fig. 13-4). The most efficient configuration creates turbulence by passing blood between fibers and oxygen within fibers. Arterial PCO_2 is controlled by gas flow rate, and PO_2 is controlled by the fraction of inspired oxygen (FIO_2) produced by an air-oxygen blender. Modern membrane oxygenators add up to 470 mL of O_2 and remove up to 350 mL CO_2 per minute at 1 to 7 L of flow with priming volumes of 220 to 560 mL and resistances of 12 to 15 mm Hg per liter blood flow. Most units combine a venous reservoir, heat exchanger, and hollow fiber membrane oxygenator into one compact unit.

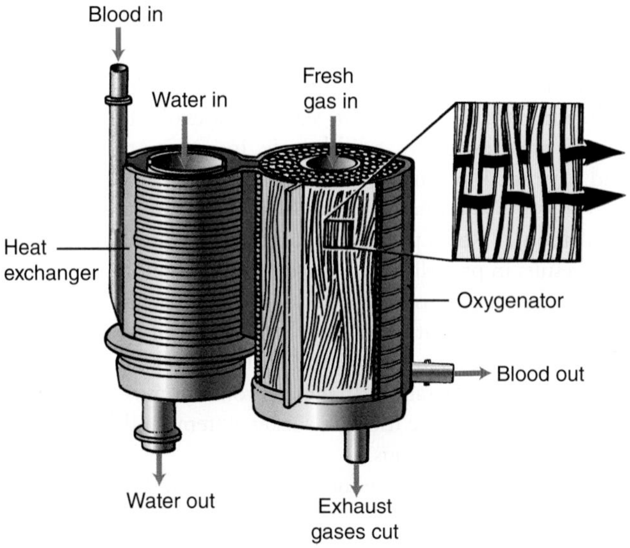

FIGURE 13-4 Diagram of a hollow fiber membrane oxygenator and heat exchanger unit. Blood enters the heat exchanger first and flows over water-cooled or water-warmed coils and then enters the oxygenator to pass between woven strands of hollow fibers. Oxygen enters one end of the bundles of hollow fibers and exits at the opposite end. The hollow fiber bundles are potted at each end to separate the blood and gas compartments. Oxygen and carbon dioxide diffuse in opposite directions across the aggregate large surface of the hollow fibers.

Oxygen and CO_2 diffuse across thin silicone membranes, which are made into envelopes and wound around a spool to produce a spiral coil oxygenator. Gas passes through the envelope and blood passes between the coil windings. Because of protein leakage that frequently occurs with hollow fiber membranes after 8 to 12 hours of use, these spiral coil silicone membranes have been preferred for the prolonged perfusions (days) used in long-term respiratory and cardiac support of extracorporeal membrane oxygenation or "ECMO" systems. More recently, however, the development of polymethylpentene oxygenators have combined the benefit of efficient small surface area hollow fiber oxygenators without the detrimental plasma leakage seen with polypropylene, and have allowed these membranes to be used with both CPB and ECMO.

Other membranes feature a very thin (0.05 μm), solid membrane on the blood side of a highly porous support matrix. This membrane reduces the risk of gas emboli and plasma leakage during prolonged CPB, but may impair transfer of volatile anesthetics.[58]

Flow regulators, flow meters, gas blender, oxygen analyzer, gas filter, and moisture trap are parts of the oxygenator gas supply system used to control the ventilating gases within membrane oxygenators. Often an anesthetic vaporizer is added, but care must be taken to prevent volatile anesthetic liquids from destroying plastic components of the perfusion circuit.

Bubble oxygenators are obsolete in the United States, but may still be used elsewhere for short-term CPB because of low cost and efficiency. Because each bubble presents a new foreign surface to which blood elements react, bubble oxygenators cause progressive injury to blood elements and entrain more gaseous microemboli.[59] In bubble oxygenators, venous blood drains directly into a chamber into which oxygen is infused through a diffusion plate (sparger). The sparger produces thousands of small (approximately 36 μm) oxygen bubbles within blood. Gas exchange occurs across a thin film at the blood-gas interface around each bubble. Carbon dioxide diffuses into the bubble and oxygen diffuses outward into blood. Small bubbles improve oxygen exchange by effectively increasing the surface area of the gas-blood interface,[60] but are difficult to remove. Large bubbles facilitate CO_2 removal. Bubbles and blood are separated by settling, filtration, and defoaming surfactants in a reservoir. Bubble oxygenators add 350 to 400 mL oxygen to blood and remove 300 to 330 mL CO_2 per minute at flow rates from 1 to 7 L/min.[56] Priming volumes are less than 500 mL. Commercial bubble oxygenators incorporate a reservoir and heat exchanger within the same unit and are placed upstream to the arterial pump.

Oxygenator malfunction requiring change during CPB occurs in 0.02 to 0.26% of cases,[61-63] but the incidence varies between membrane oxygenator designs.[64] Development of abnormal resistant areas in the blood path is the most common cause,[63] but other problems include leaks, loss of gas supply, rupture of connections, failure of the blender, and deteriorating gas exchange. Blood gases need to be monitored to ensure adequate CO_2 removal and oxygenation. Heparin coating may reduce development of abnormally high resistance areas.[62]

Heat Exchangers

Heat exchangers control body temperature by heating or cooling blood passing through the perfusion circuit. Hypothermia is frequently used during cardiac surgery to reduce oxygen demand or facilitate operative exposure with brief periods of circulatory arrest. Because gases are more soluble in cold than in warm blood, rapid rewarming of cold blood within the circuit or the body may cause formation of bubble emboli.[65] Most membrane oxygenator units incorporate a heat exchanger upstream to the oxygenator to minimize this potential problem. Blood should not be heated above 40°C to prevent denaturation of plasma proteins, and the temperature gradient between the body and the perfusion circuit remains within 10°C to prevent bubble emboli. The heat exchanger may be supplied by hot and cold tap water, but separate heater/cooler units with convenient temperature-regulating controls are preferred. Leakage of water into the blood path can cause hemolysis and malfunction of heater/cooler units may occur.[61]

Separate heat exchangers are needed for cardioplegia. The simplest system uses bags of precooled cardioplegia solution; however, commonly cardioplegia fluid is circulated through a dedicated heat exchanger or tubing coils placed in an ice or warm water bath.

Pumps

Most heart-lung machines use two types of pumps, although roller pumps can be used exclusively (Table 13-1). Centrifugal pumps are usually used for the primary perfusion circuit for safety reasons and for a possible reduction in injury to blood elements, although this remains controversial and unproven.[66]

Centrifugal pumps (Fig. 13-5) consist of a vaned impeller or nested, smooth plastic cones, which when rotated rapidly, propel blood by centrifugal force.[67] An arterial flowmeter is required to determine forward blood flow, which varies with the speed of rotation and the afterload of the arterial line. Unless a check valve is used,[68] the arterial line must be clamped to prevent backward flow when the pump is off. Centrifugal blood pumps generate up to 900 mm Hg of forward pressure, but only 400 to 500 mm Hg of negative pressure and, therefore, less cavitation and fewer gaseous microemboli. They can pump small amounts of air, but become "deprimed" if more than 30 to 50 mL of air enters the blood chamber. Centrifugal pumps are probably superior for temporary extracorporeal cardiac assist devices and left heart bypass, and for generating pump-augmented venous return.

Roller pumps consist of a length of 1/4- to 5/8-inch (internal diameter) polyvinyl, silicone, or latex tubing, which is compressed by two rollers 180° apart, inside a circular raceway. Forward flow is generated by roller compression and flow rate depends upon the diameter of the tubing, rate of rotation (RPM), the length of the compression raceway, and completeness of compression or "occlusion." Compression is adjusted before use to be barely nonocclusive against a standing column of fluid that produces 45 to 75 mm Hg back pressure.[69]

TABLE 13-1: Roller Versus Centrifugal Pump

	Roller pump	Centrifugal pump
Description	Nearly occlusive	Nonocclusive
	Afterload independent	Afterload sensitive
Advantages	Low prime volume	Portable, position insensitive
	Low cost	Safe positive and negative pressure
	No potential for backflow	Adapts to venous return
	Shallow sine-wave pulse	Superior for right or left heart bypass
		Preferred for long-term bypass
		Protects against massive air embolism
Disadvantages	Excessive positive and negative pressure	Large priming volume
	Spallation	Requires flowmeter
	Tubing rupture	Potential passive backward flow
	Potential for massive air embolism	Higher cost
	Necessary occlusion adjustments	
	Requires close supervision	

Hemolysis and tubing wear are minimal at this degree of compression.[69] Flow rate is determined from calibration curves for each pump for different tubing sizes and rates of rotation. Roller pumps are inexpensive, reliable, safe, insensitive to after-load, and have small priming volumes, but can produce high negative pressures and microparticles shed from compressed tubing (spallation).[70] Roller pumps are vulnerable to careless operation that results in propelling air; inaccurate flow calibration; back-flow when not in use if rollers are not sufficiently occlusive; excessive pressure with rupture of connections if arterial inflow is obstructed; tears in tubing; and changing roller compression settings during operation. In general roller pumps rather than centrifugal pumps are used for sucker systems and for delivering cardioplegic solutions.

Centrifugal pumps produce pulseless blood flow and standard roller pumps produce a sine wave pulse around 5 mm Hg. The arterial cannula dampens the pulse of pulsatile pumps, and it is difficult to generate pulse pressures above 20 mm Hg within the body during full CPB.[71] To date no one has conclusively demonstrated the need for pulsatile perfusion during short- or long-term CPB or circulatory assistance.[72]

Complications that may occur during operation of either type of pump include loss of electricity; loss of the ability to control pump speed, which produces "runaway pump" or

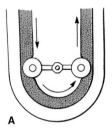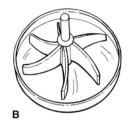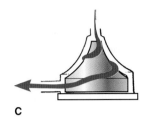

FIGURE 13-5 Diagrams of blood pumps. (A) Roller pump with two rollers, 180° apart. The compression of the rollers against the raceway is adjustable and is set to be barely nonocclusive. Blood is propelled in the direction of rotation. (B) The impeller pump uses vanes mounted on a rotating central shaft. (C) The centrifugal pump uses three rapidly rotated, concentric cones to propel blood forward by centrifugal force.

"pump creep" when turned off; loss of the flow meter or RPM indicator; rupture of tubing in the roller pump raceway; and reversal of flow by improper tubing in the raceway. A means to manually provide pumping in case of electrical failure should always be available.

Filters and Bubble Traps

MICROEMBOLI

During clinical cardiac surgery with CPB the wound and the perfusion circuit generate gaseous and biologic and non-biologic particulate microemboli (<500 μm diameter).[23,73,74] Microemboli produce much of the morbidity associated with cardiac operations using CPB (see section "Organ Damage" later in this chapter). Gaseous emboli contain oxygen or nitrogen and may enter the perfusate from multiple sources and pass through other components of the system.[12,15] Potential sources of gas entry include stopcocks, sampling and injection sites,[74] priming solutions, priming procedures, intravenous fluids, vents, the cardiotomy reservoir, tears or breaks in the perfusion circuit, loose pursestring sutures (especially during augmented venous return),[12] rapid warming of cold blood,[65] cavitation, oxygenators, venous reservoirs with low perfusate levels,[15] and the heart and great vessels. Bubble oxygenators produce many gaseous emboli; membrane oxygenators produce very few.[55,56] Aside from technical errors (open stopcocks, empty venous reservoir, air in the heart) the cardiotomy reservoir is the largest source of gaseous emboli in membrane oxygenator perfusion systems.

Blood produces a large number of particulate emboli related to thrombus formation (clots), fibrin, platelet and platelet-leukocyte aggregation, hemolyzed red cells, cellular debris, and generation of chylomicrons, fat particles, and denatured proteins.[75] Stored donor blood is also an important source of blood-generated particles.[76] Other biologic emboli include atherosclerotic debris and cholesterol crystals and calcium particles dislodged by cannulation, manipulation for exposure, or the surgery itself. Both biologic and nonbiologic particulate emboli are aspirated from the wound. Bits of muscle, bone, and fat are mixed with suture material, talc, glue, and dust and aspirated into the cardiotomy reservoir.[76,77] Materials used in manufacturing, spallated material, and dust may also enter the perfusate from the perfusion circuit[76] if it

is not first rinsed by recirculating saline through a prebypass microfilter, which is discarded.

In vivo microemboli larger than 100 μm are detected by transcranial Doppler ultrasound,[78] fluorescein angiography,[55] TEE, and retinal inspection. In the circuit, microemboli are monitored by arterial line ultrasound[79] or monitoring screen filtration pressure. Microfilter weights and examination, histology of autopsy tissues, and electron particle size counters of blood samples[76] verify microemboli beyond the circuit.

PREVENTION AND CONTROL OF MICROEMBOLI

Table 13-2 outlines sources of microemboli. Major methods include using a membrane oxygenator and cardiotomy reservoir filter; minimizing and washing blood aspirated from the field[80]; and preventing air entry into the circuit and using left ventricular vents when the heart is opened.[81,82]

The brain receives 14% of the cardiac output and is the most sensitive organ for microembolic injury.[83] Strategies to selectively reduce microembolism to the brain include reducing $PaCO_2$ to cause cerebral vasoconstriction[84]; hypothermia[85];

TABLE 13-2: Major Sources of Microemboli

Gas	Foreign	Blood
Bubble oxygenators	Atherosclerotic debris	Fibrin
Air entry into the circuit	Fat, fat droplets	Free fat
Residual air in the heart	Fibrin clot	Aggregated chylomicrons
Loose purse-string sutures	Cholesterol crystals	Denatured proteins
Cardiotomy reservoir	Calcium particles	Platelet aggregates
Rapid rewarming	Muscle fragments	Platelet-leukocyte aggregates
Cavitation	Tubing debris, dust	Hemolyzed red cells
	Bone wax, talc	Transfused blood
	Silicone antifoam	
	Glue, Surgicel	
	Cotton sponge fiber	

placing aortic cannulas downstream to the cerebral vessel[36,74]; and using special aortic cannulas with[22,23,30] or without[19] special baffles or screens designed to prevent cannula-produced cerebral atherosclerotic emboli.

Two types of blood microfilters are available for use within the perfusion circuit: depth and screen.[86,87] Depth filters consist of packed fibers or porous foam, have no defined pore size, present a large, tortuous, wetted surface, and remove microemboli by impaction and absorption. Screen filters are usually made of woven polyester or nylon thread, have a defined pore size, and filter by interception. Screen filters vary in pore size and configuration and block most air emboli; however, as pore size decreases, resistance increases. As compared with no filter, studies indicate that all commercial filters effectively remove gaseous and particulate emboli.[88,89] Most investigations find that the Dacron wool depth filter is most effective, particularly in removing microscopic and macroscopic air. Pressure differences across filters vary between 24 and 36 mm Hg at 5 L/min flow. Filters cause slight hemolysis and tend to trap some platelets; nylon filters may also activate complement.[86]

The need for microfilters in the cardiotomy suction reservoir is universally accepted,[77] and most commercial units contain an integrated micropore filter. The need for a filter in the cardioplegia delivery system, however, remains debatable,[90] and although almost always used, the requirement of an arterial line filter is unsettled.[87] In vitro studies demonstrate that an arterial filter reduces circulating microemboli[89] and clinical studies are confirmatory.[89] However, these filters do not remove all microemboli generated by the extracorporeal circuit.[12,74,77] When bubble oxygenators are used, studies show equivocal or modest reductions in microemboli[55,91] and neurologic outcome markers.[91] In contrast, membrane oxygenators produce far fewer microemboli and when used without an arterial filter, the numbers of microemboli are similar to those found with bubble oxygenators plus arterial line filters.[87]

Although the efficacy of arterial line microfilters remains unsettled, their use is almost universal[92]; and although they are effective bubble traps, they do increase cost, occasionally obstruct during use, are difficult to de-air during priming, and require a small bypass line and valved purge line to remove any air.

Other sources of biologic microemboli may be more important. Cerebral microemboli are most numerous during aortic cannulation,[93,94] application and release of aortic clamps,[94] and at the beginning of cardiac ejection after open heart procedures.[95] Furthermore, as compared with perfusion microemboli, surgically induced emboli are more likely to cause postoperative neurologic deficits.[96]

LEUKOCYTE-DEPLETING FILTERS

Leukocyte-depleting filters are discussed later in this chapter and have been recently reviewed.[97] These filters reduce circulating leukocyte counts in most studies,[98] but fail to produce convincing evidence of clinical benefit.[99]

Tubing and Connectors

The various components of the heart-lung machine are connected by polyvinyl tubing and fluted polycarbonate connectors. Medical grade polyvinyl chloride (PVC) tubing is universally used because it is flexible, compatible with blood, inert, nontoxic, smooth, nonwettable, tough, transparent, resistant to kinking and collapse, and can be heat sterilized. To reduce priming volume, tubing connections should be short. To reduce turbulence, cavitation, and stagnant areas, the flow path should be smooth and uniform without areas of constriction or expansion. Wide tubing improves rheology, but also increases priming volume. In practice 1/2- to 5/8-inch (internal diameter) tubing is used for most adults, but until a compact, integrated, complete heart-lung machine can be designed and produced as a unit, the flow path will produce some turbulence. Loose tubing connections can be sources of air intake or blood leakage and so all connections must be secure. For convenience and safety, most tubing and connectors are prepackaged and disposable.

Heparin-Coated Circuits

Heparin can be bound to blood surfaces of all components of the extracorporeal circuit by ionic or covalent bonds. The Duraflo II heparin coating ionically attaches heparin to a quaternary ammonium carrier (alkylbenzyl dimethylammonium chloride), which binds to plastic surfaces (Edwards Lifesciences, Irvine, CA). Covalent attachment is produced by first depositing a polyethylenimine polymer spacer onto the plastic surface, to which heparin fragments bind (Carmeda Bioactive Surface, Medtronic, Inc., Minneapolis, MN). Ionic-bound heparin slowly leaches, but this is irrelevant in clinical cardiac surgery. The use of heparin-coated circuits during CPB has spawned an enormous literature[100-102] and remains controversial largely because studies are contaminated by patient selection, reduced doses of systemic heparin, and washing or discarding field-aspirated blood.[102] To date, there is no irrefutable and credible evidence that heparin-coated perfusion circuits reduce the need for systemic heparin or reduce bleeding or thrombotic problems associated with CPB. Although the majority of studies indicate that heparin coatings reduce concentrations of C3a and C5b-9,[103] the inflammatory response to CPB is not reduced and the evidence for clinical benefit is not convincing.[104]

Other more recently developed and available surface modifications and coatings[101] include a phosphorylcholine coating,[105] surface-modifying additives,[106] and a trillium biopassive surface[107] as well as other proprietary substances. While many in vitro and even in vivo studies imply multiple benefits from these coatings by reductions in various inflammatory mediators and in the stimulation of the coagulation cascade, there have been no blinded randomized trials demonstrating any measurable benefit in patient outcomes. Clearly additional investigation in this area is desirable.

Cardiotomy Reservoir and Field Suction

Blood aspirated from the surgical wound may be directed to the cardiotomy reservoir for defoaming, filtration, and storage before it is added directly to the perfusate. A sponge impregnated with a surfactant removes bubbles by reducing surface tension at the blood interface and macro, micro, or combined filters remove particulate emboli. Negative pressure is generated by either a roller pump or vacuum applied to the rigid outer shell of the reservoir. The degree of negative pressure and blood level must be monitored to avoid excessive suction or introducing air into the perfusate.

The cardiotomy suction and reservoir are major sources of hemolysis, particulate and gaseous microemboli, fat globules, cellular aggregates, platelet injury and loss, thrombin generation, and fibrinolysis.[73,77,108] Air aspirated with wound blood contributes to blood activation and destruction and is difficult to remove because of the high proportion of nitrogen, which is poorly soluble in blood. High suction volumes and admixture of air are particularly destructive of platelets and red cells.[108] Commercial reservoirs are designed to minimize air entrainment and excessive injury to blood elements. Air and microemboli removal are also facilitated by allowing aspirated blood to settle within the reservoir before it is added to the perfusate.

An alternative method for recovering field-aspirated blood is to dilute the blood with saline and then remove the saline to return only packed red cells to the perfusate. Two types of centrifugal cell washers automate the process. Intermittent centrifugation (eg, Haemonetics Cell Saver, Meomonetics Corp., Braintree, MA) removes air, thrombin, and many biologic and nonbiologic microemboli from the aspirate at the cost of discarding plasma. Continuous centrifugation (eg, Fresenius/Terumo CATS, Elkton, MD) in addition removes fat and activated leukocytes.[109] A third alternative is to discard all field-aspirated blood, although most surgeons would find this practice unacceptable if it increased allogeneic blood transfusion. Increasingly, field-aspirated blood is recognized as a major contributor to the thrombotic, bleeding, and inflammatory complications of CPB.

Venting the Heart

If the heart is unable to contract, distention of either ventricle is detrimental to subsequent contractility.[110] Right ventricular distention during cardiac arrest or ventricular fibrillation is rarely a problem, but left ventricular distention can be insidious in that blood can enter the flaccid, thick-walled chamber from multiple sources during this period. During CPB, blood escaping atrial or venous cannulas and from the coronary sinus and thebesian veins may pass through the unopened right heart into the pulmonary circulation. This blood plus bronchial arterial and venous blood, blood regurgitating through the aortic valve, and blood from undiagnosed abnormal sources (patent foramen ovale, patent ductus, etc.) may distend the left ventricle unless a vent catheter is used (Fig. 13-6). During CPB bronchial blood and noncoronary

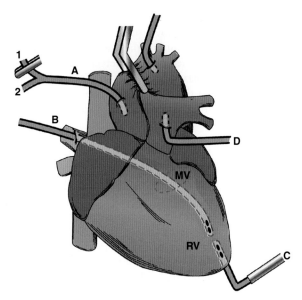

FIGURE 13-6 Diagram shows locations used to vent (decompress the heart). (A) Aortic root vent, which can also be used to administer cardioplegic solution after the ascending aorta is clamped. (B) A catheter placed in the right superior pulmonary vein/left atrial junction can be passed through the mitral valve into the left ventricle. (C) Direct venting of the left ventricle at the apex. (D) Venting the main pulmonary artery, which decompresses the left atrium because pulmonary veins lack valves.

collateral flow average approximately 140 ± 182 and 48 ± 74 mL/min, respectively.[111]

There are several methods for venting the left heart during cardiac arrest. Although it was used commonly in the past, few surgeons in the modern era vent the left ventricular apex directly because of inconvenience and myocardial injury. Most often a multihole, soft-tip catheter (8-10 French) is inserted into the junction of the right superior pulmonary vein and left atrium (see Fig. 13-6) or left atrial appendage and may or may not be passed into the left ventricle. Others prefer to place a small suction catheter into the pulmonary artery.[112] The ventricle can also be vented by passing a catheter retrograde across the aortic valve when working on the mitral valve. Vent catheters are drained to the cardiotomy reservoir by a roller pump, vacuum source, or gravity drainage,[113] but must be carefully monitored for malfunction. If connected to a roller pump, the system should be carefully tested before use to ensure proper operation. Although inspection and palpation may detect ventricular distention, TEE monitoring or direct measurements of left atrial or pulmonary arterial pressures are more reliable. The heart is no longer vented for most myocardial revascularization operations, but the ventricle must be protected from distention.[114] If the heart cannot remain decompressed during distal anastomoses, a vent should be inserted. Often the cardioplegia line inserted into the aortic root is used for venting when not used for cardioplegia.[115]

The most common and serious complication of left heart venting is residual air when the heart is filled and begins to contract. De-airing maneuvers and TEE are important methods for ensuring removal of all residual air. In addition, many surgeons aspirate the ascending aorta via a small metal or plastic cannula to detect and remove any escaping air as the heart begins to eject.[116] Bleeding, atrial perforation, mitral valve injury, and direct injury to the myocardium are other complications associated with left ventricular vents.

Cardioplegia Delivery Systems

Cardioplegic solutions contain 8 to 20 mEq/L potassium, magnesium, and often other components that are infused into the aortic root proximal to the aortic cross clamp, or retrograde into the coronary sinus to arrest the heart in diastole. The carrier may be crystalloid or blood and is infused at temperatures around 4 or 37°C, depending upon surgeon's preference. Normothermic cardioplegia must be delivered almost continuously to keep the heart arrested while cold cardioplegia may be infused intermittently. Cardioplegic solutions are delivered through a separate perfusion system that includes a reservoir, heat exchanger, roller pump, bubble trap, and perhaps microfilter (see Fig. 13-2). Temperature and infusion pressure are monitored. The system may be completely independent of the main perfusion circuit or it may branch from the arterial line. The system also may be configured to vent the aortic root when not delivering cardioplegia.

Antegrade cardioplegia is delivered through a small cannula in the aortic root or via cannulas directly into the coronary ostia when the aortic valve is exposed. Retrograde cardioplegia is delivered through a cuffed catheter inserted into the coronary sinus.[117] Proper placement of the retrograde catheter is critical, but not difficult, and is verified by palpation, TEE, color of the aspirated blood, or pressure waveform of a catheter pressure sensor.[118] Complications of retrograde cardioplegia include rupture or perforation of the sinus, hematoma, and rupture of the catheter cuff.[119]

Hemoconcentrators (Hemofiltration/ Ultrafiltration)

Hemoconcentrators, like oxygenators, contain one of several available semipermeable membranes (typically hollow fibers) that transfer water, electrolytes (eg, potassium), and molecules up to 20 kDa out of the blood compartment.[120] Hemoconcentrators may be connected to either venous or arterial lines or a reservoir in the main perfusion circuit, but require high pressure in the blood compartment to effect fluid removal. Thus a roller pump is needed unless connected to the arterial line. Suction may or may not be applied to the air side of the membrane to facilitate filtration. Up to 180 mL/min of fluid can be removed at flows of 500 mL/min.[121] Hemoconcentrators conserve platelets and most plasma proteins as compared with centrifugal cell washers, and may allow greater control of potassium

concentrations than diuretics.[122] Aside from cost, disadvantages are few and adverse effects are rare.[121]

Perfusion Monitors and Safety Devices

Table 13-3 lists monitors and safety devices that are commonly used during CPB. *Pressure in the arterial line* between pump and arterial line filter is monitored continuously to instantly detect any increased resistance to arterial inflow into the patient. This pressure should be higher than radial arterial pressure because of resistance of the filter (if used) and cannula. The arterial pressure monitor may be connected to an audible alarm or the pump switch to alert the perfusionist to dangerous increases in the arterial line pressure.

An *arterial line flowmeter* is essential for centrifugal pumps and may be desirable to confirm flow calculations with roller pumps as well.

In-line devices are available to continuously measure *blood gases, hemoglobin/hematocrit,* and *some electrolytes.*[123] Placed within the venous line, these devices permit continuous assessment of oxygen supply and demand.[124] In the arterial line the devices offer better control of blood gases.[125] The need for these devices is unproved and because reliability is still uncertain, use may distract operative personnel and spawn unnecessary laboratory measurements.[126] The use of

TABLE 13-3: Safety Devices and Procedures

Device or procedure

Low venous blood level alarm with pump cut-off
High arterial line pressure alarm with pump cut-off
Macrobubble detector with pump cut-off
Arterial line filter
Prebypass recirculation/filtration
Oxygen supply filter
In-line venous oxygen saturation
In-line arterial oxygen saturation
Oxygenator gas supply oxygen analyzer
One-way valved intracardiac vent lines
Batteries in heart-lung machine
Alternate dedicated power supply
Electrical generator
Back-up arterial pump head
Back-up heater-cooler
Back-up oxygen supply
Emergency lighting
Prebypass activated clotting time
Activated clotting time during cardiopulmonary bypass
Prebypass check list
Written protocols
Log of perfusion incidents
Log of device failures

automated analyzers by the perfusion team in the operating room is an alternative if frequent measurement of blood gases, hematocrit, and electrolytes is desirable.[123]

The *flow and concentration of oxygen* entering the oxygenator should be monitored.[127] Some teams also monitor exit gases to indirectly estimate metabolic activity and depth of anesthesia.[127] Some manufacturers recommend monitoring the *pressure gradient across membrane oxygenators*, which may be an early indication of oxygenator failure, although it is a rare event.[62-64]

Temperatures of the water entering heat exchangers must be monitored and carefully controlled to prevent blood protein denaturation and gaseous microemboli.[65] During operations using deep hypothermia, changes in venous line temperatures reflect rates of temperature change in the patient, and monitoring arterial inflow temperature helps prevent brain hyperthermia during rewarming.

A *low-level sensor* with alarms on the venous reservoir and a bubble detector on the arterial line are additional safety devices sometimes used. A *one-way valve* is recommended in the purge line between an arterial filter/bubble trap and cardiotomy reservoir to prevent air embolism. Ultrasound transducers imbedded in the arterial perfusion tubing distal to the filter are now available to monitor low-level air entry into the circulation. Valves in the venous and vent lines protect against retrograde air entry into the circulation or in the arterial line to prevent inadvertent exsanguination.[68]

Automatic data collection systems are available for preoperative calculations and to process and store data during CPB.[128] Computer systems for operating CPB are in development.[129]

CONDUCT OF CARDIOPULMONARY BYPASS

The Perfusion Team

Although the surgeon is directly responsible for the outcome of the operation, he or she needs a close working relationship with both the anesthesiologist and the perfusionist. These three principals must communicate freely, often, and candidly. Their overlapping and independent responsibilities relevant to CPB are best defined by written policies that include protocols for various types of operations and emergencies and by periodic multidisciplinary conferences. This teamwork is not unlike the communication advocated for the cockpit crew of commercial and military aircraft.

The surgeon determines the planned operation, target perfusion temperatures, methods of cardioplegia, cannulations, and anticipated special procedures. During operation the surgeon communicates the procedural steps involved in connecting and disconnecting the patient to CPB and interacts with the other principals to coordinate perfusion management with surgical exposure and working conditions. The perfusionist is responsible for setting up and priming the heart-lung machine, performing safety checks, operating the heart-lung machine, monitoring the conduct of bypass, monitoring

anticoagulation, adding prescribed drugs, and maintaining a written perfusion record.

The anesthesiologist monitors the operative field, anesthetic state and ventilation of the patient, the patient's physiology, and conduct of perfusion. A vigilant anesthesiologist is the safety officer and often "troubleshooter" of these complex procedures and along with the surgeon is in the best position to anticipate, detect, and correct deviations from desired conditions. In addition the anesthesiologist provides TEE observations before, during, and immediately after bypass.

Assembly of Heart-Lung Machine

The perfusionist is responsible for setting up and preparing the heart-lung machine and all associated components necessary for the proposed operation. Most perfusionists use commercial, sterile, preprepared customized tubing packs that are connected to the various components that constitute the heart-lung machine. This dry assembly takes about 10 to 15 minutes, and a dry system can be kept in standby for up to 7 days. Once the system is primed with fluid, which takes about 15 minutes, it should be used within 8 hours to prevent malfunction of the oxygenator. After assembly, the perfusionist conducts a safety inspection and completes a written prebypass checklist.

PRIMING

Traditional adult ECP circuits require 1.5 to 2.0 L of balanced electrolyte solution such as lactated Ringer's solution, Normosol-A, or Plasma-Lyte. Before connections are made to the patient, the prime is recirculated through a micropore filter to remove any residual particulate matter or air. In the average-sized adult, the priming volume represents approximately 30 to 35% of the patient's blood volume and reduces the hematocrit to about two-thirds of the preoperative value. In smaller patients or in the presence of peroperative anemia, banked blood may be added to the prime volume to raise the hematocrit to a predetermined minimum (eg, 25% or more), to achieve an acceptable resultant hematocrit once CPB has been initiated. There is no consensus regarding the optimal hematocrit during CPB; most perfusates have hematocrits between 20% and 25% when used with moderate hypothermia (25-32°C). Dilution reduces perfusate viscosity, which is not a problem during clinical CPB, but also reduces oxygen-carrying capacity; mixed venous oxygen saturations less than 60% usually prompt either transfusion or increased pump flow.[124] Sometimes 12.5 to 50 g of mannitol is added to stimulate diuresis and possibly minimize postoperative renal dysfunction.

Efforts to avoid the use of autologous blood include reducing the priming requirement of the machine by using smaller diameter and shorter tubing lengths and operating the machine with minimal perfusate in the venous and cardiotomy reservoirs. This latter practice increases the risk of air embolism, the risk of which can be reduced by using collapsible reservoirs and reservoir level sensors that stop

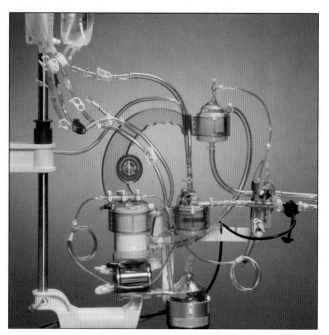

FIGURE 13-7 Typical miniature closed cardiopulmonary bypass circuit that uses coated surfaces to reduce coagulation and inflammation and removes the venous reservoir and excess tubing to reduce hemodilution.

the pump. In recent years, smaller, more compact circuits have been designed to reduce the prime volume and subsequent hemodilution, reducing transfusion requirements and platelet consumption.[130] Many of these circuits have totally removed the venous reservoir and used a variety of coated surfaces in an attempt to reduce hemodilution, avoid points of stasis and minimize activation of inflammation and coagulation cascades. A typical such mini-circuit is pictured in Fig. 13-7.

Autologous blood prime is another technique to minimize hemodilution, which displaces and then removes crystalloid prime by draining blood volume from the patient into the circuit just before beginning CPB.[131] This method reduces perfusate volume, but phenylephrine may be required to maintain stable hemodynamics.[131] The method reduces transfusions and does not affect clinical outcome.

The use of colloids (albumin, gelatins, dextrans, and hetastarches) in the priming volume is controversial.[132] Although their use clearly minimizes the decrease in colloid osmotic pressure[133] and may reduce the amount of fluid entering the extracellular space, any impact on clinical outcome remains unproved. Prospective clinical studies have failed to document significant clinical benefits with albumin,[133] which is expensive and may have adverse effects.[134] Hetastarch may contribute to postoperative bleeding.[135] McKnight et al. found no influence of prime composition on postoperative nitrogen balance.[136] Because of possible adverse effects, including neurologic deficits, the addition of glucose and/or lactate to the prime is generally avoided.[137,138]

Anticoagulation and Reversal

Porcine heparin (300-400 units/kg IV) is administered before arterial or venous cannulas are inserted, and CPB is not started until anticoagulation is confirmed by either an activated clotting time (ACT) or the Hepcon test. Although widely used, bovine heparin is more antigenic in inducing antiplatelet IgG antibodies than is porcine heparin.[139] Although the distribution of intravenously administered heparin has been shown to be extremely rapid,[140] in general, the anticoagulation effect is measured about 3 minutes after heparin administration. However, groups differ in the minimum ACT that is considered safe for CPB. The generally accepted minimum for ACT before initiation of CPB is greater than or equal to 400 seconds; however, many groups recommend 480 seconds[141] because heparin only partially inhibits thrombin formation during CPB. More recently, in an attempt to reduce surgical bleeding, some centers have advocated accepting lower ACTs in the 300 range. Although early unpublished results may suggest that this can be done safely, it is still not generally accepted. Outside the United States, where aprotinin is still available, it is important to measure ACT with kaolin as opposed to celite, because celite may artifactually and erroneously increases the ACT. Failure to achieve a satisfactory ACT may result from either inadequate heparin dosage or low concentrations of antithrombin. If a total of 500 units/kg of heparin fails to adequately prolong ACT, antithrombin III should be administered to the patient either as fresh-frozen plasma or as recombinant antithrombin III when available[142] to increase antithrombin concentrations to overcome "heparin resistance." Antithrombin III is a necessary cofactor that binds circulating thrombin; heparin accelerates this reaction a thousandfold. See Thrombosis and Bleeding for management of patients with suspected or proved heparin-induced antiplatelet IgG antibodies and alternative anticoagulants to heparin.

During CPB, ACT or the Hepcon test is measured every 30 minutes. If ACT goes below the target level, more heparin is given. As a general rule, one-third of the initial total heparin bolus required for adequate anticoagulation is given every hour even when the ACT is within the normal range. The Hepcon test titrates the heparin concentration and is more reproducible than ACT, but ACT provides satisfactory monitoring of anticoagulation. Although excessively high concentrations of heparin (ACT > 1000 seconds) may cause remote bleeding away from operative sites, low concentrations increase circulating thrombin concentrations and risk clotting within the ECP circuit.

After the patient has successfully weaned from CPB and remains stable, 1 mg of protamine is given for each 100 units of heparin given in the initial bolus dose, but not to exceed 3 mg/kg. The heparin-protamine complex activates complement and may causes acute hypotension, which may be attenuated by the administration of calcium (2 mg/1 mg protamine). Once the administration of protamine has begun, it is generally recommended that the use of cardiotomy suction into the reservoir is discontinued because of the risk of generating clot within the circuit and losing the potential for emergency support should the patient become unstable. Rarely, protamine may cause an anaphylactic reaction in patients with antibodies to protamine insulin.[143] This severe reaction may require urgently placing the patient back on CPB, although it may also be treating with resuscitation using epinephrine and immediate discontinuation of the protamine infusion. Neutralization of heparin is usually confirmed by an ACT or Hepcon test and more protamine (50 mg) is given if either test remains prolonged or bleeding is a problem. *Heparin rebound* is a term used to describe a delayed heparin effect because of release of tissue heparin after protamine is cleared from the circulation, particularly from heparin deposited in adipose tissues, and seen more often in obese patients. Although protamine is a mild anticoagulant at higher doses, one or two supplemental 25- to 50-mg doses can be given empirically if heparin rebound is suspected, or if the ACT remains elevated. It is also noted that the ACT can be elevated in the presence of significant thrombocytopenia, despite the full reversal of heparin. As a rule, the heart-lung machine should be available for unexpected decompensation and the need for urgent return to CPB until the wound is closed, the drapes are removed, and at many centers until the patient leaves the operating room.

Initiation of Cardiopulmonary Bypass

Once the appropriate cannulation has occurred and adequate anticoagulation has been confirmed, CPB is initiated at the surgeon's request with concurrence of the anesthesiologist and perfusionist. As the venous return enters the machine, the perfusionist progressively increases arterial flow while monitoring the patient's blood pressure and volume levels in all reservoirs. Six observations are critical:

1. The venous drainage is adequate for the desired flow
2. The pressure in the arterial line is acceptable
3. The arterial blood is adequately oxygenated
4. The systemic arterial pressure is acceptable
5. The systemic venous pressure is acceptable
6. The heart is adequately decompressed

Once full stable CPB is established for at least 2 minutes, lung ventilation is discontinued, perfusion cooling may begin, and the aorta may be clamped for arresting the heart. Just as is seen with initiation of dialysis, it is not uncommon to see some vasodilation and early hypotension as the patient is first exposed to the artificial surfaces, particularly the oxygenator. This can usually be managed by the perfusionist with increased flows until the vasodilation resolves, although occasionally vasopressors such as neosynephrine may be transiently required.

Cardioplegia

Antegrade blood or crystalloid cardioplegia is administered directly into the aortic root at 60 to 100 mm Hg pressure proximal to the aortic cross-clamp by a dedicated cardioplegia roller pump (see Fig. 13-2). Blood entering the right atrium from the coronary sinus is captured by the right atrial or unsnared caval catheters. If the caval snares are tightened, the right atrium should be vented to prevent right ventricular distention. Many surgeons choose to monitor myocardial temperature and administer cardioplegia to cool the myocardium to a specific temperature range. Others deliver a specific amount of cardioplegia, or monitor the electrical activity to determine the delivered volume. With appropriate delivery of antegrade cardioplegia, the heart should usually arrest within 30 to 60 seconds, and failure to do so may indicate problems with delivery of the solution or unrecognized aortic regurgitation. Some surgeons monitor myocardial temperature or pH via direct needle sensors.[144]

The usual flow of retrograde cardioplegia is 200 to 400 mL/min at coronary sinus pressures between 30 and 50 mm Hg.[145] Higher pressures may injure the coronary venous system[119]; low pressures usually indicate inadequate delivery owing to malposition of the catheter or leakage around the catheter cuff, but may also indicate a tear in the coronary sinus. Induction of electrical arrest is slower (2-4 minutes) than with antegrade delivery, and retrograde cardioplegia may provide incomplete protection of the right ventricle.[117]

Key Determinants of Safe Perfusion

The following offers rational guidelines for management of CPB, which uses manipulation of temperature, hematocrit, pressure, and flow rate to adequately support cellular metabolism during nonphysiologic conditions.

BLOOD FLOW RATE

Under normal circumstances, basal cardiac output is determined by oxygen consumption, which is approximately 250 mL/min. It is impractical to measure oxygen consumption while on CPB, so a generally accepted flow rate at 35 to 37°C with a hematocrit of 25% is approximately 2.4 L/min/m² in deeply anesthetized and muscle-relaxed patients. Hemodilution reduces blood oxygen content from approximately 20 to 10 to 12 mL/dL; consequently, flow rate must increase over resting normal cardiac output or oxygen demand must decrease. The resistance of venous catheters, turbulence, and loss of physiologic controls of the vasculature may also effect venous return and limit maximum pump flow.

Hypothermia reduces oxygen consumption by a factor of 0.5 for every 10°C decrease in temperature. However, at both normothermia and hypothermia maximal oxygen consumption falls with decreasing flow as described in the following equation:

$$VO_2 = 0.44 \, (Q - 62.7) + 71.6.$$

This relationship at various temperatures is depicted in Figure 13-8. For this reason Kirklin and Barratt-Boyes[146] recommend that flows be reduced only to levels that permit at least 85% of maximal oxygen consumption. At 30°C this flow rate in adults is approximately 1.8 L/min/m²; at 25°C, 1.6 L/min/m²; and at 18°C, 1.0 L/min/m².

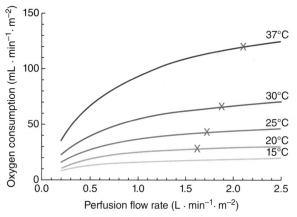

FIGURE 13-8 Nomogram relating oxygen consumption to perfusion flow rate and temperature. The small xs indicate clinical flow rates used by Kirklin and Barratt-Boyes. (Reproduced with permission from Kirklin JW, Barratt Boyes BG: *Cardiac Surgery*, 3rd ed. New York: Churchill Livingstone; 2003.)

As long as mean arterial pressure remains above 50 to 60 mm Hg (ie, above the autoregulatory range), cerebral blood flow is preserved even if systemic flow is less than normal. However, there is a hierarchal reduction of flow to other organs as total systemic flow is progressively reduced. First skeletal muscle flow falls, then abdominal viscera and bowel, and finally renal blood flow.

PULSATILE FLOW

Theoretical benefits of pulsatile blood flow include increased transmission of energy to the microcirculation, which reduces critical capillary closing pressure, augments lymph flow, and improves tissue perfusion and cellular metabolism. Theoretically, pulsatile flow reduces vasocontrictive reflexes and neuroendocrine responses and may increase oxygen consumption, reduce acidosis, and improve organ perfusion. However, despite extensive investigation no one has convincingly demonstrated a benefit of pulsatile blood flow over nonpulsatile blood flow for short- or long-term CPB.[71,147] Two studies reported the association of pulsatile flow with lower rates of mortality, myocardial infarction, and low cardiac output syndrome,[148] but others failed to detect clinical benefits.[149]

Pulsatile CPB can reproduce the normal pulse pressure within the body, but is expensive, complicated, and requires a large-diameter aortic cannula. Higher nozzle velocities increase trauma to blood elements,[150] and pulsations may damage micromembrane oxygenators.[151] Thus for clinical CPB, nonpulsatile blood flow is an acceptable, nonphysiologic compromise with few disadvantages.

ARTERIAL PRESSURE

Systemic arterial blood pressure is a function of flow rate, blood viscosity (hematocrit), and vascular tone. Perfusion of the brain is normally protected by autoregulation, but

autoregulation appears to be lost somewhere between 55 and 60 mm Hg during CPB at moderate hypothermia and a hematocrit of 24%.[84,152] Cerebral blood flow may still be adequate at lower arterial pressures,[153] but the only prospective randomized study found a lower combined major morbidity/mortality rate when mean arterial pressure was maintained near 70 mm Hg (average 69 ± 7) rather than below 60 (average 52).[154] In older patients, who may have vascular disease[155] and/or hypertension, mean arterial blood pressure is generally maintained between 70 and 80 mm Hg at 37°C. Higher pressures are undesirable because collateral blood flow to the heart and lungs increases blood in the operative field.

Hypotension during CPB may be the result of low pump flow, aortic dissection, measurement error, or vasodilatation. Phenylephrine is most often used to elevate blood pressure, but arginine vasopressin (0.05-0.1 unit/min) has more recently been introduced. If anesthesia is adequate, hypertension can be treated with nitroprusside, an arterial dilator, or nitroglycerin, which predominantly dilates veins and pulmonary vessels.

HEMATOCRIT

The ideal hematocrit during CPB remains controversial. Low hematocrits reduce blood viscosity and hemolysis, reduce oxygen-carrying capacity, and reduce the need for autologous blood transfusion. In general, viscosity remains stable when percent hematocrit and blood temperature (in degrees Celsius) are equal (ie, viscosity is constant at hematocrit 37%, temperature 37°C, or at hematocrit 20%, temperature 20°C). Hypothermia reduces oxygen consumption and permits perfusion at 26 to 28°C with hematocrits between 18% and 22%, but at higher temperatures limits on pump flow may not satisfy oxygen demand.[156,157] Hill[158] found that hematocrit during CPB did not affect either hospital mortality or neurologic outcome, but DeFoe observed[159] increasing hospital mortality with hematocrits below 23% during CPB; thus the issue remains unresolved.[160] However, higher hematocrits (25-30%) during CPB appear justified[157] in view of the increasing safety of autologous blood transfusion, improved neurologic outcomes with higher hematocrits in infant cardiac surgery,[161] and more frequent operations near normothermia in older sicker patients.

TEMPERATURE

The ideal temperature for uncomplicated adult cardiac surgery is also an unsettled question.[157] Until recently, nearly all operations reduced body temperature to 25 to 30°C during CPB to protect the brain, support hypothermic cardioplegia, permit perfusion at lower flows and hematocrits, and increase the safe duration of circulatory arrest in case of emergency. Hypothermia, however, interferes with enzyme and organ function, aggravates bleeding, increases systemic vascular resistance, delays cardiac recovery, lengthens duration of bypass, increases the risk of cerebral hyperthermia, and is associated with higher levels of depression and anxiety postoperatively.[162] Because the embolic risk of cerebral injury often is greater than perfusion risk, perfusion at higher temperatures (33-35°C), or "tepid" CPB, is recommended, in part because detrimental high blood temperatures are avoided during rewarming.[163] Increasingly, efforts are made to avoid cerebral hyperthermia during and after operation, and one study suggests improved neuropsychometric outcomes if patients are rewarmed to only 34°C.[164]

PH/PCO$_2$ MANAGEMENT

There are two strategies for managing pH/PCO$_2$ during hypothermia: pH stat and alpha stat. During deep hypothermia and circulatory arrest (see the following) there is increasing evidence that pH-stat management may produce better neurologic outcomes during pediatric cardiac surgery.[161] Alpha stat may be better in adults.[165] pH stat maintains temperature-corrected pH 7.40 at all temperatures and requires the addition of CO$_2$ as the patient is cooled. Alpha stat allows the pH to increase during cooling so that blood becomes alkalotic. Cerebral blood flow is higher, and pressure is passive and uncoupled from cerebral oxygen demand with pH stat. With alpha stat, cerebral blood flow is lower, autoregulated, and coupled to cerebral oxygen demand.[166]

ARTERIAL PaO$_2$

PaO$_2$ should probably be kept above 150 mm Hg to assure complete arterial saturation. Whether or not high levels (ie, >200 mm Hg) are detrimental has not yet been determined.

GLUCOSE

Although Hill[158] found no relationship between blood glucose concentrations during CPB and adverse neurologic outcome, others have been concerned that hyperglycemia (>180 mg/dL) aggravates neurologic injury[138] and other morbidity/mortality,[167] and recently many studies have documented the importance of tight glucose control in the prevention of infection, neurologic injury, renal and cardiac complications, as well as a reduction in ICU length of stay and overall mortality.[168]

Patient Monitors

Systemic arterial pressure is typically monitored by radial, brachial, or femoral arterial catheter. Central venous pressure is routinely monitored by a jugular venous catheter. Routine use of a Swan-Ganz pulmonary arterial catheter is controversial and not necessary for uncomplicated operations in low-risk patients.[169] During CPB the pulmonary artery catheter should be withdrawn into the main pulmonary artery to prevent lung perforation and suture ensnarement.

TRANSESOPHAGEAL ECHOCARDIOGRAPHY

A comprehensive TEE examination[170] is an important monitor during most applications of CPB[171] to assess catheter and vent insertion and location[117,172,173]; severity of regional atherosclerosis[33]; myocardial injury, infarction, dilatation, contractility, thrombi, and residual air; undiagnosed anatomic abnormalities[170]; valve function after repair or replacement; diagnosis of dissection[41,174]; and adequacy of de-airing at the end of CPB.[175]

TEMPERATURE

Bladder or rectal temperature is usually used to estimate temperature of the main body mass, but does not reflect brain temperature.[176] Esophageal and pulmonary artery temperatures may be affected by local cooling associated with cardioplegia. The jugular venous bulb temperature is considered the best surrogate for brain temperature, but is more cumbersome to obtain.[177] Nasopharyngeal or tympanic membrane temperatures are more commonly used, but tend to underestimate jugular venous bulb temperature during rewarming by 3 to 5°C.[178] During rewarming, arterial line temperature correlates best with jugular venous bulb temperature.[179]

NEUROPHYSIOLOGIC MONITORING

Neurophysiologic monitoring during CPB is becoming more commonly used in both adult and pediatric perfusion, particularly in preparation for deep hypothermic circulatory arrest. However, its full efficacy and impact on outcomes has not yet been fully established as a necessary component of CPB, and remains under investigation. Techniques being investigated include jugular venous bulb temperature and saturation, transcranial Doppler ultrasound, near-infrared transcranial reflectance spectroscopy (NIRS), and the raw or processed electroencephalogram (EEG).[180]

ADEQUACY OF PERFUSION

During CPB oxygen consumption (VO$_2$) equals pump flow rate multiplied by the difference in arterial (CaO$_2$) and venous oxygen content (CVO$_2$). For a given temperature, maintaining VO$_2$ at 85% predicted maximum during CPB assures adequate oxygen delivery (see Fig. 13-8).[146] Oxygen delivery (DO$_2$) equals pump flow multiplied by CaO$_2$ and should be greater than 250 mL/min/m^2 during normothermic perfusion.[156] Mixed venous oxygen saturation (SVO$_2$) assesses the relationship between DO$_2$ and VO$_2$; values less than 60% indicate inadequate oxygen delivery. Because of differences in regional vascular tone, higher SVO$_2$ does not assure adequate oxygen delivery to all vascular beds.[181] Metabolic acidosis (base deficit) or elevated lactic acid levels may indicate inadequate perfusion, even in the face of "normal" SVO$_2$ measurements.

URINE OUTPUT

Urine output is usually monitored but varies with renal perfusion, temperature, composition of the pump prime, diuretics, absence of pulsatility, and hemoconcentration. Urine production is reassuring during CPB and oliguria requires investigation.

GASTRIC TONOMETRY AND MUCOSAL FLOW

These Doppler and laser measurements gauge splanchnic perfusion but are rarely used clinically.

Weaning from Cardiopulmonary Bypass

Before stopping CPB the patient is rewarmed to 34 to 36°C, the heart is defibrillated if necessary, and the lungs are reexpanded and ventilated. The cardiac rhythm is monitored, and hematocrit, blood gases, acid-base status, and plasma electrolytes are reviewed. If the heart has been opened, TEE is recommended for detection and removal of trapped air before the heart is allowed to eject. Caval catheters are adjusted to ensure unobstructed venous return to the heart. If the need for inotropic drugs is anticipated, these are started at low flow rates. Vent catheters are removed, although sometimes an aortic root vent is placed on gentle suction to remove undiscovered air.

Once preparations are completed, the surgeon, anesthesiologist, and perfusionist begin to wean the patient off CPB. The perfusionist gradually occludes the venous line to allow filling of the right heart and ejection through the lungs to the left side, while simultaneously reducing pump input as cardiac rate and rhythm, arterial pressure and pulse, and central venous pressure are monitored and adjusted. Initially blood volume within the pump is kept constant, but as pump flow approaches zero, volume is added or removed from the patient to produce arterial and venous pressures within the physiologic ranges. During weaning, cardiac filling and contractility is often monitored by TEE, and intracardiac repairs and regional myocardial contractility are assessed. Pulse oximetry saturation near 100%, end-tidal CO_2 greater than 25 mm Hg, and mixed venous oxygen saturation higher than 65% confirm satisfactory ventilation and circulation. When cardiac performance is satisfactory and stable, all catheters and cannulas are removed, protamine is given to reverse the heparin, and blood return from the surgical field is discontinued.

Once the patient is hemodynamically stable, as determined by surgeon and anesthesiologist, and after starting wound closure, the perfusate may be returned to the patient in several ways. The entire perfusate may be washed and returned as packed cells, excess fluid may be removed by a hemoconcentrator, or the perfusate, which still contains heparin, can be gradually pumped into the patient for hemoconcentration by the kidneys. Occasionally some of the perfusate must be bagged and given later. The heart-lung machine should not be completely disassembled until the chest is closed and the patient is ready to leave the operating room.

SPECIAL TOPICS

Special Applications of Extracorporeal Perfusion

Reoperations, surgery of the descending thoracic aorta, and minimally invasive procedures may be facilitated by surgical incisions other than midline sternotomy. These alternative incisions often require alternative methods for connecting the patient to the heart-lung machine. Some alternative applications of CPB are presented in the following.

RIGHT THORACOTOMY

Anterolateral incisions through the fourth or fifth interspaces provide easy access to the cavae and right atrium, adequate access to the ascending aorta, as well as exposure to the left atrium and mitral valve, but no direct access to the left ventricle. Adequate exposure of the ascending aorta is available for cross-clamping, aortotomy, and administration of cardioplegia by retracting the right atrial appendage. De-airing the left ventricle (eg, after mitral valve repair) is more difficult. External pads facilitate defibrillation.

LEFT THORACOTOMY

Lateral or posterolateral incisions in the left chest are used for a variety of operations. Venous return may be captured by cannulating the pulmonary artery via a stab wound in the right ventricle, or by retrograde cannulation of the left pulmonary artery or cannulation of the left iliac or femoral vein. With iliac or femoral cannulation, venous return may be augmented by threading the cannula into the right atrium using TEE guidance.[182] The descending thoracic aorta or left subclavian, iliac, or femoral arteries are accessible for arterial cannulation.

LEFT HEART BYPASS

Left heart bypass uses the beating right heart to pump blood through the lungs to provide gas exchange.[183] An oxygenator is not used and intake cannulation sites are exposed through a left thoracotomy. The left superior pulmonary vein-left atrial junction is an excellent cannulation site for capturing blood. The left atrial appendage can also be used, but may be more friable and therefore more difficult with which to work. The apex of the left ventricle is infrequently used because of the potential for myocardial injury. The tip of the intake catheter must be free in the left atrium and careful technique is required to avoid air entry during cannulation and perfusion. The extracorporeal circuit typically consists only of tubing and a centrifugal pump and does not include a reservoir, heat exchanger, or bubble trap. This reduces the thrombin burden and may permit reduced or no heparin if anticoagulation poses an additional risk (eg, in acute head injury). Otherwise, full heparin doses are recommended. The reduced perfusion circuit precludes the ability to add or sequester fluid, adjust temperature, or intercept systemic air emboli. Intravenous volume expanders may be needed to maintain adequate flows; temperature usually can be maintained without a heat exchanger.[184]

Full left heart bypass may be employed for left-sided coronary artery surgery by draining all of the pulmonary venous return out of the left atrium and leaving no blood for left ventricular ejection. If the heart fibrillates, blood can still passively pass through the right heart and lungs, but often an elevated central venous pressure is required.[185]

Partial left heart bypass is identical in configuration and cannulation to full left heart bypass and is used to facilitate surgery on the descending thoracic aorta. This accomplishes two goals by providing perfusion to the lower body beyond the aortic clamps, as well as allowing the perfusionist to remove preload as needed by increasing the flow, thereby controlling the perfusion pressure in the proximal aorta, preventing both hypotension, as well as hypertension and potential LV strain. The patient's left ventricle supplies blood to the aorta proximal to aortic clamps, and the circuit supplies blood to the distal body. Typically about two-thirds normal basal cardiac output (ie, 1.6 L/min/m^2) is pumped to the lower body. Arterial pressure is monitored proximal (radial or brachial) and distal (right femoral, pedal) to the aortic clamps. Blood volume in the body and circuit is assessed by central venous pressure and TEE monitoring of chamber dimensions. Management is more complicated because of the single venous circulation and separated arterial circulations.[183]

PARTIAL CARDIOPULMONARY BYPASS

Partial CPB with an oxygenator is also used to facilitate surgery of the descending thoracic aorta. After left thoracotomy, systemic venous and arterial cannulas are placed as described in the preceding. The perfusion circuit includes a reservoir, pump, oxygenator, heat exchanger, and bubble trap. The beating left ventricle supplies the upper body and heart, so lungs must be ventilated and upper body oxygen saturation should be independently monitored. Blood flow to the separate upper and lower circulations must be balanced as described for partial left heart bypass.

FULL CARDIOPULMONARY BYPASS

Full CPB with peripheral cannulation is used when access to the chest is dangerous because of proximity of the heart, vital vessels (eg, mammary arterial graft), or pathologic condition (eg, ascending aortic mycotic aneurysm) abutting the anterior chest wall.[3] The patient is supine and a complete ECP circuit is prepared and primed. Venous cannulas may be inserted into the right atrium via the iliac or femoral vessels and/or the right jugular vein. The iliac, femoral, or axillary subclavian arteries may be used for arterial cannulation. Initiation of CPB decompresses the heart, but profound cooling is usually deferred to keep the heart beating and decompressed until the surgeon can insert a vent catheter, unless the conduct and complexity of the operation dictate deep hypothermic circulatory arrest (DHCA) prior to dividing the sternum.

FEMORAL VEIN TO FEMORAL ARTERY BYPASS

Femoral vein to femoral artery bypass with full CPB is used to initiate bypass outside the operating room for emergency circulatory assistance,[3] supportive angioplasty,[186] intentional (aneurysm repair) or accidental hypothermia. Femoral vessel cannulation is occasionally used during other operations to facilitate control of bleeding (eg, cranial aneurysm, tumor invading the IVC) or ensure oxygenation (eg, lung transplantation, upper airway reconstruction).

CANNULATION FOR MINIMALLY INVASIVE (LIMITED ACCESS) SURGERY

Off-pump coronary artery bypass (OP-CAB) describes construction of coronary arterial bypass grafts on the beating heart without CPB. Minimally invasive direct CAB (MID-CAB) refers to coronary arterial bypass grafting with or without CPB through small, strategically placed incisions. Peripheral cannulation sites, described above, may be used, but often central cannulation of the aorta, atrium, or central veins is accomplished using specially designed or smaller cannulas placed through the operative incision or through a separate small incisions in the chest wall.[187] Venous return may be augmented by applying negative pressure (see discussion of venous cannulation above); often soft tipped arterial catheters are used to minimize arterial wall trauma.[20]

The Port-Access System provides a means for full CPB, cardioplegia administration, and aortic cross-clamping without exposing the heart and can be used for both valvular and coronary arterial operations.[173] Through the right internal jugular vein separate transcutaneous catheters are inserted into the coronary sinus for retrograde cardioplegia and the pulmonary artery for left heart venting. A multilumen catheter is inserted through the femoral artery and using TEE and/or fluoroscopy is positioned in the ascending aorta for arterial pump inflow, for balloon occlusion of the ascending aorta, and administration of antegrade cardioplegia into the aortic root. Venous return is captured by a femoral venous catheter advanced into the right atrium. The system allows placement of small skin incisions directly over the parts of the heart that require surgical attention.

Minimally invasive surgery using CPB is associated with potential complications that include perforation of vessels or cardiac chambers, aortic dissection, incomplete de-airing, systemic air embolism, and failure of the balloon aortic clamp. Because CO_2 is heavier than air and more soluble in blood, the surgical field is sometimes flooded with CO_2 at 5- to 10-L/min flow to displace air when the heart is open. The intra-aortic balloon occluder can leak, prolapse through the aortic valve, or move distally to occlude arch vessels. For safety the position of the occluding balloon is closely monitored by TEE, bilateral radial arterial pressures, and one of the following: transcranial Doppler ultrasound, cerebral near-infrared spectroscopy, or EEG.[188]

Deep Hypothermic Circulatory Arrest

Deep hypothermic circulatory arrest is commonly used for operations involving the aortic arch, a heavily calcified or porcelain aorta, thoracoabdominal aneurysms, pulmonary thromboendarterectomy, selected uncommon cardiovascular and neurologic procedures,[189] and certain complex congenital heart procedures. The technology involves reducing body temperature to less than 20°C, arresting the circulation for a short period, and then rewarming to 37°C. Deep hypothermia reduces cerebral oxygen consumption (Fig. 13-9), and attenuates release of toxic neurotransmitters and reactive oxidants during ischemia and reperfusion.[190]

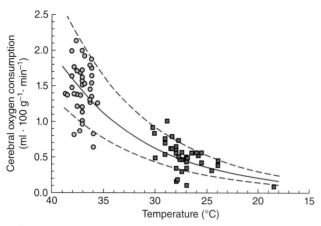

FIGURE 13-9 Relation between cerebral oxygen consumption and nasopharyngeal temperature during CPB at 2 L/min/m². (Data from Croughwell N, Smith LR, Quill T et al: The effect of temperature on cerebral metabolism and blood flow in adults during cardiopulmonary bypass, *J Thorac Cardiovasc Surg.* 1992 Mar;103(3):549-554.)

Because perfusion cooling produces differential temperatures within both the body and brain,[176] more than one temperature is customarily monitored. Bladder, pulmonary artery, esophageal, or rectal temperatures are used to estimate body temperature. Nasopharyngeal and tympanic membrane temperatures are imperfect surrogates for mean brain temperature. Most surgical teams cool to either EEG silence, jugular venous saturation greater than 95%, or for at least 30 minutes before stopping circulation at nasopharyngeal or tympanic membrane temperatures below 20°C. Caloric exchange is proportional to body mass, rate of perfusion, and temperature differences between patient and perfusate; however, rates of perfusion cooling and rewarming are restricted (see the section on heat exchangers). Perfusion cooling is usually supplemented by surface cooling using hypothermia blankets and/or packing the head in ice. Hyperthermia is avoided by keeping arterial inflow temperature below 37°C during rewarming, and by avoiding gradients greater than 10°C between the inflow blood temperature and the lowest monitored body temperature.

Changes in temperature affect acid-base balance, which must be monitored and managed during deep hypothermia. The pH-stat protocol (CO_2 is added to maintain temperature corrected blood pH at 7.4) may be preferred over the alpha-stat protocol, which allows cold blood to become alkalotic. Compared with alpha-stat, pH-stat increases the rate and uniformity of brain cooling,[191,192] slows the rate of brain oxygen consumption by 30 to 40% at 17°C,[192] and improves neurologic outcomes in animal models[161,193] and in infants,[194] but not necessarily in adults.[195] Hyperglycemia appears to increase brain injury and is avoided during deep hypothermia.[196] The value of high-dose corticosteroids or barbiturates remains unproved.

The safe duration of circulatory arrest during deep hypothermia is unknown. In adults arrest times as short as 25 minutes are associated with poor performance on neuropsychologic tests of fine motor function and memory.[197]

Ergin et al.[198] found duration of arrest was a predictor of temporary neurologic dysfunction, which correlated with long-term neuropsychologic deficits.[199] At 18°C, cerebral metabolism and oxygen consumption are 17 to 40% of normothermia[200] and abnormal encephalographic patterns and cerebrovascular responses can be detected after 30 minutes of circulatory arrest.[200] Most investigators,[201] but not all[202] report increased mortality and adverse neurologic outcomes after 40 to 65 minutes of circulatory arrest in adults. Most surgeons try to keep the period of arrest at less than 45 minutes and, if the operation allows, many perfuse for 10 to 15 minutes between serial arrest periods of 10 to 20 minutes. (For more details on DHCA, see Chapter 14.)

Antegrade and Retrograde Cerebral Perfusion

Antegrade cerebral perfusion is used in lieu of DHCA or as a supplement. Once the body has been appropriately cooled as for DHCA, the cerebral vessels can be cannulated separately and perfused together by a single pump[203] or perfused collectively after a graft with a side branch is sewn to the top of the aortic arch from which the innominate, left carotid, and left subclavian arteries originate. Separate perfusion of separately cannulated vessels is rarely done. Perfusion is usually provided by a separate roller pump that receives blood from the arterial line. Line pressure is monitored and a microfilter may or may not be used. The cerebral vessels are collectively perfused with cold blood between 10 and 18°C and at approximate flows of 10 mL/kg/min; perfusion pressures are usually restricted to 30 to 70 mm Hg, though individual protocols vary widely.[204] The adequacy of cerebral perfusion can be assessed by monitoring jugular venous saturation or near-infrared spectroscopy. Selective antegrade cerebral perfusion risks dislodging atheromatous emboli or causing air embolism, cerebral edema, or injury from excessive perfusion pressure.

Retrograde cerebral perfusion (RCP) was initially introduced in 1980 as emergency treatment for massive air embolism.[205] Later, Ueda et al. introduced continuous RCP for cerebral protection as an adjunct to DHCA during aortic surgery.[206] During RCP and DHCA the SVC is perfused at pressures usually between 25 and 40 mm Hg, temperatures between 8 and 18°C, and flows between 250 and 400 mL/min from a sideport off the arterial line, which is clamped downstream from the sideport. Some surgeons advocate much higher pressures and flows to compensate for runoff and have not shown detrimental effects.[207] A snare is usually placed around the superior caval catheter cephalad to the azygous vein to reduce runoff. The IVC may or may not be occluded.[208]

Retrograde cerebral perfusion has been widely and safely used,[207,209] but its effectiveness in protecting the brain is not clear.[210] The method can wash out some particulate emboli entering from arteries, which is a major cause of brain injury after aortic surgery.[211] However, it is not clear how adequately and completely all regions of the brain are perfused.[210] Lin et al.[209] found cortical flows to be only 10% of control values.

RCP slows but does not arrest the decrease in cerebral oxygen saturation[203,207] and the decay in amplitude of somatosensory evoked potentials.[212] Other clinical and animal studies have suggested RCP provides some cerebral protection over DHCA alone.[207,209] A few studies report that antegrade cerebral perfusion provides better protection than the retrograde technique.[203]

Complications and Risk Management

Life-threatening incidents can occur in 0.4 to 2.7% of operations with CPB and the incidence of serious injury or death is between 0.06% and 0.08% (Table 13-4).[61,92] Massive air embolism, aortic dissection, dislodgement of cannulas, and clotting within the circuit during perfusion are the principal causes of serious injury or death. Malfunctions of the heat exchanger, oxygenator, pumps, and electrical supply are the most common threatening incidents related to equipment. Others include premature takedown or clotting within the perfusion circuit.

MASSIVE AIR EMBOLISM

The incidence of massive air embolism is between 0.003% and 0.007% with 50% of outcomes adverse.[61,92] Air can enter any component of the perfusion circuit at any time during an operation if the integrity of the circuit is broken.[213] Stopcocks, connections, vent catheters, empty reservoirs, pursestring sutures, cardioplegia infusion catheters, and unremoved air in opened cardiac chambers are the most common sources of air emboli. Uncommon sources include oxygenator membrane leaks, residual air in the circuit after priming, reversal of flow in venous, vent or arterial lines, and unexpected inspiration by the patient during cannula removal.

Massive air embolism during perfusion is a catastrophe, and management guidelines are evolving.[14,205,213] Perfusion should stop immediately and clamps should be placed on both venous and arterial lines. Air in the circuit should be rapidly removed by recirculation and entrapment of all air in a reservoir or bubble trap. The patient should be immediately placed in steep Trendelenburg position and blood and air at the site of entry should be aspirated until no air is retrieved. TEE should be rapidly employed to search for air, but perfusion must resume promptly depending upon body temperature to prevent ischemic brain damage. Cooling to deep hypothermia should be considered to protect the brain and other organs while air is located and removed. As soon as possible, retrograde perfusion of the brain should be undertaken while the aortic arch is simultaneously aspirated with the patient in steep Trendelenburg position. Corticosteroids and/or barbiturates may be considered. Depending upon circumstances and availability, hyperbaric oxygen therapy may be helpful if patients can be treated within 5 hours of operation.[214]

RISK MANAGEMENT

Minimizing risks of ECP requires strict attention to personnel training, preparation and training for emergencies, equipment function, and record keeping.[14] All members of the operative team must be trained, certified, and recertified in their respective roles and participate in continuing education programs. A policy manual for the perfusion team and written protocols should be developed and continuously updated for various types of operations and emergencies. Emergency kits are prepared for out-of-operating-room (OR) crises. Adequate supplies are stocked in designated locations with sufficient inventory to support any operation or emergency for a specified period. An inventory of supplies is taken and recorded at regular intervals. Checklists are prepared and used for setting up the perfusion system and connecting to the patient. Equipment is inspected at regular intervals; worn, loose, or outdated parts are replaced; and preventive maintenance is provided and documented. New equipment is thoroughly checked before use and instructions are thoroughly digested by all user personnel. Safety alarms are optional; none replace the vigilance and attention of all OR personnel during an operation. Complete, signed written records are required for every perfusion; adverse events are recorded in a separate log and reviewed by the entire OR team. A continuous quality assurance program is desirable.[215]

During the procedure communication must be open among the surgeon, anesthetist, and perfusionist to

⊙ TABLE 13-4: Adverse Incidents Involving Cardiopulmonary Bypass

	Incidence (events/1000)	Death or serious injury (%)*
Protamine reaction	1.3	10.5
Thrombosis during cardiopulmonary bypass	0.3-0.4	2.6-5.2
Aortic dissection	0.4-0.8	14.3-33.1
Dislodgment of cannula	0.2-1.6	4.2-7.1
Rupture of arterial connection	0.2-0.6	0-3.1
Gas embolism	0.2-1.3	0.2-8.7
Massive systemic gas embolism	0.03-0.07	50-52
Electrical power failure	0.2-1.8	0-0.6
Pump failure	0.4-0.9	0-3.5
Heater-cooler problems	0.5-3	0
Replace oxygenator during cardiopulmonary bypass	0.2-1.3	0-0.7
Other oxygenator problems	0.2-0.9	0
Urgent re setup after takedown	2.9	13
Early unplanned cessation of cardiopulmonary bypass	0.2	0-0.7

*Percentage of incidents that resulted in death or serious injury. Data derived from references 94 and 151.

coordinate activites. Statements are verbally acknowledged. Distractive conversations are discouraged. The entire OR team is committed to a zero-error policy, which can only be achieved by discipline and attention to details.[216]

THROMBOSIS AND BLEEDING

Response of Humoral and Cellular Elements of Blood to Extracorporeal Circulation

Within the body the endothelial cell, the only surface in contact with circulating blood, simultaneously maintains the fluidity of blood and the integrity of the vascular system. This remarkable cell maintains a dynamic equilibrium by producing anticoagulants to maintain blood in a fluid state and generating procoagulant substances to enhance gel formation when perturbed. Blood proteins circulate as inert zymogens, which convert to active enzymes when stimulated. Likewise, blood cells remain quiescent until activated to express surface receptors and release proteins and enzymes involved in coagulation and inflammation. The continuous exposure of heparinized blood to the perfusion circuit and to cell tissues and fluid constituents of the wound during clinical cardiac surgery produces an intense thrombotic stimulus that involves both the tissue factor (TF) pathway (extrinsic coagulation pathway) in the wound and the contact and intrinsic coagulation pathways in the perfusion circuit. Thrombin is continuously generated and circulated despite massive doses of heparin in all applications of ECP.[217] This powerful enzyme along with TF from the wound and many other cytokines also activate an inflammatory reaction, which can damage tissues and ultimately produce cell death by necrosis or apoptosis.

Initial Reactions in the Perfusion Circuit

When heparinized blood contacts any biomaterial, plasma proteins are instantly adsorbed (<1 second) onto the surface to form a *monolayer* of selected proteins.[218] Different biomaterials have different intrinsic surface activities for each plasma protein. The physical and chemical compositions of the *biomaterial surface* determine the intrinsic surface activity of the biomaterial. Thus intrinsic surface activity differs among biomaterial surfaces, plasma proteins, and different bulk concentrations of plasma proteins. The composition of the protein monolayer is specific for the biomaterial and various concentrations of proteins in the plasma, but the topography of the adsorbed protein layer may not be uniform across the surface of the biomaterial.[219] Thus it is not possible to predict the "thrombogenicity" of any biomaterial except by trial and error.

On most biomaterial surfaces fibrinogen is selectively adsorbed, but the adsorbed concentration of fibrinogen and

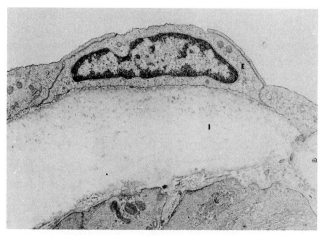

FIGURE 13-10 Electron micrograph of a rabbit endothelial cell (E), the only known nonthrombogenic surface. Note the overlapping junctions with neighboring endothelial cells. Endothelial cells rest on the internal elastic lamina (I), which abut medial smooth muscle cells. The vessel lumen is at the top. (Reproduced with permission from Colman RW, Hirsh J, Marder VJ, et al: *Hemostasis and Thrombosis: Basic Principles and Clinical Practice*, 2nd ed. Philadelphia: Lippincott Williams & Wilkins; 1987.)

other proteins may change over time.[220] The complexity of blood-biomaterial interactions is further compounded by the fact that adsorbed proteins often undergo limited conformational changes[221] that may expose "receptor" amino acid sequences that are recognized by specific blood cells or bulk plasma proteins.

Thus, heparinized blood does not directly contact biomaterial surfaces in ECP circuits, but contacts monolayers of densely packed, immobile plasma proteins arranged in undefined mosaics that differ between locations and possibly across time. All biomaterial surfaces, including heparin-coated surfaces, are *procoagulant*[222]; only the endothelial cell is truly nonthrombogenic (Fig. 13-10).

Anticoagulation

ECP and CPB are not possible without anticoagulation; the large procoagulant surface quickly overwhelms natural circulating anticoagulants—antithrombin, proteins C and S, TF pathway inhibitor, and plasmin—to produce thrombin and thrombosis within the circuit. Thrombin is produced in ECP systems with small surface areas and high-velocity flow,[223] but thrombosis may not be apparent if other procoagulants (eg, addition of blood from wounds) are absent. Generation of thrombin varies widely between applications of extracorporeal technology, but this powerful and potentially dangerous enzyme is produced whenever blood contacts a nonendothelial cell surface (Fig. 13-11).

During CPB and OHS high concentrations of heparin (3-4 mg/kg, initial dose) are needed to maintain the fluidity of blood. Heparin has both advantages and

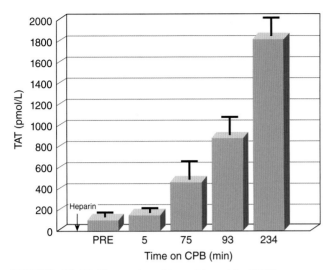

FIGURE 13-11 Plasma thrombin-antithrombin (TAT) measurements of thrombin generation during CPB and clinical cardiac surgery of varying duration. (Data from Brister SJ, Ofosu FA, Buchanan MR: Thrombin generation during cardiac surgery: is heparin the ideal anticoagulant? *Thromb Haemost.* 1993 Aug 2;70(2):259-262.)

disadvantages; the most notable advantages are parenteral use, immediate onset of action, and rapid reversal by protamine or recombinant platelet factor 4.[224] Heparin does not directly inhibit coagulation, but acts by accelerating the actions of the natural protease, antithrombin.[225] Heparin-catalyzed antithrombin, however, does not inhibit thrombin bound to fibrin[226] or factor Xa bound to platelets within clots[227]; thus, heparin only partially inhibits thrombin in vivo. Antithrombin primarily binds thrombin; its action on factors Xa and IXa is much slower. Heparin inhibits coagulation at the end of the cascade after nearly all other coagulation proteins have been converted to active enzymes. In addition, heparin to varying degrees activates several blood constituents: platelets,[228] factor XII,[229] complement, neutrophils, and monocytes.[230] Thrombin concentrations cannot be measured in real time and only insensitive, indirect methods are available to regulate heparin anticoagulation in the operating room.[231]

Heparin is also associated with some clinical idiosyncrasies. In some patients recent, prolonged parenteral heparin may reduce antithrombin concentrations and produce *heparin resistance*.[232] Insufficient antithrombin may also occur because of insufficient synthesis or increased consumption in cachectic patients and patients with advanced liver or renal disease. The deficiency in antithrombin prevents heparin from prolonging ACTs to therapeutic levels. In these patients fresh-frozen plasma or recombinant antithrombin is needed to increase plasma antithrombin concentrations to inhibit thrombin. *Heparin rebound* is a delayed anticoagulant effect after protamine neutralization because of the rapid metabolism of protamine and delayed seepage of heparin into the circulation from lymphatic tissues and other deposits. Heparin is also associated with an allergic response

in some patients that produces heparin-induced thrombocytopenia (HIT) with or without thrombosis (HITT). Lastly, heparin only partially suppresses thrombin formation during CPB and all applications of extracorporeal perfusion and mechanical circulatory and respiratory assistance despite doses two to three times those used for other indications (see Fig. 13-11).[217]

Potential safe alternatives for heparin during ECP include low-molecular-weight heparin, recombinant hirudin (lepirudin), and the organic chemical, argatroban (Texas Biotechnology Corp.). All have important drawbacks and are approved for use in HIT and in patients with circulating IgG anti-heparin–PF4 complex antibodies (see the following). Low-molecular-weight heparins have long half-lives in plasma (4-8 hours), require antithrombin as a cofactor, primarily inhibit factor Xa, and are not reversible by protamine.[233] Recombinant hirudin (lepirudin) is a direct inhibitor of thrombin, is effective rapidly, does not have an effective antidote, is monitored by the partial thromboplastin time, is cleared by the kidney, and has a relatively short half-life in plasma (40 minutes).[234] This drug has been successfully used during CPB and OHS, but in many instances bleeding after bypass has been troublesome and substantial. A newer drug is a semisynthetic bivalent thrombin inhibitor composed of 12 amino acids from hirudin.[235] This drug, bivalirudin (angiomax), has a shorter half-life than hirudin and therefore may be safer. Argatroban is also a direct thrombin inhibitor with rapid onset of action and short plasma half-life (40-50 minutes).[236] Argatroban is metabolized in the liver and is without an antidote, but can be monitored with partial thromboplastin times or ACTs. At present there growing experience with the use of argatroban and bivalirudin as alternative anticoagulant when heparin cannot be used.[237]

Heparin-Associated Thrombocytopenia, Heparin-Induced Thrombocytopenia, and Heparin-Induced Thrombocytopenia and Thrombosis

Heparin-associated thrombocytopenia (HAT) is a benign, nonimmune, 5 to 15% decrease in platelet count that occurs within a few hours to 3 days after heparin exposure. HIT and heparin-induced thrombocytopenia and thrombosis (HITT) are different manifestations of the same immune disease. Heparin binds to platelets in the absence of an antibody and releases small amounts of platelet factor 4 (as occurs in HAT). PF4 avidly binds heparin to form a heparin-PF4 (H-PF4) complex, which is antigenic in some people. In these individuals IgG antibodies to the *H-PF4 complex* are produced within 5 to 15 days after exposure to heparin and continue to circulate for approximately 3 to 6 months.[238] *IgG-anti-H-PF4 antibodies* plus *H-PF4 complexes* form *HIT complexes*, which unite IgG Fc terminals to platelet Fc receptors (Fig. 13-12). This binding strongly stimulates platelets to release more PF4.[239] A self-perpetuating, accelerating cascade of platelet activation, release,

Pathogenesis of HIT

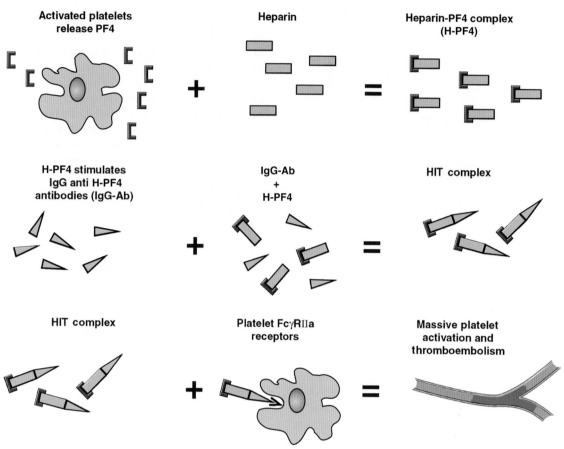

FIGURE 13-12 The generation of HIT complexes. Read each horizontal group of three left to right beginning at top left. See text for full explanation.

and aggregation ensues. Since platelet granules contain several procoagulatory proteins (eg, thrombin, fibronectin, factor V, fibrinogen, von Willebrand factor), release also activates coagulation proteins to generate thrombin.

The intensity of the immune reaction varies between patients, but also varies by the indications for heparin use. Patients who do not have conditions that activate platelets have a low incidence of HIT after administration of heparin, because few PF4 molecules are available to form H-PF4 complexes. Large doses of heparin are given and huge numbers of platelets are activated during CPB. Thus after CPB, 50% of patients have IgG anti-H-PF4 antibodies; 2% have immune heparin-induced thrombocytopenia; and approximately 1% develop HITT.[240] Because IgG antibodies are transient, a second heparin exposure 6 months after HIT is not likely to produce HIT or HITT,[239] but will stimulate production of new IgG antibodies to the H-PF4 complex. The danger is a second heparin exposure when IgG anti-H-PF4 antibodies are still circulating.

IgG anti-H-PF4 antibodies are detected in two ways. The serotonin release test detects the release of radioactive serotonin from normal platelets washed by the patient's serum.[241] An enzyme immunoassay measures IgG anti-H-PF4 antibodies directly. Both assays are equally sensitive in patients with clinical HIT, but the enzyme immunoassay is more sensitive in detecting IgG anti-H-PF4 antibodies in patients without other evidence of the disease.[242]

The clinical presentation of HIT may be insidious. If the platelet count was originally normal, the earliest sign is an abrupt decrease of at least 50% in platelet count (to <150,000/µL) in a patient who has had exposure to heparin within the past 5 to 15 days. This event is a preoperative stop sign for elective cardiac operations. After CPB, platelet counts less than 80,000/µL should trigger an order to stop all heparin, including heparin flushes, and obtain daily platelet counts. The patient should be thoroughly examined for deep vein thrombosis, extremity ischemia, stroke, myocardial infarction, or any evidence of intravascular thrombosis using ultrasound and appropriate radiographic technology. Any evidence of vascular thrombosis should prompt a plasma sample for IgG anti-H-PF4 antibodies. A positive antibody test confirms the diagnosis of HIT in patients with thrombocytopenia and HITT in those with either venous or arterial thrombosis or both. It is important to stress that HIT or HITT is a clinical diagnosis, and a positive antibody test is *not* required before stopping heparin.

Once the diagnosis of HIT or HITT is suspected, management must focus on prevention of further intravascular thrombosis. Bleeding is rarely the problem; intravascular thrombosis is. Neither heparin nor platelet transfusions should be given; platelet transfusions only add more PF4 if heparin and IgG anti-H-PF4 antibodies are still circulating. If heparin is proven absent from the circulation, platelet transfusions may be used very cautiously if the patient has significant nonsurgical bleeding. Surgical measures to reopen thrombosed large arteries are usually futile because the platelet-rich thrombus (white clot) often extends into small arteries and arterioles.

Modern management also includes full anticoagulation with recombinant hirudin (lepirudin), argatroban, or possibly bivalirudin to prevent further extension of thrombosis or development of clinical intravascular thrombosis. This may occur in 40 to 50% of patients with HIT who are treated only with heparin cessation.[243] At present there is little experience with argatroban in cardiac surgical patients with HITT, but the drug is a direct thrombin inhibitor, has attractive pharmokinetics, and is approved for patients with HITT.[244] Full anticoagulation with hirudin or bivalirudin in fresh postoperative cardiac surgical patients is recommended, but the safety zone between bleeding and thrombosis is narrow. The patient must be carefully monitored for pericardial tamponade and signs of hidden bleeding. Hirudin is monitored by a PTT and the range used is similar to that with intravenous heparin. Dose must be reduced in patients with renal failure because the kidney clears the drug. Argatroban is sometimes a better choice, but it should be remembered that it is difficult to manage in the presence of liver disease because it is metabolized in that organ. In most patients oral anticoagulation with warfarin is started at the same time as intravenous hirudin.

Emergency or urgent OHS with CPB using hirudin is possible in patients with circulating IgG anti-HPF4 antibodies. The therapeutic level of drug should be between 3.5 and 4.5 µg/mL during CPB.[245] Greinacher recommends bolus doses of 0.25 mg/kg IV and 0.2 mg/kg in the priming volume followed by an infusion of 0.5 mg/min until 15 minutes before stopping CPB. At that time 5 mg of hirudin is added to the perfusate to prevent clotting within the heart-lung machine. Bivalirudin has been compared to heparin and found to be comparable related to post op bleeding.[246]

Coagulation and Extracorporeal Perfusion: Thrombin Generation

Generation of thrombin during CPB and other applications of extracorporeal circulatory technology is the cause of the thrombotic and bleeding complications associated with ECP. Theoretically, if thrombin formation could be completely inhibited during ECP, the consumptive coagulopathy, which consumes coagulation proteins and platelets and causes bleeding complications, would not occur.

Thrombin generation and the fibrinolytic response primarily involve the extrinsic and intrinsic coagulation pathways, the contact and fibrinolytic plasma protein systems, and platelets, monocytes, and endothelial cells.

CONTACT SYSTEM

The contact system includes four primary plasma proteins—factor XII, prekallikrein, high-molecular-weight kininogen (HMWK), and C-1 inhibitor and is activated during CPB and clinical cardiac surgery.[247] This system is involved in complement and neutrophil activation and the inflammatory response to ECP, but is not involved in thrombin formation in vivo.

INTRINSIC COAGULATION PATHWAY

The intrinsic coagulation pathway probably does not generate thrombin in vivo, but does initiate thrombin formation when blood contacts nonendothelial cell surfaces such as perfusion circuits.[248]

EXTRINSIC (TISSUE FACTOR) COAGULATION PATHWAY

The extrinsic coagulation pathway is the major coagulation pathway in vivo and is a major source of thrombin generation during CPB and clinical cardiac surgery.[249,250] Exposure of blood to TF by direct contact in the wound or by wound blood aspirated into the ECP circuit initiates the extrinsic coagulation pathway.[251] TF is a cell-bound glycoprotein that is constitutively expressed on the cellular surfaces of fat, muscle, bone, epicardium, adventia, injured endothelial cells, and many other cells except pericardium.[252] Plasma TF associated with wound monocytes is a second source of TF and may be an important source during CPB and clinical cardiac surgery.[253]

COMMON COAGULATION PATHWAY

Factor Xa is the gateway protein of the common coagulation pathway. Factor Xa slowly cleaves prothrombin to α-thrombin, the active enzyme, and a fragment, F1.2, and is the major pathway producing thrombin.[251] F1.2 is a useful marker of the reaction.

THROMBIN

Thrombin is a powerful enzyme that accelerates its own formation by several feedback loops.[254] Thrombin is the major activator of factor XI and the exclusive activator of factor VIII in the intrinsic pathway. Thrombin is a secondary activator of factor VII, but once formed may be the most important activator in the wound.

Thrombin has both procoagulant and anticoagulant properties.[254] Thrombin is the enzyme that cleaves fibrinogen to fibrin and in the process creates two fragments, fibrinopeptides A and B. Thrombin activates platelets via the platelet thrombin receptor and thus may be the major agonist for platelets both in the wound and in the perfusion circuit. Thrombin also activates factor XIII to cross-link fibrin to an insoluble form and attenuate fibrinolysis.

Thrombin also stimulates the production of anticoagulants. Surface glycosaminoglycans, such as heparan sulfate, inhibit thrombin and coagulation via antithrombin. Thrombin stimulates endothelial cells to produce tissue plasminogen activator, t-PA, which is the major enzyme that cleaves plasminogen to plasmin, and initiates fibrinolysis.

THROMBIN GENERATION DURING EXTRACORPOREAL PERFUSION

All applications of ECP and exposure of blood to nonendothelial cell surfaces generate thrombin.[217] F1.2 is a protein fragment that is formed when prothrombin is cleaved to thrombin; thus F1.2 is a measure of thrombin generation but not of thrombin activity. F1.2 and thrombin-antithrombin (TAT) complex increase progressively during clinical cardiac surgery with CPB, during applications of circulatory assist devices[255] and during extracorporeal life support (ECLS) (Fig. 13-13). The amount of thrombin produced seems to vary with the intensity of the stimuli for thrombin production and may vary with age, comorbid disease, and clinical health of the patient. Complex cardiac surgery that requires several hours of CPB produces more F1.2 than short procedures with minimal exposure of circulating blood to the wound.[256] Thrombin generation varies with the amount and type of anticoagulant used; surface area of the blood-biomaterial interface; duration of exposure to the surface; turbulence, stagnation, and cavitation within perfusion circuits; and to a lesser degree temperature and the "thromboresistant" characteristics of biomaterial surfaces.[257]

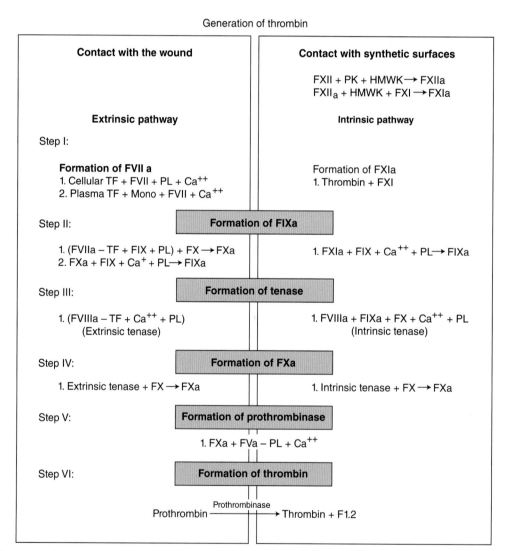

FIGURE 13-13 Steps in the generation of thrombin in the wound and in the perfusion circuit via the extrinsic, intrinsic, and common coagulation pathways. PK, prekallikrein; HMWK, high-molecular-weight kininogen; Ca^{2+}, calcium ion; PL, cellular phospholipid surface; TF, tissue factor; Mono, monocyte. Activated coagulation proteins are indicated by the suffix -a.

For many years blood contact with the biomaterials of the perfusion circuit was thought to be the major stimulus to thrombin formation during CPB and OHS. Increasing evidence indicates that the wound is the major source of thrombin generation during CPB and clinical cardiac surgery. This understanding has encouraged development of strategies to reduce the amounts of circulating thrombin during clinical cardiac surgery by either discarding wound blood[258] or exclusively salvaging red cells by centrifugation and washing in a cell saver. The reduced thrombin formation in the perfusion circuit has also supported strategies for reducing the systemic heparin dose during first-time coronary revascularization procedures using heparin-bonded circuits.[259] Although there is no good evidence that heparin-bonded circuits reduce thrombin generation, there is strong evidence that discarding wound plasma or limiting exposure of circulating blood to the wound (eg, less bleeding in the wound) does reduce the circulating thrombin burden.[260]

Cellular Procoagulants and Anticoagulants

PLATELETS

Platelets are activated by thrombin, contact with the surface of nonendothelial cells, heparin, and platelet-activating factor produced by a variety of cells during all applications of extracorporeal perfusion and/or recirculation of anticoagulated blood that has been exposed to a wound. Circulating thrombin and platelet contact with surface-adsorbed fibrinogen in the perfusion circuit are probably the earliest and strongest agonists. Circulating thrombin, although rapidly inhibited by antithrombin, is a powerful agonist and binds avidly to two specific thrombin receptors on platelets: PAR-1 and GPIb α.[261] As CPB continues, complement, plasmin, hypothermia, epinephrine, and other agonists also activate platelets and contribute to their loss and dysfunction.

The initial platelet reaction to agonists is shape change. Circulating discoid platelets extend pseudopods, centralize granules, express GPIb and GPIIb/IIIa receptors,[262] and secrete soluble and bound P selectin receptors from alpha granules.[263] GPIIb/IIIa ($\alpha_{IIb} \beta3$) receptors almost instantaneously bind platelets to exposed binding sites on the α- and γ-chains on surface-adsorbed fibrinogen (Fig. 13-14),[264] but the rough surfaces accumulate more platelets than smooth surfaces. Platelet adhesion and aggregate formation reduce the circulating platelet count, which is already reduced by dilution with pump priming solutions.

Plasma fibrinogen forms bridges between platelets expressing GPIIb/IIIa receptors to produce circulating platelet aggregates. Platelet bound P-selectin binds platelets to monocytes and neutrophils to form aggregates.[265] During ECP the circulating platelet pool is reduced by dilution, adhesion, aggregation, destruction, and consumption. The platelet mass consists of a reduced number of morphologically normal platelets, platelets with pseudopod formation, new and larger platelets released from megakaryocytes, partially and completely degranulated platelets. Most of the circulating platelets appear structurally normal, but bleeding times increase and remain prolonged for several hours after protamine.[266] The functional state of the circulating intact platelet during and early after CPB is reduced, but it is not clear whether this functional defect is intrinsic or extrinsic to the platelet. Flow cytometry studies of circulating intact platelets show little change in platelet membrane receptors.[267]

MONOCYTES

In the wound with calcium present, monocytes associate with plasma TF to rapidly accelerate the conversion of factor VII to factor VIIa.[268] This association is specific for monocytes as the reaction is essentially nil for platelets, neutrophils, and lymphocytes—and does not occur if monocytes, plasma TF, or factor VII is not present. The major sources of TF in the

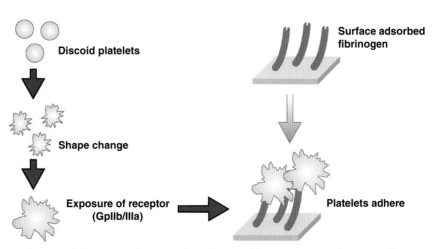

FIGURE 13-14 Adhesion of activated platelets binding to surface-adsorbed fibrinogen via GPIIb/IIIa ($\alpha_{IIb} \beta3$) receptors. The same receptors bind plasma fibrinogen molecules to form platelet aggregates.

wound are the combination of monocytes, plasma TF, and cell-bound TF.

Endothelial Cells

Endothelial cells, charged with maintaining the fluidity of circulating blood and the integrity of the vascular system, are activated during CPB and clinical cardiac surgery by thrombin, C5a, IL-1, and TNF-α.[269] Endothelial cells produce both procoagulants and anticoagulants. Procoagulant activities of endothelial cells include expression of TF and production of a host of procoagulant proteins.[270] Anticoagulant activities of endothelial cells include the production of tissue plasminogen activator (t-PA), heparin sulfate, TF inhibitor protein, prostacyclin, nitric oxide, and adenosine.[271]

Fibrinolysis

Circulating thrombin activates endothelial cells to produce tissue plasminogen activator (t-PA), which binds avidly to fibrin.[272] Endothelial cells are the principal source of t-PA.[273] The combination of t-PA, fibrin, and plasminogen cleaves plasminogen to plasmin; plasmin cleaves fibrin. This reaction produces the protein fragment, D-dimer, which is a useful marker of fibrinolysis, and a marker of thrombin activity because fibrin is cleaved from fibrinogen by thrombin.[274]

Fibrinolysis is controlled by native protease inhibitors, α2-antiplasmin, α2-macroglobulin, and plasminogen activator inhibitor-1.[274] Alpha 2-antiplasmin rapidly inhibits unbound plasmin, preventing the enzyme from circulating, but poorly inhibits plasmin bound to fibrin.

Consumptive Coagulopathy

Simultaneous and ongoing thrombin formation and fibrinolysis are by definition a consumptive coagulopathy[275] and is present in all applications of ECP. In the normal state the fluidity of blood and the integrity of the vascular system are established and maintained by an equilibrium between procoagulants favoring clot and anticoagulants favoring liquidity (Fig. 13-15A). Blood contact with ECP systems and the wound disrupts this equilibrium to produce a massive procoagulant stimulus that overwhelms natural anticoagulants; therefore, an exogenous anticoagulant, heparin, is required for nearly all applications of ECP (Fig. 13-15B). Exceptions are only possible in applications that produce a relatively weak procoagulant stimulus and a minimal thrombin burden that can be contained by natural anticoagulants. Surgeons must realize that any blood exposure to nonendothelial cell surfaces, including prosthetic heart valves, produces a procoagulant stimulus whether or not a clot is produced. Except for the healthy endothelial cell, no nonthrombogenic surface exists.

This concept of an equilibrium between procoagulants and anticoagulants is helpful in managing the thrombotic and bleeding complications associated with all applications of ECP. During ECP procoagulant stimuli, manifested by thrombin formation that is not measurable in real time, must

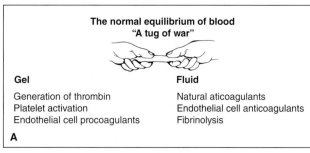

FIGURE 13-15 (A) The balance between procoagulant and anticoagulant forces that produces an equilibrium allows blood to circulate. (B) During CPB and OHS (open heart surgery) the normal equilibrium is disturbed by changes in both procoagulants and anticoagulants. Imbalance of procoagulants risks thrombosis; an imbalance of anticoagulants risks bleeding.

be balanced by *either* increased anticoagulation or a reduction in the thrombin burden to maintain equilibrium. After ECP, anticoagulants must be inhibited to avoid excessive bleeding. During consumptive coagulopathy, coagulation proteins and platelets are consumed and may become too deficient to generate thrombin and fibrin-platelet clots. In cardiac surgical patients many additional variables affect the coagulation equilibrium and impact the availability of coagulation proteins and functional platelets. These variables include the quantity of blood in contact with the wound; surface area of the perfusion system; duration of perfusion; circulating anticoagulants; and to lesser degrees temperature and the rheology and biomaterials of the perfusion system. Patient factors also affect the coagulation equilibrium; these include age, infection, history or presence of cardiogenic shock, massive blood losses and transfusions, platelet coagulation deficiencies, fibrinolysis, liver disease, cachexia, reoperation, and hypothermia.

Management of Bleeding

The cornerstone of bleeding management is meticulous surgical hemostasis during all phases of an operation. The surgical techniques, topical agents, and customary drugs used do not need reiteration for trained surgeons. Most cardiac surgical operations involving CPB are accompanied by net blood losses between 200 and 600 mL. Reoperations; complex procedures; prolonged (>3 hours) CPB; and patient factors listed above may be associated with excessive and ongoing blood losses. Most surgeons use an antifibrinolytic, such as tranexamic acid or epsilon amino caproic acid, to reduce fibrinolysis in prolonged or complex operations. Problem patients who bleed excessively after heparin neutralization require an attempt to rebalance procoagulants and anticoagulants to near normal, pre-CPB concentrations.

The most useful tests in the operating room are an ACT or a protamine titration test to assess the presence of heparin; prothrombin time to uncover deficiency in the extrinsic coagulation pathway; and platelet count. If heparin is neutralized, the partial thromboplastin time may be measured to assess possible deficiency of coagulation proteins. Other tests such as measurements of fibrinogen, template bleeding time, and the thromboelastograph are controversial and/or difficult to obtain. Platelet counts below 80,000 to 100,000/μL should initiate platelet transfusions in bleeding patients, except those with IgG anti-H-PF4 antibodies, to add functioning platelets to the mass of partially dysfunctional platelets.

Measurements of F1.2 and D-dimer are two tests that can be very helpful and probably should be made available on an emergency basis in hospitals that perform complex procedures and offer mechanical circulatory and respiratory assistance. F1.2 measures thrombin formation by factor Xa, and if absent or low, there may be a deficiency in the concentrations of coagulation proteins; fresh-frozen plasma is needed. If F1.2 and D-dimer (a measurement of fibrinolytic activity) are both elevated, thrombin is being formed and an antifibrinolytic (tranexamic acid or epsilon amino caproic acid) is needed to neutralize plasmin. If both markers or F1.2 remain elevated

after the antifibrinolytic drug, this indicates continuing thrombin generation, and the cause (eg, infection usually) should be aggressively treated with antibiotics. Some thrombin is needed to stop bleeding, but excessive thrombin production feeds the consumptive coagulopathy. As with diffuse intravascular coagulopathy,[275] no guaranteed therapeutic recipe is known; success requires patience, persistence, and judicious use of platelets, antifibrinolytics, specific clotting factors, and replacement transfusions to rebalance the coagulation equilibrium at near normal concentrations of the constituents.

THE INFLAMMATORY RESPONSE
Primary Blood Constituents
COMPLEMENT

The complement system constitutes a group of more than 30 plasma proteins that interact to produce powerful vasoactive anaphylatoxins, C3a, C4a, and C5a, and the terminal complement cytotoxic complex, C5b-9.[276] Complement is activated by three pathways, but only the classical and alternative pathways are involved in CPB. Direct contact between heparinized blood and the synthetic surfaces of the ECP circuit activates the contact plasma proteins and the classical complement pathway. Activation of C1, possibly by activated factor XIIa, sequentially activates C2 and C4 to form C4b2a (classical C3 convertase) that cleaves C3 to form C3a and C3b (Fig. 13-16).

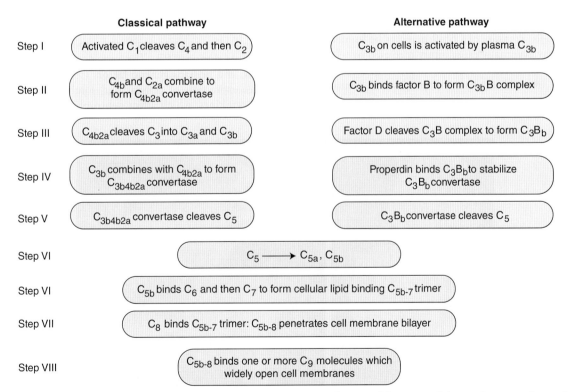

	Classical pathway	Alternative pathway
Step I	Activated C_1 cleaves C_4 and then C_2	C_{3b} on cells is activated by plasma C_{3b}
Step II	C_{4b} and C_{2a} combine to form C_{4b2a} convertase	C_{3b} binds factor B to form $C_{3b}B$ complex
Step III	C_{4b2a} cleaves C_3 into C_{3a} and C_{3b}	Factor D cleaves C_3B complex to form C_3B_b
Step IV	C_{3b} combines with C_{4b2a} to form C_{3b4b2a} convertase	Properdin binds C_3B_b to stabilize C_3B_b convertase
Step V	C_{3b4b2a} convertase cleaves C_5	C_3B_b convertase cleaves C_5

Step VI	$C_5 \longrightarrow C_{5a}, C_{5b}$
Step VI	C_{5b} binds C_6 and then C_7 to form cellular lipid binding C_{5b-7} trimer
Step VII	C_8 binds C_{5b-7} trimer: C_{5b-8} penetrates cell membrane bilayer
Step VIII	C_{5b-8} binds one or more C_9 molecules which widely open cell membranes

FIGURE 13-16 Steps in activation of the classical and alternative complement pathways and formation of the membrane attack complex, C5b-9. (Data from Walport MJ: Complement. *NEJM* 2001; 344:1058; and Volkankis JE, Frank ME: *The Human Complement System in Health and Disease.* New York: Marcel Dekker; 1998.)

Generation of C3b activates the alternative pathway, which involves factors B and D in the formation of C3bBb, which is the alternative pathway C3 convertase that cleaves C3 to form C3a and C3b (see Fig. 13-16). Whereas the classical pathway proceeds in sequential steps, the alternative pathway contains a feedback loop that greatly amplifies cleavage of C3 by membrane-bound C3 convertase to membrane-bound C3b and C3a. During CPB complement is largely activated by the alternative pathway.[277]

The complement system is activated at three different times during CPB and cardiac surgery: during blood contact with nonendothelial cell surfaces[278] and wound exudate-containing tissue factor[279]; after protamine administration and formation of the protamine-heparin complex[280]; and after reperfusion of the ischemic, arrested heart.[281] CPB and myocardial reperfusion activate complement by both the classical and alternative pathways; the heparin-protamine complex activates complement by the classical pathway.

The two C3 convertases effectively merge the two complement pathways by producing C3b, which activates C5 to C5a and C5b (see Fig. 13-16). C3a and C5a are potent vasoactive anaphylatoxins. C5a, which avidly binds to neutrophils and therefore is difficult to detect in plasma, is the major agonist. C3b acts as an opsonin, which binds target cell hydroxyl groups and renders them susceptible to phagocytic cells expressing specific receptors for C3b.[282,283] C5b is the first component of the terminal pathway that ultimately leads to formation of the membrane attack complex, C5b-9. In prokaryotic cells like erythrocytes, C5b-9 creates transmembrane pores, which cause death by intracellular swelling after loss of the intracellular/interstitial osmotic gradient. In eukaryotic cells, deposits of C5b-9 may not be immediately lethal but may eventually cause injury mediated by release of arachidonic acid metabolites (thromboxane A2, leukotrienes) and oxygen free radicals by macrophages and neutrophils, respectively.[284]

NEUTROPHILS

Neutrophils are strongly activated during CPB (Fig. 13-17).[285] The principal agonists are kallikrein and C5a produced by the contact and complement systems. Neutrophils are recruited to localized areas of injury or inflammation by chemokines, complement proteins (C5a), IL-1β, TNF-α, and adhesion molecules. During CPB thrombin stimulates endothelial cell production of platelet activating factor (PAF).[286] Thrombin and PAF cause rapid expression of P-selectin by endothelial cells.[287] Regional vasoconstriction mediated by PAF reduces blood flow rates within local vascular beds to allow neutrophils to marginate near endothelial cell surfaces. P-selectin weakly binds to neutrophils[288]; selectin binding causes the slowly passing neutrophils to roll and eventually stop (Fig. 13-18).[289] Stronger adherence is produced by intracellular adhesion molecule-1 (ICAM-1) expressed on endothelial cells, which binds β2 neutrophil integrins, principally CD11b/CD18. These adhesion molecules from the immunoglobulin superfamily completely stop neutrophils and the process of transmigration begins in response to chemoattractants and cytotoxins produced in the extravascular space.[290] This trafficking is strongly regulated by IL-8 produced by neutrophils, macrophages, and other cells.[291]

Using pseudopods and following the scent of complement proteins (C5a, C3b) and IL-8, neutrophils arrive at the scene of inflammation to begin the process of phagocytosis and release of cytotoxins. Organs and tissues experience periods of ischemia followed by reperfusion (lung, heart, brain) during CPB, and as a result express adhesion receptors and reactive oxidants, and are sources of neutrophil chemoattractants.[292] Neutrophils vary considerably among individuals in expression of adhesive receptors[293] and responsiveness to chemoattractants during CPB. The presence of diabetes, oxidative stress, and perhaps genetic factors (see the following) influences expression of cellular and soluble adhesive receptors and cytokines, which affect neutrophil adhesion and release

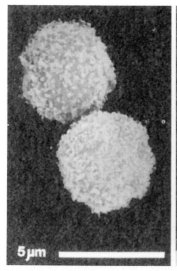
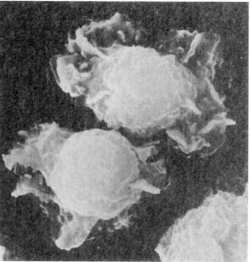

FIGURE 13-17 Scanning electron micrographs of resting neutrophils (*left*) and 5 seconds after exposure to a chemoattractant. (Reproduced with permission from Baggiolini M: Chemokines and leukocyte traffic, *Nature* 1998 Apr 9;392(6676):565-568.)

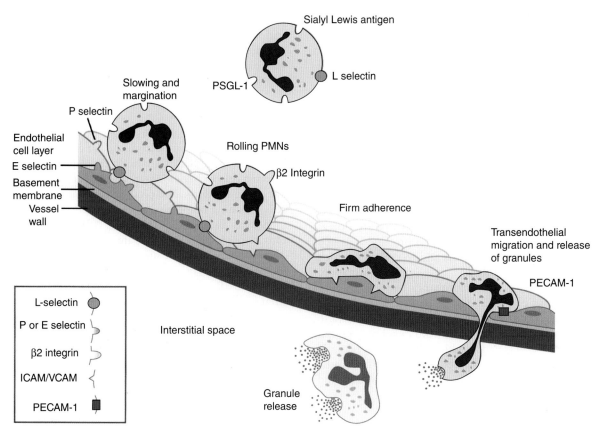

FIGURE 13-18 Mechanism of arrest and transmigration of neutrophils into the interstitial space. Neutrophils constitutively express L-selectin, which binds to endothelial cell glycoprotein ligands. Simultaneously, early response cytokines stimulate endothelial cells to rapidly express P-selectin and later E-selectin receptors, which weakly bind neutrophil PSGL-1 ligands. Marginated neutrophils, which are slowed by local vasoconstriction and reduced blood flow, lightly adhere to endothelial cells via selectin expression and begin to roll. Neutrophils activated by C5a, kallikrein, and early response cytokines express β2 CD11b and c receptors, which bind firmly to cytokine-activated endothelial cell intergrins, ICAM-1, and VCAM-1. Once arrested, L-selectins are shed and PECAM receptors on endothelial cell surfaces mediate neutrophil transmigration through endothelial cell junctions, led by chemoattractants into the interstitial space.

of granule contents. Neutrophils contain a potent arsenal of proteolytic and cytotoxic substances. Azurophilic granules contain lysozyme, myeloperoxidase, cationic proteins, elastase, and collagenases.[294] Activated neutrophils, in a "respiratory burst," also produce cytotoxic reactive oxygen and nitrogen intermediates including superoxide anion, hydrogen peroxide, hydroxyl radicals, singlet oxygen molecules. Finally, neutrophils produce arachidonate metabolites, prostaglandins, leukotrienes, and platelet-activating factor. During CPB these vasoactive and cytotoxic substances are produced and released into the extracellular environment and circulation. Circulation of these substances mediates many of the manifestations of the "whole body inflammatory response" or "systemic inflammatory response syndrome" (SIRS) associated with CPB and clinical cardiac surgery.[295]

MONOCYTES

Monocytes and macrophages (tissue monocytes) are relatively large, long-lived cells that are involved in both acute and chronic inflammation. Monocytes respond to chemical signals, are mobile, phagocytize microorganisms and cell fragments, produce and secrete chemical mediators, participate in the immune response, and generate cytotoxins.[296] Monocytes are activated during CPB and have a major role in thrombin formation. Monocytes also produce and release many inflammatory mediators during acute inflammation, including proinflammatory cytokines, reactive oxygen and nitrogen intermediates, and prostaglandins.

ENDOTHELIAL CELLS

Endothelial cells are activated during CPB and OHS by a variety of agonists.[297] The principal agonists for endothelial cell activation during CPB are thrombin, C5a, and the cytokines IL-1β and TNF-α. IL-1β and TNF-α induce the early expression of P-selectin and the later synthesis and expression of E-selectin, which are involved in the initial stages of neutrophil and monocyte adhesion. The two cytokines also induce expression of ICAM-1 and Vascular Cell Adhesion Molecule-1 (VCAM-1), which firmly bind neutrophils and monocytes to the endothelium and initiate leukocyte trafficking to the extravascular space (see Fig. 13-18). Experimentally ICAM-1 is upregulated during CPB in pulmonary vessels[298] and there is evidence that selectins are upregulated during CPB and in myocardial ischemia-reperfusion sequences. IL-1β and TNF-α induce endothelial cell production of the chemotactic proteins IL-8 and MCP-1, and induce production of PGI2 (prostacyclin) by the cyclooxygenase pathway and NO by NO synthase. These two vasodilators reduce shear stress and increase vascular permeability and therefore enhance leukocyte adhesion and transmigration.

PLATELETS

Platelets are probably initially activated during CPB by thrombin, which is the most potent platelet agonist. Plasma epinephrine, PAF, vasopressin, from other cells, and internally generated thromboxane A2 contribute to activation as CPB continues. Platelets possess several protease-activated receptors to most of these agonists and to collagen, which has an important role in adhesion and thrombus formation. Platelets contribute to the inflammatory response by synthesis and release of eicosanoids[299]; serotonin from dense granules; chemokines; and other proteins.[300] Platelets also produce and release acid hydrolases from membrane-bound lysozymes. Platelet-secreted cytokines may be particularly involved in the inflammatory response to CPB because of strong activation of platelets in both the wound and perfusion circuit.

Other Mediators of Inflammation

ANAPHYLATOXINS

The anaphylatoxins C3a, C4a, and C5a are bioactive protein fragments released by cleavage of complement proteins C3, C4, and C5. These fragments have potent proinflammatory and immuno-regulatory functions and contract smooth muscle cells, increase vascular permeability, serve as chemoattractants, and in the case of C5a, activate neutrophils and monocytes.[301] Anaphylatoxins contribute to increased

pulmonary vascular resistance, edema, and neutrophil sequestration and an increase in extravascular water during CPB. The duration of postoperative ventilation directly correlates with plasma C3a concentrations.[302] C3a and C5a are important mediators in ischemia/reperfusion injuries.

CYTOKINES

Cytokines are small, cell-signaling peptides produced and released into blood or the extravascular environment by both blood and tissue cells. Cytokines stimulate specific receptors on other cells to initiate a response in that cell. All blood leukocytes and endothelium produce cytokines, but many tissue cells including fibroblasts, smooth muscle cells, and cardiac monocytes also produce cytokines.[303] IL-1β and TNF-α are early response cytokines that are produced by macrophages. These proteins stimulate surrounding cells to produce chemokines. The main anti-inflammatory cytokine observed during CPB is IL-10, which inhibits the production of chemokines from leukocytes.[304] Proinflammatory cytokines increase during and after cardiac surgery using CPB with peak concentrations occurring 12 to 24 hours after CPB[305] (Fig. 13-19). Some of the variation in measurements between studies also may be caused by patient factors such as age, left ventricular function, and genetic factors.[306]

REACTIVE OXIDANTS

Neutrophils, monocytes, and macrophages produce reactive oxidants, which are cytotoxic inside the phagosome, but act as cytotoxic mediators of acute inflammation outside. Four enzymes generate a large menu of reactive oxidants: NADPH (nicotinamide adenine dinucleotide phosphate) oxidase, super-oxide dismutase, nitric oxide synthase, and myeloperoxidase.[307] The four products produced by these enzymes, O_2, H_2O_2, NO, and HOCL, generate all reactive oxidants from nonenzymatic reactions with other molecules or ions.

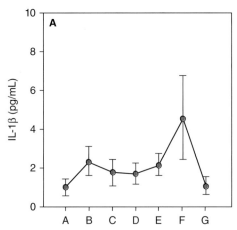
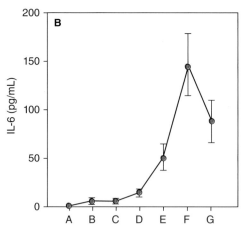

FIGURE 13-19 Changes in IL-1β (A) and IL-6 (B) in 30 patients who had elective first-time myocardial revascularization. Letters on x-axis represent the following events: (A) induction of anesthesia; (B) 5 minutes after heparin; (C) 10 minutes after starting CPB; (D) end of CPB; (E) 20 minutes after protamine; (F) 3 hours after CPB; (G) 24 hours after CPB. (Adapted with permission from Steinberg JB, Kapelanski DP, Olson JD, et al: Cytokine and complement levels in patients undergoing cardiopulmonary bypass, *J Thorac Cardiovasc Surg*. 1993 Dec;106(6):1008-1016.)

ENDOTOXINS

Endotoxins, including lipopolysaccharides, and fragments of bacteria that are powerful agonists for complement, neutrophils, monocytes, and other leukocytes.[308] Endotoxins have been detected during CPB and after aortic cross-clamping.[309] Sources include contaminants within sterilized infusion solutions, the bypass circuit, and possibly the gastrointestinal tract owing to changes in microvascular intestinal perfusion, which may translocate bacteria.[310]

METALLOPROTEINASES

CPB induces the synthesis and release of matrix metalloproteinases,[311] which are one of the four major classes of mammalian proteinases. These proteolytic enzymes have a major role in degradation of collagens and proteins in the pathogenesis of atherosclerosis and postinfarction left ventricular remodeling. The significance and possible injury produced by activation of these interstitial degradation enzymes over the long term remain to be determined.

Control of the Acute Inflammatory Response to Cardiopulmonary Bypass

OFF-PUMP CARDIAC SURGERY

Myocardial revascularization without either CPB or cardioplegia reduces the acute inflammatory response, but does not prevent it.[312] The response to surgical trauma, myocardial ischemia, manipulation of the heart, pericardial suction, heparin, protamine, other drugs, and anesthesia activates the extrinsic clotting system and produces an increase in the markers of acute inflammation, C3a, C5b-9, proinflammatory cytokines (TNF-α, IL-6, IL-9), neutrophil elastase, and reactive oxidants, but the magnitude of the response is significantly less than that observed with CPB.[313] Although it has not been shown that the attenuated acute inflammatory response directly reduces organ dysfunction, elderly patients, and those with reduced renal and pulmonary function often tolerate off-pump surgery with less morbidity and mortality than patients created with CPB.[314]

PERFUSION TEMPERATURE

Release of mediators of inflammation is temperature sensitive. Normothermic CPB increases the release of cytokines and other cellular and soluble mediators of inflammation,[312] whereas hypothermia reduces production and release of these mediators until rewarming begins.[315] Perfusion at tepid temperatures between 32 and 34°C is a reasonable compromise for many operations requiring 1 to 2 hours of CPB.[316]

PERFUSION CIRCUIT COATINGS

Ionic- or covalent-bonded heparin perfusion circuits are the most widely used surface coatings and are often combined with reduced doses of systemic heparin in first-time myocardial revascularization patients.[317] It is well established that heparin is an agonist for platelets, complement, factor XII, and leukocytes, but there is no reproducible evidence that heparin coating either produces a nonthrombogenic surface or reduces activation of the clotting cascade.[318] Clinical trials that have combined heparin-coated circuits with reduced systemic heparin and exclusion of field-aspirated blood from the perfusion circuit have demonstrated significant clinical benefits[319] (Fig. 13-20). New surface coatings are being developed or undergoing clinical studies.[320] In clinical trials these surface coatings significantly reduced platelet loss and granule release, and reduced markers of thrombin generation.[320,321] PMEA (poly-2-methylethylacrylate) is another manufactured surface coating designed to reduce surface adsorption of plasma proteins. Laboratory studies show reduced surface adsorption of fibrinogen and reduced bradykinin and thrombin generation in pigs.[321] Clinical studies show significant reductions in C3a, C4D, and neutrophil elastase, but ambivalent effects on IL-6 and platelets.[322]

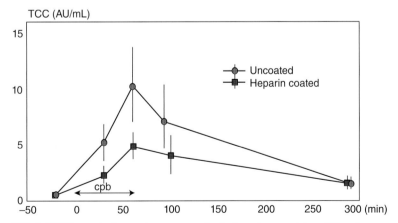

FIGURE 13-20 Changes in C5b-9 (TCC) terminal complement complex in heparin coated (n = 15) and uncoated (n = 14) perfusion circuits during myocardial revascularization. The two curves are significantly different by ANOVA (*p* = .004). (Reproduced with permission from Videm V, Mollnes TE, Fosse E, et al: Heparin-coated cardiopulmonary bypass equipment. I. Biocompatibility markers and development of complications in a high-risk population, *J Thorac Cardiovasc Surg*. 1999 Apr;117(4):794-802.)

MODIFIED ULTRAFILTRATION

Modified ultrafiltration to remove intravascular (and extra-vascular) water and inflammatory substances has produced improved results in adults and children.[323,324] Dialysis during CPB in adults may be beneficial in removing water, potassium, and protein wastes in patients with renal insufficiency.

COMPLEMENT INHIBITORS

The sequential activation cascade with convergence of the classical and alternative pathways at C3 offers many opportunities for inhabitation by recombinant proteins. Using a humanized, recombinant antibody to C5 (h5G1.1-scFv), Fitch et al. demonstrated that generation of C5b-9 was completely blocked in a dose-response manner (Fig. 13-21) and that neutrophil and monocyte CD11b/CD18 expression was attenuated in patients during and for several hours after clinical cardiac surgery using CPB.[325] Large-scale clinical trials

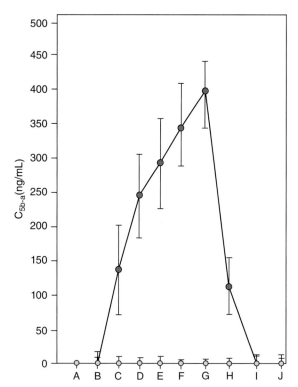

FIGURE 13-21 Inhibition of C5b-9, complement terminal attack complex, with placebo (solid circles) and 2 μg/kg of h5G1.1-scFv (open circles) during clinical cardiac surgery with CPB. Letters on x-axis represent the following events: (A) before heparin; (B) 5 minutes after drug; (C) 5 minutes after cooling to 28°C; (D) after beginning rewarming; (E) 5 minutes after reaching 32°C; (F) 5 minutes after reaching 37°C; (G) 5 minutes after CPB; (H) 2 hours after CPB; (I) 12 hours after CPB; (J) 24 hours after CPB. HcG1.1-scFv completely inhibited formation of the C5b-9 terminal attack complex. (Data from Fitch JC, Rollins S, Matis L, et al: Pharmacology and biological efficacy of a recombinant, humanized, single-chain antibody C5 complement inhibitor in patients undergoing coronary artery bypass graft surgery with cardiopulmonary bypass, *Circulation.* 1999 Dec 21-28;100(25):2499-2506.)

that have followed have shown significant improvements in morbidity and mortality.[326]

Other complement recombinant protein inhibitors have been developed and are under active investigation because of the importance of this plasma protein system in CPB, ischemia/reperfusion, and injuries that summon the acute inflammatory response. Although any effective and safe inhibitor is welcome, C3 may be a better target for inhibition because both activation pathways are blocked at the point of convergence and because C3 concentrations in plasma are 15 times greater than C5.[327]

GLUCOCORTICOIDS

Many investigators have used glucocorticoids to suppress the acute inflammatory response to CPB and clinical cardiac surgery, but beneficial effects in adult patients have been inconsistent.[328] Steroids reduce release of rapid-response cytokines, TNF-α, and IL-1β from macrophages, enhance release of IL-10, and suppress expression of endothelial cell selectins and neutrophil integrins.[329] Clinical results from a few randomized trials are conflicting: One study observed earlier extubation and reduced shivering,[330] but another found increased blood glucose levels and delayed extubation.[331] A recent large meta-analysis found that low-dose corticosteroids reduced atrial fibrillation incidence, and decreased ICU and hospital length of stay without increasing infectious complications.[332]

ORGAN DAMAGE

Cardiopulmonary bypass can preempt normal reflex and chemoreceptor control of the circulation, initiate coagulation, activate blood cells, release circulating cell-signaling proteins, generate vasoactive and cytotoxic substances, and produce a variety of microemboli. Venous pressure can be elevated, plasma colloid osmotic pressure is reduced, flow is nonpulsatile, and temperature is manipulated. Tissues and organs may suffer from regional malperfusion that is independent of physiologic controls, and is caused by microemboli, increased interstitial water, and perfusion with a variable amount of cytotoxic substances. Reversible and irreversible cell injury may occur, but damage is diffusely distributed throughout the entire body as individual cells or small groups of cells are affected. Ischemia-reperfusion injury augments damage to the heart and on occasion to other organs. Amazingly, the body is able to withstand and for the most part repair the cellular damage, although some abnormalities may appear later. This section summarizes the reversible and permanent organ damage produced by CPB and complements the preceding two sections of this chapter and the chapter on ischemia and reperfusion (see Chapter 3).

Mechanisms

Cardiac output during CPB is carefully monitored and synchronized with temperature and hemoglobin concentration to ensure that the entire body is adequately supplied with oxygen (see earlier section on ECP systems). Excessive hemodilution reduces oxygen delivery,[333] and hemoglobin concentrations significantly below 8 g/L cause organ dysfunction at temperatures above 30°C.[334] However, regional hypoperfusion is not monitored; is independent of reflex and chemoreceptor controls; and is influenced by the inflammatory response, which produces circulating vasoactive substances. Regional perfusion is also influenced by acid-base relationships during cooling and may affect postoperative organ function. Alpha-stat management (pH increases during cooling) decreases cerebral perfusion during hypothermia; pH stat (pH 7.40 is maintained by adding CO_2) improves organ perfusion but may increase embolic injury.[335] Temperature differences within the body and within organs produce regional temperature-perfusion mismatch,[336] which can precipitate regional hypoperfusion and acidosis caused by inadequate oxygen delivery.

The inflammatory response produces the cytotoxic compounds and activated neutrophils and monocytes that can and do destroy organ and tissue cells. These agents directly access the specialized cells of every organ by passing between endothelial cell junctions to reach the interstitial compartment. Reduced plasma colloid osmotic pressure, elevated venous pressure, and widened endothelial cell junctions[337] increase the volume of the interstitial space during CPB in proportion to the duration of bypass, magnitude of the dissection, transfusions, and other factors. In prolonged complicated perfusions the interstitial compartment may increase 18 to 33%,[338] but intracellular water does not increase during CPB.

Microemboli are defined as particles less than 500 μm in diameter. They enter the circulation during CPB from a variety of sources.[339] Table 13-2 summarizes sources of gas, foreign, and blood-generated microemboli, which are more fully discussed earlier. Air entry into the perfusion circuit produces the most dangerous gas emboli because nitrogen is poorly soluble in blood and is not a metabolite. Carbon dioxide is rapidly soluble in blood and is sometimes used to flood the surgical field to displace air. Foreign emboli, largely generated in the surgical wound, reach the circulation from the surgical field via the cardiotomy reservoir. The cardiotomy reservoir is the primary source of foreign emboli and the major source of blood-generated emboli, particularly fat emboli.[340] Extensive activation and physical damage to blood elements produce a wide variety of emboli, which tend to increase with the duration of perfusion.[335]

Strategies for Reducing Microemboli

Although discussed in earlier sections, the principal methods for reducing circulating microemboli deserve emphasis and include the following: adequate anticoagulation; membrane oxygenator; washing blood aspirated from the surgical wound[341]; filtering the cardiotomy reservoir; secure pursestring sutures around cannulas; strict control of all air entry sites within the perfusion circuit; removal of residual

TABLE 13-5: Minimizing Microemboli
Membrane oxygenator, centrifugal arterial pump
Cardiotomy reservoir filter (≤40 μm)
Arterial line filter/bubble trap (≤40 μm)
Keep temperature differentials ≤8-10 °C
Prime with carbon dioxide flush; recirculate with saline and filter (5 μm)
Prevent air entry into the circuit
Snug purse-string sutures
Three-way stopcocks on all sampling ports
Meticulous syringe management
Adequate cardiotomy reservoir volume (for debubbling)
Avoid excessive suction on vents
One-way valved purge lines for bubble traps
Use transesophageal echocardiography to locate trapped intracardiac air; de-air thoroughly
Wash blood aspirated from the surgical field
Prevent thrombus formation with adequate anticoagulation
Assess inflow cannulation site by epiaortic ultrasound imaging
Cannulate distal aorta or axillary artery
Consider use of special aortic cannulas

air from the heart and great vessels; avoidance of atherosclerotic emboli; and selective filtration of cerebral vessels (Table 13-5).[342,343]

Many intraoperative strategies are available to reduce cerebral atherosclerotic embolization. These include routine epicardial echocardiography of the ascending aorta to detect both anterior and posterior atherosclerotic plaques and find sites free of atherosclerosis for placing the aortic cannula.[344] Recently, special catheters with or without baffles or screens have been developed to reduce the number of atherosclerotic emboli that reach the cerebral circulation.[345] In patients with moderate or severe ascending aortic atherosclerosis a single application of the aortic clamp as opposed to partial or multiple applications is strongly recommended and has been shown to reduce postoperative neuronal and neurocognitive deficits in a large clinical series.[346] Retrograde cardioplegia is preferred over antegrade cardioplegia in these patients to avoid a sandblasting effect of the cardioplegic solution.[347] No aortic clamp may be safe or even possible in some patients with severe atherosclerosis or porcelain aorta. If intracardiac surgery is required in these patients, deep hypothermia may be used with or without graft replacement of the ascending aorta. If only revascularization is needed, pedicled single or sequential arterial grafts,[348] T or Y grafts from a pedicled mammary artery,[349] or vein grafts anastomosed to arch vessels can be used.

In-depth or screen filters are essential for cardiotomy reservoirs and are usually used in arterial lines. The efficacy of arterial line filters is controversial because screen filters with a pore size less than 20 microns cannot be used because of flow resistance across the filter. However, air and fat emboli can pass through filters although 20 micron screen filters more effectively trap microemboli than larger sizes.[350]

Cardiac Injury

It is difficult to separate postoperative cardiac dysfunction from injury owing to CPB, ischemia/reperfusion, direct surgical trauma, the disease being treated, and maladjustment of preload and afterload to myocardial contractile function. The heart, like all organs and tissues, is subject to microemboli, protease and chemical cytotoxins, activated neutrophils and monocytes, and regional hypoperfusion during CPB before and after cardioplegia or fibrillatory arrest. However, the heart is protected from CPB for at least one half of the case when the aorta is cross-clamped. Some degree of myocardial "stunning" during the period coronary blood flow is interrupted is inevitable,[351] as is some degree of reperfusion injury after ischemia. Both myocardial edema and distention of the flaccid cardioplegic heart during aortic cross-clamping[352] reduce myocardial contractility. Lastly, if myocardial contractility is weak, excessive preload or high afterload during weaning from CPB increases ventricular end-diastolic volume, myocardial wall stress, and oxygen consumption. Thus postoperative performance of the heart depends upon many variables and not just the injuries produced by CPB.

Neurologic Injury

The brain is the effecter organ for all behavior, innate, and learned. It is the monarch of blood flow and will shut down all other vascular systems to preserve its own supply. Conversely, dysfunction in other organs can adversely affect brain function. It monitors other organ systems and is acutely sensitive and responsive to both the external and internal environment. Thus, even small injuries to the brain may produce symptomatic, functional losses that would not be detectable or important in other organs. Regional hypoperfusion, edema, microemboli, circulating cytotoxins or subtle changes in blood glucose, insulin, or calcium may result in changes in cognitive function, ranging from subtle to profound. A small 2-mm infarct may cause a disruption of behavioral patterns, physiologic and physical function changes can pass unnoticed, be accepted, and dismissed, or profoundly compromise the patient's quality of life. Move the lesion half a centimeter and the same volume lesion may result in a catastrophic stroke. Thus the brain is the most sensitive organ exposed to damage by CPB and also the organ that, with the heart, is most important to protect.

ASSESSMENT

Routine assessment of neurologic injury that occurs in the setting of cardiac surgery is not done for most patients because of the priority of the cardiac lesion as well as costs in time and money. General neurologic examinations by members of the surgical team or individuals lacking specialized training are not adequate to rule out subtle neurologic injuries, and this is the principal reason that the incidence of stroke, or neurologic or neuropsychological injury varies widely in the surgical literature.[353]

The most obvious neurologic abnormalities are paresis, loss of vital brain functions such as speech, vision, comprehension, or coma. These are commonly lumped under the general heading of stroke. Disorders of awareness or consciousness can include coma, delirium, and confusion, but transitory episodes of delirium and confusion are often dismissed as caused by anesthesia or medications. More subtle losses are determined by comparison of preoperative and postoperative performances using a standard battery of neuropsychological tests prepared by a group of neuropsychologists. A neuropsychological examination is basically an extension of the neurologic examination with a much greater emphasis on higher cortical function. Dysfunction is objectively defined as a deviation from the expected, relative to a large population. For example, although performing at a 95 IQ level is in the normal range, it is low for a physician, and a search for a neurologic impairment would be triggered by such a poor performance. A 20% decline in two or more of these tests, compared with the patient's own baseline, suggests a neuropsychological deficit that should be followed until resolved or not resolved.[354] In studies involving long-term follow-up the inclusion of a control group of unoperated patients with the same disease and similar demographics helps define the causes of neuropsychological decline that occurs later than 3 to 6 months after surgery.[355]

Computed axial tomograms (CAT) or magnetic resonance imaging (MRI) scans are essential for the definitive diagnosis of stroke, delirium, or coma. Preoperative imaging is usually not necessary when new techniques such as diffusion-weighted MRI imaging, MRI spectroscopy, or MRI angiography are used to assess possible new lesions after operation.[356] Biochemical markers of neurologic injury after cardiac surgery are relatively nonspecific and inconclusive. Neuron-specific enolase (NSE) is an intracellular enzyme found in neurons, normal neuroendocrine cells, platelets, and erythrocytes.[357] S-100 is an acidic calcium-binding protein found in the brain.[358] The beta dimer resides in glial and Schwann cells. Both S-100 and NSE increase in spinal fluid with neuronal death and may correlate with stroke or spinal cord injury after CPB.[359] However, plasma levels are contaminated by aspiration of wound blood into the pump and hemolysis and are often elevated after prolonged CPB in patients without otherwise detectable neurologic injury.[360] Newer blood-borne biochemical markers such as Tau have been identified, but as of yet have not been shown to be diagnostic for subtle neurologic injury.

POPULATIONS AT RISK

Advancing age increases the risk of stroke or cognitive impairment in the general population, and surgery, regardless of type, increases the risk still higher.[361] In 1986, Gardner and colleagues reported the risk of stroke during CABG surgery to be directly related to age.[362] A European study compared 321 elderly patients without surgery to 1218 patients who had noncardiac surgery and found a 26% incidence of cognitive dysfunction 1 week after operation and a 10% incidence at 3 months.[363] Between 1974 and 1990 the number of patients

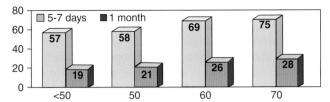

FIGURE 13-22 Effect of age by decade on neuropsychologic outcome after CABG. Abnormal neuropsychologic outcomes at 1 week and 1 month postoperative are more common with advancing age. Percentages of patients with deficits on two or more tests are shown (n = 374). (Reproduced with permission from Hammon JW Jr, Stump DA, Kon ND, et al: Risk factors and solutions for the development of neurobehavioral changes after coronary artery bypass grafting, *Ann Thorac Surg* 1997 Jun;63(6):1613-1618.)

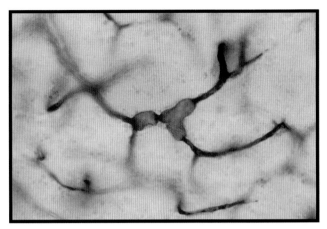

FIGURE 13-23 Small capillary and arterial dilatations (SCADs) in cerebral vessels in a patient who expired 48 hours after CABG using cardiopulmonary bypass. (Alkaline phosphatase-stained celloidin section, 100 μm thick: ×100.)

undergoing cardiac surgery over age 60 and over age 70 increased twofold and sevenfold, respectively[364] (Fig. 13-22). Genetic factors also influence the incidence of cognitive dysfunction after cardiac surgery.[365] The incidence of cognitive dysfunction at 1 week after cardiac surgery is approximately double that of noncardiac surgery.

As the age of cardiac surgical patients' increases, the number with multiple risk factors for neurologic injury also increases. Hypertension and diabetes occur in approximately 55% and 25% of cardiac surgical patients, respectively.[366] Fifteen percent have carotid stenosis of 50% or greater, and up to 13% have had a transient ischemic attack or prior stroke. The total number of MRI atherosclerotic lesions in the brachiocephalic vessels adds to the risk of stroke or cognitive dysfunction,[367] as does the severity of atherosclerosis in the ascending aorta as detected by epiaortic ultrasound scanning.[368] Palpable ascending aortic atherosclerotic plaques markedly increase the risk of right carotid arterial emboli as detected by Doppler ultrasound.[369] The incidence of severe aortic atherosclerosis is 1% in cardiac surgical patients less than 50 years old and is 10% in those aged 75 to 80.[370]

MECHANISMS OF INJURY

The three major causes of neurologic dysfunction and injury during cardiac surgery are microemboli, hypoperfusion, and a generalized inflammatory reaction, which can occur in the same patient at the same time for different reasons. The vast majority of intraoperative strokes are caused by the embolization of atherosclerotic material from the aorta and brachiocephalic vessels. This occurs as a result of manipulation of the heart and major thoracic vasculature as well as dislodgement of atheromata from shearing forces directed at the walls of vessels from inflow CPB cannulae.[371] The use of a no-touch technique for CABG where patients with aortic atherosclerosis have no manipulation of the aorta and all arterial grafting have produced the best results in avoiding emboli.[386] Microemboli are distributed in proportion to blood flow[20]; thus reduced cerebral blood flow reduces microembolic injury but increases the risk of hypoperfusion.[372] During CPB both alpha-stat acid-base management and phenylephrine reduce cerebral injury in adults, probably by causing cerebral vessel

vasoconstriction and reducing the number of microemboli.[373] Air, atherosclerotic debris, and fat are the major types of microemboli causing brain injury in clinical practice, and all cause neuronal necrosis by blocking cerebral vessels.[374] Massive air embolism causes a large ischemic injury, but gaseous cerebral microemboli may directly damage endothelium in addition to blocking blood flow.[375] The identification of unique small capillary arteriolar dilatations (SCADs) in the brain associated with fat emboli[376] (Fig.13-23) raises the possibility that these emboli not only block small vessels, but also release cytotoxic free radicals, which may significantly increase the damage to lipid-rich neurons.

Anemia and elevated cerebral temperature increase cerebral blood flow but may cause inadequate oxygen delivery to the brain,[377] however, these conditions are easily avoided during clinical cardiac surgery. Although some investigators speculate that normothermic and/or hyperthermic CPB cause cerebral hypoperfusion,[378] experimental studies indicate that cerebral blood flow increases with temperature. Brain injuries associated with this practice are more likely due to increased cerebral microemboli, which produce larger lesions at higher cerebral temperatures.[376]

NEUROPROTECTIVE STRATEGIES

Recommended conditions for protecting the brain during CPB include mild hypothermia (32-34°C) and hematocrit above 25%.[161] Temporary increases in cerebral venous pressure caused by SVC obstruction and excessive rewarming above blood temperatures of 37°C should be avoided.[379] A randomized study in which patients were mildly rewarmed to 35°C core temperature demonstrated improved neurocognitive outcomes over patients rewarmed to 37°C. Mean perfusion pressure (MPP) appears to have an effect on neurological outcome. Gold et al. randomized 248 patients to low (50-60 mm Hg) or high (80-100 mm Hg) MPP. The incidence of neurologic injury in the high pressure group was significantly reduced.[380] Either jugular venous bulb oxygen saturation or near-infrared cerebral oximetry are recommended for monitoring cerebral perfusion in patients who may be at high risk for cerebral injury.[381]

Barbiturates reduce cerebral metabolism by decreasing spontaneous synaptic activity and provide a definite neuroprotective effect during clinical cardiac surgery using CPB.[382] Unfortunately, these agents delay emergence from anesthesia and prolong intensive care unit stays. NMDA (*N*-methyl-D-aspartate) antagonists, which are effective in animals, provide mild protection compared with control patients, but have a high incidence of neurologic side effects.[383] A small study demonstrated a neuroprotective effect of lidocaine, but this beneficial effect has not been reproduced.[384] Thus corticosteroids are the only drugs with potential neuroprotective effects that have significant evidence for a positive effect on outcomes.[332]

Off-pump myocardial revascularization theoretically avoids many of the causes of cerebral injury owing to CPB, but, as noted, many causes of neuronal injury are independent of CPB and related to atherosclerosis and air entry sites into the circulation. Nonrandomized measurements of carotid emboli by Doppler ultrasound indicate fewer emboli and slightly improved neurocognitive outcomes in high-risk patients who have off-pump surgery.[385] Clinical trials of off-pump versus on-pump patients have demonstrated a lower stroke rate in off-pump patients who were treated with all arterial grafting and a no-touch surgical technique.[386]

PROGNOSIS

Patients with intraoperative stroke or those who develop stroke symptoms in the first week after surgery often improve in direct relation to the lesion size and location on imaging studies. Neuropsychologic deficits that are present after 3 months are almost always permanent.[386] Assessments after that time are confounded by development of new deficits, particularly in aged patients.[387,388]

The difficulty of separating intraoperative brain injury from that which occurs in the early or late postoperative period has been recently addressed by a reanalysis of data published earlier. The authors tracked specific neuropsychological deficits that persisted unchanged for 6 months (persistent deficits) and separated them from new deficits that appeared after surgery[389] (Fig. 13-24). Using this technique it is possible to accurately measure surgical brain injury and design techniques to eliminate this important cause of morbidity. Late follow-up studies should include a control group with similar risk factors but not having cardiac operations.[390] This technique demonstrated similar outcomes in surgical and nonsurgical controls at 3 years, putting to rest the previous fear that surgical patients had recurrent neurocognitive deficits and were thus at greater risk for poor long-term outcomes. In a recent study, a group of surgical patients who were evaluated with preoperative and postoperative neuropsychological studies had rigid control of cardiovascular risk factors.[391] They demonstrated no delayed or late cognitive decline offering hope that aggressive medical therapy can compliment skillful surgery in preventing neurological injury.

Lung Injury

Patient factors and the separate effects of operation and CPB combine to compromise lung function early after operation. Chronic smoking and emphysema are the most common patient factors, but muscular weakness, chronic bronchitis, occult pneumonia, preoperative pulmonary edema, and unrelated respiratory disease are other contributors to

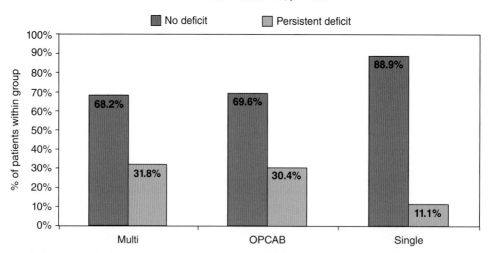

Persistent neurobeavioral deficits at 6 months
Fisher's exact test, p = 0.061

FIGURE 13-24 Neurobehavioral deficits at 6 months after coronary artery bypass surgery. Note that an intraoperative strategy utilizing a single cross clamp results in fewer persistent neuropsyscological deficits than multiple cross clamp or off pump coronary artery bypass (OPCAB). (Data from Hammon JW, Stump DA, Butterworth JF, et al: Coronary artery bypass grafting with single cross-clamp results in fewer persistent neuropsychological deficits than multiple clamp or off-pump coronary artery bypass grafting, *Ann Thorac Surg*. 2007 Oct;84(4):1174-1178.)

postoperative pulmonary dysfunction. Incisional pain, lack of movement, shallow respiratory sighs, increased work of breathing, reduced pulmonary compliance, weak cough, increased pulmonary arterial-venous shunting, and interstitial edema, to some degree, are consequences of anesthesia and any operation. CPB significantly adds to this injury.

During CPB the lungs are supplied by the bronchial arteries and pulmonary arterial blood flow may be absent or minimal. Whether or not alveolar cells suffer an ischemic/reperfusion injury is unclear, but the lungs are subject to many insults that combine to increase pulmonary capillary permeability and interstitial lung water. Hemodilution, reduced plasma oncotic pressure, and temporary elevation of left atrial or pulmonary venous pressure during CPB or during weaning from CPB increase extravascular lung water.[392] Microemboli and circulating cellular, vasoactive, and cytotoxic mediators of the inflammatory response reach the lung via bronchial arteries during CPB and with resumption of the pulmonary circulation during weaning.[393,394] These agents increase pulmonary capillary permeability, perivascular edema, and bronchial secretions, and perhaps cause observed changes in alveolar surfactant.[395] The combination of increased interstitial lung water and bronchial secretions, altered surfactant, patient factors, and the consequences of operation reduces pulmonary compliance and functional residual capacity and increases the work of breathing.[396] All of these changes combine to enhance regional atelectasis, increase susceptibility to infection, and increase the physiologic arterial-venous shunt, which reduces systemic arterial PaO_2.

Postoperative respiratory care is based on restoring normal pulmonary capillary permeability and interstitial lung volume; preventing atelectasis; reinflating atelectatic segments; maintaining normal arterial blood gases; and preventing infection and facilitating removal of bronchial mucus. Improved postoperative respiratory care, an understanding of the mechanisms of lung injury during CPB, and efforts to prevent or control the causes of injury[397] have markedly reduced the incidence of pulmonary complications in recent years. (See Chapter 16 for a more detailed discussion of postoperative care.)

Acute respiratory distress syndrome (ARDS) is a rare complication of lung injury during CPB and is usually caused by intrabronchial bleeding from traumatic injury by the endotracheal tube or pulmonary artery catheter or to extravasation of blood into alveoli from acute increases in pulmonary venous pressure or severe pulmonary capillary toxic injury.[398]

Renal Injury

As with other organs, the preoperative health of the kidneys is a major factor in the ability of that organ to withstand the microembolic, cellular, and regional malperfusion injuries caused by extracorporeal circulation. Risk factors include previous renal injury, increased age, and complex disease or cardiac operation.[399] The incidence of acute renal failure requiring dialysis after CPB is remarkably low, averaging 1%; however, the incidence increases to 5% with complex operations.

Some degree of renal injury is inevitable during CPB and post-perfusion proteinuria occurs in all patients.[400] Renal blood and plasma flow, creatinine clearance, free water clearance, and urine volume decrease without hemodilution.[401] Hemodilution attenuates most of these functional changes and also reduces the risk of hemoglobin precipitation in renal tubules if plasma-binding proteins become saturated with free hemoglobin during extracorporeal perfusion. Hemoglobin is toxic to renal tubules and precipitation can block both blood and urine flow to the tubules. Hemodilution dilutes plasma hemoglobin; improves flow to the outer renal cortex; improves total renal blood flow; increases creatinine, electrolyte, and water clearance; and increases glomerular filtration and urine volume.[402]

Perioperative periods of low cardiac output and/or hypotension added to the microembolic, cellular, and cytotoxic injuries of CPB and to any preoperative renal disease are the major cause of postoperative renal failure.[403] Low cardiac output reduces renal perfusion pressure and causes angiotensin II production and renin release, which further decrease renal blood flow. Kidneys, already compromised by preoperative disease and the CPB injury, are particularly sensitive to ischemic injury secondary to low cardiac output and hypotension. Thus perioperative management includes efforts to maximize cardiac output using dopamine or dobutamine if necessary, avoiding renal arterial vasoconstrictive drugs, providing adequate crystalloid infusions to maintain urine volume, and alkalinizing urine to minimize precipitation of tubular hemoglobin if excessive hemolysis has occurred.

If perioperative low cardiac output and hypotension do not occur, the normal kidney has sufficient functional reserve to provide adequate renal function during and after operation. The appearance of oliguric renal failure is ominous and usually requires dialysis, which is generally permanent if required for more than 2 weeks. Oliguric renal failure markedly increases morbidity and mortality by approximately eightfold.

Injury to the Gastrointestinal Organs

LIVER INJURY

Although subjected to microemboli, cytotoxins, and regional malperfusion during CPB, the enormous functional reserve and reparative processes of the normal liver nearly always overcome the injury without consequences. Often liver enzymes are mildly elevated, and 10 to 20% of patients are mildly jaundiced. Persistent and rising bilirubin 2 or more days after CPB may precede development of liver failure and is associated with increased morbidity and mortality.[404] Catastrophic liver failure, however, occurs in patients with overwhelming sepsis, oliguric renal failure, anesthetic or drug toxicity, or after a prolonged period of low cardiac output or an episode of hemorrhagic shock and multiple blood transfusions and is uniformly fatal. The liver usually is involved in patients who develop multiorgan failure and is often presaged by sudden hypoglycemia.

PANCREATIC INJURY

Less than 1% of patients develop clinical pancreatitis after CPB, but approximately 30% develop a transitory, asymptomatic increase in plasma amylase and/or lipase.[405] A history of recurrent pancreatitis, perioperative circulatory shock or hypotension, excessively prolonged CPB, and continuous, high doses of inotropic agents are risk factors for developing postoperative pancreatitis.[406] Experimentally and clinically, high doses of calcium increase intracellular trypsinogen activation and histologic evidence of pancreatitis.[407] Fulminant pancreatits is very rare, but is often fatal.

STOMACH AND GUT INJURY

CPB at adequate flow rates does not decrease splanchnic blood flow.[408] Risk factors for gastrointestinal complications include advanced age, emergency surgery, prolonged CPB, postoperative low cardiac output or shock, prolonged vasopressor therapy, and elevated preoperative systemic venous pressure.[409]

CPB decreases gastric pH, which declines further after operation. Before the advent of H2 blockers and regular use of antacids, duodenal and/or gastric erosion, ulcer, and bleeding were frequent complications after clinical cardiac surgery and were associated with mortality that approached 33 to 50%.[410] These complications are now uncommon.

Several days to 1 week after operation very elderly patients rarely may develop mesenteric vasculitis or severe mesenteric vasoconstriction in response to vasopressors that proceeds to small bowel ischemia and/or infarction. New onset abdominal pain with a silent, rigid abdomen and abrupt rise in white count may be the only signs of this catastrophic complication, which is frequently fatal. If suspected before infarction, infusion of papaverine or alternative vasodilators directly into the mesenteric arteries may prevent or limit subsequent infarction.

The role of CPB in the etiology of gastrointestinal complications is not completely known. If the complications listed in the preceding develop, an increase in the morbidity and mortality may be expected.[411]

REFERENCES

1. Gravlee GP, Davis RF, Kurusz M, Utley JR: *Cardiopulmonary Bypass: Principles and Practice*, 2nd ed. Philadelphia, Lippincott Williams & Wilkins, 2000.
2. Arom KV, Ellestad C, Grover FL, Trinkle JK: Objective evaluation of the efficacy of various venous cannulas. *J Thorac Cardiovasc Surg* 1981; 81:464.
3. Merin O, Silberman S, Brauner R, et al: Femoro-femoral bypass for repeat open-heart surgery. *Perfusion* 1998; 13:455.
4. Winter FS: Persistent left superior vena cava: survey of world literature and report of thirty additional cases. *Angiology* 1954; 5:90.
5. Hasel R, Barash PG: Dilated coronary sinus on pre-bypass echocardiography. *J Cardiothorac Vasc Anesth* 1996; 10:430.
6. Shahian DM: Retrograde coronary sinus cardioplegia in the presence of persistent left superior vena cava. *Ann Thorac Surg* 1992; 54:1214.
7. Yokota M, Kyoku I, Kitano M, et al: Atresia of the coronary sinus orifice: fatal outcome after intraoperative division of the drainage left superior vena cava. *J Thorac Cardiovasc Surg* 1989; 98:30.
8. Toomasian JM, McCarthy JP: Total extrathoracic cardiopulmonary support with kinetic assisted venous drainage: experience in 50 patients. *Perfusion* 1998; 13:137.
9. Taketani S, Sawa Y, Massai T, et al: A novel technique for cardiopulmonary bypass using vacuum system for venous drainage with pressure relief valve: an experimental study. *Artif Organs* 1998; 22:337.
10. Humphries K, Sistino JJ: Laboratory evaluation of the pressure flow characteristics of venous cannulas during vaccum-assisted venous drainage. *J Extracorp Tech* 2002; 34:111.
11. Willcox TW, Mitchell SJ, Gorman DF: Venous air in the bypass circuit: a source of arterial line emboli exacerbated by vacuum-assisted venous drainage. *Ann Thorac Surg* 1999; 68:1285.
12. Willcox TW: Vacuum-assisted venous drainage: to air or not to air, that is the question: has the bubble burst? *J Extracorp Tech* 2002; 34:24.
13. Davila RM, Rawles T, Mack MJ: Venoarterial air embolus: a complication of vacuum-assisted venous drainage. *Ann Thorac Surg* 2001; 71:1369.
14. Hessel EA II: Cardiopulmonary bypass equipment, in Estafanous FG, Barash PG, Reves JG (eds): *Cardiac Anesthesia: Principles and Clinical Practice*, 2nd ed. Philadelphia, Lippincott Williams & Wilkins, 2001; p 335.
15. Jones TJ, Deal DD, Vernon JC, et al: How effective are cardiopulmonary bypass circuits at removing gaseous microemboli? *J Extracorp Tech* 2002; 34:34.
16. Ambesh SP, Singh SK, Dubey DK, Kaushik S: Inadvertent closure of the superior vena cava after decannulation: a potentially catastrophic complication after termination of bypass [letter]. *J Cardiothorac Vasc Anesth* 1998; 12:723.
17. Brodman R, Siegel H, Lesser M, Frater R: A comparison of flow gradients across disposable arterial perfusion cannulas. *Ann Thorac Surg* 1985; 39:225.
18. Galletti PM, Brecher GA: *Heart-lung Bypass*. New York, Grune & Stratton, 1962.
19. Weinstein GS: Left hemispheric strokes in coronary surgery: implication for end-hole aortic cannulas. *Ann Thorac Surg* 2001; 71:128.
20. Muehrcke DD, Cornhill JF, Thomas JD, Cosgrove DM: Flow characteristics of aortic cannulae. *J Card Surg* 1995; 10:514.
21. Joubert-Hubner E, Gerdes A, Klarproth P, et al: An in-vitro evaluation of aortic arch vessel perfusion characteristics comparing single versus multiple stream aortic cannulae. *Eur J Cardiothorac Surg* 1999; 15:359.
22. Cook DJ, Zehr KJ, Orszulak TA, Slater JM: Profound reduction in brain embolization using an endoaortic baffle during bypass in swine. *Ann Thorac Surg* 2002; 73:198.
23. Reichenspurner H, Navia JA, Benny G, et al: Particulate embolic capture by an intra-aortic filter device during cardiac surgery. *J Thorac Cardiovasc Surg* 2000; 119:233.
24. Gerdes A, Hanke T, Sievers H-H: In vivo hydrodynamics of the Embol-X cannula. *Perfusion* 2002; 17:153.
25. Harringer W: Capture of a particulate embolic during cardiac procedures in which aortic cross-clamp is used. *Ann Thorac Surg* 2000; 70:1119.
26. Banbury MK, Cosgrove DM 3rd: Arterial cannulation of the innominate artery. *Ann Thorac Surg* 2000; 69:957.
27. Mills NL, Everson CT: Atherosclerosis of the ascending aorta and coronary artery bypass: pathology, clinical correlates, and operative management. *J Thorac Cardiovasc Surg* 1991; 102:546.
28. Beique FA, Joffe D, Tousignant G, Konstadt S: Echocardiographic-based assessment and management of atherosclerotic disease of the thoracic aorta. *J Cardiothorac Vasc Anesth* 1998; 12:206.
29. Blauth CI, Cosgrove DM, Webb BW, et al: Atheroembolism from the ascending aorta. *J Thorac Cardiovasc Surg* 1992; 103:1104.
30. Murphy DA, Craver JM, Jones EL, et al: Recognition and management of ascending aortic dissection complicating cardiac surgical operations. *J Thorac Cardiovasc Surg* 1983; 85:247.
31. Davila-Roman VG, Kouchoukos NT, Schechtman KB, Barzilai B: Atherosclerosis of the ascending aorta is a predictor of renal dysfunction after cardiac operations. *J Thorac Cardiovasc Surg* 1999; 117:111.
32. Davila-Roman V, Phillips K, Davila R, et al: Intraoperative transesophageal echocardiography and epiaortic ultrasound for assessment of atherosclerosis of the thoracic aorta. *J Am Coll Cardiol* 1996; 28:942.
33. Konstadt SN, Reich DL, Quintana C, Levy M: The ascending aorta: how much does transesophageal echocardiography see? *Anesth Analg* 1994; 78:240.

34. Gaudino M, Glieca F, Alessandrini F, et al: The unclampable ascending aorta in coronary artery bypass patients: a surgical challenge of increasing frequency. *Circulation* 2000; 102:1497.

35. Byrne JG, Aranki SF, Cohn LH: Aortic valve operations under deep hypothermic circulatory arrest for the porcelain aorta: "no-touch" technique. *Ann Thorac Surg* 1998; 65:1313.

36. Grossi EA, Kanchuger MS, Schwartz DS, et al: Effect of cannula length on aortic arch flow: protection of the atheromatous aortic arch. *Ann Thorac Surg* 1995; 59:710.

37. McLeskey CH, Cheney FW: A correctable complication of cardiopulmonary bypass. *Anesthesiology* 1982; 56:214.

38. Watson BG: Unilateral cold neck. *Anaesthesia* 1983; 38:659.

39. Magner JB: Complications of aortic cannulation for open-heart surgery. *Thorax* 1971; 26:172.

40. Gott JP, Cohen CL, Jones EL: Management of ascending aortic dissections and aneurysms early and late following cardiac operations. *J Card Surg* 1990; 5:2.

41. Troianos CA, Savino JS, Weiss RL: Transesophageal echocardiographic diagnosis of aortic dissection during cardiac surgery. *Anesthesiology* 1991; 75:149.

42. Lees MH, Herr RH, Hill JD, et al: Distribution of systemic blood flow of the rhesus monkey during cardiopulmonary bypass. *J Thorac Cardiovasc Surg* 1971; 61:570.

43. Svensson LG: Editorial comment: autopsies in acute Type A aortic dissection, surgical implications. *Circulation* 1998; 98:II-302.

44. Hendrickson SC, Glower DD: A method for perfusion of the leg during cardiopulmonary bypass via femoral cannulation. *Ann Thorac Surg* 1998; 65:1807.

45. Gates JD, Bichell DP, Rizzu RJ, et al: Thigh ischemia complicating femoral vessel cannulation for cardiopulmonary bypass. *Ann Thorac Surg* 1996; 61:730.

46. Van Der Salm TJ: Prevention of lower extremity ischemia during cardiopulmonary bypass via femoral cannulation. *Ann Thorac Surg* 1997; 63:251.

47. Carey JS, Skow JR, Scott C: Retrograde aortic dissection during cardiopulmonary bypass: "nonoperative" management. *Ann Thorac Surg* 1977; 24:44.

48. Sabik JF, Lytle BW, McCarthy PM, Cosgrove DM: Axillary artery: an alternative site of arterial cannulation for patients with extensive and peripheral vascular disease. *J Thorac Cardiovasc Surg* 1995; 109:885.

49. Neri E, Massetti M, Capannini G, et al: Axillary artery cannulation in type A aortic dissection operations. *J Thorac Cardiovasc Surg* 1999; 118:324.

50. Whitlark JD, Sutter FP: Intrathoracic subclavian artery cannulation as an alternative to the femoral or axillary artery cannulation [letter]. *Ann Thorac Surg* 1998; 66:296.

51. Golding LAR: New cannulation technique for the severely calcified ascending aorta. *J Thorac Cardiovasc Surg* 1985; 90:626.

52. Coselli JS, Crawford ES: Femoral artery perfusion for cardiopulmonary bypass in patients with aortoiliac artery obstruction. *Ann Thorac Surg* 1987; 43:437.

53. Orenstein JM, Sato N, Arron B, et al: Microemboli observed in deaths following cardiopulmonary bypass surgery: silicone antifoam agents and polyvinyl chloride tubing as source of emboli. *Hum Pathol* 1982; 13:1082.

54. Schonberger JPAM, Everts PAM, Hoffman JJ: Systemic blood activation with open and closed venous reservoirs. *Ann Thorac Surg* 1995; 59:1549.

55. Blauth CI, Smith PL, Arnold JV, et al: Influence of oxygenator type on the prevalence and extent of micro-emboli retinal ischemia during cardio-pulmonary bypass: assessment by digital image analysis. *J Thorac Cardiovasc Surg* 1990; 99:61.

56. Pearson DT: Gas exchange; bubble and membrane oxygenators. *Semin Thorac Cardiovasc Surg* 1990; 2:313.

57. Drinker PA, Bartlett RH, Bialer RM, Noyes BS Jr: Augmentation of membrane gas transfer by induced secondary flows. *Surgery* 1969; 66:775.

58. Wiesenack C, Wiesner G, Keyl C, et al: In vivo uptake and elimination of isoflurane by different membrane oxygenators during cardiopulmonary bypass. *Anesthesiology* 2002; 97:133.

59. Clark RE, Beauchamp RA, Magrath RA, et al: Comparison of bubble and membrane oxygenators in short and long term perfusions. *J Thorac Cardiovasc Surg* 1979; 78:655.

60. Hammond GL, Bowley WW: Bubble mechanics and oxygen transfer. *J Thorac Cardiovasc Surg* 1976; 71:422.

61. Jenkins OF, Morris R, Simpson JM: Australasian perfusion incident survey. *Perfusion* 1997; 12:279.

62. Wahba A, Philipp A, Behr R, Birnbaum DE: Heparin-coated equipment reduces the risk of oxygenator failure. *Ann Thorac Surg* 1998; 65:1310.

63. Fisher AR: The incidence and cause of emergency oxygenator change-overs. *Perfusion* 1999; 14:207.

64. Svenmarker S, Haggmark S, Jansson E, et al: The relative safety of an oxygenator. *Perfusion* 1997; 12:289.

65. Geissler HJ, Allen JS, Mehlhorn U, et al: Cooling gradients and formation of gaseous microemboli with cardiopulmonary bypass: an echocardiographic study. *Ann Thorac Surg* 1997; 64:100.

66. Moen O, Fosse E, Broten J, et al: Difference in blood activation related to roller/centrifugal pumps and heparin coated/uncoated surfaces in a cardiopulmonary bypass model circuit. *Perfusion* 1996; 11:113.

67. Leschinsky BM, Zimin NK: Centrifugal blood pumps—a brief analysis: development of new designs. *Perfusion* 1991; 6:115.

68. Kolff J, McClurken JB, Alpern JB: Beware centrifugal pumps: not a oneway street, but a dangerous siphon! *Perfusion* 1990; 5:225.

69. Bernstein EF, Gleason LR: Factors influencing hemolysis with roller pumps. *Surgery* 1967; 61:432.

70. Uretzky G, Landsburg G, Cohn D, et al: Analysis of microembolic particles originating in extracorporeal circuits. *Perfusion* 1987; 2:9.

71. Wright G: Hemodynamic analysis could resolve the pulsatile blood flow controversy [current review]. *Ann Thorac Surg* 1994; 58:1199.

72. Edmunds LH Jr: Pulseless cardiopulmonary bypass. *J Thorac Cardiovasc Surg* 1982; 84:800.

73. Pearson DT: Micro-emboli: gaseous and particulate, in Taylor KM (ed): *Cardiopulmonary Bypass: Principles and Management*. Baltimore, Williams & Wilkins, 1986: p 313.

74. Borger MA, Feindel CM: Cerebral emboli during cardiopulmonary bypass: effect of perfusionist interventions and aortic cannulas. *J Extracorp Tech* 2002; 34:29.

75. Lee WH Jr, Krumhaar D, Fonkalsrud EW, et al: Denaturation of plasma proteins as a cause of morbidity and death after intracardiac operations. *Surgery* 1961; 50:1025.

76. Liu J-F, Su Z-F, Ding W-X: Quantitation of particle microemboli during cardiopulmonary bypass: experimental and clinical studies. *Ann Thorac Surg* 1992; 54:1196.

77. Brooker RF, Brown WR, Moody DM, et al: Cardiotomy suction: a major source of brain lipid emboli during cardiopulmonary bypass. *Ann Thorac Surg* 1998; 65:1651.

78. Ringelstein EB, Droste DW, Babikian VL, et al: Consensus on microembolus detection by TCD. *Stroke* 1998; 29:725.

79. Wright G, Furness A, Haigh S: Integral pulse frequency modulated ultrasound for the detection and quantification of gas microbubbles in flowing blood. *Perfusion* 1987; 2:131.

80. Kincaid E, Jones T, Stump D, et al: Processing scavenged blood with a cell saver reduces cerebral lipid microembolization. *Ann Thorac Surg* 2000; 70:1296.

81. Hammon JW, Stump DA, Hines M, et al: Prevention of embolic events during coronary artery bypass graft surgery. *Perfusion* 1994; 9:412.

82. Hammon JW, Stump DA, Kon ND, et al: Risk factors and solutions for the development of neurobehavioral changes after coronary artery bypass grafting. *Ann Thorac Surg* 1997; 63:1613.

83. Edmunds LH Jr: Thromboembolic complications of current cardiac valvular prostheses. *Ann Thorac Surg* 1982; 34:96.

84. Plochl W, Cook DJ: Quantification and distribution of cerebral emboli during cardiopulmonary bypass in the swine: the impact of $PaCO_2$. *Anesthesiology* 1999; 90:183.

85. Cook DJ, Plochl W, Orszulak TA: Effect of temperature and $PaCO_2$ on cerebral embolization during cardiopulmonary bypass in swine. *Ann Thorac Surg* 2000; 69:415.

86. Berman L, Marin F: Micropore filtration during cardiopulmonary bypass, in Taylor KM (ed): *Cardiopulmonary Bypass: Principles and Management*. Baltimore, Williams & Wilkins, 1986; p 355.

87. Joffe D, Silvay G: The use of microfilters in cardiopulmonary bypass. *J Cardiothorac Vasc Anesth* 1994; 8:685.

88. Ware JA, Scott MA, Horak JK, Solis RT: Platelet aggregation during and after cardiopulmonary bypass: effect of two different cardiotomy filters. *Ann Thorac Surg* 1982; 34:204.

89. Gourlay T: The role of arterial line filters in perfusion safety. *Perfusion* 1988; 3:195.

90. Munsch C, Rosenfeldt F, Chang V: Absence of particle-induced coronary vasoconstriction during cardioplegic infusion: is it desirable to use a microfilter in the infusion line? *J Thorac Cardiovasc Surg* 1991; 101:473.

91. Pugsley W, Klinger L, Paschalie C, et al: The impact of micro-emboli during cardiopulmonary bypass on neurological functioning. *Stroke* 1994; 25:1393.

92. Mejak BL, Stammers A, Raush E, et al: A retrospective study of perfusion incidents and safety devices. *Perfusion* 2000; 15:51.

93. Sylivris S, Levi C, Matalanis G, et al: Pattern and significance of cerebral microemboli during coronary artery bypass grafting. *Ann Thorac Surg* 1998; 66:1674.

94. Grocott HP, Croughwell ND, Amory DW, et al: Cerebral emboli and serum S-100-B during cardiac operation. *Ann Thorac Surg* 1998; 65:1645.

95. Milsom FP, Mitchell SJ: A dual-vent left heart de-airing technique markedly reduces carotid artery microemboli. *Ann Thorac Surg* 1998; 66:785.

96. Clark RE, Brillman J, Davis DA, et al: Microemboli during coronary artery bypass grafting: genesis and effects on outcome. *J Thorac Cardiovasc Surg* 1995; 109:249.

97. Morris SJ: Leucocyte reduction in cardiovascular surgery. *Perfusion* 2001; 11:371.

98. Gu YJ, deVries AJ, Voa P, et al: Leukocyte depletion during cardiac operations: a new approach through the venous bypass circuit. *Ann Thorac Surg* 1999; 67:604.

99. Hurst T, Johnson D, Cujec B, et al: Depletion of activated neutrophils by a filter during cardiac valve surgery. *Can J Anaesth* 1997; 44:131.

100. Mahoney CB: Heparin-bonded circuits: clinical outcome and costs. *Perfusion* 1998; 13:1892.

101. Hsu L-C: Heparin-coated CPB circuits: current status. *Perfusion* 2001; 16:417.

102. Edmunds LH Jr, Stenach N: The blood-surface interface, in Gravlee GP, Davis RF, Kurusz M, Utley JR (eds): *Cardiopulmonary Bypass: Principles and Practice*, 2nd ed. Media, PA, Williams & Wilkins, 2000; p 149.

103. Videm V, Mollnes TE, Fosse E, et al: Heparin-coated cardiopulmonary bypass equipment, I: biocompatibility markers and development of complications in a high-risk population. *J Thorac Cardiovasc Surg* 1999; 117:794.

104. Wildevuur CRH, Jansen DGM, Bezemer PD, et al: Clinical evaluation of Duraflo II heparin treated extracorporeal circuits. *Eur J Cardiothorac Surg* 1997; 11:616.

105. DeSomer F, VanBelleghem Y, Cases F, et al: Phosphorylcholine coating offers natural platelet preservation during CPB. *Perfusion* 2002; 17:39.

106. Ereth MH, Nuttall GA, Clarke SH, et al: Biocompatibility of trillium biopassive surface-coated oxygenator versus un-coated oxygenator during CPB. *J Cardiothorac Vasc Anesth* 2001; 15:545.

107. Gu YJ, Boonstra PW, Rijnsburger AA, et al: Cardiopulmonary bypass circuit treated with surface-modifying additives: a clinical evaluation of blood compatibility. *Ann Thorac Surg* 1998; 65:1343.

108. Edmunds LH Jr, Saxena NH, Hillyer P, Wilson TJ: Relationship between platelet count and cardiotomy suction return. *Ann Thorac Surg* 1978; 25:306.

109. Kincaid EH, Jones TJ, Stump DA, et al: Processing scavenged blood with a cell saver reduces cerebral lipid microembolism. *Ann Thorac Surg* 2000; 70(4):1296.

110. Downing SW, Edmunds LH Jr: Release of vasoactive substances during cardiopulmonary bypass. *Ann Thorac Surg* 1992; 54:1236.

111. Baile EM, Ling IT, Heyworth JR, et al: Bronchopulmonary anastomotic and noncoronary collateral blood flow in humans during cardiopulmonary bypass. *Chest* 1985; 87:749.

112. Little AG, Lin CY, Wernley JA, et al: Use of the pulmonary artery for left ventricular venting during cardiac operations. *J Thorac Cardiovasc Surg* 1984; 87:532.

113. Casha AR: A simple method of aortic root venting for CABG [letter]. *Ann Thorac Surg* 1998; 66:608.

114. Olinger GM, Bonchek LI: Ventricular venting during coronary revascularization: assessment of benefit by intraoperative ventricular function curves. *Ann Thorac Surg* 1978; 26:525.

115. Salomon NW, Copeland JG: Single catheter technique for cardioplegia and venting during coronary artery bypass grafting. *Ann Thorac Surg* 1980; 29:88.

116. Marco JD, Barner HB: Aortic venting: comparison of vent effectiveness. *J Thorac Cardiovasc Surg* 1977; 73:287.

117. Clements F, Wright SJ, deBruijn N: Coronary sinus catheterization made easy for port-access minimally invasive cardiac surgery. *J Cardiothorac Vasc Anesth* 1998; 12:96.

118. Aldea GS, Connelly G, Fonger JD, et al: Directed atraumatic coronary sinus cannulation for retrograde cardioplegia administration. *Ann Thorac Surg* 1992; 54:789.

119. Panos AL, Ali IS, Birnbaum PL, et al: Coronary sinus injuries during retrograde continuous normothermic blood cardioplegia. *Ann Thorac Surg* 1992; 54:1132.

120. Journois D, Israel-Biet E, Pouard P, et al: High volume, zero-balance hemofiltration to reduce delayed inflammatory response to cardiopulmonary bypass in children. *Anesthesiology* 1996; 85:965.

121. Boldt J, Zickmann B, Fedderson B, et al: Six different hemofiltration devices for blood conservation in cardiac surgery. *Ann Thorac Surg* 1991; 51:747.

122. High KM, Williams DR, Kurusz M: Cardiopulmonary bypass circuits and design, in Hensley FA Jr, Martin DE (eds): *A Practical Approach to Cardiac Anesthesia*, 2nd ed. Boston, Little, Brown, 1995; p 465.

123. Stammers AH: Monitoring controversies during cardiopulmonary bypass: how far have we come? *Perfusion* 1998; 13:35.

124. Baraka A, Barody M, Harous S, et al: Continuous venous oximetry during cardiopulmonary bypass: influence of temperature changes, perfusion flow and hematocrit level. *J Cardiothorac Anesth* 1990; 4:35.

125. Pearson DT: Blood gas control during cardiopulmonary bypass. *Perfusion* 1988; 31:113.

126. Mark JB, Fitzgerald D, Fenton T, et al: Continuous arterial and venous blood gas monitoring during cardiopulmonary bypass. *J Thorac Cardiovasc Surg* 1991; 102:431.

127. Kirson LE, Goldman JM: A system for monitoring the delivery of ventilating gas to the oxygenator during cardiopulmonary bypass. *J Cardiothorac Vasc Anesth* 1994; 8:51.

128. Berg E, Knudsen N: Automatic data collection for cardiopulmonary bypass. *Perfusion* 1988; 3:263.

129. Beppu T, Imai Y, Fukui Y: A computerized control system for cardiopulmonary bypass. *J Thorac Cardiovasc Surg* 1995; 109:428.

130. Castiglioni A, Verzini A, Pappalardo F, et al: Minimally invasive closed circuit versus standard extracorporeal circulation for aortic valve replacement. *Ann Thorac Surg* 2007; 83:586-591.

131. Rosengart T, DeBois W, O'Hara M, et al: Retrograde autologous priming for cardiopulmonary bypass: a safe and effective means of decreasing hemodilution and transfusion requirements. *J Thorac Cardiovasc Surg* 1998; 115:426.

132. Boldt J: Volume therapy in cardiac surgery: does the kind of fluid matter? *J Cardiothorac Vasc Anesth* 1999; 13:752.

133. Hoeft A, Korb H, Mehlhorn U, et al: Priming of CPB with human albumin or ringer lactate: effect on colloid osmotic pressure and extravascular lung water. *Br J Anaesth* 1991; 66:77.

134. Cochrane Injuries Group Albumin Reviews: Human albumin administration in critically ill patients: systemic review of randomized controlled trials. *BMJ* 1998; 317:235.

135. Wilkes MM, Navickis RJ, Sibbald WJ: Albumin versus hydroxyethyl starch in CPB surgery: a meta-analysis of post-operative bleeding. *Ann Thorac Surg* 2001; 72:527.

136. McKnight CK, Holden MJ, Pearson DT, et al: The cardiopulmonary bypass pump priming fluid and nitrogen balance after open heart surgery in adults. *Perfusion* 1986; 1:47.

137. McKnight CK, Elliott MJ, Pearson DT, et al: The effect of four different crystalloid bypass pump priming fluids upon the metabolic response to cardiac operations. *J Thorac Cardiovasc Surg* 1985; 90:97.

138. Lanier WL: Glucose management during cardiopulmonary bypass: cardiovascular and neurologic implications. *Anesth Analg* 1991; 72:423.

139. Francis JL, Palmer GJ III, Moroose R, Drexler A: Comparison of bovine and porcine heparin in heparin antibody formation after cardiac surgery. *Ann Thorac Surg* 2003; 75(1):15-16.

140. Heres EK, Speight K, Benckart D, et al: The clinical onset of heparin is rapid. *Anesth Analg* 2001; 92:1391-1395.

141. Bull BS, Huse WM, Brauer FS, et al: Heparin therapy during extracorporeal circulation: the use of a drug response curve to individualize heparin and protamine dosage. *J Thorac Cardiovasc Surg* 1975; 69:685.

142. Levy JH, Despotis GJ, Szlam F, et al: Recombinant human transgenic antithrombin in cardiac surgery: a dose finding study. *Anesthesiology* 2002; 96:1095.

143. Weiss ME, Nyhan D, Peng Z, et al: Association of protamine IgE and IgG antibodies with life-threatening reactions to intravenous protamine. *New Engl J Med* 1989; 320:886.

144. Khabbaz KR, Zankoul F, Warner KG: Intraoperative metabolic monitoring of the heart, II: online measurement of myocardial tissue pH. *Ann Thorac Surg* 2001; 72:S2227.

145. Ikonomidis JS, Yau IM, Weisel RD, et al: Optimal flow rates for retrograde warm cardioplegia. *J Thorac Cardiovasc Surg* 1994; 107:510.

146. Kirklin JW, Barrett-Boyes BE: *Cardiac Surgery*, 2nd ed. New York, Wiley, 1993; Ch. 2.

147. Taylor KM, Bain WH, Maxted KJ, et al: Comparative studies of pulsatile and nonpulsatile bypass, I: pulsatile system employed and its hematologic effects. *J Thorac Cardiovasc Surg* 1978; 75:569.

148. Taylor KM, Bain WH, Davidson KG, Turner MA: Comparative clinical study of pulsatile and non-pulsatile perfusion in 350 consecutive patients. *Thorax* 1982; 37:324.

149. Shaw PJ, Bates D, Cartlige NEF: Analysis of factors predisposing to neurological injury in patients undergoing coronary bypass operations. *QJM* 1989; 72:633.

150. Rees W, Schiessler A, Schulz F, et al: Pulsatile extra-corporeal circulation: fluid-mechanic considerations. *Perfusion* 1993; 8:459.

151. Gourlay T, Taylor KM: Pulsatile flow and membrane oxygenators. *Perfusion* 1994; 9:189.

152. Sugurtekin H, Boston US, Cook DJ: Bypass flow, mean arterial pressure, and cerebral perfusion during cardiopulmonary bypass in dogs. *J Cardiothorac Vasc Anesth* 2000; 14:25.

153. Hill SE, van Wermeskerken GK, Lardenoye J-WH, et al: Intraoperative physiologic variables and outcome in cardiac surgery, part I: in-hospital mortality. *Ann Thorac Surg* 2000; 69:1070.

154. Gold JP, Charlson MR, Williams-Russa P, et al: Improvements of outcomes after coronary artery bypass: a randomized trial comparing intraoperative high versus low mean arterial pressure. *J Thorac Cardiovasc Surg* 1995; 110:1302.

155. Hartman GS, Yao F-S, Bruefach M, et al: Severity of aortic atheromatous disease diagnosed by transesophageal echocardiography predicts stroke and other outcomes associated with coronary artery surgery: a prospective study. *Analg Anesth* 1996; 83:701.

156. Liam B-L, Plöchl W, Cook DJ, et al: Hemodilution and whole body oxygen balance during normothermic cardiopulmonary bypass in dogs. *J Thorac Cardiovasc Surg* 1998; 115:1203.

157. Cook DJ: Optimal conditions for cardiopulmonary bypass. *Semin Cardiothorac Vasc Anesth* 2001; 5:265.

158. Hill SE, Van Wermesker, Ken GK, et al: Intraoperative physiologic variables and outcome in cardiac surgery, part I: in-hospital mortality. *Ann Thorac Surg* 2000; 69:1070.

159. DeFoe GR, Ross CS, Olmstead EM, et al: Lowest hematocrit on bypass and adverse outcomes associated with coronary artery bypass grafting. *Ann Thorac Surg* 2001; 71:769.

160. Groom RC: High or low hematocrits during cardiopulmonary bypass for patients undergoing coronary artery bypass graft surgery? An evidence-based approach to the question. *Perfusion* 2002; 17:99.

161. Jonas RA: Optimal pH strategy for hypothermic circulatory arrest [editorial]. *J Thorac Cardiovasc Surg* 2001; 121:204.

162. Khatri P, Babyak M, Croughwell ND, et al: Temperature during coronary artery bypass surgery affects quality of life. *Ann Thorac Surg* 2001; 71:110.

163. Engleman RM, Pleet AB, Hicks R, et al: Is there a relationship between systemic perfusion temperature during coronary artery bypass grafting and extent of intraoperative ischemic central nervous system injury? *J Thorac Cardiovasc Surg* 2000; 119:230.

164. Nathan HJ, Wells GA, Munson JL, Wozny D: Neuroprotective effect of mild hypothermia in patients undergoing coronary artery surgery with cardiopulmonary bypass. A randomized trial. *Circulation* 2001; 104(suppl I):I-85.

165. Stephan H, Weyland A, Kazmaier S, et al: Acid-base management during hypothermic cardiopulmonary bypass does not affect cerebral metabolism but does affect blood flow and neurologic outcome. *Br J Anaesth* 1992; 69:51.

166. Murkin JM, Farrar JK, Tweed WA, et al: Cerebral autoregulation and flow/metabolism coupling during cardiopulmonary bypass: rhe influence of $PaCO_2$. *Anesth Analg* 1987; 66:825.

167. Van den Berghe G, Wouters P, Weekers F, et al: Intensive insulin therapy in critically ill patients. *New Engl J Med* 2001; 345:1359.

168. Shine TS, Uchikado M, Crawford CC, Murray MJ: Importance of perioperative blood glucose management in cardiac surgical patients. *Asian Cardiovasc Thorac Annals* 2007; 15:534-538.

169. Bernard GR, Sopko G, Cerra F, et al: National Heart Lung and Blood Institute and Food and Drug Administration Workshop Report: Pulmonary Artery Catheterization and Clinical Outcomes (PACC). *JAMA* 2000; 283:2568.

170. Shanewise JS, Cheung AT, Aronson S, et al: ASE/SCA guidelines for performing a comprehensive intraoperative multiplane transesophageal echocardiography examination: recommendation of the American Society of Echocardiography council for intraoperative echocardiography and the Society of Cardiovascular Anesthesiologists task force for certification in perioperative echocardiography. *Anesth Analg* 1999; 99:870.

171. Lucina MG, Savage RM, Hearm C, Kraenzler EJ: The role of transesophageal echocardiography on perfusion management. *Semin Cardiothorac Vasc Anesth* 2001; 5:321.

172. Paul D, Hartman GS: Foley balloon occlusion of the atheromatous ascending aorta: the role of transesophageal echocardiography. *J Cardiothorac Vasc Anesth* 1998; 12:61.

173. Siegel LC, St Goar FG, Stevens JH, et al: Monitoring considerations for Port-Access cardiac surgery. *Circulation* 1997; 96:562.

174. Yamada E, Matsumura M, Kimura S, et al: Usefulness of transesophageal echocardiography in detecting changes in flow dynamics responsible for malperfusion phenomena observed during surgery of aortic dissection. *Am J Cardiol* 1997; 79:1149.

175. Tingleff J, Joyce FS, Pettersson G: Intraoperative echocardiographic study of air embolism during cardiac operations. *Ann Thorac Surg* 1995; 60:673.

176. Stone JG, Young WL, Smith CR, et al: Do standard monitoring sites reflect true brain temperature when profound hypothermia is rapidly induced and reversed? *Anesthesiology* 1995; 82:344.

177. Rumana CS, Gopinath SP, Uzura M, et al: Brain temperature exceeds systemic temperature in head-injured patients. *Crit Care Med* 1998; 26:562.

178. Johnson RZ, Fox MA, Grayson A, et al: Should we rely on nasopharyngeal temperature during cardiopulmonary bypass? *Perfusion* 2002; 17:145.

179. Nussmeier NA, personal communication, 2002.

180. Stump DA, Jones JJ, Rorie KD: Neurophysiologic monitoring and outcomes in cardiovascular surgery [review article]. *J Cardiothorac Vasc Anesth* 1999; 13:600.

181. McDaniel LB, Zwischenberger JM, Vertrees RA, et al: Mixed venous oxygen saturation during cardiopulmonary bypass poorly predicts regional venous saturation. *Anesth Analg* 1994; 80:466.

182. Wenger R, Bavaria JE, Ratcliffe M, Edmunds LH Jr: Flow dynamics of peripheral venous catheters during extracorporeal membrane oxygenator (ECMO) with a centrifugal pump. *J Thorac Cardiovasc Surg* 1988; 96:478.

183. Hessel EA II: Bypass techniques for descending thoracic aortic surgery. *Semin Cardiothorac Vasc Anesth* 2001; 5:293.

184. Ireland KW, Follette DM, Iguidbashian J, et al: Use of a heat exchanger to prevent hypothermia during thoracic and thoracoabdominal aneurysm repairs. *Ann Thorac Surg* 1993; 55:534.

185. Edmunds LH Jr, Austen WG, Shaw RS, Kosminski S: Clinical and physiologic considerations of left heart bypass during cardiac arrest. *J Thorac Cardiovasc Surg* 1961; 41:356.

186. Hedlund KD, Dattilo R: Supportive angioplasty [letter]. *Perfusion* 1990; 5:297.

187. Toomasian JM: Cardiopulmonary bypass for less invasive procedures. *Perfusion* 1999; 14:279.

188. Grocott HP, Smith MS, Glower DC, Clements FM: Endovascular aortic balloon clamp malposition during minimally invasive cardiac surgery. *Anesthesiology* 1998; 88:1396.

189. Young WL, Lawton MT, Gupta DF, Hashimoto T: Anesthetic management of deep hypothermic circulatory arrest for cerebral aneurysm surgery. *Anesthesiology* 2002; 96:497.

190. Soong WAL, Uysal S, Reich DL: Cerebral protection during surgery of the aortic arch. *Semin Cardiothorac Vasc Anesth* 2001; 5:286.

191. Hiramatsu T, Miura T, Forbess JM, et al: pH strategies and cerebral energetics before and after circulatory arrest. *J Thorac Cardiovasc Surg* 1995; 109:948.

192. Kurth CD, O'Rourke MM, O'Hara IB: Comparison of pH-stat and alpha stat cardiopulmonary bypass on cerebral oxygenation and blood flow in relation to hypothermic circulatory arrest in piglets. *Anesthesiology* 1998; 98:110.

193. Sakamoto T, Zurakowski D, Duebener LF, et al: Combination of alpha-stat strategy and hemodilution exacerbates neurologic injury in a survival piglet model with deep hypothermic circulatory arrest. *Ann Thorac Surg* 2002; 73:180.

194. Jonas RA, Bellinger DC, Rappaport LA et al: Relation of pH-strategy and development outcome after hypothermic circulatory arrest. *J Thorac Cardiovasc Surg* 1993; 106:362.

195. Hindman BJ: Choice of α-stat or pH-stat management and neurologic outcomes after cardiac surgery: it depends. *Anesthesiology* 1998; 98:5.

196. Ekroth R, Thompson RJ, Lincoln C, et al: Elective deep hypothermia with total circulatory arrest: changes in plasma creatine kinase BB, blood glucose, and clinical variables. *J Thorac Cardiovasc Surg* 1989; 97:30.

197. Reich DL, Uysal S, Sliwinski M, et al: Neuropsychological outcome following deep hypothermia circulatory arrest in adults. *J Thorac Cardiovasc Surg* 1999; 117:156.

198. Ergin MA, Galla JD, Lansman SL, et al: Hypothermic circulatory arrest in operations on the thoracic aorta. *J Thorac Cardiovasc Surg* 1994; 107:788.

199. Ergin MA, Uysal S, Reich DL, et al: Temporary neurological dysfunction after deep hypothermic circulatory arrest: a clinical marker of long term functional deficit. *Ann Thorac Surg* 1999; 67:1886.

200. Mezrow CK, Midulla PS, Sadeghi AM, et al: Quantitative electroencephalography: a method to assess cerebral injury after hypothermic circulatory arrest. *J Thorac Cardiovasc Surg* 1995; 109:925.

201. Newberger JW, Jonas RA, Wernovsky G, et al: A comparison on the peri-operative neurologic defect of hypothermic circulatory arrest versus low flow cardiopulmonary bypass in infant heart surgery. *New Engl J Med* 1993; 329:1057.

202. Grabenwoger M, Ehrlich M, Cartes-Zumelzu F, et al: Surgical treatment of aortic arch aneurysms in profound hypothermia and circulatory arrest. *Ann Thorac Surg* 1997; 64:1067.

203. Higami T, Kozawa S, Asada T, et al: Retrograde cerebral perfusion versus selective cerebral perfusion as evaluated by cerebral oxygen saturation during aortic arch reconstruction. *Ann Thorac Surg* 1999; 67:1091.

204. Kazui T, Kimura N, Yamada O, Komatsu S: Surgical outcome of aortic arch aneurysms using selective cerebral perfusion. *Ann Thorac Surg* 1994; 57:904.

205. Mills NL, Ochsner JL: Massive air embolism during cardiopulmonary bypass: causes, prevention, and management. *J Thorac Cardiovasc Surg* 1980; 80:708.

206. Ueda Y, Miki S, Kusuhara K, et al: Surgical treatment of aneurysm or dissection involving the ascending aorta and aortic arch, utilizing circulatory arrest and retrograde cerebral perfusion. *J Cardiovasc Surg* 1990; 31:553.

207. Ganzel BL, Edmonds HL Jr, Pank JR, Goldsmith LJ: Neurophysiologic monitoring to assure delivery of retrograde cerebral perfusion. *J Thorac Cardiovasc Surg* 1997; 113:748.

208. DeBrux J-L, Subayi J-B, Pegis J-D, Dillet J: Retrograde cerebral perfusion: anatomic study of the distribution of blood to the brain. *Ann Thorac Surg* 1995; 60:1294.

209. Lin PJ, Chang GH, Tan PPC, et al: Prolonged circulatory arrest in moderate hypothermia with retrograde cerebral perfusion: is brain ischemic? *Circulation* 1996; 95 (suppl II):II-166.

210. Murkin JM: Retrograde cerebral perfusion: is the brain really being perfused? [editorial]. *J Cardiothorac Vasc Anesth* 1998; 12:249.

211. Kouchoukos NT: Adjuncts to reduce the incidence of embolic brain injury during operations on the aortic arch. *Ann Thorac Surg* 1994; 57:243.

212. Cheung AT, Bavaria JE, Weiss SJ, et al: Neurophysiologic effects of retrograde cerebral perfusion used for aortic reconstruction. *J Cardiothorac Vasc Anesth* 1998; 12:252.

213. Kurusz M, Butler BD, Katz J, Conti VR: Air embolism during cardiopulmonary bypass. *Perfusion* 1995; 10:361.

214. Ziser A, Adir Y, Lavon H, Shupof A: Hyperbaric oxygen therapy for massive arterial air embolism during cardiac operations. *J Thorac Cardiovasc Surg* 1999; 117:818.

215. Pedersen T, Kaargen AL, Benze S: An approach toward total quality assurance in cardiopulmonary bypass: which data to register and how to assess perfusion quality. *Perfusion* 1996; 11:39.

216. Palanzo DA: Perfusion safety: past present and future. *J Cardiothorac Vasc Anesth* 1997; 11:383.

217. Brister SJ, Ofosu FA, Buchanan MR: Thrombin generation during cardiac surgery: is heparin the ideal anticoagulant? *Thromb Haemost* 1993; 70:259.

218. Uniyal S, Brash JL: Patterns of adsorption of proteins from human plasma onto foreign surfaces. *Thromb Haemost* 1982; 47:285.

219. Horbett TA: Proteins: structure, properties, and adsorption to surfaces, in Ratner BD, Hoffman AS, Schoen FJ, and Lemons JE (eds): *Biomaterials Science: An Introduction to Materials in Medicine*. San Diego, Academic Press, 1996; p 133.

220. Horbett TA: Principles underlying the role of adsorbed plasma proteins in blood interactions with foreign materials. *Cardiovasc Pathol* 1993; 2:137S.

221. Brash JL, Scott CF, ten Hove P, et al: Mechanism of transient adsorption of fibrinogen from plasma to solid surfaces: role of the contact and fibrinolytic systems. *Blood* 1988; 71:932.

222. Edmunds LH Jr, Stenach N: The blood-surface interface, in Gravlee GP, Davis RF, Kurusz M, Utley JR (eds): *Cardiopulmonary Bypass: Principles and Practice*, 2nd ed. Media, PA, Williams & Wilkins, 2000; p 149.

223. Edmunds LH Jr: Blood activation in mechanical circulatory assist devices. *J Congestive Heart Failure Circ* 2000; 1(supp l):141.

224. Bernabei AF, Gikakis N, Maione T, et al: Reversal of heparin anticoagulation by recombinant platelet factor 4 and protamine sulfate in baboons during cardiopulmonary bypass. *J Thorac Cardiovasc Surg* 1995; 109:765.

225. Rosenberg RD, Edelberg M, Zhang L: The heparin-antithrombin system: a natural anticoagulant mechanism, in Colman RW, Hirsh J, Marder VJ, et al (eds): *Hemostasis and Thrombosis: Basic Principles and Clinical Practice*. Philadelphia, JB Lippincott, 2001; p 711.

226. Weitz JI, Hudoba M, Massel D, et al: Clot-bound thrombin is protected from inhibition by heparin-antithrombin III-independent inhibitors. *J Clin Invest* 1990; 86:385.

227. Eisenberg PR, Siegel JE, Abendschein DR, Miletich JP: Importance of factor Xa in determining the procoagulant activity of whole-blood clots. *J Clin Invest* 1993; 91:1877.

228. Khuri S, Valeri CR, Loscalzo J, et al: Heparin causes platelet dysfunction and increases fibrinolysis before the institution of cardiopulmonary bypass. *Ann Thorac Surg* 1995; 60:1008.

229. Sobel M, McNeill PM, Carlson PL, et al: Heparin inhibition of von Willebrand factor-dependent platelet function in vitro and in vivo. *J Clin Invest* 1991; 87:1878.

230. Kirklin JK, Chenoweth DE, Naftel DC, et al: Effects of protamine administration after cardiopulmonary bypass on complement, blood elements, and the hemodynamic state. *Ann Thorac Surg* 1986; 41:193.

231. Shore-Lesserson L, Gravlee GP: Anticoagulation for cardiopulmonary bypass, in Gravlee GP, Davis RF, Kurusz M, Utley JR (eds): *Cardiopulmonary Bypass: Principles and Practice*. Philadelphia, Lippincott Williams & Wilkins, 2000; p 435.

232. Dietrich W, Spannagl M, Schramm W, et al: The influence of preoperative anticoagulation on heparin response during cardiopulmonary bypass. *J Thorac Cardiovasc Surg* 1991; 102:505.

233. Hirsh J, Levine MN: Low molecular weight heparin. *Blood* 1992; 79:1.

234. Stringer KA, Lindenfeld J: Hirudins: antithrombin anticoagulants. *Ann Pharmacother* 1992; 26:1535.

235. Gladwell TD: Bivalirudin: a direct thrombin inhibitor. *Clin Ther* 2002; 1:38.

236. Swan SK, St. Peter JV, Lanbrecht LJ, Hursting MJ: Comparison of anticoagulant effects and safety of argatroban and heparin in healthy subjects. *Pharmacotherapy* 2000; 20:756.

237. Beiderlinden M, Treschan TA, Gorlinger K, et al: Argatroban anticoagulation in critically ill patients. *Ann Pharmacother* 2007; 42:421.

238. Warkentin TE, Kelton JG: Temporal aspects of heparin-induced thrombocytopenia. *New Engl J Med* 2001; 344:1286. Cohn_Ch12_p0283-0330.indd 325 8/26/11 2:58:30 PM 326 Part 2/Perioperative/Intraoperative Care

239. Horne DK: Nonimmune heparin-platelet interactions: implications for the pathogenesis of heparin-induced thrombocytopenia, in Warkentin TE, Greinacher A (eds): *Heparin-Induced Thrombocytopenia*. New York, Marcel Dekker, 2001; p 137.

240. Lee DH, Warkentin TE: Frequency of heparin-induced thrombocytopenia, in Warkentin TE, Greinacher A (eds): *Heparin-Induced Thrombocytopenia.* New York, Marcel Dekker, 2001; p 87.

241. Warkentin TE, Greinacher A: Laboratory testing for heparin-induced thrombocytopenia, in Warkentin TE, Greinacher A (eds): *Heparin-Induced Thrombocytopenia.* New York, Marcel Dekker, 2001; p 231.

242. Warkentin TE, Greinacher A: Laboratory testing for heparin-induced thrombocytopenia, in Warkentin TE, Greinacher A (eds): *Heparin-Induced Thrombocytopenia.* New York, Marcel Dekker, 2001; p 231.

243. Wallis DE, Workman KL, Lewis BE, et al: Failure of early heparin cessation as treatment for heparin-induced thrombocytopenia. *Am J Med* 1999; 106:629.

244. Nuttall GA, Oliver WJ Jr, Santrach PJ, et al: Patients with a history of type II heparin-induced thrombocytopenia with thrombosis requiring cardiac surgery with cardiopulmonary bypass: a prospective observational case series. *Anesth Analg* 2003; 96:344.

245. Greinacher A: Recombinant hirudin for the treatment of heparin-induced thrombocytopenia, in Warkentin TE, Greinacher A (eds): *Heparin-Induced Thrombocytopenia.* New York, Marcel Dekker, 2001; p 349.

246. Dyke CM, Smedira NG, Koster A, et al: A comparison of bivalirudin to heparin with protamine reversal in patients undergoing cardiac surgery with cardiopulmonary bypass: the EVOLUTION-ON study. *J Thorac Cardiovasc Surg* 2006; 131(3):533.

247. Colman RW: Contact activation pathway: inflammatory, fibrinolytic, anticoagulant, antiadhesive and antiangiogenic activities, in Colman RW, Hirsh J, Marder VJ, et al (eds): *Hemostasis and Thrombosis: Basic Principles and Practice.* Philadelphia, Lippincott Williams & Wilkins, 2001; p 103.

248. Sundaram S, Gikakis N, Hack CE, et al: Nafamostat mesilate, a broad spectrum protease inhibitor, modulates cellular and humoral activation in simulated extracorporeal circulation. *Thromb Haemost* 1996; 75:76.

249. Boisclair MD, Lane DA, Philippou H, et al: Mechanisms of thrombin generation during surgery and cardiopulmonary bypass. *Blood* 1993; 82:3350.

250. Chung JH, Gikakis N, Rao AK, et al: Pericardial blood activates the extrinsic coagulation pathway during clinical cardiopulmonary bypass. *Circulation* 1996; 93:2014.

251. Jenny NS, Mann KG: Thrombin, in Colman RW, Hirsh J, Marder VJ, et al (eds): *Hemostasis and Thrombosis: Basic Principles and Practice.* Philadelphia, Lippincott Williams & Wilkins, 2001; p 171.

252. Drake TA, Morrissey JH, Edginton TS: Selective cellular expression of tissue factor in human tissues. *Am J Pathol* 1989; 134:1087.

253. Hattori T, Khan MMH, Coleman RW, Edmunds LH: Plasma tissue factor plus activated peripheral mononuclear cells activate Factors VII and X in cardiac surgical wounds. *JACC* 2005; 46(4):707.

254. Hirsh J, Colman RW, Marder VJ, et al: Overview of thrombosis and its treatment, in Colman RW, Hirsh J, Marder VJ, et al (eds): *Hemostasis and Thrombosis: Basic Principles and Practice.* Philadelphia, Lippincott Williams & Wilkins, 2001; p 1071.

255. Spanier T, Oz M, Levin H, Weinberg A, et al: Activation of coagulation and fibrinolytic pathways in patients with left ventricular assist devices. *J Thorac Cardiovasc Surg* 1996; 112:1090.

256. Ovrum E, Holen EA, Tangen G, et al: Completely heparinized cardiopulmonary bypass and reduced systemic heparin: clinical and hemostatic effects. *Ann Thorac Surg* 1995; 60:365.

257. Rubens FD, Labow RS, Lavallee GR, et al: Hematologic evaluation of cardiopulmonary bypass circuits prepared with a novel block copolymer. *Ann Thorac Surg* 1999; 67:696.

258. Aldea GS, O'Gara P, Shapira OM, et al: Effect of anticoagulation protocol on outcome in patients undergoing CABG with heparin-bonded cardiopulmonary bypass circuits. *Ann Thorac Surg* 1998; 65:425.

259. Despotis GJ, Joist JH, Hogue CW, et al: More effective suppression of hemostatic system activation in patients undergoing cardiac surgery by heparin dosing based on heparin blood concentrations rather than ACT. *Thromb Haemost* 1996; 76:902.

260. Tabuchi N, Haan J, Boonstra PW, van Oeveren W: Activation of fibrinolysis in the pericardial cavity during cardiopulmonary bypass. *J Thorac Cardiovasc Surg* 1993; 106:828.

261. Coughlin SR, Vu T-K H, Hung DT, Wheaton VI: Characterization of a functional thrombin receptor. *J Clin Invest* 1992; 89:351.

262. Michelson AD, MacGregor H, Barnard MR, et al: Reversible inhibition of human platelet activation by hypothermia in vivo and in vitro. *Thromb Haemost* 1994; 71:633.

263. Weerasinghe A, Taylor KM: The platelet in cardiopulmonary bypass. *Ann Thorac Surg* 1998; 66:2145.

264. Rinder CS, Bonnert J, Rinder HM, et al: Platelet activation and aggregation during cardiopulmonary bypass. *Anesthesiology* 1991; 74:388.

265. Gluszko P, Rucinski B, Musial J, et al: Fibrinogen receptors in platelet adhesion to surfaces of extracorporeal circuit. *Am J Physiol* 1987; 252:H615.

266. Zilla P, Fasol R, Groscurth P, et al: Blood platelets in cardiopulmonary bypass operations. *J Thorac Cardiovasc Surg* 1989; 97:379.

267. Kestin AS, Valeri CR, Khuri SF, et al: The platelet function defect of cardiopulmonary bypass. *Blood* 1993; 82:107.

268. Khan MMH, Hattori T, Niewiarowski S, Edmunds LH, Coleman RW: Truncated and microparticle-free soluble tissue factor bound to peripheral monocytes preferentially activate factor VII. *Thromb Haemost* 2006; 95:462.

269. Steinberg JB, Kapelanski DP, Olson JD, Weiler JM: Cytokine and complement levels in patients undergoing cardiopulmonary bypass. *J Thorac Cardiovasc Surg* 1993; 106:1008.

270. Saadi S, Platt JL: Endothelial cell responses to complement activation, in Volankis JE, Frank MM (eds): *The Human Complement System in Health and Disease.* New York, Marcel Dekker, 1998; p 335.

271. Vane JR, Anggard EE, Botting RM: Regulatory functions of the vascular endothelium. *New Engl J Med* 1990; 323:27.

272. Levin EG, Marzec U, Anderson J, et al: Thrombin stimulates tissue plasminogen activator from cultured human endothelial cells. *J Clin Invest* 1984; 74:1988.

273. Francis CW, Marder VJ: Physiologic regulation and pathologic disorders of fibrinolysis, in Colman RW, Hirsh J, Marder VJ, et al: *Hemostasis and Thrombosis: Basic Principles and Practice.* Philadelphia, Lippincott Williams & Wilkins, 2001; p 975.

274. Bachmann F: Plasminogen-plasmin enzyme system, in Colman RW, Hirsh J, Marder VJ, et al: *Hemostasis and Thrombosis: Basic Principles and Practice.* Philadelphia, Lippincott Williams & Wilkins, 2001; p 275.

275. Feinstein DI, Marder VJ, Colman RW: Consumptive thrombohemorrhagic disorders, in Colman RW, Hirsh J, Marder VJ, et al: *Hemostasis and Thrombosis: Basic Principles and Practice.* Philadelphia, Lippincott Williams & Wilkins, 2001; p 1197.

276. Walport MJ: Complement. *New Engl J Med* 2001; 344:1058.

277. Fung M, Loubser PG, Ündar A, et al: Inhibition of complement, neutrophil, and platelet activation by an anti-factor D monoclonal antibody in simulated cardiopulmonary bypass circuits. *J Thorac Cardiovasc Surg* 2001; 122:113.

278. van Oeveren W, Kazatchkine MD, Descamps-Latscha B, et al: Deleterious effects of cardiopulmonary bypass: a prospective study of bubble versus membrane oxygenation. *J Thorac Cardiovasc Surg* 1985; 89:888.

279. Chenoweth DE, Cooper SW, Hugli TE, et al: Complement activation during cardiopulmonary bypass: evidence for generation of C3a and C5a anaphylactoxins. *New Engl J Med* 1981; 304:497.

280. Cavarocchi NC, Schaff HV, Orszulak TA, et al: Evidence for complement activation by protamine-heparin interaction after cardiopulmonary bypass. *Surgery* 1985; 98:525.

281. Weisman HF, Bartow T, Leppo MK, et al: Recombinant soluble CR1 suppressed complement activation, inflammation, and necrosis associated with reperfusion of ischemic myocardium. *Trans Assoc Am Phys* 1990; 103:64.

282. Walport MJ: Complement. *New Engl J Med* 2001; 344:1058.

283. Moat NE, Shore DF, Evans TW: Organ dysfunction and cardiopulmonary bypass: the role of complement and complement regulatory proteins. *Eur J Cardiothorac Surg* 1993; 7:563.

284. Moat NE, Shore DF, Evans TW: Organ dysfunction and cardiopulmonary bypass: the role of complement and complement regulatory proteins. *Eur J Cardiothorac Surg* 1993; 7:563.

285. Dreyer WJ, Smith CW, Entman ML: Neutrophil activation during cardiopulmonary bypass. *J Thorac Cardiovasc Surg* 1993; 105:763.

286. Fantone JC: Cytokines and neutrophils: neutrophil-derived cytokines and the inflammatory response, in Remick DG, Friedland JS (eds): *Cytokines in Health and Disease,* 2nd ed. New York, Marcel Dekker, 1997; p 373.

287. Warren JS, Ward PA: The inflammatory response, in Beutler E, Coller BS, Lichtman MA, et al: *Williams Hematology,* 6th ed. New York, McGraw-Hill, 2001; p 67.

288. Yang J, Furie BC, Furie B: The biology of P-selectin glycoprotein ligand-1: its role as a selectin counterreceptor in leukocyte-endothelial and leukocyte-platelet interaction. *Thromb Haemost* 1999; 81:1.

289. Springer TA: Traffic signals for lymphocyte circulation and leukocyte migration: the multistep paradigm. *Cell* 1994; 76:301.

290. Asimakopoulos G, Taylor KM: Effects of cardiopulmonary bypass on leukocyte and endothelial adhesion molecules. *Ann Thorac Surg* 1998; 66:2135.

291. Smith WB, Gamble JR, Clarklewis I, Vadas MA: Chemotactic desensitization of neutrophils demonstrates interleukin-8 (IL-8)-dependent and IL-8-independent mechanisms of transmigration through cytokine-activated endothelium. *Immunology* 1993; 78:491.

292. Hayashi Y, Sawa Y, Ohtake S, et al: Peroxynitrite formation from human myocardium after ischemia-reperfusion during open heart operation. *Ann Thorac Surg* 2001; 72:571.

293. Ilton MK, Langton PE, Taylor ML, et al: Differential expression of neutrophil adhesion molecules during coronary artery surgery with cardiopulmonary bypass. *J Thorac Cardiovasc Surg* 1999; 118:930.

294. Borregaard N, Cowland JB: Granules of the human neutrophilic polymorphonuclear leukocyte. *Blood* 1997; 89:3503.

295. Blackstone EH, Kirklin JW, Stewart RW, et al: The damaging effects of cardiopulmonary bypass, in Wu KK, Roxy EC (eds): *Prostaglandins in Clinical Medicine: Cardiovascular and Thrombotic Disorders.* Chicago, Yearbook Medical Publishers, 1982; p 355.

296. Chung JH, Gikakis N, Drake TA, et al: Pericardial blood activates the extrinsic coagulation pathway during clinical cardiopulmonary bypass. *Circulation* 1996; 93:2014.

297. Vane JR, Anggard EE, Botting RM: Regulatory functions of the vascular endothelium. *New Engl J Med* 1990; 323:27.

298. Dreyer WJ, Burns AR, Phillips SC, et al: Intercellular adhesion molecule-1 regulation in the canine lung after cardiopulmonary bypass. *J Thorac Cardiovasc Surg* 1998; 115:689.

299. Funk CD: Platelet eicosanoids, in Colman RW, Hirsh J, Marder VJ, et al (eds): *Hemostasis and Thrombosis: Basic Principles and Practice.* Philadelphia, Lippincott Williams & Wilkins, 2001; p 533.

300. Fukami MH, Holmsen H, Kowalska A, Niewiarowski S: Platelet secretion, in Colman RW, Hirsh J, Marder VJ, et al (eds): *Hemostasis and Thrombosis: Basic Principles and Practice.* Philadelphia, Lippincott Williams & Wilkins, 2001; p 559.

301. Ember JA, Jagels MA, Hugli TE: Characterization of complement anaphylatoxins and their biological responses, in Volankis JE, Frank MM (eds): *The Human Complement System in Health and Disease.* New York, Marcel Dekker, 1998; p 241.

302. Steinberg JB, Kapelanski DP, Olson JD, Weiler JM: Cytokine and complement levels in patients undergoing cardiopulmonary bypass. *J Thorac Cardiovasc Surg* 1993; 106:1008.

303. Pizzo SV, Wu SM: a-Macroglobulins and kinins, in Colman RW, Hirsh J, Marder VJ, et al (eds): *Hemostasis and Thrombosis: Basic Principles and Practice.* Philadelphia, Lippincott Williams & Wilkins, 2001; p 367.

304. Powrie F, Bean A, Moore KW: Interleukin-10, in Remick DG, Friedland JS (eds): *Cytokines in Health and Disease,* 2nd ed. New York, Marcel Dekker, 1997; p 143.

305. Frering B, Philip I, Dehoux M, et al: Circulating cytokines in patients undergoing normothermic cardiopulmonary bypass. *J Thorac Cardiovasc Surg* 1994; 108:636.

306. Drabe N, Zünd G, Grünenfelder J, et al: Genetic predisposition in patients undergoing cardiopulmonary bypass surgery is associated with an increase of inflammatory cytokines. *Eur J Cardiothorac Surg* 2001; 20:609.

307. Babior BM: Phagocytes and oxidative stress. *Am J Med* 2000; 109:33.

308. Kharazmi A, Andersen LW, Baek L, et al: Endotoxemia and enhanced generation of oxygen radicals by neutrophils from patients undergoing cardiopulmonary bypass. *J Thorac Cardiovasc Surg* 1989; 98:381.

309. Nilsson L, Kulander L, Nystrom S-O, Eriksson O: Endotoxins in cardiopulmonary bypass. *J Thorac Cardiovasc Surg* 1990; 100:777.

310. Neuhof C, Wendling J, Friedhelm D, et al: Endotoxin and cytokine generation in cardiac surgery in relation to flow mode and duration of cardiopulmonary bypass. *Shock* 2001; 16:39.

311. Smith EEJ, Naftel DC, Blackstone EH, Kirklin JW: Microvascular permeability after cardiopulmonary bypass. *J Thorac Cardiovasc Surg* 1987; 94:225.

312. Menasché PH: The systemic factor: the comparative roles of cardiopulmonary bypass and off-pump surgery in the genesis of patient injury during and following cardiac surgery. *Ann Thorac Surg* 2001; 72:S2260.

313. Ascione R, Lloyd CT, Underwood MJ: Inflammatory response after coronary revascularization with and without cardiopulmonary bypass. *Ann Thorac Surg* 2000; 69:1198.

314. Cleveland JC Jr, Shroyer LW, Chen AY, et al: Off-pump coronary artery bypass grafting decreases risk-adjusted mortality and morbidity. *Ann Thorac Surg* 2001; 72:1282.

315. Menasché P, Peynet J, Heffner-Cavaillon N, et al: Influence of temperature on neutrophil trafficking during clinical cardiopulmonary bypass. *Circulation* 1995; 92(suppl II): II-334.

316. Menasché P: The inflammatory response to cardiopulmonary bypass and its impact on postoperative myocardial function. *Curr Opin Cardiol* 1995; 10:597.

317. Øvrum E, Tangen G, Øystese R, et al: Comparison of two heparin-coated extracorporeal circuits with reduced systemic anticoagulation in routine coronary artery bypass operations. *J Thorac Cardiovasc Surg* 2001; 121:324.

318. Gorman RC, Ziats NP, Gikakis N, et al: Surface-bound heparin fails to reduce thrombin formation during clinical cardiopulmonary bypass. *J Thorac Cardiovasc Surg* 1996; 111:1.

319. Aldea GS, O'Gara P, Shapira OM, et al: Effect of anticoagulation protocol on outcome in patients undergoing CABG with heparin-bonded cardiopulmonary bypass circuits. *Ann Thorac Surg* 1998; 65:425.

320. Wendel HP, Ziemer G: Coating-techniques to improve the hemocompatibility of artificial devices used for extracorporeal circulation. *Eur J Cardiothorac Surg* 1999; 16:342.

321. Gunaydin S, Farsak B, Kocakulak M, et al: Clinical performance and biocompatibility of poly (2-methoxyethylacrylate) coated extracorporeal circuits. *Ann Thorac Surg* 2002; 74:819.

322. Ninomiya M, Miyaji K, Takamoto S: Poly (2-methoxyethy-lacrylate)-coated bypass circuits reduce perioperative inflammatory response. *Ann Thorac Surg* 2003; 75:913.

323. Naik SK, Knight A, Elliot M: A prospective randomized study of a modified technique of ultrafiltration during pediatric open-heart surgery. *Circulation* 1991; 84(suppl III):III-422.

324. Luciani GB, Menon T, Vecchi B, et al: Modified ultrafiltration reduces morbidity after adult cardiac operations: a prospective, randomized clinical trial. *Circulation* 2001; 104(suppl I):I-253.

325. Fitch JCK, Rollins S, Matis L, et al: Pharmacology and biological efficacy of a recombinant, humanized, single-chain antibody C5 complement inhibitor in patients undergoing coronary artery bypass graft surgery with cardiopulmonary bypass. *Circulation* 1999; 100:2499.

326. Carrier M, Menasche P, Levy M, et al: Inhibition of complement activation by pexelizumab reduces death in patients undergoing combined valve replacement and coronary bypass surgery. *J Thorac Cardiovasc Surg* 2006; 131:352.

327. Chai PJ, Nassar R, Oakeley AE, et al: Soluble complement receptor-1 protects heart, lung, and cardiac myofilament function from cardiopulmonary bypass damage. *Circulation* 2000; 101:541.

328. Paparella D, Yau TM, Young E: Cardiopulmonary bypass induced inflammation: pathophysiology and treatment update. *Eur J Cardiothorac Surg* 2002; 21:232.

329. Cronstein BN, Kimmel SC, Levin RI, et al: A mechanism for the antiinflammatory effects of corticosteroids: the glucocorticoid receptor regulates leukocyte adhesion to endothelial cells and expression of endothelial-leukocyte adhesion molecule 1 and intercellular adhesion molecule 1. *Proc Natl Acad Sci USA* 1992; 89:9991.

330. Harig F, Hohenstein B, von der Emde J, Weyand M: Modulating IL-6 and IL-10 levels by pharmacologic strategies and the impact of different extracorporeal circulation parameters during cardiac surgery. *Shock* 2001; 16:33.

331. Yared JP, Starr NJ, Torres FK, et al: Effects of single dose, postinduction dexamethasone on recovery after cardiac surgery. *Ann Thorac Surg* 2000; 69:1420.

332. Ho KM, Tan JA: Benefits and risks of corticoid prophylaxis in adult cardiac surgery. *Circulation* 2009; 119:1853.

333. Levy JH, Hug CC: Use of cardiopulmonary bypass in studies of the circulation. *Br J Anaesth* 1988; 60:35S.

334. Carson JL, Poses RM, Spence RK, et al: Severity of anaemia and operative mortality and morbidity. *Lancet* 1988; 1:727.

335. Stump DA, Brown WR, Moody DM, et al: Microemboli and neurologic dysfunction after cardiovascular surgery. *Semin Cardiothorac Vascular Anesth* 1999; 3:47.

336. Stone JG, Young WL, Smith CR, et al: Do standard monitoring sites reflect true brain temperature when profound hypothermia is rapidly induced and reversed? *Anesthesiology* 1995; 82:344.

337. Smith EEJ, Naftel DC, Blackstone EH, Kirklin JW: Microvascular permeability after cardiopulmonary bypass. *J Thorac Cardiovasc Surg* 1987; 94:225.

338. Pacifico AD, Digerness S, Kirklin JW: Acute alterations of body composition after open intracardiac operations. *Circulation* 1970; 41:331.

339. Edmunds LH Jr, Williams W: Microemboli and the use of filters during cardiopulmonary bypass, in Utley JR (ed): *Pathophysiology and Techniques of Cardiopulmonary Bypass*, vol II. Baltimore, Williams & Wilkins, 1983; p 101.

340. Brooker RF, Brown WR, Moody DM, et al: Cardiotomy suction: a major source of brain lipid emboli during cardiopulmonary bypass. *Ann Thorac Surg* 1998; 65:1651.

341. Kincaid EH, Jones TJ, Stump DA, et al: Processing scavenged blood with a cell saver reduces cerebral lipid microembolization. *Ann Thorac Surg* 2000; 70:1296.

342. Reichenspurner H, Navia JA, Benny G, et al: Particulate embolic capture by an intra-aortic filter device during cardiac surgery. *J Thorac Cardiovasc Surg* 2000; 119:233.

343. Cook DJ, Zehr KJ, Orszulak TA, Slater JM: Profound reduction in brain embolization using an endoaortic baffle during bypass in swine. *Ann Thorac Surg* 2002; 73:198.

344. Barzilai B, Marshall WG Jr, Saffitz JE, et al: Avoidance of embolic complications by ultrasonic characterization of the ascending aorta. *Circulation* 1989; 80:1275.

345. Reichenspurner H, Navia JA, Benny G, et al: Particulate embolic capture by an intra-aortic filter device during cardiac surgery. *J Thorac Cardiovasc Surg* 2000; 119:233.

346. Hammon JW, Stump DA, Butterworth JE, et al: Single cross clamp improves six month cognitive outcome in high risk coronary bypass patients. *J Thorac Cardiovasc Surg* 2006; 131:114.

347. Loop FD, Higgins TL, Panda R, et al: Myocardial protection during cardiac operations: decreased morbidity and lower cost with blood cardioplegia and coronary sinus perfusion. *J Cardiovasc Surg* 1992; 104:608.

348. Sundt TM, Barner HB, Camillo CJ, et al: Total arterial revascularization with an internal thoracic artery and radial artery T graft. *Ann Thorac Surg* 1999; 68:399.

349. Tector AJ, Amundsen S, Schmahl TM, et al: Total revascularization with T grafts. *Ann Thorac Surg* 1994; 57:33.

350. Jones TJ, Deal DD, Vernon JC, et al: The propagation of entrained air during cardiopulmonary bypass is affected by circuit design but not by vacuum assisted venous drainage. *Anesth Analg* 2000; 90:39.

351. Braunwald E, Kloner RA: The stunned myocardium: prolonged, postischemic ventricular dysfunction. *Circulation* 1982; 66:1146.

352. Downing SW, Savage EB, Streicher JS, et al: The stretched ventricle: myocardial creep and contractile dysfunction after acute nonischemic ventricular distention. *J Thorac Cardiovasc Surg* 1992; 104:996.

353. Newman S: The incidence and nature of neuropsychological morbidity following cardiac surgery. *Perfusion* 1989; 4:93.

354. Murkin JM, Stump DA, Blumenthal JA, et al: Defining dysfunction: group means versus incidence analysis-a statement of consensus. *Ann Thorac Surg* 1997; 64:904.

355. Selnes OA, Grega MA, Bailey MM, et al: Neurocognitive outcomes 3 years after coronary artery bypass graft surgery: a controlled study. *Ann Thorac Surg* 2007; 84:1885.

356. Baird A, Benfield A, Schlaug G, et al: Enlargement of human cerebral ischemic lesion volumes measured by diffusion-weighted magnetic resonance imaging. *Ann Neurol* 1997; 41:581.

357. Maragos PJ, Schmechel DE: Neuron-specific enolase, a clinically useful marker for neurons and neuroendocrine cells. *Annu Rev Neurol Sci* 1987; 10:269.

358. Zimmer DB, Cornwall EH, Landar A, Song W: The S-100 protein family: history, function, and expression. *Brain Res Bull* 1995; 37:417.

359. Johnsson P, Blomquist S, Luhrs C, et al: Neuron-specific enolase increases in plasma during and immediately after extracorporeal circulation. *Ann Thorac Surg* 2000; 69:750.

360. Anderson RE, Hansson LO, Liska J, et al: The effect of cardiotomy suction on the brain injury marker S100 beta after cardiopulmonary bypass. *Ann Thorac Surg* 2000; 69:847.

361. Shaw PJ, Bates D, Cartlidge NE, et al: Neurologic and neuropsychological morbidity following: major surgery: comparison of coronary artery bypass and peripheral vascular surgery. *Stroke* 1987; 18:700.

362. Gardner TJ, Horneffer PJ, Manolio TA, et al: Stroke following coronary artery bypass surgery: a ten year study. *Ann Thorac Surg* 1985; 40:574.

363. Moller JT, Cluitmans P, Rasmussen LS, et al: Long-term postoperative cognitive dysfunction in the elderly ISPOCD study. ISPOCD investigators, International Study of Post-Operative Cognitive Dysfunction. *Lancet* 1998; 351:857.

364. Jones EL, Weintraub WS, Craver JM, et al: Coronary bypass surgery: is the operation different today? *J Thorac Cardiovasc Surg* 1991; 101:108.

365. Tardiff BE, Newman MF, Saunders AM, et al: Preliminary report of a genetic basis for cognitive decline after cardiac operations. *Ann Thorac Surg* 1997; 64:715.

366. Weintraub WS, Wenger NK, Jones EL, et al: Changing clinical characteristics of coronary surgery patients: differences between men and women. *Circulation* 1993; 88:79.

367. Goto T, Baba T, Yoshitake A, et al: Craniocervical and aortic atherosclerosis as neurologic risk factors in coronary surgery. *Ann Thorac Surg* 2000; 69:834.

368. Wareing TH, Davila-Roman VG, Daily BB, et al: Strategy for the reduction of stroke incidence in cardiac surgical patients. *Ann Thorac Surg* 1993; 55:1400.

369. Stump DA, Kon NA, Rogers AT, et al: Emboli and neuropsychologic outcome following cardiopulmonary bypass. *Echocardiography* 1996; 13:555.

370. Tuman KJ, McCarthy RJ, Najafi H, et al: Differential effects of advanced age on neurologic and cardiac risks of coronary operations. *J Thorac Cardiovasc Surg* 1992; 104:1510.

371. Lata A, Stump D, Deal D, et al: Cannula design reduces particulate and gaseous emboli during cardiopulmonary bypass for coronary artery bypass grafting. *J Cardiac Surg* (in press).

372. Jones TJ, Stump DA, Deal D, et al: Hypothermia protects the brain from embolization by reducing and redirecting the embolic load. *Ann Thorac Surg* 1999; 68:1465.

373. Murkin JM, Farrar JK, Tweed WA, et al: Cerebral autoregulation and flow/metabolism coupling during cardiopulmonary bypass: the role of PaCO$_2$. *Anesth Analg* 1987; 66:665.

374. Stump DA, Brown WR, Moody DM, et al: Microemboli and neurologic dysfunction after cardiovascular surgery. *Semin Cardiothorac Vascular Anesth* 1999; 3:47.

375. Helps SC, Parsons DW, Reilly PL, et al: The effect of gas emboli on rabbit cerebral blood flow. *Stroke* 1990; 21:94.

376. Moody DM, Brown WR, Challa VR, et al: Efforts to characterize the nature and chronicle the occurrence of brain emboli during cardiopulmonary bypass. *Perfusion* 1995; 9:316.

377. Cook DJ, Oliver WC, Orsulak TA, et al: Cardiopulmonary bypass temperature, hematocrit, and cerebral oxygen delivery in humans. *Ann Thorac Surg* 1995; 60:1671.

378. Martin TC, Craver JM, Gott MP: Prospective, randomized trial of retrograde warm-blood cardioplegia: myocardial benefit and neurological threat. *Ann Thorac Surg* 1994; 59:298.

379. Nathan HJ, Wells GA, Munson JL, Wozny D: Neuroprotective effect of mild hypothermia in patients undergoing coronary artery surgery with cardiopulmonary bypass. *Circulation* 2001; 104(suppl I):I-85.

380. Gold JP, Charlson ME, Williams-Russo P, et al: Improvement if outcomes after coronary artery bypass: a randomized trial comparing intraoperative high versus low mean arterial pressure. *J Thorac Cardiovasc Surg* 1995; 110:1302.

381. Brown R, Wright G, Royston D: A comparison of two systems for assessing cerebral venous oxyhaemoglobin saturation during cardiopulmonary bypass in humans. *Anesthesia* 1993; 48:697.

382. Nussmeier N, Arlund C, Slogoff S: Neuropsychiatric complications after cardiopulmonary bypass: cerebral protection by a barbiturate. *Anesthesiology* 1986; 64:165.

383. Arrowsmith JE, Harrison MJG, Newman SP, et al: Neuroprotection of the brain during cardiopulmonary bypass: a randomized trial of remacemide during coronary artery bypass in 171 patients. *Stroke* 1998; 29:2357.

384. Mitchell SJ, Pellet O, Gorman DF, et al: Cerebral protection by lidocaine during cardiac operations. *Ann Thorac Surg* 1999; 67:1117.

385. Diegeler A, Hirsch R, Schneider F, et al: Neuromonitoring and neurocognitive outcome in off-pump versus conventional coronary bypass operation. *Ann Thorac Surg* 2000; 69:1162.

386. Moss E, Puskas JD, Thourani VH, et al: Avoiding aortic clamping during coronary artery bypass grafting reduces postoperative stroke. *J Thorac Cardiovasc Surg* 2015; 149:75-80.

387. Newman MF, Kirchner JL, Phillips-Bute B, et al: Longitudinal assessment of neurocognitive function after coronary artery bypass grafting. *New Engl J Med* 2001; 344:395-402.

388. Vermeer SE, Longstreth Jr WT, Koudstaal PJ: Silent brain infarcts: a systematic review. *Lancet Neurol* 2007; 6:611.

389. Hammon JW, Stump DA, Butterworth JE, et al: CABG with single cross clamp results in fewer persistent neuropsychological deficits than multiple clamp or OPCAB. *Ann Thorac Surg* 2007; 84:1174.

390. Selnes OA, Grega MA, Borowicz LM, et al: Cognitive outcomes three years after coronary bypass surgery: a comparison of on-pump coronary bypass surgery and nonsurgical controls. *Ann Thorac Surg* 2005; 79:1201.

391. Mullges W, Babin-Ebell J, Reents W, Toyka KV: Cognitive performance after coronary bypass grafting: a follow-up study. *Neurology* 2002; 59:741.

392. Maggart M, Stewart S: The mechanisms and management of non-cardiogenic pulmonary edema following cardiopulmonary bypass. *Ann Thorac Surg* 1987; 43:231.

393. Allardyce D, Yoshida S, Ashmore P: The importance of microembolism in the pathogenesis of organ dysfunction caused by prolonged use of the pump oxygenator. *J Thorac Cardiovasc Surg* 1966; 52:706.

394. Tonz M, Mihaljevic T, von Segesser LK, et al: Acute lung injury during cardiopulmonary bypass: are the neutrophils responsible? *Chest* 1995; 108:1551.

395. McGowan FX, del Nido PJ, Kurland G, et al: Cardiopulmonary bypass significantly impairs surfactant activity in children. *J Thorac Cardiovasc Surg* 1993; 106:968.

396. Oster JB, Sladen RN, Berkowitz DE: Cardiopulmonary bypass and the lung, in Gravlee GP, Davis RF, Kurusz M, Utley JR (eds): *Cardiopulmonary Bypass: Principles and Practice.* Philadelphia, Lippincott Williams & Wilkins, 2000; p 367.

397. Cogliati AA, Menichetti A, Tritapepe L, et al: Effects of three techniques of lung management on pulmonary function during cardiopulmonary bypass. *Acta Anaesth Belg* 1996; 47:73.

398. Sirivella A, Gielchinsky I, Parsonnet V: Management of catheter-induced pulmonary artery perforation: a rare complication in cardiovascular operations. *Ann Thorac Surg* 2001; 72:2056.

399. Zanardo G, et al: Acute renal failure in the patient undergoing cardiac operation: prevalence, mortality rate, and main risk factors. *J Thorac Cardiovasc Surg* 1994; 107:1489.

400. Utley JR: Renal function and fluid balance with cardiopulmonary bypass, in Gravlee GP, Davis RF, Utley JR (eds): *Cardiopulmonary Bypass: Principles and Practice.* Baltimore, Williams & Wilkins, 1993; p 488.

401. Clyne DH, Kant KS, Pesce AJ, et al: Nephrotoxicity of low molecular weight serum proteins: physicochemical interactions between myoglobin, hemoglobin, Bence Jones proteins and Tamm-Horsfall mucoprotein. *Curr Prob Clin Biochem* 1979; 9:299.

402. Abel RM, Buckley MJ, Austen WG, et al: Etiology, incidence and prognosis of renal failure following cardiac operations: results of a prospective analysis of 500 consecutive patients. *J Thorac Cardiovasc Surg* 1976;71:32.

403. Mangano C, et al: Renal dysfunction after myocardial revascularization: risk factors, adverse outcomes and hospital resource utilization. The Multicenter Study of Perioperative Ischemia Research Group. *Anesth Analg* 1998; 1:3.

404. Ryan TA, Rady MY, Bashour CA, et al: Predictors of outcome in cardiac surgical patients with prolonged intensive care stay. *Chest* 1997; 112:1035.

405. Rattner DW, Gu Z-Y, Vlahakes GJ, et al: Hyperamylasemia after cardiac surgery. *Ann Surg* 1989; 209:279.

406. Fernandez-del Castillo C, Harringer W, Warshaw AL, et al: Risk factors for pancreatic cellular injury after cardiopulmonary bypass. *New Engl J Med* 1991; 325:382.

407. Mithofer K, Fernandes-del Castillo C, Frick TW, et al: Acute hypercalcemia causes acute pancreatitis and ectopic trypsinogen activation in the rat. *Gastroenterology* 1995; 109:239.

408. Mori A, Watanabe K, Onoe M, et al: Regional blood flow in the liver, pancreas and kidney during pulsatile and nonpulsatile perfusion under profound hypothermia. *Jpn Circ J* 1988; 52:219.

409. Shangraw RE: Splanchnic, hepatic and visceral effects, in Gravlee GP, Davis RF, Utley JR (eds): *Cardiopulmonary Bypass: Principles and Practice.* Baltimore, Williams & Wilkins, 1993; p 391.

410. Fiddian-Green RG, Baker S: Predictive value of the stomach wall pH for complications after cardiac operations: comparison with other monitoring. *Crit Care Med* 1987; 15:153.

411. Diaz-Gomez JL, Nutter B, Xu M, et al: The effect of postoperative gastrointestinal complications in patients undergoing coronary bypass surgery. *Ann Thorac Surg* 2010; 90:109.

14

Transfusion Therapy and Blood Conservation

Andreas R. de Biasi • William J. DeBois • O. Wayne Isom • Arash Salemi

Concurrent with the development of cardiac surgery in the 1950s as a means of correcting congenital heart defects came the need for large-volume blood transfusions. In the 1960s and 1970s, the introduction of valve prostheses and direct grafting of coronary arteries also made the repair of acquired heart diseases a possibility. These landmarks, along with the early liberal use of allogeneic blood transfusion therapy, led to rapid growth of our field.

Historically, open-heart surgery has been associated with large transfusion requirements. Some reports suggest that up to 70% of this patient population requires blood transfusions, resulting in an average of 2 to 4 donor exposures per patient.[1,2] It has been reported that cardiac surgery consumes about 20% of the available blood supply in the United States, with similar figures observed worldwide.[3] These relatively high rates of transfusions are mostly attributable to cardiopulmonary-bypass-induced phenomena: coagulopathy, platelet dysfunction, and red cell hemolysis all occur to varying degrees as a result of the cardiopulmonary bypass (CPB) circuit.[4-6] Other mechanisms for bleeding include inherited and acquired disorders (including platelet dysfunctions, coagulation factor deficiencies, and derangements leading to excessive fibrinolysis) of numerous etiologies.[7] While common transfusion reactions such as urticaria and fever are easily managed and largely benign, rarer complications like transfusion-related acute lung injury (TRALI) pose serious risks to patients (eg, the mortality rate for TRALI in critically ill populations ranges from 35–58%[8,9]) and provide further impetus for the avoidance of blood product transfusions when at all possible.

Although life-threatening hemorrhage is an obvious absolute indication for blood products, many transfusions are also given to improve oxygen-carrying capacity and to avoid or reverse end-organ ischemia. Despite the potential benefits of transfusing blood to maintain end-organ oxygenation, there is a surprising lack of evidence to support the liberal use of blood transfusions in cardiac surgery. In fact, there is a growing literature base demonstrating that transfusions are associated with an increased risk of both morbidity and mortality.[10-12] For example, red blood cell (RBC) transfusions have been associated with longer intensive care unit lengths of stay as well as with worse short- and long-term survival.[13-15] A large prospective study identified RBC transfusion as the strongest independent predictor of all-cause morbidity and mortality following isolated coronary artery bypass grafting (CABG) and that each unit of blood transfused posed an additive risk for adverse outcomes.[16]

Concerns over the negative consequences of blood transfusions are not new. As cardiac surgery grew as a discipline in the 1970s, investigators concomitantly noted an increasing incidence of transfusion-transmitted hepatitis; this public health concern first alerted patients and physicians to the concept of blood conservation. The emergence of the human immunodeficiency virus (HIV) a decade later further heightened interest in this area. Considering (1) the increased awareness of blood-borne infectious diseases, (2) the ever-present shortage of available blood donors, (3) the costs of blood products to both patients and institutions, (4) the needs of special populations like Jehovah's Witnesses, and (5) the inherent risks from transfusions, a greater effort was made to perform open-heart procedures without blood transfusions, even in high-risk patients. Additionally, randomized trials showing that lower hemoglobin thresholds were tolerated in both critically ill and cardiac surgical patients further contributed to decreasing transfusions and to the acceptance of some degree of anemia in our patients.[17-19]

As we will discuss, advances in preoperative screening and patient optimization; improvements in surgical techniques and shorter operative times; the use of perioperative pharmacologics and other technologies designed to curtail blood loss; and the aforementioned tolerance of lower hematocrits, especially on bypass, have allowed for extensive procedures to be routinely performed without significant blood loss and with fewer transfusions.

Comprehensive blood conservation programs that combine such elements (analogous to the use of care bundles in the critical care setting) are likely the most effective strategy in decreasing patients' exposure to allogeneic blood. In 1991, Ovrum and colleagues established the effectiveness of the simple "core" approach to blood conservation in a cohort of 121 consecutive elective CABG patients –the authors achieved a transfusion rate of 4.1% and required only 0.06 RBC units per patient.[20] Later that year, the same group applied these principles to a larger group of 500 elective CABG patients, obtaining similar low rates of transfusion (2.4% of patients) and demonstrating that an impressive 96% of patients received no allogeneic blood products; the authors concluded their multimodal six-step blood conservation program was simple, safe, and cost effective.[21] More recently, Van der Linden and colleagues developed a blood conservation program that employed a standardized transfusion policy and algorithm-driven protocols aimed at minimizing perioperative blood loss.[22] Using this strategy, the group reported a 53% decrease in RBC utilization and a 46% decrease in the number of patients receiving any blood products, without a significant difference in postoperative hemoglobin; moreover, their strategy was also shown to be safe and cost effective.[22] It should be noted that the success of such multidisciplinary programs is not limited to large teaching institutions, as similar results have been shown in the community setting.[23]

BLOOD CONSERVATION: PREOPERATIVE CONSIDERATIONS

Identification of Patients at Risk of Bleeding or of Requiring Transfusion

An important first step in mitigating bleeding and transfusion requirements is to identify those patients most at risk for blood loss and/or for needing blood product replacement. Five factors have been identified that are consistently associated with increased rates of RBC transfusions in cardiac surgery: low preoperative hemoglobin and/or hematocrit, advanced patient age, female sex, renal insufficiency, and surgery urgency.[24] Additional risk factors include a personal and/or family history of any excessive bleeding or the presence of a documented bleeding disorder; preoperative antiplatelet or anticoagulation therapy (eg, aspirin, clopidogrel, warfarin); insulin-dependent diabetes mellitus; decreased left ventricular function; anticipated long CPB time; and type of surgery (with complex valvular and aortic surgeries conferring the greatest risks).[25] Current Society of Thoracic Surgery/Society of Cardiovascular Anesthesiologists (STS/SCA) blood conservation guidelines recommend obtaining preoperative hematocrits and platelet counts to aid risk prediction, as abnormalities in these variables are amenable to intervention; preoperative bleeding time may also be determined in high-risk patients, especially those on preoperative antiplatelet agents.[26] Of note, preoperative screening of the intrinsic coagulation system is not recommended unless there is a clinical history of a prior bleeding diathesis.[26]

Awareness of the above-listed risk factors is important as the recognition of specific risks should guide subsequent preoperative patient management with the intent of optimizing a given patient's risk profile. We will in turn discuss three such preoperative management issues: medication cessation, increasing preoperative RBC mass, and preoperative autologous donation.

Managing Medications Contributing to Bleeding and Transfusion Risks

The regular, preoperative use of antiplatelet medications like aspirin and clopidogrel have been associated with increased perioperative blood loss as well as with the need for blood products in cardiac surgery patients—as such, a thorough understanding of current guidelines pertaining to their use prior to cardiac surgery is requisite. With the advent of newer anticoagulants (eg, direct thrombin inhibitors, direct factor Xa inhibitors), insight into what to do about these drugs must be assimilated with knowledge of older, well-established guidelines on the cessation of traditional vitamin K antagonists. Table 14-1 lists some of the more commonly encountered of these drugs.

ASPIRIN

Aspirin irreversibly inhibits cyclooxygenase-1 and -2, leading to decreased formation of thromboxane A_2 and ultimately to inhibited platelet aggregation. The ability of aspirin to irreversibly induce this qualitative platelet defect has led to its widespread use as a thromboprophylaxing agent in many cardiovascular disease states (eg, coronary artery disease, carotid artery stenosis, after prosthetic valve insertion, or CABG); as such, aspirin is a very frequently encountered drug in our patient population. Current guidelines state that it is reasonable to discontinue aspirin prior to cardiac surgery only in purely elective patients not having acute coronary syndromes.[26]

ADENOSINE DIPHOSPHATE RECEPTOR INHIBITORS

These antiplatelet drugs (clopidogrel, prasugrel, ticagrelor, and ticlopidine) inhibit the $P2Y_{12}$ subtype of platelet adenosine diphosphate (ADP) receptors, thus causing irreversible platelet inhibition (of note, ticagrelor is an allosteric antagonist, making its ADP blockage reversible). Members of this class of drugs are frequently used in combination with other antiplatelet agents like aspirin as part of dual antiplatelet therapies for acute coronary syndromes and for thromboprophylaxis in those with stents and/or cerebrovascular disease. ADP receptor inhibitors are felt to confer greater bleeding and transfusion risks than aspirin; as such, guidelines recommend discontinuation of these agents as few as 3 days prior to cardiac surgery (with specific timing determined by a given drug's half-life of elimination).[26] Point-of-care (POC, discussed later) testing assessing platelet responsiveness to clopidogrel, specifically, may be used to identify those nonresponders who are candidates for early operative coronary revascularization and who may thus not require a preoperative cessation period.[26]

TABLE 14-1: Antiplatelet Agents and Anticoagulants

Drug	Mechanism	Binding	Half-life
Aspirin	Acetylation of COX-1 and -2 enzymes, resulting in inhibition of TXA_2 formation, thereby inhibiting platelet aggregation.	Irreversible	15-20 min
ADP Receptor Inhibitors			
Clopidogrel (Plavix)	Inhibits the $P2Y_{12}$ subtype of platelet ADP receptors, thus preventing GP IIb/IIIa receptor complex activation, thereby reducing platelet activation and aggregation.	Irreversible	6 h
Prasugrel (Effient)	Inhibits the $P2Y_{12}$ subtype of platelet ADP receptors, thus preventing GP IIb/IIIa receptor complex activation, thereby reducing platelet activation and aggregation.	Irreversible	7 h
Ticagrelor (Brilinta)	Inhibits the $P2Y_{12}$ subtype of platelet ADP receptors, thus preventing GP IIb/IIIa receptor complex activation, thereby reducing platelet activation and aggregation.	Reversible	7 h
Ticlopidine (Ticlid)	Inhibits the $P2Y_{12}$ subtype of platelet ADP receptors, thus preventing GP IIb/IIIa receptor complex activation, thereby reducing platelet activation and aggregation.	Irreversible	13 h
GP IIb/IIIa Inhibitors			
Abciximab (ReoPro)	Monoclonal anti-GP-IIb/IIIa antibody, resulting in steric hindrance, thus inhibiting platelet aggregation.	Noncompetitive	30 min
Eptifibatide (Integrilin)	Cyclic heptapeptide inhibitor of GP IIb/IIIa receptor, thus interferes with platelet aggregation.	Reversible	2.5 h
Tirofiban (Aggrastat)	Non-peptide inhibitor of GP IIb/IIIa receptor, thus interferes with platelet aggregation.	Reversible	2 h
Unfractionated Heparin	Complexes with AT III, accelerating the thrombin-inactivating function of AT III by 1000- to 4000-fold.	Reversible	1.5 h
Warfarin	Inhibits hepatic synthesis of vitamin K-dependent coagulation factors (II, VII, IX, and X as well as proteins C and S).	Competitive	20-60 h
Novel Oral Anticoagulants			
Dabigatran (Pradaxa)	Direct thrombin inhibitor; inhibits coagulation via prevention of thrombin-mediated effects.	Reversible	12-17 h
Apixaban (Eliquis)	Direct factor Xa inhibitor, thus inhibits conversion of prothrombin to thrombin, thereby preventing platelet activation and fibrin formation.	Reversible	12 h
Edoxaban (Savaysa)	Direct factor Xa inhibitor, thus inhibits conversion of prothrombin to thrombin, thereby preventing platelet activation and fibrin formation.	Reversible	6-11 h
Rivaroxaban (Xarelto)	Direct factor Xa inhibitor, thus inhibits conversion of prothrombin to thrombin, thereby preventing platelet activation and fibrin formation.	Reversible	5-9 h

ADP, adenosine diphosphate; AT, antithrombin; COX, cyclooxygenase; GP, glycoprotein; TXA_2, thromboxane A_2.

GLYCOPROTEIN IIb/IIIa INHIBITORS

Members of this drug class (eg, abciximab, eptifibatide, tirofiban) prevent platelet aggregation via inhibition of glycoprotein (GP) IIb/IIIa receptors on the surface of platelets; these agents are frequently used during percutaneous coronary interventions and in the treatment of acute coronary syndromes. Like the other previously mentioned high-intensity antiplatelet drugs, GP IIb/IIIa inhibitors are associated with increased bleeding after cardiac operations; as such, these medications should be stopped prior to surgery in order to decrease minor and major bleeding events.[26] Exact timing again depends on the half-life of each agent in question.

It should be noted that unfractionated heparin is the notable exception to the cessation recommendations pertaining to the high-intensity antithrombotic drugs outlined by the STS/SCA guidelines: unfractionated heparin is the only agent which can either be discontinued shortly before operation or not at all.[26]

VITAMIN K ANTAGONISTS

Vitamin K antagonists are anticoagulants that reduce hepatic production of coagulation factors II, VII, IX, and X as well as of proteins C and S—all of which depend on vitamin K for their synthesis. Warfarin, the most widely encountered of these drugs, is used both in the prophylaxis and treatment of thromboembolic disorders (eg, venous or pulmonary clots, prosthetic valve thrombosis); warfarin is similarly used in atrial fibrillation and can serve as an adjunct to reduce systemic embolic risks after myocardial infarction. According to recent guidelines produced by the European Association for Cardio-Thoracic Surgery, patients on warfarin prior to cardiac surgery should be managed in a similar manner to those undergoing major noncardiac surgery.[27] That is, warfarin should be discontinued 2 to 4 days before surgery and patients at higher risk of thrombosis should be bridged with intravenous heparin once the international normalized ratio becomes subtherapeutic.[27]

NOVEL ORAL ANTICOAGULANTS: DIRECT THROMBIN INHIBITORS AND DIRECT FACTOR XA INHIBITORS

Although novel oral anticoagulants (NOACs) belonging to the direct thrombin inhibitor (eg, dabigatran) and direct factor Xa inhibitor (rivaroxaban, apixaban, edoxaban) classes are currently not indicated for patients with mechanical valves, their ease of use and their lack of a monitoring requirement (as compared to warfarin) have increased the popularity of these drugs for patients requiring long-term anticoagulation for nonvalvular reasons. Current guidelines regarding the perioperative use of NOACs recommend these drugs be discontinued 2 to 5 days prior to procedures with a high risk of bleeding, including major abdominal, cardiovascular, and thoracic operations.[28,29] Since the diminution of the anticoagulant effects of NOACs is predictable after their cessation, bridging is typically not required after NOACs are stopped.

The management of patients on NOACs requiring emergency surgery is complicated by the fact that these agents have no specific antidote. In this setting, surgery should be deferred for at least 12 hours if at all possible; given NOACs' short half-lives, this should allow for some mitigation of bleeding risk.[30] If delaying surgery is not possible, expert opinion suggests the use of oral activated charcoal or hemodialysis; prophylactic administration of fresh frozen plasma (FFP) or prothrombin complex concentrates (PCCs, discussed below) is not recommended in the absence of major bleeding.[30]

HERBAL SUPPLEMENTS AND COMPLEMENTARY MEDICINE

The use of herbal supplements and complementary medicine has seemingly exploded in popularity recently and warrants mentioning since many of these naturopathic treatments can have profound hematologic effects. Herbs, such as thyme and rosemary have been shown to have a direct inhibitory effect on platelets.[31] Fish oil, an omega-3 polyunsaturated fatty acid, may affect platelet aggregation and/or vitamin K-dependent coagulation factors. Omega-3 fatty acids may lower thromboxane A$_2$ within platelets as well as decrease factor VII levels,[32] while garlic, ginger, and *Gingko biloba* have all been associated with platelet-dysfunction-induced bleeding.[33] Given the many possible antiplatelet and anticoagulant

effects of such alternative medicines, not to mention their myriad interactions (both known and unknown) with other drugs, it is therefore prudent to inquire about any supplements patients may be taking prior to cardiac surgery. It is our practice to have patients stop all such remedies 7 days prior to surgery.

Increasing Preoperative Red Blood Cell Mass

Increasing RBC mass prior to surgery is another component of blood conservation, as decreased preoperative hemoglobin or hematocrit levels have been shown to be powerful predictors of the need for transfusion as well as significant risk factors for early and late mortality.[25,34] Such optimization necessitates diagnosing and treating preoperative anemia. Since iron-deficiency anemia is common in the cardiac surgery population, iron supplementation can restore hemoglobin concentrations to adequate levels (eg, 13 g/dL or above), thereby decreasing transfusion risk.

The use of recombinant human erythropoietin (EPO) has been studied as an additional means of improving RBC mass in anemic patients preparing to undergo cardiac surgery. A meta-analysis examining such preoperative EPO administration demonstrated that its use prior to cardiac surgery was associated with a significant reduction in the risk of exposure to allogeneic blood.[35] While there are some concerns that chronic EPO use may carry an increased risk of thrombotic complications, a recent randomized, blinded trial of preoperative high-dose EPO of short duration showed a 56% decrease in the relative risk of exposure to blood products in patients undergoing off-pump CABG following preoperative EPO versus those not given EPO; no adverse effects were observed.[36] The contemporary STS/SCA guidelines state that it is reasonable to use preoperative EPO and iron several days prior to cardiac surgery in patients with anemia, in those who refuse transfusion (eg, Jehovah's Witness), or in patients who are at high risk for postoperative anemia.[26]

Preoperative Autologous Blood Donation

Preoperative autologous blood donation (PABD) remains an option at selected centers for minimizing patient exposures to allogeneic blood. Although this technique has been in practice since the 1960s, its use in cardiac surgery did not achieve widespread acceptance until the 1980s, when the rise of HIV led to increased interest in PABD as a way of reducing allogeneic transfusions. Unfortunately, the acuity of most cardiac operations precludes the routine use PABD as there must be sufficient time between donation and surgery to allow for the regeneration of the patient's RBC mass. In general, this time is a minimum of 2 weeks per unit of blood donated. What is more, patients must have enough reserve to tolerate the ensuing transient anemia, further limiting PABD's utility. PABD is only an option for the elective, stable preoperative patient;

additionally, there are numerous relative contraindications to PABD, including the presence of left main disease, critical aortic stenosis, congestive heart failure, severe coronary artery disease with ongoing ischemia, active endocarditis, and baseline anemia.

Most of the randomized studies evaluating PABD involve small sample sizes and level A evidence of its benefits are lacking[37]; nevertheless, a recent case-control study examining the technique showed a lower incidence of allogeneic transfusions among those patients who donated preoperatively compared to those who did not (but 20% of the donated blood products were discarded postoperatively).[38] As such, the most recent STS/STA guidelines do not directly endorse PABD; they mention PABD only in the context of EPO use, wherein the guidelines state EPO additionally may be considered to restore RBC volume in patients undergoing PABD.[26] For reasons of practicality and cost effectiveness, PABD has largely been supplanted by numerous perioperative blood conservation strategies, which we discuss in the next section.

BLOOD CONSERVATION: PERIOPERATIVE STRATEGIES
Cardiopulmonary Bypass Considerations

Numerous CPB techniques have been validated to reduce blood loss and to protect against transfusions during and after cardiac surgery. These strategies, which we discuss in turn, require coordination between the operating surgeon and perfusionist and constitute another vital component of any comprehensive blood conservation program.

ACUTE NORMOVOLEMIC HEMODILUTION

Acute normovolemic hemodilution (ANH) involves the removal of 1 to 2 units of whole blood (target hematocrit of 25–30%) from the patient immediately before, or during, surgery (but prior to CPB initiation) while simultaneously replacing it with crystalloid or colloid to maintain normovolemia. The theoretical basis for ANH (also known referred to as intraoperative autologous donation) is that this lowering of the hematocrit results in fewer RBCs being lost when the patient subsequently bleeds during the course of the operation. Moreover, the removed blood is spared the effects of hemodilution from CPB and is shielded from the inflammatory response of blood cells to the bypass circuit. The collected blood—rich in valuable components (eg, platelets, coagulation factors)—is then infused back to the patient after separation from CPB and heparin reversal.

The amount of blood that an individual patient is capable of donating via ANH depends strictly on the patient's own physiologic parameters, estimated blood volume (based on height-weight nomograms), and hematocrit. Figure 14-1 is our nomogram for allowable ANH blood drainage—this conservatively estimates the volume of blood that can be removed to achieve a hematocrit of 24% or greater (based on a 1000 mL CPB prime volume).

ANH is relatively contraindicated in patients with preoperative anemia, unstable angina, and those with ejection fractions less than 30%.[37] Additionally, evidence supporting its use is conflicting: a few prospective studies showed a significant decrease in allogeneic blood product use,[39,40] others showed no benefit from ANH,[41,42] while a meta-analysis and review found only a modest benefit.[43] Contemporary guidelines state that ANH may be considered as part of a multipronged approach to blood conservation in selected (ie, nonanemic) patients, but note that its usefulness is not well-established.[26,44]

RETROGRADE AUTOLOGOUS PRIMING

Low hematocrits during CPB were shown to have detrimental effects on end-organ function and cognitive outcomes.[45-49] In retrograde autologous priming (RAP), the CPB circuit is primed with the patient's own whole blood, thereby minimizing circuit-induced hemodilution (which results from crystalloid priming) and ideally reducing the subsequent need for allogeneic transfusions. Specifically, blood from the aorta is allowed to flow retrogradely through the arterial arm of the bypass circuit, displacing portions of the crystalloid prime. Once the desired prime volume is displaced, a similar procedure can be applied to the venous line (so-called venous antegrade priming) to remove additional crystalloid from the circuit.

RAP was shown to reduce hemodilution and allogeneic transfusions (as compared to conventional CPB priming) in a large, retrospective study[50] as well as in a recent meta-analysis[51]; however, the latter showed that RAP had no effect on clinical outcomes like ventilator hours or length of stay.[51] RAP is currently endorsed by several societal guidelines as a method of reducing allogeneic blood transfusions during on-pump cardiac surgery.[26,44]

MINI-CIRCUITS AND VACUUM-ASSISTED VENOUS DRAINAGE

Advances in CPB circuit design have further reduced the impact of priming-induced hemodilution as well as the inflammatory responses initiated by blood-material interactions—these improvements may lessen the need for subsequent transfusions. Minimizing circuit length decreases the priming volume while also reducing the surface area of foreign material to which blood is exposed. This latter point serves to decrease the contact-dependent systemic inflammatory response, thereby reducing transcapillary leak; minimizing blood-material interactions via smaller circuits can also decrease the sheering of blood cells.[37]

Newer, so-called mini-circuits are fully closed CPB systems that also eliminate blood-air contact, as these circuits often do not use a venous reservoir; mini-circuits typically have priming volumes of less than 500 mL. Compared to conventional CPB, mini-circuits have been shown to more stably maintain hemoglobin concentrations intraoperatively, to reduce postoperative transfusion requirements, and even to improve mortality after CABG.[52-54] One potential downside

Preop hematocrit% in OR			IAD removal volume mL									
Weight kg	30%	32%	34%	36%	38%	40%	42%	44%	46%	48%	50%
40	338	361	384	406	429	451	474	496	519	541	564
45	418	446	474	502	530	558	585	613	641	669	697
50	498	531	564	598	631	664	697	730	764	797	830
55	578	616	655	693	732	770	809	847	886	924	963
60	658	701	745	789	833	877	921	964	1008	1052	1096
65	737	787	836	885	934	983	1032	1082	1131	1180	1229
70	817	872	926	981	1035	1090	1144	1199	1253	1308	1362
75	897	957	1017	1076	1136	1196	1256	1316	1375	1435	1495
80	977	1042	1107	1172	1237	1302	1368	1433	1498	1563	1628
85	1057	1127	1197	1268	1338	1409	1479	1550	1620	1691	1761
90	1136	1212	1288	1364	1439	1515	1591	1667	1742	1818	1894
95	1216	1297	1378	1459	1541	1622	1703	1784	1865	1946	2000
100	1296	1382	1469	1555	1642	1728	1814	1901	1987	2000	2000
105	1376	1468	1559	1651	1743	1834	1926	2000	2000	2000	2000
110	1456	1553	1650	1747	1844	1941	2000	2000	2000	2000	2000
115	1535	1638	1740	1842	1945	2000	2000	2000	2000	2000	2000
120	1615	1723	1831	1938	2000	2000	2000	2000	2000	2000	2000
125	1695	1808	1921	2000	2000	2000	2000	2000	2000	2000	2000
130	1775	1893	2000	2000	2000	2000	2000	2000	2000	2000	2000
135	1855	1978	2000	2000	2000	2000	2000	2000	2000	2000	2000
140	1934	2000	2000	2000	2000	2000	2000	2000	2000	2000	2000
145	2000	2000	2000	2000	2000	2000	2000	2000	2000	2000	2000
150	2000	2000	2000	2000	2000	2000	2000	2000	2000	2000	2000

Legend		Based on 70 mL/kg BV, RAP, 1000 mL dilution and 24% CPBhct
0 BAG	No IAD	
I BAG	500 mL	
2 BAGS	1000 mL	
3 BAGS	1500 mL	
4 BAGS	2000 mL	

FIGURE 14-1 Nomogram for allowable acute normovolemic hemodilution/intraoperative autologous donation.

to mini-circuits is that the introduction of air into the closed venous system risks creation of an air lock; additionally, the absence of a venous reservoir creates the potential for exsanguination after uncontrolled bleeding. Based on the results of nine randomized trials and a well-constructed meta-analysis, all of which suggested mini-circuits reduce postoperative bleeding and transfusions, the STS/STA guidelines now recommend the use of these systems for blood conservation.[26]

Many mini-circuits also incorporate vacuum-assisted venous drainage, as opposed to the gravity drainage used in conventional CPB systems. While mini-circuits using vacuum drainage may improve hemostasis and decrease blood requirements compared to regular circuits, there is some concern that the vacuum entrains air and that this can lead to increased systemic microemboli compared with gravity venous drainage. Therefore, current guidelines urge caution with respect to vacuum-assisted venous drainage but point out that this technology may provide some benefit, especially in pediatric patients.[26]

MODIFIED ULTRAFILTRATION

Another method of limiting CPB-induced hemodilution involves modified ultrafiltration (UF), wherein water and low-molecular-weight substances are filtered out of the blood

at the conclusion of a case; the resultant protein-rich concentrated whole blood is then returned to the patient. Specifically, this technique uses a special UF device added to a typical bypass system; using the existing CPB cannulae, free water as well as detrimental, pump-induced inflammatory mediators are removed from the patient's blood at the conclusion of a pump run but prior to the patient leaving the operating theater. Compared with other intraoperative UF procedures (eg, conventional UF, which runs simultaneously with CPB, or zero balance UF, in which the removed free water is replaced with a crystalloid solution), modified UF has well-established benefits in terms of mitigating hemodilution as well as reducing postoperative bleeding and blood product usage.[26] As such, the current STS/STA guidelines recommend the use of modified UF for blood conservation and for reducing postoperative blood loss in adult cardiac surgeries requiring CPB.[26]

AUTOTRANSFUSION OF CARDIOTOMY-SUCTIONED, CENTRIFUGED, OR RESIDUAL-CIRCUIT BLOOD

Salvaging extravascular blood (ie, shed blood from the operative field or residual blood in the bypass circuit) is another important element in blood conservation. Cell salvage systems have been shown to decrease the incidence of RBC transfusions in cardiac surgery[55] and may be especially useful in off-pump CABG, where cardiotomy suction is not available.[37]

Contemporary blood conservation guidelines therefore recommend intraoperative autotransfusions during CPB using blood directly from cardiotomy suction and/or recycled blood that has been centrifuged to concentrate red cells.[26,44] Additionally, consensus suggests that reinfusion of residual blood in the CPB circuit at the conclusion of a procedure is a reasonable part of a blood management program.[26]

Operative Techniques

Interest in minimally invasive techniques for cardiac surgery continues to grow. At their core, these advanced procedures are intended to lessen the extent of the surgical insult, which, in turn, can translate into reduced blood loss and the avoidance of transfusions. Operations performed without CPB, via transcatheter or endovascular approaches, or through minithoracotomies (MTs) are becoming increasingly prevalent in cardiac surgery and have been studied with respect to their ability to conserve blood.

OFF-PUMP CABG

A number of well-designed studies have shown that patients undergoing off-pump CABG have reduced transfusion requirements as compared to patients undergoing CABG on CPB,[56-58] have fewer reoperations for bleeding,[57] and are less coagulopathic postoperatively.[58] As is the case with mini-circuits, these benefits from off-pump surgery stem from the avoidance of CPB-induced hemodilution and inflammation. While the current STS/STA blood conservation guidelines recommend off-pump CABG as a reasonable means of blood conservation,[26] recent evidence suggesting that graft patency is reduced in off-pump CABG patients has tempered some of the earlier excitement surrounding this technique.[56,59]

OTHER MINIMALLY INVASIVE APPROACHES

Numerous other minimally invasive surgical procedures have emerged over the last decade. These techniques are still evolving and many have not been subjected to rigorous, prospective study. Nevertheless, promising lines of evidence are beginning to emerge showing that several of these new cardiac operations may have the potential to curb blood loss and to reduce transfusion risks. For example, thoracic endovascular aortic repair (TEVAR) is increasingly being used to repair various descending aortic lesions and has been demonstrated to reduce transfusions and reoperations for bleeding as compared to open aortic surgery.[60] The use of TEVAR in selected patients was therefore added as a recommendation in the most recent STS/STA blood conservation guidelines.[26] Transcatheter aortic valve replacement (TAVR) allows for the replacement of stenotic aortic valves in high-risk patients using a sternum-sparing, endovascular approach. Although

TAVR has been associated with higher rates of vascular complications, major bleeding events occurred less often with this technique as compared to surgical aortic valve replacement (AVR).[61] Accordingly, the incidence of transfusions following TAVR was also shown to be less than with surgical AVR.[62-64]

Bleeding can also be minimized by forgoing full sternotomy in favor of smaller thoracic incisions. For instance, both the aortic and mitral valves can be approached via a small right anterior thoracotomy (ie, MT). AVR performed through MT has been shown to reduce blood loss as compared to sternotomy-based AVR[65]; similarly, mitral valve replacement (MVR) via MT was demonstrated to reduce RBC transfusion volumes as compared to MVR performed via traditional sternotomy.[66] Although current International Society for Minimally Invasive Cardiothoracic Surgery (ISMICS) guidelines do not go so far as to recommend such MT approaches outright, they point out that the ability of MTs to reduce allogeneic blood exposures should be considered when balancing the risks and benefits of these newer procedures.[44]

Topical Hemostatic Agents

Surgical bleeding (ie, bleeding from suture lines or anastomoses) accounts for over half of all cases taken back to the operating room due to postoperative blood loss.[67] As a result, numerous topical hemostatic agents have been developed to reduce or prevent surgical bleeding when used as adjuncts to conventional suturing techniques. The limited efficacy of older topical agents such as oxidized cellulose and microfibrillar collagen has led to the introduction of newer products with novel applicator systems, some of which can directly activate the clotting cascade. We briefly describe some of the more commonly encountered of these products, although evidence-based comparisons between these agents are largely lacking. Table 14-2 comprehensively summarizes most of the currently available topical agents.

Fibrin sealants (Tisseel [Baxter Healthcare Corp., Deerfield, IL, USA], Beriplast [CSL Bering, King of Prussia, PA, USA], and Hemaseel [Haemacure Corp., Montreal, QB, Canada]) comprised of freeze-dried human fibrinogen, clotting proteins, fibronectin, and bovine thrombin or bovine aprotinin have been widely used in cardiac surgery; a systematic review on their use suggested that fibrin sealants are efficacious in decreasing the need for allogeneic transfusions.[68] However, these products are quite immunogenic and can lead to an unacceptably high incidence of anaphylaxis[69]; recent reports of myocardial injury secondary to acute coronary bypass graft thrombosis[70] and of mechanical aortic valve dysfunction[71] following the use of fibrin sealants have led some to further caution against using these agents in such procedures.

FloSeal (Baxter Healthcare Corp.) is a bovine-derived gelatin matrix cross-linked with a human-derived thrombin solution, which when applied, activates the clotting cascade and simultaneously forms a nondisplacing hemostatic plug. Unlike other fibrin sealants, FloSeal requires blood as a fibrinogen source; the product is biocompatible and reabsorbed in 6 to 8 weeks. Compared to a Gelfoam-thrombin control,

TABLE 14-2: Topical Hemostatic Agents Recommended by the Society of Thoracic Surgeons/Society of Cardiovascular Anesthesiologists Blood Conservation Clinical Practice Guidelines.[26]

Agent	Commercial name	Composition	Mechanism of action	Class of recommendation
Oxidized regenerated cellulose for wound compression	Surgicel, Oxycel	Oxidized cellulose	Accelerate clotting by platelet activation followed by swelling and wound compression. Some bacteriostatic properties.	Class IIb
Microfibrillar collagen	Avitene, Colgel, Helitene	Bovine collagen shredded into fibrils	Collagen activates platelets causing aggregation, clot formation, and wound sealing.	Class IIb
Combined compression and sealant topical agent	Recothrom or Thrombin JMI added to USP porcine Gelfoam, Costasis, FloSeal	Bovine fibrillar collagen or bovine gelatin combined with thrombin and mixed with autologous plasma	Activation of platelet-related clotting followed by swelling and wound compression. Recombinant thrombin has potential safety advantage. Combination of compression and sealant agents.	Class IIb
Fibrin sealants ("fibrin glue")	Tisseel, Beriplast, Hemaseel, Crosseal	Source of fibrinogen and thrombin mixed with antifibrinolytics combined at anastomotic sites	Fibrin matrix serves to seal the wound. Contains either aprotinin or tranexamic acid.	Class IIb
Synthetic cyanoacrylate polymers	Omnex	Polymers of 2 forms of cyanoacrylate monomers	Seals wounds without need for intact clotting mechanism.	Class IIb
Synthetic polymers of polyethylene glycol	CoSeal, DuraSeal	Polymers of polyethylene glycol cross link with local proteins	Polymers and proteins form matrix sealant.	Class IIb
Sealant mixture of bovine albumin and glutaraldehyde	BioGlue	Albumin and glutaraldehyde dispensed in 2-syringe system	Sealant created without need for intrinsic clotting system by denaturation of albumin. Safety concerns because of glutaraldehyde toxicity.	Class IIb
Large surface area polysaccharide hemospheres	Arista, HemoStase	Plant-based polysaccharides with a very large surface area	Rapidly dehydrate blood by concentrating serum proteins, platelets, and other blood elements on the surface of contact.	Class IIb
Chitin-based sealants	Celox, HemCon, Chitoseal	Naturally occurring polysaccharide polymer	Chitin forms clots in defibrinated or heparinized blood by a direct reaction with the cell membranes of erythrocytes. Probably induces local growth factors.	Class IIb
Antifibrinolytic agents in solution	Trasylol, tranexamic acid	Antifibrinolytic agents dissolved in saline	Limit wound-related generation of plasmin.	Class IIa

Reproduced with permission from Ferraris VA, Brown JR, et al: 2011 update to the Society of Thoracic Surgeons and the Society of Cardiovascular Anesthesiologists blood conservation clinical practice guidelines. Society of Thoracic Surgeons Blood Conservation Guideline Task Force, *Ann Thorac Surg*. 2011 Mar;91(3):944-982.

FloSeal proved more effective in stopping arterial suture line bleeding within 10 minutes in cardiac surgery patients, especially before protamine reversal.[72]

BioGlue (CryoLife Inc., Kennesaw, GA, USA) is a biologic glue approved initially for use in the repair of aortic dissections. This product consists of a glutaraldehyde solution and a separate bovine serum albumin solution that are mixed at the time of use via a dual-cartridge, single-nozzle dispenser.

The resultant flexible mechanical seal forms within 2 minutes, independent of the body's clotting mechanism. Both observational and randomized studies have demonstrated Bio-Glue significantly decreased anastomotic bleeding in cardiac, aortic, and peripheral vascular procedures as compared with a standard surgical control.[73,74]

Current STS/STA guidelines state that topical hemostatic agents may be considered to provide local hemostasis at anastomotic sites as part of a multimodal blood management program.[26] As those guidelines point out, despite the widespread use of such products in cardiac surgery, no single topical preparation has emerged as a clear frontrunner, highlighting the need for randomized controlled trials of these agents.[26]

Antifibrinolytic Agents

Antifibrinolytic prophylaxis has been well-studied in cardiac surgery and currently is centered around two drugs: the lysine analogs tranexamic acid (TA) and epsilon-aminocaproic acid (EACA). These agents bind to plasminogen and inhibit its binding to fibrin, thereby impairing fibrinolysis. A third antifibrinolytic drug, aprotinin, is a bovine-derived serine protease inhibitor of the fibrinolytic enzyme, plasmin. While aprotinin has long been confirmed to decrease bleeding rates and transfusion requirements as compared to placebo, aprotinin was removed from market in 2007 over concerns regarding renal toxicity[75,76] and because of higher mortality in aprotinin-treated patients in a randomized, prospective trial comparing that drug with TA and EACA.[77]

TRANEXAMIC ACID

Although TA and EACA share similar mechanisms of action, the significant difference between the two agents is that TA is roughly 10 times more potent than EACA. Several meta-analyses have highlighted the benefits of TA in decreasing postoperative transfusion requirements,[78,79] the most recent of which demonstrated significant decreases in RBC transfusions and in repeat surgery rates for bleeding when comparing TA use with controls.[80] No sufficiently powered, randomized controlled trial exists, however, comparing the effects of TA administration versus placebo on transfusion requirements. Of note, concerns over TA's safety profile (seizure risk, in particular) as well as debates on dosing strategies for this drug continue. Nevertheless, the use of TA is a class I recommendation in the current STS/SCA blood conservation guidelines for reducing total blood loss and for decreasing the number of patients who require blood transfusions during cardiac procedures.[26]

EPSILON-AMINOCAPROIC ACID

Introduced to cardiac surgery in 1962,[81] EACA remains the most commonly used antifibrinolytic agent in the United States. EACA has repeatedly been shown to result in decreased postoperative RBC blood loss and in transfusion rates similar to those observed for aprotinin (when compared to placebo).[82-85] Loading doses from 50 to 150 mg/kg followed by infusions from 25 to 30 mg/kg/h allow plasma EACA levels to be maintained at greater than 130 μg/mL, the minimum concentration needed to suppress plasmin activity.[25] Like TA, EACA is indicated for blood conservation by the contemporary STS/SCA guidelines.[26]

POSTOPERATIVE CONCERNS AND MANAGEMENT

Blood conservation does not stop at the conclusion of the cardiac surgery; rather, through the coordinated efforts of both the surgical and intensivist teams, various postoperative strategies—transfusion triggers, POC testing, the use of novel blood products, etc.—can be employed to minimize further bleeding and to avoid unnecessary hemodilution and RBC transfusions. Perhaps the most central issue in this postoperative blood conservation paradigm concerns the seemingly straightforward question of "when do we transfuse a patient?"

Transfusion Triggers

The literature indicates that the anesthetized patient on full CPB at moderate hypothermia can safely tolerate a hematocrit as low as 15%, with the exception of patients at risk for decreased cerebral oxygen delivery—namely, those with a history of stroke, diabetes, or cerebrovascular disease.[86] These latter patients can tolerate a hematocrit as low as 18% when using moderate hypothermia.[87] Once the patient is warm and being weaned from CPB, these percentage points are raised by 2% each (17% and 20%, respectively) because the relative protective effects of hypothermia are no longer present. In our institution, once the patient is off CPB, our practice is to reinfuse all (or as much as possible) remaining blood in the CPB circuit to the patient and then to give all available cell salvage blood, including any blood remaining in the CPB circuit that was not initially given back to the patient; next, any blood collected from ANH, and finally, PABD blood if available. Then and only then, if the hematocrit remains unsatisfactorily low, does the patient receive allogeneic blood. Of course, the issue becomes: what does "unsatisfactorily low" mean?

Unfortunately, data to support postoperative transfusion decisions in cardiac surgery are sparse. Since a given patient's unique clinical situation (eg, volume status, hemodynamics, surgical extent, ongoing bleeding, and mixed venous oxygen saturation) is likely the most important factor in weighing his or her need for transfusion, it would be impossible to assign a single transfusion trigger that can universally be applied to all patients. However, based upon the results of numerous case series, several nonrandomized observational studies, a handful of prospective randomized clinical trials, and expert opinions, consensus now exists that helps guide us in the transfusion decision-making process.[26,88]

It is widely accepted (and as outlined by the current STS/SCA guidelines) that RBC transfusions to improve oxygen transport when a hemoglobin level is greater than 10 g/dL are almost never of benefit, whereas most patients with hemoglobin levels less than 7 g/dL do indeed stand to benefit from transfusion.[26,88] Two studies in particular formed much the basis for this understanding: in 1999, a multicenter randomized trial of Transfusion Requirements in Critical Care (TRICC) enrolled 838 critically ill patients and randomized them to either a restrictive (transfuse if hemoglobin < 7 g/dL) or a liberal (transfuse if hemoglobin < 10 g/dL) transfusion strategy.[89] The 30-day mortality rates, though better in the restrictive strategy group, did not reach statistical significance; however, myocardial infarction and pulmonary edema occurred less frequently under the restrictive strategy.[89] A subgroup analysis, which looked at younger patients (age < 55) and patients who were less acutely ill (APACHE score < 20) showed significantly lower mortality rates with the restrictive strategy.[89] Patients with known, significant cardiac disease had comparable mortality rates regardless of the transfusion strategy used.[89]

A second, more recent randomized trial examined appropriate transfusion triggers in cardiac surgical procedures specifically: the Transfusion Requirements After Cardiac Surgery (TRACS) trial randomized 502 patients who had undergone cardiac surgical procedures with the use of CPB to restrictive (maintain hematocrit ≥ 24%) versus liberal (maintain hematocrit ≥ 30%) transfusion strategies.[19] The primary, composite end point of 30-day mortality and in-hospital major morbidity was comparable between both strategies.[19] In the restrictive strategy group, there was a 60% diminution in the number of transfused units.[19] Furthermore, RBC transfusions were again found to be an independent risk factor for mortality.[19]

The contemporary STS/SCA blood conservation guidelines therefore state RBC transfusion is reasonable when hemoglobin levels are below 6 g/dL, as they can be life-saving.[26] Moreover, transfusion is reasonable in most postoperative patients whose hemoglobin is less than 7 g/dL, even though little high level evidence supports this recommendation.[26]

Point-of-Care Testing

Traditional laboratory-based testing of blood (eg, complete blood counts, coagulation profiles) helps guide rational transfusion practices. Yet, some of these assays may be limited by processing times that are quite long relative to the acuity of many postsurgical cardiac patients. Hence, various POC tests have been developed that seek to optimize and expedite patient management. The proposed advantages of POC testing include (1) the targeting of transfusion therapies according to specific coagulation abnormalities, (2) the rapid identification of patients who could benefit from pharmacologic therapy to decrease bleeding, and (3) the identification of a surgical source for excessive bleeding in the setting of normal test results.[25]

The use of thromboelastography (TEG) or rotational thromboelastometry (ROTEM) to assess whole-blood coagulation, platelet function, and fibrinolytic activity has gained popularity in cardiac surgery (Fig.14-2).[90] However, as the recent ISMICS consensus statement points out, despite some evidence that TEG/thromboelastometry may reduce blood subcomponent transfusions, results have been largely heterogeneous and no benefits have been shown with respect to clinically relevant outcomes.[44] As such, evidence remains too premature to recommend POC technologies for routine use in blood conservation following cardiac surgery.

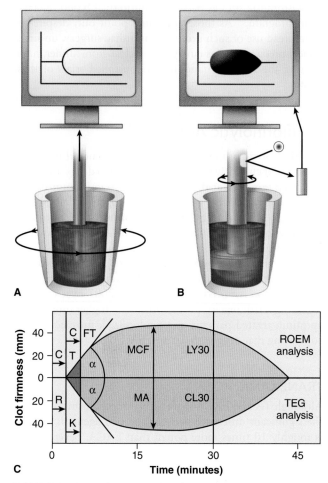

FIGURE 14-2 Working principles of thromboelastography and rotational thromboelastometry.[90] Thromboelastography (TEG) and rotational thromboelastometry (ROTEM) assess viscoelastic changes in clotting whole blood under low shear conditions after the addition of a specific coagulation activator to a sample of blood. The main end point of TEG and ROTEM is the determination of the blood's viscoelasticity, referred as amplitude (for TEG) and clot firmness (for ROTEM). Specifically, the viscoelastic (tensile) force between the blood-containing cup and the immersed pin results from the interaction between activated platelet glycoprotein IIb/IIIa receptors and polymerizing fibrin during endogenous thrombin generation and fibrin degradation by fibrinolysis. In TEG (A), the cup holding the blood sample is rotating, whereas the torsion wire is fixed. In ROTEM (B), the cup is fixed, whereas the pin is rotating. Changes in torque are detected electromechanically in TEG and optically in ROTEM. The computer-processed signal is then presented as a tracing. (C) Shows typical tracings from TEG (lower tracing) and ROTEM (upper tracing). The time course of viscoelastic changes is depicted as additional parameters that reflect the rate and stability of clot formation; the values of these parameters can then guide clinical decision-making. (Reproduced with permission from Bolliger D, Seeberger MD, Tanaka KA: Principles and practice of thromboelastography in clinical coagulation management and transfusion practice, *Transfus Med Rev.* 2012 Jan;26(1):1-13.)

Novel Blood Products

Two newer, novel blood products—recombinant activated factor VII (rFVIIa) and PCCs—have garnered considerable attention but their roles in cardiac surgery and blood conservation may not yet be widely understood by practicing surgeons. We therefore close this chapter with brief discussions of these two products.

RECOMBINANT ACTIVATED FACTOR VII

Endogenous activated factor VII plays a central role in coagulation; rFVIIa is nearly identical to the endogenous form of this factor and works by both tissue-factor-dependent and—independent mechanisms to generate thrombin.[91] The rFVIIa is approved by the Food and Drug Administration for the management of bleeding in patients with hemophilias A and B and in patients with congenital factor VII deficiency. The off-label use of rFVIIa in cardiac surgery has surged in recent years, where it is used to treat refractory intraoperative and/or postoperative hemorrhage.

However, the results of studies examining the use of this novel agent in cardiac surgery (mainly nonrandomized studies, case reports, and small case series) have been mixed. As such, a randomized controlled clinical trial was recently undertaken to assess the dose-escalating safety and efficacy of rFVIIa in postoperative cardiac surgical patients with refractory bleeding.[92] When used at either a low or high dose (40 or 80 μg/kg, respectively), rFVIIa was associated with significantly lower bleeding rates and allogeneic transfusions than was placebo.[92] The authors concluded that this therapy was effective for refractory bleeding but that the study was ultimately underpowered to speak to this blood product's safety profile.[92] A recent comprehensive review of 35 randomized clinical trials using rFVIIa for all off-label indications sought to address this question of safety and demonstrated a significantly higher incidence of arterial thrombotic events with rFVIIa versus placebo (5.5 vs 3.2%, respectively).[93]

Current blood conservation guidelines state that rFVIIa may be considered for the management of intractable nonsurgical bleeding that is otherwise unresponsive to conventional hemostatic therapies.[26,44] Yet, the routine, prophylactic use of rFVIIa in cardiac surgery cannot be endorsed for reasons of cost, due limited data on its efficacy, and because of concerns for increased risk of serious adverse events with this blood product.

PROTHROMBIN COMPLEX CONCENTRATES

PCCs are plasma-derived concentrates of vitamin K-dependent coagulation factors (II, VII, IX, X, and proteins C and S); several PCC products are currently available. PCCs are useful for the rapid reversal of oral anticoagulants; in a randomized trial of cardiac surgical patients, PCC reversed oral anticoagulation safely, more quickly, and with decreased bleeding compared to reversal with FFP.[94] PCCs are also beginning to be studied for the treatment of post-CPB coagulopathy and early results suggest that PCC use may decrease subsequent FFP and platelet transfusion requirements[95]—though these promising preliminary results have yet to be validated in larger, randomized controlled clinical trials.

KEY POINTS

- There is little evidence to support the routine, liberal use of blood transfusions in cardiac surgery.
- Comprehensive blood conservation programs are the most effective strategy in decreasing patients' exposures to allogeneic blood.
- Blood conservation should be approached in a multidisciplinary fashion using a team that includes members from surgery, anesthesiology, nursing, perfusion, blood banking, and quality improvement.
- Preoperative strategies for minimizing bleeding risks and transfusion requirements include: the identification of high-risk patients; appropriately stopping medications that contribute to coagulopathy; and increasing preoperative red cell mass with iron supplementation, erythropoietin, and/or PABD.
- The use of CPB techniques that reduce blood loss and protect against transfusions should be maximized—these include: ANH with the subsequent reinfusion of drained autologous blood, retrograde autologous priming, and the utilization of mini-circuits and modified UF.
- Antifibrinolytic drugs and topical hemostatic agents are important adjuncts to blood conservation.
- A patient's unique clinical situation, rather than rigid transfusion triggers, should guide postoperative blood utilization.
- The incorporation of new surgical techniques, novel agents and blood products, and evolving technologies into blood conservation programs must be based on evidence from well-designed clinical trials.

REFERENCES

1. Belisle S, Hardy JF: Hemorrhage and the use of blood products after adult cardiac operations: myths and realities. *Ann Thorac Surg* 1996; 62:1908.
2. Goodnough LT, Despostis GJ, Hohue CW, et al: On the need for improved transfusion indicators in cardiac surgery. *Ann Thorac Surg* 1995; 60:473.
3. Speiss BD: Transfusion and outcome in heart surgery. *Ann Thorac Surg* 2002; 74:986.
4. Woodman RC, Harker LA: Bleeding complications associated with cardiopulmonary bypass. *Blood* 1990; 76:1680.
5. Boyle EM, Verrier VD, Spiess BD: The procoagulant response to injury. *Ann Thorac Surg* 1997; 64:S16.
6. Hunt BJ, Parratt RN, Segal HC, et al: Activation of coagulation and fibrinolysis during cardiothoracic operations. *Ann Thorac Surg* 1998; 65:712.
7. Despotis G, Avidan M, Eby C: Prediction and management of bleeding in cardiac surgery. *J Thromb Haemost* 2009; 7(Suppl 1):111.
8. Gajic O, Rana R, Winters JL, et al: Transfusion-related acute lung injury in the critically ill: prospective nested case-control study. *Am J Respir Crit Care Med* 2007; 176:886.
9. Vlaar AP, Binnekade JM, Prins D, et al: Risk factors and outcome of transfusion-related acute lung injury in the critically ill: a nested case-control study. *Crit Care Med* 2010; 38:771.
10. Surgenor SD, Kramer RS, Olmstead EM, et al: The association of perioperative red blood cell transfusions and decreased long-term survival after cardiac surgery. *Anesth Analg* 2009; 108:1741.
11. Whitson BA, Huddleston SJ, Savik K, et al: Risk of adverse outcomes associated with blood transfusion after cardiac surgery depends on the amount of transfusion. *J Surg Res* 2010; 158:20.
12. Veenith T, Sharples L, Gerrard C, et al: Survival and length of stay following blood transfusion in octogenarians following cardiac surgery. *J Anesth* 2010; 65:331.

13. Koch CG, Li L, Duncan AI, et al: Transfusion in coronary artery bypass grafting is associated with reduced long-term survival. *Ann Thorac Surg* 2006; 81:1650.
14. Murphy GJ, Reeves BC, Rogers CA, et al: Increased mortality, postoperative morbidity, and cost after red blood cell transfusion in patients having cardiac surgery. *Circulation* 2007; 116:2544.
15. Scott BH, Seifert FC, Grimson R: Blood transfusion is associated with increased resource utilisation, morbidity and mortality in cardiac surgery. *Ann Card Anaesth* 2008; 11:15.
16. Koch CG, Li L, Duncan AI, et al: Morbidity and mortality risk associated with red blood cell and blood-component transfusion in isolated coronary artery bypass grafting. *Crit Care Med* 2006; 34:1608.
17. Hébert PC, Wells G, Blajchman MA, et al: A multicenter, randomized, controlled clinical trial of transfusion requirements in critical care. Transfusion Requirements in Critical Care Investigators, Canadian Critical Care Trials Group. *N Engl J Med* 1999; 340:409.
18. Lacroix J, Hébert PC, Hutchison JS, et al: Transfusion strategies for patients in pediatric intensive care units. *N Engl J Med* 2007; 356:1609.
19. Hajjar LA, Vincent JL, Galas FR, et al: Transfusion requirements after cardiac surgery: the TRACS randomized controlled trial. *JAMA* 2010; 304:1559.
20. Ovrum E, Holen EA, Linstein MA: Elective coronary artery bypass without allogeneic blood transfusion. *Scand J Thorac Cardiovasc Surg* 1991; 25:13.
21. Ovrum E, Holen EA, Abdelnoor M, et al: Conventional blood conservation techniques in 500 consecutive coronary artery bypass operations. *Ann Thorac Surg* 1991; 51:500.
22. Van der Linden P, De Hert S, Daper A, et al: A standardized multidisciplinary approach reduces the use of allogeneic blood products in patients undergoing cardiac surgery. *Can J Anaesth* 2001; 48:894.
23. Brevig J, McDonald J, Zelinka ES, et al: Blood transfusion reduction in cardiac surgery: multidisciplinary approach at a community hospital. *Ann Thorac Surg* 2009; 87:532.
24. Shehata N, Naglie G, Alghamdi AA, et al: Risk factors for red cell transfusion in adults undergoing coronary artery bypass surgery: a systematic review. *Vox Sang* 2007; 93:1.
25. Nalla BP, Freedman J, Hare GM, et al: Update on blood conservation for cardiac surgery. *J Cardiothorac Vasc Anesth* 2012; 26:117.
26. Society of Thoracic Surgeons Blood Conservation Guideline Task Force, Ferraris VA, Brown JR, et al: 2011 update to the Society of Thoracic Surgeons and the Society of Cardiovascular Anesthesiologists blood conservation clinical practice guidelines. *Ann Thorac Surg* 2011; 91:944.
27. Dunning J, Versteegh M, Fabbri A, et al: Guideline on antiplatelet and anticoagulation management in cardiac surgery. *Eur J Cardiothorac Surg* 2008; 34:73.
28. Sie P, Samama CM, Godier A, et al: Surgery and invasive procedures in patients on long-term treatment with direct oral anticoagulants: thrombin or factor-Xa inhibitors. Recommendations of the Working Group on Perioperative Haemostasis and the French Study Group on Thrombosis and Haemostasis. *Arch Cardiovasc Dis* 2011; 104:669.
29. Heidbuchel H, Verhamme P, Alings M, et al: EHRA practical guide on the use of new oral anticoagulants in patients with non-valvular atrial fibrillation: executive summary. *Eur Heart J* 2013; 34:2094.
30. Lai A, Davidson N, Galloway SW, et al: Perioperative management of patients on new oral anticoagulants. *Br J Surg* 2014; 101:742.
31. Junichiro Y, Path FRC, Yamada K, et al: Testing various herbs for antithrombotic effect. *Nutrition* 2005; 21:580.
32. Buckley MS, Goff AD, Knapp WE: Fish oil interaction with warfarin. *Ann Pharmacother* 2004; 38:50.
33. Valli G, Giardina E: Benefits, adverse effects and drug interactions of herbal therapies with cardiovascular effects. *J Am Coll Cardiol* 2002; 39:1083.
34. Kilic A, Whitman GJ: Blood transfusions in cardiac surgery: indications, risks, and conservation strategies. *Ann Thorac Surg* 2014; 97:726.
35. Alghamdi AA, Albanna MJ, Guru V, et al: Does the use of erythropoietin reduce the risk of exposure to allogeneic blood transfusion in cardiac surgery? A systematic review and meta-analysis. *J Cardiovasc Surg* 2006; 21:320.
36. Weltert L, D'Alessandro S, Nardella S, et al: Preoperative very short-term, high-dose erythropoietin administration diminishes blood transfusion rate in off-pump coronary artery bypass: a randomized blind controlled study. *J Thorac Cardiovasc Surg* 2010; 139:621.
37. Varghese R, Myers ML: Blood conservation in cardiac surgery: let's get restrictive. *Semin Thorac Cardiovasc Surg* 2010; 22:121.
38. Martin K, Keller E, Gertler R, et al: Efficiency and safety of preoperative autologous blood donation in cardiac surgery: a matched-pair analysis in 432 patients. *Eur J Cardiothorac Surg* 2010; 37:1396.
39. Kochamba GS, Pfeffer TA, Sintek CF, et al: Intraoperative autotransfusion reduces blood loss after cardiopulmonary bypass. *Ann Thorac Surg* 1996; 61:900.
40. Jalali A, Naseri MH, Chalian M, et al: Acute normovolaemic haemodilution with crystalloids in coronary artery bypass graft surgery: a preliminary survey of haemostatic markers. *Acta Cardiol* 2008; 63:335.
41. Höhn L, Schweizer A, Licker M, et al: Absence of beneficial effect of acute normovolemic hemodilution combined with aprotinin on allogeneic blood transfusion requirements in cardiac surgery. *Anesthesiology* 2002; 96:276.
42. Casati V, Speziali G, D'Alessandro C, et al: Intraoperative low-volume acute normovolemic hemodilution in adult open-heart surgery. *Anesthesiology* 2002; 97:367.
43. Segal JB, Blasco-Colmenares E, Norris EJ, et al: Preoperative acute normovolemic hemodilution: a meta-analysis. *Transfusion* 2004; 44:632.
44. Menkis AH, Martin J, Cheng DC, et al: Drug, devices, technologies, and techniques for blood management in minimally invasive and conventional cardiothoracic surgery: a consensus statement from the International Society for Minimally Invasive Cardiothoracic Surgery (ISMICS) 2011. *Innovations (Phila)* 2012; 7:229.
45. DeFoe GR, Ross CS, Olmstead EL, et al: Lowest hematocrit on bypass and adverse outcomes associated with coronary artery bypass surgery. *Ann Thorac Surg* 2001; 71:769.
46. Habib RH, Zacharias A, Schwann TA, et al: Adverse effects of low hematocrit during cardiopulmonary bypass in the adult: should current practice be changed? *J Thorac Cardiovasc Surg* 2003; 125:1438.
47. Swaminathan M, Philips-Bute BG, Conlon PJ, et al: The association of lowest hematocrit during cardiopulmonary bypass with acute renal injury after coronary artery bypass surgery. *Ann Thorac Surg* 2003; 76:784.
48. Karkouti K, Beattie WS, Wijeysundera DN, et al: Hemodilution during cardiopulmonary bypass is an independent risk factor for acute renal failure in adult cardiac surgery. *J Thorac Cardiovasc Surg* 2005; 129:391.
49. Loor G, Li L, Sabik JF III, et al: Nadir hematocrit during cardiopulmonary bypass: end-organ dysfunction and mortality. *J Thorac Cardiovasc Surg* 2012; 144:654.
50. Vandewiele K, Bové T, De Somer FM, et al: The effect of retrograde autologous priming volume on haemodilution and transfusion requirements during cardiac surgery. *Interact Cardiovasc Thorac Surg* 2013; 16:778.
51. Sun P, Ji B, Sun Y, et al: Effects of retrograde autologous priming on blood transfusion and clinical outcomes in adults: a meta-analysis. *Perfusion* 2013; 28:238.
52. Remadi JP, Marticho P, Butoi I, et al: Clinical experience with the mini-extracorporeal circulation system: an evolution or a revolution? *Ann Thorac Surg* 2004; 77:2172.
53. Kofidis T, Baraki H, Singh H, et al: The minimized extracorporeal circulation system causes less inflammation and organ damage. *Perfusion* 2008; 23:147.
54. Puehler T, Haneya A, Philipp A, et al: Minimized extracorporeal circulation system in coronary artery bypass surgery: a 10-year single-center experience with 2243 patients. *Eur J Cardiothorac Surg* 2011; 39:459.
55. Vermeijden WJ, van Klarenbosch J, Gu YJ, et al: Effects of cell-saving devices and filters on transfusion in cardiac surgery: a multicenter randomized study. *Ann Thorac Surg* 2015; 99:26.
56. Shroyer AL, Grover FL, Hattler B, et al: On-pump versus off-pump coronary-artery bypass surgery. *N Engl J Med* 2009; 361:1827.
57. Brewer R, Theurer PF, Cogan CM, et al: Morbidity but not mortality is decreased after off-pump coronary artery bypass surgery. *Ann Thorac Surg* 2014; 97:831.
58. Puskas JD, Williams WH, Duke PG, et al: Off-pump coronary artery bypass grafting provides complete revascularization with reduced myocardial injury, transfusion requirements, and length of stay: a prospective randomized comparison of two hundred unselected patients undergoing off-pump versus conventional coronary artery bypass grafting. *J Thorac Cardiovasc Surg* 2003; 125:797.
59. Parolari A, Alamanni F, Polvani G, et al. Meta-analysis of randomized trials comparing off-pump with on-pump coronary artery bypass graft patency. *Ann Thorac Surg* 2005; 80:2121.
60. Cheng D, Martin J, Shennib H, et al: Endovascular aortic repair versus open surgical repair for descending thoracic aortic disease: a systematic review and meta-analysis of comparative studies. *J Am Coll Cardiol* 2010; 55:986.

61. Smith CR, Leon MB, Mack MJ, et al: Transcatheter versus surgical aortic-valve replacement in high-risk patients. *N Engl J Med* 2011; 364:2187.

62. D'Errigo P, Barbanti M, Ranucci M, et al: Transcatheter aortic valve implantation versus surgical aortic valve replacement for severe aortic stenosis: results from an intermediate risk propensity-matched population of the Italian OBSERVANT study. *Int J Cardiol* 2013; 167:1945.

63. Papadopoulos N, Schiller N, Fichtlscherer S, et al: Propensity matched analysis of longterm outcomes following transcatheter based aortic valve implantation versus classic aortic valve replacement in patients with previous cardiac surgery. *J Cardiothorac Surg* 2014; 9:99.

64. Nagaraja V, Raval J, Eslick GD, et al: Transcatheter versus surgical aortic valve replacement: a systematic review and meta-analysis of randomised and non-randomised trials. *Open Heart* 2014; 1:e000013.

65. Brown ML, McKellar SH, Sundt TM, et al: Ministernotomy versus conventional sternotomy for aortic valve replacement: a systematic review and meta-analysis. *J Thorac Cardiovasc Surg* 2009; 137:670.

66. Cheng DC, Martin J, Lal A, et al: Minimally invasive versus conventional open mitral valve surgery: a meta-analysis and systematic review. *Innovations (Phila)* 2011; 6:84.

67. Hall TS, Sines JC, Spotnitz AJ: Hemorrhage related reexploration following open heart surgery: the impact of pre-operative and post-operative coagulation testing. *Cardiovasc Surg* 2002; 10:146.

68. Carless PA, Anthony DM, Henry DA: Systematic review of the use of fibrin sealant to minimize perioperative allogeneic blood transfusion. *Br J Surg* 2002; 89:695.

69. Schlag G, Seifert J: Fibrin sealant, aprotinin, and immune response in children undergoing operations for congenital heart disease. *J Thorac Cardiovasc Surg* 1998; 116:1082.

70. Lamm P, Adelhard K, Juchem G, et al: Fibrin glue in coronary artery bypass grafting operations: casting out the Devil with Beelzebub? *Eur J Cardiothorac Surg* 2007; 32:567.

71. Birmingham B: TEE diagnosis of mechanical AVR dysfunction associated with biological glue. *Anesth Analg* 2001; 93:1627.

72. Oz MC, Cosgrove DM III, Badduke BR, et al: Controlled clinical trial of a novel hemostatic agent in cardiac surgery. The Fusion Matrix Study Group. *Ann Thorac Surg* 2000; 69:1376.

73. Passage J, Jalali H, Tam RK, et al: BioGlue Surgical Adhesive—An appraisal of its indications in cardiac surgery. *Ann Thorac Surg* 2002; 74:432.

74. Coselli JS, Bavaria JE, Fehrenbacher J, et al: Prospective randomized study of a protein-based tissue adhesive used as a hemostatic and structural adjunct in cardiac and vascular anastomotic repair procedures. *J Am Coll Surg* 2003; 197:243.

75. Karkouti K, Beattie WS, Dattilo KM, et al: A propensity score case-control comparison of aprotinin and tranexamic acid in high-transfusion-risk cardiac surgery. *Transfusion* 2006; 46:327.

76. Mangano DT, Tudor IC, Dietzel C, et al: The risk associated with aprotinin in cardiac surgery. *N Engl J Med* 2006; 354:353.

77. Fergusson DA, Hébert PC, Mazer CD, et al: A comparison of aprotinin and lysine analogues in high-risk cardiac surgery. *N Engl J Med* 2008; 358:2319.

78. Laupacis A, Fergusson D: Drugs to minimize perioperative blood loss in cardiac surgery: meta-analyses using perioperative blood transfusion as the outcome. The International Study of Peri-operative Transfusion (ISPOT) Investigators. *Anesth Analg* 1997; 85:1258.

79. Levi M, Cromheecke ME, de Jonge E, et al: Pharmacological strategies to decrease excessive blood loss in cardiac surgery: a meta-analysis of clinically relevant endpoints. *Lancet* 1999; 354:1940.

80. Ngaage DL, Bland JM: Lessons from aprotinin: is the routine use and inconsistent dosing of tranexamic acid prudent? Meta-analysis of randomised and large matched observational studies. *Eur J Cardiothorac Surg* 2010; 37:1375.

81. Gans H, Krivit W: Problems in hemostasis during open heart surgery. III. Epsilon amino caproic acid as an inhibitor of plasminogen activator activity. *Ann Surg* 1962; 155:268.

82. Munoz JJ, Birkmeyer NJ, Birkmeyer JD, et al: Is epsilon-aminocaproic acid as effective as aprotinin in reducing bleeding with cardiac surgery? A meta-analysis. *Circulation* 1999; 99:81.

83. Chauhan S, Gharde P, Bisoi A, et al: A comparison of aminocaproic acid and tranexamic acid in adult cardiac surgery. *Ann Card Anaesth* 2004; 7:40.

84. Carless PA, Moxey AJ, Stokes BJ, et al: Are antifibrinolytic drugs equivalent in reducing blood loss and transfusion in cardiac surgery? A meta-analysis of randomized head-to-head trials. *BMC Cardiovasc Disord* 2005; 5:19.

85. Brown JR, Birkmeyer NJ, O'Connor GT: Meta-analysis comparing the effectiveness and adverse outcomes of antifibrinolytic agents in cardiac surgery. *Circulation* 2007; 115:2801.

86. Fang WC, Helm RE, Krieger KH, et al: Impact of minimum hematocrit during cardiopulmonary bypass on mortality in patients undergoing coronary artery surgery. *Circulation* 1997; 96:II194.

87. Beall AC Jr, Yow EM Jr, Bloodwell RD, et al: Open-heart surgery without blood transfusion. *Arch Surg* 1967; 94:567.

88. Society of Thoracic Surgeons Blood Conservation Guideline Task Force, Ferraris VA, Ferraris SP, et al: Perioperative blood transfusion and blood conservation in cardiac surgery: the Society of Thoracic Surgeons and The Society of Cardiovascular Anesthesiologists clinical practice guideline. *Ann Thorac Surg* 2007; 83(5 Suppl):S27.

89. Hebert PC, Wells G, Blajchman MA, et al: A multicenter, randomized, controlled clinical trial of transfusion requirements in critical care. Transfusion Requirements in Critical Care Investigators, Canadian Critical Care Trials Group. *N Engl J Med* 1999; 340:409.

90. Bolliger D, Seeberger MD, Tanaka KA: Principles and practice of thromboelastography in clinical coagulation management and transfusion practice. *Transfus Med Rev* 2012; 26:1.

91. Lisman T, De Groot PG: Mechanism of action of recombinant factor VIIa. *J Thromb Haemost* 2003; 1:1138.

92. Gill R, Herbertson M, Vuylsteke A, et al: Safety and efficacy of recombinant activated factor VII: a randomized placebo-controlled trial in the setting of bleeding after cardiac surgery. *Circulation* 2009; 120:21.

93. Levi M, Levy JH, Andersen HF, et al: Safety of recombinant activated factor VII in randomized clinical trials. *N Engl J Med* 2010; 363:1791.

94. Demeyere R, Gillardin S, Arnout J, et al: Comparison of fresh frozen plasma and prothrombin complex concentrate for the reversal of oral anticoagulants in patients undergoing cardiopulmonary bypass surgery: a randomized study. *Vox Sang* 2010; 99:251.

95. Song HK, Tibayan FA, Kahl EA, et al: Safety and efficacy of prothrombin complex concentrates for the treatment of coagulopathy after cardiac surgery. *J Thorac Cardiovasc Surg* 2014; 147:1036.

96. Bennett-Guerrero E, Zhao Y, O'Brien SM, et al: Variation in use of blood transfusion in coronary artery bypass graft surgery. *JAMA* 2010; 304:1568.

97. Likosky DS, FitzGerald DC, Groom RC, et al: Effect of the perioperative blood transfusion and blood conservation in cardiac surgery clinical practice guidelines of the Society of Thoracic Surgeons and the Society of Cardiovascular Anesthesiologists upon clinical practices. *Anesth Analg* 2010; 111:316.

Deep Hypothermic Circulatory Arrest

Bradley G. Leshnower • Edward P. Chen

15

Surgical therapy for aortic arch disease involves partial or complete replacement of the arch with great vessel reimplantation during a period of time when native cerebral blood flow is temporarily interrupted. In its original description, this interval of suspended cerebral perfusion required the cessation of blood flow to the entire body and was labeled hypothermic circulatory arrest (HCA). HCA employs the use of systemic hypothermia to protect the brain and visceral organs during the ischemic period, and provides a bloodless operative field to facilitate arch reconstruction. Since the initial report of the use of HCA for aortic arch replacement, cerebral protection, and circulation management techniques have evolved to enable safe, reproducible arch reconstruction with excellent neurologic outcomes.[1]

HCA traces its beginnings to the work of Bigelow who demonstrated a role for hypothermia in cardiac surgery in a canine model.[2] John Lewis used systemic hypothermia at 28°C combined with venous inflow occlusion to perform the first successful atrial septal defect repair. He subsequently described the use of profound systemic hypothermia (9°C) with one hour of circulatory arrest without any evidence of central nervous system injury to treat an adult with ovarian carcinoma.[3,4] Systemic hypothermia was temporarily abandoned with the arrival of the cardiopulmonary bypass machine, but was rediscovered and used in isolated reports of arch replacement in the 1960s.[5,6] However, it was the translational research of Dr. Randall Griepp, who applied lessons learned from his canine laboratory models to successfully repair aortic arch aneurysms using HCA, that ushered in the modern era of aortic arch surgery.[1]

BASIC PRINCIPLES

For the purposes of clarity throughout this chapter, the use of HCA without adjunctive cerebral perfusion will be termed as "HCA alone". The classification system in Table 15-1 will be used to describe varying degrees of hypothermia used for HCA Table 15-1. Deep hypothermic circulatory arrest (DHCA) and moderate hypothermic circulatory arrest (MHCA) are the two levels of HCA that will be primarily focused upon throughout the subsequent text.

Cerebral Metabolism and Blood Flow

Comprehension of HCA mandates a fundamental understanding of cerebral metabolism and blood flow. The metabolic rate and energy requirements of the brain are approximately 7.5 times the metabolism of non-nervous system tissues. The brain depends upon the aerobic process of glycolysis for energy and is estimated to have only a 2-minute supply of glucose stored as glycogen in neurons at any time. The brain is intolerant of ischemia and in that setting quickly resorts to anaerobic metabolism for energy production. Once adenosine triphosphate (ATP) stores are depleted, basic cellular ionic pumps fail and calcium accumulates in the intracellular space. This leads to irreversible neuronal injury.[7]

In order to support the high cerebral metabolic rate, the body provides approximately 60 mg of glucose and 3.5 mL of oxygen per 100 mg of brain tissue per minute. This translates to a cerebral blood flow of 750 to 900 mL/min or 15% of resting cardiac output under normothermic conditions.[7] The autoregulatory capacity of the cerebral microcirculation ensures constant flow rates in normotensive individuals within a mean arterial blood pressure range of 60 to 140 mm Hg. This level of perfusion maintains a ratio of cerebral blood flow to metabolism of 20:1. However, several physiologic variables including temperature, pH, and hematocrit can modulate cerebral blood flow.[8]

Since oxygen is vital to brain metabolism, measurement of the cerebral metabolic rate for oxygen ($CMRO_2$) provides important comparative information regarding the metabolic state of the brain. Hypothermia has been shown to exponentially reduce cerebral metabolism. Systemic hypothermia at 20°C reduces the $CMRO_2$ to 76% of its baseline, and deeper hypothermia to 15°C reduces $CMRO_2$ to 84% of baseline values (Table 15-2).[9] In contrast to the $CMRO_2$, hypothermia reduces cerebral blood flow in a linear fashion. As the core body temperature decreases to 22°C, the cerebral microcirculation loses its ability to autoregulate and cerebral blood flow becomes dependent upon mean arterial pressure.[10] Loss of autoregulation translates into an uncoupling of cerebral blood flow and metabolism. This produces excess or "luxury" perfusion of the brain, and the ratio of cerebral blood flow to

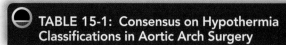

TABLE 15-1: Consensus on Hypothermia Classifications in Aortic Arch Surgery

Category	Nasopharyngeal temperature
Profound hypothermia	≤14°C
Deep hypothermia	14.1-20°C
Moderate hypothermia	20.1-28°C
Mild hypothermia	28.1-34°C

Reproduced with permission from Yan TD, Bannon PG, Bavaria J, et al: Consensus on hypothermia in aortic arch surgery, *Ann Cardiothorac Surg.* 2013 Mar;2(2):163-168.

metabolism increases to a ratio of 75:1. The significance of luxury perfusion is unclear. Potential beneficial effects of luxury perfusion include a quicker, more homogenous cooling of the brain; however, potential detrimental effects include the development of brain edema and exposure to an increased embolic load.[8]

The most clinically accessible method of assessing cerebral metabolism is the measurement of cerebral electrical activity, which can be monitored by electroencephalography (EEG). Systemic cooling diminishes cerebral electrical activity and electrocerebral or EEG silence indicates maximal cerebral metabolic suppression. Many aortic centers use complete EEG silence during the cooling period as a reliable and safe measure of adequate cerebral suppression, indicating that it is safe to initiate HCA.

pH Management

As stated previously, cerebral blood flow is impacted by temperature and the acid-base status of the blood. Two different strategies are used during HCA to manage pH. Alpha-stat pH management maintains normal acidemia and blood gases in 37°C (normothermic) blood. This optimizes cellular enzyme activity and preserves cerebral autoregulation. In

TABLE 15-2: Measurement of the Cerebral Metabolic Rate for Oxygen (CMRO$_2$) Provides Important Comparative Information Regarding the Metabolic State of the Brain

Temperature (°C)	Cerebral metabolic rate (% of base line)	Safe duration of HCA (min)
37	100	5
30	56 (52-60)	9 (8-10)
25	37 (33-42)	14 (12-15)
20	24 (21-29)	21 (17-24)
15	16 (13-20)	31 (25-38)
10	11 (8-4)	45 (36-62)

Reproduced with permission from McCullough JN, Zhang N, Reich DL, et al: Cerebral metabolic suppression during hypothermic circulatory arrest in humans, *Ann Thorac Surg.* 1999 Jun;67(6):1895-1899.

alpha-stat management, the pH is allowed to change as the blood temperature decreases, and the blood becomes more alkaline and hypocapneic. Such conditions cause a shift of the oxyhemoglobin dissociation curve to the left, which increases the affinity of hemoglobin for oxygen. The net effect is that in deep hypothermia, oxygen bound to hemoglobin is less available to be released to the tissues, and the fraction of oxygen dissolved in blood represents the major source of oxygen to the tissues.

The alternative strategy is pH-stat management, which maintains a normal pH at hypothermia by adding CO$_2$ to the blood during cooling. Supplementary CO$_2$ causes cerebral vasodilatation and eliminates the autoregulatory capacity of the cerebral microvasculature. This results in an increase in cerebral blood flow and an uncoupling of cerebral blood flow from cerebral metabolism. Due to the supplementary CO$_2$, at deep hypothermia, the oxyhemoglobin dissociation curve is shifted to the right, which decreases the affinity of hemoglobin to oxygen and increases the delivery of oxygen to the tissues. Under pH-stat management, the blood becomes acidotic and hypercapneic when the blood temperature is rewarmed to 37°C.

Studies comparing the two strategies have been conducted in both large animals and humans. The majority of human studies contain small numbers of patients who underwent either adult cardiac or congenital heart procedures that did not utilize circulatory arrest. The adult studies are composed of patients undergoing coronary artery bypass grafting under moderate-to-mild levels of hypothermia (26-32°C). Conclusions from the adult studies indicate superior outcomes with alpha-stat management. The animal and pediatric studies contain data conducted under deep hypothermia with either low flow cardiopulmonary bypass or circulatory arrest. Outcomes in these studies were superior with pH-stat management.[11]

The mechanisms of intraoperative brain injury differ between adults and children. Adults are prone to suffer embolic injury secondary to risk factors for vasculopathy (eg, hypertension, atherosclerosis, diabetes mellitus). Children undergoing repair of complex congenital heart disease are more susceptible to global ischemic injury from prolonged periods of low flow or circulatory arrest. Therefore, alpha-stat management may be more optimal in adults, where the preservation of cerebral autoregulation enables the microvasculature to adjust to areas of stenoses and any disproportionate distribution of flow. Conversely, children may benefit from the global cerebral vasodilatation associated with pH-stat management to augment blood flow during prolonged low flow states.[11-13]

Pathogenesis of Brain Injury During HCA

It is well recognized that there are two different types of brain injury observed in patients treated with HCA: (1) permanent neurologic dysfunction (PND) and (2) temporary neurologic dysfunction (TND). PND, commonly referred to as stroke, manifests clinically as a focal neurologic deficit secondary to an embolism of particulate matter or air/gas bubbles causing vascular occlusion resulting in an ischemic cerebral infarct. Risk factors for PND in patients undergoing HCA include atheromatous disease involving both the ascending aortic and the site of arterial cannulation for cardiopulmonary bypass.[14-16] The axillary artery has been shown to provide the lowest risk of stroke in patients undergoing HCA operations.[16] Other neuroprotective strategies to reduce the risk of embolic stroke include the use of epiaortic ultrasound to guide the site of arterial cannulation and aortic cross clamping, and the addition of antegrade or retrograde cerebral perfusion (RCP).

TND is a reversible, diffuse subtle injury which is attributed to inadequate cerebral protection.[17] Patients with TND can experience confusion, agitation, delirium, prolonged obtundation, orparkinsonism without localizing signs in the immediate postoperative period. Brain imaging in this clinical setting with computed tomography or magnetic resonance imaging is negative. TND is the clinical manifestation of a global cerebral ischemic injury that results in necrotic and/or apoptotic neuronal cell death.

Necrotic cell death following HCA occurs due to a failure to meet minimum cerebral cellular metabolic and oxygen requirements. In this instance, cellular stores of ATP are exhausted and the cell converts to anaerobic metabolism. The lack of ATP also causes a failure of the Na^+/K^+ pump which has a multitude of consequences including cellular swelling, depolarization of the cell membrane, opening of voltage sensitive Ca^{2+} channels and a massive influx of calcium into the cytoplasm. Accumulation of intracellular calcium activates proteases and lipases that disrupt the cellular membrane and results in cell lysis and death. Histologically, cellular necrosis is characterized by pyknotic nuclei, swollen eosinophilic cytoplasm, and the presence of an inflammatory reaction. Risk factors for neuronal cell necrosis following HCA include inadequate levels of hypothermia, the presence of electrocerebral activity at the time of circulatory arrest, and prolonged duration (>40 minutes) of HCA without cerebral perfusion.[18-20]

The second type of cell death observed in patients after HCA with inadequate cerebral protection is apoptosis. Apototic cell death is an energy-dependent process that occurs despite adequate stores of cellular energy. It represents a sublethal ischemic injury that results in the activation of specific genes, receptors and enzymes that break down the cell in a programmed manner.[21] Morphologically it is characterized by nuclear karyorrhexis, and margination of chromatin in the nucleus with minimal cytoplasmic or inflammatory changes. Apoptosis is a highly sophisticated and complex process that has not yet been fully characterized, and a detailed description is beyond the scope of this chapter. Fundamentally, it is a carefully regulated process that leads to the generation of caspases which initiate a proteolytic cascade in which one caspase activates other caspases and leads to rapid cell death.[22] Multiple animal models of DHCA have demonstrated apoptotic cell death beginning within hours of reperfusion and continuing as long as 72 hours after DHCA.[23,24]

Ischemia and hypoxia can initiate cell death through a third mechanism related to excessive neuronal stimulation and hyperactivity. Once the brain converts to anaerobic metabolism, lactate is produced. The inability of the neuronal cells to utilize lactate as an energy source, combined with the lack of blood flow during HCA, results in the accumulation of lactate and a drop in intracellular pH. The development of intracellular acidosis has a multitude of effects including the release of the potent excitatory neurotransmitters glutamate and aspartate, and failure of the neurotransport pumps. This results in the accumulation of glutamate in the intercellular space. Glutamate in increasing concentrations becomes neurotoxic and mediates the opening of calcium channels. The end result is an influx of calcium into the cytoplasm, which initiates a lethal biochemical cascade resulting in neuronal cell death. Excitotoxicity is the term applied to this type of neuronal cell death induced by excitatory amino acids. Excitotoxicity plays an important role in both necrotic and apoptotic ischemic neuronal cell death.[18] Metabolic rates differ throughout the different regions of the brain, and foci with high metabolic rates are more sensitive to ischemia. This concept has been termed "selective vulnerability" and, applies to neurons in the hippocampus, basal ganglia and cerebellum.[25,26] Patients with TND due to inadequate cerebral protection following HCA can often display poor cognition, altered short-term memory, and fine motor deficits. Neuropsychological tests in patients undergoing HCA have demonstrated memory and fine motor deficits consistent with subtle brain injury in patients following periods of DHCA > 25 minutes.[27] This type of subtle brain injury is likely due to necrotic or apoptotic neuronal cell death in the hippocampus, basal ganglia, and cerebellum. The impact of TND is not clinically insignificant and correlates with long-term memory and motor deficits following prolonged periods of DHCA.[28]

DEEP HYPOTHERMIC CIRCULATORY ARREST

Cooling

After the initiation of cardiopulmonary bypass, systemic hypothermia is achieved by cooling the blood passing through a heat exchanger connected to the perfusion circuit. A temperature gradient (arterial inflow to venous return) that does not exceed 10°C is maintained during the cooling period to prevent the formation of gaseous emboli. The duration of the cooling period required to equilibrate blood and tissue temperatures is highly variable and is dependent upon blood flow, temperature gradient (between perfusate and organs), and tissue-specific coefficients of temperature exchange. Patient-specific variables that impact cooling include occlusive vascular disease and body mass index.

There is no consensus regarding cooling strategies for HCA. Intraoperative monitoring of time, temperature, jugular venous bulb oxygen saturation, and electroencephalographic activity can assist in the evaluation of cerebral metabolic suppression during the cooling period. Temperature is monitored in many different sites including the inflow and outflow lines of the perfusion circuit, and by probes inserted into the bladder, rectum, nasopharynx, and esophagus. If the cerebral protection strategy is HCA alone or in conjunction with RCP, then the cooling strategy should be based upon esophageal or nasopharyngeal temperatures, as these sites have been shown to closely approximate brain temperature.[29] However, if antegrade cerebral perfusion is used, bladder or rectal temperatures are more important, as visceral organ protection becomes the primary goal of hypothermia.

Generally accepted parameters that ensure sufficient cerebral metabolic suppression include cooling for a minimum of 30 minutes, a goal nasopharyngeal temperature of 18°C, a jugular venous saturation > 95%, and electrocerebral silence.[30-32] However, relying on such parameters alone as a measure of adequate metabolic suppression may not be completely adequate. In a study of 109 patients undergoing HCA, >50% of patients had not achieved electrocerebral silence at a nasopharyngeal temperature of 18°C, and approximately 25% of patients have not achieved electrocerebral silence after 30 minutes of cooling.[33] This emphasizes the need to thoroughly evaluate all available monitoring parameters prior to initiating HCA. If HCA alone is employed, topical cooling by packing the head in ice is advocated in order to minimize upward drift of intracranial temperatures during the ischemic period.[31]

Rewarming

Cerebral reperfusion and rewarming following the period of HCA is a critical phase that can exacerbate neuronal injury if not conducted properly. Following HCA, reinitiating brain reperfusion with a short period of low-pressure cold blood flow prior to rewarming is recommended. In contrast to immediate rewarming, cold reperfusion has been associated with improved cerebral perfusion, a reduction in intracranial pressure, and a decrease in cerebral edema. This strategy attenuates the adverse effects of the impaired cerebral vascular autoregulation that occurs following DHCA, and results in a reduction in brain injury.[34,35] Experimental data have also suggested that reperfusion should also be carried out with a higher hematocrit and normoglycemia. A lower hematocrit in the reperfusate (≈20%) has been shown to increase the degree of histopathologic brain injury compared to a higher (30%) hematocrit.[36] In addition to an increased oxygen carrying capacity, a higher hematocrit is thought to be beneficial due to an increase in the buffer, redox and free-radical scavenging capacity. Hyperglycemia during reperfusion has been correlated with worsening intracellular acidosis, which prevents the return of normal cellular metabolism.[37]

Oxygen delivery to the brain is particularly important during the reperfusion period as there is a mismatch between cerebral metabolism and blood flow. Cerebral vascular resistance is increased for up to 8 hours following the period of HCA. This results in a reduction in cerebral blood flow and an abnormally high extraction rate of oxygen and glucose from the blood in order to sustain cerebral metabolism.[38] It is during this period that secondary brain injury can occur with episodes of hypotension, hypoxemia, and anemia.[31] A gradient < 10°C must be maintained to prevent the formation of gas emboli, and the temperature of the perfusate should not exceed 36°C. Cerebral hyperthermia results in worse neurobehavioral outcomes and increased neuronal cell injury compared to mild hypothermia following DHCA.[39] The mechanisms behind this injury are poorly understood; however, it is likely multi-factorial and related to increases in the permeability of the blood-brain barrier and cellular metabolism in the setting of hyperthermia. The risk of this delayed neurologic injury is significant, and many high volume aortic centers advocate a period of permissive hypothermia in the intensive care unit following DHCA in an attempt to reduce this risk.[18,40]

Safe Duration of DHCA

"DHCA alone" or DHCA without adjunctive cerebral perfusion represents the simplest, most convenient form of cerebral protection. It does not require complex perfusion strategies or neuromonitoring, and is the cerebral protection strategy of choice for surgeons who infrequently perform aortic arch reconstructions. The main concern surrounding the use of DHCA alone is the duration of the circulatory arrest period.

In an attempt to provide data regarding the safe interval of circulatory arrest at different temperatures, the Mount Sinai group measured arterial and venous blood gases at various time and temperature points in 37 adults undergoing HCA. This led to the calculation of the $CMRO_2$ consumption at various temperatures. Using $CMRO_2$, the Q_{10} (a well-described physiologic variable describing the temperature-dependent decrease in cerebral metabolism), and the assumption that cerebral blood flow can be safely interrupted for 5 minutes at 37°C, a calculated safe duration of HCA was determined for a range of temperatures. Figure 15-1 demonstrates the relationship between $CMRO_2$, temperature, and the calculated safe duration of HCA.[9,18]

Although most high volume aortic centers have added adjunctive cerebral perfusion to HCA as their standard strategy of cerebral protection, some centers such as Dr. Elefteriades' group at Yale still maintain the use of DHCA alone. In a contemporary series of 394 patients undergoing elective and emergent proximal and distal thoracic aortic repairs involving arch pathology, these authors cooled to a mean bladder temperature of 19°C without the use of neuromonitoring prior to initiating HCA. This correlated to a cooling period of 30 to 35 minutes. Their overall mortality and stroke rates were 6.3% and 4.8%. The incidence of seizure and dialysis were 3.1% and 2.3%, respectively. The mean DHCA time was 31 minutes, and there was a trend toward an increased stroke risk in patients with a DHCA time exceeding 40 minutes.[30] In a series of 656 patients undergoing DHCA alone

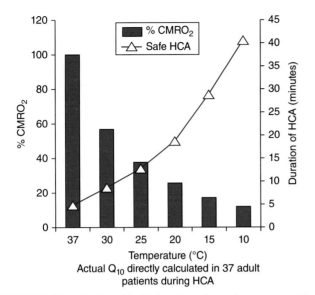

FIGURE 15-1 Limits of 'safe' duration of circulatory arrest. Q_{10} for the adult brain calculated from direct measurement of cerebral metabolic rate for oxygen ($CMRO_2$) in 37 adult patients undergoing thoracic aortic operations with DHCA. The temperature-related reduction in the metabolic rate and the calculated 'safe' periods of arrest are shown. (Data from McCullough JN, Zhang N, Reich DL, et al: Cerebral metabolic suppression during hypothermic circulatory arrest in humans, *Ann Thorac Surg.* 1999 Jun;67(6):1895-1899.)

from Dr. Crawford's Houston group, circulatory arrest times > 40 minutes were also associated with an increased risk of stroke.[41]

Based upon these data above, when using DHCA alone for the repair of aortic pathology involving the arch, cooling for 30 minutes to achieve a bladder temperature of 18°C or an esophageal/nasopharyngeal temperature of 15°C will safely provide cerebral protection for 30 minutes of circulatory arrest. When the circulatory arrest period extends beyond this duration, adjunctive cerebral perfusion should be employed.

Cerebral Perfusion

Although DCHA revolutionized aortic arch surgery, the incidence of brain injury following prolonged periods of DHCA alone was not insignificant. It was quickly recognized that complex aortic arch reconstructions requiring circulatory arrest times > 30 minutes were associated with increased rates of adverse neurologic outcomes and mortality.[30,41,42] The introduction of adjunctive cerebral perfusion as an additional method of cerebral protection had a transformative effect on the field and produced dramatic improvements in neurologic outcomes following arch reconstruction.

RETROGRADE CEREBRAL PERFUSION

RCP was first described by Mills and Ochnerin the treatment of a massive air embolus during cardiopulmonary bypass.[43] In 1990, Ueda was the first to report the use of RCP

as an adjunct to profound HCA in a series of eight patients undergoing aortic arch replacement.[44] RCP is performed by cannulating and snaring the superior vena cava, and infusing hypothermicarterial blood from the cardiopulmonary bypass circuit up the superior vena cava to perfuse the brain in a retrograde direction during the period of circulatory arrest (Fig. 15-2). Generally accepted flow rates are 300 to 500 mL/min to maintain a SVC pressure of 20 to 25 mm Hg. If performed properly, RCP will produce dark blood (suggesting cerebral oxygen extraction) flowing retrograde from the origins of the great vessels into the open aortic arch during HCA. The theoretical cerebral protection benefits of RCP are to (1) flush embolic material (gaseous and particulate) from the cerebral circulation; (2) maintain cerebral hypothermia by bathing the brain in cold blood; and (3) support cerebral metabolism by providing sufficient cerebral flow during the period of HCA.

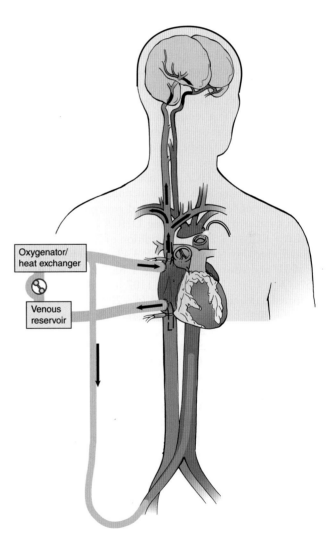

FIGURE 15-2 Schematic of retrograde cerebral perfusion (RCP). Arterial blood is perfused via the superior vena cava, with a target CVP of 25 mm Hg. Flow can be monitored through the open aortic arch. Balloon occlusion catheter can be employed to increase perfusion to body.

The proposed benefits of RCP have been extensively investigated using experimental models of HCA. RCP has been shown to significantly reduce intracranial temperatures in porcine and canine models of HCA. The maintenance of cooler temperatures resulted in a reduction of neurologic injury based upon histolopathology examinations.[45,46] RCP has also been shown to be highly effective in washing out particulate emboli from the brain using microspheres in a porcine model.[47] However, despite a large number of experiments in various animal models, the data are inconclusive regarding the capacity of RCP to provide significant cerebral blood flow. Shunting of blood away from brain capillaries occurs during profound hypothermic RCP via large venoarterial connections.[46,48-51] Cerebral blood flow can be improved with higher retrograde perfusion pressures and occlusion of the inferior vena cava; however, there is an increase in cerebral edema with histologic evidence of cerebral injury.[52] Based upon human cadaver studies, the majority of internal jugular veins have competent venous valves. In these experiments, significant retrograde cerebral blood flow was observed in <30% of cadavers, and the azygous rather than the internal jugular vein, represented the predominant pathway of flow.[53,54] Despite the unconvincing results of the cerebral blood flow data, RCP has been shown to improve metabolic support during HCA, with improved oxygen delivery, increased levels of cerebral ATP, a reduction in lactate production, and improved brain tissue oxygenation.[46,55,56]

Although human studies have also failed to conclusively demonstrate significant cerebral capillary blood flow, the addition of RCP to HCA has markedly improved clinical outcomes following arch reconstruction.[57,58] In a series of 479 patients undergoing elective and emergent arch repair, Coselli compared outcomes using DHCA (n = 189) versus DHCA + RCP (n = 290). The addition of RCP significantly reduced mortality (DHCA + RCP 3.4% vs DHCA 14.8%, $p < .001$) and stroke rates (DHCA + RCP 2.4% vs DCHA 6.5%, $p < .05$).[59] In a series of 1107 arch repairs, Estrera compared outcomes using DHCA (n = 200) versus DHCA + RCP (n = 900). For the entire series, the mortality and stroke rates were 10.4% and 2.8%, respectively. In both univariate and multivariate analyses, the addition of RCP was protective against mortality ($p < .001$) and stroke ($p = .02$). However, the incidence of TND was 15.5% with relatively short mean RCP times of 26 minutes.[60] Although this is lower than the 25% incidence of TND associated with arch reconstruction using DHCA alone,[28] it still represents a significant incidence of inadequate cerebral protection. Other groups have also reported an incidence of TND ranging from 17 to 25% with the use of DHCA + RCP.[61-63]

SELECTIVE ANTEGRADE CEREBRAL PERFUSION

DeBakey and Cooley were the first to successfully describe the use of selective antegrade cerebral perfusion (SACP) in the surgical repair of an arch aneurysm in 1957.[64] In their initial report, cannulas were placed into the right femoral and bilateral carotid arteries, and a separate pump from the main cardiopulmonary bypass machine was used to perfuse normothermic blood into the carotid arteries during the period of HCA. Despite its initial success, this method was considered complex and cumbersome, and was subsequently abandoned. SACP was later revisited in the late 1980s due to the recognition of the limitations of DHCA alone. In 1991, Bachet published a series of 54 patients undergoing open arch reconstruction in which SACP was combined with HCA for cerebral protection. The technique consisted of bilateral carotid artery cannulation and infusion of blood at temperatures of 6 to 12°C ("cold cerebroplegia") at a rate of 250 to 350 mL/min during a mean period of 22 minutes of HCA conducted at a rectal temperature of 25 to 28°C. Hospital mortality was 13% and the incidence of stroke was 1.8%.[65] One year later, Kazui reported the results of 23 arch reconstructions performed with systemic hypothermia, SACP, and lower body perfusion alone via the femoral artery. The mortality rate was 8.7% and there were no strokes. The mean SACP perfusion time was 90 minutes.[66] These two initial series provided the foundation for the use of SACP as the predominant form of cerebral protection for extended aortic arch reconstructions in the modern era.

In contrast to RCP, experimental data have confirmed the ability of SACP to provide adequate cerebral blood flow to support brain metabolism during the period of HCA. Transcranial Doppler measurements of middle cerebral artery blood flow in patients undergoing arch reconstruction have clearly demonstrated the superiority of SACP compared to RCP in providing reliable cerebral perfusion.[67] In a porcine model of HCA, Filgueiras and colleagues demonstrated the maintenance of near normal cerebral metabolism with DHCA + SACP, based upon measurements of pH and levels of cerebral metabolites. Animals undergoing DHCA + RCP or DHCA alone demonstrated a significant drop in cerebral pH during the protocol.[68] In a separate study using the same model, these same investigators demonstrated preserved cell structure upon histopathologic analysis with DHCA + SACP compared to DHCA + RCP.[69] Hagl and colleagues showed in an acute porcine model that a strategy of DHCA + SACP compared to DHCA alone is associated with improved neurophysiologic recovery, lower intracranial pressure, less cerebral edema, and reduced tissue acidosis following the circulatory arrest period.[70]

It should be recognized that the utilization of SACP changes the paradigm of circulatory arrest. Circulatory arrest, as originally described, refers to the complete interruption of the circulation and the absence of perfusion to all organs. The addition of SACP changes this concept from total body circulatory arrest to lower body circulatory arrest, as the brain, arms, and the spinal cord (via collateral circulation) are perfused. Therefore the legs and the abdominal visceral are the sole ischemic organs during the circulatory arrest period with the use of SACP.

Numerous techniques have been described for the delivery of SACP. Bilateral SACP (bSACP) involves direct cannulation of the cervical left and right common carotid arteries or the introduction of perfusion cannulas into the ostia of the

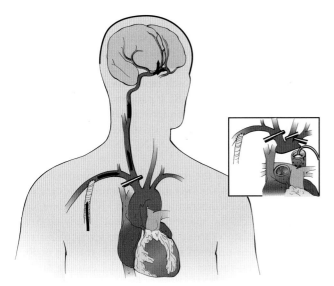

FIGURE 15-3 Schematic of right axillary artery cannulation for antegrade cerebral perfusion (ACP). Insert shows open aortic arch and ACP with occlusion of arch vessels to ensure perfusion of Circle of Willis.

innominate and left carotid arteries via the open arch at the time of HCA. The disadvantages of this latter method include the risk of introducing air or atherosclerotic emboli and cluttering the operative field with additional cannulas. At Emory, the preferred method of cerebral perfusion is unilateral SACP (uSACP) via right axillary artery cannulation. An 8-mm graft is sewn end to side to the right axillary artery prior to sternotomy and used as the arterial inflow line to initiate cardiopulmonary bypass. At the time of HCA, blood flow is decreased to 10 mL/kg/min and the base of the innominate and left common carotid arteries are occluded with vascular clamps (Fig. 15-3). Left carotid occlusion is performed to pressurize the extra cranial circulation and collateral system and minimize steal. This enables blood to flow via the right common carotid and right vertebral arteries to perfuse the brain and spinal cord. Flows are adjusted to maintain cerebral perfusion pressures of 50 to 60 mm Hg.[71] Critics of this technique argue that uSACP provides insufficient cerebral blood flow to the left cerebral hemisphere. However, both animal and clinical data have demonstrated that there is no significant difference in cerebral blood flow between uSACP and bSACP, with and without an intact circle of Willis.[72-74] Furthermore, data from a large, contemporary, propensity-matched analysis of 1097 patients undergoing arch replacement with HCA and SACP demonstrated no difference in morbidity and mortality between uSACP and bSACP. Interestingly, there was a trend toward a higher incidence of stroke in the bSACP group that was attributed to great vessel manipulation.[77]

MODERATE HYPOTHERMIA

The implementation of SACP as an adjunct to hypothermia for cerebral protection has led to a departure from the use of deep hypothermia, to the use of moderate levels of hypothermia

at the time of lower body ischemia. The rationale behind this strategy is based upon the concept that SACP has transformed total body circulatory arrest into lower body circulatory arrest. Since cerebral perfusion is maintained with cold blood throughout the period of circulatory arrest, the primary purpose of systemic hypothermia is to provide protection to the visceral organs, skeletal muscle, and spinal cord via metabolic suppression. The metabolic rate of the visceral organs and skeletal muscle is significantly less than the brain; therefore, the visceral organs require a reduced degree of hypothermia for optimal protection and are more tolerant of ischemia. As stated in the preceding sections, colder temperatures clearly correlate with a greater reduction in metabolism. However, the induction of deep hypothermia is not a benign process. It requires prolonged cardiopulmonary bypass times for cooling and rewarming which can have detrimental effects on the lungs, liver, and kidneys. Deep hypothermia has been associated with vascular endothelial dysfunction, bleeding complications, and an increased systemic inflammatory response.[75-78]

The impact of MHCA has been examined in several retrospective studies. Minatoya and colleagues evaluated the outcomes of 229 patients who received arch reconstruction with HCA + bSACP at three different temperatures: 20°C (n = 81), 25°C (n = 81), and 28°C (n = 67). Eighty-one percent of all patients received total arch replacement. There were no significant differences between the three groups with regard to the incidence of mortality, PND, or TND.[79] These authors published a subsequent review of 1007 patients undergoing elective and emergent arch reconstruction (73% total arch) comparing DHCA (<25°C)/bSACP versus MHCA (>25°C)/bSACP. Their overall mortality was 4.7% with PND and TND rates of 3.5% and 6.7%, respectively, with no differences observed between the two strategies.[80] Pacini and colleagues examined the impact of moderate hypothermia on visceral organ protection in 334 patients undergoing elective arch reconstruction with a strategy of either DHCA (<25°C)/bSACP or MHCA (>25°C)/bSACP. Overall in-hospital mortality was 4.6% and the incidence of PND and TND were 5.9% and 7.9%, respectively. The incidence of dialysis-dependent renal failure was 6.9% and there were no cases of liver failure. There was no difference in mortality, PND, TND, dialysis-dependent renal failure, or liver dysfunction between the two strategies. In a multivariate analysis of their results, cardiopulmonary bypass time > 180 minutes and deep hypothermia were predictive risk factors for renal and/or liver dysfunction.[81]

MHCA/SACP currently represents the preferred circulation management strategy for many high-volume aortic centers worldwide. At Emory, MHCA with uSACP is the standard cerebral protection method for elective and emergent hemiarch and total arch replacements. Hemiarch replacement is routinely conducted at temperatures of 28 to 29°C with mortality rates in elective and emergent cases of 4.3% and 7.7%, respectively. There is a low incidence of PND (elective 1.9%, emergent 4.6%), TND (elective 3.8%, emergent 6.2%), and dialysis-dependent renal failure (elective 2.4%, emergent 9.2%) with this technique. Mean circulatory arrest times are 23 minutes in elective cases and 33 minutes in emergent cases.[82] Total arch replacement is conducted at temperatures of 25 to 26°C for both emergent and elective cases. A recent review of 145 consecutive patients undergoing total arch replacement at Emory demonstrated an operative mortality of 9.7%. The incidence of PND, TND, and dialysis-dependent renal failure were 2.8%, 5.6%, and 2.8%, respectively. The mean duration of circulatory arrest for these patients was 55 minutes.[83] Other high volume aortic centers have reported similar outcomes confirming MHCA/SACP as a safe and effective strategy for circulation management in aortic arch surgery.[81,84-86]

COMPARISONS OF CEREBRAL PROTECTION STRATEGIES

Currently there is no consensus amongst aortic surgeons regarding the optimal method of cerebral protection during arch reconstruction. Instead, high-volume aortic centers employ a variety of different techniques using varying degrees of hypothermia with or without adjunctive cerebral perfusion. Often the method of cerebral protection is based upon the institutional bias rather than outcome data. Contemporary cerebral protection strategies are composed of multiple variables:arterial cannulation site, temperature at HCA, antegrade versus RCP, and unilateral versus bSACP. The majority of comparisons of cerebral protection strategies in the literature are essentially retrospective reviews of changes in circulation management strategies at a single institution over time. These comparisons are valuable, but limited by their retrospective nature, lack of randomization, and differences in several important variables including the extent of arch reconstruction, the temperature at HCA, antegrade versus RCP, and the percentage of emergent cases. Nevertheless, several lessons may be learned from a review of the existing literature.

Hagl reviewed the neurologic outcomes from the Mount Sinai experience of 717 patients undergoing arch replacement with different methods of cerebral protection: (1) DHCA (n = 588); (2) DHCA/RCP (n = 43); and (3) DHCA/SACP (n = 86). All patients were cooled to esophageal temperatures of 10 to 13°C. The overall incidence of PND and TND were 5.7% and 30%. In the 156 patients with HCA times > 40 minutes, there was no difference in the incidence of PND; however; DHCA/SACP significantly reduced the incidence of TND compared to the other strategies.[87] A recent retrospective review of the Japanese Adult Cardiovascular Surgery Database analyzed the outcomes of 8169 patients undergoing elective total arch replacement using either DHCA/RCP (n = 1141) or MHCA/SACP (n = 7038). The RCP group underwent HCA at 21.2°C compared to the SACP group who underwent HCA at 24.2°C. The duration of HCA was not reported in this study. In unmatched and propensity-matched analyses, there were no differences between the groups in mortality, PND, TND, or dialysis. However, it was clear that in this contemporary study, SACP was the preferred modality of cerebral perfusion amongst Japanese surgeons

for total arch replacements that required prolonged periods of HCA.[88] There is a single prospective trial comparing the impact of SACP versus RCP in the literature. Okita compared DHCA/RCP versus DHCA/SACP in 60 consecutive patients undergoing total arch replacement with a variety of different cannulation sites. RCP patients underwent HCA at 17.2°C and SACP patients underwent HCA at 22.1°C. There was no difference in mortality or stroke, but SACP significantly reduced the incidence of TND (SACP 13.3% vs RCP 33.3%, $p = .05$).[89]

The remainder of the retrospective comparisons between SACP and RCP in the literature are limited by significant differences in the temperature at which HCA is conducted. In these studies, the majority of patients receiving SACP undergo circulatory arrest at moderate levels of systemic hypothermia, as opposed to DHCA with the use of RCP. Three recurring themes emerge from the existing analyses in the literature: (1) an adjunct form of cerebral protection (SACP or RCP) is superior to DHCA alone and (2) the method of cerebral perfusion (SACP or RCP) has no impact upon the incidence of PND, however, (3) SACP significantly reduces the incidence of TND. Furthermore, most experts agree that in patients undergoing extended/complex arch reconstructions requiring prolonged periods of HCA, SACP is superior to RCP in preventing TND and is associated with improved overall neurologic outcomes.[40,90-92] The thoracic aortic surgical community recognizes the need for a prospective randomized multi-institutional trial comparing cerebral protection strategies; however, the logistics remain complicated.

Pharmacologic Adjuncts

Pharmacologic adjuncts that have been utilized to optimize cerebral protection during HCA include corticosteroids, barbiturates, and mannitol. Cardiopulmonary bypass and DHCA have been associated with a significant systemic inflammatory response, increased permeability of the blood-brain barrier and cerebral edema. Corticosteroids are a potent anti-inflammatory agent that have been shown to suppress the inflammatory response associated with DHCA. Experimental data have demonstrated that pretreatment with corticosteroids prior to cardiopulmonary bypass reduces the permeability of the blood-brain barrier, attenuates cerebral apoptosis and improves cerebral blood flow following DHCA.[93,94] At Emory our typical protocol includes the administration of 1 g of methylprednisolone following induction of anesthesia and a rapid taper of steroids over the first 72 hours of the postoperative period.

Barbiturates have been shown to reduce cerebral oxygen consumption, produce an isoelectric electroencephalogram, and minimize cerebral edema. Thiopental, the most commonly used barbiturate, is employed in several high-volume aortic centers for cerebral protection in cases requiring DHCA. The timing and dose of thiopental administration can impact its effectiveness. If administered prior to HCA, the cerebral energy state is reduced which may lead to adverse outcomes; however, its effects are considered to be advantageous when thiopental is administered during HCA. Furthermore, there is also a dose-dependent effect of barbiturates. Although low-dose barbiturates minimize cerebral metabolism, higher doses are associated with negative inotropy and sedation which could prolong the time to extubation. A recent analysis of the currently existing data did not conclusively demonstrate a cerebral protection advantage with the use of barbiturates in patients undergoing DHCA.[95,96]

Mannitol is a potent osmotic diuretic that is an established agent for reducing cerebral edema. It also possesses free oxygen radical scavenger properties and may have an anti-apoptotic effect following cerebral ischemia.[96] The impact of these three pharmacologic agents upon postoperative mortality and adverse neurologic outcomes was recently evaluated in an analysis of the German Registry for Acute Aortic Dissection Type A. Based upon univariate and multivariate analyses, steroids were the only agent that provided additional cerebral protection by reducing the risk of new postoperative PND. Both mannitol and barbiturates were associated with a significant reduction in 30-day mortality based upon the univariate analysis, but only mannitol lowered mortality in the multivariate analysis. Neither agent conferred additional neuroprotection.[96] In summary, the use of steroids and mannitol is advantageous following DHCA, while the use of thiopental cannot be recommended based upon the available data.

REFERENCES

1. Griepp RB, Stinson EB, Hollingsworth JF, Buehler D: Prosthetic replacement of the aortic arch. *J Thorac Cardiovasc Surg* 1975; 70(6):1051-1063.
2. Bigelow WG, Lindsay WK, Greenwood WF: Hypothermia; its possible role in cardiac surgery: an investigation of factors governing survival in dogs at low body temperatures. *Ann Surg* Nov 1950; 132(5):849-866.
3. Lewis FJ, Taufic M: Closure of atrial septal defects with the aid of hypothermia: experimental accomplishments and the report of one successful case. *Surgery* 1953; 33:52.
4. Niazi SA, Lewis FJ: Profound hypothermia in man: report of a case. *Ann Surg* 1958; 147(2):264-266.
5. Borst HG, Schaudig A, Rudolph W: Arteriovenous fistula of the aortic arch repair during deep hypothermia and circulatory arrest. *J Thorac Cardiovasc Surg* 1964; 3:443.
6. Lillehei CW, Todd DB, Levy MJ, et al: Partial cardiopulmonary bypass, hypothermia and total circulatory arrest: a lifesaving technique for ruptured mycotic aneurysms, ruptured left ventricle and other complicated aortic pathology. *J Thorac Cardiovasc Surg* 1969; 58:530.
7. Guyton AC and Hall JE: Cerebral blood flow, cerebrospinal fluid and brain metabolism, in Guyton AC and Hall JE (eds): *Textbook of Medical Physiology*, 11th ed. Philadelphia, PA, Elsevier Saunders, 2006; pp 761-768.
8. Harrington DK, Fragomeni F, Bonser RS: Cerebral perfusion. *Ann Thorac Surg* 2007; 83:S799-804.
9. McCullough JN, Zhang N, Reich DL, et al: Cerebral metabolic suppression during hypothermic circulatory arrest in humans. *Ann Thorac Surg* 1999; 67:1895-1921.
10. Greeley WJ, Kern FH, Ungerleider RM, et al: The effect of hypothermic cardiopulmonary bypass and total circulatory arrest on cerebral metabolism in neonates, infants, and children. *J Thorac Cardiovasc Surg* 1991; 101(5):783-794.
11. Abdul Aziz KA and Meduoye A: Is pH-stat or alpha-stat the best technique to follow in patients undergoing deep hypothermic circulatory arrest? *Interact Cardiovasc Thorac Surg* 2010; 10(2):271-282.
12. Priestley MA, Golden JA, O'Hara IB, McCann J, Kurth CD: Comparison of neurologic outcome after deep hypothermic circulatory arrest with alpha-stat and pH-stat cardiopulmonary bypass in newborn pigs. *J Thorac Cardiovasc Surg* 2001; 121(2):336-343.
13. Hickey PR: Neurologic sequelae associated with deep hypothermic circulatory arrest. *J Thorac Cardiovasc Surg* 1998; 65(6):S65-69.
14. Goldstein LJ, Davies RR, Rizzo JA, et al: Stroke in surgery of the thoracic aorta: incidence, impact, etiology and prevention. *J Thorac Cardiovasc Surg* 2001; 122(5):935-945.
15. Okada T, Shimamoto M, Yamazaki F, et al: Insights of stroke in aortic arch surgery: identification of significant risk factors and surgical implication. *Gen Thorac Cardiovasc Surg* 2012; 60(5):268-274.
16. Svensson LG, Blackstone EH, Rajeswaran J, et al: Does the arterial cannulation site for circulatory arrest influence stroke risk? *Ann Thorac Surg* 2004; 78:1274-1284.
17. Ergin MA, Griepp EB, Lansman SL, et al: Hypothermic circulatory arrest and other methods of cerebral protection during operations on the thoracic aorta. *J Card Surg* 1994; 9:525-537.
18. Ergin MA: Hypothermic circulatory arrest, in, Coselli JS and LeMaire SA (eds): *Aortic Arch Surgery Principles, Strategies and Outcomes,* 1st ed. Oxford, UK, Wiley Blackwell, 2008; pp 135-152.
19. Amir G, Ramamoorthy C, Riemer RK, Reddy VM, Hanley FL: Neonatal brain protection and deep hypothermic circulatory arrest: pathophysiology of ischemic neuronal injury and protective strategies. *Ann Thorac Surg* 2005; 80(5):1955-1964.
20. Lipton P: Ischemic cell death in brain neurons. *Physiol Rev* 1999; 79:1431-1568.
21. Thompson CB: Apoptosis in the pathogenesis and treatment of disease. *Science* 1995; 267(5203):1456-1462.
22. Elmore S: Apoptosis: a review of programmed cell death. *Toxicol Pathol* 2007; 35(4):495-516.
23. Tseng EE, Brock MV, Lange MS, et al: Glutamate excitotoxicity mediates neuronal apoptosis after hypothermic circulatory arrest. *Ann Thorac Surg* 2010; 89(2):440-445.
24. Ditsworth D, Priestley MA, Loepke AW, et al: Apoptotic neuronal cell death following deep hypothermic circulatory arrest in piglets. *Anesthesiology* 2003; 98:1119-1127.
25. Kurth CD, Priestley M, Golden J, McCann J, Raghupathi R: Regional patterns of neuronal death after deep hypothermic circulatory arrest in newborn pigs. *J Thorac Cardiovasc Surg* 1999; 118(6):1068-1077.
26. Fessatidis IT, Thomas VL, Shore DF, et al: Brain damage after profoundly hypothermic circulatory arrest: correlations between neurophysiologic and neuropathologic findings. An experimental study in vertebrates. *J Thorac Cardiovasc Surg* 1993; 106(1):32-41.
27. Reich DL, Uysal S, Silwinski M, et al: Neuropsychologic outcome after deep hypothermic circulatory arrest in adults. *J Thorac Cardiovasc Surg* 1999; 117(1):156-163.
28. Ergin MA, Uysal S, Reich DL, et al: Temporary neurological dysfunction after deep hypothermic circulatory arrest: a clinical marker of functional deficit. *Ann Thorac Surg* 1999; 67(6):1887-1890.
29. Stone GJ, Young WL, Smith CR, et al: Do standard monitoring sites reflect true brain temperature when profound hypothermia is rapidly induced and reversed? *Anesthesiology* 1995; 82:344-351.
30. Gega A, Rizzo JA, Johnson MH, et al: Straight deep hypothermic arrest: experience in 394 patients supports its effectiveness as a sole means of brain preservation. *Ann Thorac Surg* 2007; 84:759-767.
31. Greipp RB: Cerebral protection during aortic arch surgery. *J Thorac Cardiovasc Surg* 2001; 121:425-427.
32. Yan TD, Bannon PG, Bavaria JE, et al: Consensus on hypothermia in aortic arch surgery. *Ann Cardiothorac Surg* 2013; 2(2):163-168.
33. Stecker MM, Cheung, AT, Pochettino A, et al: Deep hypothermic circulatory arrest: I. Effects of cooling on electroencephalogram and evoked potentials. *Ann Thorac Surg* 2001; 71:14-21.
34. Ehrlich MP, McCullough J, Wolfe D, et al: Cerebral effects of cold reperfusion after hypothermic circulatory arrest. *J Thorac Cardiovasc Surg* 2001; 121:923-931.
35. Jonassen AE, Quaegebeur JM, Young WL: Cerebral blood flow velocity in pediatric patients is reduced after cardiopulmonary bypass with profound hypothermia. *J Thorac Cardiovasc Surg* 1995; 110:1686-1691.
36. Sakamoto T, Zurakowski D, Duebener LF, et al: Interaction of temperature with hematocrit level and pH determines safe duration of hypothermic circulatory arrest. *J Thorac Cardiovasc Surg* 2004; 128(2):220-232.

37. Anderson RV, Siegman MG, Balaban RS, Ceckler TL, Swain JA: Hyperglycemia increases cerebral intracellular acidosis during circulatory arrest. *Ann Thorac Surg* 1992; 54(6):1126-1130.

38. Mezrow CK, Gandsas A, Sadeghi AM, et al: Metabolic correlates of neurologic and behavioral injury after prolonged hypothermic circulatory arrest. *J Thorac Cardiovasc Surg* 1995; 109(5):959-975.

39. Shum-Tim D, Nagashima M, Shinoka T, et al: Postischemic hyperthermia exacerbates neurologic injury after deep hypothermic circulatory arrest. *J Thorac Cardiovasc Surg* 1998; 116:780-792.

40. Griepp RB, Bonser R, Haverich A, et al: Panel discussion: Session II-aortic arch from the aortic surgery symposium X. *Ann Thorac Surg* 2007; 83:S824-S831.

41. Svensson LG, Crawford ES, Hess KR, et al: Deep hypothermia with circulatory arrest. Determinants of stroke and early mortality in 656 patients. *J Thorac Cardiovasc Surg* 1993; 106:19-31.

42. Ehrlich MP, Ergin MA, McCullough JN, et al: Predictors of adverse outcome and transient neurologic dysfunction after ascending aorta/hemiarch replacement. *Ann Thorac Surg* 2000; 69:1755-1763.

43. Mills NL, Ochsner JL: Massive air embolism during cardiopulmonary bypass: causes, preventions, and management. *J Thorac Cardiovasc Surg* 1980; 80:708.

44. Ueda Y, Miki S, Kusuhara K, et al: Surgical treatment of aneurysm or dissection involving the ascending aorta and aortic arch, utilizing circulatory arrest and retrograde cerebral perfusion. *J Cardiovasc Surg. (Torino)* 1990; 31(5):553-558.

45. Anttila V, Pokela M, Kiviluoma K, et al: Is maintained cranial hypothermia the only factor leading to improved outcome after retrograde cerebral perfusion? An experimental study with a chronic porcine model. *J Thorac Cardiovasc Surg* 2000; 119:1021-1029.

46. Usui A, Oohara K, Liu T, et al: Comparative experimental study between retrograde cerebral perfusion and circulatory arrest. *J Thorac Cardiovasc Surg* 1994; 107(5):1228-1236.

47. Juvonen T, Weisz DJ, Wolfe D, et al: Can retrograde perfusion mitigate cerebral injury after particulate embolization? A study in a chronic porcine model. *J Thorac Cardiovasc Surg* 1998; 115(5):1142-1159.

48. Boeckxstans CJ, Flamengg WJ: Retrograde cerebral perfusion does not protect the brain in non-human primates. *Ann Thorac Surg* 1995; 60(2):319-327.

49. Ye J, Yang L, Del Rigio MR, et al: Retrograde cerebral perfusion provides limited distribution of blood to the brain: a study in pigs. *J Thorac Cardiovasc Surg* 1997; 114(4):660-665.

50. Ehrlich MP, Hagl C, McCullough JN, et al: Retrograde cerebral perfusion provides negligible flow through brain capillaries in the pig. *J Thorac Cardiovasc Surg* 2001; 122(2):331-338.

51. Razumovsky A, Tseng E, Hanley D, Baumgartner W: Cerebral hemodynamics change during retrograde brain perfusion in dogs. *J Neuroimaging* 2001; 11(2):171-178.

52. Juvonen T, Zhang N, Wolfe D, et al: Retrograde cerebral perfusion enhances cerebral protection during prolonged hypothermic circulatory arrest: a study in a chronic porcine model. *Ann Thorac Surg* 1998; 66(1):38-50.

53. Kunzil A, Zingg PO, Zund G, et al: Does retrograde cerebral perfusion via superior vena cava cannulation protect the brain? *Eur J Cardiothorac Surg* 2006; 30(6):906-909.

54. De Brux J, Subavi J, Pegis J, Pillet J: Retrograde cerebral perfusion: anatomic study of the distribution of blood to the brain. *Ann Thorac Surg* 1995; 60:1294-1298.

55. Nojima T, Magara T, Nakajima Y, et al: Optimal perfusion pressure for experimental retrograde cerebral perfusion. *J Card Surg* 1994; 9(5):548-559.

56. Safi HJ, Iliopoulos DC, Gopinath SP, et al: Retrograde cerebral perfusion during profound hypothermia and circulatory arrest in pigs. *Ann Thorac Surg* 1995; 59(5):1107-1112.

57. Lin P, Chang CH, Tan PP, et al: Prolonged circulatory arrest in moderate hypothermia with retrograde cerebral perfusion. Is brain ischemic? *Circulation* 1996; 94(9):II:169-172.

58. Yoshimura N, Ataka K, Okada M, et al: Directly visualized cerebral circulation during retrograde cerebral perfusion. *J Cardiovasc Surg (Torino)* 1996; 37(6):553-556.

59. Coselli JS, Lemaire SA: Experience with retrograde cerebral perfusion during proximal aortic surgery in 290 patients. *J Card Surg* 1997; 12(2):322-325.

60. Estrera AL, Miller III CC, Lee TY, Shah P, Safi HJ: Ascending and transverse aortic arch repair: the impact of retrograde cerebral perfusion. *Circulation* 2008; 188:S160-S166.

61. Okita Y, Takamoto S, Ando M, et al: Mortality and cerebral outcome in patients who underwent aortic arch operations using deep hypothermic circulatory arrest with retrograde cerebral perfusion: no relation of early death, stroke and delirium to the duration of circulatory arrest. *J Thorac Cardiovasc Surg* 1998; 115(1):129-138.

62. Hagl C, Ergin MA, Galla JD, et al: Neurologic outcome after ascending aorta-aortic arch operations: effect of brain protection technique in high-risk patients. *J Thorac Cardiovasc Surg* 2001; 121:1107-1121.

63. Moon MR, Sundt TM 3rd: Influence of retrograde cerebral perfusion during aortic arch procedures. *Ann Thorac Surg* 2002; 74(2):426-431.

64. DeBakey ME, Crawford ES, Cooley DA, et al: Successful resection of fusiform aneurysm of the aortic arch with replacement homograft. *Surg Gynecol Obstet* 1957; 105:657.

65. Bachet J, Guilmet D, Boudot B, et al: Cold cerebroplegia. A new technique of cerebral protection during operations on the transverse aortic arch. *J Thorac Cardiovasc Surg* 1991; 102(1):85-94.

66. Kazui T, Inoue N, Yamada O, Komatsu S: Selective cerebral perfusion during operations for aneurysms of the aortic arch: a reassessment. *Ann Thorac Surg* 1992; 53(1):109-114.

67. Tanoue Y, Tominaga R, Ochiai Y, et al: Comparative study of retrograde and selective cerebral perfusion with transcranial Doppler. *Ann Thorac Surg* 1999; 67(3):672-675.

68. Filgueiras CL, Winsborrow B, Ye J, et al: A 31p-magnetic resonance study of antegrade and retrograde cerebral perfusion during aortic arch surgery in pigs. *J Thorac Cardiovasc Surg* 1995; 110(1):55-62.

69. Filgueiras CL, Ryner L, Ye J, et al: Cerebral protection during moderate hypothermic circulatory arrest: histopathology and magnetic resonance spectroscopy of brain energetics and intracellular pH in pigs. *J Thorac Cardiovasc Surg* 1996; 112(4):1073-1080.

70. Hagl C, Khaladj N, Peterss S, et al: Hypothermic circulatory arrest with and without cold selective antegrade cerebral perfusion: impact on neurological recovery and issue metabolism in an acute porcine model. *Eur J Cardiothorac Surg* 2004; 26:73-80.

71. Halkos ME, Kerendi F, Myung R, et al: Selective antegrade cerebral perfusion via right axillary artery cannulation reduces morbidity and mortality after proximal aortic surgery. *J Thorac Cardiovasc Surg* 2009; 138:1081-1089.

72. Ye J, Dai G, Ryner LN, et al: Unilateral antegrade cerebral perfusion through the right axillary artery provides uniform flow distribution to both hemispheres of the brain: a magnetic resonance and histopathological study in pigs. *Circulation* 1999; (19 Suppl):II:309-315.

73. Urbanski PP, Lenos A, Blume JC, et al: Does anatomical completeness of the circle of Willis correlate with sufficient cross-perfusion during unilateral cerebral perfusion? *Eur J Cardiothorac Surg* 2008; 33(3):402-408.

74. Zierer A, Risteski P, El-Sayed Ahmad A, et al: The impact of unilateral versus bilateral antegrade cerebral perfusion on surgical outcomes after aortic arch replacement: a propensity-matched analysis. *J Thorac Cardiovasc Surg* 2014; 147(4):1212-1217.

75. MoraMangano CT, Neville MJ, Hsu PH, Mignea I, King J, Miller DC: Aprotinin, blood loss and renal dysfunction in deep hypothermic circulatory arrest. *Circulation* 2001; 104:276-281.

76. Cooper WA, Duarte IG, Thourani VH, et al: Hypothermic circulatory arrest causes multi-system vascular endothelial dysfunction and apoptosis. *Ann Thorac Surg* 2000; 69:696-702.

77. Livesay JJ, Cooley DA, Reul GJ, et al: Resection of aortic arch aneurysms: a comparison of hypothermic techniques in 60 patients. *Ann Thorac Surg* 1983; 36(1):19-28.

78. Qing M, Vazquez-Jimenez JF, Klosterhalfen B, et al: Influence of temperature during cardiopulmonary bypass on leukocyte activation, cytokine balance, and post-operative organ damage. *Shock* 2001; 15:372-377.

79. Minatoya K, Ogino H, Matsuda H, et al: Evolving selective cerebral perfusion for aortic arch replacement: high flow rate with moderate hypothermic circulatory arrest. *Ann Thorac Surg* 2008; 86:1827-1831.

80. Iba Y, Minatoya K, Matsuda H, et al: Contemporary open aortic arch repair with selective cerebral perfusion in the era of endovascular aortic repair. *J Thorac Cardiovasc Surg* 2013; 145(3):S72-S77.

81. Pacini D, Pantaleo A, Di Marco L, et al: Visceral organ protection in aortic arch surgery: safety of moderate hypothermia. *Eur J Cardiothorac Surg* 2014; 46(3):438-443.

82. Leshnower BG, Myung RJ, Thourani VH, et al: Hemiarch replacement at 28°C: an analysis of mild and moderate hypothermia in 500 patients. *Ann Thorac Surg* 2012; 93(6):1910-1915.

83. Leshnower BG, Kilgo PD, Chen EP: Total arch replacement using moderate hypothermic circulatory arrest and unilateral selective antegrade cerebral perfusion. *J Thorac Cardiovasc Surg* 2014; 147: 1488-1492.

84. Zierer A, Ahmad El-Sayed A, Papadopoulos N, et al: Selective antegrade cerebral perfusion and mild (28°C-30°C) systemic hypothermic circulatory arrest for aortic arch replacement: results from 1002 patients. *J Thorac Cardiovasc Surg* 2012; 144:1042-1050.

85. Khaladj N, Shrestha M, Meck M, et al: Hypothermic circulatory arrest with selective antegrade cerebral perfusion in ascending aortic and aortic arch surgery: a risk factor analysis for adverse outcome in 501 patients. *J Thorac Cardiovasc Surg* 2008; 135(4):908-914.

86. Tsai JY, Pan W, Lemaire SA, et al: Moderate hypothermia during aortic arch surgery is associated with reduced risk of early mortality. *J Thorac Cardiovasc Surg* 2013; 146(3):662-667.

87. Hagl C, Ergin MA, Galla JD, et al: Neurologic outcome after ascending aorta-aortic arch operations: effect of brain protection technique in high-risk patients. *J Thorac Cardiovasc Surg* 2001; 121:1107-1121.

88. Okie Y, Miata H, Mtomura N, et al. A study of brain protection during total arch replacement comparing antegrade cerebral perfusion versus hypothermic circulatory arrest with or without retrograde cerebral perfusion: analysis based on the Japan Adult Cardiovascular Surgery Database. *J Thorac Cardiovasc Surg* 2015; 149(2):S65-73.

89. Okita Y, Minatoya K, Tagusari O, et al: Prospective comparative study of brain protection in total aortic arch replacement: deep hypothermic circulatory arrest with retrograde cerebral perfusion or selective antegrade cerebral perfusion. *Ann Thorac Surg* 2001; 72:72-79.

90. Misfeld M, Leontyev S, Borger MA, et al: What is the best strategy for brain protection in patients undergoing aortic arch surgery? A single center experience of 636 patients. *Ann Thorac Surg* 2012; 93(5):1502-1508.

91. Usui A, Miyata H, Ueda Y, et al: Risk-adjusted and case matched comparative study between antegrade and retrograde cerebral perfusion during aortic arch surgery: based on the Japan Cardiovascular Surgery Database: the Japan Cardiovascular Surgery Database Organization. *Gen Thorac Cardiovasc Surg* 2012; 60:132-139.

92. Barnard J, Dunning J, Grossebner M, Bittar MN: In aortic arch surgery is there any benefit in using antegrade cerebral perfusion or retrograde cerebral perfusion as an adjunct to hypothermic circulatory arrest? *Interact Cardiovasc Thorac Surg* 2004; 3(4):621-630.

93. Shum-Tim D, Tchervenkov CI, Laliberte E, et al: Timing of steroid treatment is important for cerebral protection during cardiopulmonary bypass and circulatory arrest: minimal protection of pump prime methylprednisolone. *Eur J Cardiothorac Surg* 2003; 24(1):125-132.

94. Langley SM, Chai PJ, Jaggers JJ, Ungerleider RM: Preoperative high dose methylprednisolone attenuates the cerebral response to deep hypothermic circulatory arrest. *Eur J Cardiothorac Surg* 2000; 17(3):279-286.

95. Al-Hashimi S, Zaman M, Waterworth P, Bilal H: Does the use of thiopental provide added cerebral protection during deep hypothermic circulatory arrest? *Interact Cardio Vasc Thorac Surg* 2013; 17(2):392-397.

96. Kruger T, Hoffmann I, Blettner M, et al: Intraoperative neuroprotective drugs without beneficial effects? Results of the German Registry for Acute Aortic Dissection Type A (GERAADA). *Eur J Cardiothorac Surg* 2013; 44:939-946.

Myocardial Protection

*M. Salik Jahania • Roberta A. Gottlieb
• Robert M. Mentzer, Jr.*

16

Myocardial protection in the operating room refers to strategies and methods used to attenuate or prevent perioperative infarction and/or postischemic ventricular dysfunction. In the setting of an acute myocardial infarction (MI) it refers to adjuvant therapy administered before, during or after reperfusion therapy. In transplantation it refers to the methods used to preserve the donor heart. Although the clinical situations are different, the goal of protection is the same, that is, to prevent or treat myocardial stunning and infarction. The underlying pathophysiology in all three settings is the same and relates to the etiology and consequences of ischemia/reperfusion (I/R) injury. After surgery the injury may manifest as low cardiac output, hypotension, and the need for postoperative inotropic support and ultimately mechanical circulatory support. I/R injury may be reversible (stunning) or irreversible (infarction) and is differentiated by electrocardiographic abnormalities (presence of a new Q-wave), elevations in the levels of specific plasma enzymes or proteins such as creatine kinase-MB and troponin I or T and/or the presence of regional or global echocardiographic wall motion abnormalities. Depending upon the criteria used, the incidence of postoperative MI in patients undergoing coronary artery bypass grafting (CABG) with cardiopulmonary bypass (CPB) ranges between 3% and 18%.[1-4] While the majority of these are non-Q wave infarctions, they still are independently associated with adverse outcomes and prolonged aortic cross-clamp time and duration of CPB. Despite advances in techniques and cardioprotective strategies, the incidence of severe ventricular dysfunction, heart failure and death postoperatively ranges between 1% and 15%. The higher mortality rates are generally associated with high-risk patients with minimal cardiac reserve. These complications have an enormous impact on both families and society. From an economic standpoint alone, procedures for cardiovascular diseases are costly.

According to Heart Disease and Stroke Statistics–2015 Update,[5] in 2010 an estimated 954,000 percutaneous interventions (PCIs), 397,000 CABG operations, 1,029,000 diagnostic cardiac catheterizations, 97,000 defibrillator implants and 370,000 pacemaker procedures were performed on inpatients in the United States. The estimated cost was $204.4 billion. Between 2013 and 2030, medical costs of coronary heart disease alone are projected to increase by 100%. Cardiovascular disease costs more than any other diagnostic group. Therefore, a reduction in perioperative complications associated with heart surgery would have a significant impact on resource utilization and overall operative costs.[6-8] Since I/R injury is a major cause of morbidity and mortality after heart surgery, the purpose of this chapter is to review its underlying mechanisms, review the history of myocardial protection, update the reader regarding the current protective techniques and discuss new strategies under investigation.

ISCHEMIA/REPERFUSION INJURY

The etiology of perioperative myocardial necrosis and postischemic myocardial dysfunction after cardiac surgery is multifactorial. Myocardial necrosis and elevation of associated cardiac biomarkers may arise as a result of ischemia due to intrinsic coronary disease unrelated to revascularization, anesthetic factors, atrial cannulation, suturing of heart muscle, plaque rupture or platelet embolism, and graft spasm or thrombosis. Despite the considerable progress made to date, high-risk heart surgery patients including those with unstable angina, poor ventricular function, diabetes, repeat CABG, and advanced age continue to experience postoperative complications such as low cardiac output, perioperative MI and heart failure requiring prolonged intensive care. In many of these instances the complications are due to I/R injury and inadequate myocardial protection. Thus there is a compelling unmet need to develop better methods to protect the heart during surgery.

Deleterious Sequelae of Ischemia/Reperfusion

Myocardial I/R injury manifests as postischemic "stunning", which is reversible, and apoptosis and/or necrosis, which are irreversible. Myocardial stunning is an injury that lasts for hours to days despite the restoration of normal blood flow. Typically these patients require some type of temporary inotropic support in the immediate postoperative period in order to maintain an adequate cardiac output. Stunned cardiomyocytes exhibit minimal ultrastructural damage that resolves within hours to days following relief of ischemia. Apoptosis, or programed cell death, is a pattern of cell death that affects single cells. It is characterized by an intact cell membrane with blebbing, cell shrinkage, condensation of the nucleus and oligonucleosomal fragmentation of DNA. Externalization of phosphatidylserine on the outer leaflet of the plasma membrane serves as a cue for phagocytic removal of apoptotic cells by neighboring cells or professional phagocytes without inflammation. It is unclear whether apoptosis is initiated during ischemia and but manifests during reperfusion or whether it is a consequence of reperfusion, but the preponderance of evidence favors the latter.[9,10] Regardless, apoptotic cell death occurs in the infarct zone and continues to occur in the border zone subsequently. Prolonged ischemia results in necrotic cell death characterized by cell swelling, plasma membrane rupture, mitochondrial swelling and loss of cristae, and DNA degradation followed by an inflammatory response to the cellular debris. Dying cells may exhibit features of both apoptosis and necrosis, that is, both nuclear condensation and plasma membrane damage.[11-14]

Long-term Consequences

While the end result of inadequate myocardial protection is usually apparent in the immediate postoperative period, for example, low cardiac output syndrome, the full impact may not be evident for months to years. Klatte and colleagues reported that the 6-month mortality was greater in patients with increased peak creatine kinase-myocardial band (CK-MB) enzyme ratios after CABG surgery.[15] The 6-month mortality rates were 3.4%, 5.8%, 7.8% and 20% for patients with peak CK-MB ratios that were <5, 5-10, 11-20, and >20-fold higher than the upper limits of normal (UNL), respectively. In another study, Costa and colleagues[16] reported that normal postoperative CK-MB levels were observed in only 38.1% of 496 patients who underwent CABG surgery. When the CK-MB levels were stratified, the incidence of death at 30 days was 0.0%, 0.5%, 5.4%, and 7.0% when the enzyme levels were normal, 1 to 3 times higher, 4 to 5 times higher, and >5-fold higher than ULN, respectively. The 1-year mortality for these groups was 1.1%, 0.5%, 5.4%, and 10.5%. The peak postoperative cardiac enzyme level correlated significantly with worse clinical outcome. Thus, while CK-MB elevations are often dismissed as inconsequential in the setting of multivessel CABG surgery, they occur frequently and are associated with significant increases in both repeat MI and death beyond the immediate perioperative period. Consistent with this is the report by Steuer[17] and associates in which they examined postoperative serum aspartate aminotransferase and CK-MB levels and their relationship to early and late cardiac-related death in 4911 consecutive patients who underwent CABG during a 6-year period. They reported that elevated enzyme levels on the first postoperative day greatly increased the risk of early cardiac death and were associated with a 40 to 50% increased risk in late mortality at 7 years.

In a retrospective analysis Brener et al showed that CK-MB elevation was common after both percutaneous and surgical revascularization.[18] The incidence of CK-MB elevation above the normal range was 90% for CABG surgery and 38% for percutaneous coronary intervention (PCI). In a small fraction of patients the elevations exceeded 10 × ULN (6% for CABG and 5% for PCI). At 3 years follow-up the cumulative mortality was 8% for CABG and 10% for PCI. Even relatively small CK-MB elevations after interventions were associated with increased mortality over time. Similar observations were made when troponin release was used as a biomarker of myocardial injury. Lehrke et al reported in a series of 204 patients that a serum troponin-T concentration of 0.46 mcg/L or more, 48 hours after surgery was associated with a 4.9-fold increase in long-term risk of death.[19]

Finally, in one of the largest studies to date Domanski et al[20] reviewed the relationship between peak postoperative levels of biomarkers of myocardial damage and early-, intermediate- and long-term mortality reported in previously reported and randomized clinical trials and registries. A total of 18,908 patients from seven studies were included for analysis. The follow-up ranged from 3 months to 5 years. The investigators reported that, in the aggregate, even modest elevations of troponin I at the 24-hour level were prognostically significant, and any CK-MB elevation after CABG was associated with increased mortality. In short, biomarkers of myocardial injury are frequently elevated after CABG surgery and are associated with decreased short-, medium-, and long-term survival.

Intracellular Mechanisms Underlying Ischemia/Reperfusion Injury

The primary mediators of I/R injury include intracellular Ca^{2+} overload and oxidative stress induced by reactive oxygen species (ROS) generated at the onset of reperfusion[21] (Fig.16-1). The molecule nitric oxide (NO) also can interact with superoxide (O_2^-) or peroxides to generate reactive nitrogen species that are capable of inducing injury as well.[22] In addition, metabolic alterations occurring during ischemia can contribute directly and indirectly to Ca^{2+} overload and ROS formation. For example, decreased cytosolic phosphorylation potential, that is, $[ATP]/([ADP] \times [P_i])$, results in less free energy from ATP hydrolysis than is necessary to drive the energy-dependent pumps (sarcoplasmic reticulum calcium ion adenosine triphosphatase (Ca^{2+}-ATPase), the sarcolemmal Ca^{2+}-ATPase) that maintain intracellular calcium homeostasis.[23] With the onset of ischemia and the build-up of lactic acid, pH falls to as low as 6.6, resulting in proton efflux and sodium influx via the Na^+-H^+ exchanger. The driving forces for Na^+/H^+ exchange are the relative transmembrane N^+ and H^+ gradients. The activity of the exchanger is regulated by the interaction of the H^+ with a sensor site on the exchanger protein; it can be additionally modulated by phosphorylation.[24] During reperfusion the accumulated intracellular Na^+ competes with Ca^{2+} for sites on the Na^+/Ca^{2+} exchanger, effectively causing the exchanger to run in reverse, thereby exacerbating

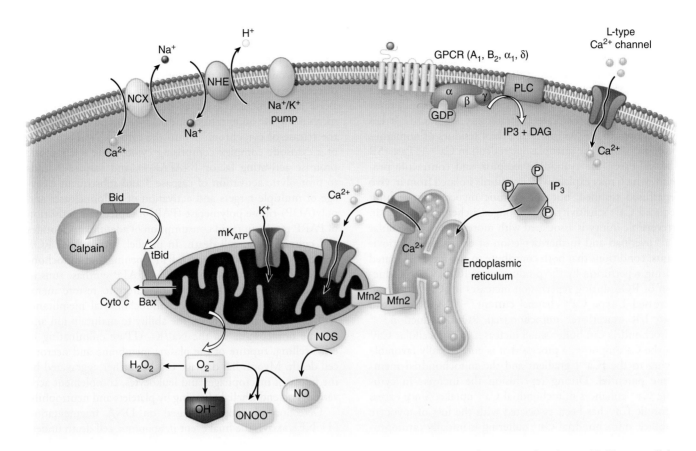

FIGURE 16-1 Myocardial alterations associated with ischemia-reperfusion injury. PKC, protein kinase C; Ca^{2+}, calcium; $[Ca^{2+}]_i$, intracellular calcium concentration; $[Na^+]_i$, intracellular sodium concentration; GPRC, G-protein coupled receptor; G_s, stimulatory G proteins; PLC, phospholipase C; IP_3 inositol trisphosphate; DAG, diacylglycerol; NHE, sodium-hydrogen exchanger; NCX, sodium-calcium exchanger; Na^+, sodium; RP, reperfusion; NO, nitric oxide; mK_{ATP} channel, mitochondrial ATP-sensitive potassium channel; mPTP, mitochondrial permeability transition pore; ER, endoplasmic reticulum; $[Ca^{2+}]_m$, intramitochondrial calcium concentration.

intracellular calcium accumulation. The elevated intracellular Ca^{2+} leads to activation of calcium-dependent proteases and phospholipases, calpain-mediated damage to myofibrillar contractile elements, gap junction dysfunction, injury of the sarcoplasmic reticulum and opening of the mitochondrial permeability transition pore (mPTP). Opening of the pore in the inner mitochondrial membrane is associated with a collapse of the membrane, uncoupling of the electron transport chain, release of cytochrome c and other proapoptotic factors, swelling of the matrix and ultimately rupture of the outer mitochondrial membrane and cell death.[25]

The metabolic changes that occur during ischemia also deplete the endogenous antioxidant defense systems of cardiac myocytes. I/R damages mitochondrial complex I generating excessive ROS (O_2^- and H_2O_2) and resulting in damage to cellular lipids, proteins and nucleic acids. Glutathione is a critical defense against oxidative stress, in which GSH (reduced glutathione) is used to repair oxidized protein thiols, generating GSSG (oxidized glutathione) system; GSH is regenerated by glutathione reductase which depends upon the nicotinamide adenine dinucleotide phosphate, reduced form: nicotinamide adenine dinucleotide phosphate (NADPH:NADP$^+$) ratio. Depletion of glutathione impairs

the ability to detoxify ROS-mediated damage to proteins.[26,27] During ischemia NADPH levels drop thereby limiting the ability to regenerate reduced glutathione. Thus, the formation of ROS during reperfusion occurs at a time when the myocyte's endogenous defense mechanisms are depressed. The NADPH:NADP$^+$ ratio is a primary determinant of the redox state of the cell, and there is evidence that the redox state plays a key role in determining the bioactivity and the redox state of NO.[22,28] In addition, there are several reports that in the absence of normal levels of its cofactors, nitric oxide synthase (NOS), itself can generate the superoxide anion.[29] Although systolic intracellular calcium concentration, $[Ca^{2+}]_i$, may decrease to normal levels early in the reperfused stunned myocardium, transient increases in $[Ca^{2+}]_i$ can result in sustained activation of protein kinase C (PKC) isoforms, calpain proteases and deoxyribonuclease II (DNase II).[30] Calpain-mediated proteolysis of contractile proteins has been implicated in the reduction of myofilament Ca^{2+} sensitivity observed in stunned myocardium.[31]

There is considerable evidence that ROS are involved in mediating myocardial stunning. Various spin-trap agents and chemical probes have demonstrated the rapid release of ROS into the vascular space during reperfusion after brief ischemia in vivo.[32] While mitochondria are a major source of intracellular ROS in cardiac myocytes, they are not the only source of ROS during I/R.[33,34] It has been shown that anti-oxidants administered before the onset of ischemia attenuate myocardial stunning in vitro and in vivo. Antioxidants administered prior to or at the onset of reperfusion may show efficacy, although there are contradictory studies.[21,35] It has been shown that ROS can attack thiol residues of numerous proteins such as the sarcoplasmic reticulum Ca^{2+} ATPase (SR Ca^{2+}-ATPase), the ryanodine receptor, and contractile proteins, which may explain why myofibrils isolated from in vivo reperfused stunned, but not necrotic myocardium, exhibit reduced Ca^{2+} sensitivity.[36,37] Prolonged ischemia resulting in irreversible injury is associated with more severe intracellular Ca^{2+} overload and further depletion of endogenous antioxidants, conditions that both contribute to and are exacerbated during reperfusion by the production of ROS. Overproduction of ROS during reperfusion increases in $[Ca^{2+}]_i$ through increased L-type Ca^{2+} channel current.[27,38,39] Ca^{2+} overload with I/R exacerbates mitochondrial ROS production.[39,40] Mitochondria can buffer small increases in intracellular Ca^{2+} via the Ca uniporter, a process that is energetically favorable owing to the $[Ca^{2+}]$ gradient and the mitochondrial membrane potential. During reperfusion the increase in cytosolic Ca^{2+} enhances mitochondrial Ca^{2+} uptake. Since excess cytosolic Ca^{2+} has been associated with the loss of myocyte viability, mitochondrial Ca^{2+} buffering is initially cardioprotective.[41] However, continued mitochondrial Ca^{2+} uptake in the face of decreased antioxidant reserves and ongoing oxidative stress ultimately triggers opening of the mitochondrial permeability transition pore, a large conductance channel that allows release of stored mitochondrial Ca^{2+}, osmotic swelling of the mitochondria, collapse of mitochondrial membrane potential and cell death. The synergistic interactions between Ca^{2+} overload and ROS formation during conditions of decreased antioxidant reserves also may explain why ROS scavengers are not very effective at reducing irreversible injury when administered at reperfusion.[42] It also possible that antioxidants employed in studies to date are not targeted to the sites where ROS are generated and mediate most of their damage. Specific mitochondrial antioxidants may be more effective.[43-45]

Broadening the Spectrum of Ischemia/Reperfusion Injury

Historically myocardial I/R injury has been characterized as either reversible or irreversible, based on staining techniques, enzyme release and histology. There is now increasing evidence that the transition from reversible to irreversible injury occurs on a continuum rather than an all-or-none phenomenon. Apoptosis depends on the availability of ATP and precedes loss of membrane integrity; however, if ATP depletion occurs rapidly, the Na^+/K^+-ATPase will be unable to regulate cell volume, resulting in plasma membrane rupture and necrotic cell death before the enzymatic processes of apoptosis are complete.[46,47] Intracellular ROS and/or intracellular

calcium overload can initiate the apoptotic program through proapoptotic BH3-only proteins Bnip3 (activated by ROS) and Bid (proteolytically activated by calpain).[48,49] (Fig. 16-2) The BH3-only proteins trigger oligomerization of Bax or Bak directly or indirectly (through interaction with antiapoptotic Bcl-2 family members, Bcl-2, Bcl-x_L, or Mcl-1), thus permeabilizing the outer mitochondrial membrane and allowing the release of cytochrome c into the cytosol.[49-51] Formation of a cytosolic complex comprising cytochrome c, apoptotic protease activating factor 1 (APAF-1), and caspase-9 leads to proteolytic activation of caspase 3 and subsequent cleavage of multiple targets and activation of endonucleases and poly(ADP)-ribose polymerase (PARP). Proteolytic activation of PARP results in rapid consumption of adenine nucleotides and culminates in cell death. In parallel, intracellular ROS and calcium overload trigger mPTP opening and mitochondrial swelling; the mitochondrial F_0-F_1 ATP synthase runs in reverse hydrolyzing ATP in a futile effort to restore membrane potential across the inner mitochondrial membrane. ATP depletion compromises the ability to maintain ion and volume homeostasis via the Na^+/K^+-ATPase culminating in cell swelling, rupture of the plasma membrane and necrotic cell death. Myocardial damage can be further aggravated by the influx of macrophages and leukocytes, complement activation, and endothelial plugging by platelets and neutrophils.

Detection of apoptosis based on DNA fragmentation (TUNEL assay), the final event in apoptotic cell death underestimates the extent of apoptosis. Detection of externalized phosphatidylserine with annexin V conjugated to a fluorescent dye allows earlier recognition of apoptosis and has been used for in vivo imaging of apoptosis in the mouse heart; however, not all cells recognized by Annexin V are irreversibly committed to cell death.[52-55] Estimates of apoptosis in I/R injury are further confounded by the fact that the apoptotic remnants are efficiently cleared by neighboring cells or professional phagocytes. Thus the magnitude and significance of apoptosis in I/R injury has remained controversial. Genetic manipulations of mice have shown that disrupting the apoptotic machinery can result in a 60 to 70% reduction in infarct size. However, attempts to mitigate apoptosis with caspase inhibitors have not resulted in substantial reductions in infarct size, possibly because interruption of the late stages of apoptosis may simply result in necrosis. As a result, many investigators have turned their attention to interventions targeting the early events in apoptosis or preventing mPTP opening and necrotic cell death. Regardless of which stage is being addressed, current cardioprotection strategies are designed to reduce cellular and subcellular ROS formation and oxidative stress to enhance the heart's endogenous antioxidant defense mechanisms and prevent intracellular Ca^{2+} overload.

CARDIOPROTECTION: HISTORICAL PERSPECTIVES

In 1883, Ringer described the antagonistic effects of calcium and potassium ions on cardiac contraction. In 1929, Hooker reported the successful resuscitation of dogs with

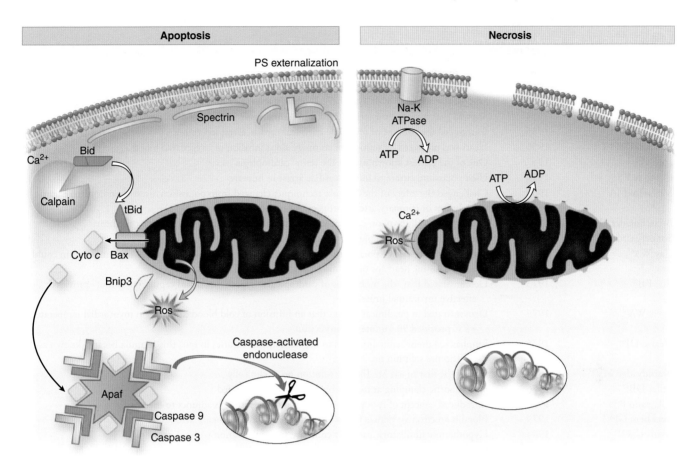

| **Apoptosis** | **Necrosis** |

FIGURE 16-2 Mechanisms of cardiomyocyte cell death following ischemia-reperfusion injury. Bax, proapoptotic family of proteins; Bcl-2, antiapoptotic protein; Ca^{2+}, calcium; ROS, reactive oxygen species; Apaf, apoptotic protease-activating factor 1; PS, phosphatidylserine; SR, sarcoplasmic reticulum. Intracellular Ca^{2+} overload during ischemia and reperfusion and reactive oxygen species (ROS) formation during reperfusion are primary mediators of cell death via apoptosis and necrosis. The mechanisms of Ca^{2+} overload and ROS formation are described in detail in the text. In the intrinsic apoptosis pathway, BH3-only proapoptotic members of the Bcl-2 family are activated by calpain or caspase 8 (Bid) or ROS (Bnip3); they interact with Bax or Bak to form pores in the outer mitochondrial membrane allowing release of cytochrome c. This interaction is opposed by the antiapoptotic Bcl-2 family members including Bcl-2, Bcl-x_L, and Mcl-1. In the cytosol, cytochrome c interacts with Apaf-1 and ATP or dATP to promote proteolytic activation of caspase 9 and the downstream executioner protease, caspase 3. Caspase 3 cleaves multiple targets, inactivating many cell survival pathways and activating endonucleases responsible for oligonucleosomal DNA fragmentation (DNA laddering). Cleavage of spectrin internal to the plasma membrane is permissive for phosphatidylserine redistribution to the external leaflet of the cell membrane, marking the dying cell for phagocytic removal by tissue macrophages or neighboring cells without an inflammatory response. In the necrotic death pathway, Ca^{2+} overload and ROS trigger opening of the mitochondrial permeability transition pore (mPTP), resulting in swelling of the matrix, disruption of the outer mitochondrial membrane, and rampant ATP hydrolysis by the ATP synthase running in reverse in a futile attempt to restore mitochondrial membrane potential. This energetic crisis leads to failure of the plasma membrane Na^+/K^+ ATPase, loss of plasma membrane integrity, and cell rupture, triggering an inflammatory response.

potassium in which ventricular fibrillation was induced by electric shock.[56,57] In 1930, Wiggers reported that injections of potassium chloride were capable of abrogating ventricular fibrillation and arrested the heart in diastole. He also demonstrated that revival of the heart was possible using calcium chloride and massage.[58] The work by Wiggers led Beck, a thoracic surgeon, to successfully apply defibrillation therapy and save a human life using this method.[59] This resulted in a surge in basic and clinical research in the field of fibrillation and defibrillation with the principles applied to cardiac surgery.

With the advent of CPB, there was a need to refine techniques to protect the heart while creating a quiescent and

bloodless field for the unhurried repair of intracardiac defects. Over the next 50 years, a variety of cardioprotective methods and techniques were introduced (Table 16-1). One of the first methodologies evolved from the concept of shielding the heart from perioperative insult using hypothermia. Bigelow and colleagues suggested using hypothermia "as a form of anesthetic" to expand the scope of surgery. The technique "might permit surgeons to operate upon the 'bloodless heart' without recourse to extra corporal pumps and perhaps allow transplantation of organs."[60] Five years later Melrose and colleagues reported another way to stop and restart the human heart reliably by injecting potassium citrate into the root of the aorta at both normal and reduced body temperatures.[61]

TABLE 16-1: Evolution of Cardioprotective Methods and Techniques

Reference	Year	Innovation
Bigelow WG[60]	1950	Studied the application of hypothermia to cardiac surgery in canines
Swan H[75]	1953	Showed that hypothermic arrest (26°C) in humans provided a bloodless field for operating
Melrose DG[61]	1955	Introduced the concept of reversible chemical cardiac arrest in canines
Lillehei CW[76]	1956	Heart was protected by retrograde coronary sinus infusion of oxygenated blood
Lam CR[77]	1957	One of the earliest known uses of the term "cardioplegia"
Gerbode F[78]	1958	Used potassium citrate to induce cardiac arrest in humans
McFarland JA[79]	1960	Challenged the safety of the Melrose technique; changed from potassium arrest to intermittent aortic occlusion or coronary artery perfusion for myocardial protection
Bretschneider HJ[65]	1964	Developed a sodium-poor, calcium-free, procaine-containing solution to arrest the heart
Sondergaard KT[80,81]	1964	Adopted Bretschneider's solution for clinical use
Gay WA[68]	1973	Credited with revival of potassium-induced cardioplegia; demonstrated that potassium solution could arrest a canine heart for 60 minutes without cellular damage
Roe BB[69]	1973	Demonstrated that "the modalities of cardioplegia, hypothermia, and capillary washout" provided effective myocardial protection
Tyers WA[62]	1974	Demonstrated in preclinical studies that an infusion of cold blood to maintain myocardial temperature <4°C provided 90 minutes of protection
Hearse DJ[66]	1975	Emphasized preischemic infusions to negate ischemic injuries in rats; this formula became known as St. Thomas solution no. 1
Braimbridge MV[67]	1975	One of the first to use St. Thomas solution no. 1 clinically
Effler DB[82]	1976	Simple aortic clamping at room temperatures recommended
Solarzano J[83]	1978	Introduced concept of retrograde coronary sinus perfusion as adjunct to myocardial protection
Buckberg GD[71]	1979	Blood is an effective vehicle for infusing potassium into coronary arteries
Akins CW[84]	1984	Hypothermic fibrillatory arrest for coronary revascularization without cardioplegia
Murry CE[85]	1986	First to report that brief periods of ischemia (preconditioning) and reperfusion enable the heart to withstand longer periods of ischemia in a canine model
Lichtenstein SV[86] Salerno TA[87]	1991	Reported warm antegrade and retrograde blood cardioplegia safe
Ikonomidis JS[88]	1995	Combined normothermic continuous retrograde cardioplegia with intermittent antegrade infusions
Teoh LK[89]	2002	Introduced concept that intermittent cross-clamp fibrillation in CABG surgery patients confers cardioprotection via ischemic preconditioning and adenosine receptor activation
Quinn DW[90]	2006	Phase II human trial demonstrated efficacy of cardioprotective effects of systemic glucose-insulin-potassium (GIK) when administered perioperatively
Mentzer Jr RM[1]	2008	Phase III myocardial protection trial demonstrated proof of concept that perioperative MI can be reduced with an intravenous infusion of a pharmacologic agent in CABG surgery patients

Soon thereafter, the clinical application of potassium citrate arrest was adopted by many centers. Interest in using the Melrose technique waned, however, with subsequent reports that potassium citrate arrest was associated with myocardial injury and necrosis. Within a short time, many cardiac surgeons shifted from using potassium-induced arrest to normothermic cardiac ischemia, that is, normothermic heart surgery performed with the aorta occluded while the patient was on CPB, intermittent aortic occlusion or coronary artery perfusion. Experimental and clinical evidence showed, however, that normothermic cardiac ischemia was associated with metabolic acidosis, hypotension and low cardiac output.[62-64] As a consequence, there was a renewed interest in discovering ways to arrest the heart. Bretschneider published the principle of arresting the heart with a low-sodium, calcium-free solution.[65] It was Hearse and colleagues however who studied the various components of cardioplegic solutions which led to the development and use of St. Thomas solution.[66] The components of this crystalloid solution were based on Ringer's solution with its normal concentrations of sodium and calcium with the addition of potassium chloride (16 mmol/L) and magnesium chloride (16 mmol/L) to arrest the heart instantly. The latter component was shown by Hearse to provide an additional cardioprotective benefit. In 1975, Braimbridge and colleagues introduced this crystalloid solution into clinical practice at St. Thomas Hospital.[67] Gay and Ebert showed experimentally that lower concentrations of potassium chloride could achieve the same degree of chemical arrest and myocardial protection afforded by the Melrose solution without the associated myocardial necrosis reported earlier.[67,68] Shortly thereafter, Roe and colleagues reported an operative mortality of 5.4% for patients who

TABLE 16-2: Components of Various Cardioplegic Solutions

	Sodium	Potassium	Magnesium	Calcium	Buffer	pH	Osmolarity (mOsm/L)	Other Components
Intracellular crystalloid CP								
Bretschneider's no. 3	12.0	10.0	4.0	0	Histidine	7.4	320	Procaine; mannitol
Bretschneider's HTK	15.0	9.0	4.0	0	Histidine	7.3	310	a-ketoglutarate; tryptophan; mannitol
Roe's	27.0	20.0	3.0	0	Tham	7.6	347	Glucose
Extracellular crystalloid CP								
del Nido solution[††]	140	5	0.75	0	Bicarbonate	7.4	375	Lidocaine; mannitol
St. Thomas no. 1	144.0	20.0	32.0	4.8	None	5.5	285	Procaine
St. Thomas no. 2	110.0	16.0	32.0	1.2	Bicarbonate	7.8	324	None
Tyer's	138.0	25.0	3.0	1.0	Bicarbonate	7.8	275	Acetate; gluconate
Blood CP[†]								
Cold Induction	118.0	18.0	1.6	0.3-0.5	± Tham	7.6-7.8	320-340	Glucose; oxygen
Warm Induction	122.0	25.0	1.6	0.15-0.25	± Tham	7.5-7.6	340-360	Glucose; oxygen; glutamate; aspartate

Composition[*]

[*]Values are expressed in milliequivalents per liter unless otherwise note.
[†]The blood cardioplegia composition when delivered in a blood to crystalloid solution ratio of 4:1. CP = Cardioplegia.
[††]History and use of del Nido cardioplegia solution at Boston Children's Hospital. Matte GS, et al. J Extra Corpor Technol. 2012.

underwent cardiac surgery with potassium-induced arrest as the primary form of myocardial protection.[69] In 1977, Tyers and colleagues demonstrated that potassium cardioplegia provided satisfactory protection in over 100 consecutive cardiac patients.[70] By the 1980s, normothermic aortic occlusion had been replaced for the most part by cold blood cardioplegia to protect the heart during cardiac surgery. The major controversy at the time was not whether cardioplegic solutions should be used, but what was the ideal composition. The chief variants consisted of (1) the Bretschneider solution (containing primarily sodium, magnesium, and procaine); (2) the St. Thomas solution (consisting of potassium, magnesium, and procaine added to Ringer's solution); and, (3) potassium-enriched solutions containing no magnesium or procaine (Table 16-2). Coincident with this controversy, another variant of cardioplegia was introduced, that is, the use of potassium-enriched blood cardioplegia.[71,72] Theoretically blood cardioplegia would be a superior delivery vehicle based on its oxygenating and buffering capacity. Ironically, Melrose and colleagues had initially used blood as the vehicle to deliver high concentrations of potassium citrate more than 20 years earlier. While hypothermia and potassium infusions remain the cornerstone of myocardial protection today, a variety of cardioprotective techniques and solutions are used

which allow patients to undergo heart operations with excellent 30-day outcomes.[73,74]

CARDIOPLEGIC TECHNIQUE

Cardioplegic surgery techniques utilize solutions containing a variety of chemical agents that are designed to arrest the heart rapidly in diastole, create a quiescent operating field and provide reliable protection against ischemia/reperfusion injury. While contemporary cardiac surgery in low-risk patients is relatively safe, patient characteristics have been changing over the past decade. In addition to coronary heart disease and poor ventricular function, patients are presenting with more comorbidities such as obesity, diabetes, renal dysfunction, peripheral vascular disease and emphysema. Despite ongoing improvements in cardioplegic techniques, low cardiac output syndrome (LCOS) still occurs after surgery and is a major factor associated with poor outcomes. In the absence of technical complications, the most common cause of postoperative LCOS is inadequate myocardial protection. For this reason, there is a real need to develop more effective strategies and novel additives to existing cardioplegic solutions. Currently there are two types of cardioplegic solutions that are used: *crystalloid cardioplegia* and *blood cardioplegia*. These solutions are administered most frequently under hypothermic conditions.

Crystalloid Cardioplegia

One of the first cardioplegic solutions used to protect the heart during surgery consisted of a cold crystalloid formulation. It was developed on the premise that its administration would protect the heart by reducing its metabolism and aid the surgeon by providing a bloodless field. Over the years a number of crystalloid cardioplegic solutions have been developed which contain different ingredients. The rationale for these ingredients has been based on the need to: (a) induce a rapid cardiac arrest using potassium or magnesium; (b) reduce energy demand and conserve ATP reserves using hypothermia; (c) maintain intracellular ionic and metabolic homeostasis; (d) lower myocardial oxygen consumption; (e) enhance anaerobic and aerobic energy production utilizing glucose and amino acids; (f) stabilize the pH using bicarbonate, phosphate, or histidine buffers; (g) stabilize cellular membranes by using steroids, oxygen free radical scavengers such as glutathione, calcium antagonists and/or procaine; (h) avoid intracellular calcium overload by providing a hypocalcemic environment and adding magnesium; and (i) prevent cellular edema by the addition of colloids such as mannitol to maintain normal oncotic pressures.

There are basically two types of crystalloid cardioplegic solutions: the intracellular type and the extracellular type.[91] Both types can be used as preservation solutions for organ transplantation. The intracellular types are characterized by absent or low concentrations of sodium and calcium. The extracellular types contain relatively higher concentrations of sodium, calcium and magnesium. Both types avoid concentrations of potassium >40 mmol/L (typical range is 10-40 mmol/L), contain bicarbonate for buffering and are osmotically balanced. Examples of various crystalloid cardioplegic solutions are shown in Table 16-2.

OPERATIVE PROCEDURE

While the degree of core cooling varies from center to center, patients undergoing CPB are cooled to between 33 and 28°C. To initiate immediate chemical arrest after cross-clamping the aorta, the solution is infused through a cardioplegic catheter inserted into the aorta proximal to the cross-clamp. The catheter may or may not be accompanied by a separate vent cannula. The cold hyperkalemic crystalloid solution is then infused (antegrade) at a volume that generally does not exceed 1000 mL. One or more infusions of 300 to 500 mL of the cardioplegic solution may be administered if there is evidence of resumption of electrical heart activity or if a prolonged ischemic time is anticipated. If myocardial revascularization is being performed, the aortic cross-clamp can be removed after completing the distal anastomoses and the heart reperfused while the proximal anastomoses are completed using a partial occlusion clamp. Alternatively, the proximal grafts can be performed after the distal grafts have been completed with the cross-clamp still in place (the single-clamp technique). Another approach is to perform the proximal aortic grafts first with a partial occlusion clamp and then cross-clamp the aorta and infuse the cardioplegic solution. When valve repair or replacement is being performed, the crystalloid cardioplegia can be administered directly into the coronary arteries via cannulation of the coronary ostia. Crystalloid cardioplegia also can be administered retrograde via a coronary sinus catheter with or without a self-inflating silicone cuff.

OUTCOMES

Although there is a concern that crystalloid cardioplegia lacks blood components and therefore has a limited oxygen carrying capacity, this has not been shown to be clinically relevant. Likewise while there is preclinical evidence that hyperkalemic crystalloid cardioplegia may damage coronary vascular endothelium and impair the ability of endothelial cells to replicate and produce endothelial derived factors, this has not been shown to be of clinical significance.[92,93] In fact, there are numerous clinical studies which demonstrate that crystalloid cardioplegia is as effective as blood cardioplegia, particularly in centers where it is the primary form of protection.[94,95]

Blood Cardioplegia

Cold blood cardioplegia, widely employed throughout the world, is the cardioplegic technique used most often in the United States. The rationale for using blood as a vehicle for hypothermic potassium-induced cardiac arrest is that it (a) provides an oxygenated environment and a method for intermittent reoxygenation of the heart during arrest; (b) limits hemodilution when large volumes of cardioplegic solution are used; (c) affords an excellent buffering capacity and osmotic properties; (d) allows for electrolyte composition and pH that are physiologic; (e) offers a number of endogenous antioxidants and free-radical scavengers; and (f) is less complex to prepare than other solutions.

Although there are a variety of formulations it is usually prepared by combining autologous blood, obtained from the extracorporeal circuit while the patient is on CPB, with a crystalloid cardioplegic solution that consists of citrate-phosphate-dextrose (CPD) buffered with tris-hydroxymethylaminomethane or bicarbonate and supplemented with potassium chloride. The CPD is used to lower the ionic calcium, and the buffer is used to maintain an alkaline pH at approximately 7.8. The final concentration of potassium used to arrest the heart is approximately 20 to 25 mEq/L. After the initial induction dose for rapid arrest, subsequent administrations may be intermittent or continuous and utilize a concentration of 8 to 10 mEq/L (the low concentration maintenance dose).[96,97] (Table 16-2)

Prior to administering blood cardioplegia, the temperature of the solution usually is lowered with a heat-exchanging coil to between 12 and 4°C. The ratio of blood to crystalloid varies among centers with the most common ratios being 8:1,

4:1, and 2:1; this in turn affects the final hematocrit of the blood cardioplegia infused. For example, if the hematocrit of the autologous blood obtained from the extracorporeal circuit is 30, these ratios would result in a blood cardioplegia with a hematocrit of approximately 27, 24, and 20, respectively.

The use of undiluted blood cardioplegia, or "miniplegia" (using a minimum amount of crystalloid additives), also has been reported to be effective. Petrucci et al studied the use of all-blood miniplegia in a clinically relevant swine preparation and compared miniplegia with crystalloid cardioplegia. They concluded that the use of all-blood miniplegia was effective or superior in the acutely ischemic heart.[98] Velez and colleagues used an acute ischemia/reperfusion canine preparation to test the hypothesis that an all-blood cardioplegia in 66:1 blood:crystalloid ratio would provide superior protection compared with a 4:1 blood cardioplegia delivered in a continuous retrograde fashion.[99] They found very little difference between the animal groups with respect to infarct size or postischemic recovery of function. This is consistent with the findings by Rousou and colleagues years earlier; that, it is the level of hypothermia that is important in blood cardioplegia not necessarily the hematocrit.[100]

With respect to efficacy, there are numerous preclinical studies and nonrandomized and randomized clinical trials that demonstrate cold blood cardioplegia is an effective way to provide excellent myocardial protection. Many of these same studies have suggested that cold blood cardioplegia is superior to cold crystalloid cardioplegia. It is important to note that other investigators have shown crystalloid cardioplegia to be as cardioprotective and cost-effective if not more so. Unfortunately, most contemporary clinical trials comparing the efficacy of blood cardioplegia with crystalloid cardioplegia have involved single-center studies, enrolled a limited number of patients, focused on a specific subset of patients and/or omitted details regarding clinical management. In 2006, Guru et al reported the results of a meta-analysis of 34 clinical trials that compared blood cardioplegia to crystalloid cardioplegia. A lower incidence of low cardiac output syndrome and CK-MB release was observed in patients administered blood cardioplegia; no difference, however, was observed in the incidence of perioperative MI or mortality.[101] Jacob et al (2008) analyzed clinical data from 15 randomized trials. Although eight of the trials reported statistically significant outcomes favoring blood cardioplegia, and five showed differences in enzyme release, the bulk of the evidence favoring one over the other was inconclusive.[95]

In 2014, Zeng performed a meta-analysis of 12 randomized control trials in which cold blood cardioplegia was compared to cold crystalloid cardioplegia.[102] The trials accounted for 2866 patients: 1357 received cold crystalloid cardioplegia; 1509 received cold blood cardioplegia. The analysis showed no significant differences in mortality risk, incidence of fibrillation or stroke. The incidence of perioperative MI was lower however in the patients receiving cold blood cardioplegia. Regardless, the authors concluded that both crystalloid and cold blood cardioplegia are safe and effective for revascularization. The limitations of the study include the inherent problems associated with meta-analyses, and mortality was assessed only at the end of 30 days.

Warm Blood Cardioplegia

The concept of using warm (normothermic) blood cardioplegia as a cardioprotective strategy dates back to the 1980s. Proponents held that warm blood cardioplegic solutions would provide nutrients and endogenous factors that were absent in crystalloid solutions, and that normothermia would avoid possible adverse consequences of hypothermia. In 1982, Rosenkranz and colleagues reported that warm induction with normothermic blood cardioplegia, followed by maintenance of arrest with multi-dose cold blood cardioplegia, resulted in better recovery of function in canines than a similar protocol using cold blood induction.[103] In 1986, Teoh and colleagues provided experimental evidence that a terminal infusion of warm blood cardioplegia before removing the cross-clamp (a "hot shot") accelerated myocardial metabolic recovery.[104] This was followed by a report in 1991 by Lichtenstein and colleagues that normothermic blood cardioplegia in humans is an effective cardioprotective approach.[86] They compared the results of 121 consecutive patients undergoing CABG surgery who received antegrade normothermic blood cardioplegia to a historical group of 133 patients who received antegrade hypothermic blood cardioplegia. The operative mortality in the warm cardioplegic group was 0.9% compared with 2.2% for the historical controls. Despite these encouraging reports, there are concerns that for any given patient, it is difficult to determine how long a warm heart can tolerate an ischemic insult if the infusion is interrupted or flow rates are reduced owing to an obscured surgical field or maldistribution of the cardioplegic solution. Another concern is the report by Martin and colleagues that warm cardioplegia is associated with an increased incidence of neurologic deficits.[52] In a prospective, randomized study conducted in 1001 patients, the efficacy of continuous warm blood cardioplegia with systemic normothermia (≥35°C) versus intermittent cold oxygenated crystalloid cardioplegia and moderate systemic hypothermia (≤28°C) were compared. While operative mortalities were similar (1.0 vs 1.6%, respectively), the incidence of permanent neurologic deficits was threefold greater in the warm blood normothermic group (3.1 vs 1.0%). Thus in this study warm blood cardioplegia offered no advantage over cold crystalloid cardioplegia in terms of myocardial protection and carried with it the risk of increased ischemic injury if the oxygen supply to the warm heart was interrupted.

In 2014, DeBryn and colleagues performed a retrospective review of a prospectively collated database to compare the relative efficacies of using either antegrade warm blood cardioplegia (32°C) or antegrade cold crystalloid cardioplegia (7°C).[105] The database included patient demographics, preoperative risk factors, operative technique, postoperative course and 30-day, in-hospital morbidity and mortality. The first 150 patients received cold crystalloid cardioplegia; the second group of 143 patients received cold blood cardioplegia.

Overall the investigators found the clinical outcome for the patients was comparable and concluded that while warm blood cardioplegia is safe; it did not confer superior protection. Thus it appears that appropriately designed protocols using intermittent antegrade warm blood cardioplegia provide clinically acceptable myocardial protection.[106-108]

Tepid Blood Cardioplegia

Both cold blood (4-10°C) and warm blood cardioplegic solutions (37°C) have temperature-related advantages and disadvantages. As a consequence, a number of studies were performed in the 1990s to determine the optimal temperature. Hayashida and colleagues were one of the first groups to study the efficacy of tepid blood (29°C) cardioplegia.[109] In this study, 72 patients undergoing CABG were randomized to receive cold (8°C) antegrade or retrograde, tepid (29°C) antegrade or retrograde, or warm (37°C) antegrade or retrograde blood cardioplegia. While protection was adequate for all three, the tepid antegrade cardioplegia was the most effective in reducing anaerobic lactate acid release during the arrest period. These authors reported similar findings when the tepid solution was delivered continuously retrograde and intermittently antegrade.[110] In contrast, Baretti et al reported in anesthetized open-chest swine placed on CPB that tepid normokalemic continuous antegrade blood cardioplegia was associated with an increased incidence of intermittent fibrillation.[111] Subsequent to this report Mallid et al, in a retrospective chart review, analyzed the effects of cold blood and warm or tepid blood cardioplegia on early and late outcomes in 6064 patients who underwent CABG surgery. In the patients receiving warm or tepid blood cardioplegia (n = 4532), the systemic temperature was maintained between 32 and 37°C. The temperature of warm blood cardioplegia was 37°C. In the tepid cardioplegia cohort the systemic temperature was allowed to drift between 32 and 34°C; the temperature of the tepid cardioplegia ranged between 28 and 30°C. In the cold blood cardioplegia cohort (n = 1532) the systemic temperature was maintained between 25 and 32°C; the temperature of the blood cardioplegia ranged between 5 and 8°C. At 5 years, actuarial survival was 91.1% in the warm cardioplegia group and 89.9% in the cold blood cardioplegia group (p = .09). While this study has all the limitations associated with a large retrospective chart review conducted over the course of a decade, the findings are consistent with the basic conclusion that current methods of cardioplegia all show similar degrees of efficacy. To date, most tepid blood cardioplegia studies have been single-center studies conducted in relatively small cohorts of patients. Whether tepid cardioplegia confers superior protection over other methods remains to be determined. For the most part, however, the current methods of cardioplegia all show similar efficacy.

Methods of Delivery

In addition to a variety of formulations and temperatures, there are also many different ways of administering the

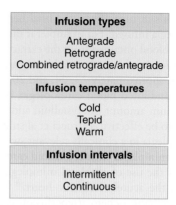

Infusion types
Antegrade
Retrograde
Combined retrograde/antegrade

Infusion temperatures
Cold
Tepid
Warm

Infusion intervals
Intermittent
Continuous

FIGURE 16-3 Methods for delivering cardioplegic solutions.

cardioplegic solutions (Fig. 16-3). As one might expect with so many options, the optimal delivery method also remains controversial. The various methods include intermittent antegrade, antegrade via the graft, continuous antegrade, continuous retrograde, intermittent retrograde, antegrade followed by retrograde and simultaneous antegrade and retrograde infusions. While all methods appear to be similarly efficacious, comparisons across trials are difficult because the studies also have differed with respect to: (1) the composition of the solution; (2) the temperature of the solution; (3) the duration of the infusion; and, (4) the infusion pressure. Additional factors that affect a surgeon's choice for delivery method include the type and complexity of the operation and the anticipated cross-clamp time.

ANTEGRADE CARDIOPLEGIA

The most widely used method of delivering cardioplegic solutions is the antegrade method. It entails infusion of the solution into the aortic root while the ascending aorta is cross-clamped. After the initiation of CPB, chemical arrest can be achieved quickly with the infusion of the solution through a catheter inserted into the aorta proximal to the cross-clamp. The catheter may or may not be accompanied by a separate vent cannula to decompress the left ventricle between infusions. The induction dose usually has a higher concentration of potassium than subsequent maintenance doses. It is infused rapidly to ensure aortic valve closure usually at a rate of 250 to 300 mL/min (10 and 15 mL/kg body weight/min). If cardiac activity persists or recurs additional infusions may be necessary. For maintenance, infusions can be administered at 15 to 20 minute intervals or as needed. Concurrent external cooling can be achieved by suffusion with cold saline (4°C).

The typical aortic root perfusion pressure is maintained between 60 mm Hg and 80 mm Hg. Adjustments in rates of administration are made to accommodate patients with hypertrophied ventricles. Intermittent maintenance doses of 300 to 500 mL of low-dose cardioplegia are administered every 15 to 20 minutes or earlier if there is evidence of resumption of electrical activity. During CABG surgery, in order to minimize cold ischemia and aortic cross clamp time, the heart can be reperfused earlier by removal of the aortic cross-clamp as soon as the distal anastomoses are completed; the proximal anastomoses are then performed using a partial occlusion clamp. Alternatively the proximal grafts can be performed after the distal grafts have been completed with the cross-clamp still in place (the single-clamp technique).

The administration of antegrade cardioplegia depends on a competent aortic valve and hence is liable to be ineffective and relatively contraindicated in patients with significant aortic valve incompetence. In such cases, antegrade cardioplegia can be administered directly into the coronary arteries via cannulation of the individual coronary ostium. This technique is used in cases requiring the opening of the ascending aorta such as in aortic valve replacement, ascending aortic aneurysm repair and aortic root replacement procedures. Coronary ostial infusion may be necessary for induction in patients with severe aortic incompetence in the presence of coronary sinus pacing leads. Potential complications include coronary dissection, unintentional selective delivery into left anterior descending or left circumflex artery due to a short left main coronary artery, and the late occurrence of coronary ostial stenosis.[112]

RETROGRADE CARDIOPLEGIA

Retrograde cardioplegia entails placement of a coronary sinus catheter with or without a self-inflating silicone cuff and infusion of the cardioplegic solution either for induction or maintenance of cardioplegia. This approach originated with a concept developed by Pratt in 1898, who suggested that oxygenated blood could be supplied to the ischemic heart via the coronary venous system.[113] Sixty years later, Lillehei and colleagues used retrograde coronary sinus perfusion to protect the heart during aortic valve surgery.[76] Today, it is an accepted method for delivering a cardioplegic solution and is used frequently as an adjunct to antegrade cardioplegia. Placement of the catheter is often facilitated by the use of catheters that are precurved and the simultaneous use of transesophageal echocardiography to guide placement. Care must be taken to avoid rupture of the coronary sinus, an uncommon but real and potentially fatal complication. This can be prevented by infusing the solution at a rate that ensures that the coronary sinus perfusion pressure does not exceed 45 to 50 mm Hg. The retrograde approach can be used for continuous or intermittent delivery of blood or crystalloid cardioplegia as well. In situations where the native coronary arteries are severely stenotic or totally occluded, the antegrade approach may result in an uneven distribution in the myocardium. In this situation retrograde infusion or infusion via the vein grafts as they are completed can be complementary. While most routine on-pump cardiac procedures can be done with good outcomes using just the antegrade technique, patients with poor ventricular function, high-risk patients requiring long aortic cross clamp times and those with occlusive coronary disease may benefit from a dual approach, that is, both antegrade and retrograde techniques. Another advantage to the retrograde technique is that it may be effective in reducing the risk of embolization from saphenous vein grafts that could occur

during antegrade perfusion for reoperative coronary artery bypass surgery. The retrograde approach also has the theoretical advantage of ensuring a more homogeneous distribution of the cardioplegic solution to regions of the heart that are poorly collateralized.

Despite these advantages, retrograde cardioplegia is not without its limitations. There are experimental and clinical studies which suggest that cardioplegia administered via the coronary sinus results in a suboptimal distribution of cardioplegia to the right ventricle. This is due in part to the anterior region of the right ventricle being poorly drained by the coronary sinus, the marked variability in venous anatomy, the frequency of coronary sinus anomalies and the Thebesian veins draining directly into the cavities of the heart. As a consequence a number of studies have been performed to evaluate not only the safety and efficacy of the retrograde approach but also to compare its efficacy to a combined antegrade/retrograde approach.[114-117] While the findings have been mixed, most of results have shown that retrograde delivery of cardioplegic solutions is safe and effective during cardiac surgery. Taking a different approach, Bhaya et al compared the efficacy of an antegrade approach with an integrated antegrade/retrograde method in patients undergoing on pump heart surgery using three-dimensional transthoracic speckle tracking echocardiography.[118] Twenty-two patients were studied one day prior to surgery and 4 to 5 days after the operation. They found that the integrated approach conferred better protection in terms of maintenance of strain parameters in segments of the septum and free wall of the left ventricular free wall and septum. These findings support the general consensus that a combined approach allows for a more reliable homogeneous distribution of cardioplegic solutions. The combined approach may be most relevant when it is anticipated that the cross-clamp time will be long and/or when the coronary artery stenoses are particularly extensive and severe.

CONTINUOUS CARDIOPLEGIA VERSUS INTERMITTENT CARDIOPLEGIA

To minimize the interruption of coronary flow during aortic cross-clamping, cardioplegia can be administered continuously using a retrograde coronary sinus catheter or cannulating the coronary ostia directly via an open aortic root. A continuous infusion, especially if it is oxygenated, has the theoretical advantage of minimizing ischemia particularly during periods of prolonged aortic cross-clamping. One of the first studies to test this assumption was by Louagie and colleagues.[119] Seventy patients undergoing CABG surgery were prospectively randomized to receive retrograde cold blood cardioplegia either intermittently (n = 35) or in a continuous fashion (n = 35). Hemodynamic measurements included right ventricular ejection fraction, cardiac output, left and right ventricular stroke work index and systemic and pulmonary vascular resistance. Coronary sinus blood samples were obtained before aortic cross-clamping and immediately after unclamping for the measurement of lactate and hypoxanthine levels; venous blood samples were collected at predetermined times to measure CK-MB and troponin levels.

Overall, they found a trend for better hemodynamics and a lower use of inotropic agents and significantly lower lactate and hypoxanthine levels in the patients who received continuous retrograde cardioplegia. On the other hand there were no differences in patient outcomes, and the CK-MB and troponin levels were comparable postoperatively. Given this was a single-center study, the surgery was performed by the same surgeon, and the relatively small sample size, it is difficult to extrapolate the findings to the general population of patients undergoing cardioplegic surgery with aortic cross-clamping. To date it remains unclear as to whether continuously administered cardioplegia is superior to intermittent cardioplegia. The major advantage of using intermittent cardioplegia is the ability to achieve and sustain a dry, quiescent operative field. Moreover, continuous cardioplegia still necessitates interruption of the surgical steps while the infusion is delivered.

Current Status of Cardioplegic Technique

In summary, controversy persists as to whether blood cardioplegia or crystalloid cardioplegia is better, which temperature is ideal and what is the best method of delivery. A survey of practice patterns in the United Kingdom in 2004 showed that 56% of all cardioplegia on-pump surgery was performed with cold blood cardioplegia; whereas, warm blood cardioplegia was used in 14% of cases.[120] In the same survey, 14% of surgeons used crystalloid cardioplegia, 21% used retrograde cardioplegia and 16% did not use any cardioplegia, preferring to use cross-clamp fibrillation only. Based on these observations and experiences in the United States, it appears that most surgeons favor cold intermittent blood cardioplegia. Nevertheless a wide spectrum of variation exists among heart centers; there is no international consensus regarding the ideal cardioplegic solution or its use.[120] Awareness of the options allows the surgeon to utilize the best approach that meets the individual needs of the patient.

Noncardioplegic Technique

Intermittent cross-clamping with fibrillation (ICCF) and systemic hypothermia with intermittent elective fibrillatory arrest are the most common forms of noncardioplegic heart surgery used today. The objective is to provide a relatively quiescent surgical field without having to arrest the heart with a cardioplegic solution.

Intermittent Aortic Cross-Clamping with Fibrillation

This technique is the earliest method developed to protect the heart during surgery and is still used at many centers. The patient is placed on CPB, the ascending aorta is cannulated and generally a dual-stage single-venous cannula is used. Often the patient is cooled to 30 to 32°C; this technique allows the surgeon to operate in a relatively quiet but not quiescent field during ventricular fibrillation. In the setting of CABG surgery, the aortic cross-clamp is removed intermittently after the

completion of each graft. The duration of fibrillation is determined by how long it takes to perform the distal anastomosis. After completion of the revascularization, the heart is defibrillated and the proximal anastomoses performed on the beating heart using an aortic partial occlusion clamp. This technique is particularly useful in patients with cold agglutinin disease, an autoimmune phenomenon in which antibody directly agglutinates human red cells at low temperatures. In these patients open heart operations with hypothermia carry the risk of red cell agglutination and may result in hemolysis, MI, renal insufficiency and cerebral damage.

As a result of increasing pressures to reduce cost and yet maintain acceptable levels of cardioprotection, there remains an interest in using this approach. There are a number of reports which indicate that satisfactory protection can be conferred using this technique. In 1992, Bonchek et al reported a large clinical series in which the advantages and safety of this technique were meticulously analyzed.[121] In this study, the authors reviewed the outcomes of the first 3000 patients at their institution who underwent primary CABG using ICCF. Preoperative risk factors, for example, age, gender, left ventricular dysfunction, preoperative use of the intra-aortic balloon pump (IABP), the urgency of operation and operative deaths were analyzed. In this series, 29% of the patients were older than 70 years of age, 27% were females, 9.7% had an ejection fraction of less than 0.30, 13% had an MI less than 1 week preoperatively and 31% had preinfarction angina in the hospital; only 26% underwent purely elective operations. Using the noncardioplegic cardioprotective technique, the authors reported an elective operative mortality rate of 0.5%, an urgent mortality rate of 1.7% and an emergency rate of 2.3%. Postoperatively, inotropic support was needed in only 6.6% of the patients, and only 1% required insertion of the IABP. It is important to note however that this was a retrospective, single-center institutional experience. The findings would have been enhanced if the analysis had included a similarly matched group of patients at the same institution in which cardioplegic arrest had been employed. Nevertheless the findings support the perspective that noncardioplegic strategies can provide satisfactory myocardial protection even in high-risk patients.

In 2002, Raco and colleagues reported their experience in 800 consecutive CABG operations performed by a single surgeon using ICCF in both elective and nonelective settings. The patients were divided into three cohorts: (1) elective; (2) urgent; and, (3) emergent. Among these cohorts the mean age, number of distal grafts and mortality among the three groups was comparable. The mortality rate in the elective, urgent and emergent groups was 0.6%, 3.1%, and 5.6%, respectively, and consistent with outcomes associated with cardioplegic surgery. Since this report reflects the experience of a single surgeon, there is the concern that the technique may not be generally applicable. Regardless, the findings do support the notion that ICCF is a safe technique for both elective and nonelective patients undergoing CABG surgery.[122-124] In 2003, Bonchek et al reported their experience in 8300 patients who underwent CABG surgery without cardioplegia. The unadjusted mortality rates in elective, urgent and emergent patients was 0.9%, 1.5%, and 4.0%, respectively. The overall mortality of 1.7%, was considerably lower than the 3.27% predicted based on the Society of Thoracic Surgeons National Database model.[125] This experience represented the work of five surgeons, three of whom had not been trained in noncardioplegic surgery; it provides additional evidence that ICCF is an effective form of cardioprotection. Evidence that the cardioprotective effects of ischemic preconditioning (IPC) may contribute to the efficacy of ICCF in the human heart has resulted in an interest in using this method of protection especially in the United Kingdom. Results in animal studies indicate that the protective effect of ICCF is blocked by protein-kinase C inhibitors and K_{ATP} channel antagonists, both of which have been implicated in the signaling pathways involved in IPC.[126] Regardless of the mechanism underlying the protection, there are numerous reports which indicate that noncardioplegic strategies such as ICCF can provide satisfactory myocardial protection even in high-risk patients.[127]

Systemic Hypothermia and Elective Fibrillatory Arrest

Elective fibrillatory arrest is another safe approach to protect the heart during noncardioplegic heart surgery. The use of systemic hypothermia (26-30°C) and maintenance of systemic perfusion pressure between 80 and 100 mm Hg are key elements. This approach is particularly applicable in the setting of the severely calcified "porcelain aorta," where clamping the aorta may be associated with increased risk of stroke and aortic dissection. Under these circumstances the distal anastomoses are performed locally occluding the coronary artery using vascular clamps or sutures. The proximal anastomoses can be completed during short periods of hypothermic circulatory arrest. Alternatively the proximal anastomoses can be based entirely on an in situ internal thoracic artery. Using this approach one can avoid manipulation of the aorta altogether. Akins and colleagues, in 1984, reported a low incidence of perioperative MI and a low hospital mortality rate in 500 consecutive patients using this technique.[84] In 1987, Akins and Carroll assessed the late results of hypothermic fibrillatory arrest in 1000 consecutive patients undergoing nonemergent CABG surgery. They concluded that the technique is effective and yields excellent event-free survival. Potential disadvantages include (1) the surgical field may be obscured as a result of existing collateral circulation; (2) ventricular fibrillation may be associated with increased muscular tone and thus compromise the surgeon's ability to position the heart for optimal exposure; (3) aortic valvular regurgitation may be exacerbated; and (4) it is generally not applicable for intracardiac procedures. An advantage with the technique is that it can be used when aortic occlusion or cardioplegic arrest is undesirable, for example, in the setting of a calcified ascending aorta. This approach can also be used in patients undergoing mitral valve surgery.[128] Imanaka et al, in 2003, published a retrospective observational study in which mitral valve surgery was performed in 27 patients with ischemic mitral regurgitation using perfused ventricular fibrillation.

Concomitant procedures included CABG in 23 patients and the Dor procedure in five patients. Surgery was performed using moderate hypothermia (~28°C) and fibrillatory arrest; flow rates on bypass were maintained at 2.4 L/min/m² and the perfusion pressure was 70 mm Hg. Among these select patients the mortality rate was 3.7%. The authors concluded that extended periods of ventricular fibrillation during hypothermic surgery can be well-tolerated without excessive morbidity and mortality and is appropriate in patients in whom aortic cross-clamping is unsuitable or the duration of cross-clamping is expected to be long.[129]

Strategies for Cardioprotection under Investigation

There are currently a number of physiological processes and pharmacological agents known to confer protection against I/R injury in the experimental setting. Several clinical trials are underway to determine the relevance of these new approaches. The purpose of this section is to review the cardioprotective strategies that are being examined and hold promise for the future.

Physiological Processes

ISCHEMIC PRECONDITIONING

"Preconditioning with ischemia is an endogenous adaptive phenomenon whereby the heart becomes more tolerant to a period of prolonged ischemia if first exposed to brief episodes of coronary artery occlusion. This adaptation to ischemia was first described by Murry and colleagues and is now referred to as *'classic,' 'first window'* or *'early phase' ischemic preconditioning (IPC)*.[85] IPC is associated with a reduction in infarct size, apoptosis, and reperfusion-associated arrhythmias and has been demonstrated in every animal species studied to date. It lasts for as long as 1 to 2 hours after the preconditioning stimulus.[130-132] It is ineffective when the sustained ischemic insult lasts for more than 3 hours; thus, protection is conferred only when the sustained ischemia is followed by timely reperfusion. Subsequent studies have revealed that this endogenous defense mechanism manifests itself in several ways. After the acute phase of preconditioning disappears, a second phase of protection appears 24 hours later and is sustained for up to 72 hours. This is referred to as the *'second window of protection,' 'late-phase' preconditioning*, or *'delayed' preconditioning*. Late phase preconditioning protects against MI and stunning unlike classic IPC which only protects against infarction."[133,134]

Cellular Mechanisms Underlying IPC. Reports of adaptation to ischemia led to major investigative efforts to elucidate the intracellular mechanism(s) underlying the heart's endogenous defenses against I/R injury. The assumption was, and still is today, that a better understanding of these mechanism(s) would lead to the development of potent new therapeutic modalities that would be more effective in treating or preventing the deleterious consequences of I/R injury.

One of the earliest hypotheses was that the primary mediator of IPC was the activation of the adenosine A_1 and/or A_3 receptors on the cardiomyocyte.[132,135] Subsequent studies have shown that in addition to adenosine, there are multiple guanine nucleotide-binding (G) protein-coupled receptors that once activated can mimic the infarct-sparing effect of ischemic preconditioning. These include bradykinin, endothelin, α_1-adrenergic, muscarinic, angiotensin II, and delta-opioid receptors (Fig. 16-4). The infusion of exogenous agents to mimic ischemic preconditioning is referred to as pharmacologic preconditioning. Exactly which of these receptors is the most important in mediating endogenous preconditioning is unknown because there appear to be species differences and redundant signaling pathways. Regardless, it is now thought that these triggers of IPC result in activation of various tyrosine kinases, isoforms of PKC, p38 mitogen-activated protein kinases and extracellular signal-regulated kinases (ERKs)]. P38 mitogen-activated protein kinases

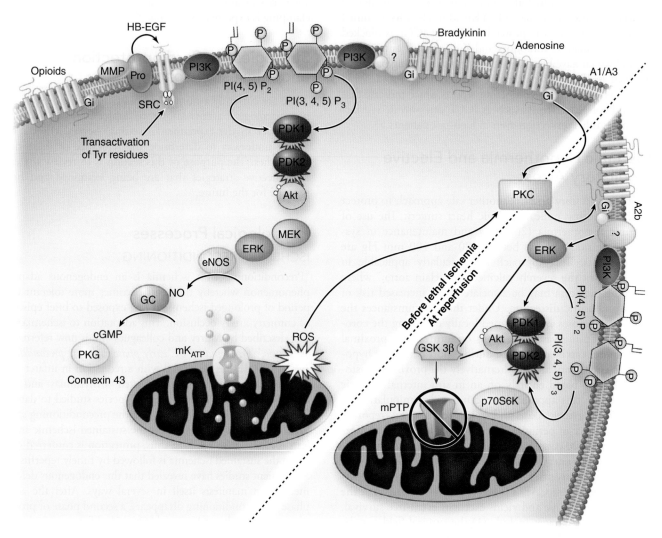

FIGURE 16-4 Signaling pathways of ischemic preconditioning (IPC). IPC, ischemic preconditioning; MMP, matrix metalloproteinases; HB-EGF, heparin-binding epidermal growth factor; Pro, Pro-HB-EGF; PI3, phosphatidylinositol 3-kinase; $PI_{4,5}P_2$, phosphatidylinositol bisphosphate; $PI_{3,4,5}$, P_3, phosphatidylinositol trisphosphate; MEK, mitogen activated protein kinase kinase; ERK, extracellular-signal regulated kinase; NO, nitric oxide; NOS, NO synthase; eNOS, endothelial NOS; GC, guanylyl cyclase; PKG, protein kinase G; PKC, protein kinase C; ROS, reactive oxygen species; mK_{ATP}, mitochondrial ATP-dependent potassium channel; p70SK6 kinase; GSK-3β, glycogen synthase kinase; mPTP mitochondrial permeability transition pore; PDK, phosphoinositide-dependent kinase. Numerous triggers (opioids, bradykinin, and adenosine) and intracellular signaling pathways are involved in the cardioprotection conferred by IPC. The signal transduction pathways are complex, interactive, and include the HB-EGF receptor, PI3K, Akt, ERK1/2, eNOS, PKG, the opening of the mK_{ATP} channel, ROS production, PKC activation, p70 S6 kinase, and GSK-3β. Possible end effectors of IPC include the opening of the mK_{ATP} channel and inhibition of the mitochondrial transition pore opening. If only a few mitochondria are affected, cytochrome c may be released and induce apoptosis and cause cell death at a later time. Recent evidence suggests a unique role for the adenosine A2b receptor when activated at the time of reperfusion. While the process of autophagy has been implicated in IPC-induced cardioprotection where and how this process interacts with the signaling pathways remains to be determined.

are a family of serine/threonine protein kinases that are responsive to various stress stimuli cytokines, include heat shock protein, and are involved in cell differentiation, apop- and autophagy. The ERK cascade couples signals from cell surface receptors to transcription factors which regulate gene expression.

Interestingly, IPC-induced cardioprotection appears to require repopulation of receptors and activation (or, in some instances, reactivation) of "pro-survival" kinases upon relief of sustained ischemia. In this regard, Hausenloy and Yellon introduced the term "Reperfusion Injury Salvage Kinase" (RISK) pathway to represent the PI3K-Akt and ERK1/2 prosurvival kinases activated at the time of reperfusion and proposed that manipulation and upregulation of the RISK pathway may represent another approach to myocardial protection.[136]

While the identity of the end effector(s) of IPC remain speculative, significant evidence has accumulated indicating that the cardiomyocyte mitochondria are key targets of conditioning-induced protection (Fig.16-4).[137,138] Specifically, inhibition of mPTP and the opening of the mitochondrial K_{ATP} (mK_{ATP}) channels have been implicated as the effectors of IPC.[139,140] Under normal conditions the mitochondrial inner membrane is impermeable to most metabolites and ions, and the mPTP is closed. While the molecular structure of the pore has yet to be determined, it is characterized by the formation of a large conductance megachannel, which is regulated by cyclophilin D in the matrix.[140a] While early investigations implicated the voltage-dependent anion channel in the outer mitochondrial membrane and the adenine nucleotide translocator (ANT) in the inner membrane in addition to cyclophilin D, genetic studies have refuted that model. Mouse models in which all ANT isoforms were deleted still exhibited mPTP opening; this was also the case for deletion of voltage-dependent anion channel (VDAC) isoforms. However, deletion of cyclophilin D resulted in hearts that were much more resistant to I/R injury, and further studies revealed that although the threshold for mPTP opening was greatly increased, it was still possible to trigger pore opening. It was concluded that cyclophilin D plays an important regulatory role in mPTP opening, but the molecular composition of the pore remains uncertain. Under conditions of stress, the mPTP may open resulting in depolarization of the inner mitochondrial membrane and an influx of water and ions into the matrix due to its high oncotic pressure. Matrix swelling expands the highly folded inner membrane but ultimately ruptures the outer membrane resulting in release of cytochrome *c* and other proapoptotic factors. Even in the absence of outer membrane rupture, loss of mitochondrial membrane potential results in ATP hydrolysis by the F_0-F_1 ATP synthase in a futile effort to restore membrane potential, thereby accelerating energy depletion.

An ATP-sensitive potassium channel in the mitochondrial inner membrane (mK_{ATP}) has been implicated on the basis of pharmacologic effects of diazoxide and pinacidil (channel openers) and 5-hydroxydecanoate and glibenclamide (channel closers). Many pharmacologic studies have demonstrated

a protective role for the putative mK_{ATP}, although its molecular composition also remains unknown. Garg and Hu have proposed that PKC activation enhances the import of plasma membrane K_{ATP} channels into mitochondria.[141] This was based on their observation that in COS-7 cells, Kir6.2 protein (a subunit of K_{ATP} channels) and channel activity increased in mitochondria after PMA treatment, and this increase was inhibited by the selective PKC inhibitor chelerythrine. Pharmacologically triggered opening of the mK_{ATP} channel has been shown to reduce calcium overload, mitochondrial ROS production, swelling, and to preserve ATP levels after ischemia/reperfusion.

While early-phase preconditioning shares many of the same signaling mechanisms with late-phase preconditioning, the most obvious difference between the two is the apparent requirement for protein synthesis in the latter. Late-phase IPC has been shown to be associated with the upregulation of various proteins including but not limited to heat-shock proteins, inducible NOS (iNOS), cyclooxygenase 2, heme-oxygenase and manganese superoxide dismutase.[142,143] There are however conflicting reports on what specific proteins are upregulated during late-phase preconditioning, which may be due to species differences as well as stimulus-specific responses.

Clinical Relevance of IPC. There is evidence that ischemic preconditioning occurs in the human being. Investigators have reported that patients experiencing angina prior to an MI have a better in-hospital prognosis and a reduced incidence of cardiogenic shock, fewer and less severe episodes of congestive heart failure and smaller infarcts as assessed by cardiac enzyme release.[144] Moreover, follow-up studies suggest that patients who have had angina prior to an infarct have better long-term survival rates.[145-147] There are also a myriad of reports that patients who undergo PCIs have an enhanced tolerance to ischemia after the first balloon inflation provided that the first balloon inflation exceeds 60 to 90 seconds.[131] Chest pain severity, regional wall motion abnormalities, ST-segment elevation, QT dispersion, lactate production and CK-MB release all have been reported to be attenuated in this setting as well.[148,149]

In patients undergoing PCI, a preconditioning-like effect has been mimicked by the administration of a variety of pharmacologic agents that are known to induce preconditioning in animal studies. For example, the administration of adenosine prior to PCI has been reported to attenuate myocardial ischemic indices during the first balloon inflation.[150] Administration of other agents, such as bradykinin and nicorandil (a K_{ATP} channel opener), also have been reported to produce similar effects.[151,152] Conversely the administration of aminophylline (a nonselective adenosine receptor antagonist), glibenclamide (a K_{ATP} channel blocker), or naloxone (an opioid receptor blocker) reportedly abolish the effects of ischemic preconditioning during PCI.[153,154] Additional studies provide evidence of delayed pharmacologic preconditioning in the clinical setting. Leesar and colleagues reported that a 4-hour intravenous infusion of nitroglycerin (an NO donor)

24 hours prior to PCI decreased ST-segment, changed and reduced chest pain during the first balloon occlusion compared with patients treated with saline vehicle.[155] An earlier report by this same group indicated that delayed preconditioning with nitroglycerin decreased exercise-induced ST-segment changes and improved exercise tolerance. Thus there are observational studies that support the hypothesis that myocardial protection conferred by ischemic preconditioning and its possible mediators in animal studies is translatable to humans. It is important to note however that classic or early ischemic preconditioning observed in animals is associated with a reduction in infarct size, but not protection against stunning, and that many of the clinical studies are either retrospective in nature or have used surrogate markers of injury as end points.

With respect to a role for IPC during cardiac surgery, numerous small trials have been conducted.[156] One of the first studies was conducted by Yellon and colleagues in patients undergoing CABG surgery.[157] Patients were subjected to a protocol that involved two cycles of 3 minutes of global ischemia. The aorta was cross-clamped intermittently and the heart was paced at 90 beats per minute to induce ischemia. This was followed by 2 minutes of reperfusion before a 10-minute period of global ischemia and ventricular fibrillation. Myocardial biopsies were obtained during the 10-minute period of global ischemia, and ATP tissue content was measured. The results showed that the ATP levels in the biopsies obtained from patients subjected to the preconditioning-like protocol were higher. However, since ATP content is not a marker of necrosis, a follow-up study was performed, and troponin T serum levels were measured. In this study the investigators reported that troponin release was attenuated in the patients subjected to the preconditioning protocol. In 2002, Teoh and colleagues reported that IPC conferred myocardial protection beyond that provided by intermittent cross-clamp fibrillation in patients undergoing CABG.[89] While other investigators reported similar findings, most of these studies have involved small numbers of patients.

In 2008, Walsh et al reported the results of a meta-analysis of the available small trials to determine the effect of IPC on patient outcomes.[156] They identified 22 eligible trials encompassing 933 patients; there were 374 patients in the IPC cohort and 402 patients served as controls. Twenty of the trials followed a protocol that involved aortic cross-clamping, and two involved coronary artery occlusion. The primary endpoint was perioperative mortality; the secondary endpoints included incidence of postoperative ventricular arrhythmias and MIs, the need for postoperative inotropic support and stroke. While the results suggested IPC was associated with a reduction in the incidence of ventricular arrhythmias, inotropic requirements and admissions to the critical care units and the incidence of perioperative MI and death was the same between the two cohorts. The investigators were appropriately cautious in the interpretation of the data considering the many caveats including bias and heterogeneity in relation to the endpoints. Given the low mortality rate in both groups,

the study was markedly underpowered to discern an effect on the primary endpoint, that is, death.

Thus despite a number of surgical studies that suggest IPC is effective in the setting of aortic cross-clamping and the administration of cardioplegia, it is important to note that the total number of patients studied to date is relatively small, and the outcomes have been limited to surrogate markers of myocardial necrosis, viz., CK-MB levels and troponin release and not definitive endpoints such as perioperative MI and death. In addition to the inherent risk of neurological complications associated with manipulation of the ascending aorta, the absence of compelling clinical outcomes may explain why IPC has not been adopted as an adjuvant approach among the myocardial protection techniques employed to date. A more promising strategy may evolve however once a better understanding of the intracellular events and effectors that confer protection have been elucidated.

Postconditioning. The phenomenon of ischemic "postconditioning" (PostCond) was first reported by Zhao et al in the canine model.[158] The term refers to rapid intermittent interruptions of blood flow in the early phase of reperfusion, that is, relief of ischemia in a stuttered or staccato manner. While the cellular mechanisms underlying PostCond are poorly defined, they appear to involve many of the same signal transduction pathways that are involved in IPC including cell surface receptor signaling, prosurvival kinases, inhibition of mPTP and activation of the mK_{ATP} channel. Although the duration and frequency of ischemia/reperfusion cycles may differ across studies, for the most part the cycles that induce PostCond are measured in seconds in smaller species and slightly longer in larger animals and humans, justifying the name "stuttering reperfusion." The reduction in infarct size appears to be comparable to that observed with IPC. Preclinical studies conducted in multiple models and species (including dog, rat, rabbit, mouse, and pig) have demonstrated a reduction in infarct size that ranges from 20 to 70%. The restoration of blood flow in a stuttering manner during early reperfusion is of major interest to clinicians since it holds particular promise for patients presenting with an acute MI. In the surgical setting PostCond could be applied in the operating room after release of the aortic cross-clamp.

Evidence that PostCond exists in humans was first reported in patients undergoing PCI. Patients receiving brief balloon inflations/deflations in the initial minutes of reperfusion during PCI exhibited smaller ST-segment changes and lower levels of total creatine kinase release compared with patients that were not subjected to stuttering reperfusion. In 2007, Darling et al conducted a retrospective chart review in patients undergoing emergent cardiac catheterization for ST segment elevation MI (STEMI).[159] The hypothesis was that outcome would be better in patients undergoing multiple balloon inflations after primary angioplasty. Patients were divided into two cohorts: those who, at the discretion of the interventional cardiologist, received one to three balloon inflations and those in whom four or more inflations were applied. In this retrospective analysis, peak CK release was less in patients requiring ≥4 inflations. In a separate study by Lønborg et al, the cardioprotective effects of PostCond in patients treated with PCI was evaluated using magnetic resonance imaging (MRI).[160] These investigators reported that mechanical PostCond appeared to be independent of the size of myocardium at risk. The findings were consistent with the concept that stuttering reperfusion confers cardioprotection during percutaneous interventions.

In the context of heart surgery, Luo reported a beneficial effect of surgical PostCond in 24 patients undergoing repair for tetralogy of Fallot at the time of aortic declamping. The postconditioning protocol consisted of aortic reclamping for 30 seconds and declamping for 30 seconds; the process was repeated twice. The intervention was reported to reduce perioperative troponin-T and CK-MB release and decreased the need for inotropic support after surgery.[161] A similar finding was reported by the same investigator in a study of adult patients undergoing valve surgery and children undergoing corrective surgery using cardioplegia. Thus there is evidence that a PostCond protocol may benefit patients undergoing heart surgery, albeit the majority of studies suggesting a beneficial effect have been conducted in the setting of percutaneous interventions. While PostCond may offer more promise than IPC in terms of clinical application, it is important to note that both are invasive in nature. Ideally, the elucidation of the cellular mechanisms underlying ischemic conditioning will lead to pharmacological approaches that would obviate the need for invasive approaches.

Remote Ischemic Preconditioning. Remote ischemic preconditioning (RIPC) is a phenomenon whereby brief ischemia of one organ or tissue confers protection on a distant naive organ or tissue against a sustained ischemia-reperfusion injury. RIPC was first described by Przyklenk and colleagues in 1993.[162] In the original study the investigators questioned whether IPC protected only heart cells exposed to brief coronary artery occlusions or was it possible that repetitive or stuttering occlusions in a remote naive vascular bed could reduce infarct size in the area subjected to prolonged ischemia. They used a canine preparation in which a branch of the circumflex coronary artery was subjected to four episodes of 5-minute occlusion and reperfusion; this was followed by 1-hour occlusion of the left anterior descending (LAD) coronary artery. After 4.5 hours of reflow, infarct size in the distribution of the LAD was measured. Indeed a marked reduction in infarct size was observed. Since then numerous other investigators have confirmed these findings, and the phenomenon has been observed in various species and with different organs. Brief occlusions of the renal and mesenteric arteries and brief restriction of blood flow to the skeletal muscle of the lower limb have also been reported to reduce myocardial infarct size.[163] As a consequence, RIPC is also referred to as inter-organ preconditioning.

Not surprisingly, multiple mechanisms trigger RIPC is signaled through neuronal signaling and multiple secreted factors (such as adenosine, bradykinin and calcitonin gene-related peptide) followed by activation of multiple kinases including p38 mitogen-activated phosphokinase (p38 MAPK), extracellular signal-regulated kinase 1/2 (ERK1/2)

and c-Jun N-terminal kinase (JNK). One way by which the remote preconditioning signal may be conveyed to the target organ is through exosomes. These membrane-bound nanoparticles contain proteins, mitochondrial RNAs (mRNAs) and microRNAs which are taken up by target cells and elicit a response.[164] As with many other cardioprotective interventions, lack of a clear understanding of the molecular basis of the phenomenon has not dampened the enthusiasm for applying the approach clinically.

One of the first studies involving surgery was conducted in 17 children undergoing congenital heart surgery with CPB.[165] Brief intermittent lower limb ischemia attenuated troponin release and the need for postoperative inotropic support. Hausenloy et al reported a similar finding in 57 patients undergoing CABG.[166] Patients were randomized to RIPC or no treatment; all patients also received cardioprotection by either intermittent cross-clamping or cardioplegia. Perioperative troponin-T release was reduced by 43% in the RIPC group. In another study involving 23 adult patients undergoing on-pump CABG surgery and cold blood cardioplegia, RIPC was associated with a 42% reduction in total troponin-T release.[167] In this study, RIPC was induced by three 5-minute cycles of right forearm ischemia by inflating a blood pressure cuff on the upper arm to 200 mm Hg with an intervening 5-minute reperfusion period; the control group had a deflated cuff placed on the upper arm for 30 minutes.

In 2013, Thielmann et al reported the results of a prospective single-center double-blind randomized controlled study in 329 CABG patients. Patients underwent surgery preceded by RIPC (n = 162) or not (n = 167). Patient demographics and perioperative data were comparable between the two groups. Postoperative troponin I levels were significantly lower in the RIPC group. At 4-year follow-up, all-cause mortality and major adverse cardiac and cerebrovascular events were less frequent; however, this did not reach significance because the study was underpowered, given the low mortality rate. This is one of the first studies to examine the clinical benefit of RIPC beyond the biochemical markers of myocardial damage. The findings parallel other studies of patients undergoing PCI electively or for ST-segment-elevation MI.[168,169] Not all studies have shown that RIPC improves clinical outcomes after surgery. To examine the effects of RIPC combined with remote ischemic PostCond (RIPostCond), Hong and colleagues prospectively randomized 1280 CABG surgery patients to receive RIPC plus RIPostCond or no conditioning.[170] The protocol consisted of four cycles of 5-minute ischemia and 5-minute reperfusion administered to the upper limb prior to initiating CPB and repeated after CPB. The primary endpoints were a reduction in major adverse events including MI, stroke and death. Treatment had no effect on mortality or the incidence of cardiac or neurological complications. Of concern, the subgroup of off-pump patients that received RIPC plus RIPostCond had an increase in composite adverse events, notably increased RBC transfusions. The impact of the study was limited by the heterogeneity of procedures and the exclusion of patients with poor ventricular function; however it did raise concern regarding clinical efficacy of RIPC and RIPostCond.

Taken altogether, these RIPC studies led to the RIPHeart Study and the ERRICA trial.

In the RIPHeart Study, the objective was to assess the efficacy of remote ischemic preconditioning (RIPC) in reducing the composite endpoint of death, MI, stroke or acute renal failure in patients undergoing CABG surgery.[170a] Patients were randomized to undergo RIPC (n=692) induced by four 5 min cycles of transient upper limb ischemia/reperfusion or a control group (n=693) receiving four cycles of blood pressure cuff inflation/deflation in an imitation arm. In this study RIPC treatment had no effect on the composite endpoint or on any of the subgroup analyses. The incidence of postoperative MI was similar for the two groups, viz., 6.8% in the RIPC arm and 9.1% in the placebo group.

The ERICCA Trial[170b] was a multicenter, sham-controlled study in which the clinical relevance of RIPC. Patients undergoing on-pump CABG with blood cardioplegia were randomized to a RIPC group (n=801) or a control group (n=811). RIPC was induced with four 5-minute inflations and deflations of a standard blood-pressure cuff on the upper arm prior to surgery. The combined endpoint was death from cardiovascular causes assessed at 12 months. In this study, RIPC had no effect on the primary endpoint or any of the secondary end points of perioperative myocardial injury. As a consequence of these studies, for now, it appears that RIPC will not become a therapeutic modality in the routine practice of cardiac surgery.

Conditioning by Stem Cells and Cell Products. While stem cells have been explored for treatment of tissue loss after MI or in the setting of chronic heart failure, most studies have focused on endpoints months to years out, based on the expectation that stem cells function by regenerating tissue. However, recent work suggests they may be beneficial in the acute setting.[171] Marbán and colleagues used cardiosphere-derived cells (CDCs) delivered via intracoronary infusion 30 minutes after onset of reperfusion in a porcine model of MI. They found that the CDC infusion resulted in lower troponin I levels at 24 hours and decreased infarct size and microvascular obstruction at 48 hours. In isolated perfused rat hearts, an infusion of mesenchymal stem cells pre-stimulated with transforming growth factor alpha (TGF-alpha) before ischemia resulted in improved functional recover and reduced inflammation and cell death.[172] A conditioned medium from human mesenchymal stem cells was shown to reduce infarct size and improve function in pigs subjected to MI.[173] The same group subsequently showed that the active component of the conditioned medium was exosomes.[174] Exosomes derived from an immortalized allogenic stem cell line offer a number of advantages for clinical development including standardization of the material, longer shelf life and availability for all patients without the need for histocompatibility matching. Thus cell therapy may be eclipsed by exosomes, and both approaches hold promise for intraoperative myocardial protection.

Autophagy. In the heart, adaptive autophagy is an endogenous protective response to cardiac stress. It plays an important

role in cardiovascular disease, neurodegeneration, and cancer. Studies are now underway to harness its cardioprotective potential and, based on this process, develop effective cardioprotective therapies to protect the heart against I/R injury. Autophagy is the process whereby a double-membrane structure called the autophagosome sequesters cytoplasmic components such as ubiquitinated protein aggregates or organelles including mitochondria, peroxisomes and endoplasmic reticulum. It is involved in degradation of long-lived proteins and the removal of excess or damaged organelles. The outer autophagosomal membrane fuses with a lysosomal membrane, resulting in degradation of the cargo by lysosomal hydrolases; the resulting macromolecules are exported to the cytosol for reuse[175] (Fig. 16-5).

One of the first studies to suggest autophagy is an adaptive process responsive to stress in the heart was the report by Decker et al in which they noted an increase in degenerating mitochondria and autophagosomes in rabbit hearts subjected to hypoxia and reoxygenation.[176] Reperfusion restored contractility, and the injured myocytes underwent a cellular repair process that involved a marked increase in lysosomal autophagy. They concluded that autophagy was part of a repair response to hypoxic stress in the heart. Upregulation of autophagy has been described in cell models of hypoxia/reoxygenation and models of I/R injury in rodents and pigs.[177-185] Hamacher-Brady et al showed that upregulation of autophagy in HL-1 myocytes protected against cell death induced by simulated ischemia reperfusion (sI/R) whereas inhibition of autophagy-enhanced cell death.[177] Dosenko et al also found that inhibition of autophagy exacerbated cell death during anoxia-reoxygenation.[178] Matsui et al showed that glucose deprivation increased the number of autophagosomes in neonatal cardiac myocytes, whereas inhibiting autophagy enhanced cell death.[179] In a porcine model of chronic myocardial ischemia and hibernating myocardium, Yan et al reported that cardiac myocytes with enhanced autophagy were not apoptotic; in contrast, apoptotic cells did not show features of autophagy.[180] Collectively these studies suggest that upregulation of autophagy promotes survival during I/R.

There is now direct evidence that autophagy plays an important role in mediating ischemic and pharmacologic preconditioning. Using HL-1 cells and adult rat cardiomyocytes, Yitzhaki et al showed that the adenosine preconditioning agent 2-chloro-N(6)-cyclopentyladenosine (CCPA) upregulated autophagy within 10 minutes of adenosine treatment and inhibition of autophagy resulted in significant loss of cytoprotection against hypoxia/reoxygenation injury. Autophagy was also shown to be important for delayed preconditioning in this cell-based model.[181] Multiple cardioprotective agents including CCPA, sulfaphenazole and chloramphenicol, as well as ischemic preconditioning, also upregulate autophagy in vivo.[182-185] Based on these findings, it appears that autophagy is an important mediator of protection in the heart.

Autophagy in the Human Heart. Delineating the role of impaired autophagy in heart patients is challenging because of the need to access tissue. One of the first studies to suggest

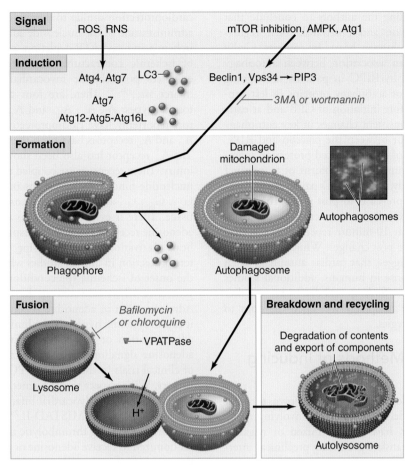

FIGURE 16-5 Cellular process of autophagy. Adapted from Gottlieb RA, Finley KD, Mentzer Jr RM: Cardioprotection requires taking out the trash. *Basic Res Cardiol* 2009; 104:169-180. I/R, ischemia/reperfusion; ROS, reactive oxygen species; RNS, reactive nitrogen species; mTor, mammalian target of rapamycin; AMPK, AMP-activated protein kinase; LC3, light chain 3-phosphatidylethanolamine; Atg1, Atg4, Atg7, Atg12, Atg16L, autophagy regulating proteins; Vps34, a class III PI3 kinase involved in vesicular trafficking, nutrient signaling, and autophagy; PIP3, phosphatidylinositol 3,4,5-trisphosphate; 3MA, 3-methyladenine. Autophagy is a dynamic adaptive process in the setting of I/R injury. The process involves the synthesis of a cup-shaped pre-autophagosomal double-membrane structure which surrounds cytoplasmic material and closes to form an autophagosome. This process is regulated by the autophagy proteins Atg4, Atg7, LC3, and the complex of Atg12-Atg5-Atg16L. The process is activated by a number of stimuli including ROS or RNS. Induction by Beclin1 and Vps34 in conjunction with other Atg proteins results in the formation of an isolation membrane to which Atg proteins are recruited. Atg12-Atg5 and LC3 proteins are involved in the expansion of the membrane. This allows the phagophore to surround and engulf damaged organelles or protein aggregates which may accumulate as a result of I/R injury. The result is the formation an autophagosome. The green insert shows autophagosomes (green puncta). This photo was obtained in a cell expressing a fusion protein of green fluorescent protein (GFP) fused to the N-terminus of LC3; the GFP-LC3 was incorporated into the double-membrane structure of the phagophore. Wortmannin and 3 MA are agents that can inhibit the initiation phase of autophagy; bafilomycin and chloroquine can inhibit the degradation phase.

that autophagy is an adaptive process in the human heart was the report by Kassiotis et al.[186] Biopsies of the left ventricle were obtained from nine patients with idiopathic dilated cardiomyopathy at the time of implantation and removal of left ventricular assist devices. Autophagy-related mRNAs and proteins were downregulated after prolonged circulatory support leading the authors to conclude that autophagy is an adaptive mechanism in the human heart. Garcia et al studied 170 patients who had undergone elective CABG and preoperatively were in normal sinus rhythm.[187] Intraoperative right atrial biopsies revealed that autophagic vesicles and lipofuscin deposits and biochemical markers of impaired autophagic flux were more commonly observed in the biopsies of the

patients who developed postoperative atrial fibrillation suggesting that loss of normal autophagic activity may increase the risk of postoperative arrhythmias. Jahania et al reported the results from 19 patients in which atrial biopsies were collected just prior to the onset of CPB and again after removal of aortic cross-clamp and weaning from CPB. Ischemic stress was associated with a significant depletion of autophagy-related proteins suggestive of a coordinated engagement of the autophagy machinery.[188] Consistent with this, Singh et al examined mRNA and protein in samples taken from right atrial appendages before cardioplegic arrest and after reperfusion.[189] I/R was associated with upregulation of several autophagy-related genes and biochemical evidence of increased autophagy, leading the authors to conclude that I/R affects gene expression and posttranslational regulation of autophagy in the human heart. In contrast, Gedik et al[190] failed to detect an association between autophagy and protection conferred by RIPC in patients undergoing CABG surgery. Analysis of autophagy proteins in left ventricular biopsies taken before initiation of CPB and at early reperfusion showed no consistent changes in key autophagy proteins either with I/R or between the placebo and RIPC cohorts, despite evidence of RIPC-induced protection manifest as a reduction in serum cardiac isoform of troponin I (cTnI). In the Jahania study, each patient's paired results were reported as a ratio from pre-CPB to post-CPB. The Gedik study reported the mean baseline (before cross-clamp) compared to the mean value at 10-minute reperfusion and may have missed individual pre-post changes. While the majority of observations to date suggest that cardiac autophagy is an active and adaptive response in humans, additional studies are needed to confirm these findings and determine whether enhancement of adaptive autophagy will open the door to new cardioprotective strategies.

Pharmacological Methods of Inducing Protection

A number of pharmacological agents are known to limit I/R injury in animal models. Clinical trials involving many of these agents, however, have yielded mixed or negative results.[191] The failure to translate promising preclinical interventions and agents into effective clinical therapies prompted the National Heart Lung and Blood Institute to convene a panel of experts in 2011 to discuss the reasons for failure and to develop a series of recommendations designed to move the field of myocardial protection forward.[192] The working group concluded that future preclinical cardioprotection studies should concentrate on relevant animal models that reflect human comorbid conditions such as atherosclerosis, hypercholesterolemia, hypertension, diabetes, and advanced age. The panel also suggested that cardioprotective candidates for future clinical development should have demonstrated efficacy in multiple independent preclinical studies involving rodent and large-animal models. Early-stage clinical trials to evaluate safety of the most promising candidates should also show efficacy based on surrogate markers. In addition to cardiac enzymes, advances in MRI make it possible to assess infarct size,[193] ischemic and pharmacologic preconditioning, postconditioning, remote postconditioning, sodium-hydrogen exchange inhibitors, adenosine analogs, and cyclosporine A have shown promise in studies using healthy young animals but have not been adequately evaluated in animal models with comorbidities such as obesity or age. The purpose of this section is to review the status of several of these treatments that have been studied clinically.

ADENOSINE

There is considerable preclinical evidence that activation of various adenosine receptor subtypes results in cardioprotection similar to that induced by IPC. Preischemic administration of the nucleoside adenosine retards the rate of ischemia-induced ATP depletion, prolongs the time to onset of ischemic contracture, attenuates myocardial stunning, enhances postischemic myocardial energetics and reduces infarct size.[194,195] There are four distinct adenosine receptor sub-types: A_1, A_{2a}, A_{2b}, and A_3. While all of the receptors reportedly have cardioprotective properties, agonists of A_1, and A_{2a} receptors have been the most widely investigated. The A_{2b} receptor has also been shown to protect against I/R injury. These receptors are coupled to heterotrimeric guanine nucleotide-binding (G) proteins in which the subtype (G_o, $G_{i\alpha2}$, $G_{i\alpha3}$, G_q, and G_s) varies according to the receptor and tissue. There is evidence that two and possibly three of the adenosine receptor subtypes are expressed in the adult human heart. Activation of the adenosine A_1 and A_{2a} receptors confers protection in animal studies when administered prior to the onset of ischemia (preconditioning); the A_{2b} receptor is protective when activated at the time of reperfusion.[196-199] Administration of adenosine is complicated by the fact that it causes systemic hypotension, limiting the use of prolonged administration or higher doses. Evidence that extracellular adenosine signaling can be protective has led to a number of clinical trials in the setting of PCI for acute MI and heart surgery. With respect to the former, two particularly intriguing ones are Acute Myocardial Infarction Study of Adenosine (AMISTAD-I) and AMISTAD-II.[200-202] In AMISTAD-I, 236 patients undergoing thrombolytic therapy for acute MI were randomized to receive adenosine or placebo within 6 hours of the onset of infarction. The primary endpoint was infarct size by technetium-^{99m} sestamibi (single-photon emission computed tomography, SPECT); secondary endpoints included myocardial salvage index and a composite endpoint comprising death, reinfarction, shock, congestive heart failure (CHF), and stroke. In this study, there was a 67% relative reduction in infarct size in patients with anterior infarction; however, there was no reduction in patients with infarcts located elsewhere. It may be easier to detect an effect on infarct size if the area at risk is larger, which is often the case when the LAD coronary artery is involved. Although there was a trend toward achieving the composite secondary endpoint, there were no significant differences in clinical outcome between the two groups. This led to the AMISTAD-II trial. In this study, 2118 patients with evolving anterior infarcts and receiving thrombolysis or primary angioplasty were randomized to receive placebo or a low or high dose of adenosine. The primary composite endpoint consisted of new CHF, first rehospitalization for CHF, or death at 6 months. In a subset of patients (n = 243), infarct size was measured by SPECT. In this study, adenosine therapy had no effect on clinical outcomes; it did demonstrate however that, as in AMISTAD-I, adenosine treatment resulted in a dose-related reduction in infarct size. At the higher dose, a 57% relative reduction in infarct size was observed. A likely explanation for the divergence between reduced infarct size and yet no effect on outcomes is that the study was underpowered to show clinical improvement. The significance of these two studies however is that for the first time there was evidence that a pharmacologic agent—specifically adenosine—could reduce infarct size when administered at reperfusion.

Other adenosine studies, however, failed to show efficacy. Desmet et al reported the effects of a high-dose intracoronary bolus of adenosine administered just prior to PCI. Patients were randomized to receive adenosine (4 mg) or placebo; infarct size was assessed using MRI. Four months later there was no evidence of infarct scar reduction or a decrease in microvascular obstruction by MRI.[203] Fokkema et al also evaluated the effect of high-dose adenosine given as intracoronary boluses on infarct size in patients with acute STEMI. Patients (n = 448) were randomized to receive placebo (n = 222) or two bolus injections of intracoronary adenosine (2 × 120 μg in 20 mL saline) (n = 226). The first bolus was administered after thrombus aspiration, and the second was given after stenting the infarct-related artery. In this study, adenosine treatment had no effect on infarct size as determined by CK and CK-MB or Thrombolysis In Myocardial Infarction (TIMI) flow.[204] A major limitation of both studies was the mode of administration. The half-life of adenosine in blood is measured in seconds; the retrospective inference is that a single or double bolus injection of adenosine is too short-lived to confer protection.[191]

With respect to adenosine and cardiac surgery, most of the studies have been relatively small as well. Fremes and colleagues reported the results of an open-label, nonrandomized CABG surgery study in which adenosine administration was combined with antegrade warm blood cardioplegia. The adenosine concentrations studied were 15, 20, and 25 μm. These investigators reported that adenosine could be added safely as a supplement to cardioplegic solutions, but it had no effect on myocardial function at the doses studied.[205] Cohen and colleagues observed a similar lack of efficacy in a phase II double-blind, placebo-controlled trial performed in patients undergoing CABG surgery. Patients were treated with placebo (saline) or warm blood cardioplegia supplemented with 15, 50, or 100 μm adenosine. These investigators found that adenosine did not alter survival, the incidence of MI or the incidence of low cardiac output syndrome. A limitation of this study was the use of low concentrations of adenosine in the setting of warm blood cardioplegia. In blood, the nucleoside is metabolized rapidly to inosine and hypoxanthine; its half-life is measured in seconds, thus limiting its potential effect.[206]

A beneficial effect was observed by Mentzer and colleagues, however, in an open-label, single-center study in which the safety, tolerance, and efficacy of high doses of adenosine were studied when added to cold blood cardioplegia in CABG surgery patients.[207] Sixty-one patients were randomized to receive standard cold blood cardioplegia or cold blood cardioplegia containing one of five adenosine doses ranging between 100 μm and 2 mm. Invasive and noninvasive studies of myocardial function were obtained sequentially after bypass. Parameters included the recording of inotropic utilization rates for the postoperative treatment of low cardiac output. Blood samples were collected for the measurement of nucleoside levels. High-dose adenosine treatment achieved a 249-fold increase in the plasma adenosine concentration and was associated with a reduction in postbypass inotropic drug utilization, improved regional wall motion and global function measured by transthoracic echocardiography.

Subsequently, Mentzer and colleagues examined the effects of high-dose adenosine treatment in 253 CABG surgery patients randomized to one of three treatment arms. This was a double-blind, placebo-controlled multicenter trial using cold blood cardioplegia. Adenosine was administered in three different doses and rates. Invasive and noninvasive measurements of ventricular performance were obtained before, during and after surgery. The study revealed a trend toward the decreased need for high-dose inotropic support and fewer perioperative MIs in the high-dose adenosine group, but it was underpowered to show an effect on any single endpoint. A post hoc composite outcome analysis revealed that patients who received high-dose adenosine were less likely to experience the composite endpoint of high-dose dopamine and epinephrine use, insertion of an intra-aortic balloon pump, MI, or death.[208]

In 2001, Wei et al[208a] initiated a prospective randomized, controlled study in 30 patients undergoing elective CABG surgery and CPB to investigate the effect of adenosine pretreatment on myocardial recovery and inflammatory response. Patients received a 7-minute infusion of adenosine prior to the initiation of CPB (n = 15); outcomes were compared to a second group of patients (n = 15) who did not receive the infusion. CPB was initiated 3 minutes after cessation of the adenosine infusion. Cold blood cardioplegic solution was infused antegrade retrograde during the period of aortic cross-clamping, and warm blood retrograde cardioplegia was administered at the end of cross-clamping. Postoperative CK-MB, perioperative leukocyte counts and various cytokines were measured. CK-MB levels were lower and the cardiac index was better in the adenosine-treated cohort. Leukocyte counts and cytokine levels were unaffected. The authors concluded that adenosine treatment was protective, but its mechanism of action was independent of effects on inflammation.

In contrast, Ahlsson et al did not detect a beneficial effect with adenosine added to cold blood cardioplegia administered continuously in patients undergoing isolated aortic valve replacement.[209] In this study, 80 patients were randomized into four groups: Group I—antegrade cardioplegia with adenosine (n = 19); Group II—antegrade cardioplegia with placebo (n = 21); Group III—retrograde cardioplegia with adenosine (n = 21); and Group IV—retrograde cardioplegia with placebo (n = 19). Adenine nucleotide content and lactate were determined from left ventricular biopsies obtained before aortic occlusion, after bolus cardioplegia, at 60 minutes of aortic occlusion and at 20 minutes after release of the aortic occlusion. CK-MB and troponin-T were measured at 1, 3, 6, 9, 12, and 24 hours after aortic occlusion. Hemodynamic profiles were obtained before surgery and 1, 8, and 24 hours after CPB. In this study, investigators observed that retrograde blood cardioplegia was associated with a higher myocardial oxygen uptake and lactate accumulation than antegrade, but the addition of adenosine to cardioplegia showed no benefit.

In summary, it is still not clear whether adenosine is beneficial in the setting of heart surgery. It is possible that this conundrum will be solved with the development of receptor-selective adenosine analogs that confer protection without causing systemic hypotension.

SODIUM-HYDROGEN EXCHANGER INHIBITORS

The sodium-hydrogen exchangers (NHEs) are a family of membrane proteins with nine isoforms that are involved in the transport of hydrogen ions in exchange for sodium ions. NHE-1 is the isoform that is expressed in the heart and most likely plays a minor role in the normal excitation-contraction coupling process. As discussed in the section, Intracellular Mechanisms of Ischemia/Reperfusion Injury, NHE-1 contributes to calcium overload and cell death. In the setting of I/R injury, NHE-1 contributes to arrhythmias, stunning, apoptosis, necrosis, postinfarction ventricular remodeling and heart failure.[210,211] In the context of heart surgery, there have been a number of small clinical trials to test whether inhibition of NHE-1 can prevent I/R injury. EXPEDITION was a phase III trial to address the safety and efficacy of NHE-1 inhibition by cariporide in the prevention of death or MI in patients undergoing CABG surgery. High-risk CABG patients (n = 5770) were randomized to receive either intravenous cariporide or placebo. The composite endpoint was assessed at 5 days, and patients were followed for up to 6 months. The incidence of postoperative MI (which had very specific criteria involving EKG changes, CK-MB elevation, with or without chest pain) in this series of patients was 18%, much higher than previously thought. The results revealed an 18.3% relative risk reduction in the incidence of death or MI at 5 days (*p* = .0002). The relative risk reduction for death or MI at day 30 and month 6 was 16.1% (*p* = .0009) and 15.7% (*p* = .0006), respectively. When MI risk was analyzed separately, the relative risk reduction was 23.8% at 5 days (*p* = .000005) and 25.6% at month 6 (*p* = .000001). This cardioprotective effect was extremely robust; however, the overall mortality rate increased at 5 days from 1.5% in the placebo group to 2.2% in the group with cariporide, which was attributed to an increase in the incidence of cerebrovascular events. Thus, while cariporide was effective in reducing the incidence of nonfatal MI, it increased the risk of death from cerebrovascular events resulting in an unacceptable safety profile. In this study the drug was administered continuously for 49 hours beginning preoperatively, although no preclinical studies had examined the necessity or possible adverse effects of prolonged administration; the preclinical studies utilized a single bolus. Nevertheless this study was significant because it was the first Phase III study in heart surgery patients to clearly demonstrate that it is possible to pharmacologically protect the heart and reduce the incidence of perioperative MI. The findings also suggest that NHE-1 inhibitors represent a new class of drugs that hold promise for reduction of MI associated with I/R injury, provided it is possible to eliminate the risk of cerebrovascular events.[1,212] It is possible that some of the newer drugs in this class may be safer.

ACADESINE

Acadesine (also known as 5-aminoimidazole-4-carboxamide-1-β-D-ribofuranoside, AICA riboside) is a purine nucleoside analog which was thought to elevate tissue levels of adenosine selectively during ischemic conditions. Numerous preclinical studies demonstrated its cardioprotective efficacy, although it is not clear whether the protective effect is due to its effects on intracellular ATP synthesis, extracellular adenosine concentrations or its ability to activate AMP-activated protein kinase (AMPK) and thereby stimulate glucose uptake and autophagy.[213,214] Early preclinical studies indicated acadesine treatment improved left ventricular wall motion after intermittent ischemia, diminished the frequency of ventricular arrhythmias during reperfusion, attenuated myocardial stunning, and preserved myocardial function after cardiac arrest and cold cardioplegia. These observations led to several clinical trials in CABG surgery patients in the 1990s. The findings however were inconclusive due in part to the fact that they were underpowered. In 2006, Mangano performed a meta-analysis on the combined data from five trials comprising more than 4000 CABG patients to determine the effects of i.v. acadesine on the prespecified perioperative outcomes of MI, stroke, and cardiac death. In these five studies, acadesine was given intravenously prior to and during surgery along with a fixed concentration included in the cardioplegia solution. The meta-analysis concluded that acadesine was effective in reducing perioperative MI, cardiac death, and combined adverse cardiovascular outcomes.[215]

Mangano et al then examined the 2-year, all-cause mortality after perioperative MI in a follow-up of the Acadesine 1024 Trial. In this analysis, patients who received acadesine and had a postreperfusion MI had a significant fourfold reduction in mortality compared to the patients who had an MI but did not receive the drug (3/46 patients vs 15/54 patients, respectively).[216] This led to a large prospective randomized trial, Reduction in Cardiovascular Events by Acadesine in Patients Undergoing CABG (RED-CABG). High-risk CABG patients were randomized to receive either acadesine or placebo prior to the induction of anesthesia. The target enrolment was 7500 patients, and the primary composite endpoint was all-cause mortality, stroke and need for mechanical support for left ventricular failure. Midway into the study, a futility analysis indicated a low probability of detecting a statistically significant difference between treatment and placebo groups; the trial was terminated after 3080 patients had been enrolled.[217] In reviewing the outcome of RED-CABG the investigators acknowledged that planning a clinical trial based on a meta-analysis carries inherent risk. While the study was intended to enroll high-risk patients (a higher event rate would make it easier to discern a beneficial effect), it turned out that many of the patients were not high risk resulting in a lower than expected event rate (the composite endpoint). Because MI was an exploratory outcome rather than a primary endpoint, enzyme levels were determined only during the first 24 hours. Despite these caveats however, the investigators concluded that acadesine treatment had no effect of all-cause mortality, nonfatal stroke or need for mechanical circulatory support. This disappointing outcome makes it unlikely that acadesine will be the subject of further clinical investigation.

GLUCOSE-INSULIN-POTASSIUM

Numerous studies have shown that glucose-insulin-potassium (GIK) infusions are effective in reducing perioperative MIs, postischemic myocardial dysfunction and atrial fibrillation in patients undergoing heart surgery.[218] Increased glycolytic flux driven by glucose and insulin supplementation increases pyruvate generation and maintains the GSH/GSSG balance. Additionally glycolytic ATP protects membranes through stimulation of the Na^+/K^+-ATPase and supports uptake of Ca^{2+} by the sarcoplasmic reticulum. Provision of K^+ improves sodium homeostasis of ischemic myocardium.

Despite a strong rationale for its application, the efficacy of GIK in the setting of heart surgery remains controversial. The use of GIK to treat patients with acute MI yielded mixed results in the 1990s. Fath-Ordoubadi and Beatt performed a meta-analysis on 1932 patients in nine small trials of GIK for acute MI and found it was beneficial. It should be noted that none of the patients underwent reperfusion therapy (thrombolysis or primary PCIs).[219] In 2003, van der Horst reported the results of a randomized open label study in which 940 patients with acute MI and eligible for angioplasty received either continuous infusion of GIK or no infusion.[220] GIK infusion had no effect on overall patient mortality, but a significant reduction in mortality was observed in the subgroup of patients without evidence of heart failure (1.2% vs 4.2%). The investigators concluded that the effect of GIK infusion in patients with heart failure was uncertain. To confirm these findings, a folstudy, GIPS-II, was initiated in 2003. The purpose was to confirm clinical benefit of GIK in STEMI patients without signs of heart failure. Patients were randomized to traditional care or additional GIK infusion. The study, however, was terminated early due to lack of efficacy. It was concluded that GIK in adjunct to reperfusion therapy in STEMI patients does not lower mortality.[221]

In follow up to the Fath-Ordoubadi and Beatt meta-analysis in 1997,[219] Mamas et al reported the results of a meta-analysis of GIK therapy for the treatment of acute MI in 2010.[222] Unlike the previous meta-analysis, this study included patients who underwent reperfusion therapy. A total of 16 randomized trials accounting for 28,373 patients were identified between 1966 and 2008. These investigators failed to find any life benefit for GIK therapy in STEMI patients. The findings were consistent with the combined subgroup analysis of GIK therapy for acute MI in the OASIS-6 and CREATE-ECLA trials which also showed that GIK infusion had no effect on key clinical endpoints.[223]

It was hypothesized that the efficacy of GIK infusions depends upon how soon it is administered after the onset of ischemia. Selker and colleagues tested this hypothesis in the IMMEDIATE Trial in 2012.[224] GIK was administered to presumed MI patients prior to hospitalization with the expectation that it would slow the progression of MI or STEMI. Secondary endpoints included the incidence of cardiac arrest, mortality and heart failure. A total of 911 patients were randomized; 59 were not enrolled because they did not give written consent on arrival at the hospital. The investigators found that MI progression did not differ between the GIK and the placebo groups, and GIK administration had no effect on 30-day survival; however, GIK was associated with a lower rate of the composite endpoint of cardiac arrest and in-hospital mortality. Moreover, infarct size was smaller in the subgroup of GIK-treated patients who underwent cardiac imaging at 30 days. The investigators concluded that early GIK therapy did not alter MI progression but had a beneficial effect on the secondary composite endpoint and called for additional studies. One-year follow-up revealed no significant differences in outcome with the exception of patients with STEMI in which the composites of cardiac arrest or 1-year mortality, and of cardiac arrest, death or rehospitalization for heart failure were significantly reduced.[225] These findings have fueled discussions over the timing of administration, target populations and overall efficacy of GIK as a cardioprotective intervention for patients with acute MI.

Bruemmer-Smith et al reported that GIK infusion during surgery had no effect on myocardial cellular damage as measured by cTnI levels 6 hours after CPB and was associated with increased hyperglycemia. Although this was a randomized, prospective, double-blind study in CABG surgery patients and the two groups were well matched for age and number of bypassed vessels, the study was most likely underpowered, given that only 42 patients were enrolled.[226] In another study, Lell et al reported on 46 patients undergoing elective off-pump CABG surgery; the patients received either normal saline or a GIK infusion for 12 hours. These investigators were also unable to demonstrate a beneficial effect on cardiac performance using the clinical measurements of cardiac index and inotropic requirements. They noted persistent hyperglycemia—a known risk factor for postoperative complications—despite the use of supplemental insulin.[227] Lazar et al[228] conducted a study in diabetic CABG patients to determine whether GIK solution with tight perioperative glycemic control was more effective than standard glycemic control and no GIK. The rationale was that GIK with tight glycemic control would optimize myocardial metabolism and improve perioperative outcomes. The preoperative patient profiles of the 141 randomized patients were similar with respect to age, sex, ejection fraction, urgency of surgery and the type of diabetes. Although the 30-day survival was comparable in both groups, the patients receiving GIK plus tight control had significantly higher cardiac indices and less need for inotropic support. There was also a lower incidence of atrial fibrillation. Follow-up data 5 years later were available in 60 of 70 GIK patients (83.3%) and in 60 of 69 placebo patients (86.9%). Survival was significantly better in the patients who received GIK; the investigators attributed these long-lasting benefits to the perioperative GIK treatment, but it might also have been due to the careful glycemic control. In another study of patients with type-2 diabetes, Barcellos et al reported their findings in 24 patients who underwent CABG surgery. Patients were administered GIK or subcutaneous insulin from the onset of anesthesia until 12 hours postoperatively. The use of GIK neither improved the cardiac index nor reduced the use of inotropic agents.[229]

In another single-center study, Quinn et al conducted a prospective, randomized, double-blind, placebo-controlled trial in 280 nondiabetic CABG surgery patients.[90] They found that GIK treatment was associated with fewer episodes of low cardiac output, less inotropic support postoperatively and a reduction in serum cardiac troponin I levels. The authors concluded that GIK is an effective, inexpensive and safe cardioprotective adjunct.[90] Rabi et al conducted a meta-analysis of 20 clinical trials to determine the effect of GIK or glucose-insulin (GI) on in-hospital mortality and atrial fibrillation (AF).[230] They found that GIK/GI failed to significantly reduce mortality or AF in patients undergoing CABG surgery. The authors discouraged the routine use of GIK/GI in patients undergoing CABG surgery until future clinical trials provided sufficient evidence to warrant the practice. Fan et al, however, came to a different conclusion in their meta-analysis of 33 randomized clinical trials.[231] This analysis involved 2113 patients: 1150 were randomized to GIK and 963 served as a control group. Most of the studies were performed in CABG patients; six trials were based on valve or combined valve/CABG operations. Twenty studies used a placebo for control and 13 used standard of care as the control. Some studies included diabetic patients; glycemic control was used in 13 trials. The insulin dose and timing of infusions varied across studies. This meta-analysis showed that GIK therapy was associated with a significant reduction in perioperative MI and inotropic support, but had no effect on all-cause mortality, postoperative atrial fibrillation or length of hospital stay.

While most studies had focused on CABG patients, Howell et al sought to evaluate the effects of GIK in patients undergoing surgery for aortic stenosis.[232] Patients with critical aortic stenosis often have left ventricular hypertrophy (LVH), which is thought to compromise myocardial protection and put them at greater risk of a poor outcome. To test the benefits of GIK in this setting, the investigators initiated a single-center, double-blind placebo-controlled study with the primary endpoint a reduction in low cardiac output syndrome. Intermittent antegrade cardioplegia using St. Thomas solution buffered in cold blood was used for myocardial protection. Left ventricular biopsies were obtained to measure posttranslational modifications of specific proteins as an indication of GIK's effect on cardioprotective signaling. Over 4 years, 217 patients were randomized to GIK (n = 110) or placebo (n = 107). The investigators found that GIK treatment was associated with higher cardiac index from the beginning of treatment until 12 hours after the removal of the cross-clamp, a significant reduction in the incidence of low cardiac output

and frequency of inotrope use 6 to 12 hours postoperatively. This was accompanied by biochemical markers consistent with cardioprotective signaling. Although the investigators had expected that hypertrophic hearts would be at greater risk for myocardial necrosis and that GIK would therapy would be associated with lower troponin levels, they found that GIK had no effect on troponin levels. This was similar to the earlier study by Quinn et al from the same institution studying CABG patients.[90] The findings suggest that GIK ameliorates myocardial stunning but not necrosis.

GIK therapy has also been examined in the setting of patients undergoing urgent off-pump CABG surgery (OPCAB) for acute MI. Shim et al (2012) reported the results of a study in which 66 patients were randomized to receive GIK infusion or placebo.[233] The primary endpoints were the highest concentrations of CK-MB and troponin-T after reperfusion and the area under the curve (AUC) of serial troponin-T measurements obtained before the operation and at 12, 24, and 48 hours after reperfusion. The secondary endpoints were troponin-T levels greater than 0.8 ng/mL, MI defined by specific criteria and composite morbidity. The investigators found that GIK therapy was associated with a significant reduction in peak concentraions of CK-MB and troponin-T and the AUC of troponin-T. However, the incidence of postoperative MI was similar for both groups as were the other secondary clincial endpoints. In contrast to the Howell study, this clinical trial of urgent OPCAB for acute coronary syndrome found GIK attenuated myocardial necrosis (troponin-T and CK-MB) but did not alter incidence of MI or composite morbidity.

Taken altogether the evidence supporting the efficacy of GIK in the setting of heart surgery is still mixed. Meta-analyses of randomized clinical trials and numerous small studies indicate it may or may not be effective in preventing postischemic ventricular dysfunction, myocardial necrosis and atrial arrhythmias. This is due in part to the many small studies that are insufficiently powered to definitively conclude that GIK is ineffective; they can only conclude that they failed to see a benefit. Additional limitations include the heavy reliance on surrogate markers of injury, inherent limitations associated with meta-analyses, variability in managing hyperglycemia, variations in the specific composition and mode of administration of GIK and inclusion of low-risk patients (which lowers the event rate and limits the chance to detect a benefit). A large randomized, multi-center clinical trial specifically designed to address these issues will be required to resolve the controversies around the use of GIK for myocardial protection during heart surgery.

CYCLOSPORINE

A major feature of reperfusion injury is the opening of the mitochondrial permeability transition pore (mPTP) which leads to necrotic cell death. For this reason preventing mPTP opening is considered a therapeutic target for I/R protection.[234-237] Cyclosporin A (CsA), Sanglifehrin A and NIM 811 act directly on cyclophilin D, a key regulator of pore opening. As Ca^{2+} and ROS trigger pore opening, other preclinical interventions have targeted those upstream modulators. mPTP opening is also suppressed at acidic intracellular pH, which has been targeted by inhibiting NHE-1 to prevent proton extrusion.[236,238] CsA has been used extensively as an immunosuppressive agent in the management of transplant patients but is also a potent inhibitor of mPTP; its efficacy has been explored in small clinical trials involving patients undergoing heart surgery or PCI for acute MI.

In 2008, Ovize's group randomized 58 patients to receive CsA (n = 30) or placebo (n = 28) immediately prior to undergoing PCI for acute STEMI.[239] The primary endpoint was myocardial necrosis measured by CK and troponin-I; for a secondary endpoint in a subgroup of 27 patients, MRI was used to assess infarct size at 5 days as determined by the area of delayed hyper-enhancement. There were no differences between groups with respect to baseline characteristics, duration of ischemia, area at risk and ejection fraction. All patients underwent stenting of the culprit lesion. The CsA group demonstrated a 40% reduction in myocardial necrosis as assessed by serial CK, although, curiously there was no difference in troponin I release. They also compared CK levels to the area at risk estimated by circumferential extent of abnormally contracting segments and found that for any given size of the area at risk, smaller infarcts were observed in the CsA-treated patients. In the subgroup of patients who were studied by MRI, hyperenhancement was significantly reduced. Ejection fraction measured by echocardiography at 3 months did not differ between the two groups. While offering promise as a novel therapeutic approach, the strength of the study's conclusions are compromised by limitations subsequently pointed out in letters to the editor of the New England Journal of Medicine where the study had been published. There were outliers in the control group with respect to CK, TnI and infarct size assessed by MRI; it was suggested that these outliers skewed the control group mean and that eliminating them would remove the significant difference between the two groups. It was also noted that in the control group 13 patients had failed thrombolytic therapy before PCI versus only five in the CsA group, which might have biased outcome.

A similar small study was performed in 78 CABG surgery patients randomized to receive an intravenous bolus of CsA (2.5 mg/kg) (n = 40) or placebo (n = 38).[240] The drug was administered after induction of anesthesia and prior to sternotomy. Perioperative infarction was assessed by serial troponin-T (cTnT) and CK-MB levels. Cold blood cardioplegia or cross-clamp fibrillation was used for cardioprotection in both groups. The two groups were similar in patient characteristics and intraoperative vessels. While CsA treatment had no effect on postoperative CK-MB or cTnT levels, the investigators found in *post hoc* analysis that in patients with longer CPB times (120 vs 70 minutes), CsA treatment was associated with reduced cTnT release. They concluded that administration of CsA prior to CABG surgery can reduce the incidence of perioperative myocardial injury in patients with longer CBP times, and the effect may be mediated by prevention mPTP opening. Concerns with this study however include the small sample size and the absence of any clinically relevant endpoints.

Subsequently, Ovize's group conducted a prospective, randomized, single-blinded, controlled study in which 61 valve surgery patients were assigned to receive an intravenous bolus of CsA (n = 30) or saline (n = 31) less than 10 minutes before aortic unclamping. The primary endpoint was the 72-hour area under the curve for cTnI release; secondary outcomes included extubation time and length of stay in the intensive care unit and hospital. After removal of the aortic cross-clamp, the need for defibrillation was the same; weaning from CPB was without incident for both groups. The CsA-treated group showed lower cTnI release (72 hours AUC) even after correcting for duration of cross-clamp time (global ischemia). There was no difference in the secondary outcomes. While this study was quite small in scope, it was exciting because the drug appeared to be effective when administered prior to reperfusion. For this reason, based on the reports that cyclosporine was effective in preventing reperfusion injury in patients undergoing PCI for AMI, coronary artery bypass surgery (CABG), and heart valve operations, the Circus trial was initiated.[241] This was a large randomized placebo, double-blind study involving patients with acute STEMI. Patients were randomized to receive intravenous cyclosporine (n = 396) or placebo (n = 395) prior to undergoing PCI revascularization for acute anterior S-T segment elevation myocardial infarction. The primary endpoint was a composite outcome comprised of death from any cause, worsening of heart failure during the initial hospitalization, re-hospitalization for heart failure, or adverse left ventricular remodeling at 1 year. In this study, cyclosporine had no effect on the incidence of the composite endpoint or any of the separate clinical components or other events, including recurrent infarction, unstable angina, and stroke. The findings in this multicenter trial highlight the importance of recognizing the limits of small single center myocardial protection studies, particularly those that rely on reductions of troponin levels as markers of myocardial injury as opposed to necrosis. At present the results of Circus trial call into question the clinical advantage of using mPTP inhibitors to protect the heart against I/R injury.

MYOCARDIAL PROTECTION DURING BEATING HEART SURGERY

In an effort to minimize complications associated with cardiopulmonary bypass such as stroke and a systemic inflammatory response, a number of coronary artery bypass graft operations are performed without cardiopulmonary bypass (off-pump: OPCAB). The assumption is that avoidance of aortic cross-clamping will be associated with a lower incidence of cerebrovascular complications and perioperative MI, lower rates of renal and respiratory failure, less postoperative bleeding, less pain and shorter length of hospitalization. There is a concern, however, that OPCAB may be associated with incomplete revascularization, a higher incidence of perioperative MI and a reduction in long-term graft patency.[242-244] While the relative benefits of OPCAB versus on-pump CABG surgery are still under investigation, as many as 20% of CABG patients undergo the procedure off-pump. Thus it is important to appreciate the principles and methods of myocardial protection as it relates to beating heart surgery.

The acceptance of OPCAB is due in part to the development and refinement of a myriad of surgical aids that allow for stabilization and local immobilization of the heart during grafting. Techniques include the temporary occlusion of the coronary artery or shunting of blood during sustained coronary artery occlusion. Since temporary occlusion of an already diseased artery may aggravate ongoing ischemia, pharmacologic agents and nonpharmacologic maneuvers are used to protect the heart during displacement required to access lateral and inferior wall vessels. Many of these interventions are designed to reduce myocardial oxygen demand at a time when supply is limited. Ischemia during temporary occlusion of a coronary artery during OPCAB may last from 6 to 25 minutes based on the surgeon's experience, quality and size of the vessel and adequacy of the exposure. Most patients with preexisting severe coronary heart disease have experienced self-limiting episodes of ischemia during daily life and may have acquired a certain degree of tolerance to the surgically induced ischemia. This tolerance has been documented using ECGs, transesophageal echocardiography and continuous mixed venous oxygen saturation (SVO_2) monitoring. In order to better understand the differences in the ischemic stress between OPCAB and on-pump CABG surgery, Chowdhury et al studied 50 patients with respect to the release pattern of various cardiac biomarkers including cardiac troponin I, heart-type fatty acid-binding protein, CK-MB, high-sensitivity C-reactive protein and myoglobin.[245] Samples were obtained at baseline and then at hourly intervals up to 72 hours after completion of the last anastomosis in the noncardioplegic OPCAB group and after release of aortic cross-clamp in the cardioplegic group. The cardioplegic group exhibited greater release of cardiac troponin I, high-sensitivity C-reactive protein and heart-type fatty acid-binding protein consistent with the fact that OPCAB surgery puts less myocardium at ischemic risk. Ventricular function as measured by transthoracic echocardiography was similar in the two groups. Schroyer et al analyzed both short-term and long-term outcomes in 2203 patients randomized to undergo either on-pump or off-pump surgery.[246] The primary endpoints included mortality and complications such as reoperation, need for new mechanical support, cardiac arrest, coma, stroke or renal failure before discharge or within 30 days of surgery. The long-term outcome consisted of the composite endpoint of death from any cause, repeat revascularization procedure or a nonfatal MI within 1 year. Secondary endpoints included graft patency and neurologic outcomes. While there were no differences at 30 days, they observed that OPCAB patients had a higher incidence of death from cardiac causes within 1 year, tended to have lower graft patency and had fewer arteries bypassed. The incidence of stroke or resource utilization was similar for both on-pump and off-pump procedures. While

OPCAB puts less myocardium at risk, it is clear that there is still a need for ischemic protection.

One approach to minimizing the risk of injury is to reduce myocardial oxygen demand using pharmacologic beta-blockade. Ultra-short-acting beta blockers such as esmolol and labetalol are frequently used to reduce inotropy and achieve negative chronotropy. Another approach is to optimize systemic mean blood pressures while reducing afterload. Calcium channel blockers such as diltiazem are used to lower blood pressure with less compromise of myocardial contractility than beta blockers. Patients who become hypertensive during the operation may benefit from intravenous nitrates to enhance coronary vasodilation and increase blood flow via collaterals. Gentle core cooling, by allowing the body temperature to drift from 35 to 36°C, and deepening the level of anesthesia are other concurrent measures that can be employed to minimize cardiac work and concomitant oxygen requirements. IPC, RIPC and volatile anesthetics with conditioning-like effects have been used in beating heart surgery in an effort to mitigate I/R injury; however, none of these have been shown to improve clinical outcomes.[247] Thus while the OPCAB approach to myocardial revascularization reduces the amount of myocardium at risk, it does not obviate the need to develop new methods to attenuate I/R injury.

Challenges of Myocardial Protection Trials

It has been difficult to translate promising cardioprotective agents identified in animal studies to the clinic. One reason may be that preclinical studies typically involve healthy young animals of a single sex. While a particular drug may show efficacy in this model, it may fail in humans when both sexes are enrolled and when the study includes patients with advanced age. Aging in itself affects numerous biological processes invoked during I/R. Furthermore, many patients may have comorbid conditions including hypertension, dyslipidemias, obesity and diabetes which may compromise the ability to mount a cardioprotective response. In support of this, preclinical studies have confirmed that obese animals show less infarct size reduction from ischemic preconditioning compared to lean animals, and it has also been reported that hypercholesterolemia interferes with ischemic preconditioning.[235] When a promising agent identified in preclinical studies advances to testing in humans, trial design is challenging. As an example of the difficulties in adapting experimental protocols to the clinical setting, agents that were shown to be protective when given prior to ischemia were much less effective when given at reperfusion which, in the case of PCI for acute MI, is the only clinically feasible approach. Clinical trials that are open-label or single-blind open the door for bias in postoperative management such as administration of inotropic support. Trials are often designed to test whether a particular agent or intervention has benefit. A far larger number of patients must be enrolled to prove the null hypothesis, that is, that the intervention has no benefit. This becomes a challenge if the endpoint, such as 30-day mortality, occurs with relatively low frequency. Given the already low early mortality associated with current surgical approaches, the size of the trial needed to test the null hypothesis becomes daunting. The study by Lehrke et al showed a clear relationship between 48-hour postoperative cTnT levels ≥0.46 μg/L and long-term (28 months) survival; it was also associated with perioperative MI, in-hospital heart failure and 30-day mortality suggesting that these short-term endpoints may be valid surrogate markers of long-term mortality.[19] A more recent meta-analysis confirmed an association between postoperative troponin release and short-term and mid-term (12-month) all-cause mortality.[248] Similar validation studies are needed for MRI assessment of infarct size and risk zone in order for this increasingly sophisticated imaging modality to become accepted as a reliable indicator of cardioprotection.[249] At present the U.S. Food and Drug Administration considers improvement in morbidity and mortality the only acceptable endpoints—rather than surrogate markers—for approval of a cardioprotective intervention. As a consequence the high cost of clinical trials has discouraged even large pharmaceutical companies from pursuing cardioprotection as a therapeutic target. In turn this has fostered the proliferation of small, single-center trials with short-term endpoints and surrogate markers that fall short of proving or disproving efficacy. Despite these considerations, cardiac surgery remains an ideal testing ground for study of cardioprotective treatments: in cardiac surgical patients it is possible to document the onset and duration of ischemia, establish the interval between onset of reperfusion and endpoint analysis and obtain MRIs before and after the ischemic stress to accurately document the volume of necrosis. This information should increase the predictive value of small clinical trials.

While considerable progress has been made in the field of myocardial protection over the past 50 years, the ideal cardioplegic solution, pharmacological intervention, technique or delivery method has yet to be determined. This is due in part to the increasing awareness of the complexity of I/R injury and the concern that surrogate markers or short-term mortality rates are only weakly predictive of durable beneficial outcomes. Myocardial stunning and necrosis remain significant challenges that impact short- and long-term outcomes; there is ongoing need to find new ways to protect the heart during cardiac surgery.

Three Billion Heartbeats

Three billion heartbeats or maybe more
Before you reach life's other shore.
When things go wrong and blood flow's blocked
The loss of muscle by the minute is clocked.
Time is essence as muscle will die
Reflected in rising troponin I.
Protect the heart, try anything!
Drugs or cells or conditioning.
Studies hold hope yet still are unclear,
But an answer grows likelier every year.

Roberta A. Gottlieb
March 20, 2015

REFERENCES

1. Mentzer RM Jr, Bartels C, Bolli R, et al: Sodium-hydrogen exchange inhibition by cariporide to reduce the risk of ischemic cardiac events in patients undergoing coronary artery bypass grafting: Results of the expedition study. *Ann Thorac Surg* 2008; 85:1261-1270.
2. Wang TK, Stewart RA, Ramanathan T, Kang N, Gamble G, White HD: Diagnosis of mi after cabg with high-sensitivity troponin t and new ecg or echocardiogram changes: Relationship with mortality and validation of the universal definition of mi. *European heart journal. Acute cardiovascular care* 2013; 2:323-333.
3. Nalysnyk L, Fahrbach K, Reynolds MW, Zhao SZ, Ross S: Adverse events in coronary artery bypass graft (cabg) trials: A systematic review and analysis. *Heart* 2003; 89:767-772.
4. Ramsay J, Shernan S, Fitch J, et al: Increased creatine kinase mb level predicts postoperative mortality after cardiac surgery independent of new q waves. *J Thorac Cardiovasc Surg* 2005; 129:300-306.
5. Mozaffarian D, Benjamin EJ, Go AS, et al: Heart disease and stroke statistics—2015 update: a report from the american heart association. *Circulation* 2015; 131:e29-322.
6. LaPar DJ, Crosby IK, Rich JB, et al: A contemporary cost analysis of postoperative morbidity after coronary artery bypass grafting with and without concomitant aortic valve replacement to improve patient quality and cost-effective care. *Ann Thorac Surg* 2013; 96:1621-1627.
7. Brown PP, Kugelmass AD, Cohen DJ, et al: The frequency and cost of complications associated with coronary artery bypass grafting surgery: results from the united states medicare program. *Ann Thorac Surg* 2008; 85:1980-1986.
8. Chen JC, Kaul P, Levy JH, et al: Myocardial infarction following coronary artery bypass graft surgery increases healthcare resource utilization. *Crit Care Med* 2007; 35:1296-1301.
9. Abbate A, De Falco M, Morales C, et al: Electron microscopy characterization of cardiomyocyte apoptosis in ischemic heart disease. *Int J Cardiol* 2007; 114:118-120.
10. Eefting F, Rensing B, Wigman J, et al: Role of apoptosis in reperfusion injury. *Cardiovasc Res* 2004; 61:414-426.
11. Verma S, Fedak PW, Weisel RD, et al: Fundamentals of reperfusion injury for the clinical cardiologist. *Circulation* 2002; 105:2332-2336.
12. Buja LM, Weerasinghe P: Unresolved issues in myocardial reperfusion injury. *Cardiovasc Pathol* 2010; 19:29-35.
13. Yellon DM, Hausenloy DJ: Myocardial reperfusion injury. *The New England journal of medicine* 2007; 357:1121-1135.
14. Rodrigo R, Prieto JC, Castillo R: Cardioprotection against ischaemia/reperfusion by vitamins c and e plus n-3 fatty acids: Molecular mechanisms and potential clinical applications. *Clin Sci (Lond)* 2013; 124:1-15.
15. Klatte K, Chaitman BR, Theroux P, et al: Increased mortality after coronary artery bypass graft surgery is associated with increased levels of postoperative creatine kinase-myocardial band isoenzyme release: Results from the guardian trial. *J Am Coll Cardiol* 2001; 38:1070-1077.
16. Costa MA, Carere RG, Lichtenstein SV, et al: Incidence, predictors, and significance of abnormal cardiac enzyme rise in patients treated with bypass surgery in the arterial revascularization therapies study (arts). *Circulation* 2001; 104:2689-2693.
17. Steuer J, Horte LG, Lindahl B, Stahle E: Impact of perioperative myocardial injury on early and long-term outcome after coronary artery bypass grafting. *Eur Heart J* 2002; 23:1219-1227.
18. Brener SJ, Lytle BW, Schneider JP, Ellis SG, Topol EJ: Association between ck-mb elevation after percutaneous or surgical revascularization and three-year mortality. *J Am Coll Cardiol* 2002; 40:1961-1967.
19. Lehrke S, Steen H, Sievers HH, et al: Cardiac troponin t for prediction of short- and long-term morbidity and mortality after elective open heart surgery. *Clin Chem* 2004; 50:1560-1567.
20. Domanski MJ, Mahaffey K, Hasselblad V, et al: Association of myocardial enzyme elevation and survival following coronary artery bypass graft surgery. *JAMA* 2011; 305:585-591.
21. Bolli R, Marban E: Molecular and cellular mechanisms of myocardial stunning. *Physiol Rev* 1999; 79:609-634.
22. Droge W: Free radicals in the physiological control of cell function. *Physiol Rev* 2002; 82:47-95.
23. Mallet RT, Bunger R: Energetic modulation of cardiac inotropism and sarcoplasmic reticulum Ca^{2+} uptake. *Biochim Biophys Acta* 1994; 1224:22-32.

24. Avkiran M, Marber MS: Na(+)/h(+) exchange inhibitors for cardioprotective therapy: Progress, problems and prospects. *J Am Coll Cardiol* 2002; 39:747-753.

25. Halestrap AP, Pasdois P: The role of the mitochondrial permeability transition pore in heart disease. *Biochim Biophys Acta* 2009; 1787:1402-1415.

26. Verbunt RJ, Van der Laarse A: Glutathione metabolism in non-ischemic and postischemic rat hearts in response to an exogenous prooxidant. *Mol Cell Biochem* 1997; 167:127-134.

27. Sharikabad MN, Hagelin EM, Hagberg IA, Lyberg T, Brors O: Effect of calcium on reactive oxygen species in isolated rat cardiomyocytes during hypoxia and reoxygenation. *J Mol Cell Cardiol* 2000; 32:441-452.

28. Gow AJ, Ischiropoulos H: Nitric oxide chemistry and cellular signaling. *J Cell Physiol* 2001; 187:277-282.

29. Xia Y, Tsai AL, Berka V, Zweier JL: Superoxide generation from endothelial nitric-oxide synthase. A Ca^{2+}/calmodulin-dependent and tetrahydrobiopterin regulatory process. *J Biol Chem* 1998; 273:25804-25808.

30. Matsumura Y, Saeki E, Otsu K, et al: Intracellular calcium level required for calpain activation in a single myocardial cell. *J Mol Cell Cardiol* 2001; 33:1133-1142.

31. Tsuji T, Ohga Y, Yoshikawa Y, et al: Rat cardiac contractile dysfunction induced by Ca^{2+} overload: possible link to the proteolysis of alpha-fodrin. *Am J Physiol Heart Circ Physiol* 2001; 281:H1286-1294.

32. Sekili S, McCay PB, Li XY, et al: Direct evidence that the hydroxyl radical plays a pathogenetic role in myocardial "stunning" in the conscious dog and demonstration that stunning can be markedly attenuated without subsequent adverse effects. *Circ Res* 1993; 73:705-723.

33. Vanden Hoek TL, Shao Z, Li C, Schumacker PT, Becker LB: Mitochondrial electron transport can become a significant source of oxidative injury in cardiomyocytes. *J Mol Cell Cardiol* 1997; 29:2441-2450.

34. Sun JZ, Tang XL, Park SW, Qiu Y, Turrens JF, Bolli R: Evidence for an essential role of reactive oxygen species in the genesis of late preconditioning against myocardial stunning in conscious pigs. *J Clin Invest* 1996; 97:562-576.

35. Li Q, Bolli R, Qiu Y, Tang XL, Murphree SS, French BA: Gene therapy with extracellular superoxide dismutase attenuates myocardial stunning in conscious rabbits. *Circulation* 1998; 98:1438-1448.

36. Xu KY, Zweier JL, Becker LC: Hydroxyl radical inhibits sarcoplasmic reticulum Ca(2+)-atpase function by direct attack on the atp binding site. *Circ Res* 1997; 80:76-81.

37. Kawakami M, Okabe E: Superoxide anion radical-triggered Ca^{2+} release from cardiac sarcoplasmic reticulum through ryanodine receptor Ca^{2+} channel. *Mol Pharmacol* 1998; 53:497-503.

38. Josephson RA, Silverman HS, Lakatta EG, Stern MD, Zweier JL: Study of the mechanisms of hydrogen peroxide and hydroxyl free radical-induced cellular injury and calcium overload in cardiac myocytes. *J Biol Chem* 1991; 266:2354-2361.

39. Thomas GP, Sims SM, Cook MA, Karmazyn M: Hydrogen peroxide-induced stimulation of l-type calcium current in guinea pig ventricular myocytes and its inhibition by adenosine A1 receptor activation. *J Pharmacol Exp Ther* 1998; 286:1208-1214.

40. Halestrap AP, Kerr PM, Javadov S, Woodfield KY: Elucidating the molecular mechanism of the permeability transition pore and its role in reperfusion injury of the heart. *Biochim Biophys Acta* 1998; 1366:79-94.

41. Delcamp TJ, Dales C, Ralenkotter L, Cole PS, Hadley RW: Intramitochondrial [Ca^{2+}] and membrane potential in ventricular myocytes exposed to anoxia-reoxygenation. *Am J Physiol* 1998; 275:H484-494.

42. Tanaka M, Richard VJ, Murry CE, Jennings RB, Reimer KA: Superoxide dismutase plus catalase therapy delays neither cell death nor the loss of the ttc reaction in experimental myocardial infarction in dogs. *J Mol Cell Cardiol* 1993; 25:367-378.

43. Effect of 48-h intravenous trimetazidine on short- and long-term outcomes of patients with acute myocardial infarction, with and without thrombolytic therapy; a double-blind, placebo-controlled, randomized trial. The emip-fr group. European myocardial infarction project–free radicals. *Eur Heart J* 2000; 21:1537-1546.

44. Smith RA, Hartley RC, Murphy MP: Mitochondria-targeted small molecule therapeutics and probes. *Antioxid Redox Signal* 2011; 15:3021-3038.

45. Hausenloy DJ, Yellon DM: Myocardial ischemia-reperfusion injury: A neglected therapeutic target. *J Clin Invest* 2013; 123:92-100.

46. Gill C, Mestril R, Samali A: Losing heart: The role of apoptosis in heart disease–a novel therapeutic target? *FASEB J* 2002; 16:135-146.

47. Elsasser A, Suzuki K, Lorenz-Meyer S, Bode C, Schaper J: The role of apoptosis in myocardial ischemia: A critical appraisal. *Basic Res Cardiol* 2001; 96:219-226.

48. Maulik N, Yoshida T, Das DK: Oxidative stress developed during the reperfusion of ischemic myocardium induces apoptosis. *Free Radic Biol Med* 1998; 24:869-875.

49. Freude B, Masters TN, Robicsek F, et al: Apoptosis is initiated by myocardial ischemia and executed during reperfusion. *J Mol Cell Cardiol* 2000; 32:197-208.

50. Kirshenbaum LA, de Moissac D: The bcl-2 gene product prevents programmed cell death of ventricular myocytes. *Circulation* 1997; 96:1580-1585.

51. Kluck RM, Bossy-Wetzel E, Green DR, Newmeyer DD: The release of cytochrome c from mitochondria: A primary site for bcl-2 regulation of apoptosis. *Science* 1997; 275:1132-1136.

52. Martin SJ, Reutelingsperger CP, McGahon AJ, et al: Early redistribution of plasma membrane phosphatidylserine is a general feature of apoptosis regardless of the initiating stimulus: Inhibition by overexpression of bcl-2 and abl. *J Exp Med* 1995; 182:1545-1556.

53. Rucker-Martin C, Henaff M, Hatem SN, Delpy E, Mercadier JJ: Early redistribution of plasma membrane phosphatidylserine during apoptosis of adult rat ventricular myocytes in vitro. *Basic Res Cardiol* 1999; 94:171-179.

54. Narayan P, Mentzer RM Jr, Lasley RD: Annexin v staining during reperfusion detects cardiomyocytes with unique properties. *Am J Physiol Heart Circ Physiol* 2001; 281:H1931-1937.

55. Hammill AK, Uhr JW, Scheuermann RH: Annexin v staining due to loss of membrane asymmetry can be reversible and precede commitment to apoptotic death. *Exp Cell Res* 1999; 251:16-21.

56. Ringer S: A further contribution regarding the influence of the different constituents of the blood on the contraction of the heart. *J Physiol* 1883; 4:29-42.

57. Hooker D: On the recovery of the heart in electric shock. *Am J Physiol* 1929-30; 91:305-328.

58. Wiggers C: Studies on ventricular fibrillation produced by electric shock. *Am J Physiol* 1929; 93:197-212.

59. Beck CS, Pritchard WH, Feil HS: Ventricular fibrillation of long duration abolished by electric shock. *J Am Med Assoc* 1947; 135:985.

60. Bigelow WG, Lindsay WK, Greenwood WF: Hypothermia; its possible role in cardiac surgery: An investigation of factors governing survival in dogs at low body temperatures. *Ann Surg* 1950; 132:849-866.

61. Melrose DG, Dreyer B, Bentall HH, Baker JB: Elective cardiac arrest. *Lancet* 1955; 269:21-22.

62. Tyers GF, Hughes HC Jr, Todd GJ, et al: Protection from ischemic cardiac arrest by coronary perfusion with cold ringer's lactate solution. *J Thorac Cardiovasc Surg* 1974; 67:411-418.

63. Colapinto ND, Silver MD: Prosthetic heart valve replacement. Causes of early postoperative death. *J Thorac Cardiovasc Surg* 1971; 61:938-944.

64. Iyengar SR, Ramchand S, Charrette EJ, Lynn RB: An experimental study of subendocardial hemorrhagic necrosis after anoxic cardiac arrest. *Ann Thorac Surg* 1972; 13:214-224.

65. Bretschneider HJ, Hubner G, Knoll D, Lohr B, Nordbeck H, Spieckermann PG: Myocardial resistance and tolerance to ischemia: Physiological and biochemical basis. *J Cardiovasc Surg (Torino)* 1975; 16:241-260.

66. Hearse DJ, Stewart DA, Braimbridge MV: Cellular protection during myocardial ischemia: the development and characterization of a procedure for the induction of reversible ischemic arrest. *Circulation* 1976; 54:193-202.

67. Braimbridge MV, Chayen J, Bitensky L, Hearse DJ, Jynge P, Cankovic-Darracott S: Cold cardioplegia or continuous coronary perfusion? Report on preliminary clinical experience as assessed cytochemically. *J Thorac Cardiovasc Surg* 1977; 74:900-906.

68. Gay WA Jr, Ebert PA: Functional, metabolic, and morphologic effects of potassium-induced cardioplegia. *Surgery* 1973; 74:284-290.

69. Roe BB, Hutchinson JC, Fishman NH, Ullyot DJ, Smith DL: Myocardial protection with cold, ischemic, potassium-induced cardioplegia. *J Thorac Cardiovasc Surg* 1977; 73:366-374.

70. Tyers GF, Manley NJ, Williams EH, Shaffer CW, Williams DR, Kurusz M: Preliminary clinical experience with isotonic hypothermic potassium-induced arrest. *J Thorac Cardiovasc Surg* 1977; 74:674-681.

71. Buckberg GD: A proposed "solution" to the cardioplegic controversy. *J Thorac Cardiovasc Surg* 1979; 77:803-815.

72. Follette DM, Mulder DG, Maloney JV, Buckberg GD: Advantages of blood cardioplegia over continuous coronary perfusion or intermittent ischemia. Experimental and clinical study. *J Thorac Cardiovasc Surg* 1978; 76:604-619.

73. Ferguson TB Jr, Hammill BG, Peterson ED, DeLong ER, Grover FL: A decade of change–risk profiles and outcomes for isolated coronary artery bypass grafting procedures, 1990-1999: A report from the sts national database committee and the duke clinical research institute. Society of thoracic surgeons. *Ann Thorac Surg* 2002; 73:480-489; discussion 489-490.

74. Mentzer RM Jr: Does size matter? What is your infarct rate after coronary artery bypass grafting? *J Thorac Cardiovasc Surg* 2003; 126:326-328.

75. Swan H, Virtue RW, Blount SG Jr, Kircher LT Jr: Hypothermia in surgery; analysis of 100 clinical cases. *Ann Surg* 1955; 142:382-400.

76. Lillehei CW, Dewall RA, Gott VL, Varco RL: The direct vision correction of calcific aortic stenosis by means of a pump-oxygenator and retrograde coronary sinus perfusion. *Dis Chest* 1956; 30:123-132.

77. Lam CR, Gahagan T, Sergeant C, Green E: Clinical experiences with induced cardiac arrest during intracardiac surgical procedures. *Ann Surg* 1957; 146:439-449.

78. Gerbode F, Melrose D: The use of potassium arrest in open cardiac surgery. *Am J Surg* 1958; 96:221-227.

79. McFarland J: Myocardial necrosis following elective cardiac arrest induced with potassium citrate. *J Thorac Cardiovasc Surg* 1960; 64:833-839.

80. Sondergaard T, Berg E, Staffeldt I, Szczepanski K: Cardioplegic cardiac arrest in aortic surgery. *J Cardiovasc Surg (Torino)* 1975; 16:288-290.

81. Sondergaard T, Senn A: [109. Clinical experience with cardioplegia according to bretschneider]. *Langenbecks Arch Chir* 1967; 319:661-665.

82. Effler DB: Editorial: The mystique of myocardial preservation. *J Thorac Cardiovasc Surg* 1976; 72:468-470.

83. Solorzano J, Taitelbaum G, Chiu RC: Retrograde coronary sinus perfusion for myocardial protection during cardiopulmonary bypass. *Ann Thorac Surg* 1978; 25:201-208.

84. Akins CW: Noncardioplegic myocardial preservation for coronary revascularization. *J Thorac Cardiovasc Surg* 1984; 88:174-181.

85. Murry CE, Jennings RB, Reimer KA: Preconditioning with ischemia: A delay of lethal cell injury in ischemic myocardium. *Circulation* 1986; 74:1124-1136.

86. Lichtenstein SV, Ashe KA, el Dalati H, Cusimano RJ, Panos A, Slutsky AS: Warm heart surgery. *J Thorac Cardiovasc Surg* 1991; 101:269-274.

87. Salerno TA, Houck JP, Barrozo CA, et al: Retrograde continuous warm blood cardioplegia: A new concept in myocardial protection. *Ann Thorac Surg* 1991; 51:245-247.

88. Ikonomidis JS, Rao V, Weisel RD, Hayashida N, Shirai T: Myocardial protection for coronary bypass grafting: The toronto hospital perspective. *Ann Thorac Surg* 1995; 60:824-832.

89. Teoh LK, Grant R, Hulf JA, Pugsley WB, Yellon DM: The effect of preconditioning (ischemic and pharmacological) on myocardial necrosis following coronary artery bypass graft surgery. *Cardiovasc Res* 2002; 53:175-180.

90. Quinn DW, Pagano D, Bonser RS, et al: Improved myocardial protection during coronary artery surgery with glucose-insulin-potassium: A randomized controlled trial. *J Thorac Cardiovasc Surg* 2006; 131:34-42.

91. Sunderdiek U, Feindt P, Gams E: Aortocoronary bypass grafting: A comparison of htk cardioplegia vs. Intermittent aortic cross-clamping. *Eur J Cardiothorac Surg* 2000; 18:393-399.

92. Parolari A, Rubini P, Cannata A, et al: Endothelial damage during myocardial preservation and storage. *Ann Thorac Surg* 2002; 73:682-690.

93. Yang Q, He GW: Effect of cardioplegic and organ preservation solutions and their components on coronary endothelium-derived relaxing factors. *Ann Thorac Surg* 2005; 80:757-767.

94. Ovrum E, Tangen G, Tollofsrud S, Oystese R, Ringdal MA, Istad R: Cold blood versus cold crystalloid cardioplegia: A prospective randomised study of 345 aortic valve patients. *Eur J Cardiothorac Surg* 2010.

95. Jacob S, Kallikourdis A, Sellke F, Dunning J: Is blood cardioplegia superior to crystalloid cardioplegia? *Interact Cardiovasc Thorac Surg* 2008; 7:491-498.

96. Allen BS BG: Myocardial management in arterial revascularization. In: G-W H, ed. *Arterial grafts for coronary artery bypass surgery.* Singapore: Springer; 1999:83-105.

97. Hayashi Y, Ohtani M, Hiraishi T, Kobayashi Y, Nakamura T: "Initial, continuous and intermittent bolus" administration of minimally-diluted blood cardioplegia supplemented with potassium and magnesium for hypertrophied hearts. *Heart Lung Circ* 2006; 15:325-331.

98. Petrucci O, Wilson Vieira R, Roberto do Carmo M, Martins de Oliveira PP, Antunes N, Marcolino Braile D: Use of (all-blood) miniplegia versus crystalloid cardioplegia in an experimental model of acute myocardial ischemia. *J Card Surg* 2008; 23:361-365.

99. Velez DA, Morris CD, Budde JM, et al: All-blood (miniplegia) versus dilute cardioplegia in experimental surgical revascularization of evolving infarction. *Circulation* 2001; 104:I296-302.

100. Rousou JA, Engelman RM, Breyer RH, Otani H, Lemeshow S, Das DK: The effect of temperature and hematocrit level of oxygenated cardioplegic solutions on myocardial preservation. *J Thorac Cardiovasc Surg* 1988; 95:625-630.

101. Guru V, Omura J, Alghamdi AA, Weisel R, Fremes SE: Is blood superior to crystalloid cardioplegia? A meta-analysis of randomized clinical trials. *Circulation* 2006; 114:I331-338.

102. Zeng J, He W, Qu Z, Tang Y, Zhou Q, Zhang B: Cold blood versus crystalloid cardioplegia for myocardial protection in adult cardiac surgery: A meta-analysis of randomized controlled studies. *J Cardiothorac Vasc Anesth* 2014; 28:674-681.

103. Rosenkranz ER, Vinten-Johansen J, Buckberg GD, Okamoto F, Edwards H, Bugyi H: Benefits of normothermic induction of blood cardioplegia in energy-depleted hearts, with maintenance of arrest by multidose cold blood cardioplegic infusions. *J Thorac Cardiovasc Surg* 1982; 84:667-677.

104. Teoh KH, Christakis GT, Weisel RD, et al: Accelerated myocardial metabolic recovery with terminal warm blood cardioplegia. *J Thorac Cardiovasc Surg* 1986; 91:888-895.

105. De Bruyn H, Gelders F, Gregoir T, et al: Myocardial protection during cardiac surgery: Warm blood versus crystalloid cardioplegia. *World Journal of Cardiovascular Diseases* 2014; 4(09):422-431.

106. Minatoya K, Okabayashi H, Shimada I, et al: Intermittent antegrade warm blood cardioplegia for cabg: Extended interval of cardioplegia. *Ann Thorac Surg* 2000; 69:74-76.

107. Franke UF, Korsch S, Wittwer T, et al: Intermittent antegrade warm myocardial protection compared to intermittent cold blood cardioplegia in elective coronary surgery—do we have to change? *Eur J Cardiothorac Surg* 2003; 23:341-346.

108. Casalino S, Tesler UF, Novelli E, et al: The efficacy and safety of extending the ischemic time with a modified cardioplegic technique for coronary artery surgery. *J Card Surg* 2008; 23:444-449.

109. Hayashida N, Ikonomidis JS, Weisel RD, et al: The optimal cardioplegic temperature. *Ann Thorac Surg* 1994; 58:961-971.

110. Hayashida N, Isomura T, Sato T, et al: Minimally diluted tepid blood cardioplegia. *Ann Thorac Surg* 1998; 65:615-621.

111. Baretti R, Mizuno A, Buckberg GD, Young HH, Baumann-Baretti B, Hetzer R: Continuous antegrade blood cardioplegia: Cold vs. Tepid. *Thorac Cardiovasc Surg* 2002; 50:25-30.

112. Onorati F, Renzulli A, De Feo M, et al: Does antegrade blood cardioplegia alone provide adequate myocardial protection in patients with left main stem disease? *J Thorac Cardiovasc Surg* 2003; 126:1345-1351.

113. Pratt FH: The nutrition of the heart through the vessels of thebesius and the coronary veins. *Am J Physiol* 1898.

114. Emery RW, Arom KV: Results with retrograde delivery of cardioplegia for myocardial protection during cardiac surgery. *J Cardiovasc Surg (Torino)* 1993; 34:123-127.

115. Bhayana JN, Kalmbach T, Booth FV, Mentzer RM Jr, Schimert G: Combined antegrade/retrograde cardioplegia for myocardial protection: A clinical trial. *J Thorac Cardiovasc Surg* 1989; 98:956-960.

116. Allen BS, Winkelmann JW, Hanafy H, et al: Retrograde cardioplegia does not adequately perfuse the right ventricle. *J Thorac Cardiovasc Surg* 1995; 109:1116-1124; discussion 1124-1116.

117. Candilio L, Malik A, Ariti C, et al: A retrospective analysis of myocardial preservation techniques during coronary artery bypass graft surgery: Are we protecting the heart? *J Cardiothorac Surg* 2014; 9:1484.

118. Bhaya M, Sudhakar S, Sadat K: Effects of antegrade versus integrated blood cardioplegia on left ventricular function evaluated by echocardiographic real-time 3-dimensional speckle tracking. *J Thorac Cardiovasc Surg* 2015; 149:877-884; e871-875.

119. Louagie YA, Jamart J, Gonzalez M, et al: Continuous cold blood cardioplegia improves myocardial protection: A prospective randomized study. *Ann Thorac Surg* 2004; 77:664-671.

120. Karthik S, Grayson AD, Oo AY, Fabri BM: A survey of current myocardial protection practices during coronary artery bypass grafting. *Ann R Coll Surg Engl* 2004; 86:413-415.

121. Bonchek LI, Burlingame MW, Vazales BE, Lundy EF, Gassmann CJ: Applicability of noncardioplegic coronary bypass to high-risk patients. Selection of patients, technique, and clinical experience in 3000 patients. *J Thorac Cardiovasc Surg* 1992; 103:230-237.

122. Raco L, Mills E, Millner RJ: Isolated myocardial revascularization with intermittent aortic cross-clamping: Experience with 800 cases. *Ann Thorac Surg* 2002; 73:1436-1439; discussion 1439-1440.

123. Boethig D, Minami K, Lueth JU, El-Banayosy A, Breymann T, Koerfer R: Intermittent aortic cross-clamping for isolated cabg can save lives and money: Experience with 15307 patients. *Thorac Cardiovasc Surg* 2004; 52:147-151.

124. Korbmacher B, Simic O, Schulte HD, Sons H, Schipke JD: Intermittent aortic cross-clamping for coronary artery bypass grafting: A review of a safe, fast, simple, and successful technique. *J Cardiovasc Surg (Torino)* 2004; 45:535-543.

125. Bonchek LI: Non-cardioplegic coronary bypass is effective, teachable, and still widely used: Letter 1. *Ann Thorac Surg* 2003; 76:660-661; author reply 661-662.

126. Fujii M, Chambers DJ: Myocardial protection with intermittent cross-clamp fibrillation: Does preconditioning play a role? *Eur J Cardiothorac Surg* 2005; 28:821-831.

127. Scarci M, Fallouh HB, Young CP, Chambers DJ: Does intermittent cross-clamp fibrillation provide equivalent myocardial protection compared to cardioplegia in patients undergoing bypass graft revascularisation? *Interact Cardiovasc Thorac Surg* 2009; 9:872-878.

128. Imanaka K, Kyo S, Ogiwara M, et al: Mitral valve surgery under perfused ventricular fibrillation with moderate hypothermia. *Circ J* 2002; 66:450-452.

129. Imanaka K, Kyo S, Ogiwara M, et al: Noncardioplegic surgery for ischemic mitral regurgitation. *Circ J* 2003; 67:31-34.

130. Raphael J: Physiology and pharmacology of myocardial preconditioning. *Semin Cardiothorac Vasc Anesth* 2010; 14:54-59.

131. Kloner RA, Jennings RB: Consequences of brief ischemia: Stunning, preconditioning, and their clinical implications: Part 2. *Circulation* 2001; 104:3158-3167.

132. Cohen MV, Baines CP, Downey JM: Ischemic preconditioning: From adenosine receptor to katp channel. *Annu Rev Physiol* 2000; 62:79-109.

133. Bolli R: The early and late phases of preconditioning against myocardial stunning and the essential role of oxyradicals in the late phase: An overview. *Basic Res Cardiol* 1996; 91:57-63.

134. Bolli R: The late phase of preconditioning. *Circ Res* 2000; 87:972-983.

135. Kin H, Zhao ZQ, Sun HY, et al: Postconditioning attenuates myocardial ischemia-reperfusion injury by inhibiting events in the early minutes of reperfusion. *Cardiovasc Res* 2004; 62:74-85.

136. Hausenloy DJ, Yellon DM: New directions for protecting the heart against ischaemia-reperfusion injury: Targeting the reperfusion injury salvage kinase (risk)-pathway. *Cardiovasc Res* 2004; 61:448-460.

137. O'Rourke B: Evidence for mitochondrial K+ channels and their role in cardioprotection. *Circ Res* 2004; 94:420-432.

138. Gomez L, Li B, Mewton N: Inhibition of mitochondrial permeability transition pore opening: Translation to patients. *Cardiovasc Res* 2009; 83:226-233.

139. Heusch G, Boengler K, Schulz R: Inhibition of mitochondrial permeability transition pore opening: The holy grail of cardioprotection. *Basic Res Cardiol* 2010; 105:151-154.

140. Gross GJ, Peart JN: Katp channels and myocardial preconditioning: An update. *Am J Physiol Heart Circ Physiol* 2003; 285:H921-930.

140a. Vianello A, Casolo V, Petrussa E, et al: The mitochondrial permeability transition pore (PTP) – an example of multiple molecular exaptation? *Biochim Biophys Acta.* 2012 Nov; 1817 (11): 2072-2086.

141. Garg V, Hu K: Protein kinase c isoform-dependent modulation of atp-sensitive K+ channels in mitochondrial inner membrane. *Am J Physiol Heart Circ Physiol* 2007; 293:H322-332.

142. Przyklenk K, Darling CE, Dickson EW, Whittaker P: Cardioprotection "outside the box"—the evolving paradigm of remote preconditioning. *Basic Res Cardiol* 2003; 98:149-157.

143. Guo Y, Bao W, Wu WJ, Shinmura K, Tang XL, Bolli R: Evidence for an essential role of cyclooxygenase-2 as a mediator of the late phase of ischemic preconditioning in mice. *Basic Res Cardiol* 2000; 95:479-484.

144. Kloner RA, Shook T, Przyklenk K, et al: Previous angina alters in-hospital outcome in timi 4. A clinical correlate to preconditioning? *Circulation* 1995; 91:37-45.

145. Anzai T, Yoshikawa T, Asakura Y, et al: Preinfarction angina as a major predictor of left ventricular function and long-term prognosis after a first q wave myocardial infarction. *J Am Coll Cardiol* 1995; 26:319-327.

146. Ottani F, Galvani M, Ferrini D, et al: Prodromal angina limits infarct size. A role for ischemic preconditioning. *Circulation* 1995; 91:291-297.

147. Tamura K, Tsuji H, Nishiue T, Tokunaga S, Iwasaka T: Association of preceding angina with in-hospital life-threatening ventricular tachyarrhythmias and late potentials in patients with a first acute myocardial infarction. *Am Heart J* 1997; 133:297-301.

148. Ishihara M, Sato H, Tateishi H, et al: Implications of prodromal angina pectoris in anterior wall acute myocardial infarction: Acute angiographic findings and long-term prognosis. *J Am Coll Cardiol* 1997; 30:970-975.

149. Kloner RA, Shook T, Antman EM, et al: Prospective temporal analysis of the onset of preinfarction angina versus outcome: An ancillary study in timi-9b. *Circulation* 1998; 97:1042-1045.

150. Leesar MA, Stoddard MF, Xuan YT, Tang XL, Bolli R: Nonelectrocardiographic evidence that both ischemic preconditioning and adenosine preconditioning exist in humans. *J Am Coll Cardiol* 2003; 42:437-445.

151. Leesar MA, Stoddard MF, Manchikalapudi S, Bolli R: Bradykinin-induced preconditioning in patients undergoing coronary angioplasty. *J Am Coll Cardiol* 1999; 34:639-650.

152. Ishii H, Ichimiya S, Kanashiro M, et al: Impact of a single intravenous administration of nicorandil before reperfusion in patients with st-segment-elevation myocardial infarction. *Circulation* 2005; 112:1284-1288.

153. Tomai F, Crea F, Gaspardone A, et al: Ischemic preconditioning during coronary angioplasty is prevented by glibenclamide, a selective atp-sensitive K+ channel blocker. *Circulation* 1994; 90:700-705.

154. Tomai F, Crea F, Gaspardone A, et al: Effects of naloxone on myocardial ischemic preconditioning in humans. *J Am Coll Cardiol* 1999; 33:1863-1869.

155. Leesar MA, Stoddard MF, Dawn B, Jasti VG, Masden R, Bolli R: Delayed preconditioning-mimetic action of nitroglycerin in patients undergoing coronary angioplasty. *Circulation* 2001; 103:2935-2941.

156. Walsh SR, Tang TY, Kullar P, Jenkins DP, Dutka DP, Gaunt ME: Ischaemic preconditioning during cardiac surgery: Systematic review and meta-analysis of perioperative outcomes in randomised clinical trials. *Eur J Cardiothorac Surg* 2008; 34:985-994.

157. Yellon DM, Alkhulaifi AM, Pugsley WB: Preconditioning the human myocardium. *Lancet* 1993; 342:276-277.

158. Zhao ZQ, Corvera JS, Halkos ME, et al: Inhibition of myocardial injury by ischemic postconditioning during reperfusion: Comparison with ischemic preconditioning. *Am J Physiol Heart Circ Physiol* 2003; 285:H579-588.

159. Darling CE, Solari PB, Smith CS, Furman MI, Przyklenk K: "Postconditioning" the human heart: Multiple balloon inflations during primary angioplasty may confer cardioprotection. *Basic Res Cardiol* 2007; 102:274-278.

160. Lonborg J, Kelbaek H, Vejlstrup N, et al: Cardioprotective effects of ischemic postconditioning in patients treated with primary percutaneous coronary intervention, evaluated by magnetic resonance. *Circ Cardiovasc Interv* 2010; 3:34-41.

161. Luo W, Li B, Lin G, Huang R: Postconditioning in cardiac surgery for tetralogy of fallot. *J Thorac Cardiovasc Surg* 2007; 133:1373-1374.

162. Przyklenk K, Bauer B, Ovize M, Kloner RA, Whittaker P: Regional ischemic "preconditioning" protects remote virgin myocardium from subsequent sustained coronary occlusion. *Circulation* 1993; 87:893-899.

163. Hausenloy DJ, Yellon DM: Remote ischaemic preconditioning: Underlying mechanisms and clinical application. *Cardiovasc Res* 2008; 79:377-386.

164. Giricz Z, Varga ZV, Baranyai T, et al: Cardioprotection by remote ischemic preconditioning of the rat heart is mediated by extracellular vesicles. *J Mol Cell Cardiol* 2014; 68:75-78.

165. Cheung MM, Kharbanda RK, Konstantinov IE, et al: Randomized controlled trial of the effects of remote ischemic preconditioning on children undergoing cardiac surgery: First clinical application in humans. *J Am Coll Cardiol* 2006; 47:2277-2282.

166. Hausenloy DJ, Mwamure PK, Venugopal V, et al: Effect of remote isch-aemic preconditioning on myocardial injury in patients undergoing coronary artery bypass graft surgery: A randomised controlled trial. *Lancet* 2007; 370:575-579.

167. Venugopal V, Hausenloy DJ, Ludman A, et al: Remote ischaemic pre-conditioning reduces myocardial injury in patients undergoing cardiac surgery with cold-blood cardioplegia: A randomised controlled trial. *Heart* 2009; 95:1567-1571.

168. Davies WR, Brown AJ, Watson W, et al: Remote ischemic precondition-ing improves outcome at 6 years after elective percutaneous coronary intervention: The crisp stent trial long-term follow-up. *Circ Cardiovasc Interv* 2013; 6:246-251.

169. D'Ascenzo F, Moretti C, Omede P, et al: Cardiac remote ischaemic preconditioning reduces periprocedural myocardial infarction for patients undergoing percutaneous coronary interventions: A meta-analysis of randomised clinical trials. *EuroIntervention* 2014; 9: 1463-1471.

170. Hong DM, Lee EH, Kim HJ, et al: Does remote ischaemic precondi-tioning with postconditioning improve clinical outcomes of patients undergoing cardiac surgery? Remote ischaemic preconditioning with postconditioning outcome trial. *Eur Heart J* 2014; 35:176-183.

170a. Meybohm P, Bein B, Brosteanu O, et al: A Multicenter Trial of Remote Ischemic Preconditioning for Heart Surgery. RIPHeart Study Collaborators. *N Engl J Med.* 2015 Oct 8; 373(15):1397-407.

170b. Hausenloy DJ, Candilio L, Evans R, et al: ERICCA Trial Investigators. Remote Ischemic Preconditioning and Outcomes of Cardiac Surgery. *N Engl J Med.* 2015 Oct 8; 373(15):1408-1417.

171. Kanazawa H, Tseliou E, Malliaras K, et al: Cellular post-condition-ing: Allogeneic cardiosphere-derived cells reduce infarct size and attenuate microvascular obstruction when administered after reper-fusion in pigs with acute myocardial infarction. *Circulation. Heart failure* 2015.

172. Herrmann JL, Wang Y, Abarbanell AM, Weil BR, Tan J, Meldrum DR: Preconditioning mesenchymal stem cells with transforming fac-tor-alpha improves mesenchymal stem cell-mediated cardioprotection. *Shock (Augusta, Ga.)* 2010; 33:24-30.

173. Timmers L, Lim SK, Arslan F, et al: Reduction of myocardial infarct size by human mesenchymal stem cell conditioned medium. *Stem cell research* 2007; 1:129-137.

174. Lai RC, Arslan F, Lee MM, et al: Exosome secreted by msc reduces myocardial ischemia/reperfusion injury. *Stem cell research* 2010; 4:214-222.

175. Gustafsson AB, Gottlieb RA: Autophagy in ischemic heart disease. *Circ Res* 2009; 104:150-158.

176. Decker RS, Wildenthal K: Lysosomal alterations in hypoxic and reoxy-genated hearts. I. Ultrastructural and cytochemical changes. *Am J Pathol* 1980; 98:425-444.

177. Hamacher-Brady A, Brady NR, Gottlieb RA: Enhancing macroautoph-agy protects against ischemia/reperfusion injury in cardiac myocytes. *J Biol Chem* 2006; 281:29776-29787.

178. Dosenko VE, Nagibin VS, Tumanovska LV, Moibenko AA: Protective effect of autophagy in anoxia-reoxygenation of isolated cardiomyocyte? *Autophagy* 2006; 2:305-306.

179. Matsui Y, Takagi H, Qu X: Distinct roles of autophagy in the heart dur-ing ischemia and reperfusion: Roles of amp-activated protein kinase and beclin 1 in mediating autophagy. *Circ Res* 2007; 100:914-922.

180. Yan L, Vatner DE, Kim SJ, et al: Autophagy in chronically ischemic myocardium. *Proc Natl Acad Sci U S A* 2005; 102:13807-13812.

181. Yitzhaki S, Huang C, Liu W, et al: Autophagy is required for precon-ditioning by the adenosine a1 receptor-selective agonist ccpa. *Basic Res Cardiol* 2009; 104:157-167.

182. Huang C, Liu W, Perry CN, et al: Autophagy and protein kinase c are required for cardioprotection by sulfaphenazole. *Am J Physiol Heart Circ Physiol* 2010; 298:H570-579.

183. Huang C, Yitzhaki S, Perry CN, et al: Autophagy induced by ischemic preconditioning is essential for cardioprotection. *J Cardiovasc Transl Res* 2010; 3:365-373.

184. Sala-Mercado JA, Wider J, Undyala VV, et al: Profound cardioprotec-tion with chloramphenicol succinate in the swine model of myocardial ischemia-reperfusion injury. *Circulation* 2010; 122:S179-184.

185. Giricz Z, Mentzer RM Jr, Gottlieb RA: Cardioprotective effects of chloramphenicol are mediated by autophagy. *J Am Coll Cardiol* 2011; 57:E1015.

186. Kassiotis C, Ballal K, Wellnitz K, et al: Markers of autophagy are down-regulated in failing human heart after mechanical unloading. *Circulation* 2009; 120:S191-197.

187. Garcia L, Verdejo HE, Kuzmicic J, et al: Impaired cardiac autophagy in patients developing postoperative atrial fibrillation. *The Journal of tho-racic and cardiovascular surgery* 2012; 143:451-459.

188. Jahania SM, Sengstock D, Vaitkevicius P, et al: Activation of the homeo-static intracellular repair response during cardiac surgery. *J Am Coll Surg* 2013; 216:719-726; discussion 726-719.

189. Singh KK, Yanagawa B, Quan A, et al: Autophagy gene fingerprint in human ischemia and reperfusion. *The Journal of thoracic and cardiovascu-lar surgery* 2014; 147:1065-1072.e1061.

190. Gedik N, Thielmann M, Kottenberg E, et al: No evidence for activated autophagy in left ventricular myocardium at early reperfusion with pro-tection by remote ischemic preconditioning in patients undergoing coro-nary artery bypass grafting. *PLoS One* 2014; 9:e96567.

191. Kloner RA: Current state of clinical translation of cardioprotective agents for acute myocardial infarction. *Circ Res* 2013; 113:451-463.

192. Schwartz Longacre L, Kloner RA, Arai AE, et al: New horizons in cardio-protection: Recommendations from the 2010 national heart, lung, and blood institute workshop. *Circulation* 2011; 124:1172-1179.

193. Berry C, Kellman P, Mancini C, et al: Magnetic resonance imaging delineates the ischemic area-at-risk and myocardial salvage in patients with acute myocardial infarction. *Circulation. Cardiovascular imaging* 2010; 3:527-535.

194. Sommerschild HT, Kirkeboen KA: Adenosine and cardioprotection during ischaemia and reperfusion—an overview. *Acta Anaesthesiol Scand* 2000; 44:1038-1055.

195. McIntosh VJ, Lasley RD: Adenosine receptor-mediated cardioprotec-tion: Are all 4 subtypes required or redundant? *J Cardiovasc Pharmacol Ther* 2012; 17:21-33.

196. Cohen MV, Downey JM: Adenosine: Trigger and mediator of cardiopro-tection. *Basic Res Cardiol* 2008; 103:203-215.

197. Eltzschig HK, Bonney SK, Eckle T: Attenuating myocardial isch-emia by targeting a2b adenosine receptors. *Trends Mol Med* 2013; 19: 345-354.

198. Przyklenk K: Role of adenosine a(2b) receptor stimulation in ischaemic postconditioning: Dawn of a new paradigm in cardioprotection. *Cardio-vasc Res* 2012; 96:195-197; discussion 198-201.

199. Muller CE, Jacobson KA: Recent developments in adenosine receptor ligands and their potential as novel drugs. *Biochim Biophys Acta* 2011; 1808:1290-1308.

200. Mahaffey KW, Puma JA, Barbagelata NA, et al: Adenosine as an adjunct to thrombolytic therapy for acute myocardial infarction: Results of a multicenter, randomized, placebo-controlled trial: The acute myocardial infarction study of adenosine (amistad) trial. *J Am Coll Cardiol* 1999; 34:1711-1720.

201. Ross AM, Gibbons RJ, Stone GW, Kloner RA, Alexander RW: A ran-domized, double-blinded, placebo-controlled multicenter trial of ade-nosine as an adjunct to reperfusion in the treatment of acute myocardial infarction (amistad-ii). *J Am Coll Cardiol* 2005; 45:1775-1780.

202. Kloner RA, Forman MB, Gibbons RJ, Ross AM, Alexander RW, Stone GW: Impact of time to therapy and reperfusion modality on the efficacy of adenosine in acute myocardial infarction: The amistad-2 trial. *Eur Heart J* 2006; 27:2400-2405.

203. Desmet W, Bogaert J, Dubois C, et al: High-dose intracoronary adenos-ine for myocardial salvage in patients with acute st-segment elevation myocardial infarction. *Eur Heart J* 2011; 32:867-877.

204. Fokkema ML, Vlaar PJ, Vogelzang M, et al: Effect of high-dose intracor-onary adenosine administration during primary percutaneous coronary intervention in acute myocardial infarction: A randomized controlled trial. *Circ Cardiovasc Interv* 2009; 2:323-329.

205. Fremes SE, Levy SL, Christakis GT, et al: Phase 1 human trial of adenos-ine-potassium cardioplegia. *Circulation* 1996; 94:II370-375.

206. Cohen G, Feder-Elituv R, Iazetta J, et al: Phase 2 studies of adenosine cardioplegia. *Circulation* 1998; 98:II225-233.

207. Mentzer RM Jr, Rahko PS, Molina-Viamonte V, et al: Safety, toler-ance, and efficacy of adenosine as an additive to blood cardioplegia in humans during coronary artery bypass surgery. *Am J Cardiol* 1997; 79: 38-43.

208. Mentzer RM Jr, Birjiniuk V, Khuri S, et al: Adenosine myocardial pro-tection: Preliminary results of a phase II clinical trial. *Ann Surg* 1999; 229:643-649; discussion 649-650.

208a. Wei M, Kuukasjarvi P, Laurikka J, Honkonen EL, Kaukinen S, Laine S, Tarkka M: Cardioprotective effect of adenosine pretreatment in coronary artery bypass grafting. *Chest* 2001 Sep; 120(3): 860-865.

209. Ahlsson A, Sobrosa C, Kaijser L, Jansson E, Bomfim V: Adenosine in cold blood cardioplegia–a placebo-controlled study. *Interact Cardiovasc Thorac Surg* 2012; 14:48-55.

210. Karmazyn M, Sostaric JV, Gan XT: The myocardial Na+/H+ exchanger: A potential therapeutic target for the prevention of myocardial ischaemic and reperfusion injury and attenuation of postinfarction heart failure. *Drugs* 2001; 61:375-389.

211. Karmazyn M, Sawyer M, Fliegel L: The Na(+)/H(+) exchanger: A target for cardiac therapeutic intervention. *Curr Drug Targets Cardiovasc Haematol Disord* 2005; 5:323-335.

212. Murphy E, Allen DG: Why did the nhe inhibitor clinical trials fail? *J Mol Cell Cardiol* 2009; 46:137-141.

213. Mullane K: Acadesine: The prototype adenosine regulating agent for reducing myocardial ischaemic injury. *Cardiovasc Res* 1993; 27:43-47.

214. Lemieux K, Konrad D, Klip A, Marette A: The amp-activated protein kinase activator aicar does not induce glut4 translocation to transverse tubules but stimulates glucose uptake and p38 mitogen-activated protein kinases α and β in skeletal muscle. *The FASEB Journal* 2003; 17:1658-1665.

215. Mangano DT: Effects of acadesine on myocardial infarction, stroke, and death following surgery. A meta-analysis of the 5 international randomized trials. The multicenter study of perioperative ischemia (mcspi) research group. *JAMA* 1997; 277:325-332.

216. Mangano DT, Miao Y, Tudor IC, Dietzel C: Post-reperfusion myocardial infarction: Long-term survival improvement using adenosine regulation with acadesine. *J Am Coll Cardiol* 2006; 48:206-214.

217. Newman MF, Ferguson TB, White JA, et al: Effect of adenosine-regulating agent acadesine on morbidity and mortality associated with coronary artery bypass grafting: The red-cabg randomized controlled trial. *JAMA* 2012; 308:157-164.

218. Bothe W, Olschewski M, Beyersdorf F, Doenst T: Glucose-insulin-potassium in cardiac surgery: A meta-analysis. *Ann Thorac Surg* 2004; 78:1650-1657.

219. Fath-Ordoubadi F, Beatt KJ: Glucose-insulin-potassium therapy for treatment of acute myocardial infarction: An overview of randomized placebo-controlled trials. *Circulation* 1997; 96:1152-1156.

220. van der Horst IC, Zijlstra F, van't Hof AW, et al: Glucose-insulin-potassium infusion inpatients treated with primary angioplasty for acute myocardial infarction: The glucose-insulin-potassium study: A randomized trial. *J Am Coll Cardiol* 2003; 42:784-791.

221. Timmer JR, Svilaas T, Ottervanger JP, et al: Glucose-insulin-potassium infusion in patients with acute myocardial infarction without signs of heart failure: The glucose-insulin-potassium study (gips)-ii. *J Am Coll Cardiol* 2006; 47:1730-1731.

222. Mamas MA, Neyses L, Fath-Ordoubadi F: A meta-analysis of glucose-insulin-potassium therapy for treatment of acute myocardial infarction. *Experimental & Clinical Cardiology* 2010; 15:e20.

223. Diaz R, Goyal A, Mehta SR, et al: Glucose-insulin-potassium therapy in patients with st-segment elevation myocardial infarction. *JAMA* 2007; 298:2399-2405.

224. Selker HP, Beshansky JR, Sheehan PR, et al: Out-of-hospital administration of intravenous glucose-insulin-potassium in patients with suspected acute coronary syndromes: The immediate randomized controlled trial. *JAMA* 2012; 307:1925-1933.

225. Selker HP, Udelson JE, Massaro JM, et al: One-year outcomes of out-of-hospital administration of intravenous glucose, insulin, and potassium (gik) in patients with suspected acute coronary syndromes (from the immediate [immediate myocardial metabolic enhancement during initial assessment and treatment in emergency care] trial). *Am J Cardiol* 2014; 113: 1599-1605.

226. Bruemmer-Smith S, Avidan MS, Harris B, et al: Glucose, insulin and potassium for heart protection during cardiac surgery. *Br J Anaesth* 2002; 88:489-495.

227. Lell WA, Nielsen VG, McGiffin DC, et al: Glucose-insulin-potassium infusion for myocardial protection during off-pump coronary artery surgery. *Ann Thorac Surg* 2002; 73:1246-1251; discussion 1251-1252.

228. Lazar HL, Chipkin SR, Fitzgerald CA, et al: Tight glycemic control in diabetic coronary artery bypass graft patients improves perioperative

outcomes and decreases recurrent ischemic events. *Circulation* 2004; 109:1497-1502.

229. Barcellos Cda S, Wender OC, Azambuja PC: Clinical and hemodynamic outcome following coronary artery bypass surgery in diabetic patients using glucose-insulin-potassium (gik) solution: A randomized clinical trial. *Rev Bras Cir Cardiovasc* 2007; 22:275-284.

230. Rabi D, Clement F, McAlister F, et al: Effect of perioperative glucose-insulin-potassium infusions on mortality and atrial fibrillation after coronary artery bypass grafting: A systematic review and meta-analysis. *The Canadian journal of cardiology* 2010; 26:178-184.

231. Fan Y, Zhang AM, Xiao YB, Weng YG, Hetzer R: Glucose-insulin-potassium therapy in adult patients undergoing cardiac surgery: A meta-analysis. *Eur J Cardiothorac Surg* 2011; 40:192-199.

232. Howell NJ, Ashrafian H, Drury NE, et al: Glucose-insulin-potassium reduces the incidence of low cardiac output episodes after aortic valve replacement for aortic stenosis in patients with left ventricular hypertrophy: Results from the hypertrophy, insulin, glucose, and electrolytes (hinge) trial. *Circulation* 2011; 123:170-177.

233. Shim JK, Yang SY, Yoo YC, Yoo KJ, Kwak YL: Myocardial protection by glucose-insulin-potassium in acute coronary syndrome patients undergoing urgent multivessel off-pump coronary artery bypass surgery. *British journal of anaesthesia* 2013; 110:47-53.

234. Halestrap AP, Clarke SJ, Javadov SA: Mitochondrial permeability transition pore opening during myocardial reperfusion–a target for cardioprotection. *Cardiovasc Res* 2004; 61:372-385.

235. Ong SB, Dongworth RK, Cabrera-Fuentes HA, Hausenloy DJ: Role of the mptp in conditioning the heart–translatability and mechanism. *Br J Pharmacol.* 2015; 172(8):2074-2084.

236. Javadov S, Karmazyn M, Escobales N: Mitochondrial permeability transition pore opening as a promising therapeutic target in cardiac diseases. *J Pharmacol Exp Ther* 2009; 330:670-678.

237. Argaud L, Gateau-Roesch O, Raisky O, Loufouat J, Robert D, Ovize M: Postconditioning inhibits mitochondrial permeability transition. *Circulation* 2005; 111:194-197.

238. Clarke SJ, McStay GP, Halestrap AP: Sanglifehrin a acts as a potent inhibitor of the mitochondrial permeability transition and reperfusion injury of the heart by binding to cyclophilin-d at a different site from cyclosporin a. *J Biol Chem* 2002; 277:34793-34799.

239. Piot C, Croisille P, Staat P: Effect of cyclosporine on reperfusion injury in acute myocardial infarction. *N Engl J Med* 2008; 359:473-481.

240. Hausenloy D, Kunst G, Boston-Griffiths E, et al: The effect of cyclosporin-a on peri-operative myocardial injury in adult patients undergoing coronary artery bypass graft surgery: A randomised controlled clinical trial. *Heart* 2014; 100:544-549.

241. Cung TT, Morel O, Cayla G, et al: Cyclosporine before PCI in patients with Acute Myocardial Infarction. *N Engl J Med.* 2015 Sep 10; 373(11):1021-1031.

242. Caputo M, Reeves BC, Rajkaruna C, Awair H, Angelini GD: Incomplete revascularization during opcab surgery is associated with reduced mid-term event-free survival. *Ann Thorac Surg* 2005; 80:2141-2147.

243. Gill IS, Higginson LA, Maharajh GS, Keon WJ: Early and follow-up angiography in minimally invasive coronary bypass without mechanical stabilization. *Ann Thorac Surg* 2000; 69:56-60.

244. Balacumaraswami L, Abu-Omar Y, Anastasiadis K, et al: Does off-pump total arterial grafting increase the incidence of intraoperative graft failure? *J Thorac Cardiovasc Surg* 2004; 128:238-244.

245. Chowdhury UK, Malik V, Yadav R, et al: Myocardial injury in coronary artery bypass grafting: On-pump versus off-pump comparison by measuring high-sensitivity c-reactive protein, cardiac troponin i, heart-type fatty acid-binding protein, creatine kinase-mb, and myoglobin release. *J Thorac Cardiovasc Surg* 2008; 135:1110-1119, 1119 e1111-1110.

246. Shroyer AL, Grover FL, Hattler B, et al: On-pump versus off-pump coronary-artery bypass surgery. *N Engl J Med* 2009; 361:1827-1837.

247. Moscarelli M, Punjabi PP, Miroslav GI, Del Sarto P, Fiorentino F, Angelini GD: Myocardial conditioning techniques in off-pump coronary artery bypass grafting. *J Cardiothorac Surg* 2015; 10:7.

248. Lurati Buse GA, Koller MT, Grapow M, Bolliger D, Seeberger M, Filipovic M: The prognostic value of troponin release after adult cardiac surgery—a meta-analysis. *Eur J Cardiothoracic Surg* 2010; 37:399-406.

249. Arai AE: Magnetic resonance imaging for area at risk, myocardial infarction, and myocardial salvage. *Journal of cardiovascular pharmacology and therapeutics* 2011; 16:313-320.

17

Postoperative Care of Cardiac Surgery Patients

Farhang Yazdchi • James D. Rawn

Mortality and morbidity in cardiac surgery have continued to decline despite increases in patient age, comorbid conditions, and procedure complexity. Much of this success can be attributed to advances in critical care. This chapter will outline some strategies and principles of modern postoperative care.

CARDIOVASCULAR CARE

Hemodynamic Assessment

Assessment and optimization of hemodynamics is a principle focus of care following cardiac surgery. Appropriate management requires knowledge of preoperative cardiac function and an appreciation of the impact of intraoperative events. The goal of postoperative hemodynamic management is the maintenance of adequate oxygen delivery to vital tissues in a way that avoids unnecessary demands on a heart recovering from the stress of cardiopulmonary bypass (CPB), ischemia, and surgery.

A basic initial hemodynamic assessment includes a review of current medications, heart rate and rhythm, mean arterial pressure (MAP), central venous pressure (CVP), and an ECG analysis to exclude ischemia and conduction abnormalities. The presence of a pulmonary artery catheter enables the measurement of pulmonary artery pressures, left-sided filling pressures (pulmonary capillary wedge pressure (PCWP)), and mixed venous oxygen saturation (MVO_2). Cardiac output (CO), as well as pulmonary and systemic vascular resistances (SVRs) can also be calculated when a PA catheter is present. CO is determined utilizing thermodilution or by using the Fick equation. CO, blood pressure (BP), and SVR are related to each other using Ohm's law (Table 17-1). Reasonable minimum goals for most patients include an MVO_2 of about 60%, MAP > 65 mm Hg, and a cardiac index (CI) > 2 L/min/m². Goals should be individualized. Patients with a history of hypertension or significant peripheral vascular disease will benefit from higher BP; patients who are bleeding or who have suture lines in fragile tissue are best served with tighter control. Strategies designed to produce a supra-normal CI or MVO_2 have failed to demonstrate a survival advantage.[1]

Failure to achieve adequate CO and end-organ oxygen delivery can be caused by many co-dependent factors. These include volume status (preload), peripheral vascular tone (afterload), cardiac pump function, heart rate and rhythm, and blood oxygen carrying capacity.

Volume status can be estimated using invasive monitoring. CVP, unless it is very low, is an unreliable indicator of left ventricular end-diastolic volume. An elevated CVP can be seen in volume overload, right heart failure, tricuspid and mitral regurgitation, pulmonary hypertension, cardiac tamponade, tension pneumothorax, and pulmonary embolism. Pulmonary artery diastolic pressure correlates with left-sided filling pressures when pulmonary vascular resistance (PVR) is normal (low). PCWP (or left atrial pressure if this is being directly measured) provides the most accurate assessment of left-sided filling pressures in the absence of significant mitral stenosis, and its correlation with pulmonary artery diastolic pressure should be noted to enable a more continuous assessment of left-sided pressures. Determination of optimum filling pressures is generally empiric. A wedge pressure of 15 mm Hg is generally adequate, but many patients can require higher pressures. Most patients arrive from the operating room with a significant net fluid gain, but much of this excess volume is extravascular due to third space and pleural cavity accumulation. Consequently, many patients are intravascularly underfilled and have on going volume requirements in the immediate postoperative period. Postoperative vasoplegia is common. Contributors include a systemic inflammatory response to CPB and the stress of surgery in addition to preoperative and perioperative medications including ACE inhibitors, calcium channel blockers, and sedatives. Urine output and bleeding are common sources of ongoing fluid loss. Hypothermia promotes vasoconstriction. As patients rewarm, changes in peripheral vascular tone contribute to labile hemodynamics which are often best treated with volume replacement.

Peripheral vascular tone needs to be sufficient to provide the patient with adequate BP; excess vasoconstriction can increase SVR and create dangerous levels of hypertension and decreased CO. Increases in afterload can be caused by medications, hypothermia, increased sympathetic output

TABLE 17-1: Common Intensive Care Values and Formulae

Early postoperative hemodynamic parameters	Expected values
Mean arterial pressure (MAP)	60-90 mm Hg
Systolic blood pressure (sBP)	90-140 mm Hg
Right arterial pressure (RAP)	5-15 mm Hg
Cardiac index (CI)	2.2-4.4 L/min/m²
Pulmonary artery wedge pressure (PAWP)	10-15 mm Hg
Systemic vascular resistance (SVR)	1400-2800 dyn-s/cm⁵

Common hemodynamic formulae	Normal values
$CO = SV \times HR$	4-8 L/min
$CI = CO/BSA$	2.2-4.0 L/min/m²
CO = cardiac output; HR = heart rate; SV = stroke volume; BSA = body surface area	
$SV = \dfrac{CO\ (L/min) \times 1000\ (mL/L)}{HR}$	60-100 mL/beat (1 mL/kg/beat)
$SVI = SV \div BSA$	33-47 mL/beat/m²
SVI = stroke volume index	
$MAP = \dfrac{DP + (SP - DP)}{3}$	70-100 mm Hg
$SVR = \dfrac{MAP - CVP}{CO} \times 80$	800-1200 dyn-s/cm⁵
CVP = central venous pressure; Ohm's law: Voltage (V) = Current (I) × Resistance (R); Resistance is directly proportional to viscosity (hematocrit) and inversely proportional to the radius to the 4th power	
$PVR = \dfrac{PAP - PCWP}{CO} \times 80$	50-250 dyn-s/cm⁵
PVR = pulmonary vascular resistance, PAP = mean pulmonary arterial pressure, PCWP = pulmonary capillary wedge pressure	
LVSWI = SVI × (MAP − PCWP) × 0.0136 (LVSWI = left ventricular stroke work index)	45-75 mg-M/beat/m²
O_2 delivery = CO (Hb × %sat)(1.39) + (PaO$_2$)(0.0031)	60-80%
1.39 is milliliters of oxygen transported per gram of serum hemoglobin (Hb); 0.0032 is solubility coefficient of oxygen dissolved in solution (mL/torr of PaO$_2$)	
A-V O_2 Difference = (1.34)(Hb) × (SaO$_2$ − SvO$_2$)	Normal Pvo$_2$ = 40 torr and SvO$_2$ = 75%
Fick Cardiac Output = $\dfrac{\text{Estimated } O_2 \text{ consumption}}{\text{A-V } O_2 \text{ difference}}$	Normal Pao$_2$ = 100 torr and SaO$_2$ = 99%
A-V = arterio-venous oxygen difference. Oxygen consumption is measured from a nomogram based on age, sex, height, height; Hb = serum hemoglobin (g/dL), SaO$_2$ = arterial oxygen saturation (%) in arterial blood, SvO$_2$ = mixed venous oxygen saturation (%) from the pulmonary artery in the absence of a shunt or calculated MvO$_2$ = (3 × SVC saturation + IVC saturation) ÷ 4, if a left-right shunt is present; 1.34 = m O_2 per gram of Hb, 10 dL/L	
Shunt Fraction = $\dfrac{Qp}{Qs} = \dfrac{(SaO_2 - Mvo_2)}{(Pvo_2 - Pao_2)}$	Normal, <5%
Qs = systemic flow (L/min); Qp = pulmonary flow (L/min)	
EF (%) = $\dfrac{\text{end-diastolic volume} - \text{end-systolic volume}}{\text{end-diastolic volume}}$	60-70%
EF = ejection fraction (an index of ventricular activity)	

(Continued)

TABLE 17-1: Common Intensive Care Values and Formulae (*Continued*)

Respiratory formulae	Normal values
$D(A - a)O_2 = (FiO_2) \times (713) - Pao_2 - (Pao_2 \div 0.8)$ $D(A - a)O_2$ = alveolar-arterial oxygen difference, taking FiO_2 (inspired oxygen into consideration); a sensitive index of efficiency of gas exchange	Suboptimal oxygenation > 350 on 100% oxygen Or Pao_2< 500 torr on 100% oxygenation

Renal and metabolic values and formulae	
$C_{CR} = \dfrac{(140 - age) \times wt\ (kg)}{72 \times Cr} \times 0.8$ (for females) Cockroft and Gault equation for creatinine clearance (C_{CR}) (an approximation to glomerular filtration rate, GFR) Or more precisely with 24 h or 2 h urine specimen: $C_{CR} = (U_{CR} \div P_{CR}) \times$ (volume/1440 min, or 120 min) U_{CR} and P_{CR} = Urinary and plasma creatinine concentrations	C_{CR} < 55 mL/min threshold below which surgical risk increases[128]

Evaluating oliguria	Prerenal	Renal
BUN/Cr	> 20:1	< 10:1
U/P creatinine	> 40	< 20
U_{osm}	> 500	< 400
U/P osmolality	> 1.3	< 1.1
Urine-specific gravity	> 1.020	1.010
U_{Na} (mEq/L)	< 20	> 40
FE_{Na}	< 1%	> 2%
Urinary sediment	Hyaline casts	Tubular epithelial casts; granular casts

BUN=urea nitrogen, serum (7-18 mg/dL)

$$FE_{Na} = \frac{U_{Na} \times P_{CR}}{P_{Na} \times U_{CR}} \times 100$$

Normal = 1-3%

FE_{Na} = fractional excretion of sodium; U and P are urinary and plasma concentrations of sodium and creatinine, respectively

Anion Gap = $(Na^+) - [(Cl^-) + (HCO_3^-)]$

Normal = 8-12

Elevated by ethanol, uremia (chronic renal failure), diabetic ketoacidosis, paraldehyde, phenformin, iron tablets, isoniazide, lactic acidosis (CN-, CO, shock), ethanol, ethylene glycol, salicylates

$C_{H2O} = V - C_{osm}$
$C_{osm} = U_{usm} \times V/P_{osm}$

P_{osm} = 275-295 mOsmol/kg

C_{H2O} = free water clearance; V = urine flow rate; P_{osm} and U_{osm} = plasma and urine osmolarity, respectively

Capillary fluid exchange (starling forces)	Edema
Net filtration pressure = $P_{net} = [(P_c - P_i) - (\pi_c - \pi_i)]$ K_f = filtration constant (capillary permeability) Net fluid flow = $(P_{net})(K_f)$ P_c = capillary pressure-tends to move fluid out of capillary P_i = interstitial fluid pressure-tends to move fluid into capillary π_c = plasma colloid oncotic pressure-tends to cause osmosis of fluid into capillary π_i = interstitial fluid colloid osmotic pressure-tends to cause osmosis of fluid out of capillary	1. High P_c; heart failure 2. Low π_c; nephritic syndrome 3. High K_f; toxins, sepsis, inflammatory cytokines 4. High π_i; lymphatic blockage

(Continued)

TABLE 17-1: Common Intensive Care Values and Formulae (*Continued*)

Prosthetic heart valves: current anticoagulation regimens (adapted from Ref. 129)	Coumadin target INR/aspirin 81 mg
AVR mechanical	2.5-3.0/yes, if high risk
AVR bioprosthetic (tissue)	2.5-3.0 (3 months) or none if aspirin used/yes
MVR mechanical	2.5-3.5 (indefinitely)/yes, if high risk
MVR bioprosthetic or MV repair	2.5-3.0 (3 months; continue 1 year if history of embolism; indefinitely if AF and LA thrombus at time of surgery)/yes, after 3 months
AVR and MVR mechanical	2.5-3.0 (indefinitely)/yes
AVR and MVT bioprosthetic (tissue)	2.5-3.0 (3 months)/yes, after 3 months
Atrial fibrillation (with any of the above)	2.5-3.0 (indefinitely)/yes

AF = atrial fibrillation; AVR = aortic valve replacement; MVR = mitral valve replacement; high risk = AF, myocardial infarction, enlarged left atrium (LA), endocardial damage, low EF, history of systemic emobolism despite adequate anticoagulation.

(including pain and anxiety) or may be secondary to hypovolemia or pump failure.

Left ventricular pump function can be influenced by levels of exogenous or endogenous inotropes, postoperative ischemic stunning or infarction, valve function, acidosis, electrolyte abnormalities, hypoxia or cardiac tamponade. Bradycardia, arrhythmias, and conduction defects can also adversely affect CO.

The oxygen carrying capacity of blood is a function of hematocrit and oxygenation. A hematocrit of 21% and oxygen saturation greater than 90% is adequate for a stable postoperative patient.

It is important not to allow the evaluation of the patient to become obscured by too many numbers or theories, and an overall assessment of the patient is always more important than any single parameter. Trends in hemodynamic parameters are usually more important than isolated values. Patients generally do well if they have warm, well-perfused extremities, a normal mental status and good urine output (>0.5 cc/kg/min). Acute changes in hemodynamic status are common postoperatively, and vigilant monitoring should enable care to be more preemptive than reactive.

Hemodynamic Management

FLUID MANAGEMENT

As emphasized previously, the goal of postoperative hemodynamic management is the maintenance of adequate end-organ perfusion without taxing the heart unnecessarily. Assessment and optimization of intravascular volume status are generally the first steps in this process. Most patients have ongoing fluid requirements in the immediate postoperative period that can be caused by persistent third spacing, warming, diuresis, vasodilation, and bleeding. Careful monitoring of fluid balance and filling pressures should guide volume resuscitation. Starling curves are highly variable; it is helpful to correlate CO and MVO_2

with changes in volume status. Patients with ventricular hypertrophy (eg, those with a history of hypertension or aortic stenosis) diastolic dysfunction or systolic anterior motion of the mitral valve usually need higher filling pressures. Patients with persistently low filling pressures despite aggressive fluid administration are usually either bleeding or vasodilated. Calculation of CO and SVR can often help sort this out. Monitoring devices that measure respiratory variation in the pulse arterial waveform have been shown to successfully predict the ability to improve CO with volume administration. In the case of significant vasodilation, judicious use of a pressor agent can help to decrease fluid requirements. Inotropic agents should not be administered for the treatment of hypovolemia. Fluid requirements can often be reduced following extubation; as decreased intrathoracic pressures will improve venous return.

The choice of an optimal resuscitation fluid has been controversial. In the acute setting, colloid infusions achieve comparable hemodynamic effects with less volume when compared to crystalloid solutions. After one hour, 80% of 1000 cc of 5% albumin solution is retained intravascularly. In situations characterized by loss of vascular endothelial integrity (ie, following CPB) albumin will redistribute into the interstitial space and increase third space fluid accumulation. One study has shown that the accumulation of extravascular pulmonary water is unaffected by the prime type or the type of fluid administered postoperatively.[2] The largest prospective randomized controlled study comparing colloid to crystalloid has been unable to demonstrate a difference in outcomes, although a subsequent subgroup analysis found increased mortality in patients who suffered brain injury who were randomized to receive colloid.[3] Albumin and hetastarch provide comparable hemodynamic benefits, although hetastarch should be avoided in bleeding or coagulopathic patients or in those with renal impairment.

Although unusual in the immediate postoperative period, volume overload is a common problem in the days following surgery. If patients have normal cardiac function they often diuresis appropriately without intervention. Conversely, volume overload is a common cause of postoperative heart failure. Diuretics and vasodilators are frequently required in patients with impaired pump function before or following surgery, or in those who receive large volumes of fluid perioperatively. Patients with impaired renal function may require renal replacement therapy (ultrafiltration, continuous veno-venous hemofiltration, or hemodialysis) to become euvolemic. Rapid diuresis accompanied by inadequate electrolyte repletion is frequently arrhythmogenic.

PHARMACOLOGIC SUPPORT

Medications are used perioperatively to provide vasoconstriction, venous and arterial vasodilation, inotropic support and treatment of arrhythmias. As summarized in Table 17-2, many of the medications commonly used have multiple actions. Selection of appropriate agents depends on accurate hemodynamic assessment.

Pressors are indicated for vasodilated patients who have normal pump function and are unresponsive to volume. These agents include α-agents (neosynephrine) and vasopressin. Methylene blue has demonstrated efficacy in vasopressor-resistant hypotension. Pressors can contribute to peripheral ischemia and vasospasm of coronary arteries and arterial conduits. Careful monitoring of extremity perfusion and

TABLE 17-2: Common ICU Scenarios and Management Strategies

Cardiac output syndromes

MAP	CVP	CO	PCW	SVR	Strategy
Normotensive	High	Low	High	Normal/High	Venodilator/diuretic/inotrope Vasodilator/iNO/iPGI$_2$
Hypertension	High	Normal	High	High	Vasodilator
Hypotension	Low	Low	Low	Normal	Volume/Inotrope/IABP
Hypotension	High	Low	High	High	α-agent
Hypotension	Normal/low	Normal/high	Normal/low	Low	

CVP = central venous pressure; CO = cardiac output; SVR = systemic vascular resistance; iNO = inhaled nitric oxide; iPGI$_2$ = inhaled prostacyclin.

Commonly used vasoactive drugs and hemodynamic effects

Pharmacological agent	HR	PCW	CI	SVR	MAP	MVO$_2$
Inotropic agents						
Dobutamine	↑↑	↓	↑	↓	↑↓	↑↔
Milrinone	↑	↓	↑	↓↓	↓	↑↓
Mixed vasoactive agents						
Epinephrine	↑↑	↑↓	↑	↑	↑	↑
Norepinephrine	↑↑	↑↑	↑	↑↑	↑↑	↑
Dopamine	↑↑	↑↓	↑	↑↓	↑↓	↑
Vasopressor agents						
Phenylephrine	↔	↑	↔	↑↑	↑↑	↑↔
Vasopressin	↔	↔	↔	↑↑	↑↑	↑↔
Methylene blue	↔	↔	↔	↑	↑	↑
Vasodilating agents						
Nitroglycerine	↑	↓↔	↔	↓	↓	↔↓
Nitroprusside	↑↑	↓↔	↔	↓↓	↓↓	↔↓
Nicardipine	↔	↔	↔	↓↓	↓↓	↔
Nesiritide	↔	↓↔	↔	↓	↓	↔

HR = heart rate; PCW = pulmonary capillary wedge; CI = cardiac index; SVR = systemic vascular resistance; MAP = mean arterial pressure; MVO$_2$ = mixed venous oxygen saturation.

(*Continued*)

TABLE 17-2: Common ICU Scenarios and Management Strategies (*Continued*)

NASPE/BPEG Pacemaker identification codes[130]

Code positions

I	II	III	IV	V
Chamber paced	Chamber sensed	Response to sensing	Programmable functions	Antitachyarrhythmia functions
V-ventricle	V-ventricle	T-triggers pacing	P-programmable rate and/or output	P-antitachyarrhythmia
A-atrium	A-atrium	I-inhibits pacing	M-multi-programmable	S-shock
D-double	D-double	D-triggers and inhibits pacing	C-communicating functions (telemetry)	D-dual (pacer and shock)
O-none	O-none	O-none	R-rate modulation	O-none
S-single chamber	S-single chamber	-	O-none	-

Postoperative mediastinal bleeding

Bleeding scenario	Diagnosis	Strategy
<50 cc/h Stable BP, coagulopathy	Post-CPB	Observation
>100 cc/h		
Hypothermic	Hypothermia	Re-warming strategies
Acute hypotension (MAP < 50 mm Hg)	(see above)	Fluid resuscitation (Aim MAP 60-65 mm Hg)
Diffuse bloody ooze		
Coagulopathy:	Borderline coagulopathy	
1. High PTT, PT		PEEP trial (5-10 cm H_2O), Coagulation screen
2. INR > 1.4	Rebound heparin effect	Heparin level; protamine
3. Low fibrinogen	Deficient clotting factors	Fresh frozen plasma
4. Platelets < $10^5/\mu L$	Deficient clotting factors	Fresh frozen plasma
5. Platelets > $10^5/\mu L$	Thrombocytopenia	Platelet pool
6. Bleeding > 10 min	Platelet dysfunction	DDAVP
7. Bleeding > 30 min (High D-dimers, evidence of fibrinolysis)	Fibrinolysis	Tranexamic acid, ε-aminocaproic acid, aprotinin
	Fibrinolysis	
>200-300 cc/h		
>200 cc/h for 4 h		
>300 cc/h for 2-3 h	Surgical bleeding	Surgical reexploration
>400 cc/h for 1 h		

DDAVP = desmopressin (synthetic vasopressin); PTT = activated partial thromboplastin time; FDP = fibrin and fibrinogen degradation products; PEEP = positive end-expiratory pressure; PT = prothrombin time; BP = blood pressure; CPB = cardiopulmonary bypass.

electrocardiographic changes is required when using these agents.

Vasodilators are indicated for hypertensive patients and for patients who are normotensive with poor pump function. Nitroglycerin and sodium nitroprusside are commonly used in the immediate postoperative period. Both have the advantage of being short acting and easy to titrate. Both can cause hypoxia by inhibiting pulmonary arterial hypoxic vasoconstriction and increasing blood flow through poorly oxygenated lung. Nitroglycerin is a stronger venodilator than an arterial dilator, and

can increase intercoronary collateral blood flow, but patients can quickly become tachyphylactic. Prolonged nitroprusside use can lead to cyanide toxicity, and methemaglobin levels must be monitored. Nicardipine is a calcium channel blocker with minimal effects on contractility or atrioventricular (AV) nodal conduction; it appears to have the efficacy of nipride without its toxicity. Nicardipine has been shown to control BP with less variability than nitroglycerine or nitroprusside and this has been found to correlate with improved outcomes. Nesiritide, or brain naturetic peptide, promotes diuresis in addition to vasodilation and may have beneficial lusitropic effects in patients with diastolic dysfunction.

Hypertension can also be treated with beta blockers. These agents work by decreasing heart rate and contractility. Esmolol is useful in the presence of labile BP because of its short half-life. Labetolol combines beta and alpha adrenergic blockade. Patients whose pump function is inotrope dependent should not receive beta blockers.

Inotropic agents are indicated when low CO persists despite optimization of fluid status (preload), vascular tone (afterload), and heart rate and rhythm. These agents include beta adrenergic agents (dobutamine) and cyclic nucleotide phosphodiesterase inhibitors (milrinone). Both of these agents increase CO by increasing myocardial contractility and by reducing afterload through peripheral vasodilation. Dobutamine is shorter acting and easier to titrate; milrinone achieves increases in CO with lower myocardial oxygen consumption. Both are arrhythmogenic and can exacerbate coronary ischemia. Both epinephrine and norepinephrine combine β and α adrenergic agonist effects; they are pressors in addition to positive inotropes. Relative α effects increase with dose. Dopamine in low doses causes splanchnic and renal vasodilation; α and β effects dominate at higher doses. Since perioperative beta blockade has been shown to improve mortality and morbidity following cardiac surgery, it seems reasonable to avoid the gratuitous use of inotropes, and efforts should be made to rapidly wean these agents when they are no longer required.

Heart Rate and Rhythm Management

Deviations from normal sinus rhythm can cause significant clinical deterioration and optimization of heart rate and rhythm is frequently an effective way to improve hemodynamic status.

PACING (SEE TABLE 17-2)

Within normal rate ranges, CO increases linearly with heart rate, and pacing is often very helpful. However, it is important to carefully monitor the response to pacing. For example, sinus bradycardia is often more effective than ventricular pacing at a more normal rate. Ventricular pacing can cause ventricular dysfunction and dys-synchrony and the loss of consistent filling from atrial contraction; ventricular pacing is often useful in acutely decreasing BP while waiting to initiate a vasodilator. If possible atrial pacing is preferred to AV pacing which is preferred to ventricular pacing. Pacing too rapidly can adversely affect cardiac performance by decreasing filling time, exacerbating ischemia or inducing heart block. Ensure that pacemakers in patients undergoing ventricular pacing can sense appropriately in order to avoid R on T and subsequent ventricular fibrillation. Internal pacemakers can often be reprogramed to improve output.

Heart block can occur following aortic, mitral and tricuspid valve surgery. It is also associated with inferior myocardial infarction and can be secondary to medications (eg, digoxin, amiodarone, calcium channel blockers, and beta blockers). If a bi-atrial trans-septal approach to the mitral valve is employed, sinus rhythm can be lost due to the division of the sinoatrial node.[4] Heart block is frequently transient. If the ventricular escape rate is absent or insufficient, pacing wire thresholds need to be carefully monitored and backup pacing methods employed (by transvenous wire, pacing pulmonary artery catheter, or external pacing pads) if needed while waiting for placement of a permanent pacemaker.

VENTRICULAR ARRHYTHMIAS

Nonsustained ventricular tachycardia (VT) is common following cardiac surgery and typically a reflection of perioperative ischemia/reperfusion injury, electrolyte abnormalities (typically hypokalemia and hypomagnesemia) or an increase in exogenous or endogenous sympathetic stimulation. Generally, nonsustained VT is more important as a symptom of an underlying cause requiring diagnosis and correction than as a cause of hemodynamic instability.

Sustained VT persisting for more than 30 seconds or associated with significant hemodynamic compromise, requires more aggressive treatment. Ongoing ischemia should be ruled out (coronary angiography may be necessary), electrolytes should be replaced and inotropes should be minimized. Beta blockers, amiodarone, and lidocaine can be useful therapies. Electrocardioversion should be employed if sustained VT causes significant compromise.

ATRIAL FIBRILLATION AND FLUTTER

Background. The incidence of postoperative atrial fibrillation (POAF) following cardiothoracic surgery is 30 to 50%,[5] and has been shown to be higher in the elderly and patients with renal impairment or chronic obstructive pulmonary disease (COPD).[6] This is associated with an increased risk of stroke, longer hospitalization, higher cost, and greater risk of long-term mortality.[7]

Prophylaxis. The incidence of POAF is 20 to 40% in coronary artery bypass graft (CABG) patients but it is generally more common in patients undergoing valve and combined procedures. POAF is typically a transient phenomenon. Use of beta blockers for the prevention of POAF is supported by the highest level of evidence. Therefore, beta blockers should be started or resumed as soon as they can be safely tolerated following cardiac surgery. Inotropic support, hemodynamic compromise, and AV block (PR interval > 0.24 ms, second or third degree block) are contraindications. Beta blockers appear to provide more effective prophylaxis when they are dosed with high frequency and titrated to produce an effect on heart rate and BP. Sotalol and amiodarone are also effective for prophylaxis but not superior. Sotalol, like other type II agents, can promote ventricular arrhythmias. Beta blockers also confer benefits other than atrial fibrillation prophylaxis, are easy to titrate, and do not have the toxicities associated with amiodarone. The postinflammatory milieu following cardiothoracic surgery may contribute to the pathogenesis of postoperative arrhythmias. For example, IL6 and C-reactive protein elevation postoperatively and atrial fibrillation (AF) have been linked. In the only randomized clinical trial in this arena atorvastatin started 7 days before cardiac surgery was associated with a >60% reduction in the incidence of postoperative AF among 200 patients undergoing CABG surgery. However, the high AF rate (~60%) in the control group of this study was not representative of the experience at most centers; this may reflect the fact that beta blockers were not administered routinely after surgery.

Treatment. There are many treatment strategies for the management of atrial fibrillation. We have developed the guidelines outlined in Table 17-1. The principle premise of this strategy is the recognition that for most patients with new onset atrial fibrillation, the arrhythmia is well tolerated and self-limited (90% of patients are in sinus rhythm within 6 to 8 weeks independent of treatment approach). The pursuit of a rate control and anticoagulation strategy typically produces outcomes comparable to a rhythm control strategy. Our prophylactic regimen begins with metoprolol 12.5 to 25 mg orally (po) four times a day and is titrated upward as tolerated.

STRATEGY FOR THE TREATMENT OF POSTOPERATIVE ATRIAL FIBRILLATION (FIG. 17-1)

A. Initial assessment: The management of atrial fibrillation should be guided by the answers to the following three questions:

1. Is the patient symptomatic? Atrial fibrillation is generally well tolerated, and over aggressive management can cause significant morbidity. Nonetheless, the first step in the management of atrial fibrillation is an assessment of its hemodynamic significance. Significant symptoms may respond to rate control alone or may require chemical or electrical cardioversion. Evidence

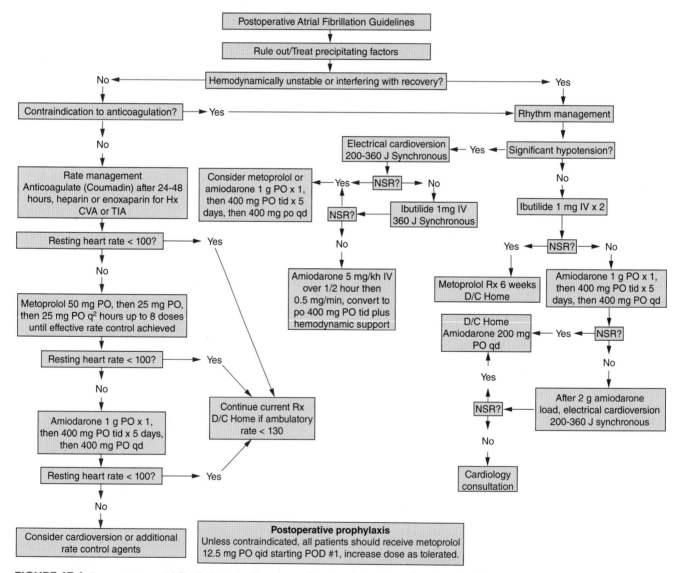

FIGURE 17-1 Postoperative atrial fibrillation guidelines. (Reproduced with permission from Maisel WH, Rawn JD, Stevenson WG: Atrial fibrillation after cardiac surgery, *Ann Intern Med.* 2001 Dec 18;135(12):1061-1073.)

of compromise includes hypotension, changes in mental status, decreased urine output, impaired peripheral perfusion, symptoms of coronary ischemia, and decreased CO or increased filling pressures.

2. **What are the precipitating factors?** Appropriate management of atrial fibrillation requires identification and treatment of potential risk factors. Atrial fibrillation can result from ischemia, atrial distension, increased sympathetic tone, electrolyte imbalances (particularly hypokalemia and hypomagnesemia precipitated by diuresis), acid-base disturbances (particularly alkalosis), sympathomimetic medications (inotropes, bronchodilators), beta blocker withdrawal, pneumonia, atelectasis, and pulmonary embolism.

3. **What are the goals of therapy?** Hemodynamic stability is the primary goal. For most patients, rate control is sufficient since 90% of patients with new onset atrial fibrillation following cardiac surgery will be in normal sinus rhythm within 6 weeks. In long-term studies of patients with chronic atrial fibrillation it has been difficult to show a benefit from rhythm control strategies.[8] Optimal target heart rates depend on many patient-specific factors. A randomized study comparing strict control (heart rate less than 80) to lenient control (heart rate less than 110) in permanent atrial fibrillation found fewer adverse events in the lenient control group.[9] Evidence of hemodynamic compromise or interference with recovery should prompt chemical or electrical cardioversion.

B. **Drug therapy:** Agents can be conveniently divided into rate control and rhythm control agents, although beta blockers are also effective in converting atrial fibrillation postoperatively. Mono drug therapy is generally better than poly drug therapy.

Rate control agents

1. **Beta blockers.** Metoprolol should be first line therapy in most patients and can be given orally or intravenously. Metoprolol should be titrated to effect with a heart rate goal typically less than 110 beats/minute at rest. The suggested treatment for new onset atrial fibrillation is 50 mg po. followed by 25 mg po every 2 to 3 hours until NSR or adequate rate control is achieved. Some patients may require oral doses over 400 mg/day.

2. **Calcium channel blockers.** Diltiazem is the agent of choice. It can be given orally starting at 30 mg po three time a day. It can also be initiated as a bolus of 0.25 mg/kg IV, followed by 0.35 mg/kg IV, followed by a continuous infusion at 5 to 15 mg/h.

3. **Digoxin** can be considered in patients with contraindications to beta blockers, in particular those with poor ejection fraction. There is evidence that it increases atrial automaticity. It has a half-life of 38 to 48 hours in patients with normal renal function, significant potential toxicity, and a narrow therapeutic range. Levels must be monitored, particularly in patients with renal insufficiency. Many agents, including amiodarone, increase its serum level.

Antiarrythmics

1. **Metoprolol**
2. **Ibutilide.** Ibutilide is given as a 1-mg intravenous bolus and repeated once if cardioversion fails to occur. Patients need to be monitored for a small but significant incidence of torsade de pointes which may be increased if given in conjunction with amiodarone.
3. **Amiodarone** can cause myocardial depression, heart block, and acute pulmonary toxicity; significant hypotension is most commonly associated with rapid bolus infusion. Significant toxicity is associated with prolonged use of amiodarone, and consideration should be given to discontinuing the drug within six weeks of surgery.
4. **Adenosine** is helpful in the treatment of supraventricular tachycardia. (It should be avoided in transplant recipients, partially revascularized patients and in patients with atrial flutter).
5. **Dronedarone.** Dronedarone is an amiodarone analog without iodine moiety in its structure, and is similar to amiodarone with regard to its structural and electrophysiological properties.[10] It has been associated with increased mortality in patients with severely depressed left ventricular function.[11,12] It appears to be less toxic but also less effective than amiodarone.[13]

C. **Electrical cardioversion:** Electrical cardioversion should be used emergently for the treatment of hemodynamically unstable atrial fibrillation. Synchronous cardioversion rather than defibrillation should be utilized to minimize the risk of precipitating ventricular fibrillation. Sedation should be used. In patients with atrial wires who are in atrial flutter, overdrive pacing can be attempted.

D. **Anticoagulation:** Patients who remain in atrial fibrillation for >24 hours or have multiple sustained episodes over this period should be started on coumadin in the absence of contraindications. Heparin (unfractionated IV or low molecular weight SQ) should be considered after 48 hours, particularly in patients with a history of stroke or TIAs or who have a low ejection fraction. Coumadin can be initiated in patients who may require permanent pacer placement as pacemakers can generally be safely placed with INR < 2. Postprocedure heparin bridging has been associated with significant rates of pocket hematoma formation.

Postoperative Ischemia and Infarction

Postoperative ischemia and infarction can be caused by inadequate intraoperative myocardial protection, kinked, spasmed or thrombosed conduits, thrombosed endarterectomized vessels, or embolization by air or atherosclerotic debris. It should be suspected in the presence of otherwise unexplained poor pump function, ST changes, new bundle branch block or complete heart block, ventricular arrhythmias or enzyme elevation. Electrocardiographic changes should be correlated with the anatomy of known atherosclerotic or revascularized territories. Air embolism preferentially involves the right coronary artery and inferior ST changes are generally present in the operating room. It typically resolves within hours. It is worth noting that nonspecific ST changes are common postoperatively and usually benign. Pericardial changes are generally characterized by diffuse concave ST elevations, accompanied by a pericardial rub and delayed in onset by at least 12 hours following surgery.

New wall motion abnormalities or mitral regurgitation diagnosed echocardiographically can help determine the hemodynamic significance of suspected ischemia or infarction. Knowledge of the quality of conduits, anastamoses, and target vessels is critical in planning management strategy (eg, there may be little to be gained and much to lose in attempting to improve flow to a small, highly diseased posterior descending artery with poor run-off). On the other hand, if significant myocardium appears at risk a timely trip to the operating room or the cardiac catheterization laboratory can dramatically improve outcomes. Ongoing ischemia should prompt consideration of standard treatment strategies including anticoagulation, beta blockade, and nitroglycerin as tolerated. Intra-aortic balloon pump placement should be considered to minimize inotrope requirements, decrease myocardial oxygen requirements and minimize infarct size.

Right Ventricular Failure and Pulmonary Hypertension

Right ventricular failure can be a particularly difficult postoperative problem. It can be caused by perioperative ischemia or infarction or by acute increases in PVR. Preexisting pulmonary hypertension is commonly caused by left-sided heart failure, aortic stenosis, mitral valve disease, and pulmonary disease. Chronic pulmonary hypertension is characterized by abnormal increased vasoconstriction and vascular remodeling.[14] Acute increases in PVR are commonly caused by acute left ventricular dysfunction, mitral valve insufficiency or stenosis, volume overload, pulmonary edema, atelectasis, hypoxia, or acidosis. Pulmonary embolism should also be considered, but it is rare in the immediate postoperative period. As the right heart fails it becomes distended, CVP increases, tricuspid regurgitation may develop, and pulmonary artery pressures and left-sided filling pressures become inadequate. Strategies for reversing this potentially fatal process begin with identifying potentially reversible etiologies. Volume status and left-sided function should be optimized. The RV has its own starling curve, and while the failing right ventricle (RV) often needs more volume to ensure adequate left-sided filling, overdistension will worsen function. Judicious use of positive end-expiratory pressure (PEEP) to recruit atelectatic lung and hyperventilation can decrease the impact of pulmonary vasoconstriction mediated by hypoxia and hypercapnia. Use of intravenous vasodilators to reduce PVR is frequently limited by systemic hypotension. Inotropes (typically milrinone which also provides vasodilation) can be beneficial. Vasopressin, unlike other pressors, appears to increase SVR more than PVR.[15] Since no intravenous vasodilator is selective for the pulmonary vasculature, topical administration can be significantly more effective in reducing PVR without causing systemic hypotension. Inhaled NO and PGI_2 have comparable efficacy. They can also improve oxygenation by shunting blood to ventilated lung.

Valve Diseases: Special Postoperative Considerations

AORTIC VALVE REPLACEMENT

The different pathophysiologies associated with aortic stenosis (primarily a pressure overload phenomenon) versus aortic insufficiency (volume overload) can result in significantly different postoperative courses.

Aortic Stenosis. Aortic stenosis can lead to the development of a hypertrophied, noncompliant left ventricle (LV). For some patients, replacement of a stenotic valve allows a ventricle conditioned to pumping against abnormally high afterload to easily achieve supranormal levels of CO and BP postoperatively. Meticulous BP control is frequently required to avoid disrupting fresh suture lines. In some patients, the degree of ventricular hypertrophy can lead to dynamic outflow obstruction; the condition is most effectively treated with volume, beta blockers, and afterload augmentation. Even without dynamic outflow obstruction, reduced compliance (diastolic dysfunction) can create significant hemodynamic compromise if the patient becomes hypovolemic or loses normal sinus rhythm (up to 30% of stroke volume can be dependent on synchrony between atria and ventricles). The placement of atrial wires in addition to ventricular wires can provide significant advantages in the event that the patient is bradycardic or experiences heart block postoperatively.

Aortic Regurgitation. The LV in a patient with aortic regurgitation is frequently dilated without significant hypertrophy and often functions poorly postoperatively. Optimization of volume, afterload, inotropy, and rhythm in these patients is often challenging.

MITRAL VALVE REPAIR/REPLACEMENT

Mitral Regurgitation. Following repair or replacement of an incompetent mitral valve, increased afterload and consequent greater wall stress unmask LV dysfunction. Frequently inotropic support and systemic vasodilation is required to reduce the afterload mismatch seen following surgery. Occasionally LV dysfunction can be the result of inadvertent suture placement compromising the circumflex coronary artery.

Mitral Stenosis. Unlike patients with mitral regurgitation, patients with mitral stenosis typically have preserved LV function. Exacerbation of preexisting pulmonary hypertension is common, however. Postoperative strategies focus on optimizing right ventricular function and decreasing PVR.

Cardiac Arrest and Cardiopulmonary Resuscitation

The incidence of cardiac arrest following cardiac surgery ranges between 0.7% and 2.9%. These patients represent a special case for application of advanced cardiac life support (ACLS) algorithms. The majority of these events happen in the immediate postoperative period when many patients are still intubated and monitored in the intensive care unit (ICU). In addition to ventricular arrhythmias, common etiologies for arrest in these patients include readily reversible causes: hypovolemia from hemorrhage, cardiac tamponade, acute hypoxia, electrolyte abnormalities, tension pneumothorax, pacing failure, and myocardial ischemia. Many of these patients develop clinical deterioration prior to the arrest which can provide clues to the mechanism of the arrest and guide therapy. Early recognition in a critical care environment, the presence of trained clinicians, patient-specific knowledge, and reversible etiologies combine to produce outcomes that are significantly better when compared to outcomes in the broader population of patients experiencing arrest. Cardiac surgery patients undergoing resuscitation in the 24 hours following surgery have survival rates up to 70%.[16,17]

The most important factors contributing to survival following cardiac arrest are prompt defibrillation and immediate, high quality, and uninterrupted chest compressions. There are special circumstances in cardiac surgery patients when chest compressions may be deferred. The European Resuscitation Council has recommended three successive (stacked) shocks for ventricular fibrillation or pulseless VT occurring in immediate postoperative cardiac surgery patients prior to chest compressions if defibrillation is immediately available.[18] Minutes matter[19] and patients at high risk for arrhythmias should have defibrillator pads placed postoperatively. Because chest compressions in the immediate postoperative period can cause myocardial injury, sternal and rib fractures, bypass graft injury, prosthetic valve dehiscence, lung injury, and hemorrhage,[20] it would be preferable to avoid compressions if return of spontaneous circulation (ROSC) can be achieved with electrical cardioversion. For asystole or severe bradycardia, pacing wires should be utilized when available prior to initiating chest compressions. Adding a ground wire in the skin can sometimes improve the capture of poorly functioning temporary pacing wires. Patients with pulseless electrical activity may respond to volume administration or pressor administration; if these interventions are ineffective, chest compressions should be initiated. Finally, if tamponade is suspected and emergency resternotomy is immediately available in the ICU, it is reasonable to minimize chest compressions and open the chest.

The efficacy of chest compressions can be monitored with preexisting arterial lines or with end-tidal CO_2 ($ETCO_2$) monitoring (quantitative waveform capnography). These techniques can also minimize interruption of chest compressions and help to identify ROSC. Systolic pressures close to 80 mm Hg or $ETCO_2 > 10$ mm Hg is considered to reflect adequate CPR. $ETCO_2 > 40$ is associated with ROSC.

If patients are not ventilated, intubation should be deferred and mask ventilation utilized until experienced personnel are available. Chest compressions should be interrupted only to insert the endotracheal tube through the vocal cords once visualized. Postoperative cardiac surgery patients are often very sensitive to increases in intrathoracic pressure and respiratory rates should be approximately 10 breaths per minute and minimal tidal volumes should be used.

Use of epinephrine should be limited and not follow standard algorithms in the resuscitation of cardiac surgery patients because of the potential for hypertension leading to suture line disruption and hemorrhage. Smaller doses may be cautiously titrated to effect. Amiodarone (300 mg IV) should be considered for persistent ventricular fibrillation or tachycardia resistant to electrical cardioversion.

Chest tubes should be placed in the mid-clavicular line in the second intercostal space if tension pneumothorax is suspected. Resternotomy should be considered if resuscitative efforts have failed to achieve ROSC within 5 to 10 minutes, particularly if tamponade is suspected. Ultrasonography can suggest, but not rule out, cardiac tamponade. Upon opening the chest, internal cardiac massage can be initiated. Clot should be evacuated, sources of bleeding identified, and bypass graft patency can be assessed.

Effective teamwork is a critical component of effective cardiopulmonary resuscitation. A call for additional help should be made if personnel resources are suboptimal. A team leader needs to be identified to manage the effort. If resources are adequate, the leader's role should be restricted to coordinating care. The leader should assign tasks after assessing a practitioner's competence to perform the assigned task. Communication should be closed loop; when team members are assigned a task they need to communicate that they understand the task and provide notification when they have completed it. The effective leader should rely on the collective knowledge of the team by actively soliciting information about the patient's condition prior to the arrest and exploring potential diagnoses and courses of action. As mentioned previously, ACLS algorithms were not developed for cardiac surgery patients specifically, and cardiopulmonary resuscitation should be performed with awareness of the special problems facing these patients postoperatively and with awareness of the specific circumstances of the patient. Knowledge of the patient's medical problems, operative details (including bleeding problems, hemodynamic instability coming off bypass, echocardiographic findings, and revascularization challenges) and postoperative course should guide strategy. Mobilization of personnel and equipment to open the chest should occur if resuscitation efforts are not immediately successful.

Training of practitioners in resuscitation is critical to optimization of outcomes. As important as knowing what to do in an emergency situation is to know how to do it. Mock codes should focus on teamwork and effective leadership in addition to focusing on issues specific to cardiac surgery patients. Required equipment should be dedicated and readily available and all members of the team should know how to access it.

BLEEDING, THROMBOSIS, AND TRANSFUSION STRATEGIES

One of the principle challenges of cardiac surgery is to achieve sufficient anticoagulation while supported on CPB without experiencing excessive bleeding postoperatively. Not surprisingly, patients undergoing off-pump CABG experience a significant reduction in postoperative bleeding and blood product transfusion requirements.[21] Excessive bleeding and its complications, including blood product transfusions, cause significant morbidity and mortality.

Preoperative Evaluation

Preoperative evaluation includes documenting a history of abnormal bleeding or thrombosis, and obtaining basic coagulation studies, a hematocrit and platelet count. A history of recent heparin exposure associated with thrombocytopenia should suggest a diagnosis of heparin-induced thrombocytopenia (HIT). Confirmation of the presence of IgG directed against platelet factor 4 (the prevalence of these antibodies in patients with previous heparin exposure can be up to 35%)[22] requires either a delay in surgery until the assay is negative (usually 3 months), or if surgery is more urgently required, alternative anticoagulation strategies (bivalirudin[23]) can be considered. Preoperative medications that can increase bleeding risk are common. Aspirin inhibits cyclooxygenase, reduces the synthesis of thromboxane-A_2, and decreases platelet aggregation. Preoperative aspirin use modestly increases postoperative bleeding, but preoperative and early postoperative use (ie, within 6 hours) is beneficial to outcome and ultimate survival.[24] Other antiplatelet agents have more profound impacts on platelet function. The glycoprotein IIb/IIIa inhibitors eptifibatide (Integrillin) and tirofiban (Aggrastat) are sufficiently short acting that surgery can be safely conducted despite recent exposure. Abciximab (Reopro) usually requires a 24 to 48-hour delay of surgery, if feasible, to avoid catastrophic bleeding. Clopidogrel (Plavix), prasugrel (effient), and ticagrelor (brilinta) inhibit the P_2Y_{12} component of platelet ADP receptors preventing ADP platelet activation. Discontinuing these agents 5 to 7 days before surgery will minimize bleeding, but they are often continued closer to the time of surgery because the risk of mortality is high from acute coronary stent occlusion, particularly in patients with recently placed drug-eluting stents. Customarily, warfarin (which inhibits the vitamin K-dependent clotting factors II, VII, IX, and X) is discontinued 4 to 7 days preoperatively to allow gradual correction of the INR. Although patients undergoing an interruption in warfarin administration frequently receive bridging anticoagulation with heparin, increasing evidence suggests that this strategy increases bleeding without preventing thromboembolism.[25,26]

Newer oral anticoagulant agents such as direct thrombin inhibitors Dabigatran (Pradaxa) and direct factor Xa inhibitors including Rivaroxaban (Xarelto), Apixaban (Eliquis), and Edoxaban (Lixiana, Savaysa) have been developed recently. The long-term efficacy and safety of these target-specific oral anticoagulants are comparable with coumadin in specific applications. The half-life of these agents is shorter, making it easier to discontinue before elective cardiac surgery. Levels can be measured by thrombin time for Dabigatran and anti-factor Xa for Apixaban. However, reversal of anticoagulant effects of these agents in an urgent situation is challenging. Antifibrinolytic agents, DDAVP, prothrombin complex concentrates (PCCs), oral activated charcoal, and hemodialysis are suggested, but there is no high-quality evidence supporting the efficacy of these interventions. There are no data to support use of rFVIIa, FFP, or cryoprecipitate for reversal.

Preoperative anemia in patients undergoing cardiac surgery is associated with increased morbidity and mortality [27,28] and increased rate of intraoperative and postoperative red blood cell transfusion. Therefore, identifying and treating reversible causes of anemia is advisable. Elective surgeries should be delayed when possible to allow optimization of preoperative hemoglobin levels with iron supplementation and vitamin B12.[29] Administration of erythropoietin has not been demonstrated to reduce the need for RBC transfusion and may actually contribute to adverse outcomes.[30] Efforts to reduce phlebotomy volumes and frequency can have a significant impact on the incidence of perioperative anemia.[31]

Intraoperative Strategies

Multiple intraoperative strategies have evolved to prevent unnecessary bleeding and blood product transfusion. Antithrombolytics Σ-aminocaproic acid (Amicar) and Tranexamic acid (Cyclokapron) inhibit plasminogen activation and limit fibrinolysis. Topical use of tranexamic acid intraoperatively prior to closure has been shown to be a simple and effective way to reduce postoperative bleeding,[32] particularly in patients with friable tissue undergoing reoperations or with previous exposure to chest irradiation.

Retrograde autologous priming of the CPB circuit involves displacing circuit prime at the initiation of CPB by draining the patient's blood both antegrade through the venous cannula and retrograde through the arterial cannula.[33] This strategy has been shown to significantly decrease the requirement for blood transfusion following CABG. The use of heparin bonded circuitry has enabled the safe use of lower anticoagulation targets while on bypass. Careful attention to hemostasis intraoperatively and avoidance of excessive use of the cell saver (which depletes platelets and clotting factors) pays dividends postoperatively.

Postoperative Bleeding

Most patients are mildly coagulopathic postoperatively, but only a minority bleeds excessively. Postoperative coagulopathy can be due to residual or rebound heparin effects following CPB, thrombocytopenia (qualitative and quantitative), clotting factor depletion, hypothermia, and hemodilution. Chest tube outputs persistently greater than 50 to 100 cc per hour or other clinical evidence of bleeding demand attention.

Strategies for avoiding postoperative hypothermia are also very important. Hypothermia ($\leq 35°C$) on arrival to the ICU is associated with delayed extubation, shivering, and increased peripheral O_2 consumption, hemodynamic instability, atrial and ventricular arrhythmias, increased SVR, and coagulopathy.

The treatment of postoperative bleeding depends initially upon making a judgment: Is bleeding surgical, coagulopathic, or both? Surgical bleeding is treated as quickly as possible by reexploration while coagulopathies can be corrected in the ICU. Coagulopathic patients demonstrate microvascular bleeding (often bleeding from wound edges and puncture sites) and rarely have significant clot formation in their chest tubes. Standard maneuvers include warming the patient, controlling BP, increasing PEEP, infusing additional Σ-aminocaproic acid, calcium gluconate and blood products. In general, blood products should not be used to correct coagulation abnormalities unless the patient is bleeding significantly. All allogeneic blood products can contribute to transfusion-related lung injury and have other adverse effects. Protamine is rarely indicated and can increase bleeding. Desmopressin (DDAVP) is a synthetic vasopressin analog which acts by increasing the concentration of Von Willebrand factor, an important mediator of platelet adhesion. It is of benefit in patients with von Willebrand's disease and in patients with severe platelet dysfunction secondary to uremia. It is sometimes used for bleeding associated with anitplatelet agents, but there is little evidence to support this practice.

Recombinant factor VIIa (rFVIIa) is a drug approved for use in hemophiliacs that has been used successfully to stop bleeding in patients with life-threatening hemorrhage after cardiac surgery. In combination with tissue factor, it activates the extrinsic coagulation system via factor X, resulting in thrombin generation and prompt correction of the PT. It has a significant risk of systemic thrombosis and should be reserved for otherwise uncontrollable bleeding.[34]

Prothrombin complex concentrates (PCCs) are indicated for the urgent reversal of acquired coagulation factor deficiency induced by vitamin K antagonist (ie, warfarin) therapy in adult patients with acute major bleeding, and can reduce the need for FFP transfusion. PCCs have less risk of graft or prosthetic valve thrombosis when compared to factor VIIa.

Mediastinal Reexploration

Reexploration should be considered when computed tomography (CT) outputs are >400 mL/h for 1 hour, >300 mL/h for 2 to 3 hours and 200 mL/h for 4 hours (Table 17-2)[35] or if signs of tamponade or hemodynamic instability develop. Tamponade should be considered in the presence of hypotension, tachycardia, elevated filling pressures, increasing inotrope requirements, pulsus paradoxus, and/or equalization of right and left atrial pressures. An echocardiogram may be useful in this situation but cannot rule out tamponade. Chest X-rays (CXRs) are a necessary element of the evaluation for bleeding, look for widening of the mediastinum or evidence of hemothorax. CXRs should be repeated on all patients with initial high chest tube output that later subsides to ensure that chest tubes have not clotted.

Autotransfusion

Autotransfusion of shed mediastinal blood remains controversial. It can be lifesaving in the presence of catastrophic bleeding. Red blood cell viability in unwashed shed mediastinal blood is comparable to that of autologous whole blood.[36] Additionally, there is evidence indicating no apparent clinical coagulopathy (low fibrinogen levels, but normal coagulation times at 1 and 24 hours) following reinfusion of shed blood.[37] This method of blood salvage is without allogeneic transfusion risks and has been shown to decrease transfusion requirements.[38] Autotransfusion should be avoided in patients with infectious endocarditis, hematologic diseases such as sickle cell or hemolysis, or if exogenous chemicals such as hemostatic agents or topical antibiotics were used during the operation.

Blood Transfusion

Recent guidelines[39] have highlighted the risks associated with blood transfusion and advocated restrictive transfusion strategies. The STS guidelines recommend transfusion for patients who have bled more than 30% of their blood volume or who are bleeding uncontrollably. In stable postoperative patients, it is recommended that transfusion be considered only if Hb falls below 7 g/dL (hematocrit < 21%). This recommendation is based, in large part, on the only significant randomized control trial examining the impact of transfusion strategies on outcome. The Canadian Critical Care Trials group found that patients randomized to a Hb target of 7 g/dL versus 10 g/dL had equivalent outcomes. Patients who were younger or less critically ill had a statistically significant improvement in survival if they received less blood.[40] Retrospective studies in cardiac surgery have shown a durable and dose-related association between transfusion and survival[41] (see Fig. 17-2). In addition, blood transfusion has been linked to an increase in postoperative infection, lung injury and prolonged intubation, myocardial ischemia and infarction, renal failure, stroke, and increased ICU length of stay, hospital length of stay, and overall cost.[42,43] A study examining patients undergoing cardiac surgery in the UK found that patients who received blood were more likely to experience death, infections, ischemic complications (myocardial infarction, stroke, and renal failure) and prolonged stays in the hospital.[44] The guidelines support transfusion above a Hb of 7 g/dL in patients with evidence of end-organ ischemia, but the evidence supporting

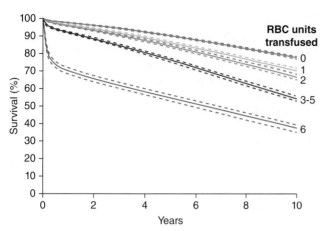

FIGURE 17-2 Survival after isolated CABG stratified by number of RBC units transfused. Increasing number of perioperative RBC transfusions results in incremental decreases in postoperative survival.[67] Solid lines are parametric estimates enclosed within dashed 68% confidence limits. RBC, red blood cell. (Reproduced with permission from Koch CG, Li L, Duncan AI, et al: Transfusion in coronary artery bypass grafting is associated with reduced long-term survival, *Ann Thorac Surg.* 2006 May;81(5):1650-1657.)

these recommendations rely almost entirely on expert consensus. In a well-designed propensity matched study, researchers compared Jehovah's witness patients (who refuse blood transfusion based on religious belief) with non-witness patients who received blood after cardiac surgery. Witnesses, who received no blood, had similar late survival compared with a matched group of cardiac surgical patients who received RBCs, and experienced fewer postoperative myocardial infarctions, a lower incidence of prolonged ventilation, less reoperation for bleeding, shorter ICU stays, and a lower hazard for in-hospital death.[45] They then compared witnesses with non-witnesses who did not receive blood and found comparable results.[46] There is little evidence supporting the belief that transfusion of stored, allogenic blood acutely improves oxygen carrying capacity. Stored blood is deficient in 2,3 DPG (and less capable of releasing oxygen to tissues) and nitric oxide; it also contains cells which are less flexible and may be more likely to occlude capillaries.

Blood transfusions have immunomodulating effects (by either alloimmunization or tolerance induction) that may increase the risk of nosocomial infections, transfusion-associated graft versus host disease, transfusion-related lung injury (TRALI), cancer recurrence, and the possible development of autoimmune diseases later in life. Furthermore, the risk of "newer" transfusion-transmitted diseases has become recognized. Proinflammatory mediators and cytokines have been associated with an increased risk of wound infection, sepsis, pulmonary and renal insufficiency.[47]

Heparin-induced Thrombocytopenia

Heparin-induced thrombocytopenia (HIT) is an immune-mediated syndrome affecting up to 3% of patients undergoing cardiac surgery. A complex of platelet factor 4 (released by

activated platelets) and heparin stimulate the production of IgG antibodies (detected by an anti-PF4 assay) which cause vigorous platelet and monocyte activation and aggregation. This process results in platelet consumption and thrombin production causing in turn a drop in platelet count and systemic thrombotic complications. These can include micro-angiopathic thrombosis in the digits, deep vein thrombosis and pulmonary embolism, and end-organ injury including stroke, renal failure, and gut ischemia. Thrombocytopenia is typical following CPB and is secondary to hemodilution, platelet destruction and aggregation. The platelet count usually reaches its nadir by the first or second postoperative day followed be a steady recovery. A second drop in platelet count of more than 30 to 50% of the postoperative peak 5 to 14 days after cardiac surgery is strongly suspicious for HIT syndrome. More rarely, patients may develop HIT earlier (within the first four postoperative days) without the characteristic postoperative rebound in platelet count. It can also occur later (weeks after hospital discharge).[48,49]

Antiplatelet antibodies are more common than thrombotic complications in patients undergoing cardiac surgery. The presence of anti-PF4 antibodies is detected utilizing an enzyme-linked immunoabsorbent assay (ELISA). The test is very sensitive (>95%) but has only a 75 to 85% specificity. A positive test occurs when optimal density (OD) values exceed 0.4. Some suggest the threshold of OD > 1 is associated with a higher likelihood of thrombotic events compared with OD values between 0.4 and 0.99.[50] The diagnosis can be confirmed with a more specific functional assay, typically, a serotonin release assay.

Once suspected, all heparin products must be discontinued, heparin-coated lines must be removed, and a direct thrombin inhibitor (bivalirudin, lepirudin, or argatroban) can be initiated. Warfarin, because it inhibits the synthesis of protein C, should be avoided initially. Bivalirudin is often the preferred thrombin inhibitor because its administration typically does not elevate the INR significantly (when compared to argatroban) making the transition to subsequent warfarin administration less complicated. Platelet transfusions can exacerbate thrombosis and are not recommended. When diagnosis is confirmed anticoagulation therapy with thrombin inhibitors should be continued until recovery of the platelet count followed by a transition to warfarin.[51,52]

RESPIRATORY CARE

Postoperative Pulmonary Pathophysiology

Patients undergoing heart surgery experience a spectrum of pulmonary dysfunction following heart surgery. The lungs become atelectatic during bypass and become edematous as a result of fluid shifts and the inflammatory response provoked by the bypass circuit. Increases are seen in the A-a gradient and pulmonary shunt fraction with a resultant decrease in compliance and impaired oxygenation. Many inflammatory mediators have been implicated. Complement is activated (C3a,

C5b-C9) and can directly damage pulmonary endothelium as well as sequester neutrophils. When activated these neutrophils release oxygen free radicals and proteases furthering injury. Macrophage cytokine production and platelet degranulation has also been demonstrated in models of bypass-induced lung injury.[53] TRALI can also exacerbate lung dysfunction.

In spite of increased knowledge of the mechanisms of injury, pharmocologic interventions have not proved effective in preventing it. To the contrary, administration of methyl-prednisolone in a randomized double-blinded study significantly increased A-a gradient and shunt fraction, decreased both static and dynamic compliance and delayed early extubation in a dose-dependent manner.[54]

Assessment on Arrival

On arrival to the intensive care unit, auscultation of the lungs should be performed to assure equal breath sounds and absence of bronchospasm. Ventilator settings should aim to minimize barotrauma and transition to a spontaneous ventilatory mode in a timely manner.[55] A review of the initial postoperative CXR should confirm proper endotracheal tube position 2 to 3 cm above the carina, proper nasogastric tube, and intravenous line placement. Clinicians should be alert for pneumothoraces, hemothoraces, and a widened mediastinum. Arterial blood gas should confirm adequate oxygenation, and absence of hypercapnea or metabolic acidosis. Arterial blood gas results should be correlated with pulse oximetry, minute ventilation, and end tidal CO_2 measurements.

Troubleshooting Hypoxia

As discussed above, oxygenation in all patients will be diminished compared to baseline. The inability to wean F_iO_2 below 50% within the first few postoperative hours should prompt a reevaluation for treatable causes. Sometimes simply replacing the pulse oximeter probe onto another finger or an earlobe will improve reported oxygen saturation. This is particularly true in patients with peripheral vasoconstriction, and more frequent ABGs may be necessary for correlation. The use of vasodilators including nitroglycerin, milrinone, sodium nitroprusside, and nicardipine can increase shunt fraction (by inhibiting hypoxic pulmonary vasoconstriction in poorly ventilated regions of the lung) enough to cause significant hypoxia. Increasing PEEP to improve alveolar recruitment is frequently beneficial.[56] Nebulizer treatments decrease bronchospasm, and repeat CXR may demonstrate pneumothorax, retained hemothorax, retained mediastinal hematoma, atelectasis, or a new infiltrate representing aspiration.

Atelectasis, particularly in the left lower lobe, is present to some degree in nearly all patients. Bibasilar atelectasis is believed to be the combined product of the prolonged supine position, and intraoperative muscle relaxation allowing upward displacement of abdominal contents and the diaphragm. This reduces functional reserve capacity by up to 1 L. On the left, this is compounded by pleurotomy for internal mammary artery take-down, compression of the left lung and decreased ventilatory tidal volumes to clear the field for IMA dissection. Lobar atelectasis, especially when associated with mucus plugging, can be improved by bronchoscopic aspiration in up to 80% of cases.[57] A prospective study comparing bronchoscopy to aggressive chest physiotherapy found the two techniques to be equally effective,[58] but only if the chest physiotherapy regimen is adhered to.

Sedation

Sedation and pain relief in cardiac surgery "fast-tracking" relies on short-acting agents including propofol, fentanyl, and midazolam. Dexmedetomidine is a highly selective α_2-adrenoreceptor agonist and has anxiolytic, sympatholytic, and analgesic effects without contributing to respiratory depression, oversedation, or delirium. It may provide myocardial protection, and has been shown to improve outcomes in cardiac surgery.[59] Hypotension and bradycardia can complicate its use.

Early Extubation

Stable patients with a normal mental status can often be extubated either in the operating room or within a few hours following arrival in the intensive care unit. Once an arterial blood gas has confirmed adequate oxygenation and ventilation, pulse oximetry and monitoring of minute ventilation or end tidal CO_2 can guide extubation, often without the need for subsequent blood gases.

Although hemodynamically unstable patients can improve following a reduction in airway pressures or extubation, a more cautious approach to early extubation should be taken in patients with preoperative pulmonary failure requiring intubation, uncompensated congestive heart failure with pulmonary edema, cardiogenic shock (including a requirement for intra-aortic balloon counterpulsion), deep hypothermic circulatory arrest, persistent hypothermia < 35.5°C; persistent hypoxia $P_aO_2{:}F_iO_2$ < 200, persistent acidosis with pH < 7.30, persistent mediastinal bleeding, or cerebrovascular accident or reduced mental status (inability to follow commands or protect airway).

Ventilator Weaning and Extubation

Prolonged mechanical ventilatory support is a source of significant morbididty and mortality. In general, every effort should be made to wean the patient from the ventilator. Minimizing barotrauma has been shown to improve outcomes both in patients with severe lung injury and in those with more normal lung function. Spontaneous ventilatory modes (pressure support) are typically better tolerated by patients and are associated with lower airway pressures. Most ventilated patients do not need to be unconscious. Oversedation can cause hypotension, delirium, and prolong intubation. Benzodiazepine infusions and prolonged propofol administration should be avoided as these agents promote delirium and accumulate.

The decision to extubate must take into account the adequacy of oxygenation and ventilation on minimal ventilatory support as well as an estimate of the patient's ability to manage secretions and protect his or her airway.[60] Finally, an assessment of the patient's ability to perform the work of breathing needs to be made. For patients unable to wean from the vent immediately following surgery, a spontaneous breathing trial (SBT) (30 minutes of spontaneous breathing with 5 cm H_2O of pressure support or unassisted breathing through a T-tube) has been shown to be the most accurate predictor of a successful extubation. Breathing trials are typically discontinued for signs of distress such as respiratory frequency > 35/min, O_2 saturation < 90%, HR > 140 bpm, SBP > 180 or <90 mm Hg, agitation, diaphoresis, or anxiety.[61] The minute ventilation V_E and maximal inspiratory pressure is significantly less predictive of successful extubation than a successful SBT.[62]

The strategy of daily or intermittent SBTs has been directly compared to weaning strategies based on stepwise reduction of the frequency of intermittent mandatory ventilation (IMV), or stepwise reduction of the level of pressure-support ventilation (PSV). Daily or intermittent SBTs lead to successful extubation 2 to 3 times earlier than either IMV or PSV weans.

Extubation Failure

Overall, approximately 5% of cardiothoracic patients require reintubation.[63] Patients with COPD have a 14% incidence,[64] while those with a past history of stroke have a 10% incidence.[65] Other risk factors include NYHA class IV functional status, renal failure, need for intra-aortic balloon counterpulsion, reduced $pO_2:F_iO_2$, reduced vital capacity, longer operating room time, a longer CPB run, and a longer initial ventilatory requirement.[66] Unfortunately for ICU patients reintubation is typically a predictor of increased length of stay and increased mortality.

Chronic Ventilation and Tracheotomy

In the early 1960s, translaryngeal intubation was associated with a prohibitively high rate of tracheal stenosis. As a result, a consensus existed that tracheotomy should be performed for patients requiring mechanical ventilation for longer than 3 days.[67] Low-pressure cuffs and soft tubes have since decreased the urgency of this intervention. A consensus subsequently evolved advocating that patients who continue to require mechanical ventilation at two weeks should undergo tracheotomy. Several trials have suggested that earlier discontinuation of mechanical ventilation and reduced complications are associated with earlier tracheotomy.[68] Tracheostomy results in reduced dead-space and airway resistance, is more comfortable for the patient, and usually allows the patient to participate more in the recovery process. It has been suggested that clinician behavior is positively affected by the presence of a tracheostomy tube; more aggressive attempts at weaning and discontinuation of mechanical support may be made because reconnecting the ventilator is easy.

Percutaneous dilatational tracheotomy (PDT) performed in the ICU has increasingly been recognized as a safe procedure. A recent randomized prospective study of medical patients projected to require more than 14 days of mechanical ventilation[69] compared two groups: PDT within 48 hours and 14 to 16 days. One hundred twenty patients were enrolled. In the early PDT group, there was a strongly significant reduction in duration of mechanical ventilation (7.6 ± 4.0 vs 17.4 ± 5.3 days, $p < .001$), incidence of pneumonia (5 vs 25%, $p < .005$), and mortality (31.7 vs 61.7%, $p < .005$). There was no difference in incidence or severity of tracheal stenosis identified in-hospital and at 10 weeks.

Pleural Effusion

Accumulation of fluid in the pleural space is common after cardiac surgery, particularly on the left side, and often resolves with time and diuresis. Contributory factors can include fluid overload, residual hematoma which can draw fluid into the pleural space, bleeding, pericardial and pleural inflammation (postpericardiotomy syndrome), atelectasis, hypoalbuminemia, pneumonia, or pulmonary embolism. Pleural effusion can cause chest pain or heaviness, shortness of breath, or hypoxia. Symptomatic effusions can be treated with thoracentesis. Nonsteroidal anti-inflammatory agents and colchicine can be used to treat postperiocardotomy syndrome. Tube thoracostomy drainage may be necessary until resolution of the inciting process. Placed utilizing the Seldinger technique, smaller diameter tubes are often better tolerated than traditional chest tubes. In contrast, a significant hemothorax may need to be evacuated surgically to avoid subsequent development of fibrothorax requiring decortication.

Pneumonia

Nosocomial pneumonias increase postoperative mortality. The incidence of ventilator associated pneumonia increases approximately 1% per day.[70] Clinical diagnosis involves identification of a new or progressive infiltrate on CXR, change in character of sputum, leukocytosis, and fever.[71] Expectorated sputum cultures are considered to be very inaccurate, and directed bronchoscopic sampling is preferred. Proper bronchoalveolar lavage requires large volumes of irrigant (>100 cc) and is infrequently performed. More commonly tracheobronchial aspiration is performed using several milliliters of normal saline. A Gram stain containing > 25 squamous epithelial cells per LPF indicates oral contamination. More than 25 neutrophils per LPF suggest infection. Quantitative culture of 10^5 to 10^6 cfu/cc ("moderate to numerous," "3 to 4+") is indicative of infection, while $\leq 10^4$ cfu/cc ("rare to few," "1 to 2+") is more suggestive of colonization. Gram-negative organisms are the most common, and should be the target of first-line empiric antibiotic coverage. Specific patient and hospital factors and culture results and sensitivities will further refine antibiotic therapy.[72]

The important role of pulmonary toilet in both the prevention and treatment of nosocomial pneumonias cannot be over emphasized. All patients should be encouraged to get out of bed and ambulate (even if attached to the ventilator), turn, cough, and deep breathe. Chest physiotherapy and bronchodilators can also provide benefits. Sterile-in line suctioning should be performed in ventilated patients to clear secretions. Nasotracheal suctioning is effective in extubated patients. Therapeutic fiberoptic bronchoscopy can also be performed.

Pulmonary Embolism

Deep venous thrombosis (DVT) and pulmonary thromboembolism (PE) are considered uncommon in the cardiac surgery population. The reported incidence of PE ranges from 0.5 to 3.5%, accounting for only 0.3 to 1.7% of perioperative deaths. This is believed to be due to large intraoperative doses of heparin, impaired platelet function post-CPB, increased use of antiplatelet agents and anticoagulants, and early ambulation. A recent autopsy study demonstrated a 52% incidence of DVT. Twenty percent of deceased cardiac surgery patients had small pulmonary emoboli,[73] and and PE was identified as the cause of death in 7%. Unfortunately, risks of bleeding and HIT make the choice of heparin DVT prophylaxis problematic. Intermittent pneumatic compression devices are effective if patients and staff are compliant with their use.

The diagnosis of PE requires a high index of suspicion, and should be considered in any postoperative patient who develops an increased PaO_2:F_iO_2 gradient, shortness of breath, or reduced exercise tolerance, particularly in the setting of a clear or unchanged CXR or thrombocytopenia consistent with HIT. Diagnosis is reliably obtained by PE-protocol thin-cut high-speed helical computed tomography of the chest,[74] although accuracy is still influenced by pretest probability.[75]

RENAL AND METABOLIC SUPPORT

Perioperative Renal Dysfunction/ Insufficiency

The new onset of renal dysfunction following cardiac surgery is correlated with significant morbidity and mortality. The incidence of acute renal failure (ARF) in CABG patients in the 1997 STS database was 3.14%, and 0.87% of these patients required dialysis.[76] Chertow studied 43,642 VA patients undergoing CABG or valve surgery.[77] The overall risk of ARF requiring dialysis was 1.1%. The mortality rate in this group was 63.7% compared with 4.3% in patients without ARF. Decreased myocardial function and advanced atherosclerosis were independent risk factors for the development of dialysis-dependent renal failure.

Patients with preoperative renal dysfunction (serum creatinine > 1.5 mg/dL) have a higher incidence of stroke, bleeding complications, dialysis, prolonged mechanical ventilation, length of stay, and death. Chertow found that preoperative renal function correlated with postoperative renal failure. The risk of ARF was 0.5%, 0.8%, 1.8%, and 4.9%

with baseline serum creatinine concentrations of <1 mg/dL, 1.0 to 1.4 mg/dL, 1.5 to 1.9 mg/dL, and 2.0 to 2.9 mg/dL, respectively. Chronic dialysis patients undergoing cardiac surgery have an 11.4% operative mortality rate, a 73% complication rate, and 32% 5-year actuarial survival rate.[78] Cardiac surgery following renal transplantation has an associated operative mortality rate of 8.8%.[79]

To optimize preoperative renal function, contrast loads should be minimized and patients should be well hydrated and receive **renoprotective** agents (eg, *N*-acetylcysteine).

Effects of Cardiopulmonary Bypass on Renal Function

Operative considerations include limiting the duration of CPB and maintenance of MAPs greater than 60 mm Hg. Additional effects of CPB include trauma to blood constituents, especially erythrocytes, with increased free hemoglobin levels and microparticle embolic insults to the kidneys. Hypothermia (during rewarming, vasodilation and hyperemia of tissue beds can result in third spacing of fluid), hemodilution (reduces viscosity of blood and plasma oncotic pressure) and ischemia reperfusion injury can influence renal function. Additionally, CPB leads to an increased release of catecholamines, hormones (rennin, aldosterone, angiotensin II, vasopressin, atrial natriuretic peptide, urodilan[80]) and inflammatory cytokines (kallikrein, bradykinin) which also affect renal function adversely. These adverse stimuli cause low renal blood flow, a decreased glomerular filtration rate and an increase in renal vascular resistance. Hypotension and pressor agents accentuate this response. Ultrafiltration is utilized in long pump runs to decrease volume overload in patients with renal dysfunction.

Independent of preoperative renal function, the primary postoperative goal is the maintenance of adequate renal perfusion pressure and a urine output greater than the 0.5 cc/kg/h. Brisk diuresis (>200 to 300 cc/h) is common following CPB. Volume replacement and maintenance of adequate BP and CO is required for adequate renal perfusion. The best measure of kidney perfusion is adequate urine output independent of diuretics. Beyond optimizing hemodynamics and avoiding nephrotoxic medications, there is no convincing evidence that treatment with diuretics, mannitol, dopamine, fenoldapam, nesiritide, or any other agent is renoprotective. This is not to say, however, that these agents are of no benefit in promoting diuresis and avoiding renal replacement therapies in the event of renal dysfunction.

Electrolyte Disturbances

CALCIUM

Levels of ionized calcium (normal, 1.1 to 1.3 mmol/L) are critical for myocardial performance and hemostasis, and involved in reperfusion injury. Hypocalcemia causes a prolonged QT interval. Postoperatively hypocalcemia is common following CPB or an episode of hemodilution, sepsis, or citrated blood transfusions. The concentration of calcium ion is greatest in the intracellular space, with small amounts in the extracellular fluid. Calcium levels bound to albumin change with the levels of serum albumin whereas ionized levels remain unchanged.

POTASSIUM

Potassium fluxes during cardiac surgery can be significant and affect cardiac automaticity and conduction. Cardioplegia, decreased urine output, decreased insulin levels, and RBC hemolysis all contribute to hyperkalemia.[81] Brisk diuresis, insulin, and alkalosis can cause hypokalemia.[82] Aggressive treatment of hypokalemia decreases the incidence of perioperative arrhythmias. Serum potassium levels and replacement protocols are an integral part of early postoperative management. Serum potassium rises logarithmically with replacement; larger quantities are required to treat significant hypokalemia.

MAGNESIUM

Magnesium (normal, 1.5 to 2 mEq/L) is the second most common intracellular cation after potassium. It is involved in endothelial cell homeostasis,[83] cardiac excitability and muscle contraction through its role as an ATP cofactor and calcium antagonist, and it is also closely involved in the regulation of intracellular potassium.[84] Following hemodilution and CPB, hypomagnesaemia is common (>70% of patients) and is associated with an increased risk of atrial fibrillation and torsade de pointes.[85]

Endocrine Dysfunction

DIABETES MELLITUS

Up to 30% of patients have diabetes (type I or II) in the cardiac surgery population. Following CPB the hormonal stress response (increased growth hormone, catecholamines, and cortisol) causes hyperglycemia (even in nondiabetics) with a decrease in insulin production; this may persist for up to 24 hours postoperatively and is exacerbated by exogenous catecholamine administration. Anthony Furnary was the first to demonstrate that moderate control of blood glucose levels with continuous insulin infusions reduces the incidence of sternal wound infection by an order of magnitude.[86] Work by Van den Berghe suggested that a more aggressive approach aimed at maintaining blood glucose levels at or below 110 mg/dL resulted in a reduction in mortality rate in critically ill patients, and guidelines were revised to encourage stricter control.[87] Subsequently, the NICE-Sugar-Study was performed to determine the optimal target range for blood glucose in critically ill patients.[88] In this study, tight control (utilizing a target of 81 to 108 mg per deciliter) was associated with a higher incidence of hypoglycemia and mortality than conventional control (utilizing a target of 180 mg/dL). The STS workforce on blood glucose management in cardiac surgery patients concluded that targets <180 mg/dL reduce mortality, morbidity, and the incidence of wound infection and improve long-term survival.

ADRENAL DYSFUNCTION

The strain of cardiac surgery activates the hypothalamic-pituitary-adrenal axis and increases plasma ACTH and cortisol levels. Subclinical adrenal insufficiency is present in up to 20% of the elderly population and can be unmasked by the stress of surgery. Perioperative stress dose steroids should be considered for patients taking exogenous steroids within 6 months of surgery. Any patient exhibiting prolonged, unexplained vasodilatory shock should be suspected of having adrenal insufficiency. Critically ill patients with normal adrenal function should have high cortisol levels. If the diagnosis is in doubt, a cosyntropin stimulation test should be performed for diagnosis. In the interim, dexamethasone may be administered IV without interfering with the test.

RELEVANT POSTOPERATIVE COMPLICATIONS

Neurological

CENTRAL NERVOUS SYSTEM

The incidence of **stroke** following cardiac surgery is procedure specific and varies between 1 and 4%. Ricotta and colleagues associated carotid stenosis (>50%), redo heart surgery, valve surgery, and prior stroke with increased postoperative neurological risk.[89] John and colleagues reviewed 19,224 patients in New York State.[90] The stroke rate was 1.4% following CABG, with a 24.8% mortality rate in that group. Multivariable logistic regression identified the following predictor variables: calcified aorta, prior stroke, age, carotid artery disease, duration of CPB, renal failure, peripheral vascular disease, smoking, and diabetes. Intraoperative factors that may cause postoperative neurologic deficits include particulate macroembolization of air, debris, or thrombus, microembolization of white blood cells, platelets, or fibrin,[91] duration of CPB,[92] cerebral hypoperfusion during nonpulsatile CPB and hypothermic circulatory arrest.[93] Because of bleeding risk, patients presenting with stroke are not candidates for intraenous thrombolytic interventions. Endovascular therapy may be beneficial in select patients with embolic occlusion if performed within 6 to 8 hours of the event, this window may be as long as 24 hours in patients with posterior circulation occlusion. If a patient is considered to be a candidate for endovascular intervention, a CT angiogram is required to define the anatomy of the vascular occlusion.

Neuropsychiatric deficits (neurocognitive dysfunction, delirium, seizures) are very common, occurring in up to 50 to 70% of patients following cardiac surgery. The cause of these neuropsychiatric disorders is uncertain and remains controversial. Although the dysfunction remains unclear, patients remain at risk for long-term cognitive decline. Van Dijk and colleagues[94] reviewed 12 cohort studies, a pooled analysis of 6 comparable studies showed 22.5% of patients to have a cognitive deficit at 2 months after operation. This may, however, be related to progression of underlying cerebrovascular disease rather than to CABG or CPB.[95]

Up to 50% of cardiac surgery patients experience delirium, particularly those with preexisting organic mental disorders, significant prior alcohol consumption, advanced age, or intracranial cerebral artery disease.[96] Perioperative medications, particularly benzodiazepines and opiates, as well as phenothiazines and anticholinergics can contribute to delerium.[97] There is increasing evidence that sedation with dexmedetomidine causes less delirium and results in improved outcomes when compared to sedation with benzodiazepines.[98] Right-sided parietal lobe lesions may present as delirium. Other causes of postoperative delirium in the cardiac intensive care patient include sleep deprivation, renal failure, hepatic failure, and thyroid abnormalities. electroencephalograms on these patients are usually abnormal, whereas in primary psychiatric diseases they are normal. Treatment involves correcting metabolic abnormalities, establishing a normal sleep-wake cycle in extubated patients, minimizing medications likely to cause delirium, and providing ventilated patients with sedation holidays.

BRACHIAL PLEXUS INJURY/PERIPHERAL NERVE INJURY

Excessive sternal retraction during a median sternotomy may cause a brachial plexus injury as the first rib may impinge the lower trunk and branches.[99] IMA harvesting may also cause damage to the brachial plexus with serious consequences.[100] Malpositioning of the upper limbs during surgery may result in a neuropraxia due to compression of the ulnar nerve.[101] Palsy or plegia of dorsiflexion and eversion of the foot can be caused by common peroneal nerve stretch or compression at the level of the head of the fibula.[102] Saphenous neuropathy (sensory changes on the medial side of the calf to the great toe) following open vein graft harvesting (less so with endoscopic harvest) is also a potential complication secondary to the avulsion of pretibial or infrapatellar branches of the nerve.[103]

Gastrointestinal

Mesenteric ischemia following cardiac surgery is infrequent but often catastrophic.[104] Risk factors include duration of bypass (hypoperfusion), use of pressor support (sympathetic vasoconstriction), use of an IABP or other sources of atherosclerotic embolism, atrial fibrillation, peripheral vascular disease, and HIT. Early surgical intervention (<6 hours) is associated with a 48% mortality rate, and this rises to 99% with delays (>6 hours) in surgical intervention. Gastrointestinal bleeding is common and can cause significant morbidity. The incidence of gastrointestinal bleeding can be reduced with the use of H_2-inhibitors, proton pump inhibitors and sucralfate.[105] Other gastrointestinal complications include pancreatitis (hyperamylasemia is present in 35 to 65% of patients and is associated with an overt pancreatitis rate of 0.4 to 3%),[106] acute acalculous cholecystitis (likely secondary to hypoperfusion or biliary stasis promoted by narcotics or parenteral nutrition[107]), dysphasia secondary to tracheal

intubation or perioperative use of TEE,[108] small or large bowel ileus (Ogilvie's syndrome is associated with long-term ventilation, narcotic use, and anticholinergic agents).[109] Preoperative liver dysfunction (noncardiac cirrhosis) is associated with a high incidence of postoperative morbidity and mortality (Child class A cirrhosis: 20% morbidity, 0% mortality; Child class B cirrhosis: 80% morbidity, 100% mortality). Although 20% of patients develop a transient hyperbilirubinemia, fewer than 1% have significant hepatocellular damage which progresses to chronic hepatitis or liver failure.[110] Liver failure associated with multisystem organ failure can lead to coagulopathy and hypoglycemia; these symptoms are generally associated with an extremely poor prognosis.

Nosocomial Infections

Ten to twenty percent of cardiac surgery patients develop a nosocomial infection. Infections may be related to the surgical wound, lung, urinary tract, invasive lines or devices, or the gastrointestinal tract. Prolonged mechanical ventilation is associated with nosocomial pneumonia. Pneumonia is second only to urinary tract infection in frequency and carries the highest mortality rate. Smokers and COPD patients are most likely to be colonized preoperatively and have a higher incidence of pulmonary infection (15.3 vs 3.6% in controls).[111]

Catheter-related infections (ie, bladder and vascular related) are common in the intensive care unit. The most common pathogens are *Staphylococcus aureus* (12%), *coagulase-negative staphylococci* (11%), *Candida albicans* (11%), *Pseudomonas aeruginosa* (10%), and *Enterococcus* sp.[112]

FEVER

Fevers are common in the intensive care setting, but are a poor indicator of postoperative bacteremia (3.2% incidence in 835 febrile CABG patients).[113] The yield of true positive bacteremia ranges from 4 to 5%, with a contamination rate ranging from 32 to 47%.[114] The incidence of false-postive blood culture resuts can be minimized by avoid blood draws from indwelling lines. Noninfectious causes of fever in cardiac surgery patients include myocardial infarction, postpericardiotomy syndrome, and drug fever. Infectious causes include wound infection, urinary tract infection, pneumonia, catheter sepsis, and loculated areas of contaminated blood accumulation (eg, pericardial, pleural, retroperitoneal, and leg wound spaces).

SEPSIS/SEPTIC SHOCK

Septic shock following cardiac surgery should prompt an agrresive search for etiology. Pathophysiologic features of sepsis include systemic inflammation, hypotension, and impaired fibrinolysis, leading to multiorgan failure, irreversible shock, and death (20 to 50% mortality has been reported).[115] MVO_2 can be abnormally high secondary to shunting and a failure to extract oxygen at the cellular level. In vasodilatory shock the maintenance of end-organ tissue perfusion is critical; this includes aggressive fluid management and vasopressin.[116] Methylene blue (which inhibits NO synthesis) has been used successfully in refractory hypotension. Bernard and colleagues[117] in the PROW/ESS study group showed a distinct survival advantage in the treatment of severe sepsis utilizing drotrecogin alfa (activated) or recombinant human-activated protein C (Zigris). These agents reduce the systemic inflammatory, procoagulant, and fibrinolytic reactions to infection. In a randomized study of 1690 patients, the mortality rate was 30.8% in the placebo group versus 24.7% in the treatment group.

WOUNDS

Delayed Sternal Closure/Sternal Infection. Complicated operations with persistent bleeding and hemodynamic instability (due to tissue edema) may preclude primary sternal closure. Delayed sternal closure allows hemodynamic stabilization, and diuresis.[118] Anderson and colleagues[119] outlined the Brigham and Women's Hospital experience: 1.7% (87 of 5177) open chests were managed with a hospital survival rate of 76%. Complications included deep sternal infection (n = 4), stroke (n = 8), and dialysis (n = 13). Multivariate analysis revealed mechanical ventricular assistance and reoperation for bleeding as independent predictors of in-hospital mortality.

Superficial and Deep Sternal Wounds. Superficial and deep sternal wound infections are significant complications of cardiac surgery. Deep sternal infection with associated mediastinitis occurs in 1 to 2% of cardiac operations, with a resultant mortality rate approaching 10%.[120] Common organisms include *Staphylococcus epidermidis*, *S. aureus* (including methicillin-resistant *S. aureus*), Corynebacterium, and enteric Gram-negative bacilli.[121] Patients predisposed to sternal infections include those with significant comorbidities (obesity, diabetes, COPD, renal dysfunction, low serum albumin), prolonged CPB, blood transfusions, reoperations, diabetics with bilateral IMA harvests,[122] and patients with hyperglycemia.[123] Simple preoperative measures such as clipping of chest hair, using Hibiclens washes, administration of adequate prophylactic antibiotics prior to skin incision, ensuring good intraoperative hemostasis without the use of bone wax, and closure with subcuticular sutures and Dermabond (topical adhesive) rather than skin staples. Effective glucose control during surgery and for at least 3 days postoperatively is associated with a significantly lower sternal wound infection rate.

Minor infections frequently respond to intravenous antibiotics, opening of the wound, and local wound care. Deeper infections require intravenous antibiotics (6 weeks); initial empiric therapy should consist of broad coverage against Gram-positive cocci and Gram-negative bacilli with the regimen adjusted when cultures (blood, mediastinal or deep sternal wound drainage) have been speciated. The mainstay of treatment is surgical exploration and extensive debridement which may require removal of the sternum with primary or secondary closure with muscle or an omental flap.[124] Postoperative vacuum-assisted closure[125] of mediastinal wounds improves wound healing and reduces hospital length of stay.

Nutrition

Preoperative debilitated or cachectic patients (ie, more than 10% weight loss over 6 months) with albumin levels of less than 3.5 g/dL[126] are exceptionally prone to complications following surgery. There is no evidence to support a role for preoperative hyperalimentation. Body mass index (a good nutritional index) of less than 15 kg/m² is associated with increased morbidity. Postoperative patients have accelerated catabolic protein losses, usually requiring 25 to 40 kcal/kg/day. Advances in immuno-nutritional pharmacology (arginine, glutamine, and n-3 fatty acids) in complex postoperative cardiac surgery patients may have a defined role in the future.[127]

REFERENCES

1. Kreter B, Woods M: Antibiotic prophylaxis for cardiothoracic operations. Meta-analysis of thirty years of clinical trials. *J Thorac Cardiovasc Surg* 1992; 104(3):590-599.
2. Gallagher JD, Moore RA, Kerns D, et al: Effects of colloid or crystalloid administration on pulmonary extravascular water in the postoperative period after coronary artery bypass grafting. *Anesth Analg* 1985; 64(8):753-758.
3. Finfer S, Bellomo R, Boyce N, et al: A comparison of albumin and saline for fluid resuscitation in the intensive care unit. *N Engl J Med* 2004; 350(22):2247-2256.
4. Garcia-Villarreal OA, Gonzalez-Oviedo R, Rodriguez-Gonzalez H, et al: Superior septal approach for mitral valve surgery: a word of caution. *Eur J Cardiothorac Surg* 2003; 24(6):862-867.
5. Echahidi N, Pibarot P, O'Hara G, Mathieu P: Mechanisms, prevention and treatment of atrial fibrillation after cardiac surgery. *J Am Coll Cardiol* 2008; 51:793-801.
6. Nisanoglu V, Erdil N, Aldemir M, et al: Atrial fibrillation after coronary artery bypass grafting in elderly patients: incidence and risk factor analysis. *Thorac Cardiovasc Surg* 2007; 55(1):32-38.
7. Villareal RP, Hariharan R, Liu BC, et al: Postoperative atrial fibrillation and mortality after coronary artery bypass surgery. *J Am Coll Cardiol* 2004; 43:742-748.
8. Wyse DG, Waldo AL, DiMarco JP, et al: A comparison of rate control and rhythm control in patients with atrial fibrillation. The Atrial Fibrillation Follow-up Investigation of Rhythm Management (AFFIRM) Investigators. *N Engl J Med* 2002; 347(23):1825-1833.
9. Van Gelder IC, Groenveld HF, Crijns HJ, et al: Lenient versus strict rate control in patients with atrial fibrillation. RACE II Investigators. *N Engl J Med* 2010; 362:1363-1373.
10. Yalta K, Turgut OO, Yilmaz MB, Yilmaz A, Tandogan I: Dronedarone: a promising alternative for the management of atrial fibrillation. *Cardiovasc Drugs Ther* 2009; 23(5):385-393.
11. Køber L, Torp-Pedersen C, McMurray JJ, et al: Increased mortality after dronedarone therapy for severe heart failure. *N Engl J Med* 2008; 358(25):2678-2687.
12. Hohnloser SH: New pharmacological options for patients with atrial fibrillation: the ATHENA trial. *Rev Esp Cardiol* 2009; 62:479-481.
13. Cook GE, Sasich LD, Sukkari SR: DIONYSOS study comparing dronedarone with amiodarone. *BMJ* 2010; 340:c285, doi: 10.1136/bmj.c285 (Published 19 January 2010).
14. Martin KB, Klinger JR, Rounds SI: Pulmonary arterial hypertension: new insights and new hope. *Respirology* 2006; 11(1):6-17.
15. Jeon Y, Ryu JH, Lim YJ, et al: Comparative hemodynamic effects of vasopressin and norepinephrine after milrinone-induced hypotension in off-pump coronary artery bypass surgical patients. *Eur J Cardiothorac Surg* 2006; 29: 952-956.

16. Dimopoulou I, Anthi A, Michalis A, Tzelepis GE: Functional status and quality of life in long-term survivors of cardiac arrest after cardiac surgery. *Crit Care Med* 2001; 29:1408-1411.

17. Anthi A, Tzelepis GE, Alivizatos P, Michalis A, Palatianos GM, Geroulanos S: Unexpected cardiac arrest after cardiac surgery: incidence, predisposing causes, and outcome of open chest cardiopulmonary resuscitation. *Chest* 1998; 113:15-19.

18. Nolan JP, Soar J, Zideman DA, et al: European Resuscitation Council guidelines for resuscitation 2010: section 1, executive summary. *Resuscitation* 2010; 81(10):1219-1276.

19. Chan PS, Krumholz HB, Nichol G, et al: American Heart Association National Registry of Cardiopulmonary Resuscitation Investigators. Delayed time to defibrillation after in-hospital cardiac arrest. *N Engl J Med* 2008; 358(1):9-17.

20. Miller AC, Rosati SF, Suffredini AF, Schrump DS: A systematic review and pooled analysis of CPR-associated cardiovascular and thoracic injuries. *Resuscitation* 2014; 85(6):724-731.

21. Puskas JD, Williams WH, Duke PG, et al: Off-pump coronary artery bypass grafting provides complete revascularization with reduced myocardial injury, transfusion requirements, and length of stay: a prospective randomized comparison of two hundred unselected patients undergoing off-pump versus conventional coronary artery bypass grafting. *J Thorac Cardiovasc Surg* 2003; 125(4):797-808.

22. Bauer TL, Arepally G, Konkle BA, et al: Prevalence of heparin-associated antibodies without thrombosis in patients undergoing cardiopulmonary bypass surgery. *Circulation* 1997; 95(5):1242-1246.

23. Koster A, Dyke C, Aldea G, et al: Bivalirudin during cardiopulmonary bypass in patients with previous or acute heparin-induced thrombocytopenia and heparin antibodies: results of the CHOOSE-ON trial. *Ann Thorac Surg* 2007; 83:572-577.

24. Mangano DT: Aspirin and mortality from coronary bypass surgery. *N Engl J Med* 2002; 347(17):1309-1317.

25. Douketis JD, Spyropoulos AC, Kaatz S, et al: Perioperative bridging anticoagulation in patients with atrial fibrillation. *N Engl J Med* 2015; 373:823-833.

26. Siegal D, Yudin J, Kaatz S, Douketis JD, Lim W, Spyropoulos AC: Periprocedural heparin bridging in patients receiving vitamin K antagonists: systematic review and meta-analysis of bleeding and thromboembolic rates. *Circulation* 2012; 126:1630-1639.

27. Ranucci M, Conti D, Castelvecchio S, et al: Hematocrit on cardiopulmonary bypass and outcome after coronary surgery in nontransfused patients. *Ann Thorac Surg* 2010; 89:11-17.

28. Kulier A, Levin J, Moser R, et al: Impact of preoperative anemia on outcome in patients undergoing coronary artery bypass graft surgery. *Circulation* 2007; 116:471-479.

29. Loor G, Koch CG, Sabik JF III, Li L, Blackstone EH: Implications and management of anemia in cardiac surgery: current state of knowledge. *J Thorac Cardiovasc Surg* 2012;144(3):538-546.

30. Unger EF, Thompson AM, Blank MJ, Temple R: Erythropoiesis-stimulating agents–time for a reevaluation. *N Engl J Med* 2010; 362:189-192.

31. Koch CG, Reineks EZ, Tang AS, et al: Contemporary bloodletting in cardiac surgical care. *Ann Thorac Surg* 2015; 99:779-784.

32. Abul-Azm A, Abdullah KM: Effect of topical tranexamic acid in open heart surgery. *Eur J Anaesthesiol* 2006; 23(5):380-384.

33. Rosengart TK, Helm RE, DeBois WJ, et al: Open heart operations without transfusion using multimodality blood conservation strategy in 50 Jehovah's Witness patients: implications for a "bloodless" surgical technique. *J Am Coll Surg* 1997; 184(6):618-629.

34. Murkin JM: A novel hemostatic agent: the potential role of recombinant activated factor VII (rFVIIa) in anesthetic practice. *Can J Anaesth* 2002; 49(10):S21-26.

35. Bojar RM: *Manual of Perioperative Care in Adult Cardiac Surgery*, 4th. ed. Malden, Blackwell Publishing, 2005.

36. Murphy GJ, Allen SM, Unsworth-White J, et al: Safety and efficacy of perioperative cell salvage and autotransfusion after coronary artery bypass grafting: a randomized trial. *Ann Thorac Surg* 2004; 77(5):1553-1559.

37. Munoz M, Garcia-Vallejo JJ, Ruiz MD, et al: Transfusion of postoperative shed blood: laboratory characteristics and clinical utility. *Eur Spine J* 2004; 13(Suppl 1):S107-113.

38. Folkersen L, Tang M, Grunnet N, Jakobsen CJ: Transfusion of shed mediastinal blood reduces the use of allogenic blood transfusion without increasing complications. *Perfusion* 2011; 26(2):145-150.

39. 2011 update to the Society of Thoracic Surgeons and the Society of Cardiovascular Anesthesiologists blood conservation clinical practice guidelines. Society of Thoracic Surgeons Blood Conservation Guideline Task Force, Ferraris VA, Brown JR, Despotis GJ, et al; Society of Cardiovascular Anesthesiologists Special Task Force on Blood Transfusion, Shore-Lesserson LJ, Goodnough LT, Mazer CD, Shander A, Stafford-Smith M, Waters J; International Consortium for Evidence Based Perfusion, Baker RA, Dickinson TA, FitzGerald DJ, Likosky DS, Shann KG: *Ann Thorac Surg* 2011; 91(3):944-982.

40. Hebert PC, Wells G, Blajchman MA, et al: A multicenter, randomized, controlled clinical trial of transfusion requirements in critical care. Transfusion Requirements in Critical Care Investigators, Canadian Critical Care Trials Group. *N Engl J Med* 11 1999; 340(6):409-417.

41. Koch CG, Li L, Duncan AI, et al: Transfusion in coronary artery bypass grafting is associated with reduced long term survival. *Ann Thorac Surg* 2006; 81:1650-1657.

42. Kumar A, Roberts D, Wood KE, et al: Duration of hypotension before initiation of effective antimicrobial therapy is the critical determinant of survival in human septic shock. *Crit Care Med* 2006; 34(6):1589-1596.

43. Rawn J: The silent risks of blood transfusion. *Current Opin Anaesthesiol* 2008; 21(5):664-668.

44. Murphy GJ, Reeves BC, Rogers CA, Rizvi SI, Culliford L, Angelini GD: Increased mortality, postoperative morbidity, and cost after red blood cell transfusion in patients having cardiac surgery. *Circulation* 2007; 116(22):2544-2552. E-pub 2007 Nov 12.

45. Pattakos G, Koch CG, Brizzio ME, et al: Outcome of patients who refuse transfusion after cardiac surgery. A natural experiment with severe blood conservation.

46. Gregory Pattakos, Colleen G. Koch, Eugene H. Blackstone: Jehovah's witnesses may not have identical outcomes with nontransfused non-witnesses after cardiac surgery—reply. *JAMA Intern Med.* 2013; 173(3):248-249.

47. Chelemer SB, Prato BS, Cox PM Jr, et al: Association of bacterial infection and red blood cell transfusion after coronary artery bypass surgery. *Ann Thorac Surg* 2002; 73(1):138-142.

48. Warkentin TE, Greinacher A, Koster A, Lincoff AM: Treatment and prevention of heparin-induced thrombocytopenia: American College of Chest Physicians Evidence-Based Clinical Practice Guidelines (8th Edition). *Chest* 2008; 133:340S-380S.

49. Warkentin TE, Kelton JG: Delayed onset heparin-induced thrombocytopenia and thrombosis. *Ann Intern Med* 2001; 135:502-506.

50. Zwicker JI, Uhl L, Huang WY, Shaz BH, Bauer KA: Thrombosis and ELISA optical density values in hospitalized patients with heparin-induced thrombocytopenia. *J Thromb Haemost* 2004; 2:2133-2137.

51. Arpally GM, Ortell TL: Clinical oractice. Heparin-induced thrombocytopenia. *N Eng J Med* 2006; 355:809-817.

52. Greinacher A: Heparin-induced thrombocytopenia. *N Eng J Med* 2015; 373:252-261.

53. Ng CS, Wan S, Yim AP, et al: Pulmonary dysfunction after cardiac surgery. *Chest* 2002; 121(4):1269-1277.

54. Chaney, MA Durazo-Arvizu, RA, et al: Cardiopulmonary support and physiology. Methylprednisolone does not benefit patients undergoing coronary artery bypass grafting and early tracheal extubation. *J Thorac Cardiovasc Surg* 2001; 121:561-569.

55. Futier E, Constantin JM, Paugam-Burtz C, et al: IMPROVE Study Group: A trial of intraoperative low-tidal-volume ventilation in abdominal surgery. *N Engl J Med* 2013; 369(5):428-437.

56. Berthelsen P, St Haxholdt O, Husum B, et al: PEEP reverses nitroglycerin-induced hypoxemia following coronary artery bypass surgery. *Acta Anesthesiologica Scand* 1986; 30:243-246.

57. Kreider ME, Lipson DA: Bronchoscopy for atelectasis in the ICU. *Chest* 2003; 124:344-350.

58. Marini JJ, Pierson DJ, Hudson LD: Acute lobar attelectasis: a prospective comparison of fiberoptic bronchoscopy and respiratory therapy. *Am Rev Respir Dis* 1979; 119:971-978.

59. Stevens RD, Burri H, Tramer MR: Pharmacologic myocardial protection in patients undergoing noncardiac surgery: a quantitative systematic review. *Anesth Analg* 2003; 97(3):623-633.

60. Epstein SK: Decision to extubate. *Intensive Care Med* 2002; 28(5):535-546.

61. Esteban A, Frutos F, Tobin MJ, et al: A comparison of four methods of weaning patients from mechanical ventilation. Spanish Lung Failure Collaborative Group. *N Engl J Med* 1995; 332(6):345-350.

62. Yang KL, Tobin MJ: A prospective study of indexes predicting the outcome of trials of weaning from mechanical ventilation. *N Engl J Med* 1991; 324(21):1445-1450.

63. Engoren M, Buderer NF, Zacharias A, et al: Variables predicting reintubation after cardiac surgical procedures. *Ann Thorac Surg* 1999; 67(3):661-665.

64. Cohen A, Katz M, Katz R, et al: Chronic obstructive pulmonary disease in patients undergoing coronary artery bypasses grafting. *J Thorac Cardiovasc Surg* 1995; 109(3):574-581.

65. Redmond JM, Greene PS, Goldsborough MA, et al: Neurologic injury in cardiac surgical patients with a history of stroke. *Ann Thorac Surg* 1996; 61(1):42-47.

66. Heffner JE: Timing tracheotomy: calendar watching or individualization of care? *Chest* 1998; 114(2):361-363.

67. Maziak DE, Meade MO, Todd TR: The timing of tracheotomy: a systematic review. *Chest* 1998; 114(2):605-609.

68. Pierson DJ: Tracheostomy and weaning. *Respir Care* 2005; 50(4):526-533.

69. Rumbak MJ, Newton M, Truncale T, et al: A prospective, randomized, study comparing early percutaneous dilational tracheotomy to prolonged translaryngeal intubation (delayed tracheotomy) in critically ill medical patients. *Crit Care Med* 2004; 32(8):1689-1694.

70. Fagon JY, Chastre J, Domart Y, et al: Nosocomial pneumonia in patients receiving continuous mechanical ventilation. Prospective analysis of 52 episodes with use of a protected specimen brush and quantitative culture techniques. *Am Rev Respir Dis* 1989; 139(4):877-884.

71. Beck KD, Gastmeier P: Clinical or epidemiologic diagnosis of nosocomial pneumonia: is there any difference? *Am J Infect Control* 2003; 31(6):331-335.

72. Baselski VS, Wunderink RG: Bronchoscopic diagnosis of pneumonia. *Clin Microbiol Rev* 1994; 7(4):533-558.

73. Rastan AJ, Gummert JF, Lachmann N, et al: Significant value of autopsy for quality management in cardiac surgery. *J Thorac Cardiovasc Surg* 2005; 129(6):1292-1300.

74. Schoepf UJ, Savino G, Lake DR, et al: The age of CT pulmonary angiography. *J Thorac Imaging* 2005; 20(4):273-279.

75. Roy PM, Colombet I, Durieux P, et al: Systematic review and meta-analysis of strategies for the diagnosis of suspected pulmonary embolism. *BMJ* 2005; 331(7511):259.

76. Bahar I, Akgul A, Ozatik MA, et al: Acute renal failure following open heart surgery: risk factors and prognosis. *Perfusion* 2005; 20(6):317-322.

77. Chertow GM, Lazarus JM, Christiansen CL, et al: Preoperative renal risk stratification. *Circulation* 1997; 95(4):878-884.

78. Franga DL, Kratz JM, Crumbley AJ, et al: Early and long-term results of coronary artery bypass grafting in dialysis patients. *Ann Thorac Surg* 2000; 70(3):813-818; discussion 819.

79. Dresler C, Uthoff K, Wahlers T, et al: Open heart operations after renal transplantation. *Ann Thorac Surg* 1997; 63(1):143-146.

80. Sehested J, Wacker B, Forssmann WG, et al: Natriuresis after cardiopulmonary bypass: relationship to urodilatin, atrial natriuretic factor, antidiuretic hormone, and aldosterone. *J Thorac Cardiovasc Surg* 1997; 114(4):666-671.

81. Weber DO, Yarnoz MD: Hyperkalemia complicating cardiopulmonary bypass: analysis of risk factors. *Ann Thorac Surg* 1982; 34(4):439-445.

82. Gennari FJ, Hypokalemia: *N Engl J Med* 1998; 339(7):451-458.

83. Shechter M, Sharir M, Labrador MJ, et al: Oral magnesium therapy improves endothelial function in patients with coronary artery disease. *Circulation* 2000; 102(19):2353-2358.

84. Agus ZS, Morad M: Modulation of cardiac ion channels by magnesium. *Annu Rev Physiol* 1991; 53:299-307.

85. England MR, Gordon G, Salem M, et al: Magnesium administration and dysrhythmias after cardiac surgery. A placebo-controlled, double-blind, randomized trial. *JAMA* 1992; 268(17):2395-2402.

86. Furnary AP, Gao G, Grunkemeier GL, et al: Continuous insulin infusion reduces mortality in patients with diabetes undergoing coronary artery bypass grafting. *J Thorac Cardiovasc Surg* 2003; 125(5):1007-1021.

87. Van den Berghe G, Wouters P, Weekers F, et al: Intensive insulin therapy in the critically ill patients. *N Engl J Med* 2001; 345(19):1359-1367.

88. The NICE-SUGAR Study Investigators, Finfer S, Chittock DR, et al: Intensive versus Conventional Glucose Control in Critically Ill Patients. *N Engl J Med* 2009; 360(13):1283-1297.

89. Ricotta JJ, Faggioli GL, Castilone A, et al: Risk factors for stroke after cardiac surgery: Buffalo Cardiac-Cerebral Study Group. *J Vasc Surg* 1995; 21(2):359-363; discussion 364.

90. John R, Choudhri AF, Weinberg AD, et al: Multicenter review of preoperative risk factors for stroke after coronary artery bypass grafting. *Ann Thorac Surg* 2000; 69(1):30-35; discussion 35-36.

91. Borger MA, Ivanov J, Weisel RD, et al: Stroke during coronary bypass surgery: principal role of cerebral macroemboli. *Eur J Cardiothorac Surg* 2001; 19(5):627-632.

92. Brown WR, Moody DM, Challa VR, et al: Longer duration of cardiopulmonary bypass is associated with greater numbers of cerebral microemboli. *Stroke* 2000; 31(3):707-713.

93. Hickey PR: Neurologic sequelae associated with deep hypothermic circulatory arrest. *Ann Thorac Surg* 1998; 65(6 Suppl):S65-69; discussion S69-70, S74-66.

94. van Dijk D, Keizer AM, Diephuis JC, et al: Neurocognitive dysfunction after coronary artery bypasses surgery: a systematic review. *J Thorac Cardiovasc Surg* 2000; 120(4):632-639.

95. McKhann GM: Neurocognitive complications after coronary artery bypass surgery. *Ann Neurol* 2005; 57(5):615-621.

96. Smith LW, Dimsdale JE: Postcardiotomy delirium: conclusions after 25 years? *Am J Psychiatry* 1989; 146(4):452-458.

97. Pisani MA, Murphy TE, Araujo KL, Slattum P, Van Ness PH, Inouye SK: Benzodiazepine and opioid use and the duration of intensive care unit delirium in an older population. *Crit Care Med* 2009; 37(1):177-183.

98. Pandharipande PP, Pun BT, Herr DL, et al: Effect of sedation with dexmedetomidine vs lorazepam on acute brain dysfunction in mechanically ventilated patients. The MENDS randomized controlled trial. *JAMA* 2007; 298(22):2644-2653.

99. Vander Salm TJ, Cutler BS, Okike ON: Brachial plexus injury following median sternotomy. Part II. *J Thorac Cardiovasc Surg* 1982; 83(6):914-917.

100. Vahl CF, Carl I, Muller-Vahl H, et al: Brachial plexus injury after cardiac surgery. The role of internal mammary artery preparation: a prospective study on 1000 consecutive patients. *J Thorac Cardiovasc Surg* 1991; 102(5):724-729.

101. Morin JE, Long R, Elleker MG, et al: Upper extremity neuropathies following median sternotomy. *Ann Thorac Surg* 1982; 34(2):181-185.

102. Vazquez-Jimenez JF, Krebs G, Schiefer J, et al: Injury of the common peroneal nerve after cardiothoracic operations. *Ann Thorac Surg* 2002; 73(1):119-122.

103. Sharma AD, Parmley CL, Sreeram G, et al: Peripheral nerve injuries during cardiac surgery: risk factors, diagnosis, prognosis, and prevention. *Anesth Analg* 2000; 91(6):1358-1369.

104. Klotz S, Vestring T, Rotker J, et al: Diagnosis and treatment of nonocclusive mesenteric ischemia after open heart surgery. *Ann Thorac Surg* 2001; 72(5):1583-1586.

105. Cook DJ, Reeve BK, Guyatt GH, et al: Stress ulcer prophylaxis in critically ill patients. Resolving discordant meta-analyses. *JAMA* 1996; 275(4):308-314.

106. Ihaya A, Muraoka R, Chiba Y, et al: Hyperamylasemia and subclinical pancreatitis after cardiac surgery. *World J Surg* 2001; 25(7):862-864.

107. Rady MY, Kodavatiganti R, Ryan T: Perioperative predictors of acute cholecystitis after cardiovascular surgery. *Chest* 1998; 114(1):76-84.

108. Hogue CW Jr, Lappas GD, Creswell LL, et al: Swallowing dysfunction after cardiac operations. Associated adverse outcomes and risk factors including intraoperative transesophageal echocardiography. *J Thorac Cardiovasc Surg* 1995; 110(2):517-522.

109. Geller A, Petersen BT, Gostout CJ: Endoscopic decompression for acute colonic pseudo-obstruction. *Gastrointest Endosc* 1996; 44(2):144-150.

110. Raman JS, Kochi K, Morimatsu H, et al: Severe ischemic early liver injury after cardiac surgery. *Ann Thorac Surg* 2002; 74(5):1601-1606.

111. Carrel TP, Eisinger E, Vogt M, et al: Pneumonia after cardiac surgery is predictable by tracheal aspirates but cannot be prevented by prolonged antibiotic prophylaxis. *Ann Thorac Surg* 2001; 72(1):143-148.

112. Gordon SM, Serkey JM, Keys TF, et al: Secular trends in nosocomial bloodstream infections in a 55-bed cardiothoracic intensive care unit. *Ann Thorac Surg* 1998; 65(1):95-100.

113. Kohman LJ, Coleman MJ, Parker FB Jr: Bacteremia and sternal infection after coronary artery bypass grafting. *Ann Thorac Surg* 1990; 49(3):454-457.

114. Badillo AT, Sarani B, Evans SR: Optimizing the use of blood cultures in the febrile postoperative patient. *J Am Coll Surg* 2002; 194(4):477-487; quiz 554-476.

115. Sands KE, Bates DW, Lanken PN, et al: Epidemiology of sepsis syndrome in 8 academic medical centers. *JAMA* 16 1997; 278(3):234-240.
116. Jochberger S, Mayr VD, Luckner G, et al: Serum vasopressin concentrations in critically ill patients. *Crit Care Med* 2006; 34(2):293-299.
117. Bernard GR, Vincent JL, Laterre PF, et al: Efficacy and safety of recombinant human activated protein C for severe sepsis. *N Engl J Med* 2001; 344(10):699-709.
118. Donatelli F, Triggiani M, Benussi S, et al: Advantages of delayed sternal closure in cardiac-compromised adult patients. *J Card Surg* 1995; 10(6):632-636.
119. Anderson CA, Filsoufi F, Aklog L, et al: Liberal use of delayed sternal closure for postcardiotomy hemodynamic instability. *Ann Thorac Surg* 2002; 73(5):1484-1488.
120. Gottlieb LJ, Beahm EK, Krizek TJ, et al: Approaches to sternal wound infections. *Adv Card Surg* 1996; 7:147-162.
121. Olsson C, Tammelin A, Thelin S: Staphylococcus aureus bloodstream infection after cardiac surgery: risk factors and outcome. *Infect Control Hosp Epidemiol* 2006; 27(1):83-85.
122. Lev-Ran O, Mohr R, Amir K, et al: Bilateral internal thoracic artery grafting in insulin-treated diabetics: should it be avoided? *Ann Thorac Surg* 2003; 75(6):1872-1877.
123. Latham R, Lancaster AD, Covington JF, et al: The association of diabetes and glucose control with surgical-site infections among cardiothoracic surgery patients. *Infect Control Hosp Epidemiol* 2001; 22(10):607-612.
124. Sjogren J, Gustafsson R, Nilsson J, et al: Clinical outcome after poststernotomy mediastinitis: vacuum-assisted closure versus conventional treatment. *Ann Thorac Surg* 2005; 79(6):2049-2055.
125. Rich MW, Keller AJ, Schechtman KB, et al: Increased complications and prolonged hospital stay in elderly cardiac surgical patients with low serum albumin. *Am J Cardiol* 15 1989; 63(11):714-718.
126. Carney DE, Meguid MM: Current concepts in nutritional assessment. *Arch Surg* 2002; 137(1):42-45.
127. Heyland DK, Novak F, Drover JW, et al: should immunonutrition become routine in critically ill patients? A systematic review of the evidence. *JAMA* 2001; 286(8):944-953.
128. Walter J, Mortasawi A, Arnrich B, et al: Creatinine clearance versus serum creatinine as a risk factor in cardiac surgery. *BMC Surg* 2003; 3:4.
129. Nagaranjan DV, Lewis PS, Botha P, Dunning J: Is addition of antiplatelet therapy to warfarin beneficial to patients with prosthetic heart valves? *Interact Cardiovasc Thorac Sur* 2004; 3:450-455.
130. Bernstein AD DJ-C, Fletcher RD, Hayes DL, et al: The revised NASPE/BPEG generic code for antibradycardia, adaptive-rate, and multisite pacing. *PACE* 2000; 25:260-264.

18

Temporary Mechanical Circulatory Support

Edwin C. McGee, Jr. • Nader Moazami

A number of ventricular assist devices (VADs) are available for acute circulatory support. As opposed to long-term VADs, which are designed primarily for bridge to transplantation or long-term support in the nontransplant patient, temporary VADs are designed to reestablish adequate organ perfusion rapidly. Patients in cardiogenic shock require early aggressive therapy. Despite relief of ischemia, inotropic drugs, and control of cardiac rhythm, some patients remain hemodynamically unstable and require some type of mechanical circulatory support in order to restore a normal cardiac output and maintain end-organ perfusion. Cardiogenic shock occurs in 2.4 to 12% of patients with acute myocardial infarction (AMI).[1] The landmark Should We Emergently Revascularize Occluded Coronaries for Cardiogenic Shock (SHOCK) trial demonstrated mortality of greater than 50% despite revascularization.[2] If instituted promptly, temporary mechanical support leads to improved survival in this group of patients.[3] The need for circulatory support in the postcardiotomy period is relatively low and has been estimated to be in the range of 0.2 to 0.6%,[4] but when it occurs, it needs to be managed effectively if the patient is to be salvaged. Additional indications for acute VADs are in chronic heart failure patients who suffer cardiovascular collapse, and severe cases of myocarditis and postpartum cardiomyopathy.

All practicing cardiac surgeons should have an understanding of current devices, and have at least one of these support systems available. Studies show that even smaller facilities that do not have advanced heart failure programs can have improved patient survival if a device can be implemented rapidly and the patient is transferred to a tertiary care facility with expanded capabilities.[5]

This chapter describes the devices currently available, indications for support, patient management, and the overall morbidity and mortality associated with temporary mechanical support. In addition, it describes some of the more promising devices that have just received approval or are currently undergoing trial. The goal of all temporary assist devices is to alleviate shock and establish an environment in which the native heart and end organs can recover. If recovery is unlikely, then a bridge to a long-term device, typically for bridging to a heart transplant, may be the best strategy. Rarely should individuals be supported directly to heart transplantation from an acute support device, because the newer generations of long-term devices typically provide more reliable support and allow for better rehabilitation in an out-of-hospital setting. It may be possible to bridge a patient who is not a transplant candidate to a long-term device, but given that these patients often are older with comorbities, bridging a patient from an acute VAD to a long-term DT pump must be done with caution.

COUNTERPULSATION

Intra-aortic balloon pumps (IABPs) are often the first line of mechanical assistance utilized for patients in cardiogenic shock. The concept of increasing coronary blood flow by counterpulsation was demonstrated by Kantrowitz and Kantrowitz in 1953 in a canine preparation and again by Kantrowitz and McKinnon in 1958 using an electrically stimulated muscle wrap around the descending thoracic aorta to increase diastolic aortic pressure.[6] In 1961, Clauss and colleagues used an external counterpulsation system synchronized to the heartbeat to withdraw blood from the femoral artery during systole and reinfuse it during diastole.[7,8] One year later, Moulopoulos and colleagues produced an inflatable latex balloon that was inserted into the descending thoracic aorta through the femoral artery and inflated with carbon dioxide.[8] Inflation and deflation were synchronized to the electrocardiogram to produce counterpulsation that reduced end-systolic arterial pressure and increased diastolic pressure. In 1968, Kantrowitz reported survival of one of three patients with postinfarction cardiogenic shock refractory to medical therapy using an IABP.[9] These pioneering studies introduced the concept of supporting the failing circulation by mechanical means.

Physiology

The major physiologic effects of the IABP are a concomitant reduction in left ventricular afterload along with an increase in coronary perfusion pressure secondary to an increase in aortic diastolic pressure.[10] Important related effects include reduction in left ventricular systolic wall tension and oxygen consumption, reduction in left ventricular end-systolic and end-diastolic volumes, reduced preload, and an increase in coronary artery and collateral vessel blood flow.[11] Cardiac output increases because of improved myocardial contractility owing to increased coronary blood flow and the reduced afterload and preload, but the IABP does not directly move or significantly redistribute blood flow.[12] IABP counterpulsation reduces peak systolic wall stress (afterload) by 14 to 19% and left ventricular systolic pressure by approximately 15%.[12] Because peak systolic wall stress is related directly to myocardial oxygen consumption, myocardial oxygen requirements are reduced proportionately. As measured by echocardiography and color-flow Doppler mapping, peak diastolic flow velocity increases by 117% and the coronary flow velocity integral increases by 87% with counterpulsation.[13] Experimentally, collateral blood flow to ischemic areas increases up to 21% at mean arterial pressures greater than 90 mm Hg.[14]

Several variables affect the physiologic performance of the IABP. The position of the balloon should be just downstream of the left subclavian artery (Fig. 18-1). Diastolic augmentation of coronary blood flow increases with proximity to the aortic valve.[15] The balloon should fit the aorta so that inflation nearly occludes the vessel. Experimental work indicates that for adults, balloon volumes of 30 or 40 mL significantly improve both left ventricular unloading and diastolic coronary perfusion pressure when compared with smaller volumes. Inflation should be timed to coincide with closure of the aortic valve,

which for clinical purposes occurs at the dicrotic notch of the aortic blood pressure trace (Fig. 18-2). Early inflation reduces stroke volume, increases ventricular end-systolic and -diastolic volumes, and increases both afterload and preload. Diastolic counterpulsation is visualized easily as a pressure curve in the arterial waveform and indicates increased diastolic perfusion of the coronary vessels (and/or bypass grafts).[16] Deflation should occur as late as possible to maintain the duration of the augmented diastolic blood pressure but before the aortic valve opens and the ventricle ejects. For practical purposes, deflation is timed to occur with the onset of the electrocardiographic R wave. Active deflation of the balloon creates a suction effect that acts to decrease left ventricular afterload (and therefore myocardial oxygen consumption).

Physiologic factors that influence the in situ hemodynamic performance of the IABP include heart rate and rhythm, mean arterial diastolic pressure, competence of the aortic valve, and compliance of the aortic wall. Severe aortic regurgitation is a contraindication to use of the IABP as a very low mean aortic diastolic pressures reduce aortic root pressure augmentation and coronary blood flow. A calcified, noncompliant aorta increases diastolic pressure augmentation but risks injury to the aortic wall. On the other hand, young patients with a highly elastic, compliant aorta may manifest decreased diastolic pressure augmentation.

For an IABP to perform optimally, a regular heart rate with an easily identified R wave or a good arterial pulse tracing with a discrete aortic dicrotic notch is required. Current

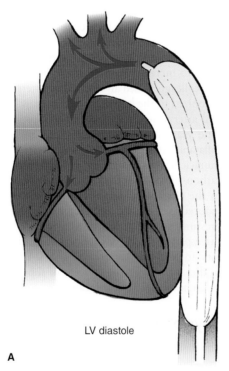
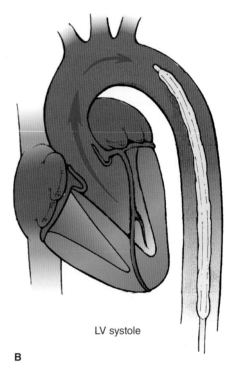

FIGURE 18-1 (A) Balloon inflation during left ventricular (LV) diastole occludes the descending thoracic aorta, closes the aortic valve, and increases proximal coronary and cerebral perfusion. (B) Balloon deflation during LV systole decreases LV afterload and myocardial oxygen demand.

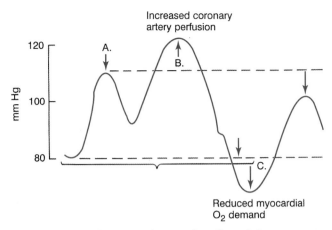

FIGURE 18-2 Illustration showing the effect of the intra-aortic balloon on aortic pressure. After ejection produces the pulse (A), inflation of the balloon increases aortic diastolic pressure (B). At end diastole, sudden deflation reduces aortic end-diastolic pressure (C) below that of an unassisted beat and reduces afterload and myocardial oxygen demand.

balloon pumps trigger off the electrocardiographic R wave or the arterial pressure tracing. Both inflation and deflation are adjustable, and operators attempt to time inflation to coincide with closure of the aortic valve and descent of the R wave. During tachycardia, the IABP usually is timed to inflate every other beat; during chaotic rhythms, the device is timed to inflate in an asynchronous fixed mode that may or may not produce a mean decrease in afterload and an increase in preload. In unstable patients, every effort is made to establish a regular rhythm, including a paced rhythm, so that the IABP can be timed properly. The newer-generation IABP consoles come with algorithms that select the most appropriate trigger mode and time inflation and deflation automatically which have been further enhanced by fiber-optic transducers at the tip of the IABP which do not require a conventional fluid-filled transducer to accurately reflect arterial pressure and are more easily timed.[17]

Indications

The traditional indications for insertion of the IABP are cardiogenic shock, uncontrolled myocardial ischemic pain, and postcardiotomy low cardiac output.[18] Additional indications for IABP have broadened to include patients with high-grade left main coronary artery stenosis, high-risk or failed percutaneous transluminal coronary angioplasty, atherectomy, or stents; patients with poorly controlled ventricular arrhythmias before or after operation; and patients with postinfarction ventricular septal defect (VSD) or acute mitral insufficiency after myocardial infarction (MI).[19] Occasionally an IABP is used prophylactically in high-risk patients with poor left ventricular function (LVF) with either mitral regurgitation or preoperative low cardiac output owing to hibernating or stunned myocardium. These patients may benefit from temporary afterload reduction in the prebypass period and during weaning from cardiopulmonary bypass.

Techniques of Insertion

The IABP usually is inserted into the common femoral artery either by the percutaneous technique or surgical cut down. A cut down is used most often during cardiopulmonary bypass when the pulse is absent. To avoid a formal cut down, a femoral artery catheter may be inserted in anticipation of IABP use in patients undergoing complex procedures who have myocardial dysfunction .The superficial femoral artery is avoided because of its smaller size and increased possibility of leg ischemia. For patients with small vessels, a 7-French catheter without a sheath is recommended to lessen the possibility of leg ischemia. The iliac and axillary arteries and, very rarely, the abdominal aorta are infrequently used alternate sites.[20,21] Direct insertion into the ascending aorta can be used intraoperatively in patients with severe aortoiliac or femoral occlusive disease that prevents passage of the balloon catheter.[22,23]

An IABP is inserted using Seldinger's technique. In the catheterization laboratory, both the guidewire and balloon are monitored by fluoroscopy, but this is not essential if not readily available. In the operating room, the guidewire and balloon are typically placed and positioned under transesophageal echocardiographic guidance.[24] The catheter can be inserted without the sheath when the size of the common femoral artery is a concern.[25]

Typically patients with an IABP receive heparin for anticoagulation, but this practice varies from center to center. The exit site of the catheter must be kept clean with antiseptics and covered in an effort to prevent local infection or septicemia.

A percutaneous IABP can be removed without exposing the femoral puncture site. The exit site is prepped and securing sutures are cut. The balloon catheter is disconnected from the pump and completely deflated using a 50-mL syringe. When the balloon is removed, the proximal artery is compressed and retrograde bleeding is allowed, which flushes any distal clot into the wound. The distal femoral artery then is compressed, and antegrade flushing then is allowed. Finally, steady nonocclusive pressure is held over the femoral puncture site. Pressure is maintained over the puncture site for 30 minutes to ensure that thrombus closes the hole. If the balloon is inserted via a cut down, the balloon preferably is removed in the operating room. The puncture site is closed with sutures. If blood flow to the lower limb is impaired after removal, a formal thromboembolectomy is required.

If the percutaneous needle punctures the iliac artery above the inguinal ligament intentionally or inadvertently in obese individuals, removal should be done through a surgical incision in the operating room because the backward slope of the pelvis makes pressure difficult to maintain after withdrawal, and substantial occult retroperitoneal bleeding may occur.

An IABP may be useful before insertion of more long-term left ventricular assist systems to optimize perfusion and right ventricular function. Use of an IABP in patients with chronic systolic heart failure as a bridge to transplantation or left ventricular assist device (LVAD) therapy is a common practice with over half of the patients being stabilized with this strategy.[26] More importantly, placement of the IABP through a graft sewn to the subclavian artery is a strategy that has allowed ambulation of the patients while waiting for the next stage of therapy with a reported success rate of 93%.[27]

In this technique, a 6-mm graft is sewn to the artery in an end-to-side manner and the shortened standard IABP sheath is inserted into this graft.[27] The IABP is then placed through a separate stab wound, or through the externalized IABP sheath and then positioned under fluoroscopy and transesophageal echocardiography (TEE). The wound over the sheath is then closed. Some groups bury the hub of the IABP sheath, but our preference is to externalize it so that if the IABP needs to be repositioned, the wound does not need to be reopened.

In patients waiting for a new heart, the presence of an IABP qualifies a patient as 1A, or the highest status, on the UNOS heart transplant waiting list.

Complications

Reported complication rates of the IABP vary between 12.9 and 29% and average approximately 20%.[28] Life-threatening complications are rare. Leg ischemia is by far the most common complication (incidence 9-25%); other complications include balloon rupture, thrombosis within the balloon, septicemia, infection at the insertion site, bleeding, false aneurysm formation, lymph fistula, lymphocele, and femoral neuropathy.[29] There is no significant difference in limb ischemia in the different types of IABPs clinically available.[28,30]

Balloon rupture occurs in approximately 1.7% of patients and usually is manifested by the appearance of blood within the balloon catheter and only occasionally by the pump alarm. Rupture may be slightly more common with transaortic insertion. Although helium usually is used to inflate the balloon, gas embolism has not been a problem. If rupture occurs, the balloon should be deflated forcibly to minimize thrombus formation within the balloon and should be promptly removed. If the patient is IABP dependent, a guidewire is introduced through the ruptured balloon, the original balloon is removed, and a second balloon catheter is inserted over the wire. If the ruptured balloon is not removed easily, a second balloon is inserted via the opposite femoral or iliac artery or through the axillary artery to maintain circulatory support.

Removal of a kinked or thrombosed ruptured balloon that cannot be withdrawn easily requires operative removal as forcibly removing a ruptured IABP which contains clot can disrupt the iliac or femoral artery upon removal and lead to uncontrollable hemorrhage. The catheter should be withdrawn as far as possible until resistance is met.

The location of the tip should be determined by x-ray or ultrasound, and an incision should be planned to expose that segment of the vascular system. The trapped balloon is removed through an arteriotomy after control of the vascular segment is obtained.

Although the incidence of clinically significant lower leg ischemia varies in from 9 to 25% of patients, up to 47% patients have evidence of ischemia during the time the IABP is used.[29] Thus, the preinsertion status of the pedal pulses should be determined and recorded before the IABP is inserted in every patient. After insertion, the circulation of the foot is followed hourly by palpating pulses or Doppler ultrasound. Foot color, mottling, temperature, and capillary refill are observed. The appearance of pain, decreased sensation, and compromised circulation indicate severe ischemia that requires restoration of the circulation to the extremity as soon as possible. There are three alternatives. If the patient is not balloon dependent, the balloon is removed immediately. In the majority of patients, this relieves the distal ischemia; a few patients require surgical exploration of the puncture site, removal of thrombus and/or emboli, and reconstruction of the femoral artery. If the patient is balloon dependent, a second balloon catheter can be introduced into the opposite femoral or iliac artery and the first is removed. Several risk factors for development of leg ischemia have emerged. Female gender, peripheral vascular disease, diabetes, cigarette smoking, advanced age, obesity, and cardiogenic shock are reported to increase the risk of ischemic complications after IABP. Because the IABP is inserted for compelling indications, identification of risk factors does not influence management, except to encourage removal of the device as soon as the cardiac status of the patient allows. In some series, longer duration of IABP counterpulsation is associated with an increased risk of complications.[29] Although most ischemic complications are the result of impairment of arterial inflow, severe atherosclerotic diseases of the descending thoracic aorta may produce embolization of atherosclerotic material. Approximately 1% of patients develop false aneurysms at the femoral puncture site either in the hospital or shortly after discharge, and rare patients develop an arteriovenous fistula. Both conditions are confirmed readily by duplex scanning.

Results

Very few complications of IABP cause death. Rare instances of bleeding (retroperitoneal or aortic), septicemia, central nervous system injury, or aortic dissection may cause or contribute to a patient's death. Mortality is higher in patients with ischemic leg complications than in those without this complication.

Without revascularization, IABP produces a marginal increase in survival, but with revascularization, both short- and long-term survival, as well as quality of life have been shown to be improved.[31] However, mortality is high in patients who receive an IABP because of the cardiac problems that led to the need for the device. Overall hospital mortality ranges from 26 to 50%.[32,33] Risk factors for hospital mortality include advanced age, female gender, high New York Heart Association (NYHA) class, preoperative nitroglycerin, operative or postoperative insertion, and transaortic insertion in one study and age and diabetes mellitus in another. A third study correlates hospital death with AMI, ejection fraction of less than 30%, NYHA class IV, and prolonged aortic cross-clamp and bypass times.[34] Time of insertion affects hospital mortality. Preoperative insertion is associated with a mortality of 18.8 to 19.6%.[18] Mortality for intraoperative insertion is 27.6 to 32.3%.[17] Postoperative IABO insertion is associated with a mortality of 39 to 40.5%. Mortality is highest at 68% for patients with pump failure, lowest at 34% for patients with coronary ischemia, and 48% for patients who had a cardiac operation. Long-term survival varies with the type of operation and is highest in patients who had cardiac transplantation or myocardial revascularization.[18] Patients who received an IABP and required valve surgery with or without revascularization have a poorer prognosis. Creswell and colleagues found 58.8% of all patients alive at 1 year and 47.2% alive at 5 years. Naunheim and associates found that nearly all survivors were in NYHA class I or II.[34] Approximately 18% of hospital survivors have some symptoms of lower extremity ischemia.

Given the overall ease of IABP insertion, excellent physiologic augmentation of coronary blood flow and left ventricular unloading, an IABP should be considered as the first line of mechanical support in patients who do not have significant peripheral vascular disease. There is some suggestion that preoperative prophylactic IABP insertion in high-risk patients (eg, left ventricular ejection fraction [LVEF] of less than 40%, unstable angina, left main stenosis of greater than 70%, or redo coronary artery bypass grafting [CABG]) can improve cardiac index, length of intensive care unit (ICU) stay, and reduce mortality.[35] However, with meticulous myocardial protection and the judicious use of inotropes, such as epinephrine and milrinone, most groups experienced in dealing with such high-risk patients do not find routine IABP insertion helpful.

According to latest 2013 ACC/AHA guidelines on ST elevation myocardial infarction (STEMI), use of MCS devices (including IABP) is reasonable in patients with STEMI who are hemodynamically unstable and require urgent CABG (Class IIa recommendation).[36] Prior to this, 2004 ACC/AHA and 2010 ESC STEMI guidelines listed specifically IABP use in cardiogenic shock as class 1B and IC recommendations, respectively, although there were no randomized trials supporting those recommendations. The IABP SHOCK II trial was a recent randomized trial of 600 patients who presented with AMI and cardiogenic shock who were to be treated with revascularization strategies. Three hundred patients received an IABP and 298 patients were treated medically. The degree of shock, and patient characteristics were similar. In this trial, there was no difference in the 30-day mortality (IABP 39.7%: control 41.3%)[37] and also no differences in adverse events, leading to downgrading in guideline recommendation class.[38]

Many surgeons consider prophylactic insertion of IABP before high-risk cardiac surgery. Although the impact of this strategy is debatable, a recent meta-analysis of randomized-controlled trials has demonstrated that in high-risk patients, prophylactic IABP insertion leads to decrease in mortality, reduces the incidence of low output cardiac syndrome and translates into shorter ICU length of stay.[39] Application of IABP in postcardiac surgery varies widely. Most surgeons consider this as the first line of mechanical circulatory support in situations of persistent hypotension or low cardiac output in the immediate postoperative phase. Again, in postcardiotomy situations, in presence of persistent low cardiac output requiring high-dose pressor and inotropic support, the impact of IABP is limited and consideration for devices that can significantly increase flow should be given.

The standard IABP has a volume of 40 cc. A 50-cc IABP has been introduced and studies show that it leads to higher augmented diastolic pressure, greater systolic unloading, and a greater reduction of pulmonary capillary wedge pressure.[40]

While an IABP can be helpful in the management of shock patients, it is important to understand that it is not the final therapy in terms of mechanical support for the failing heart. If the shock state persists, as evidence by a depressed cardiac index, then some form of direct mechanical support must be implemented so as to restore adequate end-organ perfusion. Failure to adequately treat a patient in cardiogenic shock will most assuredly result in the patient's demise.

DIRECT CIRCULATORY SUPPORT

Background

The need for acute cardiac support beyond cardiopulmonary bypass was clear from the early days of cardiac surgery. In 1966, the first successful use of a LVAD was reported after a double-valve operation by DeBakey, who used an assist device that was implanted in an extracorporeal location between the left atrium and the axillary artery.[41] The patient was supported for 10 days on the pump, eventually was discharged home, and was a long-term survivor.[41]

Ideal Device

The ideal acute support device should be capable of providing adequate flow, maximizing hemodynamics, and unloading the ventricle for patients of all sizes. Current devices have addressed the problem associated with variations in patient size by being designed as extracorporeal systems. Therefore, by virtue of having small-diameter cannulae transversing the chest, the pumps can support patients with varying body surface area. The disadvantages of such a system are the potential for driveline and mediastinal infections, as well as limiting patient mobility. In addition, the length of the cannula between the heart and the device, particularly the inflow cannula, predisposes to areas of stasis and potential thrombus generation. All current pumps require anticoagulation, which increases the ever-present threat of early postoperative bleeding. In addition, requirements for transfusion of large amounts of coagulation factors and platelets enhance the inflammatory response that is induced by surgery and is further perpetuated by the circuit. Activation of the contact and complement systems and the release of cytokines by leukocytes, endothelial cells, and macrophages further increase the potential negative and detrimental effects of use of temporary assist devices.[44] The ensuing inflammatory cascade and volume overload can have detrimental effects on the pulmonary vascular resistance and lead to right ventricular overload, often necessitating the addition of a right ventricular assist device (RVAD).

Current temporary assist devices can be configured for biventricular support as needed, provided that the lungs can support oxygenation and ventilation. In cases of acute lung injury superimposed on circulatory failure, extracorporeal life support (ECLS) can be configured with conventional or the more recent centrifugal pumps.

The clinical scenarios that lead to the need for mechanical support all require that support be instituted in an expeditious manner. Therefore, all current devices must be easily implantable. In the postcardiotomy setting with access to the great vessels, the cannulae should allow the versatility of choosing any inflow or outflow site that is clinically indicated. In an active resuscitative setting, such as cardiac arrest in the catheterization laboratory, in which time is critical and transport to the operating room often impractical, percutaneous cannulation must be an option.

At present, the ideal device does not exist. Until innovations in the field of circulatory support lead to the development of an ideal device, the currently available technology must be tailored to the specific requirements of each patient, taking into consideration the duration of support needed.

Indications for Support and Patient Selection

A wide range of indications exist for acute mechanical support, the primary goal of all being rapid restoration of the circulation and stabilization of hemodynamics. The routine use of TEE has helped greatly in assessing the etiology of cardiogenic shock by allowing evaluation of ventricular function, regional wall motion abnormalities, and valvular mechanics. In a patient with mechanical complications secondary to MI such as acute rupture with tamponade, acute papillary muscle rupture, or postinfarction VSD, emergent surgical correction may obviate the need for device support. Similarly, in the postcardiotomy setting with failure to separate from cardiopulmonary bypass, TEE may direct the surgeon to the need for additional revascularization and reparative valve surgery and successful weaning from bypass.

If echocardiography fails to reveal a surgically correctable cause for cardiogenic shock, most surgeons use hemodynamic data to consider the need for mechanical assistance. These criteria include, but are not limited to, a cardiac index of less than 2.2 L/min/m², systolic blood pressure of less than 90 mm Hg, mean pulmonary capillary wedge pressure or central venous pressure of greater than 20 mm Hg, and concomitant use of high doses of at least two inotropic agents.[42] These situations may be associated clinically with arrhythmias, pulmonary edema, and oliguria. In such circumstances, use of an IABP may be considered as the first step. In the postcardiotomy setting, the preceding hemodynamic criteria, in absence of mechanical support, are associated with a greater than 50% chance of mortality.[31] In this setting, some believe that earlier implantation of an assist device capable of supporting higher flows and allowing the heart to rest may improve results and allow for recovery of stunned myocardium.[43] Furthermore, pharmacologic agents such as the phosphodiesterase inhibitor milrinone, nitric oxide, and vasopressin have helped to optimize hemodynamics during this critical initial period, reducing the need for concomitant right ventricular support.[44,45]

Once mechanical assistance has been instituted, the stabilized patient can undergo periodic evaluation to assess native heart recovery, end-organ function, and neurologic status. If appropriate, evaluation for cardiac transplantation ensues. Patients without malignancy, severe untreated infection, or neurologic deficit and who are not at an advanced age are selected for cardiac transplantation if all other criteria are met, and there is no sign of cardiac recovery. In this subgroup, we generally transition to a chronic VAD until an organ becomes available, a strategy that has been termed "a bridge to a bridge," in that a short-term device is used to "bridge" the patient to a more durable "bridge to transplant" VAD. In patients with improvement in myocardial pump function, the devices may be weaned and removed.

DEVICES

Devices currently approved by the Food and Drug Administration (FDA) for temporary support include centrifugal pumps, roller pumps, venoarterial extracorporeal membrane oxygenation (ECLS, ECMO), the ABIOMED AB5000 Ventricle and Impella devices (ABIOMED, Danvers, MA), Thoratec Centrimag (Thoratec Inc., Pleasanton, CA), and the Thoratec paracorporeal VAD (pVAD) (Pleasanton, CA), and the TandemHeart system (CardiacAssist, Inc.). A number of other devices are undergoing investigation for short-term support.

Continuous-Flow Pumps

Two types of pumps are available commercially for extracorporeal circulation: roller pumps and centrifugal pumps. In adults, roller pumps are used rarely, if ever, for temporary circulatory support beyond routine cardiopulmonary bypass applications because of important disadvantages. Although inexpensive, roller pumps are insensitive to line pressure and require unobstructed inflow. Additionally, roller pumps may cause spallation of tubing particles and are subject to tubing failure at unpredictable times. These systems require constant vigilance and are difficult to operate for extended periods. Use of roller pumps beyond 4 to 5 hours is associated with hemolysis and, for this reason, is inappropriate for mechanical assistance that may involve several days to weeks of support.[46] Axial flow pumps, in which the pump rotor is parallel to the blood path, have entered the field of temporary support with the introduction of the Impella devices but most of the experience with temporary support devices has been with centrifugal pumps.

CENTRIFUGAL PUMPS

Centrifugal pumps are familiar assist systems because of their routine use in cardiopulmonary bypass. In these devices, the blood path is perpendicular to the rotor. Although many different pump-head designs are available, they all work on the principle of generating a rotary motion by virtue of moving blades, impellers, or concentric cones. These pumps generally can provide high flow rates with relatively modest increases in pressure. They require priming and de-airing prior to use in the circuit, and the amount of flow generated is sensitive to outflow resistance and filling pressures. The differences in design of the various commercially available pump heads are in the numbers of impellers, the shape and angle of the blades, and the priming volume. The Medtronic Bio-Pump® (Medtronic Bio-Medicus, Inc., Eden Prairie, MN), which is based on two concentric cones generating a rotary motion, has been extensively utilized in the field of acute circulatory support.[47] The pump heads are disposable, relatively cheap to manufacture, and mounted on a magnetic motorized unit that generates the power that drives the pump. Although earlier designs caused mechanical trauma to the blood elements leading to excessive hemolysis, the newly engineered pumps are less traumatic and can be used for longer periods.

The Rotoflow (Maquet Cardiovascular) is another example of a centrifugal pump that is extensively utilized in the field of acute circulatory support.

Complications. Complications with temporary mechanical assistance are high and are very similar for patients on centrifugal pump support or ECLS. The major complications reported by a voluntary registry for temporary circulatory assistance using primarily LVADs, RVADs, and biventricular assist devices (BVADs) are bleeding, persistent shock, renal failure, infection, neurologic deficits, thrombosis and emboli, hemolysis, and technical problems. Neurologic deficits occurred in approximately 12% of patients, and in Golding's experience, noncerebral emboli occurred equally often.[48] Golding also found that 13% of patients also developed hepatic failure. An autopsy study found anatomical evidence of embolization in 63% of patients, even though none had emboli detected clinically.[49]

Results. Although a meaningful comparison of results of centrifugal support from different institutions is not possible, in general, overall survival has been in the range of 21 to 41%. A voluntary registry reported the experience with 604 LVADs, 168 RVADs, and 507 BVADs; approximately 70% were with continuous-flow pumps and the remainder with pulsatile pumps.[50] There were no significant differences in the percentage of patients weaned from circulatory assistance or the percentage discharged from the hospital according to the type of perfusion circuitry. Overall, 45.7% of patients were weaned, and 25.3% were discharged from the hospital.[50] The registry also reports that long-term survival of patients weaned from circulatory support is 46% at 5 years.[50] Most of the mortality occurs in the hospital before discharge or within 5 months of discharge.

Golding reported an identical hospital survival rate for 91 patients in 1992 using only centrifugal pumps, and Noon reported that 21% of 129 patients were discharged.[49,51] Patients who received pulsatile circulatory assistance were supported significantly longer than those supported by centrifugal pumps, but there were no differences in the percentage of patients weaned or discharged. Survivors were supported an average of 3.1 days using continuous-flow pumps. Patients supported for AMI did poorly; only 11.5% survived to be discharged. Joyce reports that 42% of patients supported by Sarns impeller pumps eventually were discharged.[52]

EXTRACORPOREAL LIFE SUPPORT (ECLS/ECMO)

By the 1960s, it was clear that cardiopulmonary bypass was not suitable for patients requiring circulatory support for several days to weeks. The development of ECLS as a temporary assist device (also referred to as *extracorporeal membrane oxygenation* [ECMO]) is a direct extension of the principles of cardiopulmonary bypass and follows the pioneering efforts of Bartlett and colleagues in demonstrating the efficacy of this technology in neonatal respiratory distress syndrome.[53]

There are a number of key differences between cardiopulmonary bypass and ECLS. The most obvious difference is the duration of required support. Whereas cardiopulmonary bypass typically is employed for several hours during cardiac surgery, ECLS is designed for longer duration of support. With ECLS, lower doses of heparin are used, and reversal of heparin is not an issue. Because a continuous circuit is used, areas of stasis, such as the cardiotomy suction and venous reservoir, are not present. These differences are thought to reduce the inflammatory response and the more pronounced coagulopathy that can be seen with cardiopulmonary bypass[54] although there is generally a rapid rise of inflammatory cytokines with initiation of ECLS support.[55]

A typical ECLS circuit is demonstrated in Fig. 18-3. The system consists of the following:

1. *Hollow-fiber membrane oxygenator with an integrated heat-exchange system.* The microporous membrane provides the necessary gas-transfer capability via the micropores where there is direct blood-gas interface with minimal resistance to diffusion. By virtue of the membranes being close to each other, the diffusion distance has been reduced without a significant pressure drop across the system. Control of oxygenation and ventilation is relatively easy. Increasing

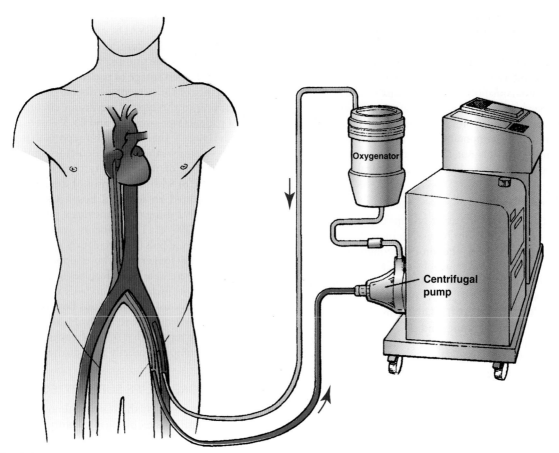

FIGURE 18-3 Percutaneous extracorporeal membrane oxygenation (ECMO) support is attained via femoral vessel access. Right atrial blood is drained via a catheter inserted into the femoral vein and advanced into the right atrium. Oxygenated blood is perfused retrograde via the femoral artery. Distal femoral artery perfusion is not illustrated.

the total gas flow rate increases CO_2 removal (increasing the "sweep") by reducing the gas-phase CO_2 partial pressure and promoting diffusion. Blood oxygenation is controlled simply by changing the fraction of O_2 in the gas supplied to the oxygenator.

2. *Centrifugal pump.* These pumps are totally nonocclusive and afterload dependent. An increase in downstream resistance, such as significant hypertension, will decrease forward flow to the body. Therefore, flow is not determined by rotational flow alone, and a flowmeter needs to be incorporated in the arterial outflow to quantitate the actual pump output. If the pump outflow should become occluded, the pump will not generate excessive pressure and will not rupture the arterial line. Similarly, the pump will not generate significant negative pressure if the inflow becomes occluded. This protects against cavitation and microembolus formation. The newer generation magnetically levitated centrifugal pumps have been also used recently in the ECLS circuit and may have less traumatic effect on the blood elements.[56]

3. *Heat exchanger.* This allows for control of blood temperature as it passes through the extracorporeal circuit. Generally, the transfer of energy occurs by circulating nonsterile water in a countercurrent fashion against the circulating blood. Use of

water as the heat-exchange medium provides an even temperature across the surface of the heat exchanger without localized hot spots. The use of a heat exchanger allows for maintenance of normothermia given the potential heal loss that can occur through the long circuit.

4. *Circuitry interfaced between the patient and the system.* The need for systemic anticoagulation on ECLS and the complications associated with massive coagulopathy and persistent bleeding during the postcardiotomy period led to the development of biocompatible heparin-bonded bypass circuits. In 1991, the Carmeda Corporation in Stockholm, Sweden, released a heparin-coating process that could be used to produce an antithrombotic surface.[57] This process was applied to extracorporeal tubing and the hollow-fiber microporous oxygenator surface.[58] Initial experience suggested that the need for systemic anticoagulation had been eliminated. In addition, heparin coating has been associated with a decrease in the inflammatory response with reduced granulocyte[59] and complement activation.[60] Bindslev and colleagues[61] and Mottaghy and colleagues[62] reported excellent hemodynamic support with minimal postoperative blood loss in experimental animals for up to 5 days. Magovern and Aranki reported similar excellent results with clinical application.[63,64]

Although these heparin-bonded circuits were initially thought to completely eliminate the need for heparinization, thrombus formation without anticoagulation remains a persistent problem. In a study of 30 adult patients with cardiogenic shock who underwent ECLS using the heparin-bonded circuits and no systemic anticoagulation, 20% of patients developed left ventricular thrombus by TEE, and an additional 6% had a visible clot in the pump head.[65] Protamine administration after starting ECLS can precipitate intracardiac clot. If the left ventricle does not eject and blood remains static within the ventricle, clot formation is more likely. Intracavitary clot is more likely in patients with MI owing to expression of tissue factor by the injured cells. Protamine may bind to the heparinized coating of the new circuit and negate an anticoagulant effect.[66]

Cannulation. The main difference between the centrifugal pump and ECLS is the presence of an in-line oxygenator. As a result, ECLS can be used for biventricular support by using central or peripheral cannulation. Intraoperatively, the most common application of ECLS has been for patients who cannot be weaned from cardiopulmonary bypass after heart surgery. In these cases, the existing right atrial and aortic cannulas can be used. An alternative strategy is to convert the system to peripheral cannulas, which potentially permits later decannulation without opening the chest.

Cannulation is accomplished by surgical cut down or percutaneous insertion. The entire vessel does not need to be mobilized, and exposure of the anterior surface of the vessels typically suffices. A purse string suture is placed over the anterior surface of the vessel. Typically, arterial cannulae of 16 to 20 French and venous cannulae of 18 to 25 French are used. The cannulation is performed under direct vision using Seldinger's technique. A stab incision is made in the skin with a no. 11 blade knife, a needle is inserted through the stab incision into the vessel, and a guidewire is advanced gently. Dilators then are passed sequentially to gently dilate the tract and the insertion point in the vessel. The cannulae then are inserted, the guidewire is removed, and a clamp is applied. For venous drainage, a long venous cannula is directed into the femoral vein to the level of the right atrium under transesophageal echocardiographic guidance.

To minimize limb complications from ischemia, one strategy is to place an 8- to 10-French perfusion cannula in the superficial femoral artery distal to the primary arterial inflow cannula to perfuse the leg (Fig. 18-4). This cannula is connected to a tubing circuit that is spliced into the arterial circuit with a Y-connector. The distal cannula directs continuous flow into the leg and significantly reduces the incidence of leg ischemia. It should be noted, however, that limb ischemia associated with long-term peripheral cannulation relates not only to arterial perfusion, but also to the relative venous obstruction that can occur with large venous lines. In such circumstances distal venous drainage can be established by splicing another small venous cannula into the circuit.

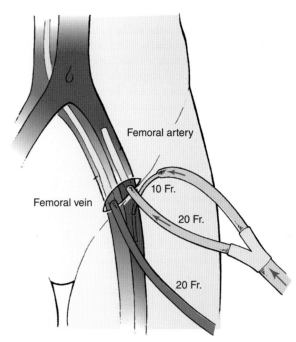

FIGURE 18-4 Surgical exposure of the femoral vessels facilitates cannulation for ECMO. A small 10-French cannula is used to perfuse the distal femoral artery.

An alternative strategy is to completely mobilize the common femoral artery and sew a 8- or 10-mm short Dacron graft to its anterior surface as a "chimney." The graft serves as the conduit for the arterial cannula. Alternatively a standard perfusion connector may be secured in the graft and hooked to the 3/8 tubing of the circuit. This strategy also allows for a more secure connection and avoids problems with inadvertent dislodgement of the cannulas because of loosening of the purse strings or tourniquets.

In general, complete percutaneous placement of arterial cannulae is avoided to prevent iatrogenic injury during insertion and ensure proper positioning of the cannula. However, when venovenous bypass is the only mode of support needed, percutaneous cannulation is performed. Surgical exposure is not necessary, and bleeding is less with this technique.

Central cannulation sometimes is indicated because of either severe peripheral vascular disease or the desire to deliver the highly oxygenated blood directly to the coronary arteries and cerebral circulation. In patients with an open chest, aortic and right atrial cannulae may be used, but our preference is to anastomose a graft to the ascending aorta and connulate the right atrium from the femoral vein. Reinforcing purse string sutures are placed and tied over rubber chokers and buttons for later tying at decannulation. The catheters are brought through the chest wall through separate stab wounds, and after bleeding is secured, the chest may be closed.

An alternative central cannulation site is the axillary artery. The most secure cannulation strategy for the axillary artery is to sew an 8- or 10-mm graft to the vessel as a "chimney." The cannula then is placed in the graft and tied securely with several circumferential sutures and zip ties. Clinicians must be vigilant for progressive arm edema, which can be controlled by partial occlusion of the distal axillary artery by vessel loop.

Once instituted, the system is simple enough to be monitored by trained ICU nurses and maintained by a perfusionist on a daily basis. Evidence of clots in the pump head requires a change. Leakage of plasma across the membrane from the blood phase to the gas phase may be a problem, gradually decreasing the efficiency of the oxygenator and increasing resistance to flow and necessitating oxygenator exchanges. Using this system, ECLS flows of 4 to 6 L/min are possible at pump speeds of 3000 to 3200 rpm. Higher pump speeds are avoided to minimize mechanical trauma to blood cells. Other means of improving flow include transfusion of blood, crystalloid, or other colloid solutions to increase the overall circulating volume.

Physiologically, ECLS will unload the right ventricle but will not unload the compromised left ventricle, even though left ventricular preload is reduced.[68] In normal hearts, the marked reduction in preload and small increase in afterload produced by the arterial inflow from the ECLS system reduce wall stress and produce smaller end-diastolic left ventricular volumes because the heart is able to eject the blood it receives. However, if the heart is dilated and poorly contracting, the increase in afterload provided by the ECLS system offsets any change in end-diastolic left ventricular volume produced by bypassing the heart. The heart remains dilated because the left ventricle cannot eject sufficient volume against the increased afterload to reduce either end-diastolic or -systolic volume. ECLS, therefore, theoretically may increase left ventricular wall stress and myocardial oxygen consumption unless the left ventricle is mechanically unloaded. If the PCWP remains high and there is evidence of pulmonary congestion, a left-sided vent, which is spliced into the venous limb of the circuit is indicated. Most groups are finding that direct LV decompression is the effective form of left-sided drainage.

As mentioned, the versatility of ECLS is that it allows rapid restoration of circulation by peripheral cannulation during active resuscitation in the setting of acute cardiac arrest, acute pulmonary embolism, or patients in cardiogenic shock, who cannot be moved safely to the operating room.

An isolated RVAD is rarely indicated in the postcardiotomy setting because, in general, these patients have global biventricular dysfunction. ECLS as an RVAD (with outflow to the pulmonary artery) may be used only in patients with good function of the left ventricle who manifest right ventricular failure and hypoxia or in patients who manifest RV failure after implantation of a long-term LVAD.

Complications. The experience in adults with ECLS for postoperative cardiogenic shock is associated with high rates of bleeding. Surgical bleeding from the chest is exacerbated by anticoagulation and the consumptive coagulopathy caused by the ECLS circuit. Even without the chest wound, bleeding was the major complication in a large study of long-term ECLS for acute respiratory insufficiency.[67] Muehrcke reported experience with ECLS using heparin-coated circuitry with no or minimal heparin.[68] The incidence of reexploration was 52% in the Cleveland Clinic experience; transfusions averaged 43 units of packed cells, 59 units of platelets, 51 units of cryoprecipitate, and 10 units of fresh-frozen plasma. Other important complications associated with ECLS using heparin-coated circuits included renal failure requiring dialysis (47%), bacteremia or mediastinitis (23%), stroke (10%), leg ischemia (70%), oxygenator failure requiring change (43%), and pump change (13%).[68] Nine of 21 patients with leg ischemia required thrombectomy and one amputation. Half the patients developed marked left ventricular dilatation, and six patients developed intracardiac clot detected by TEE. Intracardiac thrombus may form within a poorly contracting nonejecting left ventricle or atrium because little blood reaches the left atrium with good right atrial drainage. We have observed intracardiac thrombus which is related to left ventricular dysfunction and stagnant flow. In patients on temporary VADs in whom LV clot forms, the clot is removed at the time of permanent VAD implantation.

Results. The Cleveland Clinic reported their results looking at 202 adults with cardiac failure.[69] With an extended follow-up up of 7.5 years (mean 3.8 years), survival was reported to be 76% at 3 days, 38% at 30 days, and 24% at 5 years. Patients surviving 30 days had a 63% chance of being alive at 5 years, demonstrating that the high early mortality remains the Achilles heal of this technology. Interestingly, patients who were weaned or bridged to transplantation had a higher overall survival (40 and 45%, respectively). Failure to wean or bridge was secondary to end-organ dysfunction and included renal and hepatic failure and occurrence of a neurologic event while on support.

The Quadrox D oxygenator (Maquet Cardiovascular) has hollow fibers constructed of poly-methylpentene (PMP) as opposed to the standard microporous polypropylene hallow fiber oxygentators. PMP membrane oxygenerators have less plasma leakage and are as such more durable. It has demonstrated improved oxygenator durability, which has led to longer periods of support ECLS. Pokersnik and colleagues from the Cleveland Clinic Foundation compared outcomes of patients supported with ECLS from 2005 to 2010.[70] Forty-nine patients received ECMO following cardiac surgery. Patients were divided into three groups. Group 1 patients received a biomedicus pump with an affinity oxygenator, Group 2 patients received a Biomedicus pump with a Quadrox D oxygenator, and Group 3 patients received a Rotaflow pump with a Quadrox D oxygenator. Despite oxygenator durability improving markedly with the introduction of the Quadrox D (oxygenator exchange rate dropping from 64-7%), survival in the groups improved only from 27 to 33% with the newer systems. Formica and colleagues from Italy demonstrated a similar survival rate of 28% in a mixed group (n = 25) of primary and postcardiotomy cardiogenic shock patients who were placed on the Rotoflow ECLS (Maquet Cardiovascular) system which uses the Quadrox D oxygenator.[71]

NEWER DEVICES

Cardiohelp™ (Maquet Cardiovascular). Cardiohelp™ is a compact ECLS system with a low priming volume and an integrated oxygenator similar to the quadrox (Fig. 18-5). The small size of the system lends itself to transport both in and out of the hospital. Arit and colleagues reported the feasibility and effectiveness of the Cardiohelp in safely transporting patients with cardiogenic shock. From 2007 to 2010, 20 shock patients were transferred from five different hospitals while supported on Cardiohelp. The patients were treated with angioplasty (n = 2), CABG (n = 6), pulmonary embolectomy (n = 1), and permanent LVAD (n = 1) after arrival at the accepting hospital. Overall survival was 62%.[72]

TandemHeart. The TandemHeart PTVA (percutaneous ventricular assist) System (CardiacAssist, Inc., Pittsburgh, PA) has 510K FDA approval for short-term (<6 hours) mechanical support. It was envisioned for the short-term support of high-risk percutaneous interventions in the catheterization lab.[73] The device is powered by a small hydrodynamic centrifugal pump that resides in a paracorporeal location. The rotor of the pump is suspended and lubricated by a fluid interface of heparinized saline. Cannulas are introduced from the femoral vessels by either percutaneous or direct insertion techniques. Pump inflow is achieved by a novel, proprietary 21-French cannula delivered across the atrial septum. Outflow typically is directed into the common femoral artery (Fig. 18-6). Position is facilitated and confirmed by fluoroscopy and intracardiac ultrasound.[74]

As opposed to an ECLS circuit, excellent left atrial decompression is achieved as long as the inflow cannula is appropriately positioned. The device can be introduced either in the catheterization laboratory using fluoroscopy or directly in the operating room using TEE guidance. Most of the experience with the device has been in the catheterization laboratory, where it has been used extensively to facilitate high-risk

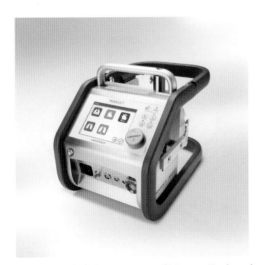

FIGURE 18-5 Cardiohelp. (Courtesy of Maquet Cardiopulmonary GmbH.)

percutaneous interventions.[75] Flows of up to 4 L are typical. With surgically implanted larger cannulae flows up to 8 L are possible.

The TandemHeart can be configured in many ways to achieve effective mechanical support. The inlet and outlet connectors to the pump are 3/8-3/8 connectors, and as such can be connected to any of a number of commercially available percutaneous or surgically implanted cannulae.

Patients with this device are typically kept in bed, given that the device is inserted through the femoral vessels. An activated clotting time (ACT) of 200 seconds is targeted while the patients are on support. The TandemHeart is a very versatile system that can be deployed and discontinued rapidly. One beneficial aspect for postcardiotomy support is that the entire device can be removed in the ICU without reopening the patient's chest. RVAD configurations with right atrial inflow and outflow to the main pulmonary artery are possible in both open[76] and percutaneous configurations.[77] Traditionally, for percutaneous RVAD, the 21-French transeptal cannula was directed into the main pulmonary artery under fluoroscopy, and a separate right atrial cannula was placed via a femoral vein.[77] While achievable, the vascular access requirements were cumbersome. The PROTEK Duo (CardiacAssist, Inc.) Cannula is a dual lumen catheter designed for veno-venous ECMO. With proper positioning, it can be configured as a single cannula percutaneous RVAD. When faced with a patient that needs biventricular support, some groups are splicing an oxygenator into the circuit and using right atrial or bi-atrial drainage. In essence such a configuration converts the assist system to ECLS circuit.[78] With transeptal drainage, the issues of left-sided congestion, which sometimes plague ECLS patients, are nonexistent.

Karr and colleagues reported 117 patients supported with the TandemHeart. Fifty-six patients (47.9%) were undergoing CPR. Thirty-day and six-month survival were 59.8% and 54.7%, respectively. The authors concluded that the TandemHeart percutaneous VAD effectively and rapidly reversed cardiogenic shock refractory to IABP and vasopressor support.[79]

Gregoric and reported the outcomes of eight patients in shock secondary to critical aortic stenosis supported with preoperative TandemHeart. Five were receiving chest compressions at the time of TandemHeart Insertion. All underwent conventional aortic valve replacement after a mean duration of support of 6 days. One patient died of postoperative sepsis. The other seven patients were discharged from the hospital and were all alive at the time of the report.[80]

Brinkman and the group at Medical City Dallas reported on the outcomes of 22 patients supported with the TandemHeart device. Mean duration of support was 6.8 days with no pump failures or pump-related neurologic events. Three patients developed bleeding and two patients had lower extremity ischemic complications. In 11 patients who were neurologically intact at the time of TandemHeart insertion, five went on to receive transplants while on TandemHeart support, three went on to permanent LVAD placement, and two patients recovered. Of 11 patients with indeterminate

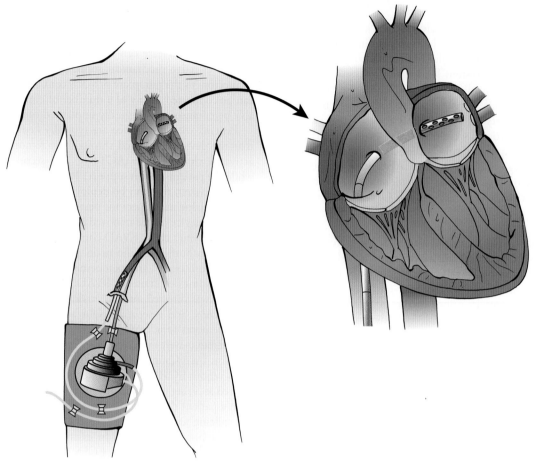

FIGURE 18-6 Transeptal inflow cannula of the TandemHeart device. (Used with permission from CardiacAssist, Inc., Pittsburgh, PA.)

neurologic status or multiorgan failure, seven died, two went on to receive permanent LVADs, one was transplanted, and one patients recovered.[81]

It should be noted that use of a TandemHeart beyond 6 hours and use with an oxygenator are off-label uses of the device. It is important to remember that when placing a long-term VAD in a patient on Tandem support, it is necessary to repair the atrial septum. Failure to do so can lead to hypoxia caused by entrainment of unoxygenated blood across the atrial septal defect created by the TandemHeart inlet cannula.

CentriMag. The CentriMag (Thoratec, Inc., Pleasanton, CA) pump is a centrifugal pump with a fully magnetically levitated impeller (Fig. 18-7).[83] Very little friction is generated and it requires only a very small priming volume. It can be configured for both right- and left-sided heart support typically with central cannulation via median sternotomy. With good cannula placement, more than 9 L of support can be achieved. It has FDA 510K approval for 6 hours of use as an LVAD and has FDA approval for use as a temporary RVAD for 30 days.

The group at the University of Minnesota reported the outcomes of 12 patients supported with CentriMag BiVADs.[83] Of 12 patients who presented in cardiogenic shock, eight

went on to receive long-term implantable VADs, two recovered, and two died. Thirty-day survival was 75% and 1-year survival was 63%.[83]

Mohamedali and colleagues reviewed the outcomes of 48 patients supported with biventricular Centrimag in shock

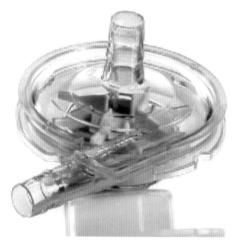

FIGURE 18-7 Thoratec CentriMag. (Used with permission from Thoratec, Inc., Pleasonton, CA.)

patients as a bridge to decision from 2008 to 2013. Thirty-day survival was 56% (27 of 48) with 9 patients explanted for recovery and 14 being transitioned to a durable LVAD.[84]

Takayama and colleagues from Columbia reported the results of 148 patients supported with CentriMag in either biventricular (67%), isolated RVAD (26%) or LVAD (8%). They reported an overall 30-day survival of 69% and 1-year survival of 49%. Failure of medical management and graft failure after heart transplantation had improved outcomes when compared to patients with postcardiotomy failure.[85]

The group at the University of Pittsburgh reported the results of using CentriMag as a temporary RVAD. The indication for RV support was postcardiotomy RV failure in seven (24%), RV failure postcardiac transplant in 10 (35%), and RV failure post-LVAD placement in 12 (41%) patients. The RVAD was able to be weaned in 43% of postcardiotomy patients, 70% of transplant patients, and 58% of LVAD patients after a mean duration of support of 8 days. The authors concluded that the CentriMag was easy to implant, provided effective support, and was easy to wean with low overall morbidity.[86]

Lazar and colleagues from the University of Rochester reported 34 patients who required CentriMag RVAD after Heartmate II insertion. The mean duration of biventricular support was 17 ± 11.9 days. Survival to discharge was not statistically different between patients receiving an isolated LVAD (95.2%) and those that required a CentriMag RVAD (88.2%). One-year survival was 87% with LVAD only compared to 77% for those requiring a temporary CentriMag RVAD (*p* = 0.03) (ATS 2013).[87]

As with similar pumps, the CentriMag can be configured with an oxygenator to create an ECLS circuit.[88] The group from Penn State compared mechanical pump function between the CentriMag pump and the much less expensive Rotoflow in a mock ECLS loop fitted with the Quadrox D and using blood and found that maximal pump flow and shut off pressure where higher in the Rotoflow than the CentriMag implying better mechanical performance. The authors concluded that it was much more economically prudent to use the Rotaflow system as it was 20 to 30 times less expensive that the CentriMag and demonstrated improved performance.[89]

AXIAL FLOW PUMPS

Impella. The Impella device is a microaxial pump, with both peripheral and central cannulation configurations available. In either case, the pump is directed across the aortic valve into the left ventricle (Fig. 18-8). The cannula portion of the device, which sits across the aortic valve, is contiguous with the integrated motor that comprises the largest diameter section of the catheter. The small diameter of the cannula is designed to allow easy co aptation of the aortic valve leaflets around it, resulting in minimal aortic valve insufficiency. Its hemodynamic support results from the design feature that provides active forward flow that increases net cardiac output, and its ability to address the needs for myocardial protection stems from simultaneously

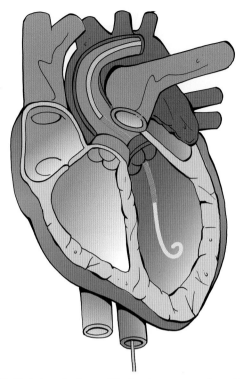

FIGURE 18-8 Impella device. (Used with permission from Abiomed, Inc, Danvers, MA.)

unloading work from the ventricle (decreasing myocardial oxygen demand) and augmenting coronary flow thereby increasing oxygen supply.[90-92]

Three versions for left ventricular support are available: 2.5 and CP that are inserted percutaneously and a 5.0 version that requires surgical approach for deployment. Typically, the catheter-pump motor is deployed across the aortic valve under fluoroscopic or echocardiographic guidance and blood is aspirated through the distal tip-inlet area from the left ventricle, and pumped into the ascending aorta at the proximal tip-outlet area of the catheter motor. The catheter has pressure transducers on each end, and effectively measures pressures on each side of the aortic valve, making it possible to adjust or reposition the device without need for additional imaging in case of catheter displacement after insertion. The Impella RP is the newest addition with the goal of providing percutaneous support for the failing right ventricle. It is deployed via the femoral vein, across pulmonary valve aspirating blood from inferior vena cava and pumping it into the pulmonary artery (Fig. 18-9). Impella R generates more than 4 L/min of flow and uses a 22F catheter.

Each of the available devices is designed for a particular application depending on the desired flow level. As with all LVADs, the actual flow depends on adequacy of blood return to the left side of the heart, which in return depends on right ventricular function, pulmonary vascular resistance, and adequate blood volume. Impella 2.5 generates up to 2.5 L/min of flow and requires a 12F catheter for insertion. Its use is now typically reserved for high risk percutaneous catheter-based

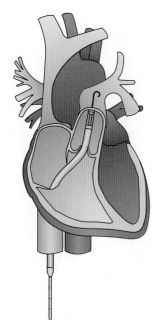

FIGURE 18-9 The Impella RP device. (Used with permission from Abiomed, Inc, Danvers, MA.)

therapies involving coronary interventions or high-risk ablation procedures.[93,94] Impella CP generates up to 4 L/min of flow and requires a 14F catheter for insertion and may be more appropriate for patients in low cardiac output state who need rapid percutaneous stabilization. If time allows for surgical access, the Impella 5.0 which generates up to 5 L/min of flow may be more appropriate. Since this device requires a 21F catheter, surgical cut down to the femoral artery, or more commonly insertion through a vascular graft sewn to the axillary artery is required for placement.

Experience with Impella 2.5 is largely with high-risk percutaneous interventions in which the device maintains hemodynamic stability during balloon inflation and stent deployment. In addition, in cases of MI it may help in reducing infarct size. In a recent prospective randomized trial, 20 patients underwent high-risk percutaneous coronary intervention (PCI) while being supported with the Impella 2.5.[93] All patients had poor LVF and had interventions on the left main or the last remaining patent conduit. Patients with recent STEMI or cardiogenic shock were excluded. The primary safety end point was the incidence of major adverse cardiac events at 30 days. The primary efficacy end point was freedom from hemodynamic compromise during intervention. The Impella 2.5 device was implanted successfully in all patients. The mean duration of circulatory support was 1.7 ± 0.6 hours (range, 0.4-2.5 hours). Mean pump flow during PCI was 2.2 ± 0.3 L/min. At 30 days, the incidence of major adverse cardiac events was 20%. (Two patients had a periprocedural MI, and two patients died at days 12 and 14.) There was no evidence of aortic valve injury, cardiac perforation, or limb ischemia. Two patients (10%) developed mild, transient hemolysis without clinical sequelae. None of the patients developed hemodynamic compromise during

PCI.[93] The more recent follow up to that study, the PROTECTII Trial[95] 452 symptomatic patients with complex 3 vessel coronary artery disease or unprotected left main and poor LVF were randomized between IABP (n-226) versus Impella 2.5 (n-226) during percutaneous intervention. Impella 2.5, as expected, provided superior hemodynamic support compared to the IABP during the intervention. However, the 30 day incidence of major adverse event was similar in both groups. Based on a substudy of PROTECT II trial in patients undergoing PCI due to three-vessel disease with impaired LVEF and MCS support, Impella 2.5 had better 90-day outcomes compared to IABP, lower rate of repeating revascularization, less readmissions and adverse events.[96]

Several studies looked at potential survival benefit of Impella systems compared to alternatives in cardiogenic shock. Based on one unadjusted retrospective comparison, there has been no difference in survival between Impella 5.0 and ECMO, while blood transfusion and arterial thrombotic events were more common in the EMCO group.[97] On the other hand, it has been suggested that Impella 5.0 improves survival in postcardiotomy shock patients with residual cardiac output of 1 L/min or more.[98]

Depending on severity, peripheral vascular disease, atherosclerosis, as well as small vessel size, are considered relative contraindications due to risk of leg ischemia, and technical difficulties in catheter placement.[99-103] Other contraindications include mechanical aortic valve, heavily calcified aortic valve, and aortic regurgitation. Some consider aortic regurgitation a relative contraindication emphasizing decreased pump efficacy as the only undesired effect.

Impella RP (Fig. 18-9) is a fairly new addition to the Impella family, with data on its use and performance still being scarce, but highlighting an expanding role of pVADs in right ventricular support.[104,105] Impella RP US clinical trial is currently underway with expected completion date June 2016 (ClinicalTrials.gov Identifier: NCT01777607).

Heartmate PHP™

The Heartmate PHP™ (Fig. 18-10) is a microaxial pump similar in concept to the Impella devices. It is designed to be placed through the femoral artery and directed across the aortic valve into the left ventricle. The pump is introduced via a 13-French introducer, which allows for percutaneous insertion. Once the pump is in the left ventricle, the segment of the catheter that houses the pump is unsheathed and expands to 24 Fr. It is then withdrawn so that it straddles the aortic valve. It is marketed as providing 4 to 5 L/min flow. It has recently received CE mark approval and as such is commercially available in Europe.

The SHIELD II (Coronary Intervention**S** in **HI**gh-Risk Pati**E**nts Using a Novel Percutaneous **L**eft Ventricular Support **D**evice) U.S. IDE Clinical Trial is a prospectice, randomized, multi-center, study comparing HeartMate PHP™ (Percutaneous Heart Pump) to the Impella® 2.5 in patients undergoing high-risk PCI. The study will randomize up to 425 patients at up to 60 sites.[106]

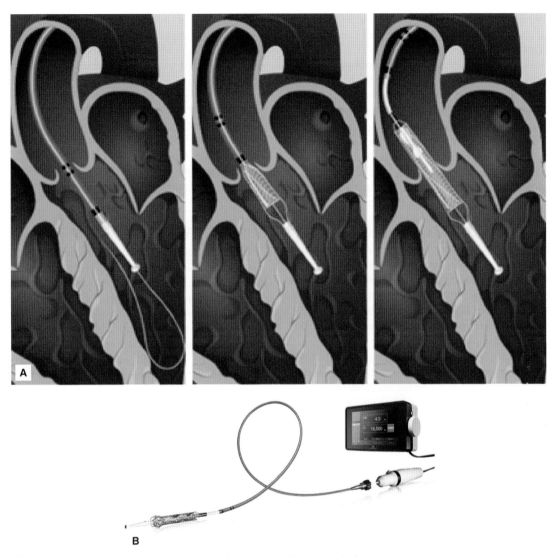

FIGURE 18-10 Thoratec PHP. (Used with permission from Thoratec, Inc., Pleasonton, CA.)

Pulsatile Pumps

ABIOMED AB VENTRICLE/AB5000

The AB5000 circulatory support system, introduced in 2004, consists of the pneumatically driven AB ventricle and the AB5000 console, which utilizes vacuum-assisted drainage. The ventricle is designed for short-to-intermediate (<3 months) support and incorporates many of the features of the ABIOCOR total artificial heart. It is driven pneumatically with valves that are constructed of Angioflex, ABIOMED's proprietary polyether-based polyurethane plastic. Inflow cannulae can be configured for atrial or ventricular placement.

Cannulation. ABIOMED cannulae are constructed from polyvinyl chloride and have a velour body sleeve that is tunneled subcutaneously. Three sizes of wire-reinforced inflow cannulas are available commercially. These include malleable

32-, 36-, and 42-French cannulas. Arterial cannulas have a precoated Dacron graft attached and are available in two sizes: a 10-mm graft for anastomosis to the smaller and lower-resistance pulmonary artery and a 12-mm graft for anastomosis to the ascending aorta.

Careful cannula insertion is important for optimal performance. The combination of the high vacuum setting and smaller cannula size can lead to hemolysis.[107] Optimal cannula placement without chamber collapse or a high-velocity jet at the inflow cannula tip must be confirmed by TEE before leaving the operating room. Anticoagulation to an ACT of 200 seconds is recommended.

Venous inflow must be unimpeded, and outflow grafts must not be kinked. In addition, careful consideration must be given to cannula position when bypass grafts cross the epicardial surface of the heart. Depending on the location of these grafts, these cannulae must be placed such that graft compression cannot occur. The three-dimensional layout of this geometry must be visualized and thought out in advance, particularly if chest closure is planned. Any graft compression will make recovery unlikely.

It is technically much easier to use cardiopulmonary bypass for placement of these cannulas, although off-pump insertion is possible and may be preferable in certain clinical situations, particularly for isolated right-sided support. A side-biting clamp typically is used on the aorta to perform the outflow anastomosis. If the patient is on cardiopulmonary bypass, the pulmonary artery anastomosis can be done without the need of a partial cross-clamp. The length of the graft is measured from the anticipated skin exit site to the site of anastomosis, and the preclotted Dacron graft is cut to an appropriate length such that there is no excessive tension or any kinking. The cutaneous exit site is planned so that approximately 2 cm of the velour cuff extends from the skin and the remainder is in the subcutaneous tunnel. The cannula is not tunneled subcutaneously until after completion of the anastomosis. For the aortic anastomosis, incorporation of a Teflon or pericardial strip helps to control suture-line bleeding. If an off pump insertion is planned, cannulae must be tunneled before anastomosis.

For atrial cannulation, a double-pledgeted purse string suture using 3-0 polypropylene is placed concentrically. Tourniquets must be secured firmly to prevent inadvertent loosening of the purse string suture and bleeding from the insertion sites. In addition, the heart, generally, is volume loaded to prevent air embolism during insertion.

For pump inflow, the 36-French malleable cannula is typically used because it provides versatility to accommodate variations in anatomy and clinical conditions. Left atrial cannulation can be achieved via the interatrial groove, the dome of the left atrium, or the left atrial appendage. The right atrial appendage provides the most hemostatic way to cannulate the right atrium because securing ligatures can be placed about the appendage and cannula to afford hemostasis. Alternatively, the body of the right ventricle or left ventricular apex may be cannulated. In the absence of left ventricular clot, the cannula can be introduced through a cruciate-shaped ventriculotomy. Ventricular cannulation offers the advantages of excellent ventricular decompression, which may enhance ventricular recovery. Bleeding in the setting of a recent MI is a consideration, but usually is not a problem if careful reinforced sutures are placed. A purse string of 00 polypropylene suture passed through a collar of bovine pericardium is a helpful hemostatic adjunct in particularly friable ventricles. Additionally, a hand-made or preordered chimney made from a preclotted graft sewn to a felt collar facilitates ventricular cannulation. A "top-hat"-type conduit is constructed and with the "brim" sewn to the left ventricle using mattress sutures. A ventriculotomy is made and a cannula is introduced through the conduit. If recovery occurs, the graft can be stapled to achieve hemostasis. It is simply removed and the site closed or converted to a more formal inlet cannulation if a long-term device must be used.

The consoles for the ABIOMED device are relatively simple to operate. The control system automatically adjusts the duration of pump diastole and systole primarily in response to changes in preload. Pump rate and flow are visible on the display monitor. With the AB5000, console vacuum is adjusted to the lowest possible setting that provides adequate flow.

Complications. A report by Anderson and colleagues looked at the outcomes of patients transferred on the ABIOMED BVS5000, which is no longer being produced, at "spoke" centers and converted to the AB5000 at "hubs." Fifty patients were studied over a 2-year period with a survival to either recovery, transplant, or destination VAD of 42%.[108]

THORATEC VENTRICULAR ASSIST DEVICE-TLC

The Thoratec pVAD (Thoratec Laboratories Corp., Pleasanton, CA) was introduced clinically in 1976 under an investigational device exemption and was approved for bridge to heart transplantation in 1995 and postcardiotomy support in 1998, respectively.

The device is a pneumatically driven pulsatile pump that contains two seamless polyurethane bladders within a rigid housing. The inlet and outlet ports contain mono-strut tilting-disk valves to provide unidirectional flow. The effective stroke volume of each prosthetic ventricle is 65 mL. The pneumatic drive console applies alternating negative and positive pressures to fill and empty each prosthetic bladder. Multiple settings can be adjusted to potentially optimize pump filling to provide univentricular (LVAD or RVAD) or biventricular support (BVAD).

Thoratec pumps reside on the upper abdominal wall and are connected to the heart with large wire reinforced cannula. The dual drive console is a large, wheeled pneumatic controller that is used early in the patient's course to optimize VAD parameters. The TLC-II driver is smaller and is approved for out-of-hospital use.

Cannulation. Device implantation typically is performed on cardiopulmonary bypass. It is important to select the cannula position and cutaneous exit sites carefully. The pump should be planned to rest on the anterior abdominal wall. Lateral placement may lead to excessive tension at the skin exit sites and prevent formation of a seal. Approximately 1.5 to 2 cm of the felt covering of the cannulas must extend beyond the skin exit site, with the remainder in the subcutaneous tunnel to promote ingrowth of tissue and create a seal. The distance between the inlet and outlet portion of the pump is 4 cm, and the distance between the inlet and outlet cannulas of the pump should be planned accordingly. The cannulae must be long enough to allow for pump connection but should be trimmed to prevent the pump from kinking when the patient sits.

The arterial cannulas are available with a 14-mm graft (for the pulmonary artery) or an 18-mm graft (for the aorta) and must be cut to length after the appropriate exit site has been selected. They come in two lengths, 15 and 18 cm, which again are selected based on the patient's anatomy and the planned exit site. The graft is generally sewn on the aorta or pulmonary artery after applying a partial-occluding clamp and sewn with 4-0 polypropylene suture with or without a strip of pericardium or Teflon felt for reinforcement. Inflow can be accomplished by cannulation of the atria or the ventricles.[109] All cannulations generally are reinforced with a double layer of pledgeted concentric purse string sutures. For atrial cannulation, a 51-French right-angled cannula is available in two lengths, 25 and 30 cm. For the left atrium, the cannula is inserted through the atrial appendage, the interatrial groove, or the superior dome of the left atrium. For right atrial cannulation, the cannula is inserted ideally into the right atrial appendage and directed toward the inferior vena cava.

Inflow cannulation of the left ventricle is preferred over left atrial cannulation[109] because it provides better drainage, higher flows, and perhaps improves the chance of myocardial recovery. Left ventricular cannulation also decreases the amount of stasis in the LV in the poorly contractile heart, which decreases thrombus formation. Atrially cannulated patients who develop thrombus are at high risk for thromboembolic complication because the ventricle usually continues to eject. Left ventricular cannulation is achieved by placing a concentric layer of pledgeted horizontal mattress sutures at the apex of the left ventricle or the acute margin of the right ventricle (superior to the posterior descending artery). The previously placed sutures are passed sequentially through the cuff, the apex of the heart is elevated, the left ventricle cored, and the cannula seated. The cannula then is inserted and secured by tying the sutures. The free end can then be directed out through the previously planned cutaneous exit site, and a tubing clamp placed to maintain hemostasis until the pump is connected. Connecting the cannulae to the pump is difficult and must be done with care. The connections to the pump have a sharp, beveled edge that should be directed carefully under gentle pressure to fit the cannulas without damaging the inner surface of the tube. In addition, if this tip bends, it may provide a nidus for thrombus formation. Gentle hand pumping can be performed to ensure complete air evacuation using an aortic vent. De-airing of pVADs is best achieved by keeping the heart full and keeping the pumps full at all time.

Complications. The complications reported for patients bridged to transplantation are similar to those reported for postcardiotomy patients. In a multicenter trial, the most common complications were bleeding in 42%, renal failure in 36%, infection in 36%, neurologic events in 22%, and multisystem organ failure in 16% of patients.[110] Similar complications have been reported from other centers.[111,112]

Results. After cardiotomy, results are similar to those obtained with ECLS and the ABIOMED BVS 5000. In a review of 145 patients with nonbridge use of the Thoratec device, 37% were weaned and 21% were discharged. More experienced centers have achieved hospital survival rates of greater than 40%.[111,112]

The Thoratec premarket approval experience for the treatment of 53 patients with postcardiotomy heart failure had an in-hospital survival of 28%. The majority of these patients were supported with a BVAD.[110] The Bad Oeynhausen group, however, has reported a 60% survival for postcardiotomy patients supported with the Thoratec device.[111,112]

During the era of large pulsatile first-generation VADs, Thoratec pVADs were the main stay of support for smaller individuals needing mechanical support, or for those needing biventricular support as a bridge to transplant. With the advent of smaller continuous flow devises such as the HeartWare HVAD that can support smaller patients and that can be configured for biventricular support, the use of the pVAD has waned. However, these devices are still available and approved for mechanical support of both ventricles and for postcardiotomy support.

Device Selection

To date, insufficient data exist to recommend one device over another for patients who require temporary mechanical support. Use of a particular device often is based on availability rather than science.

For centers with multiple devices, patient presentation and cardiopulmonary status determine the device selected. Patients undergoing cardiopulmonary resuscitation are best served by urgent femoral cannulation. This avoids the time delay of transportation and sternotomy. Patients with severe hypoxia and lung injury either from aspiration or pulmonary edema benefit from the oxygenation and lung rest provided with ECLS. In all ECLS patients, it is important to adequately lower the left atrial pressure, because hypoxia secondary to continued pulmonary venous congestion precludes weaning of the ECLS circuit. Direct venting of the left ventricle is increasing gaining favor as it not only decompresses the pulmonary bed but it also mitigates formation of LVA thrombus.

For postcardiotomy support, typically patients are supported for 48 to 72 hours while transplant evaluation is completed. Then they are transitioned to a more long-term device if myocardial recovery has failed. This approach avoids high-risk emergency heart transplantation and provides the time necessary for improved organ function.

Biventricular support is often required for fulminant myocarditis. Recovery may be possible, but often requires long-term support with a chronic device.

The TandemHeart with percutaneous transseptal left atrial drainage is a very attractive option for patients sustaining arrest in the catheterization laboratory, but required expertise with transeptal techniques. The Cardiohelp, Impella CP, may and Heart mate PHP also has a role to play in this patient population.

Patient Management

The ultimate goal is to maintain optimal perfusion of all end organs, to allow time for recovery from an acute hemodynamic insult and prevent further deterioration of organ function. Ideally, pump flow would achieve a mixed venous saturation of greater than 70%. Low-flow states can often be corrected by intravascular volume expansion. With centrifugal pumps, speed can be adjusted to control flow and allow some degree of cardiac ejection to decrease the likelihood of stasis and intracardiac thrombus formation. Increasing flow rates by using excessive pump speeds can also cause significant hemolysis. Fluid administration to expand intravascular volume is the best way to increase flow. However, right-sided heart failure also may manifest as a low-flow state in the presence of low pulmonary artery pressures. This condition usually requires the institution of right-sided circulatory support and is associated with a lower overall survival.

VENTILATORY SUPPORT

Peak inspiratory pressures are maintained below 35-cm H_2O. Inspired oxygen is set initially at 100% with a positive end-expiratory pressure of 5-cm H_2O. Fractional inspired oxygen then is decreased gradually to less than 50%, with partial pressure of oxygen maintained at between 85 and 100 mm Hg. These measures are instituted to diminish the deleterious effect of barotrauma and oxygen toxicity in the setting of lung injury.

BLEEDING/ANTICOAGULATION

Anticoagulation should be done judiciously to weigh the balance of excessive risk of bleeding against clot formation in the pump. Platelet counts decrease within the first 24 hours of support; therefore, counts are monitored every 8 hours, and platelets are transfused to maintain counts above 50,000/mm³ during routine support and above 100,000/mm³ if bleeding is present. Fresh-frozen plasma and cryoprecipitate are given to control coagulopathy and maintain the fibrinogen concentration at greater than 250 mg/dL and also replace other coagulation factors consumed by the circuit. Anticoagulation is achieved by systemic heparinization with a continuous infusion starting at 8 to 10 μg/kg/h and titrated to maintain the partial thromboplastin time at between 45 and 55 seconds once hemostasis is achieved. In most cases, heparin infusion is started within 24 hours if used in the postcardiotomy setting, but sooner in patients without a sternotomy. One must be constantly vigilant for the signs of tamponade, which is heralded by falling pump flows, falling mixed venous saturation, rising filling pressures, and falling hemoglobin. Every effort must be made to alleviate tamponade and achieve hemostasis before transferring a patient. An ambulance is far less suited to the management of tamponade or ongoing hemorrhage than is the operating room. In reality bleeding is far more of a lethal problem in the first days of support than is thromboembolism, and anticoagulation should be used judiciously.

FLUID MANAGEMENT

Patients are diuresed aggressively while on support to minimize third-space fluid accumulations. If response to diuretic therapy is suboptimal, we use continuous ultrafiltration or continuous venovenous hemodialysis. This system permits control over fluid balance that can be adjusted for volume removal and also allows for dialysis as needed.

NEUROLOGIC MONITORING

Patients are sedated with fentanyl or propofol infusion to maintain comfort. Muscle paralysis is used as needed to decrease the energy expenditure and chest wall stiffness to allow for optimal adjustment of the ventilation parameters. All patients are assessed periodically off sedation to establish neurologic function. Response to simple commands, ability to move all extremities, and spontaneous eye movements are used as gross indications of intact sensorium. A low threshold of obtaining computed tomographic scans of the head is exercised if any change is noted or index of suspicion is high.

WEANING

A weaning trial is usually attempted after 48 to 72 hours of support. It is critical not to rush weaning and to allow time for myocardial as well as end-organ recovery. The principle of weaning is common to all devices, and all have various controls available that allow reduction in flow, thereby enabling more work to be performed by the heart. Flow is reduced gradually at increments of 0.5 to 1 L/min. Adequate anticoagulation is critical during this low-flow phase to prevent pump thrombosis, and, in general, it is not recommended to reduce flow to less than 2.0 L/min for a prolonged period. We add additional heparin during this period to maintain an ACT of more than 300 seconds. With optimal pharmacologic support and continuous TEE evaluation of ventricular function, flows are reduced while monitoring systemic blood pressure, cardiac index, pulmonary pressures, and ventricular size. Maintenance of cardiac index and low pulmonary pressures with preserved LVF by echocardiography suggests that weaning is likely. A weaning failure manifests as a falling systemic blood pressure along with a drop in cardiac output and rising pulmonary artery pressures. A failed attempt at weaning should result in resumption of full flow. Absence of ventricular recovery after several weaning attempts is a poor prognostic sign. Patients who are transplant candidates undergo a full evaluation and subsequently are staged to a long-term ventricular assist device as a bridge to cardiac transplantation. We and others have found that early conversion to chronic ventricular support is beneficial and improves the low survival that is associated with cardiogenic shock, particularly in the postcardiotomy setting.

CONCLUSION

Currently a number of options exist for temporary circulatory support, and with advances in technology, the number of devices will expand. Each device has advantages and disadvantages, and to date, none satisfies all the requirements of an ideal device. We have clearly learned many lessons that should direct the development of systems and strategies that maximize survival and reduce complications. In this arena, better understanding of the host inflammatory response, appreciation of the induced derangement in the coagulation cascade, and development of systems that do not require anticoagulation should improve overall outcomes. In addition, development of therapies that alter reperfusion injury and preserve organ function is important.

Risk analysis also has taught us that patients requiring postcardiotomy support generally fit into a particular profile. Specifically, these are patients who require emergency operations, have poor ventricular reserve, are older, and have extensive atherosclerotic coronary disease and preexisting renal dysfunction. Preoperative awareness should prompt maximization of medical pharmacologic support and a readiness to implement mechanical devices early in the face of cardiac pump failure.

Use of the standard centrifugal pump gradually has fallen out of favor. Use of the Thoratec pVAD has also waned with the emergence of less morbid and more patient-friendly long-term pumps. Traditional ECLS/ECMO has seen a resurgence with smaller more compact systems like the Cardiohelp device. Other centers effectively utilize acute support devices such as the TandemHeart and CentriMag or Impella 5.0. Traditionally, transplantation after transition to long-term LVADs has been the only therapy available for patients supported with acute support devices who have not manifested recovery. Recently improved results have been reported with the use of a continuous-flow pump in stage D heart failure patients who are not transplant candidates.[113] Historically salvage rates for patients in cardiogenic shock, transitioned to destination VADs have been poor, given that typically DT patients are older with more comorbid conditions than patients being bridged to transplantation.[114] Hopefully earlier use of more effective and less morbid acute support devices can improve results in this population.

Recently a consensus statement on the use of percutaneous support devices was generated by both surgical and cardiology authors representing several societies.[3] The take home message of this important manuscript is that patients with cardiogenic shock represent a multidisciplinary challenge and acute support devices play an ever increasing role in the care of these critically ill patients.

KEY POINTS

1. Recognize cardiogenic shock in the preoperative and postoperative patient.
2. Have available at your institutions at least one of the available temporary support systems.
3. Initiate pharmacologic and first-line mechanical support (IABP) in the shock patient.
4. Attempt to treat the causative issue.
5. Recognize when these conservative methods fail, and act quickly to implement direct cardiac support to restore adequate end-organ perfusion and decompress the heart.
6. Initiate discussions with a center at which advanced heart failure therapies (transplant/long-term VAD) are possible.
7. Stabilize the patient and initiate transfer to a tertiary center for definitive therapy/weaning.

REFERENCES

1. Goldberg RJ, Gore JM, Alpert JS, et al: Cardiogenic shock after acute myocardial infarction. Incidence and mortality from a community-wide perspective, 1975 to 1988. *N Engl J Med* 1991; 325(16):1117-1122.
2. Hochman JS, Sleeper LA, Webb JG, et al: Early revascularization in acute myocardial infarction complicated by cardiogenic shock. SHOCK investigators. Should we emergently revascularize occluded coronaries for cardiogenic Shock? *N Engl J Med* 1999; 341(9):625-634.
3. Rihal CS, Naidu SS, Givertz MM, et al: 2015 SCAI/ACC/HFSA/STS Clinical Expert Consensus Statement on the use of percutaneous mechanical circulatory support devices in cardiovascular care (Endorsed by the Amercan Heart Association, the Cardiological Society of India, and Sociedad Latino Americana de Cardiologia Intervencion; Affirmation of Value by the Canadian Association of Interventional Cardiology-Association Canadienne de Cardiologie d'intervention). *J Card Fail* 2015; 21(6):499-518.
4. Smedira NG, Blackstone EH: Postcardiotomy mechanical support: risk factors and outcomes. *Ann Thorac Surg* 2001; 71(3 Suppl):S60-66; discussion S82-5.
5. Helman DN, Morales DL, Edwards NM, et al: Left ventricular assist device bridge-to-transplant network improves survival after failed cardiotomy. *Ann Thorac Surg* 1999; 68(4):1187-1194.
6. Kantrowitz A: Origins of intraaortic balloon pumping. *Ann Thorac Surg* 1990; 50(4):672-674.
7. Clauss RH, Birtwell WC, Albertal G, et al: Assisted circulation. I. The arterial counterpulsator. *J Thorac Cardiovasc Surg* 1961; 41:447-458.
8. Moulopoulos SD, Topaz S, Kolff WJ: Diastolic balloon pumping (with carbon dioxide) in the aorta—a mechanical assistance to the failing circulation. *Am Heart J* 1962; 63:669-675.
9. Kantrowitz A, Tjonneland S, Freed PS, et al: Initial clinical experience with intraaortic balloon pumping in cardiogenic shock. *JAMA* 1968; 203(2):113-118.
10. Powell WJ Jr, Daggett WM, Magro AE, et al: Effects of intra-aortic balloon counterpulsation on cardiac performance, oxygen consumption, and coronary blood flow in dogs. *Circ Res* 1970; 26(6):753-764.
11. Dunkman WB, Leinbach RC, Buckley MJ, et al: Clinical and hemodynamic results of intraaortic balloon pumping and surgery for cardiogenic shock. *Circulation* 1972; 46(3):465-477.
12. Buckley MJ, Leinbach RC, Kastor JA, et al: Hemodynamic evaluation of intra-aortic balloon pumping in man. *Circulation* 1970; 41(5 Suppl):II130-136.
13. Katz ES, Tunick PA, Kronzon I: Observations of coronary flow augmentation and balloon function during intraaortic balloon counterpulsation using transesophageal echocardiography. *Am J Cardiol* 1992; 69(19):1635-1639.
14. Weber KT, Janicki JS: Coronary collateral flow and intra-aortic balloon counterpulsation. *Trans Am Soc Artif Intern Organs* 1973; 19:395-401.
15. Weber KT, Janicki JS, Walker AA: Intra-aortic balloon pumping: an analysis of several variables affecting balloon performance. *Trans Am Soc Artif Intern Organs* 1972; 18(0):486-492.
16. Kern MJ, Aguirre FV, Tatineni S, et al: Enhanced coronary blood flow velocity during intraaortic balloon counterpulsation in critically ill patients. *J Am Coll Cardiol* 1993; 21(2):359-368.
17. Yarham G, Clements A, Morris C, et al: Fiber-optic intra-aortic balloon therapy and its role within cardiac surgery. *Perfusion* 2013; 28(2):97-102.
18. Creswell LL, Rosenbloom M, Cox JL, et al: Intraaortic balloon counterpulsation: patterns of usage and outcome in cardiac surgery patients. *Ann Thorac Surg* 1992; 54(1):11-18; discussion 18-20.
19. O'Murchu B, Foreman RD, Shaw RE, et al: Role of intraaortic balloon pump counterpulsation in high risk coronary rotational atherectomy. *J Am Coll Cardiol* 1995; 26(5):1270-1275.
20. McBride LR, Miller LW, Naunheim KS, Pennington DG: Axillary artery insertion of an intraaortic balloon pump. *Ann Thorac Surg* 1989; 48(6):874-875.
21. Blythe D: Percutaneous axillary artery insertion of an intra-aortic balloon pump. *Anaesth Intensive Care* 1995; 23(3):406-407.
22. Hazelrigg SR, Auer JE, Seifert PE: Experience in 100 transthoracic balloon pumps. *Ann Thorac Surg* 1992; 54(3):528-532.
23. Pinkard J, Utley JR, Leyland SA, Morgan M, Johnson H: Relative risk of aortic and femoral insertion of intraaortic balloon pump after coronary artery bypass grafting procedures. *J Thorac Cardiovasc Surg* 1993; 105(4):721-728.

24. Tatar H, Cicek S, Demirkilic U, et al: Exact positioning of intra-aortic balloon catheter. *Eur J Cardiothorac Surg* 1993; 7(1):52-53.

25. Phillips SJ, Tannenbaum M, Zeff RH, et al: Sheathless insertion of the percutaneous intraaortic balloon pump: an alternate method. *Ann Thorac Surg* 1992; 53(1):162-162.

26. Sintek MA, Gdowski M, Lindman BR, et al: Intra-aortic balloon counterpulsation in patients with chronic heart failure and cardiogenic shock: clinical response and predictors of stabilization. *J Card Fail* 2015; pii: S1071-9164(15)00582.

27. Tanaka A, Tuladhar SM, Onsager D, et al: The subclavian intraaortic balloon pump: a compelling bridge device for advanced heart failure. *Ann Thorac Surg* 2015 Jul 27; pii:S0003-4975(15)00926-1.

28. Patel JJ, Kopisyansky C, Boston B, et al: Prospective evaluation of complications associated with percutaneous intraaortic balloon counterpulsation. *Am J Cardiol* 1995; 76(16):1205-1207.

29. Alle KM, White GH, Harris JP, May J, Baird D: Iatrogenic vascular trauma associated with intra-aortic balloon pumping: identification of risk factors. *Am Surg* 1993; 59(12):813-817.

30. Nishida H, Koyanagi H, Abe T, et al: Comparative study of five types of IABP balloons in terms of incidence of balloon rupture and other complications: a multi-institutional study. *Artif Organs* 1994; 18(10):746-751.

31. O'Rourke MF, Norris RM, Campbell TJ, Chang VP, Sammel NL: Randomized controlled trial of intraaortic balloon counterpulsation in early myocardial infarction with acute heart failure. *Am J Cardiol* 1981; 47(4):815-820.

32. Baldwin RT, Slogoff S, Noon GP, et al: A model to predict survival at time of postcardiotomy intraaortic balloon pump insertion. *Ann Thorac Surg* 1993; 55(4):908-913.

33. Pi K, Block PC, Warner MG, Diethrich EB: Major determinants of survival and nonsurvival of intraaortic balloon pumping. *Am Heart J* 1995; 130(4):849-853.

34. Naunheim KS, Swartz MT, Pennington DG, et al: Intraaortic balloon pumping in patients requiring cardiac operations. Risk analysis and long-term follow-up. *J Thorac Cardiovasc Surg* 1992; 104(6):1654-1660.

35. Christenson JT, Schmuziger M, Simonet F: Effective surgical management of high-risk coronary patients using preoperative intra-aortic balloon counterpulsation therapy. *Cardiovasc Surg* 2001; 9(4):383-390.

36. O'Gara PT, Kushner FG, Ascheim DD, et al: 2013 ACCF/AHA guideline for the management of ST-elevation myocardial infarction: a report of the American College of Cardiology Foundation/American Heart Association Task Force on Practice Guidelines. *J Am Coll Cardiol* 2013; 61(4):e78-140.

37. Thiele H, Zeymer U, Neumann FJ, et al: Intraaortic balloon support for myocardial infarction with cardiogenic shock (IABP-SHOCK II). *N Engl J Med* 2012; 367(14):1287-1296.

38. Thiele H, Zeymer U, Neumann FJ, et al: Intra-aortic balloon counterpulsation in acute myocardial infarction complicated by cardiogenic shock (IABP-SHOCK II): final 12 month results of a randomized, open-label trial. *Lancet* 2013; 382(9905):1638-1645.

39. Pilarczyk K, Boening A, Jakob H, et al: Perioperative intra-aortic counterpulsation in high-risk patients undergoing cardiac surgery: a meta-analysis of randomized controlled trials. *Eur J Cardiothorac Surge* 2015.

40. Mulholland J, Yarham G, Clements A, et al: Mechanical left ventricular support using a 50 cc 8 Fr fibre-optic intra-aortic balloon technology: a case report. *Perfusion* 2013; 28(2):109-113.

41. DeBakey ME: Left ventricular bypass pump for cardiac assistance. Clinical experience. *Am J Cardiol* 1971; 27(1):3-11.

42. Samuels LE, Kaufman MS, Thomas MP, et al: Pharmacological criteria for ventricular assist device insertion following postcardiotomy shock: experience with the Abiomed BVS system. *J Cardiol Surg* 1999; 14(4):288-293.

43. Jett GK: Postcardiotomy support with ventricular assist devices: selection of recipients. *Semin Thorac Cardiovasc Surg* 1994; 6(3):136-139.

44. Argenziano M, Choudhri AF, Moazami N, et al: Randomized, double-blind trial of inhaled nitric oxide in LVAD recipients with pulmonary hypertension. *Ann Thorac Surg* 1998; 65(2):340-345.

45. Argenziano M, Choudhri AF, Oz MC, et al: A prospective randomized trial of arginine vasopressin in the treatment of vasodilatory shock after left ventricular assist device placement. *Circulation* 1997; 96 (9 Suppl):II-286-290.

46. Curtis JJ, Walls JT, Schmaltz RA, et al: Use of centrifugal pumps for postcardiotomy ventricular failure: technique and anticoagulation. *Ann Thorac Surg* 1996; 61(1):296-300.

47. Magovern GJ Jr: The Bio-Pump and postoperative circulatory support. *Ann Thorac Surg* 1993; 55(1):245-249.

48. Golding LA, Crouch RD, Stewart RW, et al: Postcardiotomy centrifugal mechanical ventricular support. *Ann Thorac Surg* 1992; 54(6): 1059-1063.

49. Curtis JJ, Walls JT, Boley TM, Schmaltz RA, Demmy TL: Autopsy findings in patients on postcardiotomy centrifugal ventricular assist. *ASAIO J* 1992; 38(3):M688-690.

50. Mehta SM, Aufiero TX, Pae WE Jr, Miller CA, Pierce WS: Results of mechanical ventricular assistance for the treatment of post cardiotomy cardiogenic shock. *ASAIO J* 1996; 42(3):211-218.

51. Noon GP, Ball JW, Short HD: Bio-Medicus centrifugal ventricular support for postcardiotomy cardiac failure: a review of 129 cases. *Ann Thorac Surg* 1996; 61(1):291-295.

52. Joyce LD, Kiser JC, Eales F, et al: Experience with generally accepted centrifugal pumps: personal and collective experience. *Ann Thorac Surg* 1996; 61(1):287-290.

53. Bartlett RH, Roloff DW, Custer JR, Younger JG, Hirschl RB: Extracorporeal life support: the University of Michigan experience. *JAMA* 2000; 283(7):904-908.

54. Peek GJ, Firmin RK: The inflammatory and coagulative response to prolonged extracorporeal membrane oxygenation. *ASAIO J* 1999; 45(4):250-263.

55. McIlwain IRB, Timpa JG, Kurundkar AR, et al: Plasma concentrations of inflammatory cytokines rise rapidly during ECMO-related SIRS due to the release of preformed stores in the intestine. *Lab Invest* 2008; 90(1):128-139.

56. Aziz TA, Singh G, Popjes E, et al: Initial experience with CentriMag extracorporal membrane oxygenation for support of critically ill patients with refractory cardiogenic shock. *J Heart Lung Transplant* 2010; 29(1):66-71.

57. Larm O, Larsson R, Olsson P: A new non-thrombogenic surface prepared by selective covalent binding of heparin via a modified reducing terminal residue. *Biomater Med Devices Artif Organs* 1983; 11(2-3):161-173.

58. Videm V, Mollnes TE, Garred P, Svennevig JL: Biocompatibility of extra-corporeal circulation. In vitro comparison of heparin-coated and uncoated oxygenator circuits. *J Thorac Cardiovasc Surg* 1991; 101(4):654-660.

59. Redmond JM, Gillinov AM, Stuart RS, et al: Heparin-coated bypass circuits reduce pulmonary injury. *Ann Thorac Surg* 1993; 56(3):474-478; discussion 479.

60. Videm V, Svennevig JL, Fosse E, et al: Reduced complement activation with heparin-coated oxygenator and tubings in coronary bypass operations. *J Thorac Cardiovasc Surg* 1992; 103(4):806-813.

61. Bindslev L, Gouda I, Inacio J, et al: Extracorporeal elimination of carbon dioxide using a surface-heparinized veno-venous bypass system. *ASAIO Trans* 1986; 32(1):530-533.

62. Mottaghy K, Oedekoven B, Poppel K, et al: Heparin free long-term extracorporeal circulation using bioactive surfaces. *ASAIO Trans* 1989; 35(3):635-637.

63. Magovern GJ, Magovern JA, Benckart DH, et al: Extracorporeal membrane oxygenation: preliminary results in patients with postcardiotomy cardiogenic shock. *Ann Thorac Surg* 1994; 57(6):1462-1468.

64. Aranki SF, Adams DH, Rizzo RJ, et al: Femoral veno-arterial extracorporeal life support with minimal or no heparin. *Ann Thorac Surg* 1993; 56(1):149-155.

65. Muehrcke DD, McCarthy PM, Stewart RW, et al: Complications of extracorporeal life support systems using heparin-bound surfaces. The risk of intracardiac clot formation. *J Thorac Cardiovasc Surg* 1995; 110(3):843-851.

66. von Segesser LK, Gyurech DD, Schilling JJ, Marquardt K, Turina MI: Can protamine be used during perfusion with heparin surface coated equipment? *ASAIO J* 1993; 39(3):M190-194.

67. Zapol WM, Snider MT, Hill JD, et al: Extracorporeal membrane oxygenation in severe acute respiratory failure. A randomized prospective study. *JAMA* 1979; 242(20):2193-2196.

68. Muehrcke DD, McCarthy PM, Stewart RW, et al: Extracorporeal membrane oxygenation for postcardiotomy cardiogenic shock. *Ann Thorac Surg* 1996; 61(2):684-691.

69. Smedira NG, Moazami N, Golding CM, et al: Clinical experience with 202 adults receiving extracorporeal membrane oxygenation for cardiac failure: survival at five years. *J Thorac Cardiovasc Surg* 2001; 122(1):92-102.

70. Pokersnik JA, Buda T, Bashour CA, et al: Have changes in ECMO technology impacted outcomes in adult patients developing postcardiotomy cardiogenic shock? *J Card Surg* 2012; 27(2):246-252.

71. Formica F, Avalli L, Martino A, et al: Extracorporeal membrane oxygenation with a poly-methylpentene oxygenator (Quadrox D). The experience of a single Italian centre in adult patients with refractory cardiogenic shock. *Asaio J* 2008; 54(1):89-94.

72. Arit M, Phillip A, Voelkel S, et al: Hand-held minimized extracorporeal membrane oxygenation: a new bridge to recover in patients with out-of-centre cardiogenic shock. *Eur J Cardiothorac Surg* 2011; 40(3):689-694.

73. Vranckx P, Foley DP, de Feijter PJ, et al: Clinical introduction of the TandemHeart, a percutaneous left ventricular assist device, for circulatory support during high-risk percutaneous coronary intervention. *Int J Cardiovasc Intervent* 2003; 5(1):35-39.

74. Kar B, Adkins LE, Civitello AB, et al: Clinical experience with the TandemHeart percutaneous ventricular assist device. *Tex Heart Inst J* 2006; 33(2):111-115.

75. Giaombolini C, Notaristefano S, Santucci S, et al: Percutaneous left ventricular assist device, TandemHeart, for high-risk percutaneous coronary revascularization. A single centre experience. *Acute Card Care* 2006; 8(1):35-40.

76. Takagaki M, Wurzer C, Wade R, et al: Successful conversion of Tandem Heart left ventricular assist device to right ventricular assist device after implantation of a HeartMate XVE. *Ann Thorac Surg* 2008; 86(5):1677-1679.

77. Prutkin JM, Strote JA, Stout KK: Percutaneous right ventricular assist device as support for cardiogenic shock due to right ventricular infarction. *J Invasive Cardiol* 2008; 20(7):E215-216.

78. Herlihy JP, Loyalka P, Jayaraman G, Kar B, Gregoric ID: Extracorporeal membrane oxygenation using the TandemHeart System's catheters. *Tex Heart Inst J* 2009; 36(4):337-341.

79. Kar B, Gregoric ID, Basra SS, et al: The percutaneous ventricular assist device in severe refractory cardiogenic shock. *J Am Coll Cardiol* 2011; 57(6):688-696.

80. Gregoric ID, Loyalka P, Radovancevic R, et al: TandemHeart as a rescue therapy for patients with critical aortic valve stenosis. *Ann Thorac Surg* 2009; 88(6):1822-1826.

81. Brinkman WT, Rosenthal JE, Eichhorn E, et al: Role of a percutaneous ventricular assist device in decision making for a cardiac transplant program. *Ann Thorac Surg* 2009; 88(5):1462-1466.

82. De Robertis F, Birks EJ, Rogers P, et al: Clinical performance with the Levitronix CentriMag short-term ventricular assist device. *J Heart Lung Transplant* 2006; 25(2):181-186.

83. John R, Liao K, Lietz K, et al: Experience with the Levitronix CentriMag circulatory support system as a bridge to decision in patients with refractory acute cardiogenic shock and multisystem organ failure. *J Thorac Cardiovasc Surg* 2007; 134(2):351-358.

84. Mohamedali B, Bhat G, Yost G, et al: Survival on biventricular mechanical support with CentriMag® as a bridge to decision: a single-center risk stratification. *Perfusion* 2015; 30(3):201-208.

85. Takayama H, Soni L, Kalesan B, et al: Bridge-to-decision therapy with a continuous-flow external ventricular assist device in refractory cardiogenic shock of various causes. *Circ Heart Fail* 2014; 7(5):799-806.

86. Bhama JK, Kormos RL, Toyoda Y, et al: Clinical experience using the Levitronix CentriMag system for temporary right ventricular mechanical circulatory support. *J Heart Lung Transplant* 2009; 28(9):971-976.

87. Lazar JF, Swartz MF, Schiralli MP, et al: Survival after left ventricular assist device with and without temporary right ventricular support. *Ann Thorac Surg* 2013; 96(2):2155-2159.

88. Khan NU, Al-Aloul M, Shah R, Yonan N: Early experience with the Levitronix CentriMag device for extra-corporeal membrane oxygenation following lung transplantation. *Eur J Cardiothorac Surg* 2008; 34(6):1262-1264.

89. Yulong G, Xiaowei S, McCoach R, et al: Mechanical performance comparison between RotaFlow and CentriMag centrifugal blood pumps in an adult ECLS model. *Perfusion* 2010; 25(2):71-76.

90. Burzotta F, Paloscia L, Trani C, et al: Feasibility and long-term safety of elective Impella-assisted high-risk percutaneous coronary intervention: a pilot two-centre study. *J Cardiovasc Med (Hagerstown)* 2008; 9(10):1004-1010.

91. Jurmann MJ, Siniawski H, Erb M, Drews T, Hetzer R: Initial experience with miniature axial flow ventricular assist devices for postcardiotomy heart failure. *Ann Thorac Surg* 2004; 77(5):1642-1647.

92. Meyns B, Dens J, Sergeant P, et al: Initial experiences with the Impella device in patients with cardiogenic shock. Impella support for cardiogenic shock. *Thorac Cardiovasc Surg* 2003; 51(6):312-317.

93. Dixon SR, Henriques JP, Mauri L, et al: A prospective feasibility trial investigating the use of the Impella 2.5 system in patients undergoing high-risk percutaneous coronary intervention (The PROTECT I Trial): initial U.S. experience. *JACC Cardiovasc Interv* 2009; 2(2):91-96.

94. Reddy YM, Chinitz L, Mansour M, et al: Percutaneous left ventricular assist devices in ventricular tachycardia ablation: multi center experience. *Circ Arrhythm Electrophysiol* 2014; 7(2):244-250.

95. O'Neill WW, Kleiman NS, Moses J, et al: A prospective, randomized clinical trial of hemodynamic support with Impella 2.5 versus intra-aortic balloon pump in patients undergoing high-risk percutaneous coronary intervention: the PROTECT II study. *Circulation* 2012; 126(14):1717-1727.

96. Seyfarth M, Sibbing D, Bauer I, et al: A randomized clinical trial to evaluate the safety and efficacy of a percutaneous left ventricular assist device versus intra-aortic balloon pumping for treatment of cardiogenic shock caused by myocardial infarction. *J Am Coll Cardiol* 2008; 52(19):1584-1588.

97. Lamarche Y, Cheung A, Ignaszewski A, et al: Comparative outcomes in cardiogenic shock patients managed with Impella microaxial pump or extracorporeal life support. *J Thorac Cardiovasc Surg* 2011; 142(1):60-65.

98. Siegenthaler MP, Brehm K, Strecker T, et al: The Impella Recover microaxial left ventricular assist device reduces mortality for postcardiotomy failure: a three-center experience. *J Thorac Cardiovasc Surg* 2004; 127(3):812-822.

99. de Souza CF, de Souza Brito F, De Lima VC, et al: Percutaneous mechanical assistance for the failing heart. *J Interv Cardiol* 2010; 23(2):195-202.

100. Dixon SR, Henriques JP, Mauri L, et al: A prospective feasibility trial investigating the use of the Impella 2.5 system in patients undergoing high-risk percutaneous coronary intervention (the PROTECT I trial). Initial U.S. experience. *J Am Coll Cardiol Intv* 2009; 2:91-96.

101. Ziemba EA, John R: Mechanical circulatory support for bridge to decision: which device and when to decide. *J Card Surg* 2010; 25(4):425-433.

102. Meyns B, Dens J, Sergeant P, et al: Initial experiences with the Impella device in patients with cardiogenic shock—Impella support for cardiogenic shock. *Thorac Cardiovasc Surg* 2003; 51:312-317.

103. Thiele H, Smalling RW, Schuler GC: Percutaneous left ventricular assist devices in acute myocardial infarction complicated by cardiogenic shock. *Eur Heart J* 2007; 28:2057-2063.

104. Cheung AW, White CW, Davis MK, Freed DH: Short-term mechanical circulatory support for recovery from acute right ventricular failure: clinical outcomes. *J Heart Lung Transplant* 2014; 33(8):794-799.

105. Bennett MT, Virani SA, Bowering J, et al: The use of the Impella RD as a bridge to recovery for right ventricular dysfunction after cardiac transplantation. *Innovations* 2010; 5(5):369-371.

106. HeartMate PHP [instructions for use]. Pleasanton, CA, Thoratec Corporation, 2015.

107. Samuels LE, Holmes EC, Garwood P, Ferdinand F: Initial experience with the Abiomed AB5000 ventricular assist device system. *Ann Thorac Surg* 2005; 80(1):309-312.

108. Anderson MB, Gratz E, Wong RK, Benali K, Kung RT: Improving outcomes in patients with ventricular assist devices transferred from outlying to tertiary care hospitals. *J Extra Corpor Technol* 2007; 39(1):43-48.

109. Arabia FA, Paramesh V, Toporoff B, et al: Biventricular cannulation for the Thoratec ventricular assist device. *Ann Thorac Surg* 1998; 66(6):2119-2120.

110. Farrar DJ, Hill JD: Univentricular and biventricular Thoratec VAD support as a bridge to transplantation. *Ann Thorac Surg* 1993; 55(1):276-282.

111. Korfer R, El-Banayosy A, Arusoglu L, et al: Temporary pulsatile ventricular assist devices and biventricular assist devices. *Ann Thorac Surg* 1999; 68(2):678-683.

112. Korfer R, el-Banayosy A, Posival H, et al: Mechanical circulatory support with the Thoratec assist device in patients with postcardiotomy cardiogenic shock. *Ann Thorac Surg* 1996; 61(1):314-316.

113. Slaughter MS, Rogers JG, Milano CA, et al: Advanced heart failure treated with continuous-flow left ventricular assist device. *N Engl J Med* 2009; 361(23):2241-2251.

114. Lietz K, Long JW, Kfoury AG, et al: Outcomes of left ventricular assist device implantation as destination therapy in the post-REMATCH era: implications for patient selection. *Circulation* 2007; 116(5):497-505.

ISCHEMIC
HEART DISEASE

ISCHEMIC
HEART DISEASE

Myocardial Revascularization with Percutaneous Devices

James M. Wilson • James T. Willerson

19

At its height, the success of surgical coronary revascularization spurred improvement in catheter-based technology—first for imaging quality, and later for attempted therapy. In 1974, Andreas Gruentzig completed the development of a double-lumen balloon catheter that was miniaturized for use in coronary arteries. Soon afterward, techniques for percutaneous transluminal coronary angioplasty (PTCA) expanded as technical breakthroughs were applied to subselective catheters, devices, guidewires, balloon materials, coronary stents, and circulatory support. Currently, trial evidence attests that percutaneous therapy is useful as a treatment in patients with poorly controlled angina whose anatomy does not imply a survival benefit from revascularization, and for emergency revascularization during ST-segment elevation myocardial infarction (MI). Surgical and percutaneous revascularization, however, cannot be considered equivalent.[1]

BALLOON ANGIOPLASTY

Principles

In the early balloon angioplasty era, several technical limitations restricted the use of percutaneous techniques to low-risk patients with proximal, discrete coronary artery stenoses, and procedural outcomes lacked predictability. As advances in tools and techniques were developed, higher-risk patients became candidates for percutaneous therapy. Over time, several principles for safety and success were recognized (Table 19-1).

Tools

GUIDING CATHETERS

Guiding catheters differ from diagnostic catheters in that a wire braid supports a thin catheter wall, allowing for a larger central lumen and providing enough rigidity to support the advance of subselective catheters to the distal regions of the coronary bed. The anatomy of the ascending aorta and the origin of the treated coronary artery determine which shape of guiding catheter will provide the most secure positioning (Fig. 19-1). The choice of guiding catheter often is the deciding factor for success when the arterial anatomy is challenging or when complications increase procedural difficulty. Guiding-catheter manipulation is a common cause of procedural complications that necessitate the urgent transition to coronary artery bypass surgery.

A recent innovation in guiding catheter technology is the Guideliner®. The Guideliner is a device for subselective

TABLE 19-1: Principles of Percutaneous Coronary Intervention

1. The patient's outcome is a function of age, comorbidity, and coronary morphology
2. The procedure's outcome is a function of coronary morphology and proper planning (ie, sequence and equipment choices, such as guidewires and device)
3. Proximal and distal control of the treated vessel must be maintained
   a. Choose proper guide catheter support
   b. Maintain distal wire position
   c. Keep the guide, device, and distal wire tip visible during any movement of any device
4. The needs and limits to treatment options such as devices, adjuvant medical therapy, contrast use, and circulatory support are determined by
   a. vascular access
   b. the patient's condition (eg, stable angina or acute myocardial infarction)
   c. ventricular function
   d. comorbidities such as diabetes mellitus, renal insufficiency
5. The following factors can lead to failure:
   a. Incomplete understanding of the three-dimensional anatomy of the course to be taken and lesion to be treated
   b. Unrealistic interpretation of
      i. the capacity of available techniques to achieve success
      ii. the amenability of specific anatomy to percutaneous manipulation
   c. Ignorance of or inattention to technique in subselective device movement
   d. Inattention to anticoagulation
   e. Inattention to catheter hygiene (minimizing blood and contrast stagnation within the guiding catheter or other devices)

intubation of the coronary artery branches or saphenous vein grafts; its design borrows from that of the original Palmaz-Schatz stent platform. Subselective delivery of a catheter at or beyond the origin of a lesion substantially increases the probability of successful stent delivery. Most useful in delivering stents to the obtuse marginal saphenous vein graft, the Guideliner has been used for almost every difficult anatomic variant.[2]

GUIDEWIRES

When the guiding catheter's position remains secure, the guidewire allows control of the distal vessel. Different wires vary in stiffness, coating, diameter, and design of the distal steering tip. For most procedures, the chosen wire is a 190- to 300-cm monofilament that is 0.0254 to 0.0356 cm in diameter, with either a graded tapering segment welded to the tip

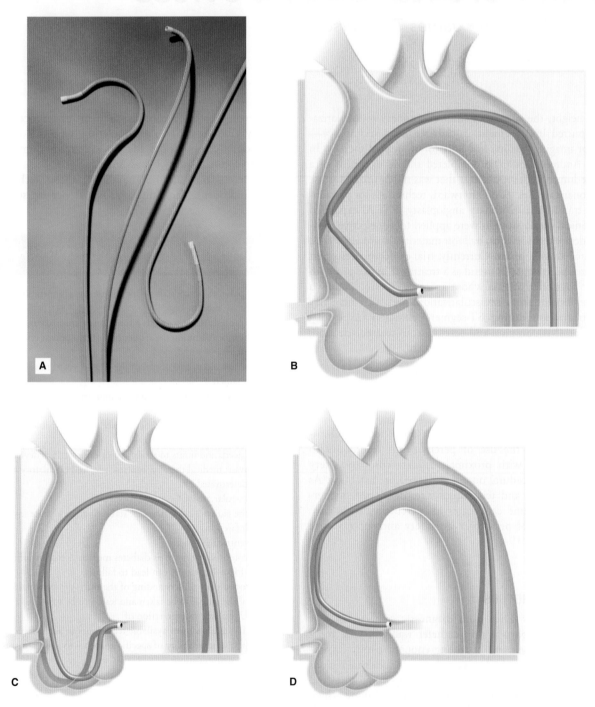

FIGURE 19-1 Commonly used guiding catheters are shown in the relaxed state (A) and as engaged with the coronary ostia in preparation for PCI: left Judkins (B), left Amplatz (C), XB (extra backup) (D), right Judkins (E), right Amplatz (F), and left coronary bypass (G). PCI = percutaneous coronary intervention. (Reprinted with permission from Cordis Corporation, a Cardinal Health company.)

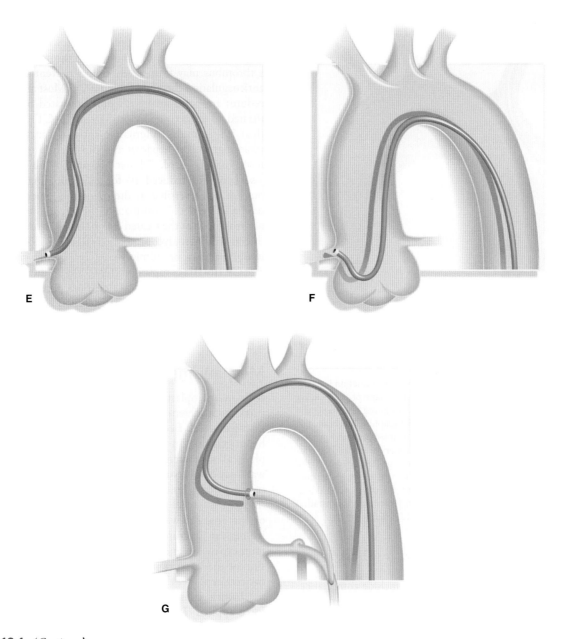

FIGURE 19-1 (*Continued*)

or a gradual taper of the monofilament. The central wire core at the tip is "plastic," or malleable, and may be shaped by the operator. In many wire designs, a wire coil wrapped around the central filament projects a blunter, less traumatic tip to the vessel that it must traverse. Generally, the softest tip is the safest tip. However, in certain situations, such as treatment of a chronic total occlusion, a stiffer wire tip with a bonded, hydrophilic coating, rather than the wire coil, is frequently most effective. Although using these stiffer, "slicker" wires increases the likelihood of crossing the lesion successfully, the wires also increase the risk of complications, such as the creation of a subintimal wire course, the induction of dissection, or the perforation of the vessel (Fig. 19-2).

TOOLS FOR LUMEN EXPANSION

Most subselective devices for coronary artery manipulation are balloon inflation catheters or something similar. Balloon catheter designs vary in the placement of the proximal opening of the central lumen. The "on the wire" design has a central lumen that extends the length of the catheter. This design affords the best trackability and capability for maneuvering through difficult anatomy, but it requires an assistant to manipulate the wire during device advance. The "monorail" design has a central lumen, extending only through the distal balloon shaft of the catheter. The remaining catheter shaft communicates only with the balloon lumen. This design,

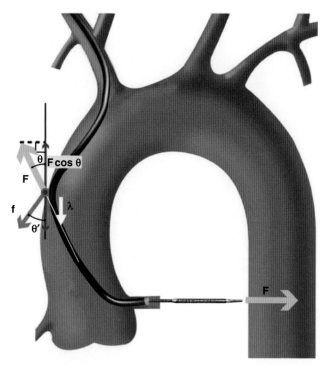

FIGURE 19-2 Support for subselective device introduction into the coronary vessels is determined primarily by the shape of the guiding catheter in relation to the anatomy of the ascending aorta and the origin of the left main coronary artery. Shown graphically, advance of the device forces the catheter backward. This movement is opposed by the alignment of the catheter with the coronary artery and by friction developing through contact between the primary curve of the catheter and the opposing wall of the aorta. (Reproduced with permission from Ikari Y, Nagaoka M, Kim JY, et al: The physics of guiding catheters for the left coronary artery in transfemoral and transradial interventions, *J Invasive Cardiol.* 2005 Dec;17(12):636-641.)

though less trackable, allows the procedure to be performed without the need for an assistant.

Properties of the angioplasty balloon include compliance, maximally tolerated pressure, profile, and friction coefficient. Compliance, or growth under pressure, and maximally tolerated pressure are a function of balloon wall thickness and material. Compliance is divided into three categories depending on the growth of the balloon under pressure: noncompliant, semicompliant, and compliant. The thin-walled, compliant balloon has the lowest deflated profile, which allows the device to pass through the most severely occluded vessels. However, the balloon may not expand uniformly or lengthen when exposed to high pressures, such as pressures in excess of 20 atm (15,200 mm Hg), which are required to dilate hard and heavily calcified stenoses or stents. A variety of balloon coatings may be used to reduce the friction coefficient or protect the lumen from abrasion (eg, from passing a stent).

ANTITHROMBOTIC THERAPY

During an angioplasty procedure, blood may stagnate in the guiding catheter or near the treated lesion when a wire or device is placed within the lumen of the target lesion. In addition, metallic components of the guidewire or other devices attract fibrinogen, thus stimulating thrombosis. Therefore, a thrombus may form easily unless prevented with intense anticoagulation therapy (Table 19-2).[3] Most angioplasty procedures are performed with unfractionated heparin (UFH) titrated to an activated clotting time (ACT) value of more than 300 seconds.[4] Alternative anticoagulants, such as low-molecular-weight heparins and direct antithrombin antagonists, may be used.[5-9] Direct thrombin inhibitors may be associated with reduced risk for major bleeding complications but are not reversible in the event that emergency surgical referral is needed.[10] Antiplatelet therapy also reduces the risk of thrombosis at the treated lesion. In addition to aspirin and thienopyridines, glycoprotein IIb/IIIa (GP IIb/IIIa) complex inhibitors may be administered in specific circumstances. The GP IIb/IIIa complex inhibitors are unique in their ability to impair platelet-platelet aggregation, regardless of the type or intensity of stimulus. Anticoagulation is titrated to a lower intensity (an ACT of 200-250 seconds) when GP IIb/IIIa inhibitors are used.

Mechanisms

Balloon angioplasty transmits increased intraluminal pressures circumferentially to the rigid intimal surface of the diseased vessel. Because atherosclerotic lesions typically are heterogeneous in their circumferential distribution and physical characteristics, the nondiseased or less diseased wall may be overstretched during balloon inflation. In most instances, the lesion segment with the greatest structural integrity is a focal point for applied stress. Adjacent regions of the vascular wall can shift, and the diseased, inelastic intima can fracture. Although this mechanism allows balloon expansion and an increase in luminal diameter, extension of the fracture into the intima-media border creates a dissection plane, the growth of which is determined by the mechanical characteristics of the lesion and the amount of force applied. If growth of the dissection plane results in significant displacement of the diseased intima, the vessel will close. This event, termed *abrupt* or *acute occlusion*, complicates about 10% of balloon angioplasty procedures. Overstretching the minimally diseased or nondiseased wall without causing plaque fracture typically results in early recoil of the treated lesion to its original state.

After balloon deflation, a small amount of thrombus accumulates, providing the stimulus and framework for colonization by inflammatory cells and myofibroblasts and the eventual, local synthesis of temporary (intimal hyperplasia) and permanent (collagen-rich) connective tissue. In addition, mechanical injury to the media and adventitia results in scar formation. The scar's contracture may reduce vessel cross-sectional area—a phenomenon termed *negative remodeling*.[11,12] During vascular healing, the encroaching intimal hyperplasia that peaks in volume at about 3 months, combined with negative remodeling, results in restenosis after 40 to 50% of balloon angioplasty procedures.[13-15]

TABLE 19-2: Adjunctive Pharmacologic Therapy for PCI

Drug	Use	Setting	Dose	Duration of effect	Duration of therapy	Complications
Aspirin	Antiplatelet	All PCI	81 mg	5-7 days	Permanent	GI bleeding
Clopidogrel	Antiplatelet	All PCI	600 mg 6 h before PCI + 75 mg/day afterward	5-7 days	6 mo-1 year	Bleeding TTP (rare)
Prasugrel[3]	Antiplatelet	All PCI	60 mg bolus + 10 mg/day	72 h	6 mo-1 year	Bleeding
Ticagrelor[3]	Antiplatelet	All PCI	180 mg bolus + 90 mg 2/2	48 h	6 mo-1 year	Bleeding Dyspnea
Abciximab	Antiplatelet	ACS	0.25 μg/kg bolus + 0.125 μg/kg/min	72 h	12 h	Bleeding Thrombocytopenia
Eptifibatide	Antiplatelet	ACS	Two 180-μg/kg boluses (10 min apart) + infusion 2 μg/kg/min	4 h	12-72 h	Bleeding
Tirofiban	Antiplatelet	ACS	0.4 μg/kg/min for 30 min, then 0.1 μg/kg/min	4 h	12-72 h	Bleeding
Heparin	Anticoagulation	All PCI	100 IU/kg *60 IU/kg	6 h	During procedure	Bleeding Thrombocytopenia Thrombosis
Bivalirudin	Anticoagulation	UFH alternative	1 mg/kg bolus + 2.5 mg/kg/h for 4 h	2 h	During procedure + 4-6 h if no clopidogrel bolus	Bleeding
Argatroban	Anticoagulation	UFH alternative	350 μg/kg bolus + 25 μg/kg/min	2 h	During procedure + 4-6 h if no clopidogrel bolus	Bleeding
Enoxaparin	Anticoagulation	UFH alternative	1 mg/kg *0.7 mg/kg	6 h	During procedure	Bleeding
Dalteparin	Anticoagulation	UFH alternative	100 IU/kg *70 IU/kg	6 h	During procedure	Bleeding
Acetylcysteine	Contrast nephropathy prophylaxis	GFR < 60 mL/min	600 mg every 12 h	Unknown	Begin 12 h before and continue for 12 h afterward	None
Verapamil/ diltiazem/ nicardipine	Vasodilator	No-/slow-reflow	0.1-0.5 mg IC	20-30 min	As needed	Hypotension Bradycardia
Nitroprusside	Vasodilator	No-/slow-reflow	30 μg IC	30-60 s	As needed	Hypotension
Adenosine	Vasodilator	No-/slow-reflow	50 μg IC	30 s	As needed	Bradycardia

*Recommended dose in conjunction with glycoprotein IIb/IIIa inhibitor therapy.
ACS = acute coronary syndrome; GFR = glomerular filtration rate; GI = gastrointestinal; IC = intracoronary; mo = month; PCI = percutaneous coronary intervention; TTP = thrombotic thrombocytopenic purpura; UFH = unfractionated heparin.

Outcomes

In approximately 2 to 10% of balloon angioplasty procedures, intimal dissection, thrombosis, and perhaps medial smooth muscle spasm combine to produce abrupt closure.[16,17] Abrupt closure may be treated successfully with repeat balloon inflation but is treated more commonly with stent implantation.[18] The specter of abrupt closure and MI or emergency bypass surgery and its complications historically has limited the application of balloon angioplasty.

In patients with stable angina, mortality from balloon angioplasty procedures is 1% at 1 month.[19] About half of the deaths are the result of a procedural complication, and most are related to low cardiac output (Table 19-3).[20] Although the incidence of restenosis (>50% diameter stenosis during follow-up) is 40 to 50% within 6 to 9 months of a PTCA procedure,[13,15,21] only 25% of patients report recurrent angina that warrants further investigation.[22] Patients with restenosis have an increased risk of MI and needing coronary artery bypass surgery.[23]

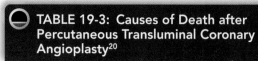

TABLE 19-3: Causes of Death after Percutaneous Transluminal Coronary Angioplasty[20]

Low-output failure	66.1%
Ventricular arrhythmias	10.7%
Stroke	4.1%
Preexisting renal failure	4.1%
Bleeding	2.5%
Ventricular rupture	2.5%
Respiratory failure	2.5%
Pulmonary embolism	1.7%
Infection	1.7%

Modified with permission from Malenka DJ, O'Rourke D, Miller MA, et al: Cause of in-hospital death in 12,232 consecutive patients undergoing percutaneous transluminal coronary angioplasty. The Northern New England Cardiovascular Disease Study Group, *Am Heart J.* 1999 Apr;137(4 Pt 1):632-638.

DEVICE-ASSISTED ANGIOPLASTY

Stents

The two failure modes of balloon angioplasty—abrupt closure and restenosis—have stimulated the development of a myriad of devices, all intended to reduce procedure-related risk, the risk of restenosis, or both. Only coronary stenting has been shown to be advantageous over balloon angioplasty alone, except in severely calcified lesions (Table 19-4). There are numerous coronary stent designs, but the majority of those in current use consist of a cylinder that is made from stainless steel (or an alloy, such as cobalt chromium) and that has been "carved," creating a so-called slotted-tube design. Stent expansion creates a series of interlocking cells, resembling a cylindrical mesh-work (Fig. 19-3). Stents are thus deformable, but when expanded, they maintain sufficient rigidity to act as scaffolding after the angioplasty balloon is deflated. Intimal disruption is contained and far less likely to propagate and occlude the treated vessel. In addition, the rigid framework left behind becomes part of the vessel wall, addressing the issue of remodeling, which is one of the mechanisms of restenosis.

Stents allow safe expansion of the vessel beyond that typically achieved with PTCA at the time of balloon expansion;

however, stent use increases the thrombotic and inflammatory responses of the vessel wall. The increased injury and a foreign-body response to stent struts result in a more intense and prolonged local inflammatory response.[24] Consequently, stent placement paradoxically exacerbates intimal hyperplasia.[25,26] If one uses the late (6 or 9 months) loss in lumen diameter after stent implantation as a measure of intimal hyperplasia, even the most modern stent designs fall within a range of about 0.8 mm—more than twice the loss incurred after PTCA (0.32 mm). As a result, with regard to restenosis after angioplasty, the impact of stenting for percutaneous coronary revascularization (PCR) is rather small in comparison with that of PTCA.[25,26] Intimal hyperplasia and restenosis risk are primarily functions of the size of the treated lumen on completion of the procedure, the length of the treated lesion, and the presence of unstable angina, hypertension, and diabetes mellitus (Table 19-5).[27-29] Long-term follow-up studies indicate that a stent that does not reocclude during the first 6 to 9 months after implantation is not subject to late, rapid disease progression.[30-34]

By reducing the likelihood of abrupt closure requiring emergency coronary artery bypass surgery and of restenosis, stent-assisted angioplasty is more effective than routine balloon angioplasty for virtually any type of coronary artery lesion. Registry data describe a risk for emergency surgery of only 0.3 to 1.1% and a procedural mortality of less than 1%.[35-38] The likelihood of procedural complications may be estimated on the basis of lesion characteristics (Table 19-6).[39] Depending on lesion characteristics and the number of lesions treated, after 1 year, 5 to 10% of patients require coronary artery bypass surgery, and 15 to 20% undergo a second percutaneous coronary intervention (PCI) procedure.[40-43] After 5 years, 10 to 15% of patients require another revascularization procedure because of the development of severe stenosis at an untreated site.[34] Diabetes increases the risk for adverse outcomes by increasing the risk of restenosis and disease progression at untreated sites.

As noted previously in the description of the guidewire, iron components of stent struts attract fibrinogen and provide a site for platelet attachment and thrombosis. The increased risk of thrombosis at the treated site persists until endothelialization is complete. As a result, more intense antithrombotic therapy is required during the procedure and for up to 1 year afterward.[44,45]

TABLE 19-4: Devices Used for Coronary Angioplasty

	Experience	Ease of use	Complications	Efficacy	Lesion type
Standard balloon angioplasty	++++	++++	+	+++	Any
Cutting balloon	+	++	++	+++	Calcified lesion, ISR, bifurcation
Rotational atherectomy	+++	+	+++	+++	Heavily calcified, nondilatable ISR
Directional atherectomy	+	+	+++	+	Bifurcation, ostial lesion
Laser atherectomy	++	++	++	++	Calcification, ISR, thrombus
Aspiration (mechanical)	++	+	+	++	Thrombus
Aspiration (manual)	+	+++	+	++	Thrombus

ISR = in-stent restenosis.

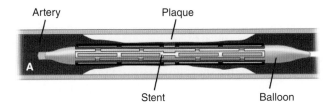

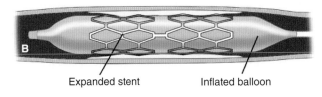

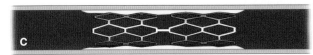

Stenting

FIGURE 19-3 The coronary stent is a metallic "meshwork" that increases its rigidity when cold worked by balloon expansion. Buttressing of the vascular wall, propagation of dissection, and early vascular recoil are reduced significantly. (Used with permission from Texas Heart Institute, www.texasheart.org.)

Stents may be used as a drug-delivery system. However, rather than simply applying a drug to the stent's surface from which it will dissipate quickly, drug delivery is controlled by using a surface polymer or by altering the design or the material used to construct the stent.[46] This drug-delivery device, called a *drug-eluting stent* (DES), allows the drug to be applied at high concentrations at the site of interest and reduces the probability of systemic toxicity.

DESs reduce the primary determinant of restenosis by 50 to 100%, as determined by measuring late lumen loss after angioplasty (Fig. 19-4). Studies that examined the efficacy of the DES resulted in the introduction of new nomenclature for the follow-up endpoints. The most useful follow-up endpoint is termed *target vessel failure* (TVF), signified by cardiac death, MI, or repeat

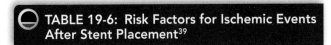

TABLE 19-6: Risk Factors for Ischemic Events After Stent Placement[39]

Strongest correlates

Nonchronic total occlusion
Degenerated SVG

Moderately strong correlates

Length ≥ 10 mm
Lumen irregularity
Large filling defect
Calcium + angle ≥ 45
Eccentric
Severe calcification
SVG age ≥ 10 years

Outcomes

Group	Definition	Death/MI/Emergency CABG (%)
Highest risk	Either of the strongest correlates	12.7
High risk	≥3 moderate correlates	8.2
Moderate risk	1-2 moderate correlates	3.4
Low risk	No risk factors	2.1

CABG = coronary artery bypass graft surgery; MI = myocardial infarction; SVG = saphenous vein graft.

revascularization of the treated vessel. One year after the procedure, the risk of TVF is reduced from 19.4 to 21% with a bare-metal stent (BMS) to 8.8 to 10% with a DES.[40,43,47]

Reduced rates of repeat intervention after DES placement have been reported for every type of lesion studied except bifurcation lesions, for which the risk of restenosis remains significant, and the risk of potentially fatal early thrombosis is as high as 3.5% (Table 19-7).[40,43,48-66] Although the use of a DES reduces the rate of failure of long-term treatment and of repeat

TABLE 19-5: Approximate Risk of Restenosis Stratified by Final Lumen Diameter and Stent Length

Final lumen diameter (mm)

Stent length (mm)	2.0	2.5	3.0	3.5	4.0
15	32%	22%	14%	8%	4%
30	42%	30%	20%	11%	7%
45	52%	39%	28%	15%	10%
60	60%	47%	35%	20%	13%

Data from de Feyter PJ, Kay P, Disco C, et al. Reference chart derived from post-stent-implantation intravascular ultrasound predictors of 6-month expected restenosis on quantitative coronary angiography, *Circulation* 1999 Oct 26;100(17):1777-1783.

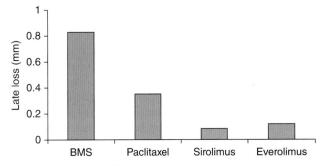

FIGURE 19-4 The effect of various stents on intimal hyperplasia in randomized trials is shown. A bare-metal stent's intimal hyperplasia thickness, or late loss, shown on the left, is compared with the late loss of drug-eluting stents shown at the right. BMS, bare-metal stent.

TABLE 19-7: The Clinical Impact of Drug-eluting Stents

Population	Endpoint	BMS (%)	DES (%)
Total[40,43]	TVF	20-24.1	9.9-10.8
Diabetes mellitus[60]	MACE 9 mo	27.2-36.3	11.3-15
Insulin-treated[53]	MACE 9 mo	31.5	19.6
Myocardial infarction[65]	TVR 8 mo	32	18
"Complex" lesions[56]	TLR 12 mo	29.8	2.4
Long lesion, small vessel[51,61,62]	MACE 9 mo	18.3-22.6	4-8
Small vessel[48]	MACE 8 mo	31.3	9.3
Bifurcation[49,50,64,66]	TVR 6 mo	13.3-38	8.6-19
Restenosis[55]	TVR 6 mo	33	8-19
Saphenous vein graft lesion[52]	MACE 6 mo	28.1	11.5

BMS = bare-metal stent; DES = drug-eluting stent; MACE = major adverse cardiac event; mo = month; TLR = target lesion revascularization; TVF = target vessel failure; TVR = target vessel revascularization.

procedures, this reduction does not translate to a reduced risk of procedure-related complications.[67] In addition, incomplete healing, a response to the eluting polymer, or both confer an increased risk of stent thrombosis that extends beyond 1 year.[68] As a result, after intervention with a first-generation DES or in a patient with acute coronary syndrome (ACS), dual antiplatelet therapy should be continued for at least 1 year in all patients and indefinitely in patients with complex lesions. Newer-generation DESs allow for more rapid reendothelialization and a slight increase in late loss without increasing the risk of in-stent restenosis. As a result, the duration of dual antiplatelet therapy can safely be reduced to less than a year. For clinically stable patients, only 6 months of dual therapy is required, which increases the number of patients who may safely receive a DES while facing the prospect of noncardiac surgery in the near future.[69]

Other Devices

PERFUSION BALLOONS

Before coronary stents came into routine use, abrupt closure owing to dissection could be treated with repeat balloon inflation and, if that was unsuccessful, with coronary artery bypass surgery. Prolonged balloon inflation generally was necessary for successfully restoring patency, but in the event of failure, transport for emergency surgery often was accompanied by severe ischemia of the treated territory. As a result, balloon catheters with a short third-lumen opening just proximal and distal to the balloon were developed. These catheters, or "perfusion balloons," allowed prolonged balloon inflation with far less ischemia and could be used to ameliorate ischemia during transport for surgery after an unsuccessful procedure. Since the introduction of the coronary stent, the use of perfusion balloons has become rare.

ATHERECTOMY

When the concept of reducing the bulk of the obstructing atheroma was first introduced, it was quite attractive.

The idea was to reduce vessel wall thickness, or "debulk," allowing balloon expansion at a lower pressure. Theoretically, with less force applied for lumen expansion, the likelihood of abrupt closure would be reduced, as would the degree of arterial injury at the time of treatment. Several devices used for debulking have been developed and studied, including directional coronary atherectomy, percutaneous transluminal rotational ablation, and laser ablation. Unfortunately, when subjected to rigorous examination, debulking devices were found to provide no substantial advantage over plain balloon angioplasty in achieving procedural success or avoiding restenosis.[70-73] Although each device has acquired a specific niche (see Table 19-4), their routine use is generally associated with an increased risk of procedural complications, including perforation and MI.[73-75]

Rotational atherectomy requires additional discussion because unlike the other types of atherectomy, it is still commonly used. The Rotablator (Boston Scientific Corporation, Natick, MA) is an olive-shaped device coated with diamond chips that is attached to an electrical motor that can rotate the device at high speeds. The device is designed to abrade a rigid atherosclerotic intima, creating microemboli that are small enough to pass through the coronary microcirculation without incident. It is also useful as an initial treatment method for very rigid, heavily calcified lesions. However, the concept of rotational atherectomy is not without shortcomings. Microembolization is likely to exacerbate ischemia and therefore is contraindicated when there are thrombotic lesions, if there is impaired microcirculatory flow associated with a recent MI, or if the treated vessel is the last remaining patent vessel. Use of this device is also associated with an increased risk of perforation in highly angulated lesions. Another recently developed form of atherectomy is the single-bladed rotational atherectomy device used for "orbital" atherectomy. This treatment's place in the PCI armamentarium has not yet been fully determined.[76]

ASPIRATION DEVICES

Several coronary aspiration devices are available to reduce the risk of distal embolization and to diminish the local concentration of prothrombotic and vasoactive substances. These devices range from a simple end-hole catheter attached to a syringe to a complex suction catheter with or without an associated mechanical disrupter. These devices forcibly extract components of the thrombus or atheroma.[77] Their use may improve flow after the treatment of thrombus-laden lesions or saphenous vein grafts (Fig. 19-5).[78]

EMBOLIC PROTECTION DEVICES

During balloon angioplasty, mechanical dissolution of thrombus (if any is present) may result in macroembolization and distal vessel occlusion. The high-pressure manipulation of an atheromatous lesion also may free cholesterol crystals and other components of the lesion, resulting in distal microembolization, thrombosis, and slow- or no-reflow phenomenon.

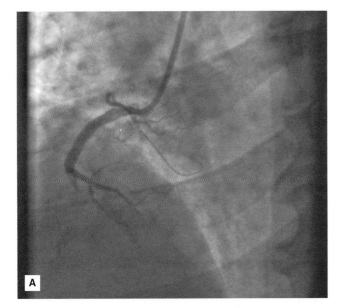

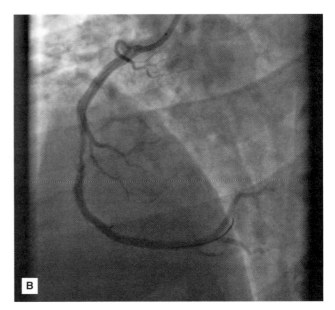

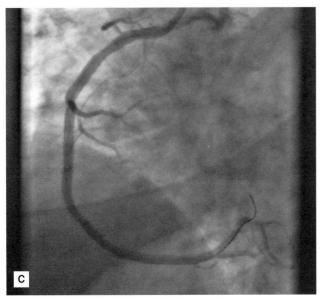

FIGURE 19-5 In a patient with ongoing inferior myocardial infarction, the right coronary artery is occluded by thrombus (A). After passage of a guidewire followed by aspiration at the site of occlusion, thrombus is withdrawn, restoring antegrade blood flow (B). A stent then is placed at the site of the culprit lesion to complete the procedure (C).

Several devices have been developed to reduce the frequency or impact of distal embolization. These devices may be placed distal or proximal to the treated lesion. Distal devices are mounted on the guidewire and use either a suspended micropore filter to trap particulate matter of 100 to 150 μm or larger or balloon occlusion of the treated vessel with posttreatment aspiration to capture embolized material. Proximally placed devices temporarily interrupt flow and aspirate the treated vessel. The PercuSurge GuardWire Plus (Medtronic, Minneapolis, MN) is a balloon occlusion and aspiration device that underwent testing in vein grafts in the Saphenous Vein Graft Angioplasty Free of Emboli Randomized trial.[79] The trial showed a 42% reduction in creatine kinase (CK) elevations and more than a 50% reduction in the no-reflow phenomenon.[79] Unfortunately, these results did not apply to patients with MI.[80]

IMAGING DEVICES

Angiography allows imaging of the coronary lumen but may be unreliable in patients with severe calcification, difficult branching patterns, or previously placed coronary stents. Furthermore, a thrombus that may increase the risk associated with PCR may go undetected by standard angiography. Therefore, several alternative imaging methods have been developed to improve diagnosis, to plan revascularization efforts, and to evaluate the success of such efforts. Angioscopy or fiber-optic imaging requires occluding the imaged vessel and perfusing it with saline. Although angioscopy is a useful tool to investigate the presence or components of thrombus within coronary vessels, it has not been a useful adjunct to PCR. In contrast, intracoronary ultrasonography has proved especially useful. Ultrasonography allows accurate determination of vessel size, luminal reduction, lesion components, and the progress of revascularization attempts. Ultrasound guidance for stent implantation is associated with a greater than 30% reduction in the need for repeat procedures.[81] Of equal importance, intracoronary ultrasonography is an invaluable research tool used to investigate the accuracy of contrast angiography and the impact of mural lesion components on complications and outcomes after angioplasty.

Optical coherence tomography uses the characteristics of light reflection to determine tissue characteristics, providing a visual representation of the interrogated artery that provides information about both anatomy and disease state. It is useful as a research tool, providing extremely accurate tissue thickness measurements, as well as spectacular anatomic images. Unfortunately, at the level of clinical care, optical coherence tomography offers little more information than intracoronary ultrasonography but increases case complexity.[82]

DEVICES THAT MEASURE LESION SEVERITY

The hemodynamic significance of coronary lesions, the appropriateness of a treatment, and the success of treatment may be determined by one of the following two means: a guidewire that measures the velocity of blood flow within coronary arteries, and a calculation of the pressure distal to a coronary lesion.

A miniaturized Doppler-equipped guidewire with a 12-MHz transducer uses a pulsed interrogation that samples 5.2 mm beyond the guidewire tip at an angle of 14° on either side. Assuming that the cross-sectional area of the interrogated vessel remains constant during all measurements, the ratio of the velocities measured reflects the ratio of blood flow between any two measurements. The most important and reliable parameter that a flow probe measures is the ratio of resting flow to vasodilated coronary flow, a value known as coronary flow reserve. When measured with the Doppler probe, the value is termed coronary velocity reserve (CVR). As a coronary lesion becomes flow limiting, attempts to normalize tissue perfusion by autoregulation result in arteriolar dilatation at rest. Therefore, the administration of an arteriolar vasodilator such as adenosine will have little additional effect on flow velocity. The absence of an appropriate increase in velocity during adenosine- or dipyridamole-induced arteriolar vasodilation produces abnormal flow reserve. A CVR less than 2.0 indicates hemodynamically significant lesions.

The CVR measurement reflects changes in flow relative to an assumed normal baseline state but is subject to error when baseline flow is abnormal. Examples of abnormal states include left ventricular (LV) hypertrophy, fibrosis, and perhaps anemia. In addition, abnormally large or small driving pressure gradients may fall outside the range of normal coronary autoregulation, altering the basal-to-hyperemic ratio. Failure to achieve arteriolar dilatation in response to adenosine or dipyridamole will produce an abnormal calculated flow reserve. Conditions that affect arteriolar dilatation include diabetes mellitus, amyloidosis, and recent caffeine or theophylline ingestion.

An alternative to flow measurement is pressure measurement proximal and distal to the lesion in question. Under normal conditions, epicardial vessels present little detectable resistance to flow. Therefore, driving pressure (P_{Ao}) and arteriolar resistance pressure (P_{RA}) determine maximal coronary blood flow. The presence of a flow-limiting coronary lesion will cause some of the driving pressure to be lost, so maximal flow will depend on the distal coronary pressure (P_d)-to-P_{RA} gradient and arteriolar resistance. Therefore, the fraction of maximal basal flow that remains possible in the presence of the lesion is

$$\dot{Q}_{lesion}/\dot{Q}_{no\ lesion} = (P_d - P_{RA}/R_{basal})/(P_{Ao} - P_{RA}/R_{basal})$$

Canceling resistance and assuming that right atrial pressure remains constant result in a very simple relationship:

$$\dot{Q}_{lesion}/\dot{Q}_{no\ lesion} = P_d/P_{Ao}$$

This ratio, called the myocardial fractional flow reserve (FFR), is obtained after the administration of adenosine. An FFR of 0.75 or less is used to identify a hemodynamically significant lesion. Routine use of FFR to ensure the necessity of PCI reduces the risk of adverse events, both immediately and 1 year after the procedure.[83]

Physicians who care for patients with coronary artery disease differ widely in their estimates of the severity of a coronary lesion. Fortunately, that conflict can be objectively resolved with FFR. Using FFR to guide revascularization decisions in most cases improves the revascularization decision, helps in assigning the patient the most appropriate care, and reduces the risk of complications and repeat procedures.[84] Absent an alternate physiologic cue for revascularization, FFR should guide the decision in all but the most obvious cases.

BRACHYTHERAPY

Before the advent of DESs, restenosis after angioplasty or stent implantation could be treated by medical therapy, repeat angioplasty, or coronary artery bypass surgery. The high frequency of restenosis led to a large population of patients with multiple treatment failures, intractable symptoms, and prohibitive contraindications to surgical treatment. Because a proportion of the cell population colonizing a treated lesion and contributing to restenosis arose from the media of the treated lesion, radiation therapy to prevent cell replication was proposed. The well-recognized dangers of high-dose, external-beam radiation limited dosing to local application, but this therapy still was seen as posing a substantial risk. Although radiation brachytherapy is a source of increased adverse events when used as a treatment for de novo coronary lesions, it has been used with some (albeit limited) success to treat refractory in-stent restenosis.[85,86]

CIRCULATORY SUPPORT

Performing a percutaneous revascularization procedure includes an obligatory period of ischemia in the treated region. The duration of ischemia may be prolonged in the event of abrupt closure or distal embolization, and

TABLE 19-8: A Score Predicting the Need for Circulatory Support[87]

Six arterial segments	LAD, D_1, S_1, OM, PLV, PDA
Score 1	Target lesion or any additional lesion with >70% diameter stenosis
Score 0.5	Subtended region is hypokinetic but has no stenosis
For a score >3	Consider IABP

D_1 = first diagonal branch; IABP = intraaortic balloon pump; LAD = left anterior descending artery; OM = obtuse marginal branch; PDA = posterior descending artery; PLV = posterior left ventricular artery; S_1 = first septal branch.

recovery may be incomplete or delayed for a period of days, as in the treatment of acute MI. For patients with depressed LV systolic function and for those in whom the treated territory is large, there is a risk for developing cardiogenic shock during and after the procedure. This risk substantially increases the possibility of acute renal failure, stroke, and death. The likelihood of shock complicating an angioplasty procedure may be predicted by using a scoring method that incorporates the extent and severity of systolic dysfunction present before the procedure and the extent that can be expected as a result of the procedure (Table 19-8).[39,87] Elective placement of an intraaortic balloon pump (IABP) is associated with a reduced risk of hypotension and major complications.[88]

The percutaneous left ventricular assist device (pLVAD) is a miniaturized axial-flow pump that is being used increasingly to support patients in shock or during high-risk angioplasty procedures.[89] The pLVAD is capable of providing up to 4 L/min of additional blood flow. The pLVAD and its variants are superior to the balloon pump in providing circulatory support and avoiding flow-related complications. However, complications at the access site and with the flow delivery limit their application to the highest-risk patients for whom we do not have an objective measure (score) to ensure benefit.[90-92]

COMPLICATIONS

In addition to abrupt closure and restenosis, there are several other potential complications of PCR that may influence the risk-to-benefit ratio for an individual patient. These complications include bleeding, vascular access-site complications, stroke, radiocontrast nephropathy (RCN), and MI owing to distal embolization.

Hemorrhage

Bleeding that necessitates transfusion or results in hemodynamic instability occurs in 0.5 to 4% of PCR procedures, depending on patient variables (eg, age, gender, presence of peripheral vascular disease), procedural variables (eg, location of femoral arteriotomy, duration), and pharmacologic

variables (eg, intensity of antithrombotic therapy).[4] Several devices have been designed to improve femoral hemostasis after sheath removal, but none has proven superior to standard compression hemostasis.[93] With the availability of lower-profile equipment, the radial artery is being used with greater frequency, which results in a reduction in bleeding and access-site complications.[94,95]

Ischemia

Stroke complicates approximately 0.18% of PCR procedures.[96] Its occurrence is associated with increased age, depressed LV ejection fraction, diabetes mellitus, saphenous vein graft intervention, and complicated or prolonged procedures requiring the placement of an IABP.[97]

The frequency with which MI complicates PCR procedures depends on the definition of MI.[98] If MI is defined as the presence of new Q wave, the incidence is 1%,[99] whereas if MI is defined as any elevation of the MB fraction of CK (CK-MB), the incidence is as high as 38%.[98] Using more stringent definitions of infarction, such as greater than 3 or 10 times the upper limit of normal, reduces the reported values to 11 to 18% or 5%, respectively.[99-101] Actually, any elevation carries prognostic significance, but elevation above three times the upper limit of normal is accepted as a definition of periprocedural MI.

Elevated markers of myocardial injury may be seen after apparently uncomplicated procedures.[98] One mechanism for such events is microscopic distal embolization. When severe, microscopic distal embolization of a coronary artery creates the angiographic appearance of slow vessel filling, it is termed *no-* or *slow-reflow*. No-reflow is seen most often during saphenous vein graft angioplasty but also may complicate rotational atherectomy and primary PCR for acute MI. Methods of quantifying abnormal flow after PCR include a subjective estimation of flow velocity, the thrombolysis in myocardial infarction (TIMI) flow rate (III, normal; II, slow; I, minimal contrast material flow beyond the treated site; and 0, no flow), and the more objective method of corrected TIMI frame count. Individual frames of the angiographic image are counted from the time of contrast material entry into the treated vessel until a predetermined distal landmark is reached. No-reflow may be a brief and self-limiting phenomenon, but when prolonged, it is associated with increased mortality.[102] Pharmacologic manipulations, including intracoronary verapamil, adenosine, and nitroprusside administration, may be used in an attempt to prevent or treat the no-reflow phenomenon (see Table 19-2).

Perforation of the coronary artery complicates 0.5% of angioplasty procedures,[103] and its frequency increases almost 10-fold when ablation devices are used (1.3% for ablation vs 0.1% for PTCA; $p < .001$). Coronary artery perforation occurs more frequently in elderly and female patients (Table 19-9).[103,104]

Pericardial tamponade is frequently but not invariably associated with coronary artery perforation. The overall incidence

⬤ **TABLE 19-9: Coronary Artery Perforations Classified by Severity**

Type	Incidence	Treatment	Mortality
I: A visible extraluminal crater without extravasation*	26%	Nonsurgical 95% of the time	Rarely fatal
II: Pericardial or myocardial blushing*	50%	Requires surgery 10% of the time	13%
III: 1-mm-diameter perforation with contrast material streaming	26%	Requires surgery or covered stent	63%

*Typically a result of improper guidewire manipulation or placement. See Fig. 19-6.
Modified with permission from Ellis SG, Ajluni S, Arnold AZ, et al: Increased coronary perforation in the new device era. Incidence, classification, management, and outcome, *Circulation* 1994 Dec;90(6):2725-2730.

of tamponade after PCI is 0.12% and doubles when ablation devices are used. Tamponade associated with PCI is recognized 55%[105] of the time during or after the procedure while the patient is still in the catheterization laboratory and 45% of the time after the patient leaves the laboratory.[100] A minority of episodes of late tamponade (13%) are associated with recognized coronary artery perforation. Tamponade requires surgical treatment in 39% of patients, is closely associated with MI complicating PCR, and carries a mortality rate of 42%.[105]

The covered stent that was developed to prevent, but failed to reduce the risk of, saphenous vein graft restenosis[106] currently is used as a rescue device after coronary artery perforation or for the treatment of coronary or saphenous vein graft aneurysms (Fig. 19-7).[107] When a covered stent is used to treat coronary artery perforation, the need for emergency surgery is reduced, as is the risk of coronary artery perforation. A small number of patients, however, still require surgery.[108]

Toxicity

Acute renal failure after exposure to radiocontrast material, or RCN, is poorly understood. Its occurrence is a function of age, congestive heart failure, hemodynamic instability, diabetes mellitus, preexisting renal insufficiency, anemia, peripheral vascular disease, and the amount of contrast material administered.[109-111] The incidence of RCN after

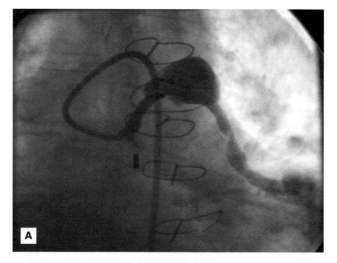

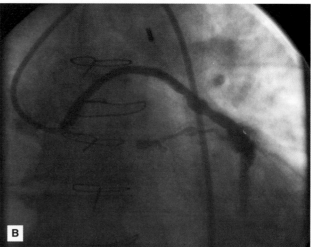

FIGURE 19-7 A large saphenous vein graft aneurysm (A) is treated with a covered stent (B).

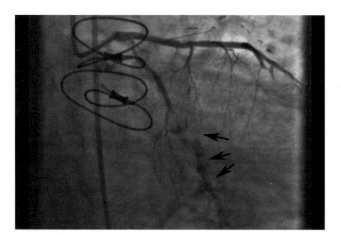

FIGURE 19-6 In cases of early saphenous vein graft closure with myocardial infarction and postinfarction angina, attempts to access the culprit native vessel with a stiff guidewire have led to coronary perforation. Shown in this injection of the left coronary artery are occlusions of the left anterior descending and left circumflex coronary arteries. Staining is seen (*arrows*) in the region of the attempted recanalization of the left circumflex coronary artery, indicating perforation (type II). The patient was treated successfully with reversal of anticoagulation and temporary occlusion of the circumflex with the PTCA balloon. PTCA, percutaneous transluminal coronary angioplasty.

coronary angiography is 5 to 6%, and the nadir of renal function occurs 3 to 5 days after the procedure.[112] Even a transient decline in renal function leads to an increased risk of ischemic cardiovascular events during follow-up, and renal failure necessitating hemodialysis is seen in about 10% of patients with RCN, increasing both short- and long-term mortality.[109,110,113]

The only methods for reducing the risk of RCN are the use of iso-osmolar contrast, volume expansion, and, perhaps, acetylcysteine administration. Using iodixanol, an iso-osmolar nonionic contrast agent, reduces the incidence of RCN after noncardiac angiography.[114] Giving four oral doses of N-acetylcysteine (600 mg each; two doses on the day before and two on the day of the procedure) to prevent RCN has had varied outcomes in several studies.[115,116] Administering crystalloid solution in volumes sufficient to maintain brisk urine flow, perhaps aided by alkalinization of urine pH, is the most effective intervention for preventing RCN by ensuring an adequate volume state.[117]

SPECIAL CIRCUMSTANCES

Acute Coronary Syndromes

Successful PTCA and stent implantation (in most instances) within the first 6 hours of ST-segment-elevation MI is at least as effective as, and perhaps more effective than, thrombolytic agents in limiting myocardial damage and improving in-hospital survival.[118-120] The routine use of coronary stents for acute MI is associated with a restenosis rate of 17% and a 6-month event-free survival of 83 to 95%.[121-124] The use of DESs reduces the risk of any adverse event from 17 to 9.4% at 300 days.[57] After failed attempts at thrombolysis or for patients with cardiogenic shock who received thrombolysis, stent revascularization increases myocardial salvage and reduces the risk of death, heart failure, or reinfarction.[125-128]

Attempts to reduce the impact of reperfusion injury have been mostly ineffective. However, one remains promising: the occlusion of mitochondrial pores, which allows the release of newly generated oxygen free radicals into the cytosol. Oxygen radicals represent a form of second messenger system inside the cell, triggering inflammatory response, prothrombotic behavior, and apoptosis. Uncoupling these responses has, historically, been the purview of statins and other cholesterol-lowering drugs. However, cyclosporine, typically considered an immunosuppressant, may also be effective in blocking mitochondrial release of oxygen radicals. The results of small, early trials are a source of enthusiasm, but confirmation in larger trials is necessary.[129]

Previous Coronary Artery Bypass

Stent implantation with the assistance of embolic protection devices is the preferred method for percutaneous treatment of occluded saphenous vein grafts.[79,126] The use of distal embolic protection reduces the risk of periprocedural MI from 14.7 to 8.6%.[79] Unfortunately, diseased grafts have a high probability of developing new lesions, reducing long-term event-free survival. After stent implantation, overall survival is 79% at 4 years, but survival free of MI or another revascularization procedure is only 29%.[130-134] DESs reduce the risk of restenosis after saphenous vein graft PCR but do not affect the likelihood of disease progression elsewhere in the diseased graft.[52]

THE FUTURE

The future of interventional cardiology lies in reducing procedural risk and extending treatment durability. For many patients, the goal of providing durable treatment success has been very nearly achieved with the introduction of DESs, an approach that has yet to be fully explored. However, a DES does not reduce procedural risk, and problems remain for patients with diffuse atherosclerosis, diabetes mellitus, bifurcation lesions, and ACSs. In cases in which it is not clear whether PCI or surgical revascularization is more likely to produce a favorable outcome, the Synergy between Percutaneous Coronary Intervention with TAXUS and Cardiac Surgery (SYNTAX) score can be used to make an objective decision.[135] The original SYNTAX score was developed to quantify—wholly on the basis of angiographic findings—the procedural risk and the odds of long-term success of revascularization by DES placement or surgical procedures. A modified version of the score includes clinical risk factors that appear to add predictive value to that of the anatomic data: LV function, renal function, and lung disease (for the latest version of the SYNTAX score calculator, see http://syntaxscore.com). Using this combined scoring method, the likely short- and long-term outcomes of both surgical and percutaneous revascularization may be compared objectively to guide the choice of revascularization method. The adoption, utilization, and regular refinement of the SYNTAX score will be difficult but necessary to match the right patient to the right treatment (Table 19-10).[136]

Ironically, the goal of reducing procedural risk has been pursued most effectively for saphenous vein graft

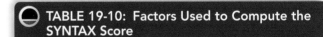

TABLE 19-10: Factors Used to Compute the SYNTAX Score

The following characteristics are used to score each coronary lesion with a diameter stenosis of ≥50% in a vessel at least 1.5 mm long:

Dominance (right or left)

Total occlusion

Trifurcation

Bifurcation

Aorto-ostial

Severe tortuosity

Length > 20 mm

Heavy calcification

Thrombus

Diffuse disease

Data from The Syntax Score. TCT2008. Syntax.

revascularization with the development of distal embolic protection devices. However, for native-vessel interventions, particularly those performed during ACSs, further advances will probably be pharmacologic rather than technical. As evidenced by observations of ischemic preconditioning, modification of myocardial energy metabolism with drugs, such as ranolazine and others, represents a means of improving the heart's ability to withstand ischemia, thus temporizing the impact of temporary vascular occlusion and macro- or micro-embolization.[137-139] In addition, inhibitors of the protein kinase family of enzymes, central to intracellular signaling, also may improve the heart's ability to withstand ischemia and reduce the severity of reperfusion injury.[129]

Local drug delivery has been met with great success in reducing the problem of restenosis. However, there are numerous methods of modifying the physiology that drives intimal hyperplasia after stent implantation. New DES platforms offer the alternative of eluting multiple drugs at different rates, thereby reducing the need for systemic medical therapy, such as prolonged dual antiplatelet therapy. In addition, complex molecules that can be absorbed by the body are being developed as stent platforms. The use of a stent that delivers antithrombotic and antiproliferative drugs could conceivably allow PCR protection from acute closure, recoil, thrombosis, and restenosis without contributing to vessel rigidity that increases the difficulty of subsequent procedures.

A growing number of patients who are surviving longer with severe multivessel coronary artery disease remain hampered by severe angina pectoris. In many instances, years of slow, steady disease progression have left extensive collateral vessels that prevent infarction and the near or complete loss of major branch vessels. These patients currently have no option for percutaneous or surgical revascularization. For this population, the use of stem cells, perhaps the most efficient producers of cytokines and growth factors in their proper sequence, has been met with early success. Direct injection of stem cells into regions of ischemic myocardium improves walking time and reduces the frequency of angina attacks.[140]

KEY POINTS

1. Percutaneous revascularization is best used to control unacceptable symptoms in patients whose anatomy suggests low procedural risk and a good probability of long-term success.
2. Stent implantation substantially improves the safety of PCI, and the use of DESs reduces the likelihood of long-term treatment failure. However, the use of DESs requires that patients be candidates for long-term, dual antiplatelet drug therapy.
3. Measurement of the FFR is crucial for determining the necessity of revascularization. In addition, its routine use for evaluating moderate lesions reduces the risk of major procedural complications compared to angiographic analysis alone.

4. When possible, all saphenous vein graft interventions should be performed with distal protection devices in place.
5. In patients who, for clinical reasons, can be treated by either percutaneous or surgical means, the modified SYNTAX score should be used to ensure an objective decision regarding the most appropriate therapy.

ACKNOWLEDGMENT

Stephen N. Palmer, PhD, ELS, and Nicole Stancel, PhD, ELS, provided editorial support for this chapter.

REFERENCES

1. Boden WE, O'Rourke RA, Teo KK, et al: Optimal medical therapy with or without PCI for stable coronary disease. *N Engl J Med* 2007; 356(15):1503-1516.
2. Pershad A, Sein V, Laufer N: GuideLiner catheter facilitated PCI—a novel device with multiple applications. *J Invasive Cardiol* 2011; 23(11):E254-259.
3. Cannon CP, Harrington RA, James S, et al: Comparison of ticagrelor with clopidogrel in patients with a planned invasive strategy for acute coronary syndromes (PLATO): a randomised double-blind study. *Lancet* 2010; 375(9711):283-293.
4. Hillegass WB, Brott BC, Chapman GD, et al: Relationship between activated clotting time during percutaneous intervention and subsequent bleeding complications. *Am Heart J* 2002; 144(3):501-507.
5. Ferguson JJ, Califf RM, Antman EM, et al: Enoxaparin vs unfractionated heparin in high-risk patients with non-ST-segment elevation acute coronary syndromes managed with an intended early invasive strategy: primary results of the SYNERGY randomized trial. *JAMA* 2004; 292(1):45-54.
6. Lincoff AM, Bittl JA, Kleiman NS, et al: Comparison of bivalirudin versus heparin during percutaneous coronary intervention (the Randomized Evaluation of PCI Linking Angiomax to Reduced Clinical Events [REPLACE]-1 trial). *Am J Cardiol* 2004; 93(9):1092-1096.
7. Lincoff AM, Kleiman NS, Kereiakes DJ, et al: Long-term efficacy of bivalirudin and provisional glycoprotein IIb/IIIa blockade vs heparin and planned glycoprotein IIb/IIIa blockade during percutaneous coronary revascularization: REPLACE-2 randomized trial. *JAMA* 2004; 292(6):696-703.
8. Madan M, Radhakrishnan S, Reis M, et al: Comparison of enoxaparin versus heparin during elective percutaneous coronary intervention performed with either eptifibatide or tirofiban (the ACTION Trial). *Am J Cardiol* 2005; 95(11):1295-1301.
9. Matthai WH Jr: Use of argatroban during percutaneous coronary interventions in patients with heparin-induced thrombocytopenia. *Semin Thromb Hemost* 1999; 25(Suppl 1):57-60.
10. Stone GW, McLaurin BT, Cox DA, et al: Bivalirudin for patients with acute coronary syndromes. *N Engl J Med* 2006; 355(21):2203-2216.
11. Liu MW, Roubin GS, King SB III: Restenosis after coronary angioplasty. Potential biologic determinants and role of intimal hyperplasia. *Circulation* 1989; 79(6):1374-1387.
12. Schwartz RS, Edwards WD, Huber KC, et al: Coronary restenosis: prospects for solution and new perspectives from a porcine model. *Mayo Clin Proc* 1993; 68(1):54-62.
13. Nobuyoshi M, Kimura T, Nosaka H, et al: Restenosis after successful percutaneous transluminal coronary angioplasty: serial angiographic follow-up of 229 patients. *J Am Coll Cardiol* 1988; 12(3):616-623.
14. Schwartz RS, Holmes DR Jr, Topol EJ: The restenosis paradigm revisited: an alternative proposal for cellular mechanisms. *J Am Coll Cardiol* 1992; 20(5):1284-1293.
15. Serruys PW, Luijten HE, Beatt KJ, et al: Incidence of restenosis after successful coronary angioplasty: a time-related phenomenon. A quantitative angiographic study in 342 consecutive patients at 1, 2, 3, and 4 months. *Circulation* 1988; 77(2):361-371.
16. Detre KM, Holmes DR Jr, Holubkov R, et al: Incidence and consequences of periprocedural occlusion. The 1985-1986 National Heart,

Lung, and Blood Institute Percutaneous Transluminal Coronary Angioplasty Registry. *Circulation* 1990; 82(3):739-750.

17. Sinclair IN, McCabe CH, Sipperly ME, et al: Predictors, therapeutic options and long-term outcome of abrupt reclosure. *Am J Cardiol* 1988; 61(14):61G-66G.

18. George BS, Voorhees WD III, Roubin GS, et al: Multicenter investigation of coronary stenting to treat acute or threatened closure after percutaneous transluminal coronary angioplasty: clinical and angiographic outcomes. *J Am Coll Cardiol* 1993; 22(1):135-143.

19. Kadel C, Vallbracht C, Buss F, et al: Long-term follow-up after percutaneous transluminal coronary angioplasty in patients with single-vessel disease. *Am Heart J* 1992; 124(5):1159-1169.

20. Malenka DJ, O'Rourke D, Miller MA, et al: Cause of in-hospital death in 12,232 consecutive patients undergoing percutaneous transluminal coronary angioplasty. The Northern New England Cardiovascular Disease Study Group. *Am Heart J* 1999; 137(4 Pt 1):632-638.

21. Holmes DR Jr, Vlietstra RE, Smith HC, et al: Restenosis after percutaneous transluminal coronary angioplasty (PTCA): a report from the PTCA Registry of the National Heart, Lung, and Blood Institute. *Am J Cardiol* 1984; 53(12):77C-81C.

22. Berger PB, Bell MR, Garratt KN, et al: Initial results and long-term outcome of coronary angioplasty in chronic mild angina pectoris. *Am J Cardiol* 1993; 71(16):1396-1401.

23. Weintraub WS, Ghazzal ZM, Douglas JS Jr, et al: Long-term clinical follow-up in patients with angiographic restudy after successful angioplasty. *Circulation* 1993; 87(3):831-840.

24. Farb A, Sangiorgi G, Carter AJ, et al: Pathology of acute and chronic coronary stenting in humans. *Circulation* 1999; 99(1):44-52.

25. Fischman DL, Leon MB, Baim DS, et al: A randomized comparison of coronary-stent placement and balloon angioplasty in the treatment of coronary artery disease. Stent Restenosis Study Investigators. *N Engl J Med* 1994; 331(8):496-501.

26. Serruys PW, de Jaegere P, Kiemeneij F, et al: A comparison of balloon-expandable-stent implantation with balloon angioplasty in patients with coronary artery disease. Benestent Study Group. *N Engl J Med* 1994; 331(8):489-495.

27. Cutlip DE, Chauhan MS, Baim DS, et al: Clinical restenosis after coronary stenting: perspectives from multicenter clinical trials. *J Am Coll Cardiol* 2002; 40(12):2082-2089.

28. de Feyter PJ, Kay P, Disco C, et al: Reference chart derived from post-stent-implantation intravascular ultrasound predictors of 6-month expected restenosis on quantitative coronary angiography. *Circulation* 1999; 100(17):1777-1783.

29. Serruys PW, Kay IP, Disco C, et al: Periprocedural quantitative coronary angiography after Palmaz-Schatz stent implantation predicts the restenosis rate at six months: results of a meta-analysis of the BElgian NEtherlands Stent study (BENESTENT) I, BENESTENT II Pilot, BENESTENT II and MUSIC trials. Multicenter Ultrasound Stent In Coronaries. *J Am Coll Cardiol* 1999; 34(4):1067-1074.

30. Choussat R, Klersy C, Black AJ, et al: Long-term (≥8 years) outcome after Palmaz-Schatz stent implantation. *Am J Cardiol* 2001; 88(1):10-16.

31. Karam C, Fajadet J, Beauchet A, et al: Nine-year follow-up of balloon-expandable Palmaz-Schatz stent in patients with single-vessel disease. *Catheter Cardiovasc Interv* 2000; 50(2):170-174.

32. Kiemeneij F, Serruys PW, Macaya C, et al: Continued benefit of coronary stenting versus balloon angioplasty: five-year clinical follow-up of Benestent-I trial. *J Am Coll Cardiol* 2001; 37(6):1598-1603.

33. Kimura T, Yokoi H, Nakagawa Y, et al: Three-year follow-up after implantation of metallic coronary-artery stents. *N Engl J Med* 1996; 334(9):561-566.

34. Laham RJ, Carrozza JP, Berger C, et al: Long-term (4- to 6-year) outcome of Palmaz-Schatz stenting: paucity of late clinical stent-related problems. *J Am Coll Cardiol* 1996; 28(4):820-826.

35. Di Sciascio G, Patti G, D'Ambrosio A, et al: Coronary stenting in patients with depressed left ventricular function: acute and long-term results in a selected population. *Catheter Cardiovasc Interv* 2003; 59(4):429-433.

36. Kornowski R, Mehran R, Satler LF, et al: Procedural results and late clinical outcomes following multivessel coronary stenting. *J Am Coll Cardiol* 1999; 33(2):420-426.

37. McGrath PD, Malenka DJ, Wennberg DE, et al: Changing outcomes in percutaneous coronary interventions: a study of 34,752 procedures in northern New England, 1990 to 1997. Northern New England Cardiovascular Disease Study Group. *J Am Coll Cardiol* 1999; 34(3):674-680.

38. Villareal RP, Lee VV, Elayda MA, et al: Coronary artery bypass surgery versus coronary stenting: risk-adjusted survival rates in 5,619 patients. *Tex Heart Inst J* 2002; 29(1):3-9.

39. Ellis SG, Guetta V, Miller D, et al: Relation between lesion characteristics and risk with percutaneous intervention in the stent and glycoprotein IIb/IIIa era: an analysis of results from 10 907 lesions and proposal for new classification scheme. *Circulation* 1999; 100(19):1971-1976.

40. Holmes DR Jr, Leon MB, Moses JW, et al: Analysis of 1-year clinical outcomes in the SIRIUS trial: a randomized trial of a sirolimus-eluting stent versus a standard stent in patients at high risk for coronary restenosis. *Circulation* 2004; 109(5):634-640.

41. Macaya C, Serruys PW, Ruygrok P, et al: Continued benefit of coronary stenting versus balloon angioplasty: one-year clinical follow-up of Benestent trial. Benestent Study Group. *J Am Coll Cardiol* 1996; 27(2):255-261.

42. Serruys PW, Unger F, Sousa JE, et al: Comparison of coronary-artery bypass surgery and stenting for the treatment of multivessel disease. *N Engl J Med* 2001; 344(15):1117-1124.

43. Stone GW, Ellis SG, Cox DA, et al: One-year clinical results with the slow-release, polymer-based, paclitaxel-eluting TAXUS stent: the TAXUS-IV trial. *Circulation* 2004; 109(16):1942-1947.

44. Mehta SR, Yusuf S, Peters RJ, et al: Effects of pretreatment with clopidogrel and aspirin followed by long-term therapy in patients undergoing percutaneous coronary intervention: the PCI-CURE study. *Lancet* 2001; 358(9281):527-533.

45. Steinhubl SR, Berger PB, Mann JT III, et al: Early and sustained dual oral antiplatelet therapy following percutaneous coronary intervention: a randomized controlled trial. *JAMA* 2002; 288(19):2411-2420.

46. Finkelstein A, McClean D, Kar S, et al: Local drug delivery via a coronary stent with programmable release pharmacokinetics. *Circulation* 2003; 107(5):777-784.

47. Serruys PW, Silber S, Garg S, et al: Comparison of zotarolimus-eluting and everolimus-eluting coronary stents. *N Engl J Med* 2010; 363(2):136-146.

48. Ardissino D, Cavallini C, Bramucci E, et al: Sirolimus-eluting vs uncoated stents for prevention of restenosis in small coronary arteries: a randomized trial. *JAMA* 2004; 292(22):2727-2734.

49. Cervinka P, Stasek J, Pleskot M, et al: Treatment of coronary bifurcation lesions by stent implantation only in parent vessel and angioplasty in sidebranch: immediate and long-term outcome. *J Invasive Cardiol* 2002; 14(12):735-740.

50. Colombo A, Moses JW, Morice MC, et al: Randomized study to evaluate sirolimus-eluting stents implanted at coronary bifurcation lesions. *Circulation* 2004; 109(10):1244-1249.

51. Degertekin M, Arampatzis CA, Lemos PA, et al: Very long sirolimus-eluting stent implantation for de novo coronary lesions. *Am J Cardiol* 2004; 93(7):826-829.

52. Ge L, Iakovou I, Sangiorgi GM, et al: Treatment of saphenous vein graft lesions with drug-eluting stents: immediate and midterm outcome. *J Am Coll Cardiol* 2005; 45(7):989-994.

53. Hermiller JB, Raizner A, Cannon L, et al: Outcomes with the polymer-based paclitaxel-eluting TAXUS stent in patients with diabetes mellitus: the TAXUS-IV trial. *J Am Coll Cardiol* 2005; 45(8):1172-1179.

54. Iakovou I, Schmidt T, Bonizzoni E, et al: Incidence, predictors, and outcome of thrombosis after successful implantation of drug-eluting stents. *JAMA* 2005; 293(17):2126-2130.

55. Kastrati A, Mehilli J, von Beckerath N, et al: Sirolimus-eluting stent or paclitaxel-eluting stent vs balloon angioplasty for prevention of recurrences in patients with coronary in-stent restenosis: a randomized controlled trial. *JAMA* 2005; 293(2):165-171.

56. Kelbaeck H: Stenting of Coronary Arteries in Non-Stress/Benestent Disease (SCANDSTENT). *Paper presented at American College of Cardiology 2005 Scientific Sessions*, 2005; Orlando, FL.

57. Lemos PA, Saia F, Hofma SH, et al: Short- and long-term clinical benefit of sirolimus-eluting stents compared to conventional bare stents for patients with acute myocardial infarction. *J Am Coll Cardiol* 2004; 43(4):704-708.

58. Moussa I, Leon MB, Baim DS, et al: Impact of sirolimus-eluting stents on outcome in diabetic patients: a SIRIUS (SIRolImUS-coated Bx Velocity balloon-expandable stent in the treatment of patients with de novo coronary artery lesions) substudy. *Circulation* 2004; 109(19):2273-2278.

59. Nakamura S, Muthusamy TS, Bae JH, et al: Impact of sirolimus-eluting stent on the outcome of patients with chronic total occlusions. *Am J Cardiol* 2005; 95(2):161-166.

60. Sabaté M: Diabetes and Sirolimus-Eluting Stent (DIABETES) trial. *Paper presented at Transcatheter Therapeutics, 2004*; Washington, D.C.

61. Schampaert E, Cohen EA, Schluter M, et al: The Canadian study of the sirolimus-eluting stent in the treatment of patients with long de novo lesions in small native coronary arteries (C-SIRIUS). *J Am Coll Cardiol* 2004; 43(6):1110-1115.

62. Schofer J, Schluter M, Gershlick AH, et al: Sirolimus-eluting stents for treatment of patients with long atherosclerotic lesions in small coronary arteries: double-blind, randomised controlled trial (E-SIRIUS). *Lancet* 2003; 362(9390):1093-1099.

63. Stone GW, Ellis SG, Cannon L, et al: Comparison of a polymer-based paclitaxel-eluting stent with a bare metal stent in patients with complex coronary artery disease: a randomized controlled trial. *JAMA* 2005; 294(10):1215-1223.

64. Tanabe K, Hoye A, Lemos PA, et al: Restenosis rates following bifurcation stenting with sirolimus-eluting stents for de novo narrowings. *Am J Cardiol* 2004; 94(1):115-118.

65. Valgimigli M, Percoco G, Malagutti P, et al: Tirofiban and sirolimus-eluting stent vs abciximab and bare-metal stent for acute myocardial infarction: a randomized trial. *JAMA* 2005; 293(17):2109-2117.

66. Yamashita T, Nishida T, Adamian MG, et al: Bifurcation lesions: two stents versus one stent—immediate and follow-up results. *J Am Coll Cardiol* 2000; 35(5):1145-1151.

67. Babapulle MN, Joseph L, Belisle P, et al: A hierarchical Bayesian meta-analysis of randomised clinical trials of drug-eluting stents. *Lancet* 2004; 364(9434):583-591.

68. Park SJ, Ahn JM, Kim YH, et al: Trial of everolimus-eluting stents or bypass surgery for coronary disease. *N Engl J Med* 2015; 372(13):1204-1212.

69. Kandzari DE, Barker CS, Leon MB, et al: Dual antiplatelet therapy duration and clinical outcomes following treatment with zotarolimus-eluting stents. *JACC Cardiovasc Interv* 2011; 4(10):1119-1128.

70. Adelman AG, Cohen EA, Kimball BP, et al: A comparison of directional atherectomy with balloon angioplasty for lesions of the left anterior descending coronary artery. *N Engl J Med* 1993; 329(4):228-233.

71. Appelman YE, Piek JJ, Strikwerda S, et al: Randomised trial of excimer laser angioplasty versus balloon angioplasty for treatment of obstructive coronary artery disease. *Lancet* 1996; 347(8994):79-84.

72. Foley DP, Melkert R, Umans VA, et al: Differences in restenosis propensity of devices for transluminal coronary intervention. A quantitative angiographic comparison of balloon angioplasty, directional atherectomy, stent implantation and excimer laser angioplasty. CARPORT, MERCATOR, MARCATOR, PARK, and BENESTENT Trial Groups. *Eur Heart J* 1995; 16(10):1331-1346.

73. Topol EJ, Leya F, Pinkerton CA, et al: A comparison of directional atherectomy with coronary angioplasty in patients with coronary artery disease. The CAVEAT Study Group. *N Engl J Med* 1993; 329(4):221-227.

74. Bittl JA, Chew DP, Topol EJ, et al: Meta-analysis of randomized trials of percutaneous transluminal coronary angioplasty versus atherectomy, cutting balloon atherotomy, or laser angioplasty. *J Am Coll Cardiol* 2004; 43(6):936-942.

75. Feld H, Schulhoff N, Lichstein E, et al: Coronary atherectomy versus angioplasty: the CAVA Study. *Am Heart J* 1993; 126(1):31-38.

76. Parikh K, Chandra P, Choksi N, et al: Safety and feasibility of orbital atherectomy for the treatment of calcified coronary lesions: The ORBIT I Trial. *Catheter Cardiovasc Interv* 2013:[E-pub ahead of print].

77. Beran G, Lang I, Schreiber W, et al: Intracoronary thrombectomy with the X-sizer catheter system improves epicardial flow and accelerates ST-segment resolution in patients with acute coronary syndrome: a prospective, randomized, controlled study. *Circulation* 2002; 105(20):2355-2360.

78. Stone GW, Cox DA, Low R, et al: Safety and efficacy of a novel device for treatment of thrombotic and atherosclerotic lesions in native coronary arteries and saphenous vein grafts: results from the multicenter X-Sizer for treatment of thrombus and atherosclerosis in coronary applications trial (X-TRACT) study. *Catheter Cardiovasc Interv* 2003; 58(4):419-427.

79. Baim DS, Wahr D, George B, et al: Randomized trial of a distal embolic protection device during percutaneous intervention of saphenous vein aorto-coronary bypass grafts. *Circulation* 2002; 105(11):1285-1290.

80. Stone GW, Webb J, Cox DA, et al: Distal microcirculatory protection during percutaneous coronary intervention in acute ST-segment elevation myocardial infarction: a randomized controlled trial. *JAMA* 2005; 293(9):1063-1072.

81. Casella G, Klauss V, Ottani F, et al: Impact of intravascular ultrasound-guided stenting on long-term clinical outcome: a meta-analysis of available studies comparing intravascular ultrasound-guided and angiographically guided stenting. *Catheter Cardiovasc Interv* 2003; 59(3):314-321.

82. Prati F, Regar E, Mintz GS, et al: Expert review document on methodology, terminology, and clinical applications of optical coherence tomography: physical principles, methodology of image acquisition, and clinical application for assessment of coronary arteries and atherosclerosis. *Eur Heart J* 2010; 31(4):401-415.

83. Tonino PA, De Bruyne B, Pijls NH, et al: Fractional flow reserve versus angiography for guiding percutaneous coronary intervention. *N Engl J Med* 2009; 360(3):213-224.

84. De Bruyne B, Fearon WF, Pijls NH, et al: Fractional flow reserve-guided PCI for stable coronary artery disease. *N Engl J Med* 2014; 371(13):1208-1217.

85. Leon MB, Teirstein PS, Moses JW, et al: Localized intracoronary gamma-radiation therapy to inhibit the recurrence of restenosis after stenting. *N Engl J Med* 2001; 344(4):250-256.

86. Waksman R, Bhargava B, White RL, et al: Intracoronary radiation for patients with refractory in-stent restenosis: an analysis from the WRIST-Crossover Trial. Washington Radiation for In-stent Restenosis Trial. *Cardiovasc Radiat Med* 1999; 1(4):317-322.

87. Ellis SG, Myler RK, King SB III, et al: Causes and correlates of death after unsupported coronary angioplasty: implications for use of angioplasty and advanced support techniques in high-risk settings. *Am J Cardiol* 1991; 68(15):1447-1451.

88. Briguori C, Sarais C, Pagnotta P, et al: Elective versus provisional intra-aortic balloon pumping in high-risk percutaneous transluminal coronary angioplasty. *Am Heart J* 2003; 145(4):700-707.

89. Thiele H, Lauer B, Hambrecht R, et al: Reversal of cardiogenic shock by percutaneous left atrial-to-femoral arterial bypass assistance. *Circulation* 2001; 104(24):2917-2922.

90. Dangas GD, Kini AS, Sharma SK, et al: Impact of hemodynamic support with Impella 2.5 versus intra-aortic balloon pump on prognostically important clinical outcomes in patients undergoing high-risk percutaneous coronary intervention (from the PROTECT II randomized trial). *Am J Cardiol* 2014; 113(2):222-228.

91. Seyfarth M, Sibbing D, Bauer I, et al: A randomized clinical trial to evaluate the safety and efficacy of a percutaneous left ventricular assist device versus intra-aortic balloon pumping for treatment of cardiogenic shock caused by myocardial infarction. *J Am Coll Cardiol* 2008; 52(19):1584-1588.

92. Thiele H, Sick P, Boudriot E, et al: Randomized comparison of intra-aortic balloon support with a percutaneous left ventricular assist device in patients with revascularized acute myocardial infarction complicated by cardiogenic shock. *Eur Heart J* 2005; 26(13):1276-1283.

93. Nikolsky E, Mehran R, Halkin A, et al: Vascular complications associated with arteriotomy closure devices in patients undergoing percutaneous coronary procedures: a meta-analysis. *J Am Coll Cardiol* 2004; 44(6):1200-1209.

94. Mann T, Cowper PA, Peterson ED, et al: Transradial coronary stenting: comparison with femoral access closed with an arterial suture device. *Catheter Cardiovasc Interv* 2000; 49(2):150-156.

95. Yadav M, Genereux P, Palmerini T, et al: SYNTAX score and the risk of stent thrombosis after percutaneous coronary intervention in patients with non-ST-segment elevation acute coronary syndromes: an ACUITY trial substudy. *Catheter Cardiovasc Interv* 2015; 85(1):1-10.

96. Wong SC, Minutello R, Hong MK: Neurological complications following percutaneous coronary interventions (a report from the 2000-2001 New York State Angioplasty Registry). *Am J Cardiol* 2005; 96(9):1248-1250.

97. Fuchs S, Stabile E, Kinnaird TD, et al: Stroke complicating percutaneous coronary interventions: incidence, predictors, and prognostic implications. *Circulation* 2002; 106(1):86-91.

98. Califf RM, Abdelmeguid AE, Kuntz RE, et al: Myonecrosis after revascularization procedures. *J Am Coll Cardiol* 1998; 31(2):241-251.

99. Stone GW, Mehran R, Dangas G, et al: Differential impact on survival of electrocardiographic Q-wave versus enzymatic myocardial infarction after percutaneous intervention: a device-specific analysis of 7147 patients. *Circulation* 2001; 104(6):642-647.

100. Brener SJ, Lytle BW, Schneider JP, et al: Association between CK-MB elevation after percutaneous or surgical revascularization and three-year mortality. *J Am Coll Cardiol* 2002; 40(11):1961-1967.

101. Briguori C, Colombo A, Airoldi F, et al: Statin administration before percutaneous coronary intervention: impact on periprocedural myocardial infarction. *Eur Heart J* 2004; 25(20):1822-1828.

102. Lee CH, Wong HB, Tan HC, et al: Impact of reversibility of no reflow phenomenon on 30-day mortality following percutaneous revascularization for acute myocardial infarction-insights from a 1,328 patient registry. *J Interv Cardiol* 2005; 18(4):261-266.

103. Ellis SG, Ajluni S, Arnold AZ, et al: Increased coronary perforation in the new device era. Incidence, classification, management, and outcome. *Circulation* 1994; 90(6):2725-2730.

104. Fasseas P, Orford JL, Panetta CJ, et al: Incidence, correlates, management, and clinical outcome of coronary perforation: analysis of 16,298 procedures. *Am Heart J* 2004; 147(1):140-145.

105. Fejka M, Dixon SR, Safian RD, et al: Diagnosis, management, and clinical outcome of cardiac tamponade complicating percutaneous coronary intervention. *Am J Cardiol* 2002; 90(11):1183-1186.

106. Schachinger V, Hamm CW, Munzel T, et al: A randomized trial of polytetrafluoroethylene-membrane-covered stents compared with conventional stents in aortocoronary saphenous vein grafts. *J Am Coll Cardiol* 2003; 42(8):1360-1369.

107. Ly H, Awaida JP, Lesperance J, et al: Angiographic and clinical outcomes of polytetrafluoroethylene-covered stent use in significant coronary perforations. *Am J Cardiol* 2005; 95(2):244-246.

108. Briguori C, Nishida T, Anzuini A, et al: Emergency polytetrafluoroethylene-covered stent implantation to treat coronary ruptures. *Circulation* 2000; 102(25):3028-3031.

109. Freeman RV, O'Donnell M, Share D, et al: Nephropathy requiring dialysis after percutaneous coronary intervention and the critical role of an adjusted contrast dose. *Am J Cardiol* 2002; 90(10):1068-1073.

110. Marenzi G, Lauri G, Assanelli E, et al: Contrast-induced nephropathy in patients undergoing primary angioplasty for acute myocardial infarction. *J Am Coll Cardiol* 2004; 44(9):1780-1785.

111. Mehran R, Aymong ED, Nikolsky E, et al: A simple risk score for prediction of contrast-induced nephropathy after percutaneous coronary intervention: development and initial validation. *J Am Coll Cardiol* 2004; 44(7):1393-1399.

112. Mueller C, Buerkle G, Buettner HJ, et al: Prevention of contrast media-associated nephropathy: randomized comparison of 2 hydration regimens in 1620 patients undergoing coronary angioplasty. *Arch Intern Med* 2002; 162(3):329-336.

113. Lindsay J, Apple S, Pinnow EE, et al: Percutaneous coronary intervention-associated nephropathy foreshadows increased risk of late adverse events in patients with normal baseline serum creatinine. *Catheter Cardiovasc Interv* 2003; 59(3):338-343.

114. Aspelin P, Aubry P, Fransson SG, et al: Nephrotoxic effects in high-risk patients undergoing angiography. *N Engl J Med* 2003; 348(6):491-499.

115. Misra D, Leibowitz K, Gowda RM, et al: Role of N-acetylcysteine in prevention of contrast-induced nephropathy after cardiovascular procedures: a meta-analysis. *Clin Cardiol* 2004; 27(11):607-610.

116. Tepel M, van der Giet M, Schwarzfeld C, et al: Prevention of radiographic-contrast-agent-induced reductions in renal function by acetylcysteine. *N Engl J Med* 2000; 343(3):180-184.

117. Kagan A, Sheikh-Hamad D: Contrast-induced kidney injury: focus on modifiable risk factors and prophylactic strategies. *Clin Cardiol* 2010; 33(2):62-66.

118. Andersen HR, Nielsen TT, Rasmussen K, et al: A comparison of coronary angioplasty with fibrinolytic therapy in acute myocardial infarction. *N Engl J Med* 2003; 349(8):733-742.

119. Ribichini F, Steffenino G, Dellavalle A, et al: Comparison of thrombolytic therapy and primary coronary angioplasty with liberal stenting for inferior myocardial infarction with precordial ST-segment depression: immediate and long-term results of a randomized study. *J Am Coll Cardiol* 1998; 32(6):1687-1694.

120. Schomig A, Kastrati A, Dirschinger J, et al: Coronary stenting plus platelet glycoprotein IIb/IIIa blockade compared with tissue plasminogen activator in acute myocardial infarction. Stent versus Thrombolysis for Occluded Coronary Arteries in Patients with Acute Myocardial Infarction Study Investigators. *N Engl J Med* 2000; 343(6):385-391.

121. Antoniucci D, Santoro GM, Bolognese L, et al: A clinical trial comparing primary stenting of the infarct-related artery with optimal primary angioplasty for acute myocardial infarction: results from the Florence Randomized Elective Stenting in Acute Coronary Occlusions (FRESCO) trial. *J Am Coll Cardiol* 1998; 31(6):1234-1239.

122. Mahdi NA, Lopez J, Leon M, et al: Comparison of primary coronary stenting to primary balloon angioplasty with stent bailout for the treatment of patients with acute myocardial infarction. *Am J Cardiol* 1998; 81(8):957-963.

123. Neumann FJ, Kastrati A, Schmitt C, et al: Effect of glycoprotein IIb/IIIa receptor blockade with abciximab on clinical and angiographic restenosis rate after the placement of coronary stents following acute myocardial infarction. *J Am Coll Cardiol* 2000; 35(4):915-921.

124. Rodriguez A, Bernardi V, Fernandez M, et al: In-hospital and late results of coronary stents versus conventional balloon angioplasty in acute myocardial infarction (GRAMI trial). Gianturco-Roubin in Acute Myocardial Infarction. *Am J Cardiol* 1998; 81(11):1286-1291.

125. Berger PB, Holmes DR Jr, Stebbins AL, et al: Impact of an aggressive invasive catheterization and revascularization strategy on mortality in patients with cardiogenic shock in the Global Utilization of Streptokinase and Tissue Plasminogen Activator for Occluded Coronary Arteries (GUSTO-I) trial. An observational study. *Circulation* 1997; 96(1):122-127.

126. Giugliano GR, Kuntz RE, Popma JJ, et al: Determinants of 30-day adverse events following saphenous vein graft intervention with and without a distal occlusion embolic protection device. *Am J Cardiol* 2005; 95(2):173-177.

127. Schomig A, Ndrepepa G, Mehilli J, et al: A randomized trial of coronary stenting versus balloon angioplasty as a rescue intervention after failed thrombolysis in patients with acute myocardial infarction. *J Am Coll Cardiol* 2004; 44(10):2073-2079.

128. Sutton AG, Campbell PG, Graham R, et al: A randomized trial of rescue angioplasty versus a conservative approach for failed fibrinolysis in ST-segment elevation myocardial infarction: the Middlesbrough Early Revascularization to Limit INfarction (MERLIN) trial. *J Am Coll Cardiol* 2004; 44(2):287-296.

129. Yellon DM, Hausenloy DJ: Myocardial reperfusion injury. *N Engl J Med* 2007; 357(11):1121-1135.

130. Brener SJ, Ellis SG, Apperson-Hansen C, et al: Comparison of stenting and balloon angioplasty for narrowings in aortocoronary saphenous vein conduits in place for more than five years. *Am J Cardiol* 1997; 79(1):13-18.

131. Eeckhout E, Goy JJ, Stauffer JC, et al: Endoluminal stenting of narrowed saphenous vein grafts: long-term clinical and angiographic follow-up. *Cathet Cardiovasc Diagn* 1994; 32(2):139-146.

132. Frimerman A, Rechavia E, Eigler N, et al: Long-term follow-up of a high risk cohort after stent implantation in saphenous vein grafts. *J Am Coll Cardiol* 1997; 30(5):1277-1283.

133. Piana RN, Moscucci M, Cohen DJ, et al: Palmaz-Schatz stenting for treatment of focal vein graft stenosis: immediate results and long-term outcome. *J Am Coll Cardiol* 1994; 23(6):1296-1304.

134. Wong SC, Baim DS, Schatz RA, et al: Immediate results and late outcomes after stent implantation in saphenous vein graft lesions: the multicenter U.S. Palmaz-Schatz stent experience. *J Am Coll Cardiol* 1995; 26(3):704-712.

135. Sianos G, Morel MA, Kappetein AP, et al: The SYNTAX Score: an angiographic tool grading the complexity of coronary artery disease. *EuroIntervention* 2005; 1(2):219-227.

136. Valgimigli M, Serruys PW, Tsuchida K, et al: Cyphering the complexity of coronary artery disease using the SYNTAX score to predict clinical outcome in patients with three-vessel lumen obstruction undergoing percutaneous coronary intervention. *Am J Cardiol* 2007; 99(8):1072-1081.

137. Kennedy JA, Kiosoglous AJ, Murphy GA, et al: Effect of perhexiline and oxfenicine on myocardial function and metabolism during low-flow ischemia/reperfusion in the isolated rat heart. *J Cardiovasc Pharmacol* 2000; 36(6):794-801.

138. Morrow DA, Givertz MM: Modulation of myocardial energetics: emerging evidence for a therapeutic target in cardiovascular disease. *Circulation* 2005; 112(21):3218-3221.

139. Tracey WR, Treadway JL, Magee WP, et al: Cardioprotective effects of ingliforib, a novel glycogen phosphorylase inhibitor. *Am J Physiol Heart Circ Physiol* 2004; 286(3):H1177-1184.

140. Perin EC, Dohmann HF, Borojevic R, et al: Improved exercise capacity and ischemia 6 and 12 months after transendocardial injection of autologous bone marrow mononuclear cells for ischemic cardiomyopathy. *Circulation* 2004; 110(11 Suppl 1):II213-218.

Myocardial Revascularization with Cardiopulmonary Bypass

20

Michael H. Kwon • George Tolis, Jr. • Thoralf M. Sundt

Coronary artery disease (CAD) remains the single largest killer of Americans, accounting for almost half a million deaths per year. It imposes a particular burden on the elderly, with more than 80% of all CAD deaths occurring in those over age 65.[1] The magnitude of this impact takes on great significance because it is expected that the number of Americans older than 65 years of age will more than double over the next four decades.[2] If you add to this aging population the anticipated increase in the prevalence of important risk factors for CAD such as diabetes mellitus (DM) and obesity, the population at risk for CAD can only be expected to increase.

Myocardial revascularization represents an effective treatment strategy shown to prolong survival. Techniques of revascularization include percutaneous coronary intervention (PCI) and coronary artery bypass graft (CABG) surgery, which can be performed with or without cardiopulmonary bypass. Current techniques for CABG can be carried out with low perioperative morbidity and mortality, with excellent long-term outcomes despite an increasing risk profile.[3] CABG surgery with cardiopulmonary bypass remains the standard by which the other techniques (ie, PCI, off-pump CABG, robotic CABG, hybrid revascularization) are measured.[4,5] It is expected that it will continue to be a cornerstone in the management of CAD in the foreseeable future.

HISTORY OF CORONARY ARTERY BYPASS GRAFTING

The modern era of myocardial revascularization with cardiopulmonary bypass began in 1954 when Dr. John Gibbon reported the development of the cardiopulmonary bypass machine.[6] An additional seminal advance occurred with the development of coronary angiography by Mason Sones at the Cleveland Clinic in 1957, which opened the door to the elective treatment of coronary atherosclerosis by means of direct revascularization.[7] Initial reports by Rene Favaloro and Donald B. Effler on their techniques to treat clinical events associated with stenotic lesions of the coronary arteries culminated in the first large series of aorto-to-coronary artery venous grafts reported in 1969.[8] Simultaneously Dudley Johnson of Milwaukee published a series of 301 patients in 1969.[9] The success of these techniques was soon demonstrated in larger series initiating the modern era of coronary artery surgery.

INDICATIONS FOR SURGICAL CORONARY REVASCULARIZATION

The practicing cardiac surgeon is confronted with no clinical question more often than, "Is coronary bypass indicated in this patient?" In brief, the indications established by the American College of Cardiology Foundation and the American Heart Association (ACCF/AHA) consensus panel are based predominantly on the results of trials comparing surgical revascularization with medical therapy for patients with chronic stable angina.[10] Three major historical trials, the Coronary Artery Surgery Study (CASS), the Veterans Administration Coronary Artery Bypass Cooperative Study Group, and the European Coronary Surgery Study (ECSS), demonstrated the greatest survival benefit of revascularization to be among those patients at highest risk of death from the disease itself as defined by the severity of angina and/or ischemia, the number of diseased vessels, and the presence of left ventricular dysfunction.[11-13] Even as the technology and methods for all manner of revascularization strategies improve, the principles established by these seminal trials continue to serve as the basis upon which the results of newer trials designed to study specific populations, clinical scenarios, and anatomic patterns of disease are compared and interpreted.

Clinical and Laboratory Assessment of Coronary Artery Disease

A surgeon's first introduction to a patient with CAD is frequently a conventional coronary angiogram. Indeed most studies of coronary revascularization have stratified risk and grouped patients according to the number and distribution of coronary lesions. For the purposes of this discussion, and in an effort to be consistent with the large body of literature upon which the current ACCF/AHA guidelines are based, "significant" stenosis is defined as ≥70% reduction in luminal diameter of a coronary artery other than the left main coronary artery (LMCA) for which ≥50% reduction is considered significant.[10] A major development in the last decade in assessing the severity of coronary disease has been the introduction of the SYNTAX score,[14] which is a pure angiographic score of severity and complexity that has recently been validated to correlate with 3-year outcomes in patients with triple vessel and/or main stem disease. It uses dedicated computer software to assign points to each lesion based on length, degree of stenosis, and relation to areas of bifurcation/trifurcation, such that the higher the overall score, the more complex the coronary disease. Although the anatomic distribution and severity of hemodynamically significant coronary lesions determines, in large part, the optimal therapy (CABG, PCI, or medical therapy), the clinical presentation and results of noninvasive studies of myocardial perfusion and function are necessary to characterize the pathophysiologic implications of the angiographic disease and its impact on prognosis and, therefore, to make a clinically appropriate recommendation. In the technological era in which we practice, the importance of the clinical history bears emphasis, particularly in an aging population. Because one of the objectives of surgery is to improve symptoms and quality of life, a thorough appreciation of the patient's functional status is a prerequisite in selecting the optimal therapeutic strategy.

The system proposed by the Canadian Cardiovascular Society for grading the clinical severity of angina pectoris is widely accepted (Table 20-1). Unfortunately, angina is a highly subjective phenomenon for both patient and physician, and prospective evaluation of the assessment of functional classification by the CCS criteria has demonstrated a reproducibility of only 73%.[15] Furthermore, there may be a strikingly poor correlation between the severity of symptoms and the magnitude of ischemia, as is notoriously the case among diabetic patients with asymptomatic "silent ischemia."

Electrocardiography (ECG), if abnormal, is helpful in assessing ischemic burden. Unfortunately, it demonstrates no pathognomonic signs in half of patients with chronic stable angina. Still the monitoring of an ECG under stress conditions is simple and inexpensive, and is therefore useful as a screening examination. Among patients with anatomically defined disease, stress ECG provides additional information about the severity of ischemia and the prognosis of the disease. The sensitivity of the test increases with age, with the severity of the patient's disease, and with the magnitude of observed ST-segment shift.[16] If ST-segment depression is greater than 1 mm, stress ECG has a predictive value of 90%, whereas a 2-mm shift with accompanying angina is virtually diagnostic.[17] Early onset of ST-segment depression and prolonged depression after the discontinuation of exercise are strongly associated with significant multivessel disease. Unfortunately, many patients cannot achieve their target heart rates owing to beta blockade or a limitation to their exercise tolerance caused by coexisting disease, decreasing the usefulness of this test in these often high-risk patients. Resting abnormalities in the ECG may also limit the predictive accuracy of the test.

Perfusion imaging with thallium-201 or a technetium-99m–based tracer may be particularly useful in patients with abnormalities on their baseline ECG. Reversible defects demonstrated by comparison of images obtained after injection of the tracer at peak stress with rest images is indicative of ischemia, and hence viability. An irreversible defect indicates a nonviable scar. The results obtained with both tracers are similar, with the average sensitivity around 90% and specificity of approximately 75%.[18] For patients unable to exercise, pharmacologic vasodilators such as adenosine or dipyridamole may be used with similar sensitivity.[19]

Echocardiographic imaging during exercise or pharmacologic stress has gained increasing popularity among cardiologists. Comparative studies have demonstrated accuracy similar to that of nuclear studies with sensitivity and specificity both around 85%.[18] Patients unable to exercise may be stressed with high-dose dipyridamole, or more commonly dobutamine at doses from 5 to 40 μg/kg/min. An initial augmentation of contractility followed by loss or "drop out" is diagnostic of ischemia (and accordingly viability), whereas failure to augment contractility at low dose suggests scar. Additionally, information regarding concomitant valvular disease may be obtained during the examination.[20]

Guidelines for Revascularization

In any discussion regarding the discrete indications for coronary revascularization, it is critical to bear in mind that the overarching goal of revascularization is to either improve

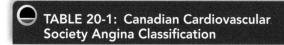

TABLE 20-1: Canadian Cardiovascular Society Angina Classification

Canadian Cardiovascular Society

Angina Classification

0 = No angina

1 = Angina only with strenuous or prolonged exertion

2 = Angina with walking at a rapid pace on the level, on a grade, or upstairs (slight limitation of normal activities)

3 = Angina with walking at a normal pace less than two blocks or one flight of stairs (marked limitation)

4 = Angina with even mild activity

symptoms, prolong survival, or, inasmuch as is inextricably tied to both of these goals, to delay and prevent the complications of coronary disease in order to provide improved quality of life over the period of prolonged survival. With this fundamental principle in mind, the guidelines for surgical revascularization established by the ACCF/AHA were significantly revised in terms of organizational structure in 2011 to reflect this understanding (Tables 20-2 and 20-3).[10] These guidelines outline the recommendations regarding whether revascularization is indicated by either CABG or PCI in comparison to medical therapy in specific subsets of patients grouped primarily by the goal of revascularization (either improvement of survival or improvement of symptoms). Indications are then only secondarily stratified by the anatomic pattern and severity of coronary lesions, taking into account the number of involved vessels, involvement of the LMCA, the proximal left anterior descending artery (LAD). Only after these two distinctions are made are the effects of baseline clinical scenario (eg, presence of diabetes, severity of left ventricular dysfunction, presence of unstable angina, non-ST elevation and ST elevation myocardial infarction [MI], and the calculated operative mortality, among others) taken into account to determine the recommendations for specific situations.[21,10] The basis for these guidelines resides in the large body of literature comparing medical therapy with CABG and PCI in patients with stable angina.

Recommendations are categorized into classes whereby Class I denotes that the benefit exceeds the risk and the procedure/treatment should be performed, Class IIa denotes that the benefit likely exceeds the risk and that it is reasonable to administer the treatment, Class IIb may be equivalent to or exceed the risk but additional studies are necessary to confirm, and that the treatment may be considered. Finally Class III represents a recommendation to not perform the procedure or treatment as it is known to have no benefit and in some cases be harmful.[10] Each recommendation is paired with a description of the strength of evidence available to support the recommendation, and ranges from Level A, denoting data derived from multiple randomized controlled trials or meta-analyses, Level B which denotes data from a single randomized trial or nonrandomized studies, and Level C which represents data from just consensus opinions from experts, case studies, and or previously established standard of care.[10]

The complexity of the guidelines reflects the overall complexity and heterogeneity of the patient population presenting with CAD. With the major components of the guidelines summarized at face value in Tables 20-2 and 20-3, this section of the chapter aims to simultaneously deepen and simplify the understanding of these guidelines by (1) providing the historical background from seminal randomized controlled trials and registry studies that provided the basis for how to assign patients with stable angina to surgical revascularization versus PCI or medical therapy, and (2) provide an update on the more recent trials that inform the current guidelines in order to provide a framework for how to approach a patient presenting with CAD today.

APPROACH TO THE LITERATURE

Before reviewing the results of the seminal trials of CABG versus medical therapy performed in the 1970s and those of newer prospectively randomized trials comparing the results of surgery with PCI and medical therapy, some limitations of these trials and of those that followed must be recognized. First, in retrospective or registry studies, it is difficult to ensure comparable patient populations by virtue of the extraordinary anatomical and physiologic complexity of CAD as well as the heterogeneity of the patient substrate. Differences in ventricular function and comorbidities such as age, diabetes, peripheral vascular disease, and pulmonary disease may have a profound impact on outcomes such as survival or quality of life. For example, caution must be exercised in interpreting the results of nonrandomized and registry reports of PCI versus surgery, because the patients subjected to the former more often have one- or two-vessel disease,[22,23] whereas the latter commonly have three-vessel or left main disease.[22,23] Attempts to correct for selection bias with statistical techniques such as propensity matching are only as valid as the parameters entered into the model. Data less tangible than gender or chronologic age, such as socioeconomic status or "physiologic age," are not easily accounted for in such analyses and yet may be a critical determinant of outcomes. Despite this limitation, retrospective and registry data provide a better glimpse of the real world of CAD. Most prospective randomized trials include only a fraction of the total population undergoing revascularization by virtue of strict entry criteria. For example, the Bypass Angioplasty Revascularization Investigators (BARI) trial entered only 5% of total patients screened.[24] Although more recent randomized controlled trials of PCI versus CABG have had better yield (41-71%), these studies have focused on specific subset populations including patients with diabetes, and those with three-vessel and/or left main coronary disease.[4,25,26] Therefore, although the prospectively randomized studies do provide objective data directly applicable to the specific patient subset represented in the study, extrapolation of the results to the more heterogeneous populations seen clinically can only be made if the implicit caveats are clearly understood. We must be mindful of the inescapable tradeoff between selection bias in registry studies and entry bias in randomized studies.

Second, as a consequence of the overrepresentation of patients at lowest risk of death in randomized trials, most are statistically underpowered with respect to survival analysis. For example, given current survival statistics, we would need approximately 2000 patients in each arm of a study to detect a 30% difference in mortality. The problem is compounded by the exclusion of the very patients for whom one would anticipate a survival advantage with adequate revascularization, such as those with depressed ventricular function. Randomized studies frequently employ softer endpoints such as angina or quality of life, or create composites of qualitatively different endpoints, such as death, stroke, and MI. Meaningful analysis is further complicated

TABLE 20-2: 2011 AHA/ACC Guidelines for CABG

Revascularization to Improve Survival Compared with Medical Therapy

Anatomic setting	Class of recommendation	LOE
Unprotected left main or complex CAD		
CABG and PCI	I—Heart Team approach recommended	C
CABG and PCI	IIa—Calculation of STS and SYNTAX scores	B
Unprotected left main*		
CABG	I	B
PCI	IIa—For SIHD when both of the following are present:	B
	• Anatomic conditions associated with a low risk of PCI procedural complications and a high likelihood of good long outcome (eg, a low SYNTAX score of ≤ 22, ostial or trunk left main CAD)	
	• Clinical characteristics that predict a significantly increased risk of adverse surgical outcomes (eg, STS-predicted risk of operative mortality ≥ 5%)	
	IIa—For UA/NSTEMI if not a CABG candidate	B
	IIa—For STEMI when distal coronary flow is TIMI flow grade < 3 and PCI can be performed more rapidly and safely than CABG	C
	IIb—For SIHD when *both* of the following are present:	B
	• Anatomic conditions associated with a low-to-intermediate risk of PCI procedural complications and an intermediate to high likelihood of good long-term outcome (eg, low-to-intermediate SYNTAX score of <33, bifurcation left main CAD)	
	• Clinical characteristics that predict an increased risk of adverse surgical outcomes (eg, moderate–severe COPD, disability from prior stroke, or prior cardiac surgery; STS-predicted risk of operative mortality > 2%)	
	III: Harm—For SIHD in patients (vs performing CABG) with unfavorable anatomy for PCI and who are good candidates for CABG	B
Three-vessel disease with or without proximal LAD artery disease		
CABG	I	B
	IIa—It is reasonable to choose CABG over PCI in patients with complex three-vessel CAD (eg, SYNTAX > 22) who are good candidates for CABG	B
PCI	IIb—Of uncertain benefit	B
Two-vessel disease with proximal LAD artery disease		
CABG	I	B
PCI	IIb	B
Two-vessel disease without proximal LAD artery disease		
CABG	IIa—With extensive ischemia	B
	IIb—Of uncertain benefit without extensive ischemia	C
PCI	IIb—Of uncertain benefit	B
One-vessel proximal LAD artery disease		
CABG	IIa—With LIMA for long-term benefit	B
PCI	IIb—Of uncertain benefit	B
One-vessel disease without proximal LAD artery involvement		
CABG	III: Harm	B
PCI	III: Harm	B
LV Dysfunction		
CABG	IIa—EF 35 to 50%	B
	IIb—EF < 35% without significant left main CAD	B
PCI	Insufficient data	
Survivors of sudden cardiac death with presumed ischemia-mediated VT		
CABG	I	B
PCI	I	C
No anatomic physiologic criteria for revascularization		
CABG	III: Harm	B
PCI	III: Harm	B

*In patients with multivessel disease who also have diabetes, it is reasonable to choose CABG (with LIMA) over PCI (Class IIa/LOE B).
CABG, coronary artery bypass graft; CAD, coronary artery disease; COPD, chronic obstructive pulmonary disease; EF, ejection fraction; LAD, left anterior descending; LIMA, left internal mammary artery; LOE, level of evidence; LV, left ventricular; PCI, percutaneous coronary intervention; SIHD, stable ischemic heart disease; STEMI, ST-elevation myocardial infarction; STS, Society of Thoracic Surgeons; SYNTAX, Synergy Between Percutaneous Coronary Intervention With Taxus and Cardiac Surgery; TIMI, Thrombolysis in myocardial infarction; UA/NSTEMI, unstable angina/non-ST-elevation myocardial infarction; UPLM, unprotected left main disease; VT, ventricular tachycardia.

TABLE 20-3: 2011 AHA/ACC Guidelines for CABG		

Revascularization to Improve Symptoms with Significant Anatomic (≥50% Left Main or ≥70% Non-Left Main CAD) or Physiological (Fractional Flow Reserve ≤ 0.80) Coronary Artery Disease

Clinical setting	Class of recommendation	LOE
≥1 significant stenoses amenable to revascularization and unacceptable angina despite GDMT		
CABG	I	A
PCI	I	A
≥1 significant stenoses and unacceptable angina in whom GDMT cannot be implemented because of medication contraindications, adverse effects, or patient preferences		
CABG	IIa	C
PCI	IIa	C
Previous CABG with ≥1 significant stenoses associated with ischemia and unacceptable angina despite GDMT		
PCI	IIa	C
CABG	IIb	C
Complex three-vessel CAD (eg, SYNTAX score > 22) with or without involvement of the proximal LAD artery and a good candidate for CABG		
CABG	IIa—CABG preferred over PCI	B
Viable ischemic myocardium that is perfused by coronary arteries that are not amenable to grafting		
Transmyocardial laser Revascularization (TMR)	IIb—TMR as an adjunct to CABG	B
No anatomic or physiologic criteria for revascularization		
CABG	III: Harm	C
PCI	III: Harm	C

CABG, coronary artery bypass graft; CAD, coronary artery disease; GDMT, guideline-directed medical therapy; PCI, percutaneous coronary intervention.

by relatively short-term follow-up in most studies. Events such as the need for subsequent revascularization and recurrence of angina characteristically occur at different time intervals after these therapies (restenosis after PCI vs graft occlusion after CABG), and an 8- to 10-year follow-up period is needed to adequately compare long-term results. Patients themselves are also generally interested in outcomes measured in years, not months.

Significant improvements in each of the treatment strategies for CAD are occurring constantly. Examples include the increased use of antiplatelet agents, angiotensin-converting enzyme inhibitors, lipid-lowering therapy, internal thoracic aortic (ITA) grafts, and drug-eluting stents (DESs). These advances, along with aggressive secondary prevention after revascularization, have steadily reduced the morbidity and mortality of CAD in all patients, making differences in the hard endpoint of survival difficult but not impossible to demonstrate for any therapy.[27] This trend will likely increase as the beneficial effect of secondary prevention becomes more widely appreciated.

Comparative Trials of Revascularization versus Medical Therapy in Stable Angina

MEDICAL THERAPY

In the decades since CABG surgery was popularized and coronary angioplasty introduced, an enormous volume of data on the results of invasive revascularization has been collected. Remarkably, almost from the outset many of these studies have been prospectively randomized. Yet in the current era there is a dearth of data concerning pharmacologic therapies for chronic CAD despite remarkable recent drug development. For example, although nitrates are unquestionably effective in relieving symptoms, the impact of long-acting nitrates on clinical outcomes has never been rigorously tested. Furthermore, there has been only one trial of beta-blocker therapy in the treatment of angina, the Atenolol Silent Ischemia Study, which demonstrated benefit for patients with mild effort induced angina or silent ischemia.[28] There remain no randomized studies examining the impact of beta blockers on survival on patients with stable angina. The only evidence for improved survival with beta-blocker use comes from one recent registry study demonstrating a statistically insignificant trend toward improved survival for post-MI patients who received beta blockers.[29] A handful of studies of combination therapy with beta blockers and calcium channel blockers have also demonstrated antianginal benefit, but again without any evidence that there is any impact on survival.[30-32]

SURGICAL VERSUS MEDICAL THERAPY

Three major randomized studies, the CASS,[12] the Veterans Administration Cooperative Study Group (VA),[13,33] and the ECSS,[34,35] as well as several other smaller randomized trials,[36-38] conducted between 1972 and 1984, provide the historical foundation for comparing the outcomes of medical and surgical therapy. Despite the limitations noted in the preceding, these studies are remarkably consistent in their major findings, and the qualitative conclusions drawn from them continue to be generalizable to current practice.

The central message from all of these studies is that the relative benefits of bypass surgery over medical therapy on survival are greatest in those patients at highest risk as defined by the severity of angina and/or ischemia, the number of diseased vessels, and the presence of left ventricular dysfunction.[39] For example, thus far, no study has shown survival benefit for CABG over medical therapy for patients with single-vessel disease not involving the proximal LAD. Accordingly, the current guidelines recommend that CABG be performed on a Class I recommendation for all unprotected left main disease,[39-41] three-vessel disease,[35,39,42-44] and two-vesseldisease with proximal LAD disease,[35,39,42-44] but only with a Class IIa recommendation for two-vessel disease without proximal LAD involvement if extensive ischemia exists,[45] and one-vessel proximal LAD disease.[10,46,47] It should be emphasized, however, that these trials involved primarily patients with moderate chronic stable angina. These conclusions may, therefore, not necessarily apply to patients with unstable angina or to those with more severe degrees of chronic stable angina.

A landmark meta-analysis by Yusuf et al, of the seven randomized trials cited in the preceding demonstrated a statistically enhanced survival at 5, 7, and 10 years, for surgically treated patients at highest risk (4.8% annual mortality) and moderate risk (2.5% annual mortality), but no evidence of a survival benefit for those patients at lowest risk.[39] The overall survival benefit at 12 years for the three large and four smaller randomized studies is shown in Fig. 20-1. Nonrandomized studies have also demonstrated a beneficial effect of surgery on survival of patients with multivessel disease and severe ischemia regardless of left ventricular function.[25-28]

Following this, between 1997 and 2004, there were three randomized controlled trials of invasive revascularization by PCI or CABG versus medical therapy. Their results make an even stronger case for revascularization. In the Asymptomatic Cardiac Ischemia Pilot (ACIP) trial, patients with anatomy amenable to CABG were randomized to angina-directed antiischemic therapy, drug therapy guided by noninvasive measures of ischemia, or revascularization by CABG or PCI.[45] At 2 years, there was a statistically significant difference in mortality of 6.6% in the angina-guided group, 4.4% in the ischemia-guided group, and 1.1% in the revascularization group. The rates of death or MI were also statistically different at 12.1%, 8.8%, and 4.7%, respectively, that is, both symptoms and survival were improved with revascularization. The Medicine, Angioplasty, or Surgery Study (MASS-II) trial randomized patients with multivessel disease among medical therapy, PCI, and CABG.[48,49] Although survival at 1 year was equivalent, freedom from additional intervention was 99.5% for surgical patients and 93.7% for medically treated patients. Reintervention was, incidentally, even higher in the PCI group than the medical group, with 86.7% free of additional intervention. Angina was superior in the CABG

group (88%) than in the PCI group (79%) or medical therapy group (46%). Meanwhile the 10-year survival rates were 74.9% with CABG, 75.1% with PCI, and 69% with MT.[49] In the Trial of Invasive versus Medical Therapy in Elderly Patients with Chronic Symptomatic Coronary-Artery Disease (TIME) study, elderly patients were studied with chronic angina. This failed to demonstrate a difference between optimized medical therapy and an invasive revascularization strategy (PCI or CABG) in terms of symptoms, quality of life, and death or nonfatal MI (20% vs 17%, p = .71). However, medically treated patients were at higher risk because of major clinical events (64% vs 26% for invasive, p < .001), which were mainly attributable to rehospitalization and revascularization.[50] In this trial of severely symptomatic elderly patients, it was encouraging that the price of an initially conservative strategy, followed by crossover to revascularization in approximately 50% of patients, was not paid for in terms of death or MI.[50]

Early historical concern over a prohibitive operative mortality among patients with impaired ventricular function has been superseded by the recognition that the survival of these patients on medical therapy was much worse than their survival with revascularization. This, coupled with ever-improving surgical techniques, such as advances in myocardial preservation and perioperative support, has made this specific subgroup the one in which the relative survival benefit of surgical therapy is the greatest. Accordingly, *left ventricular dysfunction in patients with documented ischemia is now considered an important indication*—rather than contraindication—for surgical revascularization.[10,12,39,51-53] More recently, the Surgical Treatment for Ischemic Heart failure (STICH) trial was conducted to better evaluate the effect of CABG plus optimal medical therapy to optimal medical therapy alone, an effect that the trial investigators perceived to not have been well-established by the studies referenced above considering (1) the general exclusion of patients with severe left ventricular dysfunction in the three landmark trials from the 1970s and (2) the improvements in both medical and surgical therapy that had developed since then.[53] The study of 1212 patients with an ejection fraction (EF) less than 35% and CAD amenable to CABG demonstrated a nonsignificant trend toward decreased mortality from any cause in the CABG group (36%) compared to the medical therapy group (41%). The trial has been criticized for being underpowered, and with just 56 months of mean follow-up and a large percentage of patients in the medical therapy group crossing over into the CABG group (17%) during the study period thereby potentially diminishing the statistical impact of CABG, many have interpreted this to represent evidence that the presence of left ventricular dysfunction remains an important indication to perform CABG for survival benefit. Indeed, the ACCF/AHA guidelines consider left ventricular (LV) dysfunction to represent a Class IIa recommendation for performing CABG if the EF is 35 to 50%, but only Class IIb recommendation if the EF is <35%, in part based on the results of the STICH trial.[10] In addition, recent evidence that ischemic, viable, hypokinetic myocardium (hibernating or stunned) regains

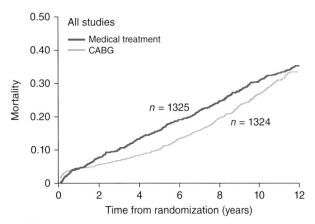

FIGURE 20-1 Survival (mortality) curves for all medically and surgically treated patients with chronic stable angina enrolled in seven prospective randomized controlled trials. (Reproduced with permission from Yusuf S, Zucker D, Peduzzi P, et al: Effect of coronary artery bypass graft surgery on survival: overview of 10-year results from randomised trials by the Coronary Artery Bypass Graft Surgery Trialists Collaboration, *Lancet.* 1994 Aug 27;344(8922):563-570.)

stronger contractile function after effective revascularization, has prompted expansion of the indications for surgical revascularization among patients with severe left ventricular dysfunction to include patients who would otherwise be considered candidates for cardiac transplantation.[54] This subject is discussed in more detail in the following.

In summary, the current guidelines recommend on the basis of a survival advantage that CABG be performed instead of medical therapy alone on a Class I recommendation for all unprotected left main disease,[39-41] three-vessel disease with or without proximal LAD involvement,[35,39,42-44] and two vessel-disease with proximal LAD disease[35,39,42-44]; with a Class IIa recommendation for two-vessel disease without proximal LAD involvement but with the presence of extensive ischemia,[45] one-vessel proximal LAD disease,[10,46,47] and moderate LV dysfunction (EF 35-50%)[39,54-57]; and with a Class IIb recommendation for two-vessel disease without proximal LAD disease or extensive ischemia,[44] and in patients with severe LV dysfunction (EF < 35%)[39,53-57] (Fig. 20-2).

Apart from affording a survival benefit, CABG is also indicated for the relief of angina pectoris and improvement in the quality of life. Between 80 and 90% of patients who are symptomatic on medical therapy become symptom-free after

CABG in the early period while approximately 60% remain symptom-free at up to 10 years.[49] This benefit extends to low-risk patients for whom survival benefit from surgery is not likely.[39] Thus, for example, whereas on the basis of a survival advantage alone CABG is only indicated for one-vessel disease if the vessel involved is the left main (Class I) or the proximal LAD (Class IIa), a symptomatic patient with single-vessel disease in any anatomic position represents a Class I, Level A indication to perform either CABG or PCI on the basis of symptom improvement (Fig. 20-2).[10,49,50,58-60] Consensus agreement by the ACC/AHA recommends on a Class IIa basis CABG is recommended for patients with at least one significant coronary lesions in any position and unacceptable angina (1) for whom guideline-directed medical therapy (GDMT) cannot be implemented because of medication contraindications, adverse effects, or patient preferences; and (2) complex three-vessel CAD (eg, SYNTAX score > 22) with or without involvement of the proximal LAD and a good candidate for CABG (CABG preferred over PCI in this situation).[10,44,61-63] Relief of symptoms appears to relate to both the completeness of revascularization and maintenance of graft patency, with the benefit of CABG diminishing with time. Recurrence of angina following CABG surgery occurs at rates of 3 to 20% per year. Although enhanced survival is reported when an ITA graft is used to the LAD, there is no significant difference in postoperative freedom from angina.[46,47] This may be because of vein graft occlusion or progression of native disease in grafted or ungrafted vessels.[13]

Unfortunately, few patients experience an advantage in work rehabilitation with surgery as compared with medical management. Generally, employment declines in both groups and is determined nearly as much by socioeconomic factors as age, preoperative unemployment, and type of job as by type of therapy or clinical factors such as postoperative angina. Notably, surgical revascularization has not been shown to reduce the incidence of nonfatal events such as MI, although this may be because of perioperative infarctions that offset the lower incidence of infarction in each study follow-up.[64,65]

PCI VERSUS MEDICAL THERAPY

PCI continues to evolve as a therapy from its historical roots as a procedure entailing balloon angioplasty alone, followed by the introduction of bare metal stents (BMSs), and subsequently DESs. Despite this evolution and the attendant reduction in overall in-stent restenosis rates in the DES era, and despite a multitude of evidence in both early and more recent trials demonstrating the ability of PCI to effectively reduce the incidence of angina compared to medical therapy in patients with stable ischemic heart disease, there remains no definitive evidence in any study to date that PCI improves survival rates or rates of subsequent MI in this patient population.[43,60,66-71]

It is worth describing the specifics of several representative studies on patients with multivessel disease. In the Randomized Intervention Treatment of Angina (RITA)–2, of 1018 patients with stable angina randomized to medicine

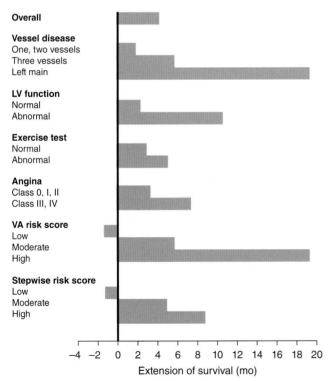

FIGURE 20-2 Extension of survival in months for various subgroups of patients with chronic stable angina treated by surgery as compared with those treated by medicine in seven prospective randomized controlled trials. (Reproduced with permission from Yusuf S, Zucker D, Peduzzi P, et al: Effect of coronary artery bypass graft surgery on survival: overview of 10-year results from randomised trials by the Coronary Artery Bypass Graft Surgery Trialists Collaboration, *Lancet*. 1994 Aug 27;344(8922):563-570.)

or PCI, one-third had two-vessel disease and 7% had three-vessel disease.[59] Perhaps surprisingly, at a median follow-up of 2.7 years, the primary endpoints of death or MI had occurred twice as often in the PCI group (6.3 vs 3.3%, $p < .02$). Surgical revascularization was required during the follow-up interval in 7.9% of the PCI group and repeat angioplasty was required in 11%. In the medical group, 23% of patients required revascularization. Angina relief and exercise tolerance were improved to a greater degree in the angioplasty group early, but this difference disappeared by 3 years. These results are echoed in the MASS-II trial, in which angina relief was superior with PCI, but rates of intervention/reintervention were actually higher in the PCI group.[48,49] This supports an initial strategy of medical therapy in patients with stable ischemic heart disease.

More recently, the COURAGE trial randomized 2287 patients with stable angina and objective evidence of ischemia to contemporary medical therapy or PCI and medical management (3% of the stents used were DESs). All patients received long-acting metoprolol, amlodipine, and/or isosorbidemononitrate, as well as lisinopril or losartan. Patients had aggressive antilipid therapy and appropriate antiplatelet therapy. The primary finding of this trial was a lack of benefit of PCI over best medical therapy for death, MI, or other major cardiovascular events.[60] Although this result has caused much controversy in the cardiology community, it is consistent with older studies.

A meta-analysis of percutaneous interventions versus medical management was published in 2005.[68] In patients with stable CAD, no benefit was found for invasive therapy in terms of death, MI, or need for subsequent revascularization. In 2014, Windecker et al performed a large scale meta-analysis of 100 trials comparing both CABG and PCI to medical therapy found that patients who received new generation everolimus- and zotarolimus-based (Resolute) DESs but not older generation DESs (sirolimus, paclitaxel, and Endeavor zotarolimus), BMSs, or balloon angioplasty alone, had reduced mortality compared to medical therapy.[71] However, given the limitations of this study, including the inclusion of only one trial comparing newer generation DESs to medical therapy and absence of individual patient data, the general consensus remains that unless and until further evidence is collected to the contrary, all patients with stable coronary disease should have a trial of optimized medical therapy before invasive intervention in the form of PCI. Accordingly there are no Class I recommendations for PCI in the setting of stable ischemic heart disease in the 2011 ACCF/AHA guildelines.[10] Based on subgroup analysis from the SYNTAX trial (discussed further in the next section), however, it is recommended on a Class IIa basis for stable ischemic heart disease patients with unprotected left main disease for benefit if they meet the following criteria: (1) anatomic conditions associated with a low risk of PCI complications and have a high likelihood of good long-term outcome; for example, low SYNTAX score ≤22, ostial or trunk left main CAD; and (2) clinical characteristics that impart a high risk of

morbidity and mortality with CABG (eg, Society of Thoracic Surgeons (STS)-predicted mortality > 5%).[72]

PCI VERSUS CABG

Randomized Studies. A number of studies comparing an initial strategy of angioplasty versus early surgery have been carried out, all with similar results. It is important to recognize that, as a rule, these studies are comparisons of treatment strategies and not head-to-head comparisons of revascularization techniques. Accordingly, crossover is permitted and endpoints are selected to determine adverse consequences of the algorithm on an "intention to treat" basis.

Most early trials of CABG versus PCI have in common that PCI was performed first in the form of balloon angioplasty alone, followed by those including BMS deployment with angioplasty. In all, over 20 randomized controlled trials comparing CABG with PCI in the form of angioplasty or BMS implantation have been conducted, and on this basis the following conclusions were made by Bravata et al[73] in a recent systematic review and cited in the establishment of the ACC/AHA 2011 guidelines:[10] (1) Survival is similar after CABG and PCI at both 1 year and 5 years, (2) incidence of MI was similar at 5 years after randomization, (3) CABG produced more effective relief from angina than with PCI at 1 and 5 years, and (4) repeat coronary revascularization was less frequent after CABG than after PCI. In other words, at least in the early era of PCI, CABG appears to have a benefit over PCI only insofar as it improves symptoms and reduces the need for repeat coronary revascularization, but without any improvement in overall survival or incidence, which reflects the results of even the earliest studies ever conducted on this topic, beginning with the 1994 Swiss trial of just 134 patients[74] and both the MASS[75,76] and MASS-II[48,49] trials. The oft-quoted BARI, Emory Angioplasty versus Surgery Trial (EAST), RITA, CABRI, and GABI multivessel PCI versus CABG surgery trials,[77-81] with only a few nonreproducible exceptions, generally support the same conclusions above.

Most of the early studies quoted above share the limitation that, in general, only a very small minority of patients undergoing revascularization at any center were entered into these trials.[82,83] Accordingly, the populations included in the trials may not be generally reflective of clinical practice. For instance, few patients in these studies had significant LV dysfunction and most randomized patients had only one- or two-vessel disease. In the RITA trial, approximately one-third of patients had single-vessel disease.[77] Among clinically eligible patients in the BARI[80,84] and EAST[81] trials, approximately two-thirds of patients were excluded on angiographic grounds that included chronic total occlusion, LMCA stenosis, diffuse disease, or other anatomical factors making PCI potentially dangerous. Consequently, these randomized trials contain only a portion of the spectrum of patients with CAD encountered clinically. Entry bias has a significant impact on the likelihood of observing an outcome difference among therapies. Because a high proportion of the randomized patients are in the low-risk group, it is possible that any potential survival benefit of CABG surgery over PCI in high- and moderate-risk groups may be masked.[83]

A second consideration in evaluating these studies is that the success of revascularization procedures depends not only on the criteria employed to define success, but also on the interpretation of those criteria by both patient and physician. In the 1985 to 1986, National Heart, Lung, and Blood Institute PCI Registry, 99% of patients were discharged alive from hospital, and 92% did not sustain a MI or require CABG surgery.[85] In the BARI trial, 99% of patients survived hospitalization and 88.6% of PCI-treated patients did not have MI or require repeat revascularization by angioplasty or surgery during the initial hospitalization.[80] Employing event-free criteria (death, MI, CABG) for the initial hospitalization, PCI can be judged successful. However, if a repeat revascularization procedure within 5 years is regarded as a negative outcome, then far fewer patients are treated successfully. Regardless, the lack of differences in mortality or MI rates permits individuals to select one or the other procedure as initial therapy without the likelihood that they will pay a price with their health.

Considering event-free survival as a more meaningful endpoint than overall survival, several more recent studies of CABG versus early era PCI (balloon angioplasty only) have demonstrated an advantage with surgery. The Argentine Randomized Trial of Coronary Angioplasty versus Bypass Surgery in Multi-vessel Disease (ERACI) trial conducted between 1988 and 1990 demonstrated no difference in death or MI, but superior event-free survival in the CABG group at 1 and 3 years.[86,87] In the French Monocentric Study, 152 patients with multivessel disease underwent PCI or CABG.[88] Again, superior event-free survival was seen in the surgical group, driven predominantly by a lesser need for subsequent revascularization. Comparing CABG to PCI with BMS implantation, Mercado et al performed a meta-analysis of the ARTS, ERATSII, MASS-II, and SOS trials that demonstrated similar rates of death, MI, or stroke at 1 year and higher repeat revascularization rates with PCI.[89] A meta-analysis of 5-year data was also recently published, confirming the 1-year results with repeat revascularization significantly more frequent after PCI than CABG (29% vs 7.9%).[90]

In large part fueled by recognition of the relatively high rates of in-stent restenosis seen with bare metal stents (22- 32% at 6 months),[91,92] many investigators had hoped that by lowering the rates of early restenosis,[67] the introduction of DESs to the PCI armamentarium might improve overall PCI outcomes and expand the indications for PCI over CABG in a wide variety of clinical scenarios. The Synergy between PCI with Taxus and Cardiac Surgery (SYNTAX) trial, assessed the optimal revascularization strategy for patients with three-vessel or left main CAD by randomizing 1800 patients to either CABG or paclitaxel-based DESs.[4] At 12 months, the rates of MI and death were similar between groups, but stroke was significantly more common in the CABG patients (2.2% vs 0.6% at 1 year). It should be noted that the CABG group had much less aggressive medical management postoperatively, including fewer patients on antiplatelet medications, which may account for some of the increase in stroke risk.

Despite the use of DESs, the rates of reintervention were still significantly higher (13.5% vs 5.9%) in the PCI group than the CABG group. Because of the lack of difference in early mortality and MI, some cardiologists have begun to suggest that left main should no longer be an indication for CABG.[93] However, others maintain that the evidence for PCI is still inadequate and that the greater freedom from reintervention with CABG suggests that CABG remains the treatment of choice for patients with left main disease.[94] Meanwhile, the SYNTAX scores themselves, which grade the severity and complexity of coronary disease according to a variety of anatomic features (extent, location, severity), were defined in post hoc analyses as low for scores ≤22, intermediate for scores 23 to 32, and high if ≥33. While the incidence of major adverse cardiac events (MACE) for patients undergoing CABG versus PCI were similar in subgroup analysis of low SYNTAX score patients, those with an intermediate or high SYNTAX score had lower incidence of MACE with CABG.[4] Furthermore, at 3-year follow-up, those with three-vessel disease had significantly lower mortality in the CABG group compared to the DES group (6.2% vs 2.9%).[63] CABG appears to be preferable to PCI for those with diffuse and complex CAD. It is on this basis that CABG is recommended over PCI on a Class IIa basis for patients those with three-vessel disease (regardless of proximal LAD involvement) in patients with SYNTAX scores > 22 who are good candidates for CABG.[10]

Notably, the SYNTAX trial also brought to light the concept of the Heart Team approach, described in the SYNTAX trial as a system in which a team consisting of a heart surgeon, an interventional cardiologist, and often the general cardiologist (if available) discuss each case and decide on the basis of mutual agreement the optimal method of revascularization in multidisciplinary fashion. The Heart Team approach, while not validated by any follow-up randomized controlled trial is recommended on a Class I basis for all patients presenting with unprotected left main or complex CAD.[10]

Since the SYNTAX trial, there have been five additional randomized controlled trials comparing CABG to PCI. Two of these trials discuss PCI with DESs in comparison to minimally invasive direct coronary artery bypass and therefore are less germane to the present discussion regarding on-pump CABG. The PRECOMBAT trial showed that PCI using DES was noninferior to CABG in UPLM at 2 years for composite endpoint and will be discussed further in the forthcoming section on left main disease.[95] Meanwhile, the CARDia trial achieved the modest goal of demonstrating that in patients with multivessel CAD and DM, PCI with the use of DES is noninferior to CABG at 1 year with respect to a composite endpoint of all-cause mortality, MI, and stroke.[96] The FREEDOM trial, which was designed similarly for a similar population but had nearly four times the study population size, demonstrated that for patients with DM and advanced CAD, CABG resulted in lower rates of the same composite endpoint compared to PCI with DES (18.7% vs 26.6%),[26] which is the first time a randomized trial of CABG versus PCI with DES has demonstrated this effect. A recent 2014 meta-analysis of six randomized trials of multivessel CAD whose goal was to accurately reflect the more modern era in which DES and arterial grafts are used more frequently in PCI and CABG, respectively, demonstrated that with a weighted average follow-up of 4.1 years, CABG was associated with significantly lower mortality, lower incidence of MI, and repeat revascularization.[97] These new findings, which now demonstrate a survival advantage and not just freedom from repeat revascularization and symptom improvement with CABG over PCI, were not available at the time of the writing of the 2011 ACCF/AHA guidelines, but have implications for the management of patients in the future if further evidence supporting the same conclusions is gathered.

Nonrandomized Database Comparisons. The information provided by randomized studies is complemented by information gleaned from large, prospectively managed, nonrandomized database studies. Such registries provide insight into the management of the sizeable population of patients who would not have been eligible for randomization. The 1994 Duke Cardiovascular Disease Databank study was one of the first large registry studies that established much of what we know today about the benefit of CABG compared to PCI insofar as it is dependent on the severity of coronary disease.[22] From a practical standpoint, in this database study and in the randomized trials, the effect of revascularization on survival depended largely on the extent of the CAD and is an example of the concept of benefit in relationship to a "gradient of risk." For the least severe (one-vessel) disease, there were no survival advantages of revascularization over medical therapy in up to 5 years of follow-up.[22] For intermediate levels of CAD severity (ie, two-vessel disease), there was a higher 5-year survival rate for patients undergoing revascularization than for those treated medically. For patients with the most-severe CAD (ie, three-vessel disease), CABG surgery provided a significant and consistent survival advantage over medical therapy. PCI appeared prognostically equivalent to medical therapy in these patients, but only a small number of patients in this subgroup underwent angioplasty. In comparing PCI with CABG surgery, PCI demonstrated a small survival advantage over CABG surgery for patients with less-severe two-vessel disease, whereas CABG surgery was superior for more severe two-vessel disease (ie, proximal LAD involvement).[22]

Several additional studies in the subsequent PCI with BMS era confirmed these findings. A study of 1999 cases from the New York State Database between 1993 and 1998 showed that a survival benefit was observed with angioplasty at 3 years for those patients with single-vessel disease not involving the LAD, whereas those with LAD or three-vessel disease had superior outcomes with surgery.[98] In a much larger CABG versus PCI registry study from the BMS era, survival was again higher among the 37,212 patients who underwent CABG than among the 22,102 patients who underwent stent placement after adjustment for known risk factors[61] (Fig. 20-3). This study has limitations of being a nonrandomized study and subject to bias; however, the surprising finding of a survival advantage apparent as early as 3 years postprocedure suggests that improvements in

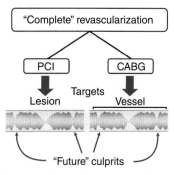

FIGURE 20-3 PCI is directed against specific culprit lesions. By bypassing diseased vessels, CABG surgery treats both culprit lesions and future culprit lesions. (Reproduced with permission from Opie LH, Commerford PJ, Gersh BJ: Controversies in stable coronary artery disease, *Lancet*. 2006 Jan 7;367(9504):69-78.)

cardiac surgical anesthetic care, myocardial protection, and intensive care management have at least matched if not surpassed advances in percutaneous technology. It is important to note that while PCI targets the culprit lesion, CABG surgery targets both the culprit lesion and potential future culprit lesions by bypassing the diseased vessel. Considering the finding that medium- and long-term clinical outcome after PCI (ie, beyond one year postprocedure) is more dependent on the progression of coronary disease in other culprit lesions than restenosis of the stented lesion,[99] this in part may explain the apparent mortality benefit derived with CABG that has persisted despite advances in stent technology that have resulted in lower restenosis rates (Fig. 20-3).[100]

In the DES era, five of six large registry studies concluded that patients undergoing CABG have lower mortality than those receiving PCI with DES.[62,101-105] In particular, the ASCERT study, upon which the Society of Thoracic Surgeons ASCERT Long-Term Survival Probability Calculator (ascertcalc.sts.org) is based, evaluated outcomes of almost 200,000 patients over the age of 65 years with multivessel disease undergoing nonemergent revascularization, and showed that although there was no difference in adjusted mortality in the CABG and PCI groups at 1 year, CABG patients had significantly lower mortality at 4 years (16.4% vs 20.8%).[104] The long-term benefit of CABG compared to PCI was independent of age, sex, diabetes, renal function, and lung disease and was evident even for patients with propensity scores most consistent with selection for PCI. Another registry study of over 105,000 propensity-matched United States Medicare beneficiaries undergoing either CABG or PCI between 1992 and 2008 showed that at 5 years, patients undergoing CABG had a higher survival rate (74.1% vs 71.9%), an effect which was more pronounced in those with diabetes, tobacco use, heart failure, and peripheral artery disease.[105]

In summary, although not void of limitations that randomized controlled trials and associated meta-analyses overcome, these large registry studies provide a more real-world picture of revascularization in actual clinical practice, and support the findings of newer randomized controlled trials that CABG confers survival benefit over PCI, especially in patients with multivessel and complex CAD, even in the era of DES use and the attendant lower rates of restenosis.

Special Circumstances

ACUTE CORONARY SYNDROMES

The acute coronary syndromes (ACS) cover a wide spectrum from ST-segment elevation MI (STEMI) with underlying coronary obstruction to Prinzmetal's or variant angina in patients with coronary vasospasm in the absence of significant underlying obstruction. The term non-ST-segment elevation (NSTEMI) ACS encompasses the entities of unstable angina, non-Q-wave MI, and postinfarction angina. They denote acute, symptomatic imbalances of the myocardial oxygen supply-demand ratio over a short time span. Prinzmetal angina, or coronary vasospasm, is diagnosed definitively by electrocardiograms obtained during the episode of pain and is treated medically. Unstable angina is not a uniform clinical entity, but comprises the spectrum of myocardial ischemia between chronic stable angina and MI, and is defined as a recent change in the severity, character, or trigger threshold of chronic stable angina or new-onset angina. Approximately 5.6 million Americans have chronic angina, and about 350,000 develop new-onset angina each year. Unstable angina develops in approximately 750,000 Americans each year and is associated with subsequent MI in approximately 10%. Postinfarction angina is defined as the presence of angina or other evidence of myocardial ischemia in a patient with a recent (1- to 2-week) Q-wave or non-Q-wave MI.

CABG in ST Elevation Myocardial Infarction. Prompt myocardial revascularization has been shown to improve outcomes compared to no reperfusion in almost all groups of patients who present after an acute STEMI. Because the degree of improvement in long-term outcomes is dependent on the time from symptom onset to revascularization,[106,107] PCI, which in general can be initiated more quickly that can CABG, is performed as the primary therapy in most cases, relegating CABG largely to a secondary position in this setting (performed in less than 5% of STEMI cases[108]). In the majority of PCI cases, the culprit lesion can be determined and successfully stented open, with subsequent improvement in myocardial ischemia. However, in certain cases where coronary disease is diffuse and not amenable to stent placement, or in the setting of complications from PCI such as coronary dissection, perforation with tamponade, stent deployment failure, or hyperacute stent closure, revascularization is either not technically possible or remains incomplete with ongoing ischemia. Emergency CABG in current practice is reserved and, in fact, recommended on a Class I basis primarily for survival benefit in the following circumstances: (1) after unsuccessful or complicated PCI with ongoing ischemia;[109] (2) mechanical complication of acute MI requiring surgery including ventricular septal defect, free wall rupture, or papillary muscle with acute mitral regurgitation;

(3) cardiogenic shock, defined as systolic blood pressure < 90 mm Hg for over 30 minutes requiring supportive measures, cardiac index ≤ 2.2 L/min/m², pulmonary capillary wedge pressure ≥ 15 mm Hg, and/or evidence of end-organ malperfusion;[106,107,110] and (4) patients with life-threatening arrhythmias in the presence of significant left main or three-vessel CAD.[10,111] The SHOCK study randomized patients to emergency revascularization versus initial medical stabilization in patients presenting with STEMI and cardiogenic shock and found that among those who were revascularized early, CABG group (36%) of patients had similar survival to those undergoing PCI despite higher rates of diabetes and complex coronary anatomy in the CABG subset.[110]

The timing of CABG after STEMI remains controversial, but overall the evidence suggests that mortality appears to peak in the 7-to-24-hour period after symptom onset. Several studies have shown that CABG with in-hospital mortality rates of 10.8% if performed within 6 hours of onset, 23.8% at 7 to 24 hours after onset, 6.7% at 1 to 3 days, 4.2% at 4 to 7 days, and 2.4% after 8 days. Another study showed that mortality was 6.1% for CABG performed within 6 hours, 50% at 7 to 23 hours, and 7.1% at 15 days or greater.[109] A reasonable approach appears to be emergency CABG within the 6-hour timeframe if possible to maximize myocardial salvage. Those who present after the 6-hour window would likely benefit from a delay of three to four days to improve survival and decrease bleeding complications.[108,109,112]

CABG in Non-ST Elevation Myocardial Infarction and Unstable Angina. The initial approach to the patient with NSTEMI ACS is pharmacologic stabilization followed by risk stratification. The latter is based on multiple clinical, demographic, and ECG variables in addition to the use of serum biomarkers. The TIMI (Thrombosis in Myocardial Infarction) risk score, which takes into account a variety of the above clinical factors, is widely used as a prognostic tool to determine in patients with unstable angina or NSTEMI the 14-day risk of all-cause mortality, new or recurrent MI, or severe recurrent ischemia requiring urgent revascularization,[113] and is often used to risk-stratify patients to a strategy of either immediate angiography, an invasive approach (angiography followed by revascularization by either PCI or CABG), or a conservative approach (initial period of medical therapy intensification). Those with hemodynamic instability, cardiogenic shock, severe LV dysfunction, persistent or recurrent angina at rest despite intensive medical therapy, mechanical complications, sustained ventricular tachycardia, and dynamic ST-T changes, are usually considered high risk irrespective of the TIMI score which does not account for these factors. Patients at intermediate or high risk (the majority) undergo early angiography with a view to revascularization. In many parts of the world, however, angiographic facilities are limited and an alternative approach based upon pharmacologic stabilization followed by mobilization and risk stratification using stress testing is employed.

In general for those undergoing angiography, the choice of PCI versus CABG is largely determined by the anatomy and specific clinical features as in the general population presenting with stable ischemic heart disease, as per the ACCF/AHA guidelines.[10]

ASYMPTOMATIC CORONARY ARTERY DISEASE

The role of revascularization either by PCI or CABG versus medical therapy in the setting of asymptomatic CAD has been studied in the ACIP trial.[114] Of 558 patients with CAD and medically controlled angina, treatment was randomized to either revascularization or medical therapy directed toward eliminating angina or eliminating ischemia during ambulatory ECG. Revascularization was more effective than medical therapy in relieving ischemia, and CABG was superior to PCI (70% freedom from ischemia vs 46%, $p < .002$). Mortality at 1 and 2 years was superior for revascularization as compared with angina-directed medical therapy, but not superior to ischemia-directed medical therapy.[45,114] The greatest benefit was among those patients with the most severe disease. Importantly, many of these patients with "silent ischemia" on ambulatory ECG monitoring did have symptomatic angina at other times and thus were not truly asymptomatic.

The documentation of ischemia, however, is critical. Several studies emphasize the flaws in the assumption that one can identify future culprit lesions in the absence of symptoms or documentation of ischemia. Among patients undergoing serial coronary arteriography who subsequently developed acute MI or unstable angina, the severity of stenosis at the time of initial angiogram is poorly predictive of the culprit lesion causing the acute ischemic syndrome.[115,116] In most cases the severity of the lesion responsible for subsequent ischemia was less than 50%, and in many patients it was not present at all on the initial angiogram, raising concern regarding the number of asymptomatic or minimally symptomatic patients undergoing angioplasty without stress testing.[117] Bech and associates have demonstrated that fractional flow reserve exceeded 0.75 in 91 of 325 patients planned for PCI without noninvasive evaluation of ischemia, and that among those patients, angioplasty had no impact on event-free survival or angina.[118]

DRUG-ELUTING STENTS

Recent progress in stent technology, particularly the introduction of DESs, has further reduced the incidence of restenosis. The use of stents has reduced adverse remodeling, and stents-eluting medications such as sirolimus, paclitaxel, or everolimus, are having a profound effect on the patterns of interventions for CAD. When compared with bare-metal stents, DES have not been shown to convey any advantage in terms of MI or mortality, but do demonstrate decreased rates of angiographic restenosis in a meta-analysis of 11 randomized trials.[67] The results of both randomized controlled trials and observational studies comparing CABG to PCI using DES are described in the preceding section, and suggest that the addition of DES, while successful in decreasing the restenosis rate inherent in BMS, the indications for PCI

and CABG have not changed.[101] Some of the most recent studies comparing these two strategies (FREEDOM trial, a meta-analysis of six randomized trials by Sipahi et al, and the ASCERT study)[26,97,104] have actually demonstrated a long-term survival benefit of CABG over PCI despite the use of DES in the PCI groups. It is important to note that because DES is associated with higher rates of in-stent thrombosis (as distinct from restenosis), patients receiving DES in general require 6 to 12 months of dual antiplatelet therapy (usually clopidogrel and aspirin) to minimize this risk.[119] Consideration for CABG or BMS should be given over DES on an individualized basis for patients in whom comorbid conditions will require withholding clopidogrel in order to perform subsequent surgery.

LEFT MAIN DISEASE

Left main CAD is present in about 5% of patients undergoing coronary angiography,[120] and when present is associated with multivessel CAD around in 70% of patients.[4,94] Significant unprotected left main disease (ie, left main disease without any preexisting distal CABGs) has been considered an indication for CABG rather than PCI for many years, but recently studies have begun to question this. A handful of registry studies[25] as well as subgroup analysis of the SYNTAX trial,[72] and finally several randomized trials of CABG versus PCI with DES[95,121] have suggested that PCI may be an acceptable method of revascularization in patients with left main disease. In a matched cohort of more than 1100 patients with unprotected left main disease, there was no difference in the rates of death or the composite outcome of death, Q-wave MI, or stroke between patients undergoing CABG or PCI despite a greater rate of target-vessel revascularization in the PCI group, including the patients who received DES.[25] The PRECOMBAT trial compared PCI using sirolimus-eluting stents to CABG in patients with left main disease and found that the risk of major adverse cardiac or cerebrovascular events (MACCE) was not significantly higher after PCI compared to CABG at two years, but did have about double the incidence of repeat revascularizations.[95] A subgroup analysis of patients in the SYNTAX trial presenting with left main disease supported these findings by showing that PCI with a paclitaxel-eluting DES did not increase the 12-month rate of MACCE in comparison to CABG, but did have a higher rate of repeat revascularization.[72] Five-year outcomes also demonstrate the same findings qualitatively.[122] However, when grouped according to SYNTAX score, while those with low or intermediate scores had similar outcomes regardless of the method of revascularization, those with high-risk scores (>32) undergoing PCI had higher incidence of MACCE than CABG patients.[72,122,123] Based primarily on this evidence, the ACCF/AHA guidelines regard PCI as a Class IIa or IIb recommendation in patients with unprotected left main disease and stable ischemic heart disease depending on how favorable the anatomy and how high the overall surgical risk (Class IIa if SYNTAX score is ≤22 and STS-predicted mortality is ≥5%, Class IIb if SYNTAX score < 33 and STS-predicted mortality > 2%).[10] PCI may be performed on a Class IIa recommendation if the patient is having unstable angina/NSTEMI and is not a CABG candidate due to high risk of operative morbidity and mortality, or in the setting of a STEMI when distal coronary flow is grade 3 and PCI can be performed more rapidly than CABG.[10] For all other instances (ie, the majority of patients), until additional data are gathered to the contrary, CABG remains the definitive Class I-recommended treatment for most patients with unprotected left main disease.[10] The EXCEL trial which is currently ongoing seeks to compare CABG to PCI using newer generation everolimus-eluting stents in patients with unprotected left main disease.

SEVERE LEFT VENTRICULAR DYSFUNCTION

Left ventricular dysfunction is a predictor of increased operative risk for most cardiac surgical procedures, and in the early days of coronary revascularization these patients were not offered CABG. Like age, however, it is also a strong predictor of poor outcome with medical therapy. Accordingly, more recently significant LV dysfunction has been considered an indication rather than contraindication to surgical revascularization. In some patients, LV function has been shown to improve—sometimes dramatically so—after revascularization, leading to the concept of "hibernating" or "stunned" myocardium.[124,125] The identification of viable myocardium, which is potentially recoverable, depends on the identification of preserved metabolic activity by positron emission tomography, cell membrane integrity by thallium-201 or technetium-99m single-photon emission computed tomography (SPECT), or dobutamine stress echocardiography.[126]

Five studies from the early era of CABG as well as several meta-analyses of these studies and others that followed showed that patients with LV systolic dysfunction (mainly mild to moderate) showed that CABG conferred improved survival in comparison to medical therapy.[39,54-57,127] In regards to severe left ventricular dysfunction, however, as mentioned above the STICH trial, showed no reduction in all-cause mortality for CABG in comparison to GDMT in patients with CAD amenable to CABG with an EF of <35%.[53] CABG did, however, demonstrate a benefit compared to medical therapy with respect to the composite endpoint of death from any cause or (1) hospitalization for heart failure, (2) hospitalization for cardiovascular access, (3) hospitalization for any cause, and (4) revascularization with PCI or CABG. In other words, event-free survival was better with CABG in this population, suggesting that with longer follow-up, an overall survival benefit might resolve. The study is being continued out to 10 years of follow-up.

The relative roles of CABG and PCI in this population are not clearly defined despite the number of randomized trials of PCI versus surgery, largely because these patients were excluded from trial entry. In an early multicenter study of patients with left ventricular dysfunction (EF < 40%), slightly more than one-fourth of the patients died in the 2 years following multivessel PCI.[128] The majority of studies comparing CABG to PCI in this population have demonstrated similar survival,[129-133] while some showed improved outcomes with

CABG.[62] Overall, aside from the STICH trial, there remains a paucity of meaningful randomized trial data informing the choice of CABG versus PCI in the setting of left ventricular dysfunction. For patients with LV dysfunction and CAD amenable to revascularization, the recommendation is to perform CABG on a Class IIa basis if the EF is slightly depressed (35-50%), and on a Class IIb basis if the EF is very low (<35%) as long as the LMCA is not involved, in which case CABG is more clearly indicated.[10] The ACCF/AHA guidelines recommend that patients in this category should have the method of revascularization tailored to clinical variables such as the presence of renal disease, diabetes, and the complexity of the coronary anatomy.[10]

CHRONIC TOTAL OCCLUSION

Chronic, totally occlusion of a coronary artery is found on up to 20% of all coronary angiograms, and of these, three-fourths have multivessel disease.[134,135] Revascularization is not possible nor attempted in 65% of patients with chronic total occlusion.[134] This population remains poorly studied in the randomized trials of multivessel PCI versus CABG as 35 to 37% of the patients excluded from the overall study were disqualified because of the presence of a chronic total occlusion of a coronary artery serving viable myocardium. Notably, the SYNTAX trial did not exclude patients with chronic total occlusion (a condition which alone contributes 10 to 15 points to the SYNTAX score), and found that complete revascularization, which has a known association with reduction in long-term mortality, MI, and repeat coronary interventions,[136] was significantly higher in patients treated with CABG compared to PCI (69% vs 49%).[4] Considering that the presence of chronic total occlusion was the most common reason for the inability to achieve complete revascularization in the PCI group, this may account for the lower rates of major adverse cardiovascular events including death in the CABG group compared to PCI.[135] However, success rates for achieving complete revascularization by PCI continue to improve as the interventional cardiology community increases its aggressiveness in using PCI to treat these lesions, as evidenced by the recent launching of at least three trials (EXPLORE, DECISION-CTO, and EURO-CTO), all designed to determine the benefit of PCI in this setting compared to medical therapy.[134] In summary, CABG surgery improves survival in patients with multivessel and complex CAD compared with PCI, in large part due to the ability of CABG to provide higher rates of complete revascularization.

THE ELDERLY

Age is a predictor of operative risk in most models, but is also a predictor of poor outcome with medical therapy in the presence of CAD. Mortality is estimated to be approximately 8 to 11% in octogenarians after CABG.[137] The Swiss Multicenter Trial of invasive versus medical therapy in the elderly (TIME) trial examined 301 patients over the age of 75 years with chronic angina and randomized them to medical therapy with or without invasive evaluation.[50] Of those undergoing angiography, two-thirds had revascularization. At the 1-year follow-up interval, there was no statistical difference in death or nonfatal MI rates. Symptoms and quality of life were also similar. However, there was a substantial increased risk of rehospitalization with revascularization in those who had medical treatment. Early interest in using off-pump CABG as a method of reducing risk in the elderly has not demonstrated any benefit in comparison to traditional on-pump CABG in two randomized controlled trials focusing specifically on patients aged 75 years and older.[138,139] A recent propensity-matched analysis of 1932 patients in this same age group showed that CABG and PCI with DES outcomes were similar at a mean follow-up interval of 1.5 years, with a higher incidence of repeat revascularization in the PCI group, similar to the conclusions drawn from studies in younger populations.[140] These data suggest that invasive evaluation should be offered to elderly people who are symptomatic only after adequate medical therapy. The choice of mode of revascularization will be particularly impacted in this group of patients by the presence of comorbidities that may increase the risk of surgical intervention, such as cerebrovascular disease, renal dysfunction, and pulmonary disease.

DIABETES MELLITUS

It has been recognized for many years that patients with DM are at higher risk following percutaneous[141] or surgical[142] revascularization. The BARI trial was the first trial large enough to identify significant differences in outcome between diabetic and nondiabetic patients. In this study, which included 353 diabetic patients, a survival benefit was observed among insulin-dependent patients undergoing CABG with an ITA, as compared with those undergoing PCI. The explanation for this is not entirely clear, although an intriguing observation is that while the incidence of subsequent MI is similar between groups, survival after MI is superior among those who have undergone surgical revascularization.[143] In fact, unlike nondiabetics, diabetics suffering spontaneous Q-wave MI were more than 10 times as likely to die with their infarction if they had been treated with PCI as compared with CABG. This survival difference was even more pronounced at 7 years with 76.4% of diabetics in the surgical arm alive as compared with 55.7% in the angioplasty arm.[144]

The physiologic basis for this difference remains a matter of speculation, although the completeness of revascularization may be a factor. Because of the significant incidence of restenosis after PCI in diabetics, Van Belle and colleagues[145] analyzed EF at 6 months and long-term cardiac mortality and morbidity among 513 diabetic patients stratified according to the presence of occlusive restenosis (n = 94), nonocclusive restenosis (n = 257), and no restenosis (n = 162). The mortality risk rose with restenosis (24% without restenosis, 35% with nonocclusive restenosis, and 59% with occlusion), and EF fell with occlusion (decrease of 4.8 ± 12.6%).

The results of the BARI trial prompted retrospective post hoc analyses of several earlier trials. The results have been variable. There was a nonsignificant trend for better survival among diabetic patients treated surgically in the EAST

trial.[146] A meta-analysis of pooled data pertaining to diabetic patients from CABRI, EAST, and RITA, however, found similar 5-year mortality rates following CABG or PCI.[147] Meanwhile, a larger meta-analysis of 10 randomized trials showed that long-term survival rates in patients with diabetes were lower in patients receiving PCI with balloon angioplasty or BMS compared to CABG.[133]

The follow-up study to BARI, BARI-2D,[148] enrolled 2368 patients with DM and stable CAD and randomized them to receive either intensive medical therapy or intensive medical therapy and prompt revascularization (CABG or PCI left to clinical judgment). At 5 years there was no difference in survival or freedom from major cardiovascular events (MI or stroke) between medical therapy and revascularization groups. This trial was not designed to compare CABG and PCI in diabetes, but rather to examine a strategy of intensive medical therapy compared with revascularization. However, in the stratum of patients who received CABG, there were fewer major cardiovascular events when compared with medical therapy (22.4 vs 30.5%, p = .002). In the stratum of patients who received PCI, there was no difference in major cardiovascular events when compared with medical therapy.

In terms of more recent randomized trials, the SYNTAX trial showed that those with higher SYNTAX scores had higher rates of repeat revascularization after PCI than after CABG.[149] More importantly, the FREEDOM trial demonstrated the most definitive and current evidence that even in the DES era, CABG confers survival benefit over PCI in diabetics with multivessel disease. It compared CABG to PCI with sirolimus- and paclitaxel-eluting stents in 1900 patients with multivessel disease and diabetes and found that 5-year rates of a composite endpoint of death from any cause, nonfatal MI, or nonfatal stroke were significantly lower in the CABG group compared to PCI (18.7 vs 26.5%)[26], supporting the results of the BARI and BARI-2D trials, but with the added caveat that the difference in outcomes was driven by a lower rate of MI and death from any cause in the CABG group.

Diabetes is a condition characterized biologically by an inflammatory, proliferative, and prothrombotic state. This may account in part for the increased risk of restenosis and occlusion. Because diabetics tend to have more diffuse disease, the importance of complete revascularization, which is more often achieved surgically that percutaneously, may be enhanced. Another explanation may have more to do with patient selection than vascular biology. It has long been recognized from the previously cited studies that the survival advantage of CABG over medical therapy is greater the more extensive the coronary disease; and more recent studies of PCI versus CABG have demonstrated similar trends. Diabetic patients tend to have more extensive disease, and in BARI diabetic patients had a higher frequency of three-vessel disease, diffuse disease, proximal LAD disease, and left ventricular dysfunction.

From a clinical standpoint with regard to patient selection for coronary revascularization and the method of revascularization, the assessment of diabetics should be made on standard principles, namely the severity and extent of coronary disease, the potential for complete revascularization, the presence or absence of left ventricular dysfunction, and the technical suitability of the lesions for PCI. The results of the aforementioned studies suggest that a preference for surgical over percutaneous revascularization remains appropriate among diabetics, especially those with complex disease and/or ventricular dysfunction. As evident from the results of the FREEDOM and SYNTAX trials, this recommendation has not changed since the introduction of DESs.

END-STAGE RENAL DISEASE

End-stage renal disease (ESRD) is a growing problem. Cardiovascular disease is the most common cause of death among those with ESRD; therefore, there will likely be high rates of revascularization required in these patients in the future. Comorbidities complicating surgical or percutaneous revascularization, such as diabetes, hypertension, and calcified vessels, are more common in patients with ESRD, increasing the risk of intervention. A study conducted by the Northern New England Consortium found dialysis-dependent patients with renal failure to be 3.1 times more likely to die after CABG after adjusting for known risk factors (OR 3.1, [2.1 to 3.7], $p < .001$).[150] They also found significantly increased rates of mediastinitis (3.6% vs 1.2%) as well as postoperative stroke (4.3% vs 1.7%). The long-term survival was also decreased with renal failure, which was found to be a highly significant predictor of mortality after adjustment.[151] Despite these risks, the prognosis without surgical correction of CAD is poor. Revascularization in patients with ESRD is associated with improved survival compared with medical management,[152-154] with some studies showing that CABG confers improved survival compared to PCI.[152,153,155-159]

Concomitant Carotid Disease

Perioperative stroke remains one of the most dreaded complications associated with CABG, and aside from the debilitating features of the stroke itself, it is associated with 21 to 23% hospital mortality.[160,161] Concomitant carotid artery disease is present in approximately 8% of patients undergoing CABG (range 2-22%, depending on the definition of stenosis, method of diagnosis, and frequency of screening).[162-165] Its presence increases the risk of perioperative stroke in some[166-169] but not all studies,[170-173] and as such, the question of whether to intervene on the carotid artery, with the goal of decreasing the perioperative as well as long-term stroke rate, has garnered significant attention in the literature. Controversy continues regarding the utility and indications for carotid endarterectomy (CEA) either before (staged), during (concomitant), or after (reverse-staged) CABG, especially in patients with asymptomatic carotid artery stenosis for whom data regarding increased risk of perioperative stroke are less wellestablished. This section will describe the relationship between extracranial carotid artery stenosis and neurologic outcomes after CABG and discuss the approach to determining whether and in what manner intervention on the carotid artery is indicated.

PERIOPERATIVE STROKE

Incidence and Causes of Perioperative Stroke. The overall incidence of perioperative stroke or TIA after CABG has been decreasing in the last two decades. Several large registry studies from prior to 2002 had estimated the incidence to be around 3%,[160,174] but recently a large registry study of almost 1.5 million patients undergoing isolated CABG between 2000 and 2009 in all STS-participating institutions has put that risk at about 1.2%.[175] The most common cause of strokes after CABG is not embolism from carotid plaques, but rather athero- or thromboembolism from complex plaques liberated from the ascending aorta as a result of direct physical manipulation inherent in the conduct of the CABG operation including cross-clamping, aortic cannulation, and the creation of proximal graft anastomoses.[176,177] Other causes include intracardiac emboli which can arise in the setting of valvular disease, atrial fibrillation, prosthetic valve implantation, suture lines, left-sided heart catheters, mural thrombus after MI, and less commonly, entrapped air. Finally, miscellaneous causes of perioperative stroke include small-vessel occlusive disease, cerebral hypoperfusion from low perfusion pressure during cardiopulmonary bypass, perioperative MI, acute arterial dissection from cannulation, and cerebral hemorrhage. Overall cardioembolic sources including those from the aorta and the aortic arch account for about 75% of perioperative strokes after CABG, while large artery stenosis, which includes carotid artery disease, accounts for 5%.[172] Although carotid disease is implicated in only a small minority of perioperative strokes, it is the one situation in which the surgeon can take definitive action to remove the pathology and in so doing, potentially also decrease the risk associated therewith.

Risk Factors for Perioperative Stroke. Age is one of the most well-established risk factors for the development of perioperative stroke. In a study from 1986, Gardner et al, showed that stroke rates increased with age, such that those younger than 45 years had stroke rates of 0.2%, rising to 3.5% for those in their 60s and 8.0% for those older than 75 years.[178] Another study in 1992 showed that stroke rates were 0.9% for those younger than 65 years but 8.9% for those older than 75 years. Other risk factors from the cardiac surgery literature include aortic calcification, renal failure, prior stroke, tobacco use, age, peripheral vascular disease, diabetes, and carotid artery disease.[161,179]

Relationship of Carotid Stenosis to Perioperative Stroke. There are several major studies dating back to the 1980s that show an increased risk of perioperative stroke after cardiac surgery in patients with significant carotid artery stenosis. In 1987, Brener and colleagues showed that among 4047 patients undergoing cardiac surgery, stroke or transient ischemic attacks (TIAs) occurred in 9.2% of patients with asymptomatic carotid artery stenosis (defined as greater than 50% luminal narrowing on carotid angiography), while those without had a stroke rate of 1.9%.[166] Faggioli and colleagues investigated this in 1990 and found similarly that those with

>75% carotid stenosis and age over 60 years, the rate of stroke was 15% versus 0.6% in patients in the same age group without carotid stenosis.[167] CEA appeared to have a protective effect; none of the patients who underwent this procedure concomitantly (19 patients) had strokes, while 14.3% (4 of 28 patients) who had carotid stenosis but did not undergo CEA developed strokes.[167] For patients 65 years or older, who are at higher risk of stroke from any cause to begin with, the degree of carotid artery stenosis was shown to affect the perioperative stroke rate such that the total neurologic event rate (stroke or TIA) was 2.5% for <50% stenosis, 7.6% for ≥50% stenosis, 109% for ≥80% stenosis, and 10.9% for unilateral occlusion.[180]

It remains unclear, however, to what extent the presence of carotid stenosis in this patient population is the direct causative element in the development of perioperative stroke, or whether its main significance is as a marker of advanced overall cardiovascular disease. Determining which of the strokes occurring in those with significant carotid stenosis actually occur ipsilaterally has given further insight into what the actual impact of performing CEA would be, especially in asymptomatic patients. Several small retrospective studies have shown that the perioperative stroke rate directly attributable to ipsilateral carotid stenosis is small in asymptomatic patients.[172,173] Li et al showed that among 18 patients with ≥50% carotid stenosis who developed perioperative stroke after CABG, only four occurred on the same side as the disease itself, and that of these four, the carotid was totally occluded in three patients, that is, not amenable to intervention. Therefore only one of 18 strokes was potentially preventable by CEA. Since 2005, there have been four studies demonstrating a 0% rate of stroke in patients with asymptomatic carotid stenosis of ≥50% (n = 156) and ≥70% (n = 42).[170,171,181,182] These data suggest, though not definitively, that at least for asymptomatic patients, the risk of perioperative stroke directly attributable to the carotid stenosis itself may be minimal, lending credence to the idea that carotid disease is perhaps more of a surrogate and that prophylactic CEA may have little benefit.

Relationship of Uncorrected Carotid Stenosis to Late Stroke.
The potential benefit of CEA in patients who have asymptomatic carotid artery disease has been shown to extend beyond the immediate perioperative period. Barnes et al showed that at 22 months following CABG in 40 patients with untreated asymptomatic carotid stenosis, the mortality rate was 10% while 17.5% had suffered a stroke.[183] One half of the patients had progression of the severity of carotid disease by noninvasive testing. Another study found that at 48 months, the risk of stroke after CABG in the setting of uncorrected significant carotid disease was 10%, that is, tenfold higher than patients who underwent combined CABG and CEA.[184] Contemporary randomized trials of surgery versus medical therapy for significant carotid stenosis have defined the late risk of carotid-related stroke in medically treated patients. In the Asymptomatic Carotid Surgery trial, actuarial risk of stroke at 5 years was

12% in medically treated patients with asymptomatic high-grade carotid stenosis.[185]

INDICATIONS FOR NONINVASIVE CAROTID TESTING
While some centers have practiced a policy of screening all patients undergoing CABG for carotid disease, studies have shown that identifying patients who are at high risk of having significant carotid disease to begin with can be screened selectively with negligible impact on the overall sensitivity. A retrospective analysis of 1421 patients undergoing CABG limited routine screening by ultrasound to only those that met the following criteria: age over 65 years, history of a stroke or TIA, and presence of a carotid bruit.[186] The investigators determined that this reduced the need for preoperative testing by 40% overall while missing only 2% of all candidates with ≥70% carotid stenosis. The ACCF/AHA issued a Class IIa recommendation that carotid artery duplex scanning should be performed for patients who have clinical features associated with a high risk of concurrent carotid artery stenosis, including age over 65 years, left main coronary stenosis, peripheral vascular disease, history of stroke or TIA, hypertension, smoking, and DM.[10]

MYOCARDIAL ISCHEMIC EVENTS IN PATIENTS AFTER CAROTID ENDARTERECTOMY
The incidence of CAD in the general population of patients undergoing CEA is high. A study from the Cleveland Clinic found that in patients studied with routine preoperative coronary angiography prior to planned CEA, only 7% had normal coronary arteries, while 28% had mild-to-moderate CAD, 30% had advanced but compensated disease, 28% had severe but correctable disease, and 7% had severe, inoperable CAD.[187] Early studies demonstrated that the risk of perioperative MI in the setting of CAD as significantly higher (4.3% compared to 0.5%).[188] Hertzer and colleagues showed that for patients undergoing CEA, MI caused more late deaths (37%) than did stroke (15%), with improved 10-year survival in the cohort of patients who had undergone incidental CABG compared to those with suspected but undocumented coronary disease (55% vs 32%).[189]

COMBINED CORONARY AND CAROTID REVASCULARIZATION

Guidelines for Combined Coronary and Carotid Revascularization.
To date, there exist no randomized trials comparing a combined or staged approach to carotid disease in asymptomatic patients to CABG alone. The CABACS trial which began in 2010 is currently ongoing and will report on the relative incidence of strokes and death from any cause by randomly assigning patients to concomitant (ie, synchronous) CEA and CABG versus CABG alone in patients with high grade carotid stenosis undergoing CABG.[190] Until then, the current guidelines from the ACCF/AHA are based on a large body of retrospective data that have not conclusively established the optimal approach

to treating this patient population. Indeed, the formal Class I recommendation is that for patients with clinically significant carotid artery disease for whom CABG is planned, a multidisciplinary team consisting of a cardiac surgery, cardiologist, neurologist, and vascular surgeon should convene and determine an individualized plan regarding whether and when to perform CEA.[10] Meanwhile, for patients with a previous TIA or stroke and a significant carotid artery lesion (≥50% stenosis), combined CABG and carotid revascularization is recommended on a Class IIa basis. The sequence and timing of intervention is determined by the relative magnitudes of cerebral and myocardial dysfunction.[10] Finally, in patients scheduled for CABG who have no history of TIA or stroke but have bilateral severe (70-99%) carotid stenosis or unilateral severe carotid stenosis with a contralateral occlusion, combined carotid revascularization is recommended on a Class IIb basis.[10]

These guideline recommendations notwithstanding, Cambria and colleagues at our institution have argued that if one accepts that (1) uncorrected carotid stenosis is associated with an increase in stroke risk for patients with severe carotid and CAD who have only isolated CABG; (2) CEA is the indicated treatment for severe symptomatic and asymptomatic carotid stenosis; (3) CAD increases the early and late risk of death for CEA patients; and (4) CABG is an indicated treatment for CAD, then the important question becomes not the indication for but the timing of the two operative procedures. It is on these grounds that some surgeons in our institution have, since the 1970s, taken an aggressive approach to patients with both CAD and carotid stenosis, with the concomitant operation used as the standard approach.

Staged versus Concomitant Carotid and Coronary Artery Operations.

The technique of performing CEA before coronary bypass grafting is referred to, by convention, as a *staged procedure*, while performing the CABG first and the CEA in delayed fashion is termed a *reverse staged procedure*. Performing both procedures under the same general anesthetic administration is a *concomitant procedure*.

On the one hand, performing CEA first might increase the risk of perioperative MI, while performing CABG first might increase the risk of perioperative stroke. If the patient does not have signs of active ischemia or hemodynamic instability, especially if the CEA can be performed safely with regional anesthesia, most agree that performing CEA first is a reasonable strategy. This argument is strengthened further in elderly patients with a history of prior stroke or TIA in whom the incidence of perioperative MI might be expected to be significantly higher. Meanwhile, for patients with active ischemia and/or hemodynamic instability secondary to coronary disease, the reversed staged procedure is sometimes favored, especially for those with asymptomatic carotid stenosis and no history of stroke or TIA. These general principles are considered on a case-by-case basis without the benefit of any randomized controlled trial data to definitively support one strategy versus the other.

The American Academy of Neurology (AAN) systematically reviewed all studies with over 50 patients comparing staged versus concomitant CEA and CABG and found that for nine studies evaluating concomitant CEA and CABG, the overall rate of stroke was 3%, while MI occurred in 2.2%, and death in 4.7%. In the one study included in this review describing staged CEA followed by CABG, the stroke rate was 1.9%, while MI occurred in 4.7%, and death in 1.6%. The AAN concluded that there was no clear general argument for one strategy versus the other based on these data.[191]

At our institution, the concomitant approach has been the standard strategy for most patients presenting with asymptomatic severe carotid stenosis and CAD amenable to CABG. Akins et al published a series of 500 patients who underwent a concomitant operation between 1979 and 2001 and found that hospital mortality was 3.6%, MI rate was 2.0%, and stroke occurred in 4.6%.[192] While 66% were neurologically asymptomatic preoperatively, 21% had prior TIAs while 13% had a prior stroke. The degree of coronary disease was relatively severe with 75% presenting with three-vessel disease and 42% presenting with significant left main disease. Three-fourths had unstable angina, and 53% had prior MI. The operation was performed either urgently or emergently in 54% of patients. In other words, the outcomes delineated above are rather favorable considering the patient population included. Of the 23 strokes that occurred, 12 were ipsilateral to the CEA and 11 were contralateral or bilateral, suggesting that this strategy may have neutralized the impact of carotid stenosis as a risk factor for stroke during CABG. The upcoming CABACS trial will, as the first randomized trial to shed light on the question of how these interventions should be sequenced, shed some light on the controversy inherent in these results, albeit on a significantly limited subset of the patients seen in actual clinical practice, that is, those undergoing elective CABG who have asymptomatic carotid stenosis.[190]

PREDICTION OF OPERATIVE RISK

Prediction of risk-adjusted outcomes permits both the surgeon and the patient to weigh the potential benefits of operation against risks of perioperative morbidity and/or mortality. The patient's comprehension of benefit versus risk is paramount to informed consent before coronary artery bypass surgery. Accurate risk-adjusted prediction of postoperative morbidity and mortality also provides an important quality improvement tool to understand and examine the variability in institutional and individual surgeon performance.

A number of cardiac surgery databases have been used to develop risk models for predicting operative morbidity and mortality in patients undergoing CABG.[21] One of the more user-friendly risk assessment tools is that provided by the STS Risk Calculator (http://www.sts.org/quality-research-patient-safety/quality/risk-calculator-and-models/risk-calculator), which provides an assessment of individual patient operative risk derived using the STS database (Table 20-4). The STS risk algorithm is proprietary and is based on data voluntarily

TABLE 20-4: Independent Variables Associated with Mortality after Isolated Coronary Artery Bypass Graft Surgery

Variable	Odds ratio	95% Confidence interval
Multiple reoperations	4.19	3.61-4.86
First reoperation	2.76	2.62-2.91
Shock	2.04	1.90-2.19
Surgery status	1.96	1.88-2.05
Renal failure/dialysis	1.88	1.80-1.96
Immunosuppressants	1.75	1.57-1.95
Insulin-dependent diabetes mellitus	1.5	1.42-1.58
Intra-aortic balloon pump use	1.46	1.37-1.55
Chronic lung disease	1.41	1.35-1.48
Percutaneous transluminal coronary angioplasty, 6 h	1.32	1.18-1.48

Data were collected from 503,478 patients undergoing isolated CABG in the United States from 1997 to 1999 from Society of Thoracic Surgeons' database. Variables are listed in decreasing order of importance.

Data from Shroyer AL, Coombs LP, Peterson ED, et al: The Society of Thoracic Surgeons: 30-day operative mortality and morbidity risk models, *Ann Thorac Surg.* 2003 Jun;75(6):1856-1864.

CABG, coronary artery bypass graft.

 TABLE 20-5: Variables Associated with Development of a Major Complication after Isolated Coronary Artery Bypass Graft Surgery

Variable	Odds ratio	95% Confidence interval
Renal failure/dialysis	2.49	2.41-2.58
Multiple reoperations	2.13	1.92-2.36
Shock	1.86	1.78-1.95
Intra-aortic balloon pump use	1.78	1.72-1.84
First reoperation	1.75	1.70-1.81
Insulin-dependent diabetes mellitus	1.59	1.54-1.64
Surgery status	1.58	1.53-1.63
Chronic lung disease	1.41	1.38-1.45
Immunosuppressants	1.34	1.26-1.43
Percutaneous transluminal coronary angioplasty < 6 h	1.33	1.23-1.43

Any major complication is defined as the composite outcome of stroke, renal failure, prolonged ventilation, mediastinitis, or reoperation. Data collected from 503,478 patients undergoing isolated CABG in the United States from 1997 to 1999 from the Society of Thoracic Surgeons' database. Variables are listed in decreasing order of importance.

Data from Shroyer AL, Coombs LP, Peterson ED, et al: The Society of Thoracic Surgeons: 30-day operative mortality and morbidity risk models, *Ann Thorac Surg.* 2003 Jun;75(6):1856-1864.

submitted by participating centers on 503,478 patients undergoing isolated CABG in the United States from 1997 to 1999; the application is available for public use.

Overall, the average risks of 30-day operative death and major complication for patients reported to the STS database undergoing CABG from 1997 to 1999 were 3.05 and 13.4%, respectively. Specific complications included stroke (1.6%), renal failure (3.5%), reoperation (5.2%), prolonged ventilation (5.9%), and sternal infection (0.63%). Risk models were developed using multivariate analysis to stratify the strength of the association from among 30 potential preoperative risk factors for mortality and major complications as shown in Tables 20-5 and 20-6. Except for deep sternal wound infection, the development of any of these complications correlated with an increased risk-adjusted operative mortality.[193]

A preliminary sense of operative mortality can be derived simply from an understanding of the core variables most predictive of risk in the aforementioned data sets. The strongest predictors of operative mortality include nonelective surgery, low EF, and prior heart surgery. Chronic comorbidities are also associated with an increased operative mortality after coronary bypass, including treated diabetes, peripheral vascular occlusive disease, chronic renal insufficiency, and chronic obstructive pulmonary disease (COPD).[21]

Patient Evaluation

Regardless of the risk model applied, there is no substitute for clinical evaluation of the patient. Unfortunately, all too often the assessment focuses disproportionately on coronary anatomy and insufficiently on the nature, duration, and severity of ischemic symptoms, as well as signs and symptoms of congestive heart failure (CHF). In addition, history of or coexisting cerebrovascular and/or peripheral vascular disease, malignancy, sternal radiation, COPD, DM, or renal and/or hepatic insufficiency can have major impact on the operative morbidity and even mortality, not all of which are captured in risk models.

Current medications and dosages with special attention to antiplatelet agents such as clopidogrel must be reviewed. Operation in the setting of recent clopidogrel use is associated with excessive bleeding and need for reoperation.[194] Most surgeons recommend 5 days from the last administered dose of clopidogrel before undertaking CABG with cardiopulmonary bypass. The same holds true for several new antiplatelet medications routinely used in clinical cardiology practice, such as prastagril as well as medications used as substitutes for warfarin in patients with atrial fibrillation (eg, dabigatran).

Physical examination of the lungs and heart should focus on the stigma of ischemic and valvular heart disease. Cardiac murmurs warrant further evaluation. Additionally, the adequacy of presternal soft tissues to permit wound closure should be considered and evidence of venous varicosities or prior vein stripping may impact plans for conduit harvest. Peripheral pulses should be documented as their presence or absence may impact from which leg to harvest the vein or

TABLE 20-6: Variables Associated with Development of a Specific Postoperative Complication

Stroke	Renal failure	Prolonged ventilation	Mediastinitis	Reoperation
Variable, odds ratio (95% confidence interval)				
PVD/CVD, 1.5 (1.44-1.56)	Renal failure/dialysis, 4.3 (4.09-4.52)	Multiple reoperations, 2.3 (2.01-2.64)	IDDM, 2.74 (2.47-3.03)	Multiple reoperations, 1.69 (1.49-1.97)
Renal failure/dialysis, 1.49 (1.37-1.62)	IDDM, 2.26 (2.16-2.37)	IABP, 2.26 (2.17-2.36)	Chronic lung disease, 1.62 (1.47-1.78)	Shock, 1.46 (1.37-1.56)
IDDM, 1.48 (1.37-1.59)	Shock, 1.6 (1.48-1.72)	First reoperation, 1.97 (1.89-2.05)	NIDDM, 1.53 (1.38-1.70)	First reoperation, 1.40 (1.33-1.47)
Previous CVA, 1.43 (1.33-1.53)	Multiple reoperations, 1.6 (1.33-1.92)	Renal failure/dialysis, 1.95 (1.86-2.04)	Immunosuppressants, 1.49 (1.18-1.89)	PTCA < 6 h, 1.42 (1.28-1.58)
Surgery status, 1.38 (1.29-1.48)	First reoperation, 1.55 (1.46-1.64)	Shock, 1.95 (1.85-2.06)	IABP, 1.43 (1.25-1.64)	Renal failure/dialysis, 1.38 (1.33-1.44)
Shock, 1.36 (1.21-1.52)	IABP, 1.54 (1.45-1.64)	Chronic lung disease, 1.67 (1.61-1.73)	Mitral insufficiency, 1.39 (1.17-1.65)	IABP, 1.36 (1.29-1.43)
NIDDM, 1.36 (1.28-1.45)	Immunosuppressants, 1.48 (1.33-1.64)	IDDM, 1.53 (1.47-1.59)	Obese female, 1.38 (1.35-1.42)	Chronic lung disease, 1.32 (1.27-1.37)
HTN, 1.30 (1.22-1.38)	PTCA < 6 h, 1.46 (1.29-1.66)	Surgery status, 1.46 (1.41-1.52)	Renal failure/dialysis, 1.27 (1.14-1.41)	Mitral insufficiency, 1.31 (1.23-1.40)

Data collected from 503,478 patients undergoing isolated CABG in the United States from 1997 to 1999 from the Society of Thoracic Surgeons' database. Variables are listed in decreasing order of importance.

CVA, cerebrovascular accident; HTN, history of hypertension; IABP, intra-aortic balloon pump; IDDM, insulin-dependent diabetes mellitus; NIDDM, non–insulin-dependent diabetes mellitus; PTCA, percutaneous transluminal coronary angioplasty; PVD/CVD, peripheral vascular disease/cardiovascular disease.

Data from Shroyer AL, Coombs LP, Peterson ED, et al: The Society of Thoracic Surgeons: 30-day operative mortality and morbidity risk models, *Ann Thorac Surg.* 2003 Jun;75(6):1856-1864.

place an intra-aortic balloon pump (IABP). A detailed neurologic examination of the ulnar, radial, and median nerves should be document in the case of planned radial artery (RA) harvest.

Diagnostic evaluation should be directed by the clinical assessment, but at a minimum should include a renal panel (creatinine), complete blood count, and chest x-ray. The ECG should be reviewed for the evidence of previous MI and conduction abnormalities. Radiologic evaluation should rule out concomitant neoplasm, active pulmonary infection, and/or ascending aorta calcification; the latter should be further assessed with a noncontrast computed tomographic (CT) scan because it will impact the location for arterial cannulation and aortic cross-clamp placement.

Hemodynamically significant coronary artery lesions on angiography are conventionally defined as those lesions with a 50% loss of arterial diameter, which is sufficient to impair coronary blood flow reserve and distal coronary pressure.[21] An assessment should be made of left ventricular function and regional wall motion abnormalities as well as the presence and degree of valvular abnormalities, including aortic stenosis and mitral regurgitation with echocardiography. Left ventriculography is not routinely performed and is reserved for patients who require direct pressure measurements of left ventricular pressures to further assess the gradient through the aortic valve. In cases where a previous sternotomy has

been performed and the internal thoracic arteries have not been utilized, their patency and integrity should be assessed at the time of cardiac catheterization since these conduits could have been injured at the time of sternal wire placement during chest closure. This becomes especially important if the saphenous veins are not available for the procedure and revascularization is dependent on the integrity of the internal thoracic artery (ITA).

It is in the surgeon's best interest to develop a good relationship with the patient and his or her significant others. Specifics including the risks, benefits, and alternatives to surgery need to be discussed to permit an informed decision. Ideally, this discussion is held in the presence of the patient's significant others, because patients often have difficulty absorbing the details of the discussion at the time related to the stress of the situation. Should the patient experience a major complication or mortality, it is often the patient's significant others with whom the surgeon will most often interact. Additionally, anticipated need for postoperative rehabilitation, as well as the time course of recovery is also of interest to all parties. A clear understanding of the expectations for the perioperative period will reduce everyone's anxiety about surgery and may promote early patient recovery. Good rapport with patients and their significant others is also the physician's best protection from litigation should untoward events occur.

BYPASS CONDUITS

Internal Thoracic Artery

The left ITA as a bypass graft to the left anterior descending coronary artery has been proven to provide superior early and late survival and better event-free survival after CABG.[46] The unparalleled long-term patency and better clinical outcomes associated with the use of the ITA make it the conduit of first choice for anastomosis to the left anterior descending coronary artery in almost all patients regardless of age, and establish an argument to use the right ITA as conduit to other targets as well.

CHARACTERISTICS

The ITA demonstrates remarkable resistance to development of atherosclerosis, which may be in part attributable to a greater resistance of its endothelium to harvest injury as compared with the saphenous vein. Under electron microscopy examination, thrombogenic intimal defects are essentially nonexistent in the ITA but are commonly detected in venous grafts.[195] Perhaps more significantly, however, is the nonfenestrated internal elastic lamina of the ITA that may inhibit cellular migration, thereby preventing initiation of intimal hyperplasia. In addition, the medial layer of the ITA is thin, with fewer smooth muscle cells and a lesser proliferative response to known mitogens such as platelet-derived growth factor and pulsatile mechanical stretch.[196,197]

The endothelium of the ITA is itself unique as well. With a significantly higher basal production of the vasodilators nitric oxide and prostacyclin, the ITA demonstrates a favorable response to pharmacologic agents commonly used in the postoperative period. For instance, the ITA shows vasodilation in response to milrinone and yet does not vasoconstrict in response to norepinephrine.[198] Furthermore, nitroglycerin causes vasodilation in the ITA, but not in the saphenous vein.[199] The endogenous secretion of such vasodilators may also have a "downstream" effect on the coronary vasculature, explaining the common observation that the native coronary vessel itself often appears relatively protected from progressive atherosclerotic disease distal to the anastomosis. Finally, the ITA exhibits remarkable remodeling over time, adapting to the demand for increased flow by often increasing in diameter over time as observed on late postoperative angiograms, a phenomenon mediated by the endothelium.[200]

SURGICAL ANATOMY OF THE INTERNAL THORACIC ARTERY

The ITA arises from the undersurface of the first portion of the subclavian artery opposite the thyrocervical trunk. The left ITA originates as a single artery in 70% of patients and as a common trunk with other arteries in 30%. In contrast, the right ITA originates as a single artery in 95% of cases.[201] At the level of the clavicle and the first rib, the ITA passes at first downward and medially behind the subclavian

vein and lateral to the innominate vein. In this area, the phrenic nerve crosses the ITA from its lateral to its medial side, before contacting the pericardium. The phrenic nerve crosses anterior to the ITA 66% of the time on the left and 74% of the time on the right.[201] It is important to keep these relations in mind to avoid phrenic nerve injury during proximal ITA harvest.

Below the first costal cartilage the ITA descends almost vertically and slightly laterally at a short distance from the margin of the sternum. The ITA lies posterior to the cartilages of the upper six ribs and the intervening internal intercostal muscles. In the upper chest there is a bare area of variable length where the ITA is covered only by the endothoracic fascia and parietal pleura. Below this level the transversus thoracis muscle covers the posterior surface of the ITA. The mean distance of the left ITA from the sternal margin at the level of the first intercostal space is 10.5 ± 3.2 mm, whereas at the level of the sixth intercostal space the distance increases to 20.0 ± 6.7 mm. The right ITA is slightly closer to the sternal margin than the left ITA. At the level of the sixth rib the ITA bifurcates into its terminal branches: the musculophrenic and superior epigastric arteries. The length of the ITA in situ ranges from 15 to 26 cm, with a mean of 20.4 ± 2.1 cm; the left ITA is slightly longer than the right.[201] A pair of internal mammary veins (venae comitantes) accompanies the ITA; at the most superior portion these veins form a single vessel, which runs medial to the artery and drains into the innominate vein.

PEDICLED HARVEST TECHNIQUE

After the sternum is divided, the left ITA is harvested using an internal mammary retractor to expose the internal mammary bed (Fig. 20-4). Excessive distraction of the sternal leaves can cause costal fractures or dislocation of the costosternal joints, resulting in severe postoperative pain as well as brachial plexus injury. The parietal pleura and loose connective tissue with accompanying fat is dissected away from the chest wall. It is our preference to enter the left pleural space widely to allow easier exposure of the ITA, especially in its most proximal aspect, and to permit the ITA to fall into a more lateral and posterior path upon wound closure, keeping the ITA medial to the lung, lateral to the pericardium, and away from the posterior table of the sternum. This makes it less susceptible to injury during potential sternal reentry in the future. Slightly rotating the operating table to the patient's left and decreasing the patient's tidal volume can aid in the visualization.

The ITA is identified lateral to the border of the sternum by inspection of the bare area or by palpation in the area of artery covered by muscle. It can be harvested using either a pedicled, semiskeletonized, or a skeletonized technique. When taken as a pedicle, the dissection plane can be started in the bare area of the ITA at the level of the third or fourth rib or at the level of the lower sternum. The intercostal space is avoided as the initial point of exposure because it contains the branch vessels. The endothoracic fascia is incised medially for

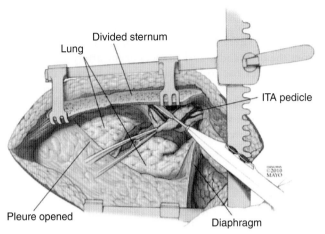

FIGURE 20-4 Internal thoracic artery (ITA) harvest. A self-retaining mammary retractor is used for exposure of the ITA bed. The left pleura is dissected away from the mammary pedicle and opened along the course of the ITA. The endothoracic fascia is incised medial and lateral to the ITA pedicle. The pedicle is carefully separated with blunt dissection from the underside of the rib. Gentle traction on the pedicle exposes arterial and venous branches at the level of the intercostal spaces; vessels are clipped on the ITA side and cauterized or clipped on the chest wall side. The proximal dissection is carried to the inferior border of the subclavian vein; the distal dissection is then carried to the level of the ITA bifurcation. The trans versus thoracis muscle must be divided to expose the ITA bifurcation. The ITA is divided after full heparinization, either at the end of harvest or just before grafting of the left anterior descending (LAD) artery. (By permission of Mayo Foundation for Medical Education and Research. All rights reserved.)

a distance of about 4 cm using the electrocautery at low setting (ie, 20). The pedicle is carefully separated from the chest wall using gentle blunt dissection with the electrocautery tip. Exposure can be enhanced by pushing the pedicle away with closed forceps or by gently grasping the fascia. The ITA is a fragile vessel and the conduit should never be grasped with the forceps. Gentle posterior traction on the pedicle allows exposure of arterial and venous branches, which should be clipped and divided.

After the pedicle has been freed for about 4 cm, the endothoracic fascia is incised laterally, allowing the pedicle to fall away from the chest wall. Dissection is continued proximally and distally to the level of the subclavian vein and ITA bifurcation. Attention should be given to avoid injury to the phrenic nerve during the proximal exposure. Once the dissection is completed, the patient is heparinized (fully or partially) and the pedicle sprayed with a papaverine solution (1 cc [30 mg] of papaverine added to 9 cc of saline). Three minutes after heparinization, the distal ITA is doubly clipped just proximal to the bifurcation and the artery divided. An atraumatic bulldog clamp is applied to the distal end of the artery and the pedicle is kept in a papaverine soaked sponge until the vessel is anastomosed to the arterial target. Alternatively, the pedicle may be left in situ and transected just before using the conduit.

SKELETONIZATION OF THE INTERNAL THORACIC ARTERY

Sternal blood flow decreases significantly after pedicled ITA harvest. Skeletonized harvest, however, reduces the degree of sternal ischemia. Two prospective randomized studies assessing sternal blood supply using bone scan with SPECT after skeletonized and pedicled harvest have demonstrated significant reduction in sternal vascularity after pedicled harvest, whereas skeletonized harvest resulted in minimal change in sternal blood supply. Multivariate analysis found harvesting technique to be the only factor responsible for postoperative sternal ischemia.[202,203]

Low rates of sternal wound infection have been reported using skeletonized bilateral ITA harvest. Matsa and associates observed a deep sternal wound infection rate of 1.7% among 765 patients undergoing bilateral skeletonized ITA harvest. Of note, sternal complications occurred in only 2.6% of 231 diabetic patients in this study, which was not significantly different from that of the nondiabetic patients.[204] In Calafiore and coworkers' review of 842 patients undergoing bilateral skeletonized ITA harvest compared with a historical nonskeletonized bilateral ITA control group, skeletonized harvest was associated with a reduced incidence of sternal wound complications (4.5%) versus pedicle harvest (1.7%). Diabetic patients in the study derived the greatest benefit from skeletonized harvest with respect to sternal wound complications: 10% in the pedicle harvest versus 2.2% in the skeletonized harvest groups.[205]

Using the skeletonized harvest technique, only the artery is mobilized, leaving the internal thoracic venous plexus intact. Although skeletonization is a technically more demanding and time-consuming procedure, it increases luminal diameter and free flow compared with a pedicled graft, and also provides a longer conduit.[206] Some surgeons have expressed concerns regarding functional integrity, vasoreactive profile, and early and long-term patency; however, several investigators have shown no difference in endothelial integrity, endothelial-dependent or neurogenic-dependent vasoreactivity between the techniques of pedicle or skeletonized harvest.[205,207,208] Furthermore, there does not appear to be any difference with respect to early and midterm patency.[209,210]

PATENCY

The superior late patency of an ITA graft to the left anterior descending coronary artery compared to a saphenous vein graft (SVG) was initially demonstrated by Barner and colleagues in the 1985.[211] Superior patency translates into improved 10-year survival (left internal thoracic artery [LITA]-to-LAD artery 82.6% vs SVG-to-LAD artery 71%) with less incidence of MI, hospitalization for cardiac events, and cardiac reoperations.[46] The superior performance of ITA grafts appears to persist in the current era despite the use of agents to improve vein graft performance. In the BARI trial the patency rates at 1 and 4 years for ITA grafts were 98 and 91% compared with vein grafts, which were 87 and 83%, respectively.[212,213] The superior patency of the ITA becomes even more prominent with longer follow-up. In an angiographic study of 1408 symptomatic post-CABG patients, patency rates for the LITA at 10 and 15 years were 95 and 88%, respectively, whereas SVG patencies were 61 and 32% at the same time intervals.[214]

Radial Artery

The use of the RA as a conduit for coronary bypass was originally described by Carpentier and associates in 1973. Spasm of the artery was common during surgery and was managed by mechanical dilation. The initial results were disappointing with 32% of grafts occluded at 2 years.[215] Accordingly, the RA was abandoned as a conduit for CABG. Acar and colleagues revived the use of the RA after several grafts, angio-graphically demonstrated to be "occluded" early postoperatively, were patent during restudy 15 years later. Acar postulated that harvest injury was responsible for the spasm/graft occlusion.[216] Proponents of the RA as a conduit have demonstrated encouraging mid- and long-term results with a pedicled harvesting technique and pharmacologic manipulation to prevent RA vasospasm.[217] As a result, this conduit has enjoyed a remarkable resurgence of interest as a supplementary arterial conduit for coronary revascularization.

CHARACTERISTICS

Histologically, the RA has a fenestrated internal elastic lamina and a thicker wall than the ITA with a higher density of myocytes in its media.[218] The RA is also more likely to have atherosclerotic changes at the time of harvest than the ITA, with 28% of RAs having some degree of demonstrable atherosclerosis, as compared with only 6% of ITAs. Whether these differences indicate that the RA will prove more susceptible to graft atherosclerosis with reduced patency is unknown.[219]

Physiologically, the RA is equally sensitive to norepinephrine as the ITA; however, given its greater muscle mass, it generates a higher force of contraction, accounting for its well-recognized propensity for spasm.[220] Fortunately, the RA also readily responds to a variety of vasodilators, including calcium channel blockers, papaverine, nitrates, and milrinone. In vitro, nitroglycerine appears to be the most effective agent for inhibiting and reversing RA spasm.[221] Additionally, nitroglycerin has been shown to be better tolerated clinically, equally effective, and less expensive than diltiazem in prophylaxis of RA spasm after CABG in a prospective randomized trial.[222]

SURGICAL ANATOMY OF THE RADIAL ARTERY

The RA originates from the brachial artery just proximal to the biceps tendon. In the proximal forearm the RA courses underneath the brachioradialis muscle. As it courses distally, it emerges from the lower surface of the muscle, becoming more superficial, and runs beneath the antebrachial fascia between the tendon of the brachioradialis muscle and the flexor carpi radialis muscle and anterior to the radius and

pronator quadratus muscle. The recurrent RA originates from the lateral aspect of the RA soon after its origin from the brachial artery. Multiple small muscular branches emerge from the deep and lateral surfaces of the artery. At the wrist the RA gives rise to the palmar carpal branch, the dorsal carpal branch, the superficial palmar branch, and the deep palm.[223] Throughout its course, the RA is accompanied by a rich plexus of venae comitantes. The average length of the RA ranges between 18 and 22 cm with an internal diameter of 2 to 3 mm.[224]

HARVEST TECHNIQUE

It is most common to consider the patient's nondominant arm for harvest, partially out of concern for the impact of even subtle neurologic changes, and partially given the convenience of harvesting the left RA simultaneously with the left ITA. The extremity of interest must have adequate ulnar collateral circulation to ensure viability of the hand. Assessment of collateral circulation is best performed via noninvasive duplex ultrasonography.[225] The RA of the dominant hand can also be harvested if needed. Tatoulis and associates reported 261 patients undergoing bilateral RA harvesting with safe functional outcomes of both extremities.[226]

The arm is prepped circumferentially and the hand wrapped in a sterile fashion. The upper extremity is placed on an arm board perpendicular to the long axis of the operating table. As shown in Fig. 20-5, a medially curved incision is made on the skin overlying the RA from a point 2 cm proximal to the styloid process of the radius to a point 2 cm distal to the elbow crease and 1 cm medial to the biceps tendon. The subcutaneous tissue is divided with the cautery. The dissection can be initiated at either end depending on the surgeon's preference. The deep fascia of the forearm is incised directly over the RA.

The RA is harvested as a pedicle with minimal manipulation using sharp dissection, diathermy, or the harmonic scalpel (our preferred method). There are data to suggest that early graft flow is superior when the harmonic scalpel is used.[227] On the proximal half of the forearm, gentle lateral retraction of the brachioradialis muscle aids exposure. At the distal end of the dissection the satellite veins are identified and divided. The proximal end of the dissection is marked by the radial recurrent artery branch and a large venous plexus in the medial aspect of the RA. It is our routine to leave the recurrent radial branch intact. The artery is divided proximally and distally and stored in a room temperature solution of lactate, nitroglycerin, and papaverine.

After the RA is removed from the forearm, hemostasis of the operative field is obtained and the arm is closed in multiple layers. A closed suction drain is placed, which we feel helps reduce postoperative seroma formation. A circumferential elastic wrap is applied. The arm is then abducted and secured to the table. Reports of endoscopic RA harvest are beginning to emerge with good functional and cosmetic results; nonetheless the impact of the technique on graft patency is unknown.[228] We have not adopted the technique.

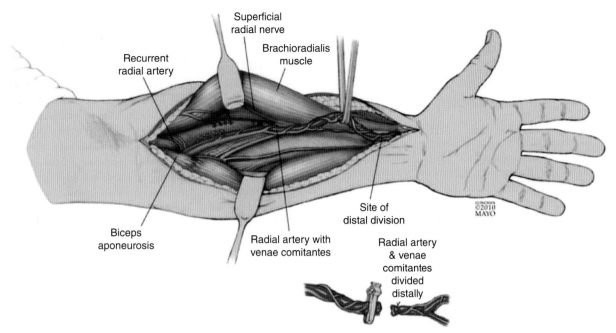

FIGURE 20-5 Radial artery harvest. A medially curved incision is made on the forearm over the artery. The deep fascia of the forearm is incised directly over the artery. The brachioradialis muscle is retracted laterally. Dissection is begun at the distal end and the satellite veins are divided. The RA is harvested as a pedicle with minimal manipulation. The proximal end of the dissection is marked by the radial recurrent branch, which is left intact. After the pedicle is free and heparin has been given, the artery is divided proximally and distally and stored in a room temperature solution of lactate, nitroglycerin, and papaverine. Hemostasis of the operative field is obtained and the arm is closed in multiple layers. A closed suction drain is placed. (By permission of Mayo Foundation for Medical Education and Research. All rights reserved.)

Two cutaneous nerves are of importance to note during RA dissection. The lateral antebrachial cutaneous nerve lies superficial to the belly of the brachioradialis muscle and runs close to its medial border. Placing the skin incision medial to the edge of the brachioradialis prevents potential injury. Damage to this nerve will produce paresthesias and numbness of the radial aspect of the volar forearm. The superficial branch of the radial nerve lies under the brachioradialis muscle and in the proximal two-thirds of the forearm runs parallel to the RA. Injury to this nerve will result in paresthesias and numbness of the thumb and the dorsum of the hand. The nerve can best be protected by avoiding excessive lateral retraction on the brachioradialis muscle.[223,229] Transient paresthesias, numbness, and thumb weakness are common and are reported by almost a third of patients after RA harvest; fortunately, the symptoms gradually resolve with time so that after 1 year only 10% of patients have residual complaints with only 1% reporting their symptoms as severe.[230-232]

The radial can also be harvested endoscopically through a small incision overlying the artery at the wrist, using a smaller size endoscope than the one normally used for endoscopic saphenous vein harvesting. A long shafted harmonic scalpel can also be used with this technique. Proponents of endoscopic RA harvesting have reported this to be a safe and effective technique, with less pain and fewer wound complications than the open surgical technique,[233] and has become the harvesting method of choice of some centers.[234]

PATENCY

Acar and associates in 1992 reported on 122 radial grafts with a 100% patency rate at 2 weeks and 93% patency at 9 months.[235] The results appear durable with reported patencies at 48 months of 89%. Several factors may affect RA graft patency, however, including both target artery runoff and competitive flow. In the prospective, randomized Radial Artery Patency Study, more severe target coronary artery stenosis was associated with lower rate of occlusion (>90% stenosis = 5.9% vs 70 to 89% stenosis = 11.8%).[236] The graft failure rate is highest if the target vessel is the right coronary artery system, but this may be related more to the coronary artery than the bypass conduit; one study showed equal patency of RA and saphenous vein bypass grafts to the right coronary artery.[237-239]

The proximal RA can be sutured to the ITA as a T- or Y-graft (composite), sutured directly to the ascending aorta, or sutured to the proximal portion or hood of a separate vein graft. In addition, a segment of vein can be interposed between the aorta and proximal RA in an end-to-end fashion. Comparisons have been made between the T- or Y-graft and direct aortic anastomosis methods. Maniar et al found at approximately 30 months follow-up, a significantly greater incidence of postoperative angiography for recurrent angina among patients with direct aortic anastomosis as compared with patients with composite anastomosis (19% vs 11%).[237] There is controversy here, however, as Jung et al found that 1-, 2-, and 5-year patency rates were significantly better with direct aortic anastomosis as compared with composite anastomosis.[240] Importantly, it appears that the overall patency of RA grafts to ideal targets may be superior to that of saphenous vein bypass grafts at 5 years, 98% versus 86%.[241]

Other Arterial Conduits

A variety of arterial conduits have been used in patients in whom no other conduits are available. The gastroepiploic artery (GEA) for the most part is utilized as an alternative conduit or as part of an all-arterial revascularization strategy. Despite the enthusiastic support of a small cohort of surgeons, the widespread use of the GEA as a coronary conduit has not been adopted, perhaps because of the increased operative time and relative difficulty required to harvest the conduit, the potential for perioperative and long-term abdominal complications, and the lack of consensus on the long-term benefit for total arterial revascularization. Anecdotal use of the ulnar, left gastric, splenic, thoracodorsal, lateral femoral circumflex and inferior epigastric arteries as coronary graft conduits has been reported in the literature. The popularity of the RA, however, has in large measure superseded these options.

Greater Saphenous Vein

The saphenous vein continues to be one of the most commonly used conduits in coronary bypass grafting. Characteristics that have solidified the greater saphenous vein as a coronary artery bypass conduit include its ease of harvest, ready availability, versatility, resistance to spasm, and thoroughly studied long-term results. Unfortunately there is a loss of clinical benefit after CABG because of time-related attrition. Accordingly, there is interest in pharmacologic strategies to maximize early and late venous graft patency.

Prospective randomized trials have shown that early aspirin administration reduces mortality after CABG. Aspirin within 48 hours after CABG also reduces early postoperative complications, including mortality, MI, stroke, renal failure, and bowel infarction.[242] More recently, it has been recognized that lipid-lowering agents reduce the progression of graft atherosclerosis.[243,244] Aggressive use of statins to achieve a low-density lipoprotein cholesterol < 100 mg/dL decrease by one-third the number of grafts affected with atherosclerosis at angiographic follow-up and also decreased the need for repeat revascularization.[243] With clear documentation of improved outcomes with these two pharmacologic strategies, systematic approaches to ensure their universal application are needed.[21]

Finally, in the future, gene therapy may allow modification of the venous vascular endothelium to avert development of intimal hyperplasia. Unfortunately, the PREVENT IV trial, testing whether short-term angiographic vein graft failure could be diminished with treatment of the saphenous vein before grafting with edifoligide (an oligonucleotide decoy that binds to and inhibits E2F transcription factors), demonstrated no impact of the treatment.[245] The concept remains a valid one, however, and gene therapy will continue to be an exciting area of investigation in the future.

HARVEST TECHNIQUE

Saphenous vein harvest can be performed with an open or endoscopic technique. Open-vein harvest can be performed with a completely opened technique or bridged technique. In the completely open technique, an extensile skin incision provides the best exposure of the vein and may allow for harvest with the least amount of surgical trauma, but that advantage comes at the risk of higher rates of wound complications and postoperative pain. Bridged skin incisions may decrease pain and wound complications but may also increase surgical manipulation of the vein conduit.

Open-vein dissection can be started either in the upper thigh, above the knee, or at the ankle (Fig. 20-6). Some

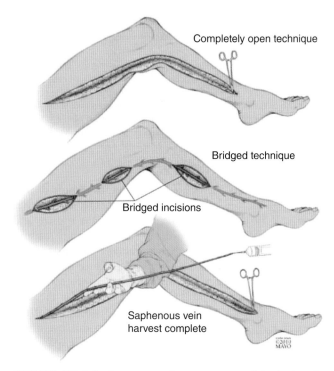

FIGURE 20-6 Saphenous vein harvest: open and bridged technique. Open technique (*top*): Dissection can be started in the upper thigh, above the knee, or at the ankle. Identification of the vein is easiest at the ankle, just above the medial malleolus. An incision is made overlying the vein and extended directly over its trajectory. The vein is dissected and all venous tributaries are ligated and divided in situ. Bridged technique (*middle*): Two- or three-step incisions are performed over the course of the vein. Dissection of the vein is carried in a similar fashion as the opened technique except that branches are divided in situ and ligated once the vein is explanted. Completed dissection (*bottom*): Once dissection is completed, the vein is ligated and divided proximally and distally. Stumps of side branches on the vein are left long and then are ligated flush with the vein, avoiding narrowing of the conduit. The vein is then gently flushed and stored in a solution of room temperature plasmalyte. The skin incisions are closed and the leg is wrapped with an elastic bandage. (By permission of Mayo Foundation for Medical Education and Research. All rights reserved.)

surgeons prefer to harvest vein from the lower leg because of a more appropriate vein caliber and wall thickness, as well as greater distance from the perineum (a potential source of infection). Others prefer to harvest vein from the thigh, arguing improved wound healing, particularly among patients with distal peripheral arterial occlusive disease. We are not aware of any data supporting one location over another. Because of the greater amount of adipose tissue present in the thigh area, wound breakdown in that location may prove more of a nuisance to treat. The fundamentals of vein harvest are to procure the conduit with a minimal amount of trauma to the vein. Specifically, the vein should not be grasped with forceps, stretched, or over-distended, because patency rates may be related to endothelial damage induced during harvest and preparation of the conduit. Identification of the vein is easiest at the ankle, just lateral to the medial malleolus.

In the completely open technique, a skin incision directly over the trajectory of the vein is made, taking care not to create skin flaps. Purposeful, directed, sharp dissection is used to free the vein from the surrounding tissue. Side branches on the vein can initially be left long. Once dissection is completed, the vein is ligated and divided proximally and distally. A blunt-tipped vein cannula is inserted into the distal end of the vein and the vein gently flushed and dilated with a room temperature solution of Plasmalyte™. The side branches can be clipped flush with the vein at this time, taking care to avoid narrowing of the conduit lumen.

When using a bridged technique, several step incisions are performed over the course of the vein. Dissection of the vein is otherwise carried out in a similar fashion as describe above. Exposure of the vein with the bridge technique may be less than optimal. Caution is necessary here to avoid excessive tension or manipulation of the conduit as an adjunct to deal with less than adequate exposure of those segments of the vein covered by a skin bridge. For all techniques of vein harvest located in the lower thigh and more distal, care should be taken to avoid trauma to the saphenous nerve, which is in close proximity to the vein. Injury to the nerve can result in debilitating postoperative neuralgia.

Endoscopic vein harvest starts with a 1.5- to 2.0-cm skin incision in the medial aspect of the extremity above the knee (Fig. 20-7). Carbon dioxide insufflation for visualization and dissection is established. Dissection is directed toward the groin region as far proximally as possible and then distally as far as needed to obtain the required length of conduit. Side branches are divided by using bipolar cauterizing scissors. Once dissection is completed, small skin punctures are made at the limits of the dissection and the vein exteriorized, ligated, and divided. The vein is removed and otherwise prepared in the standard fashion. Following skin closure, the leg is wrapped with a circumferential elastic bandage.

PATENCY

Minimally invasive harvest of the saphenous vein using an endoscopic technique is gaining popularity because it greatly reduces the wound morbidity associated with the open harvest techniques. Endoscopic harvest decreases wound

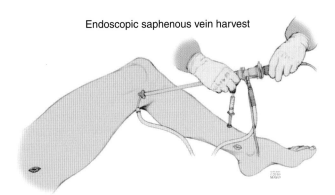

Endoscopic saphenous vein harvest

FIGURE 20-7 Endoscopic saphenous vein harvest. A 2.0-cm skin incision is made in the medial aspect of the knee. CO_2 insufflation is established. Harvesting is directed toward the groin region as far proximally as possible. Side branches are divided by using bipolar cauterizing scissors. Once dissection is completed, a small puncture is made in the groin directly over the vein and the vein is exteriorized under endoscopic guidance. After removing the vein from the leg, side branches are clipped. If any branches have been avulsed, the vein is repaired with interrupted 7-0 polypropylene sutures. (By permission of Mayo Foundation for Medical Education and Research. All rights reserved.)

complication rates and produces an improved cosmetic result, although the operative time devoted to harvest is increased as are the number of defects to the harvested conduit requiring suture repair. Initial reports showed no detrimental effects of harvest technique on vein morphology, endothelial structure or function, or graft patency.[246,247] However, in recent report of 3000 patients treated with CABG, endovascular vein harvest was associated with higher rates of vein-graft failure, death, MI, and repeat revascularization.[248]

The polar opposite to endoscopic vein harvest is the "no-touch" technique in which the vein is removed with a pedicle of surrounding tissue. The harvested vein is not distended and it is stored in heparinized blood. In a randomized study of 104 patients using this technique, the angiographic patency at 18 months was 89% for conventional versus 95% for no-touch grafts. At 8.5 years, patency rates were 76% for the conventional group versus 90% for the no-touch group. Multivariate analysis showed that the most important surgical factors for graft patency were the technique of harvesting the conduit and the vein quality. By comparison, the patency of ITA grafts was 90% in the study.[249]

Other Venous Conduits

Alternative venous conduits such as the lesser saphenous and/or upper extremity cephalic veins are usually secondary choices for conduit. If it is planned to use either of these veins, preoperative vein mapping can help guide conduit harvest. The lesser saphenous vein can be harvested in a supine position through a lateral approach by flexing the hip and medially rotating the knee or by an inferior approach with straight elevation of the extremity. A skin incision is usually started midway between the Achilles tendon and the lateral malleolus. Dissection is carried proximally up the leg to the popliteal fossa. Attention should be paid to avoid injuring the sural nerve.

The patency rate for arm veins is significantly lower than that of saphenous veins and for that reason they are considered conduits of last resort.[250] For cephalic vein harvest, the arm is prepared and positioned as during RA harvest. Incisions are placed along the medial and superior aspect of the arm. The cephalic vein is relatively thinwalled in comparison with the greater saphenous vein and is predisposed to aneurysmal dilatation.

CONDUCT OF OPERATION

Procedures are done under general anesthesia with central venous access, radial arterial lines, and pulmonary artery catheters. Transesophageal echocardiography may be helpful for identifying unsuspected intracardiac lesions or aortic atherosclerosis, and for evaluating ventricular function at the end of the procedure. If ventricular function is poor, a femoral arterial line will facilitate later placement of an IABP. We routinely use a temperature-monitoring urinary catheter. The patient is positioned in the supine position with arms tucked at the side. Care should be taken to avoid peripheral nerve complications caused by pressure injury. The lower extremities are positioned with a slight external rotation and flexion of the knees to aid with groin exposure and harvesting of saphenous vein conduits. The patient is prepared and draped to include the lower neck, the chest, and abdomen between the anterior axillary lines, and the lower extremities circumferentially. The right subclavicular area should also be widely prepped in case the axillary artery needs to be used as a source of arterial inflow.

Incisions

By far the most common approach for CABG is via median sternotomy. Cannulation for cardiopulmonary bypass, managing aortic valve insufficiency, monitoring the left ventricle for distention, and evacuating air all are easier with the midline approach. The skin incision extends from a point midway between the angle of Louis and the sternal notch to just below the tip of the xiphoid process. The scalpel is used to extend the incision through the subcutaneous tissues down to the sternum. Extensive Bovey cautery to the subcutaneous tissues should be avoided because tissue destruction here may result in increased risk of wound complication. Charcoal does not bleed, but neither does it heal.

Special attention should be devoted to identifying the middle of the sternum. The middle of the sternal periosteum is noted and marked with cautery, although we avoid scoring the periosteum continuously from notch to xiphoid as this devascularizes the periosteum unless the saw passes exactly down the line. The interclavicular ligament is divided in the sternal notch, allowing palpation of the posterior aspect of the sternal manubrium. The xiphoid process is identified and divided in the midline with heavy scissors and the midline diaphragmatic muscle attachments divided. A finger should

be inserted under the sternum to document a free space anterior to the pericardium. If there are no significant adhesions present, the sternum is divided with the oscillating saw. If the prepericardial space is adhered, the sternum should be divided using the microsagittal saw. The saphenous vein or the RA can be harvested simultaneous with the sternotomy. Once the sternum has been divided, the ITA is harvested as previously described.

Cannulation and Establishment of Cardiopulmonary Bypass

The pericardium is divided vertically down to the diaphragm and the inferior attachment of the pericardium to the diaphragm is divided transversely. The remnant of thymic tissue and pericardial fat is divided in the midline to the inferior aspect of the left innominate vein.

If the RITA will be used in situ, the fat overlying the pericardium is removed from the diaphragm inferiorly, to the innominate vein superiorly and from the left phrenic to the right phrenic nerve. This significantly increases the reach of the in situ RITA, especially if it will be used in a retro-aortic fashion for left sided targets. Although only removal of the right sided anterior pericardial fat is necessary to maximize the reach of the RITA, we have found that it is quicker and dryer to remove the entire fat pad as a block.

Pericardial retraction sutures create a pericardial cradle or well to improve exposure of the ascending aorta and right atrium. The left pericardium is divided at the level of the great vessels toward the phrenic nerve to allow the completed ITA bypass graft to fall laterally into the pleural space away from the sternum. The distal ascending aorta is inspected and palpated for soft nonatherosclerotic areas suitable for arterial cannulation, root ventilation, proximal graft anastomoses, and aortic cross-clamp placement (Fig. 20-8). In some institutions, epicardial ultrasound of the ascending aorta is performed. Now is the time to redirect the conduct of the operation should the aorta harbor areas of significant calcification, a topic of later discussion.

Systemic anticoagulation is achieved with the intravenous administration of 300 U/kg of unfractionated heparin and the adequacy of anticoagulation documented by an activated clotting time over 450 seconds. In anticipation of aortic cannulation the systolic blood pressure should be reduced to about 100 mm Hg to minimize the risk of aortic dissection. Two partial-thickness concentric diamond-shaped purse-string sutures using 2-0 braided or monofilament nonabsorbable suture (such as Ethibond™ or Prolene™, respectively) are placed in the distal ascending aorta or proximal aortic arch, leaving enough room on the ascending aorta for all necessary proximal aortic work. The size of the purse strings should be large enough to accept the aortic cannula tip, usually 20-22 French. The ends of the sutures are passed through tourniquets that will be used for tightening the purse strings and securing the cannulation site after decannulation. The aortic adventitia within the purse strings

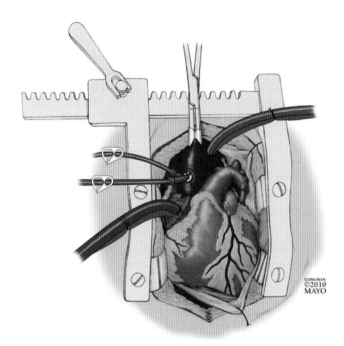

FIGURE 20-8 Cannulation. After full systemic heparinization, cannulation of the distal ascending aorta is performed with an appropriately sized curved or straight tip aortic cannula. A two-stage venous cannula is used for access to the right atrium, usually through the right atrial appendage. An aortic root cardioplegia/vent is placed. A retrograde cardioplegia cannula may be placed at the discretion of the surgeon. Patients with significant aortic regurgitation will benefit from placement of a left ventricle vent (placed via the right superior pulmonary) to avoid distention of the left ventricle during infusion of cardioplegia into the aortic root. (By permission of Mayo Foundation for Medical Education and Research. All rights reserved.)

is divided in preparation for aortotomy. The adventitia just superior to the planned aortotomy is grasped with a forceps and an aortotomy equal in size to the cannula tip is created with a no. 11 scalpel blade. Bleeding is easily controlled with slight inferior traction of the forceps on the adventitia. The aortic cannula is inserted and properly positioned, and the purse strings are tightened. The tourniquets are secured to the aortic cannula with a heavy silk tie and then the cannula is secured to the skin.

Placement of the aortic cannula can result in acute aortic dissection. Intraluminal positioning of the cannula is confirmed by watching for the cannula to fill with arterial blood. The aortic cannula is de-aired and connected to the arterial end of the pump tubing. An additional method to assess for the presence of aortic dissection is to have the perfusionist check the wave form and pressure of the arterial cannula pulse and to deliver a test infusion of 50 to 100 mL of fluid through the cannula. If an aortic dissection is present, often the test infusion will result in an increase in arterial cannula pressure.

Venous cannulation is accomplished with a two- or three-stage venous cannula inserted in the right atrial appendage. A 2-0 Ethibond or Prolene purse-string suture is placed around the tip of the right atrial appendage. The purse string should be wide enough for easy access of the

selected venous cannula. An atriotomy is made with scissors at the tip of the appendage. Small bridging fibers of muscle are divided with scissors to permit easy entry of the cannula. The venous cannula is cautiously inserted, the tip of which should lie in the inferior vena cava. The purse-string suture is tightened and the tourniquet secured to the venous cannula with a heavy silk tie. The venous line is connected to the pump tubing.

An aortic root cannula is placed in the ascending aorta and retrograde cardioplegia cannula placed in the coronary sinus via the right atrium. The patient is placed on cardiopulmonary bypass at 2.4 L/min/m² and may be perfused at normothermia or may be cooled to 34°C. Once the patient is on full bypass, flow ventilation is stopped. A left ventricle vent may be placed via the right superior pulmonary vein at this time if there is significant aortic regurgitation. Target vessels are easier to identify before cardioplegic arrest while they are fully distended in their native state. The locations of planned distal anastomoses are marked with a scalpel. The pump flow is turned down temporarily and the aortic cross-clamp applied just proximal to the arterial cannula and bypass flow returned to normal.

Cold blood cardioplegia (10 mL/kg) is administered and may be delivered antegrade, retrograde, or both, with special attention given during this time to look for evidence of aortic regurgitation such as a flaccid aorta and/or left ventricle distention. Two available options to treat significant aortic regurgitation include completion of the procedure using only retrograde cardioplegia or placement of a left ventricle vent via the right superior pulmonary vein (our preferred method). Rarely is aortic valve replacement required. Additional doses of cardioplegia (5 mL/kg) are given via the antegrade and retrograde catheters approximately every 20 minutes throughout the remainder of the cross-clamp period. Cardioplegiare dosing should be timed in such a way as not to interrupt the 'flow' of the operation.

Distal Anastomoses

LOCATION OF TARGETS AND SEQUENCE OF ANASTOMOSES

Arteriotomy sites should be chosen proximal enough to offer the largest-sized coronary target but distal enough to avoid areas of obstruction or significant atherosclerotic disease. Arteriotomies at bifurcations should be avoided. Diseased vessels with an intramyocardial course can often be localized by noting epicardial indentation, accompanying epicardial veins, or a whitish streak within the myocardium. Sharp dissection of overlying tissue is required to identify the desired target site. Often a very diseased vessel will be less diseased in the intramyocardial segment.

The LAD coronary artery can be particularly difficult to identify when it has an intramyocardial course. It can be relatively easy to inadvertently enter the right ventricular cavity while dissecting in the interventricular fat plane. If such a ventriculotomy is small, it can be closed with fine 6-0 polypropylene sutures, keeping in mind that the right ventricle is a low-pressure chamber and deep bites of myocardium are not necessary. However, if the right ventricle has been opened for a distance, it is best repaired using interrupted, pledgetted 2-0 Prolene suture (MH needle) in a horizontal mattress fashion, passing the needle under the ITA-LAD anastomosis. If difficulty is encountered in identifying an LAD artery, a fine probe may be passed retrograde via a small transverse arteriotomy into the LAD artery at the apex of the heart. The tip of the probe can be palpated in the proximal portion of the artery and cut down on appropriately. The distal arteriotomy is repaired with interrupted fine suture (7-0 or 8-0 Prolene™). The repair can be done with or without a small vein patch.

The distribution of cardioplegia is usually relatively uniform; however, the sequence of anastomoses may be planned based on ischemic regions if myocardial protection is a particular concern. Grafting the most ischemic area first, using a distal-proximal routine, will permit early antegrade delivery of cardioplegia through the graft to the area of myocardial ischemia. Alternatively, the sequence of anastomoses may be dictated by the quality of the conduit itself, matching the best conduit to the most important territories. It is customary to perform the left ITA-to-LAD artery anastomosis last to avoid tension and potential disruption of the anastomosis.

ARTERIOTOMY

The choice of the site of arteriotomy is critical. Opening into a plaque may force endarterectomy, whereas injury to the posterior wall with the knife transforms a straightforward anastomosis into a complex repair. Silastic tapes placed proximally and distally around the coronary artery may help to stabilize the vessel, a technique often employed when grafting the distal right coronary artery or when there is significant back bleeding from the opened vessel. The arteriotomy is performed with a fine scalpel blade and extended with fine Pott's scissors proximally and distally. The arteriotomy should match the conduit diameter, and should be at least 1.5 times the luminal diameter of the distal coronary artery (Fig. 20-9).

ANASTOMOTIC TECHNIQUE

The goal of the anastomosis is to join the conduit and the target vessel with precise endothelial approximation affording minimal resistance to flow. The wall of the vessel should be handled with care, avoiding endothelial injury to prevent thrombotic complications. Coronary anastomoses are typically constructed with continuous 7-0 polypropylene suture. Sutures should be evenly spaced to prevent leaks at the conclusion of the anastomosis. In order to increase anastomotic area, we prefer to bevel the conduits at approximately 30° and notch them at the heel. Anastomoses are performed with continuous suture. We prefer a continuous, parachuting technique initiated at the heel for virtually all anastomoses regardless of their configuration (ie, end-to-side vs side-to-side sequential anastomosis).

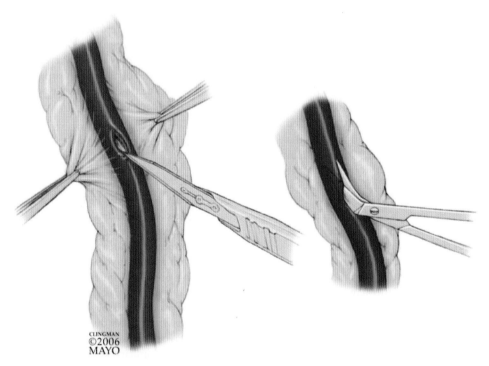

CLINGMAN
©2006
MAYO

FIGURE 20-9 Distal anastomosis: *Arteriotomy.* Arteriotomy sites should be proximal enough to offer the largest-sized coronary target, and just distal enough to avoid the area of obstruction. Intramyocardial vessels can often be localized by noting epicardial indentation, accompanying epicardial veins, or a whitish streak within the myocardium. Sharp dissection of overlying tissue is then required to identify the desired target site. The arteriotomy is then performed with a no. 11 blade. The arteriotomy is extended with fine Pott's scissors proximally and distally. The arteriotomy should match the conduit diameter, and should be at least 1.5 times the diameter of the distal coronary. (By permission of Mayo Foundation for Medical Education and Research. All rights reserved.)

Venous conduit is brought onto the field with a mosquito clamp on the adventitia at the toe of the conduit. An end-to-side anastomosis is accomplished with continuous sutures (Fig. 20-10). Starting at the 3 o'clock position on the right side of the vessel, the suture is passed outside-in on the conduit and then inside-out at the corresponding location of the target coronary vessel. Two more sutures are taken before the heel (2 and 1 o'clock positions), one directly in the heel (12 o'clock), and then two more on the left side (11 and 10 o'clock positions) of the anastomosis before parachuting the conduit down to the target vessel.

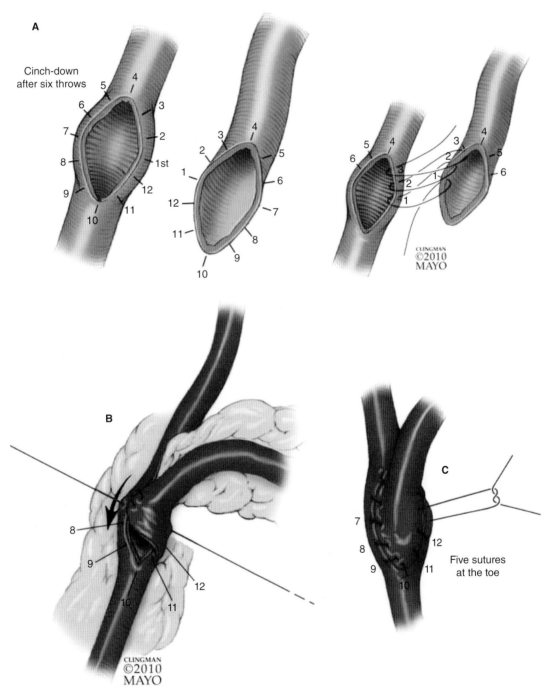

FIGURE 20-10 Distal anastomosis suture technique. (A) The conduit is beveled at 30 degrees and notched at the heel. We use a continuous, parachuting technique with 7-0 or 8-0 polypropylene suture. The conduit is brought onto the field with a mosquito clamp on the adventitia at the toe of the conduit. An end-to-side anastomosis is accomplished with 12 sutures. Starting at 3 o'clock on the right side of the vessel, the suture is passed outside-in on the conduit and then inside-out at the corresponding location of the target vessel. (B) Two more stitches are taken before the heel, one directly in the heel, and then two more on the left side of the anastomosis before parachuting the conduit down to the target vessel. (C) The anastomosis is then completed by placing another six stitches evenly spaced in the same manner for the toe. (By permission of Mayo Foundation for Medical Education and Research. All rights reserved.)

The anastomosis is continued by placing additional sutures moving in a counterclockwise fashion around the anastomosis until the other thread is encountered. The technique encourages one to move out of the heel and toe areas of the anastomosis, minimizing the risk of narrowing the outflow. Care must be taken to prevent suturing the back wall of the coronary, and the proper amount of tension on the follow-through must be provided to avoid both leakage and a purse-string effect. Just before completion of the anastomosis, a 1-mm probe is passed proximally and distally to ensure patency. To prevent anastomotic tension and torsion, pedicled conduits (ie, left ITA) can be suture-fixated to the adjacent epicardium.

Sequential grafting permits efficient use of conduit and has the potential for increased flow in the conduit. When planning sequential anastomoses, the most distal anastomosis should be to the largest target vessel with the greatest outflow potential. If the reverse situation is created, the most distal anastomosis is at increased risk for failure, given the likelihood of preferential flow to the larger more proximal anastomosis.[251,252] A clear disadvantage of sequential grafting is the reliance of two or more distal targets on a single conduit and proximal anastomosis, placing a potentially larger region of the myocardium at jeopardy.[252]

Some surgeons avoid using the ITA for sequential grafting or as a donor for composite T or Y-grafting of other conduits because of concerns of compromising critical ITA-to-LAD flow. However, several series have demonstrated successful use of the ITA for sequential grafting of stenotic diagonal coronary arteries with excellent results.[253,254] The left ITA has also been used for multiple sequential anastomoses to the circumflex territory with grafting of the right ITA to the LAD artery.[255] Sequential grafting has also been performed with the right GEA as well as the RA.[256,257]

When constructing a sequential anastomosis, it is our preference to complete the distal anastomosis first and move proximally (Fig. 20-11). We feel that this facilitates determination of optimal inter graft spacing. In the case of the LAD-diagonal graft, however, it is easier to move from proximal to distal, performing the diagonal anastomosis first. Sequential side-to-side anastomoses may be perpendicular or longitudinal. When constructing perpendicular anastomoses care must be taken not to make the arteriotomies too long, as there is risk of creating a "gull-wing" deformity and placing the graft at jeopardy. Arteriotomies in both the conduit and target are made in the direction of the long axis of the vessel. The two incisions are then aligned perpendicular to one another and the anastomosis completed, creating a diamond-shaped anastomosis. The arteriotomy for longitudinal anastomosis may be made as long as necessary without risk of distorting the conduit. Typically, the longitudinal anastomosis is begun at the heel as previously described.

Coronary Endarterectomy

Coronary endarterectomy predated CABG as a direct surgical approach to relieving coronary occlusive disease. Coronary endarterectomy has been relegated to a position of secondary importance, however, thanks to the reliable and reproducible results obtained with CABG. Recently there has been increased interest in endarterectomy techniques, because the patient population coming to CABG has a greater atherosclerotic burden owing to diabetes, hyperlipidemia, and advanced age.[258] Most commonly, the need for endarterectomy arises intraoperatively when no soft site can be identified for arteriotomy or a vessel has been inadvertently opened in an extensively diseased area not amenable to grafting. Occasionally, endarterectomy is undertaken electively in patients with diffuse and extensive coronary disease with no other choices except transplantation.

The perioperative risk of CABG with endarterectomy is higher than that for CABG alone in most studies. In a retrospective study of 1478 patients, the reported mortality rate with endarterectomy was 3.2%, which was higher than for CABG alone (2.2%). Perioperative MI rate was also higher in the endarterectomy group, 4.2% versus 3.4%. The risk of mortality appears to increase when multiple vessels require endarterectomy: single-vessel endarterectomy mortality = 1.8% versus multiple-vessel endarterectomy mortality = 5.5%.[259,260] There has been controversy regarding the risk of endarterectomy of the LAD, with some studies showing increased risk whereas others demonstrate no increased risk.[259-261]

The late results of endarterectomy are inferior to those of routine CABG, with reported 3-year patency for ITA grafts to endarterectomized LAD targets ranging from 74 to 80%.[262,263] Despite this, angina relief is remarkably good initially. Unfortunately, the rate of recurrent angina is somewhat higher than after uncomplicated CABG; reported recurrence of angina is 25% at 5 years after endarterectomy.[260,264] The reported 5-year survival following coronary endarterectomy ranges from 76 to 83%.[260,264] Among patients in whom bypass to more distal nondiseased segments is not possible, coronary endarterectomy with subsequent bypass offers a viable alternative to leaving a territory ungrafted.

TECHNIQUE

The technique of endarterectomy requires that the central core be extracted adequately in order to relieve obstruction of the branch vessels. Patency of a graft to the endarterectomized vessel depends upon the adequacy of runoff and therefore the distal endpoints of the endarterectomy core must be smoothly tapered. If the core fractures leaving behind disease in side branches, distal counter-incisions may be needed to obtain a satisfactory result.

The RCA is the vessel most often endarterectomized, usually at the level of its bifurcation. A manual eversion endarterectomy is performed after entering at the vessel approximately 1 cm proximal to the crux. A circumferential plane of dissection between the core and the adventitia is developed with a fine coronary spatula. The core is transected proximally and gently grasped with DeBakey forceps while the spatula is used to tease the adventitia away from the core. The core is regrasped hand over hand as distally

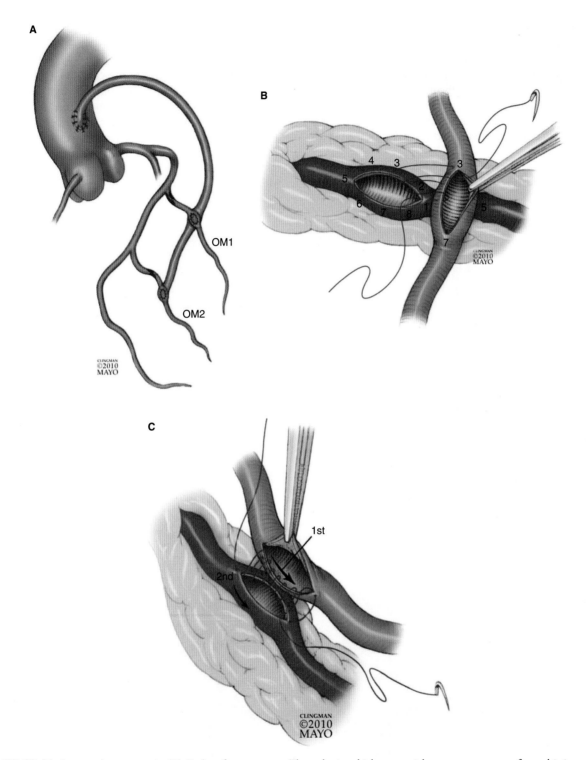

FIGURE 20-11 Sequential anastomosis. (A) Order of anastomoses: The order in which sequential anastomoses are performed is important to facilitate optimal inter graft spacing and avoid kinking. The distal anastomosis is completed first and the more proximal sequential anastomosis is performed second, except for an LAD-diagonal graft, in which the diagonal is performed first followed by the LAD. (B) Perpendicular sequential side-to-side anastomosis: Arteriotomies are made in the direction of the long axis of the coronary and the conduit. Care must be taken not to make the arteriotomies too long, because there is risk of creating a "gull-wing" deformity. The two incisions are aligned perpendicular to one another. The suture is passed starting inside-out at the apex of the target coronary and then outside-in at the mid-portion the conduit. An eight-stitch anastomosis is completed creating a diamond-shaped anastomosis. (C) Longitudinal sequential side-to-side anastomosis: The arteriotomy for longitudinal anastomosis may be made as long as necessary without risk of distorting the conduit. The anastomosis is begun at the heel and the far wall is completed open. It is then parachuted down and the front wall completed. (By permission of Mayo Foundation for Medical Education and Research. All rights reserved.)

as possible to avoid fracture. When the crux is reached, the posterior descending artery and the left ventricular branch are endarterectomized separately. If endarterectomy of the proximal segment of the RCA is needed, we prefer to use an open technique because it is difficult to obtain nice tapering of the core at the takeoff of the acute marginal branches with a retrograde eversion endarterectomy. The vessel wall is then reconstructed with a long hood created with the bypass conduit of choice.

We prefer open extended technique when the LAD is endarterectomized (Fig. 20-12). The vessel is opened as far

proximal as possible if endarterectomy is anticipated. If the vessel has been opened in its mid-portion before it is apparent that endarterectomy is necessary, we extend the incision in the adventitia proximally before developing the endarterectomy plane. Retrograde eversion endarterectomy is dangerous because branch vessels will not be opened. Once the core is separated from the adventitia, it is transected proximally at the heel and the vessel is opened beyond the takeoff of the major diagonals to permit individual eversion endarterectomy of each of the branches. The segment is reconstructed with a long hood of the conduit of choice or a vein patch into

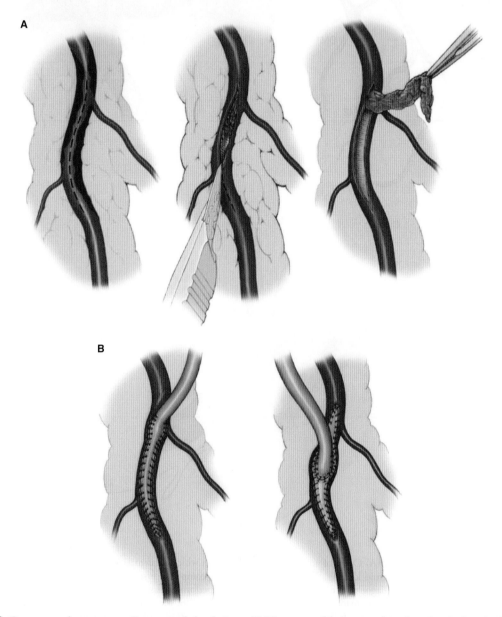

FIGURE 20-12 Coronary endarterectomy: Open extended technique. (A) The extent of disease is evaluated to plan the length of the arteriotomy and endarterectomy. The arteriotomy is performed and extended as proximal as needed before the circumferential plane of dissection between the core and the adventitia is developed with a fine coronary spatula. Once the core is separated from the adventitia, it is transected proximally at the heel and the vessel is opened beyond the takeoff of the major branches to permit individual eversion endarterectomy of each of the branches. (B) The segment is reconstructed with a long hood of the conduit of choice. The segment may be reconstructed with a vein patch into which the conduit is anastomosed. (By permission of Mayo Foundation for Medical Education and Research. All rights reserved.)

which the ITA is anastomosed. The circumflex artery is the most infrequently endarterectomized vessel. Its rapid branching pattern makes satisfactory endarterectomy difficult. We tend to begin with an eversion technique, focusing our efforts on opening the largest distal branches as much as possible.

Proximal Anastomoses

Proximal anastomoses of the saphenous vein or the RA to the aorta are performed after the distal anastomoses under the same cross-clamp clamp. Our preferred technique is to complete each respective bypass graft in a distal anastomosis-proximal anastomosis fashion. Completion of the each respective bypass graft allows antegradecardioplegia down the completed graft, aiding in myocardial protection. The single cross-clamp technique results in longer cross-clamp times than with the partial occlusion clamp method. However, the partial occlusion clamp technique requires additional aortic manipulation and although some authors have found this practice to be safe,[265] others have demonstrated that it carries a higher risk of neuropsychological deficits when compared with the single-clamp technique.[266]

ANASTOMOTIC TECHNIQUE

Once an appropriate site for aortotomy is identified, the fatty tissue overlying the aorta is removed (Fig. 20-13). An arteriotomy is created with a no. 11 blade, and a 4.0-mm punch used to create a circular aortotomy. The size of the punch may vary depending on the size of the conduit graft. The graft is measured to length with the aorta, right heart, and pulmonary artery full of blood. The graft is cut and the proximal aspect of the conduit beveled and notched at the heel. A running 5-0 polypropylene suture is used for a venous graft and a 6-0 polypropylene suture for an arterial conduit. The long axis of the graft is aligned at an appropriate angle to the ascending aorta. The anastomosis can be completed with continuous stitches. Symmetry in the spacing of sutures is paramount to obtain a hemostatic anastomosis. Free arterial grafts may also be sutured to the hood of a vein graft with continuous 7-0 Prolene suture.

COMPOSITE GRAFTS

As an alternative to proximal anastomosis to the aorta, a free graft can be anastomosed proximally to the pedicled ITA (Fig. 20-14). This technique has the theoretical advantage of providing a more physiologic arterial pressure waveform by attaching the conduit to a third-order vessel rather than to the aorta. Composite grafting is also a useful tool for the hostile, calcified ascending aorta or when there is a limited length of conduit available. It is also advantageous when there is a marked mismatch between aortic wall thickness and arterial conduit size.

A combination of composite and sequential grafting allows the opportunity to perform complete arterial revascularization with only ITA or with ITA and other arterial

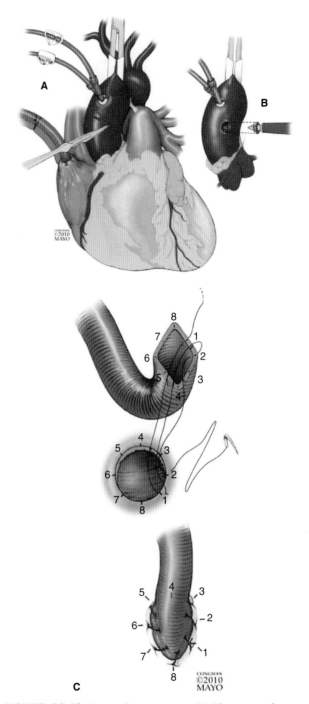

FIGURE 20-13 Proximal anastomosis. (A) The proximal anastomosis is performed using a single-clamp technique. The fatty tissue overlying the planned aortotomy site is removed. An arteriotomy is created with a no.11 blade. (B) A 4- to 5-mm aortic punch is used to create a circular aortotomy. The size of the punch will vary depending on the size of the conduit graft. (C) The proximal aspect of the conduit is beveled and then notched at the heel. A running 5-0 or 6-0 polypropylene suture is used for a venous graft and a 6-0 or 7-0 polypropylene suture for an arterial conduit. The long axis of the graft is aligned at an appropriate angle to the ascending aorta. The anastomosis can be completed with eight stitches in most cases; symmetry in the spacing between stitches is of paramount importance to ensure hemostasis. (By permission of Mayo Foundation for Medical Education and Research. All rights reserved.)

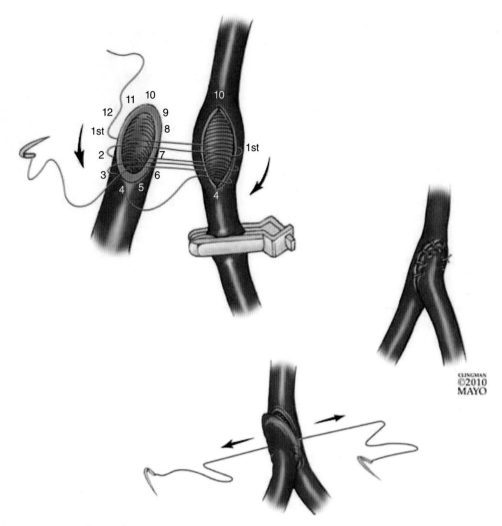

FIGURE 20-14 Composite Y-graft. Y-graft anastomotic technique: A coronary artery bypass graft (CABG) is used as a donor site for the proximal anastomosis of another conduit. An incision is created in the donor conduit. The proximal end of the recipient conduit is then anastomosed to the donor site in an end-to-side fashion as previously described for a distal anastomosis. The recipient conduit is then gently parachuted down onto the donor conduit. (By permission of Mayo Foundation for Medical Education and Research. All rights reserved.)

conduits (Fig. 20-15). Multiple configurations of Y- and T-grafts can be devised to best suit the anatomic characteristics of each patient. Some authors have advocated even using the distal segment of the LITA as a composite graft off the composite RITA to further expand the reach of a complete arterial revascularization strategy.[267] The LITA has been shown to have more than sufficient flow reserve to supply flow to the entire coronary circulation.[268] The free right ITA, the RA, or other arterial conduit can be based in this manner.

All-arterial Y-grafts are usually planned in advance and constructed before the initiation of cardiopulmonary bypass. Special care must be taken during construction of composite grafts to avoid tension, rotational torsion, or narrowing of the inflow anastomosis. Disadvantages include technical difficulty and reliance upon a single inflow source for two or more distal targets.

Management of the Atherosclerotic Ascending Aorta

Ascending aortic atherosclerosis has been consistently identified as a very important risk factor for stroke in multiple series. Routine epiaortic ultrasound should be performed to define the extent of atherosclerosis of the ascending aorta and its likelihood of embolization. Patients with severe atherosclerosis of the ascending aorta may require alternative strategies to prevent embolization of aortic atheroma. If the ascending aorta is hostile, we favor cannulation of the right axillary artery. Although most surgeons prefer to achieve axillary arterial inflow utilizing a chimney side graft, direct cannulation of the axillary artery with an appropriately designed axillary angled cannula is very safe and effective.[269] If necessary, aortic clamping may be performed in areas free of atheroma, usually in the more proximal ascending aorta.

During this time of recovery the patient is prepared for transition from supported circulation to native circulation. The aortic root vent and retrograde catheters are removed and the sites repaired with suture. The bypass grafts are checked for kinks, twists, or tension and for presence of hemostasis. The patient must be rewarmed to normothermia if cooled and the acid-base status and electrolyte abnormalities corrected. We place temporary atrial and ventricular pacing wires on all patients.

Weaning from cardiopulmonary bypass is otherwise the same as for other cardiac surgical cases. Issues particular to CABG include attention to avoid tension on the LITA from lung overinflation or overdistention of the heart, which may place all grafts on tension and disrupt anastomoses. If air has entered the heart, bubbles may pass into the aorta and down the bypass grafts causing arrhythmias and regional wall motion abnormalities. Treatment involves continued recovery on bypass and increasing the perfusion pressure as a means to drive the bubbles through the coronary circulation. Persistency of regional wall motion abnormalities may require bypass graft revision or placement of additional bypass grafts.

OUTCOMES
Operative Mortality

The risk profile of patients requiring isolated CABG in the United States changed significantly in the 1990s. Compared to previous decades, patients undergoing CABG are older, with a greater number of comorbidities, decreased left ventricular ejection fraction (LVEF), and a higher burden of atherosclerotic disease; however, early outcomes after CABG continue to improve. The STS database demonstrates that despite an increase in expected mortality from 2.6 to 3.4% (relative increase 30%) in the decade of the 1990s, the observed mortality actually decreased from 3.9 to 3.0% (relative decrease 23%).[3]

Similar observations have been made using the Veterans Affairs mandatory national database, where the unadjusted mortality rate for isolated CABG fell from 4.3% in 1989 to 2.7% in the year 2000.[271] In the private sector similar trends have been observed. In an analysis of outcomes of patients undergoing isolated CABG in the HCA system, a nationwide for-profit health care system involving 200 hospitals in 23 states, Mack and associates reported an ongoing decrease in unadjusted operative mortality among 51,353 patients, 80% of whom received CABG with cardiopulmonary bypass. In this study the operative mortality decreased from 2.9% in 1999 to 2.2% in 2002.[272]

This trend has continued throughout the first decade of the new millenium, with the observed mortality having declined to 1.9% in 2009 on the 1,297,254 patients who underwent isolated CABG during that time interval.[175] This represented a 24.4% reduction in operative mortality between 2000 and 2009.[175]

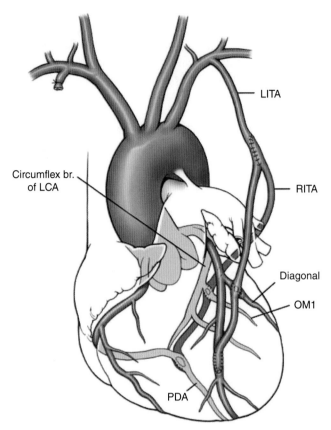

FIGURE 20-15 Total arterial revascularization: As shown, arterial revascularization can be performed using the right internal thoracic artery (RITA) off the left internal thoracic artery (LITA) as a Y-graft and liberal use of sequential grafting. (By permission of Mayo Foundation for Medical Education and Research. All rights reserved.)

Coronary revascularization can be achieved with a variety of methods. Using a "no-touch" technique, revascularization can be done using only pedicled arterial conduits, and if proximal anastomoses are required they can be based off pedicled conduits or brachiocephalic vessels. Distal anastomoses can be performed with an "on pump, beating heart" technique without aortic cross-clamping but with vessel occlusion and stabilization techniques used in off pump surgery. This does not require cooling or LV venting, two necessary features of the similar but now obsolete cold fibrillatory arrest technique. Proximal anastomoses can be performed under deep hypothermic circulatory arrest or after graft replacement of the ascending aorta if there are large mobile atheromas.[270]

Weaning from Cardiopulmonary Bypass

On completion of all anastomoses, the aortic cross-clamp is removed and a stable heart rhythm established. Some advocate allowing the heart to recover on full bypass for 10 minutes for each 60 minutes of aortic cross-clamp time.

Causes of Death

In a multicenter prospective study performed by the Northern New England Cardiovascular Disease Study Group, 384 deaths among 8641 consecutive patients undergoing isolated CABG between 1990 and 1995 were analyzed with respect to the mode of death. The mode of death was defined as the seminal event that precipitated clinical deterioration and ultimately resulted in the patient's demise. Heart failure was judged to be the primary mode of death for 65% of the patients, followed in frequency by neurologic causes (7.3%), hemorrhage (7%), respiratory failure (5.5%), and dysrhythmia (5.5%). The greatest variability in mortality rates observed across surgeons in the study was attributable to differences in rates of heart failure.[273] Cardiac causes were also identified by Sergeant and colleagues as the most common causes of death in a series 5880 patients undergoing CABG between 1983 and 1988.[274]

Operative Morbidity

MYOCARDIAL DYSFUNCTION

Postoperative myocardial dysfunction and cardiac failure after CABG may be related to preoperative ischemic injury, inadequate myocardial protection, incomplete revascularization, or postoperative graft failure. The spectrum of myocardial injury varies from subtle degrees of global myocardial ischemia to transmural infarction. The incidence of myocardial injury identified varies with the sensitivity of the method used for detection as well as the threshold set. Some studies have reported perioperative MI rates as high as 10% of patients with associated worse clinical outcomes (death, MI, or revascularization).[275]

Some elevations of cardiac-specific enzymes are ubiquitous after CABG; however, most would agree that elevations in creatinine kinase-myocardial bound (CK-MB) greater than five times the upper limit of normal (ULN) value are considered significant. In a prospective study of 2918 patients undergoing CABG, 38% of patients had a CK-MB > 5 ULN and 17% had a CK-MB > 10 ULN with an incidence of new Q-wave MI of 4.7%.[276] Troponin may be a more sensitive marker than CK-MB, but its role in large populations of CABG patients is still to be defined.[277] Prominent elevations of CK-MB and troponin have been associated with global ischemia, MI, low cardiac output, and increased operative mortality, as well as increased midterm and long-term mortality.[276,277]

Transient myocardial dysfunction necessitating low-dose inotropic support for a short period of time is also common after CABG. Significant postoperative myocardial dysfunction manifest clinically as low cardiac output syndrome may be defined by the need for postoperative inotropic support or IABP support to maintain a systolic blood pressure > 90 mm Hg or a cardiac index > 2.2 L/min. The reported incidence of low output syndrome varies depending on the defining criteria and has a reported incidence of 4 to 9%.[278,279] Low output syndrome has been shown

to be a marker for increased operative mortality by 10- to 15-fold.[280] Independent predictors of low output syndrome in order of importance include LVEF < 20%, reoperation, emergency operation, female gender, diabetes, age older than 70 years, left main disease, recent MI, and triple-vessel disease.[278]

ADVERSE NEUROLOGIC OUTCOME

Neurologic deficits after coronary surgery are divided into two types: type 1 deficits include major neurologic deficits, stupor, and coma; type 2 deficits are characterized by deterioration of intellectual function and memory. The incidence of type 1 deficits was reported to be 1.6% in a large review by the Northern New England Cardiovascular Disease Study Group with 1-, 5-, and 10-year survival rates significantly reduced in affected patients.[160] Perioperative mortality is similarly increased among those with type 1 injury at over 24%.[281] Type 2 deficits are more difficult to characterize and may be more related to the underlying atherosclerosis than to the bypass operation per se. In one nonrandomized study, there was no evidence that the cognitive test performance of CABG patients differed from that of heart healthy control groups with CAD over a 1-year period.[282]

Just like mortality rates, stroke rates have shown a decrease in incidence over the last decade (1.6% in 2000 vs 1.2 in 2009, a 26.4% decrease).[175] More extensive preoperative imaging of the aorta and its arch vessels via CT scan or ultrasound, as well as liberal usage of axillary cannulation over the last decade may be contributing to this improvement, although there is no published evidence to support this relationship.

Predictors of neurologic deficits included advanced age (≥70 years of age), and history or presence of severe hypertension. Independent predictors of type 1 deficits included proximal aortic atherosclerosis, history of prior neurologic disease, need for IABP, diabetes, unstable angina, and perioperative hypotension. Predictors of type 2 deficits included history of alcohol consumption, dysrhythmias, prior CABG, peripheral vascular disease, CHF, and perioperative hypotension. Similar predictors of adverse neurologic outcomes have been observed in other studies.[283]

DEEP STERNAL WOUND INFECTION

Deep sternal wound infection occurs in 1 to 4% of CABG patients and has historically carried a mortality rate of 25%.[284] These outcomes have dramatically improved over the past 20 years, with the latest meta-analysis reporting a 1.66% risk of mediastinitis when only one ITA is used and 2.64% when both ITAs are used.[285] When skeletonization of the ITAs is performed, these numbers drop to 1.16 and 1.48%.[285] Proven methods to reduce postoperative wound complications include the use of preoperative showers with chlorhexidine gluconate on the evening and morning before the procedure, prophylactic intranasal application of mupirocin given on the evening and the morning before the procedure and twice daily for 5 days postoperatively, hair clipping the morning of surgery, tight glycemic control, and administration of intravenous prophylactic antibiotics before skin incision.[286-288] Application of a cyanoacrylate-based microbial skin sealant may further reduce surgical site infection.[289]

Obesity and diabetes are strong independent predictors of mediastinitis. Insulin-dependent diabetic patients are especially susceptible to deep sternal wound infection.[290-292] Recent data suggest that tight glycemic control in the postoperative period decreases the risk of mediastinitis in the diabetic population.[293,294] Other preoperative variables independently associated with an increased incidence of deep sternal wound infection include reoperation, longer operative times, reexploration for bleeding, and blood transfusions.[290,291,295]

The use of bilateral ITAs had been implicated as a risk factor for sternal would complications, especially in diabetics.[296] However, this risk appears to be mitigated in part by using a skeletonized ITA harvesting technique.[297] Bilateral ITA harvest should likely be avoided in obese diabetic women, in cases of repeat sternotomy, and in patients with severe COPD, because they exhibit a higher risk of deep sternal wound infection even with skeletonization of the ITA.[204,298]

ACUTE RENAL FAILURE

Acute renal failure ensuing after CABG with cardiopulmonary bypass is an ominous event. In a prospective observational study conducted at 24 university centers in the United States, including data on 2222 CABG patients,[299] renal dysfunction not requiring dialysis occurred in 6.3%, and renal dysfunction requiring hemodialysis developed in 1.4%. Mortality was directly related to postoperative renal function. Patients with no renal dysfunction had 0.9% mortality.[299] Postoperative renal dysfunction increased mortality to 19% if no dialysis was needed and increased mortality to 63% if hemodialysis was required. Patients with large creatinine increases (>50%) after CABG surgery also have higher 90-day mortality.[300]

Independent predictors of postoperative renal dysfunction included increasing age, CHF, reoperation, DM, chronic renal insufficiency, prolonged cardiopulmonary bypass time, and low cardiac output.[299] These findings were confirmed in another series of 42,733 patients with similar incidence and mortality associated with postoperative renal dysfunction.[301] One in four patients with preoperative chronic renal insufficiency (creatinine > 1.6 mg/dL) will require renal replacement therapy post-CABG, and patients at highest risk are older than 70 years and have a baseline creatinine > 2.5 mg/dL.[302]

Continuous infusion of low-dose recombinant human B-type natriuretic peptide (nesiritide) from the start of cardiopulmonary bypass has been evaluated as a method to effectively maintain postoperative renal function. In the prospective, randomized, NAPA Trial, 272 patients with EF < 40% undergoing CABG who receive nesiritide experienced a significantly attenuated peak increase in serum creatinine and a greater urine output during the initial 24 hours after surgery. In addition, they had a shorter hospital stay and lower 180-day mortality.[303] Similar renal protective results were noted in a randomized trial using human atrial natriuretic peptide in 251 patients. The treated group had fewer postoperative complications, lower serum creatinine, and higher urinary creatinine and creatinine clearance. The maximum postoperative creatinine level and percent increase of creatinine were also significantly lower in the treatment group. No patient in the natriuretic group required hemodialysis.[304] We are awaiting further study before adopting natriuretic peptides in our routine CABG practice.

Long-term Outcomes

Long-term outcomes of surgical myocardial revascularization depend on the complex interaction of patient-related and procedure-related factors. Important patient-related factors include anatomic distribution of the CAD, the extent and severity of coronary atherosclerosis, the physiologic impact of ischemia on ventricular function at the time of the original operation, age, gender, overall health status, severity of atherosclerotic burden throughout the body, the presence and severity of associated comorbidities, development of operative complications such as stroke, and need for permanent hemodialysis. The progression rate of native coronary atherosclerosis after surgery and the development of coronary bypass graft failure are of extreme importance in the development of post-CABG angina recurrence, MI, need for reintervention, and cardiac-related mortality. Procedure-related factors that influence long-term outcomes include completeness of revascularization, myocardial protection, and selection of bypass conduits.

Sergeant and colleagues at the Gasthuiberg University Hospital of the Katholieke Universiteit (KU) Leuven, Belgium have provided several reports detailing clinical outcomes after myocardial revascularization.[305-308] From 1971 to 1993, 9600 consecutive CABG patients were prospectively followed with special attention to clinical outcomes after surgical myocardial revascularization; the investigators achieved a 99.9% complete follow-up in this cohort. Clinical outcomes prospectively followed included mortality, return of angina, MI, and coronary reintervention.[305]

Defining the return of angina as the first occurrence of angina of any intensity or duration unless it was associated on the same day with MI or death, and recording the severity of this event, was also recorded. The overall non-risk-adjusted freedom from return of angina was 95% at 1 year, 82% at 5 years, 61% at 10 years, 38% at 15 years, and 21% at 20 years. The data suggest that if followed long enough after CABG, the return of angina is almost inevitable; by 12 years one-half of operated patients had return of angina. The initial episode of recurrent angina was rated as mild in 59% of patients.[306] In the Bypass Angioplasty Revascularization Investigation (BARI) trial of 914 patients with symptomatic multivessel disease randomly assigned to receive CABG, freedom from angina was 84% at 5 and 10 years.[84]

The overall non-risk-adjusted freedom from MI after CABG at the KU Leuven was 97% at 30 days, 94% at 5 years,

86% at 10 years, 73% at 15 years, and 56% at 20 years.[308] The overall non-risk-adjusted freedom from a coronary reintervention, either PCI or reoperative CABG, was 99.7% at 30 days, 97% at 5 years, 89% at 10 years, 72% at 15 years, and 48% at 20 years (125). In the BARI trial, freedom from subsequent coronary reintervention at 10 years was 80%.[84]

Overall risk-unadjusted survival after CABG in the KU Leuven experience was 98% at 30 days, 92% at 5 years, 81% at 10 years, 66% at 15 years, and 51% at 20 years. Mortality after CABG was characterized by an initial period of high risk in the first month after surgery, then risk declined to its lowest at 1 year after the operation, and thereafter the mortality risk rose slowly and steadily for as long as the patient was followed. This slow and steady rise in the risk of death over time paralleled that of the general population when matched for sex, age, and ethnicity.[307] In the BARI trial, survival was 89% at 5 years and 74% at 10 years.[84]

The occurrence of ischemic clinical events after CABG negatively influences survival. In the KU Leuven study, overall survival was lessened by return of angina, with an observed survival of 83% at 5 years and 54% at 15 years; the more intense the severity of angina at its return, the greater its influence on survival.[306] The occurrence of MI after CABG has a greater negative effect on survival. Observed long-term survival after post-CABG infarction at the KU Leuven was 80% at 30 days, 65% at 5 years, 52% at 10 years, and 41% at 15 years.[308]

PROGRESSION OF DISEASE IN NATIVE CORONARY ARTERIES

Progression of atherosclerosis in the native coronary arteries continues after CABG. Bourassa and associates studied the progression of atherosclerosis in the native circulation 10 years after surgery and found that progression of CAD occurs in approximately 50% of nongrafted arteries.[309] The rate of progression of disease in nongrafted arteries was no different from that of grafted arteries with patent grafts; however, progression was more frequent in grafted arteries with occluded grafts. Progression of preexisting stenoses in native coronaries was more frequent than appearance of new stenoses, and it was related to the severity of the preexisting stenosis only in nongrafted arteries.

Progression of native CAD was associated with deterioration in left ventricular function. Native coronary atherosclerosis progressed at a similar rate to that of equally diseased arteries in nonoperated patients.[309] Low levels of high-density lipoprotein cholesterol and elevated levels of plasma low-density lipoprotein cholesterol correlated with native disease progression and development of new atherosclerotic lesions.[310,311] Diabetes has been related to accelerated atherosclerosis.

VEIN GRAFT FAILURE

Although the use of the saphenous vein helped popularize coronary bypass grafting, the propensity of the SVG to fail over time has been the limiting factor of the procedure. It has been reported that approximately 15% of vein grafts occlude in the first year after CABG, and by 6 and 10 years after surgery patency rates fall to approximately 75 and 60%, respectively.[197] Three entities are responsible for SVG failure: thrombosis, intimal hyperplasia, and graft atherosclerosis.

Thrombosis accounts for graft failure within the first month after CABG, and graft occlusion is found on angiography in 3 to 12% of all venous grafts. Even when performed under optimal conditions, the harvesting of venous conduits is associated with focal endothelial disruption. In particular, the high pressure distension used to overcome venospasm during harvesting causes prominent endothelial cell loss, medial damage, activation of local factors (ie, fibrinogen) influencing hemostasis. Additionally, the inherent antithrombotic properties of veins are comparatively weak. The propensity for early graft occlusion resulting from these prothrombotic effects may, on occasion, be amplified by technical factors that reduce graft flow, including intact venous valves, anastomotic stricture, or graft implantation proximal to an atheromatous segment.[197]

Intimal hyperplasia, defined as the accumulation of smooth muscle cells and extracellular matrix in the intimal compartment, is the major disease process in venous grafts between 1 month and 1 year after implantation. Nearly all veins implanted into the arterial circulation develop intimal thickening within 4 to 6 weeks, which may reduce the lumen by up to 25%. Intimal hyperplasia rarely produces significant stenosis per se; more importantly, however, is that it may provide the foundation for later development of graft atheroma.[312]

Progression of atherosclerosis in aortocoronary SVGs is frequent and represents the predominant cause of late graft failure after CABG. Vein graft atherosclerosis may begin as early as the first year, but is fully developed only after about 5 years. Ten years after surgery, 50 to 60% of SVGs will be occluded and one-half of still patent grafts will show angiographic evidence of atherosclerosis; two-thirds of these lesions will have a luminal diameter reduction of 50% or greater. Vein graft atherosclerosis is the leading cause for reintervention following CABG, more so than progression of disease in native coronary arteries.[197]

Although the risk factors predisposing to vein graft atherosclerosis are broadly similar to those recognized for native coronary disease, the pathogenic effects of these risk factors are amplified by inherent deficiencies of the vein as a conduit when transposed into the coronary arterial circulation. A multifaceted strategy aimed at prevention of vein graft disease is emerging, elements of which include continued improvements in surgical technique; more effective antiplatelet drugs; increasingly intensive risk factor modification, in particular early and aggressive lipid-lowering drug therapy; and a number of evolving therapies, such as gene transfer and nitric oxide donor administration, which target vein graft disease at an early and fundamental level. At present, a key measure is to circumvent the problem of vein graft disease by preferential selection of arterial conduits, in particular the internal mammary arteries, for coronary bypass surgery whenever possible.[197]

Extended Use of Arterial Grafting

BILATERAL INTERNAL THORACIC ARTERY GRAFT

In contrast to the easily demonstrated survival benefit conferred by an ITA graft to the LAD artery, it was more difficult to demonstrate a survival benefit to a second arterial graft. Buxton and colleagues studied 1243 patients undergoing primary CABG with bilateral ITA grafts compared with 1583 patients with single ITA grafts. This group demonstrated a 15% absolute improvement in actuarial survival rates 10 years after CABG with the use of bilateral ITA grafts, as compared with the use of a single ITA graft (10-year survival for bilateral ITA was 86 ± 3% vs 71 ± 5% for a single ITA).[312] Lytle and colleagues similarly demonstrated an improvement in survival at 12 years (79 vs 71%) as well as superior reoperation-free survival (77 vs 62%) among 2001 bilateral and 8123 single ITA graft patients.[313] The impact of selection bias in these studies is difficult to control, however, and although some surgeons have embraced bilateral ITA grafting, it still represents a small minority of cases reported to the STS database (3.8%).

COMPLETE ARTERIAL REVASCULARIZATION

The better long-term results achieved with the use of bilateral ITAs and the well-known time-related attrition in patency of venous conduits encouraged the exclusive use of arterial conduits for myocardial revascularization. Complete arterial revascularization can be achieved by a variety of strategies, including composite grafting using exclusively ITAs or secondary arterial conduits such as the RA and the GEA. The use of sequential anastomotic techniques maximizes the utilization of arterial conduits. Although technically demanding, sequential grafting can be performed safely and with excellent long-term results with reported 96% patency rates of 7.5 years of follow-up on 1150 sequential ITA anastomoses.[314]

Tector has championed complete arterial revascularization using bilateral ITAs in a T configuration with end-to-side anastomosis of one ITA as a free graft to the side of the second ITA, which is left as a pedicled graft, combined with liberal use of sequential anastomoses. In his series of 897 patients overall survival was 75%, and freedom from reintervention was 92%, 8 years after revascularization.[315] Barner has reported similar encouraging results with composite grafting using one ITA and one RA.[316] Data from randomized studies are beginning to emerge supporting improvement in early outcomes with complete arterial revascularization compared with conventional CABG. Muneretto and associates randomized 200 patients to complete arterial revascularization (left ITA to the LAD artery and composite grafts with the right ITA, RA, or both) versus conventional CABG (left ITA to the LAD artery and SVGs). In midterm follow-up (20 months) superior event-free survival (freedom from nonfatal MI, angina recurrence, graft occlusion, need for percutaneous transluminal coronary angioplasty, and late death) was demonstrable in the complete arterial revascularization patients compared to conventional CABG.[317]

The same group conducted a second randomized trial comparing complete arterial revascularization to conventional CABG (ITA to LAD artery and SVG) in 160 patients older than 70 years of age undergoing first time nonemergent CABG. Early mortality was similar, but at 16 ± 3 months, there were significantly fewer graft occlusions and recurrences of angina among the complete arterial revascularization group. Independent predictors of graft occlusion and angina recurrence were use of SVGs, diabetes, and dyslipidemia.[318] At 34 mean months of follow-up in a similar study of diabetics, the total arterial revascularization group had a lower incidence of cardiac-related events and higher graft patency rates.[319]

The most complete retrospective multicenter analysis of complete arterial revascularization versus single ITA supplemented by vein grafts compared long-term outcomes of 384 propensity matched pairs of patients.[320] It demonstrated a statistically significant survival benefit at 15 years (54 vs 41%), suggesting bilateral ITA usage should be encouraged in patients with a reasonable life expectancy.

KEY POINTS

1. Coronary artery disease (CAD) is the number one killer of Americans.
2. Coronary artery bypass is advantageous over medical therapy in patients with unprotected LMCA stenosis, complex CAD (eg, SYNTAX score > 22), three-vessel disease, two-vessel disease with proximal left anterior descending disease, two-vessel disease without proximal left anterior descending disease but with extensive ischemia, single-vessel proximal left anterior descending disease with use of an ITA graft, and in patients with left ventricular dysfunction.
3. The STS risk model for postoperative morbidity and mortality can be found on the STS web site (www.sts.org) and includes 30-day stroke and death rates of 1.6 and 3%, respectively.
4. The left internal mammary to left anterior descending CABG confers a survival advantage to coronary artery bypass patients. In the BARI trial, patency rates at 1 and 4 years were 98 and 91%, respectively.
5. Skeletonization of the internal mammary artery is associated with reduced incidence of sternal wound complications.
6. RA grafts have better 5-year patency (98 vs 86%) than SVGs.
7. Cognitive test performance of patients after CABG is no different from that of heart healthy control groups over a 1-year period.
8. Freedom from angina after CABG in the BARI trial was 84% at 5 and 10 years.
9. Bilateral compared to single internal mammary artery bypass grafting is associated with improved survival, but the benefit is not noted until about 10 years after operation.

REFERENCES

1. Roger VL, Go AS, Lloyd-Jones DM, et al: Heart disease and stroke statistics—2012 update: a report from the American Heart Association. *Circulation* 2012; 125(1):e2-e220.
2. U.S. Census Bureau: U.S. Interim Projections by Age, Sex, Race, and Hispanic Origin. http://www.census.gov/population/projections/files/summary/NP2012-T2.xls Accessed December 2014.
3. Ferguson TB Jr, Hammill BG, Peterson ED, et al: A decade of change—risk profiles and outcomes for isolated coronary artery bypass grafting procedures, 1990-1999: a report from the STS National Database Committee and the Duke Clinical Research Institute. Society of Thoracic Surgeons. *Ann Thorac Surg* 2002; 73(2):480-489; discussion 489-490.
4. Serruys PW, Morice MC, Kappetein AP, et al: Percutaneous coronary intervention versus coronary-artery bypass grafting for severe coronary artery disease. *N Engl J Med* 2009; 360(10):961-972.
5. Shroyer AL, Grover FL, Hattler B, et al: On-pump versus off-pump coronary-artery bypass surgery. *N Engl J Med* 2009; 361(19):1827-1837.
6. Gibbon JH Jr: Application of a mechanical heart and lung apparatus to cardiac surgery. *Minn Med* 1954; 37(3):171-185; passim.
7. Sones FM Jr, Shirey EK: Cine coronary arteriography. *Mod Concepts Cardiovasc Dis* 1962; 31:735-738.
8. Favaloro RG, Effler DB, Groves LK, et al: Direct myocardial revascularization with saphenous vein autograft. Clinical experience in 100 cases. *Dis Chest* 1969; 56(4):279-283.
9. Johnson WD, Flemma RJ, Lepley D Jr, et al: Extended treatment of severe coronary artery disease: a total surgical approach. *Ann Surg* 1969; 170(3):460-470.
10. Hillis LD, Smith PK, Anderson JL, et al: 2011 ACCF/AHA Guideline for Coronary Artery Bypass Graft Surgery: a report of the American College of Cardiology Foundation/American Heart Association Task Force on Practice Guidelines. *Circulation* 2011; 124(23):e652-735.
11. The European Coronary Surgery Study Group: Long-term results of prospective randomised study of coronary artery bypass surgery in stable angina pectoris. European Coronary Surgery Study Group. *Lancet* 1982; 2(8309):1173-1180.
12. Coronary artery surgery study (CASS): a randomized trial of coronary artery bypass surgery. Survival data. *Circulation* 1983; 68(5):939-950.
13. The Veterans Administra Coronary Artery Bypass Surgery Cooperative Study Group: Eleven-year survival in the Veterans Administration randomized trial of coronary bypass surgery for stable angina. The Veterans Administration Coronary Artery Bypass Surgery Cooperative Study Group. *N Engl J Med* 1984; 311(21):1333-1339.
14. Sianos G, Morel MA, Kappetein AP, et al: The SYNTAX Score: an angiographic tool grading the complexity of coronary artery disease. *EuroIntervention* 2005; 1(2):219-227.
15. Goldman L, Hashimoto B, Cook EF, et al: Comparative reproducibility and validity of systems for assessing cardiovascular functional class: advantages of a new specific activity scale. *Circulation* 1981; 64(6):1227-1234.
16. Chang JA, Froelicher VF: Clinical and exercise test markers of prognosis in patients with stable coronary artery disease. *Curr Probl Cardiol* 1994; 19(9):533-587.
17. Ribisl PM, Morris CK, Kawaguchi T, et al: Angiographic patterns and severe coronary artery disease. Exercise test correlates. *Arch Intern Med* 1992; 152(8):1618-1624.
18. Gibbons RJ, Abrams J, Chatterjee K, et al: ACC/AHA 2002 guideline update for the management of patients with chronic stable angina—summary article: a report of the American College of Cardiology/American Heart Association Task Force on practice guidelines (Committee on the Management of Patients With Chronic Stable Angina). *J Am Coll Cardiol* 2003; 41(1):159-168.
19. Ritchie JL, Bateman TM, Bonow RO, et al: Guidelines for clinical use of cardiac radionuclide imaging. Report of the American College of Cardiology/American Heart Association Task Force on Assessment of Diagnostic and Therapeutic Cardiovascular Procedures (Committee on Radionuclide Imaging), developed in collaboration with the American Society of Nuclear Cardiology. *J Am Coll Cardiol* 1995; 25(2):521-547.
20. Cheitlin MD, Armstrong WF, Aurigemma GP, et al: ACC/AHA/ASE 2003 Guideline Update for the Clinical Application of Echocardiography: summary article. A report of the American College of Cardiology/American Heart Association Task Force on Practice Guidelines (ACC/AHA/ASE Committee to Update the 1997 Guidelines for the Clinical Application of Echocardiography). *J Am Soc Echocardiogr* 2003; 16(10):1091-1110.
21. Eagle KA, Guyton RA, Davidoff R, et al: ACC/AHA 2004 guideline update for coronary artery bypass graft surgery: a report of the American College of Cardiology/American Heart Association Task Force on Practice Guidelines (Committee to Update the 1999 Guidelines for Coronary Artery Bypass Graft Surgery). *Circulation* 2004; 110(14):e340-437.
22. Mark DB, Nelson CL, Califf RM, et al: Continuing evolution of therapy for coronary artery disease. Initial results from the era of coronary angioplasty. *Circulation* 1994; 89(5):2015-2025.
23. Lenzen MJ, Boersma E, Bertrand ME, et al: Management and outcome of patients with established coronary artery disease: the Euro Heart Survey on coronary revascularization. *Eur Heart J* 2005; 26(12):1169-1179.
24. Serruys PW, Unger F, Sousa JE, et al: Comparison of coronary-artery bypass surgery and stenting for the treatment of multivessel disease. *N Engl J Med* 2001; 344(15):1117-1124.
25. Seung KB, Park DW, Kim YH, et al: Stents versus coronary-artery bypass grafting for left main coronary artery disease. *N Engl J Med* 2008; 358(17):1781-1792.
26. Farkouh ME, Domanski M, Sleeper LA, et al: Strategies for multivessel revascularization in patients with diabetes. *N Engl J Med* 2012; 367(25):2375-2384.
27. Pearson T, Rapaport E, Criqui M, et al: Optimal risk factor management in the patient after coronary revascularization. A statement for healthcare professionals from an American Heart Association Writing Group. *Circulation* 1994; 90(6):3125-3133.
28. Pepine CJ, Cohn PF, Deedwania PC, et al: Effects of treatment on outcome in mildly symptomatic patients with ischemia during daily life. The Atenolol Silent Ischemia Study (ASIST). *Circulation* 1994; 90(2):762-768.
29. Bangalore S, Steg G, Deedwania P, et al: Beta-Blocker use and clinical outcomes in stable outpatients with and without coronary artery disease. *JAMA* 2012; 308(13):1340-1349.
30. Deanfield JE, Detry JM, Lichtlen PR, et al: Amlodipine reduces transient myocardial ischemia in patients with coronary artery disease: double-blind Circadian Anti-Ischemia Program in Europe (CAPE Trial). *J Am Coll Cardiol* 1994; 24(6):1460-1467.
31. Savonitto S, Ardissiono D, Egstrup K, et al: Combination therapy with metoprolol and nifedipine versus monotherapy in patients with stable angina pectoris. Results of the International Multicenter Angina Exercise (IMAGE) Study. *J Am Coll Cardiol* 1996; 27(2):311-316.
32. Von Arnim T: Prognostic significance of transient ischemic episodes: response to treatment shows improved prognosis. Results of the Total Ischemic Burden Bisoprolol Study (TIBBs) follow-up. *J Am Coll Cardiol* 1996; 28(1):20-24.
33. Murphy ML, Hultgren HN, Detre K, et al: Treatment of chronic stable angina. A preliminary report of survival data of the randomized Veterans Administration cooperative study. *N Engl J Med* 1977; 297(12):621-627.
34. The European Coronary SurStudy Group: Prospective randomised study of coronary artery bypass surgery in stable angina pectoris. Second interim report by the European Coronary Surgery Study Group. *Lancet* 1980; 2(8193):491-495.
35. Varnauskas E: Twelve-year follow-up of survival in the randomized European Coronary Surgery Study. *N Engl J Med* 1988; 319(6):332-337.
36. Mathur VS, Guinn GA: Prospective randomized study of the surgical therapy of stable angina. *Cardiovasc Clin* 1977; 8(2):131-144.
37. Kloster FE, Kremkau EL, Ritzmann LW, et al: Coronary bypass for stable angina: a prospective randomized study. *N Engl J Med* 1979; 300(4):149-157.
38. Norris RM, Agnew TM, Brandt PW, et al: Coronary surgery after recurrent myocardial infarction: progress of a trial comparing surgical with nonsurgical management for asymptomatic patients with advanced coronary disease. *Circulation* 1981; 63(4):785-792.
39. Yusuf S, Zucker D, Peduzzi P, et al: Effect of coronary artery bypass graft surgery on survival: overview of 10-year results from randomised trials by the Coronary Artery Bypass Graft Surgery Trialists Collaboration. *Lancet* 1994; 344(8922):563-570.

40. Takaro T, Hultgren HN, Lipton MJ, et al: The VA cooperative randomized study of surgery for coronary arterial occlusive disease II. Subgroup with significant left main lesions. *Circulation* 1976; 54(6 Suppl):III107-117.
41. Caracciolo EA, Davis KB, Sopko G, et al: Comparison of surgical and medical group survival in patients with left main coronary artery disease. Long-term CASS experience. *Circulation* 1995; 91(9):2325-2334.
42. Myers WO, Schaff HV, Gersh BJ, et al: Improved survival of surgically treated patients with triple vessel coronary artery disease and severe angina pectoris. A report from the Coronary Artery Surgery Study (CASS) registry. *J Thorac Cardiovasc Surg* 1989; 97(4):487-495.
43. Dzavik V, Ghali WA, Norris C, et al: Long-term survival in 11,661 patients with multivessel coronary artery disease in the era of stenting: a report from the Alberta Provincial Project for Outcome Assessment in Coronary Heart Disease (APPROACH) Investigators. *Am Heart J* 2001; 142(1):119-126.
44. Smith PK, Califf RM, Tuttle RH, et al: Selection of surgical or percutaneous coronary intervention provides differential longevity benefit. *Ann Thorac Surg* 2006; 82(4):1420-1428; discussion 1428-1429.
45. Davies RF, Goldberg AD, Forman S, et al: Asymptomatic Cardiac Ischemia Pilot (ACIP) study two-year follow-up: outcomes of patients randomized to initial strategies of medical therapy versus revascularization. *Circulation* 1997; 95(8):2037-2043.
46. Loop FD, Lytle BW, Cosgrove DM, et al: Influence of the internal-mammary-artery graft on 10-year survival and other cardiac events. *N Engl J Med* 1986; 314(1):1-6.
47. Cameron A, Davis KB, Green G, et al: Coronary bypass surgery with internal-thoracic-artery grafts–effects on survival over a 15-year period. *N Engl J Med* 1996; 334(4):216-219.
48. Hueb W, Soares PR, Gersh BJ, et al: The medicine, angioplasty, or surgery study (MASS-II): a randomized, controlled clinical trial of three therapeutic strategies for multivessel coronary artery disease: one-year results. *J Am Coll Cardiol* 2004; 43(10):1743-1751.
49. Hueb W, Lopes N, Gersh BJ, et al: Ten-year follow-up survival of the Medicine, Angioplasty, or Surgery Study (MASS II): a randomized controlled clinical trial of 3 therapeutic strategies for multivessel coronary artery disease. *Circulation* 2010; 122(10):949-957.
50. Investigators T: Trial of invasive versus medical therapy in elderly patients with chronic symptomatic coronary-artery disease (TIME): a randomised trial. *Lancet* 2001; 358(9286):951-957.
51. Kaiser GC, Davis KB, Fisher LD, et al: Survival following coronary artery bypass grafting in patients with severe angina pectoris (CASS). An observational study. *J Thorac Cardiovasc Surg* 1985; 89(4):513-524.
52. Kirklin JW, Naftel CD, Blackstone EH, et al: Summary of a consensus concerning death and ischemic events after coronary artery bypass grafting. *Circulation* 1989; 79(6 Pt 2):I81-91.
53. Velazquez EJ, Lee KL, Deja MA, et al: Coronary-artery bypass surgery in patients with left ventricular dysfunction. *N Engl J Med* 2011; 364(17):1607-1616.
54. Tarakji KG, Brunken R, McCarthy PM, et al: Myocardial viability testing and the effect of early intervention in patients with advanced left ventricular systolic dysfunction. *Circulation* 2006; 113(2):230-237.
55. Alderman EL, Fisher LD, Litwin P, et al: Results of coronary artery surgery in patients with poor left ventricular function (CASS). *Circulation* 1983; 68(4):785-795.
56. O'Connor CM, Velazquez EJ, Gardner LH, et al: Comparison of coronary artery bypass grafting versus medical therapy on long-term outcome in patients with ischemic cardiomyopathy (a 25-year experience from the Duke Cardiovascular Disease Databank). *Am J Cardiol* 2002; 90(2):101-107.
57. Phillips HR, O'Connor CM, Rogers J: Revascularization for heart failure. *Am Heart J* 2007; 153(4 Suppl):65-73.
58. Pocock SJ, Henderson RA, Seed P, et al: Quality of life, employment status, and anginal symptoms after coronary angioplasty or bypass surgery. 3-year follow-up in the Randomized Intervention Treatment of Angina (RITA) Trial. *Circulation* 1996; 94(2):135-142.
59. Pocock SJ, Henderson RA, Clayton T, et al: Quality of life after coronary angioplasty or continued medical treatment for angina: three-year follow-up in the RITA-2 trial. Randomized Intervention Treatment of Angina. *J Am Coll Cardiol* 2000; 35(4):907-914.
60. Boden WE, O'Rourke RA, Teo KK, et al: Optimal medical therapy with or without PCI for stable coronary disease. *N Engl J Med* 2007; 356(15):1503-1516.
61. Hannan EL, Racz MJ, Walford G, et al: Long-term outcomes of coronary-artery bypass grafting versus stent implantation. *N Engl J Med* 2005; 352(21):2174-2183.
62. Hannan EL, Wu C, Walford G, et al: Drug-eluting stents vs. coronary-artery bypass grafting in multivessel coronary disease. *N Engl J Med* 2008; 358(4):331-341.
63. Kappetein AP, Feldman TE, Mack MJ, et al: Comparison of coronary bypass surgery with drug-eluting stenting for the treatment of left main and/or three-vessel disease: 3-year follow-up of the SYNTAX trial. *Eur Heart J* 2011; 32(17):2125-2134.
64. Myers WO, Schaff HV, Fisher LD, et al: Time to first new myocardial infarction in patients with severe angina and three-vessel disease comparing medical and early surgical therapy: a CASS registry study of survival. *J Thorac Cardiovasc Surg* 1988; 95(3):382-389.
65. Group, VACABSCS: Eighteen-year follow-up in the Veterans Affairs Cooperative Study of Coronary Artery Bypass Surgery for stable angina. *Circulation* 1992; 86(1):121-130.
66. Al Suwaidi J, Holmes DR Jr, Salam AM, et al: Impact of coronary artery stents on mortality and nonfatal myocardial infarction: meta-analysis of randomized trials comparing a strategy of routine stenting with that of balloon angioplasty. *Am Heart J* 2004; 147(5):815-822.
67. Babapulle MN, Joseph L, Belisle P, et al: A hierarchical Bayesian meta-analysis of randomised clinical trials of drug-eluting stents. *Lancet* 2004; 364(9434):583-591.
68. Katritsis DG, Ioannidis JP: Percutaneous coronary intervention versus conservative therapy in nonacute coronary artery disease: a meta-analysis. *Circulation* 2005; 111(22):2906-2912.
69. Kastrati A, Mehilli J, Pache J, et al: Analysis of 14 trials comparing sirolimus-eluting stents with bare-metal stents. *N Engl J Med* 2007; 356(10):1030-1039.
70. Trikalinos TA, Alsheikh-Ali AA, Tatsioni A, et al: Percutaneous coronary interventions for non-acute coronary artery disease: a quantitative 20-year synopsis and a network meta-analysis. *Lancet* 2009; 373(9667):911-918.
71. Windecker S, Stortecky S, Stefanini GG, et al: Revascularisation versus medical treatment in patients with stable coronary artery disease: network meta-analysis. *BMJ* 2014; 348:g3859.
72. Morice MC, Serruys PW, Kappetein AP, et al: Outcomes in patients with de novo left main disease treated with either percutaneous coronary intervention using paclitaxel-eluting stents or coronary artery bypass graft treatment in the Synergy Between Percutaneous Coronary Intervention with TAXUS and Cardiac Surgery (SYNTAX) trial. *Circulation* 2010; 121(24):2645-2653.
73. Bravata DM, Gienger AL, McDonald KM, et al: Systematic review: the comparative effectiveness of percutaneous coronary interventions and coronary artery bypass graft surgery. *Ann Intern Med* 2007; 147(10):703-716.
74. Goy JJ, Eeckhout E, Burnand B, et al: Coronary angioplasty versus left internal mammary artery grafting for isolated proximal left anterior descending artery stenosis. *Lancet* 1994; 343(8911):1449-1453.
75. Hueb WA, Bellotti G, de Oliveira SA, et al: The Medicine, Angioplasty or Surgery Study (MASS): a prospective, randomized trial of medical therapy, balloon angioplasty or bypass surgery for single proximal left anterior descending artery stenoses. *J Am Coll Cardiol* 1995; 26(7):1600-1605.
76. Hueb WA, Soares PR, Almeida De Oliveira S, et al: Five-year follow-op of the medicine, angioplasty, or surgery study (MASS): a prospective, randomized trial of medical therapy, balloon angioplasty, or bypass surgery for single proximal left anterior descending coronary artery stenosis. *Circulation* 1999; 100(19 Suppl):II107-113.
77. RITA trial Participants: Coronary angioplasty versus coronary artery bypass surgery: the Randomized Intervention Treatment of Angina (RITA) trial. *Lancet* 1993; 341(8845):573-580.
78. Hamm CW, Reimers J, Ischinger T, et al: A randomized study of coronary angioplasty compared with bypass surgery in patients with symptomatic multivessel coronary disease. German Angioplasty Bypass Surgery Investigation (GABI). *N Engl J Med* 1994; 331(16):1037-1043.
79. CABRI trial participants: First-year results of CABRI (Coronary Angioplasty versus Bypass Revascularisation Investigation). CABRI Trial Participants. *Lancet* 1995; 346(8984):1179-1184.
80. The BARI Investigators: Comparison of coronary bypass surgery with angioplasty in patients with multivessel disease. The Bypass Angioplasty

Revascularization Investigation (BARI) Investigators. *N Engl J Med* 1996; 335(4):217-225.

81. King SB 3rd, Barnhart HX, Kosinski AS, et al: Angioplasty or surgery for multivessel coronary artery disease: comparison of eligible registry and randomized patients in the EAST trial and influence of treatment selection on outcomes. Emory Angioplasty versus Surgery Trial Investigators. *Am J Cardiol* 1997; 79(11):1453-1459.

82. Pocock SJ, Henderson RA, Rickards AF, et al: Meta-analysis of randomised trials comparing coronary angioplasty with bypass surgery. *Lancet* 1995; 346(8984):1184-1189.

83. Sim I, Gupta M, McDonald K, et al: A meta-analysis of randomized trials comparing coronary artery bypass grafting with percutaneous transluminal coronary angioplasty in multivessel coronary artery disease. *Am J Cardiol* 1995; 76(14):1025-1029.

84. Investigators, B: The final 10-year follow-up results from the BARI randomized trial. *J Am Coll Cardiol* 2007; 49(15):1600-1606.

85. Detre K, Holubkov R, Kelsey S, et al: Percutaneous transluminal coronary angioplasty in 1985-1986 and 1977-1981. The National Heart, Lung, and Blood Institute Registry. *N Engl J Med* 1988; 318(5):265-270.

86. Rodriguez A, Boullon F, Perez-Balino N, et al: Argentine randomized trial of percutaneous transluminal coronary angioplasty versus coronary artery bypass surgery in multivessel disease (ERACI): in-hospital results and 1-year follow-up. ERACI Group. *J Am Coll Cardiol* 1993; 22(4):1060-1067.

87. Rodriguez A, Mele E, Peyregne E, et al: Three-year follow-up of the Argentine Randomized Trial of Percutaneous Transluminal Coronary Angioplasty Versus Coronary Artery Bypass Surgery in Multivessel Disease (ERACI). *J Am Coll Cardiol* 1996; 27(5):1178-1184.

88. Carrie D, Elbaz M, Puel J, et al: Five-year outcome after coronary angioplasty versus bypass surgery in multivessel coronary artery disease: results from the French Monocentric Study. *Circulation* 1997; 96(9 Suppl):II-1-6.

89. Mercado N, Wijns W, Serruys PW, et al: One-year outcomes of coronary artery bypass graft surgery versus percutaneous coronary intervention with multiple stenting for multisystem disease: a meta-analysis of individual patient data from randomized clinical trials. *J Thorac Cardiovasc Surg* 2005; 130(2):512-519.

90. Daemen J, Boersma E, Flather M, et al: Long-term safety and efficacy of percutaneous coronary intervention with stenting and coronary artery bypass surgery for multivessel coronary artery disease: a meta-analysis with 5-year patient-level data from the ARTS, ERACI-II, MASS-II, and SoS trials. *Circulation* 2008; 118(11):1146-1154.

91. Fischman DL, Leon MB, Baim DS, et al: A randomized comparison of coronary-stent placement and balloon angioplasty in the treatment of coronary artery disease. Stent Restenosis Study Investigators. *N Engl J Med* 1994; 331(8):496-501.

92. Serruys PW, de Jaegere P, Kiemeneij F, et al: A comparison of balloon-expandable-stent implantation with balloon angioplasty in patients with coronary artery disease. Benestent Study Group. *N Engl J Med* 1994; 331(8):489-495.

93. Moses JW, Leon MB, Stone GW: Left main percutaneous coronary intervention crossing the threshold: time for a guidelines revision! *J Am Coll Cardiol* 2009; 54(16):1512-1514.

94. Taggart DP, Kaul S, Boden WE, et al: Revascularization for unprotected left main stem coronary artery stenosis stenting or surgery. *J Am Coll Cardiol* 2008; 51(9):885-892.

95. Park SJ, Kim YH, Park DW, et al: Randomized trial of stents versus bypass surgery for left main coronary artery disease. *N Engl J Med* 2011; 364(18):1718-1727.

96. Kapur A, Hall RJ, Malik IS, et al: Randomized comparison of percutaneous coronary intervention with coronary artery bypass grafting in diabetic patients. 1-year results of the CARDia (Coronary Artery Revascularization in Diabetes) trial. *J Am Coll Cardiol* 2010; 55(5):432-440.

97. Sipahi I, Akay MH, Dagdelen S, et al: Coronary artery bypass grafting vs percutaneous coronary intervention and long-term mortality and morbidity in multivessel disease: meta-analysis of randomized clinical trials of the arterial grafting and stenting era. *JAMA Intern Med* 2014; 174(2):223-230.

98. Hannan EL, Racz MJ, McCallister BD, et al: A comparison of three-year survival after coronary artery bypass graft surgery and percutaneous transluminal coronary angioplasty. *J Am Coll Cardiol* 1999; 33(1):63-72.

99. Cutlip DE, Chhabra AG, Baim DS, et al: Beyond restenosis: five-year clinical outcomes from second-generation coronary stent trials. *Circulation* 2004; 110(10):1226-1230.

100. Opie LH, Commerford PJ, Gersh BJ: Controversies in stable coronary artery disease. *Lancet* 2006; 367(9504):69-78.

101. Li Y, Zheng Z, Xu B, et al: Comparison of drug-eluting stents and coronary artery bypass surgery for the treatment of multivessel coronary disease: three-year follow-up results from a single institution. *Circulation* 2009; 119(15):2040-2050.

102. Serruys PW, Onuma Y, Garg S, et al: 5-year clinical outcomes of the ARTS II (Arterial Revascularization Therapies Study II) of the sirolimus-eluting stent in the treatment of patients with multivessel de novo coronary artery lesions. *J Am Coll Cardiol* 2010; 55(11):1093-1101.

103. Park DW, Kim YH, Song HG, et al: Long-term comparison of drug-eluting stents and coronary artery bypass grafting for multivessel coronary revascularization: 5-year outcomes from the Asan Medical Center-Multivessel Revascularization Registry. *J Am Coll Cardiol* 2011; 57(2):128-137.

104. Weintraub WS, Grau-Sepulveda MV, Weiss JM, et al: Comparative effectiveness of revascularization strategies. *N Engl J Med* 2012; 366(16):1467-1476.

105. Hlatky MA, Boothroyd DB, Baker L, et al: Comparative effectiveness of multivessel coronary bypass surgery and multivessel percutaneous coronary intervention: a cohort study. *Ann Intern Med* 2013; 158(10):727-734.

106. Hochman JS, Sleeper LA, Webb JG, et al: Early revascularization and long-term survival in cardiogenic shock complicating acute myocardial infarction. *JAMA* 2006; 295(21):2511-2515.

107. Jeger RV, Urban P, Harkness SM, et al: Early revascularization is beneficial across all ages and a wide spectrum of cardiogenic shock severity: a pooled analysis of trials. *Acute Card Care* 2011; 13(1):14-20.

108. Gu YL, van der Horst IC, Douglas YL, et al: Role of coronary artery bypass grafting during the acute and subacute phase of ST-elevation myocardial infarction. *Neth Heart J* 2010; 18(7-8):348-354.

109. Filizcan U, Kurc E, Cetemen S, et al: Mortality predictors in ST-elevated myocardial infarction patients undergoing coronary artery bypass grafting. *Angiology* 2011; 62(1):68-73.

110. Hochman JS, Sleeper LA, Webb JG, et al: Early revascularization in acute myocardial infarction complicated by cardiogenic shock. SHOCK Investigators. Should We Emergently Revascularize Occluded Coronaries for Cardiogenic Shock. *N Engl J Med* 1999; 341(9):625-634.

111. Ngaage DL, Cale AR, Cowen ME, et al: Early and late survival after surgical revascularization for ischemic ventricular fibrillation/tachycardia. *Ann Thorac Surg* 2008; 85(4):1278-1281.

112. Thielmann M, Neuhauser M, Marr A, et al: Predictors and outcomes of coronary artery bypass grafting in ST elevation myocardial infarction. *Ann Thorac Surg* 2007; 84(1):17-24.

113. Antman EM, Cohen M, Bernink PJ, et al: The TIMI risk score for unstable angina/non-ST elevation MI: a method for prognostication and therapeutic decision making. *JAMA* 2000; 284(7):835-842.

114. Rogers WJ, Bourassa MG, Andrews TC, et al: Asymptomatic Cardiac Ischemia Pilot (ACIP) study: outcome at 1 year for patients with asymptomatic cardiac ischemia randomized to medical therapy or revascularization. The ACIP Investigators. *J Am Coll Cardiol* 1995; 26(3):594-605.

115. Little WC, Constantinescu M, Applegate RJ, et al: Can coronary angiography predict the site of a subsequent myocardial infarction in patients with mild-to-moderate coronary artery disease? *Circulation* 1988; 78(5 Pt 1):1157-1166.

116. Giroud D, Li JM, Urban P, et al: Relation of the site of acute myocardial infarction to the most severe coronary arterial stenosis at prior angiography. *Am J Cardiol* 1992; 69(8):729-732.

117. Topol EJ, Ellis SG, Cosgrove DM, et al: Analysis of coronary angioplasty practice in the United States with an insurance-claims data base. *Circulation* 1993; 87(5):1489-1497.

118. Bech GJ, De Bruyne B, Pijls NH, et al: Fractional flow reserve to determine the appropriateness of angioplasty in moderate coronary stenosis: a randomized trial. *Circulation* 2001; 103(24):2928-2934.

119. Levine GN, Bates ER, Blankenship JC, et al: 2011 ACCF/AHA/SCAI Guideline for Percutaneous Coronary Intervention: executive summary: a report of the American College of Cardiology Foundation/American Heart Association Task Force on Practice Guidelines and the Society for Cardiovascular Angiography and Interventions. *Circulation* 2011; 124(23):2574-2609.

120. Ragosta M, Dee S, Sarembock IJ, et al: Prevalence of unfavorable angiographic characteristics for percutaneous intervention in patients with unprotected left main coronary artery disease. *Catheter Cardiovasc Interv* 2006; 68(3):357-362.

121. Boudriot E, Thiele H, Walther T, et al: Randomized comparison of percutaneous coronary intervention with sirolimus-eluting stents versus coronary artery bypass grafting in unprotected left main stem stenosis. *J Am Coll Cardiol* 2011; 57(5):538-545.

122. Morice MC, Serruys PW, Kappetein AP, et al: Five-year outcomes in patients with left main disease treated with either percutaneous coronary intervention or coronary artery bypass grafting in the synergy between percutaneous coronary intervention with taxus and cardiac surgery trial. *Circulation* 2014; 129(23):2388-2394.

123. Mohr FW, Morice MC, Kappetein AP, et al: Coronary artery bypass graft surgery versus percutaneous coronary intervention in patients with three-vessel disease and left main coronary disease: 5-year follow-up of the randomised, clinical SYNTAX trial. *Lancet* 2013; 381(9867):629-638.

124. Braunwald E, Rutherford JD: Reversible ischemic left ventricular dysfunction: evidence for the "hibernating myocardium". *J Am Coll Cardiol* 1986; 8(6):1467-1470.

125. Dilsizian V, Bonow RO: Current diagnostic techniques of assessing myocardial viability in patients with hibernating and stunned myocardium. *Circulation* 1993; 87(1):1-20.

126. Bax JJ, Wijns W, Cornel JH, et al: Accuracy of currently available techniques for prediction of functional recovery after revascularization in patients with left ventricular dysfunction due to chronic coronary artery disease: comparison of pooled data. *J Am Coll Cardiol* 1997; 30(6):1451-1460.

127. Allman KC, Shaw LJ, Hachamovitch R, et al: Myocardial viability testing and impact of revascularization on prognosis in patients with coronary artery disease and left ventricular dysfunction: a meta-analysis. *J Am Coll Cardiol* 2002; 39(7):1151-1158.

128. Ellis SG, Cowley MJ, DiSciascio G, et al: Determinants of 2-year outcome after coronary angioplasty in patients with multivessel disease on the basis of comprehensive preprocedural evaluation. Implications for patient selection. The Multivessel Angioplasty Prognosis Study Group. *Circulation* 1991; 83(6):1905-1914.

129. O'Keefe JH Jr, Allan JJ, McCallister BD, et al: Angioplasty versus bypass surgery for multivessel coronary artery disease with left ventricular ejection fraction < or = 40%. *Am J Cardiol* 1993; 71(11):897-901.

130. Berger PB, Velianou JL, Aslanidou Vlachos H, et al: Survival following coronary angioplasty versus coronary artery bypass surgery in anatomic subsets in which coronary artery bypass surgery improves survival compared with medical therapy. Results from the Bypass Angioplasty Revascularization Investigation (BARI). *J Am Coll Cardiol* 2001; 38(5):1440-1449.

131. Brener SJ, Lytle BW, Casserly IP, et al: Propensity analysis of long-term survival after surgical or percutaneous revascularization in patients with multivessel coronary artery disease and high-risk features. *Circulation* 2004; 109(19):2290-2295.

132. Gioia G, Matthai W, Gillin K, et al: Revascularization in severe left ventricular dysfunction: outcome comparison of drug-eluting stent implantation versus coronary artery by-pass grafting. *Catheter Cardiovasc Interv* 2007; 70(1):26-33.

133. Hlatky MA, Boothroyd DB, Bravata DM, et al: Coronary artery bypass surgery compared with percutaneous coronary interventions for multivessel disease: a collaborative analysis of individual patient data from ten randomised trials. *Lancet* 2009; 373(9670):1190-1197.

134. Fefer P, Knudtson ML, Cheema AN, et al: Current perspectives on coronary chronic total occlusions: the Canadian Multicenter Chronic Total Occlusions Registry. *J Am Coll Cardiol* 2012; 59(11):991-997.

135. Strauss BH, Shuvy M, Wijeysundera HC: Revascularization of chronic total occlusions: time to reconsider? *J Am Coll Cardiol* 2014; 64(12):1281-1289.

136. Garcia S, Sandoval Y, Roukoz H, et al: Outcomes after complete versus incomplete revascularization of patients with multivessel coronary artery disease: a meta-analysis of 89,883 patients enrolled in randomized clinical trials and observational studies. *J Am Coll Cardiol* 2013; 62(16):1421-1431.

137. Alexander KP, Anstrom KJ, Muhlbaier LH, et al: Outcomes of cardiac surgery in patients > or = 80 years: results from the National Cardiovascular Network. *J Am Coll Cardiol* 2000; 35(3):731-738.

138. Houlind K, Kjeldsen BJ, Madsen SN, et al: On-pump versus off-pump coronary artery bypass surgery in elderly patients: results from the Danish on-pump versus off-pump randomization study. *Circulation* 2012; 125(20):2431-2439.

139. Diegeler A, Borgermann J, Kappert U, et al: Off-pump versus on-pump coronary-artery bypass grafting in elderly patients. *N Engl J Med* 2013; 368(13):1189-1198.

140. Hannan EL, Zhong Y, Berger PB, et al: Comparison of intermediate-term outcomes of coronary artery bypass grafting versus drug-eluting stents for patients ≥75 years of age. *Am J Cardiol* 2014; 113(5):803-808.

141. Kip KE, Faxon DP, Detre KM, et al: Coronary angioplasty in diabetic patients. The National Heart, Lung, and Blood Institute Percutaneous Transluminal Coronary Angioplasty Registry. *Circulation* 1996; 94(8):1818-1825.

142. Salomon NW, Page US, Okies JE, et al: Diabetes mellitus and coronary artery bypass. Short-term risk and long-term prognosis. *J Thorac Cardiovasc Surg* 1983; 85(2):264-271.

143. Detre KM, Lombardero MS, Brooks MM, et al: The effect of previous coronary-artery bypass surgery on the prognosis of patients with diabetes who have acute myocardial infarction. Bypass Angioplasty Revascularization Investigation Investigators. *N Engl J Med* 2000; 342(14):989-997.

144. Investigators, B: Seven-year outcome in the Bypass Angioplasty Revascularization Investigation (BARI) by treatment and diabetic status. *J Am Coll Cardiol* 2000; 35(5):1122-1129.

145. Van Belle E, Ketelers R, Bauters C, et al: Patency of percutaneous transluminal coronary angioplasty sites at 6-month angiographic follow-up: a key determinant of survival in diabetics after coronary balloon angioplasty. *Circulation* 2001; 103(9):1218-1224.

146. King SB 3rd, Kosinski AS, Guyton RA, et al: Eight-year mortality in the Emory Angioplasty versus Surgery Trial (EAST). *J Am Coll Cardiol* 2000; 35(5):1116-1121.

147. Ellis SG, Narins CR: Problem of angioplasty in diabetics. *Circulation* 1997; 96(6):1707-1710.

148. Group BDS, Frye RL, August P, et al: A randomized trial of therapies for type 2 diabetes and coronary artery disease. *N Engl J Med* 2009; 360(24):2503-2515.

149. Banning AP, Westaby S, Morice MC, et al: Diabetic and nondiabetic patients with left main and/or 3-vessel coronary artery disease: comparison of outcomes with cardiac surgery and paclitaxel-eluting stents. *J Am Coll Cardiol* 2010; 55(11):1067-1075.

150. Dacey LJ, Liu JY, Braxton JH, et al: Long-term survival of dialysis patients after coronary bypass grafting. *Ann Thorac Surg* 2002; 74(2):458-462; discussion 462-453.

151. Liu JY, Birkmeyer NJ, Sanders JH, et al: Risks of morbidity and mortality in dialysis patients undergoing coronary artery bypass surgery. Northern New England Cardiovascular Disease Study Group. *Circulation* 2000; 102(24):2973-2977.

152. Reddan DN, Szczech LA, Tuttle RH, et al: Chronic kidney disease, mortality, and treatment strategies among patients with clinically significant coronary artery disease. *J Am Soc Nephrol* 2003; 14(9):2373-2380.

153. Hemmelgarn BR, Southern D, Culleton BF, et al: Survival after coronary revascularization among patients with kidney disease. *Circulation* 2004; 110(14):1890-1895.

154. Sedlis SP, Jurkovitz CT, Hartigan PM, et al: Optimal medical therapy with or without percutaneous coronary intervention for patients with stable coronary artery disease and chronic kidney disease. *Am J Cardiol* 2009; 104(12):1647-1653.

155. Koyanagi T, Nishida H, Kitamura M, et al: Comparison of clinical outcomes of coronary artery bypass grafting and percutaneous transluminal coronary angioplasty in renal dialysis patients. *Ann Thorac Surg* 1996; 61(6):1793-1796.

156. Szczech LA, Reddan DN, Owen WF, et al: Differential survival after coronary revascularization procedures among patients with renal insufficiency. *Kidney Int* 2001; 60(1):292-299.

157. Herzog CA, Ma JZ, Collins AJ: Comparative survival of dialysis patients in the United States after coronary angioplasty, coronary artery stenting, and coronary artery bypass surgery and impact of diabetes. *Circulation* 2002; 106(17):2207-2211.

158. Ix JH, Mercado N, Shlipak MG, et al: Association of chronic kidney disease with clinical outcomes after coronary revascularization: the Arterial Revascularization Therapies Study (ARTS). *Am Heart J* 2005; 149(3):512-519.

159. Bae KS, Park HC, Kang BS, et al: Percutaneous coronary intervention versus coronary artery bypass grafting in patients with coronary artery disease and diabetic nephropathy: a single center experience. *Korean J Intern Med* 2007; 22(3):139-146.

160. Roach GW, Kanchuger M, Mangano CM, et al: Adverse cerebral outcomes after coronary bypass surgery. Multicenter Study of Perioperative Ischemia Research Group and the Ischemia Research and Education Foundation Investigators. *N Engl J Med* 1996; 335(25): 1857-1863.

161. Puskas JD, Winston AD, Wright CE, et al: Stroke after coronary artery operation: incidence, correlates, outcome, and cost. *Ann Thorac Surg* 2000; 69(4):1053-1056.

162. Bull DA, Neumayer LA, Hunter GC, et al: Risk factors for stroke in patients undergoing coronary artery bypass grafting. *Cardiovasc Surg* 1993; 1(2):182-185.

163. Kaul TK, Fields BL, Wyatt DA, et al: Surgical management in patients with coexistent coronary and cerebrovascular disease. Long-term results. *Chest* 1994; 106(5):1349-1357.

164. Qureshi AI, Alexandrov AV, Tegeler CH, et al: Guidelines for screening of extracranial carotid artery disease: a statement for healthcare professionals from the multidisciplinary practice guidelines committee of the American Society of Neuroimaging; cosponsored by the Society of Vascular and Interventional Neurology. *J Neuroimaging* 2007; 17(1): 19-47.

165. Selnes OA, Gottesman RF, Grega MA, et al: Cognitive and neurologic outcomes after coronary-artery bypass surgery. *N Engl J Med* 2012; 366(3):250-257.

166. Brener BJ, Brief DK, Alpert J, et al: The risk of stroke in patients with asymptomatic carotid stenosis undergoing cardiac surgery: a follow-up study. *J Vasc Surg* 1987; 5(2):269-279.

167. Faggioli GL, Curl GR, Ricotta JJ: The role of carotid screening before coronary artery bypass. *J Vasc Surg* 1990; 12(6):724-729; discussion 729-731.

168. D'Agostino RS, Svensson LG, Neumann DJ, et al: Screening carotid ultrasonography and risk factors for stroke in coronary artery surgery patients. *Ann Thorac Surg* 1996; 62(6):1714-1723.

169. Naylor AR, Bown MJ: Stroke after cardiac surgery and its association with asymptomatic carotid disease: an updated systematic review and meta-analysis. *Eur J Vasc Endovasc Surg* 2011; 41(5):607-624.

170. Ghosh J, Murray D, Khwaja N, et al: The influence of asymptomatic significant carotid disease on mortality and morbidity in patients undergoing coronary artery bypass surgery. *Eur J Vasc Endovasc Surg* 2005; 29(1):88-90.

171. Baiou D, Karageorge A, Spyt T, et al: Patients undergoing cardiac surgery with asymptomatic unilateral carotid stenoses have a low risk of perioperative stroke. *Eur J Vasc Endovasc Surg* 2009; 38(5):556-559.

172. Li Y, Walicki D, Mathiesen C, et al: Strokes after cardiac surgery and relationship to carotid stenosis. *Arch Neurol* 2009; 66(9):1091-1096.

173. Mahmoudi M, Hill PC, Xue Z, et al: Patients with severe asymptomatic carotid artery stenosis do not have a higher risk of stroke and mortality after coronary artery bypass surgery. *Stroke* 2011; 42(10): 2801-2805.

174. Hogue CW Jr, Barzilai B, Pieper KS, et al: Sex differences in neurological outcomes and mortality after cardiac surgery: a society of thoracic surgery national database report. *Circulation* 2001; 103(17):2133-2137.

175. ElBardissi AW, Aranki SF, Sheng S, et al: Trends in isolated coronary artery bypass grafting: an analysis of the Society of Thoracic Surgeons adult cardiac surgery database. *J Thorac Cardiovasc Surg* 2012; 143(2):273-281.

176. Barbut D, Hinton RB, Szatrowski TP, et al: Cerebral emboli detected during bypass surgery are associated with clamp removal. *Stroke* 1994; 25(12):2398-2402.

177. Likosky DS, Marrin CA, Caplan LR, et al: Determination of etiologic mechanisms of strokes secondary to coronary artery bypass graft surgery. *Stroke* 2003; 34(12):2830-2834.

178. Gardner TJ, Horneffer PJ, Manolio TA, et al: Major stroke after coronary artery bypass surgery: changing magnitude of the problem. *J Vasc Surg* 1986; 3(4):684-687.

179. John R, Choudhri AF, Weinberg AD, et al: Multicenter review of preoperative risk factors for stroke after coronary artery bypass grafting. *Ann Thorac Surg* 2000; 69(1):30-35; discussion 35-36.

180. Berens ES, Kouchoukos NT, Murphy SF, et al: Preoperative carotid artery screening in elderly patients undergoing cardiac surgery. *J Vasc Surg* 1992; 15(2):313-321; discussion 322-323.

181. Manabe S, Shimokawa T, Fukui T, et al: Influence of carotid artery stenosis on stroke in patients undergoing off-pump coronary artery bypass grafting. *Eur J Cardiothorac Surg* 2008; 34(5):1005-1008.

182. Naylor AR: Managing patients with symptomatic coronary and carotid artery disease. *Perspect Vasc Surg Endovasc Ther* 2010; 22(2):70-76.

183. Barnes RW, Nix ML, Sansonetti D, et al: Late outcome of untreated asymptomatic carotid disease following cardiovascular operations. *J Vasc Surg* 1985; 2(6):843-849.

184. Ascher E, Hingorani A, Yorkovich W, et al: Routine preoperative carotid duplex scanning in patients undergoing open heart surgery: is it worthwhile? *Ann Vasc Surg* 2001; 15(6):669-678.

185. Halliday A, Mansfield A, Marro J, et al: Prevention of disabling and fatal strokes by successful carotid endarterectomy in patients without recent neurological symptoms: randomised controlled trial. *Lancet* 2004; 363(9420):1491-1502.

186. Durand DJ, Perler BA, Roseborough GS, et al: Mandatory versus selective preoperative carotid screening: a retrospective analysis. *Ann Thorac Surg* 2004; 78(1):159-166; discussion 159-166.

187. Hertzer NR, Young JR, Beven EG, et al: Coronary angiography in 506 patients with extracranial cerebrovascular disease. *Arch Intern Med* 1985; 145(5):849-852.

188. Mackey WC, O'Donnell TF Jr, Callow AD: Cardiac risk in patients undergoing carotid endarterectomy: impact on perioperative and long-term mortality. *J Vasc Surg* 1990; 11(2):226-233; discussion 233-224.

189. Hertzer NR, Arison R: Cumulative stroke and survival ten years after carotid endarterectomy. *J Vasc Surg* 1985; 2(5):661-668.

190. Knipp SC, Scherag A, Beyersdorf F, et al: Randomized comparison of synchronous CABG and carotid endarterectomy vs. isolated CABG in patients with asymptomatic carotid stenosis: the CABACS trial. *Int J Stroke* 2012; 7(4):354-360.

191. Chaturvedi S, Bruno A, Feasby T, et al: Carotid endarterectomy—an evidence-based review: report of the Therapeutics and Technology Assessment Subcommittee of the American Academy of Neurology. *Neurology* 2005; 65(6):794-801.

192. Akins CW, Hilgenberg AD, Vlahakes GJ, et al: Late results of combined carotid and coronary surgery using actual versus actuarial methodology. *Ann Thorac Surg* 2005; 80(6):2091-2097.

193. Shroyer AL, Coombs LP, Peterson ED, et al: The Society of Thoracic Surgeons: 30-day operative mortality and morbidity risk models. *Ann Thorac Surg* 2003; 75(6):1856-1864; discussion 1864-1855.

194. Berger JS, Frye CB, Harshaw Q, et al: Impact of clopidogrel in patients with acute coronary syndromes requiring coronary artery bypass surgery: a multicenter analysis. *J Am Coll Cardiol* 2008; 52(21):1693-1701.

195. Lehmann KH, von Segesser L, Muller-Glauser W, et al: Internal-mammary coronary artery grafts: is their superiority also due to a basically intact endothelium? *Thorac Cardiovasc Surg* 1989; 37(3):187-189.

196. Cox JL, Chiasson DA, Gotlieb AI: Stranger in a strange land: the pathogenesis of saphenous vein graft stenosis with emphasis on structural and functional differences between veins and arteries. *Prog Cardiovasc Dis* 1991; 34(1):45-68.

197. Motwani JG, Topol EJ: Aortocoronary saphenous vein graft disease: pathogenesis, predisposition, and prevention. *Circulation* 1998; 97(9):916-931.

198. Gitter R, Anderson JM Jr, Jett GK: Influence of milrinone and norepinephrine on blood flow in canine internal mammary artery grafts. *Ann Thorac Surg* 1996; 61(5):1367-1371.

199. Jett GK, Arcici JM Jr, Hatcher CR Jr, et al: Vasodilator drug effects on internal mammary artery and saphenous vein grafts. *J Am Coll Cardiol* 1988; 11(6):1317-1324.

200. Gurne O, Chenu P, Buche M, et al: Adaptive mechanisms of arterial and venous coronary bypass grafts to an increase in flow demand. *Heart* 1999; 82(3):336-342.

201. Henriquez-Pino JA, Gomes WJ, Prates JC, et al: Surgical anatomy of the internal thoracic artery. *Ann Thorac Surg* 1997; 64(4):1041-1045.

202. Cohen AJ, Lockman J, Lorberboym M, et al: Assessment of sternal vascularity with single photon emission computed tomography after harvesting of the internal thoracic artery. *J Thorac Cardiovasc Surg* 1999; 118(3):496-502.

203. Lorberboym M, Medalion B, Bder O, et al: 99mTc-MDP bone SPECT for the evaluation of sternal ischaemia following internal mammary artery dissection. *Nucl Med Commun* 2002; 23(1):47-52.

204. Matsa M, Paz Y, Gurevitch J, et al: Bilateral skeletonized internal thoracic artery grafts in patients with diabetes mellitus. *J Thorac Cardiovasc Surg* 2001; 121(4):668-674.

205. Noera G, Pensa P, Lodi R, et al: Influence of different harvesting techniques on the arterial wall of the internal mammary artery graft: microscopic analysis. *Thorac Cardiovasc Surg* 1993; 41(1):16-20.

206. Calafiore AM, Vitolla G, Iaco AL, et al: Bilateral internal mammary artery grafting: midterm results of pedicled versus skeletonized conduits. *Ann Thorac Surg* 1999; 67(6):1637-1642.

207. Gaudino M, Toesca A, Nori SL, et al: Effect of skeletonization of the internal thoracic artery on vessel wall integrity. *Ann Thorac Surg* 1999; 68(5):1623-1627.

208. Gaudino M, Trani C, Glieca F, et al: Early vasoreactive profile of skeletonized versus pedicled internal thoracic artery grafts. *J Thorac Cardiovasc Surg* 2003; 125(3):638-641.

209. Athanasiou T, Crossman MC, Asimakopoulos G, et al: Should the internal thoracic artery be skeletonized? *Ann Thorac Surg* 2004; 77(6):2238-2246.

210. Raja SG, Dreyfus GD: Internal thoracic artery: to skeletonize or not to skeletonize? *Ann Thorac Surg* 2005; 79(5):1805-1811.

211. Barner HB, Standeven JW, Reese J: Twelve-year experience with internal mammary artery for coronary artery bypass. *J Thorac Cardiovasc Surg* 1985; 90(5):668-675.

212. Whitlow PL, Dimas AP, Bashore TM, et al: Relationship of extent of revascularization with angina at one year in the Bypass Angioplasty Revascularization Investigation (BARI). *J Am Coll Cardiol* 1999; 34(6):1750-1759.

213. Schwartz L, Kip KE, Frye RL, et al: Coronary bypass graft patency in patients with diabetes in the Bypass Angioplasty Revascularization Investigation (BARI). *Circulation* 2002; 106(21):2652-2658.

214. Tatoulis J, Buxton BF, Fuller JA: Patencies of 2127 arterial to coronary conduits over 15 years. *Ann Thorac Surg* 2004; 77(1):93-101.

215. Geha AS, Krone RJ, McCormick JR, et al: Selection of coronary bypass. Anatomic, physiological, and angiographic considerations of vein and mammary artery grafts. *J Thorac Cardiovasc Surg* 1975; 70(3):414-431.

216. Acar C, Ramsheyi A, Pagny JY, et al: The radial artery for coronary artery bypass grafting: clinical and angiographic results at five years. *J Thorac Cardiovasc Surg* 1998; 116(6):981-989.

217. Tatoulis J, Royse AG, Buxton BF, et al: The radial artery in coronary surgery: a 5-year experience–clinical and angiographic results. *Ann Thorac Surg* 2002; 73(1):143-147; discussion 147-148.

218. Acar C, Jebara VA, Portoghese M, et al: Comparative anatomy and histology of the radial artery and the internal thoracic artery. Implication for coronary artery bypass. *Surg Radiol Anat* 1991; 13(4):283-288.

219. Kaufer E, Factor SM, Frame R, et al: Pathology of the radial and internal thoracic arteries used as coronary artery bypass grafts. *Ann Thorac Surg* 1997; 63(4):1118-1122.

220. Chardigny C, Jebara VA, Acar C, et al: Vasoreactivity of the radial artery. Comparison with the internal mammary and gastroepiploic arteries with implications for coronary artery surgery. *Circulation* 1993; 88(5 Pt 2):II115-127.

221. Cable DG, Caccitolo JA, Pearson PJ, et al: New approaches to prevention and treatment of radial artery graft vasospasm. *Circulation* 1998; 98(19 Suppl):II15-21; discussion II21-12.

222. Shapira OM, Alkon JD, Macron DS, et al: Nitroglycerin is preferable to diltiazem for prevention of coronary bypass conduit spasm. *Ann Thorac Surg* 2000; 70(3):883-888; discussion 888-889.

223. Reyes AT, Frame R, Brodman RF: Technique for harvesting the radial artery as a coronary artery bypass graft. *Ann Thorac Surg* 1995; 59(1):118-126.

224. Shima H, Ohno K, Michi K, et al: An anatomical study on the forearm vascular system. *J Craniomaxillofac Surg* 1996; 24(5):293-299.

225. Agrifoglio M, Dainese L, Pasotti S, et al: Preoperative assessment of the radial artery for coronary artery bypass grafting: is the clinical Allen test adequate? *Ann Thorac Surg* 2005; 79(2):570-572.

226. Tatoulis J, Buxton BF, Fuller JA: Bilateral radial artery grafts in coronary reconstruction: technique and early results in 261 patients. *Ann Thorac Surg* 1998; 66(3):714-719; discussion 720.

227. Ronan JW, Perry LA, Barner HB, et al: Radial artery harvest: comparison of ultrasonic dissection with standard technique. *Ann Thorac Surg* 2000; 69(1):113-114.

228. Newman RV, Lammle WG: Radial artery harvest using endoscopic techniques. *Heart Surg Forum* 2003; 6(6):E194-195.

229. Mussa S, Choudhary BP, Taggart DP: Radial artery conduits for coronary artery bypass grafting: current perspective. *J Thorac Cardiovasc Surg* 2005; 129(2):250-253.

230. Denton TA, Trento L, Cohen M, et al: Radial artery harvesting for coronary bypass operations: neurologic complications and their potential mechanisms. *J Thorac Cardiovasc Surg* 2001; 121(5):951-956.

231. Meharwal ZS, Trehan N: Functional status of the hand after radial artery harvesting: results in 3,977 cases. *Ann Thorac Surg* 2001; 72(5):1557-1561.

232. Moon MR, Barner HB, Bailey MS, et al: Long-term neurologic hand complications after radial artery harvesting using conventional cold and harmonic scalpel techniques. *Ann Thorac Surg* 2004; 78(2):535-538; discussion 535-538.

233. Navia JL, Olivares G, Ehasz P, et al: Endoscopic radial artery harvesting procedure for coronary artery bypass grafting. *Ann Cardiothorac Surg* 2013; 2(4):557-564.

234. Patel AN, Henry AC, Hunnicutt C, et al: Endoscopic radial artery harvesting is better than the open technique. *Ann Thorac Surg* 2004; 78(1):149-153; discussion 149-153.

235. Acar C, Jebara VA, Portoghese M, et al: Revival of the radial artery for coronary artery bypass grafting. *Ann Thorac Surg* 1992; 54(4):652-659; discussion 659-660.

236. Desai ND, Cohen EA, Naylor CD, et al: A randomized comparison of radial-artery and saphenous-vein coronary bypass grafts. *N Engl J Med* 2004; 351(22):2302-2309.

237. Maniar HS, Barner HB, Bailey MS, et al: Radial artery patency: are aortocoronary conduits superior to composite grafting? *Ann Thorac Surg* 2003; 76(5):1498-1503; discussion 1503-1504.

238. Hadinata IE, Hayward PA, Hare DL, et al: Choice of conduit for the right coronary system: 8-year analysis of Radial Artery Patency and Clinical Outcomes trial. *Ann Thorac Surg* 2009; 88(5):1404-1409.

239. Tatoulis J, Buxton BF, Fuller JA, et al: Long-term patency of 1108 radial arterial-coronary angiograms over 10 years. *Ann Thorac Surg* 2009; 88(1):23-29; discussion 29-30.

240. Jung SH, Song H, Choo SJ, et al: Comparison of radial artery patency according to proximal anastomosis site: direct aorta to radial artery anastomosis is superior to radial artery composite grafting. *J Thorac Cardiovasc Surg* 2009; 138(1):76-83.

241. Collins P, Webb CM, Chong CF, et al: Radial artery versus saphenous vein patency randomized trial: five-year angiographic follow-up. *Circulation* 2008; 117(22):2859-2864.

242. Mangano DT, Multicenter Study of Perioperative Ischemia Research, G: Aspirin and mortality from coronary bypass surgery. *N Engl J Med* 2002; 347(17):1309-1317.

243. Post Coronary Artery Bypass Graft Trial, I: The effect of aggressive lowering of low-density lipoprotein cholesterol levels and low-dose anticoagulation on obstructive changes in saphenous-vein coronary-artery bypass grafts. *N Engl J Med* 1997; 336(3):153-162.

244. Hata M, Takayama T, Sezai A, et al: Efficacy of aggressive lipid controlling therapy for preventing saphenous vein graft disease. *Ann Thorac Surg* 2009; 88(5):1440-1444.

245. Alexander JH, Hafley G, Harrington RA, et al: Efficacy and safety of edifoligide, an E2F transcription factor decoy, for prevention of vein graft failure following coronary artery bypass graft surgery: PREVENT IV: a randomized controlled trial. *JAMA* 2005; 294(19):2446-2454.

246. Black EA, Guzik TJ, West NE, et al: Minimally invasive saphenous vein harvesting: effects on endothelial and smooth muscle function. *Ann Thorac Surg* 2001; 71(5):1503-1507.

247. Yun KL, Wu Y, Aharonian V, et al: Randomized trial of endoscopic versus open vein harvest for coronary artery bypass grafting: six-month patency rates. *J Thorac Cardiovasc Surg* 2005; 129(3):496-503.

248. Lopes RD, Hafley GE, Allen KB, et al: Endoscopic versus open vein-graft harvesting in coronary-artery bypass surgery. *N Engl J Med* 2009; 361(3):235-244.

249. Souza DS, Johansson B, Bojo L, et al: Harvesting the saphenous vein with surrounding tissue for CABG provides long-term graft patency comparable to the left internal thoracic artery: results of a randomized longitudinal trial. *J Thorac Cardiovasc Surg* 2006; 132(2):373-378.

250. Wijnberg DS, Boeve WJ, Ebels T, et al: Patency of arm vein grafts used in aorto-coronary bypass surgery. *Eur J Cardiothorac Surg* 1990; 4(9):510-513.

251. Christenson JT, Simonet F, Schmuziger M: Sequential vein bypass grafting: tactics and long-term results. *Cardiovasc Surg* 1998; 6(4):389-397.

252. Vural KM, Sener E, Tasdemir O: Long-term patency of sequential and individual saphenous vein coronary bypass grafts. *Eur J Cardiothorac Surg* 2001; 19(2):140-144.

253. McBride LR, Barner HB: The left internal mammary artery as a sequential graft to the left anterior descending system. *J Thorac Cardiovasc Surg* 1983; 86(5):703-705.

254. Bessone LN, Pupello DF, Hiro SP, et al: Sequential internal mammary artery grafting: a viable alternative in myocardial revascularization. *Cardiovasc Surg* 1995; 3(2):155-162.

255. Kootstra GJ, Pragliola C, Lanzillo G: Technique of sequential grafting the left internal mammary artery (LIMA) to the circumflex coronary system. *J Cardiovasc Surg (Torino)* 1993; 34(6):523-526.

256. Shapira OM, Alkon JD, Aldea GS, et al: Clinical outcomes in patients undergoing coronary artery bypass grafting with preferred use of the radial artery. *J Card Surg* 1997; 12(6):381-388.

257. Ochi M, Bessho R, Saji Y: Sequential grafting of the right gastroepiploic artery in coronary artery bypass surgery. *Ann et al Thorac Surg* 2001; 71(4):1205-1209.

258. Hallen A, Bjork L, Bjork VO: Coronary thrombo-endarterectomy. *J Thorac Cardiovasc Surg* 1963; 45:216-223.

259. Brenowitz JB, Kayser KL, Johnson WD: Results of coronary artery endarterectomy and reconstruction. *J Thorac Cardiovasc Surg* 1988; 95(1):1-10.

260. Sirivella S, Gielchinsky I, Parsonnet V: Results of coronary artery endarterectomy and coronary artery bypass grafting for diffuse coronary artery disease. *Ann Thorac Surg* 2005; 80(5):1738-1744.

261. Livesay JJ, Cooley DA, Hallman GL, et al: Early and late results of coronary endarterectomy. Analysis of 3,369 patients. *J Thorac Cardiovasc Surg* 1986; 92(4):649-660.

262. Beretta L, Lemma M, Vanelli P, et al: Coronary "open" endarterectomy and reconstruction: short- and long-term results of the revascularization with saphenous vein versus IMA-graft. *Eur J Cardiothorac Surg* 1992; 6(7):382-386; discussion 387.

263. Gill IS, Beanlands DS, Boyd WD, et al: Left anterior descending endarterectomy and internal thoracic artery bypass for diffuse coronary disease. *Ann Thorac Surg* 1998; 65(3):659-662.

264. Sundt TM 3rd, Camillo CJ, Mendeloff EN, et al: Reappraisal of coronary endarterectomy for the treatment of diffuse coronary artery disease. *Ann Thorac Surg* 1999; 68(4):1272-1277.

265. Kim RW, Mariconda DC, Tellides G, et al: Single-clamp technique does not protect against cerebrovascular accident in coronary artery bypass grafting. *Eur J Cardiothorac Surg* 2001; 20(1):127-132.

266. Hammon JW, Stump DA, Butterworth JF, et al: Coronary artery bypass grafting with single cross-clamp results in fewer persistent neuropsychological deficits than multiple clamp or off-pump coronary artery bypass grafting. *Ann Thorac Surg* 2007; 84(4):1174-1178; discussion 1178-1179.

267. Prapas SN, Anagnostopoulos CE, Kotsis VN, et al: A new pattern for using both thoracic arteries to revascularize the entire heart: the pi-graft. *Ann Thorac Surg* 2002; 73(6):1990-1992.

268. Royse AG, Royse CF, Groves KL, et al: Blood flow in composite arterial grafts and effect of native coronary flow. *Ann Thorac Surg* 1999; 68(5):1619-1622.

269. Strauch JT, Spielvogel D, Lauten A, et al: Axillary artery cannulation: routine use in ascending aorta and aortic arch replacement. *Ann Thorac Surg* 2004; 78(1):103-108; discussion 103-108.

270. Rokkas CK, Kouchoukos NT: Surgical management of the severely atherosclerotic ascending aorta during cardiac operations. *Semin Thorac Cardiovasc Surg* 1998; 10(4):240-246.

271. Grover FL, Shroyer AL, Hammermeister K, et al: A decade's experience with quality improvement in cardiac surgery using the Veterans Affairs and Society of Thoracic Surgeons national databases. *Ann Surg* 2001; 234(4):464-472; discussion 472-474.

272. Mack MJ, Brown PP, Kugelmass AD, et al: Current status and outcomes of coronary revascularization 1999 to 2002: 148,396 surgical and percutaneous procedures. *Ann Thorac Surg* 2004; 77(3):761-766; discussion 766-768.

273. O'Connor GT, Birkmeyer JD, Dacey LJ, et al: Results of a regional study of modes of death associated with coronary artery bypass grafting. Northern New England Cardiovascular Disease Study Group. *Ann Thorac Surg* 1998; 66(4):1323-1328.

274. Sergeant P, Lesaffre E, Flameng W, et al: Internal mammary artery: methods of use and their effect on survival after coronary bypass surgery. *Eur J Cardiothorac Surg* 1990; 4(2):72-78.

275. Yau JM, Alexander JH, Hafley G, et al: Impact of perioperative myocardial infarction on angiographic and clinical outcomes following coronary artery bypass grafting (from PRoject of Ex-vivo Vein graft ENgineering via Transfection [PREVENT] IV). *Am J Cardiol* 2008; 102(5):546-551.

276. Klatte K, Chaitman BR, Theroux P, et al: Increased mortality after coronary artery bypass graft surgery is associated with increased levels of postoperative creatine kinase-myocardial band isoenzyme release: results from the GUARDIAN trial. *J Am Coll Cardiol* 2001; 38(4):1070-1077.

277. Hashemzadeh K, Dehdilani M: Postoperative cardiac troponin I is an independent predictor of in-hospital death after coronary artery bypass grafting. *J Cardiovasc Surg (Torino)* 2009; 50(3):403-409.

278. Rao V, Ivanov J, Weisel RD, et al: Predictors of low cardiac output syndrome after coronary artery bypass. *J Thorac Cardiovasc Surg* 1996; 112(1):38-51.

279. Hogue CW Jr, Sundt T 3rd, Barzilai B, et al: Cardiac and neurologic complications identify risks for mortality for both men and women undergoing coronary artery bypass graft surgery. *Anesthesiology* 2001; 95(5):1074-1078.

280. Hausmann H, Potapov EV, Koster A, et al: Prognosis after the implantation of an intra-aortic balloon pump in cardiac surgery calculated with a new score. *Circulation* 2002; 106(12 Suppl 1):I203-206.

281. Dacey LJ, Likosky DS, Leavitt BJ, et al: Perioperative stroke and long-term survival after coronary artery bypass graft surgery. *Ann Thorac Surg* 2005; 79(2):532-536; discussion 537.

282. McKhann GM, Grega MA, Borowicz LM Jr, et al: Is there cognitive decline 1 year after CABG? Comparison with surgical and nonsurgical controls. *Neurology* 2005; 65(7):991-999.

283. Frye RL, Kronmal R, Schaff HV, et al: Stroke in coronary artery bypass graft surgery: an analysis of the CASS experience. The participants in the Coronary Artery Surgery Study. *Int J Cardiol* 1992; 36(2):213-221.

284. Loop FD, Lytle BW, Cosgrove DM, et al: J. Maxwell Chamberlain memorial paper. Sternal wound complications after isolated coronary artery bypass grafting: early and late mortality, morbidity, and cost of care. *Ann Thorac Surg* 1990; 49(2):179-186; discussion 186-187.

285. Dai C, Lu Z, Zhu H, et al: Bilateral internal mammary artery grafting and risk of sternal wound infection: evidence from observational studies. *Ann Thorac Surg* 2013; 95(6):1938-1945.

286. Alexander JW, Fischer JE, Boyajian M, et al: The influence of hair-removal methods on wound infections. *Arch Surg* 1983; 118(3):347-352.

287. Kaiser AB, Kernodle DS, Barg NL, et al: Influence of preoperative showers on staphylococcal skin colonization: a comparative trial of antiseptic skin cleansers. *Ann Thorac Surg* 1988; 45(1):35-38.

288. Cimochowski GE, Harostock MD, Brown R, et al: Intranasal mupirocin reduces sternal wound infection after open heart surgery in diabetics and nondiabetics. *Ann Thorac Surg* 2001; 71(5):1572-1578; discussion 1578-1579.

289. Dohmen PM, Gabbieri D, Weymann A, et al: Reduction in surgical site infection in patients treated with microbial sealant prior to coronary artery bypass graft surgery: a case-control study. *J Hosp Infect* 2009; 72(2):119-126.

290. Milano CA, Kesler K, Archibald N, et al: Mediastinitis after coronary artery bypass graft surgery. Risk factors and long-term survival. *Circulation* 1995; 92(8):2245-2251.

291. Parisian Mediastinitis Study, G: Risk factors for deep sternal wound infection after sternotomy: a prospective, multicenter study. *J Thorac Cardiovasc Surg* 1996; 111(6):1200-1207.

292. Olsen MA, Lock-Buckley P, Hopkins D, et al: The risk factors for deep and superficial chest surgical-site infections after coronary artery bypass graft surgery are different. *J Thorac Cardiovasc Surg* 2002; 124(1):136-145.

293. Zerr KJ, Furnary AP, Grunkemeier GL, et al: Glucose control lowers the risk of wound infection in diabetics after open heart operations. *Ann Thorac Surg* 1997; 63(2):356-361.

294. Furnary AP, Zerr KJ, Grunkemeier GL, et al: Continuous intravenous insulin infusion reduces the incidence of deep sternal wound infection in

diabetic patients after cardiac surgical procedures. *Ann Thorac Surg* 1999; 67(2):352-360; discussion 360-362.

295. Ottino G, De Paulis R, Pansini S, et al: Major sternal wound infection after open-heart surgery: a multivariate analysis of risk factors in 2,579 consecutive operative procedures. *Ann Thorac Surg* 1987; 44(2):173-179.

296. Gansera B, Schmidtler F, Gillrath G, et al: Does bilateral ITA grafting increase perioperative complications? Outcome of 4462 patients with bilateral versus 4204 patients with single ITA bypass. *Eur J Cardiothorac Surg* 2006; 30(2):318-323.

297. Toumpoulis IK, Theakos N, Dunning J: Does bilateral internal thoracic artery harvest increase the risk of mediastinitis? *Interact Cardiovasc Thorac Surg* 2007; 6(6):787-791.

298. Pevni D, Uretzky G, Mohr A, et al: Routine use of bilateral skeletonized internal thoracic artery grafting: long-term results. *Circulation* 2008; 118(7):705-712.

299. Mangano CM, Diamondstone LS, Ramsay JG, et al: Renal dysfunction after myocardial revascularization: risk factors, adverse outcomes, and hospital resource utilization. The Multicenter Study of Perioperative Ischemia Research Group. *Ann Intern Med* 1998; 128(3):194-203.

300. Brown JR, Cochran RP, Dacey LJ, et al: Perioperative increases in serum creatinine are predictive of increased 90-day mortality after coronary artery bypass graft surgery. *Circulation* 2006; 114(1 Suppl):I409-413.

301. Chertow GM, Levy EM, Hammermeister KE, et al: Independent association between acute renal failure and mortality following cardiac surgery. *Am J Med* 1998; 104(4):343-348.

302. Samuels LE, Sharma S, Morris RJ, et al: Coronary artery bypass grafting in patients with chronic renal failure: a reappraisal. *J Card Surg* 1996; 11(2):128-133; discussion 134-135.

303. Mentzer RM Jr, Oz MC, Sladen RN, et al: Effects of perioperative nesiritide in patients with left ventricular dysfunction undergoing cardiac surgery: the NAPA Trial. *J Am Coll Cardiol* 2007; 49(6):716-726.

304. Sezai A, Hata M, Niino T, et al: Influence of continuous infusion of low-dose human atrial natriuretic peptide on renal function during cardiac surgery: a randomized controlled study. *J Am Coll Cardiol* 2009; 54(12):1058-1064.

305. Sergeant P, Blackstone E, Meyns B: Validation and interdependence with patient-variables of the influence of procedural variables on early and late survival after CABG. K.U. Leuven Coronary Surgery Program. *Eur J Cardiothorac Surg* 1997; 12(1):1-19.

306. Sergeant P, Blackstone E, Meyns B: Is return of angina after coronary artery bypass grafting immutable, can it be delayed, and is it important? *J Thorac Cardiovasc Surg* 1998; 116(3):440-453.

307. Sergeant P, Blackstone E, Meyns B, et al: First cardiological or cardiosurgical reintervention for ischemic heart disease after primary coronary artery bypass grafting. *Eur J Cardiothorac Surg* 1998; 14(5):480-487.

308. Sergeant PT, Blackstone EH, Meyns BP: Does arterial revascularization decrease the risk of infarction after coronary artery bypass grafting? *Ann Thorac Surg* 1998; 66(1):1-10; discussion 10-11.

309. Bourassa MG, Enjalbert M, Campeau L, et al: Progression of atherosclerosis in coronary arteries and bypass grafts: ten years later. *Am J Cardiol* 1984; 53(12):102C-107C.

310. Campeau L, Enjalbert M, Lesperance J, et al: Atherosclerosis and late closure of aortocoronary saphenous vein grafts: sequential angiographic studies at 2 weeks, 1 year, 5 to 7 years, and 10 to 12 years after surgery. *Circulation* 1983; 68(3 Pt 2):II1-7.

311. Campeau L, Enjalbert M, Lesperance J, et al: The relation of risk factors to the development of atherosclerosis in saphenous-vein bypass grafts and the progression of disease in the native circulation. A study 10 years after aortocoronary bypass surgery. *N Engl J Med* 1984; 311(21):1329-1332.

312. Buxton BF, Komeda M, Fuller JA, et al: Bilateral internal thoracic artery grafting may improve outcome of coronary artery surgery. Risk-adjusted survival. *Circulation* 1998; 98(19 Suppl):II1-6.

313. Lytle BW, Blackstone EH, Loop FD, et al: Two internal thoracic artery grafts are better than one. *J Thorac Cardiovasc Surg* 1999; 117(5):855-872.

314. Dion R, Glineur D, Derouck D, et al: Long-term clinical and angiographic follow-up of sequential internal thoracic artery grafting. *Eur J Cardiothorac Surg* 2000; 17(4):407-414.

315. Tector AJ, McDonald ML, Kress DC, et al: Purely internal thoracic artery grafts: outcomes. *Ann Thorac Surg* 2001; 72(2):450-455.

316. Barner HB, Sundt TM 3rd, Bailey M, et al: Midterm results of complete arterial revascularization in more than 1,000 patients using an internal thoracic artery/radial artery T graft. *Ann Surg* 2001; 234(4):447-452; discussion 452-453.

317. Muneretto C, Negri A, Manfredi J, et al: Safety and usefulness of composite grafts for total arterial myocardial revascularization: a prospective randomized evaluation. *J Thorac Cardiovasc Surg* 2003; 125(4):826-835.

318. Muneretto C, Bisleri G, Negri A, et al: Total arterial myocardial revascularization with composite grafts improves results of coronary surgery in elderly: a prospective randomized comparison with conventional coronary artery bypass surgery. *Circulation* 2003; 108(Suppl 1):II29-33.

319. Muneretto C, Bisleri G, Negri A, et al: Improved graft patency rates and mid-term outcome of diabetic patients undergoing total arterial myocardial revascularization. *Heart Int* 2006; 2(3-4):136.

320. Buxton BF, Shi WY, Tatoulis J, et al: Total arterial revascularization with internal thoracic and radial artery grafts in triple-vessel coronary artery disease is associated with improved survival. *J Thorac Cardiovasc Surg* 2014; 148(4):1238-1243; discussion 1243-1244.

21

Myocardial Revascularization Without Cardiopulmonary Bypass

Bobby Yanagawa • Michael E. Halkos • John D. Puskas

Despite the increased prevalence of percutaneous coronary intervention (PCI) to treat coronary disease, coronary artery bypass graft (CABG) will continue to have a major role, particularly in patients with complex multivessel disease and diabetes mellitus. Currently, the majority of surgical revascularization is performed with the use of cardiopulmonary bypass (CPB), with most surgeons preferring to perform distal anastomoses on an arrested heart. Advocates of this approach cite low morbidity and mortality with outcomes that have continued to improve despite a surgical patient population with increasing comorbid conditions and more advanced and severe coronary disease.[1-3] However, complications, albeit infrequent, continue to plague a small percentage of patients undergoing CABG including stroke, renal failure, and respiratory failure. These complications occur not only because of the systemic inflammatory activation that occurs with extracorporeal circulation, but also because of the manipulation of the aorta required for cannulation, CPB, and aortic clamping. The interest in off-pump techniques was largely driven by the increased awareness of the deleterious effects of CPB and aortic manipulation.

According to the Society of Thoracic Surgeons Adult Cardiac Surgery Database (STS ACSD), off-pump CABG (OPCAB) use peaked in 2002 (23%) followed by a decline, accounting for approximately 17% of CABG cases in 2012.[4] For most surgeons, the lack of compelling evidence in large randomized controlled trials (RCTs) supporting OPCAB over conventional on-pump coronary artery bypass (ONCAB) and suggestions of more frequent incomplete revascularization have been impediments to implementing this strategy in routine practice.[1-3,5,6] Nonetheless RCTs have almost uniformly demonstrated reduced transfusion requirements, lower postoperative serum myocardial enzyme levels, and shorter length of stay. Moreover, there are many retrospective trials showing a survival benefit as well as reduced morbidity with OPCAB. Retrospective database studies have much larger sample size and include mixed-risk patients. However, inherent selection bias may limit the interpretation of these results, despite advanced statistical methodology. For individual surgeons to

consider implementing an off-pump approach, the following must be demonstrated: (1) equivalent short- and long-term patency rates; (2) complete revascularization; (3) reduced morbidity and even reduced mortality, especially in high-risk patients; and (4) cost efficiency both in the operating room and during the entire hospitalization. For certain high-risk subgroups, it would appear intuitive that avoiding the systemic effects of CPB as well as aortic manipulation would reduce the incidence of specific complications such as stroke and renal failure.

An off-pump approach is more technically challenging, with new risks not familiar to on-pump surgery. Therefore, OPCAB should be considered an advanced technique, not to be performed by all surgeons but by a select few who have trained with experts in OPCAB and who themselves perform large numbers of OPCAB procedures. Finally, there is greater appreciation that OPCAB should be performed in revascularization centers of excellence, incorporated into a comprehensive approach to revascularization, which includes minimally invasive CABG, hybrid, and total arterial revascularization.

PREOPERATIVE CONSIDERATIONS

Surgeon Experience

The adoption of OPCAB into clinical practice requires a commitment to learning a unique skill set. This is best achieved by focused training with an established OPCAB surgeon and routine adoption of OPCAB techniques such that the surgeon can employ this approach in patients likely to derive the most benefit. OPCAB surgery poses unique challenges to a surgeon who is accustomed to operating in a motionless and bloodless field. Furthermore, OPCAB requires an adept first and second assistant to provide exposure on a beating heart as well as excellent anesthesia management to maintain hemodynamics and alert the surgical team of potential hemodynamic problems. Thus, the commitment to OPCAB is usually tied to a belief that the technical challenges inherent in the procedure are worth overcoming so that the patient may benefit from the avoidance of CPB. Although the benefit may be small in low-risk patients, it is becoming apparent that certain high-risk subgroups may benefit from minimizing aortic manipulation as well as avoiding the systemic effects of CPB.

The inexperienced OPCAB surgeon embarking on the learning curve is best advised to choose his or her initial patients carefully and pay close attention to coronary anatomy and confounding patient variables. The surgeon must come to the operating room with an operative plan that is flexible enough to change as operative findings such as hemodynamic fluctuations, ischemia, or arrythmias. Early in a surgeon's experience, it is probably prudent to exclude patients with difficult lateral wall targets, especially multiple lateral wall targets, severe left ventricular dysfunction, left main disease, or other complex cases (Table 21-1). Ideal early candidates for OPCAB include those undergoing elective primary coronary revascularization with good target anatomy, preserved ventricular function, and one to three grafts with easily accessible or no lateral wall targets. As experience is gained in OPCAB, this technique can be safely and effectively applied to the vast majority of patients requiring coronary artery bypass surgery. Just as important, however, is the experience to know when it is better to use CPB in patients in whom an off-pump approach will be exceedingly difficult, impractical, or poorly tolerated.

Patient Variables

The preoperative evaluation of patients for OPCAB demands careful planning and consideration for certain risk factors. We routinely perform screening carotid duplex ultrasonography on all patients over the age of 65, smokers, those with a carotid bruit, history of transient ischemic attack or stroke, left main coronary disease, peripheral vascular disease, or history of prior carotid intervention. The remainder of the preoperative evaluation is similar to ONCAB. In patients with a

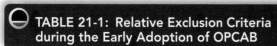

TABLE 21-1: Relative Exclusion Criteria during the Early Adoption of OPCAB

Recent myocardial infarction
More than three grafts required, especially multiple lateral
   wall targets
Difficult lateral wall targets
Intramyocardial coronary arteries
Left ventricular dysfunction
Small or diffusely diseased coronary arteries
Mild to moderate aortic or mitral regurgitation
Redosternotomy
Hemodynamically unstable
Pulmonary hypertension
Urgent/emergent cases
Left main coronary artery disease

murmur, dyspnea, a history of aortic or mitral regurgitation (MR), or ventricular dysfunction on cardiac catheterization, preoperative echocardiography is warranted. It is important to be aware of right ventricular dysfunction, valvular regurgitation, or pulmonary hypertension as positioning during OPCAB can result in dramatic changes in these parameters. Overall, the clinical condition of the patient, the urgency of the operation, and ventricular function need to be carefully assessed to determine whether an off-pump approach will be tolerated. Patients with left ventricular dysfunction from a recent infarct pose a more difficult challenge than those with chronic ventricular dysfunction, with the former being much more sensitive to cardiac manipulation and displacement and more likely to develop intraoperative arrhythmias.

Anesthesia

As in other cardiac operations, all patients require invasive monitoring with a pulmonary artery catheter, arterial line, Foley catheter, and central venous line. We use transesophageal echocardiography liberally to provide valuable information about valvular regurgitation, regional myocardial function, and pulmonary hypertension. In our experience, a well-experienced anesthesia team is essential to maintaining stable hemodynamics and ensuring a smooth and uneventful operation. Unlike ONCAB, which requires active coordination among surgeon, anesthesiologist, and perfusionist, the anesthesiologist and surgeon must work especially closely to maintain hemodynamic stability during OPCAB. Subtle changes in hemodynamic status, gradual elevation in pulmonary artery pressures, frequent boluses, or increased requirement of inotropes and vasopressors to maintain hemodynamic stability, and rhythm changes can herald cardiovascular collapse. Such an event can reliably be avoided if these changes are verbalized and discussed between anesthesiologist and surgeon preemptively. When manipulating the heart, it is important for the surgeon to communicate these abrupt maneuvers to the anesthesia team so that appropriate action can be taken and inappropriate reactions (bolusing vasopressors) avoided. Changes in table position (Trendelenburg) can provide dramatic volume changes that affect cardiac output and blood pressure. Autotransfusion of intravascular volume from the lower extremities by Trendelenburg positioning should be the first maneuver to maintain hemodynamic stability. We prefer to avoid giving massive volumes of intravenous fluids, which requires later postoperative diuresis. Instead, aggressive use of Trendelenburg positioning and judicious use of alpha-adrenergic agents provides stable hemodynamics during distal anastamoses. This includes patients with pulmonary hypertension, mild or moderate ischemic MR, or left ventricular dysfunction in which cardiac manipulation and displacement as well as regional myocardial ischemia may be poorly tolerated without inotropic support. If preload conditions have been optimized, then vasopressor agents such as norepinephrine or Neo-Synephrine may be used to assist with maintaining adequate blood pressure during distal anastomoses. In our experience, effective communication with a well-experienced anesthesiologist is of paramount importance to ensure an uneventful off-pump operation.

Maintaining normothermia is critically important and requires more effort during OPCAB procedures, because the luxury of the CPB circuit for rewarming does not exist. This usually can be accomplished by infusing intravenous fluids through warmers, warming inhalational anesthetic agents, maintaining warm room temperatures before and during the procedure, and using convective forced-air warming systems (Bair Hugger; Arizant Healthcare, Eden Prairie, MN).

Anticoagulation regimens vary according to surgeon preference. For surgeons in their early experience, a full "pump" dose of heparin is reasonable in the event that conversion to CPB becomes necessary. Some surgeons continue to implement a full dose with 400 IU/kg to maintain an activated clotting time (ACT) of greater than 400 seconds; others use a half dose or 180 IU/kg, whereas others start with 10,000 IU and administer additional doses (3000 IU every half-hour) or a heparin infusion of 100 IU/min to maintain an ACT of 300 to 400 seconds. Reversal of anticoagulation with varying doses of protamine is usually administered to facilitate hemostasis.

SURGICAL TECHNIQUE

Preparation

After the induction of anesthesia, patients are positioned, prepped, and draped in a standard fashion. At our institution, patients receive an aspirin rectal suppository (1000 mg) after induction. Aspirin 81 mg and clopidogrel (150 mg postoperatively, then 75 mg/day) are routinely administered early in the postoperative period after mediastinal drainage decreases well below 100 cc/h for 4 hours. This has not been associated with an increased risk of mediastinal reexploration.[7] Because of the absence of CPB—related coagulopathy, patients may have a relative hypercoagulable perioperative state, which theoretically may jeopardize early graft patency. For this reason, we administer aspirin preoperatively, aspirin and clopidogrel early postoperatively, and then continue dual antiplatelet therapy in the postoperative period.

Endoscopic radial artery and saphenous vein conduits are harvested simultaneously during internal mammary artery (IMA) harvest. It is our practice to administer 5000 IU of heparin before endoscopic vein harvest to minimize thrombus formation within the conduit. Concern over graft quality with endoscopic vein harvest has prompted increased vigilance in atraumatic harvest technique to ensure adequate conduits for bypass.[8] We routinely harvest skeletonized IMAs using a harmonic scalpel (Harmonic Synergy, Ethicon, Somerville, NJ). Skeletonized harvest of IMA grafts preserves sternal blood flow, leads to less postoperative dysesthesia, and may reduce sternal wound infection in higher risk patients such as those with diabetes mellitus. The Harmonic scalpel uses high-frequency mechanical vibration to cut and coagulate tissues and compared with electrocautery, minimizes surgical trauma to the sternum and reduces the risk of injury to the adjacent IMA.

After single or bilateral IMA harvest, the heparin dose is administered and the arterial conduits divided distally. The pericardium is incised in an inverted T-configuration, and then extended laterally along the diaphragm to facilitate cardiac displacement while avoiding injury to phrenic nerves. It is essential to free the left lateral pericardium from the diaphragm to allow the pericardium to be retracted to displace the heart, exposing the lateral wall of the left ventricle. We routinely dissect the left IMA distally to the bifurcation as the extra length is often necessary to avoid tension on the anastomosis during rightward displacement for lateral or inferolateral wall grafting. Dividing or removing the endothoracic fascia, skeletonizing the IMA during harvest, and dividing the left pericardium vertically toward the left phrenic nerve at the level of the pulmonary artery all provide for extra length and less tension on the anastomosis.

Several pericardial traction sutures are placed to assist with exposure and lateral displacement of the heart. To avoid compression on the right heart during lateral displacement, the right pericardium can be dissected along the diaphragm or the right pleural space opened widely to allow the heart to fall into the right chest during lateral displacement. An important traction suture is the "deep stitch," which is placed approximately two-thirds of the way between the inferior vena cava and left pulmonary vein at the point where the pericardium reflects over the posterior left atrium (Fig. 21-1). Care should be taken with placement of this suture to avoid the underlying descending thoracic aorta, esophagus, left lung, and adjacent inferior pulmonary vein. This suture should be covered with a soft rubber catheter to prevent laceration of the epicardium during retraction. Furthermore, the manual elevation and compression of the heart required to take this stitch may be poorly tolerated in patients with marginal hemodynamics or significant left main coronary artery disease. In that case,

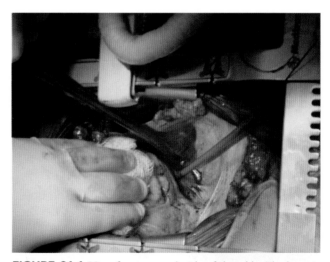

FIGURE 21-1 View from surgeon's side of the table. The heart is elevated toward the surgeon and superiorly for placement of the "deep stitch," which is placed two-thirds of the way between the inferior vena cava and inferior left pulmonary vein. With rightward retraction of the heart, the right-sided pericardial traction sutures should be relaxed to prevent compression of the right atrium and right ventricle.

grafting and reperfusion of the left anterior descending artery (LAD) should be accomplished before placing the deep pericardial traction suture.

Epiaortic Ultrasound

Epiaortic ultrasonography is used in all of our patients undergoing cardiac surgery, including OPCAB. It is a simple, noninvasive, and inexpensive tool for assessing the extent of atheromatous disease in the ascending aorta in preparation for aortic clamping or selection of an alternative clampless technique.[9] Epiaortic ultrasound has been shown to be superior to transesophageal echocardiography or palpation alone in identifying aortic atheromatous lesions, especially in the mid- to distal ascending aorta.[10-12] The 8.5-MHz linear array probe is placed inside a sterile sleeve filled with sterile saline to act as a medium between the probe and the surface of the aorta (Fig. 21-2). The information allows the surgeon to individualize placement of aortic clamps and proximal anastomotic devices to minimize the risk of atheroembolism. In our practice, for aortic atherosclerosis grades 1 to 2 (Table 21-2), we will use a side-biting clamp or promixal anastomosis device. We will not clamp or manipulate grades 3 to 5, due to the risk of embolization. Rosenberger and coworkers,[13] evaluated greater than 6000 patients with epiaortic ultrasound, suggested that the operative course was changed in 4% of patients because of the finding of aortic pathology, resulting in improved neurologic outcomes. Currently, intraoperative epiaortic ultrasound scanning is performed in only a small minority of centers. More data linking epiaortic ultrasonography to successful intraoperative decision-making and clinical outcomes should help to drive broader adoption of this promising diagnostic modality.

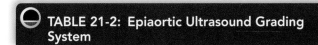

TABLE 21-2: Epiaortic Ultrasound Grading System

Epiaortic ultrasound grade of ascending aorta	Intimal thickness/severity of disease
1	Normal (<2 mm)
2	Mild (2-3 mm)
3	Moderate (3-5 mm)
4	Severe (>5 mm)
5	Mobile plaque, irrespective of thickness

Exposure

Cardiac positioners and stabilizers have greatly increased the ability to manipulate the heart with minimal hemodynamic compromise. The two systems routinely used in our institution are the Medtronic Octopus Tissue Stabilizer and Starfish or Urchin Heart Positioner (Medtronic Inc., Minneapolis, MN) and the Maquet ACROBAT stabilizer and XPOSE positioner (Maquet, Radstat, Germany). Cardiac positioning devices are frequently placed away from the apex, especially to the left of the apex, to expose the lateral wall and branches of the left circumflex coronary artery (Figs. 21-3 and 21-4). They are generally placed on the apex to expose the anterior wall (LAD territory) and inferior wall (posterior descending territory) of the heart and may be placed on the acute margin to expose the right coronary artery (RCA; Fig. 21-5). The suction-based positioning is well tolerated as the heart is not compressed, thus maintaining its functional geometry. The coronary stabilizer

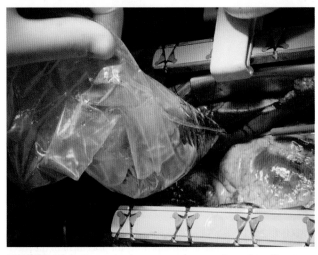

FIGURE 21-2 Epiaortic ultrasonography is performed in all patients prior to aortic manipulation. The 8.5-MHz linear array probe is placed inside a sterile sleeve filled with sterile saline to act as a medium between the probe and the surface of the aorta.

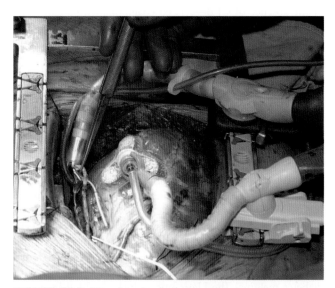

FIGURE 21-3 View from head of table. With the cardiac positioning device placed slightly away from the apex, the lateral wall can be exposed. The coronary stabilizers can then be placed to provide exposure and stabilization of obtuse marginal vessels.

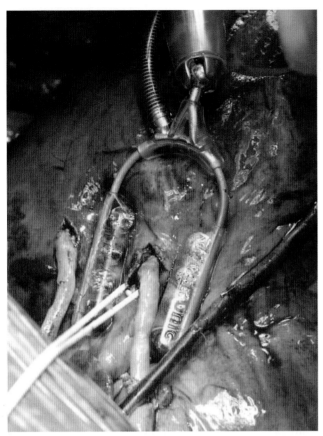

FIGURE 21-4 View from the head of table. An obtuse marginal artery is prepared for grafting. After positioning the coronary stabilizer, a silastic vessel loop is doubly passed around the proximal coronary artery to allow transient occlusion during the anastomosis.

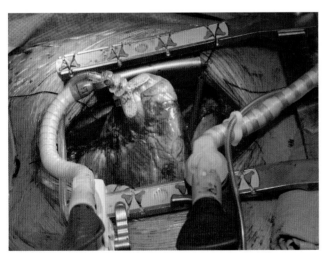

FIGURE 21-5 View from the surgeon's side of table. With cardiac positioner placed on the apex, the heart can be easily displaced to expose the inferior wall vessels. Because there is no compression used for displacement, this maneuver is usually accomplished with no hemodynamic sequelae. Note the location of the cardiac positioner and stabilizer on the surgeon's side of the retractor. Alternatively, the stabilizer can be placed on the assistant's side of the retractor. The right pericardial traction sutures are relaxed, and the "deep stitch" is retracted inferolaterally.

devices are placed with minimal tension on the epicardium to allow for an area of mechanical stabilization. The anterior wall vessels often require only the coronary stabilizer for adequate exposure. The stabilizer is positioned along the caudal aspect of the retractor toward the left, with the retractor arm placed out of the way to prevent interference during the anastomosis. For the lateral and inferior wall vessels, the cardiac positioner is usually placed on the surgeon's side at the most cephalad location of the retractor. A general rule is to put the stabilizer in the assistant's way instead of the surgeon's to prevent these devices from obstructing the surgeon's view or interfering with hand positioning during suture placement.

In addition to positioners and stabilizers, manipulating the traction sutures can greatly enhance exposure. When the "deep stitch" is retracted toward the patient's feet, it elevates the heart toward the ceiling and points the apex vertically with remarkably little change in hemodynamics. When retracted toward the patient's left side, the heart rotates from left to right, exposing the lateral wall vessels. Variable tension on this stitch will enhance exposure to both the anterior and lateral wall. The left-sided pericardial sutures should be pulled taut and the right-sided sutures completely relaxed to avoid compression on the right heart during cardiac displacement. Pericardial sutures on both the right and left sides should never be under tension simultaneously. Manipulation of the operating table can also facilitate exposure. Placing the patient in steep Trendelenburg exposes the inferior wall. Turning the table sharply toward the right will aid with exposure of the lateral wall targets. For grafting the anterior wall vessels, the "deep stitch" can be pulled toward the patient's left side and a coronary stabilizer can then be positioned to expose the target coronary artery (Fig. 21-6). Occasionally, a warm moist laparotomy pad can be placed between the heart and the posterolateral pericardium to assist with elevating the heart out of the pericardium.

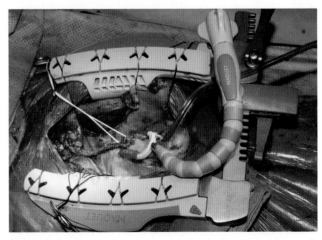

FIGURE 21-6 View from surgeon's side of table. With LAD grafting, excellent exposure can be obtained with lateral traction of the "deep stitch" and the coronary stabilizer. Note the right pericardial traction sutures are released from the retractor.

In our experience, the most common mistakes leading to suboptimal exposure are

- Incompletely freeing the left pericardium from the diaphragm
- The "deep stitch" too far from the posterior left atrium
- Not loosening the right-sided pericardial sutures during exposure of the left-sided targets
- Compressing the heart against right pericardium, sternum, or retractor
- Kinking the right ventricular outflow tract by excessive cephalad tilt of the vertical heart
- Failing to combine the techniques of deep stitch, positioning device "off-apex", elevation of the right sternal border on towels, and opening the right pleural space when needed

In preparation for distal anastomosis, a soft silastic retractor tape mounted on a blunt needle (Retract-o-tape, Quest Medical, Inc., Allen, TX) is placed widely around the proximal vessel for transient atraumatic occlusion. For inferior wall vessels, this suture can be displaced posteriorly and caudally by tying a posterior pericardial suture loosely around the retractor tape (Fig. 21-7). The pericardial retraction suture serves as a "pulley" that not only enhances coronary exposure and the surgeon's view, but also keeps this retraction stitch from interfering with the sutures during the anastomosis. The field is kept free of blood with a humidified CO_2 blower (DLP, Medtronic, Inc.), which is managed by the scrub nurse or second assistant (Fig. 21-8). To avoid injury to the coronary endothelium, the blower should be set at the minimum setting needed for exposure (<5 L CO_2) and used only when passing the needle through the vessel. Occasionally an epicardial fat retractor can be used to expose the coronary target in patients with a large amount of epicardial fat.

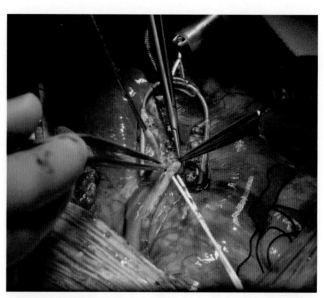

FIGURE 21-8 View from the head of the table. During the anastomosis, a humidified CO_2 blower managed by the second assistant or scrub nurse is used to expose the LAD.

Although a well-trained first assistant is necessary for providing an effortless anastomosis, the second assistant, often the scrub nurse, also plays a major role in exposure. This assistant usually stands to the right of the surgeon, and controls the CO_2 blower and the Cell Saver (Haemonetics Corp., Braintree, MA). The blower is used to keep the field free of blood and to open the target vessel and graft during suture placement. During the inferior wall or lateral wall targets, the second assistant may provide better exposure by standing to the surgeon's left. In chronically occluded vessels that have collateral and/or retrograde flow, bleeding into the field can be controlled with another retractor tape distally, a MyOcclude device (United States Surgical Corp., Norwalk, CT), or an intracoronary shunt.[14,15] We use intracoronary shunts selectively rather than routinely, as at least one study demonstrated significant endothelial injury with its use.[16] A final preparatory measure is to place temporary atrial or ventricular pacing cables before positioning the heart, particularly before RCA occlusion. As the heart is rotated toward the right, visualization of the right atrium is more difficult, so it is often prudent to place and test these cables before positioning.

Coronary Grafting

The current generation of coronary stabilizers relies on epicardial suction rather than compression to maintain epicardial tissue capture. A common mistake is to press down too hard on the epicardium, which will paradoxically cause both increased movement in the target region and impaired hemodynamics. The malleable pods of the stabilizers can be bent or manipulated in any direction to stabilize the target vessel. If there are concerns about hemodynamic stability during regional ischemia, the proximal vessel can be test occluded

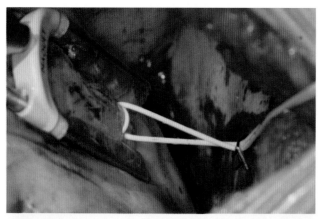

FIGURE 21-7 View from the surgeon's side of the table. For inferior vessel exposure (posterior descending or left ventricular branch) the Retract-o-tape is guided out of the surgeon's way through a "pulley" created by placing a loosely tied superficial suture in the posterior diaphragm. The Retract-o-tape can then be retracted to transiently occlude the artery.

for 2 to 5 minutes and then reperfused, providing "precon- ditioning" of the subtended myocardium. Although not used routinely, preconditioning with two cycles of 2 minutes of LAD occlusion then 3 minutes of reperfusion before the first coronary anastomosis decreased postoperative myocardial enzyme release, heart rate increase, and restored ventricular function.[17] During this time the graft can be prepared. This gives the surgeon some assurance before committing to the anastomosis by creating an arteriotomy. The anastomosis is otherwise performed in a manner identical to on-pump grafting. It is essential to continue communication with the anesthesia team so that adequate steps can be promptly taken if hemodynamic conditions deteriorate. For example, if pulmonary artery pressures begin to rise and mean arterial pressures begin to fall during a lateral wall anastomosis, sev- eral steps can be taken to avoid cardiovascular collapse: gen- tly relaxing on the cardiac positioner or coronary stabilizer, steep Trendelenburg positioning, fluid boluses, inotropes, vasopressors, or pacing. If hemodynamic conditions continue to deteriorate, the safe next step is to place an intracoronary shunt, relax the retractor tape, and release both the stabilizer and positioner, allowing the heart to recover.[15] At this point a decision must be made whether to convert "electively" to an on-pump procedure or complete the procedure off-pump. With better preparation (eg, fluids, inotropes, vasopressors, pacing, and shunt), the anastomosis can usually be com- pleted off-pump. Another option for patients at high risk for complications of CPB is the use of intra-aortic balloon coun- terpulsation for mechanical support during cardiac displace- ment and positioning.

Sequence of Grafting

Careful assessment of the cardiac catheterization is impera- tive. When planning for OPCAB, particular attention needs to be paid to the collateralizing vessel(s), intramyocardial vessels, the size of the distal targets, the degree of stenosis, the complexity of coronary disease, and the number of lat- eral wall vessels requiring grafting. The sequence of grafting is important as regional myocardial perfusion is temporar- ily interrupted during anastomosis on the beating heart. As a general rule, the collateralized vessel(s) is grafted first and the collateralizing vessel is grafted last. For example, in patients with an occluded RCA with a posterior descending artery (PDA) supplied by collaterals from the LAD, grafting the LAD first would not only leave the anterior wall isch- emic during the anastomosis, but also disrupt flow to the septum, inferior wall, and right ventricle. A more prudent approach would involve grafting the PDA first, then per- forming a proximal anastomosis to ensure adequate flow to the inferior wall while the proximal LAD is occluded during construction of the IMA-LAD anastomosis. Another sce- nario that may pose problems is a large moderately stenotic RCA. Not uncommonly, temporary occlusion will result in profound bradycardia and hypotension. The surgeon must be prepared to use an intracoronary shunt or provide temporary epicardial pacing. Additional options include a

"proximals first" approach to allow adequate regional perfu- sion after completion of each distal anastomosis.

- Perform anastomosis to completely occluded or collateral- ized vessel first
- If LAD is not a collateralizing vessel, perform LAD-LIMA anastomosis first to allow for anterior wall perfusion dur- ing lateral and inferior wall positioning
- Proximal anastomoses can be performed first to allow for perfusion of target vessels after each distal anastomosis. This can be helpful when cardiac positioning is not well tolerated
- Beware of a large RCA with moderated proximal steno- sis. Acute occlusion can cause bradycardia and hypoten- sion. Be prepared for intracoronary shunt and epicardial pacing
- Patients with moderate MR may not tolerate prolonged cardiac displacement, which can exacerbate MR, and lead to elevated PA pressures and subsequent hemodynamic deterioration. Grafting the culprit vessel causing papil- lary muscle dysfunction should be performed early in the procedure.

Proximal Anastomosis

Proximal anastomoses during OPCAB can be performed with the use of an aortic partial-occluding clamp after epi- aortic ultrasound rules out aortic atherosclerosis or a proxi- mal anastomosis device. In preparation for an aortic clamp, the systolic blood pressure is lowered (eg, <95 mm Hg), the clamp is applied and aortotomies are made with a 4.0-mm aortic punch. Proximal anastomoses are then performed using 5-0 or 6-0 polypropylene suture. Before tying down the most anterior proximal anastomosis, the clamp is released and the aorta is de-aired through the proximal anastomosis with clamps on vein grafts. After the suture is tied down, the vein grafts can be de-aired with a 25-gauge needle and clamps removed. Arterial grafts are not punctured but are allowed to bleed backward before clamp removal.

Unlike ONCAB, OPCAB provides the opportunity to minimize or completely avoid manipulation of the aorta by performing proximal anastomoses to in situ arterial grafts, or using clampless proximal anastomotic devices.[18-21] This is particularly relevant in patients with advanced aor- tic atheromatous disease detected by epiaortic ultrasound. Commercially available devices for clampless proximal anas- tomoses include the Heartstring III (Maquet Cardiovascular LLC, San Jose, CA), the PAS-Port Proximal Anastomosis System (Cardica Inc., Redwood City, CA), and the Enclose II (Vitalitec, Plymouth, MA). The Heartstring and Enclose devices create a near hemostatic seal with the inner surface of the ascending aorta that allows the creation of a hand-sewn anastomosis with a relatively bloodless field (Fig. 21-9). In contrast, the PAS-Port Proximal Anastomosis System is a fully integrated and automated system that attaches the vein graft to the aorta, instantaneously producing a reproducible anastomosis.[21-23]

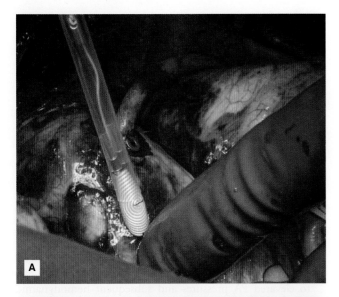

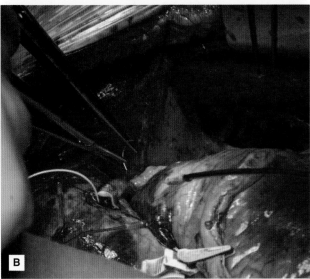

FIGURE 21-9 Proximal anastomoses can be performed without the use of an aortic clamp with either a Heartstring III (in these figures) or the PAS-Port device. The Heartstring III device requires a hand-sewn anastomosis, whereas the PAS-Port device is an automated anastomosis.

Graft Flow Measurement

We routinely quantitate graft flow using an intraoperative transit-time doppler flow meter (Medistim, Oslo, Norway). Acceptable values are flow > 15 mL/min, pulsatility index (the difference of maximum and minimum flow divided by the mean flow) <5 and diastolic fraction > 50% (for left-sided grafts). A post hoc analysis of the Veterans Affairs Randomized On/Off Bypass (ROOBY) Trial found that lower graft patency (non-FitzGibbon grade A) at 1 year was associated with low flow (<20 mL/min) or high pulsatility index (3-5 and >5) during intraoperative flow probe measurements.[24] Thus, any values outside of this range should alert the surgeon to examine the anastamoses and graft for

potential revision unless unfavorable characteristics of the conduit, native coronary artery or distal run-off can readily account for the suboptimal doppler findings.

On-Pump Beating Heart Coronary Artery Bypass

Performing beating heart coronary artery bypass with CPB support is especially useful in certain clinical scenarios such as acute coronary syndromes with cardiogenic shock or in patients with severe left ventricular dysfunction where cardiac positioning and displacement will not be tolerated.[25,26] On-pump, beating heart techniques provide hemodynamic support while avoiding aortic clamping and the global ischemic insult associated with cardioplegic arrest.[27,28] However, this is an uncommonly used technique.

Outcomes

Clinical outcomes have been compared between OPCAB and ONCAB and reported for over a decade. There is a general consensus that either approach yields excellent outcomes in low-risk patients. In select higher-risk patients, it appears in recent studies that OPCAB may reduce both morbidity and mortality. These studies can generally be divided into smaller prospective RCT and larger retrospective analyses. Prospective RCTs provide the most accurate comparison between groups and avoid surgical selection bias and confounding inherent to retrospective and observational analyses. On the other hand, retrospective and observational analyses provide much larger sample sizes with longer duration of follow-up and have included more high-risk patients, but are limited by their retrospective nature and inherent selection bias despite the use of propensity matching or other advanced statistical methodologies designed to control for confounding variables. Because of their larger size, small differences in outcomes can often be detected. Taken together, both types of studies can provide valuable information to guide clinical practice.

Operative Mortality

In the major prospective randomized large-scale, multicenter OPCAB trials, there have been no differences in operative mortality between on- and off-pump approaches. ROOBY was the first large-scale multicenter RCT comparing OPCAB and ONCAB in 2203 patients at Veterans Affairs Centers.[2] There was no difference in the short term primary composite endpoint of death or major complications before discharge or within 30 days between (OPCAB 7.0 vs ONCAB 5.6%, $p = .19$; Table 21-3). However, OPCAB was associated with higher incidence of the composite endpoint of mortality, myocardial infarction (MI) and repeat revascularization at 1 year (9.9 vs 7.4%, $p = .04$). The major criticisms of this study were insufficient surgeon experience (minimum 20 OPCAB cases; average 120 and median 50 cases), residents/trainees as

◉ TABLE 21-3: Summary of Large-Scale Randomized Controlled Trials Comparing OPCAB and ONCAB

Trial	Rooby[2]	Coronary[1,29]	Gopcabe[3]
Year	2009	2012	2013
N	2203	4752	2539
Location	18 Veterans Affairs Centers (US)	79 centers in 19 countries	12 centers (Germany)
Major patient characteristics	Patients for CABG-Only	Age ≥ 70 and 1 RF: PVD, stroke, carotid stenosis ≥ 70%, CKI; Age 60-69 years and 1 RF or age 50-59 and 2 RFs: diabetes, urgent status, LVEF ≤ 35%, recent history of smoking	Age ≥ 75 years
OPCAB experience requirement	>20 cases	2 years and >100 cases	"Expert"
Median OPCAB experience	50 cases*	—	322 cases
On-pump conversion	12.40%	7.90%	9.70%
Primary outcome	Longterm: Death, MI, stroke AKI requiring dialysis at 1 year	Death, MI, stroke, AKI requiring dialysis at 30 days; death, MI, stroke, AKI requiring dialysis, repeat revascularization at 5 years	Death, MI, AKI requiring RRT, repeat revascularization at 30 days and 1 year
30 days (OPCAB vs ONCAB)	—	9.8 vs 10.3% (p = .59)	7.8 vs 8.2% (p = .74)
1 year (OPCAB vs ONCAB)	9.9 vs 7.4% (p = .04)	12.1 vs 13.3% (p = .24)[†]	13.1 vs 14.0% (p = .48)
Average no. of grafts (OPCAB vs ONCAB)	2.9 vs 3.0 (p = .002)	3.0 vs 3.2 (p < .001)	2.7 vs 2.8 (p < .001)
Incomplete revascularization (OPCAB vs ONCAB)	17.8 vs 11.1% (p < .01)	11.8 vs 10.0% (p = .05)	34.0 vs 29.3%
1 Year graft Patency (OPCAB vs ONCAB)	82.6 vs 87.8% (p < .01)	—	—

AKI and CKI, acute and chronic kidney injury; LVEF, left ventricular ejection fraction; MI, myocardial infarction; PVD, peripheral vascular disease.
*A resident was the primary surgeon in 64% of OPCAB cases.
†Not a prespecified time point for the primary endpoint.

the primary surgeon in 64% of OPCAB cases and a relatively young and healthy male patient population, a subset that one may not expect to benefit greatly from avoidance of CPB.

The ROOBY Trial was followed by two subsequent large RCTs, the CABG Off or On Pump Revascularization Study (CORONARY)[1,29] and the German Off-Pump CABG in Elderly (GOPCABE) Trial.[3] The CORONARY study randomized 4752 high-risk patients to OPCAB versus ONCAB and is the largest international multicenter RCT to date. The co-primary endpoints were death, stroke, MI, or dialysis at 30 days and 1 year, and death, stroke, MI, dialysis, repeat revascularization at 5 years. Surgeons were required to have >2 years experience after residency training and >100 cases of OPCAB; trainees could not be the primary surgeon. The majority of patients had additive EuroSCORE 3 to 5, thus being higher risk. This trial also did not find differences between OPCAB and ONCAB in composite primary endpoint of mortality, MI and stroke neither at 30 days (9.8 vs 10.3%, p = .59) nor at 1 year (12.1 vs 13.3, p = .24). However,

there was a trend towards benefit with OPCAB for patients in higher EuroSCORE. GOPCABE was a multicenter randomized trial of 2539 high-risk patients (mean logistic EuroSCORE 8.3) ≥75 years of age comparing OPCAB versus ONCAB. Importantly, OPCAB was "routinely performed at all participating centers" and surgeons had an average 514 cases and median 322 cases with OPCAB. There was no difference in the primary endpoint, a composite risk of death, stroke, MI, repeat revascularization, or new renal replacement therapy at 30 days (7.8 vs 8.2%, p = .74) and at 1 year (13.1 vs 14.0%, p = .48).

Several registry studies powered by their large sample size were able to detect significant differences in adverse outcomes among a broad population of patients, suggesting that operative mortality may be reduced in patients undergoing OPCAB compared with ONCAB. In a study by Hannan et al,[30] 49,830 patients from the New York State registry underwent risk-adjusted analysis (Cox proportional hazard models and propensity analysis) comparing outcomes after

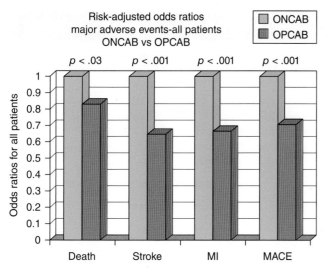

FIGURE 21-10 Risk-adjusted odds ratios for major adverse events in all patients undergoing on-pump coronary artery bypass (ONCAB) versus off-pump procedures (OPCAB). MACE = Major adverse cardiac events; MI = myocardial infarction. (Reproduced with permission from Puskas JD, Edwards FH, Pappas PA, et al: Off-pump techniques benefit men and women and narrow the disparity in mortality after coronary bypass grafting, *Ann Thorac Surg.* 2007 Nov;84(5):1447-1454.)

OPCAB versus ONCAB. In this study, OPCAB patients had significantly lower 30-day mortality (adjusted OR 0.81, 95% CI: 0.68 to 0.97, *p* = .0022). A large registry study of CABG outcomes in California demonstrated a significant reduction in propensity-adjusted operative mortality with OPCAB compared with ONCAB (2.59%, 95% CI: 2.52 to 2.67 vs 3.22%, 95% CI: 3.17 to 3.27%).[31] An intention-to-treat retrospective analysis of 42,477 patients from the STS ACSD showed a reduction in risk-adjusted operative mortality (adjusted OR 0.83, *p* = .03) as well as numerous morbidity outcomes favoring patients undergoing OPCAB (Fig. 21-10).[32] However, Chu and associates used an administrative database (Nationwide Inpatient Sample database) of 63,000 patients, and found no difference in hospital mortality between OPCAB and ONCAB (3.0 vs 3.2%, *p* = .14).[33]

Hospital Mortality in Patients Converted to On-Pump

A major complication of OPCAB is the emergent conversion to CPB support due to profound and acute hemodynamic compromise, either because of regional ischemia, valvular regurgitation from positioning, bradycardia during right-sided or inferior wall grafting, hypotension during cardiac positioning and stabilization, or intractable ventricular tachycardia/fibrillation. Such emergent conversion ("crash on pump") to ONCAB is associated with significantly higher perioperative morbidity and mortality. Several studies quote mortality specifically for converted patients ranging from 6 to 15%.[34-38] The ROOBY Trial had a 12.4% conversion rate from off- to on-pump CABG, roughly five-fold higher

than the rate reported in the STS ACSD.[32] Of these, 49.3% were elective conversions, mainly for poor visibility, whereas, 50.8% were urgent or emergent, mainly for hemodynamic instability.[39] The 1-year composite outcome of all-cause mortality, MI, and revascularization was significantly worse in the converted versus nonconverted OPCAB patients (21.1 vs 13.7%, *p* = .03). Importantly, 75% of conversions were associated with surgeons with experience of <100 OPCAB cases. Furthermore, a retrospective study of 8077 OPCAB cases used to identify risk factors for on-pump conversion confirmed surgeon experience to be the most significant multivariable predictor.[40] Importantly, there does not appear to be an increased risk of complications in patients who are *electively* converted to ONCAB.

Mid- and Long-Term Mortality

More recently, mid- and long-term follow-up data has become available in patients undergoing OPCAB.[1,3,41-46] There was no difference in 1-year mortality in the ROOBY (4.1 vs 2.9%, *p* = .15), CORONARY (5.1 vs 5.0%) or GOPCABE Trials (7.0 vs 8.0%, *p* = .38) comparing OPCAB and ONCAB. However, with sensitivity analysis, 1-year death from cardiac causes was slightly higher in the off-pump group compared with the on-pump group (2.7 vs 1.3%, *p* = .03) in ROOBY. The SMART Trial randomized 200 patients to OPCAB versus ONCAB by a single, experienced off-pump coronary surgeon.[46] In this trial, there was no difference in late survival (mean 7.5 years) (Fig. 21-11, *p* = .33), graft patency, recurrent angina nor repeat catheterization. Furthermore, a recent meta-analysis reports a trend towards improved long-term survival with ONCAB (HR 1.06; 95% CI: 1.00 to 1.13, *p* = .05) amongst all studies but there was no difference when analysis was limited to RCTs and propensity-matched studies.[47] Finally, in the observational study by Hannan et al,[30] 3-year survival was equivalent in OPCAB versus ONCAB patients (adjusted hazard ratio 1.01, 95% CI: 0.92 to 1.10, *p* = .89; unadjusted 3-year survival 89.4 vs 90.1%, log-rank test, *p* = .20). Based on these studies, it is reasonable to conclude that long-term survival after CABG is not affected by an on- or off-pump approach for the majority of patients.

Perioperative Morbidity

Large prospective and retrospective studies have consistently shown reduction in perioperative morbidities with OPCAB. In a meta-analysis of 37 randomized trials comparing OPCAB with ONCAB, OPCAB was associated with a reduced incidence of atrial fibrillation (OR 0.58; 95% CI: 0.44 to 0.77), transfusion requirements (OR 0.43; 95% CI: 0.29 to 0.65), inotrope requirements (OR 0.48; 95% CI: 0.29 to 0.65), respiratory infections (OR 0.41; 95% CI: 0.23 to 0.74), ventilation time (weighted mean difference, –3.4 hours; 95% CI: –5.1 to –1.7 hours), intensive care unit stay (OR weighted mean difference, –0.3 days; 95% CI: –0.6 to –0.1 days), and hospital stay (weighted mean difference, –1.0 days; 95% CI: –1.5 to –0.5 days).[48] Similarly, in a propensity score analysis of 548 patients,

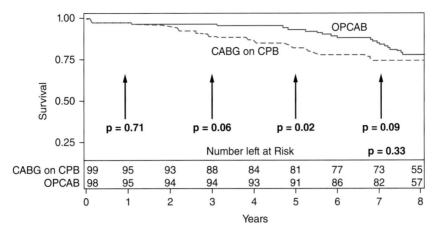

FIGURE 21-11 No difference in long-term survival comparing on-pump CABG versus OPCAB in the SMART randomized controlled trial. (Reproduced with permission from Puskas JD, Williams WH, O'Donnell R, et al: Off-pump and on-pump coronary artery bypass grafting are associated with similar graft patency, myocardial ischemia, and freedom from reintervention: long-term follow-up of a randomized trial, *Ann Thorac Surg*. 2011 Jun;91(6):1836-1842.)

OPCAB was associated with significantly lower in-hospital mortality (0.5 vs 2.9%; p = .001), incidence of stroke (0 vs 0.9%; p = .02), postoperative renal dysfunction (4.9 vs 10.8%; p = .001), pulmonary complications (10.2 vs 16.6%; p = .002), and infections (3.5 vs 6.2%; p = .03).[49]

Neurologic Outcomes

Stroke remains a significant cause of morbidity and mortality after CABG, occurring in approximately 1 to 14% of patients.[50,51] In addition, long-term survival after stroke post-CABG is negatively impacted with reductions in 1- and 5-year survival to 66% and 44% compared with 94% and 81% without stroke.[51] Recently, more attention is being focused on the observation that a large proportion of strokes is embolic in nature and occurs at the time of clamp removal.[52] Other potential sources of emboli include carotid artery disease, particulate matter aspirated from cardiotomy suction, delayed thromboembolism from clamp injuries to the ascending aortic intima or proximal anastomotic sites, or left atrial thrombi secondary to postoperative atrial fibrillation. Additional iatrogenic causes of emboli (gaseous) may include aggressive use of carbon dioxide blower devices to facilitate visualization during construction of proximal anastomoses.

It is clear that less aortic manipulation results in fewer stroke events.[53,54] Studies utilizing transcranial Doppler ultrasonography have confirmed the production of aortic emboli associated with cannulation, CPB, and application of aortic clamps.[55-57] Bowles[58] et al used transcranial Doppler ultrasonography to demonstrate production of large quantities of aortic emboli during CPB, even without manipulation of the aorta. Furthermore, Kapetanakis and colleagues[59] and Calafiore and associates[54] concluded that aortic manipulation is independently associated with an increased risk of postoperative stroke. Approaches used to decrease this embolic load include avoidance of aortic cannulation using off-pump techniques, avoidance of multiple aortic clamping, use of

clampless anastomotic devices, and a completely no-touch aortic technique.[60-62] Kim and associates[63] reported a lower incidence of postoperative stroke in patients undergoing OPCAB without any manipulation of the aorta compared with patients undergoing OPCAB with partial clamping and patients undergoing ONCAB. In 12,079 patients undergoing OPCAB, Moss et al[53] found progressively lower rates of stroke in no-touch aortic (0.6%), versus clampless facilitating device (1.2%) versus side-biting clamp (1.5%) (Fig. 21-12). Emmert et al[64] report a significantly lower incidence of stroke for OPCAB with partial occlusion clamp versus ONCAB (1.1 vs 2.4%; OR 0.35; CI: 95%: 0.17 to 0.72; p < .005) and even lower rates for OPCAB using a proximal occlusion device versus partial occlusion clamp (0.7 vs 2.3%; OR 0.39; CI: 95%: 0.16 to 0.90; p = .04) which approached that of the no-touch group (0.8%).

Large retrospective analyses[30,32,43,65-68] have demonstrated that OPCAB may be associated with a reduced incidence of stroke compared with ONCAB, but this has not been borne out in the large-scale RCTs. Hannan et al[30] reported a risk-adjusted decrease in postoperative stroke with OPCAB compared with ONCAB (adjusted OR 0.70, 95% CI: 0.57 to 0.86, p = .0006). A meta-analysis of 59 randomized trials of OPCAB versus ONCAB (N = 8961) report a 30% reduction in stroke (RR: 0.70, 95% CI: 0.49 to 0.99; Fig. 21-13).[68] Of 2468 patients in the CREDO-Kyoto Registry that underwent surgical revascularization, ONCAB was associated with higher stroke (OR 8.30, 95% CI: 2.25 to 30.7; p = .01) but only in the highest risk patient tertile (logistic EuroSCORE ≥ 6).[69] The observed reduction in postoperative stroke is likely due to lack of aortic cannulation and CPB, and possibly due to lack of aortic manipulation during proximal anastomoses. However, as mentioned, there was no difference in the rates of stroke in the large RCTs.[1-3,29] Notably, the method of construction of proximal anastomosis was left up to the surgeon and was not reported. Thus, if a significant number were performed with a side-biting clamp versus a minimal or no-touch

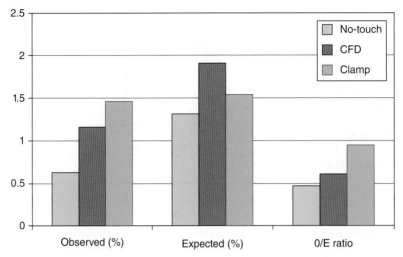

FIGURE 21-12 Stroke rate for OPCAB procedure using no-touch aortic, clampless facilitating device (CFD) and side-biting clamp. (Reproduced with permission from Moss E, Puskas JD2, Thourani VH, et al: Avoiding aortic clamping during coronary artery bypass grafting reduces postoperative stroke, *J Thorac Cardiovasc Surg.* 2015 Jan;149(1):175-180.)

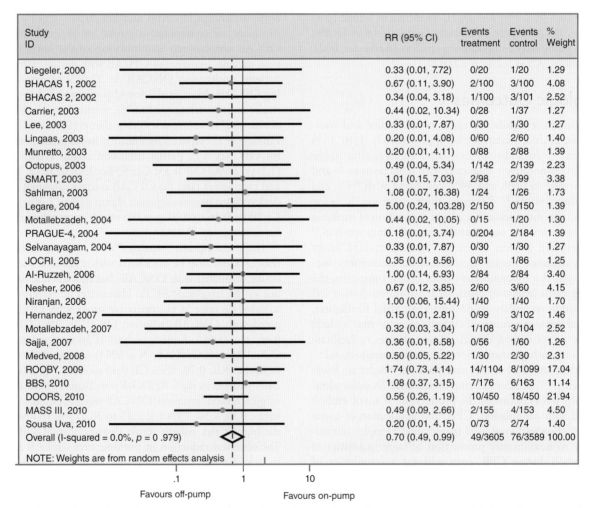

FIGURE 21-13 Forest plot for stroke. Forty-nine strokes were observed among 3605 off-pump coronary artery bypass patients compared with 76 among 3589 conventional coronary artery bypass patients, representing a 30% relative risk reduction. (Reproduced with permission from Afilalo J, Rasti M, Ohayon SM, et al: Off-pump versus on-pump coronary artery bypass surgery: an updated meta-analysis and meta-regression of randomized trials, *Eur Heart J.* 2012 May;33(10):1257-1267.)

aortic approach, the potential benefits of OPCAB with regard to postoperative stroke may have been attenuated.

Renal Failure

Preoperative renal insufficiency is a significant predictor of postoperative renal failure and mortality in patients undergoing CABG.[70] In multiple studies, OPCAB has been shown to reduce morbidity and mortality in patients with normal renal function,[71,72] those with renal dysfunction not yet on hemodialysis[73] as well as those with end-stage renal failure on dialysis.[74] In a prospective randomized trial of 116 diabetic patients with preoperative nondialysis-dependent renal insufficiency, the use of CPB was associated with a significant increase in adverse renal outcomes.[73] Two retrospective analyses, however, reported equivalent renal outcomes with either OPCAB or ONCAB.[74,75] Thus, the advantages of OPCAB to minimize or avoid renal dysfunction remain controversial.

High-Risk Patients

Several studies have documented improved outcomes in higher-risk patients undergoing OPCAB. Specifically, such higher-risk groups include women[32] and patients with left ventricular dysfunction,[77,78] ST-elevation MI,[79] prior stroke,[67] advanced age,[80] renal insufficiency,[74,81] reoperative cardiac surgery,[82,83] cirrhosis,[84] at the extremes of the BMI (<25 or >35) spectrum,[85] and in the patients with high Society of Thoracic Surgeon's predicted risk scores.[86,87] In such patients, improved end-organ perfusion, myocardial protection, limited aortic manipulation, and avoidance of systemic inflammation may explain the observed difference in major morbidity and mortality. A study of patients with left ventricular dysfunction (ejection fraction < 30%) in the STS ACSD report lower adjusted risk of death (OR 0.82), stroke (OR 0.67), major adverse cardiac events (OR 0.75), and prolonged intubation (OR 0.78) with OPCAB versus on-pump CABG.[85] Furthermore, Puskas and colleagues[87] reported that patients in the highest risk quartile had a significant reduction in hospital mortality with OPCAB compared with ONCAB (3.2 vs 6.7%, p < .0001, OR 0.45 95% CI: 0.33 to 0.63, p < .0001; Fig. 21-14). Also, as mentioned, the CORONARY Trials results showed a trend in improved outcomes for those patients in the highest EuroSCORE tertile.[1]

There is some evidence that OPCAB confers improved survival with emergent revascularization for acute coronary syndrome.[88-91] Although the safety and feasibility of OPCAB in select emergency situations has been confirmed, most surgeons today would argue against OPCAB in unstable patients.

Completeness of Revascularization, Graft Patency, and Need for Repeat Revascularization

Completeness of revascularization is critical for the success and durable benefit of CABG.[92,93] The index of completeness

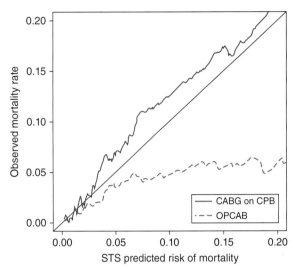

FIGURE 21-14 Regression curve comparison of observed mortality rates for off-pump coronary artery bypass grafting (OPCAB) and coronary artery bypass grafting (CABG) on cardiopulmonary bypass (CPB) across all levels of predicted risk. STS = The Society of Thoracic Surgeons. (Reproduced with permission from Puskas JD, Thourani VH, Kilgo P, et al: Off-pump coronary artery bypass disproportionately benefits high-risk patients, *Ann Thorac Surg.* 2009 Oct;88(4):1142-1147.)

of revascularization is defined as number of grafts performed divided by number deemed necessary preoperatively (number of graftable vessels with angiographically significant stenoses), which is more important than the absolute number of grafts.[94] The choice to perform a procedure off-pump should not compromise the completeness of revascularization unless the use of CPB poses obvious and significant risk for postoperative complications or mortality, which may be the case in patients with severe atherosclerotic disease of the ascending aorta. In centers that routinely perform the large majority of coronary operations without CPB, complete revascularization, even in the more difficult lateral wall territory, is routinely accomplished.

The ability to provide complete revascularization with equivalent graft patency OPCAB techniques has been challenged, to provide complete revascularization with OPCAB techniques with equivalent graft patency has been challenged, although the majority of evidence from randomized trials suggests near-equivalent revascularization.[1-3,5,6,95-97,46] In the ROOBY Trial, there were more patients with fewer grafts completed overall (2.9 vs 3.0, p = .002) and fewer than originally planned in the OPCAB group (17.8 vs 11.1%).[2] In the CORONARY Trial, there were also fewer grafts (3.0 vs 3.2, p < .001) and a trend towards higher rates of incomplete revascularization (11.8 vs 10.0%, p = .05) in the OPCAB compared to ONCAB group.[1,29] Again, in the GOPCABE Trial, OPCAB was associated with fewer grafts (2.7 vs 2.8, p < .001) and higher incomplete revascularization (34.0% vs 29.3%).[3] The DOORS Trial was a multicenter randomized trial of 900 patients ≥70 years of age, which compared OPCAB versus ONCAB with the same heparinization protocol. They also report statistically fewer grafts being performed with OPCAB (3.1 vs 2.9%, *p* = .007).[5,6] A meta-analysis of randomized trials has consistently shown a lower number of grafts per patient in off-pump versus on-pump CABG (2.6 vs 2.8, < .0001).[98] Even analysis of later trials in which surgeon experience was greater still showed fewer grafts performed off-pump versus on-pump (2.7 vs 2.9 grafts).[99] In a study of the STS ACSD by Puskas and colleagues,[32] OPCAB patients had a slightly lower index of complete revascularization than ONCAB patients. Thus, OPCAB is consistently associated with a statistically significant but small difference in absolute number of grafts performed. Given equivalent survival between OPCAB and ONCAB, whether the difference in revascularization is clinically significant is unknown.

Graft patency has been evaluated in several randomized trials, demonstrating that in experienced centers, graft patency can be equivalently excellent with either technique.[46,100] However, Shroyer et al[2] found that the overall rate of graft patency (driven by vein graft patency) was lower in the OPCAB group compared with the ONCAB group (82.6 vs 87.8%, *p* < .001). A further blinded follow-up angiographic analysis in 685 OPCAB and 685 ONCAB patients in ROOBY revealed that OPCAB was associated with lower FitzGibbon A patency for arterial conduits (85.8 vs 91.4%; *p* = .003) and saphenous vein grafts (72.7 vs 80.4%; *p* < .001).[101] As expected, ineffective revascularization was associated with greater 1-year nonfatal MI and repeat revascularization. In the DOORS Trial, OPCAB was associated with a greater incidence of graft stenosis (9 vs 5%) and occlusion (12 vs 9%) (*p* = .01), which was primarily seen in vein grafts at 6-month angiography.[5,6] Again, this may be an issue of experience. In the SMART trial, Puskas et al[46] randomized patients to either OPCAB versus on-pump CABG and demonstrated similarly excellent 1-year graft patency (93.6% for OPCAB vs 95.8% for ONCAB, *p* = .33) as well as clinical outcomes of death, stroke, MI, and reintervention. There was an increase in the rate of repeat revascularization (0.7 vs 0.2%, *p* = .01) in the CORONARY Trial, although whether this is a result of lower graft patency or greater incomplete revascularization alone is unknown.[1] A meta-analysis of 12 RCTs comparing OPCAB versus on-pump CABG showed an increased risk of graft occlusion (RR 1.35; 95% CI: 1.16 to 1.57), driven by saphenous vein graft occlusion (RR 1.41; 95% CI: 1.24 to 1.60) but not occlusion of IMA nor radial artery grafts.[102]

The New York registry data from Hannan et al[30] report that OPCAB was associated with lower in-hospital mortality and morbidity and equivalent long-term outcomes than ONCAB but greater need for repeat revascularization (93.6 vs 89.9%). However, because this was a retrospective analysis, this study was unable to differentiate whether this difference was a result of incomplete revascularization during OPCAB, reduced graft patency, or unrecognized confounding variables.

Guidelines

The 2011 ACCF/AHA Guideline for Coronary Artery Bypass Graft Surgery included two recommendations regarding OPCAB[103]: OPCAB to reduce bleeding and blood transfusion (Class IIa, Level of Evidence A) and OPCAB for patients with renal dysfunction (Class IIb, Level of Evidence B). More recently, the strength of data in support of OPCAB is recognized in the 2014 European Society of Cardiology/European Association of Cardio-Thoracic Surgery Guidelines on Myocardial Revascularization.[104] Here the recommendation is that OPCAB be performed in high-risk patients in experienced off-pump centers (Class IIa, Level of Evidence B) and in patients with ascending aortic atherosclerosis (Class I, Level of Evidence B). Furthermore, these guidelines recommend routine use of intraoperative graft flow measurements (Class IIa, Level of Evidence C).

Minimally Invasive, Robotic, and Hybrid Approaches

Widespread familiarity with off-pump techniques has facilitated the development and application of sternal-sparing minimally invasive cardiac surgery (MICS) revascularization procedures for highly selected patients. There are several different variations. A small thoracotomy has been used to accomplish LIMA harvest and off-pump bypass on the anterior wall under direct vision, known as single vessel small thoracotomy (SVST), or for multivessel, known as multivessel small thoracotomy (MVST). Thoracoscopic or robotic-assisted left IMA dissection and harvest can be followed by a direct off-pump anastomosis to the LAD (Fig. 21-15) or by a total endoscopic LIMA-LAD anastomosis; the latter is referred to as totally endoscopic CABG (TECAB). Hybrid coronary revascularization (HCR) combines a minimally invasive LIMA to LAD graft with percutaneous intervention to non–LAD targets.[105,106] The feasibility of these alternative minimally invasive approaches has been demonstrated. The use of minimally invasive techniques has generated enthusiasm in the surgical and interventional communities, and its use is expanding beyond a few select centers.

For patients with anterior single vessel disease, a SVST offers a sternal-sparing incision with the long-term patency benefit

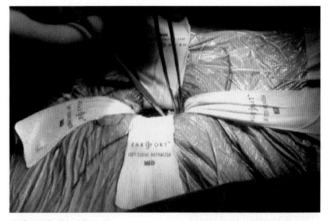

FIGURE 21-15 After endoscopic or robotic-assisted IMA harvest, a direct hand-sewn anastomosis can be performed off-pump via a left anterolateral non-rib spreading minithoracotomy.

of the LIMA graft. Blazek et al[107] show equivalent 7-year survival in 130 patients with single vessel LAD disease randomized to MIDCAB versus DES-PCI. There was no difference in the composite primary endpoint of all-cause mortality, MI, and repeat revascularization but with significantly higher repeat revascularization after PCI (HR 13.50, 95% CI: 1.76 to 103.29; $p < .001$). Moreover, a single center propensity score-matched minimally invasive direct coronary artery bypass (MIDCAB) versus DES-PCI comparison found at 10 years that DES-PCI was associated with a 2.2-fold increased risk of mortality as well as a 2.0-fold increased risk of repeat revascularization.[108] Multivessel small thoracotomy CABG offers complete revascularization with lower blood transfusion, incidence of chest wound infection, and improved postoperative physical recovery.[109] In their series of direct MVST CABG of which 75% were performed off-pump, Ruel and colleagues[110] report 92% and 100% 6-month graft patency for all grafts and for LIMA grafts, respectively.

Several experienced groups have reported successful outcomes using a robotic CABG approach.[111-113] Halkos et al[111] report 1.3% 30-day mortality, 5.2% conversion to sternotomy and 2.3% reexploration for bleeding for 307 consecutive robotic CABG procedures. For the 199 patients with predischarge follow-up angiography, LIMA-LAD patency was 95.0% and anastomotic lesions were found in only three patients. Srivastava et al[112] describe robotic multivessel CABG with bilateral IMA off-pump distal anastomoses constructed with the U-Clip Anastomotic Device (Medtronic, Minneapolis, MN). Bonaros et al[113] also present the largest experience of 500 cases of single and multivessel robotic CABG with on-pump distal anastomoses, reporting excellent results.

As described by Harskamp et al,[114] the concept of HCR stems from the hypothesis that (1) the LIMA-LAD is superior to coronary stenting and (2) contemporary DES-PCI is noninferior to venous bypass grafts used for non-LAD disease. Thus, patients with multivessel disease with a complex LAD lesion and noncomplex non-LAD lesions suitable for PCI, may be considered. Those patients with impediments to conventional CABG such as those with advanced age, frailty, obesity, lack of conduits, poor non-LAD target vessels, and porcelain aorta may be particularly suited for HCR. In the 2011 ACCF/AHA Guideline for Coronary Artery Bypass Graft Surgery, HCR is considered reasonable in patients with limitations to traditional CABG, such as heavily calcified proximal aorta or poor target vessels for CABG; lack of conduits; or unfavorable LAD artery for PCI (Class IIa, Level of Evidence B).[103] Furthermore, HCR may be reasonable as an alternative to multivessel PCI or CABG in an attempt to improve the overall risk-benefit ratio (Class IIb, Level of Evidence C). The 2014 European Society of Cardiology/European Association of Cardio-Thoracic Surgery Guidelines on Myocardial Revascularization suggests HCR for redo revascularization when lack of conduit poses a limitation to a conventional surgical approach (Class IIb, Level of Evidence C).[104]

In experienced minimally invasive revascularization centers, the major clinical outcomes of HCR are equivalent to traditional CABG.[115] Halkos et al[116] performed a propensity-matched study comparing patients with multivessel coronary disease who underwent endoscopic-assisted or robotic LIMA harvest with SVST direct LIMA-LAD grafting versus OPCAB. There was no difference in 5-year survival but there were fewer blood transfusions ($p < .001$) and more repeat revascularizations with HCR (12.2 vs 3.7%, $p < .001$). A meta-analysis of six retrospective studies found that HCR was associated with no difference in freedom from MACCE at 1 year when compared with CABG but a greater incidence of repeat revascularization (Fig. 21-16).[114] Considering that the major weakness of HCR is in-stent restenosis or thrombosis requiring repeat revascularization, young, healthy patients may benefit more from conventional CABG. In the STS ACSD, there are 950 HCR cases (0.5% of all CABG cases) between 2011 and 2013, performed in 1/3 of all cardiac centers.[117] Patients who underwent HCR had higher cardiovascular risk profiles compared with traditional CABG and after adjustment, there was no differences in the composite of in-hospital mortality and major morbidity.

Surgical Revascularization Centers of Excellence

A recurring issue in evaluation of data from RCTs comparing OPCAB versus ONCAB continues to be that of surgeon expertise. There is no doubt that OPCAB is more technically challenging for the surgeon and surgical team. Mastery of this procedure requires experience and team commitment. A review of the Nationwide Inpatient Sample Database reported a 5% decrease in the absolute probability of mortality with OPCAB between the highest and lowest volume surgeon cohorts, with the threshold for the largest improvement occurring after 50 cases/year and the lower mortality above 150 cases/year.[118] Notably, in this study, surgeons performed 105 OPCAB procedures per year (mean), which is significantly higher than the STS reported average.

As mentioned, ROOBY was criticized for lack of surgeon experience with off-pump procedures. In CORONARY and GOPCABE Trials, surgeons were considerably more experienced with off-pump procedures and in both trials, there were no differences in the primary composite endpoints. The difference in expertise was also highlighted by an OPCAB-to-ONCAB crossover rates of 12.4% for ROOBY versus 7.9% and 9.7% for CORONARY and GOPCABE, respectively.[1-3] Finally, a meta-analysis of >100,000 patients comparing OPCAB versus ONCAB by Takagi et al[119] found an increase in long-term all-cause mortality with OPCAB. But in the two largest RCTs in which expertise was defined as >2 years of experience and the completion of >100 OPCAB procedures, there was no difference in mid-term outcomes.

As such, there is increasing appreciation that OPCAB should be performed not by all surgeons at all surgical centers, but by experts in surgical revascularization at centers of excellence. To meet the technical challenges of performing successful OPCAB, young surgeons must train with established experts in surgical revascularization. Training in advanced

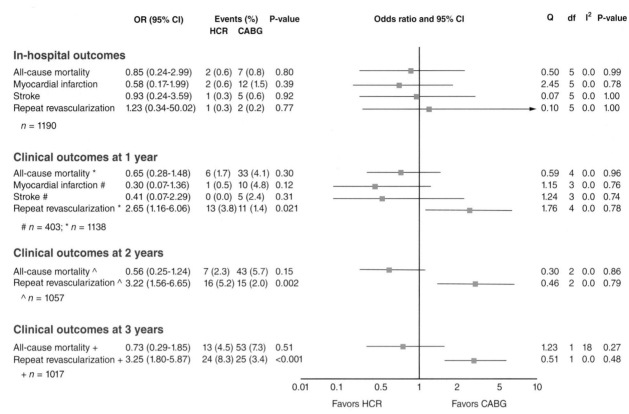

FIGURE 21-16 Forest plot for the major clinical outcomes comparing HCR versus coronary artery bypass surgery: a meta-analysis of 1190 patients. (Reproduced with permission from Harskamp RE, Bagai A, Halkos ME, et al: Clinical outcomes after hybrid coronary revascularization versus coronary artery bypass surgery: a meta-analysis of 1,190 patients, *Am Heart J.* 2014 Apr;167(4):585-592.)

surgical revascularization may include OPCAB, hybrid, total arterial, minimally invasive, and robotic revascularization. Complex revascularization cases should be referred to revascularization centers of excellence. This is a model that is well-established for cardiac surgical treatment of heart failure as well as complex valvular and aortic disease.

KEY POINTS

- The choice of OPCAB versus ONCAB requires careful attention to preoperative and intraoperative patient variables that may influence operative circumstances as well as short- and long-term morbidity and mortality.
- With the appropriate use of modern stabilizers and heart positioning devices, adequate surgeon experience and careful patient selection, equivalent completeness of revascularization and graft patency can be achieved with OPCAB.
- The quality of the anastomosis and the completeness of revascularization should not be compromised when performing off-pump anastomoses unless CPB poses excessive risk to the patient.
- Urgent or emergent conversion from OPCAB to ONCAB is associated with higher in-hospital morbidity and mortality but preemptive controlled conversion is not.

- Randomized trials have shown equivalent mortality outcomes between OPCAB and ONCAB techniques.
- In particular, low-risk patients undergoing surgical revascularization can be safely revascularized with either OPCAB or ONCAB.
- Certain high-risk groups may have better in-hospital morbidity and mortality outcomes when revascularized without the use of CPB likely due to avoidance of CPB and minimizing aortic manipulation.
- Long-term survival outcomes are equivalent in patients undergoing ONCAB or OPCAB.
- There is an improvement in resource utilization with OPCAB, including reduced transfusion requirements, shorter length of stay, less intensive care and ventilator time, and reduced cost.

REFERENCES

1. Lamy A, Devereaux PJ, Prabhakaran D, et al: Effects of off-pump and on-pump coronary-artery bypass grafting at 1 year. *N Engl J Med* 2013; 368:1179-1188.
2. Shroyer AL, Grover FL, Hattler B, et al: On-pump versus off-pump coronary-artery bypass surgery. *N Engl J Med* 2009; 361:1827-1837.
3. Diegeler A, Börgermann J, Kappert U, et al: Off-pump versus on-pump coronary-artery bypass grafting in elderly patients. *N Engl J Med* 2013; 368:1189-1198.

4. Bakaeen FG, Shroyer AL, Gammie JS, et al: Trends in use of off-pump coronary artery bypass grafting: Results from the Society of Thoracic Surgeons Adult Cardiac Surgery Database. *J Thorac Cardiovasc Surg* 2014; 148:856-853.

5. Houlind K, Kjeldsen BJ, Madsen SN, et al: On-pump versus off-pump coronary artery bypass surgery in elderly patients: results from the Danish on-pump versus off-pump randomization study. *Circulation* 2012; 125:2431-2439.

6. Houlind K, Fenger-Grøn M, Holme SJ, et al: Graft patency after off-pump coronary artery bypass surgery is inferior even with identical heparinization protocols: Results from the Danish On-pump Versus Off-pump Randomization Study (DOORS). *J Thorac Cardiovasc Surg* 2014; [Epub ahead of print].

7. Halkos ME, Cooper WA, Petersen R, et al: Early administration of clopidogrel is safe after off-pump coronary artery bypass surgery. *Ann Thorac Surg* 2006; 81:815-819.

8. Lopes RD, Hafley GE, Allen KB, et al: Endoscopic versus open vein-graft harvesting in coronary-artery bypass surgery. *N Engl J Med* 2009; 361:235-244.

9. Whitley WS, Glas KE: An argument for routine ultrasound screening of the thoracic aorta in the cardiac surgery population. *Semin Cardiothorac Vasc Anesth* 2008; 12:290-297.

10. Sylivris S, Calafiore P, Matalanis G, et al: The intraoperative assessment of ascending aortic atheroma: epiaortic imaging is superior to both transesophageal echocardiography and direct palpation. *J Cardiothorac Vasc Anesth* 1997; 11:704-707.

11. Bolotin G, Domany Y, de Perini L, et al: Use of intraoperative epiaortic ultrasonography to delineate aortic atheroma. *Chest* 2005; 127:60-65.

12. Suvarna S, Smith A, Stygall J, et al: An intraoperative assessment of the ascending aorta: a comparison of digital palpation, transesophageal echocardiography, and epiaortic ultrasonography. *J Cardiothorac Vasc Anesth* 2007; 21:805-809.

13. Rosenberger P, Shernan SK, Loffler M, et al: The influence of epiaortic ultrasonography on intraoperative surgical management in 6051 cardiac surgical patients. *Ann Thorac Surg* 2008; 85:548-553.

14. Collison SP, Agarwal A, Trehan N: Controversies in the use of intraluminal shunts during off-pump coronary artery bypass grafting surgery. *Ann Thorac Surg* 2006; 82:1559-1566.

15. Bergsland J, Lingaas PS, Skulstad H, et al: Intracoronary shunt prevents ischemia in off-pump coronary artery bypass surgery. *Ann Thorac Surg* 2009; 87:54-60.

16. Hangler H, Mueller L, Ruttmann E, et al: Shunt or snare: coronary endothelial damage due to hemostatic devices for beating heart coronary surgery. *Ann Thorac Surg* 2008; 86:1873-1877.

17. Laurikka J, Wu ZK, Iisalo P, et al: Regional ischemic preconditioning enhances myocardial performance in off-pump coronary artery bypass grafting. *Chest* 2002; 121:1183-1189.

18. Guerrieri Wolf L, Abu-Omar Y, Choudhary BP, et al: Gaseous and solid cerebral microembolization during proximal aortic anastomoses in off-pump coronary surgery: the effect of an aortic side-biting clamp and two clampless devices. *J Thorac Cardiovasc Surg* 2007; 133:485-493.

19. Medalion B, Meirson D, Hauptman E, Sasson L, Schachner A: Initial experience with the Heartstring proximal anastomotic system. *J Thorac Cardiovasc Surg* 2004; 128:273-277.

20. Akpinar B, Guden M, Sagbas E, et al: Clinical experience with the Novare Enclose II manual proximal anastomotic device during off-pump coronary artery surgery. *Eur J Cardiothorac Surg* 2005; 27:1070-1073.

21. Puskas JD, Halkos ME, Balkhy H, et al: Evaluation of the PAS-Port Proximal Anastomosis System in coronary artery bypass surgery (the EPIC trial). *J Thorac Cardiovasc Surg* 2009; 138:125-132.

22. Kempfert J, Opfermann UT, Richter M, et al: Twelve-month patency with the PAS-port proximal connector device: a single center prospective randomized trial. *Ann Thorac Surg* 2008; 85:1579-1584.

23. Fujii T, Watanabe Y, Shiono N, et al: Study of coronary artery bypass using the PAS-Port device: assessment by multidetector computed tomography. *Gen Thorac Cardiovasc Surg* 2009; 57:79-86.

24. Quin J, Lucke J, Hattler B, et al: Surgeon judgment and utility of transit time flow probes in coronary artery bypass grafting surgery. *JAMA Surg* 2014; 149:1182-1187.

25. Perrault LP, Menasche P, Peynet J, et al: On-pump, beating-heart coronary artery operations in high-risk patients: an acceptable trade-off? *Ann Thorac Surg* 1997; 64:1368-1373.

26. Izumi Y, Magishi K, Ishikawa N, Kimura F: On-pump beating-heart coronary artery bypass grafting for acute myocardial infarction. *Ann Thorac Surg* 2006; 81:573-576.

27. Rastan AJ, Eckenstein JI, Hentschel B, et al: Emergency coronary artery bypass graft surgery for acute coronary syndrome: beating heart versus conventional cardioplegic cardiac arrest strategies. *Circulation* 2006; 114:I477-I485.

28. Mizutani S, Matsuura A, Miyahara K, et al: On-pump beating-heart coronary artery bypass: a propensity matched analysis. *Ann Thorac Surg* 2007; 83:1368-1373.

29. Lamy A, Devereaux PJ, Prabhakaran D, et al: Off-pump or on-pump coronary-artery bypass grafting at 30 days. *N Engl J Med* 2012; 366:1489-1497.

30. Hannan EL, Wu C, Smith CR, et al: Off-pump versus on-pump coronary artery bypass graft surgery: differences in short-term outcomes and in long-term mortality and need for subsequent revascularization. *Circulation* 2007; 116:1145-1152.

31. Li Z, Yeo KK, Parker JP, et al: Off-pump coronary artery bypass graft surgery in California, 2003 to 2005. *Am Heart J* 2008; 156:1095-1102.

32. Puskas JD, Edwards FH, Pappas PA, et al: Off-pump techniques benefit men and women and narrow the disparity in mortality after coronary bypass grafting. *Ann Thorac Surg* 2007; 84:1447-1454.

33. Chu D, Bakaeen FG, Dao TK, et al: On-pump versus off-pump coronary artery bypass grafting in a cohort of 63,000 patients. *Ann Thorac Surg* 2009; 87:1820-1826; discussion 1826-1827.

34. Edgerton JR, Dewey TM, Magee MJ, et al: Conversion in off-pump coronary artery bypass grafting: an analysis of predictors and outcomes. *Ann Thorac Surg* 2003; 76:1138-1142.

35. Mathur AN, Pather R, Widjanarko J, et al: Off-pump coronary artery bypass: the Sudbury experience. *Can J Cardiol* 2003; 19:1261-1269.

36. Soltoski P, Salerno T, Levinsky L, et al: Conversion to cardiopulmonary bypass in off-pump coronary artery bypass grafting: its effect on outcome. *J Card Surg* 1998; 13:328-334.

37. Iaco AL, Contini M, Teodori G, et al: Off or on bypass: what is the safety threshold? *Ann Thorac Surg* 1999; 68:1486-1489.

38. Mujanovic E, Kabil E, Hadziselimovic M, et al: Conversions in off-pump coronary surgery. *Heart Surg Forum* 2003; 6:135-137.

39. Novitzky D, Baltz JH, Hattler B, et al: Outcomes after conversion in the Veterans Affairs randomized on versus off bypass trial. *Ann Thorac Surg* 2011; 92:2147-2154.

40. Chowdhury R, White D, Kilgo P, et al: Risk factors for conversion to cardiopulmonary bypass during off-pump coronary artery bypass surgery. *Ann Thorac Surg* 2012; 93:1936-1941.

41. Angelini GD, Culliford L, Smith DK, et al: Effects of on- and off-pump coronary artery surgery on graft patency, survival, and health-related quality of life: long-term follow-up of 2 randomized controlled trials. *J Thorac Cardiovasc Surg* 2009; 137:295-303.

42. Karolak W, Hirsch G, Buth K, Legare JF: Medium-term outcomes of coronary artery bypass graft surgery on pump versus off pump: results from a randomized controlled trial. *Am Heart J* 2007; 153:689-695.

43. Puskas JD, Kilgo PD, Lattouf OM, et al: Off-pump coronary bypass provides reduced mortality and morbidity and equivalent 10-year survival. *Ann Thorac Surg* 2008; 86:1139-1146.

44. Motallebzadeh R, Bland JM, Markus HS, Kaski JC, Jahangiri M: Health-related quality of life outcome after on-pump versus off-pump coronary artery bypass graft surgery: a prospective randomized study. *Ann Thorac Surg* 2006; 82:615-619.

45. Williams ML, Muhlbaier LH, Schroder JN, et al: Risk-adjusted short- and long-term outcomes for on-pump versus off-pump coronary artery bypass surgery. *Circulation* 2005; 112:I366-370.

46. Puskas JD, Williams WH, O'Donnell R, et al: Off-pump and on-pump coronary artery bypass grafting are associated with similar graft patency, myocardial ischemia, and freedom from reintervention: long-term follow-up of a randomized trial. *Ann Thorac Surg* 2011; 91:1836-1842.

47. Chaudhry UA, Harling L, Rao C, et al: Off-pump versus on-pump coronary revascularization: meta-analysis of mid- and long-term outcomes. *Ann Thorac Surg* 2014; 98:563-572.

48. Cheng DC, Bainbridge D, Martin JE, et al: Does off-pump coronary artery bypass reduce mortality, morbidity, and resource utilization when

compared with conventional coronary artery bypass? A meta-analysis of randomized trials. *Anesthesiology* 2005; 102:188-203.

49. Murzi M, Caputo M, Aresu G, et al: On-pump and off-pump coronary artery bypass grafting in patients with left main stem disease: a propensity score analysis. *J Thorac Cardiovasc Surg* 2012; 143:1382-1388.

50. Filsoufi F, Rahmanian PB, Castillo JG, et al: Incidence, topography, predictors and long-term survival after stroke in patients undergoing coronary artery bypass grafting. *Ann Thorac Surg* 2008; 85:862-870.

51. Puskas JD, Winston AD, Wright CE, et al: Stroke after coronary artery operation: incidence, correlates, outcome, and cost. *Ann Thorac Surg* 2000; 69:1053-1056.

52. Barbut D, Hinton RB, Szatrowski TP, et al: Cerebral emboli detected during bypass surgery are associated with clamp removal. *Stroke* 1994; 25:2398-2402.

53. Moss E, Puskas JD, Thourani VH, et al: Avoiding aortic clamping during coronary artery bypass grafting reduces postoperative stroke. *J Thorac Cardiovasc Surg* 2015; 149:175-180.

54. Calafiore AM, Di Mauro M, Teodori G, et al: Impact of aortic manipulation on incidence of cerebrovascular accidents after surgical myocardial revascularization. *Ann Thorac Surg* 2002; 73:1387-1393.

55. van der Linden J, Casimir-Ahn H: When do cerebral emboli appear during open heart operations? A transcranial Doppler study. *Ann Thorac Surg* 1991; 51:237-241.

56. Blauth CI: Macroemboli and microemboli during cardiopulmonary bypass. *Ann Thorac Surg* 1995; 59:1300-1303.

57. Barbut D, Yao FS, Lo YW, et al: Determination of size of aortic emboli and embolic load during coronary artery bypass grafting. *Ann Thorac Surg* 1997; 63:1262-1267.

58. Bowles BJ, Lee JD, Dang CR, et al: Coronary artery bypass performed without the use of cardiopulmonary bypass is associated with reduced cerebral microemboli and improved clinical results. *Chest* 2001; 119:25-30.

59. Kapetanakis EI, Stamou SC, Dullum MK, et al: The impact of aortic manipulation on neurologic outcomes after coronary artery bypass surgery: a risk-adjusted study. *Ann Thorac Surg* 2004; 78:1564-1571.

60. Hammon JW, Stump DA, Butterworth JF, et al: Single crossclamp improves 6-month cognitive outcome in high-risk coronary bypass patients: the effect of reduced aortic manipulation. *J Thorac Cardiovasc Surg* 2006; 131:114-121.

61. Scarborough JE, White W, Derilus FE, et al: Combined use of off-pump techniques and a sutureless proximal aortic anastomotic device reduces cerebral microemboli generation during coronary artery bypass grafting. *J Thorac Cardiovasc Surg* 2003; 126:1561-1567.

62. Mark DB, Newman MF: Protecting the brain in coronary artery bypass graft surgery. *JAMA* 2002; 287:1448-1450.

63. Kim KB, Kang CH, Chang WI, et al: Off-pump coronary artery bypass with complete avoidance of aortic manipulation. *Ann Thorac Surg* 2002; 74:S1377-1382.

64. Emmert MY, Salzberg SP, Cetina Biefer HR, et al: Total arterial off-pump surgery provides excellent outcomes and does not compromise complete revascularization. *Eur J Cardiothorac Surg* 2012; 41:e25-31.

65. Reston JT, Tregear SJ, Turkelson CM: Meta-analysis of short-term and mid-term outcomes following off-pump coronary artery bypass grafting. *Ann Thorac Surg* 2003; 76(5):1510-1515.

66. Sharony R, Grossi EA, Saunders PC, et al: Propensity case-matched analysis of off-pump coronary artery bypass grafting in patients with atheromatous aortic disease. *J Thorac Cardiovasc Surg* 2004; 127:406-413.

67. Halkos ME, Puskas JD, Lattouf OM, et al: Impact of preoperative neurologic events on outcomes after coronary artery bypass grafting. *Ann Thorac Surg* 2008; 86:504-510.

68. Afilalo J, Rasti M, Ohayon SM, et al: Off-pump vs. on-pump coronary artery bypass surgery: an updated meta-analysis and meta-regression of randomized trials. *Eur Heart J* 2012; 33:1257-1267.

69. Marui A, Okabayashi H, Komiya T, et al: Benefits of off-pump coronary artery bypass grafting in high-risk patients. *Circulation* 2012; 126:S151-157.

70. Cooper WA, O'Brien SM, Thourani VH, et al: Impact of renal dysfunction on outcomes of coronary artery bypass surgery: results from the Society of Thoracic Surgeons National Adult Cardiac Database. *Circulation* 2006; 113:1063-1070.

71. Massoudy P, Wagner S, Thielmann M, et al: Coronary artery bypass surgery and acute kidney injury—impact of the off-pump technique. *Nephrol Dial Transplant* 2008; 23:2853-2860.

72. Di Mauro M, Gagliardi M, Iaco AL, et al: Does off-pump coronary surgery reduce postoperative acute renal failure? The importance of preoperative renal function. *Ann Thorac Surg* 2007; 84:1496-1502.

73. Sajja LR, Mannam G, Chakravarthi RM, et al: Coronary artery bypass grafting with or without cardiopulmonary bypass in patients with preoperative non-dialysis dependent renal insufficiency: a randomized study. *J Thorac Cardiovasc Surg* 2007; 133:378-388.

74. Dewey TM, Herbert MA, Prince SL, et al: Does coronary artery bypass graft surgery improve survival among patients with end-stage renal disease? *Ann Thorac Surg* 2006; 81:591-598.

75. Schwann NM, Horrow JC, Strong MD 3rd, et al: Does off-pump coronary artery bypass reduce the incidence of clinically evident renal dysfunction after multivessel myocardial revascularization? *Anesth Analg* 2004; 99:959-964.

76. Asimakopoulos G, Karagounis AP, Valencia O, et al: Renal function after cardiac surgery off- versus on-pump coronary artery bypass: analysis using the Cockroft-Gault formula for estimating creatinine clearance. *Ann Thorac Surg* 2005; 79:2024-2031.

77. Youn YN, Chang BC, Hong YS, et al: Early and mid-term impacts of cardiopulmonary bypass on coronary artery bypass grafting in patients with poor left ventricular dysfunction: a propensity score analysis. *Circ J* 2007; 71:1387-1394.

78. Darwazah AK, Abu Sham'a RA, Hussein E, et al: Myocardial revascularization in patients with low ejection fraction < or =35%: effect of pump technique on early morbidity and mortality. *J Card Surg* 2006; 21:22-27.

79. Fattouch K, Guccione F, Dioguardi P, et al: Off-pump versus on-pump myocardial revascularization in patients with ST-segment elevation myocardial infarction: a randomized trial. *J Thorac Cardiovasc Surg* 2009; 137:650-656.

80. Mishra YK, Collison SP, Malhotra R, et al: Ten-year experience with single-vessel and multivessel reoperative off-pump coronary artery bypass grafting. *J Thorac Cardiovasc Surg* 2008; 135:527-532.

81. García Fuster R, Paredes F, García Peláez A, et al: Impact of increasing degrees of renal impairment on outcomes of coronary artery bypass grafting: the off-pump advantage. *Eur J Cardiothorac Surg* 2013; 44:732-742.

82. Sepehripour AH, Harling L, Ashrafian H, et al: Does off-pump coronary revascularization confer superior organ protection in re-operative coronary artery surgery? A meta-analysis of observational studies. *J Cardiothorac Surg* 2014; 9:115.

83. Dohi M, Miyata H, Doi K, et al: The off-pump technique in redo coronary artery bypass grafting reduces mortality and major morbidities: propensity score analysis of data from the Japan Cardiovascular Surgery Database. *Eur J Cardiothorac Surg* 2015; 47:299-307.

84. Gopaldas RR, Chu D, Cornwell LD, et al: Cirrhosis as a moderator of outcomes in coronary artery bypass grafting and off-pump coronary artery bypass operations: a 12-year population-based study. *Ann Thorac Surg* 2013; 96:1310-1315.

85. Keeling WB, Kilgo PD, Puskas JD, et al: Off-pump coronary artery bypass grafting attenuates morbidity and mortality for patients with low and high body mass index. *J Thorac Cardiovasc Surg* 2013; 146:1442-1448.

86. Polomsky M, He X, O'Brien SM, et al: Outcomes of off-pump versus on-pump coronary artery bypass grafting: Impact of preoperative risk. *J Thorac Cardiovasc Surg* 2013; 145:1193-1198.

87. Puskas JD, Thourani VH, Kilgo P, et al: Off-pump coronary artery bypass disproportionately benefits high-risk patients. *Ann Thorac Surg* 2009; 88:1142-1147.

88. Kerendi F, Puskas JD, Craver JM, et al: Emergency coronary artery bypass grafting can be performed safely without cardiopulmonary bypass in selected patients. *Ann Thorac Surg* 2005; 79:801-806.

89. Locker C, Mohr R, Paz Y, et al: Myocardial revascularization for acute myocardial infarction: benefits and drawbacks of avoiding cardiopulmonary bypass. *Ann Thorac Surg* 2003; 76:771-776.

90. Biancari F, Mahar MA, Mosorin M, et al: Immediate and intermediate outcome after off-pump and on-pump coronary artery bypass surgery in patients with unstable angina pectoris. *Ann Thorac Surg* 2008; 86:1147-1152.

91. Fattouch K, Guccione F, Dioguardi P, et al: Off-pump versus on-pump myocardial revascularization in patients with ST-segment elevation myocardial infarction: a randomized trial. *J Thorac Cardiovasc Surg* 2009; 137:650-656.

92. Jones EL, Weintraub WS: The importance of completeness of revascularization during long-term follow-up after coronary artery operations. *J Thorac Cardiovasc Surg* 1996; 112:227-237.

93. Synnergren MJ, Ekroth R, Oden A, et al: Incomplete revascularization reduces survival benefit of coronary artery bypass grafting: role of off-pump surgery. *J Thorac Cardiovasc Surg* 2008; 136:29-36.

94. Magee MJ, Hebert E, Herbert MA, et al: Fewer grafts performed in off-pump bypass surgery: patient selection or incomplete revascularization? *Ann Thorac Surg* 2009; 87:1113-1118.

95. Khan NE, De Souza A, Mister R, et al: A randomized comparison of off-pump and on-pump multivessel coronary-artery bypass surgery. *N Engl J Med* 2004; 350:21-28.

96. Nathoe HM, van Dijk D, Jansen EW, et al: A comparison of on-pump and off-pump coronary bypass surgery in low-risk patients. *N Engl J Med* 2003; 348:394-402.

97. Legare JF, Buth KJ, King S, et al: Coronary bypass surgery performed off pump does not result in lower in-hospital morbidity than coronary artery bypass grafting performed on pump. *Circulation* 2004; 109:887-892.

98. Puskas J, Cheng D, Knight J, et al: Off-pump versus conventional coronary artery bypass grafting: a meta-analysis and consensus statement from The 2004 ISMICS Consensus Conference. *Innovations* 2005; 1:3-27.

99. Puskas JD, Kilgo PD, Kutner M, et al: Off-pump techniques disproportionately benefit women and narrow the gender disparity in outcomes after coronary artery bypass surgery. *Circulation* 2007; 116:I192-199.

100. Magee MJ, Alexander JH, Hafley G, et al: Coronary artery bypass graft failure after on-pump and off-pump coronary artery bypass: findings from PREVENT IV. *Ann Thorac Surg* 2008; 85:494-499.

101. Hattler B, Messenger JC, Shroyer AL, et al: Off-Pump coronary artery bypass surgery is associated with worse arterial and saphenous vein graft patency and less effective revascularization: Results from the Veterans Affairs Randomized On/Off Bypass (ROOBY) trial. *Circulation* 2012; 125:2827-2835.

102. Zhang B, Zhou J, Li H, et al: Comparison of graft patency between off-pump and on-pump coronary artery bypass grafting: an updated meta-analysis. *Ann Thorac Surg* 2014; 97:1335-1341.

103. Hillis LD, Smith PK, Anderson JL, et al: 2011 ACCF/AHA Guideline for Coronary Artery Bypass Graft Surgery: executive summary: a report of the American College of Cardiology Foundation/American Heart Association Task Force on Practice Guidelines. *Circulation* 2011; 124:2610-2642.

104. Kolh P, Windecker S, Alfonso F, et al: 2014 ESC/EACTS Guidelines on myocardial revascularization: the Task Force on Myocardial Revascularization of the European Society of Cardiology (ESC) and the European Association for Cardio-Thoracic Surgery (EACTS). Developed with the special contribution of the European Association of Percutaneous Cardiovascular Interventions (EAPCI). *Eur J Cardiothorac Surg* 2014; 46:517-592.

105. Vassiliades TA Jr, Douglas JS, Morris DC, et al: Integrated coronary revascularization with drug-eluting stents: immediate and seven-month outcome. *J Thorac Cardiovasc Surg* 2006; 131:956-962.

106. Vassiliades TA, Kilgo PD, Douglas JS, et al: Clinical outcomes after hybrid coronary revascularization versus off-pump coronary artery bypass. *Innovations* 2009; 4:299-306.

107. Blazek S, Rossbach C, Borger MA, et al: Comparison of sirolimus-eluting stenting with minimally invasive bypass surgery for stenosis of the left anterior descending coronary artery: 7-year follow-up of a randomized trial. *JACC Cardiovasc Interv* 2015; 8:30-38.

108. Benedetto U, Raja SG, Soliman RF, et al: Minimally invasive direct coronary artery bypass improves late survival compared with drug-eluting stents in isolated proximal left anterior descending artery disease: a 10-year follow-up, single-center, propensity score analysis. *J Thorac Cardiovasc Surg* 2014; 148:1316-1322.

109. Lapierre H, Chan V, Sohmer B, et al: Minimally invasive coronary artery bypass grafting via a small thoracotomy versus off-pump: a case-matched study. *Eur J Cardiothorac Surg* 2011; 40:804-810.

110. Ruel M, Shariff MA, Lapierre H, et al: Results of the Minimally Invasive Coronary Artery Bypass Grafting Angiographic Patency Study. *J Thorac Cardiovasc Surg* 2014; 147:203-208.

111. Halkos ME, Liberman HA, Devireddy C, et al: Early clinical and angiographic outcomes after robotic-assisted coronary artery bypass surgery. *J Thorac Cardiovasc Surg* 2014; 147:179-185.

112. Srivastava S, Gadasalli S, Agusala M, et al: Use of bilateral internal thoracic arteries in CABG through lateral thoracotomy with robotic assistance in 150 patients. *Ann Thorac Surg* 2006; 81:800-806.

113. Bonaros N, Schachner T, Lehr E, et al: Five hundred cases of robotic totally endoscopic coronary artery bypass grafting: predictors of success and safety. *Ann Thorac Surg* 2013; 95:803-812.

114. Harskamp RE, Bagai A, Halkos ME, et al: Clinical outcomes after hybrid coronary revascularization versus coronary artery bypass surgery: a meta-analysis of 1190 patients. *Am Heart J* 2014; 167: 585-592.

115. Harskamp RE, Puskas JD, Tijssen JG, et al: Comparison of hybrid coronary revascularization versus coronary artery bypass grafting in patients ≥65 years with multivessel coronary artery disease. *Am J Cardiol* 2014; 114:224-229.

116. Halkos ME, Vassiliades TA, Douglas JS, et al: Hybrid coronary revascularization versus off-pump coronary artery bypass grafting for the treatment of multivessel coronary artery disease. *Ann Thorac Surg* 2011; 92:1695-1701.

117. Harskamp RE, Brennan JM, Xian Y, et al: Practice patterns and clinical outcomes after hybrid coronary revascularization in the United States: an analysis from the society of thoracic surgeons adult cardiac database. *Circulation* 2014; 130:872-879.

118. Lapar DJ, Mery CM, Kozower BD, et al: The effect of surgeon volume on mortality for off-pump coronary artery bypass grafting. *J Thorac Cardiovasc Surg* 2012; 143:854-863.

119. Takagi H, Umemoto T: All-Literature Investigation of Cardiovascular Evidence (ALICE) Group. Worse long-term survival after off-pump than on-pump coronary artery bypass grafting. *J Thorac Cardiovasc Surg* 2014; 148:1820-1829.

Myocardial Revascularization after Acute Myocardial Infarction

22

Deane E. Smith III • Mathew R. Williams

Acute myocardial infarction (MI) affects approximately 1.5 million individuals each year in the United States.[1] Of these patients, 30% die before reaching the hospital and another 5% die during their hospital admission.[1] Since 1998, the death rate from cardiovascular disease has declined 30.6%; however, cardiovascular disease remains the leading cause of death in the United States.[2] Prompt medical attention including transport to the hospital, diagnosis, and treatment of the MI is critical to patient survival. Over the past 40 years, many developments have led to a decrease in the overall morbidity and mortality associated with acute MI. These developments include new pharmacologic agents, advancement in interventional cardiology procedures, modifications of coronary artery bypass surgical techniques, and the development of treatment algorithms and guidelines. Despite these advances, mechanical and electrical complications such as cardiogenic shock, rupture of the ventricular septum or free wall, acute mitral regurgitation, pericarditis, tamponade, and arrhythmias continue to challenge the medical community caring for patients presenting with acute MI on a daily basis.[3] Of these complications, cardiogenic shock complicating acute MIs has the most significant impact on in-hospital mortality and long-term survival. The loss of more than 40% of functioning left ventricular mass and its accompanying systemic inflammatory response are the major causes of cardiogenic shock. Factors that impact the development of cardiogenic shock include the degree of pre-infarct ventricular dysfunction, the size of the infarcted vessel, and pathologic level of inflammatory mediators.[4,5] Revascularization of threatened myocardium offers the best chance of survival following acute coronary occlusion, but the technique and timing of revascularization continue to evolve. The available therapies that can decrease the mortality associated with acute MIs include thrombolytics, percutaneous coronary intervention (PCI), and coronary artery bypass graft (CABG) surgery.

PATHOGENESIS OF ACUTE OCCLUSION

Myocardial ischemia resulting from coronary occlusion causes ischemic zone changes from a state of active systolic shortening to one of passive systolic lengthening within 60 seconds of onset of ischemia.[6] Occlusions for less than 20 minutes usually cause reversible cellular damage and depressed function with subsequent myocardial stunning. Furthermore, reperfusion of the infarct results in variable amounts of salvageable myocardium. After 40 minutes of ischemia followed by reperfusion, 60 to 70% of the ultimate infarct is salvageable, but this decreases to approximately 10% after 3 hours of ischemia.[7,8] Evidence from animal model has also demonstrated that 6 hours of regional ischemia produces extensive transmural necrosis.[9] The exact timing in humans is more difficult to analyze because of collateral flow, which is a major determinant of myocardial necrosis in the area at risk in humans.[8] The collateral blood supply is extremely variable, especially in patients with long-standing coronary disease. In addition, collateral flow is jeopardized with arrhythmias, hypotension, or the rise of left ventricular end-diastolic pressure above tissue capillary pressure.[7] Thus, loss of collateral flow to the infarct area may lead to the cellular death of salvageable myocardium, and control of blood pressure and prevention of arrhythmias are vital during this time immediately after infarction.

Table 22-1 outlines the effects of anatomic, physiologic, and therapeutic variables on the evolution of final infarct size.

STATES OF IMPAIRED MYOCARDIUM

Infarcted Myocardium

Disruption of coronary perfusion can result in three states of impaired myocardium: infarcted, hibernating, and stunned. Each state has a unique cause of injury and carries different prognostic implications (Table 22-2). Infarcted myocardium

TABLE 22-1: Factors That Influence the Evolution and Severity of Acute Myocardial Infarction

Anatomic
  Site of lesion
  Size of myocardium at risk
  Collateral circulation
Physiologic
  Arrhythmias
  Coronary perfusion pressure
  Myocardial oxygen consumption
  Reperfusion injury
  Stunned myocardium
Therapeutic options
  Medical management
  Revascularization
  Thrombolysis
Percutaneous coronary angioplasty
  Coronary artery surgery
  Controlled reperfusion
  Buckberg solution and technique
  Mechanical circulatory support

has suffered irreversible myocardial cell death owing to prolonged ischemia and will not benefit from revascularization.

Hibernating Myocardium

Hibernating myocardium is a state of impaired myocardial and left ventricular function at rest resulting from reduced coronary blood flow and impaired coronary vasodilator reserve that can be restored to normal if a normal myocardial oxygen supply-demand relationship is reestablished.[10] Hibernating myocardium is defined as contractility-depressed myocardial function secondary to severe chronic ischemia that improves clinically immediately after myocardial revascularization. This may be acute or chronic. Carlson and associates[11] showed that hibernating myocardium was present in up to 75% of patients with unstable angina and 28% with stable angina. The entity also occurs after MI. Angina after MI commonly occurs at a distance from the area of infarction.[12]

TABLE 22-2: States of Myocardial Cells after Periods of Ischemia

Condition	Viability of cells	Cause of injury	Return of function
Infarcted	Nonviable	Prolonged ischemia	No recovery
Stunned viable	Limited ischemia	Delayed with reperfusion	Recovery
Hibernating	Viable	Ongoing ischemia	Prompt, sometimes unpredictable recovery

In fact, mortality is significantly higher in patients with ischemia at a distance (72%) compared with ischemia adjacent to the infarct zone (33%).[12] It is the hibernating myocardium that may be in jeopardy and salvageable, although its presence is usually incidental to the occurrence of the acute infarction. By distinguishing between hibernating myocardium and irreversibly injured myocardium, a more focused approach to restoring or improving blood flow to the area at risk is possible. Ventricular function often improves immediately after revascularization of appropriately selected regions.

Stunned Myocardium

Stunned myocardium is left ventricular dysfunction without cell death that occurs following restoration of blood flow after an ischemic episode. The phrase was initially coined by Braunwald and Kloner in 1982.[13] If a patient survives the insult resulting from a temporary period of ischemia followed by reperfusion, the previously ischemic areas of cardiac muscle eventually demonstrate improved contractility. Stunning can be a fully reversible process despite the severity and duration of the insult if the cells remain viable. Within 60 seconds of coronary occlusion, the ischemic zone changes from a state of active shortening to one of passive shortening. Coronary occlusions lasting less than 20 minutes provide the classic model of the stunning phenomenon.[14] The most likely mechanisms of myocardial stunning are listed in Table 22-3.[14,15]

Stunned myocardium can occur adjacent to necrotic tissue after prolonged coronary occlusion and can be associated with demand-induced ischemia, coronary spasm, and cardioplegia-induced cardiac arrest during cardiopulmonary bypass. Pathologically, these regions are edematous, and even hemorrhagic, and can clinically present as both systolic and diastolic dysfunction.[16] They also have a propensity for arrhythmias, which can lead to more extensive stunning and hypotension with subsequent infarction of these regions.

The primary distinction between stunned and hibernating myocardium is that in the former blood flow has been re-established after total occlusion whereas in the latter, coronary artery obstruction and reduced blood flow are still present.[7]

TABLE 22-3: Mechanisms of Contractile Dysfunction after Myocardial Stunning

Generation of oxygen-derived free radicals*
Excitation-contraction uncoupling due to sarcoplasmic reticulum dysfunction
Calcium overload
Insufficient energy production by mitochondria
Impaired energy use by myofibrils
Impairment of sympathetic neural responsiveness
Impairment of myocardial perfusion
Damage of the extracellular collagen matrix
Decreased sensitivity of myofilaments to calcium

*Regarded as the primary mechanism of myocardial stunning.
Adapted with permission from Bolli R: Mechanism of myocardial "stunning"
Circulation. 1990 Sep;82(3):723-738.

DIAGNOSIS OF VIABLE MYOCARDIUM

Mechanisms to identify patients with myocardial stunning and hibernation include electrocardiogram (ECG) findings, radionuclide imaging, positron emission tomography (PET), dobutamine echocardiography, and more recently magnetic resonance imaging (MRI). Thallium identifies perfusion-related defects of the myocardium and can distinguish between viable and scarred myocardium as well. However, early redistribution of thallium does not distinguish between hibernating and scarred myocardium because many segments with irreversible defects by thallium improve after reperfusion. Redistribution imaging and reinjection imaging improve the predictive value of thallium imaging in distinguishing hibernating myocardium.

PET measures the metabolic activity of myocardial cells. It has high positive and negative predictive values. It is now regarded as the best method to determine myocardial viability, particularly in patients with severe left ventricular dysfunction in whom other modalities are less accurate.[17]

Dobutamine echocardiography identifies hibernating and stunned myocardium by monitoring changes in segmental wall motion while the heart is stressed inotropically and chronotropically by dobutamine infusion. It has high specificity, sensitivity, and more importantly, positive predictive value.[18]

MRI has also been established as an effective method to assess hibernating myocardium.[19] It has been proven to accurately diagnose the degree of both acute and chronic MI and predict functional recovery.[20,21] A number of advantages exist with cardiac MRI, such as superior image resolution allowing accurate identification of transmural infarction (Fig. 22-1). By providing morphologic, functional, and metabolic information, it may ultimately supplant other modalities for the diagnosis of cardiac injury and recovery.

Finally, multislice computed tomography has been used to measure hibernating myocardium, and early data suggest it

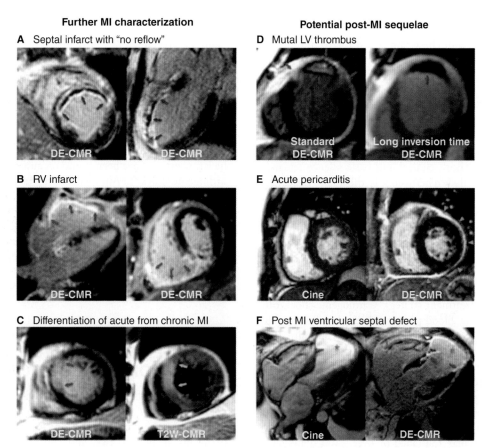

FIGURE 22-1 Cardiovascular MRI (CMR) characterization of myocardial infarction (MI) and post-myocardial infarction sequelae. Examples are shown of patients with myocardial infarction complicated by the presence of (A) microvascular damage (no reflow, *purple arrows*), and (B) right ventricular involvement (*red arrows*). (C) Acute infarcts (*red arrows*) can be differentiated from chronic infarcts by the use of T2-weighted imaging, which can show increased signal in areas of acute necrosis (*green arrows*). (D) Post-MI sequelae such as mural thrombus (*blue arrows*) can be identified by delayed-enhancement-CMR. Long-inversion-time imaging may improve detection because the image intensity of viable myocardium is gray rather than black. Thrombus is often immediately adjacent to infarcted myocardium (*red arrows*). (E) Acute pericarditis can be diagnosed by the presence of hyperenhanced pericardium (*orange arrowheads*). (F) CMR image may be used to define ventricular septal defect location (*orange stars*), extent of associated infarction (*red arrows*), and severity of shunting. (Reproduced with permission from Kim HW, Farzaneh-Far A, Kim RJ: Cardiovascular magnetic resonance in patients with myocardial infarction: current and emerging applications, *J Am Coll Cardiol.* 2009 Dec 29;55(1):1-16.)

may be a reliable and sensitive method compared with MRI, although its use in clinical practice is limited.[22]

MEDICAL MANAGEMENT OF MYOCARDIAL INFARCTION

Initial management of patients presenting with acute MI requires rapid diagnosis and assignment into the appropriate treatment algorithm. Treatment strategies should be directed toward reducing myocardial oxygen demand, maintaining circulatory support, and protecting the threatened myocardium before irreversible damage and expansion of the infarct occur.

Patients presenting with ongoing chest pain and ST-segment elevation in two contiguous leads or new left bundle branch block or anterolateral ST depression are classified as having ST-segment elevation myocardial infarction (STEMI). These patients are referred for primary revascularization, typically with fibrinolytics or percutaneous intervention in the cardiac catheterization suite, as immediately as possible assuming no contraindications exist. The other group of patients, those with non-ST-segment elevation myocardial infarction (NSTEMI), present with chest pain at rest for 10 minutes or more and ST-segment depression greater than 0.5 mm or ST-segment elevation 0.6 to 1 mm or T-wave inversions greater than 1 mm or positive troponin levels. Alternatively, there is a history of unstable angina in a patient with coronary artery disease risk factors. The initial management of these patients includes a combination of antiplatelet therapy, intravenous heparin, and other medications with a less urgent plan for cardiac catheterization. Both clinical and basic science research have demonstrated that reperfusion is the main treatment option for acute MI. Unfortunately, the majority of patients with MI receive only conservative medical management; only 40% of patients having an acute MI receive thrombolytic therapy, the most common means of reperfusion.[23]

Patients who present with STEMI can be further categorized by the presence or absence of cardiogenic shock. This distinction is important as it clearly predicts patient outcome, and it will impact treatment strategy. Cardiogenic shock can be defined as a systolic blood pressure of less than 90 mm Hg that is secondary to myocardial dysfunction. Clinically, it is associated with signs of hypoperfusion including decreased urine output, altered mental status, and peripheral vasoconstriction with cool extremities. Hemodynamic parameters consistent with cardiogenic shock include a cardiac index less than 2.2 L/min/m^2, stroke volume index less than 20 mL/m^2, mean pulmonary capillary wedge pressure greater than 18 mm Hg, and a systemic vascular resistance of over 2400 dyn-s/cm^5. These patients are defined as type IV by the Killip classification system, a widely used system to classify MIs.[24]

Shock is the most common cause of in-hospital mortality after MI.[25] The in-hospital mortality associated with cardiogenic shock has remained unchanged at approximately 80% despite the development of new treatment modalities.[26] Since 1975, the incidence of cardiogenic shock complicating

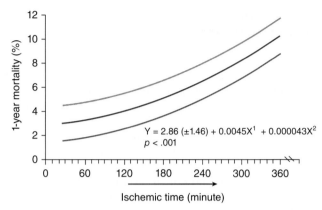

FIGURE 22-2 Relationship between time to treatment and 1-year mortality, as a continuous function, was assessed with a quadratic regression model. Dotted lines represent 95% confidence intervals of predicted mortality. (Reproduced with permission from De Luca G, Suryapranata H, Ottervanger JP, et al: Time delay to treatment and mortality in primary angioplasty for acute myocardial infarction: every minute of delay counts, *Circulation.* 2004 Mar 16;109(10):1223-1225.)

acute MIs has remained constant at 7.5%, ranging between 5 and 15% (Fig. 22-2).[25] The progressive reduction in time delay from symptom onset to treatment may account for these constant figures. Previously, patients with excessive time delays would have died before reaching the hospital or soon thereafter, as treatment delays increase 1-year mortality exponentially (Fig. 22-2).[27]

Shock is directly related to the extent of the myocardium involved, and infarctions resulting in loss of at least 40% of the left ventricle have been found on autopsy in patients with cardiogenic shock.[4,28] Autopsy findings also revealed marginal extension of the recent infarct and focal areas of necrosis in patients with cardiogenic shock.[4] Extensive three-vessel disease is usually found in individuals with cardiogenic shock, and extension of the infarct is an important determinant in those individuals.[4,28] Thus, limiting the size of the infarct and preventing its extension are the primary goals of therapeutic interventions in patients with MI.

RATIONALE FOR AGGRESSIVE MANAGEMENT OF MYOCARDIAL INFARCTION-REPERFUSION

Randomized trials have shown beneficial effects of early reperfusion within 12 hours and possibly up to 24 hours after acute MI.[11,24,26,29] Early reperfusion clearly reduces infarct size in the major areas at risk, and controlled reperfusion may even be superior. The arguments are more difficult to make for patients outside the 24-hour window; however, patients with ongoing ischemia often have ischemic border regions that are prone to arrhythmias and necrosis. In addition, these patients are at risk for prolonged periods of hypotension with resulting end-organ injury and further left ventricular dysfunction. The benefit to early revascularization may be greatest in those patients with cardiogenic shock. Even if revascularization does not appear critical, ventricular unloading with intra-aortic balloon pump (IABP) or left ventricular assist device (LVAD) may provide the bridge to recovery needed in patients dying after MI. The primary factors limiting an aggressive surgical approach are major comorbidities, which make continuation of life undesirable or unlikely, and an unclear neurologic status, especially after a period of cardiopulmonary arrest.

Although restoration of blood flow to ischemic regions is essential, the accompanying reperfusion injury initially can worsen rather than improve myocardial dysfunction. The area at risk is affected not only by reperfusion but also by the conditions of reperfusion and the composition of the reperfusate.[30] Thus, controlling reperfusion itself may aid in reducing myocardial infarct size and ventricular injury. At the cellular level, myocardial ischemia results in a change in energy production from aerobic metabolism to anaerobic metabolism. The consequences of ischemia vary from decreased adenosine triphosphate production and increased intracellular calcium to decreased amino acid precursors such as aspartate and glutamate. These changes can be reversed only by reperfusion. However, as oxygen is reintroduced into an ischemic region, oxygen free radical generation ensues with resulting cellular damage. Cellular swelling and/or contracture can lead to a "no-reflow phenomenon" that limits the recovery of some myocytes and possibly results in irreversible injury of others. The production of oxygen free radicals during ischemia, and at the time of reperfusion, is the leading mechanism proposed to explain cellular injury. Four basic types of reperfusion injury have been described: lethal cell death, microvascular injury, stunned myocardium, and reperfusion arrhythmias (Table 22-4).

Buckberg and coworkers[31-36] conducted studies of controlled reperfusion after ischemia and produced a clinical application for controlled reperfusion. The surgical strategy of controlled reperfusion includes several elements. First, extracorporeal circulation is established as expeditiously as possible with venting of the left ventricle as required. Initially, antegrade cardioplegia is delivered using either a warm Buckberg solution to rebuild adenosine triphosphate stores or cold high-potassium cardioplegia to achieve rapid diastolic arrest. Retrograde cardioplegia can be added to ensure global cooling, even in areas of active ischemia. The temperatures of the anterior and inferior walls of the ventricle are measured to ensure adequate cooling. After each distal anastomosis, cold cardioplegia is infused into each graft and the aorta at 200 mL/min over 1 minute. This is followed by retrograde infusion through the coronary sinus for 1 minute. After completion of the final distal anastomosis, warm substrate-enriched blood cardioplegia is given at 150 mL/min for 2 minutes into each anastomosis and the aorta. After removal of the aortic cross-clamp, regional blood cardioplegia is given at 50 mL/min into the graft supplying the region at risk for 18 minutes. This controlled rate of reperfusion minimizes cellular edema and myocyte damage. The proximal vein grafts are then completed, followed by reestablishment of normal blood flow. To decrease oxygen demand, the heart is allowed to beat in an empty state for 30 minutes. After this time, the patient is weaned off bypass.

Application of the Buckberg solution and technique has been shown to be effective in improving mortality rates and myocardial function after acute coronary occlusion. With ischemic times averaging 6 hours, a prevalence of multivessel disease, and cardiogenic shock, the overall mortality in patients with acute coronary occlusion who underwent surgical revascularization applying this method of reperfusion was 3.9%. Postoperative ejection fraction averaged 50%.[37] Surgical revascularization in this manner using controlled reperfusion compared favorably with percutaneous transluminal coronary angioplasty (PTCA) in several large series. These principles are reflected primarily in the surgical management of acute MI and will be outlined more specifically later in the chapter.

METHODS OF REPERFUSION

Once a patient who is a candidate for reperfusion therapy has been identified there are essentially three options available to the practitioner. They include thrombolytic therapy, primary PCI, and CABG. The intervention chosen for any particular patient will undoubtedly reflect the services that are available at the time of presentation, but they should also conform to the recommendations outlined by the ACCF/AHA guidelines including its most recent update in 2013.[38] The following is a review of the available therapies, their roles, and the data that exist to support their use.

Role of Thrombolytic Therapy

Because myocardial salvage depends on reperfusion of occluded coronary arteries, rapid dissolution of an occluding thrombus with thrombolytic therapy is an appealing intervention. Intracoronary streptokinase in patients with acute MI demonstrated that thrombolytic therapy is a safe and efficient way to achieve the desired early reperfusion.[39] Following this study, a number of multi-institutional mega-atrials showed the effectiveness of thrombolytic therapy in

---

⬤ **TABLE 22-4: Potential Types of Reperfusion Injury**

Lethal	Cell death secondary to reperfusion
Vascular	Progressive damage causes an expanding zone of "no reflow" and deterioration of coronary flow reserve during the phase of reperfusion
Reperfusion arrhythmias	Arrhythmias, mainly ventricular, that occur shortly after reperfusion
Stunned myocardium	Postischemic ventricular dysfunction

Adapted with permission from Kloner RA: Does reperfusion injury exist in humans? *J Am Coll Cardiol.* 1993 Feb;21(2):537-545.

treating acute MIs. The trial of the Italian Group for the Study of Streptokinase in Myocardial Infarction (Gruppo Italiano per lo Studio della Streptochinasi nell'Infarto Miocardio [GISSI])[40] and the Second International Study of Infarct Survival [ISIS-2][41] found a reduced hospital mortality in patients treated with streptokinase. The effectiveness of tissue-type t-PA also has been evaluated in randomized studies. The Thrombolysis in Myocardial Infarction (TIMI) study[42] and the European Cooperative Study Group[43] demonstrated the effectiveness of t-PA for the treatment of acute MI. When streptokinase and t-PA were compared, two studies failed to demonstrate any difference in mortality.[44,45] A third study, however, the Global Utilization of Streptokinase and Tissue Plasminogen Activator for Occluded Coronary Arteries (GUSTO) trial, supported the use of t-PA by demonstrating a more rapid and complete restoration of coronary flow that resulted in improved ventricular performance and reduce mortality.[46,47]

Although thrombolysis improves survival and ventricular function the patency of infarct-related arteries is reported to be between 50 and 85%.[40-47] Normal flow should be achieved in 60% of patients by today's standards. Thrombolytic therapy works well but is not without complications, including bleeding and intracranial hemorrhage.[48] Bleeding is usually minor and occurs mostly at the sites of vascular puncture. Intracranial hemorrhage and stroke rates are approximately 1%. The relative benefits of thrombolytic therapy appear to decrease as patient age increases, and a higher risk of intracranial hemorrhage in the elderly may partially account for these findings.[46,49,50] Careful selection of patients suitable for fibrinolyitc therapy is warranted, especially in an increasingly older population.

Thrombolytic therapy for patients presenting in cardiogenic shock or heart failure does not appear to improve survival in this population but may decrease the incidence of patients developing heart failure after MI.[51]

In summary, studies evaluating the effectiveness of thrombolytic therapy have demonstrated several useful points. First, survival is improved by decreasing time to reperfusion. The GUSTO trial showed that patients treated within the first hour had the greatest improvement in survival, with a 1% reduction in mortality for each hour of time saved.[46,47] Thrombolytic therapy is easy to administer in the community by trained personnel, although a significant risk of bleeding exists in certain patients. Because the time to reperfusion is a critical element in preserving myocardium, thrombolytic therapy is ideal for most communities without percutaneous interventional capabilities. The importance of these elements is evidenced by two points made in the updated ACCF/AHA guidelines. First, in the absence of contraindications, fibrinolytic therapy should be administered to patients with STEMI at non-PCI-capable hospitals when the anticipated first medical contact (FMC)-to-device time at a PCI-capable hospital exceeds 120 minutes because of unavoidable delays.[38] Second, when fibrinolytic therapy is indicated or chosen as the primary reperfusion strategy, it should be administered within 30 minutes of hospital arrival.[38]

Role of Percutaneous Coronary Intervention

Since the first reported PTCA by Gruntzig and associates[52] in 1979, the efficacy of this percutaneous intervention in the treatment of coronary artery disease has been well recognized. A number of studies have evaluated the efficacy of primary PTCA in the treatment of acute MI. The overall PTCA hospital mortality rates range from 6 to 9%.[53-56] Initial experience utilizing only balloon angioplasty was termed PTCA. One of the areas of technological advancement has been the development of new percutaneous therapies. These options include not only implantation of intracoronary stents, but also rotational atherectomy, directional atherectomy, extraction atherectomy, and laser angioplasty. In the current era, these techniques collectively are referred to as PCI. Here, we will use the term PTCA to relate data from studies limited to angioplasty, and the term PCI to accurately describe trials and studies that involve one or more of these additional techniques. This is consistent with the approach taken by the authors of 2001 ACCF/AHA Guidelines for PCI, which was a revision of the 1993 PTCA Guidelines.[57]

Several different strategies employing PCI for acute MI have been developed and examined through clinical trials. Primary, rescue, immediate, delayed, and elective PCI are options for the treatment of acute MI. Primary PCI uses percutaneous intervention as the method of reperfusion in patients presenting with acute MI. Rescue, immediate, delayed, and elective PCI are all done in conjunction with or following thrombolytic therapy. Rescue PCI is performed for recurrent angina or hemodynamic instability after thrombolytic therapy. Immediate PCI is performed in conjunction with thrombolytic therapy, and delayed PCI occurs during the intervening hospitalization. Finally, elective PCI is done following thrombolytic therapy and medical management when a positive stress test is obtained during the same hospitalization or soon thereafter.

Several studies evaluated the role of PTCA compared with thrombolytic therapy. The first study, the Primary Angioplasty in Myocardial Infarction Study Group trial in 1993, concluded that immediate PTCA without thrombolytics reduced occurrence of reinfarction and death and was associated with a lower rate of intracranial hemorrhage.[53] Since then, more than 20 studies have compared PTCA to thrombolysis. The results from these studies have consistently and conclusively demonstrated the superiority of PTCA to thrombolysis, regardless of the thrombolytic agent used. The findings include a lower short-term mortality rate, lower rates of reinfarction, reduced stroke and intracranial hemorrhage rates, and a decreased composite end point of death, reinfarction, and stroke.[58] These findings have been reconfirmed on long-term follow-up. A higher overall rate of bleeding was observed, likely because of vascular access complications. Myocardial salvage is similar for PTCA and thrombolytic therapy. However, primary PTCA may be slightly less costly than thrombolytic therapy.[54]

The use of intracoronary stents after MI has expanded as PTCA has become more prevalent. Benefits of stenting include lowered rates of restenosis and abrupt closure, and a reduced need for target revascularization after PTCA. Although the STENT-PAMI trail in 1999 using first-generation stents showed lower restenosis rates compared with thrombolysis, a trend toward higher mortality was seen, and its effectiveness as first-line therapy was questioned.[59] Composite end points of death, reinfarction, and urgent target vessel revascularization at 30 days have now been shown to be lower in subsequent studies, such as the CADILLAC, ISAR-2, and ADMIRAL trials, which employed newer-generation stents.[60-62] In these trials, a glycoprotein (GP) IIb/IIIa inhibitor, abciximab, was added to primary stenting. A significant reduction in restenosis rates with stenting plus abciximab versus PTCA alone was evident at 12-month follow-up in the CADILLAC study (41 vs 22%).[60] More recent data suggest that stenting combined with antiplatelet therapy provides superior benefit to PTCA alone. Drug-eluting stents offer the potential to lower restenosis rates even further through the use of anti-inflammatory medication delivered via the stent. More recently, patients in the STRATEGY trial treated with drug-eluting stents after acute STEMI had a significantly lower composite end point of death, reinfarction, stroke, and angiographic evidence of restenosis at 8-month follow-up compared with bare-metal stenting plus abciximab (50 vs 19%).[63] Using propensity score matching, retrospective analysis of patients post-acute MI in Massachusetts has shown a slight 2-year mortality benefit for drug-eluting stents when compared with bare-metal stents (10.7 vs 12.8%), as well as a lower need for repeat revascularization.[64] Further prospective studies are under way to determine if long-term data confirm these findings.

The optimal pharmacotherapy for these patients continues to be debated and is an area of ongoing investigation. Initial experience with heparin was believed to be improved by the addition of GP IIb/IIIa inhibitors.[65] However, routine use of GP IIb/IIIa inihibitors has fallen out favor, and current guidelines recommend limiting their use to high-risk situations. The HORIZONS-AMI (Harmonizing Outcomes with Revascularization and Stents in Acute Myocardial Infarction) trial[66,67] compared bivalirudin, a direct thrombin inhibitor, with heparin plus a GP IIb/IIIa inhibitor for use after primary PTCA with or without stenting. The data disclosed decreased 30-day major bleeding events, death from cardiac causes, and death from all causes, despite a higher 24-hour risk of stent thrombosis in the bivalirudin cohort. Interestingly the mortality benefit persisted after 3-year follow-up. Since this trial, there have been several changes in management strategy including newer antiplatelets, increased radial access, and decreased use of GPIIb/IIIa inhibitors. A similar trial comparing bivalirudin to heparin plus GP IIb/IIIa inhibitors, the EUROMAX trial, demonstrated a decrease in incidence of major bleeding at 30 days but no difference in mortality or reinfarction.[68] More recently, results of the HEAT PPCI (How Effective are Antithrombotic Therapies in Primary PPCI) trial were released. This was an open-label, randomized trial of STEMI patients which compared heparin with bivalirudin and used GP IIb/IIIa inhibitors only in

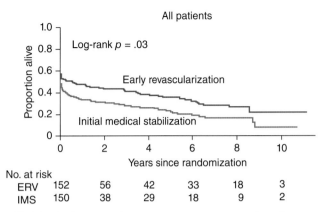

FIGURE 22-3 Revascularization rates in patients with cardiogenic shock at presentation (n = 7356). (Reproduced with permission from Babaev A, Frederick PD, Pasta DJ, et al: Trends in management and outcomes of patients with acute myocardial infarction complicated by cardiogenic shock, *JAMA* 2005 Jul 27;294(4):448-454.)

bail out situations. Heparin was associated with a significant reduction in the major cardiovascular end points of all-cause mortality, cerebrovascular accidents, reinfarction, and target vessel revascularization (5.7 vs 8.7%, $p = .01$).[69] In addition, there was no significant difference in the rate of major bleeding (3.5 vs 3.1%, $p = .59$). This study, along with others (NAPLES III, BRAVE IV), have raised significant questions regarding the benefit to using bivalirudin as opposed to heparin.[70,71]

Primary PCI may play a greater role in patients presenting in cardiogenic shock, as percutaneous interventions have become more common over the past 10 years (Fig. 22-3). The GISSI-1 and GISSI-2 trials demonstrated no benefit from intravenous thrombolysis, with morality rate of 70%.[40,44] In patients presenting in or developing cardiogenic shock after acute MI, PTCA improved survival to 40 to 60%.[72] This improvement was even greater when angioplasty was successful, as in-hospital survival rates increased to 70%. In most of these series an IABP was used in conjunction with PTCA. The SHOCK trial showed that revascularization by PTCA or CABG within 12 hours of the onset of cardiogenic shock results in improved 1- and 6-year survival rates versus medical stabilization followed by delayed revascularization (32.8 for PTCA/CABG vs 19.6% for initial medical stabilization, 6-year follow-up) in this high-risk group, particularly for those under the age of 75 years (Fig. 22-4).[11,26,29] Subgroup analysis in patients undergoing successful PTCA or with TIMI Grade 3 coronary flow after PTCA in the SHOCK trial revealed that 1-year survival was even higher, at 61%.[73] Independent predictors of mortality include age, hypotension, lower TIMI flow, and multivessel PTCA.

In conclusion, specialized centers that have 24-hour catheterization facilities can provide primary PCI as a first-line therapy for patients with acute MI. Patients with established or developing cardiogenic shock should be revascularized early by PCI rather than initial medical stabilization with thrombolytic therapy. Rescue PCI after failed thrombolytic

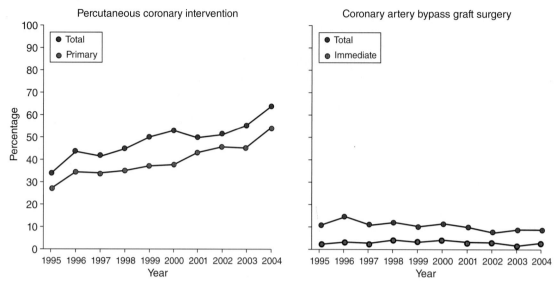

FIGURE 22-4 Survival estimates for early revascularization (n = 152) and initial medical stabilization (n = 150) groups in the SHOCK trial. Log-rank test, *p* = .03. (Reproduced with permission from Hochman JS, Sleeper LA, White HD, et al: One-year survival following early revascularization for cardiogenic shock, *JAMA*. 2001 Jan 10;285(2):190-192.)

therapy for patients with ongoing ischemia or clinical compromise is also recommended. Finally, elective PCI should be performed on patients who have recurrent or provokable angina before hospital discharge.

Role of Coronary Artery Bypass Grafting

The role of surgical revascularization in the treatment of acute MI has changed considerably over the past 30 years. During the 1980s, reports appeared recommending surgical revascularization in preference to medical therapy for acute MI.[74,75] Mortality rates under 5% were reported. Critics argued that these studies lacked randomization or consecutive entry of patients, preoperative stratification was absent, and enzyme levels were not included. Inherent bias that favored surgery in low-risk patients was believed to be the reason for the excellent outcomes.[76] At the time these reports surfaced, thrombolytic therapy and interventional cardiology were emerging as alternative options for patients with acute infarctions. With the availability of thrombolytics and PCI, large multicenter trials began looking at the efficacy and usefulness of these two techniques. Randomized trials using CABG were not done, and thus this option was never established as an alternative for acute MI. Despite this, several centers continued to use surgical revascularization to treat acute MI with excellent results. However, practical, logistic, and economic constraints relegate surgical revascularization to a third option behind thrombolytics and PCI for the primary treatment of acute MI.

There continue to be several scenarios that require emergent or urgent surgical revascularization. Failure of thrombolytics or PCI with acute occlusion may require surgical intervention. Additionally, CABG for post-infarction angina has become a critical step in the pathway of treating acute MI. Finally, surgical revascularization may be indicated in

patients with multivessel disease or left main coronary artery disease developing cardiogenic shock after MI.

Timing after Infarction

If surgical revascularization within 6 hours after the onset of symptoms is feasible, the mortality rate is improved over that of medically treated, nonrevascularized patients.[74,75] Although these early studies were not controlled and were criticized for selection bias,[76] they did demonstrate that surgical revascularization may be performed with an acceptable mortality in the presence of acute MI with improved myocardial protection, anesthesia, and surgical techniques. However, with the advent of thrombolytic therapy, PCI, and an aging population, the surgical patient we encounter today bears little resemblance to the patient population represented in these early studies.

Previous analyses of the New York State Cardiac Surgery Registry, which included every patient undergoing a cardiac operation over more than a decade in the state of New York, resulted in valuable information regarding the optimal timing of CABG in acute MI. In this large and contemporary patient population, there is a significant correlation between hospital mortality and time interval from acute MI to time of operation, particularly if CABG was performed within 1 week of acute MI. In addition, patients with transmural and nontransmural acute MI have different trends in mortality when the time course is taken into consideration. Mortality for the nontransmural group peaked if the operation was performed within 6 hours of acute MI, and then decreased precipitously (Table 22-5).[77] On the other hand, mortality for the transmural group remained high during the first 3 days before returning to baseline.[78] Multivariate analyses confirmed that CABG within 6 hours for the nontransmural group and 3 days for the transmural group were independently associated

TABLE 22-5: Comparison of Hospital Mortality with Respect to Time of Surgery—Transmural versus Nontransmural Myocardial Infarction

Time between CABG and MI	Mortality	
	Transmural MI (%)	Nontransmural MI (%)
<6 h	14	13
6-23 h	14*	6*
1-7 days	5	4
>7 days	3	3

*p < .01 nontransmural versus transmural.
Data from the New York State Cardiac Surgery Registry, which included every patient undergoing a cardiac operation in the last decade in the state of New York.

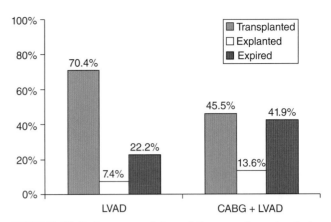

FIGURE 22-5 Outcomes of direct left ventricular assist device (LVAD) implantation versus coronary artery bypass graft (CABG) followed by LVAD implantation for cardiogenic shock. (Reproduced with permission from Dang NC, Topkara VK, Leacche M, et al: Left ventricular assist device implantation after acute anterior wall myocardial infarction and cardiogenic shock: a two-center study, *J Thorac Cardiovasc Surg*. 2005 Sep;130(3):693-698.)

with increased in-hospital mortality.[77,78] Optimal timing of CABG in patients with acute MI remains a controversial subject. Early surgical intervention has the advantage of limiting the infarct expansion and ventricular remodeling that may result in possible ventricular aneurysm and rupture.[79] However, there is the theoretical risk of reperfusion injury, which may lead to hemorrhagic infarction resulting in extension of infarct size, poor infarct healing, and scar development.[80] The data from these studies caution against early surgical revascularization, particularly within 3 days of onset, among patients with acute transmural MI.

Some have advocated the use of mechanical support to stabilize the patient and allow elective rather than emergent surgery.[81,82] Delaying CABG with "prophylactic" mechanical support in an effort to improve outcome, however, may result in placement of such support in some situations where it is unnecessary. If revascularization cannot be delayed, aggressive mechanical support (such as an LVAD) should be available because mortality is most likely a result of pump failure. Furthermore, mechanical circulatory support (MCS) has been shown to be efficacious as a bridge to ventricular recovery or transplantation for this patient cohort.[82] This approach is supported by results from a multicenter study, in which overall survival at 6 and 12 months was higher in patients who underwent direct LVAD implantation rather than revascularization followed by LVAD, in patients suffering cardiogenic shock (Fig. 22-5).[83] Although emergent cases such as structural complications and ongoing ischemia clearly cannot be delayed, nonemergent cases, particularly patients with transmural acute MI, may benefit from delay of surgery. Early surgery after transmural acute MI has a significantly higher risk and surgeons should be prepared to provide aggressive cardiac support including LVADs in this ailing population.

Risk Factors

In addition to timing of surgery as discussed, risk factors include urgency of the operation, increasing patient age, renal insufficiency, number of previous MIs, hypertension,[84]

reoperation, cardiogenic shock, depressed left ventricular function, and the need for cardiopulmonary resuscitation, left main disease, female gender, left ventricular wall motion score, need for IABP, and transmural infarction.[85] Characteristics associated with better early outcome after MI include preservation of left ventricular ejection fraction, male gender, younger patients, and subendocardial versus transmural MI.

Cardiogenic Shock

Surgical revascularization in acute MI complicated by cardiogenic shock has been shown to improve survival. Cardiogenic shock is accompanied by 80 to 90% mortality rates. The various mechanisms of cardiogenic shock in acute MI are shown in Fig. 22-6. DeWood and colleagues[86] were the first to demonstrate improved results with revascularization in patients with cardiogenic shock complicating acute MI. Patients who were stabilized with an IABP and underwent emergent surgical revascularization had survival rates of 75%. Early surgical revascularization was associated with survival rates of 40 to 88% in patients in cardiogenic shock from nonmechanical causes. Guyton and coworkers[87] reported an 88% in-hospital survival and a 3-year survival of 88%, with no late deaths reported.

Furthermore, the SHOCK trial demonstrated survival benefit in early revascularization by CABG or PTCA within 12 hours of the diagnosis of cardiogenic shock for patients of all ages.[11,29] Patients comprising the CABG cohort in the SHOCK trial had more severe disease, with higher rates of three-vessel disease, left main coronary artery disease, diabetes, and elevated mean coronary jeopardy scores than the PTCA cohort.[88] Despite this, 87.2% of these patients achieved successful and complete revascularization with CABG, compared with successful revascularization in 77.2% with PTCA and only 23.1% with complete revascularization with PTCA. Overall,

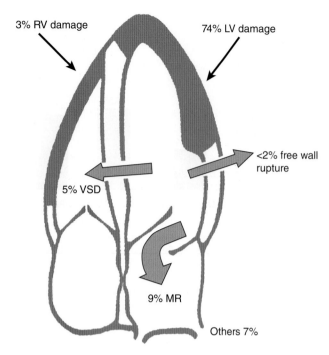

FIGURE 22-6 Mechanisms of cardiogenic shock. Apical four-chamber echo view with relative incidence of the mechanisms responsible for cardiogenic shock in the SHOCK and MILIS 4 registries. LV = left ventricle; MR = mitral regurgitation; RV = right ventricle; VSD = ventricular septal defect. (Reproduced with permission from Davies CH: Revascularization for cardiogenic shock, *QJM.* 2001 Feb;94(2):57-67.)

mortality was no different between groups at 1 year (Fig. 22-7). On subgroup analysis, patients older than age 75 years, with left main coronary disease or three-vessel disease, or with diabetes had trends toward better survival at 30 days and 1 year after CABG compared to PTCA. Thus, for patients in cardiogenic shock, surgical revascularization remains an established and viable option for select patient groups.

Advantages of Coronary Artery Bypass Grafting

Reported survival rates are similar for CABG and PCI in the treatment of acute MI. To date, there have been no large, randomized clinical trials comparing CABG with PCI and thrombolytics after MI. For patients with stable angina and elective revascularization for ischemic heart disease, a number of trials have been conducted comparing CABG with stenting.[89-92] In these studies, trends favoring CABG for multivessel disease were seen after 2 years in composite cardiac event end points, rate of reinfarction, and mortality; revascularization rates were five times higher in the stenting group.[93] Most notably, survival after CABG for two or more diseased vessels was significantly higher than stenting with 2-year follow-up in a retrospective study of the New York Cardiac Surgery Reporting System and Percutaneous Coronary Intervention Reporting System.[94] These results must be interpreted with

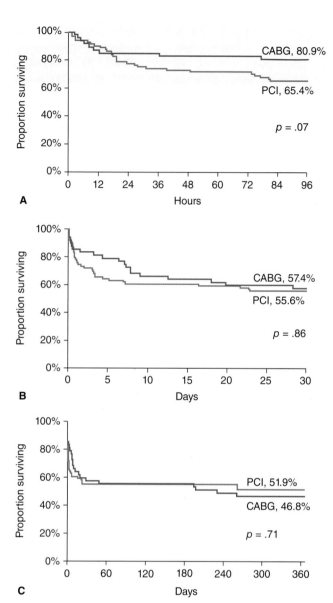

FIGURE 22-7 Kaplan-Meier survival estimates at 96 hours (A), 30 days (B), and 1 year (C) in patients treated with emergency percutaneous coronary intervention (PCI) versus emergency coronary artery bypass graft (CABG) in the SHOCK trial. (Reproduced with permission from White HD, Assmann SF, Sanborn TA, et al: Comparison of percutaneous coronary intervention and coronary artery bypass grafting after acute myocardial infarction complicated by cardiogenic shock: results from the Should We Emergently Revascularize Occluded Coronaries for Cardiogenic Shock (SHOCK) trial, *Circulation.* 2005 Sep 27;112(13):1992-2001.)

caution; however, as patients with acute infarctions less than 24 hours pretreatment were excluded. Because of the lack of prospective, randomized trials, recommendations must be based on retrospective and observational studies.

CABG does offer a few potential advantages. First, surgical revascularization is the most definitive form of treatment of the occlusion. CABG offers the longest patency of revascularized stenotic and occluded arteries; in elective cases, more than 90% of internal mammary artery grafts are patent at 10 years.

Second, CABG also offers more complete revascularization, because all vessel lesions are treated. This concept becomes especially important in patients with multivessel disease or those in cardiogenic shock, in whom remote myocardium may continue to be comprised with only "culprit vessel" revascularization and inadequate restoration of collateral flow.[95] A complete revascularization restores global myocardial perfusion to normal levels and offers the best chance for myocardial salvage. Finally, there is the opportunity for controlled reperfusion to reverse ischemic injury and reduce reperfusion injury.

Summary

Surgical revascularization following acute MI can be performed with excellent results when the timing and patient cohort are appropriate. Most patients do not need such measures and would not benefit from this aggressive form of therapy. However, patients with mechanical complications, those in cardiogenic shock, and those with post-infarction angina are likely to benefit from early CABG.

OPERATIVE TECHNIQUES FOR ACUTE MYOCARDIAL INFARCTION

Anesthesia

Anesthesia is provided by a rapid narcotics-based regimen with perfusion and surgical teams prepared to respond to catastrophic hypotension or cardiac arrest. Transesophageal echo probes are placed in these patients if possible.

Bleeding

Bleeding is a significant complication of emergency CABG and can result in further myocardial depression and pulmonary hypertension. Cytokine release induced by infusion of blood products and thromboxane A2 released as a result of cardiopulmonary bypass stimulate pulmonary hypertension, which can be catastrophic in the setting of right ventricular ischemia. Use of antifibrinolytics, such as aminocaproic acid, for re-operative, emergency, or high-risk CABG is common in many institutions.

The use of clopidogrel deserves special mention, and its expanding administration can pose unique problems for the cardiac surgeon. Clopidogrel, an oral, irreversible antagonist of the 5'-adenosine diphosphate that inhibits platelet activation and aggregation, is used extensively in patients with acute coronary syndromes and has been shown to lower cardiovascular risk by up to 20% and reduce reinfarction and stroke rates.[96,97] In addition, it is commonly given before percutaneous interventions and after intracoronary stenting to prevent thrombosis. Higher loading doses have been used with increasing efficacy against ischemic complications, which will likely expand its use in the future.[98] However, patients frequently require surgical revascularization after medical therapy or cardiac catheterization while taking

clopidogrel. The risk of bleeding after clopidogrel and cardiac surgery can be substantial. In multiple reports, the risk of reoperation for hemorrhage in patients receiving clopidogrel within 7 days of cardiac surgery was six times higher, and patients required more blood, platelet, and fresh-frozen plasma transfusions.[99,100] Because of these complication rates and the inability to reverse the drug's effect on platelets, surgery is often delayed until platelet function is restored, which may take up to 7 days, or the life of the platelets. Emergent surgery while taking clopidogrel often necessitates blood product transfusions and confers significant morbidity, and possibly mortality. Ongoing work continues in an effort to determine if current dosing regimens after acute MI can be reduced to lessen bleeding complications.

Choice of Conduits

For emergency cases, the choice of conduit should usually not differ from elective cases in most circumstances. The internal mammary artery is not associated with a higher number of complications compared with saphenous vein grafting in emergent situations and can be used in most circumstances.[101,102]

Intraoperative Considerations

Decompression of the ventricle during revascularization after acute coronary occlusion decreases muscle damage and improves functional outcome by decreasing wall tension and reducing oxygen consumption (Figs. 22-8 and 22-9).[36] In fact, ventricular decompression reduces metabolic energy consumption by 60%. Diastolic basal arrest, by avoiding the energy of contraction, is the second most important means of minimizing oxygen consumption and further reduces metabolic energy consumption by 30%. Cooling of the patient and heart has an impact on the final 10% of basal energy requirements. Reduction of myocardial energy consumption is best

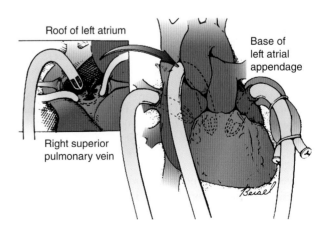

FIGURE 22-8 The inflow cannula for short-term left ventricular assist device support can be placed through the right superior pulmonary vein, the dome of the left atrium, or the left atrial appendage. Lighthouse tip cannulas allow improved venous return.

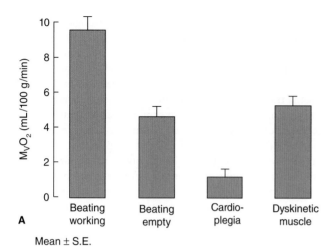

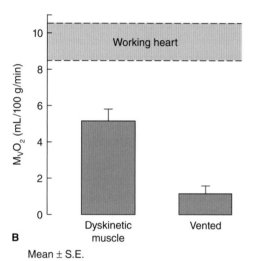

FIGURE 22-9 (A) Myocardial oxygen uptake (MvO$_2$), measured in milliliters per 100 grams per minute, in beating and working, beating and empty, and arrested hearts. Values after cardioplegia were determined both during cardiopulmonary bypass (cardioplegia) and during regional cardioplegic reperfusion in the working heart (dyskinetic muscle). Note (1) marked fall in MvO$_2$ with cardioplegia in the decompressed heart and (2) oxygen requirements of dyskinetic muscle increase fivefold over cardioplegia alone, and equal almost 55% of beating, working needs. (B) Regional oxygen uptake during selective cardioplegic reperfusion in dyskinetic and vented cardiac muscle. Stippled areas show requirements in working heart (8.5-10.5 mL/100 g/min). Note (1) high oxygen demands of dykinetic muscle and (2) marked reduction in demands when noncontracting muscle is decompressed by venting. (Reproduced with permission from Allen BS, Rosenkranz ER, Buckberg GD, et al: High oxygen requirements of dyskinetic cardiac muscle, *J Thorac Cardiovasc Surg.* 1986 Sep;92(3 Pt 2):543-552.)

achieved by early institution of cardiopulmonary bypass to maintain a high perfusion pressure. If a coronary salvage catheter has been placed across a tight coronary lesion, the catheter is left in place until just before cross-clamping. Antegrade and retrograde cardioplegia catheters are placed before cross-clamping to allow quick instillation of retrograde cardioplegia and protection of the territory supplied by the occluded or

compromised vessel. The standard Buckberg protocol is followed, including warm induction to allow regeneration of depleted adenosine triphosphate stores. If the territory at risk is to be grafted by saphenous vein, this anastomosis is performed first to allow direct instillation of cardioplegia into the territory at risk. The proximal anastomoses should be performed before removal of the cross-clamp to allow complete perfusion of the entire heart upon removal of the cross-clamp.

Although large ventricular aneurysms are treated by resection and patch, debate surrounds smaller aneurysm. If an aneurysm is resected, the defect is repaired with a patch of bovine pericardium sewn to the fibrotic rim of the endoaneurysm surface. The native left ventricular wall is closed over the patch.

Utilization of the Dor procedure (endoventricular circular patch plasty repair) in the post MI setting is another controversial subject. Some data have shown that surgical remodeling improves systolic function, ejection fraction, and intraventricular dyssynchrony, whereas other data suggest no additional benefit when the Dor procedure is added to CABG.[103-106] Further investigation is needed to definitively answer this question.

Postoperative Care

A higher incidence of complications in shock patients compared with non-shock emergencies has been reported. Guyton and associates[87] report a 47% complication rate associated with cardiogenic shock compared with 13% for patients with non-shock emergencies. This increase in complications probably reflects the preoperative condition of the patients as much as the treatment itself. Long-term follow-up in patients after emergency surgical revascularization shows that survival rates are closely correlated with postoperative ejection fraction and left ventricular size.[107,108]

USE OF THE INTRA-AORTIC BALLOON PUMP

The early use of aortic counterpulsation with an IABP demonstrated the safety but not efficacy of this device for patients in cardiogenic shock following acute MI.[109] Although survival was not improved, aortic counterpulsation did improve the myocardial oxygen requirements and myocardial energetics were reduced in patients in shock.

Over the last several decades, multiple studies have been performed to help define the role for IABP in acute MI. Early reports demonstrated that aortic counterpulsation decreased the reocclusion rate, recurrent ischemia, and need for emergency PCI in patients who had coronary patency reestablished by emergency cardiac catheterization after acute MI.[110] Prophylactic counterpulsation for 48 hours sustained patency in these patients without increasing vascular or hemorrhagic complications.[110] However, additional randomized trials have been performed which have questioned the advantage of IABP in cardiogenic shock secondary to MI.[111] Recently, the ACC/AHA guidelines have downgraded the recommendation for IABP use in cardiogenic shock from a Class I to Class IIa recommendation.[38] The IABP-Shock II Trial randomized patients with cardiogenic shock complicating acute MI who were undergoing early revascularization and optimal medical therapy to IABP versus control.[112] The 30-day outcomes showed no survival benefit with IABP support. In addition, these patients were subsequently followed for 6-month and 12-month follow-up to determine the long-term impact of IABP support. There was no significant difference in mortality, reinfarction, repeat revascularization or stroke.[113]

For patients who undergo early revascularization, the empiric addition of aortic counterpulsation with an IABP will not improve the patient's outcome; however, the IABP remains a useful adjunct for patients who are awaiting revascularization or continue to show signs of ischemia after revascularization. Placement of an IABP is also reasonable in patients who remain in cardiogenic shock despite adequate revascularization and optimal medical management if it may aid in stabilizing a patient for more definitive therapy, that is, mechanical circulatory support (MCS). The use of IABP is also effective for temporary hemodynamic stabilization in complications of acute MI, such as ventricular septal rupture,[114] acute mitral valve insufficiency,[114] post-infarct angina,[115] ventricular arrhythmias,[116] and acute heart failure following infarction.[117]

ROLE OF MECHANICAL CIRCULATORY SUPPORT

One area of ongoing development involves the use of MCS for cardiogenic shock. Mechanical assist devices augment systemic perfusion and prevent end-organ damage while resting the stunned ventricle with complete or partial pressure-volume unloading.[118] Early studies of implantable LVADs have shown that end-organ function is an early predictor of mortality. Treatment of patients before end-organ deterioration is essential to improving the odds for long-term survival. In addition to affecting end-organ function, assist devices promote "reverse remodeling" by improving myocardial contractility and calcium handling, altering the extracellular matrix, and decreasing myocardial fibrosis.[119,120] Recent studies have shown that circulatory support early after MI improves survival and offers a feasible bridge to recovery or transplantation.[82,121] Although still in its early stages, many institutions are working to develop the optimal strategy for adding MCS to their treatment algorithms for ACS. There are essentially three categories of MCS available, and the choice of type of support depends on a number of variables.

VA-ECMO is one option available for MCS in acute MI patients. Its primary use is in cardiogenic shock or cardiac arrest after acute MI, as it can often be placed rapidly and without moving the patient. There may be additional benefits to inserting cannulas under fluoroscopic-guidance while the patient is in the cath lab. Because it can be performed expeditiously, it is a useful first-line MCS therapy for these patients.

Another option available in this situation is percutaneous VADs. These include the Impella 2.5, CP or 5.0 (Abiomed Europe GmbH, Aachen, German), the TandemHeart (Cardiac Assist, Pittsburgh, PA, USA), and the Hemopump (Johnson & Johnson, Racho Cordova, CA, USA). These are also devices that can be implanted percutaneously in the cath lab to augment cardiac output in patients undergoing post-infarct PCI. The TandemHeart provides up to 4 L/min of support, producing a higher mean blood pressure and cardiac output, and lowering pulmonary capillary wedge pressure.[122] Likewise, the Impella device can provide between 2.5 L/min and 5 L/min depending on the model, and in small series, may offer superior hemodynamic support when compared with an IABP.[123]

Finally, another more invasive option for mechanical support in post-MI patients involves implantable VADs. Again, there are multiple reports utilizing different types of VADs in this particular situation. These include ABIOMED ventricular support system (Abiomed, Inc., Danvers, MA, USA), the Thoratec paracorporeal system (pVAD), the Thoratec Centrimag Blood Pump (Thoratec Corp., Pleasnaton, CA, USA), and the Syncardia ventricular support system (Syn Cardia Systems, Inc., Tucson, AZ, USA). An important consideration when selecting a device is whether there is likely to be recovery of adequate ventricular function or not. If there is an expectation of recovery, or if the plan is for surgical revascularization at the time of ventricular support, then a temporary LVAD would be the more reasonable approach. If the patient is unable to be weaned from their temporary LVAD, then a long-term device remains an option. Likewise, if the patient's ventricular function is not expected to recover, and in particular, if there are no plans for revascularization, then proceeding with a long-term LVAD may be the best course. Another factor that is part of this algorithm is whether the patient is potentially a transplant candidate or not. There are many variables which may impact the feasibility of this strategy, and some of them are exclusive of the patient's overall condition. For example, the patient's gender, size, blood type, and local allocation limitations will all impact the expected waiting times, and may preclude transplant as a viable option without long-term mechanical support. The decision-making in these instances involves a multidisciplinary team to optimize resource utilization for these patients. Enthusiasm for using mechanical support to help patients survive their acute infarcts is growing at many institutions across the country. With the development and refinement of these techniques and the ability to fit the right strategy to the right patient, we expect outcomes to improve for this group of critically ill patients. A full discussion of short-term and long-term MCS is reported in Chapters 18 and 66.

SURGICAL MANAGEMENT

The use of MCS in the setting of an acute MI is continuing to evolve. Many patients with an acute MI requiring consideration for mechanical support are in a state of uncertainty. They are by definition, unstable, and many will have already received, or will be in the process of receiving CPR. The status of their end-organ function and their neurologic function is unclear. In these situations, one option is to utilize peripheral VA-ECMO in an attempt to stabilize the patient. This can usually be done in the catheterization lab either via a percutaneous or cut-down technique. Femoral artery and venous cannulas are placed and the patient is connected to the ECMO circuit. Flow is initiated to provide as much cardiac output as possible. With adequate flow to maintain a normal cardiac output, vasoactive medications, including pressors and inotropes, can be weaned. There are several advantages to this approach. First, it allows clinicians the opportunity to assess the patient's neurologic function before embarking on a more invasive procedure or long-term support. The patient can wake up and undergo a complete neurologic evaluation while on VA-ECMO support. This is most important for patients who have received CPR prior to initiation of MCS. Second, VA-ECMO preserves, and in some cases, allows recovery of the end-organ function as patients can typically be weaned off of inotropes and pressors entirely. Again, this is an important part of the algorithm as preserved end-organ function will greatly improve the likelihood that a patient will survive the additional steps needed to bridge the patient to recovery, a long-term LVAD, or transplantation. Initiation of peripheral VA-ECMO can also decompress the heart and allow an opportunity for recovery. With the heart decompressed, there is less wall tension and stress, primarily, on the right ventricle. Although there is increased afterload on the left ventricle with VA-ECMO, there are several strategies designed to decompress the left side and allow the myocardium to recover. An in-depth discussion regarding options to assist in decompressing the left ventricle on VA-ECMO is beyond the scope of this chapter, but these options include inotropes, IABP, Impella, and surgical vents.

If patients have survived the initial event with VA-ECMO support, then they can proceed to the next step which is an evaluation for signs of myocardial recovery and a determination of the need for long-term mechanical support (Fig. 22-10). The patients have usually already received a coronary angiogram, and if feasible, an attempt at PCI. If the myocardium has recovered the patients can be weaned from ECMO and decannulated. However, if they fail to wean, then a determination of their candidacy for a long-term LVAD or transplant is made. The decision to place a long-term LVAD is influenced by many factors, but can be summarized by their score on a screening scale designed for this purpose (Table 22-6). These scores were selected to identify end-organ dysfunction (lung, liver, or kidney) and operative constraints (right-sided heart failure and bleeding). Excellent results have been reported with nearly a 90% survival if the summed scores are less than 5 points, versus 30% survival with summed scores greater than 5 points.[124] For this reason, if the total score is greater than 5 points, an attempt is made to improve end-organ function before attempting long-term LVAD insertion.

These algorithms continue to be refined as experience with mechanical support grows. Utilizing a short-term option such as VA-ECMO or a nonimplantable LVAD to stabilize the

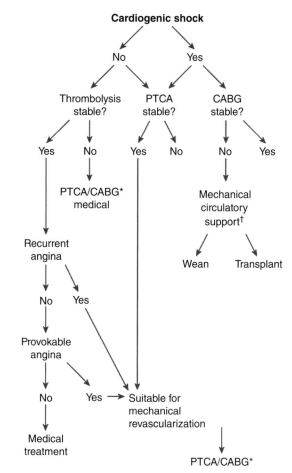

*PTCA = percutaneous transluminal coronary angioplasty; CABG = coronary artery bypass grafting. Choice of therapy is made based on the lesion(s) and comorbid factors.
†Choice of mechanical support is based on many factors (see text, along with other chapters).

FIGURE 22-10 Acute myocardial infarction algorithm.

patient, preserve their end-organs, and ensure adequate neurologic function has been an important advancement in the care of these critically ill patients. Identifying which patients will benefit most from implantation of long-term devices is an area of ongoing investigation.

TABLE 22-6: Preoperative Risk Scale for Left Ventricular Assist Device Placement*

Criteria	Points
Urine output < 30 cc/h	3
Intubated	2
Prothrombin time > 16 s	2
Central venous pressure > 16 mm Hg	2
Reoperation	1

*A combined score of >5 is associated with a 70% mortality risk.

CONSENSUS GUIDELINES

The initial evaluation and management of a patient suffering from a MI begins before the patient arrives to the hospital. First responders in the field are trained to perform the initial ECG, and initiate treatment algorithms based upon these findings and the overall condition of the patient. Throughout the literature, this point of contact marks the time of FMC, which will impact the steps that follow.

Based upon the definitions as previously stated, patients are categorized as either STEMI or NSTEMI. Patients who meet criteria for STEMI are evaluated for urgent or immediate reperfusion. Again, the approach for reperfusion will depend upon the patient's location and the medical resources available to them at their destination hospital.

The recent executive summary update to the STEMI guidelines has attempted to outline these issues (regional systems of STEMI care, reperfusion therapy, and time-to-treatment goals) with the following Class I recommendations[38]:

1. Performance of a 12-lead electrocardiogram (ECG) by emergency medical services personnel at the site of first medical contact (FMC) is recommended in patients with symptoms consistent with STEMI
2. Reperfusion therapy should be administered to all eligible patients with STEMI with symptom onset within the prior 12 hours
3. Primary PCI is the recommended method of reperfusion when it can be performed in a timely fashion by experienced operators
4. Emergency medical services transport directly to a PCI-capable hospital for primary PCI is the recommended triage strategy for patients with STEMI, with an ideal FMC-to-device time system goal of 90 minutes or less
5. Immediate transfer to a PCI-capable hospital for primary PCI is the recommended triage strategy for patients with STEMI who initially arrive at or are transported to a non-PCI-capable hospital, with an FMC-to-device time system goal of 120 minutes or less
6. In the absence of contraindications, fibrinolytic therapy should be administered to patients with STEMI at non-PCI-capable hospitals when the anticipated FMC-to-device time at a PCI-capable hospital exceeds 120 minutes because of unavoidable delays
7. When fibrinolytic therapy is indicated or chosen as the primary reperfusion strategy, it should be administered within 30 minutes of hospital arrival

An additional class IIa recommendation is as follows:

1. Reperfusion therapy is reasonable for patients with STEMI and symptom onset within the prior 12 to 24 hours who have clinical and/or ECG evidence of ongoing ischemia. Primary PCI is the preferred strategy in this population

These strategies are outlined in Fig. 22-10.

In summary, the initial decision making involves a determination of the expected time from FMC to revascularization by PCI. If the FMC-to-device time is expected to be greater than 120 minutes, then it is recommended that patients receive fibrinolytics. The next step in the algorithm was evaluated by the TRANSFER-AMI trial.[125] Here, patients who had received fibrinolytics were randomized to either standard treatment (which included rescue PCI, if required) or a strategy of immediate transfer to another hospital and PCI within 6 hours of fibrinolysis. At 30 days, patients assigned to routine early PCI had a statistically significant reduction in the incidence of the primary end point which was the composite of death, reinfarction, recurrent ischemia, new or worsening congestive heart failure, or cardiogenic shock (11.0 vs 17.2%).[125] Thus, this trial supports an aggressive approach to transferring patients for PCI even after receiving thrombolytics for an acute MI.

The same Executive Summary of STEMI Guidelines included recommendations regarding surgical therapy.[38]

Class I recommendations include:

1. Urgent CABG is indicated in patients with STEMI and coronary anatomy not amenable to PCI who have ongoing or recurrent ischemia, cardiogenic shock, severe heart failure, or other high-risk features
2. CABG is recommended in patients with STEMI at time of operative repair of mechanical defects

Class IIa recommendations include:

1. The use of mechanical circulatory support is reasonable in patients with STEMI who are hemodynamically unstable and require urgent CABG

Class IIb recommendations include:

1. Emergency CABG within 6 hours of symptom onset may be considered in patients with STEMI who do not have cardiogenic shock and are not candidates for PCI or fibrinolytic therapy

FUTURE THERAPIES AND TRENDS

Improving outcomes in patients suffering acute MI can occur through pharmacologic advances, optimization of existing practices, and application of new technology. Various medications have been described that reduce ischemic-reperfusion injury and limit infarct size in animal models, such as oxygen-derived free radical scavengers, folic acid, nitric oxide inhibitors, and others[126]; clinical study of these promising drugs will determine their efficacy. Reducing transport time to the hospital after the onset of symptoms and implementation of clinical guidelines have been the focus of many hospitals and emergency services. The increased number of local hospitals able to perform primary percutaneous interventions has meant quicker revascularization and thus improved outcomes.[27] In addition, the technology used to treat these patients continues to improve. New wires, catheters, balloons, and stents continue to be developed and improved upon compared with previous generations. Furthermore, the optimization of the medical treatment of these patients is an area of ongoing research and development. Improved antiplatelet and anticoagulation strategies are just one example. With more experience, widely available guidelines have been developed and published in an effort to standardize care for all patients across the country, regardless of where they present. This will also allow for better data collection and assessment and comparisons, and ultimately improvement in strategies.

Surgically, we continue to develop and improve our techniques for surgical revascularization. This includes advances in myocardial protection, and refinements in the cardiopulmonary bypass circuit to limit the physiologic insult of surgery. MCS has advanced greatly over the past 10 years, and pumps have become smaller, safer, less invasive, easier to use, and easier to implant. In addition, patients who remain in cardiogenic shock despite inotropes and revascularization are being identified as candidates for MCS. There is likely to be continuing review of the role of intra-aortic balloon counterpulsation in the management of STEMI with cardiogenic shock. Another area for investigation includes the optimal timing for surgical revascularization should percutaneous options fail or be unavailable. The availability of MCS backup, may allow for successful surgical revascularization and recovery in patients previously deemed not operative candidates because of their high surgical risk.

Finally, the rapidly emerging field of cellular therapy holds great promise for repair of damaged myocardium. A number of cell types, such as endothelial progenitor cells, mesenchymal stem cells, skeletal myoblasts, resident cardiac stem cells, and embryonic stem cells, are being investigated[127]; the optimal cell type, mode of delivery (intracoronary artery infusion, intravenous infusion, transendocardial injection, and transepicardial injection), and timing of administration have yet to be determined. Nevertheless, early clinical trials suggest that cellular therapy may offer benefits. One-year follow-up of 59 patients suffering acute MI in the TOPCARE-AMI trial who received either circulating progenitor cells or bone marrow-derived progenitor cells demonstrated increased cardiac function and reduced ventricular dimensions, without adverse events.[128] Precultured mesenchymal cells also offer great promise by allowing cells from an unrelated donor to be administered without the complications of an individual tissue harvest. The safety of these cells given intravenously after percutaneous revascularization in acute MI was recently published, and efficacy studies are ongoing.[129] Numerous other clinical trials are underway to address questions regarding mechanisms of benefit, cell viability, and dosing. Further randomized clinical trials will be required to establish outcome benefit.

Effective management of acute MI requires a well-coordinated plan that starts with first medical contact. Rapid diagnosis and transport to the appropriate institution in the first step. If the diagnosis is an ST-elevation MI, then the priority is reperfusion. Depending on the available resources, this will require transport to a facility with emergency-PCI capabilities. If this is not possible, then thrombolytics should be administered if there are not contraindications. If either of these options are not available, or are unsuccessful, the patient should undergo an evaluation for emergency CABG.

The initial management is the same in patients who are in cardiogenic shock; however, facilities managing these patients should have available means of providing additional support. If a reperfused patient remains in shock despite inotropes, pressors, and an IABP, consideration should be given to pursuing MCS.

REFERENCES

1. Crossman AW, D'Agostino HJ, Geraci SA: Timing of coronary artery bypass graft surgery following acute myocardial infarction: a critical literature review. *Clin Cardiol* 2002; 25:406.
2. Go AS, Mozaffarian D, Roger VL: Heart disease and stroke statistics—2013 update: a report from the American Heart Association. *Circulation* 2013; 127(1):e6-e245.
3. Goldberg RJ, Gore JM, Alpert JS, et al: Cardiogenic shock after acute myocardial infarction. *N Engl J Med* 1991; 325:1117.
4. Page DL, Caulfield JB, Kastor JA, et al: Myocardial changes associated with cardiogenic shock. *N Engl J Med* 1971; 285:133.
5. Hochman J: Cardiogenic shock complicating acute myocardial infarction: expanding the paradigm. *Circulation* 2003; 107:2998.
6. Tennant T, Wiggers CJ: Effect of coronary occlusion on myocardial contraction. *Am J Physiol* 1935; 112:351.
7. Jennings RB, Reimer KA: Factors involved in salvaging ischemic myocardium: effect of reperfusion of arterial blood. *Circulation* 1983; 68(Suppl I):I-25.
8. Schaper W: Experimental coronary artery occlusion, III: The determinants of collateral blood flow in acute coronary occlusion. *Basic Res Cardiol* 1978; 73:584.
9. Reimer KA, Jennings RB: The wavefront phenomenon of myocardial ischemic cell death, II: Transmural progression of necrosis within the framework of ischemic bed size (myocardium at risk) and collateral flow. *Lab Invest* 1979; 40:633.
10. Rahimtoola SH: The hibernating myocardium in ischemia and congestive heart failure. *Eur Heart J* 1993; 14 (Suppl A):22.
11. Carlson EB, Cowley MJ, Wolfgang TC, et al. Acute changes in global and regional rest left ventricular function after coronary angioplasty: comparative results in stable and unstable angina. *J Am Coll Cardiol* 1989; 13:1262-1269.
12. Schuster EH, Bulkley BH: Early post-infarction angina: ischemia at a distance and ischemia in the infarct zone. *N Engl J Med* 1981; 305:1101.
13. Topol EJ, Ellis SH, Califf RM, et al: Combined tissue-type plasminogen activator and prostacyclin therapy for acute myocardial infarction. *J Am Coll Cardiol* 1989; 14:877.
14. Bolli R: Mechanism of myocardial stunning. *Circulation* 1990; 82:723.
15. Marban E: Myocardial stunning and hibernation: the physiology behind the colloquialisms. *Circulation* 1991; 83:681.
16. Bolli R: Basic and clinical aspects of myocardial stunning. *Prog Cardiovasc Dis* 1998; 40:477.
17. Underwood SR, Bax JJ, vom Dahl J, et al: Imaging techniques for the assessment of myocardial hibernation. *Eur Heart J* 2004; 25:815.
18. Charney R, Schwinger ME, Cohen MV, et al: Dobutamine echocardiography predicts recovery of hibernating myocardium following coronary revascularization. *J Am Coll Cardiol* 1992; 19:176A.
19. Klein C, Nekolla SG, Bengel FM, et al: Assessment of myocardial viability with contrast-enhanced magnetic resonance imaging: comparison with positron emission tomography. *Circulation* 2002; 105:162.
20. Kim HW, Farzaneh-Far A, Kim RJ: Cardiovascular magnetic resonance in patients with myocardial infarction. *J Am Coll Cardiol* 2010; 55:1-16.
21. Gerber BL, Garot J, Bluemke DA, et al: Accuracy of contrast enhanced magnetic resonance imaging in predicting improvement of regional myocardial function in patients after acute myocardial infarction. *Circulation* 2002; 106:1083.
22. Manhken AH, Koos R, Katoh M, et al: Assessment of myocardial viability in reperfused acute myocardial infarction using 16-slice computed tomography in comparison to magnetic resonance imaging. *J Am Coll Cardiol* 2005; 45:2042.
23. Hennekens CH, O'Donnell CJ, Ridker PM, Marder VJ: Current issues concerning thrombolytic therapy for acute myocardial infarction. *J Am Coll Cardiol* 1995; 25(Suppl):18S.

24. Killip T 3rd, Kimball JT: Treatment of myocardial infarction in a coronary care unit: a two-year experience with 250 patients. *Am J Cardiol* 1972; 20:457.

25. Goldberg RJ, Gore JM, Alpert JS, et al: Cardiogenic shock after acute myocardial infarction. *N Engl J Med* 1991; 325:1117.

26. Hochman JS, Sleeper LA, Webb JG, et al: Early revascularization in acute myocardial infarction complicated by cardiogenic shock. SHOCK Investigators. Should we emergently revascularize occluded coronaries for cardiogenic shock? *N Engl J Med* 1999; 341:625.

27. De Luca G, Suryapranata H, Ottervanger JP, et al: Time delay to treatment and mortality in primary angioplasty for acute myocardial infarction. *Circulation* 2004; 109:1223.

28. Wackers FJ, Lie KI, Becker AE, et al: Coronary artery disease in patients dying from cardiogenic shock or congestive heart failure in the setting of acute myocardial infarction. *Br Heart J* 1976; 38:906.

29. Hochman JS, Sleeper LA, White HD, et al: One-year survival following early revascularization for cardiogenic shock. *JAMA* 2001; 285:190.

30. Buckberg GD: Studies of controlled reperfusion after ischemia, I. When is cardiac muscle damaged irreversibly? *J Thorac Cardiovasc Surg* 1986; 92:483.

31. Vinten-Johansen J, Buckberg GD, Okamoto F, et al: Studies of controlled reperfusion after ischemia. V. Superiority of surgical versus medical reperfusion after regional ischemia. *J Thorac Cardiovasc Surg* 1986; 92:525.

32. Vinten-Johansen J, Rosenkranz ER, Buckberg GD, et al: Studies of controlled reperfusion after ischemia. VI. Metabolic and histochemical benefits of regional blood cardioplegic reperfusion without cardiopulmonary bypass. *J Thorac Cardiovasc Surg* 1986; 92:535.

33. Allen BS, Buckberg GD, Schwaiger M, et al: Studies of controlled reperfusion after ischemia. XVI. Early recovery of regional wall motion in patients following surgical revascularization after eight hours of acute coronary occlusion. *J Thorac Cardiovasc Surg* 1986; 92:636.

34. Allen BS, Okamoto F, Buckberg GD, et al: Studies of controlled reperfusion after ischemia, XIII: Reperfusion conditions—critical importance of total ventricular decompression during regional reperfusion. *J Thorac Cardiovasc Surg* 1986; 92:605.

35. Allen BS, Okamoto F, Buckberg GD, et al: Studies of controlled reperfusion after ischemia, XII: effects of "duration" of reperfusate administration versus reperfusate "dose" on regional, functional, biochemical, and histological recovery. *J Thorac Cardiovasc Surg* 1986; 92:594.

36. Allen BS, Rosenkranz ER, Buckberg GD, et al: Studies of controlled reperfusion after ischemia. VII. High oxygen requirements of dyskinetic cardiac muscle. *J Thorac Cardiovasc Surg* 1986; 92:543.

37. Allen BS, Buckberg GD, Fontan FM, et al: Superiority of controlled surgical reperfusion versus percutaneous transluminal coronary angioplasty in acute coronary occlusion. *J Thorac Cardiovasc Surg* 1993; 105:864.

38. O'Gara PT, Kushner FG, Ascheim DD, et al: ACCF/AHA guideline for management of ST-elevation myocardial infarction: executive summary. *J Am Coll Cardiol* 2013; 61(4):485-510.

39. Rentrop P, Blanke H, Karsch KR, et al: Selective intracoronary thrombolysis in acute myocardial infarction and unstable angina pectoris. *Circulation* 1981; 63:307.

40. Gruppo Italiano per lo Studio della Streptokinasi: The effectiveness of intravenous thrombolytic treatment in acute myocardial infarction. *Lancet* 1986; 1:397.

41. ISSI-2 (Second International Study of Infarct Survival): Randomized trial of intravenous streptokinase, oral aspirin, both, or neither among 17187 cases of suspected acute myocardial infarction. *Lancet* 1988; 2:349.

42. The TIMI Study Group: Comparison of invasive and conservative strategies after treatment with intravenous tissue plasminogen activator in acute myocardial infarction. *N Engl J Med* 1989; 320:618.

43. Simons ML, Betriu A, Col J, et al: Thrombolysis with tissue plasminogen activator in acute myocardial infarction: no additional benefit from immediate percutaneous coronary angioplasty. *Lancet* 1988; 1:197.

44. Gruppo Italiano per lo Studio della Streptokinasi: GISSI-2: A factorial randomized trial of alteplase versus streptokinase and heparin versus no heparin among 12,490 patients with acute myocardial infarction. *Lancet* 1990; 336:65.

45. ISIS-3 (Third International Study of Infarct Survival): ISIS-3: A randomized comparison of streptokinase vs. tissue plasminogen activator vs. anistreplase and of aspirin plus heparin vs. aspirin alone among 41,299 cases of suspected acute myocardial infarction. *Lancet* 1993; 339:753.

46. The GUSTO Angiographic Investigators: The effects of tissue plasminogen activator, streptokinase, or both on coronary patency, ventricular function, and survival after acute myocardial infarction. *N Engl J Med* 1993; 329:1615.

47. The GUSTO Investigators: An international randomized trial comparing four thrombolytic strategies for acute myocardial infarction. *N Engl J Med* 1993; 329:673.

48. Rentrop KP: Restoration of antegrade flow in acute myocardial infarction: the first 15 years. *J Am Coll Cardiol* 1995; 25(Suppl):1S.

49. Anonymous: Indications for fibrinolytic therapy in suspected acute myocardial infarction: collaborative overview of early mortality and major morbidity results from all randomized trials of more than 1000 patients. *Lancet* 1994; 343:311.

50. Angeja BG, Rundle AC, Gurwitz JH, et al: Death or nonfatal stroke in patients with acute myocardial infarction treated with tissue plasminogen activator. *Am J Cardiol* 2001; 87:627.

51. Bates ER, Topol EJ: Limitations of thrombolytic therapy for acute myocardial infarction complicated by congestive heart failure and cardiogenic shock. *J Am Coll Cardiol* 1991; 18:1077.

52. Gruntzig AR, Senning A, Siegenthaler WE: Nonoperative dilation of coronary-artery stenosis, percutaneous transluminal coronary angioplasty. *N Engl J Med* 1979; 301(2):61-68.

53. Grines CL, Browne KF, Marco J, et al: A comparison of immediate angioplasty with thrombolytic therapy in acute myocardial infarction. *N Engl J Med* 1993;328:673.

54. Goldman L: Cost and quality of life: thrombolysis and primary angioplasty. *J Am Coll Cardiol* 1995; 25(Suppl):38S.

55. Topol EJ, Califf RM, George BS, et al: A randomized trial of immediate versus delayed elective angioplasty after intravenous tissue plasminogen activator in acute myocardial infarction. *N Engl J Med* 1987; 317:581.

56. Rogers WJ, Baim DS, Gore JM, et al: Comparison of immediate invasive, delayed invasive, and conservative strategies after tissue type plasminogen activator: results of the thrombolysis in myocardial infarction (TIMI) phase II-a trial. *Circulation* 1990; 81:1457.

57. Smith SC, Dove JT, Jacobs AK, et al: ACC/AHA guidelines for percutaneous coronary intervention (revision of the 1993 PTCA guidelines)—executive summary. *Circulation* 2001; 103:3019.

58. Keeley EC, Boura JA, Grines CL: Primary angioplasty vs. intravenous thrombolytic therapy for acute myocardial infarction. *Lancet* 2003; 361:13.

59. Grines CL, Cox DA, Stone GW, et al: Coronary angioplasty with or without stent implantation for acute myocardial infarction. Stent Primary Angioplasty in Myocardial Infarction Study Group. *N Engl J Med* 1999; 341:1949.

60. Stone GW, Grines CL, Cox DA, et al: Comparison of angioplasty with stenting, with or without abciximab, in acute myocardial infarction. *N Engl J Med* 2002; 346:957.

61. Neumann FJ, Kastrati A, Schmitt C, et al: Effect of glycoprotein IIb/IIIa receptor blockade with abciximab on clinical and angiographic restenosis rate after the placement of coronary stents following acute myocardial infarction. *J Am Coll Cardiol* 2000; 35:915.

62. Montalescot G, Barragan P, Wittenberg O, et al: Platelet glycoprotein IIb/IIIa inhibition with coronary stenting for acute myocardial infarction. *N Engl J Med* 2001; 344:1895.

63. Valgimigli M, Percoco G, Malagutti P, et al: STRATEGY Investigators: Tirofiban and sirolimuseluting stent vs. abciximab and bare-metal stent for acute myocardial infarction: a randomized trial. *JAMA* 2005; 293:2109.

64. Mauri L, Silbaugh TS, Garg P, et al: Drug-eluting or bare-metal stents for acute myocardial infarction. *N Engl J Med* 2009; 359:1330-1342.

65. DeLuca G, Suryapranata H, Stone GW, et al: Abciximab as adjunctive therapy to reperfusion in acute ST-segment elevation myocardial infarction: a meta-analysis of randomized trials. *JAMA* 2005; 293:1759-1765.

66. Mehran R, Lansky AJ, Wiztenbichler W, et al: Bivalirudin in patients undergoing primary angioplasty for acute myocardial infarction (HORIZONS-AMI): 1-year results of a randomised controlled trial. *Lancet* 2009; 374:1149-1159.

67. Stone GW, Wiztenbichler B, Guagliumi G, et al: Bivalirudin during primary PCI in acute myocardial infarction. *N Engl J Med* 2009; 358:2218-2230.

68. Steg PG, van't Hof A, Hamm CW, et al: Bivalirudin started during emergency transport for primary PCI. *N Engl J Med* 2013; 369:2207.

69. Shahzad A, Kemp I, Mars C, et al: Unfractionated heparin versus bivalirudin in primary percutaneous coronary intervention (HEAT-PPCI): an open-label, single centre, randomized controlled trial. *Lancet* 2014; 384:1849.

70. Briguori C, Visconti G, Focaccio A, et al: Novel approaches for preventing or limiting events (NAPLES III) trial: randomized comparison of bivalirudin versus unfractionated heparin in patients at high risk of bleeding undergoing elective coronary stenting through the femoral approach. Rationale and design. *Cardiovasc Drugs Ther* 2014; 28:273.

71. Schulz S, Richardt G, Laugwitz KL, et al: Prasugrel plus bivalirudin vs. clopidogrel plus heparin in patients with ST-elevation myocardial infarction. *Eur Heart J* 2014; 182:2285.

72. Lee L, Erbel R, Brown TM, et al: Multicenter registry of angioplasty therapy of cardiogenic shock: Initial and long-term survival. *J Am Coll Cardiol* 1991; 17:599.

73. Webb JG, Lowe AM, Sanborn TA, et al: Percutaneous coronary intervention for cardiogenic shock in the SHOCK Trial. *J Am Coll Cardiol* 2003; 42:1380.

74. Berg R Jr, Selinger SL, Leonard JJ, et al: Immediate coronary artery bypass for acute evolving myocardial infarction. *J Thorac Cardiovasc Surg* 1981; 81:493.

75. DeWood MA, Spores J, Berg R Jr, et al: Acute myocardial infarction: a decade of experience with surgical reperfusion in 701 patients. *Circulation* 1983; 68(Suppl II):II-8.

76. Spencer FC: Emergency coronary bypass for acute infarction: an unproved clinical experiment. *Circulation* 1983; 68(Suppl II):II-17.

77. Lee DC, Oz MC, Weinberg AD, et al: Optimal timing of revascularization: transmural versus nontransmural acute myocardial infarction. *Ann Thorac Surg* 2001; 71:1198.

78. Lee DC, Oz MC, Weinberg AD, et al: Appropriate timing of surgical intervention after transmural acute myocardial infarction. *J Thorac Cardiovasc Surg* 2003; 125:115.

79. Weiss JL, Marino N, Shapiro EP: Myocardial infarct expansion: recognition, significance and pathology. *Am J Cardiol* 1991; 68:35.

80. Roberts CS, Schoen FJ, Kloner RA: Effects of coronary reperfusion on myocardial hemorrhage and infarct healing. *Am J Cardiol* 1983; 52:610.

81. Creswell LL, Rosenbloom M, Cox JL, et al: Intraaortic balloon counterpulsation: patterns of usage and outcome in cardiac surgical patients. *Ann Thorac Surg* 1992; 54:11.

82. Chen JM, DeRose JJ, Slater JP, et al: Improved survival rates support left ventricular assist device implantation early after myocardial infarction *J Am Coll Cardiol* 1999; 33:1903.

83. Dang NC, Topkara VK, Leacche M, et al: Left ventricular assist device implantation after acute anterior wall myocardial infarction and cardiogenic shock: a two-center study. *J Thorac Cardiovasc Surg* 2005; 130:693.

84. Creswell LR, Moulton MJ, Cox JL, Rosenbloom M: Revascularization after acute myocardial infarction. *Ann Thorac Surg* 1995; 60:19.

85. Stuart RS, Baumgartner WA, Soule L, et al: Predictors of perioperative mortality in patients with unstable postinfarction angina. *Circulation* 1988; 78(Suppl I):I-163.

86. DeWood MA, Notske RN, Hensley GR, et al: Intraaortic balloon counterpulsation with and without reperfusion for myocardial infarction shock. *Circulation* 1980; 61:1105.

87. Guyton RA, Arcidi JM, Langford DA, et al: Emergency coronary bypass for cardiogenic shock. *Circulation* 1987; 76(Suppl V):V-22.

88. White HD, Assman SF, Sanborn TA, et al: Comparison of percutaneous coronary intervention and coronary artery bypass grafting after acute myocardial infarction complicated by cardiogenic shock. *Circulation* 2005; 112:1992.

89. Serruys PW, Unger F, Sousa JE, et al (Group ARTS): Comparison of coronary-artery bypass surgery and stenting for the treatment of multivessel disease. *N Engl J Med* 2001; 344:1117.

90. Rodriguez AE, Baldi J, Pereira CF, et al: Five-year follow-up of the Argentine randomized trial of coronary angioplasty with stenting versus coronary artery bypass surgery in patients with multiple vessel disease (ERACI II). *J Am Coll Cardiol* 2005; 46:582.

91. Eefting F, Nathoe H, van Dijk D, et al: Randomized comparison between stenting and off-pump bypass surgery in patients referred for angioplasty. *Circulation* 2003; 108:2870.

92. SoS Investigators: Coronary artery bypass surgery versus percutaneous coronary intervention with stent implantation in patients with multivessel coronary artery disease (the Stent or Surgery trial): a randomised controlled trial. *Lancet* 2002; 360:965.

93. Bakhai A, Hill RA, Dickson R, et al: Percutaneous transluminal coronary angioplasty with stents versus coronary artery bypass grafting for people with stable angina or acute coronary symptoms. *Cochrane Database Syst Rev* 2005; 1:1-54.

94. Hannan EL, Racz MJ, Walford G, et al: Long-term outcomes of coronary artery bypass grafting versus stent implantation. *N Engl J Med* 2005; 352:2174.

95. Gersh BJ, Frye RL: Methods of coronary revascularization—things may not be as they seem. *N Engl J Med* 2005; 352:2235.

96. CURE Study Investigators: The Clopidogrel in Unstable angina to prevent Recurrent Events (CURE) Trial Pr Programme. *Eur Heart J* 2000; 21:2033.

97. Harker LA, Boisset JP, Pilgrim AJ, et al: Comparative safety and tolerability of clopidogrel and aspirin: results from CAPRIE. CAPRIE Steering Committee and Investigators. Clopidogrel vs. Aspirin in Patients at Risk of Ischaemic Events. *Drug Saf* 1999; 21:325.

98. Dangas G, Mehran R, Guagliumi G, et al: Role of clopidogrel loading dose in patients with st-segment elevation myocardial infarction undergoing primary angioplasty. *J Am Coll Cardiol* 2009; 54:1438-1446.

99. Hongo R, Ley J, Dick S, et al: The effect of clopidogrel in combination with aspirin when given before coronary artery bypass grafting. *J Am Coll Cardiol* 2002; 40:231.

100. Kapetanakis EI, Medlam DA, Boyce SW, et al: Clopidogrel administration prior to coronary artery bypass grafting surgery: the cardiologist's panacea or the surgeon's headache? *Eur Heart J* 2005; 26:576.

101. Caes FL, Van Nooten GJ: Use of internal mammary artery for emergency grafting after failed coronary angioplasty. *Ann Thorac Surg* 1994; 57:1295.

102. Zaplonski A, Rosenblum J, Myler RK, et al: Emergency coronary artery bypass surgery following failed balloon angioplasty: role of the internal mammary artery graft. *J Cardiac Surg* 1995; 10:32.

103. Di Donato M, Sabatier M, Dor V, et al: Effects of the Dor procedure on left ventricular dimension and shape and geometric correlates of mitral regurgitation one year after surgery. *J Thorac Cardiovasc Surg* 2001; 121:91.

104. Athanasuleas CL, Buckberg GD, Stanley AWH, et al: Surgical ventricular restoration in the treatment of congestive heart failure due to postinfarction ventricular dilation. *J Am Coll Cardiol* 2004; 44:1439.

105. DiDonato MD, Toso A, Dor V, et al: Surgical ventricular restoration improves mechanical intraventricular dyssynchrony in ischemic cardiomyopathy. *Circulation* 2004; 109:2536.

106. Jones RH, Velazquez EJ, Michler RE, et al: Coronary bypass surgery with or without surgical ventricular reconstruction. *N Engl J Med* 2009; 309:1705-1717.

107. Applebaum R, House R, Rademaker A, et al: Coronary artery bypass grafting within thirty days of acute myocardial infarction. *J Thorac Cardiovasc Surg* 1991; 102:745.

108. Hochberg MS, Parsonnet V, Gielchinsky I, et al: Timing of coronary revascularization after acute myocardial infarction. *J Thorac Cardiovasc Surg* 1984; 88:914.

109. Scheidt S, Wilner G, Mueller H, et al: Intra-aortic balloon counterpulsation in cardiogenic shock. *N Engl J Med* 1973; 288:979.

110. Ohman EM, George BS, White CJ, et al: Use of aortic counterpulsation to improve sustained coronary artery patency during acute myocardial infarction. *Circulation* 1994; 90:792.

111. Ohman EM, Nanas J, Stomel RJ, et al: Thrombolysis and counterpulsation to improve survival in myocardial infarction complicated by hypotension and suspected cardiogenic shock or heart failure: results of the TACTICS trial. *J Thrombosis Thrombolysis* 2005; 19:33.

112. Thiele H, Zeymer U, Neumann FJ, et al: Intra-aortic balloon support for myocardial infarction with cardiogenic shock. *N Engl J Med* 2012; 307:1287.

113. Thiele H, Zeymer U, Neumann FJ, et al: Intra-aortic balloon counterpulsation in acute myocardial infarction complicated by cardiogenic shock (IABP-Shock II): final 12 month results of a randomized, open-label trial. *Lancet* 2013; 328:1638.

114. Mueller HS: Role of intra-aortic counterpulsation in cardiogenic shock and acute myocardial infarction. *Cardiology* 1994; 84:168.

115. Gold HK, Leinbach RC, Sanders CA, et al: Intra-aortic balloon pumping for control of recurrent myocardial ischemia. *Circulation* 1973; 47:1197.

116. Fotopoulos GD, Mason MJ, Walker S, et al: Stabilisation of medically refractory ventricular arrhythmias by intra-aortic balloon counterpulsation. *Heart* 1999; 82:96.

117. Stone GW, Ohman EM, Miller MF, et al: Contemporary utilization and outcomes of intra-aortic balloon counterpulsation in acute myocardial infarction. *J Am Coll Cardiol* 2003; 41:1940.

118. Ratcliffe MB, Bavaria JE, Wenger RK, et al: Left ventricular mechanics of ejecting postischemic hearts during left ventricular circulatory assistance. *J Thorac Cardiovasc Surg* 1991; 101:245.

119. Heerdt PM, Holmes JW, Cai B, et al: Chronic unloading by left ventricular assist device reverses contractile dysfunction and alters gene expression in end-stage heart failure. *Circulation* 2000; 102:2713.

120. Zafeiridis A, Jeevanandam V, Houser SR, et al: Regression of cellular hypertrophy after left ventricular assist device support. *Circulation* 1998; 98:656.

121. Mancini DM, Beniaminovitz A, Levin H, et al: Low incidence of myocardial recovery after left ventricular assist device implantation in patients with chronic heart failure. *Circulation* 1998; 98:2383.

122. Thiele H, Lauer B, Hambrecht R, et al: Reversal of cardiogenic shock by percutaneous left atrial-to-femoral artery bypass assistance. *Circulation* 2001; 104:2917-2922.

123. Seyfarth M, Sibbing D, Bauer I, et al: A randomized clinical trial to evaluate the safety and efficacy of a percutaneous left ventricular assist device versus intra-aortic balloon pumping for treatment of cardiogenic shock caused by myocardial infarction. *J Am Coll Cardiol* 2008; 52:1584-1588.

124. Oz MC, Pepino P, Goldstein DJ, et al: Selection scale predicts patients successfully receiving long-term, implantable left ventricular assist devices. *Circulation* 1994; 90:I-308.

125. Cantor WJ, Fitchett D, Borgundvaag B, et al: Routine early angioplasty after fibrinolysis for acute myocardial infarction. *N Engl J Med* 2009; 260:2705.

126. Moens AL, Claeys MJ, Timmermans JP, et al: Myocardial ischemia/reperfusion-injury, a clinical view on a complex pathophysiological process. *Int J Cardiol* 2005; 100:179.

127. Wollert KC, Drexler H: Clinical applications of stem cells for the heart. *Circ Res* 2005; 96:151.

128. Schachinger V, Assmus B, Britten MB, et al: Transplantation of progenitor cells and regeneration enhancement in acute myocardial infarction. Final one-year results of the TOPCARE-AMI Trial. *J Am Coll Cardiol* 2004; 44:1690.

129. Hare JM, Traverse JH, Henry TD, et al: A randomized, double-blind, placebo-controlled, dose-escalation study of intravenous adult human mesenchymal stem cell (prochymal) after acute myocardial infarction. *J Am Coll Cardiol* 2009; 54:2277-2286.

23

Minimally Invasive Myocardial Revascularization

Piroze M. Davierwala • David M. Holzhey • Friedrich W. Mohr

The term *minimally invasive coronary artery bypass grafting* (CABG) is not well defined. According to one definition, avoidance of cardiopulmonary bypass (CPB) is considered essential in decreasing the morbidity associated with conventional CABG.[1] Other authors consider median sternotomy as a potential source for morbidity, due to increased risk of deep sternal wound infection and mediastinitis and delayed return to daily activities.[2] Accordingly, a number of surgical strategies have evolved to avoid the need for extracorporeal circulation and minimize surgical access. Furthermore, eluding aortic manipulation and complete arterial revascularization are operative strategies that focus on improving short and long-term results. Likewise, it was widely recognized that conventional harvesting techniques for bypass grafts are often associated with wound-healing problems, especially in diabetic patients. As a consequence, endoscopic harvesting techniques for both, venous and radial artery grafts have been developed.

OFF-PUMP CORONARY ARTERY BYPASS (OPCAB) GRAFTING

Conventional CABG has been performed with CPB under cardioplegic arrest for decades. An empty, arrested heart, a bloodless surgical field, and an excellent exposure of all epicardial vessels have been considered to be the key factors for the success of this procedure. Excellent results and constantly declining mortality despite the ever-increasing risk profile of patients (Davierwala) have made standard CABG the "bread and butter" of our profession.[3] Anecdotal reports on the deleterious effects of CPB and systematic reports that examined the pathophysiology of extracorporeal circulation began questioning the dogma, "the pump is your friend." CPB is associated with (1) a systemic inflammatory response, (2) release of cytokines, (3) activation of the clotting cascade, (4) metabolic disturbances, and (5) microembolization among numerous other adverse effects. Although well tolerated by most patients, these effects alone or in combination may cause substantial morbidity, thus negatively affecting the results of the procedure. With an ever-aging population and increasing comorbidity, surgeons all over the world sought to further minimize the risk of CABG, and it seemed logical to question the role of CPB in CABG.

The evolution of *off-pump coronary artery bypass* (OPCAB) grafting is closely linked to the development of stabilizers that became available in the early 1990s. Initially, only pressure stabilizers were developed, but it soon became obvious that exposure of vessels on the posterolateral and inferior walls of the heart would require additional means of support. Hence, OPCAB gained greater popularity when vacuum-assisted stabilizers were introduced by the Utrecht group, which facilitated localized myocardial immobilization for all territories. Additionally, it was also recognized that OPCAB requires a team approach between the surgeon and anesthesiologist so as to prevent sudden hemodynamic changes during the procedure and to manage the same when they do occur.

Anesthesia Requirements

OPCAB is performed under general anesthesia in most centers. Incidental reports in literature demonstrate that OPCAB can also be performed under high epidural anesthesia in an awake patient breathing spontaneously.[4] Standard monitoring is used. In addition, some centers prefer continuous cardiac output measurement using the PICCO or similar methods.[5] A Swan-Ganz catheter is not always beneficial and contrarily can potentially cause arrhythmias when the heart is manipulated during the procedure. It is of utmost importance that the patient is kept warm at all times during the operation. Temperature management includes the use of a warming blanket and warm infusions, and maintaining higher the room temperatures. Volume management is essential because it is generally the preferred means to counterbalance hemodynamic changes. Exposure of the posterior wall results in severe hemodynamic compromise due to some degree of right ventricular compression under the right hemisternum, but can be treated adequately by increasing venous return by tilting the operating room table to the right in a Trendelenburg position. Excessive infusion of fluids should be avoided, especially in patients with end-stage renal disease (ESRD), as hemofiltration is not possible during surgery due to the absence of

CPB. The use of inotropes should be preferably reserved only in patients with severe hemodynamic alterations, because they invariably increase the heart rate and make grafting more difficult. A review of human factors associated with manual control and tracking revealed that a human operator can, at his or her best, track a three-dimensional motion (such as the beating heart) only up to a frequency of 1 Hz, which corresponds to a heart rate of 60 beats per minute.[6] Higher frequencies cannot be tracked; therefore the preferred heart rate should be maintained between 50 and 70 beats per minute to simplify anastomotic suturing. In case of atrial fibrillation (AF), pharmacologic reduction in the heart rate and temporary ventricular pacing using epicardial pacing wires may facilitate grafting. The use of a Cell Saver is recommended to minimize the risk of blood transfusion, which is rarely necessary. If less than 500 mL is accumulated, the blood is usually discarded in the Cell Saver.

Surgical Technique

Single or bilateral internal thoracic arteries (ITA) are harvested following a standard median sternotomy. The patient is heparinized (150-200 units/kg, ie, about half of CPB dosage). An activated clotting time (ACT) greater than 300 seconds is maintained. It may be necessary to open the right pleura in patients with severely dilated hearts, although some surgeons do it routinely to give the heart enough space during manipulation for exposure of the posterolateral wall. It avoids excessive compression of the right ventricle. Following pericardiotomy, it is advisable to hitch the left side of the pericardium onto the left sternal edge. Thereafter, the two edges of the sternum are spread out with the sternal retractor. This helps not only in rightward rotation of the heart, but also elevates the heart to a certain degree, which additionally facilitates exposure of vessels on the posterolateral wall. Subsequently, deep pericardial stay sutures are placed to further aid in exposure and manipulation of the heart. Numerous methods have been proposed for placing these sutures. Ideally, two sutures are placed deep into the pericardium (deeper than the level of the atrioventricular groove), one just medial to the inferior vena cava and the other just inferior to the left inferior pulmonary vein (Fig. 23-1). To avoid damage to the myocardium due to shearing, the sutures should be covered by plastic tubing; sponges may be used alternatively. Placement of the stay sutures should be done slowly because abrupt changes in positioning of the heart may cause undesired hemodynamic alterations or arrhythmias.

The sequence in which the grafting should be performed depends largely on the coronary anatomy and the grafting techniques used. The left anterior descending (LAD) artery is considered to be the most important target vessel and can be easily grafted without too much manipulation of the heart. Therefore, revascularization should start with an ITA graft to the LAD in most cases. A slight pull on the stay sutures easily brings the LAD into the operative field. The stabilizer is placed at the desired site of the anastomosis

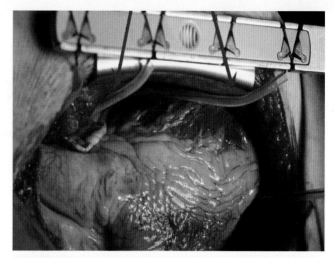

FIGURE 23-1 Setup for off-pump coronary artery bypass grafting. Placement of pericardial stay sutures.

so as to ensure adequate distance between the pods of the stabilizer and the vessel for suturing. The anterior surface of the vessel is exposed by dissecting it free from the overlying tissue. If the vessel is covered by excessive fat or muscle, low-energy cautery and clipping of epicardial veins may help to minimize bleeding from the surrounding tissue. Mechanical compression of large diagonal branches should be avoided. Vacuum stabilizers should be locked only after vacuum is applied and the stabilizer firmly holds on to the surface. Only minimal pressure will then be required to immobilize the heart. The greater the pressure exerted by the stabilizer, the greater the force with which the heart beats against it, resulting in increasing wall motion and hence the difficulty in anastomosis. Temporary occlusion of the target vessel can be achieved in many ways. Complete or partially encircling 4-0 polypropylene sutures with or without pledgets or silastic tapes are commonly used widely. The occlusion tapes or sutures should be placed at a distance of at least 5 to 10 mm from the anastomosis to avoid compression and distortion of the target vessel at the level of the anastomosis, thus allowing for safe and comfortable suturing. The suture needs to be placed deep enough in the tissue to avoid damage of the target vessel. Injury to the accompanying coronary vein should be avoided to prevent bleeding at and around the anastomotic site. Distal coronary artery occlusion should be avoided and is rarely necessary even in occluded vessels with strong backflow. A shunt can be used in the latter case. Care must be taken to avoid occluding vessels in stented areas because the occlusion sutures/tapes may bend or kink an implanted stent. The incision is usually made before the occlusion suture is tightened to ensure that the vessel is full, as it will minimize the risk of back wall injury while opening the vessel. The suture then is tightened gently until the bleeding stops. This may not be necessary in totally occluded vessels with minimal coronary blood flow. A CO_2 blower-mister is used to maintain a clear field of vision during the anastomosis by blowing away the blood flowing retrograde from septal branches or the distal coronary artery. The CO_2 flow rate should not exceed 5 L/min. Excessive blowing can produce dissection or injury to the intima of both, the graft and the coronary artery, or cause air embolism. The use of coronary artery shunts is controversial because they also may cause endothelial damage. If shunts are used, care must be taken to ensure atraumatic placement. Another option is the use of a transparent reverse thermosensitive gel (LeGoo™, Pleuromed Inc., Woburn, MA) injected at the anastomotic site after incising the coronary artery, which temporarily blocks the blood flow allowing an almost bloodfree anastomotic site. The anastomosis can then be performed without a blower-mister, shunt, or occlusion snares. The gel completely dissolves with time (after approximately 15 minutes) or with the local application of a cold sponge or gauze.[7,8]

The circumflex artery and its branches are usually grafted next, especially when a composite Y/T-grafting technique is used. Grafting the distal circumflex artery is considered to be the most challenging during OPCAB because exposure may be difficult. In patients with cardiomegaly and more importantly in those with right ventricular dilatation and dysfunction, it may be necessary to open the right pleura and divide the right-sided pericardium at the diaphragm up to the level of the inferior vena cava. This allows displacement of the heart under the right sternal edge into the right pleural cavity, thus preventing the compression of the right ventricle. Thereafter, the right coronary artery (RCA) and its branches are grafted. If the RCA is the dominant vessel and has a stenosis less than 80%, it may be necessary to use a shunt because loss of blood flow in the atrioventricular (AV) nodal artery during occlusion of the RCA can cause acute total AV block. It is therefore advisable to place and connect a temporary pacing wire before occluding such vessels.

To maximize both the short- and long-term benefits of an OPCAB procedure, composite arterial grafting is preferred. This will obviate the need for aortic clamping, which is another source for emboli and an independent predictor of stroke.[9] In fact, some authors believe that avoiding aortic manipulation is the key factor in reducing the stroke risk following CABG below that after percutaneous coronary intervention (PCI).

If aortocoronary vein or radial grafts are used, the proximal or distal anastomosis can be performed first. However, in patients with critical ischemia or hemodynamic instability, it would be beneficial to perform the proximal anastomosis initially, as it can be performed without manipulating the heart and the myocardium is revascularized as soon as the distal anastomosis is completed. It is of utmost importance to reduce the systemic blood pressure during partial clamping of the aorta to minimize the risk of embolization and aortic dissection. This can be achieved pharmacologically or mechanically by briefly compressing the inferior vena cava. This maneuver should also be repeated prior to declamping. Intraoperative graft patency control using transient-time Doppler or other imaging techniques is recommended. If the operative field is dry, heparin usually is not completely antagonized.

Postoperatively, aspirin is administered on the day of surgery, provided the patient does not bleed to muchion.

Special Situations

In patients with unstable angina, acute cardiogenic shock, or low ejection fraction (EF < 20%), the preoperative implantation of an intra-aortic balloon pump (IABP) may be useful. Alternatively, these patients can be operated on CPB without cardioplegic arrest (on-pump beating heart) to combine the advantages of preserved native coronary blood flow, decompression of the heart, and adequate organ perfusion.[13,14] Patients with AF have an irregular contraction pattern that may distract the surgeon while suturing (regular-motion patterns allow the development of coping strategies such as the "wait and see" strategy that are less effective when motion is unpredictable[5]). It may, therefore, be helpful to reduce the heart rate pharmacologically and temporarily pace the patient in a VVI mode. If AF is paroxysmal, epicardial ablation may be used for pulmonary vein isolation on the beating heart before grafting.

Results

Bakaeen et al reported recently that the number of OPCABs performed in the United States peaked in 2002 (23%) and 2008 (21%), followed by a steady decline to 17% in 2012. The last 5 years has witnessed a reduction in OPCAB rates not only in intermediate-volume centers performing between 50 and 200 cases a year, but also in high-volume centers performing >200 cases a year. They further reported that 84% of centers performed fewer than 50 off-pump cases per year, 34% of surgeons performed no off-pump operations, and 86% of surgeons performed fewer than 20 off-pump cases per year.[17] However, in some countries, especially, those with limited medical and financial resources, OPCAB still accounts for almost 80% of CABG procedures. Some units almost exclusively perform OPCAB with no patient selection. One of the major reasons for this decline is the results of several randomized controlled trials that have been unfavorable for OPCAB. The ROOBY trial reported a worse composite outcome of death and complications (9.9 vs 7.4%, $p = .04$), higher rate of incomplete revascularization (17.9 vs 11.1%; $p < .0001$), and a lower graft patency rate (82.6 vs 87.8%, $p < .01$) for OPCAB than on-pump CABG at 1 year. The Danish off-pump versus on-pump randomization study (DOORS) which included 900 patients > 70 years of age found no difference in the compound clinical endpoints between the two techniques at 30 days and 6 months.[16] However, the DOORS study group recently published a subanalysis, which revealed significantly inferior graft patency rates after OPCAB than after on-pump CABG at 6 months (79 vs 86%; $p = .01$).[17] Nevertheless, both these trials were not sufficiently powered to determine clinically relevant differences between the two techniques of surgical revascularization with respect to death, myocardial infarction, stroke, or renal failure. Sergeant and colleagues as well as Puskas and coworkers have pointed out that large cohorts of patients would be required to reveal a significant statistical difference in these outcomes between the two operative techniques.[18,19] Hence, the CORONARY trial was conducted, which randomized 4752 patients to OPCAB (2375) and on-pump CABG (2377). No differences in composite outcomes were found between groups at 30 days, 30 days to 1 year, and at 1 year after surgery.[20] Similarly, the German Off-Pump Coronary Artery Bypass Grafting in Elderly Patients (GOPCABE) study, which involved 2539 patients > 75 years of age randomized to OPCAB or on-pump CABG, showed no difference in clinical composite or individual components of death, stroke, MI, or renal replacement therapy at 30 days and 12 months between the two groups.[21] However, patients undergoing OPCAB required significantly more repeat revascularization at 30 days, which nonetheless evened out at 12 months. This finding was keeping in lieu with those of Khan et al, who reported reduced graft patency in OPCAB patients three months postoperatively.[22] Contrary to this, other studies like the SMART and Prague IV study that provide angiographic data on graft patency reveal equal patency rates for on- and off-pump bypass surgery.[23-25] This controversy concerning OPCAB has remained unresolved ever since the first reports on OPCAB regarding higher rates of incomplete revascularization[26-29] and lower graft patency[21] were published.

OPCAB does play an important role in stroke prevention, especially in patients at higher risk. A meta-analysis that involved all major randomized controlled trials comparing OPCAB with on-pump CABG between 2011 and 2010 revealed a significant 30% reduction in the occurrence of postoperative stroke with OPCAB [risk ratio (RR): 0.70]. There was no significant difference in mortality (RR: 0.90) or myocardial infarction (pooled RR: 0.89).[30] There is growing evidence that neurocognitive outcome is better and stroke rate is lower after OPCAB.[31-33] Several studies have proven CPB to be an independent predictor of adverse neurologic outcomes.[34] The embolic burden that is measured by transit-time Doppler of the medial cerebral artery is reduced significantly during OPCAB.[35-37] Neurological complications can be further reduced during OPCAB by performing the operation without aortic manipulation. In a recent retrospective analysis of 12,079 CABG patients, Moss and colleagues reported that the ratio of observed to expected stroke rate increased as the degree of aortic manipulation increased, from 0.48 in the no-touch group, to 0.61 in the clampless facilitating device group, and to 0.95 in the clamp group. Aortic clamping was independently associated with an increase in postoperative stroke compared with a no-touch technique (adjusted odds ratio (OR), 2.50; $p < .01$).[38] OPCAB has also been associated with a reduced risk of acute renal failure,[39-41] especially in high-risk patients with preoperative renal insufficiency.[42,43] A meta-analysis of 22 randomized studies involving 4819 patients affirmed these findings. OPCAB was associated with a 40% lower odds of postoperative acute kidney injury (OR 0.60; 95% confidence interval (CI) 0.43 to 0.84; $p = .003$) and a nonsignificant 33% lower odds for dialysis requirement (OR 0.67;

95% CI 0.40 to 1.12; $p = .12$) than on-pump CABG.[44] The kidney function substudy of the CORONARY trial, which enrolled 2932 patients, revealed that OPCAB reduced the risk of acute kidney injury when compared to on-pump CABG (17.5 vs 20.8%, $p = .01$); however, there was no significant difference between the two groups in the loss of kidney function at 1 year (17.1 vs 15.3%, $p = .23$).[45]

Furthermore, the incidence of postoperative AF[43,46] and blood levels of biochemical markers for myocardial injury (eg, creatinine kinase and troponin) are also reduced after OPCAB.[47-49] Blood loss is less, and transfusion rate is reduced.[19] Overall, OPCAB reduces hospital costs by 15 to 35%,[50,51] possibly owing to a decrease in the length of hospital stay and resource utilization.[50]

Most studies favor OPCAB with respect to operative and short-term mortality. A retrospective analysis of 17,969 OPCAB patients (8.8% of total) in the Society of Thoracic Surgeons database for the years 1999 and 2000 identified a significant survival advantage for OPCAB compared to on-pump CABG, as was demonstrated by risk-adjusted multivariate logistic regression analysis (OR 0.76, 95% CI 0.68 to 0.84) and conditional logistic regression of propensity-matched groups (OR 0.83, 95% CI 0.73 to 0.96).[52] Similar results have been reported from another multicenter analysis by Mack and colleagues, which included 7283 patients. Following propensity score matching and multivariate regression analysis, the use of CPB was identified as an independent predictor of mortality (OR 2.08, 95% CI 1.52 to 2.83, $p < .001$).[53] OPCAB seems to offer a survival benefit especially in high-risk populations (eg, the elderly, those with EF < 30%, and obese patients).[19,50,54,55] The International Society for Minimally Invasive Cardiac Surgery Consensus Group, in a thorough meta-analysis, published that OPCAB reduces mortality and length of stay and the incidence of postoperative myocardial infarction (MI), renal failure, AF, and transfusion rate in mixed-risk and high-risk patients[19] (Fig. 23-2). Few reports on mid-term survival showed similar outcomes for OPCAB and on-pump CABG at 2 and 4 years.[26,56]

There are limited reports comparing the long-term outcomes of OPCAB and on-pump CABG. Three major publications in the last 5 years have produced different results. The long-term follow-up of patients enrolled in the Beating Heart Against Cardioplegic Arrest Study (BHACAS 1 and 2) showed a similar likelihood of graft occlusion between OPCAB (10.6%) and on-pump CABG (11.0%) groups (OR: 1.00; $p > .99$). Similarly, no differences were noted in the hazard of death (hazard ratio (HR): 1.24) or major adverse cardiac-related events or death (HR: 0.84) between the two groups.[57] Contrarily, a large propensity-matched analysis of 5203 patients showed a similar risk of death at 30 days (OR: 0.70; $p = .31$) and up to 1 year (HR: 1.11; $p = .62$) for OPCAB and on-pump CABG, but a higher risk of death for the former at a median follow-up duration of 6.4 years (HR: 1.43; $p < .0001$).[58] A recent meta-analysis of 32 studies comparing the long-term outcomes of OPCAB and on-pump CABG concluded that OPCAB has similar mid-term

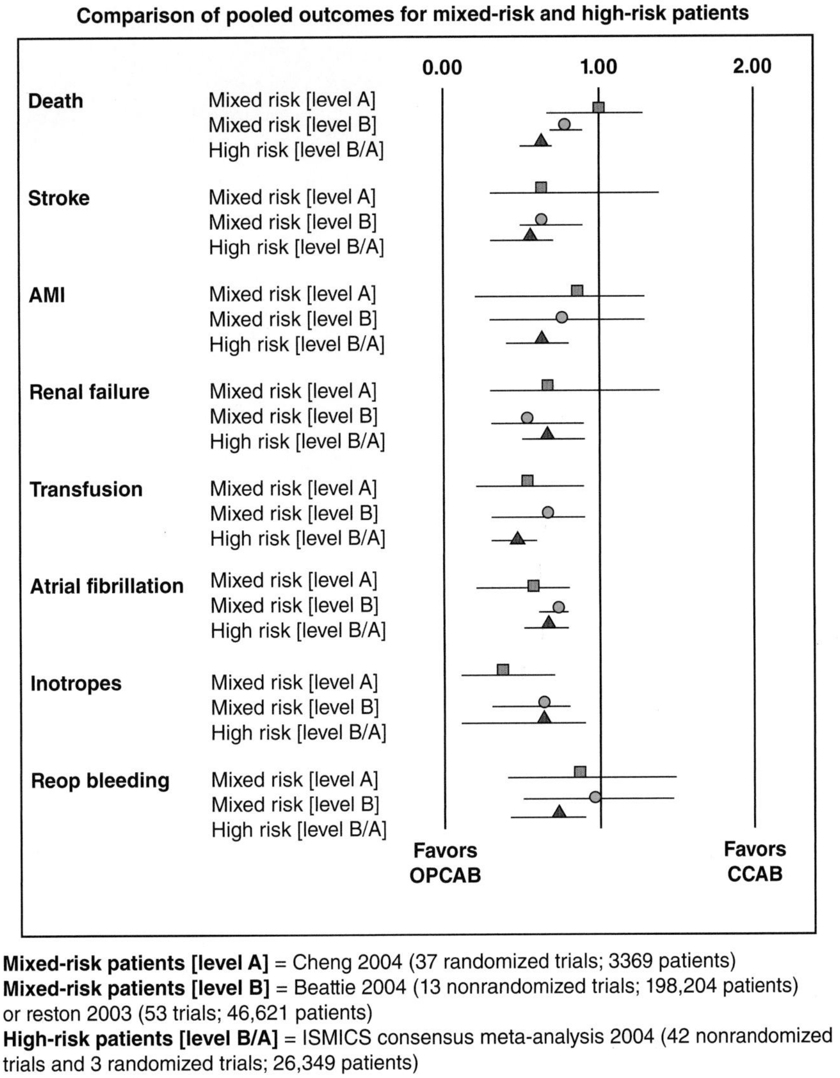

Comparison of pooled outcomes for mixed-risk and high-risk patients

Mixed-risk patients [level A] = Cheng 2004 (37 randomized trials; 3369 patients)
Mixed-risk patients [level B] = Beattie 2004 (13 nonrandomized trials; 198,204 patients)
or reston 2003 (53 trials; 46,621 patients)
High-risk patients [level B/A] = ISMICS consensus meta-analysis 2004 (42 nonrandomized
trials and 3 randomized trials; 26,349 patients)

FIGURE 23-2 Comparison of pooled outcomes for mixed-risk and high-risk patients. Square: 3369 mixed-risk patients from 37 randomized trials (level A) (Cheng 2004). Dot: 198,204 patients from 13 nonrandomized trials (level B) (Beattie 2004). Triangle: 26,349 high-risk patients from 42 nonrandomized and 3 randomized trials (level A) (ISMICS Consensus Meta-Analysis 2004). (Reproduced with permission from Puskas J, Cheng D, Knight J et al: Off-Pump versus Conventional Coronary Artery Bypass Grafting: A Meta-Analysis and Consensus Statement From The 2004 ISMICS Consensus Conference, Innovations (Phila). 2005 Fall;1(1):3-27.)

mortality and morbidity to on-pump CABG in a low-risk population. When observational studies were excluded a comparable long-term mortality was observed between the two surgical revascularization techniques.[59] To summarize, OPCAB is a technically challenging operation, which requires a prolonged learning curve compared to conventional bypass graft surgery. Some surgeons perform OPCAB almost exclusively, whereas others never use it at all. OPCAB may not be the best option for every patient or for all cardiac surgeons. It is, however, an important alternative and must be mastered with the same technical precision as conventional CABG.[60] True comparisons between OPCAB and on-pump CABG are extremely difficult even by randomized controlled trials as there are many factors such as quality of the coronary vessels anastomosed, type of conduits used, grafting techniques

(sequential, composite total arterial, venous grafts, etc), and competency and experience of the surgeons to perform OPCAB that cannot be accounted for. All the same, we have to wait for the results of long-term follow-up of large-scale, multi-institutional RCTs.

MINIMALLY INVASIVE DIRECT CORONARY ARTERY BYPASS (MIDCAB)

One of the goals of minimally invasive cardiac surgery has been to avoid sternotomy to reduce the amount of surgical trauma and avoid wound complications. Therefore, coronary artery bypass techniques on the beating heart without sternotomy were developed. The operation was termed *minimally invasive direct coronary artery bypass* (MIDCAB), and since its introduction in the mid-1990s,[61-65] it has found a widespread application. In some centers, MIDCAB is the preferred method of surgical revascularization for isolated LAD disease. In addition, MIDCAB is a valuable alternative to standard CABG or OPCAB in selected high-risk patients with multivessel disease and extensive comorbidity, who are at a prohibitively high risk for sternotomy and CPB.

Anesthesia

Standard monitoring techniques are applied, and temperature management is as described previously for OPCAB procedures. Single-lung ventilation is achieved by using a double-lumen tube or bronchus blocker to provide selective right lung ventilation. Short-acting anesthetics are used to allow early extubation.

Surgical Technique

Standard MIDCAB is usually performed through a left anterolateral minithoracotomy with the patient in a 10 to 30° right lateral position. Following a 5 to 6 cm skin incision at the level of the fifth intercostal space or the inframammary fold in females, the pectoralis muscle is displaced bluntly with minimal division of its muscle fibers (muscle-sparing approach). This decreases the likelihood of developing a lung hernia that has been sometimes reported with this approach. The chest is then usually entered one intercostal space higher than the actual incision. Excessive rib spreading must be avoided at all times to prevent dislocation or fracture. Excision of a rib is almost never necessary. LITA harvest is usually performed under direct vision, but endoscopic harvest utilizing a harmonic scalpel or telemanipulation systems has also been reported.[65-67]

The intrathoracic fascia is divided to facilitate LITA harvest, which can be performed in a pedicled or skeletonized manner, from the fifth intercostal space to the origin of the subclavian artery. Using a sceletonized technique offers the advantage of gaining more graft length, but is, of course, more time-consuming. Additional length can also be gained by dividing the mammary vein at its junction with the subclavian vein. Side branches are clipped or cauterized based on the preference of the surgeon. Heparin is administered prior to distal transsection of the graft. As in a sternotomy OPCAB, the ACT is maintained at a level greater than 300 seconds. The pericardium should be opened at a point approximately corresponding to the course of the LAD and extended to the groove between the aorta and the pulmonary artery. This will facilitate location of the target vessel in the presence of excessive epicardial fat or an intramuscular course. The target vessel is identified. To enhance exposure, one or two pericardial stay sutures may be used to position the heart. It is of utmost importance to have the anastomotic site in direct vision. Standard

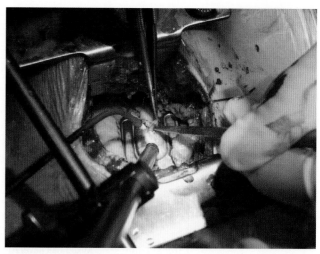

FIGURE 23-3 Minimally invasive direct coronary artery bypass. Through a muscle-sparing incision, the left anterior descending artery is easily exposed; standard pressure stabilizers are used. (Data from 1483 patients undergoing MIDCAB at the Heartcenter Leipzig.)

reusable pressure stabilizers are then used to immobilize the target vessel (Fig. 23-3). Vacuum stabilizers in general are too bulky and not required for a single anastomosis to the LAD. Proximal LAD occlusion is performed using a 4-0 pledgeted suture or vessel loops. Ischemic preconditioning is not helpful, but some surgeons use it to feel more comfortable knowing that ischemia is well tolerated. The use of shunts is rarely necessary, but they may be used based on surgeon preference, presence of significant retrograde coronary flow or evidence of ischemia or hemodynamic instability. Distal occlusion should be avoided whenever possible (99% of patients). A blower-mister is used in all cases to achieve a bloodless field. The anastomosis then is performed in a standard manner using a 7-0 or 8-0 polypropylene running suture. Finally the LITA pedicle can be fixed to the epicardial tissue. Graft patency assessment is performed routinely using transit-time Doppler flow measurements. A single chest tube is inserted into the left pleural space, and intercostal nerve blockade is applied using local anesthetics. Before closing the chest with one or two strong rib sutures, the single-lung ventilation is stopped and the left lung is inflated under direct vision of the surgeon to prevent it from causing an avulsion of the LITA and also confirm that the LITA lies perfectly without undue tension. This is facilitated by holding the LITA close to the mediastinum using the suction tip or long forceps. Extubation can be performed in the operating room or a few hours postoperatively. Antiplatelet therapy is usually administered on the day of surgery.

Results

Many papers have reported excellent results with the use of this approach. Immediate angiographic patency rates range between 94 and 98% and are thus similar to those following conventional CABG.[64,68] At 6 months, 94% patency has been reported.[69] The mid-term results published recently by Reser et al demonstrated an overall survival of 92.4 ± 0.2% and MACCE-free survival of 96.1 ± 1.7% at 24 months.[70] In our own series of 1768 patients, who underwent MIDCAB from 1996 to 2009, in-hospital mortality was 0.8% (predicted mortality by Euroscore 3.8%), and stroke rate was 0.4%. Conversion to sternotomy was necessary in 1.7%. A total of 712 patients underwent routine postoperative angiogram demonstrating a 95.5% early patency rate. Short-term target-vessel reintervention was required in 3.3% of patients. At 6-month follow-up, graft patency was 95.2% (n = 423). The 5- and 10-year survival was 88.3% (95% CI 86.6 to 89.9%) and 76.6% (95% CI 73.5 to 78.7%) (Fig. 23-4A). The corresponding freedom from MACCE and angina was 85.3% (95% CI 83.5 to 87.1%) and 70.9% (95% CI 68.1 to 73.7%) (see Fig. 23-4B).[71] These results are comparable to those of other groups.[69,72,73]

In-hospital mortality after MIDCAB is <1% and compares favorably with 1.4% mortality following off-pump single-vessel bypass and 3.6% mortality after on-pump single-vessel bypass reported in the registry of the German Society for Thoracic and Cardiovascular Surgery.[74] It is also lower than the 2.4% mortality reported from the STS database.[75] A propensity score adjusted comparison of MIDCAB versus full sternotomy revealed similar operative mortality, late survival, and need for repeat revascularization

at a mean follow-up of 6.2 years, but a lower rate of surgical site infection (2.8 vs 0.7%; p = .04).[76] Another smaller study from the UK also found MIDCAB comparable to OPCAB with regard to operative mortality, MI, stroke, reinterventions, and ICU stay. However, hospital stay was significantly lower for MIDCAB patients.[77] In general, rates of perioperative major complications such as MI and the need for target-vessel reintervention are low and comparable with standard CABG. However, due to anaortic surgery perioperative stroke is rare and considerably lower compared to conventional techniques. A few randomized trials comparing the LIMA-LAD with the MIDCAB approach to bare metal stenting for isolated proximal LAD disease have demonstrated better early patency and superior freedom from target-vessel reintervention and angina up to 5 years of follow-up in patients undergoing MIDCAB.[78-83] The 10-year results of the randomized trial conducted by our group comparing MIDCAB with bare metal stents for proximal LAD disease showed no differences in the primary composite endpoint of death, MI, and reintervention (47 vs 36%; p = .12) and hard endpoints (death and infarction) between the two revascularization modalities. However, a higher target vessel revascularization rate in the PCI group (34 vs 11%; p < .01) was observed.[84] Similar results were also reported when drug-eluting stents were compared to MIDCAB.[85] These results have been further confirmed not only by meta-analyses[86,87] but also propensity-matched data from large registries.[88]

Some studies have pointed out that the lateral approach is associated with more pain than sternotomy chiefly due to excessive rib spreading required for visualizing the LITA during harvest.[65] Rib dislocation or fracture has been reported infrequently with this approach. Direct harvesting of the LITA is regarded as being technically challenging and has been one of the main arguments used by surgeons to disregard MIDCAB as the primary operation for patients who require surgical revascularization of the LAD. Limited working space and incomplete vision are blamed for insufficient graft length, incomplete mobilization, and the occasional reports of LITA or subclavian vein injury.

MIDCAB is technically a highly demanding procedure that should be performed by surgeons who have sufficient experience in conventional and off-pump surgery. It has been shown that the complication rate of MIDCAB (viz. conversion to sternotomy, reexploration for bleeding, and reintervention on the target vessel) is significantly reduced following 100 to 150 MIDCAB procedures.[89] Therefore, it can be recommended that this operation should be performed by experienced surgeons dedicated to this technique.

Even in the era of improved outcomes following interventional procedures and lower in-stent restenosis rates with the use of drug-eluting stents,[90] MIDCAB, based on its very good long-term results,[91] will always remain an alternative revascularization strategy to PCI, especially for patients with complex ostial lesions, chronic occlusions, and in-stent restenosis of the LAD.

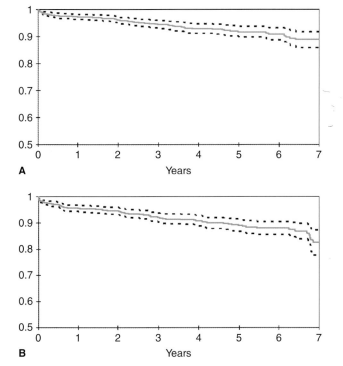

FIGURE 23-4 Kaplan-Meier (including 95% confidence interval) five-year survival curve (A) and event-free survival curve (freedom from death, myocardial infarction, stroke, freedom from angina, freedom from reintervention) (B) after minimally invasive direct coronary artery bypass. (Data from 1483 patients undergoing MIDCAB at the Heartcenter Leipzig.)

TOTAL ENDOSCOPIC CORONARY ARTERY BYPASS GRAFTING

Total endoscopic coronary artery bypass grafting (TECAB) on the beating heart is conceivably the least invasive approach for surgical revascularization. It has been well known for a long time that working through ports limits the available space to perform motions, substantially decreases the dexterity of the operator, and alters the hand-eye coordination.[92] Active assistance, an indispensable component of open surgery, is difficult in thoracoscopic procedures. The transition from limited-access cardiac surgery to endoscopic cardiac surgery therefore complicates the procedure manifold and has rendered previous attempts at endoscopic CABG using conventional endoscopic instruments impossible. To overcome some of the instrument-related limitations, computer-enhanced instrumentation systems have been developed.

Principles of Telemanipulator-Assisted Cardiac Surgery

With the use of telemanipulation devices, the operator involved in the surgery is physically away but not necessarily remote from the operation table. He sits at an *input manipulator* (surgical console, master console), from which he steers the *executing manipulator* (slave console), which is situated at the patient site. The slave console consists of all the necessary electromechanical equipment needed to operate two to three exchangeable endoscopic instruments in addition to a high definition three-dimensional endoscopic camera. Both tactile and visual information is fed back to the master console. In this way a virtual three-dimensional operative field is created, wherein the surgeon can manipulate steering handles with a perfect hand-eye coordination. The introduction of telemanipulation technology to endoscopic surgery was able to address the key performance limitations of conventional endoscopic surgery, namely, reduced articulation, monocular vision, and loss of hand-eye coordination.

Surgical Technique

Standard monitoring for cardiac surgery is used. Defibrillator pads are placed on the back and the right side of the chest. Single-lung ventilation using a double-lumen endotracheal tube or a bronchus blocker is used to ventilate only the right lung. Temperature management principles remain the same as for OPCAB surgery. After draping the instrument and camera arms, the camera and scope are calibrated, and the endostabilizer is prepared. A holding arm for the endostabilizer is mounted onto the operating table on the patient's right side, and the operating table is rotated 10 to 15° to raise the patient's left side.

After single right-lung ventilation is initiated, the camera port is inserted through the fifth intercostal space 2 cm medial to the anterior axillary line. CO_2 insufflation is used for adequate visualization and to create working space that is hemodynamically tolerated (usually 10-12 mm Hg of insufflation pressure). A 30° scope that is angled up is used for LITA harvest. The right instrument port is inserted through the third intercostal space medial to the anterior axillary line, and the left instrument port is inserted through the seventh intercostal space medial to the anterior axillary line. The instrument arms are centered for optimal range of motion by adjusting the respective setup joints, and the instruments are inserted. LITA harvest starts by division of the intrathoracic fascia covering it with low-power monopolar cautery. The LITA is dissected bluntly off the chest wall moving from the lateral to the medial aspect as a pedicle, preserving the lateral veins. Side branches are cauterized or clipped. Dissection is performed from the first intercostal space to the level of the bifurcation. The pedicle is not detached from the chest wall until the anastomosis is finally performed in order to avoid torsion of the graft. The distal end of the graft is skeletonized to facilitate suturing of the anastomosis. The pericardial fat is removed, and the mediastinal and diaphragmatic attachments to the pericardium are dissected bluntly to widen the available space. The pericardiotomy is performed through a longitudinal incision in the pericardium over the probable course of the LAD. The ideal anastomotic site is identified by the absence of visible atheromatous plaques and avoidance of proximity to bifurcations. At this point, angling the endoscope downwards may enhance visualization. After heparinization (an ACT of 300 seconds is recommended), a vascular clamp is placed across the LITA approximately 2 cm proximal to the transsection site. The LITA is clipped distally, transected, and spatulated in preparation for the anastomosis. Flow in the graft is confirmed by briefly releasing the vascular clamp. The LITA pedicle is still left attached to the chest wall in order to maintain orientation of the graft until the anastomosis is performed. A 12 mm subxyphoid cannula is inserted under endoscopic vision. Before introduction of the endostabilizer, temporary silastic occlusion tapes and a 7 cm 7-0 double-armed polypropylene suture are introduced through this port and retained in the mediastinum. Some surgeons prefer Gore-Tex sutures to avoid the memory effect of polypropylene. Alternatively, nitinol clips (U-clips) may be used. The endostabilizer then is introduced under endoscopic vision by the surgeon at the operating table (Fig. 23-5). Vacuum and saline irrigation lines are connected, and the multilink irrigator is advanced into the field of vision. The console surgeon then positions the stabilizer feet parallel to the LAD target site. After suction is applied, the feet are locked into position. After blunt dissection of the anastomotic target site, the silastic tapes are placed proximal and distal to the anastomotic site, and the LAD is temporarily occluded. After a 5 to 6 mm arteriotomy is performed, transsection of the LITA is completed, and the graft is brought in close proximity of the target site. The anastomosis is best performed by beginning in the middle of the medial edge of the incision (12 o'clock position), suturing inside-out on the LITA and out-side-in on the LAD toward and around the heel. Care has to be taken to maintain tension on the suture

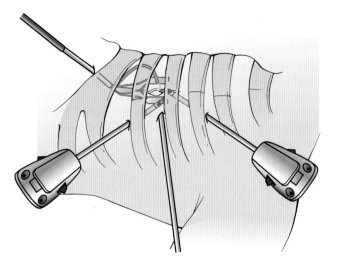

FIGURE 23-5 Setup for total endoscopic coronary artery bypass grafting. Two instrument ports, one central camera port, and a subxyphoidal port for the endostabilizer are required.

continuously. After the needles are broken off, an instrument knot is tied. The occlusion tapes and vascular clamp are released and brought out through an instrument port. The pedicle may be fixed to the epicardium by stay sutures. Graft patency can be checked by transient time Doppler flow measurements endoscopically, if a probe without a handle is available. This probe can be advanced through the stabilizer port. Alternatively, intraoperative angiography has been performed using a mobile angiography unit or modern C-arm systems when TECAB operation is performed in a hybrid suite. After the pleural space is drained under vision, the stabilizer and instruments are withdrawn, and the left lung is ventilated. A chest tube is inserted through one of the port holes. In case a four-arm system is used, the fourth arm is introduced after LITA harvest through the third intercostal space in the anterior axillary line. It may be used to provide counter traction during pericardial fat excision and pericardiotomy and to hold the pedicle during the anastomosis. The new version of the da Vinci system also allows the use of a remotely controlled stabilizer that is placed on the fourth arm and thus can be adjusted from the console.

Results

Initially, TECAB was performed on an arrested heart using the Port-Access platform with femoro-femoral CPB, endo-aortic balloon clamping, and cardioplegic arrest. CPB time and cross-clamp times were in the range of 80 to 120 and 40 to 60 minutes, respectively. The reported patency rate for the TECAB procedures on an arrested heart ranged from 95 to 100% prior to discharge and 96% at the 3-month follow-up angiography.[93-96] In addition to reporting good overall results and patency rates after TECAB, a large single-center study including 100 patients also revealed anastomotic times of 10 to 30 minutes after a long learning curve. They further acknowledged that the learning curve continues beyond 100

operations, which is even more pronounced than in MID-CAB procedures (see above).[97]

Endoscopic CABG on the beating heart is even more challenging.[93,98,99] Based on an intention-to-treat basis, the conversion rate (elective conversion to a MIDCAB procedure) in a five-center registry was 33% (37 of 117). Conversions were mostly due to calcified target vessels or the inability to locate or dissect the LAD and rarely due to other conditions such as arrhythmias or hemodynamic instability. The patency rates for completed beating-heart TECAB procedures are in the range of 92 to 94%.[75]

TECAB can be performed safely, but is currently restricted to a few indications (eg, single-vessel bypass grafting of the LAD and occasionally double-vessel grafting), but has the potential for endoscopic multivessel grafting as well.[100,101] A more commonly applied technique is an endoscopic harvesting of both ITAs and direct coronary anastomosis via a mini-thoracotomy. This yields excellent results and very short recovery times for the patients.[101,102]

Despite the use of advanced telemanipulator technology, the TECAB procedure remains technically demanding and is infrequently performed worldwide. Long operation times, extensive use of material, and operation room capacity combined with a stretched learning curve and well-established alternative minimally invasive techniques have confined TECAB to few centers and single dedicated surgeons.

MULTIPLE BYPASS GRAFTING USING MINIMALLY INVASIVE TECHNIQUES

Talking about minimally invasive surgical revascularization almost always means revascularization of the anterior wall with the left internal mammary artery. The classical MID-CAB operation is only rarely extended to graft a diagonal or even an intermediate branch as well, typically with a Y-graft using a vein or radial artery.

Recent reports have proven the feasibility of complete revascularization for multivessel disease. Bilateral internal thoracic artery harvest is possible through small incisions under direct vision or endoscopically with the help of a telemanipulator.[103] For proximal anastomoses the aorta can be mobilized and partially clamped or the internal thoracic arteries serve as sources of inflow for a radial artery or saphenous vein.

Accessibility of all areas of the heart is made possible by special stabilizers and suction retractors that allow distal anastomoses even on the beating heart. As an alternative the Heartport system for endoaortic clamping and cardioplegia can be used.

These techniques are not yet routinely used. However, the published series of patients show excellent results oftentimes superior to conventional CABG or OPCAB.[103] Lemma and coworkers reported 137 patients operated with this technique with a 1.4% incomplete revascularization and revision for bleeding. There were no conversions to sternotomy nor were there wound complications. Only two deaths occurred at a mean follow-up of 26 months. A positive stress test was reported in 4.3% of patients.[104] An angiographic patency study involving 91 patients who were prospectively enrolled to undergo minimally invasive multivessel CABG revealed a 100% patency for the LIMA-LAD graft and 92% patency for all grafts.[105] It can be assumed that these operations are performed by dedicated, experienced surgeons on selected patients. Only a more widespread application of these procedures and the treatment of a broader variety of patients together with randomized studies would bring light to their significance in the future.

HYBRID REVASCULARIZATION

The hybrid approach for patients with multivessel coronary artery disease seeks to combine the advantages of PCI and minimally invasive CABG. The principle was first described by Angelini in 1996.[106] The goal is to minimize the surgical trauma but still gain complete revascularization. The rationale is that the excellent long-term results of LIMA to LAD grafting[91,107] cannot be extended to other grafts and areas of myocardium. This is particularly true for the still commonly used venous grafts to non-LAD targets. Here PCI can potentially achieve similar long-term results, though with higher rates of reintervention. Although recent studies underline the superiority of complete surgical revascularization,[108] the avoidance of sternotomy seems to be very appealing to both patients and treating cardiologists.

However, combining the benefits of two different procedures also means adding risks inherent to each type of procedure. The drawbacks of a surgical procedure including the risk of general anesthesia and artificial ventilation are combined with an increased risk of inferior long-term outcomes after PCI resulting in higher rates of reinterventions and the possibility of eventual redo surgical multiple bypass grafting. Therefore the indication for hybrid revascularization should be discussed and agreed upon by the treating cardiologist, cardiac surgeon and, most importantly, the patient himself.

Indications for the Hybrid Approach

Current recommendations for coronary artery revascularization do not include hybrid procedures. This is due to limited availability of outcome data and a lack of randomized trials. Thus, choosing a hybrid approach is usually based on an individual decision. In all cases, the patients with multivessel disease including the proximal LAD need to be informed that the best evidence-based treatment is a sternotomy CABG procedure. However, the different reasons for choosing a hybrid approach can be summarized as follows:

- *Multimorbid or high-risk patients:* This is probably the best accepted indication and includes patients with a high risk for sternotomy such as those with skeletal anomalies like

osteogenesis imperfecta, severe osteoporosis, etc., those who are crutches- or wheel-chair-dependent, and those with a history of deep sternal wound infections following previous sternotomy. Patients with reduced life expectancy such as advanced malignancies, end-stage cardiomyopathy, advanced liver, and renal failure not amenable for transplant could also benefit from a hybrid procedure. Additionally, comorbidities that could be considered risk factors for a sternotomy and occurrence of other postoperative complications such as diabetes, severe obesity, COPD, end-stage peripheral vascular disease, porcelain aorta, and history of stroke with paraplegia might also be candidates for the hybrid approach.

- *Primary PCI of Circumflex/RCA:* Patients with acute coronary syndromes presenting with a culprit lesion in the circumflex or RCA and an additional stenosis of the LAD may undergo primary emergency PCI of the culprit lesion by the referring cardiologist. A MIDCAB procedure involving a LITA-LAD can be performed four to six weeks later. A preoperative angiogram confirming the patency of the stents should be performed prior to surgery. In the presence of an in-stent restenosis the patient can be scheduled for a standard bypass procedure.

- *Patient preference:* Some well-informed patients want to avoid a sternotomy and opt for a hybrid approach. Patients need to be informed that they might require future reinterventions including repeat target vessel revascularization or bypass surgery. Because the choice of the hybrid revascularization in these patients is not based on medical grounds, it deserves a formal discussion between the patient, interventional cardiologist, and cardiac surgeon.

Timing of the Procedures

The optimal timing and the sequence of revascularization is still controversial.[109] All three possible scenarios have inherent benefits and drawbacks:

- *PCI before CABG:* Performing PCI first is usually associated with an increased risk of bleeding at the time of surgery because of dual antiplatelet therapy. This can be avoided in stable patients who received a bare metal stent by postponing the CABG procedure for more than 4 weeks. When the interval between the two procedures is even longer, performing a preoperative check-angiogram is reasonable to exclude early in-stent restenosis.

The PCI-first strategy is most commonly used in an emergency situation, when a non-LAD culprit lesion requires primary PCI.[110]

- *CABG before PCI:* This is the most frequently used option. PCI is performed after the patient has recovered from surgery. After protection of the anterior wall the percutaneous approach for the other coronary arteries, including the left main coronary artery, is safer.[111] Additionally, the LITA-LAD graft can also be assessed.

- *Simultaneous revascularization:* The growing number of novel operating suites that provide true integration of surgical and fluoroscopic capabilities allow for complete hybrid revascularization in one session without moving the patient. After performing a standard MIDCAB/TECAB procedure the quality and patency of the bypass graft is verified and PCI of the remaining vessels is undertaken with the patient still under general anesthesia. In the rare case of a failed PCI easy and safe conversion to conventional bypass surgery is possible. Patient acceptance for this approach is high, however, good coordination and synchronization of the schedules of the cardiologist and the cardiac surgeon is required.

Results

Hybrid coronary revascularization (HCR) as a concept has been applied for almost 15 years and provides an additional approach to revascularization for patients with multivessel coronary disease. The general consensus is that hybrid integrated revascularization is feasible and safe.[112-116] Friedrich and colleagues reviewed the results of 18 studies in literature, which included 367 patients. At 6 months the LIMA stenosis rate was 2% and in-stent restenosis was 12%.[112] The large single-center series published by our group revealed a survival of 92.5% (95% CI 86.5 to 98.4%) at 1 year and 84.8% (95% CI 73.5 to 94.9%) at 5 years.[110] Eight patients died during follow-up (208 patient-years). A total of 23 patients had an angiogram for recurrent angina. One patient had an occluded LIMA bypass. Five patients showed significant in-stent-restenosis with the need for reintervention. At 1 year freedom from MACCE and angina was 85.5% (95% CI 76.9 to 94.1%) and 75.5% (95% CI 62.7 to 87.3%), respectively (Fig. 23-6).

The short-term results have been excellent.[117] Before a new therapeutic approach is routinely used, it has to be compared to well-proven standard modalities of treatment. Several controlled studies comparing the safety, feasibility, and efficacy of HCR with OPCAB have been published in the last 5 years.[118-121] However, the number of patients undergoing HCR in these studies was small and hence, conclusions drawn from such studies do not carry too much weight. A recently published meta-analysis, which included 422 patients undergoing HCR and >5000 patients undergoing OPCAB, revealed no differences in in-hospital mortality [relative risk (RR) 0.57, 95% CI 0.13 to 2.59, p = .47] or MACCE rates (RR 0.63, 95% CI 0.24 to 1.64, p = .34) between groups. Nevertheless, HCR was associated with significantly lesser length of hospitalization (RR 0.55, 95% CI 0.13 to 0.97, p = .01), length of ICU stay (RR 0.45, 95% CI 0.10 to 0.80, p < .05), intubation time (RR 0.48, 95% CI 0.13 to 0.84, p < .01) and need for red blood transfusion (RR 0.67, 95% CI 0.56 to 0.82, p < .001).[122] With regard to mid-term outcomes, Shen et al reported that mortality, MI, and stroke at 3 years after HCR were comparable to both, CABG and PCI in patients with multivessel disease.[123] However, the cumulative MACCE rate in the hybrid group (6.4%) was significantly lower than that in the PCI group (22.7%; p < .001), but similar to that in the

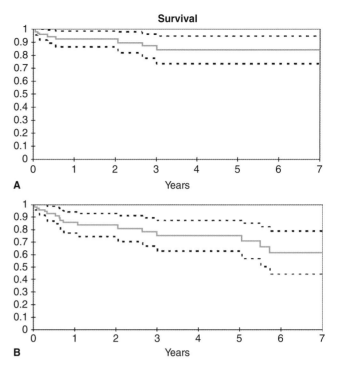

FIGURE 23-6 Kaplan-Meier (including 95% confidence interval) 5-year survival curve (A) and event-free survival curve (freedom from death, myocardial infarction, stroke, freedom from angina, freedom from reintervention) (B) after minimally invasive hybrid revascularization in 117 patients.

CABG group (13.5%; p = .14). This was chiefly driven by a higher incidence of repeat revascularization in the PCI group. But interestingly, compared with the hybrid group, repeat revascularization in the PCI group was mainly concentrated in the LAD (2 vs 10 events; p = .029), and PCI with DES for non-LAD offered a similar repeat revascularization rate in the hybrid and PCI groups (4 vs 8 events; p = .307). This clearly proves the benefit of surgical revascularization of the LAD with the LIMA. Although HCR appears to be an attractive option, especially in the elderly and those at a higher risk due to comorbidities,[124] one must keep in mind the potentially higher rate of target vessel revascularization for non-LAD vessels, especially in diabetic patients Repossini.

No randomized controlled trial comparing HCR to CABG or PCI exist, which is mandatory in the current era of evidence-based medicine. Large, multicenter RCTs are needed to compare HCR with OPCAB to identify patient populations that would benefit most from HCR. Furthermore, the strategy or the order of revascularization should also be determined through such trials.

ENDOSCOPIC CONDUIT HARVEST

To minimize the overall trauma and wound healing problems of a CABG procedure, conduit harvest should be performed endoscopically or through small incisions. There is a body of evidence indicating that while the quality of the conduit is not impaired by an endoscopic harvest, wound infections and other complications of the harvesting procedure are decreased substantially. The cosmetic advantage is obvious.

Endoscopic Saphenous Vein Harvesting

Despite the fact that arterial grafting yields better long-term results than venous grafting, and despite the increased use of the ITA and other arterial grafts, the greater saphenous vein is still frequently used for CABG. The standard longitudinal open harvesting technique of the greater saphenous vein is associated with a 2 to 25% wound complication rate (eg, dehiscence, delayed healing, infection, cellulitis, sepsis, and occasionally, limb amputation), delaying ambulation of patients, prolonging hospitalization, and causing an enormous economic burden.[125-128] In addition, open saphenous vein harvest is associated with increased postoperative and long-term pain, swelling, neuropathy, and scarring resulting in patient dissatisfaction.

Various techniques using 1 to 2 cm incisions have been described for endoscopic vein harvest. The single-incision technique involves identification of the greater saphenous vein through a 2 cm longitudinal incision at the crease of the knee posterior to the medial femoral condyle. The vein is layered free circumferentially, following which, a subcutaneous retractor or dissection cannula is introduced. An endoscope is inserted into the subcutaneous tissue. Exposure can be enhanced by insufflating CO_2. The vein is further mobilized circumferentially, and side branches are either clipped, coagulated using bipolar endoscopic cautery scissors, or vaporized using a harmonic scalpel. Whenever bipolar cautery is applied, a distance of at least 2 mm between the scissors and the vein should be maintained in order to avoid thermal damage to the graft. Proximal and distal control of the greater saphenous vein is accomplished with endoscopic application of clips or polypropylene sutures or ligation loops. With this technique, the entire length of the vein can be harvested from the sapheno-femoral junction to the medial malleolus through a single incision. The wound is closed in a standard manner, and the leg is wrapped circumferentially with crepe bandages. In experienced hands, the procedure takes between 15 and 30 minutes.[129] As with all endoscopic techniques, a learning curve is associated with endoscopic vein harvesting as well, and entails approximately 30 patients and a conversion rate ranging from 0 to 22%.

Results

The ISMICS Consensus Group reviewed the results of 1319 randomized and 8023 nonrandomized patients. In this meta-analysis, the risk of wound complications was reduced significantly by 69% with endoscopic vein harvesting compared with the open technique (OR 0.31, 95% CI 0.23 to 0.43; $p < .0001$).[130] The need for surgical intervention for wound infection also was reduced significantly (OR 0.29, 95% CI 0.12 to 0.70; $p = .007$). With regard to the incidence of moderate to severe postoperative pain, endoscopic vein harvesting

was associated with a 74% reduction when compared with the open technique (OR 0.26, 95% CI 0.12 to 0.55; $p < .0001$), and this reduction reached 90% at 4 to 6 weeks follow-up (OR 0.10, 95% CI 0.03 to 0.37; $p < .0001$). The incidence of disturbance in mobility at discharge was reduced by 69% (OR 0.31, 95% CI 0.15 to 0.65; $p = .002$).

One recent study reported worse angiographic and clinical outcomes in patients after endoscopic vein harvest.[131] Most studies, however, found no difference in the rates of myocardial infarction, recurrence of angina or reintervention, and death over the short- and mid-term follow-up.[130,132] However, the number of trials evaluating cardiac outcomes and providing angiographic data on patency rates is too limited to allow for any meaningful conclusion to be made. The few trials that assessed vascular integrity and vessel wall trauma did not find any difference between the two techniques.[133,134]

Endoscopic Radial Artery Harvest

Use of the radial artery for CABG has regained popularity over the last decade and a half. Conventional radial artery harvest involves an incision that extends from approximately 1 cm distal to the antecubital fossa up to the wrist joint, along the medial border of the brachioradialis muscle. While wound complications are reported infrequently, delayed healing of the forearm can cause severe discomfort.[135] Objective sensory loss in 10% of patients and forearm scar discomfort in 33% undergoing open radial artery harvest have been reported.[136,137] Endoscopic techniques for graft harvest have been developed subsequently.[138]

SURGICAL TECHNIQUE

Collateral circulation from the ulnar artery to the palmar arch has to be verified pre- or intraoperatively using either the standard Allen's test or modification of the test by using an arterial Doppler or pulse oximetry, especially in patients in whom the signs of visual reperfusion are doubtful. In order to prevent brachial plexus injury, the arm should not be overextended (>90°). A 2 to 3 cm incision is made 1 cm superior to the radial styloid prominence and the radial artery is identified and dissected. A subcutaneous retractor and a 5 mm, 30° endoscope are inserted into the incision. The radial artery is visualized by bluntly advancing the retractor through the subcutaneous tissue. Side branches and surrounding tissue are divided using an ultrasonic harmonic or thermowelding scalpel that is placed underneath the retractor. The fascia between the brachioradialis and flexor carpi radialis muscles is divided anterior to the radial artery with the scalpel to increase the space for insertion of the subcutaneous retractor.[139] After division of all side branches, a vessel retractor is advanced from the distal incision to verify complete isolation of the conduit. The proximal radial artery is occluded using an Endoloop" or clipped distal to the origin of the ulnar artery branch and transected with endoscopic scissors. The graft is recovered through the distal incision, and the distal end is ligated. The incision is closed in a standard manner.

RESULTS

The reported incidence of neurologic complications after standard open technique of radial artery harvest vary in the literature between 2.4 and 30% and can be related to injury of the superficial radial or the lateral antebrachial cutaneous nerves. The latter is usually not encountered in the endoscopic technique because the dissection is performed deep to the brachioradialis muscle. Superficial radial nerve injury, however, still may occur during distal dissection.[139] Endoscopic radial artery harvest is associated with a lower rate of wound infection (0-2.7%) as compared to the open technique.[129,140]

Graft patency, clinical outcomes, histological integrity, and in vitro vasoreactivity are similar to open graft harvest techniques.[141-143] Thus, endoscopic radial artery harvesting can be recommended for better patient satisfaction and fewer wound healing complications.[144]

REFERENCES

1. Jansen EW, Borst C, Lahpor JR, et al: Coronary artery bypass grafting without cardiopulmonary bypass using the octopus method: results in the first one hundred patients. *J Thorac Cardiovasc Surg* 1998; 116:60-67.
2. Vanermen H: What is minimally invasive cardiac surgery? *J Cardiac Surg* 1998; 13:268-274.
3. Yusuf S, Zucker D, Peduzzi P, et al: Effect of coronary artery bypass graft surgery on survival: overview of 10-year results from randomised trials by the coronary artery bypass graft surgery trialists collaboration. *Lancet* 1994; 344:563-570.
4. Aybek T, Kessler P, Khan MF, et al: Operative techniques in awake coronary artery bypass grafting. *J Thorac Cardiovasc Surg* 2003; 125:1394-1400.
5. Leather HA, Vuylsteke A, Bert C, et al: Evaluation of a new continuous cardiac output monitor in off-pump coronary artery surgery. *Anaesthesia* 2004; 59:385-389.
6. Falk V: Manual control and tracking—a human factor analysis relevant for beating heart surgery. *Ann Thorac Surg* 2002; 74:624-628.
7. Bouchot O, Aubin MC, Carrier M, et al: Temporary coronary artery occlusion during off-pump coronary artery bypass grafting with the new poloxamer p407 does not cause endothelial dysfunction in epicardial coronary arteries. *J Thorac Cardiovasc Surg* 2006; 132:1144-1149.
8. Mommerot A, Aubin MC, Carrier M, et al: Use of the purified poloxamer 407 for temporary coronary occlusion in off-pump cabg does not cause myocardial injury. *Innovations* 2007; 2:201-204.
9. Lev-Ran O, Braunstein R, Sharony R, et al: No-touch aorta off-pump coronary surgery: the effect on stroke. *J Thorac Cardiovasc Surg* 2005; 129:307-313.
10. Vallely MP, Potger K, McMillan D, et al: Anaortic techniques reduce neurological morbidity after off-pump coronary artery bypass surgery. *Heart Lung Circulation* 2008; 17:299-304.
11. Calafiore AM, Di Mauro M, Teodori G, et al: Impact of aortic manipulation on incidence of cerebrovascular accidents after surgical myocardial revascularization. *Ann Thorac Surg* 2002; 73:1387-1393.
12. Prapas SN, Panagiotopoulos IA, Hamed Abdelsalam A, et al: Predictors of prolonged mechanical ventilation following aorta no-touch off-pump coronary artery bypass surgery. *Eur J Cardiothorac Surg* 2007; 32:488-492.
13. Rastan AJ, Eckenstein JI, Hentschel B, et al: Emergency coronary artery bypass graft surgery for acute coronary syndrome: beating heart versus conventional cardioplegic cardiac arrest strategies. *Circulation* 2006; 114:I477-485.
14. Edgerton JR, Herbert MA, Jones KK, et al: On-pump beating heart surgery offers an alternative for unstable patients undergoing coronary artery bypass grafting. *Heart Surg Forum* 2004; 7:8-15.
15. Bakaeen FG, Shroyer AL, Gammie JS, et al: Trends in use of off-pump coronary artery bypass grafting: results from the society of thoracic surgeons adult cardiac surgery database. *J Thorac Cardiovasc Surg* 2014; 148:856-863, 864. e851; discussion 863-864.
16. Houlind K, Kjeldsen BJ, Madsen SN, et al: On-pump versus off-pump coronary artery bypass surgery in elderly patients: results from the Danish on-pump versus off-pump randomization study. *Circulation* 2012; 125:2431-2439.
17. Houlind K, Fenger-Gron M, Holme SJ, et al: Graft patency after off-pump coronary artery bypass surgery is inferior even with identical heparinization protocols: results from the Danish on-pump versus off-pump randomization study (doors). *J Thorac Cardiovasc Surg* 2014; 148:1812-1819. e1812.
18. Sergeant P, Wouters P, Meyns B, et al: Opcab versus early mortality and morbidity: an issue between clinical relevance and statistical significance. *Eur J Cardiothorac Surg* 2004; 25:779-785.
19. Puskas J, Cheng D, Knight J, et al: Off-pump versus conventional coronary artery bypass grafting: a meta-analysis and consensus statement from the 2004 ismics consensus conference. *Innovations* 2005; 1:3-27.
20. Lamy A, Devereaux PJ, Prabhakaran D, et al: Effects of off-pump and on-pump coronary-artery bypass grafting at 1 year. *N Engl J Med* 2013; 368:1179-1188.
21. Diegeler A, Borgermann J, Kappert U, et al: Off-pump versus on-pump coronary-artery bypass grafting in elderly patients. *N Engl J Med* 2013; 368:1189-1198.
22. Khan NE, De Souza A, Mister R, et al: A randomized comparison of off-pump and on-pump multivessel coronary-artery bypass surgery. *N Engl J Med* 2004; 350:21-28.
23. Puskas JD, Williams WH, Duke PG, et al: Off-pump coronary artery bypass grafting provides complete revascularization with reduced myocardial injury, transfusion requirements, and length of stay: a prospective randomized comparison of two hundred unselected patients undergoing off-pump versus conventional coronary artery bypass grafting. *J Thorac Cardiovasc Surg* 2003; 125:797-808.
24. Muneretto C, Bisleri G, Negri A, et al: Off-pump coronary artery surgery technique for total arterial myocardial revascularization: a prospective randomized study. *Ann Thorac Surg* 2003; 76:778-782; discussion 783.
25. Widimsky P, Straka Z, Stros P, et al: One-year coronary bypass graft patency: a randomized comparison between off-pump and on-pump surgery angiographic results of the prague-4 trial. *Circulation* 2004; 110:3418-3423.
26. Sabik JF, Blackstone EH, Lytle BW, et al: Equivalent midterm outcomes after off-pump and on-pump coronary surgery. *J Thorac Cardiovasc Surg* 2004; 127:142-148.
27. Czerny M, Baumer H, Kilo J, et al: Complete revascularization in coronary artery bypass grafting with and without cardiopulmonary bypass. *Ann Thorac Surg* 2001; 71:165-169.
28. Calafiore AM, Di Mauro M, Canosa C, et al: Myocardial revascularization with and without cardiopulmonary bypass: advantages, disadvantages and similarities. *Eur J Cardiothorac Surg* 2003; 24:953-960.
29. van Dijk D, Nierich AP, Jansen EW, et al: Early outcome after off-pump versus on-pump coronary bypass surgery: results from a randomized study. *Circulation* 2001; 104:1761-1766.
30. Afilalo J, Rasti M, Ohayon SM, et al: Off-pump vs. On-pump coronary artery bypass surgery: an updated meta-analysis and meta-regression of randomized trials. *Eur Heart J* 2012; 33:1257-1267.
31. Zamvar V, Williams D, Hall J, et al: Assessment of neurocognitive impairment after off-pump and on-pump techniques for coronary artery bypass graft surgery: prospective randomised controlled trial. *BMJ* 2002; 325:1268.
32. Bucerius J, Gummert JF, Borger MA, et al: Predictors of delirium after cardiac surgery delirium: effect of beating-heart (off-pump) surgery. *J Thorac Cardiovasc Surg* 2004; 127:57-64.
33. Stamou SC, Jablonski KA, Pfister AJ, et al: Stroke after conventional versus minimally invasive coronary artery bypass. *Ann Thorac Surg* 2002; 74:394-399.
34. Patel NC, Deodhar AP, Grayson AD, et al: Neurological outcomes in coronary surgery: independent effect of avoiding cardiopulmonary bypass. *Ann Thorac Surg* 2002; 74:400-405; discussion 405-406.
35. Diegeler A, Hirsch R, Schneider F, et al: Neuromonitoring and neurocognitive outcome in off-pump versus conventional coronary bypass operation. *Ann Thorac Surg* 2000; 69:1162-1166.
36. Lee JD, Lee SJ, Tsushima WT, et al: Benefits of off-pump bypass on neurologic and clinical morbidity: a prospective randomized trial. *Ann Thorac Surg* 2003; 76:18-25; discussion 25-16.

37. Scarborough JE, White W, Derilus FE, et al: Combined use of off-pump techniques and a sutureless proximal aortic anastomotic device reduces cerebral microemboli generation during coronary artery bypass grafting. *J Thorac Cardiovasc Surg* 2003; 126:1561-1567.

38. Moss E, Puskas JD, Thourani VH, et al: Avoiding aortic clamping during coronary artery bypass grafting reduces postoperative stroke. *J Thorac Cardiovasc Surg* 2015; 149:175-180.

39. Ascione R, Lloyd CT, Underwood MJ, et al: On-pump versus off-pump coronary revascularization: evaluation of renal function. *Ann Thorac Surg* 1999; 68:493-498.

40. Arom KV, Flavin TF, Emery RW, et al: Safety and efficacy of off-pump coronary artery bypass grafting. *Ann Thorac Surg* 2000; 69:704-710.

41. Bucerius J, Gummert JF, Walther T, et al: On-pump versus off-pump coronary artery bypass grafting: impact on postoperative renal failure requiring renal replacement therapy. *Ann Thorac Surg* 2004; 77:1250-1256.

42. Ascione R, Nason G, Al-Ruzzeh S, et al: Coronary revascularization with or without cardiopulmonary bypass in patients with preoperative nondialysis-dependent renal insufficiency. *Ann Thorac Surg* 2001; 72:2020-2025.

43. Weerasinghe A, Athanasiou T, Al-Ruzzeh S, et al: Functional renal outcome in on-pump and off-pump coronary revascularization: a propensity-based analysis. *Ann Thorac Surg* 2005; 79:1577-1583.

44. Seabra VF, Alobaidi S, Balk EM, et al: Off-pump coronary artery bypass surgery and acute kidney injury: a meta-analysis of randomized controlled trials. *Clin J Am Soc Nephrol* 2010; 5:1734-1744.

45. Garg AX, Devereaux PJ, Yusuf S, et al: Kidney function after off-pump or on-pump coronary artery bypass graft surgery: a randomized clinical trial. *JAMA* 2014; 311:2191-2198.

46. Athanasiou T, Aziz O, Mangoush O, et al: Does off-pump coronary artery bypass reduce the incidence of post-operative atrial fibrillation? A question revisited. *Eur J Cardiothorac Surg* 2004; 26:701-710.

47. Rastan AJ, Bittner HB, Gummert JF, et al: On-pump beating heart versus off-pump coronary artery bypass surgery-evidence of pump-induced myocardial injury. *Eur J Cardiothorac Surg* 2005; 27:1057-1064.

48. Dybdahl B, Wahba A, Haaverstad R, et al: On-pump versus off-pump coronary artery bypass grafting: more heat-shock protein 70 is released after on-pump surgery. *Eur J Cardiothorac Surg* 2004; 25:985-992.

49. Diegeler A, Doll N, Rauch T, et al: Humoral immune response during coronary artery bypass grafting: a comparison of limited approach, "off-pump" technique, and conventional cardiopulmonary bypass. *Circulation* 2000; 102:III95-100.

50. Cheng DC, Bainbridge D, Martin JE, Novick RJ: Does off-pump coronary artery bypass reduce mortality, morbidity, and resource utilization when compared with conventional coronary artery bypass? A meta-analysis of randomized trials. *Anesthesiology* 2005; 102:188-203.

51. Nathoe HM, van Dijk D, Jansen EW, et al: A comparison of on-pump and off-pump coronary bypass surgery in low-risk patients. *N Engl J Med* 2003; 348:394-402.

52. Magee MJ, Coombs LP, Peterson ED, Mack MJ: Patient selection and current practice strategy for off-pump coronary artery bypass surgery. *Circulation* 2003; 108 Suppl 1:II9-14.

53. Mack MJ, Pfister A, Bachand D, et al: Comparison of coronary bypass surgery with and without cardiopulmonary bypass in patients with multivessel disease. *J Thorac Cardiovasc Surg* 2004; 127:167-173.

54. Stamou SC, Jablonski KA, Hill PC, et al: Coronary revascularization without cardiopulmonary bypass versus the conventional approach in high-risk patients. *Ann Thorac Surg* 2005; 79:552-557.

55. Ascione R, Reeves BC, Rees K, Angelini GD: Effectiveness of coronary artery bypass grafting with or without cardiopulmonary bypass in overweight patients. *Circulation* 2002; 106:1764-1770.

56. Angelini GD, Taylor FC, Reeves BC, Ascione R: Early and midterm outcome after off-pump and on-pump surgery in beating heart against cardioplegic arrest studies (bhacas 1 and 2): a pooled analysis of two randomised controlled trials. *Lancet* 2002; 359:1194-1199.

57. Angelini GD, Culliford L, Smith DK, et al: Effects of on- and off-pump coronary artery surgery on graft patency, survival, and health-related quality of life: long-term follow-up of 2 randomized controlled trials. *J Thorac Cardiovasc Surg* 2009; 137:295-303.

58. Kim JB, Yun SC, Lim JW, et al: Long-term survival following coronary artery bypass grafting: off-pump versus on-pump strategies. *J Am Coll Cardiol* 2014; 63:2280-2288.

59. Chaudhry UA, Harling L, Rao C, et al: Off-pump versus on-pump coronary revascularization: meta-analysis of mid- and long-term outcomes. *Ann Thorac Surg* 2014; 98:563-572.

60. MacGillivray TE, Vlahakes GJ: Patency and the pump—the risks and benefits of off-pump cabg. *N Engl J Med* 2004; 350:3-4.

61. Calafiore AM, Giammarco GD, Teodori G, et al: Left anterior descending coronary artery grafting via left anterior small thoracotomy without cardiopulmonary bypass. *Ann Thorac Surg* 1996; 61:1658-1663; discussion 1664-1655.

62. Cremer J, Struber M, Wittwer T, et al: Off-bypass coronary bypass grafting via minithoracotomy using mechanical epicardial stabilization. *Ann Thorac Surg* 1997; 63:S79-83.

63. Subramanian VA, McCabe JC, Geller CM: Minimally invasive direct coronary artery bypass grafting: two-year clinical experience. *Ann Thorac Surg* 1997; 64:1648-1653; discussion 1654-1655.

64. Diegeler A, Matin M, Kayser S, et al: Angiographic results after minimally invasive coronary bypass grafting using the minimally invasive direct coronary bypass grafting (midcab) approach. *Eur J Cardiothorac Surg* 1999; 15:680-684.

65. Bucerius J, Metz S, Walther T, et al: Endoscopic internal thoracic artery dissection leads to significant reduction of pain after minimally invasive direct coronary artery bypass graft surgery. *Ann Thorac Surg* 2002; 73:1180-1184.

66. Wolf RK, Ohtsuka T, Flege JB Jr: Early results of thoracoscopic internal mammary artery harvest using an ultrasonic scalpel. *Eur J Cardiothorac Surg* 1998; 14 Suppl 1:S54-57.

67. Duhaylongsod FG, Mayfield WR, Wolf RK: Thoracoscopic harvest of the internal thoracic artery: a multicenter experience in 218 cases. *Ann Thorac Surg* 1998; 66:1012-1017.

68. Mack MJ, Magovern JA, Acuff TA, et al: Results of graft patency by immediate angiography in minimally invasive coronary artery surgery. *Ann Thorac Surg* 1999; 68:383-389; discussion 389-390.

69. Kettering K, Dapunt O, Baer FM: Minimally invasive direct coronary artery bypass grafting: a systematic review. *J Cardiovasc Surg* 2004; 45:255-264.

70. Reser D, Hemelrijck M, Pavicevic J, et al: Mid-term outcomes of minimally invasive direct coronary artery bypass grafting. *Thorac Cardiovasc Surg* 2015; 63:313-318.

71. Holzhey DM, Cornely JP, Rastan AJ, et al: Review of a 13-year single-center experience with minimally invasive direct coronary artery bypass as the primary surgical treatment of coronary artery disease. *Heart Surg Forum* 2012; 15:E61-68.

72. Calafiore AM, Di Giammarco G, Teodori G, et al: Midterm results after minimally invasive coronary surgery (last operation). *J Thorac Cardiovasc Surg* 1998; 115:763-771.

73. Mehran R, Dangas G, Stamou SC, et al: One-year clinical outcome after minimally invasive direct coronary artery bypass. *Circulation* 2000; 102:2799-2802.

74. Gummert JF, Funkat A, Krian A: Cardiac surgery in Germany during 2004: a report on behalf of the german society for thoracic and cardiovascular surgery. *Thorac Cardiovasc Surg* 2005; 53:391-399.

75. de Canniere D, Wimmer-Greinecker G, Cichon R, et al: Feasibility, safety, and efficacy of totally endoscopic coronary artery bypass grafting: multicenter European experience. *J Thorac Cardiovasc Surg* 2007; 134:710-716.

76. Raja SG, Benedetto U, Alkizwini E, et al: Propensity score adjusted comparison of midcab versus full sternotomy left anterior descending artery revascularization. *Innovations (Phila)* 2015; 10:174-178.

77. Birla R, Patel P, Aresu G, Asimakopoulos G: Minimally invasive direct coronary artery bypass versus off-pump coronary surgery through sternotomy. *Ann R Coll Surg Engl* 2013; 95:481-485.

78. Mariani MA, Boonstra PW, Grandjean JG, et al: Minimally invasive coronary artery bypass grafting versus coronary angioplasty for isolated type c stenosis of the left anterior descending artery. *J Thorac Cardiovasc Surg* 1997; 114:434-439.

79. Fraund S, Herrmann G, Witzke A, et al: Midterm follow-up after minimally invasive direct coronary artery bypass grafting versus percutaneous coronary intervention techniques. *Ann Thorac Surg* 2005; 79:1225-1231.

80. Diegeler A, Thiele H, Falk V, et al: Comparison of stenting with minimally invasive bypass surgery for stenosis of the left anterior descending coronary artery. *N Engl J Med* 2002; 347:561-566.

81. Shirai K, Lansky AJ, Mehran R, et al: Minimally invasive coronary artery bypass grafting versus stenting for patients with proximal left anterior descending coronary artery disease. *Am J Cardiol* 2004; 93:959-962.

82. Thiele H, Oettel S, Jacobs S, et al: Comparison of bare-metal stenting with minimally invasive bypass surgery for stenosis of the left anterior descending coronary artery: a 5-year follow-up. *Circulation* 2005; 112:3445-3450.

83. Reeves BC, Angelini GD, Bryan AJ, et al: A multi-centre randomised controlled trial of minimally invasive direct coronary bypass grafting versus percutaneous transluminal coronary angioplasty with stenting for proximal stenosis of the left anterior descending coronary artery. *Health Technol Assess (Winchester, England)* 2004; 8:1-43.

84. Blazek S, Holzhey D, Jungert C, et al: Comparison of bare-metal stenting with minimally invasive bypass surgery for stenosis of the left anterior descending coronary artery: 10-year follow-up of a randomized trial. *JACC Cardiovasc Interv* 2013; 6:20-26.

85. Etienne PY, D'Hoore W, Papadatos S, et al: Five-year follow-up of drug-eluting stents implantation vs minimally invasive direct coronary artery bypass for left anterior descending artery disease: a propensity score analysis. *Eur J Cardiothorac Surg* 2013; 44:884-890.

86. Deppe AC, Liakopoulos OJ, Kuhn EW, et al: Minimally invasive direct coronary bypass grafting versus percutaneous coronary intervention for single-vessel disease: a meta-analysis of 2885 patients. *Eur J Cardiothorac Surg* 2015; 47:397-406; discussion 406.

87. Deo SV, Sharma V, Shah IK, et al: Minimally invasive direct coronary artery bypass graft surgery or percutaneous coronary intervention for proximal left anterior descending artery stenosis: a meta-analysis. *Ann Thorac Surg* 2014; 97:2056-2065.

88. Hannan EL, Zhong Y, Walford G, et al: Coronary artery bypass graft surgery versus drug-eluting stents for patients with isolated proximal left anterior descending disease. *J Am Coll Cardiol* 2014; 64:2717-2726.

89. Holzhey DM, Jacobs S, Walther T, et al: Cumulative sum failure analysis for eight surgeons performing minimally invasive direct coronary artery bypass. *J Thorac Cardiovasc Surg* 2007; 134:663-669.

90. Thiele H, Neumann-Schniedewind P, Jacobs S, et al: Randomized comparison of minimally invasive direct coronary artery bypass surgery versus sirolimus-eluting stenting in isolated proximal left anterior descending coronary artery stenosis. *J Am Coll Cardiol* 2009; 53:2324-2331.

91. Holzhey DM, Jacobs S, Mochalski M, et al: Seven-year follow-up after minimally invasive direct coronary artery bypass: experience with more than 1300 patients. *Ann Thorac Surg* 2007; 83:108-114.

92. Falk V, McLoughlin J, Guthart G, et al: Dexterity enhancement in endoscopic surgery by a computer-controlled mechanical wrist. *Minim Invasive Ther Allied Technol* 1999; 8:235-242.

93. Falk V, Diegeler A, Walther T, et al: Total endoscopic off-pump coronary artery bypass grafting. *Heart Surg Forum* 2000; 3:29-31.

94. Damiano RJ Jr, Ehrman WJ, Ducko CT, et al: Initial united states clinical trial of robotically assisted endoscopic coronary artery bypass grafting. *J Thorac Cardiovasc Surg* 2000; 119:77-82.

95. Reichenspurner H, Damiano RJ, Mack M, et al: Use of the voice-controlled and computer-assisted surgical system zeus for endoscopic coronary artery bypass grafting. *J Thorac Cardiovasc Surg* 1999; 118:11-16.

96. Kappert U, Schneider J, Cichon R, et al: Wrist-enhanced instrumentation: moving toward totally endoscopic coronary artery bypass grafting. *Ann Thorac Surg* 2000; 70:1105-1108.

97. Bonatti J, Schachner T, Bonaros N, et al: Effectiveness and safety of total endoscopic left internal mammary artery bypass graft to the left anterior descending artery. *Am J Cardiol* 2009; 104:1684-1688.

98. Falk V, Diegeler A, Walther T, et al: Endoscopic coronary artery bypass grafting on the beating heart using a computer enhanced telemanipulation system. *Heart Surg Forum* 1999; 2:199-205.

99. Falk V, Diegeler A, Walther T, et al: Total endoscopic computer enhanced coronary artery bypass grafting. *Eur J Cardiothorac Surg* 2000; 17:38-45.

100. Kappert U, Cichon R, Schneider J, et al: Technique of closed chest coronary artery surgery on the beating heart. *Eur J Cardiothorac Surg* 2001; 20:765-769.

101. Srivastava S, Gadasalli S, Agusala M, et al: Use of bilateral internal thoracic arteries in cabg through lateral thoracotomy with robotic assistance in 150 patients. *Ann Thorac Surg* 2006; 81:800-806; discussion 806.

102. Subramanian VA, Patel NU, Patel NC, Loulmet DF: Robotic assisted multivessel minimally invasive direct coronary artery bypass with port-access stabilization and cardiac positioning: paving the way for outpatient coronary surgery? *Ann Thorac Surg* 2005; 79:1590-1596; discussion 1590-1596.

103. McGinn JT Jr, Usman S, Lapierre H, et al: Minimally invasive coronary artery bypass grafting: dual-center experience in 450 consecutive patients. *Circulation* 2009; 120:S78-84.

104. Lemma M, Athanasiou T, Contino M: Minimally invasive cardiac surgery-coronary artery bypass graft. *Multimed Man Cardiothorac Surg* 2013; 2013:mmt007.

105. Ruel M, Shariff MA, Lapierre H, et al: Results of the minimally invasive coronary artery bypass grafting angiographic patency study. *J Thorac Cardiovasc Surg* 2014; 147:203-208.

106. Angelini GD, Wilde P, Salerno TA, et al: Integrated left small thoracotomy and angioplasty for multivessel coronary artery revascularisation. *Lancet* 1996; 347:757-758.

107. Pick AW, Orszulak TA, Anderson BJ, Schaff HV: Single versus bilateral internal mammary artery grafts: 10-year outcome analysis. *Ann Thorac Surg* 1997; 64:599-605.

108. Serruys PW, Morice MC, Kappetein AP, et al: Percutaneous coronary intervention versus coronary-artery bypass grafting for severe coronary artery disease. *N Engl J Med* 2009; 360:961-972.

109. DeRose JJ: Current state of integrated "hybrid" coronary revascularization. *Semin Thorac Cardiovasc Surg* 2009; 21:229-236.

110. Holzhey DM, Jacobs S, Mochalski M, et al: Minimally invasive hybrid coronary artery revascularization. *Ann Thorac Surg* 2008; 86:1856-1860.

111. Mack MJ, Brown DL, Sankaran A: Minimally invasive coronary bypass for protected left main coronary stenosis angioplasty. *Ann Thorac Surg* 1997; 64:545-546.

112. Friedrich GJ, Bonatti J: Hybrid coronary artery revascularization—review and update 2007. *Heart Surg Forum* 2007; 10:E292-296.

113. Katz MR, Van Praet F, de Canniere D, et al: Integrated coronary revascularization: percutaneous coronary intervention plus robotic totally endoscopic coronary artery bypass. *Circulation* 2006; 114:I1473-I476.

114. Bonatti J, Schachner T, Bonaros N, et al: Treatment of double vessel coronary artery disease by totally endoscopic bypass surgery and drug-eluting stent placement in one simultaneous hybrid session. *Heart Surg Forum* 2005; 8:E284-E286.

115. Bonatti J, Schachner T, Bonaros N, et al: Robotic totally endoscopic coronary artery bypass and catheter based coronary intervention in one operative session. *Ann Thorac Surg* 2005; 79:2138-2141.

116. Wittwer T, Haverich A, Cremer J, et al: Follow-up experience with coronary hybrid-revascularisation. *Thorac Cardiovasc Surg* 2000; 48:356-359.

117. Halkos ME, Walker PF, Vassiliades TA, et al: Clinical and angiographic results after hybrid coronary revascularization. *Ann Thorac Surg* 2014; 97:484-490.

118. Hu S, Li Q, Gao P, et al: Simultaneous hybrid revascularization versus off-pump coronary artery bypass for multivessel coronary artery disease. *Ann Thorac Surg* 2011; 91:432-438.

119. Halkos ME, Vassiliades TA, Douglas JS, et al: Hybrid coronary revascularization versus off-pump coronary artery bypass grafting for the treatment of multivessel coronary artery disease. *Ann Thorac Surg* 2011; 92:1695-1701; discussion 1701-1702.

120. Halkos ME, Rab ST, Vassiliades TA, et al: Hybrid coronary revascularization versus off-pump coronary artery bypass for the treatment of left main coronary stenosis. *Ann Thorac Surg* 2011; 92:2155-2160.

121. Bachinsky WB, Abdelsalam M, Boga G, et al: Comparative study of same sitting hybrid coronary artery revascularization versus off-pump coronary artery bypass in multivessel coronary artery disease. *J Interv Cardiol* 2012; 25:460-468.

122. Hu FB, Cui LQ: Short-term clinical outcomes after hybrid coronary revascularization versus off-pump coronary artery bypass for the treatment of multivessel or left main coronary artery disease: a meta-analysis. *Coron Artery Dis* 2015; 26:526-534.

123. Shen L, Hu S, Wang H, et al: One-stop hybrid coronary revascularization versus coronary artery bypass grafting and percutaneous coronary intervention for the treatment of multivessel coronary artery disease: 3-year follow-up results from a single institution. *J Am Coll Cardiol* 2013; 61:2525-2533.

124. Harskamp RE, Puskas JD, Tijssen JG, et al: Comparison of hybrid coronary revascularization versus coronary artery bypass grafting in patients ≥65 years with multivessel coronary artery disease. *Am J Cardiol* 2014; 114:224-229.

125. Goldsborough MA, Miller MH, Gibson J, et al: Prevalence of leg wound complications after coronary artery bypass grafting: determination of risk factors. *Am J Crit Care* 1999; 8:149-153.

126. Allen KB, Griffith GL, Heimansohn DA, et al: Endoscopic versus traditional saphenous vein harvesting: a prospective, randomized trial. *Ann Thorac Surg* 1998; 66:26-31; discussion 31-32.

127. Bonde P, Graham A, MacGowan S: Endoscopic vein harvest: early results of a prospective trial with open vein harvest. *Heart Surg Forum* 2002; 5(Suppl 4):S378-S391.

128. Bonde P, Graham AN, MacGowan SW: Endoscopic vein harvest: advantages and limitations. *Ann Thorac Surg* 2004; 77:2076-2082.

129. Aziz O, Athanasiou T, Darzi A: Minimally invasive conduit harvesting: a systematic review. *Eur J Cardiothorac Surg* 2006; 29:324-333.

130. Cheng D, Allen K, Cohn W, et al: Endoscopic vascular harvest in coronary artery bypass grafting surgery: a meta-analysis of randomized trials and controlled trials. *Innovations* 2005; 1:61-74.

131. Lopes RD, Hafley GE, Allen KB, et al: Endoscopic versus open vein-graft harvesting in coronary-artery bypass surgery. *N Engl J Med* 2009; 361:235-244.

132. Ouzounian M, Hassan A, Buth KJ, et al: Impact of endoscopic versus open saphenous vein harvest techniques on outcomes after coronary artery bypass grafting. *Ann Thorac Surg* 89:403-408.

133. Coppoolse R, Rees W, Krech R, et al: Routine minimal invasive vein harvesting reduces postoperative morbidity in cardiac bypass procedures. Clinical report of 1400 patients. *Eur J Cardiothorac Surg* 1999; 16 Suppl 2:S61-66.

134. Crouch JD, O'Hair DP, Keuler JP, et al: Open versus endoscopic saphenous vein harvesting: wound complications and vein quality. *Ann Thorac Surg* 1999; 68:1513-1516.

135. Meharwal ZS, Trehan N: Functional status of the hand after radial artery harvesting: results in 3,977 cases. *Ann Thorac Surg* 2001; 72:1557-1561.

136. Denton TA, Trento L, Cohen M, et al: Radial artery harvesting for coronary bypass operations: neurologic complications and their potential mechanisms. *J Thorac Cardiovasc Surg* 2001; 121:951-956.

137. Tatoulis J, Royse AG, Buxton BF, et al: The radial artery in coronary surgery: a 5-year experience—clinical and angiographic results. *Ann Thorac Surg* 2002; 73:143-147; discussion 147-148.

138. Connolly MW, Torrillo LD, Stauder MJ, et al: Endoscopic radial artery harvesting: results of first 300 patients. *Ann Thorac Surg* 2002; 74:502-505; discussion 506.

139. Casselman FP, La Meir M, Cammu G, et al: Initial experience with an endoscopic radial artery harvesting technique. *J Thorac Cardiovasc Surg* 2004; 128:463-466.

140. Patel AN, Henry AC, Hunnicutt C, et al: Endoscopic radial artery harvesting is better than the open technique. *Ann Thorac Surg* 2004; 78:149-153; discussion 149-153.

141. Medalion B, Tobar A, Yosibash Z, et al: Vasoreactivity and histology of the radial artery: comparison of open versus endoscopic approaches. *Eur J Cardiothorac Surg* 2008; 34:845-849.

142. Ito N, Tashiro T, Morishige N, et al: Endoscopic radial artery harvesting for coronary artery bypass grafting: the initial clinical experience and results of the first 50 patients. *Heart Surg Forum* 2009; 12: E310-E315.

143. Bleiziffer S, Hettich I, Eisenhauer B, et al: Patency rates of endoscopically harvested radial arteries one year after coronary artery bypass grafting. *J Thorac Cardiovasc Surg* 2007; 134:649-656.

144. Nishida S, Kikuchi Y, Watanabe G, et al: Endoscopic radial artery harvesting: patient satisfaction and complications. *Asian Cardiovasc Thorac Ann* 2008; 16:43-46.

Coronary Artery Reoperations

Bruce W. Lytle • George Tolis, Jr.

24

Coronary artery reoperations are more complicated than primary operations. Patients undergoing reoperations have distinct, more dangerous pathologies; reoperations are technically more difficult to perform; and the risks are greater.[1-12] Vein graft atherosclerosis, present in most reoperative candidates, is a unique and dangerous lesion. Reoperative candidates commonly have severe and diffuse native-vessel distal coronary artery disease (CAD), a problem that has had the time to develop only because these patients did not die from their original proximal coronary artery lesions. Aortic and noncardiac atherosclerosis are also often far advanced in many reoperative candidates. Some technical hazards, including the presence of patent arterial grafts and sternal reentry, are unique to reoperations, and others, such as lack of bypass conduits and difficult coronary artery exposure, are common.

INCIDENCE OF REOPERATION

After a primary bypass operation, the likelihood of a patient undergoing a reoperation depends on patient-related variables, primary operation-related variables, adherence to strict medical control of risk factors for disease progression after bypass surgery, the possibility of alternative treatments, physician opinion about the feasibility of reoperation, and time. Studies from the Cleveland Clinic demonstrated a cumulative incidence of reoperation of 3% by 5 years, 10% by 10 years, and 25% by 20 postoperative years[13] (Fig. 24-1). Factors associated statistically with an increased likelihood of reoperation have been variables predicting a favorable long-term survival (eg, young age, normal left ventricular function [LVF], and single- or double-vessel disease), variables designating an imperfect primary operation (eg, no internal thoracic artery [ITA] graft and incomplete revascularization), and symptom status (eg, class III or IV symptoms at primary operation). Young age at primary operation and incomplete revascularization are also markers of a severe atherogenic diathesis.

Over recent decades the proportion of isolated coronary artery operations that are reoperations has decreased. In 1990, about 37% of coronary artery revascularization operations were reoperative interventions, whereas in 2002 this figure was 30%[14] (Fig. 24-2). Compared to that year, a much more dramatic decrease in reoperative coronary bypass surgery occurred during the most recent decade, with reoperative procedures representing only 4.6% of all isolated coronary bypass operations. This decrease is related in part to the more aggressive use of coronary artery interventions for patients with previous bypass surgery and probably to more effective risk factor control. Also, surgery has changed in directions that will decrease the rate of reoperation. Use of the left internal thoracic artery (LITA) to graft the left anterior descending (LAD) coronary artery decreases the risk of reoperation compared with the strategy of using only vein grafts, and the LITA-LAD graft has become a standard part of operations for coronary artery revascularization.[15] Furthermore, it now appears that use of bilateral ITA grafts decreases the likelihood of death and reoperation when compared with the single LITA-LAD strategy[16] (Fig. 24-3). The use of other arterial conduits such as the radial artery and the gastroepiploic artery in the context of total arterial revascularization may decrease the risk of reoperation further, but as yet the long-term data are insufficient to answer this question.

The patient population of reoperative candidates has evolved. Cleveland Clinic Foundation studies have shown that in the early years of bypass surgery (1967-1978), only 28% of patients underwent reoperation solely because of graft failure, and that graft failure often occurred early after the primary operation (mean postoperative interval of 28 months after primary operation). Reoperation because of the progression of atherosclerosis in nongrafted coronary arteries was common in the 1967 to 1978 time period (55% of patients).[1,2] Between 1988 and 1991, almost all patients had graft failure as at least part of the indication for reoperation (92%), but that graft failure occurred late after the primary operation at a mean interval of 116 months.[3] Today, patients undergoing reoperation usually had a successful primary operation at least 10 years previously for the treatment of multivessel CAD, and the angiographic indications

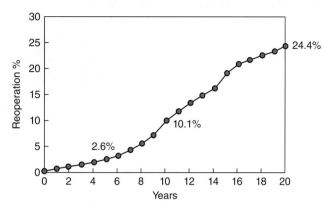

FIGURE 24-1 Study of 4000 patients who underwent bypass surgery from 1971 to 1974 showed that 25% of patients had undergone a reoperation within a period of 20 years after primary operation. (Data from Cosgrove DM, Loop FD, Lytle BW, et al: Predictors of reoperation after myocardial revascularization, *J Thorac Cardiovasc Surg*. 1986 Nov;92(5):811-821.)

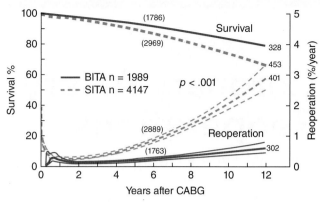

FIGURE 24-3 Comparison of survival and reoperation hazard function curves in the propensity-matched patients undergoing bilateral (BITA, n = 1989) or single ITA (SITA, n = 4147) CABG. (Reproduced with permission from Lytle BW, Blackstone EH, Loop FD, et al: Two internal thoracic artery grafts are better than one, *J Thorac Cardiovasc Surg*. 1999 May;117(5):855-872.)

for reoperation are progression of native-vessel distal CAD in combination with late graft failure caused by vein graft atherosclerosis.

GRAFT FAILURE

An understanding of the pathology and causes of saphenous vein graft (SVG) failure is important not only for an understanding of the causes of the need for reoperation, but also for understanding the dangers inherent in either the interventional or the conservative treatment of patients with previous bypass surgery. Saphenous vein to coronary artery

grafts exhibit different pathologies at different intervals after operation.[17-20] Within a few months, they often have diffuse endothelial disruptions with associated mural thrombus. The mural thrombus usually is not obstructing, and when grafts do become occluded early after operation owing to thrombosis, it may not be a result of these intimal changes, but rather may be related to hemodynamic factors. Most saphenous vein grafts examined more than 2 to 3 months after operation have developed a proliferative intimal fibroplasia. This is a concentric cellular process, and it is diffuse, extending the entire length of the graft (Fig. 24-4). It evolves with time to a more fibrous lesion. It is not friable, and although

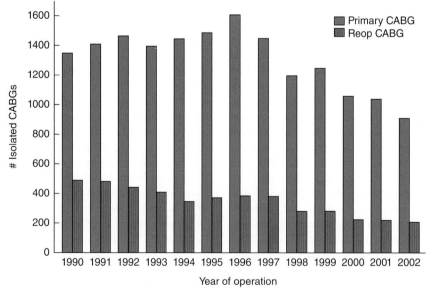

FIGURE 24-2 Study of 21,568 patients who underwent bypass surgery from 1990 to 2003 showed a steady decrease in the number of patients undergoing redo coronary artery operations. (Data from Sabik JF, Blackstone EH, Houghtaling PL, et al: Is reoperation still a risk factor in coronary artery bypass surgery? *Ann Thorac Surg*. 2005 Nov;80(5):1719-1727.)

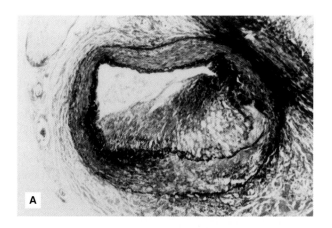

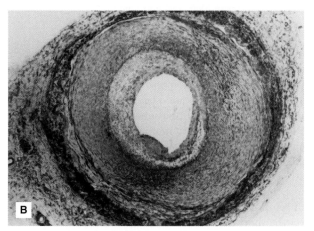

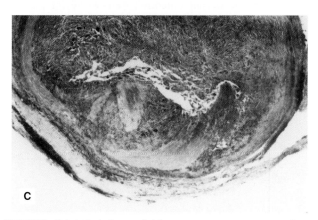

FIGURE 24-4 Pathology of (A) native coronary artery atherosclerosis, (B) vein graft intimal fibrosis, and (C) severe vein graft atherosclerosis. (Reproduced with permission from Lytle BW, Cosgrove DM: Coronary artery bypass surgery, *Curr Probl Surg* 1992 Oct:29(10):743-807.)

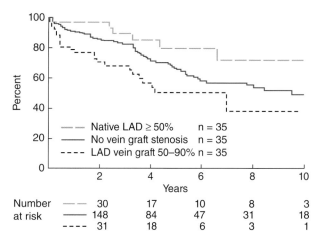

FIGURE 24-5 Patients with late stenoses in vein grafts to the LAD coronary artery had worse survival when compared with either patients with native coronary LAD stenoses or patients with no stenotic vein grafts. (Reproduced with permission from Lytle BW, Loop FD, Taylor PC, et al: Vein graft disease: the clinical impact of stenoses in saphenous vein bypass grafts to coronary arteries, *J Thorac Cardiovasc Surg.* 1992 May;103(5):831-840.)

atherosclerosis mimics that of intimal fibroplasia in that it is concentric and diffuse, although as vein graft atherosclerosis progresses, stenotic lesions may become eccentric. In addition, vein graft atherosclerosis is a superficial lesion, it is very friable, and it is often associated with overlying mural thrombus. These characteristics make it different from native-vessel coronary atherosclerosis, a process that is segmental and proximal, eccentric, encapsulated, usually not friable, and usually not associated with overlying mural thrombus. Vein graft atherosclerosis is seen in a majority of grafts explanted more than 10 years after surgery whether or not those grafts are stenotic, and atherosclerotic lesions appear to account for almost all late SVG stenoses. The extreme friability of vein graft atherosclerosis creates a substantial risk of distal coronary artery embolization during percutaneous interventions to treat stenotic lesions and during reoperations for patients with atherosclerotic vein grafts. It is also probable that spontaneous coronary artery embolization may occur from atherosclerotic grafts. In addition, atherosclerotic stenoses in vein grafts appear to predispose to graft thrombosis. Vein graft atherosclerosis appears to be an "active" event-producing lesion.

The exact incidence of late SVG stenoses and occlusions is difficult to determine even with prospective studies because death and reoperation are nonrandom events that remove patients from prospective populations available for late coronary artery angiography. However, it appears that by 10 years after operation, approximately 30% of vein grafts are totally occluded, and 30% of patent grafts exhibit some degree of stenosis or intimal irregularities characteristic of vein graft atherosclerosis.[21,22] Although vein graft atherosclerosis is not the only factor related to late SVG occlusion, it is an important one. Native-vessel stenoses distal to the insertion site of vein grafts may decrease SVG graft outflow and contribute

intimal fibroplasia involves most vein grafts, it causes stenoses or occlusions of only a few.

Vein graft atherosclerosis is a distinct pathologic process that often is recognized as early as 3 to 4 years after operation and is characterized by lipid infiltration of areas of intimal fibroplasia (Fig. 24-5). The distribution of vein graft to graft failure, but late graft occlusion usually occurs in the presence of vein graft atherosclerosis. Furthermore, when stenotic vein grafts are replaced at reoperation, the late patency rate of the new vein grafts is good.[2]

Progress has been made toward decreasing the rate of vein graft failure. The early patency rates of SVGs have been improved by the use of perioperative and long-term platelet inhibitors,[23–25] but the best data involving patients receiving platelet inhibitors indicate that the 10-year vein graft failure rate is approximately 35%. Some studies now indicate that lipid-lowering regimens decrease late vein graft disease and the risk of late cardiac events.[26,27] However, the overall level of improvement has been small.[26,27] So far, the only way known to avoid vein graft atherosclerosis is to avoid using vein grafts.

ITA grafts rarely develop late atherosclerosis, and the late attrition rate of patent ITA grafts is extremely low. Left ITA to LAD grafts have a very high late (20 years) patency rate, and for most patients, the LAD is a profoundly important coronary artery.[21,28] These factors account for the impact of the LITA-LAD graft not only in decreasing the rate of late death after primary bypass surgery, but also in decreasing the rate of reoperation.[15] Multiple ITA grafts provide incremental benefit in decreasing the risk of reoperation.[16] It is also important that ITA grafts do not develop graft atherosclerosis, and therefore do not create the risk of coronary artery embolization during reoperation. The presence of patent arterial grafts may create other technical problems during repeat surgery, but embolization is not among them.

INDICATIONS FOR REOPERATION

The randomized trials of bypass surgery versus medical management that were initiated in the 1970s provided a framework of information concerning the indications for bypass surgery, and subsequent observational studies have added substance to that framework. However, no randomized trials of medical versus surgical management pertain to patients with prior surgery. The coronary pathology of patients with previous bypass surgery is different from that of patients with only native-vessel stenoses, and we cannot assume that the natural history of, for example, triple-vessel disease based on atherosclerotic vein grafts, is equivalent to that of triple-native-vessel disease.

Two nonrandomized, retrospective studies of patients who had angiograms after bypass surgery addressed the issue of late survival.[29,30] One study showed that patients with early (fewer than 5 years after operation) stenoses in vein grafts and patients with no stenotic vein grafts had approximately the same outcomes and that these outcomes were relatively good.[29] *However, the presence of late (5 years or more after operation) stenoses in vein grafts predicted poor long-term outcomes, particularly if a stenotic vein graft supplied the LAD coronary artery. When late stenoses in LAD vein grafts were combined with other high-risk characteristics, the late survival rate was particularly dismal.* For example, patients with a 50 to 99% stenosis in an LAD vein graft combined with abnormal LVF

and triple-vessel or left main stenoses had only a 46% 2-year survival without reoperation. Patients with late stenoses in an LAD vein graft had significantly worse long-term outcomes than did patients with the LAD jeopardized by a native lesion (see Fig. 24-5). This study showed that the difference in the pathology of early (intimal fibroplasia) and late (vein graft atherosclerosis) vein graft stenoses is associated with a difference in clinical outcome and that late stenoses in vein grafts are dangerous lesions.

A second study compared the outcomes of patients with stenotic vein grafts treated with reoperation (REOP group) versus those treated with medical treatment (MED group).[30] Again, this was a nonrandomized, retrospective study, and the patients in the REOP group were older and more symptomatic, had worse LVF, and had fewer patent grafts than the patients in the MED group.

The survival of patients with early (fewer than 5 years) SVG stenoses was not different in the two groups. The operative risk for the REOP group was low (no deaths among the 59 patients) and the long-term survival was good, but late survival was just as good for the patients treated medically (Fig. 24-6). It is important to note that the patients in the REOP group were more symptomatic to start with, and at late follow-up, they were less symptomatic than the patients in the MED group. Thus, reoperation for patients with early vein graft stenosis was an effective way of relieving symptoms of angina, but it appears that patients without symptoms can be treated medically with safety, at least over the short term.

However, the overall outcomes were worse for patients with late stenoses in vein grafts, and many subgroups had improved survival rates with reoperation. By multivariate testing (Table 24-1), a stenotic (20-99%) LAD vein graft predicted late death, and performing a reoperation increased

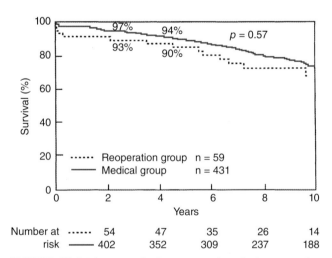

FIGURE 24-6 The survival of patients with early (<5 years after operation) stenoses in vein grafts was favorable with and without reoperation (*p* = NS). (Reproduced with permission from Lytle BW, Loop FD, Taylor AC, et al: The effect of coronary reoperation on the survival of patients with stenoses in saphenous vein to coronary bypass grafts, *J Thorac Cardiovasc Surg.* 1993 Apr;105(4):605-612.)

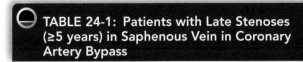

TABLE 24-1: Patients with Late Stenoses (≥5 years) in Saphenous Vein in Coronary Artery Bypass

Grafts: Multivariate model of variables influencing late survival

	p-Value	Relative risk
Variables decreasing survival		
LVF moderate/severe	.0001	2.58
Age (at catheterization)	.0001	1.04*
3VD/LMT	.0011	2.87
LAD-SVG stenosis (20-99%)	.0019	1.90
Variable increasing survival Reoperation	.0007	0.51

LVF = left ventricular function: 3VD/LMT = triple-vessel disease and/or left main stenosis.
*Per year of age.
Reproduced with permission from Lytle BW, Loop FD, Taylor AC, et al: The effect of coronary reoperation on the survival of patients with stenoses in saphenous vein to coronary bypass grafts, *J Thorac Cardiovasc Surg.* 1993 Apr;105(4):605-612.

late survival for these patients. Multivariate testing of smaller subgroups showed that the survival advantage for the REOP group was true even for patients with only class I or class II symptoms, and that reoperation still improved survival for the remaining patients when patients with stenoses in LAD vein grafts were excluded from the analysis.

Univariate comparisons for the REOP and MED subgroups of patients with stenotic LAD grafts are shown in Fig. 24-7, demonstrating the improved survival for the REOP group. When patients with stenotic LAD vein grafts were

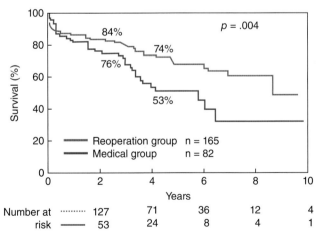

FIGURE 24-7 If patients had late (≥5 years after operation) stenoses in LAD vein grafts, they had a better survival rate (*p* = .004) with immediate reoperation than if they received initial nonoperative treatment. (Reproduced with permission from Lytle BW, Loop FD, Taylor AC, et al: The effect of coronary reoperation on the survival of patients with stenoses in saphenous vein to coronary bypass grafts, *J Thorac Cardiovasc Surg.* 1993 Apr;105(4):605-612.)

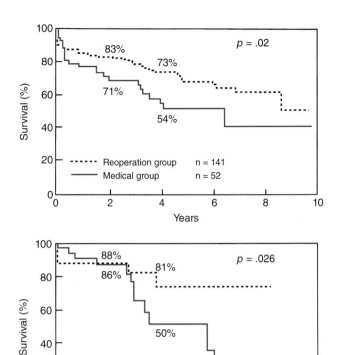

FIGURE 24-8 Patients with late stenoses in LAD vein grafts (*top*) had immediate improvement in their survival rate. Patients with moderate (20-49%) stenoses in LAD vein grafts had equivalent survival with or without reoperation for approximately 2 years, but after that point, the patients who did not have reoperation did poorly. (Reproduced with permission from Lytle BW, Loop FD, Taylor AC, et al: The effect of coronary reoperation on the survival of patients with stenoses in saphenous vein to coronary bypass grafts, *J Thorac Cardiovasc Surg.* 1993 Apr;105(4):605-612.)

subgrouped on the basis of severity of the stenotic lesions (Fig. 24-8), the patients with severely stenotic (50-99%) vein grafts obviously benefited from surgery, exhibiting a decreased risk of death even early in the follow-up period. For patients with moderate stenoses (20-49%) in LAD vein grafts, the survivals of the MED and REOP groups were equivalent for about 2 years, but after that point survival of the patients in the MED group became rapidly worse, so that by 3 to 4 years of follow-up, the survival benefit of reoperation became apparent. Although the patients in these studies did not have consistent functional testing, there is evidence that myocardial perfusion and functional studies can help to identify patients likely to benefit from reoperation. Lauer and colleagues studied 873 symptom-free postoperative patients with symptom-limited exercise thallium-201 studies and found that patients with reversible perfusion defects were more likely to die or experience major cardiac events during a 3-year follow-up.[31] Impaired exercise capacity also was strongly predictive of unfavorable outcomes.

Anatomical indications for reoperation to improve survival prognosis include: (1) atherosclerotic (late) stenoses in vein grafts that supply the LAD artery; (2) multiple stenotic vein grafts that supply large areas of myocardium; and (3) multivessel disease with a proximal LAD lesion and/or abnormal LVF based on either native-vessel lesions or stenotic vein grafts or a combination of the two pathologies. Reoperation is also effective in other anatomical situations in which severe symptoms are the indication for invasive treatment, including patients with a patent ITA to LAD graft combined with other ischemia-producing pathology and multiple early vein graft stenoses. The combination of the anatomical characteristics just noted and reversible ischemia and/or worsening LVF during stress constitutes a particularly strong indication for reoperation.

PERCUTANEOUS TREATMENT OF POSTOPERATIVE PATIENTS

Percutaneous treatments (PCTs) represent alternative anatomical treatments for postoperative patients and often are useful. The effectiveness of PCTs is related to the vascular pathology to be treated and the clinical implications of treatment failure. Today, native coronary artery stenoses often can be treated with a low restenosis rate as long as those vessels are large enough to allow intracoronary stenting. Unfortunately, many postoperative patients have very diffuse native coronary atherosclerosis that makes PCT difficult or ineffective. Also, PCT has not been as effective in the treatment of diabetic native CAD.

The rate of technologic change in interventional cardiology has been rapid, and multiple percutaneous technologies have been used to treat stenotic vein grafts. Balloon angioplasty, first-generation PCT, was relatively dangerous to perform and produced ineffective long-term revascularization, particularly when used to treat older (atherosclerotic) vein grafts.[32] Direct coronary atherectomy (DCA) increased the risk of coronary embolization at the time of the procedure without improving the restenosis rate.[33] It has been hoped that the use of intracoronary stents, particularly covered stents and drug-eluting stents (DESs), in stenotic vein grafts might provide better outcomes, and stenting does represent an improvement over balloon angioplasty.[32] The Randomized Evaluation of Polytetrafluoroethylene Covered Stent in Saphenous Vein Grafts (RECOVERS) trial, a randomized study designed to compare rates of SVG restenosis between coronary artery bypass graft (CABG) patients treated with covered stents and with bare stents, showed identical restenosis rates at 6 months of follow-up (24.2 vs 24.8%; p = .24).[34] In a nonrandomized retrospective study comparing the effects of DESs with those of bare metal stents in treating SVG stenosis, Ge and colleagues reported significant differences in in-stent stenosis between groups at 6 months of follow-up (10 vs 26%; p = .03).[35] However, other reports comparing DES with bare metal stents showed that the use of DES lowered the rate of restenosis but increased the risk of death.[36]

The kinetics of treatment failure after PCT for vein grafts are different from those for native coronary vessels. Restenosis and new stenotic lesions in vein grafts continue to appear with time, and the shoulder on the adverse outcome curve that appears at 6 months to 1 year after PCT for native vessels does not appear for vein grafts. Thus, there is still some uncertainty about the clinical impact of PCTs of stenotic vein grafts. Patients with previous bypass surgery are an extremely heterogeneous group; some subgroups are at low risk without any anatomical treatment at all, and some subgroups are at high risk without effective therapy. To date, the reported studies of PCT of SVG lesions have not included clinical risk stratifications that would allow comparison of patient survival rates.

Despite persistently high restenosis rates after percutaneous interventions, there are still many indications for their use in the treatment of patients with previous bypass surgery. Realistically, the ideal uses of PCTs are in situations in which failure of the anatomical treatment is not likely to be catastrophic as the impact of stenting on survival is unclear. These situations include symptomatic patients with: (1) early vein graft stenoses; (2) native coronary stenoses; or (3) focal late SVG stenoses in vein grafts not supplying the LAD artery. There are many patients with previous surgery who will fall into a middle ground where it is not clear whether percutaneous transluminal coronary angioplasty (PTCA) or reoperation is likely to yield the best outcome, and judgments must be made on the specific advantages and disadvantages of the treatments for those particular patients. Factors making PTCA more attractive than reoperation are listed in Table 24-2.

There are patients with postsurgical repeat ischemic syndromes and very unfavorable coronary anatomy for whom good options for anatomical treatment do not exist. For reoperative coronary surgery to be of benefit there must be bypass conduits available to construct new grafts to graftable coronary arteries that subtend substantial areas of ischemic but viable myocardium. If these conditions do not exist, surgery may not be in the interest of even a symptomatic patient. Studies of diabetic patients undergoing

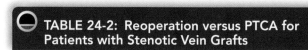

TABLE 24-2: Reoperation versus PTCA for Patients with Stenotic Vein Grafts

Factors favoring reoperation	Factors favoring PTCA
Late (≥5 years) stenoses	Early (<5 years) stenoses
Multiple stenotic vein grafts	Single stenotic vein graft
Diffusely atherosclerotic vein grafts	Other patent vein grafts
Stenotic LAD vein graft	Focal graft lesions
No patent ITA graft	Patent ITA-LAD graft
Abnormal left ventricular function	Normal left ventricular function

postsurgical repeat revascularization with PCT or surgery have shown unfavorable 10-year-survival rates.[37] Unless good coronary targets to receive bypass grafts are available, PCT may be the best choice for marginal candidates because of lower initial costs and, in some settings, lower initial mortality.

TECHNICAL ASPECTS OF CORONARY REOPERATIONS

Reoperations are more complicated than primary operations. The specific technical challenges that surgeons must recognize and solve that are unique to or more common during coronary reoperation are:

1. Sternal reentry
2. Stenotic or patent vein or arterial bypass grafts
3. Aortic atherosclerosis
4. Diffuse native-vessel coronary artery disease
5. Coronary arteries located amid old grafts and epicardial scarring
6. Lack of bypass conduits

The overall problem of myocardial protection is more difficult during reoperations, with perioperative myocardial infarction still being the most common cause of in-hospital death.[3,6] The metabolic concepts of myocardial protection in use today are valid, but the reasons that myocardial protection sometimes fails during reoperation are related to anatomical causes of myocardial infarction. These anatomical causes of perioperative myocardial infarction include injury to bypass grafts, atherosclerotic embolization from vein grafts or the aorta to distal coronary arteries, myocardial devascularization secondary to graft removal, hypoperfusion through new grafts, failure to deliver cardioplegic solution, early vein graft thrombosis, incomplete revascularization, diffuse air embolization, and technical error.[3,38–42] To be consistently successful, coronary reoperations must be designed to avoid these causes of myocardial infarction.

Preoperative Assessment

A complete understanding of the patient's native coronary and bypass graft anatomy is essential. Achieving this goal is sometimes not as easy as it sounds, particularly if the patient has had multiple previous coronary operations. If bypass grafts, venous or arterial, are not demonstrated by a preoperative coronary angiogram, it usually means that they are occluded, but it is also possible that the angiogram simply has failed to demonstrate their location. Examination of old angiograms performed before previous operations and review of previous operative records often help to illustrate the patient's coronary anatomy.

It is also important to know that graftable stenotic coronary arteries supply viable myocardium. Myocardial scar and viability can be differentiated by thallium scanning, positron-emission tomography, and stress (exercise or dobutamine) echocardiography. The intricacies of establishing myocardial viability are beyond this discussion, but it is an important issue. Before embarking on a reoperation, it makes sense to be reasonably sure that there is a matchup between the patient's graftable arteries and some viable myocardium such that grafting those arteries will provide some long-term benefits.

It is also wise to have a preoperative plan for bypass conduit selection and to document that potential bypass conduits are available. ITA angiography often is helpful. Venous Doppler studies can be used to assess the presence of greater and lesser saphenous vein segments, and arterial Doppler studies can assess the radial and inferior epigastric arteries and establish the adequacy of flow to the digits during radial artery occlusion.

Median Sternotomy Incision, Conduit Preparation, and Cannulation

Most coronary reoperations are performed through a median sternotomy. Situations associated with increased risk during a repeat median sternotomy include right ventricular or aortic enlargement, a patent vein graft to the right coronary artery, an in situ right ITA graft patent to a left coronary artery branch, an in situ left ITA graft that curls under the sternum, multiple previous operations, and difficulty reopening the sternum during a previous reoperation. In such situations, vessels for arterial (via the femoral or axillary artery) and venous access for cardiopulmonary bypass may be dissected out before sternal reentry. Alternatively, given the cannulae currently available for percutaneous access, wire access of the femoral artery and vein may be accomplished with little morbidity while providing a safety net for emergent institution of bypass if necessary. All bypass grafts except for the internal thoracic arteries may be prepared before sternal reentry in high-risk cases. Preparation of radial artery and greater and lesser saphenous vein segments can be carried out simultaneously. The most common structure injured during reentry is a bypass graft.[4]

When reopening a median sternotomy, the incision is made to the level of the sternal wires; the wires are cut anteriorly and bent back but are not removed (Fig. 24-9). An oscillating saw is used to divide the anterior table of the sternum. When the anterior table has been divided, ventilation is stopped, and the assistants elevate each side of the sternum with rake retractors while the posterior table of the sternum is divided in a caudal-cranial direction. The sternal wires that have been left in place posterior to the sternum help to protect underlying structures. Once the posterior table of the sternum has been divided with the saw, the wires are removed, and sharp dissection with scissors is used to separate each side of the sternum from underlying structures. Once the sternum has been divided, it is important that the assistants retract in an upward direction, not laterally. The right ventricle is injured more often by lateral retraction while it is still adherent to the underside of the sternum than it is by a direct saw injury.

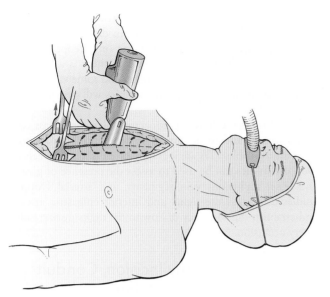

FIGURE 24-9 Leaving the sternal wires in place posteriorly helps to protect underlying structures while the posterior table of the sternum is divided with an oscillating saw. The direction of retraction with rake retractors should be anterior, not lateral.

In high-risk situations, it can be helpful to perform a small anterolateral right thoracotomy before the repeat median sternotomy. Underlying structures, such as the aorta, patent bypass grafts, and the right atrium and ventricle, can be dissected away from the sternum via this approach, and thus, with the surgeon's hand placed behind the sternum, reentry is safe. This small additional incision contributes little morbidity.

Another technique for sternal reentry in high-risk patients is to heparinize, cannulate, and initiate cardiopulmonary bypass before median sternotomy. The advantages of this strategy are that the heart can be emptied and allowed to fall away from the sternum, and cardiopulmonary bypass already has been initiated for protection if an injury does occur. The disadvantages of this approach are that extensive mediastinal dissection must be carried out in a heparinized patient, including dissection of the right internal thoracic artery if that is to be used. We rarely employ this approach except in situations in which adherence of an aortic aneurysm to the sternum or a patent right ITA-to-LAD graft creates a specific danger.

Once the sternum has been divided, the pleural cavities are entered. A general principle of dissection during reoperation is that starting at the level of the diaphragm and proceeding in a cranial direction is usually the safest approach. At the level of the diaphragm, few critical structures are injured if the wrong plane is entered. Therefore, at this point in the operation we usually dissect along the level of the diaphragm to the patient's right side until we enter the pleural cavity and then detach the pleural reflection from the chest wall in a cranial direction to the level of the innominate vein. The innominate vein is dissected away from both sides of the

sternum with scissors, a maneuver that prevents a "stretch" injury to that vein.

Once the right side of the sternum is separated from the cardiac structures, it is usually possible to prepare a right ITA graft. Once the right ITA dissection is completed to the superior border of the first rib, an incision is made in the parietal pleura to separate the proximal ITA from the area of the phrenic nerve. Thus, if the right ITA needs to be converted to a "free" graft during aortic cross-clamping, it makes division at that point easier because the proximal ITA is clearly identifiable. Although intrapericardial dissection of the left side of the heart is left until later, freeing the left side of the anterior chest wall from the underlying structures (which may include a patent ITA graft) is undertaken now. This is difficult only if there is a patent ITA graft that is densely adherent to the chest wall. Again, it is best to enter the left pleural cavity at the level of the diaphragm and proceed in a cranial direction.

The most difficult point of dissection is usually at the level of the sternal angle, where a patent ITA graft may approach the midline and be adherent to the sternum or the aorta. There are no tricks for dissecting out a patent ITA graft except for being careful. The danger to a patent left ITA graft during sternal reentry and mediastinal dissection is entirely related to the location of the graft at the time of the primary operation. Ideally, the pericardium should be divided at a primary operation, and the left ITA graft should be allowed to run posterior to the lung through the incision in the pericardium and to the LAD or circumflex artery (Fig. 24-10). When this is done, the lung will lay anterior to the left ITA, and that graft will not become adherent to the aorta or to the chest wall.

Once the left side of the chest wall is free, the left internal mammary artery (IMA) is prepared (if it has not been used at a previous operation), the sternal spreader is inserted, and the intrapericardial dissection of the aorta and right atrium is accomplished. Again, in most cases it is safest to find the correct dissection plane at the level of the diaphragm and then to continue around the right atrium to the aorta. The one situation in which this strategy may be dangerous is if an atherosclerotic vein graft to the right coronary artery lies over the right atrium. Manipulation of atherosclerotic vein grafts can cause embolization of atherosclerotic debris into coronary arteries, and it is best to employ a "no touch" technique with such grafts. If a vein graft to the right coronary artery lies in an awkward position over the right atrium, it is best to leave the right atrium alone and use the femoral vein and superior vena cava cannulation to establish venous drainage (Fig. 24-11). Once cardiopulmonary bypass has been established, the aorta has been cross-clamped, and cardioplegia has been given, the atherosclerotic vein graft then can be disconnected.

The goal of dissection of the ascending aorta is to obtain enough length for cannulation and cross-clamping and to avoid the most common error, aortic subadventitial dissection. The correct level of dissection on the aorta usually is found either by following the right atrium to the aorta in a

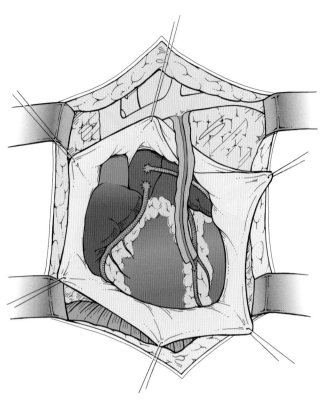

FIGURE 24-10 A patent left ITA-to-LAD graft should not pose a threat during reoperation. At a primary operation, the pericardium should be divided in a posterior direction, and the ITA graft should be placed in that incision. The ITA graft then will lie posterior to the lung and will not be pushed toward the midline by the lung or become adherent to the sternum.

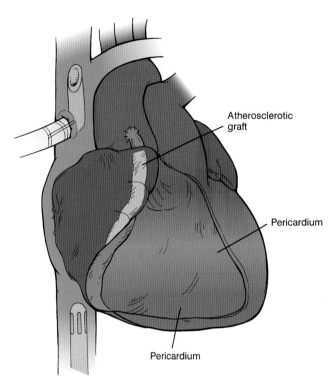

FIGURE 24-11 Manipulation of patent but atherosclerotic vein grafts should be avoided. If an atherosclerotic right coronary vein graft blocks access to the right atrium, femoral vein, and direct superior vena cava, cannulation is safer than mobilizing the vein graft so as to achieve right atrial cannulation.

caudal-to-cranial direction or by identifying the innominate vein and leaving all the tissue beneath the innominate vein on the aorta. At the level of the innominate vein, the pericardial reflection on each side of the aorta will be identifiable. Division of the pericardial reflection on the left side in a posterior direction will lead to the plane between the aorta and the pulmonary artery. Once the left side of the aorta is identified, the surgeon then may dissect posteriorly on the medial aspect of the left lung toward the hilum. The segment of tissue between these two dissection planes usually will include a patent left ITA graft, if present, and clamping that tissue will produce occlusion of the ITA graft.

When the aorta has been dissected out, heparin is given, and cannulation is undertaken. Cannulation of an atherosclerotic ascending aorta may cause atherosclerotic embolization leading to stroke, myocardial infarction, or multiorgan failure, so the ascending aorta should be studied with palpation and echocardiography to detect atherosclerosis before cannulation. Although the most widely used alternative arterial cannulation site is the femoral artery, arteriopathic patients often have severe femoral artery atherosclerosis. The axillary artery is an alternative arterial cannulation site that we have used with increasing frequency because atherosclerotic disease is usually not

present in that vessel, and its cannulation allows antegrade perfusion[44] (Fig. 24-12). If atherosclerotic disease or calcification of the aorta makes any aortic occlusion hazardous, the options are off-pump bypass surgery (see Other Options) or replacement of the aorta with axillary artery cannulation, hypothermia, and circulatory arrest. Venous cannulation usually is accomplished with a single two-stage right atrial cannula. A transatrial coronary sinus cardioplegia cannula is inserted via a right atrial purse string with the aid of a stylet, and a needle is placed in the ascending aorta for delivery of antegrade cardioplegia and for use as a vent (Fig. 24-13).

Myocardial Protection

The myocardial protection strategy used by us during most coronary artery reoperations is a combination of antegrade and retrograde delivery of intermittent cold blood cardioplegia combined with a dose of warm reperfusion cardioplegia ("hot shot") given before aortic unclamping, principles developed by Buckberg and colleagues.[45] Multiple types of cardioplegic solutions have been described, and most appear to provide a metabolic environment that effectively protects the myocardium. Because of the

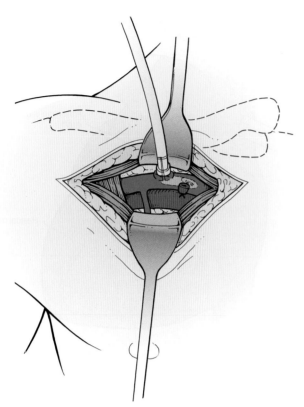

FIGURE 24-12 The axillary artery is an important alternative arterial cannulation site for patients with aortic and femoral artery atherosclerosis. A 21-gauge cannula will fit the axillary artery in most patients.

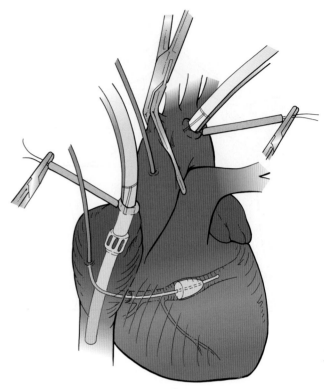

FIGURE 24-13 Standard cannulation for coronary artery reoperation includes aortic arterial cannulation, an aortic needle for antegrade delivery of cardioplegia and aortic root venting, a single two-stage venous cannula, and a transatrial coronary sinus catheter with a self-inflating balloon for delivery of retrograde cardioplegia. Cannulation is accomplished before dissection of the left ventricle.

potential anatomical challenges to cardioplegic myocardial protection during reoperations, the details of how the cardioplegic solution is delivered are very important. In most primary bypass operations, antegrade cardioplegia works well by itself. During reoperations, however, antegrade cardioplegia may not be effective for areas of myocardium that are supplied by patent in situ arterial grafts and may be dangerous because of the risk of embolization of atherosclerotic debris into the coronary arteries from old vein grafts. The delivery of cardioplegia through the coronary sinus and through the cardiac venous system to the myocardium (retrograde cardioplegia) has been a step forward in myocardial protection during reoperations.[46,47] Retrograde cardioplegia delivery avoids atheroembolism from vein grafts, can be helpful in removing atherosclerotic debris and air from the coronary artery system, and can deliver cardioplegia to areas supplied by in situ arterial grafts. The biggest disadvantage of retrograde cardioplegia is that it is not always possible to place a catheter in the coronary sinuses that will deliver cardioplegia consistently. It is important to monitor the adequacy of cardioplegia delivery by measuring the pressure in the coronary sinus, noting the distention of cardiac veins with arterial blood, the cooling of the myocardium, and the return of desaturated blood from open coronary arteries.

Cardiopulmonary bypass is begun, the perfusionist empties the heart and produces mild systemic hypothermia (34°C), and the aorta is cross-clamped. We usually initiate cardioplegia induction with aortic root cardioplegia. To induce and maintain cardioplegic protection, it is helpful to be able to occlude patent arterial grafts. If it has not yet been possible to dissect out a patent arterial graft so that it can be clamped, the systemic perfusion temperature may be decreased to 25°C until control of the graft is achieved. After antegrade cardioplegia has been given for 2 to 3 minutes, we shift to retrograde induction for another 2 to 3 minutes. Giving any antegrade cardioplegia does risk embolization from atherosclerotic vein grafts, but if these grafts have not yet been manipulated, that danger is relatively small. Once the adequacy of retrograde cardioplegia delivery has been established, it is often possible to use that route predominantly for maintenance doses.

Intrapericardial Dissection

When the heart has been arrested completely, intrapericardial dissection of the left ventricle is undertaken, starting at the diaphragm and extending out to the left of the apex of the heart. After the apex is identified, the surgeon divides the pericardium in a cranial direction on the left side of the LAD

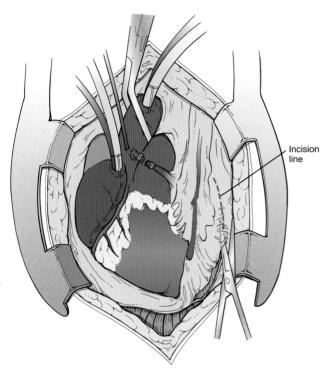

FIGURE 24-14 Division of the pericardium along the diaphragm allows the surgeon to reach a point to the left of the cardiac apex. From that point, the pericardium can be divided in a cranial direction to the left of the LAD artery, leaving a patent ITA graft in the strip of tissue overlying the LAD artery. Atherosclerotic vein grafts that are going to be replaced may be divided once a dose of antegrade cardioplegia is given.

Incision line

artery (Fig. 24-14). A patent LITA-to-LAD graft will be contained within the strip of pericardium that lies over the LAD artery. Dissection of this pedicle from the anterior aspect of the pulmonary artery will allow an atraumatic clamp to be placed across the patent ITA graft and also will allow the passage of new bypass grafts from the aorta underneath the patent ITA graft to left-sided coronary arteries. The advantages of waiting until after aortic clamping and arrest to dissect out the left ventricle are that dissection is more accurate, there is less damage to the epicardium and less bleeding, manipulation of atherosclerotic vein grafts is less likely to cause coronary embolization, and the dissection of patent ITA grafts is safer.

After the heart is dissected out completely, the coronary arteries to be grafted can be identified, the lengths that bypass conduits need to reach those vessels may be assessed, and the final operative plan can be established. The old grafts and epicardial scarring that are present during reoperations make the preoperative prediction of the lengths of conduits needed for bypass grafts quite difficult, particularly the lengths of arterial grafts, and it is wise to have some flexibility in the operative plan. Before the construction of the anastomoses, those patent but atherosclerotic vein grafts that are going to be disconnected are identified and are disconnected with a scalpel. The order of anastomosis construction that is used by the authors

is: (1) distal vein graft anastomoses; (2) distal free arterial graft anastomoses; (3) distal in situ arterial graft anastomoses; and (4) proximal (aortic) anastomoses.

Stenotic Vein Grafts

When should patent or stenotic vein grafts be replaced, and with what should they be replaced? Atherosclerosis in vein grafts is common if those grafts are more than 5 years old, and leaving them in place risks embolization of atherosclerotic debris at the time of reoperation and subsequent development of premature graft stenoses or occlusions after reoperation. On the other hand, replacement of all vein grafts extends the operation and may use up available bypass conduits.

In the past, our general rule has been to replace all vein grafts that are more than 5 years old at the time of reoperation, even if those grafts are not diseased angiographically. However, this strategy assumes that conduits are available that can replace these old grafts. Today, many patients have very limited conduits at reoperation because of the large numbers of vein grafts used at primary surgery or because of multiple previous operations. Thus, graft replacement must be individualized. Inspection of vein grafts at reoperation occasionally will identify a graft that looks normal angiographically and does not appear to have any thickening or atherosclerosis on visual inspection. Such grafts are thought to be "privileged" and often will be left alone.

Replacing old vein grafts with new vein grafts may often be accomplished by creating the new vein-to-coronary-artery anastomosis at the site of the previous distal anastomosis, leaving only 1 mm or so of the old vein in place (Fig. 24-15). If significant native-vessel stenoses have developed distal to the old vein graft, it is often best to place a new graft to the distal vessel in addition to replacing the vein graft. Many reoperative candidates have proximal occlusions of the native coronary artery system and multiple stenoses throughout the vessel, and if only new distal grafts are constructed, the proximal segments of coronary arteries and their branches that are supplied by atherosclerotic vein grafts may be jeopardized. More than one graft to a major coronary artery may be desirable during reoperation (Fig. 24-16).

Sequential vein grafts often are very helpful during reoperation because they allow more distal anastomoses and fewer proximal anastomoses. Sites for proximal anastomoses are often at a premium in the scarred reoperative aorta.

Artery-to-coronary-artery bypass grafts have many advantages during reoperations. First, they are often available. Second, the tendency of arteries to remain patent even when used as grafts to diffusely diseased coronary arteries makes them particularly applicable to reoperative candidates. Third, in situ arterial grafts do not require a proximal anastomosis. If the left ITA has not been used as a graft at a previous operation, a strong attempt should be made to use it as an in situ graft to the LAD artery. During primary operations, the right ITA usually can be crossed over as an in situ graft to left-sided vessels, but such a plan is more difficult during repeat surgery, so the right ITA is often used as a free graft.

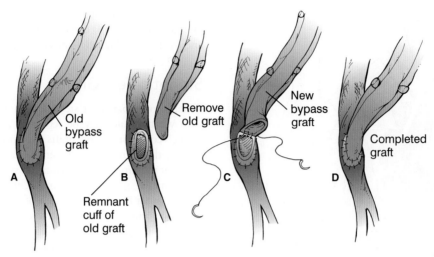

FIGURE 24-15 For patients with extensive native coronary atherosclerosis, the distal anastomotic site of an old vein graft is often the best spot for the distal anastomosis of a new graft. Only a small rim of the old graft should be left in place.

Arterial graft proximal anastomoses are a problem at reoperation because the scarring and thickening of the reoperative aorta often make direct anastomoses of arterial grafts to the aorta unsatisfactory. However, when old vein grafts become occluded, there is usually a "bubble" of the hood of the old vein graft that is not atherosclerotic and that often is a good spot for construction of a free (aorta-to-coronary-artery) arterial graft anastomosis (Fig. 24-17). In addition, if new vein grafts are performed, the hood of that new vein graft represents a favorable location for an arterial graft

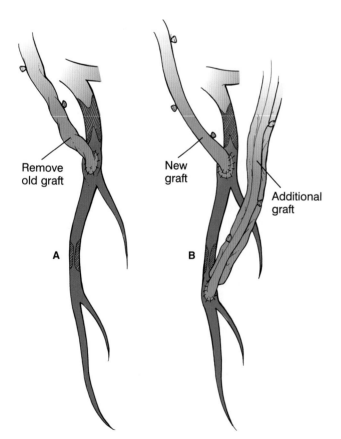

FIGURE 24-16 Extension of native-vessel coronary artery disease may indicate the placement of new distal grafts as well as replacement of diseased vein grafts supplying proximal coronary artery segments.

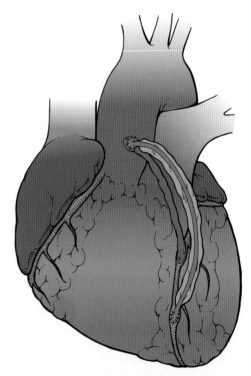

FIGURE 24-17 The hood of new or old vein grafts is often the best spot for the aortic anastomosis of free arterial grafts. Atherosclerosis rarely occurs in that "bubble" of vein.

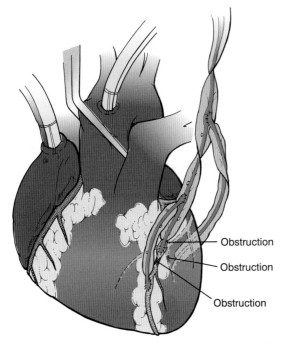

FIGURE 24-18 Composite arterial grafts can be constructed using a new or old left ITA graft as the inflow source. With its proximal anastomosis to the left ITA, a right ITA graft will easily reach the circumflex branches. Furthermore, a shorter segment of inferior epigastric artery or radial artery can be used to reach the distal LAD artery if intervening native LAD stenoses have limited the effectiveness of an old ITA graft.

anastomosis. Late angiographic data regarding this strategy are not available, but the relative freedom of the hood of vein grafts from the development of atherosclerosis means these grafts are likely to be successful.

Another effective strategy is to use either an old arterial graft or a newly constructed arterial graft for the proximal anastomosis of a free arterial graft (Fig. 24-18). Composite arterial grafts, usually using a new in situ left ITA graft at the proximal anastomotic site for a free right ITA graft, have been employed with increasing frequency, and early outcomes have been favorable.[48,49] This method is particularly useful during reoperations because it may avoid an aortic anastomosis, and less right ITA graft length is needed to reach distal circumflex arteries. Other advantages of using a previously performed patent ITA graft for the proximal anastomosis of a new arterial graft are that the old left ITA graft often has increased in size, and the preoperative angiogram has demonstrated its integrity. In situations in which the effectiveness of an LITA-to-LAD graft has been jeopardized by a distal LAD lesion, a short segment of a new arterial graft can be used to bridge that stenosis from the old arterial graft to the distal LAD artery (see Fig. 24-17).

Can an ITA graft be used to replace a vein graft during reoperation? When faced with replacing a stenotic or patent vein graft during reoperation, the surgeon has a number of options, all of which have some potential disadvantages:

1. The surgeon may leave the old vein graft in place and add an arterial graft to the same coronary vessel. The dangers of this approach are that atherosclerotic embolization from the old vein may occur during the reoperation, and competitive flow between the vein graft and the arterial graft may jeopardize the ITA graft after reoperation.

2. The surgeon may remove the old vein graft and replace it with an ITA graft. This decreases the likelihood of atherosclerotic embolization and competitive flow but risks hypoperfusion during reoperation if the arterial graft cannot supply all the flow that had been generated previously by the vein graft.

3. The surgeon may replace the old vein graft with a new vein graft. The disadvantage of this approach is a long-term one. The coronary vessel is left dependent on a vein graft.

When we examined these choices in a retrospective study of operations for patients with atherosclerotic vein grafts supplying the LAD artery, we found that the worst outcomes resulted from removing a patent (although stenotic) vein graft and replacing it with only an ITA graft.[39] This strategy was associated with a significant incidence of hypoperfusion and severe hemodynamic difficulties during reoperation that were treated effectively only by adding a vein graft to the same coronary artery. The incidence of myocardial infarction associated with leaving a stenotic vein graft in place was low. Thus, atherosclerotic embolization from an atherosclerotic vein graft is a danger, but it appears that with the use of retrograde cardioplegia, it is not commonly a major catastrophe.

Another potential disadvantage of the strategy of adding an ITA graft to a stenotic vein graft is that competition in flow from the stenotic vein graft may lead to failure of the new ITA graft. However, this is unlikely to occur as long as the stenosis in the SVG is severe.[50] Our usual approach, therefore, is to remove atherosclerotic vein grafts when replacing them with a new vein graft but leave stenotic vein grafts in place when grafting the same vessel with an arterial graft (Fig. 24-19).

Alternative arterial grafts often are very useful during reoperation. The radial artery has particular advantages during repeat surgery because it is larger and longer than other free arterial grafts. These qualities increase the range of coronary arteries that can be grafted. Early studies of radial artery grafts have shown favorable patency rates, but few long-term data currently exist. If the high patency rates that have been documented by early studies are confirmed by the tests of time, the radial artery will be used extensively during reoperations. The inferior epigastric artery often is too short to function as a separate aorta-to-coronary-artery graft during reoperation but can be extremely useful as a short composite arterial graft, as illustrated in Fig. 24-18.

The right gastroepiploic artery (RGEA) has established a good midterm graft patency rate record and often is useful during reoperation because it is an in situ graft.[51] Furthermore, it can be prepared before the median sternotomy. It is effective most often as an in situ graft to the posterior

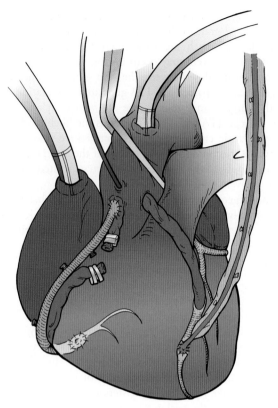

FIGURE 24-19 In this example, an atherosclerotic right coronary artery vein graft is disconnected and is replaced with a new vein graft. However, the stenotic vein graft to the LAD artery is left in place to avoid hypoperfusion, and a new ITA graft is added to the LAD artery.

descending branch of the right coronary artery or the distal LAD artery (Fig. 24-20).

The aortic anastomoses of the vein and arterial grafts are performed last during the single period of aortic cross-clamping. Sites for aortic anastomoses are often at a premium owing to previous scarring, atherosclerotic disease, or the use of Teflon felt during the primary operation, and often the locations of the previous vein graft proximal anastomoses are the best locations for the new ones. The advantages of constructing aortic anastomoses during a single period of aortic cross-clamping are that it minimizes aortic trauma and allows excellent visualization of the proximal anastomoses. In addition, if patent or stenotic vein grafts have been removed and replaced, reperfusion is not accomplished by aortic declamping until the aortic anastomoses have been completed.

The disadvantage of this approach is that it prolongs the period of aortic cross-clamping. However, our strategies for reoperation are not based on trying to minimize myocardial ischemic time. If cardioplegia can be delivered effectively, its metabolic concepts are valid, and myocardial protection is secure. Failure of myocardial protection usually is caused by anatomical events, not by metabolic failure. Once the proximal anastomosis has been constructed, a "hot shot" of substrate-enhanced blood cardioplegia is given, and the aortic cross-clamp is removed.

Other Options

Although most reoperations are performed through a median sternotomy with the use of cardiopulmonary bypass, the

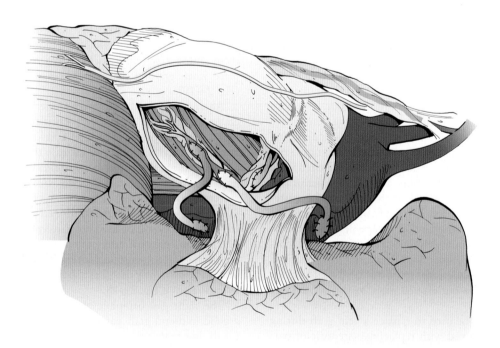

FIGURE 24-20 Circumflex vessels may be grafted through a left thoracotomy incision without cardiopulmonary bypass.

strategies of small-incision surgery and off-pump surgery that have been gaining increasing use for primary coronary artery operations also can be helpful during reoperations. Reoperations in situations in which a limited area of myocardium needs revascularization often can be accomplished through a limited incision and without the use of cardiopulmonary bypass (known as the *minimally invasive direct coronary artery bypass* [MIDCAB] *operation*). The distal LAD artery may be exposed with a small anterior thoracotomy, and the LAD or diagonal artery may be grafted with a left ITA graft. A stabilizing device usually is employed for anastomotic construction, although the intrapericardial adhesions provide some stability during reoperations. If the left ITA is not available, a segment of saphenous vein can be anastomosed to the subclavian artery and routed in a transthoracic path to the LAD artery. If the right ITA is to be used as an in situ graft to the LAD artery, a median sternotomy is indicated, but if this is the only graft, off-pump surgery usually is possible.

The lateral wall of the heart can be exposed through a left lateral thoracotomy (Fig. 24-21), and the circumflex and distal right coronary artery branches can be grafted with this approach. Often the LITA already has been used for a graft, but the descending thoracic aorta may be used as a site for the proximal anastomosis of a vein graft or a radial artery graft using a partial occluding clamp. The disadvantages of this approach are that the right ITA is difficult to use as an in situ graft, and if the circumflex vessels are deeply intramyocardial, they may be difficult to expose and isolate with the off-pump strategy.

In addition to avoiding potential complications of cardiopulmonary bypass, the "limited-area, off-pump" approach also avoids extensive dissection of the heart and possible manipulation of atherosclerotic vein grafts. The disadvantage of this approach is that most patients who are candidates for reoperation need grafts to multiple vessels in multiple myocardial areas.

Use of a median sternotomy and the off-pump strategy to graft multiple myocardial areas is now a standard approach to primary coronary revascularization and also can be used during reoperation. However, because of the need to access all areas, extensive dissection sometimes is necessary for lysis of adhesions to be able to mobilize the heart. If patients have atherosclerotic vein grafts, dissection and manipulation create the dangers of embolization of atherosclerotic debris and myocardial infarction. This problem was encountered during the early years of bypass surgery when the risks of atherosclerotic embolization were less recognized. Another disadvantage of off-pump reoperative strategies is that reoperative candidates often have very distal and diffuse CAD, which leaves intramyocardial segments as the best areas for grafting. These characteristics stress off-pump isolation and immobilization techniques. In addition, the aortic anastomoses of vein or free arterial grafts may be difficult because of aortic atherosclerosis, adhesions, or previous aortic anastomoses that may limit the application of a partial occluding clamp. On the other hand, the use of off-pump techniques may minimize aortic trauma, particularly if in situ arterial grafts can be employed to provide inflow to new grafts.

In an individual case, the disadvantages of off-pump surgery may be important or irrelevant. Surgeons who perform reoperative coronary artery surgery in a wide spectrum of situations will find both on- and off-pump strategies helpful.

RESULTS OF CORONARY ARTERY REOPERATIONS

Early Results

Coronary artery reoperations are riskier than primary operations. A study from the Society of Thoracic Surgeons (STS) database reported an in-hospital mortality rate of 6.95% associated with reoperations for the years 1991 to 1993, and in a multivariate analysis of all isolated coronary artery bypass surgery, "previous operation" was identified as a factor that increased the mortality rate.[12] At the Cleveland Clinic Foundation, the in-hospital mortality rate of a first reoperation ranged between 3 and 4% from 1967 through 1991, and the rate was 3.7% for 1663 patients having repeat surgery from 1988 through 1991.[1-3] Progress during the last decade has continued to lower this risk. In a recent report by Sabik and colleagues, the hospital mortality rate for patients undergoing reoperative CABG was reduced to 2.5% in 2002, and risk adjustment identified the comorbidity burden carried by reoperative patients as a factor that increased risk, not reoperative status itself.[14]

In the 1990s and 2000s, mortality rates from other large series range from 4.2 to 11.4%, most being around 7%.[4-9,52] In 2013, among all STS database participants the mortality rate was 3.5%, while the mortality rate for primary operations was 1.5%.

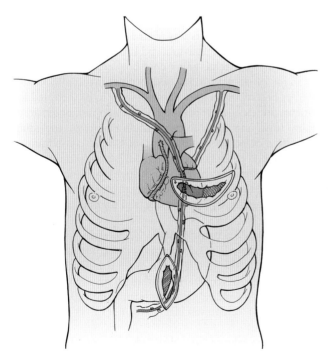

FIGURE 24-21 An in situ gastroepiploic artery (GEA) graft may be used for an on- or off-pump anastomosis to the distal LAD artery.

All these figures are two to five times higher than the rates we would expect for the risk of primary CABG. Coronary artery reoperations have been associated with a higher in-hospital mortality mostly because of an increased risk of perioperative myocardial infarction. In the Cleveland Clinic Foundation series, the cause of perioperative death was cardiovascular in 85% of cases in the most recent cohort of patients undergoing reoperation, a figure that contrasts with recent studies of primary operations, in which noncardiac causes of death have been increasingly important.[3,15] Furthermore, in the reoperative series, in-hospital mortality was associated with new perioperative myocardial infarction in 67% of cases. Multiple causes of myocardial infarction have been identified, including incomplete revascularization owing to distal CAD, vein graft thrombosis, ITA graft failure, atherosclerotic embolization from vein grafts, injury to bypass grafts, hypoperfusion from arterial grafts, preoperative myocardial infarction, and complications of PTCA.

Sternal reentry still creates risk. In a study of 1847 patients undergoing reoperation, 7% were associated with an adverse event and only previous radiation and the number of previous operations could be identified as predictors of injury. Of the 127 patients sustaining an injury, 24 (19%) experienced a major adverse outcome (stroke, myocardial infarction, or death) compared with a risk of 6.2% for those without an injury.[43]

Multiple studies of patients undergoing reoperation have identified increased age, female gender, and emergency operation as clinical variables that have a high association with in-hospital mortality. Emergency operation is a particularly strong factor. Although there is not a standard definition of *emergency*, mortality rates after emergency reoperations that have been reported range from 13 to 40%.[3,5-8] Data from the STS for the year 1997 documented a risk of 5.2% for elective reoperations, 7.4% for urgent reoperations, 13.5% for emergency reoperations, and 40.7% for "salvage" reoperations. There is clearly a major increment in risk associated with emergency reoperations, a larger increment than has existed for patients undergoing primary surgery.

Advanced age, by itself, does not increase the risk of reoperation substantially but does so when combined with other variables. In a review of 739 patients aged 70 years or older undergoing reoperation, we noted an overall in-hospital mortality rate of 7.6% and identified emergency operation, female gender, left ventricular (LV) dysfunction, creatinine concentration greater than 1.6 μg/dL, and left main coronary artery stenosis as specific factors increasing risk. For patients with none of these characteristics, the in-hospital mortality rate was only 1.5%.[53]

Specific anatomical situations, in particular, the presence of patent ITA grafts and atherosclerotic vein grafts, can increase the risk of reoperation, but with experience, these technical factors largely have been neutralized. We have never documented an increased mortality rate for patients with patent ITA grafts but have noted that the risk of ITA damage has dropped from 8% in our early experience to 3.7% more recently, an improvement almost entirely related to increased surgical experience. With proper positioning of an ITA graft at primary operation, a patent LITA-to-LAD-artery or LITA-to-circumflex-artery graft should not represent an impediment to reoperation. Situations in which a patent in situ right ITA graft crosses the midline to supply the LAD or circumflex system are more difficult and require extreme care in reoperating using a median sternotomy incision. Although these situations are uncommon and provide difficult technical challenges, the risks for these patients have not been increased.

Studies from the past noted that the presence of atherosclerotic vein grafts did increase perioperative risk. Perrault and colleagues documented mortality rates of 7, 17, and 29% for patients with one, two, or three stenotic vein grafts, respectively, and in a previous study of patients with atherosclerotic vein grafts, we noted that the presence of an atherosclerotic vein graft to the LAD artery increased in-hospital risk.[30,36] However, in our more recent study we found that atherosclerotic vein grafts did not increase mortality, although there was a nonsignificant trend toward increased risk for patients with multiple stenotic grafts.[3] The favorable results for these patients have been based on a combination of improved technology, the use of retrograde cardioplegia delivery, and increased surgeon experience.

Although arterial grafts may offer advantages at reoperation, their use may prolong an already complex operation, and the influence of arterial grafting on perioperative risk has been a concern. However, we have specifically studied this issue and found that the use of single or double ITA grafts at reoperation does not increase perioperative risk, and in fact, not having an ITA graft at either the first or second operation appeared to be a factor associated with increased in-hospital mortality.[3] Graft selection in that study was not randomized, and it is certainly possible that the increased risk for patients receiving only vein grafts was related to patient-related variables rather than surgical strategy. It does appear, however, that the use of arterial grafts does not increase risk. Except for an increased incidence of perioperative myocardial infarction, in-hospital morbidity does not seem to be increased for patients undergoing reoperation. One important observation relates to wound complications. Multiple groups, including ours, have noted an increased risk of wound complications when diabetic patients have received bilateral (simultaneous) ITA grafts. However, there does not appear to be an increased risk of wound complications for diabetic patients who receive staged ITA grafts, one at the first and another at a second operation.

Among all STS participants in 2013, when compared to primary coronary bypass, reoperative procedures appeared to be associated with an increased of major complications (17.3 vs 12.8%), risk of reoperation within 30 days (5.0 vs 3.6%). Interestingly, no additional risk of mediastinits (0.3 vs 0.2%) or permanent cerebrovascular accident (1.2 vs 1.3%) was demonstrated.

It is important to note that only the variables that can be identified and quantified are included in studies consistent enough to be identified as risk factors. For example, experience and logic dictate that severe atherosclerosis of the ascending aorta is a major risk factor, but this is rarely identified in large studies because patients do not routinely undergo echocardiography to identify the presence of aortic atherosclerosis.

Late Results

Patients who are undergoing reoperation are at a later stage in the progression of their native coronary atherosclerosis compared with the point when they underwent primary surgery, and the anatomical corrections achieved at reoperation are less perfect. Although the definition of *complete revascularization* varies widely, few reoperative candidates undergo an operation in which all diseased segments of all arteries receive bypass grafts. It is not surprising that the long-term results of reoperation have not been as favorable as the long-term results of primary operations.

The likelihood of recurrent angina after any bypass operation is related to time, but angina symptoms are more common after repeat surgery than they are after primary operation. Follow-up of our reoperative patients at a mean interval of 72 months after reoperation showed that 64% of patients were in New York Heart Association (NYHA) functional class I, although only 10% of patients had class III or class IV symptoms.[2] Weintraub and colleagues also noted at a 4-year follow-up that 41% of reoperative patients had experienced some angina.[6]

Late survival rates after reoperation are also inferior to those after primary surgery. Weintraub and colleagues noted 76% 5-year- and 55% 10-year survival rates, and our most recent follow-up study found a 10-year survival rate of 69% for in-hospital survivors (Fig. 24-22).[2,6] The predictors of late survival have varied among studies, but LV dysfunction, advanced age, and diabetes consistently have been associated with a decreased late survival rate. The variables identified by

TABLE 24-3: Factors Decreasing Late Survival after Reoperation: 1967 to 1987[2]		
Factor	*p*-Value	Relative risk
LV dysfunction	.0001	1.9
Age	.0001	1.04
Current cigarette smoking	.0001	1.6
Hypertension	.0002	1.4
Left main ≥50%	.0001	2.0
Triple-vessel disease	.0001	1.6
NYHA III/IV symptoms	.003	1.4
Peripheral vascular disease	.001	1.5
Interval > 60 months	.006	1.003
No ITA at first operation	.03	1.5

LV = left ventricular.
Data from Loop FD, Lytle BW, Cosgrove DM, et al: Reoperation for coronary atherosclerosis: changing practice in 2509 consecutive patients, *Ann Surg.* 1990 Sep;212(3):378-385.

multivariate testing as decreasing the late survival for 2429 hospital survivors of a first reoperation are listed in Table 24-3. The influence of ITA grafts on late survival has been difficult to determine for reoperations. We found a positive influence of a single ITA graft on late survival, as have others,[54] but the effect was not as dramatic as has been noted after primary operations. Weintraub and colleagues did not document an improved survival associated with ITA grafting.[6] However, there is clear evidence that usage of ITA grafts has at least partially contributed to a dramatically lower number of reoperations[55], and this could be potentially extrapolated to a positive effect of ITA grafts on late survival.

Multiple Coronary Artery Reoperations

Patients who have had more than one previous coronary artery operation are like patients undergoing first reoperations, only more so. Many patients undergoing multiple reoperations had their first procedure more than 15 years ago, and severe native-vessel disease and lack of bypass conduits are a common combination of problems. Selection criteria vary widely among institutions, but in-hospital mortality rates are increased relative to first reoperations.[10,11] Through 1993, we reoperated on 392 patients who had more than one previous bypass operation, with an in-hospital mortality rate of 8%. Over the next 10 years, this mortality rate has decreased to 5.8%.[14] Follow-up of the in-hospital survivors in the former group found late survival rates of 84% at 5 and 66% at 10 postoperative years. Thus, although the in-hospital risks were increased for these patients, the long-term outcome has been relatively favorable. Age was a major determinant of outcome. Recently, in-hospital mortality for patients younger than 70 years of age has decreased to 1 to 2%, but for patients greater than age 70, it has remained higher than 10%. Furthermore, patients greater than age 70 who did survive operation in our series had only a 50% 5-year late survival.

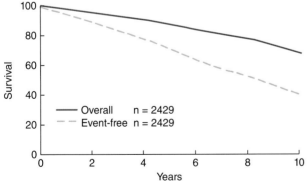

FIGURE 24-22 For 2429 hospital survivors who underwent reoperation between 1967 and 1987, the 10-year survival was 69%, and event-free survival was 41%. (Reproduced with permission from Loop FD, Lytle BW, Cosgrove DM, et al: Reoperation for coronary atherosclerosis: changing practice in 2509 consecutive patients, *Ann Surg.* 1990 Sep;212(3):378-385.)

KEY POINTS

1. Make certain the end justifies the means before performing a coronary reoperation
2. Avoid cardiac injury
3. Do not replace a patent or stenotic vein graft with an ITA graft
4. Dissect out the left side of the heart with the heart arrested
5. Use the axillary artery as an alternative cannulation site

REFERENCES

1. Lytle BW, Loop FD, Cosgrove DM, et al: Fifteen hundred coronary reoperations: results and determinants of early and late survival. *J Thorac Cardiovasc Surg* 1987; 93:847.
2. Loop FD, Lytle BW, Cosgrove DM, et al: Reoperation for coronary atherosclerosis: changing practice in 2509 consecutive patients. *Ann Surg* 1990; 212:378.
3. Lytle BW, McElroy D, McCarthy PM, et al: The influence of arterial coronary bypass grafts on the mortality of coronary reoperations. *J Thorac Cardiovasc Surg* 1994; 107:675.
4. Salomon NW, Page US, Bigelow JC, et al: Reoperative coronary surgery: comparative analysis of 6591 patients undergoing primary bypass and 508 patients undergoing reoperative coronary artery bypass. *J Thorac Cardiovasc Surg* 1990; 100:250.
5. Grinda JM, Zegdi R, Couetil JP, et al: Coronary reoperations: indications, techniques and operative results. Retrospective study of 240 coronary reoperations. *J Cardiol Surg* 2000; 41:703.
6. Weintraub WS, Jones EL, Craver JM, et al: In-hospital and long-term outcome after reoperative coronary artery bypass graft surgery. *Circulation* 1995; 92:II-50.
7. He GW, Acuff TE, Ryan WH, et al: Determinants of operative mortality in reoperative coronary artery bypass grafting. *J Thorac Cardiovasc Surg* 1995; 110:971.
8. Akins CW, Buckley MJ, Daggett WM, et al: Reoperative coronary grafting: changing patient profiles, operative indications, techniques, and results. *Ann Thorac Surg* 1994; 58:359.
9. Levy JH, Pifarre R, Schaff HV, et al: A multicenter double-blind placebo-controlled trial of aprotinin for reducing blood loss and the requirement for donor-blood transfusion in patients undergoing repeat coronary artery bypass grafting. *Circulation* 1995; 92:2236.
10. Lytle BW, Cosgrove DM, Taylor PC, et al: Multiple coronary reoperations: early and late results. *Circulation* 1989; 80:626.
11. Yau TM, Borger MA, Weisel RD, et al: The changing pattern of reoperative coronary surgery: trends in 1230 consecutive reoperations. *J Thorac Cardiovasc Surg* 2000; 120:156.
12. Edwards FH, Clark RE, Schwartz M: Coronary artery bypass grafting: The Society of Thoracic Surgeons National Database experience. *Ann Thorac Surg* 1994; 57:12.
13. Cosgrove DM, Loop FD, Lytle BW, et al: Predictors of reoperation after myocardial revascularization. *J Thorac Cardiovasc Surg* 1986; 92:811.
14. Sabik JF, Blackstone EH, Houghtaling PL, et al: Is reoperation still a risk factor in coronary artery bypass surgery? *Ann Thorac Surg* 2005; 80:1719.
15. Loop FD, Lytle BW, Cosgrove DM, et al: Influence of the internal mammary artery graft on 10-year survival and other cardiac events. *New Engl J Med* 1986; 314:1.
16. Lytle BW, Blackstone EH, Loop FD, et al: Two internal thoracic artery grafts are better than one. *J Thorac Cardiovasc Surg* 1999; 117:855.
17. Neitzel GF, Barboriak JJ, Pintar K, et al: Atherosclerosis in aortocoronary bypass grafts: morphologic study and risk factor analysis 6 to 12 years after surgery. *Arteriosclerosis* 1986; 6:594.
18. Ratliff NB, Myles JL: Rapidly progressive atherosclerosis in aortocoronary saphenous vein grafts: possible immune-mediated disease. *Arch Pathol Lab Med* 1989; 113:772.
19. Solymoss BC, Leung TK, Pelletier LC, et al: Pathologic changes in coronary artery saphenous vein grafts and related etiologic factors. *Cardiovasc Clin* 1991; 21:45.
20. Bourassa MG, Campeau L, Lesperance J: Changes in grafts and in coronary arteries after coronary bypass surgery. *Cardiovasc Clin* 1991; 21:83.
21. Lytle BW, Loop FD, Cosgrove DM, et al: Long-term (5 to 12 years) serial studies of internal mammary artery and saphenous vein coronary bypass grafts. *J Thorac Cardiovasc Surg* 1985; 89:248.
22. Fitzgibbon GM, Leach AJ, Kafka HP, et al: Coronary bypass graft fate: long-term angiographic study. *J Am Coll Cardiol* 1991; 17:1075.
23. Chesebro JH, Fuster V, Elveback LR, et al: Effect of dipyridamole and aspirin on late vein graft patency after coronary bypass operations. *New Engl J Med* 1984; 310:209.
24. Goldman S, Copeland J, Moritz T, et al: Saphenous vein graft patency 1 year after coronary artery bypass surgery and effects of antiplatelet therapy. *Circulation* 1989; 80:1190.
25. Gavaghan TP, Gebski V, Baron DW: Immediate postoperative aspirin improves vein graft patency early and late after coronary artery bypass graft surgery: a placebo-controlled, randomized study. *Circulation* 1991; 83:1526.
26. Domanski M, Tian X, Fleg J, et al: Pleiotropic effect of lovastatin, with and without cholestyramine, in the post coronary artery bypass graft (Post CABG) trial. *Am J Cardiol* 2008; 102:1023-1027.
27. Flaker GC, Warnica JW, Sacks FM, et al: Pravastatin prevents clinical events in revascularized patients with average cholesterol concentrations: Cholesterol and Recurrent Events (CARE) investigators. *J Am Coll Cardiol* 1999; 34:106.
28. Dion R, Verhelst R, Rousseau M, et al: Sequential mammary grafting: clinical, functional and angiographic assessment 6 months postoperatively in 231 consecutive patients. *J Thorac Cardiovasc Surg* 1989; 98:80.
29. Lytle BW, Loop FD, Taylor PC, et al: Vein graft disease: the clinical impact of stenoses in saphenous vein bypass grafts to coronary arteries. *J Thorac Cardiovasc Surg* 1992; 103:831.
30. Lytle BW, Loop FD, Taylor PC, et al: The effect of coronary reoperation on the survival of patients with stenoses in saphenous vein to coronary bypass grafts. *J Thorac Cardiovasc Surg* 1993; 105:605.
31. Lauer MS, Lytle B, Pashkow F, et al: Prediction of death and myocardial infarction by screening exercise-thallium testing after coronary-artery-bypass grafting. *Lancet* 1998; 351:615.
32. Brener SJ, Ellis SG, Apperson-Hansen C, et al: Comparison of stenting and balloon angioplasty for narrowings in aortocoronary saphenous vein conduits in place for more than five years. *Am J Cardiol* 1997; 79:13.
33. Holmes DR Jr, Topol EJ, Califf RM, et al: A multicenter, randomized trial of coronary angioplasty versus directional atherectomy for patients with saphenous vein bypass graft lesions. *Circulation* 1995; 91:1966.
34. Stankovic GA, Colombo A, Presbitero P, et al: Randomized evaluation of polytetrafluoroethylene-covered stent in saphenous vein grafts: the Randomized Evaluation of Polytetrafluoroethylene Covered Stent in Saphenous Vein Grafts (RECOVERS) trial. *Circulation* 2003; 108:37.
35. Ge L, Iakovou I, Sangiorgi GM, et al: Treatment of saphenous vein graft lesions with drug-eluting stents: immediate and midterm outcome. *J Am Coll Cardiol* 2005; 45:989.
36. Vermeersch P, Agostoni P, Verheye S, et al: Increased late mortality after sirolimus-eluting stents versus bare-metal stents in diseased saphenous vein grafts. Results from the randomized DELAYED RRISC trial. *J Am Coll Cardiol* 2007; 50:261-267.
37. Cole JH, Jones EL, Craver JM, et al: Outcomes of repeat revascularization in diabetic patients with prior coronary surgery. *J Am Coll Cardiol* 2002; 40:1968-1975.
38. Perrault L, Carrier M, Cartier R, et al: Morbidity and mortality of reoperation for coronary artery bypass grafting: significance of atheromatous vein grafts. *Can J Cardiol* 1991; 7:427.
39. Jain U, Sullivan HJ, Pifarre R, et al: Graft atheroembolism as the probable cause of failure to wean from cardiopulmonary bypass. *J Cardiothorac Anesth* 1990; 4:476.
40. Navia D, Cosgrove DM, Lytle BW, et al: Is the internal thoracic artery the conduit of choice to replace a stenotic vein graft? *Ann Thorac Surg* 1994; 57:40.
41. Keon WJ, Heggtveit HA, Leduc J: Perioperative myocardial infarction caused by atheroembolization. *J Thorac Cardiovasc Surg* 1982; 84:849.
42. Blauth CI, Cosgrove DM, Webb BW, et al: Atheroembolism from the ascending aorta: an emerging problem in cardiac surgery. *J Thorac Cardiovasc Surg* 1992; 103:1104.
43. Roselli EE, Pettersson GB, Blackstone EH, et al: Adverse events during reoperative cardiac surgery: frequency, characterization, and rescue. *J Thorac Cardiovasc Surg* 2008; 135:316-323.

44. Sabik JF, Lytle BW, McCarthy PM, et al: Axillary artery: an alternative site of arterial cannulation for patients with extensive aortic and peripheral vascular disease. *J Thorac Cardiovasc Surg* 1995; 109:885.

45. Partington MT, Acar C, Buckberg GD, et al: Studies of retrograde cardioplegia: II. Advantages of antegrade/retrograde cardioplegia to optimize distribution in jeopardized myocardium. *J Thorac Cardiovasc Surg* 1989; 97:613.

46. Menasche P, Kural S, Fauchet M, et al: Retrograde coronary sinus perfusion: a safe alternative for ensuring cardioplegic delivery in aortic valve surgery. *Ann Thorac Surg* 1982; 34:647.

47. Gundry SR, Razzouk AJ, Vigesaa RE, et al: Optimal delivery of cardioplegic solution for "redo" operations. *J Thorac Cardiovasc Surg* 1992; 103:896.

48. Tector AJ, Amundsen S, Schmahl TM, et al: Total revascularization with T grafts. *Ann Thorac Surg* 1994; 57:33.

49. Calafiore AM, DiGiammarco G, Teodori G, Vitolla G: Myocardial revascularization with composite arterial grafts, in Possat GF, Suma H, Alessandria F (eds): *Proceedings of the Workshop on Arterial Conduits for Myocardial Revascularization.* Rome, 1995.

50. Turner FE, Lytle BW, Navia D, et al: Coronary reoperations: results of adding an internal mammary artery graft to a stenotic vein graft. *Ann Thorac Surg* 1994; 58:1353.

51. Suma H, Wanibuchi Y, Terada Y, et al: The right gastroepiploic artery graft: clinical and angiographic midterm results in 200 patients. *J Thorac Cardiovasc Surg* 1993; 105:615.

52. Di Mauro M, Iaco AL, Contini M, et al: Reoperative coronary artery bypass grafting: analysis of early and late outcomes. *Ann Thorac Surg* 2005; 79:81.

53. Yamamuro M, Lytle BW, Sapp SK, et al: Risk factors and outcomes after coronary reoperation in 739 elderly patients. *Ann Thorac Surg* 2000; 69:464.

54. Dougenis D, Brown AH: Long-term results of reoperations for recurrent angina with internal mammary artery versus saphenous vein grafts. *Heart* 1998; 80:9.

55. ElBardissi A, Aranki S, Sheng S, et al: Trends in isolated coronary artery bypass grafting: an analysis of the Society of Thoracic Surgeons Database. *J Thorac Cardiovasc Surg* 2012; 143:273-281.

Surgical Treatment of Complications of Myocardial Infarction, Ventricular Septal Defect, Myocardial Rupture, and Left Ventricular Aneurysm

Donald D. Glower

25

Acute myocardial infarction can require surgical intervention for many reasons. Most commonly, patients may have coronary artery stenosis that may be amenable to coronary artery bypass grafting, either to halt the progress of the acute infarction, or to prevent subsequent angina, reinfarction, or death (see Chapters 20 to 25). Myocardial infarction can also result in refractory congestive heart failure and/or circulatory shock due to inability of the left and/or right ventricles to maintain the cardiovascular circulation. These patients may benefit from ventricular replacement therapy that include cardiac transplantation (see Chapter 61), extracorporeal membrane oxygenation (see Chapter 19) or placement of left and/or right ventricular assist devices (see Chapter 63). Acute myocardial infarction can have a number of other mechanical consequences that may need to be addressed surgically. These can include acute and chronic ischemic mitral regurgitation and even papillary muscle rupture (see Chapter 38) and functional tricuspid regurgitation (see Chapter 44). Three final and potentially catastrophic mechanical complications of acute myocardial infarction are addressed in this chapter and include postinfarction ventricular septal defect, cardiac rupture, and left ventricular aneurysm.

POSTINFARCTION VENTRICULAR SEPTAL DEFECT

Postmortem description of a postinfarction ventricular septal defect was first made in 1845 by Latham.[1] The first antemortem clinical diagnosis of a postinfarction ventricular septal defect was made in 1923 by Brunn.[2] Sager[3] in 1934 established specific clinical criteria for diagnosis and associated postinfarction septal rupture with coronary artery disease.

The first successful surgical repair of a postinfarction ventricular septal defect was made in 1956 by Cooley in a patient 9 weeks after the diagnosis of septal rupture.[4] The approach used was a right ventriculotomy similar to that used in patients with congenital ventricular septal defects. Thereafter the surgical mortality was sufficiently high that the strategy was to limit operation to those patients surviving for more than a month after acute septal perforation.[5] Delayed surgery also had the advantage of allowing septal healing to facilitate more secure closure of the septal rupture.[6] Heimbecker[6] described septal defect repair through a left ventriculotomy in the zone of infarction combined infarctectomy and aneurysmectomy.[7] Approaching the septal defect through the left ventricular infarct had distinct advantages of providing better exposure of the apical and inferior septum than did a right ventriculotomy. The left ventriculotomy also did not unnecessarily injure the otherwise critical right ventricle and allowed surgical remodeling of the infarcted portion of the left ventricle. Daggett et al[8] in 1977 first reported a large series of 43 patients with improved surgical outcomes using a combination of infarctectomy and prosthetic patch material. In addition to the improved results overall, Daggett et al were able to successfully treat inferoposterior septal defects that previously had been problematic.[9-11] In 1995 David described 44 patients treated with infarct excluding patches with excellent mortality of 19% and unusually low incidence of right ventricular dysfunction in two of 44 patients.[12] Today, percutaneous septal defect closure devices are evolving to have a role in selected patients,[13] and ventricular replacement therapy is finding use in some septal defect patients with extensive ventricular damage and inability to maintain end organ perfusion.[14]

Incidence

Ventricular septal defect occurs in 1 to 2% of all acute myocardial infarctions, typically 3 to 5 days after the onset of symptoms.[15] Rupture of the interventricular septum with resultant ventricular septal defect can occur as early as hours after infarction or as late as 2 weeks.[16,17] This timing correlates well with the maximal tissue necrosis from acute myocardial infarction with minimal healing having occurred. Patients with postinfarction ventricular septal defect are most likely to be men; but because women are less likely to present with transmural infarction, some suggest that women with transmural infarction are actually at somewhat higher risk of developing postinfarction ventricular septal defect. Older age and total occlusion of the infarct vessel with minimal collateralization are also associated with postinfarction ventricular septal defect. The onset of early coronary reperfusion using thrombolytics or angioplasty may have shortened the time between infarction and septal rupture in some patients, perhaps due to hemorrhagic reperfusion of the infarct. However, the overall incidence of postinfarction ventricular septal defect appears to have declined in the last two decades with the increased prevalence of early coronary perfusion and the decreased number of large, nonreperfused infarctions.[18] In the GUSTO I trial of thrombolysis for infarction due to total occlusion of a coronary vessel,[19] the median age of patients with postinfarction ventricular septal defect was 72 years with 43% of septal defect patients versus 75% of remaining patients being male, and a higher incidence of hypertension and diabetes in the septal defect group. Infarctions were anterior in 70% of septal defect patients, with 29% being inferior and 1% presenting other cardiac zones. Single vessel coronary disease was present in 50% of septal defect patients, and 57% had total occlusion of the infarct vessel with the median restenosis being 100%. Shock was present in 67% of patients, and 89% had heart failure. Thirty-day mortality was 74%, and 1-year mortality was 76% with 33% of patients undergoing bypass surgery. Survival was significantly higher for anterior infarctions (20/39 (51%)) versus inferior infarction being survival being two of 22 (9%).

Pathophysiology

Postinfarction ventricular septal defect generally involves transmural infarction of the interventricular septum with subsequent dissection of ventricular blood into the septal myocardium, resulting in a ventricular septal defect. Patients with postinfarction septal defects generally have larger infarcts involving 26% of the left ventricular wall as opposed to only 15% of the left ventricular wall in other infarction,[15] and most have single vessel disease.[20] Patients with acute postinfarction septal defect tend to have greater right ventricular infarction than other patients with acute infarction.[21] The interventricular septal defect may be large and single, as is commonly seen with anterior infarctions. On the other hand, there may be multiple defects in the septum and a serpiginous course through the septum, as is more common with inferior infarctions producing ventricular septal defects. Because of the large volume of myocardial infarction in patients with postinfarction ventricular septal defects, roughly half of septal defect patients who survive the acute phase develop ventricular aneurysms, as opposed to only 12% of acute infarction patients without ventricular septal defects developing ventricular aneurysms.[22] Roughly one-third of postinfarction ventricular septal defect patients will have some degree of mitral regurgitation due to left ventricular dilation and altered papillary and annular geometry.[23]

Once the ventricular septal defect occurs, shunting of blood from the left ventricle to the right ventricle occurs with subsequent development of left and/or right ventricular heart failure. The combination of left to right shunting along with impairment of right and/or left ventricular contractility can produce low cardiac output and cardiogenic shock with end organ malperfusion progressing to death within days to weeks. In patients with postinfarction ventricular septal defect, left ventricular muscle loss is significant enough that one-third or more of all patients may not have a survivable amount of remaining myocardium without ventricular replacement therapy.[18] Heart failure and shock are the primary causes of ultimate death. Right ventricular failure leading to shock and death is more common with inferior than anterior infarction due to more extensive right ventricular infarction along with left to right shunting.

Natural History

Without surgical intervention, the natural history of postinfarction ventricular septal defect is that nearly 25% of patients will be dead within 24 hours, 50% in one week, 65% in 2 weeks, and 80% within four weeks, with 1-year survival being 5 to 20%.[24] Those who survived the initial few days to 2 weeks tend to have smaller degrees of shunting and smaller infarctions. Spontaneous closure of the postinfarction ventricular septal defect has been seen but is quite rare.

Clinical Presentation

The typical patient with a postinfarction ventricular septal defect initially presents with a large transmural anterior myocardial infarction. Most will appear to be convalescing in the initial few days, whereupon a new systolic murmur is noted, recurrent chest pain may develop, and hemodynamics may deteriorate with onset of dyspnea, tachycardia, hypotension, and oliguria.

Diagnosis

On clinical examination, 90% of patients with postinfarction ventricular septal defect will have a new, harsh, pansystolic murmur at the left lower sternal border, usually with a palpable thrill. Chest radiographic will commonly show progressive pulmonary edema and cardiomegaly. The electrocardiogram will continue to reflect transmural myocardial infarction in the appropriate zone, with occasional transient partial atrioventricular conduction block occurring around the time of rupture. Unfortunately, no electrocardiographic findings are highly predictive or diagnostic of septal rupture itself.

The differential diagnosis of postinfarction ventricular septal defect in a patient with acute onset of congestive heart failure and a new systolic murmur several days after transmural myocardial infarction importantly involves acute ischemic mitral regurgitation with or without papillary muscle rupture. While echocardiography is the definitive means of distinguishing between these two entities, several clinical associations might lead to early suspicion of one versus the other. Septal rupture occurs most commonly in anterior infarctions, while papillary muscle rupture is more common with inferoposterior infarctions. The murmur of septal rupture tends to be greatest at the left lower sternal border with a palpable thrill in more than half of patients, while the murmur of mitral regurgitation tends to radiate towards the left axilla.

Today, echocardiography is the definitive means of making the diagnosis of postinfarction ventricular defect and differentiating it from other complications such as acute mitral regurgitation.[25] Echocardiography can also provide reasonably accurate information in terms of the location and size of the septal defect and associated ventricular wall motion abnormalities. Mitral and/or tricuspid regurgitation can be quantified along with an assessment of left ventricular and right ventricular size and contractility.

In the absence of diagnostic echocardiography, right heart catheterization or placement of a Swan-Ganz pulmonary artery catheter can be diagnostic of a significant left to right shunt inherent (1.4:1 to 8:1 or more) due to postinfarction ventricular septal defect. Right heart catheterization can provide cardiac output, central venous pressure, and pulmonary artery pressure for prognostic value and to optimize medical management. Preoperative right heart catheterization may not be needed if the diagnosis is firm based on echocardiography.

Today, many patients with postinfarction ventricular septal defect already had left heart catheterization on presentation with transmural infarction and may have already had reperfusion of the infarct vessel. If this has not been done at the time of presenting with a septal defect, then the decision to perform left heart catheterization prior to correcting the septal defect is controversial. Left heart catheterization can identify or even treat residual coronary stenoses. However, the mortality benefit from reperfusion of the infarct vessel diminishes rapidly once the patient is more than several hours into the infarction. Moreover, the relatively high incidence of single vessel disease in postinfarction ventricular septal defect patients and the risk of volume overload and nephrotoxicity from dye all suggest that the decision to perform coronary angiography after the onset of septal rupture needs to be made on a case-by-case basis.

Indications for Operation

Because of the high mortality of postinfarction ventricular septal defects and because of the progressive volume overload due to left to right shunting, postinfarction ventricular septal defects should ideally be corrected in any patient who appears to be viable. Correction of the septal defect should also be performed as soon as possible to minimize subsequent end organ damage due to heart failure and hypoperfusion. Some patients may have sufficiently poor likelihood of surviving an operation that medical and/or percutaneous therapy might be more attractive. The timing of surgery may be emergent, urgent, or delayed depending upon the patient's situation. The main reasons for delay might be to optimize the patient hemodynamically, to obtain adequate diagnostic information, and to optimize volume status as best possible in a very short period of time. Once these goals have been accomplished in a period of no more than 12 to 24 hours, further delay of surgery tends to only result in a sicker patient going to operation.[18] Exceptions might be patients with relatively small shunts and/or other overriding surgical contraindications where the septal defect might reasonably be closed on a delayed basis once the other acute conditions are sufficiently corrected. In the past, significant delays in operation simply selected out those patients likely to survive long term in either event, with many otherwise potentially salvageable patients succumbing in the interim.

Preparation for Operation

Because of the rapidly life-threatening nature of postinfarction ventricular septal defects with 50 to 60% of patients having severe congestive heart failure or low cardiac output, these patients should be managed in an intensive care setting.[26] Preoperative management has three important goals: (1) to maintain cardiac output and arterial pressure for adequate end organ perfusion, (2) to reduce systemic vascular resistance to decrease the left to right shunt, and (3) to maintain adequate coronary blood flow.[27] The surgical team should be involved immediately upon making the diagnosis of a postinfarction ventricular septal defect. Placement of an intra-aortic balloon pump should be an early intervention to achieve some of these goals by improving coronary blood flow and decreasing the left to right shunt by decreased left ventricular outflow resistance.[28]

Pharmacologic therapy for postinfarction ventricular septal defect patients includes inotropic agents to improve end organ perfusion in the face of impaired right and/or left ventricular function. In addition, intravenous diuretics are generally needed early on to treat pulmonary edema. Intravenous vasodilators such as sodium nitroprusside, nitroglycerin, or calcium-channel blockers can occasionally be helpful, but most patients are sufficiently hypotensive to not tolerate significant doses of these agents. Because these patients all have significant ventricular dysfunction that may not improve with surgery, some patients may need evaluation for mechanical ventricular replacement therapy on an acute basis. This could include extracorporeal membrane oxygenation or right and/ or left ventricular assist devices. In general, those patients receiving this type of support before operation are those who are poor candidates for surgical closure of the septal defect at the time of evaluation but in whom the end organ dysfunction is felt to be reversible. Preoperative support over a period of time could allow some healing of infarct tissue and some recovery of stunned myocardium, in addition to allowing recovery of other end organs, at the expense of the multiple risks of cardiac assist devices.[29] Postinfarction ventricular septal defect patients have an inherent risk of right to left shunting from an isolated left ventricular assist device alone. As a result, many patients might need biventricular support or at most partial left heart support.

Operative Techniques

OVERVIEW

Repair techniques for a postinfarction ventricular septal defect and can be classified based on the location of the infarct and on whether the approach of infarct excision versus exclusion is used. Infarctectomy with or without patch closure of the infarct is a technique applicable to some septal infarctions and some apical infarctions to ensure suturing to viable myocardium that will heal. Table 25-1A lists the principles of the infarctectomy as stated by Daggett.[30] Infarct exclusion potentially allows less distortion of ventricular geometry but still requires suturing to viable myocardium. Table 25-1B lists the principles of infarct exclusion has stated by David.[12] Septal defects due to apical infarction are amenable either

TABLE 25-1A: Principles of Infarctectomy Repair of Postinfarction VSD

Transinfarct approach to ventricular septal defect
 1. Thorough trimming of the left ventricular margins of the infarct back to viable muscle to prevent delayed rupture of the closure
 2. Conservative trimming of the right ventricular muscle as required for complete visualization of the margins of the defect
 3. Inspection of the left ventricular papillary muscles and concomitant replacement of the mitral valve only if there is frank papillary muscular rupture
 4. Closure of the septal defect without tension, which in most instances will require the use of prosthetic material
 5. Closure of the infarctectomy without tension with generous use of prosthetic material as indicated, and epicardial placement of the patch to the free wall to avoid strain on the friable endocardial tissue
 6. Buttressing of the suture lines with pledgets or strips of Teflon felt or similar material to prevent sutures from cutting through friable muscle

Data from Heitmiller R, Jacobs ML, Daggett WM: Surgical management of postinfarction ventricular septal rupture, *Ann Thorac Surg.* 1986 Jun;41(6):683-691.

TABLE 25-1B: Principles of Exclusion Repair of Postinfarction VSD

Transinfarct approach to ventricular septal defect
 1. No infarctectomy unless necrotic muscle along ventriculotomy is sloughing during closure
 2. Bovine pericardial patch in either an oval (anterior defect) or triangular (posterior defect) shape is sutured securely with continuous Prolene around the defect to exclude it from the LV cavity
 3. Where necessary, full-thickness bites are taken to the epicardial surface and anchored by strips of pericardium or Teflon (see text for details)
 4. An anterior patch is anchored to noninfarcted septum below the defect, then the noninfarcted endocardium of the anterolateral ventricular wall. If the infarct involves the base of the anterior muscle, full thickness anchoring bites are used
 5. A posterior patch is anchored to the mitral annulus, noninfarcted septum, and through the infarcted posterior wall along a line corresponding to the medial margin of the posteromedial papillary muscle (with full thickness anchoring)
 6. Closure of the infarctectomy using strips of pericardium or Teflon
 7. When possible, infarcted right ventricular free wall is left undisturbed during closure

Data from David TE, Dale L, Sun Z: Postinfarction ventricular septal rupture: repair by endocardial patch with infarct exclusion, *J Thorac Cardiovasc Surg.* 1995 Nov;110(5):1315-1322.

infarctectomy or exclusion techniques. Septal defects due to anterolateral infarction generally require an exclusion patch on the septum, often with primary closure of the left ventriculotomy. Septal defects due to inferior infarction generally require an exclusion patch on the septum and patch closure of the ventriculotomy.

INTRAOPERATIVE CONSIDERATIONS

Patients with postinfarction ventricular septal defects are often in cardiogenic shock, intolerant of vasodilation and needing inotropic support during the induction of anesthesia. If not already present, an intra-aortic balloon pump may be placed to ensure stability during induction. Pulmonary vasodilators and venous vasodilators should be avoided to minimize left-to-right shunting. A Swan-Ganz pulmonary artery catheter should be placed to assist postoperative inotropic management.

Median sternotomy is the incision of choice. Cardiopulmonary bypass should be to accomplished with bicaval venous drainage and bicaval isolation to avoid entraining air into the venous line given that the right heart will be open through the septal defect. Postinfarction septal defects are best repaired in the arrested heart with careful attention to good myocardial protection given the already impaired by ventricular performance in these patients.

The use of concurrent coronary bypass grafting depends upon surgical philosophy and the coronary anatomy of the each patient. Some groups argue that concurrent coronary bypass grafting and left heart catheterization can delay surgery, add unnecessary risks, and is unlikely to benefit already infarcted myocardium. The incidence of late, clinically significant, untreated coronary disease in patients receiving isolated repair of postinfarction ventricular septal defects has in fact been low in several series.[31] Others argue that concurrent bypass grafting could potentially improve myocardial protection and reduce late myocardial ischemia.

In weaning from cardiopulmonary bypass, an intra-aortic balloon pump should be used if possible. Multiple inotropes will be needed, and intravenous milrinone and inhaled nitric oxide may be of particular value. In patients who cannot be weaned from cardiopulmonary bypass using standard techniques, the use of the left and/or right ventricular assist device could be considered (see Chapter 63).[14] In postinfarction ventricular septal defect patients, one particularly needs to be cognizant of potential residual right to left shunting with resultant hypoxemia when an isolated left ventricular assist device is used.

Postoperative hemostasis can be a problem in these critically ill patients. Routine use antifibrinolytic agents such as ε-aminocaproic acid (Amicar) can be helpful. Seguin and others have recommended application of a fibrin sealant to the ventricular septum around the septal defect before formal repair,[32] followed by biological glue applied to bleeding suture lines after repair. Transfusion of appropriate blood products and isolated clotting factors may be needed, given the tissue fragility along with intolerance of ongoing bleeding or any degree of postoperative tamponade.

REPAIR OF APICAL SEPTAL RUPTURE

Daggett described the technique of apical amputation in 1970[8] where necrotic apical myocardium is resected back to left ventricle, right ventricle, and septum (Figs. 25-1A and B). The remaining apical defect is then closed using interrupted mattress sutures of 1-0 Tevdek securing the left and right ventricular walls to the interventricular septum with strips of Teflon felt outside the left ventricular wall, outside the right ventricular wall, and on either side of the interventricular septum (Figs. 25-2A and B).[8,27] After all sutures have been tied, the closure is reinforced with running suture, to ensure hemostasis.

ANTERIOR REPAIR WITH INFARCTECTOMY

Postinfarction septal defects due to anterior infarction are generally approached through a linear incision in the anterior infarct parallel to the left anterior descending artery, with infarctectomy or debridement of nonviable tissue as described by Daggett[27] (Fig. 25-3). Shumacker[33] described a plication closure of small anterior septal defects by the free anterior edge of the debrided septum to the right ventricular free wall using mattress sutures of 1-0 Tevdek over strips of felt (Fig. 25-4A).

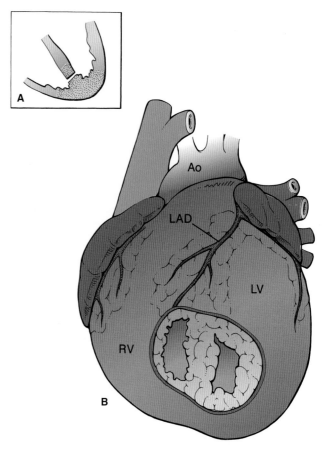

FIGURE 25-1 (A) Apical postinfarction ventricular septal defect. (B) View of the apical septal rupture, which is exposed by amputating the apex of the left and right ventricles. Ao, aorta; LAD, left anterior descending coronary artery; LV, left ventricle; RV, right ventricle; stippled region, infarcted myocardium.[27]

The transinfarct left ventriculotomy is then closed with a second row of mattress sutures buttressed with strips of Teflon felt (see Figs. 25-4B-D), followed by an outer hemostatic running suture line for ventriculotomy closure.[27,34]

In septal defects that are not small and anteriorly located, the debrided septal defect should be closed with a prosthetic patch of Dacron or bovine pericardium to reduce tension on the repair as described by Daggett[27,34] (see Fig. 25-5). After debridement of necrotic septum and left ventricular muscle, a series of pledgeted interrupted mattress sutures are placed around the perimeter of the defect (see Fig. 25-5A). Along the posterior aspect of the defect, sutures are passed through the septum from right to left. Along the anterior edge of the defect, sutures are passed from the epicardial surface of the right ventricle to the endocardial surface. All sutures are placed before the patch is inserted, and then passed through the edge of a synthetic patch, which is seated on the left side of the septum (see Fig. 25-5B). Each suture is then passed through an additional pledget and all are tied. We use additional pledgets on the left ventricular side overlying the patch (see Fig. 25-5C) to cushion each suture as it

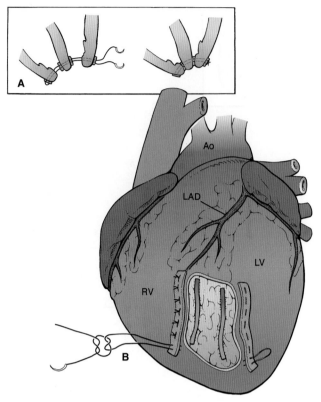

FIGURE 25-2 (A) The necrotic infarct and the apical septum have been debrided back to healthy muscle. Repair is made by approximating the left ventricle, apical septum, and right ventricle using interrupted mattress sutures of 1-0 Tevdek with buttressing strips of Teflon felt. Felt strips are used within the interior of the left and right ventricles as well as on the epicardial surface of each ventricle. (B) All sutures are placed before any are tied. A second running over-and-over suture (not shown) is used, as in left ventricular aneurysm repair, to ensure a secure hemostatic ventriculotomy closure. Ao, aorta; LAD, left anterior descending coronary artery; LV, left ventricle; RV, right ventricle.

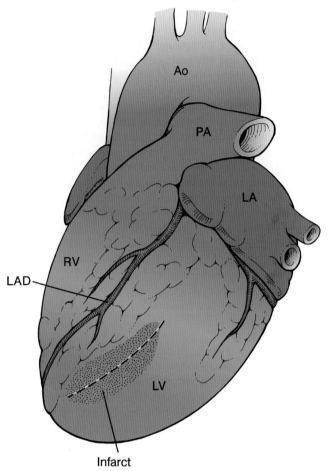

FIGURE 25-3 Transinfarct left ventricular incision to expose an anterior septal rupture. An incision (dashed line) is made parallel to the anterior descending branch of the left coronary artery (LAD) through the center of the infarct (stippled area) in the anterior left ventricle (LV). Ao, aorta; LA, left atrium; PA, pulmonary artery; RV, right ventricle.[27]

is tied down to prevent cutting through the friable muscle. The edges of the ventriculotomy are then approximated by a two-layer closure consisting of interrupted mattress sutures passed through buttressing strips of Teflon felt or bovine pericardium and a final outer running suture.[27]

POSTERIOR/INFERIOR REPAIR WITH INFARCTECTOMY

Postinfarction defects of the inferoposterior septum after inferolateral infarction have been the most challenging to repair because geometry does not lend itself to simple plication.[10,11] Daggett in 1974 described the technique of infarctectomy and patch closure which for the first time yielded reliably good results.[10] However, today many surgeons feel that the inferoposterior septal defects are particularly better suited to an exclusion technique as opposed to infarctectomy.[27] With the heart arrested and the left ventricle vented,

the heart is retracted out of the pericardial to expose the posterior descending coronary artery and the inferior infarction which may involve both ventricles (Fig. 25-6A). As described by Daggett[27,35] a transinfarct incision is made in the left ventricle, and the left ventricular portion of the infarct is excised (see Fig. 25-6B), exposing the septal defect. The left ventricular papillary muscles are inspected. If indicated, mitral valve replacement is performed through a separate conventional left atrial incision, to avoid trauma to the friable ventricular muscle. After all the infarcted left ventricular muscle has been excised, a less aggressive debridement of the right ventricle is accomplished, with the goal of resecting only as much muscle as is necessary to afford complete visualization of the defect(s). Using this technique, delayed rupture of the right ventricle has not been a problem. If the posterior septum has cracked or split from the adjacent ventricular free wall without loss of a great deal of septal tissue, then the septal rim of the posterior defect may be approximated to the edge of

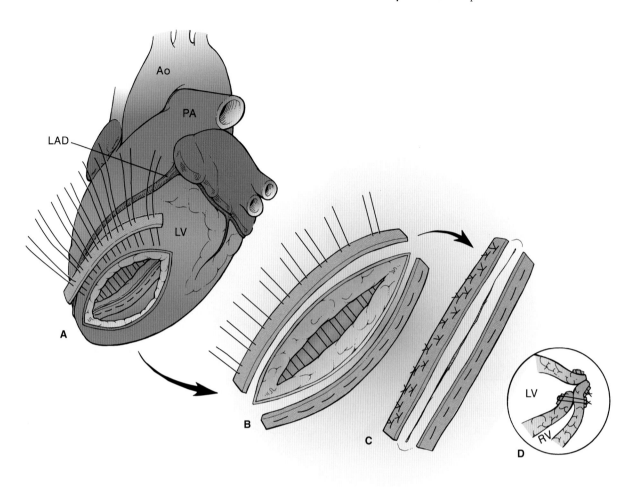

FIGURE 25-4 (A) Repair of an anterior septal rupture by plicating the free anterior edge of the septum to the right ventricular free wall with interrupted 1-0 Tevdek mattress sutures buttressed with strips of Teflon felt. (B, C, and D) The left ventriculotomy is then closed as a separate suture line, again with interrupted mattress sutures of 1-0 Tevdek buttressed with felt strips. A second running suture (not shown) is used to ensure a secure left ventriculotomy closure. Ao, aorta; LAD, left anterior descending coronary artery; LV, left ventricle; PA, pulmonary artery; RV, right ventricle. (Adapted with permission from Cohn LH (ed): Modern Techniques in Surgery: Cardiac/Thoracic Surgery. Mt. Kisco, NY: Futura; 1983.)

the diaphragmatic right ventricular free wall using mattress sutures buttressed with strips of Teflon felt or bovine pericardium (see Figs. 25-6C and D).[27,35]

Larger posterior defects require patch closure (Fig. 25-7).[27,35] Pledgeted mattress sutures are placed from the right side of the septum and from the epicardial side of the right ventricular free wall (Fig. 25-7B). All sutures are passed through the perimeter of the patch and then through additional pledgets, and are then tied (Fig. 25-7C). Thus, as in closure of large anterior defects, the patch is secured on the left ventricular side of the septum. Because direct closure of the remaining infarctectomy is rarely possible due to tension on the edges of the large defect, a Dacron prosthetic patch is generally required. Pledgeted mattress sutures are passed out through the margin of the infarctectomy (endocardium to epicardium) and then through the patch (Fig. 25-7D), which is seated on the epicardial surface of the heart. After each suture is passed through an additional pledget, all sutures are

tied (Fig. 25-7E). The cross-sectional view of the completed repair (Fig. 25-8) illustrates the restoration of relatively normal ventricular geometry, which is accomplished by the use of appropriately sized prosthetic patches.[27]

ANTERIOR AND INFEROPOSTERIOR REPAIR BY INFARCT EXCLUSION

The work of Dor and others led to the concept of ventricular endoaneurysmorrhaphy[36] or placing an intracavitary endocardial patch to exclude infarcted myocardium while maintaining ventricular geometry and thus preserving left ventricular function. David,[7] Cooley,[37] Ross[38] and others applied the infarct exclusion endocardial patch technique to repair of postinfarction ventricular septal defects, with good results in some centers but mixed results in others. The endocardial patch technique described by David[7] was felt by Daggett and others to be particularly helpful in some patients with

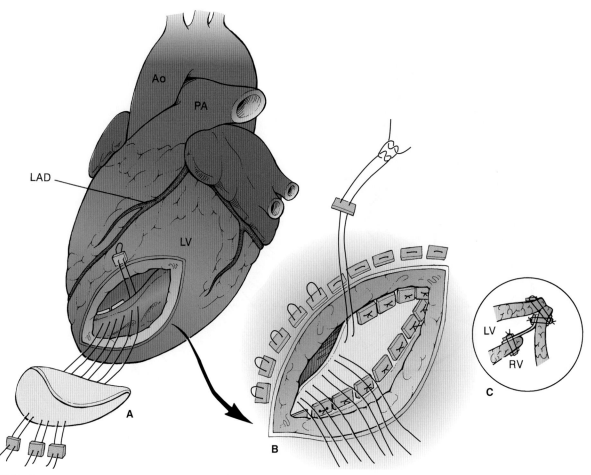

FIGURE 25-5 (A) Larger anterior septal defects require a Dacron patch, which is sewn to the left side of the ventricular septum with interrupted mattress sutures, each of which is buttressed with a pledget of Teflon felt on the right ventricular side of the septum and anteriorly on the epicardial surface of the right ventricular free wall. All sutures are placed before the patch is inserted. (B and C) Additional pledgets are placed on the left ventricular side overlying the patch to cushion each suture as it is tied down to prevent cutting through the friable muscle. Ao, aorta; LAD, left anterior descending coronary artery; LV, left ventricle; PA, pulmonary artery; RV, right ventricle. (Adapted with permission from Cohn LH (ed): Modern Techniques in Surgery: Cardiac/Thoracic Surgery. Mt. Kisco, NY: Futura; 1983.)

inferoposterior septal defects.[27] For anterior septal rupture, Daggett described the technique of David[12,39] as follows.[27]

The interventricular septum is exposed via a left ventriculotomy made through the infarct starting at the apex and extending proximally parallel to, but 1 to 2 cm away from, the anterior descending artery (Fig. 25-9A).[27,39] Stay sutures are passed through the margins of the ventriculotomy to aid in the exposure of the infarcted septum. The septal defect is located and the margins of the infarcted muscle identified. A bovine pericardial patch is tailored to the shape of the left ventricular infarction as seen from the endocardium but 1 to 2 cm larger. The patch is usually oval and measures approximately 4 × 6 cm in most patients. The pericardial patch is then sutured to healthy endocardium all around the infarct (see Fig. 25-9B). Suturing begins in the lowest and most proximal part of the noninfarcted endocardium of the septum with a continuous 3-0 polypropylene suture. Interrupted mattress sutures with felt pledgets may be used to reinforce the repair.[38,40] The patch

is also sutured to the noninfarcted endocardium of the anterolateral ventricular wall. The stitches should be inserted 5 to 7 mm deep in the muscle and 4 to 5 mm apart. The stitches in the patch should be at least 5 to 7 mm from its free margin so as to allow the patch to cover the area between the entrance and exit of the suture in the myocardium. This technique minimizes the risk of tearing muscle as the suture is pulled taut. If the infarct involves the base of the anterior papillary muscle, the suture is brought outside of the heart and buttressed on a strip of bovine pericardium or Teflon felt applied to the epicardial surface of the left ventricle. Once the patch is completely secured to the endocardium of the left ventricle, the left ventricular cavity becomes largely excluded from the infarcted myocardium. The ventriculotomy is closed in two layers over two strips of bovine pericardium or Teflon felt using 2-0 or 3-0 polypropylene sutures, as illustrated in Fig. 25-9C. No infarctectomy is performed unless the necrotic muscle along the ventriculotomy is sloughing at the time of its closure, and

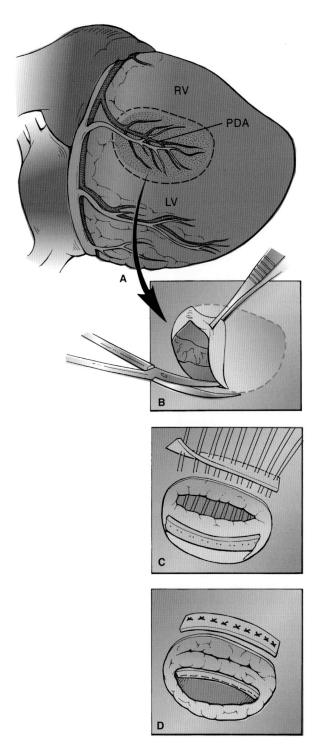

FIGURE 25-6 (A) View of an inferior infarct (stippled area) associated with posterior septal rupture. The apex of the heart is to the right. Exposure at operation is achieved by dislocating the heart up and out of the pericardial sac, and then retracting its cephalad, as in the performance of distal vein bypass and anastomosis to the posterior descending artery. (B) The inferoposterior infarct is excised to expose the posterior septal defect. Complete excision of the left ventricular portion of the infarct is important to prevent delayed rupture of the ventriculotomy repair. The free edge of the right ventricle is progressively shaved back to expose the margins of the defect clearly. (C and D) Repair of the posterior septal rupture is accomplished by approximating the edge of the posterior septum to the free wall of the diaphragmatic right ventricle with felt-buttressed mattress sutures. The repair is possible when the septum has cracked or split off from the posterior ventricular wall without necrosis of a great deal of septal muscle. The surgeon can perform repair of posterior septal rupture to best advantage by standing at the left side of the supine patient. The left ventriculotomy is then closed as a separate suture line, again with interrupted mattress sutures of 1-0 Tevdek buttressed with felt strips. A second running suture is used to ensure a secure left ventriculotomy closure (not shown). LV, posterior left ventricle; PDA, posterior descending artery; RV, diaphragmatic surface of the right ventricle. (Adapted with permission from Daggett WM: Surgical technique for early repair of posterior ventricular septum rupture, *J Thorac Cardiovasc Surg.* 1982;Aug;84(2):306-312.)

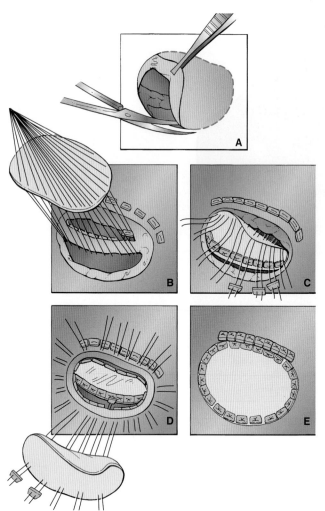

FIGURE 25-7 (A) Repair of posterior septal rupture when necrosis of a substantial portion of the posterior septum requires the use of patches. (B) Interrupted mattress sutures of 2-0 Tevdek are placed circumferentially around the defect. These sutures are buttressed with felt pledgets on the right ventricular side of the septum and on the epicardial surface of the diaphragmatic right ventricle. (C) All sutures are placed and then the Dacron patch is slid into place on the left ventricular side of the septum. The patch sutures are tied down with an additional felt pledget placed on top of the patch (left ventricular side) as each suture is tied, to cushion the tie and prevent cutting through the friable muscle. These maneuvers are viewed by Daggett et al.[27] as essential to the success of early repair of the posterior septal rupture. (D) Remaining to be repaired is the posterior left ventricular free wall defect created by infarctectomy. Mattress sutures of 2-0 Tevdek are placed circumferentially around the margins of the posterior left ventricular free wall defect. Each suture is buttressed with a Teflon felt pledget on the endocardial side of the left ventricle. With all sutures in place, a circular patch, fashioned from a Dacron graft, is slid down onto the epicardial surface of the left ventricle. An additional pledget of Teflon felt is placed under each suture (on top of the patch) as it is tied to cushion the tie and prevent cutting through the friable underlying muscle. This onlay technique of patch placement prevents the cracking of friable left ventricular muscle that occurred with the eversion technique of patch insertion. (E) Completed repair. (Adapted with permission from Daggett WM: Surgical technique for early repair of posterior ventricular septum rupture, *J Thorac Cardiovasc Surg.* 1982;Aug;84(2):306-312.)

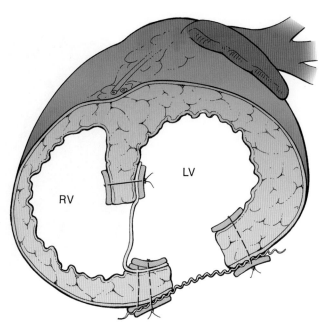

FIGURE 25-8 Cross-sectional view of the completed repair of posterior septal rupture with prosthetic patch placement of the posterior left ventricular free wall defect created by infarctectomy. LV, left ventricular cavity; RV, right ventricular cavity. (Adapted with permission from Daggett WM: Surgical technique for early repair of posterior ventricular septum rupture, *J Thorac Cardiovasc Surg.* 1982;Aug;84(2):306-312.)

even then it is minimized, because infarcted muscle will not be exposed to left ventricular pressures when the heart begins to work (see Fig. 25-9D). Alternatively, sutures can be passed through the ventricular free wall and through a tailored external patch of Teflon or pericardium (Fig. 25-10).[27]

In patients with inferoposterior septal defects, an incision is made in the inferior wall of the left ventricle 1 or 2 mm from the posterior descending artery (Fig. 25-11A).[27,39] This incision is started at the midportion of the inferior wall and extended proximally toward the mitral annulus and distally toward the apex of the ventricle. Care is taken to avoid damage to the posterolateral papillary muscle. Stay sutures are passed through the fat pad of the apex of the ventricle and margins of the ventriculotomy to facilitate exposure of the ventricular cavity. In most cases, the rupture is found in the proximal half of the posterior septum, and the posteromedial papillary muscle is involved by the infarction. A bovine pericardial patch is tailored in a triangular shape of approximately 4 × 7 cm in most patients. The base of the triangular-shaped patch is sutured to the fibrous annulus of the mitral valve with a continuous 3-0 polypropylene suture starting at a point corresponding to the level of the posteromedial papillary muscle and moving medially toward the septum until the noninfarcted endocardium is reached (see Fig. 25-11B). At that level, the suture is interrupted and any excess patch material trimmed. The medial margin of the triangular-shaped patch is sewn to healthy septal endocardium with a continuous 3-0 or 4-0 polypropylene suture taking bites the same size

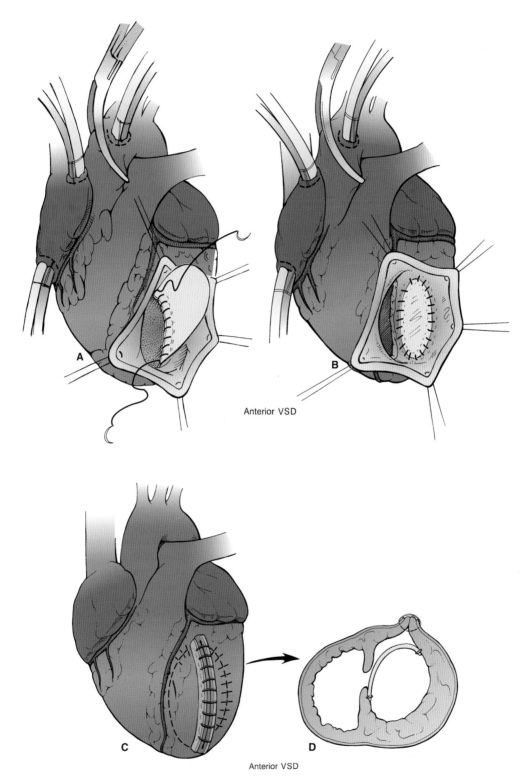

FIGURE 25-9 Repair of an anterior postinfarction ventricular septal rupture using the technique of infarct exclusion. (A) The standard ventriculotomy is made in the infarcted area of left ventricular free wall. An interior patch of Dacron, polytetrafluoroethylene, or glutaraldehyde-fixed pericardium is fashioned to replace and/or cover the diseased areas (ventricular septal defect [VSD], septal infarction, or free wall infarction). (B) The internal patch is secured to normal endocardium with a continuous monofilament suture, which may be reinforced with pledgeted mattress sutures. There is little, if any, resection of myocardium and no attempt is made to close the septal defect. Repair of an anterior postinfarction ventricular septal rupture using the technique of infarct exclusion. (C) The ventriculotomy, which is outside the pressure zone of the left ventricle, may be repaired with a continuous suture. (D) On transverse section, one can see that the endocardial patch is secured at three levels: above and below the septal rupture and beyond the ventriculotomy. (Adapted with permission from David TE, Dale L, Sun Z: Postinfarction ventricular septal rupture: repair by endocardial patch with infarct exclusion, *J Thorac Cardiovasc Surg.* 1995;Nov;110(5):1315-1322.)

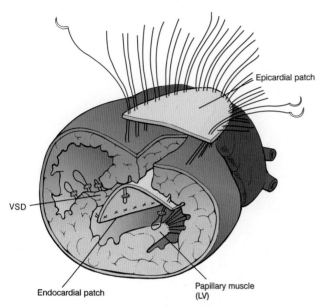

FIGURE 25-10 Repair of an anterior postinfarction ventricular septal rupture using the technique of infarct exclusion with external patching of the ventricular free wall with tailored Teflon or pericardium. LV, left ventricle; VSD, ventricular septal defect. (Adapted with permission from Cooley DA: Repair of postinfarction ventricular septal defect, *J Card Surg.* 1994;July;9(4):427-429.)

as those described for anterior defects. In this area of the septum, reinforcing pledgeted sutures may be required. The lateral side of the patch is sutured to the posterior wall of the left ventricle along a line corresponding to the medial margin of the base of the posteromedial papillary muscle. Because the posterior wall of the left ventricle is infarcted, it is usually necessary to use full-thickness bites and anchor the sutures on a strip of pericardium or Teflon felt applied on the epicardial surface of the posterior wall of the left ventricle right at the level of the posteromedial papillary muscle insertion, as shown in Fig. 25-11B. Once the patch is completely sutured to the mitral valve annulus, the endocardium of the interventricular septum, and the full thickness of the posterior wall (see Fig. 25-11C), the ventriculotomy is closed in two layers of full-thickness sutures buttressed on strips of pericardium or Teflon felt (see Fig. 25-11D). The infarcted right ventricular wall is left undisturbed. If the posteromedial papillary muscle is ruptured, mitral valve replacement is necessary.[27]

Daggett and others[27] feel that the theoretical advantages in the technique of infarct exclusion are: (1) It does not require resection of myocardium; excessive resection results in depression of ventricular function and insufficient resection predisposes to recurrence of septal rupture; (2) it maintains ventricular geometry, which enhances ventricular function; and (3) it avoids tension on friable muscle, which may diminish postoperative bleeding.

OTHER TECHNIQUES

Many have minor variants to the endocardial infarct exclusion technique have been described utilizing the principles

stated above.[41-43] Asai[44] described an approach through the right ventricle which may be appropriate for some patients but which has all of the issues with the original right ventricular approached use by Cooley and others years earlier.[4]

PERCUTANEOUS CLOSURE

Percutaneous closure of postinfarction ventricular septal defects has been performed with a number of devices, including those used to close congenital atrial or ventricular septal defects.[45-47] These devices can be placed through the systemic venous circulation into the right ventricle to access the septal defect, or through the arterial system and the left ventricle to approach the septal defect, or both. Calvert[47] reported 53 cases with percutaneous closure of postinfarction ventricular septal defects with complete shunt reduction in 23%, partial shunt reduction in 62%, and a 5-day post procedure length of stay. Percutaneous devices certainly have the theoretical advantage of avoiding cardiopulmonary bypass and the morbidity of open-heart surgery in an otherwise sick patient. However, technical issues exist with current devices, both in delivering the device to the defect (which may occur at most any location in the interventricular septum) and in obtaining a durable closure of large defects in a thick septum with poorly defined, necrotic edges. Problems have been reported with recurrent septal defects due to continued necrosis of septal tissue[48] and device migration or embolization.[46]

Results of percutaneous closure may be somewhat better 2 weeks or more after infarction, but surgical results are also better in those patients who are able to delay intervention.[45,49] Hybrid approaches have been reported where percutaneous devices were placed intraoperatively using open exposure on cardiopulmonary bypass to avoid a ventriculotomy.[50] To date, the best application of percutaneous catheter-based devices for postinfarction ventricular septal defects may be in those with recurrent or residual defects after surgical therapy.[47,51] If percutaneous closure of postinfarction ventricular septal defects can be obtained safely, even on a partial basis, the approach may have some role in palliating critically ill patients who might ultimately tolerate more definitive surgical intervention at a later date.

HIGHLIGHTS OF POSTOPERATIVE CARE

Impaired biventricular performance with low cardiac output is frequent in these patients and may require gradual weaning of inotropic support and the intra-aortic balloon pump over several days. Intravenous milrinone and inhaled nitric oxide may benefit some patients. Correction of hypoxia, hypercarbia, and acidosis can be important to maintain normal right ventricular afterload (see Chapters 12 and 18). Acute renal insufficiency and pulmonary edema are also frequent and require careful volume management, early postoperative diuresis, and the use of positive end-expiratory pressure ventilation (see Chapter 18). Ventricular and atrial arrhythmias can be poorly tolerated and can often be managed with intravenous amiodarone.

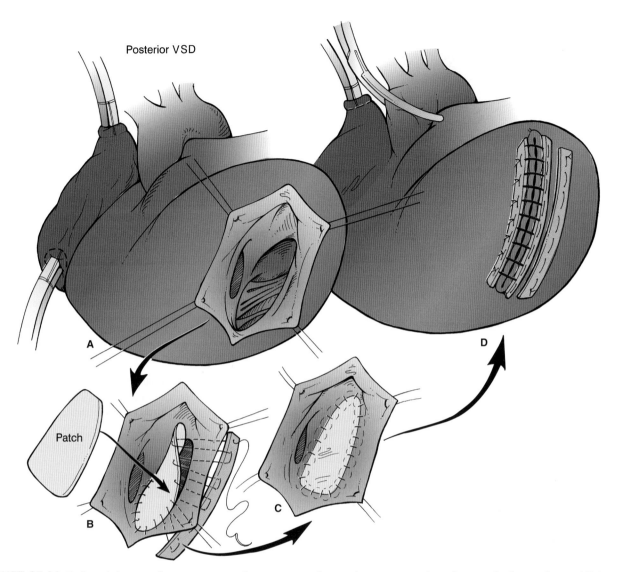

FIGURE 25-11 Endocardial repair of a posterior postinfarction ventricular septal rupture using the technique of infarct exclusion. (A) An incision is made in the inferior wall of the left ventricle 1 or 2 mm from the posterior descending artery starting at the midportion of the inferior wall and extended proximally toward the mitral annulus and distally toward the apex of the ventricle. Care is taken to avoid damage to the posterolateral papillary muscle. (B) A bovine pericardial patch is tailored in a triangular shape. The base of the triangular-shaped patch is sutured to the fibrous annulus of the mitral valve with a continuous 3-0 polypropylene suture starting at a point corresponding to the level of the posteromedial papillary muscle and moving medially toward the septum until the noninfarcted endocardium is reached. (C) The medial margin of the triangular-shaped patch is sewn to healthy septal endocardium with a continuous 3-0 or 4-0 polypropylene suture. The lateral side of the patch is sutured to the posterior wall of the left ventricle along a line corresponding to the medial margin of the base of the posteromedial papillary muscle. At this point, it is usually necessary to use full-thickness bites and anchor the sutures on a strip of pericardium or Teflon felt applied on the epicardial surface of the posterior wall of the left ventricle. (D) Once the patch is completely sutured to the mitral valve annulus, the endocardium of the interventricular septum, and the full thickness of the posterior wall, the ventriculotomy is closed in two layers of full-thickness sutures buttressed on strips of pericardium or Teflon felt. The infarcted right ventricular wall is left undisturbed. (Adapted with permission from David TE, Dale L, Sun Z: Postinfarction ventricular septal rupture: repair by endocardial patch with infarct exclusion, *J Thorac Cardiovasc Surg.* 1995;Nov;110(5):1315-1322.)

Early Results

HOSPITAL MORTALITY

Operative mortality defined as death before discharge or within 30 days of operation, ranged from 30 to 50%.[27,40,52-55] In the Massachusetts General Hospital experience of 114 patients, Daggett reported an operative mortality of 37% (Fig. 25-12A) with the risk of death falling rapidly after 1 year (see Fig. 25-12B).[27] The independent risk factors for early death were: older age, higher blood urea nitrogen (BUN), emergency surgery, higher right atrial pressure, and preoperative uses of catecholamines.[27] Inferoposterior location of the septal rupture has been associated with an increased operative mortality.[21] This has been attributed to a more technically difficult repair, the increased risk of associated mitral regurgitation, and associated right ventricular dysfunction

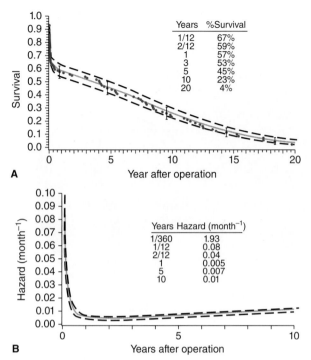

A

B

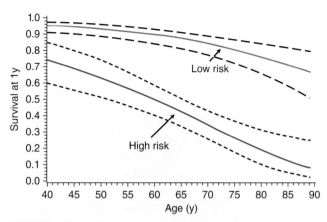

FIGURE 25-13 Nomograms (specific solutions to the multivariate equation) depicting the effect of age on risk in two different hypothetical patients. In both curves the patient was considered to have no left main disease, a blood urea nitrogen of 30 mg/dL, creatinine of 1.5 mg/dL, and no history of previous myocardial infarction. The curve for "low-risk" was solved for a patient who was not emergent and not on catecholamines. The curve for "high-risk" was for an emergent patient on inotropes. The vertical axis represents the calculated survival at 1 year.[27]

FIGURE 25-12 (A) Time-related survival after repair of postinfarction ventricular septal defect at the Massachusetts General Hospital (n = 114). Note that the horizontal axis extends to 20 years. Circles represent each death, positioned on the horizontal axis at the interval from operation to death, and actuarially (Kaplan-Meier method) along the vertical axis. The vertical bars represent 70% confidence limits (± 1 SD). The solid line represents the parametrically estimated freedom from death, and the dashed lines enclose the 70% confidence limits of that estimate. The table shows the nonparametric estimates at specified intervals. (B) Hazard function for death after repair of postinfarction ventricular septal defect (n = 114). The horizontal axis is expanded for better visualization of early risk. The hazard function has two phases, consisting of an early, rapidly declining phase, which gives way to a slowly rising phase at about 6 months. The estimate is shown with 70% confidence limits.[27]

that is an independent predictor of early mortality after posterior infarction. A short time interval between infarction and operation selects for sicker patients unable to be managed medically.

Daggett reviewed the Massachusetts General Hospital experience and concluded that patients cover a wide range of risk determined most notably by hemodynamic instability (emergency surgery and use of inotropes) (Figs. 25-13 and 25-14).[27] Daggett also concluded that a small group of high-risk patients dramatically affected the overall mortality rate, possibly explaining the tremendous variability in mortality rates between institutions with different patient selection and referral patterns, independent of surgical technique.

IN-HOSPITAL COMPLICATIONS

Daggett et al reported that the most common cause of death after repair of acute postinfarction ventricular septal defect was low cardiac output syndrome (52%), with technical failures

such as recurrent or residual septal defect and bleeding in 23%, sepsis (17%), recurrent infarction (9%), cerebrovascular complications (4%), and intractable ventricular arrhythmias.[27]

Late Results

SURVIVAL

Despite the very high early mortality rate with repair of postinfarction ventricular septal defect, mortality rates

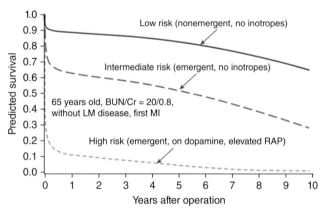

FIGURE 25-14 Nomograms (specific solutions of the multivariate equation) depicting the predicted survival in three hypothetical 65-year-old patients who present with ventricular septal defect. Each solution is for a patient who has no history of myocardial infarction and without left main coronary artery disease, blood urea nitrogen of 20 mg/dL, and creatinine of 0.8 mg/dL. The "low-risk" patient is nonemergent and not on inotropes with right atrial pressure (RAP) of 8 mm Hg. The "intermediate risk" patient is emergent and not on inotropes with RAP of 12 mm Hg. The "high-risk" patient is emergent and on inotropes with RAP of 20 mm Hg. Confidence limits have been eliminated to improve clarity.[27]

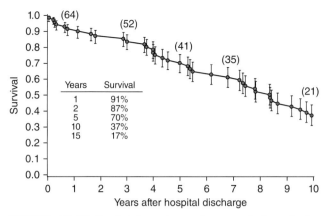

FIGURE 25-15 Survival in patients who were discharged after repair of postinfarction ventricular septal defect (Massachusetts General Hospital, n = 72). The horizontal axis is expanded and represents the time from hospital discharge to death. The depiction is otherwise similar to that seen in Fig. 25-12A.[27]

stabilized at a much lower level after about 1 year. Actuarial survival at 5 years series ranged between 40 and 60% (Fig. 25-12).[27,40,52-54] For hospital survivors, 1-, 5-, and 10-year survival have been reported at 91, 70, and 37%, respectively (Fig. 25-15).[27] The multivariable predictors of late death were: older age, previous myocardial infarction, higher creatinine, higher right atrial pressure, and the presence of left main coronary disease.[27]

SYMPTOMATIC IMPROVEMENT

Ultimately survivors also can have good functional status with Daggett reporting that 75% were in New York Heart Association functional class I, and 12.5% were class II.[9]

RECURRENT VENTRICULAR SEPTAL DEFECTS

Using echocardiography, recurrent or residual septal defects have been observed to occur in 10 to 25% of patients.[56] Large residual septal defects with a Qp:Qs > 2.0 should undergo a repair while smaller defects may be managed medically and may occasionally close spontaneously. Percutaneous approaches for these small residual septal defects have been preferred when possible. Surgical closure of late postoperative particular septal defects have been reported via a right atrial approach.[57,58]

ACUTE VENTRICULAR FREE WALL RUPTURE

Definition

Left ventricular free wall rupture is similar to rupture of the interventricular septum, except for the location of the rupture. Acute left ventricular free wall rupture is a life-threatening complication of myocardial infarction that requires early intervention. In those unusual patients who survive the initial acute, 2-week phase of ventricular free wall rupture without

diagnosis and/or therapy, this entity will ultimately evolve into a pseudoaneurysm of the left ventricular free wall. These later-phase patients have generally undergone some pericardial healing at the site of infarction, and their management more resembles that of patients with chronic true aneurysms of the left ventricle (see Chapter 26).

History

The first known case of left ventricular free wall rupture after myocardial infarction was described by William Harvey in 1647.[59] In 1765, Morgagni reported 11 postmortem cases of myocardial rupture[60] and ultimately himself later died of myocardial rupture. The first successful surgical treatment of free wall rupture of the right ventricle was reported by Hatcher in 1970.[61] FitzGibbon[62] in 1971 and Montegut[63] in 1972 reported the first successful repairs of postinfarction left ventricular free wall rupture.

Incidence

Left ventricular free wall rupture is a relatively common finding in an autopsy series of patients expiring early after acute myocardial infarction, occurring in 10 to 30% of such patients.[64,65] In clinical series of early death after acute myocardial infarction, ventricular rupture may be the second cause of death after cardiogenic shock. Postinfarction ventricular free wall rupture may be more common in elderly patients, and women, and in patients suffering their first infarction.[66] The peak incidence of postinfarction left ventricular free wall rupture occurred at a median of 5 days after infarction.[67] However, thrombolysis and early coronary perfusion may have resulted in an increased number of ventricular ruptures occurring at earlier times, as early as hours after the onset of infarction.[68] In a recent series of 1290 acute myocardial infarction patients, most of whom were reperfused, left ventricular free wall rupture occurred in 1.3%.[69] Because anterolateral infarctions are more common than inferior infarction in general, some series report the anterolateral wall as the most common sight of rupture.[64] Other series suggest that a posterolateral or inferior infarction is itself more likely to result in free wall rupture than is anterior infarction.[65]

Etiology

Acute left ventricular free wall rupture is most commonly due to acute myocardial infarction, with either blunt or penetrating trauma being another common etiology. Prior cardiac surgery, such as mitral valve replacement or transapical aortic valve replacement, can result in acute left ventricular free wall rupture.[70,71] However, once postoperative pericarditis is mature 2 weeks or more postoperatively, prior cardiac surgery is more likely to produce chronic left ventricular pseudoaneurysms instead of acute free wall rupture with tamponade. Other etiologies such as pericardial infection or cardiac tumor have rarely resulted in left ventricular free wall rupture. The treatment of acute left ventricular free wall rupture not due to infarction will be similar to that of postinfarction rupture, except that underlying coronary disease and myocardial infarction will generally be absent.

Pathophysiology

Postinfarction left ventricular free wall rupture can present on an acute, subacute, or chronic basis. *Acute* ventricular free wall rupture, in generally, results in acute pericardial tamponade, followed by shock, electromechanical dissociation, and death within a few minutes. *Subacute* rupture may initially involve a smaller ventricular wall tear which becomes partially sealed by clot and pericardial adhesions. *Chronic* left ventricular free wall rupture is by definition a left ventricular pseudoaneurysm which results when pericardial adhesions are sufficient to prevent free rupture for 2 weeks or more. Chronic left ventricular pseudoaneurysms generally have a narrow neck, contain no myocardial cells in the wall, and have a high propensity to convert to an acute rupture. On rare occasion, left ventricular free wall rupture can present with simultaneous rupture of the interventricular septum, right ventricular rupture, or rupture of a papillary muscle head.[72,73] Risk factors associated with left ventricular pseudoaneurysm in 290 patients included older age, female gender, hypertension, and inferolateral myocardial infarction.[74] The most common location for left ventricular pseudoaneurysm in these 290 patients was posteroinferior, in contrast to true left ventricular aneurysms which are more common in the anterolateral region.[74]

The pathophysiology of left ventricular free wall rupture involves initial transmural myocardial infarction followed by expansion and thinning of the infarcted wall until the elastic strength of the free wall is exceeded by the forces generated by left ventricular systole.[22,75] Transmural myocardial infarction is, in turn, associated with lack of collateral blood flow.[76] This infarct expansion and thinning results from slippage between muscle bundles and tearing of the surrounding protein matrix. Ventricular rupture may be associated with systemic hypertension which can increase infarct thinning and wall stress.[77] Thrombolysis has not had any clear positive or negative effect on the incidence of left ventricular rupture,[68,78,79] although early coronary reperfusion is associated with less transmural infarction which in turn should prevent some infarctions from turning into rupture.

Natural History

Acute left ventricular free wall rupture generally results in death within minutes of the onset of recurrent chest pain.[67,80] In an autopsy series, most patients dying from left ventricular free wall rupture died acutely.[81-83] Subacute rupture of the left ventricular free wall, in one series, was associated with a median survival time of 8 hours,[81] while another study showed that 69% of such patients died within minutes of the onset of symptoms.[84] Chronic rupture or pseudoaneurysm of the left ventricular free wall has a less well-defined prognosis. While rare patients may present with pseudoaneurysm of the

left ventricular free wall years after myocardial infarction,[85] postinfarction left ventricular pseudoaneurysm is clearly associated with a high probability of early rupture.[83,86]

Clinical Presentation

The patient with acute or subacute rupture of the left ventricular free wall generally presents with recurrent chest pain followed by a rapid, severe hemodynamic instability due to development of cardiac tamponade and resultant low cardiac output, often followed ultimately by ventricular fibrillation and/or electromechanical dissociation. Clinically these phenomena may manifest as sudden death or syncope with physical findings of hypotension, distended neck veins, pulsus paradoxus, and cardiogenic shock from the underlying cardiac tamponade. Subacute left ventricular rupture may clinically resemble infarct extension or right ventricular failure.[80] Chronic left ventricular rupture or pseudoaneurysm presents most commonly with congestive heart failure.[72,74]

Diagnosis

The primary means of diagnosing postinfarction left ventricular rupture is echocardiography. Echocardiography may show definitive evidence of a ventricular wall defect systolic and/or systolic blood flow outside the wall of the ventricle. Highly suggestive but less definitive echocardiographic findings associated with left ventricular rupture include the presence of pericardial effusion over 10 mm, echo-dense masses in a pericardial effusion, and signs of tamponade such as early diastolic collapse of the right atrium and right ventricle and increased respiratory variation in transvalvular blood flow velocities.[81,87] Aspiration of uncoagulated blood on pericardiocentesis can be suggestive of left ventricular rupture but has an incidence of false-positive and false-negative results. Aspiration of clear fluid on pericardiocentesis definitively excludes cardiac rupture.[87] Oliva[64] reported several factors associated with postinfarction left ventricular rupture in 70 consecutive patients. Some predictive value has been reported for the development of pericarditis, repetitive emesis, restlessness and agitation, recurrent or persistent ST segment elevation, and persistent T-wave changes after 48 to 72 hours.[65]

Indications for Operation

Because most patients with acute or subacute rupture of the left ventricular free wall expire within minutes to hours of onset, the diagnosis or even a high suspicion of acute left ventricular free wall rupture is itself an indication for emergent operation. At present, no acute interventional procedure is reliable in treating this catastrophic event. Chronic pseudoaneurysm of the left ventricular free wall has a significant risk of rupture and should be treated surgically.[73,88-91] Alapati[92] reported that less than 0.1% of all myocardial infarctions resulted in left ventricular pseudoaneurysm but that death occurred in the 48% patients with chronic pseudoaneurysm of the left ventricular free wall with medical therapy.

Preparation for Operation

Acute postinfarction rupture of the left ventricular wall requires a high index of suspicion and emergent surgery for survival.[84] One report suggested that emergent percutaneous intrapericardial injection of fibrin glue immediately after pericardiocentesis[93,94] may allow some patients to get to surgery. Subacute postinfarction rupture of the left ventricle similarly requires emergent surgery once the diagnosis is made without further delay for coronary angiography.[68,72] Volume resuscitation, inotropic support, intra-aortic balloon pump, and possibly pericardiocentesis may temporize the pericardial tamponade on the way to surgery.

Operative Techniques

ACUTE OR SUBACUTE FREE WALL RUPTURE

Patients being operated for postinfarction rupture of the left ventricular free wall are generally quite unstable with pericardial tamponade and recent transmural myocardial infarction. Much of the patient preparation in the operating room may be conducted while the patient is awake and minimally sedated to avoid hypotension. One should consider exposure of the femoral artery and femoral vein in the groin for rapid institution of cardiopulmonary bypass, even before median sternotomy.

Median sternotomy is the incision of choice with rapid institution of cardiopulmonary bypass, preferably from the femoral vessels. Opening the pericardium can quickly result in significant hemorrhage from the ventricular tear that may be difficult to control manually without further hemodynamic compromise until on cardiopulmonary bypass. Just a few minutes of inadequate brain perfusion can result in a poor neurologic outcome. In exceptional cases where there are no other indications for cardiopulmonary bypass such as posterior wall rupture, mitral regurgitation, ventricular septal rupture, or graftable coronary disease, good short-term results have been reported for repairing ventricular rupture without cardiopulmonary bypass[80,88] or without aortic clamping. Once on cardiopulmonary bypass, having an arrested heart with venting of the left ventricular cavity can facilitate obtaining a dry and motionless field for manipulation of friable tissue.

For repairing an acute or subacute for left ventricular free wall rupture, surgical techniques resemble those for left ventricular pseudoaneurysm repair, with the exception that the acutely or subacutely infarcted tissue is much more friable and has not had time to develop any fibrous content. Standard linear closure with large horizontal mattress sutures buttressed by two strips of Teflon felt has been reported but is limited by myocardial friability. Better results have been reported using linear closure between strips of Teflon felt, if the entire ventricular tear and surrounding infarct is covered with a plastic patch secured to the surrounding normal myocardium using a continuous polypropylene suture (Fig. 25-16).[27] A more radical approach would be to perform infarct excision and closure of the defect with either pledgeted sutures or a Dacron patch,[95] but this technique might

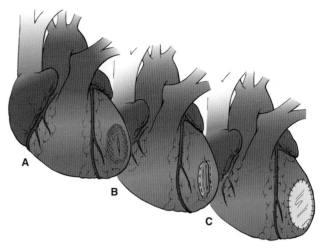

FIGURE 25-16 Technique to repair rupture of the free wall of the left ventricle. (A) Left ventricular free wall rupture. (B) A limited infarctectomy is closed with horizontal mattress sutures buttressed with two strips of Teflon felt. (C) Then the whole area is covered with a Teflon patch sutured to healthy epicardium with a continuous polypropylene suture. Alternatively, the Teflon patch can be glued to the ventricular tear and the infarcted area using a biocompatible glue. (Reproduced with permission from Buxton BF, et al: Ischemic Heart Disease Surgical Management. Philadelphia, Mosby 1999.)

best be reserved for specific indications such as the presence of a postinfarction ventricular septal defect.

Frequent reports have described using one of many biological glues to attach a patch of either Teflon felt or bovine pericardium to the ventricular tear, with or without running a polypropylene suture around the edge of the patch secured to the surrounding normal myocardium.[88] This technique has the advantage of avoiding cardiopulmonary bypass but has been reported to have some risk of late pseudoaneurysm formation.[96]

Results

The literature only contains several small series of surgical repair of acute or subacute left ventricular free wall rupture. Padró[88] reported 13 survivors and a mean follow up of 26 months using a biological glue and Teflon patch technique, without cardiopulmonary bypass in most patients. Other series have reported an operative mortality around 50%.[84,97,98]

LEFT VENTRICULAR ANEURYSM

Definition

Left ventricular aneurysm has been strictly defined as a distinct area of abnormal left ventricular diastolic contour with systolic dyskinesis or paradoxical bulging (Fig. 25-17).[99,100] Yet, a growing number of authors favor defining left ventricular aneurysm more loosely as any large area of left ventricular akinesia or dyskinesia that reduces the left ventricular ejection fraction.[101-103] This broader definition has been justified by data suggesting that the pathophysiology and treatment may

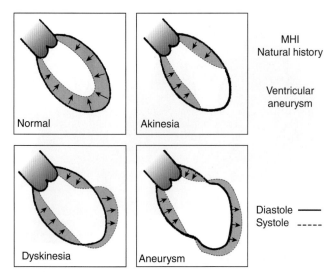

FIGURE 25-17 Diagrammatic distinction between aneurysm and other states of the left ventricle. (Reproduced with permission from Grondin P, Kretz JG, Bical O, et al: Natural history of saccular aneurysm of the left ventricle, *J Thorac Cardiovasc Surg.* 1979 Jan;77(1):57-64.)

be the same for ventricular akinesia and for ventricular dyskinesia.[102,104] However, recent studies suggest that the optimal treatment and outcomes of patients with akinetic segments versus dyskinetic segments might be different.[105,106] Intraoperatively, a left ventricular aneurysm may also be identified as an area that collapses upon left ventricular decompression.[101,104,107] True left ventricular aneurysms involve bulging of the full thickness of the left ventricular wall, whereas a false aneurysm of the left ventricle is, in fact, a rupture of the left ventricular wall contained by surrounding pericardium.

History

Left ventricular aneurysms have long been described at autopsy, but left ventricular aneurysm was not recognized to be a consequence of coronary artery disease until 1881.[108] The angiographic diagnosis of left ventricular aneurysm was first made in 1951.[108] A congenital left ventricular aneurysm was first treated surgically by Weitland in 1912 using aneurysm ligation. In 1944, Beck[109] described fasciae latae plication to treat left ventricular aneurysms. Likoff and Bailey [110] successfully resected a left ventricular aneurysm through a thoracotomy in 1955 using a special clamp without cardiopulmonary bypass. The modern treatment era began in 1958 when Cooley et al[111] successfully performed a linear repair of a left ventricular aneurysm using cardiopulmonary bypass. More geometric ventricular reconstruction or surgical ventricular restoration (SVR) techniques were subsequently devised by Stoney et al,[112] Daggett et al,[113] Dor et al,[36] Jatene,[114] and Cooley et al.[115,116] In 2009, the results of the randomized STICH trial comparing coronary bypass grafting with or without surgical ventricular restoration were published, casting some doubt on the value of repairing small aneurysms or small akinetic segments.[105]

Incidence

The incidence of left ventricular aneurysm in patients suffering from myocardial infarction has varied between 10 and 35%, depending on the definition and the methods used. Of patients undergoing cardiac catheterization in the CASS study, 7.6% had angiographic evidence of left ventricular aneurysms.[117] The absolute incidence of left ventricular aneurysms may be declining because of the increased use of thrombolytics and revascularization early after myocardial infarction.[118,119]

Etiology

More than 95% of true left ventricular aneurysms reported in the English literature result from coronary artery disease and myocardial infarction. True left ventricular aneurysms also may result from trauma,[120] Chagas' disease,[121] or sarcoidosis.[122] A very small number of congenital left ventricular aneurysms also have been reported and have been termed *diverticula* of the left ventricle.[123]

False aneurysms of the left ventricle result most commonly from contained rupture of the ventricle 5 to 10 days after myocardial infarction and often occur after circumflex coronary arterial occlusion. False aneurysm of the left ventricle also may result from submitral rupture of the ventricular wall, a dramatic event that generally occurs after mitral valve replacement with resection of the mitral valve apparatus.[124] Left ventricular pseudoaneurysm may also result from septic pericarditis[125] or any prior operation on the left ventricle, aortic annulus, or mitral annulus. Pseudoaneurysm can occur after transapical or transfemoral transcatheter aortic valve replacement (TAVR).[126]

Pathophysiology

The development of a true left ventricular aneurysm involves two principal phases: early expansion and late remodeling.

EARLY EXPANSION PHASE

The early expansion phase begins with the onset of myocardial infarction. Ventriculography can demonstrate left ventricular aneurysm formation within 48 hours of infarction in 50% of patients who develop ventricular aneurysms. The remaining patients have evidence of aneurysm formation by 2 weeks after infarction.[127]

True aneurysm of the left ventricle generally follows transmural myocardial infarction because of acute occlusion of the left anterior descending or dominant right coronary artery.

Lack of angiographic collaterals is strongly associated with aneurysm formation in patients with acute myocardial infarction and left anterior descending artery occlusion,[128] and absence of re-formed collateral circulation is probably a prerequisite for formation of a dyskinetic left ventricular aneurysm (Table 25-2). At least 88% of dyskinetic ventricular aneurysms result from anterior infarction, and the remainder follow inferior infarction.[108] Posterior infarctions that

TABLE 25-2: Factors Contributing to Left Ventricular Aneurysm Formation

Preserved contractility of surrounding myocardium
Transmural infarction
Lack of collateral circulation
Lack of reperfusion
Preserved contractility of surrounding myocardium
Elevated wall stress
Hypertension
Ventricular dilation
Wall thinning

produce a distinct dyskinetic left ventricular aneurysm are relatively unusual.[129]

In experimental transmural infarction without collateral circulation, myocyte death begins 19 minutes after coronary occlusion. Infarctions that result in dyskinetic aneurysm formation are almost always transmural and may show gross thinning of the infarct zone within hours of infarction. Within a few days, the endocardial surface of the developing aneurysm becomes smooth with loss of trabeculae and deposition of fibrin and thrombus on the endocardial surface in at least 50% of patients. Because most myocytes within the infarct are necrotic, viable myocytes often remain within the infarct zone. In a minority of patients, extravascular hemorrhage occurs in the infarcted tissue and may further depress systolic and diastolic function of involved myocardium. Inflammatory cells migrate into the infarct zone by 2 to 3 days after infarction and contribute to lysis of the necrotic myocytes by 5 to 10 days after infarction. Electron microscopy demonstrates disruption of the native collagen network several days after infarction. Collagen disruption and myocyte necrosis produce a nadir of myocardial tensile strength between 5 and 10 days after infarction, when rupture of the myocardial wall is most common. Left ventricular rupture is relatively rare after the ventricular aneurysmal wall becomes replaced with fibrous tissue.

Loss of systolic contraction in the large infarcted zone and preserved contraction of surrounding myocardium cause systolic bulging and thinning of the infarct. By Laplace's law ($T = Pr/2h$), at a constant ventricular pressure (P), increased radius of curvature (r) and decreased wall thickness (h) in the infarcted zone both contribute to increased muscle fiber tension (T) and further stretch the infarcted ventricular wall.

Relative to normal myocardium, ischemically injured or infarcted myocardium displays greater *plasticity* or *creep*, defined as deformation or stretch over time under a constant load.[130] Thus increased systolic and diastolic wall stress in the infarcted zone tends to produce progressive stretch of the infarcted myocardium (termed *infarct expansion*)[131] until healing reduces the plasticity of infarcted myocardium.

Transmural infarction without significant hibernating myocardium within the infarct region is necessary for subsequent development of a true left ventricular aneurysm. Angiographic ventricular aneurysms with evidence of hibernating myocardium (lack of Q waves or presence of uptake on technetium scan, Takotsubo cardiomyopathy, for example) may resolve over days to weeks and thus do not represent true left ventricular aneurysms by strict criteria.[132,133]

Because of increased diastolic stretch or preload and elevated catecholamines, remaining noninfarcted myocardium may demonstrate increased fiber shortening and, ultimately, myocardial hypertrophy in the presence of a left ventricular aneurysm.[134] This increased shortening and increased wall stress increase oxygen demand for noninfarcted myocardium and for the left ventricle as a whole.

In addition to increased regional wall stresses, left ventricular aneurysm can increase ventricular oxygen demand and decrease net forward cardiac output by producing a ventricular volume load because a portion of the stroke volume goes into the aneurysm instead of out of the aortic valve. Net mechanical efficiency of the left ventricle (external stroke work minus myocardial oxygen consumption) is decreased by reducing external stroke work (volume times pressure) and increasing myocardial oxygen consumption.

Left ventricular aneurysms can produce both systolic and diastolic ventricular dysfunction. Diastolic dysfunction results from increased stiffness of the distended and fibrotic aneurysmal wall, which impairs diastolic filling and increases left ventricular end-diastolic pressure.

LATE REMODELING PHASE

The remodeling phase of ventricular aneurysm formation begins 2 to 4 weeks after infarction when highly vascularized granulation tissue appears. This granulation tissue is subsequently replaced by fibrous tissue 6 to 8 weeks after infarction. As myocytes are lost, ventricular wall thickness decreases as the myocardium becomes largely replaced by fibrous tissue. In larger infarcts, the thin scar is often lined with mural thrombus.[135]

After acute myocardial infarction, animal studies show that ventricular load reduction with 8 weeks of nitrate therapy may reduce expected infarct thinning, decrease infarct stretch, and lessen hypertrophy of noninfarcted myocardium.[136] Interestingly, nitrate therapy for only 2 weeks after infarction does not prevent aneurysm formation. This observation emphasizes the importance of late remodeling from 2 to 8 weeks after infarction. Angiotensin converting-enzyme (ACE) inhibitors also reduce infarct expansion and subsequent development of ventricular aneurysm.[137] Because animal studies show that ACE inhibitors nonspecifically suppress ventricular hypertrophy, it is not clear whether suppression of the compensatory hypertrophy of surrounding myocardium is ultimately beneficial or harmful. Intravenous administration of atrial natriuretic factor for 4 weeks has improved ventricular function, dimensions, and fibrosis in rats.[138]

Lack of coronary reperfusion is probably a prerequisite for development of left ventricular aneurysm. In humans, reperfusion of the infarct vessel either spontaneously,[132] by thrombolysis,[139] or by angioplasty[140] has been associated with a lower incidence of aneurysm formation. It is speculated that coronary reperfusion as late as 2 weeks after infarction prevents aneurysm formation by improving blood flow and fibroblast migration into the infarcted myocardium. The role of delayed infarct healing in aneurysm development is supported by observations that steroids after myocardial infarction may increase the likelihood of aneurysm formation.[141]

Arrhythmias such as ventricular tachycardia may occur at any time during the development of a ventricular aneurysm, and all these patients have the substrate for reentrant conduction pathways within the heterogeneous ventricular myocardium. These pathways tend to involve border zones surrounding the ventricular aneurysm (see Chapter 57).

Natural History

The excellent prognosis of asymptomatic patients with dyskinetic ventricular aneurysms who were treated medically was demonstrated in a series of 40 patients followed for a mean of 5 years.[100] Of 18 initially asymptomatic patients, six developed class II symptoms and 12 remained asymptomatic. The 10-year survival was 90% for these patients but was only 46% at 10 years in patients who presented with symptoms (Fig. 25-18).[100]

Although an earlier autopsy series reported relatively poor survival in patients with medically managed left ventricular dyskinetic aneurysms (12% at 5 years), most recent studies report 5-year survival from 47 to 70%.[100,117,142-144] Causes of death include arrhythmia in 44%, heart failure in 33%, recurrent myocardial infarction in 11%, and noncardiac causes in 22%.[100] The natural history of patients with akinetic rather than dyskinetic left ventricular aneurysms is less well documented.[105]

Factors that influence survival with medically managed left ventricular dyskinetic aneurysm include age, heart failure score, extent of coronary disease, duration of angina, prior infarction, mitral regurgitation, ventricular arrhythmias, aneurysm size, function of residual ventricle, and left ventricular end-diastolic pressure.[100,144] Early development of

aneurysm within 48 hours after infarction also diminishes survival.[127]

In general, the risk of thromboembolism is low for patients with aneurysms (0.35% per patient-year),[142] and long-term anticoagulation is not usually recommended. However, in the 50% of patients with mural thrombus visible by echocardiography after myocardial infarction, 19% develop thromboembolism over a mean follow-up of 24 months.[145] In these patients, anticoagulation and close echocardiographic follow-up may be indicated. Atrial fibrillation and large aneurysmal size are additional risk factors for thromboembolism.

The natural history of left ventricular pseudoaneurysm is not well documented. Frank rupture of chronic left ventricular pseudoaneurysms is less common than one might expect.[89] Rupture of left ventricular pseudoaneurysms may be most likely in the acute phase or in large-sized pseudoaneurysms.[90] Left ventricular pseudoaneurysms tend to behave similarly to true aneurysms in that they may present a volume load to the left ventricle or may be a source of embolization or endocarditis. Left ventricular pseudoaneurysms after prior cardiac surgery have also been reported to compress adjacent structures such as the pulmonary artery or esophagus.

Clinical Presentation

Angina is the most frequent symptom in most series of operated patients with left ventricular aneurysm. Given that three-vessel coronary disease is present in 60% or more of these patients, the frequency of angina is not surprising.[91]

Dyspnea is the second most common symptom of ventricular aneurysm and often develops when 20% or more of the ventricular wall is infarcted. Dyspnea may occur from a combination of decreased systolic function and diastolic dysfunction.

Either atrial or ventricular arrhythmias may produce palpitations, syncope, or sudden death, or aggravate angina and dyspnea in up to one-third of patients.[91] Thromboembolism is unusual but may produce symptoms of stroke, myocardial infarction, or limb or visceral ischemia.

Diagnosis

The electrocardiogram frequently demonstrates Q waves in the anterior leads along with persistent anterior ST-segment elevation (Fig. 25-19). The chest radiograph may show left ventricular enlargement and cardiomegaly (Fig. 25-20), but the chest radiograph is not usually specific for left ventricular aneurysm.

Left ventriculography is the gold standard for diagnosis of left ventricular aneurysm. The diagnosis is made by demonstrating a large, discrete area of dyskinesia (or akinesia), generally in the anteroseptal-apical walls. Occasionally, left ventriculography also may demonstrate mural thrombus. Quantitative definition of left ventricular aneurysms has been accomplished using a centerline analysis of left ventricular wall motion on left ventriculography in the 30° right anterior oblique view.[5] Hypocontractile segments contracting more than two standard

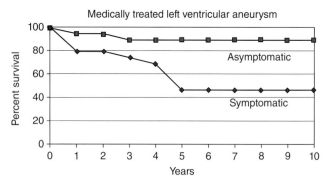

FIGURE 25-18 Survival in medically treated patients with left ventricular aneurysm based on presence (group B) or absence (group A) of symptoms. (Data from Grondin P, Kretz JG, Bical O, et al: Natural history of saccular aneurysm of the left ventricle, *J Thorac Cardiovasc Surg.* 1979 Jan;77(1):57-64.)

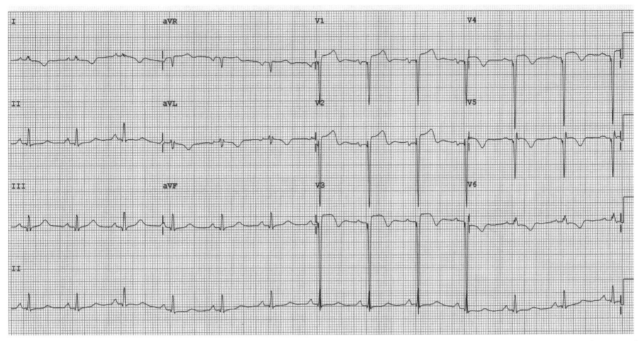

FIGURE 25-19 Electrocardiogram showing persistent ST-segment elevation with pathologic Q waves in a 72-year-old man with left ventricular aneurysm.

deviations out of normal range have also been defined as aneurysmal (Fig. 25-21).[92,102] Outward motion is termed *dyskinetic*, and remaining aneurysmal segments are termed *akinetic*. The fraction of total left ventricular circumference that is aneurysmal can thus be computed as the value %A.[103]

Two-dimensional echocardiography is also a sensitive and specific means of diagnosing left ventricular aneurysm. Echocardiography can detect mural thrombus or mitral valve regurgitation, and echocardiography can often distinguish false aneurysm from true aneurysm by demonstrating a defect in the true ventricular wall.

Magnetic resonance imaging (MRI) is the most reliable means of assessing left ventricular volume in the presence of left ventricular aneurysm[146,147] (Fig. 25-22). Magnetic resonance imaging (MRI) can accurately define left ventricular aneurysms and can detect mural thrombus.[146] Yet, distinguishing true aneurysms from pseudoaneurysms remains difficult, even with magnetic resonance imaging.[148] Gated radionuclide angiography reliably detects left ventricular aneurysms, and thallium scanning or positron emission tomography (PET) can be helpful early after infarction to differentiate a true aneurysm from hibernating myocardium with reversible dysfunction.

Indications for Operation

Because of the relatively good prognosis for asymptomatic left ventricular aneurysm,[100] no indications for repairing chronic,

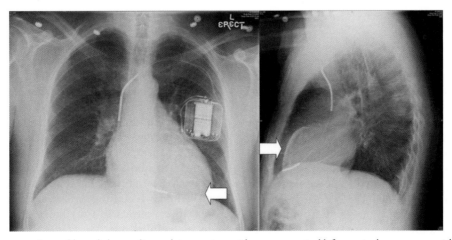

FIGURE 25-20 Posteroanterior and lateral chest radiograph in a patient with an anteroapical left ventricular aneurysm with calcification (*arrows*).

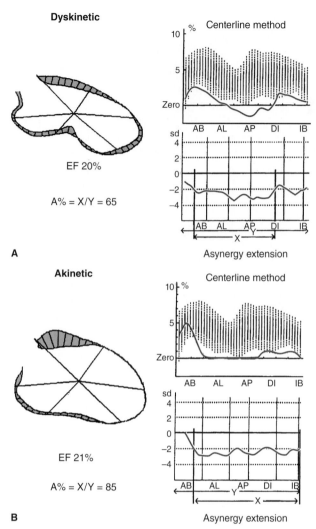

Dyskinetic

EF 20%

A% = X/Y = 65

A

Akinetic

EF 21%

A% = X/Y = 85

B

FIGURE 25-21 Examples of preoperative centerline analysis in dyskinetic (A) and akinetic (B) LV aneurysms. Vertical lines indicate the extent of asynergy. AB, anterobasal; AL, anterolateral; AP, apical; DI, diaphragmatic; EF, ejection fraction; IB, inferobasal. (Reproduced with permission from Dor V, Sabatier M, DiDonato M: Efficacy of endoventricular patch plasty in large postinfarction akinetic scar and severe left ventricular dysfunction: comparison with a series of large dyskinetic scars, *J Thorac Cardiovasc Surg.* 1998 Jul;116(1):50-59.)

asymptomatic aneurysms are established. Yet, in low-risk patients during operation for associated coronary disease, investigators report repairing large, minimally symptomatic aneurysms.[108,149] On the other hand, operation is indicated for symptoms of angina, congestive heart failure, or selected ventricular arrhythmias (see Chapter 57) (Table 25-3). For these symptomatic patients, operation offers better outcome than medical therapy.

To be worthy of operation, a dyskinetic or akinetic left ventricular aneurysm should significantly enlarge left ventricular end-systolic volume index (>80 mL/m²) and end-diastolic volume (>120 mL/m²). These volume criteria are, however, poorly defined and limited by technical difficulty

in measuring left ventricular volume in aneurysmal left ventricles. Because of data suggesting that akinetic versus dyskinetic aneurysms have similar results, Dor and others feel that dyskinesia is not a prerequisite for aneurysm repair.[102,103] Nonetheless, the only randomized trial (the STICH trial) has suggested that little benefit is obtained in terms of survival or symptoms in patients who on average have smaller, akinetic aneurysmal segments (end-systolic volume index 82 mL/m² and 50 to 56% of anterior wall involved).[105]

Operation is indicated in viable patients with contained cardiac rupture, with or without development of a false aneurysm. Because left ventricular pseudoaneurysms may have a tendency to rupture when acute or of larger size (either with or without symptoms), operation is indicated.[89-91] Similarly, congenital aneurysms have a presumed risk of rupture and should undergo repair independently of symptoms. Rarely, embolism is an indication for operation in medically treated patients at high risk for repeated thromboembolism. The role of operation in asymptomatic patients with very large aneurysms or documented expansion of aneurysms is uncertain.

Relative contraindications to operation for left ventricular aneurysm include excessive anesthetic risk, impaired function of residual myocardium outside the aneurysm, resting cardiac index less than 2.0 L/min/m², significant mitral regurgitation, evidence of nontransmural infarction (hibernating myocardium), and lack of a discrete, thin-walled aneurysm with distinct margins. Global ejection fraction may be less useful than ejection fraction of the basal, contractile portion of the heart in determining operability.[150]

Angioplasty has an uncertain role in the treatment of left ventricular aneurysms but may be indicated in patients with suitable coronary anatomy, one- or two-vessel disease, a contraindication for operation, or asymptomatic status with inducible ischemia.

Preparation for Operation

All patients being considered for operation should undergo right- and left-sided heart catheterization with coronary arteriography and left ventriculography. Patients with at least 2+ mitral regurgitation at cardiac catheterization should have echocardiography to assess the mitral valve and to look for intrinsic mitral valve disease not amenable to annuloplasty. Magnetic resonance imaging can be helpful to assess left ventricular volumes and aid in planning the size and extent of left ventricular reconstruction.[151] Patients with significant thrombus in the left ventricular cavity should ideally be treated with 4-6 weeks of anticoagulation prior to operation to avoid the risk of embolism.

Preoperative electrophysiologic study is clearly indicated in any patient with preoperative ventricular tachycardia or ventricular fibrillation. The decision to perform an electrophysiologic study in patients without preoperative ventricular arrhythmias is controversial, because the incidence of postoperative ventricular arrhythmias is low and not changed by endocardial resection at the time of operation.[108] Electrophysiologic study is frequently not helpful in patients

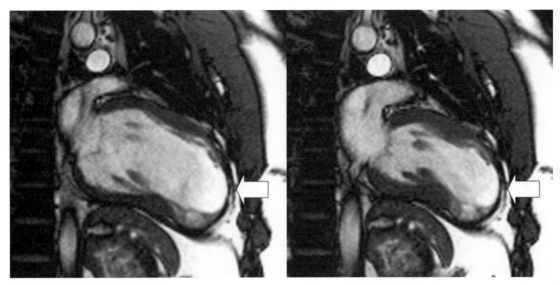

FIGURE 25-22 Magnetic resonance images of an apical left ventricular aneurysm during diastole (*left panel*) and systole (*right panel*).

with polymorphic ventricular tachycardia occurring within 6 weeks of myocardial infarction.[108]

Operative Techniques

GENERAL OPERATION

Operation for left ventricular aneurysm (aneurysmectomy, aneurysmorrhaphy, ventricular restoration) requires cardiopulmonary bypass and a balanced anesthetic technique, as generally used for coronary bypass grafting. After induction of anesthesia and endotracheal intubation, an electrocardiogram monitor, a Foley catheter, a radial arterial line, and a Swan-Ganz catheter are placed. A median sternotomy is performed, and the patient is given heparin. Saphenous vein or arterial conduits are prepared.

Cardiopulmonary bypass is begun after cannulating the ascending aorta. A single, two-stage cannula is generally adequate to cannulate the right atrium, but dual venous cannulation should be considered if the right ventricle is to be opened. Epicardial mapping is performed if necessary. The

> **TABLE 25-3: Relative Indications for Ventricular Aneurysm Operation**

Documented expansion/large size
Angina
Congestive heart failure
Arrhythmia
Rupture
Pseudoaneurysm
Congenital aneurysm
Embolism
Documented expansion/large size

left ventricle is inspected to identify an appropriate area of thinned ventricular wall. A linear vertical ventriculotomy, generally on the anterior wall 3 to 4 cm from the left anterior descending coronary artery, is made (Fig. 25-23). The left ventricle is opened (Fig. 25-24), all mural thrombus is carefully removed, and endocardial mapping is performed if necessary. A left ventricular vent is now placed through the right superior pulmonary vein-left atrial junction after mural thrombus is removed. Coronary arteries to be grafted are identified. Endocardial scar, if present, is resected, and afterwards, endocardial mapping is repeated. Body temperature is maintained at 37°C until intraoperative mapping is completed; thereafter, temperature is decreased to 28 to 32°C.

The ascending aorta is clamped, and the heart is arrested with cold anterograde and/or retrograde cardioplegic solution. Alternatively, the aorta is not clamped and the entire procedure is done during hypothermic fibrillation. The left ventricular aneurysm is repaired using one of the techniques described below. The distal coronary anastomoses are performed, followed by releasing the aortic clamp.[151] Air is removed by venting the ascending aorta and left ventricle while filling the heart and ventilating the lungs with the patient in the Trendelenburg position. The patient is rewarmed, and proximal coronary anastomoses are performed. Once normothermia is achieved, an electrophysiologic study may be repeated, if indicated. Temporary pacing wires are placed on the right atrium and right ventricle, cardiopulmonary bypass is discontinued, and heparin is reversed. The heart is decannulated, and the median sternotomy is closed with mediastinal drains after hemostasis is achieved.

Weaning from cardiopulmonary bypass frequently requires some degree of inotropic support. Typically 5 μg/kg/min of dopamine, nitroglycerin to prevent coronary spasm, and nitroprusside for afterload reduction are used. An intra-aortic balloon pump may be needed in patients with borderline ventricular function. Transesophageal echocardiography is

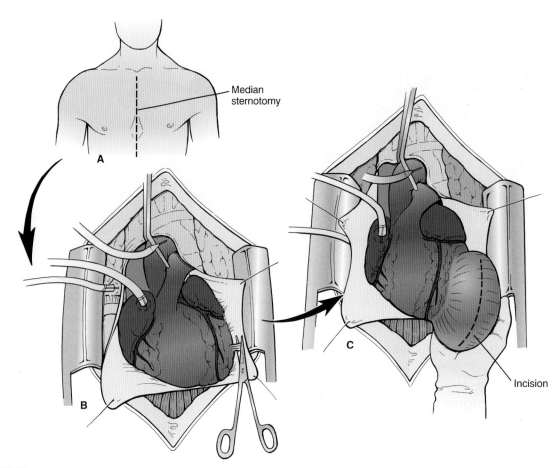

FIGURE 25-23 Technique of exposure for left ventricular aneurysm repair through a median sternotomy. The ascending aorta and right atrium are cannulated. A left ventricular vent is placed through the right superior pulmonary vein. Pericardial adhesions are divided, and the aneurysm is opened.

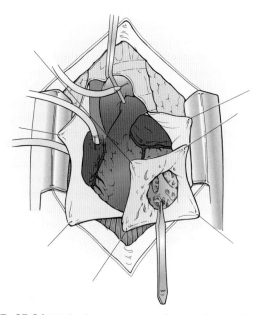

FIGURE 25-24 With the aneurysm wall opened, thrombus is removed, without injury to the papillary muscles.

useful for assessing left ventricular function and to detect residual intracardiac air.

Additional inotropic support may not increase cardiac output significantly because of abnormal ventricular compliance and may produce arrhythmias and poorly tolerated tachycardia. Hypokalemia and hypomagnesemia are corrected immediately to minimize arrhythmias. Intraoperative and postoperative ventricular ectopy is treated aggressively with intravenous lidocaine. Intravascular volume shifts are poorly tolerated in these patients because of poor ventricular compliance; therefore, rapid transfusions are avoided by meticulous hemostasis before closing. Because the left ventricle is poorly distensible, stroke volume is relatively fixed, and a resting heart rate between 90 and 115 beats per minute is not unusual to maintain a cardiac index of approximately 2.0 L/min/m².

Growing experience suggests that the ultimate size of the left ventricular cavity at the end of the procedure is critical to patient outcome.

PLICATION

Plication without opening the aneurysm is reserved for only the smallest aneurysms that do not contain mural thrombus.

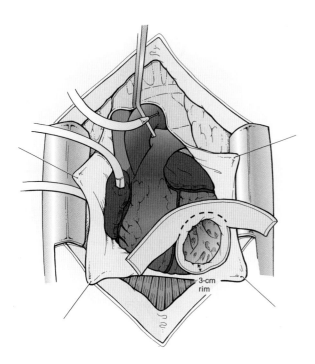

FIGURE 25-25 Linear repair. The fibrous aneurysm wall is excised, leaving a 3-cm rim of fibrous aneurysm wall attached to healthy muscle.

A two-layer suture line of 0 monofilament is placed across the aneurysm using a strip of Teflon felt on either side. The suture line is oriented to reconstruct a relatively normal left ventricular contour and does not exclude all aneurysmal tissue.

LINEAR CLOSURE

After removing all mural thrombus, the aneurysmal wall is trimmed, leaving a 3-cm rim of scar to allow reconstruction of the normal left ventricular contour (Fig. 25-25). Care is taken not to resect too much aneurysmal wall and overly reduce ventricular cavity size. A monofilament 2-0 suture may be used to reduce the neck of the aneurysm to the proper size before closure of the ventricular wall.[114] Anterior aneurysm defects are closed vertically between two external 1.5-cm strips of Teflon felt, two layers of 0 monofilament horizontal mattress sutures, and finally, two layers of running 2-0 monofilament vertical sutures with large-diameter needles (Fig. 25-26). Similar techniques can be used in less frequent posterior aneurysm resections.[152]

CIRCULAR PATCH

Inferior or posterior aneurysms generally require circular patch closure, which also can be applied to anterior aneurysms. After opening the aneurysm (Fig. 25-27) and after debridement of thrombus and aneurysm wall (Fig. 25-28), a Dacron patch is cut to be 2 cm greater in diameter than the ventricular opening. Interrupted, pledgeted 0 monofilament horizontal mattress sutures are placed through the

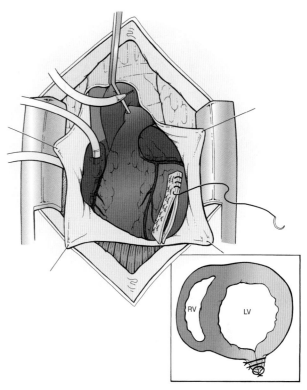

FIGURE 25-26 Linear repair. The aneurysm walls are closed in a vertical line between two layers of Teflon felt. Two layers of 0 monofilament interrupted horizontal mattress sutures are reinforced with two layers of running 2-0 monofilament sutures.

ventriculotomy rim and then through the patch, leaving the pledgets outside the ventricular cavity (Fig. 25-29). Sutures are tied, and additional interrupted sutures or a second layer of running 2-0 monofilament is placed for hemostasis.

ENDOVENTRICULAR PATCH

The endoventricular patch technique is suitable for anterior aneurysms but is less suited for inferior or posterior aneurysms,

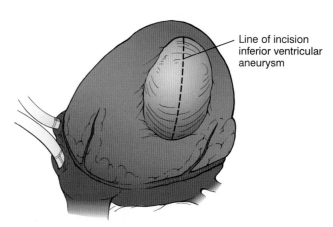

FIGURE 25-27 Circular patch repair. The aneurysm wall is incised. An inferior aneurysm is shown.

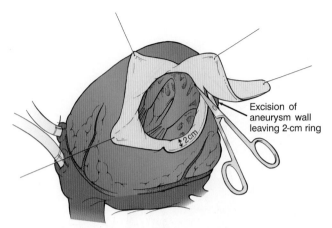

FIGURE 25-28 Circular patch repair. The aneurysmal wall is excised, leaving a 2-cm rim of fibrous aneurysmal wall attached to healthy muscle.

for which the standard (circular) patch technique is used. After debridement of thrombus, a running 2-0 polypropylene suture may be placed at the aneurysm rim to optimize left ventricular size.[4,17,50,55] Optimizing patch size and residual left ventricular cavity size can be facilitated with plastic or balloon forms (Chase Medical, Richardson, Texas) chosen to leave a left ventricular end-diastolic volume index of 50 to 60 mL/m.[100,147,153] If the remaining ventricular defect is small (<3 cm), then the ventricular wall may be closed linearly.[114] More commonly, a patch (bovine pericardium, Dacron cloth, or polytetrafluoroethylene) is cut to size sufficient to restore normal ventricular size and geometry when secured to the aneurysmal rim (Fig. 25-30). The patch is sutured to normal muscle at the aneurysmal circumference using a running 3-0 polypropylene suture that is secured with single sutures at three or four places around the patch circumference. The patch may extend onto the interventricular septum,[92,102,150] or aneurysmal septum may be plicated.[114] Interrupted 3-0

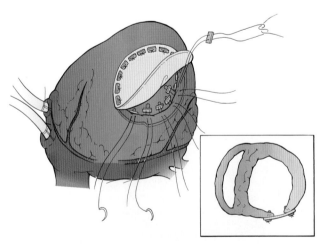

FIGURE 25-29 Circular patch repair. The aneurysmal defect is closed with a Dacron patch using interrupted 2-0 monofilament horizontal mattress sutures with reinforcing pledgets.

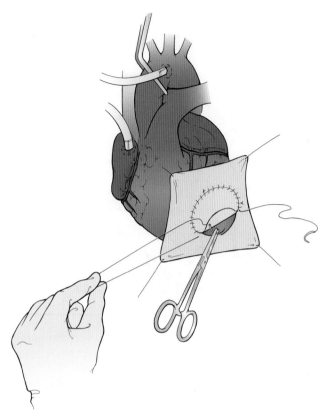

FIGURE 25-30 Endocardial patch. Without excising the aneurysm wall, the ventricular defect is closed with a Teflon felt patch using 3-0 polypropylene suture secured at three or four points along the suture line. Additional 3-0 pledgeted horizontal mattress sutures may be used to achieve hemostasis.

sutures are placed as needed to ensure good fit. Care is taken not to distort the papillary muscles. The aneurysmal rim is trimmed to allow primary closure of the native aneurysmal wall over the patch using two layers of running 2-0 monofilament suture without pledgets (Fig. 25-31).

Compared with linear and circular patch techniques, the endoventricular patch technique has technical advantages. An endoventricular patch preserves the left anterior descending artery for possible grafting and leaves no external prosthetic material to produce heavy pericardial adhesions. The technique facilitates patching the interventricular septum, and is suitable for acute infarctions when tissues are friable.[108,116,153,156]

OTHER VENTRICULAR REMODELING TECHNIQUES

In addition to the techniques listed above where left ventricular infarct tissue is excised and/or replaced with patch material, an alternative would be to alter the biological properties of the infarct scar. Remaining infarct scar (whether aneurysmal or not) can then be seeded with myoblasts or stem cells which offer the potential to restore cardiac muscle mass and contraction. This technique has been termed *cellular cardiomyoplasty*

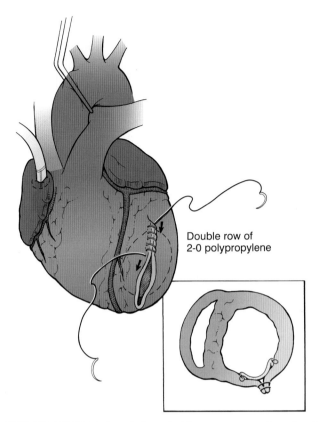

FIGURE 25-31 Endocardial patch. The aneurysm wall is closed over a Teflon patch after resecting excess aneurysm tissue. A double row of running vertical 2-0 polypropylene suture is used.

Double row of
2-0 polypropylene

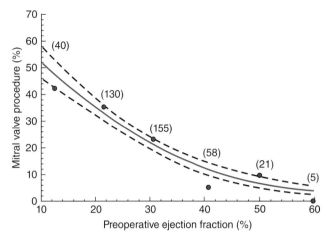

FIGURE 25-32 Prevalence of performing concomitant mitral valve procedures as a function of preoperative ejection fraction. (Reproduced with permission from Athanasuleas CL, Stanley AWHJr, Buckberg GD, et al: Surgical anterior ventricular endocardial restoration [SAVER] in the dilated remodeled ventricle after anterior myocardial infarction, *J Am Coll Cardiol.* 2001 Apr;37(5):1199-1209.)

and has been done only on a limited basis in humans.[157] In animals, cellular cardiomyoplasty has successfully improved global left ventricular performance and geometry using either myoblasts, stem cells that differentiate into myocytes, fibrocytes, or cells seeded onto a graft matrix.[158-160] Cellular cardiomyoplasty could be done by direct injection of cells at the time of coronary revascularization, or even by transcoronary or intramyocardial injection in the cardiac catheterization laboratory. Percutaneous insertion of parachute-like device into the left ventricular apex has had some early success in humans with improvement in left ventricular end-diastolic volumes and heart failure symptoms.[161,162]

CORONARY REVASCULARIZATION

Concurrent coronary revascularization is performed as in standard coronary bypass procedures. Because the endoventricular patch technique does not encroach on the left anterior descending coronary, the left internal mammary artery may be used to graft the left anterior descending coronary artery.

MITRAL REGURGITATION

The severity of mitral regurgitation should be evaluated before cardiopulmonary bypass by intraoperative transesophageal echocardiography. The need for concurrent mitral

valve operation increases as the preoperative ejection fraction decreases (Fig. 25-32).[163] The mitral valve is also inspected from below after opening the aneurysm and beginning repair of the aneurysm. Transventricular mitral valve repair may be done by placing pledgeted polypropylene sutures at both mitral commissures to reduce the circumference of the annulus.[152] This technique produces satisfactory short-term results, but long-term results are not known. Usually the mitral valve is repaired via left atriotomy after completion of the distal coronary anastomoses and before releasing the aortic crossclamp. If mitral regurgitation results from annular dilatation and systolic restriction of leaflet motion (Carpentier type IIIB), an undersized, complete, rigid mitral annuloplasty is generally done.[164]

CARDIAC TRANSPLANTATION

In symptomatic patients with sufficient depression of global left ventricular function to preclude aneurysm repair, transplantation is a reasonable alternative and may have survival and symptomatic benefit similar to ventricular aneurysm repair at a higher dollar cost.[165]

VENTRICULAR FALSE ANEURYSM

Ventricular free wall false aneurysms are repaired with the same techniques used for true ventricular aneurysms based according to the location and size of the aneurysm.[72,73,80] The circular patch technique is particularly useful in that inferior false aneurysms are common and typically have narrow necks. Usually the wall of the false aneurysm is inadequate to close over the defect. False aneurysms resulting from atrioventricular separation after mitral valve replacement generally require removal of the mitral prosthesis, repair of the neck of the aneurysm at the mitral annulus, and re-replacement of the mitral valve.[70] False aneurysms of the left ventricular apex after transapical aortic valve replacement may be directly repaired small but may require patching if large.[166]

Early Results

HOSPITAL MORTALITY

In a compilation of 3439 operations for left ventricular aneurysm between 1972 and 1987[118] and in a series of 731 ventricular restoration patients from 2002 to 2004,[167] hospital mortality was 9.9 and 9.3%, respectively, and ranged from 2 to 19%. More recent reports suggest that hospital mortality can be as low as 3 to 7% using either patch[108,116,163168,169] or linear closures.[119,149,169] The most common cause of hospital mortality is left ventricular failure, which occurs in 64% of deaths.[149]

Risk factors for hospital mortality include increased age,[118,149,163,167,169] incomplete revascularization,[149] increased heart failure class,[118,167,169-171] female gender,[118,167] emergent operation,[118] ejection fraction less than 20 to 30%,[163,169,170] concurrent mitral valve replacement,[108,118,163,167] preoperative cardiac index < 2.1 L/min/m[100,103,167] mean pulmonary artery pressure > 33 mm Hg,[103] serum creatinine > 1.8 mg/dl,[103] and failure to use the internal mammary artery.[171]

IN-HOSPITAL COMPLICATIONS

The most common in-hospital complications are shown in Table 25-4 and include low cardiac output, ventricular arrhythmias, and respiratory failure.[118,119,167-169,172] Low cardiac output may be more common in patients undergoing intraoperative mapping because of perioperative cardiac injury.[173]

LEFT VENTRICULAR FUNCTION

The preponderance of data from the last two decades have shown that left ventricular function improves in most patients undergoing operation for left ventricular aneurysm. Operation improves ejection fraction whether linear repair[104,104,174-176] or patch repair[116,163,177-181] is used (Fig. 25-33).[176] In a propensity matched series, little difference in outcome was seen between linear versus patch repair.[182] Both techniques decrease end-diastolic and end-systolic volumes[163,175,178,180] and improve exercise response[116,176] (Fig. 25-34).[176] Aneurysmal repair in general may improve diastolic filling, left ventricular diastolic compliance, left ventricular contractility, effective arterial

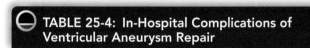

⊖ TABLE 25-4: In-Hospital Complications of Ventricular Aneurysm Repair

Low cardiac output 22-39%
Ventricular arrhythmias 9-19%
Respiratory failure 4-21%
Bleeding 4-7%
Dialysis-dependent renal failure 4%
Stroke 3-4%

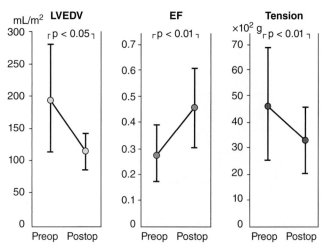

FIGURE 25-33 Effects of linear aneurysmectomy on left ventricular end-diastolic volume (LVEDV), ejection fraction (EF), and wall tension. (Reproduced with permission from Kawachi K, Kitamura S, Kawata T, et al: Hemodynamic assessment during exercise after left ventricular aneurysmectomy, *J Thorac Cardiovasc Surg*. 1994 Jan;107(1):178-183.)

elastance (Ea), and left ventricular efficiency.[134,179,180,183,184] However, recent studies have suggested little improvement or even worsening of left ventricular diastolic compliance, particularly in patients with large resections or small ventricular size or without large dyskinetic aneurysms preoperatively.[185]

Controversy remains strong regarding whether patch techniques provide results superior to those achieved with linear closures. Stoney et al[112,186] noted lower left ventricular end-diastolic pressure when more geometric reconstructions were performed. Hutchins and Brawley[187] first

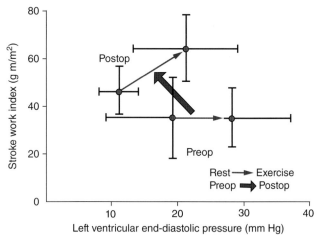

FIGURE 25-34 Relationship between stroke work index and left ventricular end-diastolic pressure. Data are shown at rest and during exercise before (preop) and after (postop) linear aneurysmectomy. Stroke work index increased only with exercise postoperatively. (Reproduced with permission from Kawachi K, Kitamura S, Kawata T, et al: Hemodynamic assessment during exercise after left ventricular aneurysmectomy, *J Thorac Cardiovasc Surg*. 1994 Jan;107(1):178-183.)

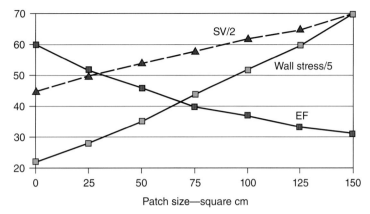

FIGURE 25-35 Computer prediction of the effects of patch size on stroke volume (SV), ejection fraction (EF), and wall stress (afterload) at a chamber pressure of 100 mm Hg. Predictions are based on data from an animal model of simulated aneurysm repair, neglecting the effects of afterload on stroke volume. Because increasing afterload in reality decreases muscle shortening, patch reconstruction can increase stroke volume only if contractile reserve is sufficient to overcome the afterload from increased ventricular size. (Data from Nicolosi AC, Weng ZC, Detwiler PW, et al: Simulated left ventricular aneurysm and aneurysm repair in swine, *J Thorac Cardiovasc Surg*. 1990 Nov;100(5):745-755.)

noted at autopsy that some patients had severe reduction and distortion of ventricular volume after linear repair. The authors proposed that a more geometric repair might avert these problems. Although no prospective studies compare results from the two procedures, several very experienced groups attribute improved symptoms, less low cardiac output, and greater improvement in ejection fraction to a switch to patch techniques.[108,116,188] In other retrospective comparisons, no differences were seen in postoperative symptoms, ejection fraction, echocardiographic ventricular dimensions, or late survival between linear and patch repairs.[175,188-191] In an animal model of simulated aneurysm repair, Nicolosi et al[185] found no difference in left ventricular systolic or diastolic function between linear and patch techniques. Two groups reported that switch to patch techniques was associated with increased operative mortality, perhaps because of excessive volume reduction,[192,193] whereas other groups found improved survival when switching from linear to patch techniques.[194] One meta-analysis has suggested that the better results with patch techniques are the result of more experience in more recent series.[188]

The durability of functional benefit from aneurysm repair remains poorly documented. In animals and humans, there is a tendency for the initial improvement in ejection fraction, ventricular volume, and filling pressures to diminish over the next 6 weeks to 12 months,[195,196] especially in patients with residual mitral regurgitation.

Although technical differences exist between patch and linear repairs, good functional results are possible with either technique. Suboptimal outcomes result from either technique when left ventricular cavitary volume is overly reduced with resultant decreased stroke volume and impaired diastolic filling.[187] Excessively small patches reduce stroke volume and impair diastolic filling, but excessively large patches reduce ejection fraction and increase wall stress (Fig. 25-35).[185]

Late Results

SURVIVAL

Survival after operation for left ventricular aneurysm is variable, largely because of differences between patient populations. Five-year survival in recent series varies between 58 and 80%,[104,170] 10-year overall survival is 34%,[170] and 10-year cardiac survival is 57%[149] (Fig. 25-36).[105,170] Cardiac causes are responsible for 57% of late deaths,[173] and most cardiac deaths result from new myocardial infarctions. In aneurysm patients randomized to medical or surgical therapy in the CASS study (most of the patients had minimal symptoms), survival was not different between medical or surgical therapy, except for patients with three-vessel disease.[144] These patients had better survival with surgery (Fig. 25-37).[144]

Preoperative risk factors for late death include age, heart failure score, ejection fraction less than 35%, cardiomegaly on chest radiograph, left ventricular end-diastolic pressure greater than 20 mm Hg, and mitral regurgitation[144,149,163,173] (Figs. 25-38, and 25-39).

The prospective, randomized STICH trial of 1000 patients with ejection fraction of 35% or less and anatomy amenable to ventricular restoration showed that, on average, left ventricular restoration techniques did not affect survival relative to coronary bypass grafting alone (Fig. 25-40).[105] However, post hoc analysis of STICH data showed that, in patients achieving postoperative left ventricular end-systolic volume index (LVESVI) of less than 70 mL/m^2, the addition of SVR to coronary bypass improved survival, while the opposite was true for patients achieving LVESVI > 70 mL/m^2.[196] The results of the STICH trial probably resulted from inclusion of relatively few patients with large, classical, dyskinetic aneurysms (mean reduction of end-systolic volume index of 16 mL/m^2 versus 48 mL/m^2 seen in classical aneurysms).[105,106] Although unproven, the net sum of evidence suggests that patients with large, classical, dyskinetic aneurysms who achieve a postoperative LVESVI

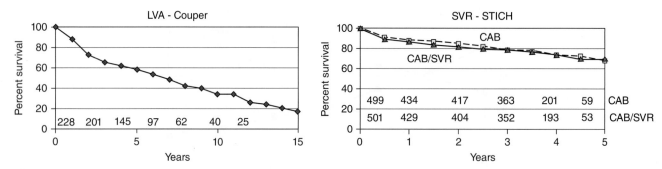

FIGURE 25-36 Survival in 303 patients undergoing left ventricular aneurysmectomy (LVA) (left panel). Survival in 1000 patients randomized to coronary bypass (CAB) or CAB and ventricular restoration (SVR) (*right panel*). (Data from Couper GS, Bunton RW, Birjiniuk V, et al: Relative risks of left ventricular aneurysmectomy in patients with akinetic scars versus true dyskinetic aneurysms, *Circulation.* 1990 Nov;82(5 Suppl):IV248-IV256.)

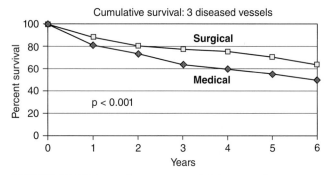

FIGURE 25-37 Survival in patients with left ventricular aneurysm and three-vessel coronary disease treated with medical or surgical therapy. (Data from Faxon DP, Myers WO, McCabe CH: The influence of surgery on the natural history of angiographically documented left ventricular aneurysm: the Coronary Artery Surgery Study, *Circulation.* 1986 Jul;74(1):110-118.)

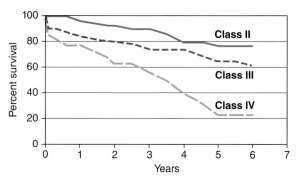

FIGURE 25-38 Effects of preoperative NYHA functional class on survival after ventricular aneurysm repair and myocardial revascularization. (Data from Vauthy JN, Berry DW, Snyder DW, et al: Left ventricular aneurysm repair with myocardial revascularization: an analysis of 246 consecutive patients over 15 years, *Ann Thorac Surg.* 1988 Jul;46(1):29-35.)

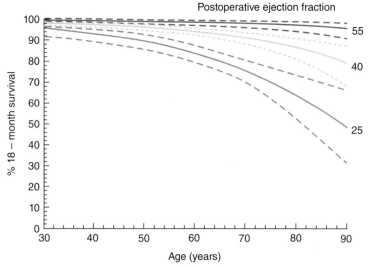

FIGURE 25-39 Nomogram of 18-month survival after ventricular restoration as a function of patient age and postoperative ejection fraction. (Reproduced with permission from Athanasuleas CL, Stanley AWHJr, Buckberg GD, et al: Surgical anterior ventricular endocardial restoration [SAVER] in the dilated remodeled ventricle after anterior myocardial infarction, *J Am Coll Cardiol.* 2001 Apr;37(5):1199-1209.)

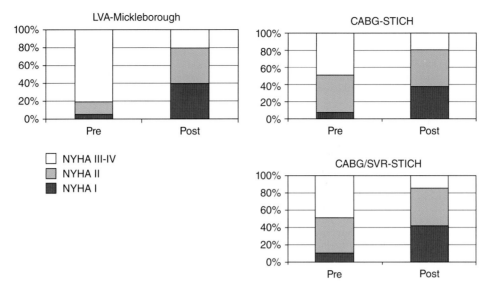

FIGURE 25-40 Preoperative (PRE) and latest follow-up (POST) symptoms of congestive heart failure (NYHA class) in patients undergoing coronary bypass alone (CABG) or CABG plus ventricular restoration (CABG/SVR) in the randomized STICH trial (*p* = 0.7 CABG versus CABG/SVR) (Data from Jones RH, Velazquez EJ, Michler RE, et al: Coronary bypass surgery with or without surgical ventricular restoration, *N Engl J Med*. 2009 Apr 23;360(17):1705-1717.)

< 70 mL/m² probably obtain more benefit from aneurysm repair than do patients with diffuse ventricular dysfunction or small akinetic segments.[106,197,198]

SYMPTOMATIC IMPROVEMENT

Studies consistently demonstrate improvement in symptoms after operation relative to preoperative symptoms[104,105,174] (Fig. 25-40). In the study of Elefteriades et al,[174] using a linear repair, mean angina class improved from 3.5 to 1.2 and mean CHF class improved from 3.0 to 1.7. In the randomized CASS study, the subset of patients with left ventricular aneurysm achieved a better heart failure class with surgical therapy than with medicine, and rehospitalization for heart failure was less common for the surgical therapy group than for the medicine group.[144] At 18 months, 85% of patients are free of rehospitalization for congestive heart failure, with rehospitalization peaking at 2 to 4 months.[163] Prucz found in a small, nonrandomized case-control study that ventricular restoration reduced hospitalization rate relative to coronary bypass alone.[199] However, the STICH trial found no benefit on average in symptoms or quality of life relative to coronary bypass alone.[105,200] (Fig 25-24) The STICH trial found that ventricular restoration significantly increased hospital cost by $14,500 or 26%.[200]

REFERENCES

1. Latham PM: *Lectures on Subjects Connected with Clinical Medicine Comprising Diseases of the Heart*. London, Longman Rees, 1845.
2. Brunn F: Diagnostik der erworbenen ruptur der kammerscheidewand des herzens. *Wien Arch Inn Med* 1923; 6:533.
3. Sager R: Coronary thrombosis: perforation of the infarcted interventricular septum. *Arch Intern Med* 1934; 53:140.
4. Cooley DA, Belmonte BA, Zeis LB, Schnur S: Surgical repair of ruptured interventricular septum following acute myocardial infarction. *Surgery* 1957; 41:930.
5. Payne WS, Hunt JC, Kirklin JW: Surgical repair of ventricular septal defect due to myocardial infarction: report of a case. *JAMA* 1963; 183:603.
6. Heimbecker RO, Lemire G, Chen C: Surgery for massive myocardial infarction. *Circulation* 1968; 11(Suppl 2):37.
7. David H, Hunter JA, Najafi H, et al: Left ventricular approach for the repair of ventricular septal perforation and infarctectomy. *J Thorac Cardiovasc Surg* 1972; 63:14.
8. Daggett WM, Burwell LR, Lawson DW, Austen WG: Resection of acute ventricular aneurysm and ruptured interventricular septum after myocardial infarction. *N Engl J Med* 1970; 283:1507.
9. Daggett WM, Buckley MJ, Akins CW, et al: Improved results of surgical management of postinfarction ventricular septal rupture. *Ann Surg* 1982; 196:269.
10. Daggett WM, Mundth ED, Gold HK, et al: Early repair of ventricular septal defects complicating inferior myocardial infarction. *Circulation* 1974; 50(Suppl 3):112.
11. Daggett WM: Surgical technique for early repair of posterior ventricular septal rupture. *J Thorac Cardiovasc Surg* 1982; 84:306.
12. David TE, Dale L, Sun Z: Postinfarction ventricular septal rupture: repair by endocardial patch with infarct exclusion. *J Thorac Cardiovasc Surg* 1995; 110:1315.
13. Calvert PA, Cockburn J, Wynne D, et al: Percutaneous closure of postinfarction ventricular septal defect: in-hospital outcomes and long-term follow-up of UK experience. *Circulation* 2014; 129:2395.
14. Samuels L, Entwistle J, Holmes E, et al: Mechanical support of the unrepaired postinfarction ventricular septal defect with the Abiomed BVS 5000 ventricular assist device. *J Thorac Cardiovasc Surg* 2003; 126:2100.
15. Hutchins GM: Rupture of the interventricular septum complicating myocardial infarction: pathological analysis of 10 patients with clinically diagnosed perforation. *Am Heart J* 1979; 97:165.
16. Selzer A, Gerbode F, Keith WJ: Clinical, hemodynamic and surgical considerations of rupture of the ventricular septum after myocardial infarction. *Am Heart J* 1969; 78:598.
17. Mann JM, Robert WC: Acquired ventricular septal defect during acute myocardial infarction: analysis of 38 unoperated necropsy patients and comparison with 50 unoperated necropsy patients without rupture. *Am J Cardiol* 1988; 62:8.

18. Morillon-Lutun S, Maucort-Boulch D, Mewton N, et al: Therapeutic management changes and mortality rates over 30 years in ventricular septal rupture complicating acute myocardial infarction. *Am J Cardiol* 2013; 112:1273.

19. Crenshaw BS, Granger CB, Birnbaum Y, et al: Risk factors, angiographic patterns, and outcomes in patients with ventricular septal defect complicating acute myocardial infarction. GUSTO-I Trial Investigators. *Circulation* 2000; 101:27.

20. Yam N, Au TW, Cheng LC: Post-infarction ventricular septal defect: surgical outcomes in the last decade. *Asian Cardiovasc Thorac Ann* 2013; 21:539.

21. Cummings RG, Reimer KA, Califf R, et al: Quantitative analysis of right and left ventricular infarction in the presence of postinfarction ventricular septal defect. *Circulation* 1988; 77:33.

22. Pfeffer MA, Braunwald E: Ventricular remodeling after myocardial infarction: clinical observations and clinical implications. *Circulation* 1990; 81:1161.

23. Miller S, Dinsmore RE, Grenne RE, Daggett WM: Coronary, ventricular, and pulmonary abnormalities associated with rupture of the interventricular septum complicating myocardial infarction. *Am J Radiol* 1978; 131:571.

24. Berger TJ, Blackstone EH, Kirklin JW: Postinfarction ventricular septal defect, in Kirklin JW, Barratt-Boyes BG (eds): *Cardiac Surgery* New York, Churchill Livingstone, 1993; p 403.

25. Smyllie JH, Sutherland GR, Geuskens R, et al: Doppler color flow mapping in the diagnosis of ventricular septal rupture and acute mitral regurgitation after myocardial infarction. *J Am Coll Cardiol* 1990; 15:1455.

26. Gaudiani VA, Miller DC, Oyer PE, et al: Post-infarction ventricular septal defect: an argument for early operation. *Surgery* 1981; 89:48.

27. Agnihotri AK, Madsen JC, Daggett WM Jr: Surgical treatment of complications of acute myocardial infarction: Postinfarction ventricular septal defect and free wall rupture, in Cohn LH (ed.): *Cardiac Surgery in the Adult*, 4th ed. New York, McGraw-Hill, 2012; p 603.

28. Gold HK, Leinbach RC, Sanders CA, et al: Intra-aortic balloon pumping for ventricular septal defect or mitral regurgitation complicating acute myocardial infarction. *Circulation* 1973; 47:1191.

29. Gregoric ID, Kar B, Mesar T, et al: Perioperative use of TandemHeart percutaneous ventricular assist device in surgical repair of postinfarction ventricular septal defect. *ASAIO J* 2014; 60:529.

30. Heitmiller R, Jacobs ML, Daggett WM: Surgical management of postinfarction ventricular septal rupture. *Ann Thorac Surg* 1986; 41:683.

31. Loisance DP, Lordez JM, Deleuze PH, et al: Acute postinfarction septal rupture: long-term results. *Ann Thorac Surg* 1991; 52:474.

32. Seguin JR, Frapier JM, Colson P, Chaptal PA: Fibrin sealant for early repair of acquired ventricular septal defect. *J Thorac Cardiovasc Surg* 1992; 104:748.

33. Shumacker H: Suggestions concerning operative management of postinfarction ventricular septal defects. *J Thorac Cardiovasc Surg* 1972; 64:452.

34. Guyton SW, Daggett WM: Surgical repair of post-infarction ventricular septal rupture, chap. installment 9, in Cohn LH (ed.): *Modern Techniques in Surgery: Cardiac/Thoracic Surgery* Mt. Kisco, Futura, 1983; p 61.

35. Hill JD, Lary D, Keith WJ, Gerbode F: Acquired ventricular septal defects: evolution of an operation, surgical technique and results. *J Thorac Cardiovasc Surg* 1975; 70:440.

36. Dor V, Saab M, Coste P, et al: Left ventricular aneurysm: a new surgical approach. *Thorac Cardiovasc Surg* 1989; 37:11.

37. Cooley DA: Repair of postinfarction ventricular septal defect. *J Card Surg* 1994; 9:427.

38. Alvarez JM, Brady PW, Ross DE: Technical improvements in the repair of acute postinfarction ventricular septal rupture. *J Card Surg* 1992; 7:198.

39. David TE, Armstrong S: Surgical repair of postinfarction ventricular septal defect by infarct exclusion. *Semin Thorac Cardiovasc Surg* 1998; 10:105.

40. Cooley DA: Postinfarction ventricular septal rupture. *Semin Thorac Cardiovasc Surg* 1998; 10:100.

41. Tashiro T, Todo K, Haruta Y, et al: Extended endocardial repair of postinfarction ventricular septal rupture: new operative technique modification of the Komeda-David operation. *J Card Surg* 1994; 9:97.

42. Usui A, Murase M, Maeda M, et al: Sandwich repair with two sheets of equine pericardial patch for acute posterior post-infarction ventricular septal defect. *Eur J Cardiothoracic Surg* 1993; 7:47.

43. Imagawa H, Takano S, Shiozaki T, et al: Two-patch technique for postinfarction inferoposterior ventricular septal defect. *Ann Thorac Surg* 2009; 88:692-694.

44. Asai T, Hosoba S, Suzuki T, et al: Postinfarction ventricular septal defect: right ventricular approach-the extended "sandwich" patch. *Semin Thorac Cardiovasc Surg* 2012; 24:59.

45. Szkutnik M, Bialkowski J, Kusa J, et al: Postinfarction ventricular septal defect closure with Amplatzer occluders. *Eur J Cardiothorac Surg* 2003; 23:323.

46. Thiele H, Kaulfersch C, Daehnert I, et al: Immediate primary transcatheter closure of postinfarction ventricular septal defects. *Eur Heart J* 2009; 30:81-89.

47. Calvert PA, Cockburn J, Wynne D, et al: Percutaneous closure of postinfarction ventricular septal defect: in-hospital outcomes and long-term follow-up of UK experience. *Circulation* 2014; 129:2395.

48. Landzberg MJ, Lock JE: Transcatheter management of ventricular septal rupture after myocardial infarction. *Semin Thorac Cardiovasc Surg* 1998; 10:128.

49. Thiele H, Kaulfersch C, Daehnert I, et al: Immediate primary transcatheter closure of postinfarction ventricular septal defects. *Eur Heart J* 2009; 30(1):81-88.

50. Lee MS, Kozitza R, Mudrick D, et al: Intraoperative device closure of postinfarction ventricular septal defects. *Ann Thorac Surg* 2010; 89:e48.

51. Maree A, Jneid H, Palacios I: Percutaneous closure of a postinfarction ventricular septal defect that recurred after surgical repair. *Eur Heart J* 2006; 27:1626.

52. Jeppsson A, Liden H, Johnson P, et al: Surgical repair of post infarction ventricular septal defects: a national experience. *Eur J Cardiothorac Surg* 2005; 27:216.

53. Deja MA, Szostek J, Widenka K, et al: Post infarction ventricular septal defect—can we do better? *Eur J Cardiothorac Surg* 2000; 18:194.

54. Dalrymple-Hay MJR, Monro JL, Livesey SA, Lamb RK: Postinfarction ventricular septal rupture: the Wessex experience. *Semin Thorac Cardiovasc Surg* 1998; 10:111.

55. Yam N, Au TW, Cheng LC: Post-infarction ventricular septal defect: surgical outcomes in the last decade. *Asian Cardiovasc Thorac Ann* 2013; 21:539.

56. Skillington PD, Davies RH, Luff AJ, et al: Surgical treatment for infarct-related ventricular septal defects. *J Thorac Cardiovasc Surg* 1990; 99:798.

57. Rousou JA, Engelman RM, Breyer RH, et al: Transatrial repair of postinfarction posterior ventricular septal defect. *Ann Thorac Surg* 1987; 43:665.

58. Filgueira JL, Battistessa SA, Estable H, et al: Delayed repair of an acquired posterior septal defect through a right atrial approach. *Ann Thorac Surg* 1986; 42:208.

59. Willius FA, Dry TJ: *A History of the Heart and Circulation*. Philadelphia, WB Saunders, 1948.

60. Morgagni JB: *The Seat and Causes of Disease Investigated by Anatomy*. London, A. Millau & T. Cadell, 1769; p 811.

61. Hatcher CR Jr, Mansour K, Logan WD Jr, et al: Surgical complications of myocardial infarction. *Am Surg* 1970; 36:163.

62. FitzGibbon GM, Hooper GD, Heggtveit HA: Successful surgical treatment of postinfarction external cardiac rupture. *J Thorac Cardiovasc Surg* 1972; 63:622.

63. Montegut FJ Jr: Left ventricular rupture secondary to myocardial infarction. *Ann Thorac Surg* 1972; 14:75.

64. Oliva PB, Hammill SC, Edwards WD: Cardiac rupture, a clinically predictable complication of acute myocardial infarction: report of 70 cases with clinicopathologic correlations. *J Am Coll Cardiol* 1993; 22:720.

65. Hutchins KD, Skurnick J, Lavendar M, et al: Cardiac rupture in acute myocardial infarction: a reassessment. *Am J Forensic Med Pathol* 2002; 23:78.

66. Herlitz J, Samuelsson SO, Richter A, Hjalmarson Å: Prediction of rupture in acute myocardial infarction. *Clin Cardiol* 1988; 11:63.

67. Batts KP, Ackermann DM, Edwards WD: Post-infarction rupture of the left ventricular free wall: clinicopathologic correlates in 100 consecutive autopsy cases. *Hum Pathol* 1990; 21:530.

68. Becker RC, Charlesworth A, Wilcox RG, et al: Cardiac rupture associated with thrombolytic therapy: impact of time to treatment in the Late Assessment of Thrombolytic Efficacy (LATE) study. *J Am Coll Cardiol* 1995; 25:1063.

69. Nozoe M, Sakamoto T, Taguchi E, et al: Clinical manifestation of early phase left ventricular rupture complicating acute myocardial infarction in the primary PCI era. *J Cardiol* 2014; 63:14.

70. Lee ME, Tamboli M, Lee AW: Use of a sandwich technique to repair a left ventricular rupture after mitral valve replacement. *Tex Heart Inst J* 2014; 41:195.

71. Pasic M, Buz S, Drews T, et al: Bleeding from the apex during transapical transcatheter aortic valve implantation: a simple solution by balloon occlusion of the apex. *Interact Cardiovasc Thorac Surg* 2014; 19:306.

72. Komeda M, David TE: Surgical treatment of postinfarction false aneurysm of the left ventricle. *J Thorac Cardiovasc Surg* 1993; 106:1189.

73. Mascarenhas DAN, Benotti JR, Daggett WM, et al: Postinfarction septal aneurysm with delayed formation of left-to-right shunt. *Am Heart J* 1991; 122:226.

74. Frances C, Romero A, Grady D: Left ventricular pseudoaneurysm. *J Am Coll Cardiol* 1998; 32:557.

75. Schuster EH, Bulkley BH: Expansion of transmural myocardial infarction: a pathophysiologic factor in cardiac rupture. *Circulation* 1979; 60:1532.

76. Hutchins GM, Bulkley BH: Infarct expansion versus extension: two different complications of acute myocardial infarction. *Am J Cardiol* 1978; 41:1127.

77. Christensen DJ, Ford M, Reading J, Castle CH: Effects of hypertension in myocardial rupture after acute myocardial infarction. *Chest* 1977; 72:618.

78. Honan MB, Harrell FE, Reimer KA, et al: Cardiac rupture, mortality and timing of thrombolytic therapy: a meta-analysis. *J Am Coll Cardiol* 1990; 16:359.

79. Westaby S, Parry A, Ormerod O, et al: Thrombolysis and postinfarction ventricular septal rupture. *J Thorac Cardiovasc Surg* 1992; 104:1506.

80. David TE: Surgery for postinfarction rupture of the free wall of the ventricle, in David TE (ed.): *Mechanical Complications of Myocardial Infarction.* Austin, TX, RG Landes, 1993; p 142.

81. Pollack H, Diez W, Spiel R, et al: Early diagnosis of subacute free wall rupture complicating acute myocardial infarction. *Eur Heart J* 1993; 14:640.

82. Feneley MP, Chang VP, O'Rourke MF: Myocardial rupture after acute myocardial infarction: ten year review. *Br Heart J* 1983; 49:550.

83. Dellborg M, Held P, Swedberg K, Vedin A: Rupture of the myocardium: occurrence and risk factors. *Br Heart J* 1985; 54:11.

84. Núñez L, de la Llana R, López Sendón J, et al: Diagnosis and treatment of subacute free wall ventricular rupture after infarction. *Ann Thorac Surg* 1982; 35:525.

85. Harper RW, Sloman G, Westlake G: Successful surgical resection of a chronic false aneurysm of the left ventricle. *Chest* 1975; 67:359.

86. Epstein JI, Hutchins GM: Subepicardial aneurysms: a rare complication of myocardial infarction. *Am J Cardiol* 1983; 75:639.

87. López-Sendón J, González A, López De Sá E, et al: Diagnosis of subacute ventricular wall rupture after acute myocardial infarction: sensitivity and specificity of clinical, hemodynamic and echocardiographic criteria. *J Am Coll Cardiol* 1992; 19:1145.

88. Padró JM, Mesa J, Silvestre J, et al: Subacute cardiac rupture: repair with a sutureless technique. *Ann Thorac Surg* 1993; 55:20.

89. Yeo TC, Malouf JF, Reeder GS, et al: Clinical characteristics and outcome in postinfarction pseudoaneurysm. *Am J Cardiol* 1999; 84:592.

90. Pretre R, Linka A, Jenni R, et al: Surgical treatment of acquired left ventricular pseudoaneurysms. *Ann Thorac Surg* 2000; 70:553.

91. Vlodaver Z, Coe JE, Edwards JE: True and false left ventricular aneurysm: propensity for the latter to rupture. *Circulation* 1975; 51:567.

92. Alapati L, Chitwood WR, Cahill J, et al: Left ventricular pseudoaneurysm: A case report and review of the literature. *World J Clin Cases* 2914; 16:90.

93. Kyo S, Ogiwara M, Miyamoto N, et al: Percutaneous intrapericardial fibrin-glue infusion therapy for rupture of the left ventricle free wall following acute myocardial infarction. *J Am Coll Cardiol* 1996; 27:327A.

94. Willecke F, Bode C, Zirlik A: Successful therapy of ventricular rupture by percutaneous intrapericardial instillation of fibrin glue: a case report. *Case Rep Vasc Med* 2013; Epub 2013 Jun 27.

95. Levett JM, Southgate TJ, Jose AB, et al: Technique for repair of left ventricular free wall rupture. *Ann Thorac Surg* 1988; 46:248.

96. Sasaki K, Fukui T, Tabata M, et al: Early pseudoaneurysm formation after the sutureless technique for left ventricular rupture due to acute myocardial infarction. *Gen Thorac Cardiovasc Surg* 2014; 62:171.

97. Pappas PJ, Cernaianu AC, Baldino WA, et al: Ventricular free-wall rupture after myocardial infarction: treatment and outcome. *Chest* 1991; 4:892.

98. Lachapelle K, deVarennes B, Ergina PL: Sutureless patch technique for postinfarction left ventricular rupture. *Ann Thorac Surg* 2002; 74:96.

99. Rutherford JD, Braunwald E, Cohn PE: Chronic ischemic heart disease, in Braunwald E (ed.): *Heart Disease: A Textbook of Cardiovascular Medicine.* Philadelphia, Saunders, 1988; p 1364.

100. Grondin P, Kretz JG, Bical O, et al: Natural history of saccular aneurysm of the left ventricle. *J Thorac Cardiovasc Surg* 1979; 77:57.

101. Buckberg GD: Defining the relationship between akinesia and dyskinesia and the cause of left ventricular failure after anterior infarction and reversal of remodeling to restoration. *J Thorac Cardiovasc Surg* 1998; 116:47.

102. Dor V, Sabatier M, DiDonato M: Efficacy of endoventricular patch plasty in large postinfarction akinetic scar and severe left ventricular dysfunction: comparison with a series of large dyskinetic scars. *J Thorac Cardiovasc Surg* 1998; 116:50.

103. DiDonato M, Sabatier M, Dor V, et al: Akinetic versus dyskinetic postinfarction scar: relation to surgical outcome in patients undergoing endoventricular circular patch plasty repair. *J Am Coll Cardiol* 1997; 29:1569.

104. Mickleborough LL, Carson S, Ivanov J: Repair of dyskinetic or akinetic left ventricular aneurysm: results obtained with a modified linear closure. *J Thorac Cardiovasc Surg* 2001; 121:675.

105. Jones RH, Velazquez EJ, Michler RE, et al: Coronary bypass surgery with or without surgical ventricular restoration. *N Engl J Med* 2009; 360:1705.

106. DiDonato M, Castelvecchio S, Kukulski T, et al: Surgical ventricular restoration: left ventricular shape influence on cardiac function, clinical status, and survival. *Ann Thorac Surg* 2009; 87:455.

107. Cox JL: Left ventricular aneurysms: pathophysiologic observations and standard resection. *Sem Thorac Cardiovasc Surg* 1997; 9:113.

108. Mills NL, Everson CT, Hockmuth DR: Technical advances in the treatment of left ventricular aneurysm. *Ann Thorac Surg* 1993; 55:792.

109. Beck CS: Operation for aneurysm of the heart. *Ann Surg* 1944; 120:34.

110. Likoff W, Bailey CP: Ventriculoplasty: excision of myocardial aneurysm. *JAMA* 1955; 158:915.

111. Cooley DA, Collins HA, Morris GC, et al: Ventricular aneurysm after myocardial infarction: surgical excision with use of temporary cardiopulmonary bypass. *JAMA* 1958; 167:557.

112. Stoney WS, Alford WC Jr, Burrus GR, et al: Repair of anteroseptal ventricular aneurysm. *Ann Thorac Surg* 1973; 15:394.

113. Daggett WM, Guyton RA, Mundth ED: Surgery for post-myocardial infarct ventricular septal defect. *Ann Surg* 1977; 86:260.

114. Jatene AD: Left ventricular aneurysmectomy: resection of reconstruction. *J Thorac Cardiovasc Surg* 1985; 89:321.

115. Cooley DA: Ventricular endoaneurysmorrhaphy: a simplified repair for extensive postinfarction aneurysm. *J Cardiac Surg* 1989; 4:200.

116. Cooley DA, Frazier OH, Duncan JM, et al: Intracavitary repair of ventricular aneurysm and regional dyskinesia. *Ann Surg* 1992; 215:417.

117. Faxon DP, Ryan TJ, David KB: Prognostic significance of angiographically documented left ventricular aneurysm from the Coronary Artery Surgery Study (CASS). *Am J Cardiol* 1982; 50:157.

118. Cosgrove DM, Lytle BW, Taylor PC, et al: Ventricular aneurysm resection: trends in surgical risk. *Circulation* 1989; 79(Suppl I):97.

119. Coltharp WH, Hoff SJ, Stoney WS, et al: Ventricular aneurysmectomy: a 25-year experience. *Ann Surg* 1994; 219:707.

120. Grieco JG, Montoya A, Sullivan HJ, et al: Ventricular aneurysm due to blunt chest injury. *Ann Thorac Surg* 1989; 47:322.

121. de Oliveira JA: Heart aneurysm in Chagas' disease. *Revista Instit Medic Trop Sao Paulo* 1998; 40:301.

122. Silverman KJ, Hutchins GM, Bulkley BH: Cardiac sarcoid: a clinicopathological study of 84 unselected patients with systemic sarcoidosis. *Circulation* 1978; 58:1204.

123. Davila JC, Enriquez F, Bergoglio S, et al: Congenital aneurysm of the left ventricle. *Ann Thorac Surg* 1965; 1:697.

124. Antunes MJ: Submitral left ventricular aneurysms. *J Thorac Cardiovasc Surg* 1987; 94:241.

125. de Boer HD, Elzenga NJ, de Boer WJ, et al: Pseudoaneurysm of the left ventricle after isolated pericarditis and Staphylococcus aureus septicemia. *Eur J Cardio-Thorac Surg* 1999; 15:97.

126. Morjan M, El-Essawi A, Anssar M, et al: Left ventricular pseudoaneurysm following transfemoral aortic valve implantation. *J Card Surg* 2013; 28:510.

127. Meizlish JL, Berger MJ, Plaukey M, et al: Functional left ventricular aneurysm formation after acute anterior transmural myocardial infarction: incidence, natural history, and prognostic implications. *N Engl J Med* 1984; 311:1001.

128. Forman MB, Collins HW, Kopelman HA, et al: Determinants of left ventricular aneurysm formation after anterior myocardial infarction: a clinical and angiographic study. *J Am Coll Cardiol* 1986; 8:1256.

129. Toker ME, Onk OA, Alsalehi S, et al: Posterobasal left ventricular aneurysms. Surgical treatment and long-term outcomes. *Tex Heart Inst J* 2013; 40:424.

130. Glower DD, Schaper J, Kabas JS, et al: Relation between reversal of diastolic creep and recovery of systolic function after ischemic myocardial injury in conscious dogs. *Circ Res* 1987; 60:850.

131. Eaton LW, Weiss JL, Bulkley BH, et al: Regional cardiac dilation after acute myocardial infarction: recognition by two-dimensional echocardiography. *N Engl J Med* 1979; 300:57.

132. Iwasaki K, Kita T, Taniguichi G, Kusachi S: Improvement of left ventricular aneurysm after myocardial infarction: report of three cases. *Clin Cardiol* 1991; 14:355.

133. Leurent G, Larralde A, Boulmier D, et al: Cardiac MRI studies of transient left ventricular apical ballooning syndrome (Takotsubo cardiomyopathy): a systematic review. *Int J Cardiol* 2009; 135:146.

134. Sakaguchi G, Young RL, Komeda M, et al: Left ventricular aneurysm repair in rats: structural, functional, and molecular consequences. *J Thorac Cardiovasc Surg* 2001; 121:750.

135. Markowitz LJ, Savage EB, Ratcliffe MB, et al: Large animal model of left ventricular aneurysm. *Ann Thorac Surg* 1989; 48:838.

136. Jugdutt BI, Khan MI: Effect of prolonged nitrate therapy on left ventricular modeling after canine acute myocardial infarction. *Circulation* 1994; 89:2297.

137. Nomoto T, Nishina T, Tsuneyoshi H, et al: Effects of two inhibitors of renin-angiotensin system on attenuation of postoperative remodeling after left ventricular aneurysm repair in rats. *J Card Surg* 2003; 18:S61.

138. Tsuneyoshi H, Nishina T, Nomoto T, et al: Atrial natriuretic peptide helps prevent late remodeling after left ventricular aneurysm repair. *Circulation* 2004; 110:II174.

139. Kayden DS, Wackers FJ, Zaret BL: Left ventricular aneurysm formation after thrombolytic therapy for anterior infarction. TIMI phase I and open label 1985–1986. *Circulation* 1987; 76(Suppl IV):97.

140. Chen JS, Hwang CL, Lee DY, et al: Regression of left ventricular aneurysm after delayed percutaneous transluminal coronary angioplasty (PTCA) in patients with acute myocardial infarction. *Int J Cardiol* 1995; 48:39.

141. Bulkley BH, Roberts WC: Steroid therapy during acute myocardial infarction: a cause of delayed healing and of ventricular aneurysm. *Am J Med* 1974; 58:244.

142. Lapeyre AC III, Steele PM, Kazimer FJ, et al: Systemic embolism in chronic left ventricular aneurysm: incidence and the role of anticoagulation. *Am J Cardiol* 1985; 6:534.

143. Benediktsson R, Eyjolfsson O, Thorgeirsson G: Natural history of chronic left ventricular aneurysm: a population based cohort study. *J Clin Epidemiol* 1991; 44:1131.

144. Faxon DP, Myers WO, McCabe CH: The influence of surgery on the natural history of angiographically documented left ventricular aneurysm: the Coronary Artery Surgery Study. *Circulation* 1986; 74:110.

145. Keren A, Goldberg S, Gottlieb S, et al: Natural history of left ventricular thrombi: their appearance and resolution in the posthospitalization period of acute myocardial infarction. *J Am Coll Cardiol* 1990; 15:790.

146. Lloyd SG, Buckberg GD, RESTORE Group: Use of cardiac magnetic resonance imaging in surgical ventricular restoration. *Eur J Cardio-Thorac Surg* 2006; 295:S216.

147. Dor V, Civaia F, Alexandrescu C, et al: The post-myocardial infarction scarred ventricle and congestive heart failure: the preeminence of magnetic resonance imaging for preoperative, intraoperative, and postoperative assessment. *J Thorac Cardiovasc Surg* 2008; 136:1405.

148. Konen E, Merchant N, Gutierrez C, et al: True versus false left ventricular aneurysm: differentiation with MR imaging—initial experience. *Radiology* 2005; 236:65.

149. Baciewicz PA, Weintraub WS, Jones EL, et al: Late follow-up after repair of left ventricular aneurysm and (usually) associated coronary bypass grafting. *Am J Cardiol* 1991; 68:193.

150. Dor V, Saab M, Coste P, Sabatier M, Montiglio F: Endoventricular patch plasties with septal exclusion for repair of ischemic left ventricle: technique, results and indications from a series of 781 cases. *Jap J Thorac Cardiovasc Surg* 1998; 46:389.

151. Akins CW: Resection of left ventricular aneurysm during hypothermic fibrillatory arrest without aortic occlusion. *J Thorac Cardiovasc Surg* 1986; 91:610.

152. Rankin JS, Hickey MSJ, Smith LR, et al: Current management of mitral valve incompetence associated with coronary artery disease. *J Cardiac Surg* 1989; 4:25.

153. Menicanti L, DiDonato M, Castelvecchio V, et al: Functional ischemic mitral regurgitation in anterior ventricular remodeling: results of surgical ventricular restoration with and without mitral repair. *Heart Failure Rev* 2004; 9:317.

154. Garatti A, Castelvecchio S, Bandera F, et al: Surgical ventricular restoration: Is there any difference in outcome between anterior and posterior remodeling? *Ann Thorac Surg* 2014; 98:S3.

155. ten Brinke EA, Klautz RJ, Steendijk P: Balloon sizing in surgical ventricular restoration: what volume are we targeting? *J Thorac Cardiovasc Surg* 2010; 140:240.

156. Cox JL: Surgical management of left ventricular aneurysms: a clarification of the similarities and differences between the Jatene and Dor techniques. *Sem Thorac Cardiovasc Surg* 1997; 9:131.

157. Menasche P, Hagege A, Scorsin M, et al: Autologous skeletal myoblast transplantation for cardiac insufficiency. First clinical case. *Arch Maladies Coeur Vaisseaux* 2001; 94:180.

158. Taylor DA, Atkins BZ, Hungspreugs P, et al: Regenerating functional myocardium: improved performance after skeletal myoblast transplantation. *Nat Med* 1998; 4:929.

159. Matsubayashi K, Fedak PW, Mickle DA, et al: Improved left ventricular aneurysm repair with bioengineered vascular smooth muscle grafts. *Circulation* 2003; 108:II219.

160. Sakakibara Y, Tambara K, Lu F, et al: Combined procedure of surgical repair and cell transplantation for left ventricular aneurysm: an experimental study. *Circulation* 2002; 106:I193.

161. Costa MA, Mazzaferri EL Jr, Sievert H, et al: Percutaneous ventricular restoration using the parachute device in patients with ischemic heart failure: three-year outcomes of the PARACHUTE first-in-human study. *Circ Heart Fail* 2014; 7:752.

162. Wechsler AS, Sadowski J, Kapelak B, et al: Durability of epicardial ventricular restoration without ventriculotomy. *Eur J Cardiothorac Surg* 2013; 44:e189.

163. Athanasuleas CL, Stanley AWH Jr, Buckberg GD, et al: Surgical anterior ventricular endocardial restoration (SAVER) in the dilated remodeled ventricle after anterior myocardial infarction. *J Am Coll Cardiol* 2001; 37:1199.

164. Wellens F, Degreick Y, Deferm H, et al: Surgical treatment of left ventricular aneurysm and ischemic mitral incompetence. *Acta Chir Belg* 1991; 91:44.

165. Williams JA, Weiss ES, Patel ND, et al: Surgical ventricular restoration versus cardiac transplantation: a comparison of cost, outcomes, and survival. *J Card Fail* 14; 547:2008.

166. Noack T, Kiefer P, Mohr FW, et al: Late left ventricular pseudoaneurysm following transfemoral transcatheter aortic valve replacement. *Eur J Cardiothorac Surg* 2014 Oct 14; pii:ezu353. [Epub ahead of print]

167. Hernandez AF, Velazquez EJ, Dullum MKC, et al: Contemporary performance of surgical ventricular restoration procedures: data from the Society of Thoracic Surgeons' national cardiac database. *Am Heart J* 2006; 152:494.

168. Dor V: Left ventricular aneurysms: the endoventricular circular patch plasty. *Sem Thorac Cardiovasc Surg* 1997; 9:123.

169. Komeda M, David TE, Malik A, et al: Operative risks and long-term results of operation for left ventricular aneurysm. *Ann Thorac Surg* 1992; 53:22.

170. Couper GS, Bunton RW, Birjiniuk V, et al: Relative risks of left ventricular aneurysmectomy in patients with akinetic scars versus true dyskinetic aneurysms. *Circulation* 1990; 82(Suppl IV):248.

171. Stahle E, Bergstrom R, Nystrom SO, et al: Surgical treatment of left ventricular aneurysm assessment of risk factors for early and late mortality. *Eur J Cardio-Thorac Surg* 1994; 8:67.

172. Silveira WL, Leite AF, Soares EC, et al: Short-term follow-up of patients after aneurysmectomy of the left ventricle. *Arquivos Bras Cardiol* 2000; 75:401.

173. Vauthy JN, Berry DW, Snyder DW, et al: Left ventricular aneurysm repair with myocardial revascularization: an analysis of 246 consecutive patients over 15 years. *Ann Thorac Surg* 1988; 46:29.

174. Elefteriades JA, Solomon LW, Salazar AM, et al: Linear left ventricular aneurysmectomy: modern imaging studies reveal improved morphology and function. *Ann Thorac Surg* 1993; 56:242.

175. Kesler KA, Fiore AC, Naunheim KS, et al: Anterior wall left ventricular aneurysm repair: a comparison of linear versus circular closure. *J Thorac Cardiovasc Surg* 1992; 103:841.

176. Kawachi K, Kitamura S, Kawata T, et al: Hemodynamic assessment during exercise after left ventricular aneurysmectomy. *J Thorac Cardiovasc Surg* 1994; 107:178.

177. David TE: Surgical treatment of mechanical complications of myocardial infarction, in Spence PA, Chitwood RA (eds): *Cardiac Surgery: State of the Art Reviews,* Vol 5. Philadelphia, Hanley and Belfus, 1991; p 423.

178. DiDonato M, Barletta G, Maioli M, et al: Early hemodynamic results of left ventricular reconstructive surgery for anterior wall left ventricular aneurysm. *Am J Cardiol* 1992; 69:886.

179. Kawata T, Kitamura S, Kawachi K, et al: Systolic and diastolic function after patch reconstruction of left ventricular aneurysms. *Ann Thorac Surg* 1995; 59:403.

180. Tanoue Y, Ando H, Fukamura F, et al: Ventricular energetics in endoventricular circular patch plasty for dyskinetic anterior left ventricular aneurysm. *Ann Thorac Surg* 2003; 75:1205.

181. Coskun KO, Popov AF, Coskun ST, et al: Surgical treatment of left ventricular aneurysm. *Asian Cardiovasc Thorac Ann* 2009; 17:490.

182. Zheng Z, Fan H, Feng W, et al: Surgery of left ventricular aneurysm: a propensity score-matched study of outcomes following different repair techniques. *Interact Cardiovasc Thorac Surg* 2009; 9:431.

183. Schreuder JJ, Castiglioni A, Maisano F, et al: Acute decrease of left ventricular mechanical dyssynchrony and improvement of contractile state and energy efficiency after left ventricular restoration. *J Thorac Cardiovasc Surg* 2005; 129:138.

184. Fantini F, Barletta G, Toso A, et al: Effects of reconstructive surgery for left ventricular anterior aneurysm on ventriculoarterial coupling. *Heart* 1999; 81:171.

185. Nicolosi AC, Weng ZC, Detwiler PW, et al: Simulated left ventricular aneurysm and aneurysm repair in swine. *J Thorac Cardiovasc Surg* 1990; 100:745.

186. Walker WE, Stoney WS, Alford WC, et al: Results of surgical management of acute left ventricular aneurysm. *Circulation* 1978; 62(Suppl II):75.

187. Hutchins GM, Brawley RK: The influence of cardiac geometry on the results of ventricular aneurysm repair. *Am J Pathol* 1980; 99:221.

188. Parolari A, Naliato M, Loardi C, et al: Surgery of left ventricular aneurysm: a meta-analysis of early outcomes following different reconstruction techniques. *Ann Thorac Surg* 2007; 83:2009.

189. Doss M, Martens S, Sayour S, et al: Long term follow up of left ventricular function after repair of left ventricular aneurysm. A comparison of linear closure versus patch plasty. *Eur J Cardio-Thorac Surg* 2001; 20:783.

190. Antunes PE, Silva R, Ferrao de Oliveira J, Antunes MJ: Left ventricular aneurysms: early and long-term results of two types of repair. *Eur J Cardio-Thorac Surg* 2005; 27:210.

191. Marchenko AV, Cherniavsky AM, Volokitina TL, Alsov SA, Karaskov AM: Left ventricular dimension and shape after postinfarction aneurysm repair. *Eur J Cardio-Thorac Surg* 2005; 27:475.

192. Vicol C, Rupp G, Fischer S, et al: Linear repair versus ventricular reconstruction for treatment of left ventricular aneurysm: a 10-year experience. *J Cardiovasc Surg* 1998; 39:461.

193. Salati M, Paje A, Di Biasi P, et al: Severe diastolic dysfunction after endoventriculoplasty. *J Thorac Cardiovasc Surg* 1995; 109:694.

194. Lundblad R, Abdelnoor M, Svennevig JL: Surgery for left ventricular aneurysm: early and late survival after simple linear repair and endoventricular patch plasty. *J Thorac Cardiovasc Surg* 2004; 128:449.

195. Ratcliffe MB, Wallace AW, Salahieh A, et al: Ventricular volume, chamber stiffness, and function after anteroapical aneurysm plication in the sheep. *J Thorac Cardiovasc Surg* 2000; 119:115.

196. Michler RE, Rouleau JL, Al-Khalidi HR, et al: Insights from the STICH trial: change in left ventricular size after coronary artery bypass grafting with and without surgical ventricular reconstruction. *J Thorac Cardiovasc Surg* 2013; 146:1139.

197. Buckberg GD, Athanasuleas CL, Wechsler AS, et al: The STICH Trial unravelled. *Eur J Heart Fail* 2010; 12:1024.

198. Rouleau JL, Michler RE, Velazquez EJ, et al: The STICH trial: evidence-based conclusions. *Eur J Heart Fail* 2010; 12:1028.

199. Prucz RB, Weiss ES, Patel ND, et al: Coronary artery bypass grafting with or without surgical ventricular restoration: a comparison. *Ann Thorac Surg* 2008; 86:806.

200. Mark DB, Knight JD, Velazquez EJ, et al: Quality of life and economic outcomes with surgical ventricular reconstruction in ischemic heart failure: results from the Surgical Treatment for Ischemic Heart Failure Trial. *Am Heart J* 2009; 157:837.

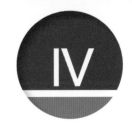

AORTIC VALVE DISEASE

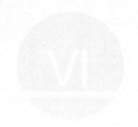

VI

AORTIC VALVE DISEASE

26

Pathophysiology of Aortic Valve Disease

Anna Brzezinski • Marijan Koprivanac • A. Marc Gillinov
• Tomislav Mihaljevic

The aortic valve (AV) is a semilunar valve positioned at the end of the left ventricular outflow tract (LVOT) between the left ventricle and aorta. Proper functioning of this valve is critical in maintaining efficient cardiac function. This chapter explores the anatomical and physiologic properties of the AV.

EMBRYOLOGIC DEVELOPMENT

Embryologic development of the AV is closely associated with development of the LVOT. In the primary heart tube, blood travels from the primitive ventricle into the bulbous cordis and out from the aortic roots. The midportion of the bulbous cordis, the conus cordis, develops into the outflow tracts of the ventricles. The distal portion of the bulbous cordis, the truncus arteriosus (TA), develops into the proximal portion of the aorta and pulmonary arteries. During the fifth week of development, pairs of opposing swellings appear in the conus cordis and TA (Fig. 26-1). These conotruncal, or bulbar, ridges grow toward each other and fuse to form the aorticopulmonary (AP) septum. The AP septum divides the conus cordis into the left and right ventricular outflow tracts and the TA into the ascending aorta and pulmonary trunk.

When partitioning of the TA is nearly completed, the AV begins to develop from three swellings of subendocardial tissue (see Fig. 26-1). Two swellings arising from the fused truncal ridges develop into the right and left AV leaflets. A third dorsal swelling develops into the posterior leaflet. These swellings are reshaped and hollowed out to form the three thin-walled cusps of the fully developed AV. The pulmonary valve develops in a similar manner.

ANATOMY

The AV separates the terminal portion of the LVOT from the aorta. The normal AV consists of three semilunar leaflets or cusps projecting outward and upward into the lumen of the ascending aorta (Fig. 26-2). The space between the free edge of each leaflet and the points of attachment to the aorta comprise the sinuses of Valsalva. Because the coronary arteries arise from two of the three sinuses, the sinuses and the respective leaflets are named the right coronary, left coronary, and posterior (noncoronary) sinuses and leaflets. The ostia of coronary arteries arise from the upper part of the sinuses, with the ostium of the left coronary artery positioned slightly higher than the ostium of the right. The leaflets are separated from one another at the aorta by the right-left, right-posterior, and left-posterior commissures (Fig. 26-3). The area adjacent to the left-posterior commissure is the fibrous continuity, which interconnects the aorta and the mitral valve annulus. The area beneath this commissure is the aortomitral curtain, which is an important anatomical landmark for root enlargement procedures. The posterior leaflet attaches above the posterior diverticulum of the LVOT and opposes the right atrial wall. The right-posterior commissure is positioned directly above the penetrating atrioventricular bundle and membranous septum. The right-left commissure opposes the posterior commissure of the pulmonary valve and the two associated aortic cusps oppose the right ventricular infundibulum. The lateral part of the left coronary sinus is the only part of the AV that is not closely related to another cardiac chamber and is in direct relationship with the free pericardial space.

The AV leaflets meet centrally along a line of coaptation, at the center of which are the thickened nodules of Arantius. Because of the semilunar shape of the leaflets, the AV does not have a true annulus in the traditional sense of a ring-like attachment. Instead, the leaflets have semilunar attachments along a hollow cylinder or cuff of tissue interconnecting the left ventricular (LV) chamber and the proximal aorta (Fig. 26-4).[1] The distal border of the cuff is the sinotubular junction, which is defined by imaginary lines connecting the commissures. The proximal border is the ventriculoarterial (VA) junction, which has both hemodynamic and anatomic parts. The hemodynamic VA junction is marked by the semilunar attachments of the leaflets, whereas the anatomic VA junction is marked by the circular attachment of the proximal aorta and the muscular and membranous ventricular septums.

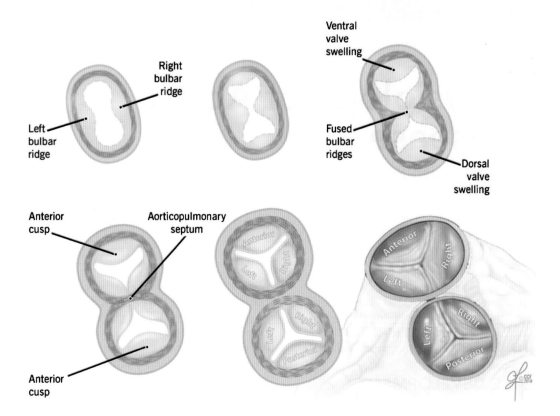

FIGURE 26-1 Schematic representation of development of the left and right ventricular outflow tracts and aortic and pulmonary valves. (*Top left*) Cross-section through the cordis showing the conotruncal ridges beginning to develop. (*Top right*) Aorticopulmonary septum forming from fusion of the conotruncal ridges and subendocardial swellings beginning to develop into the aortic and pulmonary valve leaflets. (*Bottom left*) Left and right ventricular outflow tracts separated by the aorticopulmonary septum and further development of the subendocardial swellings. (*Bottom right*) Aortic and pulmonary valves in the adult. (Reproduced with permission from Cleveland Clinic, Cleveland, OH.)

The valve leaflets consist of three layers of endothelially invested connective tissue of distinctly different density and composition. There is no demarcation between the outer layers of the aortic and ventricular sides of the leaflets and outer

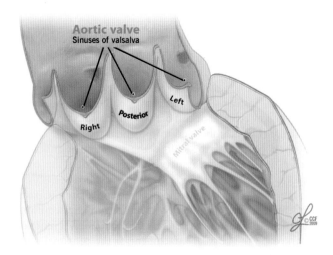

FIGURE 26-2 Anatomical relationship between the aortic valve leaflets and surrounding structures. (Reproduced with permission from Cleveland Clinic, Cleveland, OH.)

layers of the corresponding aortic and ventricular walls; that is, leaflet endothelial cells form a continuum with aortic and ventricular endothelial cells (Fig. 26-5).[2,3] Beneath the endothelium, there are extensions of the aortic intima and ventricular endocardium, termed the *arterialis* and *ventricularis*, respectively. The next layer is the lamina fibrosa, which is composed of dense collagen mostly in a circumferential pattern. Because of the thickness and density of this layer, it is the strongest layer and important for bearing the stress of diastolic pressure. The middle layer, referred to as the *spongiosa*, forms the core of the leaflets at their bases. It is made of loose connective tissue consisting of water and glycosaminoglycans with sparse fibers and cellularity. The semifluid nature of this layer gives the leaflet considerable plasticity.

MECHANICS OF MOVEMENT

The AV passively opens and closes in response to pressure differences between the left ventricle and aorta during the cardiac cycle. Pressure generated from ventricular contraction leads to valve opening, and the subsequent relatively higher pressure of the aorta leads to valve closure. The mechanical properties of the AV allow it to open with minimal transvalvular gradient and close completely with minimal flow reversal.

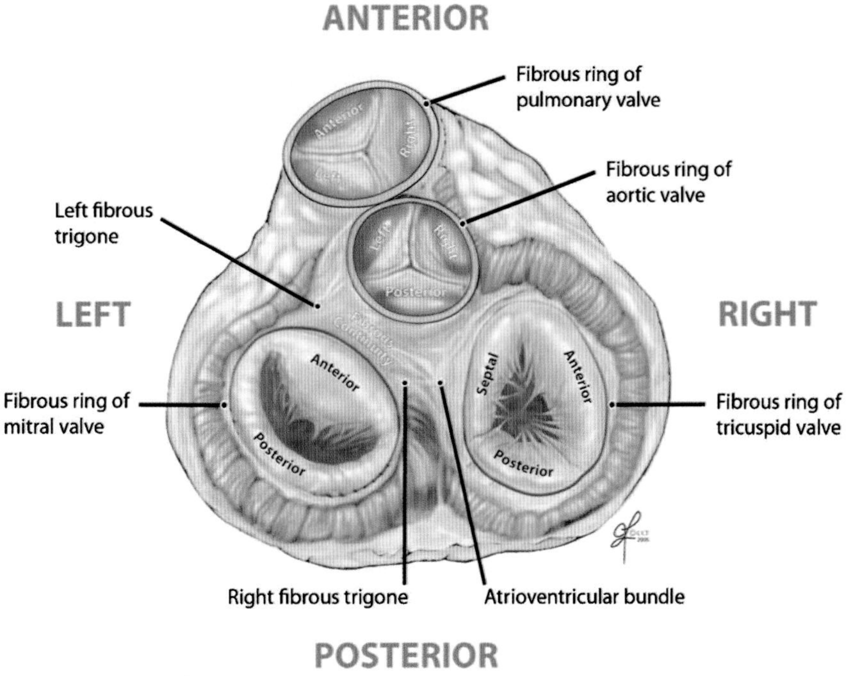

ANTERIOR

Fibrous ring of
pulmonary valve

Fibrous ring of
aortic valve

Left fibrous
trigone

LEFT

RIGHT

Fibrous ring of
mitral valve

Fibrous ring of
tricuspid valve

Right fibrous trigone

Atrioventricular bundle

POSTERIOR

FIGURE 26-3 Anatomical relationship between the aortic valve and surrounding structures. (Reproduced with permission from Cleveland Clinic, Cleveland, OH.)

Opening

Pressure differences between the aorta and the ventricle coupled with compliance of the aortic root cause aortic root dilation and constriction during the cardiac cycle. This dynamic motion of the root plays an important role in opening and closing of the AV. During late diastole, as blood fills the ventricle, a 12% expansion of the aortic root occurs 20 to 40 ms before AV opening.[4] The leaflets begin to open as a result of root dilation even before any generation of positive pressure from ventricular contraction. Root dilation alone opens the leaflets about 20%.[5] As pressure rises in the LVOT, tension across the leaflets produced from root dilation lessens. As pressure continues to rise, the pressure difference across the leaflets is minimal, and no tension is present within the leaflet.[6] This loss of tension allows the aortic root to further dilate and allows the valve to open rapidly at the beginning of ejection. Under normal circumstances, the AV presents little or no obstruction to flow because the specific gravity of the leaflets is equal to that of blood.[7] These mechanisms permit rapid opening of the valve and minimal resistance to ejection.[8]

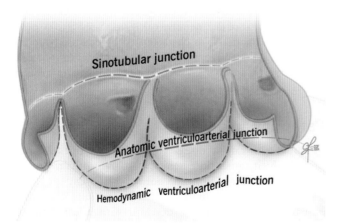

FIGURE 26-4 Schematic representation of the aortic valve cuff. The sinotubular junction marks the distal border. The ventriculoarterial junction, which has both hemodynamic and anatomic parts, marks the proximal border. (Reproduced with permission from Cleveland Clinic, Cleveland, OH.)

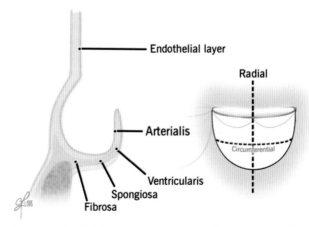

FIGURE 26-5 Schematic representation of a cross-section through the aortic valve leaflet showing the continuity of endocardial and endothelial components with the aortic valve. Inset illustrates the radial and circumferential axes of the valve leaflet. (Reproduced with permission from Cleveland Clinic, Cleveland, OH.)

Closure

Closure of the AV is an elegant mechanism, which has interested investigators since the time of Leonardo da Vinci.[9] A principal theory involved in closure is vortex theory, which recognizes the importance of the sinuses of Valsalva in valve closure.[10] As ejection occurs, blood creates small eddy currents or vortices along the aortic wall. At the end of ejection and before valve closure, these vortices fill the sinuses and balloon the leaflets away from the aortic wall toward the aortic axis. After the pressure difference across the open AV equalizes, a small flow reversal forces the leaflets completely closed. Apposition of the valve leaflets occurs briskly and the ensuing second heart sound occurs after complete closure of the AV. Upon closing, the elastic leaflets stretch and recoil to generate compression and expansion of blood. The subsequent pressure changes produce the second heart sound; the sound is not produced by physical apposition of the valve leaflets.[11]

AORTIC STENOSIS

Aortic stenosis (AS) is incomplete opening of the AV, which restricts blood flow out of the left ventricle during systole.

Prevalence and Etiology

In developed countries, AS is the most prevalent valvular heart disease in adults.[12] Observational echocardiography studies demonstrate that 2% of people 65 years of age or older have isolated calcific AS, whereas 29% exhibit age-related AV sclerosis without stenosis.[13] AS is more common in men and its prevalence increases with age.[14] In patients aged 65 to 75 years, 75 to 85 years, and greater than 85 years, the prevalence of AS is 1.3, 2.4, and 4%, respectively.[15] The most common causes of AS are acquired degenerative disease, bicuspid AV, and rheumatic heart disease.

Acquired Aortic Stenosis

The most common cause of AS is degenerative calcification of the AV, which typically occurs in septuagenarians and octogenarians. Progressive calcification, initially along the flexion lines at the leaflet bases, leads to immobilization of the cusps. The characteristic pathologic findings are discrete, focal lesions on the aortic side of the leaflets that can extend deep into the aortic annulus. The deposits may involve the sinuses of Valsalva and the ascending aorta. Although long considered to be the result of years of mechanical stress on an otherwise normal valve, it is now understood that the mechanical stress leads to proliferative and inflammatory changes, with lipid accumulation, upregulation of angiotensin-converting enzyme (ACE) activity, and infiltration of macrophages and T lymphocytes in a process similar to atherosclerosis.[16-20] The risk factors for the development of calcific AS are similar to those for atherosclerosis and include elevated serum levels of low-density lipoprotein (LDL) cholesterol, diabetes,

smoking, and hypertension.[15] Therefore, coronary artery disease is commonly present in patients with AS. Age-related AV sclerosis is associated with an increased risk of cardiovascular death and myocardial infarction (MI).

Calcific AS is also observed in a number of other conditions, including Paget's disease of bone and end-stage renal disease.[21] Ochronosis with alkaptonuria is another rare cause of AS, which also can cause a rare greenish discoloration of the AV.[22]

Bicuspid Aortic Stenosis

A calcified bicuspid AV represents the most common form of congenital AS. Bicuspid AVs are present in approximately 2% of the general population. Gradual calcification of the bicuspid AV results in significant stenosis most often in the fifth and sixth decades of life, earlier in unicommissural than bicuspid valves and earlier in men than women.[23,24] The abnormal architecture of the unicommissural or bicuspid AV induces turbulent flow, which injures the leaflets and leads to fibrosis, increased rigidity, leaflet calcification, and narrowing of the AV orifice.[25] Several genes have been associated with bicuspid AV. Mutations in the signaling and transcriptional regulator *NOTCH1* result in abnormal valve development and subsequent calcium deposition, providing a link between genetic mutations, valve morphology, and subsequent calcification associated with bicuspid AS.[26-29] Structural abnormalities in microfibrils within the AV and aortic root lead to decreased structural integrity, resulting in dilation, aneurysms, and dissection.[25,26,30]

Rheumatic Aortic Stenosis

In Western countries, rheumatic AS represents the least common form of AS in adults.[31,32] Rheumatic AS is rarely an isolated disease and usually occurs in conjunction with mitral valve stenosis.[33,34] Rheumatic AS is characterized by diffuse fibrous leaflet thickening with fusion, to a variable extent, of one or more commissures. The progression of rheumatic AS is slower than that of degenerative calcific disease.[24,35] The early stage of rheumatic AS is characterized by edema, lymphocytic infiltration, and revascularization of the leaflets, whereas the later stages are characterized by thickening, commissural fusion, and scarred leaflet edges.

Pathophysiology

In adults with calcific disease, the AV slowly thickens over time. Early, it causes little hemodynamic disturbance as the valve area is reduced from the normal 3 to 4 cm^2 to 1.5 to 2 cm^2.[24,35] Past this point, hemodynamically significant obstruction of LV outflow develops with a concomitant increase in LV pressure and lengthening of LV ejection time. The elevated LV pressure increases wall stress, which is normalized by increased wall thickness and LV hypertrophy (LVH). As it hypertrophies, the left ventricle becomes less compliant and LV end-diastolic pressure (LVEDP) increases without chamber dilatation. This reflects diastolic dysfunction and the ventricle becomes increasingly dependent on atrial systole for filling.[36] Hence, if a patient develops an atrial arrhythmia, he or she can rapidly decompensate.

Although adaptive, the concentric hypertrophy that develops has adverse consequences. LVH, increased systolic pressure, and prolonged ejection time all contribute to an increase in myocardial oxygen consumption. Increased diastolic pressure increases endocardial compression of the coronary arteries, reducing coronary flow reserve (or maximal coronary flow).[37] Prolonged ejection also results in decreased time in diastole and therefore reduced myocardial perfusion time. The increased demand of the hypertrophied ventricle and decreased delivery capacity can yield subendocardial ischemia with activity. This can result in angina and LV dysfunction. LVH also makes the heart more susceptible to ischemic injury. Severe LVH is only partly reversed by AV replacement (AVR) and is associated with decreased long-term survival even after initially successful surgery.[38]

In late stages of severe AS, the left ventricle decompensates with resulting dilated cardiomyopathy and heart failure. Cardiac output (CO) declines and the pulmonary artery pressure rises, leading to pulmonary hypertension.

Myocardial hypertrophy in patients with AS is characterized by increased gene expression for collagen I and II, and fibronectin that is associated with activation of the renin-angiotensin system.[39] Reduction in renin-angiotensin parallels regression of hypertrophy after AVR.[40] Experimental studies have indicated a role of apoptotic mechanisms in the progression to LVH and heart failure in patients with AS.[41,42] Patients who present with symptoms of congestive heart failure (CHF) have a 1-year survival of approximately 60%.[43,44]

Hemodynamics

The severity of AS can be assessed by measuring the AV orifice area (AVA), mean pressure gradient, and peak jet velocity. Effective AVA is calculated using the cross-sectional area of the LVOT (CSA_{LVOT}), flow velocity through the LVOT (VTI_{LVOT}), and AS jet velocity (VTI_{AV}) using the continuity equation, which is based on the concept that stroke volume through the LVOT and AV are equal.[45-49] The continuity equation is

$$AVA = \frac{CSA_{LVOT} \times VTI_{LVOT}}{VTI_{AV}}$$

CSA_{LVOT} is calculated using LVOT diameter (D_{LVOT}) as

$$CSA_{LVOT} = \pi \left(\frac{D_{LVOT}}{2} \right)^2$$

Valve areas of less than 1.0 cm² represent severe AS. Although the effective AVA is smaller than the anatomic AVA, it is a reliable predictor of clinical outcomes and is generally used in clinical decision making.[47,50]

The Gorlin formula, which describes the fundamental relationships linking the area of an orifice to the flow and pressure drop across the orifice, is used to calculate anatomic AVA using a Fick or thermodilution CO measurement taken during catheterization.[49,51] The Gorlin formula uses the time from AV opening to closure (SEP) as

$$AVA = \frac{CO \left(\dfrac{mL}{min} \right)}{44.3 \times HR \left(\dfrac{beats}{min} \right) \times SEP(sec) \times \sqrt{mean\ pressure\ gradient\ (mm\,Hg)}}$$

The Gorlin formula can also be used to calculate AVA from Doppler but is less favorable than the continuity equation as it underestimates the AVA in low-output states.[52,53]

In patients with AS, the transvalvular pressure gradient can be measured by simultaneous catheter pressure measurements in the left ventricle and proximal aorta. The peak-to-peak gradient, measured as the difference between peak LV pressure and peak aortic pressure, is used commonly to quantify the valve gradient.

Invasive measurements of AS severity have been largely replaced by echocardiographic measurements, which are currently the clinical standard.[47,49] The gradient can be calculated from the Doppler acquired VTI_{AV} using the Bernoulli equation as

$$Gradient = \pi\ VTI_{AV}^{2}$$

Transesophageal echocardiography (TEE) is an alternative method for assessment of AVA that uses planimetry of the systolic short-axis view of the AV (Fig. 26-6).[54] Planimetry of the valve area is challenging because the valve orifice is a complex, three-dimensional shape, and area measurements assume the valve orifice lies entirely within the image plane.

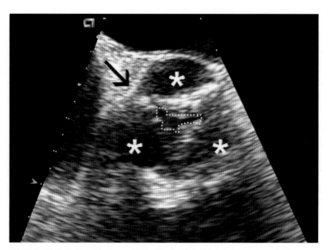

FIGURE 26-6 Transesophageal echocardiographic image of aortic stenosis resulting from severe degenerative calcification. Transverse section of the aortic root at the level of the aortic valve orifice showing the aortic ring (*arrow*), the sinuses of Valsalva (*asterisks*), and a significantly reduced aortic valve orifice area of 0.44 cm² (*dotted line*).

Thus, it is only recommended when Doppler estimation of flow velocities is unreliable.[47]

Clinical Presentation

SYMPTOMS

The cardinal symptoms of AS are angina pectoris, syncope, and symptoms of CHF (dyspnea, orthopnea, and paroxysmal nocturnal dyspnea).[55] Although the mechanisms of angina and heart failure are well understood, the mechanism of syncope is less clear. A common theory is that the augmented stroke volume that usually accompanies exercise is limited by the narrowed outflow orifice. With exercise-induced reduction in peripheral arterial resistance, blood pressure drops, leading to cerebral hypoperfusion and syncope.[56] Syncope also may be the result of dysfunction of baroreceptor mechanisms and a vasodepressor response to the increased LV systolic pressure during exercise. Besides these cardinal symptoms, patients also commonly present with more subtle symptoms, such as fatigue, decreased exercise tolerance, and dyspnea on exertion.[57]

A rare presentation of AS is gastrointestinal bleeding secondary to angiodysplasia occurring predominantly in the right colon, as well as in the small bowel or stomach. This complication arises from shear-stress-induced platelet aggregation with reduction in high-molecular-weight multimers of von Willebrand factor and increases in proteolytic subunit fragments. These abnormalities correlate with the severity of AS and are correctable by AVR.[58] Other late manifestations of severe AS include atrial fibrillation and pulmonary hypertension. Infective endocarditis can occur in younger patients with AS; it is less common in elderly patients with a severely calcified valve.

Patients who develop severe AS have a long period of asymptomatic progression in which morbidity and mortality is relatively low (Fig. 26-7).[55] Sudden death from AS before the onset of symptoms is estimated to be approximately 1% per year.[59] With the onset of symptoms, the mortality rate is 25% per year without surgical intervention.[12] Of the 35% of patients who present with angina, 50% survive for 5 years. Of the 15% who present with syncope, 50% survive for 3 years, and mean survival for those who present with CHF is 2 years.[55]

SIGNS

AS is frequently first diagnosed before symptom onset by auscultation of a murmur on physical examination. Classically, AS causes a systolic crescendo-decrescendo murmur, heard loudest at the right upper sternal border. Another sign of AS is a delayed second heart sound (S_2) because of prolongation of the systolic ejection time. S_2 also may be single when the aortic component is absent, and if the aortic component is audible, this may give rise to a paradoxical splitting of S_2.

The classic pulsus parvus (small pulse) is a sign of severe AS or decompensated AS and occurs when stroke volume and systolic and pulse pressures fall. A wide pulse pressure is also characteristic of AS. Prolongation of the ejection phase with slow rise in the arterial pressure also gives rise to the pulsus tardus (late pulse). Pulsus parvus et tardus is diagnosed by palpation.

LVH is evident as a sustained apical thrust or heave. This sign is present only when failure occurs because before failure occurs, the hypertrophy is not accompanied by dilatation, and the apical impulse is not displaced. Conversely, absence of an apical thrust (except in muscular patients, or those with emphysema or adiposity) suggests mild or moderate AS. Other physical findings of significant AS include a prominent atrial kick and prominence of the jugular venous *a* wave secondary to decreased right ventricular compliance caused by right ventricular hypertrophy.[60]

ELECTROCARDIOGRAM

Most patients with severe AS present with QRS complex or ST-T interval abnormalities reflecting LVH. Patients with a higher gradient are more likely to show a "strain" or "systolic overload" pattern. The conduction abnormalities may result from septal trauma secondary to high intramyocardial tension from hypoxic damage to the conducting fibers or from extension of valvular calcifications into the fibrous septum.

ROENTGENOGRAM

The roentgenographic characteristics of compensated AS include concentric hypertrophy of the left ventricle without cardiomegaly, poststenotic dilatation of the aorta, and calcification of the valve cusps. With decompensation, there is cardiomegaly in the posteroanterior projection and pulmonary venous congestion. It is important to recognize that a routine chest x-ray may be within normal limits in patients with hemodynamically compensated AS. The rounding of the lower-left heart border may be subtle, the poststenotic aortic dilatation may be equivocal, and the valvular calcification may be invisible on the posteroanterior view. Of equal importance, the presence of cardiomegaly in a normotensive patient with isolated AS indicates decompensated AS.

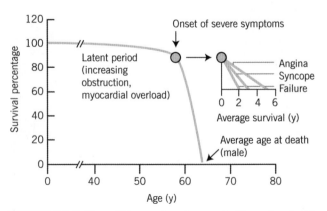

FIGURE 26-7 Natural history of aortic stenosis. (Reproduced with permission from Ross J, Braunwald E. Aortic stenosis, *Circulation.* 1968 Jul;38(1 Suppl):61-67.)

ECHOCARDIOGRAPHY

Echocardiography is the diagnostic tool of choice for confirming the diagnosis of AS and quantification of disease severity. Echocardiography is used to define: (1) the severity and etiology of AS; (2) coexisting valvular abnormalities; and (3) cardiac chamber size and function.

The development of diastolic dysfunction in patients with AS can lead to symptom development, and may increase late mortality after AVR.[38,61] Hence, the quantification of diastolic dysfunction is important in the assessment of AS. LV filling pressures can be assessed by calculating the ratio of transmitral flow velocity and annular velocity obtained at the level of the mitral annulus with tissue Doppler.[62-64] In patients with normal LV function (LVF), stress echocardiography is used to determine if symptom development during exercise is due to diastolic dysfunction.[65] Diastolic dysfunction in patients with normal LVF may cause exercise intolerance for several reasons: (1) elevated LV diastolic and pulmonary venous pressures increase the work of breathing and cause dyspnea; (2) patients with LVH exhibit a limited ability to use the Frank-Starling mechanism during exercise, resulting in a decrease in CO during exercise; and (3) elevated LV diastolic and pulmonary venous pressures result in abnormalities in the diastolic properties of the ventricle.

When AS is suspected, an initial Doppler echocardiogram can confirm the diagnosis and assess the severity. Re-examination should be performed upon change in signs or symptoms, or periodically, every 3 to 5 years for mild AS, every 1 to 2 years for moderate AS, and every 6 months to 1 year for severe AS, to identify worsening stenosis, LV dysfunction, LVH, and mitral regurgitation. Although AS is best understood as a disease continuum, severity can be graded by echocardiographic evaluation of hemodynamics. The current guidelines use definitions based on the AVA, mean pressure gradient, and peak jet velocity (Table 26-1).[49]

TABLE 26-1: Classification of Aortic Stenosis Severity

Indicator	Mild	Moderate	Severe
Aortic valve area (cm²)	>1.5	1.0-1.5	<1.0
Aortic valve area index (cm² per m²)			<0.6
Mean pressure gradient (mm Hg)	<25	25-40	>40
Peak jet velocity (m/sec)	<3.0	3.0-4.0	>4.0

Data compiled from Bonow RO, Carabello BA, Chatterjee K, de Leon AC Jr, Faxon DP, et al: 2008 focused update incorporated into the ACC/AHA 2006 guidelines for the management of patients with valvular heart disease: a report of the American College of Cardiology/American Heart Association Task Force on Practice Guidelines (Writing Committee to revise the 1998 guidelines for the management of patients with valvular heart disease). Endorsed by the Society of Cardiovascular Anesthesiologists, Society for Cardiovascular Angiography and Interventions, and Society of Thoracic Surgeons. *J Am Coll Cardiol* 2008; 52(13):e1-142.

EXERCISE TESTING

Exercise testing should be avoided in symptomatic patients with AS. Traditionally, severe AS has been regarded as a relative contraindication to exercise testing. Recent studies have indicated that quantitative exercise Doppler echocardiography can be performed safely in asymptomatic patients, including those with severe AS, and may be useful for identifying patients who at higher risk of becoming symptomatic and/or requiring AVR. Asymptomatic patients with severe AS who become symptomatic on exercise stress testing have a higher rate of cardiac death or progression to AVR.[49,66,67] Thus, patients with provoked symptoms should be considered symptomatic. Dobutamine stress echocardiography is occasionally used in severe AS, specifically to assess contractile reserve in patients with moderate to severe AS with a low AV gradient and depressed LVF.[68,69]

CARDIAC CATHETERIZATION

Although Doppler echocardiography can provide adequate anatomic and hemodynamic information for most patients, cardiac catheterization is recommended when noninvasive tests are inconclusive or there is a discrepancy between noninvasive tests and clinical findings to determine the severity of AS.[49,70] Cardiac catheterization remains the gold standard for measuring the transvalvular gradient. Left-sided heart catheterization is also used to calculate the AVA based on the Gorlin equation, as described earlier, and can provide an assessment of ejection fraction (EF) through ventriculography and information about the presence or absence of other valve lesions. Coronary artery disease is common in patients with AS and should be evaluated prior to intervention. Cardiac catheterization is indicated in patients with angina, evidence of ischemia, history of CAD, or coronary risk factors to assess coronary anatomy and evaluate the need for combined AVR and myocardial revascularization. Cardiac catheterization should also be performed in patients with epicardial CAD detected by computed tomography (CT) coronary angiography to evaluate the extent of obstruction.[49]

COMPUTED TOMOGRAPHY

CT is the only noninvasive modality that provides direct assessment of the amount of AV calcification. While CT provides the highest-resolution anatomic data of the AV, it does not provide hemodynamic data, and therefore is not recommended for the diagnosis of AS.[71] Electrocardiographically gated multidetector row CT has shown high accuracy and reproducibility in quantifying AV calcification and its progression[71,72] and estimating AVA by planimetry.[73,74] The quantification of calcification may develop into clinical applications with respect to the prognostic relevance of AV sclerosis, as well as the problem of calcification of bioprostheses after surgery. Prior to valve intervention, patients with low to intermediate probability of CAD should undergo CT coronary angiography to exclude the presence of severe obstructive CAD.[49] CT is useful preoperatively for patients undergoing transcatheter aortic valve replacement (TAVR) for measurement of the native valve annulus, leaflet length, and annular to coronary ostial distance to guide the selection of appropriate TAVR size and evaluate the prosthesis after deployment.[71,75]

MAGNETIC RESONANCE IMAGING

Cardiac magnetic resonance imaging (MRI) has emerged as an alternative noninvasive imaging modality for AS.[76] Similar to echocardiography, cardiac MRI records images throughout the cardiac cycle. Cardiac MRI uses a range of pulse sequences to assess structural heart disease. The steady-state free precession (SSFP) cine pulse sequence is commonly used in cardiac MRI and provides detailed images of AV leaflet number, leaflet thickening, valve calcification, and commissural fusion. This sequence is also useful for assessing the effects of AS, including LVH and LVF.[77] MRI is useful when acoustic windows in the echocardiogram are poor or there are discordant imaging and catheterization results.[78,79] MRI has also been used to demonstrate improvement in LVF, myocardial metabolism, and diastolic function, as well as reduced hypertrophy after AVR for AS.[80]

Management

SYMPTOMATIC PATIENTS

There is no effective medical therapy for AS. Given the biologic similarity of the calcific lesions of AS to atherosclerosis, there has been substantial effort to investigate the role of lipid-lowering agents in slowing the progression of AS, but to date prospective randomized trials have not found any benefits.[81-84] Acquired AS is considered a moderate risk condition for acquiring infective endocarditis after dental or surgical procedures, and antibiotic prophylaxis is recommended.[49,85] Management of CHF from AS has traditionally consisted of diuretics and inotropes. Beta-blockers are avoided as reduced contractility may lead to decreased CO in an overloaded ventricle. Vasodilators are avoided in AS because their administration can lead to hypotension, syncope, and reduced coronary perfusion. However, in patients with severe AS with decompensated heart failure and severe LV systolic dysfunction, vasodilators may improve cardiac function and may be used as a bridge to AVR.[49,86]

The definitive treatment for severe AS is AVR, and onset of symptoms is the primary indication for surgery. Choice of size of valve prosthesis is of substantial importance for long-term outcome. Prosthesis-patient mismatch will occur after implantation of small prosthesis, thereby increasing the residual transvalvular gradient and subsequently negatively affecting regression of LVH and coronary flow reserve, resulting in worse survival.[38,87-89]

TAVR is a viable option for treatment of severe AS in patients who are at high risk for surgical AVR. TAVR has shown superior survival to standard medical therapy and similar survival to surgical AVR but with lower periprocedural risks in the high-risk population.[90-92] It is also indicated in cases that meet an indication for AVR but have prohibitive risk for surgical approach and predicted post-TAVR survival greater than 12 months.[49,93]

Percutaneous aortic balloon dilatation is ineffective long-term since most valves tend to restenose. Currently, it is indicated as a bridge to AVR or TAVR in severely symptomatic patients with severe AS.[49,94-96]

ASYMPTOMATIC PATIENTS

As AVR has become a safer procedure and technology for assessing disease severity has improved, an identifiable high-risk subset of asymptomatic patients with severe AS has shown to benefit from AVR. While the risk of asymptomatic severe AS is low, surgery is indicated if associated with a combination of the following factors: worsening of hemodynamic parameters (LVEF < 50%, maximum aortic velocity ≥ 4 m/s, mean pressure gradient ≥ 40 mm Hg), decreased systolic opening of calcified valve, cardiac surgery for other causes, low surgical risk, and decreased exercise tolerance on exercise stress test.[49] Asymptomatic patients with an aortic jet velocity greater than 4 m/s,[57] high rates of aortic jet velocity progression and valve calcification,[97] or small AVAs and LVH[59] progress to symptom development quickly and soon require AVR. Exercise stress testing, as described earlier, is also useful to stratify high-risk patients and identify truly asymptomatic patients.

Asymptomatic patients with severe AS has significantly improved survival compared to medically managed patients.[98,99] In patients undergoing AVR for severe AS, LVH is only partly reversed and is associated with decreased long-term survival even after initially successful surgery. This suggests that intervening before development of LVH may improve outcomes.[38,100-104] Efforts have been made to better characterize asymptomatic AS patients and identify patients that would benefit from earlier AVR.[105,106] In summary, there is increasing evidence that AVR can be beneficial to a wider subset of asymptomatic patients with severe AS, but these conclusions may only apply to centers with a high volume of valve surgeries and cannot be generalized.[107,108]

AORTIC REGURGITATION

Aortic regurgitation (AR) is the diastolic reflux of blood from the aorta into the left ventricle due to failure of coaptation of the valve leaflets at the onset of diastole.

Prevalence and Etiology

AR has numerous causes, which can be grouped according to the structural components of the valve apparatus affected. AR may be caused by primary disease of the aortic leaflets and/or disease of the aortic root.

Aortic leaflet calcific degeneration, myxomatous degeneration, infective endocarditis, rheumatic disease, a bicuspid AV, and anorectic medications, such as fenfluramine and phentermine, all lead to distortion of the valve leaflets and prevent proper coaptation.[25,109-111] Aortic root dilatation caused by aortic dissection; trauma; chronic systemic hypertension; aortitis from syphilis, viral syndromes, or other systemic arteritides (eg, giant cell and Takayasu); and connective tissue disorders, such as Marfan's syndrome, Reiter's disease, Ehlers-Danlos syndrome, osteogenesis imperfecta, and rheumatoid arthritis, leads to improper leaflet coaptation and consequent AR.[112-117] AR is seen most commonly in combination with AS due to calcific or rheumatic disease in which some degree (usually mild) of AR is present. In patients with pure AR undergoing AVR, AR secondary to aortic dilation is now more common than primary valve disease.[118]

Pathophysiology

The pathophysiology of AR varies according to the onset and duration of the disease process.

ACUTE AORTIC REGURGITATION

AR that presents in the acute setting is typically caused by aortic dissection, endocarditis, or trauma. By definition, acute AR is a significant aortic incompetence of sudden onset across a previously competent AV. The blood returned to the left ventricle in diastole causes a sudden increase in LV end-diastolic volume (LVEDV) and reduces the effective or forward stroke volume. LVEDV only increases mildly (20-30%) because the ability of the left ventricle to dilate acutely is limited. This leads to a rapid increase in LVEDP. This increase is greatest in the less compliant, concentrically thickened, hypertrophic myocardium seen in those with AS or chronic systemic hypertension. Increased LVEDP results in increased mean LA and pulmonary venous pressures and produces varying degrees of pulmonary edema.[119] The rapid rise in LVEDP also blunts or abolishes the normally widened pulse pressure seen in chronic AR.[120] In the acute setting, two compensatory mechanisms attempt to maintain an effective CO: an increase in contractility attributable to the Frank-Starling mechanism and an increase in heart rate (HR). The maintenance of an appropriate effective CO depends on the adequacy of these mechanisms, especially systolic pump function.

CHRONIC AORTIC REGURGITATION

In contrast, chronic AR is a slow, insidious process, which sets in motion numerous compensatory mechanisms. The diastolic regurgitant flow in AR increases LVEDV, LVEDP, and wall stress. Adaptive signals lead to an increase in myocyte length and addition of sarcomeres in series in a pattern of remodeling known as *eccentric hypertrophy*. Typically there is a modest increase in LV wall thickness such that the ratio of wall thickness to radius is close to normal. Chamber enlargement in the setting of normal systolic function increases total stroke volume and maintains forward stroke volume (total stroke volume minus regurgitant volume).[121] The increased total stroke volume coupled with a normal to slightly elevated LVEDP is responsible for the wide pulse pressure seen

in chronic AR. Forward stroke volume in AR is increased by any physiologic change that decreases afterload or increases HR. Increasing HR increases forward stroke volume by itself, but it also decreases diastolic filling time and hence regurgitant flow time and volume. The peripheral vasodilatation and increased HR that accompany exercise increase forward stroke volume in this manner.[122] This also illustrates the physiologic basis for vasodilator therapy in the treatment of AR, and explains why bradycardia and use of negative chronotropic agents should be avoided.

As AR progresses, the hypertrophic response becomes inadequate,[123] and/or the preload reserve is eventually exhausted.[124] Thereafter, any further increase in afterload creates afterload mismatch and results in a reduction in EF. Although the hypertrophied myocardium may provide adequate compensation for many years, eventually maladaptive signals, which lead to decreased myocyte survival and fibrosis, predominate. The myocardium becomes incapable of sustaining the increased work load imposed upon it and heart failure ensues.

Myocardial ischemia in AR, which can result from both decreased coronary artery perfusion and increased myocardial oxygen demand, may lead to further impairment of LVF. The decrease in diastolic coronary perfusion that occurs with a severe reduction in aortic diastolic pressure is only partially compensated by increased coronary arterial flow during systole. In severe AR, there may even be reversal of coronary arterial flow. Superimposed CAD only exacerbates the effect of decreased diastolic coronary perfusion pressure. On the other hand, increased LV muscle mass, wall tension, and systolic ventricular pressure all contribute to increased myocardial oxygen demand. The subsequent ischemia caused by decreased perfusion and increased oxygen demand can lead to cell death and fibrosis, and chronically, can contribute to systolic dysfunction.

Clinical Presentation

SYMPTOMS

The presentation varies depending on the acuity of onset, severity of regurgitation, compliance of the ventricle and aorta, and hemodynamic conditions present at the time. Acute AR can be debilitating and life threatening if not treated emergently, whereas chronic AR is usually well tolerated for years. Severe acute AR commonly presents catastrophically with sudden cardiovascular collapse. Patients also often present with ischemic chest pain caused by decreased coronary blood flow coupled with rapidly increased myocardial oxygen consumption.

Patients with chronic, compensated AR remain asymptomatic for prolonged periods of time while the left ventricle gradually enlarges. Symptoms of heart failure, such as exertional dyspnea, orthopnea, and paroxysmal nocturnal dyspnea, usually develop gradually only after considerable ventricular hypertrophy and decompensation. Patients with severe AR may experience palpitations during emotional stress or exertion, an uncomfortable awareness of each heartbeat, especially at the ventricular apex, angina pectoris, nocturnal angina, or atypical chest pain syndromes, such as thoracic pain owing to pounding of the heart against the chest wall.[125]

SIGNS

Physical examination findings of AR vary with the chronicity of the disease process. Many of the classic findings of chronic AR are a result of the widened pulse pressure. They include a "water-hammer pulse" (Corrigan pulse), head bobbing with each heartbeat (De Musset sign), capillary pulsations in the lips and fingers (Quincke pulses), pulsus bisferiens, "pistol shot sounds" on auscultation of the femoral artery (Traube sign), pulsations of the uvula (Müller sign). Although interesting, these signs are not necessarily clinically useful. The classic auscultatory finding of AR is an immediate to early diastolic, blowing, decrescendo murmur. It is best heard with the diaphragm at the left sternal border while the patient is sitting, leaning forward, and holding respiration in deep exhalation. The murmur is often better heard along the right sternal border when AR is caused primarily by root disease.[126] When it is soft, isometric exercise, such as handgrip, can increase its intensity by increasing aortic diastolic pressure. In severe AR, the murmur may be holodiastolic. S_1 is usually soft because the mitral leaflets are close to each other at the onset of systole. S_2 is usually single because the AV does not close properly, or because LV ejection time is prolonged and P_2 is obscured by the early diastolic murmur. Other findings, if present, are associated with CHF, for example, rales and S3.[125] As discussed, the pulse pressure in acute AR is not widened; hence many of the classic signs of chronic AR are not seen in the acute setting. Instead, signs of CHF predominate.

ELECTROCARDIOGRAM

The increased LV mass in chronic AR leads to left axis deviation and increased QRS complex amplitude. A strain pattern and reduction in the total QRS complex amplitude in patients with chronic severe AR is highly predictive of severe depression of EF resulting from inadequate hypertrophy.[127] Q waves in leads I, V1, and V3 through V6 are indicative of diastolic volume overload.[128] LV conduction defects occur late in the course and are usually associated with LV dysfunction. Overall, ECG is an inaccurate predictor of AR severity.

ROENTGENOGRAM

The chest radiograph typically shows a "normal"-sized heart with pulmonary edema, although there may be some enlargement of all cardiac chambers and the main pulmonary artery. The aorta may be dilated if aortic root disease is the cause of AR. There may be signs of pulmonary emboli in AR caused by endocarditis when there is concomitant tricuspid valve endocarditis.

ECHOCARDIOGRAPHY

Echocardiography is the most useful diagnostic modality in both the initial diagnosis and continued monitoring of patients with AR. Transthoracic echocardiography (TTE) is the most commonly used imaging tool. TTE provides noninvasive assessment of the AV and aortic anatomy; the presence, severity, and etiology of regurgitation; and the size and function of the left ventricle. TEE is used when the patient's body habitus does not allow for adequate assessment with TTE and to evaluate the AV and ascending aorta in patients with suspected aortic dissection (Fig. 26-8).

Two-dimensional (2D) echocardiography with Doppler color-flow mapping has been used routinely to assess the severity of AR.[49,129-131] The color-flow jets are typically composed of three components: (1) a proximal flow convergence zone (area of acceleration into the orifice); (2) the vena contracta (the narrowest and highest-velocity region of the jet); and (3) the distal jet itself in the LV cavity. Assessment of the severity of AR is determined qualitatively by jet width and vena contracta width, and quantitatively by regurgitant volume, regurgitant fraction, and regurgitant orifice area (Table 26-2). The regurgitant orifice area is calculated by dividing the regurgitant volume by the velocity time integral of the AR jet calculated by continuous wave Doppler.[132] Measurement of LV dimensions, such as end-systolic

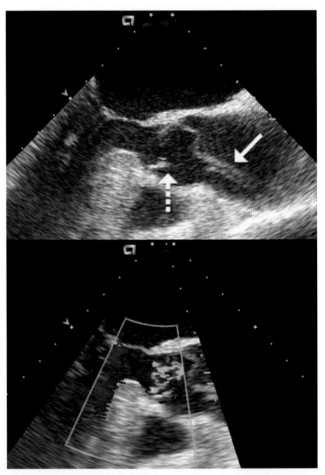

FIGURE 26-8 Transesophageal echocardiographic images of aortic regurgitation due to acute aortic dissection. (*Top*) Showing dilated annulus, prolapse of aortic valve leaflet (*dotted arrow*), and intimal flap (*solid arrow*). (*Bottom*) Color Doppler showing regurgitant flow.

TABLE 26-2: Classification of Aortic Regurgitation Severity

Indicator	Mild	Moderate	Severe
Angiographic grade	1+	2+	3-4+
Jet width	<25% LVOT	25-65% LVOT	>65% LVOT
Vena contracta width (cm)	<0.3	0.3-0.6	>0.6
Regurgitant volume (mL per beat)	<30	30-59	≥60
Regurgitant fraction (%)	<30	30-49	≥50
Regurgitant orifice area (cm²)	<0.10	0.10-0.29	≥0.30

and end-diastolic volumes and wall thickness, are useful for determining LV changes and function. Additional echocardiographic findings in AR include premature closure of the mitral valve, diastolic fluttering of the anterior mitral leaflet from regurgitant flow, and less commonly, diastolic fluttering of the posterior mitral leaflet.[133]

EXERCISE STRESS TESTING

Exercise stress testing can provide valuable information in patients with AR, especially in those whose symptoms are equivocal or difficult to assess. In the management of AR, the presence of symptoms with exercise testing is equivalent to symptoms at rest, as both circumstances warrant AVR.

CARDIAC CATHETERIZATION

Cardiac catheterization is less frequently used to assess the severity of AR. It is most commonly used during preoperative assessment of coronary anatomy in patients requiring AV repair or replacement. The amount of regurgitant flow can be determined by calculating the angiographic stroke volume minus a measured fixed stroke volume. The difference between these two measured volumes divided by the angiographic stroke volume determines the regurgitant fraction. LVEDP is measured directly and EF is estimated roughly.

COMPUTED TOMOGRAPHY

CT can be used to assess the severity of AR by measurement of the regurgitant orifice area, but currently the results are inferior to echocardiography.[134] Several studies have demonstrated the utility of CT to detect moderate and severe AR, but inaccuracies are seen with lesser degrees of AR.[135-137]

MAGNETIC RESONANCE IMAGING

With the recent advancements in MRI technology, MRI cineangiography is able to provide some of the same information provided by TTE and TEE. MRI in some aspects provides superior resolution of the valves and better quantification of regurgitant flow and LVF. The regurgitant volume

can be calculated by quantitative assessment, wherein aortic flow is subtracted from the ventricular stroke volume measured by the volumetric technique. It also can be assessed using flow mapping downstream from the AV by measuring the retrograde volume flow after valve closure. This method is more reproducible and is used more frequently for follow-up studies. However, MRI is costly, and expertise is not available in most centers. Future improvements in technology may reduce costs and increase its availability, thereby making it a standard imaging modality along with or in substitution for echocardiography.[77,138,139]

Management

Surgical options for AR are AV repair and AV replacement. AV repair is preferred due to longer durability, equal short-term- and better long-term survival, and no added risk of prosthetic valve complications. When feasible, AV repair should be attempted prior to performing AV replacement.[140,141] Patients with AR associated with ascending aortic aneurism can undergo valve-sparing aortic root replacement, also called David's procedure. Effort is made to preserve the natural AV to avoid the need for long-term anticoagulation and reduce risk of stroke.[142,143]

Medical management of patients with chronic AR and hypertension consists of calcium channel blockers or ACE inhibitors/angiotensin receptor blockers (ARBs). Beta blockers are only indicated for patients with severe AR who are not candidates for surgical intervention with symptoms or LV dysfunction.[49]

Acute AR is treated by early AV repair or replacement, depending on the etiology. With inadequate time for the left ventricle to compensate by eccentric hypertrophy, progressive CHF, tachycardia, and diminished CO occur rapidly. Vasodilators and inotropic agents, which augment forward flow and reduce LVEDP, may be helpful to manage the patient temporarily before surgery.

Compensated chronic AR is well tolerated by most patients.[144-146] Current recommendations for the management of chronic AR depend on the presence of symptoms, LVF, and LV dimensions. Patients with symptoms or EFs less than or equal to 50% should undergo AV repair or replacement.[49] Surgery is currently not recommended for patients who are asymptomatic and have normal LVF and LV dimensions, even with severe chronic AR. In asymptomatic patients with normal LVF, it is reasonable to perform surgery with an LV end-systolic dimension (LVESD) approaching 50 mm or LV end-diastolic dimension (LVEDD) approaching 65 mm if surgical risk is low.[49]

After surgery, LVEDV and LVEDP decrease significantly and with the decrease in preload, EF also decreases.[147] LV size and function eventually return to normal if the operation is timed correctly.[148-159] The best postoperative predictor of recovery in systolic function is reduction in LVEDD because the magnitude of reduction correlates well with the magnitude of increase in EF.[148] Importantly, 80% of the total reduction in LVEDD after AVR occurs within 10 to 14 days after surgery.[148,153,160] Additional changes postoperatively include regression of myocardial hypertrophy, normalization of mass-to-volume ratio, increase in diastolic coronary perfusion, and decrease in peak systolic wall stress.[148,160,161]

Despite surgery, LV dilation and/or impaired LVF may continue in some patients. The best predictors of persistent LV dilation are greater preoperative LVESD and end-diastolic radius to wall thickness ratio.[162,163] In addition to these measures, greater preoperative LVEDD and duration of LV dysfunction, and reduced EF and fractional shortening predict persistent LV dysfunction.[148,152,164-167]

Predictors for the development of future symptoms, LV dysfunction, or death include age, LVESV, LVEDV, and EF during exercise.[144,168-172] Currently, there is insufficient evidence to determine if EF during exercise is a reliable predictor because exercise EF is dependent on too many factors, such as myocardial contractility,[173] severity of volume overload,[144,173-175] and exercise-induced changes in preload and PVR.[175]

REFERENCES

1. Anderson RH, Devine WA, Ho SY, Smith A, McKay R: The myth of the aortic annulus: the anatomy of the subaortic outflow tract. *Ann Thorac Surg* 1991; 52:640-646.
2. Broom ND: The Third George Swanson Christie memorial lecture. Connective tissue function and malfunction: a biomechanical perspective. *Pathology (Phila)* 1988; 20:93-104.
3. Deck JD: Endothelial cell orientation on aortic valve leaflets. *Cardiovasc Res* 1986; 20:760-767.
4. Thubrikar M, Harry R, Nolan SP: Normal aortic valve function in dogs. *Am J Cardiol* 1977; 40:563-568.
5. Gnyaneshwar R, Kumar RK, Balakrishnan KR: Dynamic analysis of the aortic valve using a finite element model. *Ann Thorac Surg* 2002; 73:1122-1129.
6. Deck JD, Thubrikar MJ, Schneider PJ, Nolan SP: Structure, stress, and tissue repair in aortic valve leaflets. *Cardiovasc Res* 1988; 22:7-16.
7. Zimmerman J: The functional and surgical anatomy of the aortic valve. *Isr J Med Sci* 1969; 5:862-866.
8. Mercer JL: The movements of the dog's aortic valve studied by high speed cineangiography. *Br J Radiol* 1973; 46:344-349.
9. Robicsek F: Leonardo da Vinci and the sinuses of Valsalva. *Ann Thorac Surg* 1991; 52:328-335.
10. Bellhouse BJ, Reid KG: Fluid mechanics of the aortic valve. *Br Heart J* 1969; 31:391.
11. Sabbah HN, Stein PD: Investigation of the theory and mechanism of the origin of the second heart sound. *Circ Res* 1976; 39:874-882.
12. Carabello BA, Paulus WJ: Aortic stenosis. *The Lancet* 2009; 373:956-966.
13. Otto CM, Lind BK, Kitzman DW, Gersh BJ, Siscovick DS: Association of aortic-valve sclerosis with cardiovascular mortality and morbidity in the elderly. *N Engl J Med* 1999; 341:142-147.
14. Nkomo VT, Gardin JM, Skelton TN, et al: Burden of valvular heart diseases: a population-based study. *Lancet Lond Engl* 2006; 368:1005-1011.
15. Stewart BF, Siscovick D, Lind BK, et al: Clinical factors associated with calcific aortic valve disease fn1. *J Am Coll Cardiol* 1997; 29:630-634.
16. Ghaisas NK, Foley JB, O'Briain DS, et al: Adhesion molecules in non-rheumatic aortic valve disease: endothelial expression, serum levels and effects of valve replacement. *J Am Coll Cardiol* 2000; 36:2257-2262.
17. O'Brien KD, Shavelle DM, Caulfield MT, et al: Association of angiotensin-converting enzyme with low-density lipoprotein in aortic valvular lesions and in human plasma. *Circulation* 2002; 106:2224-2230.
18. Olsson M, Thyberg J, Nilsson J: Presence of oxidized low density lipoprotein in nonrheumatic stenotic aortic valves. *Arterioscler Thromb Vasc Biol* 1999; 19:1218-1222.
19. Otto CM, Kuusisto J, Reichenbach DD, Gown AM, O'Brien KD: Characterization of the early lesion of 'degenerative' valvular aortic stenosis. Histological and immunohistochemical studies. *Circulation* 1994; 90:844-853.
20. Rajamannan NM, Gersh B, Bonow RO: Calcific aortic stenosis: from bench to the bedside—emerging clinical and cellular concepts. *Heart Br Card Soc* 2003; 89:801-805.
21. Hultgren HN: Osteitis deformans (Paget's disease) and calcific disease of the heart valves. *Am J Cardiol* 1998; 81:1461-1464.
22. Hangaishi M, Taguchi J, Ikari Y, et al: Aortic valve stenosis in alkaptonuria. Images in cardiovascular medicine. *Circulation* 1998; 98:1148-1149.
23. Subramanian R, Olson LJ, Edwards WD: Surgical pathology of pure aortic stenosis: a study of 374 cases. *Mayo Clin Proc* 1984; 59:683-690.
24. Kouchoukos NT, Blackstone EH, Doty DB, Hanley FL, Karp RB: *Kirklin/Barratt-Boyes Cardiac Surgery: Morphology, Diagnostic Criteria, Natural History, Techniques, Results, and Indications.* Churchill Livingstone, 2003.
25. Fedak PWM, Verma S, David TE, et al: Clinical and pathophysiological implications of a bicuspid aortic valve. *Circulation* 2002; 106:900-904.
26. Tadros TM, Klein MD, Shapira OM: Ascending aortic dilatation associated with bicuspid aortic valve pathophysiology, molecular biology, and clinical implications. *Circulation* 2009; 119:880-890.
27. Siu SC, Silversides CK: Bicuspid aortic valve disease. *J Am Coll Cardiol* 2010; 55:2789-2800.
28. Garg V, Muth AN, Ransom JF, et al: Mutations in NOTCH1 cause aortic valve disease. *Nature* 2005; 437:270-274.
29. Mohamed SA, Aherrahrou Z, Liptau H, et al: Novel missense mutations (p.T596M and p.P1797H) in NOTCH1 in patients with bicuspid aortic valve. *Biochem Biophys Res Commun* 2006; 345:1460-1465.
30. Fedak PWM, de Sa MP, Verma S, et al: Vascular matrix remodeling in patients with bicuspid aortic valve malformations: implications for aortic dilatation. *J Thorac Cardiovasc Surg* 2003; 126:797-806.
31. Roberts WC: Anatomically isolated aortic valvular disease. The case against its being of rheumatic etiology. *Am J Med* 1970; 49:151-159.
32. Boudoulas KD, Borer JS, Boudoulas H: Etiology of valvular heart disease in the 21st century. *Cardiology* 2013; 126:139-152.
33. Roberts WC, Ko JM: Frequency by decades of unicuspid, bicuspid, and tricuspid aortic valves in adults having isolated aortic valve replacement for aortic stenosis, with or without associated aortic regurgitation. *Circulation* 2005; 111:920-925.
34. Passik CS, Ackermann DM, Pluth JR, Edwards WD: Temporal changes in the causes of aortic stenosis: a surgical pathologic study of 646 cases. *Mayo Clin Proc* 1987; 62:119-123.
35. Bonow RO, Carabello B, C. de Leon A, et al: Guidelines for the Management of Patients With Valvular Heart Disease Executive Summary A Report of the American College of Cardiology/American Heart Association Task Force on Practice Guidelines (Committee on Management of Patients With Valvular Heart Disease). *Circulation* 1998; 98:1949-1984.
36. Hess OM, Ritter M, Schneider J, et al: Diastolic stiffness and myocardial structure in aortic valve disease before and after valve replacement. *Circulation* 1984; 69:855-865.
37. Marcus ML, Doty DB, Hiratzka LF, Wright CB, Eastham CL: Decreased coronary reserve: a mechanism for angina pectoris in patients with aortic stenosis and normal coronary arteries. *N Engl J Med* 1982; 307:1362-1366.
38. Mihaljevic T, Nowicki ER, Rajeswaran J, et al: Survival after valve replacement for aortic stenosis: implications for decision making. *J Thorac Cardiovasc Surg* 2008; 135:1270-1278; discussion 1278-1279.
39. Fielitz J, Hein S, Mitrovic V, et al: Activation of the cardiac renin-angiotensin system and increased myocardial collagen expression in human aortic valve disease. *J Am Coll Cardiol* 2001; 37:1443-1449.
40. Walther T, Schubert A, Falk V, et al: Left ventricular reverse remodeling after surgical therapy for aortic stenosis: correlation to renin-angiotensin system gene expression. *Circulation* 2002; 106:I-23-26.
41. Yussman MG, Toyokawa T, Odley A, et al: Mitochondrial death protein Nix is induced in cardiac hypertrophy and triggers apoptotic cardiomyopathy. *Nat Med* 2002; 8:725-730.
42. Whelan RS, Kaplinskiy V, Kitsis RN: Cell death in the pathogenesis of heart disease: mechanisms and significance. *Annu Rev Physiol* 2010; 72:19-44.
43. Ho KK, Anderson KM, Kannel WB, Grossman W, Levy D: Survival after the onset of congestive heart failure in Framingham Heart Study subjects. *Circulation* 1993; 88:107-115.
44. Turina J, Hess O, Sepulcri F, Krayenbuehl HP: Spontaneous course of aortic valve disease. *Eur Heart J* 1987; 8:471-483.

45. Zoghbi WA, Farmer KL, Soto JG, Nelson JG, Quinones MA: Accurate noninvasive quantification of stenotic aortic valve area by Doppler echocardiography. *Circulation* 1986; 73:452-459.

46. Oh JK, Taliercio CP, Holmeset DR, et al: Prediction of the severity of aortic stenosis by Doppler aortic valve area determination: prospective Doppler-catheterization correlation in 100 patients. *J Am Coll Cardiol* 1988; 11:1227-1234.

47. Baumgartner H, Hung J, Bermejo J, et al: Echocardiographic assessment of valve stenosis: EAE/ASE recommendations for clinical practice. *Eur Heart J - Cardiovasc Imaging* 2008. doi:10.1093/ejechocard/jen303.

48. Quiñones MA, Otto CM, Stoddard M, Waggoner A, Zoghbi WA: Recommendations for quantification of Doppler echocardiography: a report from the Doppler quantification task force of the nomenclature and standards committee of the American Society of Echocardiography. *J Am Soc Echocardiogr* 2002; 15:167-184.

49. Nishimura RA, Otto CM, Bonowet RO, et al: 2014 AHA/ACC Guideline for the Management of Patients With Valvular Heart Disease: a Report of the American College of Cardiology/American Heart Association Task Force on Practice Guidelines. *J Am Coll Cardiol* 2014; 63:e57-e185.

50. Minners J, Allgeier M, Gohlke-Baerwolf C, et al: Inconsistencies of echocardiographic criteria for the grading of aortic valve stenosis. *Eur Heart J* 2008; 29:1043-1048.

51. Gorlin R, Gorlin SG: Hydraulic formula for calculation of the area of the stenotic mitral valve, other cardiac valves, and central circulatory shunts. I. *Am Heart J* 1951; 41:1-29.

52. Segal J, Lerner DJ, Miller DC, et al: When should doppler-determined valve area be better than the Gorlin formula? Variation in hydraulic constants in low flow states. *J Am Coll Cardiol* 1987; 9:1294-1305.

53. Tardif JC, Rodrigues AG, Hardy JF, et al: Simultaneous determination of aortic valve area by the Gorlin formula and by transesophageal echocardiography under different transvalvular flow conditions. Evidence that anatomic aortic valve area does not change with variations in flow in aortic stenosis. *J Am Coll Cardiol* 1997; 29:1296-1302.

54. Blumberg FC, Pfeifer M, Holmer SR, et al: Transgastric Doppler echocardiographic assessment of the severity of aortic stenosis using multiplane transesophageal echocardiography. *Am J Cardiol* 1997; 79: 1273-1275.

55. Ross J, Braunwald E: Aortic stenosis. *Circulation* 1968; 38:61-67.

56. Schwartz LS, Goldfischer J, Sprague GJ, Schwartz SP: Syncope and sudden death in aortic stenosis. *Am J Cardiol* 1969; 23:647-658.

57. Otto CM, Burwash IG, Legget ME, et al: Prospective study of asymptomatic valvular aortic stenosis. Clinical, echocardiographic, and exercise predictors of outcome. *Circulation* 1997; 95:2262-2270.

58. Vincentelli A, Susen S, Le Tourneau T, et al: Acquired von Willebrand syndrome in aortic stenosis. *N Engl J Med* 2003; 349:343-349.

59. Pellikka PA, Sarano ME, Nishimura RA, et al: Outcome of 622 adults with asymptomatic, hemodynamically significant aortic stenosis during prolonged follow-up. *Circulation* 2005; 111:3290-3295.

60. Selzer A: Changing aspects of the natural history of valvular aortic stenosis. *N Engl J Med* 1987; 317:91-98.

61. Gjertsson P, Caidahl K, Farasati M, Odén A, Bech-Hanssen O: Preoperative moderate to severe diastolic dysfunction: a novel Doppler echocardiographic long-term prognostic factor in patients with severe aortic stenosis. *J Thorac Cardiovasc Surg* 2005; 129:890-896.

62. Nagueh M, Sherif F, Middleton KJ, Kopelen HA, Zoghbi WA, Quiñones MA: Doppler tissue imaging: a noninvasive technique for evaluation of left ventricular relaxation and estimation of filling pressures. *J Am Coll Cardiol* 1997; 30:1527-1533.

63. Ommen SR, et al: Clinical utility of Doppler echocardiography and tissue Doppler imaging in the estimation of left ventricular filling pressures a comparative simultaneous Doppler-catheterization study. *Circulation* 2000; 102:1788-1794.

64. Maurer MS, Spevack D, Burkhoff D, Kronzon I: Diastolic dysfunction: can it be diagnosed by Doppler echocardiography? *J Am Coll Cardiol* 2004; 44:1543-1549.

65. Agricola E, Oppizzi M, Pisani M, Margonato A: Stress echocardiography in heart failure. *Cardiovasc Ultrasound* 2004; 2:11.

66. Amato MC, Moffa PJ, Werner KE, Ramires JA: Treatment decision in asymptomatic aortic valve stenosis: role of exercise testing. *Heart Br Card Soc* 2001; 86:381-386.

67. Das P, Rimington H, Chambers J: Exercise testing to stratify risk in aortic stenosis. *Eur Heart J* 2005; 26:1309-1313.

68. deFilippi CR, Willett DL, Brickner ME, et al: Usefulness of dobutamine echocardiography in distinguishing severe from nonsevere valvular aortic stenosis in patients with depressed left ventricular function and low transvalvular gradients. *Am J Cardiol* 1995; 75:191-194.

69. Monin J-L, Quéré JP, Monchi M, et al: Low-gradient aortic stenosis: operative risk stratification and predictors for long-term outcome: a multicenter study using dobutamine stress hemodynamics. *Circulation* 2003; 108, 319-324.

70. Nishimura RA, Carabello BA: Hemodynamics in the cardiac catheterization laboratory of the 21st century. *Circulation* 2012; 125:2138-2150.

71. Saikrishnan N, Kumar G, Sawaya FJ, Lerakis S, Yoganathan AP: Accurate assessment of aortic stenosis a review of diagnostic modalities and hemodynamics. *Circulation* 2014; 129:244-253.

72. Melina G, Scott MJ, Cunanan CM, Rubens MB, Yacoub MH: In-vitro verification of the electron beam tomography method for measurement of heart valve calcification. *J Heart Valve Dis* 2002; 11:402-407; discussion 408.

73. Alkadhi H, Wildermuth S, Plass A, et al: Aortic stenosis: comparative evaluation of 16-detector row CT and echocardiography. *Radiology* 2006; 240:47-55.

74. Shah RG, Novaro GM, Blandon RJ, et al: Aortic valve area: meta-analysis of diagnostic performance of multi-detector computed tomography for aortic valve area measurements as compared to transthoracic echocardiography. *Int J Cardiovasc Imaging* 2009; 25:601-609.

75. Delgado V, Ng AC, van de Veire NR, et al: Transcatheter aortic valve implantation: role of multi-detector row computed tomography to evaluate prosthesis positioning and deployment in relation to valve function. *Eur Heart J* 2010; 31:1114-1123.

76. Cawley PJ, Maki JH, Otto CM: Cardiovascular magnetic resonance imaging for valvular heart disease: technique and validation. *Circulation* 2009; 119:468-478.

77. Cranney GB, Lotan CS, Dean L, et al: Left ventricular volume measurement using cardiac axis nuclear magnetic resonance imaging. Validation by calibrated ventricular angiography. *Circulation* 1990; 82:154-163.

78. Caruthers SD, Lin SJ, Brown P, et al: Practical value of cardiac magnetic resonance imaging for clinical quantification of aortic valve stenosis: comparison with echocardiography. *Circulation* 2003; 108:2236-2243.

79. John AS, Dill T, Brandt RR, et al: Magnetic resonance to assess the aortic valve area in aortic stenosis: how does it compare to current diagnostic standards? *J Am Coll Cardiol* 2003; 42:519-526.

80. Beyerbacht HP, Lamb HJ, van Der Laarse A, et al: Aortic valve replacement in patients with aortic valve stenosis improves myocardial metabolism and diastolic function. *Radiology* 2001; 219:637-643.

81. Cowell SJ, Newby DE, Prescott RJ, et al: A randomized trial of intensive lipid-lowering therapy in calcific aortic stenosis. *N Engl J Med* 2005; 352:2389-2397.

82. Rossebø AB, Pedersen TR, Boman K, et al: Intensive lipid lowering with simvastatin and ezetimibe in aortic stenosis. *N Engl J Med* 2008; 359: 1343-1356.

83. Chan KL, Teo K, Dumesnil JG, Ni A, Tam J: Effect of lipid lowering with rosuvastatin on progression of aortic stenosis: results of the aortic stenosis progression observation: Measuring effects of rosuvastatin (Astronomer) trial. *Circulation* 2010; 121:306-314.

84. Moura LM, Ramos SF, Zamorano JL, et al: Rosuvastatin affecting aortic valve endothelium to slow the progression of aortic stenosis. *J Am Coll Cardiol* 2007; 49:554-561.

85. Wilson W, Taubert KA, Gewitz M, et al: Prevention of infective endocarditis: guidelines from the American Heart Association: a guideline from the American Heart Association Rheumatic Fever, Endocarditis, and Kawasaki Disease Committee, Council on Cardiovascular Disease in the Young, and the Council on Clinical Cardiology, Council on Cardiovascular Surgery and Anesthesia, and the Quality of Care and Outcomes Research Interdisciplinary Working Group. *Circulation* 2007; 116:1736-1754.

86. Khot UN, Novaro GM, Popović ZB, et al: Nitroprusside in critically ill patients with left ventricular dysfunction and aortic stenosis. *N Engl J Med* 2003; 348:1756-1763.

87. Gillinov AM, Lytle BW, Hoang V, et al: The atherosclerotic aorta at aortic valve replacement: surgical strategies and results. *J Thorac Cardiovasc Surg* 2000; 120:957-963.

88. Blais C, Dumesnil JG, Baillot R, et al: Impact of valve prosthesis-patient mismatch on short-term mortality after aortic valve replacement. *Circulation* 2003; 108:983-988.

89. Johnston DR, Soltesz EG, Vakil N, et al: Long-term durability of bioprosthetic aortic valves: implications from 12,569 implants. *Ann Thorac Surg* 2015; 99:1239-1247.

90. Kapadia SR, Leon MB, Makkar RR, et al: 5-year outcomes of transcatheter aortic valve replacement compared with standard treatment for patients with inoperable aortic stenosis (PARTNER 1): a randomised controlled trial. *Lancet* 2015. doi:10.1016/S0140-6736(15)60290-2.

91. Mack MJ, Leon MB, Smith CR, et al: 5-year outcomes of transcatheter aortic valve replacement or surgical aortic valve replacement for high surgical risk patients with aortic stenosis (PARTNER 1): a randomised controlled trial. *Lancet* 2015. doi:10.1016/S0140-6736(15)60308-7.

92. Svensson LG, Blackstone EH, Rajeswaran J, et al: Comprehensive analysis of mortality among patients undergoing TAVR: results of the PARTNER trial. *J Am Coll Cardiol* 2014; 64:158-168.

93. Leon MB, Smith CR, Mack M, et al: Transcatheter aortic-valve implantation for aortic stenosis in patients who cannot undergo surgery. *N Engl J Med* 2010; 363:1597-1607.

94. Otto CM, Mickel MC, Kennedy JW, et al: Three-year outcome after balloon aortic valvuloplasty. Insights into prognosis of valvular aortic stenosis. *Circulation* 1994; 89:642-650.

95. Ben-Dor I, Pichard AD, Satler LF, et al: Complications and outcome of balloon aortic valvuloplasty in high-risk or inoperable patients. *JACC Cardiovasc Interv* 2010; 3:1150-1156.

96. Ben-Dor I, Maluenda G, Dvir D, et al: Balloon aortic valvuloplasty for severe aortic stenosis as a bridge to transcatheter/surgical aortic valve replacement. *Catheter Cardiovasc Interv* 2013; 82:632-637.

97. Rosenhek R, Binder T, Porenta G, et al: Predictors of outcome in severe, asymptomatic aortic stenosis. *N Engl J Med* 2000; 343:611-617.

98. Pai RG, Kapoor N, Bansal RC, Varadarajan P: Malignant natural history of asymptomatic severe aortic stenosis: benefit of aortic valve replacement. *Ann Thorac Surg* 2006; 82:2116-2122.

99. Varadarajan P, Kapoor N, Bansal RC, Pai RG: Survival in elderly patients with severe aortic stenosis is dramatically improved by aortic valve replacement: results from a cohort of 277 patients aged > or =80 years. *Eur J Cardio-Thorac Surg Off J Eur Assoc Cardio-Thorac Surg* 2006; 30:722-727.

100. Orsinell DA, Aurigemma GP, Battista S, Krendel S, Gaasch WH: Left ventricular hypertrophy and mortality after aortic valve replacement for aortic stenosisA high risk subgroup identified by preoperative relation wall thickness. *J Am Coll Cardiol* 1993; 22:1679-1683.

101. Mehta RH, Bruckman D, Das S, et al: Implications of increased left ventricular mass index on in-hospital outcomes in patients undergoing aortic valve surgery. *J Thorac Cardiovasc Surg* 2001; 122:919-928.

102. Fuster RG, Argudo JA, Albarova OG, et al: Left ventricular mass index in aortic valve surgery: a new index for early valve replacement? *Eur J Cardiothorac Surg* 2003; 23:696-702.

103. Duncan AI, Lowe BS, Garcia MJ, et al: Influence of concentric left ventricular remodeling on early mortality after aortic valve replacement. *Ann Thorac Surg* 2008; 85:2030-2039.

104. Cioffi G, Faggiano P, Vizzardi E, et al: Prognostic effect of inappropriately high left ventricular mass in asymptomatic severe aortic stenosis. *Heart Br Card Soc* 2011; 97:301-307.

105. Lancellotti P, Magne J, Donal E, et al: Clinical outcome in asymptomatic severe aortic stenosis: insights from the new proposed aortic stenosis grading classification. *J Am Coll Cardiol* 2012; 59:235-243.

106. Kang D-H, Park SJ, Rim JH, et al: Early surgery versus conventional treatment in asymptomatic very severe aortic stenosis. *Circulation* 2010; 121:1502-1509.

107. Brown ML, Pellikka PA, Schaff HV, et al: The benefits of early valve replacement in asymptomatic patients with severe aortic stenosis. *J Thorac Cardiovasc Surg* 2008; 135:308-315.

108. Birkmeyer JD, Stukel TA, Siewers AE, et al: Surgeon volume and operative mortality in the United States. *N Engl J Med* 2003; 349:2117-2127.

109. Carabello BA: Progress in mitral and aortic regurgitation. *Prog Cardiovasc Dis* 2001; 43:457-475.

110. Maurer G: Aortic regurgitation. *Heart Br Card Soc* 2006; 92:994-1000.

111. Tonnemacher D, Reid C, Kawanishi D, et al: Frequency of myxomatous degeneration of the aortic valve as a cause of isolated aortic regurgitation severe enough to warrant aortic valve replacement. *Am J Cardiol* 1987; 60:1194-1196.

112. Carter JB, Sethi S, Lee GB, Edwards JE: Prolapse of semilunar cusps as causes of aortic insufficiency. *Circulation* 1971; 43:922-932.

113. Emanuel R, Ng RA, Marcomichelakis J, et al: Formes frustes of Marfan's syndrome presenting with severe aortic regurgitation. Clinicogenetic study of 18 families. *Br Heart J* 1977; 39:190-197.

114. Heppner RL, Babitt HI, Bianchine JW, Warbasse JR: Aortic regurgitation and aneurysm of sinus of Valsalva associated with osteogenesis imperfecta. *Am J Cardiol* 1973; 31:654-657.

115. Roberts WC: Aortic dissection: anatomy, consequences, and causes. *Am Heart J* 1981; 101:195-214.

116. Roldan CA: Valvular disease associated with systemic illness. *Cardiol Clin* 1998; 16:531-550.

117. Roldan CA, Chavez J, Wiest PW, Qualls CR, Crawford MH: Aortic root disease and valve disease associated with ankylosing spondylitis. *J Am Coll Cardiol* 1998; 32:1397-1404.

118. Roberts WC, Ko JM, Moore TR, Jones WH: Causes of pure aortic regurgitation in patients having isolated aortic valve replacement at a single US tertiary hospital (1993 to 2005). *Circulation* 2006; 114:422-429.

119. Rahimtoola SH: Recognition and management of acute aortic regurgitation. *Heart Dis Stroke J Prim Care Physicians* 1993; 2:217-221.

120. Reimold SC, Maier SE, Fleischmann KE, et al: Dynamic nature of the aortic regurgitant orifice area during diastole in patients with chronic aortic regurgitation. *Circulation* 1994; 89:2085-2092.

121. Grossman W, Jones D, McLaurin LP: Wall stress and patterns of hypertrophy in the human left ventricle. *J Clin Invest* 1975; 56:56-64.

122. Slørdahl SA, Piene H: Haemodynamic effects of arterial compliance, total peripheral resistance, and glyceryl trinitrate on regurgitant volume in aortic regurgitation. *Cardiovasc Res* 1991; 25:869-874.

123. Gaasch WH: Left ventricular radius to wall thickness ratio. *Am J Cardiol* 1979; 43:1189-1194.

124. Ross J: Afterload mismatch in aortic and mitral valve disease: implications for surgical therapy. *J Am Coll Cardiol* 1985; 5:811-826.

125. DeGowin RL, DeGowin EL, Brown DD, Christensen J: *Degowin & Degowin's Diagnostic Examination*. Mcgraw-Hill, 1994.

126. Otto CM, Bonow RO: *Valvular Heart Disease: A Companion to Braunwald's Heart Disease*. Elsevier Health Sciences, 2009.

127. Scognamiglio R, Fasoli G, Bruni A, Dalla-Volta S: Observations on the capability of the electrocardiogram to detect left ventricular function in chronic severe aortic regurgitation. *Eur Heart J* 1988; 9:54-60.

128. Schamroth L, Schamroth CL, Sareli P, Hummel D: Electrocardiographic differentiation of the causes of left ventricular diastolic overload. *Chest* 1986; 89:95-99.

129. Aurigemma G, Whitfield S, Sweeney A, Fox M, Weiner B: Color Doppler mapping of aortic regurgitation in aortic stenosis: comparison with angiography. *Cardiology* 1992; 81:251-257.

130. Bouchard A, Yock P, Schiller NB, et al: Value of color Doppler estimation of regurgitant volume in patients with chronic aortic insufficiency. *Am Heart J* 1989; 117:1099-1105.

131. Enriquez-Sarano M, Bailey KR, Seward JB, et al: Quantitative Doppler assessment of valvular regurgitation. *Circulation* 1993; 87:841-848.

132. Perry GJ, Helmcke F, Nanda NC, Byard C, Soto B: Evaluation of aortic insufficiency by Doppler color flow mapping. *J Am Coll Cardiol* 1987; 9:952-959.

133. Chia BL: Mitral valve fluttering in aortic insufficiency. *J Clin Ultrasound JCU* 1981; 9:198-200.

134. LaBounty TM, Glasofer S, Devereuxet RB, et al: Comparison of cardiac computed tomographic angiography to transesophageal echocardiography for evaluation of patients with native valvular heart disease. *Am J Cardiol* 2009; 104:1421-1428.

135. Feuchtner GM, Dichtl W, Mülleret S, et al: 64-MDCT for diagnosis of aortic regurgitation in patients referred to CT coronary angiography. *AJR Am J Roentgenol* 2008; 191:W1-7.

136. Feuchtner GM, Dichtl W, Schachneret T, et al: Diagnostic performance of MDCT for detecting aortic valve regurgitation. *AJR Am J Roentgenol* 2006; 186:1676-1681.

137. Jassal DS, Shapiro MD, Neilanet TG, et al: 64-slice multidetector computed tomography (MDCT) for detection of aortic regurgitation and quantification of severity. *Invest Radiol* 2007; 42:507-512.

138. Benjelloun H, Cranney GB, Kirket KA, et al: Interstudy reproducibility of biplane cine nuclear magnetic resonance measurements of left ventricular function. *Am J Cardiol* 1991; 67:1413-1420.

139. Dulce MC, Mostbeck GH, O'Sullivan M, et al: Severity of aortic regurgitation: interstudy reproducibility of measurements with velocity-encoded cine MR imaging. *Radiology* 1992; 185:235-240.

140. Kari FA, Siepe M, Sievers H-H, Beyersdorf F: Repair of the regurgitant bicuspid or tricuspid aortic valve: background, principles, and outcomes. *Circulation* 2013; 128:854-863.

141. De Meester C, Pasquet A, Gerber BL, et al: Valve repair improves the outcome of surgery for chronic severe aortic regurgitation: a propensity score analysis. *J Thorac Cardiovasc Surg* 2014; 148:1913-1920.

142. David TE, Feindel CM: An aortic valve-sparing operation for patients with aortic incompetence and aneurysm of the ascending aorta. *J Thorac Cardiovasc Surg* 1992; 103:617-621; discussion 622.

143. Svensson LG, Cooper M, Batizy LH, Nowicki ER: Simplified David reimplantation with reduction of anular size and creation of artificial sinuses. *Ann Thorac Surg* 2010; 89:1443-1447.

144. Bonow RO, Lakatos E, Maron BJ, Epstein SE: Serial long-term assessment of the natural history of asymptomatic patients with chronic aortic regurgitation and normal left ventricular systolic function. *Circulation* 1991; 84:1625-1635.

145. Ishii K, Hirota Y, Suwa M, et al: Natural history and left ventricular response in chronic aortic regurgitation. *Am J Cardiol* 1996; 78:357-361.

146. Tornos MP, Olona M, Permanyer-Miralda G, et al: Clinical outcome of severe asymptomatic chronic aortic regurgitation: a long-term prospective follow-up study. *Am Heart J* 1995; 130:333-339.

147. Boucher CA, Bingham JB, Osbakken MD, et al: Early changes in left ventricular size and function after correction of left ventricular volume overload. *Am J Cardiol* 1981; 47:991-1004.

148. Bonow RO, Dodd JT, Maron BJ, et al: Long-term serial changes in left ventricular function and reversal of ventricular dilatation after valve replacement for chronic aortic regurgitation. *Circulation* 1988; 78:1108-1120.

149. Bonow RO, Rosing DR, Maronet BJ, et al: Reversal of left ventricular dysfunction after aortic valve replacement for chronic aortic regurgitation: influence of duration of preoperative left ventricular dysfunction. *Circulation* 1984; 70:570-579.

150. Borer JS, Herrold EM, Hochreiteret C, et al: Natural history of left ventricular performance at rest and during exercise after aortic valve replacement for aortic regurgitation. *Circulation* 1991; 84:III133-139.

151. Borer JS, Rosing DR, Kent KM, et al: Left ventricular function at rest and during exercise after aortic valve replacement in patients with aortic regurgitation. *Am J Cardiol* 1979; 44:1297-1305.

152. Carabello BA, Usher BW, Hendrix GH, et al: Predictors of outcome for aortic valve replacement in patients with aortic regurgitation and left ventricular dysfunction: a change in the measuring stick. *J Am Coll Cardiol* 1987; 10:991-997.

153. Carroll JD, Gaasch WH, Zile MR, Levine HJ: Serial changes in left ventricular function after correction of chronic aortic regurgitation. Dependence on early changes in preload and subsequent regression of hypertrophy. *Am J Cardiol* 1983; 51:476-482.

154. Clark DG, McAnulty JH, Rahimtoola SH: Valve replacement in aortic insufficiency with left ventricular dysfunction. *Circulation* 1980; 61:411-421.

155. Fioretti P, Roelandt J, Sclavo M, et al: Postoperative regression of left ventricular dimensions in aortic insufficiency: a long-term echocardiographic study. *J Am Coll Cardiol* 1985; 5:856-861.

156. Gaasch WH, Andrias CW, Levine HJ: Chronic aortic regurgitation: the effect of aortic valve replacement on left ventricular volume, mass and function. *Circulation* 1978; 58:825-836.

157. Schwarz F, Flameng W, Langebartelset F, et al: Impaired left ventricular function in chronic aortic valve disease: survival and function after replacement by Björk-Shiley prosthesis. *Circulation* 1979; 60:48-58.

158. Taniguchi K, Nakano S, Hirose H, et al: Preoperative left ventricular function: minimal requirement for successful late results of valve replacement for aortic regurgitation. *J Am Coll Cardiol* 1987; 10:510-518.

159. Toussaint C, Cribier A, Cazor JL, Soyer R, Letac B: Hemodynamic and angiographic evaluation of aortic regurgitation 8 and 27 months after aortic valve replacement. *Circulation* 1981; 64:456-463.

160. Schuler G, Peterson KL, Johnson AD, et al: Serial noninvasive assessment of left ventricular hypertrophy and function after surgical correction of aortic regurgitation. *Am J Cardiol* 1979; 44:585-594.

161. Fujiwara T, Nogami A, Masaki H, et al: Coronary flow characteristics of left coronary artery in aortic regurgitation before and after aortic valve replacement. *Ann Thorac Surg* 1988; 46:79-84.

162. Gaasch WH, Carroll JD, Levine HJ, Criscitiello MG: Chronic aortic regurgitation: prognostic value of left ventricular end-systolic dimension and end-diastolic radius/thickness ratio. *J Am Coll Cardiol* 1983; 1:775-782.

163. Kumpuris AG, Quinones MA, Waggoner AD, et al: Importance of preoperative hypertrophy, wall stress and end-systolic dimension as echocardiographic predictors of normalization of left ventricular dilatation after valve replacement in chronic aortic insufficiency. *Am J Cardiol* 1982; 49:1091-1100.

164. Bonow RO, Picone AL, McIntosh CL, et al: Survival and functional results after valve replacement for aortic regurgitation from 1976 to 1983: impact of preoperative left ventricular function. *Circulation* 1985; 72:1244-1256.

165. Fioretti P, Roelandt J, Bos RJ, et al: Echocardiography in chronic aortic insufficiency. Is valve replacement too late when left ventricular end-systolic dimension reaches 55 mm? *Circulation* 1983; 67:216-221.

166. Michel PL, Lung B, Abou JS, et al: The effect of left ventricular systolic function on long term survival in mitral and aortic regurgitation. *J Heart Valve Dis* 1995; 4(Suppl 2):S160-168; discussion S168-169.

167. Stone PH, Clark RD, Goldschlager N, Selzer A, Cohn K: Determinants of prognosis of patients with aortic regurgitation who undergo aortic valve replacement. *J Am Coll Cardiol* 1984; 3:1118-1126.

168. Borer JS, Hochreiter C, Herrold EM, et al: Prediction of indications for valve replacement among asymptomatic or minimally symptomatic patients with chronic aortic regurgitation and normal left ventricular performance. *Circulation* 1998; 97:525-534.

169. Scognamiglio R, Rahimtoola SH, Fasoli G, Nistri S, Dalla Volta S: Nifedipine in asymptomatic patients with severe aortic regurgitation and normal left ventricular function. *N Engl J Med* 1994; 331:689-694.

170. Siemienczuk D, Greenberg B, Morris C, et al: Chronic aortic insufficiency: factors associated with progression to aortic valve replacement. *Ann Intern Med* 1989; 110:587-592.

171. Tarasoutchi F, Grinberg M, Spinaet GS, et al: Ten-year clinical laboratory follow-up after application of a symptom-based therapeutic strategy to patients with severe chronic aortic regurgitation of predominant rheumatic etiology. *J Am Coll Cardiol* 2003; 41:1316-1324.

172. Chaliki HP, Mohty D, Avierinos JF, et al: Outcomes after aortic valve replacement in patients with severe aortic regurgitation and markedly reduced left ventricular function. *Circulation* 2002; 106:2687-2693.

173. Shen WF, Roubin GS, Choong CY, et al: Evaluation of relationship between myocardial contractile state and left ventricular function in patients with aortic regurgitation. *Circulation* 1985; 71:31-38.

174. Greenberg B, Massie B, Bristow JD, et al: Long-term vasodilator therapy of chronic aortic insufficiency. A randomized double-blinded, placebo-controlled clinical trial. *Circulation* 1988; 78:92-103.

175. Kawanishi DT, McKay CR, Chandraratna PA, et al: Cardiovascular response to dynamic exercise in patients with chronic symptomatic mild-to-moderate and severe aortic regurgitation. *Circulation* 1986; 73:62-72.

27

Aortic Valve Replacement with a Mechanical Cardiac Valve Prosthesis

Robert W. Emery • Rochus K. Voeller • Robert J. Emery

In 1931, Paul Dudley White stated "There is no treatment for aortic stenosis." Even today the medical therapy of aortic stenosis has not significantly advanced.[1] Conversely, patients may tolerate aortic insufficiency for many years, but as the ventricle starts to dilate, a progressive downhill course begins and early operation is warranted.[2] Definitive therapy for aortic valve disease was unavailable until the advent of cardiopulmonary bypass. Innovative cardiovascular surgeons then began to develop cardiac valve prostheses. Over the subsequent 60 years,[3] the variety of prostheses that have become available for use have expanded greatly. Available aortic valve substitutes include mechanical valve prostheses, stented biologic valve prostheses, stentless biologic valve prostheses, human homograft tissue (both as isolated valve replacement and aortic root replacement), and a combination of a biologic valve utilizing a pulmonary autograft and pulmonary outflow tract replacement with heterograft prostheses (Ross procedure). Most recently, innovative transarterial/apical aortic valve replacement (TAVR) has gained approval in Europe and North America with acceptable intermediate term results.[4] Reports of the use of novel sutureless bioprosthetic valves are appearing.[5] This chapter focuses on the use of mechanical valve replacement in the aortic position.

HISTORY

In 1952, Hufnagel used an aortic valve ball and cage prosthesis heterotopically in the descending thoracic aorta to treat aortic insufficiency.[6] After the advent of cardiopulmonary bypass, initial attempts at aortic valve replacement (AVR) consisted of replacement of the individual aortic cusps with Ivalon gussets or fascialata sewn to the annulus or repair of aortic valve by bicuspidization.[7] When successful, these prostheses often calcified and results were short-lived. Shortly thereafter, surgical pioneers Starr, Braunwald, and Harkin began replacement of the aortic valve in the orthotopic position. First-generation aortic valve prostheses, the ball and cage, became the standard for AVR for over a decade (Fig. 27-1).

Many of these prostheses have remained durable for up to 40 years.[8,9] Multiple modifications ensued including changing the material of the ball from Silastic to Stellite, changes in the shape of the cage, depression of the ball occluder, the addition of cloth coating to the sewing ring and the cage, and changes in the sewing ring itself. These valves, however, required intense anticoagulation.[10] Hemodynamic performance was compromised, as there were three areas of potential outflow obstruction: the annular size of the sewing ring (the effective orifice area of the valve), the distance between the cage and the walls of the ascending aorta (particularly in the small aortic root), and obstruction to outflow by the ball itself distal to the aortic annulus. Flow patterns were also abnormal (Fig. 27-2). These problems led to the development of the next generation of aortic valve prostheses: the tilting disc valve. Innovators such as Bjork, Hall, Kastor, and Lillehei developed three models of tilting disc prostheses that became the second generation of commonly implanted aortic valve replacement devices between 1968 and 1980. The low-profile

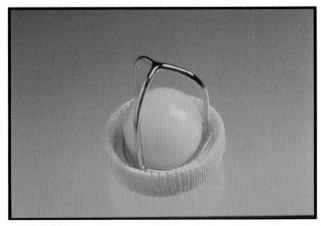

FIGURE 27-1 Prototype model of a ball and cage valve, an early Starr-Edwards model.

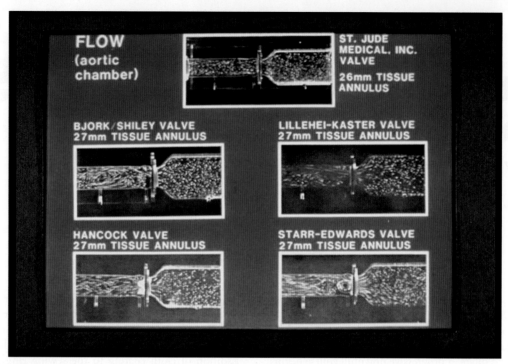

FIGURE 27-2 Prosthetic valve flow patterns utilizing the Weiting CBA-77-03 pulse duplicator with high-speed photography and resin particles. Note the laminar flow with the bileaflet aortic valve as opposed to other clinically available prostheses and the flow similarity between the bileaflet valve and the tissue valve in the lower left corner. Tilting disk valves show directional flow, stasis at the minor flow orifice, and eddy current formation distally. The ball valve demonstrates stasis beyond the ball and eddy current formation around the ball itself. Note that the ball is obstructive to outflow, as is the proximity of the ball cage to the walls of the outflow chamber. (Reproduced with permission from Emery RW, Nicoloff DM: The St. Jude Medical cardiac valve prosthesis: In vitro studies. *J Thorac Cardiovasc Surg*. 1979 Aug;78(2):269-276.)

configuration simplified surgical implantation (Fig.27-3). Problems with the tilting disc valve included stasis and eddy current formation at the minor flow orifice (see Fig. 27-2), and sticking or embolization of the leaflet, the latter leading to discontinuation of the Bjork prosthesis in spite of otherwise good long-term results.[11] The Lillehei-Kastor prosthesis evolved into the Omniscience valve, now discontinued. The Medtronic Hall valve, the third tilting disc prosthesis, is also now discontinued (Fig. 27-4A).

Kalke and Lillehei developed the first rigid bileaflet valve, but it had very limited clinical use. In 1977, the St. Jude Medical (SJM) prosthesis was developed and implanted by Nicoloff and associates (Fig. 27-4C).[3,12,13] Over the following decades, the dramatic step of a bileaflet prosthesis nearly obviated the use of all other kinds of mechanical prosthetic valves in the United States and to a large extent elsewhere. The SJM valve demonstrated low aortic gradients, minimal aortic insufficiency, and low rates of thromboembolism (TE).[12,14] Anticoagulation continued to be necessary but to a lesser extent than with previous design models.[15] Because of the low-profile design and lesser need for orientation, surgical implant was further simplified. Following the introduction of the SJM valve, several other third-generation models of bileaflet prostheses were introduced, including the Sulzer CarboMedics valve (Fig. 27-4B), the ATS Medical prosthesis (Fig. 27-4D), and the On-X prosthesis (Fig. 27-4E). Since the introduction

of the bileaflet valve, over 2 million implants on a global basis have been accomplished and extensive literature has developed. Surgeons have become more confident in earlier aortic valve replacement and guidelines for anticoagulation necessary for all mechanical valves have been developed for each generation of prosthesis at progressively decreasing target levels.[15,16]

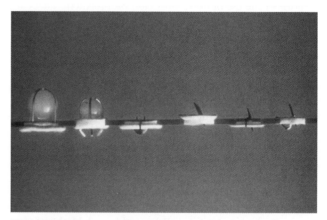

FIGURE 27-3 Low-profile prostheses simplify the surgical implant. The lowest profile is that of the bileaflet valve, and orientation of the leaflets is most commonly not necessary, as compared to tilting disc prostheses, for which the major flow orifice should be directed along the greater curvature of the aorta.

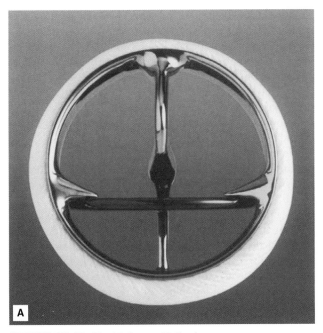

FIGURE 27-4A The Medtronic Hall valve.

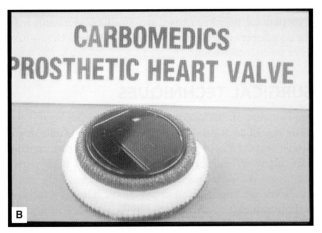

FIGURE 27-4B CarboMedics Top Hat valve.

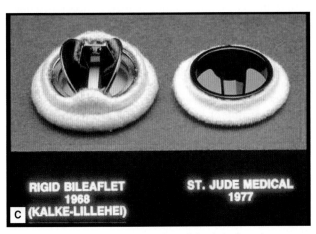

FIGURE 27-4C The original Kalke-Lillehei bileaflet valve as compared to the St. Jude Medical valve introduced nearly a decade later.

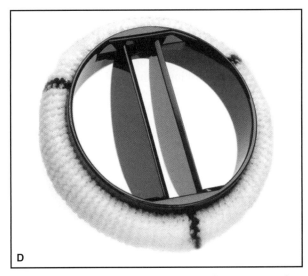

FIGURE 27-4D ATS Medical valve. Note the open pivot design maintaining leaflet insertion.

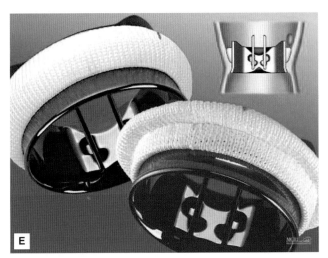

FIGURE 27-4E On-X valve. Note the flange of the inflow portion of the valve housing which seats in the left ventricular outflow tract.

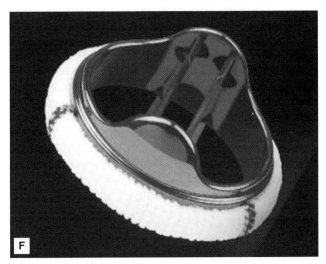

FIGURE 27-4F St. Jude Medical Regent valve.

Over the past 25 years, design and configurational changes have been made in bileaflet prostheses. The ATS Medical valve changed the "rabbit ears" pivot style of other bileaflet prostheses, incorporating a convex or open-pivot design allowing more complete washing of the moving parts of the valve and possibly a quieter valve closing.[17,18] The sewing ring of the SJM valve has changed (SJM HP) to allow a larger valve size implantation for any given tissue annulus, as has ATS Medical with its AP design. The sewing ring of the Sulzer CarboMedics valve has been modified such that this valve is implanted in a supravalvular position (top hat model). The On-X valve incorporates advanced pyrolytic carbon technology using a purer, more flexible coating to allow flanging of the inflow portion of the valve housing, better mimicking the normal flow pattern.

The most recent development in bileaflet valve design was the introduction of the SJM Regent valve (Fig. 27-4F). This valve model not only modified the sewing ring, but also redefined the external profile in a nonintrinsic structural portion of the valve, increasing the effective flow orifice area. Thus, a larger prosthesis could be implanted for any given tissue annulus diameter. This was the first mechanical prosthesis to demonstrate left ventricular mass regression across all valve sizes.[19,20] The Regent valve is seated supra-annular with only the pivot guards protruding into the aortic annulus.[21]

In spite of advances in the design and performance of AVR with a mechanical valve prosthesis, the use of mechanical aortic valves has decreased over the last decade. This is due to improvements in the longevity of bioprosthetic aortic valves, the introduction of TAVR, and the theoretical potential of valve-in-valve TAVR for failed bioprosthetic valves. More importantly, however, is the fear of chronic anticoagulation with warfarin by both patient and physician essential over the long term in patients having mechanical aortic valve prostheses.

PATIENT SELECTION

As with any medical therapy, AVR with a mechanical prosthesis is not indicated for all patients. Several prospective randomized studies have shown no difference in survival in patients having biologic or mechanical valve prostheses or among mechanical prostheses per se.[22-27] However, follow-up was limited to less than 15 years. Conversely, in other nonrandomized studies of patients followed over longer time frames, freedom from all valve-related events and from reoperation were improved in patients with mechanical valve prostheses as compared to patients with biologic prostheses.[11,28]

Most recently several publications have shown improved survival in patients having bileaflet mechanical valve prosthesis, most likely related to improved anticoagulation regimens and longer patient follow-up.[29,30] Importantly quality of life was similar to that of a biologic prosthesis, even in the elderly.[30]

While the advantages of large effective flow orifice and durability with a mechanical valve are paramount, the confounding effects resulting from the necessity for anticoagulation continue. Patients that are transient, noncompliant, or incapable of managing medications are not good candidates for long-term chronic anticoagulation, nor are those with dangerous lifestyles or hobbies.[31] Patients with higher levels of education, and those from geographic areas with a sophisticated medical infrastructure and a static population have better compliance with necessary medication, anticoagulant monitoring, and those with fewer risk factors for TE are good candidate for AVR with a mechanical valve prosthesis.[32]

Home monitoring of anticoagulation has become an important adjunct in managing international normalized ratios (INRs) in Europe, but is unfortunately lesser used in North America.

A mechanical valve prosthesis is recommended to patients having second valve reoperations regardless of the nature of the first procedure, as re-reoperative risks increase substantially.[33,34] Some studies report low mortality for reoperation of patients with failed biologic valves, but failures can occur abruptly, creating more risk.[35] Reoperative risk is also higher in those patients having combined procedures[33,36] or after prior coronary bypass.

Many surgeons have opted for an age of >70 years as the indication for bioprosthetic AVR, based on data by Akins.[33] In patients younger than 60 years of age, most would opt for a mechanical prosthesis based on prosthesis durability.[37] In the decade between 60 and 70 years of age, other factors have to be taken into account.[38,39]

SURGICAL TECHNIQUES

Implantation of mechanical valve prostheses has been previously described and is straightforward.[14] Historically, high-profile aortic valve prostheses could be difficult to implant, particularly in small aortic roots. In such cases, a hockey-stick aortotomy is used to "unroll" the aorta and expose the annulus. While the implantation of low-profile bileaflet prostheses is simpler, problems can still arise in the small aortic root. If a tilting disc prosthesis is utilized, orienting the major flow orifice toward the greater curve of the aorta is necessary. Because bileaflet prostheses are the most commonly utilized, the surgical technique for implantation of these devices is described: A midline incision and sternotomy is made and a pericardial well created. Alternatively, a right anterior thoracotomy approach with femoral cannulation may be used. A partial sternotomy is also an alternative in thin patients, creating a sternal "T" at the fourth inter-space.[40]

These alternative techniques are particularly amenable to the implantation of low-profile aortic valve prostheses. The patient is cannulated via the aorta and a single atrial venous cannula. Most commonly, retrograde cardioplegic solution is utilized and a left ventricular vent is placed via the right superior pulmonary vein to maintain a dry operative field. After cross-clamping of the aorta, a transverse aortotomy is made approximately 1 cm above the take off of the right coronary artery, slightly above the level of the sinotubular ridge (Fig. 27-5). The incision is extended three-quarters of the way around the aorta, leaving the posterior one-quarter of

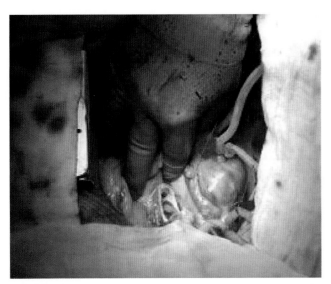

FIGURE 27-5 A transverse aortotomy has been made above the level of the sinotubular ridge. The diseased valve can readily be visualized and excised in toto.

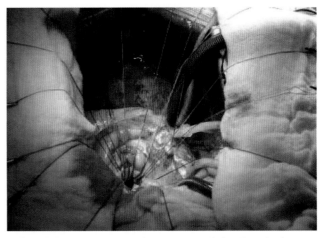

FIGURE 27-6 The annulus has been encircled with multiple interrupted pledgeted mattress sutures of 2-0 braided suture. The annulus can be readily visualized and all calcification has been extensively débrided.

the aorta intact allowing excellent visualization of the native aortic valve and annulus. The leaflets of the aortic valve are excised to the level of the annulus and the annulus is thoroughly débrided of any calcium. Extensive de-calcification will minimize the risk of paravalvular leak, particularly in newer-generation prostheses with thinner sewing rings, and allows for better seating of the valve prosthesis. Braided 2-0 sutures with pledgets are utilized. Beginning at the noncoronary commissure, the annulus is encircled with interrupted mattress sutures (Fig. 27-6) extending from the aortic to the ventricular surface (everting). Recently, a technique of placing sutures from the ventricle to the aorta has been used to place the prosthesis in a supra-annular position. Alternatively, multiple single interrupted sutures may be placed. After placement, the suture bundles are divided into two equal portions and two individual sutures placed into the sewing ring at the level of the pivot guards, orienting the pivot guard toward the ostia of the left and right coronary artery (Fig. 27-7). Next, each half of the suture bundles are inserted through the sewing ring and the prosthesis seated (Fig. 27-8).

The pivot guard sutures are tied first followed by the sutures beginning at the left coronary cusp extending to the mid-portion of the right coronary cusp. Lastly, the sutures of the noncoronary cusp are secured, seating the valve appropriately. In a small aortic root, should a valve not be able to be seated, paravalvular leak can be prevented if the unseated area of the valve is in the noncoronary cusp. External aortic sutures can be placed from outside the aorta to the valve sewing ring, securing the prosthesis and preventing paravalvular regurgitation. Because of the low-profile nature of the leaflets, opening and closing can still occur unimpeded. Leaflet motion should always be checked and the surgeon must be assured that the coronary arteries are not obstructed. The aortotomy is closed with a double layer of polypropylene suture consisting of

an underlying mattress suture and a more superficial over-and-over suture. The patient is placed in the Trendelenburg position and the heart filled with blood and cardioplegic solution, vented, and the cross-clamp removed. After resuscitation and de-airing of the heart, the procedure is completed and the patient transferred to the intensive care unit. On the first postoperative day the chest tubes are removed if output is less than 125 mL in the previous 8 hours. Following the removal of the chest tube, the patient is begun on subcutaneous heparin (5000 U every 8 hours) or low-molecular-weight heparin (1 mg per kg twice a day), and warfarin therapy started. Valve implantation can usually be accomplished in under 40 minutes of aortic cross-clamping and with cardiopulmonary bypass times of approximately 1 hour, allowing limited coagulopathic and homeopathic alterations.

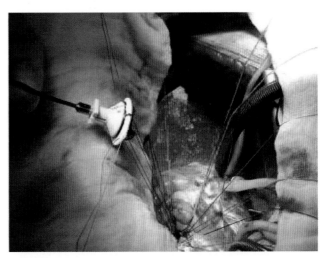

FIGURE 27-7 The pivot guard sutures have been placed aligning the pivot guards with the right and the left coronary artery.

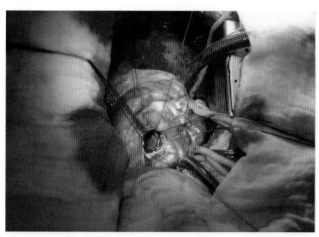

FIGURE 27-8 All sutures have been passed through the sewing ring and the valve is lowered to the aortic annulus and seated appropriately by placing gentle leverage on the valve sewing ring and traction on the suture bundles.

When coronary bypass grafting is indicated, the order of the operation changes. The diseased valve is excised, distal vein or free arterial grafts constructed, the valve is replaced, and the aortotomy closed. Proximal anastomoses are then completed, with one left untied for de-airing. The distal anastomoses of pedicled grafts (internal maxillary artery, IMA) are then completed. De-airing is accomplished through the untied proximal anastomosis.

ANTICOAGULATION

The durability and function of mechanical valve prostheses, particularly those of the modern generation, is unquestioned.[28,37,40-44] It is the process of anticoagulation that is key and drives long-term success. INR is the standard to which anticoagulation levels should be targeted.[31,45] Anticoagulation is begun slowly following removal of the chest tubes, as the danger of overshooting target INR to dangerous levels is common.[46] Current data on anticoagulant regimens indicate that a one-size-fits-all recipe is inadequate to obtain excellent long-term results.[15,32,47] Horstkotte noted that complications occur during fluctuations in the INR, and less often during steady-state levels, be they high or low.[48] When levels of INR increase, bleeding episodes become more common, and when levels of INR decrease, thromboembolic episodes become more common, both on the slope of the change. These events are opposite ends of the continuum of anticoagulation-related complications. The presence of a mechanical valve prosthesis is also not the only risk factor for TE.[32,46]

Traditional risk factors for TE listed in Table 27-1 predispose patients to thromboembolic episodes, and as such higher therapeutic INRs are warranted. Similarly, as shown in Table 27-2, nontraditional risk factors for TE will also predispose patients to embolic events.[32,46-49] Butchart has noted that the more of these risk factors patients have, the greater the

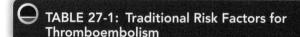

TABLE 27-1: Traditional Risk Factors for Thromboembolism

- Atrial fibrillation
- Increased left ventricular cavity size
- Regional wall motion abnormality
- Depressed ejection fraction
- Hypercoagulability
- Increased age

incidence of events and the greater the need for a higher target INR (Fig. 27-9).[19,32] Thus, it is imperative in the modern era that patient risk factors be taken into account and the INR individualized for a given patient.[15,16,47] Recommendations for INR target levels in our practice are shown in Table 27-3. These levels are more liberal than those offered by the American College of Cardiology/American Heart Association and the American College of Chest Physicians (ACCP) guidelines, but more conservative than those recommended by the European self-anticoagulation trials.[50-52] These later reports are especially relevant, because they demonstrate that a lower INR is consistent with a lower incidence of TE if patients are maintained in the therapeutic target range.[50,53] Patients with home testing were maintained in the therapeutic range a substantially greater percentage of the time than those whose status was monitored at anticoagulation clinics.[50,53] Starting self-management early after mechanical valve replacement further reduced valve-related events.[46] Puskas et al in a prospective FDA approved randomized trial substantiated theses data and showed that in patients using home INR monitoring between target INR of 1.5 and 2.0 with the addition of low-dose aspirin in these without contraindication.[16] This report documented a significantly lower risk of bleeding without a significant increase in thromboembolic events. In the United States, home testing has not become commonplace or popular. However, home testing can certainly be expected to lower the incidence of valve-related thromboembolic and bleeding events. It has been approved for reimbursement for weekly testing in patients with a mechanical valve prosthesis

TABLE 27-2: Nontraditional Risk Factors for Thromboembolism

- Cancer
- Systemic infection
- Diabetes
- Prior event
- IgA against Chlamydia pneumoniae (CP)
- Eosinophilia
- Hypertension

Data from Butchart EG, Ionescu A, Payne N, et al: A new scoring system to determine thromboembolic risk after heart valve replacement. *Circulation.* 2003 Sep 9;108 Suppl 1:II68-II74.

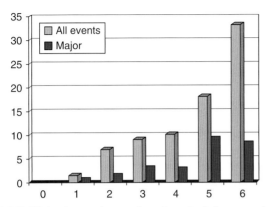

FIGURE 27-9 The correlation of number of risk factors to thromboembolic events. (Data from Butchart EG, Ionescu A, Payne N, et al: A new scoring system to determine thromboembolic risk after heart valve replacement, *Circulation*. 2003; 108(Suppl II):II-68.)

or atrial fibrillation, but only after a 3-month waiting period. Obtaining appropriate funding for access in the immediate postoperative period would be an important initiative that could acutely reduce the incidence of valve-related events.

In a report of patients followed over 25 years noted that approximately 40% of the bleeding episodes occurred in the first year following surgery. It is thus important during this initial postoperative time frame when the patient's anticoagulant levels are more likely to fluctuate, that INR be measured more frequently.[37] In the early postoperative period, INR can occasionally jump to supratherapeutic levels and result in significant bleeding events. This is an independent risk factor for mortality at 60 days.[54] Furthermore, the most important independent predictor of reduced survival is anticoagulant variability.[31] We and others therefore recommend in the early postoperative period that one proceed slowly to bring the INR to target levels while the patient is under the protection of subcutaneous enoxaparin (100 IU/kg twice a day) or heparin (5000 U every 8 hours) until the INR is therapeutic.[15,16,37,55,56] Recent data based from emerging genotype technology indicate an improved therapeutic ratio can be obtained using a pharmacogenetic algorithm for initial warfarin dosage required in transition to stable dosage.[47]

The addition of aspirin to a warfarin regimen can be expected to result in a lower incidence of TE at any given therapeutic INR with a low probability for bleeding events and so is recommended in those without contraindication.[16,57,58]

⬤ TABLE 27-3: Target INR Recommendations

1. Normal ejection fraction and cavity size, NSR: INR 1.6-2.0, ASA
2. Any single factor: INR 2.0-2.5, ASA
3. Multiple factors or atrial fibrillation: INR 2.5-3.5
4. ? Antiplatelet only

ASA, aspirin; INR, international normalized ratio; NSR, normal sinus rhythm.

An educational program to teach patients how to manage their anticoagulation is an important part of the overall operative process. Patients should be instructed on the influence of alcohol and diet on anticoagulant levels, the need for regular dosing, and the potential impact of travel and gastrointestinal illnesses on fluctuations in anticoagulant levels. Warfarin, the world's most commonly used anticoagulant, is well known to be high risk, as is insulin, yet both drugs can be managed with proper compliance and education so that the impact on lifestyle and quality of life is minimal.[10,30,59] Patient age does not appear to be a risk factor for anticoagulation[56,60-62] as long as there are no specific contraindications to anticoagulation due to the importance of regular testing cannot be overstated. The presence of a mechanical valve per se is not a risk factor for long-term neurocognitive dysfunction.[63]

Newer antithrombin agents may obviate several of the issues discussed above. These agents are showing promise in the treatment of atrial fibrillation, with a lower incidence of embolism and bleeding complications. The drugs are expensive, require multiple administrations per day, and may cause hepatic dysfunction, yet they do not require blood testing or physician visits to maintain the therapeutic effect[64] Their application to mechanical valve prostheses is as yet unknown. One trial was stopped early due to a high incidence of cerebrovascular events, but trial design has been criticized. More data are necessary.

Notably, platelet activation may be more important in the long-term therapy of an aortic prosthesis than mitral where areas of stasis predominate.[13] This is likely the reason there is no difference in the freedom from embolic events in mechanical verses biologic prosthesis over the long term.[16,28] Thus aortic valve prostheses could in theory be managed with newer strong anti-platelet therapy. Garcia-Rinaldi has tested this theory in 178 patients followed out to 7.8 years treated only with clopidogrel. Results were excellent with few bleeding episodes and minimal thromboembolic events.[65] Importantly, the authors note the majority of patients having thromboembolic events when tested for platelet inhibition were resistant to the drug or had been removed from the drug by themselves or by a physician. They stressed the importance of measurement of platelet responsiveness if only anti-platelet therapy is utilized.[60,65] A prospective randomized trial is warranted to confirm those results.

RESULTS

Outcomes from aortic valve replacement with mechanical valve prostheses vary among reports depending on the patient population. Patients with higher risk factors for TE and those with risk factors for anticoagulation will have a higher incidence of valve-related events, making meta-analyses less meaningful.[66] Older patients are at higher risk for valve-related events, particularly thromboembolic episodes, because of the greater number of risk factors that accumulate with aging.[32] The incidence of valve-related events is also determined by the intensity with which the investigators follow their patients. A higher incidence of early hemorrhagic events may also be diluted over the longer periods of follow-up.[67] Compliance is key to good long-term outcomes. Traditional and nontraditional risk factors for embolism and risk factors for anticoagulation and valve-related events must be considered.[32,46] Several trials have indicated no significant differences in events among various mechanical prostheses, but follow-up was limited.[23,25,27,68] There are, however, certain standards within which one should expect a mechanical valve to perform, and within which the medical decisions for anticoagulation must be made. The majority of valve-related morbidity is related to TE and anticoagulation-related hemorrhage (ARH).[26,29,39] The sections below deal with specific valve-related complications and acceptable current incidence.

Improvements in mechanical valve prostheses and in anti-coagulation regimens, along with maintaining and lowering target INR has led to updating of objective performance criteria (OPC) for heart valves.[69] Current criteria for events for both mechanical and biologic valves have been lowered (Table 27-4). Events including TE and perivalvular leak are similar between mechanical and bioprosthetic valves, but the OPC for hemorrhage and thrombosis is higher in mechanical valves, in spite of being quite low but prosthesis longevity favors mechanical prostheses.[69]

Valve Type

Freedom from all valve-related events over the long term is shown in Fig. 27-10. In the early follow-up period, ARH is the most common untoward event for mechanical valve prostheses. Thus, over the first 10 years of follow-up there

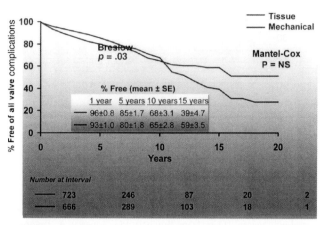

FIGURE 27-10 Freedom from all valve-related complications over 20 years. Note that in the first 10-year period of follow-up, complications related to mechanical valves exceeded those of tissue valves. The lines cross at approximately 10 years, and over the following period, complications from tissue valves were more frequent than those from mechanical valves. (Reproduced with permission from Khan SS, Trento A, DeRobertis M, et al: Twenty-year comparison of tissue and mechanical valve replacement. *J Thorac Cardiovasc Surg*. 2001 Aug;122(2):257-269.)

is a higher incidence of valve-related events in patients with mechanical prostheses as opposed to those with biologic valves.[28]

However, over the subsequent period of 10 to 20 years, the incidence of biologic valve failure changes this ratio such that the valve-related complications of biologic prostheses become more common than those with mechanical valve prostheses. In a series of aortic reoperations, Potter has noted that the time to biologic valve failure was only 7.6 years.[35] This failure rate will increase over time.[28,70] Overall, freedom from valve-related events is more strongly influenced by preexisting comorbidities than the presence of a mechanical prosthesis per se.[28,32,37,41]

Anticoagulant-related Hemorrhage

ARH is the most common valve-related event. The more intense the anticoagulation regimen, the higher the incidence of valve-related hemorrhage. Most commonly ARH will occur during fluctuations in INR values especially related to changes in warfarin dosing or medical or drug interactions.[48] The most common site for ARH is the gastrointestinal tract, the second being the central nervous system.[32] ARH also accounts for the highest incidence of patient mortality for valve-related events. Acceptable ARH rates range from 1.0 to 2.5% per patient-year in long-term reports.[11,28,37,41-44] Recent data indicate the OPC for major hemorrhage to be 1.6%.[69] The long-term reports dilute the short-term impact, as ARH risks are higher early after valve replacement.[37,44,67] With individualized and home monitored anticoagulant regimens, both related events, TE and ARH, are diminished.[50] Freedom from anticoagulation at 10 and 20 years is 75 to 80% and 65 to 70%, respectively. Importantly, one long-term

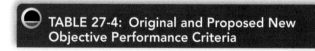

TABLE 27-4: Original and Proposed New Objective Performance Criteria

| | Mechanical valve | | Bioprosthetic valve | |
| | | Proposed new | | Proposed new |
Adverse event	Original OPC	Aortic	Original OPC	Aortic
Thromboembolism	3.0	1.6	2.5	1.5
Valve thrombosis	0.8	0.1	0.2	0.04
All hemorrhage	3.5		1.4	
Major hemorrhage	1.5	1.6	0.9	0.6
All paravalvular leak	1.2		1.2	
Major paravalvular leak	0.6	0.3	0.6	0.3
Endocarditis	1.2	0.3	1.2	0.5

OPC, objective performance criteria.
Adapted with permission from Wu YX, Burchart EG, Borer JS, Yoganathon A, Grunicemeier GL Clinical Evaluation of new Heart Valve Prosthesis: Update of Objective Performance Criteria, *Ann Thorac Surg*. 2014 Nov;98(5):1865-74.

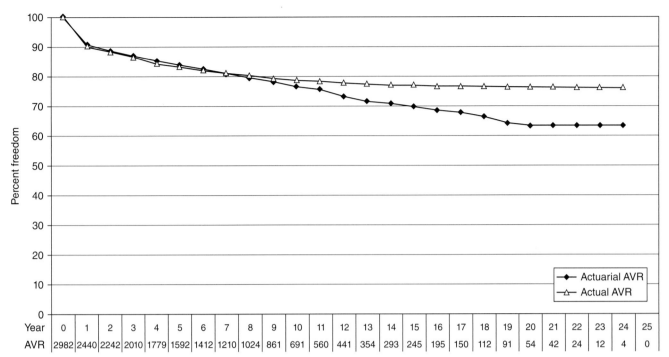

Year	0	1	2	3	4	5	6	7	8	9	10	11	12	13	14	15	16	17	18	19	20	21	22	23	24	25
AVR	2982	2440	2242	2010	1779	1592	1412	1210	1024	861	691	560	441	354	293	245	195	150	112	91	54	42	24	12	4	0

FIGURE 27-11 Kaplan-Meier curve of freedom from anticoagulation-related hemorrhage for patients having aortic valve replacement. (Reproduced with permission from Emery RW, Krogh CC, Arom DV, et al: The St. Jude Medical cardiac valve prosthesis: A 25-year experience with single valve replacement, *Ann Thorac Surg.* 2005 Mar;79(3):776-782.)

study noted that nearly 40% of all ARH that occurred over a 25-year follow-up period occurred during the first year of anticoagulation (Fig. 27-11), indicating that a slow increase to therapeutic levels, coupled with close follow-up during this early period is warranted.[15,37,54,55] Results of the European self-anticoagulation study indicate that a lower INR target is appropriate if home testing is initiated, as a greater time is spent in the therapeutic range.[50] This was recently verified by Puskas et al indicating the value of lowered target INR and the importance of home monitoring of INR.[16] Mortality more commonly occurs in relation to bleeding events than in relation to thromboembolic events.[15,37]

Thromboembolism

Thromboembolic episodes (TE) are the second most common valve-related event and are the major reason that chronic anticoagulation is warranted. Khan and associates reported in a large series of patients that the incidence of thromboembolic events between bioprostheses and mechanical prostheses are the same (Fig. 27-12), but the mechanical valve patients are on warfarin.[28] Wu et al in a meta-analysis confirms that TE rates are similar between aortic mechanical and bioprosthesis as does Puskas.[16,69] Acceptable thromboembolic rates range between 0.8 and 2.3% per patient-year.[11,28,37,41-44,70-71] Approximately one-half of these events are neurologic events, 40% are transient, and 10% peripheral.[37] Freedom from thromboembolic events at 10 and 20 years is approximately 80 to 85% and 65 to 70%, respectively.

TE is a continuous risk factor that is present throughout the life of the mechanical valve prosthesis. As patients age, risk factors for TE increase, so one must be on guard to maintain therapeutic anticoagulant levels. Changes in the target INR may be necessary as individual risks increase.

Interestingly, not all neurologic events classified historically as embolic are indeed embolic. Piper et al reported a study of patients prospectively admitted to a single institution with a neurologic event postmechanical valve replacement and intensively worked up. More than 75% were found

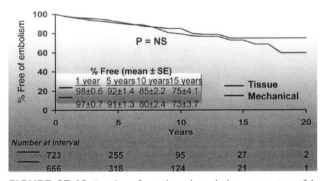

FIGURE 27-12 Freedom from thromboembolism in patients followed for 20 years. Note that there is no difference in the incidence of thromboembolic events between mechanical and tissue valves. (Reproduced with permission from Khan SS, Trento A, DeRobertis M, et al: Twenty-year comparison of tissue and mechanical valve replacement. *J Thorac Cardiovasc Surg.* 2001 Aug;122(2):257-269.)

to have intracerebral hemorrhage as the etiology of the event as opposed to embolism. These data would indicate target anticoagulant levels may be artificially high, that not all neurologic events that appear to be embolic in fact are not[72] and support efforts for lower target INR.[15,16]

Valve Thrombosis

Valve thrombosis in the aortic position is an unusual event that most commonly occurs late after valve replacement and is due to inadequate anticoagulation or noncompliance.[73,74] In bileaflet valves, thrombus formation impinging valve function occurs at the pivot guards and in the crevices of the valve. Only one bileaflet design does not have convexities into which the leaflets fit.[75]

In tilting disc valves, thrombus is most common at the minor flow orifice. The incidence of thrombosis is approximately <.3% per patient-year and freedom from valve thrombosis at 20 years is >97%.[11,28,37,41-44] Thromboses is rare in biologic valves but does occur.[69]

Prosthetic Valve Endocarditis

Prosthetic valve endocarditis is also a rare event in the modern era with prophylactic antibiotics. Approximately 60% of events occur early and are associated with staphylococci. The mortality for this event is high. The remainder appear late (>60 days). Prosthetic valve endocarditis is also a continuous variable, and patients must be cautioned to take prophylactic antibiotics for any invasive procedure. Freedom from endocarditis with mechanical valve prostheses is 97 to 98% at 20 to 25 years.[37,44]

The expected incidence is similar between mechanical and biologic valves .[69] The major reason for re-replacement of mechanical valves is endocarditis as opposed to degeneration of the prosthesis in biologic valves.[35]

Paravalvular Leak

Paravalvular leak is an operative complication and is most commonly related to implant technique but occasionally to endocarditis. With annular decalcification and closely placed sutures, these events can be minimized. The Silzone experience showed an increased incidence of paravalvular leak wherein the silver impregnated in the sewing ring not only impeded bacterial growth, but also healing of the annular ring, doubling the accepted rate of this complication.[76] The Silzone-coated sewing ring was removed from the market. There may be an anatomic predisposition to paravalvular leak in the area of the annulus extending from the right and noncoronary commissure, one-third the distance along the right coronary cusp, and two-thirds the distance to the noncoronary cusp, due to intrinsic weakness in this area of the annulus.[77] The acceptable range of paravalvular leak is approximately less than 0.1% per patient-year, with early postoperative occurrence predominating.[34,37,69]

Structural Failure

Structural failure of bileaflet aortic prostheses due to wear has not been observed or reported in long-term studies totaling more than 50,000 patient-years of follow-up. This indicates the high structural integrity of these modern aortic devices.[28,37,44] In a single study totaling 21,742 patient-years with 94% complete follow-up, there was no structural failure.[55]

Freedom from Reoperation

The long-term durability of modern mechanical valve prostheses is excellent, and a valve replacement rate of less than 2% over 25 years (Fig. 27-13) can be expected, and re-reoperation after AVR replacement is even more rare.[34] Subvalvular pannus formation is also rare with aortic bileaflet valves.[37,44] The most common reasons for prosthetic valve reimplantation are pre- and postoperative endocarditis, paravalvular leak, and valve thrombosis.

SPECIAL CIRCUMSTANCES
Technical Considerations

While the technique of implanting a mechanical valve prosthesis is very straightforward, special circumstances arise. Because of the large size of the valve housing of the St. Jude Medical Regent valve compared to the tissue annulus, entry into the aorta annulus can sometimes be difficult. Occasionally, patients have the smallest diameter of their aortic root at the sinotubular ridge. While the sizer will pass readily through the aortic annulus, seating the Regent valve itself into the annulus can sometimes be difficult and frustrating. It is important to gently rock the valve back and forth through the sinotubular ridge, tilting the valve circumferentially through the narrowest part. Once the valve is below the level of the sinotubular ridge, it will seat readily in the annulus if sizing has been correct. When tying the valve into the annulus, sutures in the pivot guards and the left and right coronary cusps should be first completed. The last sutures ligated are those of the noncoronary cusp for two reasons. It may seem like the Regent valve will not seat because of the large-sized valve housing; however, with gentle persistence seating can be completed as long as sizing has been correct. The Regent valve sits supra-annular and only the pivot guards lie inside the annulus (Fig. 27-14).

Therefore, one should leave the last sutures to be tied in the mid-part of the noncoronary cusp with the valve oriented so the leaflets are parallel to the ventricular septum.[78] With proper annular decalcification and flexibility of the annulus, we have not seen a Regent valve that has not been able to be seated properly.

Similarly, when using the On-X valve one has to be sure that the flare of the valve inflow is seated properly in the left ventricular outflow tract. Gentle manipulation and patience may be necessary. Walther and colleagues note that exact sizing requires some experience.[24]

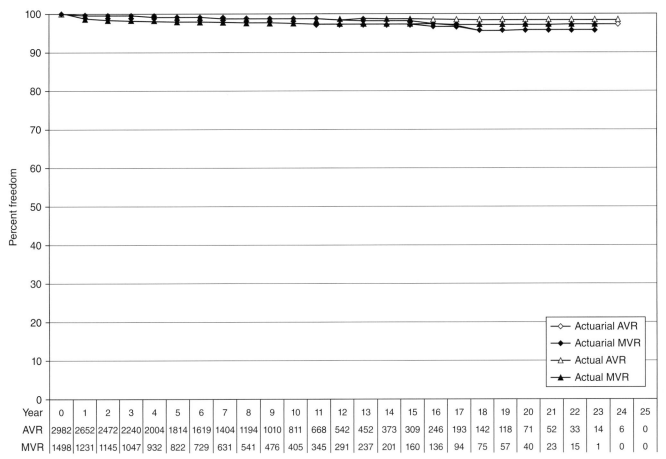

Year	0	1	2	3	4	5	6	7	8	9	10	11	12	13	14	15	16	17	18	19	20	21	22	23	24	25
AVR	2982	2652	2472	2240	2004	1814	1619	1404	1194	1010	811	668	542	452	373	309	246	193	142	118	71	52	33	14	6	0
MVR	1498	1231	1145	1047	932	822	729	631	541	476	405	345	291	237	201	160	136	94	75	57	40	23	15	1	0	0

FIGURE 27-13 Freedom from reoperations in patients having mechanical valve replacement followed over 25 years. Note that the rate of reoperation in patients with aortic valve replacement is less than 2% in over 21,000 patient-years of follow-up. (Reproduced with permission from Emery RW, Krogh CC, Arom DV, et al: The St. Jude Medical cardiac valve prosthesis: A 25-year experience with single valve replacement, *Ann Thorac Surg*. 2005 Mar;79(3):776-782.)

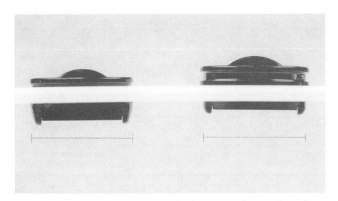

FIGURE 27-14 The St. Jude Medical Regent valve on the right as compared to the St. Jude Medical HP valve on the left. With the Regent valve only the pivot guards insert into the annulus, allowing a larger valve housing for any given tissue annulus diameter. (Reproduced with permission from Emery RW, Krogh CC, Arom DV, et al: The St. Jude Medical cardiac valve prosthesis: A 25-year experience with single valve replacement, *Ann Thorac Surg*. 2005 Mar;79(3):776-782.)

If an oversized bileaflet valve has been purposefully in a small aortic root, a bileaflet valve can be tilted and will still function without coronary obstruction as long as the highest portion of the valve is in the noncoronary cusp. Pledgeted sutures placed from outside the aorta through the sewing ring of the valve can prevent paravalvular leak, and opening and closing can still occur due to the low-profile nature of the prosthetic valve. In our review of nearly 3000 bileaflet aortic valve replacements, no annular enlarging procedures were completed.[55]

Patient-prosthesis Mismatch

Patient-prosthesis mismatch (PPM) is a concept first described by Rahimtoola and popularized by Pibarot and Dumesnil.[79,80] Unfortunately, views are varied on the importance of PPM.[81-84] This is due to the fact that virtually all contributions to the literature study mixtures of mechanical and biologic prostheses and varying types of each. In a

25-year follow-up of patients with a single-model mechanical valve prosthesis, no difference was found in overall valve-related mortality for patients who had severe PPM, moderate PPM, or insignificant PPM according the criteria described by Blais and associates.[83] This similarity in long-term survival was sustained whether the effective area was measured by in vitro (internal geometric valve area) or in vivo criteria (echo-calculated valve area) as shown in Figs. 27-15 and 27-16. This study also found no difference in valve-related events, including operative mortality, long-term cumulative mortality, ARH, TE, valve thrombosis, paravalvular leak, or diagnosis of congestive heart failure. Follow-up in this study was 94% complete and extended over 13,000 patient-years.[85] Therefore, with bileaflet mechanical valve prostheses, PPM does not appear to be an issue. This retrospective study was limited in that it did not address patient age (ie, younger vs older), patient activity, or ventricular function. Thus, it is likely that PPM is important in patients with small biologic prostheses, because as the valve leaflets stiffen, clinically significant aortic stenosis becomes prominent early in the postoperative follow-up period, affecting symptoms and survival in younger and more active patients and in those with depressed ventricular function. If one is, however, concerned about PPM, the indexed effective orifice area can be calculated for any given prosthetic valve and a determination made whether an annular enlarging procedure or a different model prosthesis with a larger effective orifice area is warranted.[86] PPM has been minimized by the new-generation Regent valve and is very rare with this prosthesis.[20,55]

Stopping Anticoagulation

Anticoagulation is recommended in all patients with mechanical valve prostheses. Limited trials have been undertaken with low-risk patients, but only after a several-month course of systemic anticoagulation. An increased incidence of valve thrombosis but with little increase in the incidence of TE has been reported in patients not taking chronic anticoagulation if antiplatelet agents are utilized.[73,87,88] One study found no significant differences in valve-related events in patients on warfarin as compared to antiplatelet therapy alone, but follow-up was limited.[89] One prospective study is currently ongoing consisting of a randomized trial of antiplatelet therapy versus warfarin after 3 months of formal anticoagulation, but the results are not yet available.[90] Certainly one can expect that highly selected patients with bileaflet mechanical valve prostheses will do well off warfarin on antiplatelet agents, but this is unproven.[21,91]

In a prospective nonrandomized trial of clopidogrel along after bileaflet aortic valve replacement, Garcia-Rinaldi et al as noted above, found thromboembolic events limited to those patients that had clopidogrel discontinued or were

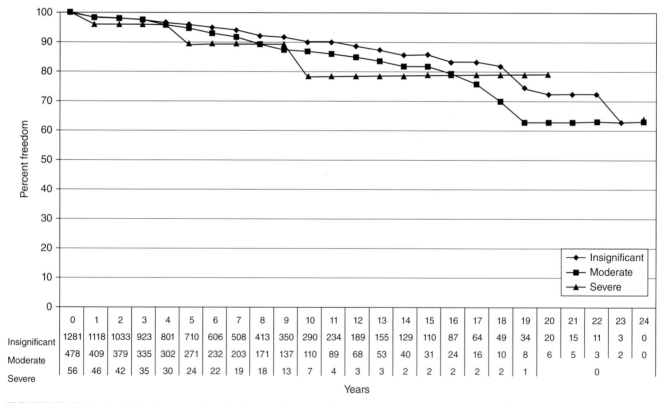

FIGURE 27-15 Kaplan-Meier determination of valve-related late mortality in patients having insignificant, moderate, or severe patient-prosthesis mismatch according to the criteria of Pibarot and colleagues. After implant of a bileaflet prosthesis, in vitro determination is calculated from the geometric flow orifice by the manufacturer. Note there is no difference in these three curves. Numbers at the bottom of the figure represent patients available for follow-up.

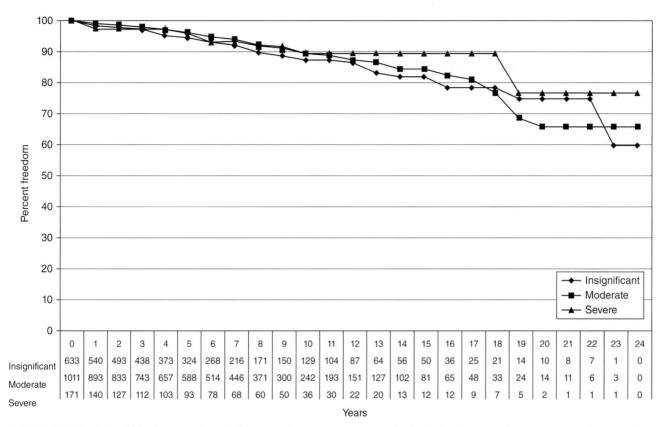

	0	1	2	3	4	5	6	7	8	9	10	11	12	13	14	15	16	17	18	19	20	21	22	23	24
Insignificant	633	540	493	438	373	324	268	216	171	150	129	104	87	64	56	50	36	25	21	14	10	8	7	1	0
Moderate	1011	893	833	743	657	588	514	446	371	300	242	193	151	127	102	81	65	48	33	24	14	11	6	3	0
Severe	171	140	127	112	103	93	78	68	60	50	36	30	22	20	13	12	12	9	7	5	2	1	1	1	0

FIGURE 27-16 Kaplan-Meier determination of valve-related late mortality in patients having insignificant, moderate, or severe patient-prosthesis mismatch by the in vivo criteria according to Blais and associates determined echocardiographically. There is no difference in the survival curves after implant of a bileaflet prosthesis. The numbers at the bottom of the graph represent patients available for follow-up.

nonresponders.[65,90] While such an approach is rational based on deductive reasoning from available data, a prospective randomized trend is required before this approach can be recommended.

When anticoagulation requires reversal electively, as for scheduled surgery, the INR is allowed to slowly drift toward normal over 5 days and the patient is admitted for intravenous heparin therapy 24 hours prior to the procedure.

Anticoagulation is restarted after the procedure with antiplatelet therapy, and subcutaneous heparin with warfarin restarted on postoperative day one. Abrupt reversal of INR in patients who have bleeding episodes may be warranted, but carries increased risk of TE. Fresh frozen plasma will gently reverse INR when necessary, but it is best to avoid the use of vitamin K. Frequent INR checks are warranted.

Following ARH episodes, when feasible, because of the high incidence of recurrent bleeding, anticoagulant therapy is withheld up to 2 weeks, using antiplatelet agents only[88] or until the source of the bleeding has been identified and definitively treated. For those patients in whom anticoagulant therapy cannot be restarted, antiplatelet therapy is warranted, but the patient should be informed of an increased incidence of TE to approximately 4% per patient-year and that of valve thrombosis to 2% per patient-year with bileaflet valves.[73,87,88,92]

Mechanical Valve Replacement in the Younger Patient

A major deterrent to mechanical valve replacement in the younger patient is the impact of long-term anticoagulation. Mechanical valves are, however, more ideal for younger patients due to their excellent durability characteristics. Most importantly, younger patients (ie, patients under the age of 50 years) are a low-risk subset for valve-related events. These individuals have very few risk factors for TE, and thus anticoagulation can be run at the lower end of the therapeutic target range, decreasing the incidence of ARH without altering the incidence of TE. In fact, many infants and children have been managed with only aspirin with quite good long-term results.[93] While this is not recommended in patients older than infancy, it is a feasible alternative. A recent study in patients under 50 years of age followed 254 patients for up to 20 years and found an exceedingly low rate of valve-related events (Table 27-5), an exceptional long-term overall survival of nearly 88%, and event-free survival probability of 92% at 19 years.[94]

Chiang et al published a propensity-based analysis of patients having AVR with a mechanical versus biologic prosthesis ages 50-69 years from the New York State database.[27] They found there was no difference in stroke or survival at up to 15 years. The patients having biologic prosthesis had

TABLE 27-5: Valve-Related Events with the St. Jude Medical Prosthetic Valve in Young Patients

Event	No. of events	Percent per patient-year	No. of deaths
Endocarditis	3	0.15	0
Paravalvular leak	6	0.30	2
Embolism	6	0.30	0
Valve thrombosis	2	0.10	0
Bleeding	6	0.10	2
Structural failure	0	0	0

Data from Emery RW, Krogh CC, Jones DJ, et al: Five-year follow up of the ATS mechanical heart valve. J He+H220art Valve Dis. 2004 Mar;13(2):231-238; Emery RW, Krogh CC, Arom DV, et al: The St. Jude Medical cardiac valve prosthesis: A 25-year experience with single valve replacement, *Ann Thorac Surg.* 2005 Mar;79(3):776-782.

a higher rate of reoperation with a 9% operative mortality. No mention is made of morbidity such as postoperative stroke or renal failure. The mortality rate is high compared to available literature.[35] Economic impact during the operative and postoperative period are also not addressed. The incidence and timing of reoperation may also be underestimated as estimates of up to one third of patients with failed bioprostheses have substantive contraindications to reoperative surgery and thus are not included in statistics for replacement of a degenerated valve. The reoperative mortality is thus be artificially low. Patients with mechanical prostheses had a significantly higher rate of ARH, but higher target INR was used compared to current recommendations.[15,16] Home anticoagulant monitoring was not utilized. Both of these factors would lower ARH incidence. The data are thus not definitive for recommending bioprosthesis for patients in this younger age group. Individual preferences and thorough discussion are thus warranted.

A further reason for implanting bioprostheses in younger patients is the feasibility and recent successes with TAVR valve-in-valve.[95,96] The experience is limited, however, and this reasoning may offer false hope as valve-in valve procedures are not effective in smaller bioprosthetic valves.[97,98]

The longest surviving patient in a series of bileaflet valve replacement patients is currently over 30 years from his procedure, which was completed in his early forties and has been without complication. The low incidence of valve-related complications in younger patients should drive a discussion of the alternative prostheses available for such individuals, especially with new aggressive and reversible antiplatelet drugs. Operative mortality increases with each succeeding procedure; therefore discussion of durability with patients becomes mandatory.[33-35] As anticoagulant regimens become further refined the incidence of ARH will be lowered, making the use of mechanical aortic valves safer.

TABLE 27-6: Considerations for Mechanical Valve Replacement

- High probability for anticoagulant use
- Need for chronic anticoagulation (any age)
- Preferences of patient
- Surgical risk for reoperation
- Age < 60 years
- Age 60-70 years with patient discussion
- Reoperations
- Good medical infrastructure

Follow-up

With the use of any valve prosthesis, long-term follow-up is a key factor. Ten years is certainly not long enough to ascertain the true durability of a biologic prosthesis. Grunkemeier reviewed several types of biologic prostheses and found that the 10-year durability was excellent, but between 12 and 18 years durability fell off and prosthetic replacement was necessary.[70] These data were echoed by Khan and colleagues and Chiang et al.[27,28] Valve-related failure of all biologic alternatives including stented prosthetic replacements, stentless prostheses, and homograft and autograft replacements have all shown long-term durability to be less than that of modern mechanical valve prostheses.

Even with some mechanical valve prostheses, durability after 10 years has not been adequate. In recommending mechanical valve replacement, one should be assured to have clinically available data on the prostheses that extend beyond 15 years, which is now available.

In conclusion, with proper selection of patients for mechanical valve replacement, one can expect excellent long-term results, long-term survival, and a low incidence of valve-related complications. Possible indications for recommending aortic valve replacement with mechanical prostheses are shown in Table 27-6.

REFERENCES

1. Carabello BA: Clinical practice. Aortic stenosis. *N Engl J Med* 2002; 346:677.
2. Tornos P, Sambola A, Permanyer-Miralda G, et al: Long-term outcome of surgically treated aortic regurgitation: influence of guideline adherence toward early surgery. *J Am Coll Cardiol* 2006; 47:1012.
3. Gott VL, Alejo DE, Cameron DE: Mechanical heart valves: 50 years of evolution. *Ann Thorac Surg* 2003; 76:S2230.
4. Pibarot P, Dumesnil JG: Valvular heart disease: changing concepts in disease management. *Circ* 2009; 119:1034.
5. Minh TH, Mazine A, Bouhour I, et al: Expanding the indication for sutureless aortic valve replacement to patients with mitral valve disease. *J Thorac Cardiovasc Surg* 2014; 148:1354.
6. Hufnagel CA, Harvey WP: The surgical correction of aortic regurgitation preliminary report. *Bull Georgetown Univ Med Cent* 1953; 6:60.
7. David TE: Aortic valve repair and aortic valve-sparing operations. *J Thorac Cardiovasc Surg* 2015; 149:9.
8. Shiono M, Sezai Y, Sezai A, et al: Long-term results of the cloth-covered Starr-Edwards ball valve. *Ann Thorac Surg* 2005; 80:204.
9. Gao G, Wu Y, Grunkemeier GL, et al: Forty-year survival with the Starr-Edwards heart valve prosthesis. *J Heart Valve Dis* 2004; 13:91.

10. Ezekowitz MD: Anticoagulation management of valve replacement patients. *J Heart Valve Dis* 2002; 11(Suppl 1):S56.

11. Oxenham H, Bloomfield P, Wheatley DJ, et al: Twenty-year comparison of a Bjork-Shiley mechanical heart valve with porcine bioprostheses. *Heart* 2003; 89:697.

12. Emery RW, Anderson RW, Lindsay WG, et al: Clinical and hemodynamic results with the St. Jude Medical aortic valve prosthesis. *Surg Forum* 1979; 30:235.

13. Emery RW, Nicoloff DM: The St. Jude Medical cardiac valve prosthesis: in vitro studies. *J Thorac Cardiovasc Surg* 1979; 78:269.

14. Nicoloff DM, Emery RW, Arom KV, et al: Clinical and hemodynamic results with the St. Jude Medical cardiac valve prosthesis. *J Thorac Cardiovasc Surg* 1982; 82:674.

15. Emery RW, Emery AM, Raikar GV, Shake JG, et al: Anticoagulation for mechanical heart valves: a role for patient based therapy. *J Thrombosis Thrombolysis* 2008; 25:18.

16. Puskas J, Gerdisch M, Nichols D, et al: Reduced antiocoagulation after mechanical aortic valve replacement: interim results for the prospective randomized on-X valve anticoagulation clinic trial randomized Food and Drug Administration Investigational Device Exemption Trail. *J Thorac Cardiovasc Surg* 2014; 147:1202.

17. Sezai A, Shiono M, Orime Y, et al: Evaluation of valve sound and its effects on ATS prosthetic valves in patients' quality of life. *Ann Thorac Surg* 2000; 69:507.

18. Emery RW, Krogh CC, Jones DJ, et al: Five-year follow up of the ATS mechanical heart valve. *J Heart Valve Dis* 2004; 13:231.

19. Bach DS, Sakwa MP, Goldbach M, et al: Hemodynamics and early clinical performance of the St. Jude Medical Regent mechanical aortic valve. *Ann Thorac Surg* 2002; 74:2003.

20. Gelsomino S, Morocutti G, Da Col P, et al: Preliminary experience with the St. Jude Medical Regent mechanical heart valve in the aortic position: early in vivo hemodynamic results. *Ann Thorac Surg* 2002; 73:1830.

21. Emery RW, Emery AM: Letter to the editor. *J Thorac Cardiovasc Surg* 2006; 131:760.

22. Hammermeister KE, Sethi GK, Henderson WG, et al: A comparison of outcomes in men 11 years after heart valve replacement with a mechanical valve or bioprosthesis. *N Engl J Med* 1993; 328:1289.

23. Autschbach R, Walther T, Falk V: Prospectively randomized comparison of different mechanical aortic valves. *Circulation* 2000; 102:III-1.

24. Walther T, Falk V, Tigges R, et al: Comparison of On-X and SJM HP bileaflet aortic valves. *J Heart Valve Dis* 2000; 9:403.

25. Masters RG, Helou J, Pipe AL, Keon WJ: Comparative clinical outcomes with St. Jude Medical, Medtronic Hall and CarboMedics mechanical heart valves. *J Heart Valve Dis* 2001; 10:403.

26. Chambers J, Roxburgh J, Blauth C, et al: A randomized comparison of the MCRI On-X and CarboMedics Top Hat bileaflet mechanical replacement aortic valves: early postoperative hemodynamic function and clinical events. *J Thorac Cardiovasc Surg* 2005; 130:759.

27. Chiang YP, Chikwa J, Moskowitz AJ, Itagaki S, Adams DH, Egorova NN: Survival and long-term outcomes following bioprothestic vs mechanical aortic valve relacement in patients ages 50-69 years. *JAMA* 2014; 312:323.

28. Khan SS, Trento A, DeRobertis M, et al: Twenty-year comparison of tissue and mechanical valve replacement. *J Thorac Cardiovasc Surg* 2001; 122:257.

29. Brown ML, Schare HV, Lahr BD, et al: Aortic valve replacement in patients aged 50 to 70 years: improved outcome with mechanical versus biologic prosthesis. *J Thorac Cardiovasc Surg* 2008; 135:878.

30. deVincentiis C, Kunkl AB, Trimarchi S, et al: Aortic valve replacement in octogenarians: is biologic valve the unique solution? *Ann Thorac Surg* 2008; 85:1296.

31 Butchart EG, Payne N, Li H, et al: Better anticoagulation control improves survival after valve replacement. *J Thorac Cardiovasc Surg* 2002; 123:715.

32. Butchart EG, Ionescu A, Payne N, et al: A new scoring system to determine thromboembolic risk after heart valve replacement. *Circulation* 2003; 108(Suppl II):II-68.

33. Akins CW, Buckley MJ, Daggett WM, et al: Risk of reoperative valve replacement for failed mitral and aortic bioprostheses. *Ann Thorac Surg* 1998; 65:1545.

34. Emery RW, Arom KV, Krogh CC, et al: Reoperative valve replacement with the St. Jude Medical valve prosthesis: long-term follow up. *J Am Coll Cardiol* 2004; 435:438A.

35. Potter DD, Sundt TM 3rd, Zehr KJ, et al: Operative risk of reoperative aortic valve replacement. *J Thorac Cardiovasc Surg* 2005; 129:94.

36. Harrington JT: My three valves. *N Engl J Med* 1993; 328:1345.

37. Emery RW, Krogh CC, Arom DV, et al: The St. Jude Medical cardiac valve prosthesis: a 25-year experience with single valve replacement. *Ann Thorac Surg* 2005; 79:776.

38. Emery RW, Arom KV, Nicoloff DM: Utilization of the St. Jude Medical prosthesis in the aortic position. *Semin Thorac Cardiovasc Surg* 1996; 8:231.

39. Emery RW, Arom KV, Kshettry VR, et al: Decision making in the choice of heart valve for replacement in patients aged 60-70 years: twenty-year follow up of the St. Jude Medical aortic valve prostheses. *J Heart Valve Dis* 2002; 11(Suppl 1):S37.

40. Bakir MD, Casselman FP, Wellens F, et al: Minimally invasive versus standard approach aortic valve replacement: a study in 506 patients. *Ann Thorac Surg* 2006; 81:1599-1604.

41. Lund O, Nielsen SL, Arildsen H, et al: Standard aortic St. Jude valve at 18 years: performance, profile and determinants of outcome. *Ann Thorac Surg* 2000; 69:1459.

42. Aagaard J, Tingleff J, Hansen CN, et al: Twelve years' clinical experience with the CarboMedics prosthetic heart valve. *J Heart Valve Dis* 2001; 10:177.

43. Butchart EG, Li H, Payne N, et al: Twenty years' experience with the Medtronic Hall valve. *J Thorac Cardiovasc Surg* 2001; 121:1090.

44. Ikonomidis JS, Kratz JM, Crumbley AJ, et al: Twenty-year experience with the St. Jude Medical mechanical valve prosthesis. *J Thorac Cardiovasc Surg* 2003; 126:200.

45. Koertke H, Korfer R: International normalized ratio self-management after mechanical heart valve replacement: is an early start advantageous? *Ann Thorac Surg* 2001; 72:44.

46. Montalescot G, Polle V, Collet JP, et al: Low molecular weight heparin after mechanical heart valve replacement. *Circulation* 2000; 101:1083.

47. International Warfarin Pharmacogenetic Consortium: Estimation of the Wargaring Dose with Clinical and Pharmacogenic Date. *N Engl J Med* 2009; 360:753.

48. Horstkotte D, Schulte H, Bircks W, Strauer B: Unexpected findings concerning thromboembolic complications and anticoagulation after complete 10-year follow-up of patients with St. Jude Medical prostheses. *J Heart Valve Dis* 1993; 2:291.

49. Butchart EG, Lewis PA, Bethel JA, Breckenridge IM: Adjusting anticoagulation to prosthesis thrombogenicity and patient risk factors. *Circulation* 1991; 84(Suppl III):III-61.

50. Koertke H, Minami K, Boethig D, et al: INR self-management permits lower anticoagulation levels after mechanical heart valve replacement. *Circulation* 2003; 108(Suppl II):II-75.

51. Bonow RO, Carabello BA, Chatterjee BA, et al: ACC/AHA 2006 guidelines for the management of patients with valvular heart disease. *J Am Coll Cardiol* 2008; 52;e1.

52. Sixth (2000) ACCP guidelines for antithrombotic therapy for prevention and treatment of thrombosis. American College of Chest Physicians. *Chest* 2001; 119(1 Suppl):1S.

53. Horstkotte D, Piper C, Wiener X, et al: Improvement of prognosis by home control in patients with lifelong anticoagulant therapy. *Ann Hematol* 1996; 72(Suppl D):AE3.

54. Koo S, Kucher N, Nguyen PL, et al: The effect of excessive anticoagulation on mortality and morbidity in hospitalized patients with anticoagulant-related major hemorrhage. *Arch Intern Med* 2004; 164:1557.

55. Emery RW, Arom KV, Krogh CC, Joyce LD: Long-term results with the St. Jude Medical aortic valve: a 25-year experience. *J Am Coll Cardiol* 2004; 435:429A.

56. Horstkotte D, Schulte HD, Bircks W, Strauer BE: Lower intensity anticoagulation therapy results in lower complication rates with the St. Jude Medical prosthesis. *J Thorac Cardiovasc Surg* 1994; 107:1136.

57. Turpie A, Gent M, Laupacis A, et al: A comparison of aspirin with placebo in patients treated with warfarin after heart valve replacement. *N Engl J Med* 1993; 329:524.

58. Massel D, Little SH: Risk and benefits of adding antiplatelet therapy to warfarin among patients with prosthetic heart valves: a meta-analysis. *J Am Coll Cardiol* 2001; 37:569.

59. Accola KD, Scott ML, Spector SD, et al: Is the St. Jude Medical mechanical valve an appropriate choice for elderly patients?: a long-term retrospective study measuring quality of life. *J Heart Valve Dis* 2006; 15:57.

60. Arom KV, Emery RW, Nicoloff DM, Petersen RJ: Anticoagulant related complications in elderly patients with St. Jude mechanical valve prostheses. *J Heart Valve Dis* 1996; 5:505.

61. Masters RG, Semelhago LC, Pipe AL, Keon WJ: Are older patients with mechanical heart valves at increased risk? *Ann Thorac Surg* 1999; 68:2169.

62. Davis EA, Greene PS, Cameron DE, et al: Bioprosthetic versus mechanical prostheses for aortic valve replacement in the elderly. *Circulation* 1996; 94(9 Suppl):II121.

63. Zimpfer D, Czerny M, Schuch P, et al: Long-term neurocognitive function after mechanical aortic valve replacement. *Ann Thorac Surg* 2006; 81:29.

64. Lip GY, Hart RG, Conway DS: Antithrombotic therapy for atrial fibrillation. *BMJ* 2002; 325:1022.

65. Garcia-Rinaldi R, Carro-Pagan C, Schaer HV, et al: Initial experience with dual antiplatelet thrombo prophylaxis with clopidogrel and aspirin in patients with mechanical aortic prosthesis. *J Heart Valve Dis* 2009; 18:617.

66. Horstkotte D: Letter to the editor. *Ann Thorac Surg* 1996; 62:1566.

67. Akins CW: Results with mechanical cardiac valvular prostheses. *Ann Thorac Surg* 1995; 60:1836.

68. David TE, Gott VL, Harker LA, et al: Mechanical valves. *Ann Thorac Surg* 1996; 62:1567.

69. Wu YX, Burchart EG, Borer JS, Yoganathon A, Grunicemeier GL: Clinical evaluation of new heart valve prosthesis: update of objective performance Criteria. *Ann Thorac Surg* 2014; 98:1865-1874.

70. Grunkemeier GL, Li HH, Naftel DC, et al: Long-term performance of heart valve prostheses. *Curr Probl Cardiol* 2000; 25:73.

71. Sawant D, Singh AK, Feng WC, et al: St. Jude Medical cardiac valves in small aortic roots: follow-up to sixteen. *J Thorac Cardiovasc Surg* 1997; 113:499.

72. Piper C, Hering D, Langer C, Horstkotte D: Etiology of stroke after mechanical heart valve replacement—results from a ten-year prospective study. *J Heart Valve Dis* 2008; 17:413.

73. Czer LS, Matloff JM, Chaux A, et al: The St. Jude valve: analysis of thromboembolism, warfarin-related hemorrhage, and survival. *Am Heart J* 1987; 114:389.

74. Durrleman N, Pellerin M, Bouchard D, et al: Prosthetic valve thrombosis: twenty-year experience at the Montreal Heart Institute. *J Thorac Cardiovasc Surg* 2004; 127:1388.

75. Van Nooten GJ, Van Belleghem Y, Caes F, et al: Lower-intensity anticoagulation for mechanical heart valves: a new concept with the ATS bileaflet aortic valve. *J Heart Valve Dis* 2003; 12:495.

76. Schaff HV, Carrel TP, Jamieson WRE, et al: Paravalvular leak and other events in silzone-coated mechanical heart valves: a report from AVERT. *Ann Thorac Surg* 2002; 73:785.

77. De Cicco G, Lorusso R, Colli A, et al: Aortic valve periprosthetic leakage, anatomic observations and surgical results. *Ann Thorac Surg* 2005; 79:1480.

78. Baudet EM, Oca CC, Roques XF, et al: A 5$^{1}/_{2}$ year experience with the St. Jude Medical cardiac valve prosthesis. Early and late results of 737 valve replacements in 671 patients. *J Thorac Cardiovasc Surg* 1985; 90:137.

79. Rahimtoola SH: The problem of valve prosthesis patient mismatch. *Circulation* 1978; 58:20.

80. Pibarot P, Dumesnil JG: Hemodynamic and clinical impact of prosthesis-patient mismatch in the aortic valve position and its prevention. *J Am Coll Cardiol* 2000; 36:1131.

81. Hanayama N, Christakis GT, Mallidi HR, et al: Patient prosthesis mismatch is rare after aortic valve replacement: valve size may be irrelevant. *Ann Thorac Surg* 2002; 73:1822.

82. Blackstone EH, Cosgrove DM, Jamieson WRE, et al: Prosthesis size and long-term survival after aortic valve replacement. *J Thorac Cardiovasc Surg* 2003; 126:783.

83. Blais C, Dumesnil JG, Baillot R, et al: Impact of valve prosthesis patient mismatch on short-term mortality after aortic valve replacement. *Circulation* 2003; 108:983.

84. Moon MR, Pasque MK, Munfakh NA, et al: Prosthesis-patient mismatch after aortic valve replacement: impact of age and body size on late survival. *Ann Thorac Surg* 2006; 81:481.

85. Emery RW, Krogh CC, Arom KV, et al: *Patient-prosthesis Mismatch: Impact on Patient Survival and Valve Related Events: A 25-year Experience with the St. Jude Medical Valve Prosthesis.* Presented at the Society of Thoracic Surgeons at the 41st Annual Meeting, San Antonio, TX. January 2005.

86. Pibarot P, Dumesnil JG: Patient-prosthesis mismatch and the predictive use of indexed effective orifice area: is it relevant? *Cardiac Surg Today* 2003; 1:43.

87. Riberiro PA, Al Zaibag M, Idris M, et al: Antiplatelet drugs and the incidence of thromboembolic complications of the St. Jude Medical aortic prosthesis in patients with rheumatic heart disease. *J Thoracic Cardiovasc Surg* 1986; 91:92.

88. Ananthasubramaniam K, Beattie JN, Rosman HS, et al: How safely and for how long can warfarin therapy be withheld in prosthetic heart valve patients hospitalized with a major hemorrhage? *Chest* 2001; 119:478.

89. Hartz RS, LoCicero J 3rd, Kucich V, et al: Comparative study of warfarin versus antiplatelet therapy in patients with a St. Jude Medical valve in the aortic position. *J Thorac Cardiovasc Surg* 1986; 92:684.

90. Garcia-Rinaldi R: Letter to the editor. *Ann Thorac Surg* 2006; 81:787.

91. Emery RW, Emery AM: Letter to the editor: reply to Garcia-Rinaldi. *Ann Thorac Surg* 2006; 81:788.

92. Cannegieter SC, Rosendaal FR, Briet E: Thromboembolic and bleeding complications in patients with mechanical heart valve prostheses. *Circulation* 1994; 89:635.

93. Cabalka AK, Emery RW, Petersen RJ: Long-term follow-up of the St. Jude Medical prosthesis in pediatric patients. *Ann Thorac Surg* 1995; 60:S618.

94. Emery RW, Erickson CA, Arom KV, et al: Replacement of the aortic valve in patients under 50 years old with the St. Jude Medical prosthesis. *Ann Thorac Surg* 2003; 75:1815.

95. Pechlivanidis K, Onorati F, Petrilli et al: In which patients is transcatheter valve replacement potentially better indicated than surgery for redo-aortic valve disease: long-term results of a 10 year surgical experience. *J Thorac Cardiovasc Surg* 2014; 148:500.

96. Bapat V, Davies W, Attia R, et al: Use of balloon expandable transcatheter valves for valve-in valve implantation in patients with degenerative stentless aortic bioprosthesis: technical condtraindications and results. *J Thorac Cardiovas Surg* 2014; 148:917-924.

97. Azadni AN, Jaussaud N, Matthews PB, et al: Transcatheter aortic valves inadequately relieve stenosis in small degenerated bioprostheses. *Interactive Cardiovasc Thorac Surg* 2010; 11:70.

98. Azadani AN, Jaussaud N, Matthews PB, et al: Aortic valva-in-valve implantation: impact of transcatheter bioprosthesis mismatch. *J Heart Valve Dis* 2009; 18:367-373.

Stented Bioprosthetic Aortic Valve Replacement

Bobby Yanagawa • Subodh Verma • George T. Christakis

28

This chapter provides an overview of aortic valve replacement (AVR) with stented bioprostheses. The *indications for aortic valve surgery* are reviewed with an emphasis on evidence-based guidelines and contemporary clinical and physiologic outcomes of aortic valve surgery with currently available stented bioprostheses.

NATURAL HISTORY AND INDICATIONS FOR OPERATION

Aortic Stenosis

NATURAL HISTORY

Aortic stenosis (AS) is primarily caused by degenerative calcification in patients over 70 years of age and bicuspid aortic valve in patients under 70 years of age in the developed world. Rheumatic valve disease is the third most common cause of AS affecting patients across the age spectrum. AS is also associated with systemic diseases such as Paget's disease of bone and end-stage renal disease. The pathogenetic mechanisms of aortic valve calcification include valvular interstitial cell transformation, inflammation and lipid accumulation, reminiscent of the pathogenesis of atherosclerotic plaques.[1] The overall incidence of calcific AS is rising with the aging population in developed countries. A population-based study of Olmstead County reported the increase in prevalence of degenerative AS and other valvulopathy in patients with age from 55 to 64 (0.6%), 65 to 74 (1.4%) and ≥75 years (4.6%; *p* < .0001, Fig. 28-1).[2]

Valvular degenerative calcification is characterized as a progressive reduction of orifice cross-sectional area caused by calcification of the cusps. The normal human aortic valve area (AVA) is between 3.0 and 4.0 cm[2] with minimal to no gradient. AS is defined as mild, moderate, severe and very severe with the corresponding AVA, mean gradients and peak jet velocities as shown (Table 28-1). In the presence of normal cardiac output, transvalvular gradient is usually greater than 50 mm Hg when the AVA is less than 1.0 cm[2].[3] A rapid increase in transvalvular gradient is seen with AVAs between 0.7 and 1.0 cm[2]. However, discordant echocardiographic parameters are not uncommon. Minners et al[4] examined 3483 echocardiographic studies with severe AVA, 25% had

less-than-severe mean gradient and 30% has less-than-severe peak velocities leaving only 40% of patients with all echocardiographic criteria consistent with severe AS. Thus, echocardiographic data require careful assessment of images and correlation with hemodynamic parameters such as preload and afterload conditions.

Hemodynamic obstruction to flow created by the reduced orifice area of the aortic valve elevates intracavitary pressures. The resultant wall stress and ischemia-induced myocardial fibrosis leads to compensatory concentric left ventricular hypertrophy (LVH) to normalize wall tension and to maintain cardiac output.[5] With progressive LVH, ventricular compliance decreases and end-diastolic pressure rises.[6] The contribution of atrial contraction to preload becomes more significant and loss of sinus rhythm to atrial fibrillation may lead to rapid progression of symptoms.

SYMPTOMATIC PATIENTS

As AS progresses to become hemodynamically significant, progressive LVH leads to the cardinal symptoms of AS, those being (1) angina, (2) syncope, and (3) dyspnea or congestive heart failure (CHF). The average AVA is 0.6 to 0.8 cm[2] at the onset of symptoms.[5] Classic natural history studies have demonstrated that average life expectancy in patients with hemodynamically significant AS is 4 years with angina, 3 years with syncope, and 2 years with CHF.[7] Symptom development in the context of AS is an absolute indication for surgical intervention.[8] Excessive delay of AVR in symptomatic patients is associated with rate of sudden death of >10% per year. Once a patient is symptomatic, average survival is less than 3 years typically from ventricular arrhythmia or CHF.[9]

ASYMPTOMATIC PATIENTS

The management of asymptomatic patients with hemodynamically significant AS remains a challenge. First, such patients should be exercised to confirm whether they are in fact asymptomatic. Symptoms on exertion will be unveiled in approximately one-third of patients during exercise testing. For truly asymptomatic patients, when considering AVR, the risk of sudden death and progressive ventricular remodeling

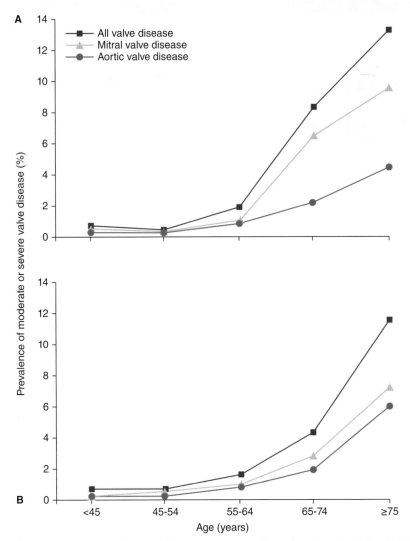

FIGURE 28-1 Prevalence of valvular heart disease by age (A) Frequency in population-based studies (N = 11,911) and (B) in the Olmsted County community (N = 16,501). (Reproduced with permission from Nkomo VT, Gardin JM, Skelton TN, et al: Burden of valvular heart diseases: a population-based study, *Lancet* 2006 Sep 16;368(9540):1005-1011.)

should be weighed against the institutional surgical outcomes or the Society of Thoracic Surgeons Adult Cardiac Surgery Database (STS ACSD) surgical mortality of 3.9%, if appropriate.[10] For uncorrected AS, the average decrease in AVA is 0.12 cm² per year, while the average increase in transvalvular pressure is often 10 to 15 mm Hg per year.[11] Overall, up to 7% of patients with asymptomatic AS experience death or

surgery 1 year after diagnosis which rises to 38% at 5 years.[12] Furthermore, freedom from death or AVR was 67% at 1 year, 56% at 2 years, and 33% at 4 years. However, the high-risk patient subset with very severe AS (jet velocity ≥ 5m/s) progressed much more rapidly with event-free survival of 64% at 1 year, 36% at 2 years, 12% at 4 years and 3% at 6 years.[13]

Early surgery in asymptomatic severe AS may limit and even reverse concentric myocardial injury and fibrosis. In high-volume centers, the operative mortality for isolated AVR is significantly lower than that reported mortality in the STS ACSD.[10] Furthermore, loss to follow up and delay from the time of symptoms to surgical referral are also of concern. For these reasons, early surgery may a reasonable strategy, particularly for young patients who are unlikely to escape the need for surgical valve replacement.

On the other hand, there is considerable variation in the rate of disease progression, there can exist a prolonged and stochastic latent period before symptoms emerge and many patients do not experience any change in gradient for several

⬤ TABLE 28-1: Classification of AS

	Mild	Moderate	Severe
AVA (cm²)	>1.5	1.5-1.0	<1.0*
Indexed AVA (cm²/m²)			<0.6
Mean Gradient (mm Hg)	<25	25-40	>40
Peak Jet Velocity (m/s)	<3.0	3.0-4.0	>4.0

*AVA < 0.6 cm² is considered very severe.

years. Sudden death is rather uncommon in the asymptomatic patient with AS and even with severe AS, the rate is less than 1% per year.[12] Furthermore, the vast majority of patients who experience sudden death will become symptomatic in the months immediately prior. In addition, early and late outcomes were similar among patients with severe AS who underwent surgery with symptoms or without.[14] Thus, watchful waiting with close clinical and echocardiographic follow up may also be considered for those with asymptomatic AS.

It is difficult to predict who will eventually need surgical intervention and to identify asymptomatic patient subsets that will benefit from an early surgical approach. As mentioned, asymptomatic patients with increases in high peak velocity jet are substantially more likely to need an operation.[13] Patients with very severe AS (AVA $\leq$ 0.75 cm^2 and jet velocity $\geq$ 4.5 m/s or mean gradient $\geq$ 50 mm Hg) have lower-mid-term all-cause mortality (2 $\pm$ 1% vs 32 $\pm$ 6%, $p < .001$) with early surgery versus conventional treatment.[15] Severe LVH (left ventricular mass [LVM] index $\geq$ 180 g/m^2) and enlarged left atrium ($\geq$5.0-cm diameter) are markers of longstanding AS and are associated with reduced survival post-AVR.[16] B-type natriuretic peptide (BNP) is released in response to increased myocardial wall stress and is a well-established marker of heart failure. Several groups have shown BNP to be a marker of symptomatic AS and an independent and objective predictor of outcome in patients with AS.[17-19] Further clinical studies will be needed to determine the clinical value of such echocardiographic measurements and biomarkers as triggers to guide the timing of surgical intervention.

LOW-GRADIENT AORTIC STENOSIS

Patients with very poor ventricular function (ejection fraction < 50%) who have severely stenotic valves but nonsevere (<40 mm Hg) transvalvular gradients or jet velocity (<4 m/s) are termed low-gradient AS (LGAS). Compromised left ventricular function in these patients may be caused by afterload mismatch created by the stenotic valve or by intrinsic cardiomyopathy, or both, particularly in the setting of chronic ischemia from diffuse coronary disease. In these patients, measurement of transvalvular gradient and valve area at rest and with positive inotropy (eg, dobutamine stress echocardiography) may distinguish cardiomyopathy versus true valvular stenosis as the most responsible diagnosis. Those patients with contractile reserve that experience an increase in valve gradient ($\geq$40 mm Hg) or jet velocity ($\geq$4 m/s) with dobutamine inotropy are considered to have *true LGAS*. An increase in augmented flow resulting in only a mild increase in transvalvular gradient but an increase in valve area by $\geq$0.2 cm^2 suggests *pseudosevere LGAS*. The lack of increase in gradient nor AVA with dobutamine suggests pseudosevere LGAS lacking contractile reserve. Severe diastolic dysfunction with EF $\geq$50% and indexed AVA $\leq$ 0.6 cm^2 but mean gradient < 40 mm Hg, jet velocity < 4 m/s and indexed stroke volume < 30 cc/m^2 is termed *paradoxical LGAS*. The latter is associated with pronounced left ventricular concentric remodeling,

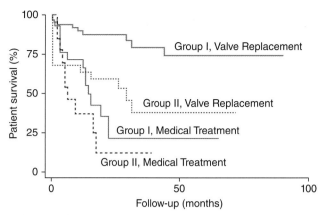

FIGURE 28-2 Kaplan-Meier survival estimates for patients with low gradient aortic stenosis with (Group 1) and without (Group 2) contractile reserve by dobutamine stress echocardiography. (Reproduced with permission from Monin JL, Quéré JP, Monchi M, et al: Low-gradient aortic stenosis: operative risk stratification and predictors for long-term outcome: a multicenter study using dobutamine stress hemodynamics. *Circulation*. 2003 Jul 22;108(3):319-324.)

moderate-to-severe diastolic dysfunction, decreased longitudinal strain and reduced stroke volume.

Patients with LGAS are a high-risk patient population with lower 5-year survival compared with those with high gradient severe AS. A retrospective study of 1154 patients with severe AS confirmed higher operative mortalities with LGAS (6.3%) and paradoxical LGAS (6.3%) compared with normal flow severe AS (1.8%).[20] However, such patients experience a significant survival benefit from valve replacement compared with medical management alone (Fig. 28-2).[21] Tribouilloy et al[22] report a high operative mortality (22%) but in survivors, an improved propensity-matched 5-year survival with AVR (65 $\pm$ 11% vs 11 $\pm$ 7%, $p = .019$). Thus, patients with LGAS should be carefully selected but can benefit from surgical AVR.

MEDICAL THERAPY

Medical therapy for afterload reduction may be beneficial in AS but there is no known medical therapy that has been shown to alter its natural history. Hypertension is associated with greater cardiovascular events and improved survival, and thus medical treatment for hypertension is reasonable.[23] Afterload reduction may be considered for patient with AS in heart failure but should be initiated and titrated cautiously as a sudden decrease in systemic vascular resistance can result in an acute reduction in cardiac output.[24] With regard to targeted therapy, three randomized controlled trials (RCTs) did not show a benefit of statins in did not halting or lowering the rate of disease progression in AS.[25-27] The importance of osteogenic processes as key mechanisms in AS has suggested potential targets for therapy but these studies are still very much in the experimental stages.[28]

INDICATIONS FOR SURGERY

In 2014, a joint task force of the American College of Cardiology (ACC) and the American Heart Association (AHA) developed evidence-based consensus guidelines for management of patients with valvular heart disease.[29] These guidelines encompass several important overarching changes since the 2006 AHA/ACC guidelines and the 2008 updates:[30,31]

1. Regarding AS and aortic regurgitation (AR), the revised guidelines include a new classification of heart valve diseases based on valve anatomy, valve hemodynamics, hemodynamic consequences, and symptoms. There are four stages with treatment recommendations for each stage: (A) at risk; (B) progressive asymptomatic; (C) severe asymptomatic (C1, with ventricular compensation; C2, with ventricular decompensation); and (D) severe symptomatic.
2. Symptomatic severe AS is subdivided into high gradient ($V_{max} \geq 4$ m/s or mean gradient ≥ 40 mm Hg), LGAS with reduced left ventricular ejection fraction (LVEF) (severe leaflet calcification with severely reduced motion, effective orifice area [EOA] ≤ 1.0 cm^2, and $V_{max} < 4$ m/s or gradient < 40 mm Hg with LVEF $< 50\%$, and EOA remaining ≤ 1.0 cm^2, but $V_{max} \geq 4$ m/s at any flow rate during dobutamine echocardiography), and paradoxical LGAS with normal LVEF (severe leaflet calcification with severely reduced motion, EOA ≤ 1.0 cm^2 and $V_{max} < 4$ m/s or gradient < 40 mm Hg with LVEF $\geq 50\%$).
3. A focus on the Heart Team approach for clinical decision-making, particularly given the availability of surgical and transcatheter interventions.
4. An integrative approach to the procedural risk, which incorporates risk scoring, frailty, major organ system dysfunction and procedural impediments.

The specific recommendations for AVR for patients with AS are shown (Table 28-2 and Fig. 28-3).[29] To summarize, AVR should be performed in all symptomatic patients with severe AS or in patients with severe asymptomatic AS who require concomitant cardiac surgery or with left ventricular dysfunction (LVD; LVEF $< 50\%$). It is reasonable to perform AVR in patients with moderate AS requiring concomitant cardiac surgery. AVR is reasonable in otherwise asymptomatic patients with very severe AS (valve area < 0.6 cm^2 and jet velocities ≥ 5 m/s), severe AS and exercise-induced symptoms, and in those with true or paradoxical LGAS. Asymptomatic patients with severe AS with rapid progression may be considered for valve replacement prior to significant ventricular decompensation or sudden death.

Aortic Regurgitation
ACUTE AORTIC REGURGITATION
Acute AR is caused by (1) acute dilatation of the aortic annulus or sinotubular junction or both, preventing adequate cusp coaptation or by (2) disruption of the valve cusps themselves. The specific causes of AR include aortic dissection, infective endocarditis, trauma, aortic cusp prolapse secondary to VSD, aortitis or arteritis (eg, syphilitic, giant cell, Takayasu) and iatrogenesis (eg, postaortic balloon valvotomy).

The heart is relatively intolerant to acute AR, as the left ventricle is unable to compensate for the sudden increase in end-diastolic volume caused by a large regurgitant volume load. A dramatic reduction in forward stroke volume ensues. In the context of a hypertrophic and poorly compliant left ventricle, hemodynamic decompensation is significantly more dramatic. Tachycardia is the initial compensatory response to acute decline in forward stroke volume. Progressive volume overload causes the left ventricular end-diastolic pressure to acutely rise above left atrial pressure resulting in early closure

⊖ TABLE 28-2: 2014 ACC/AHA Guidelines for Aortic Valve Replacement in Patients with Aortic Stenosis

Recommendation	Class	Level
AVR is recommended with severe high-gradient AS who have symptoms by history or on exercise testing (stage D1)	I	B
AVR is recommended for asymptomatic patients with severe AS (stage C2) and LVEF < 50%	I	B
AVR is indicated for patients with severe AS (stage C or D) when undergoing other cardiac surgery	I	B
AVR is reasonable for asymptomatic patients with very severe AS (stage C1, aortic velocity ≥ 5.0 m/s) and low surgical risk	IIa	B
AVR is reasonable in asymptomatic patients (stage C1) with severe AS and decreased exercise tolerance or an exercise fall in BP	IIa	B
AVR is reasonable in symptomatic patients with low-flow/low-gradient severe AS with reduced LVEF (stage D2) with a low-dose dobutamine stress study that shows an aortic velocity ≥ 4.0 m/s (or mean pressure gradient ≥ 40 mm Hg) with a valve area ≤ 1.0 cm^2 at any dobutamine dose	IIa	B
AVR is reasonable in symptomatic patients who have low-flow/low-gradient severe AS (stage D3) who are normotensive and have an LVEF ≥ 50% if clinical, hemodynamic, and anatomic data support valve obstruction as the most likely cause of symptoms	IIa	C
AVR is reasonable for patients with moderate AS (stage B) (aortic velocity 3.0 to 3.9 m/s) who are undergoing other cardiac surgery	IIa	C
AVR may be considered for asymptomatic patients with severe AS (stage C1) and rapid disease progression and low surgical risk	IIb	C

Adapted with permission from Nishimura RA, Otto CM, Bonow RO, et al: 2014 AHA/ACC guideline for the management of patients with valvular heart disease: a report of the American College of Cardiology/American Heart Association Task Force on Practice Guidelines, *J Thorac Cardiovasc Surg.* 2014 Jul;148(1):e1-e132.

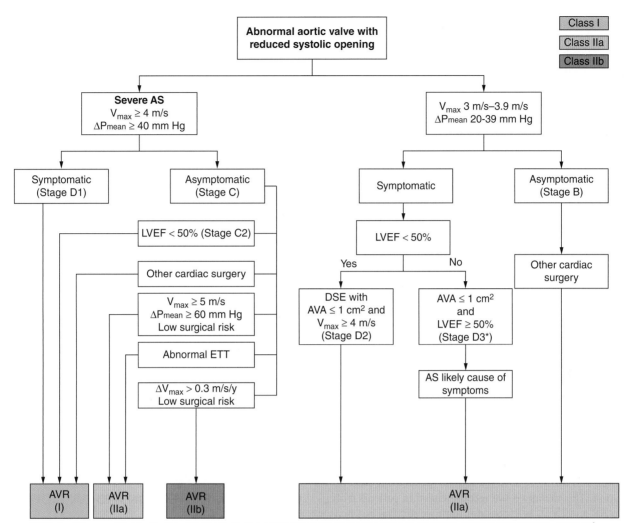

FIGURE 28-3 Indications for AVR in patients with AS. (Reproduced with permission from Nishimura RA, Otto CM, Bonow RO, et al: 2014 AHA/ACC guideline for the management of patients with valvular heart disease: a report of the American College of Cardiology/American Heart Association Task Force on Practice Guidelines, *J Thorac Cardiovasc Surg.* 2014 Jul;148(1):e1-e132.)

of the mitral valve.[32] Although this protects the pulmonary venous circulation from excessively high end-diastolic pressures, rapid progression of pulmonary edema and cardiogenic shock is unavoidable. Death secondary to progressive cardiogenic shock and malignant ventricular arrhythmias are the commonest endpoints of acute AR regardless of etiology. Thus urgent surgical treatment is warranted for all causes of hemodynamically significant acute AR.

CHRONIC AORTIC REGURGITATION

Chronic AR is caused by either slow enlargement of the aortic root or dysfunction of the valve cusps. Common causes of chronic AR include congenital abnormalities (eg, bicuspid, unicuspid, quadricuspid aortic valve), calcific cusp degeneration, rheumatic fever, endocarditis, Marfan syndrome, Ehlers-Danlos syndrome, myxomatous proliferation, osteogenesis imperfect and ankylosing spondylitis. The echocardiographic and catheter-based parameters for AR are shown (Table 28-3).

Chronic AR causes a persistent volume overload of the left ventricle. Initially, the ratio of wall thickness to chamber diameter, ejection fraction, and fractional shortening are maintained.[33] However, this volume burden eventually leads to progressive chamber enlargement without increasing

TABLE 28-3: Classification of AR

	Mild	Moderate	Severe
EROA (cm²)	>0.1	0.1-0.3	>0.3
Regurgitant fraction (%)	<30	30-50	>50
Regurgitant volume (mL)	<30	30-60	>60
Jet width (% LVOT)	<25	25-65	>65
Vena contracta (cm)	<0.3	0.3-0.6	>0.6
Angiography grade	1+	2+	3-4+

EROA, effective regurgitant orifice area; LVOT, left ventricular outflow tract.

end-diastolic pressure during the asymptomatic phase of the disease. Chamber enlargement is accompanied by adaptive eccentric hypertrophy, associated at the cellular level with sarcomere replication and elongation of myocytes. The combination of chamber dilatation and hypertrophy leads to a massive increase in left ventricular mass. A vicious cycle of chamber enlargement, continually increasing wall stress and maladaptive ventricular hypertrophy ensues. Development of interstitial fibrosis is an important pathogenic mechanism that limits further ventricular dilation elevating end-diastolic pressure and leading to left ventricular systolic dysfunction, and CHF.[34] Natural history studies of AR show that symptoms, LVD, or both develop in <6% of patients per year.[35] Progression to LVD without symptoms occurs in <4% of patients per year and sudden death occurs in <0.2% per year.[36] Independent predictors of progression to symptoms, LVD, or death in asymptomatic patients include age, left ventricular end-systolic dimension, rate of change in end-systolic dimension, and resting ejection fraction.[37] Once LVD develops, the onset of symptoms occur at a rate exceeding 25% per year.[38]

The decision to operate on patients with AR and LVD is indeed challenging since the outcomes are poor with surgery and with medical therapy. Patients with more severe LVD have decreased perioperative and late survival due to irreversible ventricular remodeling including hypertrophy and interstitial fibrosis.[39,40] Vasodilator therapy may delay progression of ventricular dysfunction by decreasing afterload thus reducing regurgitant flow. This is currently indicated in asymptomatic patients with hypertension; asymptomatic patients with severe AR, ventricular dilatation, and preserved systolic function; and for short-term hemodynamic tailoring prior to operation. This therapy is not recommended in patients with severe AR and LVD, as it does not improve survival but may be considered if such patients are considered inoperable.

INDICATIONS FOR OPERATION

A summary of the 2014 ACC/AHA Guidelines for AVR for chronic AR is presented in Table 28-4 and Fig. 28-4.[29] Symptomatic patients experience > 10% mortality per year thus

surgery is absolutely indicated.[39] Since symptoms, such as angina and dyspnea, develop only after significant ventricular decompensation has occurred, surgery is advocated prior to the symptomatic phase of the disease. Surgical intervention for asymptomatic patients is based on the identification of subtle but measurable changes in myocardial function before they become irreversible and negatively affect the patient's long-term prognosis.

CORONARY ANGIOGRAPHY AND AORTIC VALVE REPLACEMENT

Many patients requiring AVR have coexistent coronary artery disease (CAD). In North America, more than one-third of AVR procedures are accompanied with coronary artery bypass graft surgery.[10] Risk assessment for ischemic heart disease is complicated in patients with aortic valve disease since angina may be related to true ischemia from hemodynamically significant coronary lesions, or other causes such as left ventricular wall stress with subendocardial ischemia or chamber enlargement in the setting of reduced coronary flow reserve, or both.

According to the 2014 ACC/AHA Guidelines, during preoperative planning for AVR, coronary catheterization should be performed for the presence of angina, ischemia, LVD, or history of CAD; males > 40 years old; and postmenopausal women (Class I, Level of Evidence C). CT coronary angiography may be performed with low or intermediate pretest probability of CAD (Class IIa, Level of Evidence B).[29]

Technique of Operation

MYOCARDIAL PROTECTION AND CARDIOPULMONARY BYPASS

Isolated AVR is performed using a single, two-stage right atrial venous cannula and an arterial cannula into the ascending aorta for systemic perfusion of oxygenated blood. A retrograde cardioplegia cannula may be placed into the coronary sinus via the right atrium. A left ventricular vent cannula may be placed in the right superior pulmonary vein and advanced

---

⊖ **TABLE 28-4: 2014 ACC/AHA Recommendations for Aortic Valve Replacement in Chronic Severe Aortic Regurgitation**

Indication	Class	Level
AVR is indicated for symptomatic patients with severe AR regardless of LV systolic function (stage D)	I	B
AVR is indicated for asymptomatic patients with chronic severe AR and LV systolic dysfunction (LVEF < 50%) (stage C2)	I	B
AVR is indicated for patients with severe AR (stage C or D) while undergoing cardiac surgery for other indications	I	C
AVR is reasonable for asymptomatic patients with severe AR with normal LV systolic function (LVEF ≥ 50%) but with severe LV dilation (LVESD > 50 mm, stage C2)	IIa	B
AVR is reasonable in patients with moderate AR (stage B) who are undergoing other cardiac surgery	IIa	C
AVR may be considered for asymptomatic patients with severe AR and normal LV systolic function (LVEF ≥ 50%, stage C1) but with progressive severe LV dilation (LVEDD > 65 mm) if surgical risk is low	IIb	C

Adapted with permission from Nishimura RA, Otto CM, Bonow RO, et al: 2014 AHA/ACC guideline for the management of patients with valvular heart disease: a report of the American College of Cardiology/American Heart Association Task Force on Practice Guidelines, *J Thorac Cardiovasc Surg.* 2014 Jul;148(1):e1-e132.

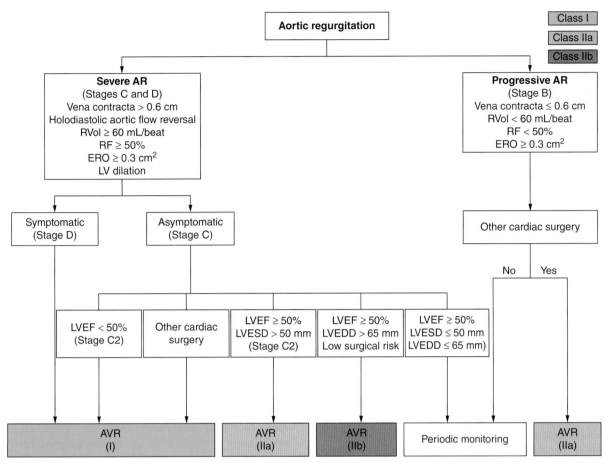

FIGURE 28-4 Indications for AVR in patients with AR. (Reproduced with permission from Nishimura RA, Otto CM, Bonow RO, et al: 2014 AHA/ACC guideline for the management of patients with valvular heart disease: a report of the American College of Cardiology/American Heart Association Task Force on Practice Guidelines, *J Thorac Cardiovasc Surg*. 2014 Jul;148(1):e1-e132.)

into the left ventricle to ensure a bloodless field and to prevent ventricular distention with aortic insufficiency. Alternatively, a vent may be placed into the pulmonary artery or directly in the left ventricular outflow tract (LVOT) via the aortotomy. Once cardiopulmonary bypass (CPB) is initiated, careful dissection of the pulmonary artery from the aorta ensures that the cross-clamp will be fully occlusive on the aorta and prevents inadvertent opening of the pulmonary artery with the aortotomy incision. Care is needed to prevent pulmonary artery injury, as this tissue is substantially more friable than the aorta.

After the cross-clamp is applied, myocardial protection is initially delivered as a single dose of high potassium blood through the ascending aorta. This will trigger prompt diastolic arrest unless there is moderate-to-severe AR in which arrest can be achieved with direct ostial or retrograde cardioplegia. Myocardial protection is maintained by continuous infusion of cold or tepid oxygenated blood cardioplegia delivered via direct cannulation of both coronary ostia after the aorta has been opened. The angiogram should be examined to rule out a short left main coronary artery, in which case, direct ostial antegrade cannulation may preferentially perfuse either the LAD or circumflex system. In the presence

of severe CAD, antegrade cardioplegia may not perfuse myocardial segments distal to significant coronary obstruction. Furthermore, direct cannulation of left main coronary artery risks endothelial injury and potential dissection or promotion of atherosclerosis development.

An alternative method of cardioprotection in aortic valve cases is retrograde cardioplegia, in either intermittent or continuous forms and utilized in isolation or in combination with antegrade cardioplegia. This is helpful in patients with significant AR or severe concomitant coronary disease. However, there are some questions regarding the quality of right ventricular perfusion using retrograde alone. If a retrograde cannula cannot be guided into the coronary sinus, conversion to bicaval cannulation will allow opening the right atrium and direct placement of the cannula into the coronary sinus. Do not place the retrograde cannula beyond the origin of the right coronary vein ostium in the coronary sinus to ensure adequate right ventricular myocardial protection.

Right ventricular myocardial protection can be a challenge for a small nondominant right coronary artery (RCA) that will not accept a direct ostial cannula. One solution is to drift the patient's temperature to 28°C with cold topical slush and frequent retrograde cardioplegia.

AORTOTOMY, VALVE EXCISION, AND DEBRIDEMENT

Once the cross-clamp has been applied and cardioplegic arrest has been achieved, the aorta is opened either with a transverse or oblique aortotomy. The low transverse aortotomy is a common approach to the aortic valve when using stented bioprostheses or mechanical valves. The aortotomy is started approximately 10 to 15 mm above the origin of the RCA and extended anteriorly and posteriorly. The initial transverse incision over the RCA may also be extended obliquely in the posterior direction into the noncoronary sinus or the commissure between the left and noncoronary cusps (Fig. 28-5). The oblique incision is often used in patients with small aortic roots, in whom root enlargement procedures may be required.

Morphology of the valve is then inspected (Fig. 28-6). The valve cusps are incised with scissors at the right cusp between the right coronary ostium and the commissure between the right and noncoronary cusps using Mayo scissors or special right-angled valve scissors (Fig. 28-7). One to two millimeters of tissue is left behind to support a sewing surface. Right cusp excision is carried first toward the left coronary cusp and then toward the noncoronary cusp and the cusp is removed as a single piece if possible. A moistened radiopaque sponge may be placed into the outflow area to catch calcific debris, which must be removed before placing the valve sutures. Thorough decalcification is then performed with a scalpel or rongeur. Debridement of all calcium deposits back to soft tissue improves seating of the prosthesis and decreases the incidence of paravalvular leak and dehiscence.

Care must be taken to prevent aortic perforation while calcific deposits are debrided from the aortic wall, particularly at the commissure between the left and noncoronary cusps,

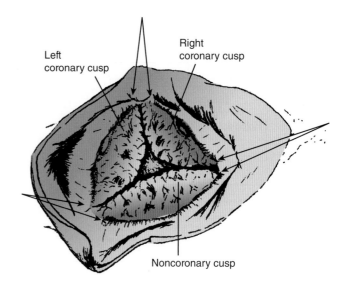

FIGURE 28-6 The exposed aortic valve.

where perforation is most likely. Several anatomic relationships must be respected during valve excision (Fig. 28-8). The bundle of His (conduction system) is located below the junction of the right and noncoronary cusps in the membranous septum. Deep debridement in this area can result in permanent heart block. The anterior leaflet of the mitral valve is in direct continuity with the left aortic valve cusp. If it is damaged during decalcification, an autologous pericardial patch can be used to repair the defect.

Once debridement is completed, the aortic root is copiously flushed with saline while the left ventricular vent is stopped. To prevent pushing debris into the left ventricle, saline in a bulb syringe is flushed through the left ventricular vent and out the aortic valve in an antegrade manner instead of retrograde through the valve. The irrigation solution is suctioned with the external wall suction and not into the cardiotomy suction.

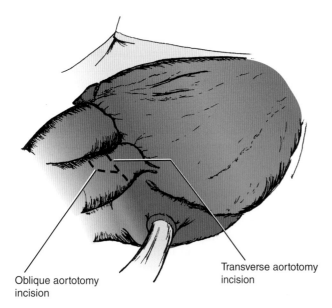

FIGURE 28-5 Exposure and aortotomy incision. A two-stage venous cannula is in place in the right atrial appendage. The aortotomy (dashed line) may be made in the transverse or oblique direction.

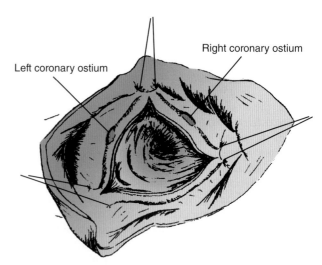

FIGURE 28-7 The aortic valve after leaflet excision.

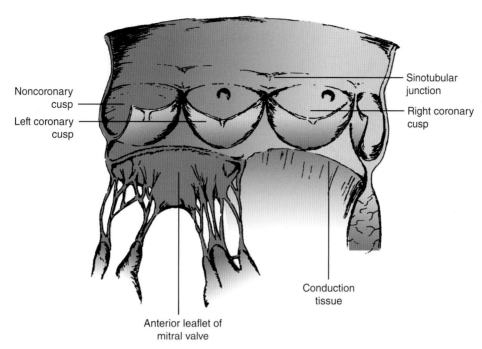

FIGURE 28-8 Anatomic relationships of the aortic valve.

VALVE IMPLANTATION

The annulus is sized with a valve-sizer designed for the selected prosthetic device. The valve is secured to the annulus using 12 to 16 double-needled interrupted 2-0 synthetic braided pledgeted sutures that are alternating in color. The pledgets can be left on the inflow/ventricular side or the outflow/aortic side of the aortic annulus (Figs. 28-9 and 28-10). Placing the pledgets on the inside of the annulus allows supra-annular placement of the valve and generally will allow implantation of as slightly larger prosthesis. If the coronary ostia are close to the annulus, supra-annular placement may only be possible along the noncoronary cusp. Mattress sutures are first placed in the three commissures and retracted to assist visualization. Some surgeons will place the commissural suture between the right and noncoronary cusps from the outside of the aorta (ie, the pledget is left on the outside of the aorta) to prevent injury to the conduction system. Pledgeted mattress sutures are then placed in a clockwise fashion typically starting in the noncoronary cusp. Sutures may be placed into the sewing ring of the prosthetic valve with each annular suture or after all annular sutures are placed. The sutures for each of the three cusps are held separately with three hemostats and retracted while the prosthesis is slid into the annulus. Sutures are then tied down in a balanced fashion alternating among the three cusps.

AORTIC CLOSURE AND DE-AIRING

The aorta is closed with a double row of synthetic 4-0 polypropylene sutures. The first suture line is started on the right side at the posterior end of the aortotomy and the double-needled suture is secured slightly beyond the incision to ensure there is no leak in this region. One end of the suture is run

as a horizontal mattress anteriorly to the midpoint of the aortotomy, and then the second end of the suture is run anteriorly, slightly superficial to the horizontal mattress suture, in an over-and-over manner. On the left side, a similar technique is

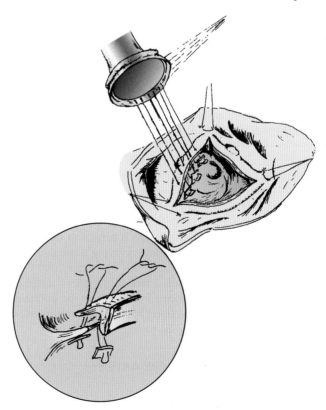

FIGURE 28-9 Placement of sutures with pledgets below the annulus.

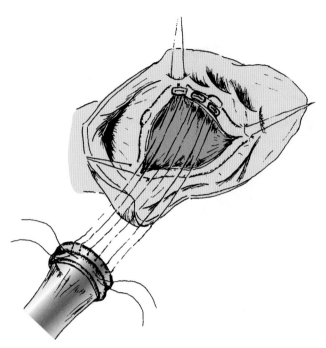

FIGURE 28-10 Placement of sutures with pledgets above the annulus.

performed, the aorta is de-aired, and the two sutures are tied to themselves and to each other at the aortotomy midpoint.

During AVR, air is entrained into the left atrium and ventricle, and aorta. This must be removed to prevent catastrophic air embolization. Immediately prior to tying the suture of the aortotomy, the heart is allowed to fill, the vent in the superior pulmonary vein is stopped, the lungs are inflated, and the cross-clamp is briefly partially opened. The influx of blood should expel most air from these cavities out of the partially open aortotomy. Closure of the aortotomy is then completed and the cross-clamp is fully removed. The cardioplegia cannula in the ascending aorta and the left ventricular vent are then placed on suction to remove any residual air as the heart begins electrical activity. A small needle (21-gauge) can be used to aspirate the apex of the left ventricle and the dome of the left atrium. To prevent air entrainment, the left ventricular vent must be removed while the pericardium is filled with saline irrigation. De-airing maneuvers are verified with visualization using transesophageal echocardiography. Vigorous shaking and careful manual compression of the heart while suctioning through the aortic vent (ie, cardioplegia tack) is helpful to remove air trapped within trabeculations. Once de-airing is complete, the aortic vent is removed. The patient is then weaned from CPB and decannulated in the standard fashion. If patients are pacemaker dependent when weaned from CPB in the operating room, it is recommended to insert atrial pacing wires to allow for synchronous atrioventricular pacing.

CONCOMITANT CORONARY ARTERY BYPASS GRAFTING

Operative technique is modified when there is concomitant CAD to optimize myocardial protection. Distal anastomoses are performed prior to AVR so that antegrade cardioplegia-may be administered through these grafts during the operation. The left internal mammary artery should be used for revascularization of the left anterior descending artery. This anastomosis is performed after the aortotomy is closed to ensure that the coronary circulation is not exposed to systemic circulation during cardioplegic arrest and to prevent trauma to the anastomosis during manipulation of the heart.

The 2014 ACC/AHA Guidelines recommend concomitant surgical revascularization for coronary stenosis ≥ 70% or left main stenosis ≥ 50% (Class IIa, Level of Evidence C).[29] The benefit of revascularization should be balanced with the increased operative mortality, which increases from 3.9 to 5.9% for combined CABG/AVR according to the STS ACSD.[10] Concomitant CABG at the time of AVR is common as reported rates were 30% in patients 51 to 60 years of age, 41% in 61 to 70 years of age and 50% in >71 years of age.[41]

CONCOMITANT ASCENDING AORTIC REPLACEMENT

The threshold for concomitant replacement of the ascending aorta at the time of AVR is an area of debate. Borger et al,[42] reviewed patients with bicuspid aortic valve undergoing AVR and report 15-year freedom from aorta-related complications was 86, 81, and 43% in patients with an aortic diameter of <4.0 cm, 4.0 to 4.4 cm, and 4.5 to 4.9 cm, respectively (Fig. 28-11). Extrapolating from these data and others to all patients with concomitant ascending aortic dilation, the current 2014 ACC/AHA Guidelines recommend aorta replacement when maximal diameter exceeds 4.5 cm for patients undergoing aortic valve surgery (Class IIa, Level of Evidence C).[29] In patients with Marfan or Loeys-Dietz Syndromes, the aortopathy is much more aggressive and a lower trigger point for replacement may be appropriate. Given the lack of data, there are currently no recommendations for concomitant

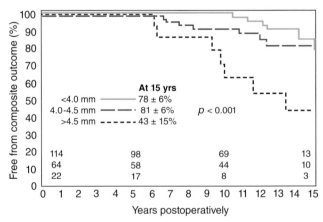

FIGURE 28-11 Freedom from ascending aortic complications for patients with a bicuspid aortic valve with an ascending aortic diameter of <4 cm, 4.0 to 4.5 cm, and 4.5 to 4.9 cm at the time of aortic valve replacement. (Reproduced with permission from Borger MA, et al: Should the ascending aorta be replaced more frequently in patients with bicuspid aortic valve disease? *J Thorac Cardiovasc Surg* 2004; Nov;128(5):677-683.)

replacement of ascending aorta when replacing a tricuspid aortic valve. Clearly the threshold should be between 4.5 and 5.5 cm. The decision is left to the surgeon and should be based on the additive risk of the procedure, patient's age, comorbidities, and overall life expectancy.

AORTIC ROOT ENLARGEMENT PROCEDURES

Detailed descriptions of aortic root enlargement procedures are presented in a later chapter. Briefly, either an anterior or posterior annular enlargement procedure may be performed in a patient with a small aortic root to allow for implantation of a larger valve. The posterior approach is the most commonly used aortic root enlargement procedure in adults and can increase the annular diameter by 2 to 4 mm. Nicks and colleagues in 1970 described a technique of root enlargement in which the aortotomy is extended downward through the noncoronary cusp, through the aortic annulus to the anterior mitral leaflet with patch augmentation.[43] In 1979, Manouguian and Seybold-Epting described a procedure extending the aortotomy incision in a downward direction through the commissure between the left and noncoronary cusps into the interleaflet triangle and into the anterior leaflet of the mitral valve with patch augmentation.[44] The anterior approach is generally used in the pediatric population. Described by Konno and colleagues in 1975, this technique, which is also known as aortoventriculoplasty, is used when more than 4 mm of annular enlargement is required.[45] Instead of a transverse incision, a longitudinal incision is made in the anterior aorta and extended to the right coronary sinus of Valsalva and then through the anterior wall of the right ventricle to open the right ventricular outflow tract. The ventricular septum is incised, allowing significant expansion of the aortic annulus and left ventricular outflow tract.

REOPERATIVE AORTIC VALVE SURGERY

Reoperative AVR may be performed for prosthetic valve-related complications or commonly for progressive AS post-CABG. Prosthetic valve-related causes include structural valve deterioration, prosthetic endocarditis, prosthesis thrombosis, or paravalvular leak. Chest reentry is the most hazardous portion of any repeat cardiac procedure. The proximity of cardiac structures to the posterior sternum must be assessed prior to redo sternotomy. This can be accomplished by lateral chest x-ray (CXR), computed tomography (CT) scan, or magnetic resonance imaging (MRI). Before making an incision, there should be blood transfusion units in the room, external defibrillator pads on the patient and the CPB pump should be primed. Femoral or axillary vessels may be exposed or CPB may be instituted through the peripheral vessels in the case of high-risk chest reentry. An oscillating saw is used to open the sternum and as little tissue as possible is dissected. Extreme caution must be employed during dissection when there are patent bypass grafts that cross the midline.

Once cardioplegic arrest is established, the old prosthesis is excised with sharp dissection. Care must be taken to count and remove all sutures and pledgets from the annulus.

Annular injuries caused while excising the prosthesis are repaired with pledgeted interrupted sutures or with a patch, typically of treated bovine pericardium. Removal of stentless prostheses may be particularly difficult. In the setting of endocarditis, aggressive debridement of all infected tissue must be performed with annular and aortic root reconstruction with pericardium when root abscesses are present.[46] Any foreign material can be seeded with bacteria, including Dacron aortic grafts, must be excised in the presence of active endocarditis as grafts can be seeded with bacteria.

In the presence of a Dacron prosthesis in the ascending aorta, chest reentry may be extremely hazardous since exsanguination will occur if the graft is inadvertently opened during dissection. To limit the systemic consequences of exsanguination at normothermia, the patient may be placed on femoro-femoral CPB and cooled to 18 to 20°C prior to chest reentry. If the Dacron graft is accidentally opened, local control of the bleeding is established and CPB is stopped. Under circulatory arrest, the graft is repaired or replaced. CPB may then be restarted. In all repeat aortic procedures, rigorous myocardial protection must be applied since these procedures often have very long ischemic times. Antegrade cold blood cardioplegia is usually employed in a continuous fashion throughout the case by selective cannulation of the coronary ostia. Retrograde cardioplegia may have benefit in the setting of patent old saphenous vein grafts.[47] More and more patients with previous cardiac surgery that require high-risk reoperative AVR are increasingly being referred to Heart Teams for consideration of transcatheter aortic valve replacement (TAVR).

PORCELAIN AORTA

Porcelain aorta is the most severe form of aortic atherosclerosis. The major risk of manipulation of a calcified aorta is atheroemboli with stroke being the most common clinical sequelae.[36] Calcified or porcelain aorta is found in approximately 1 to 2% of cases and can be diagnosed based on preoperative imaging or intraoperative assessment. A history of risk factors such as smoking, hypercholesterolemia, diabetes, hypertension, or stroke as well as imaging demonstrating ostial coronary disease, peripheral vascular disease or carotid disease should trigger a high index of suspicion for aortic atheroma. Preoperative imaging to demonstrate aortic calcification includes CXR, transthoracic echocardiogram, angiogram, CT, or MRI. Intraoperative assessment includes direct palpation, transesophageal echocardiography and epiaortic ultrasound. Of these, epiaortic ultrasound is the most sensitive modality to detect aortic calcification, particularly for soft, nonechogenic, and nonpalpable plaque components.[37]

The key strategic decisions are (1) central versus peripheral cannulation, (2) cross-clamp versus circulatory arrest, and (3) isolated AVR versus AVR and RAA. Gillinov et al[48] reported a series of patients with severe aortic calcification and AS treated with endarterectomy, replacement of ascending aorta, cross-clamp during DHCA and balloon occlusion of aorta via aortotomy with Foley catheter. Cannulation sites were aorta (34%), femoral artery (34%), axillary artery (24%), and innominate artery (8%), and all patients underwent circulatory arrest. More recently, TAVR has changed the landscape, offering an alternative to surgical valve replacement in this high-risk patient subset. In fact, porcelain aorta is the primary indication in approximately 10 to 15% of patients that undergo TAVR.[49]

POSTOPERATIVE MANAGEMENT

Special consideration must be given to the underlying pathologic changes to the ventricle during the immediate postoperative period. The severely hypertrophied, noncompliant left ventricle resulting from AS is highly dependent on sufficient preload for adequate filling. Filling pressures should be carefully titrated between 15 and 18 mm Hg with intravenous volume infusion. Subvalvular left ventricular outflow obstruction with systolic anterior wall motion of the mitral valve should be avoided. Intravenous beta-adrenergic blockade may relieve this obstruction by decreasing inotropy and chronotropy. In extreme cases reoperation and surgical myectomy may be required.

Maintenance of sinus rhythm is also essential since up to one-third of cardiac output is derived from atrial contraction in a noncompliant ventricle. Up to 10% of patients will experience low cardiac output syndrome in the immediate postoperative period. If pacing is required postoperatively, synchronous atrioventricular pacing is beneficial in preventing low cardiac output syndrome.

Complete heart block occurs in 3 to 5% of AVR patients. This complication may be due to suture placement or injury from debridement near the conduction system at highest risk inferior to the right-non commissure. Transient complete heart block caused by perioperative edema usually resolves in 4 to 6 days. After this time, insertion of a permanent pacemaker is recommended if there is no resolution.

Profound peripheral vasodilation, often seen in patients with aortic insufficiency, is treated with vasoconstrictors including alpha-adrenergic agonists or vasopressin. Adequate filling of the dilated left ventricle may also require volume infusion.

STENTED BIOPROSTHETIC AORTIC VALVEREPLACEMENT DEVICES

Stented bioprostheses may be constructed with porcine aortic valves or bovine pericardium. Over the past 40 years, advances in tissue fixation methodology and various proprietary chemical treatments have been developed to prevent extracellular matrix and calcium deposition. All heterograft valves are preserved with glutaraldehyde, which acts by cross-linking collagen fibers to reduce tissue antigenicity. Glutaraldehyde also ameliorates in vivo enzymatic degradation and causes the loss of cell viability, thereby preventing extracellular matrix turnover.[50] Glutaraldehyde fixation of porcine valves can be performed at high pressure (60 to 80 mm Hg), low pressure (0.1 to 2 mm Hg), or zero pressure (0 mm Hg). Porcine prostheses

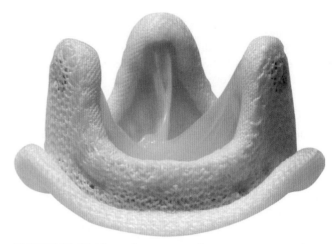

FIGURE 28-12 The Medtronic Hancock II porcine aortic prosthesis. (©Medtronic 2016.)

fixed at zero pressure retain the collagen architecture of the relaxed aortic valve cusp.[51] Pericardial prostheses are fixed in low- or zero-pressure conditions.

When comparing bioprostheses, it is important to be aware of lack of standardization in methodologies for labeling valve sizes by the different manufacturers. In general, label sizes refer to either the internal or the external diameter of the stent, not the external diameter of the sewing cuff or the maximal opening diameter of the valve leaflets. Thus, the same aortic annulus will likely fit different-sized valves from different manufacturers, depending on the convention they use and the size of their sewing cuff.

Earlier-generation Prostheses

First-generation bioprostheses were preserved with high-pressure fixation and were placed in the annular position. Second-generation prostheses are treated with low- or zero-pressure fixation. Several second-generation prostheses may also be placed in the supra-annular position, which allows placement of a slightly larger prosthesis. The Medtronic Hancock II Ultra is a porcine bioprosthesis (Medtronic, Minneapolis, MN; Fig. 28-12) and the Carpentier-Edwards Perimount (Edwards Life Sciences LLC, Irvine, CA; Fig. 28-13) is a pericardial bioprosthesis. Despite the introduction of newer-generation prostheses, some surgeons prefer implantation of Hancock II Ultra and Perimount valves because of the established long-term clinical follow up and performance of these valves.[52-56]

Third-generation Prostheses

Newer-generation prostheses incorporate zero- or low-pressure fixation with anti-mineralization processes that are designed to reduce material fatigue and calcification. Stents have become progressively thinner allowing a lower profile. Porcine valves have a lower stent post and base profile to minimize protrusion into the aortic wall and facilitate

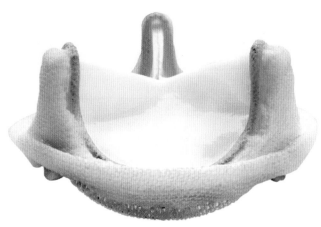

FIGURE 28-13 The Edwards Perimount pericardial aortic prosthesis. (Used with permission from Edwards Lifesciences LLC, Irvine, CA.)

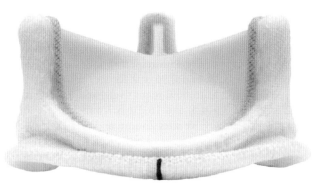

FIGURE 28-15 The Edwards Magna Ease pericardial aortic prosthesis. ((Used with permission from Edwards Lifesciences LLC, Irvine, CA.)

coronary clearance (Medtronic Mosaic Ultra; Fig. 28-14). For this reason, they are particularly favorable for tissue mitral valve replacement as the stents occupy less space in the left ventricle.

The third-generation bovine bioprostheses include the Carpentier-Edwards Magna Ease (Edwards Life Sciences LLC; Fig. 28-15), Mitroflow (Sorin, Fig. 28-16), and Trifeca (St. Jude, St. Paul, MN; Fig. 28-17). The Magna Ease is the evolution of the Perimount pericardial valve, with a narrower sewing cuff and scalloped sign for supra-annular placement. The Mitroflow Pericardial aortic prosthesis and the Trifecta are pericardial valves with the pericardium placed around the exterior of the stent, allowing for a larger opening diameter and optimal flow characteristics.

Head-to-head comparisons have been performed and despite small but significant differences in hemodynamic parameters, no valve has demonstrated improved survival nor left ventricular remodeling over another. Thalji et al[57]

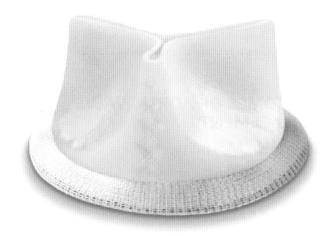

FIGURE 28-16 The Sorin Mitroflow pericardial aortic prosthesis. (Courtesy of Sorin Group, Saluggia, Italy.)

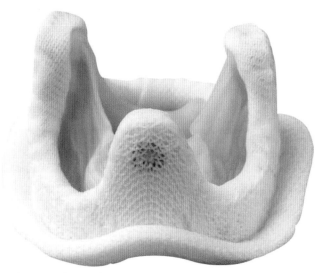

FIGURE 28-14 The Medtronic Mosaic Ultra porcine aortic prosthesis. (©Medtronic 2016.)

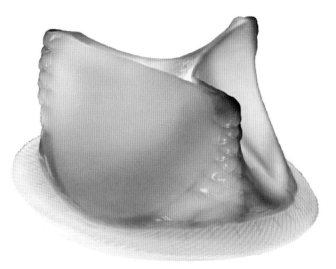

FIGURE 28-17 The St. Jude Trifecta pericardial aortic prosthesis. (Trifecta, Quartet and St. Jude Medical are trademarks of St. Jude Medical, Inc. or its related companies. Reproduced with permission of St. Jude Medical, ©2016. All rights reserved.)

performed a RCT in 241 patients with AS to receive the largest possible St. Jude Epic, Edwards Magna and Sorin Mitroflow valve. There was small but significant hemodynamic advantage for the Magna valve with respect to indexed EOA (0.93 ± 0.28, 1.04 ± 0.28, and 0.96 ± 0.26 cm²/m², p = .015 for Epic, Magna, and Mitroflow, respectively) and mean gradient (15.2 ± 5.5, 12.3 ± 4.3, and 16.2 ± 5.7 mm Hg, p < .001), primarily driven by valve sizes 23 mm and greater. However, short-term clinical outcomes and LVM regression was not different. Whether meaningful long-term clinical differences will emerge between these third-generation valves remain an open question. A retrospective comparison of Trifecta, Edwards Magna, and Magna Ease valves also found that valve type was not an independent predictor of valve area nor mean gradient overall.[58] However, for the subset of patients with small aortic roots, a 19-mm Trifecta and Mitroflow offer excellent hemodynamic properties *in vivo* and may be considered.[58,59] Dumesnil et al[60] reviewed hemodynamic properties of a range of stented bioprostheses and find comparable orifice areas with most currently available prostheses (Table 28-5).

TABLE 28-5: Mean Values for Effective Orifice Areas in Different Aortic Stented Bioprostheses

Valve type	Size (mm)						
	19	21	23	25	27	29	Ref
Mosaic	1.1	1.2	1.4	1.7	1.8	2	Dumesnil et al
Hancock II	1.2	1.3	1.5	1.6	1.6		Dumesnil et al
Perimount	1.1	1.3	1.5	1.8	2.1	2.2	Dumesnil et al
Magna*	1.3	1.7	2.1	2.3	-	-	Dumesnil et al
Biocor (Epic)*	-	1.3	1.6	1.8	-	-	Dumesnil et al
Mitroflow*	1.1	1.3	1.5	1.8	-	-	Dumesnil et al
Trifecta*	1.1	1.7	1.9	2.7	2.9	2.4	Yadlapati et al
Trifecta*	1.8	2	2.2				Levy et al

*These values are based on a limited number of patients and should thus be interpreted with caution.

Adapted with permission from Dumesnil JG, Pibarot P. The problem of severe valve prosthesis-patient mismatch in aortic bioprostheses: near extinction? *J Am Soc Echocardiogr.* 2014 Jun;27(6):598-600.

OUTCOMES OF AORTIC VALVE REPLACEMENT

Operative Mortality

Operative mortality is defined as all-cause mortality within 30 days of operation or during the same hospital admission. In 1999, the STS ACSD reviewed the results of 86,580 valve procedures to find an overall mortality of 4.3% for isolated AVR, and 8.0% for AVR with CABG.[61] Then in 2009, they again reviewed 67,292 cases of AVR between 2002 and 2006, and found an improved mortality of 3.2% for isolated AVR, and 5.6% for AVR with CABG (Table 28-6).[62] Recently, Thourani et al[63] reviewed 141,905 cases of AVR in the STS ACSD between 2002 and 2010 to show lower observed mortality rates than the STS predicted risk of mortality (PROM) in low- (1.4 vs 1.7%), medium- (5.1 vs 5.5%), and high-risk (11.8 vs 13.7%) patients groups (p < .0001). They further demonstrate a slight increase in overall operative mortality in the current surgical era (2007 to 2010) compared to previous (2002 to 2006; 2.7 vs 2.5%, p = .018) despite a significant increase

in overall STS PROM (3.05 ± 3.73% vs 2.82 ± 3.69%, p < .0001). This was attributed to lower mortality in both the moderate (5.4 vs 6.4%, p = .002) and high-risk (11.9 vs 14.4%, p = .0004) patient cohorts. It is important to note that information in this database is voluntarily submitted and includes both low-volume and high-volume centers.

Long-term Survival

There have been three major long-term RCTs comparing survival between patients receiving mechanical and bioprosthetic valves.[64-67] The 12-year results from the Edinburgh Heart Trial improved survival free from reoperation and a trend toward improved overall survival with the Bjork-Shiley mechanical prosthesis.[64] The 20-year results found no survival advantage with mechanical valves.[65] In the Veterans Affairs Trial, all-cause mortality after AVR was lower with the mechanical valve versus bioprosthesis (66 vs 79%, p = .02) at 15 years.[66] In patients ≥ 65 years after AVR, primary valve failure was not different between bioprosthetic and mechanical valves

TABLE 28-6: Frequency of Clinical Endpoints in Patients Undergoing AVR in the STS Database (2002 to 2006)

	Mort	CVA	RF	Vent	DSWI	Reop	Comp	PLOS	SLOS
N	67,292	67,292	65,828	67,292	67,292	67,292	67,292	67,292	67,292
Events	2157	1007	2774	7323	197	5369	11,706	5308	26,144
%	3.2	1.5	4.1	10.9	0.3	8	17.4	7.9	38.9

AVR, aortic valve replacement; Comp, composite adverse event (any); CVA, cerebrovascular accident (stroke); DSWI, deep sternal wound infection; Mort, mortality; PLOS, prolonged length of stay; Reop, reoperation; RF, renal failure; SLOS, short length of stay; Vent, prolonged ventilation.
Data from O'Brien SM, Shahian DM, Filardo G, et al: The Society of Thoracic Surgeons 2008 cardiac surgery risk models: part 2–isolated valve surgery, Ann Thorac Surg. 2009 Jul;88(1 Suppl):S23-S42.

(9 ± 6 vs 0%, *p* = .16). However, reoperation was higher for bioprosthetic AVR and bleeding was higher with mechanical valves. These landmark trials form the basis of our guidelines but the Bjork-Shiley single disc is no longer utilized and third generation pericardial bioprostheses are generally favored over porcine valves and the Hancock bioprostheses. Increased bioprosthetic structural deterioration in these early trials was likely influenced by the use of first-generation prostheses that are more prone to structural failure than newer generation prostheses. A more recent study of 310 patients between 55 and 70 years old randomized to either tissue or mechanical AVR showed no difference in mortality but more SVD and higher reoperation with bioprosthetic valves after 10 years (Fig. 28-18).[67] Importantly, higher bleeding events with mechanical prostheses in the VA and Edinburgh studies were not seen in the recent trial, possibly due to a lower target international normalized ratio (2-2.5).

There are several nonrandomized long-term clinical follow-up series of early generation and contemporary bioprostheses. Brennan et al[10] report long-term outcomes on 145,911 patients ≥ 65 years in the STS database undergoing AVR and AVR/CABG from 1991 to 2007 (Fig. 28-19). The

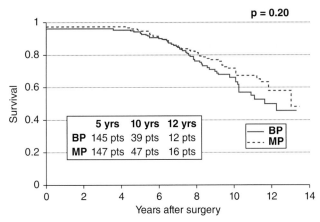

FIGURE 28-18 Overall survival of patients 55 to 70 years who received either mechanical prosthesis (MP) or biological prosthesis (BP) valves. (Reproduced with permission from Stassano P, Di Tommaso L, Monaco M, et al: Aortic valve replacement: a prospective randomized evaluation of mechanical versus biological valves in patients ages 55 to 70 years, *J Am Coll Cardiol.* 2009 Nov 10; 54(20):1862-1868.)

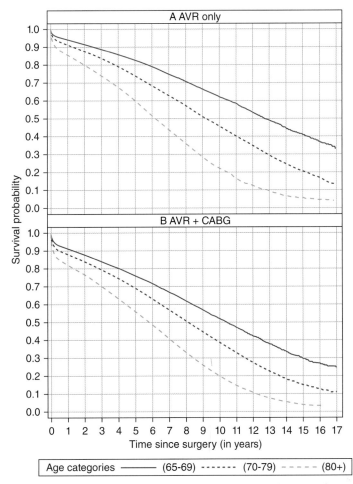

FIGURE 28-19 Long-term survival after aortic valve replacement and AVR and CABG in elderly patients between 1991 and 2007 in the STS Database. (Reproduced with permission from Brennan JM, Edwards FH, Zhao Y, et al: Developing Evidence to Inform Decisions About Effectiveness–Aortic Valve Replacement (DEcIDE AVR) Research Team. Long-term survival after aortic valve replacement among high-risk elderly patients in the United States: insights from the Society of Thoracic Surgeons Adult Cardiac Surgery Database, 1991 to 2007, *Circulation* 2012 Sep 25;126(13):1621-1629.)

TABLE 28-7: Median Survival after Isolated Aortic Valve Replacement in Elderly Patients in the STS Database between 1991 and 2007

	Isolated AVR, years			AVR+CABG, years		
	Age 65-69 years	Age 70-79 years	Age ≥80 years	Age 65-69 years	Age 70-79 years	Age ≥80 years
Overall	12.8	9.2	6.2	10.4	8.2	5.9
STS-PROM						
Low	≥10	≥10	7.3	≥10	9.5	7.2
Moderate	5.3	4.7	5	5.6	5.8	5.6
High	2.6	2.5	2.7	2.1	2.4	3.2
Lung disease						
No	≥10	≥10	6.5	≥10	9	6.3
Mild	≥10	8	5.3	9.3	7.3	5.2
Moderate	≥10	6.4	4.4	7.1	5.8	4.3
Severe	6	4.8	3.6	6.1	4.4	2.7
LVEF, %						
>30	≥10	≥10	6.3	≥10	8.6	6
≤30	9.1	6.9	4.9	7.7	5.9	5
Renal failure						
No	≥10	9.9	6.4	≥10	8.7	6.1
Yes	6	4.8	3.4	5.2	4.8	3.4
Yes/dialysis	2.5	2	0.7	1.8	1.2	1.5
Prior cardiac operations, _n_						
0	≥10	≥10	6.4	≥10	8.6	6
≥1	9.3	7.2	5.2	8.2	6.8	4.8

Adapted with permission from Brennan JM, Edwards FH, Zhao Y, et al: Developing Evidence to Inform Decisions About Effectiveness–Aortic Valve Replacement (DEcIDE AVR) Research Team. Long-term survival after aortic valve replacement among high-risk elderly patients in the United States: insights from the Society of Thoracic Surgeons Adult Cardiac Surgery Database, 1991 to 2007, _Circulation_ 2012 Sep 25;126(13):1621-1629.

median survival in patients 65 to 69, 70 to 79, and ≥80 years of age undergoing AVR was 13, 9, and 6 years, respectively (Table 28-7). Figure 28-20 shows long-term morality stratified by STS perioperative risk of mortality. Although only 5% of isolated AVR patients had a high STS perioperative risk of mortality (≥10%), their median survival was 2.5 to 2.7 years. Importantly, severe lung disease and renal failure were each associated with a ≥50% reduction in median survival. LVD and prior cardiac operation were associated with a 25% reduction in median survival.[10] The comorbidities of age, concomitant CAD, LVD, and poor functional status on middle-to-late survival after bioprosthetic AVR are additive. Other risk factors for late mortality include concomitant renal disease, female gender, concomitant cardiac or vascular procedure, and atrial fibrillation.

Valve-related Mortality

A committee of the American Association for Thoracic Surgery (AATS), STS, and European Association for Cardio-Thoracic Surgery (EACTS) has standardized prosthetic valve surgery outcomes. Valve-related mortality is defined as all deaths caused by structural valve deterioration, nonstructural valve dysfunction, valve thrombosis, embolism, bleeding event, operated valvular endocarditis, or death related to reoperation of an operated valve.[68] Sudden, unexplained, unexpected deaths of patients with an operated valve are included as valve-related mortality. Deaths caused by progressive heart failure in patients with satisfactorily functioning cardiac valves are not included. In the Hammermeister series, valve-related deaths accounted for 37% of all deaths in patients with mechanical valves and 41% of all deaths in patients with bioprostheses at 15 years.[64] Nonvalvular cardiac deaths accounted for 17 and 21% of deaths at 15 years in patients with mechanical and bioprostheses, respectively.

NONFATAL VALVE EVENTS

The joint AATS/STS/EACTS committee also defined specific guidelines for reporting outcomes on structural and nonstructural valve deterioration, valve thrombosis, embolic events, bleeding events, and prosthetic endocarditis.[68] _Structural valve deterioration_ refers to any change in function of an operated valve resulting from an intrinsic abnormality of the valve that causes stenosis or regurgitation (eg, leaflet tears, suture line disruption). _Nonstructural dysfunction_ is any abnormality

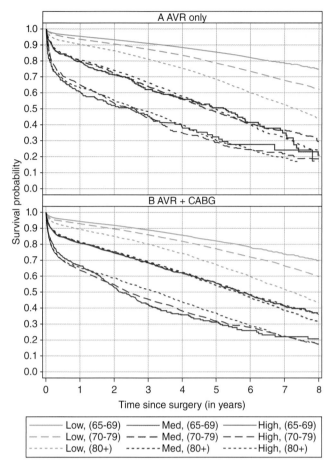

FIGURE 28-20 Long-term survival after aortic valve replacement in elderly patients between 1991 and 2007 in the STS Database stratified by STS PROM Score. (Reproduced with permission from Brennan JM, Edwards FH, Zhao Y, et al: Developing Evidence to Inform Decisions About Effectiveness–Aortic Valve Replacement (DEcIDE AVR) Research Team. Long-term survival after aortic valve replacement among high-risk elderly patients in the United States: insights from the Society of Thoracic Surgeons Adult Cardiac Surgery Database, 1991 to 2007, *Circulation* 2012 Sep 25;126(13):1621-1629.))

of an operated valve resulting in stenosis or regurgitation that is caused by factors not intrinsic to the valve itself (eg, pannus overgrowth, inappropriate sizing, or paravalvular leak). *Valve thrombosis* is any thrombus that interferes with valve function in the absence of infection. *Embolism* is any embolic event that occurs after the immediate postoperative period in the absence of infection. *Cerebral embolic events* are subclassified into *transient ischemic attacks* are short fully reversible neurologic events and *Strokes* are neurologic deficits lasting longer than >72 hours. *Bleeding event* is any episode of major internal or external bleeding that causes death, hospitalization, or permanent injury, or requires transfusion, regardless of the patient's anticoagulation status. This does not include embolic stroke followed by hemorrhagic transformation and intracranial bleed. Finally, *operated valvular endocarditis* is any infection involving an operated valve; any structural or

nonstructural valvular dysfunction, thrombosis, or embolic event associated with operated valvular endocarditis.

Structural Valve Deterioration

STENTED BIOPROSTHESES

Several large series describe long-term follow-up of first-, second-, and now third-generation stented bioprostheses (Table 28-8).[55,69-78] These series are not directly comparable since they took place in different patient populations and in different eras; however, there are some overarching results. Long-term follow-up of second-generation stented bioprostheses, including the Medtronic Hancock II porcine and Carpentier-Edwards pericardial valves show approximately 90% freedom from structural valve deterioration at 12-year follow-up. However, beyond 15-year follow-up, freedom from SVD falls rapidly in most series. In a long-term follow up of the Hancock II valve, independent predictors of reoperation due to SVD were age (odds ratio [OR]: 0.72; 95% confidence interval [CI]: 0.58 to 0.90, $p < .01$) and prosthesis-patient mismatch (OR: 1.63; 95% CI: 1.01 to 2.63; $p = .045$).[55] In large series, freedom from reoperation is approximately 95% at 5 years, 90% at 10 years, but 70% at 15 years (Table 28-8).[58-77] Notably, the freedom from SVD may be underestimated in the literature since most series report SVD by the actuarial method instead of the actual or cumulative incidence method.[79] Actuarial statistical analysis overestimates SVD in older patients since it assumes that patients who have died of other causes will continue to be at risk for SVD.

Younger patients are predisposed to premature bioprosthetic SVD.[80,81] In a younger patient cohort (age < 60 years), actuarial freedom from re-AVR was 87.4, 62.6, and 52.2% at 10, 15, and 20 years postoperatively, respectively.[56] Jamieson et al reported long-term clinical outcomes of 230 patients < 60 years old with the Carpentier-Edwards supra-annular aortic valve. Freedom from SVD at 18 years after operation was 51.0% in patients aged 51 to 60 years and 31.9% in patients < 50 years. Forcillo et al[80] report their 20-year experience in 144 patients < 60 years old (mean age 51 ± 9 years) that underwent AVR with the Edwards pericardial valves. Freedom from SVD was 84 ± 4% and 57 ± 6% at 10 and 15 years, respectively. Patients underwent reoperation for SVD at an average of 11 ± 5 years with no perioperative mortality.

Optimal Antithrombotic Therapy

Bioprosthetic valves do not require long-term anticoagulation with warfarin unless the patient is at high risk for thromboembolism or has had a thromboembolic event with their prosthesis. Stented bioprostheses have a linearized risk for thromboembolism between 0.5 and 1% per year. This risk appears to be lower in patients with stentless heterograft, allograft, or autograft valves.[83-85] Aspirin significantly decreases the risk of thromboembolism in low-risk patients with bioprostheses versus no antiplatelet therapy.[86,87] This risk is approximately the same risk of thromboembolism as fully

TABLE 28-8: Structural Deterioration of Stented Bioprosthetic Valves in the Aortic Position: Long-term Follow-up Over 10 to 20 Years

Study	Prosthesis	No. of patients	Mean age (years)	Mean follow-up (months)	Actuarial freedom from SVD (%)	Actuarial freedom from reoperation (%)
David et al	Hancock II	723	65 ± 12	68 ± 40	94 ± 2 (12 years)	89 ± 5 (12 years)
Dellgren et al	CE Pericardial	254	71 ± 9	60 ± 31	86 ± 9 (12 years)	83 ± 9 (12 years)
Poirier et al	CE Pericardial	598	65*	57.7	80 ± 5 (14 years)	72 ± 6 (14 years)
Corbineau et al	Medtronic Intact	188	72 ± 8	86.4 ± 50.4	44.2 ± 12.9 (15 years)	-
Myken et al	Biocor Porcine	1518	70.8 ± 10.9	72 ± 58.8	-	61.1% ± 8.5 (20 years)
Biglioli et al	CE Pericardial	327	67.2 ± 10.6	71.8 ± 48.8	-	52.9% ± 9.9
Sjogren et al	Mitroflow	152	79.5 ± 3.1	-	82 (10 years)	-
Une et al	Hancock II	304	49.2 ± 9.0	170.4	25.2 ± 5.0 (20 years)	25.4 ± 4.7 (20 years)
McClure et al	CE Pericardial	1000	74.1 ± 0.29	72.0 ± 43.2	82.3 (15 years)	78.3 (15 years)
Forcillo et al	CE Pericardial	2405	71 ± 9	72 ± 118	-	67 ± 4 (20 years)
Johnston et al	CE Pericardial	12,569	71 ± 11	69.6	-	55% (20 years)

CE, Carpenter-Edwards; MO, modified orifice; SA, supra-annular; SVD, structural valve deterioration.
*Values for cohort > 65 years.

anticoagulated mechanical valves, with fewer bleeding complications. Interestingly, by 15 years in the Edinburgh Heart Trial, the proportion of patients with bioprosthetic AVR on warfarin was 33%, mostly for atrial fibrillation or LVD.[65] If a patient has identified high-risk factors for thrombosis preoperatively, a mechanical prosthesis may be considered unless the risk factor is amenable to correction since formal anticoagulation with warfarin will still be necessary.

There is an immediate increased hazard function for thromboembolism before the exposed surfaces of stented bioprostheses endothelialize. In a study from the Mayo Clinic, a 41 and 3.6% per year risk of thromboembolism was reported in the interval 0-10 days and 10-90 days following bioprosthetic AVR, respectively.[86] A retrospective study of 25,656 elderly patients in the STS database report lower risk of death (relative risk [RR]: 0.80, 95% CI: 0.66 to 0.96) and embolism (RR: 0.52, 95% CI: 0.35 to 0.76) but higher risk of bleeding events (RR: 2.80, 95% CI: 2.18 to 3.60) with aspirin and warfarin versus aspirin alone in the first 3 months following bioprosthetic AVR.[87] This study revealed considerable variation in short-term anticoagulation strategies for patients with bioprosthetic AVR. There are two small prospective RCTs comparing formal anticoagulation vs antiplatelet alone postbioprosthetic AVR. In the TRAC Trial, 193 patients that underwent bioprosthetic aortic or mitral valve replacement received Triflusal (an antiplatelet agent similar to aspirin) or acenocoumarol (a vitamin K antagonist similar to warfarin). There was no difference in thromboembolic complications but greater bleeding events with anticoagulation (10 vs 3.1%, p = .048).[88] The WoA Epic Pilot Trial randomized 69 low thrombotic risk patients undergoing bioprosthetic AVR to ASA or warfarin. There was no difference in strokes (2.9 vs

2.9%, p = .99), bleeding events (2.9 vs 8.8%, p = .36).[89] The current 2014 ACC/AHA Guidelines recommend anticoagulation with warfarin (INR between 2 and 3) for the first 3 months for bioprosthetic valves (Class IIa, Level of Evidence C) then low dose aspirin as well as aspirin alone (Class IIa, Level of Evidence B).[29] The early use of anticoagulation primarily reflects the increased risk of thromboembolic events due to the lack of endothelialization of the various prosthetic materials.

Warfarin remains the only approved oral anticoagulant for patients with prosthetic valve(s). Although nonwarfarin oral anticoagulants (NOACs) have shown improved efficacy over warfarin in large trials of venous thromboembolism and nonvalvular atrial fibrillation.[90-92] The RE-ALIGN phase 2 dose-validation study comparing dabigatran versus warfarin for patients with mechanical prosthetic valves report higher stroke (5 vs 0%) and higher major bleeding (4 vs 2%) in the dabigatran group.[93] The use of NOAC for prosthetic valve anticoagulation is thus currently a class III recommendation (will cause harm; Level of Evidence B) and should not be used.[29]

Prosthesis Thrombosis

Prosthesis thrombosis is a rare but potentially devastating outcome after bioprosthetic AVR. The incidence of prosthesis thrombosis is <0.2% per year and occurs more often with mechanical prostheses.[94] Thrombolytic therapy may be used in some patients but it is often ineffective and cannot be used in the immediate postoperative period due to excessive bleeding risk. Thrombolysis is recommended in patients with left-sided thrombosis who are experiencing mild heart failure (NYHA Class I or II) or who are in severe heart failure but are considered too high risk for surgery.[29] A risk of thrombolytic therapy is cerebral or peripheral thromboembolism. Surgical treatment is recommended in severe heart failure (NYHA Class III or IV) and includes replacement of the valve or open thrombectomy, and mortality from either procedure is similar at approximately 10 to 15%. Recurrent thrombosis after de-clotting occurs in up to 40% of patients and we recommend valve replacement in virtually all patients who are managed operatively.

Prosthetic Valve Endocarditis

Prosthetic valve endocarditis (PVE) is separated into two time frames: early (<60 days postimplantation) and late (>60 days postimplantation). Early PVE is usually a sequela of perioperative bacterial seeding of the valve, either during implantation or postoperatively from wound or intravascular catheter infections. *Staphylococcus aureus, S. epidermidis,* Gram-negative bacteria, and fungal infections are common during this period.[95-98] Although most cases of late PVE are caused by septicemia from noncardiac sources, a small proportion of late cases in the first year are attributable to less virulent organisms introduced in the perioperative period, particularly *S. epidermidis.* Organisms responsible for late PVE include *Streptococcus* and *Staphylococcus* species and other organisms commonly found in native valve infectious endocarditis. All unexplained fevers should be meticulously investigated for PVE with serial blood cultures and transthoracic or transesophageal echocardiography. Transesophageal echocardiography provides more detailed anatomic information such as the presence of vegetations, abscesses, and fistulas. Transthoracic views may provide better views of the anterior portion of the valve. The annual risk of PVE in the aortic position is 0.6 to 0.9% per patient year.[95,96] The 5-year freedom from PVE is >95%.[97] Mechanical valves may have a slightly higher early hazard for PVE than stented bioprostheses.[98] However, no difference exists in risk between patients with mechanical and stented bioprosthetic prostheses after the early phase.

Outcome for patients with PVE is very poor. Invasive paravalvular infection occurs in up to 40% of cases of PVE.[96] Early PVE is associated with 30 to 80% mortality, while late PVE is associated with 20 to 40% mortality.[97] According to the 2014 ACC/AHA Guidelines, early surgeries indicated for PVE with valve dysfunction and heart failure (Class I, Level of Evidence B); paravalvular leak or partial dehiscence; presence of a new conduction defect, abscess or penetrating lesion (Class I, Level of Evidence B); persistent bacteremia and fever despite 5-7 days of appropriate antibiotic therapy (Class I, Level of Evidence B); vegetations (>10 mm); and surgery for relapsing infection (Class I, Level of Evidence C) and multiple systemic emboli with persistent vegetations (Class IIa, Level of Evidence B).[29] Notably, all fungal, and most virulent strains of *Staphylococcus aureus, Serratia marcescens,* and *Pseudomonas aeruginosa* require operation, as these organisms are highly invasive and antibiotic therapy alone is generally ineffective (Class I, Level of Evidence B).

Paravalvular Leak and Hemolysis

Paravalvular leak is uncommon when pledgeted sutures are routinely used, outside of the setting of infective endocarditis. Technical errors may result in inappropriately large gaps between sutures, leaving a small portion of the prosthesis unattached to the annulus. If paravalvular leak is sufficient to cause significant hemolysis or heart failure from acute aortic insufficiency, surgical correction should be performed (Class I, Level of Evidence B).[29] Repair can be accomplished with a few interrupted pledgeted sutures or a large defect may require valve explant, patch repair and valve reimplant. Pannus overgrowth and prosthetic structural degeneration interfering with normal valve opening and closure may also cause hemolysis severe enough to warrant reoperation. Milder cases of hemolysis may be managed conservatively by dietary supplementation with iron and folic acid, and routine measurement of hemoglobin, serum haptoglobin, and lactate dehydrogenase.

HEMODYNAMIC PERFORMANCE AND VENTRICULAR REMODELING

Left Ventricular Mass Regression

Pressure and volume overload caused by aortic valve disease leads to increased intracavitary left ventricular pressures and compensatory LVH. In severe AS, concentric ventricular hypertrophy occurs without increasing end-diastolic dimension until late in the disease process, thus maintaining the ventricular wall thickness:cavity radius ratio. On the other hand, severe AR causes volume overload with an increase in left ventricular end-diastolic volume and eccentric hypertrophy, but may not change the ratio of ventricular wall thickness to cavity radius. Both pathologies result in an increase in LVM which has a strong negative prognostic effect.[99,100] The overall goal of AVR is to alleviate the pressure and volume overload on the left ventricle, allowing myocardial remodeling and regression of LVM.

The clinical impact of LVM regression is not as well understood, despite its widespread acceptance as a measure of outcome after aortic valve surgery. In patients after AVR for isolated AS, LVM generally regresses significantly over the first 18 months and returns to normal limits.[101-102] Ventricular mass regression may continue for up to 5 years after valve replacement.[103] However, some patients never experience adequate LVM regression which can be associated with poor clinical outcome. In particular, patient-prosthesis mismatch (PPM), in which poor hemodynamic performance of a prosthesis results in poor regression of LVH, is associated with poor patient outcome.

Prosthesis-Patient Mismatch

DEFINITIONS

The term PPM has been applied to several different clinical situations. It has been used to describe absolute small valve size (ie, <21 mm), small valve size in a patient with a large body surface area, excessive transvalvular gradient postimplantation, increased transvalvular gradient with exercise, indexed EOA, and various combinations of these variables. Rahimtoola[104] originally defined PPM as a condition that occurs when the valve area of a prosthetic valve is less than the area of that patient's normal valve. Ultimately, the valve performance cannot meet the cardiac output requirements of the patient, resulting in either no relief or worsening of symptoms due to the obstructive nature of the prosthesis, which creates a residual stenosis resulting in an elevated transvalvular gradient. To varying degrees, all valve prostheses are inherently stenotic. The presence of rigid sewing rings, and in the case of stented bioprostheses, struts to hold the valve commissures, cause obstruction to outflow and will therefore cause a residual gradient despite normal prosthesis function. Patient-prosthesis mismatch is further exacerbated by annular fibrosis, annular calcification, and LVH, as seen in AS, that cause contraction of the native annulus, leading to the implantation of a smaller prosthesis. Two distinct terms are commonly used to describe the size of prosthetic valves: EOA and geometric orifice area (GOA).

EFFECTIVE ORIFICE AREA

The most commonly cited definition of PPM is a low-indexed effective orifice area (iEOA). The iEOA is calculated by dividing the echocardiographically determined EOA by the body surface area. EOA is calculated by a reconfiguration of the continuity equation:

$$EOA = (CSA_{LVOT} \times TVI_{LVOT})/TVI_{AO}$$

EOA is effective orifice area (cm^2).
CSA_{LVOT} is cross-sectional area of the LVOT (cm^2).
TVI_{LVOT} is velocity time integral of forward blood flow (cm) as derived from pulse-wave Doppler in the LVOT.
TVI_{AO} is velocity time integral of forward blood flow (cm) as derived from software integration of transvalvular continuous wave Doppler.

The EOA and mean systolic gradient of several commonly available bioprostheses are shown in Table 28-9.[105]

The EOA is a functional estimate of the minimal cross-sectional area of the transvalvular flow jet downstream of a valve and dependent on the (1) geometric area of the prosthesis, (2) shape and size of the LVOT and ascending aorta, (3) blood pressure, and (4) cardiac output. Doppler-derived EOA correlates best with catheter-derived EOA (as determined by the Gorlin formula) when the ascending aortic diameter is 4 cm, but tends to underestimate EOA in patients with smaller aortic diameters.[106] The EOA varies widely for valves from different producers. The measured EOA cannot be known for a specific valve in a specific patient until the valve has actually been implanted. Studies examining the effect of low iEOA on clinical outcomes have typically used projected iEOA using published tables of EOA derived from historical controls instead of actually measuring true in vivo postoperative EOA. Moreover, these tables have been derived from relatively small

numbers of valves in each size for each manufacturer with wide variability between studies. Nevertheless, such reference values can be helpful to predict the presence and severity of PPM for any given patient and valve. EOA correlates with postoperative valve gradients, which are not surprising considering that they are mathematically related. Echocardiographic mean and peak gradients are calculated according to the Bernoulli equation:

$$\text{Peak gradient (mm Hg)} = 4 \times (V_{AVmax}^2 - V_{LVOTmax}^2)$$
$$\text{Mean gradient (mm Hg)} = 4 \times (V_{AVmean}^2 - V_{LVOTmean}^2)$$

Several authors suggest PPM occurs at an IEOA of ≤ 0.85 cm^2/m^2 with moderate and severe PPM at an IEOA of 0.85 to 0.65 and ≤ 0.65 cm^2/m^2, respectively.[107,108] These thresholds are used in the 2009 American Society of Echocardiography/European Association of Echocardiography Guidelines.[109] Pibarot and Dumesnil[109] have redefined PPM as a condition "when the EOA of the prosthesis is too small in relation to the patient's body size, resulting in abnormally high postoperative gradients." This definition is based on the assumption that transvalvular gradients begin to rise substantially at iEOAs below this value, and that these elevated gradients result in increased left ventricular work preventing regression of LVH.

GEOMETRIC ORIFICE AREA

The GOA (also known as the internal geometric area) of the valve is the ex vivo measured maximal cross-sectional area of the valve opening that does not vary significantly between same-sized valves from the same manufacturer. It is a static measure that is known preoperatively for any given prosthesis based on manufacturer specifications or by measurement with calipers. The GOA is larger than the EOA for any given prosthesis (Figure 28-21).

CLINICAL SIGNIFICANCE

The incidence of PPM is steadily decreasing. Pibarot and Dumesnil[110] studied PPM in 1266 patients undergoing AVR and found moderate (iEOA < 0.85 cm^2/m^2) or severe (iEOA < 0.65 cm^2/m^2) PPM to be present in 38% of patients. A more recent study found moderate and severe PPM in only 15 and 6% of patients, respectively.[111] In another study, the rate of severe PPM after implantation of the Trifecta, Mitroflow, and Perimount Magna valves was 1.3% (2/150), 5.8% (44/758), and 3.2% (3/95).[105] The low contemporary incidence of PPM is likely a result of improved hemodynamic performance of newer generation bioprostheses and the increased awareness of poor outcomes with severe PPM and thus greater use of preventive strategies.[60]

There are several studies demonstrating the adverse impact of severe PPM on survival but the significance of moderate PPM still controversial.[112-118] Ruel and colleagues showed that overall survival and LVM regression was poorer in patients with PPM and LVD than those who had LVD without PPM.[115] A retrospective study of 3343 patients

TABLE 28-9: Predischarge Echocardiographic Results for 1436 Patients Who Underwent AVR with Trifecta, Mitroflow, and Magna Bioprostheses

Overall	Trifecta (n = 196)	Mitroflow (n = 1135)	Magna (n = 105)
Preop LVOT index, cm	1.18 ± 0.1	1.17 ± 0.1	1.17 ± 0.2
Postop mean grad, mm Hg	11.4 ± 4.2	16.9 ± 6.7	14.1 ± 5.4
Postop EOA, cm²	2.22 ± 0.7	1.85 ± 0.5	2.09 ± 0.5
Postop EOAI, cm²/m²	1.14 ± 0.3	0.96 ± 0.3	1.07 ± 0.3
Valve size 19 mm	(n = 23)	(n = 46)	(n = 5)
Preop LVOT index, cm	1.21 ± 0.1	1.22 ± 0.1	1.19 ± 0.1
Postop mean grad, mm Hg	15.1 ± 5.0	21.3 ± 9.1	21.4 ± 7.7
Postop EOA, cm²	1.53 ± 0.3	1.23 ± 0.3	1.26 ± 0.2
Postop EOAI, cm²/m²	0.91 ± 0.2	0.78 ± 0.3	0.76 ± 0.2
Valve size 21 mm	(n = 48)	(n = 336)	(n = 31)
Preop LVOT index, cm	1.15 ± 0.1	1.19 ± 0.1	1.23 ± 0.2
Postop mean grad, mm Hg	12.0 ± 4.1	18.4 ± 6.5	15.9 ± 5.6
Postop EOA, cm²	1.84 ± 0.4	1.52 ± 0.4	1.73 ± 0.2
Postop EOAI, cm²/m²	1.02 ± 0.3	0.87 ± 0.2	0.98 ± 0.2
Valve size 23 mm	(n = 62)	(n = 423)	(n = 32)
Preop LVOT index, cm	1.13 ± 0.1	1.15 ± 0.1	1.13 ± 0.2
Postop mean grad, mm Hg	11.2 ± 3.4	17.2 ± 6.2	14.2 ± 4.9
Postop EOA, cm²	2.23 ± 0.5	1.83 ± 0.4	2.01 ± 0.3
Postop EOAI, cm²/m²	1.12 ± 0.3	0.94 ± 0.2	1.04 ± 0.2
Valve size 25 mm	(n = 42)	(n = 262)	(n = 29)
Preop LVOT index, cm	1.21 ± 0.1	1.15 ± 0.1	1.12 ± 0.1
Postop mean grad, mm Hg	10.0 ± 3.7	14.2 ± 4.9	11.8 ± 3.6
Postop EOA, cm²	2.73 ± 0.5	2.28 ± 0.5	2.47 ± 0.5
Postop EOAI, cm²/m²	1.33 ± 0.3	1.1 ± 0.3	1.17 ± 0.2
Valve sizes 27, 29, 31 mm	(n = 18)	(n = 68)	(n = 8)
Preop LVOT index, cm	1.29 ± 0.2	1.22 ± 0.2	1.31 ± 0.2
Postop mean grad, mm Hg	8.1 ± 3.1	13.9 ± 4.8	11.3 ± 5.0
Postop EOA, cm²	3.2 ± 0.8	2.48 ± 0.5	2.8 ± 0.5
Postop EOAI, cm²/m²	1.51 ± 0.3	1.18 ± 0.3	1.33 ± 0.3

AV, Aortic valve; EOA, effective orifice area; EOAI, effective orifice area index; LVOT, left ventricular outflow tract.
Data from Ugur M, Suri RM, Daly RC, et al: Comparison of early hemodynamic performance of 3 aortic valve bioprostheses, *J Thorac Cardiovasc Surg.* 2014 Nov;148(5): 1940-1946.[105]

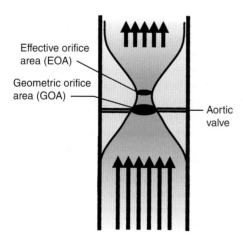

FIGURE 28-21 Diagrammatic representation of effective orifice area and geometric orifice area in relation to the left ventricular outflow tract and aortic root.

with mechanical and bioprosthetic AVR found that for the subgroup with LVD (EF < 50%), severe PPM was associated with greater 15-year mortality ($p = .049$).[117] Two meta-analyses both showed that severe PPM impact mortality and should be avoided. A meta-analysis of 34 studies including 27,186 patients found that 34.2 and 9.8% of patients undergoing AVR had moderate and severe PPM, respectively.[118] Any PPM was associated with an increase in all-cause mortality (hazard ratio [HR] = 1.34, 95% confidence interval [CI]: 1.18 to 1.51). Furthermore, moderate and severe PPM increased all-cause mortality (HR = 1.19, 95% CI: 1.07 to 1.33 and HR = 1.84, 95% CI: 1.38 to 2.45) and cardiac-related mortality (HR = 1.32, 95% CI: 1.02 to 1.71 and HR = 6.46, 95% CI: 2.79 to 14.97) (Fig. 28-22). Takagi et al[119] reviewed 24 studies revealed a 31% increase in all-cause mortality with any PPM (HR = 1.31; 95% CI: 1.16 to 1.48; $p < .00001$). Furthermore, severe PPM was associated with a 27% increase in mortality (HR = 1.27; 95% CI: 1.11 to

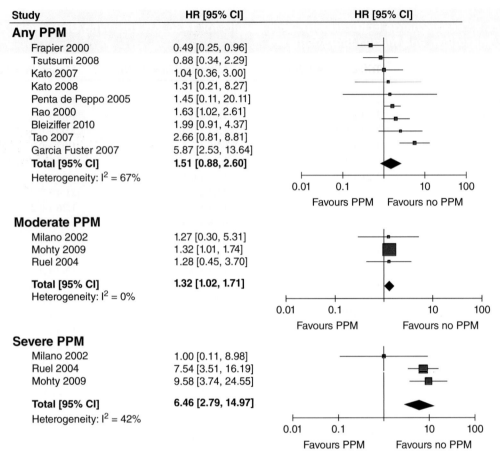

FIGURE 28-22 Pooled estimate for cardiac-related mortality: ratios demonstrate the additional hazard with prosthesis-patient mismatch in relation to a no prosthesis-patient mismatch reference group. (Reproduced with permission from Head SJ, Mokhles MM, Osnabrugge RL, et al: The impact of prosthesis-patient mismatch on long-term survival after aortic valve replacement: a systematic review and meta-analysis of 34 observational studies comprising 27 186 patients with 133 141 patient-years, *Eur Heart J* 2012 Jun;33(12):1518-29.)

1.46; *p* = .0008) but moderate PPM was not (HR 0.99; 95% CI: 0.92 to 1.07; *p* = .78). As described by Pibarot et al[120] this is explained by the fact that moderate AS is well tolerated with normal LV but not with depressed LV. Furthermore, increased hemodynamic stress from moderate PPM may beget rapid structural valve deterioration progressing to severe PPM.[121]

SMALL AORTIC ROOT

Many surgeons express concern regarding postoperative outcomes in patients with small aortic roots in whom only a very small (19 mm) valve can be implanted. However, several studies have shown no difference in LVM regression, NYHA functional class, CHF or survival with small diameter AVRs.[122-124] De Paulis et al[122] show no difference in LVM regression between patients receiving 19 and 21 mm mechanical valves versus those with 23 or 25 mm valves. Kratz et al[123] also report that small valve size was not predictive of CHF or late death. Khan et al[124] studied 19 to 23 mm Carpentier-Edwards pericardial valves and found that significant LVM regression occurred with each valve size, including 19 mm valves.

DATA SYNTHESIS

The literature is clear in that severe PPM should be avoided, particularly in those patients with poor ventricular function, but the clinical significance of less-than-severe PPM remains divided. The options to avoid PPM are implantation of a less-obstructive mechanical or stentless bioprosthesis or to perform root replacement or aortic root enlargement. Stentless prostheses in the subcoronary position may be a lower profile alternative but requires additional technical skill and cross-clamp time. Aortic root replacements or enlargement procedures require greater experience operating on the aortic root and may carry excessive mortality and wide variability in surgical outcomes even among highly experienced centers. When faced with potential PPM in the operating room, the decision to perform a more complex, higher-risk procedure must be balanced carefully with the potential benefits of implanting a larger prosthesis. Some reports have shown that transvalvular gradients in patients with lower iEOA often rise substantially with exercise.[125] Although the majority of patients undergoing AVR are elderly and unlikely to experience functional limitations from this situation, in younger, highly active patients or those with LV dysfunction, either root enlargement or stentless prostheses may provide better functional outcome with lower transvalvular gradients. In the rare circumstance of anticipated extreme mismatch (ie, iEOA < 0.6 cm^2/m^2) root enlargement is an acceptable approach in the hands of an experienced surgeon. Except in these circumstances, given the paucity of long-term data to support more complex procedures and well-documented increased risk, routine AVR with modern standard prostheses is acceptable and preferable.

PROSTHESIS SELECTION

An ideal aortic prosthesis would be simple to implant, widely available, possess long-term durability, would have no intrinsic thrombogenicity, would not have a predilection for endocarditis, and would have no residual transvalvular pressure gradient. Such a valve does not currently exist. Currently available options include mechanical valves, stented biologic heterograft valves, stentless biologic heterograft valves, allograft valves, and pulmonary autograft valves. Among these options pulmonary autograft and allograft valves are the most physiologic prostheses. They are less prone to thrombosis or endocarditis and have excellent hemodynamic characteristics.[126,127] They are most beneficial in children and younger adults. Allograft valves may also improve the results of AVR in active endocarditis.[128] Despite their potential benefits, these prostheses can be very technically demanding to implant. A further discussion of these valves is presented in subsequent chapters. The remainder of this discussion will focus on issues regarding selection of mechanical or bioprosthetic valves.

Mechanical versus Biologic Valves

When selecting between mechanical and biologic heart valves, the surgeon and patient together must balance the risks of SVD with bioprosthestic valves versus need for anticoagulation with mechanical valves. The 2014 AHA/ACC Guidelines emphasizes the importance of patient preference regarding the choice of valve prosthesis.[29]

AGE CONSIDERATIONS

Generally, patients over 70 years of age at the time of surgery should receive a biologic valve and patients under the age of 60 years should have a mechanical prosthesis to minimize the risk of structural failure requiring repeat AVR as an octogenarian. Patients between 60 and 70 represent the group in whom there is still debate regarding prosthesis selection. Those patients who have comorbidities such as severe CAD may be less likely to outlive their prosthesis and should receive a biologic valve. Having said that, there is a steady shift to greater use of bioprostheses for patients in all age cohorts, especially given the burden of anticoagulation and the potential for subsequent transcatheter valve-in-valve implantation. The STS ACSD reported a 20% absolute increase in the proportion of patients selecting bioprostheses over mechanical valves

for all patient age cohorts.[129] There was also an increase in the proportion of patients undergoing bioprosthetic AVR from 72.6% between 2002 and 2006 to 83.8% between 2007 and 2010 (p < .0001).[63] Chiang et al[130] studied 2002 propensity-matched young patient (50 to 69 years) with bioprosthetic versus mechanical AVR in New York State (1997 to 2004). As expected, they report greater 15-year reoperation rate (12.1 vs 6.9%) and lower bleeding events (6.6 vs 13.0%) bioprosthesis valves but there were no difference in 15-year actuarial survival (60.6 vs 62.1%) nor stroke events (7.7 vs 8.6%). This suggests that bioprosthetic valves offer noninferior survival without the burden of anticoagulation even for patients younger than 60 years old. As mentioned earlier, two randomized comparisons of mechanical and bioprosthetic aortic valves performed in the 1970s and one in the recent era demonstrated equivalent survival between valve types at 10 to 20 years of follow-up.[54-56] However, long-term event-free survival beyond 15 years was superior in the mechanical valve groups as the risks of reoperation and structural failures of bioprostheses became more common. A detailed and comprehensive discussion of these risks and benefits of prosthesis selection should occur with all patients and their families prior to entering the operating room.

SPECIAL PATIENT GROUPS

Patients with an absolute requirement for long-term anticoagulation such as permanent atrial fibrillation, previous thromboembolic events, hypercoagulable state, severe LVD, another mechanical heart valve in place, or intracardiac thrombus, should receive a mechanical valve regardless of age. Further considerations which may impact future patient decisions include testing for genetic variants of the *CYP2C9* and *VKORC1* genes which influence warfarin response and the use of devices to facilitate home INR monitoring.

Patients with a relative or absolute contraindication to anticoagulation, such as women of child-bearing age wishing to become pregnant, patients with bleeding disorders, those who refuse or those unreliable to take oral anticoagulation should receive a bioprosthesis. However, young patients do have a higher incidence of early SVD and need to be thoroughly counselled as such.[131] Furthermore, higher incidence of accelerated SVD (47 vs 14%, p < .05) and lower freedom from reoperation (20 vs 64%, p < .05) were reported in young women during pregnancy when compared to their nonpregnant counterparts.[132] Alternatively, implantation of mechanical prostheses in such women combined with anticoagulation using subcutaneous low-molecular weight heparin injections during the pregnancy is a possibility. The current 2014 ACC/AHA Guidelines suggest that for patients taking ≤5 mg warfarin/day to continue until delivery (Class IIa, Level of Evidence B) then switch to unfractionated heparin (UFH; Class I, Level of Evidence C). Those patients taking >5 mg warfarin/day are advised to switch to UFH or low molecular weight heparin during the first trimester (Class IIa, Level of Evidence B) and just prior to delivery (Class I, Level of Evidence C).[29]

Aortic valve prosthesis selection for patients with end-stage renal failure requiring dialysis is complicated by rapid SVD in bioprosthetic valves and dialysis-related bleeding due to anti-coagulation necessary for mechanical prostheses. A systematic review of the literature report an acceptable operative mortality, no difference in survival between bioprosthetic versus mechanical valves (HR = 1.3; 95% CI: 1.0 to 1.9, p = .09) but lower valve-related complications (OR: 0.4; 95% CI: 0.2 to 0.7, p = .002), including bleeding and thromboembolism.[133] The 2014 ACC/AHA Guidelines do not offer recommendations for valve selection in this patient subset and ultimately, the decision should be individualized balancing the risks of valve-related complications as well as the anticipated survival of the patient.

Stented versus Stentless Biologic Valves

Stentless porcine valves gained popularity in cardiac surgery due to pioneering work by Dr. Tirone David at the Toronto General Hospital in 1988.[134] Stentless valves lack obstructive stents and strut posts, thus have residual gradients that are similar to those of freehand allografts. However, their use involves a more complex operation as they are more difficult to implant and require a longer cross-clamp time. Walther and colleagues[135] performed a randomized trial comparing the ability of stented porcine and stentless porcine valves to cause regression of LVH. They showed that patients in the stentless valve group received larger valves for a given annular size and had a slightly higher degree of LVM regression. Borger et al[136] showed modestly lower mean gradients in stentless prostheses versus stented prostheses (9 vs 15 mm Hg) and LVMI (100 vs 107 g/m^2) but no difference in survival. Cheng et al[137] performed a meta-analysis of 17 randomized trials and 14 nonrandomized studies comparing stented to stentless aortic valves. They showed no difference in 2–10 year mortality (OR: 0.82, 95% CI: 0.50 to 1.33), PPM (OR: 0.30, 95% CI: 0.05 to 1.66), but stentless valves were associated with greater EOA index and lower mean gradients.

Little evidence exists regarding any incremental benefit of hemodynamic improvements afforded by stentless valves in LVM regression or clinical outcomes. Thus, the routine use of stentless bioprostheses cannot be recommended for most patients with small aortic roots based on currently available data. At this time, stentless porcine valves are most useful in younger active patients with small aortic roots who are likely to be limited by the elevated residual gradient a small stented bioprosthesis may create.

PERCUTANEOUS VALVULAR INTERVENTIONS

Percutaneous Aortic Balloon Valvotomy

As an alternative to surgical management for AS, percutaneous balaortic valvotomy may be performed.[138] Inflation of the balloon within the valve orifice can stretch the annular tissue and fracture calcified areas or open fused commissures. There is no role for valvotomy in the patient with significant AR, as this will become significantly worse after the procedure.[139,140] Balloon valvotomy is rarely successful if significant calcification is present and carries a prohibitive risk of stroke from calcific emboli.[141] The long-term outcomes of this procedure in adult patients are dismal, with restenosis usually occurring within 1 year. Prior to the TAVI era, patients with severe symptomatic AS who were too hemodynamically unstable to tolerate an operation or have comorbid illnesses, such as advanced malignancy, which contraindicate an operation, may have benefited from palliative balloon valvotomy.[142,143] Currently, this procedure may be considered to temporize a critically ill patient with AS until definitive surgery or TAVR can be performed (AHA/ACC Guidelines, Class IIb, Level of Evidence C).[29]

Transcatheter Aortic Valve Replacement (TAVR)

Surgical AVR is the gold standard treatment for aortic valve stenosis but up to one-third of patients are not candidates due to advanced age, heart failure, or other specific anatomic factors.[144] Since the first clinical description in 2002, TAVR offers an alternative to surgical AVR in select patients.[145] Currently, two commonly used valve systems are the SAPIEN 3 (Edwards Life Sciences) and the CoreValve Evolut R (Medtronic), although various other valves exist in different stages of development and evaluation (Fig. 28-23). Each valve system includes (1) the valve prosthesis, (2) the stent or frame, (3) the loading system and (4) the delivery system. The Edwards Lifesciences SAPIEN 3 (Edwards Lifesciences) is based on the perimount design with a bovine pericardial valve on a balloon-expandable stent. Whereas the CoreValve Evolut R (Medtronic) and Portico (St. Jude Medical) are porcine pericardial valves on self-expanding nitonol frames.

The approach is accomplished via a retrograde transarterial or transapical manner. The retrograde femoral approach involves femoral artery access, retrograde cannulation of the aortic valve, balloon dilatation, and device delivery. Alternatively transapical transcatheter valve delivery involves creating a small thoracotomy, direct cannulation of the left ventricular apex, and passing of a wire and stent-mounted valve under fluoroscopic and echocardiographic guidance. Both techniques require rapid ventricular pacing to ensure there is no cardiac output during device deployment. Other reported access routes include direct aortic via hemisternotomy or sternotomy, as well as retrograde via axillary, subclavian, or carotid arteries.

The PARTNER Trials have demonstrated symptom relief and survival benefit with TAVR for high-risk and prohibitive risk, nonoperative patients.[146-149] In PARTNER B, TAVI was associated with lower death or mortality at 1 year (43 vs 72%) and lower death at 2 years (43 vs 68%) compared with medical management in 358 nonoperative patients with severe symptomatic AS.[146-147] In PARTNER A, 699 patients with high-risk (operative mortality > 15% and STS PROM >10%) severe symptomatic AS were randomized to TAVR or surgical AVR. Both 1-year (24 vs 27%, NS) and 2-year mortality (34 vs 35%, NS) were not different between TAVR

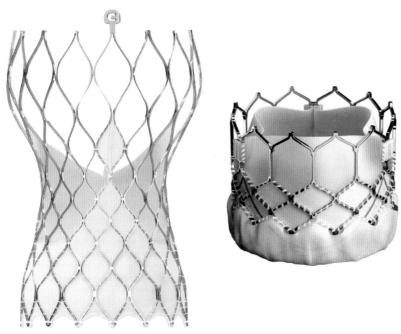

FIGURE 28-23 SCoreValve Evolut R (©Medtronic 2016) and SAPIEN 3 (Used with permission from Edwards Lifesciences LLC, Irvine, CA. Edwards, Edwards Lifesciences, Edwards SAPIEN, SAPIEN, SAPIEN XT and SAPIEN 3 are trademarks of Edwards Lifesciences Corporation).

and surgery.[148-149] In both studies TAVR was associated with higher stroke and vascular complications. Decision making between TAVR and surgery has emphasized the importance of a multidisciplinary Heart Team in the evaluation of higher risk patients (ACC/AHA Guidelines, Class I, Level of Evidence C). The composition of the Heart Team will vary between centers but should include specialists from cardiac imaging, interventional cardiology, cardiac anesthesia, and cardiac surgery. Based on the results of PARTNER Cohort B, TAVR should be considered for inoperable patients with AS and a life expectancy of >1 year (ACC/AHA Guidelines, Class I, Level of Evidence B). Based on the results of PARTNER Cohort A, TAVR is reasonable for high-risk operable patients with AS (ACC/AHA Guidelines, Class IIa, Level of Evidence B).[148,149] High-risk patients are defined as those with STS PROM > 8%, ≥2 frailty indices, compromise in 2 organ systems or possible presence of a procedure-specific impediment. Importantly, TAVR should not be offered to patients with severe comorbidities limiting life despite relief of AS (Class III, Level of Evidence B). This is a result of the lack of benefit from TAVR in the PARTNER Cohort B study subset with STS score > 15%.[147]

A nonrandomized trial of CoreValve Evolut R (Medtronic) showed comparable safety (8.4% 30-day all-cause mortality) and efficacy (99.4% implantation) with SAPIEN (Edwards Life Sciences).[150] Then the CHOICE Study randomized high-risk patients to either SAPIEN XT (Edwards Life Sciences) versus CoreValve (Medtronic) and report no difference in 30-day cardiovascular mortality (RR: 0.97; 95% CI: 0.29 to 3.25; p = .99) and lower residual aortic insufficiency (4.1 vs 18.3%; RR: 0.23; 95% CI: 0.09 to 0.58; p < .001) but higher heart block requiring permanent pacemaker with

the CoreValve (Medtronic, 37.6 vs 17.3%, p = .001).[151] The incidences of TAVR mortality and complications are consistent with that published by the large European registries France 2 and German Transcatheter Aortic Valve Interventions-Registry.[152,153]

Given the success of the PARTNER trials in high and prohibitive surgical risk patients and retrospective studies of TAVR in low and moderate risk patients, the PARTNER II (http://clinicaltrials.gov/ct2/show/NCT01314313) and SURTAVI (http://clinicaltrials.gov/show/NCT01586910) RCTs are testing the outcome of broadening the application of TAVR into intermediate risk patients with severe AS.[154]

REFERENCES

1. Selzer A: Changing aspects of the natural history of valvular aortic stenosis. *N Engl J Med* 1987; 317:91.
2. Nkomo VT, Gardin JM, Skelton TN, et al: Burden of valvular heart diseases: a population-based study. *Lancet* 2006; 368:1005.
3. Rahimtoola SH: Valvular heart disease: a perspective. *J Am Coll Cardiol* 1983; 1:199.
4. Minners J, Allgeier M, Gohlke-Baerwolf C, et al: Inconsistencies of echocardiographic criteria for the grading of aortic valve stenosis. *Eur Heart J* 2008; 29:1043-1048.
5. Braunwald E: Valvular heart disease, in Braunwald E (ed): *Braunwald: Heart Disease: A Textbook of Cardiovascular Medicine*, 6th ed. New York, WB Saunders, 2001; p 1643.
6. Hess OM, Ritter M, Schneider J, et al: Diastolic stiffness and myocardial structure in aortic valve disease before and after valve replacement. *Circulation* 1984; 69:855.
7. Horstkotte D, Loogen F: The natural history of aortic valve stenosis. *Eur Heart J* 1988; 9(Suppl E):57.
8. Lund O, Nielsen TT, Emmertsen K, et al: Mortality and worsening of prognostic profile during waiting time for valve replacement in aortic stenosis. *Thorac Cardiovasc Surg* 1996; 44:289.
9. Schwarz F, Baumann P, Manthey J, et al: The effect of aortic valve replacement on survival. *Circulation* 1982; 66:1105.

10. Brennan JM, Edwards FH, Zhao Y, et al: Developing Evidence to Inform Decisions About Effectiveness-Aortic Valve Replacement (DEcIDE AVR) Research Team. Long-term survival after aortic valve replacement among high-risk elderly patients in the United States: insights from the Society of Thoracic Surgeons Adult Cardiac Surgery Database, 1991 to 2007. *Circulation* 2012; 126:1621.

11. Otto CM, Burwash IG, Legget ME, et al: Prospective study of asymptomatic valvular aortic stenosis. Clinical, echocardiographic, and exercise predictors of outcome. *Circulation* 1997; 95:2262.

12. Rosenhek R, Binder T, Porenta G, et al: Predictors of outcome in severe, asymptomatic aortic stenosis. *N Engl J Med* 2000; 343:611.

13. Rosenhek R, Zilberszac R, Schemper M, et al: Natural history of very severe aortic stenosis. *Circulation* 2010; 121:151-156.

14. Brown ML, Pellikka PA, Schaff HV, et al: The benefits of early valve replacement in asymptomatic patients with severe aortic stenosis. *J Thorac Cardiovasc Surg* 2008; 135:308.

15. Kang DH, Park SJ, Rim JH, et al: Early surgery versus conventional treatment in asymptomatic very severe aortic stenosis. *Circulation* 2010; 121:1502-1509.

16. Beach JM, Mihaljevic T, Rajeswaran J, et al: Ventricular hypertrophy and left atrial dilatation persist and are associated with reduced survival after valve replacement for aortic stenosis. *J Thorac Cardiovasc Surg* 2014;147:362-369.e8.

17. Gerber IL, Stewart RA, Legget ME, et al: Increased plasma natriuretic peptide levels reflect symptom onset in aortic stenosis. *Circulation* 2003; 107:1884-1890.

18. Monin JL, Lancellotti P, Monchi M, et al: Risk score for predicting outcome in patients with asymptomatic aortic stenosis. *Circulation* 2009; 120:69-75.

19. Nessmith MG, Fukuta H, Brucks S, et al: Usefulness of an elevated B-type natriuretic peptide in predicting survival in patients with aortic stenosis treated without surgery. *Am J Cardiol* 2005; 96:1445-1448.

20. Clavel MA, Dumesnil JG, Capoulade R, et al: Outcome of patients with aortic stenosis, small valve area, and low-flow, low-gradient despite preserved left ventricular ejection fraction. *J Am Coll Cardiol* 2012; 60:1259.

21. Eleid MF, Sorajja P, Michelena HI, et al: Flow-gradientpatterns in severe aortic stenosis with preserve dejection fraction: clinical characteristics and predictors of survival. *Circulation* 2013; 128:1781-1789.

22. Tribouilloy C, Lévy F, Rusinaru D, et al. Outcome after aortic valve replacement for low-flow/low-gradient aortic stenosis without contractile reserve on dobutamine stress echocardiography. *J Am Coll Cardiol.* 2009;53:1865-1873.

23. Nadir MA, Wei L, Elder DH, et al: Impact of renin-angiotensin system blockade therapy on outcome in aortic stenosis. *J Am Coll Cardiol* 2011; 58:570-576.

24. Chockalingam A, Venkatesan S, Subramaniam T, et al: Safety and efficacy of angiotensin-converting enzyme inhibitors in symptomatic severe aortic stenosis: Symptomatic Cardiac Obstruction-Pilot Study of Enalapril in Aortic Stenosis (SCOPE-AS). *Am Heart J* 2004; 147:E19.

25. Rossebo AB, Pedersen TR, Boman K, et al: Intensive lipid lowering with simvastatin and ezetimibe in aortic stenosis. *N Engl J Med* 2008; 359:1343-1356.

26. Cowell SJ, Newby DE, Prescott RJ, et al: A randomized trial of intensive lipid-lowering therapy in calcific aortic stenosis. *N Engl J Med* 2005; 352:2389-2397.

27. Chan KL, Teo K, Dumesnil JG, et al: Effect of lipid lowering with rosuvastatin on progression of aortic stenosis: results of the aortic stenosis progression observation: measuring effects of rosuvastatin (ASTRONOMER) trial. *Circulation* 2010; 121:306-314.

28. Yanagawa B, Lovren F, Pan Y, et al: miRNA-141 is a novel regulator of BMP-2-mediated calcification in aortic stenosis. *J Thorac Cardiovasc Surg* 2012; 144:256-262.

29. Nishimura RA, Otto CM, Bonow RO, et al: 2014AHA/ACC Guideline for the Management of Patients with Valvular Heart Disease: a report of the American College of Cardiology/American Heart Association Task Force on Practice Guidelines. *Circulation* 2014; 129:e521-643.

30. American College of Cardiology/American Heart Association: ACC/AHA Guidelines for the Management of Patients with Valvular Heart Disease. A report of the American College of Cardiology/American Heart Association. Task Force on Practice Guidelines (Committee on Management of Patients with Valvular Heart Disease). *J Am Coll Cardiol* 1998; 32:1486.

31. Bonow RO, Carabello BA, Chatterjee K, et al: ACC/AHA 2006 Guidelines for the Management of Patients With Valvular Heart Disease: a report of the American College of Cardiology/American Heart Association Task Force on Practice Guidelines (Writing Committee to Revise the 1998 Guidelines for the Management of Patients with Valvular Heart Disease) developed in collaboration with the Society of Cardiovascular Anesthesiologists endorsed by the Society for Cardiovascular Angiography and Interventions and the Society of Thoracic Surgeons. *J Am Coll Cardiol* 2006; 48:e1.

32. Downes TR, Nomeir AM, Hackshaw BT, et al: Diastolic mitral regurgitation in acute but not chronic aortic regurgitation: implications regarding the mechanism of mitral closure. *Am Heart J* 1989; 117:1106.

33. Grossman W, Jones D, McLaurin LP: Wall stress and patterns of hypertrophy in the human left ventricle. *J Clin Invest* 1975; 56:56.

34. Starling MR, Kirsh MM, Montgomery DG, et al: Mechanisms for left ventricular systolic dysfunction in aortic regurgitation: importance for predicting the functional response to aortic valve replacement. *J Am Coll Cardiol* 1991; 17:887.

35. Bonow RO: Asymptomatic aortic regurgitation: indications for operation. *J Card Surg* 1994; 9(2 Suppl):170.

36. Bonow RO, Rosing DR, McIntosh CL, et al: The natural history of asymptomatic patients with aortic regurgitation and normal left ventricular function. *Circulation* 1983; 68:509.

37. Bonow RO, Lakatos E, Maron BJ, Epstein SE: Serial long-term assessment of the natural history of asymptomatic patients with chronic aortic regurgitation and normal left ventricular systolic function. *Circulation* 1991; 84:1625.

38. Tornos MP, Olona M, Permanyer-Miralda G, et al: Clinical outcome of severe asymptomatic chronic aortic regurgitation: a long-term prospective follow-up study. *Am Heart J* 1995; 130:333.

39. Rapaport E: Natural history of aortic and mitral valve disease. *Am J Cardiol* 1975; 35:221.

40. Bonow RO, Nikas D, Elefteriades JA: Valve replacement for regurgitant lesions of the aortic or mitral valve in advanced left ventricular dysfunction. *Cardiol Clin* 1995; 13:73-85.

41. Kvidal P, Bergström R, Hörte LG, et al: Observed and relative survival after aortic valve replacement. *J Am Coll Cardiol* 2000; 35:747-756.

42. Borger MA, David TE: Management of the valve and ascending aorta in adults with bicuspid aortic valve disease. *Semin Thorac Cardiovasc Surg* 2005; 17:143.

43. Nicks R, Cartmill T, Bernstein L: Hypoplasia of the aortic root. The problem of aortic valve replacement. *Thorax* 1970; 25:339.

44. Manouguian S, Seybold-Epting W: Patch enlargement of the aortic valve ring by extending the aortic incision into the anterior mitral leaflet. New operative technique. *J Thorac Cardiovasc Surg* 1979; 78:402.

45. Konno S, Imai Y, Iida Y, et al: A new method for prosthetic valve replacement in congenital aortic stenosis associated with hypoplasia of the aortic valve ring. *J Thorac Cardiovasc Surg* 1975; 70:909.

46. David TE: Surgical management of aortic root abscess. *J Card Surg* 1997; 12(2 Suppl):262.

47. Borger MA, Rao V, Weisel RD, et al: Reoperative coronary bypass surgery: effect of patent grafts and retrograde cardioplegia. *J Thorac Cardiovasc Surg* 2001; 121:83.

48. Gillinov AM, Lytle BW, Hoang V, et al: The atherosclerotic aorta at aortic valve replacement: surgical strategies and results. *J Thorac Cardiovasc Surg* 2000; 120:957.

49. Rodés-Cabau J, Webb JG, Cheung A, et al: Transcatheter aortic valve implantation for the treatment of severe symptomatic aortic stenosis in patients at very high or prohibitive surgical risk: acute and late outcomes of the multicenter Canadian experience. *J Am Coll Cardiol* 2010; 55:1080.

50. Hilbert SL, Ferrans VJ: Porcine aortic valve bioprostheses: morphologic and functional considerations. *J Long Term Eff Med Implants* 1992; 2:99.

51. Flomenbaum MA, Schoen FJ: Effects of fixation back pressure and antimineralization treatment on the morphology of porcine aortic biosprosthetic valves. *J Thorac Cardiovasc Surg* 1993; 105:154.

52. Chan V, Kulik A, Tran A, et al: Long-term clinical and hemodynamic performance of the Hancock II versus the Perimount aortic bioprostheses. *Circulation* 2010; 122:S10.

53. Rizzoli G, Mirone S, Ius P, et al: Fifteen-year results with the Hancock II valve: a multicenter experience. *J Thorac Cardiovasc Surg* 2006; 132:602.

54. Jamieson WR, Germann E, Aupart MR, et al: 15-year comparison of supra-annular porcine and PERIMOUNT aortic bioprostheses. *Asian Cardiovasc Thorac Ann* 2006; 14:200.

55. Une D, Ruel M, David TE. Twenty-year durability of the aortic Hancock II bioprosthesis in young patients: is it durable enough? *Eur J Cardiothorac Surg* 2014; 48:825-830.

56. Valfre C, Ius P, Minniti G, et al: The fate of Hancock II porcine valve recipients 25 years after implant. *Eur J Cardiothorac Surg* 2010; 38:141-146.

57. Thalji NM, Suri RM, Michelena HI, et al: Do differences in early hemodynamic performance of current generation biologic aortic valves predict outcomes 1 year following surgery? *J Thorac Cardiovasc Surg* 2015; 149:163-173.e2.

58. Wendt D, Thielmann M, Plicht B, et al: The new St Jude Trifecta versus Carpentier-Edwards Perimount Magna and Magna Ease aortic bioprosthesis: is there a hemodynamic superiority? *J Thorac Cardiovasc Surg* 2014; 147:1553.

59. Conte J, Weissman N, Dearani JA, et al: A North American, prospective, multicenter assessment of the Mitroflow aortic pericardial prosthesis. *Ann Thorac Surg* 2010; 90:144.

60. Dumesnil JG, Pibarot P: The problem of severe valve prosthesis-patient mismatch in aortic bioprostheses: near extinction? *J Am Soc Echocardiogr* 2014; 27:598-600.

61. Edwards FH, Peterson ED, Coombs LP, et al: Prediction of operative mortality after valve replacement surgery. *J Am Coll Cardiol* 2001; 37:885.

62. O'Brien SM, Shahian DM, Filardo G, et al: The Society of Thoracic Surgeons 2008 cardiac surgery risk models: part 2—isolated valve surgery. *Ann Thorac Surg* 2009; 88:S23.

63. Thourani VH, Suri RM, Gunter RL, et al: Contemporary real-world outcomes of surgical aortic valve replacement in 141,905 low-risk, intermediate-risk, and high-risk patients. *Ann Thorac Surg* 2015; 99:55-61.

64. Bloomfield P, Weathley J, Prescott RJ, Miller HC: Twelve-year comparison of a Bjork-Shiley mechanical valve with porcine bioprostheses. *N Engl J Med* 1991; 324:573.

65. Oxenham H, Bloomfield P, Wheatley DJ, et al: Twenty years comparison of a Bjork-Shiley mechanical heart valve with porcine bioprostheses. *Heart* 2003; 89:715.

66. Hammermeister K, Sethi GK, Henderson WG, et al: Outcomes 15 years after valve replacement with a mechanical versus a bioprosthetic valve: final report of the Veterans Affairs randomized trial. *J Am Coll Cardiol* 2000; 36:1152.

67. Stassano P, Di Tommaso L, Monaco M, et al: Aortic valve replacement: a prospective randomized evaluation of mechanical versus biological valves in patients ages 55 to 70 years. *J Am Coll Cardiol* 2009; 54:1862.

68. Akins CW, Miller DC, Turina MI, et al: Councils of the American Association for Thoracic Surgery; Society of Thoracic Surgeons; European Association for Cardio-Thoracic Surgery; Ad Hoc Liaison Committee for Standardizing Definitions of Prosthetic Heart Valve Morbidity. Guidelines for reporting mortality and morbidity after cardiac valve interventions. *J Thorac Cardiovasc Surg* 2008; 135:732.

69. David TE, Armstrong S, Sun Z: The Hancock II bioprosthesis at 12 years. *Ann Thorac Surg* 1998; 66(6 Suppl):S95.

70. Dellgren G, David TE, Raanani E, et al: Late hemodynamic and clinical outcomes of aortic valve replacement with the Carpentier-Edwards Perimount pericardial bioprosthesis. *J Thorac Cardiovasc Surg* 2002; 124:146.

71. Poirer NC, Pelletier LC, Pellerin M, Carrier M: 15-Year experience with the Carpentier-Edwards pericardial bioprosthesis. *Ann Thorac Surg* 1998; 66:S57.

72. Corbineau H, De La TB, Verhoye JP, et al: Carpentier-Edwards supra-annular porcine bioprosthesis in aortic position: 16-year experience. *Ann Thorac Surg* 2001; 71:S228.

73. Mykén PS, Bech-Hansen O: A 20-year experience of 1712 patients with the Biocor porcine bioprosthesis. *J Thorac Cardiovasc Surg* 2009; 137:76.

74. Sjögren J, Gudbjartsson T, Thulin LI: Long-term outcome of the MitroFlow pericardial bioprosthesis in the elderly after aortic valve replacement. *J Heart Valve Dis* 2006; 15:197.

75. Johnston DR, Soltesz EG, Vakil N, et al: Long-term durability of bioprosthetic aortic valves: implications from 12,569 implants. *Ann Thorac Surg* 2015 [Epub ahead of print].

76. McClure RS, Narayanasamy N, Wiegerinck E, et al: Late outcomes for aortic valve replacement with the Carpentier-Edwards pericardial bioprosthesis: up to 17-year follow-up in 1,000 patients. *Ann Thorac Surg* 2010; 89:1410-1416.

77. Forcillo J, Pellerin M, Perrault LP, et al: Carpentier-Edwards pericardial valve in the aortic position: 25-years experience. *Ann Thorac Surg* 2013; 96:486-493.

78. Biglioli P, Spampinato N, Cannata A, et al: Long-term outcomes of the Carpentier-Edwards pericardial valve prosthesis in the aortic position: effect of patient age. *J Heart Valve Dis* 2004; 13:S49.

79. Grunkemeier GL, Wu Y: Actual versus actuarial event-free percentages. *Ann Thorac Surg* 2001; 72:677.

80. Forcillo J, El Hamamsy I, Stevens LM et al: The perimount valve in the aortic position: twenty-year experience with patients under 60 years old. *Ann Thorac Surg* 2014; 97:1526-1532.

81. Vongpatanasin W, Hillis LD, Lange RA: Prosthetic heart valves. *N Engl J Med* 1996; 335:407.

82. Jamieson WR, Burr LH, Miyagishima RT, et al: Carpentier-Edwards supra-annular aortic porcine bioprosthesis: clinical performance over 20 years. *J Thorac Cardiovasc Surg* 2005; 130:994-1000.

83. O'Brien MF, Stafford EG, Gardner MA, et al: Allograft aortic valve replacement: long-term follow-up. *Ann Thorac Surg* 1995; 60(2 Suppl):S65.

84. Bodnar E, Wain WH, Martelli V, Ross DN: Long term performance of 580 homograft and autograft valves used for aortic valve replacement. *Thorac Cardiovasc Surg* 1979; 27:31.

85. Gross C, Harringer W, Beran H, et al: Aortic valve replacement: is the stentless xenograft an alternative to the homograft? Midterm results. *Ann Thorac Surg* 1999; 68:919.

86. Heras M, Chesebro JH, Fuster V, et al: High risk of thromboemboli early after bioprosthetic cardiac valve replacement. *J Am Coll Cardiol* 1995; 25:1111.

87. Brennan JM, Edwards FH, Zhao Y, et al: Early anticoagulation of bioprosthetic aortic valves in older patients: results from the Society of Thoracic Surgeons Adult Cardiac Surgery National Database. *J Am Coll Cardiol* 2012; 60:971.

88. Aramendi JI, Mestres CA, Matrinez-Leon J, et al: Triflusal versus oral anticoagulation for primary prevention of thromboembolism after bioprosthetic valve replacement (TRAC): prospective, randomized, co-operative trial. *Eur J Cardiothorac Surg* 2005; 27:854-860.

89. Colli A, Mestres CA, Castella M, et al: Comparing warfarin to aspirin (woa) after aortic valve replacement with the St. Jude Medical Epic™ heart valve bioprosthesis: results of the woa epic pilot trial. *J Heart Valve Dis* 2007; 16:667-671.

90. Connolly SJ, Ezekowitz MD, Yusuf S, et al: Dabigatran versus warfarin in patients with atrial fibrillation. *N Engl J Med* 2009; 361:1139-1151.

91. Patel MR, Mahaffey KW, Garg J, et al: Rivaroxaban versus warfarin in nonvalvular atrial fibrillation. *N Engl J Med* 2011; 365:883-891.

92. EINSTEIN Investigators, Bauersachs R, Berkowitz SD, et al: Oralrivaroxaban for symptomatic venous thromboembolism. *N Engl J Med* 2010; 363:2499-2510.

93. Eikelboom JW, Connolly SJ, Brueckmann M, et al: Dabigatran versus warfarin in patients with mechanical heart valves. *N Engl J Med* 2013; 369:1206.

94. Lengyel M, Vandor L: The role of thrombolysis in the management of left-sided prosthetic valve thrombosis: a study of 85 cases diagnosed by transesophageal echocardiography. *J Heart Valve Dis* 2001; 10:636.

95. Calderwood SB, Swinski LA, Waternaux CM, et al: Risk factors for the development of prosthetic valve endocarditis. *Circulation* 1985; 72:31.

96. Vongpatanasin W, Hillis LD, Lange RA: Prosthetic heart valves. *N Engl J Med* 1996; 335:407.

97. Blackstone EH, Kirklin JW: Death and other time-related events after valve replacement. *Circulation* 1985; 72:753.

98. Ivert TS, Dismukes WE, Cobbs CG, et al: Prosthetic valve endocarditis. *Circulation* 1984; 69:223.

99. Levy D, Garrison RJ, Savage DD, et al: Prognostic implications of echocardiographically determined left ventricular mass in the Framingham Heart Study. *N Engl J Med* 1990; 322:1561.

100. Haider AW, Larson MG, Benjamin EJ, Levy D: Increased left ventricular mass and hypertrophy are associated with increased risk for sudden death. *J Am Coll Cardiol* 1998; 32:1454.

101. Christakis GT, Joyner CD, Morgan CD, et al: Left ventricular mass regression early after aortic valve replacement. *Ann Thorac Surg* 1996; 62:1084.

102. Kuhl HP, Franke A, Puschmann D, et al: Regression of left ventricular mass one year after aortic valve replacement for pure severe aortic stenosis. *Am J Cardiol* 2002; 89:408.

103. Kennedy JW, Doces J, Stewart DK: Left ventricular function before and following aortic valve replacement. *Circulation* 1977; 56:944.

104. Rahimtoola SH: The problem of valve prosthesis-patient mismatch. *Circulation* 1978; 58:20.

105. Ugur M, Suri RM, Daly RC, et al: Comparison of early hemodynamic performance of 3 aortic valve bioprostheses. *J Thorac Cardiovasc Surg* 2014; 148:1940-1946.

106. Garcia D, Dumesnil JG, Durand LG, et al: Discrepancies between catheter and Doppler estimates of valve effective orifice area can be predicted from the pressure recovery phenomenon: practical implications with regard to quantification of aortic stenosis severity. *J Am Coll Cardiol* 2003; 41:435.

107. Yun KL, Jamieson WR, Khonsari S, et al: Prosthesis-patient mismatch: hemodynamic comparison of stented and stentless aortic valves. *Semin Thorac Cardiovasc Surg* 1999; 11(4 Suppl 1):98.

108. Dumesnil JG, Pibarot P: Prosthesis-patient mismatch and clinical outcomes: the evidence continues to accumulate. *J Thorac Cardiovasc Surg* 2006; 131:952.

109. Zoghbi WA, Chambers JB, Dumesnil JG, et al: Recommendations for evaluation of prosthetic valves with echocardiography and Doppler ultrasound: a report From the American Society of Echocardiography's Guidelines and Standards Committee and the Task Force on Prosthetic Valves. *J Am Soc Echocardiogr* 2009; 22:975-1014.

110. Pibarot P, Dumesnil JG: Hemodynamic and clinical impact of prosthesis-patient mismatch in the aortic valve position and its prevention. *J Am Coll Cardiol* 2000; 36:1131.

111. Yadlapati A, Diep J, Barnes MJ, et al: Comprehensive hemodynamic comparison and frequency of patient prosthesis mismatch between the St. Jude Medical Trifecta and Epic bioprosthetic aortic valves. *J Am Soc Echocardiogr* 2014; 27:581-589.

112. Moon MR, Lawton JS, Moazami N et al: POINT: Prosthesis-patient mismatch does not affect survival for patients greater than 70 years of age undergoing bioprosthetic aortic valve replacement. *J Thorac Cardiovasc Surg* 2009; 137:278.

113. Feindel CM: Counterpoint: aortic valve replacement: size does matter. *J Thorac Cardiovasc Surg* 2009; 137:384.

114. Rao V, Jamieson WR, Ivanov J, et al: Prosthesis-patient mismatch affects survival after aortic valve replacement. *Circulation* 2002; 102:III5.

115. Ruel M, Al-Faleh H, Kulik A, et al: Prosthesis-patient mismatch after aortic valve replacement predominantly affects patients with preexisting left ventricular dysfunction: effect on survival, freedom from heart failure, and left ventricular mass regression. *J Thorac Cardiovasc Surg* 2006; 131:1036.

116. Moon MR, Pasque MK, Munfakh NA, et al: Prosthesis-patient mismatch after aortic valve replacement: impact of age and body size on late survival. *Ann Thorac Surg* 2006; 81:481.

117. Jamieson WR, Ye J, Higgins J, et al: Effect of prosthesis-patient mismatch on long-term survival with aortic valve replacement: assessment to 15 years. *Ann Thorac Surg* 2010; 89:51.

118. Head SJ, Mokhles MM, Osnabrugge RL, et al: The impact of prosthesis-patient mismatch on long-term survival after aortic valve replacement: a systematic review and meta-analysis of 34 observational studies comprising 27 186 patients with 133 141 patient-years. *Eur Heart J* 2012; 33:1518.

119. Takagi H, Yamamoto H, Iwata K, et al: A meta-analysis of effects of prosthesis-patient mismatch after aortic valve replacement on late mortality. *Int J Cardiol* 2012; 159:150-154.

120. Pibarot P, Dumesnil JG: Valve prosthesis-patient mismatch, 1978 to 2011: from original concept to compelling evidence. *J Am Coll Cardiol* 2012; 60:1136-1139.

121. Flameng W, Herregods MC, Vercalsteren M, et al: Prosthesis-patient mismatch predicts structural valve degeneration in bioprosthetic heart valves. *Circulation* 2010; 121:2123-2129.

122. De Paulis R, Sommariva L, Colagrande L, et al: Regression of left ventricular hypertrophy after aortic valve replacement for aortic stenosis with different valve substitutes. *J Thorac Cardiovasc Surg* 1998; 116:590.

123. Kratz JM, Sade RM, Crawford FA, Jr., et al: The risk of small St. Jude aortic valve prostheses. *Ann Thorac Surg* 1994; 57:1114.

124. Khan SS, Siegel RJ, DeRobertis MA, et al. Regression of hypertrophy after Carpentier-Edwards pericardial aortic valve replacement. *Ann Thorac Surg.* 2000;69:531-535.

125. Pibarot P, Dumesnil JG: Effect of exercise on bioprosthetic valve hemodynamics. *Am J Cardiol* 1999; 83:1593.

126. Lund O, Chandrasekaran V, Grocott-Mason R, et al: Primary aortic valve replacement with allografts over twenty-five years: valve-related and procedure-related determinants of outcome. *J Thorac Cardiovasc Surg* 1999; 117:77.

127. O'Brien MF, Stafford EG, Gardner MA, et al: Allograft aortic valve replacement: long-term follow-up. *Ann Thorac Surg* 1995; 60:S65.

128. Lupinetti FM, Lemmer JH, Jr.: Comparison of allografts and prosthetic valves when used for emergency aortic valve replacement for active infective endocarditis. *Am J Cardiol* 1991; 68:637.

129. Brennan JM, Edwards FH, Zhao Y, et al: Long-term safety and effectiveness of mechanical versus biologic aortic valve prostheses in older patients: results from the Society of Thoracic Surgeons Adult Cardiac Surgery National Database. *Circulation* 2013; 127:1647.

130. Chiang YP, Chikwe J, Moskowitz AJ, et al: Survival and long-term outcomes following bioprosthetic vs mechanical aortic valve replacement in patients aged 50 to 69 years. *JAMA* 2014; 312:1323-1329.

131. North RA, Sadler L, Stewart AW, et al: Long-term survival and valve-related complications in young women with cardiac valve replacement. *Circulation* 1999; 99:2669.

132. Badduke ER, Jamieson WR, Miyagishima RT, et al: Pregnancy and childbearing in a population with biologic valvular prostheses. *J Thorac Cardiovasc Surg* 1991; 102:179.

133. Chan V, Chen L, Mesana L, et al: Heart valve prosthesis selection in patients with end-stage renal disease requiring dialysis: a systematic review and meta-analysis. *Heart* 2011; 97:2033.

134. David TE, Ropchan GC, Butany JW: Aortic valve replacement with stentless porcine bioprostheses. *J Card Surg* 1988; 3:501.

135. Walther T, Falk V, Langebartels G, et al: Prospectively randomized evaluation of stentless versus conventional biological aortic valves: impact on early regression of left ventricular hypertrophy. *Circulation* 1999; 100:II6.

136. Borger MA, Carson SM, Ivanov J, et al: Stentless aortic valves are hemodynamically superior to stented valves during mid-term follow-up: a large retrospective study. *Ann Thorac Surg* 2005; 80:2180.

137. Cheng D, Pepper J, Martin J, et al: Stentless versus stented bioprosthetic aortic valves: a systematic review and meta-analysis of controlled trials. *Innovations (Phila)* 2009; 4:61.

138. Safian RD, Berman AD, Diver DJ, et al: Balloon aortic valvuloplasty in 170 consecutive patients. *N Engl J Med* 1988; 319:125.

139. Kuntz RE, Tosteson AN, Berman AD, et al: Predictors of event-free survival after balloon aortic valvuloplasty. *N Engl J Med* 1991; 325:17.

140. Percutaneous balloon aortic valvuloplasty. Acute and 30-day follow-up results in 674 patients from the NHLBI Balloon Valvuloplasty Registry. *Circulation* 1991; 84:2383.

141. Bernard Y, Etievent J, Mourand JL, et al: Long-term results of percutaneous aortic valvuloplasty compared with aortic valve replacement in patients more than 75 years old. *J Am Coll Cardiol* 1992; 20:796.

142. Smedira NG, Ports TA, Merrick SH, Rankin JS: Balloon aortic valvuloplasty as a bridge to aortic valve replacement in critically ill patients. *Ann Thorac Surg* 1993; 55:914.

143. Cormier B, Vahanian A: Indications and outcome of valvuloplasty. *Curr Opin Cardiol* 1992; 7:222.

144. Iung B, Cachier A, Baron G, et al: Decision-making in elderly patients with severe aortic stenosis: why are so many denied surgery? *Eur Heart J* 2005; 26:2714.

145. Cribier A, Eltchaninoff H, Bash A, et al: Percutaneous transcatheter implantation of an aortic valve prosthesis for calcific aortic stenosis: first human case description. *Circulation* 2002; 106:3006.

146. Leon MB, Smith CR, Mack M, et al: Transcatheter aortic-valve implantation for aortic stenosis in patients who cannot undergo surgery. *N Engl J Med* 2010; 363:1597.

147. Makkar RR, Fontana GP, Jilaihawi H, et al: Transcatheter aortic-valve replacement for inoperable severe aortic stenosis. *N Engl J Med* 2012; 366:1696.

148. Smith CR, Leon MB, Mack MJ, et al: Transcatheter versus surgical aortic-valve replacement in high-risk patients. *N Engl J Med* 2011; 364:2187.

149. Kodali SK, Williams MR, Smith CR, et al: Two-year outcomes after transcatheter or surgical aortic-valve replacement. *N Engl J Med* 2012; 366:1686.

150. Popma JJ, Adams DH, Reardon MJ, et al: Transcatheter aortic valve replacement using a self-expanding bioprosthesis in patients With severe aortic stenosis at extreme risk for surgery. *J Am Coll Cardiol* 2014; 63:1972.

151. Abdel-Wahab M, Mehilli J, Frerker C, et al: Comparison of balloon-expandable vs self-expandable valves in patients undergoing transcatheter aortic valve replacement: the CHOICE randomized clinical trial. *JAMA* 2014; 311:1503.

152. Zahn R, Gerckens U, Grube E, et al: Transcatheter aortic valve implantation: first results from a multi-centre real-world registry. *Eur Heart J* 2011; 32:198.

153. Van Belle E, Juthier F, Susen S, et al: Postprocedural aortic regurgitation in balloon-expandable and self-expandable transcatheter aortic valve replacement procedures: analysis of predictors and impact on long-term mortality: insights from the FRANCE2 Registry. *Circulation* 2014; 129:1415.

154. Wenaweser P, Stortecky S, Schwander S, et al: Clinical outcomes of patients with estimated low or intermediate surgical risk undergoing transcatheter aortic valve implantation. *Eur Heart J* 2013; 34:1894.

29

Stentless Aortic Valve and Root Replacement

Paul Stelzer • Robin Varghese

Replacement of the aortic valve or the full aortic root can be performed using a variety of stentless valve devices. The three main options are a porcine aortic root-valve conduit (Medtronic Freestyle, Medtronic Inc., Minneapolis, MN), and the "human" valve options of the aortic homograft and the pulmonary autograft (Ross Procedure). Having reviewed the subject almost 30 years ago,[1] it is interesting to note how some things have changed but much has remained the same. Table 29-1 summarizes advantages and disadvantages of current replacement options.

HISTORICAL PERSPECTIVE

The first choice for aortic valve replacement (AVR) was the homograft aortic valve. Gordon Murray created an animal model to implant an aortic homograft valve in the descending aorta[2] and was the first to apply the concept in the human demonstrating function for up to 4 years.[3]

Duran and Gunning at Oxford described a method for orthotopic (subcoronary) implantation of an aortic homograft valve in 1962[4] and in 1962 both Donald Ross in London,[5] and Sir Brian Barratt-Boyes in Auckland,[6] did this successfully in humans.

Initially, homograft aortic valves were implanted shortly after collection.[7] This impractical method was rapidly supplanted by techniques to sterilize and preserve the valve for later use. Early methods employed beta-propiolactone[6,8] or 0.02% chlorhexidine,[9] followed by ethylene oxide or radiation exposure.[10] Some were preserved by freeze-drying.[6,10] Recognizing that the incidence of valve rupture was high in chemically treated valves, Barratt-Boyes introduced antibiotic sterilization of homografts in 1968.[11] Cryopreservation of allografts was introduced in 1975 by O'Brien and continues to be the predominant method.[12,13] Experimental use of autologous valve transplantation began in 1961 when Lower and colleagues at Stanford transposed the autologous pulmonic valve to the mitral position in dogs[14] and shortly thereafter to the aortic position.[13] Donald Ross applied this to humans, reporting in 1967 clinical experience replacing either the aortic or the mitral valve with a pulmonary autograft.[14] Nearly 20 years later the autograft was finally done in America by Elkins and Stelzer.[15] The operation came to be known as the Ross procedure. After an initial surge of interest in the 1990s (over 240 surgeons worldwide reported their experience to the Ross Procedure International Registry[16]), its use diminished in the next decade.

The porcine aortic root (Medtronic Freestyle aortic root bioprosthesis (Medtronic Inc., Minneapolis, MN)) is readily available preserved in glutaraldehyde (Fig. 29-1). Its "off the shelf" availability in a wide range of sizes make it a more flexible option compared to the homograft which is limited in both number and size by the tissue donor pool and what is available in the tissue bank. The Freestyle porcine root employed third-generation tissue technology with zero-pressure fixation and treatment with alpha amino oleic acid (AOA) which aims to decrease both leaflet and aortic wall calcification. This device first began with clinical investigation in 1992. It employed zero-pressure glutaraldehyde fixation and AOA treatment to enhance durability as a third-generation tissue valve. It was approved for clinical use in 1998. The conduit is a complete porcine aortic root with a 3-mm rim of polyester fabric along the proximal end providing additional strength for suturing.

HOMOGRAFTS

Cellular and Immunologic Aspects of Homografts

The normal living valve contains multiple viable cell types including endothelial cells, fibroblasts, and smooth muscle cells incorporated in a complex extracellular matrix. The cells and matrix elements are in a constant state of remodeling under the influence of regulatory systems that optimize the structure and function of the valve mechanism. It is understandable, therefore, that efforts to preserve homograft

TABLE 29-1: Comparison of Mechanical and Tissue Alternatives for Aortic Valve Replacement

	Mechanical	Stented bioprosthetic	Stentless bioprosthetic	Allograft	Autograft
Advantages	Long durability Easy implantation Good EOAI	Easy implantation No anticoagulation	Larger EOAI compared with stented valve. Root replacement is available option	Excellent EOAI All biologic material good for use in endocarditis	Excellent EOAI Living valve Long durability possible
Disadvantages	Anticoagulation Emboli/bleeding Noise	Durability limited Poor EOAI in small valve sizes	Durability limited More complex operative technique Harder reoperation	Complex technique Availability limited Durability limited	Complex operation Double valve or Root replacement with potential late failure of either

structure and function were translated into efforts to maintain homograft cellular viability. Radiation and chemical treatment led to very early failure and were quickly abandoned.[6,8,10,11,17] Antibiotic sterilization of homografts and storage at 4°C does not maintain cellular viability beyond a few days.[18,19] Cryopreservation became the gold standard when donor fibroblast viability was shown long after implantation.[12] Although antigenicity of the fibroblast is low and other cell types do not survive the freezing process, panel reactive antibody and donor-specific HLA I and II antibody testing is positive in 60 to 80% of homograft recipients.[20-22] The potential advantages of viability may be defeated by the detrimental effects of this immune system response. Animal studies have confirmed an immune mechanism by demonstrating that deterioration in homograft valve function is prevented by immunosuppression[23] and does not occur in T-cell-deficient rats.[24] Clinical use of immunosuppression, however, could not be justified for homograft patients.

Tissue engineering concepts led to decellularization which lyses cells and "rinses" out antigenic proteins leaving an inert matrix and intact structural framework. Preserved mechanical properties and structural integrity were demonstrated in a sheep model of such a scaffold. In addition, the empty matrix seemed to attract circulating recipient stem cells which repopulated the framework and differentiated into appropriate cell lines capable of maintaining the matrix.[25] Initial use of the decellularized aortic homograft in humans demonstrated that structural integrity could be maintained with low, stable gradients and minimal regurgitation similar to standard cryopreserved homografts.[26] The same concept has been applied to the pulmonary homograft used in the Ross operation.[27,28] The decellularized aortic homograft has been largely abandoned because of early failure rates but the decellularized pulmonary homograft has been at least as good or better than the standard pulmonary homograft when used on the right side of the heart.[29] Long-term studies are needed to determine if native cell in growth occurs reliably. A decellularized xenograft valved conduit has also been used successfully for the right ventricular outflow tract (RVOT) reconstruction with the Ross but results were poor.[30]

In summary, despite intensive investigation over decades, the relative contribution of the immune response, preservation techniques, and warm ischemia time to ultimate valve degeneration is not clear. More importantly, after consideration of the structural benefits and the immune-reaction risks, the net advantage of maintaining cellular (particularly fibroblast) viability in the homograft is not well defined.[31]

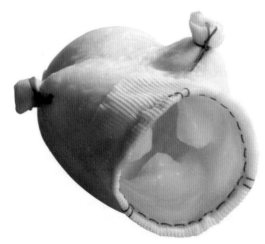

FIGURE 29-1 The Medtronic Freestyle Aortic Root Bioprosthesis. The porcine coronary arteries lie approximately 90° apart. This is in contrast to the human orientation of 140 to 160° apart.

Indications for the Porcine Xenograft (Freestyle) and Aortic Homograft

AVR with a stentless valved conduit such as the porcine root or aortic homograft has a number of advantages including excellent hemodynamic profile with low transvalvular gradients and possibly enhanced regression of left ventricular mass,[32] low risk of thromboembolism without the need for systemic anticoagulation, and low risk of prosthetic valve infection. However, these conduits are subject to structural deterioration that is inversely proportional to recipient age. Older homograft donor age may also increase rates of degeneration. Furthermore, the availability of homografts is still limited especially in the larger sizes. The strongest indication for a homograft is for treatment of active aortic valve endocarditis particularly in patients with root abscess, fistula formation, or prosthetic valve infection.[33] This is the only Class I indication for a homograft in the most recent guidelines.[34]

The porcine root is also an option in aortic valve endocarditis with root destruction requiring a root replacement with the advantage that it possesses minimal prosthetic material compared with a polyester valved-conduit graft. The pliable handling characteristics and ease of coronary reimplantation make both the homograft and porcine root a great option in root infections. The homograft is further well suited to this challenging task as it comes with the added benefits of having the attached donor mitral anterior leaflet, and the ability to reconstruct the debrided root with all biological material to minimize risk of persistent infection. The homograft's very low early hazard rate for endocarditis sets it apart from other valve alternatives.[35]

The stentless porcine root and aortic homograft are also a reasonable option in the older patient (>60 years of age) with a small aortic root. The hemodynamic advantages of the homograft translate into better relief of outflow obstruction and improved exercise tolerance. The root replacement option also eliminates the risk of coronary obstruction from

an oversized aortic prosthesis. Given its resistance to thromboembolic complications the aortic homograft can also be considered for younger patients requiring composite aortic valve or root replacement who cannot be anticoagulated. However, recent data from a prospective randomized trial would argue that most of the advantages of the homograft can be duplicated by the stentless porcine root replacement which has a significantly lower reported rate of calcification and valve dysfunction.[36]

Preoperative Evaluation

Preoperative transthoracic echocardiography (TTE) is an invaluable diagnostic tool for evaluation of the AV and associated anatomic structures. Echo measurement of the left ventricular outflow tract can accurately predict aortic annulus diameter and thus the size of the porcine root/homograft required.[37-39]

Computed tomographic angiography (CTA) or cardiac magnetic resonance (CMR) imaging can also be very useful in the evaluation of potential homograft patients particularly those with aortic root abscess (see Fig. 29-2). Coronary angiography should be employed with the standard indications but may be hazardous in patients with mobile vegetations on the aortic leaflets. Standard chest computed tomography with and without contrast should be considered in any reoperative setting to assess location of bypass grafts, proximity of vital structures to the sternum, and extent of ascending aortic or

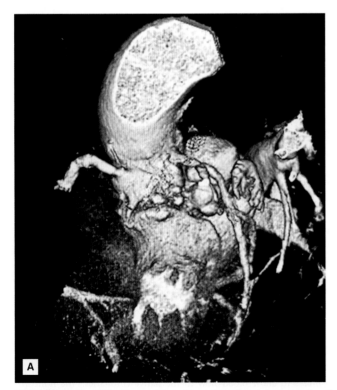
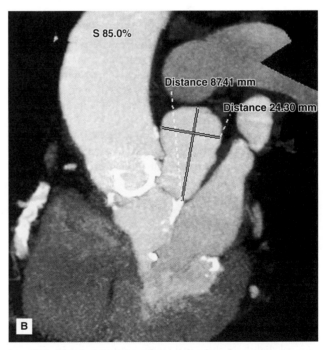

FIGURE 29-2 CTA of root abscess in setting of prosthetic aortic valve endocarditis. The abscess projects from under the valve sewing ring near the left main coronary extending over the left atrial roof under the right pulmonary artery. (A) 3D reconstruction. (B) Standard CT showing prosthetic valve outline.

arch calcification or aneurysm. Heavy calcification around the coronary ostia may preclude safe reimplantation of coronary "buttons" or even a distal subcoronary suture line.

Transesophageal echocardiography (TEE) is often necessary to establish the presence of a root abscess, but its major role is for intraoperative confirmation of the anatomy and assessment of both valve and ventricular function.

OPERATIVE TECHNIQUE

General Preparation

Routine cardiac surgical monitoring including TEE is considered standard of care. An antifibrinolytic agent such as epsilon-aminocaproic acid is helpful. A standard midline sternotomy incision provides full exposure of the heart, ease in cannulation, and access for optimal myocardial protection. Routine distal aortic cannulation and a dual stage venous cannula can usually be employed.

Unless circulatory arrest is needed, minimal systemic cooling (32°C) is adequate if the heart is maintained at 10 to 15°C using a standard insulating pad and directly monitoring the myocardial septal temperature. A combination of antegrade and retrograde cold blood cardioplegia can be used with the bulk of the protection coming from the retrograde. The open aortic root reveals coronary return from both ostia to confirm effective retrograde.

A transverse aortotomy high (1.5–2 cm) above the commissures is usually best. The diseased aortic valve is excised and the annulus is measured with cylindrical sizers. The sinotubular junction should also be evaluated for the subcoronary technique. If using the porcine root, its size can then be confirmed and the prosthesis opened and rinsed.

If using the homograft, sufficient time (20 minutes) is required to thaw the prosthesis and so a decision to use the homograft with a specific size is required prior to exposing the root and sizing it directly. Hence the measurement of the aortic annulus on TEE is essential after induction of anesthesia allowing the time to ensure that the appropriate sized conduit is available onsite.

The homograft is trimmed appropriately. In general, 3 to 4 mm of tissue proximal to the nadir of each cusp is advised for security in suture placement leaving even more for full root replacements.

Techniques of Porcine Root/Homograft Placement

SUBCORONARY IMPLANT TECHNIQUE

The subcoronary method involves two suture lines within the native root. The prosthesis is usually oriented anatomically to properly align the commissures and the coronaries. The proximal end of the prosthesis is sewn to the native annulus in a circular plane at the level of the nadir of each sinus curving upward slightly in the membranous septum to avoid injury to the conduction system. This anastomosis can be done with either interrupted or continuous sutures (see Figs. 29-3 and 29-4).

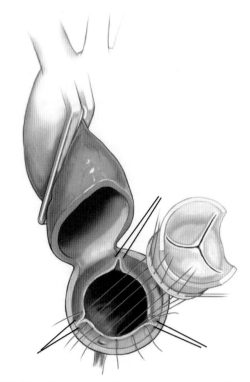

FIGURE 29-3 Subcoronary Freestyle implantation. The Freestyle is oriented anatomically and the proximal end attached in a circular plane at the level of the nadir of the recipient sinuses using either interrupted or continuous sutures. The same technique can be employed for the subcoronary homograft valve implantation.

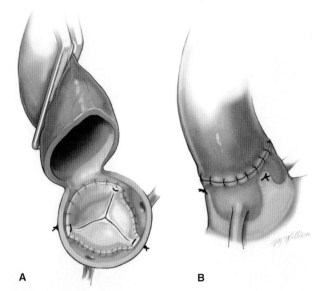

A   **B**

FIGURE 29-4 Distal Freestyle/homograft suture line. (A) The subcoronary implant is completed by tacking the aortic wall of the Freestyle/homograft to the recipient aortic wall with continuous fine polypropylene suture after trimming out the tissue in the coronary sinuses to allow blood flow to the native coronaries. The noncoronary sinus is usually left intact. (B) The aortotomy is closed in standard fashion incorporating the top of the Freestyle/homograft in the process.

The top of each commissure is tacked to the aortic wall. The right and left sinus walls are then scalloped out to a point 3 to 5 mm from the leaflets. The noncoronary sinus can also be removed but is usually left intact. A 4-0 or 5-0 polypropylene suture is started at the lowest point under each coronary ostium and a continuous suture line constructed from there up to the top of the commissure on either side. On the top of the noncoronary sinus, excess prosthetic tissue is trimmed down and tacked to the top of the aortotomy. The aortotomy is then closed with continuous 4-0 polypropylene suture incorporating the top of the prosthesis noncoronary sinus with the native aortic wall. The ascending aorta is vented as the aortic clamp is removed. TEE can quickly assess any regurgitation at this point. Distension of the ventricle should be avoided by prompt defibrillation (if necessary) and pacing if required.

Because even slight malalignment of the commissures can result in regurgitation, the subcoronary implant technique is considered more demanding than the other techniques and may have poorer long-term results.[40-44] The subcoronary technique is good for patients with small, symmetric aortic roots and sinotubular junctions, while it is a poor choice for those with dilated, asymmetric, or severely diseased roots.

Porcine Root/Homograft Cylinder: Inclusion Root Technique

The cylinder modification of the subcoronary technique was developed in an attempt to preserve the native geometry of the prosthesis inside the recipient aortic root. The proximal suture line is identical to the subcoronary method but the sinuses are not scalloped out. Instead, a buttonhole is made in the right and left sinuses in such a way as to allow the porcine root/homograft wall to be sewn to the native sinus wall around the coronary ostia. After the coronaries are secure, the distal end of the prosthesis is attached at the commissures and then incorporated circumferentially into the aortotomy closure.

Sievers and colleagues[45] and Skillington[46] have carefully described technical aspects of these operations that have proven very effective in their hands and should be reviewed by surgeons interested in using this method.

Porcine Root/Homograft Root Replacement

The root replacement technique can be used in any root and is particularly useful in small roots or in roots destroyed by endocarditis. The root replacement allows size flexibility that allows thawing an appropriate homograft without wasting clamp time. Very large roots may require commissural plication as described by Northrup.[47]

The aorta is opened transversely well above the commissures of the valve. The diseased valve is excised and annulus debrided. The aorta is transected and the coronary ostial

buttons are mobilized in standard fashion. If antegrade cardioplegia is used after this point it must be done very carefully to avoid injury to the mobilized ostia.

The homograft root is usually oriented anatomically while the porcine root is commonly oriented with the left coronary os matching that of the patient's right coronary—making matching the two roots easiest. (Porcine coronaries are closer together than human.) The proximal suture line can be constructed with either continuous or interrupted technique. Interrupted is best in difficult reoperations especially for prosthetic valve endocarditis (PVE) because it allows for very accurate, deep placement of individual stitches while distributing tension across multiple sutures. A strip of autologous (or bovine) pericardium is used to reinforce this crucial anastomosis. Polypropylene sutures of 3-0 or 4-0 are used and organization scrupulously maintained on suture guides. The homograft parachutes down as the sutures are carefully tightened (Fig. 29-5).

The Freestyle root is most often sutured with a continuous suture technique with 4-0 polypropylene begun at the right-left commissure and sewing towards oneself through the left sinus, then the noncoronary and finally the right sinus to end at the noncoronary-right commissure. The fibrous trigones and commissures of the native and homograft/Freestyle roots serve as anatomical landmarks and should match up as one proceeds around. It is recommended that the valve be sewn with the sutures kept loose during the left and noncoronary sinus suturing and the conduit parachuted down progressively. Keeping the suture line loose is essential to completing the right sinus suture line. Once all the sutures have been placed, the initially loose suture line is tightened carefully with nerve hooks and tied securely into position. Gentle tissue handling with bites 1.5 to 2 mm apart incorporating a strip of pericardium or Teflon felt is helpful in securing hemostasis at this crucial level that is virtually invisible at the end.

The coronary buttons are attached with continuous 5-0 or 6-0 polypropylene. The coronary stumps of the homograft often times are well aligned to mark locations for the new coronary ostia. For the porcine root usually the left ostium of the porcine root will line up with the left button and then one has to determine if the right ostium lines up appropriately or whether it needs to be suture ligated and another hole made for the right button. Rotating the device 120° clockwise puts the porcine left in the patient's right if that looks better. Once the buttons are completed attention can be turned to the distal anastomosis. The distal end of the conduit and the native aorta are trimmed and sewn together with continuous 4-0 polypropylene usually incorporating another strip of pericardium or felt for support. The native aorta is vented anteriorly and systemic flow rate lowered as the cross clamp is removed.

Care is taken to avoid systemic hypertension or vigorous traction on the reconstructed root to avoid bleeding. Topical hemostatic agents and biological glues may be used, but they should not be routinely necessary. Blood and blood products are not routinely required unless the

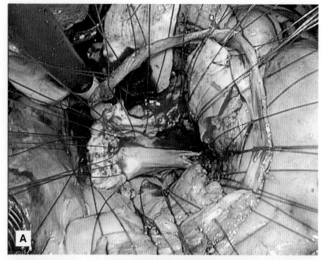

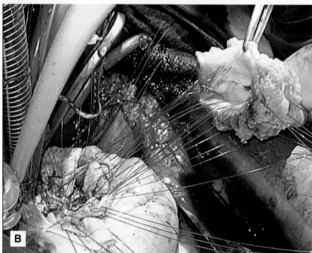

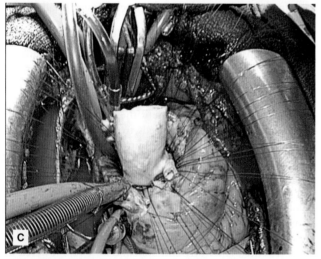

FIGURE 29-5 Homograft root replacement. (A) Interrupted 3-0 or 4-0 polypropylene sutures are placed deep in solid tissue, then passed through a pericardial strip and organization is scrupulously maintained on suture guides. (B) Sutures are then passed through the homograft from inside out. (C) The homograft parachutes down as the sutures are carefully tightened maintaining organization until each suture is tied precisely.

patient is coagulopathic or small in size with a low total blood volume.

Post Replacement Assessment

Ventricular function, regional wall motion abnormalities, and valve function may all be accurately determined with TEE. With appropriate loading conditions, moderate-to-severe aortic regurgitation (AR) warrants inspection and revision of the valve conduit. Mild AR is usually tolerated well and does not warrant reexploration.

Postoperative Management

Even mild hypertension should be avoided to prevent disruption of crucial aortic suture lines. Coagulopathic bleeding is best addressed with products targeted to specific abnormalities defined by laboratory studies.

Adequate volume replacement is required to keep the stiff ventricle of aortic stenosis (AS) filled and alpha adrenergic support is often required for the patient who is vasodilated. Atrial rhythm disturbances should be treated aggressively. Elderly patients, particularly females, with AS and diastolic dysfunction are at increased risk of morbidity and even mortality from postoperative atrial fibrillation. The increased volume loading needed to overcome the loss of atrial transport often leads to pulmonary congestion sometimes requiring reintubation and prolonged support. Forward cardiac output is impaired and renal function may deteriorate in tenuous patients. Cardioversion should be considered early in these patients and loading with intravenous amiodarone is usually indicated. Preoperative loading with amiodarone may minimize the incidence and consequences of this arrhythmia.[48]

Temporary pacing, preferably atrial as well as ventricular, should be enabled. Permanent pacing is indicated if epicardial wires become unreliable, heart block was present preoperatively, or the underlying rhythm fails to return within a week after surgery.

Stroke risk can be minimized by careful intraoperative epi-aortic ultrasound to guide or avoid cannulation and clamping of atheromatous aortic disease. TEE-guided evacuation of air is essential and flooding the field with carbon dioxide may be helpful.

Myocardial dysfunction is best prevented by careful temperature-monitored myocardial protection but long operations may still require temporary inotropic support. Caution must be used in the hyperdynamic ventricle with diastolic dysfunction. The combination of a hyperdynamic left ventricle and a dysfunctional right heart is very challenging. These patients may benefit from atrial pacing (if pacing is required), phosphodiesterase inhibitors, adequate volume replacement, and alpha agonists.

Renal insufficiency is a risk minimized by maintenance of adequate flows and pressure during bypass and generous volume administration in the early postoperative period. A thirsty patient with dry mucous membranes is a good clue that intravascular volume is still depleted. Later, diuretics are needed to encourage mobilization and excretion of this extra fluid. Hypotension should be avoided but vasopressors can have direct negative effects on renal blood flow.

Low-dose aspirin is often recommended for homograft patients, but is not necessary and formal anticoagulation with warfarin is not required at all unless dictated by other conditions. A routine predischarge echo should be done to confirm valve function, ventricular function and freedom from pericardial effusion.

Homograft Root Results

PERIOPERATIVE COMPLICATIONS

In patients without active endocarditis at the time of surgery, operative mortality in the current era is 1 to 5%.[42,49,50] The risk in experienced hands is comparable to using a stented bioprosthetic or mechanical valve. Ischemic time for a root replacement with either stentless porcine or aortic homograft is approximately 90 minutes.[51] A contemporary series of 100 consecutive aortic homografts (virtually all root replacements including 13 reoperations) demonstrated no hospital mortality with 100% survival at 1 year and 98% at 5 years.[52]

In contrast, patients with active endocarditis exhibit a higher early mortality ranging from 8 to 16%.[42,53-56] PVE (17.9-18.8%) is worse than native (2.6-10%).[53,57]

Hemorrhage, heart block, stroke, myocardial infarction, and wound complications occur with similar frequency to those of other AVRs, but early risk of endocarditis is lower with homografts than any other replacement valve.[35]

Hemodynamics and Exercise Capacity

Hemodynamic characteristics of homografts are excellent at short- and medium-term follow-up, both at rest and during exercise.[58,59] A study of 31 patients demonstrated increases in peak and mean gradients of 6.6 and 3.0 mm Hg, respectively, without a significant change in effective orifice area (EOA).[58] Importantly, the EOA of even the 17 to 19 mm homografts was 1.7 cm² and larger valves approximated the normal aortic valve areas as high as 2.7 cm² for 24 to 27 mm homografts.

The typical subcoronary homograft implant demonstrates a 1 to 2 mm Hg drop in mean transvalvular gradient over the first 6 months but with full root replacement, the hemodynamic benefit is fully realized immediately. In the randomized trial of homograft versus stentless porcine root replacement the mean gradients were only 6 ± 1 mm Hg in the stentless and 5 ± 2 mm Hg in the homografts. Only one patient in each group had mild regurgitation after 5 years.[51] These authors concluded that stentless and homograft root replacements are hemodynamically equivalent in the mid-term.

Long-term Outcomes

Long-term outcome has been shown to be technique dependent in a meta analysis of over 3000 patients (37% full root, 63% subcoronary) from 18 studies with a mean follow up of 12.5 years. Reoperation was significantly lower in the root replacement group.[60] There may have been some bias against reoperation in failing roots, where failing subcoronary implants were more readily subjected to reoperation.

The pioneering work of Mark O'Brien in Brisbane, Australia produced a huge series of homograft patients over nearly three decades with 99.3% follow-up.[50] This series demonstrated that rates of reoperation were lower in the full root patients (n = 3, 0.85%) than the subcoronary (n = 18, 3.3%). Of note, operative mortality was only 1.13% in 352 root patients.

Long-term durability was compromised by young age of recipient to the point that those under 20 years of age had a 47% rate of reoperation for structural valve degeneration at 10 years. Conversely, those over 60 had a 94% freedom from reoperation at 15 years and those between 21 and 60 had 81 to 85% freedom at 15 years. This series confirmed the very low incidence of thromboembolic phenomena (without anticoagulation) and a low but not insignificant rate of endocarditis.

Lund reported crude survival at 10 and 20 years to be 67 and 35%, respectively,[44] while Langley and O'Brien reported actuarial survival at 10, 20, and 25 years to be 81, 58, and 19%.[49,50]

Structural valve failure of homografts increases with time, and approximates 19 to 38% at 10 years and 69 to 82% at 20 years.[44,49] Freedom from repeat AVR, for any reason, parallels structural valve failure and is 86.5 and 38.8% at 10 and 20 years, respectively.[49] As heterograft tissue technology has progressed, the difference between homograft and heterograft durability has narrowed to the point of near equivalency with both showing a dramatic age-dependent relationship with youngest patients failing most rapidly.[61]

Freedom from endocarditis at 10 years is 93 to 98%,[49,50] and at 20 years 89 to 95%.[44,49,50] Freedom from thromboembolism at 15 and 20 years is 92 and 83%, respectively.[50] Thrombosis of a homograft has been reported, but in the setting of lupus anticardiolipin antibody syndrome.[62]

In patients with active endocarditis requiring AVR, results may be poorer with survival ranging from 58% at 5 years[53] to 91% at 10 years,[56] and is significantly lower in patients with PVE.[54] Of note, however, the risk of recurrent endocarditis is <4% up to 4 years postoperatively.[43,53,54,56] These results still compare favorably with alternatives so aortic homograft is considered by many to be the valve of choice for aortic valve or root replacement in patients with active endocarditis.

Stentless Porcine Root Results

Very few randomized trials exist comparing stentless and stented valves. Most data available are single-center case series outcomes or case cohort analyses comparing stentless valves to previously published stented valve outcomes. We present the current literature looking at perioperative outcomes, hemodynamics, and durability.

Perioperative Outcomes

Operative mortality defined as death during the index hospitalization or within 30 days ranges between 1.8 and 9.6%[61,62] with most experienced centers reporting operative mortalities around 3 to 5%. Many of the series that reported their mortality outcomes included patients who received concomitant coronary bypass or other valve surgery at the time of Freestyle root implantation making it difficult to compare these outcomes to isolated AVR or isolated bio-Bentall results. The predictors of operative mortality in these series included concomitant valve surgery, congestive heart failure, age, and coronary disease.[63] In a recent systematic review of the literature Sherrah and colleagues found the weighted mean for mortality to be 5.2% and 5.5% for adverse neurological events.[64]

Hemodynamics and Durability

The Freestyle stentless valve is often selected for its superior hemodynamic performance that has been demonstrated in multiple series.[65,66] A meta-analysis of 919 patients by Kunadian and colleagues demonstrated that compared with stented valves, the Freestyle exhibited a larger effective orifice area index (EOAI) and lower transvalvular gradients.[67] The weighted mean difference in aortic gradients was 3.57 mm Hg which some may argue is small; however, there was a more rapid rate of left ventricular mass regression in Freestyle valve patients although this difference disappeared at 12 months. Of note the majority of valves in this meta-analysis were implanted using the subcoronary technique as opposed to the full root replacement. Although the full root replacement technique is a longer and slightly more complicated procedure, it has been shown to yield even lower transvalvular gradients.[68]

The hemodynamic benefits of stentless valves are further exaggerated during exercise. In a study of 106 patients, Khoo and colleagues compared the hemodynamic performance of five different stentless and stented valves under rest and stress using dobutamine stress echocardiography.[69] They found the stentless bioprostheses exhibited a resting gradient of 9 mm Hg that increased to 16 mm Hg under peak stress. Conversely the stented porcine and bovine valves exhibited rest gradients of 15 and 20 mm Hg, respectively, that under peak stress increased to 29 and 30 mm Hg, respectively. Of note, the mean valve size implanted was 23 mm for the Freestyle, 23 mm for the stented porcine valve, and 21 mm for the stented bovine valve. There have been some early data to suggest that newer-generation stented valves have improved transvalvular gradients.[70]

A number of large case series have reported excellent long-term durability of the stentless porcine prosthesis. More recently Amabile and colleagues examined a cohort of 500 patients undergoing Freestyle valve implantation.[71] In this series 96% of cases were done using the modified subcoronary technique with the remaining 4% being a full root replacement. Mean age of patients was 74.5 years and 10-year actuarial survival for all-cause mortality was 44% and survival from valve-related mortality was 70%. Moreover, freedom from structural valve deterioration was 94% at 10 years yielding a cumulative incidence of structural valve deterioration of 3.7% at 10 years. When the authors examined outcomes in patients, less than 65 years at time of implantation the 10-year actuarial survival from valve-related mortality was 87%. Bach and Kon examined 15-year outcomes of the Freestyle valve in their patients with a mean age of 72 years and found a freedom from valve-related death to be 92.7%.[72] This study found the specific causes of valve-related death to include thromboembolism, endocarditis, anticoagulation-related hemorrhage, and structural valve deterioration. The results of the Freestyle valve show it has similar durability to standard stented prostheses.

Stentless Valve Reoperations

Because of extensive calcification after many years the risk at reoperation after homograft or Freestyle valve replacement can be as high as 20%.[73] The subcoronary implants may be easier in this regard because the native aortic root is preserved. The full root replacement is more of a problem. Up to about 10 years, the calcification is limited and it is theoretically possible to place a new valve inside the stentless valve annulus after removing the leaflets.[74] Ultimately, however, the conduit becomes so rigid as to preclude such an alternative and complete re-replacement of the root is required (see Fig. 29-5). The most hazardous part of this operation is related to the coronary ostial buttons which must be protected and available for use again.

Reoperation can be made easier by anticipating the need for this at the original operation. Keeping the coronary buttons large at the initial operation is one way to avoid problems with dissecting them again. The stentless valve-root should be kept as short as possible to minimize the extent of ultimately calcified wall and maximize the amount of normal aorta available for subsequent cannulation and clamping. Closing the pericardium or using a pericardial substitute can make sternal reentry safer. Careful assessment of the aorta and mediastinum on CT preoperatively can alert one to the need for early peripheral cannulation and even sternotomy under circulatory arrest.

Clamping the aorta distal to the main pulmonary artery is very useful in these cases and avoids the hazards of entering a great vessel while dissecting between them before the clamp is on. Complete excision of the calcified wall is often the best policy but leaving a little margin around each coronary ostium may make reconstruction easier. Another stentless valve is often an excellent solution because it is easier to reimplant the coronary ostia especially with the homograft, but even a Ross operation can be done in this setting as was done for the 40-year-old man (shown in Fig. 29-6).

An increasingly attractive option in the future for older patients is transcatheter valve replacement which should be well suited to the calcified stentless root as reported from Milan.[75] (see Fig. 29-7).

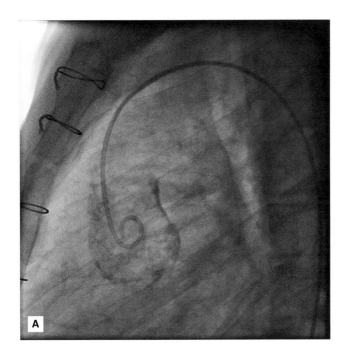

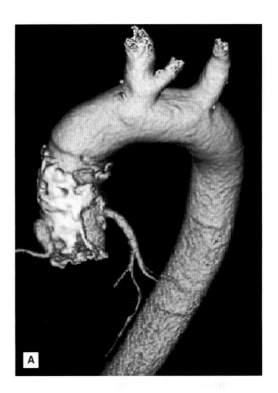

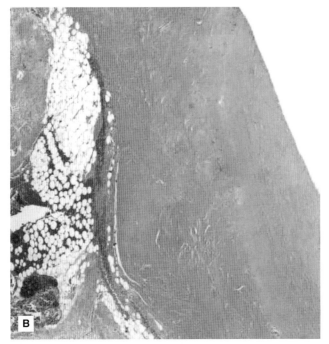

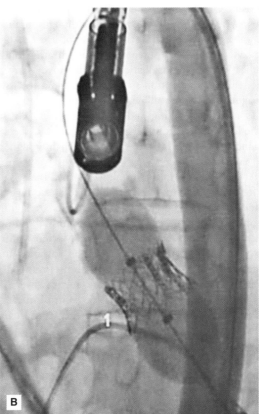

FIGURE 29-6 Calcified aortic homograft. (A) Lateral view of calcified homograft at catheterization 23 years after implantation. (B) Microscopic appearance of this homograft showing fibrosis with essentially acellular mass of collagen fibers.

PULMONARY AUTOGRAFT: ROSS PROCEDURE

Theoretical Considerations

The pulmonary autograft shares the hemodynamic advantages and antithrombotic features of the homograft but is the only valve which has the benefit of being fully viable

FIGURE 29-7 Percutaneous valve placement in calcified homograft root. (A) CTA appearance of heavily calcified homograft root. (B) Percutaneous valve being deployed in this root. (Adapted from Dainese L, Fusari M, Trabattoni P, Biglioli P: Redo in aortic homograft replacement: Transcatheter aortic valve as a valid alternative to surgical replacement. *J Thorac Cardiovasc Surg.* 2010 Jun;139(6):1656-1657.)

autologous tissue. Pulmonary leaflets have been found to have equivalent breaking strain to aortic leaflets and even higher tensile strength.[76] The living pulmonary valve demonstrates the adaptability of human biology to change in response to changing physiologic conditions. The histologic features of this adaptation have been elegantly described and illustrated.[77] The initial response is to lay down a collagen-rich support on the ventricular aspect of the leaflets. This thins out later but remains slightly thicker than normal aortic leaflets. All three layers of the leaflets, fibrosa, spongiosa, and ventricularis contain viable cells which maintain a rich extracellular matrix to support the leaflet function. Endothelial cells are transformed to become capable of smooth muscle actin production becoming more like the aortic than the pulmonary phenotype. The autograft (pulmonary artery) walls are a different story. There is rapid loss of elastin with fragmentation and loss of cellularity and increasing collagen deposition. This may reflect the need to sacrifice elasticity for strength to withstand systemic pressure.

Patient Selection

The cardinal principal in selecting patients for the Ross Procedure is that they must have a life expectancy of at least 20 to 25 years. Other simpler alternatives can be expected to give 10 to 15 years even in young patients although durability of tissue valves in patients under 35 years of age can be very limited. Active lifestyle, potential for child-bearing, and contra-indications to anticoagulation favor the Ross. Many young people seek out this option specifically to avoid the issues of anticoagulation and to allow even extreme athletic activity such as mountain biking and triathlons. Practically speaking, the ideal patient is under 50 years of age but special circumstances can extend this to 65 or even slightly higher. The improvements in tissue valves and hope for "valve-in-valve" catheter-based rescue in the future has pushed the age downward for tissue valves to relegate the Ross to the youngest ages.

The generally accepted contraindications are significant pulmonary valve disease, congenitally abnormal pulmonary valves (eg, bicuspid or quadricuspid), Marfan syndrome, other connective tissue disorders, complex coronary anomalies, and probably severe coexisting autoimmune disease, particularly if it is the cause of the aortic valve disease. Active rheumatic disease is a relative contra-indication as the autograft can be attacked early by the acute rheumatic process and lead to early failure.[78] Bacterial endocarditis is not a contraindication for the Ross procedure, though it is best used when only leaflet destruction is present or when root involvement can be reconstructed without distortion.[79]

Comorbid conditions should also be considered prior to offering this operation to any given patient. These conditions often limit life expectancy and also influence the ability of the patient to withstand this longer procedure. Poor left ventricular function, multivessel coronary disease and need for complex mitral repair are examples. Ascending aortic dilatation and aneurysm have been considered contraindications by some, but these can be easily addressed and

should be. Previous AVR or other open cardiac operations are not a contra-indication to the Ross, but all the standard considerations of reoperative surgery apply including appropriate imaging to allow safe sternal reentry.

Bicuspid aortic valves (BAVs) are the most common etiology of severe AS or regurgitation in patients under 65 years of age. Some have felt this group should not undergo the Ross procedure because of potential complications of intrinsic aortopathy which is common in BAV patients.[80] Since this is the largest group of patients potentially to benefit from the operation, it has been the quest of Ross surgeons to find ways to make the operation safe and durable in this situation. Controversy still exists as to whether primary AR is less favorable than primary AS.[81,82] The patient with AS is more likely to have a smaller annulus which is resistant to dilatation as opposed to the AR patient whose annulus is often dilated and continues to dilate if not supported. Tirone David suggests that 27 to 28 mm is the largest annulus to allow a Ross or 15 mm/m^2.[83]

There is also more of a tendency to distal aortic dilatation in the setting of AR as opposed to AS. These issues are addressable by technical modifications which will be discussed later in detail.

Preoperative Evaluation

Because most candidates for the Ross are under 50 years of age, it is not usually necessary to subject them to cardiac catheterization. CTA is an excellent tool to evaluate the entire ascending aorta and arch as well as the proximal coronary arteries. CMR can be used as well but does not give as much resolution as CTA for the coronaries. Both give excellent imaging of the entire aorta (see Fig. 29-8). TTE gives excellent assessment of the aortic valve, ventricular function, and aortic root. Approximately 1% of patients will be found to have a bicuspid pulmonary valve at surgery. Unfortunately, echo, CTA, and CMR have all been limited in their ability to define the morphology of the pulmonary valve. With proper gating, timing of contrast and attention to the pulmonary trunk, however, this can be determined fairly reliably (see Fig. 29-9).

Technique

The original description by Donald Ross involved a fully scalloped subcoronary implant of the pulmonary autograft using essentially the same technique he had used for a subcoronary homograft implant. Modifications were adopted to decrease the immediate incidence of regurgitation by maintaining the cylindrical geometry of the autograft either within the aortic root or as a complete replacement thereof. The root replacement has become the most commonly employed technique.

Full median sternotomy is usually the best incision. Aortic cannulation should be kept high and bicaval cannulation is preferable because the open RVOT is a constant source of air. Initial antegrade and then generous retrograde cold blood cardioplegia is employed insulating the heart from surrounding structures and monitoring the effectiveness of myocardial

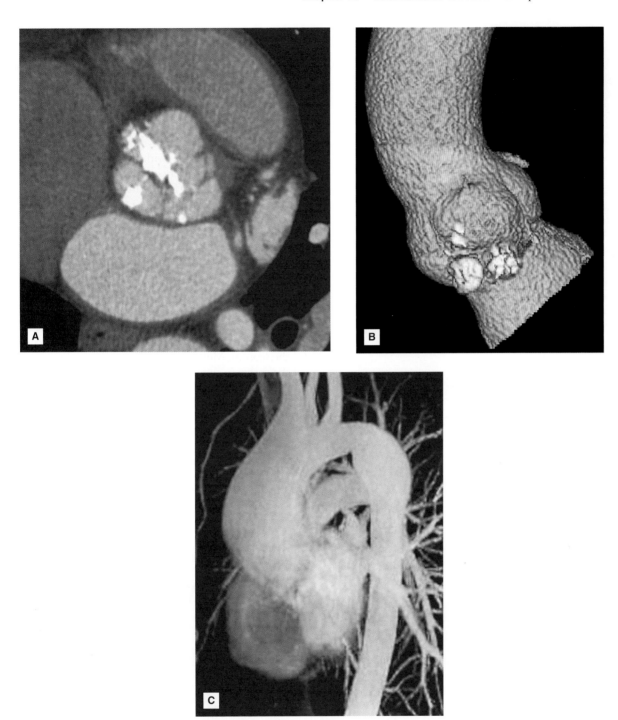

FIGURE 29-8 Preoperative imaging of the aorta. (A, B) Computed tomographic angiography. (C) Cardiac magnetic resonance.

cooling with a septal temperature probe. Traditional venting via the right superior pulmonary vein is not necessary as the open pulmonary artery serves that purpose.

Extensive dissection between the great vessels allows retraction of the aorta with an umbilical tape and keeps the cross clamp off the right pulmonary artery. After clamping the aorta, the space between the aortic and pulmonary roots is dissected until the roots are completely separated. Final

separation is often safest after the aorta is opened and coronary locations can be readily identified. The last few millimeters must be done very gently as the facing pulmonary sinus is virtually fused to the aortic root at the right-left commissure.

A rather high transverse aortotomy incision keeps all technique options open but if a subcoronary implant is planned, splitting the root down vertically into the noncoronary sinus can be employed to increase exposure. The aortic valve

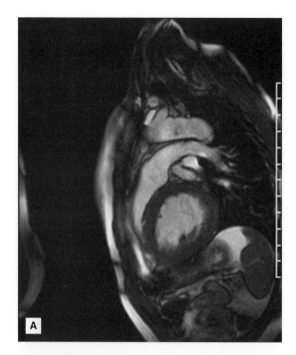

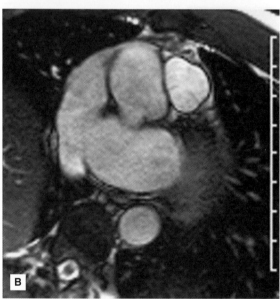

FIGURE 29-9 Evaluation of pulmonic valve by CMR. (A) Longitudinal view. (B) Cross-sectional view showing three distinct leaflets and sinuses.

pathology is inspected as well as coronary ostial positions. A stenotic valve can be excised at this point and the annulus debrided and measured. A dilated annulus can be plicated down at the posterior commissure. A subcommissural annuloplasty can be done to support a subcoronary or inclusion root procedure at this point.

Common to any of the techniques is the need to harvest the pulmonary autograft from the RVOT. The close proximity of the left coronary system and general constraints of this maneuver are obvious from the elegant anatomical casts

published by Muresian.[84] The main pulmonary artery is incised transversely just distal to the valve and the opening extended to either side taking care to avoid the left coronary. A flexible sucker can be placed in the distal PA as a vent. The pulmonic valve is inspected to make sure it is a healthy, three leaflet valve with minimal fenestrations. The remainder of the PA is divided. The adipose tissue between the back of the PA and the left main is gently dissected down to the muscle in the back of the RVOT with the cautery. The left anterior descending coronary artery can be very close to the back and the left side of the RVOT and must be protected.

The RVOT is opened with a #15 blade well below the anterior commissure as determined by palpation or by passing a suture or clamp through the muscle about 5 to 6 mm below the valve from inside out (see Fig. 29-10). The initial incision is cautiously extended until the leaflet can be clearly seen. The dissection then continues around each side leaving 3 to 4 mm of muscle cuff. Posteriorly, a natural plane can be appreciated between the right and left ventricular septal components. The septal perforators are always in the left side and can be avoided by taking only the right ventricular part of the septum. Most often they are not seen. Small branches of the coronary sinus posteriorly can be the source of annoying venous bleeding at the end so gentle administration of retrograde can identify these and allow control at this point.

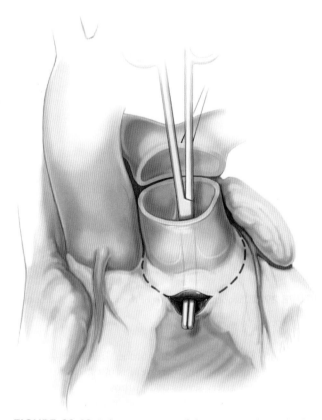

FIGURE 29-10 Pulmonary autograft harvest. A right-angle clamp can be passed through the right ventricular outflow tract muscle below the anterior commissure to assure safe beginning of the harvest incision.

The autograft is trimmed by following the curvilinear course of the leaflets on the inflow end leaving a smooth 3 to 4 mm cuff of muscle. The inflow end is measured by gently inserting cylindrical sizers. The RVOT opening can also be measured at this time. An appropriate pulmonary homograft can then be thawed.

Subcoronary Technique

If the subcoronary or inclusion cylinder technique is chosen, the operation proceeds similarly to subcoronary homograft replacement. Proximal and distal suture lines are constructed as described. Of note, the aortic root must match the autograft at both the annulus and the sinotubular junction. Accordingly, tailoring of the root with annuloplasty and/or downsizing the sinotubular junction may be required.[85] The tops of the autograft commissures must be placed at least a centimeter above the top of the natives to maintain adequate height of the new valve. The potential advantage of this technique is to preserve the native root support around the autograft which may prevent autograft dilatation and insufficiency. However, if the native aorta dilates, the autograft will do so as well.

Root Replacement Technique

In preparation for full root replacement, the aortic transection is completed and the coronary ostial buttons are dissected out and mobilized appropriately. The native noncoronary sinus and the "pillar" of tissue between the right and the left buttons are preserved for later "reinclusion" around the autograft root (Fig. 29-11). The best orientation for the autograft is determined

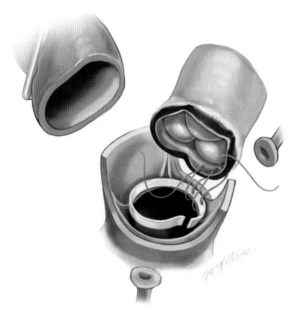

FIGURE 29-11 Proximal autograft suture line. The continuous suture technique is facilitated by leaving the sutures loose enough to easily see the leaflets to optimize depth and spacing and minimize tearing of this delicate muscle cuff. A measured strip of felt is incorporated in this suture line. Note that the noncoronary sinus tissue and the "pillar" of tissue between the coronary buttons has been preserved for later inclusion around the autograft root.

by placing it in the aortic root. Usually the bare area from the back of the PA is positioned in the left coronary sinus.

A strip of Teflon felt about 5 to 7 mm wide is cut to length around a sizer 2 mm larger than the inflow size of the autograft. The proximal autograft suture line is constructed incorporating the felt strip. This can be done with interrupted 3-0 or 4-0 simple sutures best organized on suture guides. Continuous 4-0 polypropylene can also be used beginning under the right-left commissure and working down the left sinus. The noncoronary and right sinuses follow. The sutures are left loose and slightly remote to facilitate visibility. When completed, the suture line is carefully tightened with nerve hooks and tied securely.

The coronary buttons are then reimplanted with continuous 6-0 Prolene. The position of the right coronary is always higher than anticipated, usually just at the sinotubular junction of the autograft. Occasionally, it is so high that it must be implanted in native aorta above the distal autograft suture line.

Excess pulmonary artery wall is trimmed from the autograft down to just above the commissures and very close to the tops of the coronary buttons. The native aortic wall elements that were preserved earlier are now brought up beside the autograft and shortened if necessary. If the native root was dilated or frankly aneurismal, artificial support can be employed using felt patches or vascular graft material.

The distal autograft is attached to the ascending aorta with continuous 4-0 polypropylene incorporating the natural and/or fabric support elements along with another strip of felt placing the sutures right at the tops of the commissures to establish a new sinotubular junction (see Fig. 29-12). With the aorta closed, antegrade cardioplegia can be administered to give a test of valve competence and integrity of the coronary and distal suture lines.

The pulmonary homograft is now attached to the RVOT with continuous 4-0 polypropylene. Care is taken to take long and superficial bites posteriorly over the area of the septal perforator. The distal suture line is completed with continuous 4-0 or 5-0 polypropylene. Warm blood can be administered retrograde during the last half of this suture line.

The ascending aorta is vented and the cross-clamp removed. Generous reperfusion time is recommended. Bleeding is certainly a risk with so many needle holes in delicate tissue submitted to aortic pressure. For this reason, care must be taken to avoid vigorous retraction which can cause more harm than good. Amicar is recommended as is autologous blood removal at the beginning of the operation for return at the end. Biological glues can be helpful but their use is not a substitute for accurate suture line construction.

Concomitant Aortic Surgery

Because of the recognition that patients with BAVs are at risk for late dilatation and aneurysm of the ascending aorta, one should resect any aorta >5 cm in diameter. Below 3.5 cm it is hard to justify any treatment. Between 3.5 and 4.5 cm it is reasonable to employ plication or lateral aortorrhaphy concepts to bring the aorta down to 3.5 or less.[86,87] Between

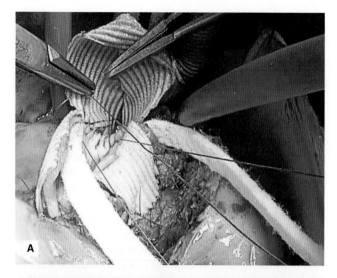

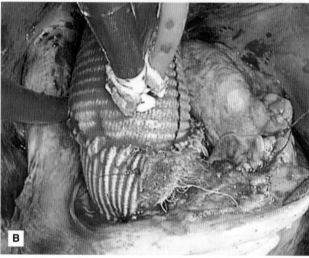

FIGURE 29-12 Fabric support of autograft wall. (A) The arterial wall of the autograft is supported by segments of vascular graft material especially when native aortic wall is intrinsically poor. The entire autograft is enclosed with a combination of native aortic wall and vascular graft material and attached to the ascending aortic graft incorporating another strip of felt. (B) Completed Ross with external fabric support and ascending aortic replacement as well.

4.5 and 5 cm special judgment is required to individualize treatment. Because the vast majority of dissection in the BAV patient begins in the ascending aorta,[88] complete resection of aneurysms up to the arch (hemiarch replacement) should be considered. This actually adds very little time to the operation if planned appropriately. The proximal end of the aortic graft is attached to the (usually reinforced) autograft root to restore aortic continuity.

Results

No discussion of the Ross Operation could be complete without a careful look back at the pioneer series of patients treated by Donald Ross.[89] The 1997 paper from this seminal source analyzed 131 hospital survivors followed for 9 to 26 years with a mean of 20 years. The technical problems that led to early reoperation with the subcoronary technique were recognized in that series and the cylinder modification adopted. Even the full root replacement method was employed as an alternative by Ross in 20 patients beginning as early as 1974.[90] Survival at 10 and 20 years was a remarkable 85 and 61%, respectively. Freedom from autograft replacement was 88 and 75%, where freedom from homograft replacement was 89 and 80% each at 10 and 20 years. Of 53 late deaths, 46 were cardiac. Importantly, of the 30 autografts that were explanted, only three had evidence of degenerative changes which was patchy and did not involve all leaflets. The remainder had completely viable structure as long as 24 years after implantation. Clearly, the transplanted pulmonary autograft is and remains a fully living valve. Homograft stenosis accounted for all but 1 of 20 late reoperations on the right side. Thromboembolic phenomena were documented in 20 patients but only one did not have another systemic risk factor for a source.

Exercise Hemodynamics of the Ross Operation

Multiple studies demonstrate the excellent hemodynamic profile offered by the autograft in the Ross operation. A comparison with normal age- and gender-matched controls showed peak gradients going from only 2 to 4 mm Hg in both groups with exercise.[91] EOAs of 3.5 cm^2 (EOAI 1.9 cm^2/m^2) did not change with exercise in either group. Full root Ross patients had better hemodynamics than subcoronary Ross patients but the difference (1.98 ± 0.57 vs 1.64 ± 0.43 cm^2/m^2) was more important statistically than it was clinically.[92] This study also documented the superiority of the Ross hemodynamics over stented and stentless valves and even over aortic homografts.

It is important to remember that the Ross operation includes RVOT reconstruction and the hemodynamics of that structure can adversely affect exercise capacity. One study documented an average resting gradient of 14 ± 10 mm Hg rising to 25 ± 22 mm Hg for the pulmonary homografts of Ross patients compared to only 3 ± 1 mm Hg at rest and 5 ± 4 mm Hg with exercise in the normal native RVOT of aortic homograft recipients.[93] The higher gradients in the RVOT may contribute to slightly lower maximal oxygen consumption compared to normal controls even though Ross patients easily exceeded 100% of predicted consumption.

Contemporary Results

There was a lot of enthusiasm for doing the Ross procedure in the 1990s which faded soon after 2000 after results were less than optimal. Those suboptimal results are at the heart of a study by Reece et al.[94] reviewing data from the STS database from 1994 through 2010 which reported a nearly threefold higher operative mortality for Ross as opposed to standard AVR after propensity matching (2.7 vs 0.9%; p = .001).

Importantly, the data available in the STS database for that time period included many of the very low volume operators (132 of 220 centers reported less than 6 total cases in this time period) and did not include any of the patients done by the highest volume surgeon in North America. They excluded 66 surgeons who only did one case in these 14 years. In addition, they noted more reexplorations for bleeding (9.4 vs 5.8%) and more renal failure (2.6 vs 0.8%) for the Ross operations. The conclusion was that the Ross could not be considered a reasonable alternative to simpler forms of AVR because of this higher rate of morbidity and mortality. These data in low volume centers are in stark contrast to results from high volume centers. Zebele and colleagues in the United Kingdom, performed a recent review of aortic valve procedures between 2000 and 2011 in children and young adults (16-30 years old) and showed a steadily decreasing trend in the use of the Ross despite an increasingly low mortality rate which reached 0% for the last 4 years of the study. The 1-year survival rate after Ross was 98.8% compared to 96.6% after AVR.[95] They concluded that the Ross operation could be done very safely in all young age groups with a lower mortality than alternatives. They observed decreased utilization of the technique but could not explain it on the basis of technical complexity or operative mortality alone. The author's own experience demonstrated a "learning curve" with three deaths in the first 30, three more in the next 178 and no deaths or reoperations for bleeding in the next 300.[96] Clearly the complexities of reoperative status, need for circulatory arrest replacement of ascending aneurysm, and concomitant mitral repair should encourage referral to an experienced surgeon if a Ross procedure is to be considered. Individualized discussion with each patient should examine the options and consider the potential risks and benefits of each. Hence it seems more appropriate using the Society for Thoracic Surgeons Database results to conclude that Ross operations should not be performed in very low-volume centers but should be referred to regional reference centers with strong experience in aortic root surgery including the Ross.

When done in experienced hands, there are solid data from four continents to support the fact that this operation can be done with only 1% mortality risk and no increase in morbidity despite the longer ischemic and perfusion times for this more complex procedure that often includes replacement or repair of the ascending aorta.[46,96-98] There is definitely a learning curve but much of that learning can be minimized by training under experienced operators.

With operative mortality now approaching that of alternative valve replacements, the long-term results are the key point in considering the Ross operation for any given patient. The comparative incidence of reoperation for structural valve deterioration with present-generation tissue valves and the continuing risks of thromboembolism and anticoagulant-related hemorrhage with modern mechanical devices must be fairly presented to patients along with the data for the Ross.

A thorough review of available series confirms that survival is extremely good after the Ross operation and approximates that of the normal age-matched population.[83,99] Combined with its low incidence of thromboembolic complications and endocarditis as well as avoidance of anticoagulation with its risks of bleeding, the Ross is a very attractive option for young people. Some of these patients will undoubtedly require further surgery, but the outcomes of subsequent surgery have also been extremely good which contributes to the long-term survival.[99,100]

Elkins reported results in 487 patients operated between 1986 and 2002.[101] Hospital mortality occurred in 19 patients (3.9%). Of 15 late deaths, none were due to reoperation but only seven were not cardiac related. Actuarial freedom from all cause mortality was 92 ± 2% at 10 years and 82 ± 6% at 16 years. There was only one documented thromboembolic event. Actuarial freedom from endocarditis was 95 ± 6% at 16 years. Of 38 patients who needed further surgery, autograft reoperation was more common than homograft reoperation. Importantly, the vast majority of these patients had bicuspid or even unicuspid morphology but their risk of reoperation was actually lower than the 9/78 three leaflet valve patients. Patients with primary AR fared significantly worse until 1996 when the institution of routine annular reduction and fixation was initiated. Subsequent results in AR were then only slightly inferior to those in AS in whom the 15-year freedom from autograft valve failure was 82 ± 6%. Technique seemed important as only 21/389 full roots required reoperation where 17/79 intra-aortic implants did. Autograft support was subsequently shown to be beneficial in the German-Dutch Ross Registry data.[102]

Incidence of Reoperation Post Ross Overall, Autograft, Homograft

PULMONARY AUTOGRAFT DYSFUNCTION

Pulmonary autograft stenosis has never been reported but the incidence of regurgitation increases with time and seems to be due to autograft or native aortic dilatation or both (Fig. 29-13). The recognition of early AR due to technical problems with intra-aortic implants led to wide-spread acceptance of the root replacement method when we reported this in 1989.[103] Unfortunately, the totally unsupported autograft as a freestanding aortic root replacement proved to have potential for dilatation with root aneurysm and AR as a result. Annular dilatation was appreciated early and addressed with annuloplasty and external fixation with fixed pericardium or prosthetic material. Dilatation at the sinus and sinotubular junction levels was not appreciated and addressed until about a decade later. Much light has been shed on this problem over the last few years. Brown found that preoperative ascending aortic dilatation, male gender, and postoperative systemic hypertension were significant in a Cox proportional hazard analysis for the development of moderate neo-AR.[104] Hypertension, particularly early postoperatively, can cause acute dilatation and damage to the delicate autograft leaflets before they have time to adapt to the systemic pressure environment. The unsupported root technique having failed in 22 of 142 patients in Rotterdam over a 17-year period, the adult Ross procedure was abandoned at Erasmus.[105] David

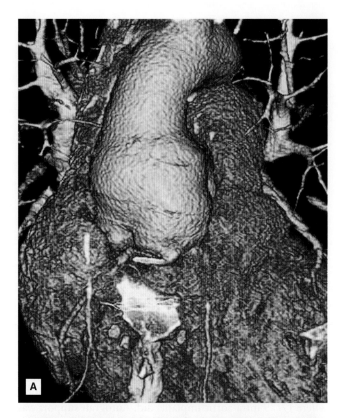

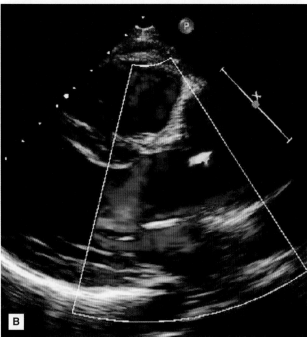

FIGURE 29-13 Dilated Ross procedure at 10 years. (A) CTA appearance. (B) Echocardiogram showing minimal central AR.

expressed concern about the potential for dilatation at multiple levels particularly in bicuspid valve patients because of a higher incidence of aortic wall pathology.[106] The data from the German-Dutch Ross Registry include 1642 adult patients

with mean follow up over 7 years.[102] There were 120 autograft reinterventions in 113 patients. The use of an unreinforced root replacement technique and preoperative pure AR were significant predictors of shorter time to reoperation. BAV had no influence on reoperation rate. A lower reoperation rate was observed in reinforced roots although this was not statistically significant from subcoronary operations.

ROOT REINFORCEMENT TECHNIQUES

In the quest to further address autograft support and prevention of late dilatation, a number of surgeons have developed techniques (in addition to those described earlier) to support the autograft. One of the more disseminated techniques is a full fabric jacket around the autograft made from vascular graft material.[107,108] The jacket is sized approximately 4 mm larger than the autograft and the autograft is sewn to the jacket at the proximal and distal ends with generous openings created for the coronary buttons. The autograft and vascular graft jacket are then sewn to the aortic annulus and distal aorta. When sewing the coronary buttons, some advocate including the jacket in this anastomosis while others have just sewn the buttons directly to the autograft wall.[109,110] Al Rashidi and colleagues reported 4.5-year results using this jacket support method in 13 patients and showed no failures and less autograft dilatation compared to patients who did not have jacket support.[111]

Other techniques similar to the ones described in this author's technique focus on supporting the annulus and STJ using felt support to fix these regions and prevent dilatation at these points (Fig. 29-12). This has been shown to decrease autograft failure in the German-Dutch Ross Registry.[102] In order to prevent proximal autograft dilatation, a number of surgeons have suggested plicating the aortic annulus and or distal aorta if they are dilated.[112]

PULMONARY HOMOGRAFT DYSFUNCTION

As part of the Ross operation, the single aortic valve operation becomes a double-valve operation also leaving the RVOT substitute at risk for future problems. The pioneer series clearly demonstrated the homograft to be superior to other alternatives of that day, but controversy remains particularly over the advantages and disadvantages of homograft viability on the right side. Although the initial hemodynamics of the cryopreserved pulmonary homografts are excellent, consistent increase in transvalvular gradients occurs within 6 to 12 months. This early increase in gradient usually stabilizes by 2 years but can be progressive in 1 to 2% of patients. An immune system response has been implicated but the mechanisms are poorly understood.[113]

Late imaging of pulmonary homografts reveals extensive calcification of the inflow end indicative of an intense scar response to the homograft muscle cuff (Fig. 29-14). Schmidtke and associates tried to minimize this with a unique trimming of the muscle and replacing it with a cuff of pericardium.[114] This proved effective over the first 2 years but failed to make a long-term difference. An intense adventitial inflammatory

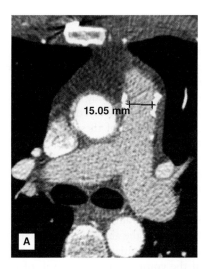

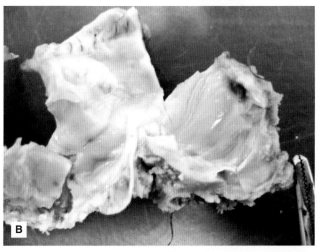

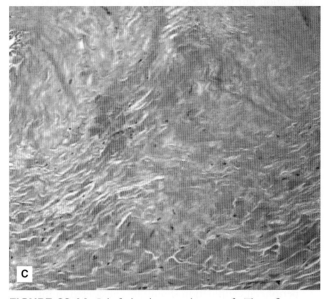

FIGURE 29.14 Calcified pulmonary homograft. The inflow anastomosis of this pulmonary homograft is markedly narrowed and calcified 16 years after a Ross procedure. Gradient was only 28 at rest but 75 mm Hg with exercise. (A) Appearance on CT scan. (B) Gross specimen at explant. (C) Microscopic showing acellular scar.

reaction with diffuse thickening along the entire homograft was described with elegant magnetic resonance imaging flow studies by Carr-White.[115] This caused extrinsic compression of the conduit portion of the homograft.

The incidence of homograft stenosis is probably 5 to 10% at 10 years. Risk factors proposed include younger donor age, shorter time of cryopreservation, and homograft size.[116] Because small size is the most consistent risk factor, oversizing helps reduce the effect of shrinkage. In a series of 338 patients in France, only three patients required isolated homograft intervention and all were treated successfully with a catheter-based valve. The low incidence was felt due to policy of oversizing and use of anti-inflammatory drugs early after surgery.[100]

Review of the homograft outcomes in the German-Dutch Ross Registry show a mean gradient of 4.7 at one month increasing to 10 by 14 years with peak gradients going from 8.4 to 18.5 mm Hg. Most of the increase comes in the first 2 years and then levels off to very slow increase. They found that smaller conduit size (mean was 26 ± 2.15 mm) was the most important risk factor with lesser impact from younger patient and donor age.[97]

Most patients tolerate peak gradients up to 50 mm Hg without symptoms so the clinical significance is less than the incidence of stenosis. In the Oklahoma series, homograft failure (reoperation or percutaneous intervention) occurred in 33 of 487 patients giving actuarial freedom from failure of 90 ± 2% at 10 years and 82 ± 4% at 16 years.[101] The advent of catheter-based valve replacement has made it possible to treat some of these patients percutaneously.[117]

Moderate or even severe homograft regurgitation may also be detected by echocardiography in as much as 10% of patients by 10 years but this lesion is well tolerated by the right ventricle in the absence of pulmonary hypertension. It is probable that most pulmonary homografts will ultimately suffer this mode of failure but the majority will last 20 to 25 years before they reach this point.

After four decades of use and research, the cryopreserved pulmonary homograft is the best RVOT substitute documented for use in the Ross procedure. Rarely, a stentless porcine bioprosthesis has been used. Tissue engineering concepts seem ideally suited to this low pressure area where a decellularized homograft or even heterograft matrix can perform nicely while providing an environment suitable for maturation of new cellular elements derived from circulating stem cells, adjacent ingrowth, or preoperative seeding. Initial clinical studies with both show promise.[30,118,119] and mid-term outcomes from the German-Dutch Ross Registry observed that decellularized homografts exhibited lower gradients than cryopreserved grafts at 6 years.[97]

Use of alternatives to the homograft has been disappointing. Stentless tissue valves have been shown to be an acceptable alternative when homografts are not available but calcification of the xenografts is worse than the homografts.[120] A large series included 73 stentless porcine devices in the pulmonary position had a 10-fold incidence of gradients over 40 mm Hg compared to homografts.[121] Tissue-engineered porcine pulmonary devices have been troubled by poor outcomes in the short term.[122]

POST ROSS REOPERATION

The prospect of reoperation after a Ross procedure has been regarded as a complex and hazardous undertaking.[105]

It is important to realize that reoperative aortic root surgery is not simple and should be done only in centers with considerable experience and volume. Redo Ross surgery is certainly in this category, perhaps more so because of the homograft in the RVOT to make things more complicated. Stulak et al. reported the Mayo Clinic experience with 56 patients requiring reoperation after a Ross most of which (43) had been done at other institutions.[123] Only one patient died (1.8%), but six patients had respiratory failure and three required ECMO support. There were four more deaths within 8 months. This experience brought them to the conclusion that patients need to be warned about potential for risky reoperative surgery in the future when they choose to have a Ross procedure in the first place.

On the other hand, the largest experience reported for reoperative surgery after Ross is from the German-Dutch Ross Registry and paints a far less ominous picture. One hundred and sixty reoperations were done on either the autograft 82, homograft 61, or both 17.[124] All patients survived short and long term. The updated series in 2012 revealed that six patients had died at 224 reoperations (2.6%) in the Registry.[125] Five of the six had endocarditis and all needed urgent or emergent surgery. There was still no mortality with elective reoperation. Emergency surgery for endocarditis is a challenging problem but this is true for any infected prosthetic root. Planned reoperation in experienced hands has lower mortality rate than many series of elective root surgery.

The availability of the bovine jugular vein with its intrinsic valve in a stent frame has become a valuable tool to treat pulmonary homograft stenosis. Initial dilatation with a balloon while demonstrating angiographic patency of the left main system is essential to avoid coronary compromise with this technique.[126]

Alsoufi and colleagues in Saudi Arabia had a predominantly young rheumatic population in which 50 of 510 patients had redo AVR at a median of 3.8 years after Ross root replacement (without support in all but 7). There was minimal root dilatation so the autograft leaflets were simply removed and a stented bioprosthesis (12) or mechanical (38) valve was placed in a standard fashion at the annulus. Follow up after the redo operations averaged 8.4 years. Only one patient required a redo root replacement in that time which made them conclude that just replacing the valve was a valid option in Ross roots less than 4 cm in diameter at the time of reoperation.[127]

The Stuttgart team did 645 Ross operations almost all freestanding roots with support. Forty-nine autograft reoperations were required in 46 patients. A David procedure was done in 18 of 35 with primarily autograft dilatation at a mean of 11 years after the original surgery. Only one of these

required further surgery within 3 years. An interesting finding that has been observed by others is that the native pulmonary valve leaflets are found to have remodeled over time to look like typical aortic valve leaflets including the development of nodules of Aranti.[128]

In Brussels where valve-sparing aortic root surgery is common, this technique was employed to save the autograft in 26 of 28 patients. Twenty of these had originally had root replacement Ross while the other six patients had an inclusion technique. Neo-aortic root dilatation was the primary reason for reoperation. Primary cusp prolapse was also treated but had unsatisfactory outcomes after repair.[129]

Concern about dissection and rupture is largely unsupported. Rupture of the autograft has never been reported. Localized dissection of the autograft does occur but does not extend across circumferential suture lines that protect the distal aorta and the coronary ostia. The wall of the autograft, though thinner than native aorta, is encased in scar tissue from the original surgery making leakage into a free pericardial space extremely unlikely.

If moderate autograft regurgitation has developed with root dilatation, a policy of waiting for symptoms or ventricular dysfunction/dilatation typically indicative for surgical intervention should be considered appropriate, not just treating a sinus dimension. If distal native aorta dilates to 5.0 cm or greater, it may be reasonable to intervene before it gets to 5.5 cm in the setting of original BAV disease. If other valve disease or coronary disease dictates operative intervention, the dilated autograft should not be ignored. If the patient had no support at the original operation and root dilatation is the primary problem, then a valve-sparing technique can be considered or a Bentall option employed. The living autograft tissue makes mobilization of the coronary buttons easier because there is no calcification but they are still more delicate than native aorta and adhesions to the adjacent pulmonary homograft can make dissection in that area difficult. A Yacoub technique[130] is suitable if the annulus was supported with a felt strip at the original operation, but a David technique is needed if the annulus is dilated and/or unsupported. Alternatively, the Yacoub can be combined with annuloplasty or independent annular support to avoid extensive dissection between the autograft and homograft.[131] Need for major leaflet revision is a marker for less durability just as it is in primary valve-sparing surgery.

Complete redo root replacement should be considered if both the leaflets and the sinuses are problematic. The living, pliable autograft makes this much easier than a redo after a homograft or stentless porcine root and perhaps even after a standard Bentall.

Safe reoperation begins with appropriate planning at the original operation where closure of the pericardium or coverage of the heart with pericardial substitute will allow safe sternal reentry. Central cannulation is almost always possible, but peripheral cannulation should be considered in multiple reoperative settings or when preoperative imaging suggests perilous reentry. Crucial to safe conduct of these operations is avoidance of the plane between the pulmonary homograft and the aorta. There is usually plenty of room distal to the pulmonary artery to clamp the aorta before this plane needs to be addressed. Coronary buttons are often very close to the distal autograft anastomosis so aortotomy at reoperation should never be proximal to this suture line. The complete spectrum of replacement options is open at reoperation including simple mechanical or stented tissue valves, subcoronary or full root stentless, aortic homograft, or Bentall operation with biologic or mechanical valved conduit. The RVOT homograft should be left alone unless grossly abnormal by preoperative evaluation. If reoperation is required for RVOT obstruction, this can be accomplished on the beating heart. The old conduit is opened longitudinally from normal right ventricular muscle to normal PA. The thick proximal scar is resected carefully and as much of the old conduit is removed as necessary to allow placement of a new homograft. The posterior wall and that facing the aorta can be left intact to avoid injury to the autograft and coronary tree.

FINAL THOUGHTS

Stentless aortic valve options provide unique advantages over stented valves. They are known for superb hemodynamics particularly in the small aortic annulus. For patients requiring replacement of the aortic root and valve, the stentless valves provide a conduit by which both issues can be addressed with one graft. Furthermore, in the setting of aortic root replacement the tissue of the stentless valve is friendlier when working with coronary button anastomoses and this is predominantly true in cases of reoperative aortic root surgery. The durability of both the homograft and Freestyle has been shown to be similar to that of the best of the stented valve options.

The stentless valve option can lead to a more complicated reoperation in either the subcoronary or full root technique and patients should be referred to expert centers where these surgeries can be done safely with low mortality and morbidity.

The Ross operation should be offered as an option for any patient under the age of 50 years with aortic valve disease and a life expectancy in excess of 20 to 25 years. Under ideal circumstances, it can be considered in the 50- to 65-year-old population where the Ross has the possibility of lasting to the end of a normal life span. Of all the substitutes for the diseased aortic valve, only the pulmonary autograft has all the biologic advantages of a truly living structure. It is delicate and demands precise implantation technique for immediate and long-term success. Appropriate aortic tailoring or support is needed in the majority of patients to prevent late autograft dilatation and dysfunction. Approximately 20% of patients will probably require additional surgery for either the neo-aortic or the neo-pulmonary aspects of this operation by 20 years but they will not require anticoagulation and will not be limited in activity or lifestyle during that time. In appropriate hands, this operation can be done very safely and is a durable and excellent choice for young active people with aortic valve disease. Compared to the virtually 100% reoperation rate at 20 years for animal tissue valves, unavoidable and ongoing risks of thromboembolic and hemorrhagic complications with mechanical valves and proven advantage

of the Ross over aortic homograft in randomized prospective trial,[132,133] the Ross is a very viable option. Long-term survival may actually be superior to any other aortic valve operation. Failure to offer this option misses an opportunity for this survival benefit.[55]

REFERENCES

1. Stelzer P, Elkins RC: Homograft valves and conduits: applications in cardiac surgery. *Curr Probl Surg* 1989; 26(6):381-452.
2. Murray G: Homologous aortic-valve-segment transplants as surgical treatment for aortic and mitral insufficiency. *Angiology* 1956; 7(5):466-471.
3. Murray G: Aortic valve transplants. *Angiology* 1960; 11:99-102.
4. Duran CG, Gunning AJ: A method for placing a total homologous aortic valve in the subcoronary position. *Lancet* 1962; 2(7254):488-489.
5. Ross DN: Homograft replacement of the aortic valve. *Lancet* 1962; 2(7254):487.
6. Barratt-Boyes BG: Homograft Aortic Valve replacement in aortic incompetence and stenosis. *Thorax* 1964; 19:131-150.
7. MD NTK, MD EHB, MD FLH, MD JKK. *Kirklin/Barratt-Boyes Cardiac Surgery: Expert Consult—Online and Print (2 Vol. Set), 4e (Kochoukas, Kirklin/Barratt-Boyes Cardiac Surgery (2 Vol. Set))*. Saunders; 2012.
8. Logrippo GA, Overhulse PR, Szilagyi DE, Hartman FW: Procedure for sterilization of arterial homografts with beta-propiolactone. *Lab Invest* 1955; 4 (3):217-231.
9. Davies H, Lessof MH, Roberts CI, Ross DN: Homograft replacement of the aortic valve: follow-up studies in twelve patients. *Lancet* 1965; 1(7392):926-929.
10. Pacifico AD, Karp RB, Kirklin JW: Homografts for replacement of the aortic valve. *Circulation* 1972; 45(1 Suppl):I36-I43.
11. Barratt-Boyes BG: Long-term follow-up of aortic valvar grafts. *Br Heart J* 1971; 33(Suppl:60-Suppl:65).
12. O'Brien MF, Stafford EG, Gardner MA, Pohlner PG, McGiffin DC: A comparison of aortic valve replacement with viable cryopreserved and fresh allograft valves, with a note on chromosomal studies. *J Thorac Cardiovasc Surg* 1987; 94(6):812-823.
13. Pillsbury RC, Shumway NE: Replacement of the aortic valve with the autologous pulmonic valve. *Surg Forum* 1966; 17:176-177.
14. Ross DN: Replacement of aortic and mitral valves with a pulmonary autograft. *Lancet* 1967; 2(7523):956-958.
15. Stelzer P, Elkins RC: Pulmonary autograft: an American experience. *J Card Surg* 1987; 2(4):429-433.
16. Oury JH, Hiro SP, Maxwell JM, Lamberti JJ, Duran CM: The Ross procedure: current registry results. *Ann Thorac Surg* 1998; 66 (6 Suppl):S162-S165.
17. Smith JC: The pathology of human aortic valve homografts. *Thorax* 1967; 22(2):114-138.
18. Armiger LC: Viability studies of human valves prepared for use as allografts. *Ann Thorac Surg* 1995; 60(2 Suppl):S118-20; discussion S120.
19. O'Brien MF, Stafford G, Gardner M, et al: The viable cryopreserved allograft aortic valve. *J Card Surg* 1987; 2(1 Suppl):153-167.
20. Hoekstra F, Witvliet M, Knoop C, et al: Donor-specific anti-human leukocyte antigen class I antibodies after implantation of cardiac valve allografts. *J Heart Lung Transplant* 1997; 16(5):570-572.
21. Shaddy RE, Hunter DD, Osborn KA, et al: Prospective analysis of HLA immunogenicity of cryopreserved valved allografts used in pediatric heart surgery. *Circulation* 1996; 94(5):1063-1067.
22. Smith JD, Ogino H, Hunt D, Laylor RM, Rose ML, Yacoub MH: Humoral immune response to human aortic valve homografts. *Ann Thorac Surg* 1995; 60(2 Suppl):S127-S130.
23. Green MK, Walsh MD, Dare A, et al: Histologic and immunohistochemical responses after aortic valve allografts in the rat. *Ann Thorac Surg* 1998; 66(6 Suppl):S216-S220.
24. Legare JF, Lee TD, Ross DB: Cryopreservation of rat aortic valves results in increased structural failure. *Circulation* 2000; 102(19 Suppl 3): III75-III78.
25. Baraki H, Tudorache I, Braun M, et al: Orthotopic replacement of the aortic valve with decellularized allograft in a sheep model. *Biomaterials* 2009; 30(31):6240-6246.

26. Zehr KJ, Yagubyan M, Connolly HM, Nelson SM, Schaff HV: Aortic root replacement with a novel decellularized cryopreserved aortic homograft: postoperative immunoreactivity and early results. *J Thorac Cardiovasc Surg* 2005; 130(4):1010-1015.

27. Brown JW, Ruzmetov M, Rodefeld MD, Turrentine MW: Right ventricular outflow tract reconstruction in Ross patients: does the homograft fare better. *Ann Thorac Surg* 2008; 86(5):1607-1612.

28. Elkins RC, Dawson PE, Goldstein S, Walsh SP, Black KS: Decellularized human valve allografts. *Ann Thorac Surg* 2001; 71(5 Suppl):S428-S432.

29. Brown JW, Ruzmetov M, Eltayeb O, Rodefeld MD, Turrentine MW: Performance of SynerGraft decellularized pulmonary homograft in patients undergoing a Ross procedure. *Ann Thorac Surg* 2011; 91(2): 416-422; discussion 422.

30. Konertz W, Dohmen PM, Liu J, et al: Hemodynamic characteristics of the matrix P decellularized xenograft for pulmonary valve replacement during the Ross operation. *J Heart Valve Dis* 2005; 14(1):78-81.

31. Armiger LC: Postimplantation leaflet cellularity of valve allografts: are donor cells beneficial or detrimental. *Ann Thorac Surg* 1998; 66(6 Suppl):S233-S235.

32. Maselli D, Pizio R, Bruno LP, Di Bella I, De Gasperis C: Left ventricular mass reduction after aortic valve replacement: homografts, stentless and stented valves. *Ann Thorac Surg* 1999; 67(4):966-971.

33. Foghsgaard S, Bruun N, Kjaergard H: Outcome of aortic homograft implantation in 24 cases of severe infective endocarditis. *Scand J Infect Dis* 2008; 40(3):216-220.

34. Svensson LG, Adams DH, Bonow RO, et al: Aortic valve and ascending aorta guidelines for management and quality measures. *Ann Thorac Surg* 2013; 95(6 Suppl):S1-66.

35. McGiffin DC, Kirklin JK: The impact of aortic valve homografts on the treatment of aortic prosthetic valve endocarditis. *Semin Thorac Cardiovasc Surg* 1995; 7(1):25-31.

36. El-Hamamsy I, Clark L, Stevens LM, Sarang Z, Melina G, Takkenberg JJ, Yacoub MH: Late outcomes following freestyle versus homograft aortic root replacement: results from a prospective randomized trial. *J Am Coll Cardiol* 2010; 55(4):368-376.

37. Greaves SC, Reimold SC, Lee RT, Cooke KA, Aranki SF: Preoperative prediction of prosthetic aortic valve annulus diameter by two-dimensional echocardiography. *J Heart Valve Dis* 1995; 4(1):14-17.

38. Moscucci M, Weinert L, Karp RB, Neumann A: Prediction of aortic annulus diameter by two-dimensional echocardiography. Application in the preoperative selection and preparation of homograft aortic valves. *Circulation* 1991; 84(5 Suppl):III76-III80.

39. Weinert L, Karp R, Vignon P, Bales A, Lang RM: Feasibility of aortic diameter measurement by multiplane transesophageal echocardiography for preoperative selection and preparation of homograft aortic valves. *J Thorac Cardiovasc Surg* 1996; 112(4):954-961.

40. Daicoff GR, Botero LM, Quintessenza JA: Allograft replacement of the aortic valve versus the miniroot and valve. *Ann Thorac Surg* 1993; 55(4):855-858; discussion 859.

41. Dearani JA, Orszulak TA, Daly RC, et al: Comparison of techniques for implantation of aortic valve allografts. *Ann Thorac Surg* 1996; 62 (4):1069-1075.

42. Lund O, Chandrasekaran V, Grocott-Mason R, et al: Primary aortic valve replacement with allografts over twenty-five years: valve-related and procedure-related determinants of outcome. *J Thorac Cardiovasc Surg* 1999; 117(1):77-90; discussion 90.

43. McGiffin DC, O'Brien MF: A technique for aortic root replacement by an aortic allograft. *Ann Thorac Surg* 1989;47(4):625-627.

44. Rubay JE, Raphael D, Sluysmans T, et al: Aortic valve replacement with allograft/autograft: subcoronary versus intraluminal cylinder or root. *Ann Thorac Surg* 1995; 60(2 Suppl):S78-S82.

45. Sievers HH, Stierle U, Charitos EI, et al: Fourteen years' experience with 501 subcoronary Ross procedures: surgical details and results. *J Thorac Cardiovasc Surg* 2010; 140(4):816-822, 822.e1.

46. Skillington PD, Mokhles MM, Takkenberg JJ, et al: Twenty-year analysis of autologous support of the pulmonary autograft in the Ross procedure. *Ann Thorac Surg* 2013; 96(3):823-829.

47. Northrup WF, Kshettry VR: Implantation technique of aortic homograft root: emphasis on matching the host root to the graft. *Ann Thorac Surg* 1998; 66(1):280-284.

48. Mitchell LB, Exner DV, Wyse DG, et al: Prophylactic oral amiodarone for the prevention of arrhythmias that begin early after revascularization,

valve replacement, or repair: PAPABEAR: a randomized controlled trial. *JAMA* 2005; 294(24):3093-3100.

49. Langley SM, McGuirk SP, Chaudhry MA, Livesey SA, Ross JK, Monro JL: Twenty-year follow-up of aortic valve replacement with antibiotic sterilized homografts in 200 patients. *Semin Thorac Cardiovasc Surg* 1999;11(4 Suppl):28-34.

50. O'Brien MF, Harrocks S, Stafford EG, et al: The homograft aortic valve: a 29-year, 99.3% follow up of 1,022 valve replacements. *J Heart Valve Dis* 2001; 10(3):334-344; discussion 335.

51. Melina G, De Robertis F, Gaer JA, Amrani M, Khaghani A, Yacoub MH: Mid-term pattern of survival, hemodynamic performance and rate of complications after medtronic freestyle versus homograft full aortic root replacement: results from a prospective randomized trial. *J Heart Valve Dis* 2004; 13(6):972-975; discussion 975.

52. Byrne JG, Karavas AN, Mihaljevic T, Rawn JD, Aranki SF, Cohn LH: Role of the cryopreserved homograft in isolated elective aortic valve replacement. *Am J Cardiol* 2003; 91(5):616-619.

53. Dearani JA, Orszulak TA, Schaff HV, Daly RC, Anderson BJ, Danielson GK: Results of allograft aortic valve replacement for complex endocarditis. *J Thorac Cardiovasc Surg* 1997; 113(2):285-291.

54. Niwaya K, Knott-Craig CJ, Santangelo K, Lane MM, Chandrasekaran K, Elkins RC: Advantage of autograft and homograft valve replacement for complex aortic valve endocarditis. *Ann Thorac Surg* 1999; 67(6):1603-1608.

55. Yacoub MH, El-Hamamsy I, Sievers HH, et al: Under-use of the Ross operation—a lost opportunity. *Lancet* 2014; 384(9943):559-560.

56. Yankah AC, Klose H, Petzina R, Musci M, Siniawski H, Hetzer R: Surgical management of acute aortic root endocarditis with viable homograft: 13-year experience. *Eur J Cardiothorac Surg* 2002; 21(2):260-267.

57. Grinda JM, Mainardi JL, D'Attellis N, et al: Cryopreserved aortic viable homograft for active aortic endocarditis. *Ann Thorac Surg* 2005; 79(3):767-771.

58. Eriksson MJ, Källner G, Rosfors S, Ivert T, Brodin LA: Hemodynamic performance of cryopreserved aortic homograft valves during midterm follow-up. *J Am Coll Cardiol* 1998; 32(4):1002-1008.

59. Hasegawa J, Kitamura S, Taniguchi S, et al: Comparative rest and exercise hemodynamics of allograft and prosthetic valves in the aortic position. *Ann Thorac Surg* 1997; 64(6):1753-1756.

60. Athanasiou T, Jones C, Jin R, Grunkemeier GL, Ross DN: Homograft implantation techniques in the aortic position: to preserve or replace the aortic root. *Ann Thorac Surg* 2006; 81(5):1578-1585.

61. Kappetein AP, Braun J, Baur LH, et al: Outcome and follow-up of aortic valve replacement with the freestyle stentless bioprosthesis. *Ann Thorac Surg* 2001; 71(2):601-607; discussion 607.

62. Mathur AN, Hourtovenko CD, Baigrie RS, Mecci SU, Ravi GD, Garg R: Stentless freestyle aortic valve/root bioprostheses: a northern Ontario community hospital perspective. *Can J Cardiol* 2000; 16(6):747-756.

63. Ennker JA, Ennker IC, Albert AA, Rosendahl UP, Bauer S, Florath I: The Freestyle stentless bioprosthesis in more than 1000 patients: a single-center experience over 10 years. *J Card Surg* 2009; 24(1):41-48.

64. Sherrah AG, Edelman JJ, Thomas SR, et al: The freestyle aortic bioprosthesis: a systematic review. *Heart Lung Circ* 2014; 23(12):1110-1117.

65. Pibarot P, Dumesnil JG, Jobin J, Cartier P, Honos G, Durand LG: Hemodynamic and physical performance during maximal exercise in patients with an aortic bioprosthetic valve: comparison of stentless versus stented bioprostheses. *J Am Coll Cardiol* 1999; 34(5):1609-1617.

66. Hanke T, Charitos EI, Paarmann H, Stierle U, Sievers HH: Haemodynamic performance of a new pericardial aortic bioprosthesis during exercise and recovery: comparison with pulmonary autograft, stentless aortic bioprosthesis and healthy control groups. *Eur J Cardiothorac Surg* 2013; 44(4):e295-e301.

67. Kunadian B, Vijayalakshmi K, Thornley AR, et al: Meta-analysis of valve hemodynamics and left ventricular mass regression for stentless versus stented aortic valves. *Ann Thorac Surg* 2007; 84(1):73-78.

68. Bach DS, Kon ND, Dumesnil JG, Sintek CF, Doty DB: Ten-year outcome after aortic valve replacement with the freestyle stentless bioprosthesis. *Ann Thorac Surg* 2005; 80 (2):480-486; discussion 486.

69. Khoo JP, Davies JE, Ang KL, Galiñanes M, Chin DT: Differences in performance of five types of aortic valve prostheses: haemodynamic assessment by dobutamine stress echocardiography. *Heart* 2013; 99(1):41-47.

70. Tasca G, Redaelli P, Riva B, De Carlini CC, Lobiati E, Gamba A: Hemodynamic comparison between Trifecta and freestyle aortic valve

during exercise in patients with small aortic root. *J Card Surg* 2015; 30(5):400-404.

71. Amabile N, Bical OM, Azmoun A, Ramadan R, Nottin R, Deleuze PH: Long-term results of Freestyle stentless bioprosthesis in the aortic position: a single-center prospective cohort of 500 patients. *J Thorac Cardiovasc Surg* 2014; 148(5):1903-1911.

72. Bach DS, Kon ND: Long-term clinical outcomes 15 years after aortic valve replacement with the Freestyle stentless aortic bioprosthesis. *Ann Thorac Surg* 2014; 97(2):544-551.

73. Sadowski J, Kapelak B, Bartus K, et al: Reoperation after fresh homograft replacement: 23 years' experience with 655 patients. *Eur J Cardiothorac Surg* 2003; 23(6):996-1000; discussion 1000.

74. Joudinaud TM, Baron F, Raffoul R, et al: Redo aortic root surgery for failure of an aortic homograft is a major technical challenge. *Eur J Cardiothorac Surg* 2008; 33(6):989-994.

75. Dainese L, Fusari M, Trabattoni P, Biglioli P: Redo in aortic homograft replacement: transcatheter aortic valve as a valid alternative to surgical replacement. *J Thorac Cardiovasc Surg* 2010; 139(6):1656-1657.

76. Gorczynski A, Trenkner M, Anisimowicz L, et al: Biomechanics of the pulmonary autograft valve in the aortic position. *Thorax* 1982; 37(7):535-539.

77. Rabkin-Aikawa E, Aikawa M, Farber M, et al: Clinical pulmonary autograft valves: pathologic evidence of adaptive remodeling in the aortic site. *J Thorac Cardiovasc Surg* 2004; 128 (4):552-561.

78. Pieters FA, Al-Halees Z, Hatle L, Shahid MS, Al-Amri M: Results of the Ross operation in rheumatic versus non-rheumatic aortic valve disease. *J Heart Valve Dis* 2000; 9 (1):38-44.

79. Oswalt JD, Dewan SJ: Aortic infective endocarditis managed by the Ross procedure. *J Heart Valve Dis* 1993; 2(4):380-384.

80. de Sa M, Moshkovitz Y, Butany J, David TE: Histologic abnormalities of the ascending aorta and pulmonary trunk in patients with bicuspid aortic valve disease: clinical relevance to the ross procedure. *J Thorac Cardiovasc Surg* 1999; 118(4):588-594.

81. Elkins RC: The Ross operation: a 12-year experience. *Ann Thorac Surg* 1999; 68(3 Suppl):S14-S18.

82. Stelzer P: Technique and results of the modified Ross procedure in aortic regurgitation versus aortic stenosis. *Adv Cardiol* 2002; 39:93-99.

83. David TE, David C, Woo A, Manlhiot C: The Ross procedure: outcomes at 20 years. *J Thorac Cardiovasc Surg* 2014; 147(1):85-93.

84. Muresian H: The Ross procedure: new insights into the surgical anatomy. *Ann Thorac Surg* 2006; 81(2):495-501.

85. Sievers H, Dahmen G, Graf B, Stierle U, Ziegler A, Schmidtke C: Midterm results of the Ross procedure preserving the patient's aortic root. *Circulation* 2003; 108(Suppl 1):II55-II60.

86. Polvani G, Barili F, Dainese L, et al: Reduction ascending aortoplasty: midterm follow-up and predictors of redilatation. *Ann Thorac Surg* 2006; 82(2):586-591.

87. Bauer M, Pasic M, Schaffarzyk R, et al: Reduction aortoplasty for dilatation of the ascending aorta in patients with bicuspid aortic valve. *Ann Thorac Surg* 2002; 73(3):720-723; discussion 724.

88. Roberts CS, Roberts WC: Dissection of the aorta associated with congenital malformation of the aortic valve. *J Am Coll Cardiol* 1991; 17(3):712-716.

89. Chambers JC, Somerville J, Stone S, Ross DN: Pulmonary autograft procedure for aortic valve disease: long-term results of the pioneer series. *Circulation* 1997; 96 (7):2206-2214.

90. Gerosa G, McKay R, Ross DN: Replacement of the aortic valve or root with a pulmonary autograft in children. *Ann Thorac Surg* 1991; 51(3):424-429.

91. Pibarot P, Dumesnil JG, Briand M, Laforest I, Cartier P: Hemodynamic performance during maximum exercise in adult patients with the ross operation and comparison with normal controls and patients with aortic bioprostheses. *Am J Cardiol* 2000; 86(9):982-988.

92. Böhm JO, Botha CA, Hemmer W, et al: Hemodynamic performance following the Ross operation: comparison of two different techniques. *J Heart Valve Dis* 2004; 13(2):174-180; discussion 180.

93. Wang A, Jaggers J, Ungerleider RM, Lim CS, Ryan T: Exercise echocardiographic comparison of pulmonary autograft and aortic homograft replacements for aortic valve disease in adults. *J Heart Valve Dis* 2003; 12(2):202-208.

94. Reece TB, Welke KF, O'Brien S, Grau-Sepulveda MV, Grover FL, Gammie JS: Rethinking the ross procedure in adults. *Ann Thorac Surg* 2014; 97(1):175-181.

95. Zebele C, Chivasso P, Sedmakov C, et al: The Ross operation in children and young adults: 12-year results and trends from the UK National Database. *World J Pediatr Congenit Heart Surg* 2014; 5(3):406-412.

96. Stelzer P, Itagaki S, Varghese R, Chikwe J: Operative mortality and morbidity after the Ross procedure: a 26-year learning curve. *J Heart Valve Dis* 2013; 22(6):767-775.

97. Sievers HH, Stierle U, Charitos EI, et al: A multicentre evaluation of the autograft procedure for young patients undergoing aortic valve replacement: update on the German Ross Registry. *Eur J Cardiothorac Surg* 2015.

98. da Costa FD, Takkenberg JJ, Fornazari D, et al: Long-term results of the Ross operation: an 18-year single institutional experience. *Eur J Cardiothorac Surg* 2014; 46(3):415-422; discussion 422.

99. Takkenberg JJ, Klieverik LM, Schoof PH, et al: The Ross procedure: a systematic review and meta-analysis. *Circulation* 2009; 119(2):222-228.

100. Juthier F, Vincentelli A, Pinçon C, et al: Reoperation after the Ross procedure: incidence, management, and survival. *Ann Thorac Surg* 2012; 93(2):598-604; discussion 605.

101. Elkins RC, Thompson DM, Lane MM, Elkins CC, Peyton MD: Ross operation: 16-year experience. *J Thorac Cardiovasc Surg* 2008; 136(3):623-630, 630.e1.

102. Charitos EI, Hanke T, Stierle U, et al: Autograft reinforcement to preserve autograft function after the ross procedure: a report from the german-dutch ross registry. *Circulation* 2009; 120(11 Suppl):S146-S154.

103. Stelzer P, Jones DJ, Elkins RC: Aortic root replacement with pulmonary autograft. *Circulation* 1989; 80(5 Pt 2):III209-III213.

104. Brown JW, Ruzmetov M, Rodefeld MD, Mahomed Y, Turrentine MW: Incidence of and risk factors for pulmonary autograft dilation after Ross aortic valve replacement. *Ann Thorac Surg* 2007; 83(5):1781-1787; discussion 1787.

105. Klieverik LM, Takkenberg JJ, Bekkers JA, Roos-Hesselink JW, Witsenburg M, Bogers AJ: The Ross operation: a Trojan horse? *Eur Heart J* 2007; 28(16):1993-2000.

106. David TE, Omran A, Ivanov J, Armstrong S, et al: Dilation of the pulmonary autograft after the Ross procedure. *J Thorac Cardiovasc Surg* 2000; 119(2):210-220.

107. Koul B, Al-Rashidi F, Bhat M, Meurling C: A modified Ross operation to prevent pulmonary autograft dilatation. *Eur J Cardiothorac Surg* 2007; 31(1):127-128.

108. Slater M, Shen I, Welke K, Komanapalli C, Ungerleider R: Modification to the Ross procedure to prevent autograft dilatation. *Semin Thorac Cardiovasc Surg Pediatr Card Surg Annu* 2005; 181-184.

109. Carrel T, Schwerzmann M, Eckstein F, Aymard T, Kadner A: Preliminary results following reinforcement of the pulmonary autograft to prevent dilatation after the Ross procedure. *J Thorac Cardiovasc Surg*. 2008; 136 (2):472-475.

110. Juthier F, Banfi C, Vincentelli A, et al: Modified Ross operation with reinforcement of the pulmonary autograft: Six-year results. *J Thorac Cardiovasc Surg* 2010; 139(6):1420-1423.

111. Al Rashidi F, Bhat M, Höglund P, Meurling C, Roijer A, Koul B: The modified Ross operation using a Dacron prosthetic vascular jacket does prevent pulmonary autograft dilatation at 4.5-year follow-up. *Eur J Cardiothorac Surg* 2010; 37(4):928-933.

112. Skillington PD, Mokhles MM, Takkenberg JJ, et al: The Ross procedure using autologous support of the pulmonary autograft: techniques and late results. *J Thorac Cardiovasc Surg* 2015; 149(2 Suppl):S46-S52.

113. Lang SJ, Giordano MS, Cardon-Cardo C, Summers BD, Staiano-Coico L, Hajjar DP: Biochemical and cellular characterization of cardiac valve tissue after cryopreservation or antibiotic preservation. *J Thorac Cardiovasc Surg* 1994; 108(1):63-67.

114. Schmidtke C, Dahmen G, Graf B, Sievers HH: Pulmonary homograft muscle reduction to reduce the risk of homograft stenosis in the Ross procedure. *J Thorac Cardiovasc Surg* 2007; 133(1):190-195.

115. Carr-White GS, Glennan S, Edwards S, et al: Pulmonary autograft versus aortic homograft for rereplacement of the aortic valve: results from a subset of a prospective randomized trial. *Circulation* 1999; 100(19 Suppl):II103-II106.

116. Raanani E, Yau TM, David TE, Dellgren G, Sonnenberg BD, Omran A: Risk factors for late pulmonary homograft stenosis after the Ross procedure. *Ann Thorac Surg* 2000; 70(6):1953-1957.

117. Boudjemline Y, Khambadkone S, Bonnet D, et al: Images in cardiovascular medicine. Percutaneous replacement of the pulmonary valve in a 12-year-old child. *Circulation* 2004; 110(22):e516.

118. Konuma T, Devaney EJ, Bove EL, et al: Performance of CryoValve SG decellularized pulmonary allografts compared with standard cryopreserved allografts. *Ann Thorac Surg* 2009; 88(3):849-54; discussion 554.

119. Ruzmetov M, Shah JJ, Geiss DM, Fortuna RS: Decellularized versus standard cryopreserved valve allografts for right ventricular outflow tract reconstruction: a single-institution comparison. *J Thorac Cardiovasc Surg* 2012; 143(3):543-549.

120. Hechadi J, Gerber BL, Coche E, et al: Stentless xenografts as an alternative to pulmonary homografts in the Ross operation. *Eur J Cardiothorac Surg* 2013; 44(1):e32-e39.

121. Miskovic A, Monsefi N, Doss M, Özaslan F, Karimian A, Moritz A: Comparison between homografts and Freestyle® bioprosthesis for right ventricular outflow tract replacement in Ross procedures. *Eur J Cardiothorac Surg* 2012; 42(6):927-933.

122. Hiemann NE, Mani M, Huebler M, et al: Complete destruction of a tissue-engineered porcine xenograft in pulmonary valve position after the Ross procedure. *J Thorac Cardiovasc Surg* 2010; 139(4):e67-e68.

123. Stulak JM, Burkhart HM, Sundt TM, et al: Spectrum and outcome of reoperations after the Ross procedure. *Circulation* 2010; 122(12):1153-1158.

124. Sievers HH, Stierle U, Charitos EI, et al: Major adverse cardiac and cerebrovascular events after the Ross procedure: a report from the German-Dutch Ross Registry. *Circulation* 2010; 122(11 Suppl):S216-S223.

125. Charitos EI, Takkenberg JJ, Hanke T, et al: Reoperations on the pulmonary autograft and pulmonary homograft after the Ross procedure: An update on the German Dutch Ross Registry. *J Thorac Cardiovasc Surg* 2012; 144(4):813-821; discussion 821.

126. Stangl K, Stangl V, Laule M: Transfemoral pulmonary valve implantation for severe pulmonary insufficiency after Ross procedure. *J Am Coll Cardiol* 2013; 61(6):e143.

127. Alsoufi B, Ahmed D, Manlhiot C, Al-Halees Z, McCrindle BW, Fadel BM: Fate of the remaining neo-aortic root after autograft valve replacement with a stented prosthesis for the failing ross procedure. *Ann Thorac Surg* 2013; 96(1):59-65; discussion 565.

128. Liebrich M, Weimar T, Tzanavaros I, Roser D, Doll KN, Hemmer WB: The David procedure for salvage of a failing autograft after the Ross operation. *Ann Thorac Surg* 2014; 98(6):2046-2052.

129. de Kerchove L, Boodhwani M, Etienne PY, et al: Preservation of the pulmonary autograft after failure of the Ross procedure. *Eur J Cardiothorac Surg* 2010; 38(3):326-332.

130. Luciani GB, Viscardi F, Pilati M, Prioli AM, Faggian G, Mazzucco A: The Ross-Yacoub procedure for aneurysmal autograft roots: a strategy to preserve autologous pulmonary valves. *J Thorac Cardiovasc Surg* 2010; 139(3):536-542.

131. Luciani GB, Lucchese G, De Rita F, Puppini G, Faggian G, Mazzucco A: Reparative surgery of the pulmonary autograft: experience with Ross reoperations. *Eur J Cardiothorac Surg* 2012; 41(6):1309-1314; discussion 1314.

132. El-Hamamsy I, Eryigit Z, Stevens LM, et al: Long-term outcomes after autograft versus homograft aortic root replacement in adults with aortic valve disease: a randomised controlled trial. *Lancet* 2010; 376(9740):524-531.

133. Aklog L, Carr-White GS, Birks EJ, Yacoub MH: Pulmonary autograft versus aortic homograft for aortic valve replacement: interim results from a prospective randomized trial. *J Heart Valve Dis* 2000; 9(2):176-188; discussion 188.

Aortic Valve Repair and Aortic Valve-Sparing Operations

Tirone E. David

30

FUNCTIONAL ANATOMY OF THE AORTIC VALVE

The aortic valve is a complex structure that is best described as a functional and anatomic unit, the aortic root. The aortic root has four components: aortoventricular junction or aortic annulus, aortic cusps, aortic sinuses, and sinotubular junction. In addition, the triangles beneath the commissures of the aortic valve, although part of the left ventricular outflow tract, are also important for valve function.

The aortic annulus unites the aortic cusps and aortic sinuses to the left ventricle. It is attached to ventricular myocardium (interventricular septum) in approximately 45% of its circumference and to fibrous structures (anterior leaflet of the mitral valve and membranous septum) in the remaining 55% (Fig. 30-1). The aortic annulus has a scalloped shape. Histologic examination of the aortic annulus reveals that it is a fibrous structure with strands attaching itself to the muscular interventricular septum and has a fibrous continuity with the mitral valve and membranous septum. The fibrous structure that separates the aortic annulus from the anterior leaflet of the mitral valve is the intervalvular fibrous body. An important structure immediately below the membranous septum is the bundle of His. The atrioventricular node lies in the floor of the right atrium between the annulus of the septal leaflet of the tricuspid valve and the coronary sinus. This node gives origin to the bundle of His, which travels through the right fibrous trigone along the posterior edge of the membranous septum to the muscular interventricular septum. At this point, the bundle of His divides into left and right bundle branches that extend subendocardially along both sides of the muscular interventricular septum.

The aortic cusps are attached to the aortic annulus in a scalloped fashion (see Fig. 30-1). The aortic cusps have a semilunar shape whereby the length of the base is approximately 1.5 times longer than the length of the free margin, as illustrated in Fig. 30-2. There are three cusps and three aortic sinuses: left, right, and noncoronary. The aortic sinuses are also referred to as sinuses of Valsalva. The left coronary artery arises from the left aortic sinus and the right coronary artery arises from the right aortic sinus. The left coronary artery orifice is closer to the aortic annulus than is the right coronary artery orifice. The highest point where two cusps meet is called the commissure, and it is located immediately below the sinotubular junction. The scalloped shape of the aortic annulus creates three triangular spaces underneath the commissures. The two triangles beneath the commissures of the noncoronary cusp are fibrous structures, whereas the triangular space beneath the commissure between the left and right cusps is mostly muscular. These three triangles are seen in Fig. 30-1. The aortic annulus evolves along three horizontal planes within a cylindrical structure. Thus, the annulus of each cusp inserts itself in the aortic root along a single horizontal plane. The sinotubular junction represents the end of the aortic root. It is an important component of the aortic root because the commissures of the aortic valve are immediately below it and changes in the diameter of the sinotubular junction affect the function of the aortic cusps.

The geometry of the aortic root and its anatomic components varies among individuals, but the geometry of these components is somewhat interrelated. For instance, the larger the aortic cusps, the larger are the diameters of the aortic annulus and sinotubular junction. The aortic cusps are semilunar (crescent shape) and their bases are attached to the annulus; the free margins extend from commissure to commissure, and the cusps coapt centrally during diastole. The size of the aortic cusps varies among individuals and within the same person, but as a rule the noncoronary cusp is slightly larger than the right and left. The left is usually the smallest of the three. Because of the crescent shape of the aortic cusps and the fact that their free margins extend from commissure to commissure, the diameter of the aortic valve orifice must be smaller than the length of the free margins. Indeed, anatomic studies of fresh human aortic roots demonstrated that the average length of the free margins of the aortic cusps was one-third longer than the diameter of the aortic orifice.

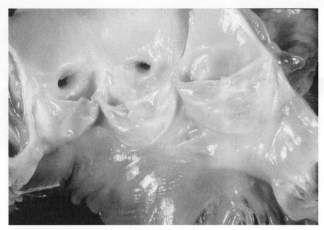

FIGURE 30-1 A photograph of a human left ventricular outflow tract and aortic root.

The diameter of the aortic annulus is 15 to 20% larger than the diameter of the sinotubular junction in children, but this relationship changes with age and the diameter of the aortic annulus is often smaller than the diameter of aortic annulus in older persons (see Fig. 30-2).

The aortic annulus, the aortic cusps, and the sinotubular junction play an important role in maintaining valve competence. On the other hand, the aortic sinuses play no role in valve competence, but they are believed to be important in minimizing mechanical stress on the aortic cusps during the cardiac cycle by creating eddies currents between the cusps and the aortic sinuses.

All components of the aortic root are very elastic and compliant in children but compliance decreases with aging as elastic fibers are replaced by fibrous tissue. Expansion and contraction of the aortic annulus during the cardiac cycle are heterogeneous probably because of its attachments to contractile myocardium as well as to fibrous structures such as the membranous septum and intervalvular fibrous body. On the other hand, the expansion and contraction of the sinotubular junction are more uniform. The aortic root also displays

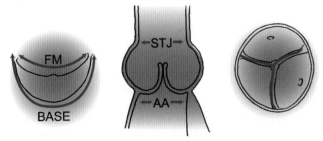

FIGURE 30-2 Geometric relationships of various components of the aortic root. The base of the aortic cusp is 1.5 times longer than its free margin. The diameter of the aortic annulus is 10 to 15% larger than the diameter of the sinotubular junction in children and young adults but it tends to become equal with aging. Three semilunar cusps seal the aortic orifice. The height of the cusps must be longer than the radius of the aortic annulus.

some degree of torsion during isovolumic contraction and ejection of the left ventricle. The movements of the aortic annulus, cusps, sinuses, and sinotubular junction also change with aging as elastic fibers are replaced by fibrous tissue.

AORTIC VALVE PATHOLOGY

Anatomically normal aortic cusps may become calcified late in life and cause aortic stenosis. This type of lesion is called dystrophic calcification, senile calcification, or degenerative calcification. The range of histopathologic lesions includes calcification, chondroid and osseous metaplasia, neorevascularization, inflammation, and lipid deposition.

Bicuspid aortic valve is estimated to occur in 0.5% to 1.5% of the population.[1] Males are affected more than females at a ratio of 4:1. There is a relatively high incidence of familial clustering, which suggests an autosomal dominant inheritance with reduced penetrance.[2] Extensive research in the genetics of bicuspid aortic valve is being presently conducted and this disorder is likely heritable.[2] Most patients with bicuspid aortic valve have three aortic sinuses and two cusps of different sizes. The larger cusp often contains a raphe instead of a commissure. The raphe extends from the mid portion of the cusp to the aortic annulus, and its insertion in the aortic root is at a lower level than the other two commissures. Bicuspid aortic valves with two aortic sinuses and no raphe are least common and called "type 0"; the most common is with one raphe and is called "type 1"; and finally with two raphes is "type 2."[3] Types 1 and 2 can be subclassified according to the fused cusps: L-R is the most common form (a raphe in between the left and right cusps). Most patients with bicuspid aortic valves have a dominant circumflex artery and a small right coronary artery. Bicuspid aortic valve may function satisfactorily until late in life when it may become calcified and stenotic.[4] It may also become incompetent, particularly in younger patients and is often associated with dilated aortic annulus and prolapsed cusp.

Other congenital anomalies of the aortic valve are the unicuspid and quadricuspid valves. Subaortic membranous ventricular septal defect can cause aortic insufficiency because of distortion of the aortic annulus and prolapse of the right cusp.

Numerous connective tissue disorders (ankylosing spondylitis, osteogenesis imperfecta, rheumatoid arthritis, Reiter's syndrome, lupus, etc.) can cause aortic insufficiency. The anorexigenic drugs phentermine and fenfluramine can also cause aortic insufficiency. Rheumatic aortic valve disease is still prevalent in developing countries and can cause aortic stenosis and/or insufficiency by causing fusion, fibrosis, and contraction of the cusps.

AORTIC ROOT AND ASCENDING AORTA PATHOLOGY

Degenerative diseases of the media with aneurysm formation are the most common disorders of the aortic root and ascending aorta. A broad spectrum of pathologic and clinical entities is grouped under degenerative disorders, and it ranges from severe degeneration of the media, which can become clinically important early in life in cases such as Loyes-Dietz syndrome, to cases of the not so important mild dilation of the ascending aorta in elderly patients. Bicuspid and unicuspid aortic valve disease often display premature degeneration of the media with dilation of the aorta. Atherosclerosis, infectious and noninfectious aortitis are other pathologic entities.

Aneurysms of the ascending aorta are often caused by cystic medial degeneration (cystic medial necrosis). Histologically, necrosis and disappearance of muscle cells in the elastic lamina, and cystic spaces filled with mucoid material are often observed. Although these changes occur more often in the ascending aorta, they may affect any portion or the entire aorta. These changes weaken the arterial wall, which dilates and forms a fusiform aneurysm. The aortic root may be involved in this pathologic process, and in patients with Marfan syndrome, the aneurysm usually begins in the aortic sinuses. A large proportion of patients with aortic root aneurysms do not fulfill the criteria of diagnosis of Marfan syndrome, but the gross appearance of the aneurysm and the histology of the arterial wall may be indistinguishable from that of Marfan syndrome. These cases are referred to as forma frusta of Marfan syndrome.

Patients with aortic root aneurysms are usually in their second or third decade of life when the diagnosis is made. These patients develop aortic insufficiency because of dilation of the sinotubular junction and/or aortic annulus (Fig. 30-3). Annuloaortic ectasia is a term used to describe dilation of the aortic annulus.

Other patients have relatively normal aortic roots but develop ascending aortic aneurysms. These patients are usually in their fifth or sixth decade of life. Finally, certain patients have extensive degenerative disease of the entire aorta and develop the so-called mega-aorta syndrome with dilation of the entire thoracic and abdominal aorta. Ascending aortic aneurysm may cause dilation of the sinotubular junction with consequent aortic insufficiency (Fig. 30-3).

Marfan Syndrome

Marfan syndrome is an autosomal dominant variably penetrant inherited disorder of the connective tissue in which cardiovascular, skeletal, ocular, and other abnormalities may be present to a variable degree. The prevalence is estimated to be around 1 in 5000 individuals. It is caused by mutations in the gene that encodes fibrillin-1 (FBN1) on chromosome 15. This is a large gene (approximately 10,000 nucleotides in the mRNA), and identification of the mutation is a complex task. More than 1000 mutations in FBN1 have been identified. The phenotype presents a highly variable degree because of varying genotype expression.

The clinical features of Marfan syndrome were thought to be a result of weaker connective tissues caused by defects in fibrillin-1, a glycoprotein, and principal component of the extracellular matrix microfibril. This concept was inadequate to explain the overgrowth of long bones, osteopenia, reduced muscular mass, and adiposity and craniofacial abnormalities often seen in Marfan syndrome.[5] Dietz and colleagues[5,6] showed in an experimental mouse with Marfan syndrome that many findings are the result of abnormal levels of activation of transforming growth factor beta (TGF-β), a potent stimulator of inflammation, fibrosis, and activation of certain matrix metalloproteinases, especially matrix metalloproteinases 2 and 9. Excess TGF-β activation in tissues correlates with failure of lung septation, development of a myxomatous mitral valve, and aortic root dilation in mice. This combination of structural microfibril matrix abnormality, dysregulation of matrix homeostasis mediated by excess TGF-β, and abnormal cell-matrix interactions is responsible for the phenotype features of the Marfan syndrome. Ongoing destruction of the elastic and collagen lamellae and medial degeneration result in progressive dilation of the aortic root, as well as a predisposition to aortic dissection from the loss of appropriate medial layer support. Loss of elasticity in the media causes increased aortic stiffness and decreased distensibility.

The diagnosis of Marfan syndrome is made on clinical grounds, and it is not always simple because of the variability in clinical expression. A multidisciplinary approach is needed to diagnose and manage patients afflicted with this syndrome. The revised Ghent criteria to diagnose Marfan syndrome is summarized in Table 30-1.[7] The most common cardiovascular features are aortic root aneurysm and mitral valve prolapse. These anatomical abnormalities may cause aortic rupture, aortic dissection, aortic insufficiency, and mitral insufficiency.

Loeys-Dietz Syndrome

Mutations in the genes encoding TGF-β receptors 1 and 2 have been found in association with a continuum of clinical

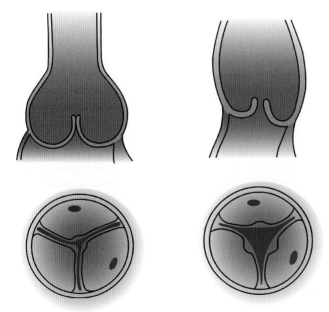

FIGURE 30-3 Dilation of the sinotubular junction causes aortic insufficiency because it displaces the commissures outward and prevents the cusps to coapt centrally.

TABLE 30-1: Revised Ghent Criteria for Diagnosis of Marfan Syndrome

In the absence of family history the diagnosis of Marfan is confirmed with:

1. Aortic root dilatation (Z ≥ 2) or dissection + ectopialentis
2. Aortic root dilatation (Z ≥ 2) or dissection + FBN1 mutation
3. Aortic root dilatation (Z ≥ 2) or dissection + systemic manifestations (≥7 points)
4. Ectopialentis + FBN1 mutation associated with aortic dissection but without aortic root dilatation or dissection

In the presence of family history of Marfan syndrome:

5. Ectopialentis + family history
6. Systemic manifestations (≥7 points) + family history
7. Aortic root dilatation (Z ≥ 2 above 20 years old or ≥3 below 20 years old) + family history

Point system for Marfan syndrome:

- Wrist and thumb sign—3 (wrist or thumb separately 1 point)
- Pectus carinatum deformity—2 (pectus excavatum or chest asymmetry separately—1)
- Hindfoot deformity—2 (plain pes planus—1)
- Pneumothorax—2
- Dural ectasia—2
- Protrusioacetabuli—2
- Reduced upper segment/lower segment ratio and increased arm/height no severe scoliosis—1
- Scoliosis or thoracolumbar kyphosis—1
- Reduced elbow extension—1
- Facial features (3/5)—1 (dolichocephaly, enophthalmos, downslanting palpebral fissures, malar hypoplasia, retrognathia)
- Skin striae—1
- Myopia > 3 diopters—1
- Mitral valve prolapse (all types)—1

(Maximum total: 20 points; score ≥ 7 indicates systemic involvement)

features. On the mild end, the mutation have been found in association with presentation similar to that of the Marfan syndrome or with familial thoracic aneurysm and dissection, and on the severe end, they are associated with a complex phenotype in which aortic dissection or rupture commonly occurs in childhood.[8] This complex phenotype is characterized by the triad of hypertelorism, bifid uvula or cleft palate, and generalized arterial tortuosity with widespread vascular aneurysm and dissection. This phenotype has been classified as Loeys-Dietz syndrome. Affected patients have a high risk of aortic dissection or rupture at an early age and at relatively small diameters. CT angiograms should be obtained from head to pelvis.

Ehlers-Danlos Syndrome

Vascular Ehlers-Danlos syndrome is a rare autosomal dominant inherited disorder of the connective tissue resulting from mutation of the COL3A1 gene encoding type III collagen. Spontaneous rupture without dissection of large- and medium-caliber arteries such as the abdominal aorta and its branches, the branches of the aortic arch, and the large arteries of the limbs accounts for most deaths. Aortic root dilation was present in 28% in a series of 71 patients with Ehlers-Danlos syndrome.[9] Aortic dissection is uncommon. Diagnosis is confirmed either by biochemical assays showing qualitative or quantitative abnormalities in type III collagen secretion or by molecular biology studies demonstrating mutation of the COL3A1 gene. Varied molecular mechanisms have been observed with different mutations in each family. No correlation has been established between genotype and phenotype. Diagnosis should be suspected in any young person presenting with arterial or visceral rupture or colonic perforation.

Other Aortic Root Aneurysm Associated with Genetic Syndromes

Aneurysm-osteoarthritis syndrome is associated with pathogenic SMAD-3 gene and is clinically characterized by aortic root aneurysm, aortic dissection, arterial aneurysms and dissection, arterial tortuosity, mitral valve prolapse, congenital cardiac defects, and osteoarthritis, soft skin, flat feet, scoliosis and recurrent hernias.[10] Aortic root aneurysms can also be associated with mutations of TGFβ-2 and with mutations of fibrillin-4 gene (FBLN4; cutis laxa syndrome).[11,12]

Other Pathologies

Familial thoracic aneurysms can be associated with mutations of various genes (TGFβ1-2, ACTA2, MLCK, SMAD3, TGF2) without systemic syndrome such as those described above. Atherosclerotic aneurysms of the ascending aorta are uncommon. They are more common in the abdominal aorta and to a lesser degree in the descending thoracic aorta. Atherosclerosis often causes irregular and saccular aneurysms of the ascending aorta rather than a more fusiform shape as seen with degenerative diseases.

Infectious aneurysms of the ascending aorta are rare. Syphilis was a common cause of aneurysm of the ascending aorta but it is seldom seen. The spirochetal infection destroys the muscular and elastic fibers of the media, which are replaced by fibrous and other inflammatory tissues. The ascending aorta is the most common site of involvement and the aneurysm is usually saccular. The wall of the ascending aorta is frequently calcified. Syphilitic aortitis also causes coronary ostial stenosis and aortic valve insufficiency. Other bacteria can also cause aneurysm of the ascending aorta.

Various types of aortitis may involve the ascending aorta. Giant cell arteritis is among the more common and it involves medium-sized arteries, but the aorta and its branches are involved in approximately 15% of the cases. The etiology is unknown. The characteristic lesion is a granulomatous inflammation of the media of large- and medium-caliber arteries such as the temporal artery. Occasionally the inflammatory process weakens the aorta leading to aneurysm formation, aortoannular ectasia, and aortic insufficiency.

Ankylosing spondylitis, Reiter's syndrome, psoriatic arthritis, and polyarteritis nodosa can cause aortic insufficiency because of annuloaortic ectasia. Behçet's disease can cause aneurysm of the ascending aorta.

NATURAL HISTORY OF AORTIC VALVE DISEASE

Aortic Stenosis

Asymptomatic patients with aortic stenosis have a good prognosis.[13] Sudden death in asymptomatic patients is uncommon. However, when symptoms develop, the prognosis becomes poor and the average survival is 2 to 3 years for patients with symptoms of angina and syncope, and 1 to 2 years for those with congestive heart failure.[14]

Aortic Insufficiency

The prognosis of symptomatic patients with aortic insufficiency is poor with death occurring within 4 years after development of angina and within 2 years after the onset of congestive heart failure.[15]

Bicuspid Aortic Valve Disease

A prospective follow-up on 642 adult patients (mean age 35 ± 9 years) with bicuspid aortic valve during a mean 9 ± 5 years in our institution revealed a late survival similar to that of the general population in spite the fact that 161 patients had an adverse event (cardiac death, aortic valve/ascending aorta surgery, dissection, or congestive heart failure).[16] Age greater than 30 years, and moderate or severe aortic stenosis or insufficiency were independent predictors of adverse event.[16] In a study from the Mayo Clinic on 212 patients (mean age 32 ± 20 years) with normal or minimally dysfunctional bicuspid aortic valve who lived in Olmsted County and followed for a mean of 15 ± 6 years revealed a 20-year survival similar to that of the general population, but the incidence of surgery on the aortic valve and/or ascending aorta was 27 ± 4% and the total adverse cardiovascular events was 42 ± 5%.[4]

Aortic Root and Ascending Aortic Aneurysms

Aortic root/ascending aortic aneurysm can cause aortic insufficiency, aortic dissection, or rupture. The transverse diameter of the aneurysm is a determinant of rupture or dissection. In a study by Coady and associates[17] on 370 patients with thoracic aneurysms (201 ascending aortic aneurysms), during a mean follow-up of 29.4 months the incidence of acute dissection or rupture was 8.8% for aneurysms less than 4 cm, 9.5% for aneurysms of 4 to 4.9 cm, 17.8% for 5 to 5.9 cm, and 27.9% for those greater than 6 cm. The median size of the ascending aortic aneurysm at the time of rupture or dissection was 5.9 cm.

In Coady's study, the growth rate ranged from 0.08 cm/year for small (<4 cm) aneurysms to 0.16 cm/year for large (8 cm) aneurysms.[17] The growth rates for chronic dissecting aneurysms were much higher than for chronic nondissecting aneurysms.

The growth rates for aortic root aneurysms may be higher than in ascending aortic aneurysms, particularly in patients with Marfan syndrome. Aortic dissection is rare in aortic root aneurysm of less than 50 mm, unless the patients have family history of aortic dissection. Without surgery, most patients with Marfan syndrome die in the third decade of their lives from complications of aortic root aneurysm such as rupture, aortic dissection, or aortic insufficiency.[18] Pregnancy in women with Marfan syndrome has two potential problems: the risk of having a child who will inherit the disorder and the risk of acute aortic dissection during the third trimester, parturition, or the first month postpartum. The offspring has a 50% risk of inheriting the syndrome.

Patients affected with Loeys-Dietz syndrome have a high risk of aortic dissection or rupture at an early age and at relatively small aortic root diameters. Surgery is recommended in adults when the aortic root exceeds 4 cm.

Patients with bicuspid aortic valve had larger aortas than patients with tricuspid aortic valve and the rate of dilation of the ascending aorta was higher (0.19 vs 0.13 cm per year, respectively) in a study by Davies et al.[19] Among patients with bicuspid aortic valve, those with aortic stenosis had a higher risk of rupture, dissection, or death.

DIAGNOSIS OF AORTIC VALVE/ROOT DISEASE

Patients with aortic stenosis remain asymptomatic for many years. Symptoms usually appear late in the course of the disease. The symptoms are: angina pectoris, syncope, and congestive heart failure. The clinical presentation of patients with aortic insufficiency is dependent on the rapidity with which aortic insufficiency develops. Patients with chronic aortic insufficiency remain asymptomatic for many years while the heart slowly enlarges. Palpitations and head pounding may occur during exertion. Angina pectoris may occur, but it is not as common as with aortic stenosis. Syncope is rare. The symptoms of congestive heart failure are usually an indication of left ventricular dysfunction. Acute aortic insufficiency is frequently associated with cardiovascular collapse, with extreme fatigue, dyspnea, and hypotension resulting from reduced stroke volume and elevated left atrial pressure. Echocardiography confirms the diagnosis of aortic valve dysfunction and provides information regarding its mechanism. Radionuclide imaging is useful in assessing the left ventricular function at rest and during exercise, valuable information in asymptomatic patients.

Most patients with aortic root aneurysm are asymptomatic and have no physical signs if the aortic valve is competent. Some patients may complain of vague chest pain. Severe chest pain is suggestive of rapid expansion or intimal tear with dissection. Echocardiography establishes the diagnosis and provides information regarding the aortic cusps. A computed tomography scan and magnetic resonance imaging of the chest are also diagnostic and it is useful to provide information regarding the thoracic aorta.

INDICATIONS FOR SURGERY

Surgeons must be familiar with the guidelines for heart valve surgery prepared by a joint committee of the ACC and AHA[20] and for surgery for aortic root and ascending aortic aneurysm set by the STS.[21]

SELECTION OF PATIENTS FOR AORTIC VALVE REPAIR

Most candidates for aortic valve repair have aortic insufficiency or normally functioning aortic valve with aortic root or ascending aortic aneurysm. Transesophageal echocardiography is the best diagnostic tool to study the aortic valve and the mechanism of aortic insufficiency. Each component of the aortic root must be carefully interrogated, and in particular the aortic cusps. The number of cusps, their thickness, the appearance of their free margins, and the excursion of each cusp during the cardiac cycle must be examined in multiple views. The lines of coaptation of the aortic cusps should be interrogated by color Doppler imaging and the direction and size of the regurgitant jets recorded in multiple views. Information regarding the morphologic features of the aortic annulus, aortic sinuses, sinotubular junction, and ascending aorta should be obtained.

The aortic cusps are the most important determinant of aortic valve repair. If the cusps are thin, mobile with smooth free margins, the feasibility of aortic valve repair is very high, including bicuspid aortic valve. Calcified or scarred and fibrotic aortic cusps preclude aortic valve repair unless autologous or xenograft glutaraldehyde fixed pericardium is used for partial excision and patch repair of the cusps.

Patients with aortic root and ascending aortic aneurysms often have normal or minimally stretched aortic cusps and reconstruction of the aortic root with preservation of the native aortic cusps is feasible. Grossly dilated aortic annulus and/or sinotubular junction are likely to have overstretched, thinned out aortic cusps with stress fenestrations along the commissural areas and may not be suitable for repair.

TECHNIQUES OF AORTIC VALVE REPAIR

Cusp Perforation

Occasionally a cusp perforation is the sole reason for aortic insufficiency. The perforation may be iatrogenic, a sequelae of healed endocarditis, or the result of resection of a papillary fibroelastoma. A simple patch of fresh or glutaraldehyde fixed autologous pericardium is adequate to correct the problem. Fresh autologous pericardium can also be used to repair small holes (<5 mm) but the patch should be larger than the defect

because it retracts during healing. We use a continuous fine polypropylene to suture the patch around the defect on the aortic side of the cusp.

Cusp Extension

Cusp augmentation has been used to repair incompetent aortic valves due to rheumatic and congenital disease. Glutaraldehyde fixed bovine or autologous pericardium has been used for this purpose.

Cusp Prolapse

Cusp prolapse is caused by elongation of the free margin. This is corrected by plication along the nodule of Arantius as illustrated in Fig. 30-4. The degree of shortening is determined by examining the other cusps and their level of coaptation.

Cusp with Stress Fenestration

Dilation of the sinotubular junction increases the mechanical stress along the free margin of the cusp near the commissures and may cause a stress fenestration with thinning and sometimes even detachment from the commissure. This type of lesion has been successfully corrected by weaving a double layer of 6-0 expanded polytetrafluoroethylene suture along the free margin of the cusp as illustrated in Fig. 30-5.

Bicuspid Aortic Valve

The most commonly performed aortic valve repair in adults is for bicuspid aortic valve with prolapse of one cusp. Although the anatomic arrangement of the bicuspid aortic valve varies, most patients have an anterior cusp attached to the interventricular septum and a posterior cusp attached to the fibrous components of the left ventricular outflow tract. The anterior

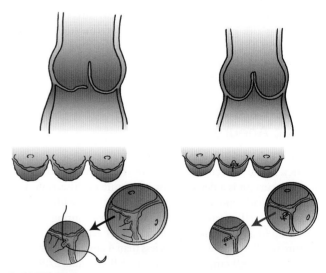

FIGURE 30-4 Repair of cusp prolapse. The free margin is shortened by plicating the area of the nodule of Arantius.

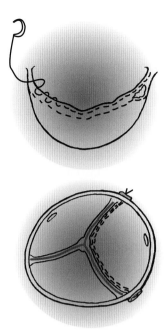

FIGURE 30-5 Reinforcement of the free margin with a double layer of 6-0 expanded polytetrafluoroethylene suture. This is often done in patients with stress fenestration.

cusp often contains a raphe at approximately where the commissure between the right and left cusps would be (Type 1, L-R). This cusp is usually the one that is elongated and prolapsed. As long as the posterior cusp is normal, repair is feasible and relatively simple. The raphe is excised and the free margin of the anterior cusp is shortened with plicating sutures as illustrated in Fig. 30-6. The lengths of the free margins of both cusps should be similar and should coapt at the same level. Suspending the arterial walls immediately above the commissures and observing the level of coaptation

of each cusp gives an estimate of the level of coaptation of the cusps.

Because most patients with incompetent bicuspid aortic valves have dilated aortic annulus, aortic valve-sparing operation may be more appropriate procedure than simple cusp repair. However, if the aortic sinuses are not aneurismal and the annulus is only mildly dilated, a reduction annuloplasty to increase the coaptation area of the cusps can be done. This is accomplished by plicating the subcommissural triangles using horizontal mattress sutures of 4-0 polypropylene with Teflon felt pledgets on the outside of the aortic root (Fig. 30-7). The suture is first passed from the outside to the inside of the aorta through the aortic annulus of both cusps 2 mm below their commissure. The same suture is passed again through the annulus and subcommissural triangle 4 or 5 mm below the first one and the ends are tied together over Teflon felt pledgets on the outside of the aorta.

AORTIC VALVE-SPARING OPERATIONS

Aortic valve-sparing operations include various procedures used to preserve the aortic cusps in patients with aortic root aneurysm or ascending aortic aneurysm with aortic insufficiency.

Ascending Aortic Aneurysm with Aortic Insufficiency

Dilation of the sinotubular junction displaces the commissures of the aortic valve outward and prevents the cusps from coapting during diastole (see Fig. 30-3). These patients are often on the sixth, seventh, or eighth decade of their lives and have ascending aortic aneurysm. The dilation of the sinotubular junction is often asymmetrical, and the commissures of

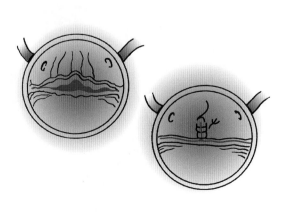

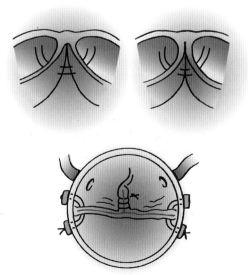

FIGURE 30-6 Repair of incompetent bicuspid aortic valve. The elongated cusp is shortened and the subcommissural triangles narrowed with sutures.

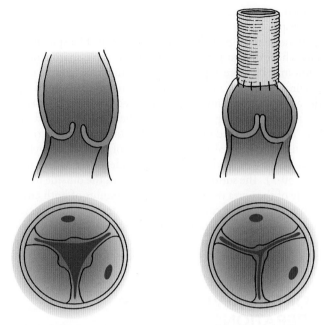

FIGURE 30-7 Dilation of the sinotubular junction causes aortic insufficiency. Correction of the dilation with a tubular Dacron graft of appropriate diameter corrects aortic insufficiency.

noncoronary aortic cusp are more affected than the other two. If the other components of the aortic root are normal, simple adjustment of the sinotubular junction restores valve competence. This is accomplished by transecting the ascending aorta 5 mm above the sinotubular junction and pulling the three commissures upward and close to each other until the cusps coapt. The three commissures form an imaginary triangle. The diameter of a circle that contains this imaginary triangle is the diameter of the graft that should be used to reconstruct the sinotubular junction. Because the aortic cusps and sinuses have different sizes, this triangle is not always equilateral and the commissures must be spaced according to the length of the free margin of each cusp. The diameter of the graft and the space between commissures are facilitated by sizing the diameter of the circle that contains all three commissures with a transparent valve sizer, such as the one used to size the aortic annulus for a stentless porcine aortic valve. Those valve sizers have three equidistant marks, and one can determine the space between the commissures by comparing to the distance between marks. The tubular Dacron graft is sutured right at the level of the sinotubular junction with a continuous 4-0 polypropylene suture (see Fig. 30-7). If after adjusting the sinotubular junction, the cusps do not coapt at the same level, one or more cusps may be elongated and the free margin has to be shortened as illustrated in Fig. 30-4. Aortic valve competence can be tested at this time by injecting cardioplegia into the graft under pressure and observing the left ventricle for distension.

If the noncoronary aortic sinus is dilated or altered by aortic dissection, a neoaortic sinus can be created by tailoring the graft with a tongue of tissue that is sutured directly to the aortic annulus as illustrated in Fig. 30-8. The height of the

neoaortic sinus of Dacron should be 3 or 4 mm more than the diameter of the graft, and the width should be 3 or 4 mm more than the estimated intercommissural distance to allow the graft to bulge and create a neoaortic sinus.

Small diameter grafts (<24 mm) should be avoided in large adult patients because they may increase left ventricular afterload, particularly if long segments of aorta are replaced such as with concomitant transverse arch replacement using the elephant trunk technique. If the estimated diameter of the sinotubular junction is less than 24 mm, a larger graft should be used and the end that is anastomosed to the aortic root to recreate the sinotubular junction should be reduced by plicating the graft in the area of the anastomosis.

Aortic Root Aneurysm

A large proportion of patients with aortic root aneurysm has normal or minimally stretched aortic cusps and an aortic valve-sparing operation is feasible. There are basically two types of aortic valve-sparing operations for patients with aortic root aneurysm: remodeling of the aortic root and reimplantation of the aortic valve.[22,23]

Remodeling of the Aortic Root

The ascending aorta is transected and the aortic root is dissected circumferentially down to the level of the aortic annulus. All three aortic sinuses are excised, leaving approximately 4 to 6 mm of arterial wall attached to the aortic annulus and around the coronary artery orifices as illustrated in Fig. 30-9. The three commissures are gently pulled vertically

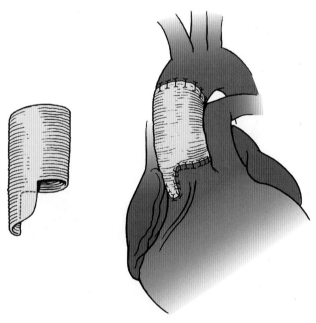

FIGURE 30-8 Correction of the sinotubular junction and replacement of the noncoronary aortic sinus.

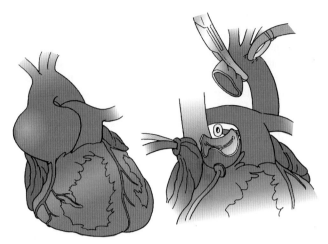

FIGURE 30-9 Remodeling of the aortic root. The aortic sinuses are excised leaving 4 to 6 mm of arterial wall attached to the aortic annulus and around the coronary arteries.

and approximated until the cusps coapt. The three commissures form a triangle and the diameter of the circle that contains that triangle is the diameter of the graft to be used for remodeling. In our experience, most grafts are 24, 26, or 28 mm in diameter. Here again, the stentless valve sizers are very useful to determine the diameter of the graft and also the distance between commissures because they may not be equidistant. The spaces in between the commissures are marked in one of the ends of the graft, and the graft is tailored to create three neoaortic sinuses (Fig. 30-10). The heights of these neoaortic sinuses should be approximately equal to the diameter of the graft. The three commissures are suspended in the graft (Fig. 30-11), which is then sutured to the remnants of the aortic wall as close as possible to aortic annulus with continuous 4-0 polypropylene sutures. The coronary arteries are reimplanted into their respective neoaortic sinuses. The aortic cusps are inspected to make sure that all three coapt at the same level and well above the nadir of the aortic annulus. If one or more cusp is prolapsing, the free margin is shortened as described previously. If one or two cusps have stress fenestrations, the free margin should be reinforced with a double layer of a fine expanded polytetrafluoroethylene suture from commissure to commissure. Aortic valve competence can be assessed by injecting cardioplegia under pressure into the reconstructed aortic root and observing the left ventricle for distension. The graft is then anastomosed to the distal ascending aorta or transverse aortic arch graft depending on the extent of the aneurysm (Fig. 30-11).

Remodeling of the aortic root may be inappropriate for patients with aortic root aneurysms associated with genetic syndromes because it has been documented that the aortic annulus may dilate postoperatively. An aortic annuloplasty along the fibrous component of the left ventricular outflow tract[18] did not prevent late dilation of the aortic annulus in patients with Marfan syndrome in our experience. Thus, reimplantation of the aortic valve may be a better operative procedure for patients with annuloaortic ectasia (Fig. 30-12)

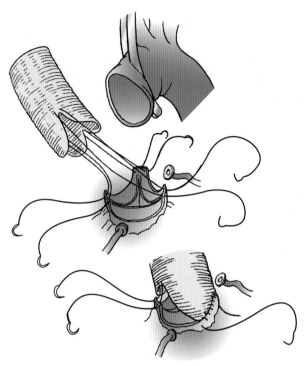

FIGURE 30-10 A graft of diameter equal to the diameter of the sinotubular junction is tailored to recreate three aortic sinuses. The three commissures are suspended into the tailored graft and the neoaortic sinuses are sutured to the aortic annulus and remnants of arterial wall.

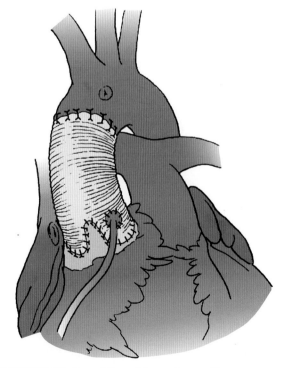

FIGURE 30-11 Remodeling of the aortic root. The coronary arteries are reimplanted into their respective neoaortic sinuses and the graft anastomosed to the distal aorta.

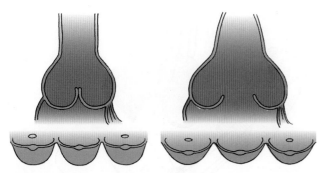

FIGURE 30-12 Annuloaortic ectasia. The subcommissural triangles of the noncoronary aortic cusps are flattened by dilation of the fibrous tissue.

because this operative procedure corrects and prevents annular dilation, whereas remodeling of the aortic root may be more suitable for patients with normal aortic annulus.

Reimplantation of the Aortic Valve

This procedure can be performed in all patients with aortic root aneurysms, but it is particularly valuable in patients with dilated aortic annulus and in acute type A aortic dissection. It is technically more demanding than remodeling of the aortic root because it requires greater knowledge of the functional anatomy of the aortic root. This is because the geometry of the aortic annulus, the aortic sinuses, the sinotubular junction, and even the aortic cusps are potentially altered during the procedure. In the original description of this procedure, the aortic valve was reimplanted into a tubular Dacron graft and

no neoaortic sinuses were created. Some investigators have suggested that the presence of the aortic sinuses is important for normal cusp motion, and potentially, cusp durability. Several modifications to the reimplantation procedure were introduced to create neoaortic sinuses. There is now a commercially available graft with sinuses of Valsalva (Vascutek Ltd. Renfrewshire, Scotland); however we have not used it because it distorts the aortic annulus because its sinuses are spherical, whereas the normal aortic annulus develops along a crescent shape on a single horizontal plane within a cylinder. However, this graft is used by many surgeons but the long-term results remain unknown.[24]

Following is a description of this procedure as we have been performing for more than two decades with excellent long-term results. The three aortic sinuses are excised as described for the remodeling procedure (see Fig. 30-9). Multiple horizontal mattress sutures of 2-0 or 3-0 polyester are passed from the inside to the outside of the left ventricular outflow tract, immediately below the nadir of the aortic annulus, through a single horizontal plane from the nadir of the left and noncoronary cusps and slightly scalloped between the subcommissural triangle of the left and right cusps and less so along the membranous septum to avoid the bundle of His as illustrated in Figure 30-13. These sutures frequently pass through right atrial wall in the area of the membranous septum and left atrial wall in the area of the sub-commissural triangle between the left and noncoronary cusps. If the fibrous portion is thin, sutures with Teflon felt pledgets should be used. A tubular Dacron graft of diameter equal to double the average height of the cusps minus 2 or 3 mm is selected and three equidistant marks placed in one

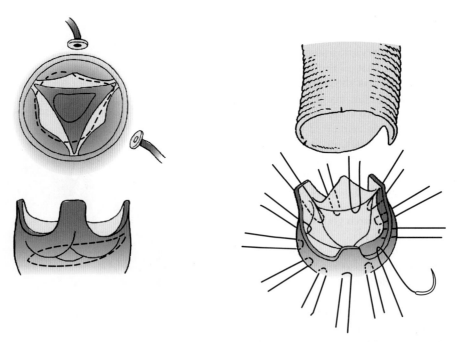

FIGURE 30-13 Reimplantation of the aortic valve. Sutures are passed below the aortic annulus in a single horizontal plane along the fibrous portion of the left ventricular outflow tract and following the scalloped shape of the aortic annulus along the muscular interventricular septum. These sutures are also passed from the inside to the outside of a tubular Dacron graft.

of its ends. A small triangular segment is cut off along the mark that corresponds to the subcommissural triangle of the left and right cusps. The sutures previously placed in the left ventricular outflow tract are now passed through the graft. The sutures should be spaced symmetrically in the graft if the aortic annulus is not dilated. If there is obvious dilation of the aortic annulus, the sutures should be spaced symmetrically along the muscular interventricular septum and around the nadirs of the aortic annulus but closer together beneath the subcommissural triangles of the noncoronary aortic cusp because that is where dilation occurs in patients with connective disorders. The sutures are then tied on the outside of the graft. Care must be exercised not to purse-string this suture line. The graft is then cut in a length of approximately 5 cm and pulled gently, and the three commissures are also pulled vertically and temporarily secured to the graft with transfixing 4-0 polypropylene sutures buttressed on small Teflon felt pledgets, but these sutures are not tied. Once all three commissures are suspended inside the graft, the commissures and the cusps are inspected to make sure they are all correctly aligned. The subcommissural triangles should also be inspected to make sure they are as narrow as the diameter of the graft allows, that is, the triangles should have a narrower base than before surgery. Next, the sutures are tied on the outside of the graft and used to secure the aortic annulus into the graft. This is accomplished by passing the suture sequentially from the inside to the outside right at the level of the annulus and from the outside to the inside at the level of the remnants of the arterial wall. We start at the level of the commissure and stop at the nadir of the aortic annulus where the sutures are tied together. The coronary arteries are reimplanted into their respective sinuses (Fig. 30-14). The coaptation of the aortic cusps is inspected and prolapse is corrected if necessary. It is important that the coaptation level is well above the aortic annulus. Creation of neoaortic sinuses are by plicating the graft at the level of the sinotubular junction and in between two commissures allows the aortic cusp to move a bit more centrally and increased its mobility as illustrated in Fig. 30-15. Valve competence can be assessed by occluding the distal graft and injecting cardioplegia under pressure. If the ventricle does not distend, no more than trace aortic insufficiency is present. The distal anastomosis is performed either to the distal ascending aorta or transverse aortic arch depending on the pathology. The graft sizes in our patients ranged from 26 to 34 mm, mean of 31 mm.

RESULTS OF AORTIC VALVE REPAIR

One of the earliest series of aortic valve repair for aortic insufficiency caused by prolapse of bicuspid aortic valve came from the Cleveland Clinic.[25] In a series of 94 patients with a mean age of 38 years, the freedom from reoperation was 84% at 7 years.[21] The only factor predictive of reoperation was residual aortic insufficiency at the time of repair.[25]

The appropriateness of aortic valve repair in patients with incompetent bicuspid aortic valve remains unclear. Competent bicuspid aortic valves appear to be durable because a large

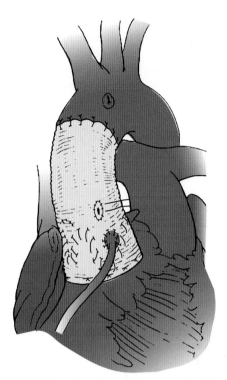

FIGURE 30-14 Reimplantation of the aortic valve. The commissures and the aortic annulus are sutured inside the graft and the coronary arteries reimplanted.

proportion of patients who require aortic valve replacement for aortic stenosis in their fifth, sixth, or seventh decades of life are found to have bicuspid aortic valves. Thus, aortic valve repair for incompetent bicuspid aortic valves is a reasonable surgical approach in young adults but the best type of repair remains to be determined. Incompetent bicuspid aortic valves

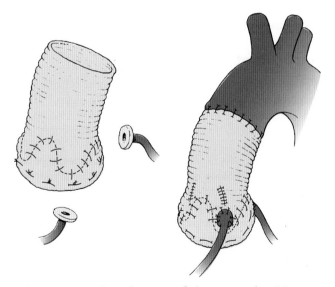

FIGURE 30-15 Reimplantation of the aortic valve. Neoaortic sinuses can be created by plicating the graft in the spaces in between the commissures at the level of the sinotubular.

are often associated with dilated aortic annulus and subcommissural plication may be inadequate to prevent future dilation and recurrent aortic insufficiency. Reimplantation of the aortic valve may provide better long-term results than simple valve repair in patients with incompetent bicuspid aortic valve and dilated aortic annulus.[26]

Ascending Aortic Aneurysm with Aortic Insufficiency

We reported our experience with aortic valve repair in patients with ascending aortic aneurysm, normal or minimally dilated aortic sinuses, and moderate or severe aortic insufficiency.[27] There were 103 patients whose mean age was 65 ± 12 years and 53% were men. The aneurysm extended into the transverse aortic arch in 60% of the patients and 20% had mega-aorta syndrome. The aortic valve repair consisted in adjusting the diameter of the sinotubular junction in all patients. In addition, repair of cusp prolapse was needed in 36 patients, and replacement of the noncoronary aortic sinus in 8. Associated procedures were: replacement of the transverse aortic arch in 62 patients, coronary artery bypass in 28, and mitral valve repair or replacement in 7. The follow-up was complete at 5.8 ± 2.3 years. There were 2 operative and 30 late deaths. The survival at 10 years was 54 ± 7%. Independent predictors of late death were transverse arch aneurysm, the use of elephant trunk technique to replace the arch and mega-aorta syndrome. Only two patients required aortic valve replacement: one for endocarditis and one for severe aortic insufficiency. The freedom from aortic valve replacement at 10 years was 98%. Only one patient developed severe and six developed moderate aortic insufficiency during the follow-up. The freedom from severe or moderate aortic insufficiency at 10 years was 80 ± 7%. These findings suggest that aortic valve repair in these patients is an excellent alternative to valve replacement and the repair remains stable in most patients during the follow-up. Late survival was suboptimal because of the extensiveness of the vascular disease.

Aortic Root Aneurysm

We reported our current experience with aortic valve-sparing operations for aortic root aneurysm in 371 patients.[28] Their mean age was 47 ± 15 years, 78% were men, 35.5% had the Marfan syndrome, 12% had type A aortic dissection, and 9% had bicuspid aortic valves. Approximately one-half of the patients had moderate or severe aortic insufficiency before surgery. The technique of remodeling of the aortic root was used in 75 patients and the reimplantation of the aortic valve in 226. The follow-up was complete at 8.9 ± 5.2 years. All patients had echocardiographic studies during the follow-up. There were 4 operative and 35 late deaths. Patients' survival at 18 years was 76.8% and approximately 10% lower than that of the general population of Ontario matched for age and gender. Age greater by 5-year increments, aortic dissection, preoperative aortic insufficiency, and left ventricular ejection fraction less than 40% were independent predictors of death.

Eighteen patients developed moderate or severe aortic insufficiency (12 reimplantation and 6 remodeling). Overall freedom from moderate or severe aortic insufficiency at 18 years was 78% and similar for both types of aortic valve-sparing operations. Ten patients required reoperation on the aortic valve (5 reimplantation and 5 remodeling) for aortic insufficiency in 8 and infective endocarditis in 2. One valve was re-repaired and 9 replaced; all patients survived reoperation. The freedom from reoperation on the aortic valve at 18 years was 94.8%. These findings suggested that aortic valve-sparing operations provide excellent long-term outcomes but there is evidence of gradual deterioration in aortic valve function during the first two decades of follow-up.

There are several other reports on long-term results of aortic valve-sparing operations with similar outcomes to those reported above but shorter follow-up.[29-31] Patients with bicuspid aortic valve seem to enjoy similar results as those with tricuspid aortic valve during the first decade of follow-up.[31,32]

Patients with aortic root aneurysm are usually on their second, third, and fourth decades of life and are frequently associated with inherited disorders such as Marfan syndrome, Loyes-Dietz syndrome, familial aneurysms, and others by the time they come to surgical attention. The aneurysm begins in the aortic sinuses and expands proximally and distally into the aortic annulus and sinotubular junction. Reimplantation of the aortic valve is ideal for these patients as well as those with incompetent bicuspid aortic and dilated aortic annulus because it corrects the annular dilatation and reshapes the aortic annulus by fixing it into the cylindrical Dacron graft. The drawback of the reimplantation procedure is that it places the aortic cusps into a noncompliant structure with consequent increase in mechanical stress on the cusps. Creation of neoaortic sinuses may reduce the mechanical stresses but it remains uncertain if improves durability.

Patients with primarily ascending aortic aneurysm may have secondarily dilated aortic sinuses but the aortic annulus remains normal. The dilatation of the aortic sinuses is often asymmetrical and the noncoronary aortic sinus is the first one to dilate, followed by the right and left. These patients are older than those with primary aortic root aneurysms and are on their fifth, sixth, and seventh decades of life. Remodeling of the aortic root is ideally suited for these patients.

Aortic valve-sparing operations are an alternative to aortic root replacement with a conduit containing a mechanical or bioprosthetic aortic valve in patients with aortic root aneurysm or ascending aortic aneurysm with dilated aortic sinuses but normal or only mildly diseased aortic cusps. When correctly performed, they provide excellent long-term results and are associated with low rates of valve-related complications. However, they are technically demanding operations and only surgeons with experience in aortic root surgery should perform them. Most failures appear to be related to technical errors.[32] The surgeon must have a sound knowledge of anatomy and pathology of the aortic valve and be able to apply the concepts of functional anatomy to create an anatomically and functionally satisfactory reconstructed aortic root.

REFERENCES

1. Movahed MR, Hepner AD, Ahmadi-Kashani M: Echocardiographic prevalence of bicuspid aortic valve in the population. *Heart Lung Circ* 2006; 15:297.
2. Prakash SK, Bossé Y, Muehlschlegel JD, et al: A roadmap to investigate the genetic basis of bicuspid aortic valve and its complications: insights from the International BAV Con (Bicuspid Aortic Valve Consortium). *J Am Coll Cardiol.* 2014; 64:832.
3. Sievers HH, Schmidtke C: A classification system for the bicuspid aortic valve from 304 surgical specimens. *J Thorac Cardiovasc Surg* 2007; 133:1226.
4. Michelena HI, Desjardins V, Avierinos JF, et al: Natural history of asymptomatic patients with normally functioning or minimally dysfunctional bicuspid aortic valve in the community. *Circulation* 2008; 117:2776.
5. Dietz HC, Loeys BL, Carta L, Ramirez F: Recent progress towards a molecular understanding of Marfan syndrome. *Am J Med Genet* 2005; 139C:4.
6. Bee KJ, Wilkes D, Devereux RB, et al: Structural and functional genetic disorders of the great vessels and outflow tracts. *Ann NY Acad Sci* 2006; 1085:256-269.
7. Loeys BL, Dietz HC, Braverman AC, et al: The revised Ghent nosology for the Marfan syndrome. *J Med Genet* 2010; 47:476.
8. Loeys BL, Chen J, Neptune ER, et al: A syndrome of altered cardiovascular, craniofacial, neurocognitive and skeletal development caused by mutations in TGFBR1 or TGFBR2. *Nat Genet* 2005; 37:275.
9. Wenstrup RJ, Meyer RA, Lyle JS, et al: Prevalence of aortic root dilation in the Ehlers-Danlos syndrome. *Genet Med* 2002; 4:112.
10. van der Linde D, van de Laar IM, Bertoli-Avella AM, et al: Aggressive cardiovascular phenotype of aneurysms-osteoarthritis syndrome caused by pathogenic SMAD-s variants. *J Am Coll Cardiol* 2012; 60:397.
11. Boileau C, Guo DC, Hanna N, et al: TGFβ2 mutations cause familial thoracic aortic aneurysms and dissections associated with mild features of Marfan syndrome. *Nat Genet* 2012; 44:916.
12. Renard M, Holm T, Veith R, et al: Altered TGFbeta signaling and cardiovascular manifestations in patients with autosomal recessive cutis laxa type I caused by fibrillin-4 deficiency. *Eur J Hum Genet* 2010; 18:895.
13. Pellika PA, Nishimura RA, Bailey KR, et al: The natural history of adults with asymptomatic hemodynamically significant aortic stenosis. *J Am Coll Cardiol* 1990; 15:1018.
14. Frank S, Johnson A, Ross J Jr: Natural history of valvular aortic stenosis. *Br Heart J* 1997; 35:41.
15. Goldschlager N, Pfeifer J, Cohn K, et al: Natural history of aortic regurgitation: a clinical and hemodynamic study. *Am J Med* 1973; 54:577.
16. Tzemos N, Terrien J, Yip J, et al: Outcomes in adults with bicuspid aortic valves. *JAMA* 2008; 300:1317.
17. Coady MA, Rizzo JA, Hammond GL, et al: Surgical intervention criteria for thoracic aortic aneurysms: a study of growth rates and complications. *Ann Thorac Surg* 1999; 67:1922.
18. Silverman DI, Burton KJ, Gray J: Life expectancy in the Marfan syndrome. *Am J Cardiol* 1995; 75:157.
19. Davies RR, Kaple RK, Mandapati D, et al: Natural history of ascending aortic aneurysms in the setting of an unreplaced bicuspid aortic valve. *Ann Thorac Surg* 2007; 83:1338-1344.
20. Nishimura RA, Otto CM, Bonow RO, et al: 2014 AHA/ACC Guideline for the Management of Patients With Valvular Heart Disease: Executive Summary: A Report of the American College of Cardiology/American Heart Association Task Force on Practice Guidelines. *Circulation.* 2014; 129:2440-2492.
21. Svensson LG, Adams DH, Bonow RO, et al: Aortic valve and ascending aorta guidelines for management and quality measures: executive summary. *Ann Thorac Surg* 2013; 95:1491.
22. David TE: Remodeling of the aortic root and preservation of the native aortic valve. *Op Tech Cardiac Thorac Surg* 1996; 1:44-56.
23. Yacoub M: Valve-conserving operation for aortic root aneurysm or dissection. *Op Tech Cardiac Thorac Surg* 1996; 1:57.
24. Cameron DE, Alejo DE, Patel ND, et al: Aortic root replacement in 372 Marfan patients: evolution of operative repair over 30 years. *Ann Thorac Surg* 2009; 87:1344.
25. Casselman FP, Gillinov AM, Akhrass R, et al: Intermediate-term durability of bicuspid aortic valve repair for prolapsing leaflet. *Eur J Cardiothorac Surg* 1999; 15:302.
26. de Kerchove L, Boodhwani M, Glineur D, et al: Valve sparing-root replacement with the reimplantation technique to increase the durability of bicuspid aortic valve repair. *J Thorac Cardiovasc Surg* 2011; 142:143.
27. David TE, Feindel CM, Armstrong S, Maganti M: Replacement of the ascending aorta with reduction of the diameter of the sinotubular junction to treat aortic insufficiency in patients with ascending aortic aneurysm. *J Thorac Cardiovasc Surg* 2007; 133:414-418.
28. David TE, Feindel CM, David CM, Manlhiot C: A quarter of century experience with aortic valve sparing operations. *J Thorac Cardiovasc Surg* 2015; 148:872.
29. Liebrich M, Kruszynski MK, Roser D, et al: The David procedure in different valve pathologies: a single-center experience in 236 patients. *Ann Thorac Surg* 2013; 95:71.
30. Kvitting JP, Kari FA, Fischbein MP: David valve-sparing aortic root replacement: equivalent mid-term outcome for different valve types with or without connective tissue disorder. *J Thorac Cardiovasc Surg* 2013; 145:117.
31. Aicher D, Langer F, Lausberg H, Bierbach B, Schäfers HJ: Aortic root remodeling: ten-year experience with 274 patients. *J Thorac Cardiovasc Surg* 2007; 134:909.
32. Oka T, Okita Y, Matsumori M, et al: Aortic regurgitation after valve-sparing aortic root replacement: modes of failure. *Ann Thorac Surg* 2011; 92:1639.

31

Surgical Treatment of Aortic Valve Endocarditis

Gösta B. Pettersson • Syed T. Hussain

The most common heart valve affected by infective endocarditis (IE) is the aortic valve. Fortunately, significant progress has been made in our understanding and management of aortic valve IE. Clinical manifestations include fever, heart murmur, splenomegaly, embolic events, and bacteremia or fungemia. Early diagnosis is extremely important because progression invariably leads to devastating complications, including acute heart failure, cerebral embolism, and death, if the infection is not treated with antibiotics, surgery, or both. Increasingly, IE has become a "surgical disease," particularly for aortic valve IE, and during the last decade, more than half of all patients have been operated on during the active phase of the disease (early surgery).[1]

EPIDEMIOLOGY

Among patients with aortic valve IE, congenitally bicuspid aortic valve is the most common predisposing lesion.[2] Other congenital abnormalities of the aortic valve predisposing to infection are degenerative calcific aortic stenosis, aortic regurgitation due to any cause, and rheumatic aortic valve disease. Occasionally, highly virulent microorganisms infect normal aortic valves. Patients with prosthetic heart valves run a constant higher risk of developing IE.

It is difficult to determine the incidence and prevalence of native aortic valve IE in the general population because the disease is continuously changing.[3,4] The annual incidence is estimated to range from 1.7 to 7.0 episodes per 100,000 person-years in North America,[5-7] and patients with prosthetic aortic valves are reported to have an incidence of 0.2 to 1.4 episodes per 100 patient-years.[8-10] Approximately 1.4% of patients undergoing aortic valve replacement develop prosthetic valve IE during the first postoperative year.[11]

The incidence of nosocomial IE is increasing because more patients are undergoing invasive procedures. IE in hemodialysis patients is fortunately relatively infrequent, but when it happens, it is associated with high mortality.[12] Dental procedures, extractions in particular, have been shown to produce bacteremia. However, daily dental flossing can also produce bacteremia in periodontally healthy individuals at a rate comparable with that caused by dental procedures for which antibiotic prophylaxis is usually given to patients with valve disease to prevent endocarditis, suggesting that prophylaxis may be futile.[13] Endoscopic procedures may also produce bacteremia. Intravenous drug users using nonsterile syringes and needles most often infect their structurally normal tricuspid valves (see "Prophylaxis of Infective Endocarditis" later in this chapter).

PATHOGENESIS AND PATHOLOGY

The key to understanding IE is appreciating the pathology progression.[6,14,15] Circulating organisms adhere and attach to areas with endocardial (valve) injury; such damaged areas often have deposition of platelets, fibrin, or clots, facilitating attachment and growth of the organisms. In 1928, Grant and colleagues[16] theorized that platelet-fibrin thrombi on the heart valve serve as a nidus for bacteria to adhere, and in 1963, Angrist and Oka[17] introduced the term *nonbacterial thrombotic endocarditis* to describe such sterile vegetations, providing experimental evidence supporting their role in the pathogenesis of endocarditis.[18] As the organism multiplies, it produces matrix material, and this, together with leukocytes and thrombotic material, accumulates in the area and forms verrucous vegetations. Formation of vegetations means formation of a biofilm, allowing the organisms protection from the host's defenses and antibiotics.

The infecting organisms produce and release virulence factors and enzymes that promote organism reproduction and survival and kill and disintegrate host tissue, primarily valve cusps and leaflets. The enzymes produced are organism specific with regard to their tissue specificity and efficiency. When tissue disintegration involves the valve annulus, the infection invades extravascular areas (invasive disease). Invasive disease develops in stages: cellulitis, abscess, abscess cavities, and finally, pseudoaneurysm formation. Invasive disease around the aortic root is generally deeper and more extensive than for any other valve because it is constantly highly pressurized. Internal fistulas, perforations, and heart block constitute specific consequences of invasion.[14] IE of the aortic valve not only causes destruction of the aortic cusps, paravalvular abscesses, and cardiac fistulas, but is also a source of systemic embolization of vegetation material.[19] Strokes and cerebral infarctions caused by embolism of vegetation material are common. An ischemic infarct may convert into a hemorrhagic infarct. However, when an infarct is hemorrhagic, there is a higher probability of a mycotic aneurysm.[20] Rupture of a mycotic aneurysm may cause devastating cerebral bleeding. Mycotic aneurysms, infarcts, and abscesses in other organs, such as the spleen, liver, kidneys, and limbs, are also common.[18] Aortic valve IE with a large vegetation that prolapses into the left ventricle and comes into contact with the anterior mitral valve leaflet causes secondary involvement of this valve (kissing lesions).[14,21] Such kissing lesions are common and manifest themselves as anterior valve leaflet pseudoaneurysms or perforations (windsock lesions).[14]

Infection of a bioprosthetic valve, porcine or pericardial, may involve the cusps, the sewing ring, or both (Fig. 31-1). Infection of aortic valve allografts and pulmonary autografts resembles that of the native aortic valves: It may begin on the aortic cusps and destroy them, causing aortic regurgitation, or it may start at old suture lines and extend into surrounding structures (Fig. 31-2). Infection of a mechanical heart valve is usually located along the sewing ring (Fig. 31-3). Endocarditis after replacement with a prosthesis frequently causes dehiscence of the prosthesis from the annulus, with consequent development of ventricular-aortic separation.

Heart block with aortic valve IE is caused by destruction of the atrioventricular node and the bundle of His. This happens when the infection invades the right atrium and the triangle of Koch (Fig. 31-2).

MICROBIOLOGY

The microbiology of aortic IE depends on whether the valve is native or prosthetic, and whether the infection is hospital or community acquired. *Staphylococcus aureus* and *Streptococcus viridans* are the most common organisms responsible for native aortic valve endocarditis.[6,22] *S. aureus* is extremely virulent. *S. viridans* and various other streptococci are not as virulent and cause an infection that often follows a more protracted course. Coagulase-negative staphylococci are also less virulent, but have emerged as an important cause of native valve IE in both the community and health care settings.[6,23]

IE caused by Gram-negative bacteria is less common, but these organisms are often resistant to many antibiotics and more difficult to treat and therefore more likely to cause complications. *Haemophilus, Actinobacillus, Cardiobacterium, Eikenella,* and *Kingella* (the HACEK group) are Gram-negative bacilli grouped together because of their characteristic fastidiousness requiring a prolonged incubation period before growth, although bacteriologic diagnostic methods have improved. Fungal IE is rare but extremely serious and very difficult to eradicate and cure. *Candida albicans* and *Aspergillus fumigatus* are the usual agents. Fungal IE is associated with large, sometimes huge, vegetations (Fig. 31-4).

The microbiology of prosthetic aortic valve IE is somewhat different from that of the native valve.[24,25] Prosthetic valve IE is classified as *early* when it occurs within the first year after surgery and *late* when it occurs after 1 year.[6] Early prosthetic valve IE is likely caused by contamination of the valve by perioperative bacteremia or contamination of the operative field at the time of implantation.[6,11,26,27] This may be particularly true when the infection is caused by coagulase-negative staphylococci and the HACEK group of bacteria. *Staphylococcus epidermidis, S. aureus,* and *Enterococcus faecalis* are more common microorganisms responsible for early prosthetic valve IE.[11,27] The sources of late prosthetic valve IE are more difficult to determine. Although streptococci and staphylococci are commonly encountered in these patients, a myriad of microorganisms can cause late prosthetic valve IE.[27] Nosocomial infections are often caused by *S. aureus* or other staphylococci.[6]

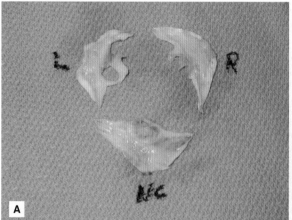
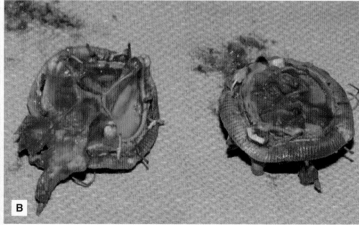

FIGURE 31-1 Native and prosthetic valve endocarditis. (A) Active aortic native valve endocarditis: Excised aortic valve cusps illustrating vegetations and disintegration, precluding valve repair. (B) Large vegetations attached on an excised aortic valve bioprosthesis in a patient with preoperative embolic stroke. (Reproduced with permission from Pettersson GB, Hussain ST, Shrestha NK, et al: Infective endocarditis: an atlas of disease progression for describing, staging, coding, and understanding the pathology, *J Thorac Cardiovasc Surg.* 2014 Apr;147(4):1142-1149.e2.)

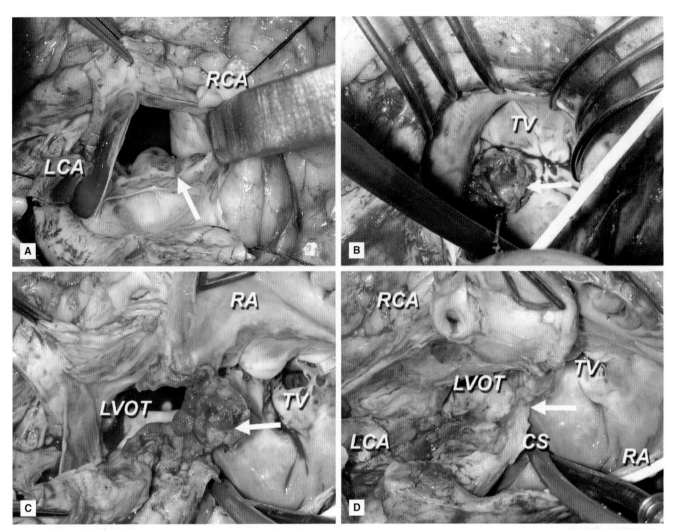

FIGURE 31-2 Allograft endocarditis with heart block. (A) Endocarditis with sepsis and heart block in patient with a history of aortic allograft root replacement. Allograft cusps are not affected, but vegetations are present on proximal aortic suture line (arrow). (B) Same patient: Cauliflower vegetation (arrow) next to atrioventricular node marking penetration into right atrium. (C) Same cauliflower vegetation (arrow) next to atrioventricular node after opening aortic and right atrial (RA) walls down to vegetation. (D) Complete removal of allograft and debridement discloses extent of peri-allograft infection, which extends from right coronary artery (RCA) counterclockwise to membranous septum and atrioventricular node (arrow). Root is ready for reconstruction. *CS,* Coronary sinus; *LCA,* left coronary artery; *LVOT,* left ventricular outflow tract; *TV,* tricuspid valve. (Reproduced with permission from Pettersson GB, Hussain ST, Shrestha NK, et al: Infective endocarditis: an atlas of disease progression for describing, staging, coding, and understanding the pathology, *J Thorac Cardiovasc Surg.* 2014 Apr;147(4):1142-1149.e2.)

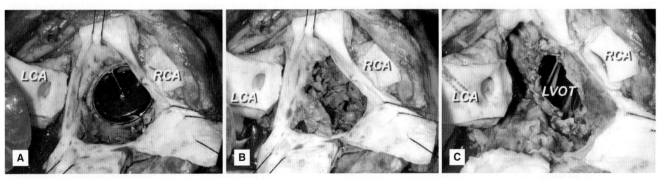

FIGURE 31-3 Mechanical prosthesis endocarditis. (A) Infected mechanical aortic valve prosthesis showing circumferential involvement of sewing ring, with some vegetations attaching on both sides of prosthesis. (B) After removal of prosthesis, the vegetations were present both above and beneath the prosthesis, and circumferential invasion is obvious. (C) Although the aortic annulus is disintegrated with atrioventricular discontinuity, the left ventricular outflow tract (LVOT) appears well preserved after debridement. LCA, Left coronary artery; RCA, right coronary artery. (Reproduced with permission from Pettersson GB, Hussain ST, Shrestha NK, et al: Infective endocarditis: an atlas of disease progression for describing, staging, coding, and understanding the pathology, *J Thorac Cardiovasc Surg.* 2014 Apr;147(4):1142-1149.e2.)

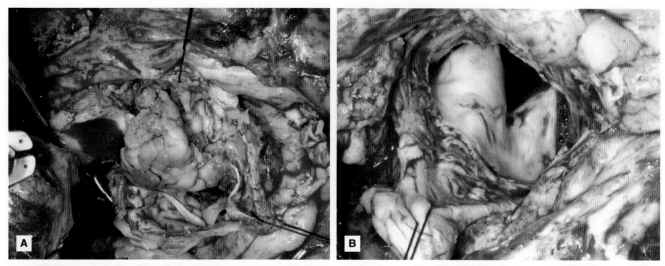

FIGURE 31-4 Fungal endocarditis. (A) Fungal endocarditis with large vegetations on aortic valve. (B) After complete debridement, no destruction or invasion is observed. (Reproduced with permission from Pettersson GB, Hussain ST, Shrestha NK, et al: Infective endocarditis: an atlas of disease progression for describing, staging, coding, and understanding the pathology, *J Thorac Cardiovasc Surg.* 2014 Apr;147(4):1142-1149.e2.)

In a small proportion of cases of aortic valve IE, no microorganism can be cultured from either the blood or surgical specimens.[6] This is called "culture-negative endocarditis," but in these cases it is important to rule out fastidious microorganisms, and every effort should be made to identify them. Valve sequencing (universal bacterial, mycobacterial, or fungal polymerase chain reaction [PCR]) is successful in identifying the causative organism in most cases.[28]

CLINICAL PRESENTATION AND DIAGNOSIS

It is helpful to classify IE as acute and subacute, because there are major differences between these two clinical presentations. Originally, before the availability of antibiotics, these concepts of acute, subacute, and chronic IE also described how long it would take patients to die. Subacute and chronic IE are caused by less virulent microorganisms, such as *S. viridans,* and the clinical course is protracted; antibiotics alone cure most cases if treatment is started before important destruction of the cusps or invasion have occurred. On the other hand, acute IE is frequently caused by a virulent and aggressive organism such as *S. aureus.* The clinical course is acute, and destruction and invasion occur fast, with antibiotics alone often failing to cure the infection.

The onset of subacute IE is usually subtle, with low-grade fever and malaise. Patients think they have the "flu," are often treated with oral antibiotics, and symptoms improve. However, in most cases the symptoms recur a few days after the antibiotics are stopped. In the majority of cases, no extracardiac source of bacteremia is identified. An aortic valve murmur is present in nearly all patients because they have preexisting aortic valve disease. Splenomegaly is common. Clubbing of the fingers and toes may develop in long-standing cases.

Skin and mucous membrane signs occur late in this form of IE. Petechiae appear on any part of the body. Small areas of hemorrhage may be seen in the ocular fundi. Hemorrhages in the nail beds usually have a linear distribution near the distal end, hence the name splinter hemorrhages. Osler nodes are acute, tender, barely palpable nodular lesions in the pulp of the fingers and toes, and bacteria have been cultured from these lesions. Embolization of large vegetation fragments may cause dramatic clinical events such as stroke, acute myocardial infarction, or splenic or hepatic infarcts. Any other organ may also be a target for an embolic event. Destruction of the aortic cusps causes aortic regurgitation and heart failure. The hematologic picture is not distinctive in subacute endocarditis. The leukocyte count is moderately elevated. Anemia without reticulocytosis develops after a few weeks in patients who are untreated. Blood cultures frequently identify the offending microorganism.

Acute IE is defined by a fulminant clinical course. A noncardiac source of bacteremia may often be identified. This form of IE can present with all the symptoms and signs described under subacute IE, but they are more severe and progress rapidly, and patients are often sicker and show signs of sepsis. Early metastatic infections are common. Two physical signs are seen only in acute IE: Janeway lesions (painless red-blue hemorrhagic lesions a few millimeters in diameter found on the palms of the hands and soles of the feet) and Roth spots (an oval pale area surrounded by hemorrhage near the optic disc). In patients with no preexisting aortic valve disease, the presentation is acute. Early extra-aortic infection and cardiac decompensation caused by severe aortic regurgitation is common. Invasion with paravalvular abscesses is also more common, and with invasion behind the central fibrous body, toward the floor of the right atrium and triangle of Koch (Fig. 31-2), the electrocardiogram may show an increased PR interval that within hours or days progresses to

---

TABLE 31-1: Modified Duke Criteria for the Diagnosis of Infective Endocarditis

Major criteria
- Blood culture positive for infective endocarditis
  Typical microorganisms consistent with infective endocarditis from two separate blood cultures: *Streptococcus viridans, S. bovis*, HACEK group, *S. aureus,* or community-acquired enterococci, in the absence of a primary focus, or Microorganisms consistent with infective endocarditis from a persistently positive blood culture, defined as follows:
  - At least two positive cultures of blood drawn >12 hours apart, or
  - All of three or a majority of >four separate cultures of blood (with the first and last samples drawn at least 1 hour apart)
  - Single positive blood culture for *Coxiella burnetii or phase I IgG* antibody titer to *C. burnetii* > 1:800
- Evidence of endocardial involvement:
  - Echocardiogram positive for infective endocarditis: TEE recommended in patients with prosthetic valves, rated at least as "possible endocarditis" by clinical criteria, or complicated endocarditis, such as endocarditis with paravalvular abscess; TTE as the first test in other patients as follows:
    - Oscillating intracardiac mass on valve or supporting structures, in the path of regurgitant jets, or on implanted material in the absence of an alternative anatomic explanation
    - Abscess
    - New partial dehiscence of prosthetic valve
  - New valvular regurgitation (worsening or changing of preexisting murmur not sufficient)

Minor criteria
- Predisposition, predisposing heart condition, or injection drug use
- Fever
- Vascular phenomena: major arterial emboli, septic pulmonary infarcts, mycotic aneurysm, intracranial hemorrhage, conjunctival hemorrhages, and Janeway lesions
- Immunologic phenomena: glomerulonephritis, Osler nodes, Roth spots, and rheumatoid factor
- Microbiologic evidence: positive blood culture but does not meet a major criterion as noted above, or serologic evidence of active infection with an organism consistent with infective endocarditis
- Echocardiographic minor criteria eliminated

Definite endocarditis = two major criteria, or one major + three minor criteria, or five minor criteria
Possible endocarditis = one major + one minor, or three minor criteria
HACEK group = Haemophilus, Actinobacillus, Cardiobacterium, Eikenella, and Kingella; IE = infective endocarditis; TEE = transesophageal echocardiography; TTE = transthoracic echocardiography
Reproduced with permission from Li JS, Sexton DJ, Mick N, et al: Proposed modifications to the Duke criteria for the diagnosis of infective endocarditis, *Clin Infect Dis.* 2000 Apr;30(4):633-638.

---

complete heart block. The blood picture is one of acute sepsis. Blood cultures often isolate the infecting agent.

Prosthetic valve IE may present as acute or subacute endocarditis.

Doppler echocardiography is ubiquitous and of fundamental importance in the diagnosis, management, and follow-up of patients with IE.[6,29] Transesophageal echocardiography (TEE) is more sensitive than transthoracic echocardiography (TTE), and multiplane is better than monoplane for diagnosing IE. The sensitivity of TTE ranges from 40 to 63% and that of TEE from 90 to 100%.[6] Echocardiography can detect vegetations as small as 1 or 2 mm, but it is more reliable in native than prosthetic valve IE. It is more useful for tissue than for mechanical valves because of the acoustic shadowing of mechanical heart valves. Echocardiography is also highly sensitive for detecting paravalvular abscesses and cardiac fistulas, but may still miss some.

Clinical investigators from Duke University proposed certain criteria for confirming or rejecting the diagnosis of IE.[29] The Duke criteria have been validated, and their limitations discussed by other investigators.[30,31] A modified version of the Duke criteria has been proposed,[31] and it is shown in Table 31-1.

TREATMENT

Appropriate antibiotic treatment is the most important aspect of the management of patients with IE.[6,22,27] Timing is important because destruction is progressive, and disintegrated cusps do not heal or regenerate. Once invasive, the infection is less likely to be cured by antibiotics alone.

Antibiotic therapy should be started soon after obtaining at least two blood cultures within a 3- to 6-hour interval taken from different peripheral sites (the modified Duke criteria have as a major criterion "At least two positive blood cultures of blood samples drawn >12 hours apart; or all of three or a majority of ≥4 separate cultures of blood [with first and last samples drawn at least 1 hour apart]"). The initial choice of antibiotics is based on clinical circumstances and the suspected source of infection. Patients who had recent dental work should receive antibiotics to counteract bacteria from the oral cavity; those who had recent urinary or colonic procedures should be treated with antibiotics that are effective against Gram-negative bacteria. Intravenous drug users are usually infected with *S. aureus* or coagulase-negative staphylococci. Once the microorganism is identified by blood cultures and its sensitivity to specific antibiotics is known, antibiotic therapy is adjusted accordingly.

Higher doses and a combination of two or three antibiotics that potentiate one another are often needed in the treatment of IE. Intravenous antibiotic therapy is continued for 6 weeks. It is difficult to eradicate infection caused by virulent microorganisms with antibiotics alone because these organisms have several mechanisms by which they avoid the patient's defense systems and resist the antibiotics, with the ability to form biofilm perhaps the most important one. Destruction of the aortic valve cusps happens rapidly and causes aortic regurgitation and congestive heart failure. These infections are usually caused by *S. aureus, Pseudomonas aeruginosa, Serratia marcescens*, or fungi.

Repeat blood cultures are performed 48 hours after starting to monitor the efficacy of antibiotic therapy. The patient must be watched closely for signs of congestive heart failure, coronary and systemic embolization, and unresponsive infection. Daily electrocardiograms and frequent echocardiograms are performed during the first 2 weeks of treatment. With any evidence of increasing aortic regurgitation, enlarging vegetations, recurrent embolism, paravalvular abscess, heart block, or poor response of clinical symptoms to antibiotics, surgery should be immediately considered. It is better to operate on patients before they develop complications, such as intractable heart failure, cardiogenic or septic shock, heart block, extensive aortic root abscesses, or stroke.

Patients with mobile vegetations larger than 10 mm are more likely to suffer serious complications, including stroke, so early surgery may be justified.[6,7,32-34] Anticoagulation is neither indicated nor effective in preventing embolization of vegetations in native or biologic valve IE; rather, it is associated with an increased risk of neurologic complications.[6]

Current guidelines for indications and timing of surgery in native and prosthetic valve IE are presented in Table 31-2. Surgical treatment should be considered in patients with signs of congestive heart failure, acute valve dysfunction, invasion with paravalvular abscess or cardiac fistulas, recurrent systemic embolization, and persistent sepsis despite adequate antibiotic therapy for more than 4 to 5 days. Approximately half of patients with IE develop severe complications that sooner or later will require an operation. In general, our recommendation is that once a surgical indication is present, surgery should not be delayed. Knowing the sensitivity of the causative organism preoperatively is important to ensure appropriate antibiotic coverage at the time of surgery. Once the patient is covered with an antibiotic to which the organism is susceptible, the penalty for operating during the active infection phase is minimized.

Preoperatively, coronary angiography is recommended in patients age 40 years or older, particularly those with at least one cardiovascular risk factor or a history of coronary artery disease or previous revascularization.[6] Exceptions to this recommendation can happen when there are large aortic vegetations that could be dislodged during catheterization, or when emergency surgery is necessary and angiography is not necessary for planning the operation.[6,32] For patients with renal dysfunction, clinical judgment should be exercised. High-resolution computed tomography (CT) imaging to diagnose coronary artery disease may be useful and acceptable in younger patients, but contrast renal toxicity remains an issue.

All patients scheduled to undergo surgery for IE should have a neurologic evaluation and a CT scan or magnetic resonance imaging of the brain performed preoperatively within a day of the operation to visualize any strokes and to determine if an infarct is ischemic or hemorrhagic. Ischemic strokes are far more common than hemorrhagic, but both are associated with increased mortality and morbidity. Hemorrhagic lesions are associated with a higher probability of mycotic aneurysms, which often require treatment before valve surgery. An angiography is needed to exclude a mycotic aneurysm and should be performed if there is bleeding and a high suspicion. Delay of the heart surgery is usually advised in patients with more serious neurologic complications; we do not operate on unconscious patients or those unable to follow simple commands until they demonstrate neurologic improvement. Patients with ischemic stroke should ideally have surgery delayed by 1 to 2 weeks and those with hemorrhagic stroke by 3 to 4 weeks.[6,7,32] The risk of delaying surgery should always be weighed against patients' hemodynamic condition.[33]

SURGICAL TREATMENT

We routinely perform surgery for aortic valve IE through a median sternotomy; intraoperative TEE is mandatory. Patients who need emergency or urgent surgery are often very sick and may be in congestive heart failure. For this reason, and because they often require complex and long surgical procedures, myocardial protection is of utmost importance. We achieve this by using initial induction with antegrade and retrograde blood cardioplegia, and repeat retrograde cardioplegia every 15 to 20 minutes. The right atrium is routinely opened to cannulate the coronary sinus directly through a purse-string suture around its orifice. We avoid unnecessary cardiac manipulation before arresting the heart.

Another important aspect of surgery for IE is minimizing residual contamination of the surgical field, instruments, drapes, and gloves with vegetations and pus. Instruments used to debride contaminated areas of the heart are discarded before reconstruction begins. In addition, local drapes, suction equipment, and surgical gloves are changed. The objective is to leave as few organisms as possible in the operative field.

The aortic valve is explored through a transverse aortotomy 1 cm or more above the right coronary artery. When the infection is limited to the cusps of the native aortic valve or a prosthetic valve, complete removal of the valve and implantation of a biologic or mechanical valve prosthesis usually resolves the problem. There is no evidence that a bioprosthesis is better than a mechanical valve in patients with active IE.[6,10,32,35] The choice of prosthesis depends on age of the patient, comorbidities, life expectancy, and compliance with anticoagulation. For native valve infection with limited localized infection, an attempt can be made to repair and preserve the valve using autologous pericardium. History of a hemorrhagic stroke is a reason to avoid a mechanical valve and its associated need for anticoagulation.

⬤ TABLE 31-2: Indications and Timing of Surgery in Native and Prosthetic Valve Infective Endocarditis

Indications	Timing*	Class	Level of evidence
Heart failure			
Aortic or mitral IE or PVE with severe acute regurgitation or valve obstruction of fistula causing refractory pulmonary edema or cardiogenic shock	Emergency	I	B
Aortic or mitral IE with severe acute regurgitation or valve obstruction and persisting heart failure or echocardiographic signs of poor hemodynamic tolerance early mitral closure or pulmonary hypertension)	Urgent	I	B
Aortic or mitral IE or severe prosthetic dehiscence with severe regurgitation and no heart failure	Elective	IIa	B
Right heart failure secondary to severe tricuspid regurgitation with poor response to diuretic therapy	Urgent/elective	IIa	C
Uncontrolled infection		I	B
Locally uncontrolled infection (abscess, false aneurysm, fistula, enlarging vegetation)	Urgent		
Persisting fever and positive blood cultures > 7-10 days not related to an extracardiac cause	Urgent	I	B
Infection caused by fungi or multiresistant organisms	Urgent/elective	I	B
PVE caused by staphylococci or Gram negative bacteria (most cases of early PVE)	Urgent/elective	IIa	C
Prevention of embolism			
Aortic or mitral IE or PVE with large vegetations (>10 mm) following one or more embolic episodes despite appropriate antibiotic therapy	Urgent	I	B
Aortic or mitral IE or PVE with large vegetations (>10 mm) and other predictors of complicated course (heart failure, persistent infection, abscess)	Urgent	I	C
Aortic or mitral or PVE with isolated very large vegetations (>15 mm†)	Urgent	Ib	C
Persistent tricuspid valve vegetations > 20 mm after recurrent pulmonary emboli	Urgent/elective	IIa	C

Class I: Evidence and/or general agreement that a given treatment or procedure is beneficial, useful, effective.
Class II: Conflicting evidence and/or divergence of opinion about the usefulness/efficacy of the given treatment or procedure.
Class IIa: Weight of evidence/opinion is in favor of usefulness efficacy.
Class IIb: Usefulness/efficacy is less well established by evidence/opinion.
Class III: Evidence of general agreement that the given treatment or procedure is not useful/effective, and in some cases may be harmful.
Level of evidence A: Data derived from multiple randomized clinical trials or meta-analyses.
Level of evidence B: Data derived from a single randomized clinical trial or large nonrandomized studies.
Level of evidence C: Consensus of opinion of the experts or small studies, retrospective studies, registries.
*Emergency surgery: Surgery performed within 24 hours, urgent surgery: within a few days, elective surgery, after at least 1 or 2 weeks of antibiotic treatment.
†Surgery may be preferred if procedure preserving the native valve is feasible.
IE, infective endocarditis: PVE, prosthetic valve endocarditis.
Reproduced with permission from Thuny F, Habib G: When should we operate on patients with acute infective endocarditis? Heart. 2010 Jun;96(11):892-897.

If the infection is invasive beyond the cusps or leaflets, radical resection of all infected tissues and foreign material (prosthesis, pledgets, and sutures) is necessary, followed by reconstruction (Fig. 31-5).[14,25,27,36,37] The pathology and anatomy of the left ventricular outflow tract (LVOT) must be well understood for complete surgical debridement and reconstruction, particularly in patients with prosthetic valve and advanced invasive aortic root IE. To reconstruct the aortic root, an aortic allograft is usually our preferred choice. Use of an allograft is no substitute for radical removal of infected tissue, as not even allografts are immune to reinfection.[37] After extensive debridement, the LVOT is almost always preserved to allow direct anastomosis to the allograft. The intervalvular fibrosa corresponding to the base of the anterior mitral valve leaflet and the two trigones on either side are the main landmarks to indicate the level of the proximal suture line. The LVOT is sized with Hegar dilators, and an allograft with an internal diameter 2 to 3 mm less than the diameter of the annulus is chosen. The coronary buttons should be well mobilized. No felt is used to support the suture lines. When patching is required, autologous pericardium is our preference, but need for patching should be uncommon! Aortic

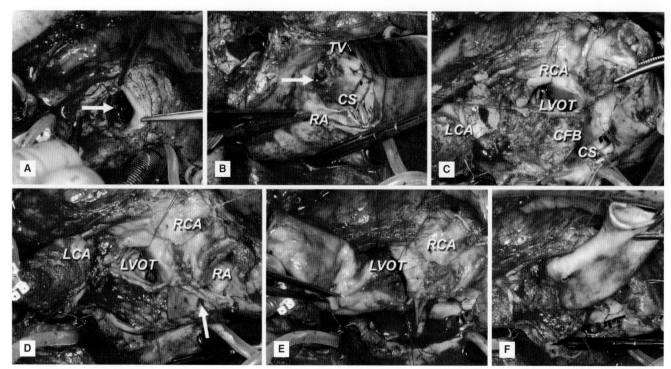

FIGURE 31-5 Prosthetic valve endocarditis with sepsis and heart block. (A) Infected mechanical prosthesis with vegetations on sewing ring (arrow). (B) Same patient with perforation visible in right atrium (RA; arrow). (C) After debridement, destruction in location of atrioventricular node is seen. This infection has worked its way around the aorta counterclockwise over an extended period, displaying a pseudoaneurysm stage anteriorly and an active cellulitis stage posteriorly and into right atrium. Left ventricular outflow tract (LVOT) is intact and ready for reconstruction. (D) After complete debridement of all infected tissue, RA is reconstructed with autologous pericardium (arrow). (E) Aortic allograft is sutured to LVOT with running monofilament suture. (F) Allograft is tied down and well seated, allowing debrided infected areas to communicate and drain to pericardium. CFB, central fibrous body; CS, coronary sinus; LCA, left coronary artery; RCA, right coronary artery; TV, tricuspid valve. (Reproduced with permission from Pettersson GB, Hussain ST, Shrestha NK, et al: Infective endocarditis: an atlas of disease progression for describing, staging, coding, and understanding the pathology, *J Thorac Cardiovasc Surg.* 2014 Apr;147(4):1142-1149.e2.)

root destruction extending into the intervalvular fibrosa or a prosthetic mitral valve is a difficult and not uncommon issue. An alternative technique some prefer when the aortic annulus is involved is patching the defect after resection of the necrotic or inflamed area, before a prosthetic valve is implanted. Use of fresh autologous pericardium to patch small defects (1 or 2 cm wide) and glutaraldehyde-fixed bovine pericardium for larger defects has been suggested.[37,38] Some surgeons also use polyester fabric to reconstruct the aortic root,[38] and a pulmonary autograft has been used as an alternative to an allograft in young patients.[39,40] Use of freestyle root replacement for complex destructive aortic valve IE has been reported as well.[41,42] Specimens are divided and sent for microbiologic and pathologic examination and also considered for PCR.

Postoperative complications are common after surgery for active IE. Septic patients may be hypotensive and may have severe coagulopathy and bleed excessively after prolonged cardiopulmonary bypass. When extensive debridement and allograft root reconstruction have been done, important surgical bleeders are controlled before protamine administration. Following protamine, the field is packed and suction is avoided, allowing adequate time (usually 20-30 minutes) for clotting to occur before additional surgical hemostasis is attempted. Antifibrinolytic agents such as aminocaproic acid

may be used in reoperations in addition to platelets, cryoprecipitate, and fresh-frozen plasma in patients with coagulopathy. Radical debridement of invasive disease with periaortic cellulitis and necrotic tissue and abscess may in itself cause heart block, for which a permanent pacemaker will be needed postoperatively. Placement of epicardial leads and implantation of the pacemaker during the operation may be considered. Multisystem organ failure may develop postoperatively. However, rapid reversal of renal dysfunction caused by immune complex glomerulonephritis has been observed. Neurologic deterioration may occur in patients with preexisting cerebral emboli.[33] Pulmonary, splenic, hepatic, and other metastatic abscesses seldom, but occasionally, require surgical treatment. Large metastatic abscesses may have to be drained, and in the case of a splenic abscess, splenectomy should be performed to avoid rupture.[6,38]

CLINICAL RESULTS

The prognosis of aortic valve IE depends largely on when and in what stage the disease is diagnosed, the offending microorganism, and how promptly it is treated.[7,22,43-46] The surgical results depend on many variables, including patient characteristics, timing of surgery,[7,44-46] whether an emergency procedure is required,[47] virulence of the organism,[43,46,48] whether the affected valve is native or prosthetic, and whether the infection has extended into and beyond the valve annulus. Until recently, patients with prosthetic aortic valve IE had a worse prognosis than patients with native aortic valve IE.[22,27,48] Nosocomial infections are associated with higher mortality than community-acquired infections.[1] The results of surgery for IE have improved significantly over time, but in-hospital mortality remains high. Variations in outcomes probably reflect variations in institution and surgeon experience in treating IE.

Operative mortality for patients with infection limited to the cusps of the aortic valve is largely dependent on the patient's clinical presentation at the time of surgery, age, and comorbidities. Most reports indicate that operative mortality for patients with noninvasive disease is under 10%.[24,27,48] Reported operative mortality is higher for prosthetic valve IE, ranging from 20 to 30%.[22,25,49] Similarly, surgery for aortic root abscess is associated with higher operative mortality.[27,49]

To provide a context for the surgery, the investigators of the International Collaboration on Endocarditis-Prospective Cohort Study (ICE-PCS), an international and multicenter database on patients with confirmed IE maintained at the Duke Clinical Research Institute, recently reported on the clinical presentation, etiology, and outcome of IE with a definite diagnosis according to Duke criteria.[22] The ICE-PCS report included a cohort of 2781 patients whose median age was 57.9 years. The IE was native in 72%, prosthetic in 21%, and pacemaker/ICD related in 7%. Approximately one-fourth of the patients had recent health care exposure. The mitral valve was infected in 41.1% and the aortic valve in 37.6%. *S. aureus* was the offending microorganism in 31.2% of all cases. Stroke was diagnosed in 16.9% and other emboli in 22.6%, congestive heart failure developed 32.2%, and paravalvular abscess occurred in 14%. Surgical treatment was common for the entire cohort (48.2%), and overall in-hospital mortality was 17.7%. Prosthetic valve IE, increasing age, pulmonary edema, *S. aureus* infection, coagulase-negative staphylococcal infection, mitral valve vegetation, and paravalvular abscess were associated with increased risk of in-hospital mortality.

In 2014, we published our current results of surgery for IE in 395 consecutive patients with isolated aortic valve active IE (Fig. 31-6).[24] One hundred sixty-three patients had native

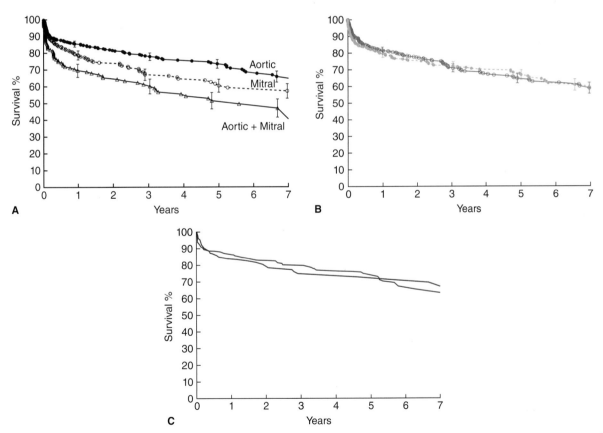

FIGURE 31-6 Survival after surgery for aortic valve endocarditis. (A) Survival after surgery for left-sided infective endocarditis (IE), stratified by the involved valve. Each *symbol* represents a death, and *vertical bars* represent the 68% confidence limits, equivalent to ±1 standard error in each figure. *Filled circles* indicate aortic valve IE alone; *open circles*, mitral valve IE alone; and *triangles*, aortic and mitral valve IE. Survival was significantly lower in the mitral and combined groups than in the isolated aortic patients (*p* < .0001). (B) Survival after surgery for native (*solid green lines*) or prosthetic (*dashed orange lines*) aortic valve IE. (C) Survival after surgery for invasive (*solid red lines*) versus noninvasive (*solid blue lines*) aortic valve IE. (Reproduced with permission from Hussain ST, Shrestha NK, Gordon SM, et al: Residual patient, anatomic, and surgical obstacles in treating active left-sided infective endocarditis, *J Thorac Cardiovasc Surg.* 2014 Sep;148(3):981-988.e4.)

valve IE and 232 prosthetic valve IE. Eight-five percent of the prosthetic valve and 44% of the native valve IE patients had invasive disease, and overall operative mortality was 7%. Survival was similar after surgery for prosthetic and native valve IE. There was also no difference in survival between those with invasive versus noninvasive IE. These excellent results reflect our improved ability to master the surgery for invasive aortic valve IE, as we are able to debride the aortic root extensively without fear and reconstruct it with an allograft.

PROPHYLAXIS OF INFECTIVE ENDOCARDITIS

The American Heart Association guidelines for prophylaxis of IE were updated in 2008.[50] Major changes in the updated recommendations include the following: (1) The committee concluded that only an extremely small number of cases of IE might be prevented by antibiotic prophylaxis for dental procedures, even if such prophylactic therapy was 100% effective. (2) IE prophylaxis for dental procedures is reasonable only for patients with underlying cardiac conditions associated with the highest risk of adverse outcome from IE. (3) For patients with these underlying cardiac conditions, prophylaxis is reasonable for all dental procedures that involve manipulation of gingival tissue or the periapical region of teeth or perforation of the oral mucosa. (4) Prophylaxis is not recommended based solely on an increased lifetime risk of acquisition of IE. (5) Administration of antibiotics solely to prevent IE is not recommended for patients who undergo a genitourinary or gastrointestinal tract procedure. These changes are intended to define more clearly when IE prophylaxis is or is not recommended and to provide more uniform and consistent global recommendations.

These new recommendations represent a dramatic shift with regard to which patients benefit and who should receive antibiotic prophylaxis for prevention of IE. However, they are "guidelines," and physicians caring for patients with organic heart valve disease should advise them according to the perceived risk of IE and potential benefit of antibiotic prophylaxis. With regard to guidelines 2 and 3 above, our recommendation is in support of prophylaxis, and we emphasize to our patients that dental extractions absolutely require prophylaxis. We continue to require "dental clearance" preoperatively for patients scheduled to undergo valve surgery.

REFERENCES

1. Hoen B, Alla F, Selton-suty C, et al: Changing profile of infective endocarditis: results of 1-year survey in France. *JAMA* 2002; 288:75-81.
2. Lamas CC, Eykyn SJ: Bicuspid aortic valve—a silent danger: analysis of 50 cases of infective endocarditis. *Clin Infect Dis* 2000; 30:336-341.
3. Moreillon P, Que YA: Infective endocarditis. *Lancet* 2004; 363:139-149.
4. Dyson C, Barnes RA, Harrison GA: Infective endocarditis: an epidemiological review of 128 episodes. *J Infect* 1999; 38:87-93.
5. Tleyjeh IM, Steckelber JM, Murad HS, et al: Temporal trends in infective endocarditis: a population-based study in Olmsted County, Minnesota. *JAMA* 2005; 293:3022-3028.
6. Habib G, Hoen B, Tornos P, et al: Guidelines on the prevention, diagnosis, and treatment of infective endocarditis (new version 2009): the Task Force on the Prevention, Diagnosis, and Treatment of Infective Endocarditis of the European Society of Cardiology (ESC). *Eur Heart J* 2009; 30:2369-2413.
7. Thuny F, Habib G: When should we operate on patients with acute infective endocarditis? *Heart* 2010; 96:892-897.
8. Chambers JC, Somerville J, Stone S, et al: Pulmonary autograft procedure for aortic valve disease: long-term results of a pioneer series. *Circulation* 1997; 96:2206-2214.
9. David TE, Ivanov J, Armstrong S, et al: Late results of heart valve replacement with the Hancock II bioprosthesis. *J Thorac Cardiovasc Surg* 2001; 121:268-277.
10. Hammermeister KE, Sethi GK, Henderson WG, et al: Outcomes 15 years after valve replacement with a mechanical versus a bioprosthetic valve: final report of the Veterans Affairs randomized trial. *J Am Coll Cardiol* 2000; 36:1152-1158.
11. Gordon SM, Serkey JM, Longworth DL, et al: Early onset prosthetic valve endocarditis: the Cleveland Clinic experience 1992-1997. *Ann Thorac Surg* 2000; 69:1388-1392.
12. McCarthy JT, Steckelberg JM: Infective endocarditis in patients receiving long-term hemodialysis. *Mayo Clin Proc* 2000; 75:1008-1014.
13. Crasta K, Daly CG, Mitchell D, et al: Bacteremia due to dental flossing. *J Clin Periodontol* 2009; 36:323-332.
14. Pettersson GB, Hussain ST, Shrestha NK, et al: Infective endocarditis: an atlas of disease progression for describing, staging, coding, and understanding the pathology. *J Thorac Cardiovasc Surg* 2014; 147:1142-1149.
15. Freedman LR: The pathogenesis of infective endocarditis. *J Antimicrob Chemother* 1987; 20(Suppl A):1-6.
16. Grant RT, Wood JR Jr, Jones TS: Heart valve irregularities in relation to subacute bacterial endocarditis. *Heart* 1928; 14:247.
17. Angrist AA, Oka M: Pathogenesis of bacterial endocarditis. *JAMA* 1963; 181:249-252.
18. Durack DT, Beeson PB, Petersdorf RG: Experimental bacterial endocarditis. 3. production and progress of the disease in rabbits. *Br J Exp Pathol* 1973; 54:142-151.
19. Mylonakis E, Calderwood SB: Infective endocarditis in adults. *N Engl J Med* 2001; 345:1318-1330.
20. Kanter MC, Hart RG: Neurologic complications of infective endocarditis. *Neurology* 1991; 41:1015-1020.
21. Piper C, Hetzer R, Korfer R, et al: The importance of secondary mitral valve involvement in primary aortic valve endocarditis: the mitral kissing vegetation. *Heart* 2002; 23:79-86.
22. Murdoch DR, Corey GR, Hoen B, et al: Clinical presentation, etiology, and outcome of infective endocarditis in the 21st century: the International Collaboration on Endocarditis–Prospective Cohort Study. *Arch Intern Med* 2009; 169:463-473.
23. Chu VH, Woods CW, Miro JM, et al: Emergence of coagulase-negative staphylococci as a cause of native valve endocarditis. *Clin Infect Dis* 2008; 46:232-242.
24. Hussain ST, Shrestha NK, Gordon SM, et al: Residual patient, anatomic, and surgical obstacles in treating active left-sided infective endocarditis. *J Thorac Cardiovasc Surg* 2014; 148:981-988.
25. David TE: The surgical treatment of patients with prosthetic valve endocarditis. *Semin Thorac Cardiovasc Surg* 1995; 7:47-53.
26. Chu VH, Miro JM, Hoen B, et al: Coagulase-negative staphylococcal prosthetic valve endocarditis—a contemporary update based on the International Collaboration on Endocarditis: prospective cohort study. *Heart* 2009; 95:570-576.
27. David TE, Gavra G, Feindel CM, et al: Surgical treatment of active infective endocarditis: a continued challenge. *J Thorac Cardiovasc Surg* 2007; 133:144-149.
28. Shrestha NK, Ledtke CS, Wang H, et al: Heart valve culture and sequencing to identify the infective endocarditis pathogen in surgically treated patients. *Ann Thorac Surg* 2015; 99:33-37.
29. Durack DT, Lukes AS, Bright DK: New criteria for diagnosis of infective endocarditis: utilization of specific echocardiographic findings. Duke Endocarditis Service. *Am J Cardiol* 1994; 96:200-209.
30. Habib G, Derumeaux G, Avierinos JF, et al: Value and limitations of the Duke criteria for the diagnosis of infective endocarditis. *J Am Coll Cardiol* 1999; 33:2023-2029.
31. Li JS, Sexton DJ, Mick N, et al: Proposed modifications to the Duke Criteria for the diagnosis of infective endocarditis. *Clin Infect Dis* 2000; 30:633-638.

32. Byrne JG, Rezai K, Sanchez JA, et al: Surgical management of endocarditis: The Society of Thoracic Surgeons clinical practice guideline. *Ann Thorac Surg* 2012; 91:2012-2019.

33. Misfeld M, Girrbach F, Etz CD: Surgery for infective endocarditis complicated by cerebral embolism: a consecutive series of 375 patients. *J Thorac Cardiovasc Surg* 2014; 147:1837-1846.

34. Thuny F, Di Salvo G, Belliard O, et al: Risk of embolism and death in infective endocarditis: prognostic value of echocardiography: a prospective multicenter study. *Circulation* 2005; 112:69-75.

35. Moon MR, Miller DC, Moore KA, et al: Treatment of endocarditis with valve replacement: the question of tissue versus mechanical prosthesis. *Ann Thorac Surg* 2001; 71:1164-1171.

36. Klieverik LM, Yacoub MH, Edwards S, et al: Surgical treatment of active native aortic valve endocarditis with allografts and mechanical prostheses. *Ann Thorac Surg* 2009; 88:1814-1821.

37. David TE, Regesta T, Gavra G, et al: Surgical treatment of paravalvular abscess: long-term results. *Eur J Cardiothorac Surg* 2007; 31:43-48.

38. Bedeir K, Reardon M, Ramlawi B: Infective endocarditis: perioperative management and surgical principles. *J Thorac Cardiovasc Surg* 2014; 147:1133-1141.

39. Pettersson G, Tingleff J, Joyce FS: Treatment of aortic valve endocarditis with the Ross procedure. *Eur J Cardiothorac Surg* 1998; 3:678-684.

40. Oswalt JD, Dewan SJ, Mueller MC, et al: Highlights of a ten-year experience with Ross procedure. *Ann Thorac Surg* 2001; 71:S332-335.

41. Heinz A, Dumfarth J, Ruttmann-Ulmer E, et al: Freestyle root replacement for complex destructive aortic valve endocarditis. *J Thorac Cardiovasc Surg* 2014; 147:1265-1270.

42. El-Hamamsy I, Stevens LM, Sarang Z, et al: Late outcomes following freestyle versus homograft aortic root replacement: results from a prospective randomized trial. *J Am Coll Cardiol* 2010; 55:368-376.

43. Miro JM, Anguera I, Cabell CH, et al: *Staphylococcus aureus* native valve endocarditis: report of 566 episodes from the International Collaboration on Endocarditis Merged Database. *Clin Infect Dis* 2005; 41:507-514.

44. Kang DH, Kim YJ, Kim SH, et al: Early surgery versus conventional treatment for infective endocarditis. *N Engl J Med* 2012; 366:2466-2473.

45. Thuny F, Beurtheret S, Mancini J, et al: The timing of surgery influences mortality and morbidity in adults with severe complicated infective endocarditis: a propensity analysis. *Eur Heart J* 2011; 32:2027-2033.

46. Ohara T, Nakatani S, Kokubo S, et al: Clinical predictors of in-hospital death and early surgery for infective endocarditis: results of CArdiac Disease REgistartion (CADRE), a nation-wide survey in Japan. *Int J Cardiol* 2013; 167:2688-2694.

47. Yankah AC, Pasic M, Klose H, et al: Homograft reconstruction of the aortic root for endocarditis with periannular abscess: a 17-year study. *Eur J Cardiothorac Surg* 2005; 28:69-75.

48. Manne MB, Shrestha NK, Lytle BW, et al: Outcomes after surgical treatment of native and prosthetic valve infective endocarditis. *Ann Thorac Surg* 2012; 93:489-494.

49. Leontyev S, Borger MA, Modi P, et al: Redo aortic valve surgery: influence of prosthetic valve endocarditis on outcomes. *J Thorac Cardiovasc Surg* 2011; 142:99-105.

50. Nishimura RA, Carabello BA, Faxon DP, et al: ACC/AHA 2008 guideline update on valvular heart disease: focused update on infective endocarditis. *J Am Coll Cardiol* 2008; 52:676-685.

32

Minimally Invasive Aortic Valve Surgery

Prem S. Shekar • Lawrence S. Lee • Lawrence H. Cohn

Aortic valve surgery started with the implantation of the Hufnagel valve in the descending thoracic aorta in 1956. Its evolution over time has culminated with the establishment of percutaneous catheter-based aortic valve replacement techniques. As a new paradigm in aortic valve replacement is ushered, there will be new challenges for the cardiac surgeons to not only maintain the efficacy and outcomes of conventional valve replacement but to provide it in a less invasive approach. Modern techniques will be measured against conventional procedures, especially in the older patients with multiple comorbidities. Minimally invasive aortic valve surgery holds promise as an effective operation with reduced pain, improved respiratory function, early recovery, and an overall reduction in trauma.

ESSENTIALS OF MINIMAL ACCESS AORTIC VALVE SURGERY

Reoperative minimal access aortic valve surgery is discussed in detail at the end of this chapter. We will first outline the known benefits and salient principles of and the essential ingredients for the conduct of primary minimal access aortic valve surgery. There are many potential benefits of minimal access aortic valve surgery:

1. It provides a cosmetically superior incision
2. There is reduced postoperative pain
3. There is faster postoperative recovery
4. There is improved postoperative respiratory function from preservation of a part of the sternum and the integrity of the costal margin
5. It can be performed with the same degree of ease and speed as a conventional operation with no difference in mortality
6. It provides access to the relevant parts of the heart and reduces dissection of other areas
7. It greatly facilitates a reoperation at a later date as the lower part of the pericardium remains closed.

There are some salient inviolate principles of minimal access aortic valve surgery:

1. Ability to safely apply a stable aortic cross-clamp
2. Ability to visualize the aortic valve completely and perform a successful replacement with the standard techniques
3. Ability to achieve the same degree of myocardial protection as through a midline sternotomy approach
4. Ability to deal with issues of the aortic root, ascending and arch of the aorta with relative ease and without the need for conversion
5. Ability to quickly convert to a standard midline sternotomy if compromising situations arise

The safety and reproducibility of minimal access aortic valve surgery depend on:

1. Availability of experienced cardiac anesthesiologists
2. Availability of transesophageal echocardiography (TEE) in every case and an experienced echocardiographer to interpret findings
3. Ability to place pulmonary artery catheters with pacing capabilities and transjugular coronary sinus catheters, if and when necessary
4. Ability to place percutaneous arterial and venous cardiopulmonary bypass canulae
5. Ability to use vacuum-assisted venous drainage on cardiopulmonary bypass
6. Availability of minimal access retractors and other relevant instruments that facilitate this operation
7. Ability to remotely monitor myocardial protection and distention by TEE
8. Availability of surgeons experienced with conventional aortic valve surgery and minimal access surgery.

APPROACHES

Whatever the surgical approach, today aortic valve replacement is done with the use of cardiopulmonary bypass and diastolic arrest of the heart. There are at least four different minimal access surgical approaches to the aortic valve:

1. Upper hemisternotomy
2. Right parasternal approach
3. Right anterior thoracotomy
4. Transverse sternotomy

The Upper Hemisternotomy Approach

This is undoubtedly the most popular of all minimal access approaches to the aortic valve.[1,2] This is performed through a 6- to 8-cm vertical midline incision over the upper part of the sternum, starting at or just above the level of the manubrio-sternal angle. The sternotomy is performed with the standard saw starting at the level of the sternal notch up to the level of the third or fourth intercostal space (Fig. 32-1). The sternotomy is then T'd off into the right or left third or fourth intercostal space using a narrow blade oscillating saw, taking care not to dive too deeply with it for risk of injuring mediastinal or pericardial structures. The decision to T into the third or fourth space can be made preoperatively with the chest x-ray being a guide to the amount of exposure that will be needed. We favor the fourth interspace because this almost always produces the ideal exposure. It is very important to ensure that the sternotomy is absolutely midline and that the midline sternotomy is not carried beyond the level of the transverse T. Failure to adhere to these principles will result in either a lateral fracture with resultant three sternal fragments or a continued lower extension of midline fracture which with retraction could result in a slow ongoing intraoperative or postoperative blood loss and also difficulty in closure. There is no need to prophylactically divide the right or left internal mammary arteries with this incision. If care is taken not to damage them, they will usually gently retract away.

A small-blade retractor spreads the sternum. The pericardium is opened in the midline (Fig. 32-2), T'd inferiorly, and at least three pericardial stay sutures are applied to either side and the needles are left on. The retractor is removed and the pericardium is tacked to the dermis of the skin and tied down. This facilitates exposure by elevating the pericardial contents

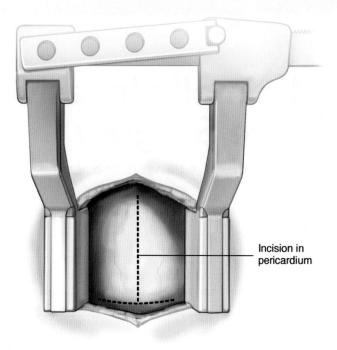

FIGURE 32-2 Midline incision in the pericardium.

forward into the operating field. The retractor is then repositioned. Care must be taken during reopening the retractor because sudden retraction with elevated cardiac structures could impede venous return, causing a sudden drop in cardiac output, and leading to acute refractory decompensation in patients with severe aortic stenosis.

We perform an epiaortic ultrasound to exclude atheromatous disease in the ascending aorta before proceeding to systemic heparinization and ascending aortic cannulation in the standard fashion. Right atrial venous cannulation is accomplished directly through the appendage (when easily accessible) (Fig. 32-3) or with a percutaneous venous cannula inserted via the right or left femoral vein. There are a variety of custom long venous canulae that are available for the same (usually 20- or 22-French), and they are inserted using the Seldinger technique. The cannula is positioned within the right atrium with the tip in the superior vena-cava using transesophageal echocardiographic guidance. The patient is then placed on cardiopulmonary bypass. We use tepid bypass with core cooling to 34 to 35°C. The need for vacuum-assisted venous drainage to facilitate this operation cannot be overemphasized.

A retrograde cardioplegia catheter can be placed in the coronary sinus via the right atrial appendage. This may require a minor adjustment to reduce the angulation of the catheter and its insertion can be facilitated by the use of transesophageal echocardiography. Alternatively, this catheter can be placed by the anesthesiologists before surgical incision via the transjugular route. Although we routinely use a transaortic left ventricular vent, a right superior pulmonary vein or a left atrial dome vent can also be easily placed via this incision.

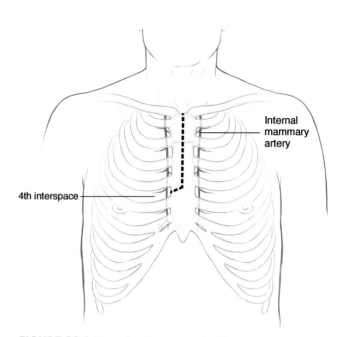

FIGURE 32-1 Upper hemisternotomy incision.

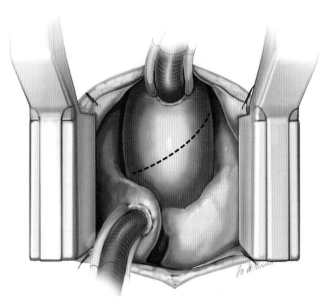

FIGURE 32-3 The pericardium has been tacked up and the patient has been canulated in the standard fashion. Oblique aortotomy has been marked.

The operation then proceeds as usual. The aorta is cross-clamped and we use 1 L of 8:1 cold blood antegrade cardioplegia. TEE is used to monitor left ventricular distention in patients who may have aortic insufficiency. Retrograde cardioplegia and additional doses of cardioplegia are administered as necessary. Standard aortic valve replacement is then carried through an oblique aortotomy (Fig. 32-4). Upon completion of the procedure, the patient is rewarmed and the aortotomy is closed. A de-airing needle is placed in the ascending aorta before removal of the aortic cross-clamp.

Almost always the heart recovers spontaneous sinus rhythm. When the heart recovers into ventricular fibrillation, it will need to be defibrillated using the external defibrillator pads placed before commencement of the operation. Defibrillation can be facilitated by turning the cardiopulmonary bypass flows down to decompress the heart and other appropriate pharmacologic maneuvers. It is usually quite difficult to introduce internal defibrillator blades through this incision, although pediatric blades can be placed successfully on occasion. Appropriate preoperative placement of external defibrillator pads are of paramount importance. The heart is de-aired using TEE guidance. In the absence of the ability to reach in and agitate the heart, a combination of ventricular filling, table positioning, and external compression is used to successfully de-air the left heart. Although this can always be successfully completed, patience may be an important tool to facilitate this. It is important remember that successful and complete de-airing does not occur until the blood has begun to circulate through the pulmonary and systemic circuits and the heart has started to eject normally.

Before emergence from bypass, pacing wires and drainage tubes will have to be placed (Fig. 32-5). It is very important to perform these placements with the heart decompressed on bypass so as to prevent injury. Invariably, there is an adequate amount of atrial and ventricular myocardium exposed to place pacing wires. We usually bring these wires out in the right inframammary area through the right-sided T. We place fluted silastic drains from a subxiphoid approach. Small incisions are made in the subxiphoid area and long grabbing forceps are used to make two retrosternal tunnels, one of which will puncture the pericardium to facilitate placement of a pericardial drain and the other will remain in the retrosternal plane. These are placed with a combination of tactile and visual control. In cases in which drains were not

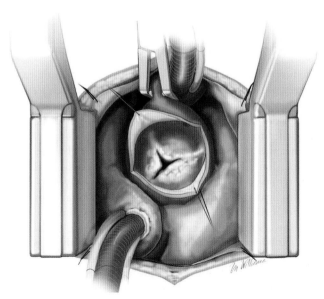

FIGURE 32-4 The aorta was opened after cross-clamping, exposing a calcified trileaflet aortic valve.

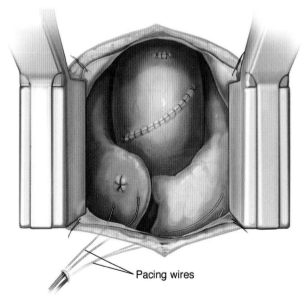

FIGURE 32-5 Theaortotomy was closed after valve replacement, and epicardial pacing wires were placed.

placed before separation from bypass and decannulation, we recommend opening the right or left pleural space and placement of transpleural drainage tubes. Placement of subxiphoid drains is not recommended after the heart is full. The wean from cardiopulmonary bypass is then performed in the standard fashion followed by decannulation and protamine administration.

The pericardium is left open. While policing the area for bleeding, some of the important sites are the coronary sinus from the placement of the retrograde catheter (which will need full sternotomy conversion for control), areas of pacing wire placement and drainage tube entry (which may or may not require conversion to full sternotomy and/or institution of bypass for visualization and control), sites of left ventricular vents, the lower edge of the sternotomy/pericardiotomy, and the internal mammary vessels on the side of the T. The sternum is closed using three or four horizontal sternal wires and an oblique wire placed between the lower intact segment of the sternum and the T'd off segment (Fig. 32-6)

Minimally invasive aortic valve replacement via the upper hemisternotomy approach was originally developed by Cosgrove and colleagues at the Cleveland Clinic[1] and soon after by Cohn and colleagues at the Brigham and Women's Hospital in Boston.[2] Johnston and Roselli[3] reported their results involving over 2300 patients undergoing minimally invasive aortic valve surgery over an 18-year period at the Cleveland Clinic, where upper hemisternotomy remains the preferred approach today for isolated aortic valve surgery. Mihaljevic and colleagues[4] from the Brigham group reported their experience with 1000 minimally invasive valve operations, of which 526 were aortic valve procedures. They reported low levels of morbidity and mortality equal to or better than conventional techniques.

Numerous authors have published their experience with the upper hemisternotomy minimal access aortic valve replacement and most report excellent outcomes. Ghanta et al[5] compared outcomes and cost of minimally invasive aortic valve replacement versus conventional surgery in a multi-institutional regional cohort. They found that 93% of minimally invasive aortic valve operations were performed via upper hemisternotomy with mortality and morbidity equivalent to the full sternotomy approach. Upper hemisternotomy was also associated with decreased ventilator time, decreased blood product use, earlier discharge, and reduced total hospital cost. Gilmanov et al[6] demonstrated excellent outcomes in 853 patients with low overall morbidity, low conversion rate, and comparable long-term survival to that of conventional aortic valve replacement. Upper hemisternotomy for aortic valve replacement has been performed safely in higher risk populations including elderly patients[7] as well as those with left ventricular dysfunction,[8,9] with morbidity and mortality comparable to conventional sternotomy techniques.

Recently, the advent of sutureless aortic prostheses has further kindled interest in minimally invasive aortic valve replacement. Dalen et al[10] reported successful implantation of a sutureless aortic valve bioprosthesis via upper hemisternotomy in 189 patients and found no difference in cross-clamp time, cardiopulmonary bypass time, early postoperative outcomes, or 2-year survival when compared to propensity score matched patients who underwent the operation with full sternotomy. Nonrandomized multicenter clinical trials in Europe also demonstrated safe and successful minimally invasive implantation of a sutureless aortic valve prosthesis through upper hemisternotomy, albeit with slightly longer operative time than with conventional sternotomy but comparable 5-year outcomes.[11]

The Right Parasternal Approach

The first foray into the world of minimal access aortic valve surgery was with use of this approach. This approach seemed to be the most logical and elegant at a time when the focus was on the morbidity of the sternotomy and surgeons were compelled to come up with this alternative.

This was performed via a vertical upper right parasternal incision. The second, third, and fourth costal cartilages were removed and the right internal mammary vessels were usually ligated and divided. It provided a similar approach to the aortic valve as an upper hemisternotomy incision described before and techniques of cannulation, cardiopulmonary bypass, myocardial protection, and valve replacement were the same. It soon gave way to the more elegant and simple upper hemisternotomy approach. One particular problem associated with the right parasternal approach was the incidence of lung herniation, which was physiologically disturbing aside from being a cosmetic disaster and

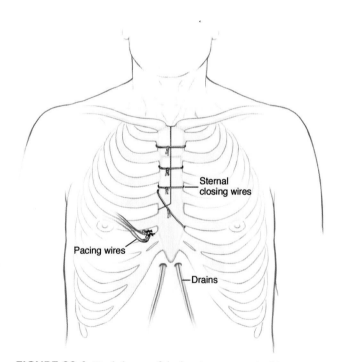

FIGURE 32-6 Final closure of the hemisternotomy incision.

often required a second operation and mesh closure of the defect.

Cohn[12] and Minale et al[13] described their experiences with the right parasternal incision for aortic valve replacement in 1998. They reported fairly low mortality and morbidity rates and had, at that time, recommended the approach for minimal access aortic valve surgery, but soon moved to a hemisternotomy approach because of occasional right lung herniation.

The Right Anterior Thoracotomy Approach

This is another method to perform minimal access primary aortic valve replacement in adults. The right anterior thoracotomy and the upper hemisternotomy are the most commonly used approaches to minimally invasive aortic valve surgery today.

This technique is usually performed via the second right intercostal space. Owing to the relatively high nature of the thoracotomy, it never reaches around to become a true anterolateral thoracotomy. One can visualize why this would be unappealing for a female patient because the incision would traverse horizontally across the upper part of the right breast, which could lead to scarring and disfigurement. This incision is carried to the right sternal edge and through this incision the right side of the aorta is easily visualized; and with appropriate strategically placed pericardial retraction sutures the area of interest could easily be moved into the operative field. Aortic and venous cannulation could be performed centrally or peripherally, although the latter may be preferable since the operative field is generally smaller and the aortic valve sits deeper within the wound with this approach than with a mini-sternotomy. The rest of the operation is fairly routine for any minimal access aortic valve surgery. Special cross-clamps may be required to facilitate this procedure.

This operation also has some relevance and indication for patients requiring isolated aortic valve surgery in whom sternotomy needs to be avoided at all costs. A unique subset of such patients is those who are disabled and routinely ambulate with the use of shoulder crutches. These patients could be made to ambulate early with the use of their crutches without the risk of sternal dehiscence by the use of this approach. Another possible subset of patients includes those with heavily irradiated or damaged sternum.

The exposure via this incision could be optimized in cases with poor exposure by extending it across the sternum with a transverse sternotomy through the manubrio-sternal angle. Reoperative aortic valve replacement is particularly difficult via this incision and the authors sincerely discourage the approach for a reoperation.

Glauber et al[14] reported their results with minimally invasive aortic valve replacement via the right anterior mini-thoracotomy approach in 138 patients and compared outcomes to a propensity-matched group undergoing full sternotomy. The right anterior mini-thoracotomy group was associated with lower incidence of blood transfusion and postoperative atrial fibrillation and shorter mechanical ventilation time and hospital length of stay, with comparable perioperative morbidity. Gilmanov et al[15] demonstrated that minimally invasive aortic valve replacement through right anterior thoracotomy can be safely performed with acceptable mortality and morbidity in octogenarians. When compared to propensity-matched patients undergoing full sternotomy, the minimal access group had shorter time to extubation and shorter hospital stay with no difference in perioperative complications or 5-year survival rates.

As with the upper hemisternotomy approach, recently several groups have reported the successful implantation of a sutureless aortic valve prosthesis through a right anterior thoracotomy approach. Vola et al[16] and Gilmanov et al[17] demonstrated in 71 and 515 patients, respectively, that minimally invasive aortic valve replacement with various sutureless prostheses can be safely and reproducibly performed via the right anterior thoracotomy incision. Both groups observed acceptable hemodynamic outcomes and low perioperative complication rates.

The Transverse Sternotomy Approach

There are anecdotal reports of this incision for minimal access aortic valve surgery.

Typically an 8- to 10-cm transverse incision is made over the manubrio-sternal angle extending onto either side. Bilateral second costal cartilages have to be excised and both internal mammary pedicles have to be ligated and divided. A transverse sternotomy is performed across the sternal angle. The retractor is placed and the sternal edges are retracted in a craniocaudal plane. Adequate exposure is obtained through this incision to permit central aortic cannulation and a routine aortic valve replacement; however, venous cannulation, retrograde coronary sinus catheter placement and vent placement (except transaortic) may have to be performed percutaneously.

For reasons that the mammary arteries are sacrificed, this incision never gained much popularity.

Lee et al,[18] De Amicis et al,[19] and Aris et al,[20] reported their small experiences with the transverse sternotomy approach and good results. However, Bridgewater et al[21] reported an unacceptably high incidence of morbidity (reexploration for bleeding, paravalvular leaks, and longer hospital stay) and mortality with this approach.

Karimov et al[22] reported a series of 85 patients who underwent an upper V-type ministernotomy in the second intercostal space with excellent results.

REOPERATIVE MINIMAL ACCESS AORTIC VALVE SURGERY

The Brigham and Women's Hospital has pioneered minimal access reoperative aortic valve replacement in patients who previously have undergone coronary artery bypass grafting or other cardiac surgery. We popularized and published our data and have since had more experience with the technique.

According to the STS database, patients requiring a reoperative aortic valve replacement after previous coronary artery bypass grafting have a mortality risk of about 8 to 12% from the procedure. The risks are associated with the performance of a reoperation in an older patient with more comorbidities and patent/diseased bypass grafts.

The Need for This Operation

1. There is a definite subgroup of patients who have undergone coronary bypass surgery who had mild or no aortic stenosis at the time of their original operation who will eventually progress to have severe aortic stenosis over time. This has sparked off a whole discussion on the management of moderate aortic stenosis with coronary artery disease[23]
2. These patients are older, sicker, and have many comorbid conditions
3. They need a simple, safe, and effective operation
4. The areas of interest are the ascending aorta and aortic root
5. Dissection of the rest of the heart and bypass grafts provide no additional benefit and are potentially harmful
6. Clipping the left internal mammary artery is not mandatory with alternative protection strategies.

Operative Strategy

Preoperatively, a computed tomogram of the chest with angiography and three-dimensional reconstruction is performed to ascertain the exact location of the old bypass grafts and their relative location to the sternum (especially the left internal mammary artery).[24] Coronary angiography and percutaneous coronary and graft intervention with drug-eluting stents are done as appropriate to optimize the revascularization as far as possible. Heart failure is controlled medically.

All patients need intraoperative transesophageal echocardiography and a pulmonary artery catheter with atrial and ventricular pacing wire placement capabilities, which should ideally be placed before incision. Accurate placement of external defibrillator pads is emphasized because internal paddles cannot be introduced in these patients.

All patients need peripheral cannulation for cardiopulmonary bypass, either right axillary or percutaneous femoral venous cannulation. Appropriate arterial line placement is needed to facilitate need for circulatory arrest and antegrade cerebral perfusion if required.[25] A standard upper hemisternotomy incision is made with a T into the right fourth intercostal space (Figs. 32-7 and 32-8). The anterior table split is performed with the use of an oscillating saw, whereas the posterior table split is performed on cardiopulmonary bypass using straight Mayo scissors starting from the top down (preferably from the assistant's side of the table). When the left internal mammary artery graft is close to the left side or the middle of the sternum, a preplanned one-third to

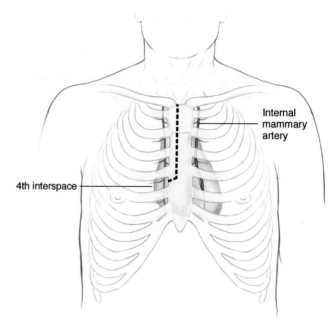

FIGURE 32-7 The upper hemisternotomy incision has been marked.

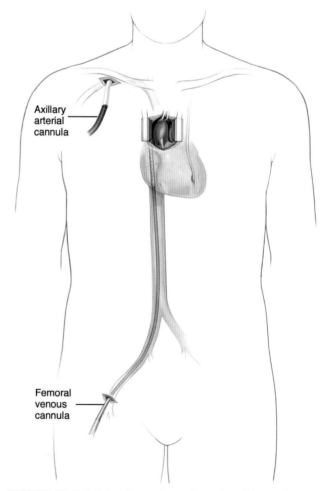

FIGURE 32-8 Peripheral cannulation for cardiopulmonary bypass.

two-thirds sternotomy to the right is performed. The right pleural space is widely opened. Only 5 to 10 mm dissection is performed underneath the left sternal edge, enough to facilitate the placement of the Kuros-Baxter® retractor. The rest of the mediastinal and aortic dissection is performed on cardiopulmonary bypass. Care is taken not to injure previous saphenous vein or radial arterial bypasses. It is not necessary to visualize the left internal mammary artery graft.

Core cooling should wait until after there is an ability to place an aortic cross-clamp. Moderate-to-deep hypothermia facilitates low flow states and reduces myocardial oxygen demand, which is important because the left internal mammary artery will continue to perfuse the heart for the duration of the operation. A retrograde coronary sinus catheter is placed through the right atrial appendage using TEE guidance. Usually, enough right atrial appendage is seen to place this catheter. Alternatively, a transjugular catheter can be placed before incision. After cross-clamping the aorta, 1 L antegrade cold blood cardioplegia is delivered through the aortic root. Thereafter, 500 cc of cold retrograde blood cardioplegia is used. Simultaneously, systemic hyperkalemia is achieved by instilling 40 mEq of potassium into the cardiopulmonary bypass. Systemic hyperkalemia will achieve diastolic arrest in the left anterior descending artery territory that is perfused by the left internal mammary artery distal to the aortic cross-clamp. All through the operation, frequent doses of antegrade (through the coronaries and grafts using perfusion canulae) and retrograde cardioplegia are delivered. Systemic hyperkalemia is maintained at a level of 6 to 7 mEq/L. This keeps the myocardium fairly quiescent during the procedure. Needless to say, heavy doses of potassium may leave the patient with severe hyperkalemia that may not be cleared in the setting of renal dysfunction. In addition to being judicious in such cases, it is imperative that the perfusion technologists be able to provide ultrafiltration as well.

The aortotomy is dictated by the location of previous bypass grafts. Although in some cases a standard oblique aortotomy can be made, most cases require a modified aortotomy such as a lazy S or a lateral vertical aortotomy (Fig. 32-9). The exposure should be adequate and an expeditious valve replacement is the key to success. We aim to keep the cross-clamp time under 60 minutes. In most cases, there will be continuous back bleeding through the left main orifice from the open left internal mammary artery graft. During debridement and suture placement in the left coronary area, the bypass flows can be reduced or briefly turned off to facilitate exposure. Rewarming is started after the valve is seated. The aortotomy is closed in the standard fashion and a de-airing needle is placed before removal of the aortic cross-clamp. The heart often recovers spontaneous sinus rhythm. Defibrillation is achieved via the external pads if required. The de-airing and wean from cardiopulmonary bypass is as described before.

Drainage tubes are always placed through the right pleural space. Subxiphoid placement is not possible and strongly

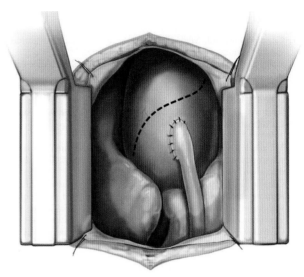

FIGURE 32-9 This is a lazy S oblique aortotomy keeping the grafts to the left.

discouraged. Rarely, when the right pleural space is completely fused, the silastic drain could be brought out in the supraclavicular area. It may be possible to place atrial pacing wires, but placement of ventricular wires is almost always quite difficult. Routine use of pulmonary artery catheter-based pacing leads is also possible. Closure is fairly standard, as described before, and care must be taken during the placement of wires on the left side of the sternum and the oblique lower wire (Fig. 32-10).

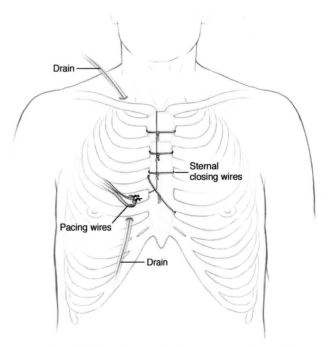

FIGURE 32-10 Final closure, also showing an occasional drainage tube in the supraclavicular space.

REFERENCES

1. Cosgrove DM 3rd, Sabik JF: Minimally invasive approach for aortic valve operations. *Ann Thorac Surg* 1996; 62(2):596-597.
2. Cohn LH, Adams DH, Couper GS, et al: Minimally invasive cardiac valve surgery improves patient satisfaction while reducing costs of cardiac valve replacement and repair. *Ann Surg* 1997; 226(4):421-426; discussion 427-428.
3. Johnston DR, Roselli EE: Minimally invasive aortic valve surgery: Cleveland Clinic experience. *Ann Cardiothorac Surg* 2015; 4(2):140-147.
4. Mihaljevic T, Cohn LH, Unic D, et al: One thousand minimally invasive valve operations: early and late results. *Ann Surg* 2004; 240(3):529-534; discussion 534.
5. Ghanta RK, Lapar DJ, Kern JA, et al: Minimally invasive aortic valve replacement provides equivalent outcomes at reduced cost compared with conventional aortic valve replacement: A real-world multi-institutional analysis. *J Thorac Cardiovasc Surg* 2015; 149:1060-1065.
6. Gilmanov D, Solinas M, Farnet PA, et al: Minimally invasive aortic valve replacement: 12-year single center experience. *Ann Cardiothorac Surg* 2015; 4(2):160-169.
7. Sharony R, Grossi EA, Saunders PC, et al: Minimally invasive aortic valve surgery in the elderly: a case-control study. *Circulation* 2003; 108(Suppl 1):II43-47.
8. Tabata M, Aranki SF, Fox JA, et al: Minimally invasive aortic valve replacement in left ventricular dysfunction. *Asian Cardiovasc Thorac Ann* 2007; 15(3):225-228.
9. Tabata M, Umakanthan R, Cohn LH, et al: Early and late outcomes of 1000 minimally invasive aortic valve operations. *Eur J Cardiothorac Surg* 2008; 33(4):537-541.
10. Dalen M, Biancari F, Rubino AS, et al: Ministernotomy versus full sternotomy aortic valve replacement with a sutureless bioprosthesis: a multicenter study. *Ann Thorac Surg* 2015; 99:524-531.
11. Shrestha M, Fischlein T, Meuris B, et al: European multicenter experience with the sutureless Perceval valve: clinical and hemodynamic outcomes up to 5 years in over 700 patients. *Eur J Cardiothorac Surg* 2015; Mar 6:1-8.
12. Cohn LH: Minimally invasive aortic valve surgery: technical considerations and results with the parasternal approach. *J Card Surg* 1998; 13(4):302-305.
13. Minale C, Reifschneider HJ, Schmitz E, Uckmann FP: Minimally invasive aortic valve replacement without sternotomy. Experience with the first 50 cases. *Eur J Cardiothorac Surg* 1998; 14(Suppl 1):S126-129.
14. Glauber M, Miceli A, Gilmanov D, et al: Right anterior minithoracotomy versus conventional aortic valve replacement: a propensity score matched study. *J Thorac Cardiovasc Surg* 2013; 145(5):1222-1226.
15. Gilmanov D, Farneti PA, Ferrarini M, et al: Full sternotomy versus right anterior minithoracotomy for isolated aortic valve replacement in octogenarians: a propensity-matched study. *Interact Cardiovasc Thorac Surg* 2015; 20(6):732-741.
16. Vola M, Albertini A, Campisi S, et al: Right anterior minithoracotomy aortic valve replacement with a sutureless bioprosthesis: early outcomes and 1-year follow-up from 2 European centers. *J Thorac Cardiovasc Surg* 2015; 149:1052-1057.
17. Gilmanov D, Miceli A, Ferrarinin M, et al: Aortic valve replacement through right anterior minithoracotomy: can sutureless technology improve clinical outcomes? *Ann Thorac Surg* 2014; 98:1585-1592.
18. Lee JW, Lee SK, Choo SJ, Song H, Song MG: Routine minimally invasive aortic valve procedures. *Cardiovasc Surg* 2000; 8(6):484-490.
19. De Amicis V, Ascione R, Iannelli G, et al: Aortic valve replacement through a minimally invasive approach. *Tex Heart Inst J* 1997; 24(4):353-355.
20. Aris A, Padro JM, Camara ML: Minimally invasive aortic valve replacement. *Rev Esp Cardiol* 1997; 50(11):778-781.
21. Bridgewater B, Steyn RS, Ray S, Hooper T: Minimally invasive aortic valve replacement through a transverse sternotomy: a word of caution. *Heart* 1998; 79(6):605-607.
22. Karimov JH, Santarelli F, Murzi M, Glauber M: A technique of an upper V-type ministernotomy in the second intercostal space. *Interact Cardiovasc Thorac Surg* 2009; 9(6):1021-1022.
23. Filsoufi F, Aklog L, Adams DH, Byrne JG: Management of mild to moderate aortic stenosis at the time of coronary artery bypass grafting. *J Heart Valve Dis* 2002; 11(Suppl 1):S45-49.
24. Gasparovic H, Rybicki FJ, Millstine J, et al: Three dimensional computed tomographic imaging in planning the surgical approach for redo cardiac surgery after coronary revascularization. *Eur J Cardiothorac Surg* 2005; 28(2):244-249.
25. Shekar PS, Ehsan A, Gilfeather MS, Lekowski RW Jr, Couper GS: Arterial pressure monitoring during cardiopulmonary bypass using axillary arterial cannulation. *J Cardiothorac Vasc Anesth* 2005; 19(5):665-666.

Percutaneous Treatment of Aortic Valve Disease

Stephanie L. Mick • Lars G. Svensson

The history of percutaneous treatment of aortic valve disease began with the work of Danish researcher, H.R. Andersen, who in the late 1980s experimented in an animal lab with a balloon-expandable stented valve.[1] The technology was later acquired by PVT Company, further developed, and later sold to Edwards. Additional early work was done by Alain Cribier[2,3] and subsequently the valve was adopted in the United States and further modified. The initial approach taken by Cribier was to insert the valve via the femoral vein, then snaking the catheter through the mitral valve and into the aortic annulus via transeptal puncture. This turned out to be a fairly cumbersome and difficult procedure with a fairly high mortality rate and an 8.1% stroke rate. At the same time, animal experiments were carried out by Michael Mack, Todd Dewey, and Lars Svensson,[4,5] using the transapical (TA) approach to insert the aortic valve. Concurrently, John Webb et al[6,7] were also developing a TA aortic valve method, and subsequently they introduced the retrograde transfemoral (TF) artery approach. This latter technique became feasible once Edwards developed a catheter that could be flexed to get around the aortic arch to access the aortic valve. At the same time the Edwards balloon-expandable valve was being developed, Medtronic introduced a nitinol-based, self-expanding percutaneous valve system, the CoreValve. Following feasibility studies,[5,8] the safety and effectiveness of both valves were established through the Placement of Aortic Transcatheter Valves (PARTNER) trial and the US CoreValve pivotal trial and both valves are currently approved by US Food and Drug Administration (FDA) for use in patients who are at extreme or high risk (owing to comorbidities or anatomical considerations) for conventional surgery in the United States.[9-11]

VALVES

At present in the United States, there are only two transcatheter valves approved for use in patients who are at extreme or high risk (owing to comorbidities or anatomical considerations) for conventional surgery.

The balloon-expandable Edwards valves consist of bovine pericardium fashioned into a trileaflet valve within a short cylindrical stent, available in sizes 23, 26, and 29 to treat annular sizes from 18 to 27 mm. There are three generations of SAPIEN valves (SAPIEN, SAPIEN XT, and SAPIEN 3) that differ by stent material and construction (Fig. 33-1) as well delivery device size (Table 33-1) and other delivery device characteristics. At the time of publication, the commercially available generation is the SAPIEN XT in the United States with the SAPIEN 3 commercially available only in Europe. However, this generation is almost certain to replace the SAPIEN XT in the United States in the coming years. The SAPIEN valves can be delivered via retrograde (eg, TF, transaortic, transcarotid, transaxillary/subclavian) and antegrade (TA) approaches. The self-expanding Medtronic CoreValve is constructed of porcine pericardium mounted in a nitinol stent that anchors within the aortic annulus and extends superiorly to anchor in the ascending aorta. It is available in sizes 23, 26, 29, and 31 to fit annulus sizes 18 to 29 mm (Fig. 33-2, Table 33-1). The CoreValve can only be delivered using retrograde approaches.

PIVOTAL TRIALS

The major landmark trials in the percutaneous treatment of aortic valve disease are the PARTNER and the CoreValve Pivotal Trials. In prospective randomized fashion, the PARTNER Trial compared balloon-expandable (SAPIEN generation) transcatheter aortic valve replacement (TAVR) with valve and medical management in inoperable (combined risk of serious morbidity or mortality exceeding at least 50% and two surgeons agreeing the patient was inoperable) patients in its IB cohort and with surgical valve replacement in high risk (Society of Thoracic Surgeons (STS) >10%) patients in its IA cohort. Likewise, the CoreValve Pivotal Trials compared self-expandable TAVR with medical and surgical treatments in similar cohorts.

Transcatheter Aortic Valve Replacement Versus Medical Therapy

In the PARTNER IB cohort, inoperable patients were randomly assigned to SAPIEN TAVR or medical management. TAVR was associated with improved 1- and 2-year mortality

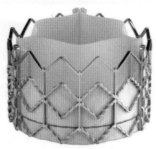 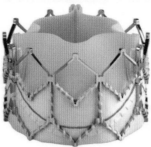 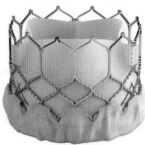

SAPIEN
Stainless steel frame
Bovine pericardium

SAPIEN XT
Cobalt-chromium frame
Bovine pericardium

SAPIEN 3
Cobalt-chromium frame
Outer skirt
Bovine Pericardium

FIGURE 33-1 Three generations of balloon-expandable Edwards SAPIEN valves. (Used with permission from Edwards Lifesciences LLC, Irvine, CA.)

(30.7% 1 year, 43.4% 2 year) compared with medical (including the use of balloon valvuloplasty) management (50.7% 1 year, 68% 2 year). The rate of the composite end point of death or repeat hospitalization was also reduced with TAVR (42.5 vs 71.6%). The stroke rate was significantly higher in the TAVR group than that in the medical therapy group at 30 days (6.7 vs 1.7%) and at 2 years (13.8 vs 5.5%).[10,12] It should be noted that TAVR improved survival in patients with an STS score of <15% but not in those with an STS score of ≥15%.[9]

These very convincing results with the balloon-expandable valve led to the conclusion that a randomized trial comparing self-expanding (CoreValve) TAVR and medical therapy could not ethically be performed. Instead, a prospective single-arm study, the CoreValve Extreme Risk US Pivotal Trial, was used to compare CoreValve TAVR to a prespecified estimate of 12-month mortality or major stroke with medical therapy (43%).[13] Nearly 500 patients underwent attempted treatment with CoreValve. In those patients, the rate of all-cause mortality or major stroke at 1 year was significantly lower

TABLE 33-1: Characteristics of Balloon-Expandable Edwards SAPIEN Valves and Self-Expanding Medtronic CoreValve

	SAPIEN	SAPIEN XT	SAPIEN 3	CoreValve EVOLUT	EVOLUT R
Frame	Stainless steel	Cobalt-chromium	Cobalt-chromium	Nitinol	Nitinol
Leaflets	Bovine pericardium	Bovine pericardium	Bovine pericardium	Porcine pericardium	Porcine pericardium
Expansion type	Balloon	Balloon	Balloon	Self-expanding (post-expansion balloon dilation possible)	Recapturable and repositionable prior to final valve release
Special features			Outer skirt to minimize paravalvular leak	Retrievable and repositionable prior to final valve release	Extended sealing skirt
Antegrade access (transapical)	+	+	+	−	−
Retrograde access (eg, transfemoral, transaortic)	+	+	+	+	+
FDA Approval	+	+	+	+	+
Annulus diameters (mm)	18-25	16-27	18-28	18-29	18-26
Valve Sizes	23, 26	20, 23, 26, 29	23, 26, 29	23, 26, 29, 31	23, 26, 29
Delivery sheath sizes	22 Fr (size 23 valve) 24 Fr (size 26 valve)	16 Fr expandable sheath (valve sizes 20, 23) 18 Fr expandable sheath (size 26 valve) 20 Fr expandable sheath (size 29 valve)	14 Fr expandable sheath (valve sizes 23, 26) 16 Fr expandable sheath (size 29 valve)	18 Fr sheath	14 Fr-equivalent System with In-Line™ Sheath

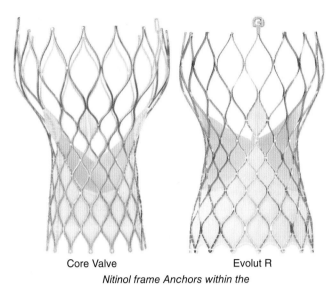

Core Valve   Evolut R
*Nitinol frame Anchors within the
aortic annulus and ascending aorta
Porcine Pericardium*

FIGURE 33-2 Two generations of Medtronic self-expanding valves. (© Medtronic 2016.)

than the prespecified expected rate (26 vs 43%), echoing the results of the PARTNER Trial.[13]

Given the known dismal prognosis of nonsurgically managed severe symptomatic aortic stenosis,[14-16] it was perhaps not surprising that aortic valve replacement was found to be associated with obviously increased survival in inoperable patients. With regard to comparison of TAVR and high-risk aortic valve replacement, the differences are subtler.

Transcatheter Aortic Valve Replacement Versus Surgery

The PARTNER Trial found similar 30-day (3.4 and 6.5%, p = .07), 1-year (24.3 and 26.8%), and 2-year (33.9 and 35.0%) mortality rates between SAPIEN TAVR and surgical valve replacement in patients at high risk for surgery randomized to either SAPIEN TAVR or surgery.

The combined stroke and transient ischemic attack rate was more frequent in the patients assigned to TAVR at 30 days (5.5% TAVR vs 2.4% surgery, p = .04) and at 1 year (8.7% TAVR vs 4.3% surgery, p = .04). The difference was of borderline significance at 2 years (11.2 vs 6.5%, p = .05). More patients undergoing TAVR reported symptom improvement at 30 days, but at 1 year, symptom improvement was similar in the two groups. At 30 days, TAVR was associated with more frequent major vascular complications (11.0 vs 3.2%) and surgery was associated with more frequent major bleeding episodes (19.5 vs 9.3%) and new-onset atrial fibrillation (16.0 vs 8.6%). The rate of new pacemaker requirement at 30 days was similar between the TAVR and surgical groups (3.8 vs 3.6%). Moderate or severe paravalvular aortic regurgitation was more common after TAVR than surgery at 30 days, 1 year, and 2 years and, importantly, was associated with increased late mortality.[10,12]

As in PARTNER, the US CoreValve High Risk Study found no difference in 30-day mortality in patients at high risk for surgery randomized to CoreValve TAVR or surgery (3.3 and 4.5%). However, unlike PARTNER, the 1-year mortality rate was lower in the CoreValve TAVR group than that in the surgical group (14.2 vs 19.1%, p < .0001 for noninferiority, p = .04 for superiority).[13,17] It is to be noted, that diabetes was more common in the surgery group compared with the TAVR cohort (45.4 vs 34.9%; p = .003), and this among other factors has led to questions about conclusions regarding the true survival benefit to TAVR over surgery in this trial.[18]

CoreValve TAVR was found to be noninferior to surgery with respect to echocardiographic indices of valve stenosis, functional status and quality of life at 1 year, and exploratory analysis suggested a reduction in the rate of major adverse cardiovascular and cerebrovascular events with TAVR. Unlike PARTNER, no increase in the risk of stroke was observed with CoreValve TAVR at 30 days (4.9% TAVR, 6.2% surgery) or 1 year (8.8% TAVR, 12.6% surgery). Major vascular complications, cardiac perforation, and permanent pacemaker implantation were more frequent after CoreValve TAVR. Life-threatening/disabling hemorrhage, acute kidney injury, and new-onset or worsening atrial fibrillation were more common after surgery.

In the PARTNER 2A trial, TAVR was studied for in intermediate risk populations. There was no difference in disabling stroke but higher risk of need for permanent pacemaker and paravalvular aortic insufficiency in TAVR than in surgical valve replacement. The FDA approved TAVR for use in intermediate risk patients in August 2016. There is interest in extending TAVR to broader, low risk populations. High-quality, randomized control trials are needed prior to such extension, and the PARTNER-3 study comparing TAVR to surgical valve replacement in low-risk patients is currently underway at the time of publication of this chapter.

COMPARISON OF CURRENTLY AVAILABLE VALVES

There is only one randomized comparison of balloon-expandable and self-expandable valves at this time. In the Comparison of Transcatheter Heart Valves in High Risk Patients With Severe Aortic Stenosis: Medtronic CoreValve versus Edwards SAPIEN XT (CHOICE) trial, 241 patients undergoing TF TAVR were randomized to either the SAPIEN XT or the CoreValve device.

The primary end point of this trial was "device success," a composite end point of four components: successful vascular access and deployment of the device with retrieval of the delivery system, correct position of the device, intended performance of the valve without moderate or severe insufficiency, and only one valve implanted in the correct anatomical location.

Owing to significantly lower residual more-than-mild aortic regurgitation with the balloon-expandable valve than with the self-expanding valve (4.1 vs 18.3%, p < .001) and less frequent need for implantation of more than one valve with the balloon-expandable valve (0.8 vs 5.8%, p = .03), the balloon-expandable SAPIEN XT valve showed a significantly higher device success rate than the self-expanding CoreValve.

Placement of a permanent pacemaker also was considerably less frequent in the balloon-expandable valve group (17.3 vs 37.6%, $p = .001$). The all-cause mortality and stroke rate at 30 days in patients receiving either valve were similar; 1 year data are pending.[19]

INSERTION OF PERCUTANEOUS VALVES: APPROACHES

Possible access routes include TF arterial, TA (not possible for CoreValve, which requires antegrade insertion), transaortic (TAo) via partial J-sternotomy or right anterior thoracotomy,[20-22] transcarotid,[23-25] and transaxillary/subclavian[26,27] approaches. Less commonly, TF-venous routes have been performed using either transseptal[28] or caval-aortic puncture.[29]

The TF approach has been favored as the first choice for patients in most institutions, owing to its ability to be performed in a completely percutaneous manner, at times without intubation and general anesthesia. In certain patients, for instance those with peripheral vascular disease and heavy arterial calcification, TA-TAVR has become an increasingly popular option, with outcomes similar to TF-TAVR after propensity score matching.[30,31] Although a significant learning curve exists,[32] we have found that the procedure can be performed with minimal morbidity and mortality. For instance, in our most recent series of TA-TAVRs, we have shown a 1.2% mortality, 4.7% renal failure, 0% stroke, and 5.9% permanent pacemaker rate.[33] This approach can even be extended to include simultaneous treatment of multiple cardiac pathologic entities, for example, percutaneous coronary intervention (PCI) and transcatheter mitral valve-in-valve implantation.[34-36]

Transfemoral Approach

The approach we have used for TF insertion is to perform all procedures in a hybrid fluoroscopy operating room with a team consisting of cardiac surgeons, interventional cardiologists, cardiac anesthesiologists, echocardiographers, perfusionists, surgical scrub nurses trained in transcatheter procedures, circulating nurses, catheterization laboratory technicians, and surgical assistants. We have found this multidisciplinary approach to facilitate rescue in the case of myocardial collapse.[37] The femoral, arterial, and venous lines are introduced percutaneously using a closure device at the end of the procedure. Thus, a venous pacing wire is inserted into the right ventricle and then two arterial wires are inserted into the groins, one for a pigtail catheter for aortography and to mark the location of the lower extent of the noncoronary sinus for valve positioning and the other for the device sheath. Typically, the patient is heparinized so the ACT is between 250 and 350 seconds. The aortic valve is crossed with a 0.035″ straight wire and generally an AL1 catheter and advanced into the left ventricle. This is then exchanged with an extra stiff wire that has been fashioned into a curved arc to minimize the risk of ventricular perforation. A balloon is then threaded over the guidewire and positioned across the aortic valve using fluoroscopy and then during rapid pacing, and breath/ventilator holding, expanded to crack the calcified aortic valve in a manner similar to balloon aortic valvuloplasty (Fig. 33-3A).

For the SAPIEN XT, as a rule, patients who need the 23 valve should have an access artery of at least 6 mm; for the size 26 valve, a 6.5 mm artery; and for a 29 valve, a 7 mm artery, depending on the tortuosity of the vessel and degree of calcification. If there is more than 90-degree angulation of the iliac arteries, then generally it would be difficult to insert the sheath unless the vessel straightens very easily with a Lunderquist wire.

Prior to inserting the valve loaded on the delivery balloon, it is checked and confirmed to be correctly oriented and is then threaded over the stiff wire and the loader pushed into the sheath and threaded across the aortic arch with the steerable catheter being flexed to get around the aortic arch and then fed down to the aortic valve. Essentially, the valve with the leading cone is fed across the valve to cross the valve and then the cone is pushed further into

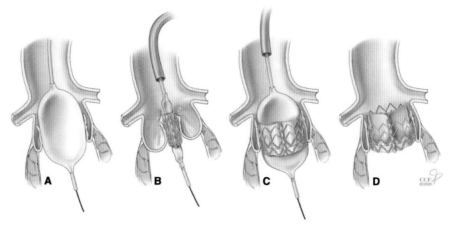

FIGURE 33-3 Transfemoral artery balloon-expandable valve insertion sequence. (Reproduced with permission from the Cleveland Clinic, Cleveland, OH.)

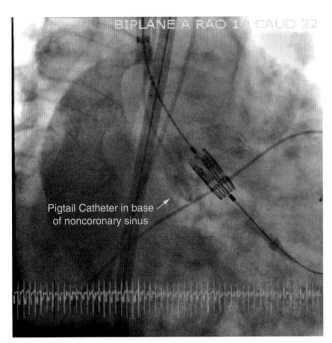

FIGURE 33-4 Positioning of balloon-expandable valve during rapid ventricular pacing. Note position of pigtail catheter at the base of the noncoronary sinus and aortography.

the ventricle so that the stent valve is free. Once the balloon is inflated, it can be expanded without limitation from the cone. We consider it very important to carefully check on the positioning of the valve across the hinged point of the native valve using both echocardiography and fluoroscopy and root injections with contrast via the pigtail catheter. The valve is positioned at the valve hinged points, approximately 60 to 70% aortic and 30 to 40% ventricular (Fig. 33-4). Once everybody agrees that the position is correct, the patient's breath is held, the heart is paced at approximately 180 beats per minute, the balloon is inflated in position and then deflated, the pacer is switched off, and ventilation is resumed (Fig. 33-3).

The most common location of perivalvular regurgitation is in the region of the noncoronary-left main leaflet commissure, probably because this is an area of less flexibility and generally calcified. Echocardiography is then used to inspect the function of the valve and aortography to confirm the lack of perivalvular leak. Thereafter, cone is first withdrawn from the left ventricle followed by removal of the catheter and sheath, and lastly the closure device is tied down at the insertion sites. We perform a completion angiogram of the access vessel in nearly all cases to rule out vascular injury (eg, dissection, occlusion, and significant extravasation).

Transapical Approach

Similar to our practice in the TF cases, we perform all TA procedures in a hybrid operating room with a multidisciplinary team. We position the patient flat supine on pillows

rather than in a traditional left thoracotomy position, so as not to interfere with the positioning of the C-arms. The ideal planes are calculated for imaging the valve with the nadir of each cusp being in the same plane from preoperative computed tomography scans.

Once the patient is positioned, she/he is prepped in the usual manner with exposure of the groin and left chest. The femoral artery and vein are exposed on the right side and the left femoral venous pacing wires are inserted. The femoral artery exposure is performed in case the patient has to be placed on cardiopulmonary bypass and also used for pigtail catheter insertion as in the TF cases.

We continue to have all of our patients undergo general anesthesia but do not use double-lumen endotracheal tubes for the TA valves. Before opening the chest, CT scan images are inspected to find the ideal place to open the left chest. Typically, the fifth intercostal space is entered and the apex of the left ventricle is palpated. Once the apex of the left ventricle has been palpated, a short piece of rib is commonly removed to expose the apex. Originally we did not do this and rather spread the ribs, but we found that some patients had severe postoperative pain as with the MIDCAB experience. We have therefore opted to resect a short piece of rib to obtain both a better exposure and less pain after surgery, particularly because many of these patients have a component of concomitant lung disease. Pericardiotomy is performed over the left ventricular (LV) apex, and heparin is administered aiming to achieve an ACT of 250 to 350. Two concentric purse string sutures reinforced with pledgets are placed as well as and a horizontal mattress suture is placed at the LV apex.

The final entry site is selected by tapping on the LV apex and then looking at the echo to make sure that the LV apex is correctly identified. This is important because the heart can be anywhere from the fourth intercostal space to the seventh or eighth intercostal space. A needle is placed into the apex, followed by soft access wire insertion in the left ventricle through the needle and directed to the aortic valve. A 12-Fr sheath is then delivered into the LV apex; then we insert a balloon-tipped Berman catheter into the left ventricle, through the aortic valve, and across the aortic arch down to the renal arteries. An extra stiff wire is then fed down to this level, the Berman catheter is removed, and the 12-Fr sheath is exchanged for the large-bore TA introduction sheath. Balloon valvuloplasty is performed through this in the same sequence with rapid pacing as for the TF approach. The valve is then loaded onto the sheath and pushed into position and the pusher is retracted into the sheath. With the valve situated approximately 60 to 70% aortic (Fig. 33-5) and with rapid pacing, the balloon is then inflated at this point. The balloon is then withdrawn into the left ventricle before stopping pacing. Both transesophageal echocardiogram (TEE) and aortic root angiography are used to confirm the position and orientation of the prosthetic valve. If all appears well, the sheath is then removed (generally under conditions of rapid pacing), the pursestring sutures are tied down, and protamine is administered.

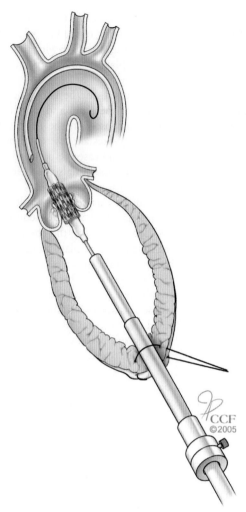

FIGURE 33-5 Transapical purse string and wire. (Reproduced with permission from the Cleveland Clinic, Cleveland, OH.)

REFERENCES

1. Andersen HR, Knudsen LL, Hasenkam JM: Transluminal implantation of artificial heart valves. Description of a new expandable aortic valve and initial results with implantation by catheter technique in closed chest pigs. *Eur Heart J* 1992; 13(5):704-708.
2. Cribier A, Eltchaninoff H, Bash A, et al: Percutaneous transcatheter implantation of an aortic valve prosthesis for calcific aortic stenosis: first human case description. *Circulation* 2002; 106(24):3006-3008.
3. Cribier A, Eltchaninoff H, Tron C, et al: Early experience with percutaneous transcatheter implantation of heart valve prosthesis for the treatment of end-stage inoperable patients with calcific aortic stenosis. *J Am Coll Cardiol* 2004; 43(4):698-703.
4. Dewey TM, Walther T, Doss M, et al: Transapical aortic valve implantation: an animal feasibility study. *Ann Thorac Surg* 2006; 82(1):11-116.
5. Svensson LG, Dewey T, Kapadia S, et al: United States feasibility study of transcatheter insertion of a stented aortic valve by the left ventricular apex. *Ann Thorac Surg* 2008; 86(1):46-54; discussion 54-55.
6. Lichtenstein SV, Cheung A, Ye J, Thompson CR, Carere RG, Pasupati S, Webb JG: Transapical transcatheter aortic valve implantation in humans: initial clinical experience. *Circulation* 2006; 114(6):591-596.
7. Webb JG, Pasupati S, Humphries K, et al: Percutaneous transarterial aortic valve replacement in selected high-risk patients with aortic stenosis. *Circulation* 2007; 116(7):755-763.
8. Leon MB, Kodali S, Williams M, et al: Transcatheter aortic valve replacement in patients with critical aortic stenosis: rationale, device descriptions, early clinical experiences, and perspectives. *Semin Thorac Cardiovasc Surg* 2006; 18(2):165-174.
9. Leon MB, Smith CR, Mack M, et al: Transcatheter aortic-valve implantation for aortic stenosis in patients who cannot undergo surgery. *N Engl J Med* 2010; 363(17):1597-1607.
10. Smith CR, Leon MB, Mack MJ, et al: Transcatheter versus surgical aortic-valve replacement in high-risk patients. *N Engl J Med* 2011; 364(23):2187-2198.
11. Adams DH, Popma JJ, Reardon MJ, et al: Transcatheter aortic-valve replacement with a self-expanding prosthesis. *N Engl J Med* 2014; 370(19):1790-1798.
12. Kodali SK, Williams MR, Smith CR, et al: Two-year outcomes after transcatheter or surgical aortic-valve replacement. *N Engl J Med* 2012; 366(18):1686-1695.
13. Popma JJ, Adams DH, Reardon MJ, et al: Transcatheter aortic valve replacement using a self-expanding bioprosthesis in patients with severe aortic stenosis at extreme risk for surgery. *J Am Coll Cardiol* 2014; 63(19):1972-1981.
14. Varadarajan P, Kapoor N, Bansal RC, Pai RG: Clinical profile and natural history of 453 nonsurgically managed patients with severe aortic stenosis. *Ann Thorac Surg* 2006; 82(6):2111-2115.
15. Iung B, Baron G, Butchart EG, et al: A prospective survey of patients with valvular heart disease in Europe: the Euro Heart Survey on Valvular Heart Disease. *Eur Heart J* 2003; 24(13):1231-1243.
16. Bonow RO, Carabello BA, Chatterjee K, et al: 2008 focused update incorporated into the ACC/AHA 2006 guidelines for the management of patients with valvular heart disease: a report of the American College of Cardiology/American Heart Association Task Force on Practice Guidelines (Writing Committee to revise the 1998 guidelines for the management of patients with valvular heart disease). Endorsed by the Society of Cardiovascular Anesthesiologists, Society for Cardiovascular Angiography and Interventions, and Society of Thoracic Surgeons. *J Am Coll Cardiol* 2008; 52(13):e1-142.
17. Adams DH, Popma JJ, Reardon MJ: Transcatheter aortic-valve replacement with a self-expanding prosthesis. *N Engl J Med* 2014; 371(10):967-968.
18. Kaul S: Transcatheter aortic-valve replacement with a self-expanding prosthesis. *N Engl J Med* 2014; 371(10):967.
19. Abdel-Wahab M, Julinda Mehilli, Christian Frerker, et al: Comparison of balloon-expandable vs self-expandable valves in patients undergoing transcatheter aortic valve replacement: the CHOICE randomized clinical trial. *JAMA* 2014; 311(15):1503-1514.
20. Okuyama K, Jilaihawi H, Mirocha J, Nakamura M, Ramzy D, Makkar R, Cheng W: Alternative access for balloon-expandable transcatheter aortic valve replacement: Comparison of the transaortic approach using right anterior thoracotomy to partial J-sternotomy. *J Thorac Cardiovasc Surg* 2014; 149(3):789-797.
21. Lardizabal JA, O'Neill BP, Desai HV, et al: The transaortic approach for transcatheter aortic valve replacement: initial clinical experience in the United States. *J Am Coll Cardiol* 2013; 61(23):2341-2345.
22. Bruschi G, De Marco F, Fratto P, et al: Direct aortic access through right minithoracotomy for implantation of self-expanding aortic bioprosthetic valves. *J Thorac Cardiovasc Surg* 2010; 140(3):715-717.
23. Thourani VH, Gunter RL, Neravetla S, et al: Use of transaortic, transapical, and transcarotid transcatheter aortic valve replacement in inoperable patients. *Ann Thorac Surg* 2013; 96(4):1349-1357.
24. Azmoun A, Amabile N, Ramadan R, et al: Transcatheter aortic valve implantation through carotid artery access under local anaesthesia. *Eur J Cardiothorac Surg* 2014; 46(4):693-698; discussion 698.
25. Rajagopal R, More RS, Roberts DH: Transcatheter aortic valve implantation through a transcarotid approach under local anesthesia. *Catheter Cardiovasc Interv* 2014; 84(6):903-907.
26. Fraccaro C, Napodano M, Tarantini G, et al: Expanding the eligibility for transcatheter aortic valve implantation the trans-subclavian retrograde approach using: the III generation CoreValve revalving system. *JACC Cardiovasc Interv* 2009; 2(9):828-833.
27. Petronio AS, De Carlo M, Bedogni F, et al: Safety and efficacy of the subclavian approach for transcatheter aortic valve implantation with the CoreValve revalving system. *Circ Cardiovasc Interv* 2010; 3(4):359-366.

28. Cohen MG, Singh V, Martinez CA, et al: Transseptal antegrade transcatheter aortic valve replacement for patients with no other access approach—a contemporary experience. *Catheter Cardiovasc Interv* 2013; 82(6):987-993.

29. Greenbaum AB, O'Neill WW, Paone G, Guerrero ME, Wyman JF, Cooper RL, Lederman RJ: Caval-aortic access to allow transcatheter aortic valve replacement in otherwise ineligible patients: initial human experience. *J Am Coll Cardiol* 2014; 63(25 Pt A):2795-2804.

30. D'Onofrio A, Salizzoni S, Agrifoglio M, et al: Medium term outcomes of transapical aortic valve implantation: results from the Italian Registry of Trans-Apical Aortic Valve Implantation. *Ann Thorac Surg* 2013; 96(3):830-835; discussion 836.

31. Johansson M, Nozohoor S, Kimblad PO, Harnek J, Olivecrona GK, Sjögren J: Transapical versus transfemoral aortic valve implantation: a comparison of survival and safety. *Ann Thorac Surg* 2011; 91(1):57-63.

32. Kempfert J, Rastan A, Holzhey D, et al: Transapical aortic valve implantation: analysis of risk factors and learning experience in 299 patients. *Circulation* 2011; 124(11 Suppl):S124-129.

33. Aguirre J, Waskowski R, Poddar K, et al: Transcatheter aortic valve replacement: experience with the transapical approach, alternate access sites, and concomitant cardiac repairs. *J Thorac Cardiovasc Surg* 2014; 148(4):1417-1422.

34. Al Kindi AH, Salhab KF, Roselli EE, et al: Alternative access options for transcatheter aortic valve replacement in patients with no conventional access and chest pathology. *J Thorac Cardiovasc Surg* 2014; 147(2):644-651.

35. Salhab KF, Al Kindi AH, Lane JH, et al: Concomitant percutaneous coronary intervention and transcatheter aortic valve replacement: safe and feasible replacement alternative approaches in high-risk patients with severe aortic stenosis and coronary artery disease. *J Card Surg* 2013; 28(5):481-483.

36. Al Kindi AH, Salhab KF, Kapadia S, et al: Simultaneous transapical transcatheter aortic and mitral valve replacement in a high-risk patient with a previous mitral bioprosthesis. *J Thorac Cardiovasc Surg* 2012; 144(3):e90-91.

37. Roselli EE, Idrees J, Mick S, Kapadia S, Tuzcu M, Svensson LG, Lytle BW: Emergency use of cardiopulmonary bypass in complicated transcatheter aortic valve replacement: importance of a heart team approach. *J Thorac Cardiovasc Surg* 2014; 148(4):1413-1416.

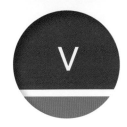

MITRAL VALVE DISEASE

V

MITRAL VALVE
DISEASE

Pathophysiology of Mitral Valve Disease

James I. Fann • Neil B. Ingels, Jr. • D. Craig Miller

34

THE NORMAL MITRAL VALVE

Anatomy

The mitral annulus is a pliable zone of discontinuous fibrous and muscular tissue that joins the left atrium and left ventricle and anchors the hinge portions of the anterior and posterior mitral leaflets.[1-3] The annulus has two major collagenous structures: (1) the right fibrous trigone, which is part of the central fibrous body and is located at the intersection of the membranous septum, the tricuspid annulus, and the aortic annulus; and (2) the left fibrous trigone, which is located near the aortic annulus under the left aortic cusp (Fig. 34-1). The anterior mitral leaflet is in direct fibrous continuity with the aortic annulus under the left and noncoronary aortic valve cusps. The posterior half to two-thirds of the annulus, which subtends the posterior leaflet, is primarily muscular with little or no fibrous tissue.[2]

The mitral valve has two major leaflets, the larger anterior (or aortic) leaflet and the smaller posterior (or mural) leaflet; the latter usually contains three or more scallops separated by fetal clefts or *subcommissures*.[4] The three posterior leaflet scallops are termed anterolateral (P1), middle (P2), and posteromedial (P3) scallops[3] (Fig. 34-2). The portions of the leaflets near the free margin on the atrial surface are called the *rough zone*, with the remainder of the leaflet surface closer to the annulus being termed the *smooth* (or *bare* or *membranous*) *zone*. The ratio of the height of the rough zone to the height of the clear zone is 0.6 for the anterior leaflet and 1.4 for the posterior leaflet because the clear zone on the posterior scallops occupies only about 2 mm.[4] The two leaflets are separated by the posteromedial and anterolateral commissures.

The histologic structure of the leaflets includes three layers: (1) the fibrosa, the solid collagenous core continuous with the chordae tendineae; (2) the spongiosa, which is on the atrial surface and forms the leaflet leading edge (it consists of few collagen fibers but has abundant proteoglycans, elastin, and mixed connective tissue cells); and (3) a thin fibroelastic covering of most of the leaflets.[2] On the atrial aspect of both leaflets, this surface (the atrialis) is rich in elastin. The ventricular side of the fibroelastic cover (the ventricularis) is much thicker and packed with elastin. The fibroelastic layers

become thickened with advancing age as a result of elaboration of more elastin and more collagen formation; accelerated similar changes also accompany progression of myxomatous (degenerative or "floppy") mitral valvular disease in young patients with Barlow syndrome. In addition to these connective tissue structures, mitral leaflets contain myocardium, smooth muscle, contractile valvular interstitial cells, and blood vessels, as well as both adrenergic and cholinergic afferent and efferent nerves.[5-10] Leaflet contractile tissue is neurally controlled and plays a role in mitral valve function.[11-14] The atrial surface of the anterior leaflet exhibits a depolarizing electrocardiogram spike shortly before the onset of the QRS complex, and the resulting contraction of leaflet muscle (which can be abolished by beta-blockade), along with contraction of smooth muscle and valvular interstitial cells, possibly aids leaflet coaptation before the onset of systole, as well as stiffens the leaflet in response to rising left ventricular (LV) pressure.[6-8,15-23]

Annular Size, Shape, and Dynamics

The average mitral annular cross-sectional area ranges from 5.0 to 11.4 cm^2 in normal human hearts (average is 7.6 cm^2).[24] The posterior annulus circumscribes approximately two-thirds of the mitral annulus. Annular area varies during the cardiac cycle and is influenced directly by both left atrial (LA) and LV contraction, size, and pressure.[25,26] Varying by 20 to 40% during the cardiac cycle, annular size increases beginning in late systole and continues through isovolumic relaxation and into diastole; maximal annular area occurs in late diastole.[25,27-29] Importantly, half to two-thirds of the total decrease in annular area occurs during atrial contraction (or *presystolic*); this component of annular area change is smaller when the PR interval is short and is abolished when atrial fibrillation or ventricular pacing is present. Annular area decreases further (if LV end-diastolic volume is not abnormally elevated) to a minimum in early to midsystole.[25-27]

The normal human mitral annulus is roughly elliptical, with greater eccentricity (ie, being less circular) in systole than in diastole.[24-26,30] In three-dimensional (3D) space, the annulus is saddle shaped (or a hyperbolic paraboloid), with

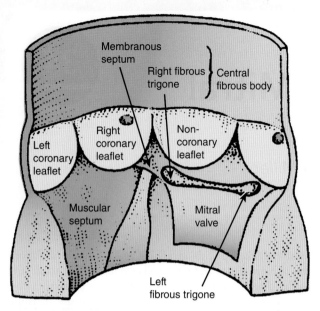

FIGURE 34-1 Diagram from a pathologic perspective with division of the septum illustrating the fibrous continuity between the mitral and aortic valves. (Reproduced with permission from Wells FC, Shapiro LM: *Mitral Valve Disease*. England: Butterworth-Heinemann; 1996.)

the highest point (farthest from the LV apex) located anteriorly in the middle of the anterior leaflet; this point is termed the *fibrosa* in the echocardiography literature and the *saddle horn* by surgeons. The low points are located posteromedially and anterolaterally in the commissures, and another less prominent high point is located directly posterior.[25,31,32] During the cardiac cycle, annular regions adjacent to the posterior leaflet move toward (during systole) and away (during diastole) from the relatively immobile anterior annulus.[25]

The mitral annulus moves upward into the left atrium in diastole and toward the LV apex during systole; the duration, average rate, and magnitude of annular displacement

correlate with (and perhaps influence) the rate of LA filling and emptying.[25,27,28,33] The annulus moves slightly during late diastole (2 to 4 mm toward the left atrium during atrial systole). This movement does not occur in the presence of atrial fibrillation. The annulus moves a greater distance (3 to 16 mm toward the LV apex) during isovolumic contraction and ventricular ejection. This systolic motion, which aids subsequent LA filling, is related to the extent of ventricular emptying and is likely driven by LV contraction.[25,28,33,34] Subsequently, the annulus moves very little during isovolumic relaxation but then exhibits rapid recoil toward the left atrium in early diastole. This recoiling increases the net velocity of mitral inflow by as much as 20%.[28,35] Annular motion can be responsible for up to 20% of LV filling and ejection.[36]

Dynamic Leaflet Motion

The posterior mitral leaflet is attached to thinner chordae tendineae than the anterior leaflet, and its motion is restrained by chordae during both systole and diastole.[4,37] Regions of both leaflets are concave toward the left ventricle during systole,[38,39] but leaflet shape is complex, and anterior leaflet curvature near the annulus is convex to the left ventricle during systole, thus resulting in a sigmoid shape.[29,31,32] Leaflet opening does not start with the free margin but rather in the center of the leaflet; leaflet curvature flattens initially and then becomes reversed (making the leaflet convex toward the left ventricle) while the edges are still approximated.[29,39] The leading edge then moves into the left ventricle (like a traveling wave), and the leaflet straightens. The leaflet edges in the middle of the valve appear to separate before those portions closer to the commissures, and posterior leaflet opening occurs approximately 8 to 40 ms later.[39,40] Early leaflet opening (e wave) is very rapid; once reaching maximum opening, the edges exhibit a slow to-and-fro movement (like a flag flapping in a breeze) until another less forceful opening impulse occurs, associated with the a wave.

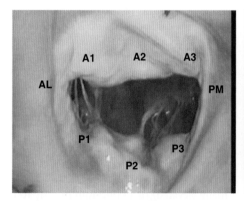

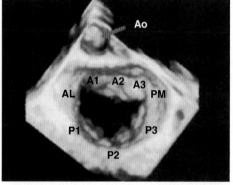

FIGURE 34-2 The operative view of the mitral valve is shown (*left*), and the corresponding "surgical view" obtained with real-time three-dimensional transesophageal echocardiography volume rendering (*right*). Images are from patient with type IIIb dysfunction (*see text*). A1, A2, A3, anterior mitral valve scallops; AL, anterolateral; P1, P2, P3, posterior mitral valve scallops; PM, posteromedial. (Reproduced with permission from O'Gara P, Sugeng L, Lang R, et al: The role of imaging in chronic degenerative mitral regurgitation, *JACC Cardiovasc Imaging*. 2008 Mar;1(2):221-237.)

Valve closure starts with the leaflet bulging toward the atrium at its attachment point to the annulus. The closure rate of the anterior leaflet is almost twice that of the posterior leaflet, thereby ensuring arrival of both cusps at their closed positions simultaneously (because the anterior leaflet is opened more widely than the posterior leaflet at the onset of ventricular systole).[40] The anterior leaflet actually arrives at the plane of the annulus in a bulged shape (concave to the ventricle), but as the closing movement proceeds and the leaflet ascends toward the atrium, this curvature appears to run through the whole leaflet, from the annulus toward the edge, in a rolling manner. The leaflet edge is the last part of the leaflet to approach the annular plane.

Chordae Tendinae and Papillary Muscles

Epicardial fibers in the left ventricle descend from the base of the heart and proceed inward at the apex to form the two papillary muscles, which are characterized by vertically oriented myocardial fibers.[41,42] The anterolateral papillary muscle usually has one major head and is a more prominent structure; the posteromedial papillary muscle can have two or more subheads and is flatter.[4] The posteromedial papillary muscle usually is supplied by the right coronary artery (or a dominant left circumflex artery in 10% of patients); the anterolateral papillary muscle is supplied by blood flow from both the left anterior descending and circumflex coronary arteries.[3,41,43]

The posteromedial and anterolateral papillary muscles give rise to chordae tendineae going to both leaflets[4,44] (Fig. 34-3). Classically, the chordae are divided functionally into three groups.[41,45] First-order chordae originate near the papillary muscle tips, divide progressively, and insert on the leading edge of the leaflets; these primary chordae prevent valve-edge prolapse during systole. The second-order chordae (including two or more larger and less branched "strut" chordae) originate from the same location and tend to be thicker and fewer in number.[4,45] They insert on the ventricular surface of the leaflets at the junction of the rough and clear zones, which is demarcated by a subtle ridge on the leaflet corresponding to the line of leaflet coaptation. The second-order chordae (including the strut chordae) serve to anchor the valve, are more prominent on the anterior leaflet, and are important for optimal ventricular systolic function. Second-order chordae may arborize from large chordae that also give rise to first-order chordae. The third-order chordae, also called *tertiary* or *basal chordae,* originate directly from the trabeculae carneae of the ventricular wall, attach to the posterior leaflet near the annulus, and can be identified by their fan-shaped patterns.[45] Additionally, distinct commissural chordae and cleft chordae exist in the commissures. In total, about 25 major chordal trunks (range 15 to 32) arise from the papillary muscles in

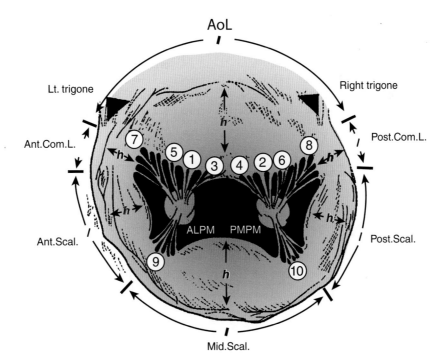

FIGURE 34-3 Mitral valve and subvalvular apparatus. ALPM, anterolateral papillary muscle; Ant.Com.L., anterior commissural leaflet; Ant.Scal., anterior scallop; AoL, aortic leaflet; h, height of leaflet; l, length of attachment of leaflet; Lt.Trigone, left fibrous trigone; Mid.Scal., middle scallop; PMPM, posteromedial papillary muscle; Post.Com.L., posterior commissural leaflet; Post.Scal., posterior scallop; Right Trigone, right fibrous trigone; 1 = anterior main chorda; 2 = posterior main chorda; 3 = anterior paramedial chorda; 4 = posterior paramedial chorda; 5 = anterior paracommissural chorda; 6 = posterior paracommissural chorda; 7 = anterior commissural chorda; 8 = posterior commissural chorda; 9 = anterior cleft chorda; 10 = posterior cleft chorda. (Reproduced with permission from Sakai T, Okita Y, Ueda Y, et al: Distance between mitral anulus and papillary muscles: anatomic study in normal human hearts, *J Thorac Cardiovasc Surg.* 1999 Oct;118(4):636-641.)

humans, equally divided between those going to the anterior and posterior leaflets; on the other end, greater than 100 smaller individual chordae attach to the leaflets.[45]

During diastole, the papillary muscles form an inflow tract. During systole, they create an outflow tract that later becomes obliterated owing to systolic thickening of the papillary muscles, thereby augmenting LV ejection by volume displacement.[42] The contribution of the papillary muscles to LV chamber volume is 5 to 8% during diastole but 15 to 30% during systole.[42,46] The anterolateral and posteromedial papillary muscles contract simultaneously and are innervated by both sympathetic and parasympathetic (vagal) nerves.[47,48] Excited synchronously with adjacent endocardium, the papillary muscles develop tension that significantly lags LV pressure and change length in concert with LV volume[49-51] (Fig. 34-4). At end of isovolumic contraction, therefore, very little papillary tension and/or contraction is available to hold the closed leaflets in place against systolic LV pressure. This has led to the suggestion that the leaflets in the closed valve are virtually self-supporting, which, in turn, has led to the following hypotheses[51]: (1) The chordae, having precise lengths and anchored by papillary tips that maintain a fixed geometric relationship to the mitral annulus, guide the leaflets into precise geometric shapes and positions at the moment of valve closure. If these initial geometric conditions are set properly at this instant (ie, the complex leaflet curvatures are set precisely and all leaflet edges are positioned precisely with respect to one another in the LV chamber), the resulting leaflet assemblage becomes a near-rigid body whose geometry is virtually independent of flow and pressure throughout systole. (2) Subsequent papillary force development, transmitted through secondary chords, contributes about 10% to the total force of LV contraction, particularly in mid-to-late systole. This may underlie the findings, originally by Lillehei and colleagues[52] but validated many times since, that clinical

outcomes are improved by chordal preservation during mitral valve replacement. (3) Papillary muscle force and shortening, continuing during and after ventricular relaxation, plays an active role in valve opening. (4) Anterior leaflet strut chords, always in tension, prevent leaflet intrusion into the outflow tract (ie, systolic anterior motion of the mitral valve) and bias leaflet motion toward closure throughout diastole.[53]

MITRAL STENOSIS

Etiology

Mitral stenosis generally is the result of rheumatic heart disease.[54-62] Nonrheumatic causes of mitral stenosis or LV inflow obstruction include severe mitral annular and/or leaflet calcification in the elderly, congenital mitral valve deformities, malignant carcinoid syndrome, neoplasm, LA thrombus, endocarditic vegetations, certain inherited metabolic diseases, and those cases related to previous commissurotomy or an implanted prosthesis.[55-59,63,64] A definite history of rheumatic fever can be obtained in only about 50 to 60% of patients; women are affected more often than men by a 2:1 to 3:1 ratio. Nearly always acquired before age 20, rheumatic valvular disease becomes clinically evident one to three decades later.

Globally, there are approximately 20 million cases of rheumatic fever, the greatest burden of which is evident as rheumatic heart disease with 282,000 new cases and 233,000 deaths annually.[60-62,65] In the United States, Western Europe, and other developed countries, the prevalence of mitral stenosis has decreased markedly. The etiologic agent for acute rheumatic fever is group A beta-hemolytic streptococcus, but the specific immunologic and inflammatory mechanisms leading to the valvulitis are less clear.[61,62,65-68] Streptococcal antigens cross react with human tissues, known as *molecular mimicry,*

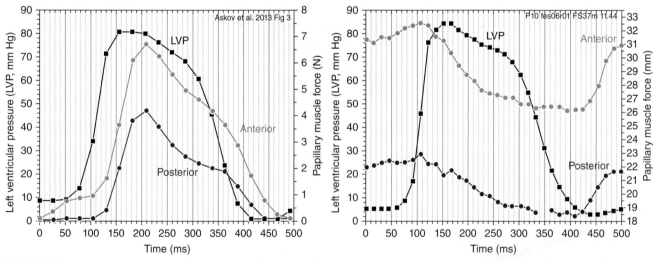

FIGURE 34-4 (Left panel) Anterior and posterior papillary muscle force in relation to LVP. (Right panel) Anterior and posterior papillary muscle length in relation to LVP. (Reproduced with permission from Ingels NB, Jr. and Karlsson M. *Mitral valve mechanics.* Linkoping Sweden: Linkoping Press; 2015.)

and may stimulate immunologic responses. Components implicated in the organism's virulence include the hyaluronic acid capsule and the antigenic streptococcal M-protein and its peptides.[61,65-67] Mimicry between streptococcal antigens and heart tissue proteins, combined with high inflammatory cytokine and low interleukin-4 production, leads to the development of autoimmune reactions and cardiac tissue damage.[61,66,67] In acute rheumatic fever and rheumatic heart disease, M-protein can cross react with cardiac myosin, which induces T-cell-mediated injury of cardiac tissue and valves.[61]

In addition to valvular involvement, rheumatic heart disease is a pancarditis affecting to various degrees the endocardium, myocardium, and pericardium[54,58,61] (Fig. 34-5). In rheumatic valvulitis, mitral valve involvement is the most common (isolated mitral stenosis is found in 40% of patients), followed by combined aortic and mitral valve disease, and least frequently, isolated aortic valve disease. Pathoanatomical characteristics of mitral valvulitis include commissural fusion, leaflet fibrosis with stiffening and retraction, and chordal fusion and shortening[59] (Fig. 34-6). Leaflet stiffening and fibrosis can be exacerbated over time by increased flow turbulence. Valvular regurgitation can develop as a result of chordal fusion and shortening. The degree of calcification varies and is more common and of greater severity in men, older patients, and those with a higher transvalvular

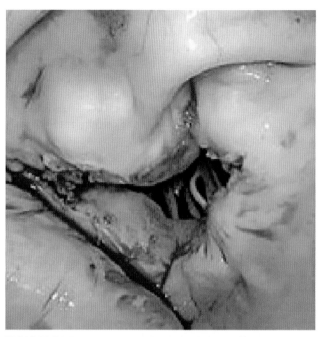

FIGURE 34-5 Intraoperative photograph of mitral stenosis as a result of rheumatic heart disease. The mitral leaflets are markedly restricted. The arrowheads point to the fused anterolateral commissure. (Used with permission from David H. Adams, MD.)

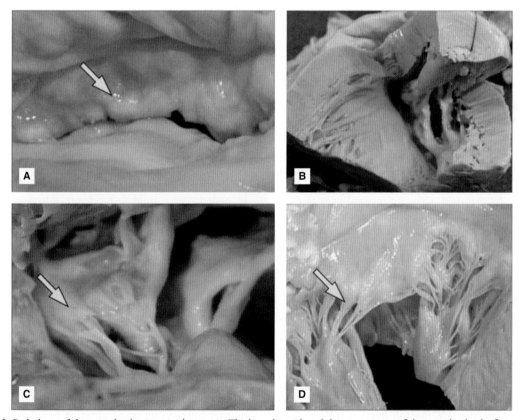

FIGURE 34-6 Pathology of the mitral valve in mitral stenosis. Thickened, rigid nodular appearance of the mitral valve leaflets viewed from the atria (A) and ventricle (B). Calcium is present in the commissure and the commissures are fused, resulting in a valve shaped like a fish mouth. Subvalvular apparatus is thick, fused, and shortened (B, C). Healthy mitral valve leaflets (D). (Reproduced with permission from Chandrashekhar Y, Westaby S, Narula J: Mitral stenosis, *Lancet*. 2009 Oct 10;374(9697):1271-1283.)

gradient.[54] In some cases, rheumatic myocarditis results in LV dilatation and progressive heart failure.

Mitral annular calcification may progress to mitral sclerosis and stenosis in the elderly or those who are dialysis dependent.[59,64] The anterior leaflet can become thick and immobile; LV inflow obstruction also results from calcification of the posterior mitral valve leaflet. Calcific protrusions into the ventricle and extension of the calcium into the leaflets further narrow the valve orifice, resulting in mitral stenosis.[59,64] In these cases, the left ventricle typically is small, hypertrophied, and noncompliant.

Hemodynamics

In patients with mitral stenosis, an early, middle, and late diastolic transvalvular gradient is present between the left atrium and ventricle; as the degree of mitral stenosis worsens, a progressively higher gradient occurs, especially late in diastole.[55,69,70] The average LA pressure in patients with severe mitral stenosis may be in the range of 15 to 20 mm Hg at rest, with a mean transvalvular gradient of 10 to 15 mm Hg.[69,70] With exercise, the LA pressure and gradient rise substantially.

Another physiologic measurement in patients with mitral stenosis is the (derived) cross-sectional valve area, which is calculated from the mean transvalvular pressure gradient and cardiac output. The transvalvular pressure gradient is a function of the square of the transvalvular flow rate; for example, doubling the flow quadruples the gradient. Mitral transvalvular flow depends on cardiac output and heart rate. An increase in heart rate decreases the duration of transvalvular LV filling during diastole; the transvalvular mean gradient increases, and consequently, so does LA pressure.[71] A high transvalvular gradient may be associated with a normal cardiac output. Conversely, if cardiac output is low, only a modest transvalvular gradient may be present.

Because of effective atrial contraction, the mean LA pressure in patients with mitral stenosis and normal sinus rhythm is lower than that in patients with atrial fibrillation.[72,73] Sinus rhythm further augments flow through the stenotic valve, thereby helping to maintain adequate forward cardiac output. The development of atrial fibrillation decreases cardiac output by 20% or more; atrial fibrillation with a rapid ventricular response can lead to acute dyspnea and pulmonary edema.[72]

Ventricular Adaptation

In patients with isolated mitral stenosis and restricted LV inflow, LV end-diastolic volume is normal or smaller than normal, and the end-diastolic pressure typically is low.[55,74,75] The peak filling rate is reduced, as is stroke volume. Cardiac output thus is diminished as a result of inflow obstruction leading to underfilling of the ventricle rather than LV pump failure.[76] During exercise, LV ejection fraction (LVEF) may increase slightly; however, LV filling is compromised by the shorter diastolic filling periods at higher heart rates, resulting in a smaller end-diastolic volume (or LV preload). Therefore,

stroke volume and a blunted increase (or even decrease) in cardiac output can occur.[75]

Approximately 25 to 50% of patients with severe mitral stenosis have LV systolic dysfunction as a consequence of associated problems (eg, mitral regurgitation, aortic valve disease, ischemic heart disease, rheumatic myocarditis or pancarditis, and myocardial fibrosis) or internal constraint of a rigid mitral valve, reduced preload, and reflex increase in afterload.[54,59,70,75] In these patients, LV end-systolic and diastolic volumes may be larger than normal. Diastolic dysfunction and abnormal chamber compliance are sometimes evident.[59] Also, because right ventricular afterload increases as pulmonary hypertension develops in these patients, right ventricular systolic performance deteriorates.[55,77]

Atrial Adaptation

In patients with mitral stenosis who are in normal sinus rhythm, the LA pressure tracing is characterized by an elevated mean LA pressure with a prominent a wave.[73] Because of the stenotic valve, coordinated LA contraction is important in maintaining adequate transvalvular flow.[73] The high LA pressure gradually leads to LA hypertrophy and dilatation, atrial fibrillation, and atrial thrombus formation.[54,75,76] The degree of LA enlargement and fibrosis does not correlate with the severity of the valvular stenosis partly because of the marked variation in duration of the stenotic lesion and atrial involvement by the underlying rheumatic inflammatory process.[75] Disorganized atrial muscle fibers are associated with abnormal conduction velocities and inhomogeneous refractory periods. Premature atrial activation owing to increased automaticity or reentry eventually may lead to atrial fibrillation, which is present in more than half of patients with either pure mitral stenosis or mixed mitral stenosis and regurgitation.[78] Major determinants of atrial fibrillation in patients with rheumatic heart disease include older age and larger LA diameter.[78]

Pulmonary Changes

In patients with mild-to-moderate mitral stenosis, pulmonary vascular resistance is not increased, and pulmonary arterial pressure may remain normal at rest, rising only with exertion or increased heart rate.[69] In severe chronic mitral stenosis with elevated pulmonary vascular resistance, pulmonary arterial pressure is elevated at rest and can approach systemic pressure with exercise. A pulmonary arterial systolic pressure greater than 60 mm Hg significantly increases impedance to right ventricular emptying and produces high right ventricular end-diastolic and right atrial pressures.

LA hypertension produces pulmonary vasoconstriction, which exacerbates the elevated pulmonary vascular resistance.[54,77] As the mean LA pressure exceeds 30 mm Hg above oncotic pressure, transudation of fluid into the pulmonary interstitium occurs, leading to reduced lung compliance. Pulmonary hypertension develops as a result of passive transmission of high LA pressure, pulmonary venous hypertension, pulmonary arteriolar constriction, and eventually, pulmonary vascular obliterative changes. Early changes in the pulmonary vascular bed may be considered protective in that the elevated pulmonary vascular resistance protects the pulmonary capillary bed from excessively high pressures. However, the pulmonary hypertension worsens progressively, leading to right-sided heart failure, tricuspid insufficiency, and occasionally, pulmonic valve insufficiency.[55,77,60]

Clinical Evaluation

Because of the gradual development of mitral stenosis, patients may remain asymptomatic for many years.[59,60,69,79,80] Characteristic symptoms of mitral stenosis eventually develop and are associated primarily with pulmonary venous congestion or low cardiac output, for example, dyspnea on exertion, orthopnea, or paroxysmal nocturnal dyspnea and fatigue. With progressive stenosis (valve area between 1 and 2 cm^2), patients become symptomatic with less effort. Correspondingly, the transmitral mean gradient is usually between 5 and 10 mm Hg at a normal heart rate.[80] The mean pressure gradient is dependent on the transvalvular flow and diastolic filling period and will vary with changes in heart rate. When mitral valve area decreases to about 1 cm^2, symptoms become more pronounced. As pulmonary hypertension and right-sided heart failure subsequently develop, signs of tricuspid regurgitation, hepatomegaly, peripheral edema, and ascites can be found.

As a result of high LA pressure and increased pulmonary blood volume, hemoptysis may develop secondary to rupture of dilated bronchial veins (or submucosal varices).[59,77,79] Over time, pulmonary vascular resistance becomes higher, and the likelihood of hemoptysis decreases. Hemoptysis also may result from pulmonary infarction, which is a late complication of chronic heart failure. Acute pulmonary edema with pink frothy sputum can occur as a result of alveolar capillary rupture.

Systemic thromboembolism, occurring in approximately 20% of patients, may be the first symptom of mitral stenosis; recurrent embolization occurs in 25% of patients.[79,81] The incidence of thromboembolic events is higher in patients with mitral stenosis or mixed mitral stenosis-mitral regurgitation than in those with pure mitral regurgitation. At least 40% of all clinically important embolic events involve the cerebral circulation, approximately 15% involve the visceral vessels, and 15% affect the lower extremities.[79,82] Embolization to coronary arteries may lead to angina, arrhythmias, or myocardial infarction; renal embolization can result in hypertension.[79] Factors that increase the risk of thromboembolic events include low cardiac output, LA dilatation, atrial fibrillation, LA thrombus, absence of tricuspid or aortic regurgitation, and the presence of echocardiographic "smoke" in the atrium, an indicator of stagnant flow. Patients with these risk factors should be anticoagulated.[79,81,82] If an episode of systemic embolization occurs in patients in sinus rhythm, infective endocarditis, which is more common in mild than in severe mitral stenosis, should be considered.

Patients with chronic mitral stenosis are often thin and frail (cardiac cachexia), indicative of longstanding low cardiac output, congestive heart failure, and inanition.[79] Heart size usually

is normal, with a normal apical impulse on chest palpation. An apical diastolic thrill may be present. In patients with pulmonary hypertension, a right ventricular lift can be felt in the left parasternal region. Auscultatory findings include a presystolic murmur, a loud S1, an opening snap, and an apical diastolic rumble.[59,79,83,84] The presystolic murmur, which occurs because of closing of the anterior mitral leaflet, is a consistent finding and begins earlier in those in sinus rhythm than in those in atrial fibrillation.[84] S1 is accentuated in mitral stenosis when the leaflets are pliable but diminished in later phases of the disease when the leaflets are thickened or calcified. As pulmonary artery pressure becomes elevated, S2 becomes prominent.[85] With progressive pulmonary hypertension, the normal splitting of S2 narrows because of reduced pulmonary vascular compliance. Other signs of pulmonary hypertension include a murmur of tricuspid and/or pulmonic regurgitation and an S4 originating from the right ventricle. Best heard at the apex, the early diastolic mitral opening snap is caused by sudden tensing of the pliable leaflets during valve opening and is absent when the leaflets are rigid or immobile.[79,83] In mild mitral stenosis, the diastolic rumble is soft and of short duration; a long or holodiastolic murmur indicates severe mitral stenosis. The intensity of the murmur does not necessarily correlate with the severity of the stenosis; indeed, no diastolic murmur may be detectable in patients with severe stenosis, calcified leaflets, or low cardiac output.[84]

On chest radiography, LA enlargement is the earliest change found in patients with mitral stenosis; it is suggested by posterior bulging of the left atrium seen on the lateral view, a double contour of the right heart border seen on the posteroanterior film, and elevation of the left main stem bronchus.[69] The overall cardiac size often is normal. Prominence of the pulmonary arteries coupled with LA enlargement may obliterate the normal concavity between the aorta and left ventricle to produce a straight left heart border. In the lung fields, pulmonary congestion may be recognized as distention of the pulmonary arteries and veins in the upper lung fields and pleural effusions. If mitral stenosis is severe, engorged pulmonary lymphatics are seen as distinct horizontal linear opacities in the lower lung fields (Kerley B lines).

The electrocardiogram is not accurate in assessing the severity of mitral stenosis and in many cases may be completely normal. In patients with severe mitral stenosis and normal sinus rhythm, LA enlargement is the earliest change (a wide notched P wave in lead II and a biphasic P wave in lead V1).[59,69,86] Atrial arrhythmias are common in patients with advanced degrees of mitral stenosis. In those with pulmonary hypertension, right ventricular hypertrophy may develop and is associated with right axis deviation, a tall R wave in V1, and secondary ST-T-wave changes; however, the electrocardiogram is not a sensitive indicator of right ventricular hypertrophy or the degree of pulmonary hypertension.[86]

Echocardiography has become the primary diagnostic method for assessing mitral valve pathology and pathophysiology.[3,59,60,80,87-89] Cross-sectional valve area and LA and LV dimensions can be quantified using two-dimensional (2D) transthoracic echocardiography (TTE).

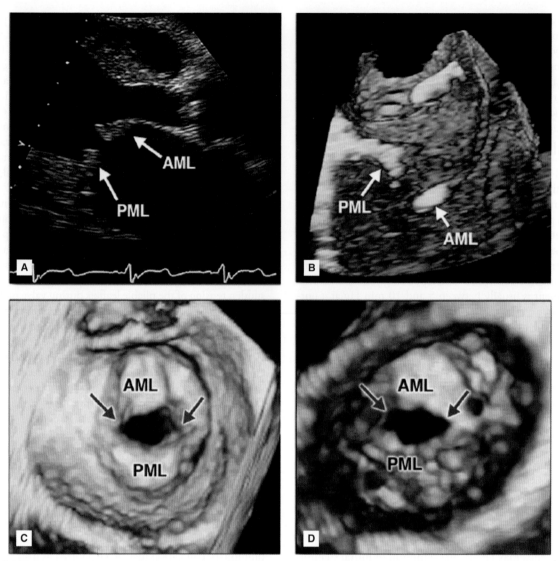

FIGURE 34-7 (A) Echocardiogram (long axis) transthoracic view of a patient with leaflet thickening and severe mitral stenosis caused by rheumatic heart disease. A thickened, stenotic valve separates an enlarged left atrium (*right*) and the left ventricle (*left*). (B) The immobility of the posterior leaflet and the doming of the anterior leaflet as typical morphological characteristics of rheumatic mitral valve disease are shown in a three-dimensional transesophageal image. The three-dimensional transesophageal images (left atrial aspect (C) and left ventricular aspect (D)) show the fusion of both commissures (red arrows). AML, anterior mitral leaflet; PML, posterior mitral leaflet. (Reproduced with permission from Wunderlich NC, Beigel R, Siegel RJ: Management of mitral stenosis using 2D and 3D echo-Doppler imaging, *JACC Cardiovasc Imaging*. 2013 Nov;6(11):1191-1205.)

Best appreciated in the parasternal long-axis view, features of rheumatic mitral stenosis include reduced diastolic excursion of the leaflets (Carpentier type IIIa leaflet motion, see below) and thickening or calcification of the valvular and subvalvular apparatus (Fig. 34-7A). M-mode findings include thickening, reduced motion, and parallel movement of the anterior and posterior leaflets during diastole. Doppler echocardiography accurately determines peak and mean transvalvular mitral pressure gradients that correlate closely with cardiac catheterization measurements.[87] To estimate mitral valve area, the pressure half-time (time required for the initial diastolic gradient to decline by 50%) has been employed; the more prolonged the half-time, the

more severe is the reduction in orifice area.[60,87] Using the pressure half-time determination, mitral valve area is equal to 220 (an empirical value) divided by the pressure half-time. Deriving mitral valve area using the pressure half-time method, however, generally has fallen out of favor. The mean mitral gradient at rest and with bicycle or supine exercise measured using Doppler echocardiography is more useful clinically than estimating mitral valve area; the simultaneous increase in right ventricular systolic pressure (estimated from continuous-wave or pulse-wave Doppler envelopes of the tricuspid regurgitation signal) during exercise is also revealing. The mitral separation index, which is the average of the maximum separation of the mitral leaflet tips in diastole in parasternal and apical four-chamber views, shows good correlation with mitral valve area measured by planimetry and pressure half-time and may be able to discriminate between hemodynamically significant and insignificant mitral stenosis.[90] Transesophageal echocardiography (TEE) is better than the transthoracic approach for visualizing details of valvular pathology, such as valve mobility and thickness, subvalvular apparatus involvement, and extent of leaflet or commissural calcification.[59,60,87,88]

Three-dimensional echocardiography facilitates spatial recognition of intracardiac structures and can evaluate cardiac valvular and congenital heart disease using both real-time 3D TTE and TEE images[60,89,91] (Fig. 34-7B-D). The addition of color-flow Doppler to 3D echocardiography provides better visualization of regurgitant lesions. Measurements of LV volume using 3D echocardiography correlate tightly with measurements obtained using both contrast ventriculography and magnetic resonance imaging (MRI). Cardiac MRI technology remains inferior to echocardiography for depiction of valvular morphology and motion.[92] Multidetector computed tomography (CT) may emerge as a technique that can evaluate both cardiac structure and function. Experience with gated multidetector CT has yielded good visualization of valve leaflet hinges, commissures, and the mitral annulus.[93]

Cardiac catheterization is not necessary to establish the diagnosis of mitral stenosis; however, it provides information regarding coronary artery status in older patients. Left-sided heart catheterization allows determination of LV end-diastolic pressure; right-sided heart catheterization is performed to measure cardiac index and the degree of pulmonary hypertension. Rarely, cardiac catheterization is used to evaluate the reversibility of severe pulmonary hypertension using pharmacologic interventions, including inhaled nitric oxide when indicated.

Postprocedure Outcome

Whereas LV systolic function is used to predict the natural history and postoperative prognosis of patients with other valvular lesions, there are few data linking LV function to outcome in patients with mitral stenosis. Not surprisingly, the best indicator is related to the degree of clinical impairment. Untreated mitral stenosis is associated with a poor prognosis once severe symptoms occur.[59] Percutaneous balloon valvuloplasty is the mainstay of treatment of mitral stenosis provided the anatomy is favorable[59,60,80] (Fig. 34-8). Generally, the technique immediately doubles mitral valve area and decreases the gradient substantially in properly selected patients with rheumatic mitral stenosis. Approximately 90% of patients improve clinically if a valve area greater than 1.5 cm^2 without significant regurgitation can be achieved.[94] Surgical intervention (eg, open mitral commissurotomy or mitral valve replacement) substantially improves functional capacity and long-term survival of patients with mitral stenosis; 67 to 90% of patients are alive at 10 years.[86,95-97]

Despite a higher operative risk for patients with severe pulmonary hypertension and right-sided heart failure, these individuals usually improve postoperatively with a reduction in pulmonary vascular pressures.[55,98] If there is not excessive scarring of the subvalvular mitral apparatus, mitral valve replacement using chordal-sparing techniques can be performed in patients with rheumatic mitral valve

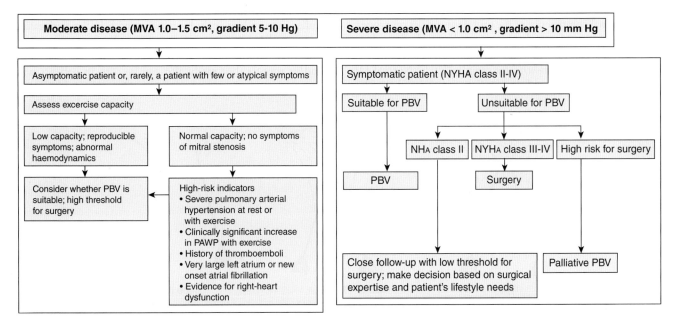

FIGURE 34-8 Treatment strategies for mitral stenosis. MVA, mitral valve area; NYHA, New York Heart Association functional class; PAWP, pulmonary artery wedge pressure; PBV, percutaneous balloon valvuloplasty. Severe mitral stenosis is rarely asymptomatic and, for such patients, we suggest use of the algorithm for assessment of patients with moderate disease. (Reproduced with permission from Chandrashekhar Y, Westaby S, Narula J: Mitral stenosis, *Lancet.* 2009 Oct 10;374(9697):1271-1283.)

disease, particularly those with mixed stenotic and regurgitant lesions; this results in a reduction in LV end-systolic and end-diastolic volumes and preservation of LV systolic pump performance.[99,100] Alternatively, the valve and the entire subvalvular apparatus have to be resected during mitral valve replacement when the disease process is very advanced and all structures are densely calcified and extremely scarred, which frequently is the case in older patients.

Summary

Mitral stenosis generally is caused by rheumatic heart disease. With worsening mitral stenosis, a progressively higher transvalvular pressure gradient develops. Mitral transvalvular flow depends on cardiac output and heart rate; an increase in heart rate decreases the duration of transvalvular filling during diastole and reduces forward cardiac output, causing symptoms. In mild-to-moderate mitral stenosis, pulmonary vascular resistance may not be elevated; pulmonary arterial pressure may be normal at rest and rise only with exercise or increased heart rate. In patients with severe mitral stenosis with elevated pulmonary vascular resistance, the pulmonary arterial pressure usually is high at rest. Characteristic symptoms of mitral stenosis are associated with pulmonary venous congestion and/or low cardiac output. Echocardiography remains the best technique for assessing mitral valve pathology. Percutaneous or surgical intervention can improve functional capacity and long-term survival of patients with mitral stenosis.

MITRAL REGURGITATION

Etiology

The functional competence of the mitral valve relies on proper, coordinated interaction of the mitral annulus and leaflets, chordae tendineae, papillary muscles, left atrium, and left ventricle, known as the *valvular-ventricular complex*.[41,101-104] Normal LV geometry and alignment of the papillary muscles and chordae tendineae permit leaflet coaptation and prevent prolapse during ventricular systole. Dysfunction of any one or more of the components of this valvular-ventricular complex can lead to mitral regurgitation. Important causes of mitral regurgitation include myxomatous degeneration ("primary" mitral regurgitation), ischemic heart disease with ischemic mitral regurgitation (IMR), dilated cardiomyopathy [for which the general term *functional mitral regurgitation* (FMR) is used], rheumatic valve disease, mitral annular calcification, infective endocarditis, congenital anomalies, endocardial fibrosis, myocarditis, and collagen-vascular disorders.[54,57,58,105-108] IMR is considered a specific subset of FMR, which is now termed "secondary" mitral regurgitation. Acute mitral regurgitation also may be the result of ventricular dysfunction from rapidly developing cardiomyopathy, such as Takotsubo cardiomyopathy, in which the mitral regurgitation is caused by LV outflow tract obstruction and systolic anterior motion of the mitral valve from apical ballooning.[109]

In general, four types of structural changes of the mitral valve apparatus may produce regurgitation: leaflet retraction from fibrosis and calcification, annular dilatation, chordal abnormalities (including rupture, elongation, or shortening), and LV systolic dysfunction with or without papillary muscle involvement.[41,110-116] Carpentier classified mitral regurgitation according to three main pathoanatomic types based on mitral leaflet motion: normal leaflet motion (type I), leaflet prolapse or excessive motion (type II), and restricted leaflet motion (type III).[110,111] Type III is further subdivided into types IIIa and IIIb based on leaflet restriction during diastole (type IIIa), as seen in rheumatic disease, or during systole (type IIIb), which is typically seen in IMR (Fig. 34-9). Mitral regurgitation with normal leaflet motion can result from annular dilatation, often secondary to LV dilatation, for example, patients with dilated cardiomyopathy or ischemic cardiomyopathy. Normal leaflet motion also includes patients with leaflet perforation due to endocarditis or a congenital cleft. Leaflet prolapse typically results from a floppy mitral valve with chordal elongation and/or rupture, but rarely also can be seen in patients with coronary artery disease who have papillary muscle elongation

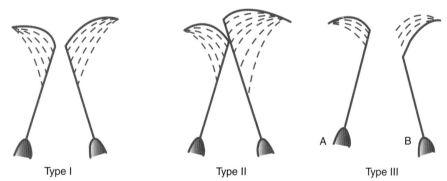

FIGURE 34-9 Carpentier's functional classification of the types of leaflet and chordal motion associated with mitral regurgitation. In type I, the leaflet motion is normal. Type II mitral regurgitation is caused by leaflet prolapse or excessive motion. Type III (restricted leaflet motion) is subdivided into restriction during diastole (A) or systole (B). Type IIIb typically is seen in patients with ischemic mitral regurgitation. The course of the leaflets during the cardiac cycle is represented by the dotted lines. (Modified with permission from Carpentier A: Cardiac valve surgery—the "French correction," *J Thorac Cardiovasc Surg.* 1983 Sep;86(3):323-337.)

or rupture. Mitral regurgitation caused by restricted leaflet motion is associated with rheumatic valve disease (types IIIa and IIIb), ischemic heart disease (IMR with type IIIb restricted systolic leaflet motion secondary to apical tethering or tenting), and dilated cardiomyopathy (type IIIb).[111,112]

MYXOMATOUS DEGENERATION

Myxomatous degeneration of the mitral valve, also known as *floppy mitral valve* or *mitral valve prolapse* and considered primary mitral regurgitation, is the most common cause of mitral regurgitation in patients undergoing surgical evaluation in the United States.[41,108,117-120] Afflicting 2 to 3% of the general population, mitral valve prolapse is both acquired (*fibroelastic deficiency* in older patients) and congenital or heritable, with excess spongy, weak fibroelastic connective tissue constituting the leaflets and chordae tendineae (*Barlow's valve* in younger patients) [54,80,108,121,122] (Fig. 34-10). Associated with connective tissue disorders, such as Marfan syndrome, Ehlers-Danlos, Loeys-Dietz syndrome, osteogenesis imperfecta, pseudoxanthoma elasticum, and aneurysm-osteoarthritis syndrome, mitral valve prolapse appears to be the result of multiple genetic pathways and can be sporadic or familial with autosomal dominant and X-linked inheritance.[108,123,124] Although three different loci on chromosomes 16, 11, and 13 (autosomal dominant) are linked to mitral valve prolapse, no specific gene has yet been incriminated.[108,123,124] Also, a locus on chromosome X cosegregates with a rare form of mitral valve prolapse called *X-linked myxomatous mitral valve dystrophy.*[108,124] Upregulation of transforming growth factor-beta and the mutations of the cytoplasmic protein filamins appear

to have a pivotal role in various pathways in the pathogenesis of mitral valve prolapse.[108] Because the dysfunctional valve is the disease, myxomatous degeneration of the mitral valve is considered primary mitral regurgitation.[80,125]

Some degree of mitral valve prolapse is seen echocardiographically in 5 to 6% of the female population.[121,126] The risk of endocarditis is increased only if valvular regurgitation is present and accompanied by a murmur. Mitral valve prolapse appears to be more widespread in women, but severe mitral regurgitation resulting from mitral valve prolapse is more common in men. Subtle signs of heart failure, usually manifest as declining stamina and fatigue, may be the presenting complaint in 25 to 40% of symptomatic patients with mitral valve prolapse. As strictly defined originally by John Barlow, "Barlow's syndrome" includes prolapse of the posterior leaflet and chest pain, and occasionally palpitations, syncope, and dyspnea; in younger patients, the initial clinical sign is a midsystolic nonejection click, which later evolves into a click followed by a late systolic murmur.[121] This latter scenario is seen typically in young patients with Barlow's valves, in which large amounts of excessive leaflet tissue and marked annular dilatation are coupled with extensive billowing of both leaflets. Because many patients have had symptoms consistent with mitral valve prolapse syndrome for many years prior to developing significant mitral regurgitation, in certain patients, beta-adrenergic receptor polymorphisms may play a role in the pathogenesis of symptoms.[127]

Pathologically, the atrial aspect of the prolapsing mitral leaflet often is thickened focally, whereas the changes on the ventricular surface of the leaflet consist of connective tissue thickening primarily on the interchordal segments with fibrous proliferation into adjacent chordae and onto the ventricular endocardium.[54,108,121,122] Histologically, elastic fiber and collagen fragmentation and disorganization are present, and acid mucopolysaccharide material accumulates in the leaflets. Myxomatous degeneration commonly involves the annulus, resulting in annular thickening and dilatation. All these changes are pronounced in young patients with Barlow's valves but can be minimal in older subjects with fibroelastic deficiency, in whom the noninvolved posterior leaflet scallops and anterior leaflet are normal and thin.[80] It is important to recognize that these two distinct varieties of mitral valve prolapse exist and can be segregated on clinical grounds, even if pathologists have difficulty discriminating between the two, because the repair techniques differ in major ways. Many centers like the Mayo Clinic encounter mainly elderly patients with coronary artery disease and fibroelastic deficiency (78% of their surgical "flail" leaflet surgical population were greater than 60 years old and/or required concomitant coronary artery bypass grafting), in whom the valvular pathology is limited, and simple repair techniques, such as the small McGoon triangular excision of the middle scallop of the posterior leaflet, are applicable and work well.[128] In contrast, other institutions may attract younger patients who have Barlow's valves or severely myxomatous mitral valves, circumstances that demand much more extensive repair techniques and different expertise.

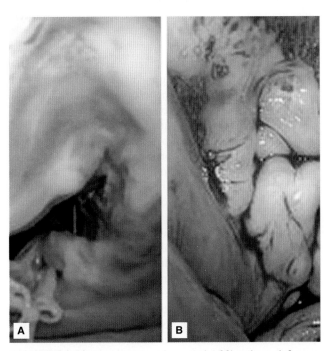

FIGURE 34-10 Intraoperative photograph of fibroelastic deficiency (A) and Barlow's disease (B). (Used with permission from David H. Adams, MD.)

Only 5 to 10% of patients with mitral valve prolapse progress to develop severe mitral regurgitation, and they can remain relatively asymptomatic for many years.[121] Mechanisms accounting for severe mitral regurgitation in those with mitral valve prolapse include annular dilatation and rupture or elongation of the first-order chordae (58%), annular dilatation without chordal rupture (19%), and chordal rupture without annular dilatation (19%).[122] Chordal rupture, probably related to defective collagen, underlying papillary muscle fibrosis or dysfunction, or bacterial endocarditis, typically is the culprit when mitral regurgitation develops acutely in patients without any previous symptoms of heart disease or suddenly becomes worse in those with known mitral valve prolapse.[41,54,56,57,106,108,129] Chordal rupture is evident in 14 to 23% of surgically excised purely regurgitant valve specimens; in 73 to 93% of these patients, the underlying pathology is degenerative or floppy mitral valves.[56,57,106] Posterior chordal rupture, usually subtending just the middle scallop, is the most frequent finding, followed by anterior chordal rupture and then combined anterior and posterior chordal rupture.[56,57,106]

FUNCTIONAL AND ISCHEMIC MITRAL REGURGITATION

FMR is the result of incomplete mitral leaflet coaptation in the setting of LV systolic dysfunction and dilatation with or without annular dilatation (eg, dilated cardiomyopathy or ischemic cardiomyopathy) and is thus now termed secondary mitral regurgitation.[80,113-116,125] LV systolic dysfunction and dilatation also may be associated with longstanding mitral regurgitation caused by severe chronic LV volume overload. Most commonly, the etiology of nonischemic cardiomyopathy is unknown or idiopathic; the second most common cause is advanced valvular disease. FMR occurs in 40% of patients with heart failure caused by dilated cardiomyopathy.[116]

IMR, a subset of FMR, is becoming widely appreciated as the population ages and more patients survive acute myocardial infarction. In those with acute infarction, IMR occurs in approximately 15% of patients with anterior wall involvement and up to 40% of patients with an inferior infarct.[56,57,130] Generally, the severity of mitral regurgitation is related to the size of the area of LV akinesia or dyskinesia. The pathophysiology of IMR can be attributed to changes in global and regional LV function or geometry, alterations in mitral annular geometry, abnormal leaflet motion and malcoaptation, increased interpapillary distance, and papillary muscle malalignment leading to apical tethering of the leaflets with restricted systolic leaflet motion (type IIIb).[110,113,114,130-139] Because of the interdependence of the elements constituting the valvular-ventricular complex in IMR, perturbation of any component, such as LV systolic function and geometry, annular geometry, leaflet motion and morphology, and papillary and chordal relationship, may result in mitral regurgitation.

Left Ventricular Systolic Function and Geometry.
Although LV dilation and dysfunction are less pronounced in the setting of inferior myocardial infarction than that

affecting the anterior wall, the incidence and severity of mitral regurgitation are greater in patients with inferior infarction.[56,57,130,132,134] Over time, as the left ventricle dilates and changes shape after the ischemic event (postinfarction remodeling), the degree of IMR progresses.[115,134,140] Geometric changes associated with ventricular remodeling, such as posteromedial papillary muscle dislocation in the lateral axis, may lead to leaflet tenting, as reflected by a larger distance from the middle of the anterior annulus (saddle horn on echocardiography) to the posteromedial papillary muscle tip, and increased annular diameter.[115,135,136,140] At the ventricular level, myocardial infarction associated with chronic IMR is associated with greater adverse perturbations in LV systolic torsion and diastolic recoil than myocardial infarction without chronic IMR.[141] These abnormalities may be linked to more LV dilatation, which possibly reduces the effectiveness of fiber shortening on torsion generation. Altered LV torsion and recoil may contribute to the "ventricular disease" component of chronic IMR, with increased gradients of myocardial oxygen consumption adversely affecting cardiac efficiency and impaired early diastolic filling.[141] Additionally, in a subacute model of IMR (less than 7 weeks), there is an equivalent increase in LV end-diastolic volume in those with mild mitral regurgitation compared to those with more severe mitral regurgitation, coupled with unchanged end-diastolic and end-systolic remodeling strains, including systolic circumferential, longitudinal, and radial strains; these findings in aggregate argue against an intracellular (cardiomyocyte) mechanism for the LV dysfunction.[142] Instead, differences in subepicardial shear strains suggest a causal role of altered interfiber interactions, and the mechanical impairment may be in extracellular matrix between the fibers and the microtubules in the cytoskeleton that couple cardiomyocyte shortening to LV wall thickening.[142]

Annular Geometry. In IMR, there may be increased mitral annular area, annular stretching and flattening (involving both anterior and posterior components of the annulus), increased septal-lateral annular dimension (also termed the *anteroposterior axis*), which is perpendicular to the line of leaflet coaptation), lateral displacement of posteromedial papillary muscle, and apically tethered posterior leaflet with restricted closing motion, any of which may contribute to leaflet malcoaptation[132,133,135,136] (Fig. 34-11). The septal-lateral annular dilatation and diminished LV systolic function determine mitral systolic tenting area, which in turn is predictive of the severity of the IMR.[132] LV dilatation and larger annular dimensions after inferior myocardial infarction require the mitral leaflets to cover more area during closing, exceeding their normal redundancy or "reserve," which is exacerbated by restricted leaflet closure (type IIIb motion) owing to apical leaflet tenting. Additionally, the distinctive saddle shape of the normal annulus, which becomes accentuated during systole, is eliminated which makes it flatter and suggests an association between maintaining the saddle shape and valvular competence.[132,143,144] Furthermore, in patients with IMR, the anterior and posterior annular perimeters and annular orifice

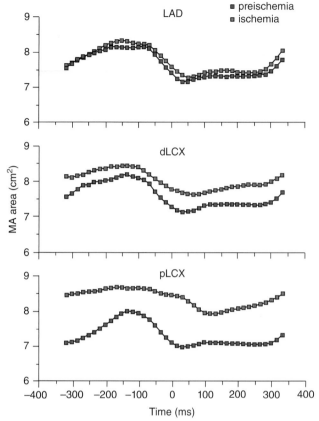

FIGURE 34-11 Average mitral annular area (in cm²) before (*blue squares*) and during (*red squares*) acute LV ischemia induced by balloon occlusion of either the LAD artery (*top*), the dLCx coronary artery (*middle*), or the pLCx coronary artery (*bottom*). A 650-ms time interval centered at end-diastole (t = 0) is shown. dLCx, distal to second obtuse marginal artery; LAD, proximal left anterior descending artery; MA, mitral annular; pLCx, proximal to second obtuse marginal artery. (Reproduced with permission from Timek TA, Lai DT, Tibayan F, et al: Ischemia in three left ventricular regions: Insights into the pathogenesis of acute ischemic mitral regurgitation, *J Thorac Cardiovasc Surg*. 2003 Mar;125(3):559-569.)

area (9.1 cm² compared with 5.7 cm² normally) are increased accompanied by an increase in the intertrigonal (anterior) annular distance and restriction of annular motion.[136]

Leaflet Motion and Morphology.

Acute IMR from proximal left circumflex artery occlusion experimentally results in delayed valve closure in early systole (termed *leaflet loitering*) and increased leaflet edge separation throughout ejection in three leaflet coaptation sites across the valve, specifically near the anterior commissure, the valve center, and near the posterior commissure.[131,133] In addition, there is lateral displacement of the central scallop of the posterior leaflet, suggesting that interscallop malcoaptation and septal-lateral annular dilatation, can contribute to IMR in certain circumstances.[139] Clinically, chronic IMR is associated with apical systolic restriction of the posterior leaflet, thereby effectively preventing competent valve closure; this restriction results in a posteriorly directed eccentric MR jet due to anterior leaflet

"pseudoprolapse." Chronic IMR is also associated with posterior leaflet displacement in the posterior direction and lateral displacement of both leaflets. When the position of each leaflet edge is assessed independently, the anterior leaflet is not displaced apically after inferior infarction, although with more time and further remodeling, apical restriction of this leaflet may occur.[135] A strong echocardiographic determinant of leaflet tenting height is the distance from the tips of the papillary muscles to the saddle horn of the anterior annulus; LV end-diastolic volume is only weakly correlated with tenting height.[145] Recent human observations have revealed that in some patients with IMR/FMR, there is growth or elongation of the leaflets associated with leaflet thickening that compensates for the larger orifice area and minimizes the amount of mitral regurgitation. In others, however, the leaflets do not become larger and cannot coapt normally across the large orifice, which causes more leaks.[146]

In the past, the leaflet morphology in patients with FMR was considered normal, but further analyses have shown the leaflets to be biochemically different, with extracellular matrix changes associated with altered cardiac dimensions.[147,148] In recipient hearts obtained at time of transplantation, mitral leaflets have up to 78% more deoxyribonucleic acid, 59% more glycosaminoglycans, 15% more collagen, but 7% less water than autopsy control leaflets.[147,148] Radially and circumferentially oriented anterior mitral leaflet strips from failing hearts are 50 to 61% stiffer and less viscous.[148] Thus, the mitral leaflets in heart failure have altered intrinsic structural properties, suggesting that the permanently distended and fibrotic tissue is unable to stretch sufficiently to cover the valve orifice and that mitral regurgitation in these patients is not purely functional.[147,148]

Papillary Muscle and Chordal Relationships.

The papillary-annular distances in the LV long axis remain relatively constant in normal hearts throughout the cardiac cycle.[114] During acute ischemia, however, these distances change, which reflects repositioning or dislocation of the papillary muscle tips with respect to the mitral annulus. This process can also contribute to apical tenting of the leaflets during systole.[110,114,135,149,150] With proximal circumflex artery occlusion and resulting IMR in an ovine model, the interpapillary distance and LV end-diastolic volume both increase. There is also increased mitral annular area and displacement of both (but predominantly the posteromedial) papillary muscle tips away from the septal annulus throughout ejection and at end-systole.[135,149] Posteromedial papillary muscle tip displacement probably results from failure of the ischemic papillary muscle to shorten during systole, lengthening of the ischemic papillary muscle over time, and dyskinesia of the ischemic LV wall subtending the papillary muscle. Since posterior papillary muscle displacement in the apical and posterior directions also occurs in sheep that did not develop substantial degrees of IMR, the additional posteromedial papillary muscle displacement in the lateral direction is a dominant factor in the development of IMR.[135] In the setting of posterolateral ischemia, a larger distance from the papillary muscle tips to the midseptal annulus is an important determinant of mitral regurgitant jet area and volume.[130,135] The nonischemic anterolateral papillary muscle may also play a role in apical leaflet restriction because this papillary muscle is displaced apically at end-systole relative to baseline. In sheep with mitral regurgitation, posteromedial papillary muscle tethering distance, papillary muscle depth, and papillary muscle angle are unchanged, and the anterolateral papillary muscle depth and papillary muscle angle decrease with decreasing ejection fraction.[149] Reduced systolic shortening of either papillary muscle in isolation, on the other hand, does not result in mitral regurgitation; thus, the previous notion that "papillary muscle dysfunction" by itself is responsible for IMR is not correct. In fact, papillary muscle dysfunction paradoxically can decrease mitral regurgitation resulting from inferobasal ischemia by reducing leaflet tethering, which improves leaflet coaptation.[151] Further insult to the LV wall underlying the papillary muscles is likely needed before valvular incompetence occurs. Acute IMR induced by experimental posterior LV ischemia is associated with chordal and leaflet tethering at the nonischemic commissural portion of the mitral valve and a paradoxical decrease of the chordal forces and relative prolapse at the ischemic commissural site.[137] Based on cardiac MRI of humans with ischemic heart disease, the loss of lateral shortening of the interpapillary muscle distance tethers the leaflet edges and impairs their systolic closure, resulting in mitral regurgitation.[150] Thus, it may be a combination of systolic annular dilatation and shape change and altered posteromedial and anterolateral papillary muscle position and motion that contributes to incomplete leaflet coaptation and IMR.

Papillary Muscle Ischemia and Rupture. Papillary muscle dysfunction in patients with ischemic heart disease has been thought to contribute to mitral regurgitation, although the significance of its role in IMR remains in question.[41,43,56,57,114,135,149,151] The papillary muscles are particularly susceptible to ischemia, more so the posteromedial papillary muscle (supplied only by the posterior descending artery in 63% of cases) than the anterolateral papillary muscle (supplied by both the left anterior descending and the circumflex arteries in 71% of cases).[41,43] Hence, myocardial infarction leading to papillary muscle dysfunction occurs more frequently with the posteromedial papillary muscle after an inferior myocardial infarction. Although papillary muscle necrosis can complicate myocardial infarction, frank rupture of a papillary muscle is rare. Total papillary muscle rupture usually is fatal as a result of severe mitral regurgitation and LV pump failure; survival long enough to reach the operating room in reasonable condition is possible with rupture of one or two of the subheads of a papillary muscle, which is associated with a lesser degree of acute mitral regurgitation. Papillary muscle rupture usually occurs 2 to 7 days after myocardial infarction; without emergency operation, approximately 50 to 75% of such patients may die within 24 hours.[152,153]

RHEUMATIC DISEASE

With decreasing incidence in the United States, rheumatic fever remains a common cause of mitral regurgitation in developing countries.[41,56-58,105-107,154] It is unknown why rheumatic fever leads to valvular stenosis in some patients and pure regurgitation in others. The pathoanatomical changes of the purely regurgitant rheumatic valve differ from those in a stenotic valve. In chronic rheumatic mitral regurgitation, the valves have diffuse fibrous thickening of the leaflets with minimal calcific deposits and relatively nonfused commissures; chordae tendineae usually are not extremely thickened or fused.[56-58] There also may be shortening of the chordae tendineae, fibrous infiltration of the papillary muscle, and asymmetric annular dilatation primarily in the posteromedial portion. During the first episodes of rheumatic fever (average age is 9 years), patients may develop acute mitral regurgitation, which is more frequently related to annular dilatation and prolapse of the anterior or posterior mitral valve leaflet.[58,154] Those with anterior leaflet prolapse tend to improve with medical management; however, those with prolapse of the posterior leaflet have a less favorable outcome and often require early surgical repair.[154]

MITRAL ANNULAR CALCIFICATION

Mitral annular calcification is a degenerative disorder that usually is confined to elderly individuals; most patients are older than 60 years of age, and women are affected more often than men.[41,64] The pathogenesis of mitral annular calcification is not known, but it appears to be a stress-induced phenomenon; annular calcification also can be associated with systemic hypertension, hypertrophic cardiomyopathy, aortic stenosis, and occasionally, advanced Barlow's disease. Other predisposing conditions include chronic renal failure and diabetes mellitus. Aortic valve calcification is an associated finding in 50% of patients with severe mitral annular calcification.

The gross appearance of mitral annular calcification may vary from small, localized calcified spicules to massive, rigid crescentic bars up to 2 cm in thickness in the annulus and leaflets.[64] Initially, calcification begins at the midportion of the posterior annulus; as the process progresses, the leaflets become upwardly deformed, stretching the chordae tendineae, and a rigid curved bar of calcium surrounding the entire posterior annulus in a horseshoe shape or even a complete ring of calcium may encircle the entire mitral orifice. The calcific deposit spurs extend into the LV myocardium and the conduction system, which can result in atrioventricular and/or intraventricular conduction defects. Annular calcification causes mitral regurgitation by displacing and immobilizing the mitral leaflets (thereby preventing their normal systolic coaptation) or impairing the presystolic sphincteric action of the annulus.[64] As the degree of mitral regurgitation worsens over time, LV volume overload can lead to heart failure. Systemic embolization can occur if the annular calcific debris is extensive and friable.

Hemodynamics

The pathophysiology of acute mitral regurgitation differs from that of chronic mitral regurgitation. Acute regurgitation may result from spontaneous chordal rupture, myocardial ischemia or infarction, infective endocarditis, or severe chest trauma.[41,129,152,153] The clinical impact of acute mitral incompetence is modulated largely by the compliance of the left atrium and the pulmonary vasculature. In a normal left atrium with a relatively low compliance, acute mitral regurgitation results in high LA pressure, which can lead rapidly to pulmonary edema. Such is not the situation in patients with chronic mitral regurgitation, in whom compensatory changes over time increase LA and pulmonary bed venous compliance such that symptoms of pulmonary congestion may not occur for many years.

With mitral regurgitation, the impedance to LV emptying is lowered because the mitral orifice is in parallel with the LV outflow tract.[41,70,155] The volume of mitral regurgitation depends on the square root of the systolic pressure gradient between the left ventricle and the atrium, the time duration of the regurgitant leak, and the effective regurgitant orifice (ERO).[41,145,156,157] The ERO is determined echocardiographically using 2D color Doppler imaging to measure the cross-sectional area of the vena contracta (narrowest width of the regurgitant jet) and the proximal isovelocity surface area (PISA), or continuous-wave Doppler measuring the ratio of regurgitant volume to regurgitant time-velocity integral.[145,158] Regurgitation into the left atrium increases LA pressure and reduces forward cardiac output. LA pressure even may remain elevated at end-diastole (transient 5- to 10-mm Hg transvalvular gradient), representing a functional gradient associated with the increased diastolic LV filling rate.

If the mitral annulus is not rigid, various diagnostic and therapeutic interventions can alter ERO. Altered loading conditions (elevated preload and afterload) and decreased contractility result in progressive LV dilatation and a larger ERO.[159] When LV size is reduced by medical management (eg, digoxin, diuretics, and most importantly, systemic arteriolar vasodilators), ERO and regurgitant volume fall.[160,161] Stress echocardiography using an inotropic drug, such as dobutamine, usually decreases ERO and the degree of mitral regurgitation in patients with FMR and IMR because the LV chamber is smaller at the beginning of systole (or end-diastole) and throughout systole secondary to enhanced LV contractility.[162]

Ventricular Adaptation

The loading conditions induced by mitral regurgitation promote more LV ejection because ventricular preload is increased and afterload is normal or decreased secondary to backward flow across the mitral valve. In terms of cardiac energetics, reduced LV impedance in patients with mitral regurgitation allows a greater proportion of contractile energy to be expended in myocardial fiber shortening than in tension development.[41,155] Because increased fiber shortening is less of a determinant of myocardial oxygen consumption than other components, such as tension (or pressure) development and heart rate, mitral regurgitation causes only small increases in myocardial oxygen consumption.[155] Reduction in developed tension as a result of lower LV systolic wall stress (LV afterload) permits the ventricle to adapt to the substantial regurgitant volume by increasing LV end-diastolic volume to maintain adequate forward output. Along with lower afterload, this increase in preload (LV end-diastolic volume or, more precisely, LV end-diastolic wall stress) allows the heart to compensate for chronic mitral regurgitation for a long time before symptoms occur.[41,163,164] A fundamental response to increased preload is augmented stroke volume and stroke work, although effective forward stroke volume may be subnormal. High LV preload eventually leads to LV dilatation and shape change, meaning more spherical remodeling, owing to replication of sarcomeres in series as a consequence of chronic elevation of LV end-diastolic wall stress.[163,164] This process is in contrast to LV hypertrophy secondary to chronic pressure overload (elevated systolic wall stress) which leads to sarcomere replication in parallel. In chronic mitral regurgitation, LV mass also increases; however, the degree of hypertrophy correlates with the amount of chamber dilatation so that the ratio of LV mass to end-diastolic volume remains in the normal range (unlike the situation in patients with LV pressure overload).[165-167] The contractile dysfunction that evolves due to chronic LV volume overload is accompanied by increased myocyte length as well as reduced myofibril content.[164,165] The basic changes thus are a combination of myofibrillar loss and the absence of significant hypertrophy in response to the progressive decrease in LV pump function. The defect is intrinsic to the myocyte *per se*, but changes in the extracellular matrix also play a role.[142,168] Conversely, in acute mitral regurgitation, the ratio of LV mass to end-diastolic volume is reduced because chamber dilatation occurs suddenly, and the LV wall becomes acutely thinned; this increase in LV end-diastolic volume is associated with sarcomere lengthening along the length-tension curve.[164]

After the initial compensatory phase, LV systolic contractility becomes progressively impaired as mitral regurgitation progresses chronically.[166-169] Because of the low impedance during systole, however, ejection-phase indexes of LV systolic function, such as ejection fraction, stroke volume, and fractional circumferential fiber shortening (%FSc), still can be normal even if LV contractile state has become depressed.[168,170,171] An ejection fraction of less than 55 to 60% or %FSc less than 28% in the presence of severe mitral regurgitation indicates an advanced degree of myocardial dysfunction. It is important to remember that all the ejection-phase indexes commonly used clinically to estimate LV pump performance, for example, ejection fraction, %FSc, cardiac output, stroke volume, stroke work, etc. are all affected by changes in LV preload and afterload.

Because of abnormal LV loading conditions in the setting of mitral regurgitation, load-independent indexes of LV contractility (eg, end-systolic elastance derived from the end-systolic pressure-volume relationship) or preload recruitable stroke work (PRSW, also termed *linearized Frank-Starling relationship*) are preferred to measure LV systolic function and mechanics.[166-169,172,173] In hypertrophied and dilated hearts, as seen in chronic mitral regurgitation, however, the utility of end-systolic elastance may be limited because of LV chamber shape and size changes. It is necessary to use the end-systolic stress-volume relationship in these circumstances. One other problem inherent in the use of end-systolic elastance or stress-volume data is that end-systole and end-ejection are dissociated in patients with mitral regurgitation. End-ejection is defined as minimum LV volume and end-systole as the instant when LV elastance reaches its maximal value. Because of this temporal dissociation of end-systole from minimal ventricular volume, end-ejection pressure-volume relations do not correlate with maximal elastance values derived using isochronal methods.[172] End-systolic dimension or LV end-systolic volume (LVESV) is less dependent on LV loading conditions than is ejection fraction, and therefore is a better measure of LV systolic contractile function. LVESV varies directly and linearly with afterload, and inversely with contractile state.[169,174-176] The larger the LVESV becomes, the worse LV contractility. Correcting LVESV for chamber geometry, LV wall thickness and afterload (end-systolic wall stress [ESS]), and body size (LV end-systolic volume index [LVESVI]) provides reliable and accurate indexes of LV systolic function that are less influenced by loading conditions and variation in patient size.[174,175] Thus, preoperative LVESV or LVESVI is a better predictor of outcome in terms of postoperative LV systolic performance and cardiac death than is LVEF, end-diastolic volume, or end-diastolic pressure.[176]

Based on load-independent indexes of LV contractility in experimental mitral regurgitation, the normalized end-systolic pressure-volume and end-systolic stress-volume relationships decline after 3 months of mitral regurgitation.[166] PRSW (the relation of stroke work to LV end-diastolic volume) and preload-recruitable pressure-volume area (the relation of stroke work to LV pressure-volume area) also fall, along with a decrease in efficiency of energy transfer from pressure-volume area to external pressure-volume work at matched LV end-diastolic volume. Furthermore, there is deterioration in ventriculoarterial coupling over time; that is, a mismatch develops between the ventricle and the total (forward and regurgitant) vascular load.[166] Although the overall (systemic plus LA) effective arterial elastance is decreased, there is a proportionally greater reduction in LV end-systolic elastance. Thus, LV systolic mechanics become impaired along with deterioration in global LV energetics and efficiency, and a mismatch develops in coupling between the left ventricle and the arterial bed.[166] Additionally, progression from acute to chronic mitral regurgitation (at 3 months) is associated with a decrease in maximum LV systolic torsional deformation from 6.3 to 4.7° and a decrease in early diastolic LV recoil from +3.8 to −1.5°.[177] Because torsion is a mechanism by which the left ventricle equalizes transmural gradients of fiber strain and oxygen demand, a decrease in systolic torsion in chronic mitral regurgitation may play a role in the inexorable and progressive decline of LV performance.[177] The left ventricle responds to decreased forward cardiac output resulting from mitral regurgitation by dilating; such dilatation equalizes the lengths of the endocardial and epicardial radii and thereby decreases systolic LV torsion. In assessing transmural 3D myocardial deformations in an ovine model of isolated mitral regurgitation, early changes in LV function at 12 weeks was evidenced by alterations in transmural strain (which may be detected before the onset of global LV dysfunction), but not by changes in B-type natriuretic peptide or PRSW.[178] The associated increase in transmural gradient of fiber strain and oxygen supply-demand imbalance results in a further decrease in forward cardiac output, leading to more LV dilatation and continuing the vicious cycle.

Diastolic inflow into the ventricle increases as total stroke volume increases during the evolution of mitral regurgitation and ventricular dilatation.[179-182] Acute mitral regurgitation enhances LV diastolic function by increasing the early diastolic filling rate and decreasing chamber stiffness. Flow across the mitral valve during early diastole is determined by the LA-LV pressure gradient, even though other factors, such as diastolic restoring forces and LV diastolic recoil (creating LV suction) during isovolumic relaxation also influence early LV filling.[179] In middle and late diastole, the lower LV chamber stiffness in patients with acute mitral regurgitation (evidenced by a shift of the LV diastolic pressure dimension or pressure-volume relationship to the right) allows the LV mean and LV end-diastolic pressures (and stresses) to remain in the normal range. In patients with chronic mitral regurgitation and preserved ejection fraction, LV chamber stiffness is also lower, similar to that during acute mitral regurgitation. Conversely, in those with impaired LV systolic function, chamber stiffness usually is normal.[181] In general, chronic mitral regurgitation causes a decrease in LV systolic contractile function but an increase in early diastolic function (as evidenced by an increase in early diastolic filling rate and a decrease in chamber stiffness).[182,183] The reduced chamber stiffness may be the result of altered ventricular geometry (more spherical shape); this shape change can exacerbate the degree of mitral regurgitation by distorting annular dimensions and dislocating the papillary muscles.[181,184] Although the LV chamber stiffness is less owing to the change in geometry, the LV myocardium may be stiffer as a result of myocyte hypertrophy and interstitial fibrosis.[181,182]

Atrial Adaptation

Regurgitant flow into the left atrium leads to progressive atrial enlargement, the degree of which does not correspond directly with the severity of mitral regurgitation.[74,155] Also, the LA v wave in mitral regurgitation does not correlate with LA volume. Compared with patients with mitral stenosis, LA size can be larger in patients with longstanding mitral regurgitation, but thrombus formation and systemic thromboembolization occur less frequently because of the absence of atrial stasis.[74,77] Atrial fibrillation occurs less often in those with mitral regurgitation than in individuals with mitral stenosis.[77]

LA compliance is an important component of the patient's overall hemodynamic status if mitral regurgitation is present.[41,128,155,185] With sudden development of mitral regurgitation from chordal rupture, papillary muscle infarction, or leaflet perforation, LA compliance is normal or reduced. The left atrium is not enlarged, but the mean LA pressure and v wave are high. Gradually, the LA myocardium becomes hypertrophied, proliferative changes develop in the pulmonary vasculature, and pulmonary vascular resistance rises. As the mitral regurgitation becomes chronic and more severe, the left atrium becomes markedly enlarged, atrial compliance is increased, the atrial wall becomes fibrotic, but LA pressure remains normal or only slightly elevated.[185] In this situation, pulmonary artery pressure and pulmonary vascular resistance usually are still in the normal range or only modestly elevated.

Pulmonary Changes

Because chronic mitral regurgitation is associated with LA enlargement and only mild elevations in LA pressure, pronounced increases in pulmonary vascular resistance usually do not develop. In patients with acute mitral regurgitation with normal or reduced LA compliance, a sudden increase in LA pressure initially elevates pulmonary vascular resistance, and occasionally acute right-sided heart failure occurs.[41,129] Pulmonary edema is seen less frequently in patients with chronic mitral regurgitation than in those with mitral stenosis because elevated LA pressure is uncommon. In patients with IMR and heart failure, however, acute pulmonary edema is associated with the dynamic changes in IMR and the resulting increase in pulmonary vascular pressure.[186] Exercise-induced changes in ERO, tricuspid regurgitant pressure gradient (estimate of pulmonary artery systolic pressure), and LVEF are independently associated with the development of pulmonary edema.[186] From the standpoint of pulmonary parenchymal function and respiratory mechanics in patients with chronic mitral regurgitation, there is a decline in vital capacity, total lung capacity, forced expiratory volume, and maximal expiratory flow at 50% vital capacity.[186] These patients also may have a positive response to methacholine challenge; this bronchial hyperresponsiveness may result from increased vagal tone owing to longstanding pulmonary congestion.

Clinical Evaluation

Patients with mild-to-moderate mitral regurgitation may remain asymptomatic for many years as the left ventricle adapts to the increased workload and maintains normal forward cardiac output. Gradually, symptoms reflecting decreased cardiac output with physical activity and/or pulmonary congestion develop insidiously, such as weakness, fatigue, palpitations, and dyspnea on exertion. If right-sided heart failure appears late in the course of the disease, hepatomegaly, peripheral edema, and ascites occur and can be associated with rapid clinical deterioration.[187,188] Conversely, acute mitral regurgitation usually is associated with marked sudden pulmonary congestion and pulmonary edema. Patients with

coronary artery disease can present with myocardial ischemia or infarction and associated mitral regurgitation. Acute papillary muscle rupture may clinically mimic the presentation of a patient with a postinfarction ventricular septal defect.[188,189]

On physical examination, the cardiac impulse in patients with mitral regurgitation is hyperdynamic and displaced laterally; the forcefulness of the apical impulse is indicative of the degree of LV enlargement. In patients with chronic mitral regurgitation, S1 usually is diminished. S2 may be single, closely split, normally split, or even widely split as a consequence of the reduced resistance to LV ejection; a common finding is a widely split S2 that results from shortening of LV systole and early closure of the aortic valve.[108,190] An S3 gallop may be appreciated from the increased transmitral diastolic flow rate during the rapid filling phase. The apical systolic murmur of mitral regurgitation can be blowing, moderately harsh, or even soft and usually radiates to the axilla and left or right sternal border and occasionally to the neck or the vertebral column.[190] With rupture of the posterior leaflet first-order chordae, the mitral regurgitation jet is directed superiorly and impinges on the atrial septum near the base of the aorta, which can produce a murmur heard best along the right sternal border and radiating to the neck.[190,191] In cases of ruptured anterior leaflet first-order chordae, the leakage is aimed laterally and toward the posterior LA wall; the murmur may be transmitted posteriorly. Although there is no correlation between the intensity of the systolic murmur and the hemodynamic severity of the mitral regurgitation, a holosystolic murmur is characteristic of more regurgitant flow. In younger patients with Barlow's valves, early in the disease process, a characteristic midsystolic click is heard followed by a late systolic murmur; as the annulus and left ventricle dilate, the murmur over time becomes holosystolic, and the midsystolic click may become inaudible.

On chest radiography, cardiomegaly indicative of LV and LA enlargement is found commonly in patients with long-standing moderate-to-severe mitral regurgitation. Chest x-ray findings of congested lung fields are less prominent in patients with mitral regurgitation than in those with mitral stenosis, but interstitial edema is seen frequently in individuals with acute mitral regurgitation and those with progressive LV failure secondary to chronic mitral regurgitation.

Changes on the electrocardiogram are not particularly useful and depend on the etiology, severity, and duration of the mitral regurgitation.[86,190] Atrial fibrillation can occur late in the natural history of the disease and usually causes sudden exacerbation of symptoms. In cases of chronic mitral regurgitation, LV volume overload leads to LA and LV dilatation, and eventually to LV hypertrophy. Electrocardiographic evidence of LV enlargement or hypertrophy occurs in one-half of patients, 15% have right ventricular hypertrophy owing to increased pulmonary vascular resistance, and 5% have combined left and right ventricular hypertrophy.[86] In those with acute mitral regurgitation, LA and/or LV dilatation may not be evident, and the electrocardiogram may be normal or show only nonspecific findings, including sinus tachycardia or ST-T-wave alterations.[86] Findings of myocardial ischemia or infarction, more commonly noted in the inferior leads, may be present when acute mitral regurgitation is related to acute inferior myocardial infarction or myocardial ischemia; in these cases, first-degree AV block is a common coexisting finding.

In the majority of individuals with mitral valve prolapse, particularly those who are asymptomatic, the resting electrocardiogram is normal.[86,126] In symptomatic patients, a variety of ST-T-wave changes, including T-wave inversion and sometimes ST-segment depression, particularly in the inferior leads, can be found.[121,126] QTc prolongation also may be seen. Arrhythmias may be observed on ambulatory electrocardiograms, including premature atrial contractions, supraventricular tachycardia, AV block, bradyarrhythmias, and premature ventricular contractions.[126] Atrial arrhythmias may be present in upward of 14% of patients, and ventricular arrhythmias are present in 30% of patients.[86,126]

TTE is the diagnostic mainstay in patients with valvular heart disease. In those with chronic mitral regurgitation, this modality is used to follow the progression of LA and LV dilatation.[3,41,89,108,192,193] Echocardiography identifies abnormalities in leaflet and chordal morphology and function, including myxomatous degeneration with or without leaflet prolapse, restricted systolic leaflet motion (as in IMR) or diastolic opening motion (as in rheumatic valve disease), lack of adequate coaptation due to annular dilatation or rheumatic valvulitis (fused subvalvular apparatus), and leaflet destruction by endocarditis[3,41,87,89,158,193] (Fig. 34-12). The degree of mitral regurgitation is assessed using 2D color Doppler echocardiography, which permits visualization of the origin, extent, direction, duration, and velocity of disturbed backward flow of the regurgitant leak.[87,158,193] Chordal rupture or elongation causing a flail leaflet is characterized by excessive motion of the leaflet backward into the left atrium beyond the normal leaflet coaptation zone. Papillary muscle rupture after myocardial infarction and annular dilatation can be visualized (Fig. 34-13). In patients with IMR or FMR, apical systolic tethering of the leaflets, tenting area and height, and leaflet opening angles can be quantitated using echocardiography[145,156,158,194] (Fig. 34-14). When the regurgitant leak is

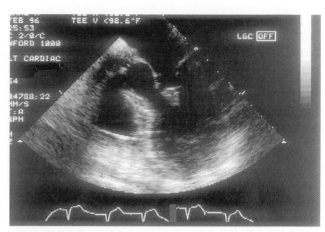

FIGURE 34-13 Echocardiogram (two-chamber view) of a patient with mitral regurgitation from ruptured papillary muscle.

caused in part or totally by annular dilatation, usually in the septal-lateral dimension, the coaptation height of the anterior and posterior leaflets can be measured.

In mitral regurgitation, ERO and regurgitant volume can be estimated quantitatively in many but not all patients using 2D color Doppler echocardiography.[145,157,158] ERO is an important predictor of outcome in a retrospective Mayo Clinic study of patients with mitral regurgitation and has been proposed as an indicator of when to proceed with mitral repair in asymptomatic patients with prolapse.[157] Accurate quantification of the degree of mitral regurgitation using ERO and regurgitant volume, however, is demanding, time consuming, fraught with error, and may not be available at all institutions. The hemodynamic magnitude or severity of the mitral regurgitation also can be estimated semiquantitatively by calculating mitral and aortic stroke volumes, with regurgitant volume being the difference between these two stroke volumes. Cardiac MRI is an accurate method to measure regurgitant volume and regurgitant fraction by comparing right- with left-sided flow.[92,195,196]

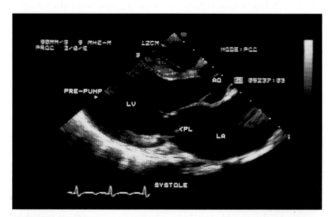

FIGURE 34-12 Echocardiogram (long-axis) of a patient with mitral regurgitation resulting from floppy mitral valve. The leaflets billow back into the left atrium during systole.

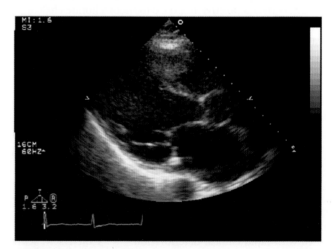

FIGURE 34-14 Echocardiogram of a patient with ischemic mitral regurgitation and apical systolic leaflet tenting.

Interest in the timing of the regurgitant leak has helped clinicians discern subtle details about the mechanism(s) responsible for the mitral regurgitation, infer information about the overall hemodynamic burden imposed by the LV volume overload, and predict the likelihood of successful and durable mitral repair.[145,156-158,194] IMR is primarily an early systolic leak, FMR occurs during early and middle systole (can be a biphasic pattern), and prolapse is associated with late systolic leaks. Although detected by pulse- and continuous-wave Doppler echocardiography for years, the timing of the mitral regurgitation also can be demonstrated using color Doppler M-mode echocardiography, which has a much faster temporal resolution (sampling frequency) than does 2D color Doppler echocardiography. Cardiac surgeons should study these color Doppler M-mode images carefully because the timing of the regurgitant leak yields important information about the mechanisms responsible for the mitral regurgitation, which in turn aids repair planning.

TTE is usually adequate to learn all that is necessary, but if high-quality TTE images cannot be obtained because of the patient's habitus or advanced emphysema, TEE provides superior image quality and can reveal additional anatomical and pathophysiologic information, including details of the valvular pathoanatomy and the mechanism, origin, direction, timing, and severity of the regurgitant leak.[3,41,108,121,158,192,193,197] TEE can detect small mitral vegetations, ruptured chordae, leaflet perforations or clefts, calcification, and other inflammatory changes and can be useful in patients with annular or leaflet calcification. TEE also is useful in patients with a previously implanted aortic valve prosthesis that can interfere with TTE assessment of mitral regurgitation owing to acoustic shadowing. Although intraoperative TEE during mitral valve repair is essential, a major limitation must always be remembered. The vascular unloading effects (vasodilatation) of general anesthesia downgrade the severity of mitral regurgitation.[198,199] The judgment about how much mitral regurgitation is present must be made on the basis of an awake TTE study when the patient has a normal ambulatory blood pressure. This concept is imperative in assessing the degree of mitral regurgitation in patients with IMR when deciding whether to add a mitral valve procedure at the time of coronary artery bypass grafting. For patients in whom the degree of mitral regurgitation has been minimized by the effects of anesthesia, intraoperative TEE provocative testing using vasoconstrictor drugs with or without volume infusion is mandatory to guide surgical decision making. Testing consists of reproducing the patient's normal awake or active ambulatory hemodynamic condition with preload challenge and afterload augmentation.[198,199] Preload challenge is performed after aortic cannulation for cardiopulmonary bypass by rapidly infusing volume from the pump until the pulmonary capillary wedge pressure reaches 15 to 18 mm Hg. If severe mitral regurgitation is not produced, LV afterload is increased by intravenous boluses of phenylephrine until the arterial systolic pressure climbs to the 150-mm Hg range. In patients undergoing coronary artery bypass grafting, if both tests are negative, or regurgitation is induced but associated with new regional LV systolic wall motion abnormalities (ie, the regurgitation is caused by

acute ischemia of viable myocardium), the valve may not require visual inspection because coronary revascularization usually is all that is necessary if the inferior wall myocardium is viable. If these tests confirm the presence of moderate-to-severe mitral regurgitation, the valve is inspected and usually is repaired at the time of coronary revascularization.

Real-time 3D echocardiography is helpful in the visual assessment of congenital and acquired valvular disease[3,108,121,194,200,201] (Fig. 34-15). In patients with mitral regurgitation, this modality is fairly accurate in elucidating the dynamic mechanisms of the regurgitant leak(s). The addition of color-flow Doppler to 3D imaging provides improved visualization and may offer improved quantitative assessment of regurgitant valvular lesions.[3,121] Additionally, 3D echocardiography provides insight into the geometric deformities of the mitral leaflets and annulus, maximum tenting site of the mitral leaflet, and quantitative measurements of mitral valve tenting and annular deformity in patients with IMR.[3,121,194,201] Real-time 3D color Doppler echocardiographic imaging provides direct measurement of vena contracta area.[3,200] The quantification of mitral regurgitant flow directly at the lesion using color Doppler echocardiography, however, has been prevented because of multiple aliasing from high flow velocities. Dealiasing of color Doppler flow at the vena contracta is feasible and appears promising for measuring severity of mitral regurgitation. This approach can be readily implemented in current systems to provide regurgitant flow volume and regurgitant fraction.[3,200]

Cardiac catheterization and coronary angiography are needed to determine coronary artery anatomy, but only in older patients with prolapse before repair and those with IMR.[41,85,163] Other techniques, such as calculating mitral regurgitant fraction (regurgitant volume determined as the difference between total LV angiographic stroke volume and the effective forward stroke volume measured by the Fick method), are limited. By measuring rest and exercise (supine bicycle) pulmonary artery pressures and cardiac output, right-sided heart catheterization can be useful occasionally to identify patients with primary myocardial disease who present with LV dilatation and relatively mild degrees of mitral regurgitation (who may not have a high likelihood of benefiting from mitral valve surgery) and those with severe mitral regurgitation who deny symptoms to see if they develop pulmonary hypertension with exercise.

Cardiac MRI can be employed to assess the cardiovascular system, including cardiac structure and function.[92,108,150,195,196,202] Specialized MRI techniques, such as phase contrast velocity mapping, planimetry, or real-time color flow, have been used to evaluate and quantify the degree of mitral regurgitation. The presence of valvular regurgitation can be determined, LV volumes and mitral regurgitant fraction estimated, and information obtained concerning mitral and coronary anatomy. Direct measurement by MRI is a promising method for assessment of the severity of mitral regurgitation; MRI planimetry of the anatomical mitral regurgitant lesion permits quantification of regurgitation with good agreement with cardiac catheterization and echocardiography.[196] Constraints of MRI, such as pacemakers or

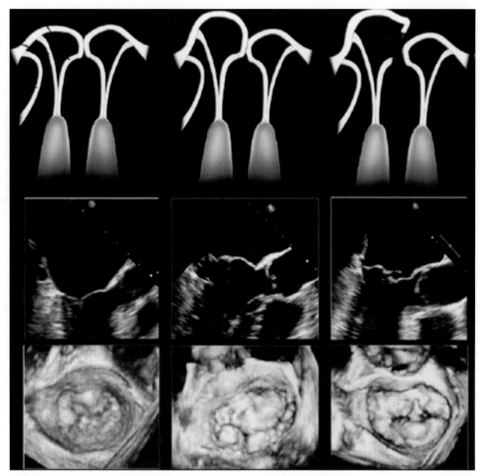

FIGURE 34-15 Intraoperative two-dimensional and three-dimensional transesophageal echocardiographic depiction of mitral valve prolapse and leaflet flail. Schematic (*upper row*) and two-dimensional and three-dimensional echocardiographic images of a patient with normal mitral valve (*left panels*), mitral valve prolapse (P1, *middle panels*), and a flail mitral valve (P2, *right panels*) as visualized with two-dimensional transesophageal echocardiography: long-axis mid-esophageal views (*middle row*) and real-time three-dimensional transesophageal echocardiographic volume rendering from the left atrial perspective (*bottom row*). (Reproduced with permission from O'Gara P, Sugeng L, Lang R, et al: The role of imaging in chronic degenerative mitral regurgitation, *JACC Cardiovasc Imaging.* 2008 Mar;1(2):221-237.)

implanted defibrillators, morbid obesity, and claustrophobia, hamper the wider use of cardiac MRI. Multidetector CT is an imaging technique that can fully evaluate both cardiac structure and function, including coronary artery anatomy; this technology has yielded good visualization of valve leaflets, commissures, and mitral annulus.[93] Limitations include image noise, requirement for a regular rhythm and a slow heart rate during imaging, time required for postprocessing data analysis, and radiation dose.

Postoperative LV Function and Surgical Outcomes

GENERAL

Successful mitral valve surgery usually is associated with clinical improvement, augmented forward stroke volume with lower total stroke volume, smaller LV end-diastolic volume, and regression of LV hypertrophy.[80,97,119,203-207] Correction of

mitral regurgitation can preserve LV contractility, particularly in patients with a normal preoperative ejection fraction who have minimal ventricular dilatation and those without significant coronary artery disease. On the other hand, in patients with LV dysfunction preoperatively, improvement in LV systolic function may not necessarily occur after operation. An LVESVI exceeding 30 mL/m^2 is associated with decreased postoperative LV function.[176,208] Thus, it is proposed that patients with chronic primary mitral regurgitation should be referred for mitral valve surgery before LVESVI exceeds 40 to 50 mL/m^2 or when LV end-systolic dimension (LVESD) reaches 4 cm or greater, consistent with the 2014 American College of Cardiology/American Heart Association (ACC/AHA) practice guidelines[80,176] (Fig. 34-16). Significant determinants of increased operative risk for mitral valve surgery include older age, higher New York Heart Association (NYHA) functional class, associated coronary artery disease, increased LV end-diastolic pressure, elevated LV end-diastolic volume index, elevated LVESD, reduced LV ESS index,

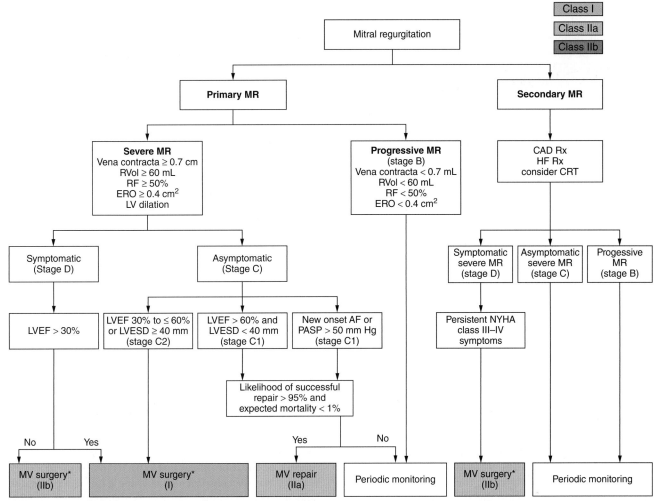

FIGURE 34-16 Indications for surgery for mitral regurgitation (MR). AF, atrial fibrillation; CAD, coronary artery disease; CRT, cardiac resynchronization therapy; ERO, effective regurgitant orifice; HF, heart failure; LV, left ventricular; LVEF, left ventricular ejection fraction; LVESD, left ventricular end-systolic dimension; MR, mitral regurgitation; MV, mitral valve; MVR, mitral valve replacement; NYHA, New York Heart Association; PASP, pulmonary artery systolic pressure; RF, regurgitant fraction; RVol, regurgitant volume; Rx, therapy. *Mitral valve repair is preferred over MVR when possible. (Reproduced with permission from Nishimura RA, Otto CM, Bonow RO, et al: 2014 AHA/ACC guideline for the management of patients with valvular heart disease: a report of the American College of Cardiology/American Heart Association Task Force on Practice Guidelines, *J Thorac Cardiovasc Surg.* 2014 Jul;148(1):e1-e132.)

depressed resting ejection fraction, decreased fractional shortening, reduced cardiac index, elevated capillary wedge or right ventricular end-diastolic pressure, concomitant operative procedures, and previous cardiac surgery.[176,208-212]

The decline in ejection fraction after mitral valve replacement for chronic mitral regurgitation historically was thought to result from an increase in LV afterload as a result of closure of the low-resistance early systolic "pop-off" into the left atrium and the surgical excision of the subvalvular apparatus. A spherical mathematical model defining the relations among LV end-diastolic dimension, systolic wall stress, and ejection fraction, demonstrated that postoperative changes in systolic stress are related directly to changes in chamber size, and LV afterload may *decrease* postoperatively if chordal-preservation valve replacement techniques are used.[213] In terms of exercise performance after surgery for nonischemic

mitral regurgitation, although patients generally report symptomatic improvement, cardiopulmonary exercise testing at 7 months may not be better than preoperatively, and abnormal neurohumoral activation persists, probably reflective of incomplete recovery of LV contractility.[214] Regarding long-term clinical outcome, risk factors portending postoperative cardiac deterioration include larger LV end-diastolic dimension, increased LVESD, increased LVESV, diminished fractional shortening, reduced LV ESS index, large LA size, decreased LV wall thickness/cavity dimension at end-systole, and associated coronary artery disease.[176,211,215-217]

PRIMARY MITRAL REGURGITATION

To evaluate the impact of the severity of regurgitation on outcomes in asymptomatic patients with primary mitral regurgitation, a Mayo Clinic study retrospectively evaluated 456 middle-aged patients with at least mild holosystolic mitral regurgitation defined echocardiographically between 1991 and 2000.[157] Baseline ejection fraction was 70%, LVESD was 3.4 ± 6 cm, LVESD was 5.6 ± 8 cm, LVESVI was 33 ± 130 mL/m², and regurgitant volume was 66 ± 40 mL/beat. At 5 years, 54% of patients had been operated on after an average of 1.2 ± 2 years of medical treatment when symptoms occurred or when worrisome echocardiographic findings were detected (based on the 1998 ACC/AHA practice guidelines). Among those who underwent a mitral valve procedure, 91% received valve repair. The patients were stratified by degree of regurgitation; mild, moderate, and severe were defined as regurgitant volumes of less than 30, 30 to 59, and 60 or more mL/beat, and ERO was defined as less than 20, 20 to 39, and 40 or greater mm², respectively. For the medically treated patients, 5-year survival compared with U.S. Census life tables was significantly inferior for those with moderate regurgitation (ERO of 20 to 39 mm², 66 vs 84%) and severe regurgitation (ERO of 40 mm² or more, 58 vs 78%).[157] The influence of ERO also held true for predicting cardiac deaths and all cardiac events. The 5-year cardiac death rate was 36% for patients with an ERO of 40 mm² or greater compared with 20% for those with an ERO of 20 to 39 mm² and only 3% for those with an ERO of less than 20 mm². Mitral valve operation was an independent determinant of fewer deaths, cardiac deaths, and cardiac events, especially in those with a larger ERO.[157] This important study, which focuses on the predictive effects of the severity of the regurgitation instead of the response of the ventricle, provides the basis for the surgical approach to asymptomatic patients with primary mitral regurgitation. On the other hand, these patient were older and most probably had prolapse due to fibroelastic deficiency; thus, these recommendations cannot safely be generalized to younger patients with Barlow's mitral valve disease or other types of mitral regurgitation.

Managed with medical therapy, mitral regurgitation from a flail leaflet is associated with high annual (6.3%) mortality rates.[120,218,219] In these patients, mitral valve repair is feasible in the large majority of patients in experienced centers and offers excellent early and late functional results.[80,119,219-221] Because fewer complications and lower operative mortality risk are associated with valve repair compared with valve replacement in this patient population, operation should be considered earlier in the natural history of the disease if the pathologic anatomy is judged favorable for valve repair.[80,111,119,120,215,218-220,222]

The 2014 AHA/ACC valve guidelines introduced several new concepts into clinical decision making for patients with mitral regurgitation.[80] The assessment of patients with mitral regurgitation now includes the following clinical stages: (A) at risk for mitral regurgitation, (B) progressive mitral regurgitation, (C) asymptomatic severe mitral regurgitation, and (D) symptomatic severe mitral regurgitation[80] (Table 34-1). For patients with primary mitral regurgitation (intrinsic leaflet disease) the degree of regurgitation is quantified with progressive regurgitation (or stage B) meaning a

vena contracta < 0.7 cm, regurgitant volume < 60 mL, regurgitant fraction < 50%, and ERO < 0.4 cm². Severe regurgitation includes a vena contracta > 0.7 cm, regurgitant volume > 60 mL, regurgitant fraction > 50%, and ERO > 0.4 cm². According to the 2014 ACC/AHA practice guidelines, all asymptomatic patients with chronic primary severe mitral regurgitation should be considered for operation if the LVEF is 30 to 60% or LVESD > 40 mm (class I evidence); asymptomatic patients in whom the LVEF > 60% and LVESD < 40 mm can be considered for early operation (class IIa evidence) if the likelihood of repair is 90% with an expected mortality of < 1% in a referent mitral surgical center[80] (Fig. 34-16). In healthier patients with LVEF greater than 63% and LVESD less than 39 mm, early mitral valve repair may also result in preserved long-term postoperative LV function.[80,223] The AHA/ACC 2014 valve guidelines for chronic secondary mitral regurgitation (FMR or IMR) have also been modified (see below).

Because many patients with chronic mitral regurgitation report no symptoms, cardiopulmonary exercise testing has been used to evaluate asymptomatic patients with primary mitral regurgitation.[224,225] In a study of asymptomatic patients with severe mitral regurgitation with a regurgitant volume of 68 mL/beat and an ERO of 35 mm², functional capacity was markedly reduced (defined as 84% or less than expected) in 19% of patients.[224] When patients with extraneous, noncardiac reasons for impaired functional capacity were excluded, 14% had a reduced functional capacity. Determinants of reduced functional capacity were impaired LV diastolic function, lower forward stroke volume, and atrial fibrillation; the impact of ERO on functional capacity was only modest.[224] Thus, it was the consequences of chronic mitral regurgitation and not the magnitude of the leak that predicted impaired functional capacity. Follow-up at 3 years revealed that 66% of patients with impaired functional capacity sustained some adverse event or required mitral surgery (vs 29% of those with normal functional capacity).[224] Consistent with the previous study, in patients with primary mitral regurgitation that underwent exercise echocardiography followed by mitral valve surgery, lower achieved metabolic equivalents were associated with worse long-term outcomes.[225] In those with preserved exercise capacity, delaying mitral valve surgery by greater than one year did not adversely affect outcomes.[225] Thus, asymptomatic patients with substantial mitral regurgitation should undergo periodic cardiopulmonary exercise testing to detect subclinical impairment in functional capacity, and repair should be recommended to those with impaired exercise capacity.

Even after mitral valve repair or replacement for chronic mitral regurgitation, some patients continue to be limited by heart failure symptoms and have suboptimal long-term postoperative outcomes. The incidence of congestive heart failure in patients who survive surgery (combined series of valve repair and valve replacement) for pure mitral regurgitation has been 23, 33, and 37% at 5, 10, and 14 years.[226] Patient survival after the first episode of congestive heart failure is dismal, being only 44% at 5 years. Causes of congestive

TABLE 34-1: Stages of Primary Mitral Regurgitation

Grade	Definition	Valve anatomy	Valve hemodynamics*	Hemodynamic consequences	Symptoms
A	At risk of MR	• Mild mitral valve prolapse with normal coaptation • Mild valve thickening and leaflet restriction	• No MR jet or small central jet area < 20% LA on Doppler • Small vena contracta < 0.3 cm	• None	• None
B	Progressive MR	• Severe mitral valve prolapse with normal coaptation • Rheumatic valve changes with leaflet restriction and loss of central coaptation • Prior IE	• Central jet MR 20 to 40% LA or late systolic eccentric jet MR • Vena contracta < 0.7 cm • Regurgitant volume < 60 mL • Regurgitant fraction < 50% • ERO < 0.40 cm² • Angiographic grade 1-2+	• Mild LA enlargement • No LV enlargement • Normal pulmonary pressure	• None
C	Asymptomatic severe MR	• Severe mitral valve prolapse with loss of coaptation or flail leaflet • Rheumatic valve changes with leaflet restriction and loss of central coaptation • Prior IE • Thickening of leaflets with radiation heart disease	• Central jet MR > 40% LA or holosystolic eccentric jet MR • Vena contracta ≥ 0.7 cm • Regurgitant volume ≥ 60 mL • Regurgitant fraction ≥ 50% • ERO ≥ 0.40 cm² • Angiographic grade 3-4+	• Moderate or severe LA enlargement • LV enlargement • Pulmonary hypertension may be present at rest or with exercise • C1 : LVEF > 60% and LVESD < 40 mm • C2: LVEF ≤ 60% and LVESD ≥ 40 mm	• None
D	Symptomatic severe MR	• Severe mitral valve prolapse with loss of coaptation or flail leaflet • Rheumatic valve changes with leaflet restriction and loss of central coaptation • Prior IE • Thickening of leaflets with radiation heart disease	• Central jet MR > 40% LA or holosystolic eccentric jet MR • Vena contracta ≥ 0.7 cm • Regurgitant volume ≥ 60 mL • Regurgitant fraction ≥ 50% • ERO ≥ 0.40 cm² • Angiographic grade 3-4+	• Moderate or severe LA enlargement • LV enlargement • Pulmonary hypertension present	• Decreased exercise tolerance • Exertional dyspnea

ERO, Effective regurgitant orifice; *IE*, infective endocarditis; LA, left atriuni/atrial; LV, left ventricular; LVEF, left ventricular ejection fraction; LVESD, left ventricular end-systolic dimension; MR, mitral regurgitation. *Several valve hemodynamic criteria are provided for assessment of MR severity, but not all criteria for each category will be present in each patient. Categorization of MR severity as mild, moderate, or severe depends on data quality and integration of these parameters in conjunction with other clinical evidence.

Reproduced with permission from Nishimura RA, Otto CM, Bonow RO, et al: 2014 AHA/ACC guideline for the management of patients with valvular heart disease: a report of the American College of Cardiology/American Heart Association Task Force on Practice Guidelines, *J Thorac Cardiovasc Surg.* 2014 Jul;148(1):e1-e132

heart failure include LV dysfunction in two-thirds of patients and valvular problems in the remaining one-third. Predictors of postoperative heart failure are lower preoperative ejection fraction, coronary artery disease, and higher NYHA functional class.[226] Importantly, preoperative functional class III/IV symptoms are associated with markedly decreased postoperative medium- and long-term survival independent of all other baseline characteristics.[227]

SECONDARY MITRAL REGURGITATION

To risk stratify patients after myocardial infarction, quantifying and staging secondary mitral regurgitation (eg, IMR) are of key importance[80,156,228-230] (Table 34-2). In a report from

the Mayo Clinic, medically managed patients who developed IMR late after myocardial infarction had a very high mortality rate (62% at 5 years) compared with those with an infarction who did not develop IMR (39% at 5 years).[156] Medium-term survival for patients with IMR and LV systolic dysfunction was inversely related to the ERO and regurgitant volume. After 5 years, the survival rate was 47% for patients with an ERO of less than 20 mm² and 29% for those with an ERO of 20 mm² or greater. Survival at 5 years was 35% when the regurgitant volume was 30 mL/beat or greater compared with 44% for those with a regurgitant volume of less than 30 mL/beat. The relative risk ratio for cardiac death for patients with IMR was 1.56 for patients with an ERO of less than 20 mm² versus 2.38 for those with an ERO of greater

TABLE 34-2: Stages of Secondary Mitral Regurgitatation

Grade	Definition	Valve anatomy	Valve hemodynamics*	Associated cardiac findings	Symptoms
A	At risk of MR	• Normal valve leaflets, chords, and annulus in a patient with coronary disease or cardiomyopathy	• No MR jet or small central jet area < 20% LA on Doppler • Small vena contracta < 0.30 cm	• Normal or mildly dilated LV size with fixed (infarction) or inducible (ischemia) regional wall motion abnormalities • Primary myocardial disease with LV dilation and systolic dysfunction	• Symptoms due to coronary ischemia or HF may be present that respond to revascularization and appropriate medical therapy
B	Progressive MR	• Regional wall motion abnormalities with mild tethering of mitral leaflet • Annular dilation with mild loss of central coaptation of the mitral leaflets	• ERO < 0.20 cm²† • Regurgitant volume < 30 mL • Regurgitant fraction < 50%	• Regional wall motion abnormalities with reduced LV systolic function • LV dilation and systolic dysfunction due to primary myocardial disease	• Symptoms due to coronary ischemia or HF may be present that respond to revascularization and appropriate medical therapy
C	Asymptomatic severe MR	• Regional wall motion abnormalities and/or LV dilation with severe tethering of mitral leaflet • Annular dilation with severe loss of central coaptation of the mitral leaflets	• ERO ≥ 0.20 cm²† • Regurgitant volume ≥ 30 mL • Regurgitant fraction ≥ 50%	• Regional wall motion abnormalities with reduced LV systolic function • LV dilation and systolic dysfunction due to primary myocardial disease	• Symptoms due to coronary ischemia or HF may be present that respond to revascularization and appropriate medical therapy
D	Symptomatic severe MR	• Regional wall motion abnormalities and/or LV dilation with severe tethering of mitral leaflet • Annular dilation with severe loss of central coaptation of the mitral leaflets	• ERO ≥ 0.20 cm²† • Regurgitant volume 30 mL • Regurgitant fraction ≥ 50%	• Regional wall motion abnormalities with reduced LV systolic function • LV dilation and systolic dysfunction due to primary myocardial disease	• HF symptoms due to MR persist even after revascularization and optimization of medical therapy • Decreased exercise tolerance • Exertional dyspnea

2D, 2-dimensional; ERO, effective regurgitant orifice; HF, heart failure; LA, left atrium: LV, left ventricular; MR, mitral regurgitation; TTE, transthoracic echocardiogram.
*Several valve hemodynamic criteria are provided for assessment of MR severity, but not all criteria for each category will be present in each patient. Categorization of MR severity as mild, moderate, or severe depends on data quality and integration of these parameters in conjunction with other clinical evidence. †The measurement of the proximal isovelocity surface area by 2D TTE in patients with secondary MR underestimates the true ERO due to the crescentic shape of the proximal convergence.
Reproduced with permission from Nishimura RA, Otto CM, Bonow RO, et al: 2014 AHA/ACC guideline for the management of patients with valvular heart disease: a report of the American College of Cardiology/American Heart Association Task Force on Practice Guidelines, *J Thorac Cardiovasc Surg.* 2014 Jul;148(1):e1-e132.

than 20 mm². Note this ERO threshold for secondary IMR if one-half the ERO threshold applied to patients with primary MR.[156,157] In those with myocardial infarction, the incidence of congestive heart failure was also high in patients with IMR.[229] At 5 years, the rate of congestive heart failure was 18% without IMR compared with 53% if IMR was present. If the ERO was less than 20 mm², the incidence of congestive heart failure was 46% compared with 68% when the ERO was 20 mm² or greater.[229]

Mitral valve repair or replacement for patients with IMR has been associated with higher operative risk (4 to 30%) than for patients with nonischemic chronic mitral regurgitation, which reflects the concomitant adverse consequences of previous myocardial infarction and ischemia.[205,206,231-237]

Coronary revascularization alone in the setting of moderate or severe IMR leaves many patients with substantial residual mitral regurgitation and heart failure symptoms.[113,238-240] Immediately postoperatively, IMR is absent or mild in 73% and severe in 6%; on the other hand, by 6 weeks, only 40% of patients have absent or mild mitral regurgitation, and 22% have severe mitral regurgitation[239] (Fig. 34-17). Because moderate IMR does not universally resolve with bypass grafting alone, it has been argued that valve repair be considered in these patients because it potentially can reduce cardiac morbidity and may improve long-term survival.[113,228,238] Conversely, some investigators have shown that for patients with moderate or moderately severe IMR, isolated coronary surgery compared to coronary revascularization combined with

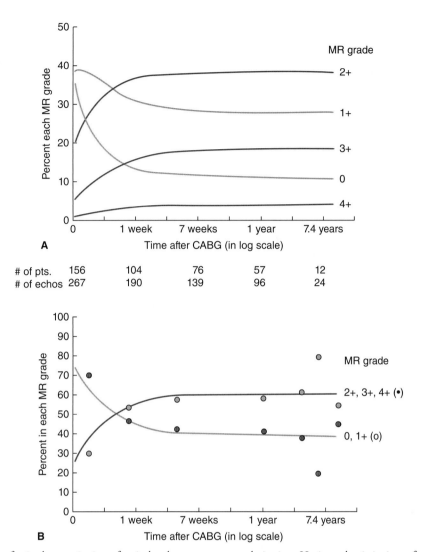

| # of pts. | 156 | 104 | 76 | 57 | 12 |
| # of echos | 267 | 190 | 139 | 96 | 24 |

FIGURE 34-17 Course of mitral regurgitation after isolated coronary revascularization. Horizontal axis is time after coronary artery bypass grafting on a logarithmic scale. 1+ is mild regurgitation, 2+ moderate, 3+ moderately severe, and 4+ severe. (A) All grades of mitral regurgitation. (B) Mitral regurgitation grades 0 or 1+ compared with 2+, 3+, or 4+. Symbols (*red circles, green circles*) represent aggregated raw echocardiographic values for mitral regurgitation grade. CABG, coronary artery bypass grafting; MR, mitral regurgitation. (Reproduced with permission from Lam BK, Gillinov AM, Blackstone EH, et al: Importance of moderate ischemic mitral regurgitation, *Ann Thorac Surg.* 2005 Feb;79(2):462-470.)

mitral annuloplasty provide similar long-term outcome with survival rates of 82 to 92% at 1 year, 40 to 75% at 5 years, and 37 to 47% at 10 years[232-234,241-243] (Fig. 34-18). Predictors of long-term mortality are older age, prior myocardial infarction, unstable angina, chronic renal failure, atrial fibrillation, absence of an internal mammary artery graft, lack of beta blocker use, lower ejection fraction, smaller LA size, global LV wall motion abnormalities, severe lateral wall motion abnormalities, ST segment elevation in the lateral leads, mitral leaflet restriction, and fewer bypass grafts.[232,234,241] In the experience of some investigators, combined mitral valve repair and coronary revascularization does not emerge as a predictor of long-term survival. Furthermore, in a recent report from the Cardiothoracic Surgical Trials Network of 301 patients with moderate IMR randomized to coronary artery bypass grafting alone or combined coronary artery bypass grafting with valve repair, the rate of death is 7.3% in and 6.7% at one year.[244] Although moderate or severe regurgitation is less common in the combined group than the coronary artery bypass group alone (11 vs 31%, respectively), the combined group had longer bypass time, longer hospital stay, and more neurologic events. Also, it is sobering that the addition of mitral valve repair does not result in a greater degree of LV reverse remodeling (measured by LVESI) at one year.[244]

To identify preoperatively those that would be more likely to benefit from isolated coronary artery bypass grafting, the Prague group evaluated 135 patients with moderate IMR undergoing isolated coronary artery bypass surgery; of these, 42% of the patients had no or mild mitral regurgitation postoperatively, whereas 47% failed to improve.[245] Preoperatively, the improvement group had significantly more viable myocardium and less dyssynchrony between papillary muscles

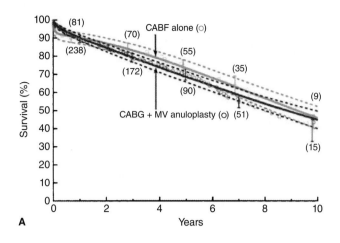

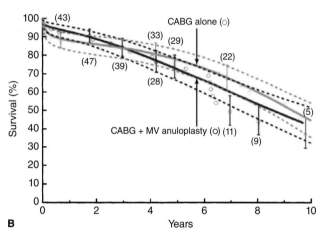

FIGURE 34-18 Survival after coronary artery bypass grafting (CABG) alone or with concomitant mitral valve (MV) annuloplasty for ischemic mitral regurgitation. Vertical bars are 68% confidence limits. Numbers in parentheses are patients alive and remaining at risk. Solid lines are parametric estimates enclosed within 68% confidence limits. (A) Unadjusted survival, based on 37 deaths after CABG alone and 92 after CABG + MV annuloplasty. (B) Propensity-matched survival, based on 19 deaths after CABG alone and 19 after CABG + MV annuloplasty. (Reproduced with permission from Mihaljevic T, Lam BK, Rajeswaran J, et al: Impact of mitral valve annuloplasty combined with revascularization in patients with functional ischemic mitral regurgitation, *J Am Coll Cardiol.* 2007 Jun 5;49(22):2191-2201.)

than the failure group. Thus, reliable improvement in moderate IMR by isolated coronary artery revascularization is likely only in patients with concomitant presence of viable myocardium and absence of dyssynchrony between papillary muscles.[245] In a pilot study of cardiac MRI in patients with IMR and ischemic cardiomyopathy, extensive scarring and severe wall motion abnormalities in the region of posterior papillary muscle correlated with recurrent mitral regurgitation after coronary artery bypass grafting and mitral annuloplasty.[246] Routinely assessing scar burden may identify patients for whom annuloplasty alone is insufficient to eliminate mitral regurgitation. Therefore, although some investigators report

that annuloplasty can be added to coronary grafting in high-risk patients without increasing early mortality, the potential benefit with respect to late survival and functional status is not proved and may be limited because of the underlying ischemic cardiomyopathy.[233-234,247]

In terms of the best type of valve surgery for patients with IMR, it is likely that the clinical condition and LV functional status are more powerful determinants of outcome than whether one undergoes repair or replacement.[231,248-252] In the Brigham and Women's Hospital experience, patients with IMR and annular dilatation who underwent valve repair and coronary revascularization had a worse long-term outcome than those who underwent valve replacement and coronary revascularization.[231] Notably, the pathophysiology or cause of the IMR was a stronger determinant of long-term survival than was the type of valve procedure. In the Cleveland Clinic experience, when patients with severe IMR underwent mitral valve surgery, undersized annuloplasty resulted in less IMR postoperatively in 70 to 85% of cases.[249] Based on propensity score analysis, they found that in the lower-risk quintiles of patients with IMR, valve repair conferred a survival advantage (58% at 5 years) over those who underwent valve replacement (36% at 5 years); however, in the highest-risk patients, late survival rates after valve repair and valve replacement were similarly poor, and valve replacement actually conferred a small survival advantage.[250] At the Laval University in Quebec, 370 patients with IMR underwent either mitral valve repair or mitral valve replacement.[251] The operative mortality was lower in the repair group (10%) compared with the replacement group (17%), but 6-year survival estimates were similar at 73 and 67%, respectively. The type of valve procedure did not emerge as a risk factor for a poor outcome. In the Italian Study on the Treatment of Ischemic Mitral Regurgitation Trial using propensity score matching analysis to evaluate surgical outcomes of patients with chronic IMR and LV dysfunction (ejection fraction less than 40%), those who underwent mitral valve repair had an 8-year survival rate of 82% compared to 80% for those undergoing mitral valve replacement.[237] Further, LV function did not improve in either group postoperatively, and mitral valve repair was a strong predictor of valve-related reoperation. The recent Cardiothoracic Surgical Trials Network multi-institutional randomized trial of 251 patients with severe IMR comparing complete rigid or semirigid ring annuloplasty with mitral valve replacement demonstrated no difference in LV reverse remodeling or survival at 12 months.[252] The rate of recurrent or residual moderate or severe IMR 6 months postoperatively was 32.6% in the annuloplasty group versus 2.3% in the MVR group.[252] Replacement provided a more durable correction of mitral regurgitation with no difference in clinical outcomes at this early follow-up period.[252] These reports emphasize the guarded prognosis of patients with severe IMR and the impact of the patient's preoperative clinical condition and LV functional status (and not the type of procedure *per se*) on outcome. Although mitral valve repair may still be preferred by some for patients with severe IMR, most surgeons today believe complete chordal-sparing mitral valve replacement is preferable to repair in the most severely ill patients and in those with certain echocardiographic characteristics such as severe bileaflet tethering. Chordal-sparing MVR certainly is more predictable and reliable.

In patients with chronic primary versus secondary mitral regurgitation, the decision to repair or replace the valve should be based on the patient's clinical status and not on whether the regurgitation is degenerative or ischemic in etiology.[235,236,253] In a Mayo Clinic study, older age, ejection fraction of 35% or less, three-vessel coronary disease, mitral valve replacement, and residual mitral regurgitation at discharge were risk factors for death. The cause of the mitral regurgitation, ischemic versus degenerative, was not a predictor of long-term survival, class III or IV congestive heart failure, or recurrent regurgitation.[235] In the Cleveland Clinic experience, analysis of the etiology of the mitral regurgitation (degenerative vs ischemic) in patients with coronary artery disease after combined mitral valve repair and coronary revascularization showed that those with IMR had more extensive coronary disease, worse ventricular function, more comorbidities, and more preoperative symptoms.[253] Unadjusted 5-year survival estimates were 64 and 82% for patients with IMR and degenerative mitral regurgitation, respectively; however, matched pairs had equivalent but poor 5-year survival rates (66 and 65%, respectively). In the Duke database of patients undergoing mitral valve repair with or without coronary artery bypass grafting, the 30-day mortality was 4.3% for those with IMR and 1.3% for nonischemic group; the 5-year survival was 56% for IMR and 84% for those with nonischemic mitral regurgitation.[236] The etiology of mitral regurgitation (ischemic vs degenerative) was not predictive of survival after annuloplasty and coronary artery grafting; importantly, the long-term outcomes were more influenced by advanced age and the number of preoperative comorbidities[236] (Fig. 34-19).

A compelling explanation for the generally poor long-term outcome of patients who undergo mitral valve repair for IMR is the presence of residual and/or recurrent mitral regurgitation postoperatively.[254-259] Persistence of mitral regurgitation after annuloplasty is due predominantly to augmented posterior leaflet apical tethering with no improvement in anterior leaflet tethering and no increase in coaptation length; higher preoperative LVED index may also predict recurrent mitral regurgitation.[256-258] In a Cleveland Clinic report of annuloplasty for IMR (95% with concomitant coronary artery bypass grafting), the proportion of patients with 0 or 1+ mitral regurgitation decreased from 71% preoperatively to 41% postoperatively, but the proportion with 3+ or 4+ residual or recurrent IMR increased from 13 to 28% during the first 6 months after repair[254] (Fig. 34-20). The temporal pattern of development of severe regurgitation was similar for those who received a partial band or a complete ring (25%), but it was substantially worse for those who received a strip of glutaraldehyde-preserved xenograft pericardium for annuloplasty (66%).[254] Others have suggested that the

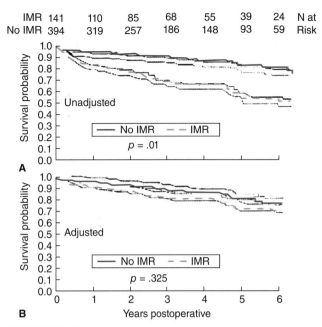

FIGURE 34-19 Survival of patients undergoing mitral valve repair with ischemic mitral regurgitation versus nonischemic mitral regurgitation before (A) and after (B) adjustment for differences in baseline patient characteristics. IMR, ischemic mitral regurgitation; NMR, nonischemic mitral regurgitation. (Reproduced with permission from Glower DD, Tuttle RH, Shaw LK, et al: Patient survival characteristics after routine mitral valve repair for ischemic mitral regurgitation, *J Thorac Cardiovasc Surg.* 2005 Apr;129(4):860-868.)

use of smaller, complete, and rigid annuloplasty rings may provide improved freedom from recurrent mitral regurgitation in patient with FMR or IMR.[260] At the Montreal Heart Institute, the operative mortality rate for those undergoing mitral valve repair for IMR was 12.3% and the 5-year survival was 68%.[261] Recurrent moderate mitral regurgitation was seen in 37%, and severe regurgitation was present in 20% at mean follow-up of 28 months. Only age and less marked preoperative posterior tethering were predictive of recurrent mitral regurgitation. Data from the Cardiothoracic Surgical Trials Network severe IMR trial demonstrated a rate of recurrence of moderate regurgitation of 26% and of severe regurgitation of 4% at 6 months after mitral valve repair.[257] The presence of inferior basal aneurysm/dyskinesis was strongly associated with recurrent regurgitation and was a better predictor of recurrence than individual measures of leaflet tethering or LV remodeling, since it integrates both leaflet tethering and LV remodeling measures.[257] The Leiden experience with the use of restrictive mitral semirigid undersized annuloplasty (mean ring size of 26 mm) in patients with FMR and heart failure demonstrated a more satisfactory 19% rate of recurrent regurgitation (grade 2-4) at a mean follow up of 2.6 years.[259] Based on their method of quantification of preoperative parameters of mitral and LV geometry using echocardiography, distal anterior leaflet tethering and posterior leaflet tethering were independent predictors of recurrent mitral regurgitation[259] (Fig. 34-21). These findings highlight

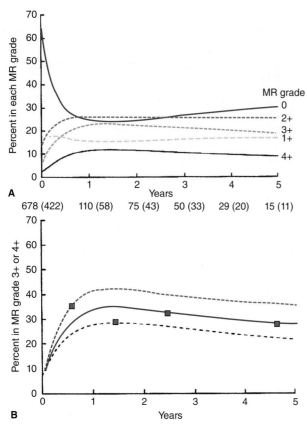

FIGURE 34-20 Progression of mitral regurgitation after surgical annuloplasty overall. (A) All grades of mitral regurgitation. Curves for each regurgitation grade represent average temporal prevalence, and they sum up to 100% at each point in time. Numbers below the horizontal axis represent echocardiograms available at various time points, with the number of patients in parentheses. (B) Prevalence of regurgitation grades 3+ or 4+. Dashed lines are 68% confidence limits of average prevalence. MR = mitral regurgitation. (Reproduced with permission from McGee EC, Gillinov AM, Blackstone EH, et al: Recurrent mitral regurgitation after annuloplasty for functional ischemic mitral regurgitation, *J Thorac Cardiovasc Surg.* 2004 Dec;128(6):916-924.)

the need for better patient selection or possibly chordal-sparing mitral valve replacement in certain patients.[254,257,259,261,262]

In brief, because mitral regurgitation is only one component of the disease, the appropriate management of patients with secondary mitral regurgitation or IMR is complicated, since restoring valve competence may not reverse the underlying pathophysiology or improve the prognosis.[80,125] For instance, in those with secondary mitral regurgitation, adverse outcomes are associated with lesser degrees of mitral regurgitation and with a smaller calculated ERO than those with primary mitral regurgitation.[80] ERO, however, may be underestimated by 2D echocardiography-derived flow convergence method due to the crescentic shape of the regurgitant orifice.[80] Importantly, the 2014 ACC/AHA valve guidelines revised the definition of severe **secondary** mitral regurgitation from an ERO of >0.4 to >0.2 cm² and a regurgitant volume of >60 to >30 ml.[80,125] However, the new guidelines present clinical challenges because 2D and 3D

echocardiography may generate disparate findings of ERO and regurgitant volume, and the nature of secondary mitral regurgitation may be dynamic depending on medical therapy (loading conditions) and after revascularization or cardiac resynchronization.[125] In terms of decision making, a rebuttal to the 2014 AHA/ACC guidelines focusing so much on ERO in patients with secondary mitral regurgitation was published in 2014 by a group of experienced echocardiographers and cardiac surgeons arguing that an integrated approach based on clinical judgment that incorporates multiple echo Doppler parameters without relying on any single parameter is best.[125] This approach would discount poor quality data (eg, ERO underestimation by PISA) and employ multiple echocardiographic variables, recognize that the definition of "severe" (ERO > 0.2 cm² and regurgitant volume > 30 mL) depends on LV size and on the LV-LA pressure gradient, and specify the quantification method (2D, PISA, planimetry, volumetric).[125]

Mitral Subvalvular Apparatus and LV Systolic Function

Originally proposed by Lillehei and colleagues in 1964, the mitral subvalvular apparatus (or valvular-ventricular complex) including chordal and papillary muscle function is important for optimal postoperative LV geometry and systolic pump function.[101-104,166,167,263-267] After mitral valve replacement with total chordal excision in the experimental and clinical settings, LV performance declines along with depression of regional and global LV elastance, dyssynergy of contraction, and dyskinesia at the papillary muscle insertion sites. Conversely, valve replacement with total or partial chordal preservation maintains LV contractile function.[101-103,183,267] Mitral valve replacement with chordal division is associated with reduced rest and exercise LVEF owing in part to an increase in LV ESS.[266] Mitral valve repair does not perturb rest and exercise ejection indexes of LV function primarily as a consequence of reducing ESS and maintaining a more ellipsoidal chamber geometry. Mitral valve replacement with complete chordal transection results in no postoperative change in LV end-diastolic volume, an increase in LVESV, an increase in ESS, and a decrease in ejection fraction.[265] Patients who undergo chordal-sparing valve replacement, on the other hand, have a smaller LV end-diastolic volume and LVESV, decreased ESS, and unchanged ejection fraction. These findings suggest that smaller chamber size, reduced systolic afterload, and preservation of ventricular contractile function act in concert to maintain ejection performance after chordal-sparing mitral valve replacement. In contrast, increased LV chamber size, increased systolic afterload, and probable reduction in LV contractile function leading to reduced ejection performance occur in patients who undergo valve replacement with chordal transection.[265]

The loss of LV systolic function after mitral valve replacement with chordal division may be caused by heterogeneity of regional LV wall stress and not local depression of regional

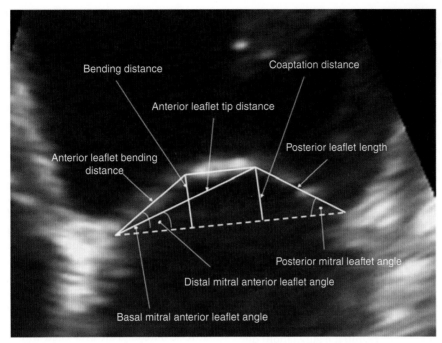

FIGURE 34-21 Method of quantification of basal mitral anterior leaflet angle, distal mitral anterior leaflet angle, and the posterior mitral leaflet angle. Measurements are depicted on echocardiographic image of the mitral valve in apical four-chamber view in mid-systole. The basal mitral anterior leaflet angle is defined as the angle between the annular plane and the basal portion of the anterior leaflet. The distal mitral anterior leaflet angle is defined as the angle between the annular plane and the anterior leaflet tip distance (which corresponds to the distance between the medial part of the mitral annulus and the coaptation point). The posterior mitral leaflet angle is defined as the angle between the annular plane and the posterior leaflet. (Reproduced with permission from Ciarka A, Braun J, Delgado V, et al: Predictors of mitral regurgitation recurrence in patients with heart failure undergoing mitral valve annuloplasty, *Am J Cardiol.* 2010 Aug 1;106(3):395-401.)

contractile function.[268] After valve replacement with chordal transection in an experimental model, outward displacement of the ventricular wall and transverse shearing deformation occurred in the LV region papillary muscle insertion during isovolumic contraction.[268] Circumferential and radial strains during ejection were maintained at the basal LV site and enhanced in the apical LV site. Chordal transection augmented regional myocardial loading at the papillary muscle insertion site; the resulting heterogeneity of regional systolic function might be the mechanism for reduced global LV function and slowed ventricular relaxation. Anterior chordal transection with mitral valve replacement caused impaired regional LV function and also impaired regional right ventricular function,[269] whereas radionuclide angiography before and after mitral valve repair showed that LVEF did not change and right ventricular ejection fraction improved. In the region of the anterolateral papillary muscle insertion, local LV contractile function deteriorated after valve replacement with chordal transection, and right ventricular apico-septal region was similarly impaired.[269]

In patients with chronic IMR, surgical division of the second-order chordae subtending the infarcted wall (usually those originating from the posteromedial papillary muscle) has been proposed to treat IMR by reducing leaflet tethering.[270-272] It is postulated that if the apical systolic tethering is eliminated, the normal redundancy of the mitral leaflet area creates better coaptation with the intact first-order

or marginal chordae preventing leaflet prolapse. Clinically, the Toronto group compared the outcomes of patients who underwent chordal-cutting mitral valve repair (n = 43) and those undergoing conventional mitral valve repair (n = 49) for IMR.[271] The reduction in tenting height before-to-after repair was similar in the two groups of patients, but those undergoing chordal cutting had a greater reduction in tenting area. The chordal-cutting group also had greater mobility of the anterior leaflet, as measured by a reduction in the distance between the free edge of the anterior mitral valve leaflet and the posterior LV wall. Additionally, those undergoing conventional mitral valve repair had a higher incidence of recurrent mitral regurgitation during 2 years of follow-up.[271] Chordal cutting did not adversely affect postoperative LVEF (10% relative increase in EF compared with 11% in the control group). The authors proposed that chordal cutting improves mitral valve leaflet mobility and reduces mitral regurgitation recurrence in patients with IMR, without any obvious deleterious effects on LV function.[271] It is known, however, that division of the chordae, especially the second-order or "strut" chordae, can impair LV systolic function.[273,274] Dividing the second-order chordae in an experimental acute ovine preparation caused regional LV systolic dysfunction near the chordal insertion sites and neither prevents nor decreases the severity of acute IMR, septal-lateral annular dilatation, leaflet tenting area, or leaflet tenting volume.[273] Cutting the anterior mitral leaflet second-order chordae alters LV chamber long-axis and subvalvular geometry, remodels end-diastolic transmural myocardial architecture in the equatorial lateral LV region, perturbs systolic transmural LV wall-thickening mechanics (thereby decreasing subendocardial "microtorsion") and wall thickening, changes systolic temporal dynamics with delayed ejection, and impairs global LV systolic function (decreased end-systolic elastance and PRSW).[274] Because of the importance of the chordae for LV structure and function, we believe that caution is necessary when considering procedures that cut second-order chordae to treat patients with IMR because of the resulting compromise in LV systolic function in ventricles that are already impaired.[273,274]

Summary

The functional competence of the mitral valve relies on the interaction of the mitral annulus and leaflets, chordae tendineae, papillary muscles, left atrium, and left ventricle. Dysfunction of any one or more components of this valvuloventricular complex can lead to mitral regurgitation. Important causes of mitral regurgitation include myxomatous degeneration and prolapse (primary mitral regurgitation) due to fibroelastic deficiency in older patients or Barlow's disease in younger subjects, ischemic heart disease with IMR (secondary mitral regurgitation), dilated cardiomyopathy leading to FMR (secondary mitral regurgitation), rheumatic valve disease, mitral annular calcification, and infective endocarditis. Four structural changes of the mitral valve apparatus may produce regurgitation: leaflet retraction from fibrosis and calcification, annular dilatation, chordal abnormalities, and LV systolic dysfunction with or without papillary muscle involvement. In IMR, changes in global and regional LV function and geometry, alterations in mitral annular geometry, abnormal leaflet (Carpentier type IIIb) motion, leaflet malcoaptation, increased interpapillary distance, and papillary muscle lateral displacement and malalignment all may result in apical tenting of the leaflets and mitral incompetence.

With mitral regurgitation, the impedance to LV emptying is lower because the mitral orifice is parallel with the LV outflow tract. Reduced LV impedance allows a greater proportion of contractile energy to be expended in myocardial fiber shortening than in tension development. After the initial compensatory phase, LV contractility becomes progressively more impaired with chronic mitral regurgitation and chronic LV volume overload. Importantly, because of the low impedance during systole, clinical indexes of systolic function, such as ejection fraction, can be normal even if depressed LV contractility is already present. LVESV is less dependent on preload than is ejection fraction and is a better measure of LV contractile reserve. Preoperative LVESV is a good predictor of postoperative outcome. Surgical mitral valve repair (or, if repair is judged not to be durable, mitral valve replacement with total chordal preservation) for chronic mitral regurgitation can preserve LV contractility, particularly in patients with a normal preoperative ejection fraction who have minimal ventricular dilatation and those without major coronary disease. In patients with impaired preoperative LV contractility,

LV systolic function may not necessarily improve after ring annuloplasty and definitely will not improve if the subvalvular apparatus and chordae are divided during mitral valve replacement.

IMR is generally associated with a higher operative risk than is nonischemic chronic mitral regurgitation. In patients with ischemic cardiomyopathy and mild mitral regurgitation, isolated coronary artery bypass grafting may suffice if the LV inferior wall is still viable. Other argue that coronary revascularization alone in the setting of moderate IMR leaves many patients with substantial residual mitral regurgitation, heart failure symptoms, and a grave prognosis. Because moderate IMR does not resolve reliably with coronary revascularization alone, valve repair should be considered because it can reduce complications and possibly improve long-term survival. Survival after mitral valve surgery and coronary artery bypass grafting is more determined by the extent of coronary artery disease and severity of preoperative LV dysfunction than by the etiology of mitral regurgitation. Because mitral regurgitation is only one component of the disease, the appropriate management of patients with IMR is complicated, since adverse outcomes are associated with lesser degrees of mitral regurgitation (a smaller ERO threshold than those with primary mitral regurgitation). The 2014 ACC/AHA practice guidelines present clinical challenges because 2D and 3D echocardiography may generate disparate findings of ERO and regurgitant volume, and the nature of secondary mitral regurgitation may be dynamic depending on loading conditions and after revascularization or resynchronization. In managing these patients, an integrated approach has been proposed that is based on clinical judgment and that incorporates multiple Doppler parameters without relying on any single parameter.

REFERENCES

1. van Gils FA: The fibrous skeleton in the human heart: embryological and pathogenetic considerations. *Virchows Arch A Pathol Anat Histol* 1981; 393:61.
2. Anderson RH, Wilcox BR: The anatomy of the mitral valve, in Wells FC, Shapiro LM (eds): *Mitral Valve Disease.* Oxford, England, Butterworth-Heinemann, 1996; p 4.
3. O'Gara P, Sugeng L, Lang R, et al: The role of imaging in chronic degenerative mitral regurgitation. *J Am Coll Cardiol Img* 2008; 1:221.
4. Ranganathan N, Lam JH, Wigle ED, et al: Morphology of the human mitral valve: II. The valve leaflets. *Circulation* 1970; 41:459.
5. Wit AL, Fenoglio J Jr, Hordof AJ, Reemtsma K: Ultrastructure and transmembrane potentials of cardiac muscle in the human anterior mitral valve leaflet. *Circulation* 1979; 59:1284.
6. Marron K, Yacoub MH, Polak JM, et al: Innervation of human atrioventricular and arterial valves. *Circulation* 1996; 94:368.
7. Ahmed A, Johansson O, Folan-Curran J: Distribution of PGP 9.5, TH, NPY, SP and CGRP immunoreactive nerves in the rat and guinea pig atrioventricular valves and chordae tendinae. *J Anat* 1997; 191:547.
8. Filip DA, Radu A, Simionescu M: Interstitial cells of the heart valves possess characteristics similar to smooth muscle cells. *Circ Res* 1986; 59:310.
9. De Biasi S, Vitellaro-Zuccarello L, Blum I: Histochemical and ultrastructural study on the innervation of human and porcine atrioventricular valves. *Anat Embryol (Berl)* 1984; 169:159.
10. Swanson JC, Davis LR, Arata K, et al: Characterization of mitral valve anterior leaflet perfusion patterns. *J Heart Valve Dis* 2009; 18:488-495.

11. Williams TH, Folan JC, Jew JY, et al: Variations in atrioventricular valve innervation in four species of mammals. *Am J Anat* 1990; 187:193.

12. Jew JY, Fink CA, Williams TH: Tyrosine hydroxylase-and nitric oxide synthase–immunoreactive nerve fibers in mitral valve of young adult and aged Fischer 344 rats. *J Auton Nerv Syst* 1996; 58:35.

13. Mulholland DL, Gotlieb AI: Cell biology of valvular interstitial cells. *Can J Cardiol* 1996; 12:231.

14. Smith RB: Intrinsic innervation of the atrioventricular and semi-lunar valves in various mammals. *J Anat* 1971; 108:115.

15. Erlanger J: A note on the contractility of the musculature of the auriculoventricular valves. *Am J Physiol* 1916; 40:150.

16. Cooper T, Sonnenblick EH, Priola DV, et al: An intrinsic neuromuscular basis for mitral valve motion, in Brewer LA (ed): *Prosthetic Heart Valves.* Springfield, IL, Charles C Thomas, 1969; Chap 2.

17. Anderson RH: The disposition and innervation of atrioventricular ring specialized tissue in rats and rabbits. *J Anat* 1972; 113:197.

18. Kawano H, Kawai S, Shirai T, et al: Morphological study on vagal innervation in human atrioventricular valves using histochemical method. *Jpn Circ J* 1993; 57:753.

19. Timek TA, Lai DTM, Dagum P, et al: Ablation of mitral annular and leaflet muscle: effects on annular and leaflet dynamics. *Am J Physiol Heart Circ Physiol* 2003; 285:H1668-H1674.

20. Wit AL, Fenoglio J Jr, Wagner BM, Bassett AL: Electrophysiological properties of cardiac muscle in the anterior mitral valve leaflet and the adjacent atrium in the dog: possible implications for the genesis of atrial dysrhythmias. *Circ Res* 1973; 32:731.

21. Rozanski GJ: Electrophysiological properties of automatic fibers in rabbit atrioventricular valves. *Am J Physiol* 1987; 253:H720.

22. Krishnamurthy G, Itoh A, Swanson JC, et al: Regional stiffening of the mitral valve anterior leaflet in the beating ovine heart. *J Biomechanics* 2009: 42:2697.

23. Itoh A, Krishnamurthy G, Swanson JC, et al: Active stiffening of mitral valve leaflets in the beating heart. *Am J Physiol Heart Circ Physiol* 2009; 296:H1766-H1773.

24. Police C, Piton M, Filly K, et al: Mitral and aortic valve orifice area in normal subjects and in patients with congestive cardiomyopathy: determination by two-dimensional echocardiography. *Am J Cardiol* 1982; 49:1191.

25. Tsakiris AG, Von Bernuth G, Rastelli GC, et al: Size and motion of the mitral valve annulus in anesthetized intact dogs. *J Appl Physiol* 1971; 30:611.

26. Tsakiris AG, Strum RE, Wood EH: Experimental studies on the mechanisms of closure of cardiac valves with use of roentgen videodensitometry. *Am J Cardiol* 1973; 32:136.

27. Davis PKB, Kinmonth JB: The movements of the annulus of the mitral valve. *J Cardiovasc Surg* 1963; 4:427.

28. Keren G, Sonnenblick EH, LeJemtel TH: Mitral annulus motion: relation to pulmonary venous and transmitral flows in normal subjects and in patients with dilated cardiomyopathy. *Circulation* 1988; 78:621.

29. Karlsson MO, Glasson JR, Bolger AF, et al: Mitral valve opening in the ovine heart. *Am J Physiol* 1998; 274:H552.

30. Roberts WC, Perloff JK: Mitral valvular disease: a clinicopathologic survey of the conditions causing the mitral valve to function abnormally. *Ann Intern Med* 1972; 77:939.

31. Levine RA, Triulzi MO, Harrigan P, Weyman AE: The relationship of mitral annular shape to the diagnosis of mitral valve prolapse. *Circulation* 1987; 75:756.

32. Levine RA, Handschumacher MD, Sanfilippo AJ, et al: Three-dimensional echocardiographic reconstruction of the mitral valve, with implications for the diagnosis of mitral valve prolapse. *Circulation* 1989; 80:589.

33. Tsakiris AG, Gordon DA, Padiyar R, et al: The role of displacement of the mitral annulus in left atrial filling and emptying in the intact dog. *Can J Physiol Pharmacol* 1978; 56:447.

34. Rushmer RF: Initial phase of ventricular systole: asynchronous contraction. *Am J Physiol* 1956; 184:188.

35. Toumanidis ST, Sideris DA, Papamichael CM, et al: The role of mitral annulus motion in left ventricular function. *Acta Cardiol* 1992; 47:331.

36. Carlhall C, Kindberg K, Wigstrom L, et al: Contribution of mitral annular dynamics to LV diastolic filling with alteration in preload and inotropic state. *Am J Physio Heart Circ Physiol* 2007; 293:H1473-H1479.

37. Rushmer R, Finlayson B, Nash A: Movements of the mitral valve. *Circ Res* 1956; 4:337.

38. Chiechi MA, Lees M, Thompson R: Functional anatomy of the normal mitral valve. *J Thorac Cardiovasc Surg* 1956; 32:378.

39. Pohost GM, Dinsmore RE, Rubenstein JJ, et al: The echocardiogram of the anterior leaflet of the mitral valve: correlation with hemodynamic and cineroentgenographic studies in dogs. *Circulation* 1975; 51:88.

40. Tsakiris AG, Gordon DA, Mathieu Y, et al: Motion of both mitral valve leaflets: a cineroentgenographic study in intact dogs. *J Appl Physiol* 1975; 39:359.

41. Fenster MS, Feldman MD: Mitral regurgitation: an overview. *Curr Probl Cardiol* 1995; 20:193.

42. Armour JA, Randall WC: Structural basis for cardiac function. *Am J Physiol* 1970; 218:1517.

43. Voci P, Bilotta F, Caretta Q, et al: Papillary muscle perfusion pattern: a hypothesis for ischemic papillary muscle dysfunction. *Circulation* 1995; 91:1714.

44. Sakai T, Okita Y, Ueda Y, et al: Distance between mitral annulus and papillary muscles: anatomic study in normal human hearts. *J Thorac Cardiovasc Surg* 1999; 118:636.

45. Lam JHC, Ranganathan N, Wigle ED, et al: Morphology of the human mitral valve: I. Chordae tendineae: a new classification. *Circulation* 1970; 41:449.

46. Ross J Jr, Sonnenblick EH, Covell JW, et al: The architecture of the heart in systole and diastole. *Circ Res* 1967; 21:409.

47. Armour JA, Randall WC: Electrical and mechanical activity of papillary muscle. *Am J Physiol* 1978; 218:1710.

48. Cronin R, Armour JA, Randall WC: Function of the in-situ papillary muscle in the canine left ventricle. *Circ Res* 1969; 25:67.

49. Askov JB, Honge JL, Jensen MO, Nygaard H, Hasenkam JM, Nielsen SL: Significance of force transfer in mitral valve-left ventricular interaction: in vivo assessment. *J Thorac Cardiovasc Surg* 2013; 145(6):1635-1641, 1641 e1631.

50. Cronin R, Armour JA, Randall WC: Function of the in-situ papillary muscle in the canine left ventricle. *Circ Res* 1969; 25(1):67-75.

51. Ingels NB Jr, Karlsson M: *Mitral Valve Mechanics,* Linkoping Press, 2015.

52. Lillehei CW, Levy MJ, Bonnabeau RC Jr: Mitral valve replacement with preservation of papillary muscles and chordae tendineae. *J Thorac Cardiovasc Surg.* 1964; 47:532-543.

53. Salisbury PF, Cross CE, Rieben PA: Chorda tendinea tension. *Am J Physiol* 1963; 205:385-392.

54. Roberts WC: Morphologic aspects of cardiac valve dysfunction. *Am Heart J* 1992; 123:1610.

55. Carabello BA: Timing of surgery in mitral and aortic stenosis. *Cardiol Clin* 1991; 9:229.

56. Waller BF, Howard J, Fess S: Pathology of mitral valve stenosis and pure mitral regurgitation, part I. *Clin Cardiol* 1994; 17:330.

57. Waller BF, Howard J, Fess S: Pathology of mitral valve stenosis and pure mitral regurgitation, part II. *Clin Cardiol* 1994; 17:395.

58. Essop MR, Nkomo VT: Rheumatic and nonrheumatic valvular heart disease: epidemiology, management, and prevention in Africa. *Circulation* 2005; 112:3584.

59. Chandrashekhar Y, Westaby S, Narula J: Mitral stenosis. *Lancet* 2009; 374:1271-1283.

60. Wunderlich NC, Beigel R, Siegel RJ: Management of mitral stenosis using 2D and 3D echo-Doppler imaging. *JACC Cardiol Img* 2013; 6: 1191-1205.

61. Seckeler MD, Hoke TR: The worldwide epidemiology of acute rheumatic fever and rheumatic heart disease. *Clin Epidemiol* 2011; 3: 67-84.

62. Carapetis JR, Steer AC, Mulholland EK, Weber M: The global burden of group A streptococcal disease. *Lancet Infect Dis* 2005; 5:685-694.

63. Khalil KG, Shapiro I, Kilman JW: Congenital mitral stenosis. *J Thorac Cardiovasc Surg* 1975; 70:40.

64. Korn D, DeSanctis RW, Sell S: Massive calcification of the mitral annulus. *N Engl J Med* 1962; 267:900.

65. Burge DJ, DeHoratious RJ: Acute rheumatic fever. *Cardiovasc Clin* 1993; 23:3.

66. Fae KC, Oshiro SE, Toubert A, et al: How an autoimmune reaction triggered by molecular mimicry between streptococcal M protein and cardiac tissue proteins leads to heart lesions in rheumatic heart disease. *J Autoimmun* 2005; 24:101.

67. Guilherme L, Cury P, Demarchi LM, et al: Rheumatic heart disease: proinflammatory cytokines play a role in the progression and maintenance of valvular lesions. *Am J Pathol* 2004; 165:1583.

68. Davutoglu V, Celik A, Aksoy M: Contribution of selected serum inflammatory mediators to the progression of chronic rheumatic valve disease, subsequent valve calcification and NYHA functional class. *J Heart Valve Dis* 2005; 14:151.

69. Hygenholtz PG, Ryan TJ, Stein SW, et al: The spectrum of pure mitral stenosis. *Am J Cardiol* 1962; 10:773.

70. Schofield PM: Invasive investigation of the mitral valve, in Wells FC, Shapiro LM (eds): *Mitral Valve Disease*. Oxford, England, Butterworth-Heinemann, 1996; p 84.

71. Braunwald E, Turi ZG: Pathophysiology of mitral valve disease, in Wells FC, Shapiro LM (eds): *Mitral Valve Disease*. Oxford, England, Butterworth-Heinemann, 1996; p 28.

72. Thompson ME, Shaver JA, Leon DF: Effect of tachycardia on atrial transport in mitral stenosis. *Am Heart J* 1977; 94:297.

73. Stott DK, Marpole DGF, Bristow JD, et al: The role of left atrial transport in aortic and mitral stenosis. *Circulation* 1970; 41:1031.

74. Kennedy JW, Yarnall SR, Murray JA, et al: Quantitative angiocardiography: relationships of left atrial and ventricular pressure and volume in mitral valve disease. *Circulation* 1970; 41:817.

75. Choi BW, Bacharach SL, Barcour DJ, et al: Left ventricular systolic dysfunction: diastolic filling characteristics and exercise cardiac reserve in mitral stenosis. *Am J Cardiol* 1995; 75:526.

76. Bolen JL, Lopes MG, Harrison DC, et al: Analysis of left ventricular function in response to afterload changes in patients with mitral stenosis. *Circulation* 1975; 52:894.

77. Schwartz R, Myerson RM, Lawrence LT, et al: Mitral stenosis, massive pulmonary hemorrhage, and emergency valve replacement. *N Engl J Med* 1966; 275:755.

78. Diker E, Aydogdu S, Ozdemir M, et al: Prevalence and predictors of atrial fibrillation in rheumatic valvular heart disease. *Am J Cardiol* 1996; 77:96.

79. Wood P: An appreciation of mitral stenosis. *BMJ* 1954; 1:1051.

80. Nishimura RA, Otto CM, Bonow RO, et al: 2014 AHA/ACC Guideline for the management of patients with valvular heart disease. *J Thorac Cardiovasc Surg* 2014; 148:e1-e132.

81. Chiang CW, Lo SK, Kuo CT, et al: Noninvasive predictors of systemic embolism in mitral stenosis. *Chest* 1994; 106:396.

82. Daley R, Mattingly TW, Holt CL, et al: Systemic arterial embolism in rheumatic heart disease. *Am Heart J* 1951; 42:566.

83. Kalmanson D, Veyrat C, Bernier A, et al: Opening snap and isovolumic relaxation period in relation to mitral valve flow in patients with mitral stenosis. *Br Heart J* 1976; 38:135.

84. Toutouzas P, Koidakis A, Velimezis A, et al: Mechanism of diastolic rumble and presystolic murmur in mitral stenosis. *Br Heart J* 1974; 36:1096.

85. Perloff JK: Auscultatory and phonocardiographic manifestations of pulmonary hypertension. *Prog Cardiovasc Dis* 1967; 9:303.

86. Goldstein MA, Michelson EL, Dreifus LS: The electrocardiogram in valvular heart disease. *Cardiovasc Clin* 1993; 23:55.

87. Kotler MN, Jacobs LE, Podolsky LA, et al: Echo-Doppler in valvular heart disease. *Cardiovasc Clin* 1993; 23:77.

88. Stoddard MF, Prince CR, Ammash NM, et al: Two-dimensional transesophageal echocardiographic of mitral valve area in adults with mitral stenosis. *Am Heart J* 1994; 127:1348.

89. Hung J, Lang R, Flachskampf F, et al: 3D echocardiography: a review of the current status and future directions. *J Am Soc Echocardiogr* 2007; 20:213-233.

90. Seow SC, Koh LP, Yeo TC: Hemodynamic significance of mitral stenosis: use of a simple, novel index by two-dimensional echocardiography. *J Am Soc Echocardiogr* 2006; 19:102.

91. Fabricius AM, Walther T, Falk V, et al: Three-dimensional echocardiography for planning of mitral valve surgery: current applicability? *Ann Thorac Surg* 2004; 78:575.

92. Han Y, Peters DC, Salton CJ, et al: Cardiovascular magnetic resonance: characterization of mitral valve prolapse. *J Am Coll Cardiol Img* 2008; 1:294-303.

93. Alkadhi H, Bettex D, Wildermuth S, et al: Dynamic cine imaging of the mitral valve with 16-MDCT: a feasibility study. *AJR* 2005; 185:636.

94. Iung B, Nicoud-Houel A, Fondard O, et al: Temporal trends in percutaneous mitral commissurotomy over a 15-year period. *Eur Heart J* 2004; 25:701-707.

95. Cohn LH, Allred EN, Cohn LA, et al: Long-term results of open mitral valve reconstruction for mitral stenosis. *Am J Cardiol* 1985; 55:731.

96. Detter C, Fischlein T, Feldmeier C, et al: Mitral commissurotomy, a technique outdated? Long-term follow-up over a period of 35 years. *Ann Thorac Surg* 1999; 68:2112.

97. Glower DD, Landolfo KP, Davis RD, et al: Comparison of open mitral commissurotomy with mitral valve replacement with or without chordal preservation in patients with mitral stenosis. *Circulation* 1998; 98:II-120.

98. Zener JC, Hancock EW, Shumway NE, et al: Regression of extreme pulmonary hypertension after mitral valve surgery. *Am J Cardiol* 1972; 30:820.

99. Chowdhury UK, Kumar AS, Mittal AB, et al: Mitral valve replacement with and without chordal preservation in a rheumatic population: serial echocardiographic assessment of left ventricular size and function. *Ann Thorac Surg* 2005; 79:1926.

100. Sugita T, Matsumoto M, Nishizawa J, et al: Long-term outcome after mitral valve replacement with preservation of continuity between the mitral annulus and the papillary muscle in patients with mitral stenosis. *J Heart Valve Dis* 2004; 13:931.

101. Hansen DE, Sarris GE, Niczyporuk MA, et al: Physiologic role of the mitral apparatus in left ventricular regional mechanics, contraction synergy, and global systolic performance. *J Thorac Cardiovasc Surg* 1989; 97:521.

102. Sarris GE, Cahill PD, Hansen DE, et al: Restoration of left ventricular systolic performance after reattachment of the mitral chordae tendineae. *J Thorac Cardiovasc Surg* 1988; 95:969.

103. Yun KL, Fann JI, Rayhill SC, et al: Importance of the mitral subvalvular apparatus for left ventricular segmental systolic mechanics. *Circulation* 1990; 82:IV-89.

104. Yun KL, Niczyporuk MA, Sarris GE, et al: Importance of mitral subvalvular apparatus in terms of cardiac energetics and systolic mechanics in the ejecting canine heart. *J Clin Invest* 1991; 87:247.

105. Hanson TP, Edwards BS, Edwards JE: Pathology of surgically excised mitral valves: one hundred consecutive cases. *Arch Pathol Lab Med* 1985; 109:823.

106. Olson LJ, Subramanian R, Ackermann DM, et al: Surgical pathology of the mitral valve: a study of 812 cases spanning 21 years. *Mayo Clin Proc* 1987; 62:22.

107. Waller BF, Morrow AG, Maron BJ, et al: Etiology of clinically isolated, severe, chronic, pure, mitral regurgitation: analysis of 97 patients over 30 years of age having mitral valve replacement. *Am Heart J* 1982; 104:188.

108. Delling FN, Vasan RS: Epidemiology and pathophysiology of mitral valve prolapse. *Circulation* 2014; 129:2158-2170.

109. Brunetti ND, Ieva R, Rossi G, et al: Ventricular outflow tract obstruction, systolic anterior motion and acute mitral regurgitation in Tako-Tsubo syndrome. *Int J Cardiol* 2008; 127:e152-e157.

110. Carpentier A: Cardiac valve surgery: the French correction. *J Thorac Cardiovasc Surg* 1983; 86:323.

111. Carpentier A, Chauvaud S, Fabiani J, et al: Reconstructive surgery of mitral valve incompetence: ten-year appraisal. *J Thorac Cardiovasc Surg* 1980; 79:338.

112. Wells FC: Conservation and surgical repair of the mitral valve, in Wells FC, Shapiro LM (eds): *Mitral Valve Disease*. Oxford, England, Butterworth-Heinemann, 1996; p 114.

113. Miller DC: Ischemic mitral regurgitation redux: to repair or to replace? *J Thorac Cardiovasc Surg* 2001; 122:1059.

114. Dagum P, Timek TA, Green GR, et al: Coordinate-free analysis of mitral valve dynamics in normal and ischemic hearts. *Circulation* 2000; 102:III-62.

115. Otsuji Y, Handschumacher MD, Liel-Cohen N, et al: Mechanism of ischemic mitral regurgitation with segmental left ventricular dysfunction: three-dimensional echocardiographic studies in models of acute and chronic progressive regurgitation. *J Am Coll Cardiol* 2001; 37:641.

116. Ngaage DL, Schaff HV: Mitral valve surgery in non-ischemic cardiomyopathy. *J Cardiovasc Surg* 2004; 45:477.

117. Olsen LJ, Subramanian R, Ackerman DM, et al: Surgical pathology of the mitral valve: a study of 712 cases spanning 21 years. *Mayo Clin Proc* 1987; 62:22.

118. Hayek E, Gring CN, Griffin BP: Mitral valve prolapse. *Lancet* 2005; 365:507.

119. David TE, Ivanov J, Armstrong S, et al: Late outcomes of mitral valve repair for floppy valves: implications for asymptomatic patients. *J Thorac Cardiovasc Surg* 2003; 125:1143.

120. Ling LH, Enriquez-Sarano M, Seward JB, et al: Early surgery in patients with mitral regurgitation due to flail leaflets. *Circulation* 1997; 96:1819.

121. Barlow JB, Pocock WA: Mitral valve prolapse, the specific billowing mitral leaflet syndrome, or an insignificant non-ejection systolic click. *Am Heart J* 1979; 97:277.

122. Roberts WC, McIntosh CL, Wallace RB: Mechanisms of severe mitral regurgitation in mitral valve prolapse determined from analysis of operatively excised valves. *Am Heart J* 1987; 113:1316.

123. Nesta F, Leyne M, Yosefy C, et al: New locus for autosomal dominant mitral valve prolapse on chromosome 13: clinical insights from genetic studies. *Circulation* 2005; 112:2022.

124. Grau JB, Pirelli L, Yu PJ, et al: The genetics of mitral valve prolapse. *Clin Genet* 2007; 72:288.

125. Grayburn PA, Carabello B, Hung J, et al: Defining "severe" secondary mitral regurgitation. *J Am Coll Cardiol* 2014; 64:2792-2801.

126. Procacci PM, Savran SV, Schreiter SL, et al: Prevalence of clinical mitral-valve prolapse in 1169 young women. *N Engl J Med* 1976; 294:1086.

127. Theofilogiannakos EK, Boudoulas KD, Gawronski BE, et al: Floppy mitral valve/mitral valve prolapse syndrome: Beta-adrenergic receptor polymorphism may contribute to the pathogenesis of symptoms. *J Cardiol* 2015; 65:434-8.

128. Enriquez-Sarano M, Schaff HV, Frye RL: Mitral regurgitation: what causes the leakage is fundamental to the outcome of valve repair. *Circulation* 2003; 108:253.

129. Roberts WC, Braunwald E, Morrow AG: Acute severe mitral regurgitation secondary to ruptured chordae tendineae. *Circulation* 1966; 33:58.

130. Kumanohoso T, Otsuji Y, Yoshifuku S, et al: Mechanism of higher incidence of ischemic mitral regurgitation in patients with inferior myocardial infarction: quantitative analysis of left ventricular and mitral valve geometry in 103 patients with prior myocardial infarction. *J Thorac Cardiovasc Surg* 2003; 125:135.

131. Glasson J, Komeda M, Daughters GT, et al: Early systolic mitral leaflet "loitering" during acute ischemic mitral regurgitation. *J Thorac Cardiovasc Surg* 1998; 116:193.

132. Srichai MB, Grimm RA, Stillman AE, et al: Ischemic mitral regurgitation: Impact of the left ventricle and mitral valve in patients with left ventricular systolic dysfunction. *Ann Thorac Surg* 2005; 80:170.

133. Timek TA, Lai DT, Tibayan F, et al: Ischemia in three left ventricular regions: insights into the pathogenesis of acute ischemic mitral regurgitation. *J Thorac Cardiovasc Surg* 2003; 125:559.

134. Enomoto Y, Gorman JH III, Moainie SL, et al: Surgical treatment of ischemic mitral regurgitation might not influence ventricular remodeling. *J Thorac Cardiovasc Surg* 2005; 129:504.

135. Tibayan FA, Rodriguez F, Zasio MK, et al: Geometric distortions of the mitral valvular-ventricular complex in chronic ischemic mitral regurgitation. *Circulation* 2003; 108:II-116.

136. Ahmad RM, Gillinov AM, McCarthy PM, et al: Annular geometry and motion in human ischemic mitral regurgitation: novel assessment with three-dimensional echocardiography and computer reconstruction. *Ann Thorac Surg* 2004; 78:2063.

137. Nielsen SL, Hansen SB, Nielsen KO, et al: Imbalanced chordal force distribution causes acute ischemic mitral regurgitation: mechanistic insights from chordae tendineae force measurements in pigs. *J Thorac Cardiovasc Surg* 2005; 129:525.

138. Levine RA: Dynamic mitral regurgitation: more than meets the eye. *N Engl J Med* 2004; 351:16.

139. Lai DT, Tibayan FA, Myrmel T, et al: Mechanistic insights into posterior mitral leaflet interscallop malcoaptation during acute ischemic mitral regurgitation. *Circulation* 2002; 106:I-40.

140. Liel-Cohen N, Guerrero JL, Otsuji Y, et al: Design of a new surgical approach for ventricular remodeling to relieve ischemic mitral regurgitation. *Circulation* 2000; 101:2756.

141. Tibayan FA, Rodriguez F, Langer F, et al: Alterations in left ventricular torsion and diastolic recoil after myocardial infarction with and without chronic ischemic mitral regurgitation. *Circulation* 2004; 110:II-109.

142. Nguyen TC, Cheng A, Langer F, et al: Altered myocardial shear strains are associated with chronic mitral regurgitation. *Ann Thorac Surg* 2007; 83:47.

143. Gorman JH III, Jackson BM, Enomoto Y, et al: The effect of regional ischemia on mitral valve annular saddle shape. *Ann Thorac Surg* 2004; 77:544.

144. Watanabe N, Ogasawara Y, Yamaura Y, et al: Mitral annulus flat-tens in ischemic mitral regurgitation: geometric differences between inferior and anterior myocardial infarction. *Circulation* 2005; 112:I-458.

145. Yiu SF, Enriquez-Sarano M, Tribouilloy C, et al: Determinants of the degree of functional mitral regurgitation in patients with systolic left ventricular dysfunction. *Circulation* 2000; 102:1400.

146. Chaput M, Handschumacher MD, Guerrero JL, et al: Mitral leaflet adaptation to ventricular remodeling: prospective changes in a model of ischemic mitral regurgitation. *Circulation* 2009; 120(Suppl 1): S-99-S-103.

147. Grande-Allen KJ, Borowski AG, Troughton RW, et al: Apparently normal mitral valves in patients with heart failure demonstrate biochemical and structural derangements. *J Am Coll Cardiol* 2005; 45:54.

148. Grande-Allen KJ, Barber JE, Klatka KM, et al: Mitral valve stiffening in end-stage heart failure: evidence of an organic contribution to functional mitral regurgitation. *J Thorac Cardiovasc Surg* 2005; 130:783.

149. Matsunaga A, Tahta SA, Duran CMG: Failure of reduction annuloplasty for functional ischemic mitral regurgitation. *J Heart Valve Dis* 2004; 13:390.

150. Kalra K, Wang Q, McIver BV, et al: Temporal changes in interpapillary muscle dynamics as an active indicator of mitral valve and left ventricular interaction in ischemic mitral regurgitation. *J Am Coll Cardiol* 2014; 64: 1867-1879.

151. Messas E, Guerrero JL, Handschumacher MD, et al: Paradoxic decrease in ischemic mitral regurgitation with papillary muscle dysfunction. *Circulation* 2001; 104:1952.

152. Kishon Y, Oh JK, Schaff HV, et al: Mitral valve operation in postinfarction rupture of a papillary muscle: immediate results and long-term follow-up in 22 patients. *Mayo Clin Proc* 1992; 67:1023.

153. LeFeuvre C, Metzger JP, Lachurie ML, et al: Treatment of severe mitral regurgitation caused by ischemic papillary muscle dysfunction: indications for coronary angioplasty. *Am Heart J* 1992; 123:860.

154. Kamblock J, N'Guyen L, Pagis B, et al: Acute severe mitral regurgitation during first attacks of rheumatic fever: clinical spectrum, mechanisms and prognostic factors. *J Heart Valve Dis* 2005; 14:440.

155. Braunwald E: Mitral regurgitation: physiologic, clinical and surgical considerations. *N Engl J Med* 1969; 281:425.

156. Grigioni F, Enriquez-Sarano M, Zehr KJ, et al: Ischemic mitral regurgitation: long-term outcome and prognostic implications with quantitative Doppler assessment. *Circulation* 2001; 103:1759.

157. Enriquez-Sarano M, Avierinos JF, Messika-Zeitoun D, et al: Quantitative determinants of the outcome of asymptomatic mitral regurgitation. *N Engl J Med* 2005; 352:875.

158. Zoghbi WA, Enriquez-Sarano M, Foster E, et al: Recommendations for evaluation of the severity of native valve regurgitation with two-dimensional and Doppler echocardiography. *J Am Soc Echocardiogr* 2003; 16:777.

159. Yoran C, Yellin EL, Becker RM, et al: Dynamic aspects of acute mitral regurgitation: effects of ventricular volume, pressure and contractility on the effective regurgitant orifice area. *Circulation* 1979; 60:170.

160. Keren G, Laniado S, Sonnenblick EH, et al: Dynamics of functional mitral regurgitation during dobutamine therapy in patients with severe congestive heart failure: a Doppler echocardiographic study. *Am Heart J* 1989; 118:748.

161. Keren G, Katz S, Strom J, et al: Dynamic mitral regurgitation: an important determinant of the hemodynamic response to load alterations and inotropic therapy in severe heart failure. *Circulation* 1989; 80:306.

162. Abe Y, Imai T, Ohue K, et al: Relation between reduction in ischaemic mitral regurgitation and improvement in regional left ventricular contractility during low dose dobutamine stress echocardiography. *Heart* 2005; 91:1092.

163. Grossman W: Profiles in valvular heart disease, in Baim DS, Grossman W (eds): *Cardiac Catheterization, Angiography and Intervention,* 5th ed. Baltimore, Williams & Wilkins, 1996; p 735.

164. Ross J Jr: Adaptations of the left ventricle to chronic volume overload. *Circ Res* 1974; 34-35:II-64.

165. Spinale FG, Ishihra K, Zile M, et al: Structural basis for changes in left ventricular function and geometry because of chronic mitral regurgitation and after correction of volume overload. *J Thorac Cardiovasc Surg* 1993; 106:1147.

166. Yun KL, Rayhill SC, Niczyporuk MA, et al: Left ventricular mechanics and energetics in the dilated canine heart: acute versus chronic mitral regurgitation. *J Thorac Cardiovasc Surg* 1992; 104:26.

167. Yun KL, Rayhill SC, Niczyporuk MA, et al: Mitral valve replacement in dilated canine hearts with chronic mitral regurgitation. *Circulation* 1991; 84:III-112.

168. Urabe Y, Mann DL, Kent RL, et al: Cellular and ventricular contractile dysfunction in experimental canine mitral regurgitation. *Circ Res* 1992; 70:131.

169. Carabello BA, Crawford FA Jr: Valvular heart disease. *N Engl J Med* 1997; 337:32.

170. Starling MR, Kirsh MM, Montgomery DG, et al: Impaired left ventricular contractile function in patients with long-term mitral regurgitation and normal ejection fraction. *J Am Coll Cardiol* 1993; 22:239.

171. Nakano K, Swindle MM, Spinale F, et al: Depressed contractile function due to canine mitral regurgitation improves after correction of the volume overload. *J Clin Invest* 1991; 87:2077.

172. Brickner ME, Starling MR: Dissociation of end systole from end ejection in patients with long-term mitral regurgitation. *Circulation* 1990; 81:1277.

173. Glower DD, Spratt JA, Snow ND, et al: Linearity of the Frank-Starling relationship in the intact heart: the concept of preload recruitable stroke work. *Circulation* 1985; 71:994.

174. Carabello BA, Nolan SP, McGuire LB: Assessment of preoperative left ventricular function in patients with mitral regurgitation: value of the end-systolic wall stress–end-systolic volume ratio. *Circulation* 1981; 64:1212.

175. Carabello BA, Williams H, Gash AK, et al: Hemodynamic predictors of outcome in patients undergoing valve replacement. *Circulation* 1986; 74:1309.

176. Borow KM, Green LH, Mann T, et al: End-systolic volume as a predictor of postoperative left ventricular performance in volume overload from valvular regurgitation. *Am J Med* 1980; 68:655.

177. Tibayan FA, Yun KL, Fann JI, et al: Torsion dynamics in the evolution from acute to chronic mitral regurgitation. *J Heart Valve Dis* 2002; 11:39.

178. Carlhall CJ, Nguyen TC, Itoh A, et al: Alterations in transmural myocardial strain: an early marker of left ventricular dysfunction in mitral regurgitation? *Circulation* 2008; 118(Suppl 1):S-256.

179. Yellin EL, Nikolic S, Frater RWM: Left ventricular filling dynamics and diastolic function. *Prog Cardiovasc Dis* 1990; 32:333.

180. Zile MR, Tomita M, Nakano K, et al: Effects of left ventricular volume overload produced by mitral regurgitation on diastolic function. *Am J Physiol* 1991; 261:H471.

181. Corin WJ, Murakami T, Monrad ES, et al: Left ventricular passive diastolic properties in chronic mitral regurgitation. *Circulation* 1991; 83:797.

182. Zile MR, Tomita M, Ishihara K, et al: Changes in diastolic function during development and correction of chronic left ventricular volume overload produced by mitral regurgitation. *Circulation* 1993; 87:1378.

183. Corin WJ, Sutsch G, Murakami T, et al: Left ventricular function in chronic mitral regurgitation: preoperative and postoperative comparison. *J Am Coll Cardiol* 1995; 25:113.

184. Sabbah HN, Kono T, Rosman H, et al: Left ventricular shape: a factor in the etiology of functional mitral regurgitation in heart failure. *Am Heart J* 1992; 123:961.

185. Braunwald E, Awe WC: The syndrome of severe mitral regurgitation with normal left atrial pressure. *Circulation* 1963; 27:29.

186. Pierard LA, Lancellotti P: The role of ischemic mitral regurgitation in the pathogenesis of acute pulmonary edema. *N Engl J Med* 2004; 351:1627.

187. Borer JS, Hochreiter C, Rosen S: Right ventricular function in severe non-ischemic mitral insufficiency. *Eur Heart J* 1991; 12:22.

188. Gray RJ, Helfant RH: Timing of surgery in valvular heart disease. *Cardiovasc Clin* 1993; 23:209.

189. Harrison MR, MacPhail B, Gurley JC, et al: Usefulness of color Doppler flow imaging to distinguish ventricular septal defect from acute mitral regurgitation complicating acute myocardial infarction. *Am J Cardiol* 1989; 64:697.

190. Perloff JK, Harvey WP: Auscultatory and phonocardiographic manifestations of pure mitral regurgitation. *Prog Cardiovasc Dis* 1962; 5:172.

191. Antman EM, Angoff GH, Sloss LJ: Demonstration of the mechanism by which mitral regurgitation mimics aortic stenosis. *Am J Cardiol* 1978; 42:1044.

192. Karalis DG, Ross JJ, Brown BM, et al: Transesophageal echocardiography in valvular heart disease. *Cardiovasc Clin* 1993; 23:105.

193. Smith MD, Cassidy JM, Gurley JC, et al: Echo Doppler evaluation of patients with acute mitral regurgitation: superiority of transesophageal echocardiography with color flow imaging. *Am Heart J* 1995; 129:967.

194. Kwan J, Shiota T, Agler DA, et al: Geometric differences of the mitral apparatus between ischemic and dilated cardiomyopathy with significant mitral regurgitation: real-time three-dimensional echocardiography study. *Circulation* 2003; 107:1135.

195. Kozerke S, Schwitter J, Pedersen EM, et al: Aortic and mitral regurgitation: quantification using moving slice velocity mapping. *J Magn Reson Imag* 2001; 14:106.

196. Buchner S, Debl K, Poschenrieder F, et al: Cardiovascular magnetic resonance for direct assessment of anatomic regurgitant orifice in mitral regurgitation. *Circ Cardiovasc Imaging.* 2008; 1:148.

197. Pieper EPG, Hellemans IM, Hamer HPM, et al: Additional value of biplane transesophageal echocardiography in assessing the genesis of mitral regurgitation and the feasibility of valve repair. *Am J Cardiol* 1995; 75:489.

198. Grewal KS, Malkowsi MJ, Piracha AR, et al: Effect of general anesthesia on the severity of mitral regurgitation by transesophageal echocardiography. *Am J Cardiol* 2000; 85:199.

199. Byrne JG, Aklog L, Adams DH: Assessment and management of functional or ischemic mitral regurgitation. *Lancet* 2000; 355:1743.

200. Plicht B, Kahlert P, Goldwasser R, et al: Direct quantification of mitral regurgitant flow volume by real-time three-dimensional echocardiography using dealiasing of color Doppler flow at the vena contracta. *J Am Soc Echocardiogr* 2008; 21:1337.

201. Ryan L P, Salgo IS, Gorman RC, Gorman JH III: The emerging role of three-dimensional echocardiography in mitral valve repair. *Semin Thorac Cardiovasc Surg* 2006; 18:126-134.

202. Hundley WG, Li HF, Willard JE, et al: Magnetic resonance imaging assessment of the severity of mitral regurgitation. *Circulation* 1995; 92:1151.

203. Suri RM, Schaff HV, Dearani JA, et al: Survival advantage and improved durability of mitral repair for leaflet prolapse subsets in the current era. *Ann Thorac Surg* 2006; 82:819.

204. DeBonis M, Lapenna E, Verzini A, et al: Recurrence of mitral regurgitation parallels the absence of left ventricular reverse remodeling after mitral repair in advanced dilated cardiomyopathy. *Ann Thorac Surg* 2008; 85:932.

205. Braun J, Bax JJ, Versteegh MIM, et al: Preoperative left ventricular dimensions predict reverse remodeling following restrictive mitral annuloplasty in ischemic mitral regurgitation. *Eur J Cardiothorac Surg* 2005; 27:847.

206. Bax JJ, Braun J, Somer ST, et al: Restrictive annuloplasty and coronary revascularization in ischemic mitral regurgitation results in reverse left ventricular remodeling. *Circulation* 2004; 110:II-103.

207. Onorati F, Santarpino G, Marturano D, et al: Successful surgical treatment of chronic ischemic mitral regurgitation achieves left ventricular reverse remodeling but does not affect right ventricular function. *J Thorac Cardiovasc Surg* 2009; 138:341.

208. Starling MR: Effects of valve surgery on left ventricular contractile function in patients with long-term mitral regurgitation. *Circulation* 1995; 92:811.

209. Wisenbaugh T, Skudicky D, Sarelli P: Prediction of outcome after valve replacement for rheumatic mitral regurgitation in the era of chordal preservation. *Circulation* 1994; 89:191.

210. Crawford MH, Souchek J, Oprian CA, et al: Determinants of survival and left ventricular performance after mitral valve replacement. *Circulation* 1990; 81:1173.

211. Levine HJ: Is valve surgery indicated in patients with severe mitral regurgitation even if they are asymptomatic? *Cardiovasc Clin* 1990; 21:161.

212. Davis EA, Gardner TJ, Gillinov AM, et al: Valvular disease in the elderly: influence on surgical results. *Ann Thorac Surg* 1993; 55:333.

213. Goldfine H, Aurigemma GP, Zile MR, et al: Left ventricular length-force-shortening relations before and after surgical correction of chronic mitral regurgitation. *J Am Coll Cardiol* 1998; 31:180.

214. LeTourneau T, deGroote P, Millaire A, et al: Effect of mitral valve surgery on exercise capacity, ventricular ejection fraction and neurohumoral activation in patients with severe mitral regurgitation. *J Am Coll Cardiol* 2000; 36:2263.

215. Salomon NW, Stinson EB, Griepp RB, et al: Patient-related risk factors as predictors of results following isolated mitral valve replacement. *Ann Thorac Surg* 1977; 24:520.

216. Michel PL, Iung B, Blanchard B, et al: Long-term results of mitral valve repair for non-ischemic mitral regurgitation. *Eur Heart J* 1991; 12:39.

217. Reed D, Abbott R, Smucker M, et al: Prediction of outcome after mitral valve replacement in patients with symptomatic chronic mitral regurgitation: the importance of left atrial size. *Circulation* 1991; 84:23.

218. Ling LH, Enriquez-Sarano M, Seward JB, et al: Clinical outcome of mitral regurgitation due to flail leaflet. *N Engl J Med* 1996; 335:1417.

219. Kang DH, Park SJ, Sun BJ, et al: Early surgery versus conventional treatment for asymptomatic severe mitral regurgitation. *J Am Coll Cardiol* 2014; 63:2398-2407.

220. Cohn LH, Couper GS, Aranki SF, et al: Long-term results of mitral valve reconstruction for regurgitation of the myxomatous mitral valve. *J Thorac Cardiovasc Surg* 1994; 107:143.

221. Deloche A, Jebara V, Relland J, et al: Valve repair with Carpentier techniques: the second decade. *J Thorac Cardiovasc Surg* 1990; 99:990.

222. Gaur P, Kaneko T, McGurk S, Rawn JD, Maloney A, Cohn LH: Mitral valve repair versus replacement in the elderly: short-term and long-term outcomes. *J Thorac Cardiovasc Surg* 2014; 148:1400-1406.

223. Kitai T, Okada Y, Shomura Y, et al: Timing of valve repair for severe degenerative mitral regurgitation and long-term left ventricular function. *J Thorac Cardiovasc Surg* 2014; 148:1978-1982.

224. Messika-Zeitoun D, Johnson BD, Nkomo V, et al: Cardiopulmonary exercise testing determination of functional capacity in mitral regurgitation physiologic and outcome implications. *J Am Coll Cardiol* 2006; 47:2521.

225. Naji P, Griffin BP, Barr T, et al: Importance of exercise capacity in predicting outcomes and determining optimal timing of surgery in significant primary mitral regurgitation. *J Am Heart Assoc* 2014; 3:e001010.

226. Enriquez-Sarano M, Schaff HV, Orszulak TA, et al: Congestive heart failure after surgical correction of mitral regurgitation. *Circulation* 1995; 92:2496.

227. Tribouilloy CM, Enriquez-Sarano M, Schaff HV, et al: Impact of preoperative symptoms on survival after surgical correction of organic mitral regurgitation. *Circulation* 1999; 99:400.

228. Bursi F, Enriquez-Sarano M, Nkomo VT, et al: Heart failure and death after myocardial infarction in the community. *Circulation* 2005; 111:295.

229. Grigioni F, Detaint D, Avierinos JF, et al: Contribution of ischemic mitral regurgitation to congestive heart failure after myocardial infarction. *J Am Coll Cardiol* 2005; 45:260.

230. Dujardin KS, Enriquez-Sarano M, Bailey KR, et al: Grading of mitral regurgitation by quantitative Doppler echocardiography: calibration by left ventricular angiography in routine clinical practice. *Circulation* 1997; 96:3409.

231. Cohn LH, Rizzo RJ, Adams DH, et al: The effect of pathophysiology on the surgical treatment of ischemic mitral regurgitation: operative and late risks of repair versus replacement. *Eur J Cardiothorac Surg* 1995; 9:568.

232. Diodato MD, Moon MR, Pasque MK, et al: Repair of ischemic mitral regurgitation does not increase mortality or improve long-term survival in patients undergoing coronary artery revascularization: a propensity analysis. *Ann Thorac Surg* 2004; 78:794.

233. Kim YH, Czer LSC, Soukiasian HJ, et al: Ischemic mitral regurgitation: revascularization alone versus revascularization and mitral valve repair. *Ann Thorac Surg* 2005; 79:1895.

234. Wong DR, Agnihotri AK, Hung JW, et al: Long-term survival after surgical revascularization for moderate ischemic mitral regurgitation. *Ann Thorac Surg* 2005; 80:570.

235. Dahlberg PS, Orszulak TA, Mullany CJ, et al: Late outcome of mitral valve surgery for patients with coronary artery disease. *Ann Thorac Surg* 2003; 76:1539.

236. Glower DD, Tuttle RH, Shaw LK, et al: Patient survival characteristics after routine mitral valve repair in ischemic mitral regurgitation. *J Thorac Cardiovasc Surg* 2005; 129:860.

237. Lorusso R, Gelsomino S, Vizzardi E, et al: Mitral valve repair or replacement for ischemic mitral regurgitation? The Italian study on the treatment of ischemic mitral regurgitation (ISTIMIR). *J Thorac Cardiovasc Surg* 2013; 145:128-139.

238. Aklog L, Filshoufi F, Flores KQ, et al: Does coronary artery bypass grafting alone correct moderate ischemic mitral regurgitation? *Circulation* 2001; 104:I-68.

239. Lam BK, Gillinov AM, Blackstone EH, et al: Importance of moderate ischemic mitral regurgitation. *Ann Thorac Surg* 2005; 79:462.

240. Grossi EA, Crooke GA, DiGiorgi PL, et al: Impact of moderate functional mitral insufficiency in patients undergoing surgical revascularization. *Circulation* 2006; 114(Suppl I):I-573.

241. Mihaljevic T, Lam BK, Rajeswaran J, et al: Impact of mitral valve annuloplasty combined with revascularization in patients with functional ischemic mitral regurgitation. *J Am Coll Cardiol* 2007; 49:2191.

242. Tolis GA Jr, Korkolis DP, Kopf GS, et al: Revascularization alone (without mitral valve repair) suffices in patients with advanced ischemic cardiomyopathy and mild-to-moderate mitral regurgitation. *Ann Thorac Surg* 2003; 74:1476.

243. Harris KM, Sundt TM III, Aeppli D, et al: Can late survival of patients with moderate ischemic mitral regurgitation be impacted by intervention on the valve? *Ann Thorac Surg* 2002; 74:1468.

244. Smith PK, Puskas JD, Ascheim DD, et al: Surgical treatment of moderate ischemic mitral regurgitation. *N Engl J Med* 2014; 371:2178-2188.

245. Penicka M, Linkova H, Lang O, et al: Predictors of improvement of unrepaired moderate ischemic mitral regurgitation in patients undergoing elective isolated coronary artery bypass graft surgery. *Circulation* 2009; 120:1474.

246. Flynn M, Curtin R, Nowicki ER, et al: Regional wall motion abnormalities and scarring in severe functional ischemic mitral regurgitation: a pilot cardiovascular magnetic resonance imaging study. *J Thorac Cardiovasc Surg* 2009; 137:1063.

247. Trichon BH, Glower DD, Shaw LK, et al: Survival after coronary revascularization, with and without mitral valve surgery, in patients with ischemic mitral regurgitation. *Circulation* 2003; 108:II-103.

248. Grossi EA, Goldberg JD, LaPietra A, et al: Ischemic mitral valve reconstruction and replacement: comparison of long-term survival and complications. *J Thorac Cardiovasc Surg* 2001; 122:1107.

249. Gillinov AM: Is ischemic mitral regurgitation an indication for surgical repair or replacement? *Heart Fail Rev* 2006; 11:231-239.

250. Gillinov AM, Wieryp PN, Blackstone EH, et al: Is repair preferable to replacement for ischemic mitral regurgitation? *J Thorac Cardiovasc Surg* 2001; 122:1125.

251. Magne J, Girerd N, Senechal M, et al: Mitral repair versus replacement for ischemic mitral regurgitation: comparison of short-term and long-term survival. *Circulation* 2009; 120(Suppl 1):S-104-S-111.

252. Acker MA, Parides MK, Perrault LP, et al: Mitral valve repair versus replacement for severe ischemic mitral regurgitation. *N Engl J Med* 2014; 370:23-32.

253. Gillinov AM, Blackstone EH, Rajeswaran J, et al: Ischemic versus degenerative mitral regurgitation: does etiology affect survival? *Ann Thorac Surg* 2005; 80:811.

254. McGee EC, Gillinov AM, Blackstone EH, et al: Recurrent mitral regurgitation after annuloplasty for functional ischemic mitral regurgitation. *J Thorac Cardiovasc Surg* 2004; 128:916.

255. Tahta SA, Oury JH, Maxwell JM, et al: Outcome after mitral valve repair for functional ischemic mitral regurgitation. *J Heart Valve Dis* 2002; 11:11.

256. Zhu F, Otsuji Y, Yotsumoto G, et al: Mechanism of persistent ischemic mitral regurgitation after annuloplasty. *Circulation* 2005; 112:I-396.

257. Kron IL, Hung J, Overbey JR, et al: Predicting recurrent MR after mitral valve repair for severe ischemic mitral regurgitation. *J Thorac Cardiovasc Surg* 2015; 149(3):752-761.

258. Lee LS, Kwon MH, Cevasco M, et al: Postoperative recurrence of mitral regurgitation after annuloplasty for functional mitral regurgitation. *Ann Thorac Surg* 2012; 94:1211-1217.

259. Ciarka A, Braun J, Delgado V, et al: Predictors of mitral regurgitation recurrence in patients with heart failure undergoing mitral valve annuloplasty. *Am J Cardiol* 2010; 106:395-401.

260. Kwon MH, Lee LS, Cevasco M, et al: Recurrence of mitral regurgitation after partial versus complete mitral valve ring annuloplasty for functional mitral regurgitation. *J Thorac Cardiovasc Surg* 2013; 146:616-622.

261. Serri K, Bouchard D, Demers P, et al: Is a good perioperative echocardiographic result predictive of durability in ischemic mitral valve repair? *J Thorac Cardiovasc Surg* 2006; 131:565.

262. Gazoni LM, Kern JA, Swenson BR, et al: A change in perspective: results for ischemic mitral valve repair are similar to mitral valve repair for degenerative disease. *Ann Thorac Surg* 2007; 84:750.

263. Lillehei CW, Levy MJ, Bonnabeau RC: Mitral valve replacement with preservation of papillary muscles and chordae tendineae. *J Thorac Cardiovasc Surg* 1964; 47:532.

264. David TE, Burns RJ, Bacchus CM, et al: Mitral valve replacement for mitral regurgitation with and without preservation of chordae tendineae. *J Thorac Cardiovasc Surg* 1984; 88:718.

265. Rozich JD, Carabello BA, Usher BW, et al: Mitral valve replacement with and without chordal preservation in chronic mitral regurgitation. *Circulation* 1992; 86:1718.

266. Tischler MD, Cooper KA, Rowen M, et al: Mitral valve replacement versus mitral valve repair: a Doppler and quantitative stress echocardiographic study. *Circulation* 1994; 89:132.

267. Pitarys CJ, Forman MB, Panayiotou H, et al: Long-term effects of excision of the mitral apparatus on global and regional ventricular function in humans. *J Am Coll Cardiol* 1990; 15:557.

268. Takayama Y, Holmes JW, LeGrice I, et al: Enhanced regional deformation at the anterior papillary muscle insertion site after chordal transection. *Circulation* 1996; 93:585.

269. Le Tourneau T, Grandmougin D, Foucher C, et al: Anterior chordal transection impairs not only regional left ventricular function but also regional right ventricular function in mitral regurgitation. *Circulation* 2001; 104:I-41.

270. Messas E, Pouzet B, Touchot B, et al: Efficacy of chordal cutting to relieve chronic persistent ischemic mitral regurgitation. *Circulation* 2003; 108:II-111.

271. Borger MA, Murphy PM, et al: Initial results of the chordal-cutting operation for ischemic mitral regurgitation. *J Thorac Cardiovasc Surg* 2007; 133:1483.

272. Szymanski C, Bel A, Cohen I, et al: Comprehensive annular and subvalvular repair of chronic ischemic mitral regurgitation improves long-term results with the least ventricular remodeling. *Circulation* 2012; 126:2720-2727.

273. Nielsen SL, Timek TA, Green GR, et al: Influence of anterior mitral leaflet second-order chordae tendineae on left ventricular systolic function. *Circulation* 2003; 103:486.

274. Rodriguez F, Langer F, Harrington KB, et al: Importance of mitral valve second-order chordae for left ventricular geometry, wall thickening mechanics, and global systolic function. *Circulation* 2004; 110:II-115.

35

Mitral Valve Repair

Dan Loberman • Paul A. Pirundini • John G. Byrne
• Lawrence H. Cohn

It can be reasonably argued that the very dawn of cardiac surgery began with a mitral valve repair. On May 20, 1923, Dr Elliot Carr Cutler (Fig. 35-1) performed the world's first successful mitral valve repair at the Peter Bent Brigham Hospital in Boston, Massachusetts.[1] Dr Cutler carried out a transventricular mitral valve commissurotomy with a neurosurgical tenotomy knife on a critically ill 12-year-old girl. His choice of instrument was likely influenced by Dr Harvey Cushing who was surgeon-in-chief at the time. A new era in surgery was introduced as well as the reality of mitral valve repair.[2] Cutler had worked assiduously on this problem in the Surgical Research Laboratories of Harvard Medical School before turning his attention to this critically ill patient. Subsequent attempts at this operation using a device to cut out a segment of the diseased mitral valve resulted in several deaths from massive mitral regurgitation and Cutler eventually abandoned the procedure.[3] Of Cutler's contemporaries, Henry Souttar of England performed a single successful transatrial finger commissurotomy in 1925, but received no further referrals.[4] After Souttar, there remained little activity in mitral valve repair until the 1940s when Dwight Harken, then the Chief of Cardiothoracic Surgery at the Peter Bent Brigham Hospital, published his groundbreaking series of valvuloplasty patients for mitral stenosis.[5] Dr Charles Bailey of Philadelphia also published a concomitant series of a similar large group of patients.[6]

That early era focused on mitral stenosis created by rheumatic heart disease, which was extremely common at the time. Surgical treatment of mitral regurgitation for prolapse was first introduced in the 1950s[7-9] but with limited success. Subsequent decades would see the visionary concepts of surgical leaders such as Alain Carpentier, Dwight McGoon, Carlos Duran, and others come to the fore as their visionary ideas for mitral valve reconstruction began to take hold and excellent results were reported. Like many other groundbreaking ideas, their concepts were met with resistance that has gradually dissipated as long-term results by these surgeons have been validated. The concept that repair of mitral regurgitation might serve to further damage a weakened left ventricle (LV) by eliminating the "pop-off" mechanism[16] of the regurgitant valve. This proved a significant barrier to referral that only in the past few decades has been overcome.

What has now become firmly established is the significant contribution to overall left ventricular function of the papillary muscle-annular interaction.[17] As a result of these contributions, mitral valve repair, if technically possible, has now become recognized as the procedure of choice for mitral valve pathology of virtually all etiologies, to the extent that mitral valve repair is always considered first in virtually any clinical situation in which the mitral valve is regurgitant.

ANATOMY OF THE MITRAL VALVE

The bicuspid mitral valve is one of the most complex structures of the human heart, its complexity lies in its multifaceted anatomy. The concept of "form follows function" is particularly applicable to the mitral valve. Because each part of the valve's anatomy is intimately related to function, there are a variety of pathways whereby regurgitation may be created. If one part of the valvular apparatus fails, regurgitation can result. There are five discrete components to the mitral valve complex: the annulus, the two leaflets (anterior and posterior), the chordae, the papillary muscles, and the LV (Fig. 35-2A).

As part of the fibrous skeleton of the heart, the annulus is the myocardial connective tissue area where the mitral valve leaflets attach to the intersection of the left atrium and LV. It is surrounded by vitally important structures that the cardiac surgeon must avoid for safe surgery: the circumflex coronary artery laterally, the coronary sinus medially, the aortic root superiorly, and the atrioventricular node superior-medially. In myxomatous disease it is the posterior annulus that usually dilates.[18] Previous dictum held that the anterior annulus does not dilate, but recent data suggest that it may dilate a limited amount.[19] Of critical importance to the surgeon are the right and left fibrous trigones. These are intimately related to the anterior annulus and are contiguous with the aortic valve curtain and must be identified during surgery. The trigones, as part of the essential structural framework of the heart, form the anchoring points for ring annuloplasty.

The anterior leaflet of the mitral valve (AML) is in continuity with the left and noncoronary cusps of the aortic valve and is located directly beneath the left ventricular outflow tract (LVOT). It is sometimes referred to as the aortic

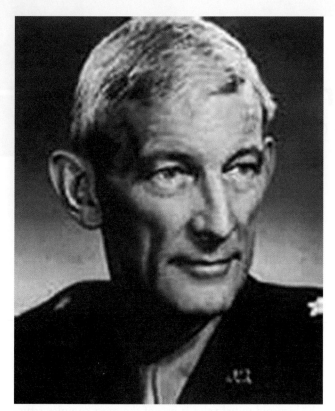

FIGURE 35-1 Elliot Carr Cutler.

leaflet. It typically accounts for approximately one-third of the circumference of the annulus, with the posterior leaflet accounting for the rest.[20] The posterior mitral valve leaflet (PML) is crescent shaped and is more commonly involved in degenerative disease. For surgical decision making and analysis, both the anterior and posterior leaflets are divided into three parts, corresponding to the three scalloped areas of each leaflet (A1, A2, A3 for the anterior leaflet; P1, P2, and P3 for the posterior leaflet; 1 refers to the leftmost, or lateral scallop; 2 the middle scallop; and 3 the rightmost, or medial scallop; Fig. 35-2B).

There are two papillary muscles, the anterolateral and the posteromedial. Each muscle is attached to the leaflets by the chordae tendinae. These chords are composed of string-like fibrous connective tissue. Primary chords are those that attach to the edge of the leaflet. Secondary chords are those that attach to the underside of the leaflets. Tertiary chords, which are only seen on the posterior mitral leaflet, are those that attach to the undersurface of the leaflet directly from the ventricular wall instead of from the papillary muscle. The papillary muscles each give off chordae to both leaflets and correspond to the anterolateral and posteromedial commissures of the mitral valve. The anterolateral papillary muscle receives blood from both the left anterior descending artery as well as the circumflex artery; the posteromedial one receives blood usually from only the posterior descending artery or a branch of the circumflex artery. Because of its single coronary blood supply, the posteromedial papillary

muscle is more susceptible to infarction and rupture than the anterolateral one.

The LV acts in concert with the papillary muscles via the chordae to pull in the leaflet edges during systole, thereby maintaining the line of coaptation and therefore valve competency. If the LV dilates from any etiology, failure of central leaflet coaptation may occur and regurgitation created. Such regurgitation in a valve with *normal leaflets but dilated annulus* is termed *functional* mitral regurgitation (MR).

MYXOMATOUS MITRAL VALVE DISEASE

Etiology and Pathophysiology

The underlying etiology of myxomatous disease is a defect in the fibroelastic connective tissue of the valvular leaflets, chordae, and annulus.[21] The myxomatous defect leads to an abnormal elongation and redundancy of valve tissue and chordae. Each particular anatomic redundancy creates mitral regurgitation in its own particular manner. Annular dilatation (Fig. 35-3) obliterates the normal coaptation line between the anterior and posterior leaflet, causing regurgitation. If primarily posterior annular dilatation occurs, there is a separation in the middle of the valve between the two leaflets and blood leaks through during ventricular contraction. Leaflet redundancy results in a movement of the redundant leaflet into the left atrium during diastole. If severe enough, that movement leads to a compromised coaptation line and MR then ensues. Elongation of the chordae also causes leaflet tissue to move into the atrium during diastole, also resulting in compromised coaptation. Ruptured or flail leaflets are often the result of systolic stresses fracturing weakened chordae, causing severe regurgitation.

Mitral regurgitation represents pure volume overload for the LV.[22] In myxomatous disease, MR is typically of the chronic compensated variety.[23] A vicious cycle is perpetuated whereby the excess volume load over time results in ventricular failure. Ventricular failure itself implies ventricular dilatation, which results in a greater degree of MR. Thus, MR begets more MR, and a downward spiral is created.[17] MR created by left ventricular failure occurs primarily by ventricular dilatation. Successful repair will result in left ventricular mass reduction.[24] Ventricular dilatation "pulls" or "tethers" the leaflets open, thereby impinging on coaptation. In degenerative disease of the mitral valve, however, the LV itself per se does not primarily cause MR in the early course of the disease.

Carpentier[10] has developed a mitral valve analysis protocol and surgical philosophy for repair of all types of valves (Fig. 35-4). Myxomatous disease has become the pathology responsible for the vast majority of patients with mitral regurgitation in the United States.[25] Currently, mitral valve prolapse, as a part of the spectrum of degenerative disease, is present in about 5% of the general population,[26] with about 10% of these patients exhibiting severe MR requiring surgery.[27] Whatever the ultimate pathologic pathway creating

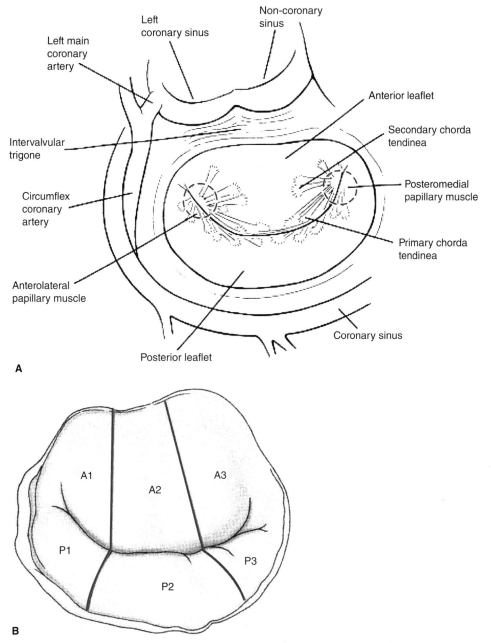

FIGURE 35-2 Surgical anatomy of the mitral valve. (A) Critical structures that the cardiac surgeon must recognize, including the circumflex coronary artery, the coronary sinus, the atrioventricular node, and aortic root. Note that the left and right trigones are superior to the commissures. (B) The conventional terminology used to describe the pathoanatomic parts of the anterior and posterior leaflets.

regurgitation, more than 95% of all degenerative disease should be amenable to successful repair.

Diagnostic Work-up and Indications for Operation

Patient presentation is typically quite varied depending on the degree of MR as well as the chronicity of the disease. Patients may be floridly symptomatic or completely asymptomatic. Symptoms can occur in different forms. Heart failure symptoms are secondary to pulmonary venous hypertension as well as fluid retention. This may include shortness of breath, limited exertional capacity, fluid overload, and in the late stage of the disease, frank heart failure. Embolization sequelae and arrhythmias form a second set of symptoms and include atrial fibrillation and increased stroke risk.[28] Additionally, regurgitation predisposes the valve to infectious endocarditis.[29] Abnormal hemodynamics create pathologic shear stresses and turbulence that generates vulnerability to infection in the valve.

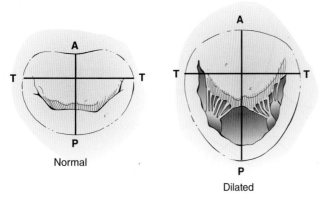

FIGURE 35-3 Annular dilatation. A, anterior; P, posterior; T, trigone.

Normal

Dilated

Evaluating MR

Key information is obtained from echocardiography: the degree of MR, associated pathophysiology, cardiac chamber dimensions, and left ventricular functional analysis. Transthoracic echocardiography is usually the first modality employed. However, if images from transthoracic echocardiography are of insufficient quality, then transesophageal echocardiography (TEE) is required. Mitral regurgitation is graded on a scale from mild to severe, with severe typically referring to a reversal of pulmonary venous blood flow in systole.[30] The methods used to determine the degree of regurgitation commonly include regurgitant volume, regurgitant fraction, and effective regurgitant orifice area.[30] Echocardiographic analysis of the MR (eg, flail leaflet, ruptured chordae, or anterior or posterior prolapse) is extremely helpful in planning the operative intervention. Other crucial information obtained by the preoperative echo includes left atrial size, ventricular function, ventricular dilatation, aortic valve function, and tricuspid valve function. A large left atrium implies chronic MR. A small LA and hyperdynamic LV implies acute MR. Ventricular function is a key component in assessing operative candidacy; a left ventricular ejection fraction below the norm of 60% indicates some degree of myocardial decompensation secondary to volume overload. Indeed, in the presence of severe MR, the ejection fraction will often decline postoperatively even if the preop ejection fraction is normal. A corollary of this fact is a normal preoperative ejection fraction does not necessarily mean normal ventricular function.

Timing of Surgery

Once pulmonary hypertension, LV dysfunction/LA dilatation or symptoms appear, the prognosis of MR worsens. Careful surveillance may result in timing of valve surgery before these negative sequelae occur.[30a] An attractive alternative strategy for treating severe chronic primary MR is to perform early mitral repair before these triggers are reached. Early mitral repair avoids the need for intensive surveillance and also obviates the possibility that patients might become lost to follow-up or delay seeing their clinician until advanced LV dysfunction has already ensued. This strategy requires expertise in clinical evaluation and cardiac imaging to evaluate severity and significance of MR.

What, precisely, are the indications for operation? In general, as surgical results improve, the indications for surgery

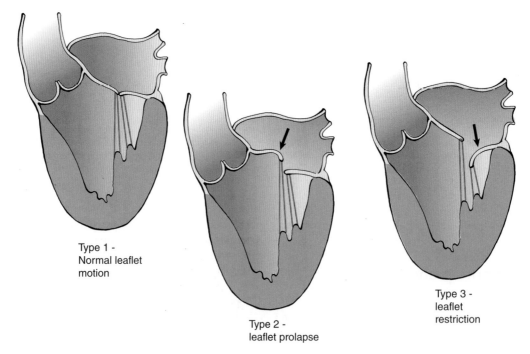

Type 1 -
Normal leaflet
motion

Type 2 -
leaflet prolapse

Type 3 -
leaflet
restriction

FIGURE 35-4 Carpentier's functional classification.

are broadening. The American Heart Association 2014 guidelines state that **"Mitral valve repair is reasonable in asymptomatic patients with chronic severe primary MR (stage C1) with preserved LV function (LVEF > 60% and LVESD 0 40 mm) in whom the likelihood of a successful and durable repair without residual MR is greater than 95% with an expected mortality rate of less than 1% when performed at a Heart Valve Center of Excellence."** Patients who would never have been considered for surgery previously are now routinely being offered repair surgery at much earlier stages of their disease. The indications for mitral valve repair have widened as the success of repair has so dramatically improved over the last several years. Better myocardial protection and cardiopulmonary bypass technology, minimally invasive incisions, increased incidence of repair, and better intensive care unit support have all contributed to the phenomenon.[31] The biggest change has been an overall broadening of the indications for mitral valve repair and lowering of the threshold for operation because of these factors,[32] even in the elderly.[33] Increasingly, asymptomatic mitral regurgitation, even without symptoms, is becoming accepted as a reasonable strategy.[34] Repair of the mitral valve, as opposed to replacement, is now accepted as the superior treatment for myxomatous mitral regurgitation. Out of a long laboratory and clinical experience have come the conclusions that repair is associated with better survival, enhanced preservation of ventricular function (by preserving the chordae and papillary muscles), and decreased late thromboembolic complications.[35-42]

For all patients with moderate-to-severe MR and moderately decreased ventricular function (left ventricular ejection fraction < 60%) valve repair is offered, because the ventricle has exhibited signs of decompensation even with a lesser degree of MR; repair in this setting is much more urgent, because severe decompensation can occur in a matter of months as left ventricular function begins to deteriorate.

The standard of care for patients with severe cardiomyopathy and severe MR is unclear presently and is one of the most controversial topics in cardiac surgery. This situation typically does not occur with myxomatous disease but rather ischemia or idiopathic cardiomyopathy and such regurgitation is functional in nature. In longstanding myxomatous disease, however, LV dysfunction may be present.

The intermediate situation of moderate mitral regurgitation and preserved ventricular function is the one in which the most judgment must be exercised. Consider the situation of a structurally normal mitral valve with moderate functional MR, but with concomitant critical aortic stenosis. The patient is to undergo an aortic valve replacement. Should the mitral valve be repaired? Perhaps not, as the moderate MR here is typically exacerbated by the patient's aortic stenosis and volume overload, and correction of the aortic stenosis and euvoluemia would likely reduce or eliminate the MR in this structurally normal valve.[39,40] However, should repair be undertaken, ring annuloplasty would be needed to correct the posterior annular dilatation. If the same situation exists, however, with a structurally abnormal valve, such as a prolapsed

P2 or markedly dilated mitral annulus in a myxomatous valve, then mitral repair should always be undertaken, because there is a structural abnormality that aortic valve replacement will not correct. What of moderate MR secondary to myxomatous disease (and not ischemia) in a patient who is to undergo coronary bypass grafting? That patient would likely be offered concomitant valve repair, because bypass grafting would not impact on the pathophysiology of the MR in this case. What of the situation of moderate-to-severe isolated MR secondary to myxomatous disease and borderline normal ventricular function? Even without symptoms of heart failure, this patient should have repair performed on an elective basis. Once left ventricular function begins to deteriorate from the normal 60 to 70% left ventricular ejection fraction, decline may be unpredictably rapid and hence intervention warranted. Increasingly, moderate ischemic, as well as degenerative, MR is thought to be detrimental for long-term survival.[41,42]

In general, no matter what the chronological age is, adequate functional status before valve repair is preferred. If symptoms of heart failure exist before surgery, optimal diuresis should be undertaken before operation. If the procedure involves coronary artery bypass grafting, the conduit status should be determined. Dental clearance on all patients should be obtained before any valvular procedure. If neurologic symptoms exist or if the patient has a history of a previous cerebrovascular disease, then preoperative carotid noninvasive studies are warranted to assess carotid arterial stenosis. All patients older than 40 years should undergo coronary angiography. Patients with MR without coronary artery disease are good candidates for smaller incisions.[43,45]

Whatever the scenario, the decision to operate and repair the valve is a decision made preoperatively as opposed to intraoperatively. Once the patient is under anesthesia, loading conditions are not physiologic and the mitral regurgitation assessed then is inevitably underestimated. Maneuvers used to "bring out the MR," such as increasing afterload with vasoactive drugs, do not reflect true physiology, but should be used in surgical decision making and may be helpful in some situations. Recent discussions of earlier referral for the treatment of MR clearly depend on a high rate of valve repair in any center.[46,47]

Operative Philosophy

Clearly, in light of elevated success rates of mitral valve repair in specialized centers but also today in all cardiac surgery programs, the patient with degenerative mitral valve disease with significant MR requires a repair procedure, rather than replacement.[49]

With the increasing numbers of trained surgeons who have absorbed the various mitral valve repair techniques and can apply them safely the percentage of valves that can be repaired and actually are repaired, is improving. Recent STS database interrogation indicates that this percentage may now be as high as 75%.[49]

Beginning in the 1980s, we have developed what we think is a simple, reproducible algorithm that can be used to repair the degenerative mitral valve in most patients. Overriding this philosophy is the belief that mitral valve repair is not an esoteric "art form" that is difficult to explain, perform, or learn. Rather, we think it is a procedure like any other that should and can be simplified, disseminated, and reproduced with success. In keeping with this philosophy, we have reduced complicated bileaflet prolapse to a competent valve with simplified and straightforward maneuvers that we have found effective with good long-term results. Our overall philosophy and technique are as follows:

1. Expose the valve well through the complete development of Sondergaard's groove, division of pericardial attachments of the superior and inferior venae cavae, and release of the left pericardial retraction stitches
2. Assess the valve through saline injection and corroborate the intraoperative findings with TEE
3. Perform basic, obvious leaflet repair procedures first (eg, quadrangular resections to the posterior leaflet)
4. Implant the annuloplasty ring sized by the height of the anterior leaflet (not the trigones or commissures)
5. Test the repair
6. Perform additional reparative procedures as needed, that is, cleft closure.

With the above maneuvers, we estimate that approximately 95% of all degenerative valves can be repaired.

Collaborative involvement with cardiac anesthesia colleagues is essential in utilizing the invaluable tool of transesophageal echocardiogram monitoring for pre- and postrepair assessment. In our clinic, standard TEE monitoring (either two- or three-dimensional) is now utilized for every patient undergoing mitral valve repair. In addition to documenting the efficacy of repair, TEE is essential in preventing and assessing the potential or persistence of systolic anterior motion (SAM) of the anterior valve.

Operative Exposure

Because the mitral valve is such a complex anatomic structure and the maneuvers involved in correcting a regurgitant valve may vary from the simple to the very complex, adequate exposure is an absolute requirement in every operative plan. This becomes more important if minimally invasive techniques are employed. Mitral valve exposure is more challenging than exposure of the aortic or tricuspid valve. Why? From the surgeon's side, the mitral valve is furthest away from the operating surgeon than any other valve. In addition, the valve in its native position naturally faces above and/or toward the surgeon's left shoulder at an oblique angle such that the surgeon does not see the valve en face.

The first critical aspect to the standard valve repair is the complete and thorough development of the Sondergaard plane reflecting the right atrium off the left atrium to the atrial septum, as depicted in Fig. 35-5. This was first described in the 1950s by the Danish surgeon Sondergaard,[50] to expose the atrial septum for noncardiopulmonary bypass treatment of atrial septal defects. In 1990, we stressed the

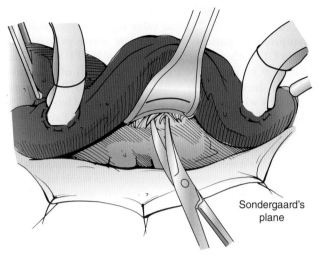

FIGURE 35-5 Dissection of Sondergaard's plane. Sondergaard's plane should be dissected at least 2 to 4 cm from the right superior pulmonary vein for adequate exposure of the mitral valve.

importance of this particular technique for exposure in mitral valve surgery.[51] Regardless of even previous procedures, it should always be possible to dissect out the groove without significant difficulty. The complete and full development of the groove is a most important aspect to obtain adequate exposure of the mitral valve. With this technique, via blunt and sharp dissection we typically have not needed any other incision for mitral valve repair or replacement, whether for primary surgery or reoperation. This incision usually brings the surgeon very close to the mitral valve. Once the right atrium is dissected off the left atrium, a generous incision in the left atrium is made, avoiding the atrial septum.

The second aspect of exposure is to bring the valve as close to an en face position to the operating surgeon as possible. Pericardial stay sutures are released on the left side. The operating table is maneuvered head up and to the left. If necessary, the left pericardium is opened and the apex of the heart moved laterally to the left pleural space. Exposure of the left trigone can be particularly challenging for stitch placement. This can be facilitated with local epicardial displacement of the midlateral LV wall medially with a spongestick (Fig. 35-6).

Cardiopulmonary Bypass

For cardiopulmonary bypass, we use a 22F percutaneous femoral vein venous catheter placed into the right atrium via the right femoral vein with TEE control. The cannula can even be advanced into the superior vena cava if desired. Because the cannula has multiple holes, is flexible and thus can still drain the inferior vena cava, this one cannula is sometimes all that is needed for drainage of both the superior and inferior vena cava. If performing a concomitant bypass procedure requiring a full sternotomy, then venous cannulation should be bicaval via the atria. One venous cannula should be placed in the superior vena cava above the right atrial/

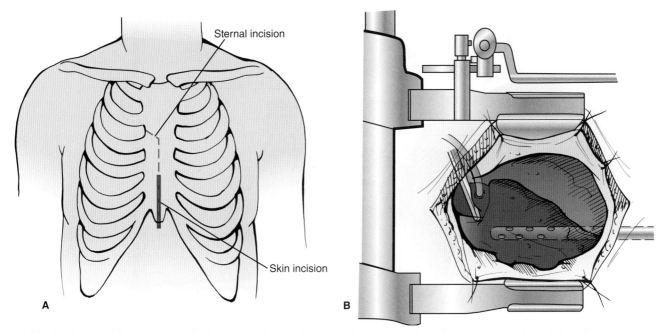

FIGURE 35-6 Minimally invasive mitral valve repair. (A) Via a 6- to 8-cm skin incision, a lower hemisternotomy through the right second interspace is performed. (B) Venous cannulation is percutaneous with vacuum assist. Aortic cannulation, cross-clamping, and cardioplegia administration are performed in the standard manner.

superior vena caval junction and the other through the lowest part of the right atrium into the mouth of the inferior vena cava. The arterial cannula should be placed directly into the distal ascending aorta.

Once on cardiopulmonary bypass, systemic temperature is allowed to drift to 34°, the ascending aorta is cross-clamped, and the heart arrested by cold blood cardioplegia. For isolated valve repair, some debate still exists regarding the use of retrograde or antegrade blood cardioplegia after cross-clamping. If there is concomitant coronary artery disease, myocardial protection in this circumstance should be antegrade and retrograde, because the coronary artery bypass graft/mitral operation presents one of the highest-risk operative settings in cardiac surgery.[36]

After the heart is arrested, the left atrium is opened well above the right superior pulmonary vein near the septum inferiorly. Retractors are placed (Fig. 35-7). The patient's bed is placed head up with a tilt to the left. A wire-reinforced suction catheter is placed in the left inferior pulmonary vein (the most dependent portion of the left atrium in this position) for drainage of collateral blood flow. Carbon dioxide is infused to minimize intracardiac air.

Alternate exposures can be obtained by the transseptal approach through the right atrium[52] or the superior septal approach.[53] The transseptal approach is a perfectly acceptable incision that allows the cardiac surgeon to be close to the mitral valve by carrying the incision through the fossa ovalis (Fig. 35-8) and up into the superior vena cava. Retraction sutures and other types of retraction devices can be utilized to expose the mitral valve exceedingly well, particularly in these minimally invasive cases. This approach may also be helpful

in patients who have had previous operations on the mitral valve or when concomitant procedures on the tricuspid valve are required.

Examination of Valve and Valve Analysis

Once exposure is obtained and a self-retaining retractor is in place, inspection of the valve is carried out. Valve analysis takes a few minutes utilizing nerve hooks, forceps, and insufflation of the ventricle with saline to determine and corroborate the pathology already diagnosed by intraoperative TEE. Valve analysis may reveal ruptured chordae or simply a prolapse of the valve with elongated chords and one or more prolapsed sections of the valve. The anterior leaflet, though frequently advertised as part of "bileaflet prolapse," often has normal length chordae and may be without specific leaflet or subvalvular pathology. Prolapse of the commissures may be found, and calcified nodules may exist that may present difficulty in mitral valve repair and may need excision. There may be healed endocarditic vegetations on one or more parts of the valve. The annulus will almost always appear to be distorted, dilated, or deformed in long-standing cases, particularly in Barlow syndrome.

Repair Strategy and Overview

After the analysis of the valve is carried out, a detailed reparative strategy can be deduced from the pathologic analysis. In a broad generalization, degenerative disease of the mitral valve creates what amounts to a PML that is too large, with or without flail segments, in an annulus that is functionally too small for the anterior leaflet. In degenerative disease, the

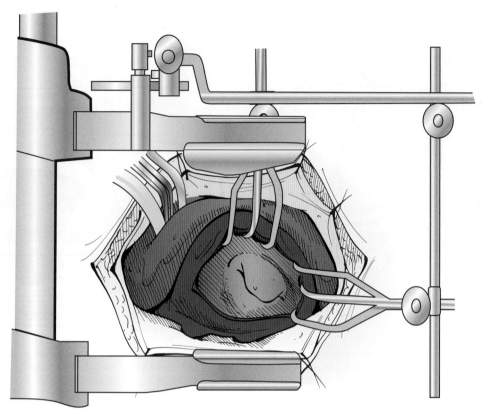

FIGURE 35-7 Minimally invasive operative exposure. After the retractors are placed, the patient is positioned with head up and the operative bed tilted to the left. Exposure is excellent.

posterior leaflet is typically pathologic, whereas the anterior leaflet usually is not.

The first principle of the repair is to reduce or obliterate the enlarged segments and to reduce the overall height of the abnormally large posterior leaflet. This reduction reconstructs the correct coaptation line with the anterior leaflet, and, just as importantly, prevents systolic anterior motion (SAM) of the anterior leaflet. If the height of the posterior leaflet is too high, it will push the anterior leaflet into the LVOT and create SAM. In general, the height of the posterior leaflet should be no more than 1 to 1.5 cm in average-sized patients once the repair is complete. The normal sections of the posterior leaflet should be used as a marker to guide the reduction of the redundant parts. Ultimately, the reconstructed posterior leaflet should appear like a "smile." Once the posterior leaflet reduction is performed, one must ensure that the anterior leaflet coapts with the subsequently reduced posterior leaflet within the correct plane using the saline test. The resulting repair should result in a coaptation line at the level of the annulus during systole. Specific methods to lower the height of the posterior leaflet and anterior leaflet will be addressed below.

A new concept of 'respect rather than resect' has become popular in recent years. Instead of resecting the leaflet segment that is flailing, this same segment is brought down back to form a coaptation line using polytetrafluoroethylene (PTFE) suture to form neochords. The excess tissue is displaced into the LV to form a new and durable coaptation

line. This approach is of value especially in small access procedures, in which implementation of more complex resection and repair can be cumbersome. Regardless of the surgeon's choice regarding whether to 'respect or resect', a prosthetic ring or band is mandatory in all repair procedures. The result of avoiding an annuloplasty ring is a significantly higher risk of recurrent moderate-to-severe mitral valve regurgitation.

A remodeling annuloplasty ring is essential for all repairs. This is a fundamental concept of Carpentier[18] and Duran,[54] both of whom developed mitral valve annuloplasty rings early in the history of mitral valve regurgitation surgery and advocated remodeling of the distorted annulus as a key principle of mitral valve repair. The annulus, after many years of regurgitation, is often deformed and in myxomatous disease, it is floppy and dilated. The best approach to conceptualize the dilated annulus in myxomatous disease is to consider it functionally too small for the anterior leaflet.

When dilated, the annulus will not provide the relatively stable support necessary for the anterior leaflet to spread out completely and thus coapt at the correct line and in the correct plane with the posterior leaflet. Rather, the floppy annulus will buckle and have an effectively smaller radius, and cause the anterior leaflet to appear as though it is "prolapsing" because the leaflet cannot spread out correctly. In reality the pathology is within the annulus. That is why we believe that oversizing the ring in degenerative disease is important. The ring then

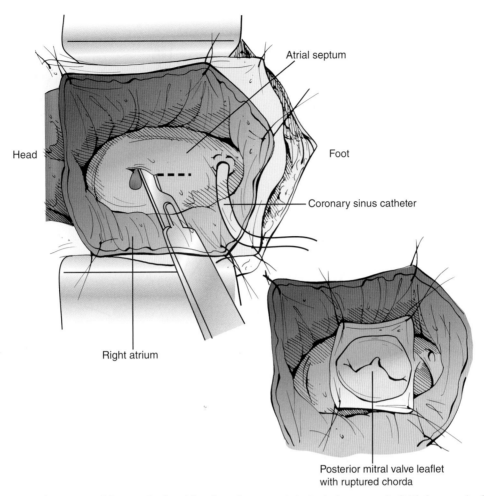

FIGURE 35-8 Transseptal exposure of the mitral valve. After the right atrium is incised, the septum is divided across the fossa ovalis, and stay sutures are placed. This incision allows very good access to the mitral valve and is an alternative to the Sondergaard plane.

recreates the relatively rigid, broad annulus that allows the anterior leaflet to spread out and coapt in the correct plane, at the correct coaptation line, without "prolapsing." A structurally sound annulus is necessary for the correct physiologic function of the anterior leaflet. Hence, our protocol is to place the annuloplasty ring after posterior leaflet repair and then reassess for any anterior or complex leaflet pathology afterward. A annular pathology often falsely gives the appearance of leaflet pathology, and by following the steps outlined above, many unnecessary procedures will be prevented.

By utilizing the two principles outlined above, the proper and necessary attention is given to the correct physiologic functioning of the valve in a manner that is surgically relevant. The height of the posterior leaflet is reduced to prevent SAM as well as to allow the correct coaptation plane. The two leaflets are made to coapt at the correct line by reinforcing the annulus with a remodeling ring. As outlined above, in our experience at the Brigham and that of others,[55] in most cases, the so-called "bileaflet prolapse" is completely eliminated by adequate posterior leaflet resection and a large remodeling annuloplasty ring without any further anterior leaflet intervention.

There is clear evidence supporting the integral and essential necessity of the ring for a lasting repair. In an early paper on mitral valve repair, we compared a repair group that had no annuloplasty ring to another group in whom a ring was implanted at the time of valve repair.[56] All valves were competent at the time of surgery, but after several years of follow-up, the rate of mitral regurgitation in the no-ring group was five times that of the ring group. Recent studies have supported the importance of ring annuloplasty.[57] Thus, a remodeling ring is critical to a long-lasting physiologic mitral valve repair.

SPECIFIC SURGICAL TECHNIQUES

Posterior Leaflet Quadrangular Resection

The most common mitral valve pathologies (approximately 80%) encountered in the myxomatous, degenerated valve are ruptured and elongated chords from the middle section of the posterior leaflet (Fig. 35-9A). In one approach limited resection of this diseased section of leaflet is shown in

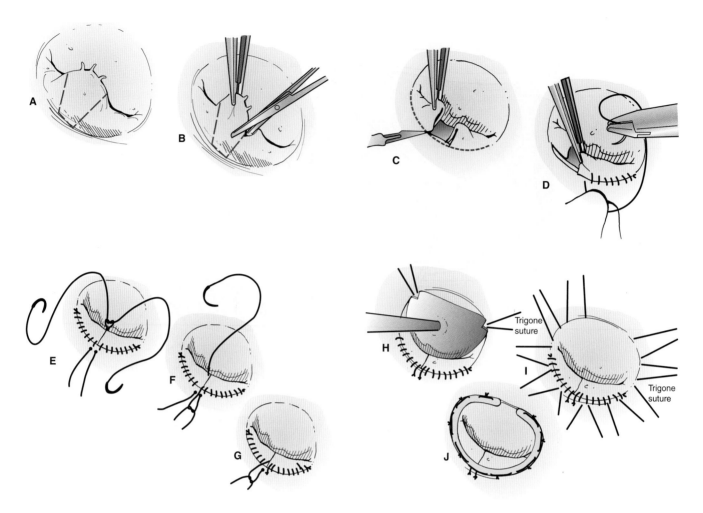

FIGURE 35-9 Repair of P2 with flail segment with ruptured chordae. (A) The classic flail P2 segment. (B) Resection of this flail segment. (C) and (D) The classic sliding valvuloplasty and advancement, in which each segment of the valve adjacent to the resected P2 segment is separated from the annulus. The valve is then reattached with the gap eliminated. At the same time, the height of the posterior leaflet is reduced. (E), (F), and (G) Completion of the classic sliding valvuloplasty. (H), (I), and (J) Placement of the annuloplasty stitches and ring placement. Sizing of the ring is done by the size of the anterior leaflet.

Fig. 35-9B. To fill the gap produced by removing the pathologic section, leaflet advancement of the remaining leaflet sections is carried out (Fig. 35-9C and D) and the cut edges of the valve are reapproximated with running monofilament suture (Fig. 35-9E, F, and G). An annuloplasty ring is then implanted (Fig. 35-9H, I, and J). This scenario is the most common pathophysiology encountered and operative strategy employed. Interestingly, recent results by Perier[58] and Lawrie[59] have reported successful results with use of only artificial PTFE chords to preserve the posterior leaflet instead of resecting it, a technique that has traditionally been applied only to the anterior leaflet.

For cardiac surgeons who perform a modest number of valve repairs, incising the posterior leaflet off the annulus may be somewhat daunting. In our own experience, a prolapsed leaflet without ruptured chordae at P2 may simply be obliterated by a few sutures to bring the leading edge of the prolapsed leaflet to the underside of the annular connection, thus reducing the height, preserving all the chords, and

accomplishing what might be done with a resection.[61] This has been termed a "folding valvuloplasty."

If the repair includes a resection of a flail segment, then some form of the leaflet advancement technique popularized by Carpentier should be employed.[60] In this technique, the two remaining sections are advanced upon each other to close the gap produced by the resected area. This includes separating each remaining segment off the annulus for a short segment. Of all the traditional techniques, this is the one that has produced some concern for surgeons who perform only moderate numbers of valve repairs because of the necessity of incising the posterior leaflet off the annulus and then reanastomosing the leaflet to the annulus.

We have evolved a simplified technique for limited PML resections in which leaflet advancement may be more easily performed, and yet still accomplish the exact same result in much less time. We have named this the "fold-over leaflet advancement." In this technique the remaining enlarged segments of P2, on either side of the elongated resected leaflet

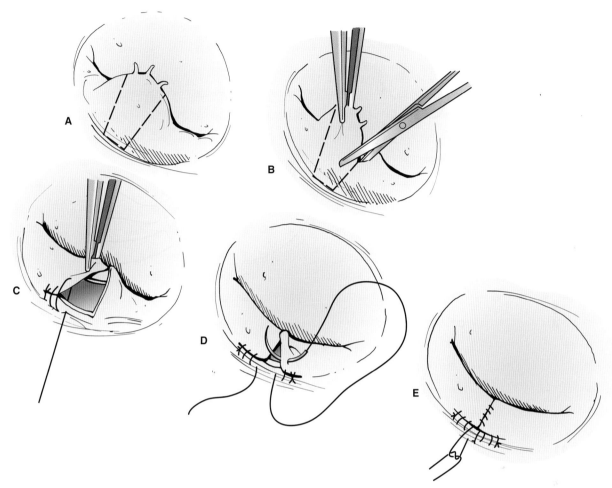

FIGURE 35-10 The fold-over leaflet advancement. Performed for a prolapsed and flail P2 segment here, the fold-over advancement accomplished the same goals as the classic sliding valvuloplasty, but with simpler surgical techniques. After resection of the flail P2 segment (B), the cut edges of each side of the resulting gap are sewn to the annulus as they are "folded down." This is done for each side of the gap for half of the original height of each side. The top halves are then sewn together (E). The result is that the leaflet gap is eliminated and the height of the leaflet reduced.

with supporting chordae, are simply folded over by a continuous polypropylene suture to the annular gap produced by the limited posterior leaflet resection, without any further incision (Fig. 35-10). The fold-over advancement accomplishes the same goals as the traditional leaflet advancement. The small gap distance, created by the small area of resected flail segment, is eliminated and the height of the posterior leaflet is reduced. We have found the fold-over advancement to be extremely effective for small resections of the posterior leaflet in any position without the necessity of incising the leaflet off the annulus.

That being stated, many situations exist with true Barlow syndrome with elongation and elevation of almost the entire posterior leaflet. In essence, the whole posterior leaflet is elongated. In these particular pathologic situations, the classic techniques are necessary. The entire posterior leaflet on both sides of the resected area, including P1 and P3, must be incised

off the annulus and careful and detailed valve advancement carried out, beginning at each commissure, with running 4-0 polypropylene (see Fig. 35-9C and D). The height of the leaflet is lowered to avoid creation of SAM and provide a good coaptation point for the anterior leaflet. Because some of these leaflets may be as high as 3 to 4 cm, if the height of the leaflet is not shortened significantly, SAM is highly likely. While performing the leaflet advancement, imbrication of PML segment areas may also be effective if there is focal enlargement at a particular area of the leaflet. This simplifies the surgical technique, reduces operative time, and achieves the same result. Multiple interrupted mattress sutures may be used.

Commissural Prolapse

As the most straightforward example of pathologic valve prolapse, chordal rupture or elongation at the anteriorlateral or

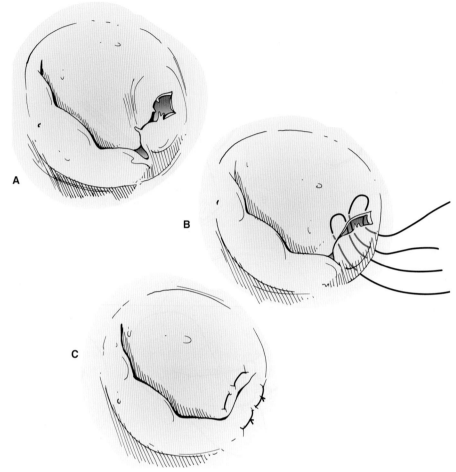

FIGURE 35-11 Commissuroplasty. Simple horizontal mattress stitches placed in the ruptured commissure eliminate regurgitation without need for further leaflet resection, even with ruptured chordae.

posteriormedial commissure provides the surgeon with the most obvious strategy of repair. Many surgeons still recommend resection of this area, but commissuroplasty is by far the most simple, direct, and efficient way to handle this particular problem. The prolapsed area is obliterated by one to three polypropylene mattress stitches (Fig. 35-11), eliminating the regurgitation at that point. A small obliteration of this area at A1 and P1 or A3 and P3 will not make any significant difference in the overall cross-sectional area of the mitral valve, so mitral stenosis is of no concern with this technique. Several other reports[62,63] have also documented this technique as an effective and long-lasting method to treat commissural prolapse.

Anterior Leaflet Prolapse

Though uncommon, true prolapse of the anterior leaflet engenders significant concern to surgeons because such pathology is associated with less successful long-term repair results than posterior leaflet pathology.[64] The height of the chordae underlying the anterior leaflet must be assessed and chords may be grossly elongated or ruptured and make the AML flail. This

problem may be addressed by a variety of techniques and the long-term follow-up on many of these techniques has been quite promising. There are four basic techniques to repair true prolapse of the anterior leaflet. They are (1) reduction of the chordal height by implantation techniques; (2) artificial PTFE chordae; (3) chordal transfer from the posterior to anterior leaflet; and (4) the edge-to-edge technique.

Resection of the Anterior Leaflet

It has been well established that the body of the anterior leaflet should be treated with great respect, and preservation of AML tissue is important. Resections can be carried out, but only as a small triangular resection for ruptured chords to reduce the bulk of a large anterior leaflet.[81] For anterior mitral valve prolapse associated with idiopathic hypertrophic subaortic stenosis, or as an alternative technique for reduction of the AML height, creation of a longitudinal periannular anterior leaflet resection with reconstruction of the leaflet has also been advocated to reduce the height of the anterior leaflet with some success.[82,83]

Chordal Shortening by Implantation into Papillary Muscles

One of the first techniques developed by Carpentier[10] of chordal shortening involves incising the papillary muscle, placing the redundant anterior leaflet chords within the muscle, and then sewing the papillary muscle over the chord, thus entrapping the chordae and shortening it (Fig. 35-12). This is a simple technique, but it has gone out of favor, as reports by Cosgrove and coworkers[65] have demonstrated that additional chordal ruptures may occur after use of this technique. They postulate that the potential sawing action of the papillary muscle on the buried chord is the cause. Other techniques of this type include papillary muscle repositioning[66] and chordal plication and free-edge (AML) remodeling.[67]

Chordal Transfer

The third technique for true anterior prolapse is chordal transfer from the posterior leaflet to the anterior leaflet. This

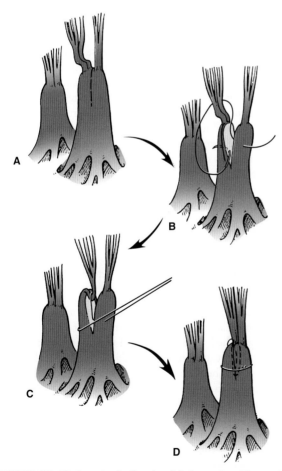

FIGURE 35-12 Anterior leaflet chordal shortening. The papillary muscle is incised and the redundant chord folded into it. The excess chord is held in place with pledgeted sutures.

was originally described by Carpentier[10] and has been popularized by the Cleveland Clinic[65] and Duran and coworkers.[72] Figure 35-13 illustrates the operative steps. A resection of the flail chordae of the anterior leaflet is carried out, and an adjacent segment of the posterior leaflet is then resected from the posterior leaflet and then transferred to the gap produced by the anterior leaflet resection. This technique has had reportedly good long-term results, but may involve both leaflets when only single leaflet pathology exists.[73]

Edge-to-Edge Technique

The edge-to-edge repair is a technique in which the anterior leaflet and posterior leaflet are sewn together at the coaptation line, producing a double-orifice mitral valve.[74] This has gained considerable popularity and even percutaneous interventional attempts to emulate this surgical maneuver are being pursued.[75] Developed by Alfieri and coworkers,[76] their theory is that with Barlow syndrome or truly redundant anterior leaflets, apposition of the midportion of the anterior leaflet to the midportion of the posterior leaflet will prevent the elevation of the anterior leaflet above the level of the posterior leaflet, thus eliminating mitral regurgitation. This technique greatly simplifies the repair of the true bileaflet prolapse and has been adopted as standard therapy for AML pathology by several groups, especially in those patients with a high probability of postrepair SAM. In particular, with anterior leaflet chordal rupture or marked elongation of the chordae to the anterior leaflet, repair consists of a single stitch carefully placed.

Figure 35-14 illustrates our technique. A figure-of-eight braided polyester suture is placed at the apposition points of the anterior and the posterior leaflet. We use this stronger suture, because there have been reports of the more commonly used polypropylene sutures rupturing. An important point of the surgical technique is our strong belief that the stitch should be placed only with myxomatous valves, so as to avoid producing mitral stenosis as has been the case with ischemic MR.[77] To ensure the adequacy of each orifice created by the edge-to-edge technique, we also measure the diameter of each orifice and confirm that it is at least 2 cm in diameter. If the orifices are less than 2 cm in diameter, the technique is abandoned. This technique is a very valuable adjunct in patients who have the potential for SAM of the mitral valve.[78,79] In fact, prevention of SAM may be the best utilization of this technique at present. In our small series of 20 patients with SAM potential, all were treated and SAM was prevented in all patients. A competent mitral valve was maintained in all at 8 years postoperatively without mitral stenosis.[78]

Medium-term results of this surgical maneuver are satisfactory and compatible with all other commonly used repair techniques, according to studies by Alfieri and coworkers,[76,80] but there have been no comparative, prospective, randomized studies comparing the classic repair techniques to this approach in the long term.

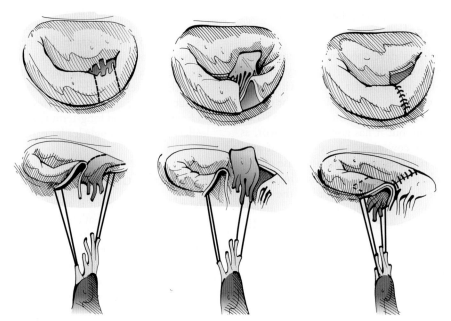

FIGURE 35-13 Chordal transfer. For an isolated flail anterior leaflet segment, first the prolapsed section of anterior leaflet is resected. An adjoining section of posterior leaflet is then resected and transposed over to the gap created by the anterior resection.

Artificial Chordae

The mitral subvalvular apparatus is a sophisticated structure that couples intact mitral valve function with support of left ventricular function. Mitral valve replacement, naturally, eliminates this important and fine connection. The use of artificial chords during mitral valve repair procedures, while "respecting rather than resecting" the mitral leaflets tissue, has the potential of restoring mitral valve anatomy and function. The goal of performing a repair while using neochords is to eliminate any regurgitation get, while preserving both leaflets and keeping the mitral annular symmetry. The use of artificial chordae for mitral valve repair, dates back to the 1960s, and during the evolution of

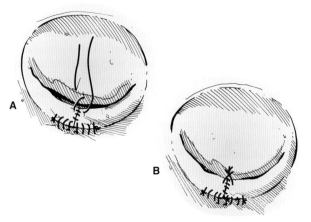

FIGURE 35-14 Edge-to-edge technique. The technique involves a braided polyester figure-of-eight stitch at apposition of A2 and P2.

this technique, a number of materials were used as artificial chordae, including silk and nylon. Today, most, if not all surgeons, use expanded polytetraflouroethylene (ePTFE) chords, and this technique is perhaps the most popular current technique for AML pathology. Originally described by Frater and Zussa,[68,69] this technique has grown in popularity over the past several years.[64,70] Lawrie[59] has also recently reported excellent results in applying PTFE neochords for the anterior and posterior leaflet repair. Duran has devised a method for more precise measurement of the correct height for these new chordal structures.[70] This technique (Fig. 35-15) involves a number of technical steps to establish a path for successful repair.

1. Attachment to the papillary muscle
2. Attachment to the leaflet
3. Length adjustment
4. Tighing of the PTFE neochord, before or after insertion of an annuloplasty ring.

We usually place a mattress suture with a pledget on the papillary muscle to which the redundant or ruptured chord has been attached. The two ends of the double-armed PTFE are then brought up through the edge of the leaflet that needs to be lowered. The critical part of this technique is determining the degree to which the leaflet is lowered and hence how tightly the stitch is tied down. This is determined by ascertaining the optimal position of the two leaflets in systole. Both the anterior and posterior leaflets should be in apposition at this point, and thus the leaflet's height in systole should be the level to which the chords are adjusted. We have used tenting of the posterior leaflet as our guide while carefully tying down the chord (Fig. 35-15B). Other techniques describe using multiple loops (David technique), using a fixed length loop

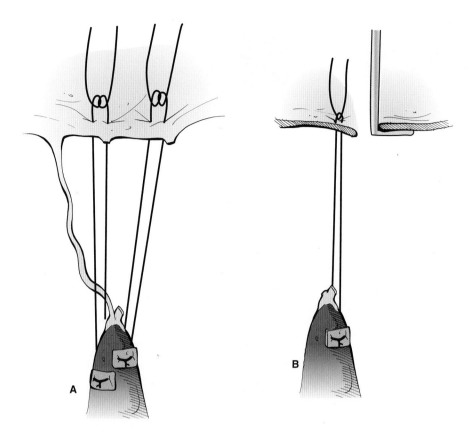

FIGURE 35-15 Artificial PTFE chords for the anterior leaflet. (A) Pledgeted PTFE stitches are placed through a papillary muscle and brought through the leading edge of the anterior leaflet. Using the tented-up posterior leaflet (B), the correct length of artificial chord is created.

technique using a caliper (von Oppell and Mohr), using a fixed length loop technique without using a caliper (Mandegar). Tam described a modification of the loop technique that involves only a single pass through the papillary muscle.

Whatever the technique employed, the end result should be that the anterior leaflet now coapts at the same level as the posterior leaflet with left ventricular contraction. Some surgeons advocate neo chordae, as opposed to leaflet resection, as the repair technique of choice for leaflet prolapse.[61]

Long-term histology results of neochord placement demonstrate that ePTFE neochords become covered with fibrous tissue as described by Bortolotti et al[93] This is consistent with our own experience demonstrated by Fig. 35-16.

SPECIAL PROBLEMS AND CONSIDERATIONS

The Calcified Annulus

Calcification, particularly of the posterior annulus, is a complicating aspect of mitral valve repair. Calcification makes repair more difficult, as stitches are more difficult to place and the risk of paravalvular leak is increased. Severe annular calcification, however, does not necessarily rule out an effective mitral valve repair. Partial or total removal of the calcified

bar may be done safely. Carpentier has promulgated removal of the entire calcified bar in radical fashion, which in essence partially detaches the LV from the left atrium.[84] Partial and selective calcification removal may also be quite effective and potentially safer.[85] Partial removal of calcium with leaflet advancement can be performed without the need for a radical debridement in many patients. Only the amount of calcium should be removed that allows adequate stitch placement and leaflet and annular flexibility. Obviously, calcification of the chordae or a substantial part of the leaflet tissue is a poor prognostic factor for long-term freedom from valve repair, and an extensively calcified valve usually indicates valve replacement.

Systolic Anterior Motion of the Mitral Valve

As mentioned above, persistent SAM of the anterior leaflet is an adverse outcome after valve repair. In this condition, the anterior leaflet obstructs the LVOT. Clearly, increased redundancy of leaflet tissue is a risk factor with a small annuloplasty ring. After repair, if the line of leaflet coaptation is displaced anteriorly, then the anterior leaflet will be displaced into the LVOT and cause LVOT obstruction.[86,87] The etiology is usually inadequate reduction of the height of the posterior leaflet, which then pushes the anterior leaflet into the LVOT. SAM

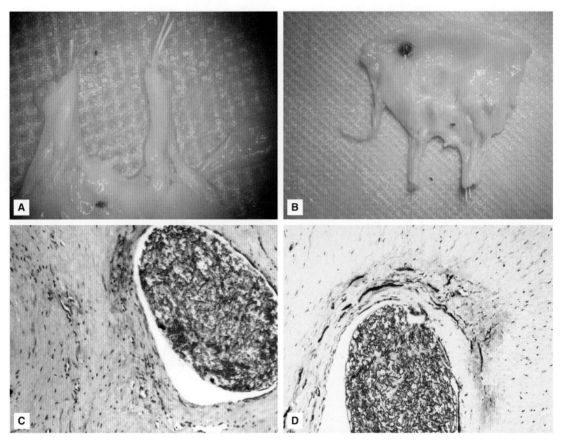

FIGURE 35-16 (A and B) Gross anatomy of an excised anterior mitral leaflet 3 years after neochordae implantation. (C) H&E stain of a neo chordae cross section. (D) Giemsa stain of the same cross section.

is particularly prevalent in patients with true bileaflet prolapse or those with extremely enlarged anterior leaflets. Thus, the PML height reduction has to be meticulously carried out, and in myxomatous valve disease, an upsizing rather than a downsizing of the mitral valve annuloplasty ring should be done. As indicated above, if the anterior leaflet is supported by a relatively small annulus, the anterior leaflet will not spread out and instead will appear to have redundant tissue above the correct plane of coaptation, predisposing to SAM.[78]

Several investigators have looked at the potential echocardiographic risk factors for SAM. Echocardiographic details that are associated with a high risk of SAM include proximity of the mitral valve coaptation point to the interventricular septum, as well as asymmetry between the anterior and posterior leaflets. If the posterior leaflet is relatively large with respect to the anterior leaflet, then SAM is potentiated. If the medial portion of A2 is larger than the medial portion of A2, then SAM is also potentiated. We look for this information before surgery and take such data into account as the repair strategy is finalized in the operating room.[78,79]

If the probability is high that SAM will occur, our practice is to use the Alfieri edge-to-edge technique to reduce such a risk after lowering the height of the posterior leaflet.[78] By forcing the coaptation line to be correct with a single stitch in the situation of high SAM probability, the probability of

SAM is reduced. Another strategy to consider in this circumstance is implantation of PTFE anterior chordae to lower the AML. That will reduce the height of the anterior leaflet, and thus further reduce the potential of SAM. In our own experience long-term competency is maintained in this group.

If SAM appears by TEE following what appears to be an excellent repair, filling the LV with fluid volume postcardiopulmonary bypass will relieve SAM in approximately 90% of patients. In rare circumstances, if an adequate reduction of the posterior leaflet has not been carried out, more posterior leaflet may have to be resected or the ring size increased. The most common alternative in our clinic is the edge-to-edge technique, as mentioned above, for situations where postrepair SAM still exists despite all techniques to reduce it.[78]

Remodeling Ring Annuloplasty

Remodeling the annulus by ring annuloplasty after mitral valve repair is essential to a complete and long-lasting repair. The remodeling concept, promulgated by Carpentier[18] and Duran[54] is that the distorted mitral annulus requires restorative structural support. There is debate on which type of ring should be used for remodeling: rigid or soft, complete or partial? It is probably not critical which type of ring is used for myxomatous valve degeneration as long as there is a relative upsizing of the ring and a secure attachment to the trigone area of the anterior mitral leaflet. There is some evidence to suggest that flexible rings may incur less possibility of SAM and that partial rings are safer with respect to SAM.[88] As none of this has been studied in a prospective randomized fashion, these opinions will continue to exist. Though we prefer the Cosgrove ring for mitral valve prolapse, our belief based on over 2000 mitral valve repairs is that the existing evidence is not compelling for any particular ring, and that the type of ring implanted is far less important than a correctly performed operation and appropriate sizing of the ring.

The technical aspects of ring implantation are important to avoid circumflex artery compromise, atrioventricular dissociation, or dehiscence of the ring. Implantation of currently available annuloplasty rings requires the placement of mattress sutures, parallel to the annulus, at the junction of the posterior leaflet and the annulus. Radially oriented bites are to be avoided because by definition they exert radial stresses and thus will pull to some extent on the circumflex artery. Bites should be deep with the needle entering the annulus, then into the left ventricular cavity, and then coming out on the atrial side again. Of paramount importance is the requirement that the plane of the needle bite should be orthogonal to the annular plane. If this is done, it is impossible for the stitch to impinge or distort the circumflex artery. That is why such bites may be made deep. Wide bites are taken such that there is not an excess number of a suture. A partial mitral ring should require approximately 9 to 15 sutures depending on the size of the annulus. The sutures are not pledgeted unless there is extreme fragility of the annular structures. Annular

integrity will of course depend on the pathology. Sutures are then passed through the fabric part of the ring. The central stabilizer frame is kept in place to maintain the ring shape while the sutures are tied down, thus preventing crimping of the cloth rings in the nonrigid or semirigid rings.

In the past decades, more than 40 mitral valve annuloplasty rings of various shapes and consistency were marketed for MR, although the effect of ring type on clinical outcome remains unclear. Until demonstrated otherwise, surgeons may choose their ring upon their judgment, tailored to specific patient needs.

Sizing is the most important aspect of ring placement. We believe that slight oversizing of the ring in myxomatous degenerated disease is appropriate. This corrects for the degenerative annulus that is functionally too small. Sizing is typically done by two techniques. Placement of aortic trigonal stitches (Fig. 35-17) allows for measurement of the intertrigonal distance. Many ring-sizing devices have notches on the rings to facilitate this. Except in rheumatic disease, we do not rely on this measurement. In myxomatous disease, the height of the anterior leaflet from the annulus to the highest point on the leaflet when it is stretched is the most important criterion for sizing, a concept originally espoused by Carpentier.[10] This height of the leaflet is the critical dimension that must be carefully measured so that during systole there is minimal redundancy that may lead to SAM. Using trigonal sizing may, in fact, downsize the ring and cause either SAM or ring dehiscence because of the huge disparity between ring size and annulus size. In our re-repair series, either improved sizing or placing the ring below the commissures were the most common

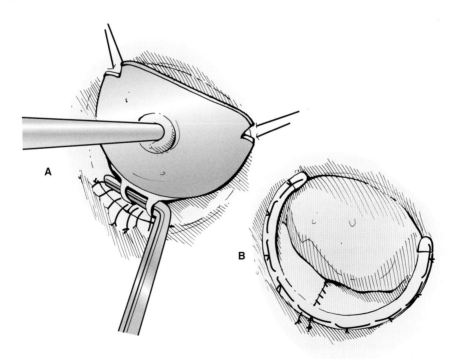

FIGURE 35-17 Ring annuloplasty sizing and insertion. The ring for degenerative disease should be slightly oversized. Sizing should be done to match the height of the anterior leaflet, not the distance between the trigones or commissures. Nine to 11 mattress sutures are usually needed.

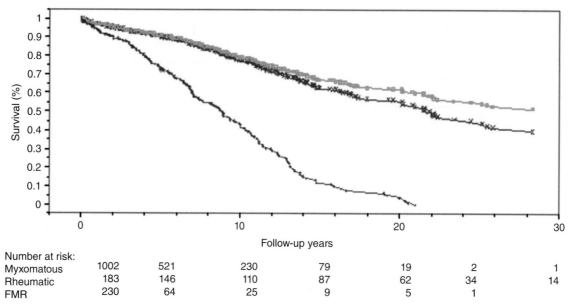

Number at risk:							
Myxomatous	1002	521	230	79	19	2	1
Rheumatic	183	146	110	87	62	34	14
FMR	230	64	25	9	5	1	

FIGURE 35-18 Etiology of mitral regurgitation determines longevity. (Reproduced with permission from DiBardino DJ, ElBardissi AW, McClure RS, et al: Four decades of experience with mitral valve repair: analysis of differential indications, technical evolution, and long-term outcome, *J Thorac Cardiovasc Surg*. 2010 Jan;139(1):76-83.)

remedies.[89] Therefore, using the sizer to evaluate anterior leaflet size is the most critical maneuver. Echocardiographic dimensions of the anterior leaflet correlate well with in vivo sizing, and calculating the anterior leaflet size by standard echocardiogram techniques is performed in every case. Deployment of a ring matching the anterior leaflet size in our experience has been most efficacious and has rarely led to SAM.[78]

Results

Based on long-term studies, the probability of a durable mitral valve repair at 10 years is greater than 90%.[42,53,56,64,90] Thromboembolic incidence is also exceedingly low; long-term anticoagulation is not required unless patients are in atrial fibrillation. Recently, we reviewed our personal operative experience (LHC) over four decades of mitral valve surgery.[91] This study has confirmed many commonly believed relationships between the etiology of MR and the durability of mitral valve repair. Etiology of regurgitation was noted to be the primary determinant of repair longevity and freedom from reoperation. Although repair of rheumatic disease was noted to ultimately require reoperation, myxomatous repair resulted in outstanding long-term freedom from recurrent MR and reoperation (Fig. 35-18).

REFERENCES

1. Brunton L, Edin MD: Preliminary note on the possibility of treating mitral stenosis by surgical methods. *Lancet* 1902; 1:352.
2. Cutler EC, Levine SA: Cardiotomy and valvulotomy for mitral stenosis: experimental observations and clinical notes concerning an operated case with recovery. *Boston Med Surg J* 1923; 188:1023.
3. Cutler EC, Beck CS: The present status of surgical procedures in chronic valvular disease of the heart: final report of all surgical cases. *Arch Surg* 1929; 18:403.
4. Souttar HS: Surgical treatment of mitral stenosis. *BMJ* 1925; 2:603.
5. Harken DE, Ellis LB, Ware PF, et al: The surgical treatment of mitral stenosis. I. Valvuloplasty. *N Engl J Med* 1948; 239:801.
6. Bailey CP: The surgical treatment of mitral stenosis (mitral commissurotomy). *Dis Chest* 1949; 15:377.
7. Davila JC, Glover RP: Circumferential suture of the mitral valve for the correction of regurgitation. *Am J Cardiol* 1958; 2:267.
8. Nichols HT: Mitral insufficiency: treatment by polar cross fusion of the mitral annulus fibrosis. *J Thorac Cardiovasc Surg* 1957; 33:102.
9. Kay EB, Mendelsohn D, Zimmerman HA: Evaluation of the surgical correction of mitral regurgitation. *Circulation* 1961; 23:813.
10. Carpentier A: Cardiac valve surgery: the "French correction." *J Thorac Cardiovasc Surg* 1983; 86:323.
11. McGoon DC: Repair of mitral insufficiency due to ruptured chordae tendineae. *J Thorac Cardiovasc Surg* 1960; 39:357.
12. Duran CG, Pomar JL, Revuelta JM, et al: Conservative operation for mitral insufficiency. Critical analysis supported by postoperative hemodynamic studies of 72 patients. *J Thorac Cardiovasc Surg* 1980; 79:326.
13. Orszulak TA, Schaff HV, Danielson GK, et al: Mitral regurgitation due to ruptured chordae tendinae. Early and late results of mitral valve repair. *J Thorac Cardiovasc Surg* 1985; 89:491.
14. Cohn LH, Couper GS, Kinchla NM, et al: Decreased operative risk of surgical treatment of mitral regurgitation with or without coronary artery disease. *J Am Coll Cardiol* 1990; 16:1575.
15. Cosgrove DM, Chavez AM, Lytle BW, et al: Results of mitral valve reconstruction. *Circulation* 1986; 74:I82.
16. Kirklin JW: Replacement of the mitral valve for mitral incompetence. *Surgery* 1972; 72:827.
17. Sarris GE, Cahill PD, Hansen DE, et al: Restoration of left ventricular systolic performance after reattachment of the mitral chordae tendineae: the importance of valvular-ventricular interaction. *J Thorac Cardiovasc Surg* 1988; 95:969.
18. Carpentier A, Deloche A, Dauptain J, et al: A new reconstructive operation for correction of mitral and tricuspid insufficiency. *J Thorac Cardiovasc Surg* 1971; 61:1.
19. McCarthy PM: Does the intertrigonal distance dilate? Never say never. *J Thorac Cardiovasc Surg* 2002; 124:1078.

20. Du Plessis LA, Marchano P: The anatomy of the mitral valve and its associated structures. *Thorax* 1964; 19:221.

21. Roberts WC: Morphologic aspects of cardiac valve dysfunction. *Am Heart J* 1992; 123:1610.

22. Wisenbaugh T, Spann JF, Carabello BA: Differences in myocardial performance and load between patients with similar amounts of chronic aortic versus chronic mitral regurgitation. *J Am Coll Cardiol* 1984; 3:916.

23. Carabello BA: Indications for mitral valve surgery. *J Cardiovasc Surg* 2004; 45:407.

24. Shyu KG, Chin JJ, Lin FY, et al: Regression of left ventricular mass after mitral valve repair of pure mitral regurgitation. *Ann Thorac Surg* 1994; 58:1670.

25. Deloche A, Jebara VA, Relland FYM, et al: Valve repair with Carpentier techniques: the second decade. *J Thorac Cardiovasc Surg* 1990; 99:990.

26. Freed LA, Levy D, Levine RA, et al: Prevalence and clinical outcome of mitral-valve prolapse. *N Engl J Med* 1999; 341:1.

27. Mills P, Rose J, Hollingsworth J, et al: Long-term prognosis of mitral-valve prolapse. *N Engl J Med* 1977; 297:13.

28. Marks AR, Choong CY, Sanfilippo AJ, et al: Identification of high-risk and low-risk subgroups of patients with mitral valve prolapse. *N Engl J Med* 1989; 320:1031.

29. Danchin N, Voiriot P, Briancon S, et al: Mitral valve prolapse as a risk factor for infective endocarditis. *Lancet* 1989; 1:743.

30. Enriquez-Sarano M, Dujardin KS, Tribouilloy CM, et al: Determinants of pulmonary venous flow reversal in mitral regurgitation and its usefulness in determining the severity of regurgitation. *Am J Cardiol* 1999; 83:535.

30a. AHA/ACC guidelines for management of valvular heart disease. *J Ame College Cardiol* 2014; 63(22).

31. Chen FY, Cohn LH: Valvular surgery in cardiomyopathy. In Baughman KL, Baumgartner WA (eds): *Treatment of Advanced Heart Disease.* New York, Taylor & Francis, 2006.

32. Stewart WJ: Choosing the "golden moment" for mitral valve repair. *J Am Coll Cardiol* 1994; 24:1544.

33. Gogbashian A, Sepic J, Soltesz EG, et al: Operative and long-term survival of elderly is significantly improved by mitral valve repair. *Am Heart J* 2006; 151:1325.

34. Kang DH, Kim JH, Rim JH, et al: Comparison of early surgery versus conventional treatment in asymptomatic severe mitral regurgitation. *Circulation* 2009; 119:797.

35. Cosgrove DM, Stewart WJ: Mitral valvuloplasty. *Curr Probl Cardiol* 1989; 14:359.

36. Sand ME, Naftel DC, Blackstone EH, et al: A comparison of repair and replacement for mitral valve incompetence. *J Thorac Cardiovasc Surg* 1987; 94:208.

37. Lawrie GM: Mitral valve repair vs. replacement: current recommendations and long-term results. *Cardiol Clin* 1998; 16:437.

38. Gillinov AM, Cosgrove DM, Blackston EH, et al: Durability of mitral valve repair for degenerative disease. *J Thorac Cardiovasc Surg* 1998; 116:734.

39. Vanden Eynden F, Bouchard D, El-Hamamsy I, Butnaru A, et al: Effect of aortic valve replacement for aortic stenosis on severity of mitral regurgitation. *Ann Thorac Surg* 2007; 83:1279.

40. Wan CK, Suri RM, Li Z, et al: Management of moderate functional mitral regurgitation at the time of aortic valve replacement: is concomitant valve repair necessary? *J Thorac Cardiovasc Surg* 2009; 137:635.

41. Enriquez-Sarano M, Avierinos JF, Messika-Zeitoun D, et al: Quantitative determinants of the outcome of asymptomatic mitral regurgitation. *N Engl J Med* 2005; 352:875.

42. Ling LH, Enriquez-Sarano M, Seward JB, et al: Clinical outcome of mitral regurgitation due to flail leaflet. *N Engl J Med* 1996; 335:1417.

43. Greelish JP, Cohn LH, Leacche M, et al: Minimally invasive mitral valve repair suggests earlier operations for mitral valve disease. *J Thorac Cardiovasc Surg* 2003; 126:365.

44. McClure RS, Cohn LH, Wiegerinck E, et al: Early and late outcomes in minimally invasive mitral valve repair: an eleven-year experience in 707. *J Thorac Cardiovasc Surg* 2009; 137:70.

45. Mihaljevic T, Cohn LH, Unic D, et al: One thousand minimally invasive valve operations: early and late results. *Ann Surg* 2004; 240:529.

46. Spencer FC, Galloway AC, Grossi EA, et al: Recent developments and evolving techniques of mitral valve reconstruction. *Ann Thorac Surg* 1998; 65:307.

47. Mohty D, Orszulak TA, Schaff HV, et al: Very long-term survival and durability of mitral valve repair for mitral valve prolapse. *Circulation* 2001; 104(Suppl I):I-1.

48. Savage EB, Ferguson TB Jr, DiSesa VJ: Use of mitral valve repair: analysis of contemporary United States experience reported to the Society of Thoracic Surgeons National Cardiac Database. *Ann Thorac Surg* 2003; 75:820.

49. Gammie JS, Sheng S, Griffith BP, et al: Trends in mitral valve surgery in the United States: results from the Society of Thoracic Surgeons Adult Cardiac Surgery Database. *Ann Thorac Surg* 2009; 87:1431.

50. Sondergaard T, Gotzsche M, Ottosen P, et al: Surgical closure of interatrial septal defects by circumclusion. *Acta Chir Scand* 1955; 109:188.

51. Larbalestier RI, Chard RB, Cohn LH: Optimal approach to the mitral valve: dissection of the interatrial groove. *Ann Thorac Surg* 1992; 54:1186.

52. Cohn LH: Mitral valve repair. *Op Techniques Thorac Cardiovasc Surg* 1998; 3:109.

53. Khonsari S, Sintek CF: Transatrial approach revisited. *Ann Thorac Surg* 1990; 50:1002.

54. Duran CG, Ubago JLM: Clinical and hemodynamic performance of a totally flexible prosthetic ring for atrioventricular valve reconstruction. *Ann Thorac Surg* 1976; 22:458.

55. Gillinov AM, Cosgrove DM 3rd, Wahi S, et al: Is anterior leaflet repair always necessary in repair of bileaflet mitral valve prolapse? *Ann Thorac Surg* 1999; 68:820.

56. Cohn LH, Couper GS, Aranki SF, et al: Long-term results of mitral valve reconstruction for regurgitation of the myxomatous mitral valve. *J Thorac Cardiovasc Surg* 1994; 107:143.

57. Gillinov AM, Tantiwongkosri K, Blackstone EH, et al: Is prosthetic annuloplasty necessary for durable mitral valve repair? *Ann Thorac Surg* 2009; 88:76.

58. Perier P: A new paradigm for the repair of posterior leaflet prolapse: respect rather than resect. *Op Techniques Thorac Cardiovasc Surg* 2005; 10:180.

59. Lawrie GM, Earle EA, Earle NR: Feasibility and intermediate term outcome of repair of prolapsing anterior mitral leaflets with artificial chordal replacement in 152 patients. *Ann Thorac Surg* 2006; 81:849.

60. Perier P, Clausnizer B, Mistraz K: Carpentier "sliding leaflet" technique for repair of the mitral valve: Early results. *Ann Thorac Surg* 1994; 57:383.

61. Tabata M, Ghanta RK, Shekar PS, Cohn LH: Early and midterm outcomes of folding valvuloplasty without leaflet resection for myxomatous mitral valve disease. *Ann Thorac Surg* 2008; 86:1288.

62. Gillinov AM, Shortt KG, Cosgrove DM 3rd: Commissural closure for repair of mitral commissural prolapse. *Ann Thorac Surg* 2005; 80:1135.

63. Aubert S, Barreda T, Acar C, et al: Mitral valve repair for commissural prolapse: surgical techniques and long term results. *Eur J Cardiothorac Surg* 2005; 28:443.

64. David TE, Ivanov J, Armstrong S, et al: A comparison of outcomes of mitral valve repair for degenerative disease with posterior, anterior, and bileaflet prolapse. *J Thorac Cardiovasc Surg* 2005; 130:1242.

65. Smedira NG, Selman R, Cosgrove DM, et al: Repair of anterior leaflet prolapse: chordal transfer is superior to chordal shortening. *J Thorac Cardiovasc Surg* 1996; 112:287.

66. Dreyfus GD, Bahrami T, Alayle N, et al: Repair of anterior leaflet prolapse by papillary muscle repositioning: a new surgical option. *Ann Thorac Surg* 2001; 71:1464.

67. Pino F, Moneta A, Villa E, et al: Chordal plication and free edge remodeling for mitral anterior leaflet prolapse repair: 8-year follow-up. *Ann Thorac Surg* 2001; 72:1515.

68. Frater RW, Vetter HO, Zussa C, et al: Chordal replacement in mitral valve repair. *Circulation* 1990; 82(5 Suppl):IV125.

69. Zussa C, Polesel E, Da Col U, et al: Seven-year experience with chordal replacement with expanded polytetrafluoroethylene in floppy mitral valve. *J Thorac Cardiovasc Surg* 1991; 108:37.

70. Duran CM, Pekar F: Techniques for ensuring the correct length of new chords. *J Heart Valve Dis* 2003; 12:156.

71. Falk V, Seeburger J, Czesla M, et al: How does the use of polytetrafluoroethylene neochordae for posterior mitral valve prolapse (loop technique) compare with leaflet resection? A prospective randomized trial. *J Thorac Cardiovasc Surg* 2008; 136:1205.

72. Duran CM: Surgical techniques for the repair of anterior mitral leaflet prolapse. *J Card Surg* 1999; 14:471.

73. Uva MS, Grare P, Jebara V, et al: Transposition of chordae in mitral valve repair: mid-term results. *Circulation* 1993; 88:35.

74. Maisano F, Torracca L, Oppizzi M, et al: The edge-to-edge technique: a simplified method to correct mitral insufficiency. *Eur J Cardiothorac Surg* 1998; 13:240.

75. Condado JA, Acquatella H, Rodriguez L, et al: Percutaneous edge-to-edge mitral valve repair: 2-year follow-up in the first human case. *Catheter Cardiovasc Intervent* 2006; 67:323.

76. Alfieri O, Maisano F, De Bonis M, et al: The double-orifice technique in mitral valve repair: a simple solution for complex problems. *J Thorac Cardiovasc Surg* 2001; 122:674.

77. Bhudia SK, McCarthy PM, Smedira NG: Edge-to-edge (Alfieri) mitral repair: results in diverse clinical settings. *Ann Thorac Surg* 2004; 77:1598.

78. Brinster DR, Unic D, D'Ambra MN, et al: Mid term results of the edge to edge technique for complex mitral repair. *Ann Thorac Surg* 2006; 81:1612.

79. Maslow AD, Regan MM, Haering JM, et al: Echocardiographic predictors of left ventricular outflow tract obstruction and systolic anterior motion of the mitral valve after mitral valve reconstruction for myxomatous valve disease. *J Am Coll Cardiol* 1999; 34:2096.

80. De Bonis M, Lorusso R, Lapenna E, et al: Similar long-term results of mitral valve repair for anterior compared with posterior leaflet prolapse. *J Thorac Cardiovasc Surg* 2006; 131:364.

81. Suri RM, Orszulak TA: Triangular resection for repair of mitral regurgitation due to degenerative disease. *Op Techniques Thorac Cardiovasc Surg* 2005; 10:194.

82. Duran CMG: Surgical techniques for the repair of anterior mitral leaflet prolapse. *J Card Surg* 1999; 14:471.

83. Chauvaud S, Jebara V, Chachques JC, et al: Valve extension with glutaraldehyde-preserved autologous pericardium. Results in mitral valve repair. *J Thorac Cardiovasc Surg* 1991; 102:171.

84. el Asmar B, Acker M, Couetil JP, et al: Mitral valve repair in the extensively calcified mitral valve annulus. *Ann Thorac Surg* 1991; 52:66.

85. Bichell DP, Adams DH, Aranki SF, et al: Repair of mitral regurgitation from myxomatous degeneration in the patient with a severely calcified posterior annulus. *J Card Surg* 1995; 10(4 Pt 1):281.

86. Lee KS, Stewart WJ, Lever HM, et al: Mechanism of outflow tract obstruction causing failed valve repair: anterior displacement of leaflet coaptation. *Circulation* 1993; 88(5 Pt 2):II24.

87. Mihaileanu S, Marino JP, Chauvaud S, et al: Left ventricular outflow obstruction after mitral repair (Carpentier's technique): proposed mechanism of disease. *Circulation* 1988; 78(3 Pt 2):78.

88. Gillinov AM, Cosgrove DM, Shiota T, et al: Cosgrove-Edwards annuloplasty system: midterm results. *Ann Thorac Surg* 2000; 69:717.

89. Shekar PS, Couper GS, Cohn LH: Mitral valve re-repair. *J Heart Valve Dis* 2005; 14:583.

90. Braunberger E, Deloche A, Berrebi A: Very long-term results (more than 20 years) of valve repair with Carpentier's techniques in nonrheumatic mitral valve insufficiency. *Circulation* 2001; 104:I-8.

91. Dibardino DJ, Elbardissi AW, McClure RS, et al: Four decades of experience with mitral valve repair: analysis of differential indications, technical evolution, and long-term outcome. *J Thoracic Cardiovasc Surg* 2010; 139:76.

92. Bitar FF, Hayek P, Obeid M: Rheumatic fever in children: a 15-year experience in a developing country. *Pediatr Cardiol* 2000; 21:119.

93. Bortolotti U, Milano AD, Frater RW: Mitral valve repair with artificial chordae: a review of its history, technical details, long term results, and pathology. *Ann Thoracic Surg* 2012; 93:684-691.

Mitral Valve Repair: Rheumatic

Javier G. Castillo • David H. Adams

36

After recovery from an initial episode of rheumatic fever, approximately 60 to 65% of patients will develop heart valve disease (rheumatic heart disease, RHD) and possibly secondary conditions such as atrial fibrillation, endocarditis, and heart failure.[1] Rheumatic heart disease is one of the leading noncommunicable diseases in developing countries with a global prevalence of up to 19.6 million in 2005 and an incidence of 282,000 new cases per year.[2]

In Western countries, economic and sociopolitical changes together with prophylactic initiatives led by the American Heart Association and the World Heart Federation contributed to eliminate rheumatic fever by the 1980s (current prevalence in the United States is 0.05/1000). Much of the morbidity and mortality due to RHD has been proven to be effectively prevented by secondary prophylaxis including long-acting penicillin, oral anticoagulants, and surgical interventions.[3] However, the costs of prophylaxis continue to burden low-income and middle-income countries as well as certain concentered populations of higher-income countries (demographic shifts due to immigration).[4] In this context, an estimated of up to 468,164 patients die each year from RHD and or its clinical complications. Interestingly, recent echocardiographic data have shown that the true prevalence of the disease is significantly higher than the current global estimate if we take into consideration subclinical RHD.[5]

Rheumatic heart disease is unarguably the most common cardiovascular disease among individuals aged <25 years worldwide, and has a peak age group of 25 to 35 years (female predominance) in developing countries[6] (Fig. 36-1). Conversely, patients with RHD in industrialized countries are either old (mostly above 50 years of age) or young immigrants. In this setting, the mitral valve is affected in 50% of patients and results in mitral regurgitation, mitral stenosis, or both.[7] In younger patients, mitral regurgitation is predominant, but mitral stenosis becomes more prevalent with age and calcification of tissues. Regurgitant mitral valves are edematous with fibrotic thickening, and annular dilatation and anterior leaflet pseudoprolapse are often seen, whereas stenotic mitral valves present with stiff, nonpliable, and severely restricted leaflets, fusion of the subvalvular apparatus and commissures and often annular calcification[8] (Fig. 36-2). Clinical assessment and two-dimensional echocardiography are paramount to detect and assess mitral stenosis, particularly in asymptomatic patients.[9]

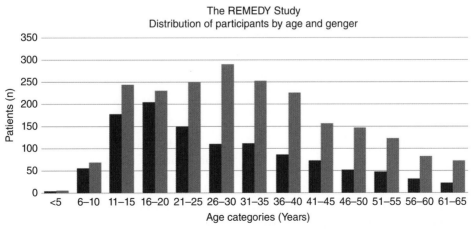

FIGURE 36-1 Age and gender distribution of 3339 children and adults with rheumatic heart disease form the REMEDY study. ((Adapted with permission from Zühlke L, Engel ME, Karthikeyan G, et al: Characteristics, complications, and gaps in evidence-based interventions in rheumatic heart disease: the Global Rheumatic Heart Disease Registry (the REMEDY study), *Eur Heart J.* 2015 May 7;36(18):1115-1122a.)

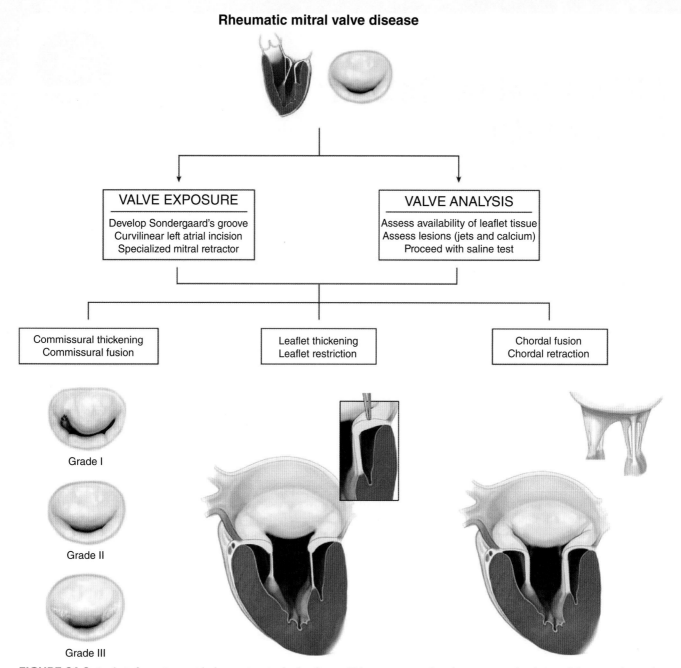

FIGURE 36-2 Analysis for patients with rheumatic mitral valve disease. Valve exposure and analysis are considered part of the repair due to their impact in achieving optimal surgical outcomes. The most common lesions encountered are commissural thickening and fusion, leaflet restriction and retraction, and chordal fusion and retraction.

PATHOPHYSIOLOGICAL IMPLICATIONS

The main consequence of RHD and more particularly rheumatic mitral valve disease (RMVD) is mitral stenosis.[10] This circumstance results in an increase of diastolic gradients across the mitral valve with invariable measurements of the mitral area due to moderate-to-severe commissural fusion. From a hemodynamic standpoint, transvalvular flow and heart rate are considered to play an important role in the perioperative management of patients with RMVD.[11] Mean mitral gradient increases in parallel with cardiac output (importance of atrial contraction) or with fast heart rates.

Increasing mitral gradients trigger left atrium enlargement due to chronic escalating left atrial pressures. This in turn favors the occurrence of atrial fibrillation leading to annular dilatation and thrombus formation. The logical rise in pulmonary artery pressure leads to pulmonary hypertension and late in the course to right ventricular hypertrophy, right ventricular dilatation, secondary tricuspid regurgitation and eventually right ventricular dysfunction (inherent surgical risk). This is important to understand why patients undergoing mitral valve repair often receive adjuvant tricuspid valve repair and a Maze procedure.[12] Finally, it is important to emphasize on the role of rhythm control therapies and central vasodilators during the preoperative period and medical optimization for surgery.

SURGICAL CONSIDERATIONS

Although mitral stenosis was the first mitral valve dysfunction treated surgically (Elliot Carr Cutler performed a closed transventricular mitral commissurotomy with a cardiovalvulotome in 1923), nowadays most of the patients with mitral valve stenosis receive a percutaneous balloon valvuloplasty unless the lesions are not amenable to balloon dilatation (or there is a high risk of embolic events), there is concomitant regurgitation, or a previous balloon valvuloplasty has failed.[13] When surgery is indicated, mitral valve repair is always preferred to mitral valve replacement due to lower perioperative mortality rates,[14,15] superior preservation of left ventricular function,[16] lower thromboembolic complications[17] and risk of endocarditis (critical in patients with deficient socio-economic conditions), and greater long-term durability.[18] This is particularly important in young patients. However, although repair rates have been shown to be near a 100% in prolapsing valves or patients with isolated annular dilatation, repair techniques are feasible in only 50 to 75% of patients with RMVD (percentage varies according to age, leaflet dysfunction and degree of calcification).[19,20] This difference is attributable to the vast spectrum of lesion complexity found in patient with RHD and therefore the need for more complex surgical techniques that often cannot guarantee long-term durability. In addition, when deciding about repair versus replacement, the evolving nature of the rheumatic process, which implies a progressive distortion of the subvalvular apparatus even beyond a successful repair, needs to be part of the equation. In this context, it is crucial to distinguish between the lesions in patients from developing countries (the histological rheumatic process is active) and that of patients from industrialized countries were the process is controlled.

From a strictly technical point of view, several aspects have recently transformed the field of mitral valve repair in patients with RMVD. The first one is introduction of polytetrafluoroethylene neochordoplasty to either replace diseased chords or reinforce leaflet segments which has significantly impacted surgical outcomes.[21] Neochordoplasty has actually replaced many of the subvalvular techniques originally described and promoted by Carpentier such as chordal shortening, chordal transfer, or papillary muscle reposition.[22] Additionally, although leaflet extension is not a new technique,[23] the relatively recent introduction of gluteraldehyde-fixed pericardium has avoided shrinkage, thickening and calcification of the autologous pericardium potentially leading to more durable results.[24]

Type I Dysfunction

Two mechanisms may lead to type I dysfunction[25] in patients with RHD. The first one is rapid left ventricular dilatation and subsequent mitral annular dilatation due to pancarditis (early stages), which often impacts left ventricular contractility due to an acute inflammatory reaction (myocarditis). The second mechanism is annular dilatation secondary to chronic atrial fibrillation. Atrial fibrillation (very common in patients with RHD) impairs atrial contraction thus increasing left atrial pressures. This in turn results in left atrial dilatation and pure mitral annular dilatation.

Type II Dysfunction

The most frequent lesions encountered leading to type II dysfunction[25] are true prolapse and pseudoprolapse of the anterior leaflet. In the setting of true prolapse of the anterior leaflet, the leaflet overrides the coaptation plane during systole resulting in mitral regurgitation. Causes of true anterior prolapse in patients with RMVD include elongation or rupture (secondary to an acute inflammatory reaction) of the chordae tendinae or papillary muscles, or secondary rupture caused by bacterial endocarditis (facilitated and exacerbated by a dysfunctional rheumatic valve as occurs in patients with severe underlying degenerative mitral valve disease).

In the setting of anterior leaflet pseudoprolapse, as opposed to true anterior leaflet prolapse, the anterior leaflet does not override the plane of coaptation during systole (minor prolapse of the free edge of A2 due to distention and posterolateral displacement of the paramedical chordae). This lesion is often found in patients with opposing dysfunction, this being a combination of type IIIb dysfunction of the posterior leaflet (restricted motion) and consequent anterior leaflet pseudoprolapse (also known as type IIa/IIIp). In this case, mitral regurgitation is secondary to the lack of coaptation between the anterior and the posterior leaflets, which permits full unfolding of the anterior leaflet (there is no coaptation surface against the posterior leaflet) without overriding the plane of coaptation or annular plane.

Type III Dysfunction

Type III is the most frequent dysfunction[25] in patients with RMVD. In the early stages of rheumatic valve involvement, mild degrees of leaflet fibrosis (incipient symmetric bileaflet restriction) might create mild mitral regurgitation and very subtle hemodynamic changes. Moreover, mitral regurgitation at this stage might be often aggravated by certain degree of annular dilatation. When the inflammatory process induces a more significant fibrotic reaction both leaflets present greater degrees of restricted motion with important hemodynamic consequences. This circumstance might certainly impede leaflet coaptation in systole leading to severe mitral regurgitation. However, in this setting, the more advanced fibrotic thickening of both leaflets as well as the fusion of both commissures and the subvalvular apparatus also impedes leaflet opening in diastole resulting in mitral stenosis. When restricted motion mainly affects valve opening during diastole owing to isolated commissural fusion or further rheumatic changes pure mitral stenosis is predominant.

MITRAL VALVE REPAIR TECHNIQUES

The use of a prosthetic-ring or prosthetic-band annuloplasty is currently a standard technique in all patients receiving mitral valve repair (obviously pediatric patients are an exception requiring biodegradable or pericardial rings or bands) regardless of the etiology of mitral valve disease.[26] Except in rare cases of pure mitral stenosis (with preserved ventricular function and mild atrial enlargement and therefore no secondary annular deformation), annular dilatation is present in the majority of patients with RMVD and mandate correction with a prosthesis size based on the surface of the anterior leaflet or on the intertrigonal distance (any discrepancy between two sizes should lead the surgeon to choose the larger size always). The use of ring annuloplasty has been shown to reduce the incidence of both mitral and tricuspid regurgitation (and subsequent reoperations) in patients with RMVD. In the setting of pure mitral stenosis with obvious annular dilatation, ring annuloplasty contributes to prevent commissural leaks by providing better surface of coaptation between both leaflets (commissurotomy might result in valve regurgitation in the presence of severe annular dilatation).

Commissurotomy

Commissural fibrosis and fusion leading to mitral valve stenosis is by far the most frequent lesion encountered in patients with RMVD. According to the severity of commissural fusion, three categories have been described: Grade I—partial fusion of the commissures with chordal preservation; Grade II—complete fusion of the commissure with preserved delineation between the anterior and the posterior leaflets; and Grade III—complete fusion of the commissures with absence of leaflet delineation and calcium deposition (Fig. 36-2).

Commissural fusion is treated by a commissurotomy (Fig. 36-3). Traction of the anterior leaflet with a nerve hook helps to identify the commissural line that delineates anterior and posterior leaflets. Subsequently, using a #11 blade, an incision is made about 5 mm from the annulus (preservation of tissue equivalent to a commissural leaflet) and extended towards the mitral orifice. The incision is then discontinued about 5 mm from the orifice and the commissural chordae are identified and isolated with a nerve hook. The incision is then carried down to the head of the papillary muscle (leaving chordae on each side of the defect) thus creating a subcommissural orifice (the papillary muscle splitting can be further completed by a fenestration). In cases of severe commissural fusion (where an aggressive commissurotomy and debridement might be required), cases of concomitant excessive annular dilatation, or in the setting of acute bacterial

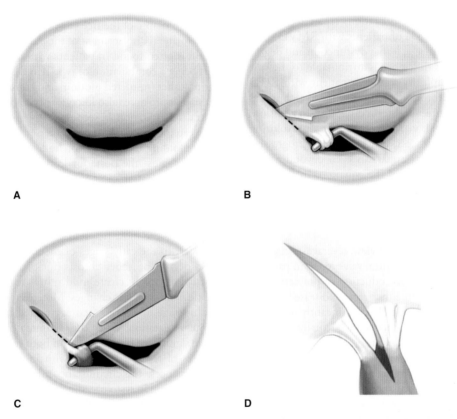

A   B

C   D

FIGURE 36-3 Commissurotomy. Commisural fusion (A) traction of the anterior leaflet with a nerve hook helps to identify the commissural line that delineates anterior and posterior leaflets (B) using a #11 blade, an incision is made about 5 mm from the annulus and carried down to the head of the papillary muscle (C) Chordae are preserved on each side of the defect creating a subcommissural orifice (D). (Adapted with permission from Carpentier A, Adams DH, Filsoufi F: Carpentier's Reconstructive Valve Surgery. St. Louis: Saunders/Elsevier; 2010.)

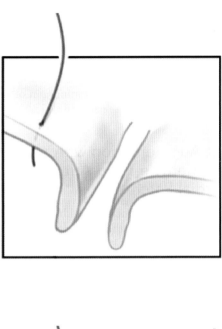
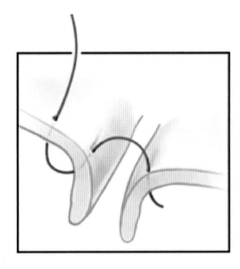
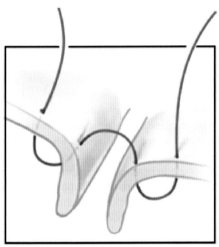
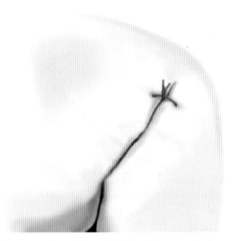

FIGURE 36-4 Carpentier's commissuroplasty "magic suture" (top). Commissural resuspension with a CV-5 double-armed polytetrafluoroethylene suture (bottom).

endocarditis (additional commissural destruction and prolapse), commissural resuspension or reconstruction might be necessary (Fig. 36-4). This is best accomplished with a "magic suture" or commisuroplasty (4-0 polypropylene sutures).

Leaflet Resuspension (Subvalvular Techniques)

Leaflet mobilization and resuspension is achieved with subvalvular techniques, mainly chordal resection and fenestration. In dramatic cases of excessive fibrosis and fusion of the subvalvular apparatus, splitting of the papillary muscle as well as resection of marginal chords and subsequent replacement (neochordoplasty) are considered valid repair options (Fig. 36-5).

Identification of secondary chordae is critical to achieve leaflet mobilization without inducing leaflet prolapse.

The secondary chordae to be resected should be identified and isolated with a nerve hook. The attachment to the papillary muscle is usually cut first (easier visualization) to subsequently expose the leaflet attachment by gentle traction. In severe cases (rarely amenable to repair), marginal chordae can be also resected as long as there is one marginal chordae every 4 mm to support the free edge of the leaflet. If this axiom is not possible, chordal replacement with polytetrafluoroethylene artificial chordae (neochordoplasty) is required (the use of artificial chordae has displaced classic techniques such as chordal transfer or chordal transposition in advanced disease). Fused marginal chordae contributing to subvalvular obstruction are not resected but fenestrated. Fenestration is usually carried down thus spilling the corresponding papillary muscle.

Finding a healthy chord in the setting of RMVD might be more than challenging, therefore techniques such as chordal

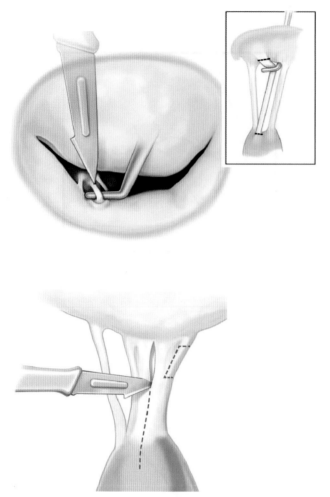

FIGURE 36-5 Subvalvular techniques include resection fo secondary chords (top) and chordal fenestrationm (bottom).

transfer, chordal transposition or the posterior leaflet flip have been abandoned. The alternative is polytetrafluoroethylene neochordoplasty (and variants such as the loop technique or the loop in loop technique), which has been increasingly used in mitral valve repair. A CV-5 double-armed polytetrafluoroethylene suture is passed and looped through the fibrous tip

of the papillary muscle. Next, the two ends of the artificial chord are passed through the leaflet margin (approximately with a 3-mm distance between them) and a two slip knots are tied (Fig. 36-4). After functional adjustment (insufflation of saline test after remodeling annuloplasty to assess the plane of coaptation and chordal height), a minimum of six knots are then completed to secure the new chord.

Leaflet Augmentation with a Gluteraldehyde-fixed Autologous Pericardial Patch

Although leaflet augmentation with autologous pericardium was introduced in the 1960s,[23] optimal results were not achieved until the late 1980s due to the introduction of gluteraldehyde fixation. Briefly, a piece of autologous pericardium (approximately 5 cm × 5 cm) is freed from adhesions, unfolded onto cardboard (secured with clips), and immersed in 0.625% buffered gluteraldehyde solution for 10 minutes. Subsequently, the patch is rinsed in saline for 10 to 15 minutes (some authors recommend different baths of 5 minutes each).[27] Fixation prevents shrinkage (stabilizes collagen cross-linkages), reduces tissue antigenicity, and minimizes enzymatic degradation and cell viability (avoidance of calcification and fibrosis).

Leaflet augmentation, most commonly of the posterior leaflet (depending on the type and extent of lesions), is performed to increase leaflet surface area in patients with type IIIa dysfunction and severe leaflet retraction (when mobilization cannot be achieved with subvalvular techniques) or to replace leaflet segments where severe calcification has led to a significant defect after resection that cannot be closed primarily. Before proceeding with leaflet augmentation, pliability of the anterior leaflet is assessed by pushing the anterior leaflet with a pair of forceps; if the leaflet rebounds into position then fibrosis probably precludes repair techniques (Fig. 36-2). The technique starts with placement of traction sutures in order to unfold the leaflet as much as possible (Fig. 36-6). Next, a transverse incision is made about 5 mm from and parallel to the annulus (the extent of the incision depends on the degree of leaflet retraction). All secondary chordae are then resected

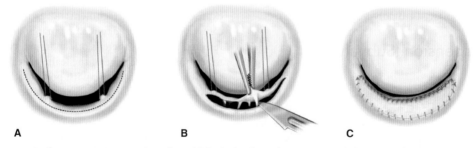

FIGURE 36-6 Posterior leaflet augmentation with a gluteraldehyde-fixed autologous pericardial patch. After placement of traction sutures, a transverse incision is made about 5 mm from and parallel to the annulus (A) secondary chordae are resected to free and resuspend the leaflet (B) A semilunar autologous pericardial patch is tailored to the leaflet defect adding a 2-mm margin for suturing (C) an oversized ring (one size larger) or classic ring is selected in order to fully accommodate the posterior leaflet.

to free and resuspend the leaflet. Finally, a semilunar autologous pericardial patch is tailored to the leaflet defect adding a 2-mm margin for suturing. The height of the patch should provide a 15-20-mm posterior leaflet. The patch is then sutured using continuous 4-0 polypropylene sutures. Interlocked bites are used on the leaflet side to prevent a potential purse-string effect. An oversized ring (one size larger) is selected in order to fully accommodate the posterior leaflet.

Pericardial patch augmentation of the anterior leaflet is similar to that of the posterior leaflet with an only particular difference, the leaflet incision might be transverse or vertical (rare occasions) depending on the leaflet morphology. The resulting opening after incision will guide our decision about the size and shape of the corresponding patch.

Decalcification Techniques

The main goal before proceeding with mitral valve repair in patients with RMVD is ensuring (as much as possible) leaflet mobility and pliability. This is achieved with a multistep repair algorithm that should be tailored to every individual patient. The initial step is to interrogate the commissures and the subvalvular apparatus. Subsequently, if the leaflets are not pliable, decalcification techniques can be applied including leaflet shaving, leaflet peeling or leaflet (cuspal) thinning. The latter should be always performed in leaflet areas amenable to a potential patch augmentation (leaflet thinning may lead to secondary windsock deformity and perforation). Calcified areas can be shaved off the leaflet and the annular hinge to facilitate leaflet excursion. Additionally, the thick fibrotic layer of tissue that accumulates on the atrial surface of the leaflet can be peeled off. Finally, if all these techniques do not compensate for leaflet retraction and scarring, leaflet extension is performed.

OUTCOMES

Mitral valve replacement has been traditionally considered as the predominant procedure for patients with RMVD, particularly if we take into account that unfortunately many patients with prolapsing valves (a mitral lesion with a near 100% repair rate) still receive mitral valve replacement.[28] However, relatively recent sophistication in reconstructive techniques has contributed to the expansion of mitral valve repair, and this has had a potential impact on outcomes regardless of disease etiology.[29] The most current series on rheumatic mitral valve repair reported an increment of the repair rate from 42 to 69% (within the same surgical group) in the last decade.[30] This represents a great improvement in comparison with previous series which have reported repair rates around 25% in experienced hands.[31] However, the literature needs to be interpreted with meticulous caution. If one analyzes the study population in every large series, can see that those with lower repair rates include a significant larger percentage of patients with mitral stenosis (more complex lesions of uncertain durability if repaired) and older patients (more likely to have subvalvular fibrosis and calcified lesions)[32] (Table 36-1).

It is well known that repair for RMVD (particularly in the setting of pure or concomitant mitral stenosis) cannot be consistent.[33] Regardless of geographical location and length of follow up, reoperation rates (when adjusted to survival) are higher in patients receiving mitral valve repair mainly due to fibrosis (particularly commissural) and calcification of the subvalvular apparatus and the disease progression.[34] Other authors have reported age and mitral regurgitation at the acute phase as significant factors for repair failure.[35] The estimated failure rate of mitral valve repair in patients with RMVD is 2 to 5% per year (vs 1 to 2% per year in patients with degenerative mitral valve disease).[30,36]

There is scarce data comparing outcomes (particularly late outcomes) after mitral valve repair to those achieved with mitral valve replacement, especially in the adult population. In this context, Shuhaiber et al conducted a systematic meta-analysis of clinical outcomes following surgical correction of mitral valve disease (including RMVD) and demonstrated consistent findings favoring a lower operative mortality in patients receiving mitral valve repair with the one exception of those patients with active RMVD (OR

TABLE 36-1: Results of Mitral Valve Repair in Adult Patients with Rheumatic Mitral Valve Disease												
Author (Reference)	Year	N	Age	I	II	III	IIa/IIIp	MS	RR	Mortality	Survival	Durability
Duran et al[33]	1994	537	32 ± 14	NA	NA	NA	NA	NA	57%	1%	90 ± 1%	81 ± 1% (R)
Yau et al[31]	2000	573	54 ± 14	NA	NA	NA	NA	85%	25%	0.7%	88 ± 1%	72 ± 1% (R)
Choudhary et al[36]	2001	818	23 ± 11	6%	5%	88%	1%	None	NA	4.0%	93 ± 1%	52 ± 3% (E)
Chavaud et al[34]	2001	951	25 ± 18	7%	33%	36%	24%	None	NA	2.0%	89 ± 2%	82 ± 2% (R)
Kumar et al[35]	2006	898	22 ± 10	NA	NA	NA	NA	54%	NA	3.6%	92 ± 1%	81 ± 5% (R)
Kim et al[32]	2010	540	49 ± 11	NA	NA	NA	NA	69%	23%	1.1%	86 ± 5%	97 ± 2% (R)
Yakub et al[29]	2013	627	32 ± 19	NA	NA	NA	NA	13%	69%	2.4%	83 ± 4%	72 ± 5% (E)

Survival and durability are estimated up to 10 years.
The absence of RR (repair rate) indicates a report on a selected patient population (mitral valve repairs were selected only).
Mortality (of mitral valve repair); MS mitral stenosis (any degree of MS including combined MS and MR; RR repair rate; (R) reoperation; freedom from reoperation; (E) echocardiographic; freedom from > moderate MR.

2.98, CI 95% 1.45 to 6.15).[37] This is consistent with generic data from the Society of Thoracic Surgeons database where mortality after isolated mitral valve replacement regardless of the dysfunction is as high as 6 versus 1.6% in patients undergoing isolated mitral valve repair.[15] In the classic study by Yau and associates from Toronto, operative mortality after risk adjustment was also reported to be worse in patients undergoing replacement (5.1 vs 0.7%).[31] Overall, in large series from experienced centers, operative mortality for patients undergoing rheumatic mitral valve repair ranges from 0.7 to 4.0%.

REFERENCES

1. Carapetis JR, Currie BJ, Mathews JD: Cumulative incidence of rheumatic fever in an endemic region: a guide to the susceptibility of the population? *Epidemiol Infect* 2000; 124(2):239-244.
2. Carapetis JR, Steer AC, Mulholland EK, Weber M: The global burden of group A streptococcal diseases. *Lancet Infect Dis* 2005; 5(11):685-694.
3. Gordis L: The virtual disappearance of rheumatic fever in the United States: lessons in the rise and fall of disease. T. Duckett Jones memorial lecture. *Circulation* 1985; 72(6):1155-1162.
4. Kaplan EL: T. Duckett Jones Memorial Lecture. Global assessment of rheumatic fever and rheumatic heart disease at the close of the century. Influences and dynamics of populations and pathogens: a failure to realize prevention? *Circulation* 1993; 88(4 Pt 1):1964-1972.
5. Roberts K, Maguire G, Brown A, et al: Echocardiographic screening for rheumatic heart disease in high and low risk Australian children. *Circulation* 2014; 129(19):1953-1961.
6. Zuhlke L, Engel ME, Karthikeyan G, et al: Characteristics, complications, and gaps in evidence-based interventions in rheumatic heart disease: the Global Rheumatic Heart Disease Registry (the REMEDY study). *Eur Heart J* 2015; 36(18):1115-22a.
7. Kassebaum NJ, Bertozzi-Villa A, Coggeshall MS, et al: Global, regional, and national levels and causes of maternal mortality during 1990-2013: a systematic analysis for the Global Burden of Disease Study 2013. *Lancet* 2014; 384(9947):980-1004.
8. Antunes MJ: Repair of rheumatic mitral valve regurgitation: how far can we go? *Eur J Cardiothorac Surg* 2013; 44(4):689-691.
9. Jain S, Mankad SV: Echocardiographic assessment of mitral stenosis: echocardiographic features of rheumatic mitral stenosis. *Cardiol Clin* 2013; 31(2):177-191.
10. Bouleti C, Iung B, Himbert D, et al: Relationship between valve calcification and long-term results of percutaneous mitral commissurotomy for rheumatic mitral stenosis. *Circ Cardiovasc Interv* 2014; 7(3):381-389.
11. Remenyi B, Wilson N, Steer A, et al: World Heart Federation criteria for echocardiographic diagnosis of rheumatic heart disease–an evidence-based guideline. *Nat Rev Cardiol* 2012; 9(5):297-309.
12. Kim GS, Lee CH, Kim JB: Echocardiographic evaluation of mitral durability following valve repair in rheumatic mitral valve disease: impact of Maze procedure. *J Thorac Cardiovasc Surg* 2014; 147(1):247-253.
13. Cohn LH: The first successful surgical treatment of mitral stenosis: the 70th anniversary of Elliot Cutler's mitral commissurotomy. *Ann Thorac Surg* 1993; 56(5):1187-1190.
14. Nishimura RA, Otto CM, Bonow RO, et al: 2014 AHA/ACC guideline for the management of patients with valvular heart disease: a report of the American College of Cardiology/American Heart Association Task Force on Practice Guidelines. *Circulation* 10 2014; 129(23):e521-643.
15. Vahanian A, Alfieri O, Andreotti F, et al: Guidelines on the management of valvular heart disease (version 2012). *Eur Heart J* 2012; 33(19):2451-2496.
16. Tribouilloy C, Rusinaru D, Grigioni F, et al: Long-term mortality associated with left ventricular dysfunction in mitral regurgitation due to flail leaflets: a multicenter analysis. *Circ Cardiovasc Imaging* 2014; 7(2):363-370.
17. Russo A, Grigioni F, Avierinos JF, et al: Thromboembolic complications after surgical correction of mitral regurgitation incidence, predictors, and clinical implications. *J Am Coll Cardiol* 25 2008; 51(12):1203-1211.
18. David TE, Ivanov J, Armstrong S, Christie D, Rakowski H: A comparison of outcomes of mitral valve repair for degenerative disease with posterior, anterior, and bileaflet prolapse. *J Thorac Cardiovasc Surg* 2005; 130(5):1242-1249.
19. Castillo JG, Anyanwu AC, El-Eshmawi A, Adams DH: All anterior and bileaflet mitral valve prolapses are repairable in the modern era of reconstructive surgery. *Eur J Cardiothorac Surg* 2014; 45(1):139-145; discussion 145.
20. Castillo JG, Anyanwu AC, Fuster V, Adams DH: A near 100% repair rate for mitral valve prolapse is achievable in a reference center: implications for future guidelines. *J Thorac Cardiovasc Surg* 2012; 144(2):308-312.
21. David TE, Armstrong S, Ivanov J: Chordal replacement with polytetrafluoroethylene sutures for mitral valve repair: a 25-year experience. *J Thorac Cardiovasc Surg* 2013; 145(6):1563-1569.
22. Zussa C, Frater RW, Polesel E, Galloni M, Valfre C: Artificial mitral valve chordae: experimental and clinical experience. *Ann Thorac Surg* 1990; 50(3):367-373.
23. Frater RW, Berghuis J, Brown AL Jr, Ellis FH Jr: The experimental and clinical use of autogenous pericardium for the replacement and extension of mitral and tricuspid value cusps and chordae. *J Cardiovasc Surg (Torino)* 1965; 6(3):214-228.
24. Vincentelli A, Zegdi R, Prat A, et al: Mechanical modifications to human pericardium after a brief immersion in 0.625% glutaraldehyde. *J Heart Valve Dis* 1998; 7(1):24-29.
25. Carpentier A: Cardiac valve surgery—the "French correction". *J Thorac Cardiovasc Surg* 1983; 86(3):323-337.
26. Carpentier AF, Lessana A, Relland JY, et al: The "physio-ring": an advanced concept in mitral valve annuloplasty. *Ann Thorac Surg* 1995; 60(5):1177-1185; discussion 1185-1186.
27. Dillon J, Yakub MA, Nordin MN, Pau KK, Krishna Moorthy PS: Leaflet extension in rheumatic mitral valve reconstruction. *Eur J Cardiothorac Surg* 2013; 44(4):682-689.
28. Gammie JS, Sheng S, Griffith BP, et al: Trends in mitral valve surgery in the United States: results from the Society of Thoracic Surgeons Adult Cardiac Surgery Database. *Ann Thorac Surg* 2009; 87(5):1431-1437; discussion 1437-1439.
29. Dillon J, Yakub MA, Kong PK, Ramli MF, Jaffar N, Gaffar IF: Comparative long-term results of mitral valve repair in adults with chronic rheumatic disease and degenerative disease: is repair for "burnt-out" rheumatic disease still inferior to repair for degenerative disease in the current era? *J Thorac Cardiovasc Surg* 2015; 149(3):771-777.
30. Yakub MA, Dillon J, Krishna Moorthy PS, Pau KK, Nordin MN: Is rheumatic aetiology a predictor of poor outcome in the current era of mitral valve repair? Contemporary long-term results of mitral valve repair in rheumatic heart disease. *Eur J Cardiothorac Surg* 2013; 44(4):673-681.
31. Yau TM, El-Ghoneimi YA, Armstrong S, Ivanov J, David TE: Mitral valve repair and replacement for rheumatic disease. *J Thorac Cardiovasc Surg* 2000; 119(1):53-60.
32. Kim JB, Kim HJ, Moon DH, et al: Long-term outcomes after surgery for rheumatic mitral valve disease: valve repair versus mechanical valve replacement. *Eur J Cardiothorac Surg* 2010; 37(5):1039-1046.
33. Duran CM, Gometza B, Saad E: Valve repair in rheumatic mitral disease: an unsolved problem. *J Card Surg* 1994; 9(2 Suppl):282-285.
34. Chauvaud S, Fuzellier JF, Berrebi A, Deloche A, Fabiani JN, Carpentier A: Long-term (29 years) results of reconstructive surgery in rheumatic mitral valve insufficiency. *Circulation* 2001; 104(12 Suppl 1):I12-15.
35. Kumar AS, Talwar S, Saxena A, Singh R, Velayoudam D: Results of mitral valve repair in rheumatic mitral regurgitation. *Interact Cardiovasc Thorac Surg* 2006; 5(4):356-361.
36. Choudhary SK, Talwar S, Dubey B, Chopra A, Saxena A, Kumar AS: Mitral valve repair in a predominantly rheumatic population. Long-term results. *Tex Heart Inst J* 2001; 28(1):8-15.
37. Shuhaiber J, Anderson RJ: Meta-analysis of clinical outcomes following surgical mitral valve repair or replacement. *Eur J Cardiothorac Surg* 2007; 31(2):267-275.

37

Surgery for Functional Mitral Regurgitation

Matthew A. Romano • Steven F. Bolling

Functional mitral regurgitation (FMR) is a complication of ischemic or dilated cardiomyopathy, occurring secondary to left ventricular (LV) geometrical distortion from tenting, inferobasilar migration, apical displacement, annular dilation and posterior leaflet restriction, and/or regional LV wall dysfunction. MR leads to a vicious cycle of LV volume overload, increased geometric distortion and progressive MR. FMR complicating congestive heart failure predicts a poor survival. Mitral surgery, to treat FMR has been undertaken with an acceptably low operative mortality. However, the exact MR surgery (repair or replacement) for which patient and what benefit, remains controversial.

Congestive heart failure is one of the world's leading causes of morbidity and mortality. As our population ages, the number of patients suffering from end-stage heart failure will continue to rise. In the United States alone, there are nearly 7 million patients suffering from heart failure. In 2012, heart failure "therapy" cost the United States over $50 billion. This total includes health care services, medications, and lost productivity. Yet of the 700,000 new congestive heart failure (CHF) patients diagnosed each year, less than 3000 are offered transplantation due to limitations of age, comorbid conditions and donor availability. Even fewer are presently served with a mechanical assist device. One of the most common (up to 50% of patients) and serious problems in cardiomyopathy is the development of functional or secondary mitral regurgitation. Functional mitral regurgitation (FMR), nonorganic mitral valve (MV) disease, may eventually affect almost all heart failure patients as a preterminal or terminal event.[1] FMR is not caused by intrinsic disease of the valve, but by left ventricular (LV) remodeling, dilation, and dysfunction leading to geometric reconfiguration of the mitroventricular apparatus, including papillary muscle displacement and annular dilation. MV leaflets become tethered, with failure of anterior-posterior leaflet coaptation, resulting in symmetric or asymmetric regurgitation.[2,3] The progressive dilatation of the left ventricle initially gives rise to FMR that begets further ventricular dilatation and more FMR. FMR is associated with poor quality of life and a reduction in long-term survival. Mitral surgery, while not addressing the underlying ventricular pathology, hopefully could interrupt this cycle of ventricular deterioration through the restoration of mitral competency.

BACKGROUND

It has been well documented that even small amounts of FMR are harmful in CHF patients. Grigioni et al[4] showed that when FMR regurgitant volume was >30 ml the 5-year survival was <35% compared to 44% for a regurgitant volumes of 1 to 29 ml and 61% for CHF patients with no MR. Bursi[5] also examined the role of FMR and its impact in CHF. CHF patients (469) were followed for mortality according to severity of their FMR. Their 5-year survival was 83% in patients with no/1+ FMR, 64% in 2+, 58% in 3+, and 46% in 4 + ($p < .0001$). The association between FMR and Major Adverse Cardiac and Cerebrovascular Events (MACCE) was strong and independent in this propensity matched analysis. A further study[6] denoted that among 303 patients post MI, ischemic MR was present in 194 (64%), and was a significant independent predictor of long-term mortality (relative risk, RR [95% confidence interval, CI] = 1.88, $p = .003$).[1] Additionally, in a study from the Duke Cardiovascular Databank,[7] 3-4+ FMR was present in 30% of 2057 HF patients with an left ventricular ejection fraction (LVEF) < 40%, and was an independent predictor of 5-year mortality (adjusted hazard ratio [95% CI] = 1.23).[2] Lastly, the Mayo Clinic[8] looked at the prognostic implications of FMR in patients with advanced systolic CHF in a heart failure clinic. Of 558 NYHA III-IV patients, those with at least moderate MR had a 5-year survival of only 27%. These studies demonstrate that FMR is not just a sign of advanced CHF, but an independent determinant of CHF death. That FMR is bad for CHF patients is supported by many other studies that show that the severity of MR impacts quality of life, as well as survival. Furthermore, there is a strong association between the presence of ischemic FMR severity and heart failure hospitalizations. However, while the presence of FMR predicts a poor prognosis in patients with left ventricular dysfunction and heart failure, unfortunately, "proof" that correction of FMR improves prognosis remains elusive.

Historically, the surgical approach to FMR was nonvalve sparing MV replacement, at a time when little was understood of the interdependence of ventricular function and the annular-papillary muscle continuity. Consequently, patients with low EF who underwent MV replacement with removal of the subvalvular apparatus had prohibitively high mortality rates. As explanation the erroneous concept of a beneficial "pop-off" effect of FMR was conceived. This idea erroneously proposed that mitral incompetence provided low-pressure relief during systolic ejection for the failing ventricle, and that removal of this effect through mitral replacement was responsible for the perioperative deterioration of ventricular function. Consequently, MV replacement in patients with heart failure and FMR was discouraged.

FMR ANATOMY

A firm understanding of the anatomy of the MV is fundamental to the surgical management of FMR. The MV apparatus consists of the annulus, leaflets, chordae tendineae, and papillary muscles as well as the entire left ventricle. These structures form a "closure cylinder" with the papillary musculature directly aligned beneath the annulus. Most importantly, the maintenance of chordal, annular, and subvalvular continuity is essential for the preservation of mitral geometric relationships, as well as ventricular twist mechanics and systolic power. MR in heart failure is not primarily related to the valve but to ventricular pathology. The degree of LV distortion reflects the degree of MR. As the ventricle fails, progressive dilatation of the LV results in outward papillary muscle migration, alteration of the closure cylinder, and thus loss of the zone of coaptation (Fig. 37-1).

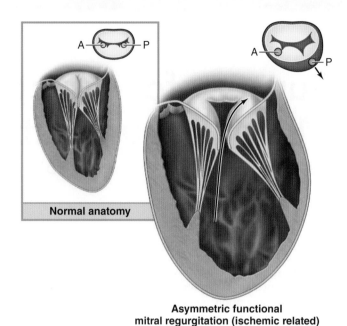

Asymmetric functional mitral regurgitation (ischemic related)

FIGURE 37-2 Asymmetric FMR noted with ischemic related LV changes due to posterior infarction.

The end result of progressive FMR and global ventricular remodeling is similar regardless of the etiology of cardiomyopathy. The primary lesion in ischemic FMR is leaflet tethering, which results from ventricular remodeling associated with an ischemic insult. Posterior-lateral and apical displacement of the papillary muscles, which correlates with a measurable "tethering distance," leads to apical tenting and restriction of the free margin of the leaflets and poor leaflet coaptation. Tethering of secondary chordae can lead to a "seagull" deformation of the anterior leaflet. Although both papillary muscles may be displaced, the posterior papillary muscle usually predominates, which leads to tethering of the "P3" leaflet segment.[9,10] This is seen in posterior infarction related to the posterior descending artery distribution and the mitral regurgitation jet is usually eccentric and posteriorly directed along the P3 area which is restricted (Fig. 37-2). In contrast, left anterior descending infarction leads to more global remodeling involving both papillary muscles, and more diffuse leaflet tethering with large central jets of mitral regurgitation. Although annular dilatation and ventricular remodeling accompanies all MR, it is usually an associated finding, as opposed to a primary causal lesion in ischemic mitral regurgitation. The degree of annular dilatation is much less in ischemic mitral regurgitation than in degenerative mitral regurgitation, which is one of the reasons that "downsizing" of the mitral ring annuloplasty may best address leaflet tethering in ischemic MV regurgitation. Conversely, FMR associated with dilated cardiomyopathies tends to have more symmetric distortion with more annular dilation than asymmetric ischemic FMR.[11,12] Because of this difference in geometric distortion, as well as patient comorbidity profiles, it may be that dilated and ischemic FMR patients should be thought of and treated in somewhat different manners.

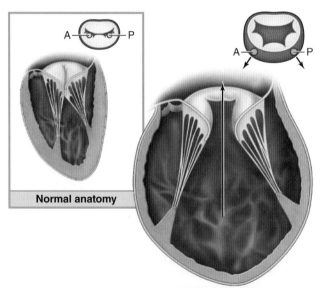

Functional mitral regurgitation

FIGURE 37-1 LV geometric distortion in FMR.

THERAPY OF FMR

Despite the underlying pathology, the goals of therapy for FMR patients are to improve symptoms and quality of life, reduce heart failure hospitalization, and, hopefully to improve survival. The therapies shown to be most effective for FMR are those directed at the underlying LV dysfunction, most importantly guideline-directed medical therapy (GDMT) for HF.[1,13-15] Cardiac resynchronization (with or without a defibrillator) if indications are met (wide QRS > 150 ms) should also be considered when appropriate.[16,17] Finally of course, coronary revascularization should be performed in patients with ischemia and myocardial viability. While all patients with FMR should receive GDMT for management of CAD, LV dysfunction and heart failure, unfortunately morbidity and mortality of patients with CHF and secondary FMR remains high. A recent study showed that among 404 FMR patients treated with GDMT, 4-year cardiac mortality occurred in 43 and 45% with moderate and severe MR, respectively, compared to only 6% with mild MR ($p = .003$).[13] Furthermore, moderate or severe FMR was also shown to be a high independent predictor of new onset HF in patients with ischemic LV dysfunction (RR = 3.2, $p = .0001$). The role of surgical MV repair or replacement is to potentially interrupt the vicious cycle of LV volume overload causing LV dilatation leading to secondary MR, which further increases LV volume overload and dilatation further increasing MR.

FMR SURGERY

The present AHA/ACC Valve Guidelines (2014) and the ESC/EACTS Guidelines[18,19] have separate guidelines for functional or secondary ischemic mitral regurgitation (FMR). As noted, these guidelines state that treating ischemia with coronary artery bypass grafting or percutaneous methods should be primarily undertaken for FMR. Additionally, all FMR patients should have guideline GDMT, with consideration for CRT, if they have a QRS greater than 150 ms. However, if the patients remain symptomatic with severe mitral regurgitation or stage D disease, they may be considered for "MV surgery" as a 2B indication. Yet, from the surgeon's perspective, while it is recommended that surgical correction of FMR should be considered exactly how to successfully correct FMR remains unclear. Currently, the most common technique to restore valve competence is placing an undersized or restrictive annuloplasty ring to reduce mitral annulus size and increase leaflet coaptation. Unfortunately, ischemic FMR may persist or recur after restrictive MV annuloplasty. Persistent or recurrent FMR in post op patients is understandably associated with unabated ventricular dilatation, an escalation of CHF symptomatology and possible reduction in long-term survival.

Surgical mitral annuloplasty improves symptoms in patients with CHF and it has been shown that mitral repair is feasible with a low mortality. Several authors have demonstrated 30-day mortality rates as low as 1 to 5% for mitral repair for MR in CHF. Recently, Geidel reported that the late results of restrictive annuloplasty in patients with FMR and advanced cardiomyopathy demonstrated a 3% 30-day mortality and 91% 12 months survival with little postoperative recurrence of significant MR. Similarly, data from Germany in transplant candidates, showed a 7% operative mortality and no difference in survival after MV repair versus transplant indicating that high risk MV surgery in patients with cardiomyopathy and FMR may offer a midterm alternative treatment for patients with drug refractory heart failure and FMR.[20-22] Perhaps, the most compelling data for the safety and efficacy of MV repair for FMR comes from the MV surgery alone arm of the prospective Acorn trial (CorCap Cardiac Support Device, a prospective, randomized, multicenter trial). The Acorn trial showed a 98% 30-day survival rate, 2% repeat reoperation, and 85% 24 months survival and significant improvements in quality of life, exercise performance, and NYHA class. Furthermore, in the MV surgery arm, improvement in LV volumes, mass, and shape was sustained out to 5 years with little recurrence of significant MR.[23]

However, the "achilles heel" of MV repair in may series of FMR is persistent, residual or recurrent MR.[24-27] It was learned that the intertrigonal distance is not stable in FMR, with dilatation occurring along, not only the insertion of the posterior leaflet, but also in the anterior portion. This intertrigonal portion dilates and although once considered to be a "measurable" standard by which to size annuloplasty rings, it is now known from a landmark paper of Hueb that this is not the case.[28] Therefore, previous methods of FMR sizing were incorrect and "undersizing" rings has become the standard for these functional MR patients. This may partly explain the operation "failing" and recurrence of mitral regurgitation in functional MR patients when using too large "classic-sized" rings or when using a partial or flexible rings.

However, despite undersizing rings, there is significant disparity in reccurence rates among FMR series. The lack of a mortality benefit may be partially explained by the absence of a durable repair. When McGee and Gillinov[24] showed no mortality benefit in FMR after mitral repair, they also noticed the rate of recurrent significant MR to be 30 to 40% at 1 year. Others have shown even higher rates of return of FMR, up to 80%.[29] This has led to an attempt to identify surgical predictors of recurrent MR and for improved surgical techniques that result in a more permanent repair.[30] In order to observe a survival benefit in these patients after mitral repair, FMR must be fixed permanently, as residual and recurrent MR may obscure or obliterate any possible survival benefit.

PREDICTORS OF RECURRENT MITRAL REGURGITATION

Many of the mechanisms of recurrent functional MR have been elucidated and include annular level and subvalvar components. Major predictors of recurrent FMR include LV size greater than 65 mm, a coaptation depth of greater than 1 cm below the annular plane and angulation of the MV apparatus, all of which indicate degree of LV distortion. In patients with a posterior leaflet angle > 45° (high posterolateral restriction) undergoing restrictive annuloplasty for ischemic MR, preoperative echo was shown to accurately predict persistence of MR and 3-year survival. Also studies show that the angle between the tip of the anterior leaflet and the annular plane is a predictor of MR recurrence. An anterior leaflet angle greater than 25 to 40° was a predictor of MR recurrence. Many have also shown LV function or degree of MR as determinants of recurrent MR while others point out the importance of both LV sphericity and tethering depth as predictors.[31-33]

One of the most important LV predictor of recurrent MR may be left ventricular end diastolic dimension (LVEDD) > 65 mm. In patients with preoperative LVEDD of 65 mm or less, restrictive mitral annuloplasty with revascularization provided a mortality benefit for ischemic mitral regurgitation and heart failure; however, when LVEDD exceeded 65 mm, outcome was poor and a different approach to CHF should be considered. Perhaps, the most important mechanistic predictor of recurrent FMR is an increased anterior-posterior or septal-lateral mitral annular diameter. This is the most significant determinant of FMR as leaflet coaptation and therefore mitral competency, is dependent upon the diameter of the MV annulus. The MV is thought to have roughly twice the amount of coaptive surface as needed. This redundancy allows for LV volume changes and explains why obligatory FMR occurs when the LVEDD approaches 65 mm. Furthermore, this may explain why FMR is evanescent. Studies of FMR reveal that decreasing filling and systemic vascular resistance lead to reduction in dynamic FMR. This is attributed to a reduction in the mitral orifice area relating to decreased LV volume and annular distension.[34]

This complex relationship between mitral annular area and leaflet coaptation may explain why an undersized "valvular" repair may help a "ventricular" problem. Three-dimensional magnetic resonance imaging and echo studies showed that the mitral annulus flattens and significantly increases its AP diameter. This CHF-related change has been shown not only in animal models, but in humans as well. Kongsaerepong et al[35] found that the strongest predictor of recurrent FMR following mitral repair was a residual large AP diameter, that is, a "too large" ring. Lastly, Spoor demonstrated that the use of flexible rings (which flex and allow the largest AP diameter) as opposed to a rigid complete ring was associated with a five times higher recurrent mitral regurgitation rate. Presently numerous rigid, complete FMR specific rings with stable AP dimension reduction are available.[10]

Interestingly, acute remodeling of the base of the heart with complete rigid, undersized rings may also play a beneficial role in FMR hearts. These disease-specific rings may reestablish an ellipsoid shape to the LV, as evidenced by the acute decreased sphericity index and LV volumes. Restoration of LV geometry is of paramount importance in CHF patients. This has been demonstrated by the Restore—MV trial. In that trial ischemic FMR patients, requiring coronary artery bypass graft (CABG) did better with a direct LV reshaping device (Coapsys), than with CABG with the addition of an undersized mitral ring, even though they had slightly more

residual MR. This study pointed out the differential effects of MR and the LV.[36] In summary, patients with predictors of failure should be considered poor candidates for FMR repair, and alternatives should be contemplated. Unfortunately, progression of ventricular disease may have the worst predictive outcome for these patients. This is not amenable by mitral repair and one must be aware that fundamentally FMR is a ventricular disease.

INDICATIONS FOR FMR SURGERY

The indications for surgery for FMR are more cautious than those for primary, degenerative MR due to the recognition that surgical outcomes are linked to underlying LV remodeling. Secondary FMR can acutely be corrected by MV surgery, however, it has never clearly been demonstrated that reducing or eliminating FMR alters the natural history or improves survival.[37,38] Moreover, whether the response to surgery is different in secondary MR due to ischemic versus nonischemic cardiomyopathy has also not been established. One-year mortality after MV surgery for severe ischemic MR (with or without CABG) is up to 17%. Therefore, the benefit of MV repair in patients with FMR and heart failure is unclear. Wu et al showed no mortality benefit in FMR patients treated with MV repair, although they did not examine the effect of recurrent mitral regurgitation. In ischemic cardiomyopathy patients, several nonrandomized studies showed that MV repair in addition to CABG for ischemic FMR did not alter long-term functional status or survival when compared with CABG alone.[16-19] Trichon demonstrated a survival advantage in ischemic cardiomyopathy patients who underwent CABG plus MV repair only compared with medical management, as there was no difference between CABG plus MV repair versus CABG alone.[6] Conversely, far more other nonrandomized studies, have demonstrated that MV repair plus CABG does improve survival compared with medical therapy or CABG alone in patients with FMR due to ischemic cardiomyopathy.[37–39]

MODERATE FMR

The first published randomized prospective FMR trial for moderate FMR was by Fattouch et al[40] This study describes 102 patients with moderate chronic ischemic MR (mean MR grade 2+ and LVEF 43%) and moderately dilated left ventricles (mean LVEDD 59 mm) that were randomized to CABG plus MV repair (n = 48) or CABG alone (n = 54). Postoperative and follow-up MR grade, NYHA class, and LV remodeling were improved in the MV repair group. That trial was not powered for mortality analysis and in-hospital and 5-year survival was not statistically different between groups. Interestingly, exercise echo at 1 year in these patients showed far better hemodynamic response and less occurrence of MR in the mitral repair group.

Reinforcing this finding, Deja published in Circulation the results of the mitral surgery arm for all patients with FMR and an EF of <35% from the STICH trial. This report of 1212 patients, showed not only a quality of life improvement, but hinted at a survival benefit from the addition of MV repair to CABG in these high risk patients.[37] Finally, Chan reported results from a randomized, prospective survival trial of CABG with or without MV repair for FMR in the RIME trial. At 1 year of follow-up, FMR patients who had the addition of MV repair had lower LV end-systolic volume index (LVESVI), brain naturetic protein (BNP) and MR grade, as well as better sphericity and exercise performance.[40] Conversely, in a recent NIH-sponsored, multicenter randomized controlled trial (RCT) conducted by the Cardiothoracic Surgery Trials Network (CTSnet), despite MV repair with CABG being significantly more effective than CABG alone in reducing or eliminating moderate ischemic MR, there were no differences at 1-year in LVESVI or rates of major adverse cardiac and cerebrovascular event.[41] Longer follow-up could reveal whether differences in residual/recurrent MR will manifest in clinical endpoints such as death and rehospitalization for heart failure. Of note, in these randomized trials of mitral repair for moderate ischemic FMR, there appears to be no operative mortality penalty for the addition of an undersized ring.[42] Given the improvements seen with MR correction in patients with only moderate MR and moderate LV dysfunction, it is tempting to hypothesize clinical benefits at longer follow up.

SEVERE FMR

There are very few randomized trials of surgery for severe FMR. Nonrandomized evidence including the meta-analysis by Vassileva et al[43] favoring mitral repair is a compilation of retrospective and single center studies. Conversely, Lorusso et al[44] demonstrated no difference in short- or long-term mortality between patients treated with MV replacement versus repair in severe FMR.

In a further study,[44] the CTSnet enrolled 251 patients with severe ischemic MR and coronary artery disease between 2009

and 2011 and randomized them to ether receive undersized MV repair (126 patients) or chord-sparing replacement (125 patients). The primary endpoint was LV reverse remodeling assessed by LVESVI measured at 12 months. At 12 months, LVESVI was 54 mL/m² in the repair group versus 60 mL/m² in the replacement group. There was no significant difference in LVESVI. The 1-year mortality rate was 14.3% in the repair group versus 17.6% in the replacement group. However, the repair group showed a significantly higher rate of recurrence of moderate or severe MR at 12 months (32.6 vs 2.3%). There were no significant differences in the rate of a MACCE, functional status or quality of life at 12 months. In this propensity-matched study MV repair was the strongest predictor of need for valve reoperation, with a recurrence of MR in surviving patients at 1 year of 32.6% and at 2 years of 46% (Fig. 37-3).[7] Interestingly, however, in a subgroup analysis of MV repair[45] patients who did not have recurrent FMR, LV reverse remodeling was significantly better than in patients who had MV replacement. Mitral repair without recurrent MR was also far better than those with a "bad" repair (ie, significant recurrence of MR) (Fig. 37-4). This may imply that a "good" FMR repair without significant recurrence is better than a replacement. However, the high recurrence rate of significant FMR is problematic. The choice of repair versus replacement remains controversial since MV repair may be associated with lower short- and intermediate-term morbidity and mortality, while at the same time MV repair of FMR is associated with high recurrence rates of moderate/severe FMR, but equal survival and CHF status.

Lastly, the role for MV repair in nonischemic cardiomyopathy patients has been less extensively studied. Bolling et al described excellent survival following MV repair in a series of cardiomyopathy patients without coronary artery disease.[20,21] Another report of idiopathic dilated cardiomyopathy patients treated with MV repair had significant resolution of mitral regurgitation and heart failure symptoms, with excellent long-term survival.[46] DeBonis et al

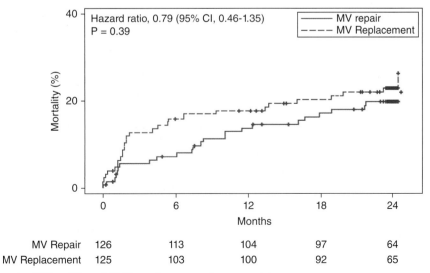

FIGURE 37-3 Survival in the CTSnet "Severe" FMR repair versus replacement trial.

LVESVI (ml/m²)	Repair	
	Recurrence	No recurrence
	62.6 ± 26.9	42.7 ± 26.4

FIGURE 37-4 Resultant reverse remodeling in the CTSnet "Severe" FMR trial: "Bad" (with recurrence of significant MR) versus "Good (no recurrence of MR).

demonstrated 81% survival at 3.5 years, with excellent freedom from MR and heart failure symptoms, in a smaller series of nonischemic FMR patients undergoing MV repair.[47] Despite these excellent outcomes, there are very little data comparing surgery to medical management in patients with nonischemic FMR.

ECHO DEFINITIONS OF FMR

When examining the reports of FMR surgery, it must be remembered, that there is disparity among the guidelines as to what constitutes moderate versus severe FMR. All the guidelines agree that EROA ≥ 0.4 cm², RgV ≥ 60 mL, and RgF ≥ 50% constitute severe *primary* MR. However, the recent ACC/AHA Guidelines on valvular heart disease propose a new definition for severe FMR at an EROA > 0.2 cm². This lower threshold accounts for the possibility that the actual EROA is larger than calculated by PISA in FMR, as well as the fact that "moderate" or more FMR in the setting of a cardiomyopathy has been associated with an adverse prognosis. However, it is not clear what to do with an FMR patient with a EROA of 0.2 cm², nor are there convincing data showing that correction of "severe" FMR at the lower threshold improves patient outcomes in FMR. Therefore, this new recommendation remains controversial.[48]

TECHNIQUES OF MITRAL SURGERY FOR FMR

For FMR operations, meticulous attention should be paid to myocardial preservation and cardiopulmonary perfusion. At the time of exposure of the MV, it can be noted that the MV appears "normal". The reduction in AP diameter and orifice area of the MV is an overcorrection and overcompensation for a disease of the ventricle. This "undersizing" of the mitral ring was first proposed by Bolling, in 1995 and has become a standard technical approach for FMR repair. When undersizing a mitral ring, it is recommended that one use numerous annular sutures, as compared to degenerative MR repairs, to distribute the workload of annular reductive force. These sutures may be put very closely together, or even on a diagonal. Some advocate the use of pledgeted sutures, or the use of an extra row or a few pledgeted reinforcement sutures posteriorly, once the ring is tied in place.

In terms of FMR ring sizing, the normal mitral annulus is roughly proportional to a patients thumb and forefinger in a circle. One must "downsize" from there. There are some who have advocated double downsizing, meaning two sizes below that measured at the time of operation; however, the vast majority of patients may be well served with a "small" 26 or 28 mm ring. Although initially in FMR patients there was concern for both systolic anterior motion of the anterior leaflet (SAM) and/or mitral stenosis from such downsizing, these have not resulted in significant clinical sequelae in long-term FMR follow-up series. However, it must be noted that some investigators have reported "functional" mitral stenosis with provocative (dobutamine) testing with undersized rings.[49]

The type of ring utilized for FMR repairs is an important technical consideration. As noted, in a landmark paper by Hueb, the fibrous portion of the mitral annulus anteriorly between the two mitral trigones dilated proportionally and as much as the posterior muscular annulus. Magne reported failure rates of up to 80% at 6 months postoperatively with large flexible and/or partial bands for FMR patients. Silberman et al[51] reported on predictors of residual and recurrent mitral regurgitation in FMR and the two largest multivariate predictors were LV size and the type of ring. In fact, the type of ring was a better predictor than LV size. That study showed that small rigid and complete rings were best for FMR. In the specific disease of FMR, large partial or incomplete rings probably do not result in a durable repair and are not favored technically. Presently, there are numerous specific small rigid and complete FMR rings with a disproportionate AP diameter dimension reduction. While none of these rings have shown clinical outcome differences between them, they are probably most favored for the repair of FMR.[51]

There are some FMR patients that should be approached with clinical caution. Silverman showed the larger the ventricle, the worst the outcome for FMR patients. This was also shown in a study from Dion which demonstrated that LVEDDs over 65 mm had a much poorer outcome than those starting at a smaller LV size. Probably, there are some ventricles that are "too far gone" and mitral repair will not be beneficial in these patients. Furthermore, patients with poor RV function and very high PA pressures should be carefully evaluated and perhaps avoided.

When coming off cardiopulmonary bypass there should be no mitral regurgitation seen on intraoperative postop transesophageal echocardiography. And not only should there be no mitral regurgitation, the zone of coaptation should be measured and should be at least 8 to 10 mm long. If this is not the case then the patient certainly has a much higher incidence of recurrence of mitral regurgitation when they are awake and removed from the unloading effects of general anesthesia.

There are other adjunct therapies that have been used for the FMR repair. In the dilated FMR MV, there are often deep clefts between P1/P, and P2/P3 which should be closed. Borger has advocated the use of lysis of secondary chords to both the anterior and posterior leaflets to allow for a longer zone of coaptation. While this method has been technically successful, there is no long-term follow-up and the effect of disrupting any chordal structures on LV function is unknown.

FMR is a ventricular disease and surgeons have tried to add adjunctive and inventive "ventricular" therapies to an undersized mitral ring, thereby directing operative therapy to the ventricle itself. Kron has advocated the use of "ring and string" by placing a Goretex traction suture in the posterior papillary muscle and bringing it up towards the annular plane. Hvass has demonstrated the use a double annular ring, placing a standard annular ring at the annulus level and then a second one of Gortex, woven around the papillary muscles to recreate the normal cylinder of closure. Many authors have reported moving papillary muscles or even sewing them together. None of these operations have had long-term follow-up. Some surgeons have advocated augmenting the anterior or the posterior leaflet with bovine pericardium to improve the length of the zone of coaptation. While these approaches increase the technical difficulty of the operation, they are certainly appealing on the basis of altering the underlying problem. Other types of ventricular therapies which have been utilized: the ACORN restriction jacket, the Coapsys ventricular tether, a silicon lifting pad behind the posterior inferior ventricular wall amongst others. None of these therapies have long-term follow-up.[52-54]

MITRAL VALVE REPLACEMENT IN FMR

Which FMR valves to replace primarily remains controversial. The recent reports in the NEJM have added to our decision-making knowledge base. Perhaps the most important is the summary paper by Lancellotti.[9] In this report the predictors of failed FMR repair are mild annular dilatation, coaptation depth more than 1 cm, reverse angulation of the posterior leaflet or LV remodeling greater than 65 mm or a LVEDV greater than 100 mm indexed. Kron has also shown in the follow-up paper to Acker (NEJM) that posterior-basilar dyskinesia or akinesia is associated with a high rate of MR recurrence, even with an undersized repair.

While which patient to replace in FMR remains controversial, there is a consensus on the technical aspects of MV replacement for FMR. MV replacement should be a total valve sparing replacement. Yun demonstrated in a randomized trial comparing partial versus complete choral sparing MV replacement, that the effects on left ventricular volume and function were much better preserved with complete versus posterior leaflet sparing. Nonvalve sparing mitral replacement should be abandoned. There are numerous techniques for total valve sparing MV replacement in FMR including anterior flip-over, in which a C-shaped incision is placed in the anterior leaflet and the entire anterior apparatus is moved posteriorly. Following appropriate valve sizing, pledgeted stitches are placed through the posterior annulus, the edge of the posterior leaflet, and the "flipped" anterior leaflet, placing both chordal apparatus and leaflets behind the MV prosthesis (Fig. 37-5). A second method of achieving total valve sparing is to remove the center of the anterior leaflet then rotating the

remaining portions of the anterior leaflet to the left and right. Valve sizing for FMR should be prudent and not "oversized". With modern MV prostheses there should not be undue worry of stenosis and overly large bulky valves may impair LV dynamics in these already poor LVs. Acker showed in severe FMR patients, a total valve sparing operative mortality of 4.2%, which was only slightly higher than the operative mortality of 1.6% mitral repair for FMR patients.

PERCUTANEOUS FMR OPTIONS

Percutaneous mitral therapy could theoretically offer improved safety as compared to surgical MV surgery and may be suited for the treatment of higher risk FMR patients. Taramasso reported a nonrandomized comparison of 91 patients undergoing surgical for FMR, and compared them against 52 patients undergoing MitraClip. All patients had severe FMR, were symptomatic despite GDMT and had ischemic or idiopathic dilated myopathies. The decision to perform surgical correction versus MitraClip therapy was based on logistic EuroSCORE and frailty. Patients were followed 18 months for surgery and 8 months for MitraClip. The surgical group underwent concomitant CABG 35%, tricuspid valve repair 25%, and atrial fibrillation ablation (26%). The MitraClip group was older, had a two-fold higher logistic EuroScore, Bigger LVs (LVEDD 70 mm vs 66 mm), and TR grade was higher. For the surgical group, in-hospital mortality was 6.6%, postoperative LOS was 11 days. No patient had predischarge MR grade ≥ 3+, and 1-year freedom from MR ≥ 3+ was excellent at 94% with 89% surviving. For the MitraClip group, in-hospital mortality was 0%, postoperative LOS was 5 days, 9.6% had predischarge MR grade ≥ 3+, and 1-year freedom from MR ≥ 3+ was 79% with 88% surviving. At 1-year follow-up, 89% of the surgery patients were NYHA Class I/II (22% NYHA Class I). In the MitraClip group at 1-year, 84% of the patients were NYHA Class I/II (48% NYHA Class I).[55] Additionally, Franzen[56] reported 6-month follow-up on 50 subjects with FMR with LVEF ≤ 25%, MR ≥ 3+ and in NYHA functional Class III or IV. After a mitralclip procedure, MR ≤ 2+ was present in 92% and 30-day and 6-month mortality was 6% and 19%. There were improvements in functional class, but only mild favorable LV remodeling at 6 months. Lastly, Aurrichio[57] described 51 symptomatic nonresponders to CRT with FMR grade ≥ 2+ treated with a Mitralclip. They reported two procedural deaths, an additional 30-day mortality of 4.2%, and a 12-month mortality of 18%. These MitraClip reports are interesting, as there are few reports of MitraClip in subjects with FMR at high surgical risk. While none of these studies were randomized, the COAPT trial (MitraClip therapy in FMR vs GDMT) is currently underway in the United States to investigate the safety and effectiveness of the MitraClip in comparison to GDMT for FMR. The primary effectiveness endpoint is heart failure rehospitalizations at 24 months. Although the trial is not powered for mortality, this endpoint will be examined. This trial will be one of the largest studies in FMR and is expected to shape future surgical and

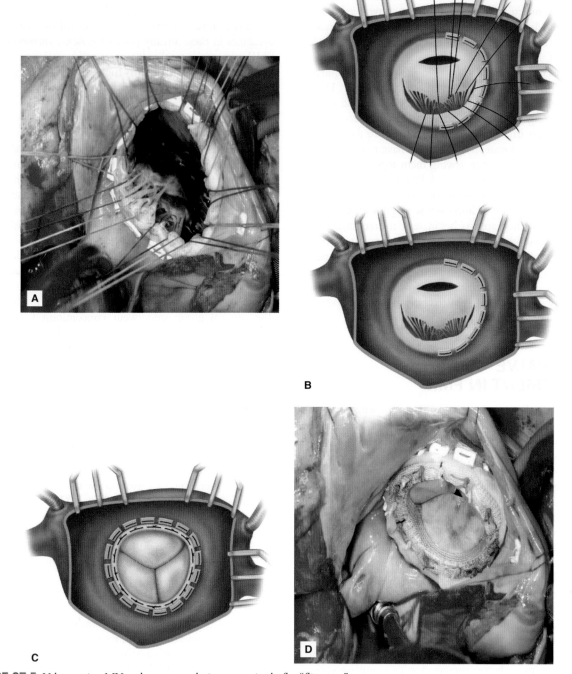

FIGURE 37-5 Valve sparing MV replacement technique: anterior leaflet "flip-over."

transcatheter FMR trials. Finally, new percutaneous devices for FMR, including annuloplasty and total mitral replacement are on the near horizon.

SUMMARY

In summary, FMR is a ventricular disease, not a valvular disease. FMR leads to a vicious cycle of LV volume overload, and progressive MR. FMR complicating CHF predicts a

poor survival. Mitral surgery, to treat FMR has been undertaken with an acceptably low operative mortality.[58] However, one must decide on specific patient factors whether or not intervention to correct FMR is warranted in CHF patients, as a clear survival impact has not been shown compared GDMT or revascularization therapy alone. If surgery is undertaken, undersizing repairs with a complete rigid ring and valve sparing replacement is recommended. While "good" mitral repair probably leads to better LV remodeling, patients identified to be at high risk for FMR recurrence after annuloplasty should have MV replacement. More complex mitral operations and percutaneous devices have shown promising results, but remain investigational. However, we do know that FMR is bad for CHF patients, and its elimination should be a therapeutic goal for these interesting and complex patients.

REFERENCES

1. Yancy CW, Jessup M, Bozkurt B, et al: 2013 ACCF/AHA guideline for the management of heart failure: a report of the American College of Cardiology Foundation/American Heart Association Task Force on Practice Guidelines. *JACC* 2013; 62:e147-239.
2. Nagasaki M, Nichimura S, Ohtaki E, et al: The echocardiographic determinants of functional mitral regurgitation differ in ischemic and non-ischemic cardiomyopathy. *Internat J of Cardiol* 2009; 108(2):171-76.
3. Dagum P, Timek TA, Green GR, et al: Coordinate-free analysis of mitral valve dynamics in normal and ischemic hearts. *Circulation* 2002; 102:III62-69.
4. Grigioni F, Enriquez-Sarano M, Zehr KJ, Bailey KR, Tajik AJ: Ischemic mitral regurgitation: long-term outcome and prognostic implications with quantitative Doppler assessment. Circulation 2001; 103:1759-1764.
5. Bursi F, Barbieri A, Grigioni F, et al: Prognostic implications of functional mitral regurgitation according to the severity of the underlying chronic heart failure: a long-term outcome study. *Eur J Heart Failure* 2010; 12(4) 382-388.
6. Trichon BH, Felker GM, Shaw LK, Cabell CH, O'Connor CM: Relation of frequency and severity of mitral regurgitation to survival among patients with left ventricular systolic dysfunction and heart failure. *AJC* 2003; 91:538-543.
7. DUKE.
8. Enriquez-Sarano M, Nkomo V, Mohty D, Avierinos JF, Chalili H: Mitral regurgitation: predictors of outcome and natural history. *Adv Cardiol* 2002; 39:133-143.
9. Lancellotti P, Moura L, Pierard LA, et al: European association of echocardiography recommendations for the assessment of valvular regurgitation. Part 2: mitral and tricuspid regurgitation (native valve disease). *Eur J Echocardiogr.* 2010; 11:307-332.
10. Thavendiranathan P, Liu S, Datta S, et al: Quantification of chronic functional mitral regurgitation by automated 3-dimensional peak and integrated proximal isovelocity surface area and stroke volume techniques using real-time 3-dimensional volume color Doppler echocardiography: in vitro and clinical validation. *Circ Cardiovasc Imaging* 2013; 6:125-133.
11. Watanabe N, Ogasawara Y, Yamaura Y, et al: Geometric differences of the mitral valve tenting between anterior and inferior myocardial infarction with significant ischemic mitral regurgitation: quantitation by novel software system with transthoracic real-time three-dimensional echocardiography. *J Am Soc Echocardiogr* 2006; 19:71-75.
12. Kwan J, Shiota T, Agler DA, et al: Real-time three-dimensional echocardiography s. Geometric differences of the mitral apparatus between ischemic and dilated cardiomyopathy with significant mitral regurgitation: real-time three-dimensional echocardiography study. *Circulation* 2003; 107:1135-1140.
13. Agricola E, Ielasi A, Oppizzi M, et al: Long-term prognosis of medically treated patients with functional mitral regurgitation and left ventricular dysfunction. *EJHF* 2009; 11:581-587.
14. Capomolla S, Febo O, Gnemmi M, et al: Beta-blockade therapy in chronic heart failure: diastolic function and mitral regurgittition improvement by carvedilol. *AHJ* 2000; 139:596-608.
15. Comin-Colet J, Sanchez-Corral MA, Manito N, et al: Effect of carvedilol therapy on functional mitral regurgitation, ventricular remodeling, and contractility in patients with heart failure due to left ventricular systolic dysfunction. *Transplant Proc* 2002; 34:177-178.
16. Cleland JG, Daubert JC, Erdmann E, et al: The effect of cardiac resynchronization on morbidity and mortality in heart failure. *New Engl J Med.* 2005; 352:1539-1549.
17. van Bommel RJ, Marsan NA, Delgado V, et al: Cardiac resynchronization therapy as a therapeutic option in patients with moderate-severe functional mitral regurgitation and high operative risk. *Circulation* 2011; 124:912-919.
18. Nishimura RA, Otto CM, Bonow RO, et al: 2014 AHA/ACC guideline for the management of patients with valvular heart disease: a report of the American College of Cardiology/American Heart Association Task Force on Practice Guidelines. *J Am Coll Cardiol* 2014; 63: e57-185.
19. Vahanian A, Alfieri O, Andreotti F, et al: ESC Committee for Practice Guidelines (CPG): Joint Task Force on the Management of Valvular Heart Disease of the European Society of Cardiology (ESC) and the European Association for Cardio-Thoracic Surgery (EACTS). Guidelines on the management of valvular heart disease (version 2012). *Eur J Cardiothorac Surg* 2012; 42(4):S1-44.
20. Bolling SF, Deeb GM, Brunsting LA, Bach DS: Early outcome of mitral valve reconstruction in patients with end-stage cardiomyopathy. *J Thorac Cardiovasc Surg* 1995; 4:676-683.
21. Bach DS, Bolling SF: Early improvement in congestive heart failure after correction of secondary mitral regurgitation in end-stage cardiomyopathy. *Am Heart J* 1995; 129:1165-1170.
22. Di Salvo TG, Acker MA, Dec GW, Byrne JG: Mitral valve surgery in advanced heart failure. *J Am Coll Cardiol* 2010; 5(4):271-282.
23. Acker MA, Jessup M, Bolling SF, et al: Mitral valve repair in heart failure: five-year follow-up from the mitral valve replacement stratum of the Acorn randomized trial. *J Thorac Cardiovasc Surg* 2011; 142(3), 569-574.
24. McGee EC Jr, Gillinov AM, Blackstone EH, et al: Recurrent mitral regurgitation after annuloplasty for functional ischemic mitral regurgitation. *J Thorac Cardiovasc Surg* 2004; 128(6):916-924.
25. Shiota M, Gillinov AM, Takasaki K, Fukuda S, Shiota T: Recurrent mitral regurgitation late after annuloplasty for ischemic mitral regurgitation. *Echocardiography* 2011; 28:161-166.
26. Crabtree TD, Bailey MS, Moon MR, et al: Recurrent mitral regurgitation and risk factors for early and late mortality after mitral valve repair for functional ischemic mitral regurgitation. *Ann Thorac Surg* 2008; 85:1537-1543.
27. De Bonis M, Bolling SF: Mitral valve surgery: wait and see vs. early operation. *Eur Heart J* 2013; 34(1):13-19a.
28. DeBonis M, Lapenna E, Verzini A, et al: Recurrence of mitral regurgitation parallels the absence of left ventricular reverse remodeling after mitral repair in advanced dilated cardiomyopathy. *Ann Thorac Surg* 2008; 85(3):932-939.
29. Hueb AC, Jatene FB, Moreira LF, Pomerantzeff PM, Kallás E, de Oliveira SA: Ventricular remodeling and mitral valve modifications in dilated cardiomyopathy: new insights from anatomic study. *J Thorac Cardiovasc Surg* 2002; 124:1216-1224.
30. Hung J, Papakostas L, Tahta SA: Mechanism of recurrent ischemic mitral regurgitation after annuloplasty: continued LV remodeling as a moving target. *ACC Curr J Rev* 2005; 14(2):83-84.
31. Gelsomino S, van Garasse L, Lucà F, et al: Impart of preoperative anterior leaflet tethering on the recurrence of ischemic mitral regurgitation and the lack of left ventricular reverse remodeling after restrictive annuloplasty *J Am Soc Echocardiogr* 2011; 23(12):1265-1275.
32. Jeno T, Sakata R, Iguro Y, Yamamoto H, Ueno T, Matsumoto K: Preoperative advanced left ventricular remodeling predisposes to recurrence of ischemic mitral regurgitation with less reverse remodeling. *J Heart Valve Dis* 2008; 17(1):36-41.
33. DiGiammarco G, Liberi R, Giancane M, et al: Recurrence of functional mitral regurgitation in patients with dilated cardiomyopathy undergoing mitral valve repair: how to predict it. *Interact Cardiovasc Thorac Surg* 2007; 6:340-44.
34. Ciarka A, Braun J, Delgado V, et al: Predictors of mitral regurgitation recurrence in patients with heart failure undergoing mitral valve annuloplasty. *Am J Cardiol* 2010; 106:395-401.
35. Kongsaerepong V, Shiota M, Gillinov AM, et al: Echocardiographic predictors of successful versus unsuccessful mitral valve repair in ischemic mitral regurgitation. *Am J Cardiol* 2006; 98(4):504-508.
36. Spoor MT, Geltz A, Bolling SF: Flexible versus nonflexible mitral valve rings for congestive heart failure: differential durability of repair. *Circulation* 2006; 114(1 Suppl):I67-71.
37. Grossi EA, Goldberg JD, LaPietra A, et al: Ischemic mitral valve reconstruction and replacement: comparison of long term survival and complications. *J Thorac Cardiovasc Surg* 2001; 122:1107-1124.

38. Deja MA, Grayburn PA, Sun B, et al: Influence of mitral regurgitation repair on survival in the surgical treatment for ischemic heart failure trial. *Circulation* 2012; 125(21): 2639-2648.

39. Milano CA, Daneshmand MA, Rankin JS, et al: Survival prognosis and surgical management of ischemic mitral regurgitation. *Ann Thorac Surg* 2008; 86:735-744.

40. Fattouch K, Sampognaro R, Speziale G, et al: The impact of moderate ischemic mitral reguritation after isolated coronary artery bypass grafting. *Ann Thorac Surg* 2010; 90(4):1187-1194.

41. Chan KM, Punjabi PP, Flather M, et al: RIME Investigators: Coronary artery bypass with or without mitral annuloplasty in moderate functional ischemic mitral regurgitiation. *Circulation* 2012; 126:2502-2510.

42. Smith PK, Puskas JD, Ascheim DD, et al: Cardiothoracic Surgical Trials Network Investigators: surgical treatment of moderate ischemic mitral regurgitation. *N Engl J Med* 2014; 371(23):2178-2188.

43. Vassileva CM, Boley T, Markwell S, Hazelrigg S: Meta-analysis of short-term and long-term survival following repair versus replacement for ischemic mitral regurgitation. *Eur J Cardiothorac Surg* 2011; 39:295-303.

44. Lorusso R, Gelsomino S, Vizzardi E, et al: Mitral valve repair or replacement for ischemic mitral regurgitation? The Italian Study on the Treatment of Ischemic Mitral Regurgitation (ISTIMIR). *J Thorac Cardiovasc Surg* 2014; 145:128-139.

45. Acker MA, Parides MK, Perrault LP, et al: CTSN: Mitral valve repair versus replacement for severe ischemic mitral regurgitation. *N Engl J Med* 2014; 370(1):23-32.

46. Kron IL, Hung J, Overby JR, et al: for the CTSN investigators: Predicting recurrent mitral regurgitation after mitral valve repair for severe ischemic mitral regurgitation. *J Thorac Cardiovasc Surg* 2014; 149(3):752–761.

47. DeBonis M, Lapenna E, Verzini A, et al: Recurrence of mitral regurgitation parallels the absence of left ventricular reverse remodeling after mitral valve repair in advanced dilated cardiomyopathy. *Ann Thorac Surg* 2008; 85:932-939.

48. Grayburn PA, Carabello B, Hung J, et al: Defining "Severe" secondary mitral regurgitation: emphasizing an integrated approach. *JACC* 2014; 64:2792-2801.

49. Magne J, Sénéchal M, Mathieu P, Dumesnil JG, Dagenais F, Pibarot P: Restrictive annuloplasty for ischemic mitral regurgitation may induce functional mutral stenosis. *J Am Coll Cardiol* 2008; 51(17):1692-1701.

50. Bothe W, Swanson JC, Ingels NB, Miller DC: How much septal-lateral mitral annular reduction do you get with new ischemic/functional mitral regurgitation annuloplasty rings? Original Research Article. *J Thorac Cardiovasc Surg* 2010; 140(1):117-121.e3.

51. Silberman S, Klutstein MW, Sabag T, et al: Repair of ischemic mitral regurgitation: comparison between flexible and rigid annuloplasty rings. *Ann Thorac Surg* 2011; 87(6):1721-1727.

52. Borger MA, Murphy PM, Alam A, et al: Initial results of the chordal-cutting operation for ischemic mitral regurgitation. *J Thorac Cardiovasc Surg* 2007; 133:1483-1492.

53. Szymanski C, Bel A, Cohen I, et al: Comprehensive annular and sub-valvular repair of chronic ischemic mitral regurgitation improves long-term results with the least ventricular remodeling. *Circulation* 2012; 126:2720-2727.

54. Bouma W, van der Horst ICC, Wijdh-den-Hamer IJ, et al: Chronic ischemic mitral regurgitation. Current treatment results and new mechanism-based surgical approaches. *Eur J Cardiothorac Surg* 2010; 37:170-185.

55. Taramasso M, Maisano F, Latib A, et al: Clinical outcomes of MitraClip for the treatment of functional mitral regurgitation. *EuroIntervention* 2014; 10(6):746-752.

56. Franzen O, van der Heyden J, Baldus S, et al: MitraClip(R) therapy in patients with end-stage systolic heart failure. *Eur J Heart Fail* 2011; 13:569-576.

57. Auricchio A, Schillinger W, Meyer S, et al: Correction of mitral regurgitation in nonresponders to cardiac resynchronization therapy by MitraClip improves symptoms and promotes reverse remodeling. *J Am Coll Cardiol* 2011; 58:2183-2189.

58. Wu AH, Aaronson KD, Bolling SF, Pagani FD, Welch K, Koelling TM: Impact of mitral valve annuloplasty on mortality risk in patients with mitral regurgitation and left ventricular systolic dysfunction. *J Am Coll Cardiol* 2005; 45(3):381-387.

Surgical Treatment of Mitral Valve Endocarditis

Gösta B. Pettersson • Syed T. Hussain

38

Mitral valve infective endocarditis (IE) is one of the more devastating complications of mitral valve disease, and if left untreated, it is universally fatal, like any other form of IE. In surgical practice, mitral valve endocarditis is usually less common than aortic valve endocarditis, with most infections occurring in native mitral valves. Although the distribution of causes of mitral valve dysfunction has changed in recent years, the overall incidence of IE has increased during the past 3 decades.[1-6] Rheumatic valve disease, which was a frequent predisposing factor to IE in the 1980s, is now rare in industrialized nations.[6-7] Predisposing factors more frequently encountered today, several of which are consequences of advances that characterize modern medicine,[1-7] include degenerative valvular disease, prosthetic valves, other intravascular prostheses and devices, hemodialysis, nosocomial infections, intravenous drug abuse, and immunosuppression. Repaired valves have a low risk of endocarditis compared with prosthetic valves. (To learn more about the epidemiology of IE, see Chapter 31.)

More effective antimicrobial agents have improved the early and long-term outcomes of patients treated for endocarditis. However, endocarditis is still associated with high rates of complications, morbidity, and mortality and frequently requires an operation for cure.[1-13] Increased experience and advances in surgical techniques have improved the success of these challenging operations.

PATHOLOGY

Native Mitral Valve Endocarditis

Native valve endocarditis (NVE) begins with endocardial injury, which allows deposition of fibrin and platelets with subsequent attachment of bacteria.[6,14] Endocardial injury may be secondary to rheumatic valvulitis or other leaflet disease, or valvular or annular calcification. Although vegetations may be seen anywhere on the leaflets or chordae, the usual site at which infective NVE of the mitral valve causes valvular destruction and invasion is the base of the atrial aspect of the mitral valve leaflets. Annular or subanular invasion is more likely to cause atrioventricular (AV) separation when the invasion site is underneath the leaflet and is exposed to high ventricular pressure. Invasion into the AV groove fat with abscess formation is more serious and difficult to radically debride and sterilize (Fig. 38-1).[15] Fortunately, mitral annular invasion more often opens toward the atrium and is therefore shallow in most cases; invasion is generally more common and deeper in aortic valve IE.[16]

Destruction of the fibrous trigones and intervalvular fibrosa between the anterior mitral valve leaflet and the aorta is usually a consequence of aortic valve endocarditis with secondary mitral involvement.[17] An infected aortic valve may seed the anterior mitral leaflet or the tensor apparatus of the mitral valve, resulting in double-valve endocarditis; the mechanism may be a large vegetation hitting and directly infecting the anterior mitral leaflet or a jet lesion from aortic regurgitation that becomes infected.[18]

Prosthetic Mitral Valve Endocarditis

Prosthetic valve endocarditis (PVE) is on the rise as the number of patients with prosthetic valves continues to increase. PVE is more common in the aortic than the mitral position.[16] This is because a majority of mitral valves are repaired, and repair is associated with a lower risk of endocarditis.

PVE within the first postoperative year is considered early endocarditis, and cases appearing more than 1 year after operation are termed late.[6,19] The risk of early PVE appears to be greatest approximately 5 weeks after valve implantation and declines thereafter.[19] The overall incidence of early PVE is 1%,[20] and the incidence of late PVE is 0.5 to 1% per year.[21-23] The type of prosthesis (mechanical vs bioprosthesis) does not influence the risk of PVE.

Early PVE is usually the result of intraoperative infection. Common portals of entry for bacteria that cause PVE are dental procedures, intravascular catheters, and skin infection.[6,24] Nosocomial infections contribute to late PVE, particularly in patients with medical comorbidities that require frequent

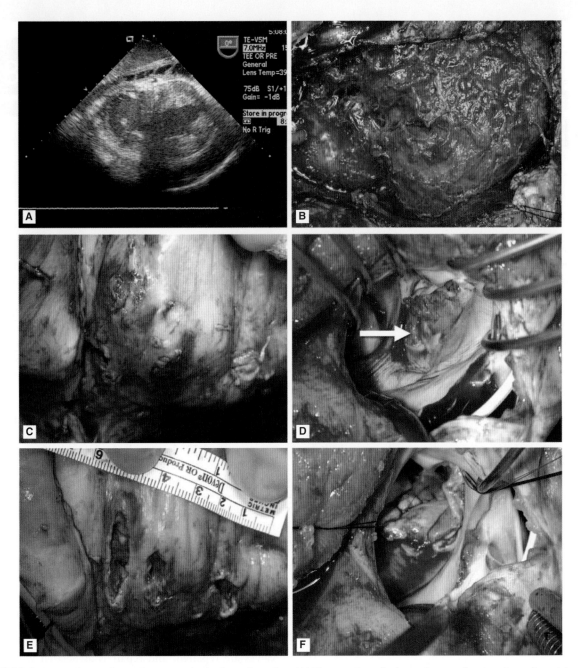

FIGURE 38-1 A case of very advanced invasive mitral valve endocarditis. (A) Transesophageal echocardiogram showing circumferential pericardial effusion with fibrin stranding posteriorly. (B) Severe hemorrhagic pericarditis. Patient was septic and not responding to adequate antibiotic therapy. (C) After peeling fibrinous capsule off heart, these multiple necrotic spots, suggesting abscesses along the AV groove, became apparent. (D) Vegetations were found on the base of P$_3$ scallops of posterior leaflet. (E) After debridement, multiple abscess cavities in the AV groove were seen to communicate with both the left atrium and pericardium. Intact coronary vessels bridge the infected groove. (F) Annulus defect and communication were closed from inside the left atrium with an autologous pericardial patch. Groove was allowed to drain to the pericardium. (Reproduced with permission from Pettersson GB, Hussain ST, Shrestha NK, et al: Infective endocarditis: an atlas of disease progression for describing, staging, coding, and understanding the pathology, *J Thorac Cardiovasc Surg* 2014 Apr;147(4):1142-1149.e2.)

hospital admissions or instrumentations (eg, hemodialysis) or immunosuppression (eg, organ transplantation).

Early PVE usually affects the sewing ring or the interface of the prosthetic valve and the annulus (often a site of clot formation). Involvement of the sewing ring starts locally but eventually becomes circumferential. Enzymatic degradation of the tissue holding the sutures results in dehiscence of the prosthesis and periprosthetic leak. Progression of the infection and invasion may lead to tissue necrosis, abscess, and pseudoaneurysm formation. Mitral PVE may extend anteriorly to the fibrous trigone or posteriorly, causing AV separation.

MICROBIOLOGY

Endocarditis of native valves is most often caused by *Streptococcus viridans, Staphylococcus aureus* or *epidermidis,* or *Enterococci*, with proportions varying according to valve (native vs prosthetic), pathology stage (noninvasive vs invasive), source of infection, patient age, and coexisting conditions.[2,3,6,24-26] *S. aureus* accounts for 25 to 30% of all infections and is also the most common organism in each major risk group, including intravenous drug users and those with intracardiac devices.[4,6,25] In our study, *S. aureus* was the most common pathogen for NVE (27.6%) and the second most common cause of PVE (22.1%), for which coagulase-negative *Staphylococcus* was most common (24.1%).[8] Among the major causative organisms, *Staphylococcus* species are most likely to be associated with invasive endocarditis (49%) and *Streptococcus* least likely (11%).[16] (IE microbiology is discussed in more detail in Chapter 31.)

DIAGNOSIS

Clinical Presentation

The diverse nature and evolving epidemiologic profile of IE ensure that it remains a diagnostic challenge.[6] The clinical presentation varies according to causative organism, preexisting cardiac disease, comorbidities, and complications. Mitral IE may present as an acute, rapidly progressive infection or as a subacute or chronic disease. Up to 90% of patients present with fever, often associated with systemic symptoms of chills, poor appetite, and weight loss.[6] Other findings include a new murmur (85%) or a change in an existing murmur. Embolic phenomena may cause petechiae, Roth spots, Osler nodes, and Janeway lesions. Embolic events occur in 20 to 50% of patients. Neurologic events develop in 20 to 40% of all patients with IE and are mainly the consequence of embolism of vegetation material, while mycotic aneurysm is much less common.[6] Splenomegaly may be present in both NVE and PVE. A high index of suspicion and low threshold of investigation to exclude IE are essential to diagnose and treat these affected patients early.

Laboratory findings include an elevated white blood cell count, anemia, and hematuria. Blood cultures from separate sites are usually positive in patients with bacterial endocarditis; two positive cultures out of three are considered diagnostic. However, cultures in patients with fastidious organisms or fungi may take more than 3 weeks to become positive, although diagnostic methods have improved. When IE is suspected, ideally three or more blood cultures should be collected before antibiotics are initiated, and at least two should be obtained immediately from different peripheral sites. Additional blood cultures should be obtained a few hours later. Unless the patient is septic, it is appropriate to hold off on starting antibiotics until an adequate number of blood cultures have been collected. Cases of IE in which blood cultures are negative (10%) may reflect either patients treated with antibiotics before the blood culture was drawn or

infections caused by fastidious organisms.[3] For cases caused by fastidious organisms, serologic testing or valve or blood polymerase chain reaction (PCR) assay can identify the pathogen 60% of the time.[3,6]

Echocardiography and Imaging Studies

The present gold-standard diagnostic modality for documenting IE is transesophageal echocardiography (TEE). Specificity for TEE is approximately 90% and sensitivity is 90 to 100%.[6] In contrast, transthoracic echocardiography (TTE) is more operator dependent, and images may be compromised by surrounding structures; it is only 50% sensitive and 90% specific for IE.[6] Echocardiography must be performed as soon as IE is suspected.[6] TTE should be performed first, but often both TEE and TTE need to be performed.[6] Echocardiographic findings of IE include vegetations, periprosthetic leakage in patients with PVE, intracardiac fistulae, and abscess cavities. The echocardiographic examination is very good at evaluating valve function, but less reliable for assessing the severity and invasiveness of the infection. A negative echocardiogram does not exclude the diagnosis of IE. In situations with strong suspicion of IE, the diagnosis may be pursued by magnetic resonance imaging (MRI). In most patients with IE, MRI will demonstrate abnormal consistency of tissue in the annulus.

Metastatic infection is a possibility, and patients with IE and abdominal symptoms should undergo computed tomography (CT) scanning to rule out splenic or hepatic abscesses. Embolic infection of viscera is typically caused by staphylococcal organisms, and the brain is the most important and frequent site for emboli.[3,6] Any neurologic deficit or abnormality should trigger investigation with CT or MRI of the brain, funduscopic examination, and occasionally cerebrospinal fluid examination. We require a CT or MRI of the brain irrespective of symptoms if the patient is going to undergo operation. Preoperative coronary angiography is indicated in all patients age 40 years or older, particularly if they have a history of coronary artery disease or previous revascularization procedures, or if coronary embolization is suspected. Clinical judgment must be exercised in patients with renal dysfunction.

Diagnostic Criteria and Their Limitations

The Duke (and modified Duke) criteria for IE, based on echocardiographic results along with clinical, microbiologic, and pathologic findings, provide high sensitivity and specificity (~80% overall) for the diagnosis of IE (Table 38-1).[27] The Duke criteria, discussed in more detail in Chapter 31, are useful for the classifying IE, but do not replace clinical judgment for diagnosing IE when blood cultures are negative or when infection affects a prosthetic valve or pacemaker lead.

TABLE 38-1: Duke Criteria for Native Valve Endocarditis and Prosthetic Valve Endocarditis

Major Criteria

Positive Blood Cultures for Infective Endocarditis

Typical microorganism for infective endocarditis from two separate blood cultures: *Streptococcus viridans, S. bovis*, and HACEK group or community-acquired *Staphylococcus aureus* or *enterococci* in the absence of a primary focus, or

Persistently positive blood cultures, defined as recovery of a microorganism consistent with infective endocarditis from:

Blood cultures drawn >12 hours apart or

All of three or most of four or more separate blood cultures, with the first and last drawn at least 1 hour apart

Evidence of Endocardial Involvement

Positive echocardiogram for infective endocarditis

Oscillating intracardiac mass on valve or supporting structures or in the path of regurgitant jets or on implanted material in the absence of an alternative anatomic explanation, abscess, new partial dehiscence of prosthetic valve, or new valvular regurgitation (increase or change in preexisting murmur not sufficient)

Minor Criteria

Predisposition: predisposing heart condition or intravenous drug use

Fever: temperature ≥38 C (100.4°F)

Vascular phenomena: major arterial emboli, septic pulmonary infarcts, mycotic aneurysm, intracranial hemorrhage, conjunctival hemorrhage, and Janeway lesions

Immunologic phenomena: glomerulonephritis, Osler nodes, Roth spots, rheumatoid factor

Microbiologic evidence: positive blood culture but not meeting major criterion as noted previously or serologic evidence of active infection with organisms consistent with infective endocarditis

Echocardiogram: consistent with infective endocarditis but not meeting major criterion as noted previously

New-onset heart failure

New conduction disturbances

HACEK group = Haemophilus spp., Actinobacillus actinomycetemcomitans, Cardiobacterium hominis, Eikenella corrodens, and Kingella kingae
Data from Pérez-Vázquez A1, Fariñas MC, García-Palomo JD, et al: Evaluation of the Duke criteria in 93 episodes of prosthetic valve endocarditis: could sensitivity be improved? *Arch Intern Med.* 2000 Apr 24;160(8):1185-1191.

INDICATIONS FOR SURGERY

Surgery plays a pivotal role in managing native mitral valve endocarditis. Indications for surgical intervention in patients with NVE and PVE are presented in Table 38-2.

Congestive heart failure is the most common indication for surgery. Our indications for surgery have gradually moved toward earlier intervention to avoid devastating complications.

The majority of patients with PVE will require surgery for cure.[6,28] Indications for surgical intervention in patients with PVE include heart failure, new heart block (much less common with mitral valve IE than aortic valve IE), ongoing sepsis, valve dehiscence, recurrent systemic embolism, relapse of infection, and fungal infection. Surgery should be considered in all cases of early PVE, because most are caused by *staphylococci* or other aggressive organisms.[6,19]

Operation for large mobile vegetations to prevent embolization in both NVE and PVE remains a controversial indication in the absence of hemodynamic compromise or other surgical indications.[6] The risk of embolism is highest during the first 2 weeks of antibiotic therapy and is related to the size and mobility of the vegetation. The decision to operate early to prevent embolism thus depends on size and mobility of vegetations, previous embolism, type of microorganism, and duration of antibiotic therapy.

Fungal mitral valve PVE is uncommon and characterized by large vegetations, and these infections are even more

 TABLE 38-2: Surgical Indications for Native Valve Endocarditis and Prosthetic Valve Endocarditis

1. Severe mitral regurgitation, with or without symptoms of congestive heart failure
2. Uncontrolled sepsis despite proper antibiotic therapy
3. Presence of an antibiotic-resistant organism
4. Fungal endocarditis or endocarditis caused by *Staphylococcus aureus* or gram-negative bacteria
5. Presence of mitral annular abscess, extension of infection to intervalvular fibrous body, or formation of intracardiac fistulas
6. Onset of a new conduction disturbance
7. Large vegetations (>1 cm), particularly those that are mobile and located on the anterior leaflet, and thus at high risk for embolic complications
8. Multiple emboli despite appropriate antibiotic therapy

difficult to cure than is PVE caused by other organisms. Lifelong oral suppressive antifungal therapy after completion of intravenous therapy is often recommended.[6]

TIMING OF SURGERY

Many patients with NVE and a majority with PVE require surgical intervention, and the challenge for the surgeon is to determine the appropriate timing of surgery.[3,6,24,29-32] It is our belief that in most cases, the operation should not be delayed once surgical indications are present. It is, however, important to know the sensitivity of the organism to ensure appropriate antibiotic coverage at the time of surgery. The presence of locally uncontrollable infection indicates a need for early surgery in patients with NVE. Early surgery is required for most patients with PVE before it is complicated by heart failure, severe prosthetic dysfunction, or abscess. Patients with PVE caused by *S. aureus* risk rapid progression and invasion. The same principle applies to PVE caused by fungal or other highly resistant organisms.[6] However, delaying surgery is usually advised in the presence of cerebral complications.[6,32,33] Before valve surgery, patients with IE should undergo careful neurologic evaluation, and all should be evaluated by head CT or MRI. The standard recommendation is that surgery should be delayed for 1 to 2 weeks in patients with non-hemorrhagic strokes, and for 3 to 4 weeks in patients with hemorrhagic strokes, to reduce the risk of further intracranial bleeding during heart surgery.[6,32] Intracranial hemorrhage in the setting of PVE has been associated with mortality as high as 28 to 69%. To exclude a mycotic aneurysm, an angiography is required. Nonhemorrhagic embolic stroke has a low risk of transformation into a hemorrhagic infarct during heparinization and cardiopulmonary bypass. The risk of worsening neurologic symptoms as a consequence of operation is time related, decreasing with increasing interval from the initial neurologic event. The risk of worsening the stroke symptoms must be weighed against the indications for surgery and the risk of additional emboli during the waiting period. If cerebral hemorrhage has been excluded by CT or MRI and neurologic damage is not severe (ie, coma), surgery can be performed with a relatively low neurologic risk (3 to 6%) and good probability of complete neurologic recovery.[6]

OPERATIVE TECHNIQUES

General Principles

Operations for endocarditis are guided by some basic principles: optimal timing of surgery as discussed above, good exposure of the valve, radical debridement, optimal choice for reconstruction of the heart and repair or replacement of the valve, and adequate postoperative antibiotic treatment. Radical debridement with removal of all infected and necrotic tissue and foreign material is difficult to accomplish in mitral cases with AV groove invasion, necrosis, and abscess formation (Fig. 38-1). Aortic root infections are much easier to lay open and debride. In addition, reconstruction after invasion of the AV groove and AV separation entails closing off the infected space and leaving it without drainage.

Native Mitral Valve Endocarditis

Intraoperative TEE should be performed in all cases to carefully evaluate the valve before commencing the procedure. For NVE, our approach is to attempt repair if feasible. Mitral valve repair can be performed provided there is sufficient remaining tissue to allow valvular reconstruction.[12,34-43] Successful repair can be achieved by an experienced surgeon in up to 80% of patients.[41] If repair is not technically feasible and valve replacement is needed, the choice of a tissue or mechanical valve is based primarily on consideration of age, life expectancy, presence of comorbidities, and compliance with anticoagulation.[7,32] Although there is some experience with the mitral valve allograft for treating mitral valve IE, it remains experimental, with too few data available to support this strategy.[44]

Operations for NVE are best conducted through a full median sternotomy. Cannulation for cardiopulmonary bypass involves arterial return via the ascending aorta and bicaval cannulation for venous drainage. It is advisable to arrest the heart before manipulating it too much. Myocardial protection is achieved using antegrade and retrograde blood cardioplegia. We have a preference for opening the right atrium and placing the retrograde cardioplegia cannula directly into the coronary sinus through a purse-string suture.

The mitral valve is exposed either via a left atriotomy through the interatrial groove or transseptally through the right atrium, which is our preference. If the left atrium is small, an extended transseptal-dome approach is used. Opening the aorta allows dual exposure and is helpful in many cases for debridement and suture placement and for avoiding unnecessary damage to the aortic valve. Once good exposure of the mitral valve is accomplished, the valve is evaluated to assess for presence of paravalvular abscesses, intracardiac fistulae, or intervalvular fibrous body/ventricular involvement. Radical resection of all necrotic tissue is performed. All grossly infected tissue is removed without too much concern for the possibility of repair. Unaffected leaflet, chordae, and papillary muscles are preserved to support the posterior annulus. Specimens are divided and sent for both pathologic and microbiologic examination and need for PCR is considered.

Anterior Leaflet Repair

Kissing lesions of the anterior mitral leaflet encountered with aortic endocarditis can be repaired with autologous pericardium.[45] A patch of pericardium is sutured to the remaining tissue of the anterior leaflet with running polypropylene suture (Fig. 38-2). More extensive destruction involving both the aortic valve and the anterior leaflet of the mitral valve can be repaired using a freestanding aortic root allograft with the anterior leaflet of the mitral valve still attached. The allograft's attached aortomitral curtain can be used to reconstruct the base of the native anterior mitral leaflet.[17]

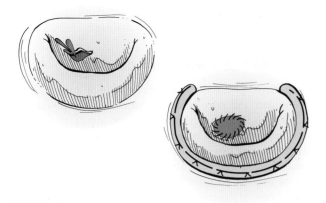

FIGURE 38-2. Repair of anterior leaflet perforation using a patch with autologous pericardium followed by annuloplasty.

Involvement of the free margin of the anterior leaflet can be managed with triangular resection. Anterior leaflet chordal rupture can be repaired with chordal transposition from the posterior leaflet or transfer of secondary chorda to the free margin of the anterior leaflet. Artificial chordae may also be used to replace ruptured anterior leaflet chordae.

Posterior Leaflet Repair

The middle scallop (P_2 segment) of the posterior leaflet is frequently affected by the infectious process. Repair can be performed with triangular or quadrangular resection of the middle scallop. A sliding repair is useful to close the gap between the remaining two scallops (Fig. 38-3). Extensive destruction of the posterior annulus requires removal of all necrotic tissue and annular reconstruction with autologous pericardium. Occasionally, repair of the annulus and the posterior leaflet can be accomplished with the same patch if chordal support to the leaflet is good. Any patch needs to be generous, and suture lines must be tension free. Running polypropylene sutures (4-0 or 5-0) are used on the entire patch. If replacement is required, a mechanical or bioprosthetic valve may then be inserted, affixing the prosthesis to the patch.[15]

Use of a prosthetic anuloplastyring in NVE may be necessary to provide a durable repair and has a low risk of reinfection.[39,40] A good and durable repair outweighs the added low risk of reinfection associated with the anuloplasty ring.

Prosthetic Valve Endocarditis

Operations for PVE are reoperations, preferably performed via a median sternotomy. A preoperative chest CT is valuable to avoid adverse events during reentry. A right anterolateral thoracotomy in the fourth intercostal space is an alternative; this approach is suggested by some as particularly useful in patients with multiple previous sternotomies, bypass grafts near the sternum, or a history of mediastinal radiation and/

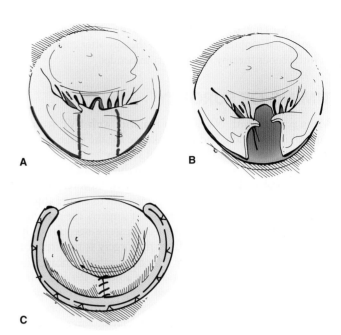

FIGURE 38-3. Quadrangular resection and sliding repair for posterior leaflet vegetation with ruptured chordae. (A, B) Segment of posterior leaflet is resected and a portion of leaflet detached from the annulus. (C) Leaflet remnants are sutured to the annulus, taking deep bites to reduce leaflet height. Leaflet edges are re-approximated in the center. Anuloplasty completes the repair.

or mediastinitis.[46,47] However, a right thoracotomy for mitral reoperations allows limited access, sometimes denies aortic clamping, and may be associated with a risk of stroke. We uniformly use sternotomy for these reoperations.

Myocardial Protection

Cardiopulmonary bypass is instituted using the ascending aorta and bicaval cannulation, and myocardial protection is achieved using antegrade and retrograde blood cardioplegia. Open direct cannulation of the coronary sinus is preferred.

Mitral Valve Exposure

Our usual approach to the mitral valve is via the right atrium and atrial septum. If the left atrium is large and adhesions modest, a standard left atriotomy may be used. Exposure may be enhanced by dividing the superior vena cava and extending the left atriotomy under the aortic root, toward the left auricle. This approach provides good exposure even when the left atrium is small. Releasing the left heart from the chest wall improves mitral valve exposure, while not doing that sometimes makes exposure very difficult. Presence of an aortic valve prosthesis also makes exposure more difficult.

Reconstruction of the Mitral Annulus

Once exposure of the mitral valve is obtained, the infected prosthesis is removed and the annulus debrided of all old suture material and pledgets. Mitral valve PVE may produce separation of the left atrium, left ventricle, and prosthesis. In these situations, the operation includes debridement of the annulus with subsequent annulus reconstruction using autologous or possibly glutaraldehyde-fixed bovine pericardium (David technique).[15,48] With this technique, a semicircular pericardial patch is used to reconstruct the annulus, with one side of the patch sutured to the endocardium of the left ventricle and the other side to the left atrium. This patch covers the cavity, which must be thoroughly debrided and sterilized before the patch is affixed. The new valve prosthesis is affixed to this reconstructed annulus (Fig. 38-4). The patch should be generous in order to minimize tension on suture lines. We look at this patch as a reinforcement of an undermined area rather than true reconstruction. The prosthesis should be implanted in such a way that there is no residual pseudo aneurysm on the ventricular side. In most situations with annular reconstruction, we use a bioprosthesis to avoid anticoagulation in the postoperative period, and have a preference for prostheses with generous soft sewing rings.

An alternative technique for mitral annular reconstruction is that described by Carpentier and colleagues.[49] This technique involves suture closure of the AV separation. Valve sutures are then placed with a large needle around this suture line with pledgets on the ventricular side. We have observed pseudoaneurysm formation after application of this technique, but still consider it useful in cases with shallow and fairly narrow AV separation.

Reconstruction of the Fibrous Trigones and Intervalvular Fibrosa

Extension of PVE into the intervalvular fibrosa/fibrous trigones may necessitate replacement of both the mitral and aortic valves. This usually occurs in the setting of PVE affecting both the aortic and mitral valves and seldom with isolated mitral valve endocarditis. Reconstruction of the intervalvular fibrosa as well as replacement of both the aortic and mitral valves are required (Fig. 38-5). In such circumstances the fibrous trigone may be reconstructed with autologous (or bovine) pericardium.[17,49-52] Perfect exposure is mandatory, whether it is provided by the extended transseptal approach or by dividing the superior vena cava and extending the left atriotomy from anterior to the right superior pulmonary vein toward the dome of the left atrium. This approach allows debridement of the aortic and mitral valves as well as the fibrous trigones. The prosthetic mitral valve is then sewn normally to the annulus posteriorly, medially, and laterally. The superior portion of the mitral valve annulus is reconstructed with a pericardial patch that supports and replaces the intervalvular fibrosa. This patch is anchored to the mitral valve annulus and the sewing ring of the prosthesis far enough back where the mitral annulus is still preserved. The patch is sandwiched between the mitral valve suture pledgets and annulus on the ventricular side. Once the mitral valve is secured in place, the aortic valve prosthesis is affixed to the aortic annulus. Posteriorly, the pericardial patch is used to

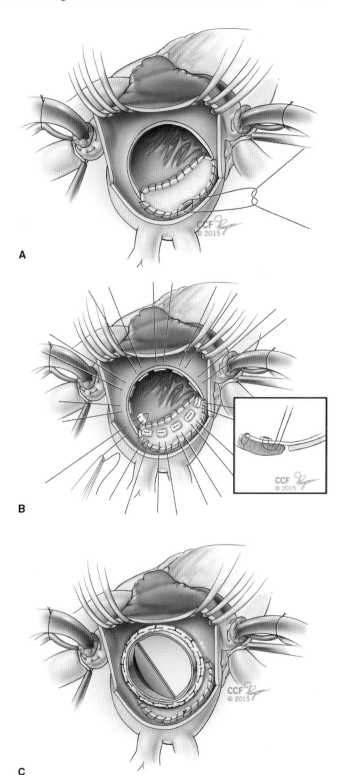

A

B

C

FIGURE 38-4 Reconstruction of mitral annulus. (A) Prosthetic valve endocarditis with posterior paravalvular abscess. The valve has been removed and the abscess debrided. A generous pericardial patch sewn to the ventricle and atrium excludes the abscess cavity and reconstructs the annulus. (B) Valve sutures are placed with the pledgets on the ventricular side. (C) A new prosthesis is affixed to the pericardial patch and annulus. (Reprinted with permission, Cleveland Clinic Center for Medical Art & Photography ©2015. All rights reserved.)

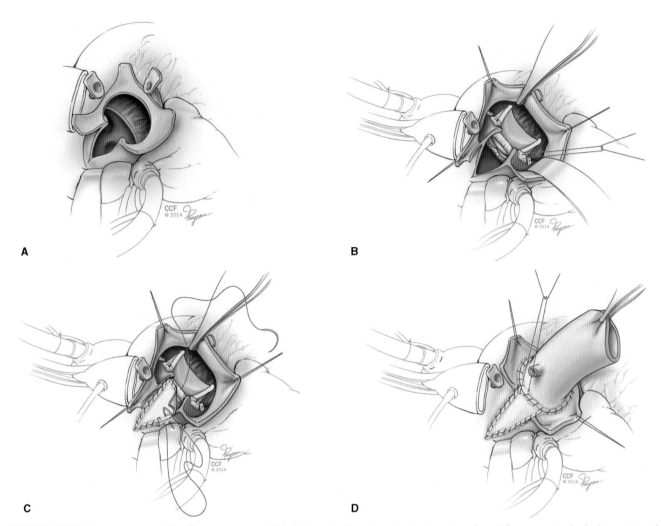

A

B

C

D

FIGURE 38-5 Reconstruction of the fibrous trigones. (A) Infection involves the mitral and aortic valves. After removing both the aortic and mitral prostheses, the divided intervalvular fibrosa converts the aortic and mitral orifices into a single large opening into the left ventricle. Notice that the planes of the mitral and aortic annuli are at right angles to each other. (B) Mitral prosthesis in place, with two-thirds of the sewing ring placed along the posterior mitral annulus and a residual defect toward the aorta anteriorly. (C) A triangular autologous pericardial patch is used to reconstruct the intervalvular fibrosa and close the roof of the left atrium. The base of the patch is sewn to the anterior third of the mitral prosthesis. (D) Implantation of an aortic allograft. The base of the allograft mitral valve is sewn to the mitral valve prosthesis and patch. It is important to pay attention to the corners by the central fibrous body and the lateral trigone in order to ensure that the corners are sealed and no sutures are under tension to avoid tears and leaks. (Reproduced with permission from Pettersson GB, Hussain ST, Ramankutty RM, et al. Reconstruction of fibrous skeleton: technique, pitfalls, and results, Multimed Man Cardiothorac Surg. 2014 Jun 18;2014.)

cover any defect in the annulus and intervalvular fibrosa, and the lateral corners are sealed. The aortic valve is then sewn to that patch.[17] Another option is aortic valve and root allograft replacement with the allograft in an anatomic position and orientation, suturing the intervalvular fibrosa/mitral valve of the allograft directly to the mitral valve prosthesis.[17]

Postoperative Antibiotic Treatment

Regardless of the mitral procedure performed, all patients with active infection receive 6 weeks of postoperative antibiotic therapy as final cure of the infection is by the antibiotics. In patients with fungal endocarditis, the intravenous treatment is followed by oral antifungal suppression for life.

RESULTS

Native Mitral Valve Endocarditis

Overall, the outcomes for patients requiring surgery for mitral valve IE are worse than for patients with aortic valve IE (Fig. 38-6).[15] This is explained by mitral IE patients being sicker as well as the fact that invasive mitral disease is surgically more difficult to deal with. Superior event-free survival, lower hospital mortality, and improved long-term survival for mitral valve repair compared with replacement have been reported (Fig. 38-7).[35-43] In our Cleveland Clinic series of 146 patients who had surgery for NVE, valve repair resulted in lower hospital mortality ($p = .008$) and better long-term survival ($p = .05$) than valve replacement.[43] Infection-free

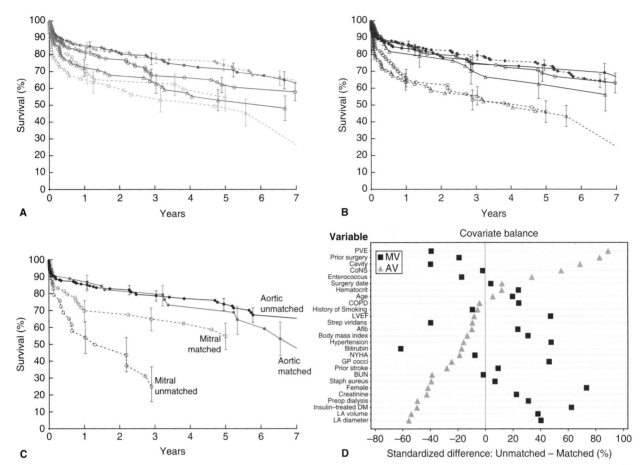

FIGURE 38-6 Survival after surgery for left-sided infective endocarditis (IE). Each *symbol* represents a death and *vertical bars* 68% confidence limits, equivalent to ± 1 standard error. *Filled circles,* aortic valve IE alone; *open circles,* mitral valve IE alone; and *triangles,* aortic and mitral valve IE. (A) Stratified by native (*solid green lines*) versus prosthetic (*dashed orange lines*) valve IE. (B) Stratified by invasive (*dashed red lines*) versus noninvasive (*solid blue lines*) IE according to valve position. (C) Stratified by propensity-matched and unmatched isolated aortic and mitral valve IE. (D) Standardized differences* between propensity matched and unmatched cases of isolated invasive mitral valve IE and isolated invasive aortic valve IE. Key: Afib, atrial fibrillation; BUN, blood urea nitrogen; CoNS, coagulase-negative staphylococci; COPD, chronic obstructive pulmonary disease; DM, diabetes mellitus; GP, Gram-positive; LA, left atrial; LVEF, left ventricular ejection fraction; NYHA, New York Heart Association; Preop, preoperative; PVE, prosthetic valve endocarditis. (Reproduced with permission from Hussain ST, Shrestha NK, Gordon SM, et al: Residual patient, anatomic, and surgical obstacles in treating active left-sided infective endocarditis, *J Thorac Cardiovasc Surg.* 2014 Sep;148(3):981-988.e4.)

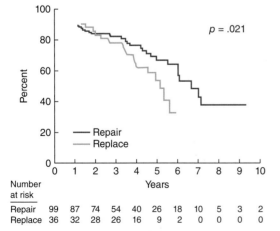

FIGURE 38-7 Event-free survival for all patients undergoing mitral valve repair or replacement. (Reproduced with permission from Muehrcke DD, Cosgrove DM 3rd, Lytle BW, et al. Is there an advantage to repairing infected mitral valves? *Ann Thorac Surg* 1997 Jun;63(6):1718-1724.)

Number at risk										
Repair	99	87	74	54	40	26	18	10	5	3	2
Replace	36	32	28	26	16	9	2	0	0	0	0

survival was also better after valve repair than replacement, with a reinfection rate of less than 1% per year.[43] The most important explanations for these excellent outcomes after valve repair are (1) less advanced disease, (2) use of less prosthetic material in the infected field, (3) better preservation of left ventricular function associated with repairing mitral valves, and (4) less sick patients. Those undergoing valve replacement were the sickest patients with the most advanced and destructive disease. The choice of prosthesis, whether bioprosthetic or mechanical, does not make a difference, as they have similar survival rates and freedom from reinfection.[32,53,54]

Prosthetic Valve Endocarditis

Despite improved antimicrobial regimens, outcomes of medical therapy alone are poor for PVE, particularly for patients with annular involvement or early endocarditis after valve surgery. PVE has been associated with a much higher operative mortality than NVE.[10,48,53] With improved understanding of the disease and better management, both medical and surgical, the results of mitral PVE now approach those of mitral NVE (Fig. 38-6).[14] Outcomes are worse for invasive mitral infection than for both invasive aortic infection and infection limited to valve cusps or leaflets, and this is true for PVE and NVE (Fig. 38-6).[14] The reason is related to the inherent mitral valve anatomy in patients with invasive disease into the AV groove, limiting our ability to perform radical debridement, sterilization, and drainage of the infected area. In addition, we lack an alternative mitral valve prosthesis that is equally optimal for IE, simple to implant, and as good as the allograft for the aortic valve. Allograft mitral valve replacement is not simple and is still experimental.[55]

REFERENCES

1. Cabell CH, Abrutyn E, Fowler VG, et al: Use of surgery in patients with native valve infective endocarditis: results from the international collaboration on endocarditis merged database. *Am Heart H* 2005; 150:1092-1098.
2. Murdroch DR, Corey GR, Hoen B, et al: Clinical presentation, etiology, and outcomes of infective endocarditis in the 21st century: the international collaboration on endocarditis-prospective study. *Arch Intern Med* 2009; 169:463-473.
3. Hoen B, Duval X: Clinical practice. Infective endocarditis. *N Engl J Med* 2013; 368:1425-1433.
4. Bashore TM, Cabell C, Fowler V Jr: Update on infective endocarditis. *Curr Probl Cardiol* 2006; 31:274-352.
5. Galve-Acebal J, Rodriguez-Bano J, Martinez-Marcos FJ, et al: Prognostic factors in left-sided endocarditis: results from the Andalusian multicenter cohort. *BMC Infect Dis* 2010; 10:17.
6. Habib G, Hoen B, Tornos P, et al: Guidelines on the prevention, diagnosis, and treatment of infective endocarditis (new version 2009). The task force on the prevention, diagnosis, and treatment of infective endocarditis of the European society of cardiology (ESC). *Eur Heart J* 2009; 30:2369-2413.
7. Bouza E, Menasalvas A, Munoz P, et al: Infective endocarditis—A prospective study at the end of the twentieth century: new predisposing conditions, new etiologic agents, and still a high mortality. *Medicine (Baltimore)* 2001; 80:298.
8. Manne MB, Shrestha NK, Lytle BW, et al: Outcomesafter surgical treatment of native and prosthetic valve infective endocarditis. *Ann Thorac Surg* 2012; 93:489-493.
9. Sabik JF, Lytle BW, Blackstone EH, et al: Aortic root replacement with cryopreserved allograft for prosthetic valve endocarditis. *Ann Thorac Surg* 2002; 74:650-659.
10. David TE, Gavra G, Feindel CM, et al: Surgical treatment of active endocarditis: a continued challenge. *J Thorac Cardiovasc Surg* 2007; 133:144-149.
11. David TE, Regesta T, Gavra G, et al: Surgical treatment of paravalvular abscess: long-term results. *Eur J Cardiothorac Surg* 2007; 31:43-48.
12. Sheikh AM, Elhenawy AM, Maganti M, et al: Outcomes for surgical intervention for isolated active mitral valve endocarditis. *J Thorac Cardiovasc Surg* 2009; 137:110-116.
13. Lytle BW, Sabik JF, Blackstone EH, et al: Reoperative cryopreserved root and ascending aorta replacement for acute aortic prosthetic valve endocarditis. *Ann Thorac Surg* 2002; 74:S1754-sa757; discussion S1792-s1799.
14. Pettersson GB, Hussain ST, Shrestha NK, et al: Infective endocarditis: an atlas of disease progression for describing, staging, coding, and understanding the pathology. *J Thorac Cardiovasc Surg* 2014; 147:1142-1149.e2.
15. David TE, Feindel CM, Armstrong S, et al: Reconstruction of the mitral annulus. A ten-year experience. *J Thorac Cardiovasc Surg* 1995; 110:1323-1332.
16. Hussain ST, Nabin NK, Gordon SM, et al: Residual patient, anatomic, and surgical obstacles in treating active left-sided infective endocarditis. *J Thorac Cardiovasc Surg* 2014; 148:981-988.
17. Pettersson GB, Hussain ST, Ramankutty RM, et al: Reconstruction of fibrous skeleton: technique, pitfalls, and results. *Multimed Man Cardiothorac Surg* Jun 18, 2014. pii: mmu004. doi: 10.1093/mmcts/mmu004. Print 2014.
18. Piper C, Hetzer R, Korfer R, et al: The importance of secondary mitral valve involvement in primary aortic valve endocarditis: the mitral kissing vegetation. *Heart* 2002; 23:79-86.
19. Gordon SM, Serkey JM, Longworth DL, et al: Early onset prosthetic valve endocarditis: the Cleveland Clinic experience 1992-1997. *Ann Thorac Surg* 2000; 69:1388-1392.
20. Agnihotri AK, McGiffin DC, Galbraith AJ, et al: The prevalence of infective endocarditis after aortic valve replacement. *J Thorac Cardiovasc Surg* 1995; 110:1708-1720.
21. Grover FL, Cohen DJ, Oprian C, et al: Determinants of the occurrence of and survival from prosthetic valve endocarditis. Experience of the Veterans Affairs Cooperative Study on Valvular Heart Disease. *J Thorac Cardiovasc Surg* 1994; 108:207-214.
22. Hammermeister KE, Sethi GK, Henderson WG, et al: A comparison of outcomes in men 11 years after heart-valve replacement with a mechanical valve or bioprosthesis. Veterans Affairs Cooperative Study on Valvular Heart Disease. *N Engl J Med* 1993; 328:1289-1296.
23. Fang G, Keys TF, Gentry LO, et al: Prosthetic valve endocarditis resulting from nosocomial bacteremia. A prospective, multicenter study. *Ann Intern Med* 1993; 119:560-567.
24. Thuny F, Grisoli D, Collart F, et al: Management of infective endocarditis: challenges and perspectives. *Lancet* 2012; 379:965-975.
25. Selton-Suty C, Celaed M, Le Moing V, et al: Preeminence of *Staphylococcus aureus* in infective endocarditis: a 1-year population-based survey. *Clin Infect Dis* 2012; 54:1230-1239.
26. Tleyjeh IM, Abdel-Latif A, Rabhi H, et al: A systematic review of population-based studies of infective endocarditis. *Chest* 2007; 132:1025-1035.
27. Li JS, Sexton DJ, Mick N, et al: Proposed modifications to the Duke criteria for the diagnosis of infective endocarditis. *Clin Infect Dis* 2000; 30:633-638.
28. Olaison L, Pettersson G: Current best practices and guidelines: indications for surgical intervention in infective endocarditis. *Infect Dis Clin North Am* 2002; 16:453.
29. Kang DH, Kim YJ, Kim SH, et al: Early surgery versus conventional treatment for infective endocarditis. *N Engl J Med* 2012; 366:2466-2473.
30. Thuny F, Beurtheret S, Mancini J, et al: The timing of surgery influences mortality and morbidity in adults with severe complicated infective endocarditis: a propensity analysis. *Eur Heart J* 2011; 32:2027-2033.
31. Ohara T, Nakatani S, Kokubo Y, et al: Clinical predictors of in-hospital death and early surgery for infective endocarditis: results of CArdiac Disease REgistration (CADRE), a nation-wide survey in Japan. *Int J Cardiol* 2013; 167:2688-2694.
32. Byrne JG, Rezai K, Sanchez JA, et al: Surgical management of endocarditis: The Society of Thoracic Surgeons clinical practice guideline. *Ann Thorac Surg* 2012; 91:2012-2019.
33. Misfeld M, Girrbach F, Etz CD: Surgery for infective endocarditis complicated by cerebral embolism: a consecutive series of 375 patients. *J Thorac Cardiovasc Surg* 2014; 147:1837-1846.
34. Dreyfus G, Serraf A, Jebara VA, et al: Valve repair in acute endocarditis. *Ann Thorac Surg* 1990; 49:706-711; discussion 712-713.
35. de Kerchove L, Vanoverschelde JL, Poncelet A, et al: Reconstructive surgery in active mitral valve endocarditis: feasibility, safety and durability. *Eur J Cardiothorac Surg* 2007; 31:592-599.
36. Shimikawa T, Kasegawa H, Matsuyama S, et al: Long-term outcomes of mitral valve repair for infective endocarditis. *Ann Thorac Surg* 2009; 88:733-739.
37. Doukas G, Oc M, Alexiou C, et al: Mitral valve repair for active culture positive infective endocarditis. *Heart* 2006; 92:361-363.
38. Feringa HH, Shaw LJ, Poldermans D, et al: Mitral valve repair and replacement in endocarditis: a systematic review of literature. *Ann Thorac Surg* 2007; 83:564-570.
39. Ruttmann E, Legit C, Poelzl G, et al: Mitral valve repair provides improved outcome over replacement in active infective endocarditis. *J Thorac Cardiovasc Surg* 2005; 130:765-771.
40. Zegdi R, Debieche M, Latremouille C, et al: Long-term results of mitral valve repair in active endocarditis. *Circulation* 2005; 111:2532-2536.

41. Feringa HH, Bax JJ, Klein P, et al: Outcome after mitral valve repair for acute and healed infective endocarditis. *Eur J Cardiothorac Surg* 2006; 29:367-373.

42. Iung B, Rousseau-Paziaud J, Cormier B, et al: Contemporary results of mitral valve repair for infective endocarditis. *J Am Coll Cardiol* 2004; 43:386-392.

43. Muehrcke DD, Cosgrove DM 3rd, Lytle BW, et al: Is there an advantage to repairing infected mitral valves? *Ann Thorac Surg* 1997; 63:1718-1724.

44. Kabbani S, Jamil H, Nabhani F, et al: Analysis of 92 mitral pulmonary autograft replacement (Ross II) operations. *J Thorac Cardiovasc Surg* 2007; 134:902-908.

45. Gillinov AM, Diaz R, Blackstone EH, et al: Double valve endocarditis. *Ann Thorac Surg* 2001; 71:1874-1879.

46. Byrne JG, Karavas AN, Adams DH, et al: The preferred approach for mitral valve surgery after CABG: right thoracotomy, hypothermia and avoidance of LIMA-LAD graft. *J Heart Valve Dis* 2001; 10:584-590.

47. Adams DH, Filsoufi F, Byrne JG, et al: Mitral valve repair in redo cardiac surgery. *J Card Surg* 2002; 17:40-45.

48. David TE: The surgical treatment of patients with prosthetic valve endocarditis. *Semin Thorac Cardiovasc Surg* 1995; 7:47-53.

49. Carpentier AF, Pellerin M, Fuzellier JF, et al: Extensive calcification of the mitral valve annulus: pathology and surgical management. *J Thorac Cardiovasc Surg* 1996; 111:718.

50. De Olivera NC, David TE, Armstrong TE, et al: Aortic and mitral valve replacement with reconstruction of intervalvular fibrosa: an analysis of clinical outcomes. *J Thorac Cardiovasc Surg* 2005; 129:286-290.

51. Kim SW, Park PW, Kim SW, et al: Long-term results of aortomitral fibrous body reconstruction with double-valve replacement. *Ann Thorac Surg* 2013; 95:635-641.

52. Davierwala PM, Binner C, Subramanian S, et al: Double valve replacement and reconstruction of the intervalvular fibrous body in patients with active infective endocarditis. *Eur J Cardiothorac Surg* 2014; 45:146-152.

53. Moon MR, Miller DC, Moore KA, et al: Treatment of endocarditis with valve replacement: the question of tissue versus mechanical prosthesis. *Ann Thorac Surg* 2001; 71:1164-1171.

54. Kaiser SP, Melby SJ, Zierer A, et al: Long-term outcomes in valve replacement surgery for infective endocarditis. *Ann Thorac Surg* 2007; 83:30-35.

55. Navia JL, Al-Ruzzeh S, Gordon S, et al: The incorporated aortomitral homograft: a new surgical option for double valve endocarditis. *J Thorac Cardiovasc Surg* 2010; 139:1077-1081.

Mitral Valve Repair for Congenital Mitral Valve Disease in the Adult

David P. Bichell • Bret Mettler

39

Isolated, non-reoperative congenital mitral valve abnormalities in adults are rare.[1,2] Mitral pathology concurrent with other cardiac anomalies is less rare. Atrial septal defect is the third commonest congenital cardiac lesion presenting in adulthood, occurring in an estimated 1/5700 persons, nearly 10% are ostium primum defects, and almost all primum defects have an associated mitral valve cleft.[3] Congenital mitral valve pathology such as arcade or parachute mitral valve very rarely present in adulthood, though the patients surviving unrepaired to adulthood may be milder forms, amenable to repair.

In contrast to the rarity of non-reoperative mitral pathology presenting in adulthood, patients needing reoperation for formerly corrected mitral pathology represent an expanding adult population. Survivors of corrective surgery in infancy and childhood add an estimated 8960 new adults cases annually to the adult congenital population in the US and there are over 1,000,000 adults living in the US today with congenital heart disease.[4] The prevalence of atrioventricular septal defect (AVSD) is 5.3 per 10,000 live births.[5] Mitral insufficiency is the principal reason for reoperation in the AVSD population. For patients undergoing an anatomic repair for complete or partial AVSD in infancy, freedom from reoperation for mitral regurgitation (MR) is 81 to 83% at 15 years, so the number of adults presenting with the need for reoperative mitral valve surgery is steadily increasing as successful infant repairs continue to accrue.[6]

PATHOPHYSIOLOGY

Normal Mitral Valve

Consideration of the normal mitral apparatus is important to the success of any repair for congenital mitral valve abnormalities. Congenital mitral valve pathology is widely variable between patients, demanding an individualized approach to each. A systematic analysis of the annular, leaflet, and subvalvar support structures informs a surgical strategy that can be tailored to the individual.

Annulus

The normal mitral valve is attached to a dynamic, saddle-shaped fibrous annulus with the horn of the saddle at the anterior annulus, and the low points of the saddle at the commissures—a shape that minimizes leaflet stress through the cardiac cycle (Fig. 39-1).[7] The annulus is dynamic through the cardiac cycle, with apical to basilar displacement of the entire annulus, annular "folding" that changes the planar versus saddle configuration of the annulus, and a 23 to 40% contraction in annular circumference between systole and diastole.[8]

Leaflets

The anterior, or aortic leaflet, occupies one-third of the annular circumference, is broader than the posterior leaflet, and is anchored in its continuity with the aortic annulus. The posterior, or mural leaflet occupies two-thirds of the annulus and is narrower than the anterior leaflet.[8] The leaflets are divided into named regions A1, P1, A2, P2, A3, P3, descriptive designations that are useful to consider in a systematic examination of the valve at repair (Fig. 39-1).

Subvalvar apparatus

All chordal leaflet support radiates from the anterolateral and posteromedial papillary muscles that are anchored on the free wall of the left ventricle, and correspond to the anterolateral and posteromedial commissures of the valve. Chordal attachments are at the free edge ("primary" or "marginal" chordae), the mid leaflet, ("secondary" or "rough zone" chordae), or closer to the hingepoint/annulus ("tertiary" or "basal" chordae).[8] Papillary muscle separation is important to normal

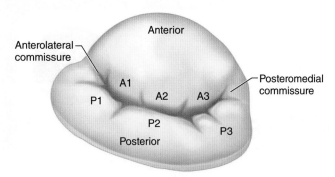

FIGURE 39-1 Descriptive anatomy of the mitral valve. The annulus is saddle-shaped, with commissures at the low points. Anterior and posterior leaflets and their subvalvar support structures are described as anterior and posterior components of 3 segments.

valve excursion, and fusion or close spacing produces functional valve stenosis.

The physiologic patterns that result from congenital dysplasias of the mitral valve defy clean categorization, as several conditions produce stenosis and insufficiency together, in variable combination. We organize our description of anatomic mitral malformations into (1) lesions predominantly causing stenosis, (2) those commonly associated with combined stenosis and regurgitation, and (3) those predominantly associated with regurgitation.

Congenital Mitral Stenosis

Ruckman and Van Praagh categorized primary congenital mitral stenosis into four basic subtypes, based on autopsy data: (1) typical, (2) hypoplastic, (3) supravalvar ring, and (4) parachute mitral valve (Fig. 39-2).[9] We will describe these categories, including a broader spectrum of supravalvar entities with supravalvar ring, and a variety of subvalvar pathologies in addition to parachute mitral valve.

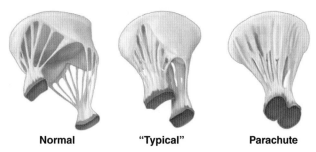

Normal   **"Typical"**   **Parachute**

FIGURE 39-2 Papillary muscle and chordal arrangement in congenital forms of mitral stenosis. LEFT: The "normal" mitral valve, with well-spaced papillary muscles, chordal support radiating from papillary muscles to their respective commissures and supporting the leaflets. Leaflets separate fully in diastole to permit optimal, unobstructed left ventricular filling. MIDDLE: The "typical" form of mitral stenosis, with normal sized annulus, closely spaced papillary muscles with inflow restriction owing to restrictive interchordal spaces and restricted leaflet mobility. RIGHT: The "parachute" deformity, with a single papillary muscle, inflow restriction at tight interchordal spaces and tethered leaflets.

Typical

In the "typical" variant of congenital valvar stenosis, the left ventricular size is normal, the mitral annulus is normal, and obstruction occurs within the valve elements themselves. The interchordal spaces are obstructed by fibrous tissue, leaflets may be thickened, chordae shortened, and papillary muscles, though distinct, are closely spaced.[9] In some cases, the chordal apparatus is nearly absent, and papillary muscle tissue may insert directly and rigidly onto the leaflet itself, greatly reducing leaflet mobility and options for repair.

Hypoplastic

The hypoplastic variant is usually associated with other left-sided abnormalities such as ventricular hypoplasia, aortic stenosis, aortic arch hypoplasia, or coarctation of the aorta. The mitral annulus itself is small, and multiple valve elements are small. Hypoplastic mitral stenosis generally produces physiology that is either lethal or requires surgical palliation in infancy, and is therefore seldom found in the adult.[9]

Supramitral Ring and other Supravalvar Pathology

Supravalvar obstruction to mitral inflow presenting in adulthood can take a variety of forms, causing inflow obstruction from a level remote from the valve (such as Cor Triatriatum), adjacent to the valve (supravalvar ring), or intimately associated with the valve (intramitral ring) (Fig. 39-3).

Cor triatriatum is embrologically distinct from true mitral valve stenosis, buts acts similarly, is encountered in the adult, and is therefore included. Cor Triatriatum is a membranous subdivision of the left atrium into two chambers—an upper chamber that receives the pulmonary veins, and a lower chamber that excludes pulmonary veins but includes the left atrial appendage. An "os" in the membrane is the portal through which all pulmonary venous return passes to the lower chamber and in turn through the mitral valve. Cor triatriatum can present with mild-to-severe restriction to mitral inflow, depending on the size of the os and the alternate pathways of left ventricular filling that may exist (Fig. 39-3).[10,11]

The true **supramitral ring** is a fibrous structure residing on the atrial side of the mitral annulus, with variable adherence to the mitral valve leaflet itself. It can produce restriction to inflow according to the size of the inflow orifice, and by restricting the movement of the leaflet itself when adherent (Fig. 39-3).

The **intramitral ring** is a thin fibrous membrane intimately associated with the leaflets and restricting leaflet excursion. The intramitral ring is always associated with subvalvar pathology (Fig. 39-3).[12]

A persistent left superior vena cava, present in 0.3 to 0.5% of population, courses across the floor of the left atrium in the supramitral area, and has been described to itself, uncommonly, produce a supravalvar obstruction.[13,14]

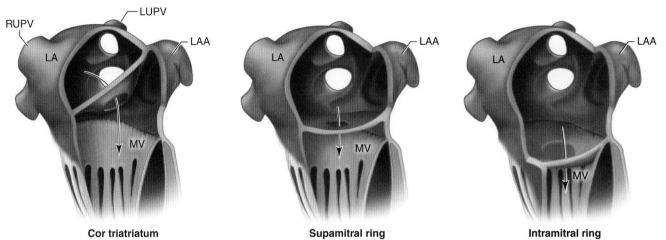

FIGURE 39-3 Congenital forms of supravalvar mitral stenosis. LEFT: Cor triatriatum is a membranous subdivision of the left atrium into two chambers. The upstream chamber contains the pulmonary veins and the downstream chamber includes the left atrial appendage. MIDDLE: The "supramitral ring" is a membranous restriction to mitral inflow that is downstream of pulmonary veins and atrial appendage, resides in close proximity to the mitral valve, sometime fused with mitral leaflet. RIGHT: The "intramitral ring" is a membranous restriction to mitral inflow that is integral with the valve leaflets themselves. RUPV, right upper pulmonary vein; LUPV, left upper pulmonary vein; LAA, Left atrial appendage; LA, left atrium; MV, mitral valve.

Parachute Mitral Valve and Other Subvalvar Pathology

There are a great variety of types of subvalvar obstruction and an understanding of the differences is important to any operative strategy to repair them.

True *"parachute mitral valve"* presenting in adulthood is very rare, with only nine published cases of isolated parachute mitral valve in adults reported over 50 years.[1] An embryologic failure in the separation of papillary muscles into two distinct columns results in parachute mitral valve, with a single papillary muscle from which all chordae radiate.[1,15] Annular and subannular restriction to mitral inflow results from thickened, shortened chordae, tethered to a single papillary origin, with tight interchordal spaces and restriction of leaflet excursion.[1] Mitral insufficiency may accompany mitral stenosis, possibly due to ischemic dysfunction of the single papillary muscle.[1] Parachute mitral valve is commonly associated with additional left heart pathology. *"Shone's"* complex is a constellation of left sided anomalies that includes a parachute mitral valve deformity, supramitral ring, subaortic stenosis, and coarctation of the aorta. The original description by John Shone in 1963 was from autopsy data from eight cases, including one adult, noting the tendency for additional left sided pathology to accompany parachute mitral valve, and the severity of disease that accounts for its rare presentation in adulthood.[15] These concomitant pathologies commonly drive the need for palliative or corrective interventions in childhood, leaving rare instances of isolated parachute mitral valve to present in adulthood.[17] *"Parachute-like mitral asymmetry"* is a similar but distinct entity where there are two distinct papillary muscles, but the anterolateral muscle is underdeveloped, short, and imparts restriction to the valve similar to that of true parachute valve.[12,17]

COMBINED MITRAL STENOSIS AND INSUFFICIENCY

Dysplasia of the mitral valve that restricts leaflet motion results in the same pathology causing both stenosis and regurgitation. Though mostly associated with stenosis, parachute mitral valve can produce regurgitation too, usually due to restricted anterior leaflet excursion. Repair may include extension of the anterior leaflet.

MITRAL ARCADE

Mitral arcade results from an embryonic failure of the elongation of mitral valve chordae. In severe cases, there are no distinct chordae and papillary muscles insert directly onto the free edge of the leaflet. The term arcade refers to the continuous band of dysplastic chordal tissue, in continuity with the mitral valve leaflet edge, that arcs between papillary muscle bases (Fig. 39-4). Papillary muscles may be indistinct or multiple. Restricted interchordal spaces and restricted leaflet mobility produce insufficiency and stenosis, often in combination.[2,12,18]

Hammock Mitral Valve

The "Hammock" mitral valve describes the appearance of a concave distortion of the posterior leaflet that results from extraneous papillary muscles and secondary chordae pulling the posterior leaflet apically and restricting its motion.[19]

Mitral arcade and Hammock mitral valve may present a combination of stenosis and insufficiency, usually associated

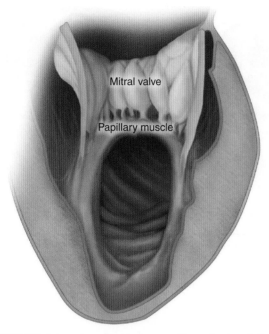

FIGURE 39-4 Mitral arcade, characterized by undeveloped chordal structures, indistinct or multiple papillary muscles, often fusing with leaflet edge to form a rigid bridge between papillary muscle bases.

with restricted excursion of the posterior leaflet, which may require augmentation as part of its repair.

Indications for Operative Intervention for Mitral Stenosis

Surgical indications for adults with congenital mitral stenosis are identical to those for acquired disease, and are detailed in the 2014 AHA/ACC consensus guidelines.[20] In brief, percutaneous balloon valvotomy is recommended for symptomatic patients with severe MS (valve inflow area of ≤1.5 cm²), if valve morphology is judged amenable to balloon palliation. Indication for surgical intervention includes severely symptomatic patients (HYHA Class III/IV) with severe mitral stenosis (≤1.5 cm²). Patients with moderate (1.6 to 2.0 cm²) to severe mitral stenosis (≤1.5 cm²) are considered for surgical intervention in the setting of concomitant cardiac surgery. Currently, there are no indications for surgical intervention in asymptomatic patients. Additional considerations at operation include resection of the left atrial appendage for patients with embolic events on anticoagulation for atrial fibrillation.[20]

REPAIR TECHNIQUES FOR CONGENITAL MITRAL STENOSIS

Fundamental to success in repair of mitral stenosis or insufficiency with restricted leaflet excursion is to create freely

mobile leaflets that permit unobstructed ventricular filling in diastole, and are sufficient in surface area and support to form a large surface area of coaptation in systole.

Supravalvar Mitral Stenosis Repair

The repair for supravalvar restriction to mitral inflow consists of a complete resection of the obstructive Cor triatriatum membrane or supravalvar mitral ring. The true supravalvar mitral ring or intramitral ring can be densely adherent to the leaflets and care must be taken to perform a complete resection of the fibroelastic membrane. Careful blunt dissection techniques establish a plane between true leaflet and membrane. Careful intraoperative assessment of additional associated mitral abnormalities must be made in addition to membrane resection.

Annular Mitral Stenosis Repair

Annular hypoplasia requires annular enlargement. Adjacent vital structures considerably limit the options to enlarge the mitral annulus. The adjacent aortic valve limits annular enlargement anteriorly, between the trigones. The His bundle limits annular enlargement rightward of the aorta, and the circumflex coronary artery lies subjacent to the posterior and leftward annular perimeter. Extensive annular resection may preclude valve repair, obligating valve replacement into the enlarged annular area or in the supra-annular position (Fig. 39-5).

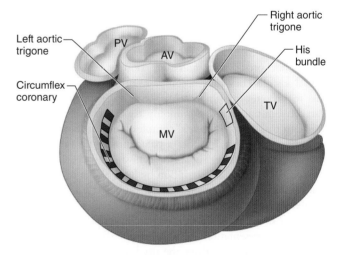

FIGURE 39-5 Surgical landmarks of the mitral valve annulus, and anatomic limitations to annular enlargement. The mitral annulus between right and left aortic trigones is tissue shared with the aortic valve annulus. Rightward of the right trigone is an area adjacent to the His bundle. Subjacent to the posterior and leftward aspect of the mitral annulus is the circumflex coronary artery.

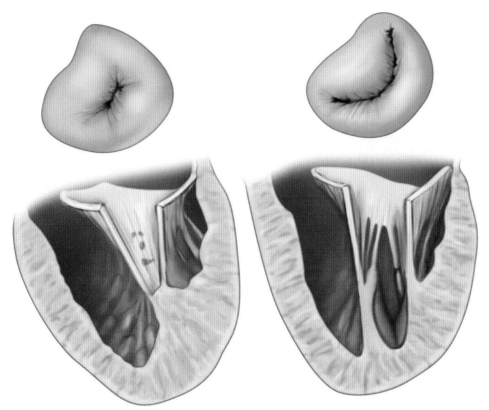

FIGURE 39-6 Parachute mitral valve, viewed en face (upper panel) and in cut-away view (lower panel). (A) Poorly developed commisures, fused chordae, leaflets tethered to a single papillary muscle. (B) After valvuloplasty consisting of the creation of commissural leaflet separation, interchordal fenestration, and the splitting if the single papillary muscle.

Subvalvar Mitral Stenosis Repair

The variant of congenital mitral stenosis classified as "typical" shares many features of parachute mitral valve, parachute-like mitral valve, hammock, and arcade. All are principally defined by subannular pathology, with normal or even dilated true annulus. The overlap between parachute mitral valve, parachute-like, arcade, and hammock has prompted the suggestion that they lie on a continuum and are not discrete entities.[21] We will describe a systematic operative approach applicable to all these lesions, with reference to specific lesions where special attention is warranted. The approach aims sequentially at all levels of restrictive valve architecture. A fibroelastic layer adherent to the leaflet is carefully dissected from the true leaflet, starting from the atrial side at the annulus and working toward the free edge, in a manner similar to that of supravalvar ring resection. Orificial restriction is relieved by commissurotomies. In the case of true parachute mitral valve, the leaflets act as a single funnel-shaped structure, and commissures are designed in "assumed" locations that radiate from the papillary muscle tip toward each trigone.[22] Restrictive interchordal spaces are opened by chordal thinning and chordal fenestration. Papilllary muscles are split where fused or closely spaced. In true parachute mitral valve, the single papillary muscle requires aggressive and complete splitting, and possibly thinning, to permit optimal separation in diastole (Fig. 39-6). Particularly referable to Hammock mitral valve, posterior leaflet restriction can be alleviated by detaching the leaflet from the annulus, reflecting it away from the annulus to expose the subvalvar pathology. This exposure permits the division of any secondary chordae or papillary attachments, and the alleviation of leaflet tethering by the separation of fused papillary muscle from the ventricular free wall (Fig. 39-7).[19] Where shortened chordae insert directly into ventricular free wall without a distinct papillary muscle, papillary-like structures can be sculpted by splitting muscle tissue away from true ventricular free wall.[22] With optimal mobilization of the leaflets, anterior and posterior leaflet height can be assessed and patch augmentation carried out as necessary to produce full leaflet mobility. Artificial chordae can be constructed to support prolapsing or unsupported portions of the rehabilitated valve.[19]

Intraoperative valve testing is performed by infusing saline into the ventricle. Intraoperative echocardiography is an essential adjunct to assure the integrity of any valve repair.

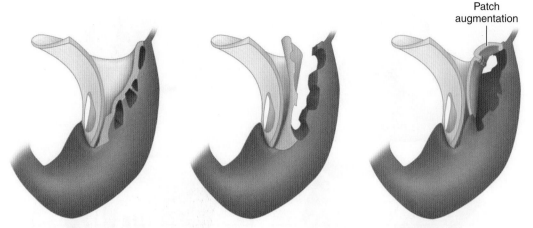

Patch augmentation

FIGURE 39-7 Repair for Hammock deformity of the mitral valve. The concave and tethered posterior leaflet (left) is detached, reflected anteriorly, and muscular attachments are divided (middle). Patch augmentation (right) further mobilizes the leaflet to permit coaptation with the anterior leaflet.

CONGENITAL MITRAL INSUFFICIENCY

Levy and Edwards classified congenital mitral insufficiency into four categories: (1) cleft leaflet (anterior or posterior), (2) anterior leaflet tissue deficiency, (3) double orifice mitral valve, and (4) anomalous mitral chordae.[23] We will organize our description of primary congenital mitral valve pathology around these major categoric headings, and further describe the growing spectrum of reoperative mitral valve pathology.

Cleft Leaflet

Mitral valve cleft can occur in isolation, but is more commonly associated with primum atrial septal defect, partial or complete AVSD. The cleft is centrally situated on the anterior leaflet, and is an inverted "V"-shaped separation of the halves of the leaflet toward the papillary muscles. While the central portion of the normal anterior leaflet has chordal support from both papillary muscles and ample leaflet surface to form a stable zone of apposition with the posterior leaflet, the cleft leaflet may suffer from insufficient leaflet material and insufficient chordal support in the central zone of apposition, producing a central regurgitant jet, and challenging the integrity of repair (Fig. 39-8).[24]

Double Orifice Mitral Valve

Double orifice mitral valve is defined as a single annulus with two complete orifices, as distinct from **duplicate mitral valve**, where there are two complete and distinct valves with complete annuli. In double orifice mitral valve, the smaller orifice is typically posteromedial, and the bridging tissue between orifices can be complete or partial.[12] though stenosis can be present, the physiologic consequence of double orifice mitral valve is predominantly insufficiency. There is frequent association with additional cardiac defects, most typically

some form of AVSD, or in combination with obstructive pathologies of the left heart.[12]

Ebstein's Malformation of the Mitral Valve

This exceedingly rare entity is characterized by MR from a posterior leaflet that is flattened against the ventricular wall and with apical annular displacement.[12]

INDICATIONS FOR OPERATIVE INTERVENTION FOR MITRAL INSUFFICIENCY

Indications for operative intervention for congenital mitral insufficiency are also identical to those for acquired disease, and are outlined in the 2014 AHA/ACC consensus guidelines.[20] In brief, mitral surgery is recommended for symptomatic patients with chronic severe MR and left

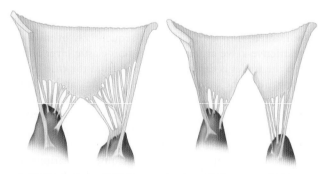

FIGURE 39-8 Leaflet and chordal arrangement of the normal mitral valve (left panel), and cleft mitral valve (right panel). With mitral cleft, leaflet tissue and chordal support may be deficient at the central zone of apposition.

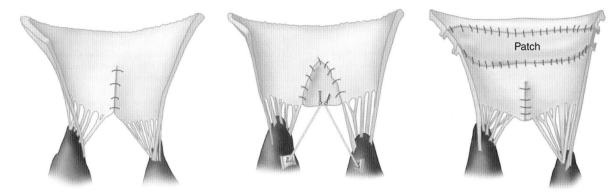

FIGURE 39-9 Strategies for repair of mitral cleft. Direct closure alone (left) may result in leaflet restriction and reduced area of apposition with the posterior leaflet. Patch augmentation of the deficient central leaflet lacks chordal support, and artificial chordae may be necessary (middle). Cleft closure with leaflet detachment near the annulus and patch augmentation (right) can improve leaflet mobility and surface area of coaptation with the posterior leaflet.

ventricular ejection fraction (LVEF) >30%, or for asymptomatic patients with chronic severe MR and LV dysfunction (LVEF 30 to 60% or LV end-systolic dimension, LVESD ≥ 40 mm). Asymptomatic patients with chronic severe MR and preserved LV function (LVEF >60%, LVESD < 40 mm) are considered for repair if judged a high likelihood of durable success, or in the setting of new onset AF, resting pulmonary hypertension (pulmonary artery pressure >50 mm Hg), or in the setting of concomitant cardiac surgery.[20]

REPAIR TECHNIQUES FOR MITRAL INSUFFICIENCY

Repair of an isolated cleft may be performed with direct closure if adequate anterior leaflet is present (Fig. 39-9). When found in association with double orifice mitral valve, complete cleft closure can result in stenosis, and valve replacement may be an only option when insufficiency persists.[12] At repair of mitral valve cleft, it is important to study the leaflet morphology to treat any deficiencies in the surface area. In those cases, simple cleft closure alone is ineffective, and leaflet augmentation should be considered in conjunction with cleft closure. The simplest augmentation for mitral cleft fills the primary inverted "V" deficiency that is central and at the zone of apposition. A wedge-shaped patch of glutaraldehyde-fixed pericardium can be used to augment the deficit directly. To prevent prolapse of the augmented central segment, chordal transfer or chordal construction can be added to the repair strategy (Fig. 39-9).[25]

In more complicated, often reoperative cases, leaflet dysplasia with deficient surface area may extend beyond the central portion of the leaflet, precluding effective repair by direct closure or central leaflet augmentation alone. Generalized deficient, dysplastic leaflet may require a radial leaflet detachment from the annulus with patch augmentation to produce or restore adequate leaflet height and mobility, and to effect competent coaptation (Fig. 39-9).[26]

Further maneuvers to improve coaptation surface at repair include posterior leaflet quadrangular resection and eccentric posterior annular reduction.[27] Posterior leaflet quadrangular resection with reduction posterior annuloplasty, chordal shortening, lengthening, and replacement techniques is discussed in detail in previous chapters.

REFERENCES

1. Hakim FA, Kendall CB, Alharthi M, et al: Parachute mitral valve in adults-a systematic overview. *Echocardiography* 2010; 275:581-586.
2. Hakim FA, Krishnaswamy C, Mookadam F: Mitral arcade in adults—a systematic overview. *Echocardiography* 2013; 303:354-359.
3. Seldon WA, Rubenstein C, Fraser AA: The incidence of atrial septal defect in adults. *Br Heart J* 1962; 24:557-560.
4. Warnes CA, Williams RG, Bashore TM, et al: ACC/AHA 2008 Guidelines for the Management of Adults With Congenital Heart Disease: A Report of the American College of Cardiology/American Heart Association Task Force on Practice Guidelines (Writing Committee to Develop Guidelines on the Management of Adults With Congenital Heart Disease) Developed in Collaboration With the American Society of Echocardiography, Heart Rhythm Society, International Society for Adult Congenital Heart Disease, Society for Cardiovascular Angiography and Interventions, and Society of Thoracic Surgeons. *J Am Coll Cardiol* 2008; 5223:e143-e263.
5. Christensen N, Andersen H, Garne E, et al: Atrioventricular septal defects among infants in Europe: a population-based study of prevalence, associated anomalies, and survival. *Cardiol Young* 2012; 2304:560-567.
6. Hoohenkerk GJF, Bruggemans EF, Koolbergen DR, et al: Long-term results of reoperation for left atrioventricular valve regurgitation after correction of atrioventricular septal defects. *Ann Thorac Surg* 2012; 933:849-55.
7. Salgo IS, Gorman JH, Gorman RC, et al: Effect of annular shape on leaflet curvature in reducing mitral leaflet stress. *Circulation* 2002; 1066:711-717.
8. Muresian H: The clinical anatomy of the mitral valve. Tubbs RS, Anderson RH, Loukas M, eds. *Clin Anat* 2009; 221:85-98.
9. Ruckman RN, van Praagh R: Anatomic types of congenital mitral stenosis: report of 49 autopsy cases with consideration of diagnosis and surgical implications. *Am J Cardiol* 1978; 424:592-601.
10. Slight RD, Nzewi OC, Buell R, et al: Cor-Triatriatum sinister presenting in the adult as mitral stenosis: an analysis of factors which may be relevant in late presentation. *Heart, Lung & Circulation* 2005; 141:8-12.
11. Saxena P, Burkhart HM, Schaff HV, et al: Surgical repair of cor triatriatum sinister: the Mayo Clinic 50-year experience. *Ann Thorac Surg* 2014; 975:1659-1663.
12. Séguéla PE, Houyel L, Acar P: Congenital malformations of the mitral valve. *Archives of Cardiovascular Diseases* 2011; 104:465-479.

13. Bjerregaard P, Laursen HB: Persistent left superior vena cava. Incidence, associated congenital heart defects and frontal P-wave axis in a pediatric population with congenital heart disease. *Acta Paediatr* 1980; 69:105-108.

14. Agnoleti G, Annecchino F, Preda L, et al: Persistence of the left superior caval vein: can it potentiate obstructive lesions of the left ventricle? *Cardiol Young* 1999; 93:285-290.

15. Shone JD, Sellers RD, Anderson RC, et al: The developmental complex of "parachute mitral valve," supravalvular ring of left atrium, subaortic stenosis, and coarctation of aorta. *Am J Cardiol* 1963; 116:714-725.

16. Davachi F, Moller JH, Edwards JE: Diseases of the Mitral Valve in Infancy: An Anatomic Analysis of 55 Cases. *Circulation* 1971; 434:565-579.

17. Oosthoek PW, Wenink AC, Wisse LJ, et al: Development of the papillary muscles of the mitral valve: morphogenetic background of parachute-like asymmetric mitral valves and other mitral valve anomalies. *J Thorac Cardiovasc Surg* 1998; 1161:36-46.

18. Layman TE, Edwards JE: Anomalous mitral arcade: a type of congenital mitral insufficiency. *Circulation* 1967: 352:389-395.

19. del Nido PJ, Baird C: Congenital mitral valve stenosis: anatomic variants and surgical reconstruction. *Semin Thorac Cardiovasc Surg* 2012; 15:69-74.

20. Nishimura RA, Otto CM, Bonow RO, et al: 2014 AHA/ACC guideline for the management of patients with valvular heart disease: executive summary: a report of the American College of Cardiology/American Heart Association Task Force on Practice Guidelines. *J Am Coll Cardiol* 2014; 6322:2438-2488.

21. Remenyi B, Gentles TL: Congenital mitral valve lesions: correlation between morphology and imaging. *Ann Pediatr Cardiol* 2012;51:3-12.

22. Delmo Walter EM, Hetzer R: Mitral valve repair in children. In Hetzer R., Rankin JS, and Yankah CA: *Mitral Valve Repair*. Heidelberg, Steinkopff, 2011:41-56.

23. Levy MJ, Edwards JE: Anatomy of mitral insufficiency. *Prog Cardiovasc Dis* 1962; 52:119-144.

24. Kanani M, Elliott M, Cook A, et al: Late incompetence of the left atrioventricular valve after repair of atrioventricular septal defects: the morphologic perspective. *J Thorac Cardiovasc Surg* 2006; 1323:640-643.

25. Artrip JH, Rumball EM, Finucane K: Repair of left atrioventricular valve cleft defects with patch augmentation. *Ann Thorac Surg* 2012; 936:2081-2083.

26. Poirier NC, Williams WG, van Arsdell GS, et al: A novel repair for patients with atrioventricular septal defect requiring reoperation for left atrioventricular valve regurgitation. *Eur J Cardiothorac Surg* 2000; 18:54-61.

27. Padala M, Vasilyev NV, Owen JW Jr, et al: Cleft closure and undersizing annuloplasty improve mitral repair in atrioventricular canal defects. *J Thorac Cardiovasc Surg* 2008; 1365:1243-1249.

40

Minimally Invasive and Robotic Mitral and Tricuspid Valve Surgery

W. Randolph Chitwood, Jr. • Barbara Robinson • L. Wiley Nifong

Minimally invasive mitral valve surgery (MIS) refers to a collection of techniques and operation-specific technologies, all of which are designed to lessen surgical trauma and improve clinical outcomes. In the last 20 years, enhanced visualization and instrumentation as well as modified perfusion and aortic occlusion methods have propelled the development of MIS operations. Cohn and Cosgrove (1996) first modified cardiopulmonary bypass techniques to enable safe, effective, minimally invasive aortic and mitral valve surgery.[1-3] Concurrently, innovative port-access methods, using endo-aortic balloon occlusion, were proven to be effective.[4,5] Thereafter, video-assisted and robotic methods were developed and applied effectively by several surgical groups.

Despite acceptance today, many surgeons initially were very critical of performing any complex valve operations through small incisions, owing to safety risks and the possibility of inferior results.[6,7] Since then many institutions worldwide have published excellent MIS comparative outcomes with traditional surgery. These showed definite clinical advantages, which included decreased blood loss and less transfusions as well as minimal postoperative care and pain. Collectively, these translated into shorter hospital stays, faster return to normal activities, less use of rehabilitation resources, and overall healthcare cost savings. Each of these advantages has been a driver for the continued development and expansion of MIS operations.

Today, replacing and repairing cardiac valves through small incisions is a standard practice. The combination of alternative sternal and thoracotomy approaches, new aortic clamping techniques, modified cardiopulmonary bypass circuits and cannulas, shafted-instruments, and three previous generations of robotic systems, all have set the stage for current minimally invasive and robotic mitral surgery, which has gained acceptance at many centers worldwide. Large institutional series as well as several meta-analyses have confirmed that MIS mitral valve surgery is safe and effective for most patients.[8-14] Although overall mitral repair rates in the United States have increased from 51% in 2000 to 62% in 2010, adoption of minimally invasive operations lags behind at less than 30% of repair cases.[15-17] In comparison, in 2015 nearly 50% of over 5000 mitral valve repairs in Germany were done minimally invasively.[18] At our center, mitral repair rates approach 100% for both MIS and robotic operations in selected patients with degenerative mitral disease.

With better understanding of the natural history of degenerative mitral valve disease, more *asymptomatic patients* now are being referred for repairs. Recent 2014 ACC/AHA (United States) and/or 2012 ESC/EACTS (European) Heart Valve Guidelines suggested that these patients should be referred only to high volume centers, having a heart team approach with a 95% chance of a repair and less than 1% operative mortality.[19,20] These same "high bar" standards now have been set for minimally invasive repairs. To this end, surgeons who plan to embark on this trek should have significant experience in repairing valves through a sternotomy as well as have a significant patient volume, a unified heart team, and full support from the operating room and hospital administration.[16]

Hopefully, this chapter will serve both as an educational tool and helpful guide for those who plan to do, or currently are doing, minimally invasive mitral and tricuspid valve surgery. Today, most surgeons have reserved the hemisternotomy for aortic valve surgery. The majority of minimally invasive mitral and tricuspid repairs are done either through a right minithoracotomy or even less invasive port access methods. Thus, this chapter will relate only to direct-vision, video-assisted (endoscopic), and robot-assisted MIS mitral/tricuspid operations performed via right thorax access.

EVOLUTION OF MITRAL VALVE REPAIR SURGERY

The First Operations

T. Lauder Brunton first suggested that the mitral valve stenosis could be treated surgically.[21] In May of 1923, Elliott Cutler performed a mitral valvulotomy in an 11-year-old girl using a tenotomy knife. Thereafter, she lived for 4.5 years. His next six patients died, and he abandoned the procedure.[22] Sir Henry Souttar performed a successful digital commissurotomy in May of 1925. His patient recovered uneventfully but he was never referred another patient for this operation.[23] Despite these early repair attempts, mitral surgery remained dormant until 1948 to 1949 when Horace Smithy, Charles Bailey Dwight Harken, and Russell Brock independently revitalized the technique of commissurotomy.[24–27] There were early successes by Lillehei and McGoon to repair degenerative mitral valves.[28,29] Other surgeons developed various annuloplasty techniques.[30,31] Some of these operations were quite successful but the development of a mitral valve replacement prosthesis eclipsed further development of repair techniques.[32,33]

Traditional Repair Success

The concept of repairing mitral valves was revived and developed by Carpentier and Duran.[34,35] Carpentier's landmark address entitled *The French Correction (1983)* made surgeons realize that most insufficient degenerative valves could be repaired and that the benefits exceeded those of a replacement.[36] His techniques were proven to yield excellent results when done through a median sternotomy. Many subsequent clinical series confirmed these benefits and repair became a standard of care in Europe and the United States, albeit slowly adopted.[37–40] The perfection of mitral repair operations done through a sternotomy laid the foundation for minimally invasive techniques to be the next wave of advancement.

Minimally Invasive Mitral Valve Surgery

The idea of MIS mitral surgery emanated during the "Heartport Era" with the development of balloon aortic occlusion devices, long-shafted instruments, and port cardiac access.[4,5] These innovations facilitated MIS greatly and encouraged surgeons to expand the development of even less invasive operations. Cohn and Cosgrove among others showed modified less invasive sternal incisions safe and efficacious when replacing and repairing mitral valves.[1–3] Later, propensity matched patient series confirmed that repair results were similar to sternotomy-based operations.[12]

The concept of operating inside the heart using *video-assisted or endoscopic vision* is not new. In November of 1923, Duff Allen and Evarts Graham planned to use a cardioscope to visualize a commissurotomy in a 31-year-old woman but were unsuccessful.[41] Harken experimented with intracardiac visualization techniques in 1943.[42] In 1958, Sakakibara predicted that valve operations could be done using endoscopic secondary vision.[43,44] Kaneko (1995) used video assistance through a sternotomy to aid in mitral repairs and commissurotomies.[45]

In February of 1996, Carpentier performed the first videoscopic minimally invasive mitral repair, which was done via a right minithoracotomy.[46] Our group performed the first camera-directed minimally invasive mitral replacement 2 months later.[47–49] Mohr, Reichenspurner, Vanermen, Hargrove, and Chitwood expanded the influence of video-directed minimally invasive mitral surgery by publishing large mitral repair series with excellent results.[8–10,14]

Robot-Assisted Mitral Valve Surgery

In 1998, Carpentier accomplished the first robotic mitral repair using a daVinci robot prototype.[50] A week later, Mohr completed seven successful robot-assisted mitral repairs with this system.[51] These operations proved that mitral repairs could be done safely using robotic telepresence alone. In 2000, Grossi performed a mitral valve leaflet repair using the Zeus robot.[52] In 1999, our group purchased the first commercial daVinci Surgical System (Intuitive Surgical, Inc., Sunnyvale, CA) in the United States and then developed additional instruments and repair techniques in our robotic laboratory. In May of 2002, under an FDA safety and efficacy clinical trial, we performed the first complete robotic mitral repair with leaflet resection and a band annuloplasty using the daVinci system.[53] This device was FDA approved for intracardiac surgery in 2002 after two clinical trials.[54] Our inaugural series of 300 patients confirmed the safety and efficacy of robot-assisted mitral valve repair.[55]

Dedicated robotic mitral valve repair referral programs have shown outcomes similar to operations done either through a sternotomy, hemisternotomy, minithoracotomy, or port only access.[56–60] The device, instrument, and maintenance costs have been challenged; however, surgeons at the Mayo and Cleveland Clinics have shown that optimized robotic care paths can render economic parity with other incisional approaches.[61,62]

ACCLIMATIZATION AND PROGRESSION

In previous book chapters, we have compared a surgeon's progression in minimally invasive valve surgery skills akin to a "Mount Everest trek." Although this analogy may be less apropos today, it does bespeak the advantages of an advancing pathway on which one can accommodate anywhere along this surgical escarpment. Embarking from a conventional median sternotomy-based operation or "base camp," surgeons can advance progressively toward less invasiveness through experience and methodological acclimatization. In this schema, entry levels of technical complexity are mastered before advancing past small-incision, direct-vision approaches (Level 1) toward more complex video-assisted/directed procedures (Level 2 or 3), and finally to completely robot-assisted operations (Level 4). With the evolution of technology and advancing surgical expertise, most established mitral repair surgeons are able to attain "comfort zones" along this trek.

This chapter shows that patient selection, preoperative screening, patient positioning, the operative setup, perfusion, and operative management are generally the *same for all of our MIS and robot-assisted operations*. This standardization should help surgeons move more rapidly through the progression of MIS operations. Major differences between direct vision and video-assisted MIS operations relate mainly to the size of the minithoracotomy. In robot-assisted operations, changes relate to instrument arm placement, instruments, and telemanipulation methods. Mitral and tricuspid valve repair techniques have been standardized for all three operative approaches.

PATIENT SELECTION

Table 40-1 shows what we consider to be an ideal mitral valve operation. Today, we have been able to achieve most of these factors: however, others remain for the future. Clearly, the die has been cast (*alea iacta est*) regarding the absolute requirement for patient safety and optimal long-lasting repairs, no matter what technique is employed. Patients who are selected for minimally invasive mitral surgery should have the same indications as outlined in either the 2014 ACC/AHA (United States) or 2012 ESC/EACTS (European) Guidelines.[19,20] At our institution, all patients with either degenerative or functional mitral insufficiency are considered for a videoscopic or robotic MIS. Asymptomatic patients are selected based on the IIa recommendations in the recent ACC/AHA guidelines.[19] Patients with significant comorbidities, and those requiring multivessel coronary revascularization, an aortic valve replacement or have a significantly dilated ascending aorta should be operated upon through a sternotomy. Operative risks, age, fragility, and mitral pathology complexity all should be considered when selecting these patients. All patients should be informed of alternative approaches, including a traditional sternotomy, and they should understand that there is a small possibility of requiring a sternal conversion. Absolute and relative *contraindications* to robotic and MIS mitral surgery

 TABLE 40-1: The Ideal Mitral Valve Repair

- Small nonrib spreading working incision
- Central antegrade cardiopulmonary perfusion
- High-definition magnified 3D vision
- Ergonomic intracardiac instrument access
- Tactile feedback
- Facile prosthesis attachment devices
- Minimal
  - Cardiopulmonary perfusion times
  - Cardiac arrest times
  - Blood product usage
  - Ventilation times
  - Intensive care requirements
  - Incision pain
  - Hospitalization
- High-quality repairs
  - Greater than 95% repairs
  - Few reoperations (<2%)
  - Operative mortality (<1%)
  - No SAM or residual leak

TABLE 40-2: Contraindications to Minimally Invasive and Robotic Mitral Valve Surgery

Absolute	Relative
Previous right thoracotomy	Previous sternotomy
Severe pulmonary dysfunction	Moderate pulmonary dysfunction
Myocardial infarction or ischemia < 30 days	Asymptomatic coronary artery disease
Coronary artery disease—requiring coronary surgery	Coronary artery disease—requiring *PCI
Severe generalized vascular disease	Limited peripheral vascular disease
Symptomatic cerebrovascular disease or stroke < 30 days	Asymptomatic cerebrovascular disease
Right ventricular dysfunction	Poor left ventricular function (*EF < 50%)
Pulmonary hypertension (fixed > 60 torr)	Pulmonary hypertension (variable > 50 mm Hg)
Significant aortic stenosis or insufficiency	Mild to moderate aortic stenosis or insufficiency
Severe mitral annular calcification	Moderate annular calcification
Severe liver dysfunction	Chest deformity (pectus or scoliosis)
Significant bleeding disorders	
Significantly dilated aortic root	

*PCI, percutaneous catheter intervention; EF, left ventricular ejection fraction

are listed in Table 40-2. Some relative contraindications can be managed by selecting alternate methods for perfusion and myocardial protection (eg, axillary artery cannulation and hypothermic ventricular fibrillation). For single vessel coronary disease, preoperative coronary stenting has obviated the need to avoid consideration for a mitral/tricuspid MIS repair.

PREOPERATIVE SCREENING

Candidates for any MIS or robot-assisted mitral operation should be screened carefully for peripheral vascular and coronary artery disease as well as pulmonary maladies. In most patients, either a computed tomographic angiogram and/or contrast coronary angiogram should be performed. Suspect patients should undergo tomographic and/or ultrasound screening for aortoiliac, carotid, and general aortic disease. Peripheral perfusion and aortic endoballoon occlusion should be avoided in patients with severe aortic atherosclerosis or a dilated ascending aorta. Pulmonary function tests should be done in heavy smokers and those having symptoms of obstructive disease. A detailed transthoracic echocardiogram should be done to define general valve pathology, ventricular function, and the presence of pulmonary hypertension. If the latter is present, a right heart catheterization may be indicated. In patients with complex disease, we perform a preoperative 3D transesophageal echocardiogram (TEE).

REPAIR PLANNING: 3D TEE STUDIES

We always develop an intraoperative "blueprint" to plan mitral and tricuspid repairs Table 40-3. After patients are anesthetized, the direction of each jet (leak) is mapped with both 2D and 3D TEE studies. The mobility and prolapse level is determined for each restricted or prolapsing segment. Leaflet segments (P_1-P_3, A_1-A_3) are measured. Next, the planar angle between the aortic and mitral valve annulus is determined. Finally, the annular diameter, outflow tract septal thickness, and coaptation point to septal (C Sept) distances are measured. Operative planning includes the avoidance of *systolic anterior motion of the anterior leaflet* (SAM). Thus, we pay special attention to the length of A_2 and P_1-P_3 heights (annulus to coapting edge). Table 40-4 shows the anatomic, operative, and dynamic features that can contribute to postoperative SAM. Preventative *structural repair measures* that may avoid this complication include: (1) implantation of a large enough ring/band, (2) reduction of the posterior leaflet height to 15 mm or less, and (3) achievement of an optimal leaflet coaptation surface (8–10 mm). The length of A_2 guides us for annuloplasty band size selection. Finally, a 3D valve model is constructed from these measurements (Fig. 40-1A–C). During the valve reconstruction, this model as well as other imaging studies can be visualized in the daVinci operating console using the Tile Pro software (Intuitive Surgical, Inc., Sunnyvale, CA). To determine the need for an adjunctive tricuspid valve repair, we quantitate the regurgitant volume and measure the annular size. We now include a tricuspid annuloplasty repair in all patients that have even moderate insufficiency with annular dilatation of more than 4 cm.

OPERATIVE MANAGEMENT: GENERAL

As mentioned before, the operative organization and management are very similar for minithoracotomy or port access

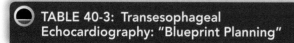

TABLE 40-3: Transesophageal Echocardiography: "Blueprint Planning"

- Degree of valve leakage
- Direction of individual leakage jets
- Lengths (mm) of A_2, and P_1, P_2, and P_3
- Annular diameter and geometry—mitral and tricuspid
- Definition of posterior leaflet clefts and interdependence
- Planar angle between mitral and aortic annulus
- Degree (mm) of leaflet segmental prolapse or restriction
- "Septal knob" thickness (mm)
- Aortic outflow tract size (mm)—coaptation to septal distance
- Reconstructed topographic mitral valve model

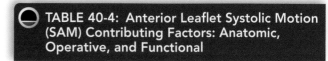

TABLE 40-4: Anterior Leaflet Systolic Motion (SAM) Contributing Factors: Anatomic, Operative, and Functional

- P_1-P_3 leaflet length > 2 cm (annulus to edge)
- A_2 leaflet length > 3 cm
- Aortomitral plane angle < 120°
- Narrow aortic outflow tract
- Thick septal "knob"
- Small annuloplasty prosthesis
- Inotropic drug support
- Under filled left ventricular

(MIS) video-assisted, direct vision, and robot-assisted mitral repairs (RMVP) and replacements. *The Atlas of Robotic Cardiac Surgery* details anesthesia management, instrument setup, and conduct of these and other operations at several well-known centers.[63] Moreover, *Cardiopulmonary Bypass and Mechanical Support: Principles and Practice* provides precise details of our method of cardiopulmonary perfusion (CPB) for all of these operations.[64] The use of endo-balloon aortic occlusion requires special attention and is detailed in these texts.

Patient Position

To help widen the right intercostal spaces (ICSs), which helps to prevent rib spreading, the right chest should be elevated by 30° using a midthorax towel roll. The right arm should be "sling" positioned inferior to the posterior axillary line. Some surgeons prefer to position the flexed right arm above the head using different forms of stabilization. At this time, anterior and posterior Zoll defibrillator pads should be placed to subtend the heart. To monitor adequate limb perfusion during CPB, we place Invos System (Somanetics, Inc., Troy, MI) oxygen saturation monitoring patches on each thigh. Standard skin preparation and draping must provide wide access to the right chest, sternum, and both groins. To facilitate transthoracic aortic clamp placement, the right chest should be prepared sterilely as far as the posterior axillary line.

Anesthesia Management

Although some surgeons prefer not to isolate the right lung, we believe that unilateral ventilation can be done safely and facilitates inspection for bleeding at the end of the operation. In the past, we deflated the lung first and then opened the pericardium with long instruments before establishing CPB. However, we now begin CPB before deflating the right lung and avoid manipulating it while heparinized. To isolate the right lung, either a double-lumen endotracheal tube or a right endobronchial blocker is used. In all of our minimally invasive cardiac surgery operations, we monitor closely cardiac dynamics and function as well as leg and brain perfusion.

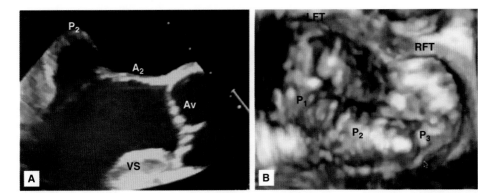
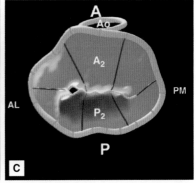

FIGURE 40-1 Preoperative transesophageal echo studies. (A) Long-axis 2D view of prolapsing P₂ leaflet segment; A₂, anterior leaflet; Av, aortic valve; VS, ventricular septum. (B) 3D view with prolapsing posterior leaflet P₂ segment; P₁ and P₂—other posterior leaflet segments; LFT, left fibrous trigone; RFT, right fibrous trigone. (C) Topographic 3D model showing prolapsing P₂ segment; A₂, anterior leaflet; AL, anterior-lateral; PM, posterior-medial; Ao, aortic valve; A, anterior; P, posterior.

Forehead patches are applied to monitor *bispectral index* (BIS, Covidien, Inc., Boulder, CO), which provides an index of cerebral perfusion and anesthetic levels.

A left radial artery catheter is placed for systemic blood pressure monitoring. If intra-aortic balloon occlusion (clamping) is planned, arterial pressures should be measured continuously in both arms. This is done to ensure that the endoballoon has not inadvertently occluded the innominate artery. Thereafter, a right internal jugular vein catheter is inserted for drug infusions and placement of a flow directed Swan–Ganz pulmonary artery catheter (Edwards Lifesciences, Irvine, CA). Using the "double stick" technique, a thin-walled (15-Fr or 17-Fr) Bio-Medicus (Medtronic, Inc., St. Paul, MN) right internal jugular venous drainage cannula is inserted under echocardiographic guidance (Fig. 40-2). Some surgeons use a single femoral venous return cannula that is passed through the right atrium into

the superior vena cava (SVC). However, to assure a dry surgical field throughout these operations, we have found that dual cannulation is more reliable. Lastly, the 3D transesophageal echo probe is positioned and detailed studies are done.

Working Incision

Today, most minimally invasive and robotic mitral/tricuspid valve operations are performed through a right fourth ICS minithoracotomy. Current visualization choices include a direct view through the incision, 2D endoscopic, or 3D robotic. However, the new Aesculap 3D EinsteinVision system (E Braun, Inc., Tuttlingen, Germany) has been compared favorably to daVinci robotic 3D visualization.[65] The *size of the working incision* usually depends on the visualization and operative methods chosen by the surgeon.

For both direct vision and 2D endoscopic MIS, a 4 to 5 cm minithoracotomy is made in the fourth ICS near the anterior axillary line. We suggest a slightly larger incision for surgeons just beginning MIS mitral surgery. For robotic operations, a smaller working incision (2 to 3 cm) is placed in the same topographic chest region. In preference to using a rib-spreading retractor, we now prefer a flexible Alexis soft tissue wound protector (Applied Medical, Inc., Rancho Santa Margarita, CA). In the past, we used the Perivue Soft Tissue retractor (Edwards Lifesciences, Inc., Irvine, CA) for nonrib spreading access. We have found that this minimizes postoperative pain and provides good working-incision exposure for either direct vision, video-assisted, or robotic minimally invasive mitral/tricuspid valve surgery. Other robotic surgeons have found that true port-access (1 to 2 cm) can be used without compromising either the operation or safety.[57–60]

Cannulation and Cardiopulmonary Perfusion

All perfusion cannulas are placed under echocardiographic guidance using the Seldinger guide-wire technique. Through a 2-cm oblique groin incision adventitial 4-0 polypropylene

FIGURE 40-2 Anesthesia preparation. TEE, transesophageal echo probe; DLET, double lumen endotracheal tube; IJ SVC, internal jugular vein to superior vena cava venous drainage cannula; IP, internal jugular vein drug infusion port; SG, internal jugular vein Swan Ganz pulmonary artery catheter.

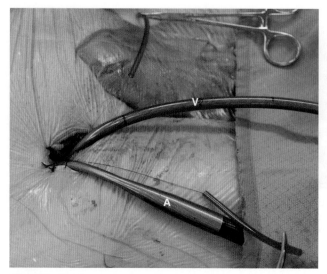

FIGURE 40-3 Cardiopulmonary bypass perfusion cannulas. Groin incision with arterial (A) and venous (V) cannulas in place for cardiopulmonary perfusion (see text for details).

oval (longitudinal) purse-string sutures are placed in both femoral vessels near the inguinal ligament. The right femoral artery is cannulated with either a 17 or 19-Fr Bio-Medicus cannula (Medtronic, Inc., Minneapolis, MN). For inferior vena caval drainage, either a 22-Fr (single stage) or a 23/25-Fr (dual stage) RAP femoral venous cannula (LivaNova, Inc., Arvada, CO) is passed into the right atrium (Fig. 40-3). In corpulent patients, we tunnel cannulas through the upper thigh subcutaneous tissue. This allows coaxial dilators and cannulas to have safer passage into vessels at a 30° to 45° angle. Vacuum-assisted venous drainage is used in all of our operations. Presently, we use Sorin S5® heart-lung machine, modified for use with a venous bag reservoir or V-Bag (Circulatory Technology, Inc., Oyster Bay, NY) and equipped with magnetic drive for Revolution centrifugal pump suction (LivaNova USA, Inc., Arvada, CO) (Fig. 40-4). Figure 40-5 Illustrates our current perfusion circuit for MIS and robotic heart surgery.

Cardiac Air Removal

Meticulous cardiac air removal is particularly important in minimally invasive valve operations. Difficulty exists in manipulating and deairing the cardiac apex, as it cannot be elevated. Also, with a right anterolateral minithoracotomy, air tends to be retained along the dorsally oriented ventricular septum and in the right pulmonary veins. Moreover, this position places the right coronary ostium in the most vulnerable position to entrap air. Continuous carbon-dioxide (CO_2) insufflation has been particularly helpful in minimizing intracardiac air and should be begun before cardiac chambers are opened. Carbon dioxide is much more soluble in blood than air and displaces it very effectively. We infuse CO_2 continuously (4-5 L/min) into the thorax, and prior to cross clamp release, ventilate both lungs vigorously to draw the gas deep

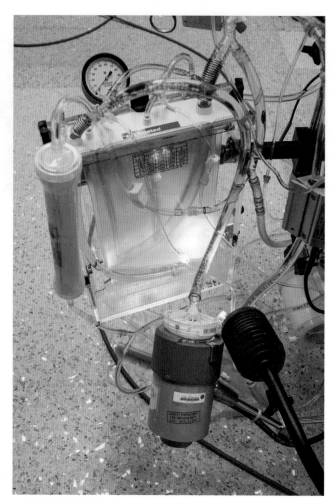

FIGURE 40-4 Cardiopulmonary bypass perfusion circuit. Venous bag reservoir or V-Bag (Circulatory Technology, Inc., Oyster Bay, NY) attached to a magnetic drive to propel the Revolution centrifugal pump suction head (LivaNova USA, Inc., Arvada, CO).

into all pulmonary veins. After atriotomy closure and following cross-clamp release, suction is applied to the aortic root vent. One can compress the right coronary artery origin during early ejection. Constant transesophageal echocardiographic monitoring is essential to assure adequate air removal before weaning from cardiopulmonary bypass.

Alternate Arterial Cannulation Techniques

Ileo-femoral and/or aortic atherosclerosis may preclude safe retrograde perfusion. To cannulate the ascending aorta directly, it is important to place two concentric pledgeted purse strings near the innominate artery origin. We use either a Biomedicus (Medtronic, Inc., Minneapolis, MN) guide-wire directed cannula or a 23-Fr Straight Shot device (Edwards Lifesciences, Irvine, CA), which is passed through the chest wall via a 10-mm trocar. If it is not feasible to cannulate the ascending aorta directly, we use the right axillary artery for

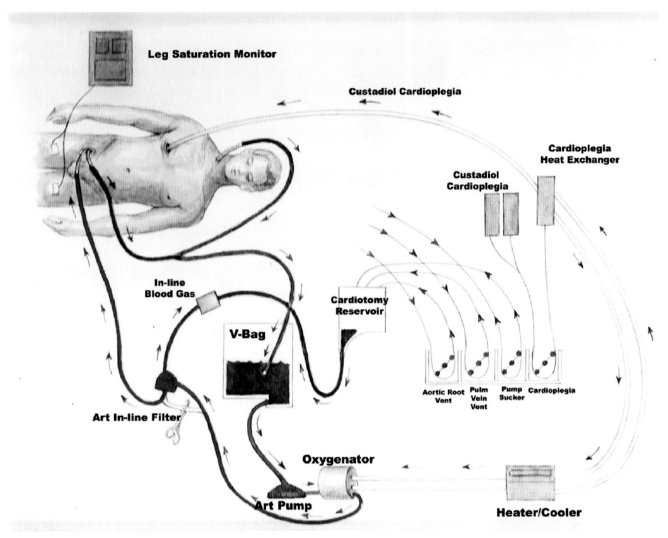

FIGURE 40-5 Cardiopulmonary bypass perfusion circuit for minimally invasive mitral surgery. Our circuit employs the venous bag reservoir pictured in Fig. 40-4. Femoral arterial and venous cannulas are inserted through a small groin incision. An internal jugular venous cannula augments return to the V-Bag reservoir. Cold Custodiol antegrade cardioplegia is delivered via an ascending aorta cannula. (Reproduced with permission from Gravlee GP, Davis RF, Hammon J, et al: *Cardiopulmonary Bypass and Mechanical Support: Principles and Practice*, 4th ed. Philadelphia: Wolter Kluwer; 2015.)

antegrade perfusion. The artery is exposed through an infraclavicular incision. An 8-mm GelSoft knitted graft (Vascutek, Terumo, Ann Arbor, MI) is sewn end-to-side to the axillary artery with 5-0 polypropylene suture. Thereafter, the graft is connected to the bypass circuit using either an appropriate size arterial cannula or a three-eighth inch pump tubing connector. Terumo also makes a PTFE graft that is annealed directly to a perfusion cannula (Fig. 40-6A and B). Alternatively, the axillary artery can be cannulated directly; however, distal arm perfusion should be monitored while the cannula is in place.

Aortic Occlusion

For aortic occlusion, we use a transthoracic cross clamp Scanlan International, Inc., St. Paul, MN as it has been proven to

be safe, reliable, economic, and simple to apply (Fig. 40-7A and B). However, a number of surgeons use the IntraClude endoballoon (Edwards Lifesciences, Irvine, CA) for aortic occlusion (Fig. 40-8). This technique has a steeper learning curve than using the clamp. The balloon position must be precise and remain stable in the ascending aorta. There is a potential for either innominate artery occlusion or intraventricular displacement. Therefore, it is essential echo monitor the balloon position throughout the operation. Also, introduction through the specialized femoral arterial cannula can limit limb perfusion. In this circumstance, the endoballoon catheter should be reinserted through the other femoral artery. Despite these concerns, this method can provide effective aortic occlusion with a simultaneous route for delivering antegrade cardioplegia and venting air.

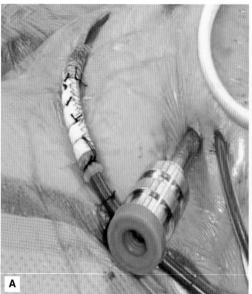
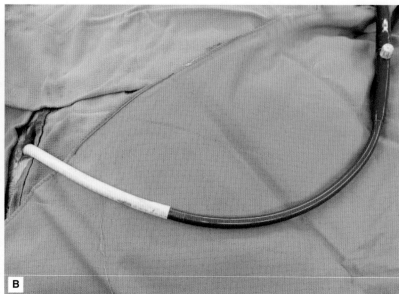

FIGURE 40-6 Axillary arterial alternate cannulation. Two methods of axillary arterial cannulation are shown. (A) An 8-mm GelSoft knitted graft (Vascutek, Terumo, Ann Arbor, MI) is sewn to the right axillary artery; a similar size arterial perfusion cannula is inserted into the graft and tied tightly in place. (B) Terumo PTFE graft that is annealed to the arterial perfusion circuit.

When applying the transthoracic aortic clamp, the posterior arm should be passed through the transverse sinus under either *direct or videoscopic vision* (Fig. 40-9A and B). The shaft of the clamp should be passed just in front of the SVC near the pericardial junction. The anterior clamp arm (tine) portion should be positioned across the aorta until it reaches the main pulmonary artery. Care must be taken not to injure the right or main pulmonary artery, left atrial appendage, left

main coronary artery, or aorta. We prefer to place the clamp with the tip directed toward the transverse aortic arch.

Myocardial Protection

As mentioned earlier, we have always used the transthoracic aortic clamp method for both minimally invasive and robot-assisted mitral valve surgery. For antegrade cardioplegia administration, a long cardioplegia-vent catheter (Medtronic, Inc., St Paul, MN) is inserted through an ascending aortic purse-string, secured, and passed either through a chest wall trocar or the working incision. We prefer a pledgeted diamond shape 4-0 PTFE purse-string suture placed distal to the right coronary artery origin near the fatty Fold of Rindfleisch (Fig. 40-10). This catheter should be inserted either under robotic, endoscopic, or direct vision.

We now use Custodiol—Bretschneider's HTK solution (Franz Köhler Chemie Bensheim GMBH, Germany) for cardioplegia as it provides much longer myocardial protection without requiring frequent reinfusions. We start with single large infusion (20 to 25 mL/kg) at 4 to 6°C, and after 1 hour give a half dose. For maximal myocardial protection, we combine antegrade cardioplegia with a systemic blood inflow temperature of 28°C. If blood cardioplegia is used, repeat administrations should be given at 15- to 30-minute intervals. Multiple cardioplegia infusions, requiring atrial retractor relaxation and repositioning, can entrain air into the aortic root. For patients having had a *previous sternotomy*, we cool systemically to 26°C and induce ventricular fibrillation by rapid pacing with a custom Swan-Ganz catheter. In patients with mild aortic insufficiency, additional intracardiac suction can be combined with dropping perfusion flow briefly for difficult suture placement.

FIGURE 40-7 Transthoracic aortic clamp. For minimally invasive mitral valve operations, the transthoracic aortic clamp (Scanlan International, Inc., St. Paul, MN) should be passed through the 3D intercostal space. (A) Transthoracic aortic clamp and (B) clamp tines with DeBakey-type teeth. (Used with permission from Scanlan International Inc., St. Paul, MN.)

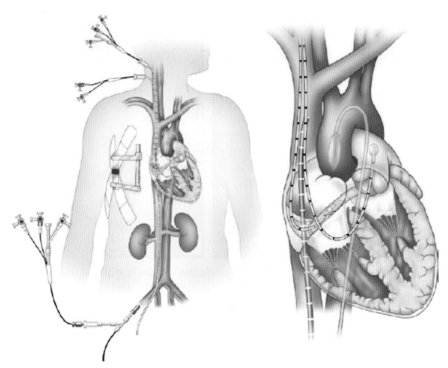

FIGURE 40-8 Endo-balloon aortic occlusion. Femoral arterial and venous perfusion cannulas have been inserted. An IntraClude endo-balloon (Edwards Lifesciences, Irvine, CA) has been passed through the femoral arterial perfusion cannula and echo-guided retrograde to the ascending aorta. A pulmonary artery vent catheter has been placed. A retrograde cardioplegia coronary sinus cannula has been inserted through the right internal jugular vein. (Reproduced with permission from Chitwood WR: Atlas of Robotic Cardiac Surgery. London: Springer-Verlag; 2014.)

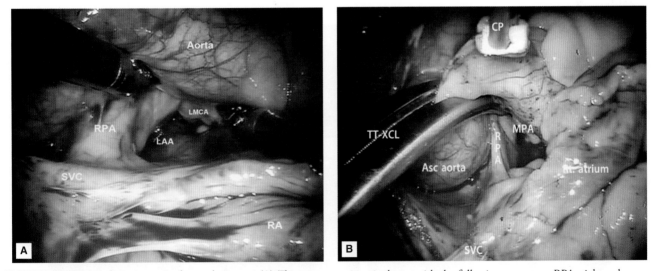

FIGURE 40-9 Transthoracic aortic clamp placement. (A) The transverse sinus is shown with the following structures: RPA, right pulmonary artery; LAA, left atrial appendage; LMCA, left main coronary artery; SVC, superior vena cava; aorta and right atrium are also shown. The correct trajectory for clamp placement from the 3D interspace, across the pericardial-SVC junction with the tip residing superior to the LAA and inferior to the RPA. (B) The transverse sinus is shown after transthoracic cross clamp (TT-XCL) placement. The clamp tip has been directed cephalically across the ascending aorta (Asc Aorta). The right pulmonary artery (RPA) and main pulmonary artery (MPA) are shown, as are the SVC and right atrium. CP denotes the cardioplegia cannula.

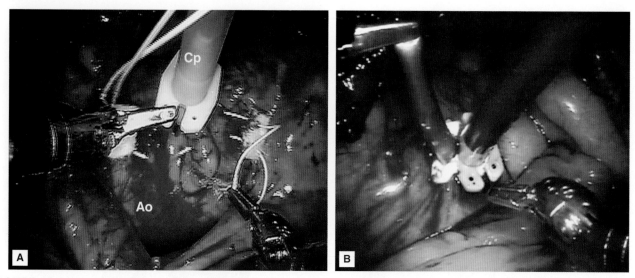

FIGURE 40-10 Cardioplegia/vent catheter insertion. (A) The cardioplegia/vent catheter (CP) has been inserted into the ascending aorta (Ao) through a 4-0 pledgeted PTFE "purse string" suture placed just distal to the right coronary artery origin in the fatty fold. (B) The cardioplegia catheter (red) has been secured in the ascending aorta with a Rummel tourniquet (blue). (Reproduced with permission from Grover FL, Mack MJ: *Master Techniques in Surgery: Cardiac Surgery.* Philadelphia: Lippincott Williams & Wilkins; 2016.)

Cardiac Exposure

After going on CPB, the pericardium is opened longitudinally 3-cm anterior to the phrenic nerve with either long shafted endoscopic or robotic instruments. Two to three well-spaced pericardial retraction sutures are placed along the inferior (dorsal) pericardial edge (Fig. 40-11A and B). We then pass the needle back through a pretied end-loop. Using a crochet hook instrument, the single suture is withdrawn laterally through the chest wall to provide cardiac exposure. Care should be taken not to stretch or directly injure the phrenic nerve.

The anterior (ventral) pericardial edge is distracted through the working incision with two sutures.

OPERATIVE MANAGEMENT: 2D VIDEO-ASSISTED MINIMALLY INVASIVE MITRAL SURGERY

Figure 40-12 shows our table arrangement for 2D video-assisted MIS mitral operations. After establishing cardiac arrest, we pass a 5-mm high-definition 2D endoscope

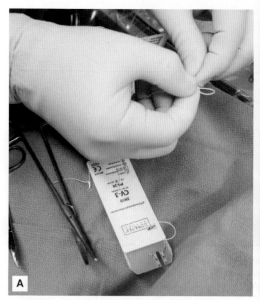
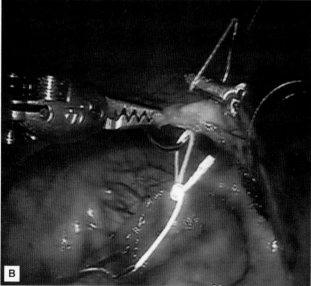

FIGURE 40-11 Suture loops: pericardal retraction/atriotomy closure. (A) Tiny PTFE loops are hand tied. These 3-0 PTFE loops are used to close the left atrium. After the suture is passed through the atriotomy tissue, the needle is passed through the loop, and the suture is tightened. This obviates the need for extracorporeal knot tying. (B) For pericardial retraction sutures, 2-0 braided suture loops are tied as in A. After the loop-suture pericardial edge fixation, the suture is passed through the lateral chest wall using a "crochet hook" instrument.

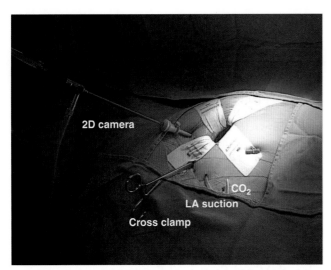

FIGURE 40-12 Video-assisted minimally invasive mitral surgery: operative setup. A 5-mm Storz videoscopic camera (2D—Camera) has been placed through a trocar inserted in the 3D intercostal space and is then attached to a table-mounted holder. The transthoracic cross clamp is shown placed through the 3D or fourth intercostal space. A nonrib spreading soft tissue retractor is shown. The CO_2 insufflation and left atrial sump suction catheters are shown. (Reproduced with permission from Grover FL, Mack MJ: *Master Techniques in Surgery: Cardiac Surgery.* Philadelphia: Lippincott Williams & Wilkins; 2016.)

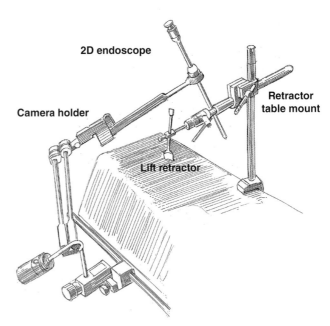

FIGURE 40-13 Video-assisted minimally invasive mitral surgery: endoscope and retractor. A table-mounted **camera holder** is shown with a **2D endoscope in position**. For mitral valve surgery, the atrial **lift retractor** is inserted through the chest wall and into the atriotomy. (Atrial Lift System, Atricure, Inc., Cincinnati, OH). Thereafter, it is supported by a fixed **retractor table mount**. (Reproduced with permission from Chitwood WR: *Atlas of Robotic Cardiac Surgery.* London: Springer-Verlag; 2014.)

(Karl Storz GmbH & Co. KG, Tuttlingen, Germany) through a third ICS trocar and attach it to a hand-positioned holder. A transthoracic atrial retractor arm (Atrial Lift System, Atricure, Inc., Cincinnati, OH) is passed through the chest wall, just medial to the sternum in the fourth interspace (Fig. 40-13). The arm is then coupled to the appropriate size blade, which is inserted into the left atrium. After minimal interatrial groove dissection, the left atriotomy should be made just medial to the right superior and inferior pulmonary veins. To lift interatrial septum and expose the mitral valve, the retractor arm is attached to a table-mounted support. This device is also used to facilitate tricuspid valve repairs.

Long-shafted instruments are used for endoscopic and direct vision MIS and provide rotational ergonomics but lack the advantage of full articulation (Fig. 40-14). Specialized knot pushers and suture cutters (Scanlan International, Inc., St. Paul, MN) greatly facilitate MIS mitral operations (Fig. 40-15). It is incumbent that needle holders have a strong grip as many positioning angles confer increased torque compared with traditional suturing methods. For suture organization, we often use Gabby-Frater suture guides (Teleflex Medical, Research Triangle, NC), placed around the working incision.

OPERATIVE MANAGEMENT: 3D ROBOT-ASSISTED MITRAL SURGERY

Heart Team Robotic Program Development

We recently published *a* consensus statement from the combined STS/AATS New Technology Committee entitled *"Pathway*

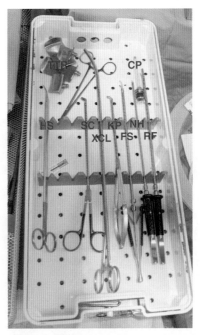

FIGURE 40-14 Video-assisted minimally invasive mitral surgery: instruments. An instrument tray for video-assisted or direct vision mitral valve surgery: TTR, transthoracic lift retractor blades; HS, heavy scissors; SC, suture cutter; XCL, transthoracic cross clamp; KP, knot pusher; FS, fine scissors; NH, needle holder; RF, Resano forceps; CP, camera port.

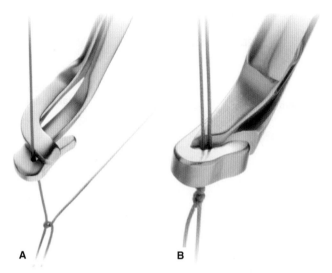

FIGURE 40-15 Knot pusher and suture cutter. (A) Minimally invasive knot pusher; (B) minimally invasive suture cutter (Scanlan International, Inc., St. Paul, MN). (Used with permission from Scanlan International Inc., St. Paul, MN.)

for surgeons and programs to establish and maintain a successful robot-assisted adult cardiac surgery program.[66] It emphasizes that an organized heart team is mandatory to develop and maintain a successful cardiac robotic surgical program. Also, our editorial entitled *"Mitral valve repair using robotic technology: Safe, effective, and durable"* provides additional helpful information and guidance for developing programs.[67]

Before beginning robot-assisted mitral and tricuspid surgery, surgeons should be accomplished at mitral repairs and preferably other minimally invasive approaches.[16] Cardiologists should fully support program development and champion participation in combined valve clinics. This cooperation encourages cardiologist and surgeons to agree upon

which patients are appropriate for a robot-assisted operation. It is important that anesthesiologists, surgeons, tableside assistants, scrub personnel, circulating nurses, and perfusionists train and work together as a unit.

Procedure training at an experience robotic valve center has been important to launch successful programs and greatly shortens the learning curve. We suggest that even skilled mitral valve referral surgeons should engage a proctor for the first operations. There are a number of experienced centers that can offer training in robotic mitral valve surgery. Our Robotic Training Center has been a mainstay for mitral valve robotic surgical training. To date, we have held 634 robotic surgery courses in all specialties. Of these, 160 were training general cardiac surgery teams with an additional 104 that were specific for robotic mitral valve repair.

The daVinci Surgical System

The daVinci surgical system (Intuitive Surgical, Inc., Sunnyvale, CA) provides operative field access with superb visualization and enhanced ergonomics, which allows surgeons to perform complex operations through small port-like incisions. Long hand-held instruments placed through a small working port have a fulcrum effect that can reverse instrument direction from that of the surgeon's hand. This factor, coupled with innate human tremor, may limit accurate suture placement and valve leaflet reconstruction. Accuracy achieved with daVinci instruments emanates from the wide freedom of instrument tip motion at the operative plane. The surgeon always has the same operating console instrument control as if they were activated directly by his or her hands.

Currently, this device is the only robotic system FDA approved to perform intracardiac surgical procedures. We have used three system generations, including the daVinci SI HD (high-definition) dual console device, which was first commercialized in 2009 (Fig. 40-16). The current daVinci XI System

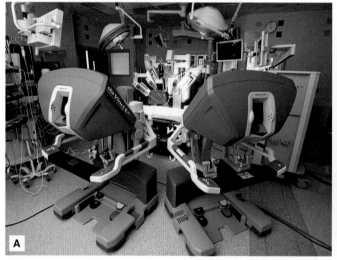
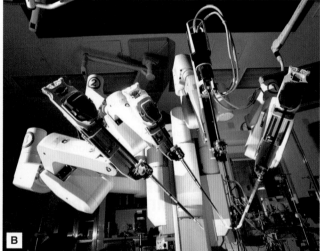

FIGURE 40-16 daVinci SI Surgical System. (A) daVinci SI dual surgeon consoles (foreground) with instrument cart in place (background) and (B) daVinci instrument cart showing with two instrument arms, a retractor arm and the 3D high-definition camera.

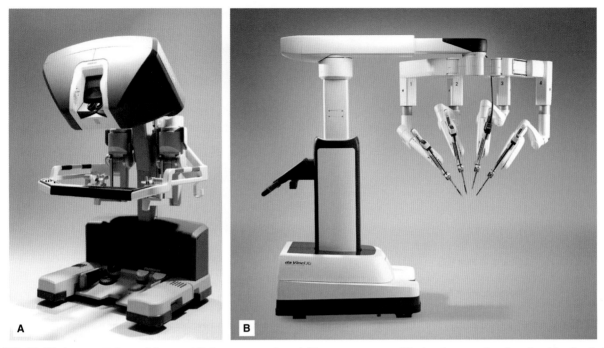

FIGURE 40-17 daVinci XI Surgical System. (A) Surgeon console and (B) instrument cart. (Used with permission from Intuitive Surgical Inc., Sunnyvale CA.)

(2014) (Fig. 40-17) has a laser targeting system that facilitates docking and instrument engagement. Moreover, 3D visualization has been improved, and the device has robotic tissue stapler capabilities.

All da Vinci systems are comprised of an operating console, an electronic vision cart, and a surgical instrument cart. For mitral/tricuspid valve surgery, the instrument cart should be positioned along the left side of the patient (Fig. 40-18). Activator arms are mobilized to gain access to right chest instrument trocars, which have been inserted through specific ICSs (Fig. 40-19). The two instrument arms, the 3D camera, and dynamic retractor are then inserted through these preplaced

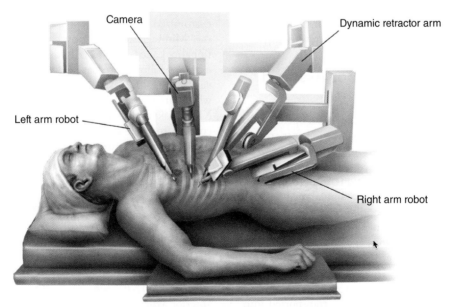

FIGURE 40-18 Robot-assisted mitral valve surgery: patient and instrument positions. The patient is positioned with a 30° lift or towel roll placed under the right shoulder with the right arm distracted to behind the chest. The robotic instrument cart should be positioned along the left side of the operating table. Activator arms are shown to be overarching the patient to gain access to pre-position instrument trocars. (Reproduced with permission from Chitwood Jr WR. Idiopathic Hypertrophic Subaortic Septal Obstruction: Robotic Trans-atrial Resection, Oper Tech Thorac Cardiovasc Surg 2012;Winter 17(4):251-260.)

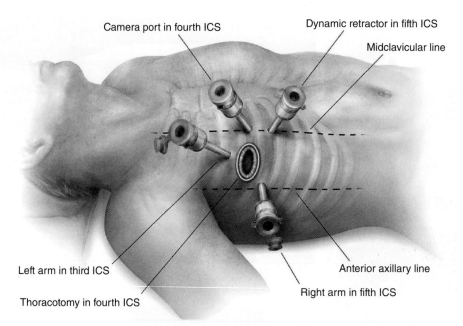

FIGURE 40-19 Robot-assisted mitral valve surgery: instrument trocar placement. Trocars have been placed in the designated intercostal spaces (ICS). (Reproduced with permission from Chitwood Jr WR. Idiopathic Hypertrophic Subaortic Septal Obstruction: Robotic Trans-atrial Resection, Oper Tech Thorac Cardiovasc Surg 2012;Winter 17(4):251-260.)

trocars. Instrument end effectors translate accurately the surgeon's hand and finger motions. A clutching mechanism enables frequent hand-position readjustments to maintain an optimal ergonomic orientation to the visual field.

Both the daVinci SI and XI have dual-console capabilities, which enable surgeon collaboration during complex cases and facilitates training. The robotic EndoWrist instruments (Intuitive Surgical, Inc., Sunnyvale, CA) have seven degrees of ergonomic freedom, and allow tremor free dexterity with both dominant and nondominant hands. This tremor filtration instills a sense of ambidexterity in the operating surgeon.

Simulation Training for Robot-Assisted Surgery

Robotic mitral repair would seem to be the ideal operation to simulate because of: (1) a single working-incision entry point, (2) instrument convergence in a limited operative environment, (3) a 3D digital mitral valve image, (4) topographic echo modeling, (5) end-effector motion freedom, and (6) a motionless arrested heart. However, simulation of actual mitral repair operations today has not been possible. Think of a future when a surgical learner could emulate the exact hand motions and instrument interactions in a simulated landscape that was an actual mitral valve repair done by an experienced surgeon. An entire digital library could be cataloged with specific pathologies. Moreover, through image fusion pathology, specific topographic "blue prints" could be transported into the simulated operative field.

Current robotic simulators have evolved to where they can be advantageous to surgeons learning robot-assisted surgery.

Figure 40-20A shows the current Mimic dV-Trainer along with the assistant surgeon simulator console, the Xperience Team Trainer (XTT). The surgeon's simulator console recapitulates realistically the telemanipulation capabilities of the daVinci SI and XI systems. The assistant trainer (Xperience Team Trainer) allows a tableside surgeon to interact with the surgical field in which the console surgeon is operating. Multiple training protocols can be developed to challenge the console and assistant surgeon to perform synchronous tasks customized for a specific operation. As seen in Fig. 40-20B, the Mimic dV-trainer now has augmented reality functionality called Maestro AR that allows trainer instruments either to follow or repeat an actual recorded surgical maneuver. Figure 40-21 shows the da Vinci backpack simulator, which attached directly to either a current daVinci SI or XI console and is integrated with the robotic software. The console surgeon performs specific training tasks using the daVinci hand controls. The daVinci backpack system and the Mimic dV-Trainer record task metrics and generate a skill report for execution accuracy, speed, and ergonomic motions. More difficult surgical tasks are provided iteratively as the surgeon gains increasing simulation experience.

Instrument Trocar Placement

Instrument trocars (see Figs. 40-19 and 40-22) are positioned as follows: (1) *left robotic arm*—3D interspace (just anterior to anterior axillary line), (2) *right robotic arm*—fifth interspace (anterior to midaxillary line), and (3) dynamic *retractor arm*—fifth interspace (midclavicular line). After tableside docking the instrument cart, the 30° endoscopic camera is passed

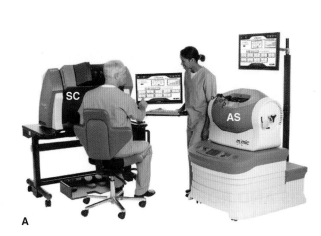

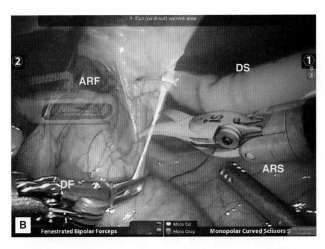

FIGURE 40-20 Robotic simulation: Mimic dV-Trainer. (A) This illustration shows the surgeon console (SC) and the assistant surgeon trainer (Xperience Team Trainer) (AS) for the Mimic dV-Trainer System. After procedure specific simulation exercises have been performed, a skill metric report is generated. (B) Augmented reality (Maestro AR function) that allows the (virtual) instruments in surgeon console trainer to either follow or repeat an actual recorded surgical maneuver. ARF, augmented reality forceps; DF, daVinci forceps; DS, daVinci scissors; ARS, augmented reality scissors. (Used with permission from Mimic Technologies, Inc., Seattle, Washington.)

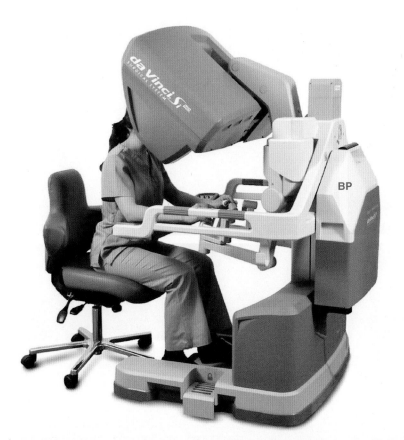

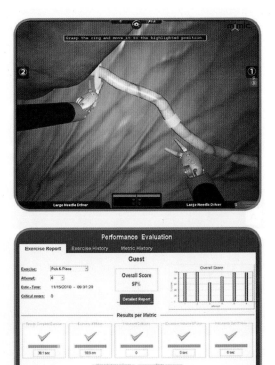

FIGURE 40-21 Robotic simulation: da Vinci Skills Simulator. The "Backpack" (BP) Skills Simulator attaches directly to either a daVinci SI or XI surgeon console. Various surgical simulated tasks challenge the surgeon and a report is generated. With advancing skills more difficult tasks are provided. (Used with permission from Intuitive Surgical Inc., Sunnyvale CA.)

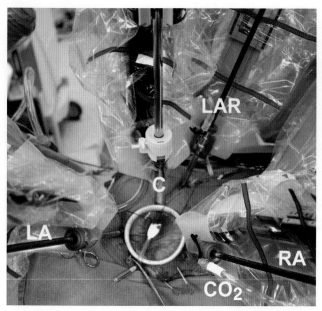

FIGURE 40-22 Robot-assisted mitral valve surgery: inserted instruments. LAR, dynamic left atrial retractor; C, 3D high-definition camera; LA, left instrument arm; RA, right instrument arm; CO_2, carbon dioxide insufflation port in the right arm trocar.

"up-looking" either through the working incision or a fourth interspace trocar, placed along the midclavicular axillary line. The camera trocar is inserted just anterior to and in the same interspace as the working incision. Robotic instruments used for mitral and tricuspid valve surgery include: Resano (8-mm) Endowrist forceps, which are deployed through the left trocar. The curved Endowrist scissors and needle holders (Suture-cut and Large) are inserted through the right port (Fig. 40-23A–D). Lastly, the dual-blade dynamic retractor is positioned in the chest before initiating CPB (Fig. 40-24).

MIS AND ROBOT-ASSISTED MITRAL/TRICUSPID VALVE REPAIR TECHNIQUES

After the da Vinci system instruments are "trocar-docked" at the operating table, CPB is begun, and the pericardium is opened and distracted laterally. We place the aortic purse-string suture and cardioplegia cannula using robotic instruments. To establish a structurally sound repair, we generally follow the operative philosophy and techniques prescribed by Carpentier.[31] However, modifications and simplifications

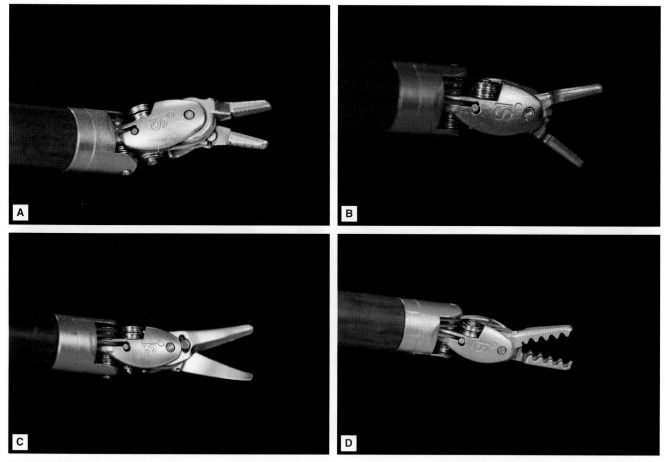

FIGURE 40-23 Robot-assisted mitral valve surgery: end-effector instruments. (A) Suture-cut needle holder; (B) large needle holder; (C) curved scissors; and (D) Resano forceps.

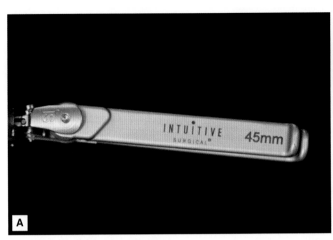
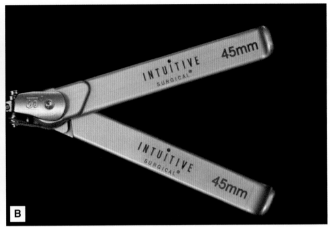

FIGURE 40-24 Robot-assisted mitral valve surgery: dynamic atrial retractor. (A) Closed position for trocar insertion and (B) open position for atrial retraction.

of these methods remain the mainstay of our repair strategy for both robot-assisted and videoscopic mitral surgery.[63] Table 40-5 shows our "Technique Toolbox" that we use for both RMVP and MIS videoscopic mitral valve repairs.

Posterior Mitral Leaflet Repair

All of our leaflet repairs are based on the preoperative echocardiographic measurements shown in Table 40-3, and from these we apply the repair techniques listed in Table 40-5. Of degenerative mitral with significant insufficiency, 80% of pathologies relate to posterior leaflet defects. Thus, a simple triangular resection often will correct isolated segmental prolapse (Fig. 40-25 A (A-E) and B).[68] We suggest first using

this method to correct isolated scallops having mid-prolapse or ruptured chords. Leaflet segments remaining longer than 2-cm can be reduced in height either using a folding plasty (Fig. 40-26A–D) or additional triangular resections.[69] In the presence of diminutive P_1 and P_2 scallops with a very large P_2, either the "haircut" resection technique (Fig. 40-27) or insertion of several PTFE neochords can be effective.[70–72] For multiple prolapsing scallops longer than 2 cm, several folding plasties can be used to create the best coaptation line. Final scallop height adjustments should be made after the annuloplasty band has been implanted. An alternative to triangular resections or folding-plasties is using multiple PTFE neochord replacements (Fig. 40-28A–D, plus insets). Native chord replacements, using either individual neochords or

⬤ TABLE 40-5: Minimally Invasive and Robotic Mitral Valve Repair "Technique Toolbox"

Posterior leaflet prolapse small segment	Posterior leaflet prolapse large segment	Anterior leaflet prolapse	Bileaflet prolapse (Barlow)	Commissure prolapse
Triangular resection	Trapezoid resection	Triangular resection (small segment)	AL—PTFE neochords PL—Multiple triangular resections	Commissure closure Alfieri stitch or "magic stitch"
PTFE neochords	PTFE neochords	PTFE neochords (large segment)	AL—PTFE neochords PL—Multiple folding-plasties	PTFE neochords
Native chord transfer	"Haircut" edge resection + Native chord transfer or PTFE neochords	Papillary folding-plasty for multiple chords	AL—PTFE neochords PL—Leaflet sliding-plasty	PL—Sliding-plasty + PTFE neochords
Leaflet folding-plasty	Leaflet folding-plasty	Combined techniques	Combined techniques	Papillary folding-plasty (elongated or multi papillary: PL and AL chords)
Interscallop cleft closure	Interscallop cleft closure	–	–	–
			AL—Anterior leaflet PL—Posterior leaflet	

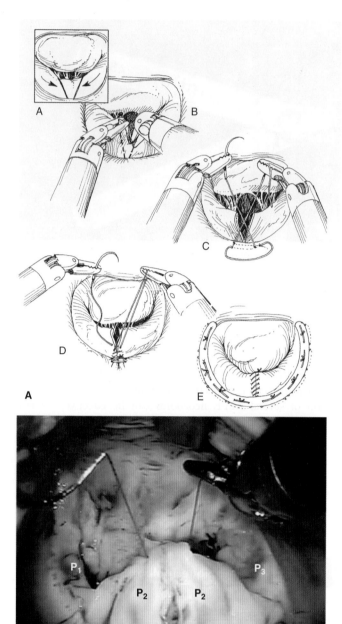

FIGURE 40-25 Mitral repair technique: posterior leaflet triangular/trapezoidal resection. (A) Trapezoidal P_2 leaflet resection; (B) triangular leaflet resection; (C and D) running suture closure; and (E) completed repair with annuloplasty band in place; (inset) after a triangular resection, reapproximated P_2 segments for interrupted suture closure.

the "Leipzig-loop" method, have been adopted widely. In severely prolapsing Barlow's valves with very elongated scallops and a great deal of redundant tissue, we still defer to a classic mid scallop (P_2) quadrangular resection with a posterior leaflet sliding-plasty (Figs. 40-29A–D and 40-30A–D). However, multiple triangular resections, folding-plasties and/

or multiple neochords may be used to repair moderately diseased Barlow's valves. All of our mitral leaflet repairs have been supported by a trigone to trigone Cosgrove annuloplasty band (Edwards Lifesciences, Inc., Irvine, CA).

Anterior Leaflet Repair

With isolated uniform anterior leaflet prolapse of less than 2 to 3 mm, we place the annuloplasty band first and then perform a saline test. Usually, this corrects a minor prolapse. When significant anterior prolapse exist, individual areas can be addressed with a local triangular resection, a secondary chord transfer or PTFE neochord replacement, or a combination of these techniques. For a large segment, anterior leaflet prolapse multiple neochords are effective as is a "flip over" chord segment transfer (Fig. 40-31A–E) from the posterior leaflet. Advancement of a chord-bearing anterior leaflet strip can be done if there is a uniform prolapse of A_2 (Fig. 40-32A–D). In elderly patients, especially with significant comorbid conditions, we may perform an ("Alfieri") edge-to-edge mid-leaflet repair, combined with an annuloplasty. We only use this repair either when reduced operative time is important or there is a significant chance of residual SAM. When a large anterior leaflet prolapsing segment is related to *multiple chords from an elongated papillary muscle*, correction can be accomplished either by muscle shortening (folding) (Fig. 40-33A–D) or insertion of several PTFE chords. We perform a saline test after each individual repair maneuver.

Commissure Repairs

In most circumstances, commissure prolapse can be corrected by: (1) closure with a Carpentier "magic" stitch (Lembert edge to edge suture) or figure of eight "Alfieri" stitch, (2) insertion of commissural PTFE chords, or (3) papillary muscle folding. The latter can shorten an elongated papillary muscle that has "seemingly" redundant chords, which are attached to both anterior and posterior leaflet edges. This should symmetrically return the prolapsing commissure to an anatomic position.

Annuloplasty Methods

Annular dilatation is present in most patients with degenerative mitral valve disease. We perform an adjunctive annuloplasty in all repairs to restore the native geometry, reduce the annular size, reinforce the repair and prevent further dilatation. Reducing the anterior-posterior annular diameter increases the leaflet coaptation surface. As mentioned before, annuloplasty band size selection is guided by our intraoperative echocardiographic derived nomogram Table 40-3. For consistency and ease of implantation, we use the Edwards Cosgrove Annuloplasty Band System (Edwards Lifesciences, Irvine Calif.) in most robotic and minimally invasive mitral repairs. Generally, a "trigone to trigone" posterior band provides optimal coaptation, while preserving a "saddle-shaped" systolic configuration.

We first place sutures through the right fibrous trigone, and continue in a clockwise direction. Previously, to

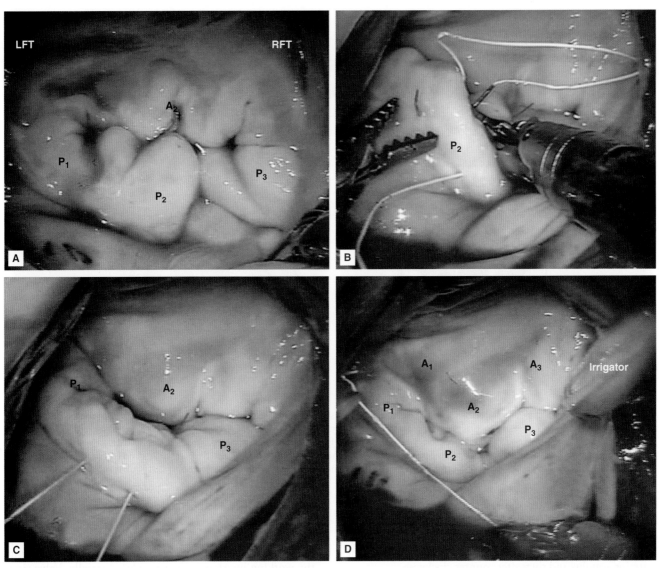

FIGURE 40-26 Mitral repair technique: posterior leaflet folding plasty. (A) Prolapsing long P$_2$ leaflet segment; LFT, left fibrous trigone; RFT, right fibrous trigone. (B) PTFE suture passed through the leaflet at the annulus, then "mattressed" back through the P$_2$ tip toward the annulus. (C) Both sutures are tightened to render an even coapting surface with the anterior leaflet (A$_2$). (D) During a saline pressure test, the PTFE suture is adjusted and tied, rendering a competent valve.

secure annuloplasty bands, we instrument tied interrupted 2-0 Ticron (Covidien, Mansfield, MA) or 2-0 Cardioflon (Peters Surgical, Paris France) sutures. The Cleveland Clinic group has shown great success in using a continuous annuloplasty band suturing technique.[73] We now prefer to use multipoint band fixation, using deep annular braded sutures (2-0 Cardioflon, Peters, Inc., Paris, France), which are secured by Cor-Knot (LSI Solutions, Inc., Victor, NY) titanium clips (Fig. 40-34A–C). After passing both suture ends through the band, they are brought through a wire loop in the applier. The suture-bearing wire loop then is withdrawn through both the applier and a titanium shim. After applying countertraction at the annuloplasty band, the device simultaneously crimps the shim and cuts the suture. The Cor-Knot device has been very effective at both speeding the operative time and providing very secure band attachment.

Tricuspid Valve Repair

Generally, we perform tricuspid repairs on the beating heart. For cardiac bicaval venous drainage, we isolate the SVC with a double-looped (Potts) umbilical tape and withdraw the IVC cannula below the liver. Alternately, the IVC can be isolated as described for the SVC. After the right atriotomy has been made, the tricuspid valve is exposed with either the stationary lift or dynamic robotic retractor. At the 2 o'clock anterior annular position, a 2-0 braded suture is placed and then passed extra corporeally through a Tri-Ad semi-rigid tricuspid

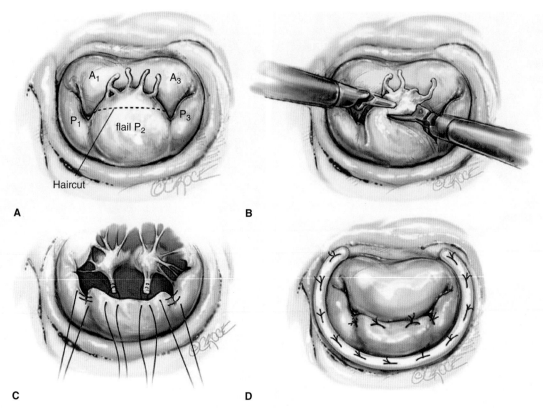

FIGURE 40-27 Mitral repair technique: "haircut" posterior leaflet plasty. (A) An extremely large flail P_2 segment is shown with many ruptured chords. Diminutive P_1 and P_2 segments preclude using a resection strategy. (B) The P_2 tip is resected horizontally to match the lengths of adjacent P_1 and P_2 segments. Remaining good P_2 chords are preserved. (C) P_1-P_2 and P_2-P_3 clefts are suture closed. Preserved chords then are reattached along the resected edge of P_2. An alternate technique is to resuspend P_2 using PTFE neochords. (D) The completed repair with a band annuloplasty. (Reproduced with permission from Chitwood WR: Haircut mitral valve repair: posterior leaflet-plasty, *Ann Cardiothorac Surg* 2015 Jul;4(4):387-392.)

annuloplasty band (Medtronic, Inc., St. Paul, MN). Then, the band is lowered to the native annulus and secured with a Core Knot titanium clip. We then continue with interrupted sutures from this first stitch, continuing clockwise along the anterior annulus and thereafter counter clockwise.

ROBOT-ASSISTED MITRAL VALVE REPLACEMENTS

Although tissue excision and suturing methods are similar in robotic mitral valve replacement operations, there are differences in the operative conduct.[74] In some rheumatic valves, leaflet and chordal excision can be difficult using the robotic technique. Current articulated instruments do not have the necessary force to cut very thick or calcified tissue. In this circumstance, we make a larger 5 to 6 cm working incision and excise the thick leaflet and chordal tissue using long manual instruments. We then place all subvalvular valve pledgeted sutures and neochords using daVinci System. Chord sparing replacements are done either by excising the anterior leaflet midportion and leaving natural chords intact or by removing them to increase the prosthesis valve size and replacing them with PTFE neochords. We attempt to preserve all native posterior leaflet chords by passing sutures through the leaflet edge and back through the annulus. In patients with a

severely calcified rheumatic valve or annulus, we may defer to either the 2D endoscopic or direct vision method for a replacement.

To organize sutures securely, guides are placed around the working incision as they are placed serially. Valve sizers are passed through the working incision, and the appropriate prosthetic valve is selected. Thereafter, extra-corporeally suture needles are passed through the prosthetic valve sewing-ring. After positioning the valve in the annulus and confirming seating, sutures are secured using the Core-Knot technique. A ventricular vent is placed and to remove residual air before closing the left atrium. Currently, for all endoscopic and robotic mitral valve operations, we use 4-0 PTFE sutures with pretied end loops to close the left atrium (see Fig. 40-11A). This technique provides a secure closure and saves operative time.

COMPLICATIONS AND PREVENTION

Patients undergoing any minimally invasive mitral/tricuspid valve operation risk the same complications that can occur with a traditional sternotomy-based procedure. Nevertheless, there are other complications that are inherent in perfusion and ventilation methods used for both MIS and robotic operations. In over 1000 robotic cardiac operations, we have never had a complication that was related directly either to the daVinci System or the robotic instruments. Our back-up plan for a system failure has always been conversion to either a direct-vision, videoscopic, or sternotomy approach.

Possible major complications with tips to prevention are listed as follows:

- *Retrograde cardiopulmonary perfusion* techniques always induce a risk of atheroembolic strokes, vena caval injury, femoral arterial complications, and retrograde aortic dissections. Careful preoperative vascular screening can minimize these problems. All cannulas should be inserted using the Seldinger technique under echocardiographic

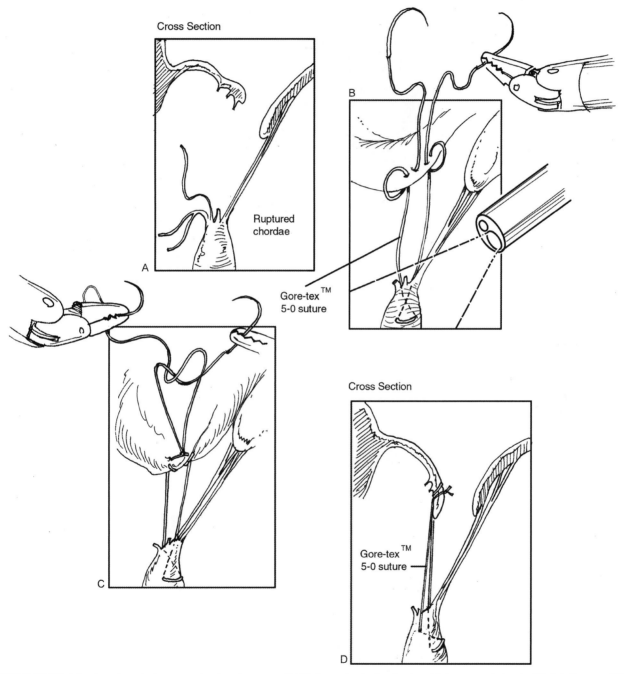

FIGURE 40-28 Mitral repair technique: neochord replacement. (A) Flail anterior leaflet from multiple ruptured chords. (B) 5-0 Gore-tex PTFE sutures are passed through the fibrous head of the corresponding papillary muscle using a tendon repair "cross stitch" configuration (W. L. Gore & Associates, Inc., Flagstaff, AZ). This precludes the need for a pledget and prevents muscle ischemia. Each suture is then passed twice through the flail leaflet edge, forming a loop hitch. (C) During saline pressure testing these loops are adjusted to provide an optimal coaptation surface. Thereafter they are tied. We suggest that final suture adjustment and tying be done after annuloplasty prosthesis placement. (D) The leaflet prolapse has been reduced to an ideal level of coaptation.

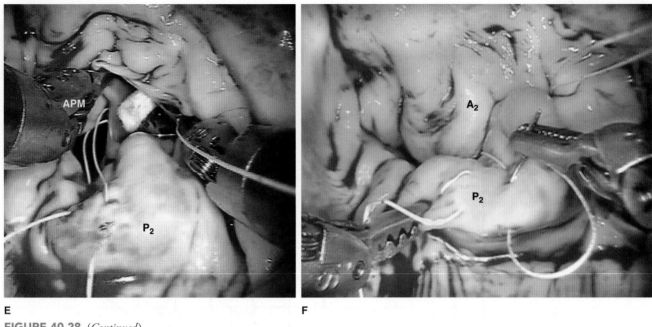

E   **F**

FIGURE 40-28 (*Continued*)

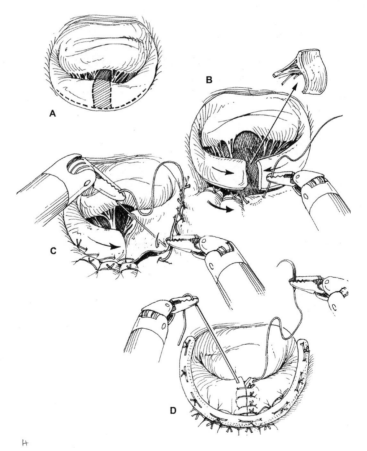

FIGURE 40-29 Mitral repair technique: posterior leaflet sliding plasty. (A) In a globally prolapsing redundant posterior leaflet, a large quadrangular resection has been performed. Thereafter, a radial periannular leaflet incision has been made on each side of the resection. (B) A number of mattress plication sutures are placed along the radial incision to reduce the annular length symmetrically. (C) Residual medial and lateral posterior leaflet tissue is advanced or "slid" centrally with a polypropylene or PTFE suture. (D) The defect between each newly approximated leaflet segment then is closed using either a running or interrupted suture technique. Finally, an annuloplasty prosthesis is implanted.

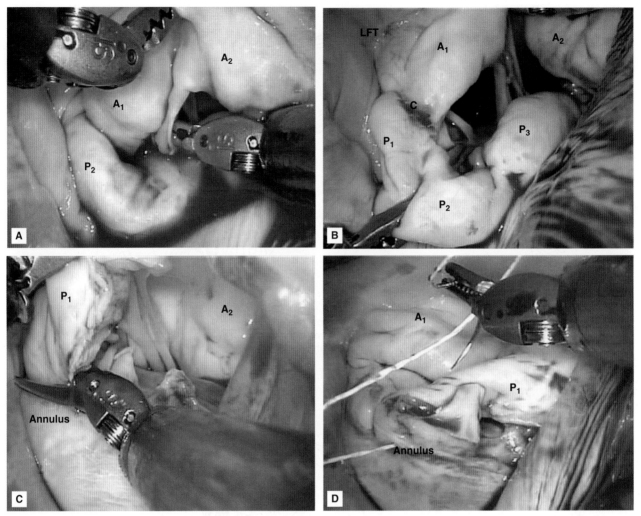

FIGURE 40-30 Mitral repair technique: posterior leaflet sliding plasty. (A and B) The entire posterior leaflet has redundant prolapsing tissue. LFT, left fibrous trigone; C, anterior commissure. (C) A large P$_2$ quadrangular resection has been performed. A radial periannulus incision has freed P$_1$ to near the anterior commissure. (D) A PTFE suture is shown "advancing/sliding" residual P$_1$ tissue centrally along the annulus to meet with the opposing P$_3$ flap. (Reproduced with permission from Chitwood WR: *Atlas of Robotic Cardiac Surgery*. London: Springer-Verlag; 2014.)

visualization. The endo-balloon should not be used in patients with mobile atheroma or diffuse aortic disease.

- *Leg ischemia during retrograde perfusion* can be avoided. We place oxygen saturation monitoring patches on both legs. With a significant decrease in cannulated leg oxygen saturation, we place we place a shunt from the CPB arterial cannula into the distal femoral artery.

- *Phrenic nerve injury* can be caused by over stretching the pericardium, cautery thermal injury, cryoablation, and/or direct instrument injury. This is a major problem in patients with compromised pulmonary function. Injury can be avoided by visualization of the nerve during instrument insertion and cautery usage. Overstretching can be avoided by making the pericardial incision at least 3-cm ventral to the nerve.

- *Unilateral pulmonary edema* is a serious complication. Short perfusion times, systemic cooling, avoiding

barotrauma, limiting blood product transfusions, and minimizing lung deflation times can reduce this risk. We also believe that low-level positive pressure and frequent alveolar recruitment, while on cardiopulmonary bypass, is beneficial.[75,76]

- *Transthoracic clamp injuries* can occur as the posterior element passes near the right pulmonary artery, left main coronary artery, and left atrial appendage. Visualization of the clamp pathway during application minimizes the chance of these complications. Pump arterial flow should be decreased during clamping. We have had no clamp related aortic dissections in any of our robot-assisted or videoscopic MIS mitral operations.

- *Right ventricular dysfunction* can be minimized. Meticulous cardiac deairing before weaning from cardiopulmonary bypass is essential. Right 30° chest elevation places the right coronary artery ostium in a perfect position

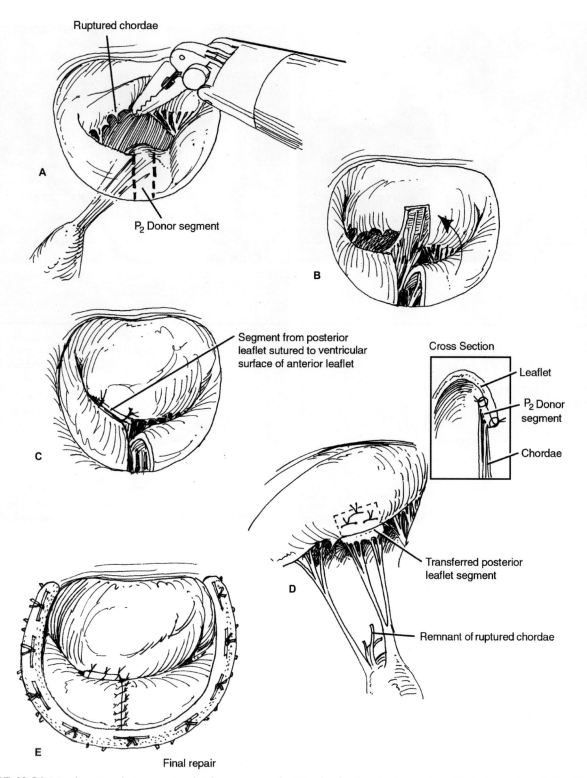

FIGURE 40-31 Mitral repair technique: native chord segment transfer. (A) A localized prolapsing portion of A_2 is shown. A small chord-bearing donor: section of posterior leaflet is selected. (B) The select area is resected and translocated while protecting intrinsic chords. This segment is "flipped over" to the prolapsing region of A_2. (C and D) The donor segment is then suture approximated to A_2; (inset) in this instance, it is attached to the posterior rough zone of A_2; and (E) the residual P_2 defect is closed, and annuloplasty prosthesis is implanted.

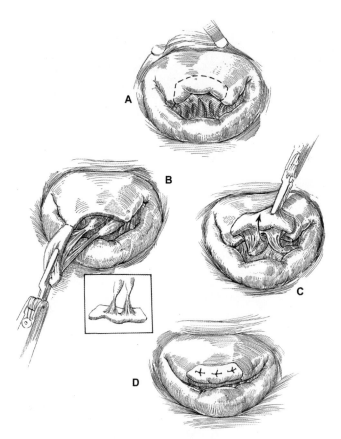

FIGURE 40-32 Mitral repair technique: anterior leaflet/chord advancement. (A) The entire A_2 is prolapsing to the same uniform level. (B) A strip of chord-bearing A_2 is transected horizontally along the coapting edge, being careful not to disrupt any chords. (C) This chord-bearing strip is advanced along the anterior surface of A_2 to the level that the prolapse is reduced to create good coaptation with P_2. (D) Using mattress sutures, the strip is attached to A_2 and annuloplasty prosthesis is implanted.

for air embolism from residual left ventricular air and/or aortic entrainment during cardioplegia infusions.

- *Left ventricular dysfunction* is a serious problem and can be avoided or minimized by selecting patients with ejection fractions of no less that 40 to 50%. If blood cardioplegia is used it must be given at 15- to 20-minute intervals. Systemic cooling (28°C) and meticulous de-airing are mandatory to maximize myocardial protection. Ventricular distention is a serious problem and can be prevented by leaving a ventricular vent after a repair or replacement.

CLINICAL OUTCOMES

Nonrobotic Minimally Invasive Mitral Valve Surgery

Many earlier observational and/or propensity-matched series have shown that direct-vision and video-assisted MIS mitral

surgery is safe with clinical results similar to operations done through a sternotomy. Four recent studies, that are cited herein, each reported over 1000 MIS mitral operations.[77–80] Nearly all of the 6179 patients were operated through a right minithoracotomy and approximately 75% underwent retrograde femoral CPB perfusion. Of these patients, the operative mortality was 0.75% and stroke rate was 1.2% (mean). Mohr et al reported the largest of these series with 2829 MIS mitral repairs.[78] Their freedom from a reoperation was 97 and 93% at 5 years and 10 years, respectively. The long-term survival was 87 and 74% at 5 and 10 years, respectively.

A recent meta-analysis from the *International Society of Minimally Invasive Cardiac Surgery* showed that versus a conventional (C) sternotomy, MIS mitral operations had less postoperative atrial fibrillation, chest tube drainage, transfusions, and infections.[13] There was no difference in the repair quality or freedom from reoperation. Moreover, operative mortality was not statistically different (1.5% C vs 1.2% MIS). Other benefits included reduced intensive care times and length of hospitalization as well as faster return to normal activity. These advantages were despite significantly longer perfusion and aortic cross clamp times. Conversely, they found more strokes (1.2% C vs 2.0% MIS), aortic dissections (0.0% C vs 0.2% MIS), and phrenic nerve injuries (0% C vs 3.0% MIS) in the MIS group. In contradistinction, the meta-analyses of Modi, Cao, and Sundermann have shown similar benefits and clinical outcomes as with traditional sternotomy operations, including strokes and operative mortality.[81–83]

The presumptive increased stroke risk with MIS has been attributed to retrograde CPB perfusion.[84–86] Most studies that impugned retrograde perfusion as the etiology of MIS strokes also included large numbers of patients who underwent endo-balloon aortic clamping. Retrograde endo-balloon catheter passage through the aorta seemingly risks cerebral atheroembolism, especially in nonscreened patients. This confounds any study that is considering the absolute relationship between retrograde perfusion and strokes. Moreover, these series did not report a vascular screening strategy and subtended the early days of MIS mitral surgery. Grossi found that there were no differences in perioperative strokes between antegrade and retrograde perfusion, if screened high-risk vascular patients were not included.[86] Atluri and Hargrove determined that in *screened patients* with retrograde CPB perfusion both endoballoon and direct aortic clamping had similar neurological events.[87] Also, Modi and Chitwood (meta-analysis) showed retrograde perfusion to be safe when patients were screened for aortic and peripheral vascular disease.[88]

Robot-Assisted Mitral Valve Surgery

Our early series (years 2000–2010) reported 540 RMVPs of which 454 patients underwent a lone mitral procedure, and 86 had a concomitant atrial fibrillation ablation.[56] In the lone repair cohort, cross clamp and CPB times averaged 116 and 153 minutes, respectively, and the operative mortality was 0.2%. Of those treated for preoperative atrial fibrillation, 96.5% were atrial fibrillation and drug free at 351 days

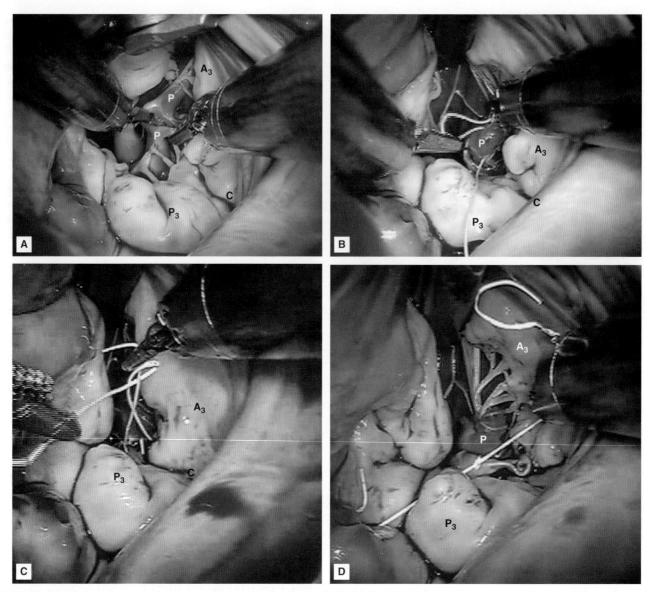

FIGURE 40-33 Mitral repair technique: papillary muscle shortening. (A) Redundant chords from the posterior papillary muscle have allowed A₃ and P₃ to create wide prolapse of the posterior commissure (C). (B) A PTFE suture has been passed through the fibrous tip of the posterior papillary muscle and then through the base. The suture should be tightened to reduce the muscle length before tying and the valve saline tested. (C and D) Thereafter, the suture is tied at the papillary muscle base.

(15–946 days). During patient follow-up, 2.9% required a re-operation for a failed repair. This study included the original FDA clinical trials and was the inaugural United States robotic mitral valve repair series.

Overall, we have performed over 1000 RMVP operations at our institution. Our single surgeon's (Dr. Chitwood) experience of 944 RMVPs (years 2000–2014) included the earlier series. For these operations, the original daVinci, the daVinci S, and the daVinci SI devices were used serially. Trento showed improving results with every device iteration, as did our group.[58] Of these patients, 675 had RMVPs alone, 321 had a concurrent maze procedure (M-RMVP) and 38 were reoperations in patients that had a prior sternotomy (Re-RMVP). For the entire series, the in-hospital mortality was 1.4%; however, for

an isolated RMVP was 0.15%. Of the entire series, 2.5% had reoperations for a failed repair, which was 1.7% for a lone RMVP. For each of these cohorts, mean CPB times were 148, 187, and 176 minutes, respectively. For RMVP and M-RMVP groups, mean aortic cross-clamp times were 108 and 128 minutes, respectively. Re-RMVP operations were done under hypothermic ventricular fibrillation (113 minutes, mean). In the RMVP patients, *major complications* included myocardial infarctions (0.9%) and strokes (0.9%). Reexplorations for bleeding were required in 2.7% of patients. There were two incidences of residual phrenic nerve palsy. Packed red cell transfusions were required in 28% of patients and 38% with any blood product. Of the RMVP patients, 56.9% were discharged within 4 days with 75.0% within 5 days. When

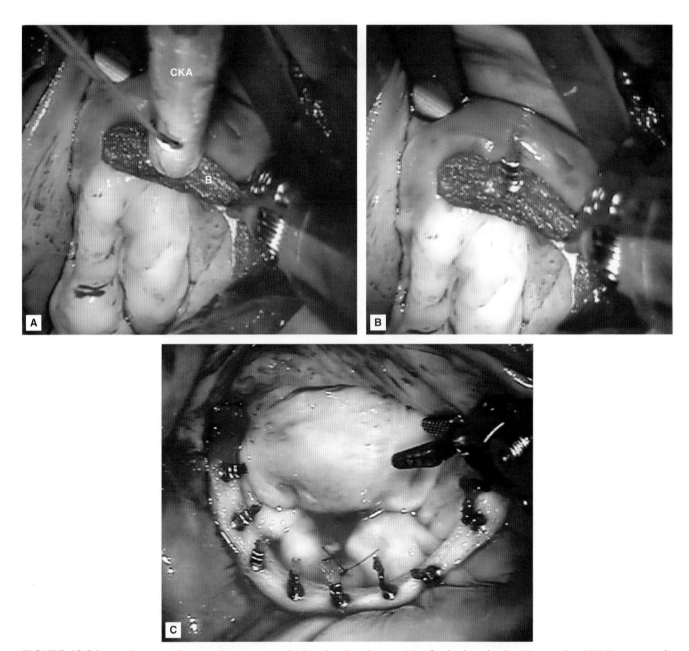

FIGURE 40-34 Mitral repair technique: Cor-Knot annuloplasty band anchoring. (A) After loading the Cor-Knot applier (CKA), a previously placed annuloplasty band (B) suture is withdrawn through a loop wire. When the wire is withdrawn, the suture transits titanium "shim," which is then crimped and the suture cut in one motion. (B) A titanium shim is shown after band approximation. (C) A completed annuloplasty band implantation using multipoint fixation Cor-Knot shims.

leaving the operating room, 97.1% of patients had no or trivial mitral regurgitation. Table 40-6 shows the complete post repair transesophageal echocardiographic data. Other large RMVP series have shown similar clinical outcomes.[57–60]

The Future

As the singer Bob Dylan said in 1964 "*The Times They Are a Changin*" and indeed they are changing …. and fast.[89,90] Long-term clinical data have established the expectation that mitral repair is the "gold" standard. Cardiology guidelines now

suggest that asymptomatic patients should be referred for surgery earlier, before atrial fibrillation, ventricular dysfunction, annular dilatation, and/or advanced valve pathology develops. Echocardiographic imaging continues to advance every year, and providing improved operative guidance. In experienced hands, minimally invasive and robotic derived repair results now parallel those of sternotomy operations. Although minimally invasive mitral surgery in the United States lags behind European centers, our younger surgeons know that the future favors even less invasive operations. Finally, the Internet and social media have given patients many more clinical choices

TABLE 40-6: Robot-Assisted Mitral Valve Repairs: N = 944 Postoperative Transesophageal Echocardiographic Studies

Residual mitral insufficiency	All patients N = 944 (%)	RMVP N = 675 (%)	C-RMVP N = 231 (%)	Re-RMVP N = 38 (%)
None	81.8	82.4	80.1	60
Trivial	15.3	15.1	16.0	36.8
Mild	2.8	2.4	3.9	2.6
Moderate	0.7	0.0	0.9	0.0
Severe	0.1	0.0	0.0	0.0

Abbreviations: C-RMVP, robotic mitral valve repair and Cryo MAZE for atrial fibrillation; Re-RMVP, robotic reoperations in patients with a prior sternotomy, RMVP, robotic mitral valve repair.
Used with permission from Edwards Lifesciences, Invine, CA.

and empowerment than in the past. They are more knowledgeable about their health care and demand to participate. Collectively, these facts seem like the "Sword of Damocles" for surgeons who scoff at the evolving mitral technology.

Advent and application of the Mitra-Clip (Abbott Vascular, Santa Clara, CA) and completion of the first Everest Trial proved that in high-risk patients, mitral regurgitation could be reduced to the point where symptoms abated. Even when some residual regurgitation remained, patients were better. This set the stage for off-pump neochord chord replacements to reduce leaflet prolapse in patients with a nondilated annulus. Transcatheter annuloplasty prostheses been developed to reduce dilatation. The story regarding treatment of ischemic mitral regurgitation is not completed, but we do know that transcatheter replacements may stabilize patients more than a repair. Heretofore, less attention was paid to the leaking "lonely" tricuspid valve. The natural history of this malady is better understood and transcatheter remedies are evolving.

Where does that leave surgeons? We are in the enviable position of being able to surgically repair mitral valves while simultaneously coopting transcatheter therapy. Owing to proven long-lasting results, surgical repair in younger patients will continue for a number of years. To be sure, if we can provide the least invasive complete repairs, based on sound engineering principles, we will prevail. Hopefully, principles set forth in this chapter comprise the entry portal to the future of mitral valve therapy.

REFERENCES

1. Navia JL, Cosgrove DM 3rd. Minimally invasive mitral valve operations. *Ann Thorac Surg* 1996;62:1542-1544.
2. Aklog L, Adams DH, Couper GS, Gobezie R, Sears S, Cohn LH. Techniques and results of direct-access minimally invasive mitral valve surgery: a paradigm for the future. *J Thorac Cardiovasc Surg* 1998;116:705-715.
3. Mihaljevic T, Cohn LH, Unic D, et al. One thousand minimally invasive valve operations: early and late results. *Ann Surg* 2004;240:529-534.
4. Pompili MF, Stevens JH, Burdon TA, et al. Port-access mitral valve replacement in dogs. *J Thorac Cardiovasc Surg* 1996;112:1268-1274.
5. Fann JI, Pompili MF, Burdon TA, et al. Minimally invasive mitral valve surgery. *Semin Thorac Cardiovasc Surg* 1997;9:320-330.
6. Baldwin JC. Editorial (con) reminimally invasive port-access mitral valve surgery. *J Thorac Cardiovasc Surg* 1998;115:563-564.
7. Cooley DA. Antagonist's view of minimally invasive heart valve surgery. *J Card Surg* 2000;15:3-5.
8. Mohr FW, Onnasch JF, Falk V, et al. The evolution of minimally invasive valve surgery–2 year experience. *Eur J Cardiothorac Surg* 1999;15:233-238.
9. Reichenspurner H, Boehm D, Reichart B. Minimally invasive mitral valve surgery using three-dimensional video and robotic assistance. *Semin Thorac Cardiovasc Surg* 1999;11235-11243.
10. Vanermen H, Farhat F, Wellens F, et al. Minimally invasive video-assisted mitral valve surgery: from Port-Access towards a totally endoscopic procedure. *J Card Surg* 2000;15:51-60.
11. McClure RS, Cohn LH, Wiegerinck E, et al. Early and late outcomes in minimally invasive mitral valve repair: an eleven-year experience in 707 patients. *J Thorac Cardiovasc Surg* 2009;137:70-75.
12. Svensson LG, Atik FA, Cosgrove DM, et al. Minimally invasive versus conventional mitral valve surgery: a propensity-matched comparison. *J Thorac Cardiovasc Surg* 2010;139:926-932.
13. Cheng DCH, Martin J, Lal A, et al. Minimally invasive versus conventional open mitral valve surgery: a meta-analysis and systematic review. *Innovations* 2011;6:84-103.
14. Modi P, Rodriguez E, Hargrove WC 3rd, Hassan A, Szeto WY, Chitwood WR, Jr. Minimally invasive video-assisted mitral valve surgery: a 12-year, 2-center experience in 1178 patients. *J Thorac Cardiovasc Surg* 2009;137:1481-1487.
15. Gammie JS, Sheng S, Griffith BP, et al. Trends in mitral valve surgery in the United States: results from the Society of Thoracic Surgeons Adult Cardiac Surgery Database. *Ann Thorac Surg* 2009;87:1431-1437.
16. Bolling SF, Li S, O'Brien SM, Brennan JM, Prager RL, Gammie JS. Predictors of mitral valve repair: clinical and surgeon factors. *Ann Thorac Surg* 2010;90:1904-1912.
17. Chatterjee S, Rankin JS, Gammie JS, et al. Isolated mitral valve surgery risk in 77,836 patients from the Society of Thoracic Surgeons database. *Ann Thorac Surg* 2013;96:1587-1594.
18. German Society for Thoracic and Cardiovascular Surgery—Annual Database Registry, 2015.
19. Joint Task Force on the Management of Valvular Heart Disease of the European Society of Cardiology (ESC); European Association for Cardio-Thoracic Surgery (EACTS), Vahanian A, et al. Guidelines on the management of valvular heart disease (version 2012). *Eur Heart J* 2012;33:2451-2496.
20. Nishimura RA, Otto CM, Bonow RO, et al. 2014 AHA/ ACC guideline for the management of patients with valvular heart disease: executive summary: a report of the American College of Cardiology/American Heart Association Task Force on Practice Guidelines. *J Am Coll Cardiol* 2014;63:2438-2488 and Circulation 2014;129:2440-2492.
21. Brunton TL. Preliminary note on the possibility of treating mitral stenosis by surgical methods. *Lancet* 1902;1:352.
22. Cutler EC, Levine SA. Cardiotomy and valvulotomy for mitral stenosis. *Boston Med Surg J* 1923;188:1023-1027.
23. Souttar HS. The surgical treatment of mitral stenosis. *Brit Med J* 1925;2:603-606.
24. Harken DE, Ellis LB, Ware PF, Norman LR. The surgical treatment of mitral stenosis. I. Valvuloplasty. *NEJM* 1948;239;801-809.

25. Bailey CP. The surgical treatment of mitral stenosis (mitral commissurotomy). *Dis Chest* 1949:15: 377-393.

26. HG, Boone JA, Stallworth JM. Surgical treatment of constrictive valvular disease of the heart. *Surg Gynecol Obstetr* 1950;90:175-192.

27. Baker C, Brock RC, Campbell M. Valvulotomy for mitral stenosis: report of six successful cases. *Br Med J*, 1950;1:1283–1293.

28. Lillehei CW, Gott VL, Dewall RA, et al. Surgical correction of pure mitral insufficiency by annuloplasty under direct vision. *J Lancet* 1957;77:446-449.

29. McGoon DC. Repair of mitral insufficiency due to ruptured chordae tendinae. *J Thorac Cardiovasc Surg* 1960;39:357-359.

30. Dávila JC. The birth of intra-cardiac surgery: a semi-centennial tribute. *Ann Thorac Surg* 1998;65:1809-1820.

31. Carpentier A, Adams DH, Filsoufi F. *Carpentier's Reconstructive valve Surgery: From Valve Analysis to Valve Reconstruction.* 2010; Saunders (Elsevier), New York.

32. Starr A, Edwards ML. Mitral replacement: clinical experience with ball valve prosthesis. *Ann Surg* 1961;154:726-740.

33. Harken DE, Soroff HS, Taylor WJ, Lefemine AA, Gupta Sk, Lunzer S. Partial and complete prosthesis in aortic insufficiency. *J Thorac Cardiovasc Surg* 1960;40:744-762.

34. Carpentier A, Deloche A, Dauptain J, et al. A new reconstructive operation for correction of mitral and tricuspid insufficiency. *J Thorac Cardiovasc Surg* 1971;61:1-13.

35. Duran CG, Pomar JL, Revuelta JM, et al. Conservative operation for mitral insufficiency: critical analysis supported by postoperative hemodynamic studies of 72 patients. *J Thorac Cardiovasc Surg* 1980;79:326-337.

36. Carpentier A. Cardiac valve surgery—the "French correction." *J Thorac Cardiovasc Surg* 1983;86:323-337.

37. David TE, Ivanov J, Armstrong S, Christie D, Rakowski H. A comparison of outcomes of mitral valve repair for degenerative disease with posterior, anterior, and bileaflet prolapse. *J Thorac Cardiovasc Surg* 2005;130:1242-1249.

38. Braunberger E, Deloche A, Berrebi A, et al. Very long-term results (more than 20 years) of valve repair with Carpentier's techniques in nonrheumatic mitral valve insufficiency. *Circulation* 2001;104(12 Suppl 1):I8-11.

39. Gillinov AM, Cosgrove DM, Blackstone EH, et al. Durability of mitral repair for degenerative disease. *J Thorac Cardiovasc Surg* 1998;116:734-743.

40. Cohn LH, Couper GS, Aranki SF, et al. Long-term results of mitral valve reconstruction for regurgitation of the myxomatous mitral valve. *J Thorac Cardiovasc Surg* 1994;107:143-150.

41. Ellis FH. *Surgery for Acquired Mitral Valve Disease.* Philadelphia: WB Saunders, p. 9, 1967.

42. Harken DE, Glidden EM. Experiments in intracardiac surgery. II. Intracardiac Visualization. *J Thorac Surg* 1943;12:566-572.

43. Sakakibara H, Ichikawa T, Hattori J. An intraoperative method for observation of cardiac septal defect using a cardioscope. *Operation* 1956;10:285-290.

44. Sakakibara H, Ichikawa T, Hattori J, et al. Direct visual operation for aortic stenosis: cardioscopic studies. *J Int Coll Surg* 1958;29:548-562.

45. Kaneko Y, Kohno T, Ohtsuka T, et al. Video-assisted observation in mitral valve surgery. *J Thorac Cardiovasc Surg* 1996;111:279-280.

46. Carpentier A, Loulmet D, Carpentier A, et al. Open heart operation under video surgery and minithoracotomy. First case (mitral valvuloplasty) operated with success. *C R Acad Sci III* 1996;319:219-223.

47. Chitwood WR, Jr, Wixon CL, Elbeery JR, et al. Video-assisted minimally invasive mitral valve surgery. *J Thorac Cardiovasc Surg* 1997;114:773-780.

48. Chitwood WR, Jr, Wixon CL, Elbeery JR, Moran JF, Chapman WHH. Video-assisted minimally invasive mitral valve surgery. *J Thorac Cardiovasc Surg* 1997;114:773-782.

49. Felger JE, Chitwood WR, Jr, Nifong LW, et al. Evolution of mitral valve surgery: toward a totally endoscopic approach. *Ann Thorac Surg* 2001;72:1203-1208.

50. Carpentier A, Loulmet D, Aupècle B, et al. Computer assisted open heart surgery. First case operated on with success. *C R Acad Sci III* 1998;321:437-442.

51. Autschbach R, Onnasch JF, Falk V, et al. The Leipzig experience with robotic valve surgery. *J Card Surg* 2000;15:82-87.

52. LaPietra A, Grossi EA, Derivaux CC, et al. Robotic-assisted instruments enhance minimally invasive mitral valve surgery. *Ann Thorac Surg* 2000;70:835-838.

53. Chitwood WR, Jr, Nifong LW, Elbeery JE, et al. Robotic mitral valve repair: trapezoidal resection and prosthetic annuloplasty with the da Vinci surgical system. *J Thorac Cardiovasc Surg* 2000;120:1171-1172.

54. Nifong LW, Chitwood WR, Pappas PS, et al. Robotic mitral valve surgery: a United States multicenter trial. *J Thorac Cardiovasc Surg* 2005;129:1395-1404.

55. Chitwood WR, Jr, Rodriguez E, Chu MW, et al. Robotic mitral valve repairs in 300 patients: a single-center experience. *J Thorac Cardiovasc Surg* 2008;136:436-441.

56. Nifong LW, Rodriguez E, Chitwood WR, Jr. 540 consecutive robotic mitral valve repairs including concomitant atrial fibrillation cryoablation. *Ann Thorac Surg* 2012;94:38-42.

57. Suri RM, Burkhart HM, Rehfeldt KH, et al. Robotic mitral valve repair for all categories of leaflet prolapse: improving patient appeal and advancing standard of care. *Mayo Clin Proc* 2011;86:838-844.

58. Ramzy D, Trento A, Cheng W, et al. Three hundred robotic-assisted mitral valve repairs: the Cedars-Sinai experience. *J Thorac Cardiovasc Surg* 2014;147:228-235.

59. Murphy DA, Moss E, Binongo J, et al. The expanding role of endoscopic robotics in mitral valve surgery: 1,257 consecutive procedures. *Ann Thorac Surg* 2015;100:1675-1681.

60. Gillinov MA, Mihaljevic T, Javadikasgari H, et al. Safety and effectiveness of robotically assisted mitral valve surgery: analysis of 1000 consecutive cases. *J Amer Coll Card.* In press. 2016.

61. Mihaljevic T, Koprivanac M, Kelava M, et al. Value of robotically assisted surgery for mitral valve disease. *JAMA Surg* 2014;149:679-686.

62. Suri RM, Thompson JE, Burkhart HM, et al. Improving affordability through innovation in the surgical treatment of mitral valve disease. *Mayo Clin Proc* 2013;88:1075-1084.

63. Chitwood WR, Jr. *Atlas of Robotic Cardiac Surgery.* New York: Springer, 2014.

64. Kypson AP, Sanderson DA, Nifong LW, et al. Cardiopulmonary bypass and myocardial protection for minimally invasive cardiac surgery. In: Gravlee GP, Davis RF, Hammon JW, et al. editors. *Cardiopulmonary Bypass and Mechanical Support: Principles & Practice.* Philadelphia: Wolters Kluwer, 2016.

65. Marie-Elisabeth S, Laufer G, Wisser W. The Endoscopic Aesculap Einstein Vision 3D System: can it compete with the daVinci System? (abstract). *AATS Mitral Valve Conclave*, 2015.

66. Rodriguez E, Nifong LW, Bonatti J, et al. Pathway for surgeons and programs to establish and maintain a successful robot-assisted adult cardiac surgery program. *Ann Thorac Surg* 2016;102:340-344.

67. Suri RM, Dearani JA, Mihaljevic T, et al. Mitral valve repair using robotic technology: safe, effective, and durable. *J Thorac Cardiovasc Surg* 2016;151:1450-1454.

68. Gazoni LM, Fedoruk LM, Kern JA, et al. A simplified approach to degenerative disease: triangular resections of the mitral valve. *Ann Thorac Surg* 2007;83:1658.

69. Cevasco M, Myers PO, Elbardissi AW, Cohn LH. Foldoplasty: a new and simplified technique for mitral valve repair that produces excellent medium-term outcomes. *Ann Thorac Surg* 2011 Nov;92(5):1634-1637.

70. Chu MW, Gersch KA, Rodriguez E, Nifong LW, Chitwood WR, Jr. Robotic "haircut" mitral valve repair: posterior leaflet-plasty. *Ann Thorac Surg* 2008;85:1460-1462.

71. David TE, Armstrong S, Ivanov J. Chordal replacement with polytetrafluoroethylene sutures for mitral valve repair: a 25-year experience. *J Thorac Cardiovasc Surg.* 2013;145:1563-1569.

72. Mihaljevic T, Pattakos G, Gillinov AM, Bajwa G, Planinc M, Williams SJ, Blackstone EH. Robotic posterior mitral leaflet repair: neochordal versus resectional techniques. *Ann Thoracic Surg* 2013;95:787-794.

73. Mihaljevic T, Jarrett CM, Gillinov AM, Blackstone EH. A novel running annuloplasty suture technique for robotically assisted mitral valve repair. *J Thorac Cardiovasc Surg* 2010;139:1343-1344.

74. Gao C, Yang M, Xiao C, et al. Robotically assisted mitral valve replacement. *J Thorac Cardiovasc Surg* 2012;143:S64-S67.

75. Keyl C, Staier K, Pingpoh C, et al. Unilateral pulmonary oedema after minimally invasive cardiac surgery via right anterolateral minithoracotomy. *Eur J Cardiothorac Surg* 2015;47(6):1097-1102.

76. Moss E, Binongo JN, Halkos MF, Murphy DA. Prevention of unilateral pulmonary edema complicating robotic mitral valve surgery. *Anna Thorac Surg* (in press), 2016.

77. Goldstone AB, Atluri P, Sezto W, et al. Minimally invasive approach provides at least equivalent results for surgical correction of mitral

regurgitation: a propensity-matched comparison. *J Thorac Cardiovasc Surg* 2013;145:748-756.

78. Davierwala PM, Seeburger J, Pfannmueller B, et al. Minimally invasive mitral valve surgery: "The Leipzig experience." *Ann Cardiothorac Surg* 2013;2:744-750.

79. Glauber M, Miceli A, Canarutto D, et al. Early and long-term outcomes of minimally invasive mitral valve surgery through right minithoracotomy: a 10-year experience in 1604 patients. *J Cardiothorac Surg* 2015;10:181.

80. Downs EA, Johnston LE, LaPar DJ, et al. Minimally invasive mitral valve surgery provides excellent outcomes without increased cost: a multi-institutional analysis. *Ann Thorac Surg* 2016;102:14-21.

81. Modi P, Hassan A, Chitwood WR, Jr. Minimally invasive mitral valve surgery: a systematic review and meta-analysis. *Eur J Cardiothorac Surg* 2008;34:943-952.

82. Cao C, Gupta S, Chandrakumar D, et al. A meta-analysis of minimally invasive versus conventional mitral valve repair for patients with degenerative mitral disease. *Ann Cardiothorac Surg* 2013;2:693-703.

83. Sündermann SH, Sromicki J, et al. Mitral valve surgery: right lateral minithoracotomy or sternotomy? A systematic review and meta-analysis. *J Thorac Cardiovasc Surg* 2014;148:1989-1995.

84. Gammie JS, Zhao Y, Peterson ED, et al. Less-invasive mitral valve operations: trends and outcomes from the Society of Thoracic Surgeons Adult Cardiac Surgery Database. *Ann Thorac Surg* 2010;9:1401-1408.

85. Bedeir K, Reardon M, Ramchandani M, Singh K, Ramlawi B. Elevated stroke risk associated with femoral cannulation during mitral valve surgery. *Semin Thorac Cardiovasc Surg* 2015;27:97-103.

86. Grossi EA, Loulmet DF, Schwartz CF, et al. Evolution of operative techniques and perfusion strategies for minimally invasive mitral valve repair. *J Thorac Cardiovasc Surg* 2012;143:S68-S70.

87. Atluri P, Goldstone AB, Fox J, Szeto WY, Hargrove WC. Port access cardiac operations can be safely performed with either endoaortic balloon or Chitwood clamp. *Ann Thorac Surg* 2014;98:1579-1583.

88. Modi p, Chitwood WR, Jr, retrograde femoral arterial perfusion and stroke risk during minimally invasive mitral valve surgery: is there cause for concern? *Ann Cardiothorac Surg* 2013;2:1-5.

89. Badhwar V, Thourani VH, Ailawadi G, Mack M. Transcatheter mitral valve therapy: the event horizon. *J Thorac Cardiovasc Surg* 2016;152:330-335.

90. Chitwood WR. Commentary: Ode to the mitral valve: "The times are a changin." *J Thorac Cardiovasc Surg* 2016;152:336.

41

Percutaneous Catheter-based Mitral Valve Repair

Mani Arsalan • J. Michael DiMaio • Michael Mack

Mitral valve repair (MVR) remains the standard of care for patients with severe valve incompetence. MVR is usually accomplished by either an open surgical (sternotomy) approach or by minimally invasive (right lateral minithoracotomy) access techniques. Recently there has been an intense interest in developing percutaneous catheter-based techniques, especially for high-risk patients.[1-4]

Although the success of transcatheter aortic valve replacement (TAVR) has been rapid, progress toward percutaneous correction of mitral regurgitation (MR) has been much more modest.[5] The success of catheter-based treatment of aortic stenosis can be attributed to a number of factors: the singular pathophysiology of the diseased valve, the aortic valve's anatomical location that allows for precise valve stent implantations at the annular level, and the successful development of delivery systems using conventional imaging techniques. The field of percutaneous MVR, however, has not progressed so rapidly for a host of reasons including the complex pathophysiology of MR with a diversity of etiologies, as well as challenges in imaging and delivery and secure anchoring of the valve without impingement on surrounding cardiac structures. These obstacles have led to slower than anticipated clinical adoption of catheter-based approaches for the treatment of MR. To understand the potential for successful therapy, it is first instructive to examine the pathophysiology of the various mechanisms of the disease.

PATHOPHYSIOLOGY OF MITRAL REGURGITATION

The mitral valve (MV) is a complex structure composed of two leaflets, a fibrous annulus with varying degrees of continuity and integrity, and a subvalvular apparatus consisting of chordae tendineae and papillary muscles attached to the wall of the left ventricle (LV). The etiology of MR can be categorized into two ways: primary also called degenerative or organic, and secondary or functional MR.

In primary MR (Carpentier Type II), the intrinsic disease is a result of leaflet degeneration, ranging from fibroelastic deficiency to an excess of connective tissue called Barlow's disease, in patients with MV prolapse. Although MR of intrinsic

disease occurs initially as isolated leaflet disease, secondary annular dilatation occurs in the majority of patients by the time that they present for treatment.

The largest proportion of patients who present with MR, however, are those with secondary MR (Carpentier Type IIIB), in which the valve is anatomically normal but has been stretched by tethering and ventricular dilatation.[6] Secondary MR is not a primary valvular pathology but is a result of a cascade of events initiated by this ventricular dilation. Ventricular dilation leads to apical and lateral distraction of the papillary muscles, which results in tethering of the mitral leaflets. This tethering causes central regurgitation secondary to failure of coaptation of the anatomically normal leaflets during systole.[7] The causes and prognosis of secondary MR are inherently different from intrinsic disease. Although annular dilatation also occurs in this disease, it is a secondary phenomenon. The principle utilized during surgical repair of secondary MR is based upon overcorrection of the annular dilatation component by performing an undersized annuloplasty to restore leaflet coaptation. To date, it is still unknown whether correcting secondary MR has any impact on the underlying pathology or affects long-term survival.[8-11]

CURRENT TRANSCATHETER APPROACHES TO THE TREATMENT OF MITRAL REGURGITATION

There is a wide spectrum of devices and approaches to manage MR from a percutaneous or transcatheter approach (Table 41-1).[12] Most catheter-based repair techniques are based on techniques that have been proven to be effective in open surgical MVR. Examples include the edge-to-edge technique, placement of artificial chords, and annular remodeling. However, the challenges in adapting these techniques to catheter-based treatment are significant and center mainly on device delivery and imaging. In contrast to open surgical therapy which employs a combination of techniques, transcatheter approaches have not yet successfully combined these different techniques, and, thus, complex pathologies are hard to correct.

TABLE 41-1: Concepts of Transcatheter Techniques for the Management of Mitral Regurgitation

Degenerative disease
   Edge-to-edge repair
   Artificial chord placement
Functional
   Edge-to-edge repair
   Coronary sinus annuloplasty
   Direct annuloplasty
   Indirect annuloplasty
   Extracardiac annuloplasty
   Mitral "spacer"
   Mitral valve replacement

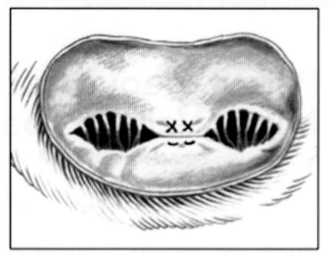

FIGURE 41-1 Concept of surgical correction of mitral regurgitation by attaching the free edges if the mitral leaflets, creating a double orifice valve.

Although many different strategies and devices have been developed, only three have received European (CE Mark) approval to date. These are the MitraClip (Abbott Vascular, Irvine, CA), NeoChord DS 1000 (NeoChord, Inc., Louis Park, MN), and Carillon Mitral Contour System (Cardiac Dimensions, Inc., Kirkland, WA). MitraClip has also received US Food and Drug Administration (FDA) approval for commercial sale in the United States, but only for patients with primary MR who are at high risk for surgical repair. Other devices are in various stages of development.

Some devices such as the MitraClip have been employed to treat both primary and secondary MR. Most, however, have been designed to treat only one etiology or the other, with the majority devoted to secondary MR because of the larger clinical need and the existence of excellent surgical repair techniques for primary disease. We will first review the procedures and devices for the management of primary mitral disease.

Primary Mitral Regurgitation

PERCUTANEOUS EDGE-TO-EDGE REPAIR

The MitraClip system is the only device with extensive clinical application, now with over 19,000 implantations worldwide. The MitraClip mimics the surgical edge-to-edge repair technique of Alfieri (Fig. 41-1).[13] The device received CE approval in 2008, and FDA approval in 2013. However, the FDA approved the MitraClip only for primary MR in high surgical risk patients and not for patients with secondary MR.

The MitraClip system is designed to allow off-pump endovascular reconstruction of the regurgitant MV. It includes a clip device (MitraClip) and a steerable guiding catheter that enables placement of the clip on the free edges of the MV leaflets. The clip ensures permanent leaflet approximation and creates a double orifice MV (Fig. 41-2). The procedure is performed percutaneously via the femoral vein with transseptal puncture in a cardiac catheterization laboratory or in a hybrid suite with echocardiographic guidance under general anesthesia. The addition of three-dimensional and X-plane echocardiography has significantly facilitated the procedure, as the improved visualization allows for more accurate MitraClip positioning (Fig. 41-3).

Without any strict recommendations from the manufacturer on type or duration of postoperative antiplatelet therapy, several anticoagulation regimens have been proposed. In the Everest I and II trials, aspirin 325 mg daily for 6 months to 1 year was implemented with 75 mg of clopidogrel daily for 1 month.[14-16] In Europe 100 mg of aspirin daily for 3 months and 75 mg of clopidogrel daily without a loading dose for 4 weeks are more commonly used.[14,17]

The primary benefit associated with the use of the MitraClip is reduction of MR with elimination of the needs for open chest surgery, cardiopulmonary bypass, and cardiac arrest. The potential risks include those associated with cardiac catheterization and transseptal puncture. The major concern regarding this technique is uncertainty regarding the efficacy of a procedure that results in a less complete correction of MR than is usually accomplished surgically. This concern is based on the knowledge that surgical edge-to-edge repair without annuloplasty is associated with a higher rate of recurrent severe regurgitation if the residual MR is greater than 1+ postoperatively.[18] Whether partial reduction of MR is sufficient to translate into ventricular reverse remodeling and, more importantly, any clinical benefit remains to be determined.[9,11] Additional concerns have been raised regarding the potential impairment of the ability to perform a subsequent surgical valve repair should this become necessary.[19-21]

There is a recent trend to implant multiple clips during a single procedure to achieve better coaptation and, thus, improved outcomes.[22] Of note, there have been very few reports of mitral stenosis necessitating intervention following MitraClip repair.[23,24] Even after multiple clip implantations in the same patient, mitral stenosis has rarely occurred.

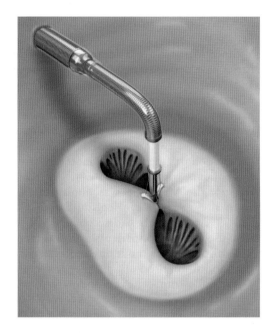
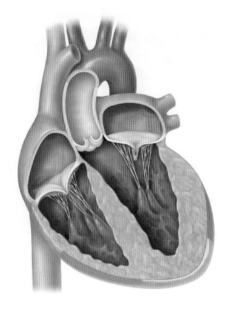
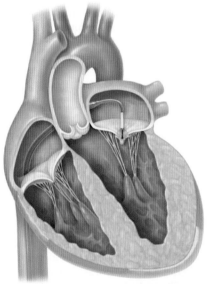
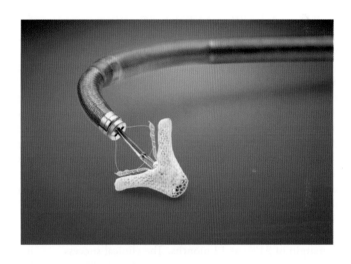
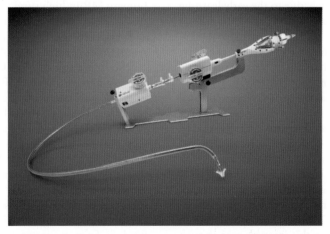

FIGURE 41-2 The Evalve MitraClip with delivery system. (© 2013 Abbott. All rights reserved. MitraClip is a trademark of the Abbott Group of Companies.)

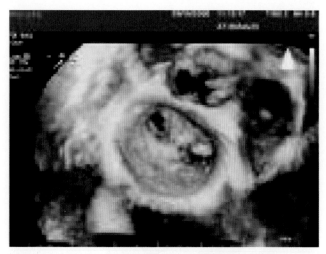

FIGURE 41-3 Three-dimensional echocardiogram demonstrating the MitraClip in position. (© 2013 Abbott. All rights reserved. Mitra-Clip is a trademark of the Abbott Group of Companies.)

MitraClip has undergone significant clinical testing. In the initial clinical feasibility trial (Everest I: Endovascular Valve Edge-to-Edge REpair STudy), 55 patients were enrolled, and both the safety and efficacy of the device were demonstrated. The pivotal Everest II trial was a multicenter randomized controlled trial to evaluate the benefits and risks of MVR using the MitraClip device compared with open MV surgery in 279 relatively low-risk patients with moderate or severe MR. It was conducted as a per-protocol analysis on a noninferiority hypothesis. Although transfusion was the major component of the composite safety endpoint in the surgical arm, the device met the safety noninferiority hypothesis criteria even if transfusion was eliminated. The primary effectiveness endpoint was determined as freedom from the combined outcome of death, MV surgery or reoperation, and MR greater than 2+ at 12 months. The trial also met the clinical success noninferiority hypothesis, which set a pre-specified margin of 31%, at 12 months. The clinical success rate in the device group was 72.4% compared with 87.8% in the control group, an absolute observed difference margin of 15.4%. However, most likely due to the early learning curve with this device, acute procedural success (MR ≤ 2+ at discharge) was achieved in only 77% of patients, and 21% required subsequent open MV surgery. Ultimately, the Everest II trial showed that the MitraClip is safer, particularly by reducing the frequency of postoperative transfusions, but not as effective in reducing MR as compared to conventional MV surgery.[25]

The EVEREST II High-Risk Registry and REALISM Continued Access Study High-Risk Arm investigated the outcome of MitraClip therapy in 351 high-risk patient with 3 to 4+ MR. MR was reduced to ≤2+ in 86% of patients at discharge.[26] Despite a mean STS-predicted operative mortality risk of 11.3 ± 7.7% for mitral replacement, the Kaplan-Meier freedom from death was 77.2% at 12 months. Freedom from MV surgery was 97.8% over this interval, even though 16.4% of patients had MR > 2+ at 12 months. This result

may have been inflated, however, by the high operative risk in these patients.

Since MitraClip was approved in Europe, several registries have demonstrated high rates of procedural success and favorable short-term outcomes. The Transcatheter Mitral Valve Interventions (TRAMI) Registry with 1064 patients (71% with secondary MR) showed that the procedure can be performed at a high success rate (95% device success) with no procedural deaths in a high-risk patient cohort (median STS mortality score 10; 69% of the patients with LVEF <50%).[27] In the ACCESS-EU registry, the MitraClip was implanted in 567 patients at 14 sites.[28] The mean logistic EuroSCORE was 23%, and 77% of patients had secondary MR. Multiple clips were used in 40% of patients. MR was reduced to ≤2+ in 91% of patients without any procedural deaths. NYHA class and 6-minute walk distance had both improved at 1-year follow-up. The European Sentinal Pilot Registry, with a similar rate of secondary MR patients (71% of 628), confirms these results while maintaining high procedural success (95.4%) and low mortality rates (in-hospital mortality 2.9%). Although the rehospitalization for heart failure was more common in the secondary MR group (25.8 vs 12.0%, p = .009), recurrence of severe MR was present only in 6% of patients at 1 year following the procedure.[29]

The current guidelines are largely influenced by the encouraging results of these clinical trials. The 2012 ESC/EACTS Valve and HF guidelines provide a class IIb (LOE C) recommendation to consider MitraClip use in symptomatic patients with both severe primary and secondary MR.[30] The patients need to be judged inoperable or at high surgical risk by a "heart team" and should have a life expectancy greater than 1 year. Patients with secondary MR additionally need to be under optimal medical therapy and cardiac resynchronization therapy, if indicated.

Despite the fact that MitraClip has CE mark approval in secondary MR and has achieved good results in the large European registries for this disease category, the FDA has approved MitraClip only for the treatment of patients with primary MR in high surgical risk patients. Thus, in the 2014 ACCF/AHA Valve guidelines, MitraClip is recommended with class IIb (LOE b) guidance for severe primary MR in symptomatic patients at prohibitive risk for MV surgery.[31]

The future role of MitraClip in the management of both primary and secondary MR remains unclear.[32] Particularly, high-risk patients with secondary MR may benefit from MitraClip therapy. Three large ongoing randomized trials (COAPT, RESHAPE-HF, and Mitra-Fr) comparing Mitra-Clip plus guideline-directed medical therapy (GDMT) versus GDMT alone in secondary MR may further elucidate the optimal role for MitraClip. The results of these trials should be available by 2017. However, even in the healthiest subgroup of patients—those with primary MR, no annular calcification, and optimal initial medical MR reduction—freedom from recurrent MR is only 60% after 9 years if annuloplasty is not performed.[33] This might be acceptable for older or high-risk patients, but not for patients who are suitable for surgery.

Leaflet Repair Using Artificial Chords

The NeoChord DS1000 device allows off-pump implantation of artificial neochordae to repair prolapsing or flail mitral leaflets. The access for this procedure is a left minithoracotomy through which a purse-string is placed at the apex of the beating heart. A delivery device that contains an infrared sensor to detect tissue supports optimal grasping of the free edge of the prolapsing leaflet. Via indirect visualization with 3D echo, a suture is passed through the grasped free edge of the leaflet. The two ends of this suture are then brought through the apex of the heart and tied on the epicardial surface (Fig. 41-4). Proper chordal length is determined by adjustment under direct transesophageal echocardiographic guidance. The chords can be appropriately lengthened or shortened based on the color jet seen on echo.

Current experience with the NeoChord DS1000 is limited to slightly more than 100 patients. The Transapical Artificial Chordae Tendinae feasibility trial showed acute procedural success in 26 out of 30 patients (86.7%), deemed as overall reduction of MR from ≥3+ to ≤2+. Four patients (13.3%) had to be converted to conventional MV repair.[34] At 30-day follow-up, only 17 patients maintained MR grade ≤2+, and four patients with recurrent MR had surgical MV repair during the 30-day follow-up. Results improved with experience: durable reduction in MR to ≤2+ at 30 days was achieved in 5 (33.3%) of the first 15 patients and 12 (85.7%) of the last 14 patients. Furthermore, the implantation of two or three chords led to an improved MR reduction, which has been similarly demonstrated in the surgical loop technique. Larger studies are needed to prove efficacy and durability of this technique. Of note, a technique to perform edge-to-edge repair with this device may be under development.

Secondary Mitral Regurgitation

MITRAL ANNULAR REMODELING TECHNIQUES

Although there is dilatation of the entire mitral annulus in patients with secondary MR, the greatest degree of dilation is in the posterior annulus and the greatest increase in dimension is in the septal-lateral (or anterior-posterior) diameter.[8,35] Therefore, secondary MR is most commonly surgically managed by reduction in the septal lateral diameter of the dilated mitral annulus by an undersized, complete, and rigid annuloplasty ring. A key element of this surgical repair includes anchoring a complete ring to the central fibrous skeleton of the heart at the fibrous trigones because anchoring the ring away from the mitral annulus in the atrial wall or in the leaflet tissue leads to less effective reduction in annular dimensions. Similarly, it has been well proven in the surgical arena that a partial posterior annuloplasty is less effective in annular reduction to treat MR.[36-38] On the other hand, correction of the septal lateral diameter by as little as 5 to 8 mm has been demonstrated to reconstitute leaflet coaptation and improve MR. Transcatheter approaches to secondary MR are based on this concept of mitral annulus remodeling to decrease the septal lateral diameter. There is no shortage of novel strategies to accomplish this goal (see Table 41-1). Some devices take advantage of the anatomical relationship between the coronary sinus and posterior mitral annulus; other devices take a more direct approach by plicating the posterior annulus; still others rely on distraction of the LV or left atrial walls to decrease the septal lateral diameter.

Coronary Sinus Annuloplasty

Its proximity to the posterior mitral annulus makes the coronary sinus an attractive access point for placement of devices to remodel the mitral annulus (Fig. 41-5).[39-43] The ease of transvenous access led to early optimism. However, variability in the anatomic relationship of the coronary sinus to the mitral annulus has made it a challenge to obtain consistent decreases in annular dimensions. Although the coronary sinus is most commonly located adjacent to the posterior annulus, it is frequently located along the free wall of the left atrium, superior to the mitral annulus therefore relying on traction on the left atrial free wall for annular remodeling.[44,45] The smallest distance between the coronary sinus and the mitral annulus is usually at the entry to the sinus. Separation of the coronary sinus from the mitral annulus is maximal at the posterolateral commissure, as demonstrated in an anatomical study by Miselli of coronary sinus anatomy in 61 human cadaver hearts.[46] In this cohort, the distance between the inferior border of the coronary sinus and the mitral annulus at the P2 and

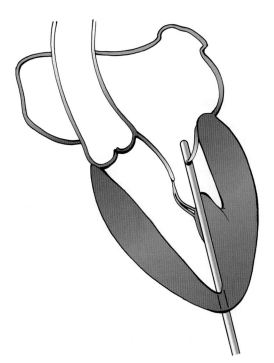

FIGURE 41-4 Placement of artificial chords from the left ventricular apex under echocardiographic guidance.

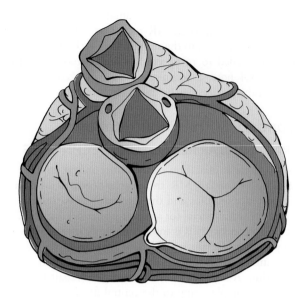

FIGURE 41-5 Concept of a posterior mitral annulus plication performed by a device placed through the coronary sinus.

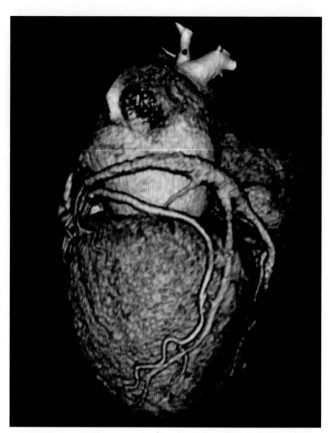

FIGURE 41-6 Example demonstrating by computerized tomography the relationships between the coronary sinus and the mitral annulus. Note the intervening circumflex coronary artery. (Reproduced with permission from Choure AJ, Garcia MJ, Hesse B, et al: In vivo analysis of the anatomical relationship of coronary sinus to mitral annulus and left circumflex coronary artery using cardiac multidetector computed tomography: implications for percutaneous coronary sinus mitral annuloplasty, *J Am Coll Cardiol.* 2006 Nov 21;48(10):1938-1945.)

P3 mitral segments averaged 9.7 mm. It is important to note that in patients with severe MR, the distance between the coronary sinus and the mitral annulus is usually much greater than in patients without severe regurgitation. In addition, the path of the circumflex coronary artery and/or its branches between the coronary sinus and mitral annulus is of significant concern. The left circumflex artery or major branches have been reported to course between the coronary sinus and the mitral annulus in up to 80% of patients (Fig. 41-6).[46] Due to all of these concerns, the Carillon Mitral Contour System, a fixed-length device designed for plication of the coronary sinus between deployable anchors placed via internal jugular access, is the only remaining device employing the coronary sinus approach. Its proximal anchor is released near the coronary sinus ostium, and its distal one is deployed near the anterior commissure, deep on the coronary sinus. In case of insufficient MR reduction, the device can be repositioned.

In the AMADEUS feasibility study, the device was successfully implanted in 30 of the 48 enrolled patients (62.5%).[47] In these patients the mitral annular diameter was significantly reduced, leading to MR reduction by at least 1 grade and improvement in functional class at 2-year follow-up. In the TITAN trial, which investigated a second-generation device, 36 of 53 patients underwent successful device implantation (67%).[48] In both studies a high number of patients (17% in the AMADEUS, 15% in the Titan trial) did not receive the device due to unwanted interaction with the left circumflex artery. In the remaining patients with unsuccessful intervention, the Carillon device was retrieved, as it did not reduce MR by at least one grade. The major adverse events rate in the two studies decreased from 13 to 1.9%, but, due to low success rates, limited reversal in LV remodeling, and lack of control groups, the results of the initial Carillon Mitral Contour System trials remain controversial.[49]

Direct Mitral Annular Remodeling

There are a number of devices designed to remodel the mitral annulus by direct plication. The Mitralign system (Mitralign, Inc., Tewksbury, MA) consists of polyester pledgets, a suture, and a stainless steel lock. A suture-based plication of the posterior annulus is placed retrograde through the aortic valve on the ventricular side of the mitral annulus. Two sutures are placed to plicate P1-P2 and P2-P3 (Fig. 41-7).[50] Sixty-one patients were enrolled in the EU study for CE mark approval which was completed in 2014. In 45 patients (73.8%), the device was implanted with improvement in MR, quality of life, and NYHA classification at 30-day follow-up.[51] A larger implant with a 50% increase in cinching distance, which may result in a stronger annulus diameter reduction and enhanced outcome, is now available, but CE mark approval is pending.

Another device, the Valtech Cardioband (Valtech, Inc., Tel Aviv, Israel), places a tensioning band with anchoring screws placed into the mitral annulus via a transseptal atrial access.[52] The tensioning band is then adjusted under echocardiographic

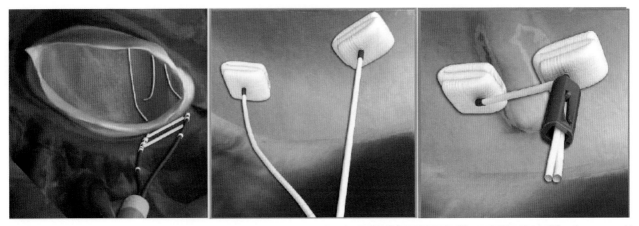

FIGURE 41-7 Plication of the posterior mitral annulus by a percutaneous transventricular approach. (© 2015 Mitralign. All rights reserved.)

guidance until the regurgitant jet disappears as leaflet coaptation is restored. Early results of a multicenter study involving 29 symptomatic patients with moderate-to-severe secondary MR showed a 100% successful implant rate and 93% acute MR reduction postoperatively with sustained results over 6 months (91% MR ≤ 2+).[53] Both 6-minute walk test and NYHA classification improved in 11 patients (37.9%) at 6-month follow-up, but improvement did not reach statistical significance. CE mark approval is still pending for the Valtech Cardioband.

Transcatheter Mitral Valve Replacement

Perhaps the most intriguing concept currently for the percutaneous treatment of secondary MR is transcatheter MV replacement (TMVR). One of the disadvantages of surgical annuloplasty for secondary MR is the recurrence of regurgitation in approximately one third of patients by one year. Even if the annuloplasty performed by a surgical or percutaneous approach leads to complete correction of MR at the time of the index procedure, the ongoing ventricular disease process may eventually cause further dilation of the ventricle. This leads to further tethering of the papillary muscles and free edges of the leaflets, resulting in return of MR some time after repair. In fact, the recurrence rate at 12 months after MVR is reported to be higher as compared to MV replacement (32.6 vs 2.3%).[54] MV replacement, instead of repair, could theoretically prevent recurrence of MR even if further left ventricular dilation occurs after the procedure because LV dilatation should not affect an implanted prosthesis.

After the TAVR evolution, rapid adoption of TMVR was anticipated. However, the development of TMVR has been delayed by the complex structure of the MV, composed of the left ventricular outflow tract, ventricular myocardium, papillary muscles, chordae, and native MV leaflets. Because the MV is a much more complex structure than the AV, many different variables must be considered during TMVR in comparison to the relatively straightforward TAVR technique. Most importantly, unlike the aortic annulus in aortic

stenosis, the mitral annulus is not calcified in MR, so there is no good anchoring zone for the implanted valve. However, the solid ring structure of a biological MV prosthesis or complete annuloplasty ring can be an ideal anchoring zone for a TAVR valve to be placed in the mitral location. Thus, in recent years, valve-in-valve (VinV) and valve-in-ring (VinR) procedures have become routine in many centers worldwide for high-risk patients. Both, VinV and VinR can be performed safely with transapical or transfemoral access.[55-59] But, without prior surgical MV or annuloplasty ring implantation, fixation of a TMVR is difficult.

Several devices have been developed to perform TMVR, of which some have recently initiated compassionate and early feasibility human trials and others have yet to initiate trials. These include the CardiAQ device (CardiAQ Valve Technologies, Inc., Winchester, MA), the Tiara device (Neovasc, Inc., Richmond, BC, Canada), the Tendyne device (Tendyne Medical, Inc., Roseville, MN), and the Fortis transapical device (Edwards Lifesciences, Irvine, CA).

The CardiAQ is a self-expanding, stent-based, bovine pericardial bioprosthesis. The device self-anchors without radial force and grabs the native MV leaflets (Fig. 41-8a). In 2012, it was the first TMVR device to reach human implantation using a transfemoral/transseptal access. After redesign, the second-generation CardiAQ device was implanted transapically in three patients 2014. The CE mark trial with 100 patients at 10 sites is anticipated to start in early 2015.[60]

The Tiara device is a self-expanding, nitinol-based, bovine pericardial bioprosthesis (Fig. 41-8b). It can be implanted transapically, facilitated by a 32F sheathless system. The device captures the native mitral leaflets and has a full atrial skirt to minimize paravalvular leak. The D shape of the valve could help to prevent LV outflow obstruction. After three successful implantations in the first-in-man (FIM) trial, the TIARA-I feasibility study started in late 2014.[61,62]

The Tendyne device is an apical, self-expanding, nitinol-based, porcine pericardial bioprosthesis with a ventricular tethering fixation system anchoring the valve to the left ventricular apex (Fig. 41-8c). It is fully retrievable and repositionable, and it is available in multiple sizes. After three patients

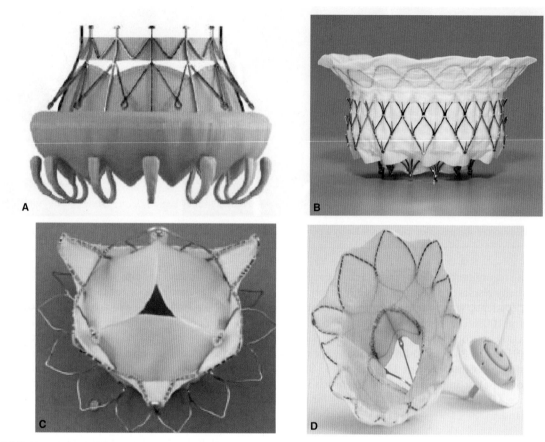

FIGURE 41-8 Transcatheter Mitral Valve Replacement devices in clinical trials. (A. Used with permission from Tiara, Neovasc Inc, Richmond, BC, Canada. B. Used with permission from Tendyne Medical, Inc., Roseville, MN. C. Used with permission from Intrepid, Medtronic Inc, Minneapolis, MN. D. Used with permission from Edwards Lifesciences LLC, Irvine, CA.)

were successfully treated under a compassionate use protocol, the device was implanted in the first patient of an early feasibility study in November 2014. The patient recovered quickly and was released from the hospital on day 5.[63]

The Fortis transapical device is composed of a cloth-covered nitinol stent with three anticalcification-treated bovine pericardial leaflets. At present, only the 29 mm size valve is available, suitable for patients with a native annular diameter (A2-P2) between 30 and 44 mm. Valve fixation is performed by two paddles that capture the mitral leaflets. An atrial flange is designed to prevent paravalvular leaks. Rapid pacing is not necessary because normal blood flow is maintained throughout the entire procedure. All seven reported implantations of the Fortis device have led to a MR Grade ≤1+. One of the patients died after a partial displacement of the valve because the posterior paddle failed to capture the posterior mitral leaflet. Enrollment for a clinical feasibility study started in August 2014.[64,65]

CONCLUSION

There are a host of unique and intriguing concepts for transcatheter treatment of MR. Although progress in the transcatheter treatment of aortic stenosis was rapid and promising,

progress with MR has been much slower due to the complex MV anatomy, the variable MR pathologies, the necessity for complex delivery systems, the limited early success in clinical trials, and the existence of an effective, established therapy (open surgery). In addition, proper trial design has proven to be challenging, with the demonstration of clinical benefit remaining particularly difficult. However, the clinical unmet need is sizable, and with a host of unique concepts under early investigation, significant progress can be expected in the near future. The MV will be one of the most interesting targets for therapeutic cardiac device innovations in the coming years.

REFERENCES

1. Feldman T: Percutaneous mitral valve repair. *J Interventional Cardiol* 2007; 20:488-494.
2. Carabello BA: The current therapy for mitral regurgitation. *J Am Coll Cardiol* 2008; 52:319-326.
3. Mack M: Fool me once, shame on you; fool me twice, shame on me! A perspective on the emerging world of percutaneous heart valve therapy. *J Thorac Cardiovasc Surg* 2008; 136:816-819.
4. Masson JB, Webb JG: Percutaneous treatment of mitral regurgitation. *Circulat Cardiovasc Interven* 2009; 2:140-146.
5. Mack MJ: Percutaneous treatment of mitral regurgitation: so near, yet so far! *J Thorac Cardiovasc Surg* 2008; 135:237-239.
6. Carpentier A: Cardiac valve surgery—the "French correction". *J Thorac Cardiovasc Surg* 1983; 86:323-337.

7. Bach DS, Bolling SF: Improvement following correction of secondary mitral regurgitation in end-stage cardiomyopathy with mitral annuloplasty. *Am J Cardiol* 1996; 78:966-969.

8. Wu AH, Aaronson KD, Bolling SF, Pagani FD, Welch K, Koelling TM: Impact of mitral valve annuloplasty on mortality risk in patients with mitral regurgitation and left ventricular systolic dysfunction. *J Am Coll Cardiol* 2005; 45:381-387.

9. Silberman S, Oren A, Klutstein MW, et al: Does mitral valve intervention have an impact on late survival in ischemic cardiomyopathy? *Israel Med Assoc J* 2006; 8:17-20.

10. Calafiore AM, Iaco AL, Gallina S, Al-Amri H, Penco M, Di Mauro M: Surgical treatment of functional mitral regurgitation. *Inter J Cardiol* 2013; 166:559-571.

11. Milano CA, Daneshmand MA, Rankin JS, et al: Survival prognosis and surgical management of ischemic mitral regurgitation. *Ann Thorac Surg* 2008; 86:735-744.

12. Fedak PW, McCarthy PM, Bonow RO: Evolving concepts and technologies in mitral valve repair. *Circulation* 2008; 117:963-974.

13. Maisano F, Torracca L, Oppizzi M, et al: The edge-to-edge technique: a simplified method to correct mitral insufficiency. *Eur J Cardiothorac Surg* 1998; 13:240-245; discussion 245-246.

14. Alsidawi S, Effat M: Peri-procedural management of anti-platelets and anticoagulation in patients undergoing Mitraclip procedure. *J Thromb Thrombolys* 2014; 38:416-419.

15. Feldman T, Wasserman HS, Herrmann HC, et al: Percutaneous mitral valve repair using the edge-to-edge technique: six-month results of the Everest Phase I Clinical Trial. *J Am Coll Cardiol* 2005; 46:2134-2140.

16. Mauri L, Garg P, Massaro JM, et al: The Everest II Trial: design and rationale for a randomized study of the Evalve Mitraclip system compared with mitral valve surgery for mitral regurgitation. *Am Heart J* 2010; 160:23-29.

17. Franzen O, Baldus S, Rudolph V, et al: Acute outcomes of Mitraclip therapy for mitral regurgitation in high-surgical-risk patients: emphasis on adverse valve morphology and severe left ventricular dysfunction. *Eur Heart J* 2010; 31:1373-1381.

18. De Bonis M, Lapenna E, Maisano F, et al: Long-term results (≤18 years) of the edge-to-edge mitral valve repair without annuloplasty in degenerative mitral regurgitation: implications for the percutaneous approach. *Circulation* 2014; 130:S19-24.

19. Dang NC, Aboodi MS, Sakaguchi T, et al: Surgical revision after percutaneous mitral valve repair with a clip: initial multicenter experience. *Ann Thorac Surg* 2005; 80:2338-2342.

20. Geidel S, Schmoeckel M: Impact of failed mitral clipping on subsequent mitral valve operations. *Ann Thorac Surg* 2014; 97:56-63.

21. Alozie A, Westphal B, Kische S, et al: Surgical revision after percutaneous mitral valve repair by edge-to-edge device: when the strategy fails in the highest risk surgical population. *Eur J Cardiothorac Surg* 2014; 46:55-60.

22. Paranskaya L, D'Ancona G, Bozdag-Turan I, et al: Percutaneous mitral valve repair with the Mitraclip system: perioperative and 1-year follow-up results using standard or multiple clipping strategy. *Catheter Cardiovasc Int* 2013; 81:1224-1231.

23. Singh K, Raphael J, Colquhoun D: A rare case of mitral stenosis after Mitraclip placement: transesophageal echocardiography findings and examination. *Anesth Analg* 2013; 117:777-779; discussion 779.

24. Cockburn J, Fragkou P, Hildick-Smith D: Development of mitral stenosis after single Mitraclip insertion for severe mitral regurgitation. *Catheter Cardiovasc Int* 2014; 83:297-302.

25. Feldman T, Foster E, Glower DD, et al: Percutaneous repair or surgery for mitral regurgitation. *N Engl J Med* 2011; 364:1395-1406.

26. Glower DD, Kar S, Trento A, et al: Percutaneous mitral valve repair for mitral regurgitation in high-risk patients: results of the Everest II Study. *J Am Coll Cardiol* 2014; 64:172-181.

27. Schillinger W, Hunlich M, Baldus S, et al: Acute outcomes after Mitraclip therapy in highly aged patients: results from the German Transcatheter Mitral Valve Interventions (TRAMI) Registry. *EuroIntervention* 2013; 9:84-90.

28. Maisano F, Franzen O, Baldus S, et al: Percutaneous mitral valve interventions in the real world: early and 1-year results from the ACCESS-EU, a prospective, multicenter, nonrandomized post-approval study of the Mitraclip therapy in Europe. *J Am Coll Cardiol* 2013; 62:1052-1061.

29. Nickenig G, Estevez-Loureiro R, Franzen O, et al: Transcatheter Valve Treatment Sentinel Registry Investigators of the ERPotESoC. Percutaneous mitral valve edge-to-edge repair: in-hospital results and 1-year follow-up of 628 patients of the 2011-2012 Pilot European Sentinel Registry. *J Am Coll Cardiol* 2014; 64:875-884.

30. Vahanian A, Alfieri O, Andreotti F, et al: Joint Task Force on the Management of Valvular Heart Disease of the European Society of C, European Association for Cardio-Thoracic S. Guidelines on the management of valvular heart disease (version 2012): the joint task force on the management of valvular heart disease of the European Society of Cardiology (ESC) and the European Association For Cardio-Thoracic Surgery (EACTS). *Eur J Cardiothorac Surg* 2012; 42:S1-44.

31. Nishimura RA, Otto CM, Bonow RO, et al: American College of Cardiology/American Heart Association Task Force on Practice Guidelines. 2014 AHA/ACC Guideline for the management of patients with valvular heart disease: a report of the American College of Cardiology/American Heart Association Task Force on Practice Guidelines. *J Am Coll Cardiol* 2014; 63:e57-185.

32. Vahanian A, Iung B: 'Edge to edge' percutaneous mitral valve repair in mitral regurgitation: it can be done but should it be done? *Eur Heart J* 2010; 31:1301-1304.

33. De Bonis M, Lapenna E, Pozzoli A, et al: Edge-to-edge surgical mitral valve repair in the era of Mitraclip: what if the annuloplasty ring is missed? *Curr Opin Cardiol* 2015.

34. Seeburger J, Rinaldi M, Nielsen SL, et al: Off-pump transapical implantation of artificial neo-chordae to correct mitral regurgitation: the tact trial (Transapical Artificial Chordae Tendinae) proof of concept. *J Am Coll Cardiol* 2014; 63:914-919.

35. Acker MA, Bolling S, Shemin R, et al: Mitral valve surgery in heart failure: insights from the acorn clinical trial. *J Thorac Cardiovasc Surg* 2006; 132:568-577, e561-564.

36. Nguyen TC, Cheng A, Tibayan FA, et al: Septal-lateral annnular cinching perturbs basal left ventricular transmural strains. *Eur J Cardiothorac Surg* 2007; 31:423-429.

37. Mihaljevic T, Lam BK, Rajeswaran J, et al: Impact of mitral valve annuloplasty combined with revascularization in patients with functional ischemic mitral regurgitation. *J Am Coll Cardiol* 2007; 49:2191-2201.

38. Ruiz CE, Kronzon I. The wishful thinking of indirect mitral annuloplasty: will it ever become a reality? *Circ Cardiovasc Interv* 2009; 2:271-272.

39. Sorajja P, Nishimura RA, Thompson J, et al: A novel method of percutaneous mitral valve repair for ischemic mitral regurgitation. *JACC Cardiovasc Interv* 2008; 1:663-672.

40. Tops LF, Kapadia SR, Tuzcu EM, et al: Percutaneous valve procedures: an update. *Curr Prob Cardiol* 2008; 33:417-457.

41. Sack S, Kahlert P, Bilodeau L, et al: Percutaneous transvenous mitral annuloplasty: initial human experience with a novel coronary sinus implant device. *Circulation Cardiovasc Interv* 2009; 2:277-284.

42. Webb JG, Harnek J, Munt BI, et al: Percutaneous transvenous mitral annuloplasty: initial human experience with device implantation in the coronary sinus. *Circulation* 2006; 113:851-855.

43. Piazza N, Bonan R: Transcatheter mitral valve repair for functional mitral regurgitation: coronary sinus approach. *J Interv Cardiol* 2007; 20:495-508.

44. Tops LF, Van de Veire NR, Schuijf JD, et al: Noninvasive evaluation of coronary sinus anatomy and its relation to the mitral valve annulus: implications for percutaneous mitral annuloplasty. *Circulation* 2007; 115:1426-1432.

45. Lansac E, Di Centa I, Al Attar N, et al: Percutaneous mitral annuloplasty through the coronary sinus: an anatomic point of view. *J Thorac Cardiovasc Surg* 2008; 135:376-381.

46. Maselli D, Guarracino F, Chiaramonti F, et al: Percutaneous mitral annuloplasty: an anatomic study of human coronary sinus and its relation with mitral valve annulus and coronary arteries. *Circulation* 2006; 114:377-380.

47. Schofer J, Siminiak T, Haude M, et al: Percutaneous mitral annuloplasty for functional mitral regurgitation: results of the carillon mitral annuloplasty device European Union Study. *Circulation* 2009; 120:326-333.

48. Siminiak T, Wu JC, Haude M, et al: Treatment of functional mitral regurgitation by percutaneous annuloplasty: results of the titan trial. *Eur J Heart Fail* 2012; 14:931-938.

49. Bach DS: Functional mitral regurgitation and transcatheter mitral annuloplasty: the carillon mitral annuloplasty device European Union Study in perspective. *Circulation* 2009; 120:272-274.

50. Siminiak T, Dankowski R, Baszko A, et al: Percutaneous direct mitral annuloplasty using the Mitralign Bident system: description of the method and a case report. *Kardiol Pol* 2013; 71:1287-1292.

51. Abizaid A. Mitralign CE Mark Study: 30-day outcome. *TCT* 2014.

52. Maisano F, La Canna G, Latib A, et al: First-in-man transseptal implantation of a "surgical-like" mitral valve annuloplasty device for functional mitral regurgitation. *JACC Cardiovasc Interv* 2014; 7:1326-1328.

53. Maisano F: Antegrade transvenous approach with the cardioband (valtech). *TCT* 2014.

54. Acker MA, Parides MK, Perrault LP, et al: Mitral-valve repair versus replacement for severe ischemic mitral regurgitation. *N Engl J Med* 2014; 370:23-32.

55. Cheung A, Webb JG, Barbanti M, et al: 5-year experience with transcatheter transapical mitral valve-in-valve implantation for bioprosthetic valve dysfunction. *J Am Coll Cardiol* 2013; 61:1759-1766.

56. Seiffert M, Conradi L, Baldus S, et al: Transcatheter mitral valve-in-valve implantation in patients with degenerated bioprostheses. *JACC Cardiovasc Interv* 2012; 5:341-349.

57. Webb JG, Wood DA, Ye J, et al: Transcatheter valve-in-valve implantation for failed bioprosthetic heart valves. *Circulation* 2010; 121:1848-1857.

58. Wilbring M, Alexiou K, Tugtekin SM, et al: Transapical transcatheter valve-in-valve implantation for deteriorated mitral valve bioprostheses. *Ann Thorac Surg* 2013; 95:111-117.

59. Descoutures F, Himbert D, Maisano F, et al: Transcatheter valve-in-ring implantation after failure of surgical mitral repair. *Eur J Cardiothorac Surg* 2013; 44:e8-15.

60. Sondergaard L: Cardiaq: design, clinical results, and next steps. *TCT* 2014.

61. Cheung A, Webb J, Verheye S, et al: Short-term results of transapical transcatheter mitral valve implantation for mitral regurgitation. *J Am Coll Cardiol* 2014; 64:1814-1819.

62. Cheung A: Neovasc tiara: design, clinical results and next steps. *TCT* 2014.

63. Grayburn PA: Tendyne transapical mitral valve replacement acute first-in human clinical results. *TCT* 2014.

64. Bapat V: Edwards Fortis: design, clinical results, and next steps. *TCT* 2014.

65. Bapat V, Buellesfeld L, Peterson MD, et al: Transcatheter mitral valve implantation (TMVI) using the Edwards Fortis device. *EuroIntervention* 2014; 10(Suppl U):U120-128.

Mitral Valve Replacement

Tsuyoshi Kaneko • Maroun Yammine • Dan Loberman • Sary Aranki

This chapter discusses the surgical indications, operative techniques, and early and late follow-up after implantation of mechanical and bioprosthetic mitral valve devices. The valves that are discussed are those that are currently (2015) approved by the Food and Drug Administration (FDA). Figure 42-1 shows the former and current FDA-approved prosthetic mechanical mitral valve devices, including the Starr-Edwards ball-and-cage valve (historical relevance only), the Omnicarbon tilting-disk valve, the Medtronic Hall tilting-disk valve, the St. Jude Medical bileaflet valve, the Carbomedics bileaflet valve, the ATS bileaflet valve, and the On-X bileaflet valve. The FDA-approved bioprosthetic valve devices are shown in Fig. 42-2 and include the Hancock II porcine valve, the Carpentier-Edwards porcine valve, the Carpentier-Edwards pericardial valve, the Mosaic porcine valve, and the Biocor porcine valve.

Heart valve prostheses are continually undergoing iterative advancement by the manufacturers; however, the ideal valve has yet to be developed. This ideal replacement prosthesis would have longevity of a mechanical prosthesis combined with the superior hemodynamic function of the native biologic tissue valve. As a result, this hypothetical ideal replacement device would not require lifetime anticoagulation and carries no risk of either thromboembolic events or valve thrombosis. Achieving this goal will require major advancements to currently available designs.

INDICATIONS FOR MITRAL VALVE REPLACEMENT

The indications for mitral valve replacement (MVR) are variable and undergoing evolution. Because of increasing use of reparative techniques, particularly for mitral regurgitation (MR), replacement or repair of a mitral valve often depends on the experience of the operating surgeon. Current indications for valve replacement pertain to the types of valve problems that are unlikely to be repaired by most surgeons or which have been shown to have poor long-term success after reconstruction. Indications are discussed according to (1) pathophysiologic states and (2) type of valve required (ie, mechanical or bioprosthetic).

MITRAL STENOSIS

Mitral stenosis (MS) is almost exclusively caused by rheumatic fever even though a definite clinical history can be obtained in only about 50% of patients. The incidence of MS has decreased substantially in the United States in the last several decades because of effective prophylaxis of rheumatic fever; nevertheless, in certain developing countries MS is still very common. Two-thirds of patients with rheumatic MS are females.

The pathologic changes associated with rheumatic valvulitis are mainly fusion of the valve leaflets at the commissures, shortening and fusion of the cordae tendineae, and thickening of the leaflets owing to fibrosis with subsequent stiffening, contraction, and calcification. Approximately 25% of patients have pure MS, but an additional 40% have combined MS and MR.[1]

Stenosis usually develops one or two decades after the acute illness of rheumatic fever with no or slow onset of symptoms until the stenosis becomes more severe. Limitation of exercise tolerance usually is the first symptom, followed by dyspnea that can progress to pulmonary edema. New-onset atrial fibrillation and the risk for thromboembolism, hemoptysis, and pulmonary hypertension are other common symptoms in patients with MS.

Besides echocardiographic imaging, the diagnostic workup of the symptomatic patient with MS should include a complete cardiac catheterization, including coronary angiography in any patient older than 40 years old. In younger patients, echocardiographic assessment of the mitral valve suffices in most symptomatic patients unless there is a history of chest pain or coronary artery disease. Typically echocardiogram establishes the extent of MS by determining valve gradients and valve area, but in complex cases cardiac catheterization with direct measurement might be more beneficial.

Recently published 2014 American Heart Association/American College of Cardiology guideline has a new staging system for MS.[2] The criteria for severe MS has changed from mitral valve area of 1.0 cm^2 or less to a mitral valve area of 1.5 cm^2, the normal native mitral valve area being 4 to 6 cm^2, and/or a diastolic half pressure time more than

150 ms. Symptomatic severe MS is considered stage D while asymptomatic severe MS is stage C. Finally, a mitral valve area of less than 1.0 cm² or diastolic half pressure time more than 220 ms is considered "very severe MS."

Currently, the first option for MS is percutaneous balloon valvuloplasty and certain anatomic characteristics allow a more successful valvuloplasty (Table 42-1).[2] The Wilkins score is used to predict the success rates of this procedure by taking into consideration valve thickness, valvular calcification, leaflet mobility, and subvalvular thickening. Each category has a score of 1 to 4 and a total score of 8 or less predicts higher success rate with balloon valvuloplasty. If the score is higher than 8, MVR is recommended.[3] Subsequently, the 2014 ACC/AHA guidelines gave class I recommendation for mitral valve surgery in severely symptomatic patients (NYHA class III/IV) with severe MS (stage D) who are not high risk for surgery and who are not candidates for previous balloon valvuloplasty or have failed a previous balloon valvuloplasty and in patients with severe MS (stage C or D) undergoing other cardiac surgery. Class IIa recommendation is given for severely symptomatic patients (NYHA class III/IV) with severe MS (stage D) provided there are other operative indications and Class IIb recommendation for patients with moderate MS (MVA 1.6-2.0 cm²) undergoing other cardiac surgery and patients with severe MS (stages C and D) who have had recurrent embolic events while receiving adequate anticoagulation. We must also mention that the degree of pulmonary artery pressure elevation secondary to MS continues to be

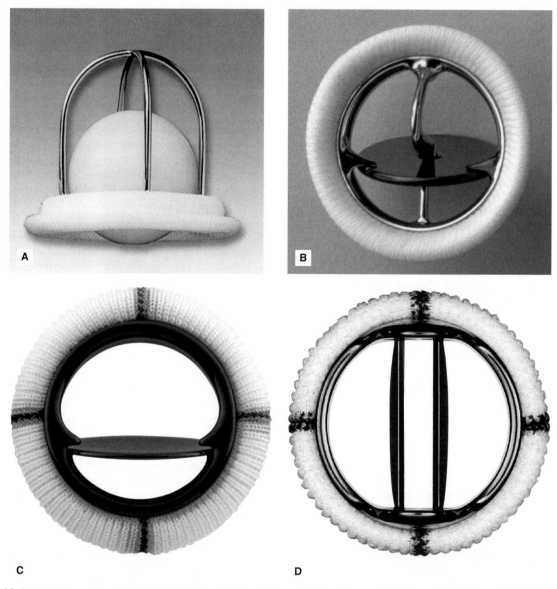

FIGURE 42-1 FDA-approved mechanical mitral valves. (A) Starr-Edwards ball-and-cage. (B) Medtronic Hall tilting-disk. (C) Omnicarbon tilting-disk. (D) St. Jude Medical bileaflet.

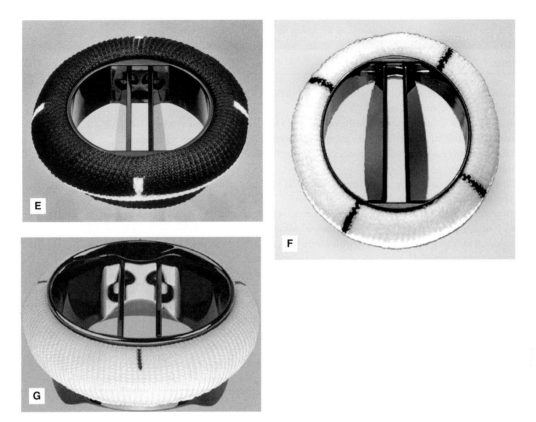

FIGURE 42-1 (*Continued*) (E) Carbomedics bileaflet. (F) ATS bileaflet. (G) On-X bileaflet.

an area of concern for the mitral valve surgeon but it has been known for more than 40 years that after MVR for MS, pulmonary artery pressure decreases within hours in most patients and decreases more gradually over weeks to months in others.[4-6]

Historically, the success with closed commissurotomy after World War II and the development of the Starr-Edwards valve in the early 1960s led to an enormous increase in operations for rheumatic mitral valve disease. It was until the 1990s that the balloon dilation of fibrotic stenotic mitral valves became increasingly common.[6-8] Open mitral commissurotomy and valvuloplasty also became an alternative for MS patients,[9,10] but some studies have shown better long-term

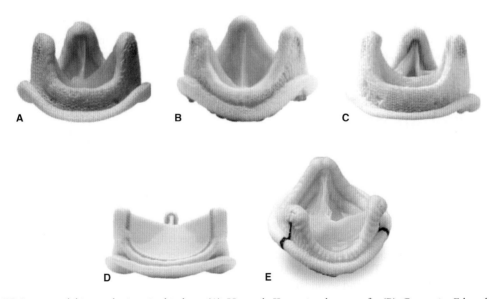

FIGURE 42-2 FDA-approved bioprosthetic mitral valves. (A) Hancock II porcine heterograft. (B) Carpentier-Edwards standard porcine heterograft. (C) Mosaic porcine heterograft. (D) Carpentier-Edwards pericardial bovine heterograft. (E) St. Jude Biocor porcine heterograft.

TABLE 42-1: Summary of Recommendations for MS Intervention

Recommendations	COR	LOE
PMBC is recommended for symptomatic patients with severe MS (MVA ≤ 1.5 cm², stage D) and favorable valve morphology in the absence of contraindications	I	A
Mitral valve surgery is indicated in severely symptomatic patients (NYHA class III/IV) with severe MS (MVA ≤ 1.5 cm², stage D) who are not high risk for surgery and who are not candidates for or failed previous PMBC	I	B
Concomitant mitral valve surgery is indicated for patients with severe MS (MVA ≤ 1.5 cm², stage C or D) undergoing other cardiac surgery	I	C
PMBC is reasonable for asymptomatic patients with very severe MS (MVA ≤ 1.0 cm², stage C) and favorable valve morphology in the absence of contraindications	IIa	C
Mitral valve surgery is reasonable for severely symptomatic patients (NYHA class III/IV) with severe MS (MVA ≤ 1.5 cm², stage D), provided there are other operative indications	IIa	C
PMBC may be considered for asymptomatic patients with severe MS (MVA ≤ 1.5 cm², stage C) and favorable valve morphology who have new onset of AF in the absence of contraindications	IIb	C
PMBC may be considered for symptomatic patients with MVA > 1.5 cm² if there is evidence of hemodynamically significant MS during exercise	IIb	C
PMBC may be considered for severely symptomatic patients (NYHA class III/IV) with severe MS (MVA ≤ 1.5 cm², stage D) who have suboptimal valve anatomy and are not candidates for surgery or at high risk for surgery	IIb	C
Concomitant mitral valve surgery may be considered for patients with moderate MS (MVA 1.6-2.0 cm²) undergoing other cardiac surgery	IIb	C
Mitral valve surgery and excision of the left atrial appendage may be considered for patients with severe MS (MVA ≤ 1.5 cm², stages C and D) who have had recurrent embolic events while receiving adequate anticoagulation	IIb	C

AF, indicates atrial fibrillation; COR, Class of Recommendation; LOE, Level of Evidence; MS, mitral stenosis; MVA, mitral valve area; NYHA, New York Heart Association; and PMBC, percutaneous mitral balloon commissurotomy.
Adapted with permission from Nishimura RA, Otto CM, Bonow RO, et al: 2014 AHA/ACC guideline for the management of patients with valvular heart disease: a report of the American College of Cardiology/American Heart Association Task Force on Practice Guidelines, *J Thorac Cardiovasc Surg.* 2014 Jul;148(1):e1-e132.

results with MVR using a mechanical valve.[11] Many patients with chronic MS now require valve replacement because the valve has developed significant dystrophic changes including marked thickening and shortening of all chordae, obliteration of the subvalvular space, agglutination of the papillary muscles, and calcification in both annular and leaflet tissue. Aggressive decalcification and heroic reconstructive techniques for these extremely advanced pathologic valves generally have produced poor long-term results; nevertheless, some surgeons still advocate aggressive repairs in this subset of patients.[12]

MITRAL REGURGITATION

The etiology of MR is very diverse and the decision to operate on patients with MR is more complex than for patients with MS, except in patients with acute ischemic MR and endocarditis in whom indications are more straightforward. The pathologic events that produce MR are related to a number of metabolic, functional, and anatomical abnormalities.[1] These can be categorized into degenerative (eg, mitral prolapse and ruptured/elongated chordae), rheumatic, infectious, and ischemic diseases of the mitral valve. The recent AHA/ACC guideline separates MR into primary MR and secondary MR and is later graded based on patient symptoms and severity of the disease.[2]

The preferred surgical approach for primary MR is mitral valve repair which is described in a different chapter in this book. Mitral valve surgery has class I recommendation for symptomatic severe MR with left ventricular ejection fraction (LVEF) over 30% or asymptomatic severe MR with decreased LVEF (30-60%). It is important to stress that depressed ejection fraction is a poor indicator of left ventricular function in patients with MR. Ejection fraction can be preserved in patients with irreversible left ventricular failure because of regurgitant flow through the valve.[13,14] Depressed cardiac function (LVEF < 40%) therefore usually indicates severe left ventricular dysfunction, and results of surgery are not as favorable in these patients as they are in those with normal ventricles.[15,16] Measurements of end-systolic volume and diameter have lately surfaced as more reliable noninvasive parameters to evaluate the status of the left ventricle and determine the optimal time for operation.[17,18] Therefore, LV end-systolic diameter over 40 mm is also considered Class I indication in patients with asymptomatic MR.

Mitral valve repair is indicated in patients with primary MR due to a degenerative prolapsing myxomatous valve especially if the prolapse is generalized and local findings that decrease the probability of a successful repair are absent.[19-23] When the probability of successful repair is low as is the case with the encounter of rheumatic MR, calcific deposits throughout the leaflet substance and shortened chordae and papillary muscles, MVR is often the most prudent operation.[24] However, good results with reconstructive surgery in this patient group have been reported.[25] In patients with endocarditis, MVR may be required because of destruction of the valve leaflets, subvalvular mechanisms and annular abscess formation. Although repair of the valve and avoidance of prosthetic material are very desirable in septic situations, the extent of the destruction may preclude repair. Therefore, MVR is required after careful debridement of the infectious tissue and reconstruction of the valve annulus.[26-28]

For secondary MR, severe secondary MR in the setting of cardiac procedure has Class IIa, and symptomatic severe secondary MR has class IIb recommendation to undergo mitral valve surgery. Recently published randomized control study that compared MVR and MV repair in patients with severe ischemic MR showed no difference in mortality and LV remodeling.[29] However, MV repair group had 33% recurrence of moderate or severe MR compared to 2% in MVR. Other specific findings that preclude satisfactory repair include restrictive valve motion from shortened, scarred papillary muscles, acutely infarcted papillary muscle, and rupture of chordae associated with extensive calcification of valve leaflets.[30-32]

CHOICE OF VALVE TYPE

Indications for Mechanical Valve Replacement

For young patients, patients in chronic atrial fibrillation who require long-term anticoagulation, and any patient who wants to minimize the chance of reoperation, a mechanical prosthetic valve should be chosen if valve replacement is required. The St. Jude Medical bileaflet valve is the most widely used prosthetic mitral valve at present because it has good hemodynamic characteristics and is easy to insert. Recent interest in the On-X mechanical valve relates primarily to the possibility for limited anticoagulation, although this remains to be borne out from current clinical trial.[33] Indications to choose one prosthetic or another vary primarily by surgeon preference and occasionally depending on the state of the annulus and whether or not there have been multiple previous operations. The most recent 2014 AHA/ACC guideline has changed its recommendation from class I recommendation of mechanical valve in age 65 years to "shared decision-making process with patients preferences and risks of reoperation."[2] There is a class IIa recommendation for mechanical valves in patients under age 60 years and either bioprostheses or mechanical prostheses for age between 60 and 70 years.

We have performed a propensity matching analysis in patients younger than 65 years who underwent MVR. Our results showed higher reoperation rate in bioprostheses group and higher survival in mechanical prostheses group (11 vs 13 years, p = .004; Fig. 42-3). Therefore, we recommend mechanical prosthesis in this patient group.[34]

Indications for Bioprosthetic Valve Replacement

Patients in any age group in sinus rhythm who wish to avoid anticoagulation may prefer a bioprosthetic valve. Recent 2014 AHA/ACC guideline gave Class I recommendation for bioprostheses in patients at any age in whom anticoagulation therapy is contraindicated, cannot be managed appropriately or is not desired. A bioprosthetic valve is preferred in patients greater than age 65 years and in sinus rhythm because these valves deteriorate more slowly in older patients.[35] In addition, some 60-year-old patients may not outlive their prosthetic valves because of coexisting comorbidities.[36,37] Specifically, patients who require combined MVR and coronary bypass grafting for ischemic MR and coronary artery disease have a significantly reduced long-term survival as compared to patients who do not have concomitant coronary artery disease.[38-43] In these individuals with little risk of reoperation, anticoagulation may better be avoided.

As 20-year results have become available for various bioprostheses, it is clear that structural valve degeneration (SVD) is the most prominent complication of these valves.[44-49] The durability of porcine mitral valves is less than that of aortic bioprostheses which is directly proportional to age.[45] Deterioration occurs within months or years in children and young adults and only gradually over years in septuagenarians and octogenarians.[44,50] Essentially, all valves implanted into patients younger than 60 years of age have to be replaced ultimately, and valve failure is prohibitively rapid in children and adults younger than 35 to 40 years of age; therefore, bioprostheses are not advisable in these age groups.[51] Nevertheless, there are still indications for mitral porcine bioprosthetic valves in young patients. In a woman who desires to become pregnant, a bioprosthesis may be used to avoid warfarin anticoagulation and fetal damage during pregnancy.[52-55]

Over the last decade several publications, mainly from European centers, reported on the use of unstented cryopreserved homografts[56-59] and stentless heterografts[60-63] for MVRs, particularly in patients with endocarditis. The prosthetic valve is transplanted so that donor papillary muscles are reattached to recipient papillary muscles and the annulus is sutured circumferentially. This technique has been shown to be safe and reproducible, but it does not always provide durable results and therefore should not be used in young patients.[60] Other reports suggest that these operations may be a feasible alternative to stented valve replacement in patients with endocarditis. Pulmonary autografts also have been used for replacing the mitral valve (Ross II procedure), but these series are small, and follow-up is relatively short.[64-66]

TRENDS IN MITRAL VALVE SURGERY

Mitral valve surgery has been in a state of constant evolution since its inception. Data regarding all cardiac surgical procedures reported to the Society of Thoracic Surgeons Adult Cardiac Surgery Database (STS ACSD) demonstrate this dynamic state as more surgeons begin to repair rather

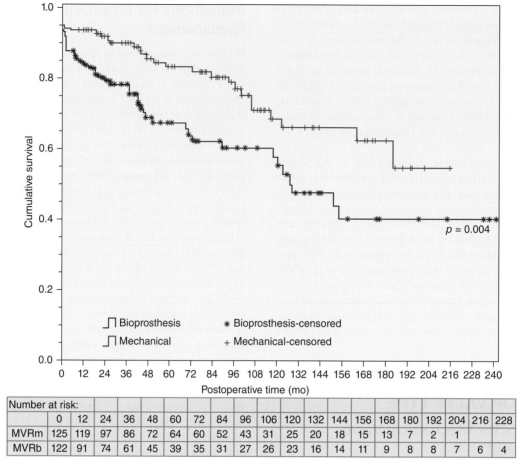

FIGURE 42-3 Comparison between bioprosthetic valve versus mechanical valve in patients under the age of 65 years who underwent mitral valve replacement. (Reproduced with permission from Kaneko T, Aranki S, Javed Q, et al: Mechanical versus bioprosthetic mitral valve replacement in patients <65 years old, *J Thorac Cardiovasc Surg.* 2014 Jan;147(1):117-126.)

than replace mitral valves. Gammie et al evaluated trends in mitral valve surgery in the United States using the STS ACSD evaluating the years between 2000 and 2007.[67] In this time period, 210,529 mitral valve procedures were performed in all settings. From the study population, 58,370 patients undergoing primary mitral valve operations were identified. Over this 7-year study time line, a 50% increase in repair rates was documented. When considering the valve replacement, a 100% increase in use of bioprosthetic devices coincided with a decline in the use of mechanical valves.

Gammie and coworkers identified clear trends with respect to patient selection as well.[67] Compared with patients undergoing mitral valve repair, those undergoing mitral replacement tended to be older, females, more likely to have multiple comorbidities (eg, diabetes mellitus, hypertension, chronic lung disease, stroke), concomitant tricuspid valve disease, MS, and were less likely to be asymptomatic. With respect to survival, overall risk adjusted mortality was lower for mitral valve repair versus replacement (OR 0.52, 95% CI: 0.45 to 0.59, $p < .0001$). The outcome with respect to choice of valve type and survival was not addressed but was felt to be confounded by patient factors that led to the initial device selection.

HEMODYNAMICS OF MITRAL VALVES DEVICES

Mechanical Prostheses

The designs of mechanical and bioprosthetic heart valves have evolved over the last five decades in an effort to develop the ideal replacement device for the pathologic mitral valve. The optimal heart valves exert minimal resistance to forward blood flow and allow only trivial regurgitant backflow as the occluder closes. The design must cause minimal turbulence and stasis in vivo under physiologic flow conditions. The valve must be durable enough to last a lifetime and must be constructed of biomaterials that are nonantigenic, nontoxic, nonimmunogenic, nondegradable, and noncarcinogenic. The valve also must have a low associated incidence of thromboembolism.

The opening resistance to blood flow is determined by the orifice diameter; the size, shape, and weight of the occluder; the opening angle; and the orientation of leaflet or disk occluders with respect to the plane of the mitral annular orifice for any given annular size. Least resistance to transvalvular blood flow during diastole for valves in the mitral position is provided by a large ratio of orifice to total annular area. A wide opening angle also improves the effective orifice area and results in decreased

TABLE 42-2: Hemodynamics of Mitral Valve Prostheses

Valve	Reference (year)	EOA (cm²) Catheterization readings					Doppler echocardiography gradient readings				
		25 mm	27 mm	29 mm	31 mm	33 mm	25 mm	27 mm	29 mm	31 mm	33 mm
Starr-Edwards	Pyle (1978)		1.4	1.4	1.9			8.0	10.0	5.0	
	Sala (1982)							7.9	6.7	5.0	
	Horskotte (1987)			1.8				6.3			
Omniscience/ Omnicarbon	Mikhail (1989)							6.1		5.4	
	Messner-Pellenc (1993)		1.9	2.2	2.0	2.0	4.3	3.6	3.5	2.0	
	Fehsk (1994)						6	6	5	6	4
	di Summa (2002)	1.7	1.9	1.6	1.9		9	4.1	5.1	5.6	
Medtronic Hall	Hall (1985)							3.0	2.7	2.0	
	Fiore (1998)						4.0	4.3	3.1	2.9	2.7
St. Jude	Chaux (1981)			2.1	2.8	3.1			1.9	1.8	1.6
	Horskotte (1987)			3.1					2.3		
	Fiore (1998)						3.0	3.3	3.8	1.5	2.5
	Hasegawa (2000)	2.6	2.5	2.4							
Carbomedics	Johnston (1992)			3.3					3.8		
	Chambers (1993)		2.1	2.1	1.8			3.9	3.3	3.3	
	Carbomedics (1993)		2.9	3.0	3.0			3.9	4.6	4.6	
	Carrier (2006)						5.3	4.9	4.6	4.4	4.9
ATS	Westaby (1996)		3	2	2	2					
	Shiono (1996)						5	6	4.5		
	Hasegawa (2000)	2.3	2.6	2.7							
	Emery (2001)						7.8	5	6	4	3
Hancock II	Johnson (1975)		1.0	2.5	1.8			12.0	5.0	5.0	
	Ubago (1982)		1.3	1.0	1.0			7.0	7.6	7.4	
	Khuri (1988)		1.5	2.0	1.8			7.0	7.0	7.0	
Carpentier-Edwards porcine	Chaitman (1979)		1.7	2.2	2.8			7.0	6.7	5.0	
	Levine (1981)			3.0	3.2				2.0	2.6	
	Pelletier (1982)		1.7	2.4	2.5			6.5	7.4	5.3	
Carpentier-Edwards pericardial	Aupart (1997)	2.6	2.7	2.6	3.1		4.1	3.0	3.0	3.0	3.1
Mosaic	Thomson (2001)			1.7 (all sizes)							
	Eichinger (2002)	2.6	1.5	1.8	2.1		4.6	3.8	4.4	2.7	
		1.1	0.9	1.0	0.9		4.2	5.8	4.8	4.0	
	Fradet (2004)										
Biocor	Rizzoli (2005)			3.1	3.3	3.6			6.7	6.2	5.4
Normal				4.6					0		
Severe stenosis				>1.0					>12		
Desired postoperative				>1.5					>10		

diastolic pressure gradients. Table 42-2 shows hemodynamic assessments of each of the FDA-approved mitral valve prostheses for the most commonly used mitral valve sizes.[68-71] The results of in vivo assessments at rest by invasive (catheterization) or non-invasive (Doppler echocardiography) techniques are tabulated.

Blood turbulence flowing across mitral valve devices results from impedance to forward or reverse flow. This impedance can be minimized by occluder design and orientation, central flow through the orifice and limited struts or pivots extending into flow areas (Fig. 42-4). Hemolysis is the product of

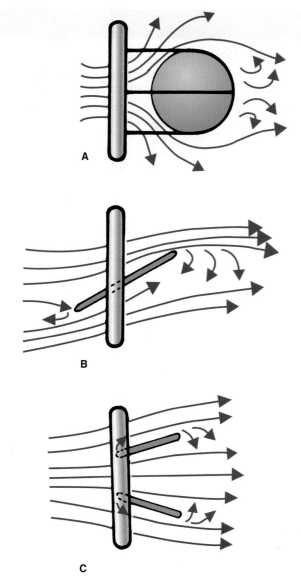

FIGURE 42-4 Flow characteristics of different mechanical valve designs. (A) Ball-and-cage. (B) Tilting-disk. (C) Bileaflet.

red blood cell destruction that is caused by cavitation and shearing stresses of turbulence, high-velocity flow, regurgitation, and mechanical damage during valve closure.[72] Areas of perivalvular blood stagnation and turbulence increase platelet aggregation, activation of the coagulation proteins, and thrombus formation.

Dynamic regurgitation is a feature of all prosthetic valves and is the sum of the closing volume during occluder closure and the leakage volume that passes through the valve while it is closed. The closing volume is a function of the effective orifice area and the time needed for closure. Leakage volume is inherent to the design of the valve and depends on the amount of time the valve remains in the closed position.[73] A small amount of regurgitant volume can be beneficial by minimizing stasis and reducing platelet aggregation; this decreases the incidence of valve thrombosis and valve-related thromboembolism.

BALL AND CAGE MECHANICAL VALVES

Starr–Edwards. Introduced in 1965, the Starr-Edwards Model 6120 was the only ball-and-cage mitral valve prosthesis approved by the FDA; however, the production was discontinued in 2007 (see Fig. 42-1A). The occluder is a barium-impregnated Silastic ball in a Stellite alloy cage that projects into the left ventricle. This valve has a large Teflon/polypropylene sewing ring that produces a relatively smaller effective orifice and larger diastolic pressure gradients than other prosthetic valves of similar annular sizes. Leakage volumes are not inherent in the ball-and-cage design, and in contrast with other mechanical valves, the presence of regurgitation may indicate a pathologic process. The central ball occluder causes lateralization of forward flow and results in turbulence and cavitation that increase the risk of hemolysis and thromboembolic complications (see Fig. 42-4A).[74-76]

MONOLEAFLET MECHANICAL VALVES

Medtronic-Hall. Tilting-disk mitral valve prostheses had better hemodynamic characteristics than ball-and-cage valves (see Fig. 42-4B) but with the development of new valve designs and technology they were taken off the market. The Medtronic Hall central pivoting-disk valve was available between 1977 and 2009 and it was based on engineering design modifications of the earlier Hall-Kaster valve[77] (see Fig. 42-1B). The opening angle of 70° produced regurgitation volumes of less than 5% of left ventricular stroke volume without significantly compromising forward flow. The disk occluder was allowed to slide out of the housing at the end of the closing cycle to provide a gap through which blood could flow to minimize stasis at the contact surfaces.[78] The large opening angle and slim disk occluder, along with a thinner sewing ring, provide improved hemodynamics with comparably larger effective orifice areas and lower mean diastolic pressure gradients for each valve size.

Omniscience-Omni Carbon. The Omniscience tilting-disk valve was first introduced in 1978 as a second-generation device derived from improvements to the design of the Lillehei-Kaster pivoting-disk valve.[79] It had a larger orifice to annular ratio, a larger opening angle of 80° and better hemodynamics compared to its predecessor. A special disk design reduced the regurgitant volume, the turbulence and the areas of stasis and shear stress. Clinical studies, however, opened a huge debate concerning this valve's hemodynamics since there was reports of a postoperative mean opening angle between 44.8°[69] and 75.9°.[80] Implicated factors causing this variation included valve sizing, orientation during implantation, and anticoagulation status.[80,81] A subsequent generation of the Omniscience valve is the all-carbon Omnicarbon monoleaflet valve that was released in 2001 in the United States but has been in clinical use in Europe since 1984 (see Fig. 42-1C). The housing material is made of pyrolytic carbon instead of titanium. As a result of this change, the incidence of thromboembolism, valvular thrombosis, and reparations was decreased significantly compared with the Omniscience valve prostheses.[82] Since 2005, however, the production of the Omnicarbon valve ended as the company decided to stop this production line.

Currently the only valve design available for implantation in the United States is the bileaflet design; it is being provided by many manufacturers.

BILEAFLET MECHANICAL VALVES

St. Jude Mechanical Valve. The unique design of the bileaflet St. Jude Medical valve was introduced in 1977, and it is currently the prosthesis used most commonly worldwide (see Fig. 42-1D). Two separate pyrolytic carbon semidisks in a pyrolytic carbon housing are attached to a Dacron sewing ring. The housing has two pivot guards that project into the left atrium. The bileaflet design produces three different flow areas through the valve orifice that provide overall a more uniform, central, and laminar flow than in the caged ball and monoleaflet tilting-disk designs. The improved flow results in less turbulence and decreased transmitral diastolic pressure gradients[73,83] (see Fig. 42-4C) at any annulus diameter size and cardiac output compared with the caged ball and single-leaflet tilting valves.[84] The favorable hemodynamics in smaller sizes makes it especially useful in children. The central opening angle is 85°, with a closing angle of 30 to 35°, which along with a thin sewing ring, provides a large effective orifice area for each valve size at the expense of greater regurgitant volumes, especially at low heart rates. Asynchronous closure of the valve leaflets in vivo also contributes to the regurgitant volume.[85] The design of this prosthesis provides excellent hemodynamic function even in small sizes in any rotational plane.[86] The antianatomical plane, however, with the central slit between the leaflets oriented perpendicular to the opening axis of the native valve leaflets decreases the potential risk of leaflet impingement by the posterior left ventricular wall.[87] Rotatable cuff designs are available on newer generation models.

Carbomedics Valve. The Carbomedics bileaflet valve was approved by the FDA in 1986 (see Fig. 42-1E). This low-profile device is constructed of pyrolytic carbon and has no pivot guards, struts, or orifice projections to decrease blood flow impedance and turbulence through the valve.[73] It has a rotatable sewing cuff design and is available with a more generous and flexible sewing cuff (the OptiForm variant) that conforms more easily to different patient anatomies and allows subannular, intraannular, or supraannular suture placement. The leaflet opening angle is 78°, which with the bileaflet design provides a relatively large effective orifice area and transvalvular diastolic pressure differences only slightly greater than the St. Jude Medical bileaflet valve. Because of its narrow closing angle and large leakage volume, the Carbomedics valve does not reduce the relatively large regurgitant volume associated with the bileaflet design. Although this valve has good hemodynamic function overall, in the mitral position, the 25-mm Carbomedics valve has a relatively high diastolic pressure gradient and large regurgitant energy loss across the valve, especially at high flows. Hemodynamic studies suggest that the Carbomedics valve should be avoided in patients with a small mitral valve orifice.[73]

Advancing the Standard (ATS) Valves. The ATS Open Pivot® bileaflet mechanical prosthesis has been in clinical use in the United States since 2000. Similar to the Carbomedics valve, the ATS valve is a low-profile bileaflet prosthesis with a pyrolytic housing and pyrolytic carbon leaflets containing graphite substrate (see Fig. 42-1F). The pivot areas are located entirely within the orifice ring, and the valve leaflets hinge on convex pivot guides on the carbon orifice ring. This design minimizes the overall height of the valve and provides a wider orifice area, and the absence of cavities in the valve ring theoretically reduces stasis or eddy currents that may develop. Valve noise, a bothersome problem for some patients, also is reduced by this design.[87] The opening angle is up to 85°, and the sewing cuff is constructed of double velour polyester fabric that is mounted to a titanium stiffening ring, which enables the surgeon to rotate the valve orifice during and after implantation.

On-X Prosthesis Valves. The On-X prosthesis was approved by the FDA in 2002. It has a bileaflet design similar to the St. Jude Medical, Carbomedics, and ATS prostheses with comparable hemodynamic performance, that is, a relatively large orifice diameter and a wide opening angle (90°) (see Fig. 42-1G). Instead of silicon-alloyed pyrolytic carbon, as used in the other mechanical prostheses, the On-X valve is made of pure pyrolytic carbon. This material is stronger and tougher than silicon-alloyed carbon and allows incorporation of hydrodynamically efficient features into the valve orifice, such as increased orifice length and a flared inlet that reduces transvalvular gradient. Early clinical results are promising and the valve produces very little hemolysis with postoperative levels of serum lactate dehydrogenase in the normal range.[88,89]

Anticoagulation for Mechanical Valves

Warfarin remains to be the mainstay of anticoagulation after mechanical valve replacement in both aortic and mitral positions.[90] The need for anticoagulation with mechanical valves has been the leading cause of people shying away from this type of valves because of the life style changes this treatment instills. In fact, this has also been a major driving force in the recently observed shift in use of the bioprosthetic valves in younger patients despite its decreased lifespan compared to mechanical valves.[90,91] Given the time needed to heparin-warfarin bridging as well as the frequent need of monitoring during Warfarin treatment, efforts are being made to find an alternative. The new oral anticoagulants (dabigatran, edoxaban, rivaroxaban ...) are promising substitutes to the warfarin therapy due to their shorter half life and the lack of need to constant monitoring.[90] Those drugs have been FDA approved for use in nonvalvular atrial fibrillation and in treatment or prevention of deep vein thrombosis/pulmonary embolism but not for anticoagulation in patients with mechanical valves. dabigatran was the only drug to be compared to warfarin in patients with mechanical valves during a phase 2 trial, the RE-ALIGN trial that was initiated in 2012.[92] Unfortunately, this trial was terminated prematurely owing to an increase in stroke, myocardial infarction and major bleeding in the dabigatran group. The FDA declared, after this study, that dabigatran is contraindicated in this patient population. In the absence of other randomized controlled studies comparing a new oral anticoagulant to warfarin in patients with mechanical valves, warfarin still holds the crown of oral anticoagulation in this patient population.

Bioprostheses

PORCINE VALVES

The porcine bioprosthetic mitral valves are designed to mimic the flow characteristics of the in situ aortic valve. The Hancock I mitral valve bioprosthesis was introduced in 1970. It has three glutaraldehyde-preserved porcine aortic valve leaflets on a polypropylene stent attached to a Dacron-covered silicone sewing ring. The design allows for central laminar flow through the valve, which tends to decrease diastolic pressure gradients and minimize turbulence.[83] The stent, however, impedes forward flow and results in relatively large diastolic pressure gradients across the bioprosthesis. The stent and the large sewing ring contribute to effective orifice areas that are smaller than those of size-matched mechanical valves (see Table 42-2).

The Hancock II porcine bioprosthesis (see Fig. 42-2A) is the more modern version of the Hancock I prosthesis. The stent is made of Delrin with a scalloped sewing ring and reduced stent profile. The leaflets are fixed in glutaraldehyde at low pressure then at high pressure for a prolonged period. To delay calcification, the leaflets are treated with sodium dodecyl sulfate.

The Carpentier-Edwards porcine valve uses a flexible stent to decrease the stress of leaflet flexion while maintaining its overall configuration (see Fig. 42-2B). The effective orifice-to-total-annulus-area ratio for the Carpentier-Edwards valve is relatively small, but exercise studies show that the effective orifice area increases significantly with increased blood flow across the valve; diastolic

gradients also increase but to a lesser degree.[70,71,93] Porcine bioprostheses in the mitral position should be avoided in patients with small left ventricles because of the possibility of ventricular rupture or left ventricular outflow obstruction caused by the large struts.[94]

The Mosaic porcine bioprosthesis is a third-generation bioprosthesis using the Hancock II stent (see Fig. 42-2C). It was introduced in the United States in 2000 and has a Delrin stent, scalloped sewing ring, and reduced stent profile. The valve tissue is pressure-free fixed with glutaraldehyde, and the prosthesis is treated with alpha-oleic acid to retard calcification.

In 2005, the FDA approved the Biocor porcine bioprosthesis (St. Jude Medical) (see Fig. 42-2E); however, it has been used and investigated for almost two decades in Europe. It belongs to the third generation of bioprostheses, and the valve tissue is pretreated in glutaraldehyde at very low pressure (<1 mm Hg), making the valve cusps less stiff with less tendency to tissue fatigue. A newer generation of this valve, the St. Jude Medical Epic valve, is identical to its precursor except that the later is treated with Linx AC ethanol-based calcium mitigation therapy.

PERICARDIAL VALVES

Previous studies indicated poor durability of pericardial valves, namely the Ionescu-Shiley valve, caused by leaflet tearing. This led to significant changes in design, including mounting of the pericardium completely within the stent, causing less leaflet abrasion and increased durability. The Carpentier-Edwards pericardial valve uses bovine pericardium as material to fabricate a trileaflet valve and that is cut, fitted, and sewn onto a flexible Elgiloy wire frame for stress reduction (see Fig. 42-2D). The tissue is preserved with glutaraldehyde with no applied pressure and the leaflets are treated with the calcium mitigation agent XenoLogiX. Compared to the Carpentier-Edwards porcine bioprosthesis, the stent profile is reduced. Long-term durability for the Carpentier-Edwards pericardial valve is strong and compared to third-generation porcine valves, valve-related complications are similar (see Discussion later in this chapter).

Hemodynamically, pericardial valves provide the best solution to flow problems. The design maximizes use of the flow area, which results in minimal flow resistance. Figure 42-5A

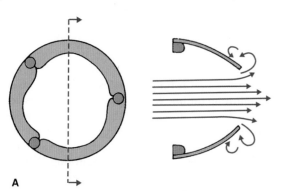
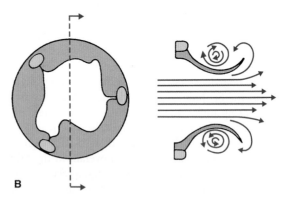

FIGURE 42-5 Flow patterns for bioprosthetic valves. (A) Pericardial bioprosthesis. (B) Porcine bioprosthesis.

shows how the cone shape of the open valve and circular valve orifice minimizes flow disturbance compared with the more irregular cone shape of the porcine valves that allow for central unimpeded flow (see Fig. 42-5B).

Structural valve deterioration is seen after long-term follow-up of patients with both porcine and pericardial bioprostheses and results in MS or MR or both. Hemodynamic studies early after operation and at 5 years reveal higher average diastolic pressure gradients and smaller effective orifice areas when compared in the same patients at the follow-up study. In some patients, these changes are sufficiently severe to require reoperation as soon as 4 to 5 years postoperatively and by 10 years the rate of primary tissue failure averages 30%. It then accelerates, and by 15 years postoperatively, the actuarial freedom from bioprosthetic primary tissue failure has ranged from 35 to 71%[44,46,48,49,68] (Table 42-3). Most of these patients show hemodynamic evidence of valvular deterioration before any clinical signs or symptoms.[71] Bioprosthetic valves have the advantage of low thrombogenicity, which must be weighed against poor long-term durability and subsequent hemodynamic deterioration and the risk of reoperation.

OPERATIVE TECHNIQUES

Preoperative Management and Anesthetic Preparation

Congestive heart failure (CHF) secondary to MS usually can be treated with aggressive diuretic therapy and sodium restriction preoperatively. If the patient is in rapid atrial fibrillation digoxin, beta blockers, and calcium channel antagonists can be used to slow down the ventricular rate. Patients with acute MR often are in cardiogenic shock, and they can be stabilized preoperatively with inotropes and arterial vasodilators to reduce systemic afterload. Intraaortic balloon counterpulsation also can be used for this purpose. Symptoms of CHF in patients with chronic MR are treated with diuretics and oral vasodilators. The vasodilators lower the peripheral vascular resistance, forward cardiac flow is hence increased and the regurgitant volume into the left atrium reduced.

Preferred anesthesia for MVR typically involves a combination of narcotic and inhalational agents. Ultimately, anesthetic management is dictated by the wide range of functional

TABLE 42-3: Freedom (Actuarial) from Structural Valve Deterioration after Mitral Valve Replacement with Bioprotheses

Valve	Reference (year)	5 y	10 y	15 y	20 y
Hancock Standard	Cohn (1989)	98%	75%	45%	
	Burdon (1992)	98%	80%	44%	
	Bortolotti (1995)	94%	73%	35%	
	Khan (1998)				65%
Hancock II	Legarra (1999)		65%		33% (18 y)
	David (2001)	100%	86%	66%	
	Rizzoli (2003)	99%	86%	60%	
	Masters (2004)		98% (8 y)		
Carpentier-Edwards porcine	Perier (1989)	89%	65%		
	Sarris (1993)	97%	60%		
	Jamieson (1995)	98%	72%	49%	
	Van Doorn (1995)	97%	71%		
	Corbineau (2001)	98%	83%	48%	
Carpentier-Edwards pericardial	Pelletier (1995)	100%	79% (8 y)		
	Takahara (1995)		84% (9 y)		
	Aupart (1997)	100%	76%		
	Marchand (1998)	98%	85% (11 y)		
	Neville (1998)	100%	78% (12 y)		
	Poirer (1998)	100%	81%		
	Bourguignon (2014)		84%	55%	24%
Mosaic	Jasinski (2000)	100% (2 y)			
	Thomson (2001)	100% (4 y)			
	Eichinger (2002)	100%			
	Fradet (2004)	100% (7 y)			
	Jamieson (2005)	98% (6 y)			
Biocor	Myken (2000)		100% (8 y)	92%	
	Rizzoli (2005)				

y indicates years.

disabilities and hemodynamic abnormalities of patients who present for MVR.[94]

Preoperative intravenous prophylactic antibiotics are administered to all patients. Monitoring should include arterial and venous lines, a urinary catheter and a pulmonary artery catheter placed before bypass to measure pulmonary pressures and cardiac output. Transesophageal echocardiography is also critical throughout the entire operation. Last but not least, temporary ventricular pacing wires are placed postoperatively, and in many instances temporary atrial pacing wires are placed for possible pacing or diagnosis of various atrial arrhythmias.

Cardiopulmonary Bypass for Mitral Valve Replacement

Cardiopulmonary bypass is instituted by placing two right-angled cannulas into the superior and inferior venae cavae. A small (22 French) plastic or metal cannula is placed directly into the superior vena cava, above the sinoatrial node. The inferior caval cannula is placed at the entrance of the inferior vena cava, low in the right atrium. These insertion sites keep the caval catheters out of the operative field and yet maintain excellent bicaval drainage. An arterial cannula is placed in the distal ascending aorta. Bypass flows are approximately 1.5 L/m² per minute, and mild hypothermia is used with vacuum-assisted suction. Myocardial protection includes antegrade and retrograde blood cardioplegia and profound myocardial hypothermia.[95] Retrograde cardioplegia is useful for all valve surgery to protect the ischemic left ventricle and help remove ascending aorta bubbles. Antegrade cardioplegia, used as an initial loading dose, is augmented by intermittent retrograde cardioplegia every 20 minutes. This provides safer delivery of cardioplegia because when the atrium is retracted during valve replacement, the aortic valve is distorted, and antegrade cardioplegia tends to fill the ventricle due to aortic regurgitation.

Exposure of the Mitral Valve

Evolution of meticulous and complicated methods of mitral valve repair and reconstruction has required optimal exposure of the mitral valve. In primary operations, median sternotomy, development of Sondergaard's plane, and incision of the left atrium close to the atrial septum provide excellent exposure[96,97] (Fig. 42-6). This incision is a ubiquitous one, and occasionally other incisions, such as the superior approach through the dome of the left atrium,[98,99] the so-called biatrial incision popularized by Guiraudon and colleagues,[100] division of the superior vena cava[101,102] and the less common but occasionally useful trans-right atrial septal incision[103] are used to obtain exposure. The trans-right atrial incision has in some studies been related to higher incidence of junctional and nonsinus rhythm postoperatively,[104] although this has not been confirmed by other studies.[78]

Intracardiac Technique

Operation entails secure fixation of a valve prosthesis to the annulus by reliable suture techniques without damage to adjacent structures or myocardium and without tissue interference with valve function. Implantation should prevent injury to anatomical structures surrounding the mitral valve annulus. Figure 42-7 shows the proximity of important cardiac structures near the mitral valve annulus. These include the circumflex coronary artery within the atrioventricular (AV) groove, the left atrial appendage, the aortic valve in continuity with the anterior mitral curtain and the AV node.

An accumulation of laboratory and clinical evidence indicates that preservation of papillary muscle-chordal attachments to the annulus is important for maintenance of left ventricular function. In patients with MS with agglutinated, fibrotic chordate, and papillary muscles, preservation of these structures probably has little effect on left ventricular dysfunction but does protect the AV groove from rupture by preserving the posterior leaflet. If fibrotic, placement of artificial Gore-Tex chordae to reattach the papillary muscles to the annulus may improve early and late preservation of cardiac output.[21] In patients with MR, however, it is important to preserve as much of the papillary muscle and annular interaction as possible. This can be achieved by a variety of techniques, as shown in Fig. 42-8. The anterior leaflet may be partially excised and brought to the posterior leaflet (see Fig. 42-8A) or can be partially excised and "furled" to the anterior annulus by a running Prolene suture[105,106] (see Fig. 42-8B).

Experimental and clinical evidence suggest that preservation of the conical shape of the ventricle is important to maintain normal cardiac output[107-110]; cutting the papillary muscles is therefore deleterious to left ventricular function because it assumes more of a globular shape. Furthermore, preservation of the posterior leaflet and chordae has dramatically reduced the incidence of perforation of the left ventricle and AV separation during MVR.[10,111,112]

Suturing techniques vary according to the type of valve that is implanted. The bioprosthetic valve is inserted preferentially with the sutures placed from ventricle to atrium (noneverting or subannular). This has been shown to be the strongest type of suturing technique to the mitral annulus and is used with this valve (Fig. 42-9A).

To ensure adequate function of bileaflet or tilting-disk valves, everting sutures (atrium to ventricle to sewing ring) should be used (see Fig. 42-9B). This technique pushes the prosthetic valve out into the center of the orifice and minimizes any tissue interference of the prosthetic valve leaflets. This is particularly important if annular-chordal attachments are preserved. Teflon-pledgeted sutures, particularly with the thin sewing rings of the currently available bileaflet and tilting-disk valves, should be used. If a bioprosthetic valve is inserted, a dental mirror is used to ensure that no annular suture is wrapped around a stent strut. A running Prolene suture for implantation of mitral valves has been advocated

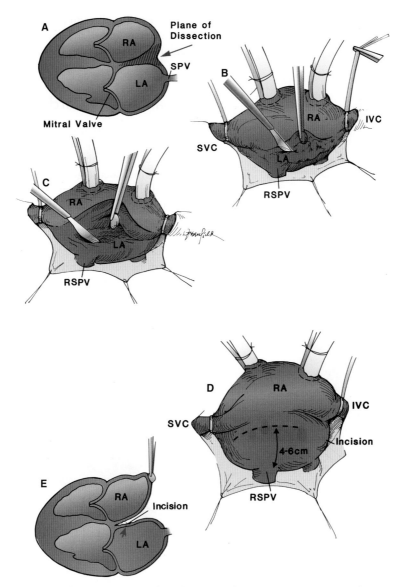

FIGURE 42-6 Exposure of the mitral valve. (A) Location of Sondergaard's plane. (B,C) Development of the interatrial plane. (D) Location of the left atrial incision. (E) Cross-sectional view.

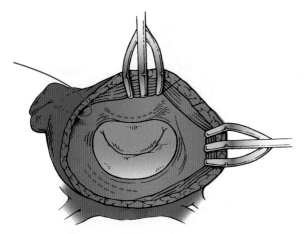

FIGURE 42-7 Location of important structures surrounding the mitral annulus. (Used with permission from David Bichell.)

by some surgeons.[113,114] This technique makes a very clean suture line with minimal knots but runs the risk of valve dehiscence if an infection occurs.[115]

Before closure, the left atrial appendage is ligated by suture or stapled to prevent clot formation in patients with chronic atrial fibrillation, enlarged left atrium, or left atrial thrombus.[116] The atrium is closed by a running Prolene suture, making sure that endocardial surfaces are approximated. If needed, a left atrial catheter can be inserted through the suture line.

ASSOCIATED OPERATIONS/PROCEDURES

Coronary bypass is the most common procedure performed with MVR and the distal anastomosis should be performed first. This reduces lifting of the heart after the rigid mitral

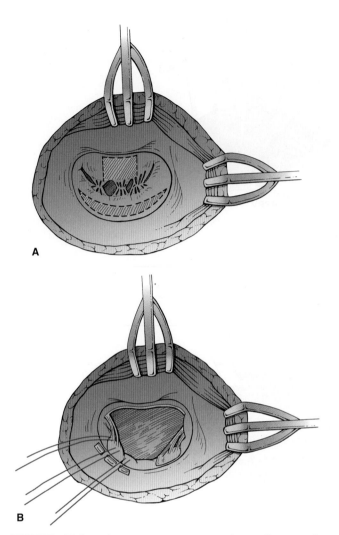

FIGURE 42-8 Techniques to maintain annular-papillary muscle continuity. (A) An ellipse is removed from the posterior leaflet, and a flap is cut from the central portion of the anterior leaflet. The anterior flap is flipped to the posterior annulus and tacked to the caudad edge of the posterior leaflet and the posterior annulus. Sutures anchoring the prosthesis include the annulus and anterior and posterior leaflet remnants to which chordae are attached. (B) The anterior leaflet is partially excised, and remnants are "furled" to the annulus by sutures used to insert the prosthesis.

valve prosthesis is in place, which can cause rupture of the myocardium or the AV groove. This also allows cardioplegia to be delivered through the bypass grafts.

Tricuspid valve repair or replacements usually are performed after replacing the mitral valve. In these cases, the mitral valve can be approached through the right atrium and a transseptal incision. After the mitral valve prosthesis is in place, the septum is closed, and the aortic cross-clamp is removed before proceeding with the tricuspid valve procedure.[117]

When both the aortic and mitral valves are replaced at the same operation, most surgeons begin with excising the aortic valve before proceeding with the mitral valve procedure. It is extremely difficult to expose the mitral annulus especially the anterior annulus with aortic prosthesis in place.

When excising the anterior mitral valve leaflet, care must be taken not to injure the aortic annulus and the intraannular region. The aortic valve then is sewn in after the mitral valve is in place.

Weaning Off Cardiopulmonary Bypass

We use transesophageal echocardiography for every valve operation and particularly for mitral valves, where excellent images can be obtained. If transesophageal echocardiography is contraindicated (eg, because of esophageal disease), direct epicardial echocardiography can be used. The echocardiograms provide information about valve and left ventricular function, possible retained material in the left atrium including thrombus and removal of intracardiac air.

A careful de-airing at the end of the operation is essential and can be completed using special maneuvers. Rewarming the patient comes next and then venous return is partially occluded and the heart is gradually volume loaded. Pulmonary artery pressures are monitored carefully and pharmacologic agents, such as amrinone or dobutamine can be used particularly for right ventricular overload.

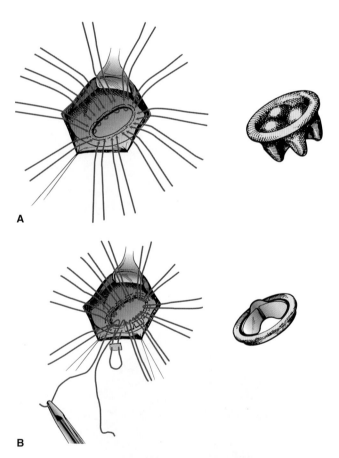

FIGURE 42-9 Suturing techniques for prosthetic mitral valve implantation. (A) Noneverting (subannular) sutures placed from ventricle to atrium for bioprosthetic or Starr-Edwards valves. (B) Everting (supraannular) sutures placed from atrium to ventricle for bileaflet or tilting-disk valves.

POSTOPERATIVE CARE

Postoperative care is directed toward the resumption of normal cardiac output, respiratory function, temperature control, electrolyte management, adequate renal flow and prophylaxis against bleeding. Patients with low cardiac output are managed with a variety of pharmacologic agents after providing adequate volume loading. Left atrial and especially pulmonary arterial catheters are of particular help in determining optimal balancing of volume loading and myocardial function in the first hours postoperatively.

In the intensive care unit, reduction in pulmonary interstitial fluid is aggressively pursued by diuretics in patients with severe pulmonary hypertension. Most patients with severe pulmonary hypertension can be extubated within 48 hours of surgery. Many patients with severe, longstanding mitral valve disease are cachectic and severely catabolic at the time of operation despite preoperative nutritional support. These patients generally require longer periods of ventilatory support owing to the lack of respiratory muscle strength. In patients with severe pulmonary hypertension and cardiac cachexia who require prolonged intubation, tracheostomy may be necessary to reduce ventilatory dead space and facilitate faster weaning and better pulmonary toilet.

Postoperative atrial arrhythmias are so common that their absence is unusual. Arrhythmias vary from rapid supraventricular tachycardias, usually atrial fibrillation, to junctional rhythm and heart block. These arrhythmias are treated by pharmacologic agents, pacemakers, or both. If rapid atrial fibrillation cannot be controlled pharmacologically and is destabilizing hemodynamically, emergency cardioversion is done to improve cardiac output. Pharmacologic management of supraventricular tachycardia usually is required but may precipitate the need for a prophylactic transvenous pacemaker if severe slowing of the heart rate occurs.

Anticoagulation is prescribed for all patients undergoing MVR with either a mechanical or bioprosthetic valve. In the first 6 weeks after operation, the incidence of atrial and other arrhythmias is high; thus, these fluctuating rhythms mandate anticoagulation even if the basic rhythm is sinus. In addition to rhythm concerns, the left atrial incisions and the possibility of stasis in the left atrial appendage justify full anticoagulation with warfarin for all patients. Some surgeons advocate immediate intravenous heparin until therapeutic warfarin doses can be reached.[118,119] Low molecular weight heparin also can be used.[120,121]

The therapeutic international normalized ratio (INR) after MVR is 2.5 to 3.5 depending on the type of valve, cardiac rhythm, and presence or absence of the aforementioned intraoperative risk factors for thromboembolism.[116,119,120] Anticoagulation levels are in the low range for patients in sinus rhythm who received tissue valves. Patients who have mechanical valves need lifelong anticoagulation. Patients who have bioprosthetic valves are evaluated at 6 to 12 weeks for cardiac rhythm abnormalities. If they are in predominantly sinus rhythm, warfarin is stopped, and one aspirin tablet is given daily indefinitely. If the patient has continuous atrial fibrillation or fluctuating rhythms, anticoagulation with warfarin is continued. Warfarin usually is started on the second postoperative day. Addition of aspirin, 80 to 150 mg daily, to the warfarin may reduce the risk of thromboembolism[122,123] and may have a role in patients with prosthetic valves.[124]

RESULTS

Early Results

The hospital mortality for MVR with and without coronary bypass grafting has decreased significantly since the inception of mitral valve surgery. The current risk (2006) of elective primary MVR with and without coronary bypass grafting is 5 to 9% in most studies (range 3.3 to 13.1%).[68] Operative (30-day) mortality is related to myocardial failure, multisystem organ failure, bleeding, respiratory failure in the chronically ill, debilitated individual, diabetes, infection, stroke, and, very rarely, technical problems.[20,40] Mortality is correlated with preoperative functional class, age, and preexisting coronary artery disease.[125]

Published results on mitral valve surgery have improved in recent years,[126] probably because of preservation of papillary muscles, preventing midventricular rupture,[111,112] and preservation of the normal geometry of the left ventricle, which aids in the maintenance of early postoperative cardiac output.[107,108,127] MVR and coronary artery bypass surgery 20 to 25 years ago had an associated mortality of about 10 to 20%.[39,128] This mortality risk also has decreased as myocardial protection has improved with the use of blood cardioplegia and retrograde methods of administration.[95,129] Some studies have indicated that the risk of combined MVR-coronary artery bypass grafting is now no greater than that of mitral valve repair with an annuloplasty ring or MVR without coronary artery bypass grafting.[107,130] Other studies have shown significantly increased morbidity and mortality with the addition of coronary artery bypass grafting.[43,131] Figures from the database of the Society of Thoracic Surgeons indicate that both reoperation and emergency operation increase operative mortality[132] (Fig. 42-10).

Late Results

FUNCTIONAL IMPROVEMENT

In more than 90% of patients after MVR, functional class improves to at least class II. A small group of patients remains in class III or IV depending on left ventricular function before surgery or other comorbidities.

SURVIVAL

The causes of late death in patients after MVR are primarily chronic myocardial dysfunction, thromboemboli and stroke, endocarditis, anticoagulant-related hemorrhage, and coronary artery disease. The extent of left ventricular dysfunction and patient age, particularly if myocardial and coronary diseases are combined, correlate with late mortality. The probability

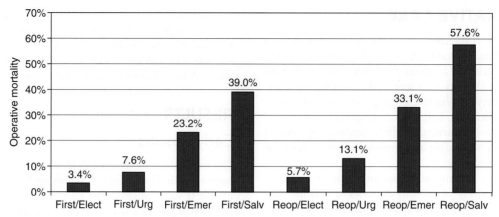

FIGURE 42-10 Operative mortality for elective, urgent, emergency, and salvage procedures for primary operations and reoperations for mitral valvular replacements. (Data from Society of Thoracic Surgeons.)

of survival after MVR at 10 years is usually around 50 to 60% (range 42 to 81%)[68] (Table 42-4). Long-term patient survival seems to be similar for patients with biologic and mechanical mitral valves.[133-135] Unlike patients with severe aortic regurgitation or aortic stenosis, arrhythmias seldom cause sudden death in patients after MVR; however, few patients die from thromboembolic stroke owing to chronic atrial fibrillation. The fact that more than 50% of patients after MVR are in chronic atrial fibrillation increases the propensity for thromboembolic stroke despite anticoagulation and for mechanical valve thrombosis if the anticoagulation protocol is altered. In addition, patients with older types of prosthetic valves who receive higher-intensity anticoagulation may develop severe anticoagulant hemorrhage.[136]

In patients with bioprosthetic valves, one of the important determinants of mortality is reoperation secondary to SVD[48,49,68] (Table 42-5). Reoperative MVR mortality has decreased significantly in the last 15 years to under 10%, even in patients who have required multiple mitral valve reoperations.[129] At the Brigham and Women's Hospital, operative mortality was less than 6% for reoperative mitral valve operations from 1990 to 1995.[129] Improved myocardial protection, earlier selection of patients for reoperation, and better perfusion techniques, including frequent femorofemoral bypass to protect the right ventricle during incision and dissection of the heart, are factors contributing to decreased mortality.[107,129,137-139]

LATE MORBIDITY

The major morbidity in patients after MVR is structural valve deterioration of a bioprosthetic valve and thromboembolism and anticoagulant hemorrhage with a mechanical prosthesis. Both valve types develop perivalvular leak and infection.

Thromboembolism. Thromboembolism is perhaps the most common complication of both biologic and mechanical mitral prostheses but is more frequent in patients with mechanical valves. Chronic atrial fibrillation and local atrial factors, discussed earlier, increase the risk of thromboembolism

in patients with mitral prostheses. A number of recent studies have summarized the thromboembolic potential of various valves (Table 42-6), and it appears that the better the valve hemodynamics, the lower is the probability of thromboemboli. The incidence of thromboemboli in currently available bileaflet and tilting-disk valves is similar to that in bioprosthetic valves—about 1.5 to 2.0% per patient-year. Thromboembolism in patients with MVR is lower in those with a small left atrium, sinus rhythm, and normal cardiac output. It is much higher in patients with a large left atrium, chronic atrial fibrillation, and the presence of intraatrial clot.[116,140] Thrombosis of a mechanical valve, once a feared complication of tilting-disk valves,[141,142] is now relatively rare unless anticoagulation is stopped for any period of time. Valve thrombosis can be treated with thrombolytic agents if the patient is not in cardiogenic shock but requires surgery if the circulation is inadequate.[143,144]

Anticoagulant Hemorrhage. Bleeding related to anticoagulation is seen most commonly in the gastrointestinal, urogenital, and central nervous systems, and usually is proportionate to the INR. The incidence of anticoagulant-related hemorrhage has decreased markedly with hemodynamic improvements in mitral valve prostheses. New valves do not require the intensity of anticoagulation of older prostheses. Patients with streamlined bileaflet or tilting-disk valves require an INR of between 2.5 and 3.5; thus, the incidence of anticoagulant hemorrhage is reduced significantly in the newer, hemodynamically improved prostheses.[145] Table 42-6 lists the incidence of anticoagulant hemorrhage with various bioprostheses and mechanical valves.

STRUCTURAL VALVE DEGENERATION

Structural valve degeneration (SVD) is the most important complication of the bioprosthetic valve. The probability of structural failure with currently available porcine valves (Hancock or Carpentier-Edwards) begins to increase 8 years after operation and reaches more than 60% at 15 years.[46,48]

TABLE 42-4: Actuarial Survival after Mitral Valve Replacement

Valve	Reference (year)	Actuarial survival				
		5 y	10 y	15 y	20 y	30 y
Starr-Edwards	Teply (1981)	78%	56%			
	Sala (1982)	78%	72%			
	Miller (1983)	71%	47%			
	Godje (1997)	85%	75%	56%	37%	23%
	Murday (2003)		57% (8 y)			
	Gao (2004)		51%		23%	8%
Omniscience/Omnicarbon	Damle (1987)	91% (4 y)				
	Peter (1993)	77% (4 y)				
	Otaki (1993)	82% (6 y)				
	Misawa (1993)	94% (3 y)				
	Thevenet (1995)		88% (9 y)			
	Iguro (1999)	88%				
	Torregrosa (1999)		81%			
	di Summa (2002)		61%			
Medtronic Hall	Vallejo (1990)	79%				
	Masters (1995)	70%	67%			
	Fiore (1998)	70%	58%			
	Butchart (2001)		58%	36%		
	Masters (2001)	75%	63%			
St. Jude	DiSesa (1989)	65% (4 y)				
	Kratz (1993)	80%	63%			
	Aoyagi (1994)	88%	81%			
	Fiore (1998)	65%	53%			
	Camilleri (2001)	89% (4 y)				
	Remadi (2001)	88%	76%	61%		
	Masters (2001)	75%	52%			
	Lim (2003)	72%				
	Murday (2003)		44% (8 y)			
Carbomedics	Bortolotti (1991)	90%	86%		39%	
	Rabelo (1991)	75% (4 y)				
	De Luca (1993)	93% (3 y)				
	Copeland (1995)	81%				
	Nistal (1996)	83%				
	Yamauchi (1996)	92%				
	Masters (2001)	76%				
	Santini (2002)	86%				
	Lim (2002)	72%				
	Soga (2002)	88%				
	Ikonamidis (2003)		61%			
	Tominaga (2005)	95%	94%			
	Kang (2005)		89%			
	Carrier (2006)	76%	59%	40%		
	Wu (2006)	74%	54%			
	Nishida (2012)		70%		40%	
On-X	Williams (2006)	87% (4 y)				
Hancock standard	Cohn (1989)	82%	60%			
	Burdon (1992)	74%	55%			
	Sarris (1993)	79%	58%			
	Khan (1998)		50%	29%	14%	

(Continued)

TABLE 42-4: Actuarial Survival after Mitral Valve Replacement (*Continued*)

Valve	Reference (year)	Actuarial survival				
		5 y	10 y	15 y	20 y	30 y
Hancock II	Legarra (1999)		65%		33% (18 y)	
	Rizzoli (2003)	72%	49%	37%		
	Masters (2004)		57% (8 y)			
	Borger (2006)		50%		6%	
Carpentier-Edwards standard	Akins (1990)	53%	45%			
	Louagie (1992)	61%	46%			
	Bernal (1995)	89%	80%			
	Pelletier (1995)	83%	62% (8 y)			
	van Doorn (1995)	75%	53%			
	Murakami (1996)		75%			
	Marchand (1998)		53% (11 y)			
Carpentier-Edwards pericardial	Takahara (1995)		59% (9 y)			
	Aupart (1997)	78%	71%			
	Marchand (1998)		53% (11 y)			
	Neville (1998)		54% (12 y)			
	Porier (1998)	84%	58%			
	Bourgignon (2014)	79%	58%	35%	17%	
Mosaic	Jasinski (2000)	100% (3 y)				
	Thomson (2001)	79% (4 y)				
	Fradet (2004)	83 (7 y)				
	Jamieson (2005)	74% (6 y)				
Biocor	Myken (2000)		55%	25%		
	Rizzoli (2005)	55%	51%			

y indicates years.

This finite durability is a major impediment to long-term success of these biologic prostheses, even though the failure rate in a patient 70 years of age or older is significantly less than in younger age groups (Table 42-7). SVD presents as MR from leaflet tear, calcific MS owing to calcification of valve leaflets or both. The appearance of a new murmur with new congestive symptoms should prompt a noninvasive investigation of the prosthesis and elective re-replacement if dysfunction is documented. SVD leading to reoperation is the cause for at least two-thirds of the reoperations in patients with bioprostheses.[137,138] The probabilities of SVD at 5, 10, and 15 years of the most commonly used biologic prostheses are shown in Table 42-3. With current quality controls, the incidence of SVD is virtually zero for bileaflet mechanical valves.

PROSTHETIC VALVE ENDOCARDITIS

Mitral valve endocarditis is considerably less common than aortic prosthetic valve endocarditis,[146] but when it occurs, it may present as septicemia, malignant burrowing infections, abscess formation, and septic emboli. With better antibiotic prophylaxis at the time of mitral surgery and improved prophylaxis for all patients having dental or other surgical procedures, the incidence of endocarditis has been reduced substantially.

The incidence of prosthetic endocarditis is highest during the initial 6 months after surgery and thereafter declines to a lower but persistent risk.[1] The probability of freedom from this morbid event is shown in Table 42-8 for both mechanical and bioprosthetic valves. Biologic and mechanical valves have a similar incidence of endocarditis, except for the initial months after valve implantation, when mechanical prostheses carry a greater risk of infection.[147]

The diagnosis of prosthetic endocarditis is made by the presence of symptoms, appearance of a new murmur, a septic embolus, or large vegetation on echocardiogram. Blood cultures usually are positive, although a small percentage of patients have culture-negative endocarditis. Echocardiograms may show a rocking motion of the prosthesis and the presence of vegetations. The most frequent organisms are still *Streptococcus* and *Staphylococcus;* the latter is usually hospital acquired. Antibiotic therapy depends on the sensitivity of the organisms, but immediate high-dose intravenous therapy must begin as soon as possible. Experience indicates that a number of patients with bioprosthetic valvular endocarditis can be "cured" of low-potency organisms such as *Streptococcus*. However, it is unlikely that antibiotics alone can sterilize more virulent mitral valve infections, particularly *Staphylococcus*. These infections usually require urgent and

TABLE 42-5: Freedom from Reoperation

Valve	Reference (year)	Actuarial freedom from reoperation		
		5 y	10 y	15 y
Hancock	Cohn (1989)	96%	79%	41%
	Perier (1989)	88%	59%	
	Bernal (1991)	92%	69%	25%
	Sarris (1993)	93%	69%	
	Khan (1998)		44%	
Hancock II	Legarra (1999)		77%	37% (18 y)
	David (2001)	98%	85%	69%
	Rizzoli (2003)	97%	88%	70%
	Borger (2006)		88%	44 (20 y)
Carpentier-Edwards standard	Perier (1989)	91%	64%	
	Jamieson (1991)	94%	64%	39%
	Sarris (1993)	91%	57% (8 y)	
	Van Doorn (1995)	95%	69%	
	Glower (1998)	94%	65%	30%
Carpentier-Edwards pericardial	Pelletier (1995)	98%	67% (8 y)	
	Murakami (1996)	100%	77%	
	Aupart (1997)		90%	
	Marchand (1998)		83% (11 y)	
	Neville (1998)		76% (12 y)	
	Poirer (1998)	99%	76%	
	Bourguignon (2014)		81%	58%
Mosaic	Jasinski (2000)	100% (3 y)		
	Eichinger (2002)	95%		
	Fradet (2004)	97% (7 y)		
Biocor	Myken (1995)			79%
	Rizzoli (2005)	95%	91%	

y indicates years.

sometimes emergent surgery because of invasion of the cardiac exoskeleton.

The indications for surgical intervention in mitral valve prosthetic endocarditis are persistent sepsis, organism, congestive failure, perivalvular leak, large vegetations, or systemic infected emboli.[27,28,148] Operative technique is similar to other mitral procedures with respect to anesthesia, monitoring, cardioplegia, left atrial incision, and exposure of the valve. Critical to successful resolution is the complete excision of the prosthetic device and debridement of all infected tissues. Surgical technique is described in a different chapter "Surgical treatment of Mitral Valve Endocarditis." Postoperative care should include at least 6 weeks of appropriate intravenous antibiotics. Hospital mortality is related primarily to ongoing sepsis, multisystem organ failure, or failure to eradicate the local infection and subsequent recurrent perivalvular leak.[149,150] Recurrence of infection depends on the type of organism and the surgeon's ability to remove all areas of infection completely. Recurrence of infection is the single most important long-term complication.

MITRAL ANNULAR CALCIFICATION

Calcification of the mitral annulus is a process commonly associated with increased age[151,152] and stress to the mitral valve apparatus.[153,154] Based on routine echocardiographic screening, the Framingham study group reported an incidence of mitral annular calcification of 2.8%[155] among the study population. Calcium deposition is most commonly observed along the posterior mitral annulus but might extend to involve the whole annulus, intervalvular fibrous body, papillary muscles and left ventricle.[154,156] Despite rare direct involvement of valve leaflets,[151] the disease process affects leaflet coaptation, restricts leaflet motion, and prevents contraction of the AV annulus.[156] Severe mitral annular calcification, by itself, is not an indication for mitral valve surgery; however, it confers high operative risks in patients undergoing mitral valve surgery due to increasing risks of developing serious complications (intractable hemorrhage, AV disruption, ventricular rupture).[156] The major challenge valve surgeons face in those operations is ensuring a strong suture line to attach the prosthesis during MVR. Sutures within the calcium deposits would almost always lead to paravalvular leaks or valve dehiscence and extensive debridement

⊖ TABLE 42-6: Incidence of Thromboembolism and Anticoagulant-Related Hemorrhage

Valve	Reference (year)	Incidence of thromboembolism (%/patient-y)	Incidence of anticoagulant-related bleeding (%/patient-y)
Starr-Edwards	Miller (1983)	5.7	3.7
	Akins (1987)	3.9	2.4
	Agathos (1993)	6.6	2.2
	Godje (1997)	1.3	0.6
Omniscience/Omnicarbon	Cortina (1986)		2.7
	Damle (1987)	2.5	
	Akalin (1992)	1.0	2.7
	Peter (1993)	1.7	0.9
	Otaki (1993)	0.7	0.0
	Misawa (1993)	1.8	0.0
	Ohta (1995)	1.1	0.8
	Thevenet (1995)	0.9	1.1
	Iguro (1999)	1.0	0.6
	Torregrosa (1999)	0.6	0.8
	di Summa (2002)	0.4	0.2
Medtronic Hall	Antunes (1988)	4.2	1.5
	Beaudet (1988)	2.1	3.2
	Akins (1991)	1.8	3.2
	Butchar (2001)	4.0	1.4
St. Jude	Czer (1990)	1.9	2.1
	Kratz (1993)	2.9	2.2
	Jegaden (1994)	1.5	0.9
	Aoyagi (1994)	1.1	0.3
	Nistal (1996)	3.7	2.8
	Camilleri (2001)	1.9	1.5
	Khan (2001)	3.0	1.9
	Ramadi (2001)	0.7	0.9
	Emery (2005)	2.8	2.7
Carbomedics	De Luca (1993)	0.8	0.0
	Copeland (1995)	0.6	1.5
	Nistal (1996)	0.9	2.8
	Yamauchi (1996)	1.6	1.5
	Jamieson (2000)	4.6	2.7
	Soga (2002)	0.8	1.3
	Santini (2002)	2.2	
	Tominaga (2005)	1.8	0.9
	Carrier (2006)	0.7	0.7
	Wu (2006)	0.5	0.4
ATS	Shiono (1996)		0.0
	Westaby (1996)	0.0	
	Emery (2004)	3.0	2.3
	Stefanitis (2005)	0.5	0.0
On-X	Laczkovics (2001)	1.8	0.0
	Moidl (2002)	1.7	1.4
	McNicholas (2006)	1.6	3.1
	Williams (2006)	1.5	1.0
Hancock standard	Cohn (1989)	2.4	0.4
	Perier (1989)	1.1	1.0
	Bortolotti (1995)	1.4	0.7
Hancock II	Rizzoli (2003)	1.7	1.1
	Borger (2006)		

(Continued)

TABLE 42-6: Incidence of Thromboembolism and Anticoagulant-Related Hemorrhage (*Continued*)

Valve	Reference (year)	Incidence of thromboembolism (%/patient-y)	Incidence of anticoagulant-related bleeding (%/patient-y)
Carpentier-Edwards Porcine	Perier (1989)	0.8	1.0
	Akins (1990)	1.4	1.2
	Jamieson (1987)	2.4	0.7
	van Doorn (1995)	1.9	
	Glower (1998)	1.7	0.7
Carpentier-Edwards Pericardial	Pelletier (1995)	1.5	0.3
	Murakami (1996)	0.6	0.0
	Aupart (1997)	0.7	1.2
	Marchand (1998)	1.2	1.0
	Neville (1998)	0.6	1.1
	Poirer (1998)	1.7	0.3
	Bourguignon (2014)	0.7	0.8
Mosaic	Fradet (2001)	1.4	1.1
	Thomson (2001)	0.2	0.9
	Eichinger (2002)	0.8	2.0
Biocor	Myken (2000)	2.1	1.1
	Rizzoli (2005)	2.0	1.1

y indicates years.

may warrant annular reconstruction hence complicating the procedure further.

Surgical exposure should not be compromised in this situation and access should always be done through a complete median sternotomy. Preoperative and intraoperative echocardiographic imaging maps the calcifications and surgeon preference dictates how to best approach the mitral valve to ensure optimal visualization of the leaflets, annulus and, if needed, the left ventricle. Previously described approaches include standard left atriotomy,[157] transseptal access,[158] and finally through aortic root and dome of left atrium if concomitant AVR is required.[156] Since the disease is limited to the annulus in most cases, adequate debridement can be enough to ensure satisfactory valve replacement. In cases of extensive annular calcifications, patch reconstruction of the annulus may be required. The long-term benefits of annular reconstruction have been extensively studied, proven to be excellent when used by surgeons of adequate expertise and subsequently strongly recommended whenever applicable.[159-161] Despite being technically demanding, this technique ensures a strong suture line and gives the option of annular enlargement to fit a larger valve. Another approach described in 1994 by Nataf and colleagues is the intraatrial insertion of the mitral prosthesis.[162] Patients undergoing this procedure benefit from minimal calcium debridement at the expense of a higher implantation of the valve which may transfer the ventricular pressure into the atrium putting the valve at risk of dehiscence. A more recent and promising technique described by Hussain and colleagues mixed the two above-mentioned techniques. It requires the sandwiching of an annular washer posteriorly from trigone to trigone between the annulus and the sewing ring of the prosthesis.[158] Annular calcium debridement in this technique is limited to minimal amounts enough to fit a

prosthesis of reasonable size. Sutures can be taken through or around the calcium deposits and the washer is subsequently attached to the left atrium with running sutures to ensure adequate seal. Authors argue that the washer technique confers a superior annular support and minimizes the risk of ventricular rupture and paravalvular leak.[158]

UNCLAMPABLE ASCENDING AORTA

Calcifications in the ascending aorta are a common finding in cardiac surgery patients with varying severity. In the majority of cases, safe sites for cannulation and cross-clamping can still be found and surgeries conducted with adequate cerebral, systemic, and coronary perfusion. Porcelain aorta represents the extreme of the aortic calcification spectrum, where the traditional cross-clamping technique cannot be applied due to the very high risks of embolization and subsequent mortality.[163-166] Affecting 2 to 5% of the overall cardiac surgery patients, porcelain aorta is being increasingly encountered with the increasing elderly population.[167-169]

Preoperative screening for porcelain aorta is not routinely done which makes it sometimes an incidental intraoperative finding that warrants a change in the whole surgical approach. There is no current uniformly applicable practice as to how to address the mitral valve.[170-172] Maintaining cerebral and coronary perfusion, while minimizing the risk of embolization, should dictate the best approach and the initial decision as to whether find a way to clamp the aorta or not. The general approach to MVR we adopt in this patient population is schemed in Fig. 42-11. In the absence of a significant aortic valve insufficiency, the preferred approach to an isolated MVR is moderate hypothermia with ventricular fibrillation without any aortic clamp.[173] It will ensure adequate valve exposure and coronary perfusion

TABLE 42-7: Freedom (Actuarial) from SVD by Age

Valve	Reference (year)	Age	Freedom from SVD		
			5 y	10 y	15 y
Hancock	Cohn (1989)	≤40		68%	
		41-69		84%	
		≥70		84%	
Hancock II	David (2001)	<65			76%
		≥65			89%
	Rizzoli (2003)	<65			82%
		≥65			92%
	Borger (2006)	<65			27% (20 y)
		≥65			59% (20 y)
Carpentier-Edwards standard	Akins (1990)	≤40		7%	
		41-50		82%	
		51-60		65%	
		61-70		79%	
		≤70		98%	
	Jamieson (1995)	≤35	79%	51%	
		36-40	99%	68%	48%
		51-64	98%	72%	42%
		65-69	98%	74%	64%
		≥70	100%	9%	90%
	Corbineau (2001)	≤35			0% (14 y)
		36-50			22% (14 y)
		51-60			34% (14 y)
		61-65			50% (14 y)
		66-70			93% (14 y)
		≥70			96% (14 y)
Carpentier-Edwards pericardial	Aupart (1997)	<60	47%		
		≥60	100%		
	Pelletier (1995)	≤59	100%	64% (8 y)	
		60-69	100%	91% (8 y)	
		≥70	100%	100% (8 y)	
	Marchand (1998)	≤60		78% (11 y)	
		61-70		89% (11 y)	
		>70		100% (11 y)	
	Neville (1998)	<60		70%	
		≥60		100%	
	Poirer (1998)	<60	100%	78%	
		60-6	100%	78%	
		≥70	100%	100%	
	Bourguignon (2014)	<65			47%
		≥65			63%
Biocor	Myken (2000)	<50			71%
		51-60			90%
		>61			100%

y indicates years.

TABLE 42-8: Prosthetic Valve Endocarditis

Valve	Reference (year)	PVE rate (%/patient-y)	Freedom from PVE at 5 y
Starr-Edwards	Miller (1983)	0.5	97%
	Akins (1987)	0.4	95%
	Agathos 1993)	0.6	
	Godje (1997)		99% (10 y)
Omniscience/Omnicarbon	Carrier (1987)	0.8	98%
	Damle (1987)	0.8	98%
	Peter (1993)	0.0	100%
	Otaki (1993)	1.5	
	Misawa (1993)	0.0	100% (3 y)
	Ohta (1995)	0.5	
	Thenevet (1995)	0.2	
	Torregrosa (1999)	0.2	99% (10 y)
	di Summa (2002)	0.0	100% (10 y)
Medtronic Hall	Keenan (1990)	0.5	98%
	Akins (1991)	0.1	100%
	Fiore (1998)		94% (10 y)
	Masters (1995)	0.1	
	Butchart (2001)	0.4	94% (10 y)
	Masters (2001)	0.6	
St. Jude	Antunes (1988)	0.5	97%
	Kratz (1993)	0.4	
	Aoyagi (1994)	0.1	100%
	Fiore (1998)		100% (10 y)
	Camilleri (2001)	0.8	
	Masters (2001)	0.4	
	Khan (2001)	0.3	
	Ikonamidis (2003)		98% (10 y)
	Emery (2005)	0.3	
Carbomedics	De Luca (1993)	0.0	100%
	Copeland (1995)	0.3	96%
	Nistal (1996)	0.0	100%
	Yamauchi (1996)	0.0	100%
	Jamieson (2000)	0.4	
	Masters (2001)	0.6	
	Santini (2002)		100%
	Soga (2002)	0.0	100%
	Tominaga (2005)	0.3	97% (10 y)
	Carrier (2006)	0.3	97% (15 y)
	Wu (2006)	0.4	98% (10 y)
ATS	Emery (2004)	0.4	
	Stefanitis (2005)	0.0	100%
On-X	Laczkovics (2001)	0.5	
	Moidl (2002)	0.7	99% (2 y)
	Williams (2006)		95% (4 y)
	McNicholas (2006)	0.0	100%
Hancock standard	Cohn (1989)		93%
	Bernal (1991)	0.3	
	Sarris (1993)		93%
	Bortolotti (1995)	0.3	

(*Continued*)

TABLE 42-8: Prosthetic Valve Endocarditis (*Continued*)

Valve	Reference (year)	PVE rate (%/patient-y)	Freedom from PVE at 5 y	
Hancock II	Legarra (1999)		97% (15 y)	
	David (2001)		91% (15 y)	
	Rizzoli (2003)	0.4	96% (15 y)	
	Masters (2004)		99% (8 y)	
	Borger (2006)		85% (20 y)	
Carpentier-Edwards porcine	Pelletier (1989)	0.4		
	Akins (1990)	1.0		
	Louagie (1992)	0.0	100%	
	Sarris (1993)		91%	
	van Doorn (1995)		97%	92% (10 y)
	Glower (1998)	0.3	97%	96% (10 y)
Carpentier-Edwards pericardial	Pelletier (1995)	0.3%	93% (10 y)	
	Murakami (1996)	0.86	94% (10 y)	
	Aupart (1997)	0.4%	97% (10 y)	
	Marchand (1998)	0.1%		
	Neville (1998)	0.6%	94% (12 y)	
	Poirer (1998)	0.3%	95% (10 y)	
	Bourguignon (2014)		95% (20 y)	
Mosaic	Jasinski (2000)		100% (3 y)	
	Fradet (2004)	0.8	98% (7 y)	
	Thomson (2001)	0.8		
	Eichinger (2002)	0.8	94%	
Biocor	Myken (2000)	0.7	93% (15 y)	
	Rizzolil (2005)		94% (8 y)	

y indicates years.

with minimal aortic manipulation.[173] It is important to keep perfusion pressure high to maintain the aortic valve closed and prevent air embolism. In patients with aortic insufficiency, many approaches have been described and include endoaortic balloon occlusion,[174,175] hypothermic fibrillation with low bypass flow[176] or replacement of the calcified ascending aorta under deep hypothermic circulatory arrest.[170]

The use of endoaortic balloon occlusion in patients with porcelain aorta has been previously described; however, it was

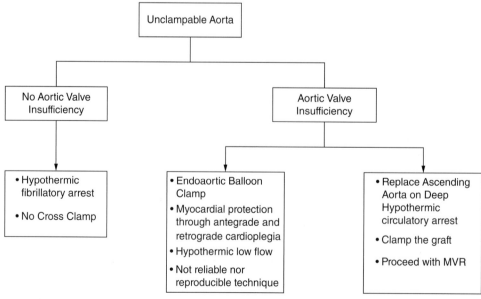

FIGURE 42-11 Approach to mitral valve replacement in patients with unclampable aorta.

abandoned by Zingone and colleagues after publishing disappointing results where the use of this device was associated with a higher than expected incidence of unfavorable events ranging from silent emboli to death.[175] The major drawback was the incomplete occlusion happening frequently and attempts to over inflate the balloon were associated with balloon protrusion.[175] Interventionists should keep in mind that if peripheral access for the balloon is sought, it should be well assessed since diffuse calcification of the femorals iliacs or descending aorta are common findings in patients with porcelain aorta.

The use of a hypothermic low flow bypass has been mostly emphasized in patients with minimal aortic valve insufficiency that worsens upon heart manipulation to obtain adequate mitral valve exposure.[174,176] It usually accompanies the previous technique to ensure the operative field does not get flooded with blood jeopardizing the practicality and diligence of the repair/replacement.

Eventually, replacement of the ascending aorta under deep hypothermic circulatory arrest came to be a preferred technique especially in patients with minimal comorbidities. It was first described in patients with porcelain aorta requiring aortic valve replacement in 1992[168] and with growing expertise, surgeons have extrapolated its applicability to mitral valve surgeries. Despite being a more invasive and radical approach, multiple studies have shown that it can be safely and effectively done.[170-172] It is not risk free and benefits need to be carefully weighed especially in elderly or patients with significant comorbidities, requiring multiple valve surgery or concomitant coronary artery bypass graft. Of specific concern is the cannulation strategy and cerebral perfusion. Arterial cannulation should be done under direct epiaortic guidance in the ascending aorta, common brachiocephalic trunk or axillary artery and the venous cannulation can be done directly into the right atrium or through the femoral vein. Cerebral perfusion can be instituted through antegrade or retrograde blood flow into the brain or not adopted at all while monitoring cerebral oxygenation indeces.[172,176]

Patient-Prosthesis Mismatch

The concept of patient-prosthesis mismatch is not new, but was first described in relationship to aortic valve replacement by Rahimtoola in 1978.[177] Since his introduction, the deleterious effects of patient-prosthesis mismatch on LV remodeling, function, and early and late survival with aortic valve replacement have been well documented. The notion of mitral valve patient prosthesis mismatch (MVPPM) in the adult was first proposed in a case report in 1981 again by Rahimtoola.[178] Most MVPPM was described in relation to pediatric mitral valve surgery, resulting in re-replacement rates approaching 30%, largely the result of somatic growth versus fixed prosthesis size. Recently, the possibility of such patient prosthesis mismatch in the mitral position has become an area of increased interest among adult cardiac surgeons. At this time, MVPPM has been studied through in vitro pulse generator analysis demonstrating that an index geometric orifice area

less than 1.3 to 1.5 cm²/m² could potentially result in any patient having a high postoperative transprosthetic gradient. Similar studies performed in the clinical arena suggest that an index effective orifice area (IEOA) less than 1.3 to 1.5 cm²/m² as measured by the continuity equation may increase the risk for MVPPM. Using this criterion, Lam and coworkers demonstrated a potential for MVPPM of roughly 32% in a recent series of 884 patients. In this population, patients at elevated risk for MVPPM measured at IEOA 1.0 to 1.25 cm²/m² were at a significantly higher risk for development of postoperative CHF than those with IEOA greater than 1.25 cm²/m². Although a weak association with CHF and pulmonary hypertension was noted, no direct correlation was found between MVPPM and the development of postoperative pulmonary hypertension.

Jamieson and coworkers recently evaluated the potential impact of MVPPM and long-term survival.[179] In contrast to prior reports, this study of nearly 2500 patients refuted the notion that MVPPM had any relation to mortality. Instead predictors of overall mortality included age, New York Heart Association III or IV, competent coronary artery disease, ventricular dysfunction, prosthesis type, body mass index, and preexisting pulmonary hypertension.

Certainly some degree of patient prosthesis mismatch may occur as a result of MVR. The surgeon should be aware of the potential for MVPPM, particularly in the setting of particularly small annulus size in patients resulting in the need for implantation of a small prosthetic device resulting in a high transprosthetic gradient. As such, foreknowledge of the devices specific IEOA may assist allowing the surgeon to choose a device that might minimize MVPPM. Unfortunately, unlike the aortic position, in which aortic root enlargement will allow for valve upsizing, the mitral position cannot be corrected as simply. As a result, in patients with particularly small mitral valve area, some degree of patient prosthesis mismatch may be unavoidable. This phenomenon remains an area of active clinical investigation.

Mitral Prosthetic Paravalvular Leak

Paravalvular leaks occur after valve replacement surgeries with an incidence of 7 to 17% in the mitral position and minimal clinical sequelae in the majority of cases.[134,180] It is estimated that only 1 to 5% of those patients develop serious clinical consequences (heart failure, endocarditis, and hemolysis) and require reintervention to modify their outcomes.[181,182] This leak arises whenever there is an incomplete seal between the prosthesis sewing ring and the mitral annulus and it has been associated with risk factors including technical (suturing technique and size and shape of the prosthesis), annular calcification, and infection.[183] Early occurrence of this leak has been linked to the technical risk factors, whereas late occurrence seem to happen as a results of suture dehiscence caused by infectious processes or suturing through annular calcifications.[183] A paravalvular leak should be therefore suspected in any patients with a new onset murmur after valve surgery or symptoms of anemia or heart failure and cardiac echocardiography is needed to confirm the finding of a systolic jet into the left atrium.

Once complications arise, patients should be evaluated for operative or transcatheter closure of the leak. Until few years ago, resternotomy was the only option available where the leak can be repaired through direct resuturing or patching or the whole valve replaced.[184-186] The main drawback of surgical reentry, however, is its association with high rate of procedure failure (12-35%) and mortality (4-13%).[187,188] The underlying disease process is still present in addition to the tissue frailty and the fact that this is a reoperation would drive surgeons away from this procedure especially in the presence of multiple comorbidities.[189] Recently, however, high-risk patients with paravalvular leak were offered an alternative percutaneous option.

Percutaneous paravalvular leak repair is a catheter-based technique during which a closure device is deployed to obliterate and seal the leak area. This procedure is not free of risk and requires advanced technical expertise in catheter-based closure-device implantations. The approach to the mitral valve can be transseptal, transaortic, and/or transapical, and the decision on the approach depends mainly on the location of the leak, the vascular access, the presence of mechanical valves, the presence of paravalvular calcification, and the size and shape of the orifice.[183,190] The optimal goal of this technique is to ensure maximal closure with minimal impingement on the valve leaflets and the challenges include the ability to adequately visualize the leak, estimate its spatial characteristics, and find the device that best suits this type of leak.[183,190-192] Angiography, transesophageal echocardiography, 3D echocardiography, and 3D-4D computed tomography angiography are available for use during this procedure to ensure best estimation of the device geometrics and flow hemodynamics.[183] In the absence of devices specifically designed for this purpose, the Amplatz family of occluder devices, commonly applied for ASD, VSD, and PDA closure, are used off-label. Two disk devices like the Amplatz Vascular plug (AVP II most used in USA and AVP III) are preferred because they hold a lower risk of embolization and are better suited for the commonly encountered geometrics of the leak.[183,192] In certain instances multiple small devices are used to close one single defect. Long-term benefits of this technique have been reported by multiple case series which included also paravalvular aortic leaks as well. These studies reported acceptable successful implantation rates (63 and 91%) as well as favorable short- and midterm outcomes in groups of very high operative risk patients.[191,193,194] Long-term mortality, however, remains very high in this patient population because of the baseline high-risk profile they have.

TRANSCATHETER TREATMENT

Introduction of transcatheter valve replacement has reshaped the treatment strategy for aortic valve replacement. In the United States, it is currently approved for aortic stenosis patients with high or prohibitive risk. Transcatheter mitral valve replacement (TMVR) has been performed by means of valve-in-valve technique.[195] This technique uses the stent of the previous bioprostheses as an anchor for the transcatheter valve; however, it not yet approved by the FDA. Some series report excellent outcome with improvement in the postprocedural gradient. This technique is commonly performed through transapical approach,[195] but other approaches via transfemoral/transseptal and transjugular are reported.[196]

There are many hurdles for the native TMVR. Currently, native mitral annulus is not rigid enough to hold the transcatheter valve. Also, the varied etiology, the complex anatomy, the difficulty in measuring the size of the valve, the exposure to increased pressure in case of paravalvular leak, the risk of left ventricular outflow tract obstruction and the excellent result of mitral valve repair are some of the difficulties that TMVR will face. Nonetheless, the technology will evolve and we may see a new transcatheter valve which will solve all these issues in the near future.

REFERENCES

1. Zipes DP, Braunwald E: *A Textbook of Cardiovascular Medicine*. Philadelphia: Saunders; 2004.
2. Nishimura RA, Otto CM, Bonow RO, et al: 2014 AHA/ACC Guideline for the Management of Patients With Valvular Heart Disease: a report of the American College of Cardiology/American Heart Association Task Force on Practice Guidelines. *Circulation* 2014; 129(23):e521-e643.
3. Wilkins GT, Weyman AE, Abascal VM, Block PC, Palacios IF: Percutaneous balloon dilatation of the mitral valve: an analysis of echocardiographic variables related to outcome and the mechanism of dilatation. *Br Heart J* 1988; 60(4):299-308.
4. Vincens JJ, Temizer D, Post JR, Edmunds LH, Jr, Herrmann HC: Long-term outcome of cardiac surgery in patients with mitral stenosis and severe pulmonary hypertension. *Circulation* 1995; 92(9 Suppl):Ii137-Ii142.
5. Li M, Dumesnil JG, Mathieu P, Pibarot P: Impact of valve prosthesis-patient mismatch on pulmonary arterial pressure after mitral valve replacement. *J Am Coll Cardiol* 2005; 45(7):1034-1040.
6. Palacios IF, Tuzcu ME, Weyman AE, Newell JB, Block PC: Clinical follow-up of patients undergoing percutaneous mitral balloon valvotomy. *Circulation* 1995; 91(3):671-676.
7. Reyes VP, Raju BS, Wynne J, et al: Percutaneous balloon valvuloplasty compared with open surgical commissurotomy for mitral stenosis. *N Engl J Med* 1994; 331(15):961-967.
8. Complications and mortality of percutaneous balloon mitral commissurotomy: a report from the National Heart, Lung, and Blood Institute Balloon Valvuloplasty Registry. *Circulation* 1992; 85(6):2014-2024.
9. Cohn LH, Allred EN, Cohn LA, Disesa VJ, Shemin RJ, Collins JJ, Jr: Long-term results of open mitral valve reconstruction for mitral stenosis. *Am J Cardiol* 1985; 55(6):731-734.
10. Glower DD, Landolfo KP, Davis RD, et al: Comparison of open mitral commissurotomy with mitral valve replacement with or without chordal preservation in patients with mitral stenosis. *Circulation* 1998; 98(19 Suppl):Ii120-123.
11. El Asmar B, Acker M, Couetil JP, et al: Mitral valve repair in the extensively calcified mitral valve annulus. *Ann Thorac Surg* 1991; 52(1):66-69.
12. Enriquez-Sarano M, Tajik AJ, Schaff HV, Orszulak TA, Bailey KR, Frye RL: Echocardiographic prediction of survival after surgical correction of organic mitral regurgitation. *Circulation* 1994; 90(2):830-837.
13. Enriquez-Sarano M, Tajik AJ, Schaff HV, et al: Echocardiographic prediction of left ventricular function after correction of mitral regurgitation: results and clinical implications. *J Am Coll Cardiol* 1994; 24(6):1536-1543.
14. Timmis SB, Kirsh MM, Montgomery DG, Starling MR: Evaluation of left ventricular ejection fraction as a measure of pump performance in patients with chronic mitral regurgitation. *Catheter Cardiovasc Interv* 2000; 49(3):290-296.

15. Kontos GJ, Jr, Schaff HV, Gersh BJ, Bove AA: Left ventricular function in subacute and chronic mitral regurgitation. Effect on function early postoperatively. *J Thorac Cardiovasc Surg* 1989; 98(2):163-169.

16. Nakano S, Sakai K, Taniguchi K, et al: Relation of impaired left ventricular function in mitral regurgitation to left ventricular contractile state after mitral valve replacement. *Am J Cardiol* 1994; 73(1):70-74.

17. Matsumura T, Ohtaki E, Tanaka K, et al: Echocardiographic prediction of left ventricular dysfunction after mitral valve repair for mitral regurgitation as an indicator to decide the optimal timing of repair. *J Am Coll Cardiol* 2003; 42(3):458-463.

18. Wisenbaugh T, Skudicky D, Sareli P: Prediction of outcome after valve replacement for rheumatic mitral regurgitation in the era of chordal preservation. *Circulation* 1994; 89(1):191-197.

19. Braunberger E, Deloche A, Berrebi A, et al: Very long-term results (more than 20 years) of valve repair with carpentier's techniques in nonrheumatic mitral valve insufficiency. *Circulation* 2001; 104(12 Suppl 1):I8-I11.

20. Cohn LH, Allred EN, Cohn LA, et al: Early and late risk of mitral valve replacement. A 12 year concomitant comparison of the porcine bioprosthetic and prosthetic disc mitral valves. *J Thorac Cardiovasc Surg* 1985; 90(6):872-881.

21. Cohn LH, Couper GS, Aranki SF, Rizzo RJ, Adams DH, Collins JJ, Jr: The long-term results of mitral valve reconstruction for the "floppy" valve. *J Card Surg* 1994; 9(2 Suppl):278-281.

22. Cosgrove DM, Chavez AM, Lytle BW, et al: Results of mitral valve reconstruction. *Circulation* 1986; 74(3 Pt 2):I82-I87.

23. Greelish JP, Cohn LH, Leacche M, et al: Minimally invasive mitral valve repair suggests earlier operations for mitral valve disease. *J Thorac Cardiovasc Surg* 2003; 126(2):365-371; discussion 371-373.

24. El Asmar B, Perier P, Couetil JP, Carpentier A: Failures in reconstructive mitral valve surgery. *J Med Liban* 1991; 39(1):7-11.

25. Chauvaud S, Fuzellier JF, Berrebi A, Deloche A, Fabiani JN, Carpentier A: Long-term (29 years) results of reconstructive surgery in rheumatic mitral valve insufficiency. *Circulation* 2001; 104(12 Suppl 1):I12-I15.

26. Alexiou C, Langley SM, Stafford H, Haw MP, Livesey SA, Monro JL: Surgical treatment of infective mitral valve endocarditis: predictors of early and late outcome. *J Heart Valve Dis* 2000; 9(3):327-334.

27. Aranki SF, Adams DH, Rizzo RJ, et al: Determinants of early mortality and late survival in mitral valve endocarditis. *Circulation* 1995; 92(9 Suppl):Ii143-Ii149.

28. Mihaljevic T, Paul S, Leacche M, et al: Tailored surgical therapy for acute native mitral valve endocarditis. *J Heart Valve Dis* 2004; 13(2):210-216.

29. Acker MA, Parides MK, Perrault LP, et al: Mitral-valve repair versus replacement for severe ischemic mitral regurgitation. *N Engl J Med* 2014; 370(1):23-32.

30. Byrne JG, Aranki SF, Cohn LH: Repair versus replacement of mitral valve for treating severe ischemic mitral regurgitation. *Coron Artery Dis* 2000; 11(1):31-33.

31. Cohn LH, Rizzo RJ, Adams DH, et al: The effect of pathophysiology on the surgical treatment of ischemic mitral regurgitation: operative and late risks of repair versus replacement. *Eur J Cardiothorac Surg* 1995; 9(10):568-574.

32. Grossi EA, Goldberg JD, LaPietra A, et al: Ischemic mitral valve reconstruction and replacement: comparison of long-term survival and complications. *J Thorac Cardiovasc Surg* 2001; 122(6):1107-1124.

33. Williams MA, van Riet S: The On-X heart valve: mid-term results in a poorly anticoagulated population. *J Heart Valve Dis* 2006; 15(1):80-86.

34. Kaneko T, Aranki S, Javed Q, et al: Mechanical versus bioprosthetic mitral valve replacement in patients <65 years old. *J Thorac Cardiovasc Surg* 2014; 147(1):117-126.

35. Jamieson WR, von Lipinski O, Miyagishima RT, et al: Performance of bioprostheses and mechanical prostheses assessed by composites of valve-related complications to 15 years after mitral valve replacement. *J Thorac Cardiovasc Surg* 2005; 129(6):1301-1308.

36. Grunkemeier GL, Jamieson WR, Miller DC, Starr A: Actuarial versus actual risk of porcine structural valve deterioration. *J Thorac Cardiovasc Surg* 1994; 108(3):709-718.

37. Peterseim DS, Cen YY, Cheruvu S, et al: Long-term outcome after biologic versus mechanical aortic valve replacement in 841 patients. *J Thorac Cardiovasc Surg* 1999; 117(5):890-897.

38. Angell WW, Pupello DF, Bessone LN, et al: Influence of coronary artery disease on structural deterioration of porcine bioprostheses. *Ann Thorac Surg* 1995; 60(2 Suppl):S276-281.

39. DiSesa VJ, Cohn LH, Collins JJ, Jr, Koster JK, Jr, Van Devanter S: Determinants of operative survival following combined mitral valve replacement and coronary revascularization. *Ann Thorac Surg* 1982; 34(5):482-489.

40. Edwards FH, Peterson ED, Coombs LP, et al: Prediction of operative mortality after valve replacement surgery. *J Am Coll Cardiol* 2001; 37(3):885-892.

41. Jones EL, Weintraub WS, Craver JM, Guyton RA, Shen Y: Interaction of age and coronary disease after valve replacement: implications for valve selection. *Ann Thorac Surg* 1994; 58(2):378-384; discussion 375-384.

42. Schoen FJ, Collins JJ, Jr, Cohn LH: Long-term failure rate and morphologic correlations in porcine bioprosthetic heart valves. *Am J Cardiol* 1983; 51(6):957-964.

43. Thourani VH, Weintraub WS, Craver JM, et al: Influence of concomitant CABG and urgent/emergent status on mitral valve replacement surgery. *Ann Thorac Surg* 2000; 70(3):778-783; discussion 774-783.

44. Burdon TA, Miller DC, Oyer PE, et al: Durability of porcine valves at fifteen years in a representative North American patient population. *J Thorac Cardiovasc Surg* 1992; 103(2):238-251; discussion 232-251.

45. Cohn LH, Collins JJ, Jr, Rizzo RJ, Adams DH, Couper GS, Aranki SF: Twenty-year follow-up of the Hancock modified orifice porcine aortic valve. *Ann Thorac Surg* 1998; 66(6 Suppl):S30-S34.

46. Corbineau H, Du Haut Cilly FB, Langanay T, Verhoye JP, Leguerrier A: Structural durability in Carpentier Edwards Standard bioprosthesis in the mitral position: a 20-year experience. *J Heart Valve Dis* 2001; 10(4):443-448.

47. Jamieson WR, Burr LH, Munro AI, Miyagishima RT: Carpentier-Edwards standard porcine bioprosthesis: a 21-year experience. *Ann Thorac Surg* 1998; 66(6 Suppl):S40-S43.

48. Khan SS, Chaux A, Blanche C, et al: A 20-year experience with the Hancock porcine xenograft in the elderly. *Ann Thorac Surg* 1998; 66(6 Suppl):S35-S39.

49. van Doorn CA, Stoodley KD, Saunders NR, Nair RU, Davies GA, Watson DA: Mitral valve replacement with the Carpentier-Edwards standard bioprosthesis: performance into the second decade. *Eur J Cardiothorac Surg* 1995; 9(5):253-258.

50. Pupello DF, Bessone LN, Hiro SP, et al: Bioprosthetic valve longevity in the elderly: an 18-year longitudinal study. *Ann Thorac Surg* 1995; 60(2 Suppl):S270-S274; discussion S275.

51. Jamieson WR, Tyers GF, Janusz MT, et al: Age as a determinant for selection of porcine bioprostheses for cardiac valve replacement: experience with Carpentier-Edwards standard bioprosthesis. *Can J Cardiol* 1991; 7(4):181-188.

52. Badduke BR, Jamieson WR, Miyagishima RT, et al: Pregnancy and childbearing in a population with biologic valvular prostheses. *J Thorac Cardiovasc Surg* 1991; 102(2):179-186.

53. Jamieson WR, Miller DC, Akins CW, et al: Pregnancy and bioprostheses: influence on structural valve deterioration. *Ann Thorac Surg* 1995; 60(2 Suppl):S282-286; discussion S287.

54. Mihaljevic T, Paul S, Leacche M, Rawn JD, Cohn LH, Byrne JG: Valve replacement in women of childbearing age: influences on mother, fetus and neonate. *J Heart Valve Dis* 2005; 14(2):151-157.

55. Sareli P, England MJ, Berk MR, et al: Maternal and fetal sequelae of anticoagulation during pregnancy in patients with mechanical heart valve prostheses. *Am J Cardiol* 1989; 63(20):1462-1465.

56. Ali M, Iung B, Lansac E, Bruneval P, Acar C: Homograft replacement of the mitral valve: eight-year results. *J Thorac Cardiovasc Surg* 2004; 128(4):529-534.

57. Deac RF, Simionescu D, Deac D: New evolution in mitral physiology and surgery: mitral stentless pericardial valve. *Ann Thorac Surg* 1995; 60(2 Suppl):S433-438.

58. Gulbins H, Kreuzer E, Uhlig A, Reichart B: Mitral valve surgery utilizing homografts: early results. *J Heart Valve Dis* 2000; 9(2):222-229.

59. Kumar AS, Choudhary SK, Mathur A, Saxena A, Roy R, Chopra P: Homograft mitral valve replacement: five years' results. *J Thorac Cardiovasc Surg* 2000; 120(3):450-458.

60. Chauvaud S, Waldmann T, d'Attellis N, et al: Homograft replacement of the mitral valve in young recipients: mid-term results. *Eur J Cardiothorac Surg* 2003; 23(4):560-566.

61. Hofmann B, Cichon R, Knaut M, et al: Early experience with a quadrileaflet stentless mitral valve. *Ann Thorac Surg* 2001; 71(5 Suppl): S323-326.

62. Lehmann S, Walther T, Kempfert J, et al: Stentless mitral valve implantation in comparison to conventional mitral valve repair or replacement at five years. *Thorac Cardiovasc Surg* 2006; 54(1):10-14.

63. Vrandecic MO, Fantini FA, Gontijo BF, et al: Surgical technique of implanting the stentless porcine mitral valve. *Ann Thorac Surg* 1995; 60(2 Suppl):S439-S442.

64. Athanasiou T, Cherian A, Ross D: The Ross II procedure: pulmonary autograft in the mitral position. *Ann Thorac Surg* 2004; 78(4):1489-1495.

65. Brown JW, Ruzmetov M, Turrentine MW, Rodefeld MD: Mitral valve replacement with the pulmonary autograft: Ross II procedure with Kabanni modification. *Semin Thorac Cardiovasc Surg Pediatr Card Surg Annu* 2004; 7:107-114.

66. Kabbani SS, Jamil H, Hammoud A, et al: The mitral pulmonary autograft: assessment at midterm. *Ann Thorac Surg* 2004; 78(1):60-65; discussion 65-66.

67. Gammie JS, Sheng S, Griffith BP, et al: Trends in mitral valve surgery in the United States: results from the Society of Thoracic Surgeons Adult Cardiac Surgery Database. *Ann Thorac Surg* 2009; 87(5):1431-1437; discussion 1437-1439.

68. Cohn LH: *Cardiac Surgery in the Adult*. New York: McGraw Hill; 2008.

69. Cordoba M AP, Martinez P, et al: *Invasive Assessment of Mitral Valve Prostheses*. New York, Futura, 1987; p 369.

70. Khuri SF, Folland ED, Sethi GK, et al: Six month postoperative hemodynamics of the Hancock heterograft and the Bjork-Shiley prosthesis: results of a Veterans Administration cooperative prospective randomized trial. *J Am Coll Cardiol* 1988; 12(1):8-18.

71. Pelletier C CB, Bonan R, Dyrda I: *Hemodynamic Evaluation of the Carpentier-Edwards Standard and Improved Annulus Bioprostheses*. New York: Yorke Medical Books; 1982.

72. Horskotte D, Loogen F, Birckson B: *Is the Late Outcome of Heart Valve Replacement Influenced by the Hemodynamics of the Heart Valve Substitute?*. New York: Springer-Verlag; 1986:55.

73. Butterfield M, Fisher J, Davies GA, Spyt TJ: Comparative study of the hydrodynamic function of the CarboMedics valve. *Ann Thorac Surg* 1991; 52(4):815-820.

74. Agathos EA, Starr A: Mitral valve replacement. *Curr Probl Surg* 1993; 30(6):481-592.

75. Miller DC, Oyer PE, Stinson EB, et al: Ten to fifteen year reassessment of the performance characteristics of the Starr-Edwards Model 6120 mitral valve prosthesis. *J Thorac Cardiovasc Surg* 1983; 85(1):1-20.

76. Murday AJ, Hochstitzky A, Mansfield J, et al: A prospective controlled trial of St. Jude versus Starr Edwards aortic and mitral valve prostheses. *Ann Thorac Surg* 2003; 76(1):66-73; discussion 64-73.

77. Hall KV: The Medtronic-Hall valve: a design in 1977 to improve the results of valve replacement. *Eur J Cardiothorac Surg* 1992; 6 Suppl 1:S64-67.

78. Mihaljevic T, Cohn LH, Unic D, Aranki SF, Couper GS, Byrne JG: One thousand minimally invasive valve operations: early and late results. *Ann Surg* 2004; 240(3):529-534; discussion 534.

79. Grunkemeier GL, Starr A, Rahimtoola SH: Prosthetic heart valve performance: long-term follow-up. *Curr Probl Cardiol* 1992; 17(6):329-406.

80. Akalin H, Corapcioglu ET, Ozyurda U, et al: Clinical evaluation of the Omniscience cardiac valve prosthesis. Follow-up of up to 6 years. *J Thorac Cardiovasc Surg* 1992; 103(2):259-266.

81. DeWall R, Pelletier LC, Panebianco A, et al: Five-year clinical experience with the Omniscience cardiac valve. *Ann Thorac Surg* 1984; 38(3):275-280.

82. Wata N, Abe T, Yamada O, et al: Comparative analysis of Omniscience and Omnicarbon prosthesis after aortic valve replacement. *Jpn J Artif Organs* 1989; 18:773.

83. Emery RW, Nicoloff DM: St. Jude Medical cardiac valve prosthesis: in vitro studies. *J Thorac Cardiovasc Surg* 1979; 78(2):269-276.

84. Nair CK, Mohiuddin SM, Hilleman DE, et al: Ten-year results with the St. Jude Medical prosthesis. *Am J Cardiol* 1990; 65(3):217-225.

85. Champsaur G, Gressier M, Niret J, et al: *When Are Hemodynamics Important for the Selection of a Prosthetic Heart Valve?* New York: Springer-Verlag; 1986.

86. D'Alessandro, Narducci C, Pucci A, et al: *The Use of Mechanical Valves in the Treatment of Valvular Heart Disease*. New York: Springer-Verlag; 1986.

87. Laub GW, Muralidharan S, Pollock SB, Adkins MS, McGrath LB: The experimental relationship between leaflet clearance and orientation of the St. Jude Medical valve in the mitral position. *J Thorac Cardiovasc Surg* 1992; 103(4):638-641.

88. Birnbaum D, Laczkovics A, Heidt M, et al: Examination of hemolytic potential with the On-X(R) prosthetic heart valve. *J Heart Valve Dis* 2000; 9(1):142-145.

89. McNicholas KW, Ivey TD, Metras J, et al: North American multicenter experience with the On-X prosthetic heart valve. *J Heart Valve Dis* 2006; 15(1):73-78; discussion 79.

90. Kaneko T, Yammine M, Aranki SF: New oral anticoagulants-what the cardiothoracic surgeon needs to know. *J Thorac Cardiovasc Surg* 2014.

91. Brown JM, O'Brien SM, Wu C, Sikora JA, Griffith BP, Gammie JS: Isolated aortic valve replacement in North America comprising 108,687 patients in 10 years: changes in risks, valve types, and outcomes in the Society of Thoracic Surgeons National Database. *J Thorac Cardiovasc Surg* 2009; 137(1):82-90.

92. Eikelboom JW, Connolly SJ, Brueckmann M, et al: Dabigatran versus warfarin in patients with mechanical heart valves. *N Engl J Med* 2013; 369(13):1206-1214.

93. Galluci V, Valfre C, Mazzucco A, et al: *Heart Valve Replacement with the Hancock Bioprosthesis: A 5- to 11-Year Follow-up*. New York: Yorke Medical Books; 1982.

94. D'Attellis N, Nicolas-Robin A, Delayance S, Carpentier A, Baron JF: Early extubation after mitral valve surgery: a target-controlled infusion of propofol and low-dose sufentanil. *J Cardiothorac Vasc Anesth* 1997; 11(4):467-473.

95. Buckberg GD: Development of blood cardioplegia and retrograde techniques: the experimenter/observer complex. *J Card Surg* 1998; 13(3):163-170.

96. Larbalestier RI, Chard RB, Cohn LH: Optimal approach to the mitral valve: dissection of the interatrial groove. *Ann Thorac Surg* 1992; 54(6):1186-1188.

97. Sondergaard T, Gotzsche H, Ottosen P, Schultz J: Surgical closure of interatrial septal defects by circumclusion. *Acta Chir Scand* 1955; 109(3-4):188-196.

98. Hirt SW, Frimpong-Boateng K, Borst HG: The superior approach to the mitral valve—is it worthwhile? *Eur J Cardiothorac Surg* 1988; 2(5):372-376.

99. Utley JR, Leyland SA, Nguyenduy T: Comparison of outcomes with three atrial incisions for mitral valve operations. Right lateral, superior septal, and transseptal. *J Thorac Cardiovasc Surg* 1995; 109(3):582-587.

100. Barner HB: Combined superior and right lateral left atriotomy with division of the superior vena cava for exposure of the mitral valve. *Ann Thorac Surg* 1985; 40(4):365-367.

101. Kon ND, Tucker WY, Mills SA, Lavender SW, Cordell AR: Mitral valve operation via an extended transseptal approach. *Ann Thorac Surg* 1993; 55(6):1413-1416; discussion 1416-1417.

102. Selle JG: Temporary division of the superior vena cava for exceptional mitral valve exposure. *J Thorac Cardiovasc Surg* 1984; 88(2):302-304.

103. Kumar N, Saad E, Prabhakar G, De Vol E, Duran CM: Extended transseptal versus conventional left atriotomy: early postoperative study. *Ann Thorac Surg* 1995; 60(2):426-430.

104. Cosgrove DM, 3rd, Sabik JF, Navia JL: Minimally invasive valve operations. *Ann Thorac Surg* 1998; 65(6):1535-1538; discussion 1538-1539.

105. David TE, Armstrong S, Sun Z: Left ventricular function after mitral valve surgery. *J Heart Valve Dis* 1995; 4 Suppl 2:S175-180.

106. Lillehei CW, Levy MJ, Bonnabeau RC, Jr: Mitral Valve Replacement With Preservation of Papillary Muscles and Chordae Tendineae. *J Thorac Cardiovasc Surg* 1964; 47:532-543.

107. Cohn LH, Couper GS, Kinchla NM, Collins JJ, Jr: Decreased operative risk of surgical treatment of mitral regurgitation with or without coronary artery disease. *J Am Coll Cardiol* 1990; 16(7):1575-1578.

108. Horskotte D, Schulte HD, Bircks W, Strauer BE: The effect of chordal preservation on late outcome after mitral valve replacement: a randomized study. *J Heart Valve Dis* 1993; 2(2):150-158.

109. Okita Y, Miki S, Ueda Y, et al: Mid-term results of mitral valve replacement combined with chordae tendineae replacement in patients with mitral stenosis. *J Heart Valve Dis* 1997; 6(1):37-42.

110. Sugita T, Matsumoto M, Nishizawa J, et al: Long-term outcome after mitral valve replacement with preservation of continuity between the

mitral annulus and the papillary muscle in patients with mitral stenosis. *J Heart Valve Dis* 2004; 13(6):931-936.

111. Karlson KJ, Ashraf MM, Berger RL: Rupture of left ventricle following mitral valve replacement. *Ann Thorac Surg* 1988; 46(5):590-597.

112. Spencer FC, Galloway AC, Colvin SB: A clinical evaluation of the hypothesis that rupture of the left ventricle following mitral valve replacement can be prevented by preservation of the chordae of the mural leaflet. *Ann Surg* 1985; 202(6):673-680.

113. Antunes MJ: Technique of implantation of the Medtronic-Hall valve and other modern tilting-disc prostheses. *J Card Surg* 1990; 5(2):86-92.

114. Cooley DA: Simplified techniques of valve replacement. *J Card Surg* 1992; 7(4):357-362.

115. Dhasmana JP, Blackstone EH, Kirklin JW, Kouchoukos NT: Factors associated with periprosthetic leakage following primary mitral valve replacement: with special consideration of the suture technique. *Ann Thorac Surg* 1983; 35(2):170-178.

116. DiSesa VJ, Tam S, Cohn LH: Ligation of the left atrial appendage using an automatic surgical stapler. *Ann Thorac Surg* 1988; 46(6):652-653.

117. Cohn LH: Tricuspid regurgitation secondary to mitral valve disease: when and how to repair. *J Card Surg* 1994; 9(2 Suppl):237-241.

118. Heras M, Chesebro JH, Fuster V, et al: High risk of thromboemboli early after bioprosthetic cardiac valve replacement. *J Am Coll Cardiol* 1995; 25(5):1111-1119.

119. Jegaden O, Eker A, Delahaye F, et al: Thromboembolic risk and late survival after mitral valve replacement with the St. Jude Medical valve. *Ann Thorac Surg* 1994; 58(6):1721-1728; discussion 1727-1728.

120. Ezekowitz MD: Anticoagulation management of valve replacement patients. *J Heart Valve Dis* 2002; 11 Suppl 1:S56-60.

121. Meurin P, Tabet JY, Weber H, Renaud N, Ben Driss A: Low-molecular-weight heparin as a bridging anticoagulant early after mechanical heart valve replacement. *Circulation* 2006; 113(4):564-569.

122. Laffort P, Roudaut R, Roques X, et al: Early and long-term (one-year) effects of the association of aspirin and oral anticoagulant on thrombi and morbidity after replacement of the mitral valve with the St. Jude medical prosthesis: a clinical and transesophageal echocardiographic study. *J Am Coll Cardiol* 2000; 35(3):739-746.

123. Yamak B, Iscan Z, Mavitas B, et al: Low-dose oral anticoagulation and antiplatelet therapy with St. Jude Medical heart valve prosthesis. *J Heart Valve Dis* 1999; 8(6):665-673.

124. Braunwald E: *Valvular Heart Diseases*. Philadelphia: Saunders; 2001.

125. Remadi JP, Bizouarn P, Baron O, et al: Mitral valve replacement with the St. Jude Medical prosthesis: a 15-year follow-up. *Ann Thorac Surg* 1998; 66(3):762-767.

126. Birkmeyer NJ, Marrin CA, Morton JR, et al: Decreasing mortality for aortic and mitral valve surgery in Northern New England. Northern New England Cardiovascular Disease Study Group. *Ann Thorac Surg* 2000; 70(2):432-437.

127. Okita Y, Miki S, Ueda Y, Tahata T, Sakai T: Left ventricular function after mitral valve replacement with or without chordal preservation. *J Heart Valve Dis* 1995; 4 Suppl 2:S181-192; discussion S183-192.

128. Arom KV, Nicoloff DM, Kersten TE, Northrup WF, 3rd, Lindsay WG: Six years of experience with the St. Jude Medical valvular prosthesis. *Circulation* 1985; 72(3 Pt 2):Ii153-Ii158.

129. Cohn LH, Aranki SF, Rizzo RJ, et al: Decrease in operative risk of reoperative valve surgery. *Ann Thorac Surg* 1993; 56(1):15-20; discussion 20-21.

130. Oury JH, Cleveland JC, Duran CG, Angell WW: Ischemic mitral valve disease: classification and systemic approach to management. *J Card Surg* 1994; 9(2 Suppl):262-273.

131. Thourani VH, Weintraub WS, Guyton RA, et al: Outcomes and long-term survival for patients undergoing mitral valve repair versus replacement: effect of age and concomitant coronary artery bypass grafting. *Circulation* 2003; 108(3):298-304.

132. STS: Society of Thoracic Surgeons: *Data Analysis of the Society of Thoracic Surgeons National Cardiac Surgery Database: The Fifth Year—January 1996*. Minneapolis: Summit Medical Systems, 1996.

133. Grossi EA, Galloway AC, Miller JS, et al: Valve repair versus replacement for mitral insufficiency: when is a mechanical valve still indicated? *J Thorac Cardiovasc Surg* 1998; 115(2):389-394; discussion 386-394.

134. Hammermeister K, Sethi GK, Henderson WG, Grover FL, Oprian C, Rahimtoola SH: Outcomes 15 years after valve replacement with a mechanical versus a bioprosthetic valve: final report of the Veterans Affairs randomized trial. *J Am Coll Cardiol* 2000; 36(4):1152-1158.

135. Sidhu P, O'Kane H, Ali N, et al: Mechanical or bioprosthetic valves in the elderly: a 20-year comparison. *Ann Thorac Surg* 2001; 71(5 Suppl):S257-260.

136. Starr A: The Starr-Edwards valve. *J Am Coll Cardiol* 1985; 6(4):899-903.

137. Cohn LH, Peigh PS, Sell J, DiSesa VJ: Right thoracotomy, femorofemoral bypass, and deep hypothermia for re-replacement of the mitral valve. *Ann Thorac Surg* 1989; 48(1):69-71.

138. Perier P, Swanson J, Takriti A, et al: *Decreasing Operative Risk in Isolated Valve Re-replacement*. New York: Yorke Medical Books; 1986.

139. Wideman FE, Blackstone EH, Kirklin JW, Karp RB, Kouchoukos NT, Pacifico AD: Hospital mortality of re-replacement of the aortic valve. Incremental risk factors. *J Thorac Cardiovasc Surg* 1981; 82(5):692-698.

140. Cohn LH, Sanders JH, Collins JJ, Jr: Actuarial comparison of Hancock porcine and prosthetic disc valves for isolated mitral valve replacement. *Circulation* 1976; 54(6 Suppl):Iii60-63.

141. Edmunds L: Thrombotic complications with the Omniscience valve. *J Thorac Cardiovasc Surg* 1989; 98:300.

142. Levantino M, Tartarini G, Barzaghi C, Grana M, Bortolotti U: Survival despite almost complete occlusion by chronic thrombosis of a Bjork-Shiley mitral prosthesis. *J Heart Valve Dis* 1995; 4(1):103-105.

143. Manteiga R, Carlos Souto J, Altes A, et al: Short-course thrombolysis as the first line of therapy for cardiac valve thrombosis. *J Thorac Cardiovasc Surg* 1998; 115(4):780-784.

144. Silber H, Khan SS, Matloff JM, Chaux A, DeRobertis M, Gray R: The St. Jude valve. Thrombolysis as the first line of therapy for cardiac valve thrombosis. *Circulation* 1993; 87(1):30-37.

145. Hering D, Piper C, Bergemann R, et al: Thromboembolic and bleeding complications following St. Jude Medical valve replacement: results of the German Experience With Low-Intensity Anticoagulation Study. *Chest* 2005; 127(1):53-59.

146. Baumgartner WA, Miller DC, Reitz BA, et al: Surgical treatment of prosthetic valve endocarditis. *Ann Thorac Surg* 1983; 35(1):87-104.

147. Calderwood SB, Swinski LA, Waternaux CM, Karchmer AW, Buckley MJ: Risk factors for the development of prosthetic valve endocarditis. *Circulation* 1985; 72(1):31-37.

148. Verheul HA, van den Brink RB, van Vreeland T, Moulijn AC, Duren DR, Dunning AJ: Effects of changes in management of active infective endocarditis on outcome in a 25-year period. *Am J Cardiol* 1993; 72(9):682-687.

149. Edwards MB, Ratnatunga CP, Dore CJ, Taylor KM: Thirty-day mortality and long-term survival following surgery for prosthetic endocarditis: a study from the UK heart valve registry. *Eur J Cardiothorac Surg* 1998; 14(2):156-164.

150. Jault F, Gandjbakhch I, Rama A, et al: Active native valve endocarditis: determinants of operative death and late mortality. *Ann Thorac Surg* 1997; 63(6):1737-1741.

151. Cammack PL, Edie RN, Edmunds LH, Jr: Bar calcification of the mitral anulus. A risk factor in mitral valve operations. *J Thorac Cardiovasc Surg* 1987; 94(3):399-404.

152. D'Cruz IA, Cohen HC, Prabhu R, Bisla V, Glick G: Clinical manifestations of mitral annulus calcification, with emphasis on its echocardiographic features. *Am Heart J* 1977; 94(3):367-377.

153. Nair CK, Sudhakaran C, Aronow WS, Thomson W, Woodruff MP, Sketch MH: Clinical characteristics of patients younger than 60 years with mitral anular calcium: comparison with age- and sex-matched control subjects. *Am J Cardiol* 1984; 54(10):1286-1287.

154. Carpentier AF, Pellerin M, Fuzellier JF, Relland JY: Extensive calcification of the mitral valve anulus: pathology and surgical management. *J Thorac Cardiovasc Surg* Vol 111. United States 1996:718-729; discussion 729-730.

155. Savage DD, Garrison RJ, Castelli WP, et al: Prevalence of submitral (anular) calcium and its correlates in a general population-based sample (the Framingham Study). *Am J Cardiol* United States 1983; 51: 1375-1378.

156. Feindel CM, Tufail Z, David TE, Ivanov J, Armstrong S: Mitral valve surgery in patients with extensive calcification of the mitral annulus. *J Thorac Cardiovasc Surg* United States 2003; 126:777-782.

157. Di Stefano S, Lopez J, Florez S, Rey J, Arevalo A, San Roman A: Building a new annulus: a technique for mitral valve replacement in heavily calcified annulus. *Ann Thorac Surg* Netherlands 2009; 87:1625-1627.

158. Hussain ST, Idrees J, Brozzi NA, Blackstone EH, Pettersson GB: Use of annulus washer after debridement: a new mitral valve replacement technique for patients with severe mitral annular calcification. *J Thorac Cardiovasc Surg* 2013; 145(6):1672-1674.

159. David TE, Feindel CM, Armstrong S, Sun Z: Reconstruction of the mitral anulus. A ten-year experience. *J Thorac Cardiovasc Surg* Vol 110. United States 1995:1323-1332.

160. Grossi EA, Galloway AC, Steinberg BM, et al: Severe calcification does not affect long-term outcome of mitral valve repair. *Ann Thorac Surg* Vol 58. United States 1994:685-687; discussion 688.

161. Ruvolo G, Speziale G, Voci P, Marino B: "Patch-glue" annular reconstruction for mitral valve replacement in severely calcified mitral annulus. *Ann Thorac Surg* Vol 63. United States 1997:570-571.

162. Nataf P, Pavie A, Jault F, Bors V, Cabrol C, Gandjbakhch I: Intraatrial insertion of a mitral prosthesis in a destroyed or calcified mitral annulus. *Ann Thorac Surg* 1994; 58(1):163-167.

163. Djaiani G, Fedorko L, Borger M, et al: Mild to moderate atheromatous disease of the thoracic aorta and new ischemic brain lesions after conventional coronary artery bypass graft surgery. *Stroke* United States 2004; 35:e356-e358.

164. Zingone B, Rauber E, Gatti G, et al: The impact of epiaortic ultrasonographic scanning on the risk of perioperative stroke. *Eur J Cardiothorac Surg* Germany 2006; 29:720-728.

165. Stern A, Tunick PA, Culliford AT, et al: Protruding aortic arch atheromas: risk of stroke during heart surgery with and without aortic arch endarterectomy. *Am Heart J* United States 1999; 138:746-752.

166. Bucerius J, Gummert JF, Borger MA, et al: Stroke after cardiac surgery: a risk factor analysis of 16,184 consecutive adult patients. *Ann Thorac Surg* 2003; 75(2):472-478.

167. Mills NL, Everson CT: Atherosclerosis of the ascending aorta and coronary artery bypass. Pathology, clinical correlates, and operative management. *J Thorac Cardiovasc Surg* 1991; 102(4):546-553.

168. Wareing TH, Davila-Roman VG, Barzilai B, Murphy SF, Kouchoukos NT: Management of the severely atherosclerotic ascending aorta during cardiac operations. A strategy for detection and treatment. *J Thorac Cardiovasc Surg* 1992; 103(3):453-462.

169. Aranki SF, Nathan M, Shekar P, Couper G, Rizzo R, Cohn LH: Hypothermic circulatory arrest enables aortic valve replacement in patients with unclampable aorta. *Ann Thorac Surg* Netherlands 2005; 80:1679-1686; discussion 1677-1686.

170. Girardi LN, Krieger KH, Mack CA, Isom OW: No-clamp technique for valve repair or replacement in patients with a porcelain aorta. *Ann Thorac Surg* Netherlands 2005; 80:1688-1692.

171. Zingone B, Rauber E, Gatti G, et al: Diagnosis and management of severe atherosclerosis of the ascending aorta and aortic arch during cardiac surgery: focus on aortic replacement. *Eur J Cardiothorac Surg* Germany 2007; 31:990-997.

172. Zingone B, Gatti G, Spina A, et al: Current role and outcomes of ascending aortic replacement for severe nonaneurysmal aortic atherosclerosis. *Ann Thorac Surg* Netherlands 2010 The Society of Thoracic Surgeons. Published by Elsevier Inc., 2010; 89:429-434.

173. Calleja F, Martinez JL, Gonzales De Vega N: Mitral valve surgery through right thoracotomy. *J Cardiovasc Surg (Torino)* 1996; 37(6 Suppl 1):49-52.

174. Greelish JP, Soltesz EG, Byrne JG: Valve surgery in octogenarians with a "porcelain" aorta and aortic insufficiency. *J Card Surg* 2002; 17(4):285-288.

175. Zingone B, Gatti G, Rauber E, Pappalardo A, Benussi B, Dreas L: Surgical management of the atherosclerotic ascending aorta: is endoaortic balloon occlusion safe? *Ann Thorac Surg* Netherlands 2006; 82:1709-1714.

176. Kasahara H, Shin H, Mori M: Cerebral perfusion using the tissue oxygenation index in mitral valve repair in a patient with porcelain aorta and aortic regurgitation. *Ann Thorac Cardiovasc Surg* Japan 2007; 13:413-416.

177. Rahimtoola SH: The problem of valve prosthesis-patient mismatch. *Circulation* 1978; 58(1):20-24.

178. Rahimtoola SH, Murphy E: Valve prosthesis—patient mismatch. A long-term sequela. *Br Heart J* 1981; 45(3):331-335.

179. Jamieson WR, Germann E, Ye J, et al: Effect of prosthesis-patient mismatch on long-term survival with mitral valve replacement: assessment to 15 years. *Ann Thorac Surg* 2009; 87(4):1135-1141; discussion 1142.

180. Ionescu A, Fraser AG, Butchart EG: Prevalence and clinical significance of incidental paraprosthetic valvar regurgitation: a prospective study using transoesophageal echocardiography. *Heart* 2003; 89(11):1316-1321.

181. Rallidis LS, Moyssakis IE, Ikonomidis I, Nihoyannopoulos P: Natural history of early aortic paraprosthetic regurgitation: a five-year follow-up. *Am Heart J* Vol 138. United States 1999:351-357.

182. Pate GE, Al Zubaidi A, Chandavimol M, Thompson CR, Munt BI, Webb JG: Percutaneous closure of prosthetic paravalvular leaks: case series and review. *Catheter Cardiovasc Interv* 2006; 68(4):528-533.

183. Kliger C, Eiros R, Isasti G, et al: Review of surgical prosthetic paravalvular leaks: diagnosis and catheter-based closure. *Eur Heart J* England 2013; 34:638-649.

184. Al Halees Z: An additional maneuver to repair mitral paravalvular leak. *Eur J Cardiothorac Surg* Germany: 2010 European Association for Cardio-Thoracic Surgery. Published by Elsevier B.V., 2011; 39:410-411.

185. Mangi AA, Torchiana DF: A technique for repair of mitral paravalvular leak. *J Thorac Cardiovasc Surg* United States 2004; 128:771-772.

186. Moneta A, Villa E, Donatelli F: An alternative technique for non-infective paraprosthetic leakage repair. *Eur J Cardiothorac Surg* England 2003; 23:1074-1075.

187. Echevarria JR, Bernal JM, Rabasa JM, Morales D, Revilla Y, Revuelta JM: Reoperation for bioprosthetic valve dysfunction. A decade of clinical experience. *Eur J Cardiothorac Surg* 1991; 5(10):523-526; discussion 527.

188. Potter DD, Sundt TM, 3rd, Zehr KJ, et al: Risk of repeat mitral valve replacement for failed mitral valve prostheses. *Ann Thorac Surg* United States 2004; 78:67-72; discussion 67-72.

189. Akins CW, Bitondo JM, Hilgenberg AD, Vlahakes GJ, Madsen JC, MacGillivray TE: Early and late results of the surgical correction of cardiac prosthetic paravalvular leaks. *J Heart Valve Dis* 2005; 14(6):792-799; discussion 800-799.

190. Kim MS, Casserly IP, Garcia JA, Klein AJ, Salcedo EE, Carroll JD: Percutaneous transcatheter closure of prosthetic mitral paravalvular leaks: are we there yet? *JACC Cardiovasc Interv* United States 2009; 2:81-90.

191. Sorajja P, Cabalka AK, Hagler DJ, Rihal CS: Percutaneous repair of paravalvular prosthetic regurgitation: acute and 30-day outcomes in 115 patients. *Circ Cardiovasc Interv* United States 2011; 4:314-321.

192. Noble S, Jolicoeur EM, Basmadjian A, et al: Percutaneous paravalvular leak reduction: procedural and long-term clinical outcomes. *Can J Cardiol* 2013; 29(11):1422-1428.

193. Sorajja P, Cabalka AK, Hagler DJ, Rihal CS: Long-term follow-up of percutaneous repair of paravalvular prosthetic regurgitation. *J Am Coll Cardiol* United States: A 2011 American College of Cardiology Foundation. Published by Elsevier Inc., 2011; 58:2218-2224.

194. Ruiz CE, Jelnin V, Kronzon I, et al: Clinical outcomes in patients undergoing percutaneous closure of periprosthetic paravalvular leaks. *J Am Coll Cardiol* United States: A 2011 American College of Cardiology Foundation. Published by Elsevier Inc., 2011; 58:2210-2217.

195. Cheung A, Webb JG, Barbanti M, et al: 5-year experience with transcatheter transapical mitral valve-in-valve implantation for bioprosthetic valve dysfunction. *J Am Coll Cardiol* 2013; 61(17):1759-1766.

196. Kaneko T, Swain JD, Loberman D, Welt FG, Davidson MJ, Eisenhauer AC: Transjugular approach in valve-in-valve transcatheter mitral valve replacement: direct route to the valve. *Ann Thorac Surg* 2014; 97(6):e161-e163.

VALVULAR HEART DISEASE (OTHER)

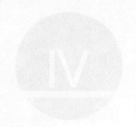

IV

VALVULAR HEART
DISEASE (OTHER)

Tricuspid Valve Disease

Richard J. Shemin • Peyman Benharash

43

The tricuspid valve consists of three leaflets (anterior, posterior, and septal), the chordae tendinea, two discrete papillary muscles, the fibrous tricuspid annulus, and the right atrial and right ventricular myocardium (Fig. 43-1A). Valve function depends on coordination of all these components. The anterior leaflet is the largest. The septal leaflet is the smallest and arises medially directly from the tricuspid annulus above the interventricular septum. Because the small septal wall leaflet is fixed and is relatively spared from annular dilation, tricuspid annular sizing has been based on the dimension of the base of the septal leaflet.[1,2] The posterior leaflet often has multiple scallops. The anterior papillary muscle provides chordae to the anterior and posterior leaflets, and the medial papillary muscle provides chordae to the posterior and septal leaflets. The septal wall gives chordae to the anterior and septal leaflets. There may be accessory chordal attachments to the right ventricular free wall and the moderator band.

Right ventricular dysfunction and dilation lead to chordal tethering contributing to loss of leaflet apposition.[2] In addition, dilation of the free wall of the right ventricle (RV) results in tricuspid annular enlargement, primarily in its anterior/posterior (mural) aspect, resulting in significant functional tricuspid regurgitation (fTR) as a result of leaflet malcoaptation[3] (Fig. 43-1B).

The tricuspid annulus has a complex three-dimensional structure, which differs from the more symmetric "saddle-shaped" mitral annulus. The tricuspid annulus is dynamic and can change markedly with loading conditions. During the cardiac cycle, there is a ~20% reduction in annular circumference (~30% reduction in annular area) with atrial systole.[4,5] This distinct shape has implications for the design and application of currently available annuloplasty rings in the tricuspid position. Most commercially available rings or bands are essentially planar except for the Edwards MC[3] annuloplasty system.

Fukuda et al.[4] studied the shape and movement of the healthy and diseased tricuspid annulus performing a real-time three-dimensional transthoracic echocardiographic study. Healthy subjects had a nonplanar, elliptical-shaped tricuspid annulus, with the posteroseptal portion being "lowest" (toward the right ventricular apex) and the anteroseptal portion the "highest" (Fig. 43-2). Patients with fTR generally had a more planar annulus, which was dilated primarily in the septal-lateral direction, resulting in a more circular and flat shape as compared with the elliptical shape in healthy subjects.[5]

CLINICAL PRESENTATION

The most common presentation of TR is secondary to cardiac valvular pathology (mostly mitral valve disease) on the left side of the heart. As pulmonary hypertension develops, leading to right ventricular dilatation, the tricuspid valve annulus will dilate. The circumference of the annulus lengthens primarily along the attachments of the anterior and posterior leaflets. The septal leaflet is fixed between the fibrous trigones, preventing lengthening (Fig. 43-1B). With progressive annular and ventricular dilatation, the chordal papillary muscle complex becomes functionally shortened, causing leaflet tethering. This combination prevents leaflet apposition, resulting in valvular incompetence.[6-9]

Eisenmenger syndrome and primary pulmonary hypertension lead to the same pathophysiology of progressive right ventricular dilatation, tricuspid annular enlargement, and valvular incompetence. A right ventricular infarction produces either disruption of the papillary muscle or a severe regional wall motion abnormality. This prevents normal leaflet apposition by a tethering effect on the leaflets. Marfan's syndrome and other variations of myxomatous disease affecting the mitral and tricuspid valves can lead to prolapsing leaflets, elongation of chordae, or chordal rupture, producing valvular incompetence.

Blunt or penetrating chest trauma may disrupt the structural components of the tricuspid valve. Dilated cardiomyopathy in the late stages of biventricular failure and pulmonary hypertension produces TR.[10-13] Infectious endocarditis can destroy leaflet tissue, mostly in drug addicts with staphylococcal infection.[14-16]

The carcinoid syndrome leads to either focal or diffuse deposits of fibrous tissue on the endocardium of valve cusps, cardiac chambers, intima of the great vessels, and coronary sinus. The white fibrous carcinoid plaques, if present on the ventricular side of the tricuspid valve cusps, adhere the leaflet

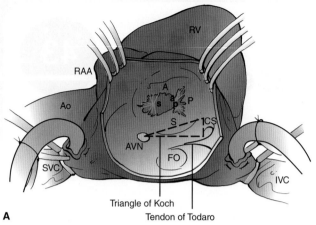

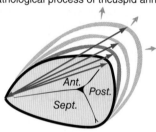

FIGURE 43-1 (A) Surgical view of the tricuspid valve complex. The tricuspid valve consists of three leaflets: anterior (A), posterior (P), and septal (S). There are two main papillary muscles, anterior (a) and posterior (p). The septal papillary muscle (s) is rudimentary, and chordae tendinea arise directly from the ventricular septum. Adjacent structures include the atrioventricular node (AVN), coronary sinus ostium (CS), and the tendon of Todaro, forming the triangle of Koch. Ao = Aorta; FO = foramen ovale; IVC = inferior vena cava; RAA = right atrial appendage; RV = right ventricle; SVC = superior vena cava. (B) Direction of progressive tricuspid valve annular dilatation. (B. Reproduced with permission from Dreyfus GD, Corbi PJ, Chan KM, et al: Secondary tricuspid regurgitation or dilatation: which should be the criteria for surgical repair? *Ann Thorac Surg.* 2005 Jan;79(1):127-132.)

tissue to the right ventricular wall, preventing leaflet coaptation.[17-19] Rheumatic disease of the tricuspid valve is always associated with mitral valve involvement, and the deformity of the tricuspid tissue results in a tricuspid valve stenosis as well as regurgitation[20] (Table 43-1).

A unique cause of TR is the result of pacemaker or defibrillator leads, which cross from the right atrium into the RV and may directly interfere with leaflet coaptation. This entity has been reported in case reports and small series but is likely more significant and prevalent than currently perceived. In a recent report by Kim et al., the effect of transtricuspid permanent pacemaker or implantable cardiac defibrillator leads on 248 subjects with echocardiograms before and after device placement was studied TR worsened by one grade or more after implant in 24.2% of subjects and that TR worsening was more common with implantable cardiac defibrillators than permanent pacemakers.[21,22]

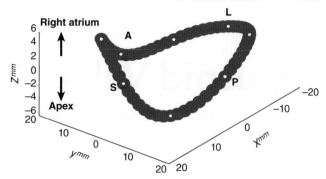

FIGURE 43-2 Three-dimensional shape of the tricuspid annulus based on a three-dimensional transthoracic echocardiographic study in healthy subjects. Note that the annulus is not planar and an optimally shaped annuloplasty ring may need to mimic this configuration. A indicates anterior; L, lateral; P, posterior; S, septal. (Reproduced with permission from Fukuda S, Saracino G, Matsumura Y, et al: Three-dimensional geometry of the tricuspid annulus in healthy subjects and in patients with functional tricuspid regurgitation: a real-time, 3-dimensional echocardiographic study, *Circulation.* 2006 Jul 4;114(1 Suppl):I492-I498.)

The current guidelines do not recommend lead extraction for patients with existing TR and transtricuspid pacing leads, because the risks of lead extraction are significant and there is potential for injury to the tricuspid valve if the lead is adherent to the valve apparatus.[23]

It has also been shown at 5 years after successful tricuspid valve repair, 42% of patients with a pacemaker had severe TR, almost double the incidence of those without pacemaker implantation.[24] This suggests removing a transtricuspid lead and replacing it with an epicardial lead at the time of tricuspid valve surgery may reduce late repair failure.

TABLE 43-1: Causes of Tricuspid Regurgitation

Primary causes (25%)
 Rheumatic
 Myxomatous
 Ebstein anomaly
 Endomyocardial fibrosis
 Endocarditis
 Carcinoid disease
 Traumatic (blunt chest injury, laceration)
 Iatrogenic (pacemaker/defibrillator lead, RV biopsy)
Secondary causes (75%)
 Left heart disease (LV dysfunction or value disease) resulting in
  pulmonary hypertension
 Any cause of pulmonary hypertension (chronic lung disease,
  pulmonary thromboembolism, left to right shunt)
 Any cause of RV dysfunction (myocardial disease, RV ischemia/
  infarction)

RV, right ventricular; LV, left ventricular.

Tricuspid Regurgitation

Patients with TR have the presenting symptoms of fatigue and weakness related to a reduction in cardiac output. Atrial fibrillation is common. Jugular vein distention is found, especially during inspiration, when a physiologic increase in venous return is accentuated. Right-sided heart failure leads to ascites, congestive hepatosplenomegaly, pulsatile liver, pleural effusions, and peripheral edema. In the late stages, these patients are wasted with cachexia, cyanosis, and jaundice. Hepatic cardiac cirrhosis can develop in neglected cases.

Echocardiography is routinely used to assess the severity of TR in clinical practice. The exam is performed in an integrative manner using color Doppler flow mapping of the direction and size of the TR jet. In addition, the morphology of continuous wave Doppler recordings across the valve and pulsed wave Doppler of the hepatic veins can be used.[25]

Serial assessments of TR must be interpreted within the clinical context, because functional mitral regurgitation (MR) severity can be affected by multiple factors, such as volume status (preload) and afterload. Right ventricular shape is complex as compared with the left ventricle, appearing crescent shaped in cross-section and triangular when viewed en face.[26] Right ventricular function can be assessed quantitatively in the four-chamber view by measuring the end-diastolic and end-systolic area to calculate the fractional area change of the RV.[27] Although right ventricular chamber dimensions may be obtained during echocardiography, magnetic resonance imaging is emerging as an improved technique for assessing right ventricular diastolic and systolic volumes.[28] More recently, the tricuspid annular peak systolic excursion, or apical movement of the annulus as measured on echocardiography, as been validated as a sensitive measure of RV function.[29] Other echocardiographic findings include a shift in the atrial septum to the left and paradoxical septal motion, consistent with right ventricular diastolic overload. Pulsed Doppler and color-flow studies help to identify systolic right ventricular to right atrial flow with inferior vena cava and hepatic vein flow reversal. Contrast-enhanced echocardiography can be useful, with a rapid saline bolus injection producing microcavities that are visible on echo, demonstrating to-and-fro motion across the valve orifice and reversal into the inferior vena cava and hepatic veins. Possible ASD or patent foramen ovale should be sought. Endocarditis vegetations are clearly visible on echocardiography. The valve may be destroyed, and septic pulmonary emboli are a common feature. The tricuspid valve in carcinoid syndrome is thickened with retracted leaflets fixed in a semiopen position throughout the cardiac cycle.[29-34]

Tricuspid Stenosis

Tricuspid stenosis (TS) is most commonly rheumatic. It is extremely rare to have isolated TS because some degree of TR will be present.[35-37] Mitral valve disease coexists with occasional involvement of the aortic valve. The third still have a significant prevalence of rheumatic mitral and tricuspid valvular disease. The anatomical features are similar to those of mitral stenosis, with fusion and shortening of the chordae and leaflet thickening. Fusion along the free edges and calcific deposits on the valve are found late in the disease. The preponderance of cases is in young women.

The diastolic gradient between the right atrium and RV is significantly elevated even at 2 to 5 mm Hg mean pressure. As the right atrial pressure increases, venous congestion leads to distention of the jugular veins, ascites, pleural effusion, and peripheral edema. Over time, the right atrial wall thickens, and the atrial chamber dilates.

Clinical features are consistent with reduced cardiac output producing the symptoms of fatigue and malaise. Significant liver engorgement produces right upper quadrant tenderness with a palpable liver with a presystolic pulse. Ascites produces increased abdominal girth. Significant peripheral edema or anasarca can develop. Severe TS may mask or reduce the pulmonary congestion of mitral stenosis owing to reduced blood flow to the left side of the heart. The low output state of the patient is prominent.

Echocardiography reveals the diagnostic features of diastolic doming of the thickened tricuspid valve leaflets, reduced leaflet mobility, and a reduced orifice of flow. The Doppler flow pattern across the tricuspid valve has a prolonged slope of antegrade flow.

Functional Tricuspid Regurgitation

Secondary tricuspid regurgitation, also called fTR, may become worse over time, leading to severe symptoms, biventricular heart failure, and death.[24] IA large retrospective echocardiographic analysis of 5223 Veterans Administration patients by Nath et al. showed that independent of echo-derived pulmonary artery systolic pressure, left ventricular ejection fraction, inferior vena cava size, and right ventricular size and function, survival was worse for patients with moderate and severe TR than for those with no TR.[38]

Pulmonary arterial hypertension from any cause is known to be associated with the development of secondary tricuspid regurgitation. However, not all patients with pulmonary hypertension develop significant tricuspid regurgitation, and the mechanisms of secondary TR are multifactorial.

Mutlak and colleagues[39] studied 2139 subjects with mild (<50), moderate (50-69), or severe (≥70) elevations in pulmonary artery systolic pressure. In their analysis, increasing PASP was independently associated with greater degrees of TR (odds ratio, 2.26 per 10 mm Hg increase). However, many patients with high PASP had only mild TR (mild TR in 65.4% of patients with PASP 50-69 mm Hg and in 45.6% of patients with PASP ≥ 70 mm Hg). Other factors, such as atrial fibrillation, pacemaker leads, and right heart enlargement, were also importantly associated with TR severity. The authors concluded that the cause of TR in patients with pulmonary hypertension is only partially related to an increase in transtricuspid pressure gradient. It remains unproved if surgical annuloplasty, in the setting of pulmonary hypertension, alters the natural course of right ventricular dilation and recurrent TR.

Thus, functional tricuspid incompetence is progressive. Surgical treatment of left-sided valvular lesions is not always adequate to resolve or prevent progressive TR. This is particularly true when pulmonary hypertension persists.

SURGICAL EXPOSURE

Tricuspid valve annuloplasty performed with either mitral and/or aortic valve operations is accomplished either through a full or partial lower sternotomy approach or less invasive right minithoracotomy exposure with mitral valve procedures. Bicaval venous cannulation with caval snares is essential to isolate the right atrium. The cannula can be placed conventionally via the right atrium or less invasively via the femoral vein. A superior vena cava cannula can be inserted via the internal jugular vein.

Left-sided valve repair or replacement (mitral and/or aortic) is performed under blood cardioplegic arrest with antegrade and/or retrograde administration, moderate systemic hypothermia, and optional surface cooling. The mitral valve can be exposed through a left atrial incision posterior to the intraatrial septum or through a right atrial and transseptal incision (Fig. 43-3). The transseptal incision is particularly useful when there is an aortic valve prosthesis, when a mitral and tricuspid valve procedure is required or in a reoperation.

After completing the mitral valve procedure and deairing maneuvers, the aorta is vented and unclamped. Attention can be turned to the tricuspid valve during rewarming and cardiac reperfusion. Using the beating heart technique, the caval snares are tightened around the venous drainage cannula and a right atriotomy is performed to expose the tricuspid valve. Misplacement of a suture potentially adversely affecting the cardiac conduction system can be assessed immediately and corrected.

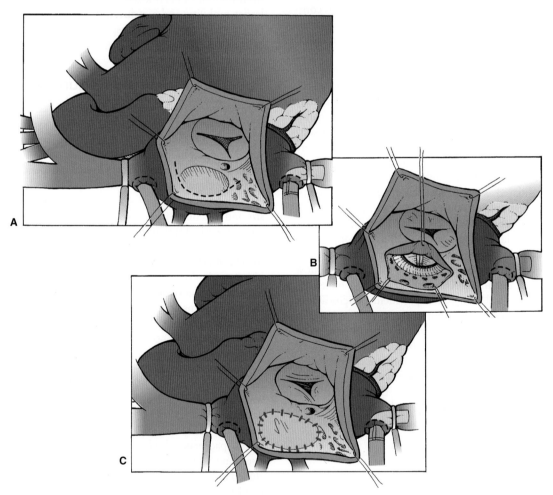

FIGURE 43-3 (A) The superior and inferior venae cavae are cannulated, an oblique atriotomy incision is made, and stay sutures are placed on the right atrial wall to aid exposure. For transatrial exposure of the mitral valve, an incision is placed in the fossa ovale and extended superiorly through the interatrial septum. The superior aspect of the septal incision is extended, if necessary, into the dome of the left atrium behind the aorta. (B) Stay sutures in the interatrial septum are used for retraction. Use of retractors is avoided to prevent injury to the AV node. The mitral prosthesis is implanted in an anti anatomic orientation. (C) The interatrial septum is closed primarily or by using a pericardial patch with a continuous 4-0 Prolene suture.

In the reoperative setting, with a dilated RV adherent or close to the sternum, It is prudent to expose of the femoral artery and vein for rapid cannulation in the case of injury to the RA or RV during sternal reentry. It is also recommended to establish fem-fem bypass prior to sternotomy to decompress the RA and RV allowing a safer sternotomy to be performed.

Approaching the tricuspid valve through a right minithoracotomy has the advantage of avoiding adhesions and possible injury to the RV during sternotomy. Femoral vein and internal jugular vein cannulae are positioned outside the right atrium and confirmed by echo. Caval snares below the cannula tips ensure venous drainage. Coronary sinus return is controlled by a sucker in its ostium.

If the operation includes the mitral valve, exposure can be simplified by using a right atrial incision and transseptal approach. If atrial fibrillation is present, a Maze procedure can be added to the technical maneuvers.

ANNULOPLASTY TECHNIQUES

Techniques to deal with a dilated tricuspid valve annulus with normal leaflets and chordal structures include plication of the posterior leaflet's annulus (bicuspidization), partial purse-string reduction of the anterior and posterior leaflet annulus (DeVega-style techniques), and rigid or flexible rings or bands placed to reduce the annular size and achieve leaflet coaptation (Fig. 43-4). Preoperative and intraoperative echocardiograms are valuable assessment tools to help the surgeon understand the structure and function of the valve.[30-34]

The degree of pulmonary hypertension, right ventricular dilatation, and systolic function, coupled with the size of the right atrium, must be factored into the surgical decision-making process. The classical technique of inserting a finger via a purse-string suture, into the right atrium to palpate the tricuspid valve and withdrawing the fingertip 2 to 3 cm from the valve orifice, so as to access the force of the regurgitant jet is of historical importance in the current era of cardiac surgery. The intraoperative transesophageal echocardiogram (TEE) allows the surgeon to access the degree of tricuspid regurgitation and look for reversal of flow in the inferior cava. Assessment of the repair with TEE under appropriate loading conditions ensures leaving the operating room with confidence that the repair is functioning satisfactorily.

Classic surgical teaching has been that in patients with minimal right atrial enlargement and +1 to +2 regurgitation, TR will resolve once left-sided valve lesions are addressed. Recent literature, however, has documented the variability in the resolution of TR after dealing effectively with the left-sided valvular lesions.

The pathologic process of fTR requires an understanding that the tricuspid annulus is a component of both the tricuspid valve and the right ventricular myocardium. For the tricuspid valve to leak, the tricuspid annulus and therefore the RV must be dilated. Without dilation of these structures, there is little chance that TR can occur.

Dilation of the tricuspid annulus occurs in the anterior and posterior directions (see Fig. 43-1B) corresponding to the free wall of the RV. In addition to tricuspid dilatation, the degree of TR is also directly related to three important factors: the preload, afterload, and right ventricular function. Thus, TR is difficult to assess accurately because these dynamic factors can interfere with the observed severity of regurgitation. Therefore, significant TR may not be detected echocardiographically despite considerable dilatation of the tricuspid valve annulus.

An understanding of these important fundamental concepts seem to contradict current practice regarding the management of secondary TR, which focuses on assessment of the severity of TR and advocates treatment of the primary lesion

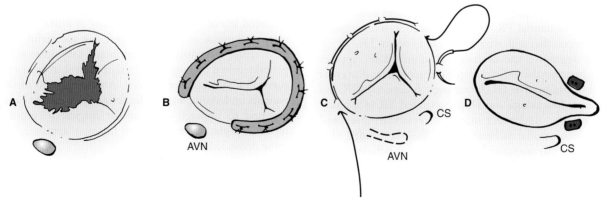

FIGURE 43-4 Predominant surgical repair techniques for functional tricuspid regurgitation (TR) in the presence of a dilated annulus. (A) Dilated tricuspid annulus with abnormal circular shape, failure of leaflet coaptation, and resultant TR. (B) Rigid or flexible annuloplasty bands are used to restore a more normal annular size and shape (ovoid), thereby reducing or eliminating TR. The open rings spares the atrioventricular node (AVN), reducing the incidence of heart block. (C) DeVega suture annuloplasty partially plicate the annulus reducing annular circumference and diameter. (D) Suture bicuspidalization is performed by placement of a mattress suture from the anteroposterior to the posteroseptal commissure along the posterior annulus. CS = Coronary sinus.

alone (ie, mitral valve disease). Treatment of the mitral valve lesion alone only reduces the RV afterload, but does not correct tricuspid annular dilatation, RV preload, and function. Once the tricuspid annulus is dilated, its size cannot return to normal spontaneously, and it may in fact continue to dilate further. This explains why some patients require a second operation for TR years after the initial mitral valve surgery. The reoperative risks in this setting are very high owing to poor myocardial function and difficulty with sternal reentry with a dilated RV.

Tricuspid annular dilatation is the primary mechanism in the development of fTR. Dreyfus and colleagues postulated that annular size may be a more reliable indicator of late outcomes than the degree of TR. Moreover, successful treatment of functional (secondary) tricuspid valve pathology may necessitate the correction of tricuspid annular dilatation in addition to mitral valve surgery even when TR is mild.

Over a 12-year period, these authors performed tricuspid valve repair for secondary tricuspid valve dilatation irrespective of the severity of TR because secondary tricuspid dilatation may or not be accompanied by TR. Tricuspid annular dilatation can be measured objectively, whereas TR can vary according to the preload, afterload, and right ventricular function.

Dreyfus and colleagues prospectively studied more than 300 patients to determine whether surgical repair of the tricuspid valve, based on tricuspid dilatation alone rather than TR, could lead to potential benefits.[40] Tricuspid annuloplasty was performed only if the tricuspid annular diameter was greater than twice the normal size (≥70 mm) regardless of the grade of regurgitation. Patients in Group 1 (163 patients, 52.4%) received mitral valve repair (MVR) alone. Patients in Group 2 (148 patients, 47.6%) received MVR plus tricuspid annuloplasty. Tricuspid regurgitation increased by more than two grades in 48% of the patients in Group 1 and in only 2% of the patients in Group 2 ($p < .001$).

The authors concluded that remodeling annuloplasty of the tricuspid valve based on tricuspid dilatation improved functional status irrespective of the grade of regurgitation. Considerable tricuspid dilatation can be present even in the absence of substantial TR. Tricuspid dilatation is an ongoing disease process that will, with time, lead to severe TR.[40]

More aggressive use of tricuspid annuloplasty appears to help improve the early postoperative course and prevent residual or progressive TR. Increasingly functional MR and TR coexist. Matsunaga and Duran analyzed TR in a group of patients who underwent successful revascularization and MVR for functional ischemic MR. They concluded that fTR is frequently associated with functional ischemic MR. After MVR, close to 50% of patients have residual TR that increases over time. The annular size may become the objective criteria, regardless of the degree of TR, to determine the need for a tricuspid annuloplasty.[41]

Special note should be taken in assessing the foramen ovale for patency. A patent foramen should always be sutured closed, reducing the possibility of paradoxical embolism or arterial desaturation from right-to-left shunting.

Surgical Repair of the TV

The main surgical approaches to rectify fTR (occurring in the presence of a dilated annulus with normal leaflets and chordal structures) involve rigid or flexible annular bands (open or closed), which are used to reduce annular size and achieve leaflet coaptation, as with mitral valve disease. Another less commonly used technique involves posterior annular bicuspidalization. This surgical technique places a pledget-supported mattress suture from the anteroposterior commissure to the posteroseptal commissure along the posterior annulus. This is based on prior studies by Deloche et al.[42] that showed posterior annulus dilation occurs in fTR and that a focal posterior tricuspid annuloplasty can be effective in selected cases. Other approaches include edge-to-edge (Alfieri-type) repairs as described by Castedo et al.[43,44] and partial purse-string suture techniques to reduce the anterior and posterior portions of the annulus (DeVega-style techniques; see Fig. 43-4). DeVega and flexible annuloplasty bands appear to have a lower freedom from recurrent TR than rigid annuloplasty rings.[24,45-47]

In the absence of simultaneous tricuspid valve repair, the prevalence of TR in the postoperative period after mitral valve surgery depends to some degree on the mechanism of MR. Matsuyama et al.[48] reported in a study of 174 patients that only 16% of patients who underwent nonischemic (ie, degenerative) mitral valve surgery without tricuspid valve surgery developed 3 to 4+ TR at 8-year follow-up. Conversely, TR appears to be far more prevalent in patients undergoing MVR for functional ischemic MR. In the series by Matsunaga et al.[49] 30% of patients undergoing MVR for functional ischemic MR had at least moderate TR before surgery. In the postoperative period, the prevalence of at least moderate TR increased over time, from 25% at less than 1 year, 53% at 1 to 3 years, and 74% at greater than 3 years of follow-up.

Significant residual tricuspid valve insufficiency contributes to a poor postoperative result, even after successful MVR. King et al.[50] studied patients requiring subsequent tricuspid valve surgery after mitral valve surgery. They had high early and late mortality. The authors encouraged a policy of liberal use of tricuspid annuloplasty at initial mitral valve surgery. Surgical series have shown that successful tricuspid valve repair (primarily when combined with other valve surgeries) resulted in a significant improvement in recurrent TR, survival, and event-free survival. Accordingly, 50 to 67% of patients undergoing surgery for mitral valve disease have been reported to undergo concomitant surgical tricuspid valve repair or replacement (although this may approach 80% in some dedicated centers).[45,51,52]

Specific Techniques

BICUSPIDIZATION

After the caval snares are tightened, the right atrium is opened via an oblique incision. Exposure and assessment of all aspects of the tricuspid valve structure should be performed before choosing the technique of annuloplasty. Suture plication to

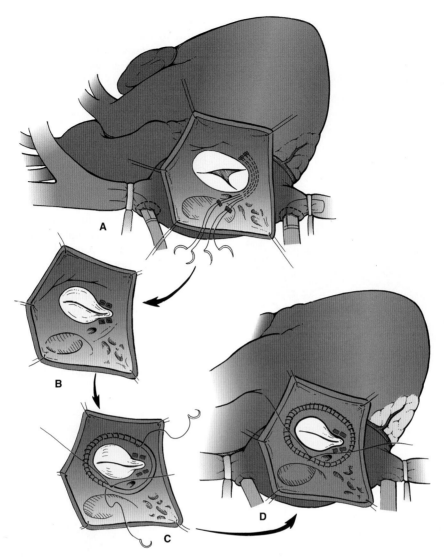

FIGURE 43-5 (A) Tricuspid valve bicuspidization is accomplished by plicating the annulus along the posterior leaflet. Two concentric, pledgeted 2-0 Ethibond sutures are used. (B) The sutures are tied, obliterating the posterior leaflet, effectively creating a bicuspid AV valve. Saline is injected into the RV to test the competency of the repair. (C) As an option to support the bicuspidization repair, a flexible ring may be placed. Prior to ring implantation, measuring the intertrigonal distance determines the annular size. As an option, the ring can be inserted using a continuous 4-0 Prolene suture. Care is taken to avoid the AV node. (D) As another option, the ring can be implanted above the coronary sinus.

deal with mild dilatation of the annulus is accomplished by placing pledgeted mattress sutures from the center of the posterior leaflet to the commissure between the septal and posterior leaflets. A second suture often is necessary to further reduce the annulus, ensuring proper leaflet coaptation while providing an adequate orifice for flow. An annuloplasty ring can be inserted to further support the annular reduction (Fig. 43-5).

DeVega TECHNIQUE

The DeVega technique also can be employed for mild-to-moderate annular dilatation.[53] This technique employs a 2-0 Prolene, Gortex, or Dacron polyester suture placed at the junction of the annulus and right ventricular free wall,

running from the anteroseptal commissure to the postero-septal commissure. The second limb of the suture is placed through a pledget and run parallel and close to the first suture line in the same clockwise direction, placing it through a second pledget at the posteroseptal commissure. The suture is tightened, producing a purse-string effect and reducing the length of the anterior and posterior annulus to provide adequate leaflet coaptation and orifice of flow (Fig. 43-6).

The judgment regarding the degree of annular reduction has varied from the guideline of being able to insert two and one-half to three fingerbreadths snugly through the valve orifice to using the ring annuloplasty sizers designed for the tricuspid valve. An annuloplasty sizer, chosen by measuring the intertrigonal distance, can be used as a template while tying the pursestring suture to achieve the proper degree

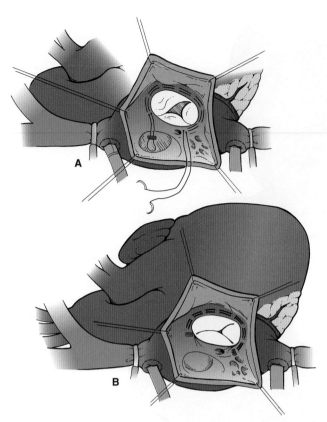

FIGURE 43-6 (A) A modified DeVega annuloplasty technique is shown. A single pledgeted 2-0 Prolene suture is placed. Care is taken to avoid the area of the AV node. (B) The suture is tied, completing the annuloplasty. Injecting saline into the RV using a bulb syringe and compressing the pulmonary artery tests the valve for competency.

of reduction. The DeVega and suture plication techniques should be reserved for mild annular reductions and situations in which the structural integrity of the annulus is not absolutely necessary for long-term success (ie, fTR expected to resolve over time). In these situations, the annuloplasty provides a competent tricuspid valve during the early postoperative course while the heart remodels after surgical treatment of the left-sided valvular lesions.[54-56]

RINGS AND BANDS

Significant degrees of annular reduction requiring durability are best accomplished with rigid rings (eg, Carpentier-Edwards and MC3), flexible rings (eg, Duran), or flexible bands (eg, Cosgrove annuloplasty system, and Medtronic Tri-Ad Adams annulopasty ring). The length of the base of the septal leaflet (ie, the intertrigonal distance) determines the size of the ring or band. These devices avoid suture placement in the region of the atrioventricular (AV) node (apex of the triangle of Koch) to avoid postoperative conduction problems. The mattress sutures are placed circumferentially, with wider bites on the annulus and smaller corresponding bites through the fabric of the ring or band, producing annular plication mostly along the length of the posterior leaflet. The

result allows the tricuspid valve orifice to be occluded primarily by the leaflet tissue of the anterior and septal leaflets. Overly aggressive annular reduction can lead to ring dehiscence owing to excessive tension on the tenuous tricuspid valve annular tissue[57,58] (Fig. 43-7).

A recent review of a 790-patient series for the durability and risk factors for failure of a repair was reported by McCarthy and colleagues.[59] The authors reported that TR one week after annuloplasty was 3+ or 4+ in 14% of patients. Regurgitation severity remained stable over time with the Carpentier-Edwards ring ($p = .7$), increased slowly with the Cosgrove-Edwards band ($p = .05$), and rose more rapidly with the DeVega ($p = .002$) and Peri-Guard ($p = .0009$) procedures. Risk factors for worsening regurgitation included higher preoperative regurgitation grade, poor left ventricular function, permanent pacemaker, and repair type other than ring annuloplasty. Right ventricular systolic pressure, ring size, preoperative New York Heart Association (NYHA) functional class, and concomitant surgery were not risk factors. Tricuspid reoperation was rare (3% at 8 years), and hospital mortality after reoperation was 37%. The authors concluded that tricuspid valve annuloplasty did not consistently eliminate functional regurgitation, and over time, regurgitation increased importantly after Peri-Guard and DeVega

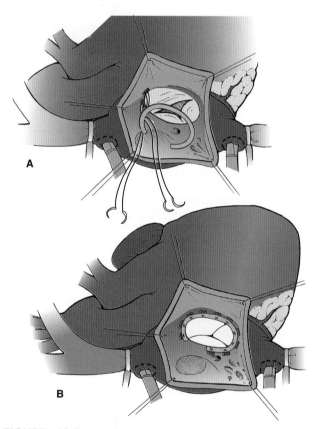

FIGURE 43-7 (A) The Carpentier-Edwards ring annuloplasty is shown. A sizer measuring the intertrigonal distance was used to determine the ring size. Multiple interrupted, pledgeted 2-0 Ethibond sutures are placed at the atrioannular junction. All sutures are inserted before seating the ring. (B) The valve is seated and the sutures are tied.

annuloplasty techniques. Therefore, these repair techniques should generally be abandoned and transtricuspid pacing leads be replaced with epicardial ones.

INTRAOPERATIVE ASSESSMENT OF THE REPAIR

Assessment of tricuspid valve competence after the annuloplasty requires filling the RV with saline and observing leaflet coaptation. This assessment is best performed with the heart beating and the pulmonary artery occluded to allow right ventricular volume to generate enough intracavitary pressure to close the tricuspid valve tightly. If the result appears inadequate, downsizing the ring or ring replacement should be performed. Final assessment is by TEE examination after completely weaning from cardiopulmonary bypass with appropriate volume and afterload adjustment.

TRICUSPID VALVE REPLACEMENT

The technique for secure fixation of a tricuspid valve is with pledgeted mattress sutures using an everting suture technique for mechanical valves and either a supra-annular or an intraannular technique for a bioprosthesis. The tricuspid valve septal and posterior leaflets are left in place, preserving the subvalvular structures and helping to avoid injury to the conduction system (Fig. 43-8). Often there is concern that the anterior leaflet could billow and obstruct the right ventricular outflow tract. The central portion of the leaflet can be excised and still preserve the chordal attachments.

Tricuspid valve replacement with a homograft is more complex. Homograft tissue consists of cadaveric mitral valve apparatus.[60-62] Sizing is performed by measuring the intratrigonal distances. Fixation of the papillary muscles is either intracavity (RV) or through the wall of the RV. This requires judgment and experience to gauge proper chordal length. The annulus is run with a monofilament suture-line. An annuloplasty ring is inserted to prevent dilatation and ensure adequate leaflet coaptation.

Special care is necessary in suture placement to avoid conduction disturbances. Suture placement and tying with the heart beating allow for immediate detection of rhythm disturbances. Similar to mitral valve replacement, leaflet and chordal preservation should be performed, or Gore-Tex suture should used as artificial chordae to maintain annular papillary muscle continuity.

A recent report documented the use of a stentless porcine valve in endocarditis in which the commissural posts were anchored to the right ventricular septal, anterior, and posterior walls. Orientation is critical to be sure that the right ventricular outflow tract is straddled by two of the commissural posts.[63] Low profile mitral bioprosthesis should be chosen.

Carpentier techniques for MVR can be applied to the tricuspid valve. Traumatic disruptions, occasionally endocarditis with healed lesions and perforations, or the rare myxomatous valve can be repaired. Pericardial patching of perforations, partial leaflet resections of the anterior (limited)

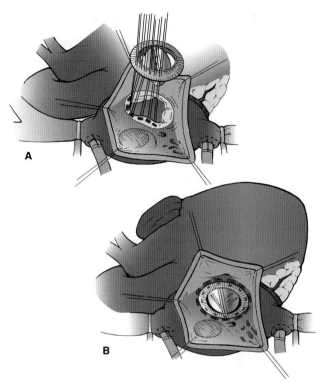

FIGURE 43-8 (A) Tricuspid valve replacement is performed with a St. Jude Medical valve. The native leaflets are left in situ, and the pledgeted 2-0 Ethibond sutures are passed through the annulus and the edges of the leaflets. (B) The valve is seated, and the sutures are tied. The subvalvular apparatus is visualized to ensure that there is no impingement of the prosthetic valve leaflets. The valve can be rotated if necessary to prevent leaflet contact with tissue.

or posterior (extensive) leaflets, chordal transfer, artificial Gore-Tex chordae, Alfieri suture and ring annuloplasty are standard techniques used to produce competent valves and avoid replacement.[64-66]

ENDOCARDITIS

In extensive infections, total excision of the tricuspid valve is possible if pulmonary pressures and the pulmonary vascular resistance are not elevated.[66-68] Blood flows passively through the right side of the heart to the lungs. After eradication of the infection, a second-stage procedure with valve replacement can be performed months to years later.

In patients with tricuspid valve endocarditis due to intravenous drug use, the second-stage valve insertion should be performed preferably after controlling the drug dependence or curing the accompanying addiction. Late survival and reinfection are correlated directly with continued drug use. Patients with less severe endocarditis can have one-stage procedures with prosthetic replacement or localized leaflet excision and repair.[69,70] Homograft tissue often is versatile for partial or total tricuspid valve repair or replacement but has the limitations of availability, technical difficulty, and limited follow-up. The stentless aortic porcine valve is a novel option.[63,64]

PROSTHETIC VALVE CHOICE

The choice of prosthesis follows an algorithm similar to that used for valve replacement in other cardiac valve positions. The patient's age, anticoagulation considerations, childbearing wishes, and social issues are all factors in valve choice. The previously reported poor results with mechanical valves in the tricuspid position were mainly due to valve thrombosis. Most of these reports were during the era of cage-ball and tilting-disk prostheses.[71] Reports with the St. Jude bileaflet valve have provided encouraging data, allowing the surgeon to recommend a mechanical valve with confidence to younger patients who do not have a contraindication to anticoagulation.[72-78]

This strategy will avoid the not uncommon situation in the past in which patients received a bioprosthetic on the right side and a mechanical prosthesis on the left. Bioprostheses, both porcine and of pericardial tissue, have functioned well in the tricuspid position.[79-82] Compared to the mitral position, bioprosthetic valves in the tricuspid position exhibit longer durability with a longer duration of freedom from structural valve dysfunction.[83]

Table 43-2 summarizes multiple reports from the literature. The reports either compare bioprosthetic and mechanical valves in the tricuspid position or present follow-up of bioprosthetic valves alone. The bioprostheses, either porcine or pericardial valves, have excellent freedom from degeneration and re-replacement for structural valve degeneration. In 1984, Cohen and colleagues reported on six simultaneously implanted and then explanted valves from the mitral and tricuspid positions. Degenerative changes were less extensive for the bioprosthetic valves in the tricuspid position than in the mitral position. However, thrombus and pannus formation (interpreted as organized thrombotic material) were observed more frequently in the tricuspid position.[83]

At 9 years, Nakano's review of the Carpentier-Edwards bovine pericardial valve reported a freedom from structural degeneration of 100% and nonstructural dysfunction of 72.8%.[81] The cause of nonstructural dysfunction was pannus formation on the ventricular side of the cusps. Often subclinical, echocardiographic follow-up after 5 years reveals up tp a 35% incidence of this anatomical finding.

Guerra reported similar changes in simultaneously explanted porcine valves.[84] The tricuspid position had less structural tissue degeneration and calcification than the mitral position. The report described the presence of pannus on the ventricular side of the cusps and interference with cusp pliability and function.

Nakano's 2001 report of bioprosthetic tricuspid valves reported an 18-year freedom from reoperation of 63%.[80] Freedom from structural deterioration was 96%, and nonstructural dysfunction was 77%. Reoperation, replacing previously placed bioprosthetic valves occurred in 12 of 58 survivors. In 6 of the 12 patients, the primary indication for reoperation was tricuspid dysfunction, and 7 of the 12 had pannus formation on the ventricular side of the cusps (Fig. 43-9). This rate of degeneration and the subclinically high incidence of pannus formation, often eventually leading to reoperation, are concerning.

Bioprosthetic valves in the tricuspid position require close echocardiographic follow-up. Possible anticoagulation of bioprosthetic valves in the tricuspid position can reduce the incidence of pannus formation. The reported data in the literature categorize pannus formation as nonstructural degeneration; therefore, clinical surgeons should be aware of future reports following this potentially serious clinical problem.

It is always possible to place large bioprosthetic or mechanical valves in the tricuspid position. Prostheses with more than a 27-mm internal diameter do not have clinically significant gradients. Therefore, hemodynamic performance is rarely an issue for tricuspid valve replacement. The data demonstrate excellent results with modern bileaflet mechanical valves. Series comparing bioprosthetic and mechanical valves have been consistent in demonstrating equality during the period of follow-up. The development of thrombus on a bileaflet valve can be treated successfully with thrombolysis.

A recent review by Filsoufi and a meta-analysis of biologic or mechanical prostheses in the tricuspid position both conclude that there is no survival benefit of a bioprosthesis over a mechanical valve[85-87] (Fig. 43-10). Some patients with mitral valve disease and TR undergoing surgery do not require surgical treatment of the tricuspid valve. Guidelines to identify these patients are poorly developed. Experience has shown that careful observation of the patient preoperatively is quite valuable. Absence of tricuspid valve regurgitation during periods of good medical control, absence of TR by TEE at the time of operation, minimal elevation of pulmonary vascular resistance, and absence of right atrial enlargement are helpful findings that permit the surgeon to replace the mitral valve confidently without performing an annuloplasty or replacement of the tricuspid valve. If unrepaired, reassessment of the tricuspid valve by TEE after weaning from cardiopulmonary bypass is essential. TEE assessment of residual TR under anesthesia can be misleading if the loading conditions are different from the conditions in an awaken patient.

If TR persists and elevated right atrial pressures greater than left atrial pressures are encountered with an underfilled, well-contracting left ventricle, tricuspid repair should be performed. A patent foramen ovale with interatrial shunting must be identified and closed surgically. Hemodynamically, when right atrial pressure is greater than left atrial pressure, the foramen may open, leading to systemic desaturation from a right-to-left shunt.

Temporary right ventricular dysfunction caused by RCA air embolism often requires a brief return to cardiopulmonary bypass, repeat of deairing maneuvers, elevation of the systemic blood pressures, TEE evaluation for residual intracavity air, and a search for the characteristic echogenic brightness in the myocardial distribution of the RCA confirming the suspicion of air embolism. Treatment should include 10 to 15 minutes of cardiopulmonary bypass support and reweaning from cardiopulmonary bypass, with inotropic support, elevated blood pressure, and reassessment of the TR and cardiac function.

TABLE 43-2: Reports of Bioprosthetic and Mechanical Valves in the Tricuspid Position

Reference	Series dates	Patients (no.)	Operative mortality — Bioprosthesis (B)	Operative mortality — Mechanical (M)	Death — Overall (A)	Death — B	Death — M	Death — A	Structural degeneration — B	Structural degeneration — M	Structural degeneration — A	Nonstructural degeneration — B	Nonstructural degeneration — M	Nonstructural degeneration — A	Tricuspid reoperation — B	Tricuspid reoperation — M	Tricuspid reoperation — A
Nakano[74]	1979-1992	39		8%			55% @14 y;		100%			72%				100% @14 y	
Nakano[79]	1978-1995	98	15%			77% @5 y; 69% @10 y; And 18 y			98% @5 y; 96% @18 y			99% @5 y; 82% @10 y; 77% @18 y*		97% @5 y; 76% @10 y; 63% @18 y			
Ratnatunga[77]	1966-1997	425	19%	16%	17%	71% @1 y; 62% @5 y; 48% @10 y	74%; 58%; 34%	72%; 60%; 43%						99% @1 y; 98% @10 y;		98%	
Glower[70]	1972-1993	129			27% (14% 1st Operation)	56% @5 y; 48% @10 y; 31% 14 y								96% @5 y; 93% @10 y; 49% @14 y		97%	
Ohata[81]	1984-1998	88	7%			88% @5 y; 81% @10 y; 69% 14 y			100% @14 y			†		@14 y			
Van Nooton[69]	1967-1987	146			16%			74% @5 y; 23% @10 y									
Singh[72]	1981-1984	14		8%			50% @10 y										

Actuarial freedom from

(Continued)

TABLE 43-2: Reports of Bioprosthetic and Mechanical Valves in the Tricuspid Position (Continued)

Reference	Series dates	Patients (no.)	Operative mortality		Actuarial freedom from													
			Bioprosthesis (B)	Mechanical (M)	Death				Structural degeneration			Nonstructural degeneration			Tricuspid reoperation		
					Overall (A)	B	M	A	B	M	A	B	M	A	B	M	A
Munro[75]	1975-1992	94	15%	14%	14%				97% @5,7 y, and 10 y	100%						97%	87%
Kaplan[70]	1980-2000	122			25%	55% @20 y	68% @20 y	65% @20 y	90% @20 y	97%[‡] @20 y							
Scully[71]	1975-1993	60			27%		50% @15 y										

*Thick fibrous pannus in 35% of survivors; freedom from nonstructural valve dysfunction at 18 years = 24%.
†Thick pannus noted in reoperative case.
‡Freedom from deterioration, endocarditis, leakage, and thromboembolism 93% @20 y.
y indicates years.

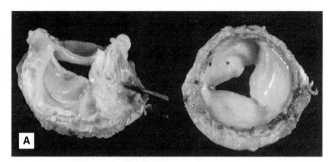

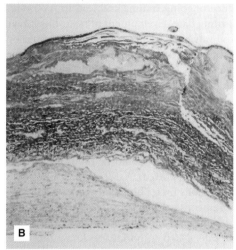

FIGURE 43-9 (A) Fibrous pannus observed 8 years after implantation of a Carpentier-Edwards pericardial valve. (B) Photomicrograph of a pericardial leaflet. The bottom of the leaflet has pannus, a dense fibrous tissue on the ventricular side. (Reproduced with permission from Nakano K, Ishibashi-Ueda H, Kobayashi J, et al: Tricuspid valve replacement with bioprostheses: long-term results and causes of valve dysfunction, *Ann Thorac Surg.* 2001 Jan;71(1):105-9.)

Bioprosthetic valves have the safety feature of not developing thrombosis or requiring anticoagulation. Bioprostheses are being considered in younger patients since percutaneous valve in valve treatment for structural deterioration is being performed with excellent results. When choosing the size of the bioprostheses, it is important to consider the size of the valve to insure the percutaneous valve-in-valve option is feasible.

CONCLUSION

Historical clinical experience has demonstrated that up to 20% of patients undergoing mitral valve replacement receive a tricuspid annuloplasty, but less than 2% require replacement. Traditionally, the surgeon's clinical judgment and experience have guided the approach to tricuspid surgery, ultimately leading to variability in reported clinical data. The accuracy of these decisions can be enhanced by assessment of risk factors for persistent or progressive tricuspid valve regurgitation. Recent studies have taught us that our ability to make these judgments is flawed and unpredictable.

We have learned about the dilated tricuspid valve annulus, the progression of TR in spite of successful left-sided surgery, and the unpredictable resolution of pulmonary hypertension. Failure to improve can have adverse impacts on late morbidity, mortality, and residual or progressive TR. Therefore, the current recommendation is to pursue aggressively tricuspid annuloplasty with remodeling rings or bands.

Older studies showed patients undergoing a tricuspid valve annuloplasty during a mitral valve replacement have more advanced disease than those having mitral valve replacement alone. This is evidenced by the elevation in operative mortality (approximately 12 vs 3%) and the progressive increased hazard of late death (5-year survival of 80 vs 70%) despite good valve function. However, these patients achieved good functional results (NYHA Class 1-2). It is unknown what the survival and functional result would have been if tricuspid repair had not been performed in these patients, but one presumes that it would have been worse. In the current era, adding an annuloplasty can have minimal adverse impact in the perioperative period and seems to confer long-term benefit.

The durability of simple annuloplasty techniques such as bicuspidization and the DeVega technique has been

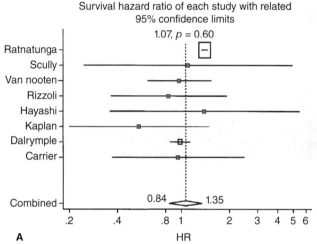

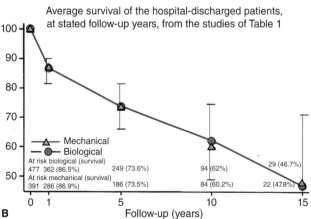

FIGURE 43-10 Meta-analysis of bioprosthetic vs mechanical valves replacing the tricuspid valve. (A) Survival hazard. (B) Survival curve of hospital survivors.

satisfactory when employed only for mild-to-moderate degrees of fTR with successful resolution of pulmonary hypertension after the mitral valve operation. Extensive experience with the tricuspid annuloplasty using the Duran, Carpentier-Edwards, and MC³ rings or bands have resulted in an 85% freedom from moderate-to-severe TR at 6 years. The subsequent requirement for tricuspid reoperation is very low. Inadequate resolution of the mitral disease and persistent pulmonary hypertension with right ventricular dilatation and dysfunction are the major predictors of poor late results.

The American College of Cardiology/American Heart Association 2014 Practice Guidelines for the surgical management of patients with TR (Table 43-3)[88] are driven by the individual patient's clinical status and the cause of their tricuspid valve abnormality. The guidelines state that the timing of surgical intervention for TR remains controversial, as do the surgical techniques. At present, surgery on the tricuspid valve for significant TR should occur at the time of mitral valve surgery, as TR does not reliably resolve after mitral valve surgery. TR associated with dilatation of the tricuspid annulus should be repaired, to prevent tricuspid annular dilation progressing and producing severe TR.[89-96]

Patients requiring tricuspid and mitral valve replacement have operative mortalities from 5 to 10% by current standards. Actuarial survival rates are 55% at 10 years (Fig. 43-10A, B). Advanced right ventricular failure or arrhythmia causes late death. Patients who need valve replacement for endocarditis comprise a unique subgroup with the additional risk for death owing to sepsis, reinfection, and the complications related to drug addiction.

Complete heart block can occur immediately postoperatively owing to damage to the conduction system during mitral and tricuspid valve surgery. This complication can be minimized intraoperatively by performing the tricuspid valve procedure on the perfused beating heart, as described earlier. Late heart block remains a persistent risk with a 25% actuarial incidence at 10 years for patients with mitral and tricuspid prostheses. The presence of two rigid prosthetic sewing rings can produce ongoing trauma and lead to AV node dysfunction over time. Late development of heart block rarely occurs after mitral valve replacement and tricuspid annuloplasty.

The surgical treatment of tricuspid valve disease presents the surgeon with challenges requiring clinical and intraoperative judgment. Following the principles presented in this chapter, appropriate decisions should lead to optimal clinical outcomes. The data support the safe use of mechanical bileaflet prostheses in select patients. A lingering concern is the pannus formation on the ventricular side of bioprosthetic cusps. This observation should be followed closely as future clinical series are reported.

Many surgeons prefer bioprosthetic valves. More recently, with percutaneous valve in valve re-replacement strategies for degenerated stented bioprostheses, this option should gain increasing safety. It is important to know the valve internal diameter to be sure a valve-in-valve option will be available for the patient.

REFERENCES

1. Yiwu L, Yingchun C, Jianqun Z, Bin Y, Ping B: Exact quantitative selective annuloplasty of the tricuspid valve. *J Thorac Cardiovasc Surg* 2001; 122: 611-614.
2. Cohn LH: Tricuspid regurgitation secondary to mitral valve disease: when and how to repair. *J Card Surg* 199; 9:237-241.
3. Ewy G: Tricuspid valve disease, in Alpert JS, Dalen JE, Rahimtoola SH (eds): *Valvular Heart Disease*, 3rd ed. Philadelphia, Lippincott Williams & Wilkins, 2000; pp 377-392.
4. Fukuda S, Saracino G, Matsumura Y, et al: Three-dimensional geometry of the tricuspid annulus in healthy subjects and in patients with functional tricuspid regurgitation: a real-time, 3-dimensional echocardiographic study. *Circulation* 2006; 114(Suppl):I-492-I-498.
5. Ton-Nu TT, Levine RA, Handschumacher MD, et al: Geometric determinants of functional tricuspid regurgitation: Insights from 2-dimensional echocardiography. *Circulation* 2006; 114(2):143-149.
6. Cohen ST, Sell JE, McIntosh CL, et al: Tricuspid regurgitation in patients with acquired, chronic, pure mitral regurgitation: I. Prevalence, diagnosis, and comparison of preoperative clinical and hemodynamic features in patients with and without tricuspid regurgitation. *J Thorac Cardiovasc Surg* 1987; 94:481.
7. Cohen SR, Sell JE, McIntosh CL, et al: Tricuspid regurgitation in patients with acquired, chronic, pure mitral regurgitation: II. Nonoperative management, tricuspid valve annuloplasty, and tricuspid valve replacement. *J Thorac Cardiovasc Surg* 1987; 94:488.
8. Tei C, Pilgrim JP, Shah PM, et al: The tricuspid valve annulus: study of size and motion in normal subjects and in patients with tricuspid regurgitation. *Circulation* 1982; 66:665.
9. Ubago JL, Figueroa A, Ochotcco A, et al: Analysis of the amount of tricuspid valve annular dilation required to produce functional tricuspid regurgitation. *Am J Cardiol* 1983; 52:155.
10. Come PC, Riley MF: Tricuspid annular dilatation and failure of tricuspid leaflet coaptation in tricuspid regurgitation. *Am J Cardiol* 1985; 55:599.

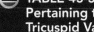

TABLE 43-3: 2014 ACC/AHA Guidelines Pertaining to the Surgical Management of Tricuspid Value Disease/Regurgitation

Class I

Tricuspid value repair is beneficial for severe TR in patients MV disease requiring MV surgery. *(Level of evidence: B)*

Class IIa

1. Tricuspid value replacement or annuloplasty is reasonable for severe primary TR when symptomatic. *(Level of evidence: C)*
2. Tricuspid value replacement is reasonable for severe TR secondary to disease/abnormal tricuspid value leaflets not amenable to annuloplasty or repair. *(Level of evidence: C)*

Class IIb

Tricuspid annuloplasty may be considered for less than severe TR in patients undergoing MV surgery when there is pulmonary hypertension or tricuspid annular dilatation. *(Level of evidence: C)*

Class III

1. Tricuspid value replacement or annuloplasty is not indicated in asymptomatic patients with TR whose pulmonary artery systolic pressure is less than 60 mm Hg in the pressure of a normal MV. *(Level of evidence: C)*
2. Tricuspid value replacement or annuloplasty is not indicated in patients with mild primary TR. *(Level of evidence: C)*

ACC, indicates American College of Cardiology; AHA, American Heart Association; TR, tricuspid regurgitation; and MV, mitral value.

11. Waller BF, Moriarty AT, Able JN, et al: Etiology of pure tricuspid regurgitation based on annular circumference and leaflet area: analysis of 45 necropsy patients with clinical and morphologic evidence of pure tricuspid regurgitation. *J Am Coll Cardiol* 1986; 7:1063.

12. Miller MJ, McKay RG, Ferguson JJ, et al: Right atrial pressure-volume relationships in tricuspid regurgitation. *Circulation* 1986; 73:799.

13. Morrison DA, Ovit T, Hammermeister KE, et al: Functional tricuspid regurgitation and right ventricular dysfunction in pulmonary hypertension. *Am J Cardiol* 1988; 62:108.

14. Atbulu A, Holmes RJ, Asfaw I: Surgical treatment of intractable right-sided infective endocarditis in drug addicts: 25 years' experience. *J Heart Valve Dis* 1993; 2:129.

15. Bayer AS, Blomquist IK, Bello E, et al: Tricuspid valve endocarditis due to *Staphylococcus aureus*. *Chest* 1988; 93:247.

16. Tanaka M, Abe T, Hosokawa ST, et al: Tricuspid valve *Candida* endocarditis cured by valve-sparing debridement. *Ann Thorac Surg* 1989; 48:857.

17. Robiolio PA, Rigolin VH, Harrison JK, et al: Predictors of outcome of tricuspid valve replacement in carcinoid heart disease. *Am J Cardiol* 1995; 75:485.

18. Ohri SK, Schofield JB, Hodgson H, et al: Carcinoid heart disease: early failure of an allograft valve replacement. *Ann Thorac Surg* 1994; 58:1161.

19. Lundin I, Norheim I, Landelius J, et al: Carcinoid heart disease: relationship of circulating vasoactive substances to ultrasound-detectable cardiac abnormalities. *Circulation* 1988; 77:264.

20. Fujii S, Funaki K, Denzunn N: Isolated rheumatic tricuspid regurgitation and stenosis. *Clin Cardiol* 1966; 9:353.

21. Kim JB, Spevack DM, Tunick PA, et al: The effect of transvenous pacemaker and implantable cardioverter defibrillator lead placement on tricuspid valve function: an observational study. *J Am Soc Echocardiogr* 2008; 21:284-287.

22. Taira K, Suzuki A, Fujino A, et al: Tricuspid valve stenosis related to subvalvular adhesion of pacemaker lead: a case report. *J Cardiol* 2006; 47:301-306.

23. Love CJ, Wilkoff BL, Byrd CL, et al: Recommendations for extraction of chronically implanted transvenous pacing and defibrillator leads: indications, facilities, training: North American Society of Pacing and Electrophysiology Lead Extraction Conference Faculty. *Pacing Clin Electrophysiol* 2000; 23:544-551.

24. McCarthy PM, Bhudia SK, Rajeswaran J, et al: Tricuspid valve repair: durability and risk factors for failure. *J Thorac Cardiovasc Surg* 2004; 127:674-685.

25. Zoghbi WA, Enriquez-Sarano M, Foster E, et al: Recommendations for evaluation of the severity of native valvular regurgitation with two-dimensional and Doppler echocardiography. *J Am Soc Echocardiogr* 2003; 16:777-802.

26. Lorenz CH, Walker ES, Morgan VL, Klein SS, Graham TP Jr: Normal human right and left ventricular mass, systolic function, and gender differences by cine magnetic resonance imaging. *J Cardiovasc Magn Reson* 1999; 1:7-21.

27. Zornoff LA, Skali H, Pfeffer MA, et al: Right ventricular dysfunction and risk of heart failure and mortality after myocardial infarction. *J Am Coll Cardiol* 2002; 39:1450-1455.

28. Nesser HJ, Tkalec W, Patel AR, et al: Quantitation of right ventricular volumes and ejection fraction by three-dimensional echocardiography in patients: comparison with magnetic resonance imaging and radionuclide ventriculography. *Echocardiography* 2006; 23:666-680.

29. Rudski LG, Lai WW, Afilalo J, et al: Guidelines for the echocardiographic assessment of the right heart in adults: a report from the American Society of Echocardiography endorsed by the European Association of Echocardiography, a registered branch of the European Society of Cardiology, and the Canadian Society of Echocardiography. *J Am Soc Echocardiogr* 2010; 23:685-713.

30. Child JS: Improved guides to tricuspid valve repair: two-dimensional echocardiographic analysis of tricuspid annulus function and color flow imaging of severity of tricuspid regurgitation. *J Am Coll Cardiol* 1989; 14:1275.

31. Wong M, Matsumura M, Kutsuzawa S, et al: The value of Doppler echocardiography in the treatment of tricuspid regurgitation in patients with mitral valve replacement. *J Thorac Cardiovasc Surg* 1990; 99:1003.

32. Czer LSC, Maurer G, Bolger A, et al: Tricuspid valve repair, operative and follow-up evaluation by Doppler color flow mapping. *J Thorac Cardiovasc Surg* 1989; 98:101.

33. DeSimone R, Lange R, Saggau W, et al: Intraoperative transesophageal echocardiography for the evaluation of mutual, aortic and tricuspid valve repair. *Eur J Cardiothorac Surg* 1992; 6:665.

34. Maurer G, Siegel RJ, Czer LSC: The use of color-flow mapping for intra-operative assessment of valve repair. *Circulation* 1991; 84:I-250.

35. Gibson R, Wood P: The diagnosis of tricuspid stenosis. *Br Heart J* 1955; 17:552.

36. Keefe JF, Wolk MJ, Levine HJ: Isolated tricuspid valvular stenosis. *Am J Cardiol* 1970; 25(2):252-257.

37. Roberts WC, Sullivan MF: Combined mitral valve stenosis and tricuspid valve stenosis: morphologic observations after mitral and tricuspid valve replacements or mitral replacement and tricuspid valve commissurotomy. *Am J Cardiol* 1986; 58:850.

38. Nath J, Foster E, Heidenreich PA: Impact of tricuspid regurgitation on long-term survival. *J Am Coll Cardiol* 2004; 43:405-409.

39. Mutlak D, Aronson D, Lessick J, et al: Functional tricuspid regurgitation in patients with pulmonary hypertension: is pulmonary artery pressure the only determinant of regurgitation severity? *Chest* 2009; 135:115-121.

40. Dreyfus GD, Corbi PJ, Chan KMJ, Toufan Bahrami T: Secondary tricus-pid regurgitation or dilatation: which should be the criterion for surgical repair? *Ann Thorac Surg* 2005; 79:127.

41. Matsunaga A, Duran CM: Progression of tricuspid regurgitation after repaired functional ischemic mitral regurgitation. *Circulation* 2005; 112:I-453.

42. Deloche A, Guerinon J, Fabiani JN, et al: Anatomical study of rheumatic tricuspid valve diseases: application to the various valvuloplasties [in French]. *Ann Chir Thorac Cardiovasc* 1973; 12:343-349.

43. Castedo E, Canas A, Cabo RA, Burgos R, Ugarte J: Edge-to-edge tricuspid repair for redeveloped valve incompetence after DeVega's annuloplasty. *Ann Thorac Surg* 2003; 75:605-606.

44. Castedo E, Monguio E, Cabo RA, Ugarte J: Edge-to-edge technique for correction of tricuspid valve regurgitation due to complex lesions. *Eur J Cardiothorac Surg* 2005; 27:933-934.

45. Tang GH, David TE, Singh SK, et al: Tricuspid valve repair with an annuloplasty ring results in improved long-term outcomes. *Circulation* 2006; 114(Suppl):I-577-I-581.

46. DeVega NG: La anuloplastia selective, reguable y permanente. *Rev Esp Cardiol* 1972; 25:6-9.

47. Ghanta RK, Chen R, Narayanasamy N, et al: Suture bicuspidization of the tricuspid valve versus ring annuloplasty for repair of functional tricuspid regurgitation: midterm results of 237 consecutive patients. *J Thorac Cardiovasc Surg* 2007; 133:117-126.

48. Matsuyama K, Matsumoto M, Sugita T, et al: Predictors of residual tricuspid regurgitation after mitral valve surgery. *Ann Thorac Surg* 2003; 75:1826-1828.

49. Matsunaga A, Duran CM: Progression of tricuspid regurgitation after repaired functional ischemic mitral regurgitation. *Circulation* 2005; 112(Suppl):I-453-I-457.

50. King RM, Schaff HV, Danielson GK, et al: Surgery for tricuspid regurgitation late after mitral valve replacement. *Circulation* 1984; 70(Suppl): I-193-I-197.

51. Singh SK, Tang GH, Maganti MD, et al: Midterm outcomes of tricuspid valve repair versus replacement for organic tricuspid disease. *Ann Thorac Surg* 2006; 82:1735-1741.

52. Silver MD, Lam JH, Ranganathan N, Wigle ED: Morphology of the human tricuspid valve. *Circulation* 1971; 43:333-348.

53. Cohn L: Tricuspid regurgitation secondary to mitral valve disease: when and how to repair. *J Card Surg* 1994; 9(Suppl):237.

54. Duran CM, Kumar N, Prabhakar G, et al: Vanishing DeVega annuloplasty for functional tricuspid regurgitation. *J Thorac Cardiovasc Surg* 1993; 106:609.

55. Chidambaram M, Abdulali SA, Baliga BG, et al: Long-term results of DeVega tricuspid annuloplasty. *Ann Thorac Surg* 1987; 43:185.

56. Carpentier A, Deloche A, Dauptain J, et al: A new reconstructive operation for correction of mitral and tricuspid insufficiency. *J Thorac Cardiovasc Surg* 1971; 61:1.

57. Brugger JJ, Egloff L, Rothlin M, et al: Tricuspid annuloplasty: results and complications. *Thorac Cardiovasc Surg* 1982; 30:284.

58. Gatti G, Maffei G, Lusa A, et al: Tricuspid valve repair with Cosgrove-Edwards annuloplasty system: early clinical and echocardiographic results. *Ann Thorac Surg* 2001; 72:764.

59. McCarthy PM, Bhudia SK, Rajeswaran J, et al: Tricuspid valve repair: durability and risk factors for failure. *J Thorac Cardiovasc Surg* 2004; 127:67.

60. Pomar JI, Mestres CA, Pate JC, et al: Management of persistent tricuspid endocarditis with transplantation of cryopreserved mitral homografts. *J Thorac Cardiovasc Surg* 1994; 107:1460.

61. Hvass U, Baron F, Fourchy D, et al: Mitral homografts for total tricuspid valve replacement: comparison of two techniques. *J Thorac Cardiovasc Surg* 2001; 3:592.

62. Katz NM, Pallas RS: Traumatic rupture of the tricuspid valve: repair by chordal replacements and annuloplasty. *J Thorac Cardiovasc Surg* 1986; 91:310.

63. Cardarelli MG, Gammie JS, Brown JM, et al: A novel approach to tricuspid valve replacement: the upside down stentless aortic bioprosthesis. *Ann Thorac Surg* 2005; 80:507.

64. Sutlic Z, Schmid C, Borst HG: Repair of flail anterior leaflets of tricuspid and mitral valves by cusp remodeling. *Ann Thorac Cardiovasc Surg* 1990; 50:927.

65. Doty JR, Cameron DE, Elmaci T, et al: Penetrating trauma to the tricuspid valve and ventricular septum: delayed repair. *Ann Thorac Surg* 1999; 67:252.

66. Arbulu A, Asfaw I: Tricuspid valvulectomy without prosthetic replacement. *J Thorac Cardiovasc Surg* 1981; 82:684.

67. Arbulu A, Thoms NW, Wilson RI: Valvulectomy without prosthetic replacement: a lifesaving operation for tricuspid Pseudomonas endocarditis. *J Cardiovasc Surg (Torino)* 1972; 74:103.

67a. Walther T, Falk V, Schneider J, et al: Stentless tricuspid valve replacement. *Ann Thorac Surg* 1999; 68:1858.

68. Arbulu A, Holmes RJ, Asfaw I: Tricuspid valvulectomy without replacement: twenty years' experience. *J Thorac Cardiovasc Surg* 1991; 102:917.

69. Turley K: Surgery of right-sided endocarditis: valve preservation versus replacement. *J Card Surg* 1989; 4:317.

70. Van Nooten G, Caes F, Tacymans Y, et al: Tricuspid valve replacement: postoperative and long-term results. *J Thorac Cardiovasc Surg* 1995; 110:672.

71. Kaplan M, Kut MS, Demirtas MM, et al: Prosthetic replacement of tricuspid valve: bioprosthetic or mechanical. *Ann Thorac Surg* 2002; 73:467.

72. Scully HE, Armstrong CS: Tricuspid valve replacement: fifteen years of experience with mechanical prostheses and bioprostheses. *J Thorac Cardiovasc Surg* 1995; 109:1035.

73. Singh AK, Feng WC, Sanofsky SJ: Long-term results of St. Jude Medical valve in the tricuspid position. *Ann Thorac Surg* 1992; 54:538.

74. Kaplan M, Kut MS, Demirtas MM, et al: Prosthetic replacement of tricuspid valve: bioprosthetic or mechanical. *Ann Thorac Surg* 2002; 73:467.

75. Nakano K, Koyanagi H, Hashimoto A, et al: Tricuspid valve replacement with the bileaflet St. Jude Medical valve prosthesis. *J Thorac Cardiovasc Surg* 1994; 108:888.

76. Munro AI, Jamieson WRE, Tyers FO, et al: Tricuspid valve replacement: porcine bioprostheses and mechanical prostheses. *Ann Thorac Surg* 1995; 59:S470.

77. Ohata T, Kigawa I, Tohda E, et al: Comparison of durability of bioprostheses in tricuspid and mitral positions. *Ann Thorac Surg* 2001; 71:S240.

78. Ratnatunga C, Edwards M-B, Dore C, et al: Tricuspid valve replacement: UK heart valve registry midterm results comparing mechanical and biological prostheses. *Ann Thorac Surg* 1998; 66:1940.

79. Glower DD, White WD, Smith LR, et al: In-hospital and long-term outcome after porcine tricuspid valve replacement. *J Thorac Cardiovasc Surg* 1995; 109:877.

80. Nakano K, Ishibashi-Ueda H, Kobayashi J, et al: Tricuspid valve replacement with bioprostheses: long-term results and causes of valve dysfunction. *Ann Thorac Surg* 2001; 71:105.

81. Nakano K, Eishi K, Kosakai Y, et al: Ten-year experience with the Carpentier-Edwards pericardial xenograft in the tricuspid position. *J Thorac Cardiovasc Surg* 1996; 111:605.

82. Ohata T, Kigawa I, Yamashita Y, et al: Surgical strategy for severe tricuspid valve regurgitation complicated by advanced mitral valve disease: long-term outcome of tricuspid valve supra-annular implantation in eighty-eight cases. *J Thorac Cardiovasc Surg* 2000; 120:280.

83. Cohen SR, Silver MA, McIntosh CL, Roberts WC: Comparison of late (62 to 104 months) degenerative changes in simultaneously implanted and explanted porcine (Hancock) bioprosthesis in the tricuspid and mitral positions in six patients. *Am J Cardiol* 1984; 53:1599.

84. Guerra F, Bortolotti U, Thiene G, et al: Long-term performance of the Hancock porcine bioprosthesis in the tricuspid position: a review of 45 patients with 14 visit follow-up. *J Thorac Cardiovasc Surg* 1990; 99:838.

85. Filsoufi F, Anyanwu AC, Salzberg SP, et al: Long-term outcomes of tricus-pid valve replacement in the current era. *Ann Thorac Surg* 2005; 80:845.

86. Solomon NAG, Lim CH, Nand P, Graham KJ: Tricuspid valve replacement: bioprosthetic or mechanical valve? *Asian Cardiovasc Thorac Ann* 2004; 12:143.

87. Rizzoli G, Vendramin I, Nesseris G, et al: Biological or mechanical prostheses in tricuspid position? A meta-analysis of intrainstitutional results. *Ann Thorac Surg* 2004; 77:1607.

88. Nishimura RA, Otto CM, Bonow RO, et al: ACC/AHA 2014 guidelines for the management of patients with valvular heart disease: a report of the American College of Cardiology/American Heart Association Task Force on Practice Guidelines. *J Thorac Cardiovasc Surg* 2014; 148(1):e1-e132.

89. Aoyagi S, Tanaka K, Hara H, et al: Modified De Vega's annuloplasty for functional tricuspid regurgitation: early and late results. *The Kurume Med J* 1992; 39:23-32.

90. Fukuda S, Song JM, Gillinov AM, et al: Tricuspid valve tethering predicts residual tricuspid regurgitation after tricuspid annuloplasty. *Circulation* 2005; 111:975-979.

91. Holper K, Haehnel JC, Augustin N, Sebening F: Surgery for tricuspid insufficiency: long-term follow-up after De Vega annuloplasty. *Thorac Cardiovasc Surg* 1993; 41:1-8.

92. Minale C, Lambertz H, Nikol S, Gerich N, Messmer BJ: Selective annuloplasty of the tricuspid valve: two-year experience. *J Thorac Cardiovasc Surg* 1990; 99:846-851.

93. Paulis RD, Bobbio M, Ottino G, DeVega N: The De Vega tricuspid annuloplasty: perioperative mortality and long term follow-up. *J Cardiovasc Surg (Torino)* 1990; 31:512-517.

94. Peltola T, Lepojarvi M, Ikaheimo M, Karkola P: De Vega's annuloplasty for tricuspid regurgitation. *Ann Chir Gynaecol* 1996; 85:40-43.

95. Kirklin JW, Barratt-Boyes BG (eds): *Cardiac Surgery*, vol. 1, 2nd ed. New York, Churchill-Livingstone, 1992; p 598.

96. Rogers JH, Bolling SF: The tricuspid valve: current perspective and evolving management of tricuspid regurgitation. *Circulation* 2009; 119:2718-2725.

44

Multiple Valve Disease

Hartzell V. Schaff • Rakesh M. Suri

Pathologic changes in the cardiac valves requiring surgical correction of more than one valve can result from rheumatic heart disease, degenerative valve diseases, infective endocarditis, and a number of other miscellaneous causes. Further, valve dysfunction may be primary; that is, a direct result of a disease process, or secondary; that is, caused by cardiac enlargement and/or pulmonary hypertension. Surgical management is influenced both by the underlying cause of valve dysfunction and, when valves are involved secondarily, by the anticipated response to replacement or repair of the primary valve lesion. In addition, the consequences of various combinations of diseased valves on left and right ventricular geometry and function frequently are different from the remodeling as a result of single-valve disease. This chapter addresses pathophysiologic considerations in multivalvular heart disease, surgical techniques, and management of commonly encountered etiologies.

Repair of multiple lesions was necessary even in the early development of operative management of valvular heart disease (Table 44-1). The first triple-valve replacement during a single operation was reported in 1960, and simultaneous replacement of all four valves was reported in 1992.[1]

Experience from clinical practice indicates that multiple valve disease requiring surgical correction occurs in a few common combinations. As seen in Table 44-2, multiple procedures account for approximately 15% of all operations on cardiac valves; 80% of these operations involve the aortic and mitral positions. Replacement of the mitral and tricuspid valves (with or without aortic replacement) accounts for 20% of operations. Only rarely is the combination of aortic and tricuspid disease encountered.

PATHOPHYSIOLOGY OF MULTIPLE VALVE DISEASE

Valvular regurgitation may result from the pathologic process affecting the valve directly or may be secondary to alterations in ventricular morphology caused by other valve lesions; this secondary or functional regurgitation affects the atrioventricular valves. In some patients, secondary valvular regurgitation may be expected to improve with repair or replacement of the primarily diseased valve. In other patients, the secondary disease process may have advanced to the stage that valve function will not improve following correction of the primary lesion, and thus simultaneous surgical correction should be considered.

Primary Aortic Valve Disease with Secondary Mitral Regurgitation

Isolated aortic valve lesions can cause secondary regurgitation of the mitral valve and rarely, the tricuspid valve. Severe aortic valve stenosis with or without left ventricular dilatation frequently is associated with some degree of mitral valve regurgitation. In one series, 67% of patients with severe aortic valve stenosis had associated mitral valve leakage.[2] When the mitral valve is structurally normal, its regurgitation would be expected to improve with relief of left ventricular outflow obstruction;[4] mild mitral valve regurgitation may, at times resolve almost completely after aortic valve replacement. Improvement in mitral valve regurgitation results from both decreased undergoing intraventricular pressure and ventricular remodeling.[5] If mitral valve regurgitation is severe, some degree of persistent regurgitation is expected after aortic valve replacement, and mitral valve annuloplasty may be required. In contrast, with aortic valve stenosis and mitral valve regurgitation associated with a structurally abnormal mitral valve, repair or replacement of the mitral valve usually is necessary. A recent report alleges that moderate MR has an adverse impact on survival in elderly patients undergoing aortic valve replacement and suggests that those with intrinsic mitral valve disease should be considered for concurrent correction.[6]

Thus determination of the morphology and pathophysiologic severity of each valve lesion is critically important in planning surgical management, and preoperative and

TABLE 44-1: History of Multiple Valve Operations

Event	Year	Institution
Staged mitral then tricuspid commissurotomy	1952	Doctor's Hospital, Philadelphia, PA[164]
Simultaneous mitral and tricuspid commissurotomy	1953	Cleveland, OH[156]
Simultaneous mitral commissurotomy and aortic valvuloplasty using cardiopulmonary bypass	1956	University of Minnesota, Minneapolis, MN[157]
Simultaneous mitral and aortic valve replacement	1961	St. Francis General Hospital, Pittsburgh, PA[121]
Simultaneous triple-valve replacement	1963	University of Oregon, Portland, OR
Simultaneous quadruple-valve replacement	1992	Mayo Clinic, Rochester, MN[165]

Source: Data from Acker M, Hargrove WC, Stephenson LW: Multiple valve replacement, *Cardiol Clin* 1985; 3:425-430.

intraoperative echocardiographic studies are necessary in all patients suspected of having multiple valve disease. Often, transthoracic echocardiography can define the etiology of mitral and tricuspid valvular regurgitation. When valve regurgitation is entirely secondary, the mitral valve leaflets will appear thin and freely mobile, without prolapsing segments. Mitral (and tricuspid) valve regurgitation secondary to rheumatic disease is readily identified when leaflets are thickened and chordae are shortened; fibrosis of these structures restricts leaflet mobility. Leaflet prolapse with or without ruptured chordae tendineae also may cause atrioventricular valve regurgitation.

Transesophageal echocardiography images the heart from a retrocardiac position, which avoids interference from interposed ribs, lungs, and subcutaneous tissue. A high-frequency (5-MHz) transducer is employed, which yields better resolution than that of images obtained with routine transthoracic imaging with 2.25- to 3.5-MHz transducers.[7] Thus transesophageal echocardiography provides the best image of the mitral and tricuspid valves and may be obtained preoperatively. Intraoperative transesophageal Doppler echocardiography should be employed in all patients having valve repair or replacement, and the technique is especially important for assessment of response of MR to relief of left ventricular outflow obstruction.[8] In some cases, preoperative left ventriculography may help to quantify left atrioventricular valve leakage. Right ventricular angiocardiography also can be useful in determining the degree of tricuspid valve dysfunction, but it is rarely employed in current practice.[9]

Tricuspid Valve Regurgitation Secondary to Other Valvular Disease

Secondary tricuspid valve regurgitation commonly is associated with rheumatic mitral valve stenosis, and the exact cause is unknown.[10,11] Some authors believe that secondary tricuspid valve regurgitation is a result of pulmonary artery hypertension and right ventricular dilatation.[12] As with the mitral valve, tricuspid valve annular dilatation in those with severe TR is asymmetric. Most enlargement occurs in the annulus subtended by the free wall of the right ventricle, and there is little dilation of the annulus adjacent to the septal leaflet of the tricuspid valve.[13,14] Although pulmonary artery hypertension with secondary enlargement of the right ventricle and tricuspid valve annulus may be an important contributing factor in secondary tricuspid regurgitation (TR), it is not the sole mechanism. For example, congenital heart lesions such as tetralogy of Fallot produce

TABLE 44-2: Prevalence of Multiple Cardiac Valve Replacement According to Institution

	University of Alabama	Mayo Clinic	Texas Heart Institute	University of Oregon	Percentage of all Valve Surgery (11,026 cases)	Percentage of Multiple Valve Surgery (1662 cases)
Years involved	1967-1976	1963-1972	1962-1974	1960-1980		
Total number of all valve operations	2555	2166	4170	2135		
All multiple valve procedures	383 (15%)	437 (20%)	541 (13%)	301 (14%)	15 (1662)	100
M-A	298 (11.6%)	320 (14.7%)	459 (11%)	253 (11.8%)	12 (1330)	80
M-A-T	40 (1.6%)	55 (2.5%)	55 (2.5%)	48 (2.2%)	2 (198)	12
M-T	41 (1.6%)	58 (2.5%)	26 (0.6%)	—	1.5 (125)	8
A-T	4 (0.1%)	4 (0.2%)	1 (0.02%)	—	0.1 (9)	5

M, mitral valve; A, aortic valve; T, tricuspid valve.
Source: Data from Acker M, Hargrove WC, Stephenson LW: Multiple valve replacement, *Cardiol Clin* 1985; 3:425-430.

systemic pressure in the right ventricle, yet severe tricuspid valve regurgitation rarely is seen in these patients. Similarly, important tricuspid valve regurgitation is uncommon in children with ventricular septal defects who have enlargement of the right ventricle associated with variable degrees of pulmonary hypertension.

Furthermore, clinical experience suggests that other mechanisms must play a role in development of secondary tricuspid valve regurgitation. Patients who have had mitral valve replacement for rheumatic mitral valve stenosis may develop regurgitation of their native tricuspid valve years after initial operation, and many patients have only modest elevation of pulmonary artery pressure.[15,16] Recent evidence points to a progressive immunologic process in rheumatic valve disease, which can lead to severe TR many years after successful percutaneous or surgical management of the mitral valve.[17]

It is useful to classify secondary mitral and tricuspid valve regurgitation as mild, moderate, and severe.[14] Usually, patients with mild tricuspid valve regurgitation do not have clinical signs and symptoms of right-sided heart failure. Also, mild TR demonstrated by preoperative echocardiography may appear even less severe in the operating room under general anesthesia. In most instances, mild secondary TR does not require intervention.

Patients with echocardiographic evidence of significant regurgitation who do not have symptoms or have their symptoms controlled by medical treatment are managed with a DeVega suture annuloplasty or a partial-ring annuloplasty.[18] Patients with severe secondary TR and clinical evidence of right-sided heart failure (eg, pulsatile liver, distended neck veins, and peripheral edema with or without ascites) are most frequently managed by concomitant ring annuloplasty or tricuspid valve replacement.[19]

The degree of pulmonary hypertension may influence surgical management of secondary tricuspid valve regurgitation. Kaul et al[20] grouped 86 patients with functional TR in association with rheumatic mitral valve disease according to the degree of pulmonary hypertension. One group had severe pulmonary hypertension (mean pulmonary pressure 78 mm Hg), and a second group had moderate pulmonary hypertension (mean pulmonary artery pressure 41 mm Hg). Patients with moderate pulmonary hypertension preoperatively had more advanced right-sided heart failure and right ventricular dilatation, and many of these patients continued to have tricuspid valve regurgitation following mitral valve surgery without tricuspid valve surgery. The patients with severe pulmonary hypertension all showed regression of TR, and 28% had complete resolution following mitral valve surgery without operation on the tricuspid valve.

The difficulty with interpretation and generalization of current literature guiding management of secondary functional TR is the significant heterogeneity in both patient disease substrate and surgical procedure performed. The incidence of severe late TR has been reported to be approximately 68% up to 30 years following mitral replacement for rheumatic disease.[21] The risk of significant late secondary TR is as high as

74% 3 years following repair of ischemic MR.[22] The most frequently identified risk factors for TR progression from these series include older age, female gender, rheumatic etiology, atrial fibrillation, the absence of a Maze operation.[21-24] Therefore, most would agree that correction of moderate or greater TR at the time of surgery for rheumatic mitral disease is indicated to prevent the development of symptoms associated with TR progression.[25] Less clear however is whether long-term survival is improved by such intervention.[24] Recent evidence suggests that remodeling annuloplasty in the patients with tricuspid annular dilatation (≥70 mm) at the time of mitral repair significantly decreases the risk of subsequent functional deterioration compared with those having tricuspid valve repair.[26] Furthermore, reliance on tricuspid annular dilation alone as suggested by Dreyfus et al[26] has recently been challenged.[27]

In contrast, although mitral valve prolapse is the most frequent cause of MR in the developed world, there are few reports addressing the incidence and fate of functional TR following successful mitral valve repair. Recent data suggest that moderate or less functional TR does not progress as aggressively following repair of leaflet prolapse as in rheumatic or ischemic mitral disease subsets.[28,29] Outcomes following isolated mitral valve repair or replacement for degenerative MR with less than severe coexistent functional TR at Mayo Clinic support the notion that risk of TR progression is low after MVr or MVR for MV prolapse. The authors recommend timely MV surgery before the development of left atrial dilatation or pulmonary hypertension, which would be expected to decrease the risk of TR progression during follow-up. Current indications for concomitant tricuspid valve repair under these circumstances include: (1) moderately severe or severe TR, (2) right-sided heart failure symptoms with moderate or severe TR, (3) moderate TR with one of the followings: primary tricuspid valve disease, structural abnormalities of the tricuspid valve (including impingement of the tricuspid leaflets by pacemaker leads), a dilated right atrium and right ventricle, severe pulmonary hypertension, or atrial fibrillation.[19]

A long-term outcome study of the prognostic impact of isolated TR confirmed that the presence of a mild-to-moderate isolated TR was not associated with a survival difference in comparison to those with trivial regurgitation, even after multivariable adjustment ($p = .34$).[30] (In summary, asymptomatic, less-than-moderate functional TR associated with degenerative mitral valve disease is unlikely to progress or impact survival following successful mitral valve repair.)

VALVE SELECTION FOR MULTIPLE VALVE REPLACEMENT

When multiple valve replacement is confined to the left ventricle, replacement valves are generally chosen from the same class with respect to the need for anticoagulation and projected longevity. There are no theoretical or practical advantages to use of a tissue valve and a mechanical valve for mitral and aortic valve replacement, and studies show no reduction in the risk of thromboembolism, valve-related morbidity, or late death.[31,32]

In addition, a lower reoperation rate is reported for patients with two mechanical valves in the left ventricle compared with patients with one mechanical and one tissue valve.[31]

For tricuspid valve replacement, alone or in conjunction with other valve procedures, use of a bioprosthesis may have advantages in regard to minimizing risk of valve thrombosis.[33,34] Furthermore, there are few hemodynamic considerations in selecting a tricuspid prosthesis; the greater hemodynamic efficiency of mechanical valves compared with bioprostheses rarely is an issue in atrioventricular valve replacement, especially the tricuspid valve, in which the annulus diameter in adults is often 33 mm or more. In vitro studies demonstrate only minimal hemodynamic improvement with atrioventricular valves larger than 25 mm.[35]

SURGICAL METHODS

Aortic and Mitral Valve Replacement

CANNULATION

Arterial inflow is established by cannulation of the distal ascending aorta near the pericardial reflection just to the left of the origin of the innominate artery (Fig. 44-1A). Venous cannulation is simplified by using a two-stage cannula in the right atrium for venous return. Individual cannulation of the superior and inferior venae cavae is reserved for operations that require right atrial or ventricular incisions (Fig. 44-2A). Provisions for intraoperative autotransfusion are used routinely, and antifibrinolytic drugs such as aprotinin or epsilon-aminocaproic acid (Amicar) may be useful, especially in reoperations, in which pericardial adhesions may worsen bleeding.[36]

CARDIOPLEGIA

If the aortic valve is competent, myocardial protection during aortic cross-clamping is achieved by initial infusion of cold (4 to 8°C) blood cardioplegia through a tack vent placed in the aorta proximal to the clamp. The volume of cardioplegia needed to achieve diastolic arrest and uniform hypothermia depends on the heart size and the presence of aortic valve regurgitation. Generally, the initial volume of cardioplegia required for hearts with multiple valve disease is higher than that required for coronary revascularization because of myocardial hypertrophy. For patients without cardiac enlargement, we infuse approximately 10 mL/kg of body weight, whereas 15 mL/kg of body weight is used for patients with significant degrees of myocardial hypertrophy. Repeat infusions of 400 mL of cardioplegia are given directly into the coronary ostia at 20-minute intervals during aortic occlusion. We use custom-designed, soft-tipped coronary perfusion catheters to minimize the potential for trauma to the coronary ostia during intubation and infusion.[37]

If aortic valve regurgitation is moderate or severe, cardioplegia is infused directly into the coronary ostia. Initial aortotomy is facilitated by emptying the heart using suction on an aortic tack vent and temporarily reducing the cardiopulmonary bypass flow rate to maximize venous return. Some surgeons prefer retrograde infusion of cardioplegia,[38] and if this method is used, even larger volumes are necessary because of non-nutritive flow through the coronary venous system and variation in coronary venous anatomy.[39,40]

PROCEDURE

After cardioplegia, the aortic valve is inspected through an oblique aortotomy extended into the noncoronary aortic sinus (see Fig. 44-1B). Aortic valve regurgitation caused by cuspal perforation or prolapse of a congenitally bicuspid valve often can be repaired,[41] but the decision for or against aortic valve repair should take into consideration whether or not a mitral valve prosthesis will be needed. For example, even though aortic valve repair might seem technically possible, prosthetic replacement may be the best option for a patient who requires mitral valve replacement and will be maintained on warfarin for long-term anticoagulation.

Severe calcification of the valve, whether it is bicuspid or tricuspid, necessitates replacement;[42] therefore, the cusps are excised and annular calcium debrided carefully. The aortic annulus then is calibrated; experience has shown that subsequent replacement of the mitral valve usually reduces the aortic annular diameter by shortening the circumference that is in continuity with the attachment of the anterior mitral valve leaflet. Therefore, we routinely identify (but do not break the sterile packaging of) two aortic prostheses: one corresponds to the calibrated dimension, and the other is the next size smaller. Final selection of the aortic prosthesis is made after mitral valve replacement or repair.

Although exposed first, the aortic valve usually is replaced after mitral valve repair or insertion of the mitral valve prosthesis. Sutures placed in the portion of the aortic valve annulus that is continuous with the anterior leaflet of the mitral valve pull the anterior leaflet superiorly toward the left ventricular outflow area and thus hinder exposure of this area as viewed through the left atriotomy.

If the aortic annulus is small, it can be enlarged with a patch of pericardium.[43] This technique increases annular diameter by 2 to 4 mm or more, and only rarely are more radical techniques necessary.[44-46] Another maneuver to accommodate as large a prosthesis as possible is to place the necessary sutures for the mitral valve repair or replacement but not secure the mitral prosthesis until the aortic valve is implanted. This eliminates downsizing of the aortic prosthesis but does not compromise insertion of sutures in the superior portion of the mitral valve annulus.

After removal of the aortic valve, the right atrial cannula is repositioned, and the mitral valve is exposed through an incision posterior to the interatrial groove (see Fig. 44-1B). The presence or absence of thrombi in the left atrium is noted, and the mitral valve is inspected. When there is rheumatic disease of the aortic valve, the mitral valve almost always will be involved to some extent. If aortic valve replacement is necessary, the surgeon should have a low threshold for replacing a diseased mitral valve because scarring and fibrosis of the rheumatic process are progressive, and mitral valve

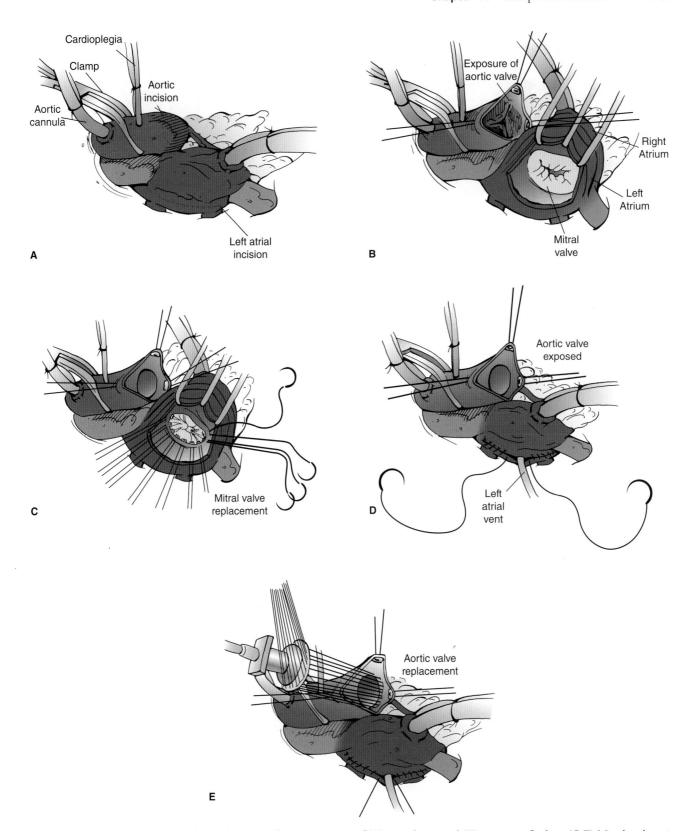

FIGURE 44-1 Aortic and mitral valve replacements showing sequence of (A) cannulation and (B) exposure of valves. (C-E) Mitral and aortic valve replacements showing the sequence of replacement of the mitral and aortic valves.

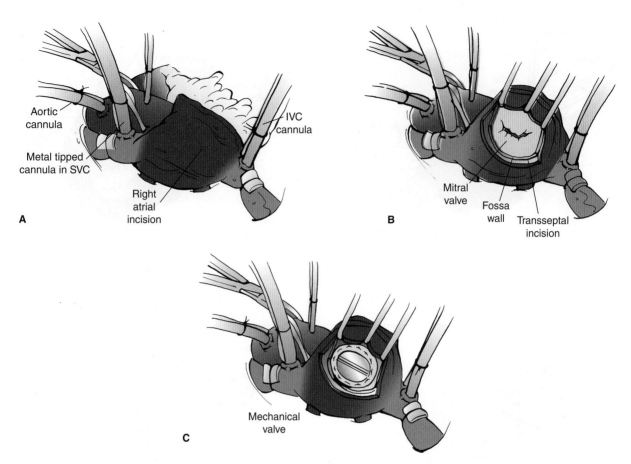

FIGURE 44-2 Combined mitral valve and tricuspid valve operation. The panels illustrate (A) cannulation, (B) transseptal incision, and (C) combined mitral valve and tricuspid valve operation: mitral replacement. (Superior vena cava snare not shown.)

repair (commissurotomy for stenosis or leaflet repair and annuloplasty for regurgitation) is less durable than repair for degenerative disease.[47-49] In contrast, when aortic valve replacement is necessary because of calcification of a bicuspid valve or senescent calcification, repair of mitral valve regurgitation owing to degenerative causes can be expected to give predictably good long-term results. Repair of the mitral valve is described in Chapter 41.

In preparation for replacement, the anterior leaflet of the mitral valve is excised, and when possible, a portion of the posterior leaflet with its chordal attachments is preserved to maintain left ventricular papillary muscle-annular continuity.[50-52] Some surgeons make a special effort to preserve the anterior leaflet and its chordal attachments, believing that this has a further beneficial effect on ventricular performance.[53] The mitral prosthesis is implanted using interrupted mattress sutures of 2-0 braided polyester reinforced with felt pledgets, which can be situated on the atrial or ventricular side of the valve annulus (see Fig. 44-1C). The leaflets of mechanical valves should be tested for free mobility following valve seating.

When atrial fibrillation is present preoperatively, we obliterate the left atrial appendage by oversewing its orifice from within the left atrium or ligating it externally. The left

atriotomy is closed from each end with running polypropylene sutures. Vent tubing is inserted through the partially closed left atriotomy and left in place while the aortic valve is being replaced (see Fig. 44-1D).

After appropriate exposure, the aortic prosthesis is sewn in place with interrupted 2-0 polyester mattress sutures backed with felt pledgets, and the aortotomy is closed, usually with two layers of 4-0 polypropylene. Any remaining air is evacuated from the heart with the usual maneuvers, and a tack vent in the ascending aorta is placed on suction as the aortic clamp is removed. The vent is removed from the left atrium, and closure of the left atriotomy is secured.

In patients with annuloaortic ectasia, the mitral valve sometimes can be visualized and replaced through the enlarged aortic annulus.[54]

Aortic Valve Replacement and Mitral Valve Repair

Intraoperative transesophageal echocardiography is useful in assessing the degree of MR and, importantly, in identifying the cause of valve leakage. When mitral valve regurgitation is only moderate and leaflet morphology is normal, we expect mitral valve function to improve following relief of

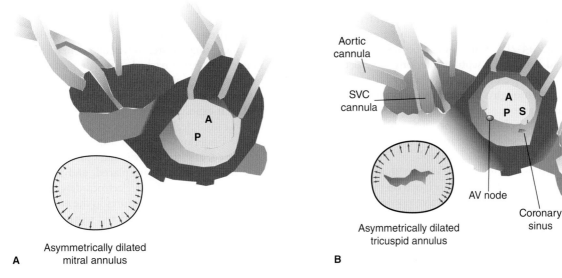

FIGURE 44-3 (A) Mitral valve repair and (B) tricuspid valve repair using a partial-ring annuloplasty. (Superior and inferior venae cavae snares not shown.)

severe aortic stenosis. In all other instances, the valve should be inspected directly to determine the need for repair or replacement.

Sternotomy, cannulation, and assessment of the aortic valve proceed as described previously. When there is no indication of tricuspid valve disease and no other right atrial procedures are planned, venous return is obtained through a single two-staged cannula (Fig. 44-3A). Specific techniques of mitral valve repair depend on operative findings.[55] Localized prolapse of a portion of the posterior leaflet with or without ruptured chordae usually is managed by triangular excision of that segment and repair with continuous 4-0 polypropylene suture.[56] Ruptured chordae to the anterior leaflet are replaced with 4-0 or 5-0 polytetrafluoroethylene (PTFE) sutures inserted into papillary muscle and through the free edge of the prolapsing leaflet.[57]

Almost all leaflet repairs are supplemented with a posterior annuloplasty. Interrupted 2-0 braided polyester mattress sutures are placed along the posterior circumference of the annulus ending at the right and left fibrous trigones (see Fig. 44-3A). Sutures then are spaced evenly through a flexible 6.0- to 6.5-cm–long partial ring; this standard length can be obtained by using a flexible 63-mm posterior annuloplasty band.[49,58] Following annuloplasty, competence of the mitral valve is tested by filling the ventricle with saline or blood; the atrium then is closed, and the aortic valve prosthesis is sewn into place.

Mitral Valve Replacement and Tricuspid Valve Replacement or Repair

In most instances, tricuspid valve regurgitation is caused by annular dilatation.[59] The severity of tricuspid valve leakage can be determined by transesophageal echocardiography before bypass and by digital exploration of the right atrium just before venous cannulation. Under general anesthesia,

changes in blood volume and cardiac output can cause significant fluctuation in the amount of regurgitation, and most often the severity of tricuspid valve leakage is lessened in the immediate prebypass period.

The patient's clinical condition must be correlated with echocardiographic findings and intraoperative assessment of the tricuspid valve. Patients with an enlarged, pulsatile liver, peripheral edema, and jugular venous distention are likely to require tricuspid valvuloplasty following mitral valve replacement or repair. Patients without the stigmata of right-sided heart failure usually have less severe valve leakage, and tricuspid valve function may improve without direct repair or replacement after left-sided valvular lesions are corrected.

The decision for repair or replacement of functional tricuspid valve regurgitation at the time of mitral valve replacement is important because the risk of subsequent reoperation is high. In our earlier experience, operative mortality was 25% in patients who required later reoperation for tricuspid valve regurgitation. Further, TR progresses in 10 to 15% of patients after replacement of rheumatic mitral valves.[60] Therefore, we maintain a liberal policy for annuloplasty or prosthetic replacement at initial operation.[61]

PROCEDURE

For operations on the tricuspid valve, insertion of a Swan-Ganz catheter is optional; if one is used, the catheter is withdrawn from the right heart chambers during inspection and assessment of the tricuspid valve. We prefer direct cannulation of the inferior and superior venae cavae.[62] After commencement of cardiopulmonary bypass and cardioplegia, the cavae are snared around the venous cannulae, and the interatrial septum and tricuspid valve are exposed through a right atriotomy (see Fig. 44-2A). A decision for repair or replacement of the tricuspid valve is made, and the necessary prosthesis is identified.

When the tricuspid valve is also addressed, we tend to expose the mitral valve through an incision in the interatrial septum, which crosses the fossa ovalis and can be extended superiorly (see Fig. 44-2B). Care should be taken during retraction to avoid tearing the septum inferiorly toward the coronary sinus and triangle of Koch. Alternatively, the mitral valve can be exposed through a standard left atriotomy posterior to the interatrial groove.

After repair or replacement of the mitral valve (see Fig. 44-2C), the septal or left atrial incision is closed, and the tricuspid valve is repaired or replaced. For tricuspid valve repair, we use either the DeVega method or ring annuloplasty.[12,18,63,64] Both techniques are based on the observation that the anterior and posterior valve portions of the tricuspid valve annulus are more prone to dilatation than the septal leaflet portion of the annulus, as described previously. When ring annuloplasty is indicated, we prefer a flexible device such as the Cosgrove-Edwards prosthesis[65] or a partial Duran ring (see Fig. 44-3B). The use of a partial ring avoids placement of sutures in the annulus near the penetrating bundle of His and reduces risk of injury to conduction tissue. There have been conflicting reports regarding the superiority of DeVega procedure versus prosthetic annuloplasty in improving freedom from recurrent TR.[66-68]

Minimally Invasive Approaches

Although addressed elsewhere in this textbook, minimally invasive approaches to primary and reoperative left- and right-sided valvular heart disease have been proposed. Various cannulation and cardioplegia techniques have been described as determined by the pattern of valve disease and patient anatomy.[69a,b]

Tricuspid Valve Replacement and Pulmonary Valve Replacement for Carcinoid Heart Disease

If there is no involvement of the mitral and aortic valves,[59,70] tricuspid and pulmonary valve replacement usually can be performed without the need for aortic occlusion and cardioplegic arrest. It is important to exclude the presence of a patent foramen ovale to eliminate the risk of air entering the left atrium, and if a defect in the atrial septum is identified, it is closed using a brief period of aortic occlusion. In the past, our strategy for patients with carcinoid heart disease was to replace the tricuspid valve and excise the diseased pulmonary valve.

Subsequent experience has suggested that right ventricular function is better preserved with a competent pulmonary valve, so we now favor pulmonary valve replacement rather than valvectomy.[71] Tricuspid valve replacement always is indicated, and it is usually necessary only to remove the anterior leaflet. A recent review of 200 patients with carcinoid heart disease at our institution demonstrated that prognosis has improved in the current era and that valve

replacement surgery was independently associated with prolonged survival.[72]

Carcinoid disease produces fibrosis and retraction of the leaflets, so anchoring sutures (interrupted mattress sutures of 2-0 braided polyester backed with felt pledgets) can be inserted into the remaining septal and posterior leaflets. We prefer to position the pledgets on the ventricular side of the valve annulus. If exposure is difficult, a brief period of aortic clamping and cardioplegic arrest is used during placement of sutures in the posterior and septal leaflets; the aortic cross-clamp is removed, and the heart is allowed to beat rhythmically. The remaining sutures are placed, and all sutures are secured with observation of the electrocardiogram. If atrioventricular block develops, the sutures in the area of the penetrating bundle of His are removed and reinserted in a more superficial location.

Pulmonary valve replacement is performed through a longitudinal incision across the valve annulus onto the outflow portion of the right ventricle. We prefer to insert the prosthetic valve using a continuous 3-0 polypropylene suture, anchoring the sewing ring to the native valve annulus for approximately two-thirds of the valve annulus and then anteriorly to a pericardial patch that is used routinely to augment the valve annulus and facilitate closure of the pulmonary artery and right ventricle.

Triple-Valve Replacement

Operative preparation is similar to that described previously. Usually left-sided valvular lesions are corrected before tricuspid valve procedures. Again, if there is aortic valve regurgitation, the aortotomy is performed first, and cardioplegia is administered; simultaneously, we snare the cavae and open the right atrium. After excision of the aortic valve and calibration of the annulus, the interatrial septum is incised, and the mitral valve is repaired or replaced. Next, the aortic valve is implanted, and after closure of the aortotomy and septotomy, the tricuspid valvuloplasty or prosthetic replacement can be performed without aortic cross-clamping.[73]

RHEUMATIC HEART DISEASE AFFECTING MULTIPLE VALVES

As shown in Table 44-3, rheumatic valvulitis is a common cause of multiple valve disease. Autopsy studies show that almost all patients with rheumatic heart disease have some involvement of the mitral valve, although it is not always evident clinically.[74] The percentages of multiple valve involvement in two autopsy studies of patients with rheumatic heart disease are shown in Table 44-4.

Forty-seven percent of those studied had involvement of more than one valve. Mitral and aortic valve disease was the most common combination and was present in 34% of patients; the second most common combination was mitral, aortic, and tricuspid valve disease (9%). A recent report has suggested that all four valves might be involved with the rheumatic process.[75]

TABLE 44-3: Reports of Operations for Multiple Valve Disease, Showing the High Incidence of Rheumatic Heart Disease

Study	Patients (no.)	Patients with rheumatic heart disease, % (no.)
Combined mitral and aortic replacement[150]	86	100 (86)
Combined mitral and aortic replacement[129]	92	100 (92)
Combined mitral and aortic replacement with tricuspid repair[62]	109	98 (107)
Triple-valve replacement[152]	48	100 (48)
Combined mitral and aortic replacement[101]	54	85 (46)
Multiple valve procedures[134]	50	86 (43)
Triple-valve replacement[33]	91	100 (91)
Combined mitral and aortic replacement[133]	65	80 (52)
Mitral replacement and tricuspid surgery[15]	32	81 (26)
Combined mitral and aortic replacement[160]	166	64 (106)
Mitral and aortic procedures[80]	124	100 (124)
Multiple valve procedures[166]	102	100 (102)
Combined mitral and aortic replacement[167]	33	82 (27)
Mitral and aortic regurgitation[168]	39	67 (26)
Mitral and aortic stenosis[88]	32	100 (32)
Mitral and aortic stenosis[86]	141	100 (141)

TABLE 44-4: Results of Autopsy Series (1910-1937) Showing Multiple Valve Involvement in 996 Patients with Rheumatic Heart Disease

Valve lesion at autopsy	Clawson[169]	Cooke and White[170]	Percentage of 996 patients studied
All combinations	321	147	47
M-A	221	100	32
M-A-T	52	35	9
M-T	31	7	4
M-A-T-P	14	5	2
A-T	2	0	0.2
A-M-P	1	0	0.1

A, aortic valve; M, mitral valve; T, tricuspid valve; P, pulmonary valve.
Source: Modified with permission from Acker M, Hargrove WC, Stephenson LW: Multiple valve replacement, *Cardiol Clin* 1985; 3:425-430.

TABLE 44-5: Patients with Rheumatic Mitral Stenosis Undergoing Valvotomy with Clinical Evidence of Multiple Valve Disease

Valve lesion at surgery	Patients (no.)	Percentage of 1000 patients with rheumatic mitral stenosis
All combinations	127	12.7
M-A	121	12.1
M-T	6	0.6

A, aortic valve; M, mitral valve; T, tricuspid valve. Does not include patients with tricuspid regurgitation.
Source: Modified with permission from Ellis LB, Harken DE, Black H: A clinical study of 1000 consecutive cases of mitral stenosis two to nine years after mitral valvuloplasty, *Circulation*. 1959 Jun;19(6):803-820.

Long-term follow-up of children with rheumatic heart disease suggests that approximately 50% of patients have multivalvular involvement.[76,77] In a study of patients undergoing mitral valvotomy for rheumatic mitral stenosis (Table 44-5), 13% had clinical evidence of other rheumatic valve stenosis or regurgitation. Most of these patients had associated rheumatic aortic disease.[78]

Rheumatic heart disease can cause valve stenosis, regurgitation, or a combination of lesions. The percentages of 290 patients with specific valvular lesions from four studies of multiple valve disease are shown in Table 44-6. Mixed lesions producing stenosis and regurgitation were encountered most commonly in both aortic and mitral valves.

Rheumatic Mitral Stenosis with Rheumatic Aortic Regurgitation

Approximately 10% of patients with rheumatic mitral valve stenosis also have rheumatic aortic regurgitation.[79,80] Clinical and laboratory characteristics of patients with mitral stenosis and aortic regurgitation are summarized in Table 44-7.

PATHOPHYSIOLOGY

In patients with mitral valve stenosis and aortic valve regurgitation, decreased cardiac output minimizes the classic signs of aortic regurgitation (eg, waterhammer pulse, head bobbing, and visibly pulsating capillaries). Also, concomitant mitral stenosis reduces left ventricular volume overload, which is a characteristic of isolated aortic regurgitation.[81] The underfilling of the left ventricle characteristic of mitral stenosis is offset by overfilling secondary to aortic valve regurgitation. Pulmonary artery hypertension characteristic of mitral stenosis usually is present.

OPERATIVE DECISION-MAKING

Patients with rheumatic mitral stenosis and rheumatic aortic regurgitation of more than a mild degree usually require replacement of both valves. Aortic valve repair is

TABLE 44-6: Hemodynamic Classification in Patients Undergoing Multiple Valve Surgery for Rheumatic Valvular Disease

	Combined mitral and aortic surgery[80]	Triple-valve replacement[152]	Combined mitral and aortic replacement[167]	Triple-valve replacement[33]	Totals
Number in study	124	48	27	91	290
MS	53% (66)	19% (9)	30% (8)	22% (20)	35.5% (103/290)
MR	47% (58)	10% (5)	52% (14)	12% (11)	30.3% (88/290)
MS/MR	—	71% (34)	19% (5)	66% (169)	34.1% (99/290)
AS	53% (66)	10% (5)	44% (12)	10% (9)	31.7% (92/290)
AR	47% (58)	35% (17)	41% (11)	33% (30)	40% (116/290)
AS/AR	—	54% (26)	15% (4)	57% (52)	28.3% (82/290)

AR, aortic regurgitation; AS, aortic stenosis; MR, mitral regurgitation; MS, mitral stenosis.

possible using techniques such as cuspal extension with glutaraldehyde-treated bovine or autologous pericardium[82] or the Trussler technique.[83] Although early results with cuspal extension have been good, inexorable progression of valve fibrosis may necessitate later prosthetic replacement for many patients.[84]

Preoperative transthoracic and intraoperative transesophageal echocardiography aids in assessing function of the aortic valve in patients requiring surgery for mitral stenosis. At operation, the degree of ventricular filling and amount of aortic root distention with infusion of cardioplegia are clues to important aortic valve regurgitation. As stated previously, if mitral valve replacement is necessary, serious consideration should be given to replacement of the aortic valve when there is moderate or worse leakage owing to rheumatic valvulitis.

Great care should be exercised to avoid ventricular distention if ventricular fibrillation occurs before aortic clamping. If ventricular fibrillation develops, distention of the heart can be prevented by inserting a left ventricular vent and compressing the heart manually. Also, even mild or moderate degrees of aortic regurgitation can complicate cardioplegia delivery through the proximal aorta.

TABLE 44-7: Characteristics of Patients with Combined Mitral Stenosis and Aortic Regurgitation

Mitral stenosis and aortic regurgitation	Terzaki et al[80]
Number of patients	26
Symptom of dyspnea	100% (26)
Electrocardiographic evidence of LVH	62% (16)
Roentgenographic evidence of LVH	54% (14)
Symptom of angina	23% (6)
Aortic diastolic pressure >70 mm Hg	46% (12)
Elevated LVEDP	38% (10)

LVEDP, left ventricular end-diastolic pressure; LVH, left ventricular hypertrophy.

Rheumatic Mitral Stenosis with Rheumatic Aortic Stenosis

PATHOPHYSIOLOGY

In contrast to isolated mitral stenosis, in which ventricular function frequently is preserved, the combination of mitral and aortic stenosis is associated with ventricular hypertrophy and diastolic dysfunction. The pressure load from the aortic stenosis causes a concentric hypertrophy with a small, noncompliant ventricular cavity.[80] Mitral stenosis compromises the ventricle's ability to maintain cardiac output (in contrast to isolated aortic stenosis, in which cardiac output is maintained).[85,86] The decrease in cardiac output minimizes the signs and symptoms of aortic stenosis and may make the diagnosis of aortic stenosis difficult.[87] Other hemodynamic parameters are similar to those of isolated mitral stenosis, for example, elevation of left atrial and pulmonary arterial pressures.[86,88]

OPERATIVE DECISION-MAKING

Although mitral valve stenosis sometimes can be treated effectively with valvuloplasty, commissurotomy for rheumatic aortic stenosis is indicated rarely. Thus, for patients with both aortic and mitral valve stenoses caused by rheumatic heart disease, we favor prosthetic replacement with mechanical prostheses if patients can manage long-term anticoagulation. If aortic valve stenosis is only mild and the decision is made not to replace the aortic valve at the time of mitral valve replacement, then the patient should be followed carefully, because more than 50% will develop moderate to severe disease by 15 years postoperatively.[89] The combination of aortic stenosis and mitral stenosis may present unique problems for the surgeon. First, concentric hypertrophy of the left ventricle may displace the mitral valve orifice anteriorly, producing poor exposure through a standard atriotomy; several maneuvers and alternative incisions are described for patients in whom mitral valve exposure is difficult.[87,90-94] Also, the small left ventricular cavity may impinge on struts of a stent-mounted bioprosthesis. There is also the potential for left ventricular outflow obstruction from high-profile prostheses in the mitral position in patients with aortic and mitral valve stenoses and small left ventricular cavity size.

Rheumatic Mitral Regurgitation with Rheumatic Aortic Regurgitation

PATHOPHYSIOLOGY

The combination of mitral and aortic valve regurgitation produces severe volume overload of the left ventricle. The reduction of impedance to ejection allows the ventricle to empty further, reducing ventricular wall tension with a resulting increase in the velocity of shortening.[95] Chronic volume overload increases stroke volume and distention of the left ventricle so that a larger stroke volume can be achieved with less myocardial fiber shortening than in normal hearts.[80] Patients who respond to increased volume load by left ventricular dilatation appear to tolerate surgical correction better than patients with left ventricular hypertrophy owing to an increased pressure load.[80] Patients with aortic valve regurgitation have augmented stroke volume to maintain an adequate cardiac output, but when MR coexists, part of the augmented stroke regurgitates into the left atrium and pulmonary veins. For this reason, when aortic regurgitation is severe, concomitant MR greatly reduces systemic cardiac output and can produce severe pulmonary congestion.[96]

OPERATIVE DECISION-MAKING

As stated previously, aortic valves involved with rheumatic disease usually require replacement. When the mitral valve also has rheumatic involvement, we replace the mitral valve at the time of aortic valve operation. After the aortic valve is excised, the mitral valve is inspected visually if it is suspected of being diseased or the degree of regurgitation is severe.

MYXOMATOUS AND PROLAPSING VALVE DISEASE AFFECTING MULTIPLE VALVES

Myxomatous degeneration is the most common etiology of MR requiring surgical correction in North America, and myxomatous aortic valve disease with annular dilatation is perhaps the most common cause of aortic regurgitation.[97-99] Most cases of isolated mitral or aortic valve prolapse are not associated with known connective tissue disorders.

TABLE 44-8: Incidence of Echocardiographic Evidence of Aortic Valve Prolapse in Patients with Mitral Valve Prolapse

	Ogawa et al[104]	Rippe et al[103]	Mardelli et al[171]	Total
Number of patients with MVP	50	400	75	525
Aortic valve prolapse	24% (12)	3% (11)	20% (15)	7% (38/525)
Aortic regurgitation	16% (8)	1% (4)	—	3% (12/450)
Aortic and mitral valve replacement	2% (1)	—	—	2% (1/50)

MVP, mitral valve prolapse. Number of patients in parentheses.

However, the coexistence of both mitral and aortic valvular prolapse together frequently can be seen in patients with connective tissue diseases such as Marfan's syndrome, Ehlers-Danlos syndrome, osteogenesis imperfecta, and others.[96]

Aortic valve regurgitation in patients with Marfan's syndrome is caused by progressive enlargement of the sinus portion of the aorta and the aortic valve annulus, that is, annuloaortic ectasia.[100,101] The principal causes of MR in patients with Marfan's syndrome are mitral annular dilatation, floppy or prolapsing leaflets, and mitral annular calcification.[101] The pathologic lesion in Marfan's syndrome is cystic medial necrosis, which is characterized by degeneration of elastic fibers and infrequent cysts.[101] Alterations in the synthesis and cellular secretion of fibrillin are responsible for the phenotypic characteristics of many patients with Marfan's syndrome.[102] Some patients have myxomatous cardiovascular lesions and annuloaortic ectasia without the other clinical characteristics of Marfan's syndrome.

Two-dimensional echocardiographic studies show that the frequency of aortic valve prolapse in patients with mitral valve prolapse varies between 3 and 24%[103,104] (Table 44-8). In one necropsy study, the frequency of MR in Marfan patients with aortic aneurysms (most with aortic regurgitation) was 54% (7 of 13).[101] About 17% of patients who undergo surgery for myxomatous aortic valve require surgical correction of MR (Table 44-9).

TABLE 44-9: Frequency of Mitral Valve Procedures in Patients Undergoing Aortic Valve Repair or Replacement for Myxomatous Degeneration, Prolapse, or Root Dilation

	David[172]	Gott et al[173]	Shigenobu et al[97]	Agozzino et al[100]	Bellitti et al[99]	Total
All aortic surgery	18	270	13	69	25	395
Number requiring concomitant mitral surgery	3 (17%)	36 (13%)	5 (38%)	16 (23%)	3 (12%)	73 (16%)

Although multiple valve involvement with myxomatous degeneration usually manifests as MR in combination with aortic regurgitation, in some cases, all four valves may be involved.[105] It is not clear whether the underlying pathology of isolated mitral valve prolapse is the same as the cardiovascular lesions that occur in Marfan's syndrome and other multiple-floppy-valve syndromes.[106,107]

Diagnosis, Signs, and Symptoms

Signs and symptoms of aortic and mitral valve regurgitation are reviewed in the section on rheumatic valvular disease. In addition to complete evaluation of the aortic and mitral valves and proximal aorta, patients with Marfan's syndrome should have assessment of the descending aorta for aneurysm or chronic dissection.

Operative Decision-Making

If annuloaortic ectasia is not present, patients with mitral and aortic valve regurgitation caused by myxomatous degeneration are candidates for repair of both valves. The aortic valve is inspected initially, and the decision for repair or prosthetic replacement is made depending on cuspal morphology. If tissue is sturdy and there is little prolapse or prolapse is limited to one cusp, repair can be undertaken with commissural narrowing and cusp resuspension. Often, aortic valve regurgitation is central, and simply narrowing the annulus by commissural plication restores valvular competence. Outcome of repair of both mitral and aortic valves has been good in terms of patient survival and freedom from valve-related complications, but reoperation is necessary in 35% of patients 10 years after the initial procedure; patients with most severe aortic valve regurgitation have an increased risk of late reoperation.[108] If tissue is attenuated, or if multiple cusps have severe prolapse, the valve is replaced.

In most instances, patients with Marfan's syndrome and aortic regurgitation require composite replacement of the aortic valve and ascending aorta.[109] Occasionally, moderate aortic regurgitation can be repaired at the time of aortic replacement by suspending the aortic valve inside a tube graft or remodeling the sinus portion of the aorta.[110] Even if the aortic valve is replaced with a composite graft and mechanical valve, the surgeon should favor repair of associated mitral regurgitation.[111] Gillinov and colleagues reported that valvuloplasty is possible in approximately 80% of patients with MR and Marfan's syndrome and that 5 years postoperatively 88% of patients are free of significant mitral valve insufficiency.[112]

Myxomatous Mitral Regurgitation with Tricuspid Regurgitation

Myxomatous degeneration also may involve the tricuspid valve, and presentation of mitral and tricuspid valve regurgitation owing to degenerative disease is not uncommon. In one study, 54% of patients with mitral valve prolapse also had tricuspid valve prolapse; however, most of these patients did not have significant regurgitation.[96] As with TR associated with rheumatic mitral disease, preoperative and intraoperative echocardiography is important in evaluating tricuspid disease in patients with myxomatous mitral regurgitation. In contrast with rheumatic disease, myxomatous mitral and tricuspid regurgitation almost always lends itself to valve repair.

SENILE CALCIFIC AORTIC VALVE DISEASE WITH MULTIPLE VALVE INVOLVEMENT

Unlike aortic stenosis caused by rheumatic disease, in which associated mitral valve disease is common, senile calcific aortic stenosis usually presents as an isolated lesion. Although the combination of mitral valve disease and senile calcific aortic stenosis is uncommon, senile aortic calcification is a frequent cause of aortic valve stenosis.[98] The incidence of senile calcific aortic disease has increased steadily in the last 20 years. Therefore, although mitral valve disease associated with calcific aortic stenosis is less common than that seen with rheumatic disease of the aortic valve, as the incidence of calcific aortic stenosis increases, so does the likelihood of encountering patients with disease of both valves.

Patterns of Multiple Valve Involvement with Calcific Aortic Stenosis

CALCIFIC AORTIC STENOSIS WITH INFECTIVE ENDOCARDITIS OF THE MITRAL VALVE

Stenotic aortic valves frequently are sites of infective endocarditis. As discussed in the section on endocarditis, the mitral valve may become involved with infective endocarditis by common abscess, by verrucous extension, or from a jet lesion, and infection may cause mitral valve aneurysm, perforation, and/or chordae disruption.[113] Management of these patients usually requires aortic valve replacement and assessment of the mitral valve at the time of operation. Vegetations of the mitral valve sometimes can be removed and perforations patched if the remaining tissue is sturdy and appears healthy.

CALCIFIC AORTIC STENOSIS WITH FUNCTIONAL MITRAL VALVE DISEASE

Senile calcification of the aortic valve may lead to mixed stenosis and regurgitation,[98] and the volume load from regurgitation may lead to left ventricular dilatation and secondary MR of an otherwise normal mitral valve.[98] MR secondary to aortic valvular disease is discussed in the section on pathophysiology of multiple valve disease.

CALCIFIC AORTIC STENOSIS WITH CALCIFICATION OF THE MITRAL VALVE

Degenerative calcification is an age-related process usually affecting the aortic and mitral valves. In a study of patients older than 75 years of age, one-third had degenerative aortic

TABLE 44-10: Comparison of Early Outcome between Patients having Multiple Valve Surgery for Infective Endocarditis and Patients having Multiple Valve Surgery for other Reasons[9,106]

	Class II	Class III	Class IV
Multiple valve procedures for infective endocarditis	20% (15)	33% (3)	20% (5)
Multiple valve procedures for other causes	16% (25)	12% (25)	36% (25)

Operative mortality is expressed as percentage, and numbers of patients are in parentheses.

or mitral calcification.[96] About 25 to 50% of patients with calcific aortic stenosis have calcification of the mitral valve annulus. Generally, patients with associated mitral annular calcification are older, have more severe aortic stenosis, and are more often female when compared with patients with aortic stenosis without mitral annular calcification.[114] Mills reported 17 patients undergoing mitral valve replacement for valvular disease related to severe annular calcification. Four of these patients also had concomitant aortic valve replacement.[115] Mitral annular calcification may exist in the setting of rheumatic or myxomatous disease.[116] These patients may have increased incidence of conduction defects,[117] aortic outflow murmurs, coronary artery disease,[118] and stroke.[119] Mitral repair or replacement is facilitated in some circumstances by removal of the annular calcium bar and pericardial reconstruction.[120]

Table 44-10 compares New York Heart Association (NYHA) class-matched groups that had multiple valve procedures for infective endocarditis and for other reasons.

CARCINOID HEART DISEASE AFFECTING MULTIPLE VALVES

Valvular heart disease develops in about 50% of patients with carcinoid tumors; patients with primary carcinoid tumor in the small intestine are more likely to have carcinoid heart disease than those with carcinoid tumors in other locations.[1] In most cases, the tricuspid and pulmonary valves are involved. We have offered valvular surgery to patients with severe symptoms of right-sided heart failure caused by carcinoid heart disease whose systemic carcinoid symptoms are controlled by octreotide and/or hepatic dearterialization.[121] Patients who are being considered for complete resection of hepatic metastases after control of the primary tumor are also candidates for extirpation of cardiac disease and valve replacement. A recent review of 200 patients with carcinoid heart disease from our institution revealed that survival has improved over the past decade. Multivariate analysis indicated that valve replacement surgery was associated with a risk reduction of 0.48.[70]

Diagnosis, Signs, and Symptoms

Jugular venous distention with v-waves (from TR) and a-waves (from tricuspid stenosis) can be evident. Right ventricular enlargement can produce a pericardial lift. Most patients have murmurs from the tricuspid and pulmonary valves.[121] Patients often demonstrates ascites and liver enlargement as a result of either right-sided heart failure or hepatic metastases or both. Therefore, these findings are not necessarily indicative of severe tricuspid valve regurgitation.

The electrocardiogram of patients with carcinoid heart disease often shows low voltage (85%), right bundle-branch block (42%), and evidence of right atrial enlargement (35%).[1,121] The chest x-ray characteristically shows cardiomegaly (69%), pleural effusions (58%), and pleural thickening (35%).[121]

Echocardiography

Echocardiographic findings of carcinoid heart disease include thickening and reduced motion of the tricuspid valve leaflets; the pulmonic valve cusps may be thickened and retracted. Fusion of the pulmonary valve commissures results in a stiff fibrotic ring that may cause a stricture in the entire pulmonary orifice. Pulmonary regurgitation and stenosis both may be present.[122]

Invasive Studies

Cardiac catheterization is not necessary unless ischemic symptoms or a history of myocardial infarction suggests coronary artery disease.

Pathophysiology

Carcinoid heart disease results from deposition of plaques on the endocardium of the valves and atria; this usually occurs on the right side of the heart. However, plaques can develop on the mitral and aortic valves when there is carcinoid tumor in the lungs or in the presence of intracardiac shunting that bypasses the lungs. Valves are damaged by exposure to circulating substances released from carcinoid tumors such as serotonin and bradykinin. Both these components are inactivated by the lungs and the liver; the relationship between tumor location and the location of cardiac lesions is summarized in Table 44-11.[123] The plaques usually deposit on the downstream side of the cardiac valves, causing adherence of the leaflet to the underlying structures and producing functional regurgitation. Carcinoid plaque deposition also may constrict the valve annulus and produce stenosis.[1]

The dominant functional lesion of carcinoid heart disease is tricuspid valve regurgitation; the valve is fixed in a semiopen position so that some degree of stenosis is present. Fibrosis and plaque deposition also affect the pulmonary valve, causing mixed stenosis and regurgitation, which increases the degree of TR.[1]

TABLE 44-11: A Comparison of Venous Drainage, Presence of Liver Metastases, and Carcinoid Plaque Location in Relation to Location of Primary Carcinoid Tumor[174]

Tumor location	Venous drainage	Liver metastases	Plaque location
Gut	Portal	Yes	Right-sided
Ovary	Systemic	No	Right-sided
Bronchial	Pulmonary	No	Left-sided

Operative Decision-Making

TIMING OF OPERATION

The primary indications for surgery are increasing symptoms of congestive failure with objective evidence of valvular disease.[124] Again, it should be noted that some of the signs of right-sided heart failure, such as peripheral edema, ascites, and hepatomegaly, can be caused by the primary disease. Another indication for operation may be progressive right ventricular enlargement in the absence of symptoms. In a small series of carcinoid patients, right ventricular size and function did not correlate with operative or late mortality.[121] Currently, we employ exercise testing to provide an objective assessment of the functional status and a guideline to the timing of cardiac surgery. If the primary cause for debilitation is right-sided heart failure, it is reasonable to offer valve replacement even though the prognosis may be guarded.[125]

Tricuspid Valve Operation

The tricuspid valve always requires replacement, and in our earlier experience, we used mechanical prostheses because of the possibility of carcinoid plaque formation on a bioprosthesis. However, review of our patients and those reported previously shows little difference in patient survival with mechanical or tissue valves. Bioprostheses are selected for patients who have liver dysfunction that would complicate anticoagulation with Coumadin and those who will undergo subsequent hepatic resection or hepatic artery embolization.

Pulmonary Valve Options

As stated previously, we now advise valve replacement rather than excision when the pulmonary valve is involved.

Management of the carcinoid syndrome during and early after operation is critically important, and this has been simplified greatly by treatment with long-acting octreotide; this is supplemented intraoperatively with intravenous administration of short-acting octreotide when there is evidence of flushing and vasodilatation.[126] Preoperative steroids and antihistamines also can be used to prevent adverse effects from tumor-released mediators.[126,127] We usually give octreotide, 500 μg intravenously, before induction of anesthesia, with additional intravenous doses given as needed at the onset

TABLE 44-12: Rare Causes of Multiple Valve Disease Requiring Surgery

Disease	Valves replaced or repaired
Methysergide/ergotamine toxicity[96]	Aortic and mitral
Fenfluramine-phentermine[175]	Left and right heart valves
Ergot-derived dopamine agonists[176]	Left and right heart valves
3,4 Methylenedioxymethamphetamine (Ecstasy)[177]	Mitral and tricuspid
Radiation injury[174,178]	Mitral and tricuspid
Q-fever endocarditis[179]	Aortic and mitral
Ectodermal anhydrotic dysplasia[180]	Aortic and mitral
Maroteaux-Lamy syndrome (mucopolysaccharidosis type VI)[181]	Aortic and mitral
Werner syndrome (adult progeria)[182]	Aortic and mitral
Blunt trauma[183]	Mitral and tricuspid
Lymphoma[184]	Aortic and mitral
Relapsing polychondritis[185]	Aortic and mitral
Systemic lupus erythematosus[186]	Mitral and tricuspid
Secondary hyperparathyroidism[187]	Aortic and mitral
Urticarial vasculitis syndrome (HUVS) with Jaccoud hands deformity[188]	Aortic and mitral

and termination of cardiopulmonary bypass. Postoperatively, octreotide is continued, and the dose is adjusted according to the severity of the flushing and vasodilatation. Aprotinin, a kallikrein inhibitor, may mitigate the effects of substances released by carcinoid tumors during anesthesia and reduce intraoperative and postoperative bleeding.[126]

RARE CAUSES OF MULTIPLE VALVE DISEASE

Table 44-12 lists some rare causes of multiple heart valve disease that require surgical correction.

RESULTS OF MULTIPLE VALVE SURGERY

Long- and Short-Term Mortality

Survival following multiple valve surgery has improved along with refinements in myocardial protection; for example, mortality for multiple valve operations performed using normothermic ischemic arrest was approximately 40%;[128] the use of cardioplegic arrest reduced operative risk by three-fourths.[80,128,129] In recent reports,[130] operative mortality (30-day mortality or hospital mortality) ranges from about 6 to 17% (Table 44-13, part A). The 5-year actuarial survival is 60 to 88% (see Table 44-13, part B), and the 10-year actuarial survival is 43 to 81% (see Table 44-13, part C).

TABLE 44-13: Summary of Morbidity and Mortality Following Multiple Valve Surgery

	DVR	MVR	AVR	*p* value	Valve type	Reference
A. Operative mortality (percent)	5.6				Various*	Teoh et al[132]
	5.9	4.3	2	—	SJM	Horstkotte et al[144]
	6.3	5.2	3.1	—	SJM	Smith et al[189]
	6.5				SJM	Armenti et al[129]
	7.2	4.7	3.9	—	SJM	Aoyagi et al[165]
	8.0	—	—	—	SJM	Emery et al[190]
	8.2	4.3	2.4	—	SJM	Ibrahim et al[191]
	10				Hancock II	David et al[192]
	10.5				C-E	Jamieson et al[193]
	10.8	11.3	7.8	—	Sorin Disc	Milano et al[194]
	10.8				Various*	Galloway et al[130]
	11.6	7.5	5.1	—	C-E	Bernal et al[139]
	15.5	—	—	—	Various	Leavitt et al[195]
	17.5				Various*	Mattila et al[134]
B. 5-Year actuarial survival (percent)	88	88	91	N.S.	SJM	Aoyagi et al[165]
	86	86	94	MVR or DVR < AVR *p* < .05	<SJM	Smith et al[189]
	78				Various*	Galloway et al[130]
	75				C-E	Bernal et al[139]
	73				Hancock II	David et al[192]
	70				C-E	Jamieson et al[193]
	62				MIPB	Lemieux et al[196]
	61	65	75	DVR < MVR or AVR *p* < .01	SJM	Khan et al[128]
	60				SJM	Armenti et al[129]
	****	****	****	DVR < AVR or MVR *p* < .006	B-S	Alvarez et al[136]
C. 10-Year actuarial survival (percent)	81	80	81	N.S.	SJM	Aoyagi et al[165]
	72	78	85	—	SJM	Horstkotte et al[144]
	60	59	71	N.S.	SJM	Ibrahim et al[191]
	55	63	65	—	B-S	Orszulak et al[197]
D. Thromboembolism (percent per patient-year)	0.3	0.3	0.6	—	SJM	Smith et al[189]
	0.79	1.6	1.3	—	SJM	Nakano et al[198]
	1.3	1.1	1.0	N.S.	SJM	Aoyagi et al[165]
	2.1				Various*	Mattila et al[134]
	2.1	1.2	1.3	N.S.	Sorin Disc	Milano et al[194]
	4.5				Various*	Mullany et al[62]
	4.6				SJM	Armenti et al[129]
	4.6	4.3	2.1	—	B-S	Orszulak et al[197]
	5.0	4.4	2.4	—	SJM	Ibrahim et al[191]
	6.6	5.1	3.7	—	SJM	Horstkotte et al[144]
E. 10-Year freedom from thromboembolism (percent)	89	92	91	—	C-E pericardial	Pelletier et al[199]
	89	89	94	N.S.	SJM	Aoyagi et al[165]
	89	83	—	—	C-E	van Doorn et al[200]
	86	88	80	—	Hancock II	David et al[192]
	77	79	87	—	B-S	Orszulak et al[197]
	ξ	ξ	ξ	N.S.	B-S	Alvarez et al[136]

(Continued)

TABLE 44-13: Summary of Morbidity and Mortality Following Multiple Valve Surgery (*Continued*)

	DVR	MVR	AVR	*p* value	Valve type	Reference
F. Anticoagulation-related	0.1	0.2	0.1	—	SJM	Nakano et al[198]
hemorrhage (percent per	0.5	0.3	0.4	—	SJM	Aoyagi et al[165]
patient-year)	0.9	0.9	0.9	N.S.	Sorin Disc	Milano et al[194]
	1.2				SJM	Armenti et al[129]
	1.2	0.7	0.2	—	SJM†	Horstkotte et al[144]
	4.5	2.1	1.2	—	SJM‡	Horstkotte et al[144]
	ξ	ξ	ξ	DVR > AVR or MVR *p* < .05	B-S	Alvarez et al[136]
G. Endocarditis (percent per	0.2	0.06	0.21	—	St. Jude	Nakano et al[198]
patient-year)	0.3	0.03	0.4	—	St. Jude	Aoyagi et al[165]
	2.1				Various*	Mattila et al[134]
	2.5				SJM	Armenti et al[129]
	ξ	ξ	ξ	DVR > AVR or MVR *p* < .05	B-S	Alvarez et al[136]
H. 8-, 10-, and 15-year freedom	77	79	87	—	C-E pericardial	Pelletier et al[199]
from structural deterioration	59.6	70.8		—	C-E	van Doorn et al[200]
for bioprostheses (percent)	44	33	62	*p* < .03	C-E	Bernal et al[145]
	38	58	80	DVR < MVR, AVR *p* < .05	MP	Pomar et al[141]

*Includes some patients with concomitant tricuspid procedures.
†dR INR 1.75 2.75.
‡INR 4 = 6.
ξResults reported graphically.
Comparisons to isolated aortic and mitral valve procedures from the same series are included when available. If statistical analysis between the results of multiple and single valve procedures was reported, the p values are included. If a series was limited to a single valve type, it is listed.
AVR, isolated aortic valve replacement; B-S, Björk-Shiley; C-E, Carpentier-Edwards; DVR, double-valve replacement; MIPB, medtronic intact porcine bioprosthesis; MP, mitroflow pericardial; MVR, isolated mitral valve replacement; N.S., not statistically significant; SJM, St. Jude Medical.

Risk factors identified for morbidity and mortality following multiple valve surgery include advanced NYHA class,[131-133] advanced age,[131-135] current or prior myocardial revascularization,[134] ejection fraction,[131] presence of coronary artery disease,[131,132] aortic stenosis,[136] elevated pulmonary artery pressure,[134] TR,[136] and diabetes mellitus.[134]

Clearly, operative mortality is influenced by patient selection,[133] and comparisons among studies are of limited value.[133] Causes of death after multiple valve surgery are low cardiac output,[133,136-139] myocardial infarction,[134] technical failure,[139] multiple-organ failure,[34] ventricular rupture,[101,134,137] and mechanical obstruction of the prosthetic leaflet.[101,138] Comparisons of late survival between patients having multiple valve versus single-valve replacement are inconsistent. Some studies show poorer survival[132] after multiple valve replacement, and others report no significant difference in survival.[34,125,128,135-140] The discrepancy in these results may be because the majority of deaths in many reports are secondary to progression of coronary artery disease and noncardiac causes rather than valve-related issues.[129,131] The presence of coronary artery disease and concomitant coronary artery surgery increases mortality following multiple valve surgery.[134,141,142]

Some causes of early death following multiple valve surgery are perhaps less common today owing to changes in practice.

In a necropsy study from 1963 to 1985 of patients who died early following double-valve replacement, prosthetic valve dysfunction secondary to mechanical interference was evident in almost 50%, and ventricular rupture had occurred in 15% of patients.[101] Most of these patients received Starr-Edwards caged-ball prosthetic valves. Mechanical failure of low-profile tilting-disk prostheses that are in current use is rare, and early valve-related death with this type of prosthesis is very unusual.[34,132,133,143] The current practice of preserving the posterior leaflet and chordal attachments of the mitral valve during prosthetic replacement may decrease the chance of ventricular disruption.[144]

Thromboembolism

Thromboembolic rates following multiple valve replacement are shown in Table 44-13, part D, and range from 1 to 7% per patient-year for double-valve replacement. Ten years postoperatively, freedom from thromboembolic events ranges from 77 to 89% (see Table 44-13, part E). Although the data presented in Table 44-13, part D, along with other sources,[145] do not indicate significant differences between single-valve replacement and multiple valve replacement, some reports suggest that both mechanical[146] and bioprosthetic[147] valves have an increased risk of thromboembolism in the mitral position.

This risk is present early (90 days after operation) in patients undergoing multiple valve replacement that includes a bioprosthetic mitral valve.[147]

Anticoagulation-Related Hemorrhage

Rates of anticoagulant-related hemorrhage following multiple valve replacement, as with single-valve surgery, depend on target international normalization ratio (INR).[148] Risks of hemorrhage are reported to be 0.1 to 4.5% per patient-year following multiple valve surgery (see Table 44-13, part F). Alvarez et al reported a significantly higher rate of anticoagulant-related hemorrhage following multiple valve replacement than following single-valve replacement.[136]

Prosthetic Valve Infective Endocarditis

Rates of infective endocarditis following multiple valve surgery range from 0.2 to 2.5% per patient-year, as shown in Table 44-13, part G. In comparison with isolated valve surgery, Alvarez et al reports that prosthesis infection is more frequent following double-valve replacement than following either isolated aortic ($p < .05$) or mitral valve replacement ($p < .001$).[136]

Valve Performance

Rates of bioprosthetic structural deterioration relate to valve position; tissue valves appear to fail earlier in the mitral position than in the aortic position. When multiple valve replacements include the mitral valve, the rates of deterioration are similar[149] or even worse than[145] isolated mitral valve replacement (see Table 44-13, part H).

COMPARISON OF BIOPROSTHETIC VALVES TO MECHANICAL VALVES

Comparisons of outcomes of patients with two or more mechanical prostheses with those of patients with two or more bioprostheses show similar rates of thromboembolism,[28,148] but freedom from operation favors those with multiple mechanical valves.[31,150,151] As might be expected, anticoagulation-related hemorrhage is less in patients with two bioprosthetic valves,[150,152] but there is no clear advantage of one prosthesis over the other in terms of early and late mortality.[31,150,152]

Results of Tricuspid Valve Procedures with Other Valve Procedures

RESULTS OF MITRAL AND TRICUSPID VALVE OPERATIONS

Reported operative mortality following mitral valve replacement and tricuspid valve repair or replacement is approximately 12 to 15%,[153] and 65 to 75% of patients are alive 5 years postoperatively.[134,153] Outlook for patients with lesser degrees of TR at the time of mitral valve replacement is good; 5-year actuarial survival for patients with TR who do not have tricuspid valve repair or replacement is 80 to 84%, and 10-year survival is 62 to 77%.[154]

Triple-Valve Surgery

The median age of 8021 triple-valve patients studied in the STS ACSD was 67 years; 60% were women; 4488 (56%) had NYHA class III to IV symptoms; and mean ejection fraction was 50%. The frequency of mitral valve repair increased over the period of the study from 13 to 41%. Tricuspid valve repair also became more frequent over time from 86 to 96%. The incidence of early death declined from 17 to 9%. Importantly, the performance of mitral and tricuspid valve repair (vs replacement) diminished the likelihood of postoperative death.[155]

Double-Valve Replacement

In North America, mortality for mitral and tricuspid replacement was 16.8% (n=1,130). For patients having mitral valve repair and tricuspid valve replacement (n=216) mortality was 10.2%, and for patients undergoing mitral valve replacement and tricuspid valve repair (n=11,448) mortality was 10.2%. Operative risk of combined mitral and tricuspid valve repair was 8.0% (n=8,262).[155a] Independent predictors of mortality were age, renal failure with dialysis, emergency status, second or more reoperations, later surgical date, and valve repair. The authors suggested that expanding efforts to repair mitral and tricuspid valves in patients requiring double-valve surgery appear warranted.

Rates of thromboembolism in patients with double-valve replacements are reported to be 5% per patient-year.[62]

Other Results

The operative mortality for double re-replacement is about 10 to 20%.[132,156] Incidence of postoperative ventricular arrhythmias is higher in patients having combined valve surgery than in those having single-valve surgery.[157] Hemolysis may be more common with multiple valve disease or following multiple valve replacement.[158,159]

The incidence of perivalvular leak following multiple valve surgery is about 4% per patient-year and may be more frequent following multiple valve surgery than following single-valve surgery.[138,140]

When multiple valve surgery is combined with myocardial revascularization, the morbidity and mortality are 12 to 24%.[141,160] Early death in this group of patients is associated with prolonged perfusion time, the need for postoperative inotropic support, and high blood loss.[165]

Triple-valve surgery via a right thoracotomy has been reported.[161,162] Proposed benefits include quicker return to normal activity, a shorter mechanical ventilation time, and less blood loss. The ability to disseminate the techniques necessary for the performance of this procedure in the general cardiac surgical community will need to be further explored.[163]

REFERENCES

1. Knott-Craig CJ, Schaff HV, Mullany CJ, et al: Carcinoid disease of the heart: surgical management of 10 patients. *J Thorac Cardiovasc Surg* 1992; 104:475.

2. Schulman DS, Remetz MS, Elefteriades J, et al: Mild mitral insufficiency is a marker of impaired left ventricular performance in aortic stenosis. *J Am Coll Cardiol* 1989; 13:796.

3. Thourani VH, Suri RM, Rankin JS, et al: Does mitral valve repair offer an advantage over replacement in patients undergoing aortic valve replacement? *Ann Thorac Surg* 2014; 98(2):598-603.

4. Christenson JT, Jordan B, Bloch A, et al: Should a regurgitant mitral valve be replaced simultaneously with a stenotic aortic valve? *Texas Heart Inst J* 2000; 27:350.

5. Harris KM, Malenka DJ, Haney MF, et al: Improvement in mitral regurgitation after aortic valve replacement. *Am J Cardiol* 1997; 80:741.

6. Barreiro CJ, Patel ND, Fitton TP, et al: Aortic valve replacement and concomitant mitral valve regurgitation in the elderly: impact on survival and functional outcome. *Circulation* 2005; 112:I-443.

7. Freeman WK, Seward JB, Khandheria BK, et al: *Transesophageal Echocardiography*. Boston, Little Brown, 1994.

8. Nowrangi SK, Connolly HM, Freeman WK, et al: Impact of intra-operative transesophageal echocardiography among patients undergoing aortic valve replacement for aortic stenosis. *J Am Soc Echocardiogr* 2001; 14:863.

9. McGrath L, Gonzalez-Lavin L, Bailey B, et al: Tricuspid valve operations in 530 patients: twenty-five-year assessment of early and late phase events. *J Thorac Cardiovasc Surg* 1990; 99:124.

10. Farid L, Dayem MK, Guindy R, et al: The importance of tricuspid valve structure and function in the surgical treatment of rheumatic mitral and aortic disease. *Eur Heart J* 1992; 13:366.

11. Pellegrini A, Colombo T, Donatelli F, et al: Evaluation and treatment of secondary tricuspid insufficiency. *Eur J Cardiothorac Surg* 1992; 6:288.

12. Carpentier A, Deloche A, Hannia G, et al: Surgical management of acquired tricuspid valve disease. *J Thorac Cardiovasc Surg* 1974; 67:53.

13. Wilson WR, Danielson GK, Giuliani ER, et al: Cardiac valve replacement in congestive heart failure due to infective endocarditis. *Mayo Clin Proc* 1979; 54:223.

14. Cohn LH: Tricuspid regurgitation secondary to mitral valve disease: when and how to repair. *J Cardiol Surg* 1994; 9:237.

15. King RM, Schaff HV, Danielson GK, et al: Surgery for tricuspid regurgitation, late after mitral valve replacement. *Circulation* 1984; 70:193.

16. Izumi C, Iga K, Konishi T: Progression of isolated tricuspid regurgitation late after mitral valve surgery for rheumatic mitral valve disease. *J Heart Valve Dis* 2002; 11:353.

17. Henein MY, O'Sullivan CA, Li W, et al: Evidence for rheumatic valve disease in patients with severe tricuspid regurgitation long after mitral valve surgery: the role of 3D echo reconstruction. *J Heart Valve Dis* 2003; 12(5):566-572.

18. DeVega NG: La anuloplastia selectiva reguable y permanente. *Rev Esp Cardiol* 1972; 25:6.

19. Shinn SH, Schaff HV: Evidence-based surgical management of acquired tricuspid valve disease. *Nat Rev Cardiol* 2013; 10(4):190-203.

20. Kaul TK, Ramsdale DR, Mercer JL: Functional tricuspid regurgitation following replacement of the mitral valve. *Int J Cardiol* 1991; 33:305.

21. Porter A, Shapira Y, Wurzel M, et al: Tricuspid regurgitation late after mitral valve replacement: clinical and echocardiographic evaluation. *J Heart Valve Dis* 1999; 8(1):57-62.

22. Matsunaga A, Duran CM: Progression of tricuspid regurgitation after repaired functional ischemic mitral regurgitation. *Circulation* 2005; 112 (9 Suppl):I453-457.

23. Kim HK, Kim YJ, Kim KI, et al: Impact of the maze operation combined with left-sided valve surgery on the change in tricuspid regurgitation over time. *Circulation* 2005; 112 (9 Suppl):I14-19.

24. Je HG, Song H, Jung SH, et al: Impact of the maze operation on the progression of mild functional tricuspid regurgitation. *J Thorac Cardiovasc Surg* 2008; 136(5):1187-1192.

25. Kwak JJ, Kim YG, Kim MK, et al: Development of tricuspid regurgitation late after left-sided valve surgery: a single-center experience with long-term echocardiographic examinations. *Am Heart J* 2008; 155(4):732-737.

26. Dreyfus GD, Corbi PJ, Chan KM, Bahrami T: Secondary tricuspid regurgitation or dilatation: which should be the criterion for surgical repair? *Ann Thorac Surg* 2005; 79:127.

27. Chan V, Burwash IG, Lam BK, et al: Clinical and echocardiographic impact of functional tricuspid regurgitation repair at the time of mitral valve replacement. *Ann Thorac Surg* 2009; 88(4):1209-1215.

28. Rajbanshi BG, Suri RM, Nkomo VT et al: Influence of mitral valve repair versus replacement on the development of late functional tricuspid regurgitation. *J Thorac Cardiovasc Surg* 2014; 148(5):1957-1962.

29. Topilsky Y, Nkomo VT, Vatury O, et al: Clinical outcome of isolated tricuspid regurgitation. *JACC Cardiovasc Imaging* 2014; 7(12):1185-1194.

30. Calafiore AM, Gallina S, Iaco AL, et al: Mitral valve surgery for functional mitral regurgitation: should moderate-or-more tricuspid regurgitation be treated? A propensity score analysis. *Ann Thorac Surg* 2009; 87(3):698-703.

31. Bortolotti U, Milano A, Testolin L, et al: Influence of type of prosthesis on late results after combined mitral-aortic valve replacement. *Ann Thorac Surg* 1991; 52:84.

32. Brown PJ, Roberts CS, McIntosh CL, et al: Relation between choice of prostheses and late outcome in double-valve replacement. *Ann Thorac Surg* 1993; 55:631.

33. Gersh BJ, Schaff HV, Vatterott PJ, et al: Results of triple valve replacement in 91 patients: perioperative mortality and long-term follow-up. *Circulation* 1985; 72:130.

34. Kawano H, Oda T, Fukunaga S, et al: Tricuspid valve replacement with the St Jude Medical valve: 19 years of experience. *Eur J Cardiothorac Surg* 2000; 18:565.

35. Struber M, Campbell A, Richard G, et al: Hydrodynamic performance of carbomedics valves in double valve replacement. *J Heart Valve Dis* 1994; 3:667.

36. Levi M, Cromheecke ME, de Jonge E, et al: Pharmacological strategies to decrease excessive blood loss in cardiac surgery: a meta-analysis of clinically relevant endpoints. *Lancet* 1999; 354:1940.

37. Tyner JJ, Hunter JA, Najafi H: Postperfusion coronary stenosis. *Ann Thorac Surg* 1987; 44:418.

38. Talwalkar NG, Lawrie GM, Earle N: Can retrograde cardioplegia alone provide adequate protection for cardiac valve surgery? *Chest* 1999; 115:1359.

39. Villanueva FS, Spotnitz WD, Glasheen WP, et al: New insights into the physiology of retrograde cardioplegia delivery. *Am J Physiol* 1995; 268:H1555.

40. Ruengsakulrach P, Buxton BF: Anatomic and hemodynamic considerations influencing the efficiency of retrograde cardioplegia. *Ann Thorac Surg* 2001; 71:1389.

41. Fraser CD, Jr, Wang N, Mee RB, et al: Repair of insufficient bicuspid aortic valves. *Ann Thorac Surg* 1994; 58:386.

42. Cosgrove DM, Ratliff NB, Schaff HV, Eards WD: Aortic valve decalcification: history repeated with a new result. *Ann Thorac Surg* 1994; 49:689.

43. Piehler JM, Danielson GK, Pluth JR, et al: Enlargement of the aortic root or annulus with autogenous pericardial patch during aortic valve replacement: long-term follow-up. *J Thorac Cardiovasc Surg* 1983; 86:350.

44. Ross DB, Trusler GA, Coles JG, et al: Successful reconstruction of aorto-left atrial fistula following aortic valve replacement and root enlargement by the Manouguian procedure. *J Cardiol Surg* 1994; 9:392.

45. de Vivie ER, Borowski A, Mehlhorn U: Reduction of the left-ventricular outflow-tract obstruction by aortoventriculoplasty: long-term results of 96 patients. *Thorac Cardiovasc Surg* 1993; 41:216.

46. Manouguian S: [A new method for patch enlargement of hypoplastic aortic annulus: an experimental study (author's translation).] *Thoraxchir Vaskulare Chir* 1976; 24:418.

47. Skoularigis J, Sinovich V, Joubert G, Sareli P: Evaluation of the long-term results of mitral valve repair in 254 young patients with rheumatic mitral regurgitation. *Circulation* 1994; 90:II-167.

48. Enriquez-Sarano M, Tajik AJ, Schaff HV, et al: Echocardiographic prediction of survival after surgical correction of organic mitral regurgitation. *Circulation* 1994; 90:830.

49. Enriquez-Sarano M, Schaff HV, Orszulak TA, et al: Valve repair improves the outcome of surgery for mitral regurgitation: a multivariate analysis. *Circulation* 1995; 91:1022.

50. Liao K, Wu JJ, Frater RW: Comparative evaluation of left ventricular performance after mitral valve repair or valve replacement with or without chordal preservation. *J Heart Valve Dis* 1993; 2:159.

51. David TE: Papillary muscle-annular continuity: is it important? *J Cardiol Surg* 1994; 9:252.

52. Suzuki N, Takanashi Y, Tokuhiro K, et al: Mitral valve replacement with and without chordal preservation in patients with chronic mitral regurgitation: mechanisms for differences. *Circulation* 1992; 86:1718.

53. Wasir H, Choudhary SK, Airan B, et al: Mitral valve replacement with chordal preservation in a rheumatic population. *J Heart Valve Dis* 2001; 10:84.

54. Crawford ES, Coselli JS: Marfan's syndrome: combined composite valve graft replacement of the aortic root and transaortic mitral valve replacement. *Ann Thorac Surg* 1988; 45:296.

55. Seccombe JF, Schaff HV: Mitral valve repair: current techniques and indications, in Franco L, Verrier ED (eds): *Advanced Therapy in Cardiac Surgery*. Hanover, PA, Sheridan Press, 1999; p 220.

56. Suri R, Orszulak T: Triangular resection for repair of mitral regurgitation due to degenerative disease. *Op Tech Thorac Cardiovasc Surg* 2005; 10:194.

57. Phillips MR, Daly RC, Schaff HV, et al: Repair of anterior leaflet mitral valve prolapse: chordal replacement versus chordal shortening. *Ann Thorac Surg* 2000; 69:25.

58. Odell JA, Schaff HV, Orszulak TA: Early results of a simplified method of mitral valve annuloplasty. *Circulation* 1995; 92:150.

59. Acar C, Perier P, Fontaliran F, et al: Anatomical study of the tricuspid valve and its variations. *Surg Radiol Anat* 1990; 12:229.

60. Izumi C, Iga K, Konishi T: Progression of isolated tricuspid regurgitation late after mitral valve surgery for rheumatic mitral valve disease. *J Heart Valve Dis* 2002; 11:353.

61. King RM, Schaff HV, Danielson GK, et al: Surgical treatment of tricuspid insufficiency late after mitral valve replacement. *Circulation* 1983; 68:III.

62. Mullany CJ, Gersh BJ, Orszulak TA, et al: Repair of tricuspid valve insufficiency in patients undergoing double (aortic and mitral) valve replacement: perioperative mortality and long-term (1 to 20 years) follow-up in 109 patients. *J Thorac Cardiovasc Surg* 1987; 94:740.

63. Duran CG, Ubago JL: Clinical and hemodynamic performance of a totally flexible prosthetic ring for atrioventricular valve reconstruction. *Ann Thorac Surg* 1976; 22:458.

64. Kay JH, Maselli-Capagna G, Tsuji HK: Surgical treatment of tricuspid insufficiency. *Ann Surg* 1965; 162:53.

65. McCarthy JF, Cosgrove DM: Tricuspid valve repair with the Cosgrove-Edwards annuloplasty system. *Ann Thorac Surg* 1997; 64:267.

66. McCarthy PM, Bhudia SK, Rajeswaran J, et al: Tricuspid valve repair: durability and risk factors for failure. *J Thorac Cardiovasc Surg* 2004; 127(3):674-685.

67. Morishita A, Kitamura M, Noji S, et al: Long-term results after De Vega's tricuspid annuloplasty. *J Cardiovasc Surg* (Torino) 2002; 43(6):773-777.

68. Tang GH, David TE, Singh SK, et al: Tricuspid valve repair with an annuloplasty ring results in improved long-term outcomes. *Circulation* 2006; 114 (1 Suppl):I577-581.

69a. Karimov JH, Bevilacqua S, Solinas M, Glauber M: Triple heart valve surgery through a right antero-lateral minithoracotomy. *Int Cardiovasc Thorac Surg* 2009; 9(2):360-362.

69b. Meyer SR, Szeto WY, Augoustides JG, et al: Reoperative mitral valve surgery by the port access minithoracotomy approach is safe and effective. *Ann Thorac Surg* 2009; 87(5):1426-1430.

70. Connolly HM, Schaff HV, Mullany CJ, et al: Surgical management of left-sided carcinoid heart disease. *Circulation* 2001; 104:I-36.

71. Connolly HM, Schaff HV, Larson RA, et al: Carcinoid heart disease: impact of pulmonary valve replacement on right ventricular function and remodeling. *Circulation* 2001; 104:II-685.

72. Moller JE, Pellikka PA, Bernheim AM, et al: Prognosis of carcinoid heart disease: analysis of 200 cases over two decades. *Circulation* 2005; 112:3320.

73. Kirklin J, Barratt-Boyes B: Combined aortic and mitral valve disease with and without tricuspid valve disease, in Kirklin J W, Barratt-Boyes B (eds): *Cardiac Surgery*. New York, Wiley, 1993; p 431.

74. Roberts WC, Virmani R: Aschoff bodies at necropsy in valvular heart disease. *Circulation* 1978; 57:803.

75. Jai Shankar K, Jaiswal PK, Cherian KM: Rheumatic involvement of all four cardiac valves. *Heart* 2005; 91:e50.

76. Bland EF, Jones TD: Rheumatic fever and rheumatic heart disease: a 20-year report on 1000 patients followed since childhood. *Circulation* 1951; 4:836.

77. Wilson MG, Lubschez R: Longevity in rheumatic fever. *JAMA* 1948; 121:1.

78. Ellis LB, Harken DE, Black H: A clinical study of 1000 consecutive cases of mitral stenosis two to nine years after mitral valvuloplasty. *Circulation* 1959; 19:803.

79. Kern MJ, Aguirre F, Donohue T, et al: Interpretation of cardiac pathophysiology from pressure waveform analysis: multivalvular regurgitant lesions. *Cathet Cardiovasc Diagn* 1993; 28:167.

80. Terzaki AK, Cokkinos DV, Leachman RD, et al: Combined mitral and aortic valve disease. *Am J Cardiol* 1970; 25:588.

81. Gash AK, Carabello BA, Kent RL, et al: Left ventricular performance in patients with coexistent mitral stenosis and aortic insufficiency. *J Am Coll Cardiol* 1984; 67:148.

82. Grinda JM, Latremouille C, Berrebi AJ, et al: Aortic cusp extension valvuloplasty for rheumatic aortic valve disease: midterm results. *Ann Thorac Surg* 2002; 74:438.

83. Liuzzo JP, ShinYT, Lucariello R, et al: Triple valve repair for rheumatic heart disease. *J Cardiol Surg* 2005; 20:358.

84. Prabhakar G, Kumar N, Gometza B, et al: Triple-valve operation in the young rheumatic patient. *Ann Thorac Surg* 1993; 55:1492.

85. Katznelson G, Jreissaty RM, Levinson GE, et al: Combined aortic and mitral stenosis: a clinical and physiological study. *Am J Med* 1960; 29:242.

86. Uricchio JF, Sinha KP, Bentivoglio L, et al: A study of combined mitral and aortic stenosis. *Ann Intern Med* 1959; 51:668.

87. Kumar N, Saad E, Prabhakar G, et al: Extended transseptal versus conventional left atriotomy: early postoperative study. *Ann Thorac Surg* 1995; 60:426.

88. Honey M: Clinical and haemodynamic observations on combined mitral and aortic stenoses. *Br Heart J* 1961; 23:545.

89. Choudhary SK, Talwar S, Juneja R, et al: Fate of mild aortic valve disease after mitral valve intervention. *J Thorac Cardiovasc Surg* 2001; 122:583.

90. Larbalestier RI, Chard RB, Cohn LH: Optimal approach to the mitral valve: dissection of the interatrial groove. *Ann Thorac Surg* 1992; 54:1186.

91. Barner HB: Combined superior and right lateral left atriotomy with division of the superior vena cava for exposure of the mitral valve. *Ann Thorac Surg* 1992; 54:594.

92. Smith CR: Septal-superior exposure of the mitral valve: the transplant approach. *J Thorac Cardiovasc Surg* 1992; 103:623.

93. Couetil JP, Ramsheyi A, Tolan MJ, et al: Biatrial inferior transseptal approach to the mitral valve. *Ann Thorac Surg* 1995; 60:1432.

94. Brawley RK: Improved exposure of the mitral valve in patients with a small left atrium. *Ann Thorac Surg* 1980; 29:179.

95. Urschel CW, Covell JW, Sonnenblick EH, et al: Myocardial mechanics in aortic and mitral valvular regurgitation: the concept of instantaneous impedance as a determinant of the performance of the intact heart. *J Clin Invest* 1968; 47:867.

96. Boucher C: Multivalvular heart disease, in Eagle K, Haber E, DeSanctis R, et al (eds): *The Practice of Cardiology*, 2nd ed. Boston, Little, Brown, 1989; p 765.

97. Shigenobu M, Senoo Y, Teramoto S: Results of surgery for aortic regurgitation due to aortic valve prolapse. *Acta Med Okayama* 1988; 42:343.

98. Dare AJ, Veinot JP, Edwards WD, et al: New observations on the etiology of aortic valve disease: a surgical pathologic study of 236 cases from 1990. *Hum Pathol* 1993; 24:1330.

99. Bellitti R, Caruso A, Festa M, et al: Prolapse of the floppy aortic valve as a cause of aortic regurgitation: a clinicomorphologic study. *Int J Cardiol* 1985; 9:399.

100. Agozzino L, de Vivo F, Falco A, et al: Non-inflammatory aortic root disease and floppy aortic valve as cause of isolated regurgitation: a clinicomorphologic study. *Int J Cardiol* 1994; 45:129.

101. Roberts WC, Sullivan MF: Clinical and necropsy observations early after simultaneous replacement of the mitral and aortic valves. *Am J Cardiol* 1986; 58:1067.

102. Milewicz DM, Pyeritz RE, Crawford ES, et al: Marfan syndrome: defective synthesis, secretion, and extracellular matrix formation of fibrillin by cultured dermal fibroblasts. *J Clin Invest* 1992; 89:79.

103. Rippe LM, Angoff G, Sloss LJ: Multiple floppy valves: an echocardiographic syndrome. *Am J Med* 1979; 66:817.

104. Ogawa S, Hayashi J, Sasaki H, et al: Evaluation of combined valvular prolapse syndrome by two-dimensional echocardiography. *Circulation* 1982; 65:174.

105. Tomaru T, Uchida Y, Mohri N, et al: Postinflammatory mitral and aortic valve prolapse: a clinical and pathological study. *Circulation* 1987; 76:68.

106. Gillinov AM, Blackstone EH, White J, et al: Durability of combined aortic and mitral valve repair. *Ann Thorac Surg* 2001; 72:20.

107. Gott VL, Cameron DE, Alejo DE, et al: Aortic root replacement in 271 Marfan patients: a 24-year experience. *Ann Thorac Surg* 2002; 73:438.

108. David TE: Aortic valve-sparing operations for aortic root aneurysm. *Semin Thorac Cardiovasc Surg* 2001; 13:291.

109. Bozbuga N, Erentug V, Kirali K, et al: Surgical management of mitral regurgitation in patients with Marfan syndrome. *J Heart Valve Dis* 2003; 12:717.

110. Gillinov AM, Hulyalkar A, Cameron DE, et al: Mitral valve operation in patients with the Marfan syndrome. *J Thorac Cardiovasc Surg* 1994; 107:724.

111. Fernicola DJ, Roberts WC: Pure mitral regurgitation associated with a malfunctioning congenitally bicuspid aortic valve necessitating combined mitral and aortic valve replacement. *Am J Cardiol* 1994; 74:619.

112. Mills NL, McIntosh CL, Mills LJ: Techniques for management of the calcified mitral annulus. *J Cardiol Surg* 1986; 1:347.

113. Utley JR, Mills J, Hutchinson JC, et al: Valve replacement for bacterial and fungal endocarditis: a comparative study. *Circulation* 1973; 3:42.

114. Lakier JB, Copans H, Rosman HS, et al: Idiopathic degeneration of the aortic valve: a common cause of isolated aortic regurgitation. *J Am Coll Cardiol* 1985; 5:347.

115. Nair CK, Aronow WS, Sketch MH, et al: Clinical and echocardiography characteristics of patients with mitral annular calcification: comparison with age- and sex-matched control subjects. *Am J Cardiol* 1983; 51:992.

116. Kim HK, Park SJ, Suh JW, et al: Association between cardiac valvular calcification and coronary artery disease in a low-risk population. *Coronary Artery Dis* 2004; 15:1.

117. Kizer JR, Wiebers DO, Whisnant JP, et al: Mitral annular calcification, aortic valve sclerosis, and incident stroke in adults free of clinical cardiovascular disease: The Strong Heart Study. *Stroke* 2005; 36:2533.

118. Feindel CM, Tufail Z, David TE, et al: Mitral valve surgery in patients with extensive calcification of the mitral annulus. *J Thorac Cardiovasc Surg* 2003; 126:777.

119. Buchbinder NA, Roberts WC: Left-sided valvular active infective endocarditis: a study of forty-five necropsy patients. *Am J Med* 1972; 53:20.

120. Mathew J, Addai T, Anand A, et al: Clinical features, site of involvement, bacteriologic findings, and outcome of infective endocarditis in intravenous drug users. *Arch Intern Med* 1995; 155:1641.

121. Propst JW, Siegel LC, Stover EP: Anesthetic considerations for valve replacement surgery in a patient with carcinoid syndrome. *J Cardiothorac Vasc Anesth* 1994; 8:209.

122. Neustein SM, Cohen E, Reich D, et al: Transoesophageal echocardiography and the intraoperative diagnosis of left atrial invasion by carcinoid tumour. *Can J Anaesth* 1993; 40:664.

123. Cartwright RS, Giacobine JW, Ratan RS, et al: Combined aortic and mitral valve replacement. *J Thorac Cardiovasc Surg* 1963; 45:35.

124. Connolly HM: Carcinoid heart disease: medical and surgical considerations. *Cancer Control* 2001; 8:454.

125. Stephenson LW, Edie RN, Harken AH, et al: Combined aortic and mitral valve replacement: changes in practice and prognosis. *Circulation* 1984; 69:640.

126. Sakamoto Y, Hashimoto K, Okuyama H, et al: Long-term results of triple-valve procedure. *Asian Cardiovasc Thorac Ann* 2006; 14:47.

127. LaSalle CW, Csicsko JF, Mirro MJ: Double cardiac valve replacement: a community hospital experience. *Ind Med* 1993; 86:422.

128. Khan S, Chaux A, Matloff J, et al: The St Jude medical valve: experience with 1000 cases. *J Thorac Cardiovasc Surg* 1994; 108:1010.

129. Armenti F, Stephenson LW, Edmunds LH, Jr.: Simultaneous implantation of St Jude Medical aortic and mitral prostheses. *J Thorac Cardiovasc Surg* 1987; 94:733.

130. Galloway A, Grossi E, Bauman F, et al: Multiple valve operation for advanced valvular heart disease: results and risk factors in 513 patients. *J Am Coll Cardiol* 1992; 19:725.

131. Fiore AC, Swartz MT, Sharp TG, et al: Double-valve replacement with Medtronic-Hall or St Jude valve. *Ann Thorac Surg* 1995; 59:1113.

132. Teoh KH, Christakis GT, Weisel RD, et al: The determinants of mortality and morbidity after multiple-valve operations. *Ann Thorac Surg* 1987; 43:353.

133. Donahoo JS, Lechman MJ, MacVaugh H 3rd: Combined aortic and mitral valve replacement: a 6-year experience. *Cardiol Clin* 1985; 3:417.

134. Mattila S, Harjula A, Kupari M, et al: Combined multiple-valve procedures: factors influencing the early and late results. *Scand J Thorac Cardiovasc Surg* 1985; 19:33.

135. He G, Acuff T, Ryan W, et al: Aortic valve replacement: determinants of operative mortality. *Ann Thorac Surg* 1994; 57:1140.

136. Alvarez L, Escudero C, Figuera D, et al: The Bjork-Shiley valve prosthesis: analysis of long-term evolution. *J Thorac Cardiovasc Surg* 1992; 104:1249.

137. Jegaden O, Eker A, Delahaye F, et al: Thromboembolic risk and late survival after mitral valve replacement with the St Jude medical valve. *Ann Thorac Surg* 1994; 58:1721.

138. Copeland J 3rd: An international experience with the Carbo-Medics prosthetic heart valve. *J Heart Valve Dis* 1995; 4:56.

139. Bernal JM, Rabasa JM, Cagigas JC, et al: Valve-related complications with the Hancock I porcine bioprosthesis: a twelve- to fourteen-year follow-up study. *J Thorac Cardiovasc Surg* 1991; 101:871.

140. Loisance DY, Mazzucotelli JP, Bertrand PC, et al: Mitroflow pericardial valve: long-term durability (see comments). *Ann Thorac Surg* 1993; 56:131.

141. Pomar JL, Jamieson WR, Pelletier LC, et al: Mitroflow pericardial bioprosthesis: clinical performance to ten years. *Ann Thorac Surg* 1995; 60:S305.

142. Cannegieter SC, Rosendaal FR, Briet E: Thromboembolic and bleeding complications in patients with mechanical heart valve prostheses (review). *Circulation* 1994; 89:635.

143. Heras M, Chesebro JH, Fuster V, et al: High risk of thromboembolism early after bioprosthetic cardiac valve replacement. *J Am Coll Cardiol* 1995; 25:1111.

144. Horstkotte D, Schulte HD, Bircks W, et al: Lower intensity anticoagulation therapy results in lower complication rates with the St Jude medical prosthesis. *J Thorac Cardiovasc Surg* 1994; 107:1136.

145. Bernal JM, Rabasa JM, Lopez R, et al: Durability of the Carpentier-Edwards porcine bioprosthesis: role of age and valve position. *Ann Thorac Surg* 1995; 60:S248.

146. Brown PJ, Roberts CS, McIntosh CL, et al: Late results after triple-valve replacement with various substitute valves. *Ann Thorac Surg* 1993; 55:502.

147. Hamamoto M, Bando K, Kobayashi J, et al: Durability and outcome of aortic valve replacement with mitral valve repair versus double valve replacement. *Ann Thorac Surg* 2003; 75:28.

148. Munro AI, Jamieson WR, Burr LH, et al: Comparison of porcine bioprostheses and mechanical prostheses in multiple valve replacement operations. *Ann Thorac Surg* 1995; 60:S459.

149. Pellegrini A, Colombo T, Donatelli F, et al: Evaluation and treatment of secondary tricuspid insufficiency. *Eur J Cardiothorac Surg* 1992; 6:288.

150. Kaul TK, Ramsdale DR, Mercer JL: Functional tricuspid regurgitation following replacement of the mitral valve. *Int J Cardiol* 1991; 33:305.

151. Kara M, Langlet MF, Blin D, et al: Triple valve procedures: an analysis of early and late results. *Thorac Cardiovasc Surg* 1986; 34:17.

152. Macmanus Q, Grunkemeier G, Starr A: Late results of triple valve replacement: a 14-year review. *Ann Thorac Surg* 1978; 25:402.

153. Cohn L, Aranki S, Rizzo R, et al: Decrease in operative risk of reoperative valve surgery. *Ann Thorac Surg* 1993; 56:15.

154. Konishi Y, Matsuda K, Nishiwaki N, et al: Ventricular arrhythmias late after aortic and/or mitral valve replacement. *Jpn Circ J* 1985; 49:576.

155. Suri RM, Thourani VH, Englum BR, et al: The expanding role of mitral valve repair in triple valve operations: contemporary North American outcomes in 8021 patients. *Ann Thorac Surg* 2014; 97(5):1513-1519; discussion 1519.

155a. Rankin JS, Thourani VH, Suri RM, et al: Associations between valve repair and reduced operative mortality in 21,056 mitral/tricuspid double valve procedures. *Eur J Cardiothorac Surg* 2013 Sep;44(3):472-476.

156. Page RD, Jeffrey RR, Fabri BM, et al: Combined multiple valve procedures and myocardial revascularisation. *Thorac Cardiovasc Surg* 1990; 38:308.

157. Trace HD, Bailey CP, Wendkos MH: Tricuspid valve commissurotomy with one-year follow-up. *Am Heart J* 1954; 47:613.

158. Brofman BL: Right auriculoventricular pressure gradient with special reference to tricuspid stenosis. *J Lab Clin Med* 1953; 42:789.

159. Lillehei CW, Gott VL, DeWall RA, et al: The surgical treatment of stenotic and regurgitant lesions of the mitral and aortic valves by direct utilization of a pump oxygenator. *J Thorac Surg* 1958; 35:154.

160. Aberg B: Surgical treatment of combined aortic and mitral valvular disease. *Scand J Thorac Cardiovasc Surg* 1980; 25:1.

161. Elmahdy HM, Nascimento FO, Santana O, Lamelas JJ: Outcomes of minimally invasive triple valve surgery performed via a right anterior thoracotomy approach. *Heart Valve Dis* 2013; 22(5):735-739.

162. Lio A, Murzi M, Solinas M, Glauber MJ: Minimally invasive triple valve surgery through a right minithoracotomy. *Thorac Cardiovasc Surg* 2014; 148(5):2424-2427. (doi:10.1016/j.jtcvs.2014.06.094. No abstract available.)

163. Rankin JS, Thourani VH, Suri RM et al: Associations between valve repair and reduced operative mortality in 21,056 mitral/tricuspid double valve procedures. *Eur J Cardiothorac Surg* 2013; 44(3):472-476; discussion 476-477.

164. Skoularigis J, Essop M, Skudicky D, et al: Valvular heart disease: frequency and severity of intravascular hemolysis after left-sided cardiac valve replacement with Medtronic Hall and St Jude medical prostheses, and influence of prosthetic type, position, size and number. *Am J Cardiol* 1993; 71:587.

165. Aoyagi S, Oryoji A, Nishi Y, et al: Long-term results of valve replacement with the St Jude Medical valve. *J Thorac Cardiovasc Surg* 1994; 108:1021.

166. West PN, Ferguson TB, Clark RE, et al: Multiple valve replacement: changing status. *Ann Thorac Surg* 1978; 26:32.

167. Lemole GM, Cuasay R: Improved technique of double valve replacement. *J Thorac Cardiovasc Surg* 1976; 71:759.

168. Shine KI, DeSanctis RW, Sanders CA, et al: Combined aortic and mitral incompetence: clinical features and surgical. *Am Heart J* 1968; 76:728.

169. Clawson BJ: Rheumatic heart disease: an analysis of 796 cases. *Am Heart J* 1940; 20:454.

170. Cooke WT, White PD: Tricuspid stenosis with particular reference to diagnosis and prognosis. *Br Heart J* 1941; 3:141.

171. Mardelli TJ, Morganroth J, Naito M, et al: Cross-sectional echocardiographic identification of aortic valve prolapse (abstract). *Circulation* 1979; 60:II-204.

172. David TE: Aortic valve repair in patients with Marfan syndrome and ascending aorta aneurysms due to degenerative disease. *J Cardiol Surg* 1994; 9:182.

173. Gott VL, Gillinov AM, Pyeritz RE, et al: Aortic root replacement: risk factor analysis of a seventeen-year experience with 270 patients. *J Thorac Cardiovasc Surg* 1995; 109:536.

174. Schoen FJ, Berger BM, Guerina NG: Cardiac effects of noncardiac neoplasms (review). *Cardiol Clin* 1984; 2:657.

175. Connolly HM, Crary JL, McGoon MD, et al: Left and right heart valves: valvular heart disease associated with fenfluramine-phentermine. *New Engl J Med* 1997; 337:581-588.

176. Pritchett AM, Morrison JF, Edwards WD, et al: Left and right heart valves: valvular heart disease in patients taking pergolide. *Mayo Clin Proc* 2002; 77:1280-1286.

177. Droogmans S, Cosyns B, D'Haenen H, et al: Mitral and tricuspid: possible association between 3,4-methylenedioxymethamphetamine abuse and valvular heart disease. *Am J Cardiol* 2007; 100:1442-1525.

178. Raviprasad GS, Salem BI, Gowda S, et al: Radiation-induced mitral and tricuspid regurgitation with severe ostial coronary artery disease: a case report with successful surgical treatment [review]. *Cathet Cardiovasc Diagn* 1995; 35:146.

179. Blanche C, Freimark D, Valenza M, et al: Heart transplantation for Q fever endocarditis. *Ann Thorac Surg* 1994; 58:1768.

180. Rozycka CB, Hryniewiecki T, Solik TA, et al: Mitral and aortic valve replacement in a patient with ectodermal anhydrotic dysplasia: a case report. *J Heart Valve Dis* 1994; 3:224.

181. Tan C, Schaff H, Miller F, et al: Clinical investigation: valvular heart disease in four patients with Maroteaux-Lamy syndrome. *Circulation* 1992; 85:188.

182. Carrel T, Pasic M, Tkebuchava T, et al: Aortic homograft and mitral valve repair in a patient with Werner's syndrome. *Ann Thorac Surg* 1994; 57:1319.

183. Pellegrini RV, Copeland CE, DiMarco RF, et al: Blunt rupture of both atrioventricular valves. *Ann Thorac Surg* 1986; 42:471.

184. Gabarre J, Gessain A, Raphael M, et al: Adult T-cell leukemia/lymphoma revealed by a surgically cured cardiac valve lymphomatous involvement in an Iranian woman: clinical, immunopathological and viromolecular studies. *Leukemia* 1993; 7:1904.

185. Lang LL, Hvass U, Paillole C, et al: Cardiac valve replacement in relapsing polychondritis: a review. *J Heart Valve Dis* 1995; 4:227.

186. Ames DE, Asherson RA, Coltart JD, et al: Systemic lupus erythematosus complicated by tricuspid stenosis and regurgitation: successful treatment by valve transplantation. *Ann Rheum Dis* 1992; 51:120.

187. Fujise K, Amerling R, Sherman W: Rapid progression of mitral and aortic stenosis in a patient with secondary hyperparathyroidism. *Br Heart J* 1993; 70:282.

188. Palazzo E, Bourgeois P, Meyer O, et al: Hypocomplementemic urticarial vasculitis syndrome, Jaccoud's syndrome, valvulopathy: a new syndromic combination. *J Rheumatol* 1993; 20:1236.

189. Smith JA, Westlake GW, Mullerworth MH, et al: Excellent long-term results of cardiac valve replacement with the St Jude Medical valve prosthesis. *Circulation* 1993; 88:II-49.

190. Emery RW, Emery AM, Krogh C, et al: The St. Jude Medical cardiac valve prosthesis: long-term follow up of patients having double valve replacement. *J Heart Valve Dis* 2007; 16(6):634-640.

191. Ibrahim M, O'Kane H, Cleland J, et al: The St Jude Medical prosthesis: a thirteen-year experience. *J Thorac Cardiovasc Surg* 1994; 108:221.

192. David TE, Armstrong S, Sun Z: The Hancock II bioprosthesis at ten years. *Ann Thorac Surg* 1995; 60:S229.

193. Jamieson WR, Burr LH, Tyers GF, et al: Carpentier-Edwards supraannular porcine bioprosthesis: clinical performance at twelve years. *Ann Thorac Surg* 1995; 60:S235.

194. Milano A, Bortolotti U, Mazzucco A, et al: Heart valve replacement with the Sorin tilting-disk prosthesis: a 10-year experience. *J Thorac Cardiovasc Surg* 1992; 103:267.

195. Leavitt BJ, Baribeau YR, DiScipio AW, Northern New England Cardiovascular Disease Study Group, et al: Outcomes of patients undergoing concomitant aortic and mitral valve surgery in northern New England. *Circulation* 2009; 120 (11 Suppl):S155-162.

196. Lemieux MD, Jamieson WR, Landymore RW, et al: Medtronic intact porcine bioprosthesis: clinical performance to seven years. *Ann Thorac Surg* 1995; 60:S258.

197. Orszulak TA, Schaff HV, DeSmet JM, et al: Late results of valve replacement with the Bjork-Shiley valve (1973 to 1982) (see comments). *J Thorac Cardiovasc Surg* 1993; 105:302.

198. Nakano K, Koyanagi H, Hashimoto A, et al: Twelve years' experience with the St Jude Medical valve prosthesis. *Ann Thorac Surg* 1994; 57:697.

199. Pelletier LC, Carrier M, Leclerc Y, et al: The Carpentier-Edwards pericardial bioprosthesis: clinical experience with 600 patients. *Ann Thorac Surg* 1995; 60:S297.

200. van Doorn C, Stoodley K, Saunders N, et al: Mitral valve replacement with the Carpentier-Edwards standard bioprosthesis: performance into the second decade. *Eur J Cardiothoracic Surg* 1995; 9:253.

Valvular and Ischemic Heart Disease

Kevin D. Accola • Clay M. Burnett

Recently, there have been exciting developments involving new technologies for the surgical treatment of valvular heart disease associated with coronary artery disease (CAD). Interventional therapies for coronary artery obstruction have been extended to multivessel disease with hybrid procedures (targeted percutaneous interventions staged with limited access surgical coronary bypass surgery) and continues to change the number and nature of patients referred for surgery.[1] Similarly, the surgical treatment of structural valvular heart disease has continued to expand with advances in techniques for repair, as well as total valve replacement and valve-sparing repair options for both aortic and mitral valve abnormalities.[2] Most recently, bioprosthetic valve manufacturing advances in regard to calcium mitigation, tissue processing, and hemodynamically superior prosthetic valve stent designs have improved prosthetic valve durability, thereby broadening the valve replacement options for young and old alike.[3] The advent of transcatheter valve replacement (TAVR procedures) has also quickly become a commercial reality and has proven to be safe and efficacious in numerous studies. The stunning early success of the TAVR approach has allowed this remarkable new option to become commonplace in many institutions in hospitals around the world.[4] Most importantly, perhaps, is that transcatheter valvular interventions have provided very high-risk patients, such as the elderly or those with a myriad of threatening comorbidities, a viable new option to consider.

There are numerous issues the surgeon must consider when planning treatment strategies in the patient with combined valvular and CAD. It is uncommon for today's surgeon to see a patient with simple aortic or mitral valvular disease who also has straightforward proximal CAD. Indeed, it is more often a patient presents with complex, acute valvular/ventricular pathology, with superimposed diffuse, CAD. The prevalence of presurgical interventional options means that patients now undergo more aggressive medical therapy and multiple intracoronary dilation attempts before being referred for surgical evaluation. As a result, they are often referred at an older age and with more complex comorbidities, with more diffuse disease, persistent dysrhythmias, and worsening ventricular function. This older, sicker cohort of patients now referred for surgery are understandably at much higher risk for postoperative morbidity and mortality than in previous eras. Consequently, contemporary surgeons often face difficult therapeutic dilemmas that usually requires a more flexible, systematic, and thoughtful approach. In fact, current decision-making is more often a result of multidisciplinary heart teams, utilizing broad, evidence-based data as a foundation for complex medical decisions.[5]

The pathophysiologic combination and interaction between valvular heart disease and associated CAD is complex. Progressive valvular heart disease clearly impacts ventricular function. The additional impact of CAD has synergistic potential to further affect ventricular morphology and physiology. In particular, the deterioration in contractile strength caused by myocardial infarction and subsequent regional wall motion injury causes progressive distortion of ventricular shape as the infarcted muscle compensates through tissue remodeling. Loss of contractile strength and remodeling after ischemic injury eventually leads to cavitary dilation, with resulting effects not only on ventricular function, but also on mitral valve performance. As valvular and subvalvular elements lose their important geometric relationships, functional valvular incompetence develops. In patients with valvular heart disease, coronary obstructions may be symptomatic or asymptomatic, but the decision to intervene surgically is often made regardless of the presence of ischemic symptoms, in order to have a protective effect toward the additive pathophysiology of concomitant cardiac diseases.

Under most circumstances, surgeons attempt to treat both valvular and CAD simultaneously. However, a combined approach leads to a prolonged and potentially complicated procedure. Accordingly, the increased risks of a combined operation demand a defined and focused operative strategy. Historically, combined coronary artery and valve operations have had an increased risk for early and late mortality compared to operations for isolated valvular heart disease (Fig. 45-1). This complexity increases the need for careful preoperative assessment of myocardial function and an understanding of the impact on ventricular function of the changing afterload and pre-load associated with valve surgery. Therefore, in adult patients with combined valvular and

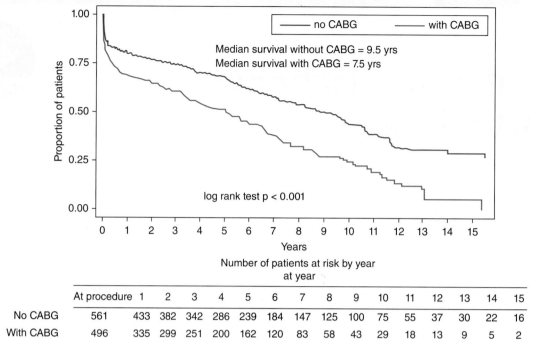

FIGURE 45-1 Long-term survival of DVS patients with or without concomitant CABG. (Reproduced with permission from Leavitt BJ, Baribeau YR, DiScipio AW, et al: Outcomes of patients undergoing concomitant aortic and mitral valve surgery in northern new England, *Circulation.* 2009 Sep 15;120(11 Suppl):S155-S162.)

ischemic heart disease, the assessment of intrinsic left ventricular function assumes paramount importance during the initial consultative process. Clinical signs and symptoms of left ventricular failure should be diligently sought. In addition to history, physical examination, and routine laboratory tests, preoperative echocardiography is mandatory. Intraoperative transesophageal echocardiography (TEE) is used to correlate preanesthetic imaging and is utilized for accurate planning of all valvular interventions, and has become standard of care in most institutions. Immediately after weaning from cardiopulmonary bypass support, intraoperative TEE is carefully reviewed by the surgeon, anesthesiologist, and imaging team to evaluate the repair. If necessary, resumption of cardiopulmonary bypass support can then be done to perform additional repair efforts; the post-bypass TEE is critical for this evaluation, and requires a commitment from the entire team to be sure that the reparative efforts are optimal before the operation is terminated.

It is also important preoperatively to attempt to distinguish heart failure resulting from valvular disease from myocardial dysfunction owing to coronary ischemia. Myocardial viability assessment may be useful in eliciting ventricular size and functional changes that are exacerbated under stress conditions and may help delineate the underlying pathology, especially of the mitral valve. At cardiac catheterization, in addition to coronary artery angiography, left ventricular end-diastolic pressure and pulmonary pressures measurements may yield additional information about left- and right ventricular function and supplement noninvasive assessments of valve function and coronary anatomy. In centers where it

is available, positron emission tomography (PET) scans and other radioisotope imaging studies can help determine the viability of myocardium with potential reversible ischemia.[6] These assessments are critically important before embarking on concomitant valve and coronary artery surgery; both for determining the operative risk, as well as planning the scope and extent of the surgical approach.

The assessment of valve pathology is covered in detail in previous chapters on isolated valvular heart disease. As has been noted, coronary angiography is not mandatory in all patients with valvular pathology who are about to undergo valve surgery. However, given the prevalence of CAD in aging Western populations, coronary angiography is usually performed in all patients greater than 40 years of age, and selects younger patients with suggestive symptoms or significant risk factors. More recently, patients felt to be at low risk for coronary occlusive disease may be adequately screened with coronary computed tomographic angiography.[7]

Because of the wide pathophysiologic spectrum of valvular and CAD, several frequently encountered valve and coronary artery combinations are considered in this chapter, including: (1) aortic stenosis (AS) with CAD, including strategies for moderate AS, (2) aortic regurgitation plus CAD, (3) mitral regurgitation plus CAD, (4) mitral stenosis plus CAD, (5) AS and mitral regurgitation plus CAD, and (6) aortic regurgitation and mitral regurgitation plus CAD.

Patients may have combined pathology of stenosis and insufficiency, but to avoid unproductive complexity, and because one lesion usually dominates, the somewhat arbitrary categorization noted above will be maintained during the ensuing discussion. For each entity, the clinical presentation, the pathophysiology of the disease state and its correction, the operative and management approach, short- and long-term results are discussed. Today's surgeon must also be familiar with evolving hybrid techniques, such as staged coronary artery stenting and percutaneous aortic valve replacement (AVR) in the management of patients with combined valve and CAD.[8] Since these new innovative strategies are rapidly gaining acceptance as appropriate options in highly select patients, this chapter will also briefly review some of the more common hybrid approaches where applicable.[9-12]

AORTIC STENOSIS AND CORONARY ARTERY DISEASE

Aortic stenosis is one of the more frequently encountered valvular lesions in adult populations and will continue to increase in prevalence due to our aging population. Degenerative calcific AS is most common in patients in their sixties, seventies, and eighties[13-15] and often is associated with CAD.[16] This disease combination is usually gratifying to treat because the response to surgical relief of AS and coronary artery obstructions is significant, immediate, and relatively durable.

Clinical Presentation

Patients with AS are asymptomatic initially due to compensatory mechanisms within the left ventricle. Eventually patients can present with angina pectoris, congestive heart failure, syncope, or some combination of these as the stenosis progresses and the compensatory mechanisms begin to fail. When significant coronary artery obstruction is present, in addition to valvular obstruction, angina pectoris is almost always manifest. However, angina pectoris can occur in the absence of significant coronary artery obstructions due to insufficient diastolic coronary flow across a severely stenotic valve. Identifying symptoms of myocardial ischemia or congestive heart failure in patients with concomitant AS and significant CAD is generally straightforward. Accurate discrimination of subtle neurologic symptoms, such as syncope, presyncope, transient ischemic symptoms, or orthostatic hypotension, may be more difficult to elicit, and careful questioning regarding transient symptomatology is required. Symptoms suggestive of carotid artery obstruction should be sought and appropriately evaluated with carotid artery ultrasound and Doppler scanning, since the murmur of AS often radiates into the neck and can obscure the detection of bruits.

Prominent findings on physical examination include the typical late-packing mid-systolic crescendo murmur heard in the aortic area, radiating into the right neck. Signs of congestive heart failure with rales on chest auscultation or peripheral extremity edema may be present in later stages. The electrocardiogram may show left ventricular strain and increased QRS height due to left ventricular hypertrophy. If the patient has suffered a recent or remote myocardial infarction, then typical ischemic electrocardiographic changes may also be present. The echocardiogram usually shows calcified and immobile aortic valve leaflets producing a contracted aortic orifice with the resultant compensatory hypertrophied left ventricle. Evidence of calcifications extending into the sinuses of Valsalva and/or the left ventricular outflow tract should be carefully evaluated. Significant acceleration of trans-valvular flow velocities, estimates of reduced outflow areas, and flow turbulence with Doppler confirms the reduced outflow area. The transaortic valvular gradient also can be determined at catheterization and is often helpful, though modern m-mode echocardiography and Doppler imaging analysis has supplanted catheter gradient assessments in many hospitals due to correlated accuracy.

The preoperative evaluation of patients with AS, CAD, and poor ventricular function is complicated. Patients with poor ventricular function often generate relatively low transaortic valve gradients. This renders the calculation of valve area for the assessment of critical AS less accurate. In those cases where poor cardiac output from left ventricular failure leads to a less-than-expected gradient across the left ventricular outflow tract, the morphologic demonstration of valve immobility and heavy leaflet calcification is an important confirmatory sign that hemodynamically significant AS is present. Fortunately, even in the presence of a low gradient, if echocardiographic signs of significant valve stenosis are present, and if left ventricular intracavitary pressure exceeds 120 mm Hg in systole, mortality rates for valve replacement are acceptable, and the clinical response to surgery is typically good.[17] In stark contrast, however, a poorly contractile, thinned-out left ventricle with low transvalvular gradients in the presence of low intracavitary systolic pressures, usually suggests that the operation carries high risks, and due to inadequate ventricular reserve, may be of very limited benefit. On the other hand, a poorly contractile ventricle that has normal, or even increased wall thickness, will usually recover significant contractile force if a substantial amount of reversible ischemic myocardium is demonstrated, and if the degree of AS is significant. In addition to ventricular function, other important determinants of the risks and advisability of surgery include patient age, functional status (ie, "frailty index"), presence of previous cardiac operations, and the presence of other comorbidities that affect end-organ function, especially renal and pulmonary function.

Pathophysiology

Aortic stenosis produces impairment of left ventricular emptying during systole, which ultimately is the source of all the symptoms and signs of AS. Most patients with AS have hypertrophied and thick-walled left ventricles to overcome the obstructive valve orifice. Contractile function is initially good, and ejection fraction is usually maintained because of these compensatory mechanisms for some time. In later stages of the disease, the ventricle begins to fail due to persistently severe afterload resistance, with enlargement

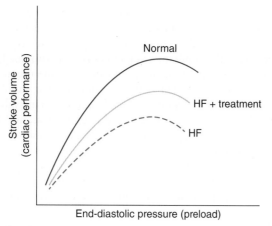

FIGURE 45-2 Starling curve of heart failure.

and global diminution of contractile function as the patient progress up the Starling curve of heart failure (Fig. 45-2). At any stage of the disease, the additional presence of critical coronary artery obstruction can cause specific regional wall motion abnormalities that may be exacerbated by stenosis of the aortic valve. Significant three-vessel CAD may itself lead to temporary global ventricular dysfunction, which may be reversible with revascularization apart from any valve replacement effects.

In patients with critical AS and good ventricular function, valve replacement immediately reduces left ventricular afterload. Because most patients with AS have thick-walled hypertrophied ventricles, intraoperative subendocardial ischemia may be more difficult to avoid during aortic cross-clamping and subsequent cardioplegic arrest. Although revascularization should not decrease left ventricular contractility, and should actually improve it long-term, some myocardial stunning with a temporary decrease in global and regional left ventricular contractility inevitably results from the surgical procedure.[18-21] This, of course, assumes even more important pathophysiologic significance in patients with poor ventricular function preoperatively. Diastolic dysfunction may also occur postoperatively, causing a less compliant left ventricle. The most extreme example of this was the so-called "stone heart"[22] that occasionally plagued early cardiac surgery pioneers who first attempted AVR surgery. Fortunately, modern myocardial preservation strategies have eliminated this feared complication through the liberal use of antegrade and retrograde delivery techniques and more physiologic cardioplegic solutions that optimally protects myocardial cellular integrity and tissue function.

Postoperatively, patients usually enjoy a dramatic improvement in symptoms. Relief of left ventricular outflow obstruction immediately leads to enhanced cardiac output and perfusion of vital organs. In addition, left ventricular remodeling and regression of hypertrophy usually occurs over time.[21] Simultaneous correction of myocardial ischemia can lead to improved subendocardial perfusion, as well as recruitment of formerly hibernating myocardium. The optimal final result is regression of hypertrophied ventricular mass, improved

diastolic relaxation, balanced transmyocardial coronary perfusion, and elimination of left ventricular outflow obstruction, culminating in recovery of normal ventricular function.

Moderate Aortic Stenosis and Coronary Artery Disease

Symptomatic, severe AS is universally agreed to benefit from AVR at the time of coronary revascularization, but the management of patients with CAD and either mild or moderate AS continues to remain a matter of controversy. The earliest debates centered on the anticipated risks of a future reoperation, particularly in a population of advanced age, versus the risks of imposing on a patient a more complex initial operation with subsequent lifelong prosthetic valve concerns that may not be immediately necessary. Given the relatively reduced 10-year survival in advanced age patients undergoing cardiac surgery, valve durability was not considered to be a central factor limiting the success of a combined initial AVR/coronary artery bypass graft (CABG) strategy. Thus, the initial opinion favored a liberal AVR/CABG combination approach in patients with moderate AS, as the reoperative risks were considered the more dangerous of the two options. However, the early STS data base for AVR/CABG outcomes clearly showed a mortality nearly double that for isolated CABG (6-7% and 2-3%, respectively)[23] challenging the belief that initial combined valve-CAD operations were generally safer in terms of primary mortality and morbidity risks. Moreover, as experience with reoperations has grown, more recent studies demonstrate much lower risks of reoperation for AVR in post-CABG patients that rival levels similar to initial AVR/CABG procedures.[24] In fact, the lowered risks of redo sternotomy for primary AVR after previous CABG (6-7%) has now shifted the debate from one of concerns over the risks of reoperation, to predicting the incremental progression in AS if it is withheld at the initial CAD surgery.[25-27]

Although there is no clearly identified method of predicting valvular progression, and surgical expertise is critical in formulating a surgical strategy and timing of intervention, estimates of the rate of progression of AS may help provide support for valve replacement, even without hemodynamically critical disease.[28] For instance, it has been established that the rate of valvular progression is more rapid if the valve is heavily calcified, and if the patient has advanced atherosclerotic systemic disease or renal failure.[25] Studies also demonstrate that age and valvular gradient at the time of diagnosis are important criteria to consider.[27] Verhoye et al[29] found that using echocardiography on a serial basis, AVR is recommended to be added to the revascularization procedure for younger patients (<70 years) if their peak gradient is >25-30 mm Hg, on the assumption of reasonable longevity and the probability AS would bear future symptoms. In older patients (>80 years), competing causes of mortality rationally increases the thresholds for concomitant replacement, and AVR is added only if their peak gradient exceeds 50 mm Hg, as longevity is often related to other factors before AS progression occurs.[25] Furthermore, studies show that reoperation for AVR after CABG rarely occurs within 5 years of CABG.[26] Consequently, from a survival standpoint, little is gained from adding AVR to patients >80 to 85 years of age at the time of coronary revascularization unless the valve is symptomatic or has severe, but incidentally identified hemodynamics.[25,26] In certain extremely high-risk cohorts, a multidisciplinary team may decide on a "hybrid" approach, utilizing percutaneous coronary artery stenting for major coronary artery obstruction, followed by percutaneous AVR (TAVR).[30-32]

Despite the recent trend outlined above favoring isolated CABG when concomitant moderate AS exits, there is also evidence that favors concomitant valve replacement in some patients with moderate AS who are referred for surgical myocardial revascularization.[33-36] In one study,[33] survival rates at both 1 year and 8 years were superior for patients who underwent valve replacement for moderate AS (gradient >30 mm Hg or gradient <40 mm Hg with valve area between 1.0 and 1.5 cm²). One-year survival was 90% in those having valve replacement compared to 85% in patients having CABG alone. Similarly, 8-year survival (55 vs 39%) was statistically significantly better ($p < .001$). Although this data may reveal some bias in healthier patients receiving concomitant AVR/CABG than their more chronically ill peers who were felt not to tolerate more extensive surgery and were only offered isolated CABG, it remains true that this dichotomy of patient groups is commonly seen in clinical practice. Thus, support for both strategies is rational and expected, and can be used to maintain a flexible approach when faced with moderate AS and severe CAD in patients of wide-ranging clinical conditions.[25-29]

In summary, given the absence of convincing data that unilaterally supports an operative strategy for the treatment of moderate AS, at the time of surgical coronary revascularization, it is best to individualize patient selection carefully, relative to surgeon and institutional expertise and practice. Significant patient comorbidities, and risk/benefit assessment, including an accurate estimate of expected rehabilitation potential (particularly in frail, elderly candidates), must be contemplated. Review of the initial and recent data and strategies derived from both experience, as well as available relevant data demonstrates that a flexible and individualized approach is warranted to yield the best patient outcomes.

Operative Management

Monitoring for surgery of the aortic valve and coronary arteries includes catheters and measurements that have become standard for most cardiac surgical operations. These include an arterial line (usually in the radial artery for blood pressure and blood gases) and an optional pulmonary artery catheter for measurement of pulmonary artery pressures, and cardiac output by thermodilution, with optical sensors for continuous estimation of mixed venous oxygen saturation. While the pulmonary artery catheter has a balloon at its tip, occlusion wedge pressure is rarely measured in the perioperative period because of the danger of pulmonary artery rupture. Particularly useful information

is provided by continuous measurement of mixed venous oxygen saturation. Of late, use of arterial flow or central venous monitoring devices, along with TEE, provides satisfactory estimates of continuous cardiac outputs and monitoring of volume management. This has significantly reduced our reliance on traditional, but more invasive, pulmonary artery catheters.

The perfusion setup is standard and similar to that for isolated coronary artery bypass. A single aortic cannula is ordinarily placed in the distal ascending aorta. A single two-stage venous cannula is placed via the right atrial appendage with its tip positioned in the inferior vena cava. After establishment of cardiopulmonary bypass, the patient is usually cooled to 32 to 34°C, during which time a left ventricular vent is positioned via the right superior pulmonary vein. With the heart well emptied, the aortic cross-clamp is applied during a temporary reduction in pump flow. Thereafter, the heart is arrested with cold (4°C) potassium crystalloid or blood cardioplegia. Low aortotomy incisions are recommended for maximal visibility, with the incision directed toward the noncoronary sinus if annular or root enlargement is anticipated. After valve excision, implant techniques according to each surgeon's preference is performed. In situations of low-lying coronary ostia, suture techniques may need to be varied to prevent ostial compression. Prior to closure, the valve and coronary ostia are carefully reinspected a final time for clearance and embolic debris, and the aorta is closed. Deairing maneuvers are routine, and TEE aids assurance of complete removal, as well as early detection of proper prosthetic function.

A combination of antegrade and retrograde cardioplegia is optimal. The initial dose of cardioplegia (15 mL/kg) is typically split into a two-thirds antegrade and one-third retrograde dose, with subsequent doses of 200 to 300 mL cardioplegia delivered via the retrograde catheter every 20 minutes throughout the duration of cardiac arrest during the operation. This is particularly convenient because retrograde cardioplegia can be given even after the aortic root is opened without disrupting exposure or flow of the operation. In patients with significant left ventricular hypertrophy, light ventricular and inferior septal protection by retrograde cardioplegia perfusion alone may be inadequate. Handheld direct antegrade perfusion directly into the coronary ostia may be helpful.

The combination of aortic valve disease and CAD in patients has historically been accepted to be a marker of significantly reduced longevity.[37] In the elderly, with reduced life expectancies, bioprosthetic valve durability remains the valve of choice, particularly when associated with concomitant CAD.[38] Currently, with the advent of new bioprosthetic valve technology with calcium mitigation processing, and proven structural longevity, there is a trend toward increased tissue valve utilization.[39,40] As a result, many younger age patients considering the obligation of lifelong anticoagulation and the improvements in valve design and durability are opting to receive bioprosthetic valves instead of mechanical prostheses.

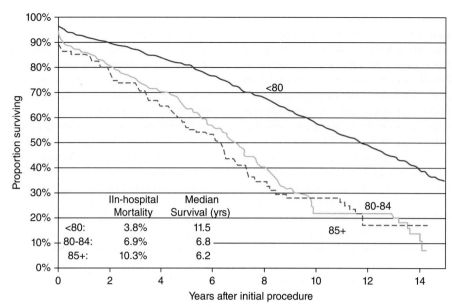

FIGURE 45-3 Adjusted survivorship by age among patients undergoing AVR + CABG. (Reproduced with permission from Likosky DS, Sorensen MJ, Dacey LJ. et al. Long-term survival of the very elderly undergoing aortic valve surgery, *Circulation* 2009 Sep 15;120(11 Suppl):S127-S133.)

Results

Early hospital mortality after concomitant AVR and CABG ranges from approximately 2 to 10%. In earlier studies, but more recent studies suggest that modern operative management reveals very similar outcomes and mortality risks in patients having isolated AVR and those having combine AVR/CABG[26,35,36,48,42-47] Higher mortality is observed in patients with more severe symptoms of heart failure and impaired ventricular function preoperatively, as well as the elderly or other patients with numerous comorbidities. The most frequent causes of operative death are low-output cardiac failure, myocardial infarction, and arrhythmia. Incremental risk factors for hospital death include patient age, functional class, diffuse CAD, and poor preoperative ventricular function. In a number of studies, late survival has ranged from 60 to 80% at 5 years and 50 to 75% at 8 years postoperatively (Fig. 45-3).[33,42-47] By multivariate analysis, risk factors for reduced late survival include older age, cardiac enlargement, and more severe preoperative clinical symptoms. The use of a mechanical prosthesis at valve replacement has been associated with similar long-term survival though lower long-term event-free survival.[39] Nonetheless, many elderly patients still have acceptable results following relief of AS, even those undergoing redo valve surgery that is combined with coronary revascularization.[47] As discussed previously, choice of valve type is a complex issue that takes on even more importance in combined valve-coronary artery surgery. A frank discussion of the advantages and drawbacks of each valve option continues to be an important component of the preoperative evaluation and planning for this type of surgery. In some circumstances, consideration of alternative procedures such as coronary artery stenting followed by percutaneous valve replacement may be indicated and necessary in otherwise inoperable or extreme risk patients.[5,8,49]

AORTIC REGURGITATION AND CORONARY ARTERY DISEASE

Significant isolated aortic regurgitation occurs less often in older populations, though it may be associated with AS when the valve becomes immobile. Aortic valvular regurgitation is also less often encountered with significant CAD than in patients with AS. Most series of patients undergoing AVR and CABG include a relatively small number (10 to 25%) of patients with aortic insufficiency as compared to AS.[36,42-44] Although the operative management of patients with aortic regurgitation and CAD is similar to that previously described, aortic insufficiency produces different pathophysiologic effects that have implications for perioperative management. Moreover, the presence of an incompetent aortic valve introduces nuances to the intraoperative management and myocardial protection of these patients, primarily due to preoperative ventricular decompensation.

Clinical Presentation

Patients with aortic regurgitation and CAD usually present in one of three ways. The aortic regurgitation may be asymptomatic and detected incidentally during evaluation for symptomatic coronary disease. Second, the patient may be asymptomatic, yet a routine physical examination reveals a murmur of aortic insufficiency that leads to cardiac evaluation and detection of coronary disease. Finally, patients may present relatively late in the course of valvular heart disease with congestive heart failure caused by decompensation of the volume-overloaded left ventricle from long-standing insufficiency or with superimposed ischemic ventricular damage from combined CAD. Insufficiency of the aortic valve may also occur with dilatation of the ascending aorta that often involves with the coronary sinuses, particularly in patients with bicuspid valvular anatomy. Patients, therefore, may present within a broad spectrum of clinical signs and symptoms ranging from no symptoms and essentially normal physiology, to classic ischemic syndromes and severe congestive heart failure. The physical signs also depend on the nature of the presentation. In general, all patients with significant aortic insufficiency have an audible early diastolic regurgitant murmur. In late stages, rales and peripheral edema and other advanced signs of congestive heart failure usually occur with a prominent diastolic murmur.

The preoperative evaluation of a patient with aortic insufficiency and CAD is no different from that previously described for patients with AS and ischemic heart disease. Echocardiography is particularly useful in detecting aortic regurgitation because a physiologically significant murmur can be difficult to detect. In addition, echocardiography gives important information regarding both ventricular contractile function and ventricular size. Because many patients with aortic regurgitation are usually asymptomatic until marked left ventricular dilation occurs, careful evaluation for changes in ventricular size or function is important. The presence of these changes may constitute an indication to proceed with surgical intervention in the absence of significant symptoms.

Pathophysiology

Aortic regurgitation increases left ventricular preload and causes left ventricular dilatation. Dilatation does not occur acutely; however, patients with acute aortic insufficiency are often severely symptomatic owing to a sudden increase in left ventricular end-diastolic pressure and a dramatic decrease in net forward cardiac output. Global left ventricular dysfunction caused by CAD also can contribute to left ventricular dilatation. Valve replacement relieves some of the preload but does not immediately result in improved left ventricular contractility. Revascularization of ischemic, hibernating myocardium in patients with AR and severe CAD may produce more immediate improved contractility as compared to patients with long-standing isolated aortic valvular insufficiency.[48,50]

The indications for surgery in aortic regurgitation are reviewed in depth in the section on aortic valve disease. When CAD is also present, ischemic regional wall motion abnormalities can usually be distinguished from severe, global ventricular dilatation due to severe aortic valvular insufficiency. In patients with symptomatic AR who also have diffuse three-vessel CAD, however, assigning the primary cause of global left ventricular dysfunction to either ischemia or acute valvular-related ventricular dilatation is difficult. Attempting to distinguish between the relative impact of either valvular insufficiency or CAD on ventricular function is of paramount importance in the preoperative assessment and risk stratification of these patients. This is because regional wall abnormalities due to CAD are more likely to immediately improve after myocardial revascularization, as compared to patients with global, severe ventricular dilation caused by long-standing AR. In difficult cases, an evaluation of myocardial viability (with thallium or PET scanning) may be helpful in evaluating candidates for surgery. Decisions about timing of aortic valve surgery in the presence of CAD are different from those in cases of isolated valvular disease, with the usual result that the valve is replaced earlier in the course of the valvular disease due to the pressing nature of symptomatic myocardial ischemia.

Operative Management

The operation is conducted in a similar fashion to that described for AS and CAD. However, in the presence of significant aortic valvular insufficiency, antegrade cardioplegia in the aortic root is often less effective because a large portion of the cardioplegia solution leaks into the left ventricle due to valvular incompetence. As a result, retrograde cardioplegia through the coronary sinus is strongly recommended. However, since retrograde cardioplegia is recognized to be less effective in protecting right ventricular myocardium due to inconsistent venous anatomy, periodic delivery of antegrade cardioplegia using handheld catheters is advised. Technical operative details are essentially the same as those outlined earlier for AS operations.

Considerations in weaning from cardiopulmonary bypass are somewhat different from those described for AS. Patients with aortic regurgitation are more likely to have dilated ventricles that poorly tolerate increases in afterload. TEE has proved invaluable in successfully managing adjustments in preload and afterload during weaning from cardiopulmonary bypass. In patients with volume-overloaded ventricles caused by aortic insufficiency, vasodilatory inotrope infusions, such as milrinone and dobutamine, have an important role because they provide both inotropic support and ventricular unloading. In some circumstances, use of an intraaortic balloon pump may be necessary and beneficial in patients with marginal functional reserve. In rare instances, mechanical circulatory assistance with a ventricular assist device is required. Its use is generally reserved for younger patients without comorbid conditions in whom prompt improvement in ventricular function is anticipated.

Results

Early results after operation for aortic regurgitation and CAD include an expected hospital mortality rate of less than 10%.[36,42,48] Incremental risk factors for hospital death are similar to those described previously, with advanced age and poor ventricular function, combined with the presence of diffuse CAD, having the greatest impact. Late survival after this operation is similar to that for AS and CAD (Fig. 45-3).[48] Despite the impression that patients with aortic insufficiency and CAD do not do as well as those with AS, aortic insufficiency has not been an independent risk factor for early or late mortality.[48] As expected, recovery of ventricular ejection fraction does have a favorable impact on late mortality. Although some improvement of function can occur with elimination of the volume overload and revascularization in patients with combined valvular and CAD, when ventricular dilatation and dysfunction occur in the setting of chronic aortic regurgitation, these often are irreversible changes. Overall, recovery of ejection fraction and ventricular function in patients with aortic insufficiency is less when compared with AS when both are corrected in the later stages of the disease process. This observation is the primary reason that valve replacement is recommended for aortic valvular insufficiency before irreversible changes in ventricular morphology and function have occurred. However, although failure of recovery of ventricular function in this setting may have an impact on long-term survival, even patients with late stage aortic valvular insufficiency should tolerate valve replacement surgery.

MITRAL REGURGITATION AND CORONARY ARTERY DISEASE

Successful management of patients with mitral regurgitation and CAD remains one of the most challenging and controversial topics in adult cardiac surgery.[51] This group of patients tends to be complex, and their surgical care is accomplished at higher risk.[52-57] This is almost certainly because of the complex interaction between the left ventricle and that of the mitral valvular apparatus. Normal mitral valve function depends on healthy supporting ventricular muscle to maintain proper alignment. Similarly, normal ventricular function depends on competence of the mitral valve. Abnormal valve function due to CAD occurs because of the impact of ischemia on the mitral valve apparatus, damaging subvalvular structural integrity including papillary muscle involvement. Remodeling of ischemic zones eventually leads to ventricular dilatation, and subsequent annular geometry.[58] Therefore, there is a unique, amplifying potential when CAD and mitral valve disease coexist, making patient management with this combination of pathophysiology more complicated, and the surgical management potentially more difficult.

In patients with preserved ventricular function, the pathophysiology and management strategies are not significantly different from those for treatment of isolated mitral regurgitation or CAD. Patients with acute onset of mild or moderate mitral insufficiency, in the presence of global ventricular dysfunction secondary to severe CAD, can be safely treated by coronary revascularization alone.[59] If it becomes necessary to include mitral valve annuloplasty to myocardial revascularization, the operation becomes more complex and longer.[60,61] Therefore, as described previously, a carefully conceived operative plan with special attention to myocardial preservation is important. However, the more interesting problems are in those patients with mitral insufficiency and CAD who do not have normal ventricular function. Often these patients present with recurrent ischemia, in addition to

previous myocardial infarction, that culminates with resultant regional wall motion abnormalities that produces mitral insufficiency.[62]

Clinical Presentation

The spectrum of clinical presentation ranges from patients who are asymptomatic to those who are moribund in cardiogenic shock. The degree of mitral insufficiency involved can widely vary from mild insufficiency when associated with a limited ischemic event causing minor segmental wall motion abnormalities, to severe regurgitation and global left ventricular failure from acute ischemic rupture of a papillary muscle. Patients who present with acute syndromes are often related to myocardial infarction and demonstrate the sudden development of mitral insufficiency. These patients are extremely ill when they present in congestive heart failure, often presenting in profound cardiogenic shock. Management of these patients can be difficult and challenging. When faced with extreme mitral insufficiency and cardiogenic shock, immediate IABP support should be instituted for cardiac support and to provide valuable mechanical afterload reduction of the acutely injured left ventricle.

Findings on physical examination obviously relate to the nature of the presentation, and can range from signs of mild mitral insufficiency to severe congestive failure and cardiogenic shock. An electrocardiogram may show evidence of acute or chronic ischemia, and all patients should undergo echocardiography. TEE should be available for intraoperative use. Transesophageal echocardiogram is particularly useful because it gives information in regard to valvular function, left ventricular geometry and contractility, ventricular wall thickness, and associated regional wall motion abnormalities. Also the status of the other valves, particularly the tricuspid, can be quickly assessed to determine if they may require surgical attention as well. Cardiac catheterization is performed in these patients for the same reasons outlined for patients with aortic valve disease.

Pathophysiology

A detailed understanding of the pathophysiology of functional mitral insufficiency is important for planning the operative approach. Limited regional wall motion abnormalities involving the papillary muscle and adjacent ventricular wall can produce dynamic changes that produce corresponding insufficiency of specific mitral valve regions. More global ventricular dysfunction from CAD can produce ventricular dilatation with profound mitral annular dilatation and progressive mitral insufficiency. The jet of ischemic mitral regurgitation typically is centrally or posteriorly directed on ECHO. Mitral regurgitation increases left ventricular preload and decreases afterload at the expense of cardiac output. Ischemic damage causes ventricular dilatation with decreased contractility and an increase in left ventricular filling pressures. These combined lesions cause synergistic decompensation, chronically leading to pulmonary hypertension with secondary tricuspid regurgitation. Cardiac output may be very low, especially in patients with acute mitral insufficiency. Mitral insufficiency may occur in association with CAD, but often the CAD is the cause of functional mitral insufficiency. The pathophysiology of ischemic mitral insufficiency results in tethering or retraction of the valve leaflets, annular dilatation, geometric displacement of the subvalvular apparatus, or some combination of all of these. Correction of mitral insufficiency either by valve repair or valve replacement produces an instantaneous increase in left ventricular afterload. The ventricle no longer has the low-impedance left atrial chamber into which to eject blood and must overcome systemic afterload in systole. Even when myocardial ischemia is reversible, recruitment of hibernating myocardium may take time. These factors, in combination with the sudden increase in left ventricular afterload, contribute to the difficulty and increased risk of managing this entity. Secondary right ventricular failure may occur because pulmonary hypertension, if present, does not decrease immediately after mitral valve repair or replacement, and CAD also may affect right ventricular function.

Symptomatic CAD in the presence of moderate or severe insufficiency in the setting of regional wall motion abnormally is the usual indicators for combined surgery. As noted, patients with acute illnesses may be in extremis and may benefit from temporizing measures.[63] Ventricular dysfunction is not a contraindication to surgery, especially if it is caused by reversible ischemia. Patients with global, irreversible, and severely dilated cardiomyopathy with severe mitral insufficiency, however, should not be operated on because the ventricle tolerates the increase in overload poorly and results are unsatisfactory. Severe diffuse CAD in which complete revascularization cannot be accomplished is a significant indication of extreme risk, as well. Estimation of the viability of the myocardium and demonstration of reversible ischemia using thallium or PET scanning therefore are important in stable patients. Left atrial enlargement in long-standing mitral valve insufficiency is common, and patients often present with atrial fibrillation. This condition also contributes to the reduction in cardiac output and ablation of the arrhythmia at the time of surgery may confer addition benefit.

Operative Management

Preoperative decision strategies in patients with mitral regurgitation and CAD remains controversial.[64,65] The decision for the necessity of associated mitral valve intervention in this setting becomes critical because if moderate insufficiency is left untreated, the patient may be compromised. However, mitral regurgitation in the presence of acute CAD with regional ventricular decompensation that is caused by reversible myocardial ischemia can improve with isolated revascularization.[66] In many instances, however, residual significant mitral valve regurgitation may remain. It is important, therefore, to distinguish organic from functional mitral insufficiency as well as acute mitral insufficiency from ischemia as opposed to a more chronic mitral valvular pathology secondary to previous

ischemia and subsequent wall motion abnormality. Intraoperative TEE is an essential tool for assessment of mitral valve function in this setting, though the vasodilator effects of general anesthesia and subsequent decrease in afterload may minimize the appearance of the insufficiency.[65] Patients with no preoperative congestive heart failure, normal left atrial dimensions, normal pulmonary pressures, and mild to moderate mitral insufficiency by TEE after induction of anesthesia typically do not need mitral valve intervention.[66,67] Many of these patients will appear to have more mitral regurgitation and higher pulmonary pressures at catheterization or when they are ischemic than when they are under anesthesia. Furthermore, although mitral valve repair improves mitral valve regurgitation volume, it does not infer late mortality advantages over revascularization alone in large studies.[67] Complete myocardial revascularization alone may suffice for milder forms of initial valvular insufficiency (Fig. 45-4).

Despite a lack of consensus on the prognostic value of concomitant mitral valve repair at the time of revascularization, several recent studies suggest that the quality of modern surgical results justifies a more aggressive approach to valve repair in patients with moderate mitral insufficiency and CAD.[51,63-65,67,68] Most patients with ventricular enlargement and annular dilation secondary to CAD with functional mitral insufficiency determined to be significant may be managed with annuloplasty alone.[69] Restricted leaflet motion is frequently a complication of ischemic changes in ventricular shape and resultant papillary muscle displacement.[70] In patients with calcification, extensive fibrosis of the posterior leaflet, or severely restricted posterior leaflet motion, mitral valve replacement is warranted. Historically, results of mitral repair and CABG are superior to those of mitral valve replacement when repair is technically possible. Anesthetic considerations are similar to those described previously, although it must be recognized that these patients are generally quite compromised. As suggested earlier, intraoperative TEE is particularly important in this group of patients for pre- and postoperative assessment of valve and ventricular function. Setup for cardiopulmonary bypass is similar to that described earlier. The most common incision providing access to the mitral

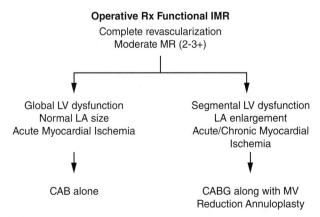

Operative Rx Functional IMR
Complete revascularization
Moderate MR (2-3+)

Global LV dysfunction
Normal LA size
Acute Myocardial Ischemia

Segmental LV dysfunction
LA enlargement
Acute/Chronic Myocardial Ischemia

CAB alone

CABG along with MV Reduction Annuloplasty

FIGURE 45-4 Complete myocardial revascularization alone may suffice for milder forms of initial valvular insufficiency.

valve is in the wall of the left atrium anterior to the right pulmonary veins. Preparative dissection (Sondegaard's maneuver) of the interatrial groove (Waterston's groove) facilitates exposure using this incision. Alternative approaches for valve exposure and their advantages have been described elsewhere.

As noted, patients with papillary muscle rupture caused by infarction usually require valve replacement. Some surgeons have reported success with reimplantation of the papillary muscle, but this strategy is risky in these patients because the operation must be both expeditious and effective. Multiple attempts to achieve mitral valve competence in this group of critically ill patients are poorly tolerated. A reimplanted, infarcted papillary muscle does not necessarily restore mitral valve competence and also may be subject to early or late breakdown.

As in combined aortic valve and coronary artery surgery, distal graft anastomoses are performed first. At this point, after the atrium has been opened, it may be prudent to undertake an arrhythmia ablation procedure in selected patients with atrial fibrillation. Radiofrequency or cryoablation probes can be used to create a standard lesion set within the left atria, as described in Chapter 55. The left atrial appendage should be oversewn. Valve repair or replacement is then carried out, followed by performance of the mammary artery anastomosis. Proximal graft anastomoses can be done either after release of the cross-clamp in place.

Weaning from cardiopulmonary bypass is similar to that in patients with aortic insufficiency and CAD. Again, in this group of patients, afterload reduction using pharmacologic agents such as dobutamine and milrinone may be indicated. There should be a low threshold for insertion of the intraaortic balloon postoperatively. Many of these patients, particularly when emergent, have severely compromised ventricular hemodynamics and may be quite tenuous for hours to days after surgery.

Strict attention must be paid to right ventricular function and intraoperative right ventricular myocardial protection in this group of patients. Right ventricular failure must be anticipated and correctly diagnosed and managed. The presence of a falling systemic blood pressure and cardiac output with rising pulmonary artery pressure, pulmonary capillary wedge pressure, and controlled venous pressure should prompt a search for right ventricular failure.

Results

Hospital mortality for this group of patients is higher than that for most other forms of acquired heart disease. Early mortality rates range from 3% in good-risk patients to 60% in the sickest patients.[64,65,67,68,71,72] The higher mortality is seen in patients with acute ischemic mitral valve disease and severe ventricular dysfunction who require emergency surgery. Incremental risk factors for early death include age, functional class, ventricular function, elevated pulmonary pressures, and cardiogenic shock. Late survival in patients with this entity is 55 to 85% at 5 years and 30 to 45% at 10 years (Fig. 45-5).[52-57,66,72-74]

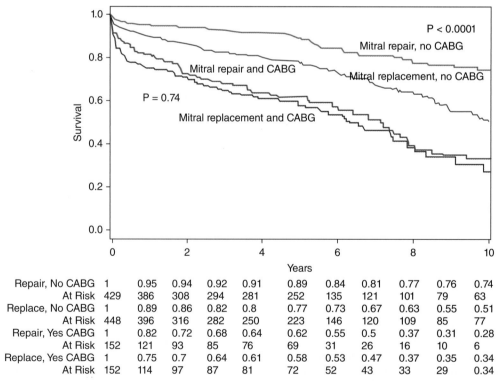

Repair, No CABG	1	0.95	0.94	0.92	0.91	0.89	0.84	0.81	0.77	0.76	0.74
At Risk	429	386	308	294	281	252	135	121	101	79	63
Replace, No CABG	1	0.89	0.86	0.82	0.8	0.77	0.73	0.67	0.63	0.55	0.51
At Risk	448	396	316	282	250	223	146	120	109	85	77
Repair, Yes CABG	1	0.82	0.72	0.68	0.64	0.62	0.55	0.5	0.37	0.31	0.28
At Risk	152	121	93	85	76	69	31	26	16	10	6
Replace, Yes CABG	1	0.75	0.7	0.64	0.61	0.58	0.53	0.47	0.37	0.35	0.34
At Risk	152	114	97	87	81	72	52	43	33	29	0.34

FIGURE 45-5 Survival, mitral valve repair versus replacement, with and without CABG. (Reproduced with permission from Thourani VH1, Weintraub WS, Guyton RA, et al: Outcomes and long-term survival for patients undergoing mitral valve repair versus replacement: effect of age and concomitant coronary artery bypass grafting, *Circulation*. 2003 Jul 22;108(3):298-304.)

In general, patients who survive surgery have good relief of symptoms, although recurrent mitral insufficiency remains an issue for some patients who have undergone restrictive annuloplasty.[66] The risk factors for this complication remain incompletely identified, although abnormal ventricular morphology and regional function appear to play a role. Significant risk factors for late death include preoperative functional class, residual postoperative left ventricular dysfunction, and diffuse myocardial ischemia.

MITRAL STENOSIS AND CORONARY ARTERY DISEASE

Patients with mitral stenosis and CAD usually have good left ventricular function and often are a relatively straightforward group of patients to care for because the mitral stenosis does not subject the left ventricle to abnormal hemodynamic loads. CAD may cause unexpected left ventricular dysfunction, but this is unusual, unless weakness, global ischemia coexists. A common concern in mitral stenosis patients is postoperative right ventricular dysfunction because pulmonary hypertension, with its potential to produce right ventricular failure and tricuspid insufficiency, is often encountered in patients with severe mitral stenosis.

Clinical Presentation

As implied earlier, mitral stenosis is usually the dominant lesion in patients with mitral stenosis and CAD; therefore, symptoms are typically caused by the valvular lesion. Patients usually present with shortness of breath, orthopnea, and fatigue, despite normal left ventricular function. Atrial fibrillation is a common presenting symptom with mitral stenosis due to left atrial dilatation. Patients with mitral stenosis and CAD infrequently have angina as a presenting symptom. The electrocardiogram may show evidence of right ventricular strain and hypertrophy. TEE confirms the diagnosis of mitral stenosis and usually shows a small left ventricle with preserved contractile function. The right ventricle may be enlarged and hypertrophied. Cardiac catheterization further confirms the diagnosis by showing a gradient across the mitral valve. Other important information gleaned from invasive catheterization includes a measurement of the pulmonary artery pressures and central venous pressure. The degree of pulmonary hypertension is a marker of the severity and duration of mitral stenosis and alerts the surgeon to the potential for right ventricular failure postoperatively. An elevated central venous pressure is a potential sign that right ventricular decompensation has already occurred. Coronary angiography should be done in all patients with angina pectoris, and as noted before, in any patient greater than age 40 years in whom mitral valve surgery is anticipated.

Pathophysiology

Unlike the other entities described, mitral stenosis and CAD do not have significantly synergistic pathologic effects on the heart. CAD usually has more profound effects on the left ventricle, since left ventricular mass remains reasonably protected in patients with mitral stenosis until late in the disease. The right ventricle is the chamber most vulnerable to the effects of long-standing mitral stenosis due to increased transpulmonary pressure gradients. However, even with right ventricular hypertension, the potential impact of CAD on right ventricular function in adults is usually not prohibitive. In circumstances involving patients with diffuse CAD and significant ischemic cardiomyopathy, the risks of surgery are elevated, primarily because of global ventricular ischemic dysfunction.

The indications for surgery, not surprisingly, are usually determined by the severity of the mitral stenosis. Patients with significant heart failure symptoms and low cardiac output from mitral stenosis whose calculated valve area is less than 1 cm² should have a mitral valve operation, and associated bypass grafting if significant CAD is present. Patients with significant CAD but only mild mitral stenosis may arise, and these patients are well managed with CABG and mitral commissurotomy, if technically feasible. Another alternative in patients considered high risk for surgery, is the staged approach of percutaneous revascularization with stents and balloon mitral valvuloplasty. The number of patients suitable for the latter procedure is relatively small and thus far there are no definitive data supporting this kind of hybrid transcatheter approach to these lesions. These clinical situations are best managed within a multidisciplinary team on an individualized, patient-by-patient basis.[5]

Operative Management

Monitoring, perfusion setup, and operative sequence are identical to those described for treatment of mitral regurgitation and CAD. TEE is useful to assess both the feasibility of mitral commissurotomy (or more extensive mitral repair) and the postoperative results of attempted valvuloplasty. In most patients with mitral stenosis, however, valve replacement is required because of irreversible calcific and fibrotic damage to the leaflets and subvalvular apparatus. A biological prosthesis is used most often due to a preponderance of advanced age patients, even if the majority of patients have chronic atrial fibrillation from left atrial enlargement. Although long-term anticoagulation is indicated in these patients, use of a biologic valve allows less aggressive anticoagulation regimens in patients often burdened with other comorbidities, and who are judged to be at significant risk for chronic anticoagulation. Particular attention must be directed to preservation of the right ventricle at regular intervals during the operation. In practice, this means that initial and subsequent doses of cardioplegia should be given antegrade, as well as retrograde, because the latter approach usually offers variable distribution of cardioplegia to the right ventricle, proximal inferior septal, and inferior left ventricular regions.

TEE is also an important adjunct in monitoring both right and left ventricular function postoperatively. The early differentiation between left and right ventricular failure is facilitated by the use of this modality during weaning from cardiopulmonary bypass. If inotropic drugs are required, their selection should be based, in part, on the consideration that pulmonary hypertension and right ventricular failure might be important components of the clinical syndrome. Drugs such as isoproterenol, dobutamine, and especially milrinone (the latter often in combination with norepinephrine or other catecholamines to counteract profound peripheral vasodilatory effects from phosphodiesterase inhibition) may be indicated for their combined beneficial effects on right ventricular contractility and pulmonary vascular resistance. Judicious use of inotropic drugs and careful administration of fluid are usually sufficient to restore adequate cardiac output. The intraaortic balloon is rarely indicated in these patients because right ventricular problems predominate. Temporary support with either a right ventricular assist device or ECMO for acute pulmonary failure may be employed if the above measures are inadequate. Once the acute postcardiotomy failure resolves dramatic decreases in pulmonary artery pressures and subsequent recovery of right ventricular function allows for removal of extraordinary support.

Results

Early mortality after combined surgery for mitral stenosis and CAD is approximately 8%.[44-46] This is not significantly different from results of surgery in lower-risk patients with mitral regurgitation and CAD. Long-term probability of survival is approximately 50% at 7 years and in one series was not significantly different from that for patients with ischemic mitral insufficiency.[54-56] Interestingly, long-term survival of patients with myxoid degeneration of the mitral valve and CAD (65%) was significantly better than survival of the patients with rheumatic or ischemic mitral valve disease and CAD in at least one series.[52] As implied, rheumatic valve pathology is a risk factor for late death, as is poor preoperative left ventricular function and the presence of ventricular arrhythmias. Interestingly, the use of a bioprosthesis without anticoagulants confers both a survival advantage and an event-free survival advantage in these patients These data lend support to the hypothesis that biologic valves may be appropriate for mitral replacement in older patients and those with CAD, whose expected life span may be shorter than the anticipated durability of the replacement device.[37]

AORTIC STENOSIS, MITRAL REGURGITATION, AND CORONARY ARTERY DISEASE

Patients with AS, mitral regurgitation, and CAD often present with AS as the predominant lesion. It is important to note that functional mitral regurgitation may improve after relief of AS with concomitant reduction in left ventricular systolic pressure. If the mitral valve is not intrinsically diseased, it may not require surgical intervention.[75]

Clinical Presentation

Patients with these diseases often present identically with patients with AS and CAD, but may do so earlier because of the combined valvular lesions. Angina, congestive heart failure, and syncope may be presenting symptoms alone or together. It is relatively uncommon for symptoms resulting from mitral insufficiency to be predominant. Echocardiography is an extremely important tool in this disease combination. Careful evaluation of the mitral valve, often using TEE, is necessary to determine the degree of intrinsic mitral valve disease, because improvement in mitral insufficiency is expected after AVR and relief of left ventricular outflow obstruction.[72] It is critical to determine whether or not the mitral valve has anatomical abnormalities that might not reverse with aortic surgery alone.[73,76] Cardiac catheterization is required, as it is for the other disease entities described.

Pathophysiology

Aortic stenosis increases left ventricular afterload and therefore can contribute to increasing the amount of mitral regurgitation. Because the combined lesions may cause patients to present earlier in the course of the disease, the left ventricle may be better preserved in this setting than in patients with isolated mitral insufficiency and CAD. Also as noted, the mitral valve may not be structurally diseased. Because of earlier presentation, pulmonary hypertension and subsequent right ventricular failure and tricuspid valve incompetence are usually not prominent features. Because relief of outflow obstruction helps left ventricular function immediately, these patients often do quite well.

The indications for surgery are usually the same as for AS and CAD. Critical AS, when documented, requires valve replacement; if significant CAD is present, CABGs are also done in the sequence previously described. Mitral valve repair is almost always appropriate with annular remodeling when mitral insufficiency is moderate to severe and reparable anatomical abnormalities of the valve are detected. End-stage ventricular dysfunction with ventricular dilatation and myocardial thinning are the primary cardiac contraindications to surgery.

Operative Management

Anesthesia and perfusion setup are identical to those described for mitral valve and coronary artery surgery. Intraoperative transesophageal echocardiographic monitoring again plays an important role because the intraoperative assessment of mitral valve structure and function before and after bypass is critical. The choice of valve for aortic replacement is the same as described previously. In most situations, however, bioprosthetic valves should be considered, especially if the mitral valve is to be repaired.

Under almost all circumstances in which anatomical abnormalities of the mitral valve are detected, or in which mitral insufficiency is severe, mitral valve repair should be considered. Annuloplasty remodeling may be all that is required if the mitral insufficiency results from annular dilatation and the insufficiency is symmetric and central. More complex disease may require more extensive repair, or even replacement of the mitral valve. When the decision is made not to operate on the mitral valve, TEE is done to assess residual mitral valve dysfunction following AVR and coronary artery bypass surgery. If moderate or severe mitral regurgitation remains, the valve should be repaired or replaced. This is technically more difficult after the aortic valve has been replaced, because the prosthesis in the aortic position hinders exposure of the mitral valve. Therefore, every effort must be made to assess mitral valvular morphology and function before starting cardiopulmonary bypass, and preferably prior to the induction of anesthesia.

As in the other entities described, distal graft anastomoses are performed first (Fig. 45-6). After these grafts are completed, the aorta is opened and the aortic valve is resected with appropriate annular debridement. Replacement of the aortic valve, however, is deferred until after the mitral valve operation because sutures used for mitral valve repair or replacement may become disrupted during later debridement of the aortic valve annulus. After resection of the aortic valve, the atrium is opened and the mitral operation is performed. The atrium is closed with a vent across the mitral valve. The aortic valve is then replaced and the aorta is closed. The internal mammary artery graft is done last. Proximal graft anastomoses can be done with the aortic cross-clamp in place. It is conceivable that at some point in the future high risk patients with this combination of lesions may undergo catheter-based coronary revascularization, catheter-based AVR, and catheter-based mitral valve repair particularly in high-risk patients.[77,78]

As noted, this group of patients may have preserved ventricular function, and weaning from cardiopulmonary bypass is often straightforward. Inotropic drugs and intraaortic balloon counter pulsation are used as indicated.

Results

Early hospital mortality is 12 to 16%[77,81] Not surprisingly, predictors of early death include severe mitral regurgitation, lower ejection fraction with more severe symptoms of heart failure, and the presence of severe triple-vessel CAD. Late survival is approximately 60% at 72 months. Multivariate predictors of late mortality include advanced symptoms of heart failure and increased severity of mitral insufficiency.

AORTIC AND MITRAL REGURGITATION AND CORONARY ARTERY DISEASE

Relatively few patients have insufficiency of both the aortic and mitral valves combined with CAD. Those patients who do usually have rheumatic heart disease and present early in the course of the valvular heart disease. Aortic regurgitation may be the predominant valve pathology in a patient with simultaneous significant CAD. The mitral valve pathology may be secondary to left ventricular dilatation from the aortic lesion and/or from ischemia resulting from the coronary obstructions. Morphologic mitral valve disease may not be present. Because of the interaction of the valve and coronary pathologies, assessment of left ventricular contractility may be difficult for the reason that both preload and afterload are altered. In addition, the presence of reversible ischemia may obscure accurate measurement of ventricular function and reserve. Therefore, assessment of myocardial viability in these patients is often important.

Clinical Presentation

Most patients with this combination of cardiac lesions present with congestive heart failure. It is unusual to see a patient who has significant insufficiency of both the aortic and mitral valves present with angina as the primary symptom. Typical murmurs of aortic and mitral insufficiency are present, and the patient may have other signs of chronic congestive heart failure, including rales and peripheral edema. If myocardial infarction is a significant component of the pathophysiology and presentation of the disease, evidence of it may be seen on electrocardiogram and echocardiogram. On echocardiography, patients may have regional wall motion abnormalities if infarction has occurred, as well as global ventricular dilatation and dysfunction from the combined valvular lesions and/or diffuse CAD. Cardiac catheterization defines the coronary anatomy and helps to assess the severity of the valvular insufficiency and ventricular dysfunction. Accurate assessment of true left ventricular function is difficult in this entity. Mitral insufficiency may abnormally inflate visual measurements of ejection fraction because the ventricle can eject into the low-pressure pulmonary venous circuit. The misleading ejection fraction, with increased preload volumes due to insufficient aortic and mitral valves, when combined with the potential contribution of dysfunctional ischemic myocardium, make it very difficult to get an accurate estimation of preoperative left ventricular function. Thallium or PET scans may be useful to assess areas of dysfunctional myocardium that may be viable. Transesophageal ECHO may be extremely helpful, with special attention to left ventricular dimensions and bi-valvular anatomy.

Pathophysiology

Symptoms and signs of left ventricular failure develop as the left ventricle dilates. In patients with rheumatic disease with both valves intrinsically damaged, ischemic disease may be minimal. In the setting of patients with aortic regurgitation and significant ischemia, mitral regurgitation is more likely to be secondary to both of these processes, and valve repair should be possible. Correction of aortic regurgitation reduces preload, whereas correction of mitral insufficiency increases afterload. The chronically dilated myopathic ventricle may not have sufficient reserves to maintain adequate output under these circumstances. Higher postoperative preload may need to be maintained while afterload is reduced. Any

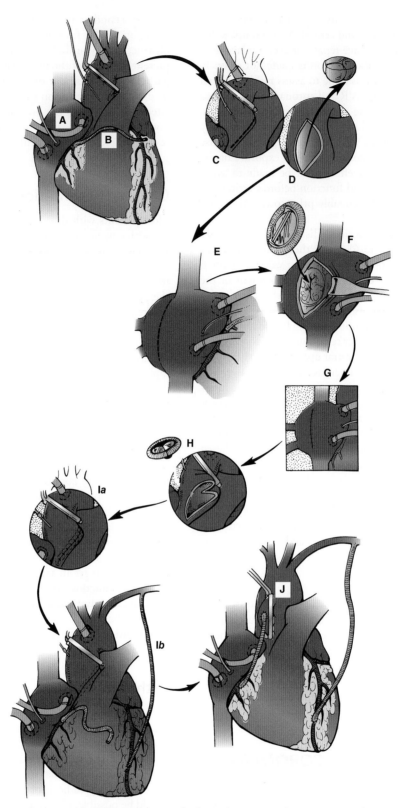

FIGURE 45-6 Operative sequence for aortic valve replacement, mitral valve replacement, and coronary artery bypass grafting. (A) Cannulation with cross-clamping of the aorta and administration of antegrade and retrograde cardioplegia. (B) Distal graft anastomoses are performed. (C) Aortotomy with standard oblique incision. (D) The aortic valve is resected but not replaced. (E) Standard left atriotomy after dissection in the interatrial groove. (F) Mitral valve repair or replacement with the prosthesis of choice. (G) Closure of the left atriotomy. (H) Aortic valve replacement with prosthesis of choice. (Ia and b) Closure of aortotomy and performance of distal anastomosis with the internal mammary artery. (J) Proximal graft anastomoses are performed. In this illustration, a partially occluding clamp has been applied to the aorta.

additional contractility as a result of revascularization should improve output further. However, because of the multiple, uncontrollable variables that inhibit preoperative assessment of ventricular function, prediction of expected improvement after this operation is difficult.

This consideration is extremely important, since patients with severe and irreversible ischemic myocardial disease and poor ventricular function will not do well with operative treatment. Therefore, preoperative assessments of myocardial viability and reversible ischemia are critical. It is also important to assess whether organic mitral valve disease is present. The best results in these patients are in those in whom no mitral operation, or at most annuloplasty, is required.

OPERATIVE MANAGEMENT

Details of the operative technique are similar to those described previously. Because of the presence of aortic insufficiency, retrograde cardioplegia must be used in conjunction with handheld ostial cannulas to deliver cardioplegia antegrade. For the reasons enunciated, excellent myocardial protection is important in these patients. TEE is required in the operating room for the assessment of mitral valve function. Residual 1+ to 2+ mitral regurgitation may be acceptable in certain patients because relief of aortic regurgitation can be expected to reduce ventricular size, which may lead to improvement of mitral regurgitation as the ventricle remodels with time. Similarly, myocardial revascularization also may lead to ultimate improvement in ventricular and mitral valve function in those with mild mitral valve insufficiency.

In weaning from cardiopulmonary bypass, afterload reduction is extremely important because of the large preoperative volume overload of the heart. Drugs that reduce ventricular afterload, including vasodilators and inotropic drugs such as milrinone, may be particularly appropriate. The intraaortic balloon pump may be needed and helpful in the perioperative care of these difficult patients.

Results

Early hospital mortality in this group of patients may be high, and if myocardial failure is severe, overall mortality rates exceed the range already noted for double-valve and coronary artery surgery.[23,79,81] Important determinants of risk in these patients are the familiar ones. In several series, predictors of hospital death and late events included severe mitral regurgitation, lower ejection fraction, more severe symptoms of congestive heart failure, and severe triple-vessel CAD.[80]

REFERENCES

1. Byrne JG, Leacche M, Vaughan DE, Zhao DX: Hybrid cardiovascular procedures. *JACC Cardiovasc Interv* 2008; 1:459.
2. Badiu C, Voss B, Dorfmeister M, et al: Valve-sparing root replacement: where are the limits? *Tex Heart Inst J* 2011; 38(6):661-662.
3. Chang H, Kim S, Kim K-H, et al: Combined anti-calcification treatment of bovine pericardium with amino compounds and solvents. *Interact Cardiovasc Thorac Surg* 2011; 12(6):903-907.
4. Guyton R: The Placement of Aortic (PARTNER) trial. The surgeon's perspective: celebration and concern. *Circulation* 2012; 125:3237-3239.
5. Holmes DR, Rich JB, Zoghbi WA, et al: The heart team of cardiovascular care. *J Am Coll Cardiol* 2013; 61(9):903-907.
6. Beanlands R, Ruddy T, PARR Investigators : the degree of recovery of left ventricular function. *J Am Coll Cardiol* 2002; 40(10):1735-1743.
7. Giustino G, Chieffo A, Spagnolo P, et al: TCT 296 routine screening of coronary artery disease with computed tomography coronary angiography in place of invasive coronary angiography in patients undergoing transcatheter aortic valve implantation. *J Am Coll Cardiol* 2014;64(11.5):doi:10.1016/j.jacc.2014.07.341.
8. Guy TS, Brzezinski M, Stechert MM, Tseng E: Robotic mammary artery harvest and anastomotic device allows minimally invasive mitral valve repair and coronary bypass. *J Card Surg* 2009; 24:170.
9. Piazza N, Serruys PW, de Jaegere P: Feasibility of complex coronary intervention in combination with percutaneous aortic valve implantation in patients with aortic stenosis using percutaneous left ventricular assist device (TandemHeart). *Catheter Cardiovasc Interv* 2009; 73:161.
10. Peels JO, Jessurun GA, Boonstra PW, et al: Hybrid approach for complex coronary artery and valve disease: a clinical follow-up study. *Neth Heart J* 2007; 15:327.
11. Harris KM, Pastorius CA, Duval S, et al: Practice variation among cardiovascular physicians in management of patients with mitral regurgitation. *Am J Cardiol* 2009; 103:255.
12. Lu JC, Shaw M, Grayson AD, et al: Do beating heart techniques applied to combined valve and graft operations reduce myocardial damage? *Interact Cardiovasc Thorac Surg* 2008; 7:111.
13. Davis EA, Gardner TJ, Gillinov AM, et al: Valvular disease in the elderly: influence on surgical results. *Ann Thorac Surg* 1993; 55:333.
14. Freeman WK, Schaff HV, O'Brien PC, et al: Cardiac surgery in the octogenarian: perioperative outcome and clinical follow-up. *J Am Coll Cardiol* 1991; 18:29.
15. Boning A, Burger S, Fraaund S, et al: Should the aortic valve be replaced in patients with mild aortic stenosis admitted for coronary surgery? *Thorac Cardiovasc Surg* 2008; 56:467.
16. Shahle E, Bergstrom R, Nystrom SO, Hansson HE: Early results of aortic valve replacement with or without concomitant coronary artery bypass grafting. *Scand J Thorac Cardiovasc Surg* 1991; 25:29.
17. Dumesnil J, Pibarot P, Carabello, B: Paradoxical low flow and/or low gradient severe aortic stenosis despite preserved left ventricular ejection fraction; implications for diagnosis and treatment. *Eur Heart J* 2010; 31:281-289.
18. Ren JF, Panidis IP, Kotler MN, et al: Effect of coronary bypass surgery and valve replacement on left ventricular function: assessment by intraoperative two-dimensional echocardiography. *Am Heart J* 1985; 103:281.
19. Braunwald E, Kloner RA: The stunned myocardium: prolonged postischemic ventricular dysfunction. *Circulation* 1982; 66:1146.
20. Braunwald E: The stunned myocardium: newer insights into mechanisms and clinical applications. *J Thorac Cardiovasc Surg* 1990; 100:310.
21. Marban E: Myocardial stunning and hibernation: the physiology behind the colloquialisms. *Circulation* 1991; 83:681.
22. Cooley PA, Reul GJ, Wakash DC: Ischemic myocardial contracture ("stone heart"). A complication of cardiac surgery. *Isrj Med Sci* 1975; 11(2-3):203-210.
23. The Society of Thoracic surgeons. Adult cardiac surgery database, executive summary, 10 years STS report. http://www.sts.org/sites/default/files/documents/pdf/ndb2010/1stHharvestExecutiveSummary%5B1%5D.
24. La Par D, Yang Z, Stakenborg G, et al: Outcomes of reoperation: aortic valve replacement after previous sternotomy. *J Thorac Cardiovas Surg* 2010; 139(2):263-272.
25. Smith WT IV, Ferguson T, Ryan T, et al: Should coronary artery bypass graft surgery patients with mild or moderate aortic stenosis undergo concomitant aortic valve replacement? A decision analysis approach to the surgical dilemma. *J Am Coll Cardiol* 2004; 44(6):1241-1247.
26. Sareyyupoglu B, Sundt TM, Schaff HV, et al: Management of mild aortic stenosis at the time of coronary artery pass surgery: should the valve be replaced? *Ann Thorac Surg* 2009; 88(4):1224-1231.
27. Nassimiha D, Aronow WS, Ahn C, et al: Rate of progression of valvular aortic stenosis in patients > or = 60 years of age. *Am J Cardiol* 2001; 87:807-809.

28. Carabello B: Controversies in cardiovascular medicine: aortic valve replacement should be operated on before symptom onset. *Circulation* 2012; 126:112-117.

29. Verhoye JP, Merliclo F, Sami IM, et al: Aortic valve replacement for aortic stenosis after previous coronary artery bypass grafting: could early reoperation be prevented? *J Heart Valve Dis* 2006; 15:474-478.

30. Alcalai R. Viola N, Mosseri M, et al: The value of percutaneous coronary intervention in aortic valve stenosis in coronary artery disease. *Am J Med* 2007; 120(2):155.

31. Peels J, Boonstrel PW, Ebels T, et al: Hybrid approach for complex coronary artery and valve disease: a clinical follow up study. *Neth Heart J* 2007; 15(10):327-328.

32. Brinster DR, Byrne M, Rogers CD: Effectiveness of same day percutaneous coronary intervention followed by minimally invasive aortic valve replacement for aortic stenosis and moderate coronary artery disease ("hybrid approach"). *Am J Cardiol* 2006; 98:1501-1503.

33. Pereira JJ, Balaban K, Lauer MS, et al: Aortic valve replacement in patients with mild or moderate aortic stenosis and coronary bypass surgery. *Am J Med* 2005; 118:735.

34. Gillinov AM, Garcia MJ: When is concomitant aortic valve replacement indicated in patients with mild to moderate stenosis undergoing coronary revascularization? *Curr Cardiol Rep* 2005; 7:101.

35. Lytle BW, Cosgrove DM, Gill CC, et al: Aortic valve replacement combined with myocardial revascularization. Late results and determinants of risk for 471 in-hospital survivors. *J Thorac Cardiovasc Surg* 1988; 95(3):402-414.

36. Morris JJ, Schaff HV, Mullany CJ, et al: Determinants of survival and recovery of left ventricular function after aortic valve replacement. *Ann Thorac Surg* 1993; 56:22.

37. Jones EL, Weintraub WS, Craver JM, et al: Interaction of age and coronary disease after valve replacement: implications for valve selection. *Ann Thorac Surg* 1994; 58:378.

38. Shinn SH, Oh S-S, et al: Short and long-term results of triple valve surgery: a single center experience. *J Korean Med Sci* 2009; 24(5): 818-823.

39. Accola KD, Scott ML, Spector SD, Is the St. Jude Medical mechanical valve an appropriate choice for elderly patients?: A long-term retrospective study measuring quality of life. *J Heart Valve Dis* 2006; 15(1):57.

40. Accola KD, Scott ML, Palmer GJ, et al: Surgical management of aortic valve disease in the elderly: a retrospective comparative study of valve choice using propensity score analysis. *J Heart Valve Dis* 2008; 17(4):355-364.

41. Dagenais F, Mathieu P, Doyle D, et al: Moderate aortic stenosis in coronary artery bypass grafting patients more than 70 years of age: to replace or not to replace? *Ann Thorac Surg* 2010; 90(5):1495-1499.

42. Kay PH, Nunley D, Grunkemeier GL, et al: Ten-year survival following aortic valve bypass as a risk factor: a multivariate analysis of coronary replacement. *J Cardiovasc Surg* 1986; 27:494.

43. Mullany CJ, Elveback LR, Frye FL, et al: Coronary artery disease and its management: influence on survival in patients undergoing aortic valve replacement. *J Am Coll Cardiol* 1987; 10:66.

44. Kirklin JK, Nartel DC, Blackstone EH, et al: Risk factors for mortality after primary combined valvular and coronary artery surgery. *Circulation* 1989; 79(Suppl I):I-1180.

45. Karp RB, Mills N, Edmunds LH Jr: Coronary artery bypass grafting in the presence of valvular disease. *Circulation* 1989; 79(Suppl I):I-I182.

46. Tsai TP, Matloff JM, Chaux A, et al: Combined valve and coronary artery bypass procedures in septuagenarians and octogenarians: results in 120 patients. *Ann Thorac Surg* 1986; 42:681.

47. Bridgewater B, Kinsman R, Walton P, et al: The 4th European association for cardiothoracic surgery adult cardiac surgery data base report. *Interact Cardiovasc Thorac Surg* 2011; 12:4-5.

48. Gunay R, Sensozy Kayacioglu I, et al: Is the aortic valve pathology type different for early and late mortality in concomitant aortic valve replacement and coronary artery bypass surgery? *Interact Cardiovasc Thorac Surg* 2009; 9(4):634.

49. Pedersen WR, Klaassen PJ, Pedersen CW, et al: Comparison of outcomes in high-risk patients > 70 years of age with aortic valvuloplasty and percutaneous coronary intervention versus aortic valvuloplasty alone. *Am J Cardiol* 2008; 101:1309.

50. Maganti M, Rao V, Armstrong S, et al: Redo valvular surgery in elderly patients. *Ann Thorac Surg* 2009; 87:521.

51. Lam BK, Gillinov AM, Blackstone EH, et al: Importance of moderate ischemic mitral regurgitation. *Ann Thorac Surg* 2005; 79:462.

52. Andrade IG, Cartier R, Panisi P, et al: Factors influencing early and late survival in patients with combined mitral valve replacement and myocardial revascularization and in those with isolated replacement. *Ann Thorac Surg* 1987; 44:607.

53. Lytle BW, Cosgrove DM, Gill CC, et al: Mitral valve replacement combined with myocardial revascularization: early and late results for 300 patients, 1970 to 1983. *Circulation* 1985; 71:1179.

54. Ashraf SS, Shaukat N, Odom N, et al: Early and late results following combined coronary bypass surgery and mitral valve replacement. *Eur J Cardiothorac Surg* 1994; 8:57.

55. Szecsi J, Herrijgers P, Sergeant P, et al: Mitral valve surgery combined with coronary bypass grafting: multivariate analysis of factors predicting early and late results. *J Heart Valve Dis* 1994; 3:236.

56. Crabtree TD, Bailey MS, Moon MR, et al: Recurrent mitral regurgitation and risk factors for early and late mortality after mitral valve repair for functional ischemic mitral regurgitation. *Ann Thorac Surg* 2008; 85:1537.

57. Sheikh KH, Bengtson JR, Rankin JS, et al: Intraoperative transesophageal Doppler color flow imaging used to guide patient selection and operative treatment of ischemic mitral regurgitation. *Circulation* 1991; 84:594.

58. Bax JJ, Braun J, Somer ST, et al: Restrictive annuloplasty and coronary revascularization in ischemic mitral regurgitation results in reverse left ventricular remodeling. *Circulation* 2004; 110:II103.

59. Cohn LH, Kowalker W, Bhatia S, et al: Comparative morbidity of mitral valve repair versus replacement for mitral regurgitation with and without coronary artery disease. *Ann Thorac Surg* 1988; 45:284.

60. Geidel S, Lass M, Osstermeyer J: Restrictive mitral valve annuloplasty for chronic ischemic mitral regurgitation: a 5-year clinical experience with the physio ring. *Heart Surg Forum* 2008; 11:E225.

61. Akins CW, Buckley MJ, Daggett WM, et al: Myocardial revascularization with combined aortic and mitral valve replacements. *J Thorac Cardiovasc Surg* 1985; 90:272.

62. Gelsomino S, Lorusso R, De Cicco G, et al: Five-year echocardiographic results of combined undersized mitral ring annuloplasty and coronary artery bypass grafting for chronic ischemic mitral regurgitation. *Eur Heart J* 2008; 29:231.

63. Ho PC, Nguyen ME: Multivessel coronary drug-eluting stenting alone in patients with significant ischemic mitral regurgitation: a 4-year follow up. *J Invasive Cardiol* 2008; 20:41.

64. Dion R: Ischemic mitral regurgitation: when and how should it be corrected? *J Heart Valves* 1993; 2:536.

65. Aklog L, Filsoufi F, Flores KQ, et al: Does coronary artery bypass grafting alone correct moderate ischemic mitral regurgitation? *Circulation* 2001; 75:I-I68.

66. Milano CA, Daneshmand MA, Rankin JS, et al: Survival prognosis and surgical management of ischemic mitral regurgitation. *Ann Thorac Surg* 2008; 86:735.

67. Benedetto U, Roscitano MG, Fiorani B, et al: Does combined mitral valve surgery improve survival when compared to revascularization along in patients with ischemic mitral regurgitation? A meta-analysis on 2479 patients. *J. Cardiovasc Med* 2009; 10(2):109-114.

68. Filsoufi F, Aklog L, Byrne JG, et al: Current results of combined coronary artery bypass grafting and mitral annuloplasty in patients with moderate ischemic mitral regurgitation. *J Heart Valve Dis* 2004; 13:747.

69. Accola KD, Scott ML, Thompson PA, et al: Midterm outcomes using the physio ring in mitral valve reconstruction: experience in 492 patients. *Ann Thorac Surg* April 2005; 79:1276-1283.

70. Cox JL, Buckberg GD: Ventricular shape and function in health and disease. *Semin Thorac Cardiovasc Surg* 2001; 13:298.

71. Diodato MD, Moon MR, Pasque MK, et al: Repair of ischemic mitral regurgitation does not increase mortality or improve long-term survival in patients undergoing coronary artery revascularization: a propensity analysis. *Ann Thorac Surg* 2004; 78:794.

72. Kay PH, Nunley DL, Grunkemeier GL, et al: Late results of combined mitral valve replacement and coronary bypass surgery. *J Am Coll Cardiol* 1985; 5:29.

73. Chiappini B, Minuti U, Gregorini R, et al: Early and long-term outcome of mitral valve repair with a Cosgrove band combined with coronary revascularization in patients with ischemic cardiomyopathy and moderate-severe mitral regurgitation. *J Heart Valve Dis* 2008; 17:396.

74. Sirivella S, Gielchinsky I: Results of coronary bypass and valve operations for valve regurgitation. *Asian Cardiovasc Thorac Ann* 2007; 5:396.

75. Wan CK, Suri RM, Li Z, Orszulak TA, et al: Management of moderate functional mitral regurgitation at the time of aortic valve replacement: is concomitant mitral valve repair necessary? *J Thorac Cardiovasc Surg* 2009; 137:635.

76. Cohn LH, Couper GS, Kinchla NM, Collins JJ Jr: Decreased operative risk of surgical treatment of mitral regurgitation with or without coronary artery disease. *J Am Coll Cardiol* 1990; 16:1575.

77. Masson JB, Webb JG: Percutaneous mitral annuloplasty. *Coron Artery Dis* 2009; 20:183.

78. Davidson MJ, Cohn LG: Surgeons' perspective on percutaneous valve repair. *Coron Artery Dis* 2009; 20:192.

79. Johnson WD, Kayser KL, Pedraza PM, Brenowitz JB: Combined valve replacement and coronary bypass surgery: results in 127 operations stratified by surgical risk factors. *Chest* 1986; 90:338.

80. Flameng WJ, Herijgers P, Szecsi J, et al: Determinants of early and late results of combined valve operations and coronary artery bypass grafting. *Ann Thorac Surg* 1996; 61(2):621-628.

Reoperative Valve Surgery

46

Julius I. Ejiofor • John G. Byrne • Marzia Leacche

The number of patients undergoing reoperation for valvular heart disease is increasing and will continue to increase as the general population ages.[1] These reoperations most commonly involve structural deterioration of a bioprosthesis or progression of native-valve disease after nonvalve cardiac surgery. Structural failure of a biologic valve should be considered a part of the natural evolution of tissue valves and should be fully appreciated by both the surgeon and the patient prior to implantation.[2] Reoperations are technically more difficult than primary operations because of adhesions around the heart with an associated risk of reentry, the presence of more advanced cardiac pathology, and the existence of more frequent comorbidities such as pulmonary hypertension. Perhaps most importantly, reoperative valve replacement operations often are performed in functionally compromised patients who tolerate complications poorly or who have little reserve.[3] As a consequence of these and other factors, reoperative valve surgery historically has been associated with a considerably higher operative mortality than primary valve surgery, particularly in patients who have had multiple prior replacements.[4] In the modern era, however, with the use of alternative surgical approaches and advanced perioperative care, there has been significant improvement in outcomes.[5-9]

Reductions in operative risk and postoperative morbidity after reoperative valve surgery have been made in the past few years through advances in myocardial protection, as well as alternative perfusion strategies such as the proper use of deep hypothermic cardiac arrest.[10] In addition, use of peripheral cannulation techniques to institute cardiopulmonary bypass (CPB) has become a relatively standard practice in reoperative cases.[11-13] Early institution of CPB prior to reentry prevents injury to the right ventricle (RV) or patent coronary artery bypass grafts during reoperative sternotomy.

Successful replacement of degenerated cardiac valves usually results in symptomatic and hemodynamic improvement. In this regard, improvements in valve design have mitigated but not eliminated primary bioprosthetic failure.[14-16] As such, the risk of re-replacement for bioprosthetic failure remains a significant factor to be considered in the selection of valve type for implantation.[17]

MECHANICAL VERSUS BIOLOGIC VALVES

The most appropriate valve substitute for an individual patient remains a source of much controversy. This choice should be adapted to each individual patient depending on age, life expectancy, life style, valve size, and cardiac as well as noncardiac comorbidities.[18] Some studies comparing the long-term outcomes between biologic and mechanical aortic valve prostheses have yielded similar results with regard to overall valve-related complications.[19-22] However, most recent large studies have documented that anticoagulant-related bleeding with mechanical valves must be balanced against life expectancy and the risk of biologic valve re-replacement.[23-25] Bioprosthetic valves are known to undergo a time-dependent process of structural deterioration that results in freedom of reoperation of 80% at 15 years.[20] Consequently, structural degeneration of a bioprosthesis is the most frequent indication for reoperation in patients with tissue valves.[19,26]

Despite this, recently improved durability of tissue valves, as well as the availability of stentless valves and homografts, has led to surgeons placing bioprostheses in progressively younger age groups.[18,27-30] Contributing to this trend, many patients do not want to accept the risk of anticoagulant-related hemorrhage associated with mechanical valves: major events 0.5% per patient-year and minor events 2 to 4% per patient-year.[31] In addition, new concepts of valve-in-valve (VinV) interventions are suggesting to patients that there may be re-replacement of bioprosthetic valves in the future.

Mechanical prostheses usually are selected for younger recipients because of their proven durability over time. However, the risk of anticoagulant-related bleeding, as well as thromboembolic events (TEs), in these valves is not trivial and depends on valve design, structural materials, and host-related interactions.[31] In a 12-year comparison of Bjork-Shiley versus porcine valves, Bloomfield et al documented severe bleeding complications in 18.6 versus 7.1%, respectively.[32] Moreover, although endocarditis, dehiscence, perivalvular leak, and pannus formation are associated with both biologic and mechanical valves, acute prosthetic thrombosis is exclusively a complication of mechanical valves.[33,34] In considering mechanical valve durability, these associated risks cannot be ignored and must be weighed against the anticipated rate of tissue-valve failure and the need for reoperation.

RISK FACTORS IN REOPERATIVE VALVE SURGERY

In evaluating patients for reoperative valve surgery, certain factors are associated with added risk. For example, Husebye et al, in a review of their 20-year experience[17] with reoperative valve surgery, found specific issues to carry higher risk (see Table 46-1). Overall operative mortality was 7% for the second and 14% for the third reoperation. Operative mortality for the first reoperation (n = 530 patients) was 5.9% in the aortic position and 19.6% in the mitral position. In the aortic position, operative mortality was 2.4% for New York Heart Association (NYHA) class I, 1.6% for NYHA class II, 6.3% for NYHA class III, and 20.8% for NYHA class IV emphasizing the significance of early referral. Regarding the urgency of surgery, the mortality for elective mitral valve reoperations was 1.4%; for urgent procedures, 8%; and for emergency procedures, 37.5%. Based on these findings, the authors have recommended that referral for reoperation be made when valve dysfunction is first noted, that is, before a significant decrement in myocardial function.[17] Similarly, Jones et al reviewed their experience with first heart valve reoperations in 671 patients between 1969 and 1998.[6] Their overall operative mortality for first-time heart valve reoperation was 8.6%, similar to the results published by Lytle et al[35] (10.9%), Cohn et al[4] (10.1%), Akins et al[36] (7.3%), Pansini et al[2] (9.6%), and Tyers et al[37] (11.0%). In the Jones and colleagues series, mortality increased from 3.0% for reoperation on a new valve site to 10.6% for prosthetic valve dysfunction or periprosthetic leak; mortality was highest (29.4%) for associated endocarditis or valve thrombosis. Concomitant coronary artery bypass grafting (CABG) carried a higher associated mortality (15.4%) than when it was not required (8.2%). Among the 336 patients requiring re-replacement of prosthetic valves, mortality was 26.1% for re-replacement of a mechanical valve

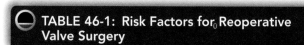

TABLE 46-1: Risk Factors for Reoperative Valve Surgery

Advanced age

Impaired ejection fraction (EF), congestive heart failure (CHF), or advanced preoperative functional class (NYHA)

Urgency of operation or unstable status preoperatively

Preoperative shock

Concomitant coronary artery bypass graft (CABG) or the presence of previous bypass grafts

Prosthetic valve endocarditis

Surgery for perivalvular leaks, valve thrombosis, or prosthetic dysfunction

Renal dysfunction

Chronic obstructive pulmonary disease (COPD)

compared with 8.6% for re-replacement of a tissue valve. The authors concluded through multivariable analysis that significant predictors of mortality were year of reoperation, patient age, indication, concomitant CABG, and the replacement of a mechanical valve rather than a tissue valve.[6]

PREOPERATIVE IMAGING IN REOPERATIVE VALVE SURGERY

Reoperative cardiac surgery is associated with higher morbidity and mortality than the first operation[38-40] partially related to the risk of surgical reentry. The main technical concern during surgical reentry is the risk of lethal injury to vital structures such as the aorta, RV, and patent coronary artery bypass grafts. The key to mitigating the risk of reentry is via careful planning of the surgical approach. This starts with knowing the exact proximity of the RV, aorta, and prior grafts to the posterior sternal table. The standard preoperative coronary angiography and chest x-ray is usually uninformative about the precise anatomic relationship of these vital structures with the sternum.

Retrospective electrocardiographic (ECG)-gated multidetector computed tomographic (MDCT) scanning has arisen as the modality of choice to assess not only the heart's location in relation to the sternum, but also graft's location and patency.[41-43] Use of ECG-gated MDCT meticulously evaluates the structures of interest to the surgeon, including sternum, mediastinal structures, bypass grafts, and their relationship to each other.[44-46] At our institution, all reoperative cardiac surgeries are preceded by a preoperative cardiac computed tomography (CT) scan assessment. For patients with prior valvular (non-CABG) surgeries in which assessment of bypass graft is not necessary, noncontrast CT scan is adequate. In 2010, the Appropriate Use Criteria of the American College of Cardiology rated this application of cardiac CT as an appropriate use of this technology.[45,47]

Preoperative CT scan will lead to a modification of surgical approach in 20% of patients undergoing redo cardiac surgery.[41,44] For example, if CT shows a distended RV adherent to the posterior sternum, it might be prudent to initiate CPB prior to attempting sternal reentry. In high-risk redo patients, MDCT is associated with a higher adoption of preventive maneuvers aimed at mitigating the risk of reentry.[48] There is evidence that preoperative MDCT reduces the risk associated with redo cardiac surgery[49] as well as shorter perfusion and cross-clamp time, shorter intensive care unit stays, and less frequent perioperative myocardial infarction (MI).[50]

REOPERATIVE AORTIC VALVE SURGERY

Historically, aortic valve surgery typically involved the placement of a mechanical valve. In the past, there were only a few generally accepted indications to use a bioprosthesis for primary, isolated aortic valve replacement (AVR): (1) the presence of well-established contraindications to anticoagulation, (2) the inability to monitor prothrombin levels adequately, and (3) patients whose survival was limited and more dependent on nonvalve-related issues.[18,26] In recent years, however, the use of biologic valves in the aortic position has become more common.[24,51]

As mentioned, reoperations are technically demanding, and many patients present in a poor functional state that further increases their mortality, in some series up to 19%.[32,52,53] Generally, optimal planning for reoperation prior to deterioration to NYHA class III to IV levels and before unfavorable comorbid conditions have arisen is imperative to ensure good outcomes.[9] Following these guidelines in the modern era, elective re-replacement of malfunctioning aortic bioprostheses can be performed with results similar to those of the primary operation.[18,23,54] The Mayo Clinic, for example, recently reviewed its experience with 162 reoperative AVRs. Early mortality for reoperative AVR was not statistically different from that for primary AVR.[55] In light of recent lower operative mortality in reoperative valve surgery, a more conservative approach toward issues such as "prophylactic" AVR in patients with asymptomatic mild-to-moderate aortic stenosis (AS) at the time of CABG also may be more appropriate.[56]

In evaluating the reoperative patient, the presence of concomitant coronary artery disease and pulmonary hypertension has been shown consistently to be independent risk factors.[18] Patients with these risk factors therefore need careful surveillance once the probability of bioprosthetic dysfunction begins increasing (ie, 6 to 10 years after implantation).[16] Regarding valve surveillance and timing of reoperation, the following variables are relevant to the clinical management of patients with an aortic bioprosthesis: a history of endocarditis before the first operation, perioperative infectious complications, coronary artery disease acquired after the first operation, an increase in pulmonary artery pressure, and a decrease in left ventricular function during the interoperative interval.[18] Proper timing of the reoperation therefore is paramount because duration of clinical signs with a dysfunctional aortic bioprosthesis may be misleading. This is further supported by the fact that the need for emergency reoperation is the most ominous risk factor and consistently yields a high early mortality rate of 25 to 44%.[57]

Reoperative Aortic Valve Surgery after Prior Coronary Revascularization

Reoperative valve surgery in patients with a prior patent left internal thoracic artery (LITA) to left anterior descending (LAD) graft is challenging for surgeons because of specific considerations for myocardial protection and prevention of patent graft injury. Unlike mitral valve surgery or CABG, in which cross-clamping of the aorta may be optional, aortic valve surgery mandates aortic cross-clamp unless hypothermic circulatory arrest is used. As such reoperative AVR in patients with a patent LITA graft presents a unique challenge of myocardial protection.

The incidence of LITA injury in the literature varies from 5 to 9%[58-61] and is associated with a 40% risk of perioperative MI[59] and 50% mortality rate.[62-64] This high morbidity and mortality rate warrants a preoperative decision concerning the most appropriate and safe surgical approach.

This is an area of recent controversy. The most traditional approach involves resternotomy, dissection of the LITA graft, and occlusion of the patent graft with a small bulldog and then aortic cross-clamping. This strategy has the advantage of short CPB time, maximizing uniform myocardial protection without cardioplegia washout but with an obvious risk of LITA injury during dissection. Efforts to reduce the risk of LITA injury have led to the "no-dissection" surgical technique in which the graft is left unclamped with use of deep hypothermic cardioplegic arrest.[58,65-67] In this approach, the LITA graft is not dissected and myocardial protection is achieved by using moderate-to-deep hypothermic cardioplegic arrest. This has the advantage of minimizing (but not eliminating) graft injury and its main disadvantage is that an unclamped LITA graft can lead to poor/uneven myocardial protection because of cardioplegia washout from the LITA territory. Another disadvantage is poor visualization due to continuous flow through the LITA. Other less utilized and studied approaches involve supraclavicular or endovascular control of the patent LITA graft.[68,69]

It is worth mentioning that another strategy of handling patent LITA grafts involves deep hypothermic circulatory arrest without controlling the graft or aortic cross-clamping. This technique is occasionally indicated in patients with "porcelain" aortas.[70]

All these concerns reiterate the importance of meticulous preoperative assessment and planning, to determine the optimal surgical approach for each individual patient. The "no-dissection" technique with hypothermic cardioplegia is a preferred approach for redo AVR in patients with patent LITA graft. Several studies have documented the safety of this method without any increased risk of perioperative mortality.[58,65-67]

Approaches and Techniques

CONVENTIONAL RESTERNOTOMY

The evolution of cardiac surgery through the last few decades has led to the popularization of various surgical approaches. Thoracotomy, for example, once was used extensively to gain access to mediastinal structures. Then median sternotomy became the standard approach. In reoperative cases, however, repeating the sternotomy carries definite surgical risks. Before proceeding with a resternotomy, the relationship between certain anterior mediastinal structures (eg, the RV and the aorta) and the posterior aspect of the sternum must be assessed carefully.[71] As described above, a CT scan with or without contrast is now the modality of choice.[41,43,62]

Exposure of the femoral vessels and preparation for emergency femoral-femoral CPB should be performed before resternotomy. In cases of heightened concern for RV-graft injury or in cases in which a left internal mammary artery

(LIMA) graft is patent, the surgeon should consider the use of CPB before chest reentry. Sternal wires from the previous operation should be undone carefully but left in place as a posterior safeguard during initial sternal division. An oscillating (not reciprocating) bone saw can be used to divide the anterior sternal table. An Army-Navy retractor, placed inferiorly in-line with the sternotomy can be used to stent open the wound during opening of the posterior table. Most authors recommend dividing the posterior table using a combination of scissors and anterolateral rake retraction.[62,71,72] Following this, bilateral pleural spaces should be entered inferiorly, followed by careful dissection of other mediastinal structures. The pericardial dissection plane can be developed by starting at the cardiophrenic angle and advancing slowly cephalad and laterally on the surface of the right side of the heart. Cephalad dissection should start with freeing the innominate vein before spreading the retractor to avoid its injury. Further dissection then is carried down to the superior vena cava (SVC), being careful to note the location of the right phrenic nerve. An area of consistently dense adhesions is the right atrial appendage, and caution should be used here. In addition, great care should be taken to avoid "deadventializing" the aorta. The area where the aorta apposes the pulmonary artery is another site of potential injury.

Repairing small ventricular or atrial lacerations should not be attempted before releasing the tension of the surrounding adhesions. Repair of great vessel injuries or severe RV injuries is best done on CPB.[71] Severe active hemorrhage during a second sternotomy usually is caused by adherence of the heart or great vessels to the posterior sternum. Prevention of this complication by interposition of pericardium or other mediastinal tissue at the time of the first operation has been suggested but has debatable relevance.[62] The incidence of resternotomy hemorrhage is between 2 and 6% per patient reoperation.[73-75] In a report of 552 patients who had undergone reoperative prosthetic valve surgery, 23 patients (4%) had complications related directly to sternal opening.[17] Of these, five patients had injury to the right atrium, seven patients had lacerated RVs, nine patients had injuries to the aorta, and two patients had a previously placed coronary artery graft divided. Nineteen of the 23 complications occurred during a first reoperation. Overall, there were two operative deaths related to resternotomy. The first death involved division of a previously placed coronary artery graft during reentry. The second death was caused by laceration of the aorta with subsequent exsanguination.[17] Of note, prior use of a right internal mammary artery (RIMA) graft can be particularly challenging because it frequently crosses the midline, and extreme caution must be used in first dissecting out this vessel.

Macmanus et al reviewed their experience with 100 patients undergoing repeat median sternotomy.[74] Eighty-one patients had one repeat sternotomy, whereas the others had undergone multiple sternotomies. All had had a previous valve procedure and were reoperated on for progressive rheumatic valvular disease or for complications related to the prosthesis. Complications included hemorrhage during reentry in eight patients, postoperative hemorrhage in

two, seroma in four, and dehiscence, wound infection, and hematoma in one patient each. There was one operative death directly related to resternotomy hemorrhage.[74] When major hemorrhage does occur on sternal reentry, attempts at resternotomy should be abandoned, and the chest should be reapproximated by pushing toward the midline. The patient should be heparinized immediately while obtaining femoral arterial and venous cannulation. Blood loss from the resternotomy should be aspirated with cardiotomy suction and returned to the pump. Once bypass has been established, core cooling should be commenced with anticipation of the need for circulatory arrest. Once cool, flow rates can be reduced briefly for less than a minute, and the remaining sternal division can be completed, followed by direct repair of the underlying injury.[62] Anticipating the possibility of this scenario, we frequently expose peripheral cannulation sites prior to beginning a resternotomy. In cases of heightened concern for RV or graft injury, or in patients with a patent LIMA to LAD artery graft, CPB and cardiac decompression may be initiated *before* sternal reentry. After safe sternal entry, the patient may be weaned from bypass for further dissection of adhesions to avoid prolonged pump times.

MINIMALLY INVASIVE REOPERATIVE AORTIC VALVE REPLACEMENT

Reoperative procedures are challenging owing to diffuse mediastinal and pericardial adhesions. A large incision that increases the operative exposure also has been associated with a higher risk of injury to cardiac structures and coronary artery bypass grafts and results in greater bleeding with its associated transfusion requirements.[76-79] A smaller incision with a limited sternotomy, on the other hand, reduces the area of pericardiolysis, thus mitigating these effects. The intact lower sternum that remains also preserves the integrity of the caudal chest wall, thereby enhancing sternal stability and promoting earlier extubation.[80,81] *Minimally invasive* valve procedures gradually have become more accepted as new technologies and instrumentation have been developed.[80] Reoperative procedures in which there is risk for graft injury are an area where minimally invasive strategies may be of direct benefit.[82,83] Our surgical approach in reoperative AVR is shown in Fig. 46-1.[80] In our series of patients, peripheral cannulation sites were exposed or cannulated before beginning the partial upper resternotomy. An external defibrillator is placed on the patient before draping for anticipated defibrillation as necessary. Transesophageal echocardiography (TEE) was used in every patient. A partial upper resternotomy was carried out to the third or fourth intercostal space depending on the estimated position of the aortic valve as documented by CT scan/TEE and then was "T'd to the right."[84] The oscillating saw was used to divide the anterior sternal table, whereas the straight Mayo scissors, under direct visualization, was used to divide the posterior sternal table. In the setting of a patent LIMA-LAD graft or other anterior coronary artery bypass grafts, patients were placed on CPB before partial resternotomy. Mediastinal dissection was limited

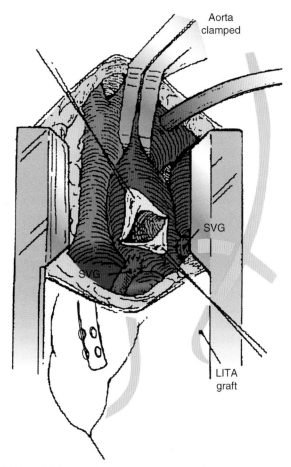

Aorta
clamped

SVG

SVG

LITA
graft

FIGURE 46-1 Partial upper resternotomy for reoperative AVR. The previous sternotomy incision is exposed to the third or fourth intercostal space depending on the position of the aortic valve, as documented by TEE. After dissection of the ascending aorta, paying particular attention to the position of coronary artery bypass grafts and their proximal anastomoses, cannulation is carried out. In this figure, the ascending aorta and innominate vein are cannulated. Frequently, however, other cannulation sites are required owing to space limitations in the chest. The ascending aorta is cross-clamped, and the aortic valve re-replacement is conducted in a standard fashion. (Reproduced with permission from Byrne JG, Karavas AN, Adams DH, et al: Partial upper re-sternotomy for aortic valve replacement or re-replacement after previous cardiac surgery, *Eur J Cardiothorac Surg.* 2000 Sep;18(3):282-286.)

to only the ascending aorta as was necessary for clamping and aortotomy. The right atrium was dissected only if it was cannulated. Although intrathoracic cannulation was preferred, we frequently used peripheral cannulation to avoid clutter in the chest. Retrograde cardioplegia, if necessary, was delivered via a transjugular coronary sinus catheter or with right atrial placement under TEE guidance. Vacuum assistance of venous drainage was used in the majority of patients. Once on CPB, all patients were systemically cooled to 20 to 25°C. Patients with patent LIMA-LAD grafts were cooled routinely to 20°C for additional myocardial protection and in so doing avoided the need and potential hazard of dissecting out the LIMA for clamping in an attempt to avoid cardioplegia washout. If flow

from the patent LIMA-LAD graft led to significant blood flow out of the coronary ostium and obscured the operative field, pump flows were turned down temporarily to allow visualization. Venting was accomplished by placing a pediatric vent through the aortic annulus. The aortic valve surgery then was performed based on patient indications. While closing the aortotomy, intracardiac air was removed by insufflating the lungs and decreasing flows on CPB. Carbon dioxide was used and flooded the operative field. Patients also were tilted from side to side to help with de-airing, and the ascending aortic vent was left open until separation from CPB. Temporary epicardial pacing wires were placed on the anterior surface of the RV while the heart was decompressed and before the aortic cross-clamp was removed. Two 32 French right-angled submammary chest tubes then were placed through the right pleural space, one angled medially into the mediastinum and one angled posterior into the pleural space. Decannulation and closure then were performed in the standard manner.

With our increasing experience in minimally invasive reoperative AVR, we have refined our technique as an alternative to conventional full resternotomy.[80] Technical details of the partial upper resternotomy approach are presented in Table 46-2. By following these guidelines, we have yet to

---

TABLE 46-2: Twelve Technical Details for Successful Aortic Valve Replacement After Previous Cardiac Surgery by Use of Partial Upper Resternotomy

1. Routine exposure of peripheral cannulation sites prior to partial upper resternotomy
2. Placement of Zoll (Zoll, Inc., Burlington, MA) defibrillator pads before prepping
3. Use of intraoperative transesophageal echocardiography for air removal and inspection of valve
4. In patients with patent left internal mammary artery to left anterior descending coronary artery (LIMA-LAD) graft, peripheral cannulation, and cardiopulmonary bypass (CPB) established before partial upper resternotomy
5. Mediastinal dissection limited to ascending aorta for clamping and aortotomy and atrium (RA), only if RA is cannulated
6. Use of peripheral cannulation to avoid clutter in the chest
7. Use of vacuum assistance on CPB
8. Use of retrograde cardioplegia (CP) delivered by transjugular retrograde CP catheter in addition to antegrade CP
9. Cooling to at least 25°C in all patients primarily for myocardial protection; if a patent LIMA-LAD graft is present, cooling to 20°C without isolation and clamping LIMA graft
10. If visualization is poor because of LIMA-LAD collaterals flowing from coronary ostia, temporary low flows on CPB to improve visualization
11. Venting with a pediatric vent placed through the aortic annulus
12. Placement of temporary pacing wires on the right ventricular free wall before aortic clamp removal

Reproduced with permission from Byrne JG, Karavas AN, Adams DH, et al: Partial upper re-sternotomy for aortic valve replacement or re-replacement after previous cardiac surgery, *Eur J Cardiothorac Surg.* 2000 Sep;18(3):282-286.

convert any patient to a full resternotomy. CT scan and/or TEE are helpful in locating the level of the aortic valve and determining the proximity of the aorta to the posterior aspect of the sternum.[84] Also, extension of the sternal incision laterally on both sides through the intercostal spaces helps to later reapproximate the sternum. We have tried to limit mediastinal and pericardial dissection primarily to the aorta, believing that this is the principal reason for decreased bleeding and transfusion requirements postoperatively.[80,82,85,86] The RV, which often is attached to the sternum, does not need to be dissected. Also, injuries to patent but atherosclerotic vein grafts can be reduced with this "no touch" technique.[87]

Arterial and venous cannulation sites can vary considerably, reflecting the individual choice of the operating surgeon and the sufficiency of intrathoracic space. Possible cannulation sites, other than standard ones, include the axillary artery, innominate vein, and percutaneous femoral vein.[13,88] Innominate vein or percutaneous femoral vein cannulation, as well as the use of TEE to place the retrograde cardioplegia catheter, has been extremely helpful in minimizing dissection of the right atrium. At present, we consider this approach to be useful for isolated, elective reoperative aortic valve surgery.[80]

REOPERATIVE AORTIC VALVE REPLACEMENT AFTER HOMOGRAFT/ROOT/ALLOGRAFT

AVR with homografts and autografts was performed increasingly because of excellent freedom from thromboembolism, resistance to infection, and reasonable hemodynamic performance.[27] Although improved durability of current tissue valves has slowed this trend, autografts and, to a lesser degree, homografts remain popular in younger patients owing to durability and, in the case of autografts, the potential for growth.[30,89] Consequently, many patients will require aortic valve re-replacement for structural degeneration of their homograft or autograft valve.[90] It is expected that about one-third of patients younger than 40 years of age will require aortic valve re-replacement within 12 years of homograft placement. This is owing primarily to calcification and structural valve degeneration. As such, the issue of homograft or autograft durability is particularly pertinent in this subgroup of younger patients who are expected to live beyond 15 years from the time of operation.[89]

The incidence of patients with homografts or autografts in need of a second valve operation is expected to increase owing to the aforementioned recent popularity and availability of these conduits. Also, there is varied opinion as to the optimal surgical method of primary homograft AVR, with increased rates of aortic insufficiency (AI) in patients with the subcoronary implantation technique. Importantly, the selected technique of primary homograft operation may have relevance at reoperation because calcification or aneurysmal dilatation of the homograft may pose surgical challenges at reoperation. Despite these challenges, Sundt and others[29,91,92] have documented the feasibility of aortic valve re-replacement after full-root replacement with a homograft. In our own series of 18 patients, full-root, mini-root, and subcoronary techniques all were amenable to valve re-replacement.[27]

How to best approach the reoperative root scenario and which valve to reimplant, however, have been debated. At one extreme, Hasnat et al documented the results of 144 patients who underwent a *second* aortic homograft replacement with a hospital mortality rate of only 3.5%.[90] Although Kumar et al, in a multivariate analysis of reoperative aortic valve surgery, did not show that a previous homograft added significant risk,[93] the technical aspects of reoperative AVR in this patient population consistently have been found to be challenging owing to the heavy calcific degeneration that invariably occurs. With this in mind, and owing to the typical absence of the need for a second root operation, we and others[94] believe that a more simplified approach to reoperative aortic valve surgery in patients with previously placed homografts may be optimal. Our approach has been to perform aortic valve re-replacement using a mechanical valve or, less commonly, a stented xenograft while reserving a second homograft and root operation for specific indications such as endocarditis, associated root pathology, or a very young patient with contraindications to a mechanical valve.

An open valve-in-homografgt approach involves resection of the degenerated or infected aortic homograft leaflets and a new valve is seated within the aortic homograft valve annulus without a need for root reconstruction.[95] The procedure is done via a median sternotomy, which is preceded by peripheral cannulation for CPB via femoral vein and artery or right axillary artery. The heart is dissected out, CPB is initiated, the patient is fibrillated and cross-clamped; antegrade (and occasional retrograde) cardioplegia is initiated.[95] The aorta is opened between the homograft root and the ascending aorta. If there is heavy calcification, a vertical or S-shaped aortotomy is made. The homograft leaflets are resected and the calcified annulus debrided with careful endarterectomy of the proximal ascending aorta. The endarterectomy is carried out starting at the annulus and coming up to allow stitches on in the softer aorta.[95] The valve prosthesis (bioprosthetic or mechanical) is then sized and implanted using interrupted noneverting 2.0 Ethibond (Ethicon, Somerville, NJ) pledgeted sutures. The valve is then seated and the sutures tied and cut. The aorta is then closed with a running 3-0 Prolene (Ethicon) suture. The cross-clamp is removed and the heart defibrillated into normal sinus rhythm.[95]

Homograft re-replacement nonetheless is performed but it is much less common, and hospital mortality varies widely across many centers, ranging between 2.5 and 50%.[29,91,92] David and colleagues, for example, recently reviewed their experience with root operations in 165 patients who previously had undergone cardiac surgery. Of these, 28 had a previous root operation. Overall, 12 operative (7%) and 20 late deaths (12%) occurred.[96] Variations in sample size, valve selection, surgical techniques, and patient factors, as well as the experience of the surgeons, may account for these wide differences.

AORTIC VALVE BYPASS SURGERY

Aortic valve bypass (AVB) surgery, also known as apical aortic conduit surgery, is an alternative for high-risk and "inoperable" reoperative patients with AS. It has been used in patients with reduced LV function,[97] porcelain aorta,[98] severe patient prosthetic mismatch,[99] excessive comorbidities, and vulnerable functional grafts[100] leading to prohibitive risk for conventional reoperative AVR. AVB surgery works by shunting blood from the apex of the left ventricle to the descending aorta through a surgically placed valve conduit (Fig. 46-2). This approach avoids cross-clamping, cardioplegic arrest, potentially CPB,[101] debridement of the native valve, and injury to patent grafts because the procedure is performed through the left chest. Patient-prosthesis mismatch is also unlikely as the indexed effective orifice area (EOAi) is the sum of the valves in both the native position and conduit.

Contraindications to this procedure include moderate AI. Relative contraindications include a heavily diseased descending aorta or significant mitral valve regurgitation. However, Gammie et al showed that the degree of mitral regurgitation (MR) is reduced after placement of the conduit and moderate MR patients are still considered.

The procedure[102,103] is performed using a left ventricular apical connector with a silicon sewing ring and a heart valve (typically a stentless porcine valve with the coronaries over sewn) sewn to a Dacron graft at the beginning of the procedure. An 8-mm side branch off the Dacron graft may be used for direct inflow from the CPB machine if performed on pump. The patient is positioned in the right lateral decubitus position with a double lumen endotracheal tube. TEE is used

to exclude apical thrombus, calcification of the descending aorta, and ensure proper conduit positioning. If going on bypass an arterial and venous cannula are place in groin. A fifth- to sixth-intercostal space thoracotomy is performed and the apex of the heart and descending thoracic aorta exposed. The valve conduit with apical connector is then oriented with connector aimed at the apex of the heart. After heparinization the distal anastomosis is performed after placement of a partial occluding clamp on the descending thoracic aorta. The clamp is removed and hemostasis achieved. Stentless valve competency will prevent blood flow out of the apical connector. The pericardium is then opened and tacked up and a mark is made 1 to 2 cm lateral to the true apex of the left ventricle: 2-0 monofilament pledgeted sutures are used in an interrupted fashion around this marked area with deep bites of nearly full thickness. These are then taken through the sewing ring of the apical connector. If CPB is to be initiated, it is done at this time. The patient is placed in steep Trendelenburg position and the ventricle is then paced at 200 beats/min to reduce ventricular ejection. A hole is made in the marked apical area and a 14 French Foley catheter is placed into the left ventricle. Tension is placed on the Foley catheter and a coring knife is used to remove a plug of apical myocardium. A coring knife 85% of the diameter of the apical connector is selected to ensure a proper fit and optimize hemostasis. The Foley catheter is then removed and the apical connector is placed in the left ventricle. The sutures are tied down. The graft is de-aired and the chest is closed. When complete blood flow from the left ventricle travels out of the native valve and the conduit where it will primarily travel distally in the aorta with some flow in the retrograde direction. Studies have shown that approximately one-third of the flow travels out the native valve, whereas two-thirds travel out the conduit.[100] The procedure has been shown to be highly efficacious, dropping the mean aortic valve gradients in one study from 43 to 10 mm.[100] The durability of the apical aortic conduit procedure is also apparent, with some patients now more than 25 years out from their operations.

TRANSCATHETER AORTIC VALVES

The PARTNER trial was the first prospective randomized control study evaluating the safety and efficacy of transcatheter AVR (TAVR) in high-risk patients (cohort B) and "prohibitive" risk patients with severe AS. The study showed that in this "prohibitive" risk cohort, TAVR was better compared to medical therapy and in the high-risk cohort (cohort A) was noninferior to surgical AVR (SAVR).[104,105] Shortly after the successful results of the PARTNER trial was published in 2010, the US Food and Drug Administration approved TAVR. This ushered in the era of TAVR in the United States.

Today, the two types of TAVR approved in the United State are the Edwards SAPIEN XT (Edwards Lifesciences, Inc.[Irvine, CA]) and the Medtronic CoreValve (Medtronic, Inc., Minneapolis, MN). The Edwards SAPIEN XT uses a balloon-expandable stainless steel alloy tubular frame

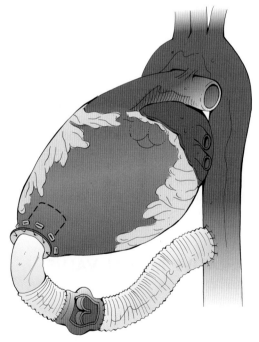

FIGURE 46-2 Apical aortic conduit. Aortic valve bypass surgery performed via left thoracotomy avoids sternotomy in difficult reoperative cases. (Reproduced with permission from Gammie JS, Krowsoski LS, Brown JM, et al: Aortic valve bypass surgery: midterm clinical outcomes in a high-risk aortic stenosis population, *Circulation* 2008 Sep 30;118(14):1460-1466.)

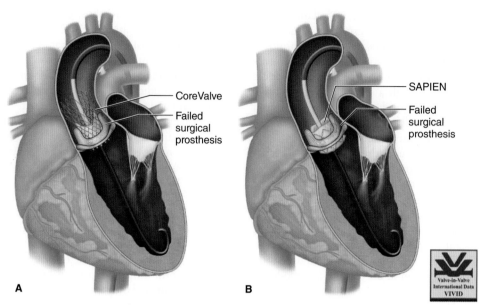

FIGURE 46-3 Transcatheter aortic valve-in-valve implantation in failed surgical bioprosthesis. (A) Showing the self-expandable CoreValve device and (B) the Balloon-expandable SAPIEN device. (Reproduced with permission from Dvir, D. In Aortic Valve-in-Valve: Insights from the Global Registry on stented vs. stentless bioprostheses, Transcatheter Cardiovascular Therapeutics (TCT), Washington D.C. 2014.)

within leaflets constructed from bovine pericardium while the Medtronic CoreValve uses a self-expanding nitinol (nickel-titanium alloy that is malleable at low temperature but rigid at body temperature) frame.[106] These devices can be implanted via percutaneous routes (transfemoral or sub-clavian/axillary), direct transapical or direct aortic access. For more on percutaneous AVR see Chapter 33.

Transcatheter Aortic Valve-in-Valve Implantation

The wide success of TAVR in patients with severe native aortic valve stenosis has led to its application beyond native aortic valve disease. This initially led to several reports of off-label TAV implantation within failed surgically inserted bioprosthetic valves (VinV).[107-110] VinV was first reported by Wenaweser et al in 2007[111] and it has garnered widespread use. A VinV procedure involves percutaneous implantation of a valve inside an already implanted bioprosthetic valve (Fig. 46-3) and it is an alternative to open surgery in high-risk patients with a degenerate aortic bioprosthesis.

VinV implantation is relatively new, but technology and experience with its application are growing exponentially. The Valve-in-Valve International Data (VIVID) registry was established in 2010 to collect data on VinV procedures from 55 centers around the world. They recently published the outcomes of 459 high-risk patients who underwent VinV implantation, the largest series to date.[112] They reported a 30-day operative mortality of 7.6%, a 1.7% major stroke rate, and an 83.2% overall 1-year survival. Of those who survived to 1-year, 92.3% had good functional status (NYHA class I/II).

Although these initial results of VinV implantation are promising, it does come with a distinct set of technical challenges and early results have been marred by unique safety concerns. These safety concerns include device malposition, ostial coronary occlusion, and elevated postprocedural gradients.[113] The VIVID registry reported a high device malposition rate of 15.3%; a 3.5% rate of ostial coronary obstruction; and a 28.4% rate of postprocedural high gradients (mean ≥ 20 mmHg).[113]

Another area of uncertainty is the long-term durability of VinV implantation. There are currently no long-term data on this relatively new procedure with most studies only stating 1-year survivals.[112-114]

Conventional open redo AVR is still considered the standard of care for patients with failed implanted valves. Although VinV is appealing as an alternative for high-risk, "inoperable" patients, long-term follow-up data will be necessary to establish the true role of VinV implantation for failed, degenerate bioprosthesis.

REOPERATIVE MITRAL VALVE SURGERY

Fundamental to a flawless surgical procedure is excellent and consistent exposure of the mitral valve.[115] Historically, the mitral valve has been exposed through a variety of surgical approaches, including median sternotomy, right thoracotomy, left thoracotomy, and transverse sternotomy.[116] The median sternotomy and right thoracotomy will be discussed in detail in the following; however, a brief description of the other approaches is warranted.

The *left* thoracotomy has been used in recent years to gain access to the mitral valve in situations in which a right thoracotomy is precluded (eg, mastectomy/radiation or pleurodesis). This incision is made through the fourth intercostal space, and the left pleural cavity is entered in the standard fashion.[116] Surgery is performed under fibrillatory arrest or with the beating-heart technique. Of importance, the mitral valve orientation is noted to be upside down with this approach, with the posterior annulus found anteriorly.[117] Thompson and colleagues recently reported their experience with the beating-heart left thoracotomy approach for reoperative mitral valve surgery. Of the 125 patients undergoing this technique, 86% were in NYHA class III or IV, and 28% had undergone two or more sternotomies. Thirty-day mortality was 6.4% with low complication rates.[118] Although occasionally useful, this approach provides limited access to the other cardiac chambers as well as poor visibility. This left-sided approach is rarely needed and typically reserved for patients in whom reoperative sternotomy or right thoracotomy is considered unacceptable. A bilateral anterior thoracotomy (ie, transverse sternotomy) carried out through the fourth intercostal space also has been described.[117,119] Rarely used today, this incision transects the sternum transversely, requiring ligation of both internal mammary arteries.

Regardless of the actual approach, once CPB has been established and the heart exposed, there are several incisions that can be employed to view the underlying mitral valve. The standard left atriotomy begins with blunt dissection of the interatrial groove (ie, Sondergaard's groove), allowing the right atrium to be retracted medially and anteriorly (see Fig. 46-4). The right superior pulmonary vein at its junction with the left atrium then is exposed, and the left atrium is opened at the midpoint between the right superior pulmonary vein insertion and the interatrial groove. This incision is extended longitudinally both superiorly and inferiorly to give enough exposure of the mitral valve. Care must be taken to avoid inadvertent injury to the posterior wall of the left atrium, and when closing, one must avoid including the posterior wall of the right pulmonary vein. The right atrial transseptal approach has become popular in recent years, especially in reoperative valve surgery. After opening the right atrium, the interatrial septum is incised starting at the fossa ovalis and moving vertically upward for a few centimeters (Figs. 46-5 and 46-6). This technique is especially helpful in reoperative surgery because it minimizes the amount of dissection required. Superior biatrial atriotomy, left ventriculotomy, and aortotomy all have been well described[15,76,115,116,120,121] as approaches to the mitral valve; each one has varying advantages and disadvantages.

Approaches and Techniques

RESTERNOTOMY

Resternotomy is still a common approach in reoperative mitral valve surgery. In many cases, this incision provides full and adequate exposure. This is especially true when concomitant procedures are necessary. However, reoperative median

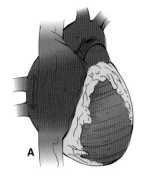
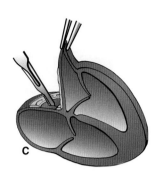
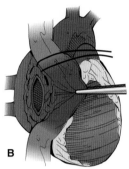

FIGURE 46-4 Sondergaard's groove approach. The left atrium enlarges to the right, increasing visualization from the right thoracotomy approach. The interatrial groove (Sondergaard's groove) is dissected approximately 1-cm deep, down to the left atrial wall. The purse-string suture is placed in the nondissected area. This prevents tearing of the dissected left atrial wall when the suture is tied down. Sagittal view shows location of the mitral valve in relation to the atriotomy. (Reproduced with permission from De DH, Pessella AT: Closed mitral commissurotomy utilizing right thoracotomy approach, *Asian Cardiovasc Thorac Ann* 2000;June:8(2):192-194.)

sternotomy has known risks, including injury to or embolism from prior grafts, sternal dehiscence, excessive hemorrhage, and inadvertent cardiac injury.[122] Patients with valvular heart disease may be especially prone to these complications because atrial dilatation can result in significant cardiomegaly, atrial thinning, and adherence of the heart to the posterior sternum. As discussed, patients undergoing prosthetic valve reoperation have a 4% incidence of complications directly related to sternal reentry that can result directly in intraoperative death.[17,35] Resternotomy also has been noted to be particularly hazardous in the presence of patent internal mammary grafts. Injury to a patent LIMA graft has an associated mortality rate approaching 50%.[62,84] Furthermore, manipulation of patent but diseased saphenous vein grafts can result in embolization into the native coronary circulation with resulting morbidity and mortality.[122,123] Patients with previous AVRs can have difficult exposure of the mitral valve owing to anterior fixation and probably are best served by an anterolateral thoracotomy approach. In general, in the setting of reoperative surgery, the resternotomy is likely to be the most dangerous part of the operation.[124] In this situation, we also have employed techniques that avoid resternotomy, such as right thoracotomy.

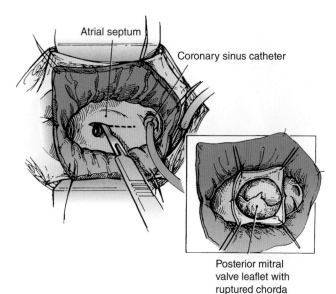

FIGURE 46-5 Atrial incision through the fossa ovalis. When the right atrium is incised, an incision is made in the atrial septum through the fossa ovalis. Retraction sutures on both the right atrium and the atrial septum of 2-0 silk then are used to elevate the septum and to keep the left atrium open. The mitral valve then will be exposed (*inset*). (Reproduced with permission from with permission from Byrne JG, Mitchell ME, Adams DH, et al: Minimally invasive direct access mitral valve surgery, *Semin Thorac Cardiovasc Surg.* 1999 Jul;11(3):212-222.)

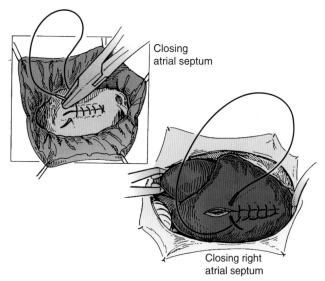

FIGURE 46-6 Closure. In the transseptal approach, the atria septum is approximated with running 4-0 Prolene sutures and is left open until the aortic cross-clamp is removed and the air is evacuated. The left ventricle should be filled with fluid before removal of the cross-clamp to help dislodgment of intraventricular air. Once the cross-clamp has been removed, air is evacuated vigorously from the left atrium through the septum or the left atrium itself, and the sutures are tied. The right atrium is then closed with running 4-0 Prolene sutures in two layers. TEE has been very important in helping to monitor the clearing of air from the intracardiac structures. We consider it mandatory in the minimally invasive technique, in which access to the entire cardiac structure is limited. (Reproduced with permission from with permission from Byrne JG, Mitchell ME, Adams DH, et al: Minimally invasive direct access mitral valve surgery, *Semin Thorac Cardiovasc Surg.* 1999 Jul;11(3):212-222.)

RIGHT THORACOTOMY

The right anterolateral thoracotomy approach was one of the first surgical approaches to the mitral valve, and it has become a safe alternative to resternotomy for mitral valve replacement[10,62,125,126] (see Fig. 46-5). This approach provides excellent exposure of the valves (mitral and tricuspid) with minimal need for dissection within the pericardium. In our recent experience with this approach,[124,127-131] operations were performed in the supine position with the right side of the chest slightly elevated. We routinely prepped and draped the right groin to allow femoral cannulation, if necessary. Preoperative and intraoperative TEE was performed in all patients, as well as standard intraoperative cardiac monitoring and a pacing Swan-Ganz catheter. A 5-cm right anterolateral thoracotomy was made, and the chest was entered through the bed of the fourth or fifth rib.[131] Adhesions of the right lung to the chest wall or pericardium were divided by electrocautery. The pericardium was entered anterior to the phrenic nerve. Arterial cannulation was achieved peripherally via the femoral artery. Peripheral cannulation was mostly via the femoral artery and this route was utilized if by TEE the atheroma grade of the descending aorta or arch is less than grade III. However, if the atheroma grade is greater than III, arterial cannulation is done via the right axillary artery. Venous cannulation was performed via the femoral vein with the tip of the cannula positioned between the SVC and the right atrium. In cases requiring tricuspid valve surgery, an additional SVC cannula is used while the femoral venous cannula is advanced at the IVC into the right atrium. After systemic heparinization, CPB is initiated with vacuum-assisted drainage. Patients were then cooled to 28°C to induce fibrillatory arrest. If spontaneous arrest did not occur with cooling, the pacing Swan-Ganz catheter was used to pace rapidly the ventricle into fibrillation. Care is used to avoid left ventricular ejection by keeping the left ventricle empty (ie, maintaining laminar, nonpulsatile arterial line tracing). In the absence of AI, aortic cross-clamping usually was not required. Regurgitant flow through the aortic valve occasionally required temporary low pump flow at appropriate temperatures to avoid cerebral injury.[131] The mitral valve was then approached through the left atrium directly by dissection of the intra-atrial (Sondergaard's) groove (see Fig. 46-4) or through the right atrium via the atrial septum (see Fig. 46-6). As the valve procedure was completed, rewarming was initiated (Fig. 46-7). Carbon dioxide (CO_2) can be continuously insufflated into the chest throughout the procedure to displace intracardiac air which reduces the time spent de-airing. In addition, perfusing blood via a cannula (eg, the left ventricular vent) positioned across the mitral valve and into the left ventricle will serve to displace residual air. A left atrial sump sucker was used to maintain a clear operative field. Upon completion of the procedure, patients then were placed in the Trendelenburg position and de-airing ascertained under TEE guidance. When core temperatures reached 37°C, the patient was weaned from CPB. Closure then was routine and at the conclusion of the procedure, patients were returned to the supine position.

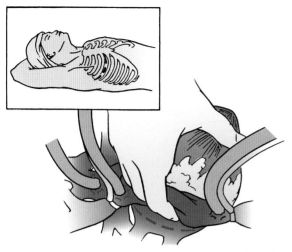

FIGURE 46-7 Right anterolateral thoracotomy through the fourth intercostal space and standard left atriotomy. (Reproduced with permission from with permission from Balasundaram SG, Duran C: Surgical approaches to the mitral valve, *J Card Surg.* 1990 Sep;5(3):163-169.)

The use of a small right anterior thoracotomy, femorofemoral bypass, and deep hypothermia has increased since our initial report in 1989.[132] Reduced blood use and decreased risk of LIMA or cardiac structural injury during sternal reentry make it a desirable approach for many complicated mitral reoperations. Deep hypothermia (~20°C) and low-flow femorofemoral bypass perfusion, without the necessity of aortic cross-clamping, provide adequate myocardial protection.[133] CPB times, blood loss, blood product usage, and LIMA injury rates have been lower in reoperative patients undergoing right thoracotomy than in those with resternotomy.[35,118,120,129,133-136]

Certain issues must be considered before the right thoracotomy approach is entertained. Patients who require simultaneous CABG generally will require a median sternotomy, although isolated right-sided grafting may be performed with a thoracotomy. Simultaneous replacement of the aortic valve is difficult from a thoracotomy approach and generally should be performed through a resternotomy. Significant AI can make effective perfusion on CPB difficult because, after opening the left atrium, blood will be returned to the pump via the cardiotomy suction. Unless the ascending aorta is clamped, effective end-organ perfusion will not be achieved. Also, in the setting of AI, exposure of the mitral valve may be difficult owing to this regurgitant flow into the surgical field. Left ventricular distension and myocardial stretch injury also can occur with fibrillatory arrest in patients with and occasionally without AI. Patients with greater than minimal AI therefore should be either excluded from a right thoracotomy approach or expected to require aortic cross-clamping either with traditional clamping or rarely with balloon occlusion with delivery of cardioplegia and aortic root venting. Significant right pleural disease, especially scarring in the right hemithorax, previously has been a relative contraindication to a right thoracotomy, although our series includes two patients

with a previous right thoracotomy who did not represent an overwhelming challenge.[137]

Our experience with 90 patients undergoing reoperative mitral valve surgery via a minimally invasive right thoracotomy without aortic cross-clamping showed excellent results.[136] In that series, the 2% operative mortality was lower than the STS-predicted mortality of 7%. Three patients developed acute renal failure postoperatively with one patient requiring new hemodialysis. One patient (1%) developed a postoperative stroke and no patient suffered a postoperative MI.[136] This study confirmed that the minimally invasive right thoracotomy technique was safe and effective in reducing operative mortality in reoperative mitral valve surgery.[136]

Minimally Invasive/Port Access Right-Sided Techniques

An alternative approach to reoperative mitral valve is with minimally invasive or port access techniques.

Some authors have noted that the distance to the mitral valve with the right thoracotomy approach at times can be limiting. Chitwood and colleagues recently reported use of a minithoracotomy aided by the voice-activated robotic camera AESOP.[138] Vleissis and Bolling also reported 22 patients who underwent a "minimally invasive" right thoracotomy approach to the atrioventricular valves.[139] The procedures performed included mitral valve repair (n = 12), mitral valve replacement (n = 5), prosthetic mitral valve re-replacement (n = 4), repair of a perivalvular leak (n = 3), tricuspid valve repair (n = 5), and closure of an atrial septal defect (n = 7). Mean bypass time was 109 minutes with a mean fibrillatory time of 62 minutes. Operative mortality in this group was 0%, and none of the patients experienced a wound complication. At follow-up, all reoperative patients thought that their recovery from this approach was more rapid and less painful than their original sternotomy.[139] Burfeind et al recently reviewed Duke University's experience with the port access technique.[140] In their series of 60 patients, a 6 cm right anterolateral thoracotomy was used with standard port access technique. Forty-five percent of patients underwent cardiac arrest with the Endo Clamp technique, whereas ventricular fibrillation was used in 55% of patients. Femoral cannulation was used in all patients. When compared with concurrent cohorts of patients undergoing reoperative sternotomy or right anterolateral thoracotomy, patients undergoing the port access technique had lower mortality and decreased transfusion requirements but significantly longer CPB times. Although similar results have been found by other groups, one should be mindful of the potential hazards of the port access technique, namely, EndoClamp migration.[141-144]

Additional Techniques of Reoperative Mitral Surgery

A less common indication for reoperative mitral valve surgery but one that can be challenging is periprosthetic leak. The incidence of perivalvular leak for both mechanical and biologic valves is about 0 to 1.5% per patient-year. Of note, perivalvular leak is slightly more common with mechanical than with tissue valves, possibly owing to differences in suture technique for each and sewing ring characteristics. The regurgitant flow across the perivalvular area frequently leads to hemolysis and, through denuding of the endocardium, endocarditis.

In evaluating patients with a periprosthetic leak, an assessment of valve function is important. If the valve itself is competent, direct repair of the leak avoids the hazards of valve replacement. Although pledgeted suturing may be attempted for smaller leaks, fibrotic tethering of surrounding tissue and the size of the defect may require a bovine or autologous pericardial patch. In cases of significant dehiscence or associated valvular dysfunction, removal of the valve is necessary. Replacement in this situation, however, is prone to leak recurrence because the annulus is partially intact, often calcified, and otherwise less than ideal for suture placement. In these cases, a bovine pericardial skirt can be fashioned and sewn to the sewing ring of the valve. Annular sutures then are placed in a typical fashion through the sewing ring, and the valve is seated. A running suture then can be used to sew this skirt to the left atrium (Fig. 46-8).

An additional risk of reoperative mitral valve replacement is atrioventricular disruption. Care must be used in removing the original valve sewing ring because it is frequently "socked in," and inadvertent removal of excessive annular tissue may occur. Any evidence of disruption of the posterior annulus necessitates patch repair with pericardium (autologous or bovine) before placement of annular sutures.[145] When faced with less than ideal annular tissue, and in an attempt to ensure stability, bites must not be overly aggressive in depth. Left circumflex injury can occur and will lead to significant morbidity and mortality (Fig. 46-9). When removal of the old sewing ring will result in severe annular disruption, the ring may be left in place and used as a "neoannulus" for suturing.

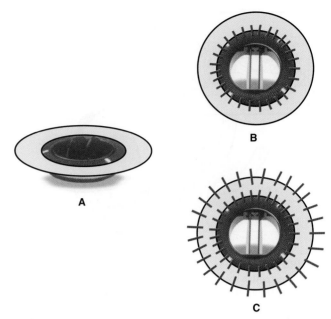

FIGURE 46-8 Pericardial skirt. Bovine pericardium can be fashioned as a skirt (A) and sewn to the sewing ring of the mitral prosthesis (B). Standard annular valve sutures are then taken through the sewing ring, the valve is seated, and the skirt is sewn to the left atrium with running technique (C). (Carbomedics mechanical valve shown.)

The benefits of preservation of the subvalvular apparatus have been clearly demonstrated during first-time mitral valve replacement.[146] Aside from improved contractile function, disruption of the posterior mitral annulus is avoided. David and colleagues found that preservation of the subvalvular apparatus is also important in reoperative patients.[147] Of 513 reoperative mitral valve replacements, preservation of the posterior subvalvular apparatus was accomplished in 103 (21%) patients, with anterior and posterior preservation occurring in 31 patients (6%). Gore-Tex neochordal construction was performed in 135 reoperative mitral valve replacement

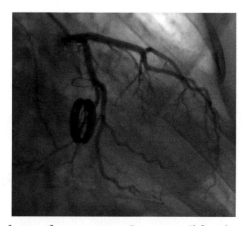 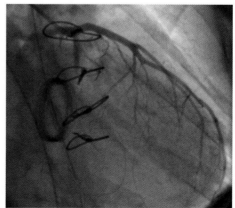

FIGURE 46-9 Left circumflex artery injury. Preoperative (*left*) and postoperative (*right*) angiograms demonstrating excessive depth of annular sutures leading to left circumflex occlusion.

patients (26%). Perioperative mortality occurred in 3.6% of redo patients with a preserved subvalvular apparatus (native tissue and/or Gore-Tex reconstruction) versus 13.3% of redo patients without preservation (*p* < .001). Attempts at preservation of the subvalvular apparatus in reoperative mitral valve patients therefore should be considered.

REOPERATIVE TRICUSPID VALVE SURGERY

The need for reoperative tricuspid valve surgery most frequently occurs in high-risk patients. In a recent series of tricuspid valve replacements (TVR) by Filsoufi et al,[148] 72% (n = 58) were reoperations. The overall operative mortality in this group was 22% (n = 18). Risk factors for mortality included urgent/emergent status, age greater than 50 years, functional etiology, and elevated pulmonary artery pressure. Of the 60 survivors, 26 (43%) died during follow-up. The authors concluded that patients requiring TVR are at high risk, frequently at end-stage functional class. As such, serious consideration of the risks should occur before embarking on such procedures (Table 46-3).

Tricuspid valve endocarditis is most commonly the result of seeding of the tricuspid valve leaflets during sustained bacteremia.[149] Continued sepsis despite antibiotic therapy, heart failure owing to tricuspid insufficiency, and recurrent multiple pulmonary emboli are indications to intervene surgically in tricuspid valve endocarditis. Complete excision of the tricuspid valve (without subsequent replacement) was first advocated by Arbulu et al.[149] From an infectious disease standpoint, this surgical approach has the obvious advantage of complete extirpation of the infected tissue and avoids placement of any prosthetic material. Although it is tolerated initially, the extirpation procedure inevitably leads to late-onset right-sided failure in the majority of patients.[149-151] In a 20-year follow-up of the originally reported series of 55 patients with intractable right-sided endocarditis who underwent tricuspid valvectomy without replacement, two patients (4%) died in the postoperative period owing to right-sided failure. Six patients (11%) required prosthetic valve insertion 2 days to 13 years later for medically refractory right-sided heart failure. Of those who underwent reoperation (n = 6), four (66%) died. As such, severe hepatic congestion and the need for reoperative valve replacement have made this approach (without replacement) untenable to some practitioners. An alternative treatment option is to perform valvectomy followed by delayed valve replacement 3 to 9 months later.[152]

FINAL POINTS

1. Reoperative valve surgery most commonly involves structural valve deterioration of a bioprosthesis or progression of native valve disease after nonvalve surgery.
2. Bioprosthetic valves are known to undergo a time-dependent process of structural deterioration that results in a freedom of reoperation of 80% at 15 years.

⬤ **TABLE 46-3: Technical Considerations for Reoperative Valve Surgery**

Consider reoperation before decline in functional status (NYHA class). Assess RV/aortic proximity to sternum preoperatively with CT scan

Consider alternate approaches (especially with patent bypass grafts)
　　Right thoracotomy for reoperative MVR
　　Mini-sternotomy for reoperative AVR

Consider alternate cannulation techniques to gain safe entry, eg, femoral, axillary

Address the LIMA-LAD graft if present
　　Dissect it out and clamp it, or
　　Cool and ignore it

Consider ease of implantation in valve choice, eg, mechanical in homograft

Use "no-touch" technique of bypass grafts

Use a conservative myocardial protection strategy
　　Antegrade and retrograde
　　Systemic cooling
　　Warm induction/final dose ("hot shot")

If using hypothermic fibrillatory arrest, beware of AI leading to LV distension and/or obscuring operative field

Place external defibrillator pads

Consider the use of antifibrinolytic agents, eg, Amicar

---

3. Major risk factors in reoperative valve surgery include advanced age, impaired ejection fraction, congestive heart failure, urgency of operation, preoperative shock, concomitant coronary artery bypass surgery or presence of previous bypass grafts, prosthetic valve endocarditis, surgery for perivalvular leaks, valve thrombosis, or prosthetic dysfunction, renal dysfunction, chronic obstructive pulmonary disease, and pulmonary hypertension.
4. ECG-gated MDCT scanning is the preferred modality for preoperative assessment of vital structures in reoperative valve surgery.
5. Reoperative valve surgery after prior CABG with patent LITA graft presents unique challenges and the decision regarding intraoperative management of the patent graft must be made during the preoperative planning phase.
6. Reoperative aortic valve surgery after homograft or root replacement can be difficult and should be simplified by replacement with a mechanical valve when possible. Reoperative root operations should be avoided if not indicated.
7. AVB surgery is an alternative for reoperative AVR in extremely difficult reoperative cases.
8. TAVR is now an established technique of reoperative valve replacement in high-risk patients and VinV implantation is the next frontier of percutaneous valve implantation.
9. The right thoracotomy approach to reoperative mitral and tricuspid valves provides excellent exposure with minimal need for dissection while also avoiding prior

bypass grafts. Significant AI and the need for bypass grafting preclude this approach when aortic clamping and cardioplegic myocardial arrest are used.

10. Most commonly, periprosthetic leaks should be patched, rather than treated with valve replacement if the valve is functioning normally.

11. Reoperative tricuspid valve surgery occurs in high-risk patients with pulmonary hypertension with variable degrees of right heart failure. As such, this operation should be carefully considered.

REFERENCES

1. Fremes SEM, Goldman BSM, Ivanov JR, Weisel RDM, David TEM, Salerno TM: Valvular surgery in the elderly. *Circulation* 1989; 80(3):I-77-90.

2. Pansini S, Ottino G, Forsennati PG, et al: Reoperations on heart valve prostheses: an analysis of operative risks and late results. *Ann Thorac Surg* 1990; 50(4):590-596.

3. Kirsch M, Nakashima K, Kubota S, Houel R, Hillion ML, Loisance D: The risk of reoperative heart valve procedures in Octogenarian patients. *J Heart Valve Dis* 2004; 13(6):991-996.

4. Cohn LH, Aranki SF, Rizzo RJ, et al: Decrease in operative risk of reoperative valve surgery. *Ann Thorac Surg* 1993; 56(1):15-20.

5. Weerasinghe A, Edwards MB, Taylor KM: First redo heart valve replacement: a 10-year analysis. *Circulation* 1999; 99(5):655-658.

6. Jones JM, O'Kane H, Gladstone DJ, et al: Repeat heart valve surgery: risk factors for operative mortality. *J Thorac Cardiovasc Surg* 2001; 122(5):913-918.

7. Cohn LH: Evolution of redo cardiac surgery: review of personal experience. *J Cardiac Surg* 2004; 19(4):320-324.

8. Wauthy P, Goldstein JP, Demanet H, Deuvaert FE: Redo valve surgery nowadays: what have we learned? *Acta Chir Belg* 2003; 103(5):475-480.

9. O'Brien MF, Harrocks S, Clarke A, Garlick B, Barnett AG: Experiences with redo aortic valve surgery. *J Cardiac Surg* 2002; 17(1):35-39.

10. Cohn LH, Peigh PS, Sell J, DiSesa VJ: Right thoracotomy, femorofemoral bypass, and deep hypothermia for re-replacement of the mitral valve. *Ann Thorac Surg* 1989; 48(1):69-71.

11. Jones RE, Fitzgerald D, Cohn LH: Reoperative cardiac surgery using a new femoral venous right atrial cannula. *J Cardiac Surg* 1990; 5(3):170-173.

12. Aranki SF, Adams DH, Rizzo RJ, et al: Femoral veno-arterial extracorporeal life support with minimal or no heparin. *Ann Thorac Surg* 1993; 56(1):149-155.

13. Bichell DP, Balaguer JM, Aranki SF, et al: Axilloaxillary cardiopulmonary bypass: a practical alternative to femorofemoral bypass. *Ann Thorac Surg* 1997; 64(3):702-705.

14. Cohn LH, Koster JK Jr, VandeVanter S, Collins JJ Jr: The in-hospital risk of rereplacement of dysfunctional mitral and aortic valves. *Circulation* 1982; 66(2 Pt 2):I153-156.

15. Antunes MJ, Sanches MF, Fernandes LE: Antibiotic prophylaxis and prosthetic valve endocarditis. *J Heart Valve Dis* 1992; 1(2):201-205.

16. Turina J, Hess OM, Turina M, Krayenbuehl HP: Cardiac bioprostheses in the 1990s. *Circulation* 1993; 88(2):775-781.

17. Husebye DG, Pluth JR, Piehler JM, et al: Reoperation on prosthetic heart valves. An analysis of risk factors in 552 patients. *J Thorac Cardiovasc Surg* 1983; 86(4):543-552.

18. Vogt PR, Brunner-LaRocca H, Sidler P, et al: Reoperative surgery for degenerated aortic bioprostheses: predictors for emergency surgery and reoperative mortality. *Eur J Cardiothorac Surg* 2000; 17(2):134-139.

19. Cohn LH, Couper GS, Aranki SF, Kinchla NM, Collins JJ Jr: The long-term follow-up of the Hancock Modified Orifice porcine bioprosthetic valve. *J Cardiac Surg* 1991; 6(4 Suppl):557-561.

20. Starr A, Grunkemeier GL: The expected lifetime of porcine valves. *Ann Thorac Surg* 1989; 48(3):317-318.

21. Myken PS, Caidahl K, Larsson P, Larsson S, Wallentin I, Berggren HE: Mechanical versus biological valve prosthesis: a ten-year comparison regarding function and quality of life. *Ann Thorac Surg* 1995; 60(2 Suppl):S447-452.

22. Milano A, Guglielmi C, De Carlo M, et al: Valve-related complications in elderly patients with biological and mechanical aortic valves. *Ann Thorac Surg* 1998; 66(6 Suppl):S82-87.

23. Barwinsky J, Cohen M, Bhattacharya S, Kim S, Teskey J: Bjork-Shiley cardiac valves long term results: winnipeg experience. *Can J Cardiol* 1988; 4(7):366-371.

24. Birkmeyer NJ, Marrin CA, Morton JR, et al: Decreasing mortality for aortic and mitral valve surgery in Northern New England. Northern New England Cardiovascular Disease Study Group. *Ann Thorac Surg* 2000; 70(2):432-437.

25. Peterseim DS, Cen YY, Cheruvu S, et al: Long-term outcome after biologic versus mechanical aortic valve replacement in 841 patients. *J Thorac Cardiovasc Surg* 1999; 117(5):890-897.

26. Borkon AM, Soule LM, Baughman KL, et al: Aortic valve selection in the elderly patient. *Ann Thorac Surg* 1988; 46(3):270-277.

27. Byrne JG, Karavas AN, Aklog L, et al: Aortic valve reoperation after homograft or autograft replacement. *J Heart Valve Dis* 2001; 10(4):451-457.

28. Kouchoukos NT: Aortic allografts and pulmonary autografts for replacement of the aortic valve and aortic root. *Ann Thorac Surg* 1999; 67(6):1846-1848; discussion 1853.

29. Albertucci M, Wong K, Petrou M, et al: The use of unstented homograft valves for aortic valve reoperations. Review of a twenty-three-year experience. *J Thorac Cardiovasc Surg* 1994; 107(1):152-161.

30. O'Brien MF, McGiffin DC, Stafford EG, et al: Allograft aortic valve replacement: long-term comparative clinical analysis of the viable cryopreserved and antibiotic 4 degrees C stored valves. *J Cardiac Surg* 1991; 6(4 Suppl):534-543.

31. Edmunds LH Jr: Thrombotic and bleeding complications of prosthetic heart valves. *Ann Thorac Surg* 1987; 44(4):430-445.

32. Bloomfield P, Wheatley DJ, Prescott RJ, Miller HC: Twelve-year comparison of a Bjork-Shiley mechanical heart valve with porcine bioprostheses. *N Engl J Med* 1991; 324(9):573-579.

33. Deviri E, Sareli P, Wisenbaugh T, Cronje SL: Obstruction of mechanical heart valve prostheses: clinical aspects and surgical management. *J Am Coll Cardiol* 1991; 17(3):646-650.

34. Rizzoli G, Guglielmi C, Toscano G, et al: Reoperations for acute prosthetic thrombosis and pannus: an assessment of rates, relationship and risk. *Eur J Cardiothorac Surg* 1999; 16(1):74-80.

35. Lytle BW, Cosgrove DM, Taylor PC, et al: Reoperations for valve surgery: perioperative mortality and determinants of risk for 1,000 patients, 1958-1984. *Ann Thorac Surg* 1986; 42(6):632-643.

36. Akins CW, Buckley MJ, Daggett WM, et al: Risk of reoperative valve replacement for failed mitral and aortic bioprostheses. *Ann Thorac Surg* 1998; 65(6):1545-1551.

37. Tyers GF, Jamieson WR, Munro AI, et al: Reoperation in biological and mechanical valve populations: fate of the reoperative patient. *Ann Thorac Surg* 1995; 60(2 Suppl):S464-468; discussion S468-469.

38. Salomon NW, Page US, Bigelow JC, Krause AH, Okies JE, Metzdorff MT: Reoperative coronary surgery. Comparative analysis of 6591 patients undergoing primary bypass and 508 patients undergoing reoperative coronary artery bypass. *J Thorac Cardiovasc Surg* 1990; 100(2):250-259; discussion 259-260.

39. Weintraub WS, Jones EL, Craver JM, Grosswald R, Guyton RA: In-hospital and long-term outcome after reoperative coronary artery bypass graft surgery. *Circulation* 1995; 92(9 Suppl):Ii50-57.

40. Yau TM, Borger MA, Weisel RD, Ivanov J: The changing pattern of reoperative coronary surgery: trends in 1230 consecutive reoperations. *J Thorac Cardiovasc Surg* 2000; 120(1):156-163.

41. Aviram G, Sharony R, Kramer A, et al: Modification of surgical planning based on cardiac multidetector computed tomography in reoperative heart surgery. *Ann Thorac Surg* 2005; 79(2):589-595.

42. Dobell AR, Jain AK: Catastrophic hemorrhage during redo sternotomy. *Ann Thorac Surg* 1984; 37(4):273-278.

43. Gilkeson RC, Markowitz AH, Ciancibello L: Multisection CT evaluation of the reoperative cardiac surgery patient. *Radiographics: a review publication of the Radiological Society of North America, Inc* 2003; 23 Spec No:S3-17.

44. Gasparovic H, Rybicki FJ, Millstine J, et al: Three dimensional computed tomographic imaging in planning the surgical approach for redo cardiac surgery after coronary revascularization. *Eur J Cardiothorac Surg* 2005; 28(2):244-249.

45. Maluenda G, Goldstein M, Weissman G, Weigold WG, Desai M, Taylor A: The role of cardiac CT prior to reoperative cardiac surgery. *Curr Cardiovasc Imaging Rep* 2013; 6(3):221-227.

46. Schlosser T, Konorza T, Hunold P, Kuhl H, Schmermund A, Barkhausen J: Noninvasive visualization of coronary artery bypass grafts using 16-detector row computed tomography. *J Am Coll Cardiol* 2004; 44(6):1224-1229.

47. Taylor AJ, Cerqueira M, Hodgson JM, et al: ACCF/SCCT/ACR/AHA/ASE/ASNC/NASCI/SCAI/SCMR 2010 Appropriate use criteria for cardiac computed tomography. A Report of the American College of Cardiology Foundation Appropriate Use Criteria Task Force, the Society of Cardiovascular Computed Tomography, the American College of Radiology, the American Heart Association, the American Society of Echocardiography, the American Society of Nuclear Cardiology, the North American Society for Cardiovascular Imaging, the Society for Cardiovascular Angiography and Interventions, and the Society for Cardiovascular Magnetic Resonance. *J Cardiovasc Comput Tomogr* 2010; 4(6):407:e401-433.

48. Kamdar AR, Meadows TA, Roselli EE, et al: Multidetector computed tomographic angiography in planning of reoperative cardiothoracic surgery. *Ann Thorac Surg* 2008; 85(4):1239-1245.

49. Khan NU, Yonan N: Does preoperative computed tomography reduce the risks associated with re-do cardiac surgery? *Interact Cardiovasc Thorac Surg* 2009; 9(1):119-123.

50. Maluenda G, Goldstein MA, Lemesle G, et al: Perioperative outcomes in reoperative cardiac surgery guided by cardiac multidetector computed tomographic angiography. *Am Heart J* 2010; 159(2):301-306.

51. Birkmeyer NJ, Birkmeyer JD, Tosteson AN, Grunkemeier GL, Marrin CA, O'Connor GT: Prosthetic valve type for patients undergoing aortic valve replacement: a decision analysis. *Ann Thorac Surg* 2000; 70(6):1946-1952.

52. Cohn LH, Collins JJ, DiSesa VJ, et al: Fifteen-year experience with 1678 Hancock porcine bioprosthetic heart valve replacements. *Ann Surg* 1989; 210(4):435-442.

53. Jamieson WR, Munro AI, Miyagishima RT, Allen P, Burr LH, Tyers GF: Carpentier-Edwards standard porcine bioprosthesis: clinical performance to seventeen years. *Ann Thorac Surg* 1995; 60(4):999-1006.

54. Gaudiani VA, Grunkemeier GL, Castro LJ, Fisher AL, Wu Y: The risks and benefits of reoperative aortic valve replacement. *Heart Surg Forum* 2004; 7(2):E170-173.

55. Potter DD, Sundt TM, Zehr KJ, et al: Operative risk of reoperative aortic valve replacement. *J Thorac Cardiovasc Surg* 2005; 129(1):94-103.

56. Phillips BJ, Karavas AN, Aranki SF, et al: Management of mild aortic stenosis during coronary artery bypass surgery: an update, 1992-2001. *J Card Surg* 2003; 18(6):507-511.

57. Bortolotti U, Guerra F, Magni A, et al: Emergency reoperation for primary tissue failure of porcine bioprostheses. *Am J Cardiol* 1987; 60(10):920-921.

58. Byrne JG, Karavas AN, Filsoufi F, et al: Aortic valve surgery after previous coronary artery bypass grafting with functioning internal mammary artery grafts. *Ann Thorac Surg* 2002; 73(3):779-784.

59. Gillinov AM, Casselman FP, Lytle BW, et al: Injury to a patent left internal thoracic artery graft at coronary reoperation. *Ann Thorac Surg* 1999; 67(2):382-386.

60. Odell JA, Mullany CJ, Schaff HV, Orszulak TA, Daly RC, Morris JJ: Aortic valve replacement after previous coronary artery bypass grafting. *Ann Thorac Surg* 1996; 62(5):1424-1430.

61. Vohra HA, Pousios D, Whistance RN, et al: Aortic valve replacement in patients with previous coronary artery bypass grafting: 10-year experience. *Eur J Cardiothorac Surg* 2012; 41(3):e1-6.

62. Dobell AR, Jain AK: Catastrophic hemorrhage during redo sternotomy. *Ann Thorac Surg* 1984; 37(4):273-278.

63. Ivert TS, Ekestrom S, Peterffy A, Welti R: Coronary artery reoperations. Early and late results in 101 patients. *Scand J Thorac Cardiovasc Surg* 1988; 22(2):111-118.

64. Lytle BW, McElroy D, McCarthy P, et al: Influence of arterial coronary bypass grafts on the mortality in coronary reoperations. *J Thorac Cardiovasc Surg* 1994; 107(3):675-682; discussion 682-683.

65. Kaneko T, Nauta F, Borstlap W, McGurk S, Rawn JD, Cohn LH: The "no-dissection" technique is safe for reoperative aortic valve replacement with a patent left internal thoracic artery graft. *J Thorac Cardiovasc Surg* 2012; 144(5):1036-1040.

66. Park CB, Suri RM, Burkhart HM, et al: What is the optimal myocardial preservation strategy at re-operation for aortic valve replacement in the presence of a patent internal thoracic artery? *Eur J Cardiothorac Surg* 2011; 39(6):861-865.

67. Smith RL, Ellman PI, Thompson PW, et al: Do you need to clamp a patent left internal thoracic artery-left anterior descending graft in reoperative cardiac surgery? *Ann Thorac Surg* 2009; 87(3):742-747.

68. Fuzellier JF, Metz D, Poncet A, Saade YA: Endovascular control of patent internal thoracic artery graft in aortic valve surgery. *Ann Thorac Surg* 2005; 79(2):e17-18.

69. Kuralay E, Cingoz F, Gunay C, et al: Supraclavicular control of patent internal thoracic artery graft flow during aortic valve replacement. *Ann Thorac Surg* 2003; 75(5):1422-1428; discussion 1428.

70. Shanmugam G: Aortic valve replacement following previous coronary surgery. *Eur J Cardiothorac Surg* 2005; 28(5):731-735.

71. Ban T, Soga Y: [Re-sternotomy]. *Nihon Geka Gakkai Zasshi*. 1998; 99(2):63-67.

72. Elami A, Laks H, Merin G: Technique for reoperative median sternotomy in the presence of a patent left internal mammary artery graft. *J Card Surg* 1994; 9(2):123-127.

73. English TA, Milstein BB: Repeat open intracardiac operation. Analysis of fifty operations. *J Thorac Cardiovasc Surg* 1978; 76(1):56-60.

74. Macmanus Q, Okies JE, Phillips SJ, Starr A: Surgical considerations in patients undergoing repeat median sternotomy. *J Thorac Cardiovasc Surg* 1975; 69(1):138-143.

75. Wideman FE, Blackstone EH, Kirklin JW, Karp RB, Kouchoukos NT, Pacifico AD: Hospital mortality of re-replacement of the aortic valve. Incremental risk factors. *J Thorac Cardiovasc Surg* 1981; 82(5):692-698.

76. Aklog L, Adams DH, Couper GS, Gobezie R, Sears S, Cohn LH: Techniques and results of direct-access minimally invasive mitral valve surgery: a paradigm for the future. *J Thorac Cardiovasc Surg* 1998; 116(5):705-715.

77. Cosgrove DM, 3rd, Sabik JF: Minimally invasive approach for aortic valve operations. *Ann Thorac Surg* 1996; 62(2):596-597.

78. Cosgrove DM, Sabik JF, Navia JL: Minimally invasive valve operations. *Ann Thorac Surg* 1998; 65(6):1535-1538.

79. Hearn CJ, Kraenzler EJ, Wallace LK, Starr NJ, Sabik JF, Cosgrove DM: Minimally invasive aortic valve surgery: anesthetic considerations. *Anesth Analg* 1996;83(6):1342-1344.

80. Byrne JG, Karavas AN, Adams DH, et al: Partial upper re-sternotomy for aortic valve replacement or re-replacement after previous cardiac surgery. *Eur J Cardiothorac Surg* 2000; 18(3):282-286.

81. Machler HE, Bergmann P, Anelli-Monti M, et al: Minimally invasive versus conventional aortic valve operations: a prospective study in 120 patients. *Ann Thorac Surg* 1999; 67(4):1001-1005.

82. Byrne JG, Aranki SF, Couper GS, Adams DH, Allred EN, Cohn LH: Reoperative aortic valve replacement: partial upper hemisternotomy versus conventional full sternotomy. *J Thorac Cardiovasc Surg* 1999; 118(6):991-997.

83. Tam RK, Garlick RB, Almeida AA: Minimally invasive redo aortic valve replacement. *J Thorac Cardiovasc Surg* 1997; 114(4):682-683.

84. Gundry SR, Shattuck OH, Razzouk AJ, del Rio MJ, Sardari FF, Bailey LL: Facile minimally invasive cardiac surgery via ministernotomy. *Ann Thorac Surg* 1998; 65(4):1100-1104.

85. Byrne JG, Karavas AN, Cohn LH, Adams DH: Minimal access aortic root, valve, and complex ascending aortic surgery. *Curr Cardiol Rep* 2000;2(6):549-557.

86. Luciani GB, Casali G, Santini F, Mazzucco A: Aortic root replacement in adolescents and young adults: composite graft versus homograft or autograft. *Ann Thorac Surg* 1998;66(6 Suppl):S189-S193.

87. Byrne JG, Aranki SF, Cohn LH: Aortic valve operations under deep hypothermic circulatory arrest for the porcelain aorta: "no-touch" technique. *Ann Thorac Surg* 1998;65(5):1313-1315.

88. Zlotnick AY, Gilfeather MS, Adams DH, Cohn LH, Couper GS: Innominate vein cannulation for venous drainage in minimally invasive aortic valve replacement. *Ann Thorac Surg* 1999; 67(3):864-865.

89. McGiffin DC, Galbraith AJ, O'Brien MF, McLachlan GJ, Naftel DC, Adams P, et al: An analysis of valve re-replacement after aortic valve replacement with biologic devices. *J Thorac Cardiovasc Surg* 1997;113(2):311-318.

90. Hasnat K, Birks EJ, Liddicoat J, et al: Patient outcome and valve performance following a second aortic valve homograft replacement. *Circulation* 1999; 100(19 Suppl):Ii42-47.

91. Sundt TM, 3rd, Rasmi N, Wong K, Radley-Smith R, Khaghani A, Yacoub MH: Reoperative aortic valve operation after homograft root replacement: surgical options and results. *Ann Thorac Surg* 1995;60 (2 Suppl):S95-S99; discussion S100.

92. Yacoub M, Rasmi NR, Sundt TM, et al: Fourteen-year experience with homovital homografts for aortic valve replacement. *J Thorac Cardiovasc Surg* 1995; 110(1):186-193.

93. Kumar P, Athanasiou T, Ali A, et al: Re-do aortic valve replacement: does a previous homograft influence the operative outcome? *J Heart Valve Dis* 2004; 13(6):904-912.

94. Sadowski J, Kapelak B, Bartus K, et al: Reoperation after fresh homograft replacement: 23 years' experience with 655 patients. *Eur J Cardiothorac Surg* 2003; 23(6):996-1000.

95. Khalpey Z, Borstlap W, Myers PO, et al: The valve-in-valve operation for aortic homograft dysfunction: a better option. *Ann Thorac Surg* Vol 94. Netherlands: 2012 The Society of Thoracic Surgeons. Published by Elsevier Inc; 2012:731-735; discussion 735-736.

96. David TE, Feindel CM, Ivanov J, Armstrong S: Aortic root replacement in patients with previous heart surgery. *J Card Surg* 2004;19(4):325-328.

97. Matsushita T, Kawase T, Tsuda E, Kawazoe K: Apicoaortic conduit for the dilated phase of hypertrophic obstructive cardiomyopathy as an alternative to heart transplantation. *Interact Cardiovasc Thorac Surg* 2009;8(2):232-234.

98. Hirota M, Oi M, Omoto T, Tedoriya T: Apico-aortic conduit for aortic stenosis with a porcelain aorta; technical modification for apical outflow. *Interact Cardiovasc Thorac Surg* 2009;9(4):703-705.

99. Chahine JH, El-Rassi I, Jebara V: Apico-aortic valved conduit as an alternative for aortic valve re-replacement in severe prosthesis-patient mismatch. *Interact Cardiovasc Thorac Surg* 2009;9(4):680-682.

100. Gammie JS, Krowsoski LS, Brown JM, et al: Aortic valve bypass surgery: midterm clinical outcomes in a high-risk aortic stenosis population. *Circulation* 2008; 118(14):1460-1466.

101. Vassiliades TA Jr: Off-pump apicoaortic conduit insertion for high-risk patients with aortic stenosis. *Eur J Cardiothorac Surg* 2003; 23(2):156-158.

102. CTSNet.org. Left ventricular apico-aortic conduit. http://www.ctsnet.org/sections/clinicalresources/videos/vg2008_luckraz_left_ventric.html., 2008.

103. CTSNet.org. Aortic Valve Bypass Surgery: Beating Heart Therapy for Aortic Stenosis. STSA Surgical Motion Picture 2008 Annual Meeting. 2008.

104. Leon MB, Smith CR, Mack M, et al: Transcatheter aortic-valve implantation for aortic stenosis in patients who cannot undergo surgery. *N Engl J Med* 2010; 363(17):1597-1607.

105. Makkar RR, Fontana GP, Jilaihawi H, et al: Transcatheter aortic-valve replacement for inoperable severe aortic stenosis. *N Engl J Med* 2012; 366(18):1696-1704.

106. Horne A Jr, Reineck EA, Hasan RK, Resar JR, Chacko M: Transcatheter aortic valve replacement: historical perspectives, current evidence, and future directions. *Am Heart J* 2014; 168(4):414-423.

107. Gotzmann M, Mugge A, Bojara W: Transcatheter aortic valve implantation for treatment of patients with degenerated aortic bioprostheses—valve-in-valve technique. *Catheterization Cardiovasc Interventions: Official J Soc Cardiac Angiogr Interventions.* 2010; 76(7):1000-1006.

108. Kempfert J, Van Linden A, Linke A, et al: Transapical off-pump valve-in-valve implantation in patients with degenerated aortic xenografts. *Ann Thorac Surg* 2010; 89(6):1934-1941.

109. Khawaja MZ, Haworth P, Ghuran A, et al: Transcatheter aortic valve implantation for stenosed and regurgitant aortic valve bioprostheses CoreValve for failed bioprosthetic aortic valve replacements. *J Am Coll Cardiol* 2010; 55(2):97-101.

110. Rodes-Cabau J, Dumont E, Doyle D, Lemieux J: Transcatheter valve-in-valve implantation for the treatment of stentless aortic valve dysfunction. *J Thorac Cardiovasc Surg* 2010; 140(1):246-248.

111. Wenaweser P, Buellesfeld L, Gerckens U, Grube E: Percutaneous aortic valve replacement for severe aortic regurgitation in degenerated bioprosthesis: the first valve in valve procedure using the Corevalve Revalving system. *Catheterization Cardiovasc Interventions: Official J Soc Cardiac Angiography Interventions.* 2007; 70(5):760-764.

112. Dvir D, Webb JG, Bleiziffer S, et al: Transcatheter aortic valve implantation in failed bioprosthetic surgical valves. *JAMA* 2014; 312(2):162-170.

113. Dvir D, Webb J, Brecker S, et al: Transcatheter aortic valve replacement for degenerative bioprosthetic surgical valves: results from the global valve-in-valve registry. *Circulation* 2012; 126(19):2335-2344.

114. Bapat V, Asrress KN: Transcatheter valve-in-valve implantation for failing prosthetic valves. *EuroIntervention: J EuroPCR in Collaboration with the Working Group on Interventional Cardiology of the European Society of Cardiology.* 2014; 10(8):900-902.

115. McCarthy JF, Cosgrove DM: Optimizing mitral valve exposure with conventional left atriotomy. *Ann Thorac Surg* 1998; 65(4):1161-1162.

116. Balasundaram SG, Duran C: Surgical approaches to the mitral valve. *J Card Surg* 1990;5(3):163-169.

117. Saunders PC, Pintucci G, Bizekis CS, et al: Vein graft arterialization causes differential activation of mitogen-activated protein kinases. *J Thorac Cardiovasc Surg* 2004; 127(5):1276-1284.

118. Thompson MJ, Behranwala A, Campanella C, Walker WS, Cameron EWJ: Immediate and long-term results of mitral prosthetic replacement using a right thoracotomy beating heart technique. *Eur J Cardiothorac Surg* 2003; 24(1):47-51.

119. Brawley RK: Improved exposure of the mitral valve in patients with a small left atrium. *Ann Thorac Surg* 1980; 29(2):179-181.

120. Bonchek LI: Mitral valve reoperation. *Ann Thorac Surg* 1991; 51(1):160-160.

121. Praeger PI, Pooley RW, Moggio RA, Somberg ED, Sarabu MR, Reed GE: Simplified method for reoperation on the mitral valve. *Ann Thorac Surg* 1989; 48(6):835-837.

122. Keon WJ, Heggtveit HA, Leduc J: Perioperative myocardial infarction caused by atheroembolism. *J Thorac Cardiovasc Surg* 1982; 84(6):849-855.

123. Grondin CM, Pomar JL, Hebert Y, et al: Reoperation in patients with patent atherosclerotic coronary vein grafts. A different approach to a different disease. *J Thorac Cardiovasc Surg* 1984; 87(3):379-385.

124. Byrne JG, Aranki SF, Adams DH, Rizzo RJ, Couper GS, Cohn LH: Mitral valve surgery after previous CABG with functioning IMA grafts. *Ann Thorac Surg* 1999; 68(6):2243-2247.

125. Londe S, Sugg WL: The challenge of reoperation in cardiac surgery. *Ann Thorac Surg* 1974; 17(2):157-162.

126. Tribble CG, Killinger WA, Harman PK, Crosby IK, Nolan SP, Kron IL: Anterolateral thoracotomy as an alternative to repeat median sternotomy for replacement of the mitral valve. *Ann Thorac Surg* 1987; 43(4):380-382.

127. Adams DH, Filsoufi F, Byrne JG, Karavas AN, Aklog L: Mitral valve repair in redo cardiac surgery. *J Card Surg* 2002; 17(1):40-45.

128. Byrne JG, Hsin MK, Adams DH, et al: Minimally invasive direct access heart valve surgery. *J Card Surg* 2000; 15(1):21-34.

129. Byrne JG, Karavas AN, Adams DH, et al: The preferred approach for mitral valve surgery after CABG: right thoracotomy, hypothermia and avoidance of LIMA-LAD graft. *J Heart Valve Dis* 2001; 10(5):584-590.

130. Byrne JG, Mitchell ME, Adams DH, Couper GS, Aranki SF, Cohn LH: Minimally invasive direct access mitral valve surgery. *Semin Thorac Cardiovasc Surg* 1999; 11(3):212-222.

131. Umakanthan R, Leacche M, Petracek MR, et al: Safety of minimally invasive mitral valve surgery without aortic cross-clamp. *Ann Thorac Surg* Netherlands 2008; 85:1544-1549; discussion 1549-1550.

132. Cohn LH, Peigh PS, Sell J, DiSesa VJ: Right thoracotomy, femorofemoral bypass, and deep hypothermia for re-replacement of the mitral valve. *Ann Thorac Surg* 1989;48(1):69-71.

133. Holman WL, Goldberg SP, Early LJ, et al: Right thoracotomy for mitral reoperation: analysis of technique and outcome. *Ann Thorac Surg* 2000; 70(6):1970-1973.

134. Berreklouw E, Alfieri O: Revival of right thoracotomy to approach atrio-ventricular valves in reoperations. *Thorac Cardiovasc Surg* 1984; 32(5):331-333.

135. Braxton JH, Higgins RS, Schwann TA, et al: Reoperative mitral valve surgery via right thoracotomy: decreased blood loss and improved hemodynamics. *J Heart Valve Dis* 1996; 5(2):169-173.

136. Umakanthan R, Petracek MR, Leacche M, et al: Minimally invasive right lateral thoracotomy without aortic cross-clamping: an attractive alternative to repeat sternotomy for reoperative mitral valve surgery. *J Heart Valve Dis* 2010; 19(2):236-243.

137. Steimle CN, Bolling SF: Outcome of reoperative valve surgery via right thoracotomy. *Circulation* 1996;94(9 Suppl):Ii126-Ii128.

138. Bolotin G, Kypson AP, Reade CC, et al: Should a video-assisted mini-thoracotomy be the approach of choice for reoperative mitral valve surgery? *J Heart Valve Dis* 2004; 13(2):155-158.

139. Vleissis AA, Bolling SF: Mini-reoperative mitral valve surgery. *J Card Surg* 1998; 13(6):468-470.

140. Burfeind WR, Glower DD, Davis RD, Landolfo KP, Lowe JE, Wolfe WG: Mitral surgery after prior cardiac operation: port-access versus sternotomy or thoracotomy. *Ann Thorac Surg* 2002;74(4):S1323-S1325.

141. Greco E, Barriuso C, Castro MA, Fita G, Pomar JL: Port-access cardiac surgery: from a learning process to the standard. *Heart Surg Forum* 2002; 5(2):145-149.

142. Onnasch JF, Schneider F, Falk V, Walther T, Gummert J, Mohr FW: Minimally invasive approach for redo mitral valve surgery: a true benefit for the patient. *J Card Surg* 2002; 17(1):14-19.

143. Schneider F, Falk V, Walther T, Mohr FW: Control of endoaortic clamp position during port-access mitral valve operations using transcranial Doppler echography. *Ann Thorac Surg* 1998; 65(5):1481-1482.

144. Trehan N, Mishra YK, Mathew SG, Sharma KK, Shrivastava S, Mehta Y: Redo mitral valve surgery using the port-access system. *Asian Cardiovasc Thorac Ann* 2002; 10(3):215-218.

145. Yoshikai M, Ito T, Murayama J, Kamohara K: Mitral annular reconstruction. *Asian Cardiovasc Thorac Ann* 2002; 10(4):344-345.

146. Hansen DE, Cahill PD, DeCampli WM, et al: Valvular-ventricular interaction: importance of the mitral apparatus in canine left ventricular systolic performance. *Circulation* 1986; 73(6):1310-1320.

147. Borger MA, Yau TM, Rao V, Scully HE, David TE: Reoperative mitral valve replacement: importance of preservation of the subvalvular apparatus. *Ann Thorac Surg* 2002; 74(5):1482-1487.

148. Filsoufi F, Anyanwu AC, Salzberg SP, Frankel T, Cohn LH, Adams DH: Long-term outcomes of tricuspid valve replacement in the current era. *Ann Thorac Surg* 2005; 80(3):845-850.

149. Arbulu A, Holmes RJ, Asfaw I: Surgical treatment of intractable right-sided infective endocarditis in drug addicts: 25 years experience. *J Heart Valve Dis* 1993; 2(2):129-137.

150. Khonsari S, Sintek C: *Cardiac Surgery: Safeguards and Pitfalls in Operative Technique*, 4 ed. Philadelphia, Lippincott Williams & Williams, 2008.

151. Yee ES, Ullyot DJ: Reparative approach for right-sided endocarditis. Operative considerations and results of valvuloplasty. *J Thorac Cardiovasc Surg* 1988; 96(1):133-140.

152. Greelish JP, Cohn LH, Leacche M, et al: Minimally invasive mitral valve repair suggests earlier operations for mitral valve disease. *J Thorac Cardiovasc Surg* 2003; 126(2):365-371.

SURGERY OF THE
GREAT VESSELS

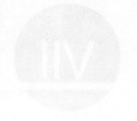

Aortic Dissection

Ravi K. Ghanta • Carlos M. Mery • Irving L. Kron

Thoracic aortic dissection occurs when an intimal tear allows redirection of blood flow from the aorta (true lumen) through the intimal defect into the media of the aortic wall (false lumen). A dissection plane that separates the intima from the overlying adventitia forms within the media. The acute form of aortic dissection is often rapidly lethal; whereas, those surviving the initial event go on to develop a chronic dissection with more protean manifestations. The purpose of this chapter is to review the etiology and pathogenesis of aortic dissection, examine current diagnostic algorithms, and provide detailed descriptions of contemporary surgical techniques for treatment. Additional information regarding follow-up and the subsequent management of these patients is presented to provide a comprehensive understanding of a clinical entity that has challenged physicians and surgeons for centuries.

HISTORY

Sennertus is credited with the first description of the dissection process, but the earliest detailed descriptions of the clinical entity appeared in the seventeenth and eighteenth centuries, during which time Maunoir named the process aortic "dissection." Laennec defined the propensity of the chronically dissected aorta to become aneurysmal. Aortic dissection was exclusively a postmortem diagnosis until the first part of the twentieth century, but in 1935 Gurin attempted surgical intervention with the first aortic fenestration procedure to treat malperfusion syndrome.[1] In 1949, Abbott and Paulin advanced surgical treatment by theoretically preventing aortic rupture by wrapping the aorta with cellophane. Other attempts at surgical treatment over the years met with limited clinical success, although certain concepts regarding surgical management are still in use today.[2] With the advent of cardiopulmonary bypass, DeBakey et al forever altered the natural history of aortic dissection by successfully performing primary surgical repair using techniques not remarkably different from contemporary procedures.[3] Investigators such as Wheat et al made substantial contributions by defining physiologically based medical management algorithms to complement surgical correction.[4] There is still considerable controversy regarding surgical versus medical treatment of certain forms of acute thoracic aortic dissection.

CLASSIFICATION

The classification systems used for aortic dissection are based on the location and extent of dissection. The particular type is then subclassified based on the timing of dissection. Acute dissection has traditionally been used to describe presentation within the first 2 weeks, whereas the term *chronic* is reserved for those patients presenting at more than 2 months after the initial event. The more recently added subacute designation is sometimes used to describe the period between 2 weeks and 2 months.

Two classification systems are most frequently used in clinical practice: the DeBakey and the Stanford systems (Fig. 47-1). The DeBakey system differentiates patients based on the location and extent of aortic dissection.[5] The advantage of this system is that four different groups of patients with different forms of aortic dissection emerge. This structure provides the greatest opportunity for subsequent comparative research. In contrast, the Stanford system proposed by Daily et al is a functional classification system.[6] All dissections that involve the ascending aorta are grouped together as type A, regardless of the position of the primary tear or the distal extent of the dissection. Proponents of the simpler Stanford system contend that the clinical behavior of patients with aortic dissection is essentially determined by involvement of the ascending aorta. Critics, however, suggest that individual patients in the type A classification may be quite different from one another depending on the distal extent. Drawing clinical conclusions from such a potentially heterogeneous patient population has inherent limitations. However, because of its simplicity, practicality, and widespread use, the Stanford system is used throughout this chapter.

INCIDENCE

Aortic dissection is the most frequently diagnosed lethal condition of the aorta. Dissection occurs nearly three times as frequently as rupture of abdominal aortic aneurysm in the

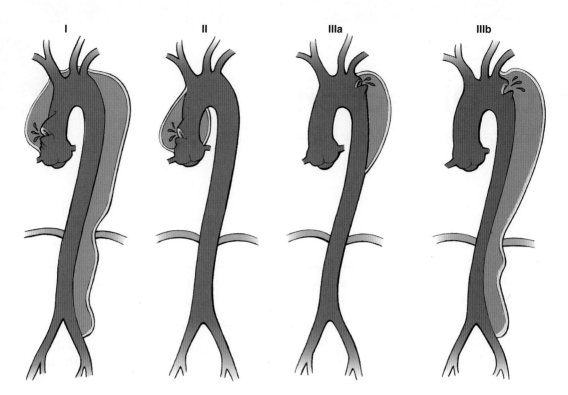

FIGURE 47-1 Classification of aortic dissection. DeBakey type I and Stanford type A include dissections that involve the proximal aorta, arch, and descending thoracic aorta. DeBakey type II only involves the ascending aorta; this dissection is included in the Stanford type A. DeBakey type III and Stanford type B include dissections that originate in the descending thoracic and thoracoabdominal aorta regardless of any retrograde involvement of the arch. These are subdivided into subtypes a and b, depending on abdominal aortic involvement.

United States.[7] There is an estimated worldwide prevalence of 0.5 to 2.95 per 100,000 per year; the prevalence ranges from 0.2 to 0.8 per 100,000 per year in the United States, resulting in roughly 2000 new cases per year.[8] These figures are only an estimate. In one autopsy series, the antemortem diagnosis was made in only 15% of patients, revealing that many immediately fatal events go undiagnosed.[9] Clinically, type A dissections occur with an overall greater frequency (Table 47-1).

ETIOLOGY AND PATHOGENESIS

Several hypotheses exist regarding the etiology of the intimal disruption (primary tear) that permits aortic blood flow to create a cleavage plane within the media of the aortic wall. This was originally viewed as a consequence of a biochemical abnormality within the media on which normal mechanical forces in the aorta acted to create an intimal tear. The link between the abnormal media, termed *cystic medial necrosis* or *degeneration*, and the primary tear has not been scientifically established. In fact, medial degeneration is found in only a minority of patients with acute aortic dissection, and most are children.[10] This theory has lost support over the years.

Alternatively, there are data supporting a relationship between aortic dissections and intramural hematoma. Advocates of this theory suggest that bleeding from vasa vasorum into the media creates a mass that results in localized areas

TABLE 47-1: Clinical Characteristics of Patients Presenting with Acute Type A and B Thoracic Aortic Dissections

	Type A	Type B
Frequency	60-75%	25-40%
Sex (M:F)	1.7-2.6:1	2.3-3:1
Age (years)	50-56	60-70
Hypertension	+ +	+ + +
Connective tissue disorder	+ +	+
Pain		
Retrosternal	+ + +	+, −
Interscapular	+, −	+ + +
Syncope	+ +	+ −
Cerebrovascular accident	+	−
Congestive heart failure	+ ̄	−
Aortic valve regurgitation	+ +	+, −
Myocardial infarction	+	−
Pericardial effusion	+, −	+ + +
Pleural effusion	+, −	+, −
Abdominal pain	+, −	+, −
Peripheral pulse deficit	Upper and lower extremities	Lower extremities

of increased stress in the intima during diastole. These areas then permit intimal disruption. In fact, between 10 and 20% of patients thought to have acute aortic dissection are found to have intramural hematoma, suggesting that it may be a precursor to dissection.[11] Penetrating atherosclerotic ulcers have been implicated as the source of intimal disruption in some cases; thus many centers treat penetrating ulcers of the ascending aorta similar to true dissections.[12] Although it may apply to certain patients, enthusiasm for the penetrating ulcer mechanism causing all dissections has waned. The pattern of atherosclerotic involvement of the thoracic aorta resulting in penetrating ulcer and the frequency of dissection throughout the aorta do not support this theory.

Although no single disorder is responsible for aortic dissection, several risk factors have been identified that can damage the aortic wall and lead to dissection (Table 47-2). These include direct mechanical forces on the aortic wall (ie, hypertension, hypervolemia, derangements of aortic flow) and forces that affect the composition of the aortic wall (ie, connective tissue disorders or direct chemical destruction). Hypertension is the mechanical force most often associated with dissection and is found in greater than 75% of cases.[8] Although the role of increased strain on the aortic wall is intuitive, the mechanism by which hypertension actually leads to dissection is unclear. Similarly, hypervolemia, high cardiac output, and an abnormal hormonal milieu certainly contribute to the increased incidence of dissection in pregnancy, but the mechanism is unclear. Atherosclerosis is not a risk factor for aortic dissection except in preexisting aneurysms or in the case of atherosclerotic ulceration. Iatrogenic trauma

to the aortic intima may result in dissection. Catheterization procedures, aortic root and femoral artery cannulation for cardiopulmonary bypass, aortic cross-clamping, surgical procedures performed on the aorta (aortic valve replacement and aortocoronary bypass grafting), and placement of intra-aortic balloon pumps have all been reported to result in dissection. Aortic transection as a result of trauma rarely results in excessive dissection and deserves differentiation from the process of aortic dissection. This process is usually limited to the aortic isthmus and in addition to the risk of rupture may present as a circular prolapse of the intima and media producing aortic obstruction referred to as "pseudocoarctation" (Fig. 47-2).

Once a cleavage plane exists in the media, the aortic wall floating within the lumen is termed the *dissection flap* and is composed of the aortic intima and partial-thickness media. The primary tear is usually greater than 50% of the circumference of the aorta. Full aortic circumference is rarely involved, but may carry a worse prognosis. The primary tear in type A dissection is usually located on the right anterior aspect of the ascending aorta and follows a somewhat predictable course, spiraling around the arch and into the descending thoracic and abdominal aorta on the left and posteriorly. The dissection may propagate in a retrograde fashion for a variable distance as well to involve the coronary ostia; this occurs in roughly 11% of all dissections.[11] Myocardial ischemia or aortic rupture into the pericardium is the cause of death in as many as 80% of mortalities from acute dissection. Often the distal false lumen communicates with the true lumen through one or more fenestrations within the dissection flap. The false lumen may also end blindly in as many as 4 to 12% of patients, in which case blood in the false lumen frequently thromboses. The false lumen may also penetrate the adventitia, causing rupture and death. Regardless of whether the true and false lumens communicate, perfusion of aortic side branches may be compromised by the dissection,

---

⬤ **TABLE 47-2: Risk Factors for Type A and B Thoracic Aortic Dissection**

Hypertension
Connective tissue disorders
Ehlers-Danlos syndrome
Marfan's disease
Turner's syndrome
Cystic medial disease of aorta
Aortitis
Iatrogenic
Atherosclerosis
Thoracic aortic aneurysm
Bicuspid aortic valve
Trauma
Pharmacologic
Coarctation of the aorta
Hypervolemia (pregnancy)
Congenital aortic stenosis
Polycystic kidney disease
Pheochromocytoma
Sheehan's syndrome
Cushing's syndrome

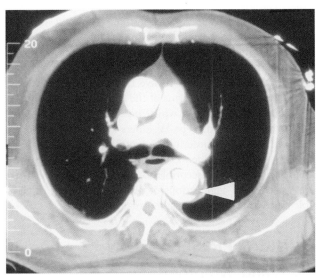

FIGURE 47-2 Axial image of CT arteriogram showing a nearly circumferential dissection flap (*arrowhead*) as a result of acute traumatic aortic dissection.

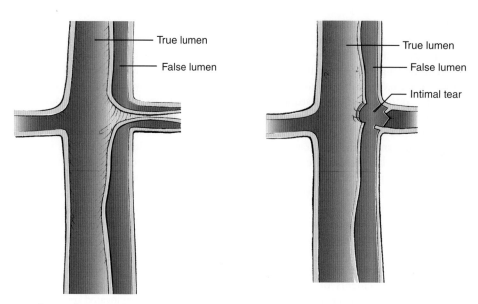

FIGURE 47-3 Diagram of aortic dissection. (A) An intact dissection membrane compresses the true lumen and causes malperfusion of a branch artery. (B) Rupture of the dissection membrane that may or may not restore blood flow to the branch.

resulting in end-organ ischemia (Fig. 47-3). If these acute complications are avoided, the weakened outer aortic wall, composed of partial media and the adventitia, may dilate over time, resulting in aneurysm formation. This evolving dilatation is the reason for operation in the majority of chronic dissections regardless of type.

The remaining adventitia provides most of the tensile strength of the aortic wall with minimal contribution from the media. The media is composed of concentrically arranged smooth muscle interposed with connective tissue proteins such as collagen, elastin, and fibrillin within the ground substance. Abnormal constituents of the media, as in certain connective tissue disorders such as Marfan's disease and Ehlers-Danlos syndrome, are associated with aortic dissection. Marfan's syndrome is an autosomal dominant inherited disorder in which a point mutation in the fibrillin-1 gene (FBN1) located on the long arm of chromosome 15 results in an abnormal media. The incidence of Marfan's syndrome is approximately 1 per 5000 live births.[13] There are, however, many incomplete forms of the disease, and as many as 25% may be sporadic in which no known fibrillin abnormalities are observed. Type IV Ehlers-Danlos syndrome is a connective tissue disorder of the proα1(III) chain of type III collagen with an incidence of 1 in 5000.[14] The structurally abnormal media is susceptible to dissection. Of note, there are also familial aggregations of dissection without discernable biochemical or genetic abnormalities.[7]

CLINICAL PRESENTATION

Signs and Symptoms

As many as 40% of patients suffering from acute aortic dissection die immediately. Those surviving the initial event may be stabilized with medical management, and it is these patients in whom subsequent therapeutic intervention on aortic dissection has altered the natural history of the disease. The clinical outcome is eventually determined by dissection type and timing of presentation, patient-related factors, and the quality and experience of the individuals and institution providing care.

The initial evaluation of a stable patient with suspected aortic dissection includes a detailed history and physical examination focusing on those elements likely to rule in the diagnosis. Most importantly, the diagnosis of aortic dissection requires a high level of suspicion. Up to 30% of patients ultimately diagnosed with acute dissection are first thought to have another diagnosis. Aortic dissection should always be considered in the setting of severe, unrelenting chest pain, which is present in most patients. Patients usually have no previous episodes of similar pain, which often causes anxiety. Pain is usually located in the midsternum for ascending aortic dissection, while in the interscapular region for descending thoracic aortic dissection (see Table 47-1). The location of maximum pain tends to change as the dissection extends in an antegrade or retrograde direction. Such "migratory pain" should arouse clinical suspicion. The character of the pain is often described as "ripping" or "tearing." The pain is constant with greatest intensity at the onset. Although painless dissection has been described, it usually occurs in the setting of an existing aneurysm in which the pain of a new dissection may not be differentiated from chronic aneurysm pain. Patients may also present with signs or symptoms related to malperfusion of the brain, limbs, or visceral organs. These findings confuse the true diagnosis, as the obvious signs of ischemia distract the historian from a less apparent initial episode of pain.

Elements of the past medical history such as primary hypertension, presence of aneurysmal disease of the aorta, or familial connective tissue disorders are useful as risk factors to help establish the diagnosis. Illicit drug use is an increasingly important predisposition to ascertain during the initial evaluation. The differential diagnosis of chest pain as a result of aortic dissection includes diagnoses such as myocardial ischemia, aortic aneurysm, acute aortic regurgitation, pericarditis, musculoskeletal pain, and pulmonary embolus. It is essential to consider aortic dissection in each case, as specific therapy (eg, thrombolytic therapy for acute myocardial infarction) may impact the survivability of acute dissection.

Patients suffering acute dissection appear ill. Tachycardia is usually accompanied by hypertension in the setting of baseline essential hypertension and increased catecholamine levels from pain and anxiety. Hypotension and tachycardia may result from aortic rupture, pericardial tamponade, acute aortic valve regurgitation, or even acute myocardial ischemia with involvement of the coronary ostia. An abnormal peripheral vascular examination is present in a minority of patients with acute aortic dissection, but when present an abnormal pulse exam may indicate the type of dissection. Absence of pulses in the upper extremity suggests ascending aortic involvement, whereas pulse deficits in the lower extremities speak to involvement of the distal aorta. These findings are subject to change as the dissection progresses or reentry into the true lumen occurs. Auscultation of the heart may reveal a diastolic murmur consistent with acute aortic regurgitation or an S3, indicating left heart volume overload. Physical exam findings such as jugular venous distention and a pulsus paradoxus are signs of pericardial tamponade that should be identified in any unstable patient to initiate the correct diagnostic and treatment algorithms. Unilateral loss of breath sounds, usually the left, may indicate hemothorax as a result of aortic leak or rupture with hemothorax. Alternatively, a pleural effusion may exist secondary to pleural inflammation related to the dissection. This finding requires additional evaluation before treatment.

A complete central and peripheral neurologic exam is critical in that abnormalities are present in up to 40% of acute type A dissections. Involvement of the brachiocephalic vessels with loss of brain perfusion may result in transient syncope or stroke. Syncope may also result from rupture into the pericardium and is an ominous sign. Stroke rarely

improves with restoration of blood flow and may even cause hemorrhage and brain death, yet surgery is indicated in such patients. Fortunately, stroke is a presenting feature in fewer than 5% of patients with acute type A dissection. Loss of perfusion to intercostals or lumbar arteries may result in spinal cord ischemia and paraplegia. Peripheral nerve ischemia as a result of malperfusion may yield findings similar to spinal cord malperfusion and should be discerned as these patients often improve with restoration of blood flow. Acute aortic dissection may also cause superior vena cava syndrome, vocal cord paralysis, hematemesis, Horner's syndrome, hemoptysis, and airway compression as a result of local compression and mass effect.

Malperfusion of aortic branch vessels may occur from the coronary ostia to the aortic bifurcation and may dominate the presentation of certain patients. Although autopsy series yield a greater percentage of patients with evidence of malperfusion, clinical series reveal that dissection is not infrequently complicated by malperfusion of at least one organ system (Table 47-3).[15] Compression of the true lumen by the false lumen is the mechanism by which aortic branch vessel occlusion occurs in the majority of cases. Branch vessels may also be completely sheared off the true lumen and perfused to various degrees by the false lumen.

Chronic aortic dissection is usually asymptomatic. It may be incidentally discovered following an asymptomatic acute dissection, most often in patients with a preexisting aortic aneurysm. Some patients eventually require surgical treatment for chronic dissection and most do so as a result of aneurysmal dilatation of a chronically dissected aortic segment. Presenting complaints often include intermittent, dull chest pain, or even severe skeletal pain from erosion into the bony thorax with large or rapidly expanding aneurysms. Aortic insufficiency may develop with chronic type A dissection and present with typical features of congestive failure, including fatigue, dyspnea, and mild, dull chest pain. Infrequently, chronic dissection may result in paralysis/paraplegia from loss of vital intercostal arteries or even distal embolization of thrombus or atheroma from the false lumen. Malperfusion syndrome is an uncommon presentation for patients with chronic dissection given the likelihood that the true and false lumens communicate.

Diagnostic Studies

Routine diagnostic studies including blood tests, chest x-ray, and electrocardiogram (ECG) should be obtained, but are often not sufficient to establish the diagnosis of acute aortic dissection. ECG often reveals no ischemic changes. Obvious ischemic changes are present in up to 20% of acute type A dissections, whereas only nonspecific repolarization abnormalities are present in nearly one-third of patients with coronary ostial involvement. The ECG may also reveal left ventricular hypertrophy in those patients with long-standing hypertension. The chest x-ray is abnormal in 60 to 90% of patients with acute dissection (Fig. 47-4). Although most patients have at least one, if not several abnormal findings,

⊖ **TABLE 47-3: Frequency and Location of Malperfusion in Acute Type A and B Thoracic Aortic Dissection**

Vascular system	Frequency (%)
Renal	23-75
Extremities (upper and lower)	25-60
Mesenteric	10-20
Coronary	5-11
Cerebral	3-13
Spinal	2-9

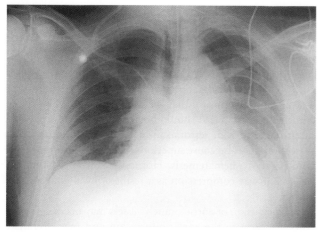

FIGURE 47-4 Plain chest x-ray exhibiting many features of acute type A dissection, such as a widened mediastinum, rightward tracheal displacement, irregular aortic contour with loss of the aortic knob, an indistinct aortopulmonary window, and a left pleural effusion.

a normal chest x-ray does not rule out the diagnosis. Blood should be drawn and sent for complete blood count, serum and electrolytes, creatine kinase with myocardial isoenzymes, troponin, and blood type and screen. These tests obtained at the time of initial observation are usually unremarkable. There is frequently a mild to moderate leukocytosis. Anemia may result from sequestration of blood or hemolysis. Liver function tests, serum creatinine, myoglobin, and lactic acid may all be abnormal in the setting of certain malperfusion syndromes.

Diagnostic Imaging

Diagnostic imaging is essential to clarify the anatomy of an acute aortic dissection, regardless of clinical certainty of diagnosis or the acuity of the patient. The diagnosis should be made rapidly with minimal distress for the patient. Two imaging modalities currently meet these criteria and are used to diagnose acute aortic dissection: computed tomography (CT) and echocardiography. Magnetic resonance imaging (MRI) and aortography, with or without intravascular ultrasound (IVUS), are used to diagnose acute aortic dissection but are second-line modalities for various reasons. The benefits, disadvantages, and diagnostic accuracy of each are useful when choosing the most appropriate study for a particular clinical situation (Table 47-4). Each test provides disruption, reentry points, whether there is flow or thrombus in the false lumen, status of the aortic valve, the presence and nature of myocardial ischemia, and brachiocephalic and aortic branch vessel involvement. Specific data may be necessary for operative planning and subsequent management to define the imaging study most appropriate for a particular patient. In a recent review, an average of 1.8 imaging studies was used to diagnose correctly acute aortic dissection.[9]

Helical CT scanning is widely available and is now the most frequently used test to diagnose acute aortic dissection. It requires intravenous contrast medium that may limit its

TABLE 47-4: Sensitivity and Specificity of Various Imaging Modalities Useful for the Diagnosis of Thoracic Aortic Dissection

Imaging study	Sensitivity (%)	Specificity (%)
Aortography	80-90	88-93
Computed tomography	90-100	90-100
Intravascular ultrasound	94-100	97-100
Echocardiography		
Transthoracic	60-80	80-96
Transesophageal	90-99	85-98
Magnetic resonance imaging	98-100	98-100

use in certain clinical situations but generates images familiar to most practitioners and has a high sensitivity and specificity. This technique can be performed quickly, fulfilling the requirements for use in the early management of acute dissection. Additional structures such as the pleural and pericardial spaces are imaged. When performed and formatted as an arteriogram, aortic branch vessels may also be evaluated: Involvement of the brachiocephalic vessels is identified with nearly 96% accuracy. The diagnosis of dissection requires two or more channels separated by a dissection flap (Fig. 47-5). For operative planning, a CT scan with arterial phase contrast of the chest, abdomen, and pelvis to the level of the femoral arteries is ideal. Transaxial two-dimensional images can be reconstructed to display three-dimensional images of the aorta that not only aid in diagnosis but also are useful for operative planning.

Transesophageal echocardiography (TEE) is currently the second most frequently used study for making the diagnosis of

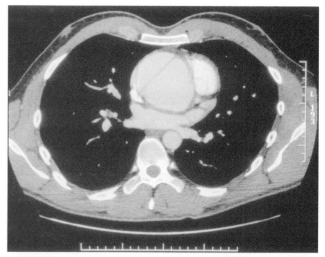

FIGURE 47-5 Axial image of CT arteriogram of acute type A dissection showing a dissection flap in the mid-ascending aorta.

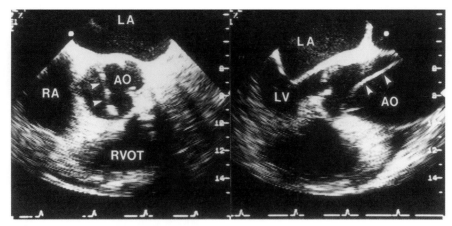

FIGURE 47-6 Transesophageal echocardiogram showing the dissection membrane (*arrowheads*) in the short (*left panel*) and long (*right panel*) views of a type A dissection.

acute aortic dissection. It is widely available, requires no intravenous contrast or radiation, and generates dynamic images of the aorta from which the diagnosis can be made (Fig. 47-6). It requires operator expertise both to acquire the necessary images and to conduct the examination safely. Although the safest setting in which to perform TEE is the operating room under general anesthesia, it can be performed in a monitored setting using topical anesthesia and light sedation. Patient comfort is paramount in this situation as rupture has been reported during difficult studies and a complete examination of the entire aorta is necessary to exclude the diagnosis of acute dissection. Absolute contraindications to TEE include esophageal abnormalities such as varices, stricture, or tumor. A full stomach or recent meal is a relative contraindication, but recognition of these conditions permits safe examination with few complications in the vast majority of patients. Criteria for making the diagnosis of acute aortic dissection include visualization of an echogenic surface separating two distinct lumens, repeatedly, in more than one view, and that can be differentiated from normal surrounding cardiac structures. The true lumen is identified by expansion during systole and collapse during diastole. Communication of the false lumen is found by identifying distal tears in the flap and flow in the false lumen with the addition of color Doppler. Similarly, the absence of flow indicates false lumen thrombosis. TEE additionally may provide high-quality images of the aortic valve and pericardial space. The coronary ostia are directly evaluated and regional left ventricular function may be assessed to identify myocardial ischemia indirectly. Color flow Doppler reliably quantifies aortic regurgitation and may be used to assess for additional valvular abnormalities. The pericardium and pleural space are also visualized and therefore effusions may be identified.

Transthoracic echocardiography (TTE) provides images of the ascending aorta and sections of the aortic arch that may yield the diagnosis but with much less sensitivity than transesophageal imaging. As such, transthoracic imaging may prove useful but is generally insufficient to establish reliably the diagnosis. Transthoracic evaluation is additionally limited by patient-related factors including body habitus,

emphysema, and mechanical ventilation. A negative transthoracic study should be complemented by a transesophageal study, which provides greater detail of the entire aorta.

Aortography was the first study used to diagnose acute dissection in 1939 and until recently was considered the gold standard for diagnosis. It is an invasive test requiring nephrotoxic contrast media in which the aorta is visualized in multiple two-dimensional projections. The diagnosis of dissection depends on visualization of the intimal flap, two distinct lumens, or compression of the true lumen by flow through an adjacent false lumen (Fig. 47-7). Indirect signs of

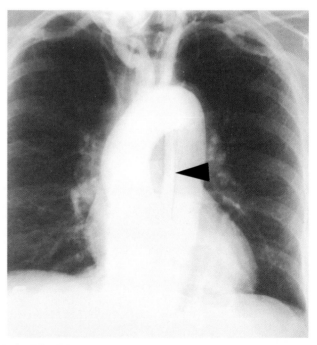

FIGURE 47-7 Aortogram of acute type B dissection illustrating differential contrast enhancement of the true and false lumens in the descending thoracic aorta. The intimal flap (*arrowhead*) can be seen separating the two lumens.

dissection include the presence of branch vessel abnormalities and abnormal intimal contour on injection of the false lumen. The status of the aortic valve may be evaluated and coronary angiography in the setting of type A dissections is possible only with this diagnostic test. However, coronary angiography is not recommended given that the coronary ostia are involved in 10 to 20% of acute type A dissections and are easily evaluated at the time of surgery. Coronary atherosclerosis is present in 25% of all patients with acute aortic dissection, but even in those patients repair of the dissection should take precedence. Aortography is sometimes useful in acute type B dissections with evidence of mesenteric ischemia or oliguria and in type A dissections with signs of malperfusion because catheter-based intervention may be possible. Aortography can have a high false-negative rate secondary to thrombosis of one lumen or when contrast equally opacifies each lumen, impairing distinction of a separate true and false lumen.[9] The diagnosis of intramural hematoma may also be difficult given the absence of intimal disruption, whereas penetrating atherosclerotic ulcer is usually easily visualized. Visualization of the dissection variants is best accomplished with either CT scanning or MRI (Figs. 47-8 and 47-9). One major limitation to the use of aortography in the acute setting is the need for skilled personnel. The time required to assemble this team varies with each institution, rendering aortography less useful when compared with other immediately available diagnostic tests. Aortography also requires arterial access, which can be painful and precipitate rupture or dissection extension.

IVUS is a catheter-based imaging tool that provides dynamic imaging of the aortic wall and an intimal flap in patients with aortic dissection. It is particularly useful in delineating the proximal and distal extent of dissection and

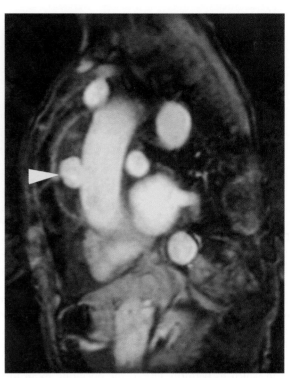

FIGURE 47-9 Sagittal contrast-enhanced MRI of penetrating atherosclerotic ulcer of the ascending aorta (*arrowhead*).

for identifying the true and false lumens in questionable cases during aortography. High-resolution images of the normal three-layered aortic wall are differentiated to identify the abnormally thin wall adjacent to the false lumen. Because the aortic wall itself is imaged, intramural hematoma and penetrating atherosclerotic ulcers may also be identified. Currently, as an isolated imaging study, it is time consuming and requires skilled personnel, as with aortography, and generally is not useful as an initial study in the acute setting. It may be most useful in combination with aortography when the initial imaging studies are negative, yet there remains a high clinical suspicion of dissection.

MRI and the newer contrast-enhanced magnetic resonance angiography (MRA) generate superior images reliably demonstrating aortic dissection (Fig. 47-10). MRI/MRA offers detailed anatomy as CT does but does not require radiation. Moreover, MRI may be particularly useful in pregnant patients. Dissection is identified as an intraluminal membrane separating two or more channels (Fig. 47-11). MRI provides detailed images of the entire aorta, the pericardium, and pleural spaces similar to those obtained with CT. Cine imaging may also be used to evaluate left ventricular function, the status of the aortic valve, and flow in aortic branch vessels as well as flow in the false lumen. It is, however, not widely available and the presence of ferromagnetic metal contraindicates its use. Another disadvantage of MRI is that artifact is identified in up to 64% of studies, which underscores the need for expert radiologic interpretation of the images. These factors account for its infrequent use in the acute setting.

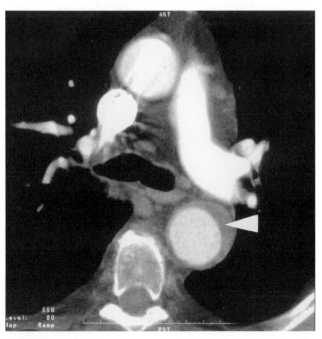

FIGURE 47-8 Axial image from a CT arteriogram showing an intramural hematoma of the descending thoracic aorta (*arrowhead*).

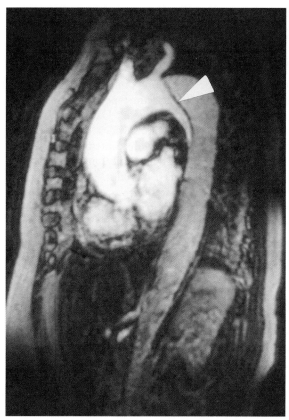

FIGURE 47-10 Sagittal contrast-enhanced MRI of a chronic type B dissection. The dissection flap (*arrowhead*) is clearly identified and the false lumen appears to extend the entire length of the thoracic and abdominal aorta (*darker posterior lumen*).

Diagnostic Strategy

The evaluation of suspected acute aortic dissection begins with a determination of the clinical likelihood that the diagnosis is correct and an evaluation of the hemodynamic stability of the patient. The unstable patient with a high suspicion for acute aortic dissection should be transferred immediately to the operating room. Medical management may be initiated as soon as the diagnosis is suspected. It is our practice to intubate and mechanically ventilate such patients while essential monitoring lines are placed. A TEE is then performed. If TEE fails to reveal acute aortic dissection, a hemodynamically unstable patient will then have a protected airway and invasive monitoring lines for subsequent evaluation of alternative diagnoses and continued resuscitation. If acute dissection is suspected despite a negative TEE, CT arteriogram (CTA) or aortography (potentially with IVUS) is the next study of choice.

Clinically stable patients permit a more detailed history and physical examination with imaging decisions tailored to specific aspects of the presentation. At the University of Virginia, all stable patients with a suspected dissection are evaluated with a CTA, as this study is definitive and provides valuable anatomic information for procedural planning. If dissection is identified on other studies, such

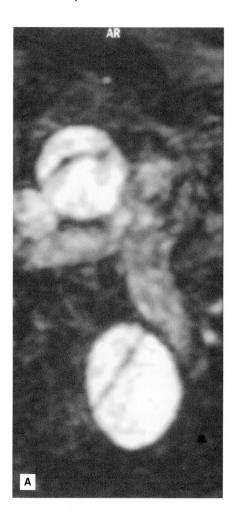

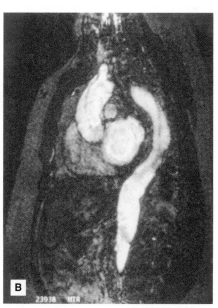

FIGURE 47-11 Axial (A) and sagittal (B) contrast-enhanced MRI of a chronic type A dissection.

as a TTE, our preference is to obtain a CTA of the chest, abdomen, and pelvis provided the patient is stable prior to proceeding to the operating room. Detailed anatomic information from CTA is valuable for operative planning and postoperative management, especially in cases with abdominal malperfusion.

Diagnostic imaging of chronic aortic dissection is usually performed for surveillance, but may also be necessary in patients with symptoms attributable to dissection and for operative planning. Routine follow-up for acute dissection occurs on a scheduled basis and is usually done with either CT or MRI. We prefer CT scanning for patients with normal renal function and no contrast allergy because CT is usually the original imaging study obtained during the acute dissection. The improved accuracy that comes with comparing similar studies combined with the availability, cost, and patient satisfaction makes CT favorable for this purpose. MRI is used mostly as a follow-up study for patients with renal insufficiency, but is the study of choice to provide precise anatomical detail for operative planning. TTE is useful to follow chronic type A dissection when there is aortic insufficiency. It can provide cross-sectional images of the ascending aorta, but generating images useful for comparison to previous studies is highly dependent on the skill of the operator. For that reason, we use echocardiography to follow patients with aortic insufficiency but also obtain a CT scan to assess ascending aortic diameter. Aortography is used primarily for operative planning. Patients older than 50 years and those with risk factors for coronary artery disease routinely undergo coronary arteriography before operation, and images of the aorta are obtained at that time. Aortography is especially useful to determine the origin of aortic branch vessels for operative planning when noninvasive imaging is inadequate (Fig. 47-12).

MANAGEMENT OF ACUTE TYPE A AORTIC DISSECTION

Natural History

Acute type A aortic dissection is impressively morbid. Fifty percent of patients suffering acute type A aortic dissection are dead within 48 hours if untreated.[16] Data such as these suggest that acute type A dissection carries a "1% per hour" mortality for missed diagnoses. More contemporary data reveal a different prognosis such that medical management may be considered in certain high-risk groups. In one such study in octogenarians, type A dissection was managed medically in 28% of patients for various reasons with a 58% in-hospital mortality.[8] Regardless, because of the extreme mortality with medical management, patients surviving acute type A aortic dissections must be aggressively diagnosed and treated with surgical intervention.

Initial Medical Management

The high morbidity of acute type A aortic dissection dictates that management should precede confirmation of diagnosis in highly suspicious cases. The initial patient encounter centers on making the diagnosis while identifying factors that require immediate treatment. The site of this initial evaluation and resuscitation is determined primarily by the hemodynamic stability of the patient. The unstable patient belongs in the operating room, whereas a more detailed diagnostic approach and subsequent management can be undertaken in stable patients. Therefore, the hypotensive patient, whether from hemorrhagic shock or tamponade, requires the aforementioned evaluation and resuscitation on transfer to the operating room. It is preferable to avoid procedures such as TEE

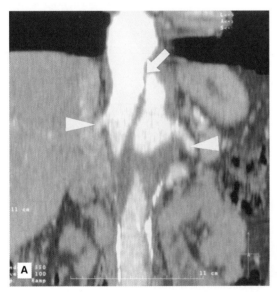
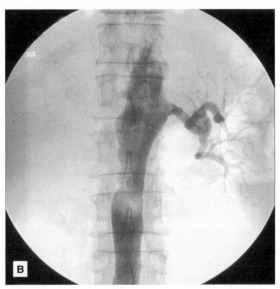

FIGURE 47-12 Coronal view of contrast-enhanced MRI (A) demonstrating chronic type B dissection with renal arteries (*arrowheads*) separated by the dissection flap (*arrow*). Aortogram (B) of the same patient revealing that each renal artery is perfused exclusively by either the true or false lumen. Such tests are often complementary and may influence surgical strategy.

or central line placement on an awaken patient outside the operating room because hypertension resulting from patient discomfort may precipitate aortic rupture or propagation of dissection. However, as in any patient with potential aortic rupture, anesthetic induction remains dangerous in patients compensating for impaired preload, whether from pericardial fluid or hypovolemia. The operating room must be prepared for prompt decompressive pericardiotomy and/or initiation of cardiopulmonary bypass.

In the hemodynamically stable patient, blood pressure is measured in both arms and both legs. These dissections can propagate in either direction, but proximal propagation can quickly destabilize the situation. In general, the goals of hypertension management in acute aortic dissection, regardless of anatomy, are twofold.[4] First, transmural aortic wall stress is diminished by decreasing the systolic blood pressure, which reduces the possibility of rupture. Second, shear stress on the aorta is decreased by minimizing the rate of rise of aortic pressure to decrease the likelihood of dissection propagation, so-called anti-impulse therapy. Specifically, the immediate goal for this situation remains to achieve a target systolic blood pressure between 90 and 110 mm Hg with a target heart rate of less than 60 beats per minute.

Pain control is important to reduce catecholamine release and decrease the risk of rupture. Therefore, therapy begins with pain control using narcotic analgesics. The drugs most commonly used for anti-impulse therapy are beta-blockers and peripheral vasodilators. In most cases, beta-blockers such as esmolol should be used first because adequate heart rate control may be difficult if the blood pressure is controlled by peripheral vasodilators first and because vasodilators may increase ventricular ejection and aortic shear stress if used unopposed. Short-acting beta-blockers should be titrated to a heart rate less than 60 beats per minute. After beta-blocker treatment has been initiated, vasodilators such as sodium nitroprusside are used for further blood pressure control. Sodium nitroprusside is a direct arterial vasodilator with a short onset and duration of action, which makes it ideal to achieve rapidly the target systolic blood pressure. Loading doses for esmolol and sodium nitroprusside should be avoided to prevent hypotension. Alternative beta-1 blocking drugs such as propranolol or metoprolol, and the combined alpha- and beta-blocker labetalol are appropriate in the subacute phase. Calcium channel blockers may be necessary to reduce systolic blood pressure in those patients with a contraindication to beta-blocker use. A commonly used alternative to nitroprusside is nicardipine. This is also a calcium channel-blocker devoid of any cardiac effects which is easily titrated to a goal blood pressure.

Operative Indications

The goals of surgery in acute type A dissection are to prevent or treat an aortic catastrophe while restoring blood flow to the true lumen of the aorta. Aortic catastrophe includes aortic rupture into the pericardium or pleural space, dissection and occlusion of the coronary ostia, and progression

TABLE 47-5: Operative Indications for Acute and Chronic Type A and B Thoracic Aortic Dissection

Dissection type	Operative indication
Acute	
Type A	Presence
Type B	Failure of medical management (persistent or recurrent pain, medically uncontrolled hypertension)
	Expanding aortic diameter
	Progressive dissection
	Impending or actual rupture
	Malperfusion
Chronic	Impending or actual rupture
	Symptoms related to dissection (congestive heart failure, angina, aortic regurgitation, stroke, pain)
	Malperfusion
	Aneurysm ≥ 5.5 cm (type A), ≥6.5 cm (type B)
	Aortic expansion > 1 cm/year

to aortic valvular incompetence. The presence of ascending aortic involvement is therefore an indication for operative management in all but the highest-risk patients (Table 47-5). The difficulty arises in determining which patients are at high risk and which additional factors should affect the management algorithm. Patient age, for example, is not regarded as an absolute contraindication to surgery. However, this factor should be considered given the relative worse outcomes of operative treatment for acute type A dissection for patients greater than 80 years of age. Neurologic status at the time of presentation can also affect the decision to operate. Although most agree that obtunded or comatose patients are unlikely to improve with surgical repair, complications such as stroke or paraplegia at the time of presentation are not contraindications to surgical correction. It must be acknowledged that dissection repair will most likely not improve neurologic condition, and may even make it worse. Neither the distal extent nor the thrombosis of the false lumen obviates the need for surgical repair because the risk of developing an aortic catastrophe remains. Similarly, patients with subacute type A dissection who present or are referred after 2 weeks of dissection onset require operation. Scholl et al demonstrated that these patients have avoided the early complications of dissection and may safely undergo elective operation rather than emergency repair.[17]

Important surgical considerations for Type A aortic dissection include extent of aortic repair, establishment of cardiopulmonary bypass, temperature management, cerebral protection, myocardial protection, and management of aortic insufficiency and end-organ perfusion during and after completion of surgery. Technical considerations for establishment of cardiopulmonary bypass, cerebral protection, and temperature management are discussed in depth below. An important component to any surgical strategy includes identification and correction of end-organ malperfusion. Patients who present with abdominal pain or tenderness and lactic acidosis may require additional endovascular procedures, such as fenestration or mesenteric stenting either immediately after or in select cases, prior to, ascending aortic repair.

ANESTHESIA AND MONITORING

Anesthesia used during the repair of aortic dissections is often narcotic based with inhalational agents for maintenance. Single-lumen endotracheal tubes are used for procedures performed through a median sternotomy, whereas double-lumen endotracheal tubes are useful but not mandatory for procedures performed through a left thoracotomy. Monitoring lines often include central venous access with a pulmonary artery catheter and one or more arterial pressure monitoring lines specific to the operation performed. Preparation must be made for all possibilities in these cases, most importantly for the possible need for hypothermic circulatory arrest. Arterial monitoring should be tailored to both the anatomy of the dissection and the method of cannulation. One or two radial arterial lines and at least one femoral line may be required to ensure adequate perfusion of the upper and lower body. If antegrade cerebral perfusion via a right axillary or innominate artery cannulation is planned, right arterial line placement (in addition to femoral and/or left radial) is useful to measure perfusion pressure. All patients require a TEE probe. Core body temperature is monitored in the bladder using a Foley catheter and in the esophagus using a nasopharyngeal probe. A wide skin preparation to include the axillary and femoral arteries is essential to provide all possible cannulation options.

Neurologic monitoring is available, but its utility remains controversial even in elective cases. Advocates of both cerebral and spinal cord monitoring argue that these monitors are able to detect injury to neurons before irreversible cellular injury.[18] Thus, this warning allows for detection of imminent injury and subsequent evasion of injury. Opponents argue that there is a significant learning curve and that the injury has already occurred once these monitors can identify ischemic neurologic changes. The optimal type of monitoring depends on the location of the dissection and the resultant details of required vascular control. Manipulation of the ascending aorta and arch can affect cerebral perfusion. In these cases, transcranial Doppler (TCD) or near-infrared spectroscopy (NIRS) has been used. Intraoperative TCD monitoring is used to identify malpositioned cannulas or document the need for adjustment of retrograde perfusion.[19] Opponents of TCD argue difficulty with low baseline flow and poor signal in patients with thick temporal bones, which confuses interpretation of the results and the response to them. Continuous noninvasive NIRS can be used to monitor cerebral oxygenation, marker of cerebral blood flow. Although the role of NIRS in aortic dissection has not been elucidated, advocates extrapolate use from studies on carotid endarterectomy and coronary bypass.

NIRS can be used for identification of regional oxygenation changes during the case, which may be particularly useful during normothermic periods of these cases.[18] Somatosensory evoked potentials (SSEP) is argued to be useful in identifying neurologic injury ranging anywhere from the peripheral nerve to the brain. These studies may even identify ischemic cerebral injury during hypothermic circulatory arrest earlier than electroencephalography (EEG).[20] SSEP can also be useful in the detection of spinal cord ischemia to identify crucial spinal cord vasculature requiring reimplantation. The use of SSEP at some centers has led to reduced intraoperative and postoperative paraplegia in retrospective studies.[21] Neurologic monitoring remains a relatively new technology that is operator dependent, but probably is useful in experienced hands.

HEMOSTASIS

Open aortic dissection repair is commonly associated with significant blood loss caused by weak tissues and coagulopathy from bleeding or hypothermia. Strict blood conservation is an important aspect of the operation. At least one cell-saver device should be available. Packed red blood cells, platelets, and fresh-frozen plasma should be in the operating room at the start of the operation. Coagulopathy as a result of the preoperative status of the patient, cardiopulmonary bypass, and deep hypothermic circulatory arrest contribute to excessive blood loss. Antifibrinolytic drugs can be useful hemostatic adjuncts. Patients will often require transfusion of fresh-frozen plasma, platelets, and possibly cryoprecipitate. Fibrin glues and hemostatic materials such as Surgicel and Gelfoam are useful as systemic coagulopathy is corrected.

CARDIOPULMONARY BYPASS

Cannulation for type A dissection repair requires thoughtful evaluation of the dissection anatomy while taking into consideration the extent of the repair to be undertaken. The crucial point is to provide arterial flow into the true lumen of the aorta with proof of sufficient end-organ perfusion, in particular as dynamic flaps may alter perfusion. Some flexibility regarding arterial access should be exercised. In certain situations, a patient may require multiple cannulation sites to perfuse adequately the entire body. Various options for cannulation exist, but the optimal choice of cannulation in aortic dissection requires tailoring to the combination of surgeon preference with dissection anatomy.

Venous cannulation remains relatively straightforward. Venous cannulation is obtained commonly through the right atrium using a two-stage venous cannula, whereas bicaval cannulation is used for certain cases in which retrograde cerebral perfusion is used during hypothermic circulatory arrest. A left ventricular vent is necessary in the setting of aortic valve incompetence and is easily placed through the right superior pulmonary vein or rarely through the left ventricular apex wall. Cardioplegia is administered in a retrograde fashion through a coronary sinus catheter with additional protection via direct cannulation of the undissected coronary ostia.

Arterial cannulation requires a much more thoughtful process. Right axillary artery, femoral artery, and direct ascending aortic cannulation are the three most common techniques. The optimal site of cannulation should be tailored based on the combined goals of surgery and the specific anatomy of the patient, with contingency plans for evidence of malperfusion.

Historically, femoral cannulation was the site of choice for arterial cannulation for type A dissection. The most favorable side of femoral cannulation has been debated in the past, but as long as there is perfusion into the true lumen, the side most likely does not matter. Reports from the University of Virginia, among others, have also shown that the dissected ascending aorta itself can be cannulated safely with echocardiographic guidance.[22] This technique involves confirming access to the true lumen of the aorta with echocardiography of the descending aorta. Then, using the Seldinger technique, a percutaneous cannula can be properly positioned. Direct cannulation should be avoided through areas with evidence of hematoma. Proper perfusion of the true lumen must be confirmed with ultrasound or echocardiography. A potential salvage maneuver involves cannulation of the ventricular apex with advancement of the cannula though the aortic valve and into the true lumen of the aorta. This technique also requires confirmation of true lumen perfusion. Aortic cannulation of either the dissection area or the apex mandates cannulation of the graft after repair in most cases.

Increasingly, the right axillary artery is being utilized for cannulation during dissection repair and is the first choice cannulation site at many institutions.[23] The right axillary artery provides direct access to the right carotid artery for selective antegrade perfusion. This can be done by sewing a graft to the artery or directly cannulating it. However, direct axillary cannulation appears to cause more morbidity than graft cannulation, including further dissection, brachial plexus injury, and limb ischemia. Axillary cannulation may be suboptimal in cases in which the axillary, right common carotid, or innominate artery are dissected. Similar techniques have been described in cannulation approaches to the innominate artery.

No matter the preferred site of arterial cannulation, the surgeon must be cognizant of whole body perfusion. Patients that are not cooling properly or show other signs of malperfusion may require more than one arterial cannulation sites for cardiopulmonary bypass. Routine confirmation of blood flow in the carotids as well as the descending aorta can be critical to avoid malperfusion.

CEREBRAL PROTECTION

Type A dissection repair involving the arch disrupts blood flow to the brachiocephalic arteries during a period of circulatory arrest. Cerebral protection during that period is critical to neurologic outcome. Cerebral protection is optimized through deep hypothermia with or without potential neuroprotective adjuncts. Straight hypothermia during circulatory arrest was the first method used to perform operations on the aortic arch and remains an effective method for shorter procedures. Two alternative primary end points for cooling are employed: goal temperature or EEG silence.

The published temperature goals vary widely, namely anywhere from 14 to 32°C. The ischemic tolerance of the brain improves with colder temperatures. However, cooling to a temperature below 14°C can result in a form of nonischemic brain injury and is therefore not recommended. The neurologic protection from straight hypothermic circulatory arrest can be very good, especially for short ischemic times. Most data suggest that straight hypothermic circulatory arrest up to 20 minutes is safe. However, increased ischemic time is directly related to increased incidence of neurologic deficits.[24] Proponents of straight hypothermic circulatory arrest have suggested in elective patients that longer times can be used safely without significant adverse cognitive outcomes but circulatory arrest should be limited to as short a time as possible.[25]

For these cases, temperature is being used as a proxy for metabolic function. Unfortunately, nasopharyngeal and tympanic temperature may be imperfect estimates of brain temperature. Moreover, temperature does not directly relate to neurologic activity. For these reasons, some groups use EEG silence to determine the appropriate point at which to discontinue cooling and perfusion. The patients are cooled until EEG silence is obtained. After 5 minutes at this temperature, the circulatory arrest period can be initiated, usually at a temperature between 15 and 22°C. Using this technique, the group from the University of Pennsylvania achieved EEG silence in 90% of patients after 45 minutes of cooling and had a postoperative stroke rate of less than 5%.[26] As a result, in the absence of EEG monitoring, they cool for at least 45 minutes in almost all cases to optimize brain protection. Although EEG is attractive in theory, it is not always available when patients with dissections are taken to the operating room. We typically cool for 45 minutes to achieve a goal temperature of 18 to 21°C.

Continued cerebral perfusion during the period of circulatory arrest is an alternative technique for cerebral protection, especially for circulatory arrest times greater than 20 minutes. Utilizing cerebral perfusion, some groups have moved progressively to more moderate hypothermia (24-28°C) during dissection repair.[27] Cerebral blood flow may be delivered in a either retrograde or antegrade fashion. The technique for retrograde cerebral perfusion depends on the venous cannulation strategy. If bicaval cannulation is used, reversing flow through the superior vena caval cannula with a proximally placed tourniquet is simple and effective. Use of retrograde flow with dual-stage venous cannulation requires placement of a retrograde "coronary sinus" catheter into the superior vena cava through a pursestring suture. The superior vena cava is then occluded with an umbilical tape to direct flow toward the head. Retrograde cerebral perfusion has the added benefit of flushing atherosclerotic material and air from the brachiocephalic vessels. A flow rate necessary to produce a superior vena caval pressure of 15 to 25 mm Hg is considered optimal.

Selective antegrade cerebral perfusion has gained popularity, particularly when extended aortic arch surgery is planned.

This can be performed by clamping the base of the innominate artery with a right axillary or innominate arterial cannulation, allowing for cerebral perfusion via the right carotid artery. This also can be performed once the aortic arch is open by encircling the innominate artery with a vessel occluder and cannulating the lumen with a retrograde "coronary sinus" cannula. Bilateral antegrade perfusion can be performed by similarly cannulating the left carotid artery lumen. With the left subclavian artery occluded, flow rates are slowly increased to achieve perfusion pressures of 50 to 70 mm Hg at the desired circulatory arrest temperature. These cannulae are then removed just before completing the anastomosis of the brachiocephalic vessels to the vascular graft, at which time cardiopulmonary bypass may be reinstituted.

A few basic principles apply to all approaches. During cooling on cardiopulmonary bypass, a maximum temperature gradient between perfusate and patient of less than 10°C is ideal. The head is then packed in ice to maintain a low brain temperature. To ensure maximal protection, the goal temperature should be maintained for 5 minutes before initiation of hypothermic circulatory arrest. Similarly, the body should be reperfused for 5 minutes at the colder temperature before beginning the rewarming process. Rewarming too early can exacerbate neurologic injury. Rewarming proceeds without exceeding a 10°C perfusate-patient temperature gradient to at least 37°C as core body temperature often falls briefly after cessation of active warming and separation from cardiopulmonary bypass.

Pharmacologic adjuncts are believed by some to decrease metabolic rate with hopes of reducing injury. Although methylprednisolone continues to be used in these cases by many, barbiturate administration during cooling has fallen mostly out of favor. If used, methylprednisolone should be given early, as the steroid effects require incorporation into the cell nucleus. Others give lidocaine and magnesium before the arrest period to stabilize the neuronal cell membrane. Furosemide and mannitol can be administered to initiate diuresis and promote free radical scavenging after circulatory arrest. The results of all these techniques are not fully substantiated yet.

OPERATIVE TECHNIQUE

The exposure for procedures performed on the ascending aorta and proximal arch is through a median sternotomy. This can be modified with supraclavicular, cervical, or trapdoor incisions to gain exposure to the brachiocephalic vessels or descending thoracic aorta. When dissecting the distal arch, it is important to identify and protect both the left vagus nerve with its recurrent branch and the left phrenic nerve. Replacement of the ascending aorta in type A dissections is best performed by an open distal anastomosis technique if the arch is involved (30%) or if arch involvement is unknown. Once the patient is placed on cardiopulmonary bypass and cardioplegia catheters are in place, the mid ascending aorta is clamped, producing cardiac arrest via administration of antegrade and/ or retrograde cardioplegic solution. The dissected ascending aorta proximal to the clamp is then opened. Evaluation and

surgical correction of the aortic valve is ideally performed at this time while systemic cooling continues. If the dissection does not involve the aortic root, the aorta is transected 5 to 10 mm distal to the sinotubular ridge. When the dissection involves the sinotubular ridge, the proximal aorta is reconstructed by reuniting the dissected aortic layers between one or two strips of Teflon felt using either 3-0 or 4-0 Prolene suture. Safi et al use a technique of interrupted pledgeted horizontal mattress sutures as compared with the felt sandwich technique.[28] In their experience, this provides superior stabilization and decreases the potential for subsequent aortic stenosis. The University of Pennsylvania has described aortic reconstruction using felt as a neomedia giving a stable platform to sew the graft to otherwise friable tissue.[26,29]

Once the temperature reaches 18 to 21°C, perfusion is discontinued during a brief period of circulatory arrest. When using antegrade or retrograde cerebral perfusion, the selected perfusion is initiated at this time. The aortic clamp is released and the intima of the aortic arch is inspected and repaired accordingly (Fig. 47-13). If the intima is intact, the distal anastomosis is performed and the graft is cannulated, deaired, and clamped for resumption of cardiopulmonary bypass with systemic warming. If the intima of the arch is violated, then a hemiarch reconstruction is performed (Fig. 47-14). We have only rarely found it necessary to perform a complete arch resection for an acute dissection. If a complex aortic root procedure is required, it is often useful to repair the aortic root with one vascular graft and use a separate graft to create the distal aortic anastomosis. The two grafts are then measured, cut, and anastomosed to provide the correct length and orientation for aortic replacement.

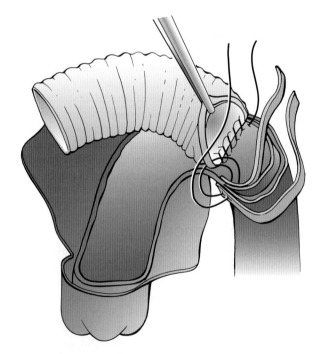

FIGURE 47-13 The false lumen of the distal aorta is closed and the aortic wall is reconstructed with inside and outside felt strips.

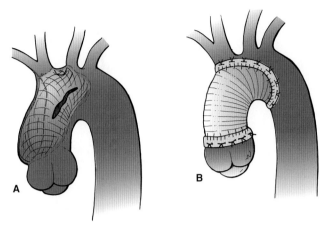

FIGURE 47-14 (A) The type A dissection extends into the proximal aortic arch. (B) The distal dissected aortic wall is reconstructed with inside and outside felt strips to replace part of the arch and ascending aorta.

If the ascending aorta cannot be cross-clamped or the surgeon prefers not to clamp the dissected aorta, the patient is first cooled to 18 to 21°C with subsequent circulatory arrest. The distal aortic reconstruction is performed first in this circumstance, at which time the graft is cannulated and proximally clamped with resumption of cardiopulmonary bypass and systemic rewarming. Cannulation of the graft for antegrade systemic perfusion and rewarming is associated with improved neurologic outcomes compared with retrograde perfusion and should be performed whenever possible. Proximal ascending aortic repair is completed during the

period of rewarming. Because a cross-clamp is not applied with this technique, the left ventricle must be decompressed once fibrillation starts during systemic cooling to prevent distention and irreversible myocardial injury. In cases of severe aortic insufficiency, ventricular distension may occur despite appropriately positioned vent catheters. In this, manual cardiac decompression or aortic cross-clamping will be required.

An alternative to the open distal technique is possible when the dissection is limited to the ascending aorta or the proximal arch away from the origin of the brachiocephalic vessels. Antegrade arterial perfusion is achieved through distal arch or right subclavian artery cannulation; retrograde perfusion via cannulation of a femoral artery has traditionally provided acceptable results. An aortic cross-clamp is applied tangentially just proximal to the innominate artery. The ascending aorta is resected to include the inferior aspect of the arch. The layers of the dissected aorta proximal to the clamp are then reunited if necessary and the ascending aorta replaced with an appropriately sized, beveled vascular graft. The proximal reconstruction and anastomosis may then be created and the entire procedure performed without requiring deep hypothermia and circulatory arrest.

Isolated dissection of the aortic arch is rare. Classified as a type A dissection, it requires resection of the arch at the site of intimal disruption and aortic replacement. Surgical management of the brachiocephalic vessels is determined by the integrity of the adjacent intima. If intact, the brachiocephalic vessels are reimplanted as a Carrel patch into a vascular graft after repair (Fig. 47-15). If the dissection involves individual

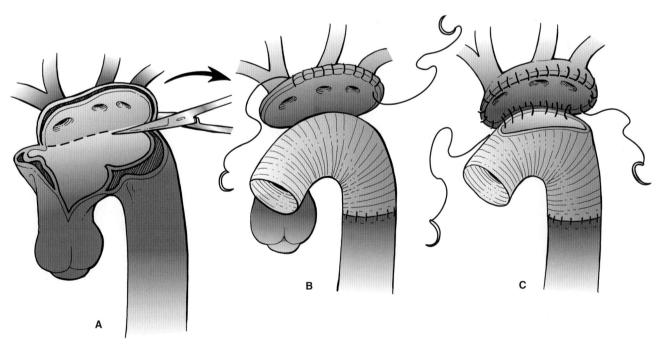

FIGURE 47-15 Brachiocephalic vessels can be reattached to an arch graft as a unit if the inner cylinder of origin of each vessel remains intact. (A) The arch vessels are excised as a unit from the superior surface of the dissected aortic arch. (B) The separated layers of the brachiocephalic patch are reunited using inner and outer felt strips and continuous suture. (C) A corresponding hole is cut in the aortic graft and the continuous brachiocephalic unit is sutured into place.

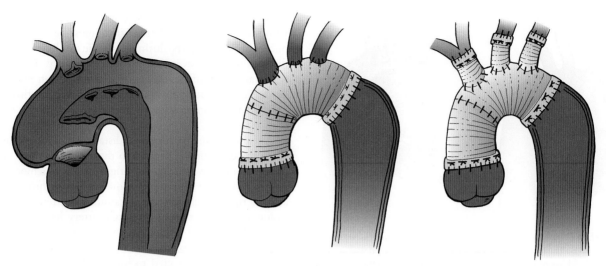

FIGURE 47-16 The brachiocephalic vessels are separated from the true lumen by the dissected false lumen (*left panel*). If individual brachioce-phalic vessels are also damaged beyond repair, short interposition grafts are added to reconnect each artery to the aortic graft (*right panel*).

vessels, each may require repair and reimplantation individu-ally into the graft used for arch replacement (Fig. 47-16).

Aortic root dissection often fails to violate the intima of the coronary ostia. Repair of the ascending aorta at the sino-tubular junction is therefore sufficient to reunite the aortic root layers and provide uninterrupted coronary blood flow. Minimal disruption of the coronary ostial intima should be repaired primarily with 5-0 or 6-0 Prolene suture. If, how-ever, the ostium is circumferentially dissected and an aortic root replacement is necessary, an aortic button should be excised and the layers reunited with running 5-0 Prolene suture, glue, or both. Coronary buttons are then reimplanted into the vascular graft or to a separate 8-mm vascular graft as part of a Cabrol repair (Fig. 47-17). Aortocoronary bypass

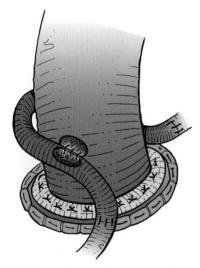

FIGURE 47-17 Illustration showing the attachment of the coro-nary ostia to the graft using the Cabrol technique. The ends of a 60-mm Dacron graft are sewn end to end to each coronary ostium. A side-to-side anastomosis is made between the intercoronary tube graft and the aortic graft.

grafting is performed only when the coronary ostium is not reconstructable and as a last resort.

Acute type A dissection is complicated by aortic valve insufficiency in up to 75% of patients. Fortunately, preserva-tion of the native valve is successful nearly 85% of the time. The mechanism of aortic insufficiency in most cases is the loss of commissural support of the valve leaflets. This is repaired using pledgeted 4-0 Prolene sutures to reposition each of the commissures at the sinotubular ridge (Fig. 47-18). The dis-sected aortic root layers are then reunited using 3-0 Prolene suture and either one or two strips of Teflon felt to recreate the sinotubular junction and reform the sinuses of Valsalva. Aortic valve preservation must always be performed using intraop-erative TEE to assess the valve postoperatively. No more than mild aortic insufficiency should be present. In addition to commissural resuspension, techniques exist to spare the aortic valve and replace the aortic root in acute type A dissection, but the experience is early and the number of patients few. This topic is covered in greater detail in the section on sur-gical techniques for chronic type A dissection. If the aortic valve cannot be spared, replacement of the ascending aorta and valve should be performed using a composite valve graft or homograft. The composite valve graft is implanted using horizontal mattress 2-0 Tycron sutures to encircle the annulus and to seat the valved conduit (Fig. 47-19). The previously excised and reconstituted coronary buttons are reimplanted into the vascular graft with running 5-0 Prolene suture (Fig. 47-20). The left coronary button is implanted first, at which time the graft is clamped and placed under pressure to define the proper orientation and position of the right coronary button. The aortic homograft is similarly implanted using horizontal mattress 2-0 Tycron sutures, except that a generous margin of aortic root below the coronary buttons is retained for a second hemostatic suture line of running 4-0 Prolene. This is an ideal solution for individuals who have a contraindication to anticoagulation or for young females. The Ross procedure (pulmonary autograft) is not applicable

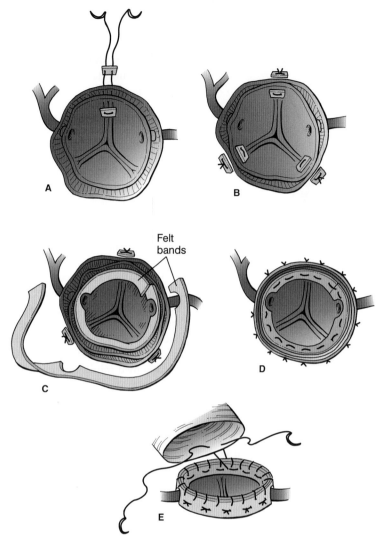

FIGURE 47-18 Resuspension and preservation of the native aortic valve in a type A dissection. (A) The dissected layers are approximated at each commissure with double-pledgeted mattress sutures. (B) The aortic valve commissures are completely resuspended. (C) Thin felt strips (8- to 10-mm wide) are placed inside and outside from the circumference of the aorta. The coronary ostia are not compromised. (D) The aortic walls are sandwiched between the felt strips with a horizontal mattress. (E) A vascular graft is sutured to the reconstructed proximal aorta.

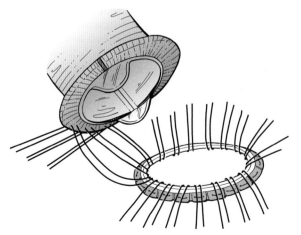

FIGURE 47-19 Everting 2-0 pledgeted mattress sutures are placed shoulder to shoulder around the aortic annulus to anchor a composite graft containing a St. Jude prosthesis.

in those patients with connective tissue disorders and not recommended in acute dissection.

Some centers have extended repairs into the descending thoracic aorta utilizing thoracic aortic endografts to potentially decrease the risk of malperfusion, reduce distal aortic aneurysmal degeneration and rupture, and decrease late distal aortic reoperation.[30,31] This hybrid repair, commonly referred to as a "frozen elephant trunk," is performed during the circulatory arrest period. A guidewire is introduced into the open true lumen and positioned in the mid-descending aorta. An endograft is then introduced over the guidewire, positioned under direct vision just distal to the left subclavian artery, and then deployed. The proximal extent of the endograft is then secured with suture to the native aorta. Institutions with hybrid operating rooms with integrated fluoroscopy may also utilize fluoroscopy to guide final endograft placement. They may also perform completion angiography and correct

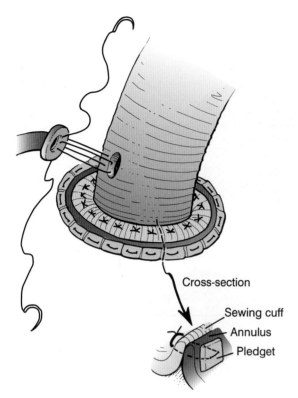

FIGURE 47-20 The coronary ostia are attached to the graft by the button technique using continuous 5-0 polypropylene suture.

Cross-section

Sewing cuff
Annulus
Pledget

any distal malperfusion with endovascular fenestration and peripheral arterial stenting. At present these techniques are not widely performed and techniques are evolving.

POSTOPERATIVE MANAGEMENT

Invasive hemodynamic monitoring is used to ensure adequate end-organ perfusion with a target systolic blood pressure between 90 and 110 mm Hg. Early postoperative blood pressure control begins with adequate analgesia and sedation using narcotics and sedative/hypnotic agents. The patient should, however, be allowed to emerge from general anesthesia briefly for a gross neurologic examination. The patient is then sedated for a period to ensure continued hemodynamic stability and facilitate hemostasis. Coagulopathy is aggressively treated with blood products and antifibrinolytic agents as necessary, and by warming the patient. Hematocrit, platelet count, coagulation studies, and serum electrolytes are obtained and corrected as necessary. An ECG and chest radiograph are used to assess for abnormalities and to serve as baseline studies. A full physical exam, including complete peripheral vascular exam, is performed on arrival. Despite adequate repair of the dissection, perfusion of the false lumen may persist; therefore, malperfusion syndrome remains possible. If an abdominal malperfusion syndrome is suspected postoperatively, this should be aggressively evaluated with ultrasound and subsequent angiography if positive. A strong clinical suspicion is enough to warrant this evaluation given the consequences of failed recognition. Exploratory

laparotomy should be performed early if bowel ischemia is suspected. The patient can be extubated once extubation criteria are met if the patient has been hemodynamically stable without excessive bleeding and the results of a neurologic exam are normal. Management is routine from that point forward.

LONG-TERM MANAGEMENT

Surviving the operation for acute dissection represents the beginning of a lifelong requirement for meticulous medical management and continued close observation. It has been estimated that replacement of the ascending aorta for type A dissection obliterates flow in the distal false lumen in fewer than 10% of patients. As a result, the natural history of repaired dissection may involve dilatation and potential rupture of the chronically dissected distal aorta. This was the reason for the late death in nearly 30% of DeBakey's original series in 1982 and is currently the leading cause of late death following surgical repair.[32] Often a multidrug antihypertensive regimen including beta-blocking agents is required to maintain systolic blood pressure below 120 mm Hg. There are some data indicating that blood pressure control within a narrow range may alter the natural history of chronic dissection by diminishing the rate of aneurysmal dilatation. The long-term durability of the aortic valve after supracoronary reconstruction is quite good with freedom from aortic valve replacement of 80 to 90% at 10 years. Progressive aortic insufficiency of the native valve is possible and should be followed with TEE in some patients.

Follow-up diagnostic imaging is required to monitor aortic diameter in patients after repair. Spiral CTA and MRI are the imaging studies of choice. MRI and ultrasound are useful in patients with renal insufficiency and those requiring only imaging of the abdominal aorta. Echocardiography is useful for imaging the ascending aorta and provides additional information regarding the aortic valve. It is important to recognize the resolution limitations of each imaging modality and inherent imprecision of comparing different imaging modalities to evaluate changes. In general, measurements should be made at the same anatomical level with respect to reproducible anatomical structures (ie, the sino-tubular ridge, proximal to the innominate or left subclavian arteries or at the diaphragmatic hiatus). It is important to recognize that the false lumen should be included in measurements of aortic diameter whether it is perfused or not. Three-dimensional reconstruction of spiral CT and MRI scans minimizes the error introduced by aortic eccentricity when comparing imaging studies and has simplified following this patient population. The current recommendations are to obtain a baseline study before hospital discharge and at 6-month intervals during the first year. If the aortic diameter remains unchanged at 1 year, studies are obtained yearly. Aortic enlargement of more than 0.5 cm within a 6-month period and greater eccentricity on comparison of three-dimensional reconstruction images are high-risk changes for which the interval is decreased to 3 months if surgery is not indicated.

Results

The operative mortality for repair of acute type A aortic dissection has fallen since DeBakey's original 40% mortality was reported in 1965. Improved ICU and floor care of these patients, earlier recognition of dissection through improved imaging modalities, development of hemostatic vascular graft material, more effective hemostatic agents, and improvements in the safety of cardiopulmonary bypass are likely responsible. In the last two decades, most centers consistently report an operative mortality for acute type A dissection of between 10 and 30%. The high early mortality in acute dissection parallels the number of patients who present profoundly hypotensive and in shock. The mode of death is stroke, myocardial ischemia/heart failure, aortic rupture, or malperfusion in most cases.

The International Registry of Acute Aortic Dissections (IRAD) recently reported on the results of 526 patients with acute type A aortic dissection who underwent surgical treatment in 18 large tertiary centers.[33] Surgery in these patients included replacement of the ascending aorta in 92%, aortic root in 32%, partial arch in 23%, complete arch in 12%, and descending aorta in 4%. Overall in-hospital mortality was 25%; 31% for hemodynamically unstable patients; and 17% for stable patients. Causes of death were aortic rupture (33%), neurologic complications (14%), visceral ischemia (12%), tamponade (3%), or nonspecified (42%).

Age is not an absolute contraindication to surgical treatment of type A aortic dissections. However, operative mortality increases with age. Retrospective series show that operative mortality increases from 20 to 30% for patients younger than 75 years of age to greater than 45 to 50% for those 80 years or older.[34]

The published results for long-term survival following surgically treated acute type A aortic dissection over the last decade is roughly 71 to 89% at 5 years and between 54 and 66% at 10 years.[35-37] Survival for patients who are discharged alive from the hospital after surgical repair of type A aortic dissection carries a survival rate of 96% at 1 year and 91% at 3 years.[38]

MANAGEMENT OF ACUTE TYPE B AORTIC DISSECTION

Type B aortic dissections account for approximately 40% of all acute aortic dissections.[8] Their natural course is more benign than that of acute type A dissections.

Most patients with acute type B aortic dissections survive the acute and subacute phases with medical management alone. Approximately 20 to 30% of patients present with complicated type B dissection, which require urgent operative (surgical or endovascular) intervention. Complicated dissection can be defined as imminent or actual aortic rupture, aortic expansion, hemodynamic instability, persistent pain despite medical management, drug-resistant hypertension, and malperfusion syndrome.[8,39] The most frequent causes of

death in acute type B dissection are aortic rupture and visceral malperfusion.

The relative success with medical management has relegated surgical treatment for acute type B dissections to patients with complicated dissections or those with progression of the disease (see Table 47-5). Medical therapy of uncomplicated type B aortic dissection confers a relatively good short-term prognosis with in-hospital survival of approximately 90%.[39] Medical management in these patients has survival rates of approximately 85% at 1 year and 71% at 5 years.[40]

On the contrary, patients with complicated dissections that require open surgical intervention have a 30-day mortality of approximately 30%.[8] More recently though, endovascular techniques have been used in these complicated dissections with reduced perioperative mortality and morbidity. Endovascular treatment of acute type B dissections was first described in 1999 by Dake et al[41] and Nienaber et al.[42] As endovascular treatment of complicated dissections has expanded, the results have improved, with studies now reporting a mortality of around 5%.[43]

Medical Management

Historically, the mortality of open surgical approaches for type B aortic dissections exceeded 50%, whereas medical management carried a mortality risk of 30% or less. Therefore, medical management has played a pivotal role in the management of these patients. Medical management is identical to that described in the initial management of the acute type A aortic dissection. The goals are control of the heart rate and blood pressure to decrease the shear stress on the aorta and limit expansion of the false lumen and propagation of the dissection.

Medical management initially requires an adequate airway and intravenous access. Patients with suspected or confirmed type B aortic dissection should be admitted to the intensive care unit for close monitoring. Pain control is important to reduce catecholamine release and is best achieved with narcotic medications, in particular morphine sulfate. Management is initiated with beta-blockers such as esmolol or propranolol.[9] These medications should be titrated to achieve optimal blood pressure (ie, systolic pressure of 100 to 120 mm Hg) and heart rate while allowing for adequate renal, gut, and brain perfusion. Heart rate control to a goal of less than 60 bpm has been shown to decrease the risk of secondary adverse events such as aortic expansion, recurrent dissection, and aortic rupture.[44]

Vasodilators such as sodium nitroprusside can be used as an adjunct to beta-blockers if blood pressure is still not adequately controlled. Vasodilators can increase the force of ventricular ejection and aortic shear stress and should therefore be only used concurrently with beta-blockade. Calcium channel blockers can also be used to control blood pressure, especially in patients intolerant to beta-blockers. However, their use has not been appropriately studied in patients with aortic dissection. Patients with normal or decreased low blood pressure at presentation, without evidence of cardiac tamponade or heart failure, may benefit from judicious intravenous volume administration.

Once the patient with uncomplicated type B aortic dissection has been stabilized, blood pressure medications should be transitioned to an oral regimen. The patient can then be discharged from the hospital with close follow-up, including imaging and clinical assessment in 3 months and every 6 months thereafter.

Operative Indications

Operative management of acute type B aortic dissection, either by endovascular or by open surgical techniques, is currently limited to the prevention or relief of life-threatening complications.[9,45] Operative treatment is indicated for patients with persistent or recurrent pain, medically uncontrolled hypertension, rapidly expanding aortic diameter, progression of dissection despite maximal medical management, signs of impending or actual aortic rupture (ie, periaortic or mediastinal hematoma), or malperfusion to limbs, kidneys, or gut (see Table 47-5).

Endovascular Therapy

GENERAL CONSIDERATIONS

Given the poor outcomes of open surgical approaches, endovascular therapy has transitioned to the frontline of therapy

for complicated type B dissections. Endovascular treatments can include placement of thoracic endovascular graft prostheses, endovascular creation of flap fenestrations, and/or placement of uncovered stents in affected branch vessels to treat malperfusion. Because of the relative simplicity and recent improvements in outcomes, endovascular grafts have become the preferred endovascular technique for treatment of aortic dissections.

The goals of endovascular graft therapy in complicated acute aortic dissection are to restore flow to the true lumen and perfusion to the distal aorta and branch vessels. Coverage of the primary tear is frequently necessary to achieve these goals, especially if the tear is in the proximal descending aorta. Obliteration of the false lumen is desirable as well because it improves the prognosis, but it is not always possible. Endoluminal treatment of these cases usually requires coverage of the entire descending thoracic aorta because of the presence of multiple tears in the intima. The optimal outcome occurs when the prosthesis covers the primary tear, reapposes the dissected layers of the aorta, and prevents blood flow into the false lumen, therefore leading to thrombosis of the false lumen, expansion of the true lumen, and restoration of branch vessel patency (Fig. 47-21).

An alternative technique used to treat branch malperfusion from aortic dissection is percutaneous fenestration with or without stenting of the malperfused branch vessels. According to this technique, a communication is created between the true and the false aortic lumens so as to

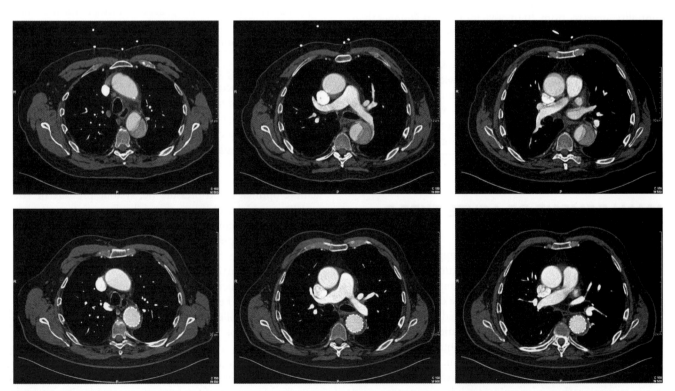

FIGURE 47-21 Endovascular stent grafting in a 77-year-old male with an acute type B aortic dissection. *Upper panel:* CTA at initial presentation showing a long dissection flap involving the descending thoracic aorta. *Lower panel:* CTA on the same patient one year after placement of an endovascular stent graft showing aortic remodeling with obliteration of the false lumen. (Used with permission from John Kern.)

provide flow to both of them. Percutaneous fenestration is performed by pulling an inflated balloon or a fenestration knife through the dissection flap to create communication between both lumens. An uncovered stent can then be placed in the true lumen at the region of the affected branch vessel or vessels to alleviate dynamic obstruction (occlusion of the branch by prolapse of the dissection flap into the branch vessel).[46] If static obstruction (extension of the dissection into

the branch vessel with reduction of the true lumen) is also present, a stent is deployed directly into the branch vessel (Fig. 47-22). The major limitation of percutaneous fenestration for treatment of aortic dissection when compared with endovascular grafting is that it does not induce thrombosis of the false lumen. False lumen thrombosis has been shown to induce aortic remodeling and decrease the long-term risk of aortic dilatation and rupture.[47]

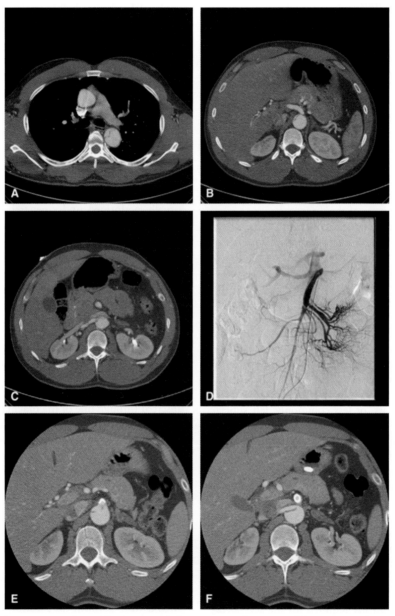

FIGURE 47-22 Endovascular treatment of visceral ischemia with fenestration and stenting of the aortic true lumen and the superior mesenteric artery (SMA) on a 40-year-old man with type B aortic dissection. (A) Near-total aortic true lumen collapse of the proximal descending aorta. (B) Dynamic compromise of the celiac artery origin. (C) Collapsed true lumen and dissection flap within the SMA suggesting both dynamic and static obstructions of this vessel. (D) Angiogram showing the dissection flap extending into the SMA. (E, F) Follow-up imaging at 1 month after percutaneous fenestration, true lumen stenting of the aorta at the level of the celiac artery, and placement of a stent into the SMA shows a patent fenestration tear in the dissection flap and a patent vessel. (Reproduced with permission from from Patel HJ, Williams DM, Meerkov M, et al: Long-term results of percutaneous management of malperfusion in acute type B aortic dissection: implications for thoracic aortic endovascular repair, *J Thorac Cardiovasc Surg.* 2009 Aug;138(2):300-308.)

Percutaneous fenestration and stenting can also be used as an adjunct to endovascular grafting when closure of the primary tear fails to improve distal malperfusion. Another technique that can be used to improve malperfusion after endovascular grafting is the PETTICOAT (provisional extension to induce complete attachment) technique.[48] According to this technique, a bare metal stent is placed as a distal extension of the previously implanted stent graft in order to expand the true lumen.

PREOPERATIVE PLANNING

The endovascular treatment of aortic dissections requires meticulous preoperative planning. The anatomy of the aorta and the actual dissection should be studied in detail with the use of imaging technology.

Preoperative imaging for endovascular repair of aortic dissections is accomplished with either computed tomographic arteriogram (CTA) or MRA. Three-dimensional sagittal and coronal reconstructions are useful to assess details of the anatomy of the aorta. Preoperative imaging allows the surgeon to size the aorta for selection of the device, ascertain the presence of adequate proximal and distal landing zones for adequate apposition of the graft, and assess the femoral and iliac vessels to plan the delivery of the device.

The left subclavian artery may be occluded in certain situations without the need for revascularization. Exclusion of the left subclavian artery without concomitant revascularization should be avoided in patients with a patent left internal mammary artery coronary bypass, those with an incomplete posterior cerebral circulation, a dominant left vertebral vessel, or a stenosed or occluded right vertebral artery.[49] Left subclavian revascularization should also be considered in those patients in whom a long segment of the aorta is being covered or those with a history of prior aortic surgeries because of the increased risk of spinal ischemia. Left subclavian revascularization is usually accomplished with the creation of a left carotid to subclavian bypass, or less commonly, left subclavian artery transposition. To assess the cerebral circulation, a head and neck CTA should be performed preoperatively in every patient in whom left subclavian exclusion is a possibility. In our experience, the left subclavian artery is covered in approximately 50% of the cases, with 25% of these patients requiring revascularization because of concerns of cerebral circulation or arm claudication.[50]

Adequate vascular access for delivery of the device is an important requirement for endovascular therapy of the aorta. Both iliofemoral systems are evaluated preoperatively with CTA or MRA with particular attention to size, tortuosity, and presence of calcification that may preclude safe delivery of the device. The minimum size required for the access vessels is determined by the outer diameter of the introducer sheath. Current devices require insertion through a vessel of at least 6 to 8 mm in diameter (equivalent to ~20 French delivery device). When the femoral vessels have an adequate caliber, no tortuosity, and minimal calcification, total percutaneous access is possible, using automated percutaneous closure devices to seal the entry point. Alternatively, an open

approach to control the common femoral arteries may be used. If the caliber of the femoral vessels is not appropriate for insertion of the device, retro-peritoneal exposure of the iliac artery with placement of a 10-mm tube graft may be necessary as a surgical conduit for insertion of the device.

Endovascular stenting of the aorta is associated with a risk of paraplegia in recent series of 0 to 3.4%.[39,51] Preoperative insertion of a lumbar catheter for drainage of cerebrospinal fluid (CSF) may decrease the risk of permanent paraplegia. In our institutions, we perform selective preoperative placement of lumbar catheters at the discretion of the surgeon, taking into account the region and length of planned aortic exclusion, and previous history of aortic surgery.[49] If there is no evidence of paraplegia postoperatively, these drains are usually discontinued 48 to 72 hours after surgery.

Operative Technique

The endovascular stenting procedure can be performed either in the angiography suite or an operating room with advanced imaging capabilities. At our institutions, the procedure is performed in the angiography suite by a team of cardiovascular surgeons and interventional radiologists. The procedure is usually performed under general anesthesia, although local or epidural anesthesia can also be used, depending on the comorbidities and clinical status of the patient. Monitoring lines are placed, including a radial arterial line in the right upper extremity. A lumbar drain for CSF drainage is placed preoperatively at the discretion of the surgeon, as stated. Antibiotic prophylaxis is administered.

In most cases, bilateral iliofemoral arterial access is used for the procedure. The larger side with less calcification and tortuosity is chosen for the delivery of the device. The other side is used for percutaneous insertion of a 5 French pigtail catheter for diagnostic contrast injection. If only one side is appropriate for use, the diagnostic pigtail catheter may be inserted through one of the brachial arteries.

If there is significant calcification of the vessel or the surgeon does not feel comfortable with the use of a percutaneous vascular closure device, the femoral artery is surgically exposed and controlled. In our experience, approximately 20% of patients have femoral vessels of an inadequate caliber to accommodate the delivery device. In these patients, a flank incision is performed and the retroperitoneal common iliac artery is exposed. A 10-mm polyester surgical conduit is then anastomosed to the common iliac artery and used as access for delivery of the device.

The pigtail catheter is inserted percutaneously and advanced to the arch of the aorta. Aortography or IVUS is then used to confirm the location of the catheter within the true lumen, define the anatomy, localize the entry tear, and create a roadmap for the procedure. The confirmation of the device being in the true lumen cannot be overemphasized. Many centers use only IVUS for these procedures. From these images, the decision is made regarding the site of deployment. The left subclavian artery may need to be covered to ensure an adequate proximal landing zone and completely exclude the primary tear. The proximal landing zone is usually visualized best at a fluoroscopic angle of approximately 45 to 75 degrees left anterior oblique (LAO).

A super-stiff wire is then inserted through a sheath placed into the iliofemoral vessel previously chosen for device delivery, and advanced into the aortic arch. The patient is heparinized to an ACT of greater than or equal to 200 seconds. The appropriate sheath is advanced into the abdominal aorta under direct fluoroscopic visualization. The device is then advanced to the selected point of delivery. Placement of the sheath and the device into the aorta are probably the most dangerous parts of this procedure. Before the deployment of the device, blood pressure and heart rate should be pharmacologically controlled so as to avoid undue strain on the heart and migration of the endograft on deployment. The device is then deployed. The optimal placement of the prosthesis is confirmed by angiography or IVUS. Although the device may need to be ballooned for full opening and apposition to the aortic wall, this maneuver has inherent risks given the weakness of the aortic wall and the pressure required to expand the stent grafts.

It is important to confirm the correct placement of the device, the absence of endoleaks, and the resolution of malperfusion to branch vessels at the end of the procedure. For this purpose, an angiogram is performed through the diagnostic pigtail catheter. If there is evidence of persistent malperfusion, adjunctive therapies should be considered such as percutaneous fenestration or deployment of additional bare-metal stents on the distal aspect of the prosthesis to expand the true lumen (PETTICOAT technique). Branch vessel stenting may also be necessary to relieve static obstruction.[46] In case of a ruptured dissection, the endovascular prosthesis should cover both the site of the primary tear and the site of rupture. Furthermore, in patients with significant hemothorax the dissection should be treated before draining the chest, as this may be tamponading the rupture.

Surgical Therapy

GENERAL CONSIDERATIONS

Open surgical intervention for type B aortic dissections is performed under general anesthesia with narcotic and inhalational agents. Double-lumen endotracheal intubation allows for lung isolation, which is critical in exposure of the thoracic aorta. Central venous access, right radial and femoral arterial lines, and in selected cases a pulmonary artery catheter, are inserted before the procedure. Core body temperature is usually measured with the use of a temperature probe in the Foley catheter and/or an esophageal probe. Antibiotic prophylaxis is administered.

Spinal cord ischemia resulting in paraplegia or paraparesis is a recognized complication of acute dissection repair that may be partially preventable and even reversible. The incidence of spinal cord ischemia is between 19 and 36% after repair of acute type B dissection.[52,53] Whereas various strategies exist to prevent spinal cord ischemia during repair of a chronic dissection, very few are feasible in the acute setting.

Pharmacologic agents such as steroids, free radical scavengers, vasodilators, and adenosine are promising adjuncts to prevent spinal cord ischemia but presently have little to no proven clinical utility. We presently use left atrial to femoral artery bypass and reimplant key intercostals arteries and selectively use CSF drainage as outlined by Safi et al.[54]

OPERATIVE TECHNIQUE

The patient is positioned in right lateral decubitus. The pelvis is canted posteriorly to allow access to both femoral vessels. A posterolateral thoracotomy in the fourth intercostal space provides sufficient access to the aorta; notching the fifth and sixth ribs posteriorly can facilitate wider exposure of the thorax. A thoracoabdominal incision may be required to access the abdominal aorta in the case of visceral malperfusion. This may be performed through either a transperitoneal or a retroperitoneal approach. The left hemidiaphragm is divided in a radial fashion while marking adjacent sites on each side of the division with metal clips for later reapproximation.

The ideal open acute type B aortic dissection repair involves replacement of as little of the descending thoracic aorta as necessary. The extent of replacement rarely exceeds the proximal third, which includes the primary tear in most cases. Such a strategy optimizes perfusion of the spinal cord by preserving more intercostals arteries.[52] This point is controversial, however, and some groups advocate replacement of the entire thoracic aorta. Any less extensive aortic replacement leaves dissected aorta with the potential for late aneurysmal dilation when there is perfusion of the false lumen. The ideal strategy to minimize spinal cord malperfusion yet resect all involved aorta has not been proved.

Once the thoracic aorta has been exposed, the operation continues with division of the mediastinal pleura between the left subclavian and the left common carotid arteries. It is essential that the left vagus and recurrent laryngeal nerves are identified and preserved during the course of the dissection. The left subclavian artery is encircled with an umbilical tape and Rummel tourniquet. Ultimately, the entire distal arch must be free enough to place an aortic clamp between the left common carotid and left subclavian arteries. Next, the proximal descending thoracic aorta is circumferentially mobilized, dividing intercostal arteries in the segment to be excised.

The formerly popular "clamp and sew" technique used for repair of acute type B dissection has largely been replaced by the use of partial left heart bypass. To institute left heart bypass, the left inferior pulmonary vein is dissected and a 4-0 Prolene pursestring suture placed posteriorly for cannulation. Arterial cannulation sites for this technique include the distal thoracic aorta for limited dissections of the proximal descending thoracic aorta or the femoral artery for those extending into the abdomen. It is important to assure that distal perfusion during cannulation is directed into the true lumen. Following the administration of 100 U/kg of intravenous heparin, 14 French cannulae are inserted into the left inferior pulmonary vein and either a normal-appearing area of descending thoracic aorta or percutaneously into either femoral artery. Bypass is then initiated with flow rates between 1 and 2 L/min.

The left subclavian artery is controlled and vascular clamps are placed on the aorta proximal to the left subclavian artery and distally on the mid-thoracic aorta. Right radial artery pressure is measured to maintain proximal aortic systolic pressure between 100 and 140 mm Hg and mean femoral artery pressure greater than 60 mm Hg.[53] The aorta is then opened longitudinally and bleeding from intercostals arteries is controlled by suture ligation. Transection of the aorta distal to the origin of the left subclavian artery provides a site for the proximal anastomosis. This is performed using 3-0 Prolene suture and may require external reinforcement with Teflon felt strips.

The graft inclusion technique is another procedure in which the posterior aspect of the proximal aorta is not fully transected. The proximal anastomosis is then created to the intact posterior aspect of the aorta. We do not recommend this technique because one cannot be certain of including all layers of the aorta in the anastomosis.

The size of the vascular graft is based on the diameter of the distal aorta and beveled to match the aorta proximally. This anastomosis may include the origin of the left subclavian to treat dissection in this vessel. A separate 6- to 8-mm Dacron graft can be used if there is intimal disruption involving the proximal segment of the left subclavian artery. Once the proximal anastomosis is completed, the proximal clamp is released and repositioned on the vascular graft to inspect the anastomosis. The distal anastomosis is then completed, the clamps are released, and partial left heart bypass is terminated. Percutaneously placed femoral artery cannulae 14 French or smaller may be removed without direct repair of the vessel. When cannulae 15 French or larger are required, open surgical repair of the femoral arteriotomy is indicated.

Rupture of the thoracic aorta before or during repair is a catastrophic event often leading to operative death. Successful management requires immediate cannulation of the femoral artery and vein for cardiopulmonary bypass and eventual deep hypothermic circulatory arrest. Assisted venous drainage through the femoral vein is often adequate, but direct cannulation of the right ventricle through the pulmonary artery may also be performed. A left atrial vent is placed through the left inferior pulmonary vein once the heart begins to fibrillate; the left ventricle may be vented as well directly through the apex. Once the nasopharyngeal temperature reaches 15°C, the vent is occluded and cardiopulmonary bypass is stopped. The head is placed down and the aorta opened for repair under circulatory arrest. The distal aorta should be clamped to minimize blood loss. Once the proximal anastomosis is performed, the proximal clamp is moved onto the graft and the graft cannulated to resume cardiopulmonary bypass.

Malperfusion of intra-abdominal viscera or lower extremities may be apparent at the time of presentation or may follow surgical repair of aortic dissections. Proximal repair of the dissection is a standard treatment and may be sufficient to treat the malperfusion syndrome. However, if malperfusion

presents or persists after surgical repair, percutaneous or surgical fenestration may be necessary. As specified, percutaneous fenestration is accomplished by using a balloon or a percutaneous knife to create a communication between the false and the true lumens. Surgical fenestration is performed through a midline laparotomy or left flank incision to provide exposure of the infrarenal aorta (Fig. 47-23). Occasionally, fenestration of intra-abdominal aortic branch vessels may be required if the intima is violated beyond the ostia. If the dissection flap cannot be completely excised, the distal vessel layers must be reunited. Consideration should be given to patch angioplasty to prevent narrowing when closing smaller vessels. In the event that perfusion is not reestablished, extra-anatomic bypass may be required.

Obstruction of the terminal aorta or malperfusion of the lower extremities following operative repair is best treated with percutaneous fenestration. Surgical fenestration remains an option if percutaneous techniques fail to reestablish blood flow. In the event that surgical fenestration fails, the best solution is femoral-femoral bypass grafting in the setting of unilateral malperfusion or axilla-femoral and femoral-femoral bypass if bilateral lower extremity malperfusion exists.

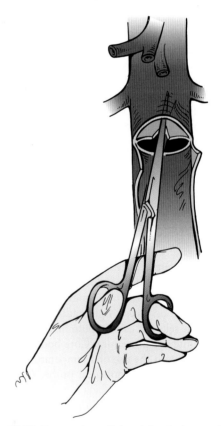

FIGURE 47-23 Fenestration of the abdominal aorta for visceral malperfusion. A transverse incision is made into the aorta, preferably into a nondissected aorta. The proximal dissection membrane is incised and then excised to decompress the false lumen as far proximally as possible. The dissected layers are reconstructed with Teflon felt or glue and the aortotomy is closed directly.

Results

Medical management remains the mainstay of treatment for acute uncomplicated type B aortic dissections. Early medical management alone is an adequate treatment in approximately 68 to 85% of patients presenting with acute type B dissection and leads to a 30-day survival rate of 89 to 93%.[39,55] The long-term outcomes of medical management are not as favorable. In the IRAD series, only 78% of 189 patients discharged alive from the hospital after medical management of type B dissections were alive at 3 years.[38] Predictors of follow-up mortality were female gender, history of prior aneurysm, history of atherosclerosis, in-hospital renal failure, pleural effusion, and in-hospital hypotension or shock. In a separate series of patients, 87% of patients managed medically were alive at 5 years, with 25% of patients requiring aortic-related interventions.[56] Similarly, in a series of 122 patients with type B aortic dissections managed medically over 36 years, Umana et al reported survival rates of 85% at 1 year and 71% at 5 years, with reoperation rates of 14% at 5 years.[40]

These outcomes have prompted some authors to consider operative treatment of uncomplicated dissections in an attempt to prevent long-term aortic-related complications. The rationale for this consideration also comes from the fact that endovascular stenting induces thrombosis of the false lumen in 75% of cases[43] and false lumen patency is associated with long-term aortic-related complications and mortality.[57]

Xu et al recently reported a series of 63 patients with type B aortic dissections (59 uncomplicated) treated with endovascular grafting.[58] The authors delayed the intervention in uncomplicated patients until 2 weeks after presentation so as to allow fibrosis and increased stability of the intimal flap. The perioperative mortality was only 3% with morbidity including stroke in one patient, renal failure in two, and retrograde aortic dissection in two. No patients developed paraplegia. Complete thrombosis of the false lumen was achieved in 98% of patients at 1 year, and the 4-year survival was nearly 90%.

Two European randomized clinical trials have been designed to answer the question of whether uncomplicated type B dissections should be treated with endovascular grafting or with medical management alone. The results of the first trial, the INSTEAD (INvestigation of STEnt Grafts in Aortic Dissection) trial, have been recently published.[59] This trial randomized 140 patients with subacute or chronic type B aortic dissection (>14 days but <1 year) to either elective stent graft placement or optimal medical management alone. Survival was not significantly different between both groups with 2-year survival rates of 96 and 89% after optimal medical therapy and endovascular stenting, respectively. There were also no differences in the rates of a combined end point, including aortic-related deaths or reinterventions. Complete thrombosis of the false lumen was more common among patients with endovascular stenting (91% with stenting vs 19% with medical management). Aortic expansion to greater than 6 cm was also more common in the group with medical management, requiring crossover to stent grafting in 16% of cases and conversion to open surgery in 4%. All crossover

patients had uneventful outcomes and no deaths. Therefore, the trial supported the use of optimal medical management for treatment of uncomplicated type B aortic dissections and reserving endovascular interventions for those patients that develop complications or other indications for intervention. A recent landmark analysis of the INSTEAD trial, however, demonstrated that at 5 years aorta associate mortality was decreased with endovascular stenting (6.9 vs 19.3%).[60] The second trial, the ADSORB (Acute Uncomplicated Aortic Dissection Type B) trial has been designed to study patients with acute uncomplicated dissection (<14 days) by randomizing them to optimal medical management or endovascular stenting.[61] In 61 randomized patients, endovascular stenting increased true lumen size, decreased false lumen size, and reduced overall aortic diameter.[62] These short- and mid-term results appear to support that endovascular stenting is safe and potentially leads to favorable aortic remodeling in uncomplicated dissections. At present, medical management remains the standard of care for *uncomplicated* type B aortic dissection, however indications for endovascular stenting remains evolving. Longer term data are required to determine the utility and timing of intervention in uncomplicated type B aortic dissection.

Approximately 20% of patients with acute type B aortic dissection present with complications requiring intervention.[39] In the past, surgical intervention was the only therapy available for these patients. The development of endovascular techniques has provided an additional treatment option that is now preferred in the majority of cases.

Surgical treatment of aortic dissection was traditionally poised with dismal outcomes. Even though morbidity and mortality remain high, outcomes from surgical management have improved over the last few decades, from as high as 50% in the 1960s to as low as 13% in more recent times.[63] In a series of 76 patients treated emergently with surgery for acute complicated type B aortic dissection including 22% patients with aortic rupture, Bozinovski and Coselli reported an in-hospital mortality of 22% with a risk of stroke of 7%, paraplegia of 7%, and renal failure of 20%.[64] Similarly, as part of the IRAD series, 82 patients surgically treated for acute type B aortic dissection had an in-hospital mortality of 29% with a risk of stroke of 9%, paraplegia of 5%, and acute renal failure of 8%.[65]

Because of the unfavorable outcomes of open surgical therapy for acute complicated type B aortic dissection, endovascular therapies have been increasingly used in this patient population. Table 47-6 summarizes the current experience with endovascular therapy for treatment of type B aortic dissections.[39,41,42,46,50,51,58,66-74]

A recent meta-analysis of 39 studies involving 609 patients using endovascular repair of aortic dissections between 1999 and 2004 showed a procedural success of 98% with emergency surgical conversion of 1%. In-hospital complications occurred in 14% of patients including neurological complications in 3%, retrograde dissection in 2%, and a perioperative mortality of 5%.[43] Survival rates at 2 years were 89% with a risk of aortic rupture at follow-up of 2%.

TABLE 47-6: Selected Retrospective Series with Endovascular Treatment of Type B Aortic Dissection

Study	N	Type of dissection	Technique	Technical success (%)	Perioperative mortality (%)	Morbidity	Permanent paraplegia (%)	Endoleak (%)	Median follow up (month)	Long-term survival (%)	False lumen thrombosis (%)
Böckler, 2009[51]	54	Acute and chronic	Stent graft	93	11	19	0		32	66	60% complete, 13% partial
Dake, 1999[41]	19	Acute	Stent graft	100	16	21	0	15	13	79	79% complete, 21% partial
Dialetto, 2005[74]	28	Acute	Stent graft	100	11		0		18	86	
Duebener, 2004[73]	10	Acute	Stent graft	90	20	50	10		25	80	
Fattori, 2008[39]	66	Acute	65% stent graft, 35% fenestration	94% stent graft, 50% fenestration	10.6	20.8	3.4				
Hutschala, 2002[72]	9	Acute	Stent graft	100	0	11	0		3		22% complete, 78% partial
Khoynezhad, 2009[71]	28	Acute	Stent graft	90	11		0	28	36	78	88% complete, 12% partial
Kische, 2009[70]	171	Acute and chronic	Stent graft	98	5	17	1.7	29	22	81	
Nathanson, 2005[69]	40	Acute and chronic	Stent graft	95	2.5	38	2.5	2.5	20	85	79
Nienaber, 1999[42]	12	Chronic	Stent graft	100	0	0	0		12	100	100
Nienaber, 2002[68]	127	Acute	Stent graft	100	1.6	3	0.8		28	97	
Palma, 2002[67]	70	Acute	Stent graft	93	5.7	31.4	0		29	91	
Patel, 2009[46]	69	Acute	Fenestration and/or branch stenting	96	17.4	21.7	2.9*		42	64	—
Pitton, 2008[66]	13	Acute	Stent graft	100	15	31	7.7*		13	66	
Siefert, 2008[50]	34	Acute and chronic	Stent graft	100	0	11.7	0	38%		86	
Xu, 2006[58]	63	Acute and chronic	Stent graft	95	3.2	19	0		12	90	98

*Patients presented preoperatively with paraplegia.

Most of these studies have used endografts, rather than percutaneous fenestrations, as the endovascular treatment of choice. In one of the largest series of percutaneous fenestration for treatment of type B aortic dissection, Patel et al reports the experience from the University of Michigan from 1997 to 2008.[46] During this period, 69 patients with type B aortic dissection and malperfusion by angiography were treated with endovascular flap fenestration and/or branch vessel stenting. Overall technical success for flow restoration was 96% with an early mortality of 17%. Complications included stroke in 4%, acute renal failure requiring dialysis in 14%, and permanent spinal cord ischemia in two patients that presented initially with paraplegia from their dissection. However, despite these encouraging outcomes all-cause mortality at follow-up was as high as 36% with 7% risk of aortic rupture, likely related to the obligate persistence of the false lumen as part of the fenestration procedure.

Despite the multiple isolated series reporting outcomes after different treatment strategies for acute type B aortic dissection, there are currently no randomized controlled trials addressing this issue. The most recent retrospective report by IRAD comparing the different strategies included 571 patients with acute complicated or uncomplicated type B aortic dissection between 1996 and 2005. Of these, 390 patients (68%) were treated medically and 125 required intervention for complicated dissection; 59 (10%) underwent open surgical procedures and 66 (11%) had endovascular treatment with either stent grafts or percutaneous fenestration. In-hospital mortality was significantly higher for patients that underwent surgery (34%) when compared to those that had endovascular procedures (11%) (Fig. 47-24). In-hospital complications

occurred in 40% of patients undergoing surgical treatment and in 21% of those undergoing endovascular therapy. These findings remained true even after comparing patients with similar comorbidities. Interestingly, in-hospital mortality was similar for those patients that underwent endovascular therapy and those that were treated medically, and significantly better than in those that underwent surgery. The low mortality risk of patients treated medically is obviously related to the fact that most of these patients presented with uncomplicated disease and were deemed eligible for medical management. However, the data suggest that endovascular therapies may improve outcomes of patients with *complicated* type B aortic dissection to the rate of those with uncomplicated dissections managed medically. The data have to be interpreted with caution though, because part of these findings may be associated to selection bias in treatment modality based on patient characteristics not accounted for, or in differing treatment strategies in different institutions.

MANAGEMENT OF CHRONIC AORTIC DISSECTION

Chronic type A dissection develops in patients who fail to undergo immediate surgical treatment of the acute dissection. Patients with chronic type B aortic dissection include those that have been successfully managed medically after an acute dissection and those with repaired type A aortic dissections that have retained segments of dissected descending thoracic aorta.

Patients with a history of acute aortic dissection, especially those with retained dissected segments, require close surveillance indefinitely. Our preference for follow-up imaging in patients with normal renal function and no contrast allergy is CTA. CTA provides good imaging, is cost effective, and is usually the technique used for the original acute dissection, making it ideal for longitudinal comparison of studies. MRA is utilized mostly as a follow-up study for patients with renal insufficiency but is the study of choice to provide precise anatomical detail for operative planning.

Many patients treated for aortic dissection, especially those with persistent communication between true and false lumens, can progress to develop aneurysmal dilatation of the aorta. They carry similar risk for aortic rupture that of atherosclerotic aneurysms. Chronic dissections have an annual rate of expansion of 0.9 to 7.2 mm per year.[75-77] Despite appropriate medical management and close follow-up, approximately 20 to 40% of patients have aortic enlargement during follow up.[75,78] This number is probably even higher in those patients with connective tissue disorders. In one study of 50 patients over a period of 40 months, 18% had fatal rupture and another 20% underwent surgical repair because of symptoms or aneurysm enlargement, emphasizing the need for diligent follow-up care.[75] Risk factors for rupture of chronic type B dissection include older age, chronic obstructive pulmonary disease (COPD), and hypertension. Chronic beta-blocker treatment reduces the rate of aortic

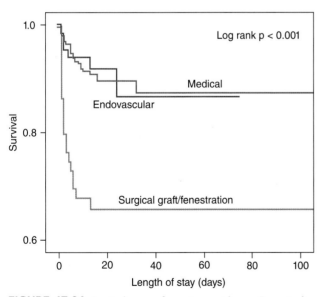

FIGURE 47-24 Survival curves for patients with type B aortic dissection managed with medical, endovascular, or surgical treatment according to the IRAD. (Reproduced with permission from Fattori R, Tsai TT, Myrmel T, et al: Complicated acute type B dissection: is surgery still the best option? A report from the International Registry of Acute Aortic Dissection, *JACC Cardiovasc Interv.* 2008 Aug;1(4):395-402.)

dilatation as well as the incidence of dissection-related hospital admissions and procedures.[78]

The presence of a patent false lumen is a significant predictor of aortic enlargement and is associated with a higher incidence of aortic-related complications and death.[57,76] In a study of 101 patients followed after medical management for type B uncomplicated dissections, the most important risk factors for aortic enlargement were a maximum aortic diameter of 4 cm or more and a patent false lumen.[79]

Operative Indications

The operative indications for chronic type A and B dissection are shown in Table 47-5. Chronic type A dissection is rarely symptomatic yet a minority of patients will present with chest pain as a result of aneurysm expansion or heart failure related to aortic regurgitation. Chronic type B dissection may present with intermittent dull chest or back pain, or infrequently, with malperfusion syndrome. Although each of these findings is an indication for intervention, the most common indications for operative management are aneurysmal dilatation of the aorta, rapid expansion, or aortic rupture. The size criteria for intervention in aortic dissection are controversial, but the one generally used is similar to that for general thoracic aortic aneurysms. Based on these criteria, aortic intervention is indicated at a size of 5.5 cm for type A dissections and 6.5 cm for type B dissections, or slightly less if there is a family history or physical stigmata of a connective tissue disorder.[80] Similarly, aortic expansion greater than 1 cm per year should be considered an indication for repair.

Recent retrospective studies from Japan have shown that patients with aortic diameters greater than or equal to 4 cm and a patent false lumen have a high likelihood of aortic-related complications (up to 50% in 6 months).[79,81] Based on these findings, it has been suggested that these patients should be considered for early repair depending on their operative risk. This issue is controversial and further studies are required before making more definitive recommendations.

Techniques for Chronic Type A Aortic Dissection

Chronic type A dissection, with or without aneurysmal enlargement, is treated using similar operative techniques described for acute dissection. The particular operation performed depends on the specific pathology involving the aortic root, status of the aortic valve, distal extent of dissection, and brachiocephalic vessel involvement. The pathology of each of these components can be very different in a chronic dissection as compared with the acute process. These differences underlie the need for surgical techniques appropriate to each unique abnormality. In general, the ascending aorta is replaced using a vascular graft to include the entire diseased segment as in acute dissection, but surgical treatment of the aortic valve and creation of the distal anastomosis differ.

Whereas the aortic valve can be repaired in most cases of acute type A dissection by simple commissural resuspension, the rate of aortic valve replacement is much higher in patients with chronic dissection. Preservation of the aortic valve is complicated by morphologic changes in the valvular apparatus such as leaflet elongation and annuloaortic ectasia, which render the valve irreparable in as many as 50% of cases. More severe grades of preoperative aortic regurgitation portend a lower probability of valve preservation. In cases in which the aortic valve cannot be preserved with simple commissural reattachment, three options exist to treat aortic insufficiency: composite root replacement, aortic valve replacement with separate ascending aortic replacement, and finally, valve-sparing aortic root repair. The technical aspects of composite valve-graft repair were covered under the surgical management of acute type A dissection. Separate aortic valve and ascending aortic replacement are appropriate when there is an operative indication to repair the ascending aorta in the setting of a normal aortic root and structural aortic valve disease. Note that this operation is not appropriate for patients with connective tissue disease. In this situation, aortic root replacement is required.

Several methods for aortic valve preservation have been described for cases affecting the aortic root. One such technique is performed by reimplanting the valve commissures into an appropriately sized vascular graft, which is secured to the left ventricular outflow tract using multiple horizontal mattress sutures.[82] Another elegant yet time-consuming technique requires resection of the sinuses of Valsalva leaving a 5-mm rim of aorta circumferentially around the leaflets.[83] Scallops are then created in the vascular graft to resuspend the commissures and remodel the aortic root. David et al advocate Teflon felt reinforcement of the aortic annulus to prevent late annular dilatation and recurrent aortic insufficiency for the remodeling technique.[84] The mid-term outcome of such operations revealed a freedom from reoperation rate of 97 to 99% at 5 years and a 5-year survival for the aortic dissection subgroup of 84%. Cochran and Kunzelman devised a similar technique to recreate the sinuses of Valsalva, which may be more important than previously recognized and contribute to improved long-term valve durability.[85] Such data in patients with chronic dissection are lacking. These techniques appear appropriate for patients with Marfan disease and in those with congenitally bicuspid aortic valves.

Treatment of the distal aorta in chronic type A dissection is somewhat controversial. Some advocate obliteration of flow in the false lumen with distal aortic repair, whereas others purposely maintain flow into both the true and false lumen using distal resection of the intimal flap. Those who reunite the chronically dissected aortic layers to perfuse only the true lumen maintain that false lumen perfusion continues through distal reentry tears in greater than 50% of cases. There is a theoretical concern that important side branches arise exclusively from the false lumen and perfusion may be interrupted with this technique. Our practice at the University of Virginia is to resect the distal chronic dissection flap as far as possible to obviate such concerns. The distal anastomosis is therefore made to the outer wall of the aorta, which has been strengthened over time. Malperfusion of the brachiocephalic vessels as a result of chronic type A dissection is treated with resection of the dissection flap from the arch. Infrequently, the chronic dissection flap extends into more distal branch vessels and may present as transient ischemic attacks or stroke. In such cases it is often necessary to resect the dissection flap into the branch vessel or reunite the layers distally before reimplantation.

Infrequently, chronic type A dissection results in extensive aneurysmal dilatation of the aorta extending from the ascending aorta through the arch and into the descending thoracic aorta. Surgical treatment of such extensive disease has traditionally been performed as a staged procedure in which the ascending aorta and arch are replaced first through a sternotomy. The second stage of the so-called elephant trunk procedure is performed 6 weeks later through a left thoracotomy for replacement of the descending aorta using a second vascular graft. Originally described by Borst et al, this technique has been used extensively with good results.[86] In some cases, the aorta distal to the left subclavian artery may be so large as to preclude the use of a two-stage repair. Kouchoukos et al have described a single-stage repair performed through a bilateral anterior thoracotomy in which the arch is repaired first during a brief period of circulatory arrest. Right subclavian and femoral artery cannulation for cardiopulmonary bypass provide proximal and distal perfusion during the subsequent ascending and descending aortic replacement. The hospital mortality was 6.2% and there were no adverse neurologic outcomes in the small series.[87] Postoperative and long-term management of these cases are identical to the acute repairs, but with an emphasis on monitoring for evidence of malperfusion.

Techniques for Chronic Type B Aortic Dissection

ENDOVASCULAR THERAPY

Endovascular therapy has been recently used for management of chronic type B aortic dissections[42,50,51,58,69,70] (see Table 47-6). The goal of endovascular therapy is to seal any dissection entry points, promote thrombosis of the false lumen, induce aortic remodeling, and prevent further aneurysmal dilatation, rupture, or malperfusion.

The general considerations, preoperative assessment, and operative technique for endovascular therapies in chronic dissection are similar to the ones described for acute type B dissection. Although percutaneous fenestrations may be used in cases of malperfusion, most chronic dissections require treatment for aneurysmal dilatation and aortic expansion because of the persistence of a false lumen, an obligate consequence of fenestrations. Therefore, the endovascular treatment of choice for most chronic dissections is endovascular grafting. Because of the increased risk of spinal malperfusion, lumbar drainage for spinal protection is used liberally in chronic dissections.

Preoperative planning with CTA or MRA is important to define the anatomy and plan the deployment of the endovascular graft. Multiple connections between the true and the false lumen may be identified in chronic dissections. It is important to seal all entry points with the endovascular graft to depressurize the false lumen. Follow-up imaging and close surveillance after the endovascular procedure are necessary.

SURGICAL THERAPY

The purpose of surgical intervention in chronic aortic dissection is to replace all segments of dissected aorta at risk for rupture and prevent the possibility of subsequent malperfusion syndrome. The conduct of the operation including surgical approach, monitoring lines required, anesthetic technique, and cardiopulmonary bypass is similar to that described for acute dissections. Greater emphasis is placed on methods of spinal cord protection.

The incidence of paraplegia after repair of thoracoabdominal aneurysms resulting from aortic dissection is reportedly as high as 25%.[88] Both mechanical and pharmacologic interventions have been advocated over the last decade to reduce this risk. Partial left heart bypass alone for replacement of the thoracic aorta above the level of T9 can reduce paraplegia rate between 5 and 8%.[89] We routinely use a lumbar drain for aneurysms extending below T9.[54] Reimplanting intercostals and lumbar arteries between T9 and L1 can be an important adjunct.[90] The aortic cross-clamp is sequentially moved distally to perfuse branches as they are reimplanted. The combination of distal perfusion, CSF drainage, and reimplanting large intercostal and lumbar arteries has significantly reduced the incidence of paraplegia at our institutions. Additional techniques used for spinal cord protection include measurement of sensory and motor evoked potentials, regional epidural cooling, and the use of a variety of pharmacologic agents for cellular protection.

The techniques used for replacement of the descending thoracic aorta are identical to those described for treatment of acute type B dissection. The extent of resection, however, for chronic type B dissection is usually greater with the goal to remove all dissected aorta at risk for rupture or symptoms. Usually these operations can be performed through the left chest, but more extensive aneurysms or cases of visceral malperfusion require a thoracoabdominal incision or a staged repair. The proximal anastomosis is ideally made to undissected normal aorta but infrequently the distal arch is involved, which requires alteration in surgical strategy.

As mentioned, we prefer the combination of partial left heart bypass and CSF drainage for spinal cord protection. Sites for cannulation are the left inferior pulmonary vein and the left femoral artery or descending thoracic aorta. Depending on location and extent of aneurysm, the distal arch is mobilized first. The area between the left common carotid and left subclavian artery is circumferentially dissected, and the left subclavian artery is independently controlled. Partial left heart bypass is then initiated. Ideally, clamps are placed between the left subclavian and left common carotid arteries and on the aorta distal to the involved segment. If the entire descending thoracic aorta is diseased, the clamp is placed on the mid-thoracic aorta to perform the proximal anastomosis first. The aorta is opened and small intercostal arteries are oversewn. The proximal anastomosis is made to normal aorta whenever possible with running 3-0 Prolene; 4-0 Prolene is used if the tissue is fragile. The clamp is moved distally onto the graft to inspect the proximal anastomosis and achieve hemostasis. Several centimeters of the dissection flap is then resected from the lumen of the distal aorta and the distal anastomosis created to the adventitia of the chronic dissection. In more extensive thoracoabdominal disease, the clamp is progressively moved distal as intercostal arteries below T7 to L2 and visceral vessels are reimplanted (Fig. 47-25). Bypass is terminated and the operation completed.

Full cardiopulmonary bypass with deep hypothermic circulatory arrest may be necessary in cases in which the proximal anastomosis cannot be safely or adequately performed with a clamp in the usual position.

RESULTS

The operative mortality for chronic type A dissections is between 4 and 17%.[90,91] The stroke rate after repair is 4%, with early neurologic complications occurring in 9%.[28] Regular follow-up of the aortic valve is necessary when the native valve is preserved at the initial operation. This is best performed using TTE on a yearly basis. Early reports indicated that nearly 20% of patients require reoperation secondary to progressive aortic regurgitation. The most recent data from David et al, however, reveal a 90 ± 4% 5-year freedom from severe or moderate aortic insufficiency in patients with aortic root aneurysm and 98 ± 2% in patients with ascending aortic aneurysm following valve-sparing operation.[84]

The perioperative mortality after surgical treatment of chronic type B dissections has been reported to be as low as 10% with a rate of permanent paraplegia of 9%.[28] Long-term survival for type A and B chronic dissections is similar with rates at 1, 5, 10, and 15 years after surgery of 78, 60, 45, and 27%, respectively.[92] Approximately one-third of deaths

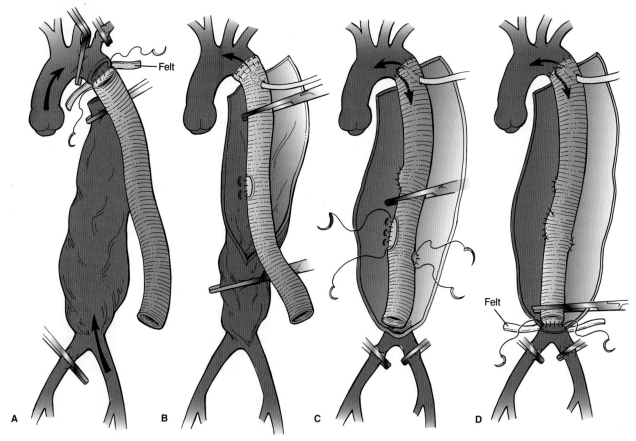

FIGURE 47-25 Replacement of the thoracoabdominal aorta. (A) A left femoral cannula perfuses the lower body and viscera while the heart continues to eject. The arch is transected near or at the left subclavian and any dissection involving the proximal cuff is repaired. (B) The clamp is moved down and a second arterial cannula is inserted into the proximal graft to perfuse the upper body and heart. The anterior wall of the dissection is incised longitudinally and bleeding intercostals of the upper six pairs are oversewn. A group of lower intercostal arteries above the celiac axis is sutured to the graft. (C) The clamp is moved down and the distal aortic clamp is moved to the left common iliac artery. A patch of aorta containing the celiac, superior mesenteric, and right renal artery is sewn into the graft. The left renal artery is sutured separately to the graft. (D) The proximal clamp is moved below the visceral anastomoses and the distal aortic anastomosis is made to the aortic bifurcation.

are cardiac-related, and at least 15% of deaths are related to complications or extension of the aortic dissection.

Recently, endovascular therapies have been used for management of chronic type B aortic dissections. The outcomes cited in Table 47-6 are similar to the outcomes after endovascular treatment of acute dissections. Although the results of these studies look promising, this topic needs to be studied further before recommendations or indications of endovascular repair in chronic type B dissections are elucidated.

CONCLUSION

Considerable improvement in the treatment of patients with acute and chronic aortic dissection has occurred over the last 50 years. The management of aortic dissections will continue to evolve as improved medical, endovascular, and surgical techniques are refined. At the present time, surgical therapy remains the standard of care for acute type A aortic dissections. Uncomplicated type B dissections should continue to be treated with optimal medical management and close surveillance until further studies define whether "prophylactic" endovascular repair will play a role in these patients. The treatment of acute complicated type B dissections has significantly evolved over the last few years, with endovascular therapies now providing an alternative to surgical therapy. The long-term outcomes of endovascular treatment are still unclear but appear to be promising. Patients undergoing operative intervention for aortic dissection will undoubtedly benefit from the novel basic and clinical research taking place in the areas of spinal cord and cerebral protection, strategies for cardiopulmonary bypass, improved vascular graft and endograft technology, and procedures for preservation of the aortic valve. Such progress may even permit advancement in our greatest remaining clinical challenge, those patients who are hemodynamically unstable following aortic dissection.

REFERENCES

1. Gurin D: Dissecting aneurysms of the aorta: diagnosis and operative relief of acute arterial obstruction due to this cause. *NY State J Med* 1935; 35:1.
2. Abbott OA: Clinical experiences with the application of polythene cellophane upon the aneurysms of the thoracic vessels. *J Thorac Surg* 1949; 18:435-461.
3. DeBakey ME, Cooley DA, Creech JO: Surgical considerations of dissecting aneurysm of the aorta. *Ann Surg* 1955; 14:24.
4. Wheat MW Jr, Palmer RF, Bartley TD, Seelman RC: Treatment of dissecting aneurysms of the aorta without surgery. *J Thorac Cardiovasc Surg* 1965; 50:364-373.
5. Beall AC Jr, Lewis JM, Weibel J, Crawford ES, DeBakey ME: Angiographic evaluation of the vascular surgery patient. *Surg Clin North Am* 1966; 46:843-862.
6. Daily PO, Trueblood HW, Stinson EB, et al: Management of acute aortic dissections. *Ann Thorac Surg* 1970; 10:237-247.
7. Coady MA, Rizzo JA, Goldstein LJ, Elefteriades JA: Natural history, pathogenesis, and etiology of thoracic aortic aneurysms and dissections. *Cardiol Clin* 1999; 17:615-635; vii.
8. Hagan PG, Nienaber CA, Isselbacher EM, et al: The International Registry of Acute Aortic Dissection (IRAD): new insights into an old disease. *JAMA* 2000; 283:897-903.
9. Erbel R, Alfonso F, Boileau C, et al: Diagnosis and management of aortic dissection. *Eur Heart J* 2001; 22:1642-1681.
10. Larson EW, Edwards WD: Risk factors for aortic dissection: a necropsy study of 161 cases. *Am J Cardiol* 1984; 53:849-855.
11. Coady MA, Rizzo JA, Elefteriades JA: Pathologic variants of thoracic aortic dissections. Penetrating atherosclerotic ulcers and intramural hematomas. *Cardiol Clin* 1999; 17:637-657.
12. Sundt TM: Intramural hematoma and penetrating atherosclerotic ulcer of the aorta. *Ann Thorac Surg* 2007; 83:S835-841; discussion S846-850.
13. Robinson PN, Booms P: The molecular pathogenesis of the Marfan syndrome. *Cell Mol Life Sci* 2001; 58:1698-1707.
14. Callewaert B, Malfait F, Loeys B, De Paepe A: Ehlers-Danlos syndromes and Marfan syndrome. *Best Pract Res Clin Rheumatol* 2008; 22:165-189.
15. Cambria RP, Brewster DC, Gertler J, et al: Vascular complications associated with spontaneous aortic dissection. *J Vasc Surg* 1988; 7:199-209.
16. Anagnostopoulos CE, Prabhakar MJ, Kittle CF: Aortic dissections and dissecting aneurysms. *Am J Cardiol* 1972; 30:263-273.
17. Scholl FG, Coady MA, Davies R, et al: Interval or permanent nonoperative management of acute type A aortic dissection. *Arch Surg* 1999; 134:402-405; discussion 405-406.
18. Kohl BA, McGarvey ML: Anesthesia and neurocerebral monitoring for aortic dissection. *Semin Thorac Cardiovasc Surg* 2005; 17:236-246.
19. Estrera AL, Garami Z, Miller CC 3rd, et al: Cerebral monitoring with transcranial Doppler ultrasonography improves neurologic outcome during repairs of acute type A aortic dissection. *J Thorac Cardiovasc Surg* 2005; 129:277-285.
20. Stecker MM, Cheung AT, Pochettino A, et al: Deep hypothermic circulatory arrest: II. Changes in electroencephalogram and evoked potentials during rewarming. *Ann Thorac Surg* 2001; 71:22-28.
21. Schepens M, Dossche K, Morshuis W, et al: Introduction of adjuncts and their influence on changing results in 402 consecutive thoracoabdominal aortic aneurysm repairs. *Eur J Cardiothorac Surg* 2004; 25:701-707.
22. Reece TB, Tribble CG, Smith RL, et al: Central cannulation is safe in acute aortic dissection repair. *J Thorac Cardiovasc Surg* 2007; 133:428-434.
23. Etz CD, Plestis KA, Kari FA, et al: Axillary cannulation significantly improves survival and neurologic outcome after atherosclerotic aneurysm repair of the aortic root and ascending aorta. *Ann Thorac Surg* 2008; 86:441-446; discussion 446-447.
24. Ergin MA, Griepp EB, Lansman SL, et al: Hypothermic circulatory arrest and other methods of cerebral protection during operations on the thoracic aorta. *J Card Surg* 1994; 9:525-537.
25. Gega A, Rizzo JA, Johnson MH, et al: Straight deep hypothermic arrest: experience in 394 patients supports its effectiveness as a sole means of brain preservation. *Ann Thorac Surg* 2007; 84:759-766; discussion 766-757.
26. Bavaria JE, Pochettino A, Brinster DR, et al: New paradigms and improved results for the surgical treatment of acute type A dissection. *Ann Surg* 2001; 234:336-342; discussion 342-333.
27. Comas GM, Leshnower BG, Halkos ME, et al: Acute type a dissection: impact of antegrade cerebral perfusion under moderate hypothermia. *Ann Thorac Surg* 2013; 96(6):2135-2141.
28. Safi HJ, Miller CC 3rd, Reardon MJ, et al: Operation for acute and chronic aortic dissection: recent outcome with regard to neurologic deficit and early death. *Ann Thorac Surg* 1998; 66:402-411.
29. Rylski B, Bavaria JE, Milewski RK, et al: Long-term results of neomedia sinus valsalva repair in 489 patients with type a aortic dissection. *Ann Thorac Surg* 2014; 98(2):582-588; discussion 588-589.
30. Roselli EE, Rafael A, Soltesz EG, Canale L, Lytle BW: Simplified frozen elephant trunk repair for acute debakey type I dissection. *J Thorac Cardiovasc Surg* 2013; 145(3 Suppl):S197-201.
31. Preventza O, Cervera R, Cooley DA, et al: Acute type I aortic dissection: traditional versus hybrid repair with antegrade stent delivery to the descending thoracic aorta. *J Thorac Cardiovasc Surg* 2014; 148(1):119-125.
32. DeBakey ME, McCollum CH, Crawford ES, et al: Dissection and dissecting aneurysms of the aorta: twenty-year follow-up of five hundred twenty-seven patients treated surgically. *Surgery* 1982; 92:1118-1134.
33. Trimarchi S, Nienaber CA, Rampoldi V, et al: Contemporary results of surgery in acute type A aortic dissection: The International Registry of Acute Aortic Dissection experience. *J Thorac Cardiovasc Surg* 2005; 129:112-122.
34. Piccardo A, Regesta T, Zannis K, et al: Outcomes after surgical treatment for type A acute aortic dissection in octogenarians: a multicenter study. *Ann Thorac Surg* 2009; 88:491-497.

35. Driever R, Botsios S, Schmitz E, et al: Long-term effectiveness of operative procedures for Stanford type a aortic dissections. *J Card Surg* 2004; 19:240-245.

36. Ehrlich MP, Ergin MA, McCullough JN, et al: Results of immediate surgical treatment of all acute type A dissections. *Circulation* 2000; 102:III248-III252.

37. Kallenbach K, Oelze T, Salcher R, et al: Evolving strategies for treatment of acute aortic dissection type A. *Circulation* 2004; 110:II243-249.

38. Tsai TT, Evangelista A, Nienaber CA, et al: Long-term survival in patients presenting with type A acute aortic dissection: insights from the International Registry of Acute Aortic Dissection (IRAD). *Circulation* 2006; 114:I350-I356.

39. Fattori R, Tsai TT, Myrmel T, et al: Complicated acute type B dissection: is surgery still the best option? A report from the International Registry of Acute Aortic Dissection. *JACC Cardiovasc Interv* 2008; 1:395-402.

40. Umana JP, Lai DT, Mitchell RS, et al: Is medical therapy still the optimal treatment strategy for patients with acute type B aortic dissections? *J Thorac Cardiovasc Surg* 2002; 124:896-910.

41. Dake MD, Kato N, Mitchell RS, et al: Endovascular stent-graft placement for the treatment of acute aortic dissection. *N Engl J Med* 1999; 340:1546-1552.

42. Nienaber CA, Fattori R, Lund G, et al: Nonsurgical reconstruction of thoracic aortic dissection by stent-graft placement. *N Engl J Med* 1999; 340:1539-1545.

43. Eggebrecht H, Nienaber CA, Neuhauser M, et al: Endovascular stent-graft placement in aortic dissection: a meta-analysis. *Eur Heart J* 2006; 27:489-498.

44. Kodama K, Nishigami K, Sakamoto T, et al: Tight heart rate control reduces secondary adverse events in patients with type B acute aortic dissection. *Circulation* 2008; 118:S167-170.

45. Tsai TT, Nienaber CA, Eagle KA: Acute aortic syndromes. *Circulation* 2005; 112:3802-3813.

46. Patel HJ, Williams DM, Meerkov M, et al: Long-term results of percutaneous management of malperfusion in acute type B aortic dissection: implications for thoracic aortic endovascular repair. *J Thorac Cardiovasc Surg* 2009; 138:300-308.

47. Rodriguez JA, Olsen DM, Lucas L, et al: Aortic remodeling after endografting of thoracoabdominal aortic dissection. *J Vasc Surg* 2008; 47:1188-1194.

48. Nienaber CA, Kische S, Zeller T, et al: Provisional extension to induce complete attachment after stent-graft placement in type B aortic dissection: the PETTICOAT concept. *J Endovasc Ther* 2006; 13:738-746.

49. Adams JD, Garcia LM, Kern JA: Endovascular repair of the thoracic aorta. *Surg Clin North Am* 2009; 89:895-912, ix.

50. Siefert SA, Ailawadi G, Thompson RB, et al: Is limited stent grafting a viable treatment option in type B aortic dissections? 55th Annual Meeting, Southern Thoracic Surgical Association. Austin, TX; 174.

51. Bockler D, Hyhlik-Durr A, Hakimi M, Weber TF, Geisbusch P: Type B aortic dissections: treating the many to benefit the few? *J Endovasc Ther* 2009; 16(Suppl 1):I80-90.

52. Coselli JS, LeMaire SA, de Figueiredo LP, Kirby RP: Paraplegia after thoracoabdominal aortic aneurysm repair: is dissection a risk factor? *Ann Thorac Surg* 1997; 63:28-35; discussion 35-26.

53. Cunningham JN Jr, Laschinger JC, Spencer FC: Monitoring of somatosensory evoked potentials during surgical procedures on the thoracoabdominal aorta. IV. Clinical observations and results. *J Thorac Cardiovasc Surg* 1987; 94:275-285.

54. Safi HJ, Hess KR, Randel M, et al: Cerebrospinal fluid drainage and distal aortic perfusion: reducing neurologic complications in repair of thoracoabdominal aortic aneurysm types I and II. *J Vasc Surg* 1996; 23:223-228; discussion 229.

55. Estrera AL, Miller CC, Goodrick J, et al: Update on outcomes of acute type B aortic dissection. *Ann Thorac Surg* 2007; 83:S842-845; discussion S846-850.

56. Schor JS, Yerlioglu ME, Galla JD, et al: Selective management of acute type B aortic dissection: long-term follow-up. *Ann Thorac Surg* 1996; 61:1339-1341.

57. Bernard Y, Zimmermann H, Chocron S, et al: False lumen patency as a predictor of late outcome in aortic dissection. *Am J Cardiol* 2001; 87:1378-1382.

58. Xu SD, Huang FJ, Yang JF, et al: Endovascular repair of acute type B aortic dissection: early and mid-term results. *J Vasc Surg* 2006; 43:1090-1095.

59. Nienaber CA, Rousseau H, Eggebrecht H, et al: Randomized comparison of strategies for type B aortic dissection: the INvestigation of STEnt Grafts in Aortic Dissection (INSTEAD) trial. *Circulation* 2009; 120:2519-2528.

60. Nienaber CA, Kische S, Rousseau H, et al: Endovascular repair of type b aortic dissection: long-term results of the randomized investigation of stent grafts in aortic dissection trial. *Circ Cardiovasc Interv* 2013; 6(4):407-416.

61. Tang DG, Dake MD: TEVAR for acute uncomplicated aortic dissection: immediate repair versus medical therapy. *Semin Vasc Surg* 2009; 22:145-151.

62. Brunkwall J, Kasprzak P, Verhoeven E, et al: Endovascular repair of acute uncomplicated aortic type B dissection promotes aortic remodelling: 1 year results of the adsorb trial. *Eur J Vasc Endovasc Surg* 2014; 48(3):285-291.

63. Miller DC, Mitchell RS, Oyer PE, et al: Independent determinants of operative mortality for patients with aortic dissections. *Circulation* 1984; 70:I153-I164.

64. Bozinovski J, Coselli JS: Outcomes and survival in surgical treatment of descending thoracic aorta with acute dissection. *Ann Thorac Surg* 2008; 85:965-970; discussion 970-961.

65. Trimarchi S, Nienaber CA, Rampoldi V, et al: Role and results of surgery in acute type B aortic dissection: insights from the International Registry of Acute Aortic Dissection (IRAD). *Circulation* 2006; 114:I357-I364.

66. Pitton MB, Herber S, Schmiedt W, et al: Long-term follow-up after endo-vascular treatment of acute aortic emergencies. *Cardiovasc Intervent Radiol* 2008; 31:23-35.

67. Palma JH, de Souza JA, Rodrigues Alves CM, et al: Self-expandable aortic stent-grafts for treatment of descending aortic dissections. *Ann Thorac Surg* 2002; 73:1138-1141; discussion 1141-1132.

68. Nienaber CA, Ince H, Petzsch M, et al: Endovascular treatment of thoracic aortic dissection and its variants. *Acta Chir Belg* 2002; 102:292-298.

69. Nathanson DR, Rodriguez-Lopez JA, Ramaiah VG, et al: Endoluminal stent-graft stabilization for thoracic aortic dissection. *J Endovasc Ther* 2005; 12:354-359.

70. Kische S, Ehrlich MP, Nienaber CA, et al: Endovascular treatment of acute and chronic aortic dissection: midterm results from the Talent Thoracic Retrospective Registry. *J Thorac Cardiovasc Surg* 2009; 138:115-124.

71. Khoynezhad A, Donayre CE, Omari BO, et al: Midterm results of endovascular treatment of complicated acute type B aortic dissection. *J Thorac Cardiovasc Surg* 2009; 138:625-631.

72. Hutschala D, Fleck T, Czerny M, et al: Endoluminal stent-graft placement in patients with acute aortic dissection type B. *Eur J Cardiothorac Surg* 2002; 21:964-969.

73. Duebener LF, Lorenzen P, Richardt G, et al: Emergency endovascular stent-grafting for life-threatening acute type B aortic dissections. *Ann Thorac Surg* 2004; 78:1261-1266; discussion 1266-1267.

74. Dialetto G, Covino FE, Scognamiglio G, et al: Treatment of type B aortic dissection: endoluminal repair or conventional medical therapy? *Eur J Cardiothorac Surg* 2005; 27:826-830.

75. Juvonen T, Ergin MA, Galla JD, et al: Risk factors for rupture of chronic type B dissections. *J Thorac Cardiovasc Surg* 1999; 117:776-786.

76. Sueyoshi E, Sakamoto I, Hayashi K, Yamaguchi T, Imada T: Growth rate of aortic diameter in patients with type B aortic dissection during the chronic phase. *Circulation* 2004; 110:II256-II261.

77. Hata M, Shiono M, Inoue T, et al: Optimal treatment of type B acute aortic dissection: long-term medical follow-up results. *Ann Thorac Surg* 2003; 75:1781-1784.

78. Genoni M, Paul M, Jenni R, et al: Chronic beta-blocker therapy improves outcome and reduces treatment costs in chronic type B aortic dissection. *Eur J Cardiothorac Surg* 2001; 19:606-610.

79. Marui A, Mochizuki T, Mitsui N, et al: Toward the best treatment for uncomplicated patients with type B acute aortic dissection: a consideration for sound surgical indication. *Circulation* 1999; 100:II275-II280.

80. Coady MA, Rizzo JA, Hammond GL, et al: What is the appropriate size criterion for resection of thoracic aortic aneurysms? *J Thorac Cardiovasc Surg* 1997; 113:476-491; discussion 489-491.

81. Kato M, Bai H, Sato K, et al: Determining surgical indications for acute type B dissection based on enlargement of aortic diameter during the chronic phase. *Circulation* 1995; 92:II107-II112.

82. David TE, Feindel CM: An aortic valve-sparing operation for patients with aortic incompetence and aneurysm of the ascending aorta. *J Thorac Cardiovasc Surg* 1992; 103:617-621; discussion 622.

83. Yacoub MH, Gehle P, Chandrasekaran V, et al: Late results of a valve-preserving operation in patients with aneurysms of the ascending aorta and root. *J Thorac Cardiovasc Surg* 1998; 115:1080-1090.

84. David TE, Armstrong S, Ivanov J, et al: Results of aortic valve-sparing operations. *J Thorac Cardiovasc Surg* 2001; 122:39-46.

85. Cochran RP, Kunzelman KS: Methods of pseudosinus creation in an aortic valve-sparing operation for aneurysmal disease. *J Card Surg* 2000; 15:428-433.

86. Borst HG, Walterbusch G, Schaps D: Extensive aortic replacement using "elephant trunk" prosthesis. *Thorac Cardiovasc Surg* 1983; 31:37-40.

87. Kouchoukos NT, Masetti P, Rokkas CK, Murphy SF, Blackstone EH: Safety and efficacy of hypothermic cardiopulmonary bypass and circulatory arrest for operations on the descending thoracic and thoracoabdominal aorta. *Ann Thorac Surg* 2001; 72:699-707; discussion 707-698.

88. Panneton JM, Hollier LH: Dissecting descending thoracic and thoracoabdominal aortic aneurysms: Part II. *Ann Vasc Surg* 1995; 9:596-605.

89. Coselli JS, LeMaire SA: Left heart bypass reduces paraplegia rates after thoracoabdominal aortic aneurysm repair. *Ann Thorac Surg* 1999; 67:1931-1934; discussion 1953-1958.

90. Safi HJ, Miller CC 3rd, Carr C, et al: Importance of intercostal artery reattachment during thoracoabdominal aortic aneurysm repair. *J Vasc Surg* 1998; 27:58-66; discussion 66-68.

91. Sabik JF, Lytle BW, Blackstone EH, et al: Long-term effectiveness of operations for ascending aortic dissections. *J Thorac Cardiovasc Surg* 2000; 119:946-962.

92. Fann JI, Smith JA, Miller DC, et al: Surgical management of aortic dissection during a 30-year period. *Circulation* 1995; 92:II113-II121.

Ascending and Arch Aortic Aneurysms

Chase R. Brown • *Joseph E. Bavaria* • *Nimesh D. Desai*

The Greek physician Galen first described superficial false aneurysms arising from venesection in the antecubital fossa and in gladiators injured during battle in the second century A.D.[1] Antyllos, during the same time period, distinguished between true and false aneurysms and attempted surgical treatment with proximal and distal ligation, opening of the aneurysmal sac, and removal of its contents.[2]

The French physician Jean Francois Fernel, in 1542, described aneurysms, "in the chest, or about the spleen and mesentery where a violent throbbing is frequently observable."[3] In 1543, Andeas Versalius described a thoracic aortic aneurysm. In the late 1500s, Ambroise Paré described a death by a ruptured thoracic aortic aneurysm and either Fernel or Paré proposed that syphilis played a causative role in some aortic aneurysms.[1] In 1760, Morgagni reported the first cases of aortic dissection and in 1773, Alexander Monro described three coats of the arterial wall, and the destruction of the wall in the formation of true and false aneurysms.[1]

Peripheral arterial ligation was developed in the 1800s by John Hunter, who demonstrated safe and reproducible means of ligating certain peripheral arteries.[4] Innovative measures used to cause thrombosis of aneurysms included the insertion of long segments of wire[5] with the application of an electric current,[6] and wrapping of aneurysms with cellophane or other irritating materials.[7,8]

In 1888, Rudolph Matas introduced obliterative endoaneurysmorrhaphy in which stitches placed from within the aneurysm sac obliterated the arterial openings.[9] This allowed closure of large aneurysms that would have been difficult to ligate externally. Recognizing the importance of maintaining arterial continuity for certain aneurysms, he subsequently devised techniques of restorative or reconstructive endoaneurysmorrhaphy, in which diseased segments of the aneurysm wall were resected and the remaining vessel wall was reconstructed to reestablish flow.[10] The number of aneurysms to which these techniques could be applied, however, was very limited. The broad application of surgical treatment for major arterial aneurysms would have to await the development of satisfactory conduits and the techniques to insert them.

The first report of a descending aortic repair was described by Cooley and DeBakey in 1952. The technique involved lateral resection and aortography performed on a saccular aneurysm without cardiopulmonary bypass (CPB).[11] In 1956, Cooley and DeBakey performed replacement of the ascending aorta with a segment of homograft with CPB.[12] Polyester cloth grafts were introduced by DeBakey, who discovered it in a Houston department store, and it soon became the artificial conduit of choice for aortic replacement.[13] Technical improvements in graft replacements included the impregnation of polyester grafts with albumin, collagen, or gelatin, which has greatly reduced the blood loss through the grafts.[14]

Wheat et al in 1964, resected the ascending aorta and entire aortic root except for the aortic tissue surrounding the coronary arteries.[15] They then performed a mechanical valve insertion and fashioned the proximal tube graft to accommodate the coronary arteries, which were left in situ. The first composite aortic root replacement was performed by Bentall and De Bono in 1963 to treat an ascending aortic aneurysm in a patient with Marfan syndrome (MFS) who had severe thinning of the aortic wall in the sinus segment.[16] The original technique involved hand sewing a Starr #13 mechanical prosthesis to a preclotted graft (Fig. 48-1). An inclusion-type technique with aortic wrap in which the coronary buttons were left in situ and anastomosed to holes made in the graft was performed. Due to concerns about coronary malposition, in 1981, Cabrol et al described the use of an 8 to 10 mm Dacron graft to attach to independently mobilized coronary artery buttons.[17] Techniques eventually evolved to the current method of individual coronary button reimplantation as described by Kouchoukos and Karp with end-to-end anastomoses as opposed to the inclusion technique which tended to be prone to pseudoaneurysm formation.[18]

SURGICAL ANATOMY

The aortic root is in extension of the left ventricular outflow tract and that provides the scaffolding for the elements of the

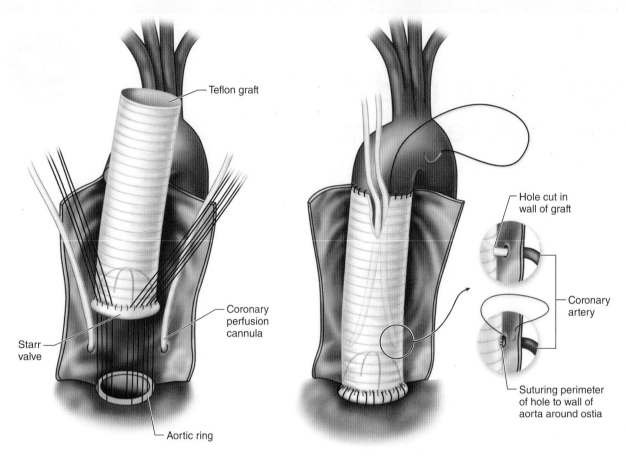

FIGURE 48-1 The original root replacement operation as described by Bentall and De Bono. (Reproduced with permission from Bentall H, De Bono A: A technique for complete replacement of the ascending aorta, Thorax 1968 Jul;23(4):338-339.)

aortic valve and connects to the descending aorta. Its components include the aortic valve cusps, the sinuses of Valsalva, the aortic annulus and subcommissural triangles, and the sinotubular junction (Fig. 48-2).[19] The aortic valve cusps attach to the aortic annulus at hinge point following a semilunar

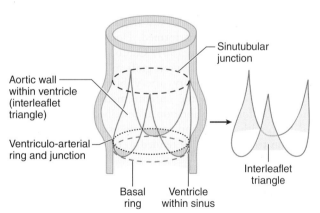

FIGURE 48-2 Aortic Root Geometry. (Reproduced with permission from Sutton JP 3rd, Ho SY, Anderson RH. The forgotten interleaflet triangles: a review of the surgical anatomy of the aortic valve, *Ann Thorac Surg* 1995 Feb;59(2):419-427.)

contour being a three-pointed crown type arrangement not a circular or oval ring. The annular tissue itself is typically 50 to 60% fibrous tissue along the hinge point between the aortic and mitral valves as well as the membranous portion of the septum, and the remainder is muscular. Small projections of collagen anchor the aortic root to the ventricular muscle.[20] The apices of the attachments of the cusps to the aortic annulus are known as commissures and the most superior aspect of the commissures interrelates with the sinotubular junction. The sinotubular junction is a ridge which marks the beginning of the ascending aorta. The sinotubular junction diameter is typically 15 to 20% smaller than annular diameter in younger patients.[21] With aging, the sinotubular junction diameter becomes larger. When the sinotubular junction is more than 10% larger than the annular diameter there is frequently resultant aortic insufficiency as the leaflets were no longer coapt due to displacement of the commissures.

Between the sinotubular junction and the aortic annulus are expanded segments of the aorta referred to as the sinuses of Valsalva. The sinuses form a cloverleaf rather than circular alignment when viewed in cross-section (Fig. 48-3).[22] Dilatation of the aortic sinuses and annulus is referred to as aortoannular ectasia. Each sinus is named for its corresponding coronary artery (right, left, and noncoronary).

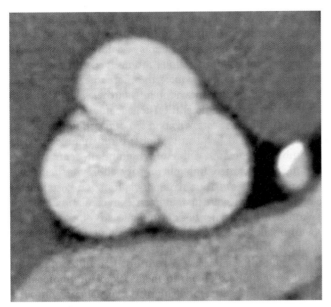

FIGURE 48-3 Anatomy of the aortic root from a Cardiac Gated CT Angiogram. Note the "cloverleaf" orientation of the sinuses.

The noncoronary sinus is anatomically related to the left and right atria as well as the transverse sinus. The left coronary sinus anatomically relates to the left atrium and the right coronary sinus is related to the right atrium and right ventricle. The subcommissural triangle between the right and noncoronary arteries is anatomically related to the conduction system within the membranous septum as well as the septal leaflet of the tricuspid valve. The left and noncoronary subcommissural triangles are related to the anterior leaflet of the mitral valve. The ascending aorta starts at the level of the sinotubular junction and ascends to the level of the takeoff of the innominate artery.

PATHOPHYSIOLOGY

The ascending aorta histologically contains a high proportion of compliant elastic tissue allowing it to serve as a reservoir and that stores kinetic energy from the systolic pulse wave as it expands and uses it to maintain flow during diastole via elastic recoil. The ascending aorta is a three layered structure composed of a smooth intimal layer composed of a single layer of endothelial cells adhered to a basal lamina; a medial layer composed of layers of elastin sheets, collagen, smooth muscle cells, and extracellular matrix; and an outer layer of adventitial tissue which includes the vasa vasorum and nerves.[23] The elastin content of the aorta decreases distally and in the abdominal aorta is less than half of that in the ascending aorta.[24] The principle biologic causes of aneurysm formation in the ascending aorta are related to degenerative processes in the elastic media, as compared to primarily atherosclerotic changes in the descending and abdominal aortas.[25]

Ascending aortic aneurysm formation is the result of several biologic and mechanical mechanisms. Disruption of the balance between homeostatic mechanisms within the aortic wall including elastic and collagen elements, proteoglycans, proteolytic enzymes and their inhibitors, and inflammatory mediators causes a spectrum of aortic pathology which manifests in the final pathway as aortic enlargement eventually leading to rupture or dissection. Fragmentation of the extracellular matrix of the aortic media occurs due to matrix-degrading enzymes such as matrix metalloproteinases and cathepsin groups.[26-30] Matrix metalloproteinases comprise a family of proteases that are capable of degrading virtually all components of the extracellular milieu and perform a variety of tasks necessary for normal homeostasis, including maintenance of the dynamic integrity of the extracellular structure within the arteries.[26-28] Aneurysms form as elastic layers fragment, smooth muscle cells become dysfunctional, and eventually elastic and smooth muscle components are replaced with a cystic appearing mucoid material (Fig. 48-4).[31] This process is referred to as cystic medial degeneration. The term cystic medial necrosis has also been applied to this condition but has been largely

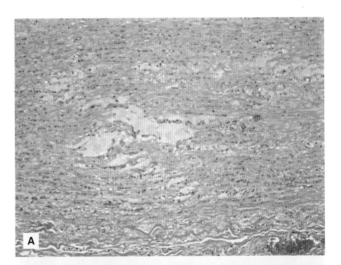

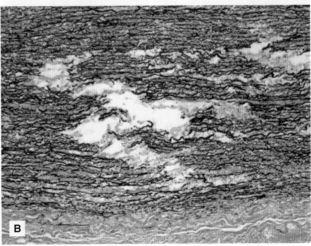

FIGURE 48-4 Cystic Medial Degeneration with (A) pools of glycosaminoglycans with 25% transmural extent and (B) associated loss of elastic fibers.

abandoned as there is no true necrotic process involved. To a lesser extent, mild degeneration of the aortic wall is common with advanced age and is responsible for the slow dilation of the ascending aorta with age. Smoking tends to exacerbate this degeneration.[32]

Mechanical changes to aortic wall characteristics such as alterations in cross-sectional symmetry, compliance, and stress-strain relationships likely predate dilatation. The Young-Laplace relationship describes the relationship between aortic diameter and wall tension where increases in aortic wall diameter lead to increases in wall stress at similar pressures (tension = pressure × radius). Changes in aortic wall compliance, broadly defined as the change in volume of the vessel with a change in pressure, lead to increased stress applied to the aortic wall during the systolic impulse and further exacerbate the biologic derangements leading to aneurysm formation.[33] The coupling between mechanical forces on the arterial wall and the biochemical changes leading to aneurysm formation (mechano-transduction) are not yet clearly elucidated.

Degenerative aortic aneurysms cause asymmetric enlargement of the ascending aorta as the segment of aorta along the inner curvature is adherent to the pulmonary artery.[34] Hence, there is significant rightward and anterior displacement of the aortic wall (Fig. 48-5). This causes a relative elongation of

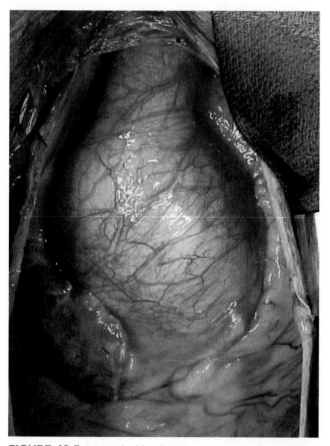

FIGURE 48-5 Massively dilated aortic root in a Marfan syndrome patient. Note the severe dilation of the aortic annulus and relative sparing of the proximal arch.

the ascending aorta in an asymmetric fashion which tends to push the heart into a horizontal arrangement. This also causes a significant change in the orientation of the aortic valve annulus to more oblique arrangement.[34] Aneurysmal widening will typically involve the aorta to the level of the sinotubular junction and frequently involves the noncoronary sinus to a lesser extent.[35] This widening at the level of the sinotubular junction is responsible for aortic insufficiency in these cases and frequently placement of tube graft to the sinotubular junction will resolve significant central aortic insufficiency. The left and noncoronary sinuses are fairly normal in these cases. The noncoronary aortic valve cusp may be elongated along its free margin in order to compensate for the asymmetric enlargement of the noncoronary sinus.

SPECIFIC ETIOLOGIES

Marfan Syndrome

MFS is an autosomal dominant syndrome with complete penetrance. Up to 25% of Marfan cases are from sporadic dictation in the overall incidence is one per 3000 to 10,000 live births.[36] Traditionally it is thought to have been caused by alterations in the gene (FBM1) coding the aortic wall protein fibrillin-1 leading to elastin derangement, medial degeneration, and aneurysm formation.[37,38] More recently, homology between fibrillin-1 molecules and latent transforming growth factor (TGF) beta binding proteins has led investigators to infer that altered sequestration of the latent form of TGF beta in the extracellular matrix may increase TGF beta activity which negatively impacts smooth muscle development and the extracellular matrix.[39] Approximately 80% of patients with MFS develop aortic root aneurysms and nearly half develop mitral regurgitation.[40] The clinical manifestations of MFS involve multiple organ systems as it is a systemic disease. Diagnosis has traditionally been made using the Ghent criteria, although it is now made definitively using genotyping.[41] Anatomically, MFS results in severe aortoannular ectasia and can have massively dilated sinuses and aortic annulus (Fig. 48-5).

More recently, reports have shown that the use of angiotensin-converting enzyme inhibitors can prolong the life expectancy of smooth muscle cells in the aortic tissue of Marfan patients via an angiotensin-2 type II receptor blockade mechanism which may antagonize TGF beta.[42] This has led to the clinical application of the angiotensin receptor blocker losartan as a prophylactic therapy to diminish aortic degeneration and aneurysm formation, which has been shown in animal models to be effective when given in the early stages of the disease.[43] A small clinical study of 18 pediatric patients also showed decreased aortic growth rate with treatment of losartan.[44]

Loeys-Deitz Syndrome

Loeys-Deitz syndrome (LDS) is a more recently described autosomal dominant syndrome.[45] Rather than a fibrillin-1 defect, however, there is a mutation in TGF beta receptors 1 and 2. Characteristics of LDS include cleft palate, bifid uvula, scoliosis, orbital hypertelorism, pectus deformities, developmental abnormalities, and congenital heart defects including persistent patent ductus arteriosus and atrial septal defects.[45] Patients may phenotypically have characteristics that overlapped between LDS and MFS.[46] Histologically, it is associated with increased medial collagen and a subtle but diffuse form of elastic fiber fragmentation and extracellular matrix deposition.[47] LDS has a more rapid clinical course than MFS and prophylactic aortic root replacement or reimplantation is often recommended at younger ages and with smaller aortic dimensions.

Ehlers-Danlos Syndrome

Ehlers-Danlos syndrome is caused by either sporadic mutation or inherited autosomal dominant trait resulting in a connective tissue disorder derived from defective type III collagen synthesis. The type IV variant of the Ehlers-Danlos syndrome is associated with spontaneous arterial rupture. Most commonly this occurs in the mesenteric or carotid arteries. However, spontaneous rupture of the descending aorta and aortic arch has been described.[48] The arterial wall of these patients is extremely thin and friable. Ascending aortic involvement may occur as a consequence of retrograde extension of a primary brachiocephalic branch pathology.

Familial Thoracic Aortic Aneurysms and Dissections

Approximately 20% of patients with thoracic aortic aneurysms have a first-degree relative with an aortic aneurysm.[49] These families often exhibit strong tendencies for thoracic aortic aneurysm formation without any clearly definable syndromic connective tissue disorder such as MFS or LDS. Grouped together as familial thoracic aortic aneurysms and dissections (FTAAD), mutations in ACTA2, SMAD3, TGFBR1, TGFBR2, TGFB2, and MYH11 have been identified to predispose patients to thoracic aortic aneurysms and dissections in an autosomal dominant manner. These mutations result in incomplete penetrance, variable expression, and variable age of aneurysm onset.[49-55] Genetic testing for patients and family members with multiple first- and second-degree relatives and suspected FTAAD is available. New evidence suggests that these patients are at increased risk for earlier rupture and dissection at diameters less than 5 cm, as seen in patients with LDS and MFS. Genetic testing has the opportunity to stratify these patients and identify those at greatest risk for rupture.

Infectious and Inflammatory Etiologies

Infections and systemic inflammatory disorders can occasionally cause damage to the wall of the ascending aorta leading to aneurysm formation. Frequently, despite high-quality preoperative imaging and even with intraoperative tissue pathology, it is not possible to distinguish definitively between the different possible etiologies.

Ascending aortic aneurysms caused by infection are extremely uncommon. Such mycotic ascending aortic aneurysms are frequently related to concomitant left-sided valvular endocarditis. Most common organisms include, in order of decreasing frequency, *Staphylococcus aureus*, *S. epidermidis*, Salmonella, and Streptococcus.[56] In cases of atherosclerotic aneurysm, if there is intraluminal clot in the ascending aorta, transient bacteremia may lead to infected clot leading to a mycotic aneurysm.[57]

Syphilis, caused by the spirochete *Treponema pallidum*, was the predominant cause of ascending aortic aneurysms in the pre-antibiotic era and accounted for 5 to 10% of all cardiovascular deaths.[58] Typically syphilitic aortitis involves the thoracic aorta with a particular predilection for the ascending aorta, likely due to its rich vascular and lymphatic supply. The pathologic process involves a multifocal lymphoplasmacytic infiltrate of the vasa vasorum leading to degeneration of the medial elastic fibers. The intima develops wrinkles, ridges, and plaques described as a "tree bark" appearance.[59] Inflammation around the coronary artery ostia may lead to high-grade proximal occlusions. The inflammatory process may be either patchy or diffusely involve a large section of aorta. Once established, treatment of syphilis with antibiotics does not reverse the vascular lesions.

Other systemic arteritis conditions may also produce ascending aortic aneurysms. Takayasu's arteritis, associated with inflammation of the vasa vasorum, medial necrosis and may also have intimal changes similar to syphilis. It is typically seen in females between 15 to 30 years of age and frequently involves occlusive lesions to major branch vessels of the arch.[60] While syphilis aortitis often leads to rapid aneurysmal degeneration, this is much less common in Takayasu's aortitis, occurring only in 15% of cases.[61] Giant cell arteritis is a systemic arteritis that occurs in elderly patients, most commonly affecting the temporal artery. It is also more common in females and is also associated with polymyalgia rheumatica. Giant cell arteritis is an inflammatory process with inflammatory infiltration with lymphocytes, plasma cells, and histiocytes. There is variable presence of giant cells.[62] Aortitis leading to aortic aneurysm may also be associated rarely with Behçet's disease, rheumatoid arthritis, sarcoidosis, ankylosing spondylitis, lupus erythematosus, and Wegener's granulomatosis.

Bicuspid Aortopathy

Bicuspid aortic valve is a complex familial syndrome with a male predominance of 3:1.[63] It is also associated with Turner syndrome. There is a 9% prevalence of bicuspid aortic valve disease in first-degree relatives of patients with bicuspid aortic valve disease.[64] More than half of the patients with aortic coarctation have an associated bicuspid aortic valve.[65] Several genetic defects have been implicated in the formation of bicuspid aortic valve disease however no single genetic etiology has been derived. Aortic dilatation is frequently associated with bicuspid aortic valve disease; however, the mechanism for this occurring is not well delineated. Originally thought to be a sequela of post-stenotic dilatation, aortic aneurysm formation in patients with bicuspid aortic valve may occur without any significant aortic stenosis although there is clearly flow perturbation in the proximal sinuses of Valsalva and descending aorta in patients with bicuspid aortic valve.[66] Recent investigation has shown that embryologically, the aortic valve and ascending aorta arise from the neural crest cells implicating a potential common mechanism for the development of a bicuspid aortic valve and subsequent aneurysm formation.[67] The aortic wall in the patients with bicuspid aortic valve disease shows increased elastic fragmentation, fibrillin-1 deficiency, matrix disruption, increased levels of matrix metallic proteinases, and smooth muscle cell apoptosis.[67-72]

Fazel and colleagues using a cluster-type analysis identified four distinct patterns of aortic dilatation including aortic root alone (13%), ascending aorta alone (10%), ascending aorta and proximal transverse arch (28%), and aortic root, ascending aorta, and proximal transverse arch (45%) (Fig. 48-6).[73] This study suggests that for younger patients, definitive treatment of bicuspid aortic valve disease with aortic dilatation requires strategies that address the aortic root, ascending aorta, and proximal transverse hemi-arch. It is advisable to perform an aggressive hemi-arch resecting all aortic tissue along the lesser curve to the level of the subclavian artery take-off in younger bicuspid aortic valve patients to eliminate as much of the diseased aorta as possible. However, total arch replacement with brachiocephalic branch reimplantation is rarely necessary as the aneurysmal component rarely involves the distal aspect of the transverse arch.

Isolated Sinus of Valsalva Aneurysm

Aneurysms of the sinuses of Valsalva (SVA) that occur as isolated lesions are rare abnormalities caused by either a congenital defect in the continuity between the medial layer of the affected sinus and the aortic valve annulus or, less commonly, acquired causes such as endocarditis, syphilis, tuberculosis, focal dissection, iatrogenic causes.[74] They are more common in males and may be associated with subaortic stenosis, ventricular septal defects, and aortic insufficiency. In over 90% of cases, they involve the right coronary sinus (Fig. 48-7).[75,76] The noncoronary sinus of the second most common location and these aneurysms are extremely uncommon in a left coronary sinus. They are generally asymptomatic until they rupture when they usually cause intracardiac shunts. Right sinus of Valsalva aneurysms typically rupture into the right ventricle, effectively causing a hemodynamic defect similar to a ventricular septal defect. Aneurysms of the noncoronary sinus typically rupture into the right atrium and the left coronary sinus rupture into the pulmonary artery or left ventricle. Occasionally an unruptured left

coronary sinus of Valsalva aneurysm may compress the left main coronary artery.[76]

CLINICAL PRESENTATION

Symptoms

Most ascending aortic aneurysms are asymptomatic when diagnosed, being incidentally noted on chest x-ray or echocardiogram. Anterior chest pain is the most frequent symptom. The pain may be acute in onset signifying impending rupture or a chronic gnawing pain from compression of the overlying sternum. Occasionally signs of superior vena cava (SVC) or airway compression are present. Hoarseness resulting from stretch injury of the left recurrent laryngeal nerve suggests involvement of the distal aortic arch or proximal descending thoracic aorta. Less commonly, aneurysms of the ascending aorta or aortic root can rupture into the right atrium or the SVC, presenting with high-output cardiac failure or bleed into the lungs with ensuing hemoptysis. Acute dissection of the ascending aorta presents with severe tearing pain in over 75% of patients.[77]

Physical Examination

Physical examination is often unremarkable. If there is related aortic insufficiency, a widened pulse pressure or diastolic murmur may be present. If dilation is isolated to the ascending aorta, however, the aneurysm can reach large dimensions without producing physical findings. A thorough vascular examination should be carried out to look for any concomitant peripheral vascular disease, carotid disease, or abdominal aortic aneurysm. Abdominal aortic aneurysms may be present in 10 to 20% of patients with atherosclerotic involvement of an ascending aortic aneurysm.[78]

DIAGNOSTIC STUDIES

Electrocardiogram

With significant aortic insufficiency, left ventricular hypertrophy or strain is evident. Patients with generalized atherosclerosis may show evidence of concomitant coronary artery disease or previous myocardial injury.

Chest Radiography

Many asymptomatic ascending aortic aneurysms are first detected on chest x-ray. The enlarged ascending aorta produces a convex contour of the right superior mediastinum (Fig. 48-8A). In the lateral view, there is loss of the retrosternal air space (Fig. 48-8B). Aneurysms confined to the aortic root can be obscured by the cardiac silhouette and may not be evident on chest radiograph.[79]

Echocardiography

Transesophageal echocardiography (TEE) is a portable diagnostic tool that accurately detects and differentiates between

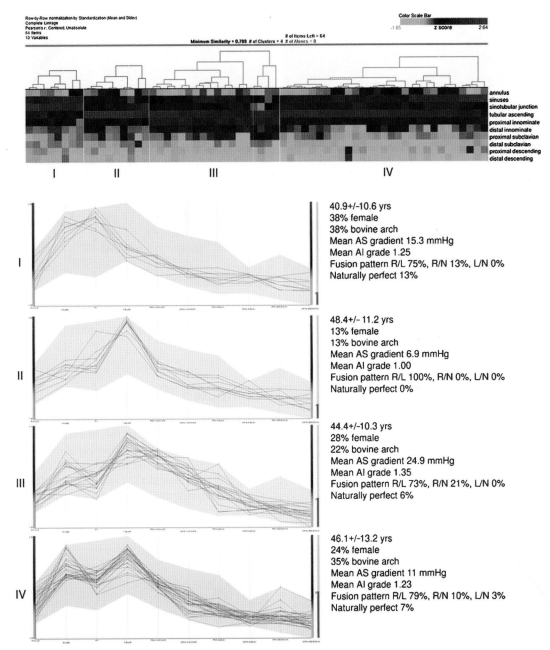

FIGURE 48-6 Patterns of aortic pathology in bicuspid aortopathy patients using hierarchal clustering methodology. The top panel shows a "heat map" in which each column represents a patient and each row represents aortic diameters that have been color coded according to the calculated within-patient z scores on a continuous scale shown on the top right corner of the panel. Cluster I patients had predominant involvement of the aortic root (n = 8). Cluster II patients had predominant involvement of the tubular portion of the ascending aorta (n = 9). Cluster III patients had involvement of the tubular portion of the ascending aorta and the transverse arch (n = 18). Cluster IV patients had diffuse involvement of the thoracic aorta with dilation extending from the aortic root to the midtransverse arch (n = 29). The 4 clusters are shown again in the bottom 4 panels, which depict the metric aortic diameters across the thoracic aorta for each individual patient. The clinical data for each cluster are summarized to the right of each cluster panel. AS, Aortic stenosis; AI, aortic insufficiency. (Reproduced with permission from Fazel SS, Mallidi HR, Lee RS, et al: The aortopathy of bicuspid aortic valve disease has distinctive patterns and usually involves the transverse aortic arch, *J Thorac Cardiovasc Surg.* 2008 Apr;135(4):901-907.)

ascending aortic aneurysms, dissections, and intramural hematoma (Fig. 48-9).[80-82] TEE is an invasive imaging modality and carries a small risk of esophageal perforation, respiratory compromise, and hemodynamic instability. Imaging of the distal ascending aorta is obscured on TEE by air in the tracheobronchial tree, with up to 40% of its distal extent not well visualized, although this is somewhat mitigated with the use of modern multiplanar probes.[83] Although somewhat

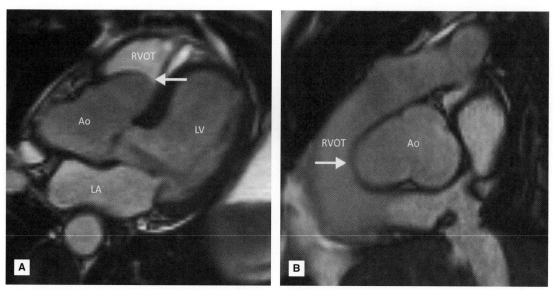

FIGURE 48-7 Contrast MR showing three-chamber view (A) and the aortic valve plane (B) demonstrate a right SVA protruding into the right ventricular outflow tract (arrows). There is an associated turbulent jet of aortic regurgitation. LA, left atrium; LV, left ventricle; Ao, aorta; RVOT, right ventricular outflow tract. (Reproduced with permission from Brandt J, Jögi P, Lührs C. Sinus of Valsalva aneurysm obstructing coronary arterial flow: case report and collective review of the literature. *Eur Heart J*. 1985 Dec;6(12):1069-73.)

operator dependent, TEE provides a reliable technique to measure the annular, sinus, sinotubular junction, and ascending dimensions. It is uniquely well suited to examine the most proximal aspects of the aortic root, which are often blurred by motion artifact on computed tomography (CT) scans. Transthoracic echocardiography is far less reliable but may be useful for assessing the severity of aortic regurgitation.

Computed Tomography

Contrast-enhanced CT is the most widely used noninvasive technique for imaging the thoracic aorta. CT scanning provides rapid and precise evaluation of the ascending aorta in regards to size, extent, and location of the disease process (Fig. 48-10). CT scanning detects areas of calcification, and modern scanner accurately identifies dissections and mural thrombus.[81]

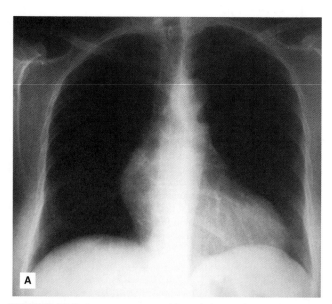
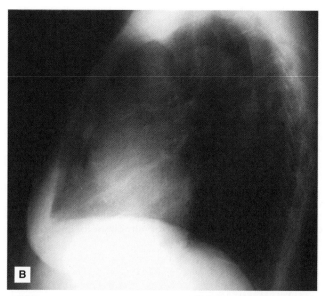

FIGURE 48-8 Posteroanterior and lateral chest radiograph of a patient with an ascending aortic aneurysm. The posteroanterior view (A) shows convexity of the right mediastinum, and the lateral view (B) shows loss of the normal retrosternal air space. (Reproduced with permission from Downing SW, Kouchokos NT: Ascending aortic aneurysm, in Edmunds LH Jr (ed): *Cardiac Surgery in the Adult*. New York, McGraw-Hill, 1997; p 1163.)

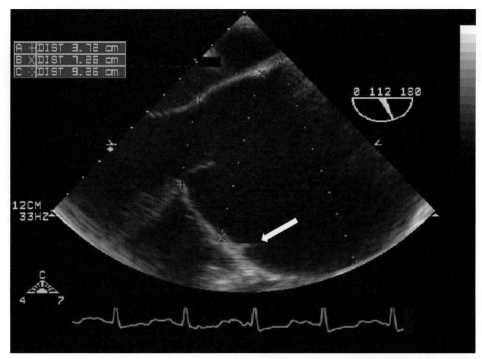

FIGURE 48-9 Transesophageal echocardiogram of a massive aortic root aneurysm with dissection (arrow).

CT scan technology has evolved with multidetector scanners such that the entire thoracic aorta can be evaluated on one breath-hold and the distance between axial slices can be as small as 0.5 mm. Three-dimensional volume rendering is a highly useful tool for determining true in-plane aortic diameters and the proximal and distal extent of aortic disease relative to the arch vessels, which can aid the surgeon in operative planning

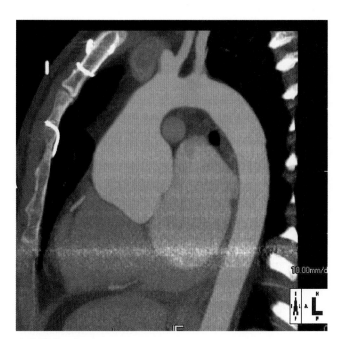

FIGURE 48-10 CT angiogram of an enlarged aortic root in a Marfan patient.

(Fig. 48-11). Ideally, the entire thoracic and abdominal aorta should be examined for evidence of concomitant aneurysm disease in the arterial tree. Gating to the electrocardiogram during image acquisition eliminates the motion artifact that may be seen in the most proximal aspects of the aortic root and can also allow for assessment of the coronary arteries.[85] The main disadvantage of CT scans is the need for contrast solution for optimal resolution, which may be contraindicated in those patients with renal insufficiency or a history of a dye allergy. Noncontrast CT scans allow for assessment of aortic diameters but cannot identify dissection flaps or other acute pathologies.

Magnetic Resonance Imaging

Magnetic resonance imaging (MRI) can provide axial and three-dimensional reconstruction of the ascending aorta with the avoidance of iodinated contrast agents and radiation exposure. Contrast-enhanced MR angiography with gadolinium allows more precise measurements of the aorta and its major branches with images comparable to conventional angiography (Fig. 48-12).[86] MRI scanners are relatively unsuitable for those patients connected to mechanical ventilators or hemodynamic monitoring equipment. MRI is more expensive, less readily available, and requires significantly more acquisition time than CT scanning and is used less frequently.

NATURAL HISTORY

Elective aortic replacement is used as a means to prophylactically prevent aortic catastrophe such as dissection and rupture which carry high mortality. Recent data from the International

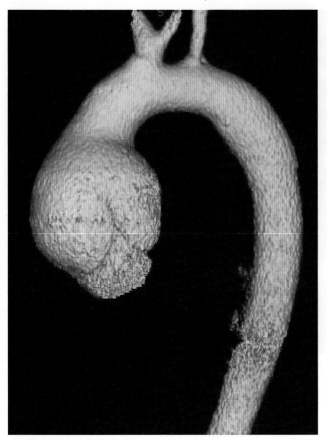

FIGURE 48-11 3D reconstruction of an aortic root aneurysm in a Marfan patient.

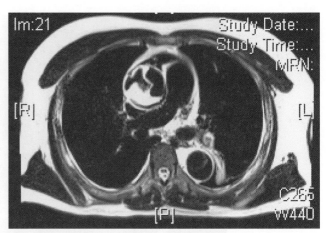

FIGURE 48-12 MR angiogram (without contrast) depicting an acute type A dissection. The partially thrombosed false lumen is denoted by the arrow.

Registry of Acute Aortic Dissections (IRAD) show an operative mortality for emergent type A aortic dissection repair of 26%, although this is generally lower in more experienced centers.[87] Bickerstaff et al examined the natural history of 72 patients that were diagnosed with aortic aneurysms and

did not undergo surgery.[88] Over a 5-year follow-up period, 74% of patients experienced aortic rupture or dissection (Fig. 48-13). Of these 94% died. The overall 5-year survival was only 13% in untreated aneurysm patients compared with 75% in control patients without aortic aneurysms.

Traditionally, the most important criterion for ascending aortic replacement on an elective basis is maximal aortic diameter. In natural history studies by Coady et al, patients with 3.5 to 3.9 cm aortic aneurysms were very unlikely to rupture within 3 to 4 years, and each incremental 1 cm increase from this point increased rupture risk (Fig. 48-14).[89] Patients with aneurysms greater than 5 cm showed substantially higher dissection and rupture risk within the first year. Using a logistic regression model, they found that the aneurysm with maximal diameter of 6.0 to 6.9 cm had a 4.3 times greater increased risk of rupture or dissection then an aneurysm that is 4.0 to 4.9 cm in diameter. Growth rates for aortic aneurysms less than 4 cm are about 0.1 cm per year and this increases gradually as aortic

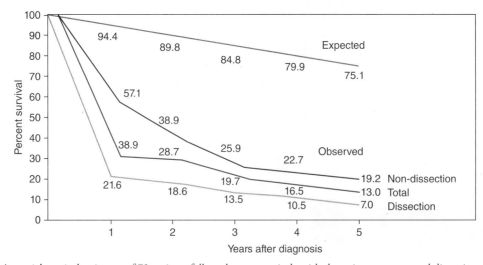

FIGURE 48-13 Actuarial survival estimates of 72 patients followed nonoperatively with thoracic aneurysms and dissections.

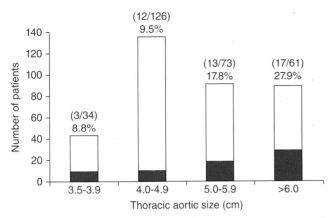

FIGURE 48-14 The incidence of acute dissection or rupture of thoracic aneurysms according to size. The height of the column corresponds to the total number of patients and the blue area to the proportion of patients who suffered complications of dissection or rupture. (Reproduced with permission from Coady MA, Rizzo JA, Hammond GL, et al: What is the appropriate size criterion for resection of thoracic aortic aneurysms? *J Thorac Cardiovasc Surg* 1997; 113:476.)

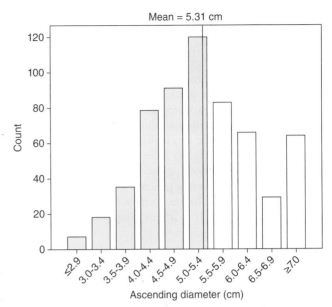

FIGURE 48-16 Distribution of aortic size at time of presentation with acute type A aortic dissection (cm). (Reproduced with permission from Pape LA, Tsai TT, Isselbacher EM, et al: Aortic diameter >or = 5.5 cm is not a good predictor of type A aortic dissection: observations from the International Registry of Acute Aortic Dissection (IRAD), *Circulation*. 2007 Sep 4;116(10):1120-1127.)

size increases up to 0.4 cm per year.[90,91] Uncontrolled hypertension, smoking, and presence of connective tissue disorders are associated with more rapid aortic growth.[90] Patients with MFS are at particularly high risk for rupture or dissection of smaller sizes and dissection is frequently seen with a maximal ascending aortic dimension of less than 5 to 6 cm (Fig. 48-15).[92] Strikingly the average age of death for untreated patients with MFS is 32 years, with complications of the aortic root being responsible for 60 to 80% of these deaths.[93] Marfan's patients with a family history of early dissection or rupture are at the highest risk for aortic catastrophe occurring at smaller dimensions.[94]

Although size clearly correlates with rupture risk, it is important to note that many aortic dissections occur in ascending aortas that are less than 5.5 cm in diameter. In the IRAD registry, over 59% of 591 enrolled patients with acute type A aortic dissections had maximum aortic dimensions less than 5.5 cm and 40% were less than 5.0 cm (Fig. 48-16).[95]

As the understanding of the biologic mechanisms behind aortic aneurysm formation improves, in the future, serum biologic markers and sensitive imaging techniques that can detect subtle changes in aortic strain characteristics or compliance may provide more accurate identification of the high-risk aorta.

MEDICAL TREATMENT OF PROXIMAL AORTIC ANEURYSMS

Therapies designed to limit the growth of aortic aneurysms are targeted at mechanisms either to diminish stress on the aortic wall or to prevent deleterious degenerative biochemical changes. In general, patients with aortic aneurysms should avoid high intensity isometric exercise such as weight lifting as aortic pressures may increase rapidly and exert significant stress on the aortic wall. Weight lifting restriction should be less than 1/3 to 1/2 of the patient's body weight. Additionally exercises with rapid bursts of acceleration and deceleration such as basketball may place excess of stress of aortic wall.

Anti-impulse therapies are the mainstay treatment for thoracic aortic aneurysms. Due to their negative chronotropic and inotropic effects, beta blockers are typically used as a first line treatment.[96] The primary goals of beta blocker therapy are to decrease the overall blood pressure and to decrease the change in aortic pressure over time (dP/dT) to diminish the stress applied to the aorta in systole thereby limiting damage to the media layer. The rationale for using beta blockers was initially established with an ex vivo plastic model of

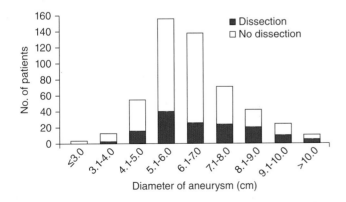

FIGURE 48-15 Diameter of the aneurysm in 524 adult patients with Marfan Syndrome, according to the Presence of Aortic Dissection.

aortic dissection by Wheat et al in which a tear created in an artificial intimal layer of rubber cement in the plastic tubing propagated less when the pulse pressure was artificially flattened, while variation of mean blood pressure and flow rates had no effect.[97] Studies performed on turkeys, which are uniquely prone to aortic dissection, showed that the combination of sodium nitroprusside and propanolol were effective at preventing rupture, while lowering blood pressure with nitroprusside alone was ineffective and may have actually increased dP/dT due to reflex sympathetic stimulation causing increased chronotropy and inotropy.[98] In a landmark study by Shores et al, young patients with MFS randomized to a regimen of beta blocker therapy had significantly less aortic dilatation over a 10-year follow-up period (Fig. 48-17)

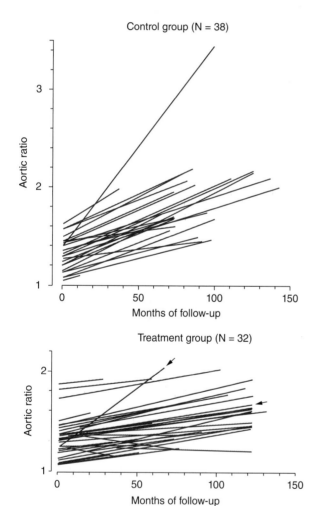

FIGURE 48-17 Changes in the Aortic ratio in the propranolol-treated group and untreated controls. Aortic ratio is ratio of the diameter of the aorta measured in a patient to the diameter expected in a subject with the same body-surface area and age. ine indicates the length of follow-up. One patient in the control group had an exceptional aortic ratio (>3.4) at 100 months. Two patients in the treatment group (arrows) did not comply with propranolol therapy. (Reproduced with permission from Palmer RF and Wheat MW Jr: Treatment of dissecting aneurysms of the aorta, *Ann Thorac Surg* 1967 Jul;4(1):38-52.)

and also had a lower incidence of a composite end point of death, congestive heart failure, aortic dissection, severe regurgitation, or aortic root surgery versus controls.[99] These results have been extrapolated to a wider variety of patients with ascending aortic aneurysms in whom beta blockade is used extensively.

INDICATIONS FOR SURGERY

Non-Elective Indications

Any new onset of acute dissection, rupture, or intramural hematoma generally warrants immediate surgery. The presence of symptoms of chest pain in patients with ascending aortic aneurysms greater than 4.5 to 5 cm is a sign of impending rupture and should also be managed operatively with expediency. Acute severe congestive heart failure secondary to root dilatation and loss of sinotubular junction either from rapid aneurysm expansion or from chronic dissection also warrants early operative management, although aggressive diuresis and cardiac optimization for 1 to 2 days prior to surgery are frequently helpful.

Elective Indications

Despite the limitations of size criteria, decisions to intervene are still largely decided based on maximal aortic diameter and growth rate. For degenerative aneurysms in the absence of connective tissue disorders or other cardiac pathology, elective repair is reasonable at an absolute maximal diameter of 5.5 cm.[100] Growth rate of greater than 1 cm per year is generally accepted as a strong indication to proceed with surgery for degenerative aneurysms regardless of diameter.[101] Some groups have also advocated the use of normalized aortic dimensions to body size to provide a more accurate reflection of the aneurysm dimension for an individual patient.[102]

The aortic ratio is calculated as measured diameter divided by predicted diameter for a given age and body surface area. Using this method, elective replacement is warranted at an aortic ratio of 1.5 in an asymptomatic patient without a connective tissue disorder or other complicating factors.[103] This leads to intervention at a size of only 4.8 to 5.0 cm in an adult less than 40 years of age with a body surface area of 2 m².[104] Because the ascending aorta normally increases in size with age, the diameter for intervention would be higher in a patient more than 40 years old.

Special Considerations

Patients with MFS are at higher risk for rupture and the ascending aorta should be replaced prophylactically at a diameter of 4.5 cm or an aortic ratio of 1.3 to 1.4.[103,104] Patients with Loeys-Dietz rupture at a smaller dilation than in MFS and should be electively repaired at 4.2 cm.[105] Among patients with bicuspid aortic valves, there remains ongoing debate. The 2013 Society of Thoracic Surgeons Clinical Practice guidelines suggest 5.0 cm (4.5 cm if there is a family history of aortic dissection) whereas the ACC/AHA Valve guidelines recommend 5.5 cm (5.0 cm for a family history of aortic dissection or rapid aortic growth greater than 5 mm/year).[106,107] In the setting of connective tissue disorders, bicuspid aortic valve or chronic dissection, a growth rate of greater than 0.5 cm per year should warrant repair. A chronically dissected aorta, which the external aortic wall is supported only by the residual outer third of the medial and advential layers, should be replaced when aortic diameters reach 4.5 cm or a ratio of 1.3 to 1.4 due to the intrinsic weakness of the aortic wall.[103,108] Pseudoaneurysms, which are frequently from previous aortic suture lines, should be repaired upon diagnosis due to high rupture risk related to their extremely thin walls.

In younger patients, where aortic root reimplantation is preferred to avoid life-long anticoagulation, earlier repair may prevent the development of aortic valve cusp pathology and improve the chances of successful repair. Among patients undergoing aortic valve replacement who have ascending aortic aneurysms, Prenger et al reported a 27% incidence of aortic dissection if the aorta was greater than 5 cm versus 0.6% incidence if aortic size was normal.[109] In general, in the setting of other cardiac surgery, ascending aortas with a maximal dimension of 5.0 cm or a ratio of 1.5 should be replaced.[103,109]

PREOPERATIVE PREPARATION

Nearly one-third of patients undergoing surgery for thoracic aortic disease have chronic obstructive pulmonary disease.[110] Patients with suspect pulmonary function should have spirometry and room air arterial blood gases. Smoking cessation, antibiotic treatment of chronic bronchitis, and chest physiotherapy may prove beneficial in elective situations. Normal renal function should be ensured with the appropriate blood work, and abnormal results should prompt further investigation. Because unaddressed severe carotid disease is a risk factor for stroke during ascending aortic operations, patients over the age of 65 should have duplex imaging of their carotids.[111] Younger patients with peripheral vascular disease, extensive coronary artery disease, carotid bruits, or history suspicious for cerebral ischemia should be investigated as well. CT or MRI of the thoracic and abdominal aorta is usually indicated. Coronary angiography should be performed in all patients to evaluate for significant coronary atherosclerosis and lesions with greater than 50 to 60% stenosis should be bypassed. Coronary angiography also helps define the coronary anatomy to identify anomalous or intramural coronary arteries which may complicate root replacement.[112]

OPERATIVE MANAGEMENT
Monitoring and Anesthesia

All procedures are performed using central venous access and a pulmonary artery catheter. Location of arterial line for blood pressure monitoring should be discussed with the anesthesia team preoperatively although generally right radial is preferred. Nasopharyngeal and bladder temperature monitors are used. Bilateral near infrared spectroscopy (NIRS) is employed to provide real-time estimation of cerebral saturation though out the bypass run.[113] Precipitous drops in cerebral saturations are managed with increasing perfusion pressure and hematocrit to the cerebral circulation. In circulatory arrest cases, EEG monitoring is also employed to ensure EEG silence during interruption of cerebral circulation.

TEE plays a critical role in diagnosis, particularly of degree of aortic insufficiency and sinus segment and sinotubular junction anatomy that is not well assessed by CT angiography. It is also critical for hemodynamic management separating from CPB.

Anesthesia management includes fentanyl 25 to 50 μg/kg, midazolam 0.1 to 0.2 mg/kg, isoflurane 0.5 to 1.5%, pancuronium 0.1 to 0.2 mg/kg, and end-tidal concentration in CO_2. Aminocaproic acid is dosed initially as an intravenous bolus of 5 g, followed by a maintenance intravenous infusion of 1 g/h and stopped within 2 hours of patient admission to the intensive care unit. Pharmacologic adjuncts in circulatory arrest cases include 1 g of methylprednisolone, 1 g of magnesium sulfate, 2.5 mg/kg of lidocaine, and 12.5 g of mannitol.[114]

Myocardial Protection

Typically, 1 L of cold blood hyperkalemic cardioplegia (4°C) is given antegrade into the aortic root. A left ventricular vent is employed to prevent distension. In cases of severe aortic insufficiency, the aorta is opened and the coronary ostia are cannulated directly with handheld cannula. A temperature probe is placed through the anterior myocardium into the septum and a myocardial temperature of 6 to 8°C is achieved. Retrograde cardioplegia is administered at least every 20 minutes and continuously when possible. It is important to give cardioplegia immediately prior to commencing circulatory arrest and at its conclusion.

Circulation Management

Cannulation strategies vary significantly with individual pathology and the modern cardiovascular surgeon must be proficient in several different techniques. With experience, ascending aortas as large as 7 cm may be directly cannulated. This can be done with the traditional stab-technique or using a Seldinger technique over a wire in thin-walled aortas. In aneurysms which terminate prior to the innominate artery, the transverse arch is easily directly cannulated. In cases where antegrade cerebral perfusion is required, either the ascending aorta may be cannulated directly if using selective direct perfusion cannulas or the right axillary artery may be employed. Right axillary artery cannulation, which has grown in popularity in recent years, should be performed through an 8 or 10 mm Dacron graft anastomosed end-to side to the axillary artery as there is risk of dissection from direct cannulation of this friable artery. In some instances, femoral artery cannulation can be employed, but should be avoided in patients with atheroma in the thoracic aorta by CT scan or TEE. A standard two-stage venous cannula is used unless performing concomitant mitral or tricuspid surgery.

DEEP HYPOTHERMIC CIRCULATORY ARREST AND CEREBRAL PROTECTION

The use of deep hypothermic circulatory arrest (DHCA) was first described in conjunction with cardiac operations in the 1960s.[115] In the 1970s, there was renewed interest in DHCA after its successful use during repair of complex congenital defects.[116] Later, Greipp and Stinson reported the first case series using DHCA during arch aneurysm repairs and supported its efficacy in cerebral protection.[117] As interest in DHCA continued to grow; investigators, using dog models, illustrated how profound cerebral hypothermia dramatically decreased cerebral metabolism.[118-120] As knowledge of DHCA physiology increased, it promoted the development of new techniques such as antegrade and retrograde cerebral perfusion (RCP) and allowed for more complex aortic aneurysm repairs.

There are two basic mechanisms that lead to ischemic cerebral injury during repair of proximal aortic aneurysms. While the stroke is one of the most common postoperative complications of aortic aneurysm repairs, its risk is not associated with duration of DHCA.[121] Rather, stroke risk is associated with plaque, clot, and the artheromatous burden in the aortic arch and brachiocephalic vessels.[122,123] The second type of brain injury is temporary neurological dysfunction (TND) and is characterized by confusion, agitation, obtundation, and even transient parkinsonism. Studies suggest that TND results from inadequate cerebral protection during DHCA. In 200 adults who underwent DHCA, 19% of patients had clinical symptoms of TND, which correlated significantly with age and the duration of DHCA (33 min in patients without TND and 47 min in those with TND).[122] Furthermore, in patients with advanced age, DHCA duration longer than 25 minutes was an independent risk factor for long-term neurocognitive impairment, specifically for worse performance on fine motor and memory testing.[124] It is posited that due to its high metabolic demand, the hippocampus is acutely sensitive to hypoperfusion, which may be the reason for memory impairment and cognitive dysfunction after DHCA.[125] Nonetheless, while TND does occur in some patients, clinical studies in adults after DHCA have demonstrated that a safe period of arrest is about 30 minutes at 15°C and 40 minutes at 10°C, after which cerebral anoxia occurs.[126]

Cooling and Rewarming During Deep Hypothermic Circulatory Arrest

Data from Cheung et al have shown that only 60% of subjects undergoing DHCA achieve EEG silence at a core temperature of 18°C or a cooling time of 30 minutes.[127] In cases where EEG monitoring is not available, a safer technique is to cool for a minimum of 50 minutes, at which point 100%

of patients will have EEG silence.[128] Cooling is performed maintaining less than a 2 to 3°C gradient between arterial inflow temperature and venous return temperature to ensure even cooling. Nasopharyngeal temperature and bladder temperature which correlate with intracranial temperature and core body temperature, respectively, are also monitored during cooling to guide initiation of arrest.

During rewarming, the bladder, nasopharyngeal, and the systemic perfusion temperatures are monitored. The perfusion is kept at a gradient of not more than 10°C above the nasopharyngeal temperature. This ensures that oxygen demand will not exceed oxygen supply during the interval of cerebral vasoconstriction after DHCA.[129-131] Avoiding high perfusate temperatures is important and should not exceed 37°C. The bladder temperature which is raised from 32 to 34°C represents the core body temperature and will lag considerably behind the nasopharyngeal temperature. Monitoring bladder temperature helps to ensure uniform rewarming and minimize rebound hypothermia after CPB.

Cerebral Protection Techniques: Historical Perspective

In the 1980s, mounting evidence suggested that DHCA alone was neither efficacious nor safe for the long durations of cross-clamp time and arrest required for repairing extensive, complex proximal aortic aneurysms. This necessitated the need to develop novel techniques. While first reported in 1957 by Debakey during his early aortic arch aneurysm repairs, selective antegrade cerebral perfusion (ACP) was used. The setup involved multiple pumps and bilateral cannulation of the subclavian and carotid arteries. However, this ACP technique had difficulty in uniformly perfusing separate vascular beds simultaneously,[65] and resulted in high mortality rates and was quickly abandoned. It was later recognized that using ACP in combination with DHCA improved outcomes compared to DHCA alone.[132,133] In 1986, Kazui et al described his first approach with selective ACP.[134] His results from 1990 to 1999 showed that 220 patients underwent total arch replacement with ACP and DHCA with 12.7% in-hospital mortality and 3.3% permanent stroke rate, a significant improvement from only DHCA alone. Later in 2003, Di Eusanio demonstrated efficacy with ACP and DHCA in further reducing both risk of stroke and TND. In a multicenter trial, 580 patients underwent partial and total aortic arch replacement, the risk of permanent stroke and TND was 3.8 and 5.6%, respectively, with an overall mortality of 8.7%.[135] These results were only possible because of the introduction and refinement of the antegrade and retrograde cerebral protection techniques.

Antegrade Cerebral Perfusion Techniques

Used routinely by many centers, antegrade cerebral perfusion is primarily beneficial over RCP in situations where the expected circulatory arrest time is greater than 35 to 45 minutes.

Common strategies include direct cannulation of the cerebral vessels with balloon-tip catheters as described by Kazui or by right axillary cannulation.[136] When performing direct arch vessel cannulation it is advisable to use balloon tip catheters which have individual pressure-monitoring lines so the true perfusion pressures can be monitored to avoid cerebral hypertension. Right radial artery monitoring may also be helpful. Perfusion is typically performed at 10 cc/kg/min and mean pressures are maintained at 40 to 70 mm Hg. Perfusate temperature should approximate the core temperature. Optimal protection is gained by direct perfusion of all three arch branches, not just the left common carotid and innominate arteries.

Axillary cannulation is performed via cut down to the right axillary artery with a 8 to 10 mm Dacron graft sewn on in an end-side fashion (Fig. 48-18A,B). The graft is ligated

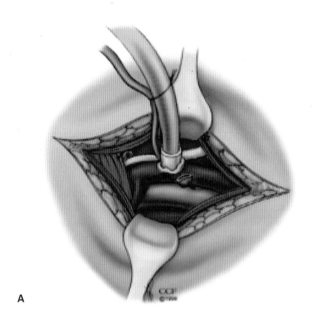

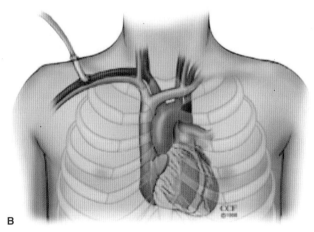

FIGURE 48-18 (A) Direct cannulation of axillary artery with right-angle arterial cannula (note division of crossing vein). (B) Cannulation of axillary artery with a side graft. A straight arterial cannula is inserted into graft. (Reprinted with permission, Cleveland Clinic Center for Medical Art & Photography ©2016. All rights reserved.)

at the end of the procedure. Given the fragility of the axillary artery, few surgeons cannulate it directly. As with direct cerebral vessel perfusion, perfusion pressure is maintained at 10 cc/kg/min and mean pressures are 40 to 70 mm Hg. The innominate artery is either snared or clamped at its origin. While antegrade cerebral perfusion via this method is rapid and effective, it only provides unilateral perfusion and contralateral ischemia may still occur. To maintain adequate cerebral perfusion pressure and eliminate the effect of arterial-arterial collaterals stealing flow, ideally the left common carotid and subclavian artery origins are controlled as well with additional selective cerebral catheters.[137]

Retrograde Cerebral Perfusion Techniques

RCP is an alternate technique that provides retrograde perfusion to the brain via the venous circulation. While the nutritive flow of RCP is questionable, it provides cooling and excellent de-airing of the cerebral circulation. For RCP, a 24 Fr wire reinforced cannula is placed cephalad to the azygous vein in the SVC and secured with a caval tape. RCP with oxygenated blood is adjusted to maintain a right internal jugular venous pressure of 25 mm Hg, a flow rate of 200 to 300 cc/min, with the patient in an approximately 10-degree Trendelenberg position.[127] Minimal exsanguination into the pump is performed upon cessation of bypass to facilitate later deairing. RCP may be initiated via a Y-connection to the arterial line or from the cardioplegia system through a high pressure stopcock that can connect to the Y-connection between the SVC and right atrial cannulas. RCP may be interrupted for variable periods of time during deep hypothermia as required by various surgical maneuvers. The temperature of the retrograde perfusate is maintained at 12 to 18°C. After completion of aortic arch anastomoses, air is removed from the aorta and graft by allowing it to fill by RCP. After arch deairing, a cross-clamp is placed across the ascending aortic graft, and standard CPB with antegrade cerebral perfusion, that is, antegrade graft perfusion, is reinstituted for the final repair and rewarming. Our practice is to always reestablish antegrade flow via direct cannulation of the ascending graft using either a prefabricated 8 or 10 mm sidearm or by placing a purse-string suture in the graft and directly cannulating it.

An Algorithmic Approach to Decision-Making for Proximal Aortic Aneurysms

Choice of procedure when managing ascending or arch aortic aneurysms is predicated on a detailed understanding of individual patient anatomy and pathophysiology. The potential operative decisions include whether to replace the aortic valve, aortic sinuses, ascending aorta, or aortic arch. Any combination of these procedures is theoretically possible. A systematic approach to evaluate the aorta and aortic root begins with determining if there is a suspicion for connective tissue disorder. Patients with MFS, Ehlers-Danlos syndrome, LDS, bicuspid valve-related aortopathy, or strong family history of aortic dissection or rupture should generally be treated more aggressively by replacing the sinus segment, ascending aorta, and proximal arch as late reintervention is more likely in this group.[138] Proximal reconstruction in these patients may be accomplished by either root replacement or a valve-sparing root reimplantation procedure.[139]

The next step is to determine the pathology of the aortic valve. Moderate or worse aortic stenosis with or without insufficiency generally requires replacement while the management of pure aortic insufficiency is more complex. Aortic insufficiency caused solely by dilatation of the sinotubular junction, typically from an atherosclerotic aneurysm in an elderly patient, may be full addressed with tube graft replacement of the ascending aorta alone with anastomosis to the sinotubular junction (Fig. 48-19). Care must be taken in this instance to appropriately size the graft to within 10% of the annular dimension to allow full coaptation of the aortic valve leaflets.[140] The sinus segment must also be closely interrogated. If it is particularly thin or aneurysmal this should be replaced. Normal dimensions of the sinus of Valsalva are typically 30 to 32 mm when the aortic annulus measures 23 to 24 mm and the sinotubular junction measures 24 to 25 mm.[141] If there are aneurysmal sinuses and annular dilatation, that is, aortoannular ectasia, but the leaflets appear fairly normal, then a valve-sparing aortic valve reimplantation is often feasible (Fig. 48-20). Technical details of this procedure are discussed in a previous chapter. If the annulus

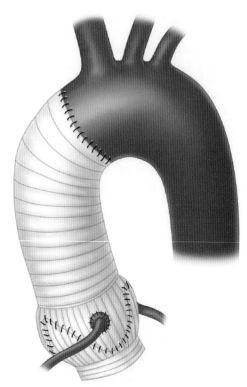

FIGURE 48-20 Valve-sparing aortic root reimplantation using a Dacron graft with a premade Sinus of Valsalva segment.

or sinusus are dilated and the leaflets are abnormal and not repairable, root replacement is performed. Prosthesis options include prefashioned composite mechanical root prostheses, sewing a stented tissue valve to a conduit, or using a porcine bioroot. Prosthesis selection is based on several competing factors including the elevated hazard for structural deterioration of biologic prostheses in younger patients, anticoagulant-related complications with mechanical prostheses, complexity and difficulty of performing future redo root replacements for bioprosthetic failure, and the growing trend toward the avoidance of warfarin in younger patients. The innovation of transcatheter valves, which have the potential to extend the life of a biologic root prosthesis without repeat sternotomy, has generated interest in using these prostheses in younger patients.[142] Pulmonary autografts may also be used as root replacements, but their practicality in aneurysm patients is somewhat limited as degenerative aneurysms tend to occur in older patients who would not benefit from the durability of the pulmonary autograft. Younger aneurysm patients, who could potentially benefit, frequently have bicuspid pathology or connective tissue disorders that may lead to early valve failure. Bicuspid patients have been shown to have significant histologic arterial wall derangements including the cystic medial necrosis, elastic fragmentation, and changes in the smooth muscle cell orientation in the autograft root.[143]

In patients where there is an isolated dilatation of the noncoronary sinus in degenerative aneurysms with preserved sinus dimensions in the coronary sinuses, the noncoronary

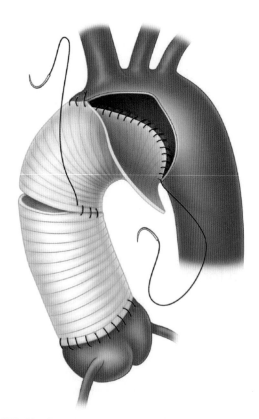

FIGURE 48-19 Replacement of the ascending aorta and transverse arch with an aggressive hemiarch anastomosis.

sinus may be individually excised and a "tongue" of the ascending aortic graft is used to reconstruct this sinus with the rest of the graft anastomosed above the native annulus, that is, a Yacoub-type remodeling procedure isolated to the noncoronary sinus.[144] Such a procedure carries the risk of late dilatation or suture-line disruption as the remaining aortic tissue is often thin and weak. It is also possible to perform an isolated noncoronary sinus reimplantation as described by David and Feindel.[145] Unless operative risk is prohibitive, it is preferential to perform a full root replacement or reimplantation in such patients rather than treat only one sinus.

In cases where the aortic valve needs to be replaced due to leaflet pathology, the sinus segment is not aneurysmal and there is an ascending aneurysm, a modified Wheat procedure with replacement of the aortic valve and placement of a tube graft to the sinotubular junction is used (Fig. 48-21).[15] This approach is especially useful in elderly patients who have mild-to-moderate sinus segment dilatation but a root replacement carries significant extra perioperative risk and the likelihood of future proximal reoperation is negligible.

Distal repair may be done as either a total arch, hemiarch, open distal, or clamped distal anastomosis. Aneurysmal extension into the proximal aortic arch is a common variant and is well treated with an aggressive hemi-arch. Resection of the ascending aorta to the innominate artery on the greater curve and to the level of the subclavian take-off on the lesser curve provides excellent protection from future aneurysmal

degeneration of the arch (Fig. 48-21). While clamped techniques for the distal anastomosis are suitable for isolated root pathologies such as complex endocarditis repair, in aneurysm cases it is preferable to excise the cross-clamped portion of aorta and perform an open distal anastomosis.

Total arch replacement with or without elephant trunk (ET) extension is typically reserved for patients with full arch aneurysms extending into the descending thoracic aorta or mega-aorta syndrome. The key decision point when determining the aggressiveness of the arch operation is to determine whether the open proximal operation will completely treat the pathology or if further intervention of the distal arch/descending aorta is required. If open intervention of the distal aorta is anticipated, creation of an ET anastomosis will prevent the need for circulatory arrest in the second stage. If thoracic endovascular aortic repair (TEVAR) is anticipated, creation of a 3 to 4 cm Dacron landing zone for TEVAR placement by forward mobilization of the cerebral vessels is a simpler approach than ET and avoids the difficulty of cannulating the free-floating ET for TEVAR. These approaches as well as debranching and hybrid approaches are described later in this chapter.

ASCENDING AORTIC REPLACEMENT: SPECIFIC OPERATIVE TECHNIQUES

After the aortic cross-clamp is applied and cardioplegic arrest is achieved as described above, the ascending aorta is transected about 1 cm below the clamp and resected to the level of the sinotubular junction. The aorta is carefully freed from the pulmonary artery using low-energy electrocautery. Using a metric sizer, the diameter of the sinotubular junction that provides adequate leaflet coaptation is determined and this should be within 10% of the annular diameter. The aortic valve is inspected to ensure that it is trileaflet and free from significant calcification or leaflet pathology. If the aortic valve is to be replaced, this is performed at this point using standard techniques. An appropriate size graft is then anastomosed to the sinotubular junction using a running 4-0 polypropylene. The external aspect may be reinforced with Teflon felt if the aorta appears especially thin and a root replacement is not feasible. In cases of acute dissection individual pledgeted sutures are placed at upper aspects of the commissures to resuspend the aortic valve and Teflon felt is placed inside between the dissected layers to form a robust neomedia that can hold sutures.

Composite Root Replacement

Aortic root replacement involves excision of the entire ascending aorta to the native valve annulus with mobilization of coronary buttons and placement of a composite valve and polyester graft conduit into the annulus. After cross-clamping and administration of cardioplegia, the ascending aorta is resected to the level of the sinotubular junction. The sinuses are mobilized off of the pulmonary arteries and

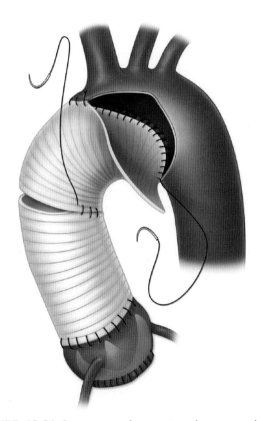

FIGURE 48-21 Separate ascending aortic replacement and aortic valve replacement with retention of the native sinus segment.

right ventricle and the coronary buttons are mobilized as described below. Unless a root reimplantation procedure is being performed, excessive proximal mobilization of the root is unnecessary.

The aortic valve leaflets are excised. The annular dimension is sized and an appropriately sized prosthesis is selected. Mechanical composite prostheses come prefabricated with either a polyester straight tube graft or artificial neo-sinuses created by changing the orientation of the polyester in the sinus segment. If a tissue valve is desired, a polyester graft that is either straight or has neo-sinuses is anastomosed with a running 3-0 or 4-0 polypropylene suture to an appropriately sized stented tissue valve. If using a Dacron graft with neo-sinuses, this should be sewn 3 to 4 mm below the start of the neo-sinus segment. The valve sutures must pass through both the valve sewing ring and the Dacron graft to ensure hemostasis.

The composite prosthesis may be placed with either pledgeted everting (ie, "intraannular") mattress sutures with pledgets on the outside of the annulus or in a "supra-annular" configuration with pledgets on the ventricular side of the annulus. Typically, the everting technique is used as it is hemostatic and strong. Implanting the root with pledgets on the ventricular side requires less mobilization of the sinuses which may be advantageous in certain situations and may allow for a slightly larger prosthesis. When implanting a mechanical prosthesis, the everting technique is preferred as it is less prone to pannus formation which may interfere with valve function. Care must be taken with either technique to not shorten the mitral valve anterior leaflet with excessively large bites with the annular sutures along the left and noncoronary sinuses. Polyester, braided 2-0 sutures with a larger needle than used for aortic valve replacement are employed.

Once the valve-conduit is tied down, the coronary buttons are anastomosed using 5-0 prolene sutures as described below (Fig. 48-22). Pressurization of the new root by inserting a catheter into the proximal graft, running cardioplegia, and clamping the graft distally after de-airing the neoroot allows assessment of all suture lines.

Implantation of stentless bioroots, homograft roots, pulmonary autografts, and valve-sparing procedures is discussed in previous chapters.

Management of Coronary Arteries

Mobilization of the coronary artery buttons in root operations remains the most technically demanding and least forgiving aspect of root operations. The left main button is mobilized after the aorta has been fully dissected from the pulmonary artery. It is frequently useful to work from the inside of the aorta outward, gently scoring the dissection plane with low intensity electrocautery. Generally, 1 to 2 cm of freedom of motion in all directions is required for adequate mobilization. Care must be taken mobilizing the right coronary artery to ensure the right ventricle is not inadvertently entered. Application of retrograde and direct

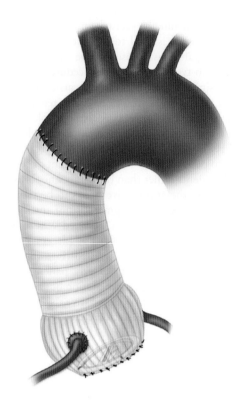

FIGURE 48-22 Composite root replacement with a mechanical prosthesis.

antegrade cardioplegia into the coronaries after mobilization will identify any small branch disruptions or major injuries while they are still repairable.

When anastomosing the left coronary button to the aortic graft, if a graft with premade sinuses of Valsalva is used, the button is typically sewn at or below the level of the equator of the sinus segment. The right coronary, which is more likely to kink as the right ventricle pushes it cephalad once the heart fills, is sewn at or above the level of the equator. When using a straight graft, some surgeons will determine the final position of the right coronary button after completing the graft-to-graft anastomosis, filling the heart, and briefly removing the cross-clamp. When separating from bypass, if there are new gross wall motion abnormalities, coronary artery injury or kinking should be immediately suspected. Our preference in these situations is to immediately bypass the affected territory rather than attempt to salvage a friable coronary button. For a right-sided problem, a bypass graft to the right coronary artery will typically resolve the problem expediently.

In complex endocarditis, dissection, severe calcification, or reoperative cases, coronary artery buttons may be too damaged or immobile to directly attach to the graft. In such situations, a Cabrol-type coronary anastomosis, where the coronary ostia are anastomosed to an 8 to 10 mm Dacron grafts in a "moustache" configuration may be employed (Fig. 48-23). Alternatively, segments of reversed saphenous vein can be used as interposition grafts. Typically these grafts are 3 to 5 cm in length, are anastomosed fairly high on the

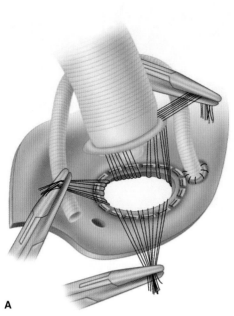

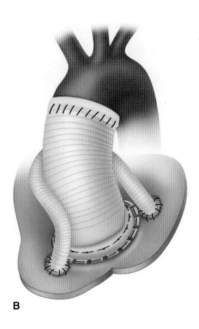

FIGURE 48-23 Classic Cabrol technique for coronary reimplantation. (A) An 8- to 10-mm Dacron tube graft is anastomosed end-to-end to the aortic tissue surrounding the left and right coronary ostia. (B) An opening is made in the mid-portion of the coronary graft and in an appropriate position in the aortic graft and an anastomosis is formed. The modified Cabrol technique involves the formation of individual coronary buttons allowing the small-caliber Dacron graft to be sewn to the full thickness of the aortic tissue surrounding the coronary ostia. (Reproduced with permission from Edmunds LH: *Cardiac Surgery in the Adult*. New York: McGraw-Hill; 1997.)

aortic graft, and follow a gentle s-shaped curve to prevent kinking. In cases of right coronary button problems, proximal ligation and bypass to the main right coronary artery is another alternative.

Distal Anastomosis

Distal reconstruction is performed as a clamped or open anastomosis. In aneurysm cases, open distal techniques which eliminate all diseased aorta and the weakened cross-clamp site are routinely employed. Circulatory arrest techniques as previously described are employed. Distal anastomoses are performed with a beveled polyester graft using a running 4-0 polypropylene suture. The distal anastomosis is performed as an "on-lay" type anastomosis with the graft invaginated into the distal aorta. This pushes the graft material into the native aorta when the aorta is pressurized and prevents leaks. In cases of extremely friable aorta, Teflon felt placed along the outer aspect may also be beneficial but does not substitute for a proper "on-lay" technique.

ENDOVASCULAR APPROACHES FOR THE ASCENDING AORTA

Advances in the design of highly flexible and low profile thoracic aortic stent grafts have generated an interest in using these devices for the ascending aorta in patients who are otherwise not reasonable risk surgical candidates. Key design requirements for ascending aortic stent grafts include a high

degree of flexibility and conformability, short graft lengths, no exposed bare metal, and long delivery systems as most TEVAR delivery systems will not reach the proximal ascending aorta from the femoral artery. Alternative approaches for access sites for the stent graft include axillary artery, carotid artery, and perhaps most promising, transapical. Graft lengths are more critical in the ascending aorta than in the thoracic aorta as the distance between sinotubular junction and/or coronary ostia and the take-off of the innominate artery is typically shorter than 10 cm, and is therefore shorter than most thoracic devices. The antegrade transapical technique may also offer potential advantage by limiting the distance between the sheath and the device thereby minimizing potential for device migration during deployment, as is seen in transapical deployment of transcatheter aortic valves. Stent graft placement has been described to treat focal ascending aneurysms in nonoperative candidates (Fig. 48-24).[146,147]

AORTIC ARCH REPLACEMENT: SPECIFIC OPERATIVE TECHNIQUES

There has been a diversity of surgical approaches across institutions on how best to repair aortic arch aneurysms. Originally reported in 1960s, the first arch aneurysm repair was completed by using an "island technique" and anastomosing the supra-aortic vessels to the aortic graft. It was not until the twenty-first century that novel approaches were developed that limited cerebral ischemia and the duration of CPB

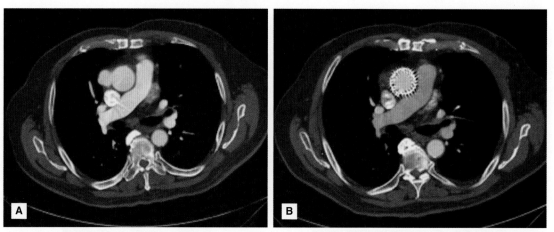

FIGURE 48-24 Placement of a covered stent graft in the ascending aorta to treat a pseudoaneurysm after previous cardiac surgery. Preoperative CT angiogram (A) demonstrates a saccular pseudoaneurysm in the ascending aorta after previous coronary artery bypass graft. Postoperative CT angiogram (B) demonstrates exclusion of pseudoaneurysm with no evidence of endoleak. (Reproduced with permission from Szeto WY, Moser WG, Desai ND, et al: Transapical deployment of endovascular thoracic aortic stent graft for an ascending aortic pseudoaneurysm, *Ann Thorac Surg* 2010; 89(2):616-618.)

time. In 2000, Kazui et al developed an integrated branched arch graft that contained three fixed limbs for anastomosing the great vessels and a side arterial cannulation limb for CPB.[134] In 2002, Speilvogel et al described the technique of debranching the great vessels from the arch and anastomosing them to a trifurcated graft that could then be sewed to the main aortic graft.[148] These techniques improved patient outcomes by decreasing the duration of DHCA, improving cerebral protection, and excluding the diseased aorta from the anastomosis, as was necessary with the island technique. More recently, with the advancements in endovascular device technology, hybrid approaches are available that combine debranching procedures and stent grafts in a single-staged repair. These hybrid approaches have even further reduced CPB and DHCA time.

OPEN TECHNIQUES

Branched Arch Grafts (Kazui Technique)

The branched aortic arch graft is prefabricated graft with 3 branches for the great vessels and an additional side branch for systemic perfusion.[134] This technique (Fig. 48-25A-H) begins with systemic cooling and initiation of DHCA. The aortic arch is opened and the brachiocephalic vessels are transected distal to their origins and selective ACP catheters are inserted into the innominate and left common carotid arteries, while the left subclavian artery is clamped (Fig. 48-25B). Then the distal anastomosis of the graft is first performed on the descending aorta (Fig. 48-25C). After this is completed, antegrade systemic circulation is started from the side branch of the graft (Fig. 48-25D). Next, the left subclavian artery is reimplanted to the graft and perfused (Fig. 48-25E). The proximal anastomosis is then finished (Fig. 48-25F), and attention is turned toward the anastomosis of the left carotid and left innominate arteries to the branched graft (Fig. 48-25G,H).

The aorta is de-aired, cross-clamp is released, and the side branch for CPB is ligated.

Since clot and atheroma in the aorta develop more often at the origin of the brachiocephalic vessels, manipulation of these arteries increases the risk of stroke after aortic arch repair. One benefit of this technique is that brachiocephalic vessels are transected distal to their origins before the resection of the aortic arch, preventing embolization and decreasing stroke risk. Depending on the extent of aneurysmal disease, this operation can be completed in one or two stages. For concomitant descending thoracic aneurysmal disease, an ET graft can be completed during the arch replacement as an easy setup for the second stage, which could include an endovascular option or smaller left thoracotomy approach. However, one limitation of this technique is that the cerebral branches of the graft are short and fixed to the graft. This decreases options to tailor the graft based on the patient's exact anatomy.

Debranching Graft Techniques

Several types of debranching grafts are available on the market to repair aortic arch aneurysms. One of the first grafts used was a double-Y or trifurcated graft that could be anastomosed to the main aortic body graft during the operation (Fig. 48-26). However, other grafts currently available have the branched limbs pre-anastomosed to the aortic graft. While stylistically different, the generalized debranching concepts presented are similar.

In the debranching approach, the aorta is cross-clamped proximal to the innominate artery and CPB is initiated via the axillary artery. While the patient is being cooled to core hypothermia, the proximal aorta is opened and a multibranched limb graft or tube graft is anastomosed to the sinotubular junction. If aortic valve and/or root pathology is present, surgical repair can be completed while the patient is cooled.

Once hypothermia is reached, ACP is initiated via axillary artery cannulation. Attention is then turned toward the distal aortic arch and the main body of the graft is anastomosed to healthy, nonaneurysmal aorta. At this point, the distal clamp is removed and CPB is reinitiated either down the side limb of the graft or via direct cannulation of the aortic body graft. ACP is continued via axillary cannulation and selective perfusion catheters may be used for bilateral ACP until the left subclavian, left carotid, and innominate arteries are each anastomosed to the three graft limbs, respectively. After debranching is completed, the proximal aortic reconstruction is de-aired and the patient is decannulated from CPB.

In case of a laterally displaced left subclavian artery from the aortic aneurysm, a left subclavian to carotid artery (LSCA) bypass can be completed 2 to 4 days before the debranching procedure. After a LSCA bypass, the debranching procedure only needs to be executed for the innominate artery and left carotid artery (Fig. 48-27).

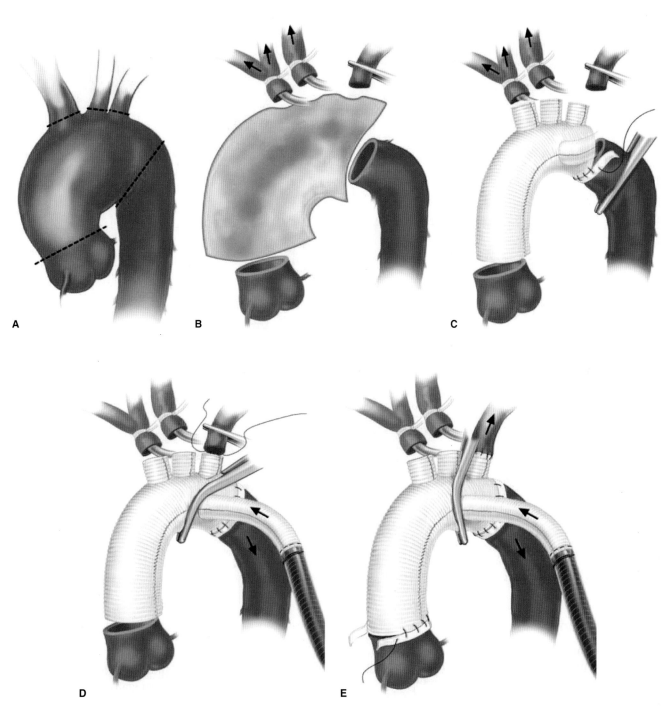

FIGURE 48-25 (A-H). Branched Arch Graft (Kazui) Technique. (*Continued*)

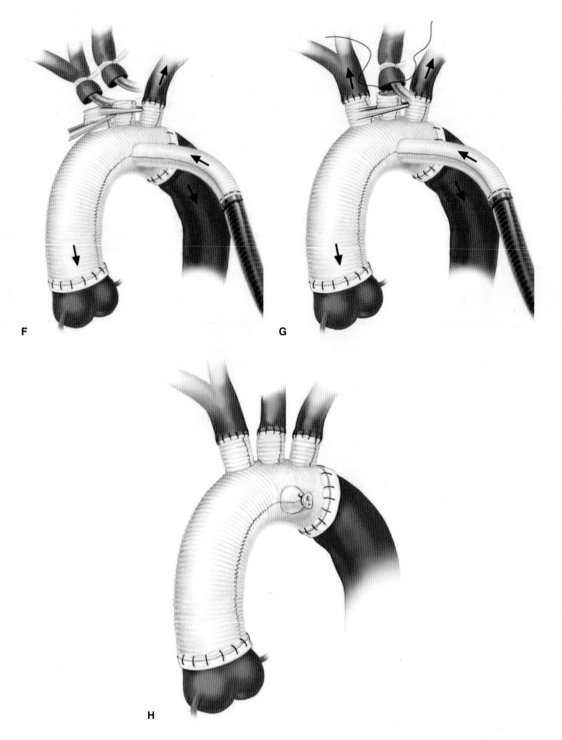

FIGURE 48-25 (F-H). Kazui Technique using a four branch graft for total arch replacement.

Elephant trunk

The elephant trunk (ET) is part of a two staged approach to treat arch aneurysms with extensive pathology distal to the left subclavian artery. First used in the 1980s by Borst et al, the benefit of the ET is it provides a platform for an easier second stage operation to treat distal aortic aneruysms and dissections with either an open or an endovascular repair.[149] Open repairs with an ET graft make for technically easier operations with smaller incisions and less cross-clamp time. Furthermore, it creates a proximal landing zone within the diseased distal aorta to place a stent graft.

Figure 48-28A-J illustrates the total arch replacement with a trifurcated graft and ET technique. Similar to as described above, right axillary cannulation is created to initiate CPB (Fig. 48-28B) and the aorta is cross-clamped proximal to the innominate artery (Fig. 48-28C). Once DHCA is reached the innominate, left carotid, and left subclavian arteries are anastomosed to the trifurcated graft and ACP is initiated from the right axillary artery, restoring perfusion to the brain and upper extremities (Fig. 48-28D,E). Attention is then turned toward the distal aorta. It is important to protect the left recurrent laryngeal nerve, so a suitable cuff of aortic tissue adjacent to the nerve is preserved. Studies demonstrate that the ET technique decreases the risk for laryngeal nerve injury during extensive aortic arch and descending aortic aneurysm repairs.[149,150] Next the proximal end of the ET graft is invaginated in itself and the midportion of the graft is anastomosed to the distal aorta with Teflon felt reinforcement (Fig. 48-28F). The origins of the left carotid and subclavian arteries are then oversewn. The proximal end of the anastomosis is then pulled out of the ET and can be anastomosed to the sinutubular junction, or as in Fig. 48-28G,H, the distal end of the graft from the aortic root repair. If a graft-to-graft anastomosis is required, it is necessary to bevel each graft end to maintain proper curvature (Fig. 48-28G). Next, the trifurcated graft limb remains clamped and is anastomosed to the proximal aspect of the aortic graft (Fig. 48-28E). Once the clamp is removed from the trifurcated limb, full myocardial

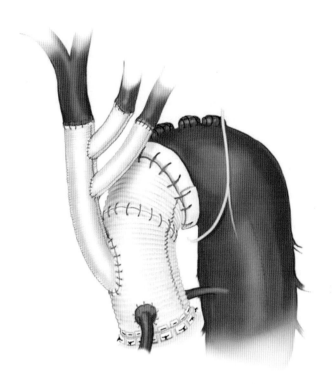

FIGURE 48-26 Trifurcated graft used to debranch the innominate, left carotid, and left subclavian arteries.

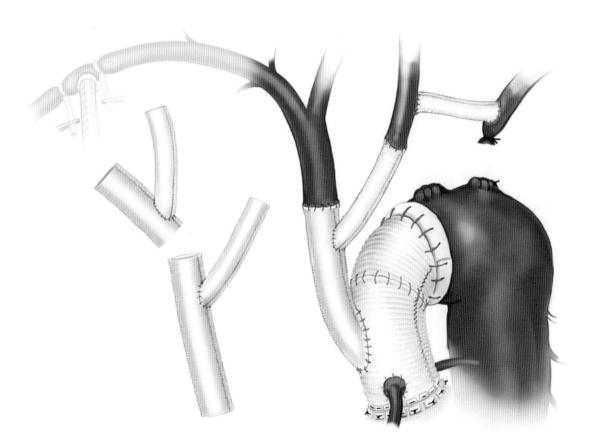

FIGURE 48-27 In case of a laterally displaced left subclavian artery from the aortic aneurysm, a left subclavian artery to carotid artery (LSCA) bypass can be completed.

and systemic perfusion is restored (Fig. 48-28J). With the stage 1 repair complete, the patient can then undergo the stage 2 procedure at another time with either an endovascular graft or open repair through a left thoracotomy. Nonetheless, while ET sets up for a convenient, easier stage 2 procedure, it is not without complications and pitfalls. Complications include kinking of the graft, spinal cord ischemia, peripheral thromboembolism, and visceral malperfusion.[151-153]

Arch First Technique

The "arch first" technique was described by Kouchoukos and Rokkas as an additional approach to treat aortic arch and proximal descending aortic aneurysm disease.[154] This single stage repair is performed via bilateral anterior thoracotomies providing excellent exposure of the aortic arch and descending aorta. One significant pitfall to this approach is it requires sacrificing both internal mammary arteries. Figure 48-29A-G illustrates the "arch first" technique. First, the heart and arch are exposed by bilateral thoracotomies in the fourth interspace with a transverse sternotomy. CPB is initiated via right axillary artery cannulation. While the patient is cooled, the great vessels are exposed with great attention to preserve the recurrent and phrenic nerves. The most distal aspect of the descending aortic aneurysm is mobilized. Once the DHCA is initiated, the innominate, left carotid, and left subclavian arteries are transected and clamped. Then both the proximal and the distal aorta are transected (Fig. 48-29B). The distal aorta can be clamped and lower body perfusion can be established via a femoral artery. As described in the Kazui technique, a four-branched graft is used and the great vessels are anastomosed starting with the left subclavian artery and moving proximally (Fig. 48-29C,D). After these anastomoses are completed, the brachiocephalic arteries can be flushed off to remove emboli (Fig. 48-29E). The graft body is then clamped both proximally and distally to reestablish cerebral and upper body perfusion (Fig. 48-29F). Next, the systemic perfusion from the femoral artery is discontinued and the distal anastomosis is completed. Systemic circulation is then started via the sidearm graft. Finally, the proximal aortic anastomosis is finished to complete the repair and clamps are removed (Fig. 48-29G). Kouchoukos et al reported on 46 "arch first"

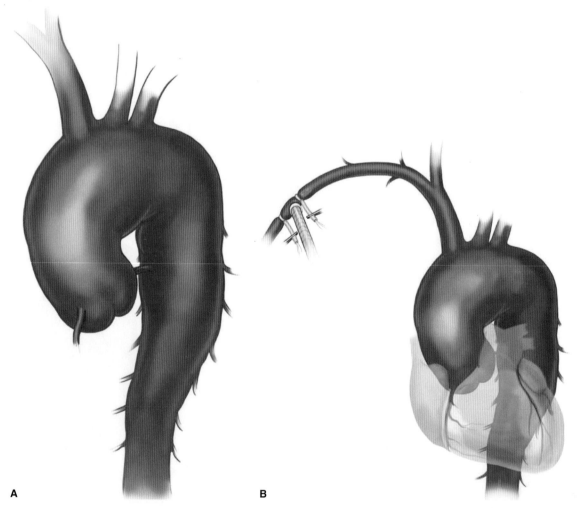

A   **B**

FIGURE 48-28 Total arch replacement using trifurcated graft and elephant trunk technique for atherosclerotic aorta. (A) Ascending and arch aneurysm. (B) Right axillary artery cannulation.

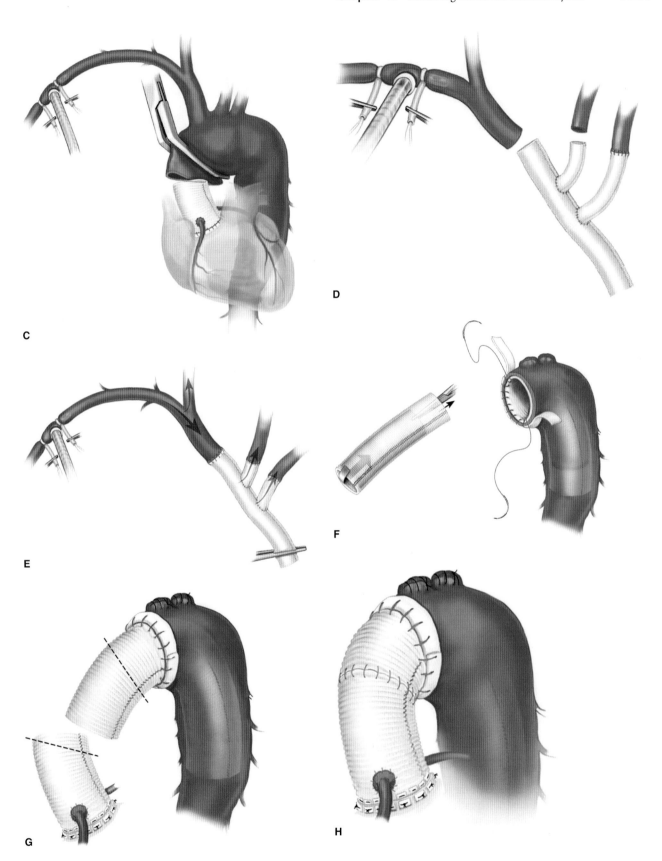

FIGURE 48-28 (*Continued*) (C) Proximal root reconstruction. (D) Trifurcated graft to the innominate, left carotid, and left subclavian arteries. (E) Antegrade cerebral perfusion from right axillary artery. (F) Invagination of the proximal part of the elephant trunk graft into the distal aspect and anastomosis of the graft to distal aorta. (G-H) Beveling the both grafts and graft to graft anastomosis.

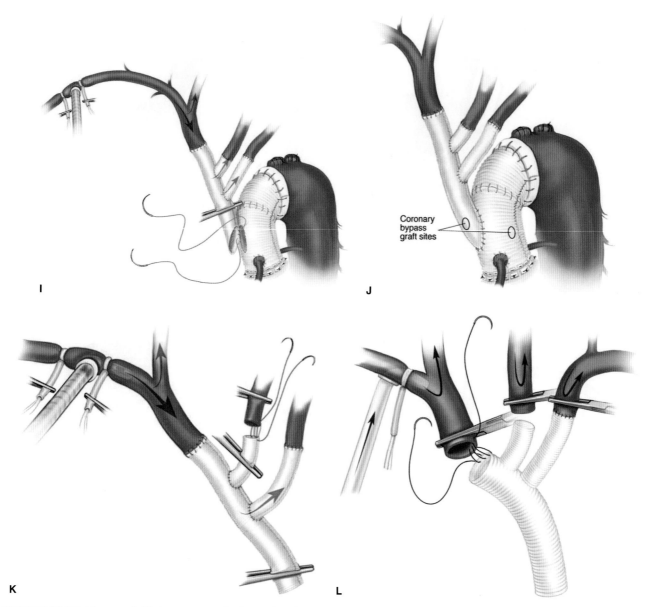

FIGURE 48-28 (*Continued*) (I) Anastomosis of trifurcated graft to ascending aortic graft. (J) Completed aortic arch repair. (K-L) Alternative sequence of brachiocephalic reconstruction to minimize DHCA.

procedures with a hospital mortality of 6.5%. There were no reports of permanent neurological events but 13% of patients developed clinical signs of TND.[154]

HYBRID TECHNIQUES

Hybrid arch procedures that combine open cerebral debranching with concomitant antegrade endovascular stent placement have emerged over the previous decade as a novel treatment option for aortic arch aneurysms. The benefit of this technique significantly limits the duration of cross-clamp time and cerebral ischemia and is beneficial in older patients with a high comorbidity indices.[155] The three key concepts to this approach are to (1) debranch the cerebral vessels (2)

reconstruct the ascending aorta to create a landing zone (Zone 0) for an endovascular stent graft, and (3) deploy an antegrade stent graft from Zone 0 to healthy distal aorta to exclude the arch aneurysm.

To grasp these concepts, an appreciation of landing zone classification is crucial. Thoracic aortic landing zones can be divided into five anatomic regions (Fig. 48-30).

- Zone 0: ascending aorta to the innominate artery
- Zone 1: between the innominate and the left carotid artery
- Zone 2: between the left carotid and left subclavian
- Zone 3: beyond the left subclavian and along the curved portion of the distal arch
- Zone 4: straight portion of the distal arch starting at the level of T4

and needs reconstruction of the distal landing zone (Zone 0) with a proximal landing zone below the diaphragm.

In a Type 1 hybrid arch, a debranching procedure is performed to bypass the cerebral vessels and involves an end-to-side anastomosis of a four-branched graft to the ascending aorta. This can often be completed with a side-biting clamp and done off CPB. After the debranching is performed, an endovascular stent graft is deployed antegrade via a separate side branch of the multibranched graft with distal landing zone in the native ascending aorta at Zone 0 under fluoroscopic guidance.

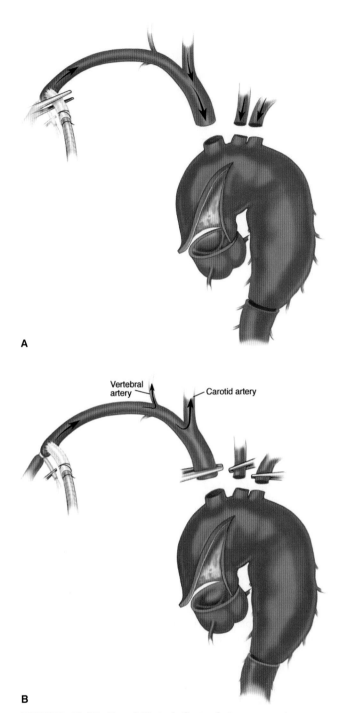

FIGURE 48-29 (A and B) Arch first technique to repair an aortic arch and proximal descending aortic aneurysm via bilateral thoracotomies.

Based on these zones, we have previously proposed a classification system for aortic arch pathology for hybrid repairs.[156] As seen in Fig. 48-31, a Type 1 hybrid arch has a suitable (nonaneurysmal) proximal aortic Zone 0 and distal Zone 2/3 landing zones for a stent graft. A Type 2 hybrid arch needs reconstruction of the Zone 0 landing zone but has a suitable landing zone in Zones 2 and 3. A Type 3 hybrid arch represents a mega-aorta

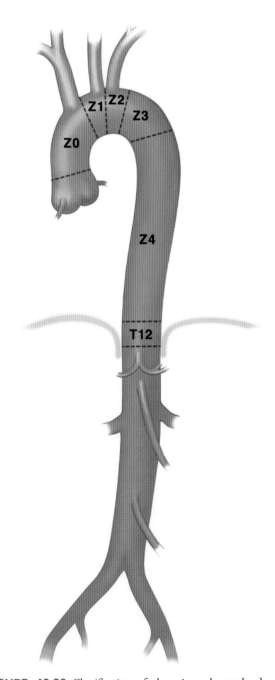

FIGURE 48-30 Classification of thoracic endovascular landing zones.

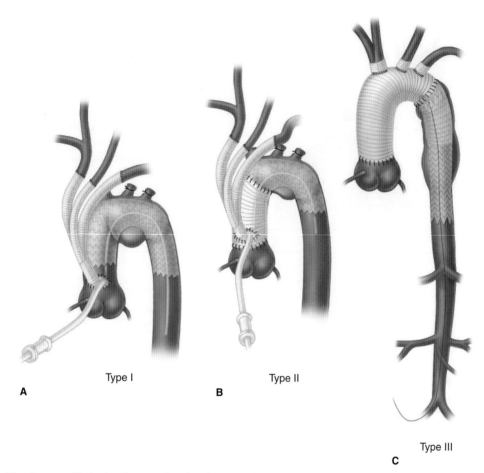

FIGURE 48-31 Classification of hybrid arch repairs based on location of aortic aneurysms. (A) Type 1 hybrid arch has a suitable aortic Zone 0 and distal Zone 2/3 landing zones for a stent graft. (B) A Type 2 hybrid arch needs reconstruction of the zone 0 landing zone but has a suitable landing zone in zones 2/3. (C) A Type 3 hybrid arch represents a mega-aorta and needs reconstruction of the landing zone (zone 0) with the other landing zone in the below the diaphragm.

A Type 2 hybrid arch does not have a proximal landing zone in Zone 0 due to ascending aortic pathology. Therefore, this repair involves replacement of the ascending aorta and debranching of the cerebral vessels so a stent graft can be deployed to exclude the arch aneurysm. A multibranched tube graft is used to replace the ascending aorta and the cerebral vessels are bypassed. DHCA may be necessary if a hemiarch anastomosis is required. After the graft is anastomosed, the stent graft is deployed antegrade via a separate side branch of the multibranched graft and landed distally in Zone 0 within the graft.

A Type 3 hybrid arch is a mega-aorta with diffuse proximal and distal aortic aneurysmal disease. This requires replacement of the ascending aorta and debranching as previously described for a Type 2 hybrid arch. The distal anastomosis of the graft is completed in the aneurysmal aorta but will be later excluded after the stent graft is deployed. Again, the stent graft is deployed antegrade via a side branch in the multibranched graft with the distal landing zone at Zone 0 in the graft and the proximal landing zone in the distal aorta.

Figure 48-32 shows a Type 1 hybrid arch repair for a Zone 2/3 descending aortic aneurysm. For this repair, there is a suitable proximal and distal landing zone to exclude the aneurysm after the great vessels are debranched. To complete this repair, CPB is initiated and a side-bitting clamp is placed on the aorta. It is best to utilize CPB so the side-biting clamp is not directly placed on the pulsatile ascending aorta. The main trunk of the trifurcated graft is anastomosed to the aorta. Next, the left subclavian artery is clamped and transected. The proximal stump is oversewn and the artery is then anastomosed to a limb of the trifurcated graft at which point perfusion is restored. In a similar fashion, the left carotid and innominate arteries are anastomosed to the remaining limbs of the trifurcated graft (Fig. 48-32A). An endovascular stent graft can then be deployed antegrade through a side branch to exclude the aneurysm. If the left subclavian anatomy is difficult on preoperative imaging, one approach would be to first perform a left subclavian to left carotid artery bypass (Fig. 48-32B). It is also possible to perform an intraoperative extra-anatomic bypass to the left axillary artery by tunneling the graft through the first or second intercostal space (Fig. 48-32C).

While hybrid repairs are technically easier, require less cross-clamp and require less DHCA time, there are several

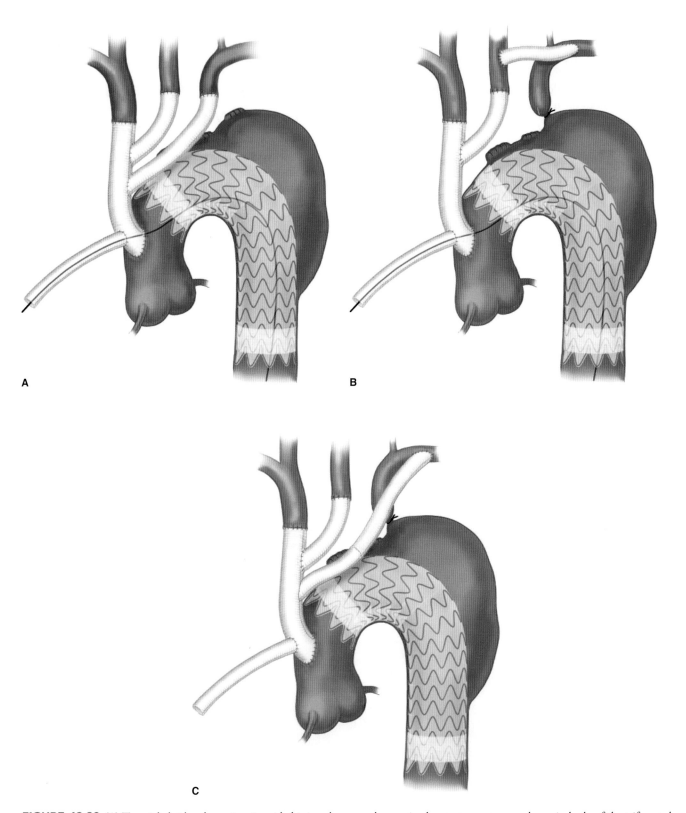

FIGURE 48-32 (A) Type 1 hybrid arch repair using side-bitting clamp on the proximal aorta to anastomose the main body of the trifurcated graft. The great vessels are then debranched with the limbs of the trifurcated graft. An endovascular stent graft is then deployed antegrade through a side limb. (B) Left subclavian to left carotid artery bypass for difficult left subclavian anatomy. (C) Intraoperative extra-anatomic bypass to the left axillary artery by tunneling the graft through the first or second intercostal space for difficult subclavian anatomy.

pitfalls. Complications consist of embolic stroke, type 1 endoleaks, and stent migration. In a systemic review of hybrid arch repairs of 1886 patients, there was a pooled perioperative mortality rate of 10.8%, stroke rate of 7%, and spinal cord ischemia of 7%.[157] Endoleaks are unique to hybrid operations in comparison to open techniques and have an incidence up to 15% in some reports.

COMPLETE ENDOVASCULAR AORTIC ARCH REPAIRS

Complete endovascular repair of aortic arch aneurysms remains in its infancy. Several techniques have been employed comprising custom fenestrated grafts, chimney/snorkle techniques, and in situ double branched graft fenestrations.[158,159] While the literature abounds with case reports and small series, no large studies exist to demonstrate long-term efficacy.

Figure 48-33A-C demonstrates an endovascular approach to an arch aneurysm and reveals the single chimney technique. This repair involves a staged operation by first completing a left subclavian to carotid artery transposition and a left carotid to innominate artery transposition (Fig. 48-33B). While transpositions are not always feasible due to anatomical variability, a left subclavian to carotid artery bypass and a left carotid to innominate artery bypass could equally have been completed. After several days, a stent graft is deployed retrograde from a femoral artery and landed proximally in Zone 0/1 with the fenestration at the innominate artery. The right axillary or right carotid artery can then be accessed to deploy a retrograde stent into the innominate fenestration. The advantage of this approach is CPB and DHCA are unnecessary. However, while studies have demonstrated feasibility with total endovascular aortic arch repair, the rates of stroke, type 1 endoleaks, need for secondary interventions, and early conversions to open repairs are high.[158-160] Patient selection is critical and these approaches are for patients at too high of a risk for the open, gold standard repair.

ADDITIONAL CONSIDERATIONS
Concomitant Mitral Surgery

Mitral valve disease is frequently encountered in patients with aortic aneurysms. This is particularly true for patients with MFS, in whom the incidence approaches 30%.[161] Patients who have evidence of moderate-to-severe mitral regurgitation should undergo mitral valve repair at the time of aortic replacement. Gillinov et al reported results of mitral valve repair in patients with MFS, many of whom also had simultaneous replacement of the aortic root.[162] They observed an 88% actuarial rate of freedom from significant mitral regurgitation at 5 years. A fairly liberal approach to mitral valve intervention is warranted in aortic root replacement patients as reoperation for late mitral regurgitation may be particularly technically difficult. Additionally, care must be taken when taking the annular stitches along the aortomitral continuity to avoid shortening the anterior leaflet of the mitral valve.

Aortic Wrapping and Reduction Aortoplasty

Reduction ascending aortoplasty and aortic wrapping are less common techniques to address ascending aortic aneurysms typically reserved for patients undergoing concomitant aortic valve replacement but who are deemed too high risk for either composite root or ascending aortic replacement or who have ascending aortic dimensions less than the recommendations for replacement as a prophylactic measure to prevent aneurysm formation. Reduction aortoplasty involves excision of a segment of the ascending aorta to achieve a normal radial maximal dimension. It may be performed either with

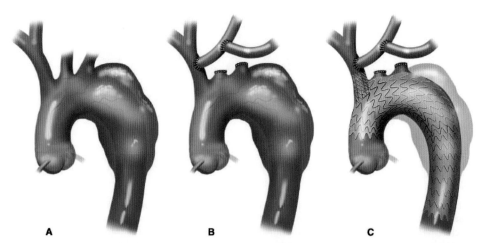

A   **B**   **C**

FIGURE 48-33 An endovascular approach to exclude an arch aneurysm using the single chimney technique and fenestrated graft. (A) A type 1 hybrid arch. (B) A left subclavian to carotid artery transposition and a left carotid to innominate artery transposition. (C) Retrograde endovascular stent graft from the femoral artery and an antegrade stent placed into the innominate artery from the right axillary or right carotid artery.

a side-biting aortic clamp, cross-clamped or with open technique depending on the length of aortoplasty and technique used.[163-165] The excised segment may be taken in the long axis of the aorta down to the sinotubular junction (true reduction annuloplasty) or lesser plication techniques. External reinforcement can also be performed in conjunction with reduction aortoplasty. Concerns regarding this technique include dehiscence or aortic rupture at the suture line, which is constantly under tension from the radial force on the aortic wall during systole.

Aortic wrapping of girdling is performed either by itself or in conjunction with reduction aortoplasty. Wrapping has been performed with cellophane, polyester grafts and meshes, polytetrafluoroethylene (PTFE), and other materials. Neri et al described two patients required reoperation because of development of false aneurysms following aortic valve replacement with aortoplasty and wrapping.[166] The unwrapped parts of the ascending aorta in both patients appeared normal; conversely, the aortic wall underlying the wrap was severely atrophic, a phenomenon previously reported with abdominal aneurysms that were wrapped without aortoplasty. In a larger series by Cohen et al, among 102 patients who underwent aortic wrapping with a polyester mesh followed for a median of 4.7 years, there were no instances of major aortic complications and an average aneurysm growth of 2.6 mm over the follow-up period.[167]

REOPERATIVE CONSIDERATIONS

Reoperative surgery on the ascending aorta and aortic root can be particularly challenging but is becoming more frequent in experienced centers. Increased use of tissue aortic valves in younger patients, biologic porcine or composite pericardial roots, and homografts in past few decades suggest that many patients may require reoperative root intervention. Additionally, root replacement may be required after the development of ascending aortic aneurysms in bicuspid patients who have previously undergone aortic valve replacement only. Indications for reoperation include aortic insufficiency, development of aneurysms or dissections in remaining segments of the thoracic aorta, false aneurysms, prosthetic valve dysfunction, infection or thrombosis, or degeneration of biologic prostheses.

Reentry is usually accomplished with a repeat sternotomy incision, although for complex arch operations involving the proximal descending aorta, a thoracosternotomy approach may be required.[168] In cases of massive ascending aortic aneurysm, adhesion of the aorta to the posterior table of the sternum or contained ruptures and exposure of alternative cannulation site such as the right axillary artery or femoral artery are necessary. Massive aortic hemorrhage upon sternal entry should be locally controlled by forcibly reapproximating the sternum, heparinizing the patient, instituting peripheral CPB, and cooling to deep hypothermia such that the sternal reentry can be completed under lower flow conditions with active pump-suction in the operative field. If entering the aorta on reentry is felt to be inevitable, starting CPB and

cooling prior to sternotomy may be a superior strategy. In cases of moderate-to-severe aortic insufficiency, venting of the left ventricle prior to cardiac fibrillation is mandatory and can be accomplished by a small left anterior thoracotomy incision and direct venting of the apex.

Cross-clamping in the reoperative scenario may also be hazardous as previous graft material may cause severe adhesions to the pulmonary artery making the dissection of a clamping site difficult. Previous use of a porcine root prosthesis or left-sided bypass grafts makes this dissection particularly difficult. If the pulmonary artery is inadvertently entered, patching with a pericardial substitute is usually necessary.

Mobilization of the coronary arteries is frequently difficult and creation of a Cabrol-type anastomosis, interposition grafts, or bypass grafts are frequently necessary. Previous coronary bypass grafts should be reimplanted, and frequently, interposition vein grafts are required to accomplish this. Direct cardioplegia administration down bypass grafts is preferred but avoided when there is diffuse vein graft disease.[169] Retrograde cardioplegia is extremely helpful in this circumstance.

In cases of reoperation for failed porcine bioroots, root replacement is preferable to simple aortic valve implantation within the porcine root as there is a higher likelihood for valve dehiscence due to the degenerative nature of the root tissue.[170] If aortic valve implantation into a porcine root is being performed, all of the aortic valve implantation sutures must traverse the native aortic root tissue, not just the porcine tissue.

OPERATIVE COMPLICATIONS
Bleeding

Woven Dacron grafts impregnated with collagen or gelatin are relatively impervious to blood and have reduced blood loss following replacement of the ascending aorta compared with knitted grafts. Precise suturing with careful attention to avoid torque on the suture needles while constructing anastomoses is critical to avoid the inevitable needle-hole bleeding at the end of the surgery. Tension must be avoided at the sites of coronary reimplantation, as this is a frequent site of bleeding. The modified Cabrol method or an interposition graft should be used when any tension is present. The inclusion technique of graft insertion is associated with an increased incidence of bleeding and pseudoaneurysm formation and has largely been abandoned. In very friable aortas, Teflon felt may be used to reinforce the suture line on the outside of the anastomosis in which a thin strip of felt is slipped into the suture line as it is tightened. Alternatively, it may be sewn to the inside, outside, or both sides of the native aorta with a running polypropylene stitch prior to sewing the graft.

In cases of refractory coagulopathy, the anastomosis can be wrapped tightly with a small segment of polyester graft or Teflon felt to reduce tension on the suture line and reduce needle-hole bleeding (Fig. 48-34). Blood transfusion can be avoided in a significant number of patients with the use of blood conservation

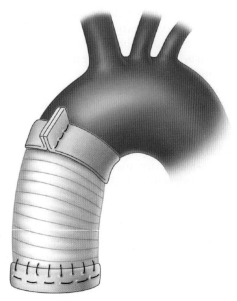

FIGURE 48-34 Suture line bleeding may be effectively controlled with a circumferential wrap of the anastomosis with a strip of Teflon felt or Dacron. (Reproduced with permission from Edmunds LH: *Cardiac Surgery in the Adult.* New York: McGraw-Hill; 1997.)

techniques such as Cell Savers, autologous blood donation, plateletpheresis, the reinfusion of chest tube drainage, and the use of antifibrinolytics such as aminocaproic acid and tranexamic acid. Since the removal of the antifibrinolytic agent aprotinin from the market due to concerns regarding renal dysfunction and mortality, bleeding has anecdotally become more common. Activated human recombinant factor VII may be helpful as a last resort when treating refractory bleeding that does not respond to any other therapies, although this may induce unanticipated thrombosis in arterial structures.[171]

In cases of ongoing postoperative hemorrhage, expedient return to the operating room for reexploration is preferable to massive transfusion or tamponade. Postoperative bleeding requiring reexploration ranges from 2.4 to 11.1%.[172,173]

Stroke

Neurologic injury following proximal aortic surgery remains a significant cause of morbidity and mortality. Embolization of atherosclerotic debris or thrombus from the ascending aorta and arch produces focal neurologic deficits. Diffuse injury can be attributed to microemboli of air or cellular debris, insufficient or uneven cooling, and a prolonged circulatory arrest period. After circulatory arrest periods exceeding 40 minutes the incidence of stroke greatly increases.[174] Profound hypothermia may itself be injurious to the central nervous system without associated circulatory arrest.[175]

Stroke due to embolization is diminished when the aorta is evaluated via epiaortic ultrasound or other imaging modality to detect atherosclerotic plaques and thrombus.[176] This allows appropriate adjustments to be made in clamping and cannulation strategies. Resumption of antegrade circulation through the graft once the distal aortic anastomosis is complete, rather than retrograde via the femoral vessels, after a period of circulatory arrest avoids embolization of distal aortic debris. Patients with severe carotid artery occlusive disease are at increased risk of stroke during ascending aortic procedures, and patients older than 65, those with peripheral vascular disease, or those with pertinent histories should be evaluated.[177]

Patients with new postoperative strokes should be rapidly evaluated by the consultant neurology service and undergo early brain imaging. New embolic events should be managed aggressively with induced hypertension once intracranial hemorrhage has been ruled out.

Pulmonary Dysfunction

CPB is known to cause alterations in pulmonary function as evidenced by changes in alveolar-arterial oxygen gradients, pulmonary vascular resistance, pulmonary compliance, and intrapulmonary shunting. Usually these changes are subclinical, but a full-blown adult respiratory distress-like syndrome is reported in 0.5 to 1.7% of patients following CPB.[178-180] The specific cause is the subject of much investigation and debate, but it is generally accepted that exposure of blood elements to the foreign surface of the cardiopulmonary circuit results in the activation of inflammatory cells and the complement cascade resulting in pulmonary injury.[181] The duration of CPB, urgency of the procedure, and general condition of the patient may roughly correlate with the occurrence and severity of pulmonary dysfunction, but it can be unpredictable.

Treatment is supportive, with early diagnosis and treatment of any subsequent pulmonary infections. Ten to eighteen percent of patients require prolonged mechanical ventilation. Preventive measures may include preoperative optimization of pulmonary function, minimization of pump time, judicious use of blood products, heparin-coated bypass circuits, and leukocyte depletion.[182]

Myocardial Dysfunction

Transient myocardial dysfunction following complex aortic surgery requiring inotropic support is common with 18 to 25% of patients requiring more than 6 hours of inotropic support.[183,184] Meticulous attention should be paid to integrated myocardial protection with cold blood cardioplegia administered frequently in antegrade and retrograde fashions. This is particularly important in patients with significant left ventricular dilatation seen with aortic insufficiency or hypertrophy seen with aortic stenosis. Maintenance of high perfusion pressures after removal of cross-clamp optimizes myocardial perfusion during the critical reperfusion period. Optimization of right ventricular function with afterload reducing agents such as milrinone or inhaled prostaglandins while weaning from CPB is vital for maintaining adequate left ventricular filling in cases of severe diastolic dysfunction or ventricular hypertrophy. Postoperative myocardial infarction, reported in up to 2.5% of cases, may be related to technical problems with coronary reimplantation.[185]

Perioperative Mortality

Contemporary surgical series on ascending aortic disease using modern grafting techniques and methods of cerebral and myocardial protection report hospital mortality rates of 1.7 to 17.1%.[185-189] Comparison of outcomes is difficult, however, because of heterogeneity of patients. Some series do not include dissection, and the proportion of emergent operations, reoperations, and arch replacements is highly variable. The common causes of early death are cardiac failure, stroke, bleeding, and pulmonary insufficiency.[185,186]

Emergent operation after the onset of acute dissection or rupture is the highest risk factor for early death. Risk of death following elective intervention is increased by increasing New York Heart Association classification, increasing age, prolonged CPB time, dissection, previous cardiac surgery, and need for concomitant coronary revascularization.[188,189]

LATE COMPLICATIONS

Late Mortality

Reported actuarial survival, like early mortality, is variable and dependent on the patient cohort. Survival rates are 81 to 95% at 1 year, 73 to 92% at 5 years, 60 to 73% at 8 to 10 years, and 48 to 67% at 12 to 14 years.[190-193] Predictors of late mortality include elevated New York Heart Association class, requirement for arch reconstruction, MFS, and extent of distal disease.[194-197] The most common cause of late death is cardiac, but distal aortic disease accounted for 32% of late deaths in one series.[198]

Reoperation

Reoperations occur due to pseudoaneurysm formation, valve thrombosis, endocarditis or graft infection, progression of disease in the native valve or remaining aortic segments, or degeneration of a bioprosthesis. Reported mortality for reoperative ascending aortic surgery varies between 4 and 22%.[199,200]

Freedom from reoperation is 86 to 90% at 9 to 10 years (Fig. 48-35).[201,202] Predictors of late reoperation have included MFS, the inclusion cylinder technique, and chronic dissection.[203] Surveillance of patients who have undergone previous aortic surgery to minimize the need for urgent reoperations and appropriate resection of all diseased aortic tissue at the time of original operation improves outcomes. Up to 60% of reoperations occur due to inadequate repair during the initial operation.[204] This is due to failure to resect the most distal aspects of aneurysmal disease by performing a clamped distal anastomosis or failure to adequately address root pathology with full root replacement. Previous inclusion-type anastomotic techniques were associated with higher rates of early reoperation due to pseudoaneurysm formation (Fig. 48-36).[205]

MFS patients are particularly prone to requiring reoperation (Fig. 48-37).[206] Gott et al reviewed the experience with root replacement at 10 surgical centers in 675 Marfan patients between 1968 and 1996.[207] The 30-day mortality was 3.3%,

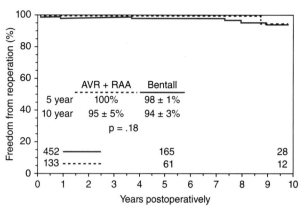

FIGURE 48-35 Long term freedom from reoperation following full aortic root replacement and separate ascending aortic and valve replacemnt. (Reproduced with permission from Sioris T, David TE, Ivanov J, et al: Clinical outcomes after separate and composite replacement of the aortic valve and ascending aorta, *J Thorac Cardiovasc Surg* 2004 Aug;128(2):260-5.)

but was only 1.5% for elective repair. Emergency surgery resulted in a 30-day mortality of nearly 12%. The survival rate was 93% at 1 year, 84% at 5 years, 75% at 10 years, and 59% at 20 years. Complications related to the residual thoracic aorta and arrhythmias were the leading causes of death. The most frequent late complication was thromboembolism. Advanced New York Heart Association class at the time of original operation was the only predictor of late death.

Graft infection

Graft infections are reported in up to 0.9 to 6% of patients following surgery of the thoracic aorta and are associated

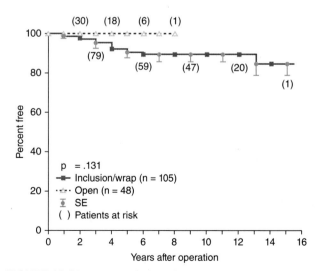

FIGURE 48-36 Long term freedom from reoperation for pseudoaneurysm of the aortic or coronary ostial suture lines by operative technique (inclusion or open). (Reproduced with permission from Kouchoukos NT, Wareing TH, Murphy SF, et al: Sixteen-year experience with aortic root replacement: Results of 172 operations, *Ann Surg* 1991 Sep;214(3):308-18.)

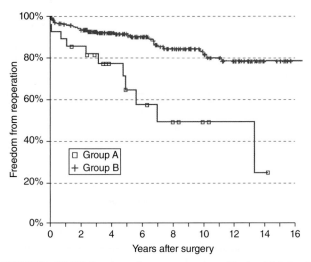

FIGURE 48-37 Freedom from reoperation (Kaplan-Meier) of patients with Marfan syndrome [Group A] versus those without fibrillinopathic etiologies [Group B]. (Reproduced with permission from Detter C, Mair H, Klein HG, et al: Long-term prognosis of surgically-treated aortic aneurysms and dissections in patients with and without Marfan syndrome, *Eur J Cardiothorac Surg* 1998; Apr;13(4):416-423.)

with a very high (25-75%) mortality rate.[208-210] Most graft infections occur in the first month after operation and are frequently associated with wound infections. They may occur years later in cases of associated valve endocarditis or bacteremia from indwelling catheters or other systemic infections. The major infectious agents are *Staphylococcus aureus*, *S. epidermidis*, and Pseudomonas.[211] The ascending aortic graft may be particularly vulnerable because of proximity to the wound and poor natural tissue coverage. For this reason, full coverage of the ascending graft material with the pericardial fat pad is advisable in all cases. This serves to isolate the graft from the sternum should it become infected.

Patients frequently present with persistent fevers and elevated white cell count. CT or MRI may demonstrate air or fluid collections around the graft. There may be associated pseudoaneurysms, fistula, anastomotic leak, hemolysis, and embolism. Nuclear imaging techniques may be helpful but can be nonspecific for infection versus normal postoperative inflammation.[212] TEE may show valvular vegetations or abscesses.

Ideally, treatment of the stable patient begins with intravenous antibiotics to control septicemia and often clear blood cultures prior to reoperation. In extremely high-risk patients, where reoperative mortality is prohibitive, life-long suppressive antibiotics may be acceptable. Surgical treatment of infected ascending aortic grafts, as described by Hargrove and Edmunds, includes removal of all infected prosthetic material, aggressive tissue debridement, local irrigation, systemic antibiotic therapy, replacement of the infected conduit, and utilization of autologous tissue to surround the graft and obliterate dead space.[213] Aortic homograft may potentially be more resistant to repeat infection. Greater omentum may be also brought up through the diaphragm as a vascularized pedicle to wrap around the aortic graft and isolate it from

the sternum. Concomitant sternal infections should be managed with aggressive debridement, sterilization with vacuum-assisted wound drainage, and delayed flap reconstruction. In severe cases, open continuous antibiotic wound irrigation for several days can assist clearing the infection.[214] Long-term antibiotics should be continued intravenously for at least 6 weeks and suppressive oral antibiotics may be indicated over the long-term thereafter.

REFERENCES

1. Elkin DC: Aneurysms following surgical procedures. *Ann Surg* 1948; 127:769-779.
2. Bergqvist D: Historical aspects on aneurysmal disease. *Scand J Surg* 2008; 97(2):90-99.
3. Hajdu SI: A note from history: the first pathology book and its author. *Ann Clin Lab Sci* 2004 Spring; 34(2):226-227.
4. Cooper A: *Lectures on the Principles and Practice of Surgery*, 2nd ed. London, FC Westley, 1830; p 110.
5. Moore C: On a new method of procuring the consolidation of fibrin in certain incurable aneurysms. *Med Chir Trans* (London) 1864; 47:129.
6. Matas R: Surgery of the vascular system, in Matas R (ed): *Surgery, Its Principles and Practice*, Vol. 5. Philadelphia, WB Saunders, 1914.
7. Harrison P, Chandy J: A subclavian aneurysm cured by cellophane fibrosis. *Ann Surg* 1943; 118:478.
8. Poppe J, De Oliviera H: Treatment of syphilitic aneurysms by cellophane wrapping. *J Thorac Surg* 1946; 15:186.
9. Matas R: An operation for the radical cure of aneurism based upon arteriorrhaphy. *Ann Surg* 1903; 37:161.
10. Matas R: Endo-aneurismorrhaphy. *Surg Gynecol Obstet* 1920; 30:456.
11. Cooley DA, De Bakey ME: Surgical considerations of intrathoracic aneurysms of the aorta and great vessels. *Ann Surg* 1952; 135:660.
12. Cooley DA, DeBakey ME: Resection of the entire ascending aorta in fusiform aneurysm using cardiac bypass. *JAMA* 1956; 162:1158.
13. Westaby S, Cecil B: Surgery of the thoracic aorta, in Westaby S (ed): *Landmarks in Cardiac Surgery*. Oxford, Isis Medical Media, 1997; p 223.
14. Kadoba K, Schoen FJ, Jonas RA: Experimental comparison of albumin-sealed and gelatin-sealed knitted Dacron conduits. Porosity control, handling, sealant resorption, and healing. *J Thorac Cardiovasc Surg* 1992; 103(6):1059-1067.
15. Wheat MWJ, Wilson JR, Bartley TD: Successful replacement of the entire ascending aorta and aortic valve. *JAMA* 1964; 188:717.
16. Bentall H, De Bono A: A technique for complete replacement of the ascending aorta. *Thorax* 1968; 23:338.
17. Cabrol C, Pavie A, Gandjbakhch I, et al: Complete replacement of the ascending aorta with reimplantation of the coronary arteries: new surgical approach. *J Thorac Cardiovasc Surg* 1981; 81:309.
18. Kouchoukos NT, Karp RB: Resection of ascending aortic aneurysm and replacement of aortic valve. *J Thorac Cardiovasc Surg* 1981; 81(1):142-143.
19. Sutton JP 3rd, Ho SY, Anderson RH: The forgotten interleaflet triangles: a review of the surgical anatomy of the aortic valve. *Ann Thorac Surg* 1995; 59(2):419-427.
20. Hokken RB, Bartelings MM, Bogers AJ, Gittenberger-de Groot AC: Morphology of the pulmonary and aortic roots with regard to the pulmonary autograft procedure. *J Thorac Cardiovasc Surg* 1997; 113(3):453-461.
21. Maselli D, Montalto A, Santise G, Minardi G, Manzara C, Musumeci F: A normogram to anticipate dimension of neo-sinuses of valsalva in valve-sparing aortic operations. *Eur J Cardiothorac Surg* 2005; 27(5):831-835.
22. Otani K, Takeuchi M, Kaku K, et al: Assessment of the aortic root using real-time 3D transesophageal echocardiography. *Circ J* 2010; 74(12):2649-2657.
23. Nejjar I, Pieraggi MT, Thiers JC, Bouissou H: Age-related changes in the elastic tissue of the human thoracic aorta. *Atherosclerosis* 1990; 80(3):199-208.
24. Greenwald SE. Ageing of the conduit arteries. *J Pathol* 2007; 211(2):157-172.

25. Halloran BG, Davis VA, McManus BM, Lynch TG, Baxter BT: Localization of aortic disease is associated with intrinsic differences in aortic structure. *J Surg Res* 1995; 59(1):17-22.

26. Wilson WR, Anderton M, Choke EC, Dawson J, Loftus IM, Thompson MM: Elevated plasma MMP1 and MMP9 are associated with abdominal aortic aneurysm rupture. *Eur J Vasc Endovasc Surg* 2008; 35(5):580-584.

27. Geng L, Wang W, Chen Y, et al: Elevation of ADAM10, ADAM17, MMP-2 and MMP-9 expression with media degeneration features CaCl₂-induced thoracic aortic aneurysm in a rat model. *Exp Mol Pathol* 2010; 89(1):72-81.

28. Sheth RA, Maricevich M, Mahmood U: In vivo optical molecular imaging of matrix metalloproteinase activity in abdominal aortic aneurysms correlates with treatment effects on growth rate. *Atherosclerosis* 2010; 212(1):181-187.

29. Jones JA, Ruddy JM, Bouges S, et al: Alterations in membrane type-1 matrix metalloproteinase abundance after the induction of thoracic aortic aneurysm in a murine model. *Am J Physiol Heart Circ Physiol* 2010; 299(1):H114-124.

30. Liu J, Sukhova GK, Yang JT, et al: Cathepsin L expression and regulation in human abdominal aortic aneurysm, atherosclerosis, and vascular cells. *Atherosclerosis* 2006; 184(2):302-311.

31. Homme JL, Aubry MC, Edwards WD, et al: Surgical pathology of the ascending aorta: a clinicopathologic study of 513 cases. *Am J Surg Pathol* 2006; 30(9):1159-1168.

32. Cohen JR, Sarfati I, Wise L: The effect of cigarette smoking on rabbit aortic elastase activity. *J Vasc Surg* 1989; 9(4):580-582.

33. Okamoto RJ, Xu H, Kouchoukos NT, Moon MR, Sundt TM 3rd: The influence of mechanical properties on wall stress and distensibility of the dilated ascending aorta. *J Thorac Cardiovasc Surg* 2003; 126(3): 842-850.

34. Grande KJ, Cochran RP, Reinhall PG, Kunzelman KS: Stress variations in the human aortic root and valve: the role of anatomic asymmetry. *Ann Biomed Eng* 1998; 26:534-545.

35. Agozzino L, Ferraraccio F, Esposito S, et al: Medial degeneration does not involve uniformly the whole ascending aorta: morphological, biochemical and clinical correlations. *Eur J Cardiothorac Surg* 2002; 21:675-682.

36. Judge DP, Dietz HC: Marfan's syndrome. *Lancet* 2005; 366:1965-1976.

37. Hollister DW, Godfrey M, Sakai LY, Pyeritz RE: Immunohistologic abnormalities of the microfibrillar-fiber system in the Marfan syndrome. *N Engl J Med* 1990; 323(3):152-159.

38. Dietz HC, Cutting GR, Pyeritz RE, et al: Marfan syndrome caused by a recurrent de novo missense mutation in the fibrillin gene. *Nature* 1991; 352(6333):337-339.

39. Mizuguchi T, Collod-Beroud G, Akiyama T, et al: Heterozygous TGFBR2 mutations in Marfan syndrome. *Nat Genet* 2004; 36(8):855-860.

40. Marsalese DL, Moodie DS, Vacante M, et al: Marfan's syndrome: natural history and long-term follow-up of cardiovascular involvement. *J Am Coll Cardiol* 1989; 14:422.

41. Keane MG, Pyeritz RE: Medical management of Marfan syndrome. *Circulation* 2008; 117(21):2802-2813.

42. Nagashima H, Sakomura Y, Aoka Y, et al: Angiotensin II type 2 receptor mediates vascular smooth muscle cell apoptosis in cystic medial degeneration associated with Marfan's syndrome. *Circulation* 2001;104(12 Suppl 1):I282-I287.

43. Habashi JP, Judge DP, Holm TM, et al: Losartan, an AT1 antagonist, prevents aortic aneurysm in a mouse model of Marfan syndrome. *Science* 2006; 312(5770):117-121.

44. Brooke BS, Habashi JP, Judge DP, Patel N, Loeys B, Dietz HC 3rd: Angiotensin II blockade and aortic-root dilation in Marfan's syndrome. *N Engl J Med* 2008; 358(26):2787-2795.

45. Loeys BL, Chen J, Neptune ER, et al: A syndrome of altered cardiovascular, craniofacial, neurocognitive and skeletal development caused by mutations in TGFBR1 or TGFBR2. *Nat Genet* 2005; 37(3):275-281.

46. Van Hemelrijk C, Renard M, Loeys B: The Loeys-Dietz syndrome: an update for the clinician. *Curr Opin Cardiol* 2010; 25(6):546-551.

47. Maleszewski JJ, Miller DV, Lu J, Dietz HC, Halushka MK: Histopathologic findings in ascending aortas from individuals with Loeys-Dietz syndrome (LDS). *Am J Surg Pathol* 2009; 33(2):194-201.

48. Shields LB, Rolf CM, Davis GJ, Hunsaker JC 3rd: Sudden and unexpected death in three cases of Ehlers-Danlos syndrome type IV. *J Forensic Sci* 2010; 55(6):1641-1645.

49. Guo DL, Papke CL, Tran-Fadulu V, et al: Mutations in smooth muscle alpha-actin (ACTA2) cause coronary artery disease, stroke, and

50. Moyamoya disease, along with thoracic aortic disease. *Am J Hum Genet* 2009; 84(5):617-627.

50. van de Laar IM, Oldenburg RA, Pals G, et al: Mutations in SMAD3 cause a syndromic form of aortic aneurysms and dissections with early-onset osteoarthritis. *Nat Genet* 2011; 43(2):121-126.

51. Milewicz DM, Carlson AA, Regalado ES: Genetic testing in aortic aneurysm disease: PRO. *Cardiol Clin* 2010; 28(2):191-197.

52. Kontusaari S, Tromp G, Kuivaniemi H, Romanic AM, Prockop DJ: A mutation in the gene for type III procollagen (COL3A1) in a family with aortic aneurysms. *J Clin Invest* 1990; 86(5):1465-1473.

53. Keramati AR, Sadeghpour A, Farahani MM, Chandok G, Mani A: The non-syndromic familial thoracic aortic aneurysms and dissections maps to 15q21 locus. *BMC Med Genet* 2010; 11:143.

54. Wang L, Guo DC, Cao J, et al: Mutations in myosin light chain kinase cause familial aortic dissections. *Am J Hum Genet* 2010; 87(5):701-707.

55. Pannu H, Fadulu VT, Chang J, et al: Mutations in transforming growth factor-beta receptor type II cause familial thoracic aortic aneurysms and dissections. *Circulation* 2005; 112(4):513-520.

56. Lee JH, Burner KD, Fealey ME, et al: Prosthetic valve endocarditis: clinicopathological correlates in 122 surgical specimens from 116 patients (1985-2004). *Cardiovasc Pathol* 2011; 20(1):26-35.

57. Feigl D, Feigl A, Edwards JE: Mycotic aneurysms of the aortic root: a pathologic study of 20 cases. *Chest* 1986; 90:553.

58. Tavora F, Burke A: Review of isolated ascending aortitis: differential diagnosis, including syphilitic, Takayasu's and giant cell aortitis. *Pathology* 2006; 38(4):302-308.

59. Kuniyoshi Y, Koja K, Miyagi K, et al: A ruptured syphilitic descending thoracic aortic aneurysm. The characteristic findings on computed tomography for the etiological diagnosis of aneurysm. *Ann Thorac Cardiovasc Surg* 1998; 4(2):99-102.

60. Tavora F, Burke A: Review of isolated ascending aortitis: differential diagnosis, including syphilitic, Takayasu's and giant cell aortitis. *Pathology* 2006; 38(4):302-308.

61. Matsumura K, Hirano T, Takeda K, et al: Incidence of aneurysms in Takayasu's arteritis. *Angiology* 1991; 42(4):308-315.

62. Austen WB, Blennerhasset JB: Giant cell aortitis causing an aneurysm of the ascending aorta and aortic regurgitation. *N Engl J Med* 1964; 272:80.

63. Warnes CA: Sex differences in congenital heart disease: should a woman be more like a man? *Circulation* 2008; 118(1):3-5.

64. Huntington K, Hunter AG, Chan KL: A prospective study to assess the frequency of familial clustering of congenital bicuspid aortic valve. *J Am Coll Cardiol* 1997; 30(7):1809-1812.

65. Lewin MB, Otto CM: The bicuspid aortic valve: adverse outcomes from infancy to old age. *Circulation* 2005; 111(7):832-834.

66. Guntheroth WG, Spiers PS: Does aortic root dilatation with bicuspid aortic valves occur as a primary tissue abnormality or as a relatively benign poststenotic phenomenon? *Am J Cardiol* 2005; 95(6):820.

67. Jain R, Engleka KA, Rentschler SL, et al: Cardiac neural crest orchestrates remodeling and functional maturation of mouse semilunar valves. *J Clin Invest* 2010 Dec 13; pii: 44244. doi: 10.1172/JCI44244.

68. Nataatmadja M, West M, West J, et al: Abnormal extracellular matrix protein transport associated with increased apoptosis of vascular smooth muscle cells in Marfan syndrome and bicuspid aortic valve thoracic aortic aneurysm. *Circulation* 2003; 108(Suppl 1):II329-334.

69. LeMaire SA, Wang X, Wilks JA, et al: Matrix metalloproteinases in ascending aortic aneurysms: bicuspid versus trileaflet aortic valves. *J Surg Res* 2005; 123(1):40-48.

70. Fedak PW, de Sa MP, Verma S, et al: Vascular matrix remodeling in patients with bicuspid aortic valve malformations: implications for aortic dilatation. *J Thorac Cardiovasc Surg* 2003; 126(3):797-806.

71. Matthias Bechtel JF, Noack F, Sayk F, et al: Histopathological grading of ascending aortic aneurysm: comparison of patients with bicuspid versus tricuspid aortic valve. *J Heart Valve Dis* 2003; 12(1):54-59; discussion 59-61.

72. Bonderman D, Gharehbaghi-Schnell E, Wollenek G, Maurer G, Baumgartner H, Lang IM: Mechanisms underlying aortic dilatation in congenital aortic valve malformation. *Circulation* 1999; 99(16):2138-2143.

73. Fazel SS, Mallidi HR, Lee RS, et al: The aortopathy of bicuspid aortic valve disease has distinctive patterns and usually involves the transverse aortic arch. *J Thorac Cardiovasc Surg* 2008; 135(4):901-907.

74. Feldman DN, Roman MJ: Aneurysms of the sinuses of Valsalva. *Cardiology* 2006; 106(2):73-81.

75. Goldberg N, Krasnow N: Sinus of Valsalva aneurysms. *Clin Cardiol* 1990; 13(12):831-836.

76. Brandt J, Jögi P, Lμhrs C: Sinus of Valsalva aneurysm obstructing coronary arterial flow: case report and collective review of the literature. *Eur Heart J* 1985; 6(12):1069-1073.

77. Collins JS, Evangelista A, Nienaber CA, et al: International Registry of Acute Aortic Dissection (IRAD). Differences in clinical presentation, management, and outcomes of acute type A aortic dissection in patients with and without previous cardiac surgery. *Circulation* 2004; 110(11 Suppl 1):II237-242.

78. Crawford ES, Svensson LG, Coselli JS, et al: Surgical treatment of aneurysm and/or dissection of the ascending aorta, transverse aortic arch, and ascending aorta and transverse aortic arch: factors influencing survival in 717 patients. *J Thorac Cardiovasc Surg* 1989; 98:659.

79. Guthaner DF: The plain chest film in assessing aneurysms and dissecting hematomas of the thoracic aorta, in Taveras JN, Ferrucci JT (eds): *Radiology: Diagnosis-Imaging-Intervention.* Philadelphia, JB Lippincott, 1994.

80. Wiet SP, Pearce WH, McCarthy WJ, Joob AW, Yao JS, McPherson DD: Utility of transesophageal echocardiography in the diagnosis of disease of the thoracic aorta. *J Vasc Surg* 1994; 20(4):613-620.

81. Penco M, Paparoni S, Dagianti A, et al: Usefulness of transesophageal echocardiography in the assessment of aortic dissection. *Am J Cardiol* 2000; 86(4A):53G-56G.

82. Bossone E, Evangelista A, Isselbacher E, et al: International Registry of Acute Aortic Dissection Investigators: Prognostic role of transesophageal echocardiography in acute type A aortic dissection. *Am Heart J* 2007; 153(6):1013-1020.

83. Konstadt SN, Reich DL, Quintana C, Levy M: The ascending aorta: how much does transesophageal echocardiography see? *Anesth Analg* 1994; 78:240.

84. Chung JH, Ghoshhajra BB, Rojas CA, Dave BR, Abbara S: CT angiography of the thoracic aorta. *Radiol Clin North Am* 2010; 48(2):249-264, vii.

85. Chartrand-Lefebvre C, Cadrin-Chênevert A, Bordeleau E, et al: Coronary computed tomography angiography: overview of technical aspects, current concepts, and perspectives. *Can Assoc Radiol J* 2007; 58(2):92-108.

86. Bonnichsen CR, Sundt Iii TM, Anavekar NS, et al: Aneurysms of the ascending aorta and arch: the role of imaging in diagnosis and surgical management. *Expert Rev Cardiovasc Ther* 2011; 9(1):45-61.

87. Hagan PG, Nienaber CA, Isselbacher EM, et al: The International Registry of Acute Aortic Dissection (IRAD): new insights into an old disease. *JAMA* 2000; 283(7):897-903.

88. Bickerstaff LK, Pairolero PC, Hollier LH, et al: Thoracic aortic aneurysms: a population-based study. *Surgery* 1982; 92(6):1103-1108.

89. Coady MA, Rizzo JA, Hammond GL, et al: What is the appropriate size criterion for resection of thoracic aortic aneurysms? *J Thorac Cardiovasc Surg* 1997; 113:476.

90. Masuda Y, Takanashi K, Takasu J, et al: Expansion rate of thoracic aortic aneurysms and influencing factors. *Chest* 1992; 102:461.

91. Hirose Y, Hamada S, Takamiya M, et al: Aortic aneurysms: growth rates measured with CT. *Radiology* 1992; 185:249.

92. Gott VL, Greene PS, Alejo DE, et al: Replacement of the aortic root in patients with Marfan's syndrome. *N Engl J Med* 1999; 340:1307.

93. Murdoch JL, Walker BA, Halpern BL, Kuzma JW, McKusick VA: Life expectancy and causes of death in the Marfan syndrome. *N Engl J Med* 1972; 286(15):804-808.

94. Marsalese DL, Moodie DS, Vacante M, et al: Marfan's syndrome: natural history and long-term follow-up of cardiovascular involvement. *J Am Coll Cardiol* 1989; 14:422.

95. Pape LA, Tsai TT, Isselbacher EM, et al: International Registry of Acute Aortic Dissection (IRAD) Investigators: Aortic diameter > or = 5.5 cm is not a good predictor of type A aortic dissection: observations from the International Registry of Acute Aortic Dissection (IRAD). *Circulation* 2007; 116(10):1120-1127.

96. Palmer RF, Wheat Jr MW: Treatment of dissecting aneurysms of the aorta. *Ann Thorac Surg* 1967; 4:38-52.

97. Wheat Jr M, Palmer RF, Barley TD, et al: Treatment of dissecting aneurysms of the aorta without surgery. *J Thorac Cardiovasc Surg* 1965; 50:364-373.

98. Simpson CF, Boucek RJ: The B-aminopropionitrile fed turkey: a model for detecting potential drug action on arterial tissue, *Cardiovasc Res* 1983; 17(1):26-32.

99. Shores J, Berger KR, Murphy EA, et al: Progression of aortic dilatation and the benefit of long-term beta-adrenergic blockade in Marfan's syndrome. *N Engl J Med* 1994; 330(19):1335-1341.

100. Patel HJ, Deeb GM: Ascending and arch aorta: pathology, natural history and treatment. *Circulation* 2008; 118:188-195.

101. Dapunt OE, Galla JD, Sadeghi AM, et al: The natural history of thoracic aortic aneurysms. *J Thorac Cardiovasc Surg* 1994; 107(5):1323-1332.

102. Davies RR, Gallo A, Coady MA, et al: Novel measurement of relative aortic size predicts rupture of thoracic aortic aneurysms. *Ann Thorac Surg* 2006; 81(1):169-177. Erratum in: *Ann Thorac Surg* 2007 Dec; 84(6):2139.

103. Ergin MA, Spielvogel D, Apaydin A, et al: Surgical treatment of the dilated ascending aorta: when and how? *Ann Thorac Surg* 1999; 67:1834.

104. Baumgartner WA, Cameron DE, Redmond JM, et al: Operative management of Marfan syndrome: the Johns Hopkins experience. *Ann Thorac Surg* 1999; 67:1859.

105. Hiratzka LF, Bakris GL, Beckman JA, Bersin RM, Carr VF, Casey Jr DE: American College of Cardiology Foundation/American Heart Association Task Force on Practice Guidelines, American Association for Thoracic Surgery, American College of Radiology, American Stroke Association, Society of Cardiovascular Anesthesiologists, Society for Cardiovascular Angiography and Interventions, Society of Interventional Radiology, Society of Thoracic Surgeons, Society for Vascular Medicine, et al: 2010 ACCF/AHA/AATS/ACR/ASA/SCA/SCAI/SIR/STS/SVM guidelines for the diagnosis and management of patients with Thoracic Aortic Disease: a report of the American College of Cardiology Foundation/American Heart Association Task Force on Practice Guidelines, American Association for Thoracic Surgery, American College of Radiology, American Stroke Association, Society of Cardiovascular Anesthesiologists, Society for Cardiovascular Angiography and Interventions, Society of Interventional Radiology, Society of Thoracic Surgeons, and Society for Vascular Medicine. *Circulation* 2010; 121(13):266-369.

106. Nishimura RA, Otto CM, Bonow RO, et al: 2014 AHA/ACC guideline for the management of patients with valvular heart disease: a report of the American College of Cardiology/American Heart Association Task Force on Practice Guidelines. *J Thorac Cardiovasc Surg* 2014; 148(1):1-132.

107. Svensson LG, Adams DH, Bonow RO, et al: Aortic valve and ascending aorta guideline for management and quality measures: executive summary. *Ann Thorac Surg* 2013; 95(4):1491-1505.

108. Borger MA, Preston M, Ivanov J, et al: Should the ascending aorta be replaced more frequently in patients with bicuspid aortic valve disease? *J Thorac Cardiovasc Surg* 2004; 128(5):677-683.

109. Prenger K, Pieters F, Cheriex E: Aortic dissection after aortic valve replacement: incidence and consequences for strategy. *J Card Surg* 1994; 9(5):495-498; discussion 498-499.

110. Crawford ES, Svensson LG, Coselli JS, Safi HJ, Hess KR: Surgical treatment of aneurysm and/or dissection of the ascending aorta, transverse aortic arch, and ascending aorta and transverse aortic arch: factors influencing survival in 717 patients. *J Thorac Cardiovasc Surg* 1989; 98:659.

111. Berens ES, Kouchoukos NT, Murphy SF, et al: Preoperative carotid artery screening in elderly patients undergoing cardiac surgery. *J Vasc Surg* 1992; 15:313.

112. O'Blenes SB, Feindel CM: Aortic root replacement with anomalous origin of the coronary arteries. *Ann Thorac Surg* 2002; 73(2):647-649.

113. Murkin JM: NIRS: a standard of care for CPB vs. an evolving standard for selective cerebral perfusion? *J Extra Corpor Technol* 2009; 41(1):P11-114.

114. Appoo JJ, Augoustides JG, Pochettino A, et al: Improving Clinical Outcomes through Clinical Research Investigators: Perioperative outcome in adults undergoing elective deep hypothermic circulatory arrest with retrograde cerebral perfusion in proximal aortic arch repair: evaluation of protocol-based care. *J Cardiothorac Vasc Anesth* 2006; 20(1):3-7.

115. Borst HG, Schaudig A, Rudolph W: Arteriovenous fistula of the aortic arch: repair during deep hypothermia and circulatory arrest. *J Thorac Cardiovasc Surg* 1964; 48:443-447.

116. Barratt-Boyes BG, Simpson M, Neutze JM: Intracardiac surgery in neonates and infants using deep hypothermia with surface cooling and limited cardiopulmonary bypass. *Circulation* 1971; 43:I25-30.

117. Griepp RB, Stinson EB, Hollingsworth JF, Buehler D: Prosthetic replacement of the aortic arch. *J Thorac Cardiovasc Surg* 1975; 70:1051-1063.

118. Michenfelder JD, Theye RA: Hypothermia: effect on canine brain and whole-body metabolism. *Anesthesiology* 1968; 29:1107-1112.

119. Michenfelder JD, Milde JH: The relationship among canine brain temperature, metabolism, and function during hypothermia. *Anesthesiology* 1991; 75:130-136.[PubMed: 2064037]

120. Mault JR, Ohtake S, Klingensmith ME, et al: Cerebral metabolism and circulatory arrest: effects of duration and strategies for protection. *Ann Thorac Surg* 1993; 55:57-63; discussion 4.

121. Svensson L, Crawford E, Hess K, et al: Deep hypothermia with circulatory arrest. Determinants of stroke and early mortality in 656 patients. *J Thorac Cardiovasc Surg* 1993; 106:19-28.

122. Ergin MA, Galla JD, Lansman SL, et al: Hypothermic circulatory arrest in operations on the thoracic aorta. Determinants of operative mortality and neurologic outcome. *J Thorac Cardiovasc Surg* 1994; 107:788-799.

123. Hagl C, Ergin MA, Galla JD, et al: Neurologic outcome after ascending aorta-aortic arch operations: effect of brain protection technique in high-risk patients. *J Thorac Cardiovasc Surg* 2001; 121:1107-1121.

124. Reich DL, Uysal S, Sliwinski M, et al: Neuropsychologic outcome after deep hypothermic circulatory arrest in adults. *J Thorac Cardiovasc Surg* 1999; 117:156-163.

125. Ergin MA, Uysal S, Reich DL, et al: Temporary neurological dysfunction after deep hypothermic circulatory arrest: a clinical marker of long-term functional deficit. *Ann Thorac Surg* 1999; 67:1887-1890; discussion 91-94.

126. McCullough JN, Zhang N, Reich DL, et al: Cerebral metabolic suppression during hypothermic circulatory arrest in humans. *Ann Thorac Surg* 1999; 67:1895-1899; discussion 919-921.

127. Cheung AT, Bavaria JE, Pochettino A, Weiss SJ, Barclay DK, Stecker MM: Oxygen delivery during retrograde cerebral perfusion in humans. *Anesth Analg* 1999; 88(1):8-15.

128. Stecker MM, Cheung AT, Pochettino A, Kent GP, Patterson T, Weiss SJ, Bavaria JE: Deep hypothermic circulatory arrest: I. Effects of cooling on electroencephalogram and evoked potentials. *Ann Thorac Surg* 2001; 71(1):14-21.

129. Mezrow CK, Midulla PS, Sadeghi AM, et al: Quantitative electroencephalography: a method to assess cerebral injury after hypothermic circulatory arrest. *J Thorac Cardiovasc Surg* 1995; 109:925-934.

130. Midulla PS, Gandsas A, Sadeghi AM, et al: Comparison of retrograde cerebral perfusion to antegrade cerebral perfusion and hypothermic circulatory arrest in a chronic porcine model. *J Cardiac Surg* 1994; 9:560-574; discussion 75.

131. Mezrow CK, Gandsas A, Sadeghi AM, et al: Metabolic correlates of neurologic and behavioral injury after prolonged hypothermic circulatory arrest. *J Thorac Cardiovasc Surg* 1995; 109:959-975.[PubMed: 7739258].

132. Frist W, Baldwin JC, Starnes VA, et al: A reconsideration of cerebral perfusion in aortic arch replacement. *Ann Thorac Surg* 1986; 42: 273-281.

133. Bachet J, Guilmet D, Goudot B, et al: Cold cerebroplegia. A new technique of cerebral protection during operations on the transverse aortic arch. *J Thorac Cardiovasc Surg* 1991; 102:85-93; discussion 4.

134. Kazui T, Washiyama N, Muhammad BA, et al: Total arch replacement using aortic arch branched grafts with the aid of antegrade selective cerebral perfusion. *Ann Thorac Surg* 2000; 70:3-8; discussion 9.

135. Di Eusanio M, Schepens MA, Morshuis WJ, et al: Brain protection using antegrade selective cerebral perfusion: a multicenter study. *Ann Thorac Surg* 2003; 76:1181-1189.

136. Sabik JF, Nemeh H, Lytle BW, et al: Cannulation of the axillary artery with a side graft reduces morbidity. *Ann Thorac Surg* 2004; 77:1315.

137. Kazui T: Which is more appropriate as a cerebral protection method-unilateral or bilateral perfusion? *Eur J Cardiothorac Surg* 2006; 29(6):1039-1040.

138. Donaldson RM, Ross DN: Composite graft replacement for the treatment of aneurysms of the ascending aorta associated with aortic valvular disease. *Circulation* 1982; 66(2 Pt 2):I116-121.

139. Volguina IV, Miller DC, LeMaire SA, et al: Aortic Valve Operative Outcomes in Marfan Patients study group: Valve-sparing and valve-replacing techniques for aortic root replacement in patients with Marfan syndrome: analysis of early outcome. *J Thorac Cardiovasc Surg* 2009; 137(5):1124-1132.

140. David TE, Feindel CM, Armstrong S, Maganti M: Replacement of the ascending aorta with reduction of the diameter of the sinotubular junction to treat aortic insufficiency in patients with ascending aortic aneurysm. *J Thorac Cardiovasc Surg* 2007; 133(2):414-418.

141. Burman ED, Keegan J, Kilner PJ: Aortic root measurement by cardiovascular magnetic resonance: specification of planes and lines of measurement and corresponding normal values. *Circ Cardiovasc Imaging* 2008; 1(2):104-113.

142. Kapetanakis EI, Maccarthy P, Monaghan M, Wendler O: Trans-apical aortic valve implantation in a patient with stentless valve degeneration. *Eur J Cardiothorac Surg* 2010; 39:1051-1053.

143. de Sa M, Moshkovitz Y, Butany J, David TE: Histologic abnormalities of the ascending aorta and pulmonary trunk in patients with bicuspid aortic valve disease: clinical relevance to the ross procedure. *J Thorac Cardiovasc Surg* 1999; 118(4):588-594.

144. Westaby S, Saito S, Anastasiadis K, Moorjani N, Jin XY: Aortic root remodeling in atheromatous aneurysms: the role of selected sinus repair. *Eur J Cardiothorac Surg* 2002; 21(3):459-464.

145. David TE, Feindel CM: An aortic valve-sparing operation for patients with aortic incompetence and aneurysm of the ascending aorta. *J Thorac Cardiovasc Surg* 1992; 103(4):617-621.

146. Szeto WY, Moser WG, Desai ND, et al: Transapical deployment of endovascular thoracic aortic stent graft for an ascending aortic pseudoaneurysm. *Ann Thorac Surg* 2010; 89(2):616-618.

147. Roselli EE, Idrees J, Greenberg RK, Johnston DR, Lytle BW: Endovascular stent grafting for ascending aorta repair in high-risk patients. *J Thorac Cardiovasc Surg* 2015; 149(1):144-151.

148. Spielvogel D, Strauch JT, Minanov OP, Lansman SL, Griepp RB: Aortic arch replacement using trifurcated graft and selective cerebral antegrade perfusion. *Ann Thorac Surg* 2002; 74(5):1810-1814.

149. Borst HG, Walterbusch G, Schaps D: Extensive aortic replacement using "elephant trunk" prosthesis. *Thorac Cardiovasc Surg* 1983; 31:37-40.

150. Kuki S, Taniguchi K, Masai T, Endo S: A novel modification of elephant trunk technique using a single four-branched arch graft for extensive thoracic aortic aneurysm. *Eur J Cardiothorac Surg* 2000; 18:246-248.

151. Ius F, Hagl C, Haverich A, Pichlmaier M: Elephant trunk procedure 27 years after Borst: what remains and what is new? *Eur J Cardiothorac Surg* 2011; 40(1):1-11.

152. Toda K, Taniguchi K, Masai T, Takahashi T, Kuki S, Sawa Y: Arch aneurysm repair with long elephant trunk: a 10-year experience in 111 patients. *Ann Thorac Surg* 2009; 88:16-22.

153. Etz C, Plestis KA, Kari FA, et al: Staged repair of thoracic and thoracoabdominal aortic aneurysms using the elephant trunk technique: a consecutive series of 215 first stage and 120 complete repairs. *Eur J Cardiothorac Surg* 2008; 34:605-615.

154. Kouchoukos NT, Mauney MC, Masetti P, Castner CF: Single-stage repair of extensive thoracic aortic aneurysms: experience with the arch-first technique and bilateral anterior thoracotomy. *J Thorac Cardiovasc Surg* 2004; 128:669-676.

155. Milewski RK, Szeto WY, Pochettino A, et al: Have hybrid procedures replaced open aortic arch reconstruction in high-risk patients? A comparative study of elective open arch debranching with endovascular stent graft placement and conventional elective open total and distal aortic arch reconstruction. *J Thorac Cardiovasc Surg* 2010; 140:590-597.

156. Szeto WY, Bavaria JE, Bowen FW, et al: The hybrid total arch repair: brachiocephalic bypass and concomitant endovascular aortic arch stent graft placement. *J Card Surg* 2007; 22:97-102; discussion 103-104.

157. Cao P, De Rango P, Czerny M, et al: Systematic review of clinical outcomes in hybrid procedures for aortic dissections and other arch diseases. *J Thorac Cardiovasc Surg* 2012; 144:1286-1300.

158. Moulakakis KG, Mylonas SN, Dalainas I, et al: The chimney-graft technique for preserving supra-aortic branches: a review. *Ann Cardiothorac Surg* 2013; 2:339-346.

159. Haulon S, Greenberg RK, Spear R, et al: Global experience with an inner branched arch endograft. *J Thorac Cardiovasc Surg* 2014; 148(4):1709-1716.

160. O'Callaghan A, Mastracci TM, Greenberg RK, Eagleton MJ, Bena J, Kuramochi Y. Outcomes for supra-aortic branch vessel stenting in the treatment of thoracic aortic disease. *J Vasc Surg* 2014; 60:914-920.

161. Byers PH: Disorders of collagen biosynthesis and structure, in Schriver CR, Beaudet AL, Sly WS, Valle D (eds): *The Metabolic Basis of Inherited Diseases*. New York, McGraw-Hill, 1995; p 4029.

162. Gillinov AM, Hulyalkar A, Cameron DE, et al: Mitral valve operation in patients with the Marfan syndrome. *J Thorac Cardiovasc Surg* 1994; 107:724.

163. Gill M, Dunning J: Is reduction aortoplasty (with or without external wrap) an acceptable alternative to replacement of the dilated ascending aorta? *Interact Cardiovasc Thorac Surg* 2009; 9(4):693-697.

164. Bauer M, Pasic M, Schaffarzyk R, et al: Reduction aortoplasty for dilatation of the ascending aorta in patients with bicuspid aortic valve. *Ann Thorac Surg* 2002; 73:720-724.

165. Barnett M, Fiore A, Vaca K, Milligan T, Barner H: Tailoring aortoplasty for repair of fusiform ascending aortic aneurysm. *Ann Thorac Surg* 1995; 59:497-501.

166. Neri E, Massetti M, Tanganelli P, et al: Is it only a mechanical matter? Histologic modifications of the aorta underlying external banding. *J Thorac Cardiovasc Surg* 1999; 118(6):1116.

167. Cohen O, Odim J, De la Zerda D, et al: Long-term experience of girdling the ascending aorta with Dacron mesh as definitive treatment for aneurysmal dilation. *Ann Thorac Surg* 2007; 83(2):S780-784.

168. Ohata T, Sakakibara T, Takano H, Ishizaka T: Total arch replacement for thoracic aortic aneurysm via median sternotomy with or without left anterolateral thoracotomy. *Ann Thorac Surg* 2003; 75:1792-1796.

169. Borger MA, Rao V, Weisel RD, et al: Reoperative coronary bypass surgery: effect of patent grafts and retrograde cardioplegia. *J Thorac Cardiovasc Surg* 2001; 121(1):83-90.

170. Thiene G, Valente M: Achilles' heel of stentless porcine valves. *Cardiovasc Pathol* 2007; 16(5):257.

171. Zangrillo A, Mizzi A, Biondi-Zoccai G, et al: Recombinant activated factor VII in cardiac surgery: a meta-analysis. *J Cardiothorac Vasc Anesth* 2009; 23(1):34-40.

172. Jault F, Nataf P, Rama A, et al: Chronic disease of the ascending aorta: surgical treatment and long-term results. *J Thorac Cardiovasc Surg* 1994; 108:747.

173. Lewis CT, Cooley DA, Murphy MC, et al: Surgical repair of aortic root aneurysms in 280 patients. *Ann Thorac Surg* 1992; 53:38.

174. Milewski RK, Pacini D, Moser GW, et al: Retrograde and antegrade cerebral perfusion: results in short elective arch reconstructive times. *Ann Thorac Surg* 2010; 89(5):1448-1457.

175. Svensson LG: Brain protection. *J Card Surg* 1997; 12:326.

176. Royse AG, Royse CF: Epiaortic ultrasound assessment of the aorta in cardiac surgery. *Best Pract Res Clin Anaesthesiol* 2009; 23(3):335-341.

177. Kouchoukos NT: Adjuncts to reduce the incidence of embolic brain injury during operations on the aortic arch. *Ann Thorac Surg* 1994; 57:243.

178. Asimakopoulos G, Smith PL, Ratnatunga CP, Taylor KM: Lung injury and acute respiratory distress syndrome after cardiopulmonary bypass. *Ann Thorac Surg* 1999; 68:1107.

179. Milot J, Perron J, Lacasse Y, Létourneau L, Cartier PC, Maltais F: Incidence and predictors of ARDS after cardiac surgery. *Chest* 2001; 119(3):884-888.

180. Kaul TK, Fields BL, Riggins LS, Wyatt DA, Jones CR, Nagle D: Adult respiratory distress syndrome following cardiopulmonary bypass: incidence, prophylaxis and management. J Cardiovasc Surg (Torino). 1998; 39(6):777-781.

181. Nieman G, Searles B, Carney D, et al: Systemic inflammation induced by cardiopulmonary bypass: a review of pathogenesis and treatment. *J Extra Corpor Technol* 1999; 31(4):202-210.

182. Redmond JM, Gillinov AM, Stuart RS, et al: Heparin-coated bypass circuits reduce pulmonary injury. *Ann Thorac Surg* 1993; 56:474.

183. Kouchoukos NT, Wareing TH, Murphy SF, Perrillo JB: Sixteen-year experience with aortic root replacement: results of 172 operations. *Ann Surg* 1991; 214:308.

184. Schachner T, Vertacnik K, Nagiller J, Laufer G, Bonatti J: Factors associated with mortality and long time survival in patients undergoing modified Bentall operations. *J Cardiovasc Surg (Torino)* 2005; 46(5):449-455.

185. Okita Y, Ando M, Minatoya K, et al: Early and long-term results of surgery for aneurysms of the thoracic aorta in septuagenarians and octogenarians. *Eur J Cardiothorac Surg* 1999; 16:317.

186. Fleck TM, Koinig H, Czerny M, et al: Impact of surgical era on outcomes of patients undergoing elective atherosclerotic ascending aortic aneurysm operations. *Eur J Cardiothorac Surg* 2004; 26:342.

187. Gott VL, Gillinov AM, Pyeritz RE, et al: Aortic root replacement: risk factor analysis of a seventeen-year experience with 270 patients. *J Thorac Cardiovasc Surg* 1995; 109:536.

188. Cohn LH, Rizzo RJ, Adams DH, et al: Reduced mortality and morbidity for ascending aortic aneurysm resection regardless of cause. *Ann Thorac Surg* 1996; 62:463.

189. Mingke D, Dresler C, Stone CD, Borst HG: Composite graft replacement of the aortic root in 335 patients with aneurysm or dissection. *Thorac Cardiovasc Surg* 1998; 46:12.

190. Estrera AL, Miller CC 3rd, Huynh TT, et al: Replacement of the ascending and transverse aortic arch: determinants of long-term survival. *Ann Thorac Surg* 2002; 74:1058.

191. Ergin MA, Spielvogel D, Apaydin A, et al: Surgical treatment of the dilated ascending aorta: when and how? *Ann Thorac Surg* 1999; 67:1834.

192. Gott VL, Gillinov AM, Pyeritz RE, et al: Aortic root replacement: risk factor analysis of a seventeen-year experience with 270 patients. *J Thorac Cardiovasc Surg* 1995; 109:536.

193. Taniguchi K, Nakano S, Matsuda H, et al: Long-term survival and complications after composite graft replacement for ascending aortic aneurysm associated with aortic regurgitation. *Circulation* 1991; 84:III3.

194. Lewis CT, Cooley DA, Murphy MC, et al: Surgical repair of aortic root aneurysms in 280 patients. *Ann Thorac Surg* 1992; 53:38.

195. Raudkivi PJ, Williams JD, Monro JL, Ross JK: Surgical treatment of the ascending aorta: fourteen years' experience with 83 patients. *J Thorac Cardiovasc Surg* 1989; 98:675.

196. Jault F, Nataf P, Rama A, et al: Chronic disease of the ascending aorta: surgical treatment and long-term results. *J Thorac Cardiovasc Surg* 1994; 108:747.

197. Bhan A, Choudhary SK, Saikia M, et al: Surgical experience with dissecting and nondissecting aneurysms of the ascending aorta. *Indian Heart J* 2001; 53:319.

198. Crawford ES, Svensson LG, Coselli JS, et al: Surgical treatment of aneurysm and/or dissection of the ascending aorta, transverse aortic arch, and ascending aorta and transverse aortic arch: factors influencing survival in 717 patients. *J Thorac Cardiovasc Surg* 1989; 98:659.

199. Silva J, Maroto LC, Carnero M, et al: Ascending aorta and aortic root reoperations: are outcomes worse than first time surgery? *Ann Thorac Surg* 2010; 90(2):555-560.

200. Szeto WY, Bavaria JE, Bowen FW, et al: Reoperative aortic root replacement in patients with previous aortic surgery. *Ann Thorac Surg* 2007; 84(5):1592-1598; discussion 1598-1599.

201. Detter C, Mair H, Klein HG, et al: Long-term prognosis of surgically-treated aortic aneurysms and dissections in patients with and without Marfan syndrome. *Eur J Cardiothorac Surg* 1998; 13:416.

202. Sioris T, David TE, Ivanov J, Armstrong S, Feindel CM: Clinical outcomes after separate and composite replacement of the aortic valve and ascending aorta. *J Thorac Cardiovasc Surg* 2004; 128(2):260-265.

203. Ng SK, O'Brien MF, Harrocks S, McLachlan GJ: Influence of patient age and implantation technique on the probability of re-replacement of the homograft aortic valve. *J Heart Valve Dis* 2002; 11(2):217-223.

204. Luciani GB, Casali G, Faggian G, Mazzucco A: Predicting outcome after reoperative procedures on the aortic root and ascending aorta. *Eur J Cardiothorac Surg* 2000; 17:602.

205. Kouchoukos NT, Wareing TH, Murphy SF, Perrillo JB: Sixteen-year experience with aortic root replacement: results of 172 operations. *Ann Surg* 1991; 214:308.

206. Svensson LG, Blackstone EH, Feng J, et al: Are Marfan syndrome and marfanoid patients distinguishable on long-term follow-up? *Ann Thorac Surg* 2007; 83(3):1067-1074.

207. Gott VL, Greene PS, Alejo DE, et al: Replacement of the aortic root in patients with Marfan's syndrome. *N Engl J Med* 1999; 340:1307.

208. Lytle BW, Sabik JF, Blackstone EH, Svensson LG, Pettersson GB, Cosgrove DM 3rd: Reoperative cryopreserved root and ascending aorta replacement for acute aortic prosthetic valve endocarditis. *Ann Thorac Surg* 2002; 74(5):S1754-1757; S1792-9.

209. Coselli JS, Crawford ES, Williams TW Jr, et al: Treatment of postoperative infection of ascending aorta and transverse aortic arch, including use of viable omentum and muscle flaps. *Ann Thorac Surg* 1990; 50:868.

210. Nakajima N, Masuda M, Ichinose M, Ando M: A new method for the treatment of graft infection in the thoracic aorta: in situ preservation. *Ann Thorac Surg* 1999; 67:1994.

211. Coselli JS, Koksoy C, LeMaire SA: Management of thoracic aortic graft infections. *Ann Thorac Surg* 1999; 67:1990.

212. Keown PP, Miller DC, Jamieson SW, et al: Diagnosis of arterial prosthetic graft infection by indium-111 oxine white blood cell scans. *Circulation* 1982; 66:I130.

213. Hargrove WC 3rd, Edmunds LH Jr: Management of infected thoracic aortic prosthetic grafts. *Ann Thorac Surg* 1984; 37:72.

214. Ninomiya M, Makuuchi H, Naruse Y, Kobayashi T, Sato T: Surgical management of ascending aortic graft infection. No-sedation-technique for open mediastinal irrigation. *Jpn J Thorac Cardiovasc Surg* 2000; 48(10):666-669.

Descending and Thoracoabdominal Aortic Aneurysms

Joseph S. Coselli • Kim de la Cruz • Ourania Preventza • Scott A. LeMaire

Treating aneurysms that arise from the aortic segments distal to the left subclavian artery poses challenges that are distinct from those presented by aneurysms of the more proximal ascending and arch segments. The distal aortic segments comprise the descending thoracic aorta, which extends from the left subclavian artery to the diaphragm within the chest, and the abdominal segment that extends from the diaphragm to the iliac bifurcation. The diaphragm divides the thoracic aorta from the abdominal aorta.

An aortic aneurysm that is limited to the chest (distal to the left subclavian artery) is classified as a descending thoracic aortic aneurysm (DTAA). An aortic aneurysm that traverses the diaphragm and extends into both the chest and the abdomen to any degree is considered a thoracoabdominal aortic aneurysm (TAAA) (Fig. 49-1). Aneurysms in these locations can be extensive and can involve many or all of the aortic branch vessels. In the last decade there have been substantial changes regarding the treatment of distal aortic aneurysms because of the emergence of thoracic endovascular aortic repair (TEVAR) and its near dominance in DTAA repair. Although open repair remains the standard of care for TAAAs, it is now selectively used for DTAAs. Modern critical care and continually refined surgical adjuncts for organ protection have made the outcomes of surgical repair better than they were in previous decades, but operative treatment of DTAA and TAAA continues to represent a significant clinical challenge to the cardiovascular surgeon.

PATHOGENESIS

The etiology of DTAA and TAAA has changed over time. Whereas tertiary syphilis was the most common cause of thoracic aneurysms in the early 1900s, other causes are more prevalent today. Well-established causes of DTAA and TAAA include medial degeneration, atherosclerosis, aortic dissection, connective tissue disorders, aortitis (eg, Takayasu arteritis), aortic coarctation, infection, and trauma. As our understanding of genetics increases, and as more advanced genetic testing becomes available, classification systems are likely to evolve to include more molecular factors. Perhaps partly because of improved screening for aneurysmal disease and the increasing age of the population, it is certain that the incidence and prevalence of thoracic aortic aneurysms are increasing over time.[1]

The most common types of aneurysms of the descending and thoracoabdominal aorta today are grouped into the category of atherosclerotic aneurysms. Unfortunately, although this term may be descriptive, it may not accurately describe the mechanism of aneurysmal changes. Although atherosclerosis and aortic aneurysms share common risk factors and frequently coexist, thoracic aortic aneurysms are primarily the result of age-related medial degeneration, which is characterized by changes in elastin and collagen that reduce aortic integrity and tensile strength. Subsequent aortic enlargement and aneurysm formation provide fertile ground for superimposed intimal atherosclerosis and further degeneration of the aortic wall. The usual histologic changes in the aging aorta include elastin fragmentation, fibrosis with increased collagen deposition, and medial degeneration.[2] As with most aneurysmogenic processes, medial degeneration usually causes diffuse, fusiform aortic dilatation. In some cases, medial degeneration produces discrete saccular aneurysms along the descending thoracic aorta; however, saccular aneurysms are more commonly associated with aortic infection (see below). Additionally, saccular aneurysms may be superimposed on or coexist with more generalized, fusiform aneurysmal disease of the thoracoabdominal aorta.

Risk factors for aortic dissection and aortic aneurysm overlap to a great extent, but once an aorta becomes dissected, the dissection itself becomes an independent risk factor for subsequent dilation and aneurysmal changes. Two of the DeBakey types of aortic dissection involve the distal aorta: type I, in

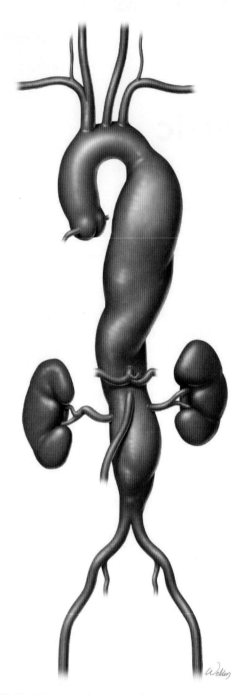

FIGURE 49-1 Drawing depicting a thoracoabdominal aortic aneurysm. (Printed with permission from Baylor College of Medicine.)

which nearly the entire length of the aorta is dissected, and type III, in which the dissection is limited to varying portions of the distal aorta, and the proximal aorta is unaffected. Aortic dissections occur in the medial layer separating the intima from the adventitia; blood flows through the true aortic lumen and through one or more false lumen channels that can form at various points along the aorta. This process weakens the outer aortic wall, making it prone to progressive aneurysmal dilatation (Fig. 49-2).

In survivors of DeBakey type I dissection, the persistence of a pressurized false lumen has been associated with subsequent distal aneurysm formation, need for intervention, and increased mortality.[3] In an attempt to thrombose the false channel and thereby decrease the risk of late aneurysm formation, endovascular strategies have been developed to exclude segments of the false lumen in both acute (≤2 weeks since onset)[4] and chronic[5] aortic dissection. Such approaches are dependent on a variety of factors, including the extent of aortic dissection; downstream portions of the false lumen—those without endovascular obliteration—continue to be pressurized and may perfuse upstream portions in a retrograde fashion.

Penetrating aortic ulcers and intramural hematomas are two variants of aortic dissection that can occur in the descending and abdominal aortic segments. Penetrating aortic ulcers are disrupted atherosclerotic plaques that can penetrate the aortic wall, leading to classic dissection or rupture. Intramural hematomas are collections of blood within the aortic wall that occur without an intimal tear; growth of the hematoma can result in classic dissection.

Genetic mutations or defects can give rise to defective components of the aortic extracellular matrix, leading to aortic aneurysm and dissection. Aortic aneurysms that occur in patients with these genetic disorders can be a part of a named syndrome, accompanied by a constellation of extra-aortic symptoms, or they may be part of a heterogeneous group of familial thoracic aortic aneurysms and dissections that occur in isolation. In a national registry of genetically triggered thoracic aortic aneurysms, Marfan syndrome is the most common genetic cause of aortic aneurysms (36%).[6] Marfan syndrome is a connective tissue disorder that results

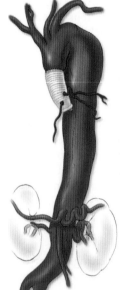
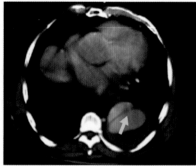

FIGURE 49-2 Drawing and computed tomography image of a thoracoabdominal aortic aneurysm caused by dilatation of the false lumen in a patient with chronic aortic dissection.

from a fibrillin-1 (FBN1) gene mutation; the altered fibrillin leads to aberrant signaling of transforming growth factor beta (TGF-β) and other events that lead to the deposition of extensive amounts of mucopolysaccharides in the aortic extracellular matrix and fragmentation of elastic fibers. The aorta in Marfan syndrome patients is prone to dissection, which is the most common cause of DTAAs and TAAAs in these patients.[7,8] Other syndromes that are infrequently encountered during DTAA and TAAA repairs include vascular Ehlers-Danlos, aneurysms-osteoarthritis, and Loeys-Dietz. Like Marfan syndrome, Loeys-Dietz syndrome is an autosomal dominant disorder that is linked to an alteration in TGF-β signaling. First described in 2005, Loeys-Dietz is a particularly aggressive aortic disorder, characterized by vascular tortuosity, and a greater propensity for rupture at smaller aortic diameters than in patients with Marfan syndrome. Recently, four types of Loeys-Dietz have been identified, each associated with a mutation in a particular gene: transforming growth factor (TGF)-beta receptor I (*TGFBR1*), TGF-beta receptor II (*TGFBR2*), decapentaplegic homolog 3 (*SMAD3*), and transforming growth factor beta 2 ligand (*TGFB2*).[9]

Both chronic, nonspecific aortitis and systemic autoimmune disorders—such as Takayasu arteritis, giant cell arteritis (temporal arteritis), and rheumatoid aortitis—can cause destruction of the aortic media and progressive aneurysm formation. Although Takayasu arteritis usually causes obstructive lesions related to severe intimal thickening, the associated medial destruction can result in aneurysmal dilatation.

Aneurysms involving the upper descending thoracic aorta can develop in patients with congenital aortic coarctation. These aneurysms may occur concomitantly with unrepaired native coarctation or years after any manner of coarctation repair, including endovascular repair.[10,11] The postrepair aneurysms appear to be more common in patients who have had balloon angioplasty than in those who underwent surgery; this is speculated to be due to the rupture of elastic fibers during dilatation.[11]

Infection can produce a saccular "mycotic" aneurysm in a localized area of the aortic wall that has been damaged by the infectious process. For unknown reasons, such mycotic aneurysms tend to occur along the lesser curvature of the transverse aortic arch or in the upper abdominal aorta adjacent to the origins of the visceral branches. In such cases, only a portion of the aortic circumference is affected; consequently, localized weakening causes a diverticular or saccular outpouching. Common causative organisms include *Staphylococcus aureus*, *Staphylococcus epidermidis*, *Salmonella*, and *Streptococcus*,[12] and more than one pathogen may be present. Although uncommon, when a distal mycotic aneurysm is suspected, urgent evaluation is warranted; mycotic saccular aneurysms tend to be unpredictable, often have periods of rapid growth, and rupture more readily than fusiform aneurysms caused by medial degeneration.[13]

Each of the disease processes described above causes aneurysms through progressive degeneration and dilatation of the aortic wall. In contrast, pseudoaneurysms of the thoracic aorta form as the result of chronic leaks through discrete defects in the aortic wall. These leaks are initially contained by surrounding tissue; the accumulation of organized thrombus and the associated fibrosis forms the wall of the pseudoaneurysm. Pseudoaneurysms can develop after aortic surgery, endovascular aortic repair, invasive imaging, or from primary defects in the aortic wall. Unrepaired blunt and penetrating injuries are the other common cause of aortic pseudoaneurysms. Chronic traumatic pseudoaneurysms typically develop in the proximal descending thoracic aorta after blunt aortic injuries; the management of these lesions is covered in detail in a subsequent chapter.

NATURAL HISTORY

An untreated aneurysm in the thoracic and thoracoabdominal aorta can progress to dissection, rupture, or both if given enough time. A dissected aorta that was originally of normal caliber will tend to dilate and become aneurysmal. The causes and genetics of these aneurysms vary, but there are commonalities in the mechanical and pathophysiologic aspects of their formation and development. Understanding these processes will help surgeons determine the timing and the nature of the operative intervention needed.

An aneurysm is defined as a permanent dilation of an artery to at least 1.5 times its normal diameter at a given location.[14] However, the normal aortic diameter is perhaps more difficult to define because it varies by the patient's age, gender, and body size. Even when adjusted for age and body surface area, mean aortic size is significantly smaller in women than in men; on average, aortic diameter is 2 to 3 mm greater in men than in women. In the community-based Framingham Heart Study, computed tomography studies from 3431 adults, at least 35 years old, were analyzed by age, gender, and body surface area. At the descending thoracic aorta, the average aortic diameter was 25.8 mm for men and 23.1 mm for women; at the infrarenal abdominal aorta, it was 19.3 mm for men and 16.7 mm for women; and at the lower abdominal aorta, it was 18.7 mm for men and 16.0 mm for women.[15] In this study, aortic enlargement was strongly correlated with male gender, advancing age, and increased body surface area—for men ≥ 65 years old and with a large body surface area (≥2.1), the mean descending thoracic aortic diameter increased by 4.5 to 30.3 mm; and for women ≥ 65 years and with a large body surface area (≥1.9), this increased by 4.0 to 27.1 mm. Notably, body surface area is a better predictor of aortic size than height or weight, particularly in patients less than 50 years of age.[16]

The descending thoracic aorta has a slightly higher rate of expansion over time than the ascending aorta and is noted to average 1 to 4 mm/year.[17] The rate is not constant, and it increases as the diameter increases. A dissection in an otherwise small aneurysm can lead to a sudden increase in the rate of growth; likewise, a chronically dissected aorta tends to dilate at a faster rate than a nondissected one. The relationship among pressure, vessel diameter, and vessel wall tension is described by Laplace's law. As the luminal diameter increases, there is increasing wall tension, which in turn contributes to the cycle of progressive dilatation. Unfortunately, as the dilation progresses, the wall tension eventually becomes too great for the maximally stretched aortic wall. A tear can occur within the intimal and medial layers, resulting in a dissection that propagates down the length of the aorta, or a tear can penetrate the full thickness of the aortic wall, resulting in contained or free rupture. The aortic size at which this event occurs is determined by several factors, including the presence or absence of a connective tissue disorder, the presence and severity of hypertension, and the patient's body size. In a large series of patients, Elefteriades and colleagues[18] have shown that in the thoracic aorta, there is a sharp increase in the incidence of aortic complications at aneurysmal diameters greater than 6 cm, with a 14% combined risk of rupture, dissection, and death. In a population-based study, the 5-year risk of rupture doubled from 16% for aneurysms 4 to 5.9 cm in diameter to 31% in aneurysms 6 cm or more in diameter.[19]

CLINICAL PRESENTATION AND DIAGNOSIS

At the time of diagnosis, patients with DTAAs and TAAAs are commonly asymptomatic. For example, Panneton and Hollier[20] reported that degenerative TAAAs are asymptomatic in roughly 43% of patients. In asymptomatic patients, DTAAs and TAAAs are often discovered when imaging studies are performed to evaluate unrelated problems. For example, computed tomography scans may indicate aortic dilatation, and chest radiographs may show widening of the descending thoracic aortic shadow, which may be outlined by a rim of calcification outlining the dilated aneurysmal aortic wall (Fig. 49-3). Aneurysmal calcium may also be seen in the upper abdomen on standard radiograms.

Although DTAAs and TAAAs remain asymptomatic for long periods of time, most ultimately produce a variety of symptoms before they rupture. Degenerative TAAAs produce symptoms in approximately 57% of patients; 9% of patients present with rupture.[20] The most frequent symptom is back pain between the scapulae. When the aneurysm is large in the region of the aortic hiatus, pressure on adjacent structures may cause mid-back and epigastric pain. Other potential signs and symptoms related to compression or erosion of adjacent organs include stridor, wheezing, cough, hemoptysis, dysphagia, and gastrointestinal obstruction or bleeding. Hoarseness results from traction on the vagus nerve as the distal aortic arch expands and causes recurrent laryngeal nerve paralysis. Thoracic or lumbar vertebral body erosion (Fig. 49-4) causes back pain, spinal instability, and neurologic deficits from spinal cord compression; mycotic aneurysms have a peculiar propensity to destroy vertebral bodies. Additionally, neurologic symptoms, including paraplegia, paraparesis, or both, may result from thrombosis of intercostal and lumbar arteries. This is most frequently seen with acute aortic dissection, which may occur primarily or be superimposed on medial degenerative fusiform aneurysmal

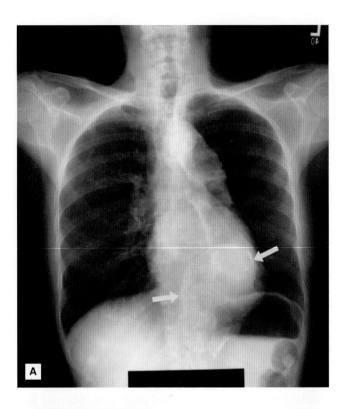

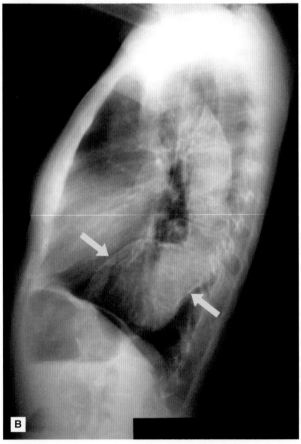

FIGURE 49-3 Chest radiographs in (A) posteroanterior and (B) lateral projections showing the calcified wall (arrows) of a thoracoabdominal aortic aneurysm.

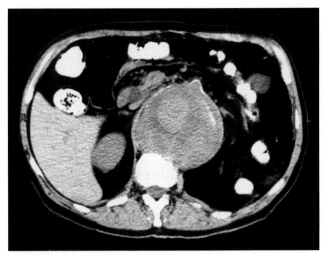

FIGURE 49-4 Computed tomography image of a large thoracoabdominal aortic aneurysm that has caused erosion of the adjacent vertebral body.

disease. Thoracic aortic aneurysms, like aneurysms in other locations, may produce distal emboli of clot or atheromatous debris that gradually obliterate and thrombose visceral, renal, or lower-extremity branches.

Imaging technology is critical in diagnosis and determining anatomic details for operative planning. Computed tomography (CT) scanning and magnetic resonance angiography (MRA) enable clinicians to obtain excellent images without the potential morbidity or cost associated with angiography. CT scanning is widely available and can image the entire thoracic and abdominal aorta, major branch vessels, and virtually all adjacent organs. Computer programs can construct sagittal, coronal, and oblique images, as well as three-dimensional reconstructions, from CT data. Contrast-enhanced CT scanning (Figs. 49-2, 49-4, and 49-5) also provides information about the aortic lumen, intraluminal thrombus, presence of aortic dissection, intramural hematoma, mediastinal or retroperitoneal hematoma, aortic rupture, and periaortic fibrosis associated with inflammatory aneurysms.[21] CT angiography with multiplanar reconstruction is especially useful for planning endovascular procedures. Advantages of CT include being less expensive and somewhat quicker to perform than MRA and, at present, the wider availability of CT expertise. Also, CT can be used with patients who have implanted ferromagnetic prostheses or other devices, which can cause injury in patients undergoing MRA. The chief advantages of MRA are that it does not expose the patient to ionizing radiation and that it reveals disease within the aortic wall, including intramural hemorrhage. The gadolinium-based contrast agents used in MRA were once considered to be safer for patients with renal insufficiency than CT contrast media. Ironically, reports have associated the use of certain gadolinium-based contrast agents with nephrogenic

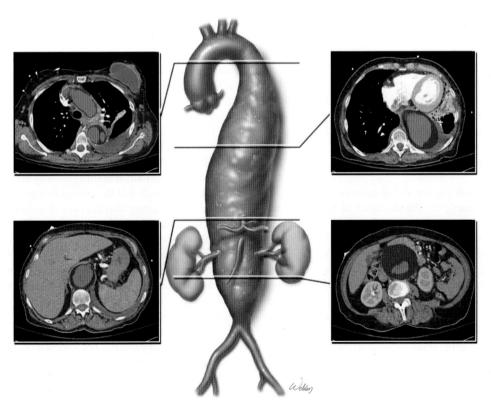

FIGURE 49-5 Drawing and contrast-enhanced computed tomography images of a degenerative extent II thoracoabdominal aortic aneurysm with extensive intraluminal thrombus.

systemic fibrosis (NSF)—a scleroderma-like fibrotic process that can affect not only the skin but also internal organs—in patients with renal insufficiency.[22] The current recommendation is to avoid using such agents in patients with advanced renal failure (ie, with a glomerular filtration rate < 30 mL/min) or in patients who are dialysis-dependent.[23]

Ongoing improvements in noninvasive imaging modalities have substantially reduced the role of catheter aortography in assessing thoracic aortic aneurysms. However, catheter aortography remains useful in situations where noninvasive methods are not feasible—for example, when artifact or heavy calcification obscures the area of interest. Anterior, posterior, oblique, and lateral views provide detailed information about branch vessels. The risks posed by aortography include renal toxicity from the large volumes of contrast material required to adequately fill large aneurysms. There is also a risk of embolization from laminated thrombus secondary to manipulation of intraluminal catheters. Furthermore, angiography underestimates the size of an aneurysm in areas of laminated thrombus. Nonetheless, angiography can be helpful in patients with suspected renal or visceral ischemia, aortoiliac occlusive disease, horseshoe kidney, or peripheral aneurysms.

DETERMINING APPROPRIATE TREATMENT

Whenever possible, patients with known aortic disease (ie, patients with previous aortic dissection, prior aortic repair, or abnormal aortic diameter) are regularly followed by an imaging surveillance protocol to monitor the possible development of distal aortic aneurysm. For this and other incidental findings, once an aneurysm involving the descending thoracic or thoracoabdominal aorta has been discovered, precise determination of the extent and severity of disease is the critical next step toward clarifying the specific diagnosis, determining the appropriate treatment, and, when repair is indicated, planning the appropriate intervention.

Indications for Operation

In asymptomatic patients, the decision to consider surgical repair is based primarily on the diameter of the aneurysm. To prevent fatal rupture, current guidelines recommend elective operation when the aortic diameter exceeds 5.5 cm in cases of chronic dissection and 6 cm in cases of degenerative aneurysm. In patients with connective tissue disorders, such as Marfan syndrome and related disorders, the diameter-based threshold for operation is lowered. Although guidelines specify a rapid dilatation rate for only the proximal aorta, indicating repair when expansion exceeds 0.5 cm/year, it is not unreasonable to apply this threshold to the distal aorta as well.[24] Nonoperative management—which consists of strict blood pressure control, cessation of smoking, and at least yearly surveillance with imaging studies—is appropriate for asymptomatic patients who have small aneurysms. Symptomatic patients, however, are at increased risk of rupture and

warrant expeditious evaluation and urgent aneurysm repair, even when the abovementioned threshold diameters have not been reached. The onset of new pain in a patient with a known aneurysm is particularly concerning and often heralds significant expansion, leakage, or impending rupture. Malperfusion caused by chronic dissection is also an indication for TAAA repair. Degenerative DTAAs and TAAAs with superimposed acute dissection are especially prone to rupture and are therefore treated with emergent repair.

Endovascular Considerations

Since 2005, when a TEVAR device was approved by the US Food and Drug Administration (FDA) to treat DTAA, indications for TEVAR have expanded, and TEVAR devices are now approved for treating all lesions of the descending thoracic aorta—acute or chronic aortic dissection, penetrating aortic ulcer, and blunt trauma—with suitable anatomy. In contrast, custom-manufactured fenestrated or branched endovascular repair of TAAA remains experimental in the United States with ongoing clinical trials.[25] Although endovascular repairs are covered in detail in a subsequent chapter, all patients in our practice are evaluated for possible endovascular intervention, and an individualized surgical option best suited for the patient is selected. Appropriate anatomy is also critical for successful endovascular repair. Landing zones that have inadequate length, excessive angulation, extensive intraluminal thrombus, dissection in the proximal landing zone, or severe vessel calcification will not allow secure endograft fixation, precluding endovascular repair. Two important factors to consider when deciding between open and endovascular aneurysm repair are the patient's physiologic reserve and vascular anatomy.[26] Open repairs have well-documented outcomes and excellent long-term durability, and they allow repair of aneurysms with complex anatomy. However, the patients must have considerable physiologic reserve to undergo and recover from these procedures.

Hybrid, off-label approaches that combine open and endovascular repair have been selectively used to repair DTAAs and TAAAs. A common type of hybrid DTAA repair involves extending the proximal landing zone by rerouting the left subclavian artery such that the endograft may cover the ostia of the left subclavian artery; this has been done in fairly large numbers of patients and is thought to add little risk and protect against the risk of stroke.[27] Additionally, a traditional open "elephant trunk" repair—which leaves a small section of replacement graft floating in the descending thoracic aorta after replacing the aortic arch—can be subsequently combined with TEVAR, either as part of the initial repair or in a subsequent procedure (see following section). Hybrid "elephant trunk" procedures involve landing the proximal portion of the endograft in the trunk, but this approach is not widely used. In contrast, "frozen elephant trunk" procedures (performed in a single stage) are now commonly performed in Europe, especially for the treatment of acute DeBakey type I dissections, with the use of several readily available hybrid devices. The ultimate goal of this approach is to thrombose the false lumen to prevent additional late aortic complications.[28] In the United States, there are several versions of this approach, including the antegrade placement of the endograft in the proximal descending thoracic aorta after proximal hemiarch repair.[29]

Hybrid TAAA approaches typically involve open visceral bypass grafting, which is performed to secure organ perfusion, and followed by stent-graft coverage of the entire aneurysm, including visceral and other branch-vessel ostia. However, a recent approach to hybrid TAAA repair involves replacing the visceral portion of aorta with a multibranched graft in an open fashion (such as in an extent III or IV repair) and repairing the more proximal section of the descending thoracic aorta with a stent graft that is then secured to the proximal section of the multibranched graft.[30] Although hybrid TAAA procedures are somewhat less invasive than open TAAA repair, they have not yet yielded a substantial decrease in morbidity and mortality rates, and patient fitness must again be considered in order to obtain an optimal outcome.[31]

Other off-label approaches to TAAA repair include the use of parallel grafts (also called "chimney," "sandwich," or "snorkel" approaches); a large diameter endograft is used to cover the aneurysm, and a small diameter stent is run parallel to the main endograft and into branching arteries so that they are perfused. In select patients with substantial comorbidities, parallel endovascular repair remains an option; however, because published reports describe only small patient series,[25] it is difficult to judge the utility of this approach. The same is true for the multilayer modulator stent, which is now being used for TAAA repair outside the United States, because only short-term data are available.[32]

Endovascular descending thoracic aortic repair is widespread, and its use to treat degenerative aneurysm should be strongly considered when feasible per current US guidelines.[24] Furthermore, recent 5-year evidence from the INSTEAD-XL randomized trial of 140 patients with uncomplicated chronic aortic dissection who underwent either optimal medical therapy or TEVAR with optimal medical therapy suggests that TEVAR substantially improves late aortic-specific survival and delays disease progression.[5] Data suggest that, in general, endovascular repair of the descending thoracic aorta is associated with less early mortality and morbidity than open repair,[33,34] and TEVAR is less likely to be affected by whether the repair is performed at a high-volume or low-volume center,[35] even in cases of rupture.[36] However, the early survival benefit may be lost within a few years after repair, because 5-year survival is similar between those with open and endovascular Medicare cohorts[37] or is worse after endovascular repair.[38,39] There also appears to be a greater need for reintervention after TEVAR than after open DTAA repair.[39-41] Of interest, emerging evidence suggests that different aortic pathologies (degenerative aneurysm vs chronic dissection vs acute dissection) are associated with different modes of repair failure after TEVAR.[42,43]

Because endovascular aortic repair has become substantially more common in recent years and the indications for its use have evolved, these devices are increasingly encountered in subsequent open operations. Complications after endovascular repair may result from progression of the aneurysmal process to an adjacent portion of the aorta that is not amenable to further endovascular treatment, progressive dilation of the treated segment owing to persistent endoleak, infection of the endovascular device, or device migration. In certain cases, endovascular devices do not incorporate into the aneurysm thrombus and aortic intima in the way that conventional Dacron grafts incorporate into the periadventitial tissue. Explantation of the endovascular device and open graft replacement of the thoracic aorta can be accomplished with relatively good success.[44-46] In the absence of infection, salvaging the device or portions of the device is also possible. Although we have applied the aortic cross-clamp to a proximal aortic segment with an endovascular stent graft in place and repaired a distal segment in an open fashion, in cases in which the stent graft encroaches on the aortic arch, it may not be possible to place a cross-clamp, and hypothermic circulatory arrest may be needed. Suturing an existing stent graft to a standard Dacron graft in a hemostatic fashion is also feasible, particularly if the surrounding aortic tissue can be incorporated into the suture line. Notably, endovascular aortic repair in patients with connective tissue disorders is not supported by current US guidelines;[24] however, selective use as bridge to open repair or to treat late complications of open repair may be an appropriate strategy.[47,48]

PREOPERATIVE EVALUATION

In each patient, the indications for operation discussed above are weighed against the risks posed by surgical intervention.[49,50] The Crawford classification of TAAA (Fig. 49-6) permits standardized reporting of the extent of aortic involvement, thereby allowing appropriate risk stratification, choice of specific treatment modalities according to the extent of the aneurysm, and a type-specific determination of the risks for neurologic deficits and other morbidities and mortality associated with TAAA repair. Extent I TAAA repairs involve replacing most or all of the descending thoracic aorta and the upper abdominal aorta. Extent II repairs involve most or all of the descending thoracic aorta and extend into the infrarenal abdominal aorta. Extent III repairs involve the distal half or less of the descending thoracic aorta and varying portions of the abdominal aorta. Extent IV repairs involve most or all of the abdominal aorta. In general, less extensive distal aortic repair (DTAA, extents III and IV TAAA) tend to pose less operative risk than more extensive distal aortic repair (extents I and II TAAA), although patient-specific disease, such as having a heavy atherosclerotic burden, can increase risk in lesser repairs.

Most commonly, patients with DTAA and TAAA meeting criteria for repair are in their mid-to-late 60s. Younger patients tend to include those patients with connective tissue disorders or chronic aortic dissection. Additionally, there appears to be substantial differences in patient characteristics by extent of repair. Regarding our comprehensive TAAA experience,[51] about 10% of TAAA patients have a connective tissue disorder; however, this increases to 17% in extent II repairs and decreases to 5% in extent IV TAAA repair. Chronic aortic

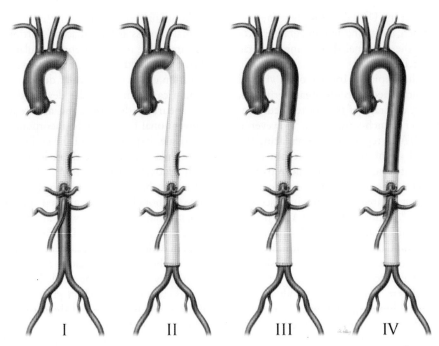

FIGURE 49-6 The Crawford classification of thoracoabdominal aortic aneurysm repairs. (Printed with permission from Baylor College of Medicine.)

dissection is present in nearly a third of patients; this proportion is increased in extent I and II repairs (39 and 44%, respectively) and decreased in extent III and IV repairs (19 and 11%, respectively). Furthermore, while roughly a quarter of TAAA patients have had a prior distal aortic repair, this rate is increased in extent III and IV repairs (42 and 36%)—this speaks to the progressive nature of repair in extents III and IV, as many of these prior repairs were abdominal aortic repairs.

An adequate preoperative assessment of physiologic reserve is critical in evaluating operative risk. Many patients have significant comorbidities; chronic pulmonary obstructive disease, coronary artery disease, hypertension, cerebrovascular disease, and peripheral vascular disease are all relatively common in TAAA repair. Chronic elevated serum creatinine levels (>3.0 mg/dL) are relatively uncommon in patients undergoing TAAA repair, and affect 3% of patients in our experience.[51] Unless they require emergency operation, patients undergo a thorough preoperative evaluation with emphasis on cardiac, pulmonary, and renal function.

Cardiac Status

Impaired myocardial contractility and reduced coronary reserve are common among elderly patients who undergo aortic reconstruction. Patients need substantial cardiac reserve in order to tolerate clamping of the thoracic aorta. Given the prevalence of preoperative cardiac disease and the physiologic strain of aortic clamping, it is not surprising that cardiac complications are a major cause of postoperative mortality. Reports indicate that cardiac disease has been responsible for 49% of early deaths and 34% of late deaths after TAAA repair, attesting to the importance of careful preoperative cardiac evaluation.[20,52]

Several imaging techniques are useful in preoperative screening for cardiac disease. Transthoracic echocardiography is noninvasive and can satisfactorily evaluate both valvular and biventricular function. Dipyridamole-thallium myocardial scanning identifies regions of myocardium that are reversibly ischemic, and it is more practical than exercise testing in this generally elderly population, whose exercise capacity is often limited by concurrent lower-extremity peripheral vascular disease. In patients with evidence of reversible ischemia on noninvasive studies, and in those with a significant history of angina or an ejection fraction of 30% or less, cardiac catheterization and coronary arteriography are performed. Patients who have asymptomatic aneurysms and severe coronary artery occlusive disease (ie, significant left main, proximal left anterior descending, or triple-vessel coronary artery stenosis) undergo myocardial revascularization before aneurysm repair. In appropriate patients, percutaneous transluminal angioplasty is carried out before surgery. If clamping proximal to the left subclavian artery is anticipated in patients in whom the left internal thoracic artery has been used as a coronary artery bypass graft, a left-carotid-to-subclavian bypass is typically necessary to prevent cardiac ischemia when the aortic clamp is applied.[53]

Renal Status

Preoperative renal insufficiency has been a major risk factor for early mortality throughout the history of TAAA repair.[49,54] It was among the predictive variables selected in Svensson et al's[54] multivariable analysis of Crawford's complete experience with TAAA surgery in 1509 patients treated between 1960 and 1991. Patients with severely impaired renal function who are not receiving long-term hemodialysis frequently require temporary hemodialysis early after operation and are clearly at increased risk for postoperative complications.

Although patients are not rejected as surgical candidates on the basis of renal function, careful assessment of renal function aids in estimating perioperative risk and adjusting treatment strategies accordingly. Renal function is assessed preoperatively by measuring serum electrolytes, blood urea nitrogen, and creatinine. Kidney size and perfusion can be evaluated by using the imaging studies obtained to assess the aorta. Patients who have poor renal function secondary to severe proximal renal artery occlusive disease are revascularized at operation by renal arterial endarterectomy, stenting under direct vision, or bypass grafting, with the expectation that renal function will stabilize or improve.[52]

Because of the nephrotoxic effects of vascular contrast agents, surgery is delayed (if possible) for 24 hours or longer after CT scanning or aortography has been performed. This is especially important in patients with preexisting renal impairment. Strategies to reduce the risk of contrast-induced nephropathy include periprocedural administration of acetylcysteine and intravenous hydration. If renal insufficiency occurs or worsens after contrast administration, the surgical procedure is postponed until renal function returns to baseline or is satisfactorily stabilized.

Pulmonary Status

Pulmonary complications are the most common form of postoperative morbidity in patients who undergo DTAA and TAAA repairs. Most patients undergo pulmonary function screening with arterial blood gases and spirometry. Patients with an FEV_1 greater than 1.0 and a PCO_2 less than 45 mmHg are satisfactory surgical candidates. In suitable patients, borderline pulmonary function frequently is improved by smoking cessation, progressive treatment of bronchitis, weight loss, and a general exercise program that the patient follows for a period of 1 to 3 months before operation. However, surgery is not withheld from patients with symptomatic aortic aneurysms and poor pulmonary function. In such patients, preservation of the left recurrent laryngeal nerve, phrenic nerve, and diaphragmatic function is particularly important.

OPEN SURGICAL REPAIR

Anesthetic Strategies

Coordination among the surgeon, anesthesiologist, and perfusionist is critical during a DTAA or TAAA repair procedure. Management of hemodynamics during aortic clamping and unclamping, blood volume management, anticoagulation and hemostasis, and proper lung management occur in real time, with anticipation and preparation by the anesthesia team. Swan-Ganz catheters are routinely used for hemodynamic monitoring. The arterial catheter is placed in the right radial artery whenever the left subclavian artery flow may be interrupted during aortic clamping. A large-bore central venous line is necessary for volume return. We reinfuse filtered, unwashed whole blood from the cell saver through a rapid infusion system during periods of substantial blood loss, such as when the aorta is opened. With careful scavenging of shed blood and meticulous surgical hemostasis, operations without the use of blood and blood products are frequently possible. However, when coagulopathy does occur after the cross-clamp is released, rapid replacement of blood components with fresh frozen plasma, platelets, and cryoprecipitate is necessary. Single lung ventilation, usually by a double-lumen endobronchial tube, is necessary for exposure, although this may not be critical in extent IV TAAA repairs. The lung is handled minimally during anticoagulation to prevent lung hematoma and contusion. Deflating the left lung reduces retraction trauma to the lung, improves exposure, and alleviates the risk of cardiac compression. When motor evoked potentials are used for spinal cord monitoring, muscle paralytics must be avoided. Sodium bicarbonate solution is routinely infused to prevent acidosis during aortic cross-clamping, and mannitol can be given before cross-clamping to enhance renal perfusion. Proximal blood pressure, afterload, and cardiac performance are closely monitored by Swan-Ganz catheter and transesophageal echocardiography probe when necessary and are aggressively maintained.

Surgical Adjuncts for Organ Protection

Organ ischemia is a major source of the morbidity related to DTAA and TAAA repair. We currently employ a multimodal approach (Table 49-1) that is primarily based on the extent of repair in an attempt to maximize organ protection during these operations (Fig. 49-7).[55] The rationale for and details of several important strategies are discussed below.

HEPARIN

Potential benefits of heparinization include preserving the microcirculation and preventing embolization. Additionally,

TABLE 49-1: Current Strategy for Spinal Cord and Visceral Protection During Descending and Thoracoabdominal Aortic Aneurysm Repair

All extents
- Moderate heparinization (1 mg/kg)
- Permissive mild hypothermia (32-34°C, nasopharyngeal)
- Aggressive reattachment of segmental arteries, especially between T8 and L1
- Perfusion of renal arteries with 4°C solution when possible
- Sequential aortic clamping when possible

Extent I and II thoracoabdominal repairs
- Cerebrospinal fluid drainage
- Left heart bypass during proximal anastomosis
- Selective perfusion of celiac axis and superior mesenteric artery during intercostal and visceral anastomoses

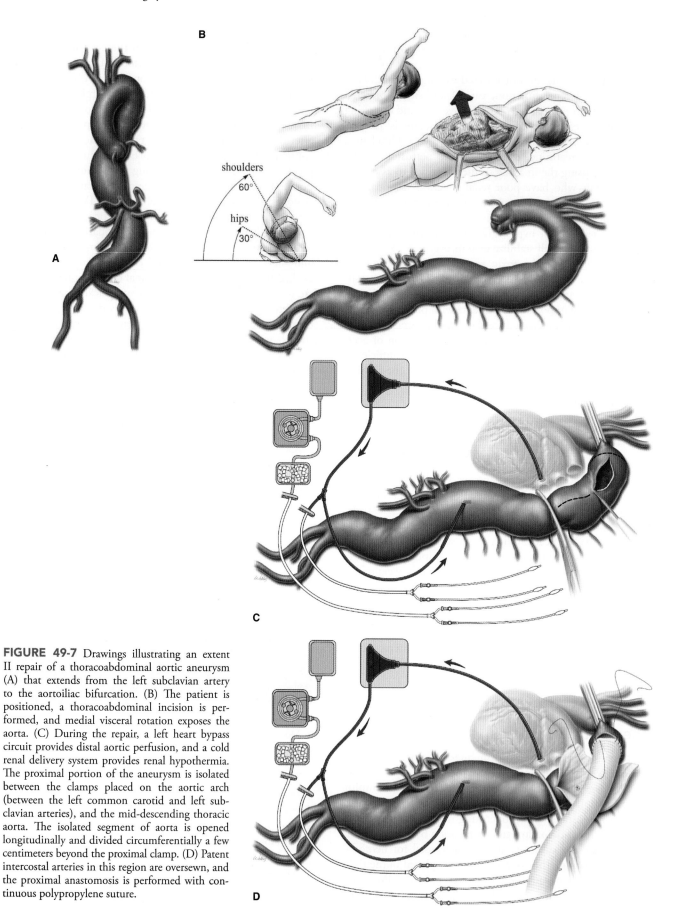

FIGURE 49-7 Drawings illustrating an extent II repair of a thoracoabdominal aortic aneurysm (A) that extends from the left subclavian artery to the aortoiliac bifurcation. (B) The patient is positioned, a thoracoabdominal incision is performed, and medial visceral rotation exposes the aorta. (C) During the repair, a left heart bypass circuit provides distal aortic perfusion, and a cold renal delivery system provides renal hypothermia. The proximal portion of the aneurysm is isolated between the clamps placed on the aortic arch (between the left common carotid and left subclavian arteries), and the mid-descending thoracic aorta. The isolated segment of aorta is opened longitudinally and divided circumferentially a few centimeters beyond the proximal clamp. (D) Patent intercostal arteries in this region are oversewn, and the proximal anastomosis is performed with continuous polypropylene suture.

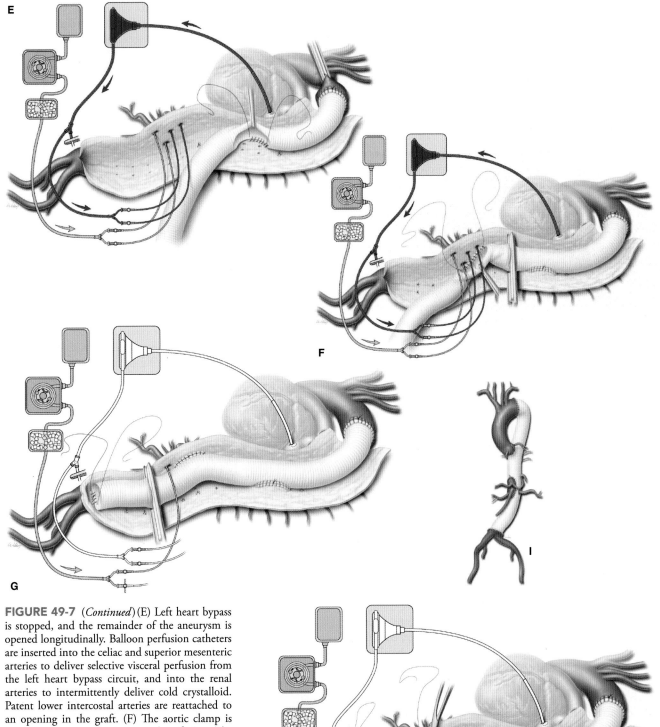

FIGURE 49-7 (*Continued*) (E) Left heart bypass is stopped, and the remainder of the aneurysm is opened longitudinally. Balloon perfusion catheters are inserted into the celiac and superior mesenteric arteries to deliver selective visceral perfusion from the left heart bypass circuit, and into the renal arteries to intermittently deliver cold crystalloid. Patent lower intercostal arteries are reattached to an opening in the graft. (F) The aortic clamp is repositioned to restore intercostal perfusion. The celiac axis, superior mesenteric, and right renal arteries are reattached to an opening in the side of the graft. (G) The aortic clamp is repositioned to restore visceral and right renal perfusion. The distal anastomosis is performed with continuous polypropylene suture at the level of the aortic bifurcation. (H) The mobilized left renal artery is reattached. (I) The completed extent II thoracoabdominal aortic aneurysm repair is shown. (Printed with permission from Baylor College of Medicine).

by inhibiting the clotting cascade, the use of heparin may help to reduce the incidence of disseminated intravascular coagulation.

Heparin (1 mg/kg) is administered intravenously before aortic clamping or the start of left heart bypass (LHB). After this small heparin dose is administered, the activated clotting time generally ranges from 220 to 270 seconds.

HYPOTHERMIA

Hypothermia decreases the metabolic demand of tissues and is protective during ischemic states. The protective effects of hypothermia on the spinal cord are well accepted. We routinely use mild passive systemic hypothermia during DTAA and TAAA repairs. The patient's temperature is allowed to drift down to a nasopharyngeal temperature of 32 to 33°C. After the aortic repair, rewarming can be accomplished by irrigating the thoracic and abdominal cavities with warm saline.

Profound systemic hypothermia on full cardiopulmonary bypass is an operative strategy for organ protection. Kouchoukos and colleagues[56-58] have reported that hypothermic cardiopulmonary bypass with circulatory arrest can safely and substantially protect against paralysis and renal, cardiac, and visceral organ system failure during operations on the thoracic and thoracoabdominal aorta. Despite these protective effects, many clinicians avoid using this approach, principally because of the associated risks of coagulopathy, pulmonary dysfunction, and massive fluid shift. We use hypothermic circulatory arrest selectively when the aneurysm anatomy precludes safe proximal clamping.

LEFT HEART BYPASS

Disruption of blood flow to the spinal cord and abdominal viscera contributes significantly to the development of ischemic complications. Conversely, maintaining flow through spinal and visceral arteries during all or part of the anatomic repair should reduce the duration of organ ischemia and prevent associated morbidity. Borst et al[59] found that using LHB for distal perfusion during DTAA and TAAA repair effectively unloads the proximal circulation during aortic occlusion and maintains adequate perfusion of distal vital organs, thereby reducing early mortality and renal failure. Further, combined distal perfusion and aggressive reattachment of distal intercostal arteries decreased the risk of spinal cord damage.

Typically used during the proximal aortic anastomosis, LHB is achieved by establishing a temporary bypass from the left atrium to either the distal descending thoracic aorta (usually a few centimeters proximal to the origin of the celiac axis) or the femoral artery (most commonly the left), with a closed-circuit in-line centrifugal pump (Fig. 49-7C). The left atrial cannula is placed via an opening in the inferior pulmonary vein (Fig. 49-7C). When we first began using LHB, cannulation of the distal descending thoracic aorta (usually at the level of the diaphragm) was used solely as an alternative to femoral artery cannulation in patients with femoral or iliac artery occlusive disease. However, because this technique causes few complications and eliminates the

need for femoral artery exposure and repair, distal aortic cannulation has become our preferred approach. Careful examination of CT or MR images assists selection of an appropriate site for direct aortic cannulation. Areas with intraluminal thrombus (Fig. 49-4) are avoided because cannulation could lead to distal embolization. Bypass flows are adjusted to maintain normal proximal arterial and venous filling pressures. Flows between 1500 and 2500 mL/min are generally used. LHB facilitates rapid adjustment of proximal arterial pressure and cardiac preload, thereby reducing the need for pharmacologic intervention. Because LHB effectively unloads the left ventricle, it is useful in patients with suboptimal cardiac reserve.

SPINAL CORD PROTECTION

Paraplegia remains an index complication specific to both distal aortic surgery and endovascular repair. Historically, rates for spinal cord deficits (paraplegia or paraparesis) have been as high as 30% for extent II aortic replacements.[54] Although the mechanism of developing paraplegia following spinal cord ischemia as part of open aortic repair is imperfectly understood, it is generally associated with interrupted distal aortic blood flow following proximal aortic clamping and the intraoperative loss of intercostal and lumbar arteries; additional factors include the role of the left subclavian and hypogastric arteries in perfusing the spinal cord (which tends to vary by patient), reperfusion injury, and the possible dissemination of embolic debris.[60,61] With modern operative techniques and spinal adjuncts, paraplegia rates in aortic centers are currently 1 to 5%.[44,56,62,63] Because multiple adjuncts are used in combination and are continuously evolving,[64] it is difficult to attribute the improvements in outcome to one technique.

Cerebrospinal Fluid Drainage. The drainage of cerebrospinal fluid (CSF) in the context of aortic surgery for spinal cord protection was tested in animal models in the early 1960s.[65] The rationale for CSF drainage was that it would enhance spinal perfusion by decreasing the pressure on the cord during aortic cross-clamping. Today, its use is widespread and specifically recommended by current US practice guidelines during both open and endovascular repairs in patients at high risk of developing paraplegia (Class I recommendation, level of evidence B).[24] In our study of 145 patients who underwent extent I or II TAAA repair, patients were randomly assigned to receive CSF drainage or no CSF drainage. Postoperatively, paraplegia or paraparesis developed in 9 patients (13%) in the control group but in only 2 patients (2.6%) in the CSF drainage group ($p = .03$).[66] Although the safety of CSF drainage has been shown clinically,[67] known risks include intracranial bleeding, perispinal hematoma, meningitis, and spinal headaches.[68]

We routinely use CSF drainage in patients undergoing Crawford extent I or II TAAA repairs because of the higher risks of paraplegia in these extensive TAAA repairs. We selectively use CSF drainage during less extensive repairs, such as

DTAA or extent III or IV TAAA repairs, depending upon the individual risk factors involved; for example, we would use CSF drainage in a redo aortic operation in which the spinal collateral is compromised and a long cross-clamp time is anticipated because of the complex configuration of the aneurysm. The intrathecal catheter is placed through the second or third lumbar space preoperatively after induction of anesthesia and is maintained 1 to 2 days postoperatively in the intensive care unit. The catheter allows both monitoring of the CSF pressure and therapeutic drainage of the fluid. The CSF is allowed to drain passively from the catheter and can be aspirated with a closed collection system as needed to keep the CSF pressure between 8 and 10 mm Hg during the operation and between 10 and 12 mm Hg during the early postoperative period. Once the patients are awake and neurologic examinations confirm that they are able to move their legs, the CSF pressures are allowed to rise to a higher range of 15 to 18 mm Hg. To prevent intracranial hemorrhage, we avoid draining more than 25 mL per hour.

Left Heart Bypass for Spinal Protection. LHB appears to provide the greatest benefit to patients who undergo the more extensive repairs. Our own retrospective review of 1250 consecutive extent I or extent II TAAA repairs found that using LHB (in 666 cases) reduced the incidence of spinal cord deficits only in patients who underwent extent II repairs.[69] In patients who underwent extent I repairs, the incidence of paraplegia was similar in the LHB and no-LHB groups, even though the LHB group had significantly longer aortic clamp times. This finding suggests that, by providing spinal cord protection, LHB gives the surgeon more time to create secure anastomoses. A propensity-score analysis of 387 of our patients who underwent DTAA repair with (n = 46) or without (n = 341) LHB during the construction of the proximal anastomosis found no effect of LHB on postoperative paraplegia and paraparesis rates.[70] Because patients who undergo extensive TAAA repairs (extents I and II) are at greatest risk of postoperative paraplegia or paraparesis, we routinely use LHB to provide distal aortic perfusion during the proximal portion of the aortic repair.

Segmental Artery Reattachment and Sequential Graft Clamping. Because of the often tenuous nature of the blood supply to the spinal cord, we take an aggressive approach to reattaching patent segmental arteries. Intimal atherosclerosis, particularly in medial degenerative fusiform aneurysms, obliterates many intercostal and lumbar arteries and complicates matters anatomically. Pairs of patent segmental arteries from T8 to L1 are selectively reattached as patches to one or more openings made in the graft (Fig. 49-7E). Large arteries with little or no back-bleeding are considered particularly important. When none of these arteries is patent, endarterectomy of the aortic wall and removal of calcified intimal disease can be considered as a means of identifying arteries suitable for reattachment. Infrequently, a small-diameter graft may be used to facilitate bypass reattachment of selected arteries. After intercostal arteries are

reattached, the proximal clamp is often moved down the graft to restore intercostal perfusion. Sequential clamping restores perfusion to the proximal branch vessels and will decrease the ischemic time to the spinal cord. However, this benefit needs to be weighed against the additional time needed to control the potential bleeding from the proximal aortic anastomosis, the intercostal patch, and the collateral intercostal and lumbar branches that often results when the clamp is moved below the intercostal patch. In addition, the possibility of dislodging emboli that could lodge in branching arteries and create localized ischemia should be considered. The reattachment of intercostal arteries appears most significant in extent II TAAA repair; recently, we identified such reattachment independently predicted a 54% reduction in the risk of developing permanent paraplegia in such repairs.[51]

Spinal Cord Monitoring. Somatosensory evoked potential (SSEP), motor evoked potential (MEP), and near-infrared spectroscopy (NIRS) monitoring have been used for intraoperative assessment of spinal cord function. MEP monitoring involves electrical excitation of the motor cortex or motor neurons and measuring the amplitude of the resulting motor response in the peripheral muscles of the arms and legs. Monitoring MEPs allows real-time assessment of spinal cord motor function and was approved for this use during surgical TAAA repair by the FDA in 2003. Because the motor function of the anterior horn of the spinal cord is more susceptible than the posterior horn to ischemia and infarction, MEP changes are a sensitive indicator of spinal cord ischemia and are predictive of adverse neurological events. In contrast, SSEP monitoring is less sensitive because the sensory pathways on the dorsal horn are more resistant to injury and are sometimes spared when ischemic injury occurs. Irreversible loss of either MEPs or SSEPs is predictive of immediate neurologic deficit on recovery.[60] Less is known about the effectiveness of NIRS as applied to distal aortic repair, but it appears to have promising sensitivity and response time.[60,71] Importantly, monitoring MEPs precludes the use of neuromuscular paralytic agents during repair, adding complexity to anesthetic management. Although we have used MEP monitoring in the past for extent II and other selective TAAA repairs, we no longer use this approach in part because of the risk of false positive results; however, in expert hands, this remains a valuable approach.[72]

Regional Spinal Hypothermia. Regional spinal cord hypothermia can be accomplished by direct infusion of cold perfusate into the epidural or intrathecal space and by intravascular cold perfusion of isolated thoracic aortic segments (with the expectation that the intercostal vessels will deliver the cold perfusate to the spinal cord). A series of 337 TAAA repairs reported by Cambria and colleagues[73] showed that, in patients who underwent extent I, II, or III TAAA repairs, the incidence of spinal cord ischemic injury was reduced from 19.8 to 10.6% after the introduction of epidural cooling at their institution in 1993. Using an epidural catheter containing cold saline, Inoue et al[74] demonstrated its effectiveness in reducing epidural temperature in a leporine model; in clinical application, it was used in 37 distal aortic repairs without any postoperative spinal cord deficits.[75] A similar technique, cold perfusion into isolated aortic segments, has been tested in animal models to show that cord temperature and, consequently, the extent of ischemic spinal cord injury can be effectively reduced by this method.[76]

Collateral Network Concepts. Collateral network concepts refute the existence of dominant intercostal and lumbar arteries (eg, the artery of Adamkiewicz) and imply that reattaching select intercostal arteries is largely unnecessary;[77] instead, the network of small arteries that perfuse the spinal cord may readily remodel following ischemic insult to provide sufficient perfusion of the spinal cord.[78] Efforts to further develop this approach have led to emerging endovascular-spinal-cord preconditioning techniques by selectively coiling segmental arteries to promote remodeling and better tolerate subsequent open distal aortic repair.[79] Staged distal aortic repair is also being developed as a method to facilitate remodeling of the spinal cord between repairs, and porcine models showed this to be effective at preventing paraplegia after extensive aortic repair if the two stages were separated by 7 days.[80] While staged repair may prove difficult in extensive open distal aortic repairs, this approach is not dissimilar from current approaches to extensive distal aortic dissection—typically only the dilated section is repaired, and thus, often a DTAA or an extent I repair is followed by an extent III or IV repair.[62]

Rescue Measures for Spinal Cord Deficit. Postoperative management remains critical to spinal cord protection. Adequate blood pressure, preload, and cardiac inotropic state are carefully maintained to keep spinal perfusion sufficient. In the absence of postoperative bleeding, blood pressure should be kept near its preoperative baseline level. Delayed paraplegia can arise hours to days after aortic surgery.[81] In the immediate postoperative period, strategies to reverse paraplegia and paraparesis include inducing systemic hypertension; placing a CSF drain, if one is not already present; decreasing CSF pressure; administering cardiac inotropes, mannitol, or steroids; correcting anemia; and preventing fever. Recovery from paraplegia is possible, but if cord function does not return promptly after these measures are taken, such a recovery is not likely.

RENAL PROTECTION

Postoperative renal failure after DTAA and TAAA remains an important complication and is predictive of mortality.[82] Although distal aortic perfusion with LHB provides renal perfusion during proximal anastomosis, the ability to provide continued renal protection is valuable. Our approach to renal protection for repair of TAAA has evolved from the results of two of our randomized clinical trials.[83,84] Once the renal vessels are exposed during distal repair, the renal arteries can be directly perfused with cold (4°C) perfusate (Fig. 49-7E). Our current technique is to provide an initial

bolus of 200 to 300 mL of cold crystalloid perfusate that is administered to each kidney, followed by the intermittent infusion of 100 to 150 mL per kidney, which is delivered every 10 to 15 minutes until arterial flow is restored. The volume and frequency of perfusate delivery are adjusted to avoid fluid overload or hypothermia (a systemic temperature of 32°C is targeted). First, we reported on a group of patients who underwent Crawford extent II TAAA repair with LHB and who were randomly assigned to receive either renal artery perfusion of cold LR solution for renal cooling or to isothermic blood perfusion from the LHB circuit. Multivariate analysis confirmed that cold crystalloid perfusion was independently protective against acute renal dysfunction.[84] Second, we reported on a group of patients who underwent Crawford extent II or III TAAA repair and compared the outcomes of cold blood to cold crystalloid for renal protection. Although we found no significant difference between patients regarding renal failure or early death, a trend toward less paraplegia was observed in the cold crystalloid group.[83] Wynn and colleagues[85] were able to demonstrate the effectiveness of moderate systemic hypothermia and cold (4°C) renal perfusion using a similar approach in a retrospective review of 455 patients who underwent TAAA repair. Among aortic centers, there is considerable variation in perfusate; some centers have shifted from lactated Ringer's solution to histidine-tryptophan-ketoglutarate (HTK) solution.[86] Current US aortic guidelines recommend the use of cold renal perfusion (class IIB, level of evidence B).[24] Other groups continue to selectively perfuse the renal arteries with blood from the LHB circuit.

VISCERAL PROTECTION

Similarly, distal aortic perfusion by LHB provides flow to the mesenteric branches during the initial portion of a TAAA repair. Once the visceral origins are exposed, selective visceral perfusion can be delivered through separate balloon perfusion catheters that are placed within the origins of the celiac and superior mesenteric arteries; these catheters are attached to the LHB circuit via a Y-line from the arterial perfusion line (Fig. 49-7C). This system provides oxygenated blood to the abdominal viscera while the intercostal and visceral branches are being reattached to the graft (Figs. 49-7E-F). Reducing hepatic ischemia in this fashion may decrease the risk of postoperative coagulopathy, and reducing bowel ischemia may decrease the risk of bacterial translocation.

Operative Techniques

INCISIONS AND AORTIC EXPOSURE

Aneurysms limited to the descending thoracic aorta are approached through a full posterolateral thoracotomy (Fig. 49-8A). In most cases, the left pleural space is entered through the sixth intercostal space; however, if the aneurysm predominantly involves the upper portion of the descending thoracic aorta, the fifth intercostal space provides better access to the distal aortic arch. Exposure of the distal descending

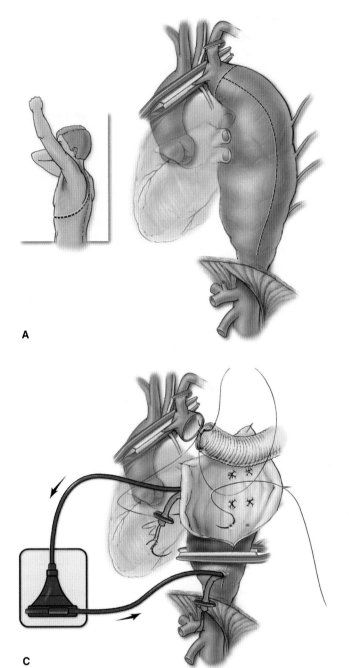

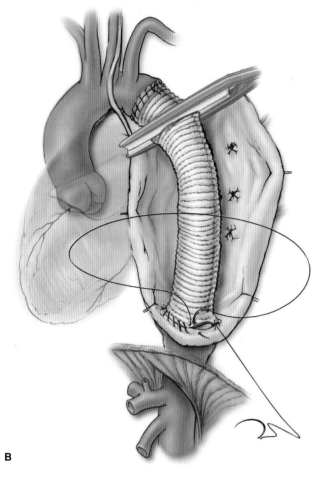

FIGURE 49-8 Drawings illustrating techniques for repairing a descending thoracic aortic aneurysm. (A) In the clamp-and-sew technique, the operation is performed through a posterolateral thoracotomy (inset). Clamps are placed on the aortic arch (between the left common carotid and left subclavian arteries) and the left subclavian artery (using a bulldog clamp). The aorta is opened longitudinally and divided circumferentially a few centimeters beyond the proximal clamp. (B) After the proximal anastomosis is completed, the aortic clamp is repositioned onto the graft, flow is restored to the left subclavian artery, and the remainder of the aneurysm is opened longitudinally. An open distal anastomosis completes the repair. (C) As an alternative to the clamp-and-sew technique, left heart bypass can be used to provide distal aortic perfusion during the repair.

thoracic aorta is enhanced by dividing the costal margin without dividing the diaphragm.

The full thoracoabdominal incision extends from the left posterior chest (between the scapula and the spine), crosses the costal margin, and traverses obliquely to the umbilicus. The length and level varies according to the anatomy of the aneurysm. The incision is gently curved as it crosses the costal margin to reduce the risk of tissue necrosis at the apex of the lower portion of the musculoskeletal tissue flap (Fig. 49-9A). Stabilized on a bean bag, the patient is placed in a modified right lateral decubitus position with the shoulders placed at 60° to 80° and the hips rotated to 30° to 40° from

horizontal. In extent I and II repairs, which require access to the left subclavian artery and distal arch in the upper chest, our standard approach is through the sixth intercostal space. Rarely, the upper or lower ribs may be divided posteriorly to achieve additional proximal or distal exposure, respectively. For extent III aneurysm repairs, entering through the seventh or eighth intercostal space will allow adequate access. Extent IV aneurysms are approached via a straight oblique incision through the ninth or tenth interspace (Fig. 49-9B). Ending the incision distally at the level of the umbilicus will allow access to the aortic bifurcation. The incision can be extended toward the pubis if iliac aneurysms also require repair.

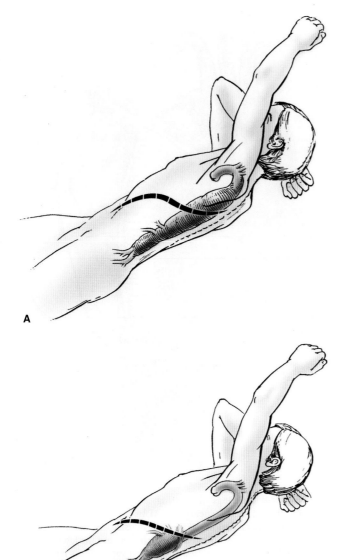

A

B

FIGURE 49-9 Drawings of the typical incisions used in thoracoabdominal aortic aneurysm repairs. (A) A curvilinear incision is used to approach the aorta in extents I, II, and III thoracoabdominal aneurysm repairs. (B) A straighter, oblique incision is used to approach extent IV thoracoabdominal aortic aneurysm repairs.

For thoracoabdominal access, the diaphragm is divided partially or completely in a circular fashion to protect the phrenic nerve and to preserve as much diaphragm as possible. The crus of the diaphragm is divided at the hiatus, and a 3- to 4-cm rim of diaphragmatic tissue is left posterolaterally on the chest wall to facilitate closure when the operation is complete. Below the diaphragm, the retroperitoneum is entered lateral to the left colon, and medial visceral rotation is performed to expose the aorta. A dissection plane is developed anterior to the psoas muscle, and the left kidney, left colon,

spleen, and left ureter are retracted anteriorly and to the right. The abdominal aortic segment is approached transperitoneally; opening the peritoneum permits direct inspection of the abdominal viscera and its blood supply after aortic reconstruction is completed. An entirely retroperitoneal approach can be used in patients with a "hostile abdomen," that is, patients with multiple prior abdominal operations or a history of extensive adhesions, peritonitis, or both.

The left renal artery is identified but generally does not require mobilization. The aorta is approached laterally to avoid injury to the mesenteric vessels and the abdominal organs. Commonly, a large lumbar branch of the left renal vein courses posteriorly around the aorta. This branch may be ligated and divided as needed. An anomalous retroaortic left renal vein is occasionally encountered and should be preserved. If the retroaortic renal vein or its tributaries require division for exposure, direct reanastomosis or interposition grafting to the inferior vena cava can be performed if the left kidney appears congested and shows distended collaterals.

PROXIMAL ANASTOMOSIS

For DTAA and extent I and II TAAA repairs, options for establishing proximal control include applying a proximal aortic clamp distal to the left subclavian artery; applying an aortic clamp between the left subclavian and the left carotid artery and applying a separate bulldog clamp to the left subclavian artery; applying an aortic clamp to an existing graft during an elephant trunk operation; or open anastomosis under hypothermic circulatory arrest with full cardiopulmonary bypass when an aortic clamp cannot be safely applied. The decision is based on the anatomy of the aneurysm. We use aortic clamping distal to the left subclavian artery whenever possible, although others have advocated using circulatory arrest routinely.[56]

In aneurysms suitable for aortic clamping, the distal aortic arch is gently mobilized by dividing the remnant of the ductus arteriosus. The vagus and recurrent laryngeal nerves are identified. The vagus nerve may be divided below the recurrent nerve to provide additional mobility, thereby protecting the recurrent nerve from injury. Preserving the recurrent laryngeal nerve is particularly important in patients with chronic obstructive pulmonary disease and reduced pulmonary function. If the aneurysm encroaches upon the left subclavian artery, clamping proximal to the left subclavian artery should be anticipated; the left subclavian artery is then circumferentially mobilized to enable placement of a bulldog clamp.

After heparin is administered, the proximal clamp is applied to the proximal descending thoracic aorta or the distal transverse aortic arch between the left common carotid and left subclavian arteries (Figs. 49-7B and 49-8A). When LHB is used, it is initiated at a flow rate of 500 mL/min just before the proximal aorta is clamped. After the proximal clamp is applied, LHB flow is increased to 2 L/min and a second distal aortic clamp is placed between T4 and T7 (Fig. 49-7C). After the aorta is opened, patent upper intercostal arteries are oversewn (Fig. 49-8C). In cases of chronic dissection, the septum between the true and false lumens is completely removed. The aorta is transected 2 to 3 cm beyond the proximal clamp and is separated from the esophagus to allow the surgeon to place full-thickness sutures in the aortic wall without injuring the esophagus. A 22- or 24-mm, gelatin-impregnated woven Dacron graft is used in most patients. The proximal anastomosis is performed with continuous polypropylene suture (Fig. 49-7D). Most anastomoses are made with 3-0 polypropylene suture; however, in patients with particularly fragile aortic tissues, such as patients with acute aortic dissection or Marfan syndrome, 4-0 polypropylene sutures are commonly used. Felt strips are generally not used; instead, intermittent polypropylene mattress sutures with felt pledgets are used to reinforce selected portions of the anastomoses. The use of surgical adhesives is avoided in these operations.

Open Anastomosis Under Hypothermic Circulatory Arrest.

In repairs of large aneurysms at the distal arch or aneurysms with enormous size, contained rupture, or in redo operations in which safe dissection and clamping are not possible, an alternative strategy is total cardiopulmonary bypass with hypothermic circulatory arrest. Arterial inflow is established by placing a cannula in the distal aorta or the femoral artery, depending on patient-specific factors. Venous drainage is usually established by inserting a long, multiholed cannula into the left femoral vein and advancing it into the right atrium with transesophageal echocardiographic guidance. The left atrium or left ventricle can be vented via a right-angled sump cannula placed in the left pulmonary vein to prevent cardiac distension. Total cardiopulmonary bypass is initiated, and the patient is cooled to electrocerebral silence. Circulatory arrest is initiated, and the aneurysm is opened. Direct antegrade cerebral perfusion into the left carotid artery can be accomplished via a separate balloon catheter arising from the arterial limb of the circuit. An open proximal anastomosis is performed. After this anastomosis is completed, a Y-limb from the arterial line is connected to a side branch of the graft. The graft is deaired and clamped, pump flow to the upper body is resumed, and the remainder of the aortic repair is performed.

Elephant Trunk Repairs.

A staged operative procedure is preferred in patients who present with extensive aneurysmal disease involving the ascending aorta, aortic arch, and descending thoracic or thoracoabdominal aorta (Fig. 49-10A). When the DTAA or TAAA is not causing symptoms and is not substantially larger than the ascending aorta, the proximal aortic repair is performed first. This allows treatment of valvular and coronary artery occlusive disease during the first operation.

Our current preference for reconstruction of the innominate, left carotid, and left subclavian artery is separate end-to-end anastomoses with a branched trifurcated graft (Fig. 49-10B). The bypass to the left subclavian artery during the first stage is not critical, and the left subclavian artery origin

can remain intact on the native aorta. The aorta itself can be replaced with a skirted elephant trunk graft, which facilitates the distal aortic anastomosis to aneurysmal tissue, because the skirt accommodates any size discrepancy between the graft and native aorta. The proximal aortic anastomosis is placed to the supravalvar ascending aorta, and the distal skirt anastomosis can be placed fairly anteriorly on the aortic arch at the level of the innominate artery, facilitating hemostasis. The proximal end of the trifurcated graft is then anastomosed to an opening in the mid-ascending aspect of the aortic graft. The distal aortic anastomosis later becomes unimportant when the elephant trunk anastomosis to the descending aorta is completed at the second stage (Fig. 49-10D). The presence of the elephant trunk graft within the descending aorta allows secure clamping of even very large aneurysms distal to the left subclavian artery. If the left subclavian artery was not bypassed during the arch vessel reconstruction, a side branch from the descending aorta can be anastomosed to the subclavian artery from the left chest during the second stage. During the second stage repair, an ultrasound probe may be used to identify the distal end of the elephant trunk before incision.

Reversed Elephant Trunk Repairs.

Conversely, in patients with similarly extensive aneurysmal disease who present with a DTAA or TAAA that has ruptured, causes symptoms (eg, back pain), or is considerably larger than the ascending aorta (Fig. 49-11A), the DTAA or TAAA is treated during the initial operation, and the ascending aorta and transverse aortic arch are repaired in a second procedure. During this "reversed" elephant trunk repair (Fig. 49-11B), a portion of the proximal end of the aortic graft is inverted down into the lumen during the first operation and is later used to facilitate second-stage repair of the ascending and transverse aortic arch.[87]

INTERCOSTAL PATCH ANASTOMOSIS AND COMPLETION OF THE DTAA REPAIR

After the proximal anastomosis is completed, LHB is discontinued and the distal aortic clamp is removed. The remainder of the aneurysm is opened longitudinally to its distal extent (Fig. 49-7E). The blood in the open aorta is scavenged via cell saver and returned as whole blood by a rapid infuser system. When intraluminal thrombus is present, it is evacuated by hand. If the aneurysm was clamped proximal to the left subclavian artery, the aortic clamp is moved down onto the graft and the left subclavian artery clamp is removed; this restores blood flow to the left vertebral artery and to spinal collaterals. For repairs that extend to the diaphragm or beyond, patent lower intercostal arteries are selected and reattached to an opening cut in the side of the graft. If the aortic tissue is particularly friable, a separate, 8-mm graft can be attached in an end-to-end fashion to the selected intercostal vessels. In DTAA repairs, the distal anastomosis is then performed (Fig. 49-8B) as an open distal anastomosis. For aneurysms arising from chronic dissections, the membrane between the true and false lumen is fenestrated distally to ensure that both lumens are perfused.

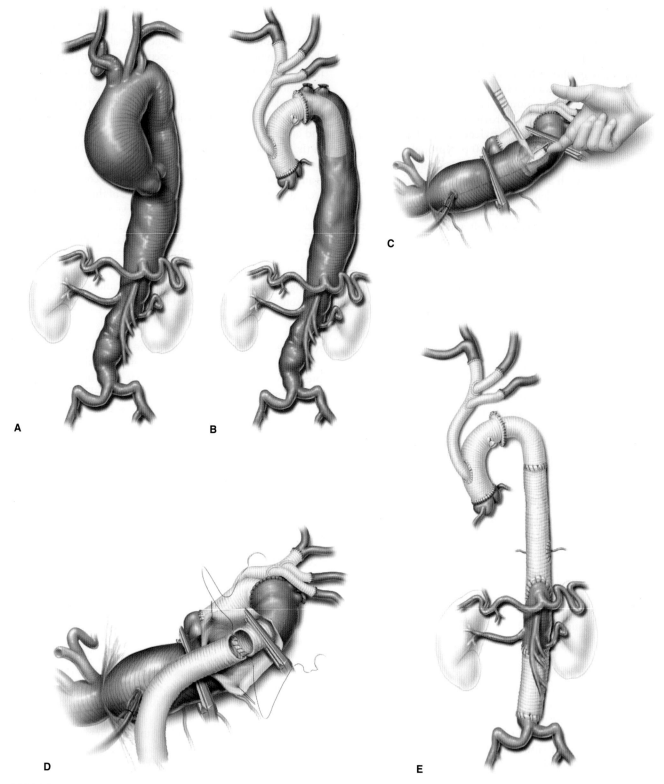

FIGURE 49-10 Drawings illustrating the two-stage elephant trunk repair of an extensive aneurysm (A) involving the ascending, transverse arch, and entire thoracoabdominal aorta. (B) The first stage includes graft replacement of the ascending aorta and transverse aortic arch. A segment of the graft (the elephant trunk) is left suspended within the aneurysmal descending thoracic aorta. (C) During the second stage, the elephant trunk is retrieved and (D) used for the proximal anastomosis. (E) The completed repair includes reattachment patches for a pair of intercostal arteries and the visceral arteries. (Figures B-D reproduced with permission from Baylor College of Medicine. Figure E reproduced with permission from LeMaire SA, Price MD, Parenti JL, et al: Early outcomes after aortic arch replacement by using the Y-graft technique, *Ann Thorac Surg.* 2011 Mar; 91(3):700-707.)

VISCERAL BRANCH VESSEL ANASTOMOSES

In patients with TAAAs, after the descending thoracic aortic repair is completed, the remainder of the aneurysm is opened longitudinally (Fig. 49-7E). This incision runs posterior to the origin of the left renal artery and continues to the distal extent of the aneurysm. When present, the remaining dissecting membrane is excised. The origins of the visceral and renal branches are identified. Cold perfusate is intermittently delivered to the renal arteries via balloon catheters. In patients receiving LHB, balloon cannulas are also placed in the celiac and superior mesenteric arteries so that selective visceral perfusion can be delivered from the pump circuit. Subsequently, the celiac, superior mesenteric, and renal arteries are reattached. In extent I repairs, the reattachment of the visceral arteries is often incorporated into a beveled distal anastomosis

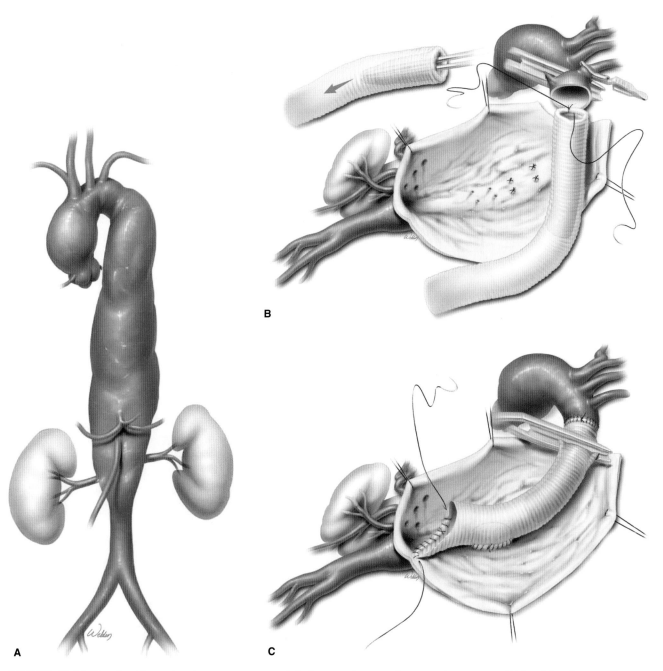

FIGURE 49-11 Drawings illustrating the two-stage reversed elephant trunk repair of an extensive aneurysm (A) involving the ascending, transverse arch, and thoracoabdominal aorta. (B) The first stage involves graft replacement of the thoracoabdominal aorta. The proximal portion of the graft is invaginated, and the folded edge is used to create the proximal anastomosis. (C) After reattachment of intercostal arteries, a beveled distal anastomosis is performed behind the visceral ostia.

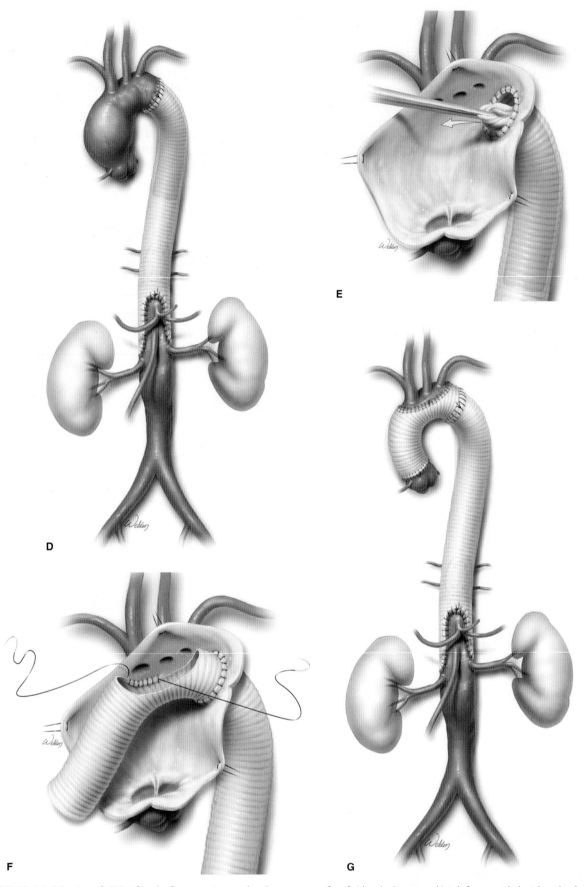

D

E

F

G

FIGURE 49-11 (*Continued*) (D) After the first stage is completed, a segment of graft (the elephant trunk) is left suspended within the descending thoracic aortic graft. (E) During the second stage, the elephant trunk is retrieved through the open aortic arch and (F) used to replace the arch and ascending aorta, (G) which completes the repair.

(Fig. 49-11C), but in extent II and III repairs, the visceral artery origins are reattached to one or more oval openings in the graft (Fig. 49-7F). Commonly, the origin of the left renal artery is displaced laterally and is best attached to a separate opening in the graft (Fig. 49-7H). Patients with genetic disorders such as Marfan or Loeys-Dietz syndrome are prone to aneurysms involving their visceral reattachment patch; a multibranched graft enables separate bypasses to each of the vessels, thereby minimizing the amount of remaining aortic tissue and reducing the risk of recurrent aneurysms. Multibranched grafts are also useful in patients with large aneurysms that have caused wide displacement of the celiac, superior mesenteric, and renal arterial ostia (Fig. 49-12). Visceral artery stenosis is typically encountered in at least 25% of cases and necessitates endarterectomy (if anatomically suitable), stenting, or interposition bypass grafting.[54,88]

DISTAL AORTIC AND ILIAC ANASTOMOSES

When the TAAA extends below the renal arteries, a distal anastomosis is performed near the aortic bifurcation (Fig. 49-7H). In patients with iliac artery aneurysms, a bifurcation graft is sewn onto the end of the straight graft; the graft's limbs are then anastomosed to the common iliac, external iliac, or common femoral artery, depending on the extent of disease. The right limb of the bifurcation graft is tunneled retroperitoneally into the pelvis near the right iliac artery. Exposure of the left iliac artery is more straightforward from the left retroperitoneal incision. As needed for stenosis or extensive calcification, endarterectomy may be performed or stents may be used under direct vision to repair one or both iliac arteries.

CLOSURE

After all clamps are removed, heparin is reversed with protamine sulfate. Hemostasis is achieved by surgically

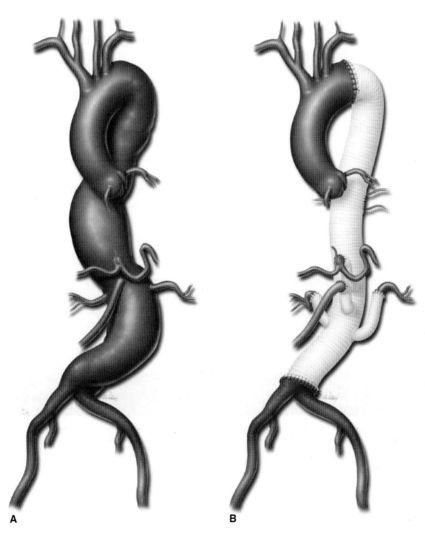

A   **B**

FIGURE 49-12 Drawings showing (A) a thoracoabdominal aortic aneurysm with wide displacement of the celiac, superior mesenteric, and both renal arterial ostia. (B) The aorta has been replaced with a multibranched graft that facilitates separate reattachment of each of the visceral arteries. (Printed with permission from Baylor College of Medicine.)

reinforcing the anastomoses and administering blood products as necessary. The renal, visceral, and peripheral circulations are assessed. To ensure that renal function is adequate, blue dye is administered intravenously, and transit time to urine output is measured. The bowel, spleen, and liver are all assessed for adequacy of perfusion. The spleen is examined for capsular injury; if a splenic hematoma is present, the spleen is removed to avoid postoperative bleeding and hypotension. The aneurysm wall is then loosely wrapped around the aortic graft. Two posteriorly located thoracic drainage tubes and a closed-suction retroperitoneal drain are placed before closure. The diaphragm is closed with continuous polypropylene suture; postoperative disruption of the diaphragmatic repair is exceedingly rare.

EARLY POSTOPERATIVE CARE

Postoperative blood pressure management is critical and must be balanced between hypertension (which can cause bleeding) and hypotension (which can lead to paraplegia/paraparesis). Because aortic anastomoses are often extremely fragile during the early postoperative period, even brief episodes of hypertension may disrupt suture lines and cause severe bleeding or pseudoaneurysm formation. In most cases, we use nitroprusside, intravenous β-antagonists, and intravenous calcium-channel blockers to keep the mean arterial blood pressure between 80 and 90 mm Hg. In patients with severely friable aortic tissue, such as those with Marfan syndrome, we use a target range of 70 to 80 mm Hg.

OUTCOMES

Since 1986, we have performed open surgical repair of 4040 DTAAs and TAAAs. Combined hospital and 30-day operative mortality was 7.1% (n = 286). Complications that are commonly associated with an increased risk of death include paraplegia, renal failure, respiratory failure, cardiac events, and bleeding. The incidence of paraplegia and paraparesis in our series was 4.8% (n = 195), paraplegia alone was 2.7% (n = 111), and the incidence of renal failure necessitating

hemodialysis was 5.7% (n = 231). The rate of return to the operating room for bleeding has been 3.5% in our experience (n = 142). Our most recent data (from 2009 to 2015), which reflect the results of our current organ-protection strategies, are shown in Table 49-2; for the majority of postoperative complications, operative risk varies by the extent of repair.

Pulmonary complications following distal aortic repair are quite common, affecting more than a third of patients and tending to occur more frequently after extensive repair (extents I and III TAAA repair) than less extensive repair (extent IV TAAA repair). Of note, vocal cord paralysis can contribute to respiratory complications; it should be suspected in patients with postoperative hoarseness and confirmed by direct examination. This complication can be treated effectively by direct cord medialization (ie, type 1 thyroplasty) or by polytetrafluoroethylene injection. In general, younger patients (≤50 years) tend to have far fewer postoperative complications than older patients; however, extensive TAAA repair (extent II TAAA) in the elderly (>80 years) should be cautioned as patients do quite poorly.[89]

SURVEILLANCE FOR ADDITIONAL AORTIC DISEASE

Patients who have undergone DTAA or TAAA repair remain at risk for developing new aneurysms in other aortic segments or in reattachment patches; this is especially true for patients with residual distal aortic dissection. Progressive weakening of aortic tissue at suture lines can lead to pseudoaneurysm formation—this late risk tends to be more pronounced in patients with uncontrolled hypertension or connective tissue disorder. If concerning symptoms develop (such as any ischemic complications or sudden onset of pain), patients should be made aware that they should seek urgent treatment. To detect new aortic disease before life-threatening complications occur, we recommend that all patients undergo annual CT or MR imaging of the chest and abdomen. This strategy of lifelong surveillance is especially important in patients with genetic disorders.[8] Subsequent aortic repairs can be performed with surprisingly low mortality and morbidity risk, particularly when done electively.[90]

TABLE 49-2: Results of 705 Contemporary (2009-2015) Open Descending Thoracic or Thoracoabdominal Aortic Aneurysm Repairs-Baylor College of Medicine

Extent of repair	No. of patients	30-day deaths	Paraplegia*	Stroke*	Renal Failure*
DTAA	51	2 (4%)	2 (4%)	1 (2%)	1 (2%)
TAAA I	161	5 (3%)	3 (2%)	4 (3%)	8 (5%)
TAAA II	226	16 (7%)	11 (5%)	4 (2%)	22 (10%)
TAAA III	118	4 (3%)	10 (8%)	0	16 (14%)
TAAA IV	149	5 (3%)	4 (3%)	3 (2%)	8 (5%)
Total	705	32 (5%)	30 (4%)	12 (2%)	55 (8%)

DTAA, descending thoracic aortic aneurysm; TAAA, thoracoabdominal aortic aneurysm.
*Discharged as a persistent impairment or present at time of early death.

ACKNOWLEDGMENTS

The authors thank Joseph Huh, MD, for his substantial contribution to the chapter published in the 4th edition of the textbook, on which this updated chapter is based; Scott A. Weldon, MA, CMI, and Carol P. Larson, BS, AMI, for their outstanding medical illustrations; and Stephen N. Palmer, PhD, ELS, Susan Y. Green, MPH, Eric K. Rachlin, and D'Arcy Wainwright for invaluable editorial support.

REFERENCES

1. Olsson C, Thelin S, Stahle E, et al: Thoracic aortic aneurysm and dissection: increasing prevalence and improved outcomes reported in a nationwide population-based study of more than 14,000 cases from 1987 to 2002. *Circulation* 2006; 114(24):2611-2618.

2. Kohn JC, Lampi MC, Reinhart-King CA: Age-related vascular stiffening: causes and consequences. *Front Genet* 2015; 6:112.

3. Fattouch K, Sampognaro R, Navarra E, et al: Long-term results after repair of type a acute aortic dissection according to false lumen patency. *Ann Thorac Surg* 2009; 88(4):1244-1250.

4. Moulakakis KG, Mylonas SN, Dalainas I, et al: Management of complicated and uncomplicated acute type B dissection. A systematic review and meta-analysis. *Ann Cardiothorac Surg* 2014; 3(3):234-246.

5. Nienaber CA, Kische S, Rousseau H, et al: Endovascular repair of type B aortic dissection: long-term results of the randomized investigation of stent grafts in aortic dissection trial. *Circ Cardiovasc Interv* 2013; 6(4):407-416.

6. Song HK, Bavaria JE, Kindem MW, et al: Surgical treatment of patients enrolled in the national registry of genetically triggered thoracic aortic conditions. *Ann Thorac Surg* 2009; 88(3):781-787; discussion 787-788.

7. Song HK, Kindem M, Bavaria JE, et al: Long-term implications of emergency versus elective proximal aortic surgery in patients with Marfan syndrome in the Genetically Triggered Thoracic Aortic Aneurysms and Cardiovascular Conditions Consortium Registry. *J Thorac Cardiovasc Surg* 2012; 143(2):282-286.

8. LeMaire SA, Carter SA, Volguina IV, et al: Spectrum of aortic operations in 300 patients with confirmed or suspected Marfan syndrome. *Ann Thorac Surg* 2006; 81(6):2063-2078; discussion 2078.

9. MacCarrick G, Black JH, 3rd, Bowdin S, et al: Loeys-Dietz syndrome: a primer for diagnosis and management. *Genet Med* 2014; 16(8):576-587.

10. Preventza O, Livesay JJ, Cooley DA, et al: Coarctation-associated aneurysms: a localized disease or diffuse aortopathy. *Ann Thorac Surg* 2013; 95(6):1961-1967; discussion 1967.

11. Hu ZP, Wang ZW, Dai XF, et al: Outcomes of surgical versus balloon angioplasty treatment for native coarctation of the aorta: a meta-analysis. *Ann Vasc Surg* 2014; 28(2):394-403.

12. Brown SL, Busuttil RW, Baker JD, et al: Bacteriologic and surgical determinants of survival in patients with mycotic aneurysms. *J Vasc Surg* 1984; 1(4):541-547.

13. Jaffer U, Gibbs R: Mycotic thoracoabdominal aneurysms. *Ann Cardiothorac Surg* 2012; 1(3):417-425.

14. Johnston KW, Rutherford RB, Tilson MD, et al: Suggested standards for reporting on arterial aneurysms. Subcommittee on Reporting Standards for Arterial Aneurysms, Ad Hoc Committee on Reporting Standards, Society for Vascular Surgery and North American Chapter, International Society for Cardiovascular Surgery. *J Vasc Surg* 1991; 13(3):452-458.

15. Rogers IS, Massaro JM, Truong QA, et al: Distribution, determinants, and normal reference values of thoracic and abdominal aortic diameters by computed tomography (from the Framingham Heart Study). *Am J Cardiol* 2013; 111(10):1510-1516.

16. Pearce WH, Slaughter MS, LeMaire S, et al: Aortic diameter as a function of age, gender, and body surface area. *Surgery* 1993; 114(4):691-697.

17. Coady MA, Rizzo JA, Hammond GL, et al: Surgical intervention criteria for thoracic aortic aneurysms: a study of growth rates and complications. *Ann Thorac Surg* 1999; 67(6):1922-1926; discussion 1928-1953.

18. Elefteriades JA: Natural history of thoracic aortic aneurysms: indications for surgery, and surgical versus nonsurgical risks. *Ann Thorac Surg* 2002; 74(5):S1877-S1880; discussion S1878-1892.

19. Clouse WD, Hallett JW, Jr, Schaff HV, et al: Improved prognosis of thoracic aortic aneurysms: a population-based study. *J Am Med Assoc* 1998; 280(22):1926-1929.

20. Panneton JM, Hollier LH: Nondissecting thoracoabdominal aortic aneurysms: part I. *Ann Vasc Surg* 1995; 9(5):503-514.

21. Weinbaum FI, Dubner S, Turner JW, et al: The accuracy of computed tomography in the diagnosis of retroperitoneal blood in the presence of abdominal aortic aneurysm. *J Vasc Surg* 1987; 6(1):11-16.

22. Jalandhara N, Arora R, Batuman V: Nephrogenic systemic fibrosis and gadolinium-containing radiological contrast agents: an update. *Clin Pharmacol Ther* 2011; 89(6):920-923.

23. Thomsen HS: How to avoid nephrogenic systemic fibrosis: current guidelines in Europe and the United States. *Radiol Clin North Am* 2009; 47(5):871-875, vii.

24. Hiratzka LF, Bakris GL, Beckman JA, et al: 2010 ACCF/AHA/AATS/ACR/ASA/SCA/SCAI/SIR/STS/SVM guidelines for the diagnosis and management of patients with thoracic aortic disease: a report of the American College of Cardiology Foundation/American Heart Association Task Force on Practice Guidelines, American Association for Thoracic Surgery, American College of Radiology, American Stroke Association, Society of Cardiovascular Anesthesiologists, Society for Cardiovascular Angiography and Interventions, Society of Interventional Radiology, Society of Thoracic Surgeons, and Society for Vascular Medicine. *Circulation* 2010; 121(13):e266-369.

25. Orr N, Minion D, Bobadilla JL: Thoracoabdominal aortic aneurysm repair: current endovascular perspectives. *Vasc Health Risk Manag* 2014; 10:493-505.

26. Greenberg RK, Clair D, Srivastava S, et al: Should patients with challenging anatomy be offered endovascular aneurysm repair? *J Vasc Surg* 2003; 38(5):990-996.

27. Patterson BO, Holt PJ, Nienaber C, et al: Management of the left subclavian artery and neurologic complications after thoracic endovascular aortic repair. *J Vasc Surg* 2014; 60(6):1491-1497 e1491.

28. Shrestha M, Bachet J, Bavaria J, et al: Current status and recommendations for use of the frozen elephant trunk technique: a position paper by the Vascular Domain of EACTS. *Eur J Cardiothorac Surg* 2015; 47(5):759-769.

29. Preventza O, Cervera R, Cooley DA, et al: Acute type I aortic dissection: traditional versus hybrid repair with antegrade stent delivery to the descending thoracic aorta. *J Thorac Cardiovasc Surg* 2014; 148(1):119-125.

30. Ghanta RK, Kern JA: Staged hybrid repair for extent II thoracoabdominal aortic aneurysms and dissections. *Oper Tech Thorac Cardiovasc Surg* 2014; 19(2):238-251.

31. Moulakakis KG, Mylonas SN, Antonopoulos CN, et al: Combined open and endovascular treatment of thoracoabdominal aortic pathologies: a systematic review and meta-analysis. *Ann Cardiothorac Surg* 2012; 1(3):267-276.

32. Sultan S, Sultan M, Hynes N: Early mid-term results of the first 103 cases of multilayer flow modulator stent done under indication for use in the management of thoracoabdominal aortic pathology from the independent global MFM registry. *J Cardiovasc Surg (Torino)* 2014; 55(1):21-32.

33. Hughes K, Guerrier J, Obirieze A, et al: Open versus endovascular repair of thoracic aortic aneurysms: a Nationwide Inpatient Sample study. *Vasc Endovascular Surg* 2014; 48(5-6):383-387.

34. Gopaldas RR, Huh J, Dao TK, et al: Superior nationwide outcomes of endovascular versus open repair for isolated descending thoracic aortic aneurysm in 11,669 patients. *J Thorac Cardiovasc Surg* 2010; 140(5):1001-1010.

35. Patel VI, Mukhopadhyay S, Ergul E, et al: Impact of hospital volume and type on outcomes of open and endovascular repair of descending thoracic aneurysms in the United States Medicare population. *J Vasc Surg* 2013; 58(2):346-354.

36. Gopaldas RR, Dao TK, LeMaire SA, et al: Endovascular versus open repair of ruptured descending thoracic aortic aneurysms: a nationwide risk-adjusted study of 923 patients. *J Thorac Cardiovasc Surg* 2011; 142(5):1010-1018.

37. Conrad MF, Ergul EA, Patel VI, et al: Management of diseases of the descending thoracic aorta in the endovascular era: a Medicare population study. *Ann Surg* 2010; 252(4):603-610.

38. Goodney PP, Travis L, Lucas FL, et al: Survival after open versus endovascular thoracic aortic aneurysm repair in an observational study of the Medicare population. *Circulation* 2011; 124(24):2661-2669.

39. von Allmen RS, Anjum A, Powell JT: Outcomes after endovascular or open repair for degenerative descending thoracic aortic aneurysm using linked hospital data. *Br J Surg* 2014; 101(10):1244-1251.

40. Gillen JR, Schaheen BW, Yount KW, et al: Cost analysis of endovascular versus open repair in the treatment of thoracic aortic aneurysms. *J Vasc Surg* 2015; 61(3):596-603.

41. van Bogerijen GH, Patel HJ, Williams DM, et al: Propensity adjusted analysis of open and endovascular thoracic aortic repair for chronic type B dissection: a twenty-year evaluation. *Ann Thorac Surg* 2015; 99(4):1260-1266.

42. Patterson B, Holt P, Nienaber C, et al: Aortic pathology determines mid-term outcome after endovascular repair of the thoracic aorta: report from the Medtronic Thoracic Endovascular Registry (MOTHER) database. *Circulation* 2013; 127(1):24-32.

43. Scali ST, Beck AW, Butler K, et al: Pathology-specific secondary aortic interventions after thoracic endovascular aortic repair. *J Vasc Surg* 2014; 59(3):599-607.

44. LeMaire SA, Price MD, Green SY, et al: Results of open thoracoabdominal aortic aneurysm repair. *Ann Cardiothorac Surg* 2012; 1(3):286-292.

45. Roselli EE, Abdel-Halim M, Johnston DR, et al: Open aortic repair after prior thoracic endovascular aortic repair. *Ann Thorac Surg* 2014; 97(3):750-756.

46. Canaud L, Alric P, Gandet T, et al: Open surgical secondary procedures after thoracic endovascular aortic repair. *Eur J Vasc Endovasc Surg* 2013; 46(6):667-674.

47. Schwill S, LeMaire SA, Green SY, et al: Endovascular repair of thoracic aortic pseudoaneurysms and patch aneurysms. *J Vasc Surg* 2010; 52(4):1034-1037.

48. Preventza O, Mohammed S, Cheong BY, et al: Endovascular therapy in patients with genetically triggered thoracic aortic disease: applications and short- and mid-term outcomes. *Eur J Cardiothorac Surg* 2014; 46(2):248-253.

49. Coselli JS, LeMaire SA, Miller CC, III, et al: Mortality and paraplegia after thoracoabdominal aortic aneurysm repair: a risk factor analysis. *Ann Thorac Surg* 2000; 69(2):409-414.

50. LeMaire SA, Miller CC, III, Conklin LD, et al: A new predictive model for adverse outcomes after elective thoracoabdominal aortic aneurysm repair. *Ann Thorac Surg* 2001; 71(4):1233-1238.

51. Coselli JS, LeMaire SA, Preventza O, et al: Outcomes of 3309 Thoracoabdominal Aortic Aneurysm Repairs. *J Thorac Cardiovasc Surg* 2016; 151(5):1323-1338.

52. Svensson LG, Crawford ES, Hess KR, et al: Thoracoabdominal aortic aneurysms associated with celiac, superior mesenteric, and renal artery occlusive disease: methods and analysis of results in 271 patients. *J Vasc Surg* 1992; 16(3):378-389; discussion 389-390.

53. Jones MM, Akay M, Murariu D, et al: Safe aortic arch clamping in patients with patent internal thoracic artery grafts. *Ann Thorac Surg* 2010; 89(4):e31-32.

54. Svensson LG, Crawford ES, Hess KR, et al: Experience with 1509 patients undergoing thoracoabdominal aortic operations. *J Vasc Surg* 1993; 17(2):357-368; discussion 368-370.

55. MacArthur RG, Carter SA, Coselli JS, et al: Organ protection during thoracoabdominal aortic surgery: rationale for a multimodality approach. *Semin Cardiothorac Vasc Anesth* 2005; 9(2):143-149.

56. Kouchoukos NT, Kulik A, Castner CF: Outcomes after thoracoabdominal aortic aneurysm repair using hypothermic circulatory arrest. *J Thorac Cardiovasc Surg* 2013; 145(3 Suppl):S139-141.

57. Kouchoukos NT, Kulik A, Castner CF: Open thoracoabdominal aortic repair for chronic type B dissection. *J Thorac Cardiovasc Surg* 2015; 149(2 Suppl):S125-129.

58. Kouchoukos NT, Scharff JR, Castner CF: Repair of primary or complicated aortic coarctation in the adult with cardiopulmonary bypass and hypothermic circulatory arrest. *J Thorac Cardiovasc Surg* 2014; 149(2 Suppl):S83-5.

59. Borst HG, Frank G, Schaps D: Treatment of extensive aortic aneurysms by a new multiple-stage approach. *J Thorac Cardiovasc Surg* 1988; 95(1):11-13.

60. Etz CD, Weigang E, Hartert M, et al: Contemporary spinal cord protection during thoracic and thoracoabdominal aortic surgery and endovascular aortic repair: a position paper of the vascular domain of the European Association for Cardio-Thoracic Surgery. *Eur J Cardiothorac Surg* 2015; 47(6):943-957.

61. Tanaka H, Minatoya K, Matsuda H, et al: Embolism is emerging as a major cause of spinal cord injury after descending and thoracoabdominal aortic repair with a contemporary approach: magnetic resonance findings of spinal cord injury. *Interact Cardiovasc Thorac Surg* 2014; 19(2):205-210.

62. Coselli JS, Green SY, Zarda S, et al: Outcomes of open distal aortic aneurysm repair in patients with chronic DeBakey type I dissection. *J Thorac Cardiovasc Surg* 2014; 148(6):2986-2993 e2981-2982.

63. Pujara AC, Roselli EE, Hernandez AV, et al: Open repair of chronic distal aortic dissection in the endovascular era: implications for disease management. *J Thorac Cardiovasc Surg* 2012; 144(4):866-873.

64. Von Aspern K, Luehr M, Mohr FW, et al: Spinal cord protection in open- and endovascular thoracoabdominal aortic aneurysm repair: critical review of current concepts and future perspectives. *J Cardiovasc Surg (Torino)* 2015; 56(5):745-749.

65. Miyamoto K, Ueno A, Wada T, et al: A new and simple method of preventing spinal cord damage following temporary occlusion of the thoracic aorta by draining the cerebrospinal fluid. *J Cardiovasc Surg (Torino)* 1960; 1:188-197.

66. Coselli JS, LeMaire SA, Köksoy C, et al: Cerebrospinal fluid drainage reduces paraplegia after thoracoabdominal aortic aneurysm repair: results of a randomized clinical trial. *J Vasc Surg* 2002; 35(4):631-639.

67. Estrera AL, Sheinbaum R, Miller CC, et al: Cerebrospinal fluid drainage during thoracic aortic repair: safety and current management. *Ann Thorac Surg* 2009; 88(1):9-15.

68. Youngblood SC, Tolpin DA, LeMaire SA, et al: Complications of cerebrospinal fluid drainage after thoracic aortic surgery: a review of 504 patients over 5 years. *J Thorac Cardiovasc Surg* 2013; 146(1):166-171.

69. Coselli JS: The use of left heart bypass in the repair of thoracoabdominal aortic aneurysms: current techniques and results. *Semin Thorac Cardiovasc Surg* 2003; 15(4):326-332.

70. Coselli JS, LeMaire SA, Conklin LD, et al: Left heart bypass during descending thoracic aortic aneurysm repair does not reduce the incidence of paraplegia. *Ann Thorac Surg* 2004; 77(4):1298-1303; discussion 1303.

71. Etz CD, von Aspern K, Gudehus S, et al: Near-infrared spectroscopy monitoring of the collateral network prior to, during, and after thoracoabdominal aortic repair: a pilot study. *Eur J Vasc Endovasc Surg* 2013; 46(6):651-656.

72. Jacobs MJ, Mess W, Mochtar B, et al: The value of motor evoked potentials in reducing paraplegia during thoracoabdominal aneurysm repair. *J Vasc Surg* 2006; 43(2):239-246.

73. Cambria RP, Clouse WD, Davison JK, et al: Thoracoabdominal aneurysm repair: results with 337 operations performed over a 15-year interval. *Ann Surg* 2002; 236(4):471-479.

74. Inoue S, Mori A, Shimizu H, et al: Combined use of an epidural cooling catheter and systemic moderate hypothermia enhances spinal cord protection against ischemic injury in rabbits. *J Thorac Cardiovasc Surg* 2013; 146(3):696-701.

75. Shimizu H, Mori A, Yoshitake A, et al: Thoracic and thoracoabdominal aortic repair under regional spinal cord hypothermia. *Eur J Cardiothorac Surg* 2014; 46(1):40-43.

76. Tetik O, Islamoglu F, Yagdi T, et al: An intraaortic solution trial to prevent spinal cord injury in a rabbit model. *Eur J Vasc Endovasc Surg* 2001; 22(2):175-179.

77. Etz CD, Halstead JC, Spielvogel D, et al: Thoracic and thoracoabdominal aneurysm repair: is reimplantation of spinal cord arteries a waste of time? *Ann Thorac Surg* 2006; 82(5):1670-1677.

78. Griepp RB, Griepp EB: Spinal cord protection in surgical and endovascular repair of thoracoabdominal aortic disease. *J Thorac Cardiovasc Surg* 2015; 149(2 Suppl):S86-90.

79. Etz CD, Debus ES, Mohr FW, et al: First-in-man endovascular preconditioning of the paraspinal collateral network by segmental artery coil embolization to prevent ischemic spinal cord injury. *J Thorac Cardiovasc Surg* 2015; 149(4):1074-1079.

80. Bischoff MS, Scheumann J, Brenner RM, et al: Staged approach prevents spinal cord injury in hybrid surgical-endovascular thoracoabdominal aortic aneurysm repair: an experimental model. *Ann Thorac Surg* 2011; 92(1):138-146; discussion 146.

81. Wong DR, Coselli JS, Amerman K, et al: Delayed spinal cord deficits after thoracoabdominal aortic aneurysm repair. *Ann Thorac Surg* 2007; 83(4):1345-1355; discussion 1355.

82. Schepens MA, Kelder JC, Morshuis WJ, et al: Long-term follow-up after thoracoabdominal aortic aneurysm repair. *Ann Thorac Surg* 2007; 83(2):S851-855; discussion S852-890.

83. LeMaire SA, Jones MM, Conklin LD, et al: Randomized comparison of cold blood and cold crystalloid renal perfusion for renal protection during thoracoabdominal aortic aneurysm repair. *J Vasc Surg* 2009; 49(1):11-19; discussion 19.

84. Köksoy C, LeMaire SA, Curling PE, et al: Renal perfusion during thoracoabdominal aortic operations: cold crystalloid is superior to normothermic blood. *Ann Thorac Surg* 2002; 73(3):730-738.

85. Wynn MM, Acher C, Marks E, et al: Postoperative renal failure in thoracoabdominal aortic aneurysm repair with simple cross-clamp technique and 4 degrees C renal perfusion. *J Vasc Surg* 2015; 61(3):611-622.

86. Tshomba Y, Kahlberg A, Melissano G, et al: Comparison of renal perfusion solutions during thoracoabdominal aortic aneurysm repair. *J Vasc Surg* 2014; 59(3):623-633.

87. Coselli JS, LeMaire SA, Carter SA, et al: The reversed elephant trunk technique used for treatment of complex aneurysms of the entire thoracic aorta. *Ann Thorac Surg* 2005; 80(6):2166-2172; discussion 2172.

88. LeMaire SA, Jamison AL, Carter SA, et al: Deployment of balloon expandable stents during open repair of thoracoabdominal aortic aneurysms: a new strategy for managing renal and mesenteric artery lesions. *Eur J Cardiothorac Surg* 2004; 26(3):599-607.

89. Aftab M, Songdechakraiwut T, Green SY, et al: Contemporary outcomes of open thoracoabdominal aortic aneurysm repair in octogenarians. *J Thorac Cardiovasc Surg* 2014; 149(2 Suppl):S134-41.

90. Coselli JS, Poli de Figueiredo LF, LeMaire SA: Impact of previous thoracic aneurysm repair on thoracoabdominal aortic aneurysm management. *Ann Thorac Surg* 1997; 64(3):639-650.

50

Endovascular Therapy for the Treatment of Thoracic Aortic Disease

Susan D. Moffatt-Bruce • R. Scott Mitchell

Patients with thoracic aortic disease pose many challenges. Frequently, these patients are older and present with multiple comorbidities. Additionally, the posterior location of the descending thoracic aorta requires a large thoracotomy incision, with its own inherent morbidity.

The modern surgical treatment of thoracic aortic disease began in the 1950s, when successful treatment utilizing segmental resection and graft replacement was first reported by Swan, Lam, DeBakey, and Etheridge.[1-3] Soon thereafter, DeBakey and Cooley reported the first successful repair of an ascending aortic aneurysm using cardiopulmonary bypass.[4] Cardiopulmonary bypass and commercially available tube grafts were the mainstays of our surgical armamentarium for the next 30 years. Improved diagnostic capabilities, surgical techniques, and perioperative care have resulted in improved outcomes, even as the risk profile has worsened.[5,6] In an effort to limit the morbidity of these operations,[7,8] endovascular techniques emerged as an attractive alternative. Originally devised for high-risk patients, and following on developments directed toward aneurysms of the abdominal aorta, thoracic endovascular stent-graft technology has rapidly evolved. Although originally intended for repair of atherosclerotic thoracic aortic aneurysms,[9–11] thoracic stent-graft applications have been expanded to the treatment of multiple pathologies, including acute and chronic aortic dissections, penetrating atherosclerotic aortic ulcers, and thoracic aortic trauma.[12-19] Results have steadily improved, and long-term durability has been encouraging; however, the necessity for long-term follow-up remains,[20-22] with obvious financial implications.

HISTORY

Endovascular stent-graft technology, initially targeting the abdominal aortic aneurysm, was introduced by Parodi.[23] Balloon-expandable stents, sewn inside the ends of a vascular tube graft, were placed within the aneurysmal aorta, excluding the aneurysm sac. Simultaneously, at Stanford University Medical Center, a collaborative effort between interventional radiologists and cardiovascular surgeons proved highly synergistic and resulted in a homemade thoracic stent graft.

Self-expanding Gianturco Z stents (Cook Company, Bloomington, IN) were fastened together and covered with a woven Dacron graft (Meadox-Boston Scientific, Natick, MA; Fig. 50-1), and then compressed into a 28-French introducer sheath. The first homemade thoracic graft was implanted in the descending thoracic aorta in 1992 after Institutional Review Board (IRB) approval was obtained. Subsequently, a high-risk trial was approved for patients with thoracic aortic aneurysms who were deemed nonsurgical candidates.[24] Thirteen such patients were treated utilizing stent grafts, customized-designed for each patient. Placement of these stents was successful in all patients, with complete thrombosis of the aneurysm sac reported in 12 of the 13 patients. At 1 year, there were no deaths, paraplegia, strokes, or distal embolization.

Feasibility having been established, IRB approval was obtained for a subsequent trial of 103 patients, 60% of whom were deemed unfit for conventional open surgical repair.[25] Using the same "homemade" first-generation stent graft, complete aneurysm thrombosis was achieved in 83% of patients. Thirty-day mortality was 9% and was significantly associated with a history of cerebral vascular accidents and myocardial infarctions. Major perioperative morbidities included paraplegia in three patients, cerebrovascular accidents in seven patients, and respiratory insufficiency in 12 patients. Actuarial survival was 81% at 1 year and 73% at 2 years. Given the high-risk nature of this patient population, these first-generation results were deemed satisfactory. It was, however, recognized that mortality and morbidity occurred frequently and that long-term follow-up was necessary to establish the long-term efficacy. Subsequently, in 2004, mid-term results were reported for these initial 103 patients treated with first-generation stent grafts.[26] Overall actuarial survival was dismal; 82, 49, and 27% at 1, 5, and 8 years, respectively.

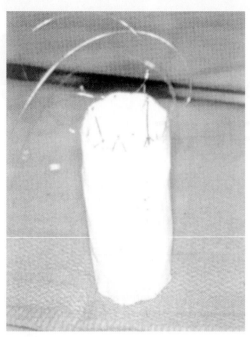

FIGURE 50-1 First-generation stent graft assembled from articulated Z stents and covered with a woven Dacron tube graft.

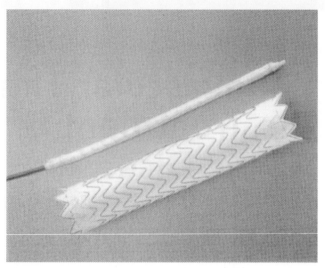

FIGURE 50-2 Second-generation commercially manufactured thoracic aortic stent graft. The thoracic Excluder TAG system by W.L. Gore contains a thin-walled PTFE graft covered by a nitinol exoskeleton.

However, for potentially operable candidates, survival was 93 and 78% at 1 and 5 years, respectively, as contrasted to a 74 and 31% survival at 1 and 5 years, respectively, in those patients deemed inoperable. Late rupture in 11 patients reinforced the mandate for continued lifelong follow-up.

This technology was extended to the treatment of complicated acute type B aortic dissections, as reported by Dake and associates in the *New England Journal of Medicine* in 1999.[27] Again, utilizing these first-generation homemade devices, stent grafts were placed across the primary entry tear, successfully excluding false lumen perfusion. Distal malperfusion was corrected, and false lumen thrombosis within the chest occurred in 79% of patients. Early mortality was 16%, which largely reflected very late referral. Favorable clinical results persisted out to a mean follow-up of 13 months.

TECHNICAL DEVELOPMENT

Homemade stent-graft devices persisted for another 10 years, as commercial development was slow to evolve. Homemade devices were made in 10, 15, and 20 cm lengths, with diameters from 23 to 36 mm. Two-centimeter proximal and distal landing zones were recommended, and stent grafts were oversized to approximately 10 to 15%. These grafts were then loaded into 28-French delivery sheaths, which were advanced into the descending thoracic aorta, usually through a femoral artery cutdown. In addition to small iliofemoral vessels, additional anatomic constraints of these early first-generation stent grafts, which precluded either delivery or secure fixation, included acute angulation of the distal arch, a severe sigmoid-like tortuosity through the diaphragmatic crura, and excessive mural thrombus.

The advent of this new stent-graft technology required a new terminology for endoleaks, which allowed the aneurysmal sac to remain pressurized. Type I endoleaks occur at the proximal (A) or distal (B) attachment sites and signify a failure to achieve a hemostatic seal at these implant sites. Type II endoleaks denote a communication between a branch vessel and the excluded aneurysm sac, and are commonly seen with back-bleeding intercostal vessels. Type III endoleaks occur at graft to graft junctions, and Type IV endoleaks are characterized by increase in aneurysm sac size in the absence of an identifiable endoleak, variously referred to as endotension.

In 2005 and 2006, commercially produced stent grafts became available. Initially, the Gore Excluder TAG system (W.L. Gore, Sunnyvale, CA) was approved (Fig. 50-2), followed shortly thereafter by the Medtronic Talent Graft (Medtronic, Sunrise, FL) and the Cook Zenith (Cook Company, Bloomington, IN). These second- and third-generation endoprostheses addressed many of the deficiencies of the early homemade devices. The delivery systems have become increasingly smaller in diameter and more flexible. The exoskeleton has to provide high column strength and ductility and be compression- and kink-resistant. Nitinol is used predominantly, covered by either Dacron or polytetrafluoroethylene (PTFE) graft material.

EARLY RESULTS

In January 2005, the phase II multicenter trial of the Gore Excluder TAG thoracic endoprosthesis was reported.[28] This multicenter, prospective, nonrandomized trial was conducted at 17 sites and compared the results of stent-graft repair of descending thoracic aortic aneurysms in 140 patients, with the results of open repair in 94 patients. Strict inclusion and

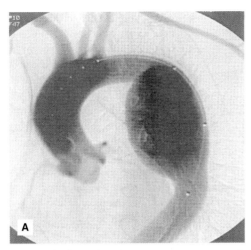
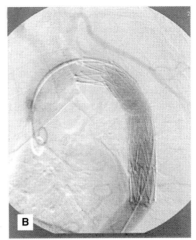

FIGURE 50-3 (A) Angiogram of a descending thoracic aortic aneurysm suitable for stent-graft repair. (B) Angiogram illustrating successful exclusion of the aneurysm sac with a thoracic stent graft.

exclusion criteria were defined in an attempt to ensure comparability of both groups. Follow-up computed tomography (CT) scans were obtained at 1, 6, 12, and 24 months. For stent-graft patients, operative blood loss, renal failure, paraplegia, and mortality rates were all significantly less than for the open repair group (Fig. 50-3). Interestingly, stroke rates were approximately equal in both groups. ICU stay and total hospital stay and time to return to normal activity were approximately 50% shorter for the stent-graft group than for those with open repair. Although stent-graft patients had reduced aneurysm-related mortality out to 2 years (3% vs 10%), interestingly, all-cause mortality was similar between groups at 2 years, similar to the results of recent randomized trials in abdominal aortic aneurysm stent grafts.

THORACIC AORTIC ANEURYSMS

Approximately 50% of all thoracic aortic aneurysms are located in the descending aorta; these aneurysms commonly arise at the level of the left subclavian artery and are often atherosclerotic in nature.[29] The size–rupture correlation has been demonstrated through the natural history of these aneurysms, as reported by Clouse and associates, using the Olmstead County database, in which thoracic aortic aneurysms have an overall 5-year rupture risk of 30%.[30] The Mount Sinai group has identified clinical variables that predict the risk for rupture, including increasing age, presence of chronic obstructive pulmonary disease, maximal thoracic and abdominal aneurysm diameter, and presence of pain.[31] The Yale Aortic Diseases Group has documented rupture and dissection of thoracic aortic aneurysms at a median diameter of 7.2 cm.[6] The Yale Group also reported the mean rate of rupture or dissection as 2% per year for smaller aneurysms, 3% for aneurysms 5.0 to 5.9 cm, and 6.9% for aneurysms 6.0 cm and larger.[32] Open surgical graft replacement has been the traditional mainstay of treatment for these patients, and mortality rates of 5 to 10 % have been reported from experienced centers.[33,34] Similarly,

paraplegia rates have decreased to the 3 to 8% range, with increasing risk associated with increased extent of resection, emergency operation, and renal dysfunction. Utilization of distal circulatory support and cerebral spinal fluid drainage was protective.[35-38] However, in an ever-increasingly elderly population with multiple comorbidities, endovascular repair has become increasingly attractive, especially for patients with favorable anatomy.

Technological progress has also been very enabling. Smaller and more flexible delivery systems have assured access in most patients. Coverage of the left subclavian artery to create a satisfactory proximal landing zone has been frequently employed with few complications. Preoperative left subclavian-to-carotid transposition needs to be entertained only for extensive thoracic coverage, diminutive right vertebral artery, impaired perfusion of both left subclavian and hypogastric arteries, and for patients with previously repaired abdominal aortic aneurysms. Patients considered at high risk for paraplegia should receive a spinal drain preoperatively and hypotension assiduously avoided. Increasingly, percutaneous access is sufficient, even in obese patients. Lastly, much like abdominal aortic aneurysms, endograft technology can be very efficient for the management of ruptured thoracic aortic aneurysms.

THORACIC AORTIC DISSECTION

Perhaps the greatest impact of this endovascular technology has been on the treatment of thoracic aortic dissections. Previously, open repair of complicated acute type B aortic dissections, defined as those dissections with rupture or impending rupture, rapid expansion, or malperfusion syndromes, was associated with high mortalities. Endovascular repair, because of its ability to cover the primary entry tear, thus redirecting flow into the true lumen and eliminating "dynamic malperfusion"; also allows treatment of "static malperfusion" during the same interventional setting.

Uncovered stents placed in branch vessel orifices occluded by an intimal flap are remarkably effective for these malperfused organ systems.[39-42]

For uncomplicated acute type B aortic dissections, there is increasing enthusiasm for prophylactic placement of stent grafts to allow aortic remodeling during the acute and subacute phases. Conventional medical therapy successes may still fail in the late follow-up due to aneurysmal expansion of the false lumen. Early stent-graft intervention, if it could be achieved with low morbidity and mortality, could allow positive aortic remodeling in the stented aorta, avoiding these very problematic late aneurysmal complications. Given the likely development of disease-specific stents, ideally, a covered segment in the proximal portions and uncovered stents for the more distal aorta, prophylactic stent grafting in the subacute stage could allow positive aortic remodeling for the entire thoracic aorta (Fig. 50-4).[27] Hopefully, genetic risk factors which place patients at increased risk for late aneurysmal changes could be identified, which would allow targeting those patients who would most benefit from such a prophylactic intervention.

Chronic aortic dissections are more problematic. Frequently, these patients are much older, with very large aneurysmal components, and multiple communications between true and false lumens. Open surgical repair has been associated with significant morbidity and mortality. Unfortunately, since the dissection frequently extends into the abdomen, and because of multiple fenestrations between the true and false lumens, exclusion of false lumen filling is difficult. Although aneurysmal dilation frequently involves only the proximal descending thoracic aorta, it is unknown whether endograft coverage of the entire thoracic aorta to the level of the celiac artery will be sufficient to provoke false lumen thrombosis. Recent publication of a select series by Hughes and the Duke aortic group has documented good results with low morbidity by stent grafting from the left subclavian artery to the celiac axis.[43] Complete exclusion of a patent false lumen distally, especially in the absence of multibranch grafts, can be very problematic, even with snorkel and chimney grafts and occluder devices. New technical advances should provide more tools to address these very problematic patients. Roselli and the Cleveland Clinic group recently reported surgical

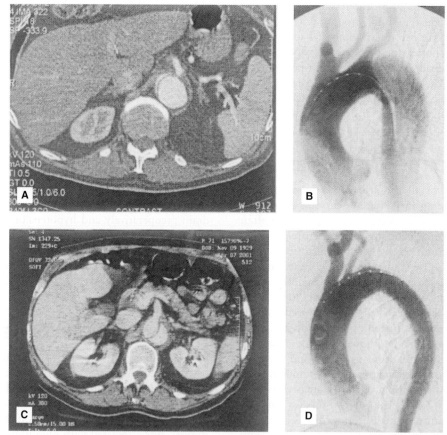

FIGURE 50-4 (A) Intravenous contrast-enhanced CT scan of the upper abdomen demonstrating an aortic dissection with compression of the true lumen. (B) Angiogram of the thoracic aorta demonstrating a type B dissection involving the descending thoracic aorta. (C) CT scan of the abdomen, and (D) angiogram of the descending thoracic aorta after stent-graft implantation into the true lumen in the proximal descending thoracic aorta.

and endovascular experience in this very challenging group of patients, highlighting the competing risks of death and intervention.[44]

PENETRATING ATHEROSCLEROTIC ULCERS AND INTRAMURAL HEMATOMAS

Intramural hematoma (IMH) of the aorta is attracting growing interest as a variant of aortic dissection.[45] The exact pathophysiology is not well understood. Although by definition, pure IMH likely occurs from hemorrhage into the media from the vasa vasorum, many maintain that an intimal disruption is present in all cases.

Certainly, in the absence of any intimal disruption, there would be no indication for stent-graft repair. IMH, however, is often associated with or even precipitated by penetrating atherosclerotic ulcers (PAUs) of the descending thoracic aorta. Therefore, covering the PAU with a stent graft may limit the progression of the IMH and allow healing to occur.[46-48] Unfortunately, even with successful stent-graft implantation using both first- and second-generation grafts, retrograde aortic dissection, new ulcer formation, and endoleaks have been noted in a significant percentage of patients, emphasizing the diffuse and severe nature of this disease.[49-52]

The Stanford group has reported their mid-term results treating PAU of the descending thoracic aorta, with an average of 51 months of follow-up[19] (Fig. 50-5). Using both

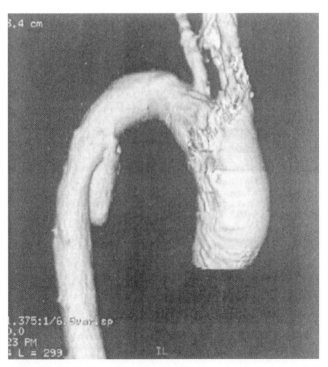

FIGURE 50-5 Three-dimensional CT scan of a giant penetrating ulcer involving the descending thoracic aorta that is perfectly suited to treatment with a thoracic stent graft.

first- and second-generation commercial devices, 26 patients were treated, 14 of whom were deemed nonoperative candidates. The primary success rate was 92%, with actuarial survival estimates of 85, 76, and 70% at 1, 3, and 5 years, respectively. Perioperative mortality was 12%. Increasing aortic diameter and female gender were determinants of treatment failure. These risk factors reflect the importance of careful patient selection based on anatomical criteria and clinical factors. In addition, long-term follow-up with serial CT angiography is necessary to detect late complications.

THORACIC AORTIC TRAUMA

Aortic injuries secondary to nonpenetrating trauma are frequently lethal lesions, with 80 to 90% of patients dying in the hour after the accident.[53] Urgent surgical graft replacement of the aorta has been the conventional treatment, but these patients frequently have other major injuries, including closed head injuries, pulmonary contusions, myocardial contusions, and other solid organ injuries, which may limit options for surgical repair. Thoracic endografts would appear to be an invaluable addition to our surgical armamentarium. Initially, however, all available stent grafts were too large to be utilized inside the smaller aortas of these younger patients. Fortunately, smaller stent grafts, as well as tapered stent grafts, have become available, greatly facilitating repair of these traumatic injuries.[54-58]

Blunt aortic injuries have been classified in an SVS classification system. Class I injury involves only an intimal laceration with no other radiographic changes. Type II injury includes an intimal laceration and mild intramural hemorrhage without significant compromise of the vessel lumen or expansion of the adventitial diameter. Extent III denotes an intramural hemorrhage, sufficient to cause an increase in aortic diameter and compression of the intimal lumen, the classical pseudo-aneurysm. Class IV denotes rupture or impending rupture. For Class I and II injuries, most authors recommend no acute treatment, with repeat imaging in 24 to 48 hours. When anatomically feasible, stent-graft coverage for Class III and IV injuries has become the procedure of choice, limiting stent-graft length to that necessary to cover the injured area. Endografts longer than 15 cm may be associated with an increased risk of paraplegia. For type II injuries noted to progress and for type III injuries, delayed repair may be elected in a stable patient to allow recovery from other injuries. With an Extent III injury and with the necessity for permissive hypertension in the treatment of a closed head injury, early intervention may be warranted (Fig. 50-6). In patients for whom permissive hypertension is desirable, that is, patients with closed head injuries, early stent-graft placement may be indicated. Otherwise, for stable type III or minimally progressive Extent II injuries, delayed stent-graft placement may be most effective, allowing interval recovery from polytrauma. There is little data demonstrating the durability of these stent grafts in past 5 years, but it is expected that interval surveillance will allow safe and timely reintervention if necessary.

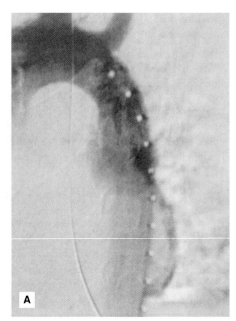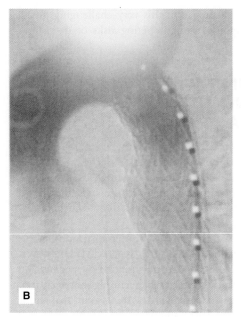

FIGURE 50-6 (A) Thoracic angiogram demonstrating a contained rupture of the descending thoracic aorta in a trauma victim. (B) Thoracic angiogram revealing repair of the aortic rupture with a thoracic stent graft.

FUTURE DIRECTIONS

Despite the many advances in the field of endovascular surgery, stent grafting of the thoracic aorta remains in a developmental phase.[20,59] Newer stent-graft technologies had been slow to become available in the United States, especially compared to China and Japan. Unibranch grafts may allow more proximal repairs into the aortic arch, and multibranch and fenestrated grafts may allow complex repair of thoracoabdominal aortic aneurysms. There are currently many new stent-graft and interventional technologies in the pipeline, which will facilitate aortic repairs in the future. Disease-specific endografts and combinations will also likely become available, further enabling endovascular repair.

Finally, it is important that these patients be followed longitudinally. Early success is no long-term guarantee, as we have seen even totally thrombosed aortic aneurysm sacs elongate with a late appearance of type I endoleaks. Serial imaging may allow timely reintervention, but obviously does incur added expense.

Diseases of the thoracic aorta pose a significant challenge to the surgeon because of complexity of the disease and the characteristics of an ever-aging patient population. Current literature supports increasing application of endovascular technology in well-suited patients, but further follow-up and additional trials may be necessary to further refine the exact role of endovascular repair for the future.

REFERENCES

1. Swan H, Maaske C, Johnson M, Grover R: Arterial homografts II. Resection of thoracic aortic aneurysm using a stored human arterial transplant. *Arch Surg* 1950; 61:732.

2. Lam CR, Aram HH: Resection of a descending thoracic aorta for aneurysm: a report of the use of a homograft in a case and an experimental study. *Ann Surg* 1951; 134:743.

3. DeBakey ME, Cooley DA: Successful resection of aneurysm of thoracic aorta and replacement by graft. *J Am Med Assoc* 1953; 152:673.

4. Cooley DA, DeBakey ME: Resection of entire ascending aorta in fusiform aneurysm using cardiac bypass. *J Am Med Assoc* 1956; 162:1158.

5. Coady MA, Rizzo JA, Goldstein LJ, Elefteriades JA: Natural history, pathogenesis, and etiology of thoracic aortic aneurysms and dissections. *Cardiol Clin North Am* 1999; 17:615.

6. Coady MA, Rizzo JA, Elefteriades JA: Developing surgical intervention criteria for thoracic aortic aneurysm. *Cardiol Clin North Am* 1999; 17:827.

7. Gillum RF: Epidemiology of aortic aneurysm in the United States. *J Clin Epidemiol* 1995; 48:1289.

8. Hagan PG, Nienaber CA, Isselbacher EM, et al: The International Registry of Acute Aortic Dissection. New insights into an old disease. *J Am Med Assoc* 2000; 283:897.

9. Volodos NL, Karpovich IP, Troyan VI, et al: Clinical experience of the use of self-fixing synthetic prosthesis for remote endoprosthetics of the thoracic and the abdominal aorta and iliac arteries through the femoral artery and as intraoperative endoprosthesis for aorta reconstruction. *VASA* 1991; 33(Suppl):93.

10. Ruiz CE, Zhang HP, Douglas JT, et al: A novel method for treatment of abdominal aortic aneurysms using percutaneous implantation of a newly designed endovascular device. *Circulation* 1995; 91:2470.

11. Chuter TAM: Stent-graft design: the good, the bad and the ugly. *Cardiovasc Surg* 2002; 10:7.

12. Umana JP, Mitchell RS: Endovascular treatment of aortic dissections and thoracic aortic aneurysms. *Semin Vasc Surg* 2000; 13:290.

13. Nienaber CA, Fattori R, Lund G, et al: Nonsurgical reconstruction of thoracic aortic dissection by stent-graft placement. *New Engl J Med* 1999; 340:1539.

14. Mitchell RS: Endovascular solution for diseases of the thoracic aorta. *Cardiol Clin North Am* 1999; 17:815.

15. Tokui T, Shimono T, Kato N, et al: Less invasive therapy using endovascular stent graft repair and video-assisted thoracoscopic surgery for ruptured acute aortic dissection. *Jpn Thorac Cardiovasc Surg* 2000; 48:603.

16. Buffolo E, da Fonseca JHP, de Souza JAM, Alves CMR: Revolutionary treatment and aneurysms and dissections of descending aorta: the endovascular approach. *Ann Thorac Surg* 2002; 74:S1815.

17. Kato N, Dake MD, Miller DC, et al: Traumatic thoracic aortic aneurysm: treatment with endovascular stent-grafts. *Radiology* 1997; 205:657.

18. Kasirajan K, Marek J, Langsfeld M: Endovascular management of acute traumatic thoracic aneurysm. *J Trauma* 2002; 52:357.

19. Demers P, Miller C, Mitchell RS, et al: Stent-graft repair of penetrating atherosclerotic ulcers in the descending thoracic aorta: mid-term results. *Ann Thorac Surg* 2004; 77:81.

20. Gleason TG: Thoracic aortic stent grafting: is it ready for prime time? *J Thorac Cardiovasc Surg* 2006; 131:16.

21. Nienaber CA, Erbel R, Ince H: Nihil nocere on the rocky road to endovascular stent-graft treatment. *J Thorac Cardiovasc Surg* 2004; 127:620.

22. Mitchell RS, Dake MD, Semba CP, et al: Endovascular stent-graft repair of thoracic aortic aneurysms. *J Thorac Cardiovasc Surg* 1996; 111:1054.

23. Parodi JC, Palmaz, JC, Barone HD: Transfemoral intraluminal graft implantation for abdominal aortic aneurysms. *Ann Vasc Surg* 1991; 5:491.

24. Dake MD, Miller DC, Semba CP, et al: Transluminal placement of endovascular stent-grafts for the treatment of descending thoracic aortic aneurysms. *New Engl J Med* 1994; 331:1729.

25. Mitchell RS, Miller DC, Dake MD, et al: Thoracic aortic aneurysm repair with an endovascular stent graft: the "first generation". *Ann Thorac Surg* 1999; 67:1971.

26. Demers P, Miller DC, Mitchell RS, et al: Midterm results of endovascular repair of descending thoracic aortic aneurysms with first-generation stent grafts. *J Thorac Cardiovasc Surg* 2004; 127:664.

27. Dake MD, Kato N, Mitchell RS, et al: Endovascular stent-graft placement for the treatment of acute aortic dissection. *New Engl J Med* 1999; 340:1546.

28. Makaroun MS, Dillavou ED, Kee ST, et al: Endovascular treatment of thoracic aortic aneurysms: results of the phase II multicenter trial of the GORE TAG thoracic endoprosthesis. *J Vasc Surg* 2005; 41:1.

29. Pressler V, McNamara JJ: Thoracic aortic aneurysm. *J Thorac Cardiovasc Surg* 1980; 79:489.

30. Clouse WD, Hallett JW, Schaff HV, et al: Improved prognosis of thoracic aortic aneurysms: a population-based study. *J Am Med Assoc* 1998; 280:1926.

31. Jovoenen T, Ergin MA, Galla JD, et al: Prospective study of the natural history of thoracic aortic aneurysms. *Ann Thorac Surg* 1999; 63:551.

32. Davies RR, Goldstein LJ, Coady MA, et al: Yearly rupture or dissection rates for thoracic aortic aneurysms: simple prediction based on size. *Ann Thorac Surg* 2002; 73:17.

33. Svensson LG, Crawford ES, Hess KR, et al: Variables predictive of outcome in 832 patients undergoing repairs of the descending thoracic aorta. *Chest* 1993; 104:1248.

34. Kouchoukos NT, Masetti P, Rokkas CK, et al: Safety and efficacy of hypothermic cardiopulmonary bypass and circulatory arrest for operations on the descending thoracic and thoracoabdominal aorta. *Ann Thorac Surg* 2001; 72:699.

35. Estrera AL, Rubenstein FS, Miller CC, et al: Descending thoracic aortic aneurysm: surgical approach and treatment using the adjuncts cerebrovascular fluid drainage and distal aortic perfusion. *Ann Thorac Surg* 2001; 72:482.

36. Gharagozloo F, Neville RF, Cox JL: Spinal cord protection during surgical procedures on the descending thoracic and thoracoabdominal aorta: a critical overview. *Semin Thorac Cardiovasc Surg* 1998; 10:25.

37. Griepp RB, Ergin MA, Galla JD, et al: Minimizing spinal cord injury during repair of descending thoracic and thoracoabdominal aneurysms: the Mount Sinai approach. *Semin Thorac Cardiovasc Surg* 1998; 10:57.

38. Rokkas CK, Kouchoukos NT: Profound hypothermia for spinal cord protection in operations on the descending thoracic and thoracoabdominal aorta. *Semin Thorac Cardiovasc Surg* 1998; 10:57.

39. Elefteriades JA, Lovoulos CJ, Coady MA, et al: Management of descending aortic dissection. *Ann Thorac Surg* 1999;67; 67:2002.

40. Fann JI, Sarris GE, Mitchell RS, et al: Treatment of patients with aortic dissection presenting with peripheral vascular complications. *Ann Surg* 1990; 212:705.

41. Umana JP, Lai DT, Mitchell RS, et al: Is medical therapy still the optimal treatment strategy for patients with acute type B aortic dissections? *J Thorac Cardiovasc Surg* 2002; 124:896.

42. Nienaber CA, Zannetti S, Barbieri B, et al: INvestigation of STEnt in patients with type B Aortic Dissection: design of the INSTEAD trial—A prospective multicenter, European randomized trial. *Am Heart J* 2005; 149:592.

43. Hughes CC, Ganapathi AM, Englum BR, et al: Thoracic endovascular aortic repair for chronic DeBakey IIIB aortic dissection. *Ann Thorac Surg* 2014; 98:2092.

44. Roselli EE: TEVAR versus open surgery for type-B chronic dissection. *J Thorac Cardiovasc Surg* 2014; 11:028.

45. Coady MA, Rizzo JA, Elefteriades JA: Pathologic variants of thoracic aortic dissections: penetrating artherosclerotic ulcers and intramural hematomas. *Cardiol Clin North Am* 1999; 17:637.

46. Nienaber CA, Richartz BM, Rehders T, et al: Aortic intramural hematoma: natural history and predictive factors for complications. *Heart* 2004; 90:372.

47. Song JK, Kim HS, Kang DH, et al: Different clinical features of aortic intramural hematoma versus dissection involving the ascending aorta. *J Am Coll Cardiol* 2001; 37:1604.

48. Ganaha F, Miller DC, Sugimoto K, et al: Prognosis of aortic intramural hematoma with and without penetrating atherosclerotic ulcer: a clinical and radiological analysis. *Circulation* 2002; 106:342.

49. Sailer J, Peloschek P, Rand T, et al: Endovascular treatment of aortic type B dissection and penetrating ulcer using commercially available stent-grafts. *Am J Roentgenol* 2001; 177:1365.

50. Kos X, Bouchard L, Otal P, et al: Stent-graft treatment of penetrating thoracic aortic ulcers. *J Endovasc Ther* 2002; 9:SII25.

51. Brittenden J, McBride K, McInnes G, et al: The use of endovascular stents in the treatment of penetrating ulcers of the thoracic aorta. *J Vasc Surg* 1999; 30:946.

52. Murgo S, Dussaussois L, Golzarian J, et al: Penetrating atherosclerotic ulcer of the descending thoracic aorta: treatment by endovascular stent-graft. *Cardiovasc Intervent Radiol* 1998; 21:454.

53. Parmley LF, Mattingly TW, Manion WC, et al: Nonpenetrating traumatic injury to the aorta. *Circulation* 1958; 17:1086.

54. Razzouk AJ, Gundry SR, Wang N, et al: Repair of traumatic aortic rupture: a 25-year experience. *Arch Surg* 2000; 135:913.

55. Tatou E, Steinmetz E, Jazayeri S, et al: Surgical outcome of traumatic rupture of the thoracic aorta. *Ann Thorac Surg* 2000; 69-70.

56. Iannelli G, Piscione F, Tommaso LD, et al: Thoracic aortic emergencies: impact of endovascular surgery. *Ann Thorac Surg* 2004; 77:591.

57. Rousseau H, Dambrin C, Marcheix B, et al: Acute traumatic aortic rupture: a comparison of surgical and stent-graft repair. *J Thorac Cardiovasc Surg* 2005; 129:1050.

58. Doss M, Wood JP, Balzer J, et al: Emergency endovascular interventions for acute thoracic aortic rupture: four-year follow-up. *J Thorac Cardiovasc Surg* 2005; 129:645.

59. Mitchell RS: Stent grafts for the thoracic aorta: a new paradigm? *Ann Thorac Surg* 2002; 74:S1818.

Trauma to the Great Vessels

Tom P. Theruvath • Claudio J. Schonholz • John S. Ikonomidis

51

Injury to the aorta and great vessels of the thorax may occur secondary to penetrating or blunt trauma. The management strategy involves control of immediate hemorrhage with prevention of distal malperfusion or pseudoaneurysm development and rupture. Blunt thoracic aortic injury (BTAI) is the most common thoracic vascular injury and is the second leading cause of death in the United States from nonpenetrating trauma. Its incidence is estimated at 7500 to 8000 cases per year.[1] In 75 to 90% of cases, death occurs at the accident scene, typically in those with four or more serious injuries in addition to their aortic transection.[2] Current data suggest that approximately 4% of patients die during transport from the scene, and an additional 19% die during the initial trauma evaluation.[3] A meta-analysis in 2011 reported that in-hospital mortality of patients managed nonoperatively was as high as 46%, whereas mortality was 9% in patients treated by endovascular repair and 19% for open repair.[4] After aortic transection at the isthmus, aortic disruption at the base of the innominate artery is the most common site of injury, followed by the base of the left subclavian artery, and the base of the left carotid. Central venous structures are rarely injured with blunt trauma, but this can occur with penetrating trauma.[5] Traditionally, open surgical repair of these injuries has proved effective. Since the first endovascular thoracic aortic device became commercially available in the United States in 2005, the treatment of BTAI has rapidly evolved as high-volume trauma centers applied the principles of endovascular aneurysm repair to BTAI in an off-label manner. With the growing shift from open repair to thoracic endovascular aortic repair (TEVAR) as the primary treatment in patients with BTAI, outcomes have improved with significantly reduced mortality and morbidity, including procedure-related paraplegia.[6] This chapter describes the traumatic injuries to the thoracic aorta and its brachiocephalic branch vessels. The mechanism, clinical presentation, and treatment strategies are presented. The emphasis is directed to endovascular strategies which have emerged as the most commonly utilized intervention in blunt aortic and brachiocephalic branch vessel trauma.

The chapter is divided into the ascending, arch, and descending zones and both open surgical and endovascular approaches are described with regard to the specific zones.

GENERAL CONSIDERATIONS

Zonal Divisions of the Thoracic Aorta

In order to facilitate international correspondence and a clinically more useful system with regard to anatomical identification of the thoracic aorta, an "anatomical endograft landing zone map" was advocated at the First International Summit on Thoracic Aortic Endografting held in Tokyo in 2001.[7] We suggest using this landing zone map to classify not only the proximal deployment site of an endograft but also extent of open surgical repairs. In 2002, this landing zone map was expanded to include the position of the distal end of the endograft. Since then, the map (Fig. 51-1) has achieved consensus as the standardized anatomical definition to evaluate outcomes.[8] On a more personal notation, we refer to the aortic root as the "double-0" site.

Clinical Presentation

Patients presenting to the emergency department with injury to a great vessel should be evaluated according to standard advanced trauma life support (ATLS) protocols. Those suffering blunt trauma are often hemodynamically stable; therefore, a high index of suspicion for intrathoracic vascular disruption must be based on the mechanism and constellation of related injuries. In addition to high-speed collisions involving automobiles or motorcycles, crush injuries and falls often have sufficient force to rupture a thoracic vessel.[9-12] There are often clues evident in the initial evaluation of a trauma patient that can suggest aortic disruption. In contrast to blunt injury to the arch vessels, patients sustaining descending thoracic aortic rupture are often hemodynamically stable on presentation at the emergency department. Although patients may complain

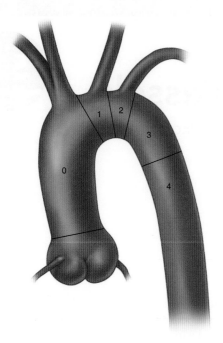

FIGURE 51-1 Zonal divisions of the thoracic aorta.

of dyspnea or back pain and display differential blood pressures in the upper versus lower extremities, specific signs or symptoms of aortic rupture have been identified in less than 50% of cases. Complete de-gloving injury may result in intussusception of the aortic media into the descending thoracic aorta, with resultant "pseudocoarctation" and subsequently variable degrees of distal malperfusion (Fig. 51-2). Commonly associated complaints include neck and chest pain, and physical examination may reveal ecchymosis across the chest and neck from the seatbelt shoulder harness.[13,14]

Physical examination findings concerning for rupture of a great vessel include supraclavicular swelling or bruit, diminished pulse in the ipsilateral upper extremity, neck hematoma with or without tracheal deviation, acute Horner's syndrome, and an acute superior vena cava-like syndrome.[11,14-16] In a stable patient with evidence of a stab or gunshot wound located between the mid clavicular lines or in zone I of the neck, great vessel penetration should be suspected.[17] A precordial bruit suggesting arteriovenous fistula (AVF) formation may be noted in up to 30% of patients.[18] Penetrating distal subclavian injuries may demonstrate pulsatile bleeding during initial evaluation.[19] More commonly, patients suffering penetrating injury to the chest or neck will be hemodynamically unstable on arrival to the emergency department, possibly with evidence of cardiac tamponade, and those *in extremis* should undergo emergent thoracotomy. Hypotensive patients may proceed directly to the operating room without diagnostic imaging; the mortality of patients presenting with hypotension is nearly three times greater than that of stable patients.[18,19] Therefore, an organized, efficient, and effective evaluation of these patients is necessary to prevent unnecessary loss of life.

Classification System for Traumatic Aortic Injury

The classification scheme for grading the severity of BTAI has been widely accepted and is shown in Fig. 51-3.[20] Grade I demonstrates an intimal tear or flap. Grade II demonstrates an intramural hematoma without significant change in the external contour of the aorta. Grade III demonstrates a contained pseudoaneurysm with extension beyond the normal contours of the aorta. Grade IV involves full-thickness aortic injury with extravasation. The Society of

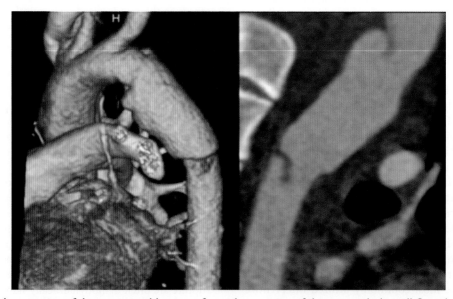

FIGURE 51-2 Pseudocoarctation of the aorta caused by circumferential transection of the aorta with the wall flap telescoping into the distal aorta. Blood flow between the proximal and distal aortic segments is maintained by the surrounding adventitia alone.

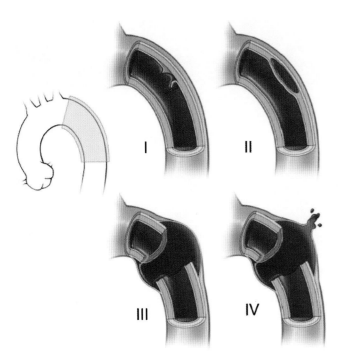

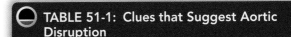
TABLE 51-1: Clues that Suggest Aortic Disruption

History
   Motor vehicle crash >50 km/h
   Motor vehicle crash into fixed barrier
   No seatbelt
   Ejection from vehicle
   Broken steering wheel
   Motorcycle or airplane crash
   Pedestrian hit by motor vehicle
   Falls greater than 3 m
   Crush or cave-in injuries
   Loss of consciousness
Physical signs
   Hemodynamic shock (systolic blood pressure < 90 mm Hg)
   Fracture of sternum, first rib, clavicle, scapula, or multiple ribs
   Steering wheel imprint on chest
   Cardiac murmurs
   Hoarseness
   Dyspnea
   Back pain
   Hemothorax
   Unequal extremity blood pressures
   Paraplegia or paraparesis

FIGURE 51-3 Classification system for blunt thoracic aortic injury (BTAI). The different grades of BTAI are shown: Grade I—intimal tear/flap, Grade II—intramural hematoma, Grade III—pseudoaneurysm, Grade IV—rupture.

Vascular Surgery guidelines recommend TEVAR for grade II through IV BTAIs, given that grade I injuries typically heal spontaneously.

Initial Evaluation

A multitrauma patient should be evaluated according to standard ATLS protocols regardless of whether aortic disruption is suspected. The primary and secondary survey, routine radiographs, and hemodynamic stabilization must be completed before the team can begin investigating specific injuries. The first step in diagnosing a blunt traumatic aortic injury is identifying the at-risk patient. Motor vehicle collisions, falls from height, explosions, and crush injuries have the impact and deceleration forces required to cause aortic transection; therefore these patients should undergo imaging directed at ruling out this potentially fatal injury.[21-24] Operative management of intracranial space-occupying lesions and intra-abdominal hemorrhage takes priority over nonbleeding aortic injuries. Hemodynamically unstable patients with signs of exsanguinating hemorrhage should go directly to the operating room for control of hemorrhage, and transesophageal ultrasound may be used to evaluate for aortic injury. Ninety-five percent of patients with aortic disruption have associated injuries. Data accrued from a trial which included approximately 50 trauma centers across the United States and Canada, the American Association for the Surgery of Trauma

(AAST) trial,[25] demonstrated that current advancements in emergency medical resuscitation in the field have provided more patients the opportunity to reach the hospital and receive aggressive definitive care. There are often clues evident in the initial evaluation in these patients that can suggest aortic disruption (Table 51-1).

CHEST X-RAY

In the majority of trauma patients, a supine chest radiograph is obtained as part of the initial evaluation, and the constellation of grossly widened mediastinum, hemothorax, and transient hemodynamic instability on arrival appear to be predictive of early in-hospital death from BTAI.[26] During the evaluation of a blunt trauma patient, an anteroposterior chest radiograph is routinely obtained and ought to be examined for one of the 15 signs that have been associated with aortic rupture (Table 51-2).[27] Widening of the mediastinum to a width exceeding 25% of the total chest width, obliteration of the aortic knob, apical pleural capping, and fractures of the sternum, scapula, clavicle, or first rib are some of the most common findings (Fig. 51-4). None of these signs have demonstrated sufficient sensitivity or specificity to effectively rule out aortic injury, however, and up to 40% of patients with aortic rupture have had chest x-ray findings interpreted as normal.[22,23,28-32] When abnormalities are identified, however, they can aid the practitioner in determining which patients require aggressive imaging to definitively rule out an aortic injury.

TABLE 51-2: Chest X-ray Findings Associated with Blunt Aortic Disruption

Widened mediastinum (>8.0 cm)

Mediastinum-to-chest width ratio >0.25

Tracheal shift to the patient's right

Blurred aortic contour

Irregularity or loss of the aortic knob

Left apical cap

Depression of the left main bronchus

Opacification of the aortopulmonary window

Right deviation of the nasogastric tube

Wide paraspinal lines

First rib fracture

Any other rib fracture

Clavicle fracture

Pulmonary contusion

Thoracic spine fracture

Data from Cook AD, Klein JS, Rogers FB, et al: Chest radiographs of limited utility in the diagnosis of blunt traumatic aortic laceration, *J Trauma*. 2001 May; 50(5):843-847.

COMPUTED TOMOGRAPHY

In the typical hemodynamically stable blunt trauma patient, head and abdominopelvic computed tomography (CT) should be conducted to identify closed-head or intra-abdominal injury. Those with an abnormal chest x-ray or a traumatic mechanism consistent with aortic injury should undergo helical CT scan of the chest with intravenous contrast at this time. Since its introduction in the early 1990s, CT has become the screening tool of choice at most medical institutions to detect traumatic aortic rupture due to its availability, speed, and ease of interpretation. Additionally, sensitivities and negative predictive values nearing 100% have

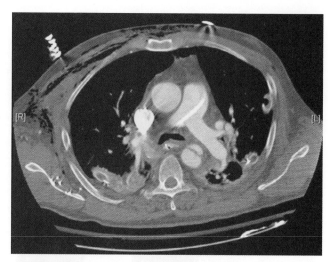

FIGURE 51-5 Helical computed tomography scan of the chest in a 30-year-old male after a high-speed motor vehicle collision demonstrating an intimal flap in the proximal descending thoracic aorta and periaortic hematoma.

been reported for volumetric helical or spiral CT.[22,23,32-35] Normal aorta portrays homogeneous enhancement, while filling defects, contrast extravasation, intimal flaps, periaortic hematoma, pseudoaneurysm, and mural thrombi may suggest the presence of an aortic injury (Fig. 51-5).[34] Moreover, the enhanced resolution of CT imaging has allowed identification of minimal aortic injuries, such as small intimal flaps with minimal or no mediastinal changes, that may be safely managed with anti-impulse therapy.[23,34,36]

TRANSESOPHAGEAL ECHOCARDIOGRAPHY

Transesophageal echocardiography (TEE) has become a valuable tool in cardiothoracic surgery due to its ability to image the entire descending thoracic aorta along with portions of the ascending aorta arch and its portability. In unstable blunt trauma patients requiring laparotomy, TEE can be utilized to evaluate the descending aorta for evidence of rupture, such as a mural flap or a thickened vessel wall concerning for mural thrombus. Multiplanar TEE probes permit acquisition of cross-sectional images at different angles along a single rotational axis. The typical 5- or 7-MHz transducer permits adequate resolution of structures as small as 1 to 2 mm. Doppler mapping of turbulent blood flow near a vessel wall abnormality may be suggestive of blunt aortic disruption, and time-resolved imaging allows evaluation of the movement of anatomic structures, thereby enhancing the ability to define the physiologic consequences of such abnormalities. Chronic atheromatous disease of the aorta can complicate obtaining and interpreting TEE images; therefore observation of multiple-related signs of injury, such as mural flap with a surrounding mediastinal hematoma, is more reliable. A disadvantage of TEE, and potential inhibitor to its widespread use as a screening tool for aortic injury, is its operator-dependent nature with sensitivities as low as 63% documented for this modality.[37] A prospective comparison of imaging techniques

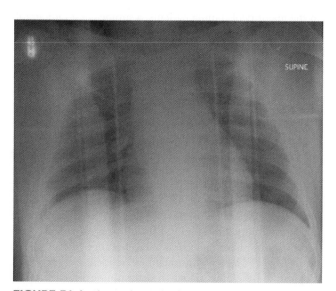

FIGURE 51-4 Chest radiograph of an 18-year-old male victim of a motor vehicle collision showing a widened mediastinum.

for diagnosis of blunt aortic trauma reported, however, sensitivity and specificity of 93 and 100% for TEE compared to 73 and 100% for helical CT.[35] Thoracoscopy has also been used to evaluate traumatic hemothoraces, however with experienced practitioners intraoperative TEE has superb sensitivity and specificity for aortic transection.[38,39] TEE is more invasive than helical CT, but overall the associated risk is low. Contraindications include concomitant injury to the cervical spine, oropharynx, esophagus, or maxillofacial structures.[35]

MAGNETIC RESONANCE ANGIOGRAPHY

Vascular structures are well imaged by magnetic resonance angiography (MRA), particularly the thoracic aorta, and its utility in the diagnosis and follow-up of complex aortic disease including aortic dissections and aneurysms is firmly established.[40-42] The time required to capture images inhibits the utility of MRA in the acute evaluation of a trauma patient, however it may be effective in posttherapeutic surveillance of traumatic thoracic injuries.

AORTOGRAPHY

Aortography may be useful when helical CT or TEE fail to definitively identify or adequately characterize an aortic injury. The role of aortography in evaluating blunt thoracic injuries was firmly established prior to the advent of noninvasive, sophisticated imaging techniques, and it may still be considered the gold standard. In experienced hands its sensitivity and specificity both approach 100%.[43] Intra-arterial digital subtraction is most often used because it allows rapid generation of images (Fig. 51-6). In the past, intravenous digital subtraction was used as well. After injecting intravenous

contrast, time-delayed images of the arch and descending aorta were obtained, and although this technique greatly decreased the duration of the procedure, it was abandoned because the diagnostic accuracy for aortic disruption was less than 70%.[40] With the availability and speed of helical CT, aortography is now rarely used for diagnosis, but routinely utilized for endovascular stent graft placement. This intervention requires a highly trained team of endovascular specialists and can be time-consuming; therefore trauma patients with additional life or limb threatening injuries should be otherwise stabilized before entering the endovascular suite. Rates of exsanguination and death of up to 10% have previously been reported during diagnostic aortography, but this incidence has decreased significantly as endovascular proficiency has improved.[40,44,45] In fact, complication rates attributed directly to aortography are low, but patients may suffer contrast reactions, contrast nephropathy, groin hematomas, or femoral artery pseudoaneurysms. False-positive studies are usually attributed to atheromata or ductal diverticula.

Decision to Repair Versus Expectant Management

Uniformly, hemodynamically unstable blunt trauma patients should bypass diagnostic imaging and be taken to the operating room immediately. During a damage control exploratory laparotomy or thoracotomy, TEE may be conducted to diagnose contained aortic rupture.[35] Operative repair of the aorta should not be attempted at this time, however, as this group of patients benefit from immediate transfer to the intensive care unit for further resuscitation. Once hemodynamic stability is achieved, anti-impulse therapy with beta-blockade should be initiated to minimize aortic wall stress. Hemodynamically stable patients diagnosed with blunt aortic injury, and lacking severe associated injuries requiring interventions, warrant immediate repair. Treatment of all nonlife-threatening injuries should be delayed until after definitive aortic repair. As such, delayed management has demonstrated to be safe and effective in carefully selected patients with severe associated injuries or comorbidities.[46-57] Patients with thoracic, intraperitoneal or retroperitoneal hemorrhage, or intracranial bleeding that cause mass effect should be managed with aggressive anti-impulse therapy to minimize the risk of aortic rupture while these injuries are addressed.[55] The goal of anti-impulse therapy should be to maintain a systolic blood pressure less than 120 mm Hg and/or a mean arterial pressure less than 80 mm Hg.[23] The aortic insult should also be monitored by TEE during surgical repair of concomitant injuries, and routinely imaged with CT during the delayed management period. The mortality rate of patients awaiting aortic repair has ranged from 30 to 50%, but the majority of deaths have not been related to the aortic injury.[49,50,55] In the AAST trial, those presenting in extremis or with evidence of free aortic rupture were excluded, and the mortality rate of patients with associated injuries that precluded initial aortic repair was 55%.[25] Therefore, evidence supports operative delay

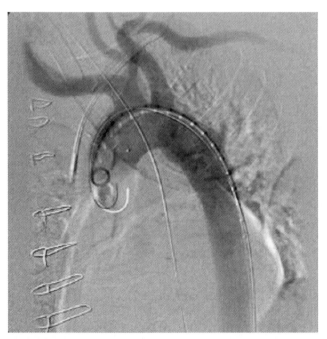

FIGURE 51-6 Digital subtraction arteriogram of an acute traumatic aortic disruption near the isthmus.

or even nonoperative management in select patients with blunt aortic injury who may be considered poor operative candidates. Even in carefully selected patient with BTAIs deliberate nonoperative management has been shown to be a reasonable alternative in the polytrauma patient.[58] Anti-impulse therapy with beta-blockers should be initiated in patients proceeding directly to the operating room for aortic repair, as well as in those selected for delayed repair, to reduce blood pressure and thereby reduce aortic wall stress.[23,24,59] In-hospital aortic rupture rates have been reduced through aggressive beta-blockade without adversely affecting the outcome of associated injuries.[23]

THE ASCENDING AORTA

Mechanism of Injury

Descending thoracic aortic transection is the most common vascular injury resulting from blunt thoracic force. The ascending aorta and arch vessels, however, may also be disrupted, commonly leading to dissection or pseudoaneurysm formation.[11,14] Mechanistically, the transmission of force through the thoracic cavity from blunt injury is believed to cause torsion of the ascending aorta, leading to disruption of the wall with an associated shearing effect on the heart.[60] Additionally, a water-hammer effect is described in which an aortic occlusion at the diaphragm occurs with impact and a high pressure wave is reflected back to the ascending aorta and aortic arch.[61]

Operative Repair

Pseudoaneurysm of the ascending aorta should be repaired using cardiopulmonary bypass. Femorofemoral or axillofemoral cannulation and commencement of cardiopulmonary bypass before sternotomy may decompress the ascending aorta and decrease the risk of pseudoaneurysm rupture on opening the chest.[16] After entering the pericardium, the pseudoaneurysm should be carefully mobilized, if possible, to gain proximal and distal control. Depending on the nature and extent of the injury, repair may be conducted by primary repair, patch angioplasty, or prosthetic replacement of aortic segment. If aortic valve insufficiency is encountered, prosthetic valve replacement may be warranted.[62] Occasionally, deep hypothermic circulatory arrest is required, especially if proximal and distal control cannot be comfortably obtained or the pseudoaneurysm extends into the proximal aortic arch. This will allow for excision of the pseudoaneurysm and closure of the aortic defect with a prosthetic patch.[60] As with descending thoracic aortic injuries, a delay in operative management may be considered in hemodynamically stable patients with associated injuries at high risk for bleeding, especially intracranial lesions.[60] The application of this delayed approach depends on the nature of the ascending aortic injury. For instance, it must be a discrete lesion without evidence of circumferential involvement or compromised adjacent structures. Safe observation entails maintaining a mean arterial pressure less than 80 mm Hg

and cerebral perfusion pressure greater than 50 mm Hg, typically through short-acting intravenous beta-blockade.[63] Conservative management must be accompanied by regular assessment of the aortic lesion through serial CT scans of the thorax and a low threshold for operative intervention if enlargement of the pseudoaneurysm is identified.[63]

Endovascular Interventions

Several studies have reported safety and effectiveness of TEVAR of the descending aorta, but the role of TEVAR for treating ascending aortic pathology is less well known. Especially the role of ascending TEVAR (or A-TEVAR) in the setting of trauma has not been evaluated and reported to date. Only a small number of studies have described outcomes with this approach.[64-66] The reported experience demonstrates that endovascular repair of the ascending aorta is technically feasible in settings of chronic aneurysms or acute aortic dissections and can be accomplished with promising early results. Currently there are no commercially available endovascular devices specifically designed to treat the ascending aorta. Compared with TEVAR of the descending thoracic aorta, endovascular therapy for the ascending aorta is challenged by more complex pathology, hemodynamic characteristics, and anatomy. As such, the proximity of the aortic valve and coronary arteries to the ascending aorta makes it particularly challenging to obtain seal and fixation within the proximal landing zone. Thus far the only intervention is the open surgical approach via median sternotomy and cardiopulmonary bypass as described in the previous section.

THE AORTIC ARCH BRANCH VESSELS

Mechanism of Injury

The pathogenesis of blunt innominate artery rupture has been postulated to be the result of anteroposterior compression of the mediastinum between the sternum and vertebrae, displacing the heart posteriorly and to the left, thereby increasing the curvature of the aortic arch and increasing tension on all of its outflow vessels.[67] Hyperextension of the cervical spine with head rotation provides additional tension on the right carotid artery, which is transmitted to the innominate artery, and can lead to rupture.[67] The left carotid artery undergoes stretching injury with rapid deceleration, producing an intimal tear and subsequent dissection.[11] Additional mechanisms of carotid artery injury include hyperflexion of the neck to cause compression between the mandible and cervical spine, basilar skull fracture transecting the artery, and strangulation injury.[11] Blunt subclavian artery injuries are more common in the middle and distal third of the artery and are theorized to be caused by downward forces fracturing the first rib with the anterior scalene acting as a fulcrum so that the subclavian artery is pinched between the first rib and clavicle.[9] The abrupt deceleration of the shoulder, owing to the seatbelt shoulder harness, is also believed to cause subclavian artery shearing injuries.[9]

Operative Repair

INNOMINATE ARTERY

The innominate artery is the second most common site of thoracic vascular injury following blunt trauma. In a review of 117 reported cases of blunt innominate artery rupture, 83% were in the proximal vessel, 3% were in the middle, 9% were distal, and the remaining injuries involved multiple sections.[10] The most common finding was disruption of the intima and media with pseudoaneurysm formation (Fig. 51-7).[10] Although primary repair may be possible in some cases, surgical repair of an innominate artery rupture has traditionally been performed by a prosthetic aorto-innominate bypass graft from the aortic arch to healthy distal vessels through a full or upper median sternotomy with extension of the incision along the anterior border of the right sternocleidomastoid as necessary.[17,68] Operative repair of a penetrating innominate artery injury is approached in the same manner.[17] The entire length of the innominate artery should be mobilized to achieve distal control and the pericardium opened to gain proximal control at the level of the aortic arch.[69] After systemic administration of heparin, a partial occlusion clamp is applied to the aortic arch and the proximal anastomosis of the prosthetic graft performed end-to-side with polypropylene suture.[69] Depending on the location and extent of the injury, the distal end-to-end anastomosis may involve only the innominate artery or a Y-graft may be required to reconstruct the proximal portions of the right carotid and right subclavian arteries individually.[10] The origin of the innominate artery should then be fully exposed and oversewn with pledgeted nonabsorbable sutures.[69] Healthy patients typically tolerate temporary innominate artery occlusion caused by adequate collateral flow through the contralateral carotid and vertebral arteries.[69] Cerebral protection, cardiopulmonary bypass, electroencephalogram monitoring, hypothermia with circulatory arrest, or carotid shunting (for stump pressure < 50 mm Hg) should be employed in patients with neurologic abnormalities or suspicion of a contralateral carotid artery injury.[68,69] Long-term patency of prosthetic aorto-innominate artery bypass grafts has been reported to be greater than 96% at 10 years.[70]

CAROTID ARTERY

Therapeutic management of blunt carotid artery injury must be directed at preventing cerebral ischemia and surgical intervention should be weighed against observation and anticoagulation.[71] Small intimal flaps may resolve, whereas larger flaps can lead to thrombosis and therefore require anticoagulation to prevent thromboembolism.[72] Arterial dissection may progress to luminal narrowing, placing the patient at risk for thrombosis, and anticoagulation therapy is especially important in patients with bilateral carotid artery dissection owing to the morbidity and mortality associated with bilateral thrombosis.[73] When operative intervention is indicated because of pseudoaneurysm formation (Fig. 51-8), the surgeon may bypass the lesion, but reconstruction or ligation of the artery can also be employed.[11] Open repair of an intrathoracic carotid artery injury should occur through a median sternotomy with extension along the anterior border of the ipsilateral sternocleidomastoid muscle as necessary to gain adequate exposure.[18] After gaining proximal and distal control, arterial repair may be accomplished by primary repair or interposition grafting with saphenous vein or prosthetic material.[18]

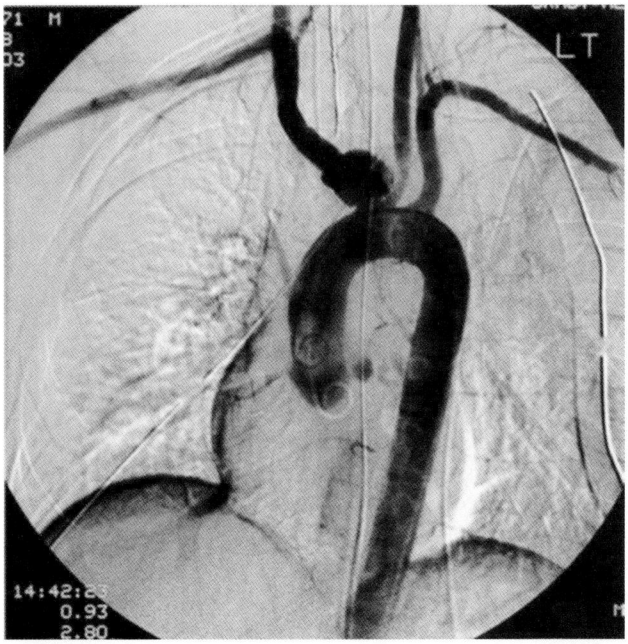

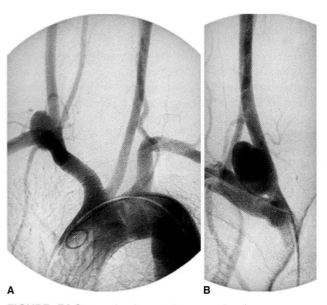

FIGURE 51-7 Arteriogram showing rupture of proximal segment of innominate artery and pseudoaneurysm at the site of rupture. (Reproduced with permission of Symbas JD, Halkos ME, Symbas PN: Rupture of the innominate artery from blunt trauma: current options for management, *J Card Surg* 2005 Sep-Oct;20(5):455-459.)

A   **B**

FIGURE 51-8 Digital subtraction angiography demonstrating a wide-necked pseudoaneurysm at the base of the right common carotid artery. Slide A is a left anterior oblique view with an aortic arch injection. Slide B shows the right anterior oblique view with innominate artery injection. (Reproduced with permission from Simionato F, Righi C, Melissano G, et al: Stent-graft treatment of a common carotid artery pseudoaneurysm, *J Endovasc Ther*. 2000 Apr;7(2):136-140.)

SUBCLAVIAN ARTERY

Injury to the subclavian artery, from blunt or penetrating trauma, carries a mortality rate of 5 to 30% resulting from the inability to obtain adequate hemorrhagic control through direct pressure.[74,75] Additionally, because of the close proximity of the trachea, esophagus, subclavian vein, and brachial plexus, subclavian artery injuries are associated with 40% morbidity.[74] Operative exposure may be achieved by median sternotomy, limited sternotomy, supraclavicular incision, infraclavicular incision, thoracotomy, or a combination of these depending on the location of the injury.[76] Left-sided lesions are often managed through an anterolateral thoracotomy with either an infraclavicular or supraclavicular counter incision; however, some surgeons perform a median sternotomy for a proximal injury.[9,76] Right-sided injuries, on the other hand, require median sternotomy with supraclavicular extension.[9] In cases in which the defect involves a long segment of the subclavian artery, a portion of the clavicle may be resected to optimize exposure, although this procedure carries considerable postoperative morbidity.[19,76] Once establishing proximal and distal control of the subclavian artery, the damaged arterial segment may be excised and arterial reconstruction accomplished with an interposition graft using a saphenous vein or prosthetic material.[9] In cases in which minimal arterial debridement is required, primary repair is often attained.[77] Ligation of the subclavian artery may be performed on critically ill patients unable to tolerate an extensive operative repair, and minimal short-term morbidity in the affected limb has been reported.[19,76,77] When planning operative repair of the subclavian artery, concomitant injuries to nearby structures such as the subclavian vein and brachial plexus should be considered.

Endovascular Interventions

Arteriography is considered the gold standard for diagnosis and characterization of an intrathoracic vascular injury, and as endovascular stent technology and surgeon proficiency continue to advance, arteriography may become the preferred method of treatment in hemodynamically stable patients. The literature is currently populated with small case series and case reports documenting the feasibility of this approach and minimal short-term morbidity and mortality, but very little long-term data exist. Similar to other minimally invasive techniques, endovascular management of a traumatic injury to an intrathoracic vessel can provide an opportunity for patients to avoid sternotomy or thoracotomy and the associated pain, prolonged recovery time, and infection risk.[78,79] An analysis of endovascular versus open procedures in the National Trauma Database revealed a survival advantage for endovascular repair when controlling for injury severity score, associated injuries, and age.[80] Widespread application of endovascular techniques to manage great vessel trauma in hemodynamically stable patients is constrained by lesion anatomy. With regard to accessing the injury, the relationship of the vascular defect to the aortic arch is rarely an issue because brachial and carotid artery approaches, with or without a concomitant femoral approach, are increasingly

employed.[79] However, the likelihood that the adjacent healthy vessel segments will provide adequate landing zones and the preservation of branch vessels are important considerations.[81] Therefore, critical assessment of each individual lesion is required to assure appropriate use of this technology. Common endovascular modalities such as bare-metal or covered stents (stent grafts) and coil embolization have been employed in vascular trauma. Stent grafts were not commercially available before 2000; therefore, case reports published in that timeframe described use of home-made devices in which the surgeon affixed autologous tissue, expanded polytetrafluoroethylene (ePTFE), or polyester to a bare-metal stent and then repackaged the device for endovascular deployment across an AVF or pseudoaneurysm.[82] There are currently a number of self-expandable and balloon-expandable stent grafts approved for coronary or peripheral vascular interventions that have been successfully used in the aortic arch vessels, specifically the wall-stent endoprosthesis (Boston Scientific, Natick, MA), the Gore Viabahn endoprosthesis (W.L. Gore & Associates, Flagstaff, AZ), and the Jostent stent-graft coronary or peripheral (Abbott Vascular, Redwood City, CA).[83]

INNOMINATE ARTERY

Stable patients who have suffered either a blunt or penetrating injury to the innominate artery have benefited from endovascular repair with a stent graft, without reported complications.[13,78,84-86] One technical consideration when approaching an innominate artery pseudoaneurysm is whether the distal landing zone of the stent graft will occlude the carotid artery. This situation can potentially be avoided by realignment of the guidewire such that the orifice of the subclavian artery is covered instead, a lesion that is typically asymptomatic owing to the extensive collateralization of the upper extremity around the shoulder.[78,87] Alternatively, if the stent graft must traverse the origin of the right common carotid, a subclavian-carotid bypass may be performed before deployment.[78] Appropriate follow-up for these endovascular repairs has yet to be defined, but biannual duplex ultrasound examinations or CT scans have been proposed. The duration of antiplatelet therapy after stent graft deployment is also unclear; however, the majority of patients are discharged from the hospital on daily aspirin therapy with or without Plavix (Bristol-Myers Squibb, Princeton, NJ).[13,88,89]

CAROTID ARTERY

Trauma to the intrathoracic carotid artery is rare, but cases of successful stent-graft exclusion of pseudoaneurysms have been reported.[90-96] Embolic risk should be considered when assessing whether the lesion is suitable for endovascular intervention, and many surgeons advocate for delayed stenting of carotid injuries to minimize arterial manipulation and the potential embolic sequelae.[97] Safely anticoagulating the trauma patient with concomitant intracranial or solid organ injuries can be difficult, but maintaining a partial thromboplastin time between 40 and 50 seconds has been shown to effectively cover carotid artery injuries without significantly increasing the bleeding risk.[73] Full heparinization is vital during the stent-graft deployment procedure, however, and should be followed by antiplatelet therapy with Plavix for at least 2 weeks with subsequent conversion to lifelong aspirin therapy.[91] Although patients should be monitored for alterations in neurologic function as a marker of stent stenosis or occlusion, serial duplex ultrasounds ought to be employed to identify subclinical luminal narrowing.[97]

SUBCLAVIAN ARTERY

Endovascular repair of subclavian artery injuries has been relatively well described in the literature because of the obvious benefits of this procedure compared with the morbidity of open subclavian artery exposure.[83,87,94,98-104] Stent grafts have effectively treated pseudoaneurysms, lacerations, AVFs, and complete transections of the subclavian artery and theoretically reduce the incidence of brachial plexus injury since dissection of the traumatized field has been eliminated.[81,101,105] An interventional consideration unique to the subclavian artery has been the presence of branch vessels that may be covered by the stent graft and provide a source for endoleak. If contralateral vertebral artery patency and antegrade flow have been visualized, these branch vessels may often be coil embolized.[81] If the vertebral artery cannot be safely occluded, however, a vertebral-carotid transposition should be completed before deployment of the stent graft.[104] Alternatively, stent-graft repair of the subclavian artery may cover an internal thoracic artery that has been used as a pedicled graft for coronary artery bypass grafting, placing the patient at risk for significant cardiac ischemia. Postprocedure antiplatelet therapy has consisted of Plavix for 1 to 3 months followed by lifelong aspirin therapy.[104] Repetitive compression of the stent graft between the clavicle and first rib over the lifespan of a young trauma patient creates the risk of stent fracture (Fig. 51-9). Therefore, long-term follow-up with serial imaging is required.[87] Both stenosis and stent fracture, although often asymptomatic, have been treated with balloon dilation and deployment of an additional stent such that open intervention may still be avoided.[81,102]

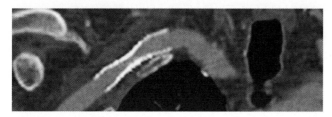

FIGURE 51-9 Balloon-expandable stent-graft 8 months after deployment demonstrating signs of compression between the clavicle and the first rib. (Reproduced with permission from Schoder M, Cejna M, Holzenbein T, et al: Elective and emergent endovascular treatment of subclavian artery aneurysms and injuries, *J Endovasc Ther.* 2003 Feb;10(1):58-65.)

THE DESCENDING THORACIC AORTA

Mechanism of Injury

Traumatic aortic disruptions typically occur in motor vehicle drivers, passengers, or pedestrians hit by vehicles.[25,106,107] Alcohol or other substance abuse is involved in greater than 40% of these motor vehicle accidents.[107] Patients ejected from the vehicle are twice as likely to sustain traumatic aortic injury, and seatbelt use can decrease this risk fourfold.[107] Overall, seatbelts have been demonstrated to be more effective than airbags at preventing blunt aortic injury, and aortic rupture of both the ascending and descending aorta has been attributed to the deployment of an airbag.[108-110] Falls from significant height, crush injuries, and airplane accidents have also caused aortic rupture.[22,25,106,111] The pathogenesis of aortic transection remains controversial and no integrated understanding of these forces has been achieved. The "whiplash" theory proposes that a combination of traction, torsion, shear, and bursting forces interact owing to differential deceleration of tissues within the mediastinum, thereby causing adequate stress to rupture the aorta at the isthmus.[107,112-116] The ligamentum arteriosum, the left main stem bronchus, and the paired intercostal arteries limit aortic mobility. Investigations have shown that displacement of the aorta in a longitudinal direction may cause a tear at the isthmus.[114] Alternatively, the "osseous pinch" mechanism has been proposed based on quantifiable thoracic compression.[117,118] With this mechanism, anterior thoracic osseous structures (manubrium, first rib, and clavicular heads) rotate posteriorly and inferiorly and may impact the vertebral column, pinching the aortic isthmus and proximal descending thoracic aorta.[118] This pinch is theorized to cause shearing of the aorta and some clinical data do support the osseous pinch mechanism.[119] Overall, diversity among the direction and magnitude of forces generated by a blunt traumatic event in patients suffering descending thoracic aortic rupture have prohibited identification of a single pathogenetic mechanism. Traumatic aortic disruptions in the descending thoracic aorta occur most commonly at the aortic isthmus, and an autopsy series identified 54% at this site, with 8% in the ascending aorta, 2% in the arch, and 11% in the distal descending aorta.[120] In those who survive, the periadventitial tissues around the isthmus appear to provide protection against free rupture and allow time for transfer to a hospital; consequently, surgical case series have reported 84 to 97% of aortic ruptures occurring at the isthmus.[25,121-125] The strength of the aortic wall is in its adventitial layer, and despite the increased incidence of transection at the aortic isthmus, there is no evidence to suggest that the adventitia in this area is deficient.[126] Additionally, the structure of the aortic wall surrounding the transection has not demonstrated any defect and atherosclerotic disease does not play a role in this injury.[106,107,120] The transverse transection caused by blunt aortic trauma typically involves all three layers of the wall and the edges may be separated by several centimeters.[106,120] Occasionally, noncircumferential or partial aortic wall disruptions have been described, particularly posteriorly, and under these circumstances intramural hematomas and focal dissections may occur.[106,120,127]

Operative Strategies

BTAI has traditionally undergone open repair with interposition graft placement, and this approach has proved to be safe, effective, and durable, thereby establishing it as the standard with which new repair strategies should be compared. Mortality after an open repair has been approximated at 20%, and the morbidity rate may be as high as 14%, largely attributable to the incidence of spinal cord ischemia.[128] The popularity of endovascular stent grafting (EVSG) or TEVAR of traumatic aortic disruptions has grown immensely in the current era because of expected decreases in operating room time, complication rate, morbidity, and mortality.[129,130] A prospective, nonrandomized, multicenter trial of endovascular aortic repair using Valiant Captivia for BTAI (RESCUE) reports on 50 patients with BTAI. These patients were enrolled between April 2010 and January 2012. All-cause mortality within 1 year was 12%. There were no conversions to open repair. There were no device-related adverse events. This study demonstrated that TEVAR has favorable early midterm outcomes in the treatment of BTAI. The authors conclude that TEVAR remains the treatment modality of choice; however, the longevity of the stent grafts in this patient population has yet to be established.[129] As such this approach is particularly attractive in multitrauma patients, and several institution series have reported good short-term outcomes.[131-139] Many anatomical details must be considered when pursuing TEVAR for traumatic aortic rupture in a young, otherwise healthy patient with a normal-caliber thoracic aorta. The landing zones may not coincide with those expected when the commercially available stent graft was designed for the treatment of aneurysm disease; therefore, successful placement of the stent graft relies on individual surgeon ingenuity and long-term durability of these repairs remains unknown.[129] TEVAR techniques continue to evolve, however, and are not uniformly applicable; therefore, surgeons treating thoracic aortic disruption must be comfortable with conventional open repair techniques.

OPEN REPAIR

The major controversy regarding open operative repair of blunt aortic trauma involves spinal cord protection. Some still report safety and efficacy with a "clamp-and-sew" technique, whereas the majority of surgeons have successfully reduced the historical 10% paraplegia rate through some form of lower body perfusion to minimize spinal cord and visceral organ ischemia.[25,121,123-125,140,141]

ARTERIAL SUPPLY TO THE SPINAL CORD

Blood supply to the spinal cord relies on three longitudinal arteries, the anterior spinal artery located in the anterior-median position and supplying 75% of the spinal cord, and the paired posterior spinal arteries located near the nerve roots. Segmental intercostal and lumbar arteries originating from the posterior aspect of the aorta supply a series of unpaired

radicular arteries that subsequently contribute flow to the anterior spinal artery. The vertebral arteries also provide radicular branches to supply the anterior spinal artery; therefore, in addition to the risk of cord ischemia during aortic cross-clamp at the isthmus and associated paraplegia rates, clamping proximal to the left subclavian compromises flow into the left vertebral and further threatens the integrity of the spinal cord. The posterior spinal arteries are supplied by smaller radicular arteries that originate from the aorta at nearly every spinal level. The largest and most significant radicular artery, typically originating at the level of T10 and entering the vertebral column at the first lumbar vertebrae, is the arteria radicularis magna (or artery of Adamkiewicz) and this vessel is essential for spinal cord perfusion in nearly 25% of patients.

AORTIC CROSS-CLAMP

Some groups report low paraplegia rates exclusively using a "clamp-and-sew" technique; however, these results are not widely reproducible and rely on cross-clamp times of less than 30 minutes.[124] Because of its simplicity, this technique may be preferentially employed by the noncardiothoracic surgeon confronted with repair of a blunt aortic injury. Fragility of the aortic wall, anatomical distortion by the periaortic hematoma, and extension of the defect into the left subclavian artery pose significant obstacles and the average cross-clamp time reported in the literature is 41 minutes.[125] Paraplegia rates are greatly reduced and may even approach zero when extracorporeal lower body perfusion techniques are paired with short cross-clamp times (Tables 51-3, 51-4, and Fig. 51-10).[25,140-142]

ADJUVANT PERFUSION TECHNIQUES

Elective repair of thoracic or thoracoabdominal aneurysms allows employment of several techniques to minimize spinal cord ischemia, but the preoperative preparation required to monitor somatosensory evoked potentials, provide lumbar cerebrospinal fluid drainage, or achieve epidural cooling is typically not available in the trauma setting.[141,143-145] Hypothermic circulatory arrest techniques have been successfully applied to injuries involving the arch, but are not

TABLE 51-3: Incidence of Postoperative Paraplegia in Relation to Surgical Management: Meta-analysis

Operative technique	Patients, n	Paraplegia, %	Clamp time, minutes
No shunt	443	19.2	31.8
Passive shunt	424	11.1	46.8
CPB*	490	2.4	47.8
Partial bypass†	71	1.4	39.5

*CPB, cardiopulmonary bypass with oxygenator and heparin.
†Partial bypass, partial left heart, or femoral vein to artery without systemic heparin.
Data from von Oppell UO, Dunne TT, De Groot KM, et al: Spinal cord protection in the absence of collateral circulation: meta-analysis of mortality and paraplegia, *J Card Surg.* 1994 Nov;9(6):685-691.

TABLE 51-4: Incidence of Postoperative Paraplegia in Relation to Surgical Management: AAST Prospective Trial		
Operative technique	Patients, n	Paraplegia, %
Bypass	134	4.5*
Gott shunt	4	0
Full bypass	22	4.5
Partial bypass	39	7.7
Centrifugal pump	69	2.9†
Clamp and sew	73	16.4*,†

*p < .004, bypass versus clamp and sew.
†p < .01, centrifugal pump versus clamp and sew.
Data from Fabian TC, Richardson JD, Croce MA, et al. Prospective study of blunt aortic injury: Multicenter Trial of the American Association for the Surgery of Trauma, *J Trauma.* 1997 Mar;42(3):374-380.

practical when partial bypass systems are employed.[146,147] The system used by any one group should be routine; however, it is important to be well versed in the various lower body perfusion systems because distinct circumstances may require alterations in practice. Intra-arterial blood pressure monitoring of both the upper and lower limbs should be performed with a goal perfusion pressure of 60 to 70 mm Hg.[148] Systemic heparinization poses a significant risk of hemorrhage in the trauma patient, particularly in those with severe lung or intracranial injuries. Use of a centrifugal pump with heparin-bonded tubing and active partial left heart bypass or use of a heparin-bonded passive shunt is an option that does not require systemic heparinization.[148,149] Alternatively, safe use of partial left heart bypass with full systemic heparinization has been reported as well.[150,151] For partial left heart bypass, pump inflow is established by cannulating the left atrium through the left inferior pulmonary vein using a small single- or dual-stage cannula (Fig. 51-11). Pulmonary

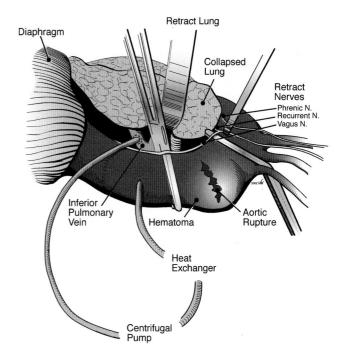

FIGURE 51-11 Diagram showing a typical setup for partial left heart bypass in a patient with aortic disruption at the isthmus.

venous cannulation near its confluence with the left atrium has demonstrated a lower complication rate than cannulation of the left atrial appendage.[152] Arterial cannulation may occur through the distal descending aorta or the femoral artery. Distal aortic cannulation has the advantage of convenience and speed. Partial left heart bypass serves several purposes: (1) to unload the left heart and control proximal hypertension at the time of cross-clamping; (2) to maintain lower body perfusion; (3) to allow rapid infusion of volume; and (4) to control (remove) intravascular volume. Lower body mean arterial pressure should be maintained

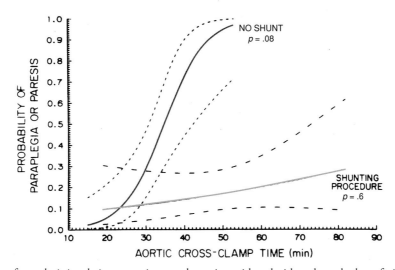

FIGURE 51-10 Probability of paraplegia in relation to aortic cross-clamp time with and without lower body perfusion in patients with traumatic aortic disruption at the isthmus. (Reproduced with permission from Katz NM, Blackstone EH, Kirklin JW, et al: Incremental risk factors for spinal cord injury following operation for acute traumatic aortic transection, *J Thorac Cardiovasc Surg.* 1981 May;81(5):669-674.)

at 60 to 70 mm Hg and this can typically be accomplished with a perfusion flow rate of 2 to 3 L/min. Mean arterial pressures from 70 to 80 mm Hg are generated in the upper body by the native heart and ventricular arrhythmias remain a significant risk. The pump reservoir and/or cell saver are employed to return blood from the field and a heat exchanger can be used to maintain core temperatures above 35°C. If the system is used without systemic heparinization, however, heat exchangers and oxygenators should be removed from the circuit to minimize surface area and thrombotic risks.

In full or partial cardiopulmonary bypass, a long venous catheter with multiple side holes may be introduced through the left common femoral vein and placed in the right atrium with a guidewire. Alternatively, direct right atrial cannulation at the inferior vena cava-right atrial junction may be accomplished from a left thoracotomy by simple, transverse, inferior pericardiotomy below the left phrenic nerve. Right atrial-femoral arterial bypass has also been used with or without an oxygenator-like partial left heart bypass. A partial arterial oxygen pressure of 40 mm Hg has been reported in non-oxygenated circuits, a level shown to be sufficient for lower body tissue oxygenation when the hemoglobin is maintained at 10 g/dL.[153] In cases of aortic arch injury, full cardiopulmonary bypass is beneficial.[154,155] Partial or complete bypass may be established before entering the chest by pursuing right femoral venous to arterial bypass, a technique particularly advantageous when a concomitant right lung contusion inhibits oxygenation. In cases of aortic arch transection in proximity to the innominate or left common carotid, anterior exposure via sternotomy or thoracosternotomy may offer better exposure for total arch replacement under deep hypothermic circulatory arrest (HCA).[154,155] Use of HCA in trauma patients poses significant bleeding risks; therefore, aortic injuries requiring this technique may be appropriate for anti-impulse therapy and a delay in repair until other concomitant injuries have been addressed. Additionally, aortic valvular insufficiency must be ruled out. When HCA is used within the left chest, the left ventricle should be vented through the left atrium. A passive (Gott) shunt has been described where the proximal and distal ends of a heparin-coated polyvinyl tube are placed in the ascending aorta or arch and the descending aorta or femoral artery, respectively. Ventricular cannulation had been used in the past; however, it was abandoned because of a high rate of ventricular dysrhythmias, reduced shunt flows, and a higher rate of paraplegia.[156,157] Flow through this fixed tube is dependent on a pressure gradient and this inability to control flow is the main disadvantage of the Gott shunt.[157] Moreover, it offers no left ventricular unloading or loading advantage, as partial bypass systems do; therefore, blood pressure control is left to pharmacology alone.

Operative Techniques

The patient is positioned in the right lateral decubitus position with the left groin prepped for arterial and venous access.

A right radial arterial line is preferred to avoid losing arterial pressure tracing if occlusion of the left subclavian artery is required during the repair. Use of a pulmonary arterial catheter is optional. Selective ventilation of the right lung is required. A standard fourth interspace posterolateral thoracotomy with or without fifth rib notching usually provides excellent exposure to the aortic isthmus and proximal descending aorta. The incision should be long enough to facilitate dissection of the descending aorta below the level of the inferior pulmonary vein and dissection of the arch of the aorta between the left common carotid and left subclavian arteries. In a patient with a prior left thoracotomy, the associated scarring offers both an advantage and disadvantage to the patient. The adhesions between the lung and mediastinum help contain the rupture, making it less likely to exsanguinate. Dissection near the isthmus or tear should be avoided until both proximal and distal aortic control is established. Depending on the stability of the patient, lower body perfusion can be established before aortic exposure by gaining access to the left groin. If cannulation is planned in the chest, the left inferior pulmonary vein-left atrial junction is dissected and cannulated, in addition to arterial cannulation of the distal descending thoracic aorta or left common femoral vein. Excessive compression or traction of the lung should be avoided, particularly when dissecting out the aortic arch, because the left pulmonary artery may be easily disrupted at this location. Distal control is obtained first, usually by fairly simple passage of a blunt instrument or finger around the descending aorta at the distal margin of the hematoma. Care must be taken not to avulse intercostal arterial branches with this maneuver. The subclavian artery is isolated next. Great care is taken to avoid injury to either the phrenic or vagus nerves as they pass over the aortic arch, which can be difficult because they are often obscured by the hematoma. They should be reflected off the aorta with the overlying pleura and retracted medially by attaching stay sutures to the pleura just lateral to the vagus nerve. Loops around the nerves themselves should be avoided, as even stretch of these nerves can result in paresis. This reflection exposes the arch of the aorta between the left common carotid and left subclavian arteries, which is the point needed for proximal aortic control in the majority of cases. Inferiorly, the vagus nerve and its branching left recurrent laryngeal nerve are reflected medially as well. This exposes the ligamentum arteriosum, which can be sharply divided, but usually this step is not required. Careful dissection is then undertaken between the left common carotid artery and left subclavian artery using a combination of sharp and gentle finger dissection to completely encircle the aortic arch with an umbilical tape. As with distal aortic control, the periaortic hematoma facilitates this dissection considerably. There should be no dissection distal to either the left subclavian or the ligamentum in order to avoid free disruption of the hematoma. Lower body perfusion is initiated, and once systemic blood pressure is stabilized the left subclavian artery is clamped (if necessary) followed by the proximal aorta. With modern imaging techniques, it is usually possible to predict, to the millimeter, exactly where the aortic tear is in order to avoid involving it in the proximal clamp. The distal aorta is clamped last. Traumatic aortic disruptions that occur in close proximity (<1 cm) from the left subclavian artery portend a higher mortality risk and greater operative difficulty than injuries further away from the left subclavian ostium.[154] Upper and lower body pressures are stabilized with the bypass circuit to maintain upper body mean arterial pressures of 70 to 80 mm Hg and a lower body pressure of 60 to 70 mm Hg with flows of 2 to 3 L/min. The periaortic hematoma is then entered, and the edges of the transected aorta are identified. Usually the aorta is completely transected, and the edges are separated by 2 to 4 cm.[106,120] Less frequently, the transection is partial. Some authors advocate primary repair at this point.[156,158] However, we advocate placing a short interposition graft after debridement of the torn edges in all cases.[151,159,160] Collagen-coated woven polyester grafts or gelatin-impregnated grafts are used most commonly. Use of intraluminal prostheses has been abandoned by most groups.[161] Grafts are sewn using a running polypropylene suture with the proximal anastomosis performed first, followed by the distal. Generous amounts of adventitial tissue are included in each bite. If the proximal anastomosis is done under HCA, cardiopulmonary bypass and reperfusion of the arch should be reinstituted immediately after completion of the proximal anastomosis for optimal neurocerebral protection. This requires cannulation of the graft just beyond the proximal anastomosis (branched grafts are useful here for recannulation), and then the distal anastomosis is completed using a dual arterial-inflow perfusion setup perfusing the arch and lower body simultaneously. The left subclavian can either be incorporated into the proximal anastomosis or grafted separately as appropriate. If it is discovered that the tear extends above the proximal aortic clamp, an attempt can be made to dissect more proximally and place a second clamp provided the left common carotid artery is not compromised. If this is not possible, the best recourse is to cannulate the aortic arch in addition to the distal arterial cannula, commence full cardiopulmonary bypass through both arterial routes, and perform the proximal anastomosis during a brief period of profound HCA. We cool to 20°C and use cerebral protection adjuncts, including packing the head in ice and 15 mg/kg sodium thiopental intravenously. One must be prepared to vent the left ventricular apex if distention occurs as a result of cooling induced ventricular fibrillation. A continuous short-axis view by transesophageal echocardiography is very useful is this circumstance. If the aorta is already ruptured with bleeding into the hemithorax, proximal aortic dissection between the left carotid and subclavian arteries is rapidly performed, and a cross-clamp quickly applied. The descending aorta is then clamped below the injury, and the hematoma opened. No attempt is made to establish lower body perfusion, but every attempt is made at maintaining adequate mean arterial pressure during clamping. The aortic repair is done as expeditiously as possible to minimize clamp time. Repair sutures are placed accordingly after clamps are removed. Hemostasis is achieved after continuity of the aorta is re-established. Occasionally, the aortic tear will extend into the left subclavian orifice. In this case the proximal clamp may have to partially or totally occlude the left common carotid. The left subclavian

can then be completely detached from the aorta, the proximal anastomosis completed, and the clamp then moved distally onto the graft. The left subclavian is then reattached to the aortic graft with an interposition graft after completing the distal aortic anastomosis. The left subclavian interposition graft is fashioned with an end-to-end anastomosis distally and an end-to-side anastomosis proximally.

Endovascular Stent Grafting/Thoracic Endovascular Aortic Repair

Use of endovascular techniques to treat abdominal aortic aneurysms began in 1991 and has subsequently been expanded to degenerative thoracic aortic aneurysms. In trauma patients with blunt aortic injury, this technology was initially applied to patients considered extremely high risk for open repair, such as those with a head injury, abdominal visceral injury, or severe pulmonary contusions.[53,54,137,162] The safety and efficacy of this procedure has since been demonstrated and EVSG is considered the preferred method of treatment by many groups.[52,131,132,134-139,162-170] Theoretical advantages of stent grafting include avoidance of thoracotomy, one-lung ventilation, the systemic effects of cardiopulmonary bypass, aortic cross-clamping, and spinal cord ischemia, which should decrease perioperative mortality and complications.[6,129,132,134,135,137-139,162,171-175]

In patients with stable aortic injuries (grade II or III), the timing of intervention is usually dictated by the severity of associated nonaortic injuries. With proper anti-impulse control, delayed management of BTAI until life-threatening nonaortic injuries have been treated has been shown to be a safe and beneficial approach.[47,176] The optimal timing of aortic repair has continued to evolve as the treatment of BTAI has shifted from open aortic repair to TEVAR. The minimally invasive nature of TEVAR has allowed for earlier aortic repair in stable patients, emergent treatment of unstable patients, and easier concomitant management of both aortic and nonaortic injuries. In patients without other serious injuries, the trend has been to treat grade II or III injuries within 24 hours of admission to avoid progression to rupture (grade IV) and the potential deleterious effects of aggressive impulse control in certain patient populations.

Several anatomical considerations must be addressed when deciding whether a patient is a candidate for TEVAR of a blunt aortic transection. A proximal landing zone of at least 1.5 cm is considered necessary to achieve a reliable seal, raising the concern of left arm ischemia if the left subclavian artery needs to be covered; however, this has not been observed.[136,165] In the rare case of symptomatic left arm ischemia, elective carotid to subclavian bypass may be performed.[165] A recent study from Texas demonstrated no statistically significant difference in physical health scores between left subclavian artery coverage and uncovered TEVAR for traumatic aortic injury and hence coverage of the left subclavian artery appears safe and does not impair normal activities.[166] The left subclavian artery origin is also a good marker for an area of acute angulation of the proximal descending aorta and the wall stents used in early TEVAR procedures often became distorted in this region.[177,178] Newer flexible stents have overcome this issue. Additionally, the graft diameter should be oversized 10 to 20% for appropriate seating.[133,136] The size of the chosen graft will determine the route of placement. Early procedures used grafts designed as extension cuffs for abdominal aortic grafts, and these devices had delivery systems 65 cm in length, necessitating iliac or distal aortic access.[133,138] Those frequently reported in the literature include the Gore Excluder (W.L. Gore and Associates, Flagstaff, AZ), AneuRx (Medtronic, Santa Rosa, CA), and Zenith (Cook, Inc., Indianapolis, IN). These cuff diameters range from 18 to 28 mm, and the lengths range from 3.3 to 3.75 cm, necessitating placement of several cuffs to achieve adequate coverage.[79] Commercially available thoracic aortic stent grafts have been designed for treatment of aneurysm disease. Therefore, the diameters are often too large for the otherwise healthy aorta encountered in a patient with traumatic aortic transection. The Gore TAG (W.L. Gore and Associates, Flagstaff, AZ) fits vessels 23 to 37 mm, and the Talent Valiant (Medtronic, Santa Rosa, CA) may be applied to vessels 20 to 42 mm in diameter, excluding a large percentage of blunt aortic transection victims.[177] The ideal device for repair of traumatic aortic injury would be 16 to 40 mm in diameter, be available in 5-, 10-, and 15-cm lengths, and conform to a 90-degree curvature without deformation. Additionally, the delivery system should be distally flexible and approximately 80 to 90 cm in length.[79] A recent study by Canaud and colleagues compared the conformability of the four commercially available thoracic devices with increasing aortic arch angulation and oversizing. All second-generation devices performed significantly better than their respective predecessors. Both the Valiant and the C-TAG devices performed well, with complete wall apposition and arch angulation up to 140° and 120°, respectively.[179]

Patients who will undergo TEVAR for traumatic aortic disruption should be positioned supine in a hybrid operating room/angiosuite or conventional operating room table with fluoroscopic capabilities. General endotracheal anesthesia is typically employed. Conversion to open repair is rare, but has occurred because of postdeployment stent migration; therefore, the operative team must be prepared for rapid conversion.[180] Retrograde aortic access is accomplished percutaneously or by cutdown on the femoral or iliac artery depending on the chosen stent graft. A floppy tipped J-wire should be advanced into the aorta under fluoroscopic guidance with subsequent placement of marked catheter. An aortogram should be obtained in steep left anterior oblique projection to clearly visualize the arch. The details of the aortic injury and device measurements are obtained from a computed tomography angiography (CTA) during operative planning, but the intraoperative aortogram is vital to confirming appropriate anatomy for TEVAR and selection of the correct device. Additionally, the length of graft coverage is determined by this intraoperative image. Deployments of stent grafts have been successful with and without administration of systemic heparin (Fig. 51-12).[181] Intravascular ultrasound may be a useful adjunct when determining coverage length

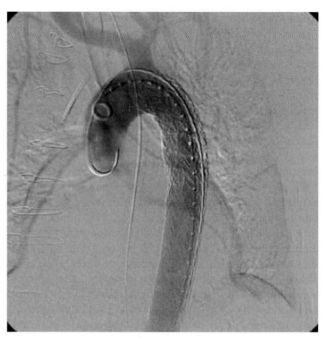

FIGURE 51-12 Endovascular stent graft repair of a blunt traumatic aortic injury demonstrating coverage of the left subclavian artery.

and graft diameter.[182,183] Based on the proximity to the aortic injury, the left subclavian artery may need to be covered, and if covered, it may need to be embolized and bypassed or transposed to the left common carotid artery to ensure a proximal graft seal and avoid problems of ischemia to the left arm or vertebrobasilar system.[138,184-186] Despite whether single or multiple graft devices have been deployed, successful exclusion of the pseudoaneurysm has been accomplished in 90 to 100% of patients reported in the literature.[136-138,187] Decreased operating room time, diminished physiologic derangement and hypothermia, decreased transfusion rates, and shorter intensive care unit and overall hospital stays have been documented in series directly comparing open and endovascular repair of blunt traumatic aortic injury.[137,138,180] Procedure-related paraplegia and mortality rates are also markedly reduced to nearly zero.[137,138,180] Long-term surveillance is recommended to evaluate for endoleak, stent migration, or delayed pseudoaneurysm formation with annual CTA. The optimal follow-up strategy is evolving as imaging technology continues to improve. Also long-term experience grows. In general, CTA is utilized at 1, 3, and 12 months. The individual follow-up strategy is usually tailored to the patient. In the absence of endoleak or endograft collapse or migration on those initial studies, repeat imaging is usually performed every 3 to 5 years.

The Future

With the development of newer-generation devices leading to improved outcomes and less endograft-related complications, TEVAR has established itself as the primary treatment for most patients with thoracic aortic injuries. Future iterations of devices should include shorter lengths and smaller and more precise deployment mechanisms. The potential ability to redeploy the same endograft will make this a very adaptable technique. The use of TEVAR in traumatically injured patients continues to evolve, and TEVAR has supplanted open surgical repair as the primary treatment for BTAIs in most centers. Since the release of the Society of Vascular Surgery clinical guidelines,[4] many issues have been resolved. Other problems associated with TEVAR for thoracic aortic injuries are evolving as this chapter is being written, with improved newer-generation devices. Soon enough, a time will come where most interventions for treatment of acute injuries to the aorta and its great vessels are undertaken by TEVAR with open surgical techniques being discussed in historical chapters.

REFERENCES

1. Smith RS, Chang FC: Traumatic rupture of the aorta: still a lethal injury. *Am J Surg* 1986; 152:660-663.
2. Teixeira PG, Inaba K, Barmparas G, et al: Blunt thoracic aortic injuries: an autopsy study. *J Trauma* 2011; 70:197-202.
3. Arthurs ZM, Starnes BW, Sohn VY, Singh N, Martin MJ, Andersen CA: Functional and survival outcomes in traumatic blunt thoracic aortic injuries: an analysis of the National Trauma Databank. *J Vasc Surg* 2009; 49:988-994.
4. Lee WA, Matsumura JS, Mitchell RS, et al: Endovascular repair of traumatic thoracic aortic injury: clinical practice guidelines of the Society for Vascular Surgery. *J Vasc Surg* 2011; 53:187-192.
5. Ruddy JM, Ikonomidis JS: Trauma to the great vessels, in Cohn LH, (ed.): *Cardiac Surgery In The Adukt*. The McGraw-Hill Companies, Inc., 2012.
6. Azizzadeh A, Charlton-Ouw KM, Chen Z, et al: An outcome analysis of endovascular versus open repair of blunt traumatic aortic injuries. *J Vasc Surg* 2013; 57:108-114; discussion 15.
7. Mitchell RS, Ishimaru S, Ehrlich MP, et al: First International Summit on Thoracic Aortic Endografting: roundtable on thoracic aortic dissection as an indication for endografting. *J Endovasc Ther* 2002; 9(Suppl 2):II98-105.
8. Ishimaru S: Endografting of the aortic arch. *J Endovasc Ther* 2004; 11(Suppl 2):II62-71.
9. Cox CS Jr, Allen GS, Fischer RP, et al: Blunt versus penetrating subclavian artery injury: presentation, injury pattern, and outcome. *J Trauma* 1999; 46:445-449.
10. Hirose H, Moore E: Delayed presentation and rupture of a posttraumatic innominate artery aneurysm: case report and review of the literature. *J Trauma* 1997; 42:1187-1195.
11. Kraus RR, Bergstein JM, DeBord JR: Diagnosis, treatment, and outcome of blunt carotid arterial injuries. *Am J Surg* 1999; 178:190-193.
12. Symbas PJ, Horsley WS, Symbas PN: Rupture of the ascending aorta caused by blunt trauma. *Ann Thorac Surg* 1998; 66:113-117.
13. Miles EJ, Blake A, Thompson W, Jones WG, Dunn EL: Endovascular repair of acute innominate artery injury due to blunt trauma. *Am Surg* 2003; 69:155-159.
14. Stover S, Holtzman RB, Lottenberg L, Bass TL: Blunt innominate artery injury. *Am Surg* 2001; 67:757-759.
15. Pretre R, Chilcott M, Murith N, Panos A: Blunt injury to the supra-aortic arteries. *Br J Surg* 1997; 84:603-609.
16. Pretre R, LaHarpe R, Cheretakis A, et al: Blunt injury to the ascending aorta: three patterns of presentation. *Surgery* 1996; 119:603-610.
17. Fulton JO, De Groot MK, von Oppell UO: Stab wounds of the innominate artery. *Ann Thorac Surg* 1996; 61:851-853.
18. Buchan K, Robbs JV: Surgical management of penetrating mediastinal arterial trauma. *Eur J Cardiothorac Surg* 1995; 9:90-94.
19. Lin PH, Koffron AJ, Guske PJ, et al: Penetrating injuries of the subclavian artery. *Am J Surg* 2003; 185:580-584.
20. Azizzadeh A, Keyhani K, Miller CC 3rd, Coogan SM, Safi HJ, Estrera AL: Blunt traumatic aortic injury: initial experience with endovascular repair. *J Vasc Surg* 2009; 49:1403-1408.
21. Williams JS, Graff JA, Uku JM, Steinig JP: Aortic injury in vehicular trauma. *Ann Thorac Surg* 1994; 57:726-730.
22. Demetriades D, Gomez H, Velmahos GC, et al: Routine helical computed tomographic evaluation of the mediastinum in high-risk blunt trauma patients. *Arch Surg* 1998; 133:1084-1088.
23. Fabian TC, Davis KA, Gavant ML, et al: Prospective study of blunt aortic injury: helical CT is diagnostic and antihypertensive therapy reduces rupture. *Ann Surg* 1998; 227:666-676; see also discussion pp. 76-77.
24. Nagy K, Fabian T, Rodman G, Fulda G, Rodriguez A, Mirvis S: Guidelines for the diagnosis and management of blunt aortic injury: an EAST Practice Management Guidelines Work Group. *J Trauma* 2000; 48:1128-1143.
25. Fabian TC, Richardson JD, Croce MA, et al: Prospective study of blunt aortic injury: Multicenter Trial of the American Association for the Surgery of Trauma. *J Trauma* 1997; 42:374-380; see also discussion pp. 80-83.
26. Simon BJ, Leslie C: Factors predicting early in-hospital death in blunt thoracic aortic injury. *J Trauma* 2001; 51:906-910; discussion 11.
27. Cook AD, Klein JS, Rogers FB, Osler TM, Shackford SR: Chest radiographs of limited utility in the diagnosis of blunt traumatic aortic laceration. *J Trauma* 2001; 50:843-847.
28. Gavant ML, Menke PG, Fabian T, Flick PA, Graney MJ, Gold RE: Blunt traumatic aortic rupture: detection with helical CT of the chest. *Radiology* 1995; 197:125-133.
29. Gundry SR, Burney RE, Mackenzie JR, et al: Assessment of mediastinal widening associated with traumatic rupture of the aorta. *J Trauma* 1983; 23:293-299.
30. Kram HB, Appel PL, Wohlmuth DA, Shoemaker WC: Diagnosis of traumatic thoracic aortic rupture: a 10-year retrospective analysis. *Ann Thorac Surg* 1989; 47:282-286.
31. Mattox KL: Fact and fiction about management of aortic transection. *Ann Thorac Surg* 1989; 48:1-2.
32. Parker MS, Matheson TL, Rao AV, et al: Making the transition: the role of helical CT in the evaluation of potentially acute thoracic aortic injuries. *AJR Am J Roentgenol* 2001; 176:1267-1272.
33. Dyer DS, Moore EE, Ilke DN, et al: Thoracic aortic injury: how predictive is mechanism and is chest computed tomography a reliable screening tool? A prospective study of 1,561 patients. *J Trauma* 2000; 48:673-682; see also discussion pp. 82-83.
34. Gavant ML: Helical CT grading of traumatic aortic injuries. Impact on clinical guidelines for medical and surgical management. *Radiol Clin North Am* 1999; 37:553-574, vi.
35. Vignon P, Boncoeur MP, Francois B, Rambaud G, Maubon A, Gastinne H: Comparison of multiplane transesophageal echocardiography and contrast-enhanced helical CT in the diagnosis of blunt traumatic cardiovascular injuries. *Anesthesiology* 2001; 94:615-622; discussion 5A.
36. Malhotra AK, Fabian TC, Croce MA, Weiman DS, Gavant ML, Pate JW: Minimal aortic injury: a lesion associated with advancing diagnostic techniques. *J Trauma* 2001; 51:1042-1048.
37. Saletta S, Lederman E, Fein S, Singh A, Kuehler DH, Fortune JB: Transesophageal echocardiography for the initial evaluation of the widened mediastinum in trauma patients. *J Trauma* 1995; 39:137-141; see also discussion pp. 41-42.
38. Feliciano DV, Rozycki GS: Advances in the diagnosis and treatment of thoracic trauma. *Surg Clin North Am* 1999; 79:1417-1429.
39. Graeber GM, Jones DR: The role of thoracoscopy in thoracic trauma. *Ann Thorac Surg* 1993; 56:646-648.
40. Eddy AC, Nance DR, Goldman MA, et al: Rapid diagnosis of thoracic aortic transection using intravenous digital subtraction angiography. *Am J Surg* 1990; 159:500-503.
41. Nienaber CA, von Kodolitsch Y, Brockhoff CJ, Koschyk DH, Spielmann RP: Comparison of conventional and transesophageal echocardiography with magnetic resonance imaging for anatomical mapping of thoracic aortic dissection. A dual noninvasive imaging study with anatomical and/or angiographic validation. *Int J Card Imaging* 1994; 10:1-14.
42. Nienaber CA, von Kodolitsch Y, Nicolas V, et al: The diagnosis of thoracic aortic dissection by noninvasive imaging procedures. *New Engl J Med* 1993; 328:1-9.

43. Sturm JT, Hankins DG, Young G: Thoracic aortography following blunt chest trauma. *Am J Emerg Med* 1990; 8:92-96.

44. Kram HB, Wohlmuth DA, Appel PL, Shoemaker WC: Clinical and radiographic indications for aortography in blunt chest trauma. *J Vasc Surg* 1987; 6:168-176.

45. LaBerge JM, Jeffrey RB: Aortic lacerations: fatal complications of thoracic aortography. *Radiology* 1987; 165:367-369.

46. Cook J, Salerno C, Krishnadasan B, Nicholls S, Meissner M, Karmy-Jones R: The effect of changing presentation and management on the outcome of blunt rupture of the thoracic aorta. *J Thorac Cardiovasc Surg* 2006; 131:594-600.

47. Di Eusanio M, Folesani G, Berretta P, et al: Delayed management of blunt traumatic aortic injury: open surgical versus endovascular repair. *Ann Thorac Surg* 2013; 95:1591-1597.

48. Hirose H, Gill IS, Malangoni MA: Nonoperative management of traumatic aortic injury. *J Trauma* 2006; 60:597-601.

49. Holmes JH, Bloch RD, Hall RA, Carter YM, Karmy-Jones RC: Natural history of traumatic rupture of the thoracic aorta managed nonoperatively: a longitudinal analysis. *Ann Thorac Surg* 2002; 73:1149-1154.

50. Kwon CC, Gill IS, Fallon WF, et al: Delayed operative intervention in the management of traumatic descending thoracic aortic rupture. *Ann Thorac Surg* 2002; 74:S1888-1891; see also discussion pp. S92-98.

51. Langanay T, Verhoye JP, Corbineau H, et al: Surgical treatment of acute traumatic rupture of the thoracic aorta a timing reappraisal? *Eur J Cardiothorac Surg* 2002; 21:282-287.

52. Pacini D, Angeli E, Fattori R, et al: Traumatic rupture of the thoracic aorta: ten years of delayed management. *J Thorac Cardiovasc Surg* 2005; 129:880-884.

53. Reed AB, Thompson JK, Crafton CJ, Delvecchio C, Giglia JS: Timing of endovascular repair of blunt traumatic thoracic aortic transections. *J Vasc Surg* 2006; 43:684-688.

54. Rousseau H, Dambrin C, Marcheix B, et al: Acute traumatic aortic rupture: a comparison of surgical and stent-graft repair. *J Thorac Cardiovasc Surg* 2005; 129:1050-1055.

55. Symbas PN, Sherman AJ, Silver JM, Symbas JD, Lackey JJ: Traumatic rupture of the aorta: immediate or delayed repair? *Ann Surg* 2002; 235:796-802.

56. Wahl WL, Michaels AJ, Wang SC, Dries DJ, Taheri PA: Blunt thoracic aortic injury: delayed or early repair? *J Trauma* 1999; 47:254-259; see also discussion pp. 9-60.

57. Hemmila MR, Arbabi S, Rowe SA, et al: Delayed repair for blunt thoracic aortic injury: is it really equivalent to early repair? *J Trauma* 2004; 56:13-23.

58. Caffarelli AD, Mallidi HR, Maggio PM, Spain DA, Miller DC, Mitchell RS: Early outcomes of deliberate nonoperative management for blunt thoracic aortic injury in trauma. *J Thorac Cardiovasc Surg* 2010; 140:598-605.

59. Williams MJ, Low CJ, Wilkins GT, Stewart RA: Randomised comparison of the effects of nicardipine and esmolol on coronary artery wall stress: implications for the risk of plaque rupture. *Heart* 2000; 84:377-382.

60. Carter YM, Karmy-Jones R, Aldea GS: Delayed surgical management of a traumatic aortic arch injury. *Ann Thorac Surg* 2002; 73:294-296.

61. Brinkman WT, Szeto WY, Bavaria JE: Overview of great vessel trauma. *Thorac Surg Clin* 2007; 17:95-108.

62. Pretre R, Faidutti B: Surgical management of aortic valve injury after nonpenetrating trauma. *Ann Thorac Surg* 1993; 56:1426-1431.

63. Maggisano R, Nathens A, Alexandrova NA, et al: Traumatic rupture of the thoracic aorta: should one always operate immediately? *Ann Vasc Surg* 1995; 9:44-52.

64. Preventza O, Henry MJ, Cheong BY, Coselli JS: Endovascular repair of the ascending aorta: when and how to implement the current technology. *Ann Thorac Surg* 2014; 97:1555-1560.

65. Roselli EE, Idrees J, Greenberg RK, Johnston DR, Lytle BW: Endovascular stent grafting for ascending aorta repair in high-risk patients. *J Thorac Cardiovasc Surg* 2015;149(1):144-151.

66. Vallabhajosyula P, Gottret JP, Bavaria JE, Desai ND, Szeto WY: Endovascular repair of the ascending aorta in patients at high risk for open repair. *J Thorac Cardiovasc Surg* 2014.

67. Graham JM, Feliciano DV, Mattox KL, Beall AC Jr: Innominate vascular injury. *J Trauma* 1982; 22:647-655.

68. Symbas JD, Halkos ME, Symbas PN: Rupture of the innominate artery from blunt trauma: current options for management. *J Card Surg* 2005; 20:455-459.

69. Hirose H, Gill IS: Blunt injury of proximal innominate artery. *Ann Thorac Cardiovasc Surg* 2004; 10:130-132.

70. Kieffer E, Sabatier J, Koskas F, Bahnini A: Atherosclerotic innominate artery occlusive disease: early and long-term results of surgical reconstruction. *J Vasc Surg* 1995; 21:326-336; see also discussion pp. 36-37.

71. Sanzone AG, Torres H, Doundoulakis SH: Blunt trauma to the carotid arteries. *Am J Emerg Med* 1995; 13:327-330.

72. Sawchuk AP, Eldrup-Jorgensen J, Tober C, et al: The natural history of intimal flaps in a canine model. *Arch Surg* 1990; 125:1614-1616.

73. Fabian TC, Patton JH Jr, Croce MA, Minard G, Kudsk KA, Pritchard FE: Blunt carotid injury. Importance of early diagnosis and anticoagulant therapy. *Ann Surg* 1996; 223:513-522; see also discussion pp. 22-25.

74. Abouljoud MS, Obeid FN, Horst HM, Sorensen VJ, Fath JJ, Chung SK: Arterial injuries of the thoracic outlet: a ten-year experience. *Am Surg* 1993; 59:590-595.

75. Aksoy M, Tunca F, Yanar H, Guloglu R, Ertekin C, Kurtoglu M: Traumatic injuries to the subclavian and axillary arteries: a 13-year review. *Surg Today* 2005; 35:561-565.

76. McKinley AG, Carrim AT, Robbs JV: Management of proximal axillary and subclavian artery injuries. *Br J Surg* 2000; 87:79-85.

77. Graham JM, Mattox KL, Feliciano DV, DeBakey ME: Vascular injuries of the axilla. *Ann Surg* 1982; 195:232-238.

78. du Toit DF, Odendaal W, Lambrechts A, Warren BL: Surgical and endovascular management of penetrating innominate artery injuries. *Eur J Vasc Endovasc Surg* 2008; 36:56-62.

79. Hoffer EK: Endovascular intervention in thoracic arterial trauma. *Injury* 2008; 39:1257-1274.

80. Reuben BC, Whitten MG, Sarfati M, Kraiss LW: Increasing use of endovascular therapy in acute arterial injuries: analysis of the National Trauma Data Bank. *J Vasc Surg* 2007; 46:1222-1226.

81. du Toit DF, Strauss DC, Blaszczyk M, de Villiers R, Warren BL: Endovascular treatment of penetrating thoracic outlet arterial injuries. *Eur J Vasc Endovasc Surg* 2000; 19:489-495.

82. Becker GJ, Benenati JF, Zemel G, et al: Percutaneous placement of a balloon-expandable intraluminal graft for life-threatening subclavian arterial hemorrhage. *J Vasc Interv Radiol* 1991; 2:225-229.

83. Schonholz CJ, Uflacker R, De Gregorio MA, Parodi JC: Stent-graft treatment of trauma to the supra-aortic arteries. A review. *J Cardiovasc Surg (Torino)* 2007; 48:537-549.

84. Blattman SB, Landis GS, Knight M, Panetta TF, Sclafani SJ, Burack JH: Combined endovascular and open repair of a penetrating innominate artery and tracheal injury. *Ann Thorac Surg* 2002; 74:237-239.

85. Chandler TA, Fishwick G, Bell PR: Endovascular repair of a traumatic innominate artery aneurysm. *Eur J Vasc Endovasc Surg* 1999; 18:80-82.

86. Gifford SM, Deel JT, Dent DL, Seenu Reddy V, Rasmussen TE: Endovascular repair of innominate artery injury secondary to air rifle pellet: a case report and review of the literature. *Vasc Endovascular Surg* 2009; 43:301-305.

87. Arthurs ZM, Sohn VY, Starnes BW: Vascular trauma: endovascular management and techniques. *Surg Clin North Am* 2007; 87:1179-1192, x-xi.

88. Huang CL, Kao HL: Endovascular management of post-traumatic innominate artery transection with pseudo-aneurysm formation. *Catheter Cardiovasc Interv* 2008; 72:569-572.

89. Axisa BM, Loftus IM, Fishwick G, Spyt T, Bell PR: Endovascular repair of an innominate artery false aneurysm following blunt trauma. *J Endovasc Ther* 2000; 7:245-250.

90. Saket RR, Razavi MK, Sze DY, Frisoli JK, Kee ST, Dake MD: Stent-graft treatment of extracranial carotid and vertebral arterial lesions. *J Vasc Interv Radiol* 2004; 15:1151-1156.

91. Simionato F, Righi C, Melissano G, Rolli A, Chiesa R, Scotti G: Stent-graft treatment of a common carotid artery pseudoaneurysm. *J Endovasc Ther* 2000; 7:136-140.

92. Uflacker R, Schonholz C, Hannegan C, Selby JB: Carotid artery angioplasty and stenting: interventional radiology point of view. *J S C Med Assoc* 2006; 102:117-121.

93. Schonholz C, Krajcer Z, Carlos Parodi J, et al: Stent-graft treatment of pseudoaneurysms and arteriovenous fistulae in the carotid artery. *Vascular* 2006; 14:123-129.

94. du Toit DF, Leith JG, Strauss DC, Blaszczyk M, Odendaal Jde V, Warren BL: Endovascular management of traumatic cervicothoracic arteriovenous fistula. *Br J Surg* 2003; 90:1516-1521.

95. Archondakis E, Pero G, Valvassori L, Boccardi E, Scialfa G: Angiographic follow-up of traumatic carotid cavernous fistulas treated with

endovascular stent graft placement. *AJNR Am J Neuroradiol* 2007; 28:342-347.

96. Saatci I, Cekirge HS, Ozturk MH, et al: Treatment of internal carotid artery aneurysms with a covered stent: experience in 24 patients with mid-term follow-up results. *AJNR Am J Neuroradiol* 2004; 25:1742-1749.

97. Hershberger RC, Aulivola B, Murphy M, Luchette FA: Endovascular grafts for treatment of traumatic injury to the aortic arch and great vessels. *J Trauma* 2009; 67:660-671.

98. Hilfiker PR, Razavi MK, Kee ST, Sze DY, Semba CP, Dake MD: Stent-graft therapy for subclavian artery aneurysms and fistulas: single-center mid-term results. *J Vasc Interv Radiol* 2000; 11:578-584.

99. Marin ML, Veith FJ, Cynamon J, et al: Initial experience with transluminally placed endovascular grafts for the treatment of complex vascular lesions. *Ann Surg* 1995; 222:449-465; see also discussion pp. 65-69.

100. Marin ML, Veith FJ, Panetta TF, et al: Transluminally placed endovascular stented graft repair for arterial trauma. *J Vasc Surg* 1994; 20:466-472; see also discussion pp. 72-73.

101. Parodi JC, Schonholz C, Ferreira LM, Bergan J: Endovascular stent-graft treatment of traumatic arterial lesions. *Ann Vasc Surg* 1999; 13:121-129.

102. Patel AV, Marin ML, Veith FJ, Kerr A, Sanchez LA: Endovascular graft repair of penetrating subclavian artery injuries. *J Endovasc Surg* 1996; 3:382-388.

103. Sanchez LA, Veith FJ, Ohki T, et al: Early experience with the Corvita endoluminal graft for treatment of arterial injuries. *Ann Vasc Surg* 1999; 13:151-157.

104. Schoder M, Cejna M, Holzenbein T, et al: Elective and emergent endovascular treatment of subclavian artery aneurysms and injuries. *J Endovasc Ther* 2003; 10:58-65.

105. White R, Krajcer Z, Johnson M, Williams D, Bacharach M, O'Malley E: Results of a multicenter trial for the treatment of traumatic vascular injury with a covered stent. *J Trauma* 2006; 60:1189-1195; see also discussion pp. 95-96.

106. Parmley LF, Mattingly TW, Manion WC, Jahnke EJ Jr: Nonpenetrating traumatic injury of the aorta. *Circulation* 1958; 17:1086-1101.

107. Greendyke RM: Traumatic rupture of aorta; special reference to automobile accidents. *JAMA* 1966; 195:527-530.

108. Brasel KJ, Quickel R, Yoganandan N, Weigelt JA: Seat belts are more effective than airbags in reducing thoracic aortic injury in frontal motor vehicle crashes. *J Trauma* 2002; 53:309-312; see also discussion p. 13.

109. deGuzman BJ, Morgan AS, Pharr WF: Aortic transection following air-bag deployment. *New Engl J Med* 1997; 337:573-574.

110. Dunn JA, Williams MG: Occult ascending aortic rupture in the presence of an air bag. *Ann Thorac Surg* 1996; 62:577-578.

111. Pezzella AT: Blunt traumatic injury of the thoracic aorta following commercial airline crashes. *Tex Heart Inst J* 1996; 23:65-67.

112. Gotzen L, Flory PJ, Otte D: Biomechanics of aortic rupture at classical location in traffic accidents. *Thorac Cardiovasc Surg* 1980; 28:64-68.

113. Marsh CL, Moore RC: Deceleration trauma. *Am J Surg* 1957; 93:623-631.

114. Sevitt S: The mechanisms of traumatic rupture of the thoracic aorta. *Br J Surg* 1977; 64:166-173.

115. Stapp JP: Human tolerance to deceleration. *Am J Surg* 1957; 93:734-740.

116. Lundevall J: Traumatic rupture of the aorta, with special reference to road accidents. *Acta Pathol Microbiol Scand* 1964; 62:29-33.

117. Cohen AM, Crass JR, Thomas HA, Fisher RG, Jacobs DG: CT evidence for the "osseous pinch" mechanism of traumatic aortic injury. *AJR Am J Roentgenol* 1992; 159:271-274.

118. Crass JR, Cohen AM, Motta AO, Tomashefski JF Jr, Wiesen EJ: A proposed new mechanism of traumatic aortic rupture: the osseous pinch. *Radiology* 1990; 176:645-649.

119. Javadpour H, O'Toole JJ, McEniff JN, Luke DA, Young VK: Traumatic aortic transection: evidence for the osseous pinch mechanism. *Ann Thorac Surg* 2002; 73:951-953.

120. Feczko JD, Lynch L, Pless JE, Clark MA, McClain J, Hawley DA: An autopsy case review of 142 nonpenetrating (blunt) injuries of the aorta. *J Trauma* 1992; 33:846-849.

121. Cowley RA, Turney SZ, Hankins JR, Rodriguez A, Attar S, Shankar BS: Rupture of thoracic aorta caused by blunt trauma. A fifteen-year experience. *J Thorac Cardiovasc Surg* 1990; 100:652-660; see also discussion pp. 60-61.

122. Kieny R, Charpentier A: Traumatic lesions of the thoracic aorta. A report of 73 cases. *J Cardiovasc Surg (Torino)* 1991; 32:613-619.

123. Razzouk AJ, Gundry SR, Wang N, del Rio MJ, Varnell D, Bailey LL: Repair of traumatic aortic rupture: a 25-year experience. *Arch Surg* 2000; 135:913-918; see also discussion p. 9.

124. Sweeney MS, Young DJ, Frazier OH, Adams PR, Kapusta MO, Macris MP: Traumatic aortic transections: eight-year experience with the "clamp-sew" technique. *Ann Thorac Surg* 1997; 64:384-387; see also discussion pp. 7-9.

125. von Oppell UO, Dunne TT, De Groot MK, Zilla P: Traumatic aortic rupture: twenty-year metaanalysis of mortality and risk of paraplegia. *Ann Thorac Surg* 1994; 58:585-593.

126. Butcher HR Jr: The elastic properties of human aortic intima, media and adventitia: the initial effect of thromboendarterectomy. *Ann Surg* 1960; 151:480-489.

127. Katz S, Mullin R, Berger RL: Traumatic transection associated with retrograde dissection and rupture of the aorta: recognition and management. *Ann Thorac Surg* 1974; 17:273-276.

128. Carter Y, Meissner M, Bulger E, et al: Anatomical considerations in the surgical management of blunt thoracic aortic injury. *J Vasc Surg* 2001; 34:628-633.

129. Khoynezhad A, Donayre CE, Azizzadeh A, White R: One-year results of thoracic endovascular aortic repair for blunt thoracic aortic injury (RESCUE trial). *J Thorac Cardiovasc Surg* 2014.

130. Yamane BH, Tefera G, Hoch JR, Turnipseed WD, Acher CW: Blunt thoracic aortic injury: open or stent graft repair? *Surgery* 2008; 144:575-580; see also discussion pp. 80-82.

131. Faneyte IF, Goslings JC, van Lienden KP, Idu MM: Penetrated descending thoracic aorta after blunt chest trauma: successful endovascular repair. *J Trauma* 2009; 66:E36-38.

132. Karmy-Jones R, Ferrigno L, Teso D, Long WB 3rd, Shackford S: Endovascular repair compared with operative repair of traumatic rupture of the thoracic aorta: a nonsystematic review and a plea for trauma-specific reporting guidelines. *J Trauma* 2011; 71:1059-1072.

133. Karmy-Jones R, Hoffer E, Meissner MH, Nicholls S, Mattos M: Endovascular stent grafts and aortic rupture: a case series. *J Trauma* 2003; 55:805-810.

134. Klima DA, Hanna EM, Christmas AB, et al: Endovascular graft repair for blunt traumatic disruption of the thoracic aorta: experience at a non-university hospital. *Am Surg* 2013; 79:594-600.

135. Nor Elina NS, Naresh G, Hanif H, Zainal AA: Thoracic Endovascular Aortic Repair (TEVAR) in traumatic high-velocity blunt injury to thoracic aorta. *Med J Malaysia* 2013; 68:239-244.

136. Orford VP, Atkinson NR, Thomson K, et al: Blunt traumatic aortic transection: the endovascular experience. *Ann Thorac Surg* 2003; 75:106-111; see also discussion pp. 11-12.

137. Ott MC, Stewart TC, Lawlor DK, Gray DK, Forbes TL: Management of blunt thoracic aortic injuries: endovascular stents versus open repair. *J Trauma* 2004; 56:565-570.

138. Peterson BG, Matsumura JS, Morasch MD, West MA, Eskandari MK: Percutaneous endovascular repair of blunt thoracic aortic transection. *J Trauma* 2005; 59:1062-1065.

139. Powers WF 4th, Kane PN, Kotwall CA, Clancy TV, Hope WW: Endovascular repair of traumatic thoracic aortic injuries at a level II trauma center. *Am Surg* 2013; 79:E91-92.

140. Crestanello JA, Zehr KJ, Mullany CJ, et al: The effect of adjuvant perfusion techniques on the incidence of paraplegia after repair of traumatic thoracic aortic transections. *Mayo Clinic Proc* 2006; 81:625-630.

141. von Oppell UO, Dunne TT, De Groot KM, Zilla P: Spinal cord protection in the absence of collateral circulation: meta-analysis of mortality and paraplegia. *J Card Surg* 1994; 9:685-691.

142. Katz NM, Blackstone EH, Kirklin JW, Karp RB: Incremental risk factors for spinal cord injury following operation for acute traumatic aortic transection. *J Thorac Cardiovasc Surg* 1981; 81:669-674.

143. Black JH, Davison JK, Cambria RP: Regional hypothermia with epidural cooling for prevention of spinal cord ischemic complications after thoracoabdominal aortic surgery. *Semin Thorac Cardiovasc Surg* 2003; 15:345-352.

144. Laschinger JC, Cunningham JN Jr, Nathan IM, Krieger K, Isom OW, Spencer FC: Intraoperative identification of vessels critical to spinal cord blood supply—use of somatosensory evoked potentials. *Curr Surg* 1984; 41:107-109.

145. McCullough JL, Hollier LH, Nugent M: Paraplegia after thoracic aortic occlusion: influence of cerebrospinal fluid drainage. Experimental and early clinical results. *J Vasc Surg* 1988; 7:153-160.

146. Kouchoukos NT, Masetti P, Rokkas CK, Murphy SF, Blackstone EH: Safety and efficacy of hypothermic cardiopulmonary bypass and circulatory arrest for operations on the descending thoracic and thoracoabdominal aorta. *Ann Thorac Surg* 2001; 72:699-707; see also discussion p. 8.

147. Peltz M, Douglass DS, Meyer DM, et al: Hypothermic circulatory arrest for repair of injuries of the thoracic aorta and great vessels. *Interact Cardiovasc Thorac Surg* 2006; 5:560-565.

148. Szwerc MF, Benckart DH, Lin JC, et al: Recent clinical experience with left heart bypass using a centrifugal pump for repair of traumatic aortic transection. *Ann Surg* 1999; 230:484-490; see also discussion pp. 90-92.

149. Hess PJ, Howe HR Jr, Robicsek F, et al: Traumatic tears of the thoracic aorta: improved results using the Bio-Medicus pump. *Ann Thorac Surg* 1989; 48:6-9.

150. Fullerton DA: Simplified technique for left heart bypass to repair aortic transection. *Ann Thorac Surg* 1993; 56:579-580.

151. Merrill WH, Lee RB, Hammon JW Jr, Frist WH, Stewart JR, Bender HW Jr: Surgical treatment of acute traumatic tear of the thoracic aorta. *Ann Surg* 1988; 207:699-706.

152. Karmy-Jones R, Carter Y, Meissner M, Mulligan MS: Choice of venous cannulation for bypass during repair of traumatic rupture of the aorta. *Ann Thorac Surg* 2001; 71:39-41; see also discussion p. 2.

153. Turney SZ: Blunt trauma of the thoracic aorta and its branches. *Semin Thorac Cardiovasc Surg* 1992; 4:209-216.

154. Carter YM, Karmy-Jones RC, Oxorn DC, Aldea GS: Traumatic disruption of the aortic arch. *Eur J Cardiothorac Surg* 2001; 20:1231.

155. Leshnower BG, Litt HI, Gleason TG: Anterior approach to traumatic mid aortic arch transection. *Ann Thorac Surg* 2006; 81:343-345.

156. Schmidt CA, Wood MN, Razzouk AJ, Killeen JD, Gan KA: Primary repair of traumatic aortic rupture: a preferred approach. *J Trauma* 1992; 32:588-592.

157. Verdant A, Page A, Cossette R, Dontigny L, Page P, Baillot R: Surgery of the descending thoracic aorta: spinal cord protection with the Gott shunt. *Ann Thorac Surg* 1988; 46:147-154.

158. McBride LR, Tidik S, Stothert JC, et al: Primary repair of traumatic aortic disruption. *Ann Thorac Surg* 1987; 43:65-67.

159. Hilgenberg AD, Logan DL, Akins CW, et al: Blunt injuries of the thoracic aorta. *Ann Thorac Surg* 1992; 53:233-238; see also discussion pp. 8-9.

160. Wallenhaupt SL, Hudspeth AS, Mills SA, Tucker WY, Dobbins JE, Cordell AR: Current treatment of traumatic aortic disruptions. *Am Surg* 1989; 55:316-320.

161. Ablaza SG, Ghosh SC, Grana VP: Use of a ringed intraluminal graft in the surgical treatment of dissecting aneurysms of the thoracic aorta. A new technique. *J Thorac Cardiovasc Surg* 1978; 76:390-396.

162. Dunham MB, Zygun D, Petrasek P, Kortbeek JB, Karmy-Jones R, Moore RD: Endovascular stent grafts for acute blunt aortic injury. *J Trauma* 2004; 56:1173-1178.

163. Czermak BV, Waldenberger P, Perkmann R, et al: Placement of endovascular stent-grafts for emergency treatment of acute disease of the descending thoracic aorta. *AJR Am J Roentgenol* 2002; 179:337-345.

164. Lachat M, Pfammatter T, Witzke H, et al: Acute traumatic aortic rupture: early stent-graft repair. *Eur J Cardiothorac Surg* 2002; 21:959-963.

165. Mattison R, Hamilton IN Jr, Ciraulo DL, Richart CM: Stent-graft repair of acute traumatic thoracic aortic transection with intentional occlusion of the left subclavian artery: case report. *J Trauma* 2001; 51:326-328.

166. McBride CL, Dubose JJ, Miller CC 3rd, et al: Intentional left subclavian artery coverage during thoracic endovascular aortic repair for traumatic aortic injury. *J Vasc Surg* 2015; 61:73-79 e1.

167. Murphy EH, Dimaio JM, Dean W, Jessen ME, Arko FR: Endovascular repair of acute traumatic thoracic aortic transection with laser-assisted in-situ fenestration of a stent-graft covering the left subclavian artery. *J Endovasc Ther* 2009; 16:457-463.

168. Patterson BO, Holt PJ, Nienaber C, Fairman RM, Heijmen RH, Thompson MM: Management of the left subclavian artery and neurologic complications after thoracic endovascular aortic repair. *J Vasc Surg* 2014; 60:1491-1498 e1.

169. Si Y, Fu W, Liu Z, et al: Coverage of the left subclavian artery without revascularization during thoracic endovascular repair is feasible: a prospective study. *Ann Vasc Surg* 2014; 28:850-859.

170. Singh MJ, Rohrer MJ, Ghaleb M, Kim D: Endoluminal stent-graft repair of a thoracic aortic transection in a trauma patient with multiple injuries: case report. *J Trauma* 2001; 51:376-381.

171. Khoynezhad A, Azizzadeh A, Donayre CE, Matsumoto A, Velazquez O, White R: Results of a multicenter, prospective trial of thoracic endovascular aortic repair for blunt thoracic aortic injury (RESCUE trial). *J Vasc Surg* 2013; 57:899-905 e1.

172. Adams JD, Kern JA: Blunt thoracic aortic injury: Current issues and endovascular treatment paradigms. *Endovascular Today* 2014; September 2014:38-42.

173. Asaid R, Boyce G, Atkinson N: Endovascular repair of acute traumatic aortic injury: experience of a level-1 trauma center. *Ann Vasc Surg* 2014; 28:1391-1395.

174. Canaud L, Marty-Ane C, Ziza V, Branchereau P, Alric P: Minimum 10-year follow-up of endovascular repair for acute traumatic transection of the thoracic aorta. *J Thorac Cardiovasc Surg* 2014.

175. Echeverria AB, Branco BC, Goshima KR, Hughes JD, Mills JL Sr: Outcomes of endovascular management of acute thoracic aortic emergencies in an academic level 1 trauma center. *Am J Surg* 2014; 208:974-980.

176. Demetriades D, Velmahos GC, Scalea TM, et al: Blunt traumatic thoracic aortic injuries: early or delayed repair—results of an American Association for the Surgery of Trauma prospective study. *J Trauma* 2009; 66:967-973.

177. Borsa JJ, Hoffer EK, Karmy-Jones R, et al: Angiographic description of blunt traumatic injuries to the thoracic aorta with specific relevance to endograft repair. *J Endovasc Ther* 2002; 9(Suppl 2):II84-91.

178. Kato N, Dake MD, Miller DC, et al: Traumatic thoracic aortic aneurysm: treatment with endovascular stent-grafts. *Radiology* 1997; 205:657-662.

179. Canaud L, Cathala P, Joyeux F, Branchereau P, Marty-Ane C, Alric P: Improvement in conformability of the latest generation of thoracic stent grafts. *J Vasc Surg* 2013; 57:1084-1089.

180. Andrassy J, Weidenhagen R, Meimarakis G, Lauterjung L, Jauch KW, Kopp R: Stent versus open surgery for acute and chronic traumatic injury of the thoracic aorta: a single-center experience. *J Trauma* 2006; 60:765-771; see also discussion pp. 71-72.

181. Bent CL, Matson MB, Sobeh M, et al: Endovascular management of acute blunt traumatic thoracic aortic injury: a single center experience. *J Vasc Surg* 2007; 46:920-927.

182. Greenberg R: Treatment of aortic dissections with endovascular stent grafts. *Semin Vasc Surg* 2002; 15:122-127.

183. Herold U, Piotrowski J, Baumgart D, Eggebrecht H, Erbel R, Jakob H: Endoluminal stent graft repair for acute and chronic type B aortic dissection and atherosclerotic aneurysm of the thoracic aorta: an interdisciplinary task. *Eur J Cardiothorac Surg* 2002; 22:891-897.

184. Czerny M, Zimpfer D, Fleck T, et al: Initial results after combined repair of aortic arch aneurysms by sequential transposition of the supra-aortic branches and consecutive endovascular stent-graft placement. *Ann Thorac Surg* 2004; 78:1256-1260.

185. Gorich J, Asquan Y, Seifarth H, et al: Initial experience with intentional stent-graft coverage of the subclavian artery during endovascular thoracic aortic repairs. *J Endovasc Ther* 2002; 9(Suppl 2):II39-43.

186. Rehders TC, Petzsch M, Ince H, et al: Intentional occlusion of the left subclavian artery during stent-graft implantation in the thoracic aorta: risk and relevance. *J Endovasc Ther* 2004; 11:659-666.

187. Marcheix B, Dambrin C, Bolduc JP, et al: Endovascular repair of traumatic rupture of the aortic isthmus: midterm results. *J Thorac Cardiovasc Surg* 2006; 132:1037-1041.

52

Pulmonary Embolism and Pulmonary Thromboendarterectomy

Stuart W. Jamieson • Michael M. Madani

Pulmonary embolism (PE) results in at least 630,000 symptomatic episodes in the United States yearly, making it about half as common as acute myocardial infarction, and three times as common as cerebrovascular accidents.[1] Acute PE is the third most common cause of death (after heart disease and cancer). Estimates of PE are probably low because approximately 75% of autopsy-proved PE are not detected clinically[2] and in 70 to 80% of the patients in whom the primary cause of death was PE, premortem diagnosis was completely unsuspected.[3,4] Of all hospitalized patients who develop PE, 12 to 21% die in the hospital, and another 24 to 39% die within 12 months.[5-7] Thus, approximately 36 to 60% of patients who survive the initial episode live beyond 12 months, and may present later in life with a wide variety of symptoms.

In addition, approximately 2.5 million Americans develop deep vein thrombosis (DVT) each year, and more than 90% of clinically detected pulmonary emboli are associated with lower extremity DVT. However, in two-thirds of patients with DVT and PE, the DVT is asymptomatic.[8-10]

For the most part, DVT and acute PE are managed medically. Cardiac surgeons rarely become involved in management of acute PE, unless it is in a hospitalized patient who survives a massive embolus that causes life-threatening acute right heart failure with low cardiac output, with a large clot burden. On the other hand, the mainstay of treatment for patients with chronic pulmonary thromboembolic disease[11] is the surgical removal of the disease by means of pulmonary thromboendarterectomy. Medical management for this condition is only palliative, and surgery by means of transplantation is an inappropriate use of resources with outcomes inferior to thromboendarterectomy.

DEEP VEIN THROMBOSIS

Deep vein thrombosis primarily affects the veins of the lower extremity or pelvis. It is most common in hospitalized patients but may occur in ambulatory patients outside the hospital.[12,13] The process may involve superficial as well as deep veins, but superficial venous thrombosis does not generally propagate beyond the saphenofemoral junction and therefore very rarely causes PE.[9,14,15] Venous thrombosis of the upper extremity is almost always associated with trauma, indwelling catheters, or other pathologic states and is an uncommon cause of PE, but can be fatal. Pulmonary emboli that do not originate from the deep venous system of the legs, pelvis, or arms are thought to come from a diseased right atrium or ventricle or retroperitoneal and hepatic systems.[12,13]

Pathogenesis

In 1856, Rudolf Virchow made the association between DVT and PE and suggested that the causes of DVT were related to venous stasis, vein wall injury, and hypercoagulopathy. This triad of etiologic factors remains relevant today and is supported by an ever-growing body of evidence.

Immobilization is by far the most important cause of venous stasis in hospitalized patients. Injections of contrast material in foot veins require up to 1 hour to clear from the venous valves in the soleus muscle of immobilized patients.[16] Venous stasis may also be produced by mechanical obstruction of proximal veins, by low cardiac output, by venous dilatation, and by increased blood viscosity.[17] Some pelvic tumors, bulky inguinal adenopathy, the gravid uterus, previous caval or iliac venous disease, and elevated central venous pressures from cardiac causes also enhance venous stasis.

The role of vein wall injury is less clear because DVT often begins in the absence of mechanical trauma. Recent work shows that subtle vein wall injuries may occur during operation in veins remote from the operative field.[18,19] In animals, endothelial cell tears have been found at junctions of small veins with larger veins at remote sites during hip replacement (Fig. 52-1).

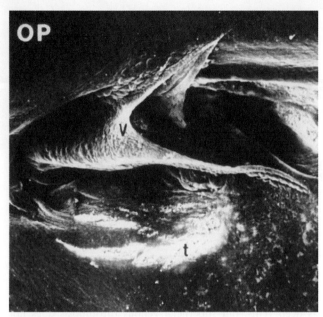

FIGURE 52-1 Scanning electron photomicrograph of a canine jugular vein after total hip replacement with significant operative venous dilatation. An endothelial cell tear (t) is visible near a valve cusp (V). (Reproduced with permission from Cometra AJ, Stewart GJ, White JV: Combined dihydroergotamine and heparin prophylaxis of postoperative deep vein thrombosis: proposed mechanism of action, *Am J Surg* 1985 Oct 8;150(4A):39-44.)

Three uncommon familial deficiencies associated with venous thrombosis are seen in antithrombin, protein C, and protein S. Antithrombin is a natural plasma protease that inhibits thrombin after it is formed, and to a lesser extent before it is formed. Antithrombin is also the cofactor that is accelerated 1000-fold by heparin. Protein C is a potent inhibitor of factor V and platelet-bound factor VII and requires protein S as a cofactor for anticoagulant activity. Both protein C and S are vitamin-K–dependent zymogens that are activated by thrombin and accelerated by thrombomodulin produced by endothelial cells.[20,21]

A much more common coagulation deficiency, resulting from a mutation of factor V (factor V Leiden) that prevents its degradation by protein C, has been described and is present in approximately 6 to 7% of study populations of Swedes and North American males.[22-24] Both the homozygous and heterozygous mutants are strongly associated with venous thrombosis and PE but are not associated with manifestations of arterial thrombosis.[24,25]

The presence of the lupus anticoagulant, which is an acquired IgG or IgM antibody against prothrombinase, increases the likelihood of venous thrombosis by poorly understood mechanisms.[25] The disease may be associated with lupus-like syndromes, immunosuppression, or intake of specific drugs, such as procainamide.

Risk Factors for Deep Vein Thrombosis

Table 52-1 presents a list of major risk factors for the development of DVT or PE. Previous thromboembolism, older age,

TABLE 52-1: Major Risk Factors for Venous Thromboembolism

Previous venous thromboembolism	Age over 45 years
Major hip or knee surgery	Bed rest 7 days or longer
Recent major surgery	Cancer
Congestive heart failure	Paralysis of lower extremity
Pelvis, hip, or leg fracture	Multiple trauma
High-dose estrogen therapy	

immobilization for more than 1 week, orthopedic surgery of the hip or knee, recent surgery, multiple trauma, and cancer are strong risk factors. In patients with a history of venous thromboembolism the risk of developing a new episode during hospitalization is nearly eight times that of someone without a history.[9,26-29] Up to 10% of patients with a first episode of DVT or PE and up to 20% of those with a recurrent event develop a new episode of venous thromboembolism within 6 months.[30]

The incidence of DVT and PE increases exponentially with age (Fig. 52-2). Males are at greater risk than females. Prolonged bed rest or immobility from any cause are major risk factors. Although usually other risk factors are present, the incidence of autopsy-proved venous thrombosis rises from 15 to 80% in patients at bed rest for more than 1 week.[30,31]

The incidence of venous thromboembolism increases threefold in patients who have operations for cancer.[9] Of particular interest to cardiac surgeons and cardiologists is the observation that clinically silent DVT develops during hospitalization in nearly 50% of patients after myocardial revascularization.[32]

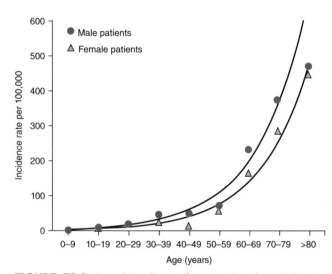

FIGURE 52-2 Annual incidence of venous thromboembolism in the United States stratified for age. Males have a significantly higher incidence rate of venous thromboembolism than females. Both curves fit an exponential function.

A follow-up study[33] found that the incidence of PE in hospital after coronary arterial bypass operations was 3.2% and hospital mortality in patients with PE was 18.7%. Interestingly, valvular surgery was not associated with the development of PE. In a retrospective study of 5694 patients who had open heart surgery, Gillinov and colleagues found the risk of PE proved by V/Q scan (20 patients), angiography (four patients), or autopsy (eight patients) was 0.56% within 60 days. The mortality was 34% in patients with PE.[34]

Diagnosis

Approximately two-thirds of patients with DVT do not have clinical symptoms;[9] therefore, the diagnosis depends on a high degree of clinical suspicion and a variety of objective diagnostic tests. Venography remains the most reliable test for detecting thrombus in calf veins, but is invasive, not suitable for serial studies, and the contrast material may be thrombogenic if allowed to remain within the deep venous system.[10]

The most popular noninvasive test, which can be done at the bedside, is a combination of ultrasound and color flow Doppler mapping, widely referred to as *duplex scanning*. The method does not detect fresh thrombi directly but infers the presence of clot by flow patterns and the inability to compress the vessel in specific locations.[10] In the hands of skilled examiners duplex scanning is highly accurate for the detection of thrombus in popliteal, deep femoral, and superficial femoral veins and has a sensitivity between 89 and 100% against venography in symptomatic patients. Magnetic resonance imaging (MRI) is a noninvasive method that can image the entire venous system, including upper extremity veins and mediastinum.[35] Against MRI duplex scanning has a sensitivity of 70% for pelvic veins and a specificity of nearly 100%.[36] Impedance plethysmography assesses volume changes in the leg after occlusion of the vein with calf electrodes and a thigh cuff. It is clinically useful in symptomatic patients but has relatively low sensitivity and specificity in asymptomatic patients and calf thrombosis.[36] Injection of iodine 125-labeled fibrinogen with subsequent leg scanning is a sensitive test for detecting calf vein thrombus but does not detect iliofemoral vein thrombosis. The combination of these two tests improves sensitivity and specificity, but in most hospitals duplex scanning, venography, and MRI have superseded both tests.

Prophylaxis

The prevalence of DVT, its strong association with PE, and the identification of risk factors in the pathogenesis of the disease provide the basis and rationale for prophylactic measures that are recommended in patients with two or more major risk factors, such as age over 40 years and major surgery.[9] Innocuous measures such as compression stockings probably should be prescribed more often and be used in most nonambulating patients in the hospital. Intermittent pneumatic compression is more expensive and more cumbersome but is effective. Both methods reduce the incidence of DVT after general surgery to approximately 40% of control patients.[9] Low-dose subcutaneous heparin and low-molecular-weight heparin given once a day reduce the incidence of DVT to approximately 35 and 18% of controls, respectively.[9,31,37] The reduction in PE with subcutaneous standard heparin or low-molecular-weight heparin is similar.[31,37]

Calf vein DVT that does not propagate has a low risk of PE, and controversy exists as to whether or not these patients should be anticoagulated.[15] Of patients who have DVT diagnosed in hospital without PE, the probability of clinically diagnosed PE within the next 12 months is 1.7%.[5] If PE occurs, the probability of recurrent PE is 8.0%.[5] Six months of warfarin anticoagulation is recommended for patients who have DVT with or without PE, as prophylaxis against recurrent disease.[38]

PULMONARY EMBOLISM

Pathology and Pathogenesis

The only firm attachment of leg thrombus is at the site of origin, usually a venous saccule or venous valve pocket.[26] The degree of organization within the thrombus varies, but recent clots are more likely to migrate than older thrombi that are more firmly attached to the vessel wall.

Detached venous thrombi are carried in the bloodstream through the right heart into the pulmonary circulation. In autopsy series the percentage of emboli that obstruct two or more lobar arteries (major) ranges between 25 and 67% of all emboli;[39] but this figure varies with the thoroughness of the examination. In clinical trials based on angiographic data the percentage of major emboli is similar and ranges from 30 to 64%.[40] The majority of pulmonary emboli lodge in the lower lobes,[12] and are slightly more common in the right lung than the left. This is probably the result of relative flow to those areas of the lung. Soon after reaching the lungs emboli become coated with a layer of platelets and fibrin.[12]

Simple mechanical obstruction of one or more pulmonary arteries does not entirely explain the often devastating hemodynamic consequences of major or massive emboli. Humoral factors, specifically serotonin, adenosine diphosphate (ADP), platelet-derived growth factor (PDGF), thromboxane from platelets coating the thrombus, platelet-activating factor (PAF), and leukotrienes from neutrophils are also involved.[41,42] Anoxia and tissue ischemia downstream from the emboli inhibit endothelium-derived relaxing factor (EDRF) production and enhance release of superoxide anions by activated neutrophils. The combination of these effects contributes to increased pulmonary vasoconstriction.[41]

Natural History

The mortality of a large, untreated PE is 18 to 33%, but can be reduced to about 8% if diagnosed and treated.[7,43,44] Seventy-five to ninety percent of patients who die of pulmonary emboli do so within the first few hours of the primary event.[45] In patients who have sufficient cardiopulmonary reserve and right ventricular strength to survive the initial few hours, autolysis of emboli occurs over the next few days and weeks.[46] On average, approximately 20% of the clot disappears by 7 days, and complete resolution may occur by 14 days.[44,46,47] For many patients, up to 30 days are needed to dissolve small emboli and up to 60 days for massive clots.[48] As the natural fibrinolytic system dissolves the embolic mass, the available cross-sectional area of the pulmonary arterial tree progressively increases, and pulmonary vascular resistance and right ventricular afterload decreases. In the vast majority of patients, pulmonary emboli continue to resolve and thus an immediate interventional therapy, particularly surgical embolectomy, is not necessary for survival except in a minority of patients.

In an unknown but small percentage of patients with acute PE the clot will not lyse, and chronic thromboembolic obstruction of the pulmonary vasculature develops. The reasons for failure of emboli to dissolve are unknown. Patients often are asymptomatic until symptoms of dyspnea, exercise intolerance, or right heart failure develop, mostly secondary to the pulmonary hypertension that ensues. Asymptomatic patients may have partial or complete chronic thrombotic occlusion of one or more segmental or lobar arteries. Symptomatic patients usually have more than 40% of their pulmonary vasculature obstructed by organized and fresh thrombi; however, significant pulmonary hypertension can develop in patients despite lesser degrees of vascular obstruction.

Clinical Presentation

Acute PE usually presents suddenly. Symptoms and signs vary with the extent of blockage, the magnitude of the humoral response, and the pre-embolus reserve of the cardiac and pulmonary systems of the patient.[49] Symptoms and signs vary widely, and in autopsy series of proven emboli only 16 to 38% of patients were diagnosed during life.[39]

The acute disease is conveniently stratified into minor, major (submassive), or massive embolism on the basis of hemodynamic stability, arterial blood gases, and lung scan or angiographic assessment of the blocked pulmonary arteries.[40,49,50] Most pulmonary emboli are minor. These patients present with sudden, unexplained anxiety, tachypnea or dyspnea, pleuritic chest pain, cough, and occasionally streak hemoptysis.[39,45,50] Examination may reveal tachycardia, rales, low-grade fever, and sometimes a pleural rub. Heart sounds and systemic blood pressure are often normal; sometimes the pulmonary second sound is increased. Interestingly less than one-third of the patients will have evidence of clinical DVT.[39] Room air arterial blood gases indicate a PaO_2 between 65 and 80 torr and a normal $PaCO_2$ around 35 torr.[45] Pulmonary angiograms show less than 30% occlusion of the pulmonary arterial vasculature.

Major PE is associated with dyspnea, tachypnea, dull chest pain, and some degree of hemodynamic instability

manifested by tachycardia, mild to moderate hypotension, and elevation of the central venous pressure.[45,50] Some patients may present with syncope rather than dyspnea or chest pain. In contrast to massive PE, patients with major embolism (at least two lobar pulmonary arteries obstructed) are hemodynamically stable and have adequate cardiac output.[40] Room air blood gases reveal moderate hypoxia (PaO_2 <65, >50 torr) and mild hypocarbia ($PaCO_2$ <30 torr).[50] Echocardiograms may show right ventricular dilatation. Pulmonary angiograms indicate that 30 to 50% of the pulmonary vasculature is blocked.

Massive PE is truly life-threatening and it causes hemodynamic instability.[40] It is usually associated with occlusion of more than 50% of the pulmonary vasculature, but may occur with much smaller occlusions, particularly in patients with preexisting cardiac or pulmonary disease. The diagnosis is clinical, not anatomical. Patients develop acute dyspnea, tachypnea, tachycardia, and diaphoresis; and sometimes may lose consciousness. Both hypotension and low cardiac output (<1.8 L/m^2/min) are present. Cardiac arrest may occur. Neck veins are distended; central venous pressure is elevated, and a right ventricular impulse may be present. Room air blood gases show severe hypoxia (PaO_2 < 50 torr), hypocarbia ($PaCO_2$ < 30 torr), and sometimes acidosis.[40,45,50] Urine output falls; peripheral pulses are decreased and perfusion is poor.

Diagnosis

The clinical diagnosis of acute major or massive PE is wrong in 70 to 80% of patients who subsequently have angiography.[49,51] Even in postoperative patients and those with additional major risk factors for DVT, differentiation of major or massive PE from acute myocardial infarction, aortic dissection, septic shock, and other catastrophic states is difficult and uncertain.

The chest film may be normal but usually shows some combination of parenchymal infiltrate, atelectasis, and pleural effusion. A zone of hypovascularity or a wedged-shaped pleural-based density raises the possibility of PE. Usually, the ECG shows nonspecific T-wave or ST segment changes with PE. A minority of patients with massive embolism (26%) may show evidence of cor pulmonale, right axis deviation, or right bundle branch block.[49] An echocardiogram showing right heart dilatation raises the possibility of major or massive PE. A Swan-Ganz catheter generally shows pulmonary arterial desaturation (PaO_2 < 25 torr), but usually does not show pulmonary hypertension over 40 mm Hg because of low cardiac output and cor pulmonale (the unprepared right ventricle cannot generate pulmonary hypertension).

Ventilation-perfusion (V/Q) scans will provide confirmatory evidence, but these studies may be unreliable because pneumonia, atelectasis, previous pulmonary emboli, and other conditions may cause a mismatch in ventilation and perfusion and mimic positive results. In general, negative V/Q scans essentially exclude the diagnosis of clinically significant PE. V/Q scans usually are interpreted as high, intermediate, or low probability of PE to emphasize the lack of specificity but high sensitivity of the test (Fig. 52-3). Pulmonary angiograms provide the most definitive diagnosis, but collapse of the circulation may not allow time for this procedure, and pulmonary angiograms should not be performed if the patient's circulation cannot be stabilized by pharmacologic or mechanical means.[52,53]

MRI and CT angiography are better noninvasive methods for the diagnosis of pulmonary emboli and provide specific information regarding flow within the pulmonary vasculature.[54] Unfortunately, these methods are expensive, somewhat time consuming, and not widely available. Furthermore, they are not generally suitable for hemodynamically unstable patients. Transthoracic (TTE) or transesophageal (TEE) echocardiography with color flow Doppler mapping can provide reliable information about the presence or absence of major thrombi obstructing right-sided chambers or the main pulmonary artery. More than 80% of patients with clinically significant PE have abnormalities of right ventricular volume or contractility, or acute tricuspid regurgitation by TTE (Fig. 52-4).[55] In some patients,

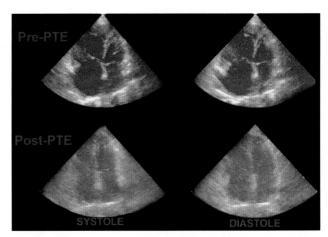

FIGURE 52-4 Appearance of echocardiography before and after the operation. The top pictures represent pre-PTE and bottom pictures represent post-PTE. Note the shift of the intraventricular septum toward the left in the systole before the operation, together with the relatively small left atrial and left ventricular chambers. After the operation, the septum has normalized, and the right-sided chambers are no longer massively enlarged. LA, left atrium; LV, left ventricle; PTE, pulmonary thromboendarterectomy; RA, right atrium; RV, right ventricle.

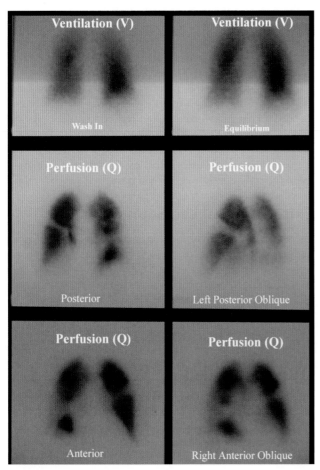

FIGURE 52-3 Anterior and posterior views from a radionuclide perfusion scan in a patient with chronic thromboembolic disease. Note the large punched out defects.

abnormal flow patterns can be discerned in major pulmonary arteries during TEE.

Management of Acute Major Pulmonary Embolism

For the purposes of this chapter, major or submassive PE is defined as an acute episode that causes hypoxia and mild hypotension (systolic arterial pressure > 90 mm Hg), but does not cause cardiac arrest or sustained low cardiac output and cardiogenic shock. By definition there is sufficient time in these patients to definitely establish the diagnosis and to attempt pharmacologic therapy and possibly remove the embolic material by catheter suction.

The first priority after sudden collapse of any patient is to establish adequate ventilation and circulation. The first may require intubation and mechanical ventilation. Pharmacologic agents, including cardiovascular pressors and vasoactive agents, are then used to help stabilize the patient's hemodynamics. If the patient's circulation can be stabilized, intravenous heparin is started with an initial bolus of 70 U/kg followed by 18 to 20 U/kg/h if there are no contraindications. Heparin will prevent propagation and formation of new thromboemboli, but does not dissolve the existing clot. In most instances the patient's own fibrinolytic system lyses fresh thrombi over a period of days or weeks.[46]

The addition of lytic therapy, that is, streptokinase, urokinase, or recombinant tissue plasminogen activator (rt-PA), increases the rate of lysis of fresh thrombi and is recommended in patients with a stable circulation and no contraindications. This increases the rate of lysis of fresh pulmonary clots over that of heparin alone during treatment,[56] but there is little difference in the amount of residual thrombus between the two treatments at 5 days or thereafter.[57-60] There is also no statistical difference in mortality or in the incidence of recurrent PE, but more recent experience shows a trend toward better results with thrombolytic therapy because of a more rapid reduction in right ventricular afterload and dysfunction.[56] Furthermore, there are no data that indicate that thrombolysis reduces the subsequent development of chronic pulmonary thromboembolism and pulmonary hypertension. Compared with Heparin therapy alone, thrombolytic agents carry a higher risk of bleeding complications, and despite precautions, bleeding complications occur in approximately 20% of patients.[56,61,62]

Mechanical removal of pulmonary thrombi is possible by a catheter device inserted under local anesthesia into the femoral (preferred) or jugular vein.[50,63-66] Successful extraction of clot with meaningful reduction in pulmonary arterial pressure varies between 61 and 84%.[64,66]

Management of Acute Massive Pulmonary Embolism

If the circulation cannot be stabilized at survival levels within several minutes or if cardiac arrest occurs after a massive PE, time becomes of paramount importance. Eleven percent of patients with fatal PE die within the first hour, 43 to 80% within 2 hours, and 85% within 6 hours.[67] To a great extent, circumstances and the timely availability of necessary equipment and personnel determine therapeutic options. A decision to treat medically in an effort to stabilize the circulation at a survival level may preempt life-saving surgery, but also may make surgery unnecessary. The relative infrequency of treatment opportunities in massive PE, mitigating factors, and the lack of clear criteria for prescribing medical or surgical therapy leave the management of massive PE unsettled.

When surgery is not immediately available, in patients who may not be surgical candidates, or in whom an alternate diagnosis seems more likely, emergency extracorporeal life support (ECLS) using peripheral cannulation is an attractive alternative.[68,69] In prepared institutions ECLS can be instituted rapidly outside the operating room. ECLS compensates for acute cor pulmonale and hypoxia and sustains the circulation until the clot partially lyses, pulmonary vascular resistance falls, and pulmonary blood flow becomes adequate.

Emergency Pulmonary Thromboembolectomy

Emergency pulmonary thromboembolectomy is indicated for suitable patients with life-threatening circulatory insufficiency, but should not be done without a definitive diagnosis because a clinical diagnosis of PE is often wrong.[47,58,65,70] If a patient has been taken directly to the operating room without a definitive diagnosis, TEE and color Doppler mapping can confirm or refute the diagnosis in the operating room. TEE will indicate increased right ventricular volume, poor right ventricular contractility, and tricuspid

regurgitation, which are strongly associated with massive PE and acute cor pulmonale.[71] Echocardiographic detection of a large clot trapped within the right atrium or ventricle in a hemodynamically compromised patient with massive acute PE is another indication for emergency pulmonary thromboembolectomy.[72-74]

A midline sternotomy incision is used and cardiopulmonary bypass is initiated. The heart may be electrically fibrillated or arrested with cold cardioplegic solution. The main pulmonary artery is then opened 1 to 2 cm downstream to the valve, and the incision is extended into the proximal left pulmonary artery. Forceps and suction catheters are used to remove the clot from the left pulmonary artery and behind the aorta to the right pulmonary artery. If necessary the right pulmonary artery can also be exposed and opened between the aorta and superior vena cava to allow better exposure in the distal segments. If a sterile pediatric bronchoscope is available, the surgeon can use this instrument to locate and remove thrombi in tertiary and quaternary pulmonary vessels. Alternatively, the pleural spaces are entered, and each lung is gently compressed to dislodge small clots into larger vessels and suctioned out. Greenfield recommends placement of an inferior vena caval filter before closing the chest.[10,66,75,76] European surgeons generally clip the intrapericardial vena cava at the end of pulmonary thromboembolectomy to prevent migration of large clots into the pulmonary circulation.[74] However, this clip increases venous pressure and stagnant flow in the lower half of the body and causes considerable morbidity in more than 60% of patients.[72,74,75]

Anticoagulation for 6 months is recommended for most patients with PE, but an inferior vena caval filter is recommended for patients with contraindications to anticoagulation or with recurrent PE, or those who will require pulmonary thromboendarterectomy. The cone-shaped Greenfield filter is the one most widely used and is associated with a lifetime recurrent embolism rate of 5% and has a 97% patency rate.[77]

Extracorporeal Life Support

The wider availability of long-term extracorporeal perfusion (termed *extracorporeal life support*, ECLS) using peripheral vessel cannulation to stabilize the circulation offers a compromise position because most massive pulmonary emboli will dissolve in time. ECLS can be implemented outside the operating room within 15 to 30 minutes by an equipped team of trained personnel.[68,69]

ECLS should not be needed beyond 1 to 2 days because clot lysis proceeds rapidly. Once pulmonary vascular resistance is adequately reduced, ECLS should be discontinued in the operating room as the femoral vessels will need to be surgically repaired because of the need for heparin and long-term anticoagulation.

Results

Mortality rates for emergency pulmonary thromboembolectomy vary widely between 40 and 92%.[66,72-75,78]

Results are best if cardiopulmonary bypass is used to support the circulation during pulmonary arteriotomy.[73] The eventual outcome depends largely upon the preoperative condition and circulatory status of the patient. If cardiac arrest occurs and external massage cannot be stopped without ECLS, the mortality ranges between 45 and 75%. Without cardiac arrest mortality ranges between 8 and 36%.[72-74] ECLS instituted during cardiac resuscitation is associated with survival rates between 43 and 56%.[70,72] Recurrent embolism is uncommon,[75,79] and approximately 80% of survivors maintain normal pulmonary arterial pressures and exercise tolerance. In these patients postoperative angiograms are normal or show less than 10% obstructed vessels. A minority of patients have 40 to 50% of the pulmonary vessels obstructed and have significantly reduced exercise tolerance and pulmonary function.[79]

CHRONIC THROMBOEMBOLIC PULMONARY HYPERTENSION

Incidence

The incidence of pulmonary hypertension caused by chronic PE is even more difficult to determine than that of acute PE. Twenty-five years ago, it was estimated that there were more than 500,000 survivors per year of acute *symptomatic* episodes of acute pulmonary embolization in the United States alone.[11,76,80] The population has increased since then, and of course many cases of PE are asymptomatic. The incidence of chronic thrombotic occlusion in the population depends on what percentage of patients fails to resolve acute embolic material. One estimate is that chronic thromboembolic disease develops in only 0.5% of patients with a clinically recognized acute PE.[76] If these figures are correct and counting only patients with symptomatic acute pulmonary emboli, approximately 2500 individuals would progress to chronic thromboembolic pulmonary hypertension (CTEPH) in the United States each year. However, because most patients diagnosed with chronic thromboembolic disease have no antecedent history of acute embolism, the true incidence of this disorder is probably much higher; we estimate on the order of five to ten times this number.

Regardless of the exact incidence or the circumstances, it is clear that acute embolism and its chronic relation, fixed chronic thromboembolic occlusive disease, are both much more common than generally appreciated and are seriously underdiagnosed. Houk and colleagues[81] in 1963 reviewed the literature of 240 reported cases of chronic thromboembolic obstruction of major pulmonary arteries but found that only six cases had been diagnosed correctly before death. Calculations extrapolated from mortality rates and the random incidence of major thrombotic occlusion found at autopsy would support a postulate that more than 100,000 people in the United States currently have pulmonary hypertension that could be relieved by operation.

Pathology and Pathogenesis

Although most individuals with chronic pulmonary thromboembolic disease are unaware of a past thromboembolic event and give no history of DVT, the origin of most cases of unresolved pulmonary emboli are from acute embolic episodes. Why some patients have unresolved emboli is not certain, but a variety of factors must play a role, alone or in combination.

The volume of acute embolic material may simply overwhelm the lytic mechanisms. Total occlusion of a major arterial branch may prevent lytic material from reaching, and therefore dissolving, the embolus completely. Repetitive emboli may not be able to be resolved. The emboli may be made of substances that cannot be resolved by normal mechanisms (already well-organized fibrous thrombus, fat, or tumor). The lytic mechanisms themselves may be abnormal, or some patients may actually have a propensity for thrombus or a hypercoagulable state. In addition, there are other special circumstances. Chronic indwelling central venous catheters and pacemaker leads are sometimes associated with pulmonary emboli. More rare causes include tumor emboli; tumor fragments from stomach, breast, and kidney malignancies have been demonstrated to cause chronic pulmonary arterial occlusion. Right atrial myxomas may also fragment and embolize.

After the clot becomes wedged in the pulmonary artery, one of two processes occurs:[82]

1. Organization of the clot proceeds to canalization, producing multiple small endothelialized channels separated by fibrous septa (ie, bands and webs) or
2. Complete fibrous organization of the fibrin clot without canalization may result, leading to a solid mass of dense fibrous connective tissue totally obstructing the arterial lumen.

As previously described and discussed, in addition to the embolic material, a propensity for thrombosis or a hypercoagulable state may be present in a few patients. This abnormality may result in spontaneous thrombosis within the pulmonary vascular bed, encourage embolization, or be responsible for proximal propagation of thrombus after an embolus. But, whatever the predisposing factors to residual thrombus within the vessels, the final genesis of the resultant pulmonary vascular hypertension may be complex. With the passage of time, the increased pressure and flow as a result of redirected pulmonary blood flow in the previously normal pulmonary vascular bed can create a vasculopathy in the small precapillary blood vessels similar to the Eisenmenger's syndrome.

Factors other than the simple hemodynamic consequences of redirected blood flow are probably also involved in this process. For example, after a pneumonectomy, 100% of the right ventricular output flows to one lung, yet little increase in pulmonary pressure occurs, even with follow-up to 11 years.[83] In patients with thromboembolic disease, however, we frequently detect pulmonary hypertension even when less than 50% of the vascular bed is occluded by thrombus. It thus appears that sympathetic neural connections, hormonal changes, or both might initiate pulmonary hypertension in the initially unaffected pulmonary vascular bed. This process can occur with the initial occlusion either being in the same or the contralateral lung.

Regardless of the cause, the evolution of pulmonary hypertension as a result of changes in the previously unobstructed bed is serious, because this process may lead to an inoperable situation. Consequently, with accumulating experience in patients with thrombotic pulmonary hypertension, we have increasingly been inclined toward early operation so as to avoid these changes.

Clinical Presentation

Chronic thromboembolic pulmonary hypertension is a frequently under-recognized but treatable cause of pulmonary hypertension. There are no signs or symptoms specific for chronic thromboembolism. The most common symptom associated with thromboembolic pulmonary hypertension, as with all other causes of pulmonary hypertension, is exertional dyspnea. This dyspnea is characteristically out of proportion to any abnormalities found in clinical examination.

Nonspecific chest pains or tightness occur in approximately 50% of patients with more severe pulmonary hypertension. Hemoptysis can occur in all forms of pulmonary hypertension and probably results from abnormally dilated vessels distended by increased intravascular pressures. Peripheral edema, early satiety, and epigastric or right upper quadrant fullness or discomfort may develop as the right heart fails (cor pulmonale). Some patients with chronic pulmonary thromboembolic disease present with right heart failure after a relatively small PE, superimposed on chronic disease.

The physical signs of pulmonary hypertension are the same no matter what the underlying pathophysiology. Initially the jugular venous pulse is characterized by a large A-wave. As the right heart fails, the V-wave becomes predominant. The right ventricle is usually palpable near the lower left sternal border, and pulmonary valve closure may be audible in the second intercostal space. Occasional patients with advanced disease are hypoxic and slightly cyanotic. Clubbing is an uncommon finding.

The second heart sound is often narrowly split and varies normally with respiration; P2 is accentuated. A sharp systolic ejection click may be heard over the pulmonary artery. As the right heart fails, a right atrial gallop usually is present, and tricuspid insufficiency develops. Because of the large pressure gradient across the tricuspid valve in pulmonary hypertension, the murmur is high pitched and may not exhibit respiratory variation. These findings are quite different from those usually observed in tricuspid valvular disease. A murmur of pulmonic regurgitation may also be detected.

Pulmonary function tests reveal minimal changes in lung volume and ventilation; patients generally have normal or slightly restricted pulmonary mechanics. Diffusing capacity

(DLCO) is often reduced and may be the only abnormality on pulmonary function testing. Pulmonary arterial pressures are elevated and suprasystemic pulmonary pressures are not uncommon. Resting cardiac outputs are lower than the normal range, and pulmonary arterial oxygen saturations are reduced. Most patients are hypoxic; room air arterial oxygen tension ranges between 50 and 83 torr, the average being 65 torr.[84] CO_2 tension is slightly reduced and is compensated by reduced bicarbonate. Dead space ventilation is increased. Ventilation-perfusion studies show moderate mismatch with some heterogeneity among various respirator units within the lung and correlate poorly with the degree of pulmonary obstruction.[85]

Diagnosis

To ensure accurate diagnosis in patients with chronic pulmonary thromboembolism, a standardized evaluation is recommended for all patients who present with unexplained pulmonary hypertension. This workup includes a chest radiograph, which may show either apparent vessel cutoffs of the lobar or segmental pulmonary arteries or regions, or oligemia suggesting vascular occlusion. The central pulmonary arteries are enlarged, and the right ventricle may also be enlarged without enlargement of the left atrium or ventricle (Fig. 52-5). Despite these classic findings, many patients present with a relatively normal chest radiograph, even in

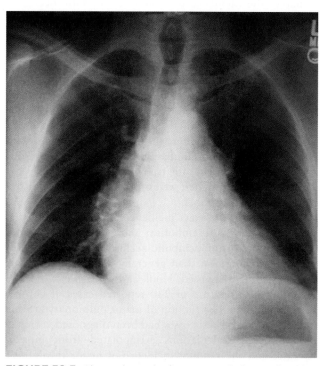

FIGURE 52-5 Chest radiograph of a patient with chronic thromboembolic pulmonary disease, and evidence of pulmonary hypertension. Note the enlarged right atrium and right ventricle, disparity of size between the left and right pulmonary arteries, and the hypoperfusion in several areas of the lung fields.

the setting of high degrees of pulmonary hypertension. The electrocardiogram demonstrates findings of right ventricular hypertrophy (right axis deviation, dominant R-wave in V1). Pulmonary function tests are necessary to exclude obstructive or restrictive intrinsic pulmonary parenchymal disease as the cause of pulmonary hypertension.

The ventilation-perfusion lung scan is the essential test for establishing the diagnosis of unresolved pulmonary thromboembolism. An entirely normal lung scan excludes the diagnosis of both acute or chronic, unresolved thromboembolism. The usual lung scan pattern in most patients with pulmonary hypertension either is relatively normal or shows a diffuse nonuniform perfusion.[84,85-87] When subsegmental or larger perfusion defects are noted on the scan, even when matched with ventilatory defects, pulmonary angiography is appropriate to confirm or rule out thromboembolic disease.

Currently, pulmonary angiography still remains the gold standard for the diagnosis of CTEPH. Organized thromboembolic lesions do not have the appearance of the intravascular filling defects seen with acute pulmonary emboli, and experience is essential for the proper interpretation of pulmonary angiograms in patients with unresolved, chronic embolic disease. Organized thrombi appear as unusual filling defects, webs, or bands, or completely thrombosed vessels that may resemble congenital absence of the vessel[87] (Fig. 52-6). Organized material along the wall of a recanalized vessel produces a scalloped or serrated luminal edge. Because of both vessel wall thickening and dilatation of proximal vessels, the contrast-filled lumen may appear relatively normal in diameter.

Distal vessels demonstrate the rapid tapering and pruning characteristic of pulmonary hypertension (see Fig. 52-6).

Pulmonary angiography should be performed whenever there is a possibility that chronic thromboembolism is the etiology of pulmonary hypertension. Many thousands of angiograms in pulmonary hypertensive patients have now been performed at our institution without mortality.

In addition to pulmonary angiography, patients over 40 undergo coronary arteriography and other cardiac investigation as necessary. If significant disease is found, additional cardiac surgery is performed at the time of pulmonary thromboendarterectomy.

Medical Treatment

Chronic anticoagulation represents the mainstay of a medical regimen. This is primarily used to prevent future embolic episodes, but also serves to limit the development of thrombus in regions of low flow within the pulmonary vasculature. Inferior vena caval filters are used routinely to prevent recurrent embolization. If caval filtration and anticoagulation fail to prevent recurrent emboli, immediate thrombolysis may be beneficial, but lytic agents are incapable of altering the chronic component of the disease.

Right ventricular failure is treated with diuretics and vasodilators, and although some improvement may result, the effect is generally transient because the failure is owing to a mechanical obstruction and will not resolve until the obstruction is removed. Similarly, the prognosis is unaffected by medical therapy,[88,89] which should be regarded as only supportive.

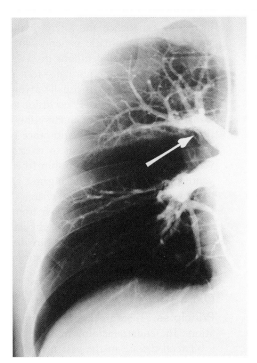
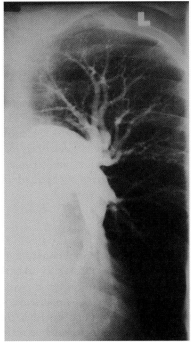

FIGURE 52-6 Right and left pulmonary angiograms demonstrate enlarged pulmonary arteries, poststenotic dilatation of vessels, lack of filling to the periphery in many areas, and abrupt cutoffs of branches. The arrow points to intraluminal filling defects representative of a web or band.

Because of the bronchial circulation, pulmonary embolization seldom results in tissue necrosis. Surgical endarterectomy therefore will allow distal pulmonary tissue to be used once more in gas exchange.

The only other surgical option for these patients is transplantation. However, transplantation is not appropriate for this disease because of the mortality and morbidity rates of patients on the waiting list, the higher risk of the operation, and the contrasted survival rate (approximately 80% at 1 year at experienced centers for transplantation vs more than 95% for pulmonary endarterectomy). Furthermore, pulmonary endarterectomy is considered to be permanently curative, and the issues of a continuing risk of rejection and immunosuppression are not present.

Natural History

The natural history of CTEPH is dismal, and nearly all patients die of progressive right heart failure.[11] Because of the insidious onset, the diagnosis is usually made relatively late in the progression of the disease when dyspnea and/or early symptoms of right heart failure develop and pulmonary hypertension is severe (>40 mm Hg mean). In Riedel's series of 13 patients, nine died a mean of 28 months after the diagnosis of right heart failure.[11] Seven of the 13 had recurrent episodes of fresh emboli demonstrated by new perfusion defects or by autopsy. The severity of pulmonary hypertension at the time of diagnosis inversely correlates with duration of survival.[11]

Pulmonary Thromboendarterectomy

Although there were previous attempts, Allison et al[90] did the first successful pulmonary "thromboendarterectomy" through a sternotomy using surface hypothermia, but only fresh clots were removed. Since then, there have been many occasional surgical reports of the surgical treatment of chronic pulmonary thromboembolism,[91-94] but most of the surgical experience in pulmonary endarterectomy has been reported from the UCSD Medical Center. Braunwald commenced the UCSD experience with this operation in 1970, which now totals more than 3500 cases. The operation described in the following pages, using deep hypothermia and circulatory arrest, is the standard procedure and has now been adopted by other major centers.

INDICATIONS

When the diagnosis of thromboembolic pulmonary hypertension has been firmly established, the decision for operation is based on the severity of symptoms and the general condition of the patient. Early in the pulmonary endarterectomy experience, Moser and colleagues[92] pointed out that there were three major reasons for considering thromboendarterectomy: hemodynamic, alveolo-respiratory, and prophylactic. The hemodynamic goal is to prevent or ameliorate right ventricular compromise caused by pulmonary hypertension. The respiratory objective is to improve respiratory function by the removal of a large ventilated but unperfused physiologic dead space, regardless of the severity of pulmonary hypertension. The prophylactic goal is to prevent progressive right ventricular dysfunction or retrograde extension of the obstruction, which might result in further cardiorespiratory deterioration or death.[92] Our subsequent experience has added another prophylactic goal: the prevention of secondary arteriopathic changes in the remaining patent vessels.[87]

Most patients who undergo operation are within New York Heart Association (NYHA) class III or IV. The ages of the patients in our series have ranged from 3 to 85 years. A typical patient will have a severely elevated pulmonary vascular resistance (PVR) level at rest, the absence of significant comorbid disease unrelated to right heart failure, and the appearances of chronic thrombi on angiogram that appear to be relatively in balance with the measured PVR level. Exceptions to this general rule, of course, occur.

Although most patients have a PVR level in the range of 800 dynes/sec/c^{-5} and pulmonary artery pressures less than systemic, the hypertrophy of the right ventricle that occurs over time makes pulmonary hypertension to suprasystemic levels possible. Therefore many patients (approximately 20% in our practice) have a level of PVR in excess of 1000 dynes/sec/cm^{-5} and suprasystemic pulmonary artery pressures. There is no upper limit of PVR level, pulmonary artery pressure, or degree of right ventricular dysfunction that excludes patients from operation.

We have become increasingly aware of the changes that can occur in the remaining patent (unaffected by clot) pulmonary vascular bed subjected to the higher pressures and flow that results from obstruction in other areas. Therefore, with the increasing experience and safety of the operation, we offer surgery to symptomatic patients whenever the angiogram demonstrates thromboembolic disease. A rare patient might have a PVR level that is normal at rest, although elevated with minimal exercise. This is usually a young patient with total unilateral pulmonary artery occlusion and unacceptable exertional dyspnea because of an elevation in dead space ventilation. Operation in this circumstance is performed not only to reperfuse lung tissue, but to re-establish a more normal ventilation perfusion relationship (thereby reducing minute ventilatory requirements during rest and exercise), and also to prevent the chronic arterial changes associated with long-term exposure to pulmonary hypertension, thus preserving the integrity of the contralateral circulation.

If not previously implanted, an inferior vena caval filter is routinely placed several days in advance of the operation.

OPERATION

Principles. There are several guiding principles for the operation. The endarterectomy must be bilateral because this is a bilateral disease in the vast majority of our patients, and for pulmonary hypertension to be a major factor, both pulmonary vasculatures must be substantially involved. The only reasonable approach to both pulmonary arteries is therefore through a median sternotomy incision. Historically, there were many reports of unilateral operation, and perhaps this is still performed occasionally in inexperienced centers, through a thoracotomy. However, the unilateral approach ignores the disease on the contralateral side, subjects the patient to hemodynamic jeopardy during the clamping of the pulmonary artery, does not allow good visibility because of the continued presence of bronchial blood flow, and exposes the patient to a repeat operation on the contralateral side. In addition, collateral channels develop in chronic thrombotic hypertension not only through the bronchial arteries but also from diaphragmatic, intercostal, and pleural vessels. The dissection of the lung in the pleural space via a thoracotomy incision can therefore be extremely bloody. The median sternotomy incision, apart from providing bilateral access, avoids entry into the pleural cavities, and allows the ready institution of cardiopulmonary bypass.

Cardiopulmonary bypass is essential to ensure cardiovascular stability when the operation is performed and to cool the patient to allow circulatory arrest. Excellent visibility is required, in a bloodless field, to define an adequate endarterectomy plane and then follow the pulmonary endarterectomy specimen deep into the subsegmental vessels. Because of the copious bronchial blood flow usually present in these cases, periods of circulatory arrest are necessary to ensure perfect visibility. Again, there have been sporadic reports of the performance of this operation without circulatory arrest. However, it should be emphasized that although endarterectomy is possible without circulatory arrest, a complete endarterectomy is not. We always initiate the procedure without circulatory arrest, and a variable amount of dissection is possible before the circulation is stopped, but never complete dissection. The circulatory arrest periods are limited to 20 minutes, with restoration of flow between each arrest. With experience, the endarterectomy usually can be performed with a single period of circulatory arrest on each side.

A true endarterectomy in the plane of the media must be accomplished. It is essential to appreciate that the removal of visible thrombus is largely incidental to this operation. Indeed, in most patients, no free thrombus is present; and on initial direct examination, the pulmonary vascular bed may appear normal. The early literature on this procedure indicates that thrombectomy was often performed without endarterectomy, and in these cases the pulmonary artery pressures did not improve, often with the resultant death of the patient.

Preparation and Anesthetic Considerations.
Much of the preoperative preparation is common to any open heart procedure. Routine monitoring for anesthetic induction includes a surface electrocardiogram, cutaneous oximetry, and radial and pulmonary artery pressures. After anesthetic induction a femoral artery catheter, in addition to a radial arterial line, is also placed. This provides more accurate measurements during rewarming and on discontinuation of cardiopulmonary bypass because of the peripheral vasoconstriction that occurs

after hypothermic circulatory arrest. It is generally removed in the intensive care unit when the two readings correlate.

Electroencephalographic recording is performed to ensure the absence of cerebral activity before circulatory arrest is induced. The patient's head is enveloped in a cooling jacket, and cerebral cooling is begun after the initiation of bypass. Temperature measurements are made of the esophagus, tympanic membrane, urinary catheter, rectum, and blood (through the Swan-Ganz catheter). If the patient's condition is stable after the induction of anesthesia, up to 500 mL of autologous whole blood is withdrawn for later use, and the volume deficit is replaced with crystalloid solution.

Surgical Technique.
After a median sternotomy incision, the pericardium is incised longitudinally and attached to the wound edges. Typically the right heart is enlarged, with a tense right atrium and a variable degree of tricuspid regurgitation. There is usually severe right ventricular hypertrophy, and with critical degrees of obstruction, the patient's condition may become unstable with the manipulation of the heart.

Anticoagulation with heparin (400 U/kg, intravenously) is administered to prolong the activated clotting time beyond 400 seconds. Full cardiopulmonary bypass is instituted with high ascending aortic cannulation and two caval cannulae. These cannulae must be inserted into the superior and inferior vena cavae sufficiently to enable subsequent opening of the right atrium if necessary. A temporary pulmonary artery vent is placed in the midline of the main pulmonary artery 1 cm distal to the pulmonary valve. After cardiopulmonary bypass is initiated, surface cooling with both the head jacket and the cooling blanket is begun. The blood is cooled with the pump-oxygenator. During cooling a 10°C gradient between arterial blood and bladder or rectal temperature is maintained.[93] Cooling generally takes 45 minutes to an hour. When ventricular fibrillation occurs, an additional vent is placed in the left atrium through the right superior pulmonary vein to prevent distention from the large amount of bronchial arterial blood flow that is common with these patients.

It is most convenient for the primary surgeon to stand initially on the patient's left side. During the cooling period, some preliminary dissection can be performed, with full mobilization of the right pulmonary artery from the ascending aorta. The superior vena cava is also fully mobilized. The approach to the right pulmonary artery is made medial, not lateral, to the superior vena cava. All dissection of the pulmonary arteries takes place intrapericardially, and neither pleural cavity should be entered. An incision is then made in the right pulmonary artery from beneath the ascending aorta out under the superior vena cava and entering the lower lobe branch of the pulmonary artery just after the take-off of the middle lobe artery (Fig. 52-7). The incision stays in the center of the vessel and continues into the lower rather than the middle lobe artery.

Any loose thrombus, if present, is now removed, to obtain good visualization. It is most important to recognize, however, that first, an embolectomy without subsequent endarterectomy is quite ineffective and, second, that in most

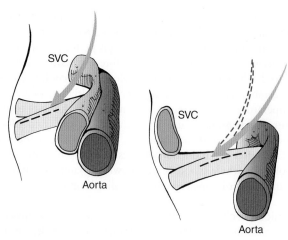

FIGURE 52-7 Recommended surgical approach on the right side. This approach, medial to the superior vena cava (SVC), and between the SVC and aorta, provides a direct view into the right pulmonary artery. Note that an approach on the lateral side of the SVC will only provide a restricted view, and should be avoided.

patients with chronic thromboembolic hypertension, direct examination of the pulmonary vascular bed at operation generally shows no obvious embolic material. Therefore, to the inexperienced or cursory glance, if fresh thrombus is not present the pulmonary vascular bed may well appear normal even in patients with severe chronic embolic pulmonary hypertension.

If the bronchial circulation is not excessive, the endarterectomy plane can be found during this early dissection. However, although a small amount of dissection can be performed before the initiation of circulatory arrest, it is unwise to proceed unless perfect visibility is obtained, because the development of a correct plane is essential.

There are four broad types of pulmonary occlusive disease related to thrombus that can be appreciated, and we use the following classification[87,94]: Type I disease (approximately 15% of cases of thromboembolic pulmonary hypertension) (Fig. 52-8) refers to the situation in which major vessel clot is present and readily visible on the opening of the pulmonary arteries. All central thrombotic material has to be completely removed before the endarterectomy. In type II disease (approximately 55% of our cases; Fig. 52-9), no major vessel thrombus can be appreciated. In these cases only thickened intima can be seen, occasionally with webs, and the endarterectomy plane is raised in the main, lobar, or segmental vessels. Type III disease (approximately 30% of our cases; Fig. 52-10) presents the most challenging surgical situation. The disease is very distal and confined to the segmental and subsegmental branches. No occlusion of vessels can be seen initially. The endarterectomy plane must be carefully and painstakingly raised in each segmental and subsegmental branch. Type III disease is most often associated with presumed repetitive thrombi from indwelling catheters (such as pacemaker wires) or ventriculo-atrial shunts. It may also represent "burnt-out" disease, where the thrombotic obstruction developed years before, and has since resolved in many areas, but intrinsic

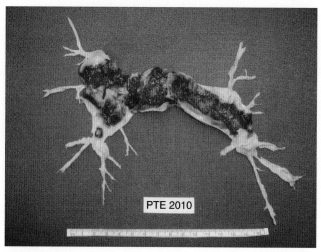

FIGURE 52-8 Surgical specimen removed from a patient showing evidence of some fresh and some old thrombus in the main and both right and left pulmonary arteries. Note that simple removal of the gross disease initially encountered on pulmonary arteriotomy will not be therapeutic, and any meaningful outcome involves a full endarterectomy into all the distal segments.

vessel disease now contributes to the pulmonary hypertension. Type IV disease (Fig. 52-11) does not represent primary thromboembolic pulmonary hypertension and is inoperable. In this entity there is intrinsic small-vessel disease, although secondary thrombus may occur as a result of stasis. Small-vessel disease may be unrelated to thromboembolic events ("primary" pulmonary hypertension) or occur in relation to thromboembolic hypertension as a result of a high flow or high pressure state in previously unaffected vessels similar to the generation of Eisenmenger's syndrome. We believe that there may also be sympathetic "cross-talk" from an affected contralateral side or stenotic areas in the same lung.

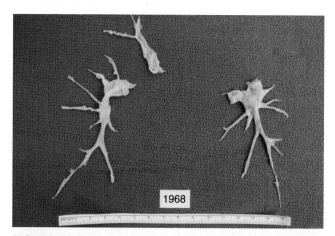

FIGURE 52-9 Specimen removed in a patient with type II disease. Both pulmonary arteries have evidence of chronic thromboembolic material. Note the distal tails of the specimen in each branch. Full resolution of pulmonary hypertension is dependent on complete removal of all the distal tails.

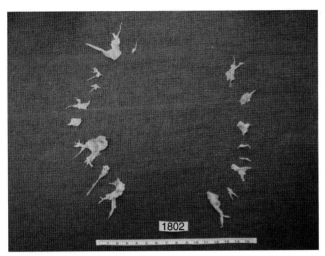

FIGURE 52-10 Specimen removed from a patient with type III disease. Note that the disease is distal, and the plane was raised at each segmental level.

When the patient's temperature reaches 20°C, the aorta is cross-clamped and a single dose of cold cardioplegic solution (1 L) is administered. Additional myocardial protection is obtained by the use of a cooling jacket. The entire procedure is now performed with a single aortic cross-clamp period with no further administration of cardioplegic solution.

A modified cerebellar retractor is placed between the aorta and superior vena cava. When blood obscures direct vision of the pulmonary vascular bed, thiopental is administered (500 mg-1 g) until the electroencephalogram becomes isoelectric. Circulatory arrest is then initiated, and the patient is exsanguinated. All monitoring lines to the patient are turned off to prevent the aspiration of air. Snares are tightened

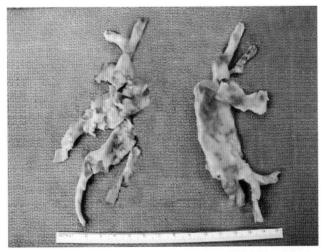

FIGURE 52-11 Note the absence of distal "tails" in this specimen removed from a patient with surgical classification type IV. All "tails" are replaced by "trousers." No clinical benefit was obtained from this procedure and the patient's postoperative hemodynamics was not improved, despite what appears to be an impressive endarterectomy specimen. The patient had primary pulmonary hypertension.

around the cannulae in the superior and inferior vena cavae. With experience it is rare that one 20-minute period for each side is exceeded. Although retrograde cerebral perfusion has been advocated for total circulatory arrest in other procedures, it is not helpful in this operation because it does not allow a completely bloodless field, and with the short arrest times that can be achieved with experience, it is not necessary.

Any residual loose, thrombotic debris encountered is removed. Then, a microtome knife is used to develop the endarterectomy plane posteriorly, because any inadvertent egress in this site could be repaired readily, or simply left alone. Dissection in the correct plane is critical because if the plane is too deep the pulmonary artery may perforate, with fatal results, and if the dissection plane is not deep enough, inadequate amounts of the chronically thromboembolic material will be removed. The plane should only be sought in the diseased parts of the artery; this often requires the initial dissection to begin quite distally.

The ideal layer is marked with a pearly white plane, which strips easily. There should be no residual yellow plaque. If the dissection is too deep, a reddish or pinkish color indicates the adventitia has been reached. A more superficial plane should be sought immediately.

Once the plane is correctly developed, a full-thickness layer is left in the region of the incision to ease subsequent repair. The endarterectomy is then performed with an eversion technique, using a specially developed dissection instrument (Jamieson aspirator, Fehling Corp.). Because the vessel is partly everted and subsegmental branches are being worked on, a perforation here will become completely inaccessible and invisible later. This is why absolute visualization in a completely bloodless field provided by circulatory arrest is essential. It is important that each subsegmental branch is followed and freed individually until it ends in a "tail," beyond which there is no further obstruction.

Once the right-sided endarterectomy is completed, circulation is restarted, and the arteriotomy is repaired with a continuous 6-0 polypropylene suture. The hemostatic nature of this closure is aided by the nature of the initial dissection, with the full thickness of the pulmonary artery being preserved immediately adjacent to the incision.

The surgeon now moves to the patient's right side. The pulmonary vent catheter is withdrawn, and an arteriotomy is made either from the site of the pulmonary vent hole or adjacent to it, out laterally beneath the pericardial reflection, and again into the lower lobe, but avoiding entry into the left pleural space. Additional lateral dissection does not enhance intraluminal visibility, may endanger the left phrenic nerve, and makes subsequent repair of the left pulmonary artery more difficult (Fig. 52-12). There is often a lymphatic vessel encountered on the left pulmonary artery at the level of the pericardial reflection ("Jamieson's lymphatic"), and it is wise to clip this before it being divided with the pulmonary artery incision.

The left-sided dissection is virtually analogous in all respects to that accomplished on the right. By the time the circulation is arrested once more it will have been

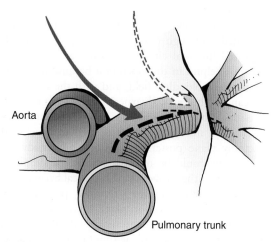

FIGURE 52-12 Surgical approach on the left side. The incision in the left pulmonary artery begins in the midpoint of the main pulmonary trunk, at the insertion site of the pulmonary artery vent. This incision provides better visibility than a more distal approach (*dotted line and arrow*). Care must be taken to avoid injury to the phrenic nerve.

reinitiated for at least 10 minutes, by which time the venous oxygen saturations are in excess of 90%. The duration of circulatory arrest intervals on the left side are again limited to 20 minutes.

After the completion of the endarterectomy, cardiopulmonary bypass is reinstituted and warming is commenced. Methylprednisolone (500 mg, intravenously) and mannitol (12.5 g, intravenously) are administered, and during warming a 10°C temperature gradient is maintained between the perfusate and body temperature, with a maximum perfusate temperature of 37°C. If the systemic vascular resistance level is high, nitroprusside is administered to promote vasodilatation and warming. The rewarming period generally takes approximately 90 to 120 minutes but varies according to the body mass of the patient.

When the left pulmonary arteriotomy has been repaired, the pulmonary artery vent is replaced. The right atrium is then opened and examined. Any intra-atrial communication is closed. Although tricuspid valve regurgitation is invariable in these patients and is often severe, tricuspid valve repair is not performed unless there is independent structural damage to the tricuspid valve itself. Right ventricular remodeling occurs within a few days, with the return of tricuspid competence. If other cardiac procedures are required, such as coronary artery or mitral or aortic valve surgery, these are conveniently performed during the systemic rewarming period. Myocardial cooling is discontinued once all cardiac procedures have been concluded. The left atrial vent is removed, and the vent site is repaired. All air is removed from the heart, and the aortic cross-clamp is removed.

When the patient has rewarmed, cardiopulmonary bypass is discontinued. Dopamine hydrochloride is generally administered at renal doses, and other inotropic agents and vasodilators are titrated as necessary to sustain acceptable hemodynamics. The cardiac output is generally high, with a low systemic vascular resistance. Temporary pacing wires are placed.

Despite the duration of extracorporeal circulation, hemostasis is readily achieved, and blood products are generally unnecessary. Wound closure is routine. A vigorous diuresis is usual for the next few hours, also a result of the previous systemic hypothermia.

POSTOPERATIVE CARE

Meticulous postoperative management is essential to the success of this operation. All patients are mechanically ventilated overnight, and subjected to a maintained diuresis with the goal of reaching the patient's preoperative weight within 24 hours. Although much of the postoperative care is common to more ordinary open-heart surgery patients, there are some important differences.

A higher minute ventilation is often required early after the operation to compensate for the temporary metabolic acidosis that develops after the long period of circulatory arrest, hypothermia, and cardiopulmonary bypass. Tidal volumes higher than those normally recommended after cardiac surgery are therefore generally used to obtain optimal gas exchange. The maximum inspiratory pressure is maintained below 30 cm of water if possible. Extubation should be performed on the first postoperative day, whenever possible.

Diuresis. Patients have considerable positive fluid balance after operation. After hypothermic circulatory arrest, patients initiate an early spontaneous aggressive diuresis for unknown reasons, but this may in part be related to the increased cardiac output related to a now lower PVR level, and improved RV function. This diuresis should be augmented with diuretics, however, with the aim of returning the patient to the preoperative fluid balance within 24 hours of operation. Because of the increased cardiac output, some degree of systemic hypotension is readily tolerated. Fluid administration is minimized, and the patient's hematocrit level should be maintained above 30% to increase oxygen-carrying capacity and to reduce the likelihood of the pulmonary reperfusion phenomenon.

Arrhythmias. The development of atrial arrhythmias, at approximately 10%, is no more common than that encountered in patients who undergo other types of non valvular heart surgery. When a small atrial septal defect or persistent foramen ovale is closed this is done with a small inferior atrial incision directly over the fossa ovalis, away from the conduction system of the atrium or its blood supply. The siting and size of this incision may be helpful in the reduction of the incidence of these arrhythmias.

Transfusion. Despite the requirement for the maintenance of an adequate hematocrit level, with careful blood conservation techniques used during operation, transfusion is required in a minority of patients.

Inferior Vena Caval Filter and Anticoagulation. A Greenfield filter is usually inserted before operation, to minimize recurrent PE after pulmonary endarterectomy. However, if this is not possible, it can also be inserted at the time of operation. If the device is to be placed at operation, radiopaque markers should be placed over the level of the spine corresponding to the location of the renal veins to allow correct positioning. Postoperative venous thrombosis prophylaxis with intermittent pneumatic compression devices is used, and the use of subcutaneous heparin is begun on the evening of surgery. Anticoagulation with warfarin is begun as soon as the pacing wires and mediastinal drainage tubes are removed, with a target international normalized ratio (INR) of 2.5 to 3.

COMPLICATIONS

Aside from complications that are associated with open heart and major lung surgery (arrhythmias, atelectasis, wound infection, pneumonia, mediastinal bleeding, etc.), there are complications specific to this operation. These include persistent pulmonary hypertension, reperfusion pulmonary response, and neurologic disorders related to deep hypothermia.

Persistent Pulmonary Hypertension. The decrease in PVR level usually results in an immediate and sustained restoration of pulmonary artery pressures to normal levels, with a marked increase in cardiac output. In a few patients, an immediately normal pulmonary vascular tone is not achieved, but an additional substantial reduction may occur over the next few days because of the subsequent relaxation of small vessels and the resolution of intraoperative factors such as pulmonary edema. In such patients, it is usual to see a large pulmonary artery pulse pressure, the low diastolic pressure indicating good runoff, yet persistent pulmonary arterial inflexibility still resulting in a high systolic pressure.

There are a few patients in whom the pulmonary artery pressures do not resolve substantially. If the operation has been performed as described in the preceding, using circulatory arrest, and ensuring that all distal disease is removed, this will be the result of type IV disease. We do operate on some patients with severe pulmonary hypertension but equivocal embolic disease. Despite the considerable risk of attempted endarterectomy in these patients, because transplantation is the only other avenue of therapy, there may be a point when it is unlikely that a patient will survive until a donor is found. In our most recent 1000 patients, the majority of perioperative deaths were directly attributable to the problem of inadequate relief of pulmonary artery hypertension. This was a diagnostic rather than an operative technical problem. Attempts at pharmacologic manipulation of high residual PVR levels with sodium nitroprusside, epoprostenol sodium, or inhaled nitric oxide are generally not effective. Because, if the operation has been performed thoroughly, there will be no further resolution, it is not appropriate to use mechanical circulatory support or extracorporeal membrane oxygenation in these patients if they deteriorate subsequently.

The "Reperfusion Response." A specific complication that occurs in many patients to some degree is localized pulmonary edema, or the "reperfusion response." Reperfusion response or reperfusion injury is defined as a radiologic opacity seen in the lungs within 72 hours of pulmonary endarterectomy. This unfortunately loose definition may therefore encompass many other causes, such as fluid overload and infection.

True reperfusion injury that directly adversely impacts the clinical course of the patient now occurs in approximately 10% of patients. In its most dramatic form, it occurs soon after operation (within a few hours) and is associated with profound desaturation. Edema-like fluid, sometimes with a bloody tinge, is suctioned from the endotracheal tube.[95] Frank blood from the endotracheal tube, however, signifies a mechanical violation of the blood airway barrier that has occurred at operation and generally stems from a technical error, though we have seen some cases where significant blood in the airway was the result of a technically good operation, but reperfusion of a known infarcted area of the lung with subsequent cavity formation. This complication should be managed, if possible, by identification of the affected area by bronchoscopy and balloon occlusion of the affected lobe until coagulation can be normalized.

One common cause of reperfusion pulmonary edema is persistent high pulmonary artery pressures after operation when a thorough endarterectomy has been performed in certain areas, but there remains a large part of the pulmonary vascular bed affected by type IV change. In this situation all pulmonary artery flow is directed toward the endarterectomized areas. However, the reperfusion phenomenon is often encountered in patients after a seemingly technically perfect operation with complete resolution of high pulmonary artery pressures. In these cases the response may be one of reactive hyperemia, after the revascularization of segments of the pulmonary arterial bed that have long experienced no flow. Other contributing factors may include perioperative pulmonary ischemia and conditions associated with high permeability lung injury in the area of the now denuded endothelium. Fortunately, the incidence of this complication is much less common now in our series, probably as a result of the more complete and expeditious removal of the endarterectomy specimen that has come with the large experience over the last decade.

Management of the "Reperfusion Response". Early measures should be taken to minimize the development of pulmonary edema by diuresis, maintenance of hematocrit levels, and the early use of peak end-expiratory pressure. Once the capillary leak has been established, however, treatment is supportive because reperfusion pulmonary edema will eventually resolve if satisfactory hemodynamics and oxygenation can be maintained. Careful management of ventilation and fluid balance is required. The hematocrit is kept high (32-36%), and the patient undergoes aggressive diuresis, even if this requires ultrafiltration. The patient's ventilatory status may be dramatically position sensitive. The fraction of inspired oxygen (FIO$_2$) level is kept as low as is compatible with an oxygen saturation of 90%. A careful titration of positive end-expiratory pressure is carried out, with a progressive transition from volume to pressure-limited inverse ratio ventilation and the acceptance of moderate hypercapnia.[95] The use of steroids is discouraged because they are generally ineffective and may lead to infection. Infrequently, inhaled nitric oxide at 20 to 40 parts per million can improve the gas exchange. On occasion we have used extracorporeal perfusion support (extracorporeal membrane oxygenator or extracorporeal carbon dioxide removal) until ventilation can be resumed satisfactorily, usually after 7 to 10 days. However, the use of this support is limited to patients who have benefited from hemodynamic improvement, but are suffering from significant reperfusion response. Extracorporeal devices should not be used if there is no evidence or hope of subsequent hemodynamic improvement, because it will not play a role in improving irreversible pulmonary pressures and carries mortality close to 100%.

Delirium. Early in the pulmonary endarterectomy experience (before 1990), there was a substantial incidence of postoperative delirium. A study of 28 patients who underwent pulmonary endarterectomy showed that 77% experienced the development of this complication.[96,97] Delirium appeared to be related to an accumulated duration of circulatory arrest time of more than 55 minutes; the incidence fell to 11% with significantly shorter periods of arrest time.[96-98] With the more expeditious operation that has come with our increased experience, postoperative confusion is now encountered no more commonly than with ordinary open heart surgery.

RESULTS

More than 3500 pulmonary thromboendarterectomy have been performed at UCSD Medical Center since 1970. Almost all of these cases have been completed since 1990, when the surgical procedure was modified as described earlier in this chapter. The mean patient age in our group is 54 years, with a range of 3 to 85 years. There is a very slight male predominance. In nearly one-third of the cases, at least one additional cardiac procedure was performed at the time of operation. Most commonly, the adjunct procedure was closure of a persistent foramen ovale or atrial septal defect (26%) or coronary artery bypass grafting (8%).[87]

Hemodynamic Results. A reduction in pulmonary pressures and resistance to normal levels and a corresponding improvement in pulmonary blood flow and cardiac output are generally immediate and sustained.[98,99] In general, these changes can be assumed to be permanent. Whereas before the operation, more than 95% of the patients are in NYHA functional class III or IV; at 1 year after the operation, 95% of patients remain in NYHA functional class I or II.[99,100] In addition, echocardiographic studies have demonstrated that, with the elimination of chronic pressure overload, right ventricular geometry rapidly reverts toward normal. Right atrial

and right ventricular enlargement regresses. Tricuspid valve function returns to normal within a few days as a result of restoration of tricuspid annular geometry after the remodeling of the right ventricle, and tricuspid repair is not therefore part of the operation.

Operative Morbidity. Severe reperfusion injury was the single most frequent complication in the UCSD series, occurring in 10% of patients. Some of these patients did not survive, and other patients required prolonged mechanical ventilatory support. A few patients were salvaged only by the use of extracorporeal support and blood carbon dioxide removal. Neurologic complications from circulatory arrest appear to have been eliminated, probably as a result of the shorter circulatory arrest periods now experienced, and perioperative confusion and stroke are now no more frequent than with conventional open heart surgery. Early postoperative hemorrhage required re-exploration in 2.5% of patients, and less than half of patients required intraoperative or postoperative blood transfusion. Despite the prolonged operation, wound infections are relatively infrequent. Only 1.8% experienced the development of sternal wound complications, including sterile dehiscence or mediastinitis.

Deaths. In our experience, the overall mortality rate (30 days or in-hospital if the hospital course is prolonged) is 6% for the entire patient group, which encompasses a time span of over 35 years. The mortality rate was 9.4% in 1989 and has been less than 5% for more than 3000 patients who have undergone the operation since 1990. In our most recent experience over the last 5 years, the mortality rate has been less than 2%. With our increasing experience and many referrals, we continue to accept some patients who, in retrospect, were unsuitable candidates for the procedure (type IV disease). We also accept patients in whom we know that the entire degree of pulmonary hypertension cannot be explained by the occlusive disease detected by angiography but feel that they will be benefited by operation, albeit at higher risk. Primary causes of death are operation on patients in whom thromboembolic disease was not the cause of the pulmonary hypertension (50%) and the rare case of reperfusion pulmonary edema that progresses to a respiratory distress syndrome of long-standing, which is not reversible (25%).

LATE FOLLOW-UP

A survey of the surviving patients who underwent pulmonary endarterectomy surgery at UCSD between 1970 and 1995 formally evaluated the long-term outcome.[100] Questionnaires were mailed to 420 patients who were more than 1 year after operation. Responses were obtained from 308 patients. Survival, functional status, quality of life, and the subsequent use of medical help were assessed. Survival after pulmonary thromboendarterectomy was 75% at 6 years or more. Ninety-three percent of the patients were found to be in NYHA class I or II, compared with about 95% of the patients being in NYHA class III or IV preoperatively. Of the working population, 62% of patients who were unemployed before operation returned to work. Patients who had undergone pulmonary endarterectomy scored several quality-of-life components just slightly lower than normal individuals, but significantly higher than the patients before endarterectomy. Only 10% of patients used oxygen, and in response to the question, "How do you feel about the quality of your life since your surgery?" Seventy-seven percent replied much improved, and twenty percent replied improved. These data appear to confirm that pulmonary endarterectomy offers substantial improvement in survival, function, and quality of life, with minimal later health-care requirements.[100]

REFERENCES

1. Dalen JE, Alpert JS: Natural history of pulmonary embolism. *Prog Cardiovasc Dis* 1975; 17:259-270.
2. Landefeld CS, Chren MM, Myers A, et al: Diagnostic yield of the autopsy in a university hospital and a community hospital. *N Engl J Med* 1988; 318:1249.
3. Goldhaber SZ, Hennekens CH, Evens DA, et al: Factors associated with correct antemortem diagnosis of major pulmonary embolism. *Am J Med* 1982; 73:822-826.
4. Rubinstein I, Murray D, Hoffstein V: Fatal pulmonary emboli in hospitalized patients: an autopsy study. *Arch Intern Med* 1988; 148:1425-1426.
5. Kniffin WD Jr, Baron JA, Barrett J, et al: The epidemiology of diagnosed pulmonary embolism and deep venous thrombosis in the elderly. *Arch Intern Med* 1994; 154:861.
6. Martin M: PHLECO. A multicenter study of the fate of 1647 hospital patients treated conservatively without fibrinolysis and surgery. *Clin Invest* 1993; 71:471.
7. Carson JL, Kelley MA, Duff A, et al: The clinical course of pulmonary embolism. *N Engl J Med* 1992; 326:1240.
8. Clagett GP, Anderson FA Jr, Levine MN, et al: Prevention of venous thromboembolism. *Chest* 1992; 102:391S.
9. Anderson FA Jr, Wheeler HB: Venous thromboembolism; risk factors and prophylaxis, in Tapson VF, Fulkkerson WJ, Saltzman HA (eds): *Clinics in Chest Medicine, Venous Thromboembolism*, vol 16. Philadelphia, Saunders, 1995; p 235.
10. Greenfield LJ: Venous thrombosis and pulmonary thromboembolism, in Schwartz SI (ed): *Principals of Surgery*, 6th ed. New York, McGraw-Hill, 1994; p 989.
11. Riedel M, Stanek V, Widimsky J, Prerovsky I: Long term follow up of patients with pulmonary embolism: late prognosis and evolution of hemodynamic and respiratory data. *Chest* 1982; 81:151.
12. Sevitt S: The structure and growth of valve pocket thrombi in femoral veins. *J Clin Pathol* 1974; 27:517.
13. Philbrick JT, Becker DM: Calf deep vein thrombosis: a wolf in sheep's clothing? *Arch Intern Med* 1988; 148:2131.
14. Godleski JJ: Pathology of deep vein thrombosis and pulmonary embolism, in Goldhaber SZ (ed): *Pulmonary Embolism and Deep Venous Thrombosis*. Philadelphia, Saunders, 1985; p 11.
15. Moser KM: Venous thromboembolism. *Am Rev Resp Dis* 1990; 141:235.
16. Kakkar VV, Flan C, Howe CT, Clark MB: Natural history of postoperative deep vein thrombosis. *Lancet* 1969; 2:230.
17. Salzmen EW, Hirsh J: The epidemiology, pathogenesis, and natural history of venous thrombosis, in Colman RW, Hirsch J, Marder VJ, Salzman EW (eds): *Hemostasis and Thrombosis: Basic Principals and Clinical Practice*, 3rd ed. Philadelphia, Lippincott, 1994; p 1275.
18. Stewart GJ, Lackman JW, Alburger PD, et al: Intraoperative venous dilation and subsequent development of deep vein thrombosis in patients undergoing total hip or knee replacement. *Ultrasound Med Biol* 1990; 16:133.
19. Comerota AJ, Stewart GJ, Alburger PD, et al: Operative venodilation, a previously unsuspected factor in the cause of postoperative deep vein thrombosis. *Surgery* 1989; 106:301.
20. Comerota AJ, Stewart GJ: Operative venous dilation and its relationship to postoperative deep vein thrombosis, in Goldhaber SZ (ed): *Prevention of Venous Thromboembolism*. New York, Marcel Dekker, 1993; p 25.
21. Weiss HJ, Turitto VT, Baumgartner HR, et al: Evidence for the presence of tissue factor activity on subendothelium. *Blood* 1989; 73:968.
22. Bertina RM, Koeleman BPC, Koster T, et al: Mutation in blood coagulation factor V associated with resistance to activated protein C. *Nature* 1994; 369:64.
23. Svensson PJ, Dahlback B: Resistance to activated protein C as a basis for venous thrombosis. *N Engl J Med* 1994; 330:517.
24. Ridker PM, Hennekens CH, Lindpaintner K, et al: Mutation in the gene coding for coagulation factor V and the risk of myocardial infarction, stroke, and venous thrombosis in apparently healthy men. *N Engl J Med* 1995; 332:912.
25. Feinstein DI: Immune coagulation disorders, in Colman RW, Hirsh J, Marder VJ, Salzman EW (eds): *Hemostasis and Thrombosis: Basic Principal and Clinical Practice*, 3rd ed. Philadelphia, Lippincott, 1994; p 881.
26. Robertson BR, Pandolfi M, Nilsson IM: "Fibrinolytic capacity" in healthy volunteers at different ages as studied by standardized venous occlusion of arms and legs. *Acta Med Scand* 1972; 191:199.
27. Prins MH, Hirsh J: A critical review of the evidence supporting a relationship between impaired fibrinolysis and venous thromboembolism. *Arch Intern Med* 1991; 151:1721.
28. Wheeler HB, Anderson FA Jr, Cardullo PA, et al: Suspected deep vein thrombosis: management by impedance plethysmography. *Arch Surg* 1982; 117:1206.
29. Samama MM, Simonneau G, Wainstein JP, et al: SISIUS Study: epidemiology of risk factors of deep vein thrombosis (DVT) of the lower limbs in community practice (abstract). *Thromb Haemost* 1993; 69:763.
30. Hull R, Hirsh J, Jay R: Different intensities of anticoagulation in the long term treatment of proximal vein thrombosis. *N Engl J Med* 1982; 307:1676.
31. Collins R, Scrimgeor A, Yusuf S, et al: Reduction in fatal pulmonary embolism and venous thrombosis by perioperative administration of subcutaneous heparin. Overview of results and randomized trials in general, orthopedic, and urologic surgery. *N Engl J Med* 1988; 318:1162.
32. Reis SE, Polak JF, Hirsch DR, et al: Frequency of deep vein thrombosis in asymptomatic patients with coronary artery bypass grafts. *Am Heart J* 1991; 122:478.
33. Josa M, Siouffi SY, Silverman AB, et al: Pulmonary embolism after cardiac surgery. *J Am Coll Cardiol* 1993; 21:990.
34. Gillinov AM, Davis EA, Alberg AJ, et al: Pulmonary embolism in the cardiac surgical patient. *Ann Thorac Surg* 1992; 53:988.
35. Evans AJ, Sostman HC, Knelson M, et al: Detection of deep vein thrombosis: a prospective comparison of MR imaging with contrast venography. *Am J Roentgenol* 1993; 161:131.
36. Burk B, Sostman D, Carroll BA, Witty LA: The diagnostic approach to deep vein thrombosis, in *Venous Thromboembolism, Clinics in Chest Medicine*, vol 16. Philadelphia, Saunders, 1995; pp 253-268.
37. Hirsh J, Levine MN: Low molecular weight heparin. *Blood* 1992; 72:1.
38. Shulman S, Rhedin A-S, Lindmarker P, et al: A comparison of six weeks with six months of oral anticoagulant therapy after a first episode of venous thromboembolism. *N Engl J Med* 1995; 332:1661.
39. Goldhaber SZ: Strategies for diagnosis, in Goldhaber SZ (ed): *Pulmonary Embolism and Deep Vein Thrombosis*. Philadelphia. Saunders, 1985; p 79.
40. Hoaglang PM: Massive pulmonary embolism, in Goldhaber SZ (ed): *Pulmonary Embolism and Deep Vein Thrombosis*. Philadelphia, Saunders, 1985; p 179.
41. Malik AB, Johnson B: Role of humoral mediators in the pulmonary vascular response to pulmonary embolism, in Weir EK, Reeves JT (eds): *Pulmonary Vascular Physiology and Pathophysiology*. New York, Marcel Dekker, 1989; p 445.
42. Huval WV, Mathieson MA, Stemp LI, et al: Therapeutic benefits of 5-hydroxytryptamine inhibition following pulmonary embolism. *Ann Surg* 1983; 197:223.
43. Barritt DW, Jordan SC: Anticoagulant drugs in treatment of pulmonary embolism: Controlled Trial. *Lancet* 1960; 1:1309.
44. The urokinase pulmonary embolism trial. A national cooperative study. *Circulation* 1973; 47(Suppl II):1.
45. Bell WR, Simon TR: Current status of pulmonary thromboembolic disease: pathophysiology, diagnosis, prevention, and treatment. *Am Heart J* 1982; 103:239.
46. Dalen JE, Banas JS Jr, Brooks HL, et al: Resolution rate of pulmonary embolism in man. *N Engl J Med* 1969; 280:1194.

47. Tow DE, Wagner HN: Recovery of pulmonary arterial blood flow in patients with pulmonary embolism. *N Engl J Med* 1967; 276:1053.

48. Dalen JE, Alpert JS: Natural history of pulmonary embolism. *Prog Cardiovasc Dis* 1975; 17:259.

49. Palevsky HI: The problems of the clinical and laboratory diagnosis of pulmonary embolism. *Sem Nucl Med* 1991; 21:276.

50. Greenfield LJ, Proctor MC, Williams DM, Wakefield TW: Long term experience with transvenous catheter pulmonary embolectomy. *J Vasc Surg* 1993; 18:450.

51. Goodall RJR, Greenfield LJ: Clinical correlations in the diagnosis of pulmonary embolism. *Ann Surg* 1980; 191:219.

52. McCracken S, Bettmen S: Current status of ionic and nonionic intravascular contrast media. *Postgrad Radiol* 1983; 3:345.

53. Novelline RA, Baltarowich OH, Athanasoulis CA, et al: The clinical course of patients with suspect pulmonary embolism and a negative pulmonary arteriogram. *Radiology* 1978; 126:561.

54. Schiebler M, Holland G, Hatabu H, et al: Suspected pulmonary embolism: prospective evaluation with pulmonary MR angiography. *Radiology* 1993; 189:125.

55. Come PC: Echocardiographic evaluation of pulmonary embolism and its response to therapeutic interventions. *Chest* 1992; 101:1515.

56. Goldhaber SZ: Thrombolytic therapy in venous thromboembolism. Clinical trials and current indications, in Tapson VF, Fulkerson WJ, Saltzman HA (eds): *Clinics in Chest Medicine, Venous Thromboembolism*, vol 16. Philadelphia, Saunders, 1995; p 307.

57. Marder VJ, Sherry S: Thrombolytic therapy: current status. *N Engl J Med* 1988; 318:1585.

58. Goldhaber SZ, Haire WD, Feldstein ML, et al: Alteplase versus heparin in acute PE; randomized trial assessing right ventricular function and pulmonary perfusion. *Lancet* 1993; 341:507.

59. Tibbutt DA, Davies JA, Anderson JA, et al: Comparison by controlled clinical trial of streptokinase and heparin in treatment of life-threatening PE. *BMJ* 1974; 1:343.

60. Ly B, Arnesen H, Eie H, Hol R: A controlled clinical trial of streptokinase and heparin in the treatment of major PE. *Acta Med Scand* 1978; 203:465.

61. Levine MN: Thrombolytic therapy for venous embolism. Complications and contraindications, in Tapson VF, Fulkerson WJ, Saltzman HA (eds): *Clinics in Chest Medicine, Venous Thromboembolism*, vol 16. Philadelphia, Saunders, 1995; p 321.

62. Levine M, Hirsh J, Weitz J, et al: A randomized trial of a single bolus dosage regimen of recombinant tissue plasminogen activator in patients with acute PE. *Chest* 1990; 98:1473.

63. Gray JJ, Miller GAH, Paneth M: Pulmonary embolectomy: its place in the management of pulmonary embolism. *Lancet* 1988; 25:1441.

64. Timist J-F, Reynaud P, Meyers G, Sors H: Pulmonary embolectomy by catheter device in massive pulmonary embolism. *Chest* 1991; 100:655.

65. Tapson VF, Witty LA: Massive pulmonary embolism, in Tapson VF, Fulkerson WJ, Saltzman HA (eds): *Clinics in Chest Medicine, Venous Thromboembolism*, vol 16. Philadelphia, Saunders, 1995; p 329.

66. Mattox KL, Feldtman RW, Beall AC, De Bakey ME: Pulmonary embolectomy for acute massive pulmonary embolism. *Ann Surg* 1982; 195:726.

67. Boulafendis D, Bastounis E, Panayiotopoulos YP, Papalambros EL: Pulmonary embolectomy: answered and unanswered questions. *Int J Angiol* 1991; 10:187.

68. Kasper W, Meinterz MD, Henkel B, et al: Echocardiographic findings in patients with proved pulmonary embolism. *Am Heart J* 1986; 112:1284.

69. Stewart JR, Greenfield LS: Transvenous vena cava filtration and pulmonary embolectomy. *Surg Clin No Am* 1982; 62:411.

70. Schmid C, Zietlow S, Wagner TOF, et al: Fulminant pulmonary embolism: symptoms, diagnostics, operative technique and results. *Ann Thorac Surg* 1991; 52:1102.

71. Greenfield LJ, Zocco J, Wilk JD, et al: Clinical experience with the Kim-Ray Greenfield vena cava filter. *Ann Surg* 1977; 185:692.

72. Anderson HL III, Delius RE, Sinard JM, et al: Early experience with adult extracorporeal membrane oxygenation in the modern era. *Ann Thorac Surg* 1992; 53:553.

73. Wenger R, Bavaria JB, Ratcliff MB, Edmunds LH Jr: Flow dynamics of peripheral venous catheters during extracorporeal membrane oxygenator (ECMO) with a centrifuge pump. *J Thorac Cardiovasc Surg* 1988; 96:478.

74. Gray HH, Morgan JM, Miller GAH: Pulmonary embolectomy for acute massive pulmonary embolism: an analysis of 71 cases. *Br Heart J* 1988; 60:196.

75. Del Campo C: Pulmonary embolectomy: a review. *Can J Surg* 1985; 28:111.

76. Gulba DC, Schmid C, Borst H-G, et al: Medical compared with surgical treatment for massive pulmonary embolism. *Lancet* 1994; 343:576.

77. Clark DB: Pulmonary embolectomy has a well-defined and valuable place. *Br J Hosp Med* 1989; 41:468.

78. Soyer R, Brunet M, Redonnet JY, et al: Follow-up of surgically treated patients with massive pulmonary embolism, with reference to 12 operated patients. *Thorac Cardiovasc Surg* 1982; 30:103.

79. Benotti JR, Ockene IS, Alpert JS, Dalen JE: The clinical profile of unresolved pulmonary embolism. *Chest* 1983; 84:669-678.

80. Moser KM, Auger WF, Fedullo PF: Chronic major-vessel thromboembolic pulmonary hypertension. *Circulation* 1990; 81:1735-1743.

81. Houk VN, Hufnnagel CA, McClenathan JE, Moser KM: Chronic thrombosis obstruction of major pulmonary arteries: report of a case successfully treated by thromboendarterectomy and review of the literature. *Am J Med* 1963; 35:269-282.

82. Dibble JH: Organization and canalization in arterial thrombosis. *J Pathol Bacteriol* 1958; 75:1-4.

83. Cournad A, Rilev RL, Himmelstein A, Austrian R: Pulmonary circulation in the alveolar ventilation perfusion relationship after pneumonectomy. *J Thorac Surg* 1950; 19:80-116.

84. Kapitan KS, Buchbinder M, Wagner PD, Moser KM: Mechanisms of hypoxemia in chronic pulmonary hypertension. *Am Rev Respir Dis* 1989; 139:1149.

85. Moser KM, Daily PO, Peterson K, et al: Thromboendarterectomy for chronic, major vessel thromboembolic pulmonary hypertension: immediate and long term results in 42 patients. *Ann Int Med* 1987; 107:560.

86. Moser KM: Pulmonary vascular obstruction due to embolism and thrombosis, in Moser KM (ed): *Pulmonary Vascular Disease* New York, Marcel Dekker, 1979; p 341.

87. Jamieson SW, Kapalanski DP: Pulmonary endarterectomy. *Curr Probl Surg* 2000; 37(3):165-252.

88. Dantzker DR, Bower JS: Partial reversibility of chronic pulmonary hypertension caused by pulmonary thromboembolic disease. *Am Rev Respir Dis* 1981; 124:129-131.

89. Dash H, Ballentine N, Zelis R: Vasodilators ineffective in secondary pulmonary hypertension. *N Engl J Med* 1980; 303:1062-1063.

90. Allison PR, Dunnill MS, Marshall R: Pulmonary embolism. *Thorax* 1960; 15:273.

91. Simonneau G, Azarian R, Bernot F, et al: Surgical management of unresolved pulmonary embolism: a personal series of 72 patients [abstract]. *Chest* 1995; 107:52S.

92. Moser KM, Houk VN, Jones RC, Hufnagel CC: Chronic, massive thrombotic obstruction of the pulmonary arteries: analysis of four operated cases. *Circulation* 1965; 32:377-385.

93. Winkler MH, Rohrer CH, Ratty SC, et al: Perfusion techniques of profound hypothermia and circulatory arrest for pulmonary thromboendarterectomy. *J Extra Technol* 1990; 22:57-60.

94. Jamieson SW: Pulmonary thromboendarterectomy, in Franco KL, Putnam JB (eds): *Advanced Therapy in Thoracic Surgery*. Hamilton, Ontario, BC Decker, 1998; pp 310-318.

95. Levinson RM, Shure D, Moser KM: Reperfusion pulmonary edema after pulmonary artery thromboendarterectomy. *Am Rev Respir Dis* 1986; 134:1241-1245.

96. Wragg RE, Dimsdale JE, Moser KM, Daily PO, et al: Operative predictors of delirium after pulmonary thromboendarterectomy. A model for postcardiotomy syndrome? *J Thorac Cardiovasc Surg* 1988; 96:524-529.

97. Jamieson SW, Auger WR, Fedullo PF, et al: Experience and results of 150 pulmonary thromboendarterectomy operations over a 29 month period. *J Thorac Cardiovasc Surg* 1993; 106:116-127.

98. Moser KM, Auger WR, Fedullo PF, Jamieson SW: Chronic thromboembolic pulmonary hypertension: clinical picture and surgical treatment. *Eur Respir J* 1992; 5:334-342.

99. Fedullo PF, Auger WR, Channick RN, Moser KM, Jamieson SW: Surgical management of pulmonary embolism, in Morpurgo M (ed): *Pulmonary Embolism*. New York, Marcel Dekker, 1994; p 223-240.

100. Archibald CJ, Auger WR, Fedullo PF, et al: Long-term outcome after pulmonary thromboendarterectomy. *Am J Respir Crit Care Med* 1999; 160:523-528.

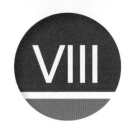

SURGERY
FOR CARDIAC
ARRHYTHMIAS

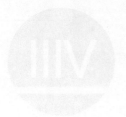

VIII

SURGERY
FOR CARDIAC
ARRHYTHMIAS

Interventional Therapy for Atrial and Ventricular Arrhythmias

Jason S. Chinitz • Robert E. Eckart • Laurence M. Epstein

Interventional therapies for the treatment of heart rhythm disorders have rapidly evolved over the past three decades, and continue to go through significant evolution. Though management options for cardiac arrhythmias were previously limited to pharmacologic therapy, the transformation and adaptation of surgical procedures to less invasive catheter-based approaches have led to a new paradigm in arrhythmia management. A fundamental understanding of diagnostic and therapeutic strategies for treating heart rhythm disorders is critical to surgical specialties exposed to these rhythm disorders.

The recording of intracardiac signals through electrodes, and subsequent stimulation of the cardiac tissue, allowed for the concept of ablation. In 1967, Durrer and associates described reproducible initiation and termination of tachycardia in a patient with atrioventricular re-entrant tachycardia (AVRT) using a bypass tract.[1] In 1969, the His bundle was first reproducibly recorded using a transvenous electrode catheter.[2] The continued advancements allowing localization of intracardiac signals led to the study of a variety of tachyarrhythmias.

The concept emerged that critical regions of cardiac tissue were necessary for the initiation and propagation of tachyarrhythmias, and that if these regions could be interrupted, the tachyarrhythmia could be cured. Once catheter-based mapping strategies were developed to localize arrhythmogenic foci, surgical excision was contemplated. In 1968, a description of such a surgical procedure for the elimination of an accessory pathway (AP) was first published.[3] This heralded an era of nonpharmacologic treatment of tachyarrhythmias.

ABLATION ACCESS

Surgical Ablation

A variety of arrhythmogenic foci and circuits were successfully mapped and ablated using surgical techniques in the 1970s.

Resection of an atrial focus felt to be responsible for an atrial tachycardia was reported in 1973.[4] Identification of reentry circuits within the atrioventricular (AV) node allowed surgical dissection to treat AV nodal re-entrant tachycardia (AVNRT) without causing complete heart block.[5] Although surgical ablation was therapeutic for a variety of tachyarrhythmias, the morbidity and mortality associated with thoracotomy and open-heart surgery limited its widespread application. Because most supraventricular tachycardias (SVTs) are not life-threatening, the risk of the procedure limited its routine adoption. Surgical ablation was therefore limited to highly symptomatic patients refractory to medical therapy.

Catheter Ablation

In order to minimize the morbidity associated with surgical ablation, a method of using a transvenous catheter for the delivery of energy directly to cardiac tissue was sought. In 1981, Scheinman and colleagues reported the first catheter-based ablation procedure, describing the ablation of the His bundle in dogs.[6] This same group performed the first closed-chest ablation procedure in a human; in a patient with atrial fibrillation (AF) and rate control refractory to medical therapy, a transvenous catheter was advanced to the His bundle region. Using a standard external direct-current (DC) defibrillator, they attached one of the defibrillator pads to the intracardiac catheter and used the second defibrillator pad as a cutaneous grounding pad. A series of DC shocks was delivered between the two pads and complete heart block, and thereby rate control, was achieved.[7]

This closed-chest catheter-based procedure was quickly adopted to treat a variety of SVTs dependent on the AV node.[8] As experience was gained and dedicated ablation catheters were developed, energy could be more precisely directed to allow ablation of APs, atrial tachycardia, single limb of AVNRT, and ventricular tachycardia (VT).

Although DC shock ablation allowed for the initiation of catheter-based ablation, it had various limitations. Because energy delivery was not titratable, such treatment had variable outcomes and complications, including massive damage to surrounding myocardium.[6,7,9] Because DC energy was delivered from the intracardiac electrode toward a cutaneous site, general anesthesia was required.

The introduction of radiofrequency (RF) energy as an ablative energy source heralded a new era in the catheter-based treatment of arrhythmias. RF energy had been used for decades by surgeons for surgical cutting and cautery and had a long history of safety and efficacy. Animal studies using RF energy for the treatment of arrhythmia were first described in 1987.[10] Intracardiac RF energy produces controlled lesions at the catheter tip using resistive heating.[11,12] RF now remains the primary energy source for catheter-based ablation, though alternative energy sources such as microwave, laser, high-intensity focused ultrasound, and cryothermal energy continue to be developed as a means to optimize patient safety and clinical outcomes.[13]

BIOPHYSICS OF ABLATION

Ablation using RF as an energy source involves the delivery of sinusoidal alternating current between the catheter tip at the endocardial surface and a large grounding pad on the skin. The current has a frequency of 350 to 700 kHz. The principal method of tissue injury with RF delivery is thermal. As the RF energy passes through the tissue at the distal electrode of the ablation catheter, resistive heating occurs at the catheter tip, and deeper tissue heating occurs through passive heat conduction, producing coagulation necrosis, and a discrete homogenous lesion. To achieve irreversible tissue injury, a tissue temperature of 50 to 58°C is required. Lesion size is proportional to the tissue temperature, size of the ablation electrode, contact force between the catheter and tissue, and duration of RF delivery.[14] If subendocardial tissue temperature exceeds 100°C, steam may form within the tissue, resulting in a rapid expansion and crater formation and an audible "pop" during ablation. Much like DC shocks, such "steam pops" can cause unpredictable injury (eg, to surrounding normal conduction tissue) as well as local tissue rupture. Contemporary RF ablation catheters have a thermistor or thermocouple that allows for automatic adjustment of the power output to achieve a preset temperature at the electrode tip-tissue interface.

With endocardial ablation, the lesions produced are limited such that some intramural and epicardial foci and arrhythmia circuits may not be reachable with standard ablation. One method to increase lesion size and depth uses the principle of limiting coagulum development by increasing the electrode-tissue interface by increasing tip size.[15,16] A limitation of larger catheter tips is that the larger surface area makes it difficult to regulate power delivery and achieve even temperatures.

Cooling the ablation catheter tip with saline irrigation, either within the catheter or external to the catheter, can also prevent coagulum formation at the tissue interface. This prevents a rise in impedance and allows for more energy delivery deep into the tissue.[17,18] Irrigated RF catheters bathe the catheter tip internally using recirculating saline or externally through a porous electrode tip. These catheters continue to use RF as an energy source, with maximization of power delivery resulting in deeper lesions with a greater volume than with standard RF.[19] Cooled epicardial RF ablation probes have been US Food and Drug Administration (FDA) approved, and transfers established catheter-based technology to a surgical approach for epicardial ablation of cardiac arrhythmias, used primarily in conjunction with other open cardiac surgical procedures.[20,21]

Because of concern about the irreversible nature of RF delivery, alternative energy sources have been developed that allow for a transient tissue injury before placement of permanent lesions. Cryoablation uses cryothermal energy delivered via a dedicated cryoablation catheter to produce gradual cooling of cardiac tissue to create local tissue damage. Hypothermia has been the preferred method of delivering linear lesions in surgical ablation. This technique uses pressurized nitrogen or nitrogen oxide flow through a catheter tip nozzle. As the gas expands beyond the obstruction, there is a temperature drop to as much as −90°C. The major advantage of cryothermal energy delivery relative to RF is its ability to deliver both transient and permanent injury to the tissue; the initial cooling phase ("Cryomapping") allows one to assess not only the impact of cryoablation on pathologic tissue (eg, anteroseptal APs, the slow limb of a dual AV node), but also the impact of potential lesion placement on nearby structures such as surrounding normal conduction tissue.[22] If the Cryomapping phase yields desirable results, then the temperature is lowered even further to a "freezing" stage. The ability to deliver reversible injury and catheter stabilization has made cryoablation increasingly popular in those cases in which the pathologic lesion is in close proximity to the AV node, and in younger patients in whom avoiding the need for pacemaker implantation is the highest priority.[23]

A second potential disadvantage to RF as an energy source is the risk of extracardiac tissue injury. For example, ablation of AF is becoming the most commonly performed electrophysiologic procedure, and is based on elimination or isolation of triggers for AF, which occur most commonly within the pulmonary veins (PVs). During catheter-based pulmonary vein isolation (PVI), ablation within the left atrium carries risks of collateral damage to surrounding structures, resulting in potentially highly morbid complications such as PV stenosis, atrioesophageal fistulas, and phrenic nerve paralysis.[24,25] As the esophagus runs adjacent to the posterior wall of the left atrium, this structure is highly vulnerable during ablation of AF. Though the rate of clinical atrioesophageal fistulas after ablation of AF is very low (around 0.04%),[26] the rate of intraoperative atrioesophageal perforation was as high as 1.3% in one open-chest series of patients undergoing linear lesions between PV ostia, to include the posterior wall overlaying the esophagus.[27] Current ablation strategies include methods to monitor for esophageal heating, such as continuous monitoring of esophageal temperature with an adjustable esophageal temperature probe.

ELECTROPHYSIOLOGY STUDY PROCEDURAL PROTOCOL

Diagnostic Electrophysiology Study

Diagnostic localization of tachyarrhythmias involves positioning catheters in strategic locations within the heart to obtain intracardiac recordings from various cardiac chambers as well as from the His bundle. Venous access is typically obtained in the bilateral femoral veins using the Seldinger technique. Catheters of 4 to 6 French in size are passed under fluoroscopic guidance into the right atrium and right ventricle, as well as positioned just across the tricuspid valve (TV) on the septum to obtain His bundle recordings. To obtain recordings of the left atrium and left ventricle (LV), a catheter is guided into the coronary sinus (CS), which passes posteriorly behind the mitral annulus and drains into the right atrium (Fig. 53-1).

Anticoagulation and Electrophysiology Studies

Direct recordings of the left heart are sometimes necessary and accomplished either by transseptal cannulation through the intra-atrial septum from the right atrium, or via a retrograde approach across the aortic valve into the LV, using catheters percutaneously placed into the femoral artery. Catheter and sheath placement within the left heart, however, imposes a risk of thrombus formation on the intracardiac catheter and

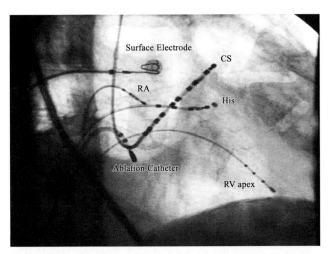

FIGURE 53-1 Radiograph in the right anterior oblique projection showing catheters positioned for a standard diagnostic electrophysiology procedure. Three nonsteerable diagnostic catheters are introduced from the inferior vena cava into the right heart. Two 4-French catheters with four electrodes are positioned in the region of the right atrial appendage (RA) and right ventricular apex (RV apex). A 5-French catheter with six electrodes is positioned across the tricuspid annulus to obtain a His bundle recording (His). A nonsteerable 6-French catheter is introduced via the right internal jugular vein into the coronary sinus (CS) to obtain left atrial and ventricular recordings. Finally, a deflectable 7-French ablation catheter is positioned in the region of the low right atrium.

at the site of ablation, with the resultant risk of stroke and thromboembolism. Animal models have determined that mural thrombus is evident in up to 50% of cases immediately after RF ablation.[10,28] In addition to the risk of mural thrombus at the site of ablation, there are mounting evidence of a systemic prothrombotic condition after RF ablation.[29,30] Therefore, during left-sided ablation, anticoagulation with intravenous heparin is typically administered throughout the procedure, and substantially reduces the thromboembolic risk. During ablation of AF, with the majority of the procedure performed within the left atrium, heparin is administered to achieve and maintain a target activated clotting time of 300 to > 400 seconds throughout the procedure.[31] Many patients undergoing ablation, particularly for AF, are on chronic systemic anticoagulation. Historically anticoagulation with warfarin was held prior to the procedure, and the patient was bridged with heparin in the periprocedural period. This strategy has now been recognized to be associated with a high incidence of bleeding complications, and now ablations are routinely performed in patients on uninterrupted therapeutic anticoagulation. In the event of procedure-related bleeding complications such as cardiac tamponade, anticoagulation can be reversed with protamine, fresh frozen plasma, and/or prothrombin complex concentrate (PCC). While most experience has been with continuous warfarin, evidence is emerging that ablations can also be safely performed in the setting of anticoagulation with the novel oral thrombin inhibitor or Factor Xa inhibitors, though clinical experience is limited and options for reversal of anticoagulation, when necessary, are still in development.[31]

Once diagnostic catheters are positioned in preparation of an electrophysiologic study, programmed electrical stimulation is performed to induce and study the tachyarrhythmia. Sometimes modulation of the autonomic nervous system is required to induce tachyarrhythmias with the infusion of atropine, isoproterenol, or epinephrine.[32] Once an optimal site for ablation is determined, a steerable ablation catheter is positioned at the target site, and energy is delivered.

At the end of the procedure, all catheters and sheaths are removed and manual pressure is applied to the access sites to achieve hemostasis. If the patient was heparinized for the procedure, sheath removal is delayed until anticoagulation reverses, either when the activated clotting time is less than 200 to 250 seconds, or after administration of protamine. The patient is placed on bed rest for 4 or more hours. Routine follow-up studies are not warranted unless required to assess for a complication. As mentioned, because of the risk of thromboembolic events, patients are frequently sent home on aspirin, thienopyridines, low-molecular-weight heparin, warfarin, or a combination of risk-appropriate antithrombotic therapies depending on the type and extent of ablation performed.

Complications Associated with Electrophysiology Studies

In referring patients for catheter ablation, it is important to weigh the risks and benefits of the procedure for the individual patient. Most tachyarrhythmias, although causing a variety of symptoms, are generally hemodynamically well tolerated and are not life-threatening. Thus awareness of the potential complications of catheter ablation is necessary before referring a patient. Complications can be divided into those involving vascular access, catheter manipulation within the heart, and ablation.

Access-related complications include pain, adverse drug reaction from anesthesia and sedation, infection, thrombophlebitis, bleeding at the site of access, hematoma, arteriovenous fistula, and pseudoaneurysm formation. Arterial damage or dissection may also result. Systemic or pulmonary thromboembolism can occur, most seriously resulting in transient ischemic attack or stroke. It is felt that performance of complex ablations while on systemic anticoagulation and with externally irrigated tipped catheters may reduce the risk of mural thrombus and thereby periprocedural embolic events. However, there may be an increased risk of access complications in a patient with therapeutic anticoagulation.[33,34]

Complications associated with placement of intracardiac catheters can be more life threatening. These include perforation of a cardiac chamber or the CS, resulting in hemopericardium, cardiac tamponade, and potentially coronary artery injury. Programmed electrical stimulation can result in the induction of hemodynamically unstable tachyarrhythmias such as VT or fibrillation. Catheter manipulation can also result in usually transient but sometimes permanent damage to valvular apparatus or the conduction of the right or left bundle branches owing to mechanical trauma.

RF delivery to cardiac tissue is associated with risk of collateral damage to intracardiac and extracardiac structures. Inadvertent ablation of the normal conduction system may result in complete heart block requiring permanent pacing. Perforation of a cardiac chamber or vascular structure can also occur with catheter manipulation or RF delivery; small perforations can often be adequately controlled with percutaneous pericardiocentesis and reversal of anticoagulation if present, however, if cardiac bleeding does not stop with these conservative measures an urgent open surgical approach is needed. Collateral damage to coronary circulation can result in myocardial infarction, heart failure, or cardiogenic shock. Phrenic nerve paralysis can occur due to ablation in proximity to the right or left phrenic nerves, which course along the pericardium. Ablation near the PVs within the left atrium can result in venous stenosis and pulmonary hypertension. Ablation in the posterior wall of the left atrium, as is routinely performed during ablation of AF, can result in damage to the esophagus, including esophageal ulcer formation and the potentially fatal complication of atrial-esophageal fistula.[35] Given these risks, a center undertaking these procedures must be prepared to urgently treat these potential complication. All operators performing electrophysiologic studies should be trained in pericardiocentesis, and certain procedures associated with higher risks of perforation should only be performed at centers with available cardiac surgeons in the event of severe complications.[36]

An 8-year prospective study published in 1996 of 3966 procedures found an overall complication rate of 3.1% for ablative and 1.1% for diagnostic procedures, with complications more likely to occur in elderly patients and those with systemic disease.[37] A more recent series evaluating ablations performed in patients across a series of age ranges identified a rate of procedural complications of 1.3%, with no significant differences between patients under 70 years of age relative to septagenarians or octogenarians.[38] Various studies have shown very low mortality rates directly attributable to the electrophysiology study.

DIAGNOSTIC ELECTROPHYSIOLOGY TECHNIQUES

A variety of techniques have been developed to elucidate the origin and mechanism of tachyarrhythmia propagation. Some of these techniques involve pacing in sinus rhythm, whereas others are performed during the tachyarrhythmia. Diagnostic studies typically involve programmed electrical stimulation with pacing at particular intervals to initiate a tachyarrhythmia, assess its response to pacing maneuvers, or terminate it.[39]

Activation mapping is used to localize the origin of various tachycardias. It involves positioning a mapping catheter in various intracardiac locations during the tachyarrhythmia, to identify a site where activation is earliest, and precedes any other intracardiac activation or corresponding surface P wave or QRS. The earliest site of activation during a focal tachycardia must by definition be the source of the tachycardia.[40,41] This technique is most useful for localizing focal atrial tachycardias, stable VT, and APs.

Entrainment mapping is used for localization of re-entrant circuits, and is often used in conjuction with activation mapping to identify targets for ablation. In entrainment mapping, pacing is performed from intracardiac sites during tachycardia and slightly faster, to penetrate the arrhythmia circuit and entrain the tachycardia when pacing from sites within the re-entrant circuit, the time from the last paced stimulus to the first return signal on the pacing electrode (called the "post-pacing interval") should equal the tachycardia cycle length. Since you are pacing from within the circuit, one cycle results in the "return" signal which is the same of the tachycardia cycle length. Pacing from sites more remote from the circuit will produce a post-pacing interval greater than the tachycardia cycle length. Because pacing is not within the circuit, the time to the "return" signal is the sum of one revolution around the circuit (the tachycardia cycle length) plus the time it takes to get to the circuit and back from the circuit. The difference between the post-pacing interval and the tachycardia cycle length can be used to determine whether sites are within the arrhythmia circuit and therefore guide ablation. This strategy is particularly useful for mapping atrial flutter, re-entrant atrial tachycardia, and scar-related VT.[42]

Pace mapping is another method used to localize the origin of a tachycardia, with particular usefulness in mapping VT or ventricular ectopy.[43] In this method, pacing is performed during sinus rhythm at various intracardiac locations, and the paced QRS morphology is compared to the

QRS morphology during tachycardia; the disparity in QRS morphologies can be assessed and the catheter repositioned until a match is obtained. At the site of tachycardia origin or myocardial exit, pacing is likely to produce a QRS morphology identical to that observed during tachycardia since the remainder of the heart is being activated in a similar manner.[44]

Mapping may also be performed based on anatomical landmarks. For example, ablation of the slow AV nodal pathway for the treatment of AVNRT is performed by ablating well-defined targets identified by fluoroscopy with or without the assistance of an electroanatomic mapping system. In common right atrial flutter, in which conduction across the cavotricuspid isthmus (CTI) is necessary to sustain the arrhythmia, anatomical landmarks are used for ablation to create a line of block between the tricuspid annulus and the inferior vena cava (IVC).[45]

In various clinical situations, a combination of these mapping techniques may be used to localize an appropriate target for ablation.

Advanced Mapping Techniques

The success of ablation is dependent on precise localization of arrhythmogenic foci and critical parts of arrhythmogenic circuits. Advanced mapping techniques have been developed as adjuncts to conventional mapping methods to improve the efficacy and safety of catheter ablation. The systems described below are useful to improve the rapidity and precision of mapping arrhythmias, while decreasing the need for fluoroscopy.

The CARTO electroanatomical mapping system (Biosense-Webster, Diamond Bar, CA) uses a magnetic field and emitted currents to localize a mapping catheter in three-dimensional space. Various locator pads placed beneath the patient's chest generate ultra-low-intensity magnetic fields in the form of spheres that decay in strength. A sensor in the catheter tip measures the relative strength and hence the distance from each of the pads, triangulating the temporal-spatial location of the catheter. For activation mapping, electrodes at the catheter tip record local electrograms, and the local activation times acquired from various mapping points are reconstructed on a three-dimensional map relative to a reference catheter, and presented on the map in a color-coded fashion. By acquiring multiple mapping points during tachycardia, the sequence of arrhythmia propagation can be reconstructed. Voltage maps can also be obtained to delineate regions of scar and diseased myocardium.[46]

Another commonly used nonflouroscopic three-dimensional electroanatomic mapping system is the EnSite system (Ensite NavX and EnSite Velocity, St. Jude Medical, St. Paul, MN), which consists of surface electrode patches applied to several places on the patient's body. To create a three-dimensional model of the chamber of interest in the heart, an electrical signal is transmitted between the patches, and the signal is sensed by the catheters within the heart; as the catheter is moved within the chamber, information from the intracardiac catheters including location, activation timing, and local electrogram amplitude is relayed to the computer system that generates the three-dimensional model. Cardiac electrical activity, including activation and voltage maps, can be superimposed on the anatomic model. The EnSite Velocity System can display the real-time position of conventional electrophysiology catheters, and can provide visualization and navigation of up to 128 electrodes on a combination of catheters.[47]

Intracardiac ultrasound catheters have had substantial benefits in improving the safety and efficacy of ablation, by providing real-time visualization of intracardiac structures. Radial array intravascular ultrasound (IVUS) (9 MHz Ultra ICE, Boston-Scientific, Natick, MA) may be positioned within the atria, allowing visualization of the interatrial septum, thereby enhancing the safety of transseptal punctures. Phased array intracardiac echocardiography (ICE) has extended the principles of IVUS for electrophysiologic use.[48] Newer ICE catheters are steerable and have Doppler capability (Acuson, AcuNav, Mountain View, CA). In addition to guiding transseptal punctures, ICE catheters allow the accurate targeting of anatomical sites such as PV ostia and papillary muscles.[49] They are also useful for imaging diagnostic and ablation catheter positions and visualization of tissue contact for optimal ablation. Additional benefit to ICE is integration with electroanatomical mapping systems to allow for non-contact real-time reconstruction of cardiac structures (CartoSound, Biosense-Webster, Diamond Bar, CA) (Fig. 53-2).

CLINICAL APPLICATIONS

Using the techniques described in the preceding sections, most focal and re-entrant tachyarrhythmias can be mapped and targeted for catheter-based ablation.

Atrioventricular Nodal Re-entrant Tachycardia

AVNRT is the most common form of SVT identified during electrophysiologic studies. This tachycardia can present at any age, although most patients who present for medical attention are in their forties and the majority are females.[50,51] Advances in catheter ablation of this tachycardia has made it a first-line therapy for those symptomatic patients not wishing to take long-term medications.[52]

AVNRT has a re-entrant mechanism using two distinct electrical pathways within the AV nodal tissue. The common pathways are known as "slow" and "fast" based on their relative conduction properties. The anatomical location of these pathways is variable but generally located within the triangle of Koch in the septal right atrium, which is bounded by the tricuspid annulus and the tendon of Todaro with the CS at the base. The apex of the triangle is the His bundle at the membranous septum where it passes through the central fibrous body. The anterior third of the triangle contains the compact AV node and the fast pathway, and the inferior and posterior portion, near the CS ostium, is the typical location for the slow pathway (Fig. 53-3).[53]

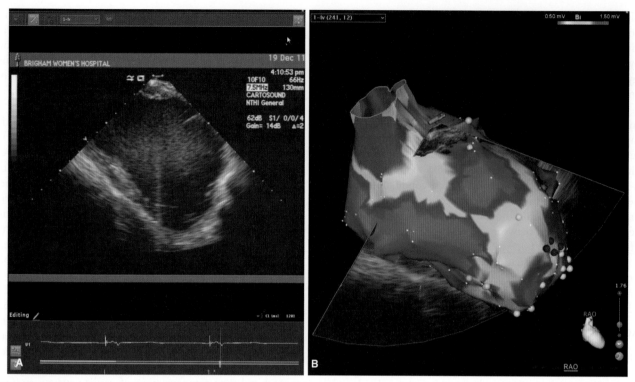

FIGURE 53-2 Integration of live intracardiac echocardiography (A) into the creation of a three-dimensional electroanatomic map of the left ventricle using the CARTO mapping system (CartoSound, Biosense-Webster, Diamond Bar, CA). (B) A voltage map of the left ventricle is shown in the RAO view, superimposed over the corresponding echocardiographic image.

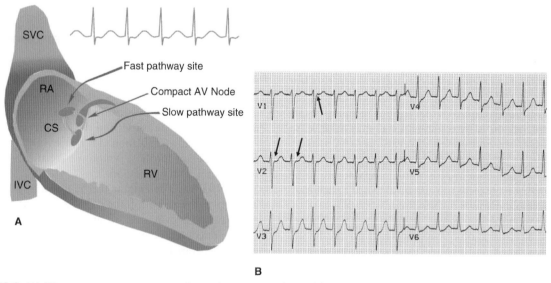

FIGURE 53-3 (A) Diagrammatic representation of typical atrioventricular nodal re-entrant tachycardia. Surface ECG shows narrow complex tachycardia with no clear P waves. The re-entrant circuit (*blue arrows*) consists of the posterior slow pathway region acting as the antegrade limb, and the anterior fast pathway region acting as the retrograde limb. The slow pathway target site is located between the coronary sinus os (CS) and the tricuspid valve annulus (TV). IVC = inferior vena cava; RA = right atrium; RV = right ventricle; SVC = superior vena cava. (B) Surface ECG showing precordial leads in AVNRT. This demonstrates that the retrograde P waves are barely discernible in some leads. In V$_1$, it forms a pseudo r′ wave (*arrow*). P waves are also visible in the terminal portions of QRS complexes in V$_2$ and V$_3$ but not in the lateral leads.

In the typical form of AVNRT, antegrade conduction from the atrium to the ventricle occurs over the slow AV nodal pathway, and the retrograde conduction through the AV node occurs over the fast pathway. Because conduction in the retrograde direction is fast, the atria and ventricle are depolarized almost simultaneously. Thus the electrocardiographic feature of this tachycardia is P waves that are inscribed within the QRS and thus not seen or barely discernible at the termination of the QRS complex.[54] The arrhythmia is usually triggered by an atrial premature complex (APC). The refractory period of the fast pathway is longer than that of the slow. Under the right conditions, the premature impulse blocks in the fast pathway and proceeds antegrade down the slow pathway, resulting in marked PR prolongation (a "jump"). Since nothing came down the fast pathway the impulse can turn around and conduct retrograde up the fast pathway resulting in an atrial echo beat. If the slow pathway has recovered the tachycardia can continue.[55] In fewer than 10% of cases, the circuit is reversed. In *atypical* AVNRT, antegrade conduction occurs over the fast pathway and retrograde conduction occurs over the slow pathway. Thus the ECG of this tachycardia shows inverted P waves in the inferior leads denoting retrograde activation of the atria with a longer RP segment owing to slower retrograde conduction.[56] Less commonly other AV nodal circuits may be present such as "slow-slow" AVNRT, using antegrade conduction down one slow pathway, and retrograde conduction utilizing another "slow pathway," with different functional and anatomic properties. These alternate AV nodal pathways occasionally have leftward extensions creating eccentric retrograde atrial activation patterns.[55]

Slow pathway ablation has a high degree of success for elimination of AVNRT, with a recurrence rate in the range of 2 to 7%. Complete AV block can occur as a complication of attempted slow pathway ablation in less than 1% (range 0 to 3%) of cases.[57] The North American Society of Pacing and Electrophysiology (NASPE) self-reported surveys on 4249 patients who underwent slow pathway ablations had success rates of greater than 96% and complication rates of less than 1%.[58,59]

Atrioventricular Re-entrant Tachycardia

About 30% of SVTs are caused by AVRT. This is a re-entrant tachycardia using the AV node and an AP. These APs are muscular bundles or remnants of conductive tissue from embryonic development that span the normally electrically inert tricuspid and mitral valve annulus and provide an independent path of conduction between the atria and the ventricles outside of the AV node. AVRT is part of the Wolff-Parkinson-White (WPW) syndrome of ventricular pre-excitation and symptomatic arrhythmias. The most common APs connect the atrium to the ventricular myocardium, but other APs may connect the atria or AV node to the His-Purkinje system. APs can conduct in the antegrade direction, retrograde direction, or both. In sinus rhythm, in patients with antegrade conduction over the AP there is preexcitation of the ventricles.

Ventricular activation is a result of "fusion" between activation over the AP and over the AV node. The degree of preexcitation is determined by the conduction velocity through the AV node and the time the sinus impulse takes to get to the AP. Preexcitation is manifested on the surface electrocardiogram by a short PR segment and slurring of the onset of the QRS, known as the delta wave. This slurring is due to slower "muscle to muscle" conduction in the ventricle from site of AP insertion. Absence of these findings does not exclude an AP. This may be due to a "latent AP" where there is antegrade conduction but the majority of the ventricle is being activated by the normal conduction system. This is most often seen in young patients with rapid AV nodal conduction and a far left lateral AP. In addition, up to 30% of AP conduct in the retrograde direction only ("concealed pathways").[60]

The term "WPW syndrome" is the combination of ventricular preexcitation on the surface ECG and symptomatic palpitations. However, it is often used to refer to any patient with an AP and SVT. Patients with WPW typically present with palpitation caused by rapid heart rate. This may be the result of AVRT or any supraventricular arrhythmia, including AF, with resulting rapid AV conduction via the AP. Associated symptoms may be mild such as palpitation and shortness of breath, or as severe as syncope and sudden death.[61,62] Sudden death is a very rare complication of rapidly conducting APs, and may be caused by ventricular fibrillation resulting from the extremely rapid ventricular activation over the AP during AF.

Indications for ablation of APs include patients with symptomatic AVRT or those with atrial tachyarrhythmias with rapid ventricular conduction who fail or do not wish to undergo medical therapy.[62] Relative indications for ablations include asymptomatic patients with "high risk" APs that are capable of rapid conduction thus posing a small risk of sudden death as the initial presentation of AF. Similarly, patients in high-risk professions, those with family history of sudden death, or those mentally distraught over their condition may be candidates for ablation.[63]

In the typical or orthodromic form of AVRT, antegrade conduction from the atrium to the ventricle occurs over the AV node and retrograde conduction occurs over the AP. In this form of AVRT, the P wave in the tachycardia follows the preceding QRS complex, resulting in a "short RP" tachycardia but often a longer RP segment on the surface ECG than seen in AVNRT (Fig. 53-4). In the rare antidromic form of AVRT, antegrade conduction occurs over the AP with retrograde conduction over the AV node, or more commonly a second AP. This results in eccentric depolarization of the ventricle, producing a wide complex tachycardia with retrograde P waves that can be easily mistaken for VT with one-to-one ventriculoatrial conduction.

An unusual form of AVRT utilizes a slowly conducting or decremental AP. Since conduction in both limbs, antegrade AV node and retrograde AP, is slow the tachycardia can be very stable and almost incessant. These tachycardias were misnamed the "permanent form of reciprocating junctional

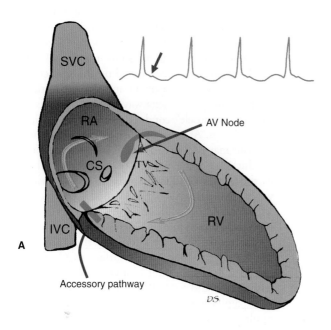

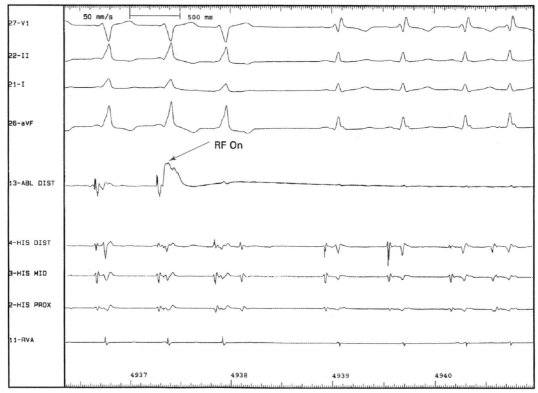

FIGURE 53-4 (A) Diagrammatic representation of atrioventricular re-entrant tachycardia. This macro re-entrant circuit (*gray arrows*) uses the AV node and an accessory pathway (AP), in this case a right lateral pathway. In orthodromic AVRT, antegrade conduction occurs over the AV node and retrograde conduction occurs over the AP. Because of the conduction delay from the His-Purkinje system through the ventricular myocardium to reach the AP, retrograde P waves are discernible after the QRS complexes (*arrow*). In antedromic AVRT, the re-entrant circuit is reversed and surface ECG shows P waves that closely precede the QRS complexes. CS = coronary sinus; IVC = inferior vena cava; RA = right atrium; RV = right ventricle; SVC = superior vena cava; TV = tricuspid valve. (B) Intracardiac recording of atrioventricular re-entrant tachycardia with termination of eccentric conduction over the accessory pathway during RF ablation. The tracing at 50-mm-per-second speed shows four surface leads (VI, II, I, and aVF) and intracardiac recording from catheters: ablation (ABL); His distal, mid, and proximal; as well as right ventricular apex (RVA). The first three beats of the tracing show evidence of eccentric conduction over an accessory pathway: short PR segment and delta wave. With onset of RF energy (RF On) from the ablation catheter positioned in the region of shortest AV conduction, conduction becomes normal within two beats, with normalization of the PR segment and loss of the delta wave.

tachycardia" or PJRT. They tend to be relatively slow (100 to 140 BPM) and can be mistaken for sinus tachycardia. On the surface ECG this is a "long RP" tachycardia with a short PR interval and inverted P waves in the inferior leads. It is important to recognize this entity as the incessant elevated heart rate can lead to a tachycardia-related cardiomyopathy. These pathways are almost always posteroseptal in location and ablation results in normalization of ejection fraction in most cases.[64]

Additional unusual APs are those that conduct slowly in the antegrade direction, connect into the specialized conduction system, and support preexcited tachycardias with a wide QRS. These are known as Mahiem pathways in which there is a slowly conducting antegrade AP connecting from the atrium to a fascicle (atriofascicular pathway) or from the AV node to a fascicle (nodofascicular pathway).

The 1998 NASPE prospective catheter ablation registry reported on 654 patients with a 94% success rate.[59] Success rates are lower (in the range of 84-88%) for septal and right free wall pathways.[65-67] Mortality rates are less than 1% and nonfatal complications occur in about 4%.[59] The major challenges of AP ablation are the location of APs near the normal conduction system and those that are epicardial in location. Ablation of pathways that are anteroseptal and midseptal in location carry a higher risk of causing complete heart block due to ablation near the compact AV node or His bundle. In these cases, alternate ablative energy sources such as cryoablation may offer a potentially safer alternative due to its ability to deliver reversible injury, permitting of the resulting effects, prior to irreversible lesion formation.[22,68,69] However, the vast majority of these pathways can be safely ablated with standard RF energy.

Atrial Tachycardia

Atrial tachycardias depend wholly on atrial tissue for initiation and maintenance of the tachycardia. Ectopic atrial tachycardia, sinoatrial nodal re-entrant tachycardia, inappropriate sinus tachycardia, atrial flutter, and AF can all be considered atrial tachycardias. Multifocal atrial tachycardia is caused by multiple foci of abnormal automaticity or triggered activity and is not amenable to curative catheter ablation.[70]

Focal atrial tachycardias, a less common type of SVT, form about 10% of all SVTs referred for electrophysiologic studies.[63] These arrhythmias are more common in patients with structural heart disease. Indications for ablation include failure or intolerance of medical therapy. Rarely, incessant tachycardias can lead to cardiomyopathy. With control of heart rate or restoration of sinus rhythm, myocardial dysfunction can be reversed, although there may be a delayed risk of sudden death that necessitates use of a defibrillator.[71-73]

Surface ECG features of focal atrial tachycardia include abnormal P wave morphology or axis that are typically close to the following QRS complexes (long RP tachycardia). Mapping and ablation of atrial tachycardias can be more difficult than ablation of other SVTs, as they can originate from anywhere in the right or left atrium, or within the interatrial septum and venous/arterial structures. Fortunately, there are specific anatomical regions that have a high incidence of foci and serve as primary targets, including the crista terminalis, atrial appendages, CS ostium, valve annuli, and pulmonary vein ostia.[74] Focal atrial tachycardia is frequently amenable to catheter ablation by targeting the site of origin of the arrhythmia, typically by identifying the earliest site of atrial activation using activation mapping. However, ablation success rates for AT are lower than that for other SVTs; the wide range of possible locations of AT origin require that the arrhythmia be present or readily inducible at the time of mapping, so that it can be localized for successful ablation. Success rates for ablation of focal AT have been reported to be 86% on average, with a recurrence rate of 8%. Complications from ablation include cardiac perforation, phrenic nerve damage, AV block, and sinus node dysfunction, with a combined incidence of 1 to 2% in experienced centers.[63]

Sinoatrial nodal reentry tachycardias occur infrequently and experience with catheter ablation of these tachycardias is more limited, however possible. As the name suggests the tachycardia is due to reentry in the tissue in and around the sinus node. The P wave morphology is identical to sinus rhythm but the tachycardia can start and stop suddenly, unlike sinus.[75]

Inappropriate sinus tachycardia is a not a well-defined disorder. It appears to result from a combination of autonomic dysfunction (when part of the postural orthostatic tachycardic syndrome, POTS) and perhaps some other endocrine and psychiatric component. While catheter ablation has been utilized as a "last resort" it is challenging because of the variability and diffuse location of sinoatrial tissue, as well as its multifactorial causes not treated by ablation.[76] Catheter ablation may be complicated by sinoatrial node dysfunction and persistent junctional escape rhythm, necessitating implantation of a pacemaker. Even if the resting heart rate is reduced with nodal modification, symptoms may continue with episodes of tachycardia. Catheter ablation is therefore generally avoided, in favor of a multidisciplinary approach, including cardiovascular, endocrinologic, and psychiatric evaluation and pharmacologic management.[77]

Atrial Flutter

Atrial flutter is a type of atrial tachycardia that uses a macro re-entrant circuit contained within the atria. A variety of natural and surgical barriers to conduction can create a re-entrant circuit within the atria. "Typical" or "isthmus dependent" atrial flutter involves a right atrial circuit, with an obligate limb in the isthmus of tissue between the IVC and the TV annulus, known as the cavotricuspid isthmus (CTI). The flutter circuit is bound anteriorly by the TV annulus, and posteriorly by the superior vena cava, crista terminalis, IVC, eustachian ridge, and CS (Fig. 53-5).[78]

In the most common form of typical, isthmus-dependent atrial flutter, the circuit transverses the right atrium in a counterclockwise manner in the frontal plane. Because the anatomy of the right atrium is elongated in a caudad-cephalad direction, a typical atrial flutter spends large portions of circuit

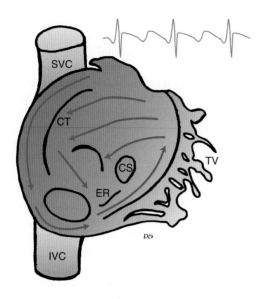

FIGURE 53-5 Diagrammatic representation of typical or counterclockwise right atrial flutter. Surface ECG shows large inverted P waves in the inferior leads. Lead III above shows 2:1 AV conduction with "sawtooth" flutter waves. The re-entrant circuit is confined to the right atrium by the tricuspid valve annulus (TV) and barriers to conduction within the right atrium. These include the superior vena cava (SVC), crista terminalis (CT), inferior vena cava (IVC), eustachian ridge (ER), and coronary sinus (CS). The isthmus between the IVC and TV is the preferred target for ablation.

activation going superior along the interatrial septum; therefore, on the surface ECG in leads II, III, and a VF, the P waves (called "flutter waves") are negative and have a sawtooth appearance. In V_1, the flutter waves are usually upright and in V_6 they are inverted. Clockwise isthmus-dependent flutter uses the same circuit but in a reversed direction, and the ECG also shows a reversed pattern with upright flutter waves in the inferior leads, and flutter waves that are negative in V_1 and upright in V_6. This surface ECG morphology is suggestive of the circuit but needs intracardiac confirmation.[79]

Catheter ablation for typical atrial flutter involves ablation in the CTI, by transecting the flutter circuit between the IVC and TV annulus. Long-term success rates for eradication of CTI-dependent atrial flutter have been reported to be approximately 87 to 95%.[80] Given high success rates and relatively infrequent complications, ablation has become the first line of therapy for recurrent typical atrial flutter. Despite successful treatment of flutter, up to one half of patients may develop de novo AF after flutter ablation during long-term follow-up, mandating careful monitoring for recurrent arrhythmias prior to cessation of anticoagulation even after successful ablation.[81,82]

Although the isthmus-dependent right atrial circuit described in the preceding is the most common type of flutter, a variety of other macro re-entrant circuits in the right and left atria are also possible, and are termed "atypical atrial flutters". These are more common in patients with underlying heart disease, or in those having previously undergone atrial ablation or cardiac surgery.[49,83-85] Mapping and ablation

of these arrhythmias are now also routinely performed. However, the success rate is somewhat lower than that for typical isthmus-dependent atrial flutter.

Incisional scars from prior cardiac surgery can be the substrate for re-entrant atrial arrhythmias.[86-88] The most common post-surgical atrial tachycardia is an atypical atrial flutter related to a lateral right atrial incision. Activation mapping typically demonstrates a circuit encircling a region of scar related to the incision. Ablation from the end of the scar to either the superior vena cava or more commonly the IVC is often curative (Fig. 53-6).[89]

Atrial arrhythmias are also common in patients who have undergone prior atrial ablation, particularly after more extensive left atrial ablation performed for persistent AF, or after a surgical Maze procedure (see below). These tachycardias may be a result of macro reentry, micro reentry, or a focal source. Common macro re-entrant circuits in these patients include typical right atrial flutter or atypical flutters encircling the mitral annulus or involving the roof of the left atrium. Re-entrant circuits may result from incomplete lines of block created during the prior intervention, or through alternative pathways such as the musculature surrounding the CS.[90] These tachycardias are often incessant and may be highly symptomatic and difficult to control with antiarrhythmic medications. Catheter ablation is therefore frequently pursued to target these recurrent arrhythmias and restore sinus rhythm. Ablation of these post-ablation arrhythmias are often delayed until 2 or 3 months after the index ablation, once the inflammatory response to the initial ablation has passed and the lesions have completely healed. During electrophysiologic study, the circuit of these arrhythmias can usually be determined using a combination of activation and entrainment mapping.[91] The main principle of ablation involves interrupting these circuits in obligate limbs, such as the left atrial roof or lateral mitral isthmus, by ablating between electrically inert anatomic barriers, such as the mitral annulus and the electrically isolated PV antrum.[92]

Atrial Fibrillation

Atrial fibrillation is the most common cardiac arrhythmia effecting upwards of 8 million Americans. AF is often highly symptomatic due to irregular and/or rapid ventricular rates and loss of AV synchrony. Patients can also be completely asymptomatic, but are still at risk of stroke, heart failure, and dilated cardiomyopathy due to prolonged periods of tachycardia.[73,93] The primary goal of pharmacologic therapy is prevention of thromboembolism in those at risk using systemic anticoagulation. Pharmacologic therapy for control of AF-related symptoms, however, has limited efficacy, carries risk of proarrhythmia and other systemic toxicities, and has not demonstrated a benefit in the reduction of stroke or mortality in large trials.[94-97] Catheter ablation of AF has consistently shown greater efficacy in maintenance of sinus rhythm than antiarrhythmic drugs and avoids long-term drug-related side effects. Ablation therefore has an expanding role in the restoration of sinus rhythm and control of AF-related symptoms,

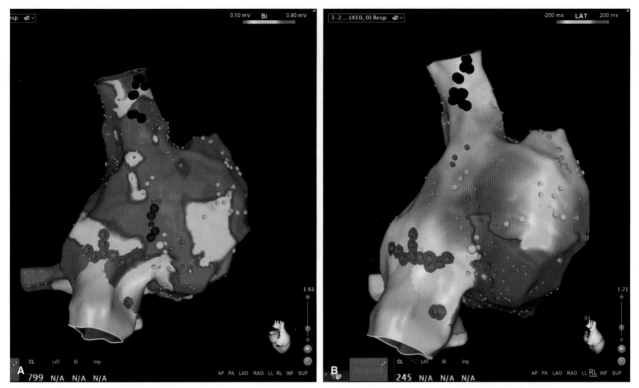

FIGURE 53-6 Electroanatomic reconstruction of the right atrium in a patient with an atypical atrial flutter following mitral valve surgery. Panel A shows a voltage map, with regions of low voltage (nonpurple regions on map), and electrically nonexcitable tissue (gray dots) representing abnormal or scarred atrial myocardium, likely related to the lateral atriotomy incision site. Panel B shows an activation map during tachycardia, demonstrating a macro re-entrant circuit around the scarred segments in the right atrium. Ablation lesions between electrically inert regions of the right atrium (red dots in panel A) terminated the tachycardia.

particularly after failure or intolerance of at least one antiarrhythmic drug trial. In patients with tachycardia-related cardiomyopathy, ablation is also often considered when medical therapy is inadequate for persistent rate control, or when restoration of sinus rhythm is the priority.[31]

The initial surgical Maze procedure was performed in 1987, and with several modifications aimed to make the procedure more tolerable, the Cox Maze III procedure has shown excellent long-term success rates, with an operative mortality of 2 to 3%.[98,99] This procedure is based on the concept that AF consists of multiple re-entrant circuits within the atria, and that creation of lines of conduction block between nonconducting atrial structures may preclude propagation of arrhythmic circuits and such that AF cannot sustain.[100] It is termed the "MAZE" in addition to creating lines of conduction block there is an attempt to avoid areas of atrial isolation and therefore promote atrial contraction in sinus rhythm. The electrical impulse from the sinus node therefore traverses a "MAZE" as it makes its way to the AV node. This procedure has been limited by the need for open-heart surgery with its mortality, morbidity, and expense, as well as post-op sinus node dysfunction requiring a pacemaker and the creation of new atrial arrhythmias. The surgical experience with the Maze procedure has led to the development of both more minimally invasive surgical approaches and a catheter-based approach.

Attempts at catheter-based left atrial or biatrial lesions for the purpose of replicating the Maze were met with limited success because of the prolonged procedure times, high risk of complications, and limited efficacy.[101] As understanding of the mechanism of AF has evolved, attempts to block propagation of atrial fibrillatory circuits have given way to attempted ablation of the fibrillatory triggers. When the identification of AF triggers arising from the PVs was first described by Haissaguerre et al. in 1998, the discipline of catheter-based ablation of AF emerged into the forefront of clinical electrophysiology. In a series of patients undergoing a left-sided catheter Maze procedure it was discovered that rapidly firing premature atrial contractions arising from the musculature of the PVs were triggering AF. Ablation of these foci eliminated AF in some patients.[102] Catheter-based ablation targeting triggers within the PVs has now gained worldwide acceptance as a therapeutic option for patients with symptomatic AF.

An early approach to PVI involved segmental isolation of each PV by mapping the location of the connecting muscular fibers.[103] This procedure has since evolved to an empiric electrical isolation of the PVs, with complete encircling of the PV antra, typically performed as ipsilateral pairs (Fig. 53-7).[104,105] In patients with paroxysmal AF, antral PVI is often sufficient to prevent recurrent AF. Ablation of additional atrial substrate is often needed to restore sinus rhythm in patients with more persistent forms of AF.[106]

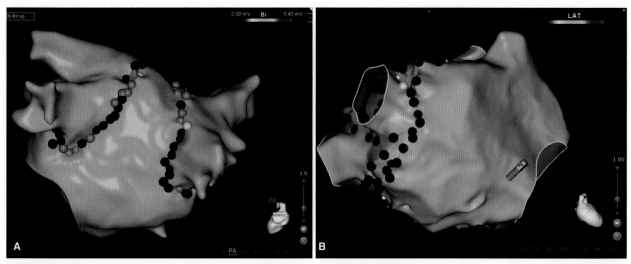

FIGURE 53-7 Electroanatomic map showing a series of radiofrequency ablation lesions (red and pink dots) encircling the pulmonary vein antra as ipsilateral pairs. Panel A: posterior-anterior view; panel B: right anterior oblique view.

Due to the high prevalence of AF in the general population, along with the increasing success of ablation, catheter ablation for AF has become one of the most commonly performed electrophysiologic procedures. However, methods for optimizing outcomes are still in evolution. Approaches beyond PVI, particularly for patients with persistent AF, continue to be evaluated. While in most patients with paroxysmal AF the arrhythmia is driven by PV triggers, as the arrhythmia becomes more persistent or occurs in more diseased atria, AF becomes maintained by arrhythmogenic atrial substrate. Those with a more permanent form of AF have been demonstrated to have either atrial scarring or structural disease in 65%. This arrhythmogenic substrate may be manifest as regions of electrical block and complex fractionated atrial electrograms (CFAEs) on intracardiac recordings, and may be targeted during catheter ablation.[106]

Whether ablation targeting additional atrial substrate, including CFAE ablation or creating additional lines of ablation to segment the atria (similar to the Maze procedure), improve ablation success is still under investigation. In randomized trials, the addition of targeting of CFAEs to a conventional PV antral isolation has not resulted in increased freedom from recurrent arrhythmia.[107,108] In a study comparing the efficacy of adding linear lesions to PVI alone, additional lines did improve the maintenance of sinus rhythm, although the results were much more apparent in those with persistent AF at baseline.[109] As discussed above, additional lines of ablation also predispose to recurrent atrial tachycardias, which have the potential to conduct rapidly and may be even more symptomatic than was the original arrhythmia. Though PVI alone may be sufficient for most patients with paroxysmal AF, those with persistent arrhythmia often require more extensive ablation to terminate AF and prevent recurrence. In all patients, targeting additional substrate in the pulmonary venous antra appears to have a beneficial role over ostial isolation alone. A recent systematic

review and meta-analysis found a highly significant lower rate of recurrent arrhythmias in patients undergoing wide antral PVI relative to segmental ostial isolation (odds ratio 0.42, $p < .00001$), including a much lower AF recurrence rate (odds ratio 0.33), despite a trend towards greater incidence of left atrial tachycardia occurrence in the wide antral circumferential ablation group.[110] In addition, ostial ablation increases the risk of PV stenosis, which is largely avoided by wide circumferential ablation.

Due to the evolving nature of AF ablation and range of techniques and experience, as well as nonuniform methods of follow-up and postoperative surveillance, accurate data regarding the efficacy and long-term outcomes of the procedure are limited. Furthermore, results are also dependent on individual patient factors, particularly the pattern of preexisting AF (universally worse outcomes in patients with persistent AF), patient comorbidities, and left atrial size. There is now strong evidence that ablation improves maintenance of sinus rhythm greater than antiarrhythmic medications. One randomized multicenter comparison of ablation versus antiarrhythmic drugs in patients with paroxysmal AF who failed at least one medication found freedom from documented symptomatic recurrence in 66% of patients treated with ablation compared to 16% of patients treated with medications at 9 months (hazard ratio 0.30, $p < .001$), as well as greater improvement in symptom severity score and quality of life in the ablation group.[111] Another meta-analysis comparing ablation to medical management in patients with paroxysmal AF found that at 1 year, ablation was associated with a 16-fold rate of freedom from recurrent AF (odds ratio, 15.78; 95% CI, 10.07-24.73) and with decreased hospitalization for cardiovascular causes (rate ratio, 0.15; 95% CI, 0.10–0.23).[112]

One-year outcomes after AF ablation, particularly in well-selected patients with paroxysmal arrhythmia, have demonstrated impressive results; the A4 trial showed at 1 year, 23%

of those randomized to antiarrhythmic drug therapy, and 89% of those randomized to ablation had no recurrence of AF.[113] A large international survey assessing global outcomes from AF, including over 20,000 ablations performed between 2003 and 2006, found that a median of 70% of patients became asymptomatic without antiarrhythmic drugs, and another 10% became asymptomatic in the presence of previously ineffective antiarrhythmic drugs over an average of 18 months of follow-up. Success rates were significantly greater for patients with paroxysmal AF (75% without antiarrhythmic drugs) than in patients with persistent or long-standing AF (63-65% without antiarrhythmic drugs).[26] A second ablation procedure is often required to achieve the quoted freedom from arrhythmia in up to 30% of patients, either from recurrent AF or due to post-ablation atrial tachycardias.[26] Most patients with arrhythmia recurrence demonstrate recovered electrical conduction into the PVs at the time of redo procedures, demonstrating the difficulty achieving durable transmural ablation lesions. Furthermore, since arrhythmias can recur asymptomatically and sporadically, it is likely that the published rates of ablation success are an underestimation of the actual rate of AF recurrence.

As AF has been associated with increased mortality in various populations, it is possible that ablation will have a positive effect on mortality, though this has not yet been proven. Trials to assess the late success and long-term outcomes of AF ablation with regard to mortality, stroke risk, and heart failure, such as the CABANA trial, are ongoing.[31]

Encouraging results for AF ablation, however, must be tempered by the rare but significant risks involved. In the worldwide survey of AF, major complications occurred in 4.5% of procedures, including cardiac tamponade, PV stenosis, diaphragmatic paralysis, thromboembolism, atrioesophageal fistula, pneumothorax or hemothorax, vascular complications, valve damage, and congestive heart failure; procedure-related death occurred in 0.15%.[26] Interestingly, the rate of major adverse effects from antiarrhythmic drug treatment (including life-threatening arrhythmias and disabling drug intolerance) has been higher than ablation-related complications in various comparisons.[111,114]

Increasing acknowledgement of the risks associated with RF ablation have led to interest in alternate approaches to PVI, with the intent of improving the permanency of lesion formation and avoiding collateral damage to extracardiac structures. One such approach may be through the use of energy-delivering balloons, which can be placed within the orifice of a PV with the goal of creating circumferential lesions around the vein ostia. Most notably, the Cryoballoon (Arctic Frost, Medtronic CryoCath, Montreal, Quebec, Canada) using cryothermal energy from a balloon-tipped catheter has been used with success for treatment of paroxysmal AF.[115] Though the Cryoballoon provides a relatively simple alternative to point-by-point RF ablation delivery and may be associated with a lower rate of cardiac perforation, with increasing experience with this tool various complications have been reported including atrioesophageal fistulas, and a higher rate of phrenic nerve palsy.[116] Initial enthusiasm for an

endocardial deflectable catheter-based high-intensity focused ultrasound balloon (ProRhythm, Ronkonkoma, NY), allowing for the development of transmural linear lesions without direct tissue contact was dampened by low clinical success, and significant morbidity and mortality.[117,118] Using endoscopic visualization, laser balloon ablation (CardioFocus, Marlborough, MA) has also demonstrated promising initial results.[119]

In elderly patients or those with severe comorbidities in whom standard treatment modalities cannot be achieved or are contraindicated, permanent rate control may be achieved through AV junction ablation and permanent pacemaker implantation, eliminating the need for aggressive pharmacologic treatment. The "Ablate and Pace" strategy is highly effective, relatively simple to perform, has been shown to improve quality of life in highly symptomatic patients, and may improve cardiac symptoms and decrease healthcare utilization when pharmacologic therapy is limited by hypotension or intolerable side effects.[120] Cessation of previously needed rate control and antiarrhythmic medications, often used in high-doses, after this procedure also generally results in immediate symptomatic improvement. This strategy is potentially problematic for many patients though, as it mandates continued anticoagulation, creates pacemaker dependence and tolerates permanent AV dyssynchrony. Patients dependent on the atrial contribution to diastole, such as those with diastolic dysfunction, may not symptomatically improve with this strategy. An additional limitation of this strategy is that right ventricular pacing promotes interventricular dyssynchrony, and may result in worsened LV function. The PAVE trial found that biventricular pacing after AV node ablation can result in better performance status (31 vs 24% above baseline in the 6-min walk test) and LV function (LV ejection fraction 46 vs 41%) at 6 months compared to right ventricular pacing.[121] This improvement with cardiac resynchronization may be even more pronounced in patients with preexisting systolic dysfunction. In a retrospective study comparing PV antral isolation versus AV node ablation and pacemaker implantation, the ablate and pace strategy was associated with a shorter procedure time with fewer complications, although there was higher rate of heart failure and continued, albeit asymptomatic, AF.[122]

A more complex technique known as AV node modification attempts to ablate certain inputs to the AV node thus slowing the ventricular rate without requiring concomitant pacemaker implantation.[123] This procedure has not been widely implemented because of the risk of inadvertent complete AV block, and a tendency for the ventricular rate to rise again in the post-ablation period.

Ventricular Tachycardia

Catheter ablation also has an important role in the treatment and prevention of VT. Greater than 90% of life-threatening ventricular arrhythmias originate in myocardium with structural abnormalities, most commonly ischemic heart disease. In these cases, regions of scarred myocardium create channels of viable tissue that support re-entrant circuits; these circuits may be mapped and targeted with ablation. Patients with nonischemic cardiomyopathy generally also have scar-related circuits related to myocardial fibrosis, however, these scars are often multifocal and located in the epicardium or midmyocardium, complicating endocardial ablation. Initial experience with surgical endocardial resection and direct surgical ablation to eliminate VT led to advancements in catheter-based ablation techniques. In patients with extensive structural abnormalities, multiple VT circuits are often present, and thus even after successful VT ablation primary therapy remains implantable cardiac defibrillators (ICDs) for prevention of sudden death. However, VT ablation is an important adjunct to reduce the arrhythmia burden and ICD shocks. According to the 2006 ACC/AHA/ESC guidelines on management of ventricular arrhythmias, VT ablation has a class I indication as an adjunctive therapy in patients with an ICD who have received multiple shocks for sustained VT that is not manageable by device reprogramming of drug therapy.[124]

Ablation for VT can be performed during ongoing VT, using activation and entrainment mapping to localize the critical isthmus supporting the re-entrant circuit, or by identifying arrhythmogenic substrate during sinus rhythm. In "substrate mapping," intracardiac electrodes are used to identify regions with abnormal myocardial substrate that represent areas of slow conduction within the region of scar that may support VT. Determination of scarred myocardium requires the use of an electroanatomic mapping system, in which the amplitude of electrograms recorded at various sites are recorded, and area with low amplitude electrograms are represented as regions of scar on a color-coded three-dimensional map. Pace-mapping allows identification of VT exit or isthmus sites by matching the QRS morphology produced by pacing during sinus rhythm to the VT morphology; pacing can also identify areas with delayed conduction that may occur when pacing from within a protected channel, such as within the VT isthmus. Ablation is performed generally within the scar at sites thought to be critical for supporting re-entrant circuits (Fig. 53-8).[125]

In experienced centers, epicardial mapping and ablation is also commonly performed when the VT substrate cannot be eradicated by endocardial ablation. Access to the pericardium is achieved via pericardial puncture from a subxiphoid

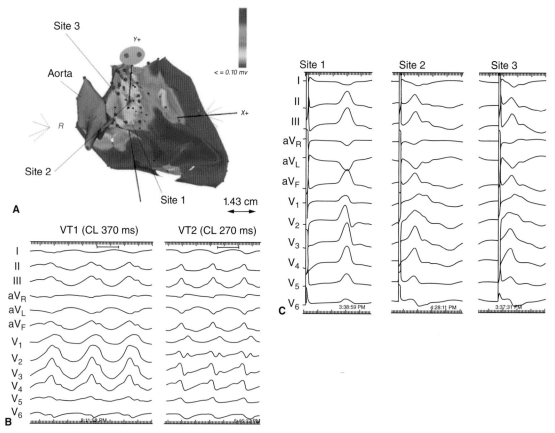

FIGURE 53-8 (A) Endocardial voltage map of the left ventricle created using a three-dimensional electroanatomic mapping system. An extensive region of low voltage representing scarred myocardium is present in the left ventricular outflow tract region. (B) Two morphologies of ventricular tachycardia were induced. (C) Pace mapping from different sites within the scar are shown. A good pace map for VT1 is observed with pacing at sites 2 and 3. A long delay between the pacing stimulus and the QRS occurs with pacing from site 1, demonstrating slow conduction away from the pacing site. A series of radiofrequency ablation lesions (red dots in panel A) across this region abolished both VT morphologies. (Reproduced with permission from Soejima K1, Stevenson WG, Sapp JL, et al: Endocardial and epicardial radiofrequency ablation of ventricular tachycardia associated with dilated cardiomyopathy: the importance of low-voltage scars, *J Am Coll Cardiol.* 2004 May 19;43(10):1834-1842.)

approach, and is often not possible in patients who have had prior cardiac surgery, particularly prior coronary artery bypass surgeries.[126] Epicardial ablation is more likely to be required in patients with nonischemic cardiomyopathy, arrhythmogenic right ventricular cardiomyopathy, and in patients who have failed initial attempts at endocardial ablation.

In large trials, success of VT ablation in patients with structural heart disease is promising, but recurrences are common. Acute procedural success is usually defined as noninducibility of any VT after ablation, while partial short-term success is defined as ablation of the clinical VT only. The Multicenter Thermacool Ventricular Tachycardia Ablation trial evaluated 231 patients with recurrent monomorphic VT, including 69% of patients with hemodynamically poorly tolerated VT, and a median of three VTs per patient; ablation acutely abolished all inducible VTs in 49% of patients, while at 6 months 53% of patients were VT-free.[127] Furthermore, ablation success is dependent on the underlying myocardial substrate and patient population. A recent prospective evaluation reported a VT-free survival at 1 year of 57% for patients with ischemic cardiomyopathy, and 40.5% for patients with nonischemic cardiomyopathy, despite complete acute procedural success achieved in 77% of patients with ischemic cardiomyopathy, and 67% of patients with nonischemic cardiomyopathy.[128] While VT is not completely abolished in all patients, the frequency of VT recurrences and associated ICD shocks may be dramatically reduced, resulting is a substantial improvement in an individual's quality of life, even when VT is not completely eradicated. In the Thermacool VT Ablation trial, among patients with at least 6 months of follow-up, VT episodes were reduced from a median of 11.5 episodes preablation, to a median of 0 postablation, and the frequency of VT was reduced by ≥75% in two-thirds of patients.[127] Complications from VT ablation include stroke, cardiac tamponade, valve damage, heart failure, AV block, vascular complications, and death. Procedure-related deaths have been reported in up to 3%, and most commonly occurs as a result of progressive ventricular arrhythmias and cardiac arrest after failed ablation. In the Thermacool study, death occurred in the electrophysiology laboratory in 4 of 231 patients. Nonfatal complications have been reported in approximately 7%.[127,129-131]

Bundle branch reentry VT is another type of VT that may occur in patients with dilated cardiomyopathy and His-Purkinje system disease. In bundle branch reentry, a macro re-entrant circuit using the conduction system occurs, most commonly with propagation antegrade down the right bundle branch and retrograde up the left bundle branch, resulting in a wide complex tachycardia with a left bundle branch block pattern. Patients typically present with palpitation, syncope, or sudden death. Treatment involves ablation of the right bundle branch to interrupt the re-entrant circuit. Long-term success is good for prevention of recurrent bundle branch reentry, however, as these patients generally have extensive ventricular structural abnormalities, other VTs may develop, and ICDs are still required even after successful ablation. In addition to other established risks of ablation, ablation within the specialized conduction system poses a risk of ablation-related heart block.[132,133]

Other cardiac disorders associated with sustained monomorphic VT include right ventricular dysplasia,[134] infiltrative disorders such as cardiac sarcoidosis[135,136] and hypertrophic cardiomyopathy.[137] Patients with prior ventricular surgery can develop incision-related VT, commonly seen in patients who have undergone repair of congenital cardiac abnormalities such as tetralogy of Fallot,[138] or after corrective valve surgery.[139]

VT that presents in patients without structural heart disease is termed *idiopathic* and represents up to 10% of all VTs that present to tertiary referral centers. In these patients, VT ablation may be curative, and long-term prognosis after ablation is good even without ICDs. Patients may be asymptomatic or present with palpitation, dizziness, or syncope. Patients may present with frequent premature ventricular contractions (PVCs), nonsustained VT, or even sustained VT. In patients with a high PVC burden (>20,000 in 24 h) a myopathy may develop that is treatable by elimination of the ventricular ectopy. Idiopathic outflow tract arrhythmias typically have a left bundle branch QRS morphology with an inferior axis; though classically described as originating in the right ventricular outflow tract, PVCs, or VT may be mapped and successfully ablated anywhere in the base of the heart, including in the regions of the aortic valve cusps or along the mitral annulus. These occur more often in women than in men, and patients typically present in their thirties to fifties.[140] While they may be responsive to medical management with beta blockers or other medications such as flecainde (if there is no underlying cardiomyopathy) they are certainly amenable to ablation. One of the biggest reasons for failure is the lack of target PVCs/tachycardia at the time of ablation.

Other idiopathic VTs may be focal or involve a micro re-entrant circuit, often using branches of the Purkinje system. Fascicular VT most often originates from the left posterior fascicle, producing a right bundle branch VT morphology with rightward, superior axis. These VTs occurs more often in men, and are classically sensitive to verapamil. Success rates for ablation of idiopathic VT are in the range of 70 to 90% with recurrence rates in the range of 15%. Complication rates are consistent with those of other ablative procedures.[27,141]

Cost-effectiveness

Several studies have shown the cost-effectiveness of catheter ablation compared with medical therapy and surgical ablation. Catheter ablation has lower procedural costs than surgical ablation and reduces the need for further medical care and emergency department visits in comparison to drug therapy. Studies from the United States, Canada, the United Kingdom, and from Australia have shown both cost savings and improvement in quality of life for those undergoing catheter-based ablation compared to medical management.[142-146]

As AF is the most common sustained arrhythmia and is associated with substantial healthcare costs related to hospitalizations and drug costs, the cost-effectiveness of catheter ablation for the treatment of AF has gained particular attention. AF ablation is associated with substantial upfront expenditures but greater efficacy in maintaining sinus rhythm, and thus likely fewer subsequent cardioversions and hospitalization costs. Initial ablation costs have been estimated at approximately $15,000, with follow-up costs after ablation ranging from $200 to $1300 annually, compared to approximately $4000 annually for patients treated with antiarrhythmic medications; total costs of the two strategies appear to converge after about 5 years of follow-up.[147] Another analysis suggested that the cost-effectiveness of a rhythm-control strategy with ablation would be most cost-effective in younger patients and patients with at least moderate risk of stroke.[148] One study performed in the United Kingdom demonstrated cost savings for ablation in combination with antiarrhythmic drug therapy compared to drug therapy alone, in large part driven by reduction in healthcare utilization rather than the mere cost of the drug itself.[149] Essentially all cost-effectiveness analyses of AF ablation thus far have calculated incremental cost-effectiveness ratios close to the value of $50,000 per quality-adjusted life year that is typically considered acceptable in the United States.[147] The cost-effectiveness calculations for ablation, however, will continue to be unreliable until the long-term outcomes of ablation with regard to mortality and morbidity are clarified. In addition the value of this procedure will continue to evolve along with the procedure itself. The development of a more reliably successful ablation procedure that only requires a single attempt would dramatically increase cost effectiveness.

FUTURE DIRECTIONS

Catheter ablation is a relatively young field and has undergone dramatic advances over the past three decades. Technologic developments focused on improving the safety and efficacy of targeted catheter ablation, using minimally invasive methods, have lead the way to a revolution in the treatment of arrhythmias. Mapping systems are rapidly evolving to provide more accurate reconstructions of intracardiac geometry and electrical activation. Integration of ICE, MRI, and CT images, fluoroscopy, and cineangiographic sequences into electroanatomic maps can support understanding of complex anatomy, and allow contextual visualization of the movement of intracardiac catheters, while minimizing fluoroscopic exposure to the operator.[150] Noncontact mapping systems are also in development to quickly reproduce cardiac activation sequences without tedious point-by-point electrogram acquisition.[151] For patients with AF, ablation techniques beyond targeting PV triggers are of great interest. Methods of mapping AF-sustaining substrate in the atria, such as electrical rotors, have been developed that use intracardiac catheters to reconstruct three-dimensional maps of AF propagation; early studies suggest that ablation targeting this substrate in addition to conventional triggers improves long-term freedom from arrhythmia.[152] Developing technology and techniques are also focusing on novel methods to more effectively and safely deliver durable ablation lesions. The recent approval of force sensing catheters in the United States has the potential to revolutionize the industry; real-time feedback of force application within the cardiac chamber during mapping and ablation supports improved ablation delivery, lesion creation, and safety. Multicenter experience using force sensing catheter for ablation of AF have shown promise that this technology will improve outcomes.[153] Integration of careful impedance monitoring into electroanatomic mapping systems provides additional feedback of local heating and lesion application.[154] New techniques are also focusing on novel methods to deliver ablation deep into tissues. Ablation of VT is sometimes limited by inability to reach arrhythmogenic substrate deep within the myocardium, such as within the interventricular septum. A novel needle-tipped ablation catheter, capable of mapping and delivering RF energy from a retractable needle, is undergoing clinical trials, and holds promise to improve ablation of deep intramyocardial substrate not reachable by traditional endocardial ablation.[155]

Remote navigation systems have been developed and are now in use to support catheter ablation of various arrhythmias. Though these tools have not replaced the value of a human operator, but do reduce operator exposure to fluoroscopy and may shorten procedural times.[156-160] The Niobe system (Stereotaxis, Inc., St. Louis, MO) is a remote magnetic navigation system that uses two externally located magnets to create a steerable field that can be used to steer the magnetically active atraumatic catheter tip (Magnetic GentleTouch Catheters, Stereotaxis). The unit can be completely controlled remotely through a small motor, and the entire system can be controlled from a shielded room by joystick and touch-screen monitors using a hands-free robotic catheter control.[161] Another robotic catheter system, Sensei (Hansen Medical, Mountain View, CA) allows catheter manipulation from a control room using a mechanical steering outer sheath through which a conventional catheter is inserted.[162] Clinical results from remote navigation for AF ablation have yet to demonstrate superiority over manual operation and frequently require crossover to manual ablation. In addition the cost of the equipment greatly reduces the cost effectiveness of the procedure.

As the left atrial appendage is the most important source of thrombi in patients with non-valvular AF,[163] percutaneous left atrial appendage occlusion devices have been developed to reduce stroke risk in patients with AF and elevated bleeding risks that preclude systemic anticoagulation. The Watchman device is nearing FDA approval. In the Watchman Left Atrial Appendage System for Embolic Protection in Patients with AF (PROTECT AF) trial, the Watchman occlusion device percutaneously implanted at the ostium of the left atrial appendage compared favorably to warfarin with regard to the composite endpoint of stroke, cardiovascular or unexplained death, or systemic embolism at a mean follow-up of 18 months.[164] With extended follow-up, it appears that most complications associated with the device occur in the early post-procedure period and decline with operator experience. Other methods of left atrial appendage closure, such as epicardial suture ligation have also been used. The lariat device is delivered via subxiphoid epicardial access, and has been used with success in various centers.

The past 40 years have seen the development of intracardiac recording, programmed stimulation, and catheter ablation. Though rapidly expanding, the field of interventional electrophysiology is still young. Tremendous advances in technology and understanding of arrhythmia mechanisms have resulted in improvement in the care, and in many cases cure, or formerly intractable arrhythmias. Similar advances have allowed these minimally invasive procedures to be performed with impressive safety. Further improvements in the interventional treatment of complex arrhythmias such as AF and VT will come with further understanding of the mechanisms underlying these arrhythmias. Future innovations in catheter design, energy delivery, and imaging techniques will continue to advance the field of electrophysiology.

REFERENCES

1. Durrer D, Schoo L, Schuilenburg RM, et al: The role of premature beats in the initiation and the termination of supraventricular tachycardia in the Wolff-Parkinson-White syndrome. *Circulation* 1967; 36(5):644-662.
2. Scherlag BJ, Lau SH, Helfant RH, et al: Catheter technique for recording His bundle activity in man. *Circulation* 1969; 39(1):13-18.
3. Cobb FR, Blumenschein SD, Sealy WC, et al: Successful surgical interruption of the bundle of Kent in a patient with Wolff-Parkinson-White syndrome. *Circulation* 1968; 38(6):1018-1029.
4. Coumel P, Aigueperse J, Perrault MA, et al: [Detection and attempted surgical exeresis of a left auricular ectopic focus with refractory tachycardia. Favorable outcome]. *Annales de cardiologie et d'angeiologie* 1973; 22(3):189-199.
5. Pritchett EL, Anderson RW, Benditt DG, et al: Reentry within the atrioventricular node: surgical cure with preservation of atrioventricular conduction. *Circulation* 1979; 60(2):440-446.
6. Gonzalez R, Scheinman M, Margaretten W, et al: Closed-chest electrode-catheter technique for His bundle ablation in dogs. *Am J Physiol* 1981; 241(2):H283-287.
7. Scheinman MM, Morady F, Hess DS, et al: Catheter-induced ablation of the atrioventricular junction to control refractory supraventricular arrhythmias. *JAMA* 1982; 248(7):851-855.
8. Gallagher JJ, Svenson RH, Kasell JH, et al: Catheter technique for closed-chest ablation of the atrioventricular conduction system. *N Engl J Med* 1982; 306(4):194-200.
9. Weber H, Schmitz L, Dische R, et al: Percutaneous intracardiac direct-current shocks in dogs: arrhythmogenic potential and pathological changes. *Eur Heart J* 1986; 7(6):528-537.
10. Huang SK, Bharati S, Graham AR, et al: Closed chest catheter desiccation of the atrioventricular junction using radiofrequency energy—a new method of catheter ablation. *J Am Coll Cardiol* 1987; 9(2):349-358.
11. Haines D: Biophysics of ablation: application to technology. *J Cardiovasc Electrophysiol* 2004; 15(10 Suppl):S2-S11.
12. Nath S, DiMarco JP, Haines DE: Basic aspects of radiofrequency catheter ablation. *J Cardiovasc Electrophysiol* 1994; 5(10):863-876.
13. Comas GM, Imren Y, Williams MR: An overview of energy sources in clinical use for the ablation of atrial fibrillation. *Semin Thorac Cardiovasc Surg* 2007; 19(1):16-24.
14. Nath S, DiMarco JP, Mounsey JP, et al: Correlation of temperature and pathophysiological effect during radiofrequency catheter ablation of the AV junction. *Circulation* 1995; 92(5):1188-1192.
15. Langberg JJ, Gallagher M, Strickberger SA, et al: Temperature-guided radiofrequency catheter ablation with very large distal electrodes. *Circulation* 1993; 88(1):245-249.
16. Otomo K, Yamanashi WS, Tondo C, et al: Why a large tip electrode makes a deeper radiofrequency lesion: effects of increase in electrode cooling and electrode-tissue interface area. *J Cardiovasc Electrophysiol* 1998; 9(1):47-54.
17. Demazumder D, Mirotznik MS, Schwartzman D: Biophysics of radiofrequency ablation using an irrigated electrode. *J Interv Card Electrophysiol* 2001; 5(4):377-389.
18. Everett THt, Lee KW, Wilson EE, et al: Safety profiles and lesion size of different radiofrequency ablation technologies: a comparison of large tip, open and closed irrigation catheters. *J Cardiovasc Electrophysiol* 2009; 20(3):325-335.
19. Dorwarth U, Fiek M, Remp T, et al; Radiofrequency catheter ablation: different cooled and noncooled electrode systems induce specific lesion geometries and adverse effects profiles. *Pacing Clin Electrophysiol: PACE* 2003; 26(7 Pt 1):1438-1445.
20. Hamner CE, Potter DD Jr, Cho KR, et al: Irrigated radiofrequency ablation with transmurality feedback reliably produces Cox maze lesions in vivo. *Ann Thorac Surg* 2005; 80(6):2263-2270.
21. Wood MA, Ellenbogen AL, Pathak V, et al: Efficacy of a cooled bipolar epicardial radiofrequency ablation probe for creating transmural myocardial lesions. *J Thorac Cardiovasc Surg* 2010; 139(2):453-458.
22. Friedman PL, Dubuc M, Green MS, et al: Catheter cryoablation of supraventricular tachycardia: results of the multicenter prospective "frosty" trial. *Heart Rhythm* 2004; 1(2):129-138.
23. Skanes AC, Dubuc M, Klein GJ, et al: Cryothermal ablation of the slow pathway for the elimination of atrioventricular nodal reentrant tachycardia. *Circulation* 2000; 102(23):2856-2860.
24. Saad EB, Marrouche NF, Saad CP, et al: Pulmonary vein stenosis after catheter ablation of atrial fibrillation: emergence of a new clinical syndrome. *Ann Intern Med* 2003; 138(8):634-638.
25. Gillinov AM, Pettersson G, Rice TW: Esophageal injury during radiofrequency ablation for atrial fibrillation. *J Thorac Cardiovasc Surg* 2001; 122(6):1239-1240.
26. Cappato R, Calkins H, Chen SA, et al: Updated worldwide survey on the methods, efficacy, and safety of catheter ablation for human atrial fibrillation. *Circ Arrhythm Electrophysiol* 2010; 3(1):32-38.
27. Mohr FW, Fabricius AM, Falk V, et al: Curative treatment of atrial fibrillation with intraoperative radiofrequency ablation: short-term and midterm results. *J Thorac Cardiovasc Surg* 2002; 123(5):919-927.
28. Goli VD, Prasad R, Hamilton K, et al: Transesophageal echocardiographic evaluation for mural thrombus following radiofrequency catheter ablation of accessory pathways. *Pacing Clin Electrophysiol: PACE* 1991; 14(11 Pt 2):1992-1997.
29. Chiang CE, Chen SA, Wu TJ, et al: Incidence, significance, and pharmacological responses of catheter-induced mechanical trauma in patients receiving radiofrequency ablation for supraventricular tachycardia. *Circulation* 1994; 90(4):1847-1854.
30. Wang TL, Lin JL, Hwang JJ, et al: The evolution of platelet aggregability in patients undergoing catheter ablation for supraventricular tachycardia with radiofrequency energy: the role of antiplatelet therapy. *Pacing Clin Electrophysiol: PACE* 1995; 18(11):1980-1990.
31. Calkins H, Brugada J, Packer DL, et al: 2012 HRS/EHRA/ECAS expert consensus statement on catheter and surgical ablation of atrial fibrillation: recommendations for patient selection, procedural techniques, patient management and follow-up, definitions, endpoints, and research trial design: a report of the Heart Rhythm Society (HRS) Task Force on Catheter and Surgical Ablation of Atrial Fibrillation. Developed in partnership with the European Heart Rhythm Association (EHRA), a registered branch of the European Society of Cardiology (ESC) and the European Cardiac Arrhythmia Society (ECAS); and in collaboration with the American College of Cardiology (ACC), American Heart Association (AHA), the Asia Pacific Heart Rhythm Society (APHRS), and the Society of Thoracic Surgeons (STS). Endorsed by the governing bodies of the American College of Cardiology Foundation, the American Heart Association, the European Cardiac Arrhythmia Society, the European Heart Rhythm Association, the Society of Thoracic Surgeons, the Asia Pacific Heart Rhythm Society, and the Heart Rhythm Society. *Heart Rhythm* 2012; 9(4):632-696 e21.
32. Lister JW, Stein E, Kosowsky BD, et al: Atrioventricular conduction in man. Effect of rate, exercise, isoproterenol and atropine on the P-R interval. *Am J Cardiol* 1965; 16(4):516-523.
33. Hussein AA, Martin DO, Saliba W, et al: Radiofrequency ablation of atrial fibrillation under therapeutic international normalized ratio: a safe and efficacious periprocedural anticoagulation strategy. *Heart Rhythm* 2009; 6(10):1425-1429.
34. Oral H, Chugh A, Ozaydin M, et al: Risk of thromboembolic events after percutaneous left atrial radiofrequency ablation of atrial fibrillation. *Circulation* 2006; 114(8):759-765.
35. Singh SM, d'Avila A, Singh SK, et al: Clinical outcomes after repair of left atrial esophageal fistulas occurring after atrial fibrillation ablation procedures. *Heart Rhythm* 2013; 10(11):1591-1597.
36. Belhassen B: A 1 per 1,000 mortality rate after catheter ablation of atrial fibrillation: an acceptable risk? *J Am Coll Cardiol* 2009; 53(19):1804-1806.

37. Chen SA, Chiang CE, Tai CT, et al: Complications of diagnostic electrophysiologic studies and radiofrequency catheter ablation in patients with tachyarrhythmias: an eight-year survey of 3,966 consecutive procedures in a tertiary referral center. *Am J Cardiol* 1996; 77(1):41-46.

38. Pedrinazzi C, Durin O, Agricola P, et al: Efficacy and safety of radiofrequency catheter ablation in the elderly. *J Interv Card Electrophysiol* 2007; 19(3):179-185.

39. Stevenson WG, Sager PT, Friedman PL: Entrainment techniques for mapping atrial and ventricular tachycardias. *J Cardiovasc Electrophysiol* 1995; 6(3):201-216.

40. Wellens HJ: Twenty-five years of insights into the mechanisms of supraventricular arrhythmias. *J Cardiovasc Electrophysiol* 2003; 14(9):1020-1025.

41. Wellens HJ, Brugada P: Mechanisms of supraventricular tachycardia. *Am J Cardiol* 1988; 62(6):10D-15D.

42. Deo R, Berger R: The clinical utility of entrainment pacing. *J Cardiovasc Electrophysiol* 2009; 20(4):466-470.

43. Joshi S, Wilber DJ: Ablation of idiopathic right ventricular outflow tract tachycardia: current perspectives. *J Cardiovasc Electrophysiol* 2005; 16 Suppl 1:S52-8.

44. Brunckhorst CB, Delacretaz E, Soejima K, et al: Identification of the ventricular tachycardia isthmus after infarction by pace mapping. *Circulation* 2004; 110(6):652-659.

45. Saoudi N, Ricard P, Rinaldi JP, et al: Methods to determine bidirectional block of the cavotricuspid isthmus in radiofrequency ablation of typical atrial flutter. *J Cardiovasc Electrophysiol* 2005; 16(7):801-803.

46. Gepstein L, Hayam G, Ben-Haim SA: A novel method for nonfluoroscopic catheter-based electroanatomical mapping of the heart. In vitro and in vivo accuracy results. *Circulation* 1997; 95(6):1611-1622.

47. Eitel C, Hindricks G, Dagres N, et al: EnSite Velocity cardiac mapping system: a new platform for 3D mapping of cardiac arrhythmias. *Expert Rev Med Devices* 2010; 7(2):185-192.

48. Bruce CJ, Friedman PA: Intracardiac echocardiography. *Eur J Echocardiogr: the journal of the Working Group on Echocardiography of the European Society of Cardiology* 2001; 2(4):234-244.

49. Beldner S, Gerstenfeld EP, Lin D, et al: Ablation of atrial fibrillation: localizing triggers, mapping systems and ablation techniques. *Minerva Cardioangiol* 2004; 52(2):95-109.

50. Akhtar M, Jazayeri MR, Sra J, et al: Atrioventricular nodal. Clinical, electrophysiological, and therapeutic considerations. *Circulation* 1993; 88(1):282-295.

51. Jazayeri MR, Hempe SL, Sra JS, et al: Selective transcatheter ablation of the fast and slow pathways using radiofrequency energy in patients with atrioventricular nodal reentrant tachycardia. *Circulation* 1992; 85(4):1318-1328.

52. Zipes DP, DiMarco JP, Gilette PC, et al: Guidelines for clinical intracardiac electrophysiological and catheter ablation procedures. A report of the American College of Cardiology/American Heart Association Task Force on Practice Guidelines (Committee on Clinical Intracardiac Electrophysiologic and Catheter Ablation Procedures), developed in collaboration with the North American Society of Pacing and Electrophysiology. *J Am Coll Cardiol* 1995; 26(2):555-573.

53. McGuire MA, Johnson DC, Robotin M, et al: Dimensions of the triangle of Koch in humans. *Am J Cardiol* 1992; 70(7):829-830.

54. Kalbfleisch SJ, el-Atassi R, Calkins H, et al: Differentiation of paroxysmal narrow QRS complex tachycardias using the 12-lead electrocardiogram. *J Am Coll Cardiol* 1993; 21(1):85-89.

55. Heidbuchel H, Jackman WM: Characterization of subforms of AV nodal reentrant tachycardia. *Europace: European pacing, arrhythmias, and cardiac electrophysiology : journal of the working groups on cardiac pacing, arrhythmias, and cardiac cellular electrophysiology of the European Society of Cardiology* 2004; 6(4):316-329.

56. Michaud GF, Tada H, Chough S, et al: Differentiation of atypical atrioventricular node re-entrant tachycardia from orthodromic reciprocating tachycardia using a septal accessory pathway by the response to ventricular pacing. *J Am Coll Cardiol* 2001; 38(4):1163-1167.

57. Kalbfleisch SJ, Strickberger SA, Williamson B, et al: Randomized comparison of anatomic and electrogram mapping approaches to ablation of the slow pathway of atrioventricular node reentrant tachycardia. *J Am Coll Cardiol* 1994 23(3):716-723.

58. Scheinman MM: North American Society of Pacing and Electrophysiology (NASPE) survey on radiofrequency catheter ablation: implications for clinicians, third party insurers, and government regulatory agencies. *Pacing Clin Electrophysiol: PACE* 1992; 15(12):2228-2231.

59. Scheinman MM, Huang S: The 1998 NASPE prospective catheter ablation registry. *Pacing Clin Electrophysiol: PACE* 2000; 23(6):1020-1028.

60. Obel OA, Camm AJ: Accessory pathway reciprocating tachycardia. *Eur Heart J* 1998; 19 Suppl E:E13-24, E50-1.

61. Prystowsky EN, Fananapazir L, Packer DL, et al: Wolff-Parkinson-White syndrome and sudden cardiac death. *Cardiology* 1987; 74 Suppl 2:67-71.

62. Santinelli V, Radinovic A, Manguso F, et al Asymptomatic ventricular preexcitation: a long-term prospective follow-up study of 293 adult patients. *Circ Arrhythm Electrophysiol* 2009; 2(2):102-107.

63. Blomstrom-Lundqvist C, Scheinman MM, Aliot EM, et al: ACC/AHA/ESC guidelines for the management of patients with supraventricular arrhythmias-executive summary: a report of the American College of Cardiology/American Heart Association Task Force on Practice Guidelines and the European Society of Cardiology Committee for Practice Guidelines (Writing Committee to Develop Guidelines for the Management of Patients with Supraventricular Arrhythmias). *Circulation* 2003; 108(15):1871-1909.

64. Kang KT, Potts JE, Radbill AE, et al: Permanent junctional reciprocating tachycardia in children: a multicenter experience. *Heart Rhythm* 2014; 11(8):1426-1432.

65. Dagres N, Clague JR, Kottkamp H, et al: Radiofrequency catheter ablation of accessory pathways. Outcome and use of antiarrhythmic drugs during follow-up. *Eur Heart J* 1999; 20(24):1826-1832.

66. Jackman WM, Wang XZ, Friday KJ, et al: Catheter ablation of accessory atrioventricular pathways (Wolff-Parkinson-White syndrome) by radiofrequency current. *N Engl J Med* 1991; 324(23):1605-1611.

67. Lesh MD, Van Hare GF, Schamp DJ, et al: Curative percutaneous catheter ablation using radiofrequency energy for accessory pathways in all locations: results in 100 consecutive patients. *J Am Coll Cardiol* 1992; 19(6):1303-1309.

68. Kardos A, Paprika D, Shalganov T, et al: Ice mapping during tachycardia in close proximity to the AV node is safe and offers advantages for transcatheter ablation procedures. *Acta Cardiol* 2007; 62(6):587-591.

69. Miyazaki A, Blaufox AD, Fairbrother DL, et al: Prolongation of the fast pathway effective refractory period during cryoablation in children: a marker of slow pathway modification. *Heart Rhythm* 2005; 2(11):1179-1185.

70. Tucker KJ, Law J, Rodriques MJ: Treatment of refractory recurrent multifocal atrial tachycardia with atrioventricular junction ablation and permanent pacing. *J Invasive Cardiol* 1995; 7(7):207-212.

71. Chiladakis JA, Vassilikos VP, Maounis TN, et al: Successful radiofrequency catheter ablation of automatic atrial tachycardia with regression of the cardiomyopathy picture. *Pacing Clin Electrophysiol: PACE* 1997; 20(4 Pt 1):953-959.

72. Corey WA, Markel ML, Hoit BD, et al: Regression of a dilated cardiomyopathy after radiofrequency ablation of incessant supraventricular tachycardia. *Am Heart J* 1993; 126(6):1469-1473.

73. Khasnis A, Jongnarangsin K, Abela G, et al: Tachycardia-induced cardiomyopathy: a review of literature. *Pacing Clin Electrophysiol: PACE* 2005; 28(7):710-721.

74. Callans DJ, Schwartzman D, Gottlieb CD, et al: Insights into the electrophysiology of atrial arrhythmias gained by the catheter ablation experience: "learning while burning, Part II". *J Cardiovasc Electrophysiol* 1995; 6(3):229-243.

75. Yusuf S, Camm AJ: The sinus tachycardias. *Nat Clin Pract Cardiovasc Med* 2005; 2(1):44-52.

76. Koplan BA, Parkash R, Couper G, et al: Combined epicardial-endocardial approach to ablation of inappropriate sinus tachycardia. *J Cardiovasc Electrophysiol* 2004; 15(2):237-240.

77. Brady PA, Low PA, Shen WK: Inappropriate sinus tachycardia, postural orthostatic tachycardia syndrome, and overlapping syndromes. *Pacing Clin Electrophysiol: PACE* 2005; 28(10):1112-1121.

78. Cabrera JA, Sanchez-Quintana D, Farre J, et al: The inferior right atrial isthmus: further architectural insights for current and coming ablation technologies. *J Cardiovasc Electrophysiol* 2005; 16(4):402-408.

79. Weinberg KM, Denes P, Kadish AH, et al: Development and validation of diagnostic criteria for atrial flutter on the surface electrocardiogram. *Ann Noninvasive Electrocardiol* 2008; 13(2):145-154.

80. Hsieh MH, Tai CT, Chiang CE, et al: Recurrent atrial flutter and atrial fibrillation after catheter ablation of the cavotricuspid isthmus: a very long-term follow-up of 333 patients. *J Interv Card Electrophysiol* 2002; 7(3):225-231.

81. Perez FJ, Schubert CM, Parvez B, et al: Long-term outcomes after catheter ablation of cavo-tricuspid isthmus dependent atrial flutter: a meta-analysis. *Circ Arrhythm Electrophysiol* 2009; 2(4):393-401.

82. Chinitz JS, Gerstenfeld EP, Marchlinski FE, et al: Atrial fibrillation is common after ablation of isolated atrial flutter during long-term follow-up. *Heart Rhythm* 2007; 4(8):1029-1033.

83. Matsuo S, Wright M, Knecht S, et al: Peri-mitral atrial flutter in patients with atrial fibrillation ablation. *Heart Rhythm* 2010; 7(1):2-8.

84. Onorati F, Esposito A, Messina G, et al: Right isthmus ablation reduces supraventricular arrhythmias after surgery for chronic atrial fibrillation. *Ann Thorac Surg* 2008; 85(1):39-48.

85. Horlitz M, Schley P, Shin DI, et al: Atrial tachycardias following circumferential pulmonary vein ablation: observations during catheter ablation. *Clinl Res Cardiol* 2008; 97(2):124-130.

86. Lukac P, Hjortdal VE, Pedersen AK, et al: Atrial incision affects the incidence of atrial tachycardia after mitral valve surgery. *Ann Thorac Surg* 2006; 81(2):509-513.

87. Lukac P, Pedersen AK, Mortensen PT, et al: Ablation of atrial tachycardia after surgery for congenital and acquired heart disease using an electroanatomic mapping system: which circuits to expect in which substrate? *Heart Rhythm* 2005; 2(1):64-72.

88. Reithmann C, Hoffmann E, Dorwarth U, et al: Electroanatomical mapping for visualization of atrial activation in patients with incisional atrial tachycardias. *Eur Heart J* 2001; 22(3):237-246.

89. Nakagawa H, Shah N, Matsudaira K, et al: Characterization of reentrant circuit in macroreentrant right atrial tachycardia after surgical repair of congenital heart disease: isolated channels between scars allow "focal" ablation. *Circulation* 2001; 103(5):699-709.

90. Ellenbogen KA, Hawthorne HR, Belz MK, et al: Late occurrence of incessant atrial tachycardia following the maze procedure. *Pacing Clin Electrophysiol: PACE* 1995; 18(2):367-369.

91. Weerasooriya R, Jais P, Wright M, et al: Catheter ablation of atrial tachycardia following atrial fibrillation ablation. *J Cardiovasc Electrophysiol* 2009; 20(7):833-838.

92. Kalman JM, Olgin JE, Saxon LA, et al: Electrocardiographic and electrophysiologic characterization of atypical atrial flutter in man: use of activation and entrainment mapping and implications for catheter ablation. *J Cardiovasc Electrophysiol* 1997; 8(2):121-144.

93. Anguera I, Brugada J, Roba M, et al: Outcomes after radiofrequency catheter ablation of atrial tachycardia. *Am J Cardiol* 2001; 87(7):886-890.

94. Corley SD, Epstein AE, DiMarco JP, et al: Relationships between sinus rhythm, treatment, and survival in the Atrial Fibrillation Follow-Up Investigation of Rhythm Management (AFFIRM) Study. *Circulation* 2004; 109(12):1509-1513.

95. Kaufman ES, Zimmermann PA, Wang T, et al: Risk of proarrhythmic events in the Atrial Fibrillation Follow-up Investigation of Rhythm Management (AFFIRM) study: a multivariate analysis. *J Am Coll Cardiol* 2004; 44(6):1276-1282.

96. Steinberg JS, Sadaniantz A, Kron J, et al: Analysis of cause-specific mortality in the Atrial Fibrillation Follow-up Investigation of Rhythm Management (AFFIRM) study. *Circulation* 2004; 109(16):1973-1980.

97. Hohnloser SH, Crijns HJ, van Eickels M, et al: Effect of dronedarone on cardiovascular events in atrial fibrillation. *N Engl J Med* 2009; 360(7):668-678.

98. Cox JL, Ad N, Palazzo T, et al: Current status of the Maze procedure for the treatment of atrial fibrillation. *Semin Thorac Cardiovasc Surg* 2000; 12(1):15-19.

99. Damiano RK, Gaynor SL, Bailey M, et al: The long-term outcome of patients with coronary disease and atrial fibrillation undergoing the Cox maze procedure. *J Thorac Cardiovasc Surg* 2003; 126(6):2016-2021.

100. Oral, H: Mechanisms of atrial fibrillation: lessons from studies in patients. *Prog Cardiovasc Dis* 2005; 48(1):29-40.

101. Zhou L, Keane D, Reed G, et al: Thromboembolic complications of cardiac radiofrequency catheter ablation: a review of the reported incidence, pathogenesis and current research directions. *J Cardiovasc Electrophysiol* 1999; 10(4):611-620.

102. Haissaguerre M, Jais P, Shah DC, et al: Spontaneous initiation of atrial fibrillation by ectopic beats originating in the pulmonary veins. *N Engl J Med* 1998; 339(10):659-666.

103. Oral H, Knight BP, Tada H, et al: Pulmonary vein isolation for paroxysmal and persistent atrial fibrillation. *Circulation* 2002; 105(9):1077-1081.

104. Pappone C, Oreto G, Rosanio S, et al: Atrial electroanatomic remodeling after circumferential radiofrequency pulmonary vein ablation: efficacy of an anatomic approach in a large cohort of patients with atrial fibrillation. *Circulation* 2001; 104(21):2539-2544.

105. Oral H, Chugh A, Good E, et al: Randomized comparison of encircling and nonencircling left atrial ablation for chronic atrial fibrillation. *Heart Rhythm* 2005; 2(11):1165-1172.

106. Elayi CS, Verma A, Di Biase L, et al: Ablation for longstanding permanent atrial fibrillation: results from a randomized study comparing three different strategies. *Heart Rhythm* 2008; 5(12):1658-1664.

107. Khaykin Y, Skanes A, Champagne J, et al: A randomized controlled trial of the efficacy and safety of electroanatomic circumferential pulmonary vein ablation supplemented by ablation of complex fractionated atrial electrograms versus potential-guided pulmonary vein antrum isolation guided by intracardiac ultrasound. *Circ Arrhythm Electrophysiol* 2009; 2(5):481-487.

108. Deisenhofer I, Estner H, Reents T, et al: Does electrogram guided substrate ablation add to the success of pulmonary vein isolation in patients with paroxysmal atrial fibrillation? A prospective, randomized study. *J Cardiovasc Electrophysiol* 2009; 20(5):514-521.

109. Gaita F, Caponi D, Scaglione M, et al: Long-term clinical results of 2 different ablation strategies in patients with paroxysmal and persistent atrial fibrillation. *Circ Arrhythm Electrophysiol* 2008; 1(4):269-275.

110. Proietti R, Santangeli P, Di Biase L, et al: Comparative effectiveness of wide antral versus ostial pulmonary vein isolation: a systematic review and meta-analysis. *Circ Arrhythm Electrophysiol* 2014; 7(1):39-45.

111. Wilber DJ, Pappone C, Neuzil P, et al: Comparison of antiarrhythmic drug therapy and radiofrequency catheter ablation in patients with paroxysmal atrial fibrillation: a randomized controlled trial. *JAMA* 2010; 303(4):333-340.

112. Piccini JP, Lopes RD, Kong MH, et al: Pulmonary vein isolation for the maintenance of sinus rhythm in patients with atrial fibrillation: a meta-analysis of randomized, controlled trials. *Circ Arrhythm Electrophysiol* 2009; 2(6):626-633.

113. Jais P, Cauchemez B, Macle L, et al: Catheter ablation versus antiarrhythmic drugs for atrial fibrillation: the A4 study. *Circulation* 2008; 118(24):2498-2505.

114. Pappone C, Augello G, Sala S, et al: A randomized trial of circumferential pulmonary vein ablation versus antiarrhythmic drug therapy in paroxysmal atrial fibrillation: the APAF Study. *J Am Coll Cardiol* 2006; 48(11):2340-2347.

115. Neumann T, Vogt J, Schumacher B, et al: Circumferential pulmonary vein isolation with the cryoballoon technique results from a prospective 3-center study. *J Am Coll Cardiol* 2008; 52(4):273-278.

116. Bhat T, Baydoun H, Asti D, et al: Major complications of cryoballoon catheter ablation for atrial fibrillation and their management. *Expert Rev Cardiovasc Ther* 2014; 12(9):1111-1118.

117. Metzner A, Chun KR, Neven K, et al: Long-term clinical outcome following pulmonary vein isolation with high-intensity focused ultrasound balloon catheters in patients with paroxysmal atrial fibrillation. *Europace: European pacing, arrhythmias, and cardiac electrophysiology: journal of the working groups on cardiac pacing, arrhythmias, and cardiac cellular electrophysiology of the European Society of Cardiology* 2010; 12(2):188-193.

118. Schmidt B, Chun KR, Metzner A, et al: Pulmonary vein isolation with high-intensity focused ultrasound: results from the HIFU 12F study. *Europace: European pacing, arrhythmias, and cardiac electrophysiology: journal of the working groups on cardiac pacing, arrhythmias, and cardiac cellular electrophysiology of the European Society of Cardiology* 2009; 11(10):1281-1288.

119. Reddy VY, Neuzil P, Themistoclakis S, et al: Visually-guided balloon catheter ablation of atrial fibrillation: experimental feasibility and first-in-human multicenter clinical outcome. *Circulation* 2009; 120(1):12-20.

120. Nattel S, Khairy P, Roy D, et al: New approaches to atrial fibrillation management: a critical review of a rapidly evolving field. *Drugs* 2002; 62(16):2377-2397.

121. Doshi RN, Daoud EG, Fellows C, et al: Left ventricular-based cardiac stimulation post AV nodal ablation evaluation (the PAVE study). *J Cardiovasc Electrophysiol* 2005; 16(11):1160-1165.

122. Hsieh MH, Tai CT, Lee SH, et al: Catheter ablation of atrial fibrillation versus atrioventricular junction ablation plus pacing therapy for elderly patients with medically refractory paroxysmal atrial fibrillation. *J Cardiovasc Electrophysiol* 2005; 16(5):457-461.

123. Williamson BD, Hummel J, Neibauer M, et al: Radiofrequency catheter modification of atrioventricular conduction to control the ventricular rate during atrial fibrillation. *N Engl J Med* 1994; 331(14):910-917.

124. Zipes DP, Camm AJ, Borggrefe M, et al: ACC/AHA/ESC 2006 Guidelines for Management of Patients with Ventricular Arrhythmias and the Prevention of Sudden Cardiac Death: a report of the American College of Cardiology/American Heart Association Task Force and the European Society of Cardiology Committee for Practice Guidelines (writing committee to develop Guidelines for Management of Patients With Ventricular Arrhythmias and the Prevention of Sudden Cardiac Death): developed in collaboration with the European Heart Rhythm Association and the Heart Rhythm Society. *Circulation* 2006; 114(10):e385-484.

125. Tedrow U, Stevenson WG: Sinus rhythm targeting of channels for ablation of postinfarction ventricular tachycardia. *Circ Arrhythm Electrophysiol* 2014; 7(1):7-9.

126. Wissner E, Stevenson WG, Kuck KH: Catheter ablation of ventricular tachycardia in ischaemic and non-ischaemic cardiomyopathy: where are we today? A clinical review. *Eur Heart J* 2012; 33(12):1440-1450.

127. Stevenson WG, Wilber DJ, Natale A, et al: Irrigated radiofrequency catheter ablation guided by electroanatomic mapping for recurrent ventricular tachycardia after myocardial infarction: the multicenter thermocool ventricular tachycardia ablation trial. *Circulation* 2008; 118(25):2773-2782.

128. Dinov B, Fiedler L, Schonbauer R, et al: Outcomes in catheter ablation of ventricular tachycardia in dilated nonischemic cardiomyopathy compared with ischemic cardiomyopathy: results from the Prospective Heart Centre of Leipzig VT (HELP-VT) Study. *Circulation* 2014; 129(7):728-736.

129. Gonska BD, Cao K, Schaumann A, et al: Catheter ablation of ventricular tachycardia in 136 patients with coronary artery disease: results and long-term follow-up. *J Am Coll Cardiol* 1994; 24(6):1506-1514.

130. Morady F, Harvey M, Kalbfleisch SJ, et al: Radiofrequency catheter ablation of ventricular tachycardia in patients with coronary artery disease. *Circulation* 1993; 87(2):363-372.

131. Stevenson WG, Khan H, Sager P, et al: Identification of reentry circuit sites during catheter mapping and radiofrequency ablation of ventricular tachycardia late after myocardial infarction. *Circulation* 1993; 88(4 Pt 1): 1647-1670.

132. Blanck Z, Dhala A, Deshpande S, et al: Bundle branch reentrant ventricular tachycardia: cumulative experience in 48 patients. *J Cardiovasc Electrophysiol* 1993; 4(3):253-262.

133. Mehdirad AA, Keim S, Rist K, et al: Long-term clinical outcome of right bundle branch radiofrequency catheter ablation for treatment of bundle branch reentrant ventricular tachycardia. *Pacing Clin Electrophysiol: PACE* 1995; 18(12 Pt 1):2135-2143.

134. Marcus FI, Fontaine G: Arrhythmogenic right ventricular dysplasia/cardiomyopathy: a review. *Pacing Clin Electrophysiol: PACE* 1995; 18(6): 1298-1314.

135. Aizer A, Stern EH, Gomes JA, et al: Usefulness of programmed ventricular stimulation in predicting future arrhythmic events in patients with cardiac sarcoidosis. *Am J Cardiol* 2005; 96(2):276-282.

136. Koplan BA, Soejima K, Baughman K, et al: Refractory ventricular tachycardia secondary to cardiac sarcoid: electrophysiologic characteristics, mapping, and ablation. *Heart Rhythm* 2006; 3(8):924-929.

137. Fujita T, et al: Increased extent of myocardial fibrosis in genotyped hypertrophic cardiomyopathy with ventricular tachyarrhythmias. *J Cardiol* 2014.

138. Khairy P, Stevenson WG: Catheter ablation in tetralogy of Fallot. *Heart Rhythm* 2009; 6(7):1069-1074.

139. Eckart RE, Hruczkowski TW, Tedrow UB, et al: Sustained ventricular tachycardia associated with corrective valve surgery. *Circulation* 2007; 116(18):2005-2011.

140. John R, Tedrow UB, Koplan BA, et al: Ventricular arrhythmias and sudden cardiac death. *Lancet* 2012; 380(9852):1520-1529.

141. Rodriguez LM, Smeets JL, Timmermans C, et al: Predictors for successful ablation of right- and left-sided idiopathic ventricular tachycardia. *Am J Cardiol* 1997; 79(3):309-314.

142. Khaykin Y, Wang X, Natale A, et al: Cost comparison of ablation versus antiarrhythmic drugs as first-line therapy for atrial fibrillation: an economic evaluation of the RAAFT pilot study. *J Cardiovasc Electrophysiol* 2009; 20(1):7-12.

143. McKenna C, Palmer S, Rodgers M, et al: Cost-effectiveness of radiofrequency catheter ablation for the treatment of atrial fibrillation in the United Kingdom. *Heart* 2009; 95(7):542-549.

144. Cheng CH, Sanders GD, Hlatky MA, et al: Cost-effectiveness of radiofrequency ablation for supraventricular tachycardia. *Ann Intern Med* 2000; 133(11):864-876.

145. Marshall DA, O'Brien BJ, Nichol G: Review of economic evaluations of radiofrequency catheter ablation for cardiac arrhythmias. *Can J Cardiol* 2003; 19(11):1285-1304.

146. Weerasooriya HR, Murdock CJ, Harris AH, et al: The cost-effectiveness of treatment of supraventricular arrhythmias related to an accessory atrioventricular pathway: comparison of catheter ablation, surgical division and medical treatment. *Aust N Z J Med* 1994; 24(2):161-167.

147. Martin-Doyle W, Reynolds MR: Is AF ablation cost effective? *J Atrial Fibrillation* 2010; 2(1):727-739.

148. Chan PS, Vijan S, Morady F, et al: Cost-effectiveness of radiofrequency catheter ablation for atrial fibrillation. *J Am Coll Cardiol* 2006; 47(12):2513-2520.

149. Rodgers M, McKenna C, Palmer S, et al: Curative catheter ablation in atrial fibrillation and typical atrial flutter: systematic review and economic evaluation. *Health Technol Assess* 2008; 12(34):iii-iv, xi-xiii, 1-198.

150. Russo MS, et al: First report of image integration of cine-angiography with 3D electro-anatomical mapping of the right ventricle in postoperative Tetralogy of Fallot. *Int J Cardiovasc Imaging* 2014.

151. Schilling RJ, Peters NS, Davies DW: Feasibility of a noncontact catheter for endocardial mapping of human ventricular tachycardia. *Circulation* 1999; 99(19):2543-2552.

152. Narayan SM, Baykaner T, Clopton P, et al: Ablation of rotor and focal sources reduces late recurrence of atrial fibrillation compared with trigger ablation alone: extended follow-up of the CONFIRM trial (Conventional Ablation for Atrial Fibrillation With or Without Focal Impulse and Rotor Modulation). *J Am Coll Cardiol* 2014; 63(17):1761-1768.

153. Natale A, Reddy VY, Monir G, et al: Paroxysmal AF catheter ablation with a contact force sensing catheter: results of the prospective, multicenter SMART-AF trial. *J Am Coll Cardiol* 2014; 64(7):647-656.

154. Anter E, Tschabrunn CM, Contreras-Valdes FM, et al: Radiofrequency ablation annotation algorithm reduces the incidence of linear gaps and reconnection after pulmonary vein isolation. *Heart Rhythm* 2014; 11(5):783-790.

155. Sapp JL, Beeckler C, Pike R, et al: Initial human feasibility of infusion needle catheter ablation for refractory ventricular tachycardia. *Circulation* 2013; 128(21):2289-2295.

156. Pappone C, Vicedomini G, Manguso F, et al: Robotic magnetic navigation for atrial fibrillation ablation. *J Am Coll Cardiol* 2006; 47(7):1390-1400.

157. Di Biase L, Fahmy TS, Patel D, et al: Remote magnetic navigation: human experience in pulmonary vein ablation. *J Am Coll Cardiol* 2007; 50(9):868-874.

158. Schmidt B, Tilz RR, Neven K, et al: Remote robotic navigation and electroanatomical mapping for ablation of atrial fibrillation: considerations for navigation and impact on procedural outcome. *Circ Arrhythm Electrophysiol* 2009; 2(2):120-128.

159. Saliba W, Reddy VY, Wazni O, et al: Atrial fibrillation ablation using a robotic catheter remote control system: initial human experience and long-term follow-up results. *J Am Coll Cardiol* 2008; 51(25): 2407-2411.

160. Di Biase L, Wang Y, Horton R, et al: Ablation of atrial fibrillation utilizing robotic catheter navigation in comparison to manual navigation and ablation: single-center experience. *J Cardiovasc Electrophysiol* 2009; 20(12):1328-1335.

161. Bradfield J, Tung R, Mandapati R, et al: Catheter ablation utilizing remote magnetic navigation: a review of applications and outcomes. *Pacing Clin Electrophysiol: PACE* 2012; 35(8):1021-1034.

162. Thomas D, Scholz EP, Schweizer PA, et al: Initial experience with robotic navigation for catheter ablation of paroxysmal and persistent atrial fibrillation. *J Electrocardiol* 2012; 45(2):95-101.

163. Holmes DR, Reddy VY, Turi ZG, et al: Percutaneous closure of the left atrial appendage versus warfarin therapy for prevention of stroke in patients with atrial fibrillation: a randomised non-inferiority trial. *Lancet* 2009; 374(9689):534-542.

164. Reddy VY, Holmes D, Doshi SK, et al: Safety of percutaneous left atrial appendage closure: results from the Watchman Left Atrial Appendage System for Embolic Protection in Patients with AF (PROTECT AF) clinical trial and the Continued Access Registry. *Circulation* 2011; 123(4):417-424.

54

Surgery for Atrial Fibrillation

Matthew C. Henn • Spencer J. Melby • Ralph J. Damiano, Jr.

Atrial fibrillation (AF) remains the most common arrhythmia in the world.[1] It is associated with significant morbidity and mortality secondary to its detrimental sequelae: (1) palpitations resulting in patient discomfort and anxiety; (2) loss of atrioventricular (AV) synchrony, which can compromise cardiac hemodynamics, resulting in various degrees of ventricular dysfunction; (3) stasis of blood flow in the left atrium, increasing the risk of thromboembolism and stroke.[2-11]

Medical treatment of AF has had many shortcomings including both the inefficacy of many of the antiarrhythmic drugs and their unwanted side effects. Because of this, interest in nonpharmacologic treatment approaches led to the development of catheter-based and surgical techniques beginning in the 1980s. Initial attempts aimed at providing rate control failed to address the detrimental hemodynamic and thromboembolic sequelae of AF. The early attempts at finding a surgical treatment culminated in the introduction of the Maze procedure in 1987, which became the surgical gold standard for decades.

The following sections describe the historical aspects and the current status of surgery for AF, including the introduction of minimally invasive techniques.

HISTORICAL ASPECTS

The Left Atrial Isolation Procedure

The first surgical procedure designed specifically to eliminate AF, the *left atrial isolation*, was described in 1980 in the laboratory of Dr. James Cox at Duke University. This approach confined AF to the left atrium, and restored the remainder of the heart to sinus rhythm (Fig. 54-1).[12] This reestablished a regular ventricular rate without requiring a permanent pacemaker. Isolating the left atrium allowed the right atrium and the right ventricle to contract in synchrony, providing a normal right-sided cardiac output. This effectively restored normal hemodynamics.

However, by confining AF to the left atrium, the left atrial isolation procedure only eliminated two of the three detrimental sequelae of AF: an irregular heartbeat and compromised cardiac hemodynamics. It did not eliminate the thromboembolic risk because the left atrium usually remained in fibrillation. This procedure never achieved clinical acceptance, and was only performed in a single patient.

Catheter Ablation of the Atrioventricular Node-His Bundle Complex

In 1982, Scheinman and coworkers introduced *catheter fulguration of the His bundle*, a procedure that controlled the irregular cardiac rhythm associated with AF and other refractory supraventricular arrhythmias.[13] This procedure electrically isolated the fibrillation to the atria. Unfortunately, ablating the bundle of His required permanent ventricular pacemaker implantation to restore a normal ventricular rate.

The shortcoming of this intervention was that it only eliminated the irregular heartbeat. Both atria remained in fibrillation, and the risk of thromboembolism persisted. AV contraction remained desynchronized, compromising cardiac hemodynamics. In addition, patients become pacemaker dependant for the remainder of their lives. Nevertheless, AV node ablation has remained a common treatment for medically refractory AF.

The Corridor Procedure

In 1985, Guiraudon and associates developed the *corridor procedure* for the treatment of AF.[14] This operation isolated a strip of atrial septum harboring both the sinoatrial (SA) node and the AV node, allowing the SA node to drive both the ventricles. This procedure effectively eliminated the irregular heartbeat associated with AF, but both atria either remained in fibrillation or developed their own asynchronous intrinsic rhythm because they were isolated from the septal "corridor." Furthermore, the atria were isolated from their respective ventricles, thereby preventing AV synchrony. The corridor procedure was abandoned because it had no effect on the hemodynamic compromise or the risk of thromboembolism associated with AF.

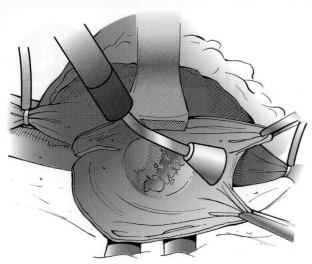

FIGURE 54-1 Standard left atriotomy, demonstrating incisions to the mitral valve annulus at both the 10 and 2 o'clock positions. The superior and inferior vena cavae are seen with tourniquets, and the pulmonary vein orifices are seen inferiorly. Cryoablation is used to complete the line of conduction block at the valve annuli. (Adapted with permission from Williams JM, Ungerleider RM, Lofland GK, Cox JL: Left atrial isolation: new technique for the treatment of supraventricular arrhythmias, *J Thorac Cardiovasc Surg.* 1980 Sep;80(3):373-380.)

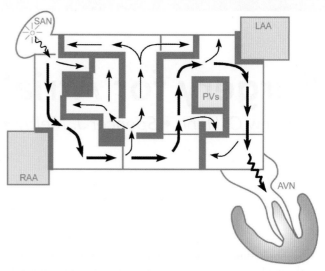

FIGURE 54-2 By creating a myriad of surgical incisions in the atria, the Maze procedure was designed to prevent atrial fibrillation. AVN = atrioventricular node; LAA = left atrial appendage; PVs = pulmonary veins; RAA = right atrial appendage; SAN = sinoatrial node. (Reproduced with permission from Cox JL, Schuessler RB, D'Agostino HJ Jr, et al: The surgical treatment of atrial fibrillation. III. Development of a definitive surgical procedure, *J Thorac Cardiovasc Surg.* 1991 Apr;101(4):569-583.)

The Atrial Transection Procedure

In 1985, Dr. James Cox and associates described the first procedure that attempted to terminate rather than simply isolate or confine AF to the atria.[15] Using a canine model, they found that a single long incision around both atria and down into the septum could terminate AF. This *atrial transection procedure* effectively prevented AF or atrial flutter in animals.[16] Although this procedure was not effective clinically and was soon abandoned, it laid the foundation for the development of the Cox-Maze procedure.

THE COX-MAZE PROCEDURE

The Maze procedure was clinically introduced in 1987 by Dr. Cox after extensive animal investigation.[16-18] The Cox-Maze procedure was originally developed to interrupt any and all macro-reentrant circuits that were felt to cause AF, thereby precluding the ability of the atrium to flutter or fibrillate (Fig. 54-2). Unlike previous procedures, the Cox-Maze procedure successfully restored both AV synchrony and sinus rhythm, thus potentially reducing the risk of thromboembolism and stroke.[19] The operation consisted of creating an array of surgical incisions across both the right and left atria. These incisions were placed so that the SA node could still direct the propagation of the sinus impulse throughout both atria. It allowed for most of the atrial myocardium to be activated, resulting in preservation of atrial transport function in animals and in most patients.[20]

The first iteration of the Maze procedure was modified because of problems with late chronotropic incompetence

and a high incidence of pacemaker implantation. The resulting Maze II procedure, however, was technically difficult to perform, and was soon replaced by the Maze III procedure (Fig. 54-3).[21,22]

The Cox-Maze III procedure—often referred to as the "cut-and-sew" Maze—became the gold standard for the surgical treatment of AF. In a long-term study of patients who underwent the Cox-Maze III procedure at our institution, 97% of the patients at late follow-up were free of symptomatic AF.[23] These excellent results have been reproduced by other groups.[24-26]

Although the Cox-Maze III procedure was effective in eliminating AF, it was technically difficult and required a lengthy period of aortic cross-clamping. This limited adoption and only a handful of cardiac surgeons still perform the cut-and-sew operation.

Over the last 15 years, the field of AF surgery was revolutionized by the introduction of a variety of ablation devices that have been used to replicate the surgical incisions on the atrium. This has made AF ablation much simpler to perform. These ablation-assisted procedures have greatly expanded the field of AF surgery and have resulted in a much wider adoption.[27] With present ablation technology, surgery can be performed with low morbidity and mortality and often through less invasive approaches.

SURGICAL ABLATION TECHNOLOGY

The development of surgical ablation technology has transformed a difficult and time-consuming operation that few surgeons were willing to perform into a procedure that is

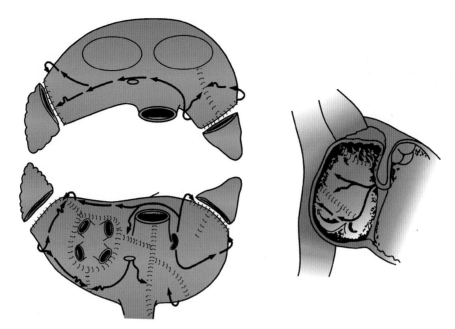

FIGURE 54-3 The lesions set of the traditional cut-and-sew Cox-Maze III procedure. (Reproduced with permission from Cox JL, Schuessler RB, D'Agostino HJ Jr, et al: The surgical treatment of atrial fibrillation. III. Development of a definitive surgical procedure, *J Thorac Cardiovasc Surg.* 1991 Apr;101(4):569-583.)

technically easier, shorter, and less invasive. Several ablation technologies exist, each with its relative advantages and disadvantages.

For an ablation technology to successfully replace surgical incisions, it must meet several criteria. First, it must reliably produce bidirectional conduction block across the line of ablation. This is the mechanism by which incisions prevent AF, by either blocking macro-reentrant or micro-reentrant circuits or isolating focal triggers. Our laboratory and others have shown that this requires a transmural lesion, as even small gaps in ablation lines can conduct both sinus and fibrillatory impulses.[28-30] Second, the ablation device must be safe. This requires a precise definition of dose-response curves to limit excessive or inadequate ablation, and potential injury to surrounding vital cardiac structures, such as the coronary sinus, coronary arteries, and valvular structures. Third, the ablation device should make AF surgery simpler and require less time to perform. This requires the device to create lesions rapidly, be simple to use, and have adequate length and flexibility. The following sections will briefly summarize the two current ablation technologies in clinical use: cryoablation and radiofrequency (RF) ablation.

Cryoablation

Cryoablation technology is unique in that it destroys myocardial tissue by freezing rather than heating. It has the benefit of preserving the myocardial fibrous skeleton and collagen structure and is thus one of the safest energy sources available. These devices work by pumping a refrigerant to the electrode tip where it undergoes transformation from a liquid to a gas phase, and in so doing absorbs heat energy from the tissue in contact with the tip. The formation of intracellular and extracellular ice crystals disrupts the cell membrane and causes cell death. There is also evidence that the induction of apoptosis plays a role in late lesion expansion. Lesion size depends on the temperature of the probe and thermal conductivity and temperature of the tissue.[31]

There are currently two commercially available sources of cryothermal energy that are being used in cardiac surgery. The older technology, based on nitrous oxide, is manufactured by AtriCure (Cincinnati, OH). More recently, devices using argon have been developed, and are currently distributed by Medtronic (Minneapolis, MN). At 1 atmosphere of pressure, nitrous oxide is capable of cooling tissue to –89.5°C, whereas argon has a minimum temperature of –185.7°C. The nitrous oxide technology has a well-defined efficacy and safety profile and is generally excellent except around the coronary arteries.[32,33] Experimental and clinical studies have shown intimal hyperplasia and coronary stenosis after cryoablation.[33-35] The potential disadvantage of cryoablation, however, is its relatively long time required to create lesions (1-3 minutes). There is also difficulty in creating lesions on the beating heart because of the "heat sink" of the circulating blood volume.[36] Furthermore, if blood is frozen during epicardial ablation on the beating heart, it may coagulate, creating a potential thromboembolic risk.

Radiofrequency Energy

RF energy has been used for cardiac ablation for many years in the electrophysiology laboratory, and was one of the first energy sources to be applied in the operating room.[37] Resistive RF energy can be delivered by either unipolar or bipolar electrodes, and the electrodes can be either dry or irrigated. With unipolar RF devices, the energy is dispersed between the electrode tip and an indifferent electrode, usually the grounding pad applied to the patient. In bipolar RF devices, alternating current is passed between two closely approximated electrodes. The lesion size depends on electrode-tissue contact area, the interface temperature, the current and voltage (power), and the duration of delivery. The depth of the lesion can be limited by char formation, epicardial fat, myocardial and endocavity blood flow, and tissue thickness.

There have been numerous unipolar RF devices developed for ablation. These include both dry and irrigated devices and devices that incorporate suction. Although dry unipolar RF has been shown to create transmural lesions on the arrested heart in animals with sufficiently long ablation times, it has not been consistently successful in humans. After 2-minute endocardial ablations during mitral valve surgery, only 20% of the in vivo lesions were transmural.[38] Epicardial ablation on the beating heart has been even more problematic. Animal studies have consistently shown that unipolar RF is incapable of creating epicardial transmural lesions on the beating heart.[39,40] Epicardial RF ablation in humans resulted in only 10% of the lesions being transmural.[41] This deficiency of unipolar RF ablation has been felt to be caused by the heat sink of the circulating blood.[42] This has led industry to examine adding both irrigation and suction to improve lesion formation. Although these additions have improved depth of penetration, there has been no unipolar RF device that has been shown by independent laboratories to be capable of creating reliable transmural lesions on the beating heart.

To overcome this problem, bipolar RF clamps were developed. With bipolar RF, the electrodes are embedded in the jaws of a clamp to focus the delivery of energy. By shielding the electrodes from the circulating blood pool, this improves and shortens lesion formation and limits collateral injury. Bipolar ablation has been shown to be capable of creating transmural lesions on the beating heart both in animals and humans with short ablation times.[43-45] Two companies (AtriCure, West Chester, OH and Medtronic, Minneapolis, MN) currently market bipolar RF devices.

Another advantage of bipolar RF energy over unipolar RF is its safety profile. A number of clinical complications of unipolar RF devices have been reported, including coronary artery injuries, cerebrovascular accidents, and esophageal perforation leading to atrioesophageal fistula.[46-49] Bipolar RF technology has virtually eliminated this collateral damage; there have been no injuries described with these devices despite extensive clinical use. The Cobra Fusion™ (AtriCure, West Chester, OH) is a new device that combines bipolar and unipolar RF into a single suction-assisted device. Early experimental results have shown consistency in creating transmural epicardial lesions on the beating heart.[50]

Other types of devices utilizing microwave, laser, and ultrasound energy have been used clinically, but limitations of each technology have led to limited use and withdrawal of these devices from the market.[42,51-55]

In summary, ablation technology has made significant progress over the past decade and has allowed for a broader application of surgical ablation. As new devices and techniques are developed, continued research investigating their effects on atrial hemodynamics, function, and electrophysiology is imperative.

SURGICAL TECHNIQUES

There are three categories of procedures that presently are performed to surgically treat AF: the Cox-Maze procedure, left atrial lesion sets, and pulmonary vein isolation (PVI). Each of these approaches is described in the following sections.

The Cox-Maze IV Procedure

The original "cut-and-sew" Cox-Maze III procedure is rarely performed today. At most centers, the surgical incisions have been replaced with lines of ablation using a variety of energy sources. At our institution, bipolar RF energy and cryoablation has been used successfully to replace most of the surgical incisions of the Cox-Maze III procedure. Our current RF ablation-assisted procedure, termed the Cox-Maze IV, incorporates the lesions of the Cox-Maze III (Fig. 54-4).[56] Our clinical results have shown that this modified procedure has significantly shortened operative time while maintaining the high success rate of the original Cox-Maze III procedure.[57,58]

The Cox-Maze IV procedure is performed on cardiopulmonary bypass with central or femoral cannulation. The operation can be done either through a median sternotomy or a less invasive (4-5 cm) right minithoracotomy. The right and left pulmonary veins (PVs) are bluntly dissected. If the patient is in AF, amiodarone is administered and the patient is electrically cardioverted. Pacing thresholds are obtained from each PV. Using a bipolar RF ablation device, the PVs are individually isolated by ablating a cuff of atrial tissue surrounding the right and left PVs. Proof of electrical isolation is confirmed after ablation by demonstrating exit block from each PV.

The right atrial lesion set is performed on the beating heart. A bipolar RF clamp is used to create most of the lesions (Fig. 54-5). A unipolar device, either cryoablation or RF energy, is used to complete the ablation lines endocardially down to the tricuspid annulus because of the difficulty of clamping in this area.

The remaining left-sided lesion set (Fig. 54-6) is performed on the arrested heart. First, the left atrial appendage is amputated and an ablation is performed through the amputated left atrial appendage into one of the left PVs. A standard left atriotomy is performed and extended inferiorly around the right inferior PV and superiorly onto the dome of the left atrium. Connecting lesions are made with the bipolar RF device into the left superior and inferior PVs and a final ablation is performed down toward the mitral annulus. Our group has shown that isolating the entire posterior left atrium with ablation lines into both left PVs resulted in a

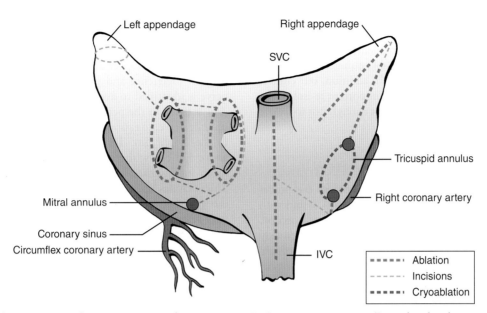

FIGURE 54-4 The Cox-Maze IV lesion sets. IVC = inferior vena cava; SVC = superior vena cava. (Reproduced with permission from Cox JL, Schuessler RB, D'Agostino HJ Jr, et al: The surgical treatment of atrial fibrillation. III. Development of a definitive surgical procedure, *J Thorac Cardiovasc Surg.* 1991 Apr;101(4):569-583.)

better drug-free freedom from AF at 6 and 12 months than a single connecting lesion.[59] Unipolar cryoablation is used to connect the lesion to the mitral annulus and complete the left atrial isthmus line.

Left Atrial Procedures

Over the past decade, there have been a number of new surgical procedures introduced in attempt to cure AF. The results have been variable and have had a wide range of success rates.[55,60-67] Various ablation technologies have been used to create a large number of different lesion patterns. All of

these procedures have generally involved some subset of the left atrial lesion set of the Cox-Maze procedure. Results have been dependent on the technology used, the lesion set, and the patient population. From a technical standpoint, all of the approaches have attempted to isolate the PVs. The importance of the rest of the left atrial Cox-Maze lesion set has also been generally established. However, Gillinov et al. published

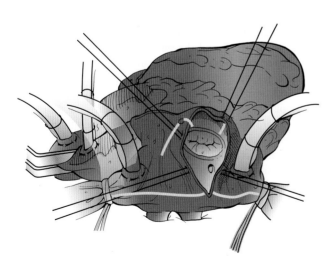

FIGURE 54-5 Illustration of the right atrial lesion set. White lines indicate bipolar RF ablation. Cryoablation is used to complete the ablation line at the tricuspid valve annulus.

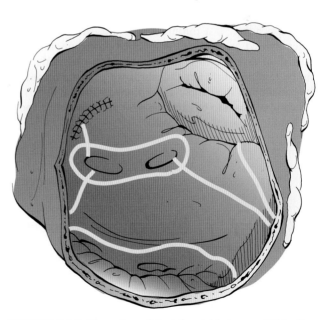

FIGURE 54-6 Illustration of the left atrial lesion set. White lines indicate RF bipolar ablation. Cryoablation is used to complete the ablation line at the mitral valve annulus.

a large series demonstrating that the omission of the left atrial isthmus lesion resulted in a significantly higher incidence of recurrent AF in patients with permanent AF.[68] To complete this lesion, it is mandatory to also ablate the coronary sinus in line with the endocardial lesion. In addition, our clinical results have shown that it is critically important to isolate the entire posterior left atrium and it is not enough just to isolate the PVs.[59]

Pulmonary Vein Isolation

PVI is an attractive therapeutic strategy because the procedure can be done without cardiopulmonary bypass and with minimally invasive techniques, using either a thoracoscopic approach or small incisions. It can also be easily and quickly added to other cardiac surgery procedures (eg, coronary bypass graft or a valve procedure). Based on the original report of Hassaiguerre, it has been well documented that the triggers for paroxysmal AF originate from the PVs in the majority of cases.[69] However, it is important to remember that up to 30% of triggers may originate outside the PVs.[70] In an attempt to increase efficacy, some investigators have added ablation of the ganglionic plexi (GP).[71-73]

The PVs can be isolated separately or as a box (Fig. 54-7). The most common approach for treatment of lone AF uses an endoscopic, port-based approach to minimize incision size and pain for the patient. At our center, bipolar RF clamps are favored to isolate the PVs, but unipolar RF, cryoablation, and HIFU devices have also been used.[53,74,75] Accumulating data suggest that a box isolation of the entire posterior left atrium is the more effective strategy.[59,76]

Patient preparation begins with double-lumen endotracheal intubation. A transesophageal echocardiogram is performed to confirm the absence of thrombus in the left atrial appendage. If a thrombus is found, the procedure is either aborted or converted to an open procedure, in which the risk of systemic thromboembolism from left atrial clot can be minimized. External defibrillator pads are placed on the patient and the patient is positioned with the right side turned upward 45 to 60° and the right arm positioned above the head to expose the right axilla.

An initial port for the thoracoscopic camera is placed at the sixth intercostal space. Under thoracoscopic vision, a small working port can then be placed in either the third or fourth intercostal space at the midaxillary line depending on surgeon preference and patient anatomy. The right phrenic nerve is identified to avoid injury to this structure. An incision is made in the pericardium, anterior and parallel to the phrenic nerve, to expose the heart from the superior vena cava to the diaphragm. Through this pericardiotomy, the space above and below the right PVs is dissected to allow enough room for insertion of a specialized thoracoscopic dissector. This includes opening into the oblique sinus and dissecting the space between the right superior PV and the right pulmonary artery. The dissector and a guiding sheath is introduced through a second port, either lateral or medial to the scope port, and guided into the space between the right superior PV and right pulmonary artery. After the dissector is carefully removed from the chest, the sheath remains in place as a guide for the insertion of the bipolar RF clamp. At this point, the patient is cardioverted into sinus rhythm so that pacing thresholds can be obtained. As with a Cox-Maze IV procedure, it is critical to document pacing thresholds from the PVs before isolation. Some surgeons also use the opportunity provided by surgical exposure to test and ablate ganglionated plexi but there are no data to support this and it is not performed at our institution.

The sheath is attached to the lower jaw of a bipolar RF clamp. The clamp is introduced into the chest, and the left atrium surrounding the PVs is clamped and ablated. After confirmation of exit block by pacing, the instruments are removed from the right chest and the right chest ports are closed.

The approach to the left chest is similar to the right. The patient is repositioned such that the left chest is elevated 45 to 60° and the left arm is held up to expose the left axilla. A port for the thoracoscopic camera is placed in the sixth intercostal space, slightly more posterior than on the right side. With thoracoscopic visualization, a left-sided working port is created in the third or fourth intercostal space. The left phrenic nerve is identified, and the pericardium is opened posterior to the course of the nerve. The ligament of Marshall is identified and divided. The dissector is then introduced through a second port, also in the sixth intercostal space. This port site is placed to allow for a straight-line introduction of the dissector around the PVs. The guiding sheath is used to position the RF clamp around the left PVs, and they are isolated. Again, conduction block is confirmed with pacing.

The procedure is not complete until the left atrial appendage has been addressed. Historically, this has been done by stapling across the base of the left atrial appendage with an endoscopic stapler. This requires careful surgical technique and attention because it can result in tears and bleeding.[77] Clip devices have been designed to address this difficulty, and they are used exclusively at our center because of their improved efficacy and safety when compared to staplers.[78,79] After ablation of the left PVs and exclusion of the left atrial appendage, the left side of the pericardium is closed.

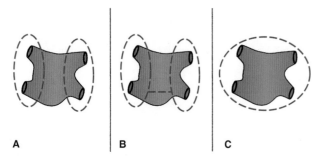

A **B** **C**

FIGURE 54-7 Diagram illustrating the methods to isolate the pulmonary veins, either separately (A), with a connecting lesion (B), or as a box isolation of the entire posterior left atrium (C).

SURGICAL RESULTS

The Cox-Maze Procedure

The Cox-Maze III procedure has had excellent long-term results. In our series at Washington University, 97% of 198 consecutive patients who underwent the procedure with a mean follow-up of 5.4 years were free from symptomatic AF. There was no difference in the cure rates between patients undergoing a stand-alone Cox-Maze procedure and those undergoing concomitant procedures.[23] Similar results have been obtained from other institutions around the world with the traditional "cut-and-sew" method.[24,26,80]

Our results from patients who underwent the Cox-Maze IV procedure have been encouraging as well. In a prospective, single-center trial from our institution, 91% of patients at the 6-month follow-up were free from AF.[43,58] The Cox-Maze IV procedure has significantly shortened the mean cross-clamp times for a lone Cox-Maze from 93 ± 34 minutes for the Cox-Maze III to 47 ± 26 minutes for the Cox-Maze IV ($p < .001$), and from 122 ± 37 minutes for a concomitant Cox-Maze III procedure to 92 ± 37 minutes ($p < .005$) in those undergoing the Cox-Maze IV procedure concomitantly with another cardiac operation.[43] A propensity analysis performed by our group has shown that there was no significant difference in the freedom from AF at 3, 6, or 12 months between the Cox-Maze III and IV groups.[58] A more recent prospective study in 100 consecutive patients who underwent the Cox-Maze IV procedure demonstrated postoperative freedom from AF at 93, 90, and 90% at 6, 12, and 24 months, respectively.[81] We also recently reported over two decades of experience at our institution with both the Cox-Maze III and Cox-Maze IV procedures. Freedom from AF was 93% and freedom from AF and AADs was 82% at a mean follow-up time of 3.6 years, while freedom from symptomatic AF was 85% at 10 years.[82]

The Cox-Maze IV procedure worked as well in patients with paroxysmal as for long-standing persistent AF. The 6-month freedom for AF was 91% in the paroxysmal group compared with 88% in the persistent group ($p = .53$). The drug-free success rate was also similar.[83] Our present series consists of 532 consecutive patients undergoing a Cox-Maze IV between January 2002 and September 2014. All patients have been followed with ECGs or prolonged monitoring. Our 12-month freedom from AF was 92%, with 82% of patients also off all antiarrhythmic drugs, while our 5-year freedom from AF was 77%, with 64% of patients also off all antiarrhythmic drugs (unpublished data).

The Cox-Maze procedure has also been very successful in reducing the incidence of stroke. In patients undergoing the Cox-Maze procedure, the preoperative incidence of neurological events has been high due to inherent risk in patients with AF. In a report from our institution, 57 out of 389 patients (14%) had experienced a neurological event before surgery. Despite this, there were only six neurological events during long-term follow-up (mean, 6.6 ± 5.0 years) in this cohort. The long-term stroke rate after the Cox-Maze procedure has been 0.2% per year despite the fact that the great majority of patients were able to discontinue anticoagulation.[84]

The Cox-Maze procedure is being increasingly used as a concomitant procedure.[27] Previous studies from our institution and others have documented high rates of restoration of sinus rhythm without increasing morbidity following concomitant procedures including coronary artery bypass, mitral valve surgery, and tricuspid valve surgery.[85-91] Surgical ablation should be considered in all patients with AF undergoing concomitant cardiac procedures, and a biatrial Cox-Maze IV lesion set is recommended in most cases. A recent study from Dr. Ad and his colleagues have shown that adding a Cox-Maze procedure to either aortic valve replacement or coronary artery bypass grafting did not increase operative morbidity or mortality.[92]

In an effort to decrease operative morbidity, a minimally invasive Cox-Maze IV lesion set has been introduced through a right minithoracotomy.[93,94] In both the stand-alone Cox-Maze IV and concomitant population, this approach has been shown to be equally effective at restoring sinus rhythm while significantly decreasing major complications, operative mortality, intensive care unit length of stay, and hospital length of stay when compared to sternotomy approach.[95]

Left Atrial Lesion Sets

A number of centers around the world have suggested performing ablation confined to the left atrium only to cure AF. This concept is supported by the fact that the majority of paroxysmal AF appears to originate around the PVs and the posterior left atrium. A left atrial lesion set typically involves PVI with a lesion to the mitral annulus as well as removal of the left atrial appendage. One advantage of avoiding right atrial lesions is a potentially lower rate of postoperative pacemaker implantation.[96] Many ablation technologies have been used to create these lesion sets with varied degrees of success.[48,60-67]

There have been no randomized trials of biatrial versus left atrial ablation only in the surgical population. Because of this, the importance of the right atrial lesions of the traditional Cox-Maze procedure is difficult to precisely determine. A meta-analysis of the published literature by Barnett and Ad revealed that a biatrial lesion set resulted in a significantly higher late freedom from AF when compared with a left atrial lesion set alone (87 vs 73%, $p = .05$).[97] This is not surprising considering the results of intraoperative mapping of patients with AF. Both our group and others have shown that AF can originate from the right atrium in 10 to 30% of cases.[97-100]

Of the specific left atrial lesions of the Cox-Maze procedure, it is difficult to determine the precise importance of each ablation line. All surgeons agree on the importance of isolating the PVs. As stated previously, work from Gillinov et al has shown the importance of the left atrial isthmus in a retrospective study.[68] Moreover, omitting the lesion to the mitral annulus leaves the patient at risk for the development of late left atrial flutter. In a rare randomized trial, Gaita and coauthors examined PVI alone versus two alternate lesion sets that both included ablation of the left atrial isthmus. In this study, normal sinus rhythm at 2-year follow-up was only seen in 20% in the PVI group versus 57% in the other groups ($p < .006$).[65]

Finally, our group has shown that isolating the entire posterior left atrium significantly improved our drug-free freedom from AF at 6 months (54 vs 79%, $p = .011$) in a retrospective analysis of our results.[59] Thus, it is our opinion that most of the left atrial Cox-Maze lesion set is needed to ensure a high success rate.

Pulmonary Vein Isolation

The results of PVI alone have been variable and have been dependent on patient selection and the energy source utilized. In the first report of surgical PVI, Wolf and colleagues reported that 91% of patients undergoing a video-assisted bilateral PVI and left atrial appendage exclusion were free from AF at three months follow-up.[101] However, this was a small study with very limited follow-up. Edgerton et al reported on 57 patients undergoing PVI with GP ablation with more thorough follow-up and found 82% of their patients with paroxysmal AF to be free from AF at 6 months, with 74% off antiarrhythmic drugs.[102]

Subsequent studies have shown encouraging results in patients with paroxysmal AF. In a study involving 21 patients with paroxysmal AF undergoing PVI with GP ablation, McClelland et al reported 88% freedom from AF at 1 year without antiarrhythmic drugs.[72] A larger, single-center trial recently reported a 65% single-procedure success at 1 year in a series of 45 patients undergoing PVI with GP ablation, including patients with persistent and paroxysmal AF.[103] A multicenter trial reported 87% normal sinus rhythm rate in a more diverse patient population, including some patients with long-standing persistent AF; however, those patients with long-standing persistent AF only had a 71% incidence of normal sinus rhythm.[104] The FAST trial, a more recent multicenter randomized trial, compared 63 patients who received linear antral PVI by way of catheter ablation and 61 patients who received bipolar RF PVI and ganglionated plexi ablation. Most patients in both groups had paroxysmal AF. At 1 year, freedom from left atrial arrhythmias >30 seconds evaluated by a 7-day Holter without antiarrhythmic drugs was 66% for surgical ablation versus 37% for catheter ablation ($p = .002$).[105]

In patients with long-standing or persistent AF, the results have been worse. In a study from Edgerton and his group, only 35% of patients were free from AF and antiarrhythmic drugs at 6 months follow-up.[106] Long-term data for PVI with ganglion plexus ablation are equally disappointing. One group reported 139 patients with up to 5 years of follow-up: freedom from AF and antiarrhythmic drugs was 52, 28, and 29% for paroxysmal, persistent, and long-standing persistent AF.[107] With concomitant procedures, the success rate of PVI is also low. Of 23 patients undergoing mitral valve surgery or coronary revascularization with concomitant PVI, only half of patients were free from AF at a follow-up of 57 ± 37 months.[108] In the setting of mitral valve disease, Tada and colleagues report only 17% freedom from AF and antiarrhythmic drugs in their series of 66 patients undergoing PVI.[109] In patients undergoing aortic valve replacement and PVI, freedoms from AF and antiarrhythmic drugs was only 50% at two years at our institution.[110]

INDICATIONS FOR SURGICAL ABLATION

The indications for surgery have been defined in a recent consensus statement.[111] These presently include (1) All symptomatic patients with documented atrial fibrillation undergoing other cardiac surgical procedures; (2) selected asymptomatic patients with atrial fibrillation undergoing cardiac surgery in which the ablation can be performed with minimal risk in experienced centers; and (3) stand-alone atrial fibrillation ablation should be considered for symptomatic patients with atrial fibrillation who either prefer a surgical approach, have failed one or more attempts at catheter ablation, or are not candidates for catheter ablation.

There is still controversy regarding the referral of patients for surgery with medically refractory, symptomatic AF in lieu of catheter ablation. In these instances, clinical decisions should be made based on the individual institution's experience with catheter and surgical ablation, the relative outcomes and risks of each in the individual patient, and patient preference. Programs involved in the surgical treatment of AF should develop a team approach to these patients, including both electrophysiologists and surgeons, to ensure appropriate selection of patients.

There are relative indications for surgery that were not included in the consensus statement. The first is a contraindication to long-term anticoagulation in patients with persistent AF and a high risk for stroke (CHADS score ≥ 2). Up to one-third of patients with AF screened for participation in clinical trials of warfarin were deemed ineligible for chronic anticoagulation, mainly because of a high perceived risk for bleeding complications.[112-114] In one study, the annual rate of intracranial hemorrhage in anticoagulated patients with AF was 0.9% per year, and the overall major bleeding complication rate was 2.3% per year.[114] The stroke rate following the Cox-Maze procedure off anticoagulation has been remarkably low, even in high-risk patients. At our institution, only 5 of 450 patients had a stroke after a mean follow-up of 6.9 ± 5.1 years. There was no difference in stroke rate in those patients with CHADS scores above or below 2.[115] This low risk of stroke after the Cox-Maze procedure has been noted in other series.[19,116,117] The decrease in stroke risk is likely due to the high cure rate, as well as the obliteration of the left atrial appendage. Surgical treatment for AF with amputation of the left atrial appendage also should be considered in patients with chronic AF who have suffered a cerebrovascular accident despite adequate anticoagulation, as these patients are at high risk for repeat neurologic events.

HYBRID ABLATIONS

Although the Cox-Maze procedure achieves high rates of success and recent technological advances have made it easier to perform through less invasive incisions, it still requires cardiopulmonary bypass. Several groups have started performing epicardial ablations with the aid of suction based RF and cryoablation probes, which can be placed through thoracoscopic ports. However, these probes do not achieve the same degree of transmurality achieved with bipolar probes.[118] This led to the idea of combining both endocardial ablation via transcatheter techniques and epicardial ablation via surgical techniques in a "hybrid" approach.

Though specific lesion sets and approaches vary greatly from institution to institution, early results are promising.[119,120] In one study, 78 consecutive patients underwent thoracoscopic hybrid ablation and 74% were free of AF off antiarrhythmic drugs without further ablations at 24 months follow-up.[121] Another group utilized a similar lesion set via a pericardioscopic hybrid approach in 101 consecutive patients, and demonstrated a freedom from AF in 66% at one year.[122] However, with increasing data on these newer procedures, important safety concerns including high rates of conversion to sternotomy and reoperation for bleeding have been reported.[123]

Though new minimally invasive and hybrid techniques have yet to be standardized, they hold promise and require continued clinical investigation to determine their precise role.

FUTURE DIRECTIONS IN AF SURGERY

The ideal surgical procedure for AF would be a minimally invasive operation that does not require cardiopulmonary bypass. Such a procedure should preserve normal atrial physiology, have minimal morbidity, and a have a high success rate. Achieving this goal will require progress in understanding the mechanism of AF in individual patients, and tailoring of treatment approaches. The surgical approach may need to be redesigned based on a better understanding of the mechanisms and the effects of surgical ablation on atrial electrophysiology.

It is now known that there are multiple different possible mechanisms of AF. Multipoint mapping is necessary to describe this complex arrhythmia.[98,100,101,124,125] Epicardial activation sequence mapping has been the traditional gold standard for mapping of AF, but is both invasive and time consuming, limiting its clinical use.[18] A newer noninvasive technique, electrocardiographic imaging (ECGI), offers a potentially useful way to describe the atrial activation sequence and determine mechanistic information from conscious patients.[126] The technique uses body surface potentials, measured by surface electrodes, and anatomical data obtained through computed tomographic scanning to indirectly calculate the surface potentials on the surface of the heart. This technique has been shown to work well for normal sinus rhythm and atrial flutter as well as ventricular arrhythmias.[127-130] This modality has also been tested in a variety of patient populations including patients with heart failure undergoing biventricular pacing therapy or heart transplant,[131] patients with different substrates of AF,[132] and patients undergoing open-heart surgery.[133] In one particular study, 26 patients with AF underwent ECGI. AF complexity (including number of wavelets, focal sites, and rotor activity)

increased with longer clinical history of AF, although the degree of complexity of nonparoxysmal AF varied widely. This highlights the coexistence of a variety of mechanisms and variable complexity among patients, which could be targeted by patient-specific ablation approaches.[132] Currently our group is testing the technique in patients with AF and mitral valve disease, with a goal of further identifying the mechanisms of AF in this population.

The information acquired from ECGI can be analyzed to determine activation sequence and frequency maps for individual patients noninvasively. Using these data, a strategy for designing patient-specific optimal lesion sets is being developed, taking into account the patient's atrial geometry, conduction velocity, and refractory period.[132,134] Previous work has demonstrated that a critical mass is necessary to maintain AF, and initial lesions could be determined by a calculation of the critical area needed to maintain AF in the individual patient.[135] This could be done using mechanistic information derived from activation data and anatomical data from a CT scan. It will also allow identification of focal sources that can then be either isolated or ablated in the electrophysiologic laboratory or operating room.

In instances in which a specific mechanism of AF cannot be defined, the goal will be to create a lesion pattern that will make the atria unable to fibrillate. Failures of the Cox-Maze III and IV procedures have been seen in patients with increasing left atrial size or long-standing AF.[116,135,136] A study performed by our laboratory on a canine model found that the probability of maintaining AF is correlated with increasing atrial tissue areas, widths, and weights, as well as the length of the effective refractory period and the conduction velocity of the tissue.[134] All of these data can be acquired noninvasively through magnetic resonance imaging scans and ECGI. Using these data may allow surgeons to design custom operations for each patient based on the mechanism of their arrhythmia and their specific atrial anatomy or electrophysiology.

Finally, the limitations of present ablation devices have impeded the development of a truly minimally invasive procedure. Unfortunately, the creation of reliable transmural lines of ablation on the beating heart has been difficult. This has been because of the heat sink of the circulating endocardial blood pool.[42] Future advances may be anticipated with devices that overcome this limitation, but the introduction of hybrid procedures in which surgeons and electrophysiologists work together to complete lines of block with avoiding cardiopulmonary bypass may also circumvent this issue and have shown early promise.

In conclusion, the development of ablation technologies has dramatically changed the field of AF surgery. The replacement of the surgical incisions with linear lines of ablation has transformed a complex, technically demanding procedure into one accessible to the majority of surgeons. More importantly, these new ablation technologies have introduced minimally invasive surgery for AF, prompting efforts to develop simpler procedures that can be performed epicardially on the beating heart. However, surgeons must remember that the

Cox-Maze procedure has excellent efficacy in these patients and can be performed using a small thoracotomy with low morbidity.[95] It is imperative for surgeons trying new procedures to carefully follow their results and publish them in peer-reviewed journals. For surgeons performing AF ablation, it is mandatory to adhere to the recently published guidelines for follow-up of patients and for determining success or failure after these procedures.[111] As we learn more about the mechanisms of AF and develop improved preoperative diagnostic technologies capable of precisely identifying mechanisms, it may become possible to tailor specific lesion sets and ablation modalities to individual patients, making the surgical treatment of AF more effective and available to an even larger population of patients.

REFERENCES

1. Andrade J, Khairy P, Dobrev D, Nattel S: The clinical profile and pathophysiology of atrial fibrillation: relationships among clinical features, epidemiology, and mechanisms. *Circ Res* 2014; 114:1453-1468.
2. Wolf PA, Benjamin EJ, Belanger AJ, Kannel WB, Levy D, D'Agostino RB: Secular trends in the prevalence of atrial fibrillation: The Framingham Study. *Am Heart J* 1996; 131:790-795.
3. Wolf PA, Abbott RD, Kannel WB: Atrial fibrillation as an independent risk factor for stroke: the Framingham Study. *Stroke; J Cerebral Circ* 1991; 22:983-988.
4. Wolf PA, Abbott RD, Kannel WB: Atrial fibrillation: a major contributor to stroke in the elderly. The Framingham Study. *Arch Intern Med* 1987; 147:1561-1564.
5. Steger C, Pratter A, Martinek-Bregel M, et al: Stroke patients with atrial fibrillation have a worse prognosis than patients without: data from the Austrian Stroke registry. *Eur Heart J* 2004; 25:1734-1740.
6. Sherman DG, Kim SG, Boop BS, National Heart, Lung and Blood Institute AFFIRM Investigators et al: Occurrence and characteristics of stroke events in the Atrial Fibrillation Follow-up Investigation of Sinus Rhythm Management (AFFIRM) study. *Arch Intern Med* 2005; 165:1185-1191.
7. Hart RG, Halperin JL, Pearce LA, and Stroke Prevention in Atrial Fibrillation I et al: Lessons from the Stroke Prevention in Atrial Fibrillation trials. *Ann Intern Med* 2003; 138:831-838.
8. Glader EL, Stegmayr B, Norrving B, et al: Large variations in the use of oral anticoagulants in stroke patients with atrial fibrillation: a Swedish national perspective. *J Intern Med* 2004; 255:22-32.
9. Cairns JA: Stroke prevention in atrial fibrillation trial. *Circulation* 1991; 84:933-935.
10. Benjamin EJ, Levy D, Vaziri SM, D'Agostino RB, Belanger AJ, Wolf PA: Independent risk factors for atrial fibrillation in a population-based cohort. The Framingham Heart Study. *JAMA* 1994; 271:840-844.
11. Laupacis A, Boysen G, Connolly S, et al: Risk factors for stroke and efficacy of antithrombotic therapy in atrial fibrillation. Analysis of pooled data from five randomized controlled trials. *Arch Intern Med* 1994; 154:1449-1457.
12. Williams JM, Ungerleider RM, Lofland GK, Cox JL: Left atrial isolation: new technique for the treatment of supraventricular arrhythmias. *J Thorac Cardiovasc Surg* 1980; 80:373-380.
13. Scheinman MM, Morady F, Hess DS, Gonzalez R: Catheter-induced ablation of the atrioventricular junction to control refractory supraventricular arrhythmias. *JAMA* 1982; 248:851-855.
14. Guiraudon G, Campbell CS, Jones DL: Combined sinoatrial node atrioventricular node isolation: a surgical alternative to His bundle ablation in patients with atrial fibrillation. *Circulation* 1985; 72.
15. Smith PK, Holman WL, Cox JL: Surgical treatment of supraventricular tachyarrhythmias. *Surg Clin North Am* 1985; 65:553-570.
16. Cox JL, Schuessler RB, D'Agostino HJ, Jr, et al: The surgical treatment of atrial fibrillation. III. Development of a definitive surgical procedure. *J Thorac Cardiovasc Surg* 1991; 101:569-583.
17. Cox JL: The surgical treatment of atrial fibrillation. IV. Surgical technique. *J Thorac Cardiovasc Surg* 1991; 101:584-592.
18. Cox JL, Canavan TE, Schuessler RB, et al: The surgical treatment of atrial fibrillation. II. Intraoperative electrophysiologic mapping and description of the electrophysiologic basis of atrial flutter and atrial fibrillation. *J Thorac Cardiovasc Surg* 1991; 101:406-426.
19. Cox JL, Ad N, Palazzo T: Impact of the maze procedure on the stroke rate in patients with atrial fibrillation. *J Thorac Cardiovasc Surg* 1999; 118:833-840.
20. Feinberg MS, Waggoner AD, Kater KM, Cox JL, Lindsay BD, Perez JE: Restoration of atrial function after the maze procedure for patients with atrial fibrillation. Assessment by Doppler echocardiography. *Circulation* 1994; 90:II285-II292.
21. Cox JL, Boineau JP, Schuessler RB, Jaquiss RD, Lappas DG: Modification of the maze procedure for atrial flutter and atrial fibrillation. I. Rationale and surgical results. *J Thorac Cardiovasc Surg* 1995; 110:473-484.
22. Cox JL: The minimally invasive Maze-III procedure. *Op Techn Thorac Cardiovasc Surg* 2000; 5.
23. Prasad SM, Maniar HS, Camillo CJ, et al: The Cox Maze III procedure for atrial fibrillation: long-term efficacy in patients undergoing lone versus concomitant procedures. *J Thorac Cardiovasc Surg* 2003; 126:1822-1828.
24. McCarthy PM, Gillinov AM, Castle L, Chung M, Cosgrove D, 3rd: The Cox-Maze procedure: the Cleveland Clinic experience. *Semin Thorac Cardiovasc Surg* 2000; 12:25-29.
25. Raanani E, Albage A, David TE, Yau TM, Armstrong S: The efficacy of the Cox/Maze procedure combined with mitral valve surgery: a matched control study. *Eur J Cardiothorac Surg* 2001; 19:438-442.
26. Schaff HV, Dearani JA, Daly RC, Orszulak TA, Danielson GK: Cox-Maze procedure for atrial fibrillation: Mayo Clinic experience. *Semin Thorac Cardiovasc Surg* 2000; 12:30-37.
27. Gammie JS, Haddad M, Milford-Beland S, et al: Atrial fibrillation correction surgery: lessons from the Society of Thoracic Surgeons National Cardiac Database. *Ann Thorac Surg* 2008; 85:909-914.
28. Inoue H, Zipes DP: Conduction over an isthmus of atrial myocardium in vivo: a possible model of Wolff-Parkinson-White syndrome. *Circulation* 1987; 76:637-647.
29. Ishii Y, Nitta T, Sakamoto S, Tanaka S, Asano G: Incisional atrial reentrant tachycardia: experimental study on the conduction property through the isthmus. *J Thorac Cardiovasc Surg* 2003; 126:254-262.
30. Melby SJ, Lee AM, Zierer A, et al: Atrial fibrillation propagates through gaps in ablation lines: implications for ablative treatment of atrial fibrillation. *Heart Rhythm* 2008; 5:1296-1301.
31. Melby SJ, Lee AM, Damiano RJ Jr.: *Advances in surgical ablation devices for atrial fibrillation.* Boston: Blackwell Futura; 2005.
32. Gage AM, Montes M, Gage AA: Freezing the canine thoracic aorta in situ. *J Surg Res* 1979; 27:331-340.
33. Holman WL, Ikeshita M, Ungerleider RM, Smith PK, Ideker RE, Cox JL: Cryosurgery for cardiac arrhythmias: acute and chronic effects on coronary arteries. *Am J Cardiol* 1983; 51:149-155.
34. Watanabe H, Hayashi J, Aizawa Y: Myocardial infarction after cryoablation surgery for Wolff-Parkinson-White syndrome. *Jpn J Thorac Cardiovasc Surg: Official Publication of the Japanese Association for Thoracic Surgery—Nihon Kyobu Geka Gakkai zasshi* 2002; 50:210-212.
35. Manasse E, Colombo P, Roncalli M, Gallotti R: Myocardial acute and chronic histological modifications induced by cryoablation. *Eur J Cardiothorac Surg* 2000; 17:339-340.
36. Aupperle H, Doll N, Walther T, et al: Ablation of atrial fibrillation and esophageal injury: effects of energy source and ablation technique. *J Thorac Cardiovasc Surg* 2005; 130:1549-1554.
37. Viola N, Williams MR, Oz MC, Ad N: The technology in use for the surgical ablation of atrial fibrillation. *Semin Thorac Cardiovasc Surg* 2002; 14:198-205.
38. Santiago T, Melo JQ, Gouveia RH, Martins AP: Intra-atrial temperatures in radiofrequency endocardial ablation: histologic evaluation of lesions. *Ann Thorac Surg* 2003; 75:1495-1501.
39. Thomas SP, Guy DJ, Boyd AC, Eipper VE, Ross DL, Chard RB: Comparison of epicardial and endocardial linear ablation using handheld probes. *Ann Thorac Surg* 2003; 75:543-548.
40. Hoenicke EM, Strange RG, Patel H, et al: Initial experience with epicardial radiofrequency ablation catheter in an ovine model: moving towards an endoscopic Maze procedure. *Surg Forum* 2000; 51:79-82.
41. Santiago T, Melo J, Gouveia RH, et al: Epicardial radiofrequency applications: in vitro and in vivo studies on human atrial myocardium. *Eur J Cardiothorac Surg* 2003; 24:481-486; discussion 486.
42. Melby SJ, Zierer A, Kaiser SP, Schuessler RB, Damiano RJ, Jr: Epicardial microwave ablation on the beating heart for atrial fibrillation: the

dependency of lesion depth on cardiac output. *J Thorac Cardiovasc Surg* 2006; 132:355-360.

43. Gaynor SL, Diodato MD, Prasad SM, et al: A prospective, single-center clinical trial of a modified Cox maze procedure with bipolar radiofrequency ablation. *J Thorac Cardiovasc Surg* 2004; 128:535-542.

44. Prasad SM, Maniar HS, Diodato MD, Schuessler RB, Damiano RJ, Jr: Physiological consequences of bipolar radiofrequency energy on the atria and pulmonary veins: a chronic animal study. *Ann Thorac Surg* 2003; 76:836-841; discussion 841-842.

45. Prasad SM, Maniar HS, Schuessler RB, Damiano RJ, Jr: Chronic transmural atrial ablation by using bipolar radiofrequency energy on the beating heart. *J Thorac Cardiovasc Surg* 2002; 124:708-713.

46. Demaria RG, Page P, Leung TK, et al: Surgical radiofrequency ablation induces coronary endothelial dysfunction in porcine coronary arteries. *Eur J Cardiothorac Surg* 2003; 23:277-282.

47. Gillinov AM, Pettersson G, Rice TW: Esophageal injury during radiofrequency ablation for atrial fibrillation. *J Thorac Cardiovasc Surg* 2001; 122:1239-1240.

48. Kottkamp H, Hindricks G, Autschbach R, et al: Specific linear left atrial lesions in atrial fibrillation: intraoperative radiofrequency ablation using minimally invasive surgical techniques. *J Am Coll Cardiol* 2002; 40:475-480.

49. Laczkovics A, Khargi K, Deneke T: Esophageal perforation during left atrial radiofrequency ablation. *J Thorac Cardiovasc Surg* 2003; 126:2119-2120; author reply 2120.

50. Saint LL, Lawrance CP, Okada S, et al: Performance of a novel bipolar/monopolar radiofrequency ablation device on the beating heart in an acute porcine model. *Innovations* 2013; 8:276-283.

51. Groh MA, Binns OA, Burton HG, 3rd, Champsaur GL, Ely SW, Johnson AM: Epicardial ultrasonic ablation of atrial fibrillation during concomitant cardiac surgery is a valid option in patients with ischemic heart disease. *Circulation* 2008; 118:S78-S82.

52. Klinkenberg TJ, Ahmed S, Ten Hagen A, et al: Feasibility and outcome of epicardial pulmonary vein isolation for lone atrial fibrillation using minimal invasive surgery and high intensity focused ultrasound. *Europace: Eur Pacing, Arrhythmias, Cardiac Electrophysiol: Journal of the Working Groups on Cardiac Pacing, Arrhythmias, and Cardiac Cellular Electrophysiology of the European Society of Cardiology* 2009; 11:1624-1631.

53. Mitnovetski S, Almeida AA, Goldstein J, Pick AW, Smith JA: Epicardial high-intensity focused ultrasound cardiac ablation for surgical treatment of atrial fibrillation. *Heart, Lung Circul* 2009; 18:28-31.

54. Nakagawa H, Antz M, Wong T, et al: Initial experience using a forward directed, high-intensity focused ultrasound balloon catheter for pulmonary vein antrum isolation in patients with atrial fibrillation. *J Cardiovasc Electrophysiol* 2007; 18:136-144.

55. Ninet J, Roques X, Seitelberger R, et al: Surgical ablation of atrial fibrillation with off-pump, epicardial, high-intensity focused ultrasound: results of a multicenter trial. *J Thorac Cardiovasc Surg* 2005; 130:803-809.

56. Damiano Jr RJ GS: Atrial fibrillation ablation during mitral valve surgery using the AtriCure device. *Op Techn Thorac Cardiovasc Surg* 2004; 9:24-33.

57. Mokadam NA, McCarthy PM, Gillinov AM, et al: A prospective multicenter trial of bipolar radiofrequency ablation for atrial fibrillation: early results. *Ann Thorac Surg* 2004; 78:1665-1670.

58. Lall SC, Melby SJ, Voeller RK, et al: The effect of ablation technology on surgical outcomes after the Cox-maze procedure: a propensity analysis. *J Thorac Cardiovasc Surg* 2007; 133:389-396.

59. Voeller RK, Bailey MS, Zierer A, et al: Isolating the entire posterior left atrium improves surgical outcomes after the Cox maze procedure. *J Thorac Cardiovasc Surg* 2008; 135:870-877.

60. Sie HT, Beukema WP, Misier AR, et al: Radiofrequency modified maze in patients with atrial fibrillation undergoing concomitant cardiac surgery. *J Thorac Cardiovasc Surg* 2001; 122:249-256.

61. Schuetz A, Schulze CJ, Sarvanakis KK, et al: Surgical treatment of permanent atrial fibrillation using microwave energy ablation: a prospective randomized clinical trial. *Eur J Cardiothorac Surg* 2003; 24:475-480; discussion 480.

62. Kondo N, Takahashi K, Minakawa M, Daitoku K: Left atrial maze procedure: a useful addition to other corrective operations. *Ann Thorac Surg* 2003; 75:1490-1494.

63. Knaut M, Spitzer SG, Karolyi L, et al: Intraoperative microwave ablation for curative treatment of atrial fibrillation in open heart surgery—the MICRO-STAF and MICRO-PASS pilot trial. MICROwave Application

in Surgical treatment of Atrial Fibrillation. MICROwave Application for the Treatment of Atrial Fibrillation in Bypass-Surgery. *Thorac Cardiovasc Surgeon* 1999; 47 Suppl 3:379-384.

64. Imai K, Sueda T, Orihashi K, Watari M, Matsuura Y: Clinical analysis of results of a simple left atrial procedure for chronic atrial fibrillation. *Ann Thorac Surg* 2001; 71:577-581.

65. Gaita F, Riccardi R, Caponi D, et al: Linear cryoablation of the left atrium versus pulmonary vein cryoisolation in patients with permanent atrial fibrillation and valvular heart disease: correlation of electroanatomic mapping and long-term clinical results. *Circulation* 2005; 111:136-142.

66. Fasol R, Meinhart J, Binder T: A modified and simplified radiofrequency ablation in patients with mitral valve disease. *J Thorac Cardiovasc Surg* 2005; 129:215-217.

67. Benussi S, Nascimbene S, Agricola E, et al: Surgical ablation of atrial fibrillation using the epicardial radiofrequency approach: mid-term results and risk analysis. *Ann Thorac Surg* 2002; 74:1050-1056; discussion 1057.

68. Gillinov AM, McCarthy PM, Blackstone EH, et al: Surgical ablation of atrial fibrillation with bipolar radiofrequency as the primary modality. *J Thorac Cardiovasc Surg* 2005; 129:1322-1329.

69. Haissaguerre M, Jais P, Shah DC, et al: Spontaneous initiation of atrial fibrillation by ectopic beats originating in the pulmonary veins. *New Engl J Med* 1998; 339:659-666.

70. Lee SH, Tai CT, Hsieh MH, et al: Predictors of non-pulmonary vein ectopic beats initiating paroxysmal atrial fibrillation: implication for catheter ablation. *J Am Coll Cardiol* 2005; 46:1054-1059.

71. Doll N, Pritzwald-Stegmann P, Czesla M, et al: Ablation of ganglionic plexi during combined surgery for atrial fibrillation. *Ann Thorac Surg* 2008; 86:1659-1663.

72. McClelland JH, Duke D, Reddy R: Preliminary results of a limited thoracotomy: new approach to treat atrial fibrillation. *J Cardiovasc Electrophysiol* 2007; 18:1289-1295.

73. Mehall JR, Kohut RM, Jr, Schneeberger EW, Taketani T, Merrill WH, Wolf RK: Intraoperative epicardial electrophysiologic mapping and isolation of autonomic ganglionic plexi. *Ann Thorac Surg* 2007; 83:538-541.

74. Geuzebroek GS, Ballaux PK, van Hemel NM, Kelder JC, Defauw JJ: Medium-term outcome of different surgical methods to cure atrial fibrillation: is less worse? *Interact Cardiovasc Thorac Surg* 2008; 7:201-216.

75. Reyes G, Benedicto A, Bustamante J, et al: Restoration of atrial contractility after surgical cryoablation: clinical, electrical and mechanical results. *Interact Cardiovasc Thorac Surg* 2009; 9:609-612.

76. Bisleri G, Rosati F, Bontempi L, Curnis A, Muneretto C: Hybrid approach for the treatment of long-standing persistent atrial fibrillation: electrophysiological findings and clinical results. *Eur J Cardiothorac Surg* 2013; 44:919-923.

77. Healey JS, Crystal E, Lamy A, et al: Left Atrial Appendage Occlusion Study (LAAOS): results of a randomized controlled pilot study of left atrial appendage occlusion during coronary bypass surgery in patients at risk for stroke. *Am Heart J* 2005; 150:288-293.

78. Salzberg SP, Gillinov AM, Anyanwu A, Castillo J, Filsoufi F, Adams DH: Surgical left atrial appendage occlusion: evaluation of a novel device with magnetic resonance imaging. *Eur J Cardiothorac Surg* 2008; 34:766-770.

79. Salzberg SP, Plass A, Emmert MY, et al: Left atrial appendage clip occlusion: early clinical results. *J Thorac Cardiovasc Surg* 2010; 139:1269-1274.

80. Arcidi JM, Jr, Doty DB, Millar RC: The Maze procedure: the LDS Hospital experience. *Semin Thorac Cardiovasc Surg* 2000; 12:38-43.

81. Weimar T, Bailey MS, Watanabe Y, et al: The Cox-maze IV procedure for lone atrial fibrillation: a single center experience in 100 consecutive patients. *J Intervent Cardiac Electrophysiol* 2011; 31:47-54.

82. Weimar T, Schena S, Bailey MS, et al: The cox-maze procedure for lone atrial fibrillation: a single-center experience over 2 decades. *Circ Arrhythm Electrophysiol* 2012; 5:8-14.

83. Aziz A, Bailey M, Patel A, et al: The type of atrial fibrillation does not influence late outcome following the Cox-Maze IV procedure. *Heart Rhythm* 2008; 5:S318.

84. Pet M, Robertson JO, Bailey M, et al: The impact of CHADS2 score on late stroke after the Cox maze procedure. *J Thorac Cardiovasc Surg* 2013; 146:85-89.

85. Stulak JM, Sundt TM, 3rd, Dearani JA, Daly RC, Orsulak TA, Schaff HV: Ten-year experience with the Cox-maze procedure for atrial fibrillation: how do we define success? *Ann Thorac Surg* 2007; 83:1319-1324.

86. Saint LL, Damiano RJ, Jr, Cuculich PS, et al: Incremental risk of the Cox-maze IV procedure for patients with atrial fibrillation undergoing mitral valve surgery. *J Thorac Cardiovasc Surg* 2013; 146:1072-1077.

87. Saint LL, Bailey MS, Prasad S, et al: Cox-Maze IV results for patients with lone atrial fibrillation versus concomitant mitral disease. *Ann Thorac Surg* 2012; 93:789-794; discussion 794-795.

88. Lawrance CP, Henn MC, Miller JR, Sinn LA, Schuessler RB, Damiano RJ, Jr: Comparison of the stand-alone Cox-Maze IV procedure to the concomitant Cox-Maze IV and mitral valve procedure for atrial fibrillation. *Ann Cardiothorac Surg* 2014; 3:55-61.

89. Damiano RJ, Jr, Gaynor SL, Bailey M, et al: The long-term outcome of patients with coronary disease and atrial fibrillation undergoing the Cox maze procedure. *J Thorac Cardiovasc Surg* 2003; 126:2016-2021.

90. Ad N, Holmes SD, Massimiano PS, Pritchard G, Stone LE, Henry L: The effect of the Cox-maze procedure for atrial fibrillation concomitant to mitral and tricuspid valve surgery. *J Thorac Cardiovasc Surg* 2013; 146:1426-1434; discussion 1434-1435.

91. Abreu Filho CA, Lisboa LA, Dallan LA, et al: Effectiveness of the maze procedure using cooled-tip radiofrequency ablation in patients with permanent atrial fibrillation and rheumatic mitral valve disease. *Circulation* 2005; 112:I20-I25.

92. Ad N, Henry L, Hunt S, Holmes SD: Do we increase the operative risk by adding the Cox Maze III procedure to aortic valve replacement and coronary artery bypass surgery? *J Thorac Cardiovasc Surg* 2012; 143:936-944.

93. Saint LL, Lawrance CP, Leidenfrost JE, Robertson JO, Damiano RJ, Jr: How I do it: minimally invasive Cox-Maze IV procedure. *Ann Cardiothorac Surg* 2014; 3:117-119.

94. Lee AM, Clark K, Bailey MS, Aziz A, Schuessler RB, Damiano RJ, Jr: A minimally invasive cox-maze procedure: operative technique and results. *Innovations* 2010; 5:281-286.

95. Lawrance CP, Henn MC, Miller JR, et al: A minimally invasive Cox maze IV procedure is as effective as sternotomy while decreasing major morbidity and hospital stay. *J Thorac Cardiovasc Surg* 2014; 148:955-961; discussion 962-962.

96. Phan K, Xie A, Tsai YC, Kumar N, La Meir M, Yan TD: Biatrial ablation vs. left atrial concomitant surgical ablation for treatment of atrial fibrillation: a meta-analysis. *Europace: Eur Pacing, Arrhythm Cardiac Electrophysiol: Journal of the Working Groups on Cardiac Pacing, Arrhythmias, and Cardiac Cellular Electrophysiology of the European Society of Cardiology* 2015; 17:38-47.

97. Barnett SD, Ad N: Surgical ablation as treatment for the elimination of atrial fibrillation: a meta-analysis. *J Thorac Cardiovasc Surg* 2006; 131:1029-1035.

98. Nitta T, Ishii Y, Miyagi Y, Ohmori H, Sakamoto S, Tanaka S: Concurrent multiple left atrial focal activations with fibrillatory conduction and right atrial focal or reentrant activation as the mechanism in atrial fibrillation. *J Thorac Cardiovasc Surg* 2004; 127:770-778.

99. Sahadevan J, Ryu K, Peltz L, et al: Epicardial mapping of chronic atrial fibrillation in patients: preliminary observations. *Circulation* 2004; 110:3293-3299.

100. Schuessler RB, Kay MW, Melby SJ, Branham BH, Boineau JP, Damiano RJ, Jr: Spatial and temporal stability of the dominant frequency of activation in human atrial fibrillation. *J Electrocardiol* 2006; 39:S7-S12.

101. Wolf RK, Schneeberger EW, Osterday R, et al: Video-assisted bilateral pulmonary vein isolation and left atrial appendage exclusion for atrial fibrillation. *J Thorac Cardiovasc Surg* 2005; 130:797-802.

102. Edgerton JR, Jackman WM, Mack MJ: Minimally invasive pulmonary vein isolation and partial autonomic denervation for surgical treatment of atrial fibrillation. *J Intervent Cardiac Electrophysiol: Int J Arrhythm Pacing* 2007; 20:89-93.

103. Han FT, Kasirajan V, Kowalski M, et al: Results of a minimally invasive surgical pulmonary vein isolation and ganglionic plexi ablation for atrial fibrillation: single-center experience with 12-month follow-up. *Circ Arrhythm Electrophysiol* 2009; 2:370-377.

104. Beyer E, Lee R, Lam BK: Point: Minimally invasive bipolar radiofrequency ablation of lone atrial fibrillation: early multicenter results. *J Thorac Cardiovasc Surg* 2009; 137:521-526.

105. Boersma LV, Castella M, van Boven W, et al: Atrial fibrillation catheter ablation versus surgical ablation treatment (FAST): a 2-center randomized clinical trial. *Circulation* 2012; 125:23-30.

106. Edgerton JR, Edgerton ZJ, Weaver T, et al: Minimally invasive pulmonary vein isolation and partial autonomic denervation for surgical

107. Zheng S, Li Y, Han J, et al: Long-term results of a minimally invasive surgical pulmonary vein isolation and ganglionic plexi ablation for atrial fibrillation. *PLoS One* 2013; 8:e79755.

108. Melby SJ, Zierer A, Bailey MS, et al: A new era in the surgical treatment of atrial fibrillation: the impact of ablation technology and lesion set on procedural efficacy. *Ann Surg* 2006; 244:583-592.

109. Tada H, Ito S, Naito S, et al: Long-term results of cryoablation with a new cryoprobe to eliminate chronic atrial fibrillation associated with mitral valve disease. *Pacing Clin Electrophysiol: PACE* 2005; 28 Suppl 1:S73-S77.

110. Henn MC, Lawrance CP, Sinn LA, et al: The effectiveness of surgical ablation in patients with atrial fibrillation and aortic valve disease. *Ann Thorac Surg* 2015.

111. Calkins H, Kuck KH, Cappato R, et al: Heart Rhythm Society Task Force on C and Surgical Ablation of Atrial F. 2012 HRS/EHRA/ECAS expert consensus statement on catheter and surgical ablation of atrial fibrillation: recommendations for patient selection, procedural techniques, patient management and follow-up, definitions, endpoints, and research trial design: a report of the Heart Rhythm Society (HRS) Task Force on Catheter and Surgical Ablation of Atrial Fibrillation. Developed in partnership with the European Heart Rhythm Association (EHRA), a registered branch of the European Society of Cardiology (ESC) and the European Cardiac Arrhythmia Society (ECAS); and in collaboration with the American College of Cardiology (ACC), American Heart Association (AHA), the Asia Pacific Heart Rhythm Society (APHRS), and the Society of Thoracic Surgeons (STS). Endorsed by the governing bodies of the American College of Cardiology Foundation, the American Heart Association, the European Cardiac Arrhythmia Society, the European Heart Rhythm Association, the Society of Thoracic Surgeons, the Asia Pacific Heart Rhythm Society, and the Heart Rhythm Society. *Heart Rhythm* 2012; 9:632-696 e21.

112. Stroke Prevention in Atrial Fibrillation Study. Final results. *Circulation* 1991; 84:527-539.

113. Rosand J, Eckman MH, Knudsen KA, Singer DE, Greenberg SM: The effect of warfarin and intensity of anticoagulation on outcome of intracerebral hemorrhage. *Arch Intern Med* 2004; 164:880-884.

114. Schaer GN, Koechli OR, Schuessler B, Haller U: Usefulness of ultrasound contrast medium in perineal sonography for visualization of bladder neck funneling—first observations. *Urology* 1996; 47:452-453.

115. Pet MA Damiano JR, Jr, Bailey MS, et al: Late stroke following the Cox-Maze procedure for atrial fibrillation: the impact of CHADS2 score on long-term outcomes. *Heart Rhythm* 2009; 6:S14.

116. Gillinov AM, Sirak J, Blackstone EH, et al: The Cox maze procedure in mitral valve disease: predictors of recurrent atrial fibrillation. *J Thorac Cardiovasc Surg* 2005; 130:1653-1660.

117. Ad N, Cox JL: The Maze procedure for the treatment of atrial fibrillation: a minimally invasive approach. *J Cardiac Surg* 2004; 19:196-200.

118. Schuessler RB, Lee AM, Melby SJ, et al: Animal studies of epicardial atrial ablation. *Heart Rhythm* 2009; 6:S41-S45.

119. Pison L, La Meir M, van Opstal J, et al: Hybrid thoracoscopic surgical and transvenous catheter ablation of atrial fibrillation. *J Am Coll Cardiol* 2012; 60:54-61.

120. Mahapatra S, LaPar DJ, Kamath S, et al: Initial experience of sequential surgical epicardial-catheter endocardial ablation for persistent and long-standing persistent atrial fibrillation with long-term follow-up. *Ann Thorac Surg* 2011; 91:1890-1898.

121. Pison L, Gelsomino S, Luca F, et al: Effectiveness and safety of simultaneous hybrid thoracoscopic and endocardial catheter ablation of lone atrial fibrillation. *Ann Cardiothorac Surg* 2014; 3:38-44.

122. Gehi AK, Mounsey JP, Pursell I, et al: Hybrid epicardial-endocardial ablation using a pericardioscopic technique for the treatment of atrial fibrillation. *Heart Rhythm* 2013; 10:22-28.

123. Je HG, Shuman DJ, Ad N: A systematic review of minimally invasive surgical treatment for atrial fibrillation: a comparison of the Cox-Maze procedure, beating-heart epicardial ablation, and the hybrid procedure on safety and efficacy dagger. *Eur J Cardiothoracic Surg* 2015.

124. Berenfeld O, Mandapati R, Dixit S, et al: Spatially distributed dominant excitation frequencies reveal hidden organization in atrial fibrillation in the Langendorff-perfused sheep heart. *J Cardiovasc Electrophysiol* 2000; 11:869-879.

125. Nattel S, Shiroshita-Takeshita A, Brundel BJ, Rivard L: Mechanisms of atrial fibrillation: lessons from animal models. *Progr Cardiovasc Dis* 2005; 48:9-28.

126. Ramanathan C, Ghanem RN, Jia P, Ryu K, Rudy Y: Noninvasive electrocardiographic imaging for cardiac electrophysiology and arrhythmia. *Nat Med* 2004; 10:422-428.

127. Wang Y, Schuessler RB, Damiano RJ, Woodard PK, Rudy Y: Noninvasive electrocardiographic imaging (ECGI) of scar-related atypical atrial flutter. *Heart Rhythm* 2007; 4:1565-1567.

128. Damiano RJ, Jr, Schuessler RB, Voeller RK: Surgical treatment of atrial fibrillation: a look into the future. *Semin Thorac Cardiovasc Surg* 2007; 19:39-45.

129. Ghanem RN, Jia P, Ramanathan C, Ryu K, Markowitz A, Rudy Y: Noninvasive electrocardiographic imaging (ECGI): comparison to intraoperative mapping in patients. *Heart Rhythm* 2005; 2:339-354.

130. Intini A, Goldstein RN, Jia P, et al: Electrocardiographic imaging (ECGI), a novel diagnostic modality used for mapping of focal left ventricular tachycardia in a young athlete. *Heart Rhythm* 2005; 2:1250-1252.

131. Desouza KA, Joseph SM, Cuculich PS, Ewald GA, Rudy Y: Noninvasive mapping of ventricular activation in patients with transplanted hearts. *J Electrocardiol* 2013; 46:698-701.

132. Cuculich PS, Wang Y, Lindsay BD, et al: Noninvasive characterization of epicardial activation in humans with diverse atrial fibrillation patterns. *Circulation* 2010; 122:1364-1372.

133. Ghosh S, Rhee EK, Avari JN, Woodard PK, Rudy Y: Cardiac memory in patients with Wolff-Parkinson-White syndrome: noninvasive imaging of activation and repolarization before and after catheter ablation. *Circulation* 2008; 118:907-915.

134. Byrd GD, Prasad SM, Ripplinger CM, et al: Importance of geometry and refractory period in sustaining atrial fibrillation: testing the critical mass hypothesis. *Circulation* 2005; 112:I7-I13.

135. Kosakai Y: Treatment of atrial fibrillation using the Maze procedure: the Japanese experience. *Semin Thorac Cardiovasc Surg* 2000; 12:44-52.

136. Gaynor SL, Schuessler RB, Bailey MS, et al: Surgical treatment of atrial fibrillation: predictors of late recurrence. *J Thorac Cardiovasc Surg* 2005; 129:104-111.

55

Surgical Implantation of Pacemakers and Automatic Defibrillators

Henry M. Spotnitz • Michelle D. Spotnitz

Pacemaker and defibrillator management is the subject of comprehensive reviews.[1-8] The efficacy and cost-effectiveness of pacemakers are widely accepted, but the appropriate role for ICD insertion[7] and biventricular pacing[5] in older patients is still in evolution. Pacemaker and ICD technology are now applicable across the entire span of human age. Pacing for heart failure and ICD prophylaxis against lethal arrhythmias are recent frontiers. Electrophysiologists dominate these areas, reflecting decreased interest by thoracic surgeons and cardiology referral patterns. However, thoracic surgeons must maintain skills as implanters in order to serve as consultants or surgeons for complex or complicated cases. This chapter reviews practical information related to pacemaker and ICD insertion and management.

A permanent pacemaker or ICD consists of leads and a generator.[2] The generator consists of a battery, a telemetry antenna, and integrated circuits. ICDs also include capacitors that store energy for high-output shocks. The power source is generally lithium iodide, but rechargeable and nuclear batteries have been used. The integrated circuits include programmable microprocessors, oscillators, amplifiers, and sensing circuits.[2] The integrated circuits employ complementary metal-oxide semiconductor (CMOS) technology, which is subject to damage by ionizing radiation. Current pacemakers and ICDs monitor and report the status of internal components, external connections, programmed settings, recent activity, and notable arrhythmias. Unfortunately, each programmer controls only the devices of its manufacturer.[4] Pacing systems compatible with magnetic resonance imaging (MRI)[2] and wireless ICDs and pacemakers are now available, and wireless telemetry is available for remote follow-up.[4]

PACEMAKERS FOR CONTROL OF BRADYCARDIA

History

Early cardiac surgery was complicated by lethal iatrogenic heart block. Transthoracic pacing with Zoll cutaneous electrodes provided an early solution. Percutaneous endocardial pacing (1959) and "permanent" pacemakers using epicardial electrodes (1960) followed.[9] Ensuing advances in bioengineering and technology have dramatically improved the quality of life for recipients. Persistent problems include lead durability, inflammatory responses to pacemaker materials, infection, device size, programmer compatibility, battery life, periodic battery replacement, and expense. *Cardiac resynchronization therapy* (CRT) for heart failure has made coronary sinus (CS) lead insertion an important technical skill.

Anatomy of Surgical Heart Block

The conduction system is vulnerable to injury during heart surgery. Complete heart block can result from suture placement during aortic, mitral, or tricuspid valve surgery, septal defect closure, or from myotomy for idiopathic hypertrophic subaortic stenosis. These lesions are mapped in Fig. 55-1. Infarction/abscess of the conduction system, inadequate myocardial protection, or trauma from retraction can also result in surgical heart block.

International Pacemaker Code

A three-letter code describes the principal pacemaker functions (Table 55-1).[10] The first letter is the chamber paced, the second the chamber sensed, and the third the algorithm integrating pacing and sensing functions. Fixed-rate ventricular and atrial pacemakers are VOO and AOO, respectively. Demand (rate-inhibited) pacers for the same chambers are VVI and AAI. VDD pacemakers pace only the ventricle but sense both atrium and ventricle. DVI indicates atrial and ventricular pacing, but only ventricular sensing. DDD is the most flexible of current designs. The suffix R after the three-letter code indicates rate responsiveness. Pacemakers capable of biventricular pacing or CRT are referred to as *CRT-P*. Biventricular pacemaker-defibrillators are called *CRT-D*.[8]

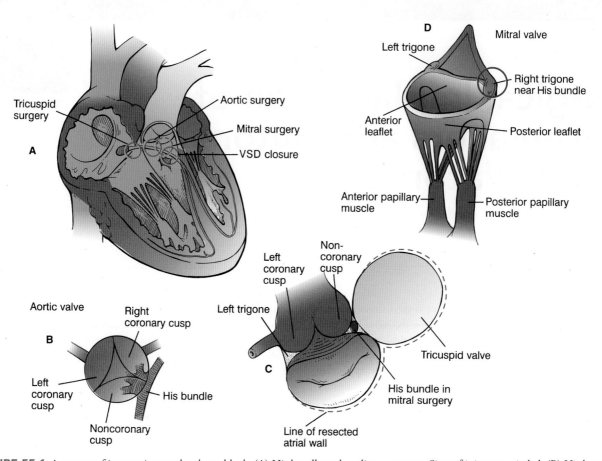

FIGURE 55-1 Anatomy of iatrogenic complete heart block. (A) His bundle and cardiac structures. Sites of injury are circled. (B) His bundle in the ventricular septum, below the noncoronary-right coronary aortic commissure. (C, D) During mitral surgery, the His bundle is on the ventricular septum anteromedial to the posterior commissure and right fibrous trigone. VSD = ventricular septal defect.

Cellular Electrophysiology

Cell membrane depolarization and repolarization provide automaticity of the cardiac chambers and conduction system. The outside of the resting myocardial cell is positive, and the interior is negative. Unipolar pacing threshold is lowest when the negative terminal (cathode) of a pacemaker is connected to the heart and the positive terminal (anode) is connected to ground. Electrogram amplitude is unaffected by polarity.[2]

Rhythm Disorders

INDICATIONS FOR PACEMAKER INSERTION

Pacemaker insertion guidelines (Table 55-2) are periodically updated. In 2008, an American College of Cardiology/American Heart Association/North American Society for Pacing and Electrophysiology (ACC/AHA/NASPE) task force revised recommendations for pacemaker and ICD insertion, further updated in 2013.[11] Any practitioner who implants arrhythmia control devices should be familiar with these guidelines. Documentation is required for billing and can be an important medical-legal issue.

Indication categories are "accepted (Class I)," "controversial (Class II)," or "not warranted (Class III)." Evidence from large randomized clinical trials is designated level A, from less stringent trials or registries, level B, and from consensus, level C. Profound sinus bradycardia or symptomatic second- or

TABLE 55-1: International Pacemaker Code

I Chamber paced	II Chamber sensed	III Pacing algorithm
A	A	T
V	V	I
D	D	D
O	O	O
S	S	—

A, atrium; D, dual (both triggered and inhibited); I, inhibited; O, none; S, single; T, triggered; V, ventricle.

TABLE 55-2: Medicare Guidelines for Cardiac Pacemaker Implantation (pre-2002)

Accepted, in symptomatic patients with chronic conditions
    Atrioventricular block
        Complete (third-degree)
        Incomplete (second-degree)
            Mobitz I
            Mobitz II
        Incomplete with 2:1 or 3:1 block
    Sinus node dysfunction (symptomatic)
        Sinus bradycardia, sinoatrial block, sinus arrest
        Bradycardia-tachycardia syndrome
Controversial
    In symptomatic patients
        Bifascicular/trifascicular intraventricular block
        Hypersensitive carotid sinus syndrome
    In asymptomatic patients
        Third-degree block
        Mobitz II
        Mobitz II atrioventricular block following myocardial
            infarction
        Congenital atrioventricular block
        Sinus bradycardia < 40 bpm with long-term necessary
            drug therapy
        Overdrive pacing for ventricular tachycardia
Not warranted
    Syncope of undetermined cause
    In asymptomatic patients
        Sinus bradycardia, sinoatrial block, or sinus arrest
        Bundle-branch blocks
        Mobitz I

Data from Epstein AE, DiMarco JP, Ellenbogen KA, et al: ACC/AHA/HRS 2008 Guidelines for Device-Based Therapy of Cardiac Rhythm Abnormalities: a report of the American College of Cardiology/American Heart Association Task Force on Practice Guidelines (Writing Committee to Revise the ACC/AHA/ NASPE 2002 Guideline Update for Implantation of Cardiac Pacemakers and Antiarrhythmia Devices): developed in collaboration with the American Association for Thoracic Surgery and Society of Thoracic Surgeons, *Circulation.* 2008 May 27;117(21):e350-e408.

third-degree heart block indicates pacemaker insertion. Sinus bradycardia justifies pacemaker insertion if simultaneous symptoms are documented by Holter or other means. Pacemakers may be appropriate for bradycardia less than 40 bpm if long-term drug therapy is necessary for supraventricular arrhythmias, ventricular tachycardia (VT), hypertension, or angina. Although new indications for arrhythmia control devices may be supported by clinical research, certification of advances by the Food and Drug Administration, insurance carriers, and regulatory agencies is often slow. Electrophysiology (EP) studies help define proper treatment.[3,11]

ATRIOVENTRICULAR BLOCK

First-degree block is prolongation of the P-R interval beyond 200 ms. First-degree block at a low atrial rate may progress to Wenckebach as the atrial rate increases. Second-degree block is incomplete dissociation of the atrial and ventricular rates, either with increasing P-R intervals and dropped beats (Wenckebach and Mobitz I, usually atrioventricular (AV) nodal block), or frequently dropped beats without progression of the P-R interval (Mobitz II, usually in the His-Purkinje system).[3] Third-degree block is complete AV dissociation, the atrial rate usually exceeding the ventricular rate. Left and right bundle-branch blocks and left anterior and posterior hemiblocks are partial conduction system blocks detected by electrocardiogram (ECG). Etiologies of AV block include ischemic injury, idiopathic fibrosis, cardiomyopathy, iatrogenic injury, AV node ablation, Lyme disease, abscess in bacterial endocarditis, and congenital lesions related to maternal lupus erythematosus and other autoimmune diseases.[3]

SINUS NODE DYSFUNCTION

Sinus node dysfunction is an intrinsic disease that can be accentuated by drugs required for ancillary conditions. The role for pacing depends on symptoms. Sinus node dysfunction is caused by coronary artery disease, cardiomyopathy, and reflex abnormalities.[3]

Reflex problems include carotid sinus hypersensitivity, vasovagal syncope, and oddities including micturition-induced and deglutition syncope. Cardioinhibitory (asystole >3 seconds) and vasodepressor (marked fall in blood pressure despite adequate heart rate) components of reflex-mediated syncope are recognized. Medical therapy is favored for vasodepressor syncope. Tilt table testing provides objective data.[3,12,13] Decisions on pacemaker insertion are based on symptoms and the duration of asystole. Pacemaker insertion is recommended for asystolic intervals greater than 3 seconds. Dual-chamber pacing (DDD or VDD) is favored for these patients, because AV synchrony increases stroke volume and decreases symptoms.[3,14]

Features of Permanent Pacing

DUAL-CHAMBER PACING AND ATRIOVENTRICULAR SYNCHRONY

In the normal heart, stroke volume is increased 5 to 15% by AV synchrony versus asynchrony.[8,14] Left ventricular hypertrophy, decreased diastolic compliance, and heart failure increase the quantitative importance of AV synchrony.[8,14] Pacing of the right ventricular apex disrupts the normal sequence of activation because depolarization spreads more slowly over the ventricular myocardium than through the conduction system.[8,14]

Recent experience emphasizes clinical relevance of the sequence of activation. Right ventricular outflow tract pacing may improve stroke volume versus apical pacing because of favorable effects on the activation sequence.[15] Disruption of activation sequence by DDD pacing reduces the ventricular-aortic gradient in some patients with idiopathic hypertrophic subaortic stenosis.[16,17] Biventricular (right ventricle [RV] apex and CS) pacing in patients with advanced cardiomyopathy and an intraventricular conduction defect improves left ventricular function by restoring simultaneous contraction of the septum and free wall, also known as cardiac resynchronization therapy (CRT).[5,18] Single-site, epicardial left ventricular pacing may provide similar benefits.[18] For temporary pacing in postoperative heart block, biventricular pacing is superior to right ventricular pacing[18] and may be useful for left ventricular dysfunction after cardiac surgery. Clinical trials suggest that biventricular pacing is superior to standard pacing for heart block.[8]

DUAL-CHAMBER PACING ALGORITHM

DDD pacemaker programming includes a lower rate, an upper rate, and AV delay. When the intrinsic atrial rate is between the upper and lower rate limits, the pacemaker tracks the atrium to maintain a 1:1 response between the right atrium and right ventricle. If the atrial rate falls to or below the lower rate limit, the atrium is paced at the lower rate limit. If the atrial rate exceeds the upper rate limit, the ventricle is paced at the upper rate limit with loss of AV synchrony, resembling a Wenckebach effect. If the patient develops atrial fibrillation, mode switching converts the pacing algorithm to VVI or VVI(R) at the lower rate limit.

Programmable AV delay defines the interval allowed between atrial and ventricular depolarization. Timing starts with the atrial electrogram or pacing stimulus and continues until the AV delay elapses. If no ventricular depolarization is detected during the delay, the ventricle is paced. *Atrial latency*, a varying delay between the atrial pacing artifact and the P wave, requires different AV delays for atrial sensing versus pacing.[4]

RATE RESPONSE TO INCREASED METABOLIC DEMAND

During high metabolic demand, cardiac output is augmented by increased ventricular contractility, venous return, and heart rate. In patients with heart block and a normal sinus exercise response, dual-chamber pacing maintains both AV synchrony and a physiologic rate response.[8] However, sinus node incompetence (no atrial rate increase with exercise) or single-chamber ventricular (VVI) pacemakers require alternate mechanisms for rate response. The letter R after the three-letter pacemaker code indicates rate responsive capability. If a sensor detects increased metabolic demand, the lower rate of the pacemaker increases within a programmable range. Body vibration or respiratory rate[8,19,20] is commonly employed to estimate demand. Other indicators are body temperature, venous oxygen saturation, QT interval, right ventricular systolic pressure, and right ventricular stroke volume. All such indicators can aberrantly increase heart rate, for example, during a bumpy car ride. Patients with sedentary life styles do not benefit from rate-responsive pacing. Adverse results of fast heart rates can include angina or infarction in patients with coronary disease.

CHOICE OF PACING TECHNIQUE

Dual-chamber pacing has become the standard of care, except in chronic atrial fibrillation. Sinus rhythm appears to be better maintained by atrial than ventricular pacing, and paroxysmal atrial fibrillation, previously problematic for DDD pacemakers, is now well handled by mode switching. Advantages of dual-chamber pacing in reflex-mediated syncope with cardioinhibitory features have also been reported. Dual-chamber pacing may not be warranted in elderly patients, except when pacemaker syndrome, hypertension, or congestive heart failure is present. VVI or VVIR pacing is appropriate for patients with bradycardia and chronic atrial fibrillation. AAIR is useful for cardiac allograft recipients with sinus arrest or sinus bradycardia. Biventricular pacing using an endocardial CS lead is recommended for symptomatic heart failure.[8]

Pacemaker Technology

EPICARDIAL VERSUS ENDOCARDIAL LEADS

Epicardial leads are generally inferior to endocardial leads in electrical characteristics and are prone to conductor fractures.[2] Steroid-eluting tips and small contact surfaces have improved epicardial leads. Epicardial pacing is more difficult at reoperative cardiac surgery, where epicardial fibrosis elevates pacing thresholds. Infected epicardial leads must be removed by thoracotomy. The epicardial approach is preferred in patients with congenital septal defects, single ventricle physiology, mechanical tricuspid valves, or venous thrombosis/occlusion.[21] During thoracotomy, insertion of endocardial leads through an atrial pursestring is a useful option.[22] Epicardial left ventricular pacing by the minimal access approach is increasing in importance, driven by a 5 to 10% technical failure rate for CS lead insertion. Approaches to DDD pacing during open-heart surgery are illustrated in Fig. 55-2. Fixed-screw, positive fixation leads are introduced via atrial pursestrings and fixed into position by axial rotation. When a tricuspid prosthesis or ring is to be inserted, a ventricular lead can be passed between the sutures securing the ring or the valve.

UNIPOLAR VERSUS BIPOLAR

Bipolar leads incorporate two insulated conductors. In unipolar systems, the patient's body is the second (anodal) conductor; a single conductor in the lead carries the negative current to the heart. Bipolar leads reduce electrical noise (oversensing) and adventitious pacing of the diaphragm or chest wall. These advantages are offset by increased engineering complexity. Bipolar leads historically were prone to breakdown of insulation or conductor fracture. This would compromise sensing, pacing, or both (Fig. 55-3). Recent bipolar leads are much improved and similar in dimensions and handling to unipolar leads (Figs. 55-4 and 55-5).[2] Technical failures of some new technology pacemaker and ICD leads emphasize the importance of advanced lead extraction.[6]

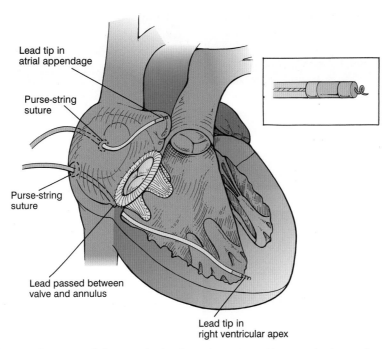

FIGURE 55-2 Endocardial pacing from epicardial approach. Atrial pursestrings provide access; leads are advanced and screwed into position guided by manual palpation. The ventricular lead is passed between the valve prosthesis and the annulus. The inset shows the tip of the endocardial screw-in lead. The coronary sinus os is also accessible.

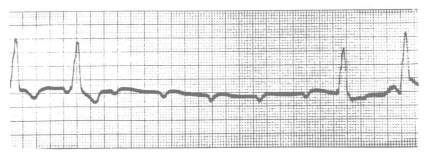

FIGURE 55-3 Telemetry from a patient with third-degree block, poor escape rhythm, a bipolar VVI pacemaker, and dizzy spells. Programming to VOO mode eliminated the pauses. The patient was discharged after lead replacement. This illustrates a life-threatening effect of oversensing. This older model pacemaker was not capable of monitoring electrograms to confirm the diagnosis.

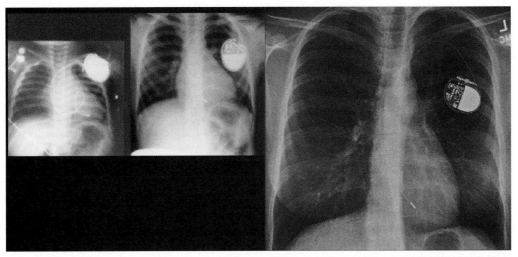

FIGURE 55-4 Positive fixation lead in x-rays demonstrating effects of growth on an intracardiac lead loop from age 1 (*left*) to age 5 (*center*) to age 14 (*right*) years.

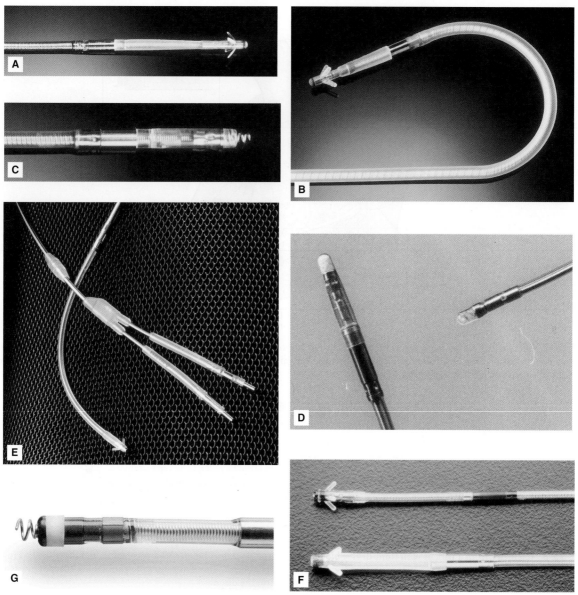

FIGURE 55-5 (A) Bipolar tined ventricular pacing lead with steroid-eluting tip. (B) Similar to (A), with J shape for atrial pacing. (C) Bisping bipolar ventricular pacing lead with retractable, screw-in tip. (D) Bipolar (*left*) and unipolar (*right*) pacing leads with fixed-screw tips. A soluble tip coating dissolves in blood and reduces snagging during insertion. These leads can be used in the atrium or ventricle. The unipolar lead was used by the author for atrial and ventricular pacing. (E) Single-pass lead for VDD pacing. (F) Current leads demonstrating progress in reduction of bipolar lead diameter. (G) Fixed-screw bipolar 7-French lead with steroid-eluting white collar at lead tip. (A, B, and C: Reproduced with permission of Medtronic, Inc.; D-G: Image provided courtesy of Boston Scientific. © 2016 Boston Scientific Corporation or its affiliates. All rights reserved.)

LEAD FIXATION

We prefer endocardial positive fixation leads, particularly in chambers with sparse trabeculation. A small wire spiral or screw holds these leads in place (Fig. 55-5G). In designs with fixed, extended screws, a soluble coating over the tip promotes venous passage. In retractable screw designs (Bisping), extension/retraction is accomplished by rotation of the pin at the lead tip. Axial clockwise rotation of screw-in leads during fixation provides tactile feedback on the firmness and security of attachment. Lead impedance provides feedback on the adequacy of tip extension and fixation.

Tined leads use miniature anchors to secure the lead tip within myocardial trabeculae (Fig. 55-5A). Tines require larger introducers than screw-in leads and are not secure in smooth-walled or dilated chambers. Nevertheless, some physicians prefer these leads.[2]

Temporary Pacing

Acute bradycardia can be treated with transthoracic pacing, temporary endocardial pacing, or chronotropic drugs, including atropine, dobutamine, or isoproterenol. Right ventricular perforation has become less prevalent with current temporary endocardial leads but must be borne in mind if hypotension develops acutely after removal of temporary wires.

Bradycardia after cardiac surgery is commonly treated with pacing via temporary atrial and ventricular epicardial wires. Problems include unfavorable evolution of right atrial (RA) or right ventricular thresholds and RA sensing. Atrial undersensing and pacemaker competition can precipitate atrial fibrillation or atrial flutter. If atrial sensing is not adequate, overdriving the atrium faster than the intrinsic rate can ameliorate competition. Reversing polarity or inserting a cutaneous ground wire under local anesthesia can improve pacing threshold. The output of the temporary pacemaker in volts or milliamps should be at least twice the threshold and should be measured daily. Ventricular undersensing in critically ill patients can result in pacing during the vulnerable period, which can precipitate VT or fibrillation.

CARDIAC OUTPUT AND PACING RATE

For patients with hemodynamic compromise following cardiac surgery, optimization of pacing rate and AV delay can affect hemodynamics by compensating for valve leaks or fixed stroke volume. Mean arterial pressure reflects cardiac output if systemic resistance is constant. Rate and timing adjustments over intervals of less than 20 seconds minimize reflex effects. Settings producing the highest sustained mean arterial pressure should also maximize cardiac output.

Pacemaker Insertion

ENVIRONMENT AND ANESTHESIA

Pacemaker and ICD surgery are now predominantly performed in EP laboratories. Whether in the operating room or EP laboratory, properly functioning equipment is essential. Infection control is critical[23]; operating room standards for air quality should be enforced. Problems calling for presence of an anesthesiologist include angina, transient cerebral ischemia, patient disorientation, lidocaine toxicity, dementia, myocardial ischemia, heart failure, anxiety, or VT. If English is not the patient's first language, a translator is helpful. Vancomycin reactions (red man syndrome), pacing-induced ventricular fibrillation (VF), air embolism, and Stokes-Adams attacks are rare emergencies that are less problematic if considered in advance. Intraoperative death can occur because of hemorrhage, pericardial tamponade, VF, heart failure, myocardial infarction, and other causes.

MONITORING

R-wave detection by an ECG monitor is inadequate for pacemaker insertion, because pacing artifacts may trigger the monitor but fail to capture. Thus, subthreshold pacing can elicit regular beeping from the monitor in an asystolic patient. Oxygen saturation monitors are optimal and beep only during blood flow. Pulse oximeters should not be placed on the same extremity as the blood pressure cuff. When monitors are unreliable, palpation by an anesthesiologist or nurse

of the temporal, facial, or radial artery pulse can detect asystole before the patient becomes symptomatic.

VENOUS ACCESS STRATEGY

Choices include which side to be employed and whether to use cutdown or percutaneous venipuncture. Approaches to the cephalic, subclavian, axillary, external jugular, and internal jugular system are useful.[6] Anatomical considerations[24] may reduce the frequency of subclavian crush (Fig. 55-6). Deep vein punctures are associated with an apparently unavoidable but low incidence of pneumothorax, hemothorax, and major venous injury. Contrast injection from an IV on the side of the implant can confirm patency and location of the target vein. Ultrasonic vessel locators may further reduce the frequency of injury.

Venous access is problematic in superior vena cava syndrome or subclavian/innominate vein obstruction/thrombosis (eg, with chronic dialysis, mediastinal tracheostomy, or multiple

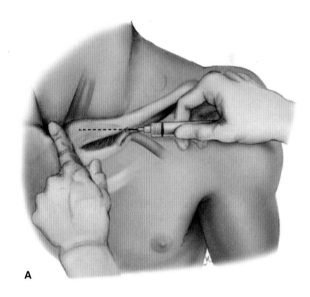

A

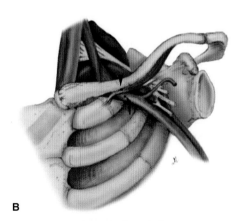

B

FIGURE 55-6 Landmarks for subclavian vein puncture. Potential complications include subclavian crush injury. (Reproduced with permission from Magney JE, Flynn DM, Parsons JA, et al: Anatomical mechanisms explaining damage to pacemaker leads, defibrillator leads, and failure of central venous catheters adjacent to the sternoclavicular joint, Pacing Clin Electrophysiol. 1993 Mar;16(3 Pt 1):445-457.)

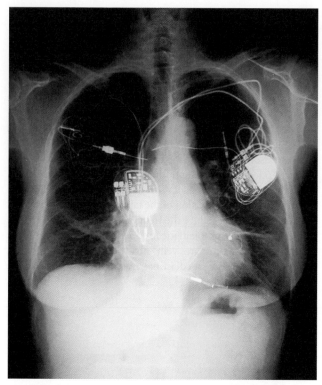

FIGURE 55-7 X-ray of a patient with very poor escape rhythm, bilateral venous obstruction, and severe exit block. A new pacing system was inserted through the right atrial appendage via right parasternal mediastinotomy. Older pacemaker programmed to backup mode and scheduled for later removal.

pacemaker leads). Access from below or transhepatically is possible,[6] but potential for bleeding, venous thrombosis, and pulmonary embolism are concerns. Right parasternal mediastinotomy with exposure of the right atrium and a Seldinger approach with small introducers and atrial pursestring sutures are useful in difficult cases[22] (Fig. 55-7). Lead extraction may permit reinsertion of leads via the extraction cannula.[6]

ANTIBIOTIC PROPHYLAXIS

Antibiotic prophylaxis is indicated for insertion of a prosthetic device.[6,23] We have used 1 g of intravenous cefazolin, but the current recommendation is 2 g. We also irrigate the operative field with a solution of 1 g of cefazolin in a liter of warm saline. Patients with prosthetic valves or a penicillin or cefazolin allergy receive vancomycin (500–1000 mg) and gentamicin (1 mg/kg). Doses are adjusted for renal function.

PACING SYSTEMS ANALYZER

Pacing thresholds and electrogram amplitudes are measured with a pacing systems analyzer. Electrogram characteristics and slew rate can be assessed, and electrogram telemetry is available from most current pacemakers. Analyzers must be serviced and tested periodically, including batteries. Any discrepancies between measurements by the analyzer and the pacemaker should be noted and related functions of the analyzer rechecked.

A skilled operator is needed to run the analyzer and record the results. If placed in a sterile bag, the analyzer can be operated by the surgeon. Manufacturer's representatives, an increasing intraoperative presence, are skilled in operation of these analyzers.

CABLES

The cables connecting the analyzer to the leads are the patient's lifeline. Even with excellent quality control, cables with open or reversed connections may be delivered to the surgical field. Errors can also occur in connecting the cables to the analyzer. Routine testing of the cables and the integrity of their connections is recommended. After passing the cables from the operating table, pacing is initiated from the analyzer at 5-V output. The connectors are then briefly touched to the subcutaneous tissue, with caution to minimize inhibition of the permanent pacemaker. Current measured in the analyzer should rise to 300 to 1000 ohms. If impedance is more than 5000 ohms, the circuit is faulty. The operation should not proceed until the problem is corrected, if impedance indicates the analyzer-cable circuit is defective. Connections to the analyzer should also be checked, because inadvertent reversal of polarity can make measured pacing thresholds inappropriately high. Disposable leads with polarized connectors have been delivered to us on occasion with the connectors reversed.

FLUOROSCOPY

Fluoroscopy is essential for transvenous device implantation, and personnel must be familiar with the equipment. Distracting problems with image orientation, rebooting, timers, brakes, and locks can be avoided by a knowledgeable team. Sudden failure of fluoroscopy at a critical point can occur. If a backup unit is not available, the options include "blind" endocardial lead insertion, epicardial insertion, or postponing the procedure. The use of low-dose and pulsed image options can prevent overheating of the fluoroscope, although image quality may be compromised. Radiation exposure or fluoroscopy time should be monitored and recorded.[6]

SURGICAL APPROACH

For routine implants, we prefer to approach from the patient's left. The fluoroscope is positioned carefully on the right to allow visualization of the apex, right atrium, and deltopectoral groove. The right arm is extended rightward on an arm board. The drapes are suspended from IV poles. The right-sided pole is caudad to the arm board. Proper positioning exposes the left clavicular region while leaving the patient adequate light and air. After skin preparation, towels aligned with the deltopectoral groove and clavicle define essential landmarks. Conscious sedation with 0.5 mg midalozam and/or 25.0 mcg of fentanyl may be useful. The region of the incision and underlying generator is infiltrated with 1% lidocaine, producing a field block. A 5- to 6-cm horizontal incision is created 4 cm beneath the clavicle, the lateral extent of the incision just reaching the deltopectoral groove. This allows the generator to be positioned away from the groove and axilla, avoiding interference with motion of the left arm at the shoulder. An alternate incision overlying the deltopectoral groove is preferred for exposure of the cephalic vein in obese patients or elderly patients with atretic veins.

VENOUS ACCESS

When the deltopectoral groove is exposed, additional anesthetic is infiltrated into the lateral margin of the pectoralis and laterally into the deltoid. The dissection proceeds into the deltopectoral groove, following the lateral edge of the pectoralis, until the cephalic vein or another venous branch is exposed. Failure to find a vein may mean the incision is too far cephalad or caudad or not lateral enough. The incision can be deepened into the subpectoral fat if necessary. If the vein is too small to pass a pacemaker lead, the curved end of the guidewire for a 7-French introducer is passed centrally. The ability to manually stiffen and extend the curve by manipulation of the tension in the guidewire is an important technical aid in tortuous veins. Hydrophilic guidewires are also useful. The method illustrated in Fig. 55-8 can be used to dilate the vein. A no. 18 Angiocath is advanced over the guidewire, and the vein is slit longitudinally, exposing larger segments more proximally. This step can be repeated until a 7 French introducer will enter the vein. If the introducer

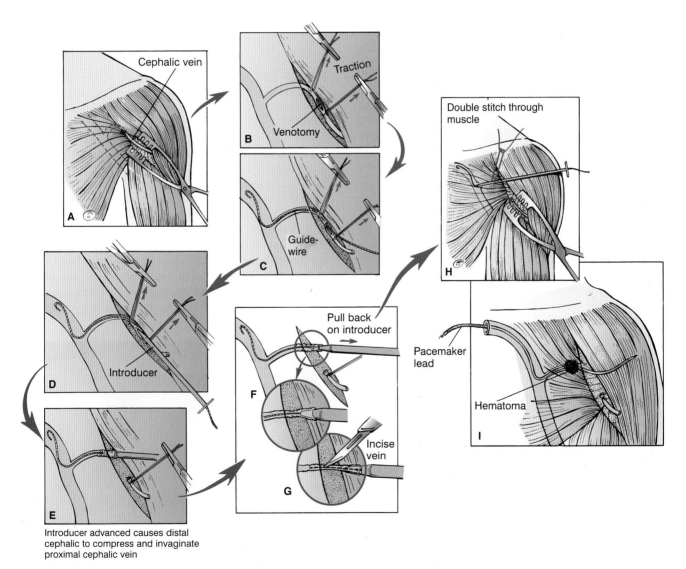

Introducer advanced causes distal cephalic to compress and invaginate proximal cephalic vein

FIGURE 55-8 Cephalic cutdown approach to small veins passing a guidewire centrally but blocking an introducer. Resistance is from entrapment of the introducer tip and inversion of the vein. This entrapment can be harnessed to split the vein. After the guidewire is advanced (C), pass a no. 18 Angiocath over the guidewire and incise the vein longitudinally (not shown). This allows the introducer tip to enter the vein (D). If the vein does not split, the introducer becomes impaled and will not advance (E). Partially pull the introducer back, stretching the impaled vein (F). Incise the exposed vein segment longitudinally with a no. 11 blade (G). Steps (D) to (G) can be repeated, if necessary, until the introducer advances centrally. A pursestring suture approximates soft tissue around the path of the introducer to achieve hemostasis (H, I).[70]

will not advance without invaginating the vein, pulling the introducer back exposes the impaled vein, which can again be longitudinally incised to allow the introducer to advance. If dual-chamber pacing is planned, a guidewire should be reinserted before the introducer is stripped away. These steps provide venous access for the duration of the procedure.[25,26] A pursestring suture in the muscle controls bleeding and stabilizes the lead(s).[27] Ultrasonic localizers may be useful at this stage, with appropriate sterile precautions. If a guidewire will not pass centrally, a no. 18 Angiocath can be advanced for angiography with iodinated contrast. Venography reduces the risk of hemo/pneumothorax during needle puncture.

RIGHT VENTRICULAR LEAD INSERTION

From the patient's left, a gentle spiral in the distal 10 cm of the stylet will guide the lead toward the tricuspid valve, right ventricle, and pulmonary artery. Advancing the lead into the pulmonary artery outside the cardiac silhouette confirms that the lead is not in the CS. For fixed-screw positive fixation leads, withdrawing the stylet 3 to 5 cm minimizes the risk of apical perforation while the lead tip is screwed into the myocardium with axial clockwise rotation. Reverse torque developing as the lead is rotated indicates the tip is in healthy myocardium and is an index of the security of fixation. We fix these leads with three consecutive 360-degree clockwise rotations of the lead shaft, and then the torque is released. This fixation sequence is repeated if necessary, until the lead is secure, with substantial reverse torque after the first 360-degree rotation. No more than three complete axial rotations are employed in any sequence. A potential problem with screw-in leads is ventricular perforation. The lead tip should be imaged during fixation looking for extra-anatomical passage along the edge of the cardiac silhouette and around the apex, tracking cephalad. If this happens, the lead should be withdrawn and repositioned. An echocardiogram should be obtained and the patient monitored for tamponade.

When the lead tip has been properly positioned, the stylet is withdrawn and thresholds are tested. Patient hyperventilation and coughing confirms fixation. The ventricular pacing threshold should be less than 0.7 V, with R-wave amplitude more than 5 mV, and impedance 400 to 1000 ohms, depending on lead design. There should be no diaphragmatic pacing at an output of 10 V.

If the lead is dislodged by hyperventilation and coughing, or thresholds are not adequate, the lead should be repositioned. A positive fixation lead can be unscrewed by counterclockwise axial rotation until it floats free. Positive fixation leads can be secured almost anywhere along the margins of the right ventricular silhouette (Fig. 55-9), including the right ventricular outflow tract (Fig. 55-10).[28] In difficult cases, we have relocated leads as many as 15 times. The geographic center of the right ventricular silhouette is not a desirable location, as it can lead to entanglement of the lead in the chordae tendineae (see Fig. 55-9).

CORONARY SINUS LEAD INSERTION

Left ventricular pacing via the CS is a valued skill since the MIRACLE trial and subsequent studies indicated that CRT

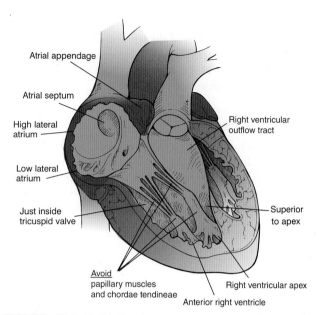

FIGURE 55-9 Useful sites for transvenous atrial and ventricular pacing using fixed-screw leads. Avoid the geographic center of the right ventricle (RV), where fixing the lead can entrap it in the chordae tendineae.

reduces symptoms of heart failure and mortality of dilated cardiomyopathy.[5] Electrophysiologists are familiar with CS entry for arrhythmia mapping; steerable mapping catheters and biplane fluoroscopy are important tools. However, the technical failure rate of CS lead insertion is 5 to 10%.[5,29] The CS orifice is usually a posterior structure near the caudal aspect of the tricuspid valve (Fig. 55-11). Locating the os in heart failure patients may be difficult, because the CS can be angulated and distorted as a result of cardiac enlargement. Transesophageal echocardiography and venography may help locate the os. CRT candidates may be prone to ventricular arrhythmias, and

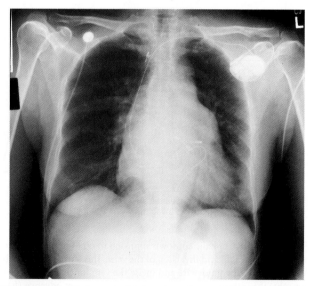

FIGURE 55-10 Screw-in lead in the right ventricular outflow tract of a patient with complete heart block after tricuspid valve replacement for Ebstein anomaly.

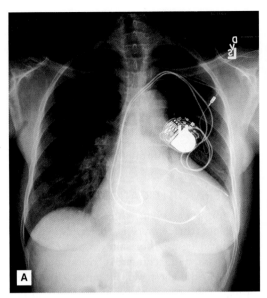
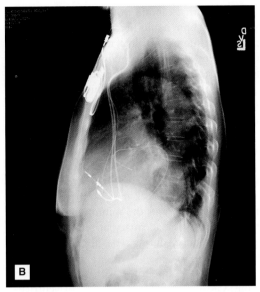

FIGURE 55-11 (A) Biventricular, CRT-P pacemaker with endocardial leads in the right atrium, right ventricle, and lateral branch of the coronary sinus (left ventricle). This patient was relieved of dobutamine dependence by addition of the left ventricular lead. (B) Lateral x-ray of the same patient. Note posterior course of the coronary sinus.

rapid defibrillation capability is desirable. Even experienced operators may require hours to insert a CS lead with present methods, although technology for both endocardial and epicardial left ventricular lead placement is improving. Over-the-wire lead designs are the most successful.

We prefer to insert the CS lead first via the cephalic approach, RA and right ventricular lead insertion after via subclavian puncture. CS lead insertion involves advancing an angled cannula into the CS, followed by CS venography and lead insertion through the cannula into a lateral CS branch. The CS cannula is then removed and stripped away without dislodging the lead. Positive fixation leads are not available. A large selection of angled CS cannulas, steerable probes, and lead designs testifies to the technical challenge.[2,5] The difficulty of CS lead insertion in heart failure patients should not be underestimated; special training is desirable. Recent availability of multielectrode CS leads is very helpful in preventing phrenic nerve pacing, a complication that can be minimized by high output test pacing.

LENGTH ADJUSTMENT

If lead length is "too short," flattening of the diaphragm during a deep breath can result in lead displacement, if "too long," a cough can force intracardiac loops that effectively shorten the lead, also potentially causing displacement. Hyperventilation by the patient under fluoroscopy helps adjust length. Vigorous coughing tests the security of lead tip fixation. This valuable feedback is lost if sedation is excessive. Minimizing sedation also promotes early detection of pacemaker syndrome.

ATRIAL LEAD INSERTION

For dual-chamber pacing, the atrial lead is introduced last. A J or S stylet shape is best for finding the atrial appendage from the left side. The S shape is also useful for passing a positive fixation

lead to the right margin of the atrium near the junction of the atrium and inferior vena cava (Fig. 55-12). P-wave amplitude is often best in this location. The atrial pacing threshold should be less than 2 V. In the presence of complete heart block, it may

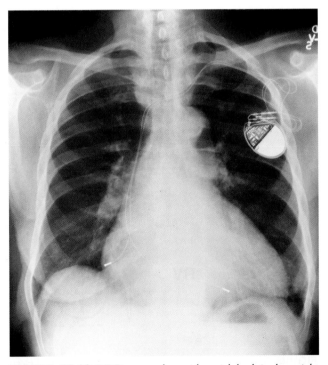

FIGURE 55-12 DDD pacemaker with atrial lead in low right atrium, advantageous after obliteration of the atrial appendage at heart surgery. This location, which requires positive fixation leads, often provides good P-wave amplitude when other sites fail. Phrenic nerve pacing must be excluded with 10-V pacing at this location.

be difficult to confirm atrial capture from the surface ECG. Pacing the atrium at 150 bpm results in rapid oscillation of the lead tip, which is visible fluoroscopically if mechanical function of the atrium is sufficient. Lead oscillation may thus be used to determine the atrial pacing threshold. This technique should only be used if the high atrial rate is not conducted to the ventricle. In patients with complete heart block, high-output atrial pacing can inhibit whatever temporary VVI pacing is supporting the patient, resulting in asystole.

The P-wave electrogram is the Achilles heel of dual-chamber pacing. If atrial sensing is not satisfactory, a DDD pacemaker will not function properly. The P-wave amplitude should ideally be greater than 2 mV. P-wave amplitude may vary during respiration, and the minimum value, not the maximum, determines the adequacy of sensing. P-wave amplitude is generally reduced during atrial fibrillation versus values in sinus rhythm.

Measurement of P-wave amplitude with unipolar leads can be confusing. Crosstalk or far-field sensing of ventricular depolarization from the atrial lead can occur, so that the signal measured through a pacemaker analyzer is not the P wave but the QRS complex. Simultaneous measurement and display of atrial and ventricular electrograms as well as the surface ECG can resolve this.

Atrial and ventricular electrogram telemetry provide valuable data. For example, inability to pace the atrium or to record atrial electrograms may indicate low-amplitude atrial fibrillation or supraventricular tachycardia invisible on the surface ECG but detectable in electrograms. Electrogram telemetry can confirm proper DDD pacing (Fig. 55-13).

GENERATOR LOCATION

We use a watertight, three-layer skin closure for primary implants, three layers in generator replacements. Dermabond can be used for skin closure. Cosmetic appearance is important, and technique is critical to optimize healing. Past injury to the chest wall or surgery/ radiotherapy for breast cancer can present a formidable technical problem. Bipolar systems facilitate optional generator placement behind the

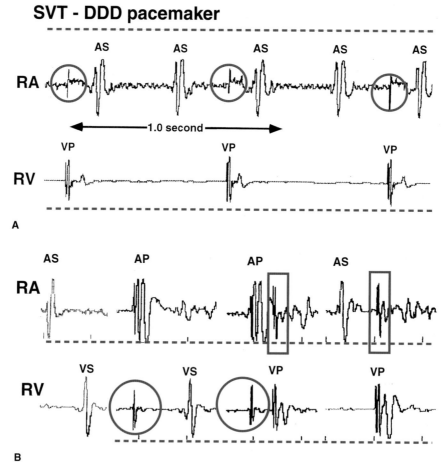

FIGURE 55-13 Right atrial (RA) and right ventricular (RV) electrograms from a unipolar DDD pacemaker during supraventricular tachycardia (SVT). Regular atrial depolarizations appear (AS) at a rate of 160 bpm. The pacemaker paces the ventricle (VP) at 80 bpm, because alternate P waves fall inside the postventricular atrial refractory period and are not detected. The circles illustrate far-field sensing of the RV pacing artifact in the RA lead. The SVT was not detected preoperatively. Once this recording was obtained, overdrive atrial pacing from the pacemaker converted the SVT to normal sinus rhythm, and normal pacemaker function returned.

pectoralis or inside the rectus sheath. Diminutive generators are available, but battery life is reduced. Innovative locations for pacemaker generators include axillary, retromammary, intrathoracic, intra-abdominal, and preperitoneal sites. These approaches are rarely indicated with present generator designs. Temporary endocardial pacing wires are removed under fluoroscopy, watching carefully for displacement of the new permanent leads.

Length of Stay after Pacemaker Implantation

AMBULATORY SURGERY

Same-day hospital discharge after pacemaker insertion is reasonable in patients who have an adequate escape rhythm and positive fixation leads. After monitoring and recovery from sedation, patients are ambulated and shown range of motion exercises for the shoulder. A chest x-ray documents lead position and rules out hemothorax, pneumothorax, or increasing heart size.

PACEMAKER-DEPENDENT PATIENTS

Lead displacement can result from technical error, struggling of demented patients, and other factors. A small percentage of lead displacement is probably unavoidable.[6,30] Patients who might suffer death or injury in the event of pacemaker failure should be observed in the hospital overnight on telemetry. However, lead displacement in our ambulatory patients has not been more frequent than in hospitalized patients. Swan-Ganz catheter removal/insertion, endomyocardial biopsy, or cardiac catheterization can displace pacemaker leads, requiring a backup pacing plan.

Pacemaker Generator Replacement

PLANNING

Complications of pacemaker generator replacement include infection, lead damage, connector problems, and asystole during the transition from the old generator to the new. Pacemaker independence at the time of initial pacemaker implant may progress to total pacemaker dependence by the time of generator replacement. Ambulatory surgery is common. As a practical matter, we do not completely reverse warfarin for pacemaker generator replacement unless lead replacement is expected.[31] Patients with leads more than 10 years old should be carefully evaluated for pacemaker dysfunction before the procedure; a Holter monitor should be obtained if lead dysfunction is suspected. Rising pacing threshold may indicate impending lead failure. The possibility of unexpected lead replacement should be discussed with the patient in advance.

BACKUP PACING

A backup temporary transvenous pacing wire can be inserted for pacemaker generator replacement, but this is rarely necessary. The output of the replacement unit must be higher than the threshold of the chronically implanted leads. This can be problematic if the expiring generator is an older type with a fixed output of 5.4 V. Lack of programmability prevents preoperative threshold testing, and the 5.4-V output is higher than possible for some current generators. The pacing threshold should be determined with a pacemaker analyzer and the replacement should be programmed to appropriate output. Before disconnecting the old generator, be sure that the pacemaker analyzer, cables, and connections are intact and personnel in the operating room are aware of the cables. Some place the analyzer in a sterile bag on the operative field. With many generators, an Allen wrench placed in the header establishes electrical continuity with the ventricular lead; the pacing threshold can then be established before disconnecting the old generator. The old generator should be kept within reach as a backup in case of trouble with the new generator, the analyzer, or the connectors. Replacement generators must be programmed unipolar or bipolar to match the indwelling lead(s).

LEAD SIZES

VS-1 or IS-1 are common lead types, both 3.5 mm in diameter. The contacts do not always line up correctly across VS-1 and IS-1 generator ports, even though the connector diameter is the same. It is important to determine in advance whether adapters are needed to bridge incompatibilities. Older 5 and 6 mm leads, increasingly rare, require special adapters or generators.

Postoperative Care

WOUND CARE

Patients are instructed to keep implant wounds dry until an office visit 7 to 10 days postoperatively. Any wound drainage at the postoperative visit is cultured, and prophylactic antibiotics are started until culture results are available. We have abandoned aspiration of the rare postoperative hematoma in favor of close observation, unless infection is an issue or spontaneous drainage occurs or appears imminent.

ANTIBIOTIC PROPHYLAXIS

Routine use of prophylactic antibiotics before dental work and other invasive procedures in pacemaker or ICD recipients is not recommended under AHA/ACC guidelines. We recommend prophylaxis for 3 months after device insertion, allowing time for the pacing leads to become endothelialized.

Testing and Follow-up

OFFICE/CLINIC VERSUS TELEPHONE

Pacemakers require periodic testing to confirm sensing and pacing function and battery reserve. Currently these functions are tested at 1- to 3-month intervals. Follow-up can be done by transtelephonic monitoring, wireless telemetry and clinic or office visits.[4] Transtelephonic monitoring alleviates transportation issues for elderly patients, but may be confusing for new subscribers. In addition to reducing travel and office visits, transtelephonic monitoring can provide 24-hour emergency service, an advantage with apprehensive or incapacitated patients. Techniques for remote management of pacemakers and ICDs are available with some current devices.

PACEMAKER PROGRAMMING

Trained, experienced personnel can do programming in the office. Manufacturer's representatives can provide valuable help and programmer upgrades. Remote pacemaker/ICD monitoring and programming are under development.

DDD pacemaker programming allows adjustment of electrogram sensitivity as well as pacing stimulus amplitude/pulse width for both the atrium and ventricle. Lower rate, upper rate, AV delay (AVD), and refractory periods for atrial and ventricular sensing are programmable. Rate responsiveness, unipolar/bipolar configuration, and many other options are also adjustable noninvasively.

We program newly inserted pacemaker stimulation amplitude 50% higher than nominal. At a 7- to 10-day

initial office visit, pacing thresholds are retested and amplitude and pulse width are adjusted to nominal levels if pacing thresholds are low. High initial output is less important with steroid-eluting leads. Details of pacemaker programming have been described elsewhere.[4-6,8] Many current pacemakers provide automated threshold adjustment, but this may function inappropriately with unipolar leads.

Most problems detected by monitoring or device interrogation can be corrected by programming. The etiology of symptoms may be elicited from real-time electrograms or stored data. Adjustments can include not only sensitivity or pacing output but also pacing mode and rate for new-onset atrial fibrillation (Fig. 55-14A) or sinus node incompetence related to medication changes (Fig. 55-14B). Reoperation is required for lead displacement or fracture (Fig. 55-15), insulation degradation (Fig. 55-3), very low sensing amplitudes, and exit block (Fig. 55-16).[30]

Pacemaker interrogation should begin with a printout of the initial settings, an invaluable reference after involved programming. Telemetry defines time-related variation in heart rate, percentage of beats sensed and paced, the quality of the electrograms, lead impedance, and battery voltage.

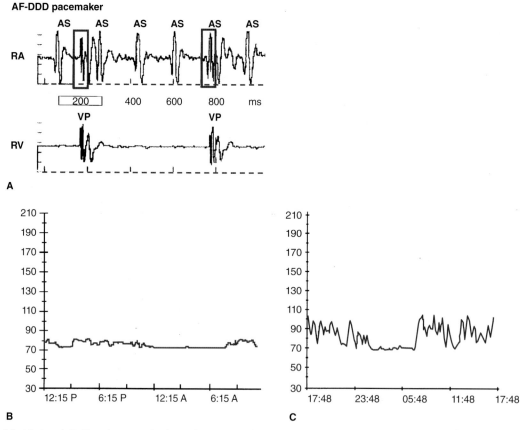

FIGURE 55-14 (A) Atrial (RA) and ventricular (RV) electrograms from unipolar DDD pacemaker during atrial fibrillation (AF). AF appears as rapid atrial depolarizations (AS). The upper rate limit and postventricular atrial refractory period of the pacemaker determine the rate at which the pacemaker stimulates the ventricle (VP). (B,C) Heart rate over 24 hours from memory of DDD pacemaker. (B) Sinus node incompetence during amiodarone therapy for paroxysmal atrial fibrillation. (C) Rate variation after activation of rate response. Patient reported improved exercise tolerance.

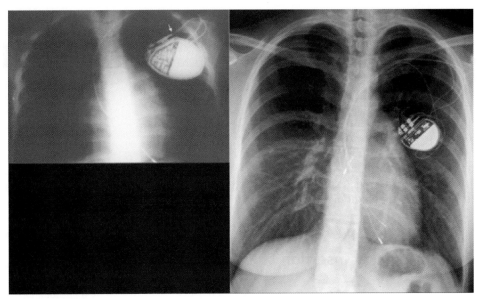

FIGURE 55-15 Unipolar lead fracture in a 3-year-old child with complete heart block, revealed by x-ray. A replacement lead was inserted and is still functioning normally 18 years later.

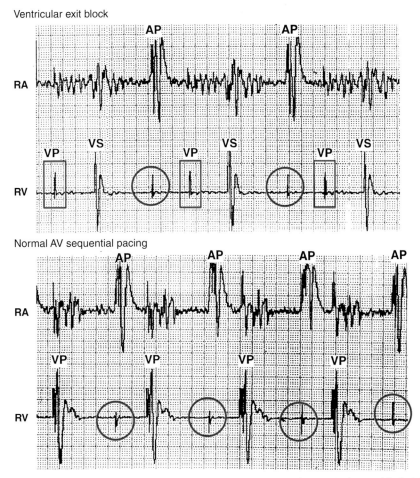

FIGURE 55-16 Right atrial (RA) and right ventricular (RV) unipolar electrograms in right ventricular exit block (*above*). Atrial (AP) and ventricular (VP) pacing are required for sinus arrest and marked first-degree atrioventricular block. Right ventricular capture is restored after RV pacing amplitude is programmed from 3.5 (*above*) to 5.4 V (*below*). Ventricular capture increases the effective heart rate, because the late, conducted ventricular electrograms (VS) in the upper tracing are sensed by the pacemaker and used to begin a new cardiac timing cycle. The circles indicate far-field sensing of the RA pacing artifact in the RV lead.

Pacing amplitude and pulse width are finely tuned for patient complaints, malfunctions on telemetry, or at 1-year follow-up visits. At least 100% safety margin is programmed on the pulse width threshold or amplitude. Parameters are adjusted to optimize patient comfort and battery life. Some pacemakers allow programmed reduction of a lower rate at night, eliminating unnecessary pacing during sleep. Very long AVD can eliminate ventricular pacing in some patients with first-degree block, but a reduction in the upper rate limit to 105 bpm may be necessary to extend AVD to 300 ms. Current pacemakers have a variety of algorithms to prevent excessive pacing in first-degree heart block, including automatic switching between AAI and DDD modes.

Complications of Pacemaker Insertion

MORTALITY

Death is a rare complication of pacemaker implantation.[30,33] Lethal problems can include lead displacement, venous or cardiac perforation, air embolism, and VT or fibrillation.[30] A review of 650 pacemaker insertions by the author between January 1984 and April 1993 revealed one perioperative death resulting from heart failure induced by general anesthesia in a child with congenital heart disease (Table 55-3).

INCIDENCE OF COMPLICATIONS

The incidence of early pacemaker complications in one recent series was 6.7 and 4.9% requiring reoperation.[30] For patients older than 65 years, comparable figures were 6.1 and 4.4%, respectively. Lead displacement, pneumothorax, and cardiac perforation were the most common complications. The incidence of late complications was 7.2%.[30] The incidence of reoperation in the author's review of 480 cases was 4.0% (see Table 55-3).

LEAD DISPLACEMENT

The incidence of endocardial lead displacement with early lead designs was more than 10%.[32] With tined and positive fixation leads this has fallen to about 2%.[6,30,32,33] The incidence of this complication was 1.5% for atrial and ventricular leads in our review (see Table 55-3). Relevant technical issues have been described. We find that positive fixation leads can be applied in unique anatomical locations with essentially no increase in lead displacement (Table 55-4).

MYOCARDIAL INFARCTION

Pacemaker insertion may become an adjunct to medical therapy of angina in patients with inoperable coronary artery disease. However, angina, myocardial infarction, or death can result when heart rate increases of 10 bpm or more accompany surgical implants.

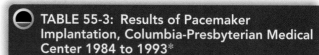

TABLE 55-3: Results of Pacemaker Implantation, Columbia-Presbyterian Medical Center 1984 to 1993*

Surgical mortality	1/616 (general anesthesia related)
Mean follow-up	884 ± 675 (SD) days (n = 480 patients, 679 leads)
Morbidity	19 Reoperations (4.0% of 480)
	4 Infections (0.8%)
	7 Lead displacements (1.5%)
	4 Exit block (0.8%)
	4 Undersensing (0.8%)
	5 Suspected right ventricular perforations
	2 Leads abandoned (chordal entrapment)
	41 Reprogrammed for dysfunction
	0 Hemothorax
	0 Pneumothorax
	1 Procedure abandoned for thoracotomy (newborn)

Characteristics at generator replacement (n = 40, 75 ± 31 months after implant)	
Pacing threshold	1.3 ± 0.5 V
	3.0 ± 1.3 mA
R-wave amplitude	8.9 ± 4.3 mV
Long-term DDD pacing	89% (1109 ± 34 days follow-up)
Causes of DDD failure	8.4% Atrial fibrillation
	2.4% Lead dysfunction

*Models 479-01 and 435-02 unipolar, positive fixation leads, Intermedics, Inc., Bellaire, TX.
Used with permission from Spotnitz HM, Mason DP, Carter YM: Unpublished observations.

TABLE 55-4: Lead Stability in Unusual Locations, Columbia-Presbyterian Medical Center 1984 to 1993*

Location	n	Displaced
Coronary sinus (to left ventricle)	2	0
Atrial conduit	1	0
Right atrium of transplant	20	0
Lateral right atrium	27	1
Right ventricular outflow—single	22	0
Right ventricular outflow—paired (ICD recipients)	11 (×2)	0
Infants—looped leads (<1 year old)	7	0
Children—looped leads	42	2
Total	132	3 (2.3%)

*Models 479-01 and 435-02 unipolar, positive fixation leads, Intermedics, Inc., Bellaire, TX.
ICD, implantable cardioverter defibrillator.
Used with permission from Spotnitz HM, Mason DP, Carter YM: Unpublished observations.

HEMOPNEUMOTHORAX

Hemopneumothorax and pericardial tamponade result from injury to the heart, lungs, arteries, or veins. Errors with the Seldinger technique can cause such injuries. In patients older than 65 years, pneumothorax has been related to subclavian puncture.[33] In our experience with more than 1000 pacemaker insertions by cephalic cutdown, hemopneumothorax did not occur. In contrast, a recent review of 1088 consecutive implants by subclavian puncture revealed a 1.8% incidence of pneumothorax.[33]

PACEMAKER SYNDROME

Loss of AV synchrony produces symptoms related to reflex effects or contraction of the atria against closed AV valves. The resulting constellation of symptoms is known as *pacemaker syndrome*.[4,8] The symptoms are quite variable, but severely affected patients may refuse pacemaker magnet testing. Symptoms are relieved immediately by conversion from VVI to dual-chamber pacing.

LEAD ENTRAPMENT

Fixed-screw pacemaker leads can become firmly entangled in chordae tendineae beneath the tricuspid valve. Possible responses include further escalation of force, lead extraction,[6,35-37] or an open procedure. Our experience with this involved three firmly entangled leads in our first 1000 implants of fixed-screw positive fixation leads. The leads were capped and abandoned rather than escalate risk. We now avoid the anatomic center of the right ventricle when implanting these leads. This problem has not recurred subsequent to this experience and presumably is avoidable with Bisping leads.

INFECTION AND EROSION

Pacemaker infection manifests as frank sepsis, fever with vegetations/inflammation, and/or purulence or drainage at the pacemaker pocket. Indolent generator erosion or cellulitis are alternate presentations. Antibiotic suppression may temporarily abolish signs of infection, but the problem usually recurs weeks or months later.[6,38,39] Negative cultures and erosion may suggest moving the device to a fresh, adjacent site, but this is usually futile. Clinical resolution of recurrent device infection almost always requires removal of all hardware and insertion of a new device in a fresh site, optimally after a device-free interval.[2,38,39] The incidence of erosion, infection, hematoma, and lead displacement early after pacemaker implantation is reduced by operator experience.[6]

PACEMAKER DYSFUNCTION

Mechanical defects in leads, lead displacement, or connection errors can cause pacemaker dysfunction. Late onset of lead dysfunction usually represents scarring at the lead—myocardial interface, changes in myocardial properties owing to tissue necrosis or drug effects, or a poor choice of lead position.

Insulation erosion can cause oversensing or, in bipolar leads, pacing failure owing to short-circuiting between the two conductors.

GENERATOR DYSFUNCTION

Electrical component failures are rare. Three pacemaker or ICD generator failures have required urgent device replacement over 10 years at our center. New pacemaker and lead designs may contain flaws that do not become apparent for many years.[2]

UNDERSENSING

Undersensing is failure to detect atrial or ventricular electrograms corresponding to P waves or R waves. The result is atrial or ventricular pacing that should have been inhibited by the unsensed beat. In a dual-chamber pacemaker, P wave undersensing may also cause failure to pace the ventricle after the P wave. Undersensing is often correctable by increasing generator sensitivity, but this can lead to oversensing. The latitude for reprogramming can be estimated by examining telemetered electrograms[2,4] (Figs. 55-17 and 55-18).

OVERSENSING

Inappropriate pacemaker inhibition or triggering may result from detection of myopotentials (muscular activity). This is most common in unipolar systems and may be correctable by programming reduced pacemaker sensitivity. External insulation erosion within the pacemaker pocket is a cause of oversensing (Fig. 55-3).

CROSSTALK AND FAR-FIELD SENSING

A deflection on the ventricular lead immediately after the atrial pacing artifact could be either premature ventricular depolarization (Fig. 55-17) or far-field sensing of an atrial depolarization (Fig. 55-13). Many pacemakers deal with this ambiguity by pacing the ventricle at a short (100 ms) AVD, an algorithm known as *safety pacing*.

Complexities of DDD programming involve blanking and refractory periods used to compensate for crosstalk or prevent retrograde AV conduction from causing pacemaker-mediated tachycardia (see the following). Crosstalk is ameliorated by bipolar lead systems.

EXIT BLOCK

Exit block is rising pacing threshold due to edema or scarring at the lead tip. Pacing threshold tends to increase over 7 to 14 days after lead insertion and stabilizes at about 6 weeks. This phenomenon is related to inflammation at the lead tip and is ameliorated by steroid-eluting leads.[2] Exit block may be overcome by programming increased amplitude or pulse width, but this shortens battery life. In unipolar systems, pacing of the chest wall and/or diaphragm may result from high generator output.

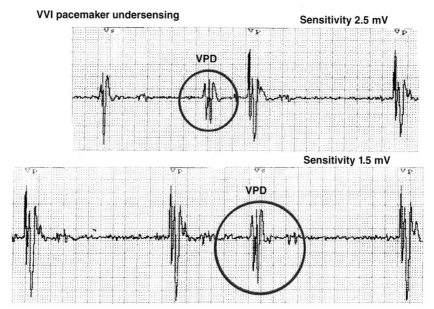

FIGURE 55-17 Undersensing of ventricular premature depolarizations (VPD) illustrated in the upper panel of electrograms obtained by telemetry from a VVI pacemaker. The amplitude of the electrograms increases, and sensing is corrected after reprogramming to increase sensitivity to P waves from 2.5 mV (*above*) to 1.5 mV (*below*).

LEAD FRACTURE

Fracture of lead insulation or conductors may be demonstrable by chest x-ray (Fig. 55-15). Lead impedance less than 300 ohms suggest an insulation break, whereas impedance more than 1000 ohms suggests conductor problems, a loose setscrew, or improper connection. High impedance also can indicate incomplete extension of the fixation coil in a Bisping lead. Telemetry may detect impending lead fracture as electrical noise during hyperventilation, coughing, bending, or arm swinging. Oversensing of this type usually mandates lead replacement or repair.

At reoperation, dysfunctional leads can be capped or removed by lead extraction techniques (Figs. 55-19 and 55-20). Lead fracture has been promoted historically by design errors, bipolar construction, certain forms of polyurethane insulation, and epicardial insertion.[1] Technical factors in fracture include ties applied to the lead without an anchoring sleeve, kinking, lead angulation, vigorous exercise programs, and subclavian crush.[6,24]

SUBCLAVIAN CRUSH

Subclavian crush is probably caused by lead entrapment between the clavicle and first rib, in the costoclavicular ligament.

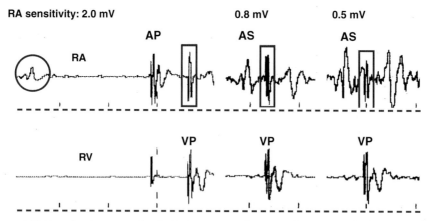

FIGURE 55-18 Right atrial (RA) and right ventricular (RV) electrograms from DDD pacemaker during correction of atrial undersensing. Amplitude of the RA electrogram increases after atrial sensitivity is increased from 2.0 mV (*left*) to 0.8 mV (*center*) to 0.5 mV (*right*). The P-wave electrogram (*circled*) is not sensed at 2.0 mV, resulting in unnecessary atrial pacing (AP). Proper sensing is restored and the size of the electrogram increases (AS) as sensitivity is increased. VP indicates ventricular pacing. Rectangles in RA tracing identify far-field sensing of the ventricular pacing artifact.

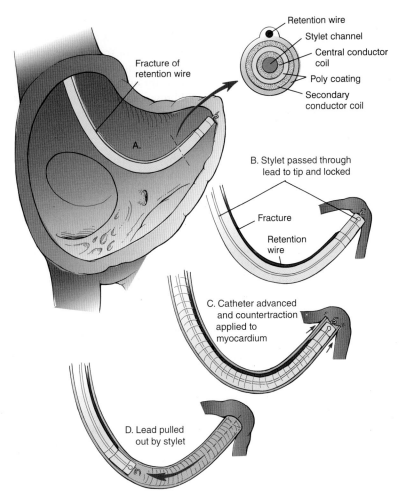

FIGURE 55-19 Byrd method of lead extraction using Cook catheters. Drawings illustrate successful removal of a Telectronics Accufix J-lead with a fractured retention wire.

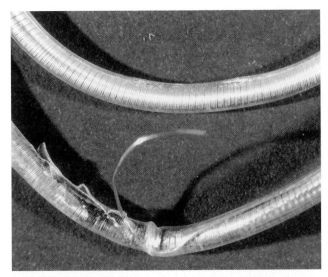

FIGURE 55-20 Telectronics Accufix atrial J-leads removed for retention wire fracture. Region of fracture appears benign in upper image. Lower image illustrates retention wire extrusion after percutaneous extraction. Extruded wire resembles a safety pin.

Stress during body movement is then thought to cause early lead failure. This pertains primarily to leads implanted by percutaneous puncture of the subclavian vein and seems to be minimized by cephalic cutdown. Techniques to minimize this problem have been described (Fig. 55-6).[6,24]

PACEMAKER-MEDIATED TACHYCARDIA

DDD pacemakers can propagate a reentrant arrhythmia, pacemaker-mediated tachycardia. This involves retrograde conduction through the AV node, initially triggered by a premature ventricular depolarization. If the pacemaker senses the retrograde atrial depolarization and paces the ventricle, a cycle is set up that can continue indefinitely at the upper rate limit of the pacemaker. Avoiding high upper rate limits and adjusting the postventricular atrial refractory period so that the pacemaker ignores atrial depolarizations for 300 to 350 ms after the QRS complex can mitigate this problem. Current pacemakers also attempt to break reentrant arrhythmias by periodic interruption of continuous high-rate pacing. Pacemaker telemetry provides notification of high-rate pacing suspicious of pacemaker-mediated tachycardia.[4]

Innovations and Special Problems

LEAD REPAIR

Repair can extend the useful life of implanted leads for years. Most repairs are done within the device pocket or in surrounding areas. Fracture or erosion of conductors or insulation can result from normal wear or active life styles. Lead dysfunction can result from vigorous exercise including situps (abdominal insulation erosion), handball (insulation/conductor erosion), and wood chopping (conductor damage).[2]

Repair kits contain silicone glue and silicone tubing or unipolar tip replacements. Possible repairs differ for unipolar and bipolar leads. Unipolar leads consist of a single conductor surrounded by insulation. Insulation breaks can be overlaid with glue and tubing. Conductor fracture can be repaired by splicing a new lead tip onto the functional segment.[41] Bipolar leads contain two conductors with two levels of insulation, one to prevent short-circuiting between the conductors and the other to prevent external current leaks and conductor-generator contact. Representative designs are shown in Figs. 55-19, 55-20, and 55-26d. External insulation repair in such leads is similar to unipolar lead repair. However, internal insulation faults require converting the lead to unipolar function and splicing on a new lead tip. Conductor fracture also can be repaired this way. The repair involves exposing and baring about 10 mm of the conductor to be preserved. The conductor to be excluded is cut back 5 to 10 mm to avoid short-circuiting. A new tip is attached to the bared conductor, using an internal setscrew, silicone glue, and ties. These repairs have been robust in our experience but are not recommended in pacemaker-dependent patients.

Unipolar and bipolar epicardial leads can also be repaired, if the break is accessible. Unipolar lead repair is similar to repair of unipolar endocardial leads. Bipolar epicardial leads generally consist of two unipolar leads connected by a Y to coaxial segments for connection. The simplest repair involves locating the unipolar segment of the good lead and splicing on a new tip. Particularly challenging is a fracture near one of the cardiac electrodes, at a point of metal fatigue. If the broken conductor is not the tip electrode, reprogramming the generator to a unipolar configuration restores function. If the cathode segment is fractured, most generators cannot be programmed to use the anode, and pacing is lost. However, function can be restored by exposing the lead, splicing a new tip on the anode, connecting that lead to generator, and capping the cathode.[41]

When exposing leads within the pocket for repairs, the electrocautery should be set as low as practical, to avoid melting external lead insulation. If cautery contacts a bare conductor, myocardial injury can render the lead useless because of exit block. Also, conduction of cautery to the myocardium can induce VF. Sharp dissection is preferred when close to friction points or angulation that promote conductor exposure.

PACEMAKER LEAD EXTRACTION

Indications for lead extraction include chronic infection or life-threatening mechanical defects.[6,35-37] Some recommend that any dysfunctional pacemaker lead should be removed, but there is little objective data to support this. Until recently, extraction of transvenous leads required external traction or thoracotomy/cardiotomy with inflow occlusion or cardiopulmonary bypass. Chronically implanted leads can be densely fibrosed to the right ventricular myocardium, vena cava, innominate vein, or subclavian vein.

Lead extraction was developed by Byrd.[35] A locking stylet is passed inside the central channel to the tip of the lead where it uncoils, allowing traction to be applied to the lead tip. Telescoping Teflon, plastic, or metal sheaths fitting the lead are passed along the lead to mobilize it. When the long sheath reaches the lead tip, counter traction is applied to the myocardium with the sheath while traction is applied to the lead tip with the locking stylet (see Fig. 55-19). Success with this technique has been greater than 90%, with a 3% chance of serious morbidity or death. Laser or radiofrequency energy can also be transmitted through specially constructed sheaths to ablate adhesions.[6,39] Technical details have been described.[6] Extraction of leads more than 10 years old is difficult and tedious. Complete removal of lead tips is inversely related to the age of the lead (Fig. 55-21A).[37]

ACCUFIX LEAD

An unusual fracture affects the Telectronics Accufix lead, a bipolar, Bisping-type atrial screw-in lead. A J shape near the tip directs the lead to the atrial appendage. A curved retention wire welded to the indifferent ring electrode near the tip and bonded to the lead body with polyurethane maintains the J-shape. Fracture and extrusion of this retention wire (Figs. 55-19 and 55-20) was associated with deaths from cardiac tamponade, related to punctures of the atrium or aorta by fractured wire. More than 45,000 of these leads were implanted, and many have been surgically extracted. Because some morbidity and mortality occurred during extraction of this lead, the manufacturer recommended conservative management. Recently, conservative management has also been recommended for a fracture tendency in the Sprint Fidelis ICD lead.[6]

ATRIAL FIBRILLATION AND MODE SWITCHING

Sinoatrial node dysfunction can involve both sinus bradycardia and paroxysmal atrial fibrillation. Early DDD pacemakers responded to atrial fibrillation by pacing at the upper rate limit. Initially DDD pacing was avoided in atrial fibrillation for this reason. The current view that atrial pacing decreases the frequency of paroxysmal atrial fibrillation, and mode switching allows DDD pacing to be used despite a history of paroxysmal atrial fibrillation. Mode switching is triggered when a programmed upper rate limit is exceeded. The pacemaker then switches to VVIR mode until the atrial rate returns to the physiologic range. Successful mode switching requires bipolar leads and high sensitivity in patients with low-amplitude atrial fibrillation. Management of atrial fibrillation in elderly people may involve fewer medications and interventions than in younger patients.[8]

DATABASE SUPPORT

Pacemaker and ICD data are needed for billing, operative notes, device tracking, programming, and follow-up. Data should be available in real time in the event of an emergency room visit involving device malfunction. Commercial and homegrown software packages are available for this. Security, audit trails, 24/7 availability, and multiuser wireless capability are important characteristics for such systems.

GENERAL SURGERY AND PACEMAKERS

General surgery in a pacemaker-dependent patient raises important questions,[42] especially when surgery requires unipolar cautery. The following must be documented: (1) model and manufacturer of the pacemaker, from pacemaker ID card, monitoring service, medical record, or x-ray appearance;[43,44] (2) magnet mode behavior and any peculiarities related to impedance sensing monitors; (3) successful testing of programmer on the pacemaker; (4) programmed parameters, polarity, battery life, and lead characteristics; (5) degree of pacemaker dependence; (6) a backup plan transthoracic pacing or chronotropic agents if the pacemaker fails; (7) reprogramming to VOO, DOO, or VVT mode intraoperatively with rate response off to prevent inhibition or pacemaker acceleration[44] by electromagnetic interference (EMI); (8) a physician to deal with any intra-operative pacemaker problem; and (9) restored pacemaker program, thresholds, and function postoperatively. Regarding pacemaker dependence, if the preoperative ECG reveals 100% pacing, the pacemaker should be reprogrammed while monitoring to determine the presence and rate of an escape rhythm. Pacemaker dependence may increase during anesthesia, with withdrawal of sympathetic stimulation. The Heart Rhythm Society has defined guidelines for perioperative management of these patients.

ELECTROCAUTERY

Manufacturers recommend against using electrocautery in pacemaker patients because of possible EMI or pacemaker damage. If electrocautery must be used, unipolar cautery is likely to cause EMI, whereas bipolar cautery is not. Unipolar pacemakers are more susceptible to EMI than bipolar units. EMI effects include (1) pacemaker oversensing, confusing EMI with a rapid heart rate. Pacemaker inhibition results but reverses when the EMI stops. (2) Pacemaker reprogramming. (3) Acceleration of impedance-sensing pacemakers to the upper rate limit. (4) Reversion to a "backup mode" or "magnet mode." (5) Permanent loss of pacing, fortunately rare.[43]

Programming sensing off and increasing the pacing rate above the intrinsic heart rate anticipated during surgery can minimize EMI pacemaker inhibition. However, if competition with spontaneous beats does occur, there is a risk of inducing of atrial fibrillation or VT. In view of this, the pacemaker should be returned to an appropriate sensing mode as soon as possible after the completion of surgery.

MAGNET MODE

A permanent magnet placed over a pacemaker closes a magnetic reed switch and initiates "magnet mode." In some pacemakers, magnet mode is VOO, eliminating all sensing. Other pacemakers convert to VOO for a few beats, then revert to the programmed function. A magnet may also induce a threshold margin test; this assesses the adequacy of the pacing margin by decreasing the pulse width in a predictable pattern.

STEROID-ELUTING LEADS

Fibrosis at the lead tip can be limited by incorporating a dexamethasone pellet that dissolves over months. This improves early pacing thresholds versus conventional leads[2] and has been particularly advantageous in epicardial leads.

ADULTS WITH CONGENITAL HEART DISEASE

Congenital heart disease may include a persistent left superior vena cava draining to the CS. This favors a right subclavian approach, although the left side can be used.[27] Preoperative echo-Doppler or angiography can define caval and CS anatomy. A left superior vena cava may dislocate the subclavian vein, increasing the risk of subclavian vein puncture and favoring cephalic cut down. Situs inversus and corrected transposition are disorienting, if undetected prior to pacemaker insertion.

Positive fixation leads are particularly useful for atrial pacing after a Mustard operation or a caval-pulmonary anastomosis and for pacing the smooth-walled "right" ventricle in corrected transposition of the great arteries.[27] A CS lead can provide ventricular pacing in some patients after Fontan surgery (Fig. 55-21). Pacing via the CS or middle cardiac vein may be useful in patients with a mechanical tricuspid valve (Fig. 55-21B).

PACING IN INFANTS AND CHILDREN

Transvenous leads in children should include an intracardiac loop to allow for growth (Figs. 55-4 and 55-15). Unipolar,

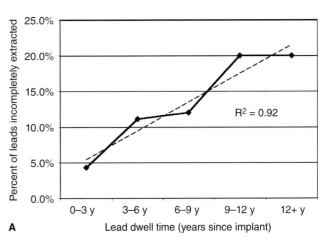

A Lead dwell time (years since implant)

FIGURE 55-21A Duration of lead implantation (Dwell Time) versus incidence of incomplete lead extraction. Incidence decreases from 23% for 12- to 25-year leads to 6% for 0- to 3-year leads. Lead fragments left behind were solid metal tips entrapped connective tissue sheath around lead. This results in tip separation, usually at the level of the innominate vein. There were no clinical complications related to retention of these lead tips.[37]

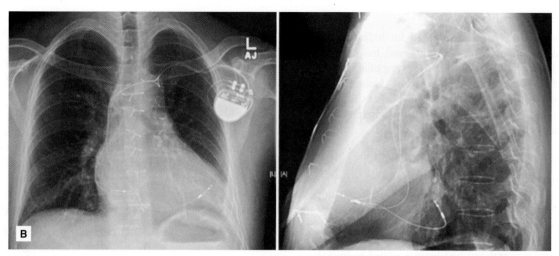

FIGURE 55-21B This 31-year-old male with sinoatrial node dysfunction and third degree heart block had previously undergone closure of atrial and ventricular septal defects, a Maze procedure, and pulmonary and tricuspid valve replacement twice, most recently with a mechanical tricuspid valve. Ventricular pacing was achieved with endocardial lead in posterior cardiac vein, avoiding thoracotomy. (Reproduced with permission from Spotnitz HM, Wang DY: Middle and posterior cardiac veins: an underused option for ventricular pacing, *J Thorac Cardiovasc Surg.* 2012 May;143(5):1223-1225.)

positive fixation leads are ideal for this purpose,[27] but other approaches have been described.[22] We prefer cephalic cutdown, with optical magnification, if needed. A flexible guidewire is passed centrally and a 7-French introducer introduces the lead. A longitudinal split of the cephalic vein facilitates advancing the introducer (Fig. 55-8). In very small infants, the external jugular vein at the thoracic inlet may be useful. A catheter introduced via the femoral vein can guide subclavian vein puncture. Thoracotomy is a third option.[22] Infants less than 6 months of age are suboptimal candidates for transvenous pacing because of limited long-term lead utility. Subpectoral generator placement in children less than 6 years old reduces infection risk.

DEMENTIA

Dementia complicates surgery under local anesthesia. Sedation can make dementia worse and exaggerate bradycardia. A demented patient's arms should be secured to prevent groping for the surgical wound. Postoperative confusion and thrashing can cause pacemaker lead displacement. An intracardiac loop decreases this hazard. A family member at the bedside may minimize patient alarm. Every effort should be made to anticipate and avoid such issues.

ARRHYTHMIA ABLATION

Arrhythmia ablation is the commonest therapeutic intervention in EP laboratories, with hundreds of thousands performed annually. Ablation procedures can result in AV block or sinus bradycardia requiring permanent pacing. Ablation in the vicinity of the AV node is particularly hazardous. Most commonly, temporary pacing supports heart rate until a permanent pacemaker can be inserted. If ventricular escape rhythm is poor, overnight observation on telemetry and high

initial pacemaker output are desirable. Alternatively, a pacemaker can be inserted and allowed to heal before ablation, if high-grade block is anticipated.

TRANSPLANT RECIPIENTS

The usual indication for pacemaker insertion in cardiac transplant recipients is sinus bradycardia or sinus arrest, managed with AAIR pacing.[45] Patients frequently outgrow the need for pacing within 2 years.[45] The surface ECG may be confusing, showing P waves from the atria of both the donor and the recipient and AV dissociation of the recipient atrium and donor ventricle. If a 1:1 ventricular response is observed with atrial pacing at 150 bpm, a ventricular lead is not essential. The atrial appendage is located toward the midline in these patients (Fig. 55-22).

IMPLANTABLE CARDIOVERTER DEFIBRILLATOR RECIPIENTS

In the early evolution of ICDs, crosstalk with pacemakers could lead to inappropriate ICD shocks or ICD undersensing of VF. Independent implantation of pacemakers and ICDs is described,[46] but with availability of integrated ICD-DDD pacemakers, such techniques are now rarely indicated.

LONG QT SYNDROME

Long QT is a genetically determined repolarization abnormality that is associated with sudden death. Recommended therapies include stellate ganglionectomy and/or adrenergic blockade.[47] In severe cases, the pacing threshold may be too high for ventricular pacing, and atrial pacing may be preferable. ICD therapy is now common, and techniques for implantation in infants have been described.

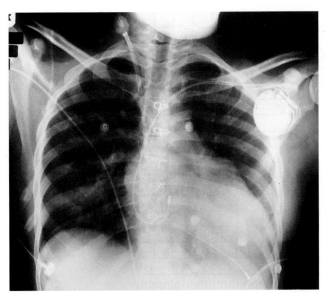

FIGURE 55-22 DDDR pacing system in a cardiac allograft recipient illustrates a shift of the atrial appendage toward the midline, characteristic of these patients.

IDIOPATHIC HYPERTROPHIC SUBAORTIC STENOSIS

Idiopathic hypertrophic subaortic stenosis (obstructive cardiomyopathy), with severe left ventricular outflow obstruction, causes angina and/or syncope. Right ventricular pacing with a short AVD preexcites the ventricle and decreases outflow gradients in some patients[16,17] (Fig. 55-23). ICD therapy is increasingly common in this population.

PERMANENT BIVENTRICULAR PACING

End-stage cardiomyopathy and heart failure progress with time, leading ultimately to cardiac transplantation, cardiac assist devices, or death. CRT is a lower cost option for class III or IV and possibly class II failure. Clinical trials demonstrate modest subjective and objective benefits of CRT in dilated cardiomyopathy with left ventricular ejection fraction less than 36% and QRS intervals greater than 120 ms.[5,18,29,34] Mortality benefits are suggested by recent trials.[5,34] Marked clinical improvement is seen in some patients (Fig. 55-11), but up to 40% of patients are nonresponders. Endocardial LV lead insertion fails in 5 to 10% of candidates, usually because of difficulty cannulating the CS. These failures often result in referrals to thoracic surgeons for epicardial lead insertion. More than 100,000 patients undergo CRT annually in the United States, which could lead to 5000 referrals yearly for epicardial lead insertion. Minimal access[48] and robotic[49] LV lead insertion have been developed. Referrals might increase if better techniques for epicardial LV lead insertion were available.

TEMPORARY BIVENTRICULAR PACING

Clinical success with CRT and the potential to increase cardiac output while reducing myocardial oxygen consumption make temporary biventricular pacing attractive for management of low-output states after cardiac surgery. Preliminary results[50,51] indicate that this approach is promising. Temporary biventricular pacing can be recommended and is readily achievable for patients in low-output states with second- or third-degree block after cardiac surgery.[18]

ATRIAL AND VENTRICULAR TACHYARRHYTHMIAS

Overdrive pacing can be effective for ventricular tachyarrhythmias, Wolff-Parkinson-White syndrome, or atrial flutter. Implantable defibrillators are under development for atrial fibrillation. Antitachycardia ventricular pacing for ventricular tachyarrhythmia has been integrated into ICD therapy. Ablation procedures are available for many supraventricular and ventricular arrhythmias.

Environmental Issues

ELECTROMAGNETIC INTERFERENCE

EMI[43] can be caused by electrocautery, cellular telephones, magnetic resonance imagers, microwaves, diathermy, arc welders, powerful radar or radio transmitters, and theft detectors in retail stores. Any defective, sparking electrical appliance or motor, electric razor, lawn mower, or electric light can be problematic. EMI is most concerning in pacemaker dependent patients and ICD recipients. Pacemaker recipients who are not pacemaker dependent will not be distressed by brief periods of pacemaker inhibition, but pacemaker-dependent patients can lose consciousness in 5 to 15 seconds. Bipolar pacing systems provide added protection against EMI. Cellular telephones should be separated by several inches from pacemaker generators, preferably on the contralateral side. ICD circuits are insulated against inappropriate firing precipitated by EMI. During surgery using unipolar cautery, the defibrillation circuit of an ICD should be temporarily disabled. MRI compatible pacemakers and defibrillators are now available but require specific facility protocols.

MECHANICAL INTERFERENCE

Lithotripsy, trauma, dental equipment, and even bumpy roads can affect pacemakers. Automobile accidents have caused pacemaker damage and disruption of pacemaker wounds. Vibration causes inappropriately high heart rates in rate-responsive units. Patients with poor escape rhythms should be discouraged from exposure to deceleration injury in contact sports, basketball, handball, downhill skiing, surfing, diving, mountain climbing, and gymnastics. Participants in these activities should realize that abrupt pacemaker failure could occur in the event of lead displacement related to trauma.

RADIOACTIVITY

The integrated circuits of current pacemakers can be damaged by radiotherapy.[2] If the pacemaker cannot be adequately shielded from the radiation field, it may be necessary to remove and replace it or move the pacing system to a remote site.

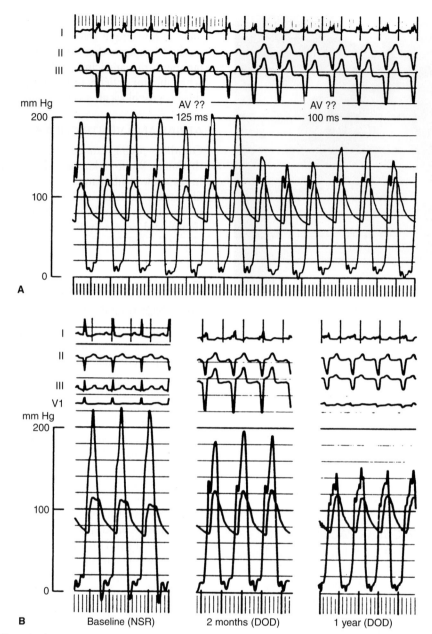

FIGURE 55-23 (A) Effect of reducing AVD in DDD pacing from 125 (*left*) to 100 ms (*right*) on left ventricular outflow gradient in idiopathic hypertrophic subaortic stenosis. (B) Effect of time and DDD pacing on left ventricular outflow gradient in idiopathic hypertrophic subaortic stenosis. (Reproduced with permission from Fananapazir L, Epstein ND, Curiel RV, et al: Long-term results of dual-chamber (DDD) pacing in obstructive hypertrophic cardiomyopathy. Evidence for progressive symptomatic and hemodynamic improvement and reduction of left ventricular hypertrophy, *Circulation* 1994 Dec;90(6):2731-2742.)

QUALITY OF LIFE

Quality of life is not a major concern for most pacemaker recipients. This preferred system involves transtelephonic monitoring, a preoperative visit, a 10-day post-operative visit, a 1-year visit to adjust output, and yearly visits unless functional problems or impending battery depletion are detected. Some recipients are never happy with their pacemakers because of body image problems, vague symptoms, or concern that life will be artificially prolonged. The value of continued pacing or generator replacement in patients with advanced debilitation is a subject of debate.[4]

IMPLANTABLE CARDIAC DEFIBRILLATORS

Background

More than 400,000 deaths in the United States each year are classified as sudden and likely to be caused by arrhythmias.[7] Michel Mirowski conceptualized the implantable defibrillator in the late 1960s. Overcoming theoretical, engineering, and financial obstacles, he participated in a successful clinical trial of his device in the early 1980s.[52] Current ICDs reflect a dramatic and expensive growth in technology. The efficacy of the ICD in prevention of sudden death is well established. Clinical trials, experience, and the passage of time emphasize survival advantages of the ICD over other modalities, including antiarrhythmic drugs and subendocardial resection.[7] The ICD is associated with the lowest sudden death mortality (1–2% per year) of any known form of therapy.[53,54] The cost of an ICD plus leads exceeds $30,000 and has increased with incorporation of CRT. Prophylactic ICD insertion for primary prevention is increasing, despite discomfort and lifestyle issues.

Clinical trials including AVID, MUSST, MADIT I and II, SCD-HeFT, and COMPANION demonstrated benefits of ICD therapy.[7,42,55-58] The CABG Patch Trial,[57] which compared coronary artery bypass graft (CABG) to CABG+ICD, and DINAMIT, which studied ICD implantation early after myocardial infarction, failed to demonstrate advantages of ICD insertion. Trials now focus on prophylactic ICD therapy, CRT-Ds and cost-effectiveness. Accumulating evidence supports prophylactic use of CRT-Ds in patients with coronary disease or dilated cardiomyopathy.[7,58] The appropriate role for prophylactic CRT-Ds is still evolving. The Heart Rhythm Society will not certify surgeons to implant ICDs unless they have passed its certification exam. Patients with prophylactic device insertion are being followed in a national registry. Information about this can be found at http://www.accncdr.com/webncdr/ICD. ICD insertion for primary prevention has doubled or tripled the number of candidates for these devices.

ICD battery life is greater than 5 years. Today's devices are highly programmable. Size and weight are similar to pacemakers of the 1970s. Lead systems have evolved from epicardial patches requiring thoracotomy to endocardial systems.[7,54,59,60] Defibrillation thresholds (DFTs) are reduced by biphasic shocks and "hot can" technology.[7] Pectoral implantation is the current standard, some deep to the pectoralis major. Abdominal implantation is now reserved for special cases (Figs. 55-24 and 55-25). Electrograms can be downloaded to expedite decisions about antiarrhythmics, prevent inappropriate shocks, and detect oversensing. Remote monitoring of ICD function is available from some manufacturers. VVI, DDD, biventricular, and anti-tachycardia pacing have been integrated into ICDs. Accelerated development has pressured the Food and Drug Administration to rapidly approve new technology. When the US Health Care Finance Administration refused in 1995 to allow Medicare reimbursement to support device development, ICD development shifted overseas.

Physiology

VT associated with ischemic cardiomyopathy is commonly a reentrant arrhythmia that may be prevented by drugs, catheter ablation, or surgical maneuvers that alter the timing and electrical attributes of the reentrant circuit. Myocardial

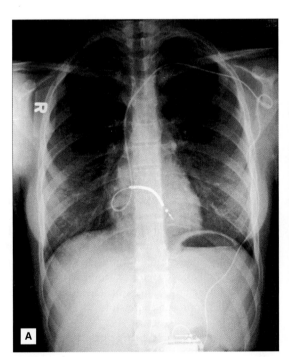
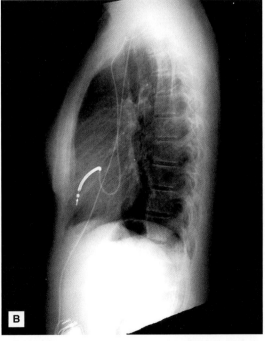

FIGURE 55-24 (A) ICD implant in 13-year-old girl with long QT syndrome. Intracardiac loop allows for growth. Strain relief loop is in the shoulder. Single-coil, screw-in lead permitted intracardiac loop. Twin-coil leads are now available. Generator is in posterior rectus sheath. (B) Lateral x-ray.

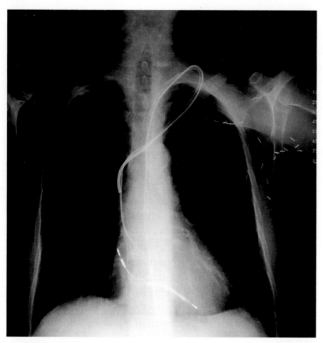

FIGURE 55-25 ICD/DDD pacemaker for VT with prior bilateral radical mastectomies. Venous access via external jugular vein. Positive fixation leads tunneled vertically in the midline, the only location on the chest wall with adequate tissue. Generator subcutaneous in abdomen. Cosmetic result acceptable to patient.

infarction creates the areas of scarring and slow conduction needed for reentry. Other forms of VT and VF involve aberrancies of automaticity related to acute myocardial ischemia, increased ventricular wall stress, and myopathic cellular injury. Some class I antiarrhythmics have been shown to increase postinfarction mortality, possibly owing to proarrhythmic effects.

Indications

Candidates for ICD insertion for secondary prevention therapy have suffered documented VT or VF in the absence of acute myocardial infarction and have been proved unsuitable for antiarrhythmic drug or surgical therapy, based on programmed electrical stimulation studies in the EP laboratory. However, many patients who suffer cardiac arrest do not have inducible VT at EP study, and many patients with a history of syncope and presyncope have inducible VT but no history of a clinical arrhythmia. Many antiarrhythmics have negative inotropic and proarrhythmic effects. Serial EP studies of drug efficacy have been discredited in clinical trials.[7]

In mid-1996 the Food and Drug Administration approved an indication for prophylactic ICD insertion based on early termination of the MADIT trial.[55] If EP studies demonstrate inducible VT in patients with nonsustained VT and a remote history of myocardial infarction, an ICD is indicated. MADIT II results support ICD insertion in all patients with a history of myocardial infarction and left ventricular ejection fraction less than 30%. Primary prevention indications include ischemic cardiomyopathy with LVEF ≤ 35% and NYHA Class II or III ≥ 40 days post MI. LVEF ≤ 30% and NYHA Class I ≥ 40 days after MI also qualifies, as does nonischemic myopathy with LVEF ≤ 35% and NYHA Class II or III.

Device Description

ICDs usually employ one bipolar lead for ventricular pacing/rate sensing and another to deliver the defibrillation current (Fig. 55-26). These are integrated into a single lead body for endocardial insertion.[7] A unipolar ventricular lead paired with an "active can" delivers the defibrillation current in some designs. Rate and waveform identify malignant rhythms for treatment. Up to 30% of ICD shocks are inappropriate, for sinus tachycardia or other supraventricular tachyarrhythmias. A bipolar atrial lead can help differentiate supraventricular arrhythmias from VT. Subcutaneous leads can be added for patients with high DFTs. Most implants are just caudad to the clavicle, but long lead lengths allow abdominal locations. Positive fixation leads are preferred.

The ICD contains a high-energy battery and a capacitor that steps up the output voltage to 600 to 800 V at 35 to 40 J. Shocks with positive and negative phases reduce DFTs. ICDs incorporate integrated circuits and a telemetry antenna. A broad range of programmable diagnostic and therapeutic functions are supported.

Surgical Procedure

PATIENT PREPARATION

Most ICD recipients are at increased mortality/morbidity risk for any surgery. Preoperative optimization of therapy for ischemia, heart failure, and systemic illnesses is critical. The mortality of ICD implantation in our program has been low since 1983, with ischemia more lethal than severe cardiomyopathy. Ischemia on stress testing mandates CABG, coronary angioplasty, intra-aortic balloon pump, or deferral of DFT testing.

SURGICAL APPROACH

Epicardial patch leads[59,60] are now rarely used. They fell into disfavor when the CABG Patch Trial demonstrated that infectious complications were more common in ICD recipients than control patients.[57] Extrapericardial ICD patches cause less fibrosis, less impairment of diastolic properties,[61,62] and less potential for graft impingement than intrapericardial patches. Biphasic waveforms, improved leads, high-output "hot can" generators, and subcutaneous leads have made the endocardial approach successful.[7]

MANUFACTURER'S REPRESENTATIVES

The complexity of current devices and a large number of spare parts, leads, and catheters have legitimized the presence of manufacturer's representatives during ICD implants.

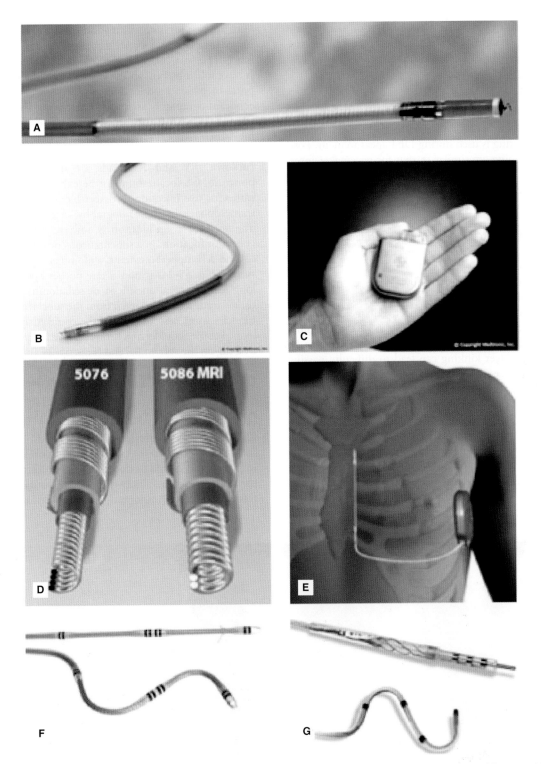

FIGURE 55-26 (A) ICD lead (9 French) with Gore-Tex-coated shocking coils. (B) ICD lead (7 French) with retractable screw. (C) ICD/pacemaker. (D) Early design MRI-compatible pacemaker leads. (E) Wireless ICD. (F) and (G) Over-the-wire multielectrode lead for coronary sinus pacing. (A, E: Image provided courtesy of Boston Scientific. © 2016 Boston Scientific Corporation or its affiliates. All rights reserved. B, C, D, F: Reproduced with permission of Medtronic, Inc.; G: Trifecta, Quartet and St. Jude Medical are trademarks of St. Jude Medical, Inc. or its related companies. Reproduced with permission of St. Jude Medical, © 2016. All rights reserved.)

This increases influence of the manufacturer on the implant and warrants oversight. CRS regulations mandate electrophysiologist oversight of DFT measurement.

TECHNIQUE

We prefer local anesthesia, conscious sedation, and unipolar cautery for endocardial ICD insertion. Invasive, radial artery pressure monitoring is used during DFT measurement. Positioning and draping are similar to that for pacemaker insertion. Adhesive defibrillation pads are added over the right breast and beneath the left scapula. Pads should not be placed directly over the site of a possible subcutaneous ICD patch or array in the lateral axilla; this can result in serious equipment damage from arcing if external defibrillation is necessary. Cefazolin or combined vancomycin/gentamicin is used for antibiotic prophylaxis.

We prefer a cephalic vein cutdown via a 6-cm incision over the deltopectoral groove. If the vein is small, a guidewire is used to insert a 9-French introducer. Enlargement of the cephalic venotomy may be helpful (Fig. 55-8). The guidewire can be left in place if a multiple-lead system is to be employed. Introducer kinking can lead to difficulty passing ICD leads. High central pressures will cause bleeding until the introducer is removed. Aligning the introducer with the course of the subclavian vein before removing the obturator minimizes this.

As the lead enters the ventricle, VT or VF may be triggered. This is less disruptive if an external defibrillator is connected and precharged, with a capable OR nurse or electrophysiologist at the controls. The ventricular lead should be advanced gently as far as possible to the apex. Positive fixation ICD

leads are best for both atrium and ventricle. Fluoroscopic and impedance checks for lead displacement are warranted during DFTs, particularly if external defibrillation is necessary. Intravenous norepinephrine is useful for blood pressure support. In patients under general anesthesia, transesophageal echocardiography is useful for monitoring LV function during DFTs. Swan-Ganz catheters are not useful for monitoring—their removal can dislodge the ICD leads.

If CRT is indicated, we insert the LV lead first, via cephalic cutdown. RV and RA leads are inserted via subclavian puncture. CS localization can be expedited by steerable EP catheters, dye injection to detect blood flow out of the CS, transesophageal echocardiography, and other techniques.[5] The left subclavian location is now the standard of care for generator location, in a subcutaneous or subpectoral pocket.

The left upper quadrant abdominal or posterior rectus sheath (Fig. 55-24) is now a rare pocket option and requires long leads, general anesthesia or sedation/local anesthesia to tunnel leads to the abdomen from the subclavian incision. The tunneler must pass anterior to the costal margin. The lead is looped at the shoulder and firmly secured against displacement by a tug on the abdominal end (Figs. 55-24 and 55-25). A limited thoracotomy may be required to add an epicardial lead for CRT if endocardial CS lead insertion fails (Fig. 55-27).

DEFIBRILLATION THRESHOLD

DFT testing was previously the standard of care but is increasingly controversial, particularly in primary prevention implants, and should be done in consultation with an electrophysiologist.[5] Vulnerability testing is a described option. DFT testing is also less important as technological advances have

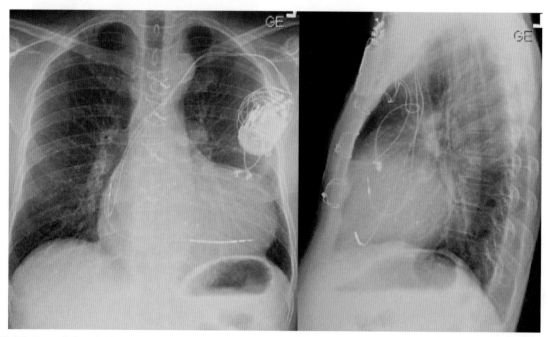

FIGURE 55-27 Epicardial LV leads inserted in 45-year-old man for treatment of congestive heart failure after two failed endocardial attempts. PM-ICD was required for complete heart block and cardiomyopathy after aortic and mitral valve replacement for bacterial endocarditis.

increased the probability of success. The DFT is the point of maximum risk in ICD insertion and is usually induced twice and reversed by the ICD to confirm a 10-J safety margin and adequate sensing of VF. Backup defibrillation is available through defibrillation pads. If the DFT is too high after optimizing RV lead location, a subcutaneous axillary patch or wire is used to distribute the defibrillation current over the posterolateral left ventricle. High-output generators and reversed shock polarity may also help. DFT testing can depress cardiac function and cause a low-output state.[5,46] The mortality of ICD insertion is about 1%. Complications include myocardial infarction, heart failure, infection, lead displacement, venous occlusion, tamponade, hemopneumothorax, and pocket hematoma.

REFRACTORY VENTRICULAR FIBRILLATION

VF may become refractory to external defibrillation as a result of iatrogenic pneumothorax, myocardial ischemia, electromechanical dissociation, and inappropriate ICD lead location. Refractory VF rarely may require open cardiac massage or cardiopulmonary bypass until a solution can be found.

POSTOPERATIVE CARE

Same day discharge or telemetry and an overnight stay are both current practice after ICD insertion for secondary prevention, and DFT testing is controversial. Pacing and sensing properties confirm lead stability before discharge. In some cases, DFTs are also retested. An ICD magnet should be available for treatment of patients with freshly implanted ICDs. The magnet is used to inhibit inappropriate shocks caused by ventricular lead displacement or supraventricular arrhythmias. Patients undergoing ICD insertion for primary prevention may be discharged on the day of surgery. We administer ciprofloxacin for 5 days after discharge to complete prophylaxis based on a historical precedent. A postoperative office visit is scheduled 7 to 14 days after implant.

SURGICAL FOLLOW-UP

At the postoperative office visit, lead position, patient symptoms, EP follow-up appointments, and the surgical site are assessed. If drainage is present, the wound is cultured and treated. For sterile drainage, ciprofloxacin or trimethoprim-sulfamethoxazole is administered for 10 days, and the patient is asked to keep the site dry until healing is complete. Refractory infection requires hospitalization and ICD removal.

DEVICE FOLLOW-UP

ICDs require outpatient EP evaluation at 1- to 3-month intervals to cycle the capacitors, confirm battery life, test pacing thresholds, and download electrograms. Data are reviewed for aborted charging cycles arrhythmias. Programming is adjusted accordingly. For any shocks reported, telemetry can confirm proper function, detect inappropriate shocks, and demonstrate electrical noise or oversensing that requires lead revision. Wireless ICD monitoring from home is now a clinical reality for some ICDs.

Late Follow-up and Generator Replacement

BATTERY DEPLETION

ICD battery life is now typically more than 60 months. Complications of generator replacement include infection, myocardial infarction, and death. Progression of heart failure and/or coronary artery disease increases the risk of replacement. Replacement is done under local anesthesia, with sedation during DFTs. DFTs may be deferred if the risk is excessive. Patients are discharged on the same day with antibiotic coverage, unless leads are replaced.

LEAD DYSFUNCTION

The incidence of lead failure increases with time. About 50% of ICD recipients have some lead revision by 10 years of follow-up.[63] Problems include lead fracture,[64] high DFTs, oversensing, undersensing, and exit block. Oversensing can be caused by insulation damage. Oversensing can be corrected by adding a transvenous rate-sensing lead, preferably of the positive-fixation type. Visible insulation damage inside the defibrillator pocket may be repairable with silicone glue, tubing, and ties.

Patch leads can fail because of conductor fracture or distortion by fibrosis. With endocardial leads, DFTs may increase as a result of cardiac enlargement, which shifts the left ventricle laterally, away from the right ventricular lead. Insertion of a subcutaneous patch or array (Fig. 55-28) and/or a high-output generator can correct high DFTs.

Additional Issues

BRIDGE TO TRANSPLANT

CRT-D therapy is increasingly common for amelioration of symptoms and protection against VT/VF in patients awaiting cardiac allografting. Cost is an important concern.

QUALITY OF LIFE

Issues include the discomfort and distress of shocks and inconvenience of outpatient visits. These are particularly trying for elderly patients. ICD generators, though shrinking in size and weight, are bulky compared with pacemakers. Many patients are elated to be rescued by their ICD from a malignant arrhythmia, but others find this distressing.[40,65,66] Many ICD patients do not comply with recommended limitations on driving automobiles.[67,68] Fortunately, the rate of driving accidents in ICD recipients is reportedly low.

COST-EFFECTIVENESS

ICD therapy is expensive, but VT/VF management in the absence of an ICD is also costly.[69] Low cost of ICD generators and leads would increase the economic appeal of ICD prophylaxis.

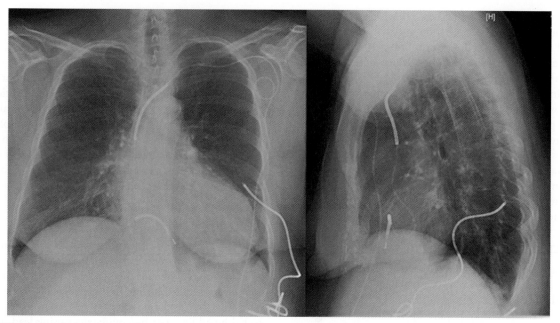

FIGURE 55-28 This illustrates posterolateral accessory lead inserted in chest wall for failure of ICD to defibrillate. Patient is 62-year-old female with prior anteroseptal myocardial infarction. ICD function was initially satisfactory, but progressive CHF and LV dilatation created excessive ICD energy requirement.

NEW TECHNOLOGY

ICDs and pacemakers that do not require endocardial leads are available or in clinical trials. Functionality of these systems is limited but valuable for selected patients.

REFERENCES

1. Ellenbogen KA, Kaszala K: *Cardiac Pacing and ICDs*, 6th ed. Chichester, West Sussex, John Wiley and Sons, 2014.
2. Kalahasty G, Kapa S, Cooper JM: Components of a pacing and ICD system: basic concepts of pacing, 6th ed. Chichester, West Sussex, John Wiley and Sons, 2014; pp 1-33.
3. John RM: Indications for permanent and temporary cardiac pacing, 6th ed. Chichester, West Sussex, John Wiley and Sons, 2014; pp 34-81.
4. Doppalapudi H, Blitzer ML, Shoenfeld MH: Follow-up of the patient with a CIED, 6th ed. Chichester, West Sussex, John Wiley and Sons, 2014; 453-503.
5. Cha YM: Cardiac resynchronization therapy, 6th ed. Chichester, West Sussex, John Wiley and Sons, 2014; 374-412.
6. Marine JE, Brinker JA: Techniques of pacemaker implantation and removal, 6th ed. Chichester, West Sussex, John Wiley and Sons, 2014; pp 150-210.
7. Gold MR, Swerdlow C: The implantable cardioverter-defibrillator, 6th ed. Chichester, West Sussex, John Wiley and Sons, 2014; pp 323-373.
8. Stambler BS, Varma N: Hemodynamics of cardiac pacing and pacing mode selection, 6th ed. Chichester, West Sussex, John Wiley and Sons, 2014; 82-133.
9. Furman S, Schwedel JB: An intracardiac pacemaker for Stokes-Adams seizures. *N Engl J Med* 1959; 261:943-948.
10. Bernstein AD, Camm AJ, Fletcher R, et al: The NASPE/BPEG generic pacemaker code for antibradyarrhythmia and adaptive rate pacing and antitachyarrhythmia devices. *Pacing Clin Electrophysiol* 1987;10(4 Pt 1): 794-799.
11. Epstein AE, DiMarco JP, Ellenbogen KA, et al: 2012 ACCF/AHA/HRS focused update incorporated into the ACCF/AHA/HRS 2008 Guidelines for Device-Based Therapy of Cardiac Rhythm Abnormalities: a report of the American College of Cardiology Foundation/American Heart Association Task Force on Practice Guidelines and the Heart Rhythm Society. *Circulation* 2013; 127(3):e283-e352.
12. Nelson SD, Kou WH, De Buitleir M, et al: Value of programmed ventricular stimulation in presumed carotid sinus syndrome. *Am J Cardiol* 1987; 60(13):1073-1077.
13. Sra JS, Jazayeri MR, Avitall B, et al: Comparison of cardiac pacing with drug therapy in the treatment of neurocardiogenic (vasovagal) syncope with bradycardia or asystole. *N Engl J Med* 1993; 328(15):1085-1090.
14. Prech M, Grygier M, Mitkowski P, et al: Effect of restoration of AV synchrony on stroke volume, exercise capacity, and quality-of-life: can we predict the beneficial effect of a pacemaker upgrade? *Pacing Clin Electrophysiol* 2001; 24(3):302-307.
15. Karpawich PP, Mital S: Comparative left ventricular function following atrial, septal, and apical single chamber heart pacing in the young. *Pacing Clin Electrophysiol* 1997; 20(8 Pt 1):1983-1988.
16. Fananapazir L, Epstein ND, Curiel RV, et al: Long-term results of dual-chamber (DDD) pacing in obstructive hypertrophic cardiomyopathy. Evidence for progressive symptomatic and hemodynamic improvement and reduction of left ventricular hypertrophy. *Circulation* 1994; 90(6):2731-2742.
17. Gadler F, Linde C, Daubert C, et al: Significant improvement of quality of life following atrioventricular synchronous pacing in patients with hypertrophic obstructive cardiomyopathy. Data from 1 year of follow-up. PIC study group. Pacing In Cardiomyopathy. *Eur Heart J* 1999; 20(14):1044-1050.
18. Berberian G, Quinn TA, Kanter JP, et al: Optimized biventricular pacing in atrioventricular block after cardiac surgery. *Ann Thorac Surg* 2005; 80(3):870-875.
19. Lau CP, Butrous GS, Ward DE, et al: Comparison of exercise performance of six rate-adaptive right ventricular cardiac pacemakers. *Am J Cardiol* 1989; 63(12):833-838.
20. Kay GN, Bubien RS, Epstein AE, et al: Rate-modulated cardiac pacing based on transthoracic impedance measurements of minute ventilation: correlation with exercise gas exchange. *J Am Coll Cardiol* 1989; 14(5):1283-1289.
21. Cohen MI, Vetter VL, Wernovsky G, et al: Epicardial pacemaker implantation and follow-up in patients with a single ventricle after the Fontan operation. *J Thorac Cardiovasc Surg* 2001; 121(4):804-811.
22. Byrd CL, Schwartz SJ: Transatrial implantation of transvenous pacing leads as an alternative to implantation of epicardial leads. *Pacing Clin Electrophysiol* 1990; 13(12 Pt 2):1856-1859.

23. Da Costa A, Kirkorian G, Cucherat M, et al: Antibiotic prophylaxis for permanent pacemaker implantation: a meta-analysis. *Circulation* 1998; 97(18):1796-1801.

24. Magney JE, Flynn DM, Parsons JA, et al: Anatomical mechanisms explaining damage to pacemaker leads, defibrillator leads, and failure of central venous catheters adjacent to the sternoclavicular joint. *Pacing Clin Electrophysiol.* 1993; 16(3 Pt 1):445-457.

25. Ong LS, Barold S, Lederman M, et al: Cephalic vein guide wire technique for implantation of permanent pacemakers. *Am Heart J* 1987; 114(4 Pt 1): 753-756.

26. Belott PH: A variation on the introducer technique for unlimited access to the subclavian vein. *Pacing Clin Electrophysiol* 1981; 4(1):43-48.

27. Spotnitz HM: Transvenous pacing in infants and children with congenital heart disease. *Ann Thorac Surg* 1990; 49(3):495-496.

28. Barin ES, Jones SM, Ward DE, et al: The right ventricular outflow tract as an alternative permanent pacing site: long-term follow-up. *Pacing Clin Electrophysiol* 1991; 14(1):3-6.

29. Leclercq C, Cazeau S, Ritter P, et al: A pilot experience with permanent biventricular pacing to treat advanced heart failure. *Am Heart J* 2000; 140(6):862-870.

30. Kiviniemi MS, Pirnes MA, Eranen HJ, et al: Complications related to permanent pacemaker therapy. *Pacing Clin Electrophysiol* 1999; 22(5):711-720.

31. Goldstein DJ, Losquadro W, Spotnitz HM: Outpatient pacemaker procedures in orally anticoagulated patients. *Pacing Clin Electrophysiol* 1998; 21(9):1730-1734.

32. Brewster GM, Evans AL: Displacement of pacemaker leads—a 10-year survey. *Br Heart J* 1979; 42(3):266-270.

33. Link MS, Estes NA 3rd, Griffin JJ, et al: Complications of dual chamber pacemaker implantation in the elderly. Pacemaker Selection in the Elderly (PASE) Investigators. *J Interv Card Electrophysiol* 1998; 2(2):175-179.

34. Cleland JG, Daubert JC, Erdmann E, et al: The effect of cardiac resynchronization on morbidity and mortality in heart failure. *N Engl J Med.* 2005; 352(15):1539-1549.

35. Wilkoff BL, Love CJ, Byrd CL, et al: Transvenous lead extraction: Heart Rhythm Society expert consensus on facilities, training, indications, and patient management: this document was endorsed by the American Heart Association (AHA). *Heart Rhythm* 2009; 6(7):1085-1104.

36. Epstein LM, Byrd CL, Wilkoff BL, et al: Initial experience with larger laser sheaths for the removal of transvenous pacemaker and implantable defibrillator leads. *Circulation* 1999; 100(5):516-525.

37. Rusanov A, Spotnitz HM: A 15-year experience with permanent pacemaker and defibrillator lead and patch extractions. *Ann Thorac Surg* 2010; 89(1):44-50.

38. Margey R, McCann H, Blake G, et al: Contemporary management of and outcomes from cardiac device related infections. *Europace* 2010; 12(1):64-70.

39. Molina JE: Undertreatment and overtreatment of patients with infected antiarrhythmic implantable devices. *Ann Thorac Surg* 1997; 63(2):504-509.

40. May CD, Smith PR, Murdock CL, et al: The impact of implantable cardioverter defibrillator on quality-of-life. *Pacing Clin Electrophysiol* 1995; 18(7):1411-1418.

41. Rusanov A, Spotnitz HM: Salvage of a failing bifurcated bipolar epicardial lead with conductor fracture. *Ann Thorac Surg* 2010; 90(2):649-651.

42. The Cardiac Arrhythmia Suppression Trial (CAST) Investigators. Preliminary report: effect of encainide and flecainide on mortality in a randomized trial of arrhythmia suppression after myocardial infarction. *N Engl J Med* 1989; 321(6):406-412.

43. Madigan JD, Choudhri AF, Chen J, et al: Surgical management of the patient with an implanted cardiac device: implications of electromagnetic interference. *Ann Surg* 1999; 230:(5):639-647.

44. Bourke ME: The patient with a pacemaker or related device. *Can J Anaesth* 1996; 43(5 Pt 2):R24-R41.

45. Raghavan C, Maloney JD, Nitta J, et al: Long-term follow-up of heart transplant recipients requiring permanent pacemakers. *J Heart Lung Transplant* 1995; 14:(6 Pt 1):1081-1089.

46. Spotnitz HM, Ott GY, Bigger JT Jr, et al: Methods of implantable cardioverter-defibrillator-pacemaker insertion to avoid interactions. *Ann Thorac Surg* 1992; 53(2):253-257.

47. Zareba W, Moss AJ: Long QT syndrome in children. *J Electrocardiol* 2001; 34 Suppl:167-171.

48. Doll N, Opfermann UT, Rastan AJ, et al: Facilitated minimally invasive left ventricular epicardial lead placement. *Ann Thorac Surg* 2005; 79(3):1023-1025.

49. DeRose JJ, Ashton RC, Belsley S, et al: Robotically assisted left ventricular epicardial lead implantation for biventricular pacing. *JACC* 2003; 41:(8):1414-1419.

50. Wang DY, Richmond ME, Quinn TA, et al: Optimized temporary biventricular pacing acutely improves intraoperative cardiac output after weaning from cardiopulmonary bypass: a substudy of a randomized clinical trial. *J Thorac Cardiovasc Surg* 2011; 141(4):1002-1008.

51. Spotnitz HM, Cabreriza SE, Wang DY, et al: Primary endpoints of the biventricular pacing after cardiac surgery trial. *Ann Thorac Surg* 2013; 96:808-815.

52. Mirowski M, Reid PR, Mower MM, et al: Termination of malignant ventricular arrhythmia with an implantable automatic defibrillator in human beings. *N Engl J Med* 1980; 303(6):322-324.

53. Zipes DP, Roberts D: Results of the international study of the implantable pacemaker cardioverter-defibrillator. A comparison of epicardial and endocardial lead systems. *Circulation* 1995; 92:(1):59-65.

54. Shahian DM, Williamson WA, Svensson LG, et al: Transvenous versus transthoracic cardioverter-defibrillator implantation. *J Thorac Cardiovasc Surg* 1995; 109(6):1066-1074.

55. Prystowsky EN, Nisam S: Prophylactic implantable cardioverter defibrillator trials: MUSTT, MADIT, and beyond. Multicenter Unsustained Tachycardia Trial. Multicenter Automatic Defibrillator Implantation Trial. *Am J Cardiol* 2000; 86(11):1214-1215, A5.

56. Bardy GH, Lee KL, Mark DB, et al for the Sudden Cardiac Death in Heart Failure Trial (SCD-HeFT) Investigators: Amiodarone or an implantable cardioverter-defibrillator for congestive heart failure. *N Engl J Med* 2005; 352(3):225-237.

57. Bigger JT for the Coronary Artery Bypass Graft (CABG) Patch Trial Investigators: Prophylactic use of implanted cardiac defibrillators in patients at high risk for ventricular arrhythmias after coronary-artery bypass graft surgery. *N Engl J Med* 1997; 337(22):1569-1575.

58. Epstein AE: Update on primary prevention implantable cardioverter-defibrillator therapy. *Curr Cardiol Rep* 2009; 11(5):335-342.

59. Spotnitz HM: Surgical approaches to ICD insertion. In: Spotnitz HM. *Research Frontiers in Implantable Defibrillator Surgery.* Austin, TX: RG Landes: 1992; 23-34.

60. Watkins L Jr, Taylor E Jr: Surgical aspects of automatic implantable cardioverter-defibrillator implantation. *Pacing Clin Electrophysiol* 1991; 14(5 Pt 2):953-960.

61. Auteri JS, Jeevanandam V, Bielefeld MR, et al: Effects of location of AICD patch electrodes on the left ventricular diastolic pressure-volume curve in pigs. *Ann Thorac Surg* 1991; 52(5):1052-1057.

62. Barrington WW, Deligonul U, Easley AR, et al: Defibrillator patch electrode constriction: an underrecognized entity. *Ann Thorac Surg* 1995; 60(4):1112-1115.

63. Mattke S, Muller D, Markewitz A, et al: Failures of epicardial and transvenous leads for implantable cardioverter defibrillators. *Am Heart J.* 1995; 130(5):1040-1044.

64. Roelke M, O'Nunain, Osswald S, et al: Subclavian crush syndrome complicating transvenous cardioverter defibrillator systems. *Pacing Clin Electrophysiol* 1995; 18(5 Pt 1):973-979.

65. Ahmad M, Bloomstein L, Roelke M, et al: Patients' attitudes toward implanted defibrillator shocks. *Pacing Clin Electrophysiol* 2000; 23(6):934-938.

66. Kohn CS, Petrucci RJ, Baessler C, et al: The effect of psychological intervention on patients' long-term adjustment to the ICD: a prospective study. *Pacing Clin Electrophysiol* 2000; 23(4 Pt 1):450-456.

67. Vijgen J, Botto G, Camm J, et al: Consensus statement of the European Heart Rhythm Association: updated recommendations for driving by patients with implantable cardioverter defibrillators. *Europace* 2009; 11(8):1097-1107.

68. Lampert R: Managing with pacemakers and implantable cardioverter defibrillators. *Circulation* 2013; 128(14):1576-1585.

69. Thijssen J, van den Akker, van Marle ME, et al: Cost-effectiveness of primary prevention implantable cardioverter defibrillator treatment: data from a large clinical registry. *Pacing Clin Electrophysiol* 2014; 37(1):25-34.

70. Spotnitz HM: *Technique of Pediatric Pacemaker Insertion.* [Quicktime]. 1992.

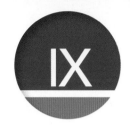

OTHER CARDIAC
OPERATIONS

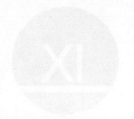

XI

OTHER CARDIAC OPERATIONS

Surgery for Adult Congenital Heart Disease

Redmond P. Burke

56

Adults with congenital heart disease now outnumber children with this malady. They constitute a growing population of survivors, with increasingly complex treatment requirements for their heart disease. Over the past two decades, the spectrum of complexity for adult congenital heart disease (ACHD) patients has evolved from late primary repairs of patients with simple lesions—including coarctation, patent ductus arteriosus, septal defects, and tetralogy of Fallot—to *n*th time reoperations on survivors of complex multistaged palliations. Significant efforts to define the optimal program resources necessary to effectively treat ACHD patients have been made worldwide,[1] yet many congenital heart patients continue to suffer from poor continuity of care as they enter adulthood. This chapter will describe several salient treatment strategies for adult patients undergoing congenital heart surgery.

REDUCING CUMULATIVE THERAPEUTIC TRAUMA

The optimal venue for ACHD treatment is unknown, and it is fair to say that no two programs are the same. The need for a coordinated and comprehensive programmatic strategy for care has been well described, and should encompass not only the lifetime of a generation of patients with congenital heart defects from fetal to adult life, but also the health of pregnant mothers with congenital heart disease who will give birth to a new generation.[2] Pregnant mothers with fetal diagnoses of congenital heart disease may be asked to undergo invasive intrauterine procedures to palliate their fetal child's heart, thus creating a new group of adult patients dealing with the trauma of congenital heart care.[3]

Our congenital heart program philosophy is to reduce the cumulative trauma of care for each patient with congenital heart disease over their lifetime. To achieve this, we discuss each adult patient referred to our program for surgery or intervention in a combined conference with participation from adult and pediatric interventional cardiologists and surgeons, dedicated cardiac intensivists, cardiac anesthesiologists, cardiac imaging specialists, and the cardiac nursing, pharmacy

and social work teams. Treatment options are selected so that the least traumatic form of effective therapy is chosen as the initial approach. Failure to achieve a good result leads to an escalation to the next least traumatic option. As an example, a patient with a secundum atrial septal defect (ASD) would be put forward for device closure, and if this failed, the patient would then be given the option of a minimally invasive surgical repair.

INFORMATION SYSTEMS

Adult congenital heart disease patients with complex lesions often have dense medical histories, stored in multimedia formats, which expose the weaknesses of current paper and electronic medical record (EMR) systems. Increasing utilization of EMRs by medical teams, and personal health records (PHRs) by patients and families, has been demonstrated to improve outcomes in some patients with chronic disease.[4] However, pediatric heart patients and their families often have not been educated about their disease, and what to expect as they transition to adulthood. The PHR could be used to enhance patients' understanding, and provide roadmaps for follow-up treatments and diagnostic studies. These information systems could also be linked to national and international registries designed to measure clinical outcomes and performance for centers treating adult congenital heart patients.[5]

The emergence of Web-based hospital EMR systems allows our cardiac team to track patients over their lifetime, and retrieve critical patient information on demand. We have also enabled our patients to access specific data fields from the EMR. We capture intraoperative endoscopic images of each congenital heart lesion, before and after repair,[6] and store these images in our EMR. We also capture and store a daily picture of each hospitalized patient. These images are reviewed in morbidity and mortality conferences, to correlate with other clinical information and imaging techniques. The operative images are reviewed prior to reoperations, to regain familiarity with the patient's anatomy.[7] The operative images from this chapter were retrieved from this online image database (Fig. 56-1).

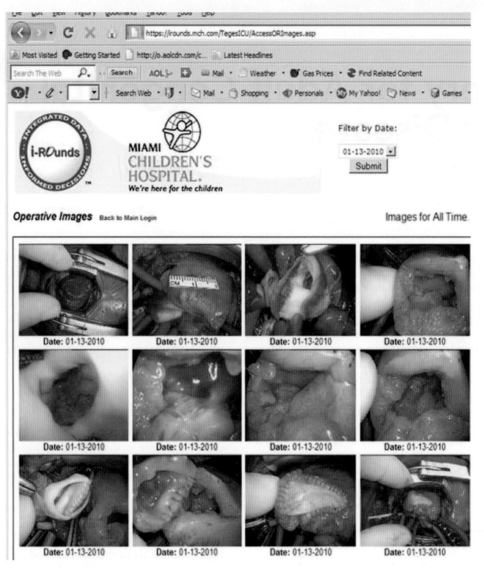

FIGURE 56-1 This is a screen image from our first electronic medical record, showing the operative images for a patient with truncus arteriosus. These images were captured in the operating room, and immediately uploaded to a Web-based EMR. These can be retrieved on demand by searching by procedure, diagnosis, or individual patient.

COMMON ADULT CONGENITAL HEART DISEASE PROCEDURES

Reoperative Sternotomy

Congenital heart procedures in adults are frequently reoperations, however, standardized protocols for reoperations in patients with acquired heart disease may not match the challenges presented by ACHD patients. Risk factors for traumatic repeat sternotomy in ACHD patients differ from those identified in patients with acquired heart disease, which often focus on dealing with patent coronary artery bypass grafts.[8] Femoral cannulation is often difficult in ACHD patients who have undergone multiple interventional catheterizations during their growth years, resulting in stenotic or occluded femoral vessels. Consequently,

we rarely use elective or emergent peripheral cannulation. Key risk factors for ACHD reoperations include retrosternal ventricular to pulmonary artery conduits, particularly if they are calcified, have multiple stents in place, or are clearly embedded in the sternum. Fusion to the sternum should be suspected when the conduit does not move with the cardiac cycle on lateral angiograms. Patients with pulmonary hypertension, right ventricular enlargement, prior sternal infections, aneurysms of the right or left ventricular outflow tracts, pectus excavatum, or aortopulmonary shunts are at increased risk, and qualify for preliminary vascular access dissection and pursestring placement. Patients with multiple risk factors may be placed on bypass to decompress the right ventricle prior to sternal division.

We excise previous sternotomy scars and remove sternal wires. The xiphoid process is removed, and cautery dissection is begun at the inferior sternal edge. The oscillating saw is used to divide the anterior sternal table. Rakes are used to elevate the two sides of the sternum and expose the retrosternal scar. Short segments of retrosternal scar are released, followed by gradual sternal division with the oscillating saw, proceeding up the sternum.

In the event of cardiac or great vessel penetration during sternotomy, when we have not already exposed vessels for cannulation, we release the sternal retractors, and immediately extend the neck incision up and to the right to expose the innominate artery and the internal jugular or high innominate vein. These vessels are cannulated through pursestrings, and bypass is initiated. In patients where venous access cannot be achieved in the suprasternal area, we dissect the inferior vena cava just above the diaphragm. This approach has been described as "simplified aortic cannulation."[9] The sternotomy is completed with the patient in Trendeleberg position. We continuously infuse carbon dioxide into the operative field during every operation to reduce the risk of air embolism, although evidence supporting this technique is not conclusive.[10]

To reduce adhesion formation, and decrease the risk of future sternotomy, we prevent cardiac dessication by covering the heart with saline-soaked gauze throughout each operation. At the completion of ACHD repairs we occasionally place antiadhesion materials to decrease retrosternal adhesions. In some centers, expanded polytetrafluoroethylene (PTFE) is routinely placed behind the sternum prior to closure.[11] Capsule formation may obscure natural tissue planes, making subsequent reoperative dissection more difficult. Bioresorbable films[12] and sheets of extracellular matrix[13] derived from pig jejunum have also been approved for use as pericardial substitutes.

Atrial Septal Defects

The advent of transcatheter device closure for ASDs has significantly changed the average complexity level of ACHD surgical case volumes. Patent foramen ovale and most secundum defects are effectively closed with devices, and are rarely referred for surgical closure in programs with effective interventional catheterization teams. Sinus venosus and primum defects, transitional and complete atrioventricular canal, common atrium, and secundum defects with deficient inferior and superior rims are referred for surgery and we repair these on cardiopulmonary bypass with bicaval cannulation and ischemic arrest.

Multiple incisional approaches have been described to improve the cosmetic result, and reduce operative trauma, after open-heart surgery. These include partial upper and lower sternotomy, transxiphoid, anterior thoracotomy, and submammary incisions. Despite the visible scar, median sternotomy may be the least traumatic incision for ACHD patients, allowing the surgeon to avoid vascular trauma from peripheral cannulation, intercostal muscle, vessel, and nerve damage, and mitigate the risk of post-thoracotomy pain syndrome. Median sternotomy

allows direct aortic control for safe, effective cannulation, decannulation, deairing, and cardioplegia administration with minimal risk of dissection. Median sternotomy also ensures direct and rapid access to the entire mediastinum, allowing surgeons to deal with unanticipated anatomic variations discovered at surgery, which are not uncommon in ACHD patients.

Our venous cannulation strategy for ASDs is bicaval, via the right atrial appendage into the superior vena cava, and down the inferior venal caval junction into the inferior vena cava. Smaller defects, which in the past might have been closed primarily, are now rarely referred for surgery, and we find that repairs are best performed with patch materials, ideally glutaraldehyde-treated pericardium. Placing the smooth surface on the left atrial side, we use running suture lines of fine polypropylene to create tension-free suture lines (Fig. 56-2A).

For sinus venosus defects, we place a right-angled cannula in the innominate vein, to enable exposure of the partial anomalous pulmonary veins entering the superior vena cava. The atrial incision is made laterally to avoid the sinus node area, and is extended superiorly to a point above the entrance of the highest anomalous vein. A native pericardial patch is used to close the atrial incision to avoid superior vena caval stenosis (Fig. 56-2B).

In patients with primum ASDs, the cleft mitral valve is routinely repaired with fine running polypropylene suture lines, approximating the line of contact between the leaflet segments. Even patients with competent valves are repaired, as late onset of cleft regurgitation is known to occur. Patients at risk for mitral stenosis, particularly those with a single papillary muscle in the left ventricle, may have their clefts left open to avoid valvar stenosis. Results for these repairs are excellent, even in patients at advanced ages.[14]

Ebstein's Anomaly

Surgery for Ebstein's anomaly can be performed in older patients at low risk and with good late outcome. The operation is comprised of tricuspid valve repair or replacement, and concomitant procedures such as ASD closure, arrhythmia surgery, and coronary artery bypass grafting.[15] Repair techniques for these patients continue to evolve. We believe the presence of an untethered and well-developed anterior tricuspid valve leaflet increases the chance of a successful repair, and have used the Cone technique in adult patients.[16] This repair requires dissection of the anterior and posterior tricuspid valve leaflets from their right ventricular attachment. The free edge of the anterior leaflet is then rotated clockwise and sutured to the septal leaflet border. This produces a cone-shaped valve, fixed distally at the right ventricular apex, and proximally at the tricuspid valve annulus. The septal leaflet is incorporated into the cone wall whenever possible, and the ASD is partially closed. Results have been good, with low mortality, significantly less tricuspid regurgitation, and improvement in functional class.

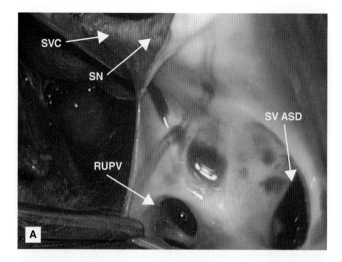

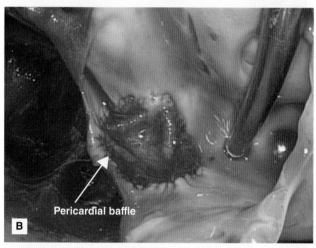

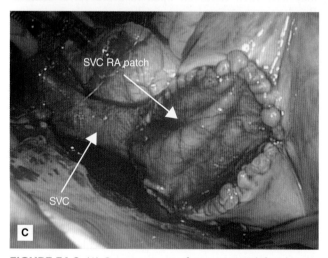

FIGURE 56-2 (**A**) Operative image of sinus venosus defect showing the pulmonary vein orifices, the superior vena cava, and the septal defect. (**B**) Operative image of two patch repair with an internal patch baffling the pulmonary veins to the left atrium, and an external patch to prevent obstruction of the superior venal caval entry into the right atrium.

Fontan Revision

In the modern era, the primary cause of death for adult patients with cyanotic lesions is arrhythmia, followed by heart failure.[17] Fontan patients may present with arrhythmia and complications related to systemic ventricular failure, protein-losing enteropathy (PLE), systemic venous pathway obstruction, and semilunar and atrioventricular valve dysfunction. Initial evaluations must focus on ensuring a completely unobstructed vascular pathway to the lungs. The different types of surgical technique historically used to create the Fontan circulation each have characteristic complications. Patients with intracardiac baffles and atriopulmonary connections may present with extreme right atrial enlargement, resulting in stagnant flow, right pulmonary vein compression, and arrhythmia.

Fontan conversion involves takedown of the previously created venous connection, and creation of an extracardiac cavopulmonary connection with a conduit. Because the extracardiac Fontan excludes the systemic veins from the heart, any catheterization procedures requiring atrial level intervention, particularly electrophysiology interventions, must be planned before conversion. We therefore plan Fontan conversions with our electrophysiology team, and frequently combine Fontan conversions with arrhythmia surgery,[18] and treatment of atrioventricular valve dysfunction. Valve repairs are often complex in these patients, and replacements are often required to achieve good hemodynamic results.[19] Results depend on the patients' underlying anatomy, right ventricular function, and pulmonary vascular resistance.[20]

We perform extracardiac Fontan procedures with bicaval cannulation, and leave the heart warm and beating whenever possible. The inferior vena cava is transected at the cavo-atrial junction under a clamp, and the cardiac end is oversewn with a running 4-0 polypropylene suture. We use a ring reinforced expanded PTFE graft from 19 to 23 mm in diameter, and leave enough length to avoid right pulmonary vein compression. The superior anastomosis to the superior vena caval junction with the right pulmonary artery is then constructed with a running 6-0 polypropylene suture. Hybrid stenting procedures, where the interventional catheterization team comes into the cardiac operating room to deploy stents, are used to treat stenoses in the retroaortic pulmonary arteries.

In patients with complex cardiac anatomy, these Fontan revision procedures may best be performed with the participation of the electrophysiology team. This ensures effective interruption or ablation of all reentrant pathways, which may not follow the patterns seen in patients with acquired heart disease and normal cardiac anatomic relationships. A variety of Maze type procedures have been described in an effort to disrupt atrial reentrant pathways. The unpredictable anatomy of the conduction tissue in ACHD patients has resulted in frequent need for pacemaker insertion. In many centers, customized pacemaker therapy has been advocated for management of patients following Fontan conversion. However, based on an experience with 120 Fontan conversion from 1994 to 2008, which began with a flexible approach to each patient's anticipated pacing needs, Tsao et al now recommend routine placement of a dual-chamber antitachycardia pacemaker with bipolar steroid-eluting leads in patients undergoing Fontan revision.[21]

Right Ventricular Outflow Tract Reconstruction

Right ventricular outflow tract (RVOT) reconstruction after previous repair of tetralogy of Fallot, double outlet right ventricle, pulmonary atresia, truncus arteriosus, and arterial switch procedures are increasingly common, as patients who underwent successful neonatal and infant repairs are returning with pulmonary insufficiency and/or stenosis, resulting in right ventricular dysfunction, exercise intolerance, arrhythmias, and sudden death.[22] The first percutaneous pulmonary valve replacement was performed by Bonhoeffer and colleagues in 2000,[23] and this therapy is increasingly available as clinical trials have demonstrated safety and efficacy, and improvement in the New York Heart Association (NYHA) functional class is evident at 1-month postprocedure.[24] This less invasive therapy has accelerated the study of ACHD patients with pulmonary valve disease who were previously followed for years to avoid the trauma of reoperation. The growing experience with transcatheter pulmonary valve insertion into previously placed RVOT homografts and conduits suggests that homograft infection is rare, and stent fractures are more common (32%), but benign. The percutaneous valves have a median maximum instantaneous gradient across the RVOT of 23 mm Hg.[25] With surgical standby, patients with rupture can be placed on emergent bypass, and undergo surgical repair with good results.[26] Indications for pulmonary valve replacement in ACHD patients are evolving, and optimal indications and timing remain unclear. Preoperative evaluation with echocardiography, magnetic resonance imaging (MRI), and cardiac catheterization are used to identify concomitant lesions, particularly patent foramen ovale, coronary anatomy, and right ventricular dimensions and function.

For patients not amenable to transcatheter pulmonary valve implantation, our standard surgical approach includes median sternotomy, bicaval cannulation, and repair on cardiopulmonary bypass with moderate hypothermia. These repairs may be performed without ischemic arrest if provocative preoperative testing (bubble test with Valsalva) is negative; however, we prefer to perform these operations with the aorta cross-clamped. We control the branch pulmonary arteries with tourniquets and place a right ventricular vent in the atrium to create a clear operative field. If a previous right ventricular incision or patch is present, this is used as a safe reentry point, and the incision is extended fare enough to inspect the right ventricle and allow resection of obstructing intracavitary muscle bundles. Pulmonary valve replacement options include pulmonary and aortic homografts, bovine

jugular vein grafts, bioprosthetic valves, and mechanical prosthetic valves.

Homografts may be selected based on appropriate size and length to match the patient's anatomy, and echocardiographic estimates of the normal pulmonary valve dimensions for that patient's weight. Conduits must be cut to the appropriate length to prevent tension (too short) and kinking (too long). We perform the distal pulmonary artery anastomosis with a running 6-0 monofilament polypropylene suture, and then trim the proximal homograft muscle cuff to match the right ventricular incision. The proximal anastomosis is constructed with a larger running suture and needle, and care is taken to avoid the left main and anterior descending coronary arteries. When these cannot be visualized due to epicardial scarring, we use intraoperative fluorescent imaging to map the coronary arteries on the surface of the right ventricle.[27] The anterior portion of the outflow tract is completed with a patch of native or bovine pericardium (Fig. 56-3).

The bovine jugular vein valve is sized and implanted in a similar way to homografts, with a distal running suture line. The proximal graft is beveled, so that a separate hood patch is not necessary. Ten years after implantation, bovine jugular vein grafts have significantly less failure, dysfunction, and explant rates, than pulmonary homografts in matched patient groups (Fig. 56-4).[28]

Bioprosthetic and mechanical valves are positioned in the RVOT at the normal pulmonary valve annulus in patients with normal right ventricular anatomy, or in a position that avoids sternal compression (more distal implantation is often necessary after repair of truncus arteriosus and pulmonary atresia). Compression of the left main coronary artery must also be considered when positioning these rigid valve rings. We have used both an interrupted horizontal mattress suture technique, and a running polypropylene suture technique for these implants. Both require that the valve suture line be constructed so that the valve orients parallel to the main

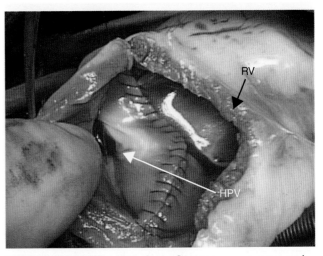

FIGURE 56-3 Right ventricular outflow tract reconstruction with a pulmonary homograft.

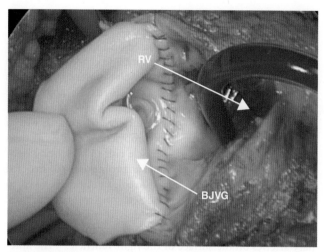

FIGURE 56-4 Right ventricular outflow tract reconstruction with a bovine jugular vein graft.

pulmonary, avoiding the tendency for the valve to aim up toward the sternum. The surgeon must also ensure that valve struts do not obstruct the branch pulmonary arteries. A patch may be used to close the main pulmonary artery and infundibulum when the implanted valve does not fit in the native outflow tract (Fig. 56-5).

Advantages and disadvantages exist for each pulmonary valve replacement option.[29] Homografts and bovine jugular veins have length and can be used to span long gaps between the right ventricle and the branch pulmonary arteries. The distal anastomosis can be configured to repair stenotic sections of the main pulmonary artery and the proximal branches. They also form suitable conduits for subsequent insertion of transcatheter pulmonary valves in the future if they become stenotic or insufficient. We try to tailor our conduit decisions to meet the implantation requirements for transcatheter pulmonary valve insertion. These evolving requirements

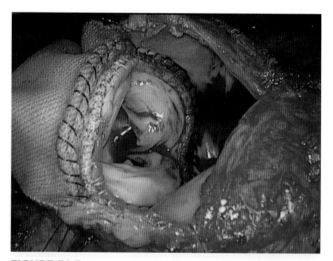

FIGURE 56-5 Reconstruction of the right ventricular outflow tract with a bioprosthetic valve using a running suture technique and an onlay patch.

are factored into our decision process in selecting a conduit during our current surgical pulmonary valve replacements. Available bioprosthetic valves are also suitable for subsequent insertion of a transcatheter valve, as the valve ring provides a stable landing zone for the transcatheter valve stent. Mechanical valves do not allow subsequent placement of a transcatheter pulmonary valve, and we no longer use them for in the pulmonary position. RVOT reconstruction can now be performed with low morbidity and mortality, and conduit options continue to expand.

Left Ventricular Outflow Tract Reconstruction

Isolated areas of left ventricular outflow tract obstruction (LVOTO) are less common in ACHD patients than in those with acquired left-sided lesions. ACHD patients with LVOTO must be evaluated for upstream and downstream stenoses, as multiple levels of obstruction are common. Patients with Shone's syndrome often undergo numerous surgical and interventional procedures over their lifetimes, and these interventions are at best palliative. Adult congenital teams must be prepared to perform primary Ross, Ross-Konno, and Konno procedures, and deal with reoperations for each of these palliations. The Ross operation is often used in pediatric patients with complex LVOTO to treat combined valvar and supravalvar lesions, avoid anticoagulation, and maintain some growth potential. These patients may require reoperations as adults to replace or repair failing neo aortic valves, and stenotic or regurgitant pulmonary valves. Follow-up of right ventricular reconstructions after Ross operations shows that 4% of patients will require conduit replacement for right ventricular dysfunction at 10 years. Conduit size less than 14 mm is an independent predictor of allograft dysfunction.[30]

Freedom from reoperation for regurgitation of the pulmonary autograft in the aortic position is quite variable, with reports from 87[31] to 96%.[30] The advent of percutaneous aortic and pulmonary valve options may increase the utilization of the Ross operation, as reinterventions on the autograft and allograft may not require reoperation. Aneurysmal dilation of the neo aortic root after the Ross operation is related to use of the root technique, and may be seen in up to 11% of patients at 7 years after surgery. Good outcomes after reoperation can be achieved, but successful repair of the autograft is more likely if the diagnosis is made early, before the neo aortic valve becomes insufficient.[32]

The Konno aortico ventriculoplasty is used to treat complex LVOTO in patients with supravalvar, valvar, and subvalvar obstruction, and may be encountered in adults who require initial treatment, or reoperations for valve malfunction or outgrown valves. The Ross-Konno, utilizing the transplanted pulmonary autograft with a ventricular septal patch or infundibular extension, has been shown to increase in size as the patients grow, making this an excellent option in small pediatric patients. In a review of 53 patients operated on from 1980 to 2004, with an average age of 19, Suri et al reported risk factors for overall mortality included NYHA class (hazard ratio 2.22, *p* = .04). The cumulative probability of aortic valve reoperation was 19% at 5 years and 39% at 10 years, occurring in 15 patients at a median of 3.8 years. Pulmonary regurgitation was detected in six patients. Pulmonary valve replacement was performed in three (6%).[33]

Reoperations after Ross, Ross-Konno, and Konno procedures may be particularly challenging. This is especially true if the RVOT has been reconstructed with a large patch covering the anterior aortic wall. Exposure of the aortic root then necessitates reentry into the right ventricle. Given the high incidence of reoperations on these patients, antiadhesion barriers are recommended.

Arrhythmia Surgery

Maintaining a functional conduction system is a crucial aspect of reducing the cumulative lifetime trauma for a congenital heart patient. Despite efforts to prevent conduction tissue injury, ACHD patients are at risk for a wide array of conduction delays, as well as atrial and ventricular tachyarrhythmias. Pacemaker and defibrillator insertion, lead extractions, and generator changes are frequently complicated in ACHD patients who may have unusual anatomic pathways and stenotic or occluded veins. Epicardial lead placements are often necessary in single ventricle patients who have limited or no venous access to the endocardium. Common indications for lead removal include pocket infection, malfunctioning leads, skin erosion, endocarditis/septicemia, vena cava thrombosis, and painful leads. Lead extraction technology is evolving, and can be safely managed as a hybrid effort with a surgeon and electrophysiologist working together. A number of lead removal catheters are available using blades or laser energy to excise embedded leads. Surgical support is necessary in the event of cardiac perforation. Outcomes are generally good, even in octegenarians,[34] with sepsis being the strongest predictor of death after pacemaker device removal.[35]

Supraventricular and ventricular arrhythmias are a major cause of morbidity and mortality in adult patients with congenital heart disease. For patients with atrial fibrillation or flutter undergoing open-heart repairs, a right-sided Maze procedure can be performed with the expectation of 93% freedom from arrhythmia, and improvement in functional class.[36]

Minimally invasive approaches to arrhythmia surgery, such as the Mini-Maze procedure, are increasingly popular in patients with acquired heart disease and arrhythmia.[37] These approaches may be difficult to accomplish in certain ACHD patients because of unusual anatomic relationships, and extensive reoperative scarring, which may limit exposure through small incisions. The Cox-Maze procedure for supraventricular arrhythmias in ACHD patients is often complex, and an alternative approach using intraoperative monopolar irrigated radiofrequency ablation (IRA) has been described with good results for patients undergoing elective cardiac surgery. Prophylactic arrhythmia surgery for patients undergoing congenital heart repairs has been considered for high risk groups, and these strategies are evolving.[38]

Hybrid Procedures

We define hybrid procedures as those using combined surgical and interventional personnel and technology during a single operation. Hybrid procedures can be performed in the catheterization laboratory, the operating room, or ideally in a hybrid procedure suite. We select the venue based on which technology is most critical for the success of a given procedure. The advent of percutaneous cardiac valve replacement and endovascular stenting reinforce the need to embrace a unified team approach for adult congenital heart patients. In those requiring interventional, surgical, and electrophysiological procedures, we attempt to integrate the procedures into a single hybrid operation, with the surgical team providing the least traumatic form of vascular access. Surgeons can also provide central vascular and direct cardiac access for sheath placement in patients with stenotic or occluded peripheral vessels, or when placing large devices in small patients. We routinely deploy aortic and pulmonary artery stents in the operating room using direct vision, video assisted cardioscopy, and angiography (Fig. 56-6).

Elective or emergent cardiopulmonary bypass support should be available on demand in the hybrid operating room, catheterization laboratory, and cardiac intensive care unit (Fig. 56-7).

Real-time consultation between surgeons and interventionalists may enhance outcomes for patients undergoing transvascular stent, device, and valve implantations. With a surgeon's input at the time of implantation, pulmonary artery stents may be positioned to facilitate subsequent operations. For example, pulmonary artery stents may be positioned more proximally to avoid damage to small distal branches at the time of reoperation. Aortic arch stent positioning can be optimized to reduce the distance down the distal arch the surgeon must dissect if reoperation is required to open a stent that cannot reach adult size. This type of planning and teamwork has proven to be useful in the emerging experience with transcatheter aortic valve replacements.[39]

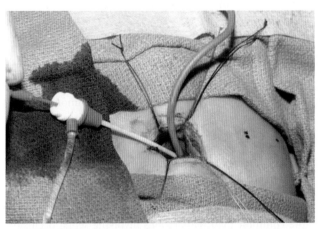

FIGURE 56-6 A hybrid procedure with surgical partial lower sternotomy and transcardiac sheath placement followed by interventional catheterization.

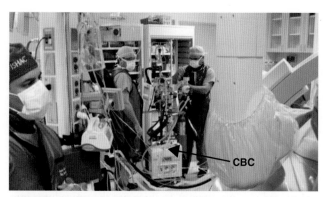

FIGURE 56-7 A cardiopulmonary bypass circuit is prepared for emergent or elective use during hybrid procedures and complex interventional catheterizations.

Coarctation of the Aorta

Primary and recurrent coarctation of the aorta in adult patients is increasingly managed percutaneously with balloon dilation and stents.[40] We provide surgical backup for these procedures in the event of device migration, dissection, or rupture, and occasionally to establish vascular access. When transcatheter therapy is not feasible, we proceed with surgical repair of adults with coarctation and aortic arch obstruction. These operations are performed through a left thoracotomy in patients with a left aortic arch, and the perfusion team is on standby for left atrial appendage to descending aortic cardiopulmonary bypass. Three general techniques can be used, including coarctation resection with end-to-end anastomosis, onlay patch enlargement with tissue or prosthetic patch, and synthetic tube interposition. Aortic mobility is limited in adult patients, and tension-free repairs most often require interposition grafts. We use subcutaneous local anesthetic infusion catheters and liposomal bupivacaine to control postoperative pain. We anticipate labile blood pressure responses in patients with long-standing hypertension. Postoperative hypertension is common and responds to sodium nitroprusside. Mortality for these procedures is rare, and at follow up 75% of patients will be normotensive without medication.[41]

INTERVENTIONAL DEVICE MANAGEMENT

Cardiac surgeons will increasingly encounter ACHD patients with intravascular devices in the aorta and pulmonary arteries, atrial[42] and ventricular septal occlusion devices, and transcatheter stented valves. Vascular stents are being effectively used in neonates and infants, with the understanding that patients will inevitably outgrow the maximum size these stents can achieve.[43] We have a growing experience with reoperations on patients who have outgrown stents in the aortic arch and the branch pulmonary arteries, and these are far more common than reoperations involving septal occlusion devices. At reoperation early after stent implantation, within 3 months or less, it may be possible to completely remove

the stent by chipping away with the cells using scissors. The stents can be collapsed inward and peeled away from the vessel wall. After 3 months, vascular ingrowth is usually substantial enough that the stent is incorporated into the vessel wall, making removal difficult and traumatic. When patients undergo reoperations to enlarge stents which have reached their maximum diameter, operative planning requires consideration of the optimal location of the longitudinal incision made to open the stent, anticipating that the stent will have to be spread open like a hot dog bun to create space for an onlay patch. This requires that every link be cut to the distal ends of the stent to avoid leaving a persistent complete ring of metal in the vessel wall (Fig. 56-8).

Stents often end close to branch points, so the distal extension of the stent incision must be planned to avoid spiral tears into smaller branch vessels, which may result in branch occlusion. Onlay patches may be constructed with native or bovine pericardium, PTFE grafts, pulmonary or aortic homografts, or extracellular matrix grafts. If the final vessel reconstruction does not achieve a full adult-sized vessel lumen, or is compressed by adjacent structures, the patched split stent is a safe landing zone for subsequent placement of an adult-sized stent. We have placed these stents immediately in the operating room as a hybrid procedure, or later, after the patched vessel has time to heal, thus reducing the risk of suture line rupture and bleeding.

Atrial septal stents are occasionally used to achieve unrestrictive flow across the atrial septum when restriction develops after previous surgical septectomy.[44] At late reoperation, these stents are firmly encased in septal tissue, and may extend into the pulmonary vein orifices. When necessary, these stents can be removed with scissor dissection, trimming the exposed metal, peeling out the embedded sections, and enucleating the ingrown scar tissue. The atrium must be inspected for full thickness tears, which are repaired with polypropylene suture.

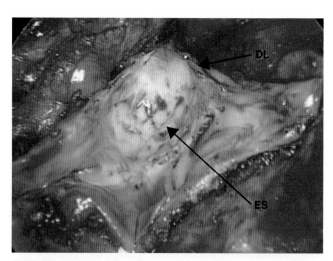

FIGURE 56-8 An operative image of reoperation on a stented pulmonary artery, requiring an incision through the front wall of the stent and through the most distal cells.

IMPROVED OUTCOMES USING CONGENITAL HEART SURGEONS TO TREAT ADULT CONGENITAL HEART DISEASE

Management guidelines for adults with congenital heart disease have been developed by the American Heart Association and the American College of Cardiology.[45] In a review of 72 US centers performing ACHD surgery, Patel and Kogon reported 2800 operations performed per year, ranging from 0 to 230 (median 28) per program. There were a median of two surgeons per program, with each surgeon averaging 20 cases per year.[46] While individual surgeon and program results will vary, patients with ACHD appear to have better outcomes when they are repaired by surgeons who primarily perform pediatric congenital heart surgery (1.87% mortality), compared to surgeons who primarily operated on acquired adult heart disease (4.84% mortality, $p < .0001$).[47] Patients with congenital heart disease are living longer. Arrhythmia remains the primary contributing cause of death for those with cyanotic lesions. Myocardial infarction is now the leading contributing cause for adults with noncyanotic congenital heart disease consistent with late survival and an increasing impact of acquired heart disease. With increasing experience and a team approach synthesizing surgery, intervention, electrophysiology, anesthesia, nursing and intensive care, adults with congenital heart disease should experience improved outcomes with less cumulative lifetime therapeutic trauma.

REFERENCES

1. Toyoda T, Tateno S, Kawasoe Y, et al: Nationwide survey of care facilities for adults with congenital heart disease in Japan. *Circ J* 2009; 73(6):1147-1150.
2. Dearani JA, Connolly HM, Martinez R, Fontanet H, Webb GD: Caring for adults with congenital cardiac disease: successes and challenges for 2007 and beyond. *Cardiol Young* 2007; 17 Suppl 2:87-96.
3. Donofrio MT, Moon-Grady AJ, Hornberger LK, et al: Diagnosis and treatment of fetal cardiac disease: a scientific statement from the American Heart Association. *Circulation* 2014; 129(21):2183-2242.
4. Winkelman WJ, Leonard KJ, Rossos PG: Patient-perceived usefulness of online electronic medical records: employing grounded theory in the development of information and communication technologies for use by patients living with chronic illness. *J Am Med Inform Assoc* 2005; 12(3):306-314.
5. Gibson PH, Burns JE, Walker H, Cross S, Leslie SJ: Keeping track of congenital heart disease-is it time for a national registry? *Int J Cardiol* 2010; 145(2):331-332.
6. Jacobs JP, Elliott MJ, Anderson RH, et al: Creating a database with cardioscopy and intra-operative imaging. *Cardiol Young* 2005; 15 Suppl 1: 184-189.
7. Burke RP, White JA: Internet rounds: a congenital heart surgeon's Web log. *Semin Thorac Cardiovasc Surg* 2004; 16(3):283-292.
8. Luciani N, Anselmi A, De GR, Martinelli L, Perisano M, Possati G: Extracorporeal circulation by peripheral cannulation before redo sternotomy: indications and results. *J Thorac Cardiovasc Surg* 2008; 136(3):572-577.
9. Knott-Craig CJ, Goldberg SP, Kirklin JK: Surgical strategy to prevent cardiac injury during reoperation in infants. *J Cardiothorac Surg* 2008; 3:10.
10. Giordano S, Biancari F: Does the use of carbon dioxide field flooding during heart valve surgery prevent postoperative cerebrovascular complications? *Interact Cardiovasc Thorac Surg* 2009; 9(2):323-326.
11. Jacobs JP, Iyer RS, Weston JS, et al: Expanded PTFE membrane to prevent cardiac injury during resternotomy for congenital heart disease. *Ann Thorac Surg* 1996; 62(6):1778-1782.
12. Okuyama N, Wang CY, Rose EA, et al: Reduction of retrosternal and pericardial adhesions with rapidly resorbable polymer films. *Ann Thorac Surg* 1999; 68(3):913-918.
13. Keane TJ, Badylak SF: The host response to allogeneic and xenogeneic biological scaffold materials. *J Tissue Eng Regen Med* 2014.
14. Horvath KA, Burke RP, Collins JJ Jr, Cohn LH: Surgical treatment of adult atrial septal defect: early and long-term results. *J Am Coll Cardiol* 1992; 20(5):1156-1159.
15. Dearani JA, Mavroudis C, Quintessenza J, et al: Surgical advances in the treatment of adults with congenital heart disease. *Curr Opin Pediatr* 2009; 21(5):565-572.
16. da Silva JP, Baumgratz JF, da Fonseca L, et al: The cone reconstruction of the tricuspid valve in Ebstein's anomaly. The operation: early and mid-term results. *J Thorac Cardiovasc Surg* 2007; 133(1):215-223.
17. Pillutla P, Shetty KD, Foster E: Mortality associated with adult congenital heart disease: trends in the US population from 1979 to 2005. *Am Heart J* 2009; 158(5):874-879.
18. Jang WS, Kim WH, Choi K, et al: The mid-term surgical results of Fontan conversion with antiarrhythmia surgery. *Eur J Cardiothorac Surg* 2014; 45(5):922-927.
19. Mavroudis C, Stewart RD, Backer CL, Deal BJ, Young L, Franklin WH: Atrioventricular valve procedures with repeat Fontan operations: influence of valve pathology, ventricular function, and arrhythmias on outcome. *Ann Thorac Surg* 2005; 80(1):29-36.
20. Mavroudis C, Deal BJ, Backer CL, et al: J. Maxwell Chamberlain Memorial Paper for congenital heart surgery. 111 Fontan conversions with arrhythmia surgery: surgical lessons and outcomes. *Ann Thorac Surg* 2007; 84(5):1457-1465.
21. Tsao S, Deal BJ, Backer CL, Ward K, Franklin WH, Mavroudis C: Device management of arrhythmias after Fontan conversion. *J Thorac Cardiovasc Surg* 2009; 138(4):937-940.
22. Gatzoulis MA, Balaji S, Webber SA, et al: Risk factors for arrhythmia and sudden cardiac death late after repair of tetralogy of Fallot: a multicentre study. *Lancet* 2000; 356(9234):975-981.
23. Lurz P, Gaudin R, Taylor AM, Bonhoeffer P: Percutaneous pulmonary valve implantation. *Semin Thorac Cardiovasc Surg Pediatr Card Surg Annu* 2009; 112-117.
24. Lurz P, Riede FT, Taylor AM, et al: Impact of percutaneous pulmonary valve implantation for right ventricular outflow tract dysfunction on exercise recovery kinetics. *Int J Cardiol* 2014; 177(1):276-280.
25. Meadows JJ, Moore PM, Berman DP, et al: Use and performance of the Melody Transcatheter Pulmonary Valve in native and postsurgical, nonconduit right ventricular outflow tracts. *Circ Cardiovasc Interv* 2014; 7(3):374-380.
26. Kostolny M, Tsang V, Nordmeyer J, et al: Rescue surgery following percutaneous pulmonary valve implantation. *Eur J Cardiothorac Surg* 2008; 33(4):607-612.
27. Vogt PR, Bauer EP, Graves K: Novadaq Spy Intraoperative Imaging System-current status. *Thorac Cardiovasc Surg* 2003; 51(1):49-51.
28. Brown JW, Ruzmetov M, Rodefeld MD, Eltayeb O, Yurdakok O, Turrentine MW: Contegra versus pulmonary homografts for right ventricular outflow tract reconstruction: a ten-year single-institution comparison. *World J Pediatr Congenit Heart Surg* 2011; 2(4):541-549.
29. Vricella LA, Kanani M, Cook AC, Cameron DE, Tsang VT: Problems with the right ventricular outflow tract: a review of morphologic features and current therapeutic options. *Cardiol Young* 2004; 14(5):533-549.
30. Brown JW, Ruzmetov M, Fukui T, Rodefeld MD, Mahomed Y, Turrentine MW: Fate of the autograft and homograft following Ross aortic valve replacement: reoperative frequency, outcome, and management. *J Heart Valve Dis* 2006; 15(2):253-259.
31. Klieverik LM, Takkenberg JJ, Bekkers JA, Roos-Hesselink JW, Witsenburg M, Bogers AJ: The Ross operation: a Trojan horse? *Eur Heart J* 2007; 28(16):1993-2000.
32. Luciani GB, Viscardi F, Pilati M, Prioli AM, Faggian G, Mazzucco A: The Ross-Yacoub procedure for aneurysmal autograft roots: a strategy to preserve autologous pulmonary valves. *J Thorac Cardiovasc Surg* 2010; 139(2):536-542.
33. Suri RM, Dearani JA, Schaff HV, Danielson GK, Puga FJ: Long-term results of the Konno procedure for complex left ventricular outflow tract obstruction. *J Thorac Cardiovasc Surg* 2006; 132(5):1064-1071.

34. Williams SE, Arujuna A, Whitaker J, et al: Percutaneous extraction of cardiac implantable electronic devices (CIEDs) in octogenarians. *Pacing Clin Electrophysiol* 2012; 35(7):841-849.

35. Hamid S, Arujuna A, Ginks M, et al: Pacemaker and defibrillator lead extraction: predictors of mortality during follow-up. *Pacing Clin Electrophysiol* 2010; 33(2):209-216.

36. Stulak JM, Dearani JA, Puga FJ, Zehr KJ, Schaff HV, Danielson GK: Right-sided Maze procedure for atrial tachyarrhythmias in congenital heart disease. *Ann Thorac Surg* 2006; 81(5):1780-1784.

37. Saltman AE, Gillinov AM: Surgical approaches for atrial fibrillation. *Cardiol Clin* 2009; 27(1):179-188, x.

38. Mavroudis C, Stulak JM, Ad N, et al: Prophylactic atrial arrhythmia surgical procedures with congenital heart operations: review and recommendations. *Ann Thorac Surg* 2015; 99(1):352-359.

39. Berlin DB, Davidson MJ, Schoen FJ: The power of disruptive technological innovation: transcatheter aortic valve implantation. *J Biomed Mater Res B Appl Biomater* 2014.

40. Noble S, Ibrahim R: Percutaneous interventions in adults with congenital heart disease: expanding indications and opportunities. *Curr Cardiol Rep* 2009; 11(4):306-313.

41. Jatene MB, Abuchaim DC, Oliveira JL Jr, et al: Outcomes of aortic coarctation surgical treatment in adults. *Rev Bras Cir Cardiovasc* 2009; 24(3):346-353.

42. Mellert F, Preusse CJ, Haushofer M, et al: Surgical management of complications caused by transcatheter ASD closure. *Thorac Cardiovasc Surg* 2001; 49(6):338-342.

43. Stanfill R, Nykanen DG, Osorio S, Whalen R, Burke RP, Zahn EM: Stent implantation is effective treatment of vascular stenosis in young infants with congenital heart disease: acute implantation and long-term follow-up results. *Catheter Cardiovasc Interv* 2008; 71(6):831-841.

44. Pedra CA, Neves JR, Pedra SR, et al: New transcatheter techniques for creation or enlargement of atrial septal defects in infants with complex congenital heart disease. *Catheter Cardiovasc Interv* 2007; 70(5):731-739.

45. Warnes CA, Williams RG, Bashore TM, et al: ACC/AHA 2008 guidelines for the management of adults with congenital heart disease: a report of the American College of Cardiology/American Heart Association Task Force on Practice Guidelines (Writing Committee to Develop Guidelines on the Management of Adults with Congenital Heart Disease). Developed in Collaboration with the American Society of Echocardiography, Heart Rhythm Society, International Society for Adult Congenital Heart Disease, Society for Cardiovascular Angiography and Interventions, and Society of Thoracic Surgeons. *J Am Coll Cardiol* 2008; 52(23):e143-e263.

46. Patel MS, Kogon BE: Care of the adult congenital heart disease patient in the United States: a summary of the current system. *Pediatr Cardiol* 2010; 31(4):511-514.

47. Karamlou T, Diggs BS, Person T, Ungerleider RM, Welke KF: National practice patterns for management of adult congenital heart disease: operation by pediatric heart surgeons decreases in-hospital death. *Circulation* 2008; 118(23):2345-2352.

57

Pericardial Disease

Eric N. Feins • Jennifer D. Walker

The pericardium envelops the heart and portions of the great vessels as a protective capsule. When incised longitudinally and transversely along the diaphragm it can be suspended to present the heart for surgical procedures. The surgical importance of the pericardium stems from its involvement in alterations of cardiac filling. When the limited space between the noncompliant pericardium and heart acutely fills with fluid, cardiac compression and tamponade may ensue. Constrictive disorders arise when inflammation and scarring cause the pericardium to shrink and densely adhere to the surface of the heart. This chapter discusses pericardial anatomy and function and describes the conditions that commonly give rise to the surgical problems of pericardial constriction and tamponade. The chapter also describes the diagnosis and therapy of these entities, the management of effusions and tamponade early and late after cardiac surgery, and the rationale for and against pericardial closure at the time of cardiac surgery.

ANATOMY AND FUNCTION

The pericardium serves two major functions. It maintains the position of the heart within the mediastinum and prevents cardiac distension by sudden volume overload. The pericardium attaches to the ascending aorta just inferior to the innominate vein and the superior vena cava (SVC) several centimeters above the sinoatrial node. The pericardial reflection encompasses the superior and inferior pulmonary veins and encircles the inferior vena cava (IVC), thereby making it possible for the surgeon to control the IVC from within the pericardium. The pericardial reflection attaches to the left atrium near the entrances of the pulmonary veins just below the atrioventricular groove (Fig. 57-1). The pericardiophrenic arteries that travel with the phrenic nerves as well as the branches of the internal mammary arteries and feeder branches directly from the aorta perfuse the pericardium. It is innervated by vagal fibers from the esophageal plexus, and the phrenic nerves course within it.

The pericardium is a conical fibroserous sac made up of two intimately connected layers. The inner layer (serous pericardium) is a transparent monolayer of mesothelial cells. The visceral portion of the serous pericardium, or epicardium, and the parietal portion, which lines the fibrous pericardial sac, are continuous. The oblique sinus lies within the venous confluence and the transverse sinus lies between the arterial (aorta and pulmonary artery) and venous reflections (dome of left atrium and SVC). Such potential spaces allow the pericardium to expand and accommodate a limited amount of fluid. Normal pericardial fluid volume is approximately 10 to 20 mL. The pericardial mesothelial cells contain dense microvilli, which are 1 μm wide and 3 μm high, and facilitate fluid and ion exchange.[1] Visceral pericardial lymphatic drainage occurs via the tracheal and bronchial mediastinal nodes, whereas lymphatic drainage of the parietal pericardium occurs via the anterior and posterior mediastinal lymph nodes.

The parietal layer, or fibrous pericardium, is composed mostly of dense parallel bundles of collagen, which render this layer relatively noncompliant. Because the pericardium is stiffer than cardiac muscle, it tends to equalize the compliance of both ventricles. By doing so, the pericardium contributes to the resting cavitary diastolic pressure of both ventricles, maximizing diastolic ventricular interaction.[2] An example of this phenomenon is the diminution of systemic arterial pressure during inspiration. Intrapericardial pressure tends to approximate pleural pressure, and varies with respiration. The negative intrathoracic pressure generated during inspiration augments right ventricular filling. The interventricular septum shifts leftward to accommodate the increase in right ventricular volume and therefore impairs left ventricular filling. Impaired left ventricular filling translates to decreased cardiac output and a slight diminution in systemic blood pressure during inspiration. This phenomenon is greatly magnified with an increase in intrapericardial pressure (eg, during acute filling of the pericardial space or circulatory volume overload), resulting in pulsus paradoxus.[3]

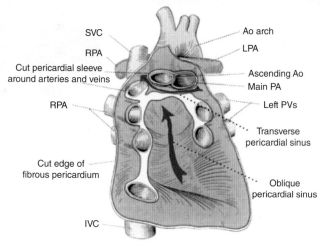

FIGURE 57-1 Pericardial attachments, reflections, and sinuses. Ao, aorta; IVC, inferior vena cava; LPA, left pulmonary artery; PA, pulmonary artery; PV, pulmonary vein; RPA, right pulmonary artery; SVC, superior vena cava.

CONGENITAL ABNORMALITIES

Most congenital abnormalities of the pericardium are asymptomatic and are often incidentally discovered at the time of surgery or investigation of unrelated problems.[4,5] They are rare, and one-third are associated with cardiac, skeletal, and pulmonary abnormalities.[6] Partial absence of the pericardium can occur and is most commonly seen on the left (70%) due to premature atrophy of the left common cardinal vein. Right-sided and complete defects of the pericardium account for 17 and 13% of these defects, respectively. The right duct of Cuvier goes on to form the SVC and ensures closure of

the right pleuropericardial membrane.[7] Accordingly, right-sided defects tend to be lethal. Magnetic resonance imaging (MRI), CT, and echocardiography are useful for evaluating patients with pericardial defects. MRI provides excellent pericardial imaging without contrast and is therefore the imaging modality of choice. CT and echocardiography are useful for evaluation of pericardial thickening and the extent and location of defects.[4] Although complete pericardial agenesis is rarely clinically significant, unilateral absence is potentially problematic because it may accentuate cardiac mobility, allowing the heart to be displaced into the pleural space with consequent incarceration of the left atrial appendage or left ventricle. Treatment may involve pericardial resection or replacement with a prosthetic patch.[6] Both therapies appear to yield good outcomes.

Pericardial cysts are the most common congenital pericardial disorder, surpassed only by lymphoma as the most prevalent of middle mediastinal masses.[8] They occur as asymptomatic incidental findings in 75% of patients; 70% occur in the right costophrenic angle and 22% in the left.[5] They do not communicate with the pericardial space and are typically unilocular, smooth, and less than 3 cm in diameter (Fig. 57-2). When present, symptoms may include chest pain, dyspnea, cough, and arrhythmias, probably owing to compression and inflammatory involvement of adjacent structures. They can also become secondarily infected.[9] Contrast CT is the imaging modality of choice for diagnosis and surveillance.[10,11] Observation with serial CT scanning in asymptomatic patients is suggested. Percutaneous aspiration is associated with a 30% recurrence rate at 3 years. Sclerosis has been reported to decrease recurrence after aspiration.[12] Indications for resection include large size, symptoms, patient concern, and question of malignancy.[8] Video-assisted

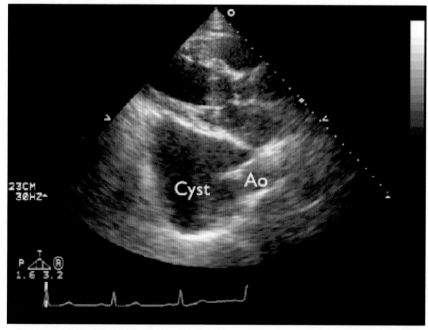

FIGURE 57-2 Transesophageal echocardiogram of large pericardial cyst.

thoracoscopy is the surgical approach most commonly used for excision. Infrasternal mediastinoscopy can be used for anterior cysts. Thoracotomy is also an acceptable technique. Surgery is the only definitive cure.[12]

PATHOPHYSIOLOGY OF PERICARDIAL COMPRESSION

Pericardial compression results from disturbance of the normal anatomical and physiologic relationships among the pericardium, pericardial cavity, and heart. Because the pericardium is relatively noncompliant and pericardial fluid noncompressible, the heart alone must compensate for acute changes in pericardial pressure. Acute volume overload within the fixed pericardial space results in a rapid, nonlinear increase in intrapericardial pressure (Fig. 57-3), producing cardiac compression.[13] The anatomic basis for pericardial compression involves either a space-occupying lesion (eg, cyst or excessive fluid) within the pericardial space or pericardial constriction.

Tamponade

Although blood in the pericardial space is the most common etiology, effusions, clot, pus, gas, or any combination of these can also produce tamponade. As fluid entering the pericardial space rapidly exceeds the pericardial reserve volume intrapericardial pressure rises abruptly. At this point, pericardial fluid volume can only increase by reducing cardiac chamber volumes. Because of its lower filling pressures, the right heart is more susceptible to compression (Fig. 57-4). The physiologic consequences are impaired diastolic filling with decreased cardiac output and increased central venous pressure.[14] Clinical manifestations include hypotension, jugular venous distention, and decreased heart sounds (Beck's triad).

To preserve cardiac output, higher pressures are required to fill the cardiac chambers, which may be partially achieved

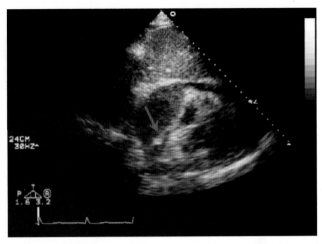

FIGURE 57-4 Transesophageal echocardiogram with right atrial inversion and cardiac tamponade.

by parallel increases in systemic and pulmonary venous pressure by vasoconstriction.[15] Other compensatory mechanisms include tachycardia, chronic pericardial stretch, and blood volume expansion.[16] The latter two mechanisms have little impact in acute tamponade. As tamponade progresses, right heart filling becomes increasingly volume dependent and limited to inspiration, when pericardial pressure is lower. Increased right ventricular filling causes it to encroach on, and impair, left ventricular filling. However, during expiration the converse is true, and left ventricular filling and output increase. This exaggeration of physiologic ventricular interdependence is the basis of pulsus paradoxus.[13]

The clinical presentation of tamponade varies widely depending on the severity of hemodynamic impairment and the degree of physiologic reserve. Rapid accumulation of as little as 100 mL of fluid in the pericardial space (eg, after a penetrating cardiac wound) may exceed the limited compliance of the parietal pericardium and produce critical tamponade. On the other hand, in chronic inflammatory conditions (eg, rheumatoid arthritis) the pericardium may compensate for large pericardial effusions, exceeding 1 L. The cardiac silhouette may appear normal in acute tamponade, but chronic pericardial distension is often obvious on plain chest radiography (Fig. 57-5), chest CT (Fig. 57-6), and echocardiography (Fig. 57-7). Low-pressure tamponade can also occur, in which a pericardial effusion is not hemodynamically significant until the patient becomes hypovolemic, typically from dehydration, blood loss, or diuretic therapy. Venous filling pressures may be normal or mildly elevated in this setting, making this diagnosis difficult.[17]

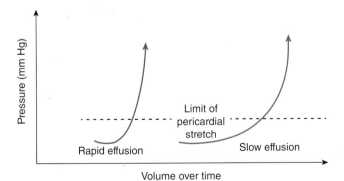

FIGURE 57-3 Relationship of pressure and volume in pericardial cavity. Normal pericardium will tolerate small amounts of fluid with a minimal increase in intrapericardial pressure. Above this small volume, small increases in volume result in large nonlinear increases in pressure. Gradual accumulation of fluid coincides with pericardial accommodation of much larger volumes of fluid up to a critical pressure.

Pericardial Constriction

A variety of conditions promote pericardial scar formation, the pathologic process underlying constrictive pericarditis (CP). As with tamponade, the physiologic basis is compromised cardiac filling leading to systemic venous congestion and low cardiac output. In contrast with tamponade, however, onset

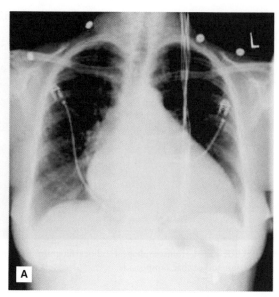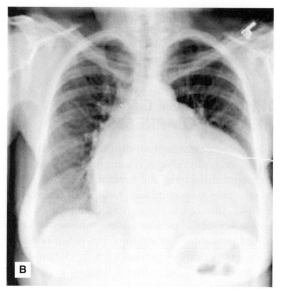

FIGURE 57-5 Slowly enlarging pericardial effusion detected on chest x-ray. (A) At discharge; (B) 3 weeks after discharge.

is often insidious and symptoms may be present for months to years.[18] Common complaints include fatigue, decreased exercise tolerance with dyspnea/orthopnea, as well as peripheral edema and ascites from hepatic congestion in advanced disease. The principal etiologies behind pericardial scar formation have shifted over time, with a declining incidence of infectious cases (eg, tuberculosis) and an increasing incidence of iatrogenic cases (eg, mediastinal radiation therapy, cardiac surgery).[19]

Pericardial constriction exerts its pathophysiologic effects by limiting cardiac filling. Unlike tamponade, in which cardiac filling is limited from the onset of diastole, pericardial constriction does not restrict filling in early diastole. Later in diastolic filling the ventricles are prevented from reaching full

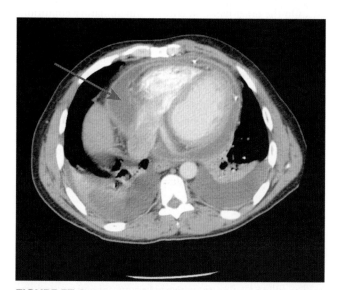

FIGURE 57-6 CT scan with large circumferential pericardial effusion and bilateral pleural effusions.

capacity as they encounter the contracted and noncompliant pericardium. As a result, 70 to 80% of diastolic filling occurs in the first 25 to 30% of diastole, after which diastolic pressures increase abruptly.[20] The ventricular free walls are then immobilized, leaving the interventricular septum as the last yielding structure; it is rapidly displaced in response to the sudden interventricular pressure differential. This produces the characteristic "septal bounce" seen echocardiographically. Other echocardiographic findings include pericardial thickening, caval plethora, and small chamber volumes. Inspiration exaggerates leftward septal deviation and reciprocal Doppler flows between the right and left sides (the echocardiographic correlate of pulsus paradoxus).

Modern axial imaging with CT (Fig. 57-8) and MRI (Fig. 57-9) are often able to visualize thickened and/or calcified pericardium, with or without coexisting effusion. Dynamic CT and MRI also demonstrate many of the physiologic features seen with echocardiography.[21] Importantly, although pericardial thickening is usually present in CP, it is possible to have CP with normal pericardial thickness, as well as pericardial thickening without CP.[22]

Prior to the modern era of echocardiography and axial imaging, the diagnosis of CP was dependent on hemodynamic tracings obtained during cardiac catheterization. The sudden increase in diastolic ventricular pressure is reflected in the dip and plateau, or "square-root" sign (Fig. 57-10). Similarly, right atrial pressure tracings reveal a steep *y* descent, which correlates with the nadir of the square-root sign. Under normal circumstances, inspiration results in a 3 to 7-mm Hg drop in right atrial pressure. The high pressure of pericardial constriction prevents the right atrium from accepting inspiratory acceleration of blood from the central veins. Instead, neck veins become distended during inspiration in patients with CP, a phenomenon known as *Kussmaul's sign*.

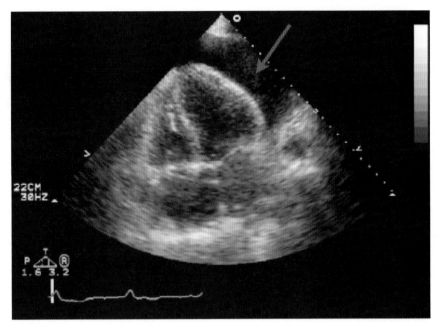

FIGURE 57-7 Transesophageal echocardiogram with very large pericardial effusion.

Catheterization can help differentiate CP from restrictive cardiomyopathy (RCM).[23,24] RCM is characterized by noncompliant ventricular muscle and diastolic dysfunction, which impede cardiac filling. RCM is caused by a variety of infiltrative or fibrosing conditions (eg, amyloidosis, sarcoidosis, radiation, and carcinoid). Although RCM may mimic many of the presenting features of CP, it is not a surgical disease and therefore must be distinguished from CP

(Table 57-1). Systolic ventricular function may be normal or near-normal in both conditions, but pulmonary and hepatic congestion are often present in RCM. Evidence of pericardial thickening (>2 mm) favors but does not confirm the diagnosis of CP over RCM. There are instances, particularly in radiation-induced CP, in which the conditions can coexist, making diagnosis challenging. Amyloidosis and other infiltrative conditions that cause RCM may demonstrate distinctive myocardial speckling on echocardiography. Endomyocardial biopsy is useful to establish the presence of one of the

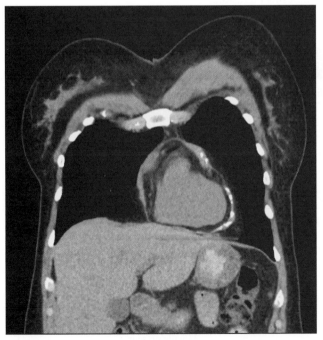

FIGURE 57-8 CT scan showing pericardial thickening and calcification.

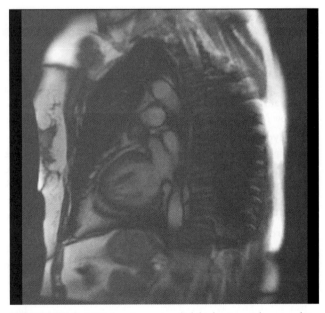

FIGURE 57-9 MRI showing pericardial thickening with pericarditis.

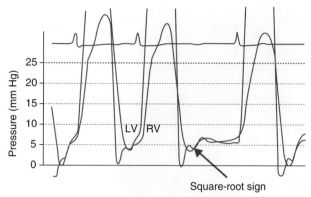

FIGURE 57-10 Square-root sign in right ventricular pressure tracing in constrictive pericarditis. (Modified with permission from Spodick DH: *The Pericardium: A Comprehensive Textbook.* New York: Marcel Dekker; 1997.)

conditions known to be associated with RCM; unfortunately, a negative biopsy does not rule it out.

In an attempt to provide additional criteria to differentiate CP from RCM, Hurrell et al measured respiratory variation of the gradient between left ventricular pressure and pulmonary capillary wedge pressure during the rapid filling phase of diastole.[25] This was done to assess the dissociation of intrathoracic and intracardiac pressures that accompanies CP. A difference of 5 mm Hg in the gradient between inspiratory and expiratory cycles had a 93% sensitivity and a 81% specificity for CP. Furthermore, increased ventricular interdependence was assessed by comparing left and right ventricular systolic pressures during respiration. Although concordant increases in left and right ventricular systolic pressure are expected during inspiration, discordant pressures are encountered during

inspiration in patients with CP. This finding has 100% sensitivity and 95% specificity for CP.

ACQUIRED ABNORMALITIES

Pericarditis, the most common pericardial disorder, has many etiologies (Table 57-2), including infectious (viral, bacterial, fungal), metabolic (uremic, drug induced), autoimmune (arthritis, thyroid), postradiation, neoplastic, traumatic, postinfarction (Dressler's syndrome, 10–15%), postpericardiotomy (5–30%), and idiopathic (Fig. 57-11). The clinical syndrome for all causes is similar. Chest pain (dull, aching, pressure, tightness) is usually present and may be associated with constitutional symptoms (eg, weakness and malaise), fever (occasionally with rigors), and other symptoms, such as cough or odynophagia. The pain may be pleuritic, and thus exacerbated by inspiration, cough, or recumbency. These patients therefore often sit up and lean forward for relief. Acute disease may become chronic. The cardinal sign of pericarditis is a pericardial rub, which may be positional and muffled because of an effusion.[26]

Electrocardiography, chest x-ray, and echocardiography are useful in making the diagnosis. The electrocardiogram may range from normal, to nonspecific ST-segment deviations, to diffuse concave elevation of the ST segments without reciprocal depressions or Q waves (Fig. 57-12). PR-segment depression may also be present. Troponin may be elevated with a normal CPK. Ventricular arrhythmias and conduction abnormalities are uncommon and if present are suggestive of an underlying cardiac abnormality. Echocardiography may reveal fibrinous thickening of the pericardium with or without a small effusion.

⊖ TABLE 57-1: Differentiation between Constrictive Pericarditis and Restrictive Cardiomyopathy

Finding	Pericardial constriction	Restrictive cardiomyopathy
Physical examination		
Pulsus paradoxus	Variable	Absent
Pericardial knock (high frequency)	Present	Absent
S3 (low frequency)	Absent	Present
Hemodynamics		
Prominent *y* descent	Present	Variable
Equalization of right and left side filling pressures	Present	Left > right
RV end-diastolic pressure/systolic pressure	>1/3	<1/3
Pulmonary hypertension	Rare	Common
Square-root sign	Present	Variable
Echocardiography		
Respiratory variation in left-right pressures/flows	Increased	Normal
Septal bounce	Present	Absent
Atrial enlargement	Variable	Biatrial
Ventricular hypertrophy	Absent	Usually present
Pericardial thickness	Increased	Normal

TABLE 57-2: Acquired Etiologies of Acute Pericarditis

Infectious

Bacterial
    Tuberculous (mycobacterial)
    Suppurative (streptococcal, pneumococcal)
Viral
    Coxsackie
    Influenza
    HIV
    Hepatitis A, B, C
    Other
Fungal
Parasitic
Other
    Rickettsial
    Spirochetal
    Spirillum
    Mycoplasma
    Infectious mononucleosis
    Leptospira
    Listeria
    Lymphogranuloma venereum
    Psittacosis

Autoimmune/Vasculitides

Rheumatoid arthritis
Rheumatic fever
Systemic lupus erythematosus
Drug-induced lupus erythematosus
Scleroderma
Sjögren's syndrome
Whipple's disease
Mixed connective tissue disease
Reiter's syndrome
Ankylosing spondylitis
Inflammatory bowel diseases
    Ulcerative colitis
    Crohn's disease
Serum sickness
Wegener's granulomatosis
Giant cell arteritis
Polymyositis
Behçet's syndrome
Familial mediterranean fever
Panmesenchymal syndrome
Polyarteritis nodosa
Churg-Strauss syndrome
Thrombohemolytic-thrombocytopenic purpura
Hypocomplementemic uremic vasculitis syndrome
Leukoclastic vasculitis
Other

Metabolic disorders

Renal failure
    Uremia in chronic or acute renal failure
    "Dialysis" pericarditis
Myxedema
    Cholesterol pericarditis
    Gout
Scurvy

Disease of contiguous structures

Myocardial infarction/cardiac surgery
    Acute myocardial infarction
    Postmyocardial infarction syndrome
    Postpericardiotomy syndrome
    Ventricular aneurysm
Aortic dissection
Pleural and pulmonary disease
    Pneumonia
    Pulmonary embolism
    Pleuritis
Malignancies of lung

Neoplastic

Primary
    Mesothelioma
    Sarcoma
    Fibroma
Secondary
    Metastatic; carcinomas, sarcomas
    Direct extension; bronchogenic, esophageal carcinomas
    Hematogenous; lymphoma, leukemia

Trauma

Penetrating
    Stab wound or gunshot wound to the chest, iatrogenic
    During diagnostic or therapeutic cardiac catheterization
    During pacemaker insertion
Radiation pericarditis

Uncertain etiologies and pathogenesis

Pericardial fat necrosis
Loeffler's syndrome
Thalassemia
Drug reactions
    Procainamide
    Hydralazine
    Others
Pancreatitis

Uncertain etiologies and pathogenesis

Sarcoidosis
Fat embolism
Bile fistula to pericardium
Wissler syndrome
PIE syndrome
Stevens-Johnson syndrome
Gaucher's disease
Diaphragmatic hernia
Atrial septal defect
Giant cell aortitis
Takayasu's syndrome
Castleman's disease
Fabry's disease
Kawasaki's disease
Degos' disease
Histiocytosis X
Campylodactyly-pleuritis-pericarditis syndrome
Farmer lung
Idiopathic

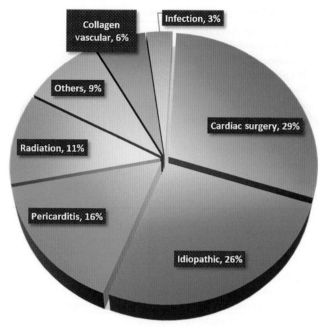

FIGURE 57-11 Etiologies and frequency of pericardial constriction.

Nonsteroidal anti-inflammatory drugs (NSAIDs) are the mainstay of treatment, although recent clinical studies support the routine use of colchine. A recent, large, multicenter randomized controlled trial (ICAP), in which patients with a first attack of pericarditis were randomized to conventional anti-inflammatories with either placebo or colchicine, demonstrated significantly reduced rates of incessant or recurrent pericarditis in those patients who received colchicine.[27] Other recent clinical trials focusing on recurrent pericarditis (CORP and CORP-2) have also demonstrated a significant benefit

with the use of colchicine.[28,29] Chronic pericardial effusion or CP may follow acute pericarditis as well as tuberculosis (TB), malignancy, radiation, rheumatoid arthritis (RA), or surgery.[26] Chronic, relapsing pericarditis that fails medical therapy can effectively be managed surgically with pericardiectomy.[30]

Infectious Pericarditis

VIRAL PERICARDITIS

Infectious pericarditis is most often viral and results from immune complex deposition, direct viral attack, or both. It is often difficult to diagnose and is therefore labeled as "idiopathic." Treatment is expectant, and symptoms generally resolve within 2 weeks. Surgical intervention is rarely required.

BACTERIAL PERICARDITIS

This is uncommon because of the availability of effective antibiotic therapy. Microorganisms may invade the pericardial space from contiguous infections in the heart (endocarditis), lung (pneumonia, abscess), subdiaphragmatic space (liver or splenic abscess), or wounds (traumatic, surgical). Hematogenous seeding may also occur in the setting of bacteremia and immune compromise.

The most common bacteria implicated are *Haemophilus influenzae*, meningococci, pneumococci, staphylococci, or streptococci.[31] Gram-negative rods, *Salmonella,* and opportunistic sources of infection must be excluded. Regardless of the source or organism, acute suppurative pericarditis is life threatening. A toxic presentation with a high fever is typical with an acute, fulminant clinical course. Purulent pericarditis with tamponade or septicemia may require acute surgical intervention via pericardial window or pericardiectomy and treatment of the inciting cause (eg, removal of foreign body

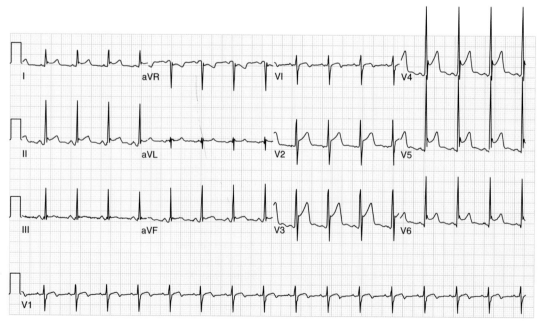

FIGURE 57-12 ECG demonstrating diffuse ST segment elevations, characteristic of pericarditis.

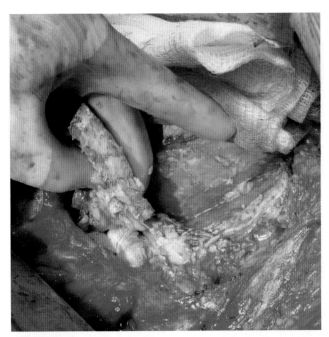

FIGURE 57-13 Intraoperative photo of a patient with septic pericarditis undergoing pericardiectomy. The pericardium is severely thickened.

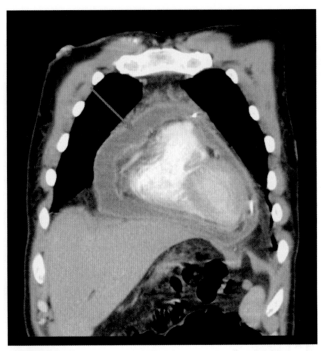

FIGURE 57-14 CT scan of chronic pericardial thickening and calcification and larger pericardial effusion in a patient with TB.

or drainage of abscess) (Fig. 57-13). In adults, pneumopyopericardium is often caused by fistula formation between a hollow viscus and the pericardium. However, invasion from contiguous foci, implantation at the time of surgery, trauma, mediastinitis, endocarditis, and subdiaphragmatic abscess can also cause this condition. Scarring with resultant pericardial constriction may require pericardiectomy. These patients have an excellent outcome when treated appropriately.[31]

TUBERCULOUS PERICARDITIS

Although the incidence of TB has significantly declined in industrialized countries, it has increased dramatically in Africa, Asia, and Latin America, accounting for 95% of all cases of active TB. This resurgence in TB reflects the increasing incidence of human immunodeficiency virus (HIV) infection.[32] The immune response to the acid-fast bacilli penetrating the pericardium induces a delayed hypersensitivity reaction with lymphokine release and granuloma formation. The cause of the exudative TB pericarditis is complement-fixing antibodies, which initiate cytolysis mediated by antimyolemmal antibodies.[32] The definitive diagnosis is established by examining the pericardium or pericardial fluid for mycobacteria.

Four pathologic states are recognized:

1. Fibrinous exudation, with robust polymorphonuclear infiltration and abundant mycobacteria.
2. Serous or serosanguineous effusions with a mainly lymphocytic exudation and foam cells (Fig. 57-14).
3. Absorption of effusion, with organization of caseating granulomas, and pericardial thickening caused by fibrin and collagen deposition and fibrosis.

4. Constrictive scarring, often with extensive calcification occurring over a period of years (Fig. 57-15 A, B).

The clinical course of TB pericarditis is variable. An effusion usually develops insidiously along with fever, night sweats, fatigue, and weight loss. Children and immunocompromised patients can have a more fulminant presentation, often demonstrating both constrictive and tamponade physiology. Despite prompt anti-TB antibiotic treatment, CP, one of the most severe sequelae, occurs in 30 to 60% of patients. Echocardiography is useful for diagnosing effusive and subacute constrictive TB pericarditis. Standard anti-TB therapy is instituted promptly. Steroids remain controversial, especially in HIV-infected patients. Based on physiology and response to therapy, immediate or interval pericardiectomy is performed to avoid chronic CP. If calcific pericarditis is present, surgery is undertaken earlier.[33]

FUNGAL PERICARDITIS

Fungal pericarditis is uncommon. *Nocardia, Aspergillus, Candida,* and *Coccidioides* are implicated, with regional specification, in the setting of immunocompromise, debilitation, HIV, severe burns, infancy, or steroid therapy. *Candida* and *Aspergillus* generate an insidious clinical picture, which may develop into tamponade or constriction. Fungi that tend to be endemic to certain geographic regions (eg, *Histoplasma*) may cause pericarditis in young, healthy, immunocompetent patients. This is usually self-limited and resolves within 2 weeks. Similarly, *Coccidioides* can infect healthy individuals in the setting of pneumonia, osteomyelitis, meningitis, or adenopathy. These

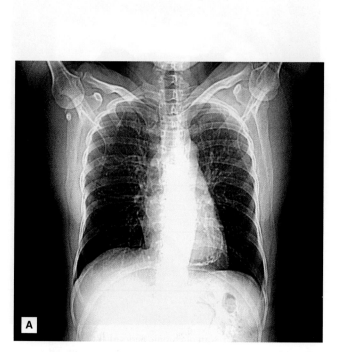

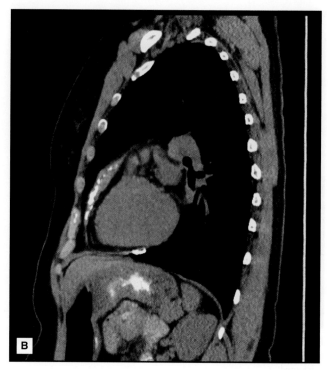

FIGURE 57-15 (A) PA CXR in patient with TB showing calcification of pericardium around LV apex. (B) CT scan of chronic pericardial thickening and calcification in patient with TB.

conditions often resolve either spontaneously or in response to antifungal therapy. Surgical intervention is not usually required in the acute setting.

Metabolic Causes of Pericarditis

Pericarditis is known to occur in the setting of renal failure, pharmacotherapy with certain drugs, autoimmune diseases (eg, rheumatoid arthritis), and hypothyroidism.

UREMIC PERICARDITIS

Uremic pericarditis was first recognized by Bright in 1836.[34] Although it is recognized that nitrogen retention (blood urea nitrogen levels generally >60 mg/dL) is required for uremic pericarditis, the inciting agent remains unknown. The clinical profile typically involves a patient with chronic renal insufficiency who develops pain, fever, and a friction rub.[35] There is usually a pericardial fluid collection, which can be exudative or transudative and is often hemorrhagic. Although the incidence of tamponade is decreasing because of the more widespread use of renal replacement therapy, it still occurs.[36] Initial therapy includes NSAIDs and aggressive dialysis. Pericardial drainage is reserved for cases of tamponade or refractory effusions (more than 2 weeks despite intensive dialysis), but the latter is the subject of debate.[37] Heparin should be administered cautiously, if at all, during dialysis because of the risk of hemorrhagic pericarditis and tamponade.[38] Pericardial effusions may also develop in this population because of a variety of conditions such as heart failure,

volume overload, and hypoproteinemia. Nonuremic pericarditis can also occur in patients on long-standing dialysis.[39] Finally, pericardial effusion increases the risk of low-pressure tamponade during dialysis by mechanisms described above.[17]

DRUG-INDUCED PERICARDITIS

Pericarditis may occur in the setting of a drug-induced hypersensitivity reaction or lupus-like syndrome.[40] Procainamide, hydralazine, isoniazid, methysergide, cromolyn, penicillin, and emetine (among others) have been associated with pericardial inflammation. Minoxidil has been associated with pericardial effusions.[41] The clinical presentation and guidelines for management are similar to those for other types of pericarditis. The inciting agent should be discontinued.

PERICARDITIS ASSOCIATED WITH RHEUMATOID ARTHRITIS

Pericarditis is common in patients with RA. Approximately half of patients with RA have pericardial effusions, and almost half of all patients with RA have significant pericardial adhesions at autopsy.[42] The condition is encountered more often with advanced RA and is thought to be caused by the higher rheumatoid factor titers seen with more severe disease. Immune complex deposition in the pericardium appears to be the inciting event underlying the inflammatory response.[43] The diagnosis is often complicated by the many clinical variants and possible concurrent diseases, such as drug-induced and viral pericarditis. Pericardial drainage is often employed early for symptomatic effusions because response to medical treatment of the underlying RA is slow and unpredictable. Pericardiectomy should be considered in patients with long-standing RA who have developed constriction.[44]

Hypothyroidism

Severe hypothyroidism produces large, clear, high-protein, high-cholesterol, and high-specific-gravity effusions in 25 to 35% of patients.[45] The effusion may precede other signs of hypothyroidism. Clinical tamponade is rare because fluid accumulation is slow. However, acute exacerbations owing to acute pericarditis, hemorrhage, or cholesterol pericarditis can induce tamponade.[46]

Radiation Pericarditis

Radiation is now the most common etiology of CP in the United States. This was first recognized in patients who received high-dose mantle radiation for Hodgkin's lymphoma in the 1960s and 1970s and developed cardiac and pericardial pathology, approximately 10 to 15 years after therapy. Radiation induces acute pericarditis, pancarditis, and accelerated coronary artery disease in a dose-dependent relationship.[47] Patients may present with a combination of pericardial constriction, RCM, valvular heart disease, and coronary artery disease with a predilection for ostial lesions.[48] When symptomatic effusions are drained, fluid should be analyzed to clarify the etiology (ie, malignancy vs radiation effect). CP can develop several years later and is best treated by pericardiectomy.[49]

Neoplastic Pericardial Disease

Secondary neoplasms of the pericardium (ie, from metastasis or adjacent infiltration) account for more than 95% of pericardial neoplastic diseases. Primary pericardial tumors are rare. Paraneoplastic effusions can also occur in response to remote tumors.[50]

The most common secondary tumors involving the pericardium in males (including both metastasis and local extension) are carcinoma of the lung (31.7%), esophagus (28.7%), and lymphoma (11.9%). In females, carcinoma of the lung (35.9%), lymphoma (17.0%), and carcinoma of the breast (7.5%) are the most common. Benign tumors are generally encountered in infancy or childhood. Malignant tumors (eg, mesotheliomas, sarcomas, and angiosarcomas) typically present in the third or fourth decade of life.[51]

In both primary and secondary tumor involvement, the clinical presentation is usually silent, and may be associated with large pericardial effusions. Tamponade can result from hemorrhage into a malignant effusion. Occasionally tumors can induce constriction because of neoplastic tissue, adhesions, or both. The role of surgery is limited to diagnosis and palliation in most cases. Large refractory effusions associated with tamponade may need surgical drainage. In such cases, a fluid sample should be submitted to confirm the presence of malignant cells or evaluate for other causes of effusion in patients with cancer because this may influence management.[52] Simple pericardiocentesis has a high failure rate, while subxiphoid drainage and percutaneous balloon pericardiotomy are only transiently effective.[53] Although extensive resection and debulking may be necessary in persistent or recurrent malignant pericardial constriction, it has only transient benefit without adjunctive chemotherapy and/or radiation therapy. There is no consensus about the optimal therapeutic approach for patients with malignant, symptomatic pericardial effusions. A recent study compared chemotherapy alone versus chemotherapy plus pericardiocentesis versus chemotherapy plus surgical pericardial window. It showed that patients undergoing a pericardial window had better response rates compared to those receiving chemotherapy alone or chemotherapy with percutaneous drainage.[54] While pericardial window has had a better/lower recurrence rate than simple pericardiocentesis, prolonged percutaneous pericardial drainage has improved recurrence rates while minimizing the morbidity associated with surgery.[55] Life expectancy of patients with malignant pericardial involvement averages less than 4 months.[56] The surgeon should individualize decisions regarding how aggressively to pursue diagnostic or therapeutic interventions.

Traumatic Pericardial Conditions

PENETRATING TRAUMA

Knives, bullets, needles, and intracardiac instrumentation are the main causes of penetrating trauma to the pericardium and heart. Tamponade is more common in stab wounds than gunshot wounds. The right ventricle is most often involved in anterior chest wounds. Because tamponade provides hemostasis and prevents exsanguination, patients with tamponade have better survival rates than those with uncontrolled hemorrhage. Diagnosis is often made on clinical grounds supplemented by ultrasonography.[57] Unstable patients should undergo thoracotomy in the emergency department. Stable patients can be explored in the operating room. The timing of induction of anesthesia is critical. Anesthetic induction can lead to hemodynamic collapse in the setting of tamponade and preload dependence. Therefore, the patient should be positioned, prepped, and draped before induction of anesthesia, in order to allow prompt opening of the chest and pericardium should hemodynamics rapidly deteriorate.

BLUNT TRAUMA

Blunt cardiac and pericardial injuries rarely occur in isolation. Trauma owing to compression (including cardiopulmonary resuscitation), blast, and deceleration can produce a spectrum of injuries ranging from cardiac contusion to cardiac rupture and pericardial laceration with herniation or luxation of the heart. Patients with pericardial rupture and cardiac herniation typically have suffered high-energy deceleration trauma and are hypotensive from associated injuries. Hypovolemia may lead to rapid decompensation because cardiac filling becomes increasingly volume dependent in the setting of tamponade. Likewise, patients may initially respond to volume resuscitation. Chest imaging may demonstrate displacement of the heart or free air or intra-abdominal organs within the pericardium. If the heart herniates into the pleura, positioning the patient with the contralateral side down may reduce the herniation. Thoracotomy is required for definitive treatment and repair of associated injuries.[58]

Acute Postinfarction Pericarditis and Dressler's Syndrome

Postinfarction pericarditis is thought to occur in almost half of patients suffering a transmural myocardial infarction (MI), although it is symptomatic in far fewer. The incidence is decreasing because of more aggressive revascularization in recent decades. Chest pain is almost universally present, and it is therefore important to distinguish the pain of pericarditis from ischemic pain by its positional and pleuritic nature. The pain of early post-MI pericarditis occurs in the first 24 to 72 hours. Dressler's syndrome is a diffuse pleuropericardial inflammation thought to have an autoimmune etiology that occurs weeks to months after infarction. A pericardial rub and effusion may be present but tamponade is rare. A pleural rub and effusion may also be present. The ECG signs of pericarditis may be obscured by those of infarction. Post-MI pericarditis is typically treated with aspirin and/or NSAIDs.[59,60] Steroids or colchicine may be used for persistent or recurrent symptoms; however, glucocorticoid use is associated with recurrence of pericarditis.[61]

Cardiac Surgery and the Pericardium

POSTINFARCTION PERICARDITIS

Postinfarction pericarditis is an important entity for the surgeon to consider in the evaluation of patients with acute coronary syndromes. To the unwary it may masquerade as post-infarction angina and prompt an unnecessarily early operation after MI. Extensive fibrinous adhesions and murky gelatinous fluid may be present in the pericardial space and obscure epicardial vessels. When the pericardium is opened late in such a patient, the surgeon should expect dense pericardial adhesions.

POSTOPERATIVE PERICARDIAL EFFUSION AND POST-PERICARDIOTOMY SYNDROME

Pericardial effusions not infrequently develop following cardiac surgery, occurring in 1 to 6% of patients. They range from small, asymptomatic, and clinically insignificant effusions to larger effusions that cause dyspnea, malaise, chest pain, or presyncope/syncope. Risk factors for the development of postoperative pericardial effusions include increased body surface area, pulmonary embolism, immunosuppression, surgery type (heart transplant, aortic aneurysm surgery), increased cardiopulmonary bypass time, urgency of surgery, and renal failure. Medical therapy for late effusions that are smaller and do not require drainage has traditionally involved NSAIDs. Some data, however, suggest that NSAID therapy is of limited benefit.[62] Management of large, symptomatic effusions involves pericardiocentesis, especially

when these are detected late (more than 7 days postoperatively). A pericardial drain is left in place for 1 to 3 days with periodic drainage. Surgical drainage can also be performed, and is generally undertaken for large effusions that develop early (within 7 days of surgery).[63] Beyond just an effusion, some patients develop Dressler's syndrome postoperatively. Although this condition is benign, it is important (and sometimes difficult) to distinguish between postoperative pericarditis and myocardial ischemia. This distinction can often be made on clinical grounds based on symptoms, hemodynamics, and ECG patterns.[64] Echocardiography or angiography may be used in borderline cases.

Prevention of postoperative pericardial effusions and post-pericardiotomy syndrome has also been studied. There may be a benefit to perioperative indomethacin for preventing pericardial effusions after aortic surgery, although the side effects of indomethacin must be considered, and further study is required before its routine perioperative use can be recommended.[65] Postoperative colchicine administration has been shown to reduce the incidence of post-pericardiotomy syndrome and pericardial effusions, and its routine use postoperatively should be considered.[66] Preoperative colchicine administration also reduces the rate of post-pericardiotomy syndrome; however, there is an increased incidence of adverse gastrointestinal side effects and drug discontinuation, which limits its beneficial effect.[67]

POSTOPERATIVE TAMPONADE

Early postoperative tamponade rarely goes undetected for long because of the high level of vigilance and close hemodynamic monitoring that attend the patient during this time. A vital feature of postoperative tamponade is that a circumferential fluid collection is not required for compromised cardiac function. Hemodynamic deterioration can occur in the setting of localized clot within the pericardium, particularly if it is impinging upon the right heart.[68] Surgeons must also be aware of the potential for late cardiac tamponade that presents after hospital discharge—often to a clinician other than the cardiac surgeon. This entity is a potentially lethal complication and occurs in 0.5 to 6% of patients after heart surgery, almost exclusively in those on anticoagulation. It is more common in younger patients following isolated valve surgery. Patients present on average 3 weeks after surgery, frequently in the setting of an elevated prothrombin time. They are often severely symptomatic, with declining exercise tolerance, dyspnea, oligo/anuria, and sometimes hypotension. Any patient on anticoagulation whose recovery takes an otherwise unexplained decline in this interval should be suspected of having late tamponade and should undergo echocardiographic examination. Nearly all patients with late tamponade respond favorably to pericardiocentesis and can safely resume anticoagulation.[69]

PERICARDIAL CLOSURE

Redo sternotomy may be more hazardous when the heart is adherent to the inner sternal table. Closing the pericardium at the time of surgery interposes a protective tissue layer between the sternum and the heart and may reduce the risks of redo sternotomy. The value of any added protection against cardiac injury on sternal reentry is limited by the relative infrequency of reoperation and the already low incidence of cardiac injury at repeat sternotomy when the pericardium is left open. On the negative side, closing the pericardium can cause kinking of bypass grafts after coronary artery bypass surgery and may result in hemodynamic compromise caused by cardiac compression. Rao et al demonstrated the adverse effects of pericardial closure on postoperative hemodynamics.[70] In this ingenious study, the pericardial edges were marked with radiopaque markers and the pericardium was closed with a running suture, the ends of which were exteriorized. After obtaining a postoperative chest x-ray that demonstrated pericardial approximation, a set of baseline hemodynamics was measured. The suture was then removed, another x-ray was taken to demonstrate distraction of the pericardial edges, and the hemodynamic measurements were repeated. Pericardial closure resulted in transient, moderate hemodynamic compromise in the first 8 hours postoperatively (Table 57-3). Although this and other studies have demonstrated adverse short-term hemodynamic consequences of pericardial closure, they have yet to report clinical evidence of worse outcomes.[71] Therefore, the risks of pericardial closure must be weighed against its potential benefits, and clinical practice should be individualized to the patient.

TABLE 57-3: Structural and Hemodynamic Changes after Pericardial Closure in Patients Undergoing Elective Isolated Coronary Artery Bypass Grafting

Parameters measured	Open pericardium	Closed pericardium	p-value
Retrosternal space at 1 week (cm)	13 ± 5	20 ± 7	.0003
Retrosternal space at 3 months (cm)	7 ± 3	14 ± 7	.0001
CI L/min/m² 1 hour postoperation	3.1 ± 0.8	2.3 ± 0.6	.003
CI L/min/m² 4 hours postoperation	3.1 ± 0.9	2.7 ± 0.7	.156
CI L/min/m² 8 hours postoperation	3.0 ± 0.8	2.8 ± 0.5	.402
LVSWI g/m/m² 1 hour postoperation	72 ± 18	52 ± 13	.002
LVSWI g/m/m² 4 hours postoperation	68 ± 17	54 ± 8	.016
LVSWI g/m/m² 8 hours postoperation	62 ± 22	52 ± 10	.087

CI, cardiac index; LVSWI, left ventricular stroke work index.

PERICARDIAL IMAGING

Multiple modalities are utilized to image the pericardium, including echocardiography, CT, and MRI. Each modality has strengths and weaknesses, and each has particular applicability to certain pericardial conditions. As such, multimodality imaging is recommended. Transthoracic echocardiography (TTE) is typically the first-line imaging test for any patient suspected of having pericardial disease. TTE is simple, cost-effective, and noninvasive. Moreover, it provides both imaging and functional/hemodynamic data. CT and/or MRI should be considered in the following circumstances[72]:

1. Acute or recurrent pericarditis with: (a) inconclusive TTE imaging, (b) failed response to NSAID therapy, (c) atypical presentation, (d) concern for CP, (e) prior trauma, (f) associated MI, neoplasm, infection, or pancreatitis.
2. Pericardial effusions that: (a) are complex with subacute tamponade requiring drainage, (b) have suspected hemopericardium, clot, malignancy, or inflammation, (c) cause regional tamponade postoperatively (TEE should also be considered).
3. Constrictive pericarditis: (a) with inconclusive TTE imaging, (b) when pericardial thickness or tissue assessment is necessary.
4. Pericardial masses to: (a) more fully characterize tissue, (b) assess for metastases, (c) evaluate for pericardial diverticulum or cyst.
5. Congenital absence of the pericardium, when pericardial morphology must be assessed.

OPERATIONS

Mediastinal Reexploration

Postoperative hemorrhage complicates approximately 3 to 5% of cardiac operations, a risk that nearly doubles in the setting of reoperations or valve surgery.[73] Common management for the postoperative cardiac surgical patient involves placing anterior and posterior mediastinal drains. Despite this, postoperative tamponade may still occur. The typical scenario involves declining chest tube output after a period of early postoperative bleeding, tachycardia, narrowed pulse pressure, increased right-sided filling pressures, oliguria, acidosis, escalating inotrope and/or vasopressor requirement, and decreased cardiac index. Echocardiography is not routinely helpful because the pericardial space and any associated thrombus may be difficult to visualize in the immediate postoperative period. Subtle echocardiographic findings have been reported, including an inspiratory increase in right ventricular end-diastolic diameter and a reciprocal decrease in left ventricular end-diastolic diameter, as well as an increase in early peak tricuspid flow velocity and reduction in flow across the mitral valve.[74,75] Because postoperative hemorrhage and tamponade can precipitate rapid deterioration, expedient mediastinal drainage is imperative. The importance of simultaneous correction of coagulopathy, hypothermia, acidosis, and hypovolemia is critical.[76] Extreme circumstances may dictate that temporizing decompression be performed in the ICU followed by definitive management in the operating room. Reported outcomes among patients explored in the ICU include perioperative survival of 85% and a sternal wound infection rate of 2%.[77]

During reexploration the first priority is to relieve tamponade by evacuating retained mediastinal blood and controlling life-threatening hemorrhage. Dramatic hemodynamic improvement is frequently observed upon chest reopening. Mediastinal reexploration is then undertaken in a thorough and methodical manner with careful attention paid to all suture lines. Complete mediastinal evaluation should be performed even if the culprit source is thought to be identified. Inspection proceeds from top down while simultaneously obtaining hemostasis; this prevents "rundown" from obscuring small sources of bleeding. Copious warm saline irrigation and judicious use of gauze packing are helpful adjuncts.

Pericardiocentesis

Pericardiocentesis is usually performed in a procedure suite under fluoroscopic, sonographic, or CT guidance. Arterial and right heart catheterizations are often performed for hemodynamic monitoring. After administration of 1% lidocaine to the skin and soft tissues of the left xiphocostal area, a 25-mL syringe is affixed to a three-way stopcock and then to an 18-gauge spinal needle. This pericardial needle is connected to an ECG V lead. Under electrocardiographic and imaging guidance, the needle is advanced from the left of the subxiphoid area aiming toward the left shoulder. ST-segment elevation may be seen on the V lead when the needle touches the epicardium. Under these circumstances, the needle is retracted slightly until ST-segment elevation disappears. Once the pericardial space is entered, a guidewire is introduced into the pericardial space. The needle is removed and a catheter is inserted into the pericardial sac over the guidewire. At our institution, a pigtail-shaped drainage catheter with an end hole and multiple side holes is used. Intrapericardial pressure is measured with pressure transducer system connected to the intrapericardial catheter. Pericardial fluid may then be removed. Symptom relief may be immediate and dramatic. In the presence of pericardial tamponade, aspiration of fluid is continued until there is clear clinical and hemodynamic improvement. If blood is withdrawn, 5 mL should be placed on a sponge to see if it clots. Clotting blood suggests that the needle has either inadvertently entered a cardiac chamber or caused epicardial injury. Defibrinated blood that has been present in the pericardial space for even a short time usually does not clot. The pericardial space is drained every 8 hours; the catheter is flushed with heparinized solution and is typically removed within 24 to 72 hours. Pneumothorax is a potential complication, and chest radiography is mandatory post-procedure.

Pericardial Window

The purpose of partial pericardial resection (window) is to drain fluid into the pleural or peritoneal compartment to prevent reaccumulation. The procedure can be performed via thoracoscopy, anterior thoracotomy, or subxiphoid incision; although each approach has its unique merits, reported outcomes among the three are relatively similar.[78,79] General anesthesia may not be tolerated by some patients in tamponade, in which case the subxiphoid approach under local anesthesia in a semirecumbent position can be employed. When the pericardium is incised, fluid will invariably drain under pressure. The excised portion of pericardium should be as large as is feasible to prevent recurrence.[80] The surgeon should remain mindful of the rare possibility of cardiac prolapse. With the transthoracic or thoracoscopic approaches, all accessible pericardium ventral to the phrenic nerve should be excised. Similarly, via the subxiphoid approach, as much diaphragmatic pericardium should be excised as possible.

Surgical pericardial window, when compared to pericardiocentesis, is a more definitive procedure with much lower recurrence rates. Complications rates have also been reported to be lower with surgery; although more recent studies demonstrate less morbidity with pericardiocentesis. This likely reflects increased experience and decreased complication rates with percutaneous techniques.[81] When considering whether to pursue percutaneous versus surgical drainage, the risks and benefits of each procedure must be weighed.

Pericardiectomy

Chronic pericardial constriction is treated by pericardial excision (Fig. 57-16). Because dense adhesions and calcification can penetrate into the myocardium, pericardial resection can be technically challenging. The procedure is usually done via median sternotomy with the capability to use cardiopulmonary bypass as needed.[33] Practice is variable, as some use cardiopulmonary bypass routinely, whereas others prefer to avoid the additional burden of coagulopathy unless absolutely necessary. Also, some surgeons prefer the countertraction provided by the filled heart, which facilitates pericardial stripping. Some surgeons use a left anterior thoracotomy, the approach taken by Edward Churchill, who reported the first pericardiectomy for CP done in the United States.[82] The objective of the procedure is to release the ventricles from the densely adherent pericardial shell. The lack of a surgical plane can make this a bloody operation, and attention must be paid to salvage and reinfusion of blood. Epicardial coronary vessels are at risk in this dissection, and particular care must be taken to avoid injuring them. The goal is to excise all anterior pericardium between the phrenic nerves and the posterior pericardium around its reflection on the venae cavae and pulmonary veins. Complete resection should restore pressure-volume loops to their normal position. Complete pericardial resection is not feasible in all cases, especially radiation-induced disease, and leaving densely adherent scar, particularly over the venae cavae and atria, may be safer.

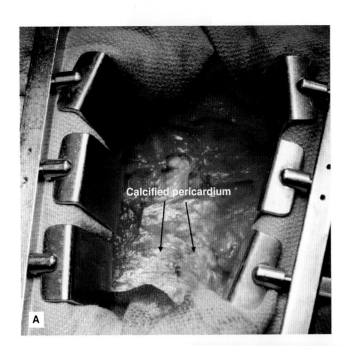

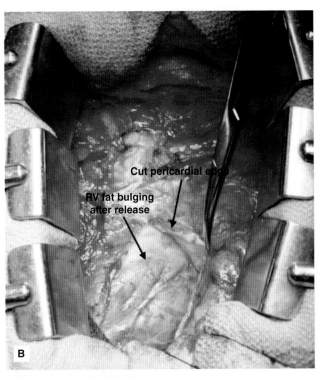

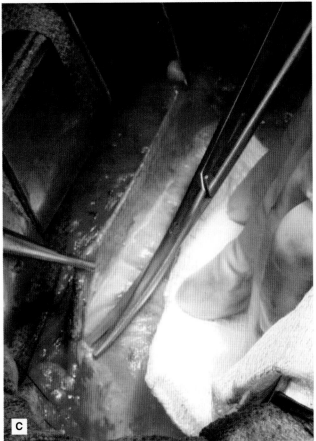

FIGURE 57-16 (A) Intraoperative photograph of TB pericardial thickening and calcification causing severe constriction. (B) Intraoperative photograph of pericardiectomy for constrictive TB pericarditis with RV free wall bulging through opening in pericardium, thick pericardial edge. (C) Adhesive pericarditis discovered incidentally in CABG patient. Technique for dividing adhesions over left ventricle and pulmonary artery.

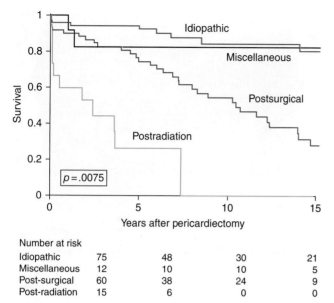

Number at risk				
Idiopathic	75	48	30	21
Miscellaneous	12	10	10	5
Post-surgical	60	38	24	9
Post-radiation	15	6	0	0

FIGURE 57-17 Kaplan-Meier curve showing a significant difference (log-rank test, p = .0075) in overall survival of patients after pericardiectomy, based on the presumed cause of constrictive pericarditis. (Reproduced with permission from Bertog S, Thambidorai S, Parakh K, et al: Constrictive pericarditis: etiology and cause-specific survival after pericardiectomy, *J Am Coll Cardiol.* 2004 Apr 21;43(8):1445-1452.)

Outcomes vary with the etiology and severity of the disease. Operative mortality has been reported as high as 10 to 20%, but is typically 5 to 6% in most contemporary series, and varies based on severity of heart failure, elevation of right atrial pressure, and comorbidities.[83-85] Although surgery alleviates or improves symptoms in most patients, long-term survival is diminished in patients who have had prior heart surgery, and particularly in patients with radiation-induced CP, in whom concurrent RCM may exist (Fig. 57-17).[86]

Waffle Procedure

In some cases of pericardial constriction patients have thickening and calcification of the epicardium (ie, visceral pericardium), and conventional pericardiectomy may not improve cardiac function. Little-to-no improvement in diastolic constriction is seen because the heart is still constricted by the thickened epicardial layer. If pericardiectomy does not result in prompt hemodynamic improvement intraoperatively, then a waffle procedure can be performed. This involves creation of intersecting longitudinal and transverse incisions through the epicardium across the entire surface of the ventricles, resulting in small islands of epicardial scar tissue (~1 cm² in size). These incisions relieve constriction and enable proper ventricular dilation/filling (Fig. 57-18). Results following a waffle procedure have been encouraging, although published data are relatively limited.[87,88]

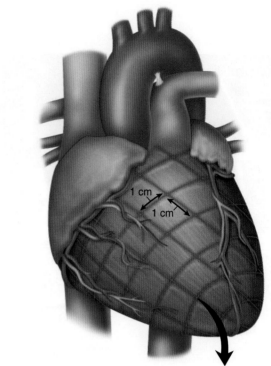

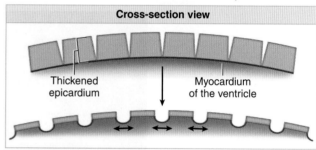

FIGURE 57-18 Waffle procedure demonstrating intersecting epicardial incisions to create small islands of epicardial scar tissue. Large epicardial vessels are preserved. The incisions allow for stretching of the epicardium and improved diastolic filling of the ventricles. (Reproduced with permission from Shiraishi M, Yamaguchi A, Muramatsu K, et al. Validation of waffle procedure for constrictive pericarditis with epicardial thickening, *Gen Thorac Cardiovasc Surg.* 2015 Jan;63(1):30-37.)

KEY POINTS

- Tamponade occurs when intrapericardial pressure impedes cardiac filling, causing increased venous pressure, decreased cardiac output, and progression to shock and death if left untreated.
- Pericardial reserve volume is limited; therefore, acute fluid accumulation can rapidly produce tamponade.
- Constrictive pericarditis, the end result of several inflammatory conditions, is characterized by a prominent *y* descent, square-root sign, septal bounce, and exaggerated respiratory variation in right- and left-sided flows; it is best treated with pericardiectomy.

- Restrictive cardiomyopathy, a myocardial disorder causing diastolic heart failure, is differentiated from pericardial constriction by the presence of pulmonary hypertension, biatrial enlargement, and ventricular thickening; it is not treated surgically.
- Patients with pericardial disease should undergo echocardiography supplemented as needed with CT and/or MRI, and catheter-based hemodynamic measurements or drainage for diagnosis.
- Acute pericarditis is often self-limited and responds to NSAIDs ± colchicine.
- The underlying disorder in secondary pericarditis can often be modified to improve the course of the pericardial disease.
- Intervention for postoperative hemorrhage and tamponade is required in less than 5% of cardiac surgeries. It should be undertaken promptly (in the ICU if necessary) with concurrent correction of coagulopathy, hypovolemia, hypothermia, and acidosis.
- Pericardiectomy is associated with decreased short- and long-term survival because of the severity of associated illnesses.

ACKNOWLEDGMENT

The authors would like to thank Mark S. Adams for the preparation of the figures, echocardiographic images, and photographs for the chapter.

REFERENCES

1. Spodick DH: The normal and diseased pericardium: current concepts of pericardial physiology, diseases and treatment. *J Am Coll Cardiol* 1983; 1:240.
2. Hammond HK, White FC, Bhargava V, et al: Heart size and maximal cardiac output are limited by the pericardium. *Am J Physiol* 1992; 263:H1675.
3. Santamore WP, Dell'Italia LJ: Ventricular interdependence: significant left ventricular contributions to right ventricular systolic function. *Prog Cardiovasc Dis* 1990; 40:298.
4. Barcin C, Olcay A, Kocaoglu M, Atac K, Kursaklioglu H: Asymptomatic congenital pericardial defect: an aspect of diagnostic modalities and treatment. Case Report. *Anadolu Kardiyol Derg* 2006; 6(4):387.
5. Spodick DH: Congenital abnormalities of the pericardium, in Spodick DH (ed): *The Pericardium: A Comprehensive Textbook.* New York, Marcel Dekker, 1997; p 65.
6. Risher WH, Rees AD, Ochsner JL, et al: Thoracoscopic resection of pericardium for symptomatic congenital pericardial defect. *Ann Thorac Surg* 1993; 56:1390.
7. Drury NE, DeSilva RJ, Hall RMO, Large SR: Congenital defects of the pericardium. *Ann Thorac Surg* 2007; 83:1552-1553.
8. Kraev A, Komanapalli B, Schipper PH, Sukumar MS: Pericardial cyst. *CTSNet* 2006; 16:1-4.
9. Barva GL, Magliani L, Bertoli D, et al: Complicated pericardial cyst: atypical anatomy and clinical course. *Clin Cardiol* 1998; 21:862.
10. Lau CL, Davis RD: The mediastinum, in *Sabiston's Textbook of Surgery,* 17th ed. Philadelphia, Elsevier, 2004; pp 1738-1739, 1758.
11. Patel J, Park C, Michaels J, Rosen S, Kort S: Pericardial cyst: case reports and a literature review. *Echocardiography* 2004; 21:269-272.
12. Weder W, Klotz HP, Segesser LV, et al: Thoracoscopic resection of a pericardial cyst. *J Thorac Cardiovasc Surg* 1994; 107:313.
13. Little WC, Freeman GL: Pericardial disease. *Circulation* 2006; 113:1622.
14. Spodick DH: Acute cardiac tamponade. *N Engl J Med* 2003; 349:684.
15. Spodick DH: Pathophysiology of cardiac tamponade. *Chest* 1998; 113:1372.
16. Reddy PS, Curtiss EI, Uretsky BF: Spectrum of hemodynamic changes in cardiac tamponade. *Am J Cardiol* 1990; 66:1487.
17. Sagrista-Sauleda J, Angel J, Sambola A, et al: Low-pressure cardiac tamponade: clinical and hemodynamic profile. *Circulation* 2006; 114:945.
18. Maisch B, Seferovic PM, Ristic AD, et al: Guidelines on the diagnosis and management of pericardial diseases executive summary: the task force on the diagnosis and management of pericardial diseases of the European society of cardiology. *Eur Heart J* 2004; 25:587.
19. Ling LH, Oh JK, Schaff HV, et al: Constrictive pericarditis in the modern era: evolving clinical spectrum and impact on outcome after pericardiectomy. *Circulation* 1999; 100:1380.
20. Myers RBH, Spodick DH: Constrictive pericarditis: clinical and pathophysiologic characteristics. *Am Heart J* 1999; 138:219.
21. Godwin C, Kesavan S, Flamm SD, Sivananthan MU: Role of MRI in clinical cardiology. *Lancet* 2004; 363:2162.
22. Talreja DR, Edwards WD, Danielson GK, et al: Constrictive pericarditis in 26 patients with histologically normal pericardial thickness. *Circulation* 2003; 108:1852.
23. Troughton RW, Asher CR, Klein AL: Pericarditis. *Lancet* 2004; 363:717.
24. Chinnaiyan KM, Leff CB, Marsalese DL: Constrictive pericarditis versus restrictive cardiomyopathy: challenges in diagnosis and management. *Cardiol Rev* 2004; 12:314.
25. Hurrell DG, Nishimura RA, Higano ST, et al: Value of dynamic respiratory changes in left and right ventricular pressures for the diagnosis of constrictive pericarditis. *Circulation* 1996; 93:2007.
26. *Pericarditis: Cardiovascular Disorders.* Merck Manual Professional. 2010; 1-9.
27. Imazio M, Brucato A, Ferrua S, et al: A randomized trial of colchicine for acute pericarditis. *N Engl J Med* 2013; 369:1522-1528.
28. Imazio M, Brucato A, Cemin R, et al: Colchicine for recurrent pericarditis (CORP): a randomized trial. *Ann Intern Med* 2011; 155:409-414.
29. Imazio M, Belli R, Brucato A, et al: Efficacy and safety of colchicine for treatment of multiple recurrences of pericarditis (CORP-2): a multicenter, double-blind, placebo-controlled, randomized trial. *Lancet* 2014; 383:2232-2237.
30. Khandaker MH, Schaff HV, Greason KL, et al: Pericardiectomy vs medical management in patients with relapsing pericarditis. *Mayo Clin Proc* 2012; 87:1062-1070.
31. Koster N, Narmi A, Anand K: Bacterial pericarditis. *Am J Med* 2009; 122-5:e1-e2.
32. Mayosi BM, Burgess LJ, Doubell AF: Tuberculous pericarditis. *Circulation* 2005; 112:3608.
33. Tirilomis T, Univerdoben S, von der Emde J: Pericardiectomy for chronic constrictive pericarditis: risks and outcome. *Eur J Thorac Cardiovasc Surg* 1994; 8:487.
34. Bright R: Tabular view of the morbid appearance in 100 cases connected with albuminous urine: with observations. *Guys Hosp Rep* 1836; 1:380.
35. Alpert MA, Ravenscraft MD: Pericardial involvement in end-stage renal disease. *Am J Med Sci* 2003; 325:228.
36. Banerjee A, Davenport A: Changing patterns of pericardial disease in patients with end-stage renal disease. *Hemodial Int* 2006; 10:249.
37. Leehey DJ, Daugirdas JT, Ing TS: Early drainage of pericardial effusions in patients with dialysis pericarditis. *Arch Intern Med* 1983; 143:1673.
38. Zakynthinos E, Theodorakopoulou M, Daniil, Z, et al: Hemorrhagic cardiac tamponade in critically ill patients with acute renal failure. *Heart Lung* 2004; 33:55.
39. Rutsky EA: Treatment of uremic pericarditis and pericardial effusion. *Am J Kidney Dis* 1987; 10:2.
40. Rheuban KS: Pericarditis. *Curr Treat Options Cardiovasc Med* 2005; 7:419.
41. Oates JA, Wilkinson GR: Principles of drug therapy, in Isselbacher KJ, Braunwald E, Wilson JD, et al (eds): *Harrison's Principles of Internal Medicine.* New York, McGraw-Hill, 1994; p 409.
42. Turesson C, Lacobsson L, Bergstrom U: Extra-articular rheumatoid arthritis: prevalence and mortality. *Rheumatology* 1999; 38:668.
43. Gulati S, Kumar L: Cardiac tamponade as an initial manifestation of systemic lupus erythematosus in early childhood. *Ann Rheum Dis* 1992; 51:179.
44. Harle P, Salzberger B, Gluck T, et al: Fatal outcome of constrictive pericarditis in rheumatoid arthritis. *Rheumatol Int* 2003; 23:312.
45. Kabadi UM, Kumar SP: Pericardial effusion in primary hypothyroidism. *Am Heart J* 1990; 120:1393.
46. Gupta R, Munyak J, Haydock T, et al: Hypothyroidism presenting as acute cardiac tamponade with viral pericarditis. *Am J Emerg Med* 1999; 17:176.

47. Stewart JR, Fajardo LF: Radiation induced heart disease: an update. *Prog Cardiovasc Dis* 1984; 27:173.

48. Lee PJ, Malli R: Cardiovascular effects of radiation therapy: practical approach to radiation induced heart disease. *Cardiol Rev* 2005; 13:80.

49. Bertog SC, Thambidorai SK, Parakh K, et al: Constrictive pericarditis: etiology and cause-specific survival after pericardiectomy. *J Am Coll Cardiol* 2004; 43:1445.

50. Spodick DH: Neoplastic pericardial disease, in Spodick DH (ed): *The Pericardium: A Comprehensive Textbook*. New York, Marcel Dekker, 1997; p 301.

51. Warren MH: Malignancies involving the pericardium. *Semin Thorac Cardiovasc Surg* 2000; 12:119.

52. Gornik HL, Gerhard-Herman M, Beckman JA: Abnormal cytology predicts poor prognosis in cancer patients with pericardial effusion. *J Clin Oncol* 2005; 23:5211.

53. Wang HJ, Hsu KL, Chiang FT, et al: Technical and prognostic outcomes of double-balloon pericardiotomy for large malignancy-related pericardial effusions. *Chest* 2002; 122:893.

54. Celik S, Lestuzzi C, Cervesato E, et al: Systemic chemotherapy in combination with pericardial window has better outcomes in malignant pericardial effusions. *J Thorac Cardiovasc Surg* 2014; 148:2288-2293.

55. Patel N, Rafique AM, Eshaghian S, et al: Retrospective comparison of outcomes, diagnostic value, and complications of percutaneous prolonged drainage versus surgical pericardiotomy of pericardial effusion associated with malignancy. *Am J Cardiol* 2013; 112:1235-1239.

56. Hazelrigg SR, Mack MJ, Landreneau RJ, et al: Thoracoscopic pericardiectomy for effusive pericardial disease. *Ann Thorac Surg* 1993; 56:792.

57. Bahner D, Blaivas M, Cohen HL, et al: AIUM Practice guideline for the performance of the Focused Assessment with Sonography for Trauma (FAST) Examination. *J Ultrasound Med* 2008; 27:313.

58. Schultz JM, Trunkey DD: Blunt cardiac injury. *Crit Care Clin* 2004; 20:57.

59. Tenenbaum A, Koren-Morag N, Spodick DH, et al: The efficacy of colchicine in the treatment of recurrent pericarditis related to postcardiac injury (postpericardiotomy and postinfarcted) syndrome: a multicenter analysis. *Heart Drug* 2004; 4:141.

60. Imazio M, Bobbio M, Cecchi E, et al: Colchicine in addition to conventional therapy for acute pericarditis: results of the COlchicine for acute PEricarditis (COPE) Trial. *Circulation* 2005; 112:2012.

61. Imazio M, Brucato A, Cumetti D, et al: Corticosteroids for recurrent pericarditis—high versus low doses: a nonrandomized observation. *Circulation* 2008; 118:667.

62. Meurin P, Tabet JY, Thabut G, et al: Nonsteroidal anti-inflammatory drug treatment for postoperative pericardial effusion: a multicenter randomized, double-blind trial. *Ann Intern Med* 2010; 152(3):137-143.

63. Ashikhmina EA, Schaff HV, Sinak LJ, et al: Pericardial effusion after cardiac surgery: risk factors, patient profiles, and contemporary management. *Ann Thorac Surg* 2010; 89:112-118.

64. Lange RA, Hillis D: Acute pericarditis. *N Engl J Med* 2004; 351:2195.

65. Inan MB, Yazicioglu L, Eryilmaz S, et al: Effects of prophylactic indomethacin treatment on postoperative pericardial effusion after aortic surgery. *J Thorac Cardiovasc Surg* 2011; 141:578-582.

66. Imazio M, Trinchero R, Brucato A, et al: COPPS Investigators. Colchicine for the prevention of the post-pericardiotomy syndrome (COPPS): a multicenter, randomized, double-blind, placebo-controlled trial. *Eur Heart J* 2010; 31(22):2749-2754.

67. Imazio M, Brucato An, Ferrazzi P, et al: Colchicine for prevention of post-pericardiotomy syndrome and postoperative atrial fibrillation: The COPPS-2 randomized clinical trial. *JAMA* 2014; 312(10):1016-1023.

68. Ionescu A: Localized pericardial tamponade: difficult echocardiographic diagnosis of a rare complication after cardiac surgery. *J Am Soc Echocardiogr* 2005; 14:220.

69. Mangi AA, Palacios IF, Torchiana DF: Catheter pericardiocentesis for delayed tamponade after cardiac valve operation. *Ann Thorac Surg* 2002; 73:1479.

70. Rao W, Komeda M, Weisel RD, et al: Should the pericardium be closed routinely after heart operations? *Ann Thorac Surg* 1999; 67:484.

71. Bittar MN, Barnard JB, Khasati N, et al: Should the pericardium be closed in patients undergoing cardiac surgery? *Interact Cardiovasc Thorac Surg* 2005; 4:151.

72. Klein AK, Abbara S, Agler DA, et al: American Society of Echocardiography clinical recommendations for multimodality cardiovascular imaging of patients with pericardial disease: endorsed by the Society for Cardiovascular Magnetic Resonance and Society of Cardiovascular Computed Tomography. *J Am Soc Echocardiogr* 2013; 26:965-1012.

73. Moulton MJ, Creswell LL, Mackey ME, et al: Reexploration for bleeding is a risk factor for adverse outcomes after cardiac operations. *J Thorac Cardiol Surg* 1996; 111:1037.

74. Gonzalez MS, Basnight MA, Appleton CP: Experimental cardiac tamponade: hemodynamic and Doppler echocardiographic reexamination of right and left heart ejection dynamics to the phase of respiration. *J Am Coll Cardiol* 1991; 18:243.

75. Appleton C, Hatle LK, Popp RL: Cardiac tamponade and pericardial effusion: respiratory variation in transvalvular flow velocities during experimental cardiac tamponade. *J Am Coll Cardiol* 1988; 11:1020.

76. Makar M, Taylor J, Zhao M, et al: Perioperative coagulopathy, bleeding, and hemostasis during cardiac surgery: a comprehensive review. *ICU Director* 2010; 1:17.

77. Fiser SM, Tribble CG, Kern JA, et al: Cardiac reoperation in the intensive care unit. *Ann Thorac Surg* 2001; 71:1888.

78. O'Brien PK, Kucharczuk JC, Marshall MB, et al: Comparative study of subxiphoid versus video-thoracoscopic pericardial "window." *Ann Thorac Surg* 2005; 80:2013.

79. Liberman M, Labos C, Sampalis JS, et al: Ten-year surgical experience with nontraumatic pericardial effusions: a comparison between the subxiphoid and transthoracic approaches to pericardial window. *Arch Surg* 2005; 140:191.

80. Georghiou GP, Stamler A, Sharoni E, et al: Video-assisted thoracoscopic pericardial window for diagnosis and management of pericardial effusions. *Ann Thorac Surg* 2005; 80:607.

81. Saltzman AJ, Paz YE, Rene AG, et al: Comparison of surgical pericardial drainage with percutaneous catheter drainage for pericardial effusion. *J Invasive Cardiol* 2012; 24(11):590-593.

82. Churchill ED: Decortication of the heart for adhesive pericarditis. *Arch Surg* 1929; 19:1447.

83. Seifert FC, Miller DC, Oesterle SN, et al: Surgical treatment of constrictive pericarditis: analysis of outcome and diagnostic error. *Circulation* 1985; 72 (3 Pt 2):II264.

84. Schwefer M, Aschenbach R, Hidemann J, et al: Constrictive pericarditis, still a diagnostic challenge: comprehensive review of clinical management. *Eur J Cardiothorac Surg* 2009; 36:502.

85. Ha JW, Oh JK, Schaff HV, et al: Impact of left ventricular function on immediate and long-term outcomes after pericardiectomy in constrictive pericarditis. *J Thorac Cardiovasc Surg* 2008; 136:1136.

86. Bertog S, Thambidorai S, Parakh K, et al: Constrictive pericarditis: etiology and cause-specific survival after pericardiectomy. *J Am Coll Cardiol* 2004; 43:1445.

87. Shiraishi M, Yamaguchi A, Muramatsu K, et al: Validation of waffle procedure for constrictive pericarditis with epicardial thickening. *Gen Thorac Cardiovasc Surg* 2015; 63:30-37.

88. Yamamoto N, Ohara K, Nie M, et al: For what type of constrictive pericarditis is the waffle procedure effective? *Asian Cardiovasc Thorac Ann* 2011; 19(2):115-118.

58

Cardiac Neoplasms

Basel Ramlawi • Michael J. Reardon

Neoplasms of the heart can be divided into primary cardiac tumors arising in the heart and secondary cardiac tumors from metastasis. Primary cardiac tumors can be further stratified into benign and malignant tumors. Between 10 and 20% of patients dying of disseminated cancer have metastatic involvement of the heart or pericardium.[1,2] Surgical resection is seldom possible or advisable for these tumors, and intervention usually is limited to drainage of malignant pericardial effusions and/or diagnostic biopsies.

The incidence of primary cardiac neoplasm ranges between 0.17 and 0.19% in unselected autopsy series.[3-5] Seventy-five percent of primary cardiac tumors are benign, and 25% are malignant.[2,6] Fifty percent of the benign tumors are myxomas, and 75% of malignant tumors are sarcomas.[2,6] The clinical incidence of these tumors is 1 in 500 cardiac surgical patients. With the exception of myxomas, most surgeons will rarely encounter primary cardiac tumors. The purpose of this chapter is to summarize useful information for the evaluation and management of patients with cardiac tumors and to provide a reference for additional study.

HISTORICAL BACKGROUND

A primary cardiac neoplasm was first described by Realdo Colombo in 1559.[7] Alden Allen Burns of Edinburgh described a cardiac neoplasm and suggested valvular obstruction by an atrial tumor in 1809.[8] A series of six atrial tumors, with characteristics we now recognize as myxoma, was published in 1845 by King.[9] In 1931, Yates reported nine cases of primary cardiac tumor and established a classification system similar to what we use today.[10] The first antemortem diagnosis of a cardiac tumor was made in 1934 when Barnes diagnosed a cardiac sarcoma using electrocardiography and biopsy of a metastatic lymph node.[11] In 1936, Beck successfully resected a teratoma external to the right ventricle,[12] and Mauer removed a left ventricular lipoma in 1951.[13] Treatment of cardiac tumors was profoundly influenced by two events: the introduction of cardiopulmonary bypass (CPB) in 1953 by John Gibbon, which allowed a safe and reproducible approach to the cardiac chambers, and the introduction of cardiac echocardiography, which allowed safe and noninvasive diagnosis of an intracardiac mass. The first echocardiographic diagnosis of an intracardiac tumor was made in 1959.[14] An intracardiac myxoma was diagnosed by angiography in 1952 by Goldberg, but attempts at surgical removal were unsuccessful.[9] A large right atrial myxoma was removed by Bhanson in 1952 using caval inflow occlusion, but the patient died 24 days later.[15] Crafoord in Sweden first successfully removed a left atrial myxoma in 1954 using CPB,[16] and Kay in Los Angeles first removed a left ventricular myxoma in 1959.[17] By 1964, 60 atrial myxomas had been removed successfully, with improved results owing to the increasing safety of CPB and use of echocardiography for detection. Operations are currently performed routinely on patients with atrial myxoma with minimal mortality.[6,18-21] Primary malignant tumors, however, continue to represent a challenge.

CLASSIFICATION

A pathologic classification is listed in Table 58-1. Mural thrombus is listed as a pseudotumor, although not really a cardiac tumor, its presentation may mimic myxoma clinically and pathologically. Most mural thrombi are associated with underlying valvular disease, myocardial infarction, dysfunction, or atrial fibrillation.[22] Mural thrombi also have been noted in hypercoagulable syndromes, particularly antiphospholipid syndrome.[23] With increasing use of long-term central catheters, we have seen several right atrial masses that were difficult to define and upon removal were mural thrombi.

Heterotopias and tumors of ectopic tissue include cystic tumors of the atrioventricular (AV) node consisting of multiple benign cysts in the region of the AV node that can cause heart block or sudden death. Most are diagnosed at autopsy, but a biopsy diagnosis of AV nodal tumor has been reported.[24] Germ cell tumors of the heart usually are teratomas, occurring within the pericardial sac, but yolk sac tumors have been described in infants and children.[25] Ectopic thyroid tissue may occur within the myocardium and is referred to as *struma cordis*. Right ventricular outflow track obstruction may be present, but most patients are asymptomatic.

Most of the remaining tumors arise in the mesenchymal, fat, fibrous, neural, or vascular cells of the heart, with myxoma

TABLE 58-1: Types of Cardiac Tumors by Pathology

Pseudotumors
  Mural thrombi
Heterotopias and tumors of ectopic tissue
  Tumors of the atrioventricular nodal region
  Teratoma
  Ectopic thyroid
Tumors of mesenchymal tissue
  Hamartoma of endocardial tissue
  Papillary fibroelastomas
Hamartomas of cardiac muscle
  Rhabdomyoma
  Histiocytoid cardiomyopathy (Purkinje cell hamartoma)
Tumors and neoplasms of fat
  Lipomatous hypertrophy, interarterial septum
  Lipoma
  Liposarcoma
Tumors and neoplasms of fibrous and myofibroblastic tissue
  Fibroma
  Inflammatory pseudotumor (inflammatory myofibroblastic tumor)
  Sarcomas (malignant fibrous histiocytoma, fibrosarcoma, leiomyosarcoma)
Vascular tumors and neoplasms
  Hemangioma
  Epithelioid hemangioendothelioma
  Angiosarcoma
Neoplasm of uncertain histogenesis
  Myxoma
Neoplasms of neural tissue
  Granular cell tumor
  Schwannoma/neurofibroma
Paraganglioma
Malignant schwannoma/neurofibrosarcoma (rare)
Malignant lymphoma
Malignant mesothelioma
Metastatic tumors to the heart

TABLE 58-2: Benign Cardiac Neoplasms in Adults

Tumor	No.	Percentage
Myxoma	118	49
Lipoma	45	19
Papillary fibroelastoma	42	17
Hemangioma	11	5
AV node mesothelioma	9	4
Fibroma	5	2
Teratoma	3	1
Granular cell tumor	3	1
Neurofibroma	2	<1
Lymphangioma	2	<1
Rhabdomyoma	1	<1
Total	241	100

Reproduced with permission from McAllister HA Jr, Fenoglio JJ Jr: Tumors of the cardiovascular system, in *Atlas of Tumor Pathology*. Washington, DC, Armed Forces Institute of Pathology; 1978, fas. 15.

representing a tumor of undetermined histogenesis. Primary cardiac lymphoma, mesothelioma, and metastatic tumors to the heart represent the remaining pathologic categories that comprise the greater part of this chapter.

PRIMARY BENIGN TUMORS

Myxoma

Myxomata comprise 50% of all benign cardiac tumors in adults and 15% of such tumors in children. Occurrence during infancy is rare (Tables 58-2 and 58-3). A vast majority of myxomas occur sporadically and tend to be more common in women.[4,21] The peak incidence is between the third and sixth decades of life, and 94% of tumors are solitary.[26] Approximately 75% occur in the left atrium[27] and 10 to 20% occur

in the right atrium. The remaining proportion are equally distributed between the ventricles.[2] The deoxyribonucleic acid (DNA) genotype of sporadic myxomas is normal in 80% of patients.[28] Myxomas are unlikely to be associated with other abnormal conditions and have a low recurrence rate.[4,27]

About 5% of myxoma patients show a familial pattern of tumor development based on autosomal dominant inheritance.[29-31] These patients and 20% of those with sporadic myxoma have an abnormal DNA genotype chromosomal pattern.[28] In contrast to the "typical" sporadic myxoma profile, familial patients are more likely to be younger, equally likely to be male or female, and more often (22%) have multicentric tumors originating from either the atrium or ventricle.[32-36] Although familial myxomas have the same histology, they have a higher recurrence rate after surgical resection (21-67%).[27,37] Approximately 20% of familial patients have associated conditions such as adrenocortical nodule hyperplasia, Sertoli cell tumors of the testes, pituitary tumors, multiple myxoid breast fibroadenomas, cutaneous myomas, and facial or labial pigmented spots.[26,37] These conditions often are described as *complex myxomas* within the group of familial myxoma.[28] A familial syndrome with autosomal X-linked inheritance characterized by primary pigmented nodular adrenocortical disease with hypercortisolism, cutaneous pigmentous lentigines, and cardiac myxoma is referred to as *Carney's complex.*[26,37]

PATHOLOGY

Both biatrial and multicentric myxomas are more common in familial disease. Biatrial tumors probably arise from bidirectional growth of a tumor originating within the atrial septum.[38] Atrial myxomas generally arise from the interatrial septum at the border of the fossa ovalis but can originate anywhere within the atrium, including the appendage.[4]

TABLE 58-3: Benign Cardiac Neoplasms in Children

Tumor	0 to 1-year-old		1 to 15-year-olds	
	Number	Percentage	Number	Percentage
Rhabdomyoma	28	62	35	45.0
Teratoma	9	21	11	14.0
Fibroma	6	13	12	15.5
Hemangioma	1	2	4	5.0
AV node mesothelioma	1	2	3	4.0
Myxoma	—	—	12	15.5
Neurofibroma	—	—	1	1.0
Total	45	100	78	100

Reproduced with permission from McAllister HA Jr, Fenoglio JJ Jr: Tumors of the cardiovascular system, in *Atlas of Tumor Pathology*. Washington, DC, Armed Forces Institute of Pathology; 1978, fas. 15.

In addition, isolated reports confirm that myxomas can arise from the cardiac valves, pulmonary artery (PA) and vein, and vena cava.[30,31] Right atrial myxomas are more likely to have broad-based attachments than left atrial tumors; they also are more likely to be calcified,[34] and thus visible on chest radiographs. Ventricular myxomas occur more often in women and children and may be multicentric.[2,39] Right ventricular tumors typically arise from the free wall, and left ventricular tumors tend to originate in the proximity of the posterior papillary muscle.

Grossly, about two-thirds of myxomas are round or oval tumors with a smooth or lobulated surface (Fig. 58-1).[21] Most are polypoid, compact, pedunculated, mobile, and not likely to fragment spontaneously.[2,4] Mobility depends on stalk length, the extent of attachment to the heart, and the amount of tumor collagen.[4] Most are pedunculated with a short, broad base, and sessile forms are unusual.[2,40] Less common villous or papillary myxomas are gelatinous and fragile and prone to fragmentation and embolization, occurring about one-third of the time.[21,41] Myxomas are white, yellow, or brown in color, and are frequently covered with thrombus.[2] Focal areas of hemorrhage, cyst formation, or necrosis may be seen in cut section. The average size is about 5 cm in diameter, but growth to 15 cm in diameter and larger has been reported.[4] Myxomatous tumors appear to grow rapidly, but growth rates vary, and occasionally, tumor growth arrests spontaneously.[4] Weights range from 8 to 175 g, with a mean between 50 and 60 g.[5]

Histologically, myxomas are composed of polygonal-shaped cells and capillary channels within an acid mucopolysaccharide matrix.[4] The cells appear singularly or in small clusters throughout the matrix, and mitoses are rare.[42,43] The matrix also contains occasional smooth muscle cells, reticulocytes, collagen, elastin fibers, and a few blood cells. Cyst, areas of hemorrhage, and foci of extramedullary hematopoiesis are also found.[37,41] Ten percent of the tumors have microscopic deposits of calcium and metastatic bone deposits, as well as sometimes glandular-like structures.[37,41] The base of the tumor contains a large artery and veins that connect with the subendocardium but do not typically extend deep beyond the subendocardium.[37] A coronary angiography in our own institution revealed a large feeding vessel and was suspected originally of being an angiosarcoma but on histology proved to be a typical benign myxoma. Myxomas tend to grow into the overlying cardiac cavity rather than into the surrounding myocardium. Myxomas arise from the endocardium and are considered derivative of the subendocardial multipotential mesenchymal cell.[44-46] This accounts for the occasional presence of hematopoietic tissue and bone in these tumors. Interestingly, myxomas have developed after cardiac trauma, including repair of atrial septal defects and trans-septal puncture for percutaneous dilatation of the mitral valve.

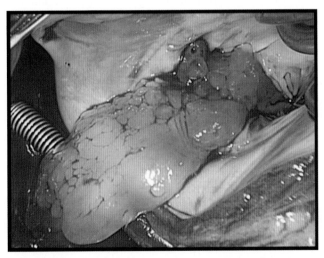

FIGURE 58-1 Large in situ left atrial myxoma as seen from the surgeon's perspective just before removal.

CLINICAL PRESENTATION

The classic clinical presentation of a myxoma is intracardiac obstruction with congestive heart failure (67%); signs of embolization (29%); systemic or constitutional symptoms of fever (19%); weight loss or fatigue (17%); and immunologic manifestations of myalgia, weakness, and arthralgia (5%).[21] Cardiac rhythm disturbances and infection occur less frequently.

Constitutional Symptoms. Nearly all myxoma patients admit to a variety of constitutional symptoms. These complaints may be accompanied by a leukocytosis, elevated erythrocyte levels and sedimentation rate, hemolytic anemia, thrombocytopenia, and elevated C-reactive protein. Immunoelectrophoresis may reveal abnormal immunoglobulin levels with increased circulating IgG.[47] The recent discovery of elevated levels of interleukin-6 in patients with myxoma has been linked to a variety of associated conditions, including lymphadenopathy, tumor metastasis, ventricular hypertrophy, and development of constitutional symptoms.[39,48,49] Other less frequent complaints include Raynaud's phenomenon, arthralgias, myalgias, erythematous rash, and clubbing of the digits.[4,50]

Possible etiologies of such varied complaints and symptoms include tumor embolization with secondary myalgias and arthralgias and elevated immunoglobulin response.[51] Circulating antibody–tumor antigen complexes with complement activation also may play a role.[43] Such symptom complexes tend to resolve following surgical resection of the tumor.[52]

Obstruction. Obstruction of blood flow in the heart is the most common cause of acute presenting symptoms. The nature of these symptoms is determined by which of the chambers is involved and the size of the tumor. Myxomas in the left atrium tend to mimic mitral disease. These produce positional dyspnea and other signs and symptoms of heart failure associated with elevated left atrial and pulmonary venous pressures. Clinically, mitral stenosis often is suspected and leads to echocardiography and diagnosis of myxoma. Syncopal episodes occur in some patients and are thought to result from temporary occlusion of the mitral orifice.[34,53] Right atrial myxomas can produce a clinical picture of right-sided heart failure with signs and symptoms of venous hypertension, including hepatomegaly, ascites, and dependent edema and can cause tricuspid valve stenosis by partially obstructing the orifice.[34,53] If a patent foramen ovale is present, right-to-left atrial shunting may occur with central cyanosis, and paradoxical embolization has been reported.[54] Large ventricular myxomas may mimic ventricular outflow obstruction. The left ventricular myxoma may produce the equivalent of subaortic or aortic valvular stenosis,[54,55] whereas right ventricular (RV) myxomas can simulate RV outflow track or pulmonic valve obstruction.

Embolization. Systemic embolization is the second most common mode of myxomatous presentation, occurring in 30 to 40% of patients.[2,4,34] Because the majority of myxomas are left-sided, approximately 50% of embolic episodes affect the central nervous system owing to both intra- and extracranial vascular obstruction. The neurologic deficits following embolization can be transient but are often permanent.[56] Specific central nervous system consequences include intracranial aneurysms, seizures, hemiparesis, and brain necrosis.[57-59] Retinal artery embolization with visual loss has occurred in some patients.[60]

Embolic myxomatous material has been found blocking iliac and femoral arteries.[61,62] Other sites of tumor embolization include abdominal viscera and the renal and coronary arteries.[63] Histologic examination of surgically removed peripheral myxoma that has embolized provides the diagnosis of an otherwise unsuspected tumor.[34] Renal artery specimens from a nephrectomy have shown viable enlarging embolic myxoma after excision of the primary tumor. Right-sided myxomatous emboli mainly obstruct PAs and cause pulmonary hypertension and even death from acute obstruction.[4,54]

Infection. Infection arising in a myxoma is a rare complication and produces a clinical picture of infectious endocarditis.[64,65] Infection increases the likelihood of systemic embolization,[4] and an infected myxoma warrants urgent surgical resection.

DIAGNOSIS

Clinical Examination. Findings at the time of clinical assessment of a patient with cardiac myxoma vary according to the size, location, and mobility of the tumor. Left atrial myxomas may produce auscultatory or clinical findings similar to mitral disease. The well-described "tumor plop" can be confused with a third heart sound,[66] occurring just after the opening snap of the mitral valve created from contact between the tumor and endocardial wall.[66] Left atrial myxomas that cause partial obstruction of left ventricular filling may result in elevated pulmonary vascular pressures with augmentation of the pulmonary component of the second heart sound.[67]

Right atrial myxomas may produce similar auscultatory findings as left atrial myxomas with the exception that they are best heard along the lower right sternal border rather than at the cardiac apex. In addition, right atrial hypertension may produce a large *a* wave in the jugular venous pulse and, when severe, may mimic superior vena caval syndrome.

Chest Radiograph and Electrocardiogram. The findings on chest roentgenogram may include generalized cardiomegaly, individual cardiac chamber enlargement, and pulmonary venous congestion. More specific rare findings are density within the cardiac silhouette caused by calcification within the tumor (see Fig. 58-3) occurring more often with right-sided myxomas.[4]

Electrocardiographic Findings. Nonspecific abnormalities such as chamber enlargement, cardiomegaly, bundle-branch blocks, and axis deviation can be found.[68] Fewer than 20% of patients have atrial fibrillation.[39] Evaluation of nonspecific electrocardiographic abnormalities occasionally leads to an incidental diagnosis of myxoma which most electrocardiograms are not helpful in establishing a diagnosis.

Echocardiography. Cross-sectional echocardiography is the most useful test employed for the diagnosis and evaluation of myxoma. The sensitivity of two-dimensional (2-D) echocardiography for myxoma is 100%, and this imaging technique largely has supplanted angiocardiography.[69] However, coronary angiography usually is performed in myxoma patients more than 40 years of age to rule out significant coronary disease. Transesophageal echocardiography (TEE) provides the best information concerning tumor size, location, mobility, and attachment.[70]

Transesophageal echocardiograms detect tumors as small as 1 to 3 mm in diameter.[71] Most surgeons obtain a transesophageal echocardiogram in the operating room before the operation (Fig. 58-2). We particularly evaluate the posterior left atrial wall, atrial septum, and right atrium, which often are not well displayed on transthoracic examination, to exclude the possibility of biatrial multiple tumors. Additionally, postoperative TEE ensures a normal echocardiogram before leaving the operating room.

Computed Tomography and Magnetic Resonance Imaging. Although myxomas have been identified using computed tomography (CT),[69,72] this modality is most useful in malignant tumors of the heart because of its ability to demonstrate myocardial invasion and tumor involvement of adjacent structures.[68] Similarly, magnetic resonance imaging (MRI) has been employed in the diagnosis of myxomas and may yield a clear picture of tumor size, shape, and surface characteristics.[68-72] MRI is particularly useful in detecting intracardiac and pericardial extension, invasion of malignant secondary tumors, and the evaluation of ventricular masses that occasionally turn out to be myxoma. Both CT and MRI detect tumors as small as 0.5 to 1.0 cm and provide information regarding the composition of the tumor.[4]

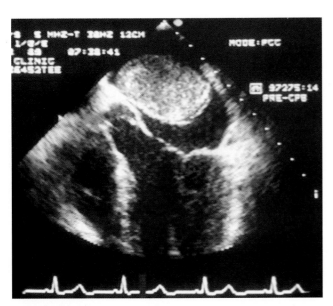

FIGURE 58-2 Transesophageal echocardiogram of a giant left atrial myxoma that does not appear attached to the mitral valve.

Neither CT nor MRI is needed for atrial myxomas if an adequate echocardiogram is available. The exception is the occasional right atrial myxoma that extends into one or both caval or tricuspid orifices. CT or MRI should be reserved for the situation in which the diagnosis or characterization of the tumor is unclear after complete echocardiographic evaluation.

SURGICAL MANAGEMENT

Surgical resection is the only effective therapeutic option for patients with cardiac myxoma and should not be delayed because death from obstruction to flow within the heart or embolization may occur in as many as 8% of patients awaiting operation.[73] A median sternotomy approach with ascending aortic and bicaval cannulation usually is employed. Manipulation of the heart before initiation of CPB is minimized in deference to the known friability and embolic tendency of myxomas. In the event of preoperative known cerebral embolization without hemorrhage, the tumor should be resected approximately seven days after the event to prevent further embolization and yet allow time for stabilization of the brain for CPB. For left atrial myxomas, the venae cavae are cannulated through the right atrial wall, with the inferior cannula placed close and laterally to the inferior vena cava (IVC)–right atrial junction. Caval snares are always used to allow opening of the right atrium, if necessary. If extensive exposure of the left atrium is needed or a malignant left atrial tumor is suspected, we mobilize and directly cannulate the superior vena cava (SVC), which allows it to be transected if necessary for additional exposure. Body temperature is allowed to drift down, but there is no attempt to induce systemic hypothermia unless the need for reduced perfusion flow is anticipated. Modern cardioplegic techniques yield a quiet operative field and protect the myocardium from ischemic injury during aortic crossclamping. CPB is started, and the aorta is clamped before manipulation of the heart.

Exposure of left atrial myxomas is maximized by using several principles from mitral valve repair surgery. The surgeon desires the right side of the heart to rotate up and the left side of the heart to rotate down. Therefore, stay sutures are placed low on the pericardium on the right side, and no pericardial stay sutures are placed on the left before placing the chest retractor. This rotates the heart for optimal exposure of both the right and, particularly, the left atrium (Fig. 58-3). For left atrial tumors, the SVC is mobilized extensively, as is the IVC–right atrial junction, allowing increased mobility and exposing the left atrial cavity. Left atrial myxomas can be approached by an incision through the anterior wall of the left atrium anterior to the right pulmonary veins (Fig. 58-4). This incision can be extended behind both cavae for greater exposure (Fig. 58-5). Exposure and removal of large tumors attached to the interatrial septum may be aided by a second incision parallel to the first in the right atrium. This biatrial incision allows easy removal of tumor attached to the fossa ovalis with a full-thickness Ro (margin-negative) excision at

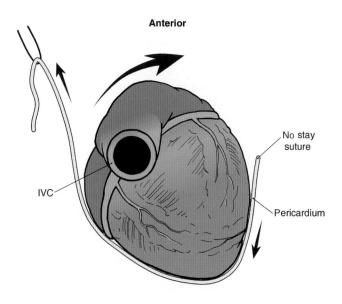

FIGURE 58-3 Rotation of the heart with pericardial stay sutures for left atrial exposure. IVC = inferior vena cava.

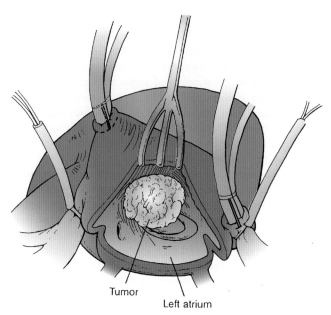

FIGURE 58-5 Left atrial atriotomy posterior to the interatrial groove to expose the left atrial tumor.

the site of attachment and easy patch closure of the atrial septum if necessary (Fig. 58-6).

Right atrial myxomas pose special venous cannulation problems, and intraoperative echocardiography may be beneficial. Both venae cavae may be cannulated directly. When low- or high-lying tumor pedicles preclude safe transatrial cannulation, cannulation of the jugular or femoral vein can provide venous drainage of the upper or lower body. In general, we always can cannulate the SVC distal enough from the right atrium to allow adequate tumor resection, but occasionally femoral venous cannula drainage has been necessary. If the tumor is large or attached near both caval orifices, peripheral cannulation of both jugular and femoral veins may be used to initiate CPB and deep hypothermia. After the aorta

is cross-clamped and the heart is arrested with antegrade cardioplegia, the right atrium may be opened widely for resection of the tumor and reconstruction of the atrium during a period of circulatory arrest if this is needed for a dry field. Resection of large or critically placed right atrial myxomas often requires careful preoperative planning, intraoperative TEE, and special extracorporeal perfusion techniques to ensure complete removal of the tumor, protection of right atrial structures, and reconstruction of the atrium. Because myxomas rarely extend deep in the endocardium, it is not necessary to resect deeply around the conduction tissue. The tricuspid valve and the right atrium, as well as the left atrium

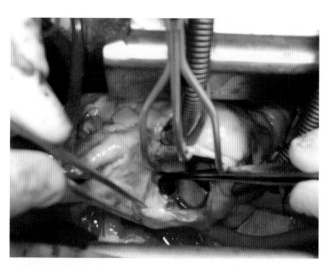

FIGURE 58-4 Left atriotomy and exposure of myxoma.

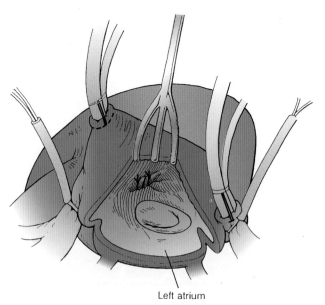

FIGURE 58-6 Repair of left atrial wall after removal of myxomas.

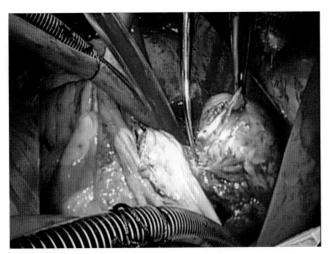

FIGURE 58-7 Giant left atrial myxoma just before removal.

and ventricle, should be inspected carefully for multicentric tumors in patients with right atrial myxoma. Regardless of the surgical approach, the ideal resection encompasses the tumor and a portion of the cardiac wall or interatrial septum to which it is attached (Fig. 58-7). Our policy is to perform a full-thickness resection whenever possible. However, partial-thickness resection of the area of tumor attachment has been performed when anatomically necessary without a noted increase in recurrence rate.[74,75]

Ventricular myxomas usually are approached through the AV valve[76] or by detaching the anterior portion of the AV valve for exposure and resection and reattachment after resection. Occasional small tumors in either outflow tract can be removed through the outflow valve.[76] If necessary, the tumor is excised through a direct incision into the ventricle, but this is unusual and the least preferred approach. It is not necessary to remove the full thickness of the ventricular wall because no recurrences have been reported with partial-thickness excisions. As with right atrial myxoma, the presence of ventricular myxoma prompts inspection for other tumors because of the high incidence of multiple tumors.

Every care should be taken to remove the tumor without fragmentation. Following tumor removal from the field, the area should be liberally irrigated, suctioned, and inspected for loose fragments. There are rare instances of distant metastases from myxoma many years after tumor resection, and these reports raise the issue of potential intraoperative dissemination of tumor.[77] Cardiotomy suction can be used during the operation, but wall suction should strictly be used during the brief time that the tumor is exposed. The low malignant potential of the vast majority of myxomas and the rarity of metastasis support the author's current policy of retaining rather than discarding blood, and we believe that most cases of metastatic implantation of myxoma represent a preoperative embolic event.

Minimally Invasive Approaches to Surgical Removal. Minimally invasive approaches are being applied with increasing frequency in all areas of cardiac surgery, and cardiac tumors are no exception. Experience is confined to benign tumors and is quite limited. Approaches have included right parasternal or partial sternotomy exposure with standard cardioplegic techniques,[78] right submammary incision with femoral–femoral bypass and nonclamped ventricular fibrillation,[79] and the right submammary port access method with antegrade cardioplegia and ascending aortic balloon occlusion.[80] Thoracoscopic techniques have been used to aid in visualization and removal of ventricular fibroelastomas[81,82] (Fig. 58-8). Myxoma removal is possible via thoracoscopy.[83] Results in this limited number of selected patients have been good, but more experience and longer follow-up are needed before this can be recommended as a standard approach.

Minimally invasive cardiac surgical (MICS) approaches are possible for myxomas and fibroelastomas in appropriate anatomic locations in the right and left atria or AV valves. A right chest (nonsternal) approach is used to gain access to the atria or the ventricles through the mitral or tricuspid valves. Fibroelastomas are also amenable to excision through a MICS approach to the aortic valve and left ventricular outflow tract (LVOT).

MICS approaches are generally performed through a limited right lateral third or fourth intercostal space (ICS) incision (5-8 cm) for exposure of the right and left atria. Exposure of the aortic valve and LVOT is achieved via an upper mini-sternotomy toward the third ICS or anterior thoracotomy with disarticulation of the third rib at the sternum.

In mini-sternotomy approaches, the patient is positioned supine with arms at the side and full exposure to the femoral and axillary spaces. In right lateral approaches, the patient is positioned supine with a bump placed vertically to elevate the right hemi-thorax; exposing the lateral ribs as well as the axillary and femoral spaces.

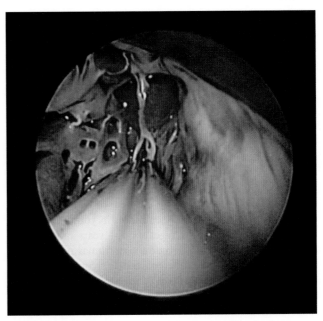

FIGURE 58-8 Thoracoscopic view of left atrial fibroelastoma.

Safe and complete CPB is essential to achieve optimal clinical outcomes. Complete tumor resection, adequate venous drainage, aortic clamping, and complete de-airing are essential for a successful result. In left-sided tumors, CPB can be safely performed via femoral vessel Selinger access (percutaneously or cut-down) and multistage venous drainage. In patients where right-sided cardiac access is necessary, a separate SVC cannula can be inserted and snared separately via the right mini-thoracotomy. Optimal venous drainage is essential for adequate visualization and RV myocardial protection. Arterial cannulation can be performed femorally, directly into the ascending aorta or via the axillary artery.

Myocardial protection in MICS procedures, similar to MICS valve surgery, is dependent on delivery of cardioplegia. Antegrade cardioplegia is usually administered directly into the ascending aorta. Retrograde cardioplegia is performed via direct catheterization of the coronary sinus (CS) through the right atrium. Alternatively, a percutaneous CS catheter can be inserted via a neck approach prior to surgery. Aortic clamping is optimally performed via standard Chitwood clamp inserted through an axillary stab. Endovascular balloon aortic occlusion may also be performed if the aortotomy is not required. Venting of the LV may be performed through direct cannulation of the LA/LV via right superior pulmonary vein or percutaneously through PA drainage (Fig. 58-37a and 58-37b).

Excellent preoperative imaging (optimally through cardiovascular magnetic resonance) is necessary to delineate tumor anatomy and involvement prior to MICS procedures and surgical planning. If performed adequately, MICS tumor resection is a viable and safe option for complete removal of tumors. With these approaches, patients may benefit from decreased transfusions, length of stay, and pain medication requirement.

Results

Removal of atrial myxomas carries an operative mortality rate of 5% or less.[21] Operative mortality is related to advanced age or disability and comorbid conditions. Excision of ventricular myxomas can carry a higher risk (approximately 10%). Our experience over the last 15 years with 85 myxomas shows no operative or hospital mortality.

Recurrence of nonfamilial sporadic myxoma is approximately 1 to 4%.[4,74,75] Many large series report no recurrent tumors.[74,83-86] The 20% of patients with sporadic myxoma and abnormal DNA have a recurrence rate estimated at between 12 and 40%.[4] The recurrence rate is highest in patients with familial complex myxomas, all of whom exhibit DNA mutation, and this is estimated to be about 22%.[4] Overall, recurrences are more common in younger patients. The disease-free interval averages about 4 years and can be as brief as 6 months.[75] Most recurrent myxomas occur within the heart, in the same or different cardiac chambers, and may be multiple.[19,34,87] Extracardiac recurrence after resection of tumor, presumably from embolization and subsequent tumor growth and local invasion, has been observed.[19,87,88] The biology of the tumor, dictated by gene expression rather than histology, may be the only reliable factor predicting recurrence. DNA testing of all patients with cardiac myxoma may prove to be the best predictor of the likelihood of recurrence.[89]

Myxomas generally classified as "malignant" are often found on subsequent review to be sarcomas with myxoid degeneration.[90] However, this issue also remains unsettled because of reports of metastatic growth of embolic myxoma fragments in the brain, arteries, soft tissue, and bones.[56,88,91-97] Symptomatic lesions of possible metastatic myxoma should be excised if feasible.[56,91]

The extent to which patients should be subjected to long-term echocardiographic surveillance after myxoma resection is not standardized. It would seem prudent to closely follow patients who are treated initially for multicentric tumors, those whose tumors are removed from unusual locations in the heart, all tumors believed to have been incompletely resected, and all tumors found to have an abnormal DNA genotype. Patients undergoing resection of tumors thought to be myxomas but with malignant characteristics at pathologic examination should have long-term, careful follow-up.

Other Benign Cardiac Tumors

As shown in Table 58-2, myxomas comprise approximately 41% of benign cardiac tumors, with three other tumors (ie, lipoma, papillary fibroelastoma, and rhabdomyoma) together contributing a similar proportion. A number of rarely encountered tumors account for the remainder.

LIPOMA

Lipomas are well-encapsulated tumors consisting of mature fat cells that may occur anywhere in the pericardium, subendocardium, subepicardium, and intra-atrial septum.[2] They may occur at any age and have no sex predilection. Lipomas are slow growing and may attain considerable size before producing obstructive or arrhythmic symptoms. Many are asymptomatic and are discovered incidentally on routine chest roentgenogram, echocardiogram, or at surgery or autopsy.[98,99] Subepicardial and parietal lipomas tend to compress the heart and may be associated with pericardial effusion. Subendocardial tumors may produce chamber obstruction. The right atrium and left ventricle are the sites affected most often. Lipomas lying within the myocardium or septum can produce arrhythmias or conduction abnormalities. Large tumors that produce severe symptoms should be resected. Smaller, asymptomatic tumors encountered unexpectedly during cardiac operation should be removed if excision can be performed without adding risk to the primary procedure. These tumors are not known to recur.

Lipomatous Hypertrophy of the Interatrial Septum

Nonencapsulated hypertrophy of the fat within the atrial septum is known as *lipomatous hypertrophy*.[2] This abnormality is more common than cardiac lipoma and is usually encountered in elderly, obese, or female patients as an incidental finding during a variety of cardiac imaging procedures.[84] Various arrhythmias and conduction disturbances have been attributed to its presence.[85,100] The main difficulty is differentiating this from a cardiac neoplasm on echocardiography.[101] After the demonstration of a mass by echocardiography, the typical T1 and T2 signal intensity of fat on MRI usually can establish a diagnosis.[102,103] Arrhythmias and heart block are considered by some as indications for resection, but data are lacking as to the long-term benefits from resection.[104]

Papillary Fibroelastoma of the Heart Valves

Papillary fibroelastomas are tumors that arise characteristically from the cardiac valves or adjacent endocardium.[105] These tumors are described as resembling sea anemones with frond-like projections in gross description (Fig. 58-9). The AV and semilunar valves are affected with equal frequency. It is now known that these are capable of producing obstruction of flow, particularly coronary ostial flow, and may embolize to the brain and produce stroke.[106-115] They are usually asymptomatic until a critical event occurs. Papillary fibroelastomas of the cardiac valve should be resected whenever diagnosed, and valve repair rather than replacement should follow the resection of these benign tumors whenever technically feasible (Fig. 58-10). Cytomegalovirus has been recovered in these tumors, suggesting the possibility of viral induction of the tumor and chronic viral endocarditis.[111]

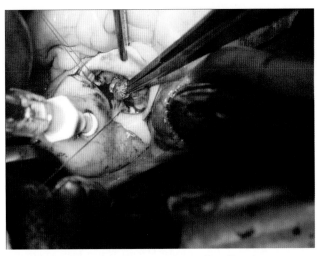

FIGURE 58-10 Surgical removal of a papillary fibroelastoma.

RHABDOMYOMA

Rhabdomyoma is the most frequently occurring cardiac tumor in children. It usually presents during the first few days after birth. It is thought to be a myocardial hamartoma rather than a true neoplasm.[116] Although rhabdomyoma appears sporadically, it is associated strongly with tuberous sclerosis, a hereditary disorder characterized by hamartomas in various organs, epilepsy, mental deficiency, and sebaceous adenomas. Fifty percent of patients with tuberous sclerosis have rhabdomyoma, but more than 50% of patients with rhabdomyoma have or will develop tuberous sclerosis.[117] More than 90% of rhabdomyomas are multiple and occur with approximately equal frequency in both ventricles.[118] The atrium is involved in fewer than 30% of patients. Pathologically, these tumors are firm, gray, and nodular and tend to project into the ventricular cavity. Micrographs show myocytes of twice normal size filled with glycogen, containing hyperchromatic nuclei and eosinophilic-staining cytoplasmic granules.[2,119] Scattered bundles of myofibrils can be seen within cells by electron microscopy.[118]

Clinical findings may mimic valvular or subvalvular stenosis. Arrhythmias, particularly ventricular tachycardia and sudden death, may be a presenting symptom.[119] Atrial tumors may produce atrial arrhythmias.[119] The diagnosis is made by echocardiography. Rarely, no intramyocardial tumor is found in a patient with ventricular arrhythmias, and the site of rhabdomyoma is located by electrophysiologic study.[119]

Early operation is recommended in patients who do not have tuberous sclerosis before 1 year of age.[86] The tumor usually is removed easily in early infancy, and some can be enucleated.[86] Unfortunately, symptomatic tumors often are both multiple and extensive, particularly in patients with tuberous sclerosis, who, unfortunately, have a dismal long-term outlook. In such circumstances, surgery offers little benefit.

FIBROMA

Fibromas are the second most common benign cardiac tumor, with more than 83% occurring in children. These tumors are

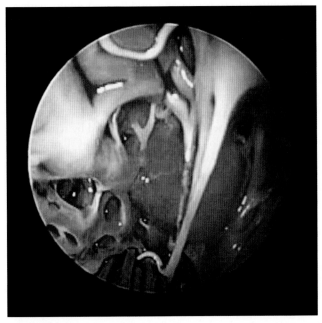

FIGURE 58-9 Additional enhanced view of an in situ left atrial fibroelastoma.

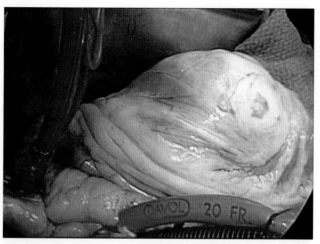

FIGURE 58-11 Left ventricular fibroma as seen from an external view of the heart.

solitary, occur exclusively within the ventricle and the ventricular septum, and affect the sexes equally. Fewer than 100 tumors have been reported, and most are diagnosed by age 2 years. These tumors are not associated with other disease, nor are they inherited. Fibromas are nonencapsulated, firm, nodular, gray-white tumors that can become bulky. They are composed of elongated fibroblasts in broad spiral bands and whirls mixed with collagen and elastin fibers. Calcium deposits or bone may occur within the tumor and occasionally are seen on roentgenography (Figs. 58-11 and 58-12).

Most fibromas produce symptoms through chamber obstruction, interference with contraction, or arrhythmias. Depending on size and location, such a tumor may interfere with valve function, obstruct flow paths, or cause

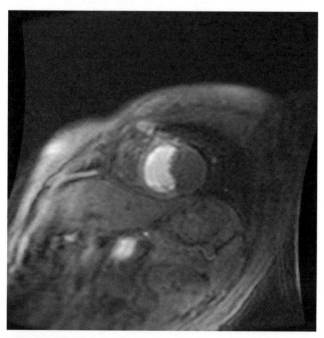

FIGURE 58-12 MRI of left ventricular fibroma.

sudden death from conduction disturbances in up to 25% of patients.[114] Intracardiac calcification on chest roentgenograms suggests the diagnosis, which is confirmed by echocardiogram.

Surgical excision is successful in some patients, particularly if the tumor is localized, does not involve vital structures, and can be enucleated.[86,120-122] However, it is not always possible to remove the tumor completely, and partial removal is only palliative, although some patients have survived many years.[86,121] Operative mortality may be high in infants. Most cases are in adolescents and adults.[186,120,121] Successful, complete excision is curative.[120,121] Children with extensive fibromas have been treated with cardiac transplantation.[122,123]

MESOTHELIOMA OF THE AV NODE

Mesothelioma of the AV node is also termed *polycystic tumor*, *Purkinje tumor*, or *conduction tumor*. It is a relatively small, multicystic tumor that arises in proximity to the AV node and may extend upward into the interventricular septum and downward along the bundle of His.[2] Mesothelioma is associated with heart block, ventricular fibrillation,[124] and sudden death. Cardiac pacing alone does not prevent subsequent ventricular fibrillation. Surgical excision has been reported.[24]

PHEOCHROMOCYTOMA

Cardiac pheochromocytomas arise from chromaffin cells of the sympathetic nervous system and produce excess amounts of catecholamines, particularly norepinephrine. Approximately 90% of pheochromocytomas are in the adrenal glands. Fewer than 2% arise in the chest. Only 32 cardiac pheochromocytomas had been reported by 1991.[125] The tumor predominantly affects young and middle-aged adults with an equal distribution between the sexes. Approximately 60% occur in the roof of the left atrium. The remainders involve the interatrial septum or anterior surface of the heart. The tumor is reddish brown, soft, lobular, and consists of nests of chromatin cells.

The patients usually present with symptoms of uncontrolled hypertension or are found to have elevated urinary catecholamines. The tumor usually is located by scintigraphy using [I131] metaiodo-benzylguanidine[126] and CT or MRI.[126] Cardiac catheterization with differential blood chamber sampling sometimes is necessary in addition to coronary angiography.[125] After the tumor is located, it should be removed using CPB with cardioplegic arrest. Patients require preanesthetic alpha and beta-blockade and careful intraoperative and immediate postoperative monitoring. Most tumors are extremely vascular, and uncontrollable operative hemorrhage has occurred.[126] Resection may require removal of the atrial and/or ventricular wall or a segment of a major coronary artery.[127] Explantation of the heart to allow resection of a large left atrial pheochromocytoma has been attempted.[128] Transplantation has been performed for unresectable tumor and complete excision produces cure.[121-123]

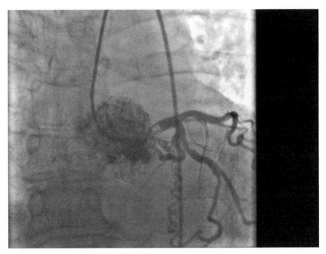

FIGURE 58-13 Paraganglioma blush of tumor during cardiac catheterization.

PARAGANGLIOMA

Paragangliomas are endocrine tumors that can secrete catecholamines. As a result, their presentation is often similar to that of pheochromocytomas. When found within the thoracic cavity, they are located most often in the posterior mediastinum. Paragangliomas typically present with atypical chest pain.[129,130] On echocardiography, they are often large and highly vascular tumors.[131] On cardiac catheterization, they may be intimately associated with the coronary arteries (Fig. 58-13).[132] Between March 2004 and October 2010, 7 male patients from our institution who underwent surgical resection of cardiac paraganglioma were retrospectively reviewed. In 5 patients, paragangliomas originated from the roof of the left atrium, and in 2 patients, they originated from the aortic root. Hospital mortality was 14%. Complete surgical resection remains the mainstay of therapy and can be curative, but carries a significant risk of intraoperative bleeding and usually requires CPB and often complex resection techniques, including cardiac autotransplantation (Fig. 58-14).

HEMANGIOMA

Hemangiomas of the heart are rare tumors (24 clinical cases reported), affect all ages, and may occur anywhere within the heart.[133,134] These are vascular tumors composed of capillaries or cavernous vascular channels. Patients usually develop dyspnea, occasional arrhythmias, or signs of right-sided heart failure.[135] Diagnosis is difficult, and echocardiography or cardiac catheterization can establish a diagnosis of cardiac tumor by showing an intracavity filling defect.[127] CT and MRI show axial T2-weighted; MRI should show a high signal mass owing to vascularity (Fig. 58-15). Coronary angiography typically shows a tumor blush and maps the blood supply to the tumor. During resection, meticulous ligation of feeding vessels is required to prevent postoperative residual arteriovenous fistulas or intracavity communications. Partial resections have produced long-term benefits.[133] Tumors rarely resolve spontaneously.[136]

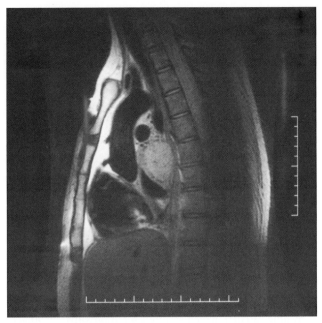

FIGURE 58-14 MRI of left atrial paraganglioma that required an autotransplant for removal.

TERATOMA

Cardiac teratoma is a rare tumor that typically presents in infants and young children.[137] About 80% of the tumors are benign.[138] These tumors are discovered by echocardiography after a variety of symptoms lead to cardiac or mediastinal evaluation. There is little experience with surgical removal, which should be possible.

CASTLEMAN TUMOR

Castleman disease is a poorly understood lymphoproliferative disorder. The disease was first described by Castleman

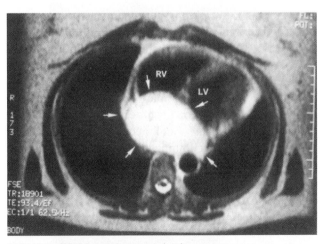

FIGURE 58-15 Axial T2-weighted magnetic resonance image showing high signal mass of left atrial hemangioma. (Reproduced with permission from Lo JJ, Ramsay CN, Allen JW, et al: Left atrial cardiac hemangioma associated with shortness of breath and palpitations, *Ann Thorac Surg* 2002 Mar;73(3):979-981.)

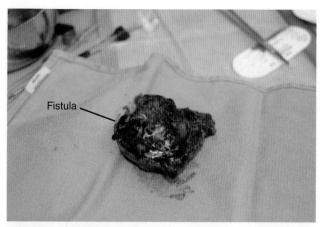

FIGURE 58-16 Castleman tumor showing fistula site indicated by insertion of a coronary probe.

and colleagues in 1956.[139] It typically presents as a solitary lesion in the mediastinum. The most common histologic type is hyaline vascular, which accounts for approximately 90% of cases and often behaves in a benign fashion. The more aggressive subgroups are the plasma and mixed-cell types, which have a more malignant behavior.[140] Patients may have a localized or multicentric disease with lymph node involvement, typically in the mediastinum. These tumors typically present as well-circumscribed masses. There have been reports of Castleman disease with myocardial and coronary artery invasion or development of a coronary pseudoaneurysm.[141] In these more aggressive cases, cardiac assist devices have been used as a bridge to recovery[141] (Figs. 58-16 and 58-17). CT imaging of the lesions reveals atypical or target-like enhancement that corresponds to various degrees of degeneration, necrosis, and fibrosis. Technetium-99m tetrofosmin and

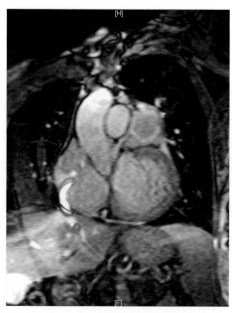

FIGURE 58-17 MRI of Castleman tumor.

[I^{123}] beta-methyliodophenyl pentadecanoic acid (BMIPP) imaging may aid in the diagnosis. On BMIPP, these tumors show reduced uptake compared with the surrounding normal myocardium.[142] Complete surgical resection is considered curative.[143]

PRIMARY MALIGNANT TUMORS

Primary cardiac malignancy is very uncommon, with only 21 surgically treated cases noted in a 25-year surgical experience from 1964 to 1969, combining the experience of two large institutions, the Texas Heart Institute and the MD Anderson Cancer Center in Houston.[144] Additional current reports from the Texas Medical Center include a series from the Methodist Debakey Heart and Vascular Center and MD Anderson Cancer Center of 27 patients selected from 1990 to 2006.[144] Approximately 25% of primary cardiac tumors are malignant, and of these, about 75% are sarcomas. McAllister's survey of cardiac tumors found the most common to be angiosarcomas (31%), rhabdomyosarcomas (21%), malignant mesotheliomas (15%), and fibrosarcomas (11%),[2] see Table 58-4.

Rather than histologic classification of cardiac sarcoma, we propose a classification system based on anatomic location. Histology does not greatly affect treatment or prognosis as much as anatomic location.[144,145] The revised classification system divides primary cardiac sarcomas into right heart sarcomas, left heart sarcomas, and PA sarcomas, and these are the categories that will be used in the discussion to follow.

Right heart sarcomas tend to metastasize early, present as bulky masses (Fig. 58-18), and are characteristically infiltrative.[145] Right heart sarcomas often occupy much of the right atrium growing largely in an outward pattern, and often avoid heart failure until the latest stage of presentation. This presentation often allows time for neoadjuvant chemotherapy

⬤ TABLE 58-4: Primary Malignant Cardiac Neoplasms in Adults

Tumor	Number	Percentage
Angiosarcoma	39	33
Rhabdomyosarcoma	24	21
Mesothelioma	19	16
Fibrosarcoma	13	11
Lymphoma	7	6
Osteosarcoma	5	4
Thymoma	4	3
Neurogenic sarcoma	3	2
Leiomyosarcoma	1	<1
Liposarcoma	1	<1
Synovial sarcoma	1	<1
Total	117	100

Reproduced with permission from McAllister HA Jr, Fenoglio JJ Jr: Tumors of the cardiovascular system, in *Atlas of Tumor Pathology*. Washington, DC, Armed Forces Institute of Pathology; 1978, fas. 15.

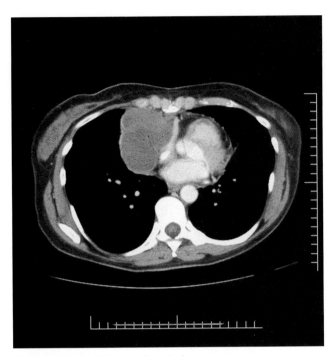

FIGURE 58-18 CT scan of a right heart tumor.

TABLE 58-5: Symptoms of Primary Malignant Cardiac Tumors

Symptom	Number	Percentage
Dyspnea	13/21	61.9
Chest pain	6/21	28
Congestive heart failure	6/21	28
Palpitations	5/321	24
Fever	3/21	14
Myalgia	2/21	10

Data from Murphy MC, Sweeney MS, Putnam JB Jr, et al: Surgical treatment of cardiac tumors: a 25-year experience, *Ann Thorac Surg* 1990 Apr;49(4):612-617.

in an attempt to shrink the tumor and sterilize the infiltrating edges to increase the chances of obtaining a resection with microscopically negative margins.

Left heart sarcomas tend to be more solid with less infiltration than right heart sarcomas and tend to metastasize later in the course of disease.[146] Left-sided sarcomas are most often located in the left atrium, and tend to grow into the wall. Diminution of blood flow quickly results in life-threatening heart failure. Neoadjuvant chemotherapy can rarely be used because of this presentation. Most left atrial sarcomas are initially clinically diagnosed as mxyomas, have a positive resection margin, rapidly recur, and require repeat resection.

Primary malignant cardiac tumors arise sporadically, showing no inherited linkage. Although they may span the entire age spectrum, they usually occur in adults more than 40 years of age. The patients usually present with symptoms of congestive heart failure, pleuritic chest pain, malaise, anorexia, and weight loss.[137,147] The most common symptom has been dyspnea[148] (Table 58-5). Some develop refractory arrhythmias, syncope, pericardial effusion, and tamponade.[148] The chest x-ray may be abnormal and even show a mass lesion, but the definite diagnosis usually is made with cardiac echocardiography.[147,149] Right atrial lesions are more frequently malignant (usually angiosarcoma) than left-sided lesions (usually myxoma but, when malignant, often malignant fibrous histiocytoma [MFH]). If malignancy is suspected, chest CT or MRI may suggest histology and provide detailed anatomy and help in staging and assessing resectability. The current status of positron-emission tomographic (PET) scans in evaluating these patients remains controversial. We perform cardiac catheterization on all patients older than 40 years of age presenting with intracardiac masses and on all patients with large right atrial masses. Malignancy may be suggested and coronary involvement suspected by tumor blush. This is not pathognomic because we have seen a large feeding vessel and tumor blush in a histologically confirmed myxoma.

Unfortunately, primary cardiac malignancy may grow to a large size before detection and involve portions of the heart not amenable to resection. Some of these patients have been considered for transplantation and will be discussed later. Otherwise, palliative medical therapy can be attempted with radiation therapy, although success in both symptom relief and longevity has been somewhat limited. Whether the tumor is primary or secondary, the decision to resect is based on tumor size and location and an absence of metastatic spread seen on complete evaluation. Unfortunately, most primary cardiac malignancies that have been referred to our center were considered to be benign initially and were resected incompletely at presentation. If malignancy is suspected or confirmed, and if the lesion appears anatomically resectable and there is no metastatic disease, then resection should be considered. If complete resection is possible, surgery provides better palliation and potentially can double survival.[150] After resection, we recommend adjuvant chemotherapy and believe that this can improve survival.[138,150] Complete resection will depend on the location of the tumor, the extent of involvement of the myocardium and/or fibrous skeleton of the heart, and histology.

Angiosarcoma

Angiosarcomas are two to three times more common in men than in women and have a predilection for the right side of the heart. Eighty percent arise in the right atrium.[148,151,152] These tumors tend to be bulky and aggressively invade adjacent structures, including the great veins, tricuspid valve, RV free wall, interventricular septum, and right coronary artery[151] (Fig. 58-19). Obstruction and right-sided heart failure are not uncommon. Pathologic examination of resected specimens demonstrates anastomosing vascular channels lined with typical anaplastic epithelial cells. Unfortunately, most of these tumors have spread by the time of presentation, usually to the lung, liver, and brain.[148] Without resection, 90% of the

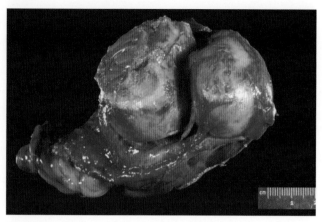

FIGURE 58-19 Pathology specimen photograph of a right atrial tumor.

patients are dead within 9 to 12 months of diagnosis despite radiation or chemotherapy.[22,148] We have seen carefully selected patients without evidence of spread on metastatic evaluation who have undergone complete surgical resection with subsequent chemotherapy (Fig. 58-20). In addition to surgical resection of the right atrium, right coronary bypass and even tricuspid valve repair or replacement may be undertaken (Fig. 58-21). We have had no hospital mortality in this small group, and most patients die from metastasis rather than recurrence at the local site.[153]

Malignant Fibrous Histiocytoma

MFH is the most common soft tissue sarcoma in adults. Its occurrence as a cardiac primary malignancy has been relatively recently accepted as a specific entity. It is characterized histologically by a mixture of spindle cells in a storiform pattern, polygonal cells resembling histiocytes, and malignant giant cells. The cell of origin is the fibroblast or histioblast.[149,154] It usually occurs in the left atrium and often mimics myxoma. In fact, every left atrial MFH referred to our institution has been previously incompletely resected when thought to represent a myxoma. The tendency to metastasize early is not as prominent as with angiosarcoma. Several reports document rapid symptomatic recurrence after incomplete resection despite chemotherapy. These patients often die of local cardiac disease before the development of metastases. We believe that if complete resection can be obtained (particularly if the malignant nature is recognized and complete resection can be done at the original operation) and adequate chemotherapy can be provided, we may improve survival in this otherwise dismal disease.

Rhabdomyosarcoma

Rhabdomyosarcomas do not evolve from rhabdomyomas and occur equally in the sexes. The tumors are multicentric in 60% of patients and arise from either ventricle. These tumors frequently invade cardiac valves or interfere with valve

function because of their intracavitary bulk. Microscopically, tumor cells demonstrate pleomorphic nuclei and spidery, wispy, streaming eosinophilic cytoplasm, usually in a muscle-like pattern.

The tumors are aggressive and may invade pericardium. Surgical excision of small tumors may be rational, but local and distant metastases and poor response to radiation or chemotherapy limit survival to less than 12 months in most of these patients.[120,137,138,150,155]

Other Sarcomas and Mesenchymal-Origin Tumors

McAllister and Fenoglio found that malignant mesotheliomas arising from the heart or pericardium and not from the surrounding pleura were the third most common malignant cardiac tumors and that fibrosarcomas were fourth.[2] However, in the two decades since their work, clinicians have rarely encountered these tumors. This apparent decrease in incidence may be related to changes in histologic criteria for classifying primary malignant neoplasms since their study.[5,133,138,148-150,155,156]

The histology of these tumors can be ambiguous and difficult. These neoplasms can resemble other sarcomas, and some might be deemed fibrous histiocytomas today. The behavior of these tumors is more important, and as with other cardiac sarcomas, resection of small tumors in the absence of known metastasis perhaps is justified, but data are scarce.[22,148,150,155] This being said, it is important to rule out more diffuse thoracic involvement with mesothelioma before considering resection of an isolated cardiac or pericardial mesothelioma. A PET scan may be considered, and any suspicious pleural thickening or effusion should be evaluated carefully both radiographically and histologically.

Myosarcoma, liposarcoma, osteosarcoma, chondromyxosarcoma, plasmacytoma, and carcinosarcoma arising from the heart all have been reported,[156-159] but by the time diagnosis is made, only palliative therapy usually can be offered, and surgery is indicated only occasionally. Regardless of therapy, it is unusual for patients with these diagnoses to survive more than a year.

Right-Sided Cardiac Sarcomas

The prognosis without surgery for right heart sarcoma is dismal, and surgical resection is the only treatment modality shown to increase survival. Complete surgical resection is complicated both by the bulky infiltrative nature of right heart sarcoma and the high incidence of metastatic disease at presentation. The author's current approach to right heart sarcomas has been to begin with neoadjuvant chemotherapy once a definitive tissue diagnosis of sarcoma is made using a right heart catheterization biopsy. Occasionally, a diagnosis of lymphoma or other tumor is made. Multidisciplinary treatment planning based on the *correct* diagnosis is imperative. After 4 to 6 rounds of chemotherapy (with repeat imaging

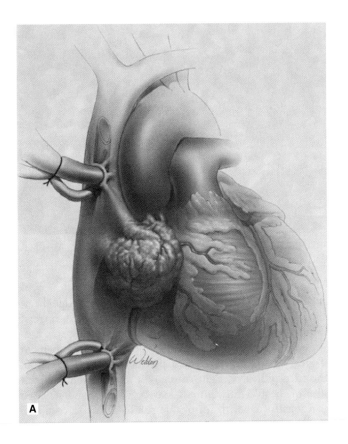
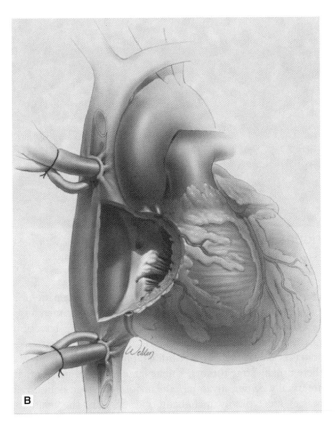
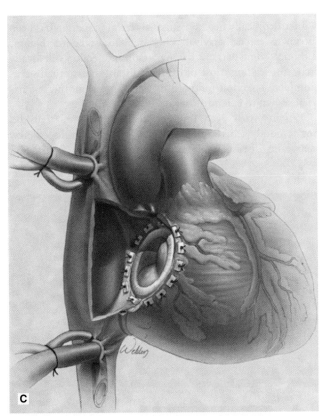
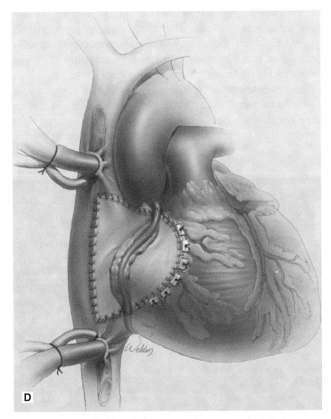

FIGURE 58-20 (A) Right atrial angiosarcoma involving right coronary artery and tricuspid valve, (B) excision of tumor with right coronary artery and tricuspid valve, (C) tricuspid valve replaced, (D) completed repair using bovine pericardium.

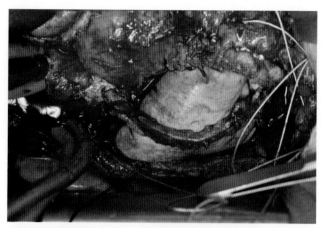

FIGURE 58-21 Right atrial angiosarcoma (final repair with right coronary artery bypass positioned over bovine pericardium).

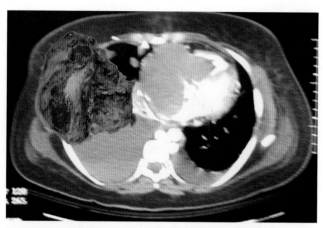

FIGURE 58-23 CT scan of a right atrial mass with the pathology specimen oriented in a similar fashion over the image.

every other cycle to assess for tumor response), the patient is evaluated for surgical resection. This treatment regimen aims to improve on the current microscopic complete resection rate of 33%. The initial diagnostic test for right heart sarcomas is transthoracic echocardiography, which rarely misses these usually large tumors. Unlike large left atrial masses that are usually benign myxomas, the majority of large right atrial masses are typically malignant (Fig. 58-22). The majority of right heart sarcomas referred to our specialty center have yet to undergo attempted resection, unlike left-sided heart tumors which are typically resected under the presumption they are benign myomas. The primary reason for local failure of a right heart sarcoma is incomplete resection, typically because of surgical hesitancy to achieve complete resection because of involvement of the right coronary artery.

Most right heart sarcomas are angiosarcomas[2] (Fig. 58-23). These tumors may occur in the right atrium (Fig. 58-24) or the right ventricle but far more commonly arise from the right atrium. They replace the right atrial wall and frequently grow into the cardiac chamber and into adjacent tissues. Right heart tumors tend to be infiltrative and form microscopic "fingers" of tumor extending beyond the margins of gross disease. Diffuse pericardial involvement, RV involvement, or encasement of great vessels or veins often precludes surgical resection. The tricuspid valve, right coronary artery, and up to about 30% of the RV muscle mass may be resected and replaced or reconstructed with reasonable risk to achieve a complete resection. Thus, all patients are evaluated preoperatively with coronary arteriography. In patients treated without surgical resection, the survival is approximately 10% at 12 months.[160] A microscopically negative surgical resection margin has been shown to extend survival[150] and remains standard therapy. Although some patients having a radical resection still locally recur, the leading cause of death is distant metastatic disease. Complete resection followed by adjuvant chemotherapy has been shown to extend survival.[150,160]

Patients with even limited metastatic disease that did not respond well to chemotherapy or who developed new metastatic disease while on treatment are not considered

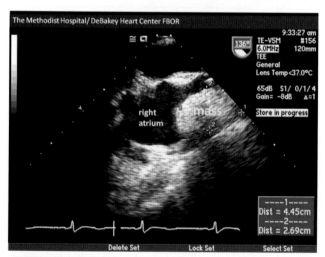

FIGURE 58-22 Transesophageal echocardiogram of a right atrial mass measuring 4.45 by 2.69 centimeters.

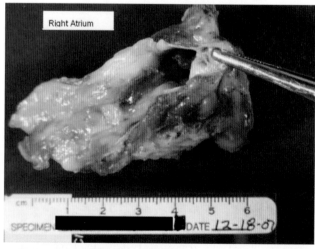

FIGURE 58-24 Right atrial sarcoma.

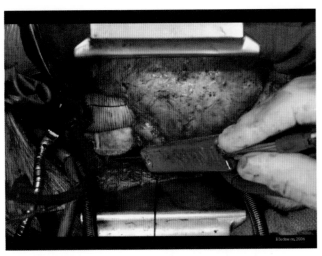

FIGURE 58-25 Bovine pericardium reconstruction of the superior vena cava (created by folding the pericardium in half and then firing an endo-GIA stapler longitudinally to form the conduit).

candidates for surgery. Patients with widely metastatic disease are not considered candidates unless palliative surgery because of severe symptoms is recommended. Every patient should be referred to oncology for potential continuation of chemotherapy after recovery from surgery.

Based on the anatomic extent of tumor and the needed margins for resection, venous cannulation for CPB must be carefully planned and individualized to each patient. Directly cannulating the high SVC for upper body drainage and

cannulating directly into the IVC at the diaphragm usually allows adequate exposure for complete inferior resection, but occasionally femoral cannulation aids in exposing the more caudal structures of the right heart. Aortic cannulation is standard, as it is distant from the tumor. The right atrium can be completely resected and replaced with bovine pericardium. If the resection involves the SVC or IVC, a vascular stapler can be used to staple lengthwise, creating a tube from bovine pericardium to recreate the vein segment (Fig. 58-25). One particular area of danger is at the right atrial junction with the root of the aorta, as overzealous resection in this area will result in damage to the fibrous skeleton of the heart, which is characteristically difficult to repair. Incomplete resection leaving gross disease rapidly leads to regrowth of the tumor and should be avoided if at all possible. When right coronary artery involvement is suspected, mobilization of the right internal mammary artery is performed at the beginning of the operation. Right ventricular wall can be simply partially replaced with bovine pericardium or incorporated into a prosthetic tricuspid valve used for valve replacement. For an illustration of the steps involved in the resection and later reconstruction of a right heart sarcoma, refer to Fig. 58-26.

Left-Sided Cardiac Sarcomas

Surgical resection is the most effective therapeutic option for patients with malignant left-sided cardiac tumors. Delay can result in death from obstruction to flow within the heart or

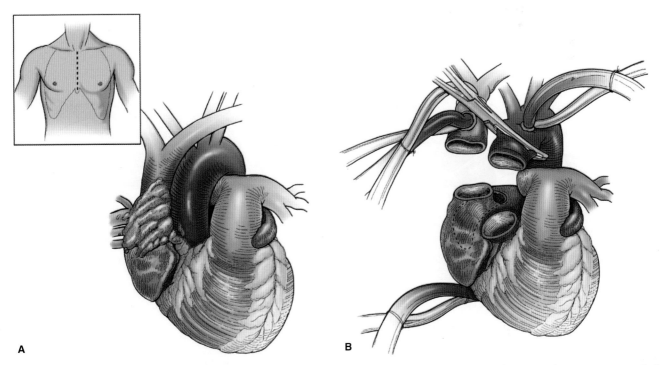

A **B**

FIGURE 58-26 (A) median sternotomy approach to a right heart sarcoma; (B) transection of the aorta, right main pulmonary artery, roof of the left atrium, and superior vena cava to rotate the right upper quadrant of the heart and allow adequate exposure for complete excision of a right heart sarcoma;

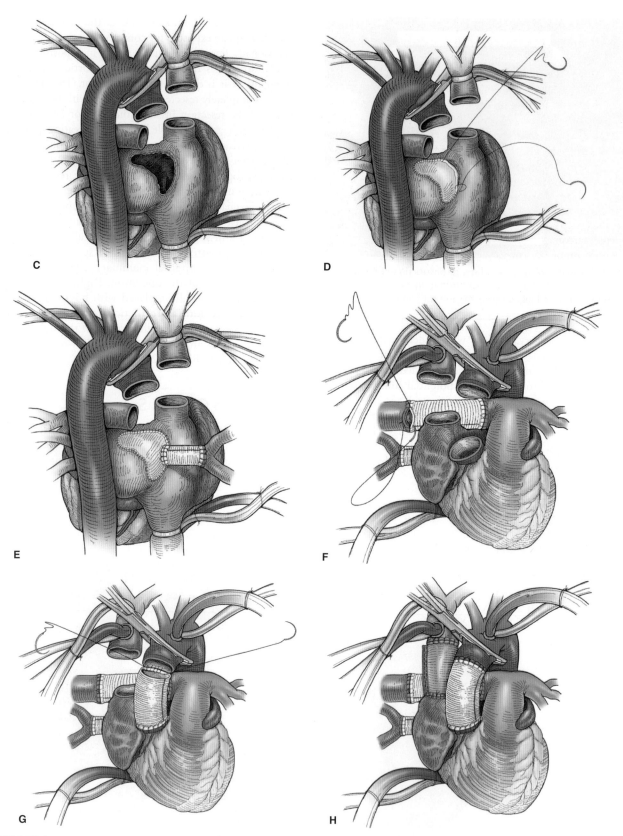

FIGURE 58-26 (*Continued*) (C) posterior view of the heart to illustrate the incisions necessary for complete removal of a right-sided cardiac sarcoma that extended into the roof of the left atrium; (D) reconstruction of the roof of the left atrium; (E) reconstruction of the pulmonary veins using a Dacron graft; (F) reconstruction from an anterior view of the right main pulmonary artery; (G) reconstruction of the aorta using a Dacron graft and a running suture; (H) complete reconstruction of the heart after radical removal of a right heart sarcoma (note the superior vena cava reconstruction with bovine pericardium folded and stapled with an endo-GIA stapler).

embolization, which may occur in as many as 8% of patients awaiting operation. The clinical presentation of patients with primary left heart sarcoma depends on the anatomic location and extent of the tumor and is not influenced by histology. Most primary left heart sarcomas are reported to occur in the left atrium, a concept supported by the author's experience; 22/24 (92%) occurred in the left atrium and 2/24 (8%) occurred in the left ventricle. Most left atrial masses seen by cardiac surgeons are mistaken to be benign myxomas. Every left atrial sarcoma patient referred to our center previously underwent resection for a presumed myxoma that was later found to be a cardiac sarcoma. Each of these cases had rapid reappearance of the left atrial tumor at the site of resection likely representing regrowth of persistent incompletely resected sarcoma. Intracavitary left ventricular tumors are very uncommon and are rarely mistaken for a simple cardiac myxoma. Heart failure caused by obstruction of intracardiac blood flow is the most common and concerning presenting symptom. Heart block from local invasion, arrhythmia, pericardial effusion, distal embolus, fever, weight loss, and malaise are also seen. The mean age of presentation is reported to be 40 years of age.[149] Transthoracic echocardiography is the most common initial diagnostic test. TEE is specifically recommended for in all left-sided cardiac tumors because of increased resolution of left-sided structures. Cardiac MRI and PET/CT scans are also obtained in patients known or suspected to have sarcoma.

Once diagnosed, primary cardiac sarcoma patients have an often dismal prognosis. When medically treated, the survival at 12 months is less than 10%.[160] Most reports in the literature are either autopsy series or individual case reports or small case series. Operative mortality usually exceeds 20%, and the mean survival is typically around 12 months.[161-163] Many published series focus on primary cardiac sarcoma in general without regard to anatomic location. The Mayo Clinic reported 34 patients over 32 years with a median survival of 12 months.[164] A combined series from the Texas Heart Institute and the MD Anderson Cancer Center reported an actuarial survival of 14% at 2 years in 21 patients over a 26-year period.[157] The authors have previously reported a combined multimodality approach, and found a median survival of 23.5 months in 27 patients over 16 years with survival of 80.9% at one year and 61.9% at two years.[147] Subsequent analyses show that histologic type does not influence survival or treatment approach.[165] The major determinant of clinical presentation and surgical approach is anatomic location. Currently, these tumors are grouped based on location, such as PA sarcomas, right heart sarcomas, or left heart sarcomas.[166]

The high rate of local recurrence and secondary resections reported in the literature[167] indicate the left atrium and ventricle present unique anatomic exposure challenges. Complete resection and reconstruction is complicated because of the left heart proximity to vital structures. Often, a surgeon's inability to adequately visualize vital structures and reconstruct leads to an inadequate resection with rapid regrowth of tumor. Typically, left atrial tumors are approached through the interatrial groove. The interatrial groove is often an adequate approach for benign tumors, but is limited for malignant tumors that are often larger and require a more generous margin of resection. We have considered complete cardiectomy and orthotopic cardiac transplantation for complete removal of these tumors. Although feasible, this approach requires the availability of a donor and postoperative immunosuppression; both of which present potential problems in cancer patients. Additionally series using orthotopic cardiac transplantation for this purpose have only shown a median survival of 12 months.[168] Left ventricular tumors can be approached through the aortic valve, the mitral valve, or through a ventriculotomy. A transaortic valve approach works nicely for benign tumors,[82] but is inadequate for malignant tumors because of their size and the amount of resection needed. A ventriculotomy through normal ventricular muscle is possible, but not ideal. The author's group adopted the approach of cardiac explantation, ex vivo tumor resection, cardiac reconstruction, and reimplantation of the heart (cardiac autotransplantation), which permits a radical tumor resection and accurate reconstruction.

CARDIAC AUTOTRANSPLANTATION

The technique of cardiac autotransplantation was introduced for cardiac tumors by Cooley in 1985 to deal with a large left atrial pheochromocytoma.[128] Although this case was not successful, it introduced the senior author (MJR) to the technique and its potential use for cardiac tumors. The author's group did the first successful cardiac autotransplant for cardiac sarcoma in 1998,[154] also reporting this for left atrial sarcoma and left ventricular sarcoma.[169] Working closely with the MD Anderson Cancer Center, the Methodist Hospital has now performed 34 cardiac auto transplants. Of the 34 patients, there were 26 primary cardiac sarcomas, 1 isolated malignant melanoma metastasis to the intracavitary left ventricle, and 7 benign cases. The benign group had no operative deaths and 100% 2-year survival. Overall 30-day, 1-year, and 2-year procedural survival was 85, 59, and 44%, respectively. For primary malignant tumors, survival at 1 and 2 years was 46 and 28%. Among patients with primary malignant tumors, 19 had isolated cardiac autotransplantation and 7 had autotransplantation plus pneumonectomy. Operative mortality (and median survival) for cardiac autotransplantation with and without pneumonectomy was 43% (55 days) and 11% (378 days), respectively. For primary sarcomas, microscopically positive or negative resection margins did not impact survival. A diagnostic algorithm for autotransplantation in cardiac tumors is included (Fig 58-37).

Cardiac autotransplantation has several fundamental differences from standard orthotopic heart transplantation.[170] In orthotopic heart transplantation, unless a domino procedure is being done, the explanted heart is not to be used and any damage to its structures is inconsequential. For a complete video of an autotransplant including replacement of the mitral valve, refer to the movie attached to this chapter. Therefore, the cardiectomy can be performed leaving a wide margin of remaining tissue to use in tailoring the heart to be implanted without regard to cutting critical structures such as the CS. Similarly, the donor heart can usually be harvested with extra tissue at its margins to be used to help tailor the implantation unlike traditional orthotopic heart transplant surgery. The heart must be excised in cardiac autotransplantation in a manner that does not damage any structures that cannot be repaired, replaced, or are vital to cardiac function. Additionally, if the heart is simply excised and reimplanted, loss of workable tissue makes reimplantation more challenging than orthotopic heart transplantation. Cannulation techniques must take into consideration planned explantation. The aorta can be cannulated distally in the transverse arch. Venous cannulation must be directly into the SVC and IVC just below the right atrial junction. This requires greater exposure and mobilization of the SVC and IVC. After commencing CPB, further mobilization of the SVC and IVC is performed until each is completely free and surround with umbilical tapes on a tourniquet. Wide mobilization of the interatrial groove and circumferential mobilization of the ascending aorta and PA follows cannulation. This facilitates both accurate excision of the heart and reimplantation. The ascending aorta is cross-clamped and antegrade cold blood potassium cardioplegia is given (10 cc/kg) to achieve cardiac arrest. The left atrium is opened at the beginning of cardioplegia, and a sump drain is placed to decompress the heart. After cardioplegia and cardiac quiescence, the left atrium is opened to confirm pathology and appropriateness of autotransplantation. The SVC first divided beyond the right atrial junction. This is followed by IVC division which should be transected near the right atrial and SVC junction. For each transection, it is important to note the rim of tissue being left behind retracts substantially toward the venous cannulae and an extraordinarily wide rim must be left or reimplantation at the IVC can be exceedingly difficult. The ascending aorta is divided about 1 cm distal to the sinotubular junction and the PA is divided just proximal to its bifurcation. The left atrium transection is then completed, dividing the atrium just anterior to the pulmonary veins and on the left side equal distant between the pulmonary veins and the mitral valve and left atrial appendage. This allows complete removal of the heart which is placed into a basin of ice slush (Fig. 58-27). The posterior left atrium is then inspected, and any tumor is widely excised (Fig. 58-28). Bovine pericardium is used for reconstruction, and the pulmonary veins may be individually reimplanted into new orifices cut in the bovine pericardium or left as a cuff, if pathology permits. The anterior left atrium can be entirely removed, including the mitral valve, leaving only a mitral annulus.

Bovine pericardial reconstruction starts with cutting a hole to match the mitral annulus opening. Mitral valve replacement using pledgeted 2-0 ticron sutures begins with pledgets placed on the left ventricular side of the annulus, passing through the annulus, through the bovine pericardium, and then through the prosthetic mitral valve. When the sutures are tied, the neo atrial wall is sealed to the valve and annulus. The anterior and posterior bovine

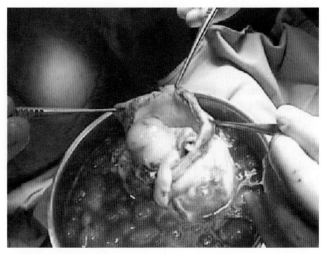

FIGURE 58-27 Ex vivo heart showing large sarcoma arising from the anterior left atrial wall.

pericardium can then be tailored by cutting darts and sewing them together before reanastomosis. Reimplantation is similar to standard cardiac transplantation, beginning with the left atrium anastomosis. The right atrium is then attached to the IVC, and then the right atrium to the SVC. If either of these anastomoses appears to be under excess tension, an interposition graft of Gore-Tex, Dacron, or crafted pericardial tube graft can be used to bridge the defect successfully (Fig. 58-29). The PA and aorta are reanastomosed in a standard fashion using Prolene suture, warm-blood potassium cardioplegia is given antegrade, and the aortic cross-clamp is removed. The procedure for left ventricular tumors is similar, and occasionally requires mitral valve excision or partial excision of the interventricular septum (Fig. 58-30). The interventricular septum can be reconstructed with bovine pericardium and valve replacement is typically done with a tissue valve. Although these patients are young, a tissue valve is often chosen to avoid anticoagulation. Issues with structural valve deterioration are of less concern because survival is counted now in years rather than decades.

Because of poor survival, lesions requiring a pneumonectomy in addition to cardiac autotransplant should be considered a contraindication to surgery. This can usually be determined preoperatively with cardiac MRI to evaluate restriction of blood flow through the pulmonary veins.

Lymphomas

Lymphomas may arise from the heart, although this is rare.[171] Most of these tumors respond to radiation and chemotherapy, and surgical resection is rarely indicated.[153] Even when complete resection is not possible, incomplete resection has been performed to relieve acute obstructive systems and, when followed with radiation and chemotherapy, has allowed for extended survival in selected patients.

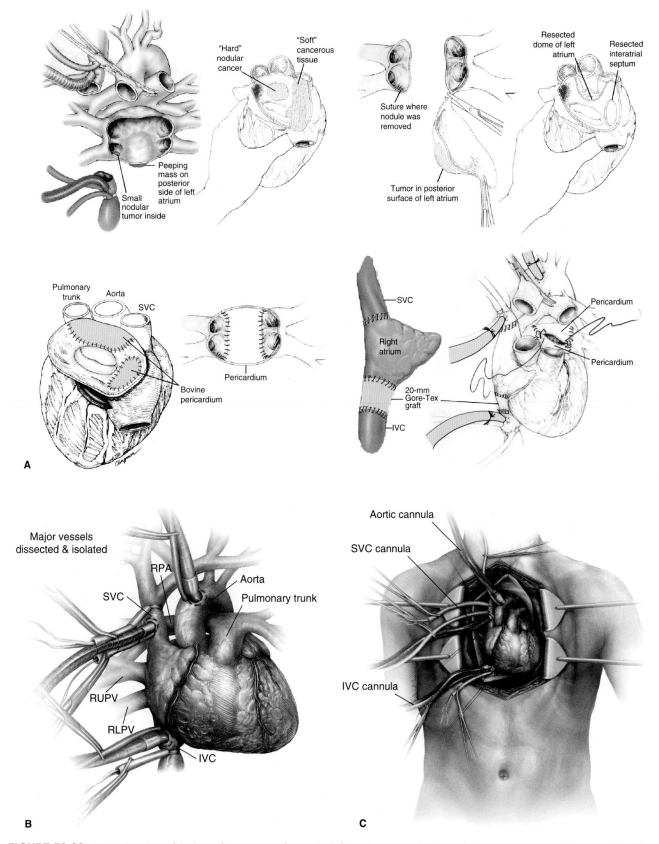

FIGURE 58-28 (A) Explanation of the heart for exposure of extensive left atrial sarcoma. (B) Cannulation strategy to optimize removal and later reimplantation of the heart (note the superior vena cava is cannulated rather than the right atrium). (C) Direct view of median sternotomy and cannulation strategy.

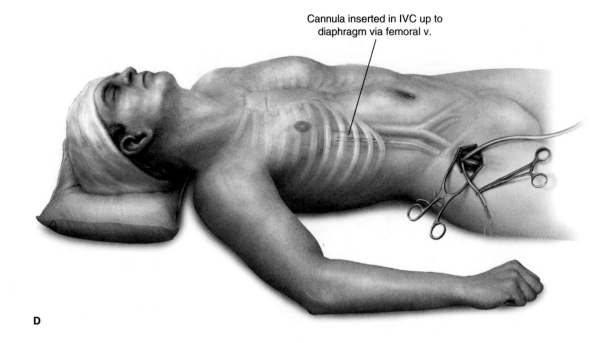

Cannula inserted in IVC up to
diaphragm via femoral v.

D

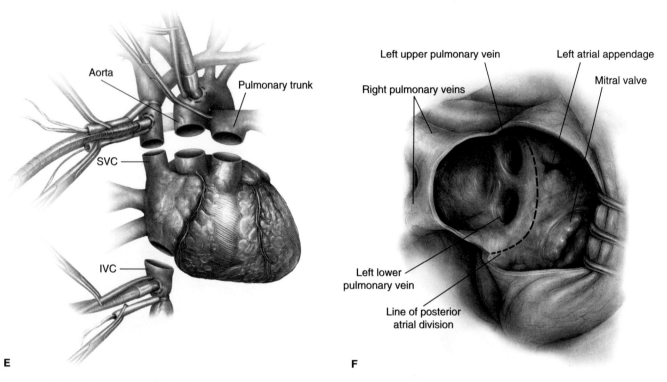

Aorta

Pulmonary trunk

SVC

IVC

Left upper pulmonary vein

Left atrial appendage

Right pulmonary veins

Mitral valve

Left lower
pulmonary vein

Line of posterior
atrial division

E   **F**

FIGURE 58-28 (*Continued*) (D) Right femoral artery cannulation to facilitate inferior vena caval reconstruction and eliminate room occupied by the cannula when the vein is to be transected and later re-connected. (E) Necessary divisions of the aorta, pulmonary artery, and cavae to begin the autotransplantation. (F) The last step in removing the heart includes separating the anterior left atrium from the pulmonary veins.

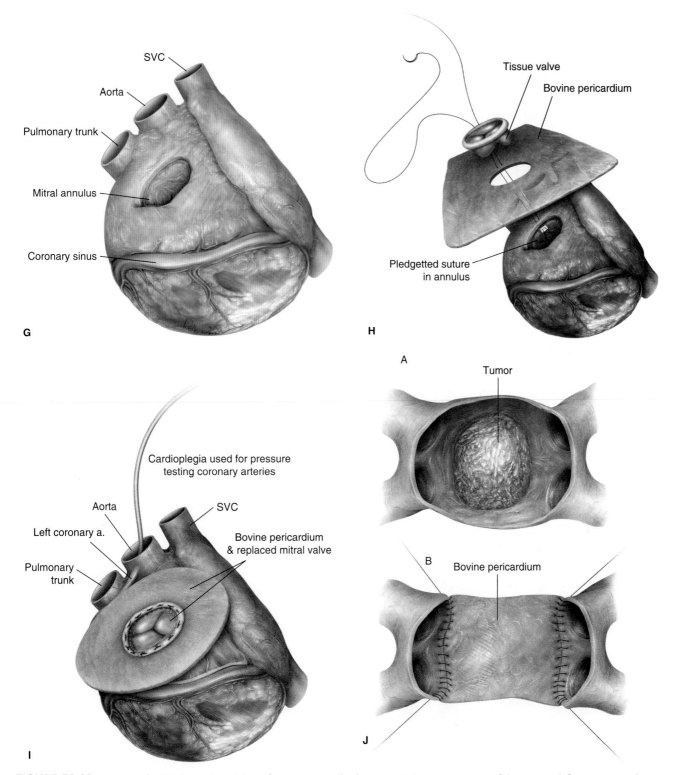

FIGURE 58-28 (*Continued*) (G) The explanted heart from an unusually clear view. (H) Reconstruction of the anterior left atrium using bovine pericardium by incorporating the pledgeted sutures through the annulus, the pericardium, and then the new valve implant, respectively. (I) Reconstruction of the anterior left atrium is complete once the sutures are tied. (J) Resection of a large posterior left atrial mass is easily completed and reconstructed with the heart explanted.

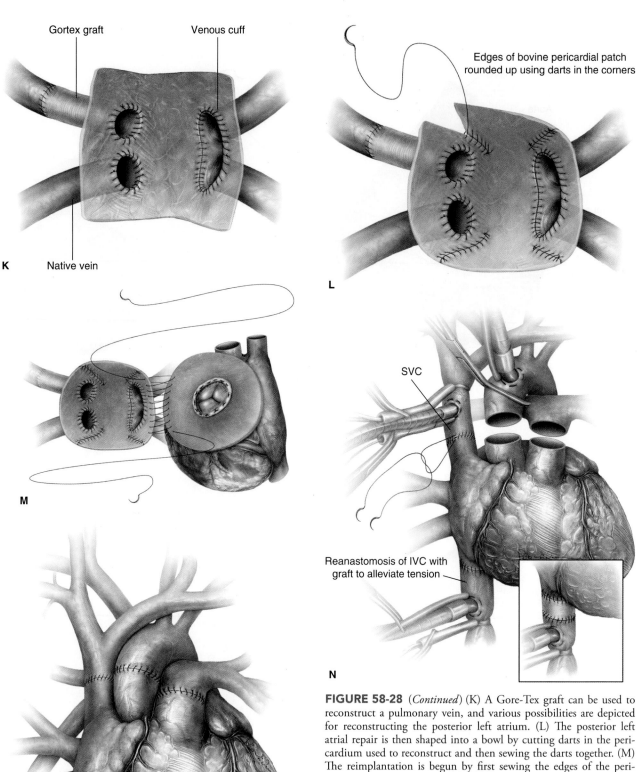

Gortex graft

Venous cuff

K Native vein

Edges of bovine pericardial patch rounded up using darts in the corners

L

M

SVC

Reanastomosis of IVC with graft to alleviate tension

N

O

FIGURE 58-28 (*Continued*) (K) A Gore-Tex graft can be used to reconstruct a pulmonary vein, and various possibilities are depicted for reconstructing the posterior left atrium. (L) The posterior left atrial repair is then shaped into a bowl by cutting darts in the pericardium used to reconstruct and then sewing the darts together. (M) The reimplantation is begun by first sewing the edges of the pericardium together (the left atrial appendage can be used as a marker for orientation). (N) Once the left atrium is reconstructed, the superior vena cava and then inferior vena cava are reconnected (please note any gaps in length can be corrected by interposing the segment with graft. (O) The completed autotransplant heart. (Figures B to O reproduced with permission from Blackmon SH, Reardon MJ: Cardiac Autotransplantation, *Oper Tech Thorac Cardiovasc Surg* 2010;Summer:15(2):147-161.)

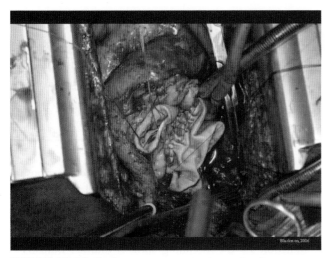

FIGURE 58-29 Cardiac reconstruction using pericardium.

Pulmonary Artery Sarcomas

Most PA sarcomas are classified. The most frequent presenting symptom is shortness of breath and peripheral edema from concomitant right-sided heart failure.[172] The diagnostic modalities of choice for both the initial evaluation and monitoring for recurrence after resection for PA sarcomas are chest CT or MRI (Figs. 58-31, 58-32, and 58-33).

PA sarcomas are very rare tumors that are often confused with acute or chronic pulmonary embolus (PE). This confusion has led to both delay in diagnosis and many being treated with a tumor thromboendarterectomy approach rather than radical resection. These tumors usually are discovered after they have grown to considerable size (Fig. 58-34). PA sarcoma can present with cough, dyspnea, hemoptysis, and chest pain that may mimic PE. Constitutional symptoms often present include fever, anemia and, weight loss which are more consistent with malignancy than PE and these mass lesions will not decrease in size with anticoagulation. These tumors tend to arise from the dorsal surface of the main PA

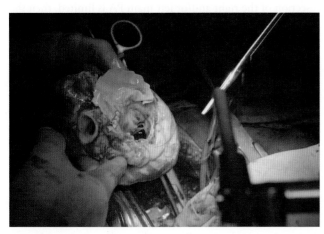

FIGURE 58-30 Explanted heart undergoing anterior left atrial reconstruction with bovine pericardium.

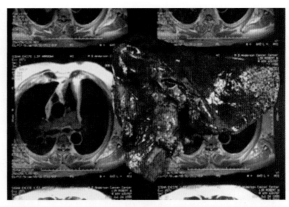

FIGURE 58-31 Pulmonary artery sarcoma as seen on a CT scan with the pathology specimen after radical removal (including pneumonectomy).

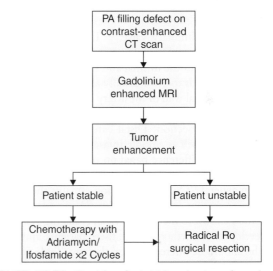

FIGURE 58-32 Algorithm for initial evaluation of a pulmonary artery sarcoma.

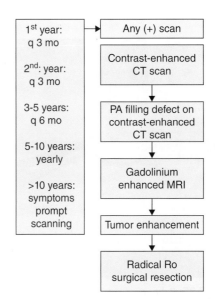

FIGURE 58-33 Postoperative evaluation algorithm for recurrent pulmonary artery sarcoma.

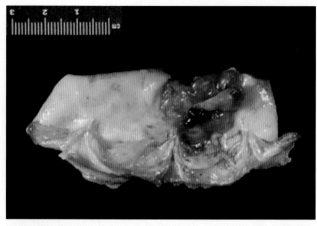

FIGURE 58-34 Pulmonary artery angiosarcoma specimen showing involvement of the pulmonary valve.

just beyond the pulmonary valve.[173] They form from multipotential mesenchymal cells from the muscle remnant of the bulbus cordis[174] in the intimal and subintimal surfaces.[165] The tumor then tends to grow distally along the artery, rarely penetrating the actual wall of the artery but rather distending it (Fig. 58-35). This characteristic is important to note when planning surgical resection. Distal extension can go to the lung parenchyma itself as emboli, infarction, or metastasis.[175] Although survival difference based on cell histology is found in limited cases, that has not been our experience in cardiac sarcoma in general.[172] Surgical resection remains the primary method of treatment in patients with PA sarcoma and the only method shown to increase survival. A staging system has been developed to further classify these patients and determine who should be offered surgical therapy (Table 58-6).

Resection often requires replacement of a portion of the pulmonary root and branch PAs using a pulmonary homograft with or without artificial graft. Pneumonectomy may

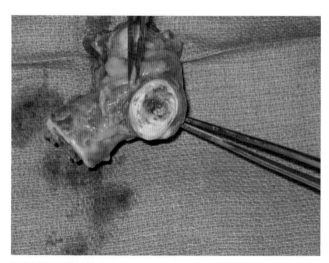

FIGURE 58-35 Pulmonary artery sarcoma demonstrating the extension of the tumor along the inside of the wall and no growth of tumor outside the arterial wall.

TABLE 58-6: Staging System for Primary Pulmonary Artery Sarcomas

Stage I	Tumor limited to the main pulmonary artery
Stage II	Tumor involving one lung plus a main pulmonary artery
Stage III	Bilateral lung involvement
Stage IV	Extrathoracic spread

be required to resect the tumor completely. Because exposure of the right main PA may require division of the aorta and possibly the SVC, we plan surgical cannulation for CPB by using dual venous cannulation with direct SVC cannulation and normal IVC cannulation via the right atrium. Arterial cannulation via the ascending aorta is routine. Both SVC and IVC are isolated with tourniquets to control blood flow into the right heart. Cardiopulmonary arrest is achieved with cold potassium blood cardioplegia. Fortunately, these tumors rarely penetrate the PA wall, allowing reasonable mobilization. The main PA has always been involved in our experience and the pulmonary valve is involved 30% of the time.[172] The main PAs can be resected out to their first branch points on each side from a median approach. In cases where one PA is relatively free and the other is involved deep into the lung, a pneumonectomy may be required. In this case, the pulmonary veins and main bronchus are dissected and divided before CPB is instituted to avoid bleeding while heparinized. The branch PAs and main PA are mobilized, CPB is instituted, and the involved main PA is divided. In such cases, the involved lung with little blood flow once resected may result in improved hemodynamics; especially after removal of tumor obstructing the contralateral PA. Once each PA has been divided or in the case of pneumonectomy the lung and main PA removed, the main PA trunk can be assessed for pulmonary valve involvement. If the pulmonary valve is involved, the entire PA trunk must be removed and replaced by a pulmonary allograft. Removal of the entire PA trunk and replacement by an allograft is similar to mobilization and replacement techniques for a Ross procedure.[175] If the resection of the right and/or left main PA is limited, then the allograft branches may be adequate to span the defect. When tumor extension is too distal for this, a Gore-Tex (ePTFE) graft can be used to interpose between the distal right PA resection point to distal left PA resection point and then implantation of the pulmonary allograft into the side of the ePTFE graft is performed. Despite the extensive nature of the resection, separation from CPB has not been difficult. The surgery relieves the patient of severe PA obstruction that is present preoperatively.

The authors have successfully resected PA sarcomas in 10 patients, three of whom required concomitant pneumonectomy. There were no in-hospital or 30-day deaths, and all patients were discharged home. Our longest survivor currently has lived more than 100 months and has no known disease. In most cases, adjuvant chemotherapy is used, even in the face of clear surgical margins. Radical PA resection is both safe and appears to prolong survival compared to minimal or palliative resection. Resection in conjunction with chemotherapy also appears to prolong survival. Currently, recommendations to record such rare tumors in a national registry may allow better analysis of long-term outcomes.

Heart Transplantation

Malignant primary cardiac tumors may grow to a large size before detection. Additionally, extensive myocardial involvement or location affecting the fibrous trigone of the heart may make complete resection impossible. Because complete resection yields better results than incomplete resection, orthotopic cardiac transplantation has been considered as a treatment option. Reports of transplantation for a number of cardiac tumors, including sarcoma,[175-178] pheochromocytoma,[171] lymphoma,[172] fibroma,[134] and myxoma have appeared. However, the long-term results are uncertain because some patients die from recurrent metastatic disease despite transplantation.[171,172,174] As of 2000, 28 patients had been reported involving orthotopic transplantation for primary cardiac tumors, and of these, 21 had malignant tumors.[174] The mean survival for patients with primary cardiac malignancy was 12 months. Although technically feasible in some cases, orthotopic transplantation is hindered by a scarcity of donor organs and coupled with an extensive recipient list of patients without cancer. In addition, the large size of the tumor when diagnosed often necessitates rapid intervention for progressive congestive heart failure. Finally, the effect of immunosuppression on any remaining malignancy is unknown. In most cases, orthotopic transplantation is reserved for unresectable benign tumors, such as cardiac fibroma.

SECONDARY METASTATIC TUMORS

Approximately 10% of metastatic tumors eventually reach the heart or pericardium, and almost every type of malignant tumor has been known to do so.[2,7] Secondary neoplasms are 20 to 40 times more common than primary.[4,175] Up to 50% of patients with leukemia develop cardiac lesions. Other cancers that commonly involve the heart include breast cancer, lung cancer, lymphoma, melanoma, and various sarcomas.[2,176,177] Metastases involving the pericardium, epicardium, myocardium, and endocardium roughly follow that order of frequency[2,7] as well (Table 58-7).

The most common means of spread, particularly for melanoma, sarcoma, and bronchogenic carcinoma, is hematogenous and ultimately via coronary arteries. In addition, metastasis can reach the heart through lymphatic channels; through direct extension from adjacent lung, breast, esophageal, and thymic tumors; and from the subdiaphragmatic vena cava. The pericardium is involved most often by direct extension of thoracic cancer; the heart is the target of hematologous and/or retrograde lymphatic metastasis.[5] Cardiac metastases rarely are solitary and nearly always produce multiple microscopic nests and discrete nodules of tumor cells[2,7] (Fig. 58-36). Cardiac metastases produce clinical symptoms in

TABLE 58-7: Metastatic Cardiac Disease

Tumor	Total (no.)	Cardiac (%)	Pericardial (%)
Leukemia	420	53.9	22.4
Melanoma	59	34.0	23.7
Lung ca	402	10.2	15.7
Sarcoma	207	9.2	9.2
Breast ca	289	8.3	11.8
Esophageal ca	65	7.7	7.7
Ovarian ca	115	5.7	7.0
Kidney ca	95	5.3	0.0
Gastric ca	3.8	3.6	3.2
Prostate ca	186	2.7	1.0
Colon ca	214	0.9	2.8
Lymphoma	75	—	14.6

Data from Kapoor AS: *Cancer and the Heart.* New York: Springer-Verlag Publishers; 1986.

only about 10% of afflicted patients.[178,179] The most common symptom is pericardial effusion or cardiac tamponade. Occasionally, patients develop refractory arrhythmias or congestive heart failure. Chest radiographs and electrocardiograms tend to show nonspecific changes, but echocardiography is particularly useful for diagnosis of pericardial effusion, irregular pericardial thickening, or intracavity masses interfering with blood flow.

Surgical therapy is limited to relief of recurrent pericardial effusions or, occasionally, cardiac tamponade. In most instances, these patients have widespread disease with limited life expectancies. Surgical therapy is directed at providing symptomatic palliation with minimal patient discomfort and hospital stay. This is most readily accomplished via subxiphoid pericardiotomy, which can be accomplished under local anesthesia if necessary with reliable relief of symptoms, a recurrence rate of about 3%, and little mortality.[177]

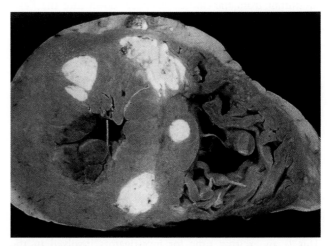

FIGURE 58-36 Hematogenous metastases within the myocardium of a patient with renal cell cancer. (Reproduced with permission from Hurst JW et al: *Atlas of the Heart.* New York: McGraw-Hill; 1988.)

Alternatively, a large pericardial window in the left pleural space can be created using thoracoscopy, but we would recommend this only under unusual circumstances.[180] This can be accomplished with minimal patient discomfort but does require general anesthesia with single-lung ventilation and may be poorly tolerated by patients with hemodynamic deterioration secondary to large effusions.

RIGHT ATRIAL EXTENSION OF SUBDIAPHRAGMATIC TUMORS

Abdominal and pelvic tumors on occasion may grow in a cephalad direction via the IVC to reach the right atrium. Subdiaphragmatic tumors are frequently renal carcinomas, although hepatic, adrenal, and uterine tumors occasionally have exhibited this behavior. Up to 10% of renal cell carcinomas invade the IVC, and nearly 40% of these reach the right atrium.[181] Radiation and chemotherapy are not effective in relieving the obstruction of blood flow. If the kidney can be fully removed, as well as the tail of the tumor thrombus, survival can approach 75% at 5 years.[96,182]

Renal cell tumors with atrial extension typically are resected with abdominal dissection to ensure resectability of the renal tumor. Initially, we performed a concomitant median sternotomy and often used CPB with hypothermic circulatory arrest when treating these patients. However, we have changed our approach and now work closely with our liver transplant surgeons who have extensive experience in the area of the retrohepatic vena cava. We have found that we can expose the vena cava up to the right atrium through an abdominal incision. With ligation of the arterial inflow, the tumor tail often shrinks below the diaphragm, and in almost all circumstances, this can be removed without the use of CPB. Occasionally venovenous bypass as used in hepatic transplantation is necessary to occlude inflow through the IVC, but this is unusual. If the tumor is too complex for this maneuver, then a median sternotomy is performed, and CPB with hypothermic circulatory arrest can be used to remove the tumor from the cardiac chambers down into the IVC. Perfusion can be restarted, followed by removal of the rest of the tumor. Although it leads to adequate exposure, significant problems with coagulopathy are often apparent after CPB and profound hypothermia.

A 5-year survival rate of 75% has been achieved following nephrectomy with resection of right atrial tumor extension.[182,183] Other subdiaphragmatic tumors with atrial extension that have been resected successfully include hepatic and adrenal carcinoma, as well gynecologic tumors.[184-188]

MOLECULAR- AND BIOLOGIC-BASED DIAGNOSIS AND THERAPY FOR CARDIAC TUMORS

This is an exciting time for investigators involved in the search for novel therapies for tumors such as many of those discussed in this chapter. A "new biology" is being developed in laboratories around the world working in these areas, and this is supplanted by the knowledge that is being obtained from the concerted Human Genome Project and the subsequent development of proteomics.[146] It is incumbent on the thoracic surgeon involved in the care of patients with cardiac tumors to have some degree of familiarity with the terms and promise of these advances because significant additional improvement in survival of many of these patients is unlikely to result from further advances in surgical technique.

Interestingly, many sarcomas demonstrate reproducible translocations that allow for the production of novel chimeric genes that may code for a variety of fusion proteins. Many of these proteins have been found to engender cellular phenotypic malignant changes, resistance to apoptosis, and unfettered growth.[181] Although not associated with cardiac involvement, the fusion proteins EWS-FL11 and EWS-ERG are noted in Ewing's sarcoma. When full-length antisense oligonucleotide constructs are used to target the mRNA of these proteins, protein expression is downregulated, and an eightfold increase in apoptosis sensitivity is noted.[189] These fusion proteins have been noted in some forms of rhabdomyosarcoma, and the most common is PAX3-FKHR. This oncoprotein combines components of two strong transcriptional activators and may increase the production of the downstream antiapoptotic protein BCL-XL. Antisense oligonucleotides directed at this oncoprotein mRNA have led to apoptosis in rhabdomyosarcoma cells.[190,191] A similar translocation and fusion protein have been noted in fibrosarcoma. This translocation [t(12;15)(p13q25)] brings together genes from chromosomes 12 and 15, which combines a transcription factor with a tyrosine kinase receptor. The resulting fusion protein is a tyrosine kinase that has oncogenic potential.[192] Reproducible translocations and fusion proteins with downstream effectors of malignant behavior have not been described for angiosarcoma, but they are actively being sought.[188] Antisense treatment has been maligned in the past owing to problems with both delivery and stability of therapeutic constructs. However, sophisticated biochemical alteration of these molecules has improved stability, and two recent solid tumor trials using antisense therapy for salvage have demonstrated positive results.[193] Additional methods of delivering antisense to tumor cells, including viral vector delivery, have been developed. Finally, in addition to antisense methods, small molecule inhibition of many of these fusion proteins should be possible.

Angiosarcoma is an obvious target for therapies based on antiangiogenesis. The weak antiangiogenic properties of interferon-alpha are presumed to be the mechanism that accounts for responses to this agent in this tumor.[194] Multiple new antiangiogenic agents are being evaluated currently in phase I and II trials, and a number of noncardiac angiosarcoma patients have been treated at our institution on this basis. We have noted several to develop stabilized disease, but no definitive data are yet published. Certainly, the use of these agents in these vascular-origin tumors is theoretically attractive.

Viral vector-mediated gene therapy has been evaluated for various sarcomas in the preclinical setting. A number of potential targets exist for these sorts of therapies. Although *p53* is not commonly mutated or absent, *mdm-2* is often overexpressed in many sarcomas, including angiosarcoma. This gene is a known oncogene that is able to directly induce cellular transformation. Importantly, when overexpressed, it binds to and inhibits *p53* activity, even though expression of *p53* may appear normal. Overexpression of *mdm-2* also has been associated with vascular endothelial growth factor (VEGF) overproduction and angiogenesis.[194] Preclinical studies of adenoviral *vector p53* transduction of sarcoma in severe combined immunodeficiency (SCID) mice have demonstrated growth delay, tumor regression, and decreases in VEGF expression.[195] Many other targets for this approach, including inhibition of nuclear factor-kappa B (NF-κB) expression using an adenoviral-dominant negative Iκ-βα construct and prodrug-mediated gene therapy using a doxorubicin prodrug and adenoviral transfer of a metabolizing enzyme in sarcoma cells, have been shown to be effective.[184] Unfortunately, the application of viral-mediated gene therapy paradigms to this tumor suffers the same problems of targeting, transgene expression durability, and immune response that are problematic for the field in general.

In regard to molecular diagnosis, there are no reproducible familial patterns for development of most malignant tumors. However, familial cardiac myxoma, rhabdomyoma, and fibroma may exhibit reproducible genetic abnormalities that lend themselves to the development of genetic testing to identify individuals at risk. Familial myxoma syndrome, or Carney complex, has been associated with mutations in the 17q24 gene *PRKAR1a* that codes for the R1 *a* regulatory subunit of cAMP-dependent protein kinase A (PKA).[195] Although not widely available, genetic diagnosis of this syndrome is now technically achievable.[196] Reproducible mutations in the *TSC-1* and *TSC-2* genes in patients with tuberous

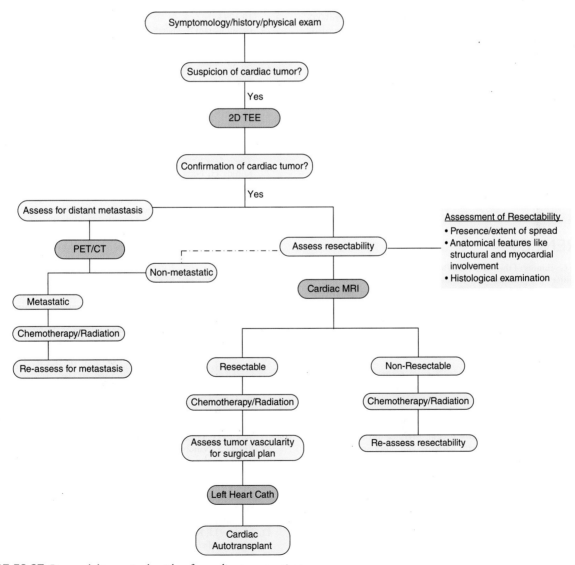

FIGURE 58-37 Proposed diagnostic algorithm for cardiac tumor patients.

sclerosis and cardiac rhabdomyoma, as well as mutations in the *PTC* gene of patients with the Gorlin syndrome and cardiac fibroma, have been noted.[197-200] It is hoped that in the near future we will be able to predict who is at particular risk for these and other cardiac tumors. This could allow for more intense surveillance, earlier detection, and a higher rate of surgical or multimodality cure for these patients.

KEY POINTS

- Complete excision and radical resection is recommended to prevent local recurrence of cardiac tumors
- All benign cardiac tumors are potentially curable with current surgical techniques
- Multimodality therapy and multidisciplinary planning should be incorporated into the care of cardiac tumor patients (Fig. 58-37)
- Cardiac sarcomas are best classified by anatomic location rather than histologic subtype, and the former dictates their presentation, treatment, and prognosis
- Right heart sarcomas tend to be more bulky, infiltrative, metastasize earlier, and are usually amenable to neoadjuvant chemotherapy
- Left heart sarcomas tend to be more solid, less infiltrative, and metastasize later
- PA sarcomas usually present with obstruction, right heart failure, and tend to grow distally within the confinement of the PA
- Cardiac tumors located in the anterior left atrial wall may require autotransplantation for complete excision of the tumor, reconstruction, and reimplantation
- Cardiac autotransplant and concomitant pneumonectomy carries an unacceptable 50% mortality rate.

REFERENCES

1. Smith C: Tumors of the heart. *Arch Pathol Lab Med* 1986; 110:371.
2. McAllister HA, Fenoglio JJ Jr: Tumors of the cardiovascular system, in *Atlas of Tumor Pathology*, Series 2. Washington, DC, Armed Forces Institute of Pathology, 1978.
3. Straus R, Merliss R: Primary tumors of the heart. *Arch Pathol* 1945; 39:74.
4. Reynen K: Cardiac myxomas. *New Engl J Med* 1995; 333:1610.
5. Wold LE, Lie JT: Cardiac myxomas: a clinicopathologic profile. *Am J Pathol* 1980; 101:219.
6. Silverman NA: Primary cardiac tumors. *Ann Surg* 1980; 91:127.
7. Columbus MR: *De Re Anatomica*, Liber XV. Venice, N Bevilacque, 1559; p 269.
8. Burns A: *Observations of Some of the Most Frequent and Important Diseases of the Heart*. London, James Muirhead, 1809.
9. Goldberg HP, Glenn F, Dotter CT, et al: Myxoma of the left atrium: Diagnosis made during life with operative and postmortem findings. *Circulation* 1952; 6:762.
10. Yates WM: Tumors of the heart and pericardium: pathology, symptomatology, and report of nine cases. *Arch Intern Med* 1931; 48:267.
11. Barnes AR, Beaver DC, Snell AMP: Primary sarcoma of the heart: report of a case with electrocardiographic and pathological studies. *Am Heart J* 1934; 9:480.
12. Beck CS: An intrapericardial teratoma and tumor of the heart: both removed operatively. *Ann Surg* 1942; 116:161.
13. Mauer ER: Successful removal of tumor of the heart. *J Thorac Surg* 1952; 3:479.
14. Effert S, Domanig E: Diagnosis of intra-auricular tumors and large thrombi with the aid of ultrasonic echography. *Dtsch Med Wochesch* 1959; 84:6.
15. Bahnson HT, Newman EV: Diagnosis and surgical removal of intracavitary myxoma of the right atrium. *Bull Johns Hopkins Hosp* 1953; 93:150.
16. Crafoord C: Panel discussion of late results of mitral commissurotomy, in Lam CR (ed): *Henry Ford Hospital International Symposium on Cardiovascular Surgery*. Philadelphia, Saunders, 1955; p 202.
17. Kay JH, Anderson RM, Meihaus J, et al: Surgical removal of an intracavity left ventricular myxoma. *Circulation* 1959; 20:881.
18. Attar S, Lee L, Singleton R, et al: Cardiac myxoma. *Ann Thorac Surg* 1980; 29:397.
19. St. John Sutton MG, Mercier LA, Giuliani ER, et al: Atrial myxomas: a review of clinical experience in 40 patients. *Mayo Clin Proc* 1980; 55:371.
20. Dein JR, Frist WH, Stinson EB, et al: Primary cardiac neoplasms: early and late results of surgical treatment in 42 patients. *J Thorac Cardiovasc Surg* 1987; 93:502.
21. Pinede L, Duhaut P, Loire R: Clinical presentation of left atrial cardiac myxoma: a series of 112 consecutive cases. *Medicine* 2001; 80:159.
22. Waller R, Grider L, Rohr T, et al: Intracardiac thrombi: frequency, location, etiology and, complications: a morphologic review, part I. *Clin Cardiol* 1995; 18:477.
23. Gertner E, Leatherman J: Intracardiac mural thrombus mimicking atrial myxoma in the antiphospholipid syndrome. *J Rheumatol* 1992; 19:1293.
24. Balasundaram S, Halees SA, Duran C: Mesothelioma of the atrioventricular node: first successful follow-up after excision. *Eur Heart J* 1992; 13:718.
25. Ali SZ, Susin M, Kahn E, Hajdu SI: Intracardiac teratoma in a child simulating an atrioventricular nodal tumor. *Pediatr Pathol* 1994; 14:913.
26. Carney JA: Differences between nonfamilial and familial cardiac myxoma. *Am J Surg Pathol* 1985; 64:53.
27. McCarthy PM, Schaff HV, Winkler HZ, et al: Deoxyribonucleic acid ploidy pattern of cardiac myxomas. *J Thorac Cardiovasc Surg* 1989; 98:1083.
28. Gelder HM, O'Brian DJ, Styles ED, et al: Familial cardiac myxoma. *Ann Thorac Surg* 1992; 53:419.
29. Kuroda H, Nitta K, Ashida Y, et al: Right atrial myxoma originating from the tricuspid valve. *J Thorac Cardiovasc Surg* 1995; 109:1249.
30. Bortolotti U, Faggian G, Mazzucco A, et al: Right atrial myxoma originating from the inferior vena cava. *Ann Thorac Surg* 1990; 49:1000.
31. King YL, Dickens P, Chan ACL: Tumors of the heart. *Arch Pathol Lab Med* 1993; 117:1027.
32. St. John Sutton MG, Mercier LA, Guiliana ER, et al: Atrial myxomas: a review of clinical experience in 40 patients. *Mayo Clin Proc* 1980; 55:371.
33. Burke AP, Virmani R: Cardiac myxoma: a clinicopathologic study. *Am J Clin Pathol* 1993; 100:671.
34. Peters MN, Hall RJ, Cooley DA, et al: The clinical syndrome of atrial myxoma. *J Am Med Assoc* 1974; 230:695.
35. Carney JA, Hruska LS, Beauchamp GD, et al: Dominant inheritance of the complex of myxomas, spotty pigmentation, and endocrine overactivity. *Mayo Clin Proc* 1986; 61:165.
36. Imperio J, Summels D, Krasnow N, et al: The distribution patterns of biatrial myxoma. *Ann Thorac Surg* 1980; 29:469.
37. McAllister HA: Primary tumors of the heart and pericardium. *Pathol Annu* 1979; 14:325.
38. Jones DR, Hill RC, Abbott AE Jr, et al: Unusual location of an atrial myxoma complicated by a secundum atrial septal defect. *Ann Thorac Surg* 1993; 55:1252.
39. Kuroki S, Naitoh K, Katoh O, et al: Increased interleukin-6 activity in cardiac myxoma with mediastinal lymphadenopathy. *Intern Med* 1992; 31:1207.
40. Reddy DJ, Rao` TS, Venkaiah KR, et al: Congenital myxoma of the heart. *Indian J Pediatr* 1956; 23:210.
41. Prichard RW: Tumors of the heart: review of the subject and report of one hundred and fifty cases. *Arch Pathol* 1951; 51:98.
42. Merkow LP, Kooros MA, Macgovern G, et al: Ultrastructure of a cardiac myxoma. *Arch Pathol* 1969; 88:390.
43. Lie JT: The identity and histogenesis of cardiac myxomas: a controversy put to rest. *Arch Pathol Lab Med* 1989; 113:724.

44. Ferrans VJ, Roberts WC: Structural features of cardiac myxomas: histology, histochemistry, and electron microscopy. *Hum Pathol* 1973; 4:111.

45. Krikler DM, Rode J, Davies MJ, et al: Atrial myxoma: a tumor in search of its origins. *Br Heart J* 1992; 67:89.

46. Glasser SP, Bedynek JL, Hall RJ, et al: Left atrial myxoma: report of a case including hemodynamic, surgical, and histologic characteristics. *Am J Med* 1971; 50:113.

47. Saji T, Yanagawa E, Matsuura H, et al: Increased serum interleukin-6 in cardiac myxoma. *Am Heart J* 1991; 122:579.

48. Senguin JR, Beigbeder JY, Hvass U, et al: Interleukin-6 production by cardiac myxoma may explain constitutional symptoms. *J Thorac Cardiovasc Surg* 1992; 103:599.

49. Buchanan RC, Cairns JA, Krag G, et al: Left atrial myxoma mimicking vasculitis: echocardiographic diagnosis. *Can Med Assoc J* 1979; 120:1540.

50. Currey HLF, Matthew JA, Robinson J: Right atrial myxoma mimicking a rheumatic disorder. *Br Med J* 1967; 1:547.

51. Byrd WE, Matthew OP, Hunt RE: Left atrial myxoma presenting as a systemic vasculitis. *Arthritis Rheum* 1980; 23:240.

52. Hattler BG, Fuchs JCA, Coson R, et al: Atrial myxomas: an evaluation of clinical and laboratory manifestations. *Ann Thorac Surg* 1970; 10:65.

53. Bulkley BH, Hutchins GM: Atrial myxomas: a fifty-year review. *Am Heart J* 1979; 97:639.

54. Panidas IP, Kotler MN, Mintz GS, et al: Clinical and echocardiographic features of right atrial masses. *Am Heart J* 1984; 107:745.

55. Meller J, Teichholz LE, Pichard AD, et al: Left ventricular myxoma: echocardiographic diagnosis and review of the literature. *Am J Med* 1977; 63:81.

56. Desousa AL, Muller J, Campbell RL, et al: Atrial myxoma: a review of the neurological complications, metastases, and recurrences. *J Neurol Neurosurg Psychiatr* 1978; 41:1119.

57. Suzuki T, Nagai R, Yamazaki T, et al: Rapid growth of intracranial aneurysms secondary to cardiac myxoma. *Neurology* 1994; 44:570.

58. Chen HJ, Liou CW, Chen L: Metastatic atrial myxoma presenting as intracranial aneurysm with hemorrhage: case report. *Surg Neurol* 1993; 40:61.

59. Browne WT, Wijdicks EF, Parisi JE, et al: Fulminant brain necrosis from atrial myxoma showers. *Stroke* 1993; 24:1090.

60. Lewis JM: Multiple retinal occlusions from a left atrial myxoma. *Am J Ophthalmol* 1994; 117:674.

61. Eriksen UH, Baandrup U, Jensen BS: Total disruptions of left atrial myxoma causing cerebral attack and a saddle embolus in the iliac bifurcation. *Int J Cardiol* 1992; 35:127.

62. Carter AB, Lowe K, Hill I: Cardiac myxomata and aortic saddle embolism. *Br Heart J* 1960; 22:502.

63. Hashimoto H, Tikahashi H, Fukiward Y, et al: Acute myocardial infarction due to coronary embolization from left atrial myxoma. *Jpn Circ J* 1993; 57:1016.

64. Rajpal RS, Leibsohn JA, Leikweg WG, et al: Infected left atrial myxoma with bacteremia simulating infective endocarditis. *Arch Intern Med* 1979; 139:1176.

65. Whitman MS, Rovito MA, Klions D, et al: Infected myxoma: case report and review. *Clin Infect Dis* 1994; 18:657.

66. Martinez-Lopez JI: Sounds of the heart in diastole. *Am J Cardiol* 1974; 34:594.

67. Harvey WP: Clinical aspects of heart tumors. *Am J Cardiol* 1968; 21:328.

68. Case records of the Massachusetts General Hospital, weekly clinicopathological exercises: Case 14-1978. *New Engl J Med* 1978; 298:834.

69. Mundinger A, Gruber HP, Dinkel E, et al: Imaging cardiac mass lesions. *Radiol Med* 1992; 10:135.

70. Ensberding R, Erbel DR, Kaspar W, et al: Diagnosis of heart tumors by transesophageal echocardiography. *Eur Heart J* 1993; 14:1223.

71. Samdarshi TE, Mahan EF 3d, Nanda NC, et al: Transesophageal echocardiographic diagnosis of multicentric left ventricular myxomas mimicking a left atrial tumor. *J Thorac Cardiovasc Surg* 1992; 103:471.

72. Bleiweis MS, Georgiou D, Brungage BH: Detection of intracardiac masses by ultrafast computed tomography. *Am J Cardiac Imag* 1994; 8:63.

73. Symbas PN, Hatcher CR Jr, Gravanis MB: Myxoma of the heart: clinical and experimental observations. *Ann Surg* 1976; 183:470.

74. McCarthy PM, Piehler JM, Schaff HV, et al: The significance of multiple, recurrent, and "complex" cardiac myxoma. *J Thorac Cardiovasc Surg* 1986; 91:389.

75. Dato GMA, Benedictus M, Dato AA, et al: Long-term follow-up of cardiac myxomas (7–31 years). *J Cardiovasc Surg* 1993; 34:141.

76. Bertolotti U, Mazzucco A, Valfre C, et al: Right ventricular myxoma: review of the literature and report of two patients. *Ann Thorac Surg* 1983; 33:277.

77. Attum AA, Johnson GS, Masri Z, et al: Malignant clinical behavior of cardiac myxomas and "myxoid imitators." *Ann Thorac Surg* 1987; 44:217.

78. Ravikumar E, Pawar N, Gnanamuthu R, et al: Minimal access approach for surgical management of cardiac tumors. *Ann Thorac Surg* 2000; 70:1077.

79. Ko PJ, Chang CH, Lin PJ, et al: Video-assisted minimal access in excision of left atrial myxoma. *Ann Thorac Surg* 1998; 66:1301.

80. Gulbins H, Reichenspurner H, Wintersperger BJ: Minimally invasive extirpation of a left-ventricular myxoma. *Thorac Cardiovasc Surg* 1999; 47:129.

81. Espada R, Talwalker NG, Wilcox G, et al: Visualization of ventricular fibroelastoma with a video-assisted thoracoscope. *Ann Thorac Surg* 1997; 63:221.

82. Walkes JC, Bavare C, Blackmon S, Reardon MJ: Transaortic resection of an apical left ventricular fibroelastoma facilitated by a thoracoscope. *J Thorac Cardiovasc* 2007; 134(3):793-794.

83. Greco E, Maestros CA, Cartanea R, Pomar JL: Video-assisted cardioscopy for removal of primary left ventricular myxoma. *Eur J Cardiothorac Surg* 1999; 16:667.

84. Reyes CV, Jablokow VR: Lipomatous hypertrophy of the atrial septum: a report of 38 cases and review of the literature. *Am J Clin Pathol* 1979; 72:785.

85. McAllister HA: Primary tumors and cysts of the heart and pericardium, in Harvey WP (ed): *Current Problems in Cardiology*. Chicago, Year Book Medical, 1979.

86. Reece IJ, Cooley DA, Frazier OH, et al: Cardiac tumors: clinical spectrum and prognosis of lesions other than classic benign myxoma in 20 patients. *J Thorac Cardiovasc Surg* 1984; 88:439.

87. Markel ML, Armstrong WF, Waller BF, et al: Left atrial myxoma with multicentric recurrence and evidence of metastases. *Am Heart J* 1986; 111:409.

88. Castells E, Ferran KV, Toledo MCO, et al: Cardiac myxomas: surgical treatment, long-term results and recurrence. *J Cardiovasc Surg* 1993; 34:49.

89. Seidman JD, Berman JJ, Hitchcock CL, et al: DNA analysis of cardiac myxomas: flow cytometry and image analysis. *Hum Pathol* 1991; 22:494.

90. Attum AA, Ogden LL, Lansing AM: Atrial myxoma: benign and malignant. *J Ky Med Assoc* 1984; 82:319.

91. Seo S, Warner TFCS, Colyer RA, et al: Metastasizing atrial myxoma. *Am J Surg Pathol* 1980; 4:391.

92. Hirsch BE, Sehkar L, Kamerer DB: Metastatic atrial myxoma to the temporal bone: case report. *Am J Otol* 1991; 12:207.

93. Kotani K, Matsuzawa Y, Funahashi T, et al: Left atrial myxoma metastasizing to the aorta, with intraluminal growth causing renovascular hypertension. *Cardiology* 1991; 78:72.

94. Diflo T, Cantelmo NL, Haudenschild DD, Watkins MT: Atrial myxoma with remote metastasis: case report and review of the literature. *Surgery* 1992; 111:352.

95. Hannah H, Eisemann G, Hiszvzynskyj R, et al: Invasive atrial myxoma: documentation of malignant potential of cardiac myxomas. *Am Heart J* 1982; 104:881.

96. Rankin LI, Desousa AL: Metastatic atrial myxoma presenting as intracranial mass. *Chest* 1978; 74:451.

97. Burton C, Johnston J: Multiple cerebral aneurysm and cardiac myxoma. *New Engl J Med* 1970; 282:35.

98. Harjola PR, Ala-Kulju K, Ketonen P: Epicardial lipoma. *Scand J Thorac Cardiovasc Surg* 1985; 19:181.

99. Arciniegas E, Hakimi M, Farooki ZQ, et al: Primary cardiac tumors in children. *J Thorac Cardiovasc Surg* 1980; 79:582.

100. Isner J, Swan CS II, Mikus JP, et al: Lipomatous hypertrophy of the interatrial septum: in vivo diagnosis. *Circulation* 1982; 66:470.

101. Simons M, Cabin HS, Jaffe CC: Lipomatous hypertrophy of the atrial septum: diagnosis by combined echocardiography and computerized tomography. *Am J Cardiol* 1984; 54:465.

102. Basu S, Folliguet T, Anselmo M, et al: Lipomatous hypertrophy of the interatrial septum. *Cardiovasc Surg* 1994; 2:229.

103. Zeebregts CJAM, Hensens AG, Timmermans J, et al: Lipomatous hypertrophy of the interatrial septum: indication for surgery? *Eur J Cardiothorac Surg* 1997; 11:785.

104. Vander Salm TJ: Unusual primary tumors of the heart. *Semin Thorac Cardiovasc Surg* 2000; 2:89.

105. Edwards FH, Hale D, Cohen A, et al: Primary cardiac valve tumors. *Ann Thorac Surg* 1991; 52:1127.

106. Israel DH, Sherman W, Ambrose JA, et al: Dynamic coronary ostial occlusion due to papillary fibroelastoma leading to myocardial ischemia and infarction. *Am J Cardiol* 1991; 67:104.

107. Grote J, Mugge A, Schfers HJ: Multiplane transesophageal echocardiography detection of a papillary fibroelastoma of the aortic valve causing myocardial infarction. *Eur Heart J* 1995; 16:426.

108. Gallas MT, Reardon MJ, Reardon PR, et al: Papillary fibroelastoma: a right atrial presentation. *Tex Heart Inst J* 1993; 20:293.

109. Grinda JM, Couetil JP, Chauvaud S, et al: Cardiac valve papillary fibroelastoma: Surgical excision for revealed or potential embolization. *J Thorac Cardiovasc Surg* 1999; 117:106.

110. Shing M, Rubenson DS: Embolic stroke and cardiac papillary fibroelastoma. *Clin Cardiol* 2001; 24:346.

111. Grandmougin D, Fayad G, Moukassa D, et al: Cardiac valve papillary fibroelastomas: clinical, histological and immunohistochemical studies and a physiopathogenic hypothesis. *J Heart Valve Dis* 2000; 9:832.

112. Mazzucco A, Bortolotti U, Thiene G, et al: Left ventricular papillary fibroelastoma with coronary embolization. *Eur J Cardiothorac Surg* 1989; 3:471.

113. Topol EJ, Biern RO, Reitz BA: Cardiac papillary fibroelastoma and stroke: Echocardiographic diagnosis and guide to excision. *Am J Med* 1986; 80:129.

114. Mann J, Parker DJ: Papillary fibroelastoma of the mitral valve: a rare cause of transient neurologic deficits. *Br Heart J* 1994; 71:6.

115. Ragni T, Grande AM, Cappuccio G, et al: Embolizing fibroelastoma of the aortic valve. *Cardiovasc Surg* 1994; 2:639.

116. Nicks R: Hamartoma of the right ventricle. *J Thorac Cardiovasc Surg* 1967; 47:762.

117. Bass JL, Breningstall GN, Swaiman DF: Echocardiographic incidence of cardiac rhabdomyoma in tuberous sclerosis. *Am J Cardiol* 1985; 55:1379.

118. Fenoglio JJ, McAllister HA, Ferrans VJ: Cardiac rhabdomyoma: a clinicopathologic and electron microscopic study. *Am J Cardiol* 1976; 38:241.

119. Garson A, Smith RT, Moak JP, et al: Incessant ventricular tachycardia in infants: Myocardial hamartomas and surgical cure. *J Am Coll Cardiol* 1987; 10:619.

120. Burke AP, Rosado-de-Christenson M, Templeton PA, et al: Cardiac fibroma: clinicopathologic correlates and surgical treatment. *J Thorac Cardiovasc Surg* 1994; 108:862.

121. Yamaguchi M, Hosokawa Y, Ohashi H, et al: Cardiac fibroma: long-term fate after excision. *J Thorac Cardiovasc Surg* 1992; 103:140.

122. Jamieson SA, Gaudiani VA, Reitz BA, et al: Operative treatment of an unresectable tumor on the left ventricle. *J Thorac Cardiovasc Surg* 1981; 81:797.

123. Valente M, Cocco P, Thiene G, et al: Cardiac fibroma and heart transplantation. *J Thorac Cardiovasc Surg* 1993; 106:1208.

124. Nishida K, Kaijima G, Nagayama T: Mesothelioma of the atrioventricular node. *Br Heart J* 1985; 53:468.

125. Jebara VA, Uva MS, Farge A, et al: Cardiac pheochromocytomas. *Ann Thorac Surg* 1991; 53:356.

126. Orringer MB, Sisson JC, Glazer G, et al: Surgical treatment of cardiac pheochromocytomas. *J Thorac Cardiovasc Surg* 1985; 89:753.

127. Cooley DA, Reardon MJ, Frazier OH, et al: Human cardiac explantation and autotransplantation: application in a patient with a large cardiac pheochromocytoma. *J Tex Heart Inst* 1985; 2:171.

128. Mirza M: Angina-like pain and normal coronary arteries: uncovering cardiac syndromes that mimic CAD. *Postgrad Med* 2005; 117:41.

129. Pac-Ferrer J, Uribe-Etxebarria N, Rumbero JC, Castellanos E: Mediastinal paraganglioma irrigated by coronary vessels in a patient with an atypical chest pain. *Eur J Cardiothorac Surg* 2003; 24:662.

130. Turley AJ, Hunter S, Stewart MJ: A cardiac paraganglioma presenting with atypical chest pain. *Eur J Cardiothorac Surg* 2005; 28:352.

131. Can KM, Pontefract D, Andrews R, Naik SK: Paraganglioma of the left atrium. *J Thorac Cardiovasc Surg* 2001; 122:1032.

132. Bizard C, Latremouille C, Jebara VA, et al: Cardiac hemangiomas. *Ann Thorac Surg* 1993; 56:390.

133. Grenadier E, Margulis T, Plauth WH, et al: Huge cavernous hemangioma of the heart: a completely evaluated case report and review of the literature. *Am Heart J* 1989; 117:479.

134. Soberman MS, Plauth WH, Winn KJ, et al: Hemangioma of the right ventricle causing outflow tract obstruction. *J Thorac Cardiovasc Surg* 1988; 96:307.

135. Weir I, Mills P, Lewis T: A case of left atrial hemangioma: echocardiographic, surgical, and morphologic features. *Br Heart J* 1987; 58:665.

136. Palmer TC, Tresch DD, Bonchek LI: Spontaneous resolution of a large cavernous hemangioma of the heart. *Am J Cardiol* 1986; 58:184.

137. Thomas CR, Johnson GW, Stoddard MF, et al: Primary malignant cardiac tumors: update 1992. *Med Pediatr Oncol* 1992; 20:519.

138. Poole GV, Meredith JW, Breyer RH, et al: Surgical implications in malignant cardiac disease. *Ann Thorac Surg* 1983; 36:484.

139. Castleman B, Iverson P, Menendez VP: Localized mediastinal lymph node hyperplasia resembling thymoma. *Cancer* 1956; 9:822.

140. Keller AR, Hochholzer L, Castleman B: Hyaline-vascular and plasma-cell types of giant lymph node hyperplasia of the mediastinum and other locations. *Cancer* 1972; 670.

141. Malaisrie SC, Loebe M, Walkes JC, Reardon MJ: Coronary pseudoaneurysm: an unreported complication of Castleman's disease. *Ann Thorac Surg* 2006; 82(1):318-320.

142. Ko SF, Wan WL, Ng SH, et al: Imaging features of atypical thoracic Castleman's disease. *Clin Imaging* 2004; 28:280.

143. Samuels LE: Castleman's disease: surgical implications. *Surg Rounds* 1997; 20:449.

144. Murphy MC, Sweeney MS, Putnam JB Jr, et al: Surgical treatment of cardiac tumors: a 25-year experience. *Ann Thorac Surg* 1990; 49:612.

145. Bakaeen F, Jaroszewski DE, Rice DC, et al: Outcomes after surgical resection of cardiac sarcoma in the multimodality treatment era. *J Cardiovasc Surg*, 2009; 137:1454-1460.

146. Blackmon SH, Patel A, Reardon MJ: Management of primary cardiac sarcomas. *Expert Rev Cardiovasc Ther.* 2008; 6(9):1217-1222.

147. Bear PA, Moodie DS: Malignant primary cardiac tumors: the Cleveland Clinic experience, 1956–1986. *Chest* 1987; 92:860.

148. Burke AP, Cowan D, Virmani R: Primary sarcomas of the heart. *Cancer* 1922; 69:387.

149. Putnam JB, Sweeney MS, Colon R, et al: Primary cardiac sarcomas. *Ann Thorac Surg* 1991; 51:906.

150. Rettmar K, Stierle U, Shiekhzadeh A, et al: Primary angiosarcoma of the heart: report of a case and review of the literature. *Jpn Heart J* 1993; 34:667.

151. Hermann MA, Shankerman RA, Edwards WD, et al: Primary cardiac angiosarcoma: a clinicopathologic study of six cases. *J Thorac Cardiovasc Surg* 1992; 102:655.

152. Wiske PS, Gillam LD, Blyden G, et al: Intracardiac tumor regression documented by two-dimensional echocardiography. *Am J Cardiol* 1986; 58:186.

153. Reardon MJ, DeFelice CA, Sheinbaum R, et al: Cardiac autotransplant for surgical treatment of a malignant neoplasm. *Ann Thorac Surg* 1999; 67:1793.

154. Miralles A, Bracamonte MD, Soncul H, et al: Cardiac tumors: clinical experience and surgical results in 74 patients. *Ann Thorac Surg* 1991; 52:886.

155. Winer HE, Kronzon I, Fox A, et al: Primary chondromyxosarcoma: clinical and echocardiographic manifestations: a case report. *J Thorac Cardiovasc Surg* 1977; 74:567.

156. Torsveit JF, Bennett WA, Hinchcliffe WA, et al: Primary plasmacytoma of the atrium: report of a case with successful surgical management. *J Thorac Cardiovasc Surg* 1977; 74:563.

157. Nzayinambaho K, Noel H, Brobet C: Primary cardiac liposarcoma simulating a left atrial myxoma. *J Thorac Cardiovasc Surg* 1985; 40:402.

158. Burke AP, Virmani R: Osteosarcomas of the heart. *Am J Surg Pathol* 1991; 15:289.

159. Neragi-Miandoab S, Kim J, Vlahakes GJ: Malignant tumours of the heart: a review of tumour type, diagnosis and therapy. *Clin Oncol (R Coll Radiol)* 2007; 19:748-756.

160. Centofani P, Di Rosa E, Deorsola L, et al: Primary cardiac tumors: early and late results of surgical treatment in 91 patients. *Ann Thorac Surg* 1999; 68:1236-1241.

161. Zhang PJ, Brooks, JS, Goldblum JR, et al: Primary cardiac sarcomas: a clinicopathologic analysis of a series with follow-up information in 17 patients and emphasis on long-term survival. *Human Pathology* 2008; 39:1385-1395.

162. Bossert Torsten B, Gummert JF, Battellini, et al: Surgical experience with 77 primary cardiac tumors. *Interact Cardiovasc Thorac Surg* 2005; 4:311-315.

163. Simpson L, Kumar SK, Okuno SH, et al: Malignant primary cardiac tumors: review of a single institution experience. *Cancer* 2008; 112(11):2440-2446.

164. Kim CH, Dancer JY, Coffey D, et al: Clinicopathologic study of 24 patients with primary cardiac sarcomas: a 10-year single institution experience. *Hum Pathol* 2008; 39:933-938.

165. Blackmon SH, Patel AR, Bruckner BA, et al: Cardiac Autotransplantation for malignant or complex primary left heart tumors. *Tex Heart Inst J* 2008; 35(3):296-300.

166. Gabelman C, Al-Sadir J, Lamberti J, et al: Surgical treatment of recurrent primary malignant tumor of the left atrium. *J Thorac Cardiovasc Surg* 1979; 77(6):914-921.

167. Gowdamarajan A, Michler RE: Therapy for primary cardiac tumors: is there a role for heart transplantation? *Curr Opin Cardiol* 2000; 15:121.

168. Reardon MJ, Walkes JC, DeFelice CA, Wojciechowski Z: Cardiac autotransplant for surgical resection of a primary malignant left ventricular tumor. *Tex Heart Inst J* 2006; 33(4):495-497.

169. Conklin LD, Reardon MJ: Autotransplantation of the heart for primary cardiac malignancy: development and surgical technique. *Tex Heart Inst J* 2002; 29(2):105-108.

170. Takagi M, Kugimiya T, Fuii T, et al: Extensive surgery for primary malignant lymphoma of the heart. *J Cardiovasc Surg* 1992; 33:570.

171. Blackmon SH, Rice DR, Correa AM, et al: Management of primary main pulmonary artery sarcomas. *Ann Thorac Surg* 2009; 87(3):977-984.

172. Baker PB, Goodwin RA: Pulmonary artery sarcomas: a review and report of a case. *Arch Pathol Lab Med* 1985; 109:35-39.

173. Schmookler BM, Marsh HB, Roberts WC: Primary sarcoma of the pulmonary trunk and/or right or left main pulmonary artery: a rare cause of obstruction to right ventricular outflow: report on two patients and analysis of 35 previously described patients. *Am J Med* 1977; 63:263-272.

174. Conklin LD, Reardon MJ: The technical aspects of the Ross procedure. *Tex Heart Inst J* 2001; 28(3):186-189.

175. Golstein DJ, Oz MC, Rose EA, et al: Experience with heart transplantation for cardiac tumors. *J Heart Lung Transplant* 1995; 14:382.

176. Baay P, Karwande SV, Kushner JP, et al: Successful treatment of a cardiac angiosarcoma with combined modality therapy. *J Heart Lung Transplant* 1994; 13:923.

177. Crespo MG, Pulpon LA, Pradas G, et al: Heart transplantation for cardiac angiosarcoma: should its indication be questioned? *J Heart Lung Transplant* 1993; 12:527.

178. Jeevanandam V, Oz MC, Shapiro B, et al: Surgical management of cardiac pheochromocytoma: resection versus transplantation. *Ann Surg* 1995; 221:415.

179. Yuh DD, Kubo SH, Francis GS, et al: Primary cardiac lymphoma treated with orthotopic heart transplantation: a case report. *J Heart Lung Transplant* 1994; 13:538.

180. Goldstein DJ, Oz MC, Michler RE: Radical excisional therapy and total cardiac transplantation for recurrent atrial myxoma. *Ann Thorac Surg* 1995; 60:1105.

181. Pillai R, Blauth C, Peckham M, et al: Intracardiac metastasis from malignant teratoma of the testis. *J Thorac Cardiovasc Surg* 1986; 92:118.

182. Aburto J, Bruckner BA, Blackmon SH, Beyer EA, Reardon MJ: Renal cell carcinoma, metastatic to the left ventricle. *Texas Heart Inst J* 2009; 36(1):48-49

183. Hallahan ED, Vogelzang NJ, Borow KM, et al: Cardiac metastasis from soft-tissue sarcomas. *J Clin Oncol* 1986; 4:1662.

184. Press OW, Livingston R: Management of malignant pericardial effusion and tamponade. *J Am Med Assoc* 1987; 257:1008.

185. Hanfling SM: Metastatic cancer to the heart: review of the literature and report of 127 cases. *Circulation* 1960; 2:474.

186. Weinberg BA, Conces DJ Jr, Waller BF: Cardiac manifestation of noncardiac tumors: I. Direct effects. *Clin Cardiol* 1989; 12:289.

187. Caccavale RJ, Newman J, Sisler GE, Lewis RH: Pericardial disease, in Kaiser LR, Daniel TM (eds): *Thorascopic Surgery*. Boston, Little, Brown, 1993; p 177.

188. Prager RL, Dean R, Turner B: Surgical approach to intracardial renal cell carcinoma. *Ann Thorac Surg* 1982; 33:74.

189. Vaislic CD, Puel P, Grondin P, et al: Cancer of the kidney invading the vena cava and heart: results after 11 years of treatment. *J Thorac Cardiovasc Surg* 1986; 91:604.

190. Shahian DM, Libertino JA, Sinman LN, et al: Resection of cavoatrial renal cell carcinoma employing total circulatory arrest. *Arch Surg* 1990; 125:727.

191. Theman TE: Resection of atriocaval adrenal carcinoma (letter). *Ann Thorac Surg* 1990; 49:170.

192. Cooper MM, Guillem J, Dalton J, et al: Recurrent intravenous leiomyomatosis with cardiac extension. *Ann Thorac Surg* 1992; 53:139.

193. Phillips MR, Bower TC, Orszulak TA, et al: Intracardiac extension of an intracaval sarcoma of endometrial origin. *Ann Thorac Surg* 1995; 59:742.

194. Tomescu O, Barr F: Chromosomal translocations in sarcomas: prospects for therapy. *Trends Mol Med* 2001; 7:554.

195. Graadt van Roggen JF, Bovee JVMG, et al: Diagnostic and prognostic implications of the unfolding molecular biology of bone and soft tissue tumors. *J Clin Pathol* 1999; 52:481.

196. Waters JS, Webb A, Cunningham D, et al: Phase I clinical and pharmacokinetic study of BCL-2 antisense oligonucleotide therapy in patients with non-Hodgkin's lymphoma. *J Clin Oncol* 2000; 18:1812.

197. Casey M, Vaughan CJ, He J, et al: Mutations in the protein kinase R1α regulatory subunit cause familial cardiac myxomas and Carney complex. *J Clin Invest* 2000; 106:R31.

198. Goldstein MM, Casey M, Carney JA, et al: Molecular genetic diagnosis of the familial myxoma syndrome (Carney complex). *Am J Med Genet* 1999; 86:62.

199. Van Siegenhorst M, de Hoogt R, Hermans C, et al: Identification of the tuberous sclerosis gene *TSC1* on chromosome 9q34. *Science* 1997; 277:805.

200. The European Chromosome 16 Tuberous Sclerosis Consortium: Identification and characterization of the tuberous sclerosis gene on chromosome 16. *Cell* 1993; 75:1305.

201. Ramlawi B, Al-Jabbari O, Blau LN, et al: Autotransplantation for the resection of complex left heart tumors. *Ann Thorac Surg* 2014; 98(3):863-868.

202. Ramlawi B, David EA, Kim MP, et al: Contemporary surgical management of cardiac paragangliomas. *Ann Thorac Surg* 2012; 93(6):1972-1976.

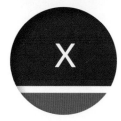

TRANSPLANT AND MECHANICAL CIRCULATORY SUPPORT

Immunobiology of Heart and Lung Transplantation

Bartley P. Griffith • Agnes Azimzadeh

59

For over 40 years, cardiac and lung transplantation have achieved remarkable one-year patient survivals beyond 90% and conditional half-lives of 13 and 7.9 years, respectively.[1] While surgeons must acquire the technical expertise to perform these often demanding surgeries, long-term graft outcomes and the recipients' well-being benefit from a multidisciplinary team well versed in the basics of the immunology of transplantation. Comfort with treating patients who receive immunosuppressive therapies, both conventional and innovative, requires familiarity with the nonsurgical language of transplantation. The goal of this enhanced chapter is to squeeze the essentials into an understandable short text. The core features of the alloresponse are presented with some specific references unique to heart and lung allografts. These include (1) histocompatibility; (2) activation of alloresponse T lymphocytes; (3) T-cell–mediated rejection (TMR); (4) antibody-mediated rejection (AMR); (5) immunosuppressive therapy; (6) surveillance for rejection; (7) immune monitoring; and (8) emerging regulators of immunity.

MAJOR HISTOCOMPATIBILITY COMPLEX

Major histocompatibility complex (MHC) molecules are a family of proteins that vary quite a lot between individuals (genetic polymorphism) and represent the molecular basis for how people's immune systems distinguish "self" from "nonself" with respect to infections and transplants. Human MHC molecules are known as human leukocyte antigens (HLA) because they are expressed at high levels on leukocytes and were first measured on peripheral blood lymphocytes. HLA are heterodimeric glycoproteins expressed on the surface of almost every cell in the human body. If recognized by an organ recipient, these proteins can trigger rejection. This is known as allorecognition.

HLA molecules on donor cells or HLA fragments, shed from thoracic organ transplants, are determined to be foreign by the immune system of the host. Intact HLA molecules expressed on the surface of cells serve two key functions in the context of transplantation. Fragments of foreign proteins, including fragments of HLA molecules, are presented in the binding groove of HLA and are recognized by T-cell receptors (TCRs) of the recipient that happen to have high affinity for that protein fragment in the context of self HLA (indirect donor antigen presentation). In addition, recipient T-cells directly recognize donor HLA as "foreign" (direct donor antigen presentation).

The genes coding for these antigens are located on the short arm of chromosome 6. This region spans over 4 million base pairs in length and encodes for over 200 genes in three regions: Class I, Class II, and Class III (Fig. 59-1). HLA owns the most polymorphic title in man as more than 5000 types have been recognized.

Classic Class I HLA proteins/antigens are HLA-A, HLA-B, and more recently HLA-C. The α-light chain is encoded in the MHC; however, the β-chain is β-2-microglobulin that is encoded on chromosome 15. When folded, the α-heavy chain contains the peptide binding region which presents peptide antigen to the T-cell. Class I antigens are constitutively expressed on nearly all cells. Expression of Class I molecules (Fig. 59-2) is upregulated on the endothelium and parenchymal cells in association with inflammation, including after ischemia and reperfusion.

Classic Class II HLA proteins/antigens are HLA-DR, HLA-DRw, HLA-DQ, and more recently HLA-DP. These proteins consist of an α-heavy chain and a β-light chain, both of which are encoded in the MHC. When folded, the α-heavy chain and β-light chain come together with each contributing part of the peptide binding region (Fig. 59-2). Class II antigens are expressed mainly on B-cell lymphocytes, activated T-cells, monocytes/macrophages, and dendritic cells. Other cell types, such as endothelial cells, may express Class II antigen expression after activation.

Each person has two different HLA genes at each HLA locus (HLA-A, B, D, etc.) HLA antigens are co-dominantly expressed on the cell surface so that each cell has two different HLA proteins for each HLA locus. HLA "haplotype" (the sequence of A, B, D genes on one chromosome) is usually inherited as a group from each parent in a Mendelian fashion. Thus, two offspring of the same parents have a 50% chance of inheriting one identical haplotype, 25% chance of inheriting two identical haplotypes, and 25% chance of

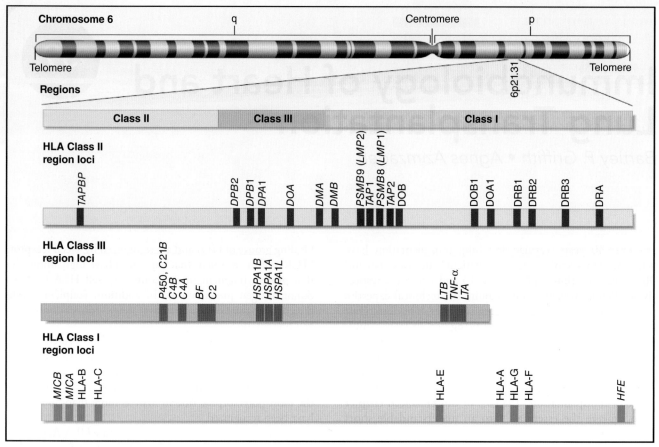

FIGURE 59-1 The major histocompatibility complex is divided into three regions or classes: Class I, Class II, and Class III.

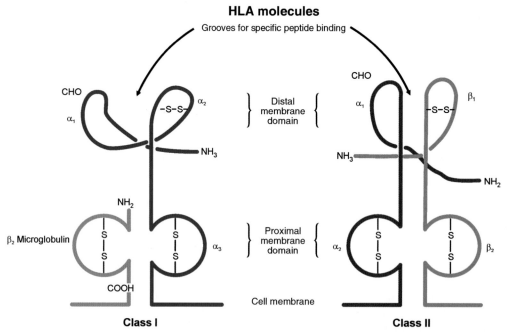

FIGURE 59-2 Class I and II HLA molecules are made up of polypeptidic chains with intrachain disulfide bonds. The α_1 and α_2 distal domains of Class I and the α_1 and β_1 domains of Class II make up the peptide binding site for alloantigen. (Adapted with permission from Haber E: *Scientific American: Introduction To Molecular Cardiology*. Philadelphia; Elsevier Health Sciences; 1995.)

having no haplotypes in common. In addition, due to the distance between these genes in the MHC, there are "hot spots" of gene recombination. Recombination in offspring occurs approximately 1 to 2% between HLA-A and C, or between HLA-B and HLA-DR, and approximately 30% between HLA-DP and HLA-DQ. Recombination accounts for most of the occasional exceptions to faithful transmission of intact parental haplotypes to their children. HLA haplotypes are found in varying frequencies across the major population groups (White, Hispanic, Black, Asian, and American Indian).

In the early days of organ transplantation, hyperacute rejection occurred due to preexisting IgM alloantibodies. Best-known examples of these are the ABO blood group IgM antibodies. While still a barrier to xenotransplantation (cross-species transplantation), blood group typing has virtually eliminated this particular cause of immediate organ destruction in allotransplantation. Of interest is the success of blood group mismatched organs in neonatal recipients before they develop IgM antibodies to blood group antigens.[2] Antibodies against blood group antigens arise between 6 and 18 months postnatal due to the presence of related carbohydrate antigens on intestinal bacteria. Today, when hyperacute rejection is seen, it is normally caused by preexisting IgG antibodies usually directed against donor HLA proteins. These antibodies are often the result of previous blood-cell transfusions (most particularly multidonor platelets due to the high HLA load) or previous pregnancies or transplants. After wide adoption of the first crossmatch technique by Patel and Terasaki in 1969, hyperacute rejection based on preexisting HLA antibodies became rare.[3] Further improvements in screening for HLA antibodies have nearly eliminated it. Of interest in 1970, against early convention, Terasaki found that HLA-mismatched kidney recipients fared as well as those zero-mismatched recipients.[4] Starzl led the use of mismatched livers first, and soon, except for bone marrow, all followed in kidney, heart, and lung transplants.[5]

While HLA mismatches seem less predictive of outcomes, those recipients who present for transplant with preformed anti-HLA antibodies (prior pregnancies or blood transfusions) or developed antibodies in responses to the mismatches have more rejection. This has led to poor survival in heart and lung recipients.[6-10] There is some evidence that posttransplant removal of these donor-specific antibodies (DSA) can improve the function of kidneys and lungs.[11,12]

ADAPTIVE IMMUNE RESPONSE: T LYMPHOCYTE

Success in heart and lung transplantation requires control over the immune response to donor HLA antigens expressed by the allograft. An adaptive response is initiated by T lymphocytes primed to donor antigens in the peripheral lymphoid tissues and are then recruited into the donor organ where those antigens are expressed. Alloreactive T lymphocytes are primed by alloantigens presented to them on donor (direct) and/or host (indirect) antigen-presenting cells

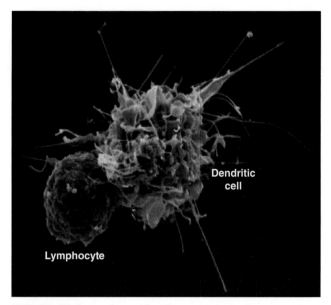

FIGURE 59-3 Dendritic cell with its typical membrane extensions engaged with T lymphocyte. (Used with permission from Institute of Cellular Therapies, Noida, UP 201303, India. www.dendriticcellresearch.com.)

(APCs) (Fig. 59-3). T-cells are the primary immune actors in the pathologic reaction to a transplanted organ. They participate in cytotoxicity and cytokine-mediated inflammation. B cells, antibodies, and macrophages contribute to the destruction of the graft via a variety of effector pathways. Ischemia/reperfusion injury of the allograft triggers innate immunity that can amplify T-cell alloresponse. Molecular modulators of innate immunity have recently been an expanding area of interest. These include cytokines, chemokines, complement, and more recently toll-like receptors (TLRs) and the inflammasome. While APCs are emphasized, B cells and natural killer (NK) cells exert influence on a host's decision to reject an allograft.[13]

T-Lymphocyte Alloactivation

A T-cell can only become triggered to proliferate and differentiate if its TCR finds a fit with foreign peptides bound in the groove of HLA molecules presented on the surface of APCs.[14] "Professional" APCs differ from other HLA-expressing cells in that they also express "co-stimulatory" molecules that efficiently stimulate activation of both the APC and the responding T-cell. These include dendritic cells, B lymphocytes, and macrophages. The peptide HLA antigen complex may be presented by resident *donor* "passenger" APCs found in the transplanted heart or lung (direct presentation) or by the *host's* APCs (indirect presentation) (Fig. 59-4). HLA-peptide antigens become the specific key that fits into a T-cell's specific TCR receptor. In the thymus, T-cells learn to enable their TCR to recognize self-HLA complexes that present endogenous peptides (positive selection). Those cells that recognize self-peptides with a high affinity are deleted

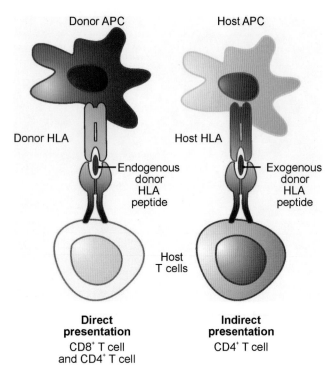

FIGURE 59-4 T cells are stimulated to proliferate when their TCR engages donor peptides processed and presented by an HLA molecule, expressed by donor or host antigen presenting cells (APCs).

(negative selection) so as to reduce the risk of their driving autoimmunity. T-cells that cannot bind self-protein HLA die from neglect. Positive selection occurs only for those T-cells whose affinity for self-protein HLA result in survival but not full proliferation. The T-cell repertoire emerging from the thymus can respond to proteins from various foreign origins (bacteria, viral, transplant). T-cells react against alloantigens because of the crossreactivity of the TCR with self and foreign HLA molecules. Host and passenger donor dendritic cells are thought to be the most efficient type of APCs for activating naive T-cells.

Pathways of Antigen Presentation to Alloreactive T-cells (Signal 1)

Donor passenger APCs transplanted with the heart or lung *directly* process endogenous HLA-derived peptides from within themselves and present them in a groove on surface Class I HLA complexes on their surfaces (Fig. 59-5A). Class I protein MHC complexes presented on the *donor-derived* APCs (key) fit into the TCR (lock) expressed by recipient CD8⁺ T-lymphocytes. This activation pathway, known as the *direct* pathway of peptide presentation, is responsible for the majority of initial T-cell activation reacting to alloantigens and thought to mediate most early events of acute cell-mediated cytotoxicity.[15]

Later alloresponses are focused on CD4⁺ T-cells because they recognize donor-specific HLA peptides presented by Class II surface molecules expressed by *recipient* APCs. These

recipient APCs gradually replace donor APCs transplanted with the heart or lungs of the donor. Host APCs trafficking through the allograft phagocytose interstitial and cellular HLA protein antigens shed from the donor graft (Fig. 59-5B). This shedding is induced when the graft is stressed by ischemia (preservation), inflammation (bacterial and viral infection), and during rejection. Donor proteins undergo endosomic proteolysis and resulting peptides are combined with Class II HLA molecules. Donor peptide Class II HLA complexes are transported to the surface of the host APC and presented *indirectly* as the "key" to the TCR complex "lock" on CD4⁺ T-cells. These T-cells then become activated by the *indirect* pathway. Because CD4⁺ T-cells provide help to donor-specific B cells, later alloresponses tend to be associated with appearance of alloantibody.[16]

In addition to the direct and indirect pathways, a third pathway of antigen presentation involves the transfer of donor cell membrane components, including donor peptide-MHC complexes, to recipient APCs. Transfer can happen by direct cell-cell contact or through the release of very small particles (exosomes) by donor cells, which fuse with recipient APC cell membranes. This process known as the *semi-direct* pathway of antigen presentation pathway leads to presentation, by recipient APCs, of the same strongly crossreactive donor MHC/peptide that drive direct presentation.[17] Finally, it is helpful to distinguish the role of these pathways in the priming versus the effector phase of immune responses.[18]

Activated dendritic cells also provide co-stimulators to the naïve T-cells that are required for a full T-cell response. Macrophages present antigens to differentiated CD4⁺ cells that activate the macrophage to promote cell-mediated immunity. B cells also serve an APC function by presenting antigens to helper T-cells. These then activate the B cell to become part of the effector humoral immune response through production of antibodies (Fig. 59-6).[19]

Pathways of T-Cell Co-Stimulation: Signal 2

In addition to activation of the T-cell by engagement of its TCR with donor peptide/MHC complexes expressed by donor or recipient APCs (**Signal 1**), several other surface molecules participate in T-cell activation. Those that enhance TCR signaling (CD4 and CD8 molecules expressed by CD4⁺ and CD8⁺ T-cells, respectively) are called **co-receptors** because they bind to part of the same HLA molecule that engages the TCR. Another group of T-cell activating surface molecules is called **co-stimulatory receptors** (**Signal 2**) (Fig. 59-7). Blockade of co-stimulatory pathways provides important new possible therapy to prolong organ transplant survival and even reach a tolerant state. Co-stimulatory receptors or ligands on T-cells recognize respective cognitive ligands or receptors presented on APCs or the graft tissue itself. The best defined **co-stimulatory receptor** and ligand pair is the constitutively expressed CD28 T-cell co-stimulatory receptor and its APC ligands B7-1 (CD80) and B7-2 (CD86). This pathway is particularly important in activation of naïve (nonmemory) T-cells. When engaged, these pairs deliver antiapoptotic signals and trigger the expression of cytokines and growth factors, including Interleukin-2 (IL-2) that encourage proliferation of alloantigen-specific CD4+ or CD8+ T-cells. If CD28 is blocked, T-cells may become anergic or apoptose. A second inducible co-stimulatory receptor for B7 molecules has been identified and termed CTLA-4 (CD152). Unlike the structurally homologous CD28, CTLA-4 appears on recently activated T-cells and is a negative regulator that promotes pathways that limit proliferation. It is efficient that the same co-stimulator (B7) can prompt initial proliferative signals via constitutive CD28 engagement and later, when CTLA-4 is induced, subsequently limit signals to the T-cell. Therapeutic targeting of this pathway with CD80 and CD86 blockade with CTLA-4-Ig-like molecules has been effective in primates and multiple clinical trials,[20] and was approved by the US Food and Drug Administration (FDA) for the prevention of acute rejection in adult kidney transplant patients in 2011. Inducible co-stimulator (ICOS) and programmed death-1 (PD-1) are more recent discoveries in the T-cell

CD28 family. When ICOS joins its ligand ICOS-L on an activated APC, it stimulates the T-cell effector response by promoting IL-4 and IL-10 production. PD-1 is the co-receptor for PD-ligands (PD-L1 and PD-L2) and, like CTLA-4, represses T-cell responses.[21]

A second family of co-stimulatory molecules belong to the tumor necrosis factor (TNF) super family.[22] The prototypic pathway is represented by the co-stimulatory receptor CD40 on APC binding to CD40 ligand (CD154) on T-cells. By reciprocal activation, CD154 on T-cells makes the APC "better" and is thought to "license" additional APCs to participate in the T-cell activation process. CD154 can also interact with CD40 expressed by CD8+ T-cells thereby providing direct help from CD4+ to CD8+ T-cells.[23] Moreover, transplantation immunobiology is influenced by the innate immunity directors against substances from microbes, including bacteria, viruses, and fungi. These substances, often nucleic acids, are called pathogen-associated molecular patterns (PAMPs). PAMPs can bind to PAMP-receptors on APCs called TLRs. This engagement has the effect of strengthening the APC

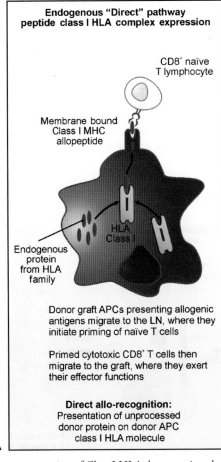

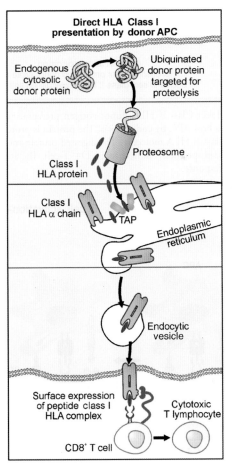

FIGURE 59-5A Direct presentation of Class I HLA donor antigen by donor APCs. Donor-derived APCs (dendritic cells within the transplant) ubiquitinate an endogenous cytosolic (donor) protein and transport it through the proteasome where it is digested. Small proteins move with transporter associated with antigen processing (TAP) into the endoplasmic reticulum where it becomes associated with Class I HLA α-chain. The protein HLA complex locates on the surface of the APC where CD8+ T-cells with TCR "locks" specific for the protein-HLA complex "keys" can associate. The association prompts CD8+ T-cell activation.

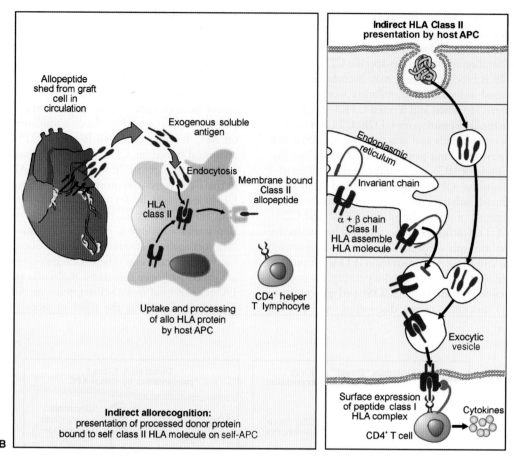

FIGURE 59-5B Indirect Class II HLA donor-antigen presentation by host APCs. Extracellular protein antigen shed from the heart or lung allograft is taken into a host APC by endocytosis. The protein is proteolyzed and transported into the Golgi. There it displaces the invariant chain held α and β-chain Class II HLA molecule. The digested protein molecule finds its specific place within the HLA molecule and is moved to the APC surface where it can specifically adhere to a CD4+ T-cell. The attached CD4+ T-cell with donor-specific TCR is stimulated to proliferate and participate in the alloresponse.

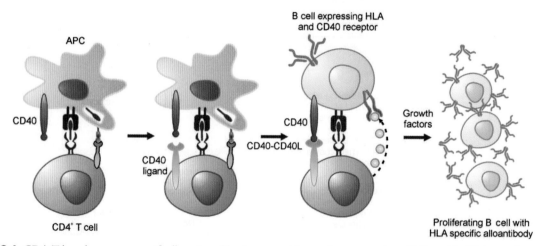

FIGURE 59-6 CD4+ T lymphocytes are specifically activated by donor peptide proteins presented on APC peptide-HLA complexes. These T-cells in turn activate B lymphocytes expressing specific HLA Class II molecules and CD40. The B cells respond to growth factors by proliferation formation of germinal centers and production of specific alloantibody.

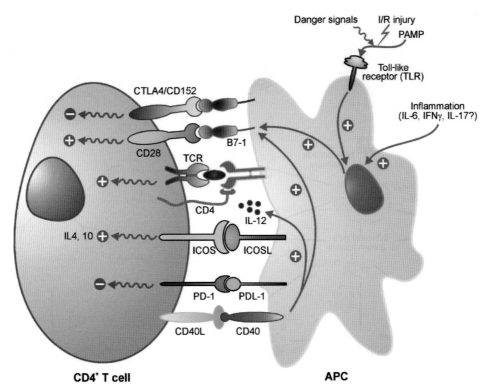

FIGURE 59-7 The process of regulating T-cell (CD4⁺ and CD8⁺) activation involves engagement of the TCR/CD4 or CD8 with the foreign protein-HLA molecule and of several co-stimulators of the co-stimulatory pathway. The constitutively expressed CD28 co-receptor drives proliferation of naïve T-cells when engaged by its ligand B7-1. Inducible CTLA-4 (CD154) co-regulator acts to regulate this process negatively along with its APC-bound B7-2 ligand. Other CD28 family co-receptors include inducible ICOS that signals for proinflammatory IL-4 and IL-10 effector responses and PD-1 that has a negative regulatory effect on the T-cell. The APC is made "better" by a reciprocal activation between T-cells and APCs and the phenomena of "licensing" in which innate receptors (PAMP—Toll receptor) stimulate B7 expression. This has the effect also on the T-cell of inducing CD40 ligand (CD154). CD40 on the APC's membrane drives additional B7 expression and elaboration of IL-12.

response, in part by increasing the expression of co-stimulatory molecules and proinflammatory cytokines, thereby strengthening signal 2.

Additional co-stimulatory molecules were recently discovered and alternative therapeutic approaches are being evaluated in experimental models.[24,25] In addition to promoting full T-cell activation, co-stimulatory signals are also crucially involved in cellular interactions between T and B cells, in which B cells receive *help* from T-cells to become fully activated and differentiate in memory B cells and antibody-producing plasma cells.

MECHANISMS OF GRAFT REJECTION

Cell-Mediated Rejection

Early cell-mediated rejection (CMR) begins with activation of CD8⁺ cells that bear TCR molecules which fit and engage donor-specific peptide-HLA Class I complexes on donor APCs. In the presence of help from CD4⁺ T-cells, they become cytolytic lymphocytes (CTLs) and directly attach to and kill graft endothelial and parenchymal cells bearing the identical donor peptide-HLA Class I complex presented to them by the APC "activators." This is known as the *direct effector pathway* (distinct from direct presentation of HLA

by donor APC) since the CD8 cell directly kills the allotarget. It is responsible for most acute CMR early (in the first few months) after transplant. In the presence of calcium, the protein perforin polymerizes onto the Class I bearing target cell and causes 16- to 20-nm pores to open in the cell membrane and allowing the CTL to release its granular content, including granzyme B and other cytotoxic molecules directly into the target cell, causing its apoptosis. Alternatively, apoptosis (programmed cell death) can also be stimulated in the target cell by interaction of the lymphocyte Fas ligand with the APO-1/Fas receptor of the target cell. Second messengers are elicited that activate endonucleases and proteases to cause fragmentation of DNA and thus organize the dissolution of the Class I bearing donor target cell (Fig. 59-8).

Unlike the CD8⁺ T-cells, the CD4⁺ T-cells primarily follow an *indirect effector pathway* (distinct from indirect presentation of HLA by recipient APC) by secreting various cytokines that drive inflammation and graft loss (Fig. 59-9). IL-2 increases the expression of its own receptors (IL-2R) on CD4⁺ T-cells, driving their proliferation and further differentiation. Activated CD4⁺ T-cells secrete additional lymphokines, including interferon-γ (IFNγ), which along with IL-2 stimulates CD8⁺ CTLs to bind to the allograft cells presenting donor MHC protein molecules. CD4⁺ T-cells are very heterogeneous. Four major categories are now recognized: Th1, Th2, Th17, and

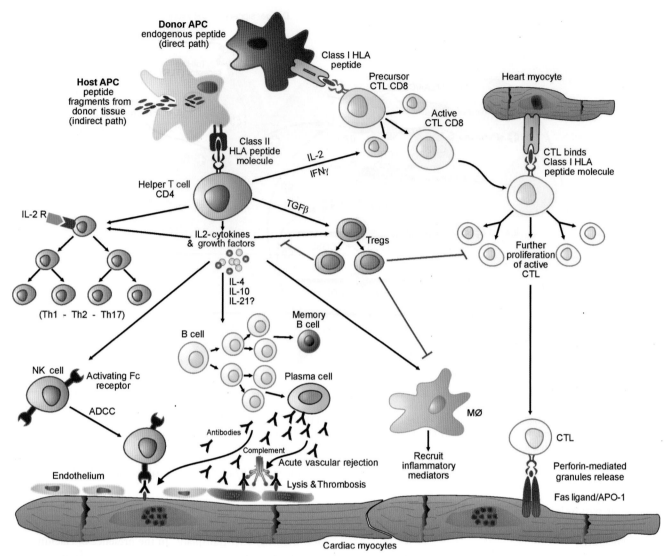

FIGURE 59-8 Complicated scheme of allograft rejection. CD8⁺ lymphocytes become activated by donor-derived dendritic cells transplanted with the allograft. These cells enter a direct alloresponse pathway by proliferating into CTLs. The CTLs recognize and attach to Class I HLA donor peptide molecules on the surface of allograft cells. They directly kill the allotarget through cell-mediated cytotoxicity by injection of proteolytic granules, creating perforin-induced membrane pores and induction of apoptosis. CD4⁺ T-cells are activated by host APCs that engulf donor protein shed from the allograft. The host APCs process the donor protein into surface-bound Class II HLA peptide molecules. The CD4 cells follow an indirect pathway in the alloresponse by proliferating and secreting growth factors plus proinflammatory cytokines. This indirect paracrine function augments CTL proliferation, attracts cellular mediators of inflammation-like macrophages and drives B cell central humoral immunity.

regulatory T-cells (Tregs). Th1 cells are the main mediators of CMR. They produce IFNγ and favor IL-12 production by macrophages. Th2 cells make IL-4, 5, and 13 and promote humoral responses. Th17 produces IL-17, a cytokine recently discovered and involved in inflammation. In conditions where the immune response is partially inhibited, Tregs develop with the ability to inhibit immune responses.

Broad Alloresponse

In severe rejection, B cells join the alloresponse when they receive help from CD4⁺ T-cells (Fig. 59-6). CD4⁺ T-cells are activated by APCs to express CD40L (CD154). Ligand B cells

expressing CD40 and MHC Class II receptors engage helper CD4⁺ T-cells and proliferate. B cells participate in the rejection of allografts by efficiently providing APC function to helper CD4⁺ T-cells and by elaboration of antibodies that (1) recognize and destroy the donor endothelial targets; (2) participate in antibody-dependent cytotoxicity (ADCC), or (3) stimulate the proliferation and migration of activated endothelial cells.[26] In the former, the endothelial antigen/antibody complexes activate the "classical" complement pathway, causing C3 and C5 to cleave, inciting inflammation (C5a) and formation of the membrane attack complex (MAC), which is comprised of C5b complexed with C6, 7, 8, and 9 (C5b-9). The MAC causes vascular cell death by inducing pores to form in the cell

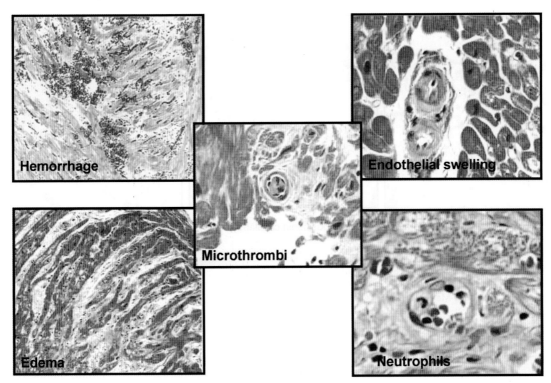

FIGURE 59-9 Histologic evidence of AMR-associated endothelial swelling, inflammation, and thrombosis accompanied by interstitial edema and hemorrhage (H&E staining). (Used with permission from SA Webber.)

membrane. When endothelial cells are activated or killed by complement, this in turn results in microvascular thrombosis and inflammation. ADCC describes the process by which antidonor IgG antibodies coating donor cells bind to the Fcγ RIII receptor of NK lymphocytes (NK cell). Cells of the innate immune system such as NK cells are also present in allografts during rejection. These may react with alloantigens because they constitutively express inhibiting receptors specific for self-HLA Class I molecules or they may engage alloantibody-bound target (donor) cells through their Fcγ receptor. NK cells can not only directly kill target cells by injecting proteolytic enzymes into their cytoplasm, but also modulate immunity by producing proinflammatory cytokines like IFNγ (Fig. 59-8).

Memory T-Cells

With improvement in immunosuppression that limits activation of naïve T-cells, donor-reactive memory cells have been recognized as a previously underappreciated risk to the allograft. This group of donor-reactive cells has an "effector memory" phenotype. This is defined by an immediate and strong recall that is less sensitive to co-stimulation blockade. Memory cells are thought to arise from heterologous immunity. This occurs when there is a resemblance between microbial antigens and donor HLA complex antigens. Some CD4+ and CD8+ cells exposed to Epstein Barr, Herpes Simplex, and cytomegalovirus (CMV) become primed to recognize allogenic HLA molecules. Memory T-cell numbers are proportionately increased following lymphoablative treatment with rabbit ATG or Alemtuzumab (anti-CD52 Ab). It is unclear

whether these memory cells are more resistant to depletion or whether they represent a conversion from naïve T-cells during repopulation. Memory CD4+ cells provide help for the alloresponse. They provide growth and proinflammatory factors that affect CD8+ T-cells and B-cell antibody production. They can illicit the proinflammatory response from nodal-bearing tissue remote from the allograft. Memory CD4+ cells recruit CD8+ cells that infiltrate the allograft across the endothelium. The memory CD8+ cells proliferate and recruit macrophages, neutrophils, and additional activated T effector cells into the donor organ.[27] To date, memory T-cells continue to evade efforts of therapeutic targeting. LFA-1 is one target that is under study for this purpose. Memory T cells are very heterogeneous and have multiple functions.

Antibody-Mediated Rejection

AMR may be defined as a form of acute graft rejection phenotypically characterized by evidence of tissue damage mediated by antigraft antibodies as effectors. The International Society for Heart and Lung Transplantation Working Group has codified specific criteria for cardiac AMR.[28,29] They include clinical evidence of DSA within the recipient, endomyocardial biopsy immunopathologic evidence of complement (specifically C4d and C3d) staining, and endothelial cell and macrophage activation (the latter assessed by CD68 staining). Similar features of AMR have been identified in the lung, although less consensus exists (Figs 59-9 and 59-10).[30]

Although B/plasma cell production of DSA is the essential pathophysiologic mechanism underlying AMR, T-cell

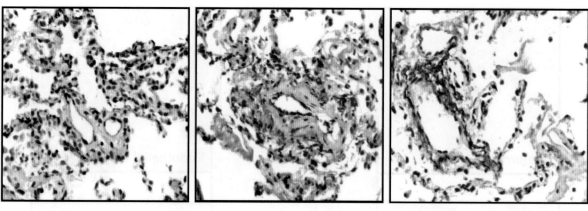

Linear, continuous, subendothelial C4d depositionin capillaries or small arterioles

Interstitium & elastic layer of the arterioles

FIGURE 59-10 Specific C4d deposition on a lung transplant allograft in a recipient with circulating HLA antibody is continuous and subendo-thelial in capillaries and small arterioles (left). Specific C4d has been seen on 31% of transbronchial biopsies in recipients with HLA-Ab. (Ionescu D.N., Transplant Immunology 15(2005) 63-68) (middle). In contrast, nonspecific staining of the interstitium and elastic layer is depicted (right). (Used with permission from K.R. McCurry, M.D.)

help directs and/or influences AMR;[31,32] consequently, AMR should not be thought of as T cell-independent. DSA may be "preformed," that is, present prior to transplantation (see discussion of crossmatching and percent reactive antibody [PRA]), or develop de novo posttransplantation. It has been shown that DSA are identified temporally prior to pathological evidence of AMR[33] and the development of anticardiac myosin immune responses.[34]

Presensitization to HLA Class I or Class II antibodies predisposes to AMR.[35] Those recipients who develop pre-sensitized antibodies, especially donor-specific, risk AMR.[36] In addition to anti-HLA antibodies, non-HLA antibodies, including those against self-antigens such as cardiac myosin, vimentin, and endothelial cells have been less often associ-ated with AMR.[37-39] Cardiac AMR occurs early (weeks to months) after transplant and, if avoided early, rarely occurs later.[40] Classically, histological diagnosis of cardiac AMR has included evidence of endothelial swelling and activation mac-rophages in the graft plus confirming immunofluorescence or immunoperoxidase staining for immunoglobulin (IgG or IgM). While absence of immunofluorescence seems reason-able to rule out AMR, capillary swelling (63%) and mac-rophage vascular adherence (30%)[41] and complement (C3d and C4d) do not. Non-AMR causes of C4d staining include organ reperfusion injury, immunosuppression, treatment with monoclonal antibodies, and viral infections.[42] The dis-tribution (diffuse vs localized) and intensity of the stains has not found a standardization for grading.

The incidence of AMR after heart or lung transplantation is uncertain due to a lack of universal screening in asymp-tomatic recipients. Symptomatic pure AMR without a com-ponent of acute cellular rejection occurs in 10 to 15% of cardiac transplant recipients, but AMR features have been reported in up to 40% of patients with acute cellular rejection (mixed rejection).[43] Clinical symptoms of cardiac AMR are those common in heart failure using echo. A >25% decrease

in ejection fraction and an increase in left ventricular mass distinguished AMR from CMR.[44] Reduced R-wave voltage-conduction abnormalities, including bundle branch block, are electrocardiographic associates.

Desensitization Therapy

Once unacceptable antigens are determined from solid-phase assay (SPA), they can be entered into the United Network for Organ Sharing (UNOS) website (www.unos.org/resources/frm_CPRA_calculator.ASP). This will provide the calculated percent reactive antibody (cPRA). If the percentage chance that any donor is acceptable for transplantation is <50%, then it is reasonable to initiate a desensitization protocol. An optimal protocol has not been established. High-dose intravenous immunoglobulin (IVIG) (2 g/kg/over 2 days q 2-4 weeks), plasmapheresis (1.5 volume exchange × 5 days), monoclonal anti-CD20 B-cell therapy (rituximab 1 g IV weekly × 4), and in the past cyclophosphamide (1 mg/kg/day) have been used in various combinations.

At UCLA, plasmapheresis, IVIG, and rituximab reduced circulatory antibody levels from 70.5 to 30.2%. Heart trans-plantation of these candidates after negative complement-dependent cytotoxicity (CDC) resulted in similar five-year outcomes to control patients and untreated but high PRA patients (81.1, 75.7, and 71.4%). Of interest, the freedom from coronary allograft vasculopathy (CAV) was 74.3, 72.7, and 76.2%, respectively.[45]

It has been agreed that patients waiting for transplantation with circulating HLA antibodies should be studied every three months, and those desensitized every two weeks after therapy. Patients on ventricular assist devices or who receive blood transfusions or with infections should be closely monitored as well. After transplantation donor-specific antibody monitor-ing is recommended at regular intervals and when a humoral rejection event is suspected. Donor-specific titers should be measured daily for 1 to 2 weeks and frequently thereafter in desensitized patients and those considered high risk for antibody response. This higher risk group of recipients is generally treated with thymoglobulin plus IVIG, plasmapheresis, and/or rituximab. Maintenance immunosuppressive therapy that has best controlled cellular and AMR includes tacrolimus, mycophenolate mofetil (MMF), and prednisone.[46]

Recent studies have demonstrated the utility of a multi-pronged approach to the treatment of DSA and AMR. The various components of this approach may suppress DSA production, deplete levels of already generated DSA, or modulate the functionality of DSA in vivo. Glucocorticoids induce B (and T) cell apoptosis,[47] while antiproliferative agents reduce B and T cell generation in the bone marrow. The anti-CD20 monoclonal Ab (mAb) rituximab depletes B cells from the circulation as well as secondary lymphoid organs; most institutional regimens for AMR treatment use rituximab.[48] Similarly, the anti-CD52 mAb alemtuzumab depletes both T and B cells, and has been used to treat AMR.[49] Although preclinical studies of anti-T cell co-stimulation agents such as belatacept (CTLA4-Ig) have shown efficacy in treating solid organ AMR,[50] little evidence is present with respect to thoracic organ AMR clinically.

The therapies above have been shown to reduce DSA and improve AMR. However, none has demonstrated consistent ability to deplete or impair plasma cells, which are generated from differentiated effector B cells are the primary source of antibody (and thus DSA) production. Recent studies have utilized the proteasome inhibitor bortezomib in the treatment of DSA/AMR,[51] with initial successes. Plasmapheresis reduces circulating general antibody and DSA levels, and is also part of most institutional regimens for the treatment of AMR.[52] Exogenous immunoglobulin (Ig) may compete with DSA for Fc receptor binding sites, impairing opsonization.[53] In addition, some amount of Ig may have anti-DSA idiotype specificity, thereby inhibiting DSA (and source B/plasma cell) activity. Finally, with respect to modulation of DSA functionality, novel complement-inhibiting drugs such as the anti-C5 mAb eculizumab have shown promise in kidney AMR, with one case report of usage for hyperacute lung allograft rejection.[54]

Coronary Allograft Vasculopathy and Chronic Cardiac Allograft Dysfunction/Rejection

Although heart transplantation continues to be the therapeutic gold standard for the management of end-stage heart disease, in terms of patient survival outcomes, functional capacity, and cardiac function, its durability is principally limited by chronic cardiac allograft dysfunction. Chronic dysfunction of the transplanted heart is at least associated with and thought to be due to acquired coronary arteriopathy.[55]

Coronary allograft vasculopathy (CAV) and resultant ischemic cardiac allograft dysfunction constitute the leading cause of allograft loss and patient mortality in heart transplant recipients after one year.[28] CAV is characterized by coronary arterial wall thickening with progressive lumen compromise, which is typically diffuse, both with respect to epicardial large vessel involvement and the presence of outflow/runoff small vessel disease.[56]

Similar to chronic lung allograft dysfunction (CLAD) in lung transplantation, a combination of allo-specific adaptive and innate immune stimuli and responses (see section on CLAD below) result in local vascular inflammation and damage of cardiac allografts. Both T and B cell responses have been implicated in the pathogenesis of CAV.[57] Endothelial cells may also function as professional Ag presenting cells and, consistent with this, inducibly express MHC Class II in the context of inflammation.[58] Thus with respect to direct alloantigen recognition, not only are antidonor HLA Class I-specific T-cells important in mediating CAV, but so too are antidonor HLA Class II-specific T-cells. In addition, antibodies directed against donor MHC and other endothelial antigens are known to be important to the development of CAV.[59-61]

Recently, it has been recognized that similarities between CAV and atherosclerotic coronary artery disease (CAD) have implications for the pathogenesis of CAV. Specifically, innate immune system-mediated vessel wall inflammation and damage is present in both settings, with resultant medial proliferation and even lipid deposition. Inflammatory signaling mediated by TLRs has been shown to facilitate CAV in experimental model systems.[62] Consistent with this, preclinical data suggest that antiproliferative agents may attenuate CAV. Sirolimus, which along with related mammalian target of rapamycin (mTOR) inhibitors are the majority of agents used in drug-eluding stents (DES), has exhibited promising results in preventing and treating CAV, either as systemic therapy[63] or in DES used for percutaneous coronary interventions (PCI) in instances of stenoses amenable to PCI.[64] In addition, the statin HMG-CoA reductase inhibitors and other drugs that regulate lipid metabolism have shown some promise in preclinical experimental studies.[65]

Chronic Lung Allograft Dysfunction and Chronic Rejection

Lung transplantation is hampered by relatively poor, long-term recipient survival, which is principally due to progressive CLAD. CLAD is due to fibrous obliteration of small airways termed obliterative bronchiolitis and the recently included restrictive allograft syndrome.[66]

Both allo-specific and nonallo-specific injurious stimuli are capable of triggering immune responses and mediate allograft damage. Allo-specific stimuli with resultant allo-specific immune responses historically have been the primary focus of immunologic investigation, and thus are the best understood.

Nonallo-specific injury may also trigger allo-specific or nonallo-specific immune responses. Infection and aspiration of gastric contents clearly induce lung injury, and some experimental studies of gastric acid-induced lung allograft injury in a unilateral lung transplant model have demonstrated disproportionate or exclusive damage to the allograft, suggestive of an allo-specific component to the immune response elicited against the generalized inflammatory stimulus. With respect to T-cell–mediated immunity, this may be due to enhanced exposure of donor MHC or MHC fragments, resulting in heightened TCR engagement and Signal 1 or inflammation-induced enhancement of expression and/or activity of co-stimulatory molecules on donor or recipient antigen-presenting cells, Signal 2. Finally, nonallo-specific injurious stimuli, such as ischemia/reperfusion injury, infection, and reflux-induced aspiration,[67] induce activation of the innate (nonadaptive) immune system. Ischemia/reperfusion injury is linked to subsequent development of CLAD, whereas the latter two mechanisms induce lung injury that is not restricted to the allograft.

Immunologic Tolerance

Generally, the T-cell repertoire is edited during T-cell development in the thymus to delete clones that are self-reactive (*central tolerance*). Mechanisms responsible for tolerance to transplant-specific HLA antigens not present in the thymus occur in the periphery (*peripheral tolerance*). These include cell death of alloreactive T-cells by apoptosis (deletion), induction of functional unresponsiveness (anergy or ignorance), and active regulation of alloimmunity by either donor-antigen–specific or nondonor-antigen–specific mechanisms (regulation). Partial anergy has been induced by exposing CD4$^+$ T-cells to MHC antigen in the absence of co-stimulation,[68] although it influences naive responses rather than those of memory. Much of the current interest has been in better understanding of a subset of CD4$^+$ T-cells called regulatory T-cells (Tregs) whose function is to suppress immune responses and to maintain tolerance of "self."[69,70] Natural Tregs develop in the thymus in response to self-antigens and are important in autoimmunity. In addition, upon antigen exposure in the periphery, CD4$^+$ T-cells can convert to a regulatory phenotype forming a population of inducible (iTregs), recently renamed peripheral Tregs (pTregs).[71] TGF-β, IL-2, and B7/CTLA-4 co-stimulation are required for nTreg production and survival. It remains to be fully elucidated how these molecules direct naïve T-cells to differentiate into effector, memory, or regulatory phenotypes under various clinically relevant circumstances. Most Tregs express the IL-2 receptor α chain (CD25) and the transcription factor Foxp3. nTregs but not pTregs are thought to express the transcription factor Helios.[70] Foxp3 is a forkhead family transcription factor important for Treg-suppressive function but is also found in activated T-cells in man and thus is not specific to identify human Tregs. Additional markers are used to identify Tregs, such as CD127 (IL-7Rα) and CD45RA. Finally, analysis of spontaneously tolerant kidney recipients has demonstrated a subset of B-cell genes associated with an upregulation of CD20 mRNA.[72]

There has been limited success in translation of laboratory rodent-based tolerance protocols in clinical practice. Freedom from immunosuppression rarely is accomplished universally in strictly controlled large animal models. Management of preexisting memory cells not inhibited by blockage of co-stimulation appears to be a major hurdle. Finally, redundant effector cell mechanisms, cytokines, and co-stimulatory pathways make single or even dual approaches seem underpowered to establish tolerance in the clinic. There has been a limited number of patients in whom tolerance was induced by a regimen, inducing a mixed allogeneic chimerism (coexistence of recipient and donor cells) for kidney allografts. However, work in the nonhuman primate model showed that even this highly tolerogenic regimen did not induce tolerance to cardiac allografts.[73] Heart and lung allografts are less easily amenable to tolerance than kidney, in other words, are more immunogenic.[74]

HLA Antibody Analysis
SEROLOGICAL TESTING

The serological lymphocytotoxic assay for antibody "screening" is based on mixing patient serum (unknown) with a panel of cells whose HLA typing is known and adding complement (or CDC assay). If antibodies are present in the patient serum that react with the cell's HLA molecules, cell death occurs due to complement activation. This method is limited to detection of antibodies represented by the panel of antigens tested and by issues of sensitivity and accuracy. The specificity of the antigen to which the antibody is reacting (HLA or non-HLA antibody) is sometimes not clear due to the presence of other proteins in the patient serum, or to the antibody isotype (IgG or IgM, etc.; some antibody isotypes do not fix complement), and the titer (low, high) is not determined. Several enhancements of this assay were developed to address these issues: (1) heat or chemical treatment of the patient serum to inactivate IgM antibodies and identify IgG antibodies which were felt to be more important to outcomes; (2) additional washes of the target cells following incubation of the patients serum to "wash off" the nonspecific reactants, and (3) addition of anti-human globulin (AHG) to the reaction to increase the detection of low titer IgG antibody (CDC-AHG method). There are other subvariations of these serological enhancements.

The antibody-screening assay consists of a "panel" of known HLA-typed cells, with each cell representing a unique set of antigen targets for the serum to react. The assay generates the "panel reactive antibody (PRA)" titer, which is reported out as a percent of the prospective donor pool that would likely be killed by the patient's serum. The result of this analysis is termed percent calculated PRA or %cPRA. The % cPRA gives a better indication of the patient's likelihood of having a compatible offer of a UNOS deceased donor organ because it is based upon actual UNOS-typed donors. The panel may consist of any number of cells; however, minimally, cells from at least 30 carefully selected individuals are needed to cover the most common HLA antigen targets. In addition to the %PRA, the specificity of the antigen targets could be identified based upon the individual cell reactions. The more different HLA antigens to which the patient is sensitized, the higher the %PRA and the less likely the patient is to have a compatible donor identified. Using conventional matching criteria, %PRA >10% and >25% have been associated with incrementally lower survival large registry reports.

Despite the use of enhancing techniques, serological antibody screening and methods of identification are not able to detect reliably low levels of HLA antibody, and are relatively poor for characterizing Class II antibody.

SOLID PHASE FLOW CYTOMETRIC ANALYSIS

With the development of polymerase chain reaction (PCR) technique in the 1990s, testing with HLA antigen proteins testing could be performed. SPA were then developed in which a specific recombinant HLA protein antigen could be bound to the "solid" surface of a plate, well and now beads.

The development of solid-phase, "microbead"-based flow cytometry assays represent a monumental improvement from the initial solid-phase enzyme-linked immunosorbent assay antibody screening and techniques for identification. The use of fluorescent dyes is foremost as report molecules, allowing detection of the antigen-antibody reactions using a flow cytometer. Fluorescent dye light emissions are several-fold more sensitive than colorimetric dyes. The detection of the antibody-antigen reaction is made using beads coated with HLA molecules. Each HLA molecule-specific bead is identified by its unique mixture of two fluorescent dye colors incorporated into the bead. A secondary antihuman antibody is conjugated to a reporter molecule, in this case, to a fluorescent dye of another color. The higher the titer of the antibody in the patient's serum, the more antibody is available to react to the antigen conjugated to the bead, and the more intense is binding of the secondary fluoresceinated antibody. The more reporter dye becomes bound to the bead complex, the more fluorescent emission is produced from the bead when analyzed by the flow cytometer. The fluorescent emission signal of each bead type is then averaged and the normalized value is reported as the "mean fluorescence intensity (MFI)" of the bead. For most laboratories, the MFI value ≥ 1000 is considered to be a positive reaction for the presence of the HLA antibody. This cutoff was derived as twice the MFI value for the negative control serum.

SPAs can now be used to classify heart and lung candidates as having no HLA antibodies, HLA antibodies without donor specificity or those with donor-specific HLA antibodies (DSA).

The HLA antigen is sourced from recombinant cell lines and is conjugated directly to the microbead, not simply captured. This allowed manufacturing of beads coated not only with the antigens of a single individual mimicking a cell ("multiantigen beads"), but also with a single HLA antigen ("single-antigen beads"). These single antigens can be further described to the exact HLA allele of that antigen. Since individuals become sensitized to the amino acid epitopes encoded by the antigen allele, microbead-based antibody analysis opened a completely new level of insight into characterizing antibodies contained in patient serum. This process is called "epitope mapping." In combination with allele-level typing of patients and potential donors, epitope mapping of antibodies can better predict outcomes of transplants in highly

sensitized patients. The flow cytometer instrument may be either a larger instrument, which can acquire data from cells or beads, or a mini-flow cytometer, which only acquires data from beads, such as a Luminex instrument (Fig. 59-11).

The results of the serum antibody test and the donor crossmatch are interpreted together as a final assessment of recipient and donor compatibility. Composite MFI values of 4000 or greater are generally predictive of a positive flow crossmatch. This composite MFI value is derived from the "sum of MFI values" and the single-antigen antibody analysis for "each" donor target antigen present, either Class I or Class II. This is a rule of thumb, as cellular expression of these target antigens varies. Most centers will post unacceptable antigens in UNOS for those single antigens with MFI values of 4000 or greater, since these single antigens alone may result in a positive flow crossmatch with donors. Based upon these MFI values, a "virtual" or *in silico* crossmatch can be reliable in predicting the actual cellular crossmatch, especially with high MFI values.

HLA Crossmatch

VIRTUAL CROSSMATCH

Practical realities of matching sensitized candidates with nonlocal donors resulted in the acceptance of the virtual crossmatch (VXM).[75,76] The VXM is a comparison of the donor HLA genotype determined by organ procurement organizations to the gene families represented by beads that bound antibody from the sensitized candidate recipient. If gene families are shared between donor and the bead, the VXM is positive. For example, a candidate with antibodies against A1, A11, and B7 by Luminex single-antigen beads would be incompatible with a donor typed as A11, A25, B55, and B57.[77] The anti-A1 antibody determined by SPA corresponds to the donor-typed A1. While currently there is no method to determine the functional characteristics of the antibodies, recently it was estimated that the positive predicative value of an incompatible VXM compared with cytotoxic crossmatch was nearly 80%. UNOS has standardized HLA molecular data typing to include HLA A, B, C, DRB1 and DQB1. Most centers refuse nonlocal donors based on an incompatible VXM and insist on a prospective CDC-AHG crossmatch for sensitized patients when possible.

Non-HLA Antibodies

It has become increasingly clear that non-HLA antibodies can cause injury in thoracic organ transplants.[78,79] About 16% of HLA antibody negative heart recipients may lose their graft to the mixed diagnosis of primary failure within 30 days of transplant.[80] SPA does not detect non-HLA antibodies, *but flow cytometry methods can detect MICA/B*. Antibodies-to-donor endothelial antigens are the largest poorly discussed group of clinically important non-HLA antibodies. These include endothelial, auto-antibodies and those to MHC Class I chain A (MICA) and B (MICB). Endothelial antigen targets may exist, constitutively or as induced auto-antigens

Purified HLA antigen is coated onto the colored microspheres

IgG antibodies in the patient serum react with the HLA A2 antigen (protein) molecules on the bead surface

Secondary anti-Human IgG antibody conjugated to fluorescent dye

Microspheres in a fluid stream

Precision fluidics align the microspheres in single file, and pass them through the lasers one at a time

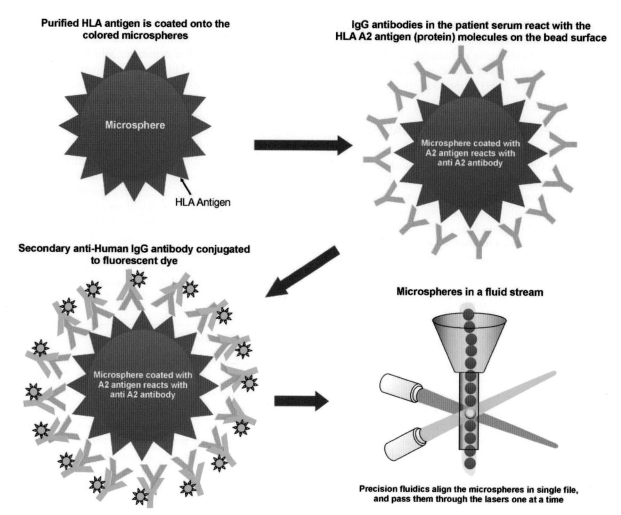

FIGURE 59-11 Solid-phase microbead-based assays for HLA antibodies have improved sensitivity and specificity of detection. Single HLA antigens from recombinant cell lines are conjugated to a colored microsphere. The bead is reacted against candidate or recipient serum resulting in the specific adherence of circulating antibody to the selected HLA antigen. The microsphere HLA-serum antibody is reacted to an antihuman IgG antibody conjugated to a fluorescent dye. The microsphere complex is channeled through a flow cytometer and mean fluorescence intensity (MFI) for the combined emitting dye is measured. (Adapted with permission from Luminex Corporation, Austin, TX.)

due to activation of the endothelium. MICA and MICB are polymorphic antigens expressed on epithelial and, to an unknown extent, on endothelial cells. MICA antibodies may occur in up to 20% of candidates and have been associated with poorer survival but not increased rejection.[80]

"Auto-antibodies" against conserved (nonpolymorphic) proteins are frequently found in the blood of thoracic transplant recipients in association with chronic rejection. Vimentin (an intracellular cytoskeletal protein found in vessel walls and activated lymphocytes), cardiac proteins (cardiac myosin), and collagen type V (expressed mainly in the lung) are among the antigens against which auto-antibodies have been described. Antivimentin antibodies form earlier than anti-HLA after transplantation and are a response in up to 30% of heart recipients to exposure of antigens mounted on the surface of damaged and activated cells.[81] Antivimentin antibodies reflect tissue injury but might also activate platelets and neutrophils.[82] Antiheart antibodies exist preoperatively

in some patients due to their primary cardiac disease. At present, it is difficult to know their true significance. Finally, IgM non-HLA antibodies are cytotoxic and can react to all leukocytes, even the patient's own. Antigen specificity is unknown as is the clinical relevance.

Gene Expression Profiling: XDx Allomap

A DNA microarray-based real-time PCR-derived biosignature for cardiac rejection has been developed by XDx, the maker of Allomap molecular expression testing. Gene expression profiling (GEP) of circulatory leukocytes measures 11 informative genes associated with ACR and scores their expression detected by PCR technology.[83] Several pathways were identified that participate in regulation of effector cell activation, trafficking and morphology, platelet activation, plus corticosteroid sensitivity. These included PDCD1 and ITGA4 for T-cell activation and migration, ILIR2 steroid-responsive gene, the decoy for IL-2, and WDR40A plus CMIR of the micro-RNA gene family. Peripheral blood samples are assigned a score with higher numbers associated with progressive risk of lack of immunological quiescence. This approach was recently randomized against surveillance endomyocardial biopsy in a multicenter trial in low-risk rejection cardiac recipients, 6 months to 5 years after transplantation.[84] The evaluation excluded recipients with a significant history of rejection, CAV, or allograft dysfunction. Results indicated 14.5% of patients profiled versus 15.3% of those surveilled by endomyocardial biopsy reached a composite endpoint of allograft loss/rejection with hemodynamic compromise, graft dysfunction due to other causes, death, or retransplantation. The low risk for rejection of the enrolled patients made interpretation to earlier and higher risk recipients problematic.[85] Other reports found that the profiled genes regulatory T-cell homeostasis and corticosteroid sensitivity can distinguish mild from moderate and severe rejection and are evident before histological, detectable rejection.[86,87] Currently, results of GEP by Allomap suggest surveillance endomyocardial biopsy in low-risk recipients may be avoided.[28,85]

Functional Activity of Immune System

A long imagined goal of selective treatment based on a quantitative assessment of the net state of immunosuppression has been approached clinically with some success. An assay from peripheral blood has been developed (Cylex, ImmuKnow, Columbia, MD) to measure the intracellular concentration of adenosine triphosphate (ATP) of activated lymphocytes. ImmuKnow measures T-cell responses by quantifying ATP activity[88] to phytohemaglutinin, a T-cell mitogen. In general, the collective studies suggest that ATP levels < 200 ng/mL correlate with an increased risk of infection.[89] In a study in 296 heart recipients spanning two weeks to 10 years posttransplant, infection in 39 recipients occurred with an average 187 + 126 ng/ATP/mL versus a steady state of 280 + 126 ng/ATP/mL. Rejection scores in eight recipients averaged 328 ng/ATP/mL and did not differ from baseline. However, three of eight with AMR scored 491 versus 280 ng/ATP/mL.[89] This assay opens the field to personalized immunosuppression that might help balance risks of infection and rejection.

IMMUNOSUPPRESSION

Outcomes following heart and lung transplantation have followed the developments in renal and transplant trials of immunosuppressants (Fig. 59-12). Early reliance on high doses of prednisone and the antimetabolic azathioprine permitted enough success for the field to advance but limited the rates of patient survival to well below current standards of more than 10 years for heart and five years for lung. This early regimen was associated with morbid infection and rapidly progressive episodes of acute rejection. Earlier, it was easy to pick out our patients by their steroid-induced Cushingoid appearances, spine and hip fractures, cataracts, and persistent hyperglycemia. Bone marrow suppression was common, and it was always a battle to achieve adequate doses of

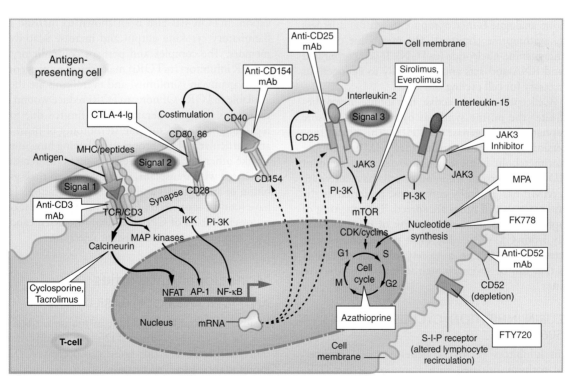

FIGURE 59-12 Individual immunosuppressive drugs and sites of action in the "Three-Signal" T-cell activation model. (Reproduced with permission from Halloran PF: Immunosuppressive drugs for kidney transplantation, *N Engl J Med.* 2004 Dec 23;351(26):2715-2729.)

azathioprine. In the early 1980s, the situation changed for the patients, and the benefits of thoracic transplantation soared with the introduction of the calcineurin inhibitor cyclosporine by Starzl and Calne. Current approaches are attempting to more selectively inhibit alloresponse by including targets of the immune active **Signal 2** pathway.

GLUCOCORTICOIDS

Prednisone is the chief oral glucocorticoid (GC) antiinflammatory. Effect is mediated by its intracellular block on nuclear factor (NF)-κB pathways.[90] This has the effect of reducing proinflammatory Th$_1$ cytokines with increase in the Th$_2$ suppressive secretome and of IL-10.[90-92] GC affects adaptive immunity by reducing the dendritic APC function, numbers of CD$^+$ cells and, at higher doses, production of anti-HLA antibody.[93,94]

Every transplant physician is aware of the heightened risk of increased infection from GC. While bacterial infections are commonly associated, GC also increases the risk of viral and protozoal-based complications. GC reduces innate immunity by effects on neutrophil adherence and trafficking, phagocytosis and expression of proinflammatory mediators.[95] Finally, GC adversely affects wound healing by reducing monocyte numbers and their entry to the wound as monocytes. Monocytes are important to healing due to their expression of growth factors and ability to phagocytose.[96,97] By limiting fibrocytes, GC further reduces wound healing.[98]

PURINE ANALOGUES: AZATHIOPRINE AND MYCOPHENOLATE MOFETIL

Early efforts in solid organ transplantation were dependent on the purine analogue 6-mercoptopure (6-MP) and its less toxic drug, azathioprine (Imuran). The metabolite of these days is 6-thioguanine nucleotide (6-TGN). It is incorporated in DNA and RNA and acts antagonistically to endogenous purines necessary for cell cycling.

MMF (Cellcept) and its active metabolite mycophenolic acid alter the purine synthesis by inhibiting inosine monophosphate dehydrogenase (IMPHD). This blocks inosine conversion to guanosine nucleotides. MMF is a more selective antimetabolic because lymphocytes are dependent on IMPHD for conversion while other cells have alternate pathways. MMF has generally come to be preferred as the rest of bone marrow and lungs are spared. The targeting of T&B lymphocytes has increased the risk of infection and particularly from CMV.[99-102] The most prominent adverse sites affected by MMF are a variety of gastrointestinal symptoms that can be severe enough to initiate a switch to azathioprine.

CALCINEURIN INHIBITION: CYCLOSPORINE A AND FK506

Calcineurin inhibitors (CNIs) impede a critical intracellular signal pathway initiated with activation of the TCR. Usually, calcineurin binds calmodulin to dephosphorylate the nuclear factor of the activated T-cells (NFAT).[103] NFAT can then translocate into the nucleus where it acts as a transcription factor for a number of immunologically important genes, including those coding for IL-2, -4, -5, TNFα and IFNγ. CNIs affect B cells indirectly by their effect on reducing T-cell help. Cyclosporine (CsA) was the first CNI to be introduced and was followed by Tacrolimus (TAC) (FK506). Both affect NFAT but bind to different immunophilins. CsA binds cyclophilins and TAC to FK-binding-proteins (FK-BPs).

CNIs can cause acute and chronic kidney injury. They reduce both tubular and glomerular function via their adverse effect on the aquaporin gene and protein production.[104] Additionally, they are associated with upregulation of renal mesangial cells and of renal fibrosis.[105,106] CNIs are also diabetogenic: they reduce the production and release of insulin and are proapoptotic to islets.[107,108] Severe neurologic complications, ranging from tremor to seizure and coma, have been associated with the use of CNIs. The cause of the neurologic side effects is likely based on multiple known neurologic interactions.[109] Other specific complications include hyperlipedemia, cholestasis, and malignancies especially skin cancer and non-Hodgkin's lymphoma.[110]

Proliferation Signal Inhibitors

mTOR INHIBITORS: SIROLIMUS, EVEROLIMUS

mTORs are proliferation signal inhibitors (PSI) that inhibit serine/threonine protein kinase which is part of multiple pathways necessary for cell activation, proliferation, and vascular endothelial growth factor production.[111,112] Immune cells with higher metabolic needs depend on mTOR activation. mTOR has also been shown to increase the proinflammatory cytokine output and increase adaptive immune memory. The complex and perhaps contradictory action of mTOR inhibitors (mTORi) make this class of agents interesting. Rapamycin (sirolimus) and everolimus are the clinically available mTORi. Of note, mTORi reduce wound healing to the extent that perioperative use is limited due to concerns regarding healing of midline sternotomy of heart transplant and particularly of the bronchus following lung implant.[113,114] Unlike other immunosuppressants, mTORi decrease tumors associated with transplant, probably due to their global inhibition of angiogenesis and cellular proliferation. These drugs have found a more secondary role as replacement or addition to lowered doses of CNIs for nephrotoxicity, cancer, neurologic complications, and resistant rejection.

Monoclonal Antibodies

ANTI-IL-2R ANTIBODY: BASILIXIMAB

Basiliximab (Simulect) is a human-mouse antibody that targets the IL-2α chain (anti-CD25). This limits the proliferation T-cell response. This agent can decrease CD25$^+$ T-cells for up to six weeks.[115] It may also affect Treg-suppressive roles as CD4$^+$/CD25$^+$/Foxp3$^+$ cells (Treg suppressive) decrease and CD4$^+$/CD25$^-$/Foxp3$^+$ cells increase.[115]

ANTI-CD20 ANTIBODY: RITUXIMAB

Rituximab depletes mature B cells by complement-mediated cytotoxicity and antibody-dependent cell toxicity. It seems also to have proapoptotic activity for B cells. This drug has been used to treat antibody-mediated allograft rejection, but its effect is at best limited. This is because it has little effect on plasma cells or mature antibody-secreting cells that do not express CD20. However, preemptive B-cell depletion at the time of transplant prevented CAV in a primate model[116] and is currently evaluated clinically (CTOT-11).

BORTEZOMIB: VELCADE

Velcade binds the catalytic site of the 26S proteasome in plasma cells. It is believed that this inhibition prevents degradation of preapoptotic factors.[117] Recently, Velcade has been approved for treatment of multiple myeloma and has been appropriated for persistent AMR of cardiac allografts. Complications include peripheral neuropathy, myelosuppression, and high incidence of varicella zoster infections. It has been successfully used with plasmapheresis to reduce cPRA in cardiac transplant candidates resistant to antibody-reducing treatment with rituximab and plasmapheresis.[118]

ANTI-CD52 ANTIBODY: ALEMTUZUMAB

Alemtuzumab (Campath) is active against CD52 which is a glycoprotein expressed by T and B lymphocytes, macrophages, monocytes, and NK cells.[119] Cell suppression can last for more than 12 months. This agent has been shown to reduce acute rejection episodes but may increase the risk of cancer.[68] It also has a tricky infection-associated profile due to its deeply and persistently suppressive effect.

CTLA4-IG: BELATACEPT

Belatacept (Nulojix) is the prototypic immunoglobulin-fusion protein. This recombinant protein is similar to the soluble form T-cell co-stimulatory receptor CTLA-4[120] and binds B7 ligands. This results in interference of Signal 2 for the CD28-B7 co-stimulation pathway. It is the only biologic used in transplantation to target specific alloimmune co-stimulation immune pathway. Signal 1 TCR activation in the absence of co-stimulation limits T-cell response and can induce T-cell anergy.[121] Belatacept succeeded Abatacept as a higher affinity construct for transplantation and was approved for acute kidney rejection in 2011.[120] This biologic was evaluated in a Phase III study of the Belatacept-based immunosuppression regimen versus cyclosporine in renal transplant recipients (BENEFIT). While renal function and blood pressure and lipid profiles were improved with Belatacept, acute rejection was more common (20% vs 7%) and worse histologically.[122] It has been proposed that memory T-cells are less controlled by co-stimulation blockade.

Polyclonal Antibodies

ANTITHYMOCYTE GLOBULIN

Antithymocyte globulin (ATG) is a polyclonal mixture of immunoglobulins (IgG) drawn from either rabbits (RATG or thymoglobulin) or horses (eATG or ATGAM). These IgG predominant preparations are based on animal immunizations with human thymocytes. They recognize multiple targets principally on T lymphocytes. Depletion of cells follows complement-based lysis, ADCC, and apoptosis.[123] Beyond depletion of T-cells, ATG also increases Tregs and depletes and impairs NKs and reduces B cells.[124] Rounding out the broad effects is ATG's interference with the uptake of antigens by DC cells.

RATG is preferred for its effectiveness in reducing rejection.[125] It is associated with an increased risk of PTLD and CMV infection due to its broadly reacting immunosuppression[126,127]

Intravenous Immunoglobulin

IVIG is made from pooled human donor IgG. It has inherent problems with supply, cost, and batch-based variability. It has become part of the regimen for treatment of AMR as it was a proven treatment for autoimmune and diverse inflammatory conditions. Its effectiveness is believed due to presence of anti-idiotypic antibodies and its ability to block complement-binding target cells and molecules.[128] The Fab-mediated antigen binding effects of IgG appear to be joined by Fc-dependent immune modulation.[129]

ACKNOWLEDGMENTS

We thank Dr. Keshava Rajagopal, Department of Surgery, University of Texas, and Dr. Debra KuKuruga, Director, HLA Laboratory of Red Cross, University of Maryland Baltimore, for their significant contributions to this chapter.

REFERENCES

1. Yusen RD, Edwards LB, Kucheryavaya AY, et al: The registry of the International Society for Heart and Lung Transplantation: thirty-first adult lung and heart-lung transplant report—2014; focus theme: retransplantation. *J Heart Lung Transplant* 2014; 33(10):1009-1024.
2. West LJ: ABO-incompatible hearts for infant transplantation. *Curr Opin Organ Transplant* 2011; 16(5):548-554.
3. Patel R, Terasaki PI: Significance of the positive crossmatch test in kidney transplantation. *New Engl J Med* 1969; 280(14):735-739.
4. Mickey MR, Kreisler M, Albert ED, et al: Analysis of HL-A incompatibility in human renal transplants. *Tissue Antigens* 1971; 1(2):57-67.
5. Starzl TE: The Puzzle People: Memoirs of a Transplant Surgeon. *University of Pittsburgh Press* 2003.
6. Angaswamy N, Saini D, Ramachandran S, et al: Development of antibodies to human leukocyte antigen precedes development of antibodies to major histocompatibility class I-related chain A and are significantly associated with development of chronic rejection after human lung transplantation. *Hum Immunol* 2010; 71(6):560-565.
7. Kaczmarek I, Deutsch MA, Kauke T, et al: Donor-specific HLA alloantibodies: long-term impact on cardiac allograft vasculopathy and mortality after heart transplant. *Exp Clin Transplant* 2008; 6(3):229-235.
8. Morales-Buenrostro LE, Castro R, Terasaki PI: A single human leukocyte antigen-antibody test after heart or lung transplantation is predictive of survival. *Transplantation* 2008; 85(3):478-481.
9. Paantjens AW, van de Graaf EA, Kwakkel-van Erp JM, et al: The induction of IgM and IgG antibodies against HLA or MICA after lung transplantation. *Pulm Med* 2011; 2011:432169.

10. Smith JD, Banner NR, Hamour IM, et al: De novo donor HLA-specific antibodies after heart transplantation are an independent predictor of poor patient survival. *Am J Transplant* 2011; 11(2):312-319.

11. Hachem RR, Yusen RD, Meyers BF, et al: Anti-human leukocyte antigen antibodies and preemptive antibody-directed therapy after lung transplantation. *J Heart Lung Transplant* 2010; 29(9):973-980.

12. Tinckam KJ, Keshavjee S, Chaparro C, et al: Survival in sensitized lung transplant recipients with perioperative desensitization. *Am J Transplant* 2015; 15(2):417-426.

13. Bromberg JS, Heeger PS, Li XC: Evolving paradigms that determine the fate of an allograft. *Am J Transplant* 2010; 10(5):1143-1148.

14. Zinkernagel RM, Doherty PC: The discovery of MHC restriction. *Immunol Today* 1997; 18(1):14-17.

15. Auchincloss H Jr, Sultan H: Antigen processing and presentation in transplantation. *Curr Opin Immunol* 1996; 8(5):681-687.

16. Benichou G, Thomson AW: Direct versus indirect allorecognition pathways: on the right track. *Am J Transplant* 2009; 9(4):655-656.

17. Afzali B, Lombardi G, Lechler RI: Pathways of major histocompatibility complex allorecognition. *Curr Opin Organ Transplant* 2008; 13(4):438-444.

18. Heeger PS: T-cell allorecognition and transplant rejection: a summary and update. *Am J Transplant* 2003; 3(5):525-533.

19. Sanchez-Fueyo A, Strom TB: Immunologic basis of graft rejection and tolerance following transplantation of liver or other solid organs. *Gastroenterology* 2011; 140(1):51-64.

20. Vincenti F, Blancho G, Durrbach A, et al: Five-year safety and efficacy of belatacept in renal transplantation. *J Am Soc Nephrol* 2010; 21(9):1587-1596.

21. Paterson AM, Vanguri VK, Sharpe AH: SnapShot: B7/CD28 costimulation. *Cell* 2009; 137(5):974-974 e1.

22. Croft M: The role of TNF superfamily members in T-cell function and diseases. *Nat Rev Immunol* 2009; 9(4):271-285.

23. Ashton-Rickardt PG: A license to remember. *Nat Immunol* 2004; 5(11):1097-1098.

24. Chen L, Flies DB: Molecular mechanisms of T cell co-stimulation and co-inhibition. *Nat Rev Immunol* 2013; 13(4):227-242.

25. Poirier N, Azimzadeh AM, Zhang T, et al: Inducing CTLA-4-dependent immune regulation by selective CD28 blockade promotes regulatory T cells in organ transplantation. *Sci Transl Med* 2010; 2(17):17ra10.

26. Zhang X, Rozengurt E, Reed EF: HLA class I molecules partner with integrin beta4 to stimulate endothelial cell proliferation and migration. *Sci Signal* 2010; 3(149):ra85.

27. Schenk AD, Nozaki T, Rabant M, et al: Donor-reactive CD8 memory T cells infiltrate cardiac allografts within 24-h posttransplant in naive recipients. *Am J Transplant* 2008; 8(8):1652-1661.

28. Mehra MR, Crespo-Leiro MG, Dipchand A, et al: International Society for Heart and Lung Transplantation Working Formulation of a standardized nomenclature for cardiac allograft vasculopathy-2010. *J Heart Lung Transplant* 2010; 29(7):717-727.

29. Berry GJ, Burke MM, Andersen C, et al: The 2013 International Society for Heart and Lung Transplantation Working Formulation for the standardization of nomenclature in the pathologic diagnosis of antibody-mediated rejection in heart transplantation. *J Heart Lung Transplant* 2013; 32(12):1147-1162.

30. McManigle W, Pavlisko EN, Martinu T: Acute cellular and antibody-mediated allograft rejection. *Semin Respir Crit Care Med* 2013; 34(3):320-335.

31. Gokmen MR, Lombardi G, Lechler RI: The importance of the indirect pathway of allorecognition in clinical transplantation. *Curr Opin Immunol* 2008; 20(5):568-574.

32. Singh N, Pirsch J, Samaniego M: Antibody-mediated rejection: treatment alternatives and outcomes. *Transplant Rev (Orlando)* 2009; 23(1):34-46.

33. Nath DS, Angaswamy N, Basha H, et al: Donor-specific antibodies to human leukocyte antigens are associated with and precede antibodies to major histocompatibility complex class I-related chain A in antibody-mediated rejection and cardiac allograft vasculopathy after human cardiac transplantation. *Hum Immunol* 2010; 71(12):1191-1196.

34. Nath DS, Ilias BH, Tiriveedhi V, et al: Characterization of immune responses to cardiac self-antigens myosin and vimentin in human cardiac allograft recipients with antibody-mediated rejection and cardiac allograft vasculopathy. *J Heart Lung Transplant* 2010; 29(11):1277-1285.

35. Nwakanma LU, Williams JA, Weiss ES, et al: Influence of pretransplant panel-reactive antibody on outcomes in 8,160 heart transplant recipients in recent era. *Ann Thorac Surg* 2007; 84(5):1556-1562; discussion 1562-1563.

36. McKenna RM, Takemoto SK, Terasaki PI: Anti-HLA antibodies after solid organ transplantation. *Transplantation* 2000; 69(3):319-326.

37. Fredrich R, Toyoda M, Czer LS, et al: The clinical significance of antibodies to human vascular endothelial cells after cardiac transplantation. *Transplantation* 1999; 67(3):385-391.

38. Jurcevic S, Ainsworth ME, Pomerance A, et al: Antivimentin antibodies are an independent predictor of transplant-associated coronary artery disease after cardiac transplantation. *Transplantation* 2001; 71(7):886-892.

39. Narayan S, Tsai EW, Zhang Q, et al: Acute rejection associated with donor-specific anti-MICA antibody in a highly sensitized pediatric renal transplant recipient. *Pediatr Transplant* 2010.

40. Hammond ME, Stehlik J, Snow G, et al: Utility of histologic parameters in screening for antibody-mediated rejection of the cardiac allograft: a study of 3,170 biopsies. *J Heart Lung Transplant* 2005; 24(12):2015-2021.

41. Hammond M, Renlund D: Cardiac allograft vascular (microvascular) rejection. *Curr Opin Organ Transplant* 2002; 7:233-239.

42. Kfoury AG, Hammond ME: Controversies in defining cardiac antibody-mediated rejection: need for updated criteria. *J Heart Lung Transplant* 2010; 29(4):389-394.

43. Almuti K, Haythe J, Dwyer E, et al: The changing pattern of humoral rejection in cardiac transplant recipients. *Transplantation* 2007; 84(4):498-503.

44. Gill EA, Borrego C, Bray BE, et al: Left ventricular mass increases during cardiac allograft vascular rejection. *J Am Coll Cardiol* 1995; 25(4):922-926.

45. Kobashigawa J, Mehra M, West L, et al: Report from a consensus conference on the sensitized patient awaiting heart transplantation. *J Heart Lung Transplant* 2009; 28(3):213-225.

46. Kobashigawa JA, Miller LW, Russell SD, et al: Tacrolimus with mycophenolate mofetil (MMF) or sirolimus vs. cyclosporine with MMF in cardiac transplant patients: 1-year report. *Am J Transplant* 2006; 6(6):1377-1386.

47. McConkey DJ, Aguilar-Santelises M, Hartzell P, et al: Induction of DNA fragmentation in chronic B-lymphocytic leukemia cells. *J Immunol* 1991; 146(3):1072-1076.

48. Sadaka B, Alloway RR, Woodle ES: Management of antibody-mediated rejection in transplantation. *Surg Clin North Am* 2013; 93(6):1451-1466.

49. Kwun J, Oh BC, Gibby AC, et al: Patterns of de novo allo B cells and antibody formation in chronic cardiac allograft rejection after alemtuzumab treatment. *Am J Transplant* 2012; 12(10):2641-2651.

50. Kim EJ, Kwun J, Gibby AC, et al: Costimulation blockade alters germinal center responses and prevents antibody-mediated rejection. *Am J Transplant* 2014; 14(1):59-69.

51. Morrow WR, Frazier EA, Mahle WT, et al: Rapid reduction in donor-specific anti-human leukocyte antigen antibodies and reversal of antibody-mediated rejection with bortezomib in pediatric heart transplant patients. *Transplantation* 2012; 93(3):319-324.

52. Glanville AR: Antibody-mediated rejection in lung transplantation: myth or reality? *J Heart Lung Transplant* 2010; 29(4):395-400.

53. Jordan SC, Toyoda M, Kahwaji J, Vo AA: Clinical aspects of intravenous immunoglobulin use in solid organ transplant recipients. *Am J Transplant* 2011; 11(2):196-202.

54. Dawson KL, Parulekar A, Seethamraju H: Treatment of hyperacute antibody-mediated lung allograft rejection with eculizumab. *J Heart Lung Transplant* 2012; 31(12):1325-1326.

55. Colvin-Adams M, Agnihotri A: Cardiac allograft vasculopathy: current knowledge and future direction. *Clin Transplant* 2011; 25(2):175-184.

56. Hofmann NP, Voss A, Dickhaus H, et al: Long-term outcome after heart transplantation predicted by quantitative myocardial blush grade in coronary angiography. *Am J Transplant* 2013; 13(6):1491-1502.

57. Yamada A, Laufer TM, Gerth AJ, et al: Further analysis of the T-cell subsets and pathways of murine cardiac allograft rejection. *Am J Transplant* 2003; 3(1):23-27.

58. Steinhoff G, Wonigeit K, Schafers HJ, et al: Sequential analysis of monomorphic and polymorphic major histocompatibility complex antigen expression in human heart allograft biopsy specimens. *J Heart Transplant* 1989; 8(5):360-370.

59. Zhang Q, Cecka JM, Gjertson DW, et al: HLA and MICA: targets of antibody-mediated rejection in heart transplantation. *Transplantation* 2011; 91(10):1153-1158.

60. Terasaki PI, Ozawa M, Castro R: Four-year follow-up of a prospective trial of HLA and MICA antibodies on kidney graft survival. *Am J Transplant* 2007; 7(2):408-415.

61. Derhaag JG, Duijvestijn AM, Damoiseaux JG, et al: Effects of antibody reactivity to major histocompatibility complex (MHC) and non-MHC alloantigens on graft endothelial cells in heart allograft rejection. *Transplantation* 2000; 69(9):1899-1906.

62. Methe H, Zimmer E, Grimm C, et al: Evidence for a role of toll-like receptor 4 in development of chronic allograft rejection after cardiac transplantation. *Transplantation* 2004; 78(9):1324-1331.

63. Topilsky Y, Hasin T, Raichlin E, et al: Sirolimus as primary immunosuppression attenuates allograft vasculopathy with improved late survival and decreased cardiac events after cardiac transplantation. *Circulation* 2012; 125(5):708-720.

64. Azarbal B, Arbit B, Ramaraj R, et al: Clinical and angiographic outcomes with everolimus eluting stents for the treatment of cardiac allograft vasculopathy. *J Interv Cardiol* 2014; 27(1):73-79.

65. Stein W, Schrepfer S, Itoh S, et al: Prevention of transplant coronary artery disease by prenylation inhibitors. *J Heart Lung Transplant* 2011; 30(7):761-769.

66. Verleden SE, Ruttens D, Vandermeulen E, et al: Restrictive chronic lung allograft dysfunction: Where are we now? *J Heart Lung Transplant* 2014.

67. Hartwig MG, Anderson DJ, Onaitis MW, et al: Fundoplication after lung transplantation prevents the allograft dysfunction associated with reflux. *Ann Thorac Surg* 2011; 92(2):462-468; discussion; 468-469.

68. Tan P, Anasetti C, Hansen JA, et al: Induction of alloantigen-specific hyporesponsiveness in human T lymphocytes by blocking interaction of CD28 with its natural ligand B7/BB1. *J Exp Med* 1993; 177(1):165-173.

69. Valujskikh A, Baldwin WM III, Fairchild, RL: Recent progress and new perspectives in studying T cell responses to allografts. *Am J Transplant* 2010; 10(5):1117-1125.

70. Shevach EM, Thornton AM: tTregs, pTregs, and iTregs: similarities and differences. *Immunol Rev* 2014; 259(1):88-102.

71. Abbas AK, Benoist C, Bluestone JA, et al: Regulatory T cells: recommendations to simplify the nomenclature. *Nat Immunol* 2013; 14(4):307-308.

72. Chesneau M, Pallier A, Braza F, et al: Unique B cell differentiation profile in tolerant kidney transplant patients. *Am J Transplant* 2014; 14(1):144-155.

73. Kawai T, Cosimi A, Spitzer T, et al: HLA-mismatched renal transplantation without maintenance immunosuppression. *N Engl J Med* 2008; 358(4):353-361.

74. Aoyama AN, CY, Millington, TM, Boskovic S, et al: Comparison of lung and kidney allografts in induction of tolerance by a mixed-chimerism approach in cynomolgus monkeys. *Transplant Proc* 2009; 41(1):429-430.

75. Bingaman AW, Murphey CL, Palma-Vargas J, Wright F: A virtual crossmatch protocol significantly increases access of highly sensitized patients to deceased donor kidney transplantation. *Transplantation* 2008; 86(12):1864-1868.

76. Stehlik J, Islam N, Hurst D, et al: Utility of virtual crossmatch in sensitized patients awaiting heart transplantation. *J Heart Lung Transplant* 2009; 28(11):1129-1134.

77. Pajaro OE, George JF: On solid-phase antibody assays. *J Heart Lung Transplant* 2010; 29(11):1207-1209.

78. Danskine A, Smith J, Stanford R: Correlation of anti-vimentin antibodies with acute and chronic rejection following cardiac transplantation. *Hum Immunol* 2002; 63(Suppl):S30-S31.

79. Suarez-Alvarez B, Lopez-Vazquez A, Gonzalez MZ, et al: The relationship of anti-MICA antibodies and MICA expression with heart allograft rejection. *Am J Transplant* 2007; 7(7):1842-1848.

80. Smith JD, Hamour IM, Banner NR, et al: C4d fixing, luminex binding antibodies - a new tool for prediction of graft failure after heart transplantation. *Am J Transplant* 2007; 7(12):2809-2815.

81. Mahesh B, Leong HS, McCormack A, et al: Autoantibodies to vimentin cause accelerated rejection of cardiac allografts. *Am J Pathol* 2007; 170(4):1415-1427.

82. Azimzadeh AM, Pfeiffer S, Wu GS, et al: Humoral immunity to vimentin is associated with cardiac allograft injury in nonhuman primates. *Am J Transplant* 2005; 5(10):2349-2359.

83. Starling RC, Pham M, Valantine H, et al: Molecular testing in the management of cardiac transplant recipients: initial clinical experience. *J Heart Lung Transplant* 2006; 25(12):1389-1395.

84. Pham MX: Teuteberg JJ, Kfoury AG, et al: Gene-expression profiling for rejection surveillance after cardiac transplantation. *New Engl J Med* 2010; 362(20):1890-1900.

85. Mehra MR, Parameshwar J: Gene expression profiling and cardiac allograft rejection monitoring: is IMAGE just a mirage? *J Heart Lung Transplant* 2010; 29(6):599-602.

86. Mehra MR, Kobashigawa JA, Deng MC, et al: Transcriptional signals of T-cell and corticosteroid-sensitive genes are associated with future acute cellular rejection in cardiac allografts. *J Heart Lung Transplant* 2007; 26(12):1255-1263.

87. Mehra MR, Kobashigawa JA, Deng MC, et al: Clinical implications and longitudinal alteration of peripheral blood transcriptional signals indicative of future cardiac allograft rejection. *J Heart Lung Transplant* 2008; 27(3):297-301.

88. Kowalski R, Post D, Schneider MC, et al: Immune cell function testing: an adjunct to therapeutic drug monitoring in transplant patient management. *Clin Transplant* 2003; 17(2):77-88.

89. Kobashigawa JA, Kiyosaki KK, Patel JK, et al: Benefit of immune monitoring in heart transplant patients using ATP production in activated lymphocytes. *J Heart Lung Transplant* 2010; 29(5):504-508.

90. Rhen T, Cidlowski JA: Antiinflammatory action of glucocorticoids—new mechanisms for old drugs. *New Engl J Med* 2005; 353(16): 1711-1723.

91. Almawi WY, Melemedjian OK, Rieder MJ: An alternate mechanism of glucocorticoid anti-proliferative effect: promotion of a Th2 cytokine-secreting profile. *Clin Transplant* 1999; 13(5):365-374.

92. Mittal SK, Sharma RK, Gupta A, Naik S: Increased interleukin-10 production without expansion of CD4+CD25+ T-regulatory cells in early stable renal transplant patients on calcineurin inhibitors. *Transplantation* 2009; 88(3):435-441.

93. Poetker DM, Reh DD: A comprehensive review of the adverse effects of systemic corticosteroids. *Otolaryngol Clin North Am* 2010; 43(4):753-768.

94. Taylor AL, Watson CJ, Bradley JA: Immunosuppressive agents in solid organ transplantation: Mechanisms of action and therapeutic efficacy. *Crit Rev Oncol Hematol* 2005; 56(1):23-46.

95. Segal BH, Sneller MC: Infectious complications of immunosuppressive therapy in patients with rheumatic diseases. *Rheum Dis Clin North Am* 1997; 23(2):219-237.

96. Atkinson JB, Kosi M, Srikanth MS, et al: Growth hormone reverses impaired wound healing in protein-malnourished rats treated with corticosteroids. *J Pediatr Surg* 1992; 27(8):1026-1028.

97. Nguyen H, Lim, J, Dresner ML, Nixon B: Effect of local corticosteroids on early inflammatory function in surgical wound of rats. *J Foot Ankle Surg* 1998; 37(4):313-318.

98. Lenco W, McKnight M, Macdonald AS: Effects of cortisone acetate, methylprednisolone and medroxyprogesterone on wound contracture and epithelization in rabbits. *Ann Surg* 1975; 181(1):67-73.

99. Laurent AF, Dumont S, Poindron P, Muller CD: Mycophenolic acid suppresses protein N-linked glycosylation in human monocytes and their adhesion to endothelial cells and to some substrates. *Exp Hematol* 1996; 24(1):59-67.

100. Moreso F, Seron D, Morales JM, et al: Incidence of leukopenia and cytomegalovirus disease in kidney transplants treated with mycophenolate mofetil combined with low cyclosporine and steroid doses. *Clin Transplant* 1998; 12(3):198-205.

101. Sollinger HW: Mycophenolate mofetil for the prevention of acute rejection in primary cadaveric renal allograft recipients. U.S. Renal Transplant Mycophenolate Mofetil Study Group. *Transplantation* 1995; 60(3):225-232.

102. Wang K, Zhang H, Li Y, et al: Safety of mycophenolate mofetil versus azathioprine in renal transplantation: a systematic review. *Transplant Proc* 2004; 36(7):2068-2070.

103. Shaw KT, Ho AM, Raghavan A, et al: Immunosuppressive drugs prevent a rapid dephosphorylation of transcription factor NFAT1 in stimulated immune cells. *Proc Natl Acad Sci U S A* 1995; 92(24):11205-11209.

104. Rinschen MM, Klokkers J, Pavenstadt H, et al: Different effects of CsA and FK506 on aquaporin-2 abundance in rat primary cultured collecting duct cells. *Pflugers Arch* 2011; 462(4):611-622.

105. Akool el S, Gauer S, Osman B, et al: Cyclosporin A and tacrolimus induce renal Erk1/2 pathway via ROS-induced and metalloproteinase-dependent EGF-receptor signaling. *Biochem Pharmacol* 2012; 83(2):286-295.

106. Lamoureux F, Mestre E, Essig M, et al: Quantitative proteomic analysis of cyclosporine-induced toxicity in a human kidney cell line and comparison with tacrolimus. *J Proteomics* 2011; 75(2):677-694.

107. Lawrence MC, Bhatt HS, Easom RA: NFAT regulates insulin gene promoter activity in response to synergistic pathways induced by glucose and glucagon-like peptide-1. *Diabetes* 2002; 51(3):691-698.

108. Ozbay LA, Smidt K, Mortensen DM, et al: Cyclosporin and tacrolimus impair insulin secretion and transcriptional regulation in INS-1E beta-cells. *Br J Pharmacol* 2011; 162(1):136-146.

109. Kasiske BL, Snyder JJ, Gilbertson DT, Wang C: Cancer after kidney transplantation in the United States. *Am J Transplant* 2004; 4(6):905-913.

110. Dandel M, Lehmkuhl HB, Knosalla C, Hetzer R: Impact of different long-term maintenance immunosuppressive therapy strategies on patients' outcome after heart transplantation. *Transpl Immunol* 2010; 23(3):93-103.

111. Powell JD, Delgoffe GM: The mammalian target of rapamycin: linking T cell differentiation, function, and metabolism. *Immunity* 2010; 33(3):301-311.

112. Wullschleger S, Loewith R, Hall MN: TOR signaling in growth and metabolism. *Cell* 2006; 124(3):471-484.

113. Azzola A, Havryk A, Chhajed P, et al: Everolimus and mycophenolate mofetil are potent inhibitors of fibroblast proliferation after lung transplantation. *Transplantation* 2004; 77(2):275-280.

114. Kuppahally S, Al-Khaldi A, Weisshaar D, et al: Wound healing complications with de novo sirolimus versus mycophenolate mofetil-based regimen in cardiac transplant recipients. *Am J Transplant* 2006; 6(5 Pt 1): 986-992.

115. Vondran FW, Timrott K, Tross J, et al: Impact of Basiliximab on regulatory T-cells early after kidney transplantation: down-regulation of CD25 by receptor modulation. *Transpl Int* 2010; 23(5):514-523.

116. Kelishadi SS, Azimzadeh AM, Zhang T, et al: Preemptive CD20+ B cell depletion attenuates cardiac allograft vasculopathy in cyclosporine-treated monkeys. *J Clin Invest* 2010; 120(4):1275-1284.

117. Bonvini P, Zorzi E, Basso G, Rosolen A: Bortezomib-mediated 26S proteasome inhibition causes cell-cycle arrest and induces apoptosis in CD-30+ anaplastic large cell lymphoma. *Leukemia* 2007; 21(4):838-842.

118. Patel J, Everly M, Chang D, et al: Reduction of alloantibodies via proteasome inhibition in cardiac transplantation. *J Heart Lung Transplant* 2011; 30(12):1320-1326.

119. Reiff A, Shaham B, Weinberg KI, et al: Anti-CD52 antibody-mediated immune ablation with autologous immune recovery for the treatment of refractory juvenile polymyositis. *J Clin Immunol* 2011; 31(4):615-622.

120. Larsen CP, Pearson, TC, Adams AB, et al: Rational development of LEA29Y (belatacept), a high-affinity variant of CTLA4-Ig with potent immunosuppressive properties. *Am J Transplant* 2005; 5(3):443-453.

121. Matzinger P: Friendly and dangerous signals: is the tissue in control? *Nat Immunol* 2007; 8(1):11-13.

122. Durrbach A, Pestana JM, Pearson T, et al: A phase III study of belatacept versus cyclosporine in kidney transplants from extended criteria donors (BENEFIT-EXT study). *Am J Transplant* 2010; 10(3):547-557.

123. Mohty M: Mechanisms of action of antithymocyte globulin: T-cell depletion and beyond. *Leukemia* 2007; 21(7):1387-1394.

124. Lopez M, Clarkson MR, Albin M, et al: A novel mechanism of action for anti-thymocyte globulin: induction of CD4+CD25+Foxp3+ regulatory T cells. *J Am Soc Nephrol* 2006; 17(10):2844-2853.

125. Hardinger KL, Rhee S, Buchanan P, et al: A prospective, randomized, double-blinded comparison of thymoglobulin versus Atgam for induction immunosuppressive therapy: 10-year results. *Transplantation* 2008; 86(7):947-952.

126. Brennan DC, Schnitzler MA: Long-term results of rabbit antithymocyte globulin and basiliximab induction. *N Engl J Med* 2008; 359(16):1736-1738.

127. Kirk AD, Cherikh WS, Ring M, et al: Dissociation of depletional induction and posttransplant lymphoproliferative disease in kidney recipients treated with alemtuzumab. *Am J Transplant* 2007; 7(11):2619-2625.

128. Kotlan B, Stroncek DF, Marincola FM: Intravenous immunoglobulin-based immunotherapy: an arsenal of possibilities for patients and science. *Immunotherapy* 2009; 1(6):995-1015.

129. Samuelsson A, Towers TL, Ravetch JV: Anti-inflammatory activity of IVIG mediated through the inhibitory Fc receptor. *Science* 2001; 291(5503):484-486.

Heart Transplantation

Richard J. Shemin • Mario Deng

The number of patients with heart failure is growing. End-stage heart failure is associated with significant morbidity, need for recurrent hospitalizations, decrease in quality of life, and increased mortality. Cardiac transplantation has evolved as an effective therapy for many of these patients. Tremendous advancements in the fields of immunosuppression, rejection, and infection have transformed what was once considered an experimental intervention into a routine treatment available worldwide.

The innovative French surgeon Alexis Carrel performed the first heterotopic canine heart transplant with Charles Guthrie in 1905. Frank Mann at the Mayo Clinic further explored the idea of heterotopic heart transplantation in the 1930s. The neck became the preferred site of implantation in early experimental animal models because of the ease of monitoring the organ, the simplicity of access to major vessels, and because the recipient's native heart could serve as a built-in cardiac assist device for the transplanted organ. Mann also proposed the concept of cardiac allograft rejection, in which biological incompatibility between donor and recipient was manifested as a leukocytic infiltration of the rejecting myocardium. In 1946, after unsuccessful attempts in the inguinal region, Vladimir Demikhov of the Soviet Union successfully implanted the first intrathoracic heterotopic heart allograft. He later demonstrated that heart-lung and isolated lung transplantation also were technically feasible.

The use of moderate hypothermia, cardiopulmonary bypass, and an atrial cuff anastomotic technique permitted Norman Shumway (Fig. 60-1) and Richard Lower at Stanford University to further explore orthotopic heart transplantation using a canine model in 1960.

The first human cardiac transplant was a chimpanzee xenograft performed at the University of Mississippi by James Hardy in 1964. Although the procedure using Shumway's technique was technically satisfactory, the primate heart was unable to maintain the recipient's circulatory load and the patient succumbed several hours postoperatively.

Despite great skepticism that cardiac transplantation ever would be performed successfully in humans, South African Christiaan Barnard surprised the world when he performed the first human-to-human heart transplant on December 3, 1967. Over the next several years, poor early clinical results led to a moratorium on heart transplantation, with only the most dedicated centers continuing experimental and clinical work in the field. The pioneering efforts of Shumway and colleagues at Stanford eventually paved the way for the reemergence of cardiac transplantation in the late 1970s.

The introduction of transvenous endomyocardial biopsy by Philip Caves in 1973 finally provided a reliable means for monitoring allograft rejection. Ultimately, however, it was the advent of the immunosuppressive agent cyclosporine that dramatically increased patient survival and marked the beginning of the modern era of successful cardiac transplantation in 1981.

Heart transplantation is now a widely accepted therapeutic option for end-stage cardiac failure; however, the annual number of transplants in the United States (approximately 2400 per year) has slowly increased since 2002, however, limited donor-organ availability remains a major limitation (from United Network for Organ Sharing [UNOS] data, through September 2012).

THE CARDIAC TRANSPLANT RECIPIENT

Recipient Selection

The evaluation of potential candidates for cardiac transplantation is performed by a multidisciplinary committee to ensure the equitable, objective, and medically justified allocation of donor organs to those patients most likely to achieve long-term benefit. It is very important to establish a mutual long-term working relationship among patient, social support system, and the entire team at the beginning of this process.

Indications and potential contraindications for cardiac transplantation are outlined in Table 60-1.[1] These inclusion and exclusion criteria can vary somewhat among transplantation centers.[1-4] The basic objective is to identify those

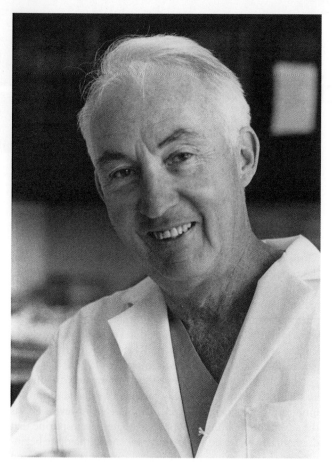

FIGURE 60-1 Norman Shumway.

relatively healthy patients with end-stage cardiac disease, refractory to other appropriate medical and surgical therapies, who possess the potential to resume a normal active life and maintain compliance with a rigorous medical regimen after cardiac transplantation.

ETIOLOGY OF END-STAGE CARDIAC FAILURE

Determination of the etiology and potential reversibility of end-stage heart failure is critical for the selection of transplant candidates. Overall, from 1982 to 2012, the indications for heart transplantation in adult recipients have been overwhelmingly ischemic heart failure and nonischemic cardiomyopathy (approximately 90%); with valvular (2-3%), adult congenital (2%), retransplantation (2%), and miscellaneous causes comprising the remainder.[5]

The perception of the irreversibility of advanced cardiac failure is changing with the growing efficacy of tailored medical therapy, high-risk revascularization procedures, and newer antiarrhythmic pharmacologic agents, as well as implantable defibrillators and biventricular pacing. Additionally, other surgical modalities, such as ventricular assist devices (VADs) and surgical ventricular restoration (SVR), have found increasing application.[6,7] Furthermore, it is

important to consider that prognosis may differ in patients with cardiomyopathy who have neither ischemic nor valvular heart disease. Caution should be exercised when judging prognosis in these patient subgroups, and a period of observation, intense pharmacologic therapy, and/or mechanical support should be undertaken before heart transplantation is considered.[4]

EVALUATION OF THE POTENTIAL CARDIAC TRANSPLANT RECIPIENT

The complexity of the recipient evaluation mandates a team approach. The initial evaluation involves a comprehensive history and physical examination because this will help to determine etiology and contraindications. Table 60-2 summarizes the cardiac transplant evaluation tests.[3] Routine hematologic and biochemical analyses and pertinent tests as illustrated by organ system are performed.[3]

For the assessment of the heart itself, in addition to routine 12-lead electrocardiogram, Holter monitor, and echocardiography, all patients should undergo cardiopulmonary exercise testing to evaluate functional capacity if disease severity allows. Peak exercise oxygen consumption measured during maximal exercise testing $\dot{V}O_{2,max}$ provides a measure of functional capacity and cardiovascular reserve, and an inverse relationship between $\dot{V}O_{2,max}$ and mortality in heart failure patients has been demonstrated.[8] Documentation of adequate effort during exercise, as evidenced by attaining a respiratory exchange ratio greater than 1.0 or achievement of an anaerobic threshold at 50 to 60% of $\dot{V}O_{2,max}$ is necessary to avoid underestimation of functional capacity.[2]

Right-sided heart catheterization should be performed at the transplanting center to evaluate the severity of heart failure (and hence the status level for transplant listing) and evaluate for the presence of pulmonary hypertension (PH). Right heart catheterization also can help guide therapy while awaiting transplantation. Coronary cineangiography should be reviewed to confirm the inoperability of coronary artery lesions in cases of ischemic cardiomyopathy. As well, either a positron emission tomographic (PET) scan, a thallium-201 redistribution study, or a cardiac magnetic resonance imaging (MRI) study should assess viability in selected patients who would be candidates for revascularization if sufficient viability is present.[2,3]

Endomyocardial biopsy should be performed on all patients in whom the etiology of heart failure is in question, especially those with nonischemic cardiomyopathies symptomatic for fewer than 6 months.[3] This can assist in therapeutic decision making and exclude diagnoses such as amyloidosis, which are considered relative contraindications to transplantation.

The neuropsychiatric assessment should be performed by persons experienced in evaluating cardiac patients to determine if organic brain dysfunction or psychiatric illness is present. An experienced social worker should assess for the presence of adequate social and financial support. At the time of listing, the transplant coordinator should ensure that the patient and family understand the peculiarities of the waiting

Indications

I. Systolic heart failure (as defined by ejection fraction <35%)
    A. Accepted etiology
        1. Ischemic
        2. Idiopathic
        3. Valvular
        4. Hypertensive
        5. Other
    B. Controversial etiology
        1. HIV infection
        2. Cardiac sarcoma
II. Intractable angina
    A. Ineffective maximal tolerated medical therapy
    B. Not a candidate for direct myocardial revascularization, percutaneous revascularization, or transmyocardial revascularization procedure
    C. Unsuccessful myocardial revascularization
III. Intractable arrhythmia
    A. Uncontrolled with pacing cardioverter defibrillator
        1. Not amenable to electrophysiology-guided single or combination medical therapy
        2. Not a candidate for ablation therapy
IV. Hypertrophic cardiomyopathy
    A. Class IV symptoms persist despite interventional therapies
        1. Alcohol injection of septal artery
        2. Myotomy and myomectomy
        3. Mitral valve replacement
        4. Maximal medical therapy
        5. Pacemaker therapy
V. Congenital heart disease in which severe fixed pulmonary hypertension is not a complication
VI. Cardiac tumor
    A. Confined to the myocardium
    B. No evidence of distant disease revealed by extensive metastatic workup
VII. Restrictive cardiomyopathy
    A. Class IV symptoms persist despite interventional therapies
    B. Amyloid (if concomitant therapy such as chemotherapy/autologous stem cell transplant feasible)

Absolute Contraindications

I. Age >65-75 years (may vary at different centers)
II. Fixed pulmonary hypertension (unresponsive to pharmacologic intervention)
    A. Pulmonary vascular resistance >4-6 Wood units
    B. Transpulmonary gradient >12-18 mm Hg
III. Systemic illness that will limit survival despite transplant
    A. Neoplasm other than skin cancer (<2-5 years disease-free survival)
    B. HIV/AIDS (CDC definition of CD4 count of <200 cells/mm^3)
    C. Systemic lupus erythematosus (SLE) or sarcoid that has multisystem involvement and is currently active
    D. Any systemic process with a high probability of recurrence in the transplanted heart
    E. Irreversible organ (eg, renal, hepatic, pulmonary) dysfunction

Potential Relative Contraindications

I. Recent malignancy
II. Chronic obstructive pulmonary disease
III. Recent and unresolved pulmonary infarction and pulmonary embolism
IV. Diabetes mellitus with end-organ damage (neuropathy, nephropathy, and retinopathy)
V. Peripheral vascular or cerebrovascular disease
VI. Active peptic ulcer disease
VII. Current or recent diverticulitis
VIII. Other systemic illness likely to limit survival or rehabilitation
IX. Severe obesity or cachexia
X. Severe osteoporosis
XI. Active alcohol, nicotine or drug abuse
XII. History of noncompliance or psychiatric illness likely to interfere with long-term compliance
XIII. Absence of psychosocial support

TABLE 60-2: Cardiac Transplant Evaluation Tests

Laboratory	Complete blood count with differential and platelet count, creatinine, blood urea nitrogen, electrolytes, liver panel, lipid panel, calcium, phosphorus, total protein, albumin, uric acid, thyroid panel, antinuclear antibodies, erythrocyte sedimentation rate (ESR), rapid plasma reagin (RPR), iron-binding tests, partial thromboplastin time, prothrombin time
	Blood type (incl. confirmatory test), IgG and IgM antibodies against cytomegalovirus, herpes simplex virus, HIV, varicella-zoster virus, hepatitis B surface antigen, hepatitis C antigen, toxoplasmosis, other titers when indicated
	Tuberculin skin test
	Prostate-specific antigen (male >50 years)
	Mammogram and Pap smear (female >40 years)
	Screening against a panel of donor antigens (panel reactive antibodies) and human leukocyte antigen phenotype
	24-hour urine for creatinine clearance and total protein, urinalysis, urine culture 1
	Baseline bacterial and fungal cultures, stool for ova and parasites if indicated
Cardiac	12-lead ECG, 24-hour Holter monitor
	Echocardiogram
	Thallium-201 imaging, positron-emission tomographic (PET) scan, or cardiac magnetic resonance imaging (MRI) to assess viability if indicated
	Exercise stress test and respiratory gas analysis with oxygen uptake measurements: peak exercise oxygen consumption $\dot{V}O_{2,max}$
	Right- and left-sided heart catheterization
	Myocardial biopsy on selected patients in whom etiology of heart failure is in question and affects treatment choice
Vascular	Peripheral vascular studies
	Carotid Doppler and duplex ultrasound 55 years
Renal	Renal ultrasound and or intravenous pyelogram if indicated
Pulmonary	Chest x-ray
	Pulmonary function tests
	Chest CT scan to evaluate abnormal chest x-ray or thoracic aorta in older patients (usually >65 years)
Gastrointestinal	Upper endoscopy/colonoscopy if indicated
	Upper gastrointestinal series and/or barium enema if indicated
	Percutaneous liver biopsy if indicated
Metabolic	Bone densitometry
Neurologic	Screening evaluation
Psychiatric	Screening evaluation
Dental	Complete dental evaluation
Physical therapy	Evaluation
Social work	Patient attitude and family support, medical insurance, and general financial resources
Transplant coordinator	Education

time, preoperative period, long-term maintenance medications, and the rules of living with the new heart. It is also of paramount importance that providers discuss the patient's preferences with regard to life support (duration and type), in case of a deterioration in his or her condition while awaiting transplant.

Indications for Cardiac Transplantation

Cardiac transplantation is reserved for a select group of patients with end-stage heart disease not amenable to optimal medical or surgical therapies. Prognosis for 1-year survival without transplantation should be less than 50%. Prediction of patient survival involves considerable subjective clinical judgment by the transplant committee because

no reliable objective prognostic criteria are available currently. Low ejection fraction (<20%), reduced $\dot{V}O_{2,max}$ (<14 mL/kg/min), arrhythmias, high pulmonary capillary wedge pressure (>25 mm Hg), elevated plasma norepinephrine concentration (>600 pg/mL), reduced serum sodium concentration (<130 mEq/dL), and N-terminal probrain natriuretic peptide (>5000 pg/mL) all have been proposed as predictors of poor prognosis and potential indications for transplantation in patients receiving optimal medical therapy.[8-11] Reduced left ventricular ejection fraction and low $\dot{V}O_{2,max}$ are widely identified as the strongest independent predictors of survival.

The indications for cardiac transplantation listing are continuously reviewed as new breakthroughs in the medical and surgical treatment of heart disease emerge.

CONTRAINDICATIONS FOR CARDIAC TRANSPLANTATION

Table 60-1 lists the traditional absolute and relative contra-indications. It should be acknowledged that strict guidelines can be problematic; therefore, each transplant program varies regarding absolute criteria based on clinical circumstances and experience. Furthermore, traditional contraindications for transplant listing are being questioned.

Age is one of the most controversial exclusionary criteria for transplantation. The upper age limit for recipients is center-specific, but emphasis should be placed on the patient's physiologic rather than chronologic age. The Official Adult Heart Transplant Report 2009 from the registry of the International Society for Heart and Lung Transplantation (ISHLT) noted that over the last 25 years, the percentage of recipients older than 60 years of age has increased steadily, approaching 25% of all heart transplants between 2002 and 2008 compared with just above 5% between 1982 and 1988.[5] Although the elderly have a greater potential for occult systemic disease that may complicate their postoperative course, some recent reports have suggested that morbidity and mortality in carefully selected older patients are comparable with those of younger recipients, and they have fewer rejection episodes than younger patients.[12,13]

Fixed PH, usually manifested as elevated pulmonary vascular resistance (PVR), is one of the few absolute contraindications to orthotopic cardiac transplantation. Fixed PH increases the risk of acute right ventricular failure when the right ventricle of the allograft is unable to adapt to significant PH in the immediate postoperative period.[14] Use of the transpulmonary gradient (TPG), which represents the pressure gradient across the pulmonary vascular bed independent of blood flow, may avoid erroneous estimations of PVR, such as those that may occur in patients with low cardiac output.[4] Some have advocated the use of PVR index (PVRI) unit, which corrects for body size.

$$PVR \text{ (Wood units)} = \frac{MPAP \text{ (mm Hg)} - PCWP \text{ (mm Hg)}}{CO \text{ (L/min)}}$$

$$PVRI \text{ (units)} = \frac{MPAP \text{ (mm Hg)} - PCWP \text{ (mm Hg)}}{CO \text{ (L/min)} \times BSA} = \frac{PVR}{BSA}$$

$$TPG \text{ (mm Hg)} = PAP \text{ (mm Hg)} - PCWP \text{ (mm Hg)}$$

where MPAP is mean pulmonary arterial pressure, PCWP is pulmonary capillary wedge pressure, CO is cardiac output, CI is cardiac index, and BSA is body surface area.

A fixed PVR greater than 5 to 6 Wood units and a TPG greater than 15 mm Hg generally are accepted as absolute criteria for rejection of a candidate.[1-4,11] Over the years, several studies have found PH to have a significant effect on posttransplant mortality using various parameters, threshold values, and follow-up periods.[15,16] However, a lack of mortality difference after heart transplantation between patients with and without preoperative PH has also been reported.[17] Perhaps more significantly, measurable parameters of PH

have been shown to improve following heart transplantation. A study of 172 patients followed for up to 15.1 years, published in 2005 from the Johns Hopkins Hospital, showed that mild to moderate pretransplantation PH (PVR = 2.5 to 5.0 Wood units) was not associated with higher mortality rate, although there was increased risk of posttransplantation PH within the first 6 months.[18] However, when the continuous variable PVR was examined, each 1 Wood unit increase in preoperative PVR demonstrated a 15% or more increase in mortality, especially within the first year, but these associations did not reach statistical significance. Severe preoperative PH (PVR ≥ 5 Wood units) was associated with death within the first year after adjusting for potential cofounders but not with overall mortality or mortality beyond the first year.

In the preoperative evaluation of the transplant recipient, if PH is discovered, an assessment of its reversibility should be performed in the cardiac catheterization laboratory.[16] Sodium nitroprusside traditionally has been used at a starting dose of 0.5 μg/kg per minute and titrated by 0.5 μg/kg per minute until there is an acceptable decline in PVR, ideally 2.5 Wood units or at least by 50%, with maintenance of adequate systemic systolic blood pressure. If sodium nitroprusside fails to produce an adequate response, other vasodilators such as adenosine, prostaglandin E$_1$ (PGE$_1$), milrinone, or inhaled nitric oxide or prostacyclin (eg, aerosolized Iloprost) may be used.[2,19] Some patients who do not respond acutely may respond to continuous intravenous inotropic therapy, and repeat catheterization can be performed after 48 to 72 hours. Intravenous B-type natriuretic peptide, eg, nesiritide (Natrecor), has shown some efficacy in refractory PH.[20] Recently, VADs are playing an important role in heart transplantation candidates with PH.[21] A period of left ventricular assist device (LVAD) support may allow for a decrease of pulmonary artery pressure secondary to unloading of the left ventricle. Patients with irreversible PH may be candidates for heterotopic heart transplantation, heart-lung transplantation, or LVAD destination therapy.[22] Use of modestly larger donor hearts for recipients with severe pretransplantation PH can provide additional right ventricular reserve.

Systemic diseases with poor prognosis and potential to recur in the transplanted heart or the potential to undergo exacerbation with immunosuppressive therapy are considered absolute contraindications for heart transplantation. Previously, any occurrence of neoplasm was a reason to exclude patients from transplantation. Currently available data do not appear to justify excluding some of these patients.[23] Most programs will consider patients who are free of disease for at least 5 years. A recent multicenter study investigated the influence of pretransplant malignancy on posttransplant recurrence and long-term survival in heart and lung transplant recipients. In this cohort, 111 recipients (lung: 37; heart: 74) with 113 pretransplant malignancies were identified. The cohort was divided into 3 groups by pretransplant cancer-free interval of <12 months, ≥12 to 60 months, and ≥60 months. Pretransplant cancer-free survival of ≥5 years was associated with the lowest recurrence at a mean follow-up of 70 ± 63 months

(6% at ≥60 months vs 26% at 12 to 60 months vs 63% at <12 months). Survival was significantly poorer in those cancer-free for <12 months, whereas there was no survival difference in the other 2 groups. Further study is warranted to determine the optimal malignancy-free period.[24] Heart transplantation for amyloid remains controversial because amyloid deposits recur in the transplanted heart. Although case reports of long-term survival can be found in the literature,[25] survival beyond 1 year tends to be reduced.[23]

Human immunodeficiency virus (HIV)-infected patients generally were excluded until a recent case series by the Columbia University Heart Transplant Group. With the newer antiretroviral drugs, the estimated 10-year survival after seroconversion exceeds 90%. In a retrospective single-center analysis of 1679 cardiac transplant patients, seven HIV-positive patients underwent heart transplantation. Five (4 men) were diagnosed with HIV before transplantation and 2 patients seroconverted after transplantation. Dilated cardiomyopathy was the indication for transplant in all patients. The 5 HIV recipients were aged 42 ± 8 years, and time after HIV seroconversion averaged 9.5 years. All underwent cardiac transplantation as high-risk candidates. The CD4 count was 554 ± 169 cells/microl, and viral load was undetectable in all patients at the time of transplantation. Two patients seroconverted to HIV-positive status at 1 and 7 years after transplant. No AIDS-defining illness was observed in any patient before or after transplant. Six patients received highly active antiretroviral therapy. Viral load remained low in the presence of immunosuppression. All patients were alive with a follow-up from transplant of 57 ± 78.9 months.[26,27]

Irreversible renal dysfunction is a contraindication to heart transplantation. A creatinine clearance of less than 50 mL/min and a serum creatinine concentration of greater than 2 mg/dL are associated with increased risk of postoperative dialysis and decreased survival following heart transplantion.[4,28] The effect of chronic kidney dysfunction (CKD) on post-HTx outcomes was recently examined in 1732 recipients. In this population, 3% were CKD stage 4 and 5 at the time of transplant, increasing to 11% at 1 year and more than 15% at 6 years after transplantation. The risk of death was significantly higher in patients with CKD 4 and 5 (hazard CKD4:1.66; CKD5:8.54; dialysis:4.07). Multiorgan transplantation was not assessed in this cohort.[29] However, patients may be considered for combined heart and kidney transplantation.

Irreversible hepatic dysfunction has implications similar to renal dysfunction.[4] If transaminase levels are more than twice their normal value and associated with coagulation abnormalities, percutaneous liver biopsy should be performed to exclude primary liver disease. This should not be confused with chronic cardiac hepatopathy, which is characterized by elevated cholestatic parameters along with little or no changes in transaminases and is potentially reversible after heart transplantation.[30] The use of MELD and MELD-XI (excluding international normalized ratio) were shown to be predictive of survival after heart transplantation and VAD. Moreover, if the MELD-XI normalized during VAD support, posttransplant survival was similar to those without prior liver dysfunction. In VAD patients with an elevated MELD-XI score, a decrease in score <17 may help identify optimal transplant candidates.[31,32]

Severe chronic bronchitis or obstructive pulmonary disease may predispose patients to pulmonary infections and may result in prolonged ventilatory support after heart transplantation. Patients who have a ratio of forced expiratory volume in 1 second to forced vital capacity (FEV_1/FVC) of less than 40 to 50% of predicted or an FEV_1 of less than 50% of predicted despite optimal medical therapy are considered poor candidates for transplantation.[2,4]

Transplantation in patients with diabetes mellitus is only contraindicated in the presence of significant end-organ damage (eg, diabetic nephropathy, retinopathy, or neuropathy).[2,4] Some centers have expanded their criteria successfully to include patients with mild to moderate end-organ damage.[33]

Active infection was a sound reason to delay transplantation before assist devices became more commonplace. Up to 48% of patients with implanted LVADs reportedly have evidence of infection. Interestingly, treatment for LVAD infection in these patients is to proceed with urgent transplantation.[34]

Other relative contraindications include severe noncardiac atherosclerotic disease, severe osteoporosis, and active peptic ulcer disease or diverticulitis, all of which may lead to increased morbidity.[2,4] Cachexia, defined as a body mass index (BMI) of less than 20 or less than 80% ideal body weight (IBW), and obesity, defined as BMI greater than 35 or greater than 140% of IBW, are associated with increased mortality after transplantation.[35] Poor nutritional status also may limit early postoperative rehabilitation. The effect of metabolic risk factors (hypertension, diabetes, obesity) was assessed in 15,960 recipients using an analysis of the UNOS Registry (1998-2008). Individually, these risk factors increased the risk of death posttransplant, with a hazard ratio of 1.10 for hypertension, 1.22 for diabetes, and 1.17 for obesity. Moreover, there was an exponential trend of increasing mortality with the addition of each risk factor, such that recipients with all 3 risk factors had a 63% increased mortality compared with recipients with none.[36]

The ultimate success of transplantation depends on the psychosocial stability and compliance of the recipient.[37] The rigorous postoperative regimen of multidrug therapy, frequent clinic visits, and routine endomyocardial biopsies demand commitment on the part of the patient. A history of psychiatric illness, substance abuse, or previous noncompliance (particularly with medical therapy for end-stage heart failure) may be sufficient cause to reject the candidacy of a patient. Lack of a supportive social system is an additional relative contraindication.

Management of the Potential Cardiac Recipient

PREFORMED ANTI-HLA ANTIBODIES

Patients with elevated levels of preformed panel reactive antibodies (PRAs) to human leukocyte antigens (HLAs) have higher rates of organ rejection and decreased survival than do patients without such antibodies.[38] Consequently, before proceeding with transplantation, many medical centers do prospective cross-matching, ie, either by flow cytometry or enzyme-linked immunosorbent assay (ELISA), to determine whether donor-specific antibodies that threaten the allograft are present. The problem has been compounded by the increased frequency of preformed reactive antibodies in patients with VADs who are awaiting cardiac transplantation.[39] Furthermore, not all antibodies are complement fixing or dangerous. Performing a prospective cross-match can be time-consuming and often it is impossible because of the unstable condition of the organ donor or travel logistics, leading to increased costs for transplantation and longer waiting times for recipients. Recently, virtual cross-matching has been used to eliminate the need for prospective tissue cross-matching. Modern laboratory techniques allow for identification and titer of antibodies. Because all donor antigens are known at the time of allocation, an assessment can be made without an actual tissue/sera assay. However, a particular patient's antibody population is dynamic and may change from the time of the antibody screen. As a result, care must be taken in patients with particularly diverse and high antibody titers. Plasmapheresis, intravenous immunoglobulins (IVIGs), cyclophosphamide, mycophenolate mofetil (MMF), and rituximab all have been used to lower the PRA levels with variable results.[2]

PHARMACOLOGIC BRIDGE TO TRANSPLANTATION

Critically compromised patients require admission to the intensive care unit for intravenous inotropic therapy. Dobutamine, a synthetic catecholamine, remains the prototype of this drug group. However, the phosphodiesterase III inhibitor milrinone is similarly effective.[40] The catecholamine dopamine is used often as a parenteral positive inotrope, but at moderate to high dose it evokes considerable systemic vasoconstriction. In candidates in whom an inotropic infusion has progressed to higher doses, combinations of dobutamine with milrinone are used. For transplant candidates dependent on inotropic infusions, eosinophilic myocarditis may develop as an allergic response to the dobutamine and may result in accelerated decline. VADs are being considered earlier, particularly as indices of nutrition decline.

MECHANICAL BRIDGE TO TRANSPLANTATION

Placement of an intraaortic balloon pump (IABP) may be necessary in patients with heart failure who are refractory to initial pharmacologic measures. Ambulatory IABP through the axillary artery has been reported in few patients as a bridge to cardiac transplantation but is not commonly used today.[41]

The landmark Randomized Evaluation of Mechanical Assistance in Treatment of Chronic Heart Failure (REMATCH) trial provided evidence that LVAD support provided a statistically significant reduction in the risk of death from any cause when compared with optimal medical management. The survival rates for patients receiving LVADs (n = 68) versus patients receiving optimal medical management (n = 61) were 52% versus 28% at 1 year and 29% versus 13% at 2 years (p = .008, log-rank test).[6,42] The extended follow-up confirmed the initial observation that LVAD therapy renders significant survival and quality-of-life benefits compared with optimal medical management for patients with end-stage heart failure. A recent systematic review of the published literature supported these findings. In the studies reviewed, implantation of an LVAD provided support for up to 390 days, with as many as 70% of patients surviving to transplantation.[43]

The total artificial heart (TAH) positioned orthotopically replaces both native cardiac ventricles and all cardiac valves. Potential advantages of this device include eliminating problems commonly seen in the bridge to transplantation with left ventricular and biventricular assist devices, such as right-sided heart failure, valvular regurgitation, cardiac arrhythmias, ventricular clots, intraventricular communications, and low blood flows. Copeland and colleagues reported that the TAH allowed for bridge to transplantation in 79% of their patients with 1- and 5-year survival rates after transplantation of 86 and 64%, respectively.[44]

Because these devices cannot be weaned, it is imperative that the patient's candidacy for transplantation be scrutinized before placement of the device. Trends toward better device durability and reduced complication rates likely will continue to improve through the development of newer, more innovative VADs, allowing destination therapy to be considered more frequently.

LIFE-THREATENING VENTRICULAR ARRHYTHMIAS

Symptomatic ventricular tachycardia (VT) and a history of sudden cardiac death are indications for placement of an automatic implantable cardioverter-defibrillator (AICD), long-term antiarrhythmic therapy with amiodarone, or occasionally, radiofrequency catheter ablation, which have been shown to improve survival.[45] Biventricular VADS and the TAH can be considered in this subgroup.

Recipient Prioritization for Transplantation

The prioritization of appropriate recipients for transplantation is based on survival and quality of life expected to be gained in comparison with maximal medical and surgical alternatives.[3] The United Network for Organ Sharing (UNOS) is a national organization that maintains organ transplantation waiting lists and allocates identified donor organs on the basis of recipients' priority status. This priority status is based on a recipient's status level (eg, IA, IB, or II), blood type, body size, and duration of time at a particular status level.[2] Geographic distance between donor and potential recipient is also taken into consideration. Highest priority is given to local status IA patients possessing the earliest listing dates. The recipient status criteria established by UNOS in 1999 are outlined in Table 60-3. In 1994, the percentage of patients awaiting transplantation for more than 2 years was 23%; this increased to 49% by 2003. From 1998 (with the

TABLE 60-3: Current Recipient Status Criteria of the United Network for Organ Sharing (UNOS)*

Status IA

A. Patients who require mechanical circulatory assistance with one or more of the following devices:
  1. Total artificial heart
  2. Left and/or right ventricular assist device implanted for 30 days or less
  3. Intraaortic balloon pump
  4. Extracorporeal membrane oxygenator (ECMO)
B. Mechanical circulatory support for more than 30 days with significant device-related complications
C. Mechanical ventilation
D. Continuous infusion of high-dose inotrope(s) in addition to continuous hemodynamic monitoring of left ventricular filling pressures
E. Life expectancy without transplant <7 days

Status IB

A. A patient who has at least one of the following devices or therapies in place:
  1. Left and/or right ventricular assist device implanted for >30 days
  2. Continuous infusion of intravenous inotropes

Status II

All other waiting patients who do not meet status Ia or Ib criteria
*UNOS Executive Order, August 1999

institution of a new status system) to 2007, the distribution of patient status at transplant changed dramatically. In 1999, the distribution was 34% (1A), 36% (1B), and 26% (2). This shifted in 2007 to 50% (1A), 36% (1B), and 14% (2).[46]

Patients considered for transplantation should be examined at least every 3 months for reevaluation of recipient status. Yearly right-sided heart catheterization is indicated for all candidates on the waiting list and in selected cases for patients rejected because of PH. Presently, there is no established method to delist patients who have stabilized on medical therapy without loss of their previously accrued waiting time.

THE CARDIAC DONOR

Donor Availability

The US Uniform Anatomic Gift Act of 1968 states that all competent individuals over the age of 18 may donate all or part of their bodies and established the current voluntary basis of organ donation practiced in the United States. To accommodate the increasing demand for organs, the original stringent criteria for donor eligibility have been relaxed, and educational campaigns have increased awareness of the need for a larger donor pool. In 1986, the Required Request Law, which required hospitals to request permission from next of kin to recover organs, was passed to encourage physician compliance in the donor request process. Future reforms will be molded by the evolving public attitude to transplantation and likely will focus on continued public and physician education.

The availability of donor organs remains the major limiting factor to heart transplantation. In the early years of heart transplantation, the number of heart transplants performed

in the United States increased steadily to a peak in 1995 of 2363 and then reached a plateau in 1998. After 1998, there was a gradual decline in heart transplants per year to a nadir of 2015 in 2004, after which the number has steadily increased to 2207 in 2007.[46] A more risk-averse approach to donor use has been discussed as contributing factor for decreased organ use.[47] Conversely, successful use of hearts with donor cardiac arrest history < 8 minutes[48] and donor cardiopulmonary resuscitation[49] has recently been reported.

Interestingly, likely owing to improved preoperative care, the death rate for patients on the waiting list for a cardiac allograft has decreased steadily.[46]

Allocation of Donor Organs

In an effort to increase organ donation and to coordinate an equitable allocation of allografts, Congress passed the National Organ Transplant Act in 1984. This act resulted in the drafting of the aforementioned Required Request Law, as well as the awarding of a federal contract to the UNOS for the development of a national organ procurement and allocation network. To facilitate transplantation, the United States is divided into 11 geographic regions.

Organs are offered to sick patients within the region in which they were donated before being offered to other parts of the country. This helps to reduce organ preservation time, improve organ quality and survival outcomes, reduce the costs incurred by the transplant patient, and increase access to transplantation.

The effect of the new UNOS broader regional algorithm for donor organ sharing that prioritizes donor heart allocation to higher-risk (status 1A and 1B) wait-listed patients was a significant reduction in waiting list mortality in status 1A and 1B patients, with no change in the waiting list mortality for lower-priority patients (status 2). Importantly posttransplant outcomes were sustained despite the higher-risk nature of the recipients.[50]

Donor Selection

Once a brain-dead individual has been identified as a potential cardiac donor, the patient undergoes a rigorous three-phase screening regimen. The primary screening is undertaken by the organ procurement agency. Information regarding the patient's age, height and weight, gender, ABO blood type, hospital course, cause of death, and routine laboratory data including cytomegalovirus (CMV), HIV, hepatitis B virus (HBV), and hepatitis C virus (HCV) serologies are collected. Cardiac surgeons and/or cardiologists perform the secondary screening, which involves further investigation in search of potential contraindications (Table 60-4), determination of the hemodynamic support necessary to sustain the donor, and review of the electrocardiogram, chest roentgenogram, arterial blood gas determination, and echocardiogram. Even when adverse donor criteria are reported, a team often is dispatched to the hospital to evaluate the donor on-site.

Although echocardiography is effective in screening for anatomical abnormalities of the heart, the use of a single echocardiogram to determine the physiologic suitability of a donor is not supported by evidence.[51] The Papworth Hospital transplant program in Great Britain increased its donor yield substantially by using a pulmonary artery catheter to guide the physiologic assessment and management of ventricular

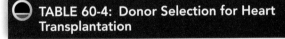

TABLE 60-4: Donor Selection for Heart Transplantation

I. Suggested criteria for cardiac donor
  A. Age <50-60
  B. Absence of the following:
    1. Prolonged cardiac arrest
    2. Prolonged severe hypotension
    3. Preexisting cardiac disease
    4. Intracardiac drug injection
    5. Severe chest trauma with evidence of cardiac injury
    6. Septicemia
    7. Extracerebral malignancy and glioblastoma
    8. Positive serologies for human immunodeficiency virus, hepatitis B (active), or hepatitis C
    9. Hemodynamic stability without high-dose inotropic support (<20 μg/kg/min of dopamine)
II. Suggested cardiac donor evaluation
  A. Past medical history and physical examination
  B. Electrocardiogram
  C. Chest roentgenogram
  D. Arterial blood gases
  E. Laboratory tests (ABO, HIV, HBV, HCV)
  F. Echocardiogram, pulmonary artery catheter evaluation, and in selected cases, coronary angiogram

dysfunction.[52] Coronary angiography is indicated in the presence of advanced donor age (traditionally for male donors >45 years of age and female donors >50 years of age). Angiography also should be performed if there is a history of cocaine use or the donor has three risk factors for coronary artery disease (CAD), such as hypertension, diabetes, smoking history, dyslipidemia, or family history of premature CAD.[51]

The final and often most important screening of the donor occurs intraoperatively at the time of organ procurement by the cardiac surgical team. Direct visualization of the heart is performed for evidence of right ventricular or valvular dysfunction, previous infarction, or myocardial contusion secondary to closed-chest compressions or blunt chest trauma. The coronary arterial tree is palpated for gross calcifications indicative of atheromatous disease. If direct examination of the heart is unremarkable, the recipient hospital is notified, and the procurement surgeons proceed with donor cardiectomy, usually in conjunction with multiorgan procurement.

Expanded Donor Criteria and Alternate Listing

As the donor shortage has worsened and the number of patients waiting for transplants has increased, one of the areas of increasing interest is the use of marginal donors for marginal recipients. For this purpose, an alternate recipient list is being used by some centers to match certain recipients who might be excluded from a standard list with marginal donor hearts that otherwise would go unused. Expanded donor criteria include the use of donors substantially smaller than the recipients, donors with coronary artery disease that may require coronary artery bypass grafting (CABG), left ventricular dysfunction, or donors from older age groups.[51] Acceptable operative mortality has been reported, and the University of California, Los Angeles (UCLA) heart transplant group has shown that alternate listing did not independently predict early or late mortality.[53]

It also appears more beneficial in terms of patient survival to receive an allograft from a donor older than 40 years of age compared to remaining on the waiting list.[54] Other high-risk donors, such as HCV-positive or HBV (core IgM-negative)-positive donors, may be appropriate in selected higher-risk recipients.[51]

Also of special interest is the effect of donor alcohol and cocaine abuse on heart transplantation. A small single-center study showed unfavorable early outcome of patients receiving hearts from alcoholic donors (>2 oz of pure alcohol daily for 3 or more months), suggesting the presence of a subclinical preoperative alcoholic cardiomyopathy and poor tolerance of rejection episodes after transplantation.[55] Because of widespread cocaine abuse, donor guidelines have declared intravenous drug abuse a "relative" contraindication for donor selection. However, the dilemma of selecting donor hearts from nonintravenous drug abusers remains an open issue. A favorable outcome for patients who received transplanted hearts obtained from nonintravenous cocaine users has been reported.[56] However, judicious use of organs from donors with a history of cocaine use is strongly advised. Specific recommendations were made in a consensus report to improve the yield of donor hearts.[51]

Management of the Cardiac Donor

Medical management of cardiac donors, an integral part of organ preservation, is complicated by the complex physiologic phenomenon of brain death and the need to coordinate procurement with other organ donor teams. Brain death is associated with an "autonomic and cytokine storm." The release of noradrenaline (norepinephrine) leads to subendocardial ischemia. Subsequent cytokine release results in further myocardial depression. This is accompanied by pronounced vasodilatation and loss of temperature control.[3] Rapid afterload reduction may be achieved with sodium nitroprusside, whereas volatile anesthetics reduce the intensity of sympathetic bursts. The initial period of intense autonomic activity is followed by loss of sympathetic tone and a massive reduction in systemic vascular resistance. Overall, brain stem death results in severe hemodynamic instability, the degree of which appears to be directly related to the severity of the brain injury and may result from vasomotor autonomic dysfunction, hypovolemia, hypothermia, and dysrhythmias.[57]

Aggressive volume resuscitation sometimes is necessary, and the use of a Swan-Ganz catheter may be crucial to guide therapy.[58] Fluid overload should be avoided to prevent postoperative allograft dysfunction caused by chamber distention and myocardial edema. Inotropic support (eg, dopamine or dobutamine, epinephrine, or norepinephrine) to maintain a mean arterial blood pressure (MAP) of 60 mm Hg or more in the presence of a central venous pressure (CVP) of 6 to 10 mm Hg is recommended.[51] ATP is depleted rapidly by exogenous catecholamine administration, and this has an adverse effect on posttransplantation cardiac function.[57] Low-dose vasopressin is being used increasingly as first-line support because, in addition to treating diabetes insipidus, it independently improves arterial blood pressure and reduces exogenous inotrope requirements in brain stem dead donors.[59] Maintenance of normal temperature, electrolyte levels, osmolarity, acid-base balance, and oxygenation is critical for optimal donor management. Central diabetes insipidus develops in more than 50% of donors because of pituitary dysfunction, and massive diuresis complicates fluid and electrolyte management.[60] The initial treatment of diabetes insipidus is aimed at correcting hypovolemia and returning the plasma sodium concentration to normal levels by fluid replacement with 5% dextrose or nasogastric water. In severe cases, intermittent treatment with the synthetic analogue 1-D-amino-8-D-arginine vasopressin (DDAVP) also may be required in addition to vasopressin infusion.[57]

Several studies have demonstrated beneficial effects of thyroid hormones and steroids on cardiac performance in brain stem dead-organ donors.[52,59,61] Recent guidelines advocate the addition of a standardized hormonal resuscitation package consisting of methylprednisolone (15 mg/kg bolus), triiodothyronine (4-μg bolus followed by infusion of 3 μg/h), and arginine vasopressin (1-unit bolus followed by 0.5-4 units/h) to the standard donor management protocol.[41] Donors also receive insulin, titrated to keep blood glucose at 120 to 180 mg/dL. Other pertinent strategies include standard ventilator management with diligent endotracheal suctioning and a thermoregulation goal of 34 to 36°C using warming blankets and lights, warm intravenous fluids, and warm inspired air. Broad-spectrum antibiotic therapy with a cephalosporin is initiated following collection of blood, urine, and tracheal aspirate for culture. The approach for management of the cardiac donor recommended at the conference entitled, Maximizing Use of Organs Recovered from the Cadaver Donor: Cardiac Recommendations, is shown in Table 60-5 and summarized in Fig. 60-2.[51]

Donor Heart Procurement

A median sternotomy is performed, and the pericardium is incised longitudinally. The heart is inspected and palpated for evidence of cardiac disease or injury. This visualization is communicated to the transplant team so the operation on the recipient can proceed timed with the expected arrival of the donor organ.

The superior and inferior venae cavae and the azygous vein are mobilized circumferentially and encircled with ties. The aorta is dissected from the pulmonary artery and isolated with umbilical tape. To facilitate access to the epigastrium by the liver procurement team, the cardiac team often then temporarily retires from the operating room table or assists with retraction. Once preparation for liver, pancreas, lung, and kidney explantation is completed, the patient is administered 30,000 units of heparin intravenously.

The azygous vein and superior vena cava (SVC) are doubly ligated (or stapled) and divided distal to the azygous vein, leaving a long segment of SVC (Fig. 60-3). The inferior vena cava (IVC) is incised and the left atrium vented either at the left atrial appendage or via a transected pulmonary vein. The aortic cross-clamp is applied at the takeoff of the innominate artery, and the heart is arrested with a single flush (1000 mL or 10-20 mL/kg) of cardioplegia solution infused proximal to the cross-clamp. Rapid cooling of the heart is achieved with copious amounts of cold saline and cold saline slush poured into the pericardial well.

After the delivery of cardioplegia, cardiectomy proceeds as the apex of the heart is elevated cephalad and any remaining intact pulmonary veins are divided.

This maneuver is modified appropriately to retain adequate left atrial cuffs for both lungs and the heart if the lungs also are being procured. While applying caudal traction to the heart with the nondominant hand, the ascending aorta is transected proximal to the innominate artery, and the pulmonary arteries are divided distal to the bifurcation (again, modification is necessary if the lungs are being procured).

More generous segments of the great vessels and SVC may be required for recipients with congenital heart disease. Alternatively, the SVC and IVC are transected, followed by the aorta and pulmonary artery. The left atrium is then divided

TABLE 60-5: Management of the Cardiac Donor

I. Conventional management, before the initial echocardiogram
  A. Adjust volume status (target central venous pressure 6-10 mm Hg)
  B. Correct metabolic perturbations, including
    1. Acidosis (target pH 7.40-7.45)
    2. Hypoxemia (target PO_2 > 80 mm Hg, O_2 saturation > 95%)
    3. Hypercarbia (target PCO_2 30-35 mm Hg)
  C. Correct anemia (target hematocrit 30%, hemoglobin 10 g/dL)
  D. Adjust inotropes to maintain mean arterial pressure at 60 mm Hg. Norepinephrine and epinephrine should be tapered off rapidly in favor of dopamine or dobutamine
  E. Target = dopamine < 10 μg/kg/min or dobutamine < 10 μg/kg/min
II. Obtain an initial echocardiogram
  A. Rule out structural abnormalities (substantial left ventricular hypertrophy, that is, IVS/PW > 13 mm, valvular dysfunction, congenital lesions)
  B. If left ventricular ejection fraction is 45%, proceed with recovery (consider aggressive management as shown below to optimize cardiac function before recovery) with final evaluation in the operating room
  C. If left ventricular ejection fraction is <45%, aggressive management with placement of a pulmonary arterial catheter and hormonal resuscitation is strongly recommended
III. Hormonal resuscitation
  A. Triiodothyronine (T3): 4-μg bolus, then continuous infusion at 3 μg/h
  B. Arginine vasopressin: 1-unit bolus, then continuous infusion at 0.5-4 units/h, titrated to a systemic vascular resistance of 800-1200 dyne/s/cm^5
  C. Methylprednisolone: 15 mg/kg bolus
  D. Insulin: 1 unit/h minimum; titrate to maintain blood sugar at 120-180 mg/dL
IV. Aggressive hemodynamic management
  A. Initiated simultaneously with hormonal resuscitation
  B. Placement of pulmonary artery catheter
  C. Duration of therapy 2 hours
  D. Adjustment of fluids, inotropes, and pressors every 15 minutes based on serial hemodynamic measurements to minimize use of beta-agonists and meet the following target (Papworth) criteria:
    1. Mean arterial pressure > 60 mm Hg
    2. Central venous pressure 4-12 mm Hg
    3. Pulmonary capillary wedge pressure 8-12 mm Hg
    4. Systemic vascular resistance 800-1200 dyne/s/cm^5
    5. Cardiac index > 2.4 L/min/m^2
    6. Dopamine < 10 μg/kg/min or dobutamine 10 μg/kg/min

Data from Zaroff JG, Rosengard BR, Armstrong WF, et al: Consensus conference report: maximizing use of organs recovered from the cadaver donor: cardiac recommendations, March 28-29, 2001, Crystal City, Va., *Circulation.* 2002 Aug 13;106(7):836-841.

as the last step. This allows for optimal division of the left atrium, particularly when lungs are recovered.

It is critically important to avoid left ventricular distention and ensure thorough cooling with ice saline.

Once the explantation is complete, the allograft is examined for evidence of a patent foramen ovale, which should be closed at that time. Any valvular anomalies are identified. The allograft then is placed in a sterile container and kept cold for transport to the recipient hospital.

Organ Preservation

Current clinical graft preservation techniques generally permit a safe ischemic period of 4 to 6 hours.[62] Factors contributing to the severity of postoperative myocardial dysfunction include insults associated with suboptimal donor management, hypothermia, ischemia-reperfusion injury, and depletion of energy stores.

A single flush of a cardioplegic or preservative solution followed by static hypothermic storage at 4 to 10°C is the preferred preservation method by most transplant centers. Crystalloid solutions of widely different compositions are available, and the debate over them speaks for the fact that no ideal solution currently exists. Depending on their ionic composition, solutions are classified as intracellular or extracellular.[62]

Intracellular solutions, characterized by moderate-to-high concentrations of potassium and low concentrations of sodium, purportedly reduce hypothermia-induced cellular edema by mimicking the intracellular milieu. Commonly used examples of these solutions include University of Wisconsin, Euro-Collins, and in Europe, Bretschneider (HTK) and intracellular Stanford solutions.

Extracellular solutions, characterized by low-to-moderate potassium and high sodium concentrations, avoid the theoretical potential for cellular damage and increased vascular resistance associated with hyperkalemic solutions. Hopkins,

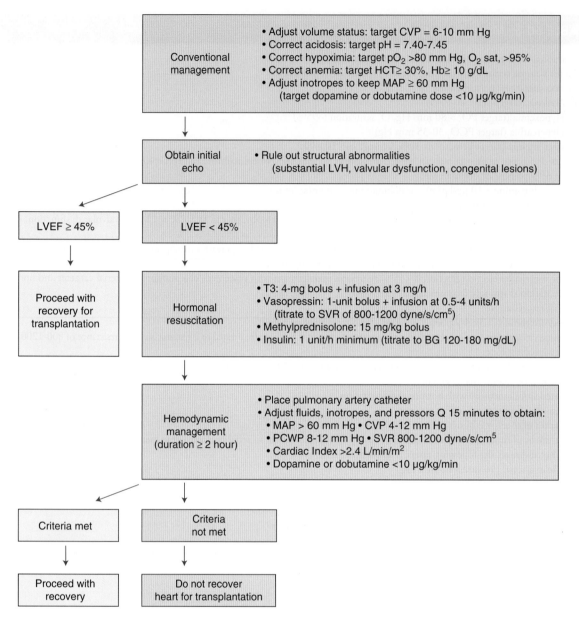

FIGURE 60-2 Recommended heart donor management algorithm. (Reproduced with permission from Zaroff JG, Rosengard BR, Armstrong WF, et al: Consensus conference report: maximizing use of organs recovered from the cadaver donor: cardiac recommendations, March 28-29, 2001, Crystal City, Va., *Circulation.* 2002 Aug 13;106(7):836-841.)

Celsior, Krebs, and St. Thomas Hospital solutions are representative extracellular cardioplegic solutions. Several comparisons of the different types of intracellular and extracellular solutions have shown variable results.[63,64] Although a plethora of pharmacologic additives has been included in cardioplegic-storage solutions, the greatest potential for future routine use may lie with impermeants, substrates, and antioxidants.[65] A number of pharmacologic and mechanical strategies for leukocyte inhibition and depletion also have been explored.[66] Potential benefits of continuous hypothermic perfusion (CHP) preservation such as uniform myocardial cooling, continuous substrate supplementation, and metabolic by-product washout are currently overshadowed by exacerbation

of extracellular cardiac edema and logistical problems inherent to a complex perfusion apparatus. Newer portable perfusion circuits are being developed, and recent studies showed reduction in oxidative stress and attenuation of DNA damage in canine heart transplant models preserved by 24-hour CHP compared with 4 hours of static preservation.[67]

In a prospective, randomized, multi-center, international, non-inferiority trial led by the University of California, Los Angeles (UCLA), the investigators hypothesized that the clinical outcomes of patients undergoing heart transplantation with donor hearts preserved on Organ Care System (OCS) versus standard cold storage are similar. This study was designed to provide data that would allow in a follow-up

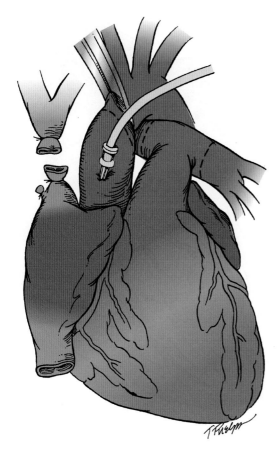

FIGURE 60-3 Donor cardiectomy.

study to test if OCS can expand the donor heart pool (by testing/improving "non-standard/marginal" donor hearts). The OC is the only clinical platform (2014) for exvivo human donor heart perfusion. It preserves the donor heart in a warm beating state during transport from the donor hospital to the recipient hospital. This study was conducted at 10 heart transplant centers in the United States and Europe. One hundred and twenty-eight patients were transplanted in the PROCEED II trial: 65 in the OCS group and 63 in the control group. With respect to the primary endpoint of 30-day patient and graft survival, the OCS group was found to be noninferior to the control group (OCS group: 94% [61/65] vs control group: 97% [61/63]). The results of secondary endpoints were similar for the two groups. Total preservation time was significantly longer in the OCS group versus control group, with a shorter cold ischemia time. Five donor hearts in the OCS group developed abnormal metabolic profile and were rejected for transplantation.[68] The clinical role of this system is yet to be determined. However, extended preservation times and better scheduling of a heart transplant are the real potential benefit of OCS preservation.

Donor-Recipient Matching

Criteria for matching potential recipients with the appropriate donor are based primarily on ABO blood group compatibility and patient size. ABO barriers should not be crossed in adult heart transplantation because incompatibility may result in fatal hyperacute rejection. Donor weight should be within 30% of recipient weight except in pediatric patients, in whom closer size matching is required. In cases of elevated PVR in the recipient (5-6 Wood units), a larger donor is preferred to reduce the risk of right ventricular failure in the early postoperative period. At UCLA we prefer a male donor for a male recipient when size and PH are an issue.

Although practices vary by transplant program, generally if the percent of PRA is greater than 10%, indicating recipient presensitization to alloantigen, a prospective negative T-cell cross-match between the recipient and donor sera is mandatory before transplantation.[32,69] A cross-match is always performed retrospectively, even if the PRA is absent or low. Retrospective studies also have demonstrated that better matching at the HLA-DR locus results in fewer episodes of rejection and infection with an overall improved survival.[70] Because of current allocation criteria and limits on ischemic time of the cardiac allograft, routine prospective HLA matching is not logistically possible.

OPERATIVE TECHNIQUES IN HEART TRANSPLANTATION

Orthotopic Heart Transplantation

OPERATIVE PREPARATION OF THE RECIPIENT

The original technique of orthotopic cardiac transplantation described by Shumway and Lower is still used commonly today. Following median sternotomy and vertical pericardiotomy, the patient is heparinized and prepared for cardiopulmonary bypass. Bicaval venous cannulation and distal ascending aortic cannulation just proximal to the origin of the innominate artery are optimal. Umbilical tape snares are passed around the superior and inferior venae cavae.

Bypass is initiated, the patient is cooled to 28°C, caval snares are tightened, and the ascending aorta is cross-clamped. The great vessels are transected above the semilunar commissures, whereas the atria are incised along the atrioventricular grooves, leaving cuffs for allograft implantation. Removal of the atrial appendages reduces the risk of postoperative thrombus formation.

Following cardiectomy, the proximal 1 to 2 cm of aorta and pulmonary artery are separated from one another with electrocautery, taking care to avoid injuring the right pulmonary artery. Continuous aspiration of pulmonary venous return from bronchial collaterals is achieved by insertion of a vent into the left atrial remnant either directly or via the right superior pulmonary vein.

Timing of donor and recipient cardiectomies is critical to minimize allograft ischemic time and recipient bypass time. Frequent communication between the procurement and transplant teams permits optimal coordination of the procedures. Ideally, the recipient cardiectomy is completed just before arrival of the cardiac allograft.

No irrevocable surgical maneuvers should be performed before one is sure of the safe arrival of the donor organ. Redo sternotomy and removal of VADs or the TAH complicates this timing and should be carefully factored into the estimated donor organ ischemic time.

IMPLANTATION

The donor heart is removed from the transport cooler and placed in a basin of cold saline. If not previously performed, preparation of the donor heart is accomplished. Electrocautery and sharp dissection are used to separate the aorta and the pulmonary artery. The left atrium is incised by connecting the pulmonary vein orifices, and excess atrial tissue is trimmed, forming a circular cuff tailored to the size of the recipient left atrial remnant (Fig. 60-4).

Implantation begins with placement of a double-armed 3-0 Prolene suture through the recipient left atrial cuff at the level of the left superior pulmonary vein and then through the donor left atrial cuff near the base of the atrial appendage (Fig. 60-5). The allograft is lowered into the recipient mediastinum atop a cold sponge to insulate it from direct thermal transfer from adjacent thoracic structures. An insulating pad is placed to protect the phrenic nerve. The suture is continued in a running fashion caudally and then medially to the inferior aspect of the interatrial septum (Fig. 60-6). The second arm of the suture is run along the roof of the left atrium and down the interatrial septum. It is important to continually assess size discrepancy between donor and recipient atria so that appropriate plication of excess tissue may be performed.

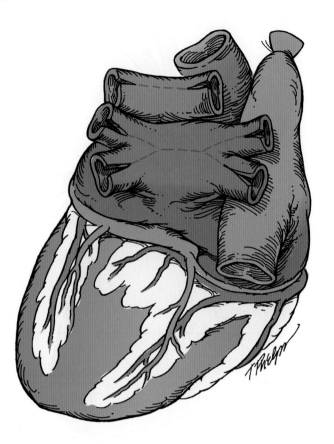

FIGURE 60-4 Donor allograft preparation for orthotopic heart transplantation. Pulmonary vein orifices joined to form left atrial cuff.

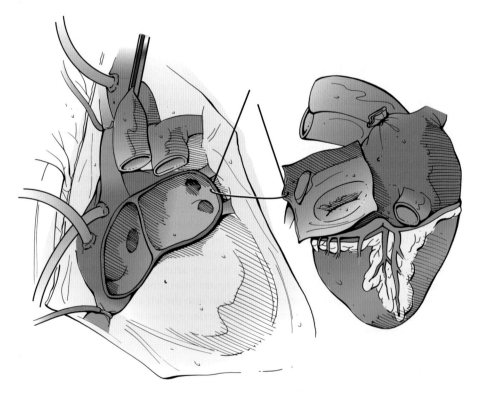

FIGURE 60-5 Implantation of allograft. First suture is placed at the level of the left superior pulmonary vein. (Reproduced with permission from Baumgartner WA, Kasper E, Reitz B, et al: *Heart and Lung Transplantation.* 2nd ed. New York: Saunders/Elsevier; 2002.)

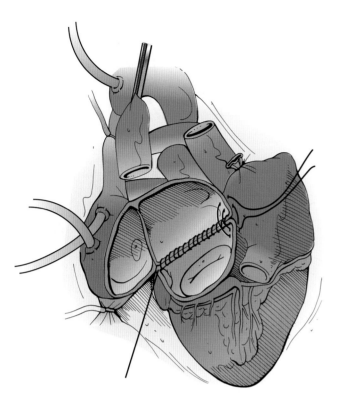

FIGURE 60-6 Implantation of allograft. Left atria anastomosis. (Reproduced with permission from Baumgartner WA, Kasper E, Reitz B, et al: *Heart and Lung Transplantation.* 2nd ed. New York: Saunders/Elsevier; 2002.)

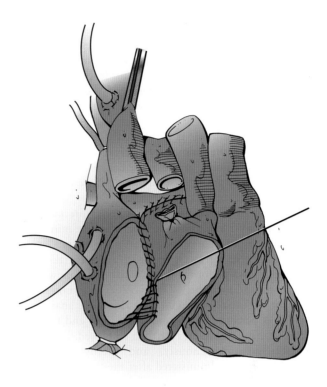

A

The left atrium is continuously irrigated with cold saline while the RA, pulmonary artery and aortic anastomosis are completed with the LA vent off. Then the two arms of suture are tied together on the outside of the heart. Constant insufflation of carbon dioxide into the mediastinum to reduce the amount of intracardiac air should be standard.

The traditional biatrial cuff technique starts with right atrial cuff anastomosis once the left atrial anastomosis is complete, a curvilinear incision is made from the inferior vena caval orifice toward the right atrial appendage of the allograft. This modification in the right atriotomy initially introduced by Barnard reduces the risk of injury to the sinoatrial (SA) node and accounts for the preservation of sinus rhythm observed in most recipients.

The tricuspid apparatus and interatrial septum are inspected. Recipients are predisposed to increased right-sided heart pressures in the early postoperative period owing to pre-existing PH and volume overload. The recovering right ventricle poorly tolerates both conditions.

To avoid refractory arterial desaturation associated with shunting, patent foramen ovale are closed. The right atrial anastomosis is performed in a running fashion similar to the left, with the initial anchor suture placed either at the most superior or inferior aspect of the interatrial septum so that the ends of the suture meet in the middle of the anterolateral wall (Fig. 60-7A,B).

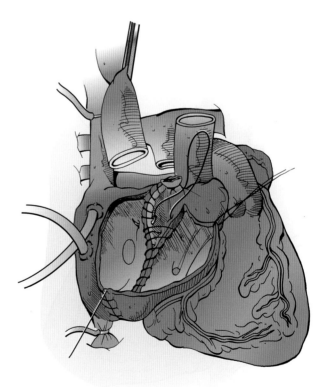

B

FIGURE 60-7 Implantation of allograft. (A) Initiation of right atrial anastomosis. (B) Completion of right atrial anastomosis. (Reproduced with permission from Baumgartner WA, Kasper E, Reitz B, et al: *Heart and Lung Transplantation.* 2nd ed. New York: Saunders/Elsevier; 2002.)

The end-to-end pulmonary artery anastomosis is next performed using a 4 or 5-0 Prolene suture beginning with the posterior wall from inside of the vessel and then completing the anterior wall from the outside (Fig. 60-8). It is crucial that the pulmonary artery ends be trimmed to eliminate any redundancy in the vessel that might cause kinking.[71]

The aortic anastomosis is performed using a technique similar to that for the pulmonary artery, except that some redundancy is desirable in the aorta because it facilitates visualization of the posterior suture line if there is bleeding (Fig. 60-9).

Like and many other centers we now prefer direct end-to-end IVC and SVC anastomoses. This technique minimizes the risk of tricuspid regurgitation or SA node injury. Care to prevent twisting or narrowing of the cava is essential. Using this technique we perform the left atrial cuff, followed by the PA, aorta and then the IVC and SVC anastomoses.

Rewarming usually is begun after the aortic anastomosis, which is performed in a standard end-to-end fashion. Routine deairing techniques are then employed. Lidocaine (100-200 mg intravenously) and methylprednisone (500-1000 mg) are administered after the atrial anastomosis. Pressure-controlled (<50 mm Hg), leucocyte-depleted,

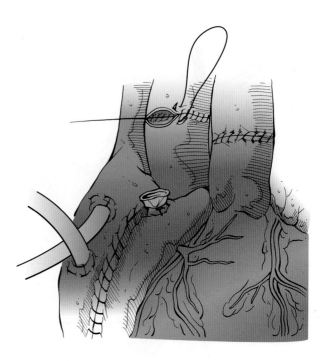

FIGURE 60-9 Implantation of allograft. Aortic anastomosis. (Reproduced with permission from Baumgartner WA, Kasper E, Reitz B, et al: *Heart and Lung Transplantation.* 2nd ed. New York: Saunders/Elsevier; 2002.)

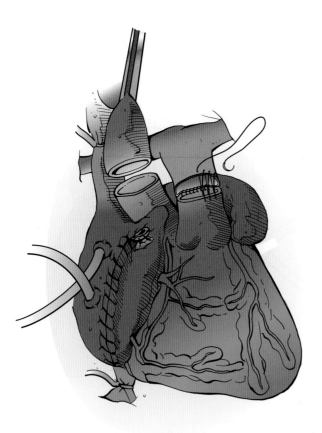

FIGURE 60-8 Implantation of allograft. Pulmonary arterial anastomosis. (Reproduced with permission from Baumgartner WA, Kasper E, Reitz B, et al: *Heart and Lung Transplantation.* 2nd ed. New York: Saunders/Elsevier; 2002.)

substrate-enhanced aspartate and glutamate warm reperfusion is given for 3 minutes followed by warm leucocyte depleted blood for 7 minutes prior to releasing the aortic cross-clamp.

The aortic cross-clamp is removed. Half of patients require electrical defibrillation. A needle vent is inserted in the ascending aorta and maintained on suction for final deairing, with the patient in steep Trendelenburg position.

Suture lines are inspected carefully for hemostasis. Inotrope infusion is initiated, and temporary pacing may be required. The patient is weaned from cardiopulmonary bypass, and the cannulae are removed. Temporary epicardial atrial and ventricular bipolar pacing wires are placed in the donor right atrium and ventricle. Following insertion of mediastinal and pleural tubes, the median sternotomy is closed in the standard fashion.

Cold-blood cardioplegia is used in many centers. An initial dose often is given following removal from the cold storage solution before implantation. A second dose, or the initial dose as given by some centers, is administered after the right atrial anastomosis or IVC anastomosis, when a bicaval technique is used.

We generally do not redose cardioplegia after the heart is removed from cold storage. However, prior to releasing the cross-clamp a warm substrate enhanced (aspartate and glutamate) reperfusion solution is administered for 4 minutes with a mean pressure of 45 to 50 mm Hg. An additional leucocyte-depleted warm blood, pressure-controlled reperfusate, is given for an additional 5 to 7 minutes.

ALTERNATIVE TECHNIQUES FOR ORTHOTOPIC HEART TRANSPLANTATION

The most commonly employed technique today is a bicaval anastomotic method. With this technique, the recipient right atrium is excised completely, leaving a left atrial cuff and a generous cuff of the IVC and SVC, respectively.

The left atrial cuff of the donor is anastomosed to the left atrial cuff of the recipient using the standard Shumway technique. The PA and aortic anastomosis are performed. Individual end-to-end anastomoses of the IVC and SVC are performed (Fig. 60-10).

Although these procedures are more technically difficult than standard orthotopic transplantation, published series using these techniques have reported shorter hospital stays, reduced postoperative dependence on diuretics, and lower incidences of atrial dysrhythmias, conduction disturbances, mitral and tricuspid valve incompetence, and right ventricular failure.[72] A single-center study comparing biatrial versus bicaval transplant showed an improved 12-month survival in the bicaval group.[73] However, an analysis of the UNOS database, including more than 11,000 patients, did not demonstrate a survival difference between patients in whom biatrial versus bicaval anastomotic techniques were used, although the bicaval technique was associated with decreased duration of hospital stay and postoperative pacemaker placement.[74]

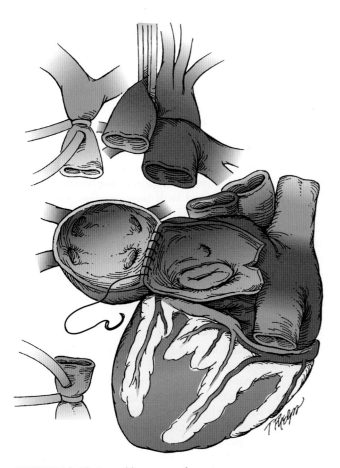

FIGURE 60-10 Bicaval heart transplantation.

Long-term outcomes and prospective, randomized studies evaluating these alternative techniques are still needed.

Heterotopic Heart Transplantation

PH and right-sided heart failure have remained the leading causes of early mortality in cardiac transplantation. This has led to an interest in heterotopic heart transplantation. Currently, heterotopic heart transplants are performed rarely but may be indicated in patients with irreversible PH or significant donor-recipient size mismatch.[22]

Heart Transplantation after VAD

Cardiac transplantation after VAD or TAH poses unique challenges. All patients should have a recent contrast chest computed tomography (CT) to identify location of cardiac structures to the sternum and the course of outflow grafts.

The femoral or axillary artery and femoral vein should be exposed for emergency cannulation before redo sternotomy. Sternal reentry should carefully dissect the heart from pleura to pleura to safely place a retractor. The initial focus is on dissection of the IVC, SVC, and aorta. Further dissection is ideal, but may require cardiopulmonary bypass. The apex and left atrium should not be manipulated before bypass as there is a risk of entraining air, particularly with axial-flow devices. Finally, before initiating bypass, the outflow graft should be clamped to prevent regurgitation through the device.

The sternotomy and lysis of adhesions can be difficult and time consuming. Timing of the dissection and the arrival of the donor heart is individualize based upon not taking any irreversible steps prior to arrival of the heart and not prolonging donor heart ischemic time for cardiectomy and device removal.

POSTOPERATIVE MANAGEMENT

Hemodynamic Management

HEART ALLOGRAFT PHYSIOLOGY

The intact heart is innervated by antagonistic sympathetic and parasympathetic fibers of the autonomic nervous system. Transplantation necessitates transection of these fibers, yielding a denervated heart with altered physiology. Devoid of autonomic input, the SA node of the transplanted allograft fires at its increased intrinsic resting rate of 90 to 110 beats per minute.[75] The allograft relies on distant noncardiac sites as its source for catecholamines; thus its response to stress (eg, hypovolemia, hypoxia, and anemia) is somewhat delayed until circulating catecholamines can exert their positive chronotropic effect on the heart. The absence of a normal reflex tachycardia in response to venous pooling accounts for the frequency of orthostatic hypotension in transplant patients.

Denervation alters the heart's response to therapeutic interventions that act directly through the cardiac autonomic nervous system.[75] Carotid sinus massage, Valsalva maneuver, and atropine have no effect on SA node firing or atrioventricular conduction. Because of depletion of myocardial catecholamine stores associated with prolonged inotropic support of the donor, the allograft often requires high doses of catecholamines. The inotropic support is often necessary for several days. In patients with pre transplant VADs the vasoplegia requires support particularly in patients who have had axial flow pumps.

ROUTINE HEMODYNAMIC MANAGEMENT

Donor myocardial performance is transiently depressed in the immediate postoperative period. Allograft injury associated with donor hemodynamic instability and the hypothermic, ischemic insult of preservation contribute to reduced ventricular compliance and contractility characteristics of the newly transplanted heart.[76]

Abnormal atrial dynamics owing to the midatrial anastomosis exacerbate the reduction in ventricular diastolic loading. An infusion of a variety of drugs such as epinephrine, norepinephrine, dobutamine and milrinone is initiated routinely in the operating room to provide temporary inotropic support.

Cardiac denervation brings in several consequences, which may include a chronotropic and inotropic supersensitivity to exogenous catecholamines.[77] Restoration of normal myocardial function usually permits the cautious weaning of inotropic support within 5 to 7 days.

Vasoplegia often requires vasopressin, norepinephrine, or neosynephrine.

RV dysfunction can be improved with inhaled nitric oxide.

EARLY ALLOGRAFT FAILURE

Early cardiac failure still accounts for up to 20% of perioperative deaths of heart transplant recipients.[78] The cause of primary graft failure may be multifactorial. The most important etiologies are myocardial dysfunction owing to donor instability, PH, ischemic injury during preservation, and occasionally acute rejection. Mechanical support with an IABP, VAD, or ECMO can be used in patients refractory to pharmacologic interventions, although this measure, as well as retransplantation, has historically been associated with increased mortality.[79,80]

Chronic right ventricular failure frequently is associated with elevated PVR, and the unprepared donor right ventricle may be unable to overcome this increased afterload. Although recipients are screened to ensure that those with irreversible PH are not considered for transplantation, right-sided heart failure remains a leading cause of early mortality. Initial management involves employing pulmonary vasodilators such as inhaled nitric oxide, nitroglycerin, or sodium nitroprusside. PH that is refractory to these vasodilators sometimes responds to PGE$_1$ or prostacyclin.[14,81] Intra-aortic balloon counterpulsation and right VADs (Centromag) also can be used in patients unresponsive to medical therapy.[82]

ECMO support for several days with an open chest has been successful to allow time for graft recovery in cases of inadequate biventricular function.

ARRHYTHMIAS

Denervation of the transplanted heart leads to loss of autonomic nervous system modulation of the heart's electrophysiologic properties. Parasympathetic denervation causes loss of basal suppression of SA node automaticity, leading to a persistent increase in resting heart rate and a loss of normal, rapid heart rate modulation. This parasympathetic loss also causes elimination of the chronotropic effects of digoxin and atropine after heart transplantation. At the same time, sympathetic denervation causes a decrease and delay in exercise- or stress-induced augmentation of SA node automaticity, resulting in a decreased maximum heart rate with exercise.[83]

Sinus or junctional bradycardia occurs in up to half of transplant recipients. Risk factors for sinus node dysfunction include prolonged organ ischemia, angiographic nodal artery abnormalities, biatrial versus bicaval anastomosis, preoperative amiodarone use, and rejection.[84] Adequate heart rate is achieved with inotropic drug infusions and/or temporary epicardial pacing. Most bradyarrhythmias resolve over 1 to 2 weeks. Theophylline has been effective in patients with bradyarrhythmias and has decreased the need for permanent pacemakers in this patient population.[85]

Atrial fibrillation, atrial flutter, and other supraventricular arrhythmias have been reported in 5 to 30% of patients after heart transplantation.[83] Individual assessment of the risk: benefit ratio for anticoagulation therapy is necessary. Supraventricular tachycardia in transplant patients should be treated in the same manner as in nontransplant patients but with lower doses. Recurrent arrhythmias from reentry circuits or defined ectopic foci often can be cured by radiofrequency ablation.

Premature ventricular complexes are generally not considered ominous. Because of their rapidly terminal nature, sustained VT and ventricular fibrillation presumably are responsible for a significant portion of the 10% of sudden and unexplained deaths in heart transplant patients.[86]

Unique aspects of common antiarrhythmic drugs reflecting the differences in their therapeutic effects in heart transplant recipients compared with nontransplant patients are shown in Table 60-6.[83] Persistence of any form of arrhythmia should warrant further investigative efforts and an aggressive search for the presence of indicators of cardiac ischemia, rejection, pulmonary pathology, or infection. If arrhythmic episodes are frequent or underlying cardiac pathology is severe, retransplantation may be considered.

SYSTEMIC HYPERTENSION

Systemic hypertension should be treated to prevent unnecessary afterload stress on the allograft. In the early postoperative period, intravenous sodium nitroprusside or nitroglycerin usually is administered. Nitroglycerin is associated with less pulmonary shunting because of a relative preservation of the pulmonary hypoxic vasoconstrictor reflex. Nicardipine infusion has been reported to control postoperative hypertension more rapidly and was superior to sodium nitroprusside in maintaining left ventricular performance immediately after

TABLE 60-6: Differences in Therapeutic Agent Effects in Heart Transplant Recipients Compared with Nontransplant Patients

Arrhythmia therapy	Differences in posttransplantation
Drugs	
AV nodal agents	
Digoxin	No effect on heart rate
β-Adrenergic antagonists	Exacerbation of exercise intolerance
Calcium channel antagonists	Accentuated slowing of SA and AV nodes; may alter cyclosporine levels
Adenosine	Accentuated slowing of SA and AV nodes
Adrenergic agonists	
Norepinephrine	Unchanged peripheral effect, slightly more inotropic and chronotropic effect
Epinephrine	Unchanged peripheral effect, slightly more inotropic and chronotropic effect
Dopamine	Unchanged peripheral effect, less inotropic effect
Dobutamine	Unchanged
Ephedrine	Unchanged peripheral effect, less inotropic effect
Neo-synephrine	Unchanged peripheral effect, no reflex bradycardia
Isoproterenol	Unchanged
Antiarrhythmic agents	
Class Ia (quinidine, disopyramide, procainamide)	No cardiac vagolytic effect
Class Ib (lidocaine, mexiletine)	None reported
Class Ic (flecainide, encainide, moricizine, propafenone)	None reported
Class III (amiodarone, sotalol, ibutilide, dofetilide)	Possible exaggerated or atypical response
Anticoagulants	
Heparin	None reported
Warfarin	None reported
Miscellaneous	
Atropine	No effect on heart rate
Methylxanthines (theophylline, aminophylline)	Possibly more chronotropic effect
Cardioversion	None reported
Radiofrequency catheter ablation	Possible differences in pathway or chamber anatomy
Electrical devices	
Pacemaker	None reported
Intracardiac defibrillator	None reported

AV, atrioventricular; SA, sinoatrial.
Reproduced with permission from Stecker EC, Strelich KR, Chugh SS, et al: Arrhythmias after orthotopic heart transplantation, *J Card Fail*. 2005 Aug;11(6):464-472.

drug infusion.[87] If hypertension persists, an oral antihypertensive can be added, if possible, to permit weaning of the parenteral agents.

Respiratory Management

The respiratory management of the cardiac transplant recipient uses the same protocols employed following routine cardiac surgery.

Renal Function

Preoperative renal insufficiency owing to chronic heart failure and the nephrotoxic effects of calcineurin inhibitors such as FK506 and cyclosporine place the recipient at increased risk of renal insufficiency. Acute calcineurin inhibitor-induced renal insufficiency usually will resolve with a reduction in dose. Continuous intravenous infusion to eliminate the wide fluctuations in levels associated with oral dosing can

be attempted. Furthermore, concurrent administration of mannitol with calcineurin inhibitors may reduce their nephrotoxicity. Most centers administer a cytolytic agent in the immediate postoperative period and delay the initiation of calcineurin inhibitor therapy.

Outpatient Follow-up

Before discharge, patients should receive comprehensive education about their medications, diet, exercise, and infection recognition. Close follow-up by an experienced transplant team is the cornerstone for successful long-term survival after cardiac transplantation. This comprehensive team facilitates the early detection of rejection, opportunistic infections, patient noncompliance, and adverse sequelae of immunosuppression. Clinic visits routinely are scheduled concurrently with endomyocardial biopsies and include physical examination, a variety of laboratory studies, chest roentgenogram, and electrocardiogram.

ACUTE REJECTION

Allo-Immunology

Cardiac allograft rejection is the normal host response to cells recognized as nonself. The vast majority of cases are mediated by the cellular limb of the immune response through an elegant cascade of events involving macrophages, cytokines, and T lymphocytes. Antibody-mediated rejection (AMR), also called *humoral rejection* or *vascular rejection*, seems less common but is also more challenging to diagnose. The highest risk factors are allografts from younger and female donors (irrespective of recipient sex). Although about 85% of episodes can be reversed with corticosteroid therapy alone,[88] rejection is still a major cause of morbidity in cardiac transplant recipients.[5,89] Therefore, key research priorities in heart transplantation over the next decade include individualized immunosuppressive therapy and investigation and management of long-term immune and nonimmune complications.[90]

Hyperacute Rejection

Hyperacute rejection results from preformed donor-specific antibodies in the recipient. ABO blood group and PRA screening have made this condition a rare complication.

The onset of hyperacute rejection occurs within minutes to several hours after transplantation, and the results are catastrophic. Gross inspection reveals a mottled or dark red, flaccid allograft, and histologic examination confirms the characteristic global interstitial hemorrhage and edema without lymphocytic infiltrate. Immunofluorescence techniques reveal deposits of immunoglobulins and complement on the vascular endothelium. Immediate plasmapheresis, IVIG, and mechanical support are immediately instituted, and retransplantation may be the only successful strategy.

Diagnosis of Acute Rejection

In the precyclosporine era, the classic clinical manifestations of acute rejection included low-grade fever, malaise, leukocytosis, pericardial friction rub, supraventricular arrhythmias, decreased voltage on ECG, low cardiac output, reduced exercise tolerance, and signs of congestive heart failure.

In the cyclosporine era, however, most episodes of rejection characteristically are insidious, and patients can remain asymptomatic even with late stages of rejection. Thus routine surveillance studies for early detection are crucial to minimize cumulative injury to the allograft.

Right ventricular endomyocardial biopsy remains the gold standard for the diagnosis of acute rejection. The most frequently used technique for orthotopic allografts is a percutaneous approach through the right internal jugular vein. Interventricular septal specimens are fixed in formalin for permanent section, although frozen sections are performed occasionally if urgent diagnosis is necessary.

Hemodynamic parameters may also be obtained with a pulmonary artery catheter. Complications are infrequent (1 to 2%) but include venous hematoma, carotid puncture,

pneumothorax, arrhythmias, heart block, and right ventricular perforation and injury to the tricuspid valve.

The exact schedule for endomyocardial biopsies varies among institutions but usually reflects the associated risk of increased rejection during the first 6 months after transplantation. Biopsies are performed initially every 7 to 10 days in the early postoperative period and eventually tapered to 3- to 6-month intervals after the first year. Suspicion of rejection warrants additional biopsies.

Evaluation of sample adequacy for the ISHLT grading scheme requires a minimum of four good endomyocardial tissue fragments, with less than 50% of each fragment being fibrous tissue, thrombus, or other noninterpretable tissues (eg, crush artifact or poorly processed fragments).[91] The pattern and density of lymphocyte infiltration, in addition to the presence or absence of myocyte necrosis in the endomyocardial biopsy, determine the severity grade of cellular rejection.[92]

Further elaboration of the pathologic features and identification of AMR have been addressed.[93] In 2004, the ISHLT Pathology Council proposed simplification of the 1990 diagnostic categories for cellular rejection to mild, moderate, and severe and identification of the histologic characteristics of AMR.[94] The new grading scale was developed to better address the challenges and inconsistencies in use of the old grading system. Tables 60-7 and 60-8 show the new 2004 ISHLT grading scale.[94]

Noninvasive studies for the diagnosis of acute rejection have been unreliable. Electrocardiographic voltage summation and E-rosette assay techniques were useful adjuncts in the early cardiac transplant experience[95]; however, they currently are of no value in patients receiving cyclosporine.[96] Attempts with signal-averaged electrocardiography,[97] echocardiography,[98] or in combination,[99] MRI,[100] technetium ventriculography,[101] and a variety of immunologic markers[102] have not provided sufficient sensitivity and specificity to warrant widespread use.[103]

⊖ TABLE 60-7: ISHLT Standardized Cardiac Biopsy Grading: Acute Cellular Rejection, 2004*

Grade 0 R[†]	No rejection
Grade 1 R (Mild)	Interstitial and/or perivascular infiltrate with up to 1 focus of myocyte damage
Grade 2 R	(Moderate) Two or more foci of infiltrate with associated myocyte damage
Grade 3 R	(Severe) Diffuse infiltrate with multifocal myocyte damage ± edema, ± hemorrhage ± vasculitis

*The presence or absence of acute antibody-mediated rejection (AMR) may be recorded as AMR 0 or AMR 1, as required (see Table 64-8).
†Where R denotes revised grade to avoid confusion with1990 scheme.
ISHLT, International Society of Heart and Lung Transplantation.
Modified with permission from Stewart S, Winters GL, Fishbein MC, et al: Revision of the 1990 working formulation for the standardization of nomenclature in the diagnosis of heart rejection, *J Heart Lung Transplant.* 2005 Nov;24(11):1710-1720.

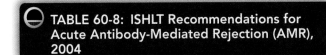

TABLE 60-8: ISHLT Recommendations for Acute Antibody-Mediated Rejection (AMR), 2004

AMR 0	Negative for acute antibody-mediated rejection
	No histologic or immunopathologic features of AMR
AMR 1	Positive for AMR
	Histologic features of AMR
	Positive immunofluorescence or immunoperoxidase staining for AMR (positive CD68, C4D)

Modified with permission from Stewart S, Winters GL, Fishbein MC, et al: Revision of the 1990 working formulation for the standardization of nomenclature in the diagnosis of heart rejection, *J Heart Lung Transplant.* 2005 Nov;24(11):1710-1720.

Peripheral blood gene expression profiling is an exciting new field.[104] The Allomap test has been FDA-cleared and widely implemented since 2006 to help rule out acute cardiac allograft rejection in stable heart transplant recipients and has led to a reduction in the use of protocol endomyocardial biopsy.[105-108]

Prophylaxis and Treatment of Acute Rejection

Baseline immunosuppression has evolved considerably over the last four decades. Current trends suggest lower use of cyclosporine A compared with tacrolimus-based calcineurinn inhibition. MMF has largely replaced imuram and remains the most commonly used adjunctive agent. Several centers are attempting to achieve a steroid-free dual immunosuppression regimen.[109]

Corticosteroids are the cornerstone for antirejection therapy. The treatment of choice for any rejection episode occurring during the first 1 to 3 postoperative months or for an episode considered to be severe is a short course (3 days) of intravenous methylprednisolone (1000 mg/day). Virtually all other episodes are treated initially with increased doses of oral prednisone (100 mg/day) followed by a taper to baseline over several weeks.[110] Although not yet universally accepted, many centers have reduced the doses of these corticosteroids successfully with reversal rates of rejection similar to traditional dosing.

Repeat endomyocardial biopsy should be performed 7 to 10 days after the cessation of antirejection therapy to assess adequacy of treatment. If the biopsy does not show significant improvement, a second trial of pulse-steroid therapy is recommended; if rejection has progressed (or if the patient becomes hemodynamically unstable), rescue therapy is indicated.

Substitution of tacrolimus for cyclosporine may obviate the need for admission in patients with steroid-refractory persistent rejection.[111] Alternatively, sirolimus may be substituted for mycophenolate or azathioprine.[112] The use of OKT3, antithymocyte globulin, and thymoglobulin generally is reserved for severe rejection with hemodynamic

compromise.[113] Methotrexate has been particularly successful in eradicating chronic low-grade rejection. Total lymphoid irradiation and photopheresis also have demonstrated success in some cases of refractory rejection.[114] Cardiac retransplantation is the ultimate therapeutic option for patients who do not respond to the aforementioned interventions. However, the results of retransplantation for rejection are dismal, and in most centers, it is no longer performed for this indication. Severe rejection with cardiogenic shock requires ECMO support during aggressive drug therapy.

Asymptomatic mild rejection (grade 1) usually is not treated but is monitored with repeat endomyocardial biopsies because only 20 to 40% of mild cases progress to moderate rejection.[115] On the other hand, the presence of myocyte necrosis (grades 3b and 4) represents a definite threat to allograft viability and is a universally accepted indication for therapy. Management of moderate rejection (grade 3a) is controversial and requires consideration of multiple variables.[116] Notably, Stoica and colleagues demonstrated that acute moderate-to-severe cellular rejection has a cumulative impact on cardiac allograft vasculopathy (CAV) onset.[117] Regardless of the biopsy results, allograft dysfunction is an indication for hospitalization, antirejection therapy, and if severe, invasive hemodynamic monitoring and inotropic support.

Antibody-Mediated Rejection

AMR, previously termed vascular rejection and humoral rejection, is mediated by the humoral limb of the immune response. Unlike acute cellular rejection, hemodynamic instability requiring inotropic support is common in patients with vascular rejection.[117] The incidence of asymptomatic AMR is higher in the first year after heart transplantation with a high recurrence rate. The more severe AMR, the lower the chances of improvement.[118]

Diagnosis requires evidence of endothelial cell swelling on light microscopy and immunoglobulin-complement deposition by immunofluorescence techniques.[119] Aggressive treatment of patients with allograft dysfunction consists of plasmapheresis, high-dose corticosteroids, heparin, IgG, and cyclophosphamide.[120] Despite these interventions, symptomatic acute vascular rejection is associated with a high mortality.[120,121] Repeated episodes of acute vascular rejection or chronic low-grade vascular rejection are believed to play a dominant role in the development of allograft coronary artery disease.[122]

INFECTIOUS COMPLICATIONS IN HEART TRANSPLANTATION
Organisms and Timing of Infections

Infection is a leading cause of morbidity and mortality in the cardiac transplant population.[5,123] The introduction of new chemoprophylactic regimens with the resultant prevention of serious disease caused by CMV has resulted in significant reductions in the number of infectious episodes and a delay in presentation after heart transplantation.[123] Patients are at greatest risk of life-threatening infections in the first 3 months

TABLE 60-9: Preliminary Nomenclature Scheme advised by ISHLT Antibody-Mediated Rejection Consensus Conference 2011

Grade pAMR 0	Negative for pathologic AMR: both histologic and immunopathologic studies are negative
pAMR 1 (H+)	pAMR 1 (H+): Histopathologic AMR alone: histological findings present and immunopathological findings negative
pAMR1 (I+)	Immunopathologic AMR alone: histological findings negative and immunopathological findings positive
pAMR 2	Pathologic AMR: Both histologic and immunopathologic findings are present
pAMR 3	Severe pathologic AMR: This category recognizes the rare cases of severe AMR with histopathologic findings of interstitial hemorrhage, capillary fragmentation, mixed inflammatory infiltrates, endothelial cell pyknosis and/or karyorrhexis and marked edema. The reported experience of the group was that these cases are associated with profound allograft dysfunction and poor clinical outcomes

ISHLT, International Society of Heart and Lung Transplantation.
Data from Berry GJ, Angelini A, Burke MM, et al: he ISHLT working formulation for pathologic diagnosis of antibody-mediated rejection in heart transplantation: evolution and current status (2005-2011), *J Heart Lung Transplant.* 2011 Jun;30(6):601-611.

after transplantation and following increases in immunosuppression for acute rejection episodes or retransplantation.[123] Table 60-10 illustrates the most common organisms causing infections in the cardiac recipient.

Preventive Measures and Prophylaxis Against Infection

Transmission of infections such as CMV, *Toxoplasma gondii*, HBV, HCV, and HIV after organ transplantation is well documented.[124] Prevention of postoperative infection begins with pretransplant screening of the donor and recipient.[125] Current suggested guidelines are outlined in Table 60-11. Perioperative and postoperative antimicrobial prophylaxes, as well as immunizations, are also outlined.

Specific Organisms Causing Infection Following Heart Transplantation

BACTERIA

Gram-negative bacilli are the most common cause of bacterial infectious complications following heart transplantation. Furthermore, *Escherichia coli* and *Pseudomonas aeruginosa* are the most prevalent organisms and usually cause urinary tract infections and pneumonias, respectively.[123] *Staphylococcus* species have been shown to cause the majority of Gram-positive-related infections.

VIRUSES

CMV remains the single most important cause of infectious disease morbidity and mortality in the heart transplant patient.[126] CMV not only results in infectious disease syndromes but also is indirectly associated with acute rejection episodes, acceleration of CAV, and posttransplant lymphoproliferative disease.[126] Furthermore, the reduction in leukocytes associated with CMV infection predisposes the patient to super-infection with

other pathogens (eg, *Pneumocystis carinii* pneumonia). Infections develop secondary to donor transmission, reactivation of latent recipient infection, or reinfection of a CMV-seropositive patient with a different viral strain.[126] Variable regimens for CMV prophylaxis with ganciclovir are being used by different centers.[127] The standard of care for symptomatic CMV disease is 2 to 3 weeks of intravenous ganciclovir (at a dose of 5 mg/kg twice daily, with dosage adjustment for renal dysfunction). For tissue-invasive disease, particularly pneumonia, many centers add anti-CMV hyperimmune globulin to this regimen.[128] Preemptive treatment strategies employ periodic surveillance using techniques such as plasma polymerase chain reaction (PCR) and CMV antigenemia, a rapid diagnostic test that detects viral protein in peripheral blood leukocytes at a significant interval before clinical disease.[129] Valganciclovir (Valcyte) is an oral prodrug of ganciclovir with a 10-fold greater bioavailability than oral ganciclovir. It has been shown to be effective for prophylaxis and preemptive treatment of CMV and allows for more convenient use.[130,131]

Although not a cure for herpes simplex or zoster viruses, acyclovir can reduce recurrences and the discomfort associated with the vesicular lesions. Epstein-Barr virus (EBV) infection may be associated with posttransplant lymphoproliferative disorders in immunocompromised hosts.[132]

FUNGI

Mucocutaneous candidiasis is common and usually can be treated with topical antifungal agents (nystatin or clotrimazole). Fluconazole is indicated for candidiasis refractory to this therapy or involving the esophagus. It is also useful for therapy of candidemia. One important caveat in the treatment of *Candida* infection with fluconazole is that certain species such as *Candida krusei* and *Candida glabrata* have a low susceptibility in vitro.[123]

Among patients undergoing heart transplantation, *Aspergillus* is the opportunistic pathogen with the highest

TABLE 60-10: Infections in Cardiac Transplant Recipients

Early infections (first month)

I. Pneumonia: Gram-negative bacilli (GNB)
II. Mediastinitis and sternal wound infections:
   Staphylococcus epidermidis
   Staphylococcus aureus
   GNB
III. Catheter-associated bacteremia:
   S. epidermidis
   S. aureus
   GNB
   Candida albicans
IV. Urinary tract infections:
   GNB
   Enterococcus
   C. albicans
V. Mucocutaneous infections:
   Herpes simplex virus (HSV)
   Candida spp.

Late infections (after first month)

I. Pneumonia:
   A. Diffuse interstitial pneumonia:
      Pneumocystis carinii
      Cytomegalovirus (CMV)*
      HSV
   B. Lobar or nodular (cavitary) pneumonia:
      Cryptococcus
      Aspergillus
      Bacteria (community-acquired, nosocomial)
      Nocardia asteroides
      Mycobacterium spp.
II. Central nervous system infections:
   A. Abscess or meningoencephalitis
      Aspergillus
      *Toxoplasma gondii**
      Meningitis
      Cryptococcus
      Listeria
III. Gastrointestinal (GI) infections:
   A. Esophagitis
      C. albicans
      HSV
   B. Diarrhea or lower GI hemorrhage
      Aspergillus
      Candida spp.
IV. Cutaneous infections:
   A. Vesicular lesions
      HSV
      Varicella-zoster
   B. Nodular or ulcerating lesions
      Nocardia
      Candida (disseminated)
      Atypical *Mycobacterium* spp.
      Cryptococcus

*Known donor-transmitted pathogens.

attributable mortality.[132] It causes a serious pneumonia in 5 to 10% of recipients during the first 3 months after transplantation. Dissemination of *Aspergillus* to the central nervous system is almost uniformly fatal.[134] Because aspergillosis is highly lethal in the immunocompromised host, even in the face of therapy, workup must be prompt and aggressive, and therapy may need to be initiated on suspicion of the diagnosis without definitive proof. Amphotericin B, itraconazole, and recently voriconazole are acceptable therapy.

PROTOZOA

In heart transplant recipients, the reported incidence of *P. carinii* pneumonia ranges from less than 1 to 10%.[135] Because the organism resides in the alveoli, bronchoalveolar lavage usually is necessary for diagnosis.[136] In the case of lung biopsy specimens, histopathologic examination is also helpful. *P. carinii* pneumonia is treated with high-dose trimethoprim-sulfamethoxazole or intravenous pentamidine.[123]

TABLE 60-11: Guidelines for Routine Screening and Prophylaxis of Infections in Heart Transplantation

I. Preoperative screening
   A. Donor
      1. Clinical assessment
      2. Serologic studies (HIV, HBV, HCV, CMV, *Toxoplasma gondii*)
   B. Recipient
      1. History and physical examination
      2. Serologic studies (HIV, HBV, HCV, CMV, *T. gondii*, herpes simplex virus, varicella-zoster virus, Epstein-Barr virus, endemic fungi)
      3. PPD (tuberculin) skin test
      4. Urine culture
      5. Stool for ova and parasites (*Strongyloides stercoralis*; center-specific)
II. Antimicrobial prophylaxis
   A. Perioperative
      1. First-generation cephalosporin (or vancomycin)
   B. Postoperative
      1. Trimethoprim-sulfamethoxazole or pentamidine (for *Pneumocystis carinii*)
      2. Nystatin or clotrimazole (for *Candida* spp.)
      3. Ganciclovir followed by acyclovir once discharged (for all patients except CMV-negative recipient and donor)
      4. Acyclovir (for herpes simplex and zoster; routine use is controversial)
      5. Standard endocarditis prophylaxis
   C. Postoperative immunizations
      1. Pneumococcal (booster every 5-7 years)
      2. Influenza A (yearly; center-specific)
      3. Exposure to measles, varicella, tetanus, or hepatitis B by a nonimmunized recipient often warrants specific immunoglobulin therapy (eg, varicella-zoster immune globulin, VZIG)

Toxoplasmosis following heart transplantation usually is the result of reactivation of latent disease in the seropositive donor heart because of the predilection of the parasite to invade muscle tissue.[137] *T. gondii* infection may be acquired from under-cooked meat and cat feces. The diagnosis is made with certainty only by histologic demonstration of trophozoites with surrounding inflammation in biopsy tissue; PCR also has been used.[138] *T. gondii* usually causes central nervous system infections and is treated with pyrimethamine with sulfadiazine or clindamycin.[123]

CHRONIC COMPLICATIONS FOLLOWING HEART TRANSPLANTATION

Cardiac Allograft Vasculopathy

Cardiac allograft vasculopathy (CAV) is a unique, rapidly progressive form of atherosclerosis in transplant recipients that is characterized in its early stages by intimal proliferation and in its later stages by luminal stenosis of epicardial branches, occlusion of smaller arteries, and myocardial infarction. Long-term survival of cardiac transplant recipients is limited primarily by the development of CAV, the leading cause of death after the first posttransplant year.[5] Angiographically detectable CAV is reported in approximately 40 to 50% of patients by 5 years after transplantation[139] Although CAV resembles atherosclerosis, there are some important differences that are illustrated in Fig. 60-11.[140] In particular, intimal proliferation is concentric rather than eccentric, and the lesions are diffuse, involving both distal and proximal portions of the coronary tree. Calcification is uncommon, and the elastic lamina remains intact.

The detailed pathogenesis of CAV is unknown, but there are strong indications that immunologic mechanisms that are regulated by nonimmunologic risk factors are the major causes of this phenomenon.[141] The immunologic mechanisms include acute rejection and anti-HLA antibodies, and some of the implicated risk factors relating to the transplant itself or the recipient are donor age, hypertension, hyperlipidemia, and preexisting diabetes. The side effects often associated with immunosuppression with calcineurin inhibitors or corticosteroids, for example, CMV infection, nephrotoxicity, and new-onset diabetes, after transplantation also play significant roles.[142-144]

It is generally believed that the initiating event of CAV is subclinical endothelial cell injury in the coronary artery of the allograft, which leads to a cascade of immunologic processes involving cytokines, inflammatory mediators, complement activation, and leukocyte adhesion molecules. These changes produce inflammation and, ultimately, thrombosis, smooth muscle cell proliferation, and vessel constriction. The initial endothelial injury may be the result of ischemia-reperfusion damage or the host-versus-graft immune response.[143,144]

CAV may begin within several weeks posttransplantation and progress insidiously at an accelerated rate to complete obliteration of the coronary lumen with allograft failure secondary to ischemia. The clinical diagnosis of CAV is difficult and complicated by allograft denervation, resulting in silent myocardial ischemia. Ventricular arrhythmias, congestive heart failure, and sudden death are commonly the initial presentation of significant CAV.[145] An annual coronary angiogram usually is performed for CAV surveillance and remains the diagnostic standard of care. Based on the current ISHLT nomenclature recommendations,[146] moderate or severe CAV 1 year after heart transplantation is associated with subsequent major adverse cardiac events.[147] Intravascular ultrasound (IVUS) is better equipped to provide important quantitative information regarding vessel wall morphology and the degree of intimal thickening.[148]

Because angiography and IVUS are invasive tests, they pose increased risks for patients. Noninvasive tests (eg, thallium scintigraphy and dobutamine stress echocardiography),

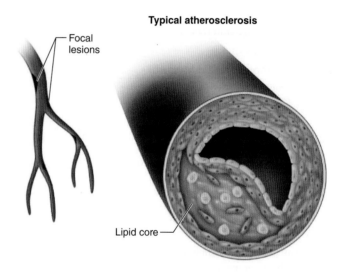

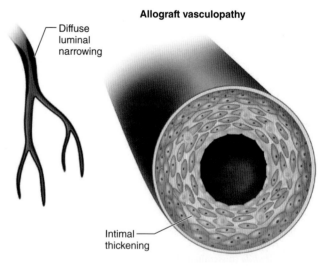

FIGURE 60-11 Schematic illustration of typical atherosclerosis and cardiac allograft vasculopathy.

however, have not been sensitive or specific enough to be a reliable screen for CAV.[149] Other possible modalities include pulse-wave tissue Doppler imaging, electron beam CT, fast CT scanning, and MRI. These modalities may replace invasive procedures in the future.

Currently, the only definitive treatment for advanced CAV is retransplantation, which has risks for the patient and poses problems associated with scarcity of donor organs.[145] Owing to the diffuse and distal nature of the disease, procedures such as stenting and angioplasty are inherently less effective than in nontransplant patients and result in a higher need for repeated procedures.[150] Therefore, prophylactic management is of paramount importance. Before transplantation, the focus should be on preventing endothelial injury at brain death, reducing cold ischemia time and improving myocardial preservation during storage and transportation.[145] Posttransplantation care focuses on empiric risk factor modification (eg, dietary and pharmacologic reduction in serum cholesterol, cessation of smoking, hypertension control, etc). Several studies have demonstrated a decrease in CAV in patients treated with a calcium channel blocker and angiotensin-converting enzyme and HMG-CoA reductase inhibitors.[151,152]

Newer immunosuppressive drugs, specifically the proliferation signal inhibitors (eg, everolimus and sirolimus), may be useful in reducing the incidence and severity of CAV and slowing disease progression.[153-157]

Renal Dysfunction

The 2009 ISHLT registry reported a significant improvement in long-term renal dysfunction in the most recent cohort of heart transplant recipients (2001 to 2007) as compared to the previous cohort (1994 to 2000). Whereas only 60% of heart transplant recipients from 1994 to 2000 were free of severe renal dysfunction (defined as a creatinine concentration of more than 2.5 mg/dL and the need for dialysis or renal transplantation) by Kaplan-Meier estimates at 10 years, recipients transplanted from 2001 to 2007 had an 11% absolute decrease in severe renal dysfunction at 5 years compared with the previous cohort.[5] Notably, the risk of death after heart transplantation is markedly increased by the development of end-stage renal failure.[158]

Cyclosporine nephrotoxicity after heart transplantation is well recognized and well documented. The improved bioavailability of cyclosporine microemulsion (Neoral) compared with the conventional formulation has led to investigations into monitoring of cyclosporine levels 2 hours after dosing (C2).[159] Neoral C2 monitoring may be a better indicator of immunosuppression efficacy than trough levels and a better measure to avoid nephrotoxicity and other cyclosporine-associated side effects.[160] Lowering cyclosporine dose may be helpful in slowing the progression of renal disease, especially with concomitant use of newer immunosuppressive regimens such as MMF and sirolimus (rapamycin).[161,162] Calcineurin-free immunosuppression is also being implemented by some centers.[163]

Hypertension

Moderate-to-severe systemic hypertension afflicts 50 to 90% of cardiac transplant recipients.[5] Peripheral vasoconstriction in combination with fluid retention seems to play the greatest role. Although the exact mechanisms are unclear, it likely involves a combination of cyclosporine-induced tubular nephrotoxicity and vasoconstriction of renal and systemic arterioles mediated by sympathetic neural activation.[164] Tacrolimus is associated with a lower incidence of hypertension than is cyclosporine.[165] No single class of antihypertensive agents has proven uniformly effective, and treatment of this refractory hypertension remains empirical and difficult. In a prospective, randomized trial, titrated monotherapy with either diltiazem or lisinopril controlled the condition in fewer than 50% of patients.[166] Diuretics should be used cautiously because the balance between edema/hypertension and volume depletion/hypotension can be tenuous in a subset of these patients. Overzealous diuresis can potentiate the apparent nephrotoxicity of cyclosporine by further reducing renal blood flow and altering cyclosporine pharmacokinetics.[167] Beta-blockers also should be used with caution because they may further blunt the heart rate response to exercise.

Malignancy

Chronic immunosuppression is associated with an increased incidence of malignancy ranging from about 4 to 18%, which is 10- to 100-fold greater than in the general population.[168] Improved graft and patient survival, owing to pharmacologic advances in the area of immunosuppressive therapy, has led to an increase in the incidence of neoplasms.[168] Malignant neoplasias have become, along with graft vasculopathy, a significant limiting factor for the long-term survival of heart transplant recipients.[5] Lymphoproliferative disorders and carcinoma of the skin are the most common malignancies found in heart transplant recipients.[168] Loss of T-lymphocyte control over EBV-stimulated B-lymphocyte proliferation appears to be the primary mechanism for the development of lymphoproliferative disorders.[169] The risk of these malignancies is increased further following monoclonal and polyclonal antibody therapy.[170,171]

Treatment options in transplantation include a reduction in immunosuppression and initiation of high-dose acyclovir (to attenuate EBV replication), in addition to conventional therapies for carcinoma (eg, chemotherapy, radiation therapy, and surgical resection), which are associated with very high risk and limited success. The role of statins and the risk of cancer were explored in a retrospective study of 255 patients who received transplants at a single center (1985-2007). The cumulative incidence of malignancy 8 years after transplantation was decreased in patients who received statins (34 vs 13%). In addition, statin use was associated with improved cancer-free and overall survival. A prospective study seems warranted, and although it was not possible for the study investigators to adjust for all confounders, these data are suggestive of improved cancer-free and overall survival in those recipients receiving statin.[172]

Other Chronic Complications

Hyperlipidemia eventually develops in the majority of recipients and is managed with dietary restrictions, exercise, and lipid-lowering agents.[173] Other complications that commonly contribute to posttransplant morbidity include osteoporosis, obesity, cachexia, and gastrointestinal complications, notably cholelithiasis.[174,175]

CARDIAC RETRANSPLANTATION

Retransplantation accounts for fewer than 3% of the cardiac transplants currently performed.[5] Primary indications for retransplantation are early graft failure, allograft coronary artery disease, and refractory acute rejection.[176,177]

The operative technique and immunosuppressive regimen are similar to those employed for the initial transplantation. Despite reduced mortality in the cyclosporine era, actuarial survival remains markedly reduced. Analysis of the ISHLT registry for retransplantations performed between 1987 and 1998 reveals survival to be 65, 59, and 55% for 1, 2, and 3 years, respectively. Intertransplant interval of 6 months or less was associated with a dismal 1-year survival of 50% in this analysis.

Conversely, when the interval between primary and retransplantation was more than 2 years, 1-year survival after retransplantation approached that of primary transplantation.[177] The 2009 ISHLT registry report indicates that the 5-year survival of retransplanted patients has increased by 15-17% with each successive decade (1982-1991, 1992-2001, 2002-2007). As well, in the most recent cohort (2002-2008), patients undergoing retransplantation at greater than 5 years from initial transplant had the same 1-year survival rate as primary transplants from the same era (86%).[5] Advanced donor age also was a predictor of increased mortality among these recipients.[177]

A recent UNOS Registry study examined risk factors associated with high risk of graft failure after retransplantation (n = 671). Older age, increasing serum creatinine, and preoperative mechanical ventilation were associated with 1-year graft failure by multivariate analysis. Each decade increase in recipient age was associated with a 20% increase in the odds of 1-year graft failure. In addition, each 1 mg/dL increase in serum creatinine increased the likelihood of graft failure by 58%.[178]

Another UNOS Registry project studied the effectiveness of bridging patients to retransplant with mechanical circulatory support. According to the UNOS Registry, 149 of 1690 retransplants were bridged with mechanical support, consisting of extracorporeal membrane oxygenation (ECMO) in 54 and a VAD in 90. Those bridged to retransplant did poorly overall, with the ECMO sub-group faring the worst. Survival

in patients who were bridged on VAD and received an allograft at least 1 year after the primary transplant was similar to those retransplant recipients who did not require VAD. However, survival was significantly worse in the bridged population who underwent retransplant within a year of the primary transplant.[179]

These data suggest that although cardiac retransplantation is associated with significant morbidity and mortality, careful selection of patients, especially those who are younger and with longer intertransplant intervals, may be associated with more favorable outcome. Nonetheless, the disparity between the demand and supply for donor hearts continues to make cardiac retransplantation an ethical dilemma.[180]

RESULTS OF HEART TRANSPLANTATION

Although no direct comparative trials have been or are likely to be performed, survival following heart transplantation remains favorable if compared with both the medical and device arms of the REMATCH trial.[2,6] The superiority of heart transplantation is more clearly evident in medium- and high-risk patients with end-stage heart failure.[181] The overall results actually are improving despite increasing risk profiles.[5,78]

The reported operative (ie, 30-day) mortality for cardiac transplantation ranges from 5 to 10%.[182] Overall 1-year survival is up to 86%.[5,78] After the steep fall in survival during the first 6 months, survival decreases at a linear rate (approximately 3.5% per year), even well beyond 15 years posttransplantation.[5] Graft failure (primary and nonspecific), multisystem organ failure, and infection account for most deaths within the first 30 days. Infection, graft failure, and acute rejection are the leading causes of death during the first year; thereafter, CAV and malignancy are the major causes of death.[5,78]

While many subgroups including patients with arrhythmogenic right ventricular cardiomyopathy, hypertrophic cardiomyopathy, restrictive cardiomyopathy (except for patients with amyloid or chemotherapy/radiation therapy), and adult congenital heart disease had comparable outcomes, posttransplant outcomes in 485 women with peripartum cardiomyopathy (PPCM) were inferior. Outcomes were examined using the UNOS Registry (1987-2010; n = 42,406). The PPCM patients were younger with a higher degree of sensitization, required higher intensity pretransplant cardiovascular support, suffered an increased graft failure and death, which may be secondary to the higher pretransplant acuity, increased rejection seen, and greater degree of sensitization.[183]

Studies examining the health-related quality of life in patients after cardiac transplantation demonstrate marked improvement, particularly in the absence of complications, and approach the general population by 10 years after transplantation.[184]

Factors affecting long-term survival were examined in several studies. In an analysis of the UNOS Registry (1987-1999), recipients surviving a minimum of 10 years (n = 9404) were identified and compared with recipients who died within 10 years (n = 10,373). Predictors of long-term survival in a multivariate model included recipient age at transplant < 55 years, shorter ischemic time, younger donor age, white race, and annual center volume > 9. Mechanical ventilation and the presence of diabetes diminished the likelihood of long-term survival.[185]

A recent study examined the influence of insurance and education on long-term survival. Medicare and Medicaid patients had lower 10-year survival (8.6 and 10.0%, respectively) than private insurance/self-pay patients. College-educated patients had 7.0% higher 10-year survival. These survival differences increased over time. Multivariable analysis demonstrated that college education decreased mortality risk by 11%, whereas Medicare and Medicaid increased the mortality risk by 18 and 33%, respectively.[186]

A recent systematic review saw a relationship between low center volume and increased mortality. The minimal acceptable transplant volume was unable to be determined; however, 10 to 12 transplants per year corresponded to the upper limit of low-volume categories that have relatively high mortality. The effect of reorganizing centers to ensure minimal target volumes was unable to be determined.[187]

The relationship between recipient risk and institutional volume on short-term mortality was studied using the UNOS Registry (2000-2010) using a previously validated recipient risk index. Institutional volume per year, defined as low (<7), medium (7-15), and high (>15) acted as a modifier on association between risk and mortality, such that high-risk recipients had improved 1-year survival when their transplants occurred at high-volume centers.[188]

Another UNOS Registry study, using mixed-effect logistic regression models, demonstrated that although 1-year mortality increases with decreasing center volume, this accounted for only 16.7% of the variability in mortality between centers. This suggests that although institutional volume may be an important predictor of outcome, other factors contribute to mortality risk that may not be encompassed by the data currently collected in the registry.[189]

Additional Insights from the United Network for Organ Sharing Database

As noted in the above sections, the recent literature on heart transplantation has seen a notable increase in clinical studies analyzing the multi-institutional UNOS open transplant cohort. This database is publically accessible and includes all heart transplants performed in the United States from October 1987 onward. The database also includes patients on the waitlist, donor information, and outcomes. As with all large administrative datasets, it is limited by potential errors in coding as well as incompletely populated variables. However, questions that had previously only been addressed using single or limited multiinstitutional data can now be investigated using this cohort of over 20,000 patients. Among those issues addressed have been the impact of

various recipient factors, on short- and long-term survival after heart transplantation. Russo and coworkers reported that uncomplicated diabetes mellitus should not preclude listing for heart transplantation due to equivalent survival with nondiabetics.[190] However, severe diabetics did have poorer survival and should be considered for destination LVAD therapy or high-risk listing. Zaidi and coworkers reported better short and intermediate survival after heart transplantation in patients with sarcoidosis compared to recipients with other diagnoses, and concluded that a diagnosis of sarcoidosis should not preclude heart transplantation.[191] Kpodonu and coworkers demonstrated that 1-year survival after heart transplant for amyloid cardiomyopathy was significantly decreased in female recipients, whereas it was comparable with other diagnoses for male recipients.[192] Nwakanma and coworkers confirmed increasing risk of rejection in the year after transplantation and decreased survival with increasing PRA levels.[193] Weiss and coworkers reported that advanced age (>60 years) was associated with acceptable long-term outcomes (>70% 5-year survival).[194] Although elderly recipients did have slightly higher rates of infection and acute renal failure, as well as a 2-day longer hospital length of stay, the survival benefit of transplantation in elderly CHF patients was compelling. Another study by Weiss and coworkers identified a potential provider bias in the listing of obese patients as potential heart transplant recipients.[195] Specifically, that obese individuals wait longer and have a lower likelihood of receiving a donor heart after listing, despite similar short-term survival.

Insights into the impact of operative technique and the use of LVADs on posttransplant survival have also been gained from the UNOS database. As noted, Weiss and coworkers reported equivalent survival after heart transplantation using biatrial versus bicaval anastomotic techniques.[74] However, they did identify that the bicaval technique was associated with a shorted hospital length of stay and decreased rates of permanent pacemaker placement. Pal and coworkers investigated status 1 patients bridged to transplant using LVADs and IV inotropes, and found that patients bridged to transplant using LVADs were, by in large, those who failed bridging with IV inotropes.[196] In contrast with International Society of Heart and Lung Transplantation data, no increase in posttransplant morbidity or mortality was found in LVAD-bridged patients compared with nonbridged status 1 patients. Shuhaiber and coworkers compared patients bridged with transplant with Novacor versus HeartMate LVADs and found no difference in 1-year survival, rates of rejection, or rates of infection.[197] However, patients bridged with Novacor LVADs demonstrated lower 5-year survival posttransplant.

Weiss and coworkers also investigated the effect of transplant center volume on long-term outcomes after heart transplantation, and reported that annual center volume is an independent predictor of short-term mortality in OHT.[198] Although the current Centers for Medicare and Medicaid Services mandate is that heart transplant centers perform 10 per year to qualify for funding, this study found that a higher cutoff resulted in better outcomes;

centers performing greater than 40 per year have a 30-day mortality less than 5%.

THE FUTURE

As a result of a series of unprecedented advances over the past decade, the clinical outcome of heart transplantation has improved dramatically. Although cardiac replacement remains the best therapeutic option for patients with end-stage heart failure, a number of challenges await future investigators to further improve survival and reduce transplant-related morbidity. A major factor limiting long-term survival of recipients is allograft rejection and the untoward effects of immunosuppression. Development of reliable, noninvasive diagnostic studies will permit more frequent evaluations for the early detection of rejection and for monitoring the effectiveness of therapy. Ultimately, this will allow more precise control of immunosuppression and, in turn, a reduction in cumulative allograft injury and infectious complications. Molecular tests and gene expression profiling could be available soon and may provide the best noninvasive option.[105,108]

Immunosuppressive strategists will continue their efforts to establish specific unresponsiveness to antigens of transplanted organs in hopes of preserving much of the recipient's immune responses. Proliferative signal inhibitors such as sirolimus and everolimus are showing promising results. Alternatively, donor organs may be made less susceptible to immunologic attack through genetic engineering techniques by altering the expression of cell membrane-bound molecules. This approach is being used currently in the pursuit of clinically applicable xenotransplant sources. Xenografts eventually may be an additional source of donor organs, although extended xenograft survival remains an elusive goal. Complicating this alternative are unresolved ethical issues concerning transgenic experimentation and the potential for transmission of veterinary pathogens to an immunosuppressed recipient.

Future improvements in organ preservation permitting extension of the storage interval will have several benefits. In addition to a modest increase in the donor pool, extension of storage times would permit better allocation of organs with respect to donor-recipient immunologic matching. Assist devices are being used currently both as a bridge to transplantation and as a destination therapy. It appears that as the technology of assist devices continues to improve, it is only a matter of time before they become a long-term solution for patients with severe congestive heart failure.

The concept of regenerating the failing heart using cardiomyocytes of different sources, autologous smooth muscle cells, and dermal fibroblasts is in the experimental stage. Lineage-negative bone marrow cells or bone marrow-derived endothelial precursor cells are also being studied to induce new blood vessel formation after experimental myocardial infarction.[199] Cardiac transplantation remains a remarkable achievement of the twentieth century and has revolutionized therapy for end-stage heart failure. Further investigations are needed to overcome the current obstacles to long-term graft function and patient survival.

REFERENCES

1. Steinman TI, Becker BN, Frost AE, et al: Guidelines for the referral and management of patients eligible for solid organ transplantation. *Transplantation* 2001; 71:1189.
2. Boyle A, Colvin-Adams M: Recipient selection and management. *Semin Thorac Cardiovasc Surg* 2004; 16:358.
3. Deng MC: Cardiac transplantation. *Heart* 2002; 87:177.
4. Costanzo MR, Augustine S, Bourge R, et al: Selection and treatment of candidates for heart transplantation: a statement for health professionals from the Committee on Heart Failure and Cardiac Transplantation of the Council on Clinical Cardiology, American Heart Association. *Circulation* 1995; 92:3593.
5. Taylor DO, Stehlik J, Edwards LB, et al: Registry of the international society for heart and lung transplantation: twenty-sixth official adult heart transplant report-2009. *J Heart Lung Transplant* 2009; 28(10):1007-1022.
6. Rose EA, Gelijns AC, Moskowitz AJ, et al: Randomized Evaluation of Mechanical Assistance for the Treatment of Congestive Heart Failure (REMATCH) Study Group: long-term mechanical left ventricular assistance for end-stage heart failure. *N Engl J Med* 2001; 345:1435.
7. Menicanti L, Di Donato M: Surgical left ventricle reconstruction, pathophysiologic insights, results and expectation from the STICH trial. *Eur J Cardiothorac Surg* 2004; 26:S42.
8. Stelken AM, Younis LT, Jennison SH, et al: Prognostic value of cardiopulmonary exercise testing using percent achieved of predicted peak oxygen uptake for patients with ischemic and dilated cardiomyopathy. *J Am Coll Cardiol* 1996; 27:345.
9. Rothenburger M, Wichter T, Schmid C, et al: Aminoterminal pro type B natriuretic peptide as a predictive and prognostic marker in patients with chronic heart failure. *J Heart Lung Transplant* 2004; 23:1189.
10. Francis GS, Cohn JN, Johnson G, et al: Plasma norepinephrine, plasma renin activity, and congestive heart failure: relations to survival and the effects of therapy in V-HeFT II. The V-HeFT VA Cooperative Studies Group. *Circulation* 1993; 87:VI40.
11. Mudge GH, Goldstein S, Addonizio LZ, et al: Twenty-fourth Bethesda Conference on Cardiac Transplantation. Task Force 3: recipient guidelines. *J Am Coll Cardiol* 1993; 22:21.
12. Laks H, Marelli D, Odim J, et al: Heart transplantation in the young and elderly. *Heart Failure Rev* 2001; 6:221.
13. Demers P, Moffatt S, Oyer PE, et al: Long-term results of heart transplantation in patients older than 60 years. *J Thorac Cardiovasc Surg* 2003; 126:224.
14. Kieler-Jensen N, Milocco I, Ricksten SE: Pulmonary vasodilation after heart transplantation: a comparison among prostacyclin, sodium nitroprusside, and nitroglycerin on right ventricular function and pulmonary selectivity. *J Heart Lung Transplant* 1993; 12:179.
15. Bourge RC, Naftel DC, Costanzo-Nordin MR, et al: Pretransplantation risk factors for death after heart transplantation: a multiinstitutional study. The Transplant Cardiologists Research Database Group. *J Heart Lung Transplant* 1993; 12:549.
16. Chen JM, Levin HR, Michler RE, et al: Reevaluating the significance of pulmonary hypertension before cardiac transplantation: determination of optimal thresholds and quantification of the effect of reversibility on perioperative mortality. *J Thorac Cardiovasc Surg* 1997; 114:627.
17. Tenderich G, Koerner MM, Stuettgen B, et al: Pre-existing elevated pulmonary vascular resistance: long-term hemodynamic follow-up and outcome of recipients after orthotopic heart transplantation. *J Cardiovasc Surg* 2000; 41:215.
18. Chang PP, Longenecker JC, Wang NY, et al: Mild vs severe pulmonary hypertension before heart transplantation: different effects on posttransplantation pulmonary hypertension and mortality. *J Heart Lung Transplant* 2005; 24:998.
19. Sablotzki A, Hentschel T, Gruenig E, et al: Hemodynamic effects of inhaled aerosolized iloprost and inhaled nitric oxide in heart transplant candidates with elevated pulmonary vascular resistance. *Eur J Cardiothorac Surg* 2002; 22:746.
20. O'Dell KM, Kalus JS, Kucukarslan S, et al: Nesiritide for secondary pulmonary hypertension in patients with end-stage heart failure. *Am J Health Syst Pharm* 2005; 62:606.
21. Salzberg SP, Lachat ML, von Harbou K, et al: Normalization of high pulmonary vascular resistance with LVAD support in heart transplantation candidates. *Eur J Cardiothorac Surg* 2005; 27:222.

22. Newcomb AE, Esmore DS, Rosenfeldt FL, et al: Heterotopic heart transplantation: an expanding role in the twenty-first century? *Ann Thorac Surg* 2004; 78:1345.

23. Sigurdardottir V, Bjortuft O, Eiskjaer H et al: Long-term follow-up of lung and heart transplant recipients with pre-transplant malignancies. *J Heart Lung Transplant* 2012; 31:1276-1280

24. Pelosi F Jr, Capehart J, Roberts WC: Effectiveness of cardiac transplantation for primary (AL) cardiac amyloidosis. *Am J Cardiol* 1997; 79:532.

25. Dubrey SW, Burke MM, Hawkins PN, et al: Cardiac transplantation for amyloid heart disease: the United Kingdom experience. *J Heart Lung Transplant* 2004; 23:1142.

26. Uriel N, Jorde UP, Cotarlan V, et al: Heart transplantation in human immunodeficiency virus-positive patients. *J Heart Lung Transplant* 2009 Jul; 28(7):667-669.

27. Koerner MM, Tenderich G, Minami K, et al: Results of heart transplantation in patients with preexisting malignancies. *Am J Cardiol* 1997; 79:988.

28. Ostermann ME, Rogers CA, Saeed I, et al: Pre-existing renal failure doubles 30-day mortality after heart transplantation. *J Heart Lung Transplant* 2004; 23:1231.

29. Thomas HL, Banner NR, Murphy CL, et al: Incidence, determinants, and outcome of chronic kidney disease after adult heart transplantation in the United Kingdom. *Transplantation* 2012; 93:1151-1157.

30. Dichtl W, Vogel W, Dunst KM, et al: Cardiac hepatopathy before and after heart transplantation. *Transpl Int* 2005; 18:697.

31. Chokshi A, Cheema FH, Schaefle KJ, et al: Hepatic dysfunction and survival after orthotopic heart transplantation: application of the MELD scoring system for outcome prediction. *J Heart Lung Transplant* 2012; 31:591-600.

32. Yang JA, Kato TS, Shulman BP, et al: Liver dysfunction as a predictor of outcomes in patients with advanced heart failure requiring ventricular assist device support: use of the Model of End-stage Liver Disease (MELD) and MELD eXcluding INR (MELD-XI) scoring system. *J Heart Lung Transplant* 2012; 31:601-610.

33. Morgan JA, John R, Weinberg AD, et al: Heart transplantation in diabetic recipients: a decade review of 161 patients at Columbia Presbyterian. *J Thorac Cardiovasc Surg* 2004; 127:1486.

34. Morgan JA, Park Y, Oz MC, et al: Device-related infections while on left ventricular assist device support do not adversely impact bridging to transplant or posttransplant survival. *ASAIO J* 2003; 49:748.

35. Lietz K, John R, Burke EA, et al: Pretransplant cachexia and morbid obesity are predictors of increased mortality after heart transplantation. *Transplantation* 2001; 72:277.

36. Kilic A, Weiss ES, Arnaoutakis GJ, et al: Identifying recipients at high risk for graft failure after heart retransplantation. *Ann Thorac Surg* 2012; 93:712-716.

37. Rivard AL, Hellmich C, Sampson B, et al: Preoperative predictors for postoperative problems in heart transplantation: psychiatric and psychosocial considerations. *Prog Transplant* 2005; 15:276.

38. Loh E, Bergin JD, Couper GS, et al: Role of panel-reactive antibody cross-reactivity in predicting survival after orthotopic heart transplantation. *J Heart Lung Transplant* 1994; 13:194.

39. McKenna D, Eastlund T, Segall M, et al: HLA alloimmunization in patients requiring ventricular assist device support. *J Heart Lung Transplant* 2002; 21:1218.

40. Aranda JM Jr, Schofield RS, Pauly DF, et al: Comparison of dobutamine versus milrinone therapy in hospitalized patients awaiting cardiac transplantation: a prospective, randomized trial. *Am Heart J* 2003; 145:324.

41. Cochran RP, Starkey TD, Panos AL, et al: Ambulatory intraaortic balloon pump use as bridge to heart transplant. *Ann Thorac Surg* 2002; 74:746.

42. Dembitsky WP, Tector AJ, Park S, et al: Left ventricular assist device performance with long-term circulatory support: lessons from the REMATCH trial. *Ann Thorac Surg* 2004; 78:2123.

43. Clegg AJ, Scott DA, Loveman E, et al: The clinical and cost-effectiveness of left ventricular assist devices for end-stage heart failure: a systematic review and economic evaluation. *Health Technol Assess* 2005; 9:1.

44. Copeland JG, Smith RG, Arabia FA, et al: CardioWest Total Artificial Heart Investigators. Cardiac replacement with a total artificial heart as a bridge to transplantation. *N Engl J Med* 2004; 351:859.

45. Ermis C, Zadeii G, Zhu AX, et al: Improved survival of cardiac transplantation candidates with implantable cardioverter defibrillator therapy: role of beta-blocker or amiodarone treatment. *J Cardiovasc Electrophysiol* 2003; 14:578.

46. Vega JD, Moore J, Murray S, et al: Heart transplantation in the United States, 1998–2007. *Am J Transplant* 2009; 9(Part 2):932-941.

47. Khush KK, Menza R, Nguyen J, Zaroff JG, Goldstein BA: Donor predictors of allograft use and recipient outcomes after heart transplantation. *Circ Heart Fail* 2013; 6:300-309.

48. Southerland KW, Castleberry AW, Williams JB, Daneshmand MA, Ali AA, Milano CA: Impact of donor cardiac arrest on heart transplantation. *Surgery* 2013; 154:312-319.

49. Quader MA, Wolfe LG, Kasirajan V: Heart transplantation outcomes from cardiac arrest-resuscitated donors. *J Heart Lung Transplant* 2013; 32:1090-1095.

50. Singh TP, Almond CS, Taylor DO, Graham DA: Decline in heart transplant wait list mortality in the United States following broader regional sharing of donor hearts. *Circ Heart Fail* 2012; 5:249-258.

51. Zaroff JG, Rosengard BR, Armstrong WF, et al: Consensus conference report: maximizing use of organs recovered from the cadaver donor: cardiac recommendations, March 28-29, 2001, Crystal City, VA. *Circulation* 2002; 106:836.

52. Wheeldon DR, Potter CD, Oduro A, et al: Transforming the "unacceptable" donor: outcomes from the adoption of a standardized donor management technique. *J Heart Lung Transplant* 1995; 14:734.

53. Laks H, Marelli D, Fonarow GC, et al: UCLA Heart Transplant Group. Use of two recipient lists for adults requiring heart transplant. *J Thorac Cardiovasc Surg* 2003; 125:49.

54. Lietz K, John R, Mancini DM, et al: Outcomes in cardiac transplant recipients using allografts from older donors versus mortality on the transplant waiting list: implications for donor selection criteria. *J Am Coll Cardiol* 2004; 43:1553.

55. Freimark D, Aleksic I, Trento A, et al: Hearts from donors with chronic alcohol use: a possible risk factor for death after heart transplantation. *J Heart Lung Transplant* 1996; 15:150.

56. Freimark D, Czer LS, Admon D, et al: Donors with a history of cocaine use: effect on survival and rejection frequency after heart transplantation. *J Heart Lung Transplant* 1994; 13:1138.

57. Smith M: Physiologic changes during brain stem death: lessons for management of the organ donor. *J Heart Lung Transplant* 2004; 23:S217.

58. Stoica SC, Satchithananda DK, Charman S, et al: Swan-Ganz catheter assessment of donor hearts: outcome of organs with borderline hemodynamics. *J Heart Lung Transplant* 2002; 21:615.

59. Rosendale JD, Kauffman HM, McBride MA, et al: Hormonal resuscitation yields more transplanted hearts, with improved early function. *Transplantation* 2003; 75:1336.

60. Harms J, Isemer FE, Kolenda H: Hormonal alteration and pituitary function during course of brain stem death in potential organ donors. *Transplant Proc* 1991; 23:2614.

61. Novitzky D, Cooper DK, Chaffin JS, et al: Improved cardiac allograft function following triiodothyronine therapy to both donor and recipient. *Transplantation* 1990; 49:311.

62. Conte JV, Baumgartner WA: Overview and future practice patterns in cardiac and pulmonary preservation. *J Card Surg* 2000; 15:91.

63. Wildhirt SM, Weis M, Schulze C, et al: Effects of Celsior and University of Wisconsin preservation solutions on hemodynamics and endothelial function after cardiac transplantation in humans: a single-center, prospective, randomized trial. *Transplant Int* 2000; 13:S203.

64. Garlicki M: May preservation solution affect the incidence of graft vasculopathy in transplanted heart? *Ann Transplant* 2003; 8:19.

65. Segel LD, Follette DM, Contino JP, et al: Importance of substrate enhancement for long-term heart preservation. *J Heart Lung Transplant* 1993; 12:613.

66. Zehr KJ, Herskowitz A, Lee P, et al: Neutrophil adhesion inhibition prolongs survival of cardiac allografts with hyperacute rejection. *J Heart Lung Transplant* 1993; 12:837.

67. Fitton TP, Barreiro CJ, Bonde PN, et al: Attenuation of DNA damage in canine hearts preserved by continuous hypothermic perfusion. *Ann Thorac Surg* 2005; 80:1812.

68. Abbas Ardehali MD, Fardad Esmailian MD, Mario Deng MD, Edward Soltesz MD, Eileen Hsich MD, Yoshifumi Naka MD, Donna Mancini MD, Margarita Camacho MD, Mark Zucker MD, Pascal Leprince MD, Robert Padera MD, Jon Kobashigawa MD, for the PROCEED II Trial Investigators: A Prospective, Randomized, Multi-center Trial of ex-vivo Donor Heart Perfusion for Human Heart Transplantation: The PROCEED II Trial. *The Lancet* 2015; 3859(9987):2577-2584.

69. Betkowski AS, Graff R, Chen JJ, et al: Panel-reactive antibody screening practices prior to heart transplantation. *J Heart Lung Transplant* 2002; 21:644.

70. Jarcho J, Naftel DC, Shroyer JK, et al: Influence of HLA mismatch on rejection after heart transplantation: a multi-institutional study. *J Heart Lung Transplant* 1994; 13:583.

71. Baumgartner WA, Reitz BA, Achuff SC: Operative techniques utilized in heart transplantations, in Achuff SC (ed): *Heart and Heart-Lung Transplantation*. Philadelphia, Saunders, 1990.

72. Milano CA, Shah AS, Van Trigt P, et al: Evaluation of early postoperative results after bicaval versus standard cardiac transplantation and review of the literature. *Am Heart J* 2000; 140:717.

73. Aziz T, Burgess M, Khafagy R, et al: Bicaval and standard techniques in orthotopic heart transplantation: medium-term experience in cardiac performance and survival. *J Thorac Cardiovasc Surg* 1999; 118:115.

74. Weiss ES, Nwakanma LU, Russell SB, et al: Outcomes in bicaval versus biatrial techniques in heart transplantation: an analysis of the UNOS database. *J Heart Lung Transplant* 2008 Feb; 27(2):178-183.

75. Cotts WG, Oren RM: Function of the transplanted heart: unique physiology and therapeutic implications. *Am J Med Sci* 1997; 314:164.

76. Tischler MD, Lee RT, Plappert T, et al: Serial assessment of left ventricular function and mass after orthotopic heart transplantation: a four-year longitudinal study. *J Am Coll Cardiol* 1992; 19:60.

77. Gerber BL, Bernard X, Melin JA, et al: Exaggerated chronotropic and energetic response to dobutamine after orthotopic cardiac transplantation. *J Heart Lung Transplant* 2001; 20:824.

78. Kirklin JK, Naftel DC, Bourge RC, et al: Evolving trends in risk profiles and causes of death after heart transplantation: a ten-year multi-institutional study. *J Thorac Cardiovasc Surg* 2003; 125:881.

79. Minev PA, El-Banayosy A, Minami K, et al: Differential indication for mechanical circulatory support following heart transplantation. *Intensive Care Med* 2001; 27:1321.

80. Srivastava R, Keck BM, Bennett LE, et al: The results of cardiac retransplantation: an analysis of the Joint International Society for Heart and Lung Transplantation/United Network for Organ Sharing Thoracic Registry. *Transplantation* 2000; 70:606.

81. Kieler-Jensen N, Lundin S, Ricksten SE, et al: Vasodilator therapy after heart transplantation: effects of inhaled nitric oxide and intravenous prostacyclin, prostaglandin E$_1$, and sodium nitroprusside. *J Heart Lung Transplant* 1995; 14:436.

82. Arafa OE, Geiran OR, Andersen K, et al: Intra-aortic balloon pumping for predominantly right ventricular failure after heart transplantation. *Ann Thorac Surg* 2000; 70:1587.

83. Stecker EC, Strelich KR, Chugh SS, et al: Arrhythmias after orthotopic heart transplantation. *J Cardiol Fail* 2005; 11:464.

84. Chin C, Feindel C, Cheng D: Duration of preoperative amiodarone treatment may be associated with postoperative hospital mortality in patients undergoing heart transplantation. *J Cardiothorac Vasc Anesth* 1999; 13:562.

85. Bertolet BD, Eagle DA, Conti JB, et al: Bradycardia after heart transplantation: reversal with theophylline. *J Am Coll Cardiol* 1996; 28:396.

86. Patel VS, Lim M, Massin EK, et al: Sudden cardiac death in cardiac transplant recipients. *Circulation* 1996; 94:II-273.

87. Kwak YL, Oh YJ, Bang SO, et al: Comparison of the effects of nicardipine and sodium nitroprusside for control of increased blood pressure after coronary artery bypass graft surgery. *J Int Med Res* 2004; 32:342.

88. Miller LW: Treatment of cardiac allograft rejection with intervenous corticosteroids. *J Heart Transplant* 1990; 9:283.

89. Sharples LD, Caine N, Mullins P, et al: Risk factor analysis for the major hazards following heart transplantation: rejection, infection, and coronary occlusive disease. *Transplantation* 1991; 52:244.

90. Shah MR, Starling RC, Schwartz Longacre L, Mehra MR: Working Group P: Heart transplantation research in the next decade—a goal to achieving evidence-based outcomes: National Heart, Lung, And Blood Institute Working Group. *J Am Coll Cardiol* 2012; 59:1263-1269.

91. Cunningham KS, Veinot JP, Butany J: An approach to endomyocardial biopsy interpretation. *J Clin Pathol* 2006; 59:121.

92. Billingham ME, Cary NRB, Hammond ME, et al: A working formulation for the standardization of nomenclature in the diagnosis of heart and lung rejection: heart rejection study group. *J Heart Lung Transplant* 1990; 9:587.

93. Rodriguez ER: International Society for Heart and Lung Transplantation. The pathology of heart transplant biopsy specimens: revisiting the 1990 ISHLT working formulation. *J Heart Lung Transplant* 2003; 22:3.

94. Stewart S, Winters GL, Fishbein MC, et al: Revision of the 1990 working formulation for the standardization of nomenclature in the diagnosis of heart rejection. *J Heart Lung Transplant* 2005; 24:1710.

95. Lower RR, Dong E, Glazener FS: Electrocardiogram of dogs with heart homografts. *Circulation* 1966; 33:455.

96. Cooper DK, Charles RG, Rose AG, et al: Does the electrocardiogram detect early acute heart rejection? *J Heart Transplant* 1985; 4:546.

97. Volgman AS, Winkel EM, Pinski SL, et al: Characteristics of the signal-averaged P wave in orthotopic heart transplant recipients. *Pacing Clin Electrophysiol* 1998; 21:2327.

98. Boyd SY, Mego DM, Khan NA, et al: Doppler echocardiography in cardiac transplant patients: allograft rejection and its relationship to diastolic function. *J Am Soc Echocardiogr* 1997; 10:526.

99. Morocutti G, Di Chiara A, Proclemer A, et al: Signal-averaged electrocardiography and Doppler echocardiographic study in predicting acute rejection in heart transplantation. *J Heart Lung Transplant* 1995; 14:1065.

100. Almenar L, Igual B, Martinez-Dolz L, et al: Utility of cardiac magnetic resonance imaging for the diagnosis of heart transplant rejection. *Transplant Proc* 2003; 35:1962.

101. Addonizio LJ: Detection of cardiac allograft rejection using radionuclide techniques. *Prog Cardiovasc Dis* 1990; 33:73.

102. Wijngaard PL, Doornewaard H, van der Meulen A, et al: Cytoimmunologic monitoring as an adjunct in monitoring rejection after heart transplantation: results of a 6-year follow-up in heart transplant recipients. *J Heart Lung Transplant* 1994; 13:869.

103. Mehra MR, Uber PA, Uber WE, et al: Anything but a biopsy: noninvasive monitoring for cardiac allograft rejection. *Curr Opin Cardiol* 2002; 17:131.

104. Horwitz PA, Tsai EJ, Putt ME, et al: Detection of cardiac allograft rejection and response to immunosuppressive therapy with peripheral blood gene expression. *Circulation* 2004; 110:3815.

105. Deng MC, Eisen HJ, Mehra RM, et al, for the CARGO Investigators: Non-invasive detection of rejection in cardiac allograft recipients using gene expression profiling. *Am J Transplant* 2006; 6:150-160.

106. Starling RC, Pham M, Valantine H, et al: Molecular Testing in the Management of Cardiac Transplant Recipients: Initial Clinical experience (Invited Editorial). *J Heart Lung Transplant* 2006; 25:1389-1395.

107. Deng MC, Elashoff B, Pham MX, et al; for the IMAGE Study Group: Utility of Gene Expression Profiling Score Variability to Predict Clinical Events in Heart Transplant Recipients. Transplantation. 2014 Mar 27; 97(6):708-714. doi: 10.1097/01.TP.0000443897.29951.cf. PMID: 24637869.

108. Pham MX, Teuteberg JJ, Kfoury AG, et al: for the IMAGE Study Group: Gene expression profiling for rejection surveillance after cardiac transplantation. *N Engl J Med* 2010; 362:1890-1900.

109. Lund LH, Edwards LB, Kucheryavaya AY et al: The Registry of the International Society for Heart and Lung Transplantation: thirtieth official adult heart transplant report—2013; focus theme: age. *J Heart Lung Transplant* 2013; 32:951-964.

110. Michler RE, Smith CR, Drusin RE, et al: Reversal of cardiac transplant rejection without massive immunosuppression. *Circulation* 1986; 74:III-68.

111. Yamani MH, Starling RC, Pelegrin D, et al: Efficacy of tacrolimus in patients with steroid-resistant cardiac allograft cellular rejection. *J Heart Lung Transplant* 2000; 19:337.

112. Radovancevic B, El-Sabrout R, Thomas C, et al: Rapamycin reduces rejection in heart transplant recipients. *Transplant Proc* 2001; 33:3221.

113. Cantarovich M, Latter DA, Loertscher R: Treatment of steroid-resistant and recurrent acute cardiac transplant rejection with a short course of antibody therapy. *Clin Transplant* 1997; 11:316.

114. Ross HJ, Gullestad L, Pak J, et al: Methotrexate or total lymphoid radiation for treatment of persistent or recurrent allograft cellular rejection: a comparative study. *J Heart Lung Transplant* 1997; 16:179.

115. Lloveras JJ, Escourrou G, Delisle MG, et al: Evolution of untreated mild rejection in heart transplant recipients. *J Heart Lung Transplant* 1992; 11:751.

116. Winters GL, Loh E, Schoen FJ, et al: Natural history of focal moderate cardiac allograft rejection: is treatment warranted? *Circulation* 1995; 91:1975.

117. Stoica SC, Cafferty F, Pauriah M, et al: The cumulative effect of acute rejection on development of cardiac allograft vasculopathy. *J Heart Lung Transplant* 2006; 25:420.

118. Michaels PJ, Espejo ML, Kobashigawa J, et al: Humoral rejection in cardiac transplantation: risk factors, hemodynamic consequences and relationship to transplant coronary artery disease. *J Heart Lung Transplant* 2003; 22:58.

119. Kfoury AG, Snow GL, Budge D et al: A longitudinal study of the course of asymptomatic antibody-mediated rejection in heart transplantation. *J Heart Lung Transplant* 2012; 31:46-51.

120. Lones MA, Czer LS, Trento A, et al: Clinical-pathologic features of humoral rejection in cardiac allografts: a study in 81 consecutive patients. *J Heart Lung Transplant* 1995; 14:151.

121. Olsen SL, Wagoner LE, Hammond EH, et al: Vascular rejection in heart transplantation: clinical correlation, treatment options, and future considerations. *J Heart Lung Transplant* 1993; 12:S135.

122. Hammond EH, Yowell RL, Price GD, et al: Vascular rejection and its relationship to allograft coronary artery disease. *J Heart Lung Transplant* 1992; 11:S111.

123. Miller LW, Naftel DC, Bourge RC, et al: Infection after heart transplantation: a multi-institutional study. *J Heart Lung Transplant* 1994; 13:381.

124. Eastlund T: Infectious disease transmission through cell, tissue, and organ transplantation: reducing the risk through donor selection. *Cell Transplant* 1995; 4:455.

125. Schaffner A: Pretransplant evaluation for infections in donors and recipients of solid organs. *Clin Infect Dis* 2001; 33:S9.

126. Rubin RH: Prevention and treatment of cytomegalovirus disease in heart transplant patients. *J Heart Lung Transplant* 2000; 19:731.

127. Merigan TC, Renlund DG, Keay S, et al: A controlled trial of ganciclovir to prevent cytomegalovirus disease after heart transplantation. *N Engl J Med* 1992; 326:1182.

128. Bonaros NE, Kocher A, Dunkler D, et al: Comparison of combined prophylaxis of cytomegalovirus hyperimmune globulin plus ganciclovir versus cytomegalovirus hyperimmune globulin alone in high-risk heart transplant recipients. *Transplantation* 2004; 77:890.

129. Egan JJ, Barber L, Lomax J, et al: Detection of human cytomegalovirus antigenemia: a rapid diagnostic technique for predicting cytomegalovirus infection/pneumonitis in lung and heart transplant recipients. *Thorax* 1995; 50:9.

130. Devyatko E, Zuckermann A, Ruzicka M, et al: Pre-emptive treatment with oral valganciclovir in management of CMV infection after cardiac transplantation. *J Heart Lung Transplant* 2004; 23:1277.

131. Wiltshire H, Hirankarn S, Farrell C, et al: Pharmacokinetic profile of ganciclovir after its oral administration and from its prodrug, valganciclovir, in solid organ transplant recipients. *Clin Pharmacokinet* 2005; 44:495.

132. Gray J, Wreghitt TG, Pavel P, et al: Epstein-Barr virus infection in heart and heart-lung transplant recipients: incidence and clinical impact. *J Heart Lung Transplant* 1995; 14:640.

133. Montoya JG, Chaparro SV, Celis D, et al: Invasive aspergillosis in the setting of cardiac transplantation. *Clin Infect Dis* 2003; 37:S281.

134. Patterson TF, Kirkpatrick WR, White M, et al: Invasive aspergillosis: disease spectrum, treatment practices, and outcomes. *Aspergillus* Study Group. *Medicine (Baltimore)* 2000; 79:250.

135. Cardenal R, Medrano FJ, Varela JM, et al: *Pneumocystis carinii* pneumonia in heart transplant recipients. *Eur J Cardiothorac Surg* 2001; 20:799.

136. Lehto JT, Anttila VJ, Lommi J, et al: Clinical usefulness of bronchoalveolar lavage in heart transplant recipients with suspected lower respiratory tract infection. *J Heart Lung Transplant* 2004; 23:570.

137. Speirs GE, Hakim M, Wreghitt TG: Relative risk of donor transmitted *Toxoplasma gondii* infection in heart, liver and kidney transplant recipients. *Clin Transplant* 1988; 2:257.

138. Cermakova Z, Ryskova O, Pliskova L: Polymerase chain reaction for detection of *Toxoplasma gondii* in human biological samples. *Folia Microbiol (Praha)* 2005; 50:341.

139. Costanzo MR, Naftel DC, Pritzker MR, et al: Heart transplant coronary artery disease detected by coronary angiography: a multi-institutional study of preoperative donor and recipient risk factors. Cardiac Transplant Research Database. *J Heart Lung Transplant* 1998; 17:744.

140. Avery RK: Cardiac-allograft vasculopathy. *N Engl J Med* 2003; 349:829.

141. Caforio AL, Tona F, Fortina AB, et al: Immune and nonimmune predictors of cardiac allograft vasculopathy onset and severity: multivariate risk factor analysis and role of immunosuppression. *Am J Transplant* 2004; 4:962.

142. Valantine H: Cardiac allograft vasculopathy after heart transplantation: risk factors and management. *J Heart Lung Transplant* 2004; 23:S187.

143. Day JD, Rayburn BK, Gaudin PB, et al: Cardiac allograft vasculopathy: the central pathogenic role of ischemia-induced endothelial cell injury. *J Heart Lung Transplant* 1995; 14:S142.

144. Hollenberg SM, Klein LW, Parrillo JE, et al: Coronary endothelial dysfunction after heart transplantation predicts allograft vasculopathy and cardiac death. *Circulation* 2001; 104:3091.

145. Kass M, Haddad H: Cardiac allograft vasculopathy: pathology, prevention and treatment. *Curr Opin Cardiol* 2006; 21:132.

146. Mehra MR, Crespo-Leiro MG, Dipchand A et al: International Society for Heart and Lung Transplantation working formulation of a standardized nomenclature for cardiac allograft vasculopathy-2010. *J Heart Lung Transplant* 2010; 29:717-727.

147. Prada-Delgado O, Estevez-Loureiro R, Paniagua-Martin MJ, Lopez-Sainz A, Crespo-Leiro MG: Prevalence and prognostic value of cardiac allograft vasculopathy 1 year after heart transplantation according to the ISHLT recommended nomenclature. *J Heart Lung Transplant* 2012; 31: 332-333.

148. Kobashigawa JA, Tobis JM, Starling RC, et al: Multicenter intravascular ultrasound validation study among heart transplant recipients: outcomes after five years. *J Am Coll Cardiol* 2005; 45:1532.

149. Smart FW, Ballantyne CM, Farmer JA, et al: Insensitivity of noninvasive tests to detect coronary artery vasculopathy after heart transplant. *Am J Cardiol* 1991; 67:243.

150. Redonnet M, Tron C, Koning R, et al: Coronary angioplasty and stenting in cardiac allograft vasculopathy following heart transplantation. *Transplant Proc* 2000; 32:463.

151. Mehra MR, Ventura HO, Smart FW, et al: Impact of converting enzyme inhibitors and calcium entry blockers on cardiac allograft vasculopathy: from bench to bedside. *J Heart Lung Transplant* 1995; 14:S246.

152. Kobashigawa JA, Katznelson S, Laks H, et al: Effect of pravastatin on outcomes after cardiac transplantation. *N Engl J Med* 1995; 333:621.

153. Mancini D, Pinney S, Burkhoff D, et al: Use of rapamycin slows progression of cardiac transplantation vasculopathy. *Circulation* 2003; 108:48.

154. Eisen HJ, Tuzcu EM, Dorent R, et al: Everolimus for the prevention of allograft rejection and vasculopathy in cardiac transplant recipients. *N Engl J Med* 2003; 349:847.

155. Mancini D, Vigano M, Pulpon LA, et al: 24-month results of a multi-center study of Certican for the prevention of allograft rejection and vasculopathy in de novo cardiac transplant recipients. *Am J Transplant* 2003; 3:550.

156. Haverich A, Tuzcu EM, Viganò M, et al: Certican in de novo cardiac transplant recipients: 24-month follow-up. *J Heart Lung Transplant* 2003; 22:S140.

157. Eisen H, Kobashigawa J, Starling RC, et al: Improving outcomes in heart transplantation: the potential of proliferation signal inhibitors. *Transplant Proc* 2005; 37:4S.

158. Senechal M, Dorent R, du Montcel ST: End-stage renal failure and cardiac mortality after heart transplantation. *Clin Transplant* 2004; 18:1.

159. Arizon del Prado JM, Aumente Rubio MD, Cardenas Aranzana M, et al: New strategies of cyclosporine monitoring in heart transplantation: initial results. *Transplant Proc* 2003; 35:1984.

160. Citterio F: Evolution of the therapeutic drug monitoring of cyclosporine. *Transplant Proc* 2004; 36:420S.

161. Angermann CE, Stork S, Costard-Jackle A: Reduction of cyclosporine after introduction of mycophenolate mofetil improves chronic renal dysfunction in heart transplant recipients: the IMPROVED multicentre study. *Eur Heart J* 2004; 25:1626.

162. Fernandez-Valls M, Gonzalez-Vilchez F, de Prada JA, et al: Sirolimus as an alternative to anticalcineurin therapy in heart transplantation: experience of a single center. *Transplant Proc* 2005; 37:4021.

163. Groetzner J, Meiser B, Landwehr P, et al: Mycophenolate mofetil and sirolimus as calcineurin inhibitor-free immunosuppression for late cardiac-transplant recipients with chronic renal failure. *Transplantation* 2004; 77:568.

164. Ventura HO, Mehra MR, Stapleton DD, et al: Cyclosporine-induced hypertension in cardiac transplantation. *Med Clin North Am* 1997; 81:1347.

165. Taylor DO, Barr ML, Radovancevic B, et al: A randomized, multi-center comparison of tacrolimus and cyclosporine immunosuppressive regimens in cardiac transplantation: decreased hyperlipidemia and hypertension with tacrolimus. *J Heart Lung Transplant* 1999; 18:336.

166. Brozena SC, Johnson MR, Ventura H, et al: Effectiveness and safety of diltiazem or lisinopril in treatment of hypertension after heart transplantation: results of a prospective, randomized multicenter trial. *J Am Coll Cardiol* 1996; 27:1707.

167. Starling RC, Cody RJ: Cardiac transplant hypertension. *Am J Cardiol* 1990; 65:106.

168. Ippoliti G, Rinaldi M, Pellegrini C, et al: Incidence of cancer after immunosuppressive treatment for heart transplantation. *Crit Rev Oncol Hematol* 2005; 56:101.

169. Hanto DW, Sakamoto K, Purtilo DT, et al: The Epstein-Barr virus in the pathogenesis of posttransplant lymphoproliferative disorders. *Surgery* 1981; 90:204.

170. Swinnen LJ, Costanzo-Nordin MR, Fisher SG, et al: Increased incidence of lymphoproliferative disorder after immunosuppression with the monoclonal antibody OKT3 in cardiac transplant recipients. *N Engl J Med* 1990; 323:1723.

171. El-Hamamsy I, Stevens LM, Carrier M, et al: Incidence and prognosis of cancer following heart transplantation using RATG induction therapy. *Transplant Int* 2005; 18:1280.

172. Frohlich GM, Rufibach K, Enseleit F et al: Statins and the risk of cancer after heart transplantation. *Circulation* 2012; 126:440-447.

173. Kirklin JK, Benza RL, Rayburn BK, et al: Strategies for minimizing hyperlipidemia after cardiac transplantation. *Am J Cardiovasc Drugs* 2002; 2:377.

174. Bianda T, Linka A, Junga G, et al: Prevention of osteoporosis in heart transplant recipients: a comparison of calcitriol with calcitonin and pamidronate. *Calcif Tissue Int* 2000; 67:116.

175. Mueller XM, Tevaearai HT, Stumpe F, et al: Gastrointestinal disease following heart transplantation. *World J Surg* 1999; 23:650.

176. Radovancevic B, McGiffin DC, Kobashigawa JA, et al: Retransplantation in 7290 primary transplant patients: a 10-year multi-institutional study. *J Heart Lung Transplant* 2003; 22:862.

177. Srivastava R, Keck BM, Bennett LE, et al: The result of cardiac retransplantation: an analysis of the joint International Society of Heart Lung Transplantation/United Network for Organ Sharing Thoracic Registry. *Transplantation* 2000; 4:606.

178. Kilic A, Weiss ES, George TJ, et al. What predicts long-term survival after heart transplantation? An analysis of 9,400 ten-year survivors. *Ann Thorac Surg* 2012; 93:699-704.

179. Khan MS, Mery CM, Zafar F, et al: Is mechanically bridging patients with a failing cardiac graft to retransplantation an effective therapy? Analysis of the United Network of Organ Sharing database. *J Heart Lung Transplant* 2012; 31:1192-1198.

180. Haddad H: Cardiac retransplantation: an ethical dilemma. *Curr Opin Cardiol* 2006; 21:118.

181. Lim E, Ali Z, Ali A, et al: Comparison of survival by allocation to medical therapy, surgery, or heart transplantation for ischemic advanced heart failure. *J Heart Lung Transplant* 2005; 24:983.

182. Luckraz H, Goddard M, Charman SC, et al: Early mortality after cardiac transplantation: should we do better? *J Heart Lung Transplant* 2005; 24:401.

183. Rasmusson K, Brunisholz K, Budge D, et al: Peripartum cardiomyopathy: post-transplant outcomes from the United Network for Organ Sharing Database. *J Heart Lung Transplant* 2012; 31:180-186.

184. Politi P, Piccinelli M, Poli PF, et al: Te n years of "extended" life: quality of life among heart transplantation survivors. *Transplantation* 2004; 78:257.

185. Kilic A, Conte JV, Shah AS, Yuh DD: Orthotopic heart transplantation in patients with metabolic risk factors. *Ann Thorac Surg* 2012; 93:718-724.

186. Allen JG, Weiss ES, Arnaoutakis GJ, et al: Insurance and education predict long-term survival after orthotopic heart transplantation in the United States. *J Heart Lung Transplant* 2012; 31:52-60.

187. Pettit SJ, Jhund PS, Hawkins NM, et al: How small is too small? A systematic review of center volume and outcome after cardiac transplantation. *Circ Cardiovasc Qual Outcomes* 2012; 5:783-790.

188. Arnaoutakis GJ, George TJ, Allen JG, et al: Institutional volume and the effect of recipient risk on short-term mortality after orthotopic heart transplant. *J Thorac Cardiovasc Surg* 2012; 143:157-167 (67e1).

189. Kilic A, Weiss ES, Yuh DD, et al: Institutional factors beyond procedural volume significantly impact center variability in outcomes after orthotopic heart transplantation. *Ann Surg* 2012; 256:616-623.

190. Russo MJ, Chen JM, Hong KN, et al: Survival after heart transplantation is not diminished among recipients with uncomplicated diabetes mellitus: an analysis of the United Network of Organ Sharing database. *Circulation.* 2006 Nov 21; 114(21):2280-2287. Epub 2006 Nov 6.

191. Zaidi AR, Zaidi A, Vaitkus PT: Outcome of heart transplantation in patients with sarcoid cardiomyopathy. *J Heart Lung Transplant* 2007; 26(7):714-717.

192. Kpodonu J, Massad MG, Caines A, Geha AS: Outcome of heart transplantation in patients with amyloid cardiomyopathy. *J Heart Lung Transplant* 2005; 24(11):1763-1765.

193. Nwakanma LU, Williams JA, Weiss ES, et al: Influence of pretransplant panel-reactive antibody on outcomes in 8,160 heart transplant recipients in recent era. *Ann Thorac Surg* 2007; 84(5):1556-1562; discussion 1562-1563.

194. Weiss ES, Nwakanma LU, Patel ND, Yuh DD: Outcomes in patients older than 60 years of age undergoing orthotopic heart transplantation: an analysis of the UNOS database. *J Heart Lung Transplant* 2008; 27(2):184-191.

195. Weiss ES, Allen JG, Russell SD, et al: Impact of recipient body mass index on organ allocation and mortality in orthotopic heart transplantation. *J Heart Lung Transplant* 2009; 28(11):1150-1157. Epub 2009 Sep 26.

196. Pal JD, Piacentino V, Cuevas AD, et al: Impact of left ventricular assist device bridging on posttransplant outcomes. *Ann Thorac Surg* 2009; 88(5):1457-1461; discussion 1461.

197. Shuhaiber J, Hur K, Gibbons R: Does the type of ventricular assisted device influence survival, infection, and rejection rates following heart transplantation? *J Card Surg* 2009; 24(3):250-255.

198. Weiss ES, Meguid RA, Patel ND, et al: Increased mortality at low-volume orthotopic heart transplantation centers: should current standards change? *Ann Thorac Surg* 2008; 86(4):1250-1259; discussion 1259-1260.

199. Orlic D, Kajstura J, Chimenti S: Bone marrow cells regenerate infarcted myocardium. *Nature* 2001; 410:701.

Lung Transplantation and Heart-lung Transplantation

Hari R. Mallidi • Jatin Anand • Robert C. Robbins

Human lung transplantation, performed as a single lung, double lung, or heart-lung bloc, has emerged as a life-saving procedure for patients with end-stage pulmonary disease. With improvement of operative techniques, organ preservation, and immunosuppressive regimens, combined heart-lung and isolated lung transplantation have become common treatments for patients with a variety of end-stage disease entities. To date, 3703 combined heart-lung transplants and 43,428 lung transplants have been reported worldwide.[1] Although the number of heart-lung transplants performed annually has declined in recent years, the number of single-lung transplantation (SLT) procedures remains stable, accompanied by a steady increase in bilateral lung transplant procedures (Fig. 61-1). Clinical progress in thoracic organ transplantation has been considerable, yet significant barriers that limit the scope of these procedures still remain. These include donor organ shortage, limited preservation techniques, graft rejection, and infectious complications. This chapter summarizes the state of the art in combined heart-lung and isolated lung transplantation.

LUNG TRANSPLANTATION

History of Lung Transplantation

In 1949, Henry Metras described many of the important technical concepts for lung transplantation, including preservation of the left atrial cuff for the pulmonary venous anastomoses and reimplantation of an aortic patch containing the origin of the bronchial arteries to prevent bronchial dehiscence.[2] Airway dehiscence was a major obstacle in experimental lung transplantation, and he proposed that preservation of the bronchial arterial supply was critical to airway healing. Unfortunately, this technique was technically cumbersome and never gained widespread popularity. In the 1960s, Blumenstock and Khan advocated transection of the transplant bronchus close to the lung parenchyma to prevent ischemic bronchial necrosis.[3] Additional surgical modifications were developed to prevent bronchial anastomotic complications, including telescoping of the bronchial anastomosis, described by Veith in 1970,[4] and coverage of the anastomosis with an omental pedicle flap, described by

the Toronto group in 1982.[5] Corticosteroids were found to be another contributor to poor bronchial healing,[6] a problem ameliorated by the introduction of cyclosporine immunosuppression. Thus, by the 1970s, the stage was set for successful lung transplantation in the human.

The first human lung transplant was described in 1963 by Hardy and colleagues at the University of Mississippi.[7] The patient, a 58-year-old man with lung cancer, survived 18 days postoperatively. Over the next two decades, nearly 40 lung transplants were performed without long-term success. In 1986, the Toronto Lung Transplant Group reported the first successful series of single-lung transplants with long-term survival.[8] Improved immunosuppression, along with careful recipient and donor selection, was pivotal to their success. For patients with bilateral lung disease, en bloc double lung replacement was introduced by Patterson in 1988 as an alternative to heart-lung transplantation with a domino procedure in which the explanted heart was offered to a second recipient with end-stage heart disease.[9] This technique was later replaced by sequential bilateral lung transplantation, described by Pasque and colleagues in 1990.[10] More recent operative innovations include living lobar transplantation, performed for the first time by Vaughn Starnes at Stanford in 1992.[11]

Lung transplantation has seen a steady growth over the past decade, with over 3800 procedures reported to the International Society for Heart and Lung Transplantation (ISHLT) registry in 2013.[1] Currently there are 153 centers reporting lung transplant data, with more than half of these performing more than 10 transplants per year. Although the number of single-lung transplants performed has been relatively stable since the mid-1990s, bilateral lung transplant procedures have shown a consistent growth in volume.[1]

Indications for Lung Transplantation

GENERAL GUIDELINES

Organ allocation for lung transplantation underwent a major change in 2005 that has significantly affected the process of recipient selection. Historically, lung allocation was determined strictly by the amount of time a patient spent on the

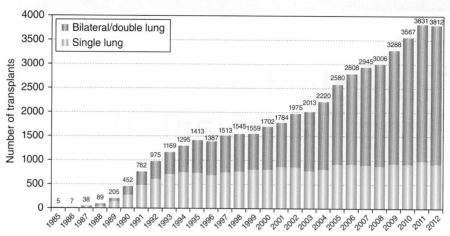

FIGURE 61-1 UNOS data representing the number of lung transplant procedures reported by year and procedure type, collected from data reported to the International Society of Heart and Lung Transplantation Registry. This figure may underestimate the total number of procedures worldwide. (Reproduced with permission from Yusen RD1, Edwards LB1, Kucheryavaya AY, et al: The registry of the International Society for Heart and Lung Transplantation: thirty-first adult lung and heart-lung transplant report—2014, *J Heart Lung Transplant.* 2014 Oct;33(10):1009-1024.)

waiting list (matching for size and blood group). Consequently, the limited supply of donor organs resulted in an increasing number of patients on the waiting list with progressively longer wait times (Fig. 61-2).[12] To address these shortcomings, the organ allocation system was revised in 2005 to prioritize medical urgency and expected outcome after transplantation. Under this system, prioritization is based on a lung allocation score (LAS) that is calculated based on the following clinical criteria: age, height, weight, lung diagnosis code, functional status, diabetes, assisted ventilation, supplemental O_2 requirement, percent predicted forced vital capacity (FVC), pulmonary artery systemic pressure, mean pulmonary artery pressure, pulmonary capillary wedge pressure, current PCO_2, highest PCO_2, lowest PCO_2, change in PCO_2, 6-minute walk distance, and serum creatinine. These values can be entered into an online calculator to derive the LAS (https://optn.transplant.hrsa.gov/resources/allocation-calculators/las-calculator/). Based on these criteria, the waitlist urgency measure (defined as the expected number of

days during the next year on the waiting list without a transplant) is subtracted from the posttransplant survival measure (defined as the expected number of days lived during the first year after transplantation) to determine the net transplant benefit. This raw allocation score is then normalized to a scale of 0 to 100 to calculate the LAS. In this scoring system, posttransplant survival is limited to 1 year because the predictive variables are only relevant in the early postoperative period.[13]

The rationale for approaching recipient selection from the perspective of transplant benefit is based on the premise that patient selection for lung transplantation must balance the anticipated survival after transplantation (currently at a median of 5 years) with projected life expectancy on the waiting list. Although waiting times have historically averaged 432 days, the institution of the LAS has reduced this period to an average of 262 days.[14] Nevertheless, mortality while on the waiting list remains at nearly 20%, so it is imperative to identify recipients as early as possible within the "transplant window."[15] Ideally, recipient evaluation should select individuals with progressively disabling pulmonary disease who still possess the capacity for full rehabilitation after transplantation. Much of the current success in lung transplantation stems from improvement in recipient selection, because early attempts were thwarted by selection of patients with prohibitive operative risk factors. Candidates should have a less than 50% 2- to 3-year predicted survival despite appropriate medical or alternative surgical strategies. Disabling symptoms prompting consideration for transplantation typically include dyspnea, cyanosis, syncope, and hemoptysis. Potential recipients are identified by their local primary physicians and referred to transplantation centers for further evaluation.

Tests required for transplant listing are reviewed in Table 61-1. Diagnostic studies that are particularly useful in evaluating potential recipients include full pulmonary function tests, an exercise performance test, electrocardiogram,

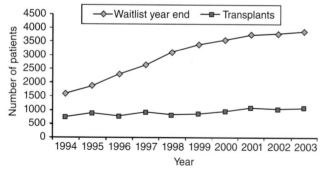

FIGURE 61-2 Between 1994 and 2003, the availability of donor organs held relatively constant, with an increasing number of patients placed on the waiting list. (Reproduced with permission from 2004 OPIN/SRTR Annual Report.)

TABLE 61-1: Typical Laboratory Tests and Studies Obtained During Recipient Evaluation for Heart-lung and Lung Transplantation

Suitability for Transplantation (Phase I)

Required Laboratory Tests and Studies

CBC with differential, platelet, and reticulocyte count

Blood type and antibody screen (ABO, Rh)

Prothrombin and activated partial thromboplastin time (PT, aPTT)

Bleeding time

Immunology panel (FANA, RF)

Electrolytes, including Mg^2

CK with isoenzymes

Serum protein electrophoresis

Urinalysis

Viral serologies

    Compromised host panel (cytomegalovirus, adenovirus, Varicella-Zoster, herpes simplex, Epstein-Barr virus)

    Hepatitis A, B, and C antibodies, Hepatitis B surface antigen (HBsAg)

    Cytomegalovirus (quantitative antibodies and IgM)

    Human immunodeficiency virus

Electrocardiogram

Chest x-ray

Studies Obtained as Indicated

Echocardiogram with bubble study

MUGA for right and left ventricular ejection fraction

Cardiac catheterization with coronary angiogram

Thoracic CT scan

Quantitative ventilation-perfusion scans

Carotid duplex

Mammogram

Colonoscopy

Sputum for Gram stain, AFB smear, KOH, and routine bacterial, mycobacterial, and fungal cultures

Required For Listing (Phase II)

HLA and DR typing

Transplant antibody

Quantitative immunoglobulins

Histoplasma, Coccidioides, and *Toxoplasma* titers

PPD

Pulmonary function tests with arterial blood gases

12-Hour urine collection for creatinine clearance and total protein

Urine viral culture

---

echocardiogram, 24-hour creatinine clearance, and liver function tests. Former smokers must undergo screening to exclude smoking-related illnesses, such as peripheral vascular disease and malignancy. A negative sputum cytology, thoracic computed tomographic (CT) scan, bronchoscopy, otolaryngologic evaluation, and carotid duplex scan are required. In addition, left heart catheterization and coronary angiography should be performed in recipient candidates who have a history of smoking.

Patients deemed suitable for transplantation during the initial evaluation are subjected to a final phase of testing (see Table 61-1). If accepted by the transplant review committee, they are listed on the national transplant registry based on LAS. Listed candidates should be seen every 3 to 6 months at the transplant center and regularly by their primary physicians, to maintain optimal medical condition. If appropriate, a period of exercise rehabilitation and nutritional modification may be initiated. Most transplant centers require patients to reside within several hours of the center by automobile or air charter.

ABO compatibilities are strictly adhered to, because isolated cases of hyperacute rejection have been reported in transplants performed across ABO barriers.[16] Donor-to-recipient lung volume matching is an important consideration. According to the 27th-30th ISHLT registry reports, taller donor heights have been shown to correlate with a lower risk for 1-year posttransplant mortality.[1,17] A range of acceptable donor heights is mandated at the time of patient listing. However, the best parameter for size matching remains controversial.

Height alone is an important predictor of lung size, yet gender affects lung size independently of height.[18] Therefore, another parameter commonly reported is the predicted total lung capacity (pTLC), which is calculated from a regression equation based on both gender and height. The pTLC of a 170-cm male is 6.5 L while that of a 170-cm female is 5.4 L, illustrating the importance of gender considerations and the utility of the pTLC.

Current ISHLT Guidelines recommend that donor pTLC should be matched to within 75 to 125% of the recipients pTLC.[19] Eberlein and colleagues evaluated a pTLC donor-to-recipient ratio (pTLC donor/pTLC recipient) in a retrospective registry study of over 10,000 patients and found an association between a high pTLC ratio (suggesting an oversized allograft) and improved survival after lung transplant.[20] The authors concluded that the pTLC ratio is an independent predictor of death in the first year after lung transplant and should therefore be carefully considered.

Preoperative comparison of donor and recipient chest tomography typically involves matching the vertical (apex to diaphragm along the midclavicular line) and transverse (level of diaphragmatic dome) radiologic dimensions. Donor lung dimensions should not be greater than 4 cm over those of the recipient. If needed, donor lungs may be downsized by lobectomy or wedge resection. As high-resolution three-dimensional CT imaging and advanced software becomes more readily available, lung-size-matching using newer technologies continues to emerge.[21]

In contrast to renal transplantation, HLA matching is not a criterion for thoracic organ allocation. Because only short ischemic times are tolerated by lung and heart-lung blocs, it is not possible to perform this tissue typing preoperatively.[22] However, several retrospective studies have been performed evaluating the influence of HLA matching on long-term graft survival and development of obliterative bronchiolitis (OB).

Wisser and colleagues examined the relationship between HLA matching and long-term survival in 78 lung transplant recipients, finding improved graft survival with matching at the HLA-B locus.[23] In a retrospective study of 74 lung transplant patients, Iwaki and coworkers also correlated matching at the HLA-B and HLA-DR loci with improved graft survival.[24] These studies suggest a relationship between HLA matching and long-term graft function.

Once an appropriate donor-recipient pairing is made, the recipient is screened for preformed antibodies against a panel of random donors. A percent reactive antibody (PRA) level greater than 25 prompts a prospective-specific crossmatch between the donor and recipient. A positive crossmatch indicates the presence of antidonor circulating antibodies in the recipient, which would likely lead to hyperacute rejection. In the event of a positive crossmatch, the donor organ cannot be accepted for that recipient.

DISEASE-SPECIFIC GUIDELINES

Common indications for lung transplantation are listed in Table 61-2, with listing criteria given in Table 61-3.

Chronic obstructive pulmonary disease (COPD) represents the most common indication for lung transplantation, accounting for 36% of lung transplants performed each year.[25] Decision making with respect to referral for transplantation and listing is based on worsening clinical deterioration as quantified by the BODE index. This predictive tool takes into account body mass index (B), degree of airflow obstruction (O), dyspnea (D, measured by the modified Medical Research Council MMRC dyspnea scale), and exercise capacity (E, measured by a 6-minute walk test).[26]

The BODE index score ranges from 0 to 10, and patients are considered for transplant with a score of 7 to 10, because median survival in this cohort is only 3 years.[26] In patients with COPD who have apically predominant emphysema, lung volume reduction surgery (LVRS) may represent an alternative strategy to postpone or eliminate the need for transplantation. Patients who have undergone pleurodesis or who have advanced disease (FEV_1 and DL_{CO} < 20% or significant pulmonary hypertension) are not eligible for LVRS.[27] Based on the National Emphysema Treatment Trial, which studied the benefit of LVRS, a cohort of transplant-eligible high-risk patients (median survival of 3 years with medical therapy) was identified in which FEV_1 was less than 20% and either DLCO less than 20% or homogeneously distributed emphysema was present.[27] The decision to perform single- versus double-lung transplantation (DLT) in a patient with COPD must take into account the patient's ability to tolerate single-lung ventilation, cardiopulmonary bypass, and the risk of ventilation-perfusion mismatch in single-lung transplant when compressive atelectasis and restriction occurs in the donor lung. Interestingly, a statistical model derived from United Network for Organ Sharing (UNOS) data between 1987 and 2004 estimated that 45% of COPD patients would gain a survival benefit of 1 year after double-lung transplant, compared with only 22% of patients who underwent single-lung transplant.[28]

Idiopathic pulmonary fibrosis (IPF) represents the second most common indication for lung transplantation worldwide, accounting for just over 20% of all lung transplants.[17] Median survival from the time of diagnosis is only 2.5 to 3.5 years, suggesting that transplant referral should be made as soon as histologic or radiographic evidence of the disease

TABLE 61-2: Indications for Lung Transplantation from January 1995 Through June 2013

Diagnosis	SLT (n = 15,321) No. (%)	BLT (n = 26,579) No. (%)	Total (n = 41,900) No. (%)
COPD/emphysema	6594 (43.0)	7078 (26.6)	13,672 (32.6)
IPF	5354 (34.9)	4825 (18.2)	10,179 (24.3)
Cystic fibrosis	234 (1.5)	6628 (24.9)	6862 (16.4)
AAT	771 (5.0)	1572 (5.9)	2343 (5.6)
IPAH	92 (0.6)	1158 (4.4)	1250 (3.0)
Sarcoidosis	280 (1.8)	776 (2.9)	1056 (2.5)
Bronchiectasis	62 (0.4)	1069 (4.0)	1131 (2.7)
LAM	138 (0.9)	302 (1.1)	440 (1.1)
Congenital heart disease	58 (0.4)	291 (1.1)	349 (0.8)
OB	105 (0.7)	351 (1.3)	456 (1.1)
Retransplant			
OB	312 (2.0)	379 (1.4)	691 (1.6)
Not OB	205 (1.3)	227 (0.9)	432 (1.0)
Interstitial pneumonitis	32 (0.3)	29 (0.2)	61 (0.3)
Cancer	7 (0.0)	29 (0.1)	36 (0.1)
Other	255 (1.7)	515 (1.9)	770 (1.8)

UNOS data from January 1995 through June 2013. AAT, A1 anti-trypsin deficiency; COPD, chronic obstructive pulmonary disease; IPAH, idiopathic pulmonary arterial hypertension; IPF, idiopathic pulmonary fibrosis; OB, obliterative bronchiolitis.
Reproduced with permission from Yusen RD, Edwards LB, Kucheryavaya AY, et al: The registry of the International Society for Heart and Lung Transplantation: thirty-first adult lung and heart-lung transplant report—2014, *J Heart Lung Transplant.* 2014 Oct;33(10):1009-1024.)

○ **TABLE 61-3: Listing Criteria Specific to the Disease Entities Commonly Evaluated for Lung Transplantation**

Chronic Obstructive Pulmonary Disease
- BODE index of 7 to 10 or at least one of the following:
  ○ History of hospitalization for exacerbation associated with acute hypercapnia (PCO_2 exceeding 50 mm Hg)
  ○ Pulmonary hypertension or cor pulmonale, or both, despite oxygen therapy
  ○ FEV_1 < 20% and either DL_{CO} < 20% or homogenous distribution of emphysema

Idiopathic Pulmonary Fibrosis
- Histologic or radiographic evidence of UIP and any of the following:
  ○ A DL_{CO} < 39% predicted
  ○ A 10% or greater decrement in FVC during 6 months of follow-up
  ○ A decrease in pulse oximetry < 88% during a 6-minute walk test
  ○ Honeycombing on HRCT (fibrosis score > 2)

Cystic Fibrosis
- FEV_1 < 30% of predicted, or rapidly declining lung function if FEV_1 > 30% (females and patients < 18 years of age have a poorer prognosis; consider earlier listing) and/or any of the following:
  ○ Increasing oxygen requirements
  ○ Hypercapnia
  ○ Pulmonary hypertension

Idiopathic Pulmonary Arterial Hypertension
- Persistent NYHA Class III or IV on maximal medical therapy
  ○ Low (350 m) or declining 6-minute walk test
  ○ Failing therapy with intravenous epoprostenol, or equivalent
  ○ Cardiac index of <2 L/min/m²
  ○ Right atrial pressure > 15 mm Hg

Sarcoidosis
- NYHA functional Class III or IV and any of the following:
  ○ Hypoxemia at rest
  ○ Pulmonary hypertension
  ○ Elevated right atrial pressure >15 mm Hg

BODE, body mass index, airflow obstruction, dyspnea, and exercise capacity; HRCT, high-resolution computed tomography; NYHA, New York Heart Association; UIP = usual interstitial pneumonitis.
Data from Kreider M, Kotloff RM: Selection of candidates for lung transplantation, *Proc Am Thorac Soc.* 2009 Jan 15;6(1):20-27.

is present. Listing a patient with IPF must take into account the fact that many patients have an indolent form of the disease, and numerous studies have identified the following risk factors for rapid decline in patients with histologic or radiographic evidence of IPF:[29]

- DLCO less than 39% of predicted
- 10% or greater decrement in FVC during a 6-month period
- Oxygen saturation less than 88% during a 6-minute walk test
- Honeycombing on CT scan

Traditionally, IPF patients have been considered for either SLT or DLT. However, recent data suggest that there may be a survival advantage for double-lung over single-lung transplant—particularly among high-risk patients (defined as LAS > 52).[30]

Cystic fibrosis (CF) is the third most common indication for lung transplant, accounting for 16% of the total number of transplants performed.[25] In these patients, bilateral sepsis mandates removal of both native lungs. In a landmark study from the Hospital for Sick Children in Toronto, Kerem and colleagues established that CF patients with an FEV_1 of less than 30% of predicted experienced a 2-year mortality rate of 50%.[31] However, subsequent risk stratification models have challenged these findings and presented conflicting data on the question of life expectancy in CF. Therefore, the current ISHLT guidelines state that an FEV_1 less than 30% should prompt a referral to a transplant center with the decision to proceed with listing dependent on other indicators of disease severity such as oxygen-dependent respiratory failure, hypercapnia, and pulmonary hypertension.[32] CF recipients should have an otolaryngologic evaluation before being placed on an active waiting list. Most of these patients require endoscopic maxillary antrostomies for sinus access and monthly antibiotic irrigation to decrease the bacterial load of the upper respiratory tract. This measure has decreased the incidence of serious posttransplant bacterial infections.[33]

Idiopathic pulmonary arterial hypertension represents 3.3% of the total lung transplantation volume worldwide.[25] Survival with this condition has improved dramatically with the institution of vasodilator therapy, with 5-year survival of 55% on epoprostenol compared with 28% among historical controls.[34] Listing for transplantation is indicated when a patient remains in NYHA Class III or IV after 3 months of therapy (often seen in the setting of declining 6-minute walk test, cardiac index of < 2 L/min/m², or right atrial pressure > 15 mm Hg).[29]

Sarcoidosis accounts for 2.6% of all lung transplants.[25] The natural course of this disease can be highly variable, but in general patients should be referred for transplant if they develop NYHA class III or IV symptoms. Impairment of exercise tolerance and hypoxemia at rest, pulmonary hypertension, or right atrial pressure greater than 15 mm Hg serve as general guidelines for listing.[32]

Less than 2% of all single- and bilateral-lung transplants are retransplantations.[25] Overall, survival is poor compared with first-time transplantation, although certain subsets of patients perform better than others. In fact, the Pulmonary Retransplant Registry has collected data from 230 patients at over 40 centers and found that 1-year survival of ambulatory, nonventilated patients undergoing retransplantation after 1991 is comparable with first-time transplants.[35]

Impact of the Lung Allocation Score

Since the introduction of the LAS in 2005, there has been a decrease in waitlist time and waitlist mortality with a concurrent increase in the number of transplants performed per year (Fig. 61-3). Although early data have suggested that the 1-year survival since introduction of the LAS has not changed, more recent data indicate that the posttransplant survival

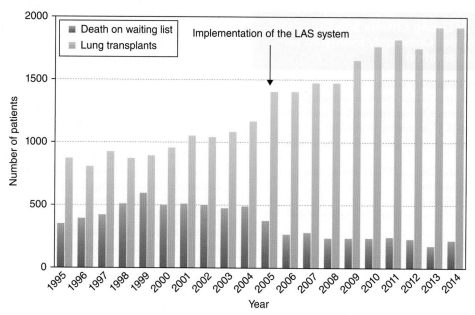

FIGURE 61-3 Since the introduction of the lung allocation score (LAS) in 2005, there has been a rise in the number of lung transplants performed each year with a concurrent decrease in the number of waiting list deaths. (Data from U.S. Department of Health and Human Services. Organ Procurement and Transplantation Network.)

beyond 1 year may be lower.[36] This is in accordance with the fact that sicker patients are being prioritized, including more that are bridged to transplantation with extracorporeal membrane oxygenation (ECMO) (Fig. 61-4). Furthermore, the most common diagnoses are also changing, with more

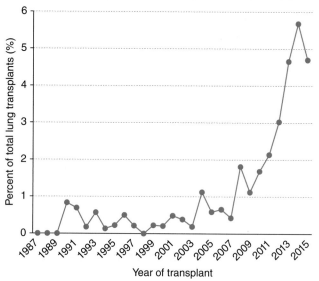

FIGURE 61-4 Percentage of patients on ECMO at the time of transplant by year. Only patients with no prior transplants were included. Figure created using the United Network for Organ Sharing (UNOS) database, based on Organ Procurement and Transplant Network (OPTN) data as of June 17, 2016. ECMO, extracorporeal membrane oxygenation.)

IPF and less COPD patients being selected for transplantation (Fig. 61-5)[1] Long-term data revealing the impact of the LAS are only recently becoming available and remain under intense investigation.

Previously, ISHLT and UNOS registries have demonstrated that DLT in COPD patients is associated with improved outcomes. Furthermore, SLT and DLT have shown similar outcomes in IPF patients. However, these data are largely from pre-LAS cohorts. In the post-LAS era, reanalysis has shown that DLT is associated with improved outcomes in both propensity-matched and unmatched cohorts of all-comers undergoing lung transplantation, as well as in analyses of patients specifically undergoing transplant for IPF.[37] For patients undergoing lung transplant for COPD, propensity-matched cohorts in the post-LAS era show similar survival whether SLT or DLT is employed.[37] These outcomes in the post-LAS era cohorts are contrary to previously published findings, and are likely explained by the fact that sicker, older patients with more comorbidities, of worse functional status, and with baseline oxygen requirements are being prioritized as a consequence of the LAS algorithm.

Analysis of post-LAS registry data in patients undergoing transplant for IPAH has revealed that those listed for transplantation have significantly worse comorbidities yet have a lower wait-list mortality and a higher incidence of transplant as compared to pre-LAS era.[38] Furthermore, those receiving double lung transplant in the post-LAS era have a survival advantage over those in the pre-LAS era while those receiving heart-lung transplant do not see the same survival advantage when compared to the pre-LAS cohort.[38] Again, these outcomes are contradictory to previously published registry analyses focused on pre-LAS cohorts.

Adult lung transplant: Major indications by year (%)

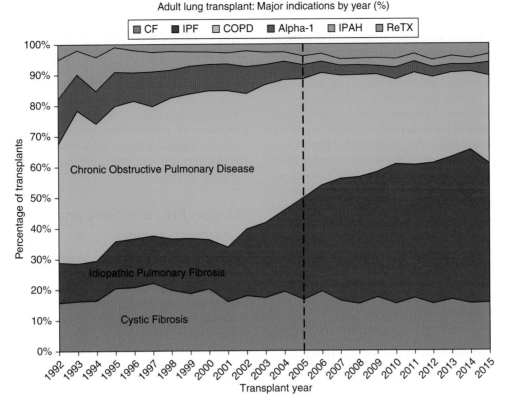

FIGURE 61-5 Major indications for lung transplantation in adults over time. Since the introduction of the lung allocation score (LAS) in 2005 (marked by the vertical dashed line), there have been more transplants for idiopathic pulmonary fibrosis (IPF) and less for chronic obstructive pulmonary disease (COPD). Figure created using the United Network for Organ Sharing (UNOS) database, based on Organ Procurement and Transplant Network (OPTN) data as of June 17, 2016. CF, cystic fibrosis; Alpha 1, Alpha 1-antitrypsin deficiency emphysema; IPAH, idiopathic pulmonary arterial hypertension; ReTX, retransplantation.)

These recent analyses help to illustrate the fact that the institution of the LAS has had a dramatic impact on lung transplantation in ways that remain largely uncharacterized. Ongoing evaluation of post-LAS cohorts with an emphasis on long-term outcomes is an area of intense focus within the lung-transplant community.

Contraindications to Lung Transplantation

There are well-established contraindications to lung transplantation (Table 61-4). In general, transplantation is an option that is restricted to patients less than 65 years old, although 9% of recipients in the first half of 2008 exceeded this cutoff.[25] Significant multisystem disease is a contraindication, although multiorgan transplants have occasionally been performed. Absolute contraindications include renal dysfunction, malignancy (bronchoalveolar carcinoma is a contraindication but not nonmelanoma skin cancer), infection with HIV, hepatitis B antigen positivity or hepatitis C infection with biopsy-proven liver disease, infection with pan-resistant respiratory flora, active or recent cigarette

TABLE 61-4: Recipient Contraindications to Lung Transplantation

Age ≥ 65 years

Significant systemic or multisystem disease (eg, peripheral or cerebrovascular disease, portal hypertension, poorly controlled diabetes mellitus)

Significant irreversible hepatic or renal dysfunction (eg, bilirubin > 3.0 mg/dL, creatinine clearance < 50 mg/mL/min)

Active malignancy

Corticosteroid therapy (>10 mg/day)

Pan-resistant respiratory flora

Cachexia or obesity (<70% or >130% ideal body weight)

Current cigarette smoking

Psychiatric illness or history of medical noncompliance

Drug or alcohol abuse

Previous cardiothoracic surgery (considered on a case-by-case basis)

Severe osteoporosis

Prolonged mechanical ventilation

HIV

HBsAg positivity or hepatitis C infection with biopsy proven liver disease smoking, drug abuse, alcohol abuse, severe psychiatric illness, noncompliance with medical care, extreme obesity, progressive unintentional weight loss, malnutrition, and absence of a consistent and reliable social support network.[29] Relative contraindications include active extrapulmonary infection, symptomatic osteoporosis, and recent history of active peptic ulcer disease. Cigarette smokers must quit smoking and remain abstinent for several months before transplantation. Patients with histories of previous thoracic surgery are evaluated on a case-by-case basis. For patients who require systemic corticosteroids, tapering to the lowest tolerable level, preferably below 10 mg/day, is critical to prevent airway healing complications. Finally, mechanical ventilation is generally considered a contraindication to transplantation; repeated studies have shown that these patients have significantly worse immediate and long-term survival after transplantation.[39] It is important that recipient candidates be educated about lifestyle modifications necessary for the success of a transplant, and willingness to comply with immunosuppression regimens and extensive posttransplant medical and surgical follow-up is mandatory.

Recipient Management After Listing

It is essential that a candidate's medical condition be optimized before transplantation. Supplemental oxygen is recommended for any patient exhibiting arterial hypoxemia, defined as either an arterial oxygen saturation less than 90% or an arterial PO_2 less than 60 mm Hg at rest, during exertion, or while asleep. Fluid balance is optimized with restriction of dietary water and salt in conjunction with diuretic therapy. Care must be taken with the use of loop diuretics, as these can incite a metabolic alkalosis that can impair the effectiveness of plasma carbon dioxide as a stimulus for breathing.

Primary pulmonary hypertension often requires the use of supplemental oxygen to prevent hypoxia-induced pulmonary vasoconstriction and secondary erythropoiesis. Pulmonary vasodilator therapy with the use of calcium channel blockers and continuous prostacyclin infusions presents another therapeutic option in the management of these patients.[40] Although these drugs exhibit potent systemic effects and must be used with caution, the response rate for calcium channel blockers is approximately 20%. Although a favorable response to short-acting vasodilators during cardiac catheterization is predictive of a successful response to calcium channel therapy, this trend is not seen in long-term prostacyclin infusion.

Interstitial lung disease in patients awaiting transplantation results from a wide variety of diffuse inflammatory processes such as sarcoidosis, asbestosis, and collagen-vascular diseases. Increases in pulmonary vascular resistance leading to right-sided heart failure are thought to arise from interstitial inflammatory infiltrates that entrap and eventually destroy septal arterioles, thus reducing the distensibility of the remaining pulmonary vessels.[41] This process, coupled with closure of peripheral bronchioles, results in arterial hypoxemia, further

aggravating pulmonary hypertension. Corticosteroids are the mainstay of treatment in this class of diseases. The adverse effects of steroids on airway healing are well established,[6,42] and mandate significant dose reductions in anticipation of transplantation.

The multisystem manifestations of CF, particularly chronic bronchopulmonary infection, malabsorption, malnutrition, and diabetes mellitus, pose difficult management problems in potential transplant recipients. These patients require aggressive chest physiotherapy, antibiotics, enteral or parenteral nutritional supplementation, and tight serum glucose control.[43]

Organ Procurement and Preservation

DONOR SELECTION

Standard criteria have been established for donor selection (Table 61-5).[44,45] Donors must have sustained irreversible brain death, but owing to the susceptibility of the lungs to edema and infection in the setting of brain death and trauma, suitable organs are often difficult to obtain (available in <20% of all organ donors).

Initial donor evaluation consists of a directed history and physical examination, chest x-ray, 12-lead ECG, arterial blood gases, and serologic screening including human immunodeficiency virus (HIV), hepatitis B surface antigen, hepatitis C antibodies, herpes simplex virus, cytomegalovirus (CMV), *Toxoplasma*, and RPR. A donor age of less than 50 years is preferred. The chest x-ray should be clear and the arterial PO_2 should exceed 140 mm Hg on an FIO_2 of 40% and 300 mm Hg on an FIO_2 of 100%. Lung compliance can be estimated by measuring peak inspiratory pressures, which should be less than 30 cm H_2O. Bronchoscopy should ensure the absence of purulent secretions or signs of aspiration. Finally, direct inspection and palpation of the lungs at explantation to verify full expansion of any atelectatic segments is an essential part of the donor organ evaluation.

Absolute contraindications to donation include prolonged cardiac arrest (30 minutes), arterial hypoxemia, active

 TABLE 61-5: Donor Selection Criteria

Age < 40 (heart-lung), <50 (lung)

Smoking history less than 20 pack-years

Arterial PO_2 of 140 mm Hg on an FIO_2 of 40% or 300 mm Hg on an FIO_2 of 100%

Normal chest x-ray

Sputum free of bacteria, fungus, or significant numbers of white blood cells on Gram and fungal staining

Bronchoscopy showing absence of purulent secretions or signs of aspiration

Absence of thoracic trauma

HIV-negative

malignancy (excluding basal cell and squamous cell carcinoma of the skin), and positive HIV status. Relative contraindications include thoracic trauma, sepsis, significant smoking history, prolonged severe hypotension (ie, <60 mm Hg for >6 hours), HBsAg or hepatitis C antibodies, multiple resuscitation attempts, and a prolonged high inotropic requirement (eg, dopamine in excess of 15 μg/kg/min for 24 hours). It is important to rule out correctable metabolic or physiologic causes of cardiac rhythm disturbances and electrocardiographic anomalies (eg, brain herniation, hypothermia, hypokalemia).

Over the last decade, there has been a trend toward liberalization of standard donor selection criteria. This strategy, initiated in response to the shortage of donor organs, is employed at a large number of transplant centers.[46-50] Donors ranging in age from 50 to 64 years have been used in thoracic transplantation with good long-term graft survival.[47] However, reports from the ISHLT document worse outcomes in recipients of lung allografts from donors older than 55 years who had ischemic times greater than 6 to 8 hours.[51] In this group of recipients, long-term survival is impaired and the risk of developing bronchiolitis obliterans is increased. Smoking history is another criterion that has been liberalized, with conventional guidelines limiting donor selection to patients with less than 20 pack-years. Modified criteria allow for a more extensive smoking history, assuming there is no evidence of COPD or other lung disease on screening tests.

Traditionally, donor lungs have been ruled out for transplantation based on evidence of infection. In that regard, prolonged ventilation before brain death and procurement has been viewed as a contraindication for organ selection. However, a positive sputum Gram stain (excluding fungus), which was once considered a basis for ruling out an organ has failed to predict the development of early pneumonia, impairment of oxygenation, or duration of mechanical ventilation in the postoperative setting.[52,53] Some groups have accepted donors with small pulmonary infiltrates on chest x-ray, although clinical correlation is necessary. Others have selectively used donor lungs in patients with PaO_2 less than 300 mm Hg on FIO_2 of 100%. Gabbay and coworkers in Australia have adopted an aggressive approach to donor management and "organ resuscitation."[48] By manipulating donors with antibiotic therapy, chest physiotherapy, careful fluid management, ventilator adjustments, and bronchial toilet, 34% of donors with an initial PaO_2 less than 300 mm Hg on FIO_2 of 100% had increases in their PaO_2, becoming acceptable donors.

Two exciting and rapidly evolving areas in the field of donor organ procurement include the use of allografts obtained from donors after cardiac death (DCD) and rehabilitation of rejected organs using ex vivo lung perfusion (EVLP).

In 2001, Steen and colleagues reported the first clinical lung transplant from a DCD donor (also known as a non-heart-beating donor). After a 54-year-old man expired from an acute myocardial infarction with failed resuscitation, his next-of-kin consented to lung donation based on the patient's prior wishes. The organ was removed and assessed ex vivo before being transplanted into a 54-year-old woman with COPD.[54] The authors reported good functional results during the first 5 months of follow-up. This landmark report not only introduced an era of DCD lung transplantation, but also the clinical application of EVLP.

Unlike an allograft obtained from a donor after brain death (DBD), lungs from a non-heart-beating donor are exposed to a prolonged period of warm-ischemic time, in which varying degrees of hypotension and shock precede organ cooling and harvest and have unknown consequence on donor organ function. EVLP began as a tool to assess the functional status of DCD lungs and ultimately evolved into a mechanism to both assess and rehabilitate the donor allografts. In 2007, Steen and colleagues reported the first use of EVLP to not only evaluate a previously rejected donor lung, but to actually rehabilitate the discarded organ until, by all conventional measures, it was deemed suitable for transplantation.[55] Again, their experiment resulted in a landmark report demonstrating good functional outcomes after EVLP was utilized to rehabilitate and transplant a rejected donor organ.

By employment of a hyperoncotic perfusate, with carefully selected components to suit the metabolic needs of the lung, Steen's group demonstrated the ability to reduce interstitial edema, improve pulmonary vascular resistance, and increase gas exchange until the donor organ met the criteria for transplantation. Others around the world, most notably Keshavjee's group in Toronto, Canada, have contributed to the immense progress in advancing the techniques for EVLP.[56,57] Multiple reports have demonstrated excellent clinical outcomes.[57-59]

With as many as 40% of the total rejected donor lungs having only minimal microbiologic, physiologic, or histologic deficiencies, there is an incredible potential for organ rescue and significant increase in the donor pool.[60] Ongoing research and long-term outcomes data are highly anticipated, yet the impact of this technology is already clinically apparent and is rapidly spreading throughout the world.

DONOR MANAGEMENT

The overriding goal in managing the thoracic organ donor is to maintain hemodynamic stability and pulmonary function. Patients suffering from acute brain injury are often hemodynamically unstable because of neurogenic shock, excessive fluid losses, and bradycardia. Donor lungs are prone to neurogenic pulmonary edema, aspiration, nosocomial infection, and contusion. Continuous arterial and central venous pressure monitoring, judicious fluid resuscitation, vasopressors, and inotropes are usually required.

Intravascular volume replacement should be limited to maintain the central venous pressure between 5 and 8 mm Hg. In general, crystalloid fluid boluses are to be avoided.

Diabetes insipidus is common in donors and requires the use of intravenous vasopressin (0.8 to 1.0 unit/h) to prevent excessive urine loss. Dopamine is the standard inotropic agent used to maintain adequate perfusion pressures, although alpha agonists (eg, phenylephrine) are often appropriate. Blood transfusions should be used sparingly to maintain a hemoglobin concentration of approximately 10 g/dL, ensuring adequate myocardial oxygen delivery. CMV-negative and leukocyte-filtered blood should be used whenever possible. Hypothermia should be avoided as it predisposes to ventricular arrhythmias and metabolic acidosis.

With regard to mechanical ventilation, F_{IO_2} values in excess of 40%, especially 100% oxygen "challenges," should be avoided, because these oxygen levels may be toxic to the denervated lung. Ventilator settings should include positive end-expiratory pressures (PEEP) between 3 and 5 cm H_2O to prevent atelectasis.

DONOR OPERATION

The donor operation is performed via a median sternotomy (Fig. 61-6A). After the sternum is divided, a standard chest retractor is placed, and both pleural spaces are opened followed by immediate inspection of the lungs and pleural spaces, particularly in cases involving trauma. The lungs are briefly deflated, and the pulmonary ligaments are divided inferiorly using electrocautery. After completely excising the thymic remnant, the pericardium is opened vertically and laterally on the diaphragm and cradled during dissection of the great vessels and trachea. The ascending aorta, pulmonary artery, and venae cavae are dissected. Umbilical tapes are placed around the ascending aorta and venae cavae (Fig. 61-6B). The pericardium overlying the trachea is incised vertically, and the trachea is encircled with an umbilical tape between the aorta and superior vena cava at the highest point possible and at least four rings above the carina (see Fig. 61-6B). The entire anterior pericardium is excised back to each hilum (Fig. 61-6C).

Approximately 15 minutes before applying the aortic cross-clamp, prostaglandin E_1 (PGE_1) is infused intravenously, initially at a rate of 20 ng/kg/min, followed by incremental increases of 10 ng/kg/min to a target rate of 100 ng/kg/min (Fig. 61-6D). During PGE_1 infusion, the mean arterial blood pressure should be maintained at or above 55 mm Hg. Ventilation is continued with a F_{IO_2} of 40% and a PEEP of 3 to 5 cm H_2O. The donor is heparinized with 30,000 units. Cannulation of the aorta and main pulmonary artery is performed, with care taken to ensure adequate flow to both branches of the pulmonary artery during pulmonary plegia.[61] The superior vena cava is ligated and a transverse incision is made across the inferior vena cava. After the heart is allowed to empty, the aortic cross-clamp is applied, and 10 mL/kg of cold crystalloid cardioplegia, commonly the Stanford formulation, is rapidly infused into the aortic root with the bag under pressure at 150 mm Hg. The inferior vena cava is incised, and the

left atrial appendage is amputated to avoid cardiac distention. Although the antegrade cardioplegia is being delivered, Perfadex (Vitrolife Inc., Englewood, CO) is rapidly flushed into the main pulmonary artery at a rate of 15 mL/kg/min for 4 minutes. Ice-cold saline or Physiosol solution (Abbott Laboratories, North Chicago, IL) is immediately poured over the heart and lungs. During the cardioplegic and Perfadex infusions, ventilation is maintained with half-normal tidal volumes of room air.

After delivery of plegic solutions, the lungs are deflated and the great vessels are divided. The heart is reflected anteriorly and a left atriotomy is performed, leaving a 2-cm cuff of atrium around the pulmonary vein orifices. Once this division is complete, the heart is removed from the chest. The lung bloc is then dissected free along the preesophageal plane above the level of the carina. The lungs are inflated and the trachea is stapled at the highest possible point. If needed, the bilateral lung bloc can be further separated into left and right lung blocs. The left atrial cuff containing the orifices of the pulmonary veins is divided in half vertically. The left and right pulmonary arteries are divided at their junction. Finally, the left mainstem bronchus is stapled near its junction with the trachea.

Once removed from the donor, grafts are wrapped in sterile gauze pads and immersed in ice-cold saline at 2 to 4°C in several sterile plastic bags placed within a sterile plastic container. This, in turn, is placed in an ice-filled chest and transported to the transplant center.

ORGAN PRESERVATION AND TRANSPORT

The principal goal of preservation is to minimize injury to the allograft from ischemia and reperfusion.[62] Ischemia-reperfusion injury is mediated by reactive oxygen species, which disrupt the homeostatic mechanisms in myocytes and endothelial cells. As receptors for leukocyte adhesion molecules are upregulated and leukocyte chemotactic factors released, an inflammatory response ensues, leading to cellular injury. Several approaches for minimizing ischemia-reperfusion injury have developed, including donor pretreatment, use of specialized preservation solutions, and recipient treatments.

Hypothermia is considered by many to be the most important method of organ preservation. It works by reducing tissue metabolic demand by up to 99%. During explantation, organs are flushed with cold plegic solutions (0 to 10°C, depending on the institution and solution employed). Organs are stored at 0 to 10°C, and during implantation they are covered with gauze soaked in saline slush or recipients are cooled through CPB.

A variety of crystalloid pulmonary artery flush solutions are used worldwide, and they can be divided into two categories based on their electrolyte compositions: intracellular and extracellular. Intracellular solutions contain moderate-to-high concentrations of potassium and little calcium and sodium. Euro-Collins, University of Wisconsin (UW), and Cardiazol are examples. Extracellular

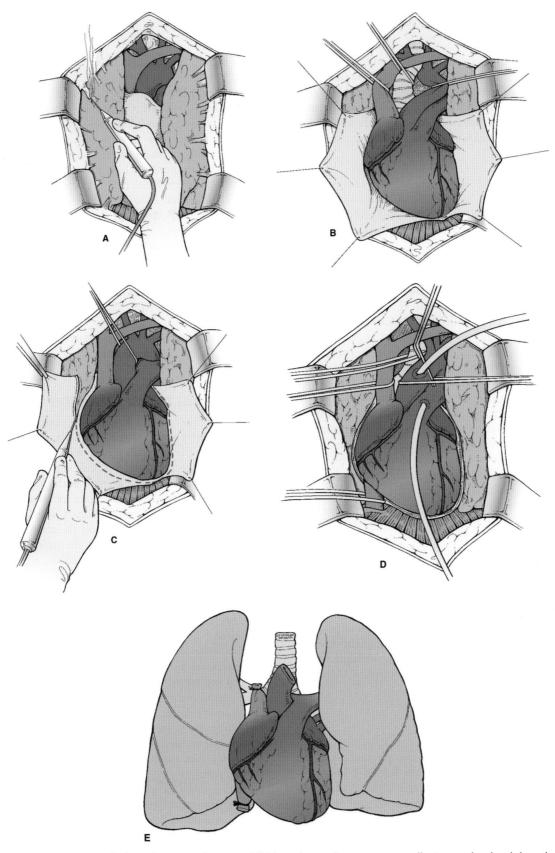

FIGURE 61-6 Donor operation for heart-lung transplantation. (A) Through a median sternotomy, adhesions are lysed and the pulmonary ligaments are divided inferiorly. (B) The pericardium is opened and cradled followed by dissection of the ascending aorta, venae cavae, pulmonary artery, and trachea. (C) The entire anterior pericardium is excised back to each hilum. (D) Cardioplegia and pulmonoplegia are infused simultaneously into the aorta and main pulmonary artery after aortic cross-clamping. Application of topical cold Physiosol follows immediately. (E) The venae cavae and aorta are divided, and the heart-lung bloc is dissected free from the esophagus and posterior hilar attachments. After the trachea is stapled and divided at the highest point possible, the entire heart-lung bloc is removed from the chest.

solutions contain high concentrations of sodium and low-to-moderate concentrations of potassium. Low-potassium dextran is an example of this type of solution (eg, Perfadex). Although Euro-Collins is the most frequently used preservation solution, there is a growing body of evidence in support of low potassium, dextran-containing extracellular solutions.[63-65]

Prostaglandins are commonly used for donor pretreatment and as an additive in pulmonary flush solutions. The administration of PGE_1 (a potent vasodilator) counteracts reflex pulmonary vasoconstriction induced by the cold flush and permits uniform distribution of perfusate throughout the lung. Studies in large animals also suggest that PGE_1 treatment may minimize reperfusion injury through its antiinflammatory properties.[66] Another commonly used pretreatment strategy is steroid treatment. Administration of intravenous methylprednisone to the donor inactivates lymphocytes, which are thought to mediate ischemic lung graft injury.

Studies suggest that lung graft function is improved when the explanted organ is inflated, 100% oxygen is used for the inflation, and transport is carried out at 10°C.[67] Research in the field of lung preservation has recently focused on the role of various flush and storage solution additives, such as antioxidants, which may act as free radical scavengers. Other additives shown to decrease reperfusion injury in research models include nitric oxide donors and phosphodiesterase inhibitors. Areas of ongoing research include the development of leukocyte depletion strategies, examining the role of gene therapy to modify donor organ susceptibility to ischemia-reperfusion injury, and the development of colloid-based perfusates.

These preservation techniques, coupled with streamlined donor and recipient protocols, have permitted procurements as far as 1000 miles from the transplant center. Extensive communication and coordination must be maintained between the organ procurement agency, donor-recipient operative teams, medical centers, and abdominal procurement teams. Worldwide, the major procurement agencies include the UNOS in the United States, Multiple Organ Retrieval in Canada, and the EURO Transplant Organization in Europe.

Recipient Operation

The recipient operation proceeds in two phases. The first is excision of the native organ(s) and the second is implantation of the allograft. Cardiopulmonary bypass is occasionally required for lung transplantation. Regardless, CPB should be available as standby at all times. In our practice, we have favored the use of CPB during bilateral lung transplantation for a variety of reasons. There is improved exposure of the hilar structures, which is particularly helpful in patients with dense adhesions and bronchial collaterals. CPB allows for early pneumonectomies without hemodynamic or respiratory instability, and ischemic time

of the second lung is substantially reduced compared with off-CPB bilateral lung transplants. Its use also prevents overperfusion of the first lung graft with the entire cardiac output. In patients with suppurative lung disease, the use of CPB facilitates careful washout of the distal trachea and proximal bronchi to prevent contamination of the first implanted lung. Others prefer to avoid CPB, as it may be associated with increased blood loss, transfusion needs, and reperfusion injury. More detailed experimental and clinical studies are needed to resolve these questions. At present, the need for CBP should be determined on a case-by-case basis.

Anesthetic monitoring includes arterial pressure monitoring, pulse oximetry, continuous electrocardiography, pulmonary artery catheter monitoring, temperature monitoring, and urine output monitoring. The use of double-lumen endotracheal tubes is particularly helpful, allowing for single-lung ventilation during certain portions of the dissection. Large-bore intravenous lines are placed for volume infusion. Transesophageal echocardiography is often performed during the procedure.

SINGLE LUNG TRANSPLANTATION

If possible, the poorer functioning lung (as determined by preoperative ventilation-perfusion scan) is selected for replacement. The patient is placed in a standard thoracotomy position with access to the groin, should CPB be needed. A posterolateral thoracotomy is made at the level of the fourth or fifth intercostal space. Adhesions are lysed and the hilar dissection performed. The pulmonary artery, the superior and inferior pulmonary veins, and the mainstem bronchus are isolated. A trial occlusion of the pulmonary artery is used to determine whether the procedure can be conducted without CPB. If the occlusion is tolerated, the pulmonary artery is ligated and divided distal to the upper lobe branch. The pulmonary veins are also ligated and divided. The mainstem bronchus is stapled and divided, and the native lung is explanted.

The donor lung is removed from its transport container and prepared for implantation. The donor bronchus is opened and secretions are aspirated and cultured. The bronchus is trimmed, leaving two cartilaginous rings proximal to the orifice of the upper lobe. Any remaining pericardial and lymphatic tissue is removed, and the left atrial cuff is trimmed as needed. The donor lung is then placed in the recipient's chest and covered with saline slush and iced laparotomy pads.

The sequence of anastomoses is a matter of preference, although most perform the deepest anastomosis (the bronchial anastomosis) first and then proceed to the more superficial ones. The bronchial anastomosis is fashioned with 4-0 polypropylene suture. We favor a continuous suture technique for the entire anastomosis, although the membranous portion can be sewn with interrupted suture. Variations on the end-to-end bronchial anastomosis include the use of a telescoping technique, in which the donor bronchus is intussuscepted into the recipient bronchus, and an omental pedicle flap is placed around the anastomosis. These techniques were developed to prevent bronchial anastomotic dehiscence but are now rarely performed.

Once the bronchial anastomosis is complete, attention is turned to the anastomoses of the pulmonary veins. A side-biting clamp is applied to the left atrium to include the pulmonary veins. The recipient pulmonary vein stumps are opened and the intervening atrial tissue is cut. This creates a cuff that is anastomosed to the donor atrial remnant using continuous 4-0 polypropylene suture. (This suture is not tied down until reperfusion.) Donor and recipient pulmonary arteries are anastomosed with 5-0 polypropylene suture. Arteries must be trimmed to an appropriate length before fashioning the anastomosis, because kinking can occur upon graft inflation if the vessels are left too long. The pulmonary artery anastomosis is then de-aired. The lung is inflated, and the pulmonary artery clamp is temporarily released to allow flushing of air through the atrial suture line. The left atrial clamp is removed to allow retrograde de-airing of the atrial anastomosis. The pulmonary venous anastomosis is then secured.

After hemostasis is ensured, apical and basal chest tubes are inserted. The ribs are reapproximated and the chest is closed in standard fashion. The double lumen endotracheal tube is exchanged for a single-lumen tube and bronchoscopy is performed to evaluate the bronchial anastomosis.

BILATERAL LUNG TRANSPLANTATION

Bilateral lung transplantation is performed as sequential single-lung transplants. Although the traditional approach to this technique has been to access the chest via bilateral anterior thoracosternotomy (clamshell) incisions, we have recently transitioned our practice to a median sternotomy approach. The lung with the least amount of function (as determined by a preoperative ventilation-perfusion scan) is removed first and replaced with an allograft as described for SLT above. Once ventilation and perfusion are established in the first allograft, the remaining lung is explanted and the second allograft is implanted. Bilateral chest tubes are placed and the chest is closed. Bronchoscopy is performed to evaluate the bronchial anastomoses.

Although single-lung transplants are usually performed off CBP, the majority of double-lung transplants are still performed on-pump. The use of CPB allows for improved exposure, shorter graft ischemic times, controlled reperfusion, and the use of leukocyte-depleting filters. As the risk of bleeding may be increased with CPB, strategies have been developed to minimize the chance of hemorrhage. These include the use of heparin-coated CPB circuits as well as the argon beam coagulator. Despite these maneuvers, there remains considerable risk associated with CPB, and many centers prefer to perform all lung transplants off-pump if possible.

Postoperative Management

GRAFT PHYSIOLOGY

Denervation of the lungs results in a diminished cough reflex and impairment of mucociliary clearance mechanisms. This predisposes recipients to pulmonary infections and necessitates aggressive postoperative pulmonary toilet.[68] Moreover, in the transplanted lung, ischemia-reperfusion injury, along with disrupted pulmonary lymphatics, may result in increased vascular permeability with varying degrees of interstitial edema.

CLINICAL MANAGEMENT IN THE EARLY POSTOPERATIVE PERIOD

Early postoperative management centers around careful fluid balance and ventilatory management. The primary objective in the immediate postoperative period is to maintain adequate perfusion and gas exchange while minimizing intravenous fluid administration, cardiac work, and barotrauma. Barotrauma and high airway pressures can compromise bronchial mucosal flow. Therefore, lower tidal volumes and flow rates may be necessary to limit peak airway pressures to less than 40 cm H_2O. After arrival in the ICU, ventilator settings are adjusted every 30 minutes to achieve an arterial PO_2 greater than 75 mm Hg on an FIO_2 of 40%, an arterial carbon dioxide pressure ($PaCO_2$) between 30 and 40 mm Hg, and a pH between 7.35 and 7.45. Pulmonary toilet with endotracheal suctioning is an effective means of reducing mucus plugging and atelectasis. Ventilatory weaning is initiated after the patient is stable, awake, and alert, with extubation typically achieved within 24 hours. Subsequent pulmonary care consists of vigorous diuresis, supplemental oxygen for several days, continued aggressive pulmonary toilet, incentive spirometry, and serial chest x-rays.

A diffuse interstitial infiltrate is often found on early postoperative chest x-rays. Previously referred to as a *reimplantation response*, this finding is better defined as graft edema owing to inadequate preservation, reperfusion injury, or early rejection.[69] It appears that the degree of pulmonary edema is inversely related to the quality of preservation. Judicious administration of fluid and loop diuretics is required to maintain fluid balance and minimize this pulmonary edema.

Early lung graft dysfunction occurs in less than 15% of transplants, and is manifest as persistent marginal gas exchange without evidence of infection or rejection.[70] This primary graft failure often results from ischemia-reperfusion injury and histologically evident as diffuse alveolar damage. Of course, technical causes of graft failure such as pulmonary venous anastomotic stenosis or thrombosis must always be considered. In cases of persistent, severe pulmonary graft dysfunction refractory to mechanical ventilatory maneuvers, ECMO[71] and inhaled nitric oxide[72] have been used successfully to stabilize gas exchange. Urgent retransplantation can also be considered if other interventions fail.

IMMUNOSUPPRESSIVE MANAGEMENT: EARLY AND LATE POSTOPERATIVE REGIMENS

Immunosuppression protocols vary from center to center. In our practice, we typically administer induction therapy of either rabbit antithymocyte globulin (RATG) at a dose of 1.5 mg/kg on POD 1, 2, 3, 5, and 7 or daclizumab at 1 mg/kg (first dose given in OR then every other week for four additional doses). For highly sensitized patients, plasmapheresis with a 1:1.5 volume exchange with fresh-frozen plasma (FFP) is performed intraoperatively, along with intravenous immunoglobulin (IVIG), which is started at 2 g/kg before releasing the cross-clamp. Methylprednisolone is given at 500 mg IV after protamine administration, and a stat retrospective crossmatch is performed.

On POD 1, T- and B-cell subset counts are performed and if the cytotoxic crossmatch is positive, RATG is given in 2 doses at 0.75 mg/kg. If the crossmatch is negative or pulmonary edema is present or expected from RATG, daclizumab is administered at 1 mg/kg and repeated every 14 days for a total of five doses. Methylprednisolone is given at 125 mg IV every 8 hours for three doses, CellCept is given at 500 mg PO BID, and Prograf is given at 0.5 mg BID and titrated to a level of 12 to 15 ng/mL. On POD 2, prednisone is started at 0.5 mg/kg PO BID. Hereafter, the patient is maintained on prednisone, Prograf, and CellCept. For sensitized patients, plasmapheresis is repeated in a 1:1.5 volume exchange with 1/2 5% albumin and 1/2 FFP. If the patient was given RATG, a second dose of 0.75 mg/kg is administered. Otherwise, IVIG 100 mg/kg is given. Plasmapheresis is repeated on POD 3 and 4, along with IVIG at 100 mg/kg. Plasmapheresis is completed on POD 5, with administration of IVIG at 1 g/kg on POD 5 and 6. A donor-specific antibody is sent before IVIG on POD 5 and after IVIG on POD 6. Finally, on POD 7 T- and B-cell subset counts are measured (and repeated weekly thereafter) along with administration of Rituximab for two doses with one dose of 375 mg/m^2 given at POD 7 and a second dose given a week later.

INFECTION PROPHYLAXIS

Antiviral and antifungal prophylaxis remain important components of the postoperative management strategy in heart-lung and lung transplant recipients. Many centers employ CMV prophylaxis with ganciclovir for any CMV-positive recipient and in any CMV-negative recipient receiving an allograft from a CMV-positive donor. Ganciclovir is typically given for a several week course, and can be associated with leukopenia. Some patients may require G-CSF if their white blood cell count falls below 4000. Fungal prophylaxis against mucosal candida infection includes use of itraconazole and nystatin swish and swallow. *Pneumocystis carinii* prophylaxis consists of trimethoprim-sulfamethoxazole or aerosolized pentamidine. In the immediate postoperative period, *Aspergillus* colonization is inhibited by the use of aerosolized amphotericin B. For *Toxoplasma*-negative recipients of grafts from *Toxoplasma*-positive patients, pyrimethamine prophylaxis is maintained for the first 6 months after transplantation.

GRAFT SURVEILLANCE: PATIENT FOLLOW-UP SCHEDULE

Routine clinical follow-up is required to monitor graft function and modify immunosuppressive regimens. Regular surveillance protocols developed to monitor graft function typically consist of serial pulmonary function tests, arterial blood gases, and bronchoscopic evaluation. Surveillance is usually conducted at 2, 4 to 6, and 12 weeks, followed by 6 months after transplantation and yearly thereafter. Transbronchial biopsies are obtained from each transplanted lung, and lavage specimens are submitted for staining (ie, Gram, fungal, acid-fast bacillus, silver), culture, and cytology. In addition to routine surveillance, follow-up is often needed to address changes in clinical status. Complications related to transplantation are many, and these must be addressed carefully and expediently to prevent long-term graft failure.

Postoperative Complications

Early morbidity and mortality after lung transplantation (within 30 days of operation or before initial discharge from hospital) are most commonly a result of primary graft failure or infection. Late mortality is most commonly caused by OB or infection.[73] Causes of death at various time points after transplantation have been compiled by the ISHLT and are presented in Fig. 61-7.

HEMORRHAGE

Perioperative hemorrhage is an infrequent but significant cause of early death in heart-lung and lung transplantation. The majority of perioperative hemorrhagic complications stem from operating in the midst of dense adhesions caused by previous operations or inflammation from chronic lung infection. As mentioned previously, meticulous attention to hemostasis is mandatory, and all available means should be used to achieve a dry field on completion of the operation.

HYPERACUTE REJECTION

ABO matching of donor and recipient has decreased the rate of hyperacute rejection. This complication, which is almost universally fatal, is mediated by preformed antibodies in the recipient that recognize antigens on the donor vascular endothelium. This humoral immune response results in activation of inflammatory and coagulation cascades, resulting in extensive thrombosis of graft vessels and subsequent graft failure.[74] To reduce the incidence of hyperacute rejection, a prospective crossmatch should be performed in recipients with a PRA greater than 25%.

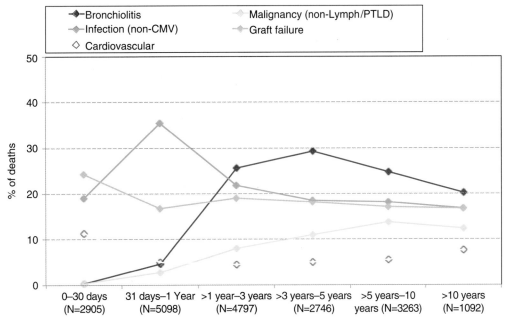

FIGURE 61-7 Causes of death at various periods after isolated lung transplantation. Infection is the major cause of death in the first year after transplant, while bronchiolitis obliterans syndrome is the major cause of death after the early post-transplant period. (Data from Yusen RD, Edwards LB, Kucheryavaya AY, et al: The registry of the International Society for Heart and Lung Transplantation: thirty-first adult lung and heart-lung transplant report—2014; focus theme: retransplantation, *J Heart Lung Transplant.* 2014 Oct;33(10):1009-1024.)

EARLY GRAFT DYSFUNCTION AND PRIMARY GRAFT FAILURE

Graft dysfunction in the first few days after transplantation is common. It is often referred to as the "reimplantation response," manifest by abnormal lung function, pulmonary edema, and pulmonary infiltrates on chest x-ray. This phenomenon is thought to be linked to ischemia and reperfusion. Other contributing factors may also include allograft contusion, inadequate preservation, or use of cardiopulmonary bypass during transplantation. Although most cases are mild and resolve with supportive care, some progress to primary graft failure. Reported rates of primary graft failure following lung transplantation range between 10 and 15%. Treatment may include the use of ECMO and inhaled nitric oxide. Unfortunately, primary graft failure is associated with a mortality of more than 60%.[70]

ACUTE REJECTION

As in cardiac transplantation, the majority of acute rejection episodes occur within the first year after transplant at a rate of 36%.[25] Despite its prevalence, death is very rarely a direct consequence of acute rejection. It is recognized, however, that the number and severity of acute rejection episodes is a risk factor for ultimately developing obliterative bronchitis (OB).

Diagnosis of acute rejection in the early posttransplant period is often based on clinical parameters. Symptoms and signs of rejection include fever, dyspnea, impaired gas exchange (manifest as a decrease in arterial Po_2), a diminished forced expiratory volume during 1 second (FEV_1, a measure

of airway flow), a fall in vital capacity (VC), and the development of characteristic bilateral interstitial infiltrates on chest x-ray (Fig. 61-8). After the first postoperative month, the chest x-ray is frequently normal during episodes of acute rejection, placing greater emphasis on other clinical parameters characteristic of rejection.

It is often difficult to distinguish between the diagnosis of acute lung rejection and pulmonary infection based on clinical findings alone. It is of paramount importance to distinguish between acute rejection and infection before initiating therapy. Fiberoptic bronchoscopy (with transbronchial parenchymal lung biopsy and bronchoalveolar lavage) is the gold standard for the diagnosis of acute lung rejection and pulmonary infection. At least five biopsy specimens are taken from the lung allografts along with bronchoalveolar lavage, which is evaluated for cytology, undergoes microbial staining, and is cultured.[75] In addition to performing bronchoscopy with transbronchial biopsy in response to changes in clinical status and graft performance, most centers maintain a schedule of surveillance biopsies for lung recipients. Interestingly, surveillance bronchoscopy reveals occult rejection or infection in 17 to 25% of transbronchial biopsy specimens from asymptomatic recipients. For patients undergoing bronchoscopy because of a change in clinical condition, 50 to 72% of biopsy specimens have shown evidence of rejection or infection. In most cases, positive biopsies directly guide successful treatment of rejection or infection.[76,77] Acute lung rejection is histologically characterized by lymphocytic perivascular infiltrates (Fig. 61-9). A grading scheme for acute lung rejection was developed by Clelland and Colin[78] and is presented in

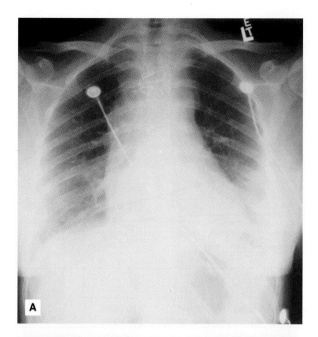

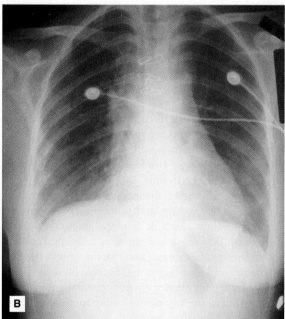

FIGURE 61-8 Acute and resolving lung rejection. (A) Chest radiograph illustrates bilateral infiltrates characteristic of acute pulmonary rejection. (B) Follow-up radiograph after pulsed methylprednisolone treatment of acute rejection demonstrating resolution of infiltrates.

Table 61-6; a similar scheme was also developed by the Lung Rejection Study Group.[75]

As in cardiac transplantation, efforts are being made to develop noninvasive ways of diagnosing early acute lung rejection. Loubeyre and coworkers at the Hôpital Cardiovasculaire et Pneumologique report an association between "ground-glass" density areas seen on high-resolution computed tomography (HRCT) and histologically confirmed

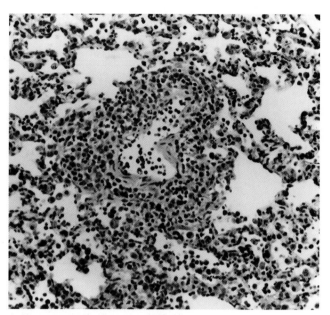

FIGURE 61-9 Moderate acute lung rejection. Moderate rejection is characterized by perivascular mononuclear cell infiltrates with extension into the adjacent alveolar septa (H&E stain; ×200).

acute lung rejection in heart-lung transplant recipients.[79] They found that ground-glass opacities on HRCT had a sensitivity of 65% for detecting lung rejection and a specificity of 85% for detecting an acute lung complication.

Treatment strategies for rejection involve augmentation of immunosuppression. At most institutions, the timing and severity of rejection episodes dictate therapy. A typical algorithm is shown in Fig. 61-10. Rejection episodes that are graded moderate or severe are treated with a "steroid pulse" (intravenous methylprednisolone 500 to 1000 mg/day for three consecutive days), followed by augmentation of the oral prednisone maintenance dose to 0.6 mg/kg/day. This maintenance dose is then tapered to 0.2 mg/kg/day over 3 to 4 weeks. Clinical and radiographic improvement

TABLE 61-6: Grading System for Acute Lung Rejection

Grade	Histologic Appearance (Transbronchial Biopsy)
0	No significant inflammation; normal specimen
1	Small, infrequent perivascular infiltrates with or without bronchiolar lymphocytic infiltrates
2	Larger, more frequent perivascular lymphocytic infiltrates with or without moderate bronchiolar lymphocytic inflammation; occasional neutrophils and eosinophils
3	Extension of infiltrates into alveolar septa and alveolar spaces with or without bronchiolar mucosal ulceration

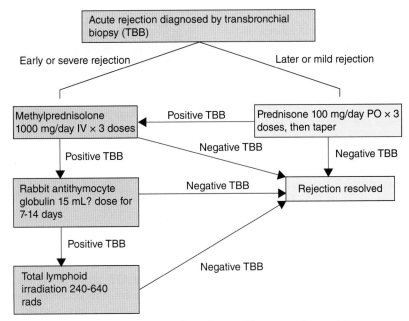

FIGURE 61-10 Typical algorithm for treating acute rejection in heart-lung and lung transplant recipients.

(see Fig. 61-8B) after steroid therapy is often dramatic, rapid, and considered confirmatory of rejection. Mild episodes are initially treated by increasing oral prednisone dose, followed by a gradual taper over 3 to 4 weeks. Transbronchial biopsies are repeated 10 to 14 days following antirejection therapy to assess efficacy. Recurrent rejection episodes may be treated by a second steroid pulse and taper. Acute rejection refractory to steroid therapy may be treated with antilymphocyte preparations. Alternatively, primary immunosuppression may be switched between cyclosporine- and tacrolimus-based therapy. Finally, in especially difficult cases of persistent rejection, total lymphoid irradiation may be useful.[80]

CHRONIC REJECTION

Chronic lung allograft rejection poses the greatest limitation to the long-term benefits of lung transplantation. Chronic lung rejection most commonly presents as OB. The onset of OB typically occurs after the first 6 months to 1 year after transplantation, with a steadily increasing incidence thereafter. Recent data demonstrate that 50% of lung recipients are diagnosed with OB by the fifth postoperative year[81] (Fig 61-11).

Transbronchial biopsies remain the "gold standard" for diagnosing OB. The sensitivity of transbronchial biopsy for

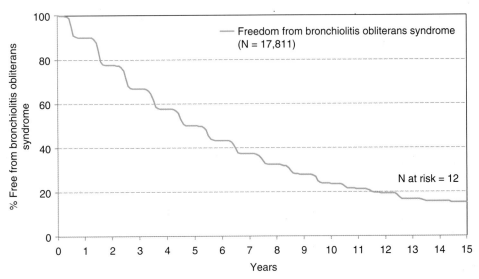

FIGURE 61-11 Adult lung transplant recipient freedom from bronchiolitis obliterans syndrome (BOS), conditional on survival to 14 days (transplant follow-ups: April 1994 to June 2013). The dashed green line shows the 95% confidence intervals. (Data from Yusen RD, Edwards LB, Kucheryavaya AY, et al: The registry of the International Society for Heart and Lung Transplantation: thirty-first adult lung and heart-lung transplant report—2014; focus theme: retransplantation, *J Heart Lung Transplant.* 2014 Oct;33(10):1009-1024.)

detecting OB has been reported between 17 and 87%.[76,82] Diagnostic yield of the biopsy procedure is related to the number of specimens taken, and current recommendations advise taking at least five specimens from each transplanted lung. Clearly, OB is a patchy process and therefore a large number of samples will be falsely negative owing to sampling error.

OB is a histologic diagnosis and is characterized by dense eosinophilic, submucosal scar tissue that partially or totally obliterates the lumen of small (2-mm) airways, particularly the terminal and respiratory bronchioles (Fig. 61-12). The physiologic consequences are decreased arterial Po_2, FEV_1, FEF_{25-75} forced expiratory flow at 25 to 75% (midrange) of lung volumes, and FEF_{50}/FVC (ratio of FEF_{50} to forced vital capacity). A characteristic "bowing" of the expiratory limb of the flow-volume loop has also been associated with OB. Clinical symptoms may be nonspecific, and include cough and dyspnea with or without exertion. The term *bronchiolitis obliterans syndrome* (BOS) was developed to refer to patients who have clinical manifestations of OB with or without proven histologic characteristics (Table 61-7). A standardized working formulation for the clinical staging of BOS was established by the ISHLT and is based on the ratio of the current FEV_1 to the best posttransplant FEV_1. Patients with a decline of 20% or greater in their FEV_1 (in the absence of infection or other process) are diagnosed with BOS, irrespective of pathologic evidence of OB.[74]

Valentine and the Stanford group reported that measurements of small airway function (ie, FEF_{25-75}, FEF_{50}/FVC) are more sensitive indicators of BOS than the FEV_1 in bilateral lung transplant recipients.[83] An FEF_{50}/FVC persistently below 0.7 for 6 consecutive weeks was the most sensitive predictor of OB. Approximately 50% of bilateral lung recipients with biopsy-proven OB developed a fall in their FEF_{50}/FVC

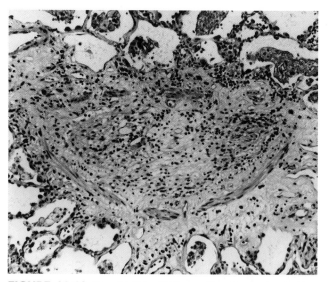

FIGURE 61-12 Bronchiolitis obliterans. Chronic airway rejection is characterized by luminal narrowing or replacement by dense eosinophilic collagenous scar tissue. Inflammatory cells may be seen in this case (H&E stain; ×150).

TABLE 61-7: Working Formulation for Bronchiolitis Obliterans Syndrome

$0_{\text{a or b}}$	No significant abnormality: FEV_1 80% of baseline
$1_{\text{a or b}}$	Mild bronchiolitis obliterans syndrome: FEV_1 66-80% of baseline
$2_{\text{a or b}}$	Moderate bronchiolitis obliterans syndrome: FEV_1 51-65% of baseline
$3_{\text{a or b}}$	Severe bronchiolitis obliterans syndrome: FEV_1 50% of baseline

a = Without pathologic evidence of obliterative bronchiolitis;
b = with pathologic evidence of obliterative bronchiolitis.

nearly 4 months before fulfilling the ISHLT working group criteria for BOS.

Experimental and clinical evidence suggests that the etiology of OB stems from the injury of the bronchial epithelium by one or more mechanisms. These include gastroesophageal reflux disease (GERD), infection (particularly CMV), chronic inflammation owing to impaired mucociliary clearance, and immunologic mechanisms.[69] These insults result in airway epithelial damage and, subsequently, an exaggerated healing response. Along with this injury, there is increased expression of major histocompatibility class II antigens in the bronchial epithelium. In a recent metaanalysis, Sharples and coworkers found that acute rejection is a risk factor for later development of OB.[84] In keeping with this finding is the association between BOS and decreased levels of immunosuppression (as may occur with noncompliance). Lymphocytic bronchitis and bronchiolitis were also closely associated with development of OB. CMV pneumonitis, other pulmonary infections, and HLA mismatching are also linked to the development of OB in small retrospective studies. Novick and coworkers reported on the relationship between OB, donor age, and graft ischemic times.[51] Using data from the ISHLT registry, they found a higher rate of OB at 3 years in recipients of grafts from donors greater than age 55 who were also subjected to 6 to 8 hours of ischemia. GERD has been recently proposed as a mechanism for the development of OB.[85] Up to 75% of patients have demonstrable postoperative reflux based on pH studies, which may result from intraoperative vagal damage, impaired cough and airway mucociliary clearance, immunosuppression, or preexisting GERD.[86] These patients have been shown to demonstrate a survival benefit as well as delayed onset of BOS after antireflux surgery in the postoperative setting.[87,88]

The current management of OB hinges on prevention, close surveillance, and immediate therapeutic intervention when patients become symptomatic or asymptomatic physiologic changes occur. Patients are encouraged to perform incentive spirometry to prevent microatelectasis of lungs that are deprived of native innervation, lack bronchial circulation, and have impaired mucociliary clearance mechanisms. Moreover, all recipients are instructed to contact their transplant center or primary care physician on development of respiratory tract symptoms so that pulmonary function tests can be performed. Any alterations in FEF_{25-75}, FEF_{50}/FVC, or specific changes in the flow-volume loop are indications for bronchoscopy with bronchoalveolar lavage and transbronchial biopsy, especially in the absence of infectious bronchitis or pulmonary edema.

Augmentation of immunosuppression is the mainstay of therapy for BOS. The prednisone dose is increased to 0.6 to 1.0 mg/kg/day and slowly tapered to 0.2 mg/kg/day while concomitantly optimizing cyclosporine and azathioprine dosing. Ganciclovir is reinstituted during treatment for those patients at risk of reactivation CMV infection, and antimicrobial therapy is directed against any organisms isolated from bronchoalveolar lavage. Follow-up pulmonary function tests are performed. Pulmonary function can be stabilized in most patients, but significant improvement is uncommon. Unfortunately, relapse rates are greater than 50% and progressive pulmonary failure or infection because of increased immunosuppression are the most common causes of death in lung transplant patients after the second year.

Retransplantation is the only option for terminal respiratory failure secondary to OB. Although survival for patients undergoing retransplantation for OB is better than for those undergoing retransplantation for other reasons, it is still worse than survival of first-time transplant recipients. Novick and coworkers recently reported results from the Pulmonary Retransplant Registry.[35] They reviewed survival rates in 237 patients who underwent pulmonary retransplantation between 1985 and 1996. At 1, 2, and 3 years after retransplantation, survival was 47, 40, and 33%, respectively. Survival was higher in nonventilated, ambulatory patients and their freedom for OB was comparable to first-time transplant recipients. The authors conclude that pulmonary retransplantation should only be performed in carefully selected recipients who have a reasonable likelihood of long-term survival.

AIRWAY COMPLICATIONS

Improvements in surgical technique and posttransplant management have resulted in a relatively low incidence of airway complications after lung transplantation. Nevertheless, up to 27% of cases are complicated by stenosis, necrosis, or dehiscence.[89] The avoidance of perioperative steroids has long been considered important in preventing airway complications. However, recent experimental and clinical evidence suggests that the detrimental effect of steroids may be overestimated.[90] The most common airway complications are partial anastomotic dehiscence and stricture. Such complications are usually diagnosed by bronchoscopy. Airway dehiscence is treated by reoperation or close observation and supportive care. Strictures are treated by balloon or bougie dilatation, often with stent placement.

INFECTION

Bacterial, viral, and fungal infections are leading causes of morbidity and mortality in lung transplantation. The rate of infection is higher in this transplant group compared with other solid organ transplant recipients. This may be related to the lung allograft's direct exposure to airway colonization and aspiration, as well as its impaired cough reflex and mucociliary clearance. The risk of infection and infection-related death peaks in the first few months after transplantation, declining to a low persistent rate thereafter. Posttransplant infections can be classified broadly into those that occur early or late after transplantation. Early infections, occurring within the first month after transplantation, are commonly bacterial (especially Gram-negative bacilli) and manifest as pneumonia, mediastinitis, urinary tract infections, catheter sepsis, and skin infections. In the late posttransplant period, opportunistic viral, fungal, and protozoan pathogens become more prevalent. The lungs, central nervous system, gastrointestinal tract, and skin are the usual sites of invasion.

Bacterial infections, particularly caused by Gram-negative bacteria, predominate during the early postoperative period. Between 75 and 97% of bronchial washings obtained from donor lungs before organ retrieval culture at least one organism.[91] Posttransplant invasive infections are frequently caused by organisms cultured from the donor. Conversely, bacterial infections developing in patients with septic lung disease, particularly CF, most commonly originate from the recipient's airways and sinuses. Treatment of bacterial infections generally involves characterization of the infective agent (eg, cultures, antibiotic sensitivities), source control (eg, catheter removal, debridement), and appropriate antibiotic regimens.

CMV infection occurs most often at 1 to 3 months after transplantation and presents either as a primary infection or reactivation of a latent infection. By definition, primary infection results when a previously seronegative recipient is infected through contact with tissue or blood from a seropositive individual. The donor organ itself is thought to be the most common vector of primary CMV infections. Reactivation infection occurs when a recipient who is seropositive prior to transplant develops clinical CMV infection during immunosuppressive therapy. Seropositive recipients are also subject to infection by new strains of CMV. Primary infection in previously seronegative recipients is generally more serious than reactivation or reinfection in seropositive patients.

Clinically, CMV infection has protean manifestations, including leukopenia with fever, pneumonia, gastroenteritis, hepatitis, and retinitis. CMV pneumonitis is the most lethal of these, with 13% mortality, and retinitis remains the most refractory to treatment. Diagnosis of CMV infection is made by direct culture of the virus from blood, urine, or tissue specimens, a fourfold increase in antibody titers from baseline, or characteristic histologic changes (ie, markedly enlarged cells and nuclei containing basophilic inclusion bodies). Most cases respond to ganciclovir and hyperimmune globulin.

CMV has been implicated as a trigger for OB[69] as well as an inhibitor of cell-mediated immunity. CMV-negative donors comprise less than 20% of the donor organ pool, and owing to organ scarcity, most transplant centers perform transplants across CMV serologic barriers using ganciclovir and/or hyperimmune globulin prophylactic protocols in CMV-positive donors and/or recipients. A study by Valantine and coworkers found that the combined use of ganciclovir and hyperimmune globulin was superior to ganciclovir alone as prophylaxis against CMV. Moreover, the ganciclovir/hyperimmune globulin cohort had longer survival at 3 years and greater freedom from OB.[92]

Invasive fungal infections peak in frequency between 10 days and 2 months after transplantation. Treatment consists of fluconazole, itraconazole, or amphotericin B. Reichenspurner and coworkers have reported that the actuarial incidence and linearized rate of fungal infections was significantly reduced in recipients who received inhaled amphotericin prophylaxis.[93]

The institution of prophylaxis with oral trimethoprim-sulfamethoxazole (or inhalational pentamidine for sulfa-allergic patients) has effectively prevented *P. carinii* pneumonia. The risk of *Pneumocystis* infection is highest during the first year after transplant. However, as infections can also occur late after transplant, most centers recommend prophylactic therapy be continued for life.

Infection prophylaxis is composed of vaccinations, perioperative broad-spectrum antibiotics, and long-term prophylactic antibiotics. Pretransplant inoculations with pneumococcal and hepatitis B vaccines, as well as DPT boosters, are recommended. All transplant recipients should receive annual influenza vaccinations. Although perioperative antibiotic regimens vary widely between transplant centers, first-generation cephalosporins (eg, cefazolin) or vancomycin are commonly used. Long-term prophylaxis typically includes nystatin mouthwash, trimethoprim-sulfamethoxazole, aerosolized amphotericin B, and antivirals such as acyclovir or ganciclovir.

NEOPLASM

Transplant recipients have a higher incidence of neoplasia than that of the general population.[94] This is undoubtedly due to chronic immunosuppression. Recipients are predisposed to a variety of tumors, including skin cancer, B-cell lymphoproliferative disorders, carcinoma in situ of the cervix, carcinoma of the vulva and anus, and Kaposi's sarcoma. On average, tumors appear approximately 5 years after transplantation.[73]

The incidence of B-cell lymphoproliferative disorders in transplant patients is a staggering 350 times greater than that of the normal age-matched population. Posttransplant lymphoproliferative disorder (PTLD) has been reported in 6% of lung transplant recipients.[95] PTLD most commonly occurs within the first year after transplantation, and is associated with Epstein-Barr virus infection. Treatment consists of reducing immunosuppression and administration of an antiviral agent such as acyclovir or ganciclovir. A response rate of 30 to 40% can be expected, and recurrence is uncommon. Chemotherapy and radiotherapy have been

used successfully in some cases. During therapy, close monitoring of the graft, along with clinical assessment of tumor status is essential.

Long-Term Results in Lung Transplantation

Pulmonary function measured by spirometry and arterial blood gases is markedly improved within several months after transplantation, with a normalization of ventilation and gas exchange after 1 to 2 years.[96] The long-term survival for lung transplant recipients reported to the Registry of the International Society for Heart and Lung Transplantation is shown in Fig. 61-13. Survival rates among transplants performed between January 1994 and June 2012 were 88% at 3 months, 80% at 1 year, 65% at 3 years, 53% at 5 years, and 32% at 10 years.[81] Survival for double lung transplant exceeds that of SLT, with the underlying indication being an important factor in the outcome between these two groups. Survival is clearly influenced by recipient age, with 1-year survival at 72% among patients older than 65 compared with 80% survival among patients less than 50.[25] Patients with COPD and IPF (who often are older with more comorbidities) tend to fare poorer than those with CF, IPAH, sarcoidosis, and A1 anti-trypsin (AAT) deficiency emphysema (as shown in Fig. 61-14). In an analysis of 10-year survivors, double-lung recipients and patients with fewer hospitalizations for rejection were found to have improved long-term survival after lung transplantation.[97,98] Operative mortality is clearly affected by center volume, with high volume centers (≥20 implants per year) having a 30-day mortality rate of just 4.1%.[97] With increasing experience with lung transplantation worldwide, both short- and long-term survival have improved over time.

HEART-LUNG TRANSPLANTATION

History of Heart-Lung Transplantation

Long before the first successful human heart-lung transplants were reported, thoracic organ transplantation flourished in the laboratory. In the 1940s, Demikhov developed the first successful method of en bloc heart-lung transplantation in dogs. In his series of 67 dogs, the longest survivor lived for 6 days postoperatively.[99] These remarkable studies demonstrated the technical feasibility of heart and lung replacement, yet remained largely unknown in the West until the 1960s. In 1953, Marcus and colleagues at the Chicago Medical School described a technique for heterotopic heart-lung grafting to the abdominal aorta and inferior vena cava in dogs.[100] Later studies in the 1960s and early 1970s examined the physiologic effect of total denervation on heart and lung function. Studies by Webb and colleagues in 1961 proved discouraging as they showed failure to resume normal spontaneous respiration following heart-lung replacement in dogs.[101] This physiologic phenomenon was confirmed by several other groups using canine models, including Lower and colleagues in 1961.[102]

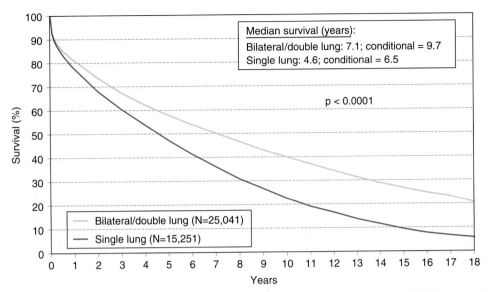

FIGURE 61-13 Kaplan-Meier survival by procedure type for adult lung transplants reported to the ISHLT registry from January 1994 through June 2012. (Data from Yusen RD, Edwards LB, Kucheryavaya AY, et al: The registry of the International Society for Heart and Lung Transplantation: thirty-first adult lung and heart-lung transplant report—2014; focus theme: retransplantation, *J Heart Lung Transplant.* 2014 Oct;33(10):1009-1024.)

Fortunately, later studies in primates by Haglin,[103] Nakae,[104] Castaneda,[105,106] and their colleagues showed that unlike dogs, primates resume a normal respiratory pattern after complete denervation with cardiopulmonary replacement. The 1970s saw the development of improved immunosuppressive medications, particularly cyclosporine, which prevented rejection of primate heart-lung allografts after transplantation. Studies from the Stanford University showed survival for well over 5 years after heart-lung allografting in primates.[107] In the 1980s, Reitz and colleagues reported a modification

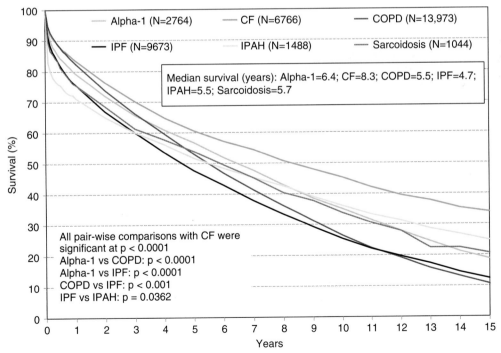

FIGURE 61-14 Kaplan-Meier survival by diagnosis for adult lung transplants reported to the ISHLT registry from January 1990 through June 2012. Alpha 1, Alpha 1-antitrypsin deficiency emphysema; CF, cystic fibrosis; COPD, chronic obstructive pulmonary disease; IPAH, idiopathic pulmonary arterial hypertension; IPF, idiopathic pulmonary fibrosis. (Data from Yusen RD, Edwards LB, Kucheryavaya AY, et al: The registry of the International Society for Heart and Lung Transplantation: thirty-first adult lung and heart-lung transplant report—2014; focus theme: retransplantation, *J Heart Lung Transplant.* 2014 Oct;33(10):1009-1024.)

to the standard technique of heart-lung replacement, using a retained portion of the right atrium for a single inflow anastomosis instead of separate caval anastomoses.[108] This technique preserved the donor sinoatrial node and eliminated the potential for caval anastomotic stenosis. These studies laid the groundwork for a clinical trial of heart-lung transplantation at the Stanford University. On March 9, 1982, Reitz and colleagues performed the first successful human heart-lung transplant in a 45-year-old woman with end-stage primary pulmonary hypertension.[109]

Indications for Heart-Lung Transplantation

Upon its introduction in 1982, heart-lung transplantation provided a life-saving therapeutic option for patients with end-stage pulmonary and cardiopulmonary disease. However, the number of heart-lung transplants performed peaked in 1990 as the techniques of SLT and DLT began to achieve improved outcomes in patients with isolated end-stage lung disease. This, combined with the donor shortage of heart-lung blocs, has restricted the procedure to patients with severe cardiopulmonary diseases (most commonly congenital heart disease with Eisenmenger's syndrome, idiopathic pulmonary arterial hypertension, and CF). Since 2003, between 75 and 86 heart-lung transplant procedures have been performed worldwide each year.[25]

The diagnostic profile of heart-lung transplant recipients reported to the Registry of the International Society for Heart and Lung Transplantation (ISHLT) is shown in Table 61-8.

⬤ TABLE 61-8: Distribution of Diagnoses Among Adult Heart-Lung Transplant Recipients

Diagnosis	No. (%)
Congenital heart disease	1178 (35.5)
Idiopathic pulmonary arterial hypertension	907 (27.4)
Cystic fibrosis	459 (13.9)
COPD disease/emphysema	141 (4.3)
Acquired heart disease	180 (5.4)
Idiopathic pulmonary fibrosis	121 (3.7)
AAT deficiency emphysema	62 (1.9)
Sarcoidosis	54 (1.6)
Retransplant:	
Not obliterative bronchiolitis	32 (1.0)
Obliterative bronchiolitis	24 (0.7)
Bronchiectasis	30 (0.9)
Obliterative bronchiolitis (not retransplant)	25 (0.8)
Other	101 (3.0)

ATT, Alpha-1 antitrypsin; COPD, chronic obstructive pulmonary disease.
ISHLT Registry patients from January 1982 through June 2013.
Reproduced with permission from Yusen RD, Edwards LB, Kucheryavaya AY, et al: The registry of the International Society for Heart and Lung Transplantation: thirty-first adult lung and heart-lung transplant report—2014, *J Heart Lung Transplant.* 2014 Oct;33(10):1009-1024.

Congenital heart disease (atrial and ventricular septal defects, patent ductus arteriosus) with secondary pulmonary hypertension (Eisenmenger's syndrome) is the most frequent indication, found in over one-third of the patients. Complex congenital heart defects that have been treated successfully with heart-lung transplantation include univentricular heart with pulmonary atresia, truncus arteriosus, and hypoplastic left heart syndrome. Data regarding the long-term survival benefit of heart-lung transplantation in patients with Eisenmenger's syndrome are mixed.[110] Some data suggest that pulmonary hypertension in these patients has a more favorable prognostic course than other types of pulmonary hypertension. There is clear evidence, however, that quality of life is improved by transplantation.[111] In patients with simpler cardiac defects, repair of the cardiac defect combined with SLT or bilateral lung transplantation is an alternative option.

Primary pulmonary hypertension with right-sided heart failure is the second most common diagnosis in heart-lung transplant recipients. Nearly one-fourths of patients in the ISHLT registry carry this diagnosis. Recently, there has been a shift toward SLT and bilateral lung transplantation in this population.[112] This new paradigm is based on the finding that normalization of pulmonary pressures following lung transplantation often allows for recovery of right heart function. However, in patients with severe right-sided heart failure and primary pulmonary hypertension, heart-lung transplantation is clearly the operation of choice.

The remainder of heart-lung transplants are performed for a variety of cardiac and pulmonary diseases. These include CF and other septic lung diseases, severe coronary artery disease (CAD) with concomitant end-stage lung disease, and primary parenchymal lung disease with severe right-sided heart failure (eg, IPF, lymphangioleiomyomatosis, sarcoidosis, and desquamative interstitial pneumonitis).

Patient Selection for Heart-Lung

As in lung transplantation, patients are stratified according to LAS with similar listing criteria and contraindications for both groups of patients. Age restrictions tend to be somewhat more selective in most centers, with an upper recipient age limit of 50 years. Most recipients for heart-lung transplantation also fall within New York Heart Association functional classes III or IV.[113] Careful attention to size matching must be carried out in the donor selection process. In a series of 82 heart-lung transplants at Papworth Hospital, Tamm and coworkers recorded recipient lung volumes posttransplantation, followed by a comparison to preoperative and predicted volumes to evaluate the influence of donor lung size and recipient underlying disease.[114] The investigators demonstrated that, by 1 year after surgery, total lung capacity (TLC) and dynamic lung volume returned to values predicted by the patient's sex, age, and height. They proposed that the simplest method of matching donor lung size to that of the recipient is to use their respective predicted TLC values. Moreover, they concluded that recipients should attain their predicted lung volumes by 1 year posttransplantation, and failure to do so suggests possible complications within the transplanted lungs.

As in lung transplantation, preoperative HLA matching is not feasible given the necessity of short ischemic times. However, histocompatibility does seem to impact on patient outcomes. Harjula and coworkers at Stanford evaluated the relationship between HLA matching and outcomes in heart-lung transplantation.[115] Among 40 heart-lung transplant recipients evaluated, they found a significant increase in graded OB with total mismatch at the HLA-A locus.

Operative Technique

PROCUREMENT

Exposure and cannulation for heart-lung blocs follows the same procedure as for lung procurement. After cross-clamp, the bloc is dissected free from the esophagus commencing at the level of the diaphragm and continuing cephalad to the level of the carina. Dissection is kept close to the esophagus, and care is taken to avoid injury to the trachea, lung, or great vessels. The posterior hilar attachments are divided. The lungs are inflated to a full normal tidal volume, and the trachea is stapled at the highest point possible with a TA-55 stapler (US Surgical, Norwalk, CT), at least four rings above the carina (Fig. 61-6E). The trachea is then divided above the staple line, and the entire heart-lung bloc is removed from the chest.

RECIPIENT IMPLANT

The recipient is positioned supine and the chest is entered through a median sternotomy. A sternal retractor is placed, and both pleural spaces are opened anteriorly from the level of the diaphragm to the level of the great vessels (Fig. 61-15A). Electrocautery is used to divide any pleural adhesions. The anterior pericardium is excised, and the lateral segments are preserved to support the heart and protect the phrenic nerves. A 3-cm border of the pericardium should be left both anterior and posterior to each phrenic nerve extending from the level of the diaphragm to the level of the great vessels (Fig. 61-15B). An alternative approach is to create posterior pericardial apertures where the pulmonary veins enter into the pericardium. A border of pericardium is left posterior to the phrenic nerves, whereas the entire remaining pericardium anterior to the phrenic nerves is left intact. After fully heparinizing the recipient, the ascending aorta is cannulated near the base of the innominate artery, and the venae cavae are individually cannulated laterally and snared. Cardiopulmonary bypass with systemic cooling to 28 to 30°C is instituted, and the heart is excised at the midatrial level. The aorta is divided just above the aortic valve, and the pulmonary artery is divided at its bifurcation (Fig. 61-15C). The left atrial remnant is then divided vertically at a point halfway between the right and left pulmonary veins.

The posterior edge of the left atrial and pulmonary venous remnant is developed in a manner allowing the left inferior and superior pulmonary veins to be displaced over into the left chest. Following division of the pulmonary ligament, the left lung is moved into the field, allowing full dissection of the posterior aspect of the left hilum, with care taken to avoid the vagus nerve posteriorly. Once this is completed, the left main pulmonary artery is divided (Fig. 61-15D), and the left main bronchus is stapled with a TA-30 stapler and divided. The same technique of hilar dissection and division is repeated on the right side (Fig. 61-15E), and both lungs are removed from the chest.

The native main pulmonary artery remnant is removed, leaving a portion of the pulmonary artery intact adjacent to the underside of the aorta (near the ligamentum arteriosus) to preserve the left recurrent laryngeal nerve. Attention is then turned to preparing the distal trachea for anastomosis. The stapled ends of the right and left bronchi are grasped and dissection is carried up to the level of the distal trachea. Bronchial vessels are individually identified and carefully ligated. Patients with congenital heart disease and pulmonary atresia or severe cyanosis secondary to Eisenmenger's syndrome may have large mediastinal bronchial collaterals that must be meticulously ligated. Perfect hemostasis is necessary in this area of the dissection, because it is obscured once graft implantation is complete. Once absolute hemostasis is achieved, the trachea is divided at the carina with a no. 15 blade. The chest is now prepared to receive the heart-lung graft.

The donor heart-lung bloc is removed from its transport container and prepared by irrigating, aspirating, and culturing the tracheobronchial tree followed by trimming of the trachea to leave one cartilaginous ring above the carina. The heart-lung graft is then lowered into the chest, passing the right lung beneath the right phrenic nerve pedicle. The left lung is then gently manipulated under the left phrenic nerve pedicle (Fig. 61-15F). The tracheal anastomosis is performed using continuous 3-0 polypropylene suture (Fig. 61-15G). The posterior membranous portion of the anastomosis is performed first, followed by completion of the anterior aspect. Ventilation is then carried out with room air at half-normal tidal volumes to inflate the lungs and reduce atelectasis. Topical cooling with a continuous infusion of cold Physiosol into both thoraces is begun. To augment endomyocardial cooling and to exclude air from the graft, a third cold, "bubble-free" line is placed directly into the left atrial appendage.

Next, the bicaval venous anastomosis is performed. The recipient inferior vena cava is anastomosed to the donor inferior vena cava-right atrial junction with a continuous 4-0 polypropylene suture. At this point, the patient is warmed toward 37°C, and the superior vena caval and aortic anastomoses are performed end-to-end with continuous 4-0 polypropylene sutures (Fig. 61-15H). After the ascending aorta and pulmonary artery are cleared of air, the aortic cross-clamp and caval tapes are removed. The left atrial catheter is removed, and the atrium is allowed to drain. The amputated left atrial stump is oversewn, and the pulmonary artery pulmonoplegia infusion site closed. The heart is defibrillated, and the patient is gradually weaned from cardiopulmonary bypass in the standard fashion. Methylprednisolone (500 mg) is administered to the recipient after heparin reversal with protamine sulfate.

PEEP at 3 to 5 cm H_2O and an FIO_2 of 40% is maintained. As in cardiac transplantation, isoproterenol

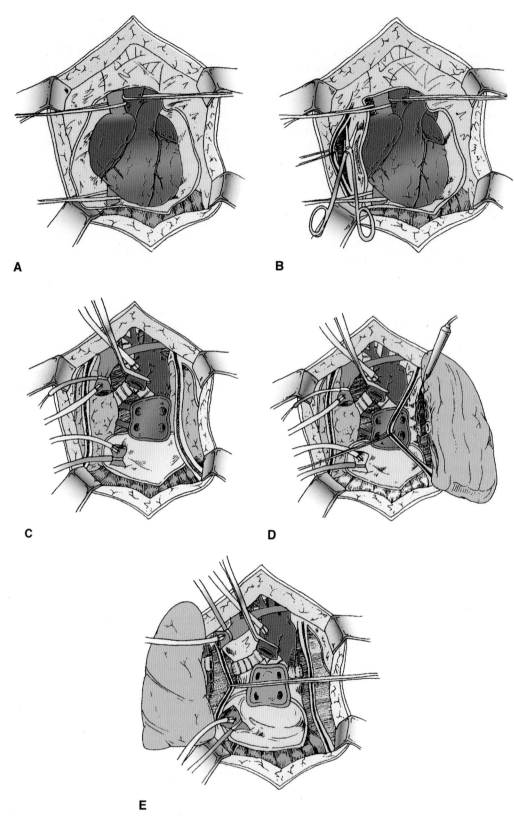

FIGURE 61-15 Recipient operation for heart-lung transplantation. (A) Through a median sternotomy, the anterior pericardium is partially removed and the ascending aorta and both venae cavae are dissected and encircled with tapes. (B) The right phrenic nerve is carefully separated from the right hilum, providing a space for inserting the right lung of the graft. (C) Cannulation for cardiopulmonary bypass consists of a cannula in the high ascending aorta and separate vena caval cannulas. Once on bypass, the native heart is excised in a manner similar to that for standard cardiac explantation. (D,E) Left and right pneumonectomies are performed by dividing the respective inferior pulmonary ligament, pulmonary artery and veins, and mainstem bronchus.

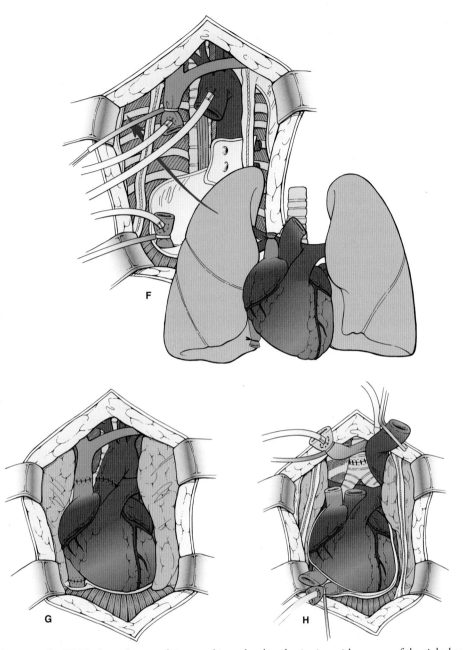

FIGURE 61-15 (*Continued*) (F) The heart-lung graft is moved into the chest beginning with passage of the right lung underneath the right phrenic nerve pedicle, followed by manipulation of the left lung beneath the left phrenic nerve pedicle. (G) The caval and aortic anastomoses are performed with a continuous 4-0 polypropylene suture. (H) The tracheal anastomosis is performed with a continuous 3-0 polypropylene suture.

(0.005 to 0.01 μg/kg/min) is usually initiated on graft reperfusion to increase the heart rate (~100-110 bpm) and to lower pulmonary vascular resistance. Temporary right atrial and ventricular pacing wires are placed. Right and left pleural "right angle" chest tubes are placed along each diaphragm, as well as a single mediastinal tube. The chest is closed in the standard fashion. Finally, the double lumen endotracheal tube is exchanged for a single lumen tube and the tracheal anastomosis is visualized by bronchoscopy before transporting the patient to the intensive care unit.

Lick and coworkers describe an interesting alternative to the standard technique in which the pulmonary hila are placed anterior to the phrenic nerves and direct caval anastomoses are used whenever feasible.[116] This modification obviates extensive dissection of the phrenic nerves and posterior mediastinum, decreasing the likelihood of phrenic and vagus nerve injury. Furthermore, the posterior mediastinum can readily be inspected for bleeding after implantation by rotating the heart-lung bloc anterior-medially while still on bypass.

Graft Physiology

For heart-lung recipients, denervation of the cardiac allograft leads to additional physiologic characteristics beyond what is seen in isolated lung transplantation. The denervated heart loses its sympathetic and parasympathetic autonomic regulation, thereby impacting on heart rate, contractility, and coronary artery vasomotor tone. The resting heart rate is generally higher due to the absence of vagal input. Respiratory sinus arrhythmia and carotid reflex bradycardia are absent. Interestingly, the denervated heart develops an increased sensitivity to catecholamines because of increased beta-adrenergic receptor density and loss of norepinephrine uptake in postganglionic sympathetic neurons.[117,118] This augmented sensitivity plays an important role in maintaining an adequate cardiac response to exercise and stress. During exercise, the recipient experiences a steady but delayed increase in heart rate, primarily because of a rise in circulating catecholamines. This initial rise in heart rate is subsequently accompanied by an immediate increase in filling pressures resulting from increased venous return. These changes lead to increased stroke volume and cardiac output sufficient to sustain activity. Although the coronary circulation's ability to dilate to meet increased myocardial oxygen demand is not eliminated in an uncomplicated heart-lung transplant, this reserve is abnormal in the presence of rejection, hypertrophy, or regional wall abnormalities.

Postoperative Management

Approximately 10 to 20% of heart-lung graft recipients experience some degree of transient sinus node dysfunction in the immediate perioperative period. This often manifests as sinus bradycardia and usually resolves within a week. The use of bicaval venous anastomoses has been reported to lower the incidence of sinus node dysfunction and improve tricuspid valve function.[119] Because cardiac output is primarily rate dependent after heart-lung transplantation, the heart rate should be maintained between 90 and 110 beats per minute during the first few postoperative days using temporary pacing or isoproterenol (0.005-0.01 μg/kg/min) as needed. Although rarely seen, persistent sinus node dysfunction and bradycardia may require a permanent transvenous pacemaker. Systolic blood pressure should be maintained between 90 and 110 mm Hg using nitroglycerin or nitroprusside for afterload reduction, if necessary. "Renal-dose" dopamine (3-5 μg/kg/min) is used frequently to augment renal blood flow and urine output. The adequacy of cardiac output is indicated by warm extremities and a urine output greater than 0.5 mL/kg/h without diuretics. Cardiac function generally returns to normal within 3 to 4 days, at which time inotropes and vasodilators can be weaned.

Nevertheless, depressed global myocardial performance is occasionally seen during the acute postoperative setting. The myocardium may be subject to prolonged ischemia, inadequate preservation, or catecholamine depletion before implantation. Hypovolemia, cardiac tamponade, sepsis,

and bradycardia are also potential contributors and should be treated expeditiously if they are present. A Swan-Ganz pulmonary artery catheter should be used in cases of persistently abnormal hemodynamics. Surveillance endomyocardial biopsies are performed at 3 months and then annually in heart-lung graft recipients.

Complications

The most common complications after heart-lung transplantation include hypertension (88.6%), renal dysfunction (28.1%), hyperlipidemia (66.4%), diabetes (20.9%), coronary artery vasculopathy (8.2%), and bronchiolitis obliterans (27.1%).[25] Common causes of death include graft failure and technical complications within the first 30 days, followed by non-CMV infections and BOS in the longer term.[25] Acute rejection remains a challenge, occurring in more than 67% of heart-lung patients within the first year between 1981 and 1994 at Stanford University.[120] Experimental and clinical evidence suggests that pulmonary and cardiac rejections occur independently of one other. Nevertheless, Higenbottam and coworkers at Papworth Hospital reported a surprisingly low diagnostic yield from routine endomyocardial biopsies in heart-lung recipients compared with functional or histologic tests of pulmonary rejection. Based on these findings, the authors concluded that transbronchial biopsy eliminates the need for routine endomyocardial biopsies in heart-lung transplant recipients.[121] These findings were supported by Sibley and coworkers at Stanford University, who demonstrated discordance between findings on endomyocardial and transbronchial biopsies during episodes of acute rejection. Endomyocardial biopsies are most often normal despite findings of pulmonary rejection on transbronchial biopsy.[76] In our practice, surveillance endomyocardial biopsies have been abandoned in patients in whom transbronchial biopsies can be reliably performed. Respiratory failure secondary OB represents a long-term complication of heart-lung transplant at a rate similar to DLT. Among heart-lung recipients with OB, Adams and coworkers at Harefield Hospital noted that retransplant survival rates were worse for those undergoing combined heart-lung replacement compared with patients who underwent isolated lung replacement.[122] The group also noted the following factors were associated with improved survival after retransplant: absence of preformed antibodies, retransplantation at least 18 months after the original transplantation, and negative preoperative sputum cultures.

Accelerated graft CAD or graft atherosclerosis is another major obstacle to long-term survival in heart-lung transplant recipients. Significant graft CAD resulting in diminished coronary artery blood flow may lead to arrhythmias, myocardial infarction, sudden death, or impaired left ventricular function with congestive heart failure. Classic angina caused by myocardial ischemia is usually not noted in transplant recipients because the cardiac graft is not innervated. Multiple etiologies for graft CAD have been proposed, all focusing on chronic, immune-mediated damage to the coronary vascular

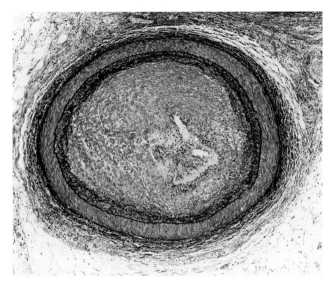

FIGURE 61-16 Cardiac graft atherosclerosis. Complete luminal obliteration by a concentric fibrointimal proliferation was observed at postmortem in this heart-lung transplant patient (Elastin von Gieson stain; ×60).

endothelium. In fact, elevated levels of antiendothelial antibodies have been correlated with graft CAD. Unlike coronary artery occlusive disease in the native heart, which tends to be a more focal process, transplant atherosclerosis is a more diffuse vascular narrowing extending symmetrically into distal branches. Histologically, transplant arteriopathy is characterized by concentric intimal proliferation with smooth muscle hyperplasia (Fig. 61-16).

Coronary angiograms are performed on a yearly basis to identify recipients with accelerated CAD. Angiography is limited, however, to assessment of luminal diameter. Intracoronary ultrasound, by contrast, can assess both

vascular wall morphology and luminal diameter, making it a more sensitive tool to detect the diffuse coronary intimal thickening typical of graft atherosclerosis. Interestingly, graft CAD occurs at a reduced incidence in heart-lung recipients compared with the cardiac transplantation population.[123] A retrospective survey at Stanford revealed 89% of heart-lung recipients were free from graft CAD at 5 years, compared with 73% of heart transplant recipients. Clinically observed risk factors for developing this condition in heart transplant recipients include donor age greater than 35 years, incompatibility at the HLA-A1, A2, and DR loci, hypertriglyceridemia (serum concentration greater than 280 mg/dL), frequent acute rejection episodes, and documented recipient CMV infection. It is not clear whether these risk factors can be extended to the heart-lung transplant population, although CMV infection has been implicated.[124] Percutaneous transluminal coronary angioplasty and coronary artery bypass grafting have been used to treat discrete proximal lesions in some cases of graft CAD. However, the only definitive therapy for diffuse graft CAD is retransplantation. Effective prevention of graft CAD will rely on development of improved immunosuppression, recipient tolerance induction, improved CMV prophylaxis, and inhibition of vascular intimal proliferation.

Infection represents another significant postoperative challenge in heart-lung transplantation. Between 1981 and 1994 at Stanford, only 20% of heart-lung transplant recipients were free from infection 3 months after transplantation. In a retrospective analysis of 200 episodes of serious infections occurring in 73 heart-lung recipients at Stanford between 1981 and 1990, Kramer and coworkers[125] found that half of all infections were caused by bacteria, whereas fungal infections accounted for only 14% of total infections. The most common viral agent was CMV, occurring primarily in the second month after transplantation and comprising 15% of

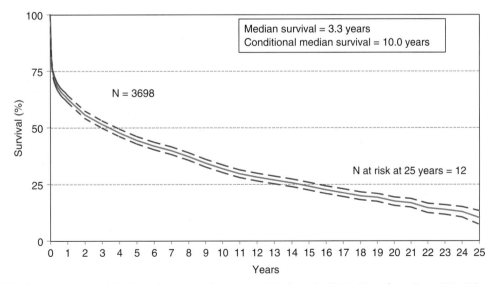

FIGURE 61-17 Kaplan-Meier survival for heart-lung transplantation, 1982 through 2012. (Data from Yusen RD, Edwards LB, Kucheryavaya AY, et al: The registry of the International Society for Heart and Lung Transplantation: thirty-first adult lung and heart-lung transplant report—2014; focus theme: retransplantation, *J Heart Lung Transplant.* 2014 Oct;33(10):1009-1024.)

all viral infections. Other viral infections (ie, herpes simplex, adenovirus, respiratory syncytial virus) were less common. Five percent of infections were attributed to *P. carinii*, typically occurring 4 to 6 months after transplantation, and 2% were caused by *Nocardia*, generally appearing after the first year. There was no significant difference in the incidence of infections between patients receiving triple-drug or double-drug (cyclosporine and prednisone) immunosuppression. Infectious mortality comprised 40% of all deaths.

Long-Term Results in Heart-Lung Transplantation

Survival rates of 72% at 3 months and 64% at 1 year have been reported in the ISHLT registry.[25] Mortality rates taper off significantly at a year posttransplant, as illustrated in Fig. 61-17. As with lung transplantation, outcomes have improved over time and are affected by recipient diagnosis.[25] Graft failure, technical complications, and non-CMV infections are all common causes of 30-day mortality, with BO and non-CMV infections impairing long-term survival.

REFERENCES

1. Yusen RD, Christie JD, Edwards LB, et al: The Registry of the International Society for Heart and Lung Transplantation: Thirtieth Adult Lung and Heart-Lung Transplant Report-2013; focus theme: age. *J Heart Lung Transplant* 2013; 32(10):965-978.
2. Metras H: Preliminary note on lung transplants in dogs. *Compte Rendue Acad Sci* 1950; 231:1176.
3. Blumenstock D, Kahn DR: Replantation and transplantation of the canine lung. *J Surg Res* 1961; 1(1):40-47.
4. Veith FJ, Richards K: Improved technic for canine lung transplantation. *Ann Surg* 1970; 171(4):553-558.
5. Lima O, Goldberg M, Peters WJ, Ayabe H, Townsend E, Cooper JD: Bronchial omentopexy in canine lung transplantation. *J Thorac Cardiovasc Surg* 1982; 83(3):418-421.
6. Lima O, Cooper JD, Peters WJ, et al: Effects of methylprednisolone and azathioprine on bronchial healing following lung autotransplantation. *J Thorac Cardiovasc Surg* 1981; 82(2):211-215.
7. Hardy JD, Webb WR, Dalton ML, Jr., Walker GR, Jr: Lung homotransplantation in man. *JAMA* 1963; 186:1065-1074.
8. Unilateral lung transplantation for pulmonary fibrosis: Toronto Lung Transplant Group. *N Engl J Med* 1986; 314(18):1140-1145.
9. Patterson GA, Cooper JD, Goldman B, et al: Technique of successful clinical double-lung transplantation. *Ann Thorac Surg* 1988; 45(6):626-633.
10. Pasque MK, Cooper JD, Kaiser LR, Haydock DA, Triantafillou A, Trulock EP: Improved technique for bilateral lung transplantation: rationale and initial clinical experience. *Ann Thorac Surg* 1990; 49(5):785-791.
11. Starnes VA, Oyer PE, Bernstein D, et al: Heart, heart-lung, and lung transplantation in the first year of life. *Ann Thorac Surg* 1992; 53(2):306-310.
12. Barr ML, Bourge RC, Orens JB, et al: Thoracic organ transplantation in the United States, 1994-2003. *Am J Transplant* 2005; 5(4 Pt 2):934-949.
13. Hachem RR, Edwards LB, Yusen RD, Chakinala MM, Alexander Patterson G, Trulock EP: The impact of induction on survival after lung transplantation: an analysis of the International Society for Heart and Lung Transplantation Registry. *Clin Transplant* 2008; 22(5):603-608.
14. Merlo CA, Weiss ES, Orens JB, et al: Impact of U.S. Lung Allocation Score on survival after lung transplantation. *J Heart Lung Transplant* 2009; 28(8):769-775.
15. Maurer JR: Patient selection for lung transplantation. *JAMA* 2001; 286(21):2720-2721.
16. Wu A, Buhler LH, Cooper DK: ABO-incompatible organ and bone marrow transplantation: current status. *Transpl Int* 2003; 16(5):291-299.
17. Christie JD, Edwards LB, Kucheryavaya AY, et al: The Registry of the International Society for Heart and Lung Transplantation: twenty-seventh official adult lung and heart-lung transplant report-2010. *J Heart Lung Transplant* 2010; 29(10):1104-1118.
18. Stocks J, Quanjer PH: Reference values for residual volume, functional residual capacity and total lung capacity. ATS Workshop on Lung Volume Measurements. Official Statement of The European Respiratory Society. *Eur Respir J* 1995; 8(3):492-506.
19. Barnard JB, Davies O, Curry P, et al: Size matching in lung transplantation: an evidence-based review. *J Heart Lung Transplant* 2013; 32(9):849-860.
20. Eberlein M, Reed RM, Maidaa M, et al: Donor-recipient size matching and survival after lung transplantation. A cohort study. *Ann Am Thorac Soc* 2013; 10(5):418-425.
21. Camargo JJ, Irion KL, Marchiori E, et al: Computed tomography measurement of lung volume in preoperative assessment for living donor lung transplantation: volume calculation using 3D surface rendering in the determination of size compatibility. *Pediatr Transplant* 2009; 13(4):429-439.
22. Hosenpud JD, Edwards EB, Lin HM, Daily OP: Influence of HLA matching on thoracic transplant outcomes. An analysis from the UNOS/ISHLT Thoracic Registry. *Circulation* 1996; 94(2):170-174.
23. Wisser W, Wekerle T, Zlabinger G, et al: Influence of human leukocyte antigen matching on long-term outcome after lung transplantation. *J Heart Lung Transplant* 1996; 15(12):1209-1216.
24. Iwaki Y, Yoshida Y, Griffith B: The HLA matching effect in lung transplantation. *Transplantation* 1993; 56(6):1528-1529.
25. Christie JD, Edwards LB, Aurora P, et al: The Registry of the International Society for Heart and Lung Transplantation: Twenty-sixth Official Adult Lung and Heart-Lung Transplantation Report-2009. *J Heart Lung Transplant* 2009; 28(10):1031-1049.
26. Celli BR, Cote CG, Marin JM, et al: The body-mass index, airflow obstruction, dyspnea, and exercise capacity index in chronic obstructive pulmonary disease. *N Engl J Med* 2004; 350(10):1005-1012.
27. Fishman A, Martinez F, Naunheim K, et al: A randomized trial comparing lung-volume-reduction surgery with medical therapy for severe emphysema. *N Engl J Med* 2003; 348(21):2059-2073.
28. Thabut G, Christie JD, Ravaud P, et al: Survival after bilateral versus single lung transplantation for patients with chronic obstructive pulmonary disease: a retrospective analysis of registry data. *Lancet* 2008; 371(9614):744-751.
29. Kreider M, Kotloff RM: Selection of candidates for lung transplantation. *Proc Am Thorac Soc* 2009; 6(1):20-27.
30. Weiss ES, Allen JG, Merlo CA, Conte JV, Shah AS: Survival after single versus bilateral lung transplantation for high-risk patients with pulmonary fibrosis. *Ann Thorac Surg* 2009; 88(5):1616-1625; discussion 1625-1616.
31. Kerem E, Reisman J, Corey M, Canny GJ, Levison H: Prediction of mortality in patients with cystic fibrosis. *N Engl J Med* 1992; 326(18):1187-1191.
32. Orens JB, Estenne M, Arcasoy S, et al: International guidelines for the selection of lung transplant candidates: 2006 update—a consensus report from the Pulmonary Scientific Council of the International Society for Heart and Lung Transplantation. *J Heart Lung Transplant* 2006; 25(7):745-755.
33. Umetsu DT, Moss RB, King VV, Lewiston NJ: Sinus disease in patients with severe cystic fibrosis: relation to pulmonary exacerbation. *Lancet* 1990; 335(8697):1077-1078.
34. Sitbon O, Humbert M, Nunes H, et al: Long-term intravenous epoprostenol infusion in primary pulmonary hypertension: prognostic factors and survival. *J Am Coll Cardiol* 2002; 40(4):780-788.
35. Novick RJ, Stitt LW, Al-Kattan K, et al: Pulmonary retransplantation: predictors of graft function and survival in 230 patients. Pulmonary Retransplant Registry. *Ann Thorac Surg* 1998; 65(1):227-234.
36. Maxwell BG, Levitt JE, Goldstein BA, et al: Impact of the lung allocation score on survival beyond 1 year. *Am J Transplant* 2014; 14(10):2288-2294.
37. Schaffer JM, Singh SK, Reitz BA, Zamanian RT, Mallidi HR: Single- vs double-lung transplantation in patients with chronic obstructive pulmonary disease and idiopathic pulmonary fibrosis since the implementation of lung allocation based on medical need. *JAMA* 2015; 313(9):936-948.

38. Schaffer JM, Singh SK, Joyce DL, et al: Transplantation for idiopathic pulmonary arterial hypertension: improvement in the lung allocation score era. *Circulation* 2013; 127(25):2503-2513.

39. Hosenpud JD, Bennett LE, Keck BM, Boucek MM, Novick RJ: The Registry of the International Society for Heart and Lung Transplantation: seventeenth official report-2000. *J Heart Lung Transplant* 2000; 19(10):909-931.

40. McLaughlin VV, Rich S: Pulmonary hypertension-advances in medical and surgical interventions. *J Heart Lung Transplant* 1998; 17(8):739-743.

41. Palevsky HI, Fishman AP: Chronic cor pulmonale. Etiology and management. *JAMA* 1990; 263(17):2347-2353.

42. Goldberg M, Lima O, Morgan E, et al: A comparison between cyclosporin A and methylprednisolone plus azathioprine on bronchial healing following canine lung autotransplantation. *J Thorac Cardiovasc Surg* 1983; 85(6):821-826.

43. Madden BP, Kamalvand K, Chan CM, Khaghani A, Hodson ME, Yacoub M: The medical management of patients with cystic fibrosis following heart-lung transplantation. *Eur Respir J* 1993; 6(7):965-970.

44. Frost AE: Donor criteria and evaluation. *Clin Chest Med* 1997; 18(2):231-237.

45. International guidelines for the selection of lung transplant candidates: The American Society for Transplant Physicians (ASTP)/American Thoracic Society(ATS)/European Respiratory Society(ERS)/International Society for Heart and Lung Transplantation(ISHLT). *Am J Respir Crit Care Med* 1998; 158(1):335-339.

46. Bhorade SM, Vigneswaran W, McCabe MA, Garrity ER: Liberalization of donor criteria may expand the donor pool without adverse consequence in lung transplantation. *J Heart Lung Transplant* 2000; 19(12):1199-1204.

47. Fischer S, Gohrbandt B, Struckmeier P, et al: Lung transplantation with lungs from donors fifty years of age and older. *J Thorac Cardiovasc Surg* 2005; 129(4):919-925.

48. Gabbay E, Williams TJ, Griffiths AP, et al: Maximizing the utilization of donor organs offered for lung transplantation. *Am J Respir Crit Care Med* 1999; 160(1):265-271.

49. Pierre AF, Sekine Y, Hutcheon MA, Waddell TK, Keshavjee SH: Marginal donor lungs: a reassessment. *J Thorac Cardiovasc Surg* 2002; 123(3):421-427; discussion 427-428.

50. Shumway SJ, Hertz MI, Petty MG, Bolman RM, 3rd: Liberalization of donor criteria in lung and heart-lung transplantation. *Ann Thorac Surg* 1994; 57(1):92-95.

51. Novick RJ, Bennett LE, Meyer DM, Hosenpud JD: Influence of graft ischemic time and donor age on survival after lung transplantation. *J Heart Lung Transplant* 1999; 18(5):425-431.

52. Weill D, Dey GC, Hicks RA, et al: A positive donor gram stain does not predict outcome following lung transplantation. *J Heart Lung Transplant* 2002; 21(5):555-558.

53. Weill D, Dey GC, Young KR, et al: A positive donor gram stain does not predict the development of pneumonia, oxygenation, or duration of mechanical ventilation following lung transplantation. *J Heart Lung Transplant* 2001; 20(2):255.

54. Steen S, Sjoberg T, Pierre L, Liao Q, Eriksson L, Algotsson L: Transplantation of lungs from a non-heart-beating donor. *Lancet* 2001; 357(9259):825-829.

55. Steen S, Ingemansson R, Eriksson L, et al: First human transplantation of a nonacceptable donor lung after reconditioning ex vivo. *Ann Thorac Surg* 2007; 83(6):2191-2194.

56. Cypel M, Yeung JC, Hirayama S, et al: Technique for prolonged normothermic ex vivo lung perfusion. *J Heart Lung Transplant* 2008; 27(12):1319-1325.

57. Cypel M, Yeung JC, Liu M, et al: Normothermic ex vivo lung perfusion in clinical lung transplantation. *N Engl J Med* 2011; 364(15):1431-1440.

58. Cypel M, Yeung JC, Machuca T, et al: Experience with the first 50 ex vivo lung perfusions in clinical transplantation. *J Thorac Cardiovasc Surg* 2012; 144(5):1200-1206.

59. Zych B, Popov AF, Stavri G, et al: Early outcomes of bilateral sequential single lung transplantation after ex-vivo lung evaluation and reconditioning. *J Heart Lung Transplant* 2012; 31(3):274-281.

60. Ware LB, Wang Y, Fang X, et al: Assessment of lungs rejected for transplantation and implications for donor selection. *Lancet* 2002; 360(9333):619-620.

61. Shigemura N, Bhama J, Nguyen D, Thacker J, Bermudez C, Toyoda Y: Pitfalls in donor lung procurements: how should the procedure be taught to transplant trainees? *J Thorac Cardiovasc Surg* 2009; 138(2):486-490.

62. Conte JV, Baumgartner WA: Overview and future practice patterns in cardiac and pulmonary preservation. *J Card Surg* 2000; 15(2):91-107.

63. Gamez P, Cordoba M, Millan I, et al: Improvements in lung preservation: 3 years' experience with a low-potassium dextran solution. *Arch Bronconeumol* 2005; 41(1):16-19.

64. Muller C, Bittmann I, Hatz R, et al: Improvement of lung preservation—from experiment to clinical practice. *Eur Surg Res* 2002; 34(1-2):77-82.

65. Wittwer T, Franke UF, Fehrenbach A, et al: Experimental lung transplantation: impact of preservation solution and route of delivery. *J Heart Lung Transplant* 2005; 24(8):1081-1090.

66. Novick RJ, Reid KR, Denning L, Duplan J, Menkis AH, McKenzie FN: Prolonged preservation of canine lung allografts: the role of prostaglandins. *Ann Thorac Surg* 1991; 51(5):853-859.

67. Kirk AJ, Colquhoun IW, Dark JH: Lung preservation: a review of current practice and future directions. *Ann Thorac Surg* 1993; 56(4):990-100.

68. Dummer JS, Montero CG, Griffith BP, Hardesty RL, Paradis IL, Ho M: Infections in heart-lung transplant recipients. *Transplantation* 1986; 41(6):725-729.

69. DeMeo DL, Ginns LC: Clinical status of lung transplantation. *Transplantation* 2001; 72(11):1713-1724.

70. Christie JD, Bavaria JE, Palevsky HI, et al: Primary graft failure following lung transplantation. *Chest* 1998; 114(1):51-60.

71. Slaughter MS, Nielsen K, Bolman RM, 3rd: Extracorporeal membrane oxygenation after lung or heart-lung transplantation. *ASAIO J* 1993; 39(3):M453-M456.

72. Adatia I, Lillehei C, Arnold JH, et al: Inhaled nitric oxide in the treatment of postoperative graft dysfunction after lung transplantation. *Ann Thorac Surg* 1994; 57(5):1311-1318.

73. Trulock EP, Edwards LB, Taylor DO, Boucek MM, Keck BM, Hertz MI: Registry of the International Society for Heart and Lung Transplantation: twenty-second official adult lung and heart-lung transplant report—2005. *J Heart Lung Transplant* 2005; 24(8):956-967.

74. Cooper JD, Billingham M, Egan T, et al: A working formulation for the standardization of nomenclature and for clinical staging of chronic dysfunction in lung allografts. International Society for Heart and Lung Transplantation. *J Heart Lung Transplant* 1993; 12(5):713-716.

75. Berry GJ, Brunt EM, Chamberlain D, et al: A working formulation for the standardization of nomenclature in the diagnosis of heart and lung rejection: Lung Rejection Study Group. The International Society for Heart Transplantation. *J Heart Transplant* 1990; 9(6):593-601.

76. Sibley RK, Berry GJ, Tazelaar HD, et al: The role of transbronchial biopsies in the management of lung transplant recipients. *J Heart Lung Transplant* 1993; 12(2):308-324.

77. Guilinger RA, Paradis IL, Dauber JH, et al: The importance of bronchoscopy with transbronchial biopsy and bronchoalveolar lavage in the management of lung transplant recipients. *Am J Respir Crit Care Med* 1995; 152(6 Pt 1):2037-2043.

78. Clelland CA, Higenbottam TW, Stewart S, Scott JP, Wallwork J: The histological changes in transbronchial biopsy after treatment of acute lung rejection in heart-lung transplants. *J Pathol* 1990; 161(2):105-112.

79. Loubeyre P, Revel D, Delignette A, Loire R, Mornex JF: High-resolution computed tomographic findings associated with histologically diagnosed acute lung rejection in heart-lung transplant recipients. *Chest* 1995; 107(1):132-138.

80. Valentine VG, Robbins RC, Wehner JH, Patel HR, Berry GJ, Theodore J: Total lymphoid irradiation for refractory acute rejection in heart-lung and lung allografts. *Chest* 1996; 109(5):1184-1189.

81. Yusen RD, Edwards LB, Kucheryavaya AY, et al: The registry of the International Society for Heart and Lung Transplantation: thirty-first adult lung and heart-lung transplant report—2014; focus theme: retransplantation. *J Heart Lung Transplant* 2014; 33(10):1009-1024.

82. Chamberlain D, Maurer J, Chaparro C, Idolor L: Evaluation of transbronchial lung biopsy specimens in the diagnosis of bronchiolitis obliterans after lung transplantation. *J Heart Lung Transplant* 1994; 13(6):963-971.

83. Valentine VG, Robbins RC, Berry GJ, et al: Actuarial survival of heart-lung and bilateral sequential lung transplant recipients with obliterative bronchiolitis. *J Heart Lung Transplant* 1996; 15(4):371-383.

84. Sharples LD, McNeil K, Stewart S, Wallwork J: Risk factors for bronchiolitis obliterans: a systematic review of recent publications. *J Heart Lung Transplant* 2002; 21(2):271-281.

85. D'Ovidio F, Keshavjee S: Gastroesophageal reflux and lung transplantation. *Dis Esophagus* 2006; 19(5):315-320.

86. Robertson AG, Shenfine J, Ward C, et al: A call for standardization of antireflux surgery in the lung transplantation population. *Transplantation* 2009; 87(8):1112-1114.

87. Davis RD, Jr., Lau CL, Eubanks S, et al: Improved lung allograft function after fundoplication in patients with gastroesophageal reflux disease undergoing lung transplantation. *J Thorac Cardiovasc Surg* 2003; 125(3):533-542.

88. Cantu E, 3rd, Appel JZ, 3rd, Hartwig MG, et al: J. Maxwell Chamberlain Memorial Paper. Early fundoplication prevents chronic allograft dysfunction in patients with gastroesophageal reflux disease. *Ann Thorac Surg* 2004; 78(4):1142-1151; discussion 1142-1151.

89. Samano MN, Minamoto H, Junqueira JJ, et al: Bronchial complications following lung transplantation. *Transplant Proc* 2009; 41(3):921-926.

90. Colquhoun IW, Gascoigne AD, Au J, Corris PA, Hilton CJ, Dark JH: Airway complications after pulmonary transplantation. *Ann Thorac Surg* 1994; 57(1):141-145.

91. Davis RD, Jr., Pasque MK: Pulmonary transplantation. *Ann Surg* 1995; 221(1):14-28.

92. Valantine HA, Luikart H, Doyle R, et al: Impact of cytomegalovirus hyperimmune globulin on outcome after cardiothoracic transplantation: a comparative study of combined prophylaxis with CMV hyperimmune globulin plus ganciclovir versus ganciclovir alone. *Transplantation* 2001; 72(10):1647-1652.

93. Reichenspurner H, Gamberg P, Nitschke M, et al: Significant reduction in the number of fungal infections after lung-, heart-lung, and heart transplantation using aerosolized amphotericin B prophylaxis. *Transplant Proc* 1997; 29(1-2):627-628.

94. Penn I: Incidence and treatment of neoplasia after transplantation. *J Heart Lung Transplant* 1993; 12(6 Pt 2):S328-336.

95. Paranjothi S, Yusen RD, Kraus MD, Lynch JP, Patterson GA, Trulock EP: Lymphoproliferative disease after lung transplantation: comparison of presentation and outcome of early and late cases. *J Heart Lung Transplant* 2001; 20(10):1054-1063.

96. Theodore J, Morris AJ, Burke CM, et al: Cardiopulmonary function at maximum tolerable constant work rate exercise following human heart-lung transplantation. *Chest* 1987; 92(3):433-439.

97. Weiss ES, Allen JG, Meguid RA, et al: The impact of center volume on survival in lung transplantation: an analysis of more than 10,000 cases. *Ann Thorac Surg* 2009; 88(4):1062-1070.

98. Weiss ES, Allen JG, Merlo CA, Conte JV, Shah AS: Factors indicative of long-term survival after lung transplantation: a review of 836 10-year survivors. *J Heart Lung Transplant* 2010; 29(3):240-246.

99. Demikhov VG: *Experimental Tansplantation of Vital Organs.* New York: Consultants Bureau; 1962.

100. Marcus E, Wong SN, Luisada AA: Homologous heart grafts; transplantation of the heart in dogs. *Surg Forum* 1951:212-217.

101. Webb WR, Deguzman V, Hoopes JE: Cardiopulmonary transplantation: experimental study of current problems. *Am Surg* 1961; 27:236-241.

102. Lower RR, Stofer RC, Hurley EJ, Shumway NE: Complete homograft replacement of the heart and both lungs. *Surgery* 1961; 50:842-845.

103. Haglin J, Telander RL, Muzzall RE, Kiser JC, Strobel CJ: Comparison of Lung Autotransplantation in the Primate and Dog. *Surg Forum* 1963; 14:196-198.

104. Nakae S, Webb WR, Theodorides T, Sugg WL: Respiratory function following cardiopulmonary denervation in dog, cat, and monkey. *Surg Gynecol Obstet* 1967; 125(6):1285-1292.

105. Castaneda AR, Zamora R, Schmidt-Habelmann P, et al: Cardiopulmonary autotransplantation in primates (baboons): late functional results. *Surgery* 1972; 72(6):1064-1070.

106. Castaneda AR, Arnar O, Schmidt-Habelman P, Moller JH, Zamora R: Cardiopulmonary autotransplantation in primates. *J Cardiovasc Surg (Torino)* 1972; 13(5):523-531.

107. Reitz BA, Burton NA, Jamieson SW, et al: Heart and lung transplantation: autotransplantation and allotransplantation in primates with extended survival. *J Thorac Cardiovasc Surg* 1980; 80(3):360-372.

108. Reitz BA, Pennock JL, Shumway NE: Simplified operative method for heart and lung transplantation. *J Surg Res* 1981; 31(1):1-5.

109. Reitz BA, Wallwork JL, Hunt SA, et al: Heart-lung transplantation: successful therapy for patients with pulmonary vascular disease. *N Engl J Med* 1982; 306(10):557-564.

110. De Meester J, Smits JM, Persijn GG, Haverich A: Listing for lung transplantation: life expectancy and transplant effect, stratified by type of end-stage lung disease, the Eurotransplant experience. *J Heart Lung Transplant* 2001; 20(5):518-524.

111. Stoica SC, McNeil KD, Perreas K, et al: Heart-lung transplantation for Eisenmenger syndrome: early and long-term results. *Ann Thorac Surg* 2001; 72(6):1887-1891.

112. Gammie JS, Keenan RJ, Pham SM, et al: Single- versus double-lung transplantation for pulmonary hypertension. *J Thorac Cardiovasc Surg* 1998; 115(2):397-402; discussion 393-402.

113. Marshall SE, Kramer MR, Lewiston NJ, Starnes VA, Theodore J: Selection and evaluation of recipients for heart-lung and lung transplantation. *Chest* 1990; 98(6):1488-1494.

114. Tamm M, Higenbottam TW, Dennis CM, Sharples LD, Wallwork J: Donor and recipient predicted lung volume and lung size after heart-lung transplantation. *Am J Respir Crit Care Med* 1994; 150(2):403-407.

115. Harjula AL, Baldwin JC, Glanville AR, et al: Human leukocyte antigen compatibility in heart-lung transplantation. *J Heart Transplant* 1987; 6(3):162-166.

116. Lick SD, Copeland JG, Rosado LJ, Arabia FA, Sethi GK: Simplified technique of heart-lung transplantation. *Ann Thorac Surg* 1995; 59(6):1592-1593.

117. Lurie KG, Bristow MR, Reitz BA: Increased beta-adrenergic receptor density in an experimental model of cardiac transplantation. *J Thorac Cardiovasc Surg* 1983; 86(2):195-201.

118. Vatner DE, Lavallee M, Amano J, Finizola A, Homcy CJ, Vatner SF: Mechanisms of supersensitivity to sympathomimetic amines in the chronically denervated heart of the conscious dog. *Circ Res* 1985; 57(1):55-64.

119. Kendall SW, Ciulli F, Mullins PA, Biocina B, Dunning JJ, Large SR: Total orthotopic heart transplantation: an alternative to the standard technique. *Ann Thorac Surg* 1992; 54(1):187-188.

120. Sarris GE, Smith JA, Shumway NE, et al: Long-term results of combined heart-lung transplantation: the Stanford experience. *J Heart Lung Transplant* 1994; 13(6):940-949.

121. Higenbottam T, Hutter JA, Stewart S, Wallwork J: Transbronchial biopsy has eliminated the need for endomyocardial biopsy in heart-lung recipients. *J Heart Transplant* 1988; 7(6):435-439.

122. Adams DH, Cochrane AD, Khaghani A, Smith JD, Yacoub MH: Retransplantation in heart-lung recipients with obliterative bronchiolitis. *J Thorac Cardiovasc Surg* 1994; 107(2):450-459.

123. Sarris GE, Moore KA, Schroeder JS, et al: Cardiac transplantation: the Stanford experience in the cyclosporine era. *J Thorac Cardiovasc Surg* 1994; 108(2):240-251; discussion 251-242.

124. Grattan MT, Moreno-Cabral CE, Starnes VA, Oyer PE, Stinson EB, Shumway NE: Cytomegalovirus infection is associated with cardiac allograft rejection and atherosclerosis. *JAMA* 1989; 261(24):3561-3566.

125. Kramer MR, Marshall SE, Starnes VA, Gamberg P, Amitai Z, Theodore J: Infectious complications in heart-lung transplantation. Analysis of 200 episodes. *Arch Intern Med* 1993; 153(17):2010-2016.

Long-term Mechanical Circulatory Support and the Total Artificial Heart

Andrew C. W. Baldwin • Courtney J. Gemmato • William E. Cohn • O. H. Frazier

Heart failure (HF) is a leading cause of death in the United States and a significant public health concern throughout the world. Results from the Framingham Heart Study suggest that the lifetime risk of developing HF for Americans over the age of 40 years is approximately 20%, and the incidence of this disease steadily increases with age.[1] An estimated 5.1 million Americans are living with HF. This figure is expected to grow significantly in the coming decades because the average age of the population is increasing, and advancements in medical therapy are allowing patients to live longer with their disease.[2,3] The economic burden of disease is also high, and total healthcare costs attributed to HF exceed $30 billion in the United States each year.[2,3] In light of the increased mortality associated with HF, strategies for managing this disease have grown increasingly sophisticated.

Treatment of advanced HF is based on three principal methodologies: medical therapy, corrective surgical intervention, and cardiac support or replacement. Appropriate medical management with antihypertensive, diuretic, vasoactive, and inotropic therapy has been shown to improve symptoms, slow the progression of disease, and (in some cases) provide survival benefits.[4] Patients with more severe disease may benefit from specific surgical interventions such as coronary revascularization, valve replacement or repair, and ventricular restoration procedures.[5,6] These procedures often pose a high risk, and surgical candidacy is typically assessed on a case-by-case basis.

Selected patients with severe HF refractory to guideline-directed medical therapy may ultimately be considered candidates for cardiac transplantation or mechanical circulatory support (MCS). Because of a relative scarcity of available donor organs for transplantation, device therapy has become an increasingly popular option for managing end-stage HF and offers documented survival benefits over medical therapy alone.[7] Whereas only 33 centers participated in the original clinical investigation (completed in 2009) of the HeartMate II

left ventricular assist device (LVAD) (Thoratec, Inc., Pleasanton, CA), a total of 145 centers are now approved for device therapy in the United States. This number will likely continue to grow as this technology and other new MCS systems become more widely accessible.[8,9]

MCS is an inclusive term that refers to any device used to assist or replace the failing heart. The options are wide-ranging and include differences in pump location (implantable vs extracorporeal), support capabilities (left, right, or biventricular), and flow characteristics (pulsatile vs continuous). This chapter will focus primarily on the available long-term options for MCS, particularly current LVADs and the total artificial heart (TAH). Although MCS is not without inherent risks, rapid advancements in technology—paired with the practical limitations of transplantation—suggest that device therapy has an important role in both the present and the future of HF surgery.

HISTORY OF MECHANICAL CIRCULATORY SUPPORT

Open heart surgery was made possible by the pioneering efforts of individuals seeking a method to provide temporary cardiopulmonary support by means of a mechanical pump oxygenator. The first successful use of cardiopulmonary bypass (CPB) was reported in 1953 by John Gibbon,[10] who used a CPB system of his own design to repair an atrial septal defect. Excessive mortality rates led some surgeons, including Gibbon himself, to abandon open heart surgery. In 1954, C. Walton Lillehei[11] reported the use of cross circulation (human-to-human perfusion), using a parent as a temporary source of cardiopulmonary support during the repair of congenital heart defects. Controversy stemming from this approach (particularly the risk of a 200% mortality rate) encouraged ongoing research in the field of mechanical support, and efforts led by Lillehei, Richard DeWall, and John Kirklin quickly led to refinements in CPB technology, resulting in improved clinical outcomes.[12] In April 1956, Denton Cooley reported the use of a modified bubble oxygenator in the repair of a postinfarction ventricular septal defect; he would perform 94 open heart procedures (primarily in children) by the end of the year.[13]

The resulting wave of open heart procedures quickly led to the observation that some patients were unable to regain sufficient cardiac function to permit withdrawal from the heart-lung machine. Anecdotal experience suggested that slow weaning (over the course of hours) allowed some hearts to successfully recover function[14] (Fig. 62-1). As a result, interest in prolonged circulatory support led to the concept of a ventricular assist device (VAD). Decades earlier, the eccentric Russian scientist Vladimir Demikhov had successfully designed and tested a device capable of maintaining the perfusion of a dog for several hours.[15] Although this breakthrough occurred in 1937, his experiments were not widely known outside the Soviet Union until years later. Throughout the 1960s, research efforts at a number of institutions were focused on the development of MCS technology. A federally funded program with this goal was established at Baylor College of Medicine, in Houston, with Michael DeBakey as its director.

The first clinical application of an LVAD was performed by DeBakey in 1963, who used the device as a temporizing measure in a patient with cardiogenic shock after aortic valve replacement. Although the pump functioned satisfactorily, the patient succumbed to pulmonary complications

4 days after its implantation. On August 8, 1966, DeBakey implanted an LVAD in a 37-year-old woman with severe HF who could not be weaned from CPB after aortic and mitral valve replacement. An extracorporeal pneumatic device, the pump routed blood from the left atrium to the right axillary artery. After 10 days of support, the patient demonstrated sufficient cardiac reserve to allow elective removal of the pump at the bedside.[14] She later returned to work, resumed normal activity, and survived for 6 years with good cardiac function before dying in an auto accident. In 1969, in an event that will be discussed later in this chapter, Cooley implanted the world's first TAH to great acclaim.[16] Despite this landmark event, effective long-term total heart replacement proved to be an elusive goal over the ensuing decades.

By the early 1970s, the complexities of immunosuppressive therapy led to waning enthusiasm for cardiac transplantation and associated MCS technology. However, research and development efforts focused on VAD therapy were continued steadily and quietly within a selected group of institutions. With support from the National Heart, Lung, and Blood Institute (NHLBI) and in collaboration with Boston-based Thermo Cardiosystems, physicians at the Texas Heart Institute began development of an abdominally positioned, pneumatically driven, pulsatile-flow LVAD. Twenty-two patients were supported by the Model 7 abdominal LVAD, including the first documented mechanical "bridge" to cardiac transplantation, performed in 1978.[17] The introduction of cyclosporine in the 1980s eventually led to renewed widespread interest in the field of transplantation and reestablished a meaningful clinical role for MCS technology. Ongoing research efforts to

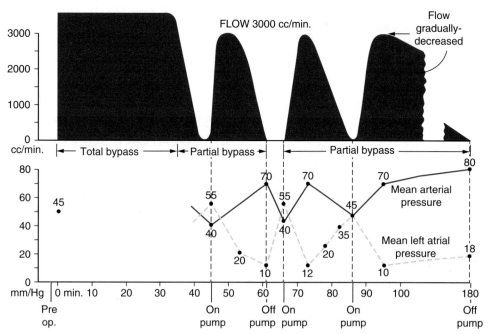

FIGURE 62-1 Correlation between cardiopulmonary bypass flows, mean arterial pressure, and left atrial pressure in a patient with left ventricular failure after aortic valve replacement. The observed efficacy of gradual weaning from cardiopulmonary bypass helped stimulate interest in mechanical circulatory support. (Reproduced with permission from DeBakey ME. Left ventricular bypass pump for cardiac assistance: clinical experience, *Am J Cardiol.* 1971 Jan;27(1):3-11.)

develop pumps capable of long-term support ultimately led to the HeartMate Implantable Pneumatic pump (Thoratec Corp; Pleasanton, CA), which became the first implantable device to be approved by the United States Food and Drug Administration (FDA) for use as a bridge to transplantation (BTT).[18,19] An electrically powered, percutaneously vented adaptation of this device, the HeartMate Extended Vented Electric (XVE) LVAD, was spawned directly by these research efforts. Upon its inaugural implantation in 1991, it became the first pump to be managed in the outpatient setting.[20]

Simultaneously, research efforts were engaged in the design of a completely different mechanism. The concept of extended nonpulsatile support was inspired by anecdotal reports concerning the use of the extracorporeal BioMedicus centrifugal-force pump (Medtronic; Minneapolis, MN) as both a temporary LVAD and an extracorporeal membrane oxygenator (ECMO). This led to a series of experimental studies that were performed by the senior author of this chapter (OHF) in the Texas Heart Institute laboratories throughout the 1980s. As a result of these efforts (and in collaboration with engineer Richard Wampler) the Hemopump, a small catheter-based, axial-flow device, was developed and successfully implanted in 1988, demonstrating the efficacy and safety of high-speed continuous-flow (CF) support[21] (Fig. 62-2). Also during this period, an association between Texas Heart Institute investigators and researcher Robert Jarvik led to the development of a long-term implantable CF pump that could be placed directly into the left ventricle.[22] The Jarvik 2000 VAD (Jarvik Heart, Inc.; New York, NY) was unique in its utilization of blood-washed bearings (previously thought to be biologically incompatible with the vascular system) and validated the clinical feasibility of axial-based CF pumps[23] (Fig. 62-3). Meanwhile, the clinical success of the Hemopump led the Nimbus Company (later absorbed by Thoratec) to develop

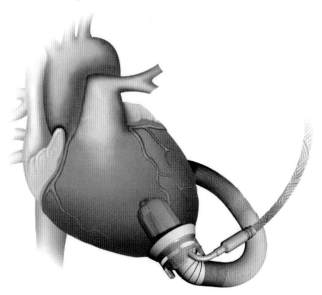

FIGURE 62-3 The Jarvik 2000 was the first left ventricular assist device to incorporate blood-washed bearings in its axial flow design. (Used with permission from Jarvik Heart, Inc.)

the HeartMate II, another implantable axial-flow device, which would eventually become the most commonly used LVAD worldwide. A final step in the development of contemporary MCS systems occurred in 1994, when collaboration between Frazier, Wampler, and financier Robert Fine led to the development of a novel CF design. Originally produced by Kriton Medical, Inc. (and later purchased by HeartWare, Inc., Framingham, MA), the HeartWare HVAD utilizes a magnetically levitated, centrifugal-flow design that permits intrapericardial placement of the discoid-shaped pump housing and can function as both a right- and left-sided VAD.[24] Within the first decade of the new millennium, all three pumps—the Jarvik 2000, the HeartMate II, and the HeartWare HVAD—saw clinical use.

Increasingly sophisticated technology and improving clinical reliability gradually led MCS to shift from an experimental endeavor to a viable treatment option. The Randomized Evaluation of Mechanical Assistance for the Treatment of Congestive Heart Failure (REMATCH) trial was designed to compare outcomes between HF patients treated with the HeartMate XVE and those treated with medical therapy alone.[7] Completed in 2001, REMATCH investigators demonstrated a nearly 50% reduction in mortality among patients with LVAD support (Fig. 62-4). By providing the first statistical evidence of a survival benefit, this study remains a landmark in the advancement of MCS therapy. Following the success of REMATCH, the HeartMate II soon became the first CF device to be approved by the FDA for both BTT indications (in 2007) and for use in patients ineligible for transplantation (2009).[25,26] The HeartWare HVAD was granted BTT status after the release of the results of the ADVANCE trial in 2010, and it is expected to receive broader approval in the near future.[27] With more pumps and

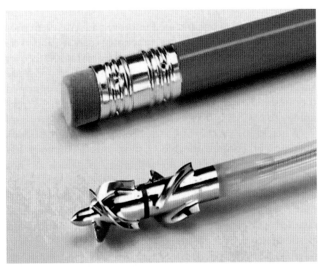

FIGURE 62-2 The catheter-based hemopump first revealed the safety and feasibility of high-speed continuous-flow circulatory support. (Used with permission from Dr. Richard Wampler.)

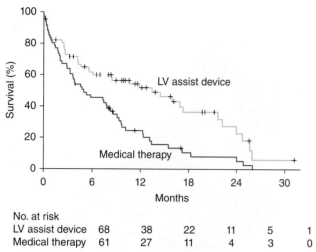

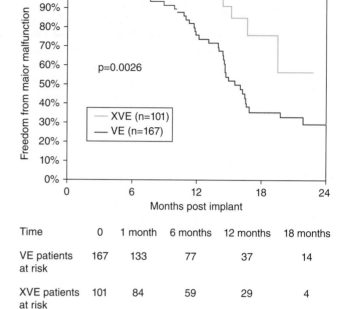

FIGURE 62-4 Kaplan-Meier survival analysis comparing end-stage heart failure patients randomized to receive either optimal medical therapy or left ventricular assist device support. The REMATCH trial researchers demonstrated a significant survival benefit for device recipients at both 1 and 2 years. (Reproduced with permission from Rose EA, Gelijns AC, Moskowitz AJ, et al: Long-term use of a left ventricular assist device for end-stage heart failure, *N Engl J Med.* 2001 Nov 15;345(20):1435-1443.)

Time	0	1 month	6 months	12 months	18 months
VE patients at risk	167	133	77	37	14
XVE patients at risk	101	84	59	29	4

FIGURE 62-5 Freedom from all major device malfunctions for the HeartMate VE and HeartMate XVE left ventricular assist devices. (Reproduced with permission from Pagani et al. Improved mechanical reliability of the HeartMate XVE Left Ventricular Assist System, *Ann Thorac Surg.* 2006 Oct;82(4):1413-1418.)

newer designs in the pipeline, options for MCS continue to grow with ever-improving outcomes.

PULSATILE VERSUS NONPULSATILE FLOW

A critical issue in the field of MCS is the physical mechanism by which flow is created. Quite logically, early efforts in device therapy sought to mimic nature's model by designing pulsatile systems. Generations of devices have utilized pneumatic compression systems, hydraulic actuators, and pusher plate technology to allow repetitive filling and forceful ejection of blood from a ventricular collection chamber. However, the engineering challenges associated with matching the simplicity and reliability of the human heart—which beats more than 40 million times each year—have been considerable.

A chief cause of late pulsatile-device failure is mechanical wear, which results from the presence of complex moving components and multiple points of contact. For example, although the HeartMate XVE represented a significant step forward, it had a relatively predictable lifespan, with a high failure rate between the first and second years of use, and few of these devices survived for more than 2 years[28] (Fig. 62-5). Pulsatility also requires a number of disadvantageous design elements to accommodate the mechanics of operation. Pneumatic systems use tunneled drivelines to communicate with an external compressor responsible for delivering (and withdrawing) pressurized air. Pusher-plate systems (such as that used for the XVE) require a mechanism to allow external venting and aspiration of air displaced by the cyclic actuation of the pump. As a result of these inescapable challenges, pulsatile pumps are generally large, complex, and vulnerable to wear.

Temporary CF technology was first adopted by Gibbon, who employed roller pumps in the design of his machine that first enabled CPB support during surgery.[10] However, early efforts to develop long-term MCS pumps focused on pulsatile blood flow to replicate natural physiology. The eventual development of CF LVADs was largely due to their associated engineering advantages, and both experimental and clinical studies quickly documented the physiologic tolerance of nonpulsatility. The technical superiority of CF devices was definitively shown in the HeartMate II Destination Therapy (DT) trial,[26] which documented improved adverse event profiles, hospital readmission rates, functional capacity, and overall survival when compared with the HeartMate XVE over a 2-year period (Table 62-1; Fig. 62-6). The widespread use and long-term efficacy of CF devices has further confirmed the important contribution of continuous blood-flow technology to MCS.

Whereas the success of CF devices has proven the body's tolerance of nonpulsatile blood flow, this technology has created a new physiology, the full effects of which are not yet known. Multiple studies have shown an association between gastrointestinal (GI) bleeding and the loss of pulsatility.[29] Histologic examination of aortic tissue samples have revealed unanticipated degeneration of smooth muscle and elastic fibers in patients supported by CF devices.[30] Ultrasonographic studies have further revealed stasis and thrombus formation representing potential sources of thromboembolism within the carotid bulb and aortic valve cusps of selected patients with nonpulsatile devices.[31] These issues present a

TABLE 62-1: Comparison of Continuous Flow and Pulsatile LVAD Outcomes and Adverse Event Profiles

Adverse Event	Continuous Flow LVAD (n = 133) No. (%)	Pulsatile Flow LVAD (n = 59) No. (%)	p Value
Pump replacement	12 (9)	20 (34)	<.001
LVAD-related infection	47 (35)	21 (36)	.01
Sepsis	48 (36)	26 (44)	<.001
Respiratory failure	50 (38)	24 (41)	<.001
Renal failure	21 (16)	14 (24)	<.001
Cardiac arrhythmia	75 (56)	35 (59)	.006
Rehospitalization	107 (94)	42 (96)	.02
Quality of Life Metric	**Score (12 months)**	**Score (12 months)**	**p Value**
Minnesota	34.1 ± 22.4	44.4 ± 23.2	.03
Kansas City	65.9 ± 20	59.1 ± 20.3	.06

LVAD, left ventricular assist device; Minnesota, Minnesota Living with Heart Failure questionnaire; Kansas City, Kansas City Cardiomyopathy Questionnaire. Adapted with permission from Slaughter et al. Advanced heart failure treated with continuous-flow left ventricular assist device, *N Engl J Med.* 2009 Dec 3;361(23):2241-2251.

significant challenge, but the engineering advantages afforded by CF pumps are considerable. These devices are smaller, more efficient, and much more durable than their pulsatile counterparts. Without the need for compliance chambers and pneumatic vents, CF pumps permit increased patient

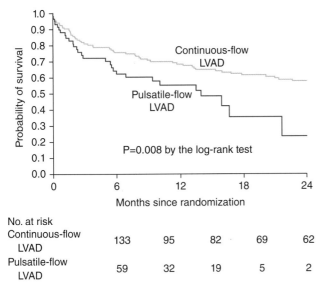

FIGURE 62-6 Kaplan-Meier survival analysis comparison of patients supported by continuous flow and pulsatile left ventricular assist devices. (Reproduced with permission from Slaughter et al. Advanced heart failure treated with continuous-flow left ventricular assist device, *N Engl J Med.* 2009 Dec 3;361(23):2241-2251.)

mobility and offer the potential for completely implantable designs. Although much more remains to be studied, CF technology represents the future of MCS.

CURRENT OPTIONS FOR MECHANICAL CIRCULATORY SUPPORT

Currently, device therapy involves a wide variety of options, obtainable through federally approved indications or investigational studies. The pumps differ in a number of important ways, including the duration of support permitted, approach to access, mechanisms of flow, and output capabilities. The most frequently used pumps and selected other devices of interest—notably all CF designs—are discussed below. A more thorough listing of currently available devices is provided in Table 62-2.

ECMO

Oxygenation of the blood by a membrane oxygenator can be achieved through the use of either veno-venous (VV) or veno-arterial (VA) ECMO. The VV option is typically used for the management of isolated respiratory failure, and it relies on the function of the native heart for systemic circulation of oxygenated blood. In contrast, through an arterial return cannula, VA ECMO allows complete cardiopulmonary support, similar to that provided by CPB. Cannulation may be central or peripheral, rendering ECMO particularly useful in both emergent and intraoperative situations. It is generally limited to periods of short-term support (measured in days).

Paracorporeal and Percutaneous Devices

A subset of devices can be inserted percutaneously or involve extracorporeal pumping components. Recent studies have shown a dramatic increase in the utilization of these short-term devices,[32] which are typically used for temporary MCS in the setting of acute cardiogenic or postcardiotomy shock. The CentriMag (Thoratec Corp.) is an extracorporeal VAD utilizing a magnetically levitated centrifugal flow impeller that can provide both right- and left-sided support (Fig. 62-7a). Access is typically gained via centrally placed CPB cannulas that can be tunneled to allow temporary chest closure. Capable of flows reaching 10 L/min, the CentriMag can also accommodate an oxygenator within the pumping circuit, permitting full cardiopulmonary support. The device is generally used for days to weeks, but support periods exceeding 30 days have been reported.[33]

The TandemHeart Percutaneous Ventricular Assist Device (pVAD) (CardiacAssist Inc.; Pittsburgh, PA) is a percutaneous device that functions as a left atriofemoral bypass. Inserted under fluoroscopic guidance, the TandemHeart has a transseptal cannula that transfers oxygenated blood from the heart to an extracorporeal, magnetically driven, centrifugal flow pump mounted on the thigh. Using a hydrodynamic

⬤ TABLE 62-2: Currently Available Options for Mechanical Circulatory Support

Device	Manufacturer	Flow type	Design	First human implant	Approval status	
					Worldwide	*United States*
Paracorporeal						
CentriMag®	Thoratec Corp. (Pleasanton, CA)	Continuous	Centrifugal	2003	CE Mark—2002	FDA 510(k)—2002 FDA IDE—2008 FDA HDE *RVAD—2008*
Percutaneous						
Impella 5.0®/CP®/ RP®	ABIOMED	Continuous	Microaxial	1999	CE Mark *5.0—2003* *CP—2012* *RP—2014*	FDA 510(k) *5.0—2009* *CP—2012* FDA HDE *RP—2015*
TandemHeart™	CardiacAssist, Inc. (Pittsburgh, PA)	Continuous	Centrifugal	2005	CE Mark—2000	FDA 510(k)—2003 FDA IDE—2012
Implantable LVADs						
HeartMate® II	Thoratec	Continuous	Axial	2000	CE Mark—2005	FDA BTT—2008 FDA DT—2010
Jarvik 2000 Flowmaker®	Jarvik Heart, Inc. (New York, NY)	Continuous	Axial	2000	CE Mark—2005	FDA IDE—2000 *BTT Trial Pending*
INCOR®	Berlin Heart GmbH (Berlin, Germany)	Continuous	Axial	2002	CE Mark—2003	—
EVAHEART®	Evaheart, Inc. (Houston, TX)	Continuous	Centrifugal	2005	CE Mark—2015 PMDA—2010	FDA IDE—2009 *BTT Trial Pending*
HVAD®	HeartWare, Inc. (Framingham, MA)	Continuous	Centrifugal	2006	CE Mark—2009	FDA BTT—2012 *DT Trial Pending*
HeartAssist 5®	ReliantHeart, Inc. (Houston, TX)	Continuous	Axial	2009	CE Mark—2013	FDA IDE—2014 *BTT Trial Pending*
HeartMate® III	Thoratec	Continuous	Centrifugal	2014	*CE Mark Pending*	FDA IDE—2014 *BTT/DT trial pending*
MVAD®	HeartWare	Continuous	Axial	2015	*CE Mark Pending*	*Awaiting FDA IDE*
Total Artificial Heart						
SynCardia TAH	SynCardia Systems, Inc. (Tucson, AZ)	Pulsatile	Pneumatic	1982	CE Mark—1999	FDA HDE—2004

CE Mark, European Union Conformité Européenne Approval; FDA, United States Food and Drug Administration; 510(k), Premarket Notification Clearance; PMA, premarket approval; IDE, investigational device exemption; HDE, humanitarian device exemption; BTT, bridge to transplant; DT, destination therapy; PMDA, Japanese Pharmaceuticals and Medical Devices Agency Approval; TAH, total artificial heart.

bearing system, the TandemHeart can provide the femoral artery with return flows reaching 4 L/min.[34]

The Impella (Abiomed; Danvers, MA) is a platform of devices based upon a catheter-mounted microaxial design conceptually similar to that of the original Hemopump (Fig. 62-7b). A percutaneous arterial catheter serves as a power source and flow conduit for the pump, and left-sided support is provided in a retrograde fashion across the aortic valve. With a maximal diameter of just 12 F (4 mm), various adaptations of the device allow flows ranging from 2.5 to 5 L/ min. A right-sided version, the Impella RP, delivers antegrade flow from the inferior vena cava to the pulmonary artery. It recently became the first percutaneous device approved by the FDA for right ventricular (RV) support.[35]

Implantable Continuous-Flow LVADs (FDA-Approved)

The HeartMate II axial-flow device is the most widely used LVAD worldwide, with more than 15,000 implants to date (Fig. 62-8a). The pump's electromagnetic motor powers a single hydrodynamically suspended impeller operating at speeds between 6000 and 15,000 rpm (although clinical operating ranges are traditionally much smaller), and capable of flows greater than 10 L/min. Most often implanted via median sternotomy, the sintered titanium pump inlet is placed within the left ventricle with an outflow graft anastomosed to the aorta. A percutaneous driveline communicates with the remainder of the system: an external device controller and two portable batteries.

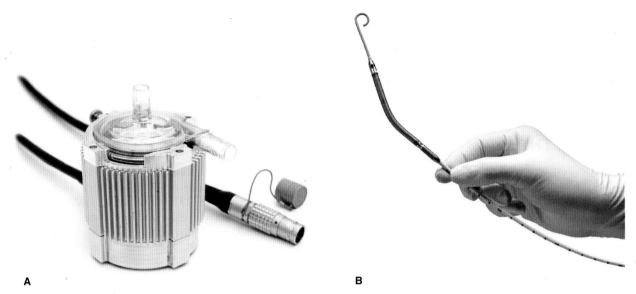

A B

FIGURE 62-7 Percutaneous ventricular assist devices. (A) The Thoratec Centrimag utilizes an extracorporeal magnetically levitated centrifugal-flow pump to provide temporary circulatory support. (Reproduced with permission from Thoratec Corporation.) (B) The Impella CP is a catheter-based pump designed to be positioned across the aortic valve and capable of producing flows as high as 4 L/min. (Reproduced with permission from ABIOMED, Inc.)

The HeartWare HVAD has a centrifugal-flow design, with a smaller and more compact profile than the HeartMate II (145 vs 375 g, respectively), integrating the ventricular inlet with the pump housing (Fig. 62-8b). The impeller is suspended via a combination of magnetic and hydrodynamic forces, and it operates at speeds ranging from 1800 to 4000 rpm, again with flows as high as 10 L/min. The flat surface of the pump body allows intrapericardial positioning and serves as an advantage for right-sided use. Like the HeartMate II, the HVAD relies on external batteries and a controller module connected to the patient by a percutaneous driveline.

A number of additional devices remain in various stages of investigational study in the United States and are likely to be more widely available in the coming years. On the

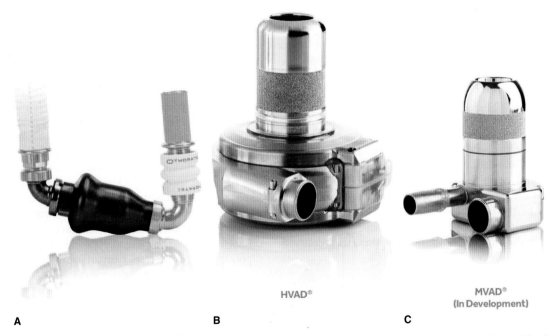

HVAD® MVAD® (In Development)

A B C

FIGURE 62-8 The HeartMate II (A) and the HeartWare HVAD (B) are the two most commonly implanted devices worldwide. While the HeartMate II utilizes an axial-flow design with an extracardiac pump housing, the centrifugal HVAD has a discoid shape designed for intrapericardial placement. Newer-generation devices, such as the HeartWare MVAD (C), reflect increasing miniaturization of mechanical circulatory support technology. (Used with permission from Thoratec Corporation [a] and HeartWare International, Inc. [b and c].)

whole, newer-generation pumps are being designed to produce excellent performance while offering a smaller profile, thus simplifying implantation and expanding potential applications to include smaller-framed and pediatric populations (Fig. 62-8c). TAH technology is discussed later in this chapter.

GOALS OF THERAPY

Before device implantation, treatment teams must designate an intended goal of therapy. Traditional categories of strategic intent represent the evolution of MCS. Originally, devices were conceived as temporizing measures while the patient awaited a transplant. The eventual inclusion of transplant-ineligible patients for device consideration required a new and separate indication, resulting in the somewhat dichotomous framework in use today. Ideally, the decision to seek device therapy should be based on the need for mechanical support rather than being indirectly affected by the patient's transplant listing status. However, the decision currently serves a critical purpose in regard to patient and device selection, timing of intervention, regulatory oversight, and data acquisition. Clinical trials aimed at seeking device approval have traditionally been designed on this model. Likewise, the United States Centers for Medicare and Medicaid Services (CMS) uses the indicated strategy for device therapy to establish a given patient's eligibility for treatment. The categories are a part of the MCS lexicon and warrant inclusion here.

Bridge to Transplantation

The original intention for MCS was to provide a "bridge" to eventual cardiac transplantation for patients awaiting a suitable donor organ. Unpredictable waitlist times and a frequently tenuous clinical condition make these patients particularly vulnerable to deterioration while awaiting a transplant. The decision to seek a BTT strategy requires consideration of estimated waitlist times, the potential for a decline in clinical status before transplantation, the patient's quality of life, and the risk of death while on the waiting list. Progressively longer waitlist times throughout the United States have resulted in the relatively standard use of BTT for the treatment of transplant-eligible patients with end-stage HF.[36] Whereas BTT remains the most common implant strategy for MCS (nearly 65% of these patients are designated as transplant candidates), the percentage of patients officially listed for a transplant at the time of device implantation has steadily declined, now totaling just 21.7%.[37]

Destination Therapy

Patients with end-stage HF who are not eligible for transplantation may benefit from MCS as a means to prolong or improve the quality of their life. The designation of destination therapy (DT) originates from the REMATCH trial, in which transplant-ineligible patients supported by MCS had better outcomes than patients supported by medical therapy alone.[7] Through this designation, patients with systemic life-threatening illnesses, malignancies, fixed pulmonary hypertension, advanced age, and morbid obesity may benefit from device therapy regardless of their transplant listing status. Designation as DT does not imply a limitation on the timeframe for treatment, as uninterrupted CF support surpassing 9 years has been reported. Over the past 7 years, the proportion of patients categorized as DT candidates at the time of implantation has steadily increased from 14.7 to 41.6%—likely as a result of increased access to FDA-approved devices for DT, as well as recognition of the possibility of reassessing the transplant status throughout the period of device support.

Bridge to Decision

The use of long-term MCS in the setting of acute hemodynamic collapse or active decompensation results in comparatively poor outcomes.[37] Short-term MCS offers the advantage of rapid and relatively less invasive access to device therapy while allowing stabilization of the patient and consideration of long-term device candidacy. Thus, patients with a myocardial infarction, myocarditis, acute cardiogenic shock, or unsuccessful percutaneous intervention can be quickly transitioned to support in anticipation of recovery, decline, or optimization before the initiation of long-term MCS.

Myocardial Reconditioning

In a selected subset of patients, a distinct improvement in ventricular function has allowed device weaning and (occasionally) deactivation. Beginning in the 1990s, studies have revealed histologic and clinical evidence of myocardial rehabilitation after periods of both pulsatile and CF device support.[38-40] Often labeled a "bridge to recovery," this phenomenon is perhaps better described as a return to medical HF therapy. A number of institutions have proposed device-weaning strategies, ranging from aggressive medical therapy using high-dose beta blockade to mechanical offloading and gradual reconditioning of the heart through systematic titration of pump speeds.[41-43] Despite promising reports, only a small percentage of patients have successfully experienced this outcome. Although little is known with certainty regarding the precise variables that govern the pace and degree of myocardial response, the potential for de-escalation of therapy supports an aggressive pursuit of weaning strategies in all patients who require device support.

Fluidity of Implantation Strategy

It is important to recognize that these designations apply only to the stated goal at the time of device implantation. Whereas regulatory guidelines mandate a proposed goal of therapy, the available choices do not reflect the reality that a patient's clinical status and transplant candidacy may change during periods of mechanical support. Although some patients may have a deteriorating clinical status or develop unexpected contraindications to transplantation, other patients—such as those with preoperative "fixed" pulmonary hypertension—may experience an improvement in conditions that originally precluded transplant listing.[44,45] The dynamic nature of device strategy is represented in reported device usage statistics, in that nearly 26% of patients initially listed for BTT were no longer listed at 1 year, and that number rose to 43.5% by 24 months. Similarly, nearly 15% of patients designated for DT at the time of device implantation were deemed eligible for transplantation by 12 months.[46] Frequent reappraisal and modification of treatment strategies corresponding to clinical status are essential for successful MCS outcomes.

INDICATIONS FOR DEVICE SUPPORT

Optimal strategies and indications for the initiation of MCS remain subjects of active investigation. Traditional hemodynamic parameters for device support continue to surface in the literature; although not absolute, these variables include blood pressure (BP) < 80 mm Hg, mean arterial pressure (MAP) < 65 mm Hg, cardiac index < 2 L/min/m², and pulmonary capillary wedge pressure (PCWP) > 20 mm Hg.[47] Strict following of hemodynamic markers can be misleading, however, as patients may present not just in acute cardiogenic shock but also with a more insidious manifestation of congestive HF. In 2013, the International Society for Heart and Lung Transplantation (ISHLT) proposed a thorough and broad-ranging compilation of recommendations for the use of MCS.[36] Although many of the proposed guidelines are limited by the relative weakness of available supporting evidence, they represent the most comprehensive and ambitious summary of consensus opinion,

and underscore the multiorgan and multidisciplinary approach to device candidacy.

In 2013, the American College of Cardiology Foundation (ACCF) and American Heart Association (AHA) released a broad slate of guidelines for the management of HF.[4] The report endorsed the use of an alternative to the traditional New York Heart Association (NYHA) staging system, emphasizing disease-specific markers rather than patient-specific symptoms (Table 62-3). The guidelines support the use of durable MCS in patients with so-called Stage D HF (refractory disease requiring specialized interventions) with reduced left ventricular ejection fraction (LVEF) as a means to both prolong survival and BTT. Although the authors refrain from further characterizing patient selection criteria, the guidelines do emphasize the perceived importance of refractory disease, reduced EF, and severe symptomatology.

In 2013, CMS released updated eligibility criteria for the use of MCS as DT in Medicare beneficiaries.[48] More specific than the ACCF/AHA guidelines, the federal standards allow the use of DT only for patients with end-stage HF (NYHA class IV) who are deemed ineligible for transplantation at the time of device implantation and who meet each of the following conditions: (a) failure to respond to optimal medical management for 45 of the last 60 days, balloon pump dependence for 7 days, or IV inotrope dependence for 14 days; (b) LVEF < 25%; and (c) measured peak oxygen consumption of <14 mL/kg/min or an inability to perform the test. The federal requirements for BTT designation are somewhat broader, mandating only that patients be listed for transplantation by an approved transplant center. However, use of a device for any purpose is permitted only if that specific device has been granted FDA approval for the chosen therapeutic goal.

The Interagency Registry for Mechanically Assisted Circulatory Support (INTERMACS) database was established in 2008 to facilitate the growth of MCS and improve patient outcomes. Paired with the registry's first report was a proposal

---

TABLE 62-3: Comparison of ACCF/AHA Stages of HF and NYHA Functional Classifications

ACCF/AHA HF stages		NYHA functional classification	
A	At high risk for HF but without structural heart disease or symptoms of HF	I	No limitation of physical activity. Ordinary physical activity does not cause symptoms of HF
B	Structural heart disease but without signs or symptoms of HF	II	Slight limitation of physical activity. Comfortable at rest, but ordinary physical activity results in symptoms of HF
C	Structural heart disease with prior or current symptoms of HF	III	Marked limitation of physical activity. Comfortable at rest, but less than ordinary activity causes symptoms of HF
D	Refractory HF requiring specialized interventions	IV	Unable to carry on any physical activity without symptoms of HF, or symptoms of HF at rest

ACCF, American College of Cardiology Foundation; AHA, American Heart Association; NYHA, New York Heart Association; HF, heart failure.
Reproduced with permission from Yancy CW, Jessup M, Bozkurt B, et al: 2013 ACCF/AHA guideline for the management of heart failure: a report of the American College of Cardiology Foundation/American Heart Association Task Force on practice guidelines, *Circulation.* 2013 Oct 15;128(16):e240-e327.

TABLE 62-4: INTERMACS Clinical Profiles of Advanced Heart Failure

Profile	Description	Timeframe for definitive intervention
1	Patient with life-threatening hypotension despite rapidly escalating inotropic support, critical organ hypoperfusion with increasing lactate levels and/or systemic acidosis. "*Crash and burn*"	Needed within hours
2	Patient with declining function despite intravenous inotropic support, may be manifest by worsening renal function, nutritional depletion, inability to restore volume balance. "*Sliding on inotropes*"	Needed within few days
3	Patient with stable blood pressure, organ function, nutrition, and symptoms on continuous intravenous inotropic support, but demonstrating repeated failure to wean owing to recurrent symptomatic hypotension or renal dysfunction. "*Dependent stability*"	Elective over a few weeks
4	Patient can be stabilized close to normal volume status but experiences frequent relapses into fluid retention, generally with high diuretic doses. Symptoms are recurrent rather than refractory. More intensive management strategies should be considered, which in some cases reveal poor compliance. "*Frequent flyer*"	Elective over weeks to months as long as treatment of episodes restores stable baseline, including nutrition
5	Patient is living predominantly within the house, performing activities of daily living and walking from room to room with some difficulty. Patient is comfortable at rest without congestive symptoms, but may have underlying refractory elevated volume status, often with renal dysfunction. "*Housebound*"	Variable, depends upon nutrition, organ function, and activity
6	Patient without evidence of fluid overload is comfortable at rest and with activities of daily living and minor activities outside the home, but fatigues after the first minutes of any meaningful activity. "*Walking wounded*"	Variable, depends upon nutrition, organ function, and activity
7	A placeholder for future specification, patients without recent unstable fluid balance, living comfortably with meaningful activity limited to mild exertion	Transplantation or circulatory support not currently indicated

Reproduced, with permission, from Stevenson LW, Couper G: On the fledgling field of mechanical circulatory support, *J Am Coll Cardiol.* 2007 Aug 21;50(8):748-751.

for a new system of classifying patients with advanced HF.[49] Seven clinical profiles were designed to establish an enhanced method for characterizing patients requiring device therapy (Table 62-4). These profiles represent a stratification of patients diagnosed with advanced HF—defined as NYHA class III and IV symptoms despite optimal therapy. By documenting the profiles of patients undergoing device implantation, INTER-MACS provides an opportunity to evaluate data and trends concerning surgical risks and indications. Clinical practice has indeed shifted since the introduction of this system, most notably through de-escalation of the preoperative clinical profile. Whereas more than 60% of patients who received device implants before 2011 were listed as having INTERMACS 1 or 2 status, the proportion of patients classified as having level 3 status has steadily increased, now representing nearly a third of all who receive implants.[8,50] Indications and guidelines continue to evolve, but these results illustrate a clear trend in the management of HF toward intervening during periods of reduced clinical acuity.

CONTRAINDICATIONS TO DEVICE SUPPORT

Relative contraindications to device therapy include irreversible major end-organ dysfunction, severe hemodynamic instability, profound coagulopathy, complex congenital anomalies, and restrictive heart disease with decreased ventricular dimensions. Because successful outcomes have nevertheless been reported in these populations, decisions should be made on a case-by-case basis in order to weigh the potential risks and benefits of intervention.[51,52] Surgery should be deferred in the presence of active infection or bacteremia to minimize the risk of bacterial device seeding; current recommendations suggest a minimum of 5 days of culture-documented clearance from infection.[36]

PREOPERATIVE EVALUATION

Once potential candidacy for device support has been determined, a thorough appraisal of perioperative risk is warranted. If at all possible, implantation of long-term MCS device should be performed electively, not under emergent circumstances. Identification of preoperative risk factors and treatment of reversible comorbidities can greatly improve patient outcomes.

Due to the importance of proper patient selection, efforts to predict early mortality after LVAD implantation have been a consistent theme in MCS research. During the era of pulsatile LVADs, several risk-evaluation scoring systems were developed with variable predictive utility. One of the most widely used of these scales, the Leitz-Miller destination therapy risk score (DTRS), was derived from a cohort of over

TABLE 62-5: Multivariable Predictors of 90-Day Mortality (HeartMate II Risk Score)

Parameter	SE	OR (95% CI)	p Value
Age (years)	0.12	1.32 (1.05-1.65)	.018
Albumin (g/dL)	0.23	0.49 (0.31-0.76)	.002
Creatinine (mg/dL)	0.20	2.10 (1.37-3.21)	<.001
INR	0.32	3.11 (1.66-5.84)	<.001
Center volume	0.34	2.24 (1.15-4.37)	.018

	Low risk	Medium risk	High risk
HMRS score	<1.58	1.58-2.48	>2.48
90-Day survival	96% (± 1%)	84% (± 2%)	71% (± 4%)

HMRS = (0.0274 × Age) − (0.723 × Alb) + (0.74 × Creat) + (1.136 × INR) + (0.807 × Vol).
*Center Volume: Yearly LVAD implant volume <15, value = "0"; Yearly volume >15, value = "1".
SE,standard error; OR, odds ratio; CI, confidence interval; INR, international normalized ratio; HMRS, HeartMate II Risk Score; Alb, albumin; Creat, creatinine; Vol, yearly device implant volume; LVAD, left ventricular assist device.
Adapted with permission from Cowger J1, Sundareswaran K, Rogers JG, et al: Predicting Survival in Patients Receiving Continuous Flow Left Ventricular Assist Devices: The HeartMate II Risk Score, *J Am Coll Cardiol.* 2013 Jan 22; 61(3):313-321.

300 HeartMate XVE patients and incorporated 9 weighted variables to estimate 90-day in-hospital mortality.[53] When systematically tested in a CF LVAD population; however, DTRS was found to provide only modest discriminatory value.[54] In contrast, the Model of End-Stage Liver Disease (MELD) has been shown to be a predictor of adverse events after implantation of both pulsatile and CF LVADs.[55] Utilizing only the creatinine level, total bilirubin level, and international normalized ratio (INR), the MELD score (and later the anticoagulation-compatible MELD-XI score) was found to correlate with overall and postoperative survival.[56] More recently, a global risk-assessment scale was developed using only CF data culled from the HeartMate II clinical trials database. The HeartMate II multivariable risk score (HMRS) utilizes five variables—patient age, albumin level, creatinine level, INR, and implanting center volume—to predict 90-day postoperative mortality[57] (Table 62-5). While similar to MELD in its direct comparison of predictive results, HMRS is more specifically designed for HF patients and may offer a modest benefit in outcome discrimination.[58] To date, no risk-assessment scale has shown absolute superiority in preoperative risk stratification, but the available models do emphasize the importance of preoperative optimization of overall end-organ function.

Operative Risk

As with any proposed cardiothoracic procedure, the surgical complexity of each case must be carefully addressed early in the evaluation process. Unfavorable anatomical scenarios—such as a history of previous sternotomies, congenital anomalies, or heavily calcified anastomotic sites—are common in this patient population and significantly escalate operative risk.

The utility of concomitant cardiac and valvular procedures is poorly understood and remains controversial. Whereas some studies have suggested that concurrent procedures are associated with diminished overall survival, consensus opinion does support intervention in specific situations.[36,59,60] Native aortic insufficiency has been shown not only to adversely affect the performance of CF pumps but also to speed the progression of valvular incompetence.[61] Although clinical practice varies, ISHLT guidelines suggest concurrent intervention for regurgitation deemed moderate or greater.[36] The presence of a mechanical prosthesis entails a prohibitive risk of thromboembolic complications and warrants surgical exclusion through ligation of the LV outflow tract, supravalvular patch closure, or a placement of a felt sandwich plug.[62-65] Tricuspid regurgitation has been implicated in the development of postoperative right-sided HF (RHF), and guidelines generally support intervention—either replacement or ring repair—for disease classified as moderate or greater.[36,66-68] The presence of mitral regurgitation (MR) does not typically necessitate surgical intervention at the time of device implantation. Whereas MR is common in patients with end-stage HF, this finding is often the result of annular distortion secondary to dilation of the left ventricle and typically improves with mechanical decompression and offloading.[69] Due to an increased risk for right-to-left shunting, atrial septal defects and patent foramen ovale (PFO) should be closed at the time of implant.[70] Unmasking of a previously undetected PFO has been reported after mechanical unloading of the left side of the heart, and this defect must be surgically or endovascularly repaired if systemic postoperative hypoxemia occurs.[69,71]

End-Organ Function

The presence of multiple medical comorbidities is a common finding in patients with end-stage HF and an ever-present challenge in the surgical management of the disease. Permanent, life-threatening comorbidities (such as preoperative dialysis dependence) are often associated with excessive perioperative risks and frequently preclude eligibility for MCS. However, improvement in end-organ function has been documented after periods of device support.[72-75] Preoperative determination of the severity of end-organ disease is a critical process, and it relies on the collective clinical judgment of the multidisciplinary treatment team.

Renal dysfunction, specifically, is strongly associated with poor outcomes after device implantation.[76,77] As a result, patients who require chronic preoperative dialysis are generally excluded from implantable MCS consideration. Additionally, multiple studies have shown a decline in postoperative survival associated with deranged markers of liver function.[78,79] While acute cardiogenic liver injury can be stabilized, elevations in bilirubin levels, aminotransferase levels, and INR warrant further workup and evaluation. Preoperative mechanical ventilation has been shown to be associated with postoperative respiratory failure, RV failure, and increased mortality.[80] An assessment of pulmonary reserve is often limited by severe cardiac dysfunction, and no specific pulmonary function criteria have been formally established for device exclusion. Impaired cognitive function or a recent history of stroke obligates a thorough neurologic and cognitive examination. Patients with significant residual deficits should undergo an occupational therapy evaluation to determine whether they possess sufficient physical dexterity to manipulate an MCS device independently.

Right Ventricular Function

Prevention and treatment of RV dysfunction is a significant challenge in the field of MCS, and postoperative RHF has long been associated with poor clinical outcomes.[37,81,82] Identification of patients at risk for RHF provides an opportunity for implementation of preoperative optimization strategies and enhanced surgical preparedness. However, methods developed thus far to predict RHF after LVAD implantation have been largely based on experience with pulsatile devices and have proven inconsistent, likely due to the variety of clinical definitions, variables, and treatment strategies.[83-86]

Despite the complex pathophysiology underlying this disease process, several recent studies have significantly improved our understanding of variables that predispose to RV dysfunction. In a retrospective analysis of the HeartMate II BTT trial, Kormos and colleagues[87] sought to identify risk factors for the development of postoperative RHF in a CF LVAD population. That study specifically identified preoperative ventilator support, an increased central venous pressure (CVP) and CVP/PCWP ratio, a decreased RV stroke work index, and elevated white blood cell and blood urea nitrogen values as significant predictors of RHF. Echocardiographic parameters have also been suggested as tools for assessing the risk of RHF after LVAD implantation. Ultrasonographic studies have implicated reduced free-wall strain, RV-to-LV diameter ratios, severity of tricuspid regurgitation, and RV EF as predictors of right-sided heart dysfunction.[88-91] Researchers at the University of Pennsylvania recently developed a risk-stratification tool to assess the preoperative likelihood for tolerance of univentricular support.[92] Although limited by its size, patient selection, and single-center design, the study identified preoperative tachycardia, elevated CVP, ventilator support, RV dysfunction, and tricuspid regurgitation as predictors of the need for biventricular support.

Thus, whereas the specific variables that may predispose patients to RHF after LVAD implantation remain unclear, certain principles have emerged to help guide patient selection and management. A consistent theme throughout the majority of these studies is an association between predictors of RHF and predictors of overall mortality.[93,94] Sicker patients—with preoperative evidence of end-organ dysfunction, hemodynamic instability, and impaired RV mechanics—are especially vulnerable to RHF after LVAD implantation. Thoughtful evaluation and preoperative consideration of these risks are paramount in surgical planning.

Multidisciplinary Assessment/Social Evaluation

Due to the comprehensive nature of device therapy and the commitment required for successful outcomes, candidates for MCS must undergo a comprehensive multidisciplinary assessment. Preoperative nutritional status should be evaluated and optimized, as studies have shown an association between cachexia and perioperative mortality rates.[95,96] A history of psychiatric illness should cause significant concern and warrants a thorough evaluation of competency and ability to adhere consistently to therapy. Routine psychosocial evaluation should be performed by qualified healthcare personnel to explore available personal, social, vocational, financial, and environmental support systems. Advanced patient age alone should not preclude device therapy.[97] Cases should be reviewed on an individual basis by a multidisciplinary committee to ensure that all concerns are addressed before surgery.

DEVICE SELECTION

Appropriate device selection is determined by a number of factors, including the patient's overall clinical condition, the indication for MCS, the proposed goal of device therapy, and relevant patient-specific considerations.

Patients with an unstable condition or acute decompensation are often best served by short-term devices that are less invasive, faster to place, and less expensive than fully implantable pumps. As a reliable and historically familiar option, VA ECMO is the procedure of choice for emergent situations in many institutions worldwide. Peripheral cannulation may be performed at the bedside, in the catheterization lab, or in the operating theater, and the presence of an oxygenator allows for full cardiopulmonary support for a period of days to weeks. Catheter-based LVADs such as the Impella and TandemHeart are used with increasing frequency for short-term LV support, particularly after high-risk coronary interventions.[32] These percutaneous devices can provide temporary support without the need for surgical access, but they are susceptible to hemolysis and positional disruption, and their use is typically limited to 1 to 2 weeks. For patients for whom more robust flows are required or percutaneous measures have failed, the CentriMag is the most frequently used temporary option. Cannulation is similar to that performed for routine CPB, and the device can be used for temporary uni- or biventricular support for up to 1 month.

Fully implantable CF LVADs are the devices of choice for patients who require long-term MCS and whose condition is stable enough to permit major surgery. Of the various options, the HeartMate II LVAD and the HeartWare HVAD are the most commonly used devices. Although they function in a similar manner, the choice between these pumps is based on factors ranging from anatomical concerns to institutional availability. In the United States, the CMS strictly mandates preoperative designation of patients as either BTT or DT candidates. Despite the fluid nature of these preimplant strategies, the HeartMate II remains the only device approved by the FDA for use in both BTT and DT patients. The HVAD, by contrast, is currently approved only for BTT in the United States, and clinical trials seeking DT approval are currently underway. No study has yet shown either pump to be superior to the other. Although the advent of smaller CF pumps has lessened the anatomical challenge of implantation, patient body habitus remains an important consideration. For example, the intrapericardial position of the HVAD makes the HeartWare device particularly appealing for smaller-framed patients.

For patients with biventricular HF, the decision to pursue uni- or biventricular MCS greatly affects the available treatment options. For patients with mild-to-moderate RHF, a CF LVAD with temporary right-sided support may be sufficient to allow RV reconditioning. In the event of failed temporary support or severe biventricular disease, dual (right and left) CF devices may be used with relative success despite the logistical complexities associated with multiple controllers and batteries. The pulsatile SynCardia TAH (SynCardia Systems; Tucson, AZ) currently is the only FDA-approved option for implantable biventricular support in patients awaiting transplantation. Although the Syncardia requires considerable intrathoracic volume displacement, it allows mobility and outpatient management by means of a portable pneumatic driver. The continued development of a fully implantable CF TAH is underway and will be discussed later in this chapter.

SURGICAL TECHNIQUE

As experience with device implantation has grown, surgical techniques have evolved to reflect lessons learned. Early in the development of LVADs, apical positioning of the inlet cannula was advocated, so as to take advantage of the longest measured span within the left ventricle. This positioning, however, often creates unfavorable angulation of the inlet toward the interventricular septum, resulting in arrhythmogenesis and mechanical obstruction of the inlet after a reduction in the LV end-diastolic dimension. Over time, a number of alternative implant strategies have been devised, ranging from a thoracotomy to subcostal incisions and from anterior to lateral pump positions.[98-100] Surgeons at our institution favor a method designed to produce a parallel orientation between the inlet cannula and the interventricular septum by placing the inlet along the diaphragmatic surface of the heart.[101,102] Although it deviates from traditional technique, this method eliminates the need for a preperitoneal pump pocket and creates a more geometrically advantageous alignment.

Whereas the technique described is specifically intended for the HeartMate II, most of the procedure is indistinguishable from implantation of other CF LVADs. Differences involving the HeartWare HVAD—the second most commonly used device worldwide—will be addressed as necessary. Essential components of the procedure include (1) positioning of the inlet cannula along the diaphragmatic aspect of the left ventricle; (2) transdiaphragmatic positioning of the HeartMate II pump housing; (3) proper sizing of the outflow graft to ensure an optimal pump position and avoidance of kinking; (4) thorough de-airing of the heart and pump circuit; and (5) titration of pump speeds under echocardiographic guidance to optimize heart function.

A vertical midline incision is made, followed by a 6-cm subxiphoid extension. A standard sternotomy is then performed with the ratchet of the sternal retractor oriented toward the patient's head to provide adequate inferior exposure. The pericardium is opened in the midline and divided along the length of the diaphragm. Both pleural cavities are entered to assist with positioning of both the pump and outflow conduit. The anterior border of the diaphragm is then incised from the midline to the apex of the heart, permitting entrance into the peritoneal cavity and adequate space for introducing the pump (Fig. 62-9a). A point of entry for the inlet cannula to traverse the diaphragm is selected to correspond with the diaphragmatic surface of the left ventricle and is marked with an electrocautery.

After systemic heparinization is achieved, the ascending aorta is cannulated distally, with consideration for potential future reoperation and transplantation. Venous cannulation is typically achieved by using a dual-stage cannula in the right atrial appendage, except in cases for which a concomitant procedure is planned—such as a tricuspid valve repair or PFO—when bicaval cannulation is preferred. In a reoperative sternotomy, the femoral vessels should be exposed to allow immediate cannulation if mediastinal dissection results in hemodynamic instability.

CPB is then initiated, and the LV apex is brought out of the chest and stabilized with an off-pump suction-cup stabilizer. For inlet placement along the diaphragmatic surface, identification of the appropriate ventriculotomy site is crucial to avoid disruption of the papillary muscles and allow the inlet to lie parallel to the interventricular septum along the short axis of the left ventricle. This is accomplished by selecting a point approximately one-third of the distance from the apex to the base of the heart (thus, anterior to the origin of the papillary muscles), with the medial edge of the sewing ring placed 0.5 to 1 cm lateral to the posterior descending artery. A coring knife—typically provided by the device manufacturer—is used to open the ventricle, with care to stay parallel to the septum and follow posteriorly in the direction of the mitral valve. The ventricular cavity is then thoroughly inspected for evidence of thrombus or potentially obstructive trabeculae.

To secure the Silastic inflow cuff of the HeartMate II, 12 braided polyester full-thickness sutures are placed circumferentially around the ventriculotomy site in a horizontal mattress fashion with broad interlocking felt pledgets. The sutures are passed through the felt sewing ring of the inflow cuff, which is then lowered into position and secured. Hemostasis around the inflow is bolstered by placing a full-thickness purse-string stitch through the pledgeted ring, using a large-caliber monofilament suture (Fig. 62-9b). The HeartWare HVAD utilizes a specialized sewing ring equipped with a locking mechanism to secure the pump in place. The HVAD sewing ring is typically placed before the ventricle is cored,

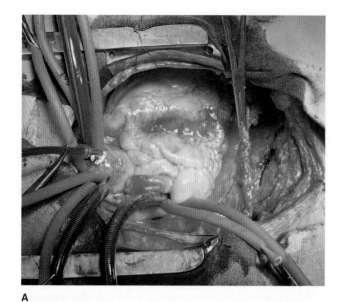

A

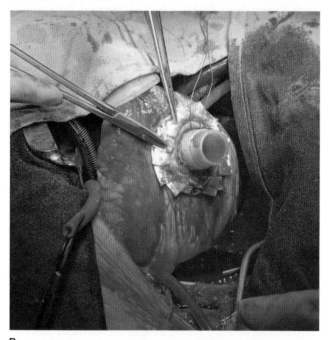

B

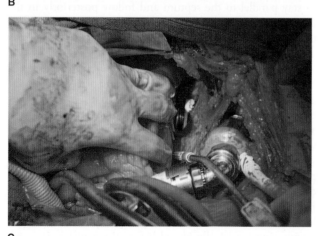

C

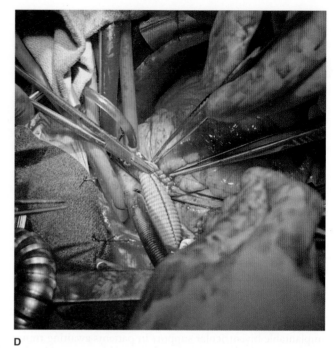

D

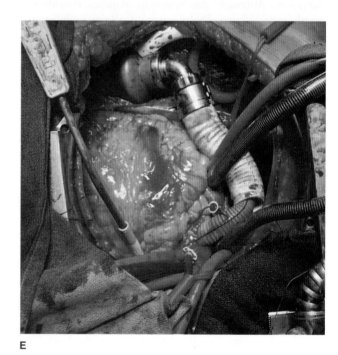

E

FIGURE 62-9 HeartMate II implantation. (A) Retraction of the diaphragm in anticipation of subdiaphragmatic pump positioning. (B) The ventricle is cored along the diaphragmatic surface of the heart—lateral to the posterior descending artery—and a pledgeted ring secures the Silastic inflow cuff. (C) Transdiaphragmatic positioning of the HeartMate II inflow cannula. (D) Anastomosis of the outflow graft to the ascending aorta, aided by a partial occluding vascular clamp. (E) Final alignment of the pump and outflow conduit. The pump housing lies beneath the diaphragm, and the outflow graft courses toward the right side of the chest. Introduction of a 19-gauge needle permits de-airing of the system.

and the ring is seated with a similar series of horizontal mattress sutures.

Next, the diaphragmatic myotomy—ample enough to admit two fingers—is completed at the previously marked location, and the pump is brought into the field after being prepared and primed on a separate table. The inlet cannula is guided through the diaphragm, inserted within the Silastic ring, and finally secured in place with two ratcheting cable ties (Fig. 62-9c). The pump housing is pulled into the abdomen until the heart lies flush with the diaphragm, and the pump is positioned above the left lobe of the liver. To protect the bowel, the body of the pump is wrapped in available omentum. The discoid shape of the HeartWare HVAD allows intrapericardial pump placement. Although the inlet is placed along the diaphragmatic aspect of the ventricle, entrance into the abdomen is not required.

Next, attention is turned to the outflow graft, which is allowed to fill, then is measured and cut in beveled fashion, with enough length to produce a gentle curve toward the right side of the chest but without excessive redundancy that might lead to kinking. After placement of a partial occluding clamp along the ascending aorta, an aortotomy is created along the anterolateral surface by sequentially firing a 4.4-mm punch. The outflow-graft anastomosis is performed in an end-to-side fashion with continuous 5-0 polypropylene suture (Fig. 62-9d). The partial occluding clamp is then removed, and the graft is de-aired while backflow is prevented by an occlusive vascular clamp.

The driveline exit site is identified two fingerbreadths below the right subcostal margin within the mid-clavicular line. A skin punch allows the introduction of a tunneling device, which is then passed behind the right rectus muscle, anteriorly to the posterior rectus sheath. The driveline is withdrawn with the tunneling device, cleaned, and connected to the device controller, with care to loop the velour-coated portion of the lead within the patient's body, as studies have shown that preservation of the velour-silicone interface beneath the level of the skin is associated with a decreased incidence of driveline infections.[103]

After thorough de-airing, the pump is started at its lowest setting (6000 rpm for the HeartMate II; 1800 rpm for the HeartWare HVAD) with a venting needle in the highest point of the outflow graft (Fig. 62-9e). CPB flows are gradually decreased while the pump speed is adjusted under transesophageal echocardiographic (TEE) guidance to optimize the chamber size, position of the interventricular septum, degree of MR, and RV function.

Protamine is administered, the cannulas are removed, and drains are placed in the mediastinum and pleural spaces. The bare portion of the outflow graft is covered with a 20-mm-diameter ringed Gore-Tex graft (Gore Medical, Newark, DE) to avoid kinking and damage during future sternal reentry. The defect in the diaphragm is partially reapproximated, and the sternum and soft tissues are closed in the standard fashion. If the patient has excessive bleeding related to severe coagulopathy, temporary chest closure may be advisable to allow correction and stabilization before delayed sternal closure is attempted.[104]

POSTOPERATIVE MANAGEMENT

Diligent and comprehensive patient care is essential for successful MCS outcomes, and proper management begins before surgery. As described earlier, careful patient selection is paramount, as is prompt identification of the most appropriate opportunity for device implantation. To minimize surgical risks, particular emphasis should be placed on the preoperative optimization of end-organ function, reversal of coagulation imbalances, correction of malnutrition, and eradication of preexisting infection. Device recipients with decompensated clinical profiles (INTERMACS levels 1 and 2) are known to experience worse outcomes than patients whose condition is comparatively stable.[37] As a result, aggressive medical management, intraaortic balloon therapy, or temporary device support is often warranted to improve the patient's hemodynamic condition before surgery. Careful planning should also include the recognition of patient-specific risks—such as the potential need for RV support—to avoid lengthy delays in the recognition and treatment of postoperative complications.

Intraoperative measures are also crucial for preventing postoperative complications. In addition to meticulous surgical technique and adequate hemostasis, judicious blood-product administration minimizes the risk of volume overload and RV failure. In the setting of profound coagulopathy, low-dose recombinant factor VIIa (NovoSeven; Novo Nordisk, Plainsboro, NJ) and four-factor prothrombin complex concentrate (Kcentra; CSL Behring GmbH, Marburg, Germany) have shown value as pharmacologic resources without causing an undue risk of device complications or thromboembolic events.[105]

Initial device setup is a critical process that occurs within the operating theater. After the pump is activated, power and flow recordings should be carefully monitored, and any suspected physical impediments to device performance, such as outflow kinking or cannula malpositioning, should be immediately identified and corrected. Intraoperative identification of optimal pump speed is a dynamic process that requires both direct visualization and TEE to assess ventricular chamber size, RV function, and interventricular septal position. The combination of CPB weaning, intravascular fluid shifts, vasoactive medications, and sternal closure can result in sudden and dramatic changes in cardiac function, and continual reassessment is required to maintain an appropriate balance between the patient and device.

Immediate postoperative management in the intensive care unit (ICU) requires an understanding of the delicate balance between pump flow, RV function, and intravascular volume status—often interpreted within the context of a volatile and complex hemodynamic milieu. Baseline comprehensive laboratory panels should be assessed immediately upon the patient's arrival in the ICU to assess acid-base status, coagulation markers, and hematologic reserves. Acidosis should be aggressively corrected and coagulopathy reversed with appropriate blood component resuscitation.

Arterial BP is principally controlled by vasoactive medications and intravascular fluid management, not pump speed.

The flows produced by CF LVADs operating at constant speed are highly dependent on the pressure differential across the pump. The resulting afterload sensitivity, particularly in centrifugal pump designs, requires careful BP titration to ensure sufficient output without causing excessive systemic pressures. Although optimal MAPs in this patient population remain unknown, our practice is to target a range of 60 to 80 mm Hg. Due to the reduction in pulse pressure created by CF LVADs, systemic arterial pressures are expressed as a single mean value and should be continuously monitored in the postoperative period. Noninvasive BP cuff measurements have been found to be unreliable in the setting of CF MCS and frequently underestimate systolic pressures. As a result, Doppler measurements have emerged as the gold-standard noninvasive modality.[106] The control of CVP is also of critical importance in the postoperative period, as excessive volume administration—a frequent obstacle in this patient population—can quickly lead to development of RV dysfunction.

Assessment of appropriate device function is based on system-specific parameters in conjunction with echocardiographic findings. Pump speed (rpm) and power expenditure (watts) are the only directly measured variables provided by the HeartMate II and HeartWare HVAD; estimated flow (L/min) is indirectly calculated and typically corresponds to changes in pump power. The pulsatility index (PI) is a parameter unique to the HeartMate II, and it is designed to indicate ventricular filling and function by interpreting changes in pump flow due to contraction of the left ventricle. Although optimal target levels are unknown, the PI can be expected to decline with increasing pump support.[69] The HeartWare HVAD provides continuous readings of pump speed, power, and flow, and it records values every 15 minutes, thus maintaining a retrievable data log for review of the preceding 30 days. Interpretation of these data recordings has shown a potential for predicting, diagnosing, and managing clinical events, including volume changes, RV dysfunction, and pump thrombosis.[107]

Any deviation in pump data warrants immediate interrogation, including assessment of hemodynamics, volume status, heart rhythm, sources of intrathoracic compression, and ventricular dimensions. Whether emergent or elective, assessment of device function is best achieved by echocardiography focused on end-diastolic dimensions, septal positioning, valvular competence, and aortic valve opening. Systematic assessment across a range of pump speeds—"speed-change" or "ramped-speed" echo—allows optimization of maintenance pump speeds by comparing functional dynamics. The preferred frequency of these studies varies among institutions; at a minimum, it should be performed in the operating room, soon after arrival in the ICU, before hospital discharge, and any time concern is raised about the adequacy of support.

Our practice is to seek early extubation, mobilization, and resumption of nutritional support. Aggressive diuresis is typically warranted for postoperative fluid offloading, and volume status is monitored using daily weights, physical findings, and hemodynamic parameters. The patient should be weaned from vasoactive and inotropic medications as tolerated. Lines and drains should be removed as early as possible to reduce the risk of postoperative infection, and strict aseptic technique is required for driveline dressing changes. An aggressive physical therapy regimen is initiated as early as possible, as is patient device training.

Management of Right Ventricular Dysfunction

After LVAD implantation, outcomes are heavily dependent on the preservation of adequate RV function. Whereas RHF is most often the result of inadequate left-sided output, the initiation of LVAD support can adversely affect RV function in several ways. The sudden increase in left-sided cardiac output and venous return requires the unsupported right ventricle to respond immediately to an increased demand. Although LVAD therapy has been shown to reduce the severity of pulmonary hypertension, this resolution may not be immediate, forcing the right ventricle to pump against a relatively high-pressure system. Furthermore, interdependence between the right and left ventricles can result in the distortion of RV and septal architecture upon unloading of the LV, leading to impaired RV contractility. In this way, initiation of device support can lead to sudden demands and strains on the right ventricle to which it cannot adequately respond.

Management personnel must be vigilant in monitoring for signs of acute RHF to allow prompt and aggressive treatment. Signs of impending or evolving RV dysfunction include increasing vasopressor requirements or hemodynamic instability, elevated or rising CVP, decreased urine output, and low mixed venous oxygen saturation (SvO_2). In 2011, Potapov and colleagues[108] suggested standardized criteria for the diagnosis of RV dysfunction that included the inability to wean from CPB, or any two of the following conditions: MAP < 55 mm Hg, CVP > 16 mm Hg, SvO_2 < 55%, LV flow rate index < 2 L/min/m², or significant inotropic dependence. In addition to hemodynamic markers, echocardiography should remain an essential component of the evaluation, allowing direct assessment of ventricular size, contractility, and septal positioning. Along with traditional signs of depressed right-sided heart function, the failure to maintain appropriate LVAD power consumption and flows in the absence of hypovolemia may suggest inability of the right ventricle to deliver sufficient volume to the pump inlet.

The majority of patients with RV dysfunction will require inotropic support, typically in the form of milrinone, dobutamine, isoproterenol, or epinephrine. Early and aggressive pharmacologic diuresis is essential to reduce RV preload, particularly in the setting of excessive volume loading and massive transfusion. Maintenance of sinus rhythm preserves the RV stroke volume and lessens myocardial strain. Although the results of studies have been contradictory, inhaled nitric oxide therapy appears to have utility in alleviating pulmonary vascular resistance and RV dysfunction through direct pulmonary arterial vasodilatory effects.[108,109] When all other management options have been exhausted, consideration of mechanical right-sided support, either temporary or permanent, is warranted.[110]

Anticoagulation

The approach to anticoagulation in patients who require long-term MCS has not yet been standardized and varies considerably between institutions. Whereas thromboembolic complications were a significant challenge for early devices, the unique textured interior surface of the HeartMate XVE resulted in the development of a neointimal blood interface that effectively eliminated the need for systemic anticoagulation.[111] The introduction of the Jarvik 2000, which utilized blood-washed bearings and a CF design, led to the widespread practice of systemic anticoagulation to reduce the perceived risk of pump thrombosis.[112] As a result, initial management strategies for CF devices involved a target INR of 2.5 to 3.5 before experience gained from the HeartMate II pivotal trial led to a suggested target range of 2 to 3 along with early postoperative heparin infusion and antiplatelet therapy in the form of aspirin and dipyridamole.[25,113]

Despite these initial recommendations, the appropriate level of anticoagulation for long-term CF support remains an area of active investigation. Studies have shown that the incidence of hemorrhagic complications is far greater than that of thrombotic events in this patient population, leading to the suggestion that a lower INR target may be appropriate.[37,114] Moreover, patients transitioned directly to warfarin without an early heparin bridge have been shown to experience reduced postoperative transfusion requirements without an increased risk of thrombotic complications.[115] Guidelines published by ISHLT recommend the initiation of heparin therapy on postoperative day 1, with warfarin and aspirin started by postoperative day 3 (target INR 2.0 to 3.0).[36] Our institution follows an alternative protocol, preferring the early introduction of warfarin and aspirin therapy (by postoperative day 1), with heparin infusion reserved for patients in whom anticoagulation remains subtherapeutic by postoperative day 4. Target INRs for this protocol are specific to the type of device, application, and presence of concomitant cardiac pathology. Standard intraoperative heparin reversal with protamine sulfate is accepted practice in most centers.

Biventricular Device Management

The concomitant use of a right-sided pump adds several complexities to device management. From a hemodynamic standpoint, determination of the appropriate balance between the two pumps can be difficult. Continuous-flow devices are principally governed by two variables: the speed of the rotor and the pressure difference across the device. As a result, the output produced by a CF pump operating at constant speed will reflect the volume of blood delivered to the inlet. This arrangement provides a degree of inherent automaticity that is advantageous when pumps are operated in series. Management of a biventricular system, therefore, requires identification of a right-sided pump speed that permits venous offloading without development of pulmonary edema—a common complication of RV assistance as a result of reduced afterload established by the low-pressure pulmonary circulation. Left-sided speeds may then be actively titrated to compensate for physiologic variations in the volume delivered to the left ventricle.

Biventricular assist device (BiVAD) support also creates a number of logistical challenges. The surgical complexity of accommodating two pump housings within the thoracic cage can be significant. Whereas the use of dual HeartMate II devices has been reported, the relatively small profile and intrapericardial pump position of the HeartWare HVAD offers a considerable advantage, making this device preferable for high-risk cases or planned biventricular support.[116-118] In our experience, the outflow conduits are best configured in opposing alignments, with the right-sided graft directed posterolaterally to allow anastomosis with the pulmonary artery trunk without interfering with the course of the LVAD graft. A further disadvantage of dual device support is the redundancy of system controllers (two) and batteries (four) required for operation. The resultant physical burden, complexity in daily use, and responsibilities for maintenance present significant challenges for long-term management of patients who require biventricular therapy.

POSTOPERATIVE OUTCOMES

Over the past 20 years, multicenter studies have documented a progressive improvement in postoperative mortality after LVAD implantation (Fig. 62-10). The landmark REMATCH trial showed a 1-year survival rate of 52% for patients randomized to receive device therapy, compared with 25% survival at 12 months for those treated with medical therapy alone.[7] Six years later, the HeartMate II BTT study showed 68% 1-year survival with CF support, a total that rose to 73% within the larger Continued Access Protocol report.[9,25] In keeping with this trend, the HeartWare ADVANCE trial results were released in 2012 and showed an 86% survival rate at 1 year, which was comparable to contemporary INTERMACS data and led to FDA approval of the HVAD for BTT indications.[27] Likely due to improved patient selection, 30-day perioperative survival has also improved during that timespan, rising from roughly 80% with the HeartMate XVE to more than 90% with contemporary devices.[53,119,120]

Analysis of the INTERMACS registry reveals several statistically significant risk factors for mortality in patients supported by CF LVADs, including severity of the preoperative clinical profile (levels 1 and 2), renal dysfunction, age over 70 years, RV dysfunction, and increased surgical complexity.[8,121] Biventricular device support is consistently associated with increased short-term mortality, although the data suggest some utility in early planned (as opposed to delayed) implementation of biventricular device therapy.[37,122] Importantly, LVAD therapy has been shown to be equivalent to transplantation in terms of 1- and 2-year mortality, and pretransplant MCS has not been shown to negatively affect outcomes for subsequent transplantation.[123,124] Quality-of-life metrics also

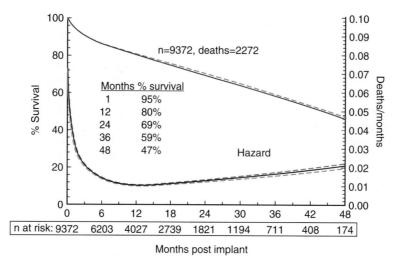

FIGURE 62-10 Actuarial survival curve for adult recipients of primary continuous-flow left ventricular support. Patients were censored at transplantation or device explantation. (Reproduced with permission from Kirklin JK, Naftel DC, Pagani FD, et al: Sixth INTERMACS annual report: a 10,000-patient database, *J Heart Lung Transplant.* 2014 Jun;33(6):555-564.)

reveal a significant improvement with LVAD therapy that is sustained through 24 months after device implantation.[37]

ADVERSE EVENTS AND DEVICE COMPLICATIONS

The implementation of device therapy is associated with specific perioperative and long-term risks for the patient. To standardize the evaluation of patient outcomes, INTERMACS has established definitions for adverse events associated with MCS. The cumulative incidence of these adverse events within the first 60 days of MCS has been reported to be as high as 89%, many such events being associated with a reduction in long-term survival[125,126] (Fig. 62-11). Implementation

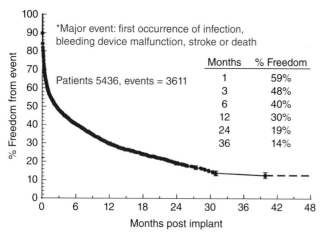

FIGURE 62-11 Actuarial freedom from major adverse events in patients supported by continuous-flow left ventricular assist devices. (Reproduced with permission from Kirklin JK, Naftel DC, Kormos RL, et al: Fifth INTERMACS annual report: risk factor analysis from more than 6,000 mechanical circulatory support patients, *J Heart Lung Transplant.* 2013 Feb;32(2):141-156.)

and management of MCS, thus, obligates a consideration of the risks associated with device therapy and an appreciation of the implications of certain events.

Perioperative Bleeding

Whereas detailed analysis is limited with regard to the currently available data registries, bleeding has historically been cited as the most common complication after LVAD implantation, and bleeding of any type (operative and late onset) is the most common adverse event recorded by INTERMACS.[25,37,126] Surgical bleeding and large-volume blood-product resuscitation has been associated with increased 30-day and 1-year mortality rates, RV dysfunction, acute lung injury, infection, and pretransplant allosensitization.[127] Reported bleeding rates were high in the early pulsatile LVAD experience, with nearly 50% of patients suffering from major bleeding complications.[81] Although the introduction of CF devices resulted in an overall improvement in outcomes, bleeding has remained a significant perioperative challenge. Early experience with the HeartMate II clinical trials showed that between 50 and 80% of patients required perioperative blood product transfusion, with 30% of patients undergoing reoperation for bleeding complications.[25,26] Single-center analyses have since revealed a modest reduction in transfusion requirements.[104,128]

Recently, the comparative analysis of different devices with regard to perioperative bleeding complications has been an area of particular interest. The HeartWare BTT trial investigators reported a lower risk of reoperation for bleeding than did the contemporary INTERMACS control group (largely comprising HeartMate II patients).[27] A single-center analysis subsequently determined that although red blood cell administration was equivalent for the two pumps, HVAD recipients required fewer blood products overall (8.3 ± 13 vs 12.6 ± 14 units) and had a lower chest-tube output than did

HeartMate II patients.[129] As a result, these studies have been used to suggest that, due to a reduction in surgical dissection, the HVAD is associated with fewer bleeding complications. However, whereas differences between pumps may indeed affect bleeding rates, these studies fail to account for wide variations in surgical approach and perioperative management that may contribute to these results. Regardless of the device used, bleeding is a significant challenge in the perioperative period.

Right-Sided Heart Failure

The identification and management of RV dysfunction has been extensively discussed. Development of RHF presents a major postoperative challenge and is strongly associated with poor clinical outcomes and increased mortality.[37,81,82] Reported criteria for the diagnosis of RV failure vary in the literature. The most commonly used definition of post-LVAD RV failure originates from the HeartMate II BTT trial, which described RV failure as the need for RV support, inotropic support for at least 14 days after implantation, or the initiation of inotropic support after 14 days of LVAD support.[9] INTERMACS utilizes considerably broader criteria for data acquisition purposes, relying primarily on signs and symptoms of elevated CVP and more specific conditions to evaluate the level of severity.[130] The reported incidence of RV failure after LVAD implantation remains highly variable, ranging from 15 to 30%.[82,87,123,126] A subset of patients with RV failure (between 8 and 10% of device recipients) will require mechanical RV support.[37,88,91,126]

Infection

Device therapy carries a significant risk of infection, primarily due to the presence of foreign material within the body and a percutaneous driveline. With early pulsatile systems, infection rates ranged from 50 to 60% during the lifetime of the pump, and more than 40% of deaths in the LVAD-supported cohort of the REMATCH trial were due to fulminant sepsis.[111,131] Although the incidence has significantly improved with the introduction of newer-generation devices, infection remains a major source of morbidity and mortality during MCS, and it is the second most reported adverse event in the INTERMACS database.[37] With regard to device comparison, the rates of driveline infection and sepsis in the original HeartMate II BTT trial were 14 and 17%, respectively, compared with 12.1 and 11.4% in the subsequent HeartWare BTT trial.[25,27] Creation of a preperitoneal pump pocket during implantation of the HeartMate II likely predisposes those patients to the development of a pump-pocket infection, which can often result in life-threatening sepsis and the need for pump exchange. As a result, our institutional preference is to avoid the need for a pump pocket by placing the pump in a subdiaphragmatic intraperitoneal position.

A review of INTERMACS data revealed percutaneous driveline infections in 9.8% of all patients supported with CF devices.[132] The mean time to development of the infection is typically greater than 6 months, implying that most such infections occur in the outpatient setting, when patients are more active and responsible for dressing care.[132-134] By 1 year, 19% of patients have developed a driveline infection, while 1 in 4 are diagnosed with a driveline infection by 2 years of CF LVAD support.[37] Whereas most patients in the INTERMACS database were treated with antibiotics alone, surgical intervention was required in 12.5% of cases.[37,132] Specific information regarding the extent of debridement is generally not reported, but vacuum-assisted closure, antibiotic bead therapy, and driveline mobilization have all been described.[135,136] Infection has been shown to adversely impact survival, increasing the 1-year mortality rate as much as 6-fold.[37,132,137] The presence of a documented device infection does not preclude transplantation.

Renal Failure

As described earlier, preoperative renal dysfunction has been shown to be strongly associated with poor outcomes after LVAD implantation.[76,77] Similarly, the development of postoperative renal failure is a significant predictor of the 1-year mortality rate after device implantation.[125] However, risk factors for postoperative renal failure are poorly understood, and indices of preoperative renal status do not appear to be strong independent predictors of such failure.[77] Although definitions vary, the incidence of postoperative renal failure ranges from 14 to 30%.[125,138,139] Factors associated with the development of this complication appear to include preoperative ventilatory support, elevated CVP, and advanced patient age. The initiation of MCS has been shown to enhance end-organ perfusion, and management options for postoperative renal failure range from supportive medical therapy to temporary or permanent renal replacement.[73] As many as 10 to 20% of patients undergoing LVAD implantation require some form of postoperative renal replacement therapy, and approximately half of that population can be expected to recover independent renal function, typically within the first month.[138,139] Development of postoperative renal failure has been shown to be associated with longer ICU stays, increased ventilator dependence, prolonged inotropic support, and a significant decline in 30-day, 3-month, and 1-year survival.[37,138]

Stroke and Neurologic Dysfunction

Despite improvements in device reliability and management strategies, stroke remains a significant source of morbidity and mortality in patients who require LVAD support. Clinically apparent strokes can result in significant functional disabilities—a particular challenge for routine device maintenance—along with impaired quality of life, significant rehabilitation needs, and decreased postevent survival. Collectively, the impact of these outcomes highlights neurologic dysfunction as a particularly feared complication of device therapy.

While strokes are typically classified under a singular adverse event heading, the disparate pathogenesis of hemorrhagic and ischemic strokes suggests the likelihood for multiple causative factors. A detailed analysis comparing stroke etiology in device patients is not yet available, but the incidence of hemorrhagic and ischemic strokes appears to be roughly equal.[26,140,141] Overall, the reported incidence of stroke among device patients in the INTERMACS database is 11% at 1 year and 17% at 2 years postimplantation.[37] Risk factors for stroke during MCS are poorly understood, and many presumed influences—including anticoagulation, atrial fibrillation, diabetes mellitus, and device type—have not been found to be statistically significant.[141] Pulsatility may play a role in the development of embolic strokes. Prolonged closure of the aortic valve has been shown to result in eddies and stasis within the aortic cusps, predisposing some patients to the formation of thrombus that can be released with later opening of the valve.[142] Similarly, some patients have developed thrombus in areas of stasis within the carotid bulb; again, such thrombus is susceptible to dislodgement after the recovery of pulsatility.[31] As a result, routine maintenance of intermittent pulsatility may provide prophylactic washout of these areas and reduce the potential for thromboembolic events. In recent studies, BP has been identified as an additional key determinant in the pathogenesis of stroke. The importance of adequate BP control in this population is suggested by the fact that patients with lower BP at hospital discharge and those receiving aggressive pharmacologic antihypertensive therapy have significantly lower rates of neurologic events.[141,143] Stroke adversely affects survival, entailing a 25% 30-day and nearly 50% 1-year mortality risk.[140,141]

Nonsurgical and Gastrointestinal Bleeding

As noted previously, bleeding of any type is the most frequent adverse event reported to INTERMACS, and late-onset spontaneous bleeding is a significant source of morbidity for patients supported by CF LVADs.[37] Researchers have consistently documented the frequency of nonsurgical (primarily GI) bleeding, particularly in older patients, and the reported incidence of this complication ranges from 18 to 30%.[144-149] GI sources account for the vast majority (70%) of nonsurgical bleeding episodes. Epistaxis, intracranial, and genitourinary episodes are progressively less common.[149] The location of GI bleeding is divided fairly evenly above and below the ligament of Treitz. Although percentages vary among studies, erosive gastritis and arteriovenous malformations (AVMs) appear to be the most frequent causative factors.[144,145,149] Whereas GI bleeding is a significant source of morbidity—principally because of more frequent hospitalizations and increased transfusion-related alloantigen exposure—no associated impact on overall mortality has been reported.

The relative frequency of GI bleeding in this patient population has led to multiple proposed explanations. Anticoagulation during long-term MCS undoubtedly exposes patients to increased bleeding risks. A comparison between nonpulsatile pumps and the pulsatile HeartMate XVE (which did not necessitate anticoagulation therapy) revealed a significant

difference in bleeding events.[29] However, the frequency of these events remains unexpectedly high, as patients supported by CF LVADs have a substantially higher risk for GI bleeding than do patients who require anticoagulation for cardiovascular disease.[147] Furthermore, bleeding events have been known to occur even without the use of anticoagulation.[150]

Some researchers have suggested that the propensity for GI bleeding may be due to an altered thrombotic physiology resulting from interaction between the device and the bloodstream. Multiple studies have shown that patients supported by CF LVADs can develop an acquired von Willebrand syndrome as a result of the proteolytic cleavage of high-molecular-weight von Willebrand factor multimers.[151-153] However, this explanation alone cannot explain the variability of bleeding events within the LVAD population, as bleeding has been shown to be nearly universal in the setting of axial-flow device support.[154]

An alternative explanation for the frequency of GI bleeding events may lie in the narrow pulse pressure created by CF support. The association between aortic stenosis and AVM formation was first described by Heyde in the 1950s, and a syndrome bearing his name was characterized over the subsequent decades.[155,156] This process is believed to result from hypoperfusion and ischemia of intestinal mucosa, leading to friable neovasculature susceptible to rupture. Application of this concept to CF MCS physiology was first suggested by Letsou and colleagues,[157] who described a series of patients supported by the Jarvik 2000. Recently, a retrospective review also documented a strong association between GI bleeding and both reduced PI and aortic valve closure, suggesting that a reduction in pulsatility may lead to increased rates of nonsurgical bleeding within the first 3 months of LVAD therapy.[149]

ISHLT guidelines suggest that anticoagulation therapy be withdrawn in the setting of clinically significant bleeding. Resumption of anticoagulation is permitted after resolution of the index bleeding event, but a reduction (or permanent cessation) of anticoagulation is justified in the case of recurrent events. When possible, pump speeds are generally reduced to allow increased native pulsatility. Endoscopic evaluation is also warranted for direct control of the bleeding source, although identification of the responsible AVM is often difficult.[36]

Pump Thrombosis and Device Malfunction

Pump thrombosis is an uncommon but potentially catastrophic complication of LVAD therapy. The HeartMate II BTT trial investigators reported an actuarial freedom from device malfunction (defined as resulting in device replacement or death) of 95% at 6 months and 93% at 1-year postimplantation, one-third of those events being attributed to primary device thrombosis.[9] This degree of reliability and durability represented a significant advance over earlier pulsatile systems, including a nearly 10-fold reduction in the need for device exchange.[158] Between 2011 and 2012, concern was raised regarding an apparent increase in the rate of pump thrombosis with the HeartMate II. A three-center collaborative study documented an increase in the incidence of pump thrombosis at 3 months from 2.2 to 8.4%; over the same timespan, a federally mandated INTERMACS review similarly described a decline in freedom from pump exchange or death at 6 months from 99 to 94%.[37,159] After extensive investigation, the cause of this discrepancy remained unclear and was likely multifactorial. More recently, however, institutional reports have suggested a reversal in the thrombosis-related trend and the HeartMate II remains the most frequently implanted device worldwide. Nevertheless, understanding the potential factors involved in device thrombosis is critical, as this complication has been shown to negatively impact overall survival.[159]

A major challenge in the prevention of thrombosis events is the complexity of the pathophysiology involved. Indeed, the term "thrombosis" has traditionally been used in a broad sense to describe not just *confirmed* thrombus within the pump housing but also *suspected* thrombus due to various nonstandardized clinical factors. In 2013, INTERMACS updated its definitions, establishing formal categories of *suspected* thrombosis (the criteria for which include hemolysis, unexplained HF symptoms, and abnormal pump parameters) and *confirmed* thrombus found on direct inspection or radiographic imaging.[130] Factors that contribute to thrombosis are likely far-ranging, and proposed mechanisms include inadequate heat dissipation at low speeds, ineffective anticoagulation strategies, surgical and anatomical considerations (such as angulation of the inlet or kinking of the outflow graft), patient-specific predisposition, and pump manufacturing and design elements.[160-162]

Despite the variable etiology of device malfunction, recent studies have led to improved methods for accurately diagnosing thrombotic events. Serum markers for hemolysis have been shown to be associated with pump thrombus formation, presumably due to the increased shear stress placed on red cells traversing the area of flow impedance. Serum-free hemoglobin (sfHg) has traditionally been used by INTERMACS for diagnostic purposes, with levels greater than 40 mg/dL indicative of significant hemolysis.[130] Recent data have shown that lactate dehydrogenase (LDH) may be a more sensitive marker than sfHg for detecting hemolysis and pump thrombosis, and subsequent INTERMACS reviews have shown a strong correlation between rising LDH levels and thrombotic events.[163] Whereas a threshold value of 600 IU/L has been proposed for diagnostic purposes (representing 2.5 times the upper limit of normal), this cutoff does not appear to be absolute, as anecdotal evidence suggests that many patients may exhibit higher LDH levels without tangible evidence of thrombosis. Other diagnostic tools, including speed-change echocardiography and three-dimensional computed tomography, also likely contribute to diagnostic accuracy.[164] Given the variability in presentation, a recent multicenter collaboration led to the development of a useful diagnostic and clinical management algorithm for patients with suspected pump thrombosis.[165]

Treatment strategies for suspected pump thrombosis are limited. Noninvasive measures, such as intravenous anticoagulation (heparin) and direct thrombin inhibitor therapy (bivalirudin or argatroban), are typically initiated early in the management process with variable independent results.[166,167] Success with thrombolytic therapy (both systemic and intraventricular) has also been reported, but this approach entails a risk of intracranial bleeding.[130,168,169] Definitive management of pump thrombosis is surgical, either through pump exchange, pump explantation, or urgent heart transplantation. Pump exchange may be performed through either a redo sternotomy or a subcostal approach, and the pump housing of the HeartMate II can be exchanged directly without disrupting the inlet or outflow conduit.[170,171] Despite the relative short-term safety of the exchange procedure, survival has been shown to decrease with each successive pump exchange, which also increases the likelihood of later infection and neurologic sequelae.[37,160] The mortality rate 6 months after transplantation or initial device replacement is similar to that for patients without a history of thrombosis.[159]

TOTAL ARTIFICIAL HEART

Whereas LVAD support has emerged as the standard of care for patients with end-stage HF, data registry analysis suggests that a sizeable percentage (typically cited as 8 to 10%) of patients will require biventricular support.[37,87,88,91] Heart transplantation has traditionally served as the gold-standard therapy for this subset of patients, but the scarcity of donor organs has led to a stagnant rate of transplantation, totaling just over 4000 procedures each year worldwide.[172] Mechanical total heart replacement is a logical and relatively inexhaustible solution to this challenge. The use of implantable BiVADs has been reported in the treatment of patients with severe biventricular HF.[116,173,174] However, available devices are designed to function independently, and logistical challenges in their implantation and management as BiVAD systems renders them cumbersome and difficult to operate. As a result, the development of a self-contained, fully implantable total heart replacement device is an important, though elusive, goal.

Early Development and Experience

The concept of replacing the human heart with a permanent or temporary mechanical device has been postulated for centuries and was first reported in the early nineteenth century by French physiologist Julien Jean Cesar Le Gallois.[175] Since that time, efforts to duplicate nature's design—including the famed collaboration between Charles Lindbergh and Alexis Carrell in the 1920s—have periodically captured the public imagination but failed to produce a reliable self-contained device.[176]

The first tangible step toward the development of a viable TAH came in 1957, when Tetsuzo Akutsu and Willem Kolff replaced the heart of a dog with an experimental pulsatile device.[177] The dog survived for several hours. Although the

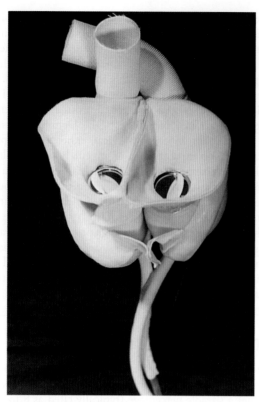

FIGURE 62-12 The Liotta total artificial heart, the first to be implanted in a human. (Courtesy Texas Heart Institute.)

pump was never tested in humans, its brief success highlighted the potential for total heart replacement. Capitalizing on a growing interest in MCS, the National Heart Institute (now termed the NHLBI) established the Artificial Heart Program in 1964, helping to fund and support research and development efforts throughout the field.

The first implantation of a TAH into a human was performed by Denton Cooley on April 4, 1969.[16] The device was placed in a 47-year-old man who could not be weaned from CPB after undergoing an LV aneurysmectomy. Designed by Domingo Liotta, the pump was a pneumatically powered, double-chambered device with Dacron-lined conduits and Wada-Cutter hingeless valves (Fig. 62-12). It was intended to support the patient only until a suitable donor heart was found. Indeed, the TAH performed adequately for 64 hours, after which the patient underwent a transplant. Despite its success, Liotta's pump was never again used clinically, but the experience showed that a TAH could be used safely and effectively for BTT.

Contemporary Options for Total Heart Replacement

SYNCARDIA TAH

In the late 1970s, under the leadership of Willem Kolff, researchers at the University of Utah began developing a TAH design that eventually evolved into what is now known

as the SynCardia TAH. The device consists of two separate, pneumatically driven pumps bound only by a Velcro patch along their adjoining walls (Fig. 62-13). Pump operation depends on the pneumatic displacement of a polyurethane diaphragm powered by an external pneumatic driver. Dacron cuffs permit atrial anastomosis after ventriculectomy, and the outflow conduits are similarly composed of woven Dacron grafts. Both components are attached to the pump housing by specialized connecting brackets. Each pump contains large-diameter SynHall valves (derived from the original Medtronic-Hall design) that regulate both inflow and outflow (27 and 25 mm, respectively) and provide minimal resistance to flow. The pneumatic drivelines are tunneled beneath the costal margin to reach the external driver, where pump rate, drive pressure, and systolic duration are controlled. The device produces a stroke volume of 70 mL and a cardiac output as high as 15 L/min.[178,179]

The earliest clinical iteration of this device, labeled the Jarvik-7, was first implanted by William DeVries in 1982, supporting a 61-year-old man with congestive HF for 112 days until he died of multiorgan failure.[180] Despite initially mixed results, clinical trials began in 1985. Over the years, the device was rebranded the Symbion, then the CardioWest TAH, and finally the SynCardia TAH.[181-183]

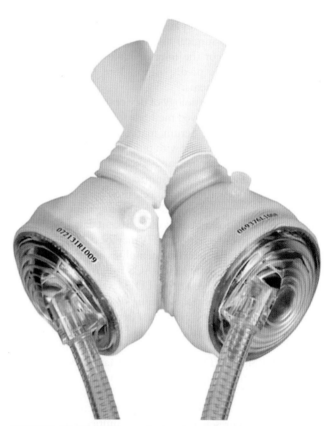

FIGURE 62-13 The Syncardia Total Artificial Heart (formerly the Jarvik-7, Symbion, and CardioWest TAH) utilizes two pneumatically driven pumps for biventricular support. (Courtesy: SynCardia Systems, Inc.)

Like many other TAHs, the SynCardia is somewhat restricted by its large size. Generally, candidates are screened for a sufficient body surface area (>1.8 m²) and for a chest anteroposterior diameter of >10 cm on computed tomography.[184] Studies have shown that the body surface area is associated with an increased risk of bleeding, infection, and overall mortality.[185] A smaller (50 mL) version of the device is currently under development. Another historic limitation of the SynCardia TAH was the inconvenience of its external components. The original console was large and relatively immobile, effectively eliminating the possibility of prolonged ambulation or outpatient management. The 2010 release of the 13-pound Freedom Driver has done much to alleviate these problems, greatly improving device portability.[186]

The SynCardia TAH is currently approved by the FDA and CMS for BTT in the treatment of biventricular failure and has been successfully used in more than 1100 patients.[187] In 2012, the device also received approval for DT use as a humanitarian exemption. Although the majority of implants have been performed for short-term support, nearly 50 patients have been supported for more than 1 year with the SynCardia, and the median duration of support is approximately 554 days. The survival-to-transplantation rate has been 72% in the long-term population. Complications have included systemic infections (35%), driveline infections (27%), thromboembolism (19%), and device malfunction (10%).[185] Survival rates are most impacted during the early postoperative period, and the vast majority of deaths occur within the first month.[188,189] Despite these limitations, the SynCardia has the potential for long-term reliable total heart replacement.

ABIOCOR TAH

The AbioCor Implantable Replacement Heart is a self-contained, single-body, electrohydraulic TAH developed by ABIOMED, Inc. (Danvers, MA) and the Texas Heart Institute.[190] The device's principal thoracic component, which is positioned orthotopically after biventriculectomy, consists of two polyurethane hydraulic pumping chambers—each flanked by trileaflet valves—that serve as artificial ventricles and function as opposing compliance chambers (Fig. 62-14). A continuous motor allows shuttling of hydraulic fluid to alternately pressurize the right and left ventricles. Active diastolic filling of the contralateral side is enabled by the negative pressure established by the hydraulic system. Unique to the design of the AbioCor is the use of radiofrequency data transmission and a transcutaneous energy transfer system designed to create a fully implantable system that can communicate with external hardware without penetrating the skin. An electronic and data component is implanted within the abdomen. The pump produces a stroke volume of 65 mL and a cardiac output as high as 12 L/min.

The AbioCor is also the only device designed to address the natural dissymmetry in native ventricular output. Management of a totally implantable pulsatile TAH system requires an understanding of the difference in stroke volumes produced by the right and left sides of the heart. The arterial blood supply to the bronchial tree (totaling 2 to 3 cc with

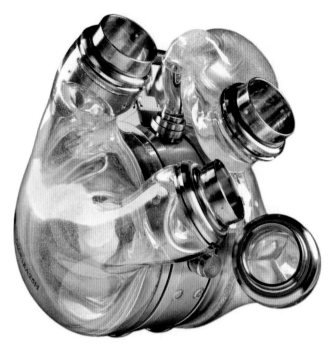

FIGURE 62-14 The AbioCor Implantable Replacement Heart. (Reproduced with permission from ABIOMED, Inc.)

each heartbeat) drains directly into the left atrium, thereby avoiding the conventional venous system and resulting in an LV output that exceeds right-sided output by 2 to 5%. Whereas this imbalance seems negligible in the short term, it accounts for as much as 250 L of blood flow each day and must be carefully considered when designing a pulsatile device responsible for producing right- and left-sided flows. To accommodate this discrepancy, the design of the AbioCor involves a right-to-left flow-balancing mechanism is designed to account for interventricular physiologic flow differences by shunting hydraulic fluid away from the right-sided pump.[191] The design functioned appropriately in both animal studies and clinical use.

With support from NHLBI, preclinical trials and extensive animal testing began at the Texas Heart Institute in 1993. In 2001, the FDA approved a phase 1 feasibility study for the device, which was first implanted in a 59-year-old man in Louisville, KY who survived for 151 days with the device.[192] Criteria for inclusion in the study were restrictive, and included the diagnosis of irreversible biventricular HF (>70% predicted 30-day mortality), with documented ineligibility for transplant. A total of 14 patients were eventually enrolled in the trial, the longest period of survival reaching 512 days. Overall survival metrics were promising, with a 71% 30-day survival rate (compared with 13% in the medical arm) and 40% survival at 2 months.[193]

A major disadvantage of this pump is its relatively large size, which limited candidacy to patients with a thoracic cage deep enough to accommodate the device. Preoperative sizing was generally performed by using three-dimensional computed tomography reconstructions, focusing primarily on anteroposterior thoracic diameter and the position of the pulmonary bifurcation.[193] Sufficient distance between the bifurcation and diaphragm was required to prevent compression of the left pulmonary veins and lower-lobe bronchus. Due to the level of anatomical complexity, a high degree of confidence with regard to sizing and fit was required before implantation was attempted. Although the AbioCor received FDA approval for use under a humanitarian device exemption in 2006, no implants have been performed since the completion of its initial feasibility study, principally due to the prohibitive economic barriers associated with its implementation.

Complexities of Mechanical Total Heart Replacement

Initial efforts to develop a viable TAH began in earnest as part of a series of bold scientific initiatives proposed by the Kennedy administration during the idealistic 1960s. Although similarly daring goals, such as manned spaceflight to the moon, were accomplished within the decade, construction of a reliable self-contained device for replacing the human heart proved to be a prohibitive technical challenge. A number of complexities, both physiologic and technologic, are to blame for the ongoing delay in realizing this objective.

From an engineering standpoint, designing a TAH presents a number of challenges, the chief of these being durability. The human heart beats more than 100,000 times each day. As a result, thin diaphragms and hydraulic actuators devised for pulsatile systems are subject to considerable mechanical wear; though capable of providing support beyond 1 year, they are unlikely to withstand the physical demands of long-term operation. Size is also a hurdle in TAH design, and the housing of biventricular volume-displacement chambers capable of producing sufficient cardiac output requires a substantial device profile that can be difficult to accommodate, even in larger patients. Moreover, portability and mobility are crucial considerations for long-term support. Pneumatic systems require drivelines for pressure venting. Even though recent efforts have reduced the size of associated equipment, compressors and power consoles can be cumbersome and limit functionality. Minimization of extracorporeal drivers, drivelines, and tethering equipment would speed postoperative recovery, minimize infectious risks, and improve overall quality of life. Remedying these concerns, however, has proved to be an immense scientific and technological undertaking.

Future Directions: the CF TAH

A quarter century of clinical experience with CF pumps has revealed the human capacity for physiologic tolerance of nonpulsatile flow and has confirmed the significant design advantages of CF devices over pulsatile TAHs. Continuous-flow devices are not only significantly smaller than pulsatile pumps but also are more anatomically appropriate thus being simpler to implant and operate. Furthermore, with few (or no) points of mechanical contact, CF designs essentially eliminate the potential for mechanical wear, resulting in a level of clinical durability far surpassing that of pulsatile systems.[194] Hemodynamically, CF pumps also appear well suited for TAH use, because (much as in the native heart) the inherent inflow sensitivity of these devices provides a degree of automaticity in responding to imbalances in right- and left-sided flows. Thus, development of a CF TAH may lead to realization of a long-awaited goal.

Over the past decade at the Texas Heart Institute, extensive research and development efforts have been dedicated to the concept of CF total heart replacement, involving both simulated models and live animal studies. To date, more than 70 calves have been implanted with paired CF VADs to provide completely nonpulsatile circulatory support. The resulting CF TAH model has revealed considerable long-term effectiveness, with more than 30 animals surviving for longer than 7 days, 8 surviving for 30 days, and 2 calves surviving for more than 90 days with nonpulsatile blood flow after CF total heart replacement.[195,196] Tolerance of this altered physiologic state is further evidenced by stable hemodynamic profiles both at rest and during treadmill exercise studies, as well as preserved hematologic and biochemical markers for end-organ function. This extensive experience with large animal models has stimulated a number of collaborative research efforts in search of a viable CF TAH design.

To this end, a novel CF TAH is currently being developed that offers tremendous potential to become a completely implantable long-term cardiac replacement device. The BiVACOR TAH, developed by BiVACOR USA in Houston, Texas, working closely with the Texas Heart Institute, is a small, compact device that utilizes a single magnetically levitated rotor to provide pulmonary and systemic blood flow without the use of bearings or valves[197] (Fig. 62-15). Impellers are mounted on each side of the rotor (which separates the right and left chambers), and its frictionless suspension permits accommodation for physiologic flow

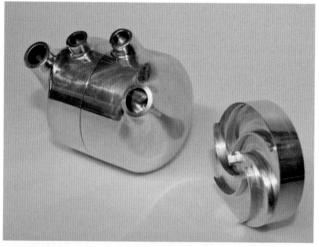

FIGURE 62-15 The BiVACOR total artificial heart employs a single moving part—a central magnetically levitated rotor—to provide compete cardiopulmonary support. (Reproduced, with permission, from BiVACOR, Inc.)

imbalances by axial displacement the rotor.[198] Also unique to the BiVACOR is the use of dynamic speed profiles to allow establishment of pulsatility in device operation.[199] Feasibility studies have been successfully performed in large animals, with a goal of human trials in the near future. A similar hydrodynamically suspended design is also in development at the Cleveland Clinic, which also has begun animal studies.[200] Thus, innovative engineering efforts and successful utilization of CF technology may soon offer the opportunity for permanent mechanical replacement of the failing human heart.

KEY POINTS

1. Continuous-flow technology has resulted in smaller, more durable MCS devices. Although the full effects of the resulting physiologic changes remain unknown, nonpulsatile blood flow is well tolerated.

2. Thoughtful patient selection and preoperative optimization of the patient's condition are crucial to ensure good outcomes after LVAD implantation.

3. Surgical considerations at the time of LVAD implantation should include careful alignment of the pump inlet and outflow conduits to minimize the risk of physical impediments to proper device function.

4. Perioperative preservation and optimization of RV function is an essential component of MCS management.

5. Due to the scarcity of available donor organs, development of a CF TAH offers the best means of providing definitive long-term treatment for patients who require total heart replacement.

REFERENCES

1. Lloyd-Jones DM, Larson MG, Leip EP, et al: Lifetime risk for developing congestive heart failure: the Framingham Heart Study. *Circulation* 2002; 106:3068-3072.

2. Heidenreich PA, Trogdon JG, Khavjou OA, et al: American Heart Association Advocacy Coordinating Committee, Stroke Council, Council on Cardiovascular Radiology and Intervention, Council on Clinical Cardiology, Council on Epidemiology and Prevention, Council on Arteriosclerosis, Thrombosis, Vascular Biology, Council on Cardiopulmonary, Critical Care, Perioperative and Resuscitation, Council on Cardiovascular Nursing, Council on the Kidney in Cardiovascular Disease, Council on Cardiovascular Surgery and Anesthesia, Interdisciplinary Council on Quality of Care and Outcomes Research: Forecasting the future of cardiovascular disease in the United States: a policy statement from the American Heart Association. *Circulation* 2011; 123:933-944.

3. National Health and Nutrition Examination Survey (NHANES): Prevalence of Common Cardiovascular and Lung Dieseases, U.S., 2007-2011. Available at: http://www.nhlbi.nih.gov/about/documents/factbook/2012/chapter4#4_5. Accessed March 17, 2015.

4. Yancy CW, Jessup M, Bozkurt B, et al: 2013 ACCF/AHA guideline for the management of heart failure: executive summary: a report of the American College of Cardiology Foundation/American Heart Association Task Force on practice guidelines. *Circulation* 2013; 128:1810-1852.

5. Deja MA, Grayburn PA, Sun B, et al: Influence of mitral regurgitation repair on survival in the surgical treatment for ischemic heart failure trial. *Circulation* 2012; 125:2639-2648.

6. Velazquez EJ, Lee KL, Deja MA, et al: Coronary-artery bypass surgery in patients with left ventricular dysfunction. *N Engl J Med* 2011; 364:1607-1616.

7. Rose EA, Gelijns AC, Moskowitz AJ, et al: Long-Term use of a left ventricular assist device for end-stage heart failure. *N Engl J Med* 2001; 345:1435-1443.

8. Kirklin JK, Naftel DC, Kormos RL, et al: Fifth INTERMACS annual report: risk factor analysis from more than 6,000 mechanical circulatory support patients. *J Heart Lung Transplant* 2013; 32:141-156.

9. Pagani FD, Miller LW, Russell SD, et al: HeartMate III: Extended mechanical circulatory support with a continuous-flow rotary left ventricular assist device. *J Am Coll Cardiol* 2009; 54:312-321.

10. Gibbon JH, Jr: Application of a mechanical heart and lung apparatus to cardiac surgery. *Minn Med* 1954; 37:171-185; passim.

11. Lillehei CW, Cohen M, Warden HE, Varco RL: The direct-vision intracardiac correction of congenital anomalies by controlled cross circulation; results in thirty-two patients with ventricular septal defects, tetralogy of Fallot, and atrioventricularis communis defects. *Surgery* 1955; 38:11-29.

12. Kirklin JW, Dushane JW, Patrick RT, et al: Intracardiac surgery with the aid of a mechanical pump-oxygenator system (Gibbon type): report of eight cases. *Proc Staff Meet Mayo Clin* 1955; 30:201-206.

13. Cooley DA, Belmonte BA, Zeis LB, Schnur S: Surgical repair of ruptured interventricular septum following acute myocardial infarction. *Surgery* 1957; 41:930-937.

14. DeBakey ME: Left ventricular bypass pump for cardiac assistance. Clinical experience. *Am J Cardiol* 1971; 27:3-11.

15. Shumacker HB, Jr: A surgeon to remember: notes about Vladimir Demikhov. *Ann Thorac Surg* 1994; 58:1196-1198.

16. Cooley DA, Liotta D, Hallman GL, Bloodwell RD, Leachman RD, Milam JD: Orthotopic cardiac prosthesis for two-staged cardiac replacement. *Am J Cardiol* 1969; 24:723-730.

17. Norman JC, Duncan JM, Frazier OH, et al: Intracorporeal (abdominal) left ventricular assist devices or partial artificial hearts: a five-year clinical experience. *Arch Surg* 1981; 116:1441-1445.

18. Frazier OH, Macris MP, Myers TJ, et al: Improved survival after extended bridge to cardiac transplantation. *Ann Thorac Surg* 1994; 57:1416-1422; discussion 1412-1421.

19. Frazier OH, Rose EA, McCarthy P, et al: Improved mortality and rehabilitation of transplant candidates treated with a long-term implantable left ventricular assist system. *Ann Surg* 1995; 222:327-336; discussion 328-336.

20. Frazier OH: First use of an untethered, vented electric left ventricular assist device for long-term support. *Circulation* 1994; 89:2908-2914.

21. Frazier OH, Nakatani T, Duncan JM, Parnis SM, Fuqua JM: Clinical experience with the Hemopump. *ASAIO Trans* 1989; 35:604-606.

22. Macris MP, Parnis SM, Frazier OH, Fuqua JM, Jr, Jarvik RK: Development of an implantable ventricular assist system. *Ann Thorac Surg* 1997; 63:367-370.

23. Jarvik RK: System considerations favoring rotary artificial hearts with blood-immersed bearings. *Artif Organs* 1995; 19:565-570.

24. Tuzun E, Roberts K, Cohn WE, et al: In vivo evaluation of the HeartWare centrifugal ventricular assist device. *Tex Heart Inst J* 2007; 34:406-411.

25. Miller LW, Pagani FD, Russell SD, et al: Use of a Continuous-Flow Device in Patients Awaiting Heart Transplantation. *N Engl J Med* 2007; 357:885-896.

26. Slaughter MS, Rogers JG, Milano CA, et al: HeartMate III: Advanced heart failure treated with continuous-flow left ventricular assist device. *N Engl J Med* 2009; 361:2241-2251.

27. Aaronson KD, Slaughter MS, Miller LW, et al: HeartWare Ventricular Assist Device Bridge to Transplant ATI: Use of an intrapericardial, continuous-flow, centrifugal pump in patients awaiting heart transplantation. *Circulation* 2012; 125:3191-3200.

28. Pagani FD, Long JW, Dembitsky WP, Joyce LD, Miller LW: Improved mechanical reliability of the HeartMate XVE left ventricular assist system. *Ann Thorac Surg* 2006; 82:1413-1418.

29. Crow S, John R, Boyle A, et al: Gastrointestinal bleeding rates in recipients of nonpulsatile and pulsatile left ventricular assist devices. *J Thorac Cardiovasc Surg* 2009; 137:208-215.

30. Segura AM, Gregoric I, Radovancevic R, Demirozu ZT, Buja LM, Frazier OH: Morphologic changes in the aortic wall media after support with a continuous-flow left ventricular assist device. *J Heart Lung Transplant* 2013; 32:1096-1100.

31. Reul JT, Reul GJ, Frazier OH: Carotid-bulb thrombus and continuous-flow left ventricular assist devices: a novel observation. *J Heart Lung Transplant* 2014; 33:107-109.

32. Stretch R, Sauer CM, Yuh DD, Bonde P: National trends in the utilization of short-term mechanical circulatory support: incidence, outcomes, and cost analysis. *J Am Coll Cardiol* 2014; 64:1407-1415.

33. Mohite PN, Zych B, Popov AF, et al: CentriMag short-term ventricular assist as a bridge to solution in patients with advanced heart failure: use beyond 30 days. *Eur J Cardiothorac Surg* 2013; 44:e310-315.

34. Kar B, Adkins LE, Civitello AB, et al: Clinical experience with the TandemHeart percutaneous ventricular assist device. *Tex Heart Inst J* 2006; 33:111-115.

35. FDA U.S. Food and Drug Administration: Impella RP System - H140001. Available at: http://www.fda.gov/MedicalDevices/ProductsandMedical-Procedures/DeviceApprovalsandClearances/Recently-ApprovedDevices/ucm433494.htm. Accessed March 19, 2015.

36. Feldman D, Pamboukian SV, Teuteberg JJ, et al: International Society for Heartand Lung Transplantation: The 2013 International Society for Heart and Lung Transplantation Guidelines for mechanical circulatory support: executive summary. *J Heart Lung Transplant* 2013; 32:157-187.

37. Kirklin JK, Naftel DC, Pagani FD, et al: Sixth INTERMACS annual report: a 10,000-patient database. *J Heart Lung Transplant* 2014; 33: 555-564.

38. Birks EJ: Molecular changes after left ventricular assist device support for heart failure. *Circ Res* 2013; 113:777-791.

39. Frazier OH, Benedict CR, Radovancevic B, et al: Improved left ventricular function after chronic left ventricular unloading. *Ann Thorac Surg* 1996; 62:675-681; discussion 672-681.

40. Scheinin SA, Capek P, Radovancevic B, Duncan JM, McAllister HA, Jr, Frazier OH: The effect of prolonged left ventricular support on myocardial histopathology in patients with end-stage cardiomyopathy. *ASAIO J* 1992; 38:M271-274.

41. Birks EJ, George RS, Hedger M, et al: Reversal of severe heart failure with a continuous-flow left ventricular assist device and pharmacological therapy: a prospective study. *Circulation* 2011; 123:381-390.

42. Drakos SG, Wever-Pinzon O, Selzman CH, et al: Magnitude and time course of changes induced by continuous-flow left ventricular assist device unloading in chronic heart failure: insights into cardiac recovery. *J Am Coll Cardiol* 2013; 61:1985-1994.

43. Frazier OH, Baldwin AC, Demirozu ZT, et al: Ventricular reconditioning and pump explantation in patients supported by continuous-flow left ventricular assist devices. *J Heart Lung Transplant* 2014; Sep 28. pii: S1053-2498(14)01350-3. doi: 10.1016/j.healun.2014.09.015. [Epub ahead of print].

44. Alba AC, Rao V, Ross HJ, et al: Impact of fixed pulmonary hypertension on post-heart transplant outcomes in bridge-to-transplant patients. *J Heart Lung Transplant* 2010; 29:1253-1258.

45. Mikus E, Stepanenko A, Krabatsch T, et al: Reversibility of fixed pulmonary hypertension in left ventricular assist device support recipients. *Eur J Cardiothorac Surg* 2011; 40:971-977.

46. Teuteberg JJ, Stewart GC, Jessup M, et al: Implant strategies change over time and impact outcomes: insights from the INTERMACS (Interagency Registry for Mechanically Assisted Circulatory Support). *JACC Heart Fail* 2013; 1:369-378.

47. Norman JC, Cooley DA, Igo SR, et al: Prognostic indices for survival during postcardiotomy intra-aortic balloon pumping. Methods of scoring and classification, with implications for left ventricular assist device utilization. *J Thorac Cardiovasc Surg* 1977; 74:709-720.

48. Centers for Medicare & Medicaid Services: Centers for Medicare & Medicaid Services. Available at: cms.gov. Accessed March 17, 2015.

49. Stevenson LW, Pagani FD, Young JB, et al: INTERMACS profiles of advanced heart failure: the current picture. *J Heart Lung Transplant* 2009; 28:535-541.

50. Kirklin JK, Naftel DC, Kormos RL, et al: The Fourth INTERMACS Annual Report: 4,000 implants and counting. *J Heart Lung Transplant* 2012; 31:117-126.

51. Shah NR, Lam WW, Rodriguez FH, 3rd, et al: Clinical outcomes after ventricular assist device implantation in adults with complex congenital heart disease. *J Heart Lung Transplant* 2013; 32:615-620.

52. Topilsky Y, Pereira NL, Shah DK, et al: Left ventricular assist device therapy in patients with restrictive and hypertrophic cardiomyopathy. *Circ Heart Fail* 2011; 4:266-275.

53. Lietz K, Long JW, Kfoury AG, et al: Outcomes of left ventricular assist device implantation as destination therapy in the post-REMATCH era: implications for patient selection. *Circulation* 2007; 116:497-505.

54. Teuteberg JJ, Ewald GA, Adamson RM, et al: Risk assessment for continuous flow left ventricular assist devices: does the destination therapy risk score work? An analysis of over 1,000 patients. *J Am Coll Cardiol* 2012; 60:44-51.

55. Matthews JC, Pagani FD, Haft JW, Koelling TM, Naftel DC, Aaronson KD: Model for end-stage liver disease score predicts left ventricular assist device operative transfusion requirements, morbidity, and mortality. *Circulation* 2010; 121:214-220.

56. Yang JA, Kato TS, Shulman BP, et al: Liver dysfunction as a predictor of outcomes in patients with advanced heart failure requiring ventricular assist device support: use of the Model of End-stage Liver Disease (MELD) and MELD eXcluding INR (MELD-XI) scoring system. *J Heart Lung Transplant* 2012; 31:601-610.

57. Cowger J, Sundareswaran K, Rogers JG, et al: Predicting survival in patients receiving continuous flow left ventricular assist devices: the HeartMate II risk score. *J Am Coll Cardiol* 2013; 61:313-321.

58. Patel CB, Cowger JA, Zuckermann A: A contemporary review of mechanical circulatory support. *J Heart Lung Transplant* 2014; 33:667-674.

59. John R, Naka Y, Park SJ, et al: Impact of concurrent surgical valve procedures in patients receiving continuous-flow devices. *J Thorac Cardiovasc Surg* 2014; 147(2):581-589; discussion 589.

60. Milano C, Pagani FD, Slaughter MS, et al: Investigators A: Clinical outcomes after implantation of a centrifugal flow left ventricular assist device and concurrent cardiac valve procedures. *Circulation* 2014; 130:S3-11.

61. Soleimani B, Haouzi A, Manoskey A, Stephenson ER, El-Banayosy A, Pae WE: Development of aortic insufficiency in patients supported with continuous flow left ventricular assist devices. *ASAIO J* 2012; 58:326-329.

62. Cohn WE, Demirozu ZT, Frazier OH: Surgical closure of left ventricular outflow tract after left ventricular assist device implantation in patients with aortic valve pathology. *J Heart Lung Transplant* 2011; 30:59-63.

63. Cohn WE, Frazier OH: The sandwich plug technique: simple, effective, and rapid closure of a mechanical aortic valve prosthesis at left ventricular assist device implantation. *J Thorac Cardiovasc Surg* 2011; 142:455-457.

64. Myers JL, Bull A, Kastl DG, Pierce WS: Fusion of prosthetic valve during left heart bypass. *J Thorac Cardiovasc Surg* 1981; 82:263-267.

65. Pelletier MP, Chang CP, Vagelos R, Robbins RC: Alternative approach for use of a left ventricular assist device with a thrombosed prosthetic valve. *J Heart Lung Transplant* 2002; 21:402-404.

66. Maltais S, Topilsky Y, Tchantchaleishvili V, et al: Surgical treatment of tricuspid valve insufficiency promotes early reverse remodeling in patients with axial-flow left ventricular assist devices. *J Thorac Cardiovasc Surg* 2012; 143:1370-1376.

67. Piacentino V, 3rd, Ganapathi AM, Stafford-Smith M, et al: Utility of concomitant tricuspid valve procedures for patients undergoing implantation of a continuous-flow left ventricular device. *J Thorac Cardiovasc Surg* 2012; 144:1217-1221.

68. Potapov EV, Schweiger M, Stepanenko A, et al: Tricuspid valve repair in patients supported with left ventricular assist devices. *ASAIO J* 2011; 57:363-367.

69. Slaughter MS, Pagani FD, Rogers JG, et al: HeartMate IICl: Clinical management of continuous-flow left ventricular assist devices in advanced heart failure. *J Heart Lung Transplant* 2010; 29:S1-39.

70. Baldwin RT, Duncan JM, Frazier OH, Wilansky S: Patent foramen ovale: a cause of hypoxemia in patients on left ventricular support. *Ann Thorac Surg* 1991; 52:865-867.

71. Nguyen DQ, Das GS, Grubbs BC, Bolman RM, 3rd, Park SJ: Transcatheter closure of patent foramen ovale for hypoxemia during left ventricular assist device support. *J Heart Lung Transplant* 1999; 18:1021-1023.

72. Farrar DJ, Hill JD: Recovery of major organ function in patients awaiting heart transplantation with Thoratec ventricular assist devices. Thoratec Ventricular Assist Device Principal Investigators. *J Heart Lung Transplant* 1994; 13:1125-1132.

73. Letsou GV, Myers TJ, Gregoric ID, et al: Continuous axial-flow left ventricular assist device (Jarvik 2000) maintains kidney and liver perfusion for up to 6 months. *Ann Thorac Surg* 2003; 76:1167-1170.

74. Radovancevic B, Vrtovec B, de Kort E, Radovancevic R, Gregoric ID, Frazier OH: End-organ function in patients on long-term circulatory support with continuous- or pulsatile-flow assist devices. *J Heart Lung Transplant* 2007; 26:815-818.

75. Sandner SE, Zimpfer D, Zrunek P, et al: Renal function after implantation of continuous versus pulsatile flow left ventricular assist devices. *J Heart Lung Transplant* 2008; 27:469-473.

76. Butler J, Geisberg C, Howser R, et al: Relationship between renal function and left ventricular assist device use. *Ann Thorac Surg* 2006; 81:1745-1751.

77. Sandner SE, Zimpfer D, Zrunek P, et al: Renal function and outcome after continuous flow left ventricular assist device implantation. *Ann Thorac Surg* 2009; 87:1072-1078.

78. Reinhartz O, Farrar DJ, Hershon JH, Avery GJ, Jr, Haeusslein EA, Hill JD: Importance of preoperative liver function as a predictor of survival in patients supported with Thoratec ventricular assist devices as a bridge to transplantation. *J Thorac Cardiovasc Surg* 1998; 116:633-640.

79. Wadia Y, Etheridge W, Smart F, Wood RP, Frazier OH: Pathophysiology of hepatic dysfunction and intrahepatic cholestasis in heart failure and after left ventricular assist device support. *J Heart Lung Transplant* 2005; 24:361-370.

80. Kormos RL, Teuteberg JJ, Siegenthaler MP, et al: 250: Pre-VAD Implant Risk Factors Influence the Onset of Adverse Events (AEs) while on a VAD. *J Heart Lung Transplant* 2009; 28:S153-S154.

81. Frazier OH, Rose EA, Oz MC, et al: HeartMate LILVAS: Multicenter clinical evaluation of the HeartMate vented electric left ventricular assist system in patients awaiting heart transplantation. *J Thorac Cardiovasc Surg* 2001; 122:1186-1195.

82. Kavarana MN, Pessin-Minsley MS, Urtecho J, et al: Right ventricular dysfunction and organ failure in left ventricular assist device recipients: a continuing problem. *Ann Thorac Surg* 2002; 73:745-750.

83. Drakos SG, Janicki L, Horne BD, et al: Risk factors predictive of right ventricular failure after left ventricular assist device implantation. *Am J Cardiol* 2010; 105:1030-1035.

84. Matthews JC, Koelling TM, Pagani FD, Aaronson KD: The right ventricular failure risk score a pre-operative tool for assessing the risk of right ventricular failure in left ventricular assist device candidates. *J Am Coll Cardiol* 2008; 51:2163-2172.

85. Ochiai Y, McCarthy PM, Smedira NG, et al: Predictors of severe right ventricular failure after implantable left ventricular assist device insertion: analysis of 245 patients. *Circulation* 2002; 106:I198-202.

86. Patel ND, Weiss ES, Schaffer J, et al: Right heart dysfunction after left ventricular assist device implantation: a comparison of the pulsatile HeartMate I and axial-flow HeartMate II devices. *Ann Thorac Surg* 2008; 86:832-840; discussion 832-840.

87. Kormos RL, Teuteberg JJ, Pagani FD, et al: HeartMate IICI: Right ventricular failure in patients with the HeartMate II continuous-flow left ventricular assist device: incidence, risk factors, and effect on outcomes. *J Thorac Cardiovasc Surg* 2010; 139:1316-1324.

88. Grant AD, Smedira NG, Starling RC, Marwick TH: Independent and incremental role of quantitative right ventricular evaluation for the prediction of right ventricular failure after left ventricular assist device implantation. *J Am Coll Cardiol* 2012; 60:521-528.

89. Kukucka M, Stepanenko A, Potapov E, et al: Right-to-left ventricular end-diastolic diameter ratio and prediction of right ventricular failure with continuous-flow left ventricular assist devices. *J Heart Lung Transplant* 2011; 30:64-69.

90. Potapov EV, Stepanenko A, Dandel M, et al: Tricuspid incompetence and geometry of the right ventricle as predictors of right ventricular function after implantation of a left ventricular assist device. *J Heart Lung Transplant* 2008; 27:1275-1281.

91. Vivo RP, Cordero-Reyes AM, Qamar U, et al: Increased right-to-left ventricle diameter ratio is a strong predictor of right ventricular failure after left ventricular assist device. *J Heart Lung Transplant* 2013; 32:792-799.

92. Atluri P, Goldstone AB, Fairman AS, et al: Predicting right ventricular failure in the modern, continuous flow left ventricular assist device era. *Ann Thorac Surg* 2013; 96:857-863; discussion 863-854.

93. Baumwol J, Macdonald PS, Keogh AM, et al: Right heart failure and "failure to thrive" after left ventricular assist device: clinical predictors and outcomes. *J Heart Lung Transplant* 2011; 30:888-895.

94. Rich JD: Right ventricular failure in patients with left ventricular assist devices. *Cardiol Clin* 2012; 30:291-302.

95. Holdy K, Dembitsky W, Eaton LL, et al: Nutrition assessment and management of left ventricular assist device patients. *J Heart Lung Transplant* 2005; 24:1690-1696.

96. Mano A, Fujita K, Uenomachi K, et al: Body mass index is a useful predictor of prognosis after left ventricular assist system implantation. *J Heart Lung Transplant* 2009; 28:428-433.

97. Adamson RM, Stahovich M, Chillcott S, et al: Clinical strategies and outcomes in advanced heart failure patients older than 70 years of age

98. El-Sayed Ahmed MM, Aftab M, Singh SK, Mallidi HR, Frazier OH: Left ventricular assist device outflow graft: alternative sites. *Ann Cardiothorac Surg* 2014; 3:541-545.

99. Riebandt J, Sandner S, Mahr S, et al: Minimally invasive thoratec HeartMate II implantation in the setting of severe thoracic aortic calcification. *Ann Thorac Surg* 2013; 96:1094-1096.

100. Umakanthan R, Haglund NA, Stulak JM, et al: Left thoracotomy HeartWare implantation with outflow graft anastomosis to the descending aorta: a simplified bridge for patients with multiple previous sternotomies. *ASAIO J* 2013; 59:664-667.

101. Frazier OH, Gregoric ID, Cohn WE: Initial experience with non-thoracic, extraperitoneal, off-pump insertion of the Jarvik 2000 Heart in patients with previous median sternotomy. *J Heart Lung Transplant* 2006; 25:499-503.

102. Gregoric ID, Cohn WE, Frazier OH: Diaphragmatic implantation of the HeartWare ventricular assist device. *J Heart Lung Transplant* 2011; 30:467-470.

103. Singh A, Russo MJ, Valeroso TB, et al: Modified HeartMate II driveline externalization technique significantly decreases incidence of infection and improves long-term survival. *ASAIO J* 2014; 60:613-616.

104. Schaffer JM, Arnaoutakis GJ, Allen JG, et al: Bleeding complications and blood product utilization with left ventricular assist device implantation. *Ann Thorac Surg* 2011; 91:740-747; discussion 747-749.

105. Bruckner BA, DiBardino DJ, Ning Q, et al: High incidence of thromboembolic events in left ventricular assist device patients treated with recombinant activated factor VII. *J Heart Lung Transplant* 2009; 28: 785-790.

106. Myers TJ, Bolmers M, Gregoric ID, Kar B, Frazier OH: Assessment of arterial blood pressure during support with an axial flow left ventricular assist device. *J Heart Lung Transplant* 2009; 28:423-427.

107. Chorpenning K, Brown MC, Voskoboynikov N, Reyes C, Dierlam AE, Tamez D: HeartWare controller logs a diagnostic tool and clinical management aid for the HVAD pump. *ASAIO J* 2014; 60:115-118.

108. Potapov E, Meyer D, Swaminathan M, et al: Inhaled nitric oxide after left ventricular assist device implantation: a prospective, randomized, double-blind, multicenter, placebo-controlled trial. *J Heart Lung Transplant* 2011; 30:870-878.

109. Argenziano M, Choudhri AF, Moazami N, et al: Randomized, double-blind trial of inhaled nitric oxide in LVAD recipients with pulmonary hypertension. *Ann Thorac Surg* 1998; 65:340-345.

110. Loforte A, Montalto A, Lilla Della Monica P, Musumeci F: Simultaneous temporary CentriMag right ventricular assist device placement in HeartMate II left ventricular assist system recipients at high risk of right ventricular failure. *Interact Cardiovasc Thorac Surg* 2010; 10:847-850.

111. Rose EA, Levin HR, Oz MC, et al: Artificial circulatory support with textured interior surfaces. A counterintuitive approach to minimizing thromboembolism. *Circulation* 1994; 90:II87-91.

112. Westaby S, Banning AP, Jarvik R, et al: First permanent implant of the Jarvik 2000 Heart. *Lancet* 2000; 356:900-903.

113. Amir O, Bracey AW, Smart FW, Delgado RM, 3rd, Shah N, Kar B: A successful anticoagulation protocol for the first HeartMate II implantation in the United States. *Tex Heart Inst J* 2005; 32:399-401.

114. Boyle AJ, Russell SD, Teuteberg JJ, et al: Low thromboembolism and pump thrombosis with the HeartMate II left ventricular assist device: analysis of outpatient anti-coagulation. *J Heart Lung Transplant* 2009; 28:881-887.

115. Slaughter MS, Naka Y, John R, et al: Post-operative heparin may not be required for transitioning patients with a HeartMate II left ventricular assist system to long-term warfarin therapy. *J Heart Lung Transplant* 2010; 29:616-624.

116. Krabatsch T, Potapov E, Stepanenko A, et al: Biventricular circulatory support with two miniaturized implantable assist devices. *Circulation* 2011; 124:S179-186.

117. Loebe M, Bruckner B, Reardon MJ, et al: Initial clinical experience of total cardiac replacement with dual HeartMate-II axial flow pumps for severe biventricular heart failure. *Methodist Debakey Cardiovasc J* 2011; 7:40-44.

118. Strueber M, Meyer AL, Malehsa D, Haverich A: Successful use of the HeartWare HVAD rotary blood pump for biventricular support. *J Thorac Cardiovasc Surg* 2010; 140:936-937.

119. Lampropulos JF, Kim N, Wang Y, et al: Trends in left ventricular assist device use and outcomes among Medicare beneficiaries, 2004-2011. *Open Heart* 2014; 1:e000109.

120. McCarthy PM, Smedira NO, Vargo RL, et al: One hundred patients with the HeartMate left ventricular assist device: evolving concepts and technology. *J Thorac Cardiovasc Surg* 1998; 115:904-912.

121. Holman WL, Kormos RL, Naftel DC, et al: Predictors of death and transplant in patients with a mechanical circulatory support device: a multi-institutional study. *J Heart Lung Transplant* 2009; 28:44-50.

122. Fitzpatrick JR, 3rd, Frederick JR, Hiesinger W, et al: Early planned institution of biventricular mechanical circulatory support results in improved outcomes compared with delayed conversion of a left ventricular assist device to a biventricular assist device. *J Thorac Cardiovasc Surg* 2009; 137:971-977.

123. Cleveland JC, Jr, Grover FL, Fullerton DA, et al: Left ventricular assist device as bridge to transplantation does not adversely affect one-year heart transplantation survival. *J Thorac Cardiovasc Surg* 2008; 136:774-777.

124. Russo MJ, Hong KN, Davies RR, et al: Posttransplant survival is not diminished in heart transplant recipients bridged with implantable left ventricular assist devices. *J Thorac Cardiovasc Surg* 2009; 138:1425-1432 e1421-1423.

125. Genovese EA, Dew MA, Teuteberg JJ, et al: Early adverse events as predictors of 1-year mortality during mechanical circulatory support. *J Heart Lung Transplant* 2010; 29:981-988.

126. Genovese EA, Dew MA, Teuteberg JJ, et al: Incidence and patterns of adverse event onset during the first 60 days after ventricular assist device implantation. *Ann Thorac Surg* 2009; 88:1162-1170.

127. Eckman PM, John R: Bleeding and thrombosis in patients with continuous-flow ventricular assist devices. *Circulation* 2012; 125:3038-3047.

128. Bunte MC, Blackstone EH, Thuita L, et al: Major bleeding during HeartMate II support. *J Am Coll Cardiol* 2013; 62:2188-2196.

129. Haglund NA, Davis ME, Tricarico NM, et al: Perioperative blood product use: a comparison between HeartWare and HeartMate II devices. *Ann Thorac Surg* 2014; 98:842-849.

130. Interagency Registry for Mechanically Assisted Circulatory Support (INTERMACS): Adverse event definitions: adult and pediatric patients.

131. Minami K, El-Banayosy A, Sezai A, et al: Morbidity and outcome after mechanical ventricular support using Thoratec, Novacor, and HeartMate for bridging to heart transplantation. *Artif Organs* 2000; 24:421-426.

132. Goldstein DJ, Naftel D, Holman W, et al: Continuous-flow devices and percutaneous site infections: clinical outcomes. *J Heart Lung Transplant* 2012; 31:1151-1157.

133. Schaffer JM, Allen JG, Weiss ES, et al: Infectious complications after pulsatile-flow and continuous-flow left ventricular assist device implantation. *J Heart Lung Transplant* 2011; 30:164-174.

134. Topkara VK, Kondareddy S, Malik F, et al: Infectious complications in patients with left ventricular assist device: etiology and outcomes in the continuous-flow era. *Ann Thorac Surg* 2010; 90:1270-1277.

135. Baradarian S, Stahovich M, Krause S, Adamson R, Dembitsky W: Case series: clinical management of persistent mechanical assist device driveline drainage using vacuum-assisted closure therapy. *ASAIO J* 2006; 52:354-356.

136. Kretlow JD, Brown RH, Wolfswinkel EM, et al: Salvage of infected left ventricular assist device with antibiotic beads. *Plast Reconstr Surg* 2014; 133:28e-38e.

137. Gordon RJ, Weinberg AD, Pagani FD, et al, Ventricular Assist Device Infection Study G: Prospective, multicenter study of ventricular assist device infections. *Circulation* 2013; 127:691-702.

138. Borgi J, Tsiouris A, Hodari A, Cogan CM, Paone G, Morgan JA: Significance of postoperative acute renal failure after continuous-flow left ventricular assist device implantation. *Ann Thorac Surg* 2013; 95:163-169.

139. Demirozu ZT, Etheridge WB, Radovancevic R, Frazier OH: Results of HeartMate II left ventricular assist device implantation on renal function in patients requiring post-implant renal replacement therapy. *J Heart Lung Transplant* 2011; 30:182-187.

140. Morgan JA, Brewer RJ, Nemeh HW, et al: Stroke while on long-term left ventricular assist device support: incidence, outcome, and predictors. *ASAIO J* 2014; 60:284-289.

141. Nassif ME, Tibrewala A, Raymer DS, et al: Systolic blood pressure on discharge after left ventricular assist device insertion is associated with subsequent stroke. *J Heart Lung Transplant* 2014.

142. Demirozu ZT, Frazier OH: Aortic valve noncoronary cusp thrombosis after implantation of a nonpulsatile, continuous-flow pump. *Tex Heart Inst J* 2012; 39:618-620.

143. Lampert BC, Eckert C, Weaver S, et al: Blood pressure control in continuous flow left ventricular assist devices: efficacy and impact on adverse events. *Ann Thorac Surg* 2014; 97:139-146.

144. Aggarwal A, Pant R, Kumar S, et al: Incidence and management of gastrointestinal bleeding with continuous flow assist devices. *Ann Thorac Surg* 2012; 93:1534-1540.

145. Demirozu ZT, Radovancevic R, Hochman LF, et al: Arteriovenous malformation and gastrointestinal bleeding in patients with the HeartMate II left ventricular assist device. *J Heart Lung Transplant* 2011; 30:849-853.

146. John R, Kamdar F, Eckman P, et al: Lessons learned from experience with over 100 consecutive HeartMate II left ventricular assist devices. *Ann Thorac Surg* 2011; 92:1593-1599; discussion 1599-1600.

147. Kushnir VM, Sharma S, Ewald GA, et al: Evaluation of GI bleeding after implantation of left ventricular assist device. *Gastrointest Endosc* 2012; 75:973-979.

148. Stulak JM, Lee D, Haft JW, et al: Gastrointestinal bleeding and subsequent risk of thromboembolic events during support with a left ventricular assist device. *J Heart Lung Transplant* 2014; 33:60-64.

149. Wever-Pinzon O, Selzman CH, Drakos SG, et al: Pulsatility and the risk of nonsurgical bleeding in patients supported with the continuous-flow left ventricular assist device HeartMate II. *Circ Heart Fail* 2013; 6:517-526.

150. Hayes HM, Dembo LG, Larbalestier R, O'Driscoll G: Management options to treat gastrointestinal bleeding in patients supported on rotary left ventricular assist devices: a single-center experience. *Artif Organs* 2010; 34:703-706.

151. Klovaite J, Gustafsson F, Mortensen SA, Sander K, Nielsen LB: Severely impaired von Willebrand factor-dependent platelet aggregation in patients with a continuous-flow left ventricular assist device (HeartMate II). *J Am Coll Cardiol* 2009; 53:2162-2167.

152. Meyer AL, Malehsa D, Bara C, et al: Acquired von Willebrand syndrome in patients with an axial flow left ventricular assist device. *Circ Heart Fail* 2010; 3:675-681.

153. Uriel N, Pak SW, Jorde UP, et al: Acquired von Willebrand syndrome after continuous-flow mechanical device support contributes to a high prevalence of bleeding during long-term support and at the time of transplantation. *J Am Coll Cardiol* 2010; 56:1207-1213.

154. Crow S, Chen D, Milano C, et al: Acquired von Willebrand syndrome in continuous-flow ventricular assist device recipients. *Ann Thorac Surg* 2010; 90:1263-1269; discussion 1269.

155. Boley SJ, Sammarteno R, Brandt LJ, Sprayregan S: Vascular ectasias of the colon. *Surg Gynecol Obstet* 1979; 149:353.

156. Heyde EC: Gastrointestinal bleeding in aortic stenosis. *N Engl J Med* 1958; 259:196-196.

157. Letsou GV, Shah N, Gregoric ID, Myers TJ, Delgado R, Frazier OH: Gastrointestinal bleeding from arteriovenous malformations in patients supported by the Jarvik 2000 axial-flow left ventricular assist device. *J Heart Lung Transplant* 2005; 24:105-109.

158. Holman WL, Naftel DC, Eckert CE, Kormos RL, Goldstein DJ, Kirklin JK: Durability of left ventricular assist devices: Interagency Registry for Mechanically Assisted Circulatory Support (INTERMACS) 2006 to 2011. *J Thorac Cardiovasc Surg* 2013; 146:437-441 e431.

159. Starling RC, Moazami N, Silvestry SC, et al: Unexpected abrupt increase in left ventricular assist device thrombosis. *N Engl J Med* 2014; 370:33-40.

160. Kirklin JK, Naftel DC, Kormos RL, et al: Interagency Registry for Mechanically Assisted Circulatory Support (INTERMACS) analysis of pump thrombosis in the HeartMate II left ventricular assist device. *J Heart Lung Transplant* 2014; 33:12-22.

161. Taghavi S, Ward C, Jayarajan SN, Gaughan J, Wilson LM, Mangi AA: Surgical technique influences HeartMate II left ventricular assist device thrombosis. *Ann Thorac Surg* 2013; 96:1259-1265.

162. Whitson BA, Eckman P, Kamdar F, et al: Hemolysis, pump thrombus, and neurologic events in continuous-flow left ventricular assist device recipients. *Ann Thorac Surg* 2014; 97:2097-2103.

163. Shah P, Mehta VM, Cowger JA, Aaronson KD, Pagani FD: Diagnosis of hemolysis and device thrombosis with lactate dehydrogenase during left ventricular assist device support. *J Heart Lung Transplant* 2014; 33:102-104.

164. Uriel N, Morrison KA, Garan AR, et al: Development of a novel echo-cardiography ramp test for speed optimization and diagnosis of device thrombosis in continuous-flow left ventricular assist devices: the Columbia ramp study. *J Am Coll Cardiol* 2012; 60:1764-1775.

165. Goldstein DJ, John R, Salerno C, et al: Algorithm for the diagnosis and management of suspected pump thrombus. *J Heart Lung Transplant* 2013; 32:667-670.

166. Sarsam SH, Civitello AB, Agunanne EE, Delgado RM: Bivalirudin for treatment of aortic valve thrombosis after left ventricular assist device implantation. *ASAIO J* 2013; 59:448-449.

167. Sylvia LM, Ordway L, Pham DT, DeNofrio D, Kiernan M: Bivalirudin for treatment of LVAD thrombosis: a case series. *ASAIO J* 2014; 60:744-747.

168. Muthiah K, Robson D, Macdonald PS, et al: Thrombolysis for suspected intrapump thrombosis in patients with continuous flow centrifugal left ventricular assist device. *Artif Organs* 2013; 37:313-318.

169. Schlendorf K, Patel CB, Gehrig T, et al: Thrombolytic therapy for thrombosis of continuous flow ventricular assist devices. *J Card Fail* 2014; 20:91-97.

170. Cohn WE, Mallidi HR, Frazier OH: Safe, effective off-pump sternal sparing approach for HeartMate II exchange. *Ann Thorac Surg* 2013; 96:2259-2261.

171. Moazami N, Milano CA, John R, et al: HeartMate III: Pump replacement for left ventricular assist device failure can be done safely and is associated with low mortality. *Ann Thorac Surg* 2013; 95:500-505.

172. Lund LH, Edwards LB, Kucheryavaya AY, et al: International Society of Heart & Lung Transplantation: The registry of the International Society for Heart and Lung Transplantation: thirty-first official adult heart transplant report–2014; focus theme: retransplantation. *J Heart Lung Transplant* 2014; 33:996-1008.

173. Frazier OH, Cohn WE: Continuous-flow total heart replacement device implanted in a 55-year-old man with end-stage heart failure and severe amyloidosis. *Tex Heart Inst J* 2012; 39:542-546.

174. Frazier OH, Myers TJ, Gregoric I: Biventricular assistance with the Jarvik FlowMaker: a case report. *J Thorac Cardiovasc Surg* 2004; 128:625-626.

175. LeGallois CJJ: Experience on the principle of life (Experience sur la principe de la vie, Paris 1812). Nancrede N, trans. Philadelphia: Thomas; 1813.

176. Lindbergh CA: An apparatus for the culture of whole organs. *J Exp Med* 1935; 62:409-431.

177. Akutsu T, Kolff WJ: Permanent substitute for valves and hearts. *Trans Am Soc Artif Intern Organs* 1958; 4:230.

178. DeVries WC: The permanent artificial heart. Four case reports. *JAMA* 1988; 259:849-859.

179. DeVries WC: Surgical technique for implantation of the Jarvik-7-100 total artificial heart. *JAMA* 1988; 259:875-880.

180. DeVries WC, Anderson JL, Joyce LD, et al: Clinical use of the total artificial heart. *N Engl J Med* 1984; 310:273-278.

181. Copeland JG: Current status and future directions for a total artificial heart with a past. *Artif Organs* 1998; 22:998-1001.

182. Copeland JG, Smith RG, Icenogle TB, Rhenman B, Williams R, Vasu MA: Early experience with the total artificial heart as a bridge to cardiac transplantation. *Surg Clin North Am* 1988; 68:621-634.

183. Johnson KE, Prieto M, Joyce LD, Pritzker M, Emery RW: Summary of the clinical use of the Symbion total artificial heart: a registry report. *J Heart Lung Transplant* 1992; 11:103-116.

184. Slepian MJ: The SynCardia temporary total artificial heart - evolving clinical role and future status. *US Cardiol* 2011; 8:39.

185. Torregrossa G, Morshuis M, Varghese R, et al: Results with SynCardia total artificial heart beyond 1 year. *ASAIO J* 2014; 60:626-634.

186. Jaroszewski DE, Anderson EM, Pierce CN, Arabia FA: The SynCardia freedom driver: a portable driver for discharge home with the total artificial heart. *J Heart Lung Transplant* 2011; 30:844-845.

187. Copeland JG, Smith RG, Arabia FA, et al: CardioWest Total Artificial Heart I: Cardiac replacement with a total artificial heart as a bridge to transplantation. *N Engl J Med* 2004; 351:859-867.

188. Copeland JG, Copeland H, Gustafson M, et al: Experience with more than 100 total artificial heart implants. *J Thorac Cardiovasc Surg* 2012; 143:727-734.

189. Kirsch ME, Nguyen A, Mastroianni C, et al: SynCardia temporary total artificial heart as bridge to transplantation: current results at la pitie hospital. *Ann Thorac Surg* 2013; 95:1640-1646.

190. Parnis SM, Yu LS, Ochs BD, Macris MP, Frazier OH, Kung RT: Chronic in vivo evaluation of an electrohydraulic total artificial heart. *ASAIO J* 1994; 40:M489-493.

191. Kung RT, Yu LS, Ochs B, Parnis S, Frazier OH: An atrial hydraulic shunt in a total artificial heart. A balance mechanism for the bronchial shunt. *ASAIO J* 1993; 39:M213-217.

192. SoRelle R: Cardiovascular news. Totally contained AbioCor artificial heart implanted July 3, 2001. *Circulation* 2001; 104:E9005-9006.

193. Dowling RD, Gray LA, Jr, Etoch SW, et al: Initial experience with the AbioCor implantable replacement heart system. *J Thorac Cardiovasc Surg* 2004; 127:131-141.

194. Westaby S, Siegenthaler M, Beyersdorf F, et al: Destination therapy with a rotary blood pump and novel power delivery. *Eur J Cardiothorac Surg* 2010; 37:350-356.

195. Cohn WE, Handy KM, Parnis SM, Conger JL, Winkler JA, Frazier OH: Eight-year experience with a continuous-flow total artificial heart in calves. *ASAIO J* 2014; 60:25-30.

196. Cohn WE, Winkler JA, Parnis S, Costas GG, Beathard S, Conger J, Frazier OH: Ninety-day survival of a calf implanted with a continuous-flow total artificial heart. *ASAIO J* 2014; 60:15-18.

197. Timms D, Fraser J, Hayne M, Dunning J, McNeil K, Pearcy M: The BiVACOR rotary biventricular assist device: concept and in vitro investigation. *Artif Organs* 2008; 32:816-819.

198. Greatrex NA, Timms DL, Kurita N, Palmer EW, Masuzawa T: Axial magnetic bearing development for the BiVACOR rotary BiVAD/TAH. *IEEE Trans Biomed Eng* 2010; 57:714-721.

199. Kleinheyer M, Timms DL, Greatrex NA, Masuzawa T, Frazier OH, Cohn WE: Pulsatile operation of the BiVACOR TAH - Motor design, control and hemodynamics. *Conf Proc IEEE Eng Med Biol Soc* 2014; 2014:5659-5662.

200. Fumoto H, Horvath DJ, Rao S, et al: In vivo acute performance of the Cleveland Clinic self-regulating, continuous-flow total artificial heart. *J Heart Lung Transplant* 2010; 29:21-26.

Tissue Engineering for Cardiac Valve Surgery

Danielle Gottlieb • *John E. Mayer*

Tissue engineering is a developing science, comprising elements of engineering and biology, whose aim is to build replacement tissues de novo, from individual cellular and structural components. The impetus for our work on tissue-engineered cardiovascular structures arises from the need to replace cardiovascular tissues that failed to develop normally during embryogenesis or have become dysfunctional as a consequence of disease. In pediatric patients, the cardiovascular structures most often afflicted by congenital anomalies involve the cardiac valves and great vessels, and the theoretical advantages of a tissue-engineered structure containing live cells are the ability to grow, remodel, and repair. Although growth potential is not a consideration for the adult population, durability of valve structures remains an important issue for bioprosthetic valves, and a tissue engineering approach offers the potential to improve durability by providing the repair and remodeling capability.

Diseases of the heart valves and large "conduit" arteries account for approximately 60,000 cardiac surgical procedures each year in the United States, and all of the currently available replacement devices have significant limitations.[1,2] Ideally, any valve or artery substitute would function like a normal valve or artery. For valves, this function includes allowing pulsatile blood flow without a transvalvar gradient or valvar regurgitation. The theoretical advantage of engineered tissue replacements is that they could also display other desirable characteristics, such as (1) durability, (2) growth (for infants and children), (3) compatibility with blood components and the absence of thrombosis or destructive inflammation, and (4) resistance to infection. None of the currently available devices, constructed from either synthetic or biologic materials, meet these criteria. Mechanical heart valves are very durable, but they require anticoagulation to reduce the risk of thrombosis and thromboembolism.[1,2] Therapeutic anticoagulation carries associated morbidity, and even among patients who receive therapeutic anticoagulation, the incidence of thromboembolic complications of mechanical heart valve replacement is not zero.[1,2] Biologic valves, whether of allograft or heterograft origin, remain subject to structural deterioration after implantation.[2-4] Neither mechanical nor biologic valves have any growth potential, and this limitation represents a major source of morbidity for pediatric patients who must undergo multiple reoperations to replace valves and/or valved conduits during the period of maximum somatic growth.

Tissue engineering is an approach based upon the hypothesis that when properly designed and fabricated, these "living" devices will simulate the biology of normal cardiovascular structures, thereby overcoming the shortcomings of currently available heart valve replacements. Of particular relevance to pediatric heart surgery is the long-term function of the engineered valve over time and the potential capacity to grow, self-repair, and remodel. This chapter summarizes some of the progress that has been made in tissue engineering research as it relates to cardiac valves and conduit arteries, and then outlines the areas where additional efforts must be focused in order to direct cardiovascular tissue engineering toward clinical utility.

NORMAL HEART VALVE BIOLOGY
Adult Valve Structure and Function

Heart valves open and close approximately 40 million times per year; this coordinated function occurs under the demands of hemodynamic forces of blood pressure and shear stress. The normal semilunar valve presents minimal resistance to opening and no pressure gradient during systolic forward flow. In diastole, the same structure is responsible for rapid and complete closure in order to prevent valve regurgitation. Semilunar valves must additionally resist pressure differences between the diastolic arterial pressure and the diastolic ventricular pressure. The atrioventricular valves must function in a comparable way, opening with minimal resistance during diastole and closing to prevent regurgitation during ventricular systole.

Like many other tissues, valve cusps are composed of cells residing within the extracellular matrix (ECM). In addition, these same cells act reciprocally on the ECM to which they are attached and receive signals from the ECM. The effects of these cellular level mechanical signals on cell phenotype and behavior have been characterized by Ingber[5,6] using the term "tensegrity" to describe the interactions between cell adhesion to ECM and the nucleus mediated by the cellular cytoskeleton. Semilunar valve cusps are thin, flexible structures with impressive microscopic and molecular complexity. Much of the strength and flexibility of normal heart valve cusps is due to the specialized proteins and polysaccharide-protein complexes of the ECM, produced by resident valve interstitial cells.[7,8] The microscopic and molecular structure of adult valves reflects the regional mechanical forces experienced by the valve cusps; valve cusp ECM is not homogeneous, and the arrangement of the ECM provides a high degree of flexibility during systole, and a high degree of strength to resist pressure loads during diastole.[7] On the surfaces, a specialized endothelium prevents thrombosis, but also acts as a transducer of mechanical force.[9,10] Beneath the endothelium, valve interstitial cells receive signals sent by the endothelium, and respond to imposed mechanical signals by secreting suitable matrix.[5,6,11]

Semilunar valve ECM is stratified into layers and its distribution is related to valve mechanics.[12] Facing the sinus of Valsalva, where eddy currents occur and diastolic pressure loads are imposed, dense collagen is found in the fibrosa layer. A middle layer of connective tissue, the spongiosa, is particularly rich in glycosaminoglycans, large complex molecules which associate with water, and this layer is thought to act as a "shock absorber," bearing largely compressive mechanical loads. The ventricularis, an elastin-rich layer facing the lumen and the flow orifice of the semilunar valve is specialized to stretch as the cusps elongate during ejection in systole. The resulting composite structure of the native semilunar valve is anisotropic, with less elasticity in the commissure to commissure direction and greater elasticity in the annulus to free edge direction. The orientation of the collagen bundles in the native semilunar valves have also been demonstrated to affect normal leaflet motion during systole and diastole.[13–15]

Valve structure and function are therefore closely related, and strategies to engineer valves are aimed to mimic normal valve structure and function, potentially at the subcellular, cellular, tissue, and whole heart valve levels.

Embryologic and Postnatal Development

Valves do not begin development as stratified tissues; as circulatory patterns evolve in fetal and postnatal life, valve morphology also changes.[12] Embryologic valve development, therefore, has relevance to tissue engineering, as a model for normal in vivo valve remodeling as programmed by gene regulatory pathways and by applied biomechanical force.

By day 15 of human embryo development, specification of myocardial and endothelial cardiac cells occurs. At day 21, formation of a linear heart tube occurs. These events are followed by rightward (dextro) looping of the heart, resulting in orientation of the cardiac chambers into their final adult positions, and opposition of two specialized segments of ECM, known as cardiac jelly.[16] The first evidence of valvulogenesis occurs in this cardiac jelly, when a subset of endothelial cells separate from the luminal surface, invade the ECM, and undergo endothelial-to-mesenchymal transformation (EMT).[17] In early fetal valve development, valve interstitial cells are highly proliferative, and reside in a glycosaminoglycan-rich, homogeneous microenvironment. Over the course of fetal development, cell proliferation slows, and production of ECM results in valve cusp elongation. During the late stages of fetal development (20 to 36 weeks of human gestation) and in early postnatal life, valve stratification into a trilaminar structure occurs, and organization and maturation of collagen fibers begins. At the time of birth, through a series of largely undefined molecular steps, changes in oxygenation and blood pressure distinguish the aortic from the pulmonary sides of the circulation.[12] Transitional neonatal circulation has been associated with a change in phenotype from activated to quiescent interstitial cells in pulmonary, but not aortic, valve cusps.[18] Valve maturation and remodeling continue during childhood; cellularity of valve interstitial cells continues to decrease into adulthood.[12] Once thought to be passive structures, increasing evidence shows cardiac valves to be dynamic organs. Mechanistically, the finding that cellular and extracellular components mature is thought to reflect the dramatic changes in flow and biomechanical loading conditions from fetal to adult life.[13,19] Further elucidation of the genetic regulatory events defining valve growth and maturation are likely to provide important information in designing biomimetic replacement devices.

ENGINEERED VALVE INPUTS

The fundamental concept of creating a tissue-engineered cardiac valve is to develop a tissue composed of living cells which will, at some point, form and remodel their own ECM and thus provide durability and growth potential. The biological and engineering challenge lies in how to provide structural organization for these cells until they are capable of forming their own mature ECM and to provide sufficient structural support and mechanical integrity until the cells form their own ECM. Therefore, the fundamental variables involved in the creation of a living "tissue-engineered" valve involve choice or manipulation of cell phenotype, induction of appropriate ECM formation by mechanical and/or biochemical signals, and provision of structural integrity and cellular organization by the scaffold until new "native" ECM formation occurs.

Approaches to tissue-engineered heart valves (TEHV) can be divided into two paradigms, based upon the type of structural scaffold employed. One approach is to use bioresorbable scaffolds (nonwoven felts, electrospun scaffolds; knitted meshes, hydrogel-based, and combinations), and the other approach involves beginning with decellularized tissue-based scaffolds. The bioresorbable scaffold approach begins with seeding cells and culturing under appropriate biomechanical conditions (static flow, pulsatile flow) and nutrient medium. With regard to tissue mechanical properties, the goal of this approach is fabrication of an adequately strong tissue with approximately constant mechanical properties, requiring that the process of scaffold degradation occurs with a reciprocal increase in ECM production. Porosity is an important characteristic of bioresorbable scaffolds as it provides a permeable framework for cell migration, nutrient supply, and waste removal. Insufficient porosity leads to nutrient deprivation and cell death. Once a sufficiently stable tissue is formed, in vivo implantation would ideally follow, placing a newly synthesized tissue, devoid of foreign elements, in the required site. An alternative approach involves use of an acellular scaffold material which can then be populated by host tissue, either by direct in-growth or seeding from the blood stream, or some combination of these two mechanisms.[20,21]

This de novo approach using cell-seeded biodegradable scaffolds is the one that has been predominantly employed in our laboratory at Children's Hospital, Boston.[23-29] This approach treats components of tissue as "building blocks," constructing valves from a variety of cell types and scaffold materials. Most in vivo studies have been carried out in the lower-pressure pulmonary circulation, which is a more tolerant system than the systemic circulation. This type of approach considers several basic questions as its foundation: (1) What cell type or combination of cell types is necessary to allow the production and maintenance of an appropriate ECM? (2) To what extent can cellular phenotype be altered, guided, or "engineered" to replicate cells found in the normal valve? (3) How can these cells be spatially organized during the development of this tissue-engineered structures until the cells in the construct produce sufficient and appropriate ECM? (4) What biochemical signals are necessary during the development of these structures to ensure proper ECM production? (5) What mechanical signals are necessary for optimal tissue development and growth? (6) Should a tissue-engineered valve construct be completely developed and have the histologic and macroscopic appearance of an adult valve prior to implantation, or can further maturation of an engineered construct occur in vivo after implantation? More recently, we have utilized acellular scaffold materials with chemical composition and fabrication processes that yield anisotropic mechanics that closely resemble those of native leaflet.[22]

Proponents of the decellularized tissue method base their approach on the premise that ECM characteristics and signals direct cell behavior, and that the closest structure to the normal valve scaffold is the normal valve ECM scaffold itself. Human aortic valve homografts are currently implanted without tissue-type matching, are found to become mostly acellular after several months in vivo, yet retain their mechanical properties for longer periods of time. As the exact features endowing the aortic valve with this improved, but still limited durability are unknown, it is hypothesized that these features are retained after ex vivo decellularization. These decellularized scaffolds can either seeded with cells prior to implantation, or implanted without seeded cells, in the expectation that appropriate circulating cell populations will populate the scaffolds in vivo. Without seeding of cells prior to implantation, however, some decellularized matrices are insufficiently endothelialized by circulating cells or ingrowth from adjacent tissues to resist surface thrombus formation in vivo.[21]

The literature of TEHV demonstrates the selection of a variety of cell types, scaffold conditions, and preconditioning regimens, and overall, methods are difficult to compare and results have been inconsistent. Systematic screening of engineered tissue elements and combinatorial approaches to building tissues have recently emerged.[30,31] A complete review of past investigations is beyond the scope of this chapter; however, a summary of the fundamental elements of synthetic, biomaterial-based TEHV will be considered in detail in the following sections. In vivo outcomes of these methods will also be considered.

Cell Origin and Phenotype

As in embryologic valvulogenesis, the "ideal" cell type for a TEHV would fulfill the function of both the valve interstitial and endothelial cells. Conceptually, these cells could be derived from fully differentiated cells capable of ECM synthesis, or from less committed, multipotent or pluripotent stem cells with the additional potential for differentiation into multiple cell types. Alternatively, two separate cell types could be potentially used to form a valve structure with valve endothelial cells on the surface and valve interstitial cells in the inner layers of the valve. The role of host cell ingrowth from adjacent tissues and/or seeding from the blood stream represent other alternative sources of cells.

The first TEHV experiments were performed with differentiated cells from artery or vein, including vascular smooth muscle cells, fibroblasts, and endothelial cells derived from the vasculature of immature animals.[20,23-25] These cells were chosen as they were readily accessible, are derived from a cardiovascular source, and can synthesize ECM proteins. A comparison of myofibroblasts from the wall of the ascending aorta with those from segments of saphenous vein revealed that the latter cells exhibit superior collagen formation and mechanical strength when cultured on biodegradable polyurethane scaffolds.[32] In our laboratory at Boston Children's Hospital TEHV based on these differentiated cells from systemic blood vessels functioned for periods of up to 4 months in vivo.[20,23] However, enhanced collagen formation may be a double-edged sword. The rapid formation of new tissue in the early culture period could give rise to an overabundance of matrix elements, leading to tissue stiffness and potential tissue contraction. Early studies with dermal fibroblasts demonstrated that valve cusps constructed from these cells developed tissue contraction, which limited the ability of valve leaflets to coapt with each other, resulting in valve regurgitation.[33] In addition to production of excessive or unfavorable types of ECM, mature cells may present a problem of senescence in long-term cell cultures in vitro, which limits the ability to quickly produce sufficient numbers of cells to seed a TEHV construct. Finally, the prospect of harvesting segments of artery from an otherwise normal peripheral circulation in order to obtain cells for a TEHV represents an undesirable clinical situation, and therefore led to a search for alternative cell sources for engineered valves.

The emergence of the field of stem cell biology has the potential to change the paradigm for candidate cell types for heart valve tissue engineering. As stem cells differentiate from their embryonic state, they lose pluripotency with each subsequent step. Multiple steps of differentiation form lineages of cells. In embryonic development, differentiation down a specific lineage occurs with biochemical signaling, occurring in a specific mechanical microenvironment.[34] How lineage specification occurs in the developing heart is currently an area of active research, with the goal of understanding the necessary cues to replicate differentiation down valve cell lineages. In normal development, differentiating cells are subject to a rapidly changing three-dimensional extracellular environment, and development is thought to occur by signals originating outside of the cell, from molecules originating in neighboring cells, and in the ECM. The importance of these mechanical interactions between cells and their immediate environment during embryonic development has been emphasized by Ingber.[6] These reciprocal interactions between cells and their environment in developing valves, the regulatory mechanisms which induce cells to secrete and respond to components of appropriate ECM, is thought to be the underlying mechanism stratifying valve cusps into their known compartments. These mechanisms are thought to be largely driven by hemodynamics in developing valves.

There is also recent evidence that stem cells with proliferative and regenerative capacities reside in many adult tissues. These stem cells are capable of not only acting locally on the tissues in which they reside, but they may also be recruited out of the circulation and enlisted in the regeneration of diverse tissues at distant sites. A recent review details emerging evidence that bone marrow-derived endothelial, hematopoietic stem and progenitor cells can also contribute to tissue vascularization during both embryonic and postnatal life.[35] Visconti and coworkers have made the intriguing observation that cardiac valve interstitial cells in mice appear to originate in the bone marrow as hematopoietic cells.[36] The idea that bone marrow contains cells capable of repairing damaged tissue has been applied to regeneration of cardiac muscle after myocardial infarction, whereby progenitor cells have been isolated from sites outside the heart, then injected back into the heart in an attempt to regain contractile function of ischemic or infarcted myocytes. Results of these trials have been equivocal, marginal, or negative, suggesting that the process of regeneration does not occur by the simple addition of multipotent cells.[37] The early experience with the SynerGraft decellularized heterograft valved conduits which were implanted in children as right ventricle-to-pulmonary artery conduits occurred with the expectation that circulating cells from the bloodstream, or ingrowth from adjacent normal tissue would repopulate the grafts and grow. In this instance, repopulation of the graft by circulating cells occurred, but did not result in adequate function or tissue growth.[38,39] Nonetheless, the progenitor cell populations represent an attractive source of cells for tissue engineering and regeneration, because they have the plasticity necessary to fulfill critical cell functions, and are potentially programmable for lineage specification.

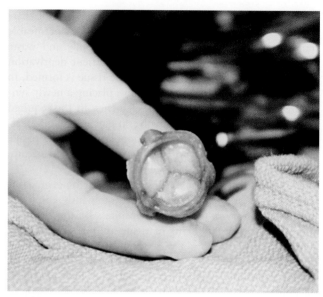

FIGURE 63-1 The tissue engineered pulmonary valve viewed from below, before implantation.

In addition, these cells can be obtained less invasively than differentiated cells.[35] Our initial experience with progenitor cells in the Mayer laboratory was gained with autologous endothelial progenitor cells (EPCs) isolated from circulating blood in lambs and seeded onto decellularized arterial segments.[20] These seeded arterial grafts were then implanted as an interposition graft in the carotid artery of the donor lamb. These grafts remained patent and functional for up to 130 days. Subsequent animal studies by Sutherland and associates used bone marrow mesenchymal stem cells (MSC) to seed a bioresorbable scaffold formed into a three-leaflet valve within a conduit (Fig. 63-1). These valved conduits were implanted as valved conduits into the main pulmonary artery of neonatal sheep, and remained in place for up to eight postoperative months.[27] This study was followed by that of Gottlieb et al, who implanted valves of similar elements into larger numbers of sheep and followed changes in function with growth of the animals using magnetic resonance imaging (MRI) and echocardiography. While the valves had trace to mild regurgitation at the time of implantation (Fig. 63-2), a loss of valve leaflets surface area was observed, which correlated with increasing valve regurgitation over time.[29] Importantly, the valve leaflets underwent a remodeling process in vivo after implantation, seen also in earlier experiments using myofibroblasts and endothelial cells from systemic arteries, and in both sets of experiments, a layered histologic appearance developed after implantation.[23,27]

Several types of progenitor cells have been used for tissue engineering applications in congenital heart disease. Cebotari and colleagues have recently reported an initial experience seeding EPCs onto homograft valves followed by implantation into two children.[40] Matsumura and associates have shown that when seeded onto a copolymer of lactic acid and ε-caprolactone, green fluorescent protein-labeled (GFP) controlling differentiation in these environments remains incompletely defined. There is evidence that EPCs are able to transdifferentiate in response to biochemical signals. Dvorin and colleagues showed that in the presence of transforming growth factor (TGF)-β1, EPCs express α-smooth muscle actin (α-SMA), after seeding on a bioresorbable copolymer scaffold.[45] This behavior is not characteristic of endothelium; SMA expression suggests a mesenchymal phenotype, and this observation is a potentially related phenomenon to EMT seen in embryologic valvulogenesis.[45] Human aortic valve endothelial cells, but not vascular endothelial cells, respond to TGF-β1 in a similar fashion, suggesting that EPCs may be suitable as a replacement for valve endothelium. Though stem cells of many types remain promising candidates for tissue engineering, their full potential will be harnessed with an understanding of their normal generative and regenerative roles in vivo.

Structural Scaffold

Although it has been possible to grow individual cell types in culture for decades, it is more difficult to induce cells to assemble or organize into complex three-dimensional structural arrangements that are found in normal tissues, and to induce cells to produce specific ECM components on demand. Implantation of engineered tissues requires that they have structural integrity at the time of implantation, and for this reason, most tissue engineers employ a scaffold that provides structural integrity, in addition to cellular material.

Given this fundamental requirement, three main strategies for development of a three-dimensional tissue have been used: (1) de novo scaffold synthesis and arrangement into a three-dimensional structure with cellularization prior to implant, (2) decellularization of a whole (usually xenograft) tissue, or (3) de novo biodegradable scaffold without preimplant cellularization.

Any scaffold for tissue engineering applications must be biocompatible and allow cells to adhere and proliferate. For congenital cardiac applications, tissue growth is our target, and therefore, the scaffold must either degrade or be remodeled in vivo. The advantage of the biopolymer approach is that the chemistry of these scaffolds allows for in vivo degradation, usually by hydrolysis.[46] The disadvantage is that heart valves are structurally complex and anisotropic; designing the structural features of the normal heart valve de novo has presented a substantial engineering challenge. The obvious advantage of the decellularization approach is that the three-dimensional complexity is largely preserved, however, there is a shortage of homograft material relative to the clinical demand, and immunogenicity remains a concern with xenografts. Perhaps most importantly, the ECM of decellularized xenografts is dense, and may prevent the penetration of seeded cells into the interstices of the matrix. In our laboratory, we have constructed trileaflet valved conduits from small intestinal submucosa and seeded them with EPCs.[26] After implantation in an ovine model, there was satisfactory short-term function, but there was no penetration of any cells into the depths of

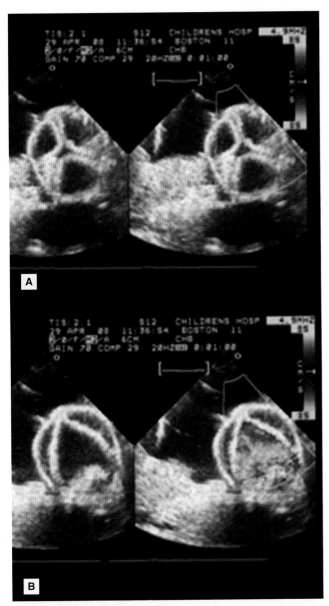

FIGURE 63-2 Representative echocardiogram images of functioning tissue engineered pulmonary valve following implantation.

cells contributed to the histogenesis of their explanted tissue-engineered vascular graft. These grafts remained patent, and explanted constructs contained GFP-labeled cells expressing both endothelial and mesenchymal markers.[33] The group at Tokyo Women's Medical College has also carried out implants of tissue-engineered vascular grafts in children with congenital heart disease using whole mononuclear cell fractions, seeded onto bioresorbable scaffolds.[41] This work is now ongoing at Yale University, due to encouraging early results.

Increasing evidence supports the idea that for cells, "geography or destination is destiny." Many cell types, including bone marrow-derived MSC exhibit surprising plasticity, and cell phenotype seems to be related to the microenvironment in which cells reside.[42-44] However, many of the factors the small intestinal submucosa scaffold. The ECM proteins, when exposed to blood components, can induce inflammation, thrombosis, and calcification, so this material has not been pursued further in our laboratory.

Our primary laboratory efforts to develop heart valves and large arteries have utilized the approach of seeding cells onto a variety of bioresorbable polymer scaffolds. Ideally, there exists an inverse relationship between scaffold degradation and ECM formation by seeded cells. Polymer degradation is related to polymer chemistry, fabrication method, and mechanism of degradation, and therefore, polymers used in tissue engineering differ in their degradation times. The first generation of scaffolds used in heart valve tissue engineering were highly porous, nonwoven felts produced from fibers of polyglycolic acid (PGA). PGA and related polymers continue to be the most widely used for multiple tissue engineering applications.[47-50] The advantage of PGA and related aliphatic polyesters, including poly-L-lactic acid (PLLA), is their safety, biocompatibility, lack of toxicity, and commercial availability. PGA has been used as the commercially available Dexon suture material since the 1970s.[51] PGA can be extruded as a fiber, which allows fabrication of nonwoven sheets with large, open pores. Open pore structures facilitate cell delivery and proliferation by allowing a large surface area for cell attachment, free diffusion of nutrients and dissolved gases, and removal of waste products of metabolism. Material properties of these nonwoven felts are well established, with reproducible hydrolytic degradation times; PGA alone degrades in 2 to 4 weeks, while the majority of fibers of the more hydrophobic PLLA degrade within 4 to 6 weeks. These scaffolds lose strength prior to losing mass, which challenges tissue engineers to seed sufficient numbers of matrix-producing cells so as to replace the scaffold strength as it is lost. Our laboratory has experimented with PGA coated with the thermoplastic polymer poly-4-hydroxybutyrate (P4HB), assembled into a trileaflet structure by attaching leaflets to a flat scaffold sheet, then wrapping the scaffold around a mandrel and heat-welding a seam of attachment. Despite promising early results using the PGA/P4HB composite, subsequent studies showed loss of structural integrity with longer periods of in vitro culture, followed by difficulties with suture retention and hemostasis in vivo. For these reasons, Sutherland and colleagues in our laboratory developed a scaffold composed of equal parts of PGA and PLLA fibers. As PGA is a stronger but more rapidly degrading polymer, and PLLA is a less strong polymer with a longer degradation time, we expected more uniform strength from the tissue when constructed from this material. The composite nonwoven felt was fabricated into a valved conduit with a trileaflet valve, and had substantially improved surgical handling characteristics.[27]

Although satisfactorily strong, polymer fiber-based scaffolds are significantly stiffer than normal valve leaflets, and with the addition of cell-secreted ECM, these constructs are notably stiff.[46] Scaffold stiffness has been shown to effect cell behavior, and tissue engineers have sought less more flexible materials.[44] Wang and colleagues at the Massachusetts Institute of Technology designed an elastic polymer with a rapid degradation time, based on sebacic acid, a derivative of castor oil. Polyglycerol sebaceate is a strong but elastomeric material, and is currently under investigation for use in heart valve tissue engineering applications.[52]

In addition to their stiffness, polymer-based scaffolds are thick, relative to normal valve leaflets. A thick scaffold leads to a nutrient gradient in culture, and many tissue engineering studies based on nonwoven materials have been limited by the lack of nutrient delivery to the deepest areas of engineered tissues. Two solutions are proposed to overcome this limitation: addition of a blood supply, and design of thinner scaffolds.

Hydrogel-based scaffolds, including collagen, alginate, agarose, gelatin, fibrin, chitosan, polyethylene glycol, hyaluronic acid, and dehydrated sheets of ECM have formed the basis of many experiments in tissue engineering. When gels become solid, cells are trapped in the cell, providing a homogeneous distribution of cells embedded in a temporary matrix. In addition, hydrogels can be laid into thin layers. A bileaflet heart valve was produced in the Tranquillo laboratory using a collagen-based scaffold seeded with dermal fibroblasts.[53] Recent advances in drug delivery technologies and microfluidics have resulted in further control of scaffold characteristics, including orchestration of scaffold polymerization with changes in temperature, pH, or exposure to light; engineering of nano- and microscale cell environments in order to direct cell distribution throughout a scaffold, and microencapsulation of growth factors and adhesion peptides on scaffolds for improved cell attachment and proliferation.[54-58]

Finally, cells and scaffold have been incorporated and directed in nanoscale fabrication techniques such as electrospinning. Still, no perfect material has been identified for heart valve tissue engineering, and in this regard, the search continues.

The complex anisotropy and three-dimensional structure of heart valves has provided another challenge for a biomimetic device. Even if the optimal scaffold material is identified, its fabrication into a three dimensionally accurate valve geometry is nontrivial. Using normal heart valve anatomy derived from computed tomography images, Sodian employed stereolithography to print a three-dimensional model for use as a mold for the thermoplastic polymer P4HB.[59] The mold was used for curing the polymer into three-dimensional valve anatomy. As improvements in imaging technology yield higher spatial and temporal resolution, anatomic definition of thin, moving, anisotropic structures in the heart such as valve leaflets will be more feasible and may be able to account for the nonuniform cellular and ECM distributions that are found in native leaflets. In addition, evolving microfabrication methods will further our ability to fabricate microscale features of valve anatomy. With defined anatomic dimensions and an understanding of outflow tract, great artery, and leaflet motion and growth, tissue engineers will have clear targets for three-dimensional fabrication of heart valve scaffolds.

Biochemical Signals

The migration and transdifferentiation of endothelial cells in the early stages of valvulogenesis (EMT) has been experimentally modeled in an ex vivo chick cardiac cushion explant system.[17] Much progress has been made to understand the signals required for the proper sequencing and execution of these early events. Vascular endothelial growth factor is one such molecule, thought to regulate EMT in an environment of adequate tissue glucose and oxygen saturation. While VEGF is secreted by endothelial cells, other important signals, such as bone morphogenetic proteins 2 and 4, are expressed by myocardium. Hyaluronic acid, a component of the ECM, is thought to regulate downstream signaling through its large, hydrated structure, which regulates ligand availability for receptor binding. Therefore, valvulogenesis is dependent in vivo upon signals from myocardium, local ECM, and endothelium.[12,34] Though very early growth of endocardial cushions and valve primordia are less understood, and late regulatory events in valve growth are poorly understood, regulators of endothelial and mesenchymal cell proliferation have been identified. These known pathways have been largely studied in isolation, and as gene regulation in organogenesis is a highly complex process, synthesis of critical gene pathway data is necessary for developing a big-picture view of required events. Current microarray technologies will yield large volumes of data, and will likely provide additional insight into the critical regulatory steps involved in valve growth. This type of information will be high yield in future generations of engineered valves.

Mechanical Signals

Identification of a suitable cell phenotype is necessary but not sufficient for engineering replacement tissues. Proper cell orientation and three-dimensional ECM microstructure are also required for tissue function; tissues demonstrate organization of cells and matrix across multiple levels of scale. In this regard, engineered tissues, like native tissues, require coordination. Hemodynamics are fundamental to the development and ongoing function of cardiovascular structures, and biomechanical signals are epigenetic regulators of tissue growth and development. Increasing evidence supports a role for endothelial cells as mechanotransducers, sending signals through the underlying ECM to the more deeply embedded valve interstitial cells.[19] Endothelial cells respond to shear stress and cyclic strains.[60] In an environment in which concentrations of soluble growth factors are held constant, endothelial cell programs can be switched between growth, differentiation, and apoptosis by varying the extent to which the cell is spread or stretched.[61] As cells are embedded in, and coupled to, their ECM serves as a vehicle through which signals must pass. Biochemical signals can be sequestered or amplified by ECM, and as cells bind to surrounding ECM via integrin receptors, the binding itself can induce phenotypic changes.[34] When human MSCs are plated onto large tissue islands that promote cell spreading, they efficiently differentiate into bone cells; when plated onto small islands, the same cells in the same culture medium differentiate into adipocytes.[61]

Clinical observations made from patients undergoing the Ross procedure has provided further evidence for the responsiveness of vascular and valve tissues to hemodynamic forces. In the Ross procedure, a pulmonary valve from the lower-pressure pulmonary circulation is transplanted into the aortic position and subjected to systemic pressure, leading to significant changes in the phenotype of valve interstitial cells, including an increase in matrix metalloproteinase activity, indicating ECM remodeling.[18]

Biophysical signaling is therefore considered fundamental to engineered tissue organization and conditioning, or training, for the in vivo environment. Mechanical forces can be applied to growing engineered tissues in a flow-loop containing tissue culture medium, known as a bioreactor. Preconditioning of tissues is thought to be important for the biology and monitoring of engineered cardiovascular tissues. Bioreactors are thought to serve two predominant purposes for engineered heart valves: first, mechanical forces influence cell phenotype and gene expression, and therefore, tissue development, and potentially, growth, are controlled by biomechanical signals. In experiments from our laboratory reported by Hoerstrup and colleagues, flow and pressure were demonstrated to increase the production of collagen in tissue-engineered semilunar valves.[23] In separate experiments, Lee and associates demonstrated the variation of ECM gene transcripts with changes in tightly controlled mechanical strains. Vascular smooth muscle cells seeded onto biodegradable scaffolds, then subjected to cyclic flexure produced more collagen and were stiffer than controls.[63] Similar findings were reproduced using MSCs, and porcine heart valves.[64,65]

In addition, since valves must not be regurgitant at the time of implantation, observation of engineered valve mechanics in a bioreactor prior to implantation has allowed investigators to monitor and predict in vivo valve function.

ENGINEERED VALVE EXPERIMENTAL OUTCOMES

Progress toward a clinically translatable engineered heart valve is not possible without in vitro study of valve development and remodeling. Developmental biology and in vitro experiments are the fundamental elements of this emerging field. However, in vivo experiments are the necessary complement to in vitro investigation, and represent the true test of engineered device function over time. The in vivo environment is more complex than can be approximated in vitro, and remodeling is dependent upon the contributions of circulating progenitor and immune cells only present in whole living organisms.

Four major implantation studies of TEHV have been undertaken using the de novo engineered approach.[23,24,29,66]

Several groups have implanted decellularized and recellularized valves into the juvenile lamb circulation,[67,68] and two major studies evaluate the growth of vascular conduits in the pulmonary circulation.[69,70] Several representative studies will be reviewed in terms of valve function, evaluation of valve/conduit growth, and observation of engineered tissue maturation.

In Vivo Valve Function, Growth and Maturation

Heart valve tissue engineering was conceptually established through proof-of-concept experiments in large animals. The first in vivo TEHV experiment involved implantation of a single leaflet into the pulmonary circulation.[20] Cells were isolated from ovine arteries and sorted into endothelial and fibroblast populations. Cells were labeled, then seeded onto PGA scaffold and subsequently implanted. Labeled cells were visualized in explanted specimens after 6 hours and after 1, 6, 7, 9, or 11 weeks. Cells produced ECM, and leaflets persisted in the circulation at all time points.

A second set of experiments involved implantation of a pulmonary valve composed of autologous ovine endothelial cells and myofibroblasts seeded on a PGA-P4HB composite scaffold.[23] After 14 days of exposure to gradually increasing flow and pressure conditions in a pulse duplicator, valves were implanted into sheep for 1 day, 4, 6, 8, 16, and 20 weeks. Valves demonstrated acceptable hemodynamics and had no evidence of thrombosis, stenosis, or aneurysm formation for up to 20 weeks. Central valvar regurgitation was noted after 16 weeks. Tissue analysis showed a layered structure with central glycosaminoglycans, collagen on the outflow surface, and elastin on the inflow surface. Elastin was detectable in the leaflets by 6 weeks in vivo. Over the 20-week study period, scaffold degradation corresponded to decreased leaflet stiffness. Histological, biochemical, and biomechanical parameters were similar to those of native pulmonary artery and leaflet tissue.

Using bone marrow-derived MSCs on a PGA/PLLA scaffold, investigators fabricated and implanted valved conduits in the pulmonary position of juvenile sheep.[27] Valves were evaluated by in vivo echocardiography; explanted tissues were analyzed by histology and immunostaining. At the time of implantation, echocardiograms demonstrated a maximum instantaneous gradient of 17.2 ± 1.33 mm Hg, with estimates of regurgitation ranging from trivial to mild. Four animals survived the immediate postoperative period. After 4 months in vivo, there were no statistically significant difference is maximum instantaneous gradient, mean gradient or effective orifice area from the time of implantation. Histologic analysis at eight postoperative months showed explanted tissue to have a layered organization, with elastin fibers identified on the inflow surface and collagen dominating the outflow surface. Glycosaminoglycans were distributed throughout the remainder of the valve. At the time of implantation, cells uniformly expressed the mesenchymal cell marker α-SMA, but at the time of valve explant, these cells were confined to

the subendothelial layer, while surface cells expressed von Willebrand factor, suggesting in vivo endothelialization of the graft. This study demonstrated the feasibility of implantation of a pulmonary valve using stem cells.

Further work in our laboratory has reproduced some of these initial findings, and studied valve function over time in larger numbers of animals.[29] Using the same scaffold material (PGA-PLLA composite nonwoven felt) and cells (MSCs), nineteen animals underwent implantation of valved conduits into the main pulmonary artery of neonatal sheep after resection of the native pulmonary leaflets. Valve function, cusp and conduit dimensions were evaluated at implantation (echocardiography), at the experimental midpoint (MRI), and at explant at 1 day; 6, 12, or 20 weeks postoperatively. At implantation, valved conduit function was excellent; maximum transvalvar pressure gradient by Doppler echocardiography was 17 mm Hg; most valved conduits showed trivial pulmonary regurgitation. At ≥12 weeks, valved conduit cusps were increasingly attenuated and regurgitant. Valved conduit diameter remained unchanged over 20 weeks. Dimensional measurements by MRI correlated with direct measurement at explant. These studies demonstrated autologous engineered valved conduits that functioned well at implantation, with subsequent monitoring of dimensions and function in real time by MRI. The valves underwent structural and functional remodeling without stenosis, but worsening pulmonary regurgitation was noted after 6 weeks.

When fibrin-based valves were implanted in sheep for 3 months, valved conduits exhibited the gross appearance of intact tissue, however, leaflets demonstrated pulmonary regurgitation due to tissue contraction.[66]

Most recent experiments have involved implantation of single electrospun anisotropic poly-carbonate urethane urea (PCUU) leaflets into the ovine pulmonary valve root without pre-implant cellularization. These studies have shown good overall valve function and repopulation of these leaflets with cells (Fig. 63-3). However, leaflet excursion did decrease with time, after implant.[71]

To date, no group has implanted valve leaflets that demonstrated in vivo growth. In many experiments, however, the microscopic structure of the valve leaflets evolved from a relatively homogeneous appearance to a layered structure. The mechanisms by which this in vivo evolution of structure and cellular activity occurs remain completely unexplored, but these observations suggest that a tissue-engineered valve may not have to be in a mature, adult form at the time of implantation into the circulation.

FUTURE DIRECTIONS

After a decade of effort toward a TEHV replacement, the clinical need for a more durable valve replacement still exists. Modes of failure of currently available heart valve replacements are well described and provide insight into strengths and weaknesses of valve designs. Though the appropriate cell source and scaffold material for heart valve tissue engineering have been areas of substantial experimental effort, the optimal

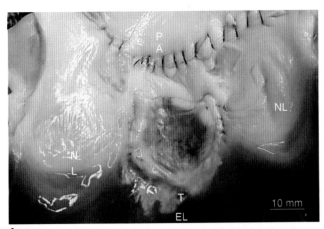

A   6 weeks explant

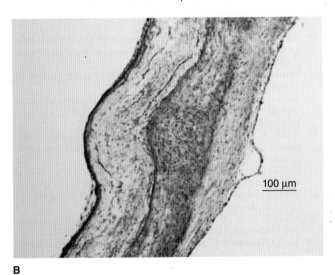

B

FIGURE 63-3 Gross section (A) and histologic section (B) of implanted tissue engineered valve leaflet after six weeks of in vivo implantation.

cell type, scaffold material, and in vitro culture conditions for a TEHV still remain unknown. Stem cells and adult progenitor cells offer promise toward this end, as they possess the capacity for self-renewal and multilineage differentiation, and therefore, growth potential. Evolving imaging technologies will allow a more complete understanding of postimplantation remodeling and growth. Though many details of in vitro preconditioning regimens are yet to be understood, bioreactor preconditioning has the potential to reduce in vitro culture times by stimulating tissue formation, and may offer a controllable environment for evaluation of valve function prior to implantation.

Complex biological events, such as heart valve development, occur through both biochemical and biophysical cues, occurring in parallel, at the cellular, tissue and organ levels. A detailed understanding of the molecular sequence of critical developmental events may allow engineering of appropriate microenvironments and three-dimensional structures

leading to the ultimate goal: a clinically translatable heart valve replacement with the capacity to grow and remain durable for a lifetime of cardiac cycles.

REFERENCES

1. Vongpatanasin W, Hillis D, Lange RA: Prosthetic heart valves. *N Engl J Med* 1996; 335:407.
2. Hammermeister KE, Sethi GK, Henderson WG, et al: Outcomes 15 years after valve replacement with a mechanical versus a bioprosthetic heart valve: final report of the veterans affairs randomized trial. *J Am Coll Cardiol* 2000; 36:1152.
3. Forbess JM, Shah AS, St. Louis JD, et al: Cryopreserved homografts in the pulmonary position: determinants of durability. *Ann Thorac Surg* 2001; 71:54.
4. Stark J, Bull C, Stajevic M, et al: Fate of subpulmonary homograft conduits: determinants of homograft failure. *J Thorac Cardiovasc Surg* 1998; 115:506.
5. Ingber DE: Mechanical signaling and the cellular response to extracellular matrix in angiogenesis and cardiovascular physiology. *Circ Res* 2002; 91:877.
6. Ingber DE: Tensegrity-based mechanosensing from macro to micro. *Prog Biophys Mol Biol* 2008; 97:163-179.
7. Rabkin-Aikawa E, Mayer JE, Jr, Schoen FJ: Heart valve regeneration, in Yannas IV (ed): *Advances in Biochemical Engineering/Biotechnology. Regenerative Medicine II.* Berlin, Springer-Verlag, 2005; p 141.
8. Schoen FJ: Aortic valve structure-functional correlations: role of elastic fibers no longer a stretch of the imagination. *J Heart Valve Dis* 1997; 6:1.
9. Davis PF: Hemodynamic shear stress and the endothelium in cardiovascular pathophysiology. *Nat Clin Pract Cardiovasc Med* 2009; 6(1):16.
10. Cummins PM, von Offenberg Sweeney N, Killeen MT, et al: Cyclic strain-mediated matrix metalloproteinase regulation within the endothelium: a force to be reckoned with. *Am J Physiol Heart Circ Physiol* 2007; 292:H28.
11. Chiquet M: Regulation of extracellular matrix gene expression by mechanical stress. *Matrix Biol* 1999; 18:417.
12. Lincoln J, Lange AW, Yutzey KE: Hearts and bones: shared regulatory mechanisms in heart, cartilage, tendon and bone development. *Dev Biol* 2006; 294(2):292.
13. Aikawa E, Whittaker P, Farber M, et al: Human semilunar cardiac valve remodeling by activated cells from fetus to adult. *Circulation* 2006; 113:1344.
14. Joyce EM, Liao J, Schoen FJ, Mayer JE, Sacks MS: Functional collagen fiber architecture of the pulmonary heart valve cusp. *Ann Thorac Surg* 2009; 87:1240-1249.
15. Hammer PE, Pacak CA, Howe RD, delNido PJ: Straightening of curved pattern of collagen fibers under load controls aortic valve shape. *J Biomech* 2014; 47:341-346.
16. Moore K, Persaud T: *The Cardiovascular System: The Developing Human.* Philadelphia, WB Saunders, 1998; p 563.
17. Armstrong EJ, Bischoff J: Heart valve development: endothelial cell signaling and differentiation. *Circ Res* 2004; 95:459.
18. Rabkin-Aikawa E, Aikawa M, Farber M, et al: Clinical pulmonary autograft valves: pathologic evidence of adaptive remodeling at the aortic site. *J Thorac Cardiovasc Surg* 2004; 128:552.
19. Butcher J, Tressel S, Johnson T, et al: Transcriptional profiles of valvular and vascular endothelial cells reveal phenotypic differences: influence of shear stress. *Arterioscler Thromb Vasc Biol* 2006; 26(1):69.
20. Shin'oka T, Bruer CK, Tanel RE, et al: Tissue engineering heart valves: valve leaflet replacement study in a lamb model. *Ann Thorac Surg* 1995; 60(Suppl 6):S-513.
21. Mendelson K, Schoen FJ: Heart valve tissue engineering: concepts, approaches, progress and challenges. *Ann Biomed Eng* 2006; 34(12):1799.
22. Bayoumi AS, D'Amore A, Cubberley A, et al: Unseeded engineered valve leaflets retain function and remodel after implant in ovine pulmonary outflow tract (abstract), Society for Heart Valve Disease, 2013, Venice, Italy.
23. Hoerstrup SP, Sodian R, Daebritz S, et al: Functional living trileaflet heart valves grown in vitro. *Circulation* 2000; 102(Suppl 3):III-44.
24. Stock UA, Nagshima M, Khalid PN, et al: Tissue engineered valved conduits in the pulmonary circulation. *J Thorac Cardiovasc Surg* 2000; 119:732.

25. Sodian R, Hoerstrup SP, Sperling JS, et al: Early in vivo experience with tissue-engineered trileaflet heart valves. *Circulation* 2000; 102(Suppl 3): III-22.

26. Matheny RG, Hutchison ML, Dryden PE, et al: Porcine small intestine submucosa as a pulmonary valve leaflet substitute. *J Heart Valve Dis* 2000; 9:769.

27. Sutherland FWH, Perry TE, Yu Y, et al: From stem cells to viable autologous semilunar heart valve. *Circulation* 2005; 111:2783.

28. Kaushal S, Amiel GE, Guleserian KJ, et al: Functional small diameter neovessels created using endothelial progenitor cells expanded ex vivo. *Nat Med* 2001; 7:1035.

29. Gottlieb D, Tandon K, Emani S, et al., In vivo monitoring of autologous engineered pulmonary valve function. *J Thorac Cardiovasc Surg* 2010;139(3):723-31.

30. Kang L, Hancock MJ, Brigham MD, et al: Cell confinement in patterned nanoliter droplets in a microwell array by wiping. *J Biomed Mater Res A* 2009; PMID 19585570.

31. Woodfield TB, Moroni L, Malda J: Combinatorial approaches to controlling cell behaviour and tissue formation in 3D via rapid-prototyping and smart scaffold design. *Comb Chem High Throughput Screen* 2009; 12(6):562.

32. Schnell AM, Hoerstrup SP, Zund G, et al: Optimal cell source for cardiovascular tissue engineering: venous vs. aortic human myofibroblasts. *J Thorac Cardiovasc Surg* 2001; 49:221.

33. Matsumura G, Miyagawa-Tomita S, Shin'oka T, et al: First evidence that bone marrow cells contribute to the construction of tissue engineered vascular autografts in vivo. *Circulation* 2003; 108:1729.

34. Combs MD, Yutzey KE: Heart valve development: regulatory networks in development and disease. *Circ Res* 2009; 105:408.

35. Rafii S, Lyden D: Therapeutic stem and progenitor cell transplantation for organ vascularization and regeneration. *Nat Med* 2003; 9:702.

36. Visconti RP, Ebihara Y, LaRue AC, et al: An in vivo analysis of hematopoietic stem cell potential: hematopoietic origin of cardiac valve interstitial cells. *Circ Res* 2006; 98:690.

37. Passier R, van Laake LW, Mummery CL: Stem-cell-based therapy and lessons from the heart. *Nature* 2008; 453(7193):322.

38. O'Brien MF, Goldstein S, Walsh S, et al: The SynerGraft valve: a new acellular, non-glutaraldehyde tissue heart valve for autologous recellularization. First experimental studies before clinical implantation. *Semin Thorac Cardiovasc Surg* 1999; 11:194.

39. Simon P, Kasimir MT, Seebacher G, et al: Early failure of the tissue engineered porcine heart valve SynerGraft in pediatric patients. *Eur J Cardiothorac Surg* 2003; 23:1002.

40. Cebotari S, Lichtenberg A, Tudorache I, et al: Clinical application of tissue engineered human heart valves using autologous progenitor cells. *Circulation* 2006; 114(Suppl I):I-132.

41. Shin'oka T, Matsumura G, Hibino N, et al: Midterm clinical result of tissue-engineered vascular autografts seeded with autologous bone marrow cells. *J Thorac Cardiovasc Surg* 2005; 129:1330.

42. Rozario T, Desimone DW: The extracellular matrix in development and morphogenesis: a dynamic view. *Dev Biol* 2010;341(1):126-40.

43. Gjorevski N, Nelson CM: Bidirectional extracellular matrix signaling during tissue morphogenesis. *Cyt Grow Fact Rev* 2009; 20(5-6):259.

44. Engler AJ, Sen S, Sweeney HL, et al: Matrix elasticity directs stem cell lineage specification. *Cell* 2006; 126:677.

45. Dvorin EL, Wylie-Sears J, Kaushal S, et al: Quantitative evaluation of endothelial progenitors and cardiac valve endothelial cells: proliferation and differentiation on poly-glycolic acid/poly-4-hydroxybutyrate scaffold in response to vascular endothelial growth factor and transforming growth factor β1. *Tissue Eng* 2003; 9:487.

46. Engelmayr GC, Sacks MS: Prediction of extracellular matrix stiffness in engineered heart valve tissues based on nonwoven scaffolds. *Biomech Model Mechanobiol* 2008; 7:309.

47. Bailey M, Wang L, Bode C, et al: A comparison of human umbilical cord matrix stem cells and temporomandibular joint condylar chondrocytes for tissue engineering temporomandibular joint condylar cartilage. *Tissue Eng* 2007; 13(8):2003.

48. Rohman G, Pettit J, Isaure F, et al: Influence of the physical properties of two-dimensional polyester substrates on the growth of normal human urothelial and urinary smooth muscle cells in vitro. *Biomaterials* 2007; 28(14):2264.

49. Roh J, Brennan M, Lopez-Soler R, et al: Construction of an autologous tissue-engineered venous conduit from bone marrow-derived vascular cells: optimization of cell harvest and seeding techniques. *J Pediatr Surg* 2007; 42(1):198.

50. Dahl S, Rhim C, Song Y, et al: Mechanical properties and compositions of tissue engineered and native arteries. *Ann Biomed Eng* 2007; 35(3):348.

51. Gao J, Niklason L, Langer R: Surface hydrolysis of poly(glycolic acid) meshes increases the seeding density of vascular smooth muscle cells. *J Biomed Mater Res* 1998; 42:417.

52. Wang Y, Ameer GA, Sheppard BJ, et al: A tough biodegradable elastomer. *Nat Biotechnol* 2002; 20:602.

53. Neidert M, Tranquillo R: Tissue-engineered valves with commissural alignment. *Tissue Eng* 2006; 12(4):891.

54. Park H, Cannizzaro C, Vunjak-novakovic G, et al: Nanofabrication and microfabrication of functional materials for tissue engineering. *Tissue Eng* 2007; 13:1867.

55. Burdick J, Kahademhosseini A, Langer R: Fabrication of gradient hydrogels using a microfluidics/photopolymerization process. *Langmuir* 2004; 20(13):5153.

56. Silva E, Mooney D: Spatiotemporal control of vascular endothelial growth factor delivery from injectable hydrogels enhances angiogenesis. *J Thromb Haemost* 2007; 5(3):590.

57. Matsumoto T, Mooney D: Cell instructive polymers. *Adv Biochem Eng Biotechnol* 2006; 102:113.

58. Bacakova L, Filova E, Kubies D, et al: Adhesion and growth of vascular smooth muscle cells in cultures on bioactive RGC peptide-carrying polylactides. *J Mater Sci Mater Med* 2007; 18(7):1317.

59. Sodian R, Fu P, Lueders C, et al: Tissue engineering of vascular conduits: fabrication of custom-made scaffolds using rapid prototyping techniques. *J Thorac Cardiovasc Surg* 2005; 53(3):144.

60. Resnick N, Junior MG: Hemodynamic forces are complex regulators of endothelial gene expression. *FASEB J* 1995; 9(10):874.

61. Ingber D: Mechanical control of tissue morphogenesis during embryological development. *Int J Dev Biol* 2006; 50:225.

62. Ingber D, Levin M: What lies at the interface of regenerative medicine and developmental biology? *Development* 2007; 134(14):2541.

63. Lee RT, Yamamoto C, Feng Y, et al: Mechanical strain induces specific changes in the synthesis and organization of proteoglycans by vascular smooth muscle cells. *J Biol Chem* 2001; 276:13847.

64. Engelmayr GC, Rabkin E, Sutherland FW, et al: The independent role of cyclic flexure in the early in vitro development of an engineered heart valve tissue. *Biomaterials* 2005; 26:175.

65. Stephens EH, Chu CK, Grande-Allen KJ: Valve proteoglycan content and glycosaminoglycan fine structure are unique to microstructure, mechanical load and age: relevance to an age-specific tissue engineered heart valve. *Acta Biomater* 2008; 4(5):1148.

66. Flanagan TC, Sachweh J, Frese J, et al: In vivo remodeling and structural characterization of fibrin-based tissue-engineered heart valves in the adult sheep model. *Tissue Eng A* 2009; 15(10):2965.

67. Hopkins RA, Jones A, Wolfinbarger L, et al: Decellularization reduces calcification while improving both durability and 1-year functional results of pulmonary homograft valves in juvenile sheep. *J Thorac Cardiovasc Surg* 2009; 137(4):907.

68. Vincentelli A, Wautot F, Juthier F, et al: In vivo autologous recellularization of a tissue-engineered heart valve: are bone marrow mesenchymal stem cells the best candidates? *J Thorac Cardiovasc Surg* 2007; 134(2):424.

69. Leyh RG, Wilhelmi M, Rebe P, et al: Tissue engineering of viable pulmonary arteries for surgical correction of congenital heart defects. *Ann Thorac Surg* 2006; 81:1466.

70. Hoerstrup SP, Cummings I, Lachat M, et al: Functional growth in tissue-engineered living, vascular grafts: follow-up at 100 weeks in a large animal model. *Circulation* 2006; 114:I-159.

71. Fan R, Bayoumi AS, Chen P, et al: Optimal elastomeric scaffold leaflet shape for pulmonary heart valve leaflet replacement. *J Biomech* 2013; 46:662-669.

Note: Page numbers followed by *f* or *t* refer to the locations of figures or tables, respectively.